The 5-Minute Clinical Consult 2023

2023

31st EDITION

The 5-Minute Clinical Consult 2023

31st EDITION

Editor-in-Chief

Frank J. Domino, MD
Professor and Director of Predoctoral Education
Department of Family Medicine and Community Health
University of Massachusetts Medical School
Worcester, Massachusetts

Associate Editors

Robert A. Baldor, MD, FAAFP
Professor and Founding Chair
Department of Family Medicine
UMass Chan Medical School-Baystate
Springfield, Massachusetts
Designated Institutional Official
Baystate Franklin Medical Center
Greenfield, Massachusetts

Kathleen A. Barry, MD
Assistant Professor
Department of Family Medicine and Community Health
Hahnemann Family Health Center
Worcester, Massachusetts

Jeremy Golding, MD, FAAFP
Professor of Family Medicine and Obstetrics & Gynecology
University of Massachusetts Medical School
Department of Family Medicine and Community Health
University of Massachusetts Memorial Health Care
Hahnemann Family Health Center
Worcester, Massachusetts

Mark B. Stephens, MD, MS, FAAFP
Interim Associate Dean for Medical Education
Professor of Family and Community Medicine
Professor of Humanities
Penn State College of Medicine
University Park, Pennsylvania

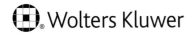 Wolters Kluwer

Philadelphia · Baltimore · New York · London
Buenos Aires · Hong Kong · Sydney · Tokyo

5MinuteConsult™

Director, Medical Practice: Rebecca Schmidt
Acquisitions Editor: Joe Cho
Content Managing Editor: Leanne Vandetty
Development Editor: Thomas Celona
Editorial Assistant: Victoria Giansante
Marketing Manager: Kirsten Watrud
Production Project Manager: Bridgett Dougherty
Design Coordinator: Stephen Druding
Manufacturing Coordinator: Beth Welsh
Prepress Vendor: Absolute Service, Inc.

31st edition

Library of Congress Cataloging-in-Publication Data available from the Publisher upon request.
ISBN-13: 978-1-9751-9155-9

shop.lww.com

This year's edition is dedicated to the steady stewards of health care who continue to battle the COVID-19 pandemic. To each of you who have stayed late, worked an extra shift, shared a meal, shared a story, and shed a tear—thank you for your dedication to doing what is right. Thank you for humbly appreciating a time when "health care heroes" were serenaded and applauded. Thank you for continuing to stand tall when (paradoxically) those same health care workers were verbally abused and confronted for continuing to do what is right. Thank you for getting vaccinated. Thank you for encouraging others to get vaccinated. Thank you for supporting science over vitriol and partisan noise. Thank you for embodying your professional oaths while never ceasing to serve others. You are noticed, and you are appreciated.

Mom, Dad, Trevor, Abby, Patty—thanks. I love you.

MARK B. STEPHENS, MD, MS, FAAFP

PREFACE

This has likely been the hardest year of your clinical career. It certainly will be one of the most memorable. Pandemic, mRNA vaccines, and public health have all had the spotlight. And yet, despite having a lifesaving vaccine and simple community-facing activities like wearing masks and distancing, deliberate misinformation has resulted in patient hesitation and death. "My own research" became a mantra for those who choose to place emotion over logic, opinion over insight. The result is our fatigue, frustration, and sadness. All the data you offer falls on deaf ears. Why?

"It is impossible to use logic to remove a thought that was placed there by emotion."

ANONYMOUS

"A point of view can be a dangerous luxury when substituted for insight and understanding."

MARSHALL MCLUHAN

What are we to do? For our patients, focus on hope.

"May your choices reflect your hopes, not your fears."

NELSON MANDELA

And for you?

"Stay positive. Always focus on how far you have come, not how far is left to go."

ANONYMOUS

"Someday we'll look back on this and it will all seem funny."

BRUCE SPRINGSTEEN

Welcome to the 2023 edition of *The 5-Minute Clinical Consult*. Your clinical practice is full of challenges and unanswered questions. Your use of this amazing tool will provide you with the answers needed to help your patients live to their fullest.

The 5-Minute Clinical Consult is here to assist in fulfilling our role as health care providers. In each patient interaction, in addition to bringing your clinical expertise, remember how your patients view you—as their advocate, someone who prioritizes their well-being unlike anyone else.

Our editorial team has collaborated with hundreds of authors so that you may deliver your patients the best care. Each topic provides you with quick answers you can trust, where and when you need them most, either in print or online at www.5MinuteConsult.com.

This highly organized content online provides you with the following:
- Differential diagnosis support from our expanded collection of algorithms
- Current evidence-based designations highlighted in each topic covering 540+ commonly encountered diseases in print, with an additional 1,500 online topics, including content from *The 5-Minute Pediatric Consult* and *The 5-Minute Sports Medicine Consult*
- FREE point-of-care CME and CE: 1/2-hour credit for every digital search
- Thousands of images to help support visual diagnosis of all conditions
- Video library of procedures, treatment, and physical therapy
- A to Z drug database from Facts & Comparisons
- Laboratory test interpretation from *Wallach's Interpretation of Diagnostic Tests*
- More than 3,000 patient handouts in English and Spanish
- ICD-10 codes and DSM-5 criteria; additionally, SNOMED codes are available online.

Our Web site, www.5MinuteConsult.com, delivers quick answers to your questions. It is an ideal resource for patient care. Integrating *The 5-Minute Clinical Consult* content into your workflow is easy and fast, and our patient education handouts can assist in helping you meet meaningful use compliance.

If you purchased the Premium Edition, your access includes 1-year FREE use of our expanded Web site; the standard edition includes a free 10-day trial! The site promises an easy-to-use interface, allowing smooth maneuverability between topics, algorithms, images, videos, and patient education materials as well as more than 1,500 online-only topics.

Evidence-based health care is the integration of the best medical information with the values of the patient and your skill as a clinician. We have updated our evidence-based medicine (EBM) content so you can focus on how to best apply it in your practice.

The algorithm section includes both diagnostic and treatment algorithms. This easy-to-use graphic method helps you evaluate an abnormal finding and prioritize treatment. They are also excellent teaching tools, so share them with the learners in your office.

This book and Web site are a source to solve problems and to help evaluate, diagnose, and treat patients' concerns. Use your knowledge, expressed through your words and actions, to address their anxiety.

The 31st edition means I have had the great fortune to help grow and support this content for half of its life. I am honored to play this role and hope to keep doing so for some years to come. I thank you, the reader, and the team at Wolters Kluwer for your support.

The 5-Minute Clinical Consult editorial team values your observations, so please share your thoughts, suggestions, and constructive criticism through our Web site: www.5MinuteConsult.com.

FRANK J. DOMINO, MD

EVIDENCE-BASED MEDICINE

WHAT IS EVIDENCE-BASED MEDICINE?

We used to treat every otitis media with antibiotics. These recommendations came about because we applied logical reasoning to observational studies. If bacteria cause an acute otitis media, then antibiotics should help it resolve sooner, with less morbidity. Yet, when rigorously studied (via a systematic review), we found little benefit to this intervention.

The underlying premise of EBM is the evaluation of medical interventions and the literature that supports those interventions in a systematic fashion. EBM hopes to encourage treatments proven to be effective and safe. And when insufficient data exist, it hopes to inform you on how to safely proceed.

EBM uses end points of real patient outcomes, morbidity, mortality, and risk. It focuses less on intermediate outcomes (bone density) and more on patient conditions (hip fractures).

Implementing EBM requires three components: the best medical evidence, the skill and experience of the provider, and the values of the patients. Should this patient be screened for prostate cancer? It depends on what is known about the test, on what you know of its benefits and harms, your ability to communicate that information, and that patient's informed choice.

This book hopes to address the first EBM component, providing you access to the best information in a quick format. Although not every test or treatment has this level of detail, many of the included interventions here use systematic review literature support.

The language of medical statistics is useful in interpreting the concepts of EBM. Below is a list of these terms, with examples to help take the confusion and mystery out of their use.

Prevalence: proportion of people in a population who have a disease (in the United States, 0.3% [3 in 1,000] people >50 years have colon cancer)

Incidence: how many *new* cases of a disease occur in a population during an interval of time; for example, "The estimated incidence of colon cancer in the United States is 104,000 in 2005."

Sensitivity: percentage of people with disease who test positive; for mammography, the sensitivity is 71–96%.

Specificity: percentage of people without disease who test negative; for mammography, the specificity is 94–97%.

Suppose you saw ML, a 53-year-old woman, for a health maintenance visit, ordered a screening mammogram, and the report demonstrates an irregular area of microcalcifications. She is waiting in your office to receive her test results, what can you tell her?

Sensitivity and specificity refer to people who are known to have disease (sensitivity) or those who are known not to have disease (specificity). But what you have is an abnormal test result. To better explain this result to ML, you need the positive predictive value.

Positive predictive value (PPV): percentage of positive test results that are truly positive; the PPV for a woman aged 50 to 59 years is approximately 22%. That is to say that only 22% of abnormal screening mammograms in this group truly identified cancer. The other 78% are false positives.

You can tell ML only 1 out of 5 abnormal mammograms correctly identifies cancer; the other 4 are false positives, but the only way to know which mammogram is correct is to do further testing.

The corollary of the PPV is the negative predictive value (NPV), which is the percentage of negative test results that are truly negative.

The PPV and NPV tests are population dependent, whereas the sensitivity and specificity are characteristics of the test and have little to do with the patient in front of you. So when you receive an abnormal lab result, especially a screening test such as mammography, understand their limits based on their PPV and NPV.

Treatment information is a little different. In discerning the statistics of randomized controlled trials of interventions, first consider an example. The Scandinavian Simvastatin Survival Study (4S) (*Lancet.* 1994;344[8934]:1383–1389) found using simvastatin in patients at high risk for heart disease for 5 years resulted in death for 8% of simvastatin patients versus 12% of those on placebo; this results in a relative risk of 0.70, a relative risk reduction of 33%, and a number needed to treat of 25.

There are two ways of considering the benefits of an intervention with respect to a given outcome. The absolute risk reduction is the difference in the percentage of people with the condition before and after the intervention. Thus, if the incidence of myocardial infarction (MI) was 12% for the placebo group and 8% for the simvastatin group, the absolute risk reduction is 4% (12% − 8% = 4%).

The relative risk reduction reflects the improvement in the outcome as a percentage of the original rate and is commonly used to exaggerate the benefit of an intervention. Thus, if the risk of MI were reduced by simvastatin from 12% to 8%, then the relative risk reduction would be 33% (4% / 12% = 33%); 33% sounds better than 4%, but the 4% is the absolute risk reduction and reflects the true outcome.

Absolute risk reduction is usually a better measure of clinical significance of an intervention. For instance, in one study, the treatment of mild hypertension has been shown to have relative risk reduction of 40% over 5 years (40% fewer strokes in the treated group). However, the absolute risk reduction was only 1.3%. Because mild hypertension is not strongly associated with strokes, aggressive treatment of mild hypertension yields only a small clinical benefit. Don't confuse relative risk reduction with relative risk.

Absolute (or attributable) risk (AR): the percentage of people in the placebo or intervention group who reach an end point; in the 4S, the absolute risk of death was 8%.

Relative risk (RR): the risk of disease of those treated or exposed to some intervention (i.e., simvastatin) divided by those in the placebo group or who were untreated

- If RR is <1.0, it reduces risk—the smaller the number, the greater the risk reduction.
- If RR is >1.0, it increases risk—the greater the number, the greater the risk increase.

Hazard ratio (HR): the probability of an event in a treatment group versus the probability of events in a control group at a given time (can be calculated at any time in the study; often applied to observational data); like RR, if HR is statistically <1.0, it reduces risk; if >1.0, it increases risk.

Relative risk reduction (RRR): the relative decrease in risk of an end point compared to the percentage of that end point in the placebo group

If you are still confused, just remember that the RRR is an overestimation of the actual effect.

Number needed to treat (NNT): This is the number of people who need to be treated by an intervention to prevent one adverse outcome. A "good" NNT can be a large number (>100) if risk of serious outcome is great. If the risk of an outcome is not that dangerous, then lower (<25) NNTs are preferred.

The NNT should be compared to a similar statistic, the number needed to harm (NNH). This is the number of people who have to be given treatment before one excess side effect or harm occurs. When the NNT is compared to the NNH, you and the patient can judge whether the benefit of the intervention is great enough to outweigh the risk of harm.

EVIDENCED-BASED GRADING

To help you interpret diagnostic and treatment recommendations within *The 5-Minute Clinical Consult*, we have graded the best information within the text and highlighted this content.

An "A" grade means the reference is from the highest quality resource, such as a systematic review. A systematic review is a summary of the medical literature on a given topic that uses strict, explicit methods to perform a thorough search of the literature and then provides a critical appraisal of individual studies, concluding in a recommendation. The most prestigious collection of systematic reviews is from the Cochrane Collaboration (www.cochrane.org).

A "B" grade means the data referenced comes from high-quality randomized controlled trials performed to minimize bias in their outcome. Bias is anything that interferes with the truth; in the medical literature, it is often unintentional, but it is much more common than we appreciate. In short, always assume some degree of bias exist in any research endeavor.

A "C" grade implies the reference used does not meet the A or B requirements; they are often treatments recommended by consensus groups (such as the American Cancer Society). In some cases, they may be the standards of care. But implicit in a group's recommendation is the bias of the author or the group that supports the reference.

BIAS

Bias is anything that interferes with the truth. There are many types of bias that should be considered by the publishers of medical information. Below describes a number of bias types that often affect our care without us knowing it is present.

Publication bias occurs when research is not published. The motivation to publish information that "didn't work" is low. It is estimated up to 40% of all medical research never gets published. When you read of an effective intervention, wonder if other studies did not show benefit and went unpublished.

Comparator bias occurs when research compares an intervention to not the standard of care. Knowing a new treatment is more effective than placebo for treating a condition is not helpful if you typically use a drug or procedure. Why not study comparing the new to the standard of care? Sometimes, the new treatment is no better than the current standard. And if a study was done to see if the new is better than the old and not published, you have an example of publication bias.

Selection bias involves choosing study populations that might be different than the average patient or just reporting a just subset of study participants from a study. Either will result in the data being skewed because it can only be applied to small subset of people.

Attrition bias and the concept of intention to treat. Attrition bias is when researchers address how a study deals with participants who do not adhere to the research protocol or drop out completely. Intention to treat analysis hopes to diminish attrition bias by statistically considering the nonadhering or dropped out patients as unsuccessfully benefiting from the intervention.

Commercial (funder) bias involves who paid for the research being done, and do they have a vested interest in the outcome. If the developer of a new drug does a large study, or a researcher has a personal financial interest in seeing a study succeed, they may consciously or unconsciously alter what is reported. The data may be accurate, but until this is studied by less vested interests, it is difficult to accept the conclusions.

A systematic review gathers all the literature on a topic, say using antibiotics to treat otitis media, and combines the data to determine if the sum of all the trials tells a different story than any single trial. The large number of participants in this type of research results in a much more statistically (and clinically) significant conclusion than any single paper.

A meta-analysis is a quantitative systematic review and demonstrates its outcomes in the form of a forest plot. The interpretation of a forest plot is to look for the diamond on the bottom. If it is totally to LEFT of the vertical line, it means risk of an outcome was reduced by the intervention. If it is fully to the RIGHT, then risk of that outcome was increased. And if the diamond touches the vertical line, it means there was no statistical influence of the intervention on the outcome.

We hope this brief introduction to EBM has been informative, clear, and helpful. If any of the information above seems unclear, or if you have a question, please contact us via www.5MinuteConsult.com.

ACKNOWLEDGMENTS

This is the 31st edition of *The 5-Minute Clinical Consult*, a comprehensive point-of-care tool to assist in the care of patients. From beginning to end, one cannot find a more current and easy-to-use collection of clinically useful content.

Developing and maintaining a book and Web site of this magnitude requires an equally broad effort from its supporting team. I wish to thank the dedication and tireless efforts of many: Rebecca Schmidt, director, medical practice; Leanne Vandetty, content managing editor; Thomas Celona, development editor; Joe Cho, acquisitions editor; and Lisa McAllister, publisher.

This 2023 edition is the direct result of the dedication and insights of our associate editors. I wish to thank Drs. Robert A. Baldor, Jeremy Golding, Mark B. Stephens, and Kathleen A. Barry for their hard work and overwhelming commitment to *The 5-Minute Clinical Consult*.

I wish to especially thank my wife, Sylvia, and my daughter, Molly, who have given greatly for this book.

The challenge of completing a book covering this broad spectrum of medicine requires insights and skills far beyond my own. Many thanks to my mentors, Bob Baldor and Mark Quirk, who have been an enormous support—always there to encourage, reassure, and impart wisdom.

Many in the academic and health care worlds are due thanks for support, insight, and friendship:

M. Diane McKee, Michele Pugnaire, Karen Rayla, Maryanne Adams, Jennifer Masoud, Phil Fournier, Erik Garcia, Jeff Stovall, Jim Comes, Leah Honor, J. Herb Stevenson, Michael Kidd, Zainab Nawab, Sanjiv and Amita Chopra, Vasilios (Bill) Chrisostomidis, James (Jay) Broadhurst, Christina Kim, Madhavi Medipally, the staff of Shrewsbury Family Medicine, Deb Huchowski, Joyce Paquette, Kate Peasha, Priscila Velez, Fanny Rodriguez, Meghan Plaza, Angie Dell'Ovo, Brittany McLean, Joseph Frappier, Mark Powicki, Steve Messineo, Jill Terrien, Susan Feeney, Rick Watson and Sara Floros, and the faculty and amazing students of the University of Massachusetts Medical School.

Medicine is a challenge I have fortunately not had to meet alone. Thanks to my parents, Frank and Angela (Jean); my brother, John, and his family, Marylou, Cate, and Jane; Frank, Mary Anne, Diane, and David Christian; the Diana and Hymie Lipschitz family; and the Bob and Ruth Pabreza family; they are responsible for who I am and my success in life.

I am blessed with the best of friends; without them, I would not be a physician. Thanks to Bob Bacic; Ron Jautz; Richard Onorato; John Horcher; Auguste Turnier; Bob Smith; Paul Saivetz; Bob and Nancy Gallinaro; Drew and Jill Grimes; Louay Toma; Laurie, Alan, Daniel, Jenny, and Matt Bugos; Alan Ehrlich; Andy Jennings; Bill Demianiuk; John and Kathleen Polanowicz; Phil and Carol Pettine; Mark and Linda Shelton; Steve Bennett; Vicki Triolo; and Bob and Laurie Jenal.

—FRANK J. DOMINO, MD

CONTRIBUTING AUTHORS

Francisca Abanyie-Bimbo, MD, MPH
Medical Epidemiologist
Division of Parasitic Diseases and
  Malaria—Malaria Branch
Centers for Disease Control and
  Prevention
Atlanta, Georgia

Zainab Abbas, MD
PGY2 Dermatology Resident
Department of Dermatology
University of Massachusetts Medical
  School
Worcester, Massachusetts

Adil Abdalla, MD
Department of Gastroenterology
CHI Health
Omaha, Nebraska

Daniel Abelev, MD
Resident Physician, PGY2
Department of Family and Community
  Medicine
Penn State Health
State College, Pennsylvania

Thomas L. Abell, MD
The Arthur M. Schoen, MD Chair in
  Gastroenterology
Department of Medicine
Division of Gastroenterology, Hepatology
  and Nutrition
University of Louisville
Louisville, Kentucky

Arabelle Abellard, MD, MSc
Resident Physician
Department of Internal Medicine
University of Illinois at Chicago/Advocate
  Christ Medical Center
Oak Lawn, Illinois

Heran Abiye, MD, BS
Resident Physician
Department of Family Medicine
HCA Medical City Arlington
Arlington, Texas

Hanadi Abou Dargham, MD
Associate Program Director
Department of Family Medicine
St. Joseph's Medical Center
Stockton, California

Ronald N. Adler, MD, FAAFP
Associate Professor
Department of Family Medicine and
  Community Health
University of Massachusetts Medical School
Worcester, Massachusetts

Radhika Agarwal, MD
Resident Physician
Department of Family Medicine
AMITA Health Saint Joseph Hospital
  Chicago
Chicago, Illinois

Faraz Ahmad, MD, MPH[†]
Assistant Clinical Professor
Department of Family and Community
  Medicine
Ohio State University
Columbus, Ohio

Hiba Ahmad, PharmD, BCOP[†]
Clinical Oncology Pharmacist
Department of Pharmacy
Yale-New Haven Hospital
New Haven, Connecticut

Aliyah Ahmed, DO
Resident Physician
Department of Family Medicine
Advocate Christ Medical Center
Oak Lawn, Illinois

Saeed Ahmed, MD
Addiction Psychiatrist
Department of Psychiatry
Rutland Regional Medical Center
Rutland, Vermont

Yasir Ahmed, MD
Cornea, Cataract & Refractive Surgeon
Houston, Texas

Yousef Ahmed, MD[†]
Undersea Medical Officer
Naval Special Warfare Group ONE
Coronado, California

Assim M. AlAbdulKader, MD, MPH,
  FAAFP
Assistant Professor and Consultant
Department of Family and Community
  Medicine
Imam Abdulrahman bin Faisal University
  College of Medicine
Dammam, Saudi Arabia

Karla M. Alba, MD
Department of Family and Community
  Medicine
University of Texas Health Science
  Center at San Antonio
San Antonio, Texas

Ahmed Aldabdob, MD
Internal Medicine
Flint, Michigan

Abdul Aleem, MD[†]
Division of Gastroenterology &
  Hepatology
Department of Internal Medicine
Lehigh Valley Health Network
Allentown, Pennsylvania

John Motley Alford, DO
Core Faculty
Department of Family Medicine
Mercy Health Anderson Hospital Family
  and Community Residency Program
Cincinnati, Ohio

Dureshahwar Ali, DO
Resident Physician
Advocate Lutheran General Hospital
Park Ridge, Illinois

Fozia Akhtar Ali, MD, FAAFP
Diplomat of American Board of Obesity
  Medicine
Associate Professor
Family and Community Medicine
  Department
UT Health San Antonio
San Antonio, Texas

Sarah Ali, MD
Department of Family Medicine
Memorial Family Medicine Residency
  Program
Sugar Land, Texas

Richard W. Allinson, MD
Associate Professor
Department of Ophthalmology
Texas A&M Health Science Center
Bryan, Texas
Baylor Scott & White Health
Waco, Texas

Lolwa Al-Obaid, MD
Resident Physician
Department of Internal Medicine
Lahey Hospital & Medical Center
Burlington, Massachusetts

Maureen Alvarado, DO
Assistant Professor/Clinical
Department of Family and Community
    Medicine
UT Health San Antonio
San Antonio, Texas

Alyce D. Alven, OD, MS
Optometrist
Baylor Scott & White Health
Waco, Texas

Alyssa Anderson, MD
Department of Family and Community
    Medicine
Penn State Health Milton S. Hershey
    Medical Center
Hershey, Pennsylvania

Kathryn E. Anderson, DO
Resident
Department of Family Medicine
Ohio State University
Columbus, Ohio

Garland E. Anderson II, MD
Associate Clinical Professor
Department of Rural Family Medicine
Louisiana State University Health
    Sciences Center New Orleans
New Orleans, Louisiana

Jessica Z. Andrade, DO
Fellow Physician
Department of Sports Medicine
University of Massachusetts Medical
    School
Worcester, Massachusetts

Pavan Annamaraju, MD
Consultant Nephrologist
BalladHealth
Abingdon, Virginia

Katyayini Aribindi, MD
Assistant Chief of Service
Division of General Medicine
McGovern Medical School
Houston, Texas

Ann M. Aring, MD, FAAFP
Associate Program Director
Department of Family Medicine
    Residency
OhioHealth Riverside Methodist Hospital
Columbus, Ohio

James J. Arnold, DO, FACOFP[†]
Director of Medical Education
96th Medical Group/Eglin Hospital
Eglin Air Force Base, Florida

Michael J. Arnold, MD[†]
Assistant Professor
Department of Family Medicine
Uniformed Services University of the
    Health Sciences
Bethesda, Maryland

Maximos Attia, MD, FAAFP
Associate Professor
Department of Family Medicine
Guthrie
Sayre, Pennsylvania

Sandra S. Augusto, MD, MPH
Assistant Professor
University of Massachusetts Chan
    Medical School
Faculty
Family Medicine Residency Program
Full Spectrum Family Medicine Clinician
    with Obstetrics
Barre Family Health Center
Department of Family Medicine and
    Community Health
University of Massachusetts
Worcester, Massachusetts

Sudeep K. Aulakh, MD, FACP, FRCPC
Director, Ambulatory Education
Baystate Internal Medicine Residency
Assistant Professor
UMass Chan Medical School-Baystate
Springfield, Massachusetts

Swati B. Avashia, MD, FAAP, FACP
Assistant Professor
Department of Population Health
Dell Medical School, The University of
    Texas at Austin
Austin, Texas

Ben Ayotte, MD
Clinical Assistant Professor
Division of Hospital Medicine
Michigan Medicine
University of Michigan
Ann Arbor, Michigan

Jennifer L. Ayres, PhD
Director of Behavioral Health Services
Family Medicine Residency Program
Dell Medical School, The University of
    Texas at Austin
Austin, Texas

Sanaa Ayyoub, MD
Endocrinologist
Dartmouth-Hitchcock
Manchester, New Hampshire

Rehan Azeem, MD
Physician
Department of UHS Family Medicine
United Health Services
Johnson City, New York

Holly L. Baab, MD
Associate Director
Family Medicine Residency
Bayfront Health
St. Petersburg, Florida

Franklyn C. Babb, MD, FAAFP
Professor
Department of Family and Community
    Medicine
Texas Tech University Health Sciences
    Center School of Medicine
Lubbock, Texas

Elisabeth L. Backer, MD
Clinical Associate Professor
Department of Family Medicine
University of Nebraska Medical Center
Omaha, Nebraska

Melissa E. Badowski, PharmD, MPH
Clinical Associate Professor
Department of Pharmacy Practice
University of Illinois at Chicago College of
    Pharmacy
Chicago, Illinois

Margo L. Bailey-Leatherwood, MD, MS
Resident
Family Medicine
Advocate Christ Medical Center
Oak Lawn, Illinois

Angela Baker, DO
Cornelius, North Carolina

Maryse Emmerencia Bakouetila, MD
Irving, Texas

Robert A. Baldor, MD, FAAFP
Professor and Founding Chair
Department of Family Medicine
UMass Chan Medical School-Baystate
Springfield, Massachusetts
Designated Institutional Official
Baystate Franklin Medical Center
Greenfield, Massachusetts

Jonathan R. Ballard, MD, MPH, MPhil, FACPM[†]
Associate Professor
Department of Family and Community Medicine
Department of Psychiatry
The Dartmouth Institute for Health Policy and Clinical Practice
Lebanon, New Hampshire
Associate Professor
Department of Community and Family Medicine
Geisel School of Medicine at Dartmouth
Hanover, New Hampshire

Kenneth A. Ballou, MD
Associate Professor of Clinical Medicine
Department of Family Medicine
University of California at Riverside School of Medicine
Riverside, California

Laurel Banach, MD
Resident Physician
Department of Family Medicine
UMass Memorial Medical Center
Worcester, Massachusetts

Huma Baqir, MD
Resident Physician
Department of Psychiatry
University at Buffalo
Buffalo, New York

Krishna Baradhi, MD
Associate Professor
Department of Nephrology
University of Oklahoma Health Sciences Center
Tulsa, Oklahoma

Elise Joyce Barney, DO
Clinical Assistant Professor
Department of Internal Medicine
University of Arizona College of Medicine
Phoenix, Arizona

John P. Barrett, MD, MPH, MS[†]
COL, MC, USA
Adjunct Associate Professor
Deputy Director
Uniformed Services University
War Related Illness and Injury Study Center
Washington DC VA Medical Center
Washington, District of Columbia

Kathleen A. Barry, MD
Assistant Professor
Department of Family Medicine and Community Health
Hahnemann Family Health Center
Worcester, Massachusetts

Rosario Bartolomeo, DO
Oak Lawn, Illinois

Khalid Bashir, MD
Assistant Professor
Department of Medicine
Creighton University
Omaha, Nebraska

Stuart H. Batten, MD[†]
Faculty Physician
Department of Family Medicine
Carl R. Darnall Army Medical Center
Fort Hood, Texas

Tricia Bautista, MD
Family Medicine Residency Program
Resident Physician
Adventist Health Hanford
Hanford, California

Maisam T. Begum, MD
Department of Family Medicine
Creighton University
Omaha, Nebraska

Venkata Raju Behara, MD
Nephrology Associates of Northern Illinois and Indiana
Section of Nephrology
Advocate Lutheran General Hospital
Park Ridge, Illinois

Paul P. Belliveau, PharmD
Professor of Pharmacy Practice
Department of Pharmacy Practice
Massachusetts College of Pharmacy and Health Sciences
Worcester, Massachusetts

Brock A. Benedict, DO
Family Physician
Department of US Army
Womack Army Medical Center
Fort Bragg, North Carolina

Rajarshi Bhadra, MD
Clinical Fellow
Department of Nephrology
University of Massachusetts Medical School
Worcester, Massachusetts

Prarthna V. Bhardwaj, MBBS
Fellow, Department of Hematology Oncology
UMass Chan Medical School-Baystate
Springfield, Massachusetts

Swagato Bhattacharyya, DO
Resident
Department of Psychiatry
Mather Hospital
Port Jefferson, New York

Siddhi Bhivandkar, MD
Department of Psychiatry
St. Elizabeth's Medical Center
Boston University
Boston, Massachusetts

Kimberly Bibb, MD
Assistant Professor
Jackson, Mississippi

Ghazaleh Bigdeli, MD, FCCP
Pulmonary Rehab Associates
Youngstown, Ohio

Laura B. Bishop, MD
Associate Professor, Associate Program Director, Attending Med-Peds Hospitalist
Department of Internal Medicine and Pediatrics Residency Program
University of Louisville
Louisville, Kentucky

Dmitry Bisk, MD
Associate Director
HonorHealth Scottsdale Osborn Family Medicine Residency Program
HonorHealth
Scottsdale, Arizona

Frances J. Boly, DO
Department of Infectious Diseases
Advocate Christ Medical Center
Oak Lawn, Illinois

Robert Bonanno, MD
Family Medicine Physician
Department of Family Medicine
Prisma Health-Upstate
Greenville, South Carolina

Curtis W. Bone, MD, MHS
Assistant Professor
Department of Family and Community Medicine
Penn State Health Milton S. Hershey Medical Center
Hershey, Pennsylvania

Teresa Bormann, MD
Site Director
Department of Family Medicine
Pierre Rural Family Medicine Residency
Pierre, South Dakota

Carley Borrelli, MD
Resident
Department of Family Medicine
Novant Health Family Medicine Residency Program
Cornelius, North Carolina

Marie L. Borum, MD, EdD, MPH[†]
Professor of Medicine
Director of the Division of
    Gastroenterology and Liver Diseases
Department of Medicine
George Washington University School of
    Medicine and Health Care Sciences
Washington, District of Columbia

Katherine E. Bouchard, DO
Department of Family Medicine
Methodist Charlton Medical Center
Dallas, Texas

Sarah Bounader, MD
University of Massachusetts Medical
    School
Worcester, Massachusetts

Stephanie M. Bouwer, DO
Resident Physician
Department of Family and Community
    Medicine
Penn State Health
State College, Pennsylvania

Andrew F. Boylan, MD
Resident
Department of Internal Medicine
George Washington University
Washington, District of Columbia

Joseph Braddock, MD
House Staff Physician PGY1
Department of Family Medicine
Creighton University School of Medicine
Omaha, Nebraska

Chandler Brandenburg, MD
Family Medicine PGY-1
Memorial Health University Medical
    Center
Savannah, Georgia

Dellyse Bright, MD
Associate Professor
Department of Family Medicine
Atrium Health Carolinas Medical Center
Charlotte, North Carolina

Ekaterina Brodski-Quigley, MD, EdM
Physician
Lancaster, Massachusetts

David T. Broome, MD
Assistant Professor
Department of Internal Medicine
Division of Metabolism, Endocrinology,
    and Diabetes
University of Michigan
Ann Arbor, Michigan

Nicholas Broughton, DO
PGY-2
Family Medicine Program
Medical City Arlington
Arlington, Texas

Kathryn M. Brown, MD, MS
Assistant Professor
Department of Family Medicine and
    Community Health
University of Minnesota
Minneapolis, Minnesota

M. Ashleigh Brown, DO
Surgical Resident
Department of General Surgery
Medical College of Georgia
Augusta University
Augusta, Georgia

Phillip Charles Brown, MD
Assistant Clinical Professor
UCLA Family Medical Department
Los Angeles, California

Michael Bruno, MD
Fellow
Division of Pediatric Cardiology
Texas Children's Hospital
Baylor College of Medicine
Houston, Texas

Daniella Davida Brutman, MD
Physician
Department of Family Medicine
AMITA Health Saint Joseph Hospital
    Chicago
Chicago, Illinois

Bonnie A. Buechel, MD, MS
Resident Physician
Department of Family and Community
    Medicine
Penn State Health Milton S. Hershey
    Medical Center
Hershey, Pennsylvania

Han Q. Bui, MD, MPH[†]
Woodbridge, Virginia

Dylan Buller, MD
Resident
Department of Urology
UConn Health
Farmington, Connecticut

Kristina Burgers, MD[†]
Family Physician
Fort Bragg, North Carolina

Liam P. Burke, MD
Assistant Professor
Department of Family Medicine and
    Community Health
University of Massachusetts Medical
    School
Worcester, Massachusetts

Sarah Burroughs, DO
Chief Resident
Department of Internal Medicine
Advocate Lutheran General Hospital
Park Ridge, Illinois

Harold J. Bursztajn, MD
Associate Professor of Psychiatry,
    Part-Time
Department of Psychiatry
Beth Israel Deaconess Medical Center
Harvard Medical School
Boston, Massachusetts

David C. Cadena Jr., MD[†]
Assistant Professor
Department of Family and Community
    Medicine
University of Texas Health Science
    Center at San Antonio
San Antonio, Texas

Boris Calderon, DO
Department of Internal Medicine
Cape Fear Valley Health System
Fayetteville, North Carolina

Angela Pauline Patawaran Calimag, MD,
    BSN, RN, MAN
Resident Physician
Department of Internal Medicine
Advocate Christ Medical Center
Oak Lawn, Illinois

Caroline R. Campbell, MD[†]
Department of General Surgery
Medical College of Georgia at Augusta
    University
Augusta, Georgia

Justin Paul Canakis, DO
Resident Doctor
Department of Internal Medicine
George Washington University
Washington, District of Columbia

Etny Raul Candelario, MD, MS
Department of Family and Community
    Medicine
University of Texas Health Science Center
San Antonio, Texas

Dana G. Carroll, PharmD, BCPS,
  CDCES, BCGP
Clinical Professor
Department of Pharmacy Practice
Auburn University Harrison School of
  Pharmacy
Tuscaloosa, Alabama

Kitty Brigitta Carter-Wicker, MD[†]
Associate Professor
Department of Family Medicine
Morehouse School of Medicine
Atlanta, Georgia

Casandra Cashman, MD, FAAFP
Assistant Director
Community East Family Medicine
  Residency Program
Indianapolis, Indiana

Jose Alejandro Castellanos, MD
Resident
Department of Family Medicine
San Joaquin General Hospital
French Camp, California

Michelle Caster, MD
Assistant Professor
Department of Family Medicine
University Hospitals
Cleveland, Ohio

Mary E. Cataletto, MD, FAAP, FCCP
Professor of Clinical Pediatrics
NYU Long Island School of Medicine
Mineola, New York

Erin Cathcart, MD, MPH
Resident Physician
Department of Family and Community
  Medicine
Penn State Health Milton S. Hershey
  Medical Center
Hershey, Pennsylvania

Jeanne M. Cawse-Lucas, MD
Associate Professor
Theodore J. Phillips Endowed Professor
  of Family Medicine
Department of Family Medicine
University of Washington
Seattle, Washington

Rachel Ceccarelli, DO, MPH
Resident Physician
Department of Family Medicine
University of Massachusetts Worcester
  Family Medicine Residency
Worcester, Massachusetts

Jan Cerny, MD, PhD[†]
Associate Professor of Medicine
Department of Medicine
Division of Hematology/Oncology
University of Massachusetts Medical
  School
Worcester, Massachusetts

Matthew Chabot, MD[†]
Worcester, Massachusetts

Joumana Chaiban, MD, MBA, FACE
Associate Professor of Medicine
Department of Internal Medicine
University of Illinois at Chicago/Advocate
  Christ Medical Center
Chicago, Illinois

Ronald G. Chambers Jr., MD, FAAFP[†]
Program Director
Department of Family Medicine
Dignity Health
Sacramento, California

Christine Chan, MD
Faculty
Hawaii Island Family Medicine Residency
Hilo, Hawaii

Molly E. Chandler, MD
Family Medicine Resident
Madigan Army Medical Center
Tacoma, Washington

Sangili Chandran, MD
Director Primary Care Sports Medicine
Advocate Christ Medical Center
Oak Lawn, Illinois
Associate Professor
Department of Family Medicine
Chicago Medical School
Roslind Franklin University of Medicine
  and Science
Chicago, Illinois

Felix B. Chang, MD, DABMA, ABIHM,
  ABIM
Director, Inpatient Service
University of Massachusetts Fitchburg
  Family Medicine Residency Program
Hospitalist, Family Medicine
University of Massachusetts Medical
  School
Worcester, Massachusetts
Hospitalist
Department of Hospital Medicine
University of Massachusetts Memorial
  Medical Group
Leominster, Massachusetts

Jennifer G. Chang, MD[†]
LtCol, USAF, MC
Department of Family Medicine Residency
96th Medical Group
Eglin Air Force Base, Florida

Juliana Chang, MD
Rheumatology Fellow
University of California, Irvine
Irvine, California

Jason Chao, MD, MS
Professor
Department of Family Medicine and
  Community Health
Case Western Reserve University and
  University Hospitals Cleveland Medical
  Center
Cleveland, Ohio

James T. Chapman, DO
PGY-2 Resident Physician
Novant Health Family Medicine
  Residency Program
Cornelius, North Carolina

Kathya M. Chartre, MD
Department of Family Medicine
AMITA Health Saint Joseph Hospital
  Chicago
Chicago, Illinois

Kimberly M. Chekan, DO, MPH
Physician
Department of Family Medicine
Novant Health Family Medicine
  Residency
Cornelius, North Carolina

Jeffrey Chen, MD
Clinical Instructor
Department of Internal Medicine
University of Texas at Houston,
  McGovern Medical School
Houston, Texas

Joseph A. Chen, MD
Resident, PGY-2
Department of Family Medicine
Tallahassee Memorial Healthcare
Tallahassee, Florida

Rensa Chen, DO
Resident Physician
Department of Family and Community
  Medicine
Penn State Health Milton S. Hershey
  Medical Center
Hershey, Pennsylvania

Tiffany Chen, DO
Resident Physician
Family and Community Medicine
    Residency Program
Mercy Health – Anderson Hospital
Cincinnati, Ohio

Ashley F. Chin, MD
Resident Physician
Department of Psychiatry
Advocate Lutheran General Hospital
Park Ridge, Illinois

Justin J. Chin, DO[†]
Capt, USAF, MC
Robins Air Force Base, Georgia

Edwin Y. Choi, MD, MS, FAAFP,
    DFPHM[†]
Associate Program Director
Department of Hospitalist Fellowship
Womack Army Medical Center
Fort Bragg, North Carolina

Lea S. Choi, DO
Resident Physician
Department of Family Medicine
Womack Army Medical Center
Fort Bragg, North Carolina

Ratnesh Chopra, MD
Assistant Professor of Medicine
University of Massachusetts Medical
    School
Worcester, Massachusetts

Sanjiv Chopra, MBBS, MACP
Professor of Medicine
Department of Beth Israel Deaconess
    Medical Center
Harvard Medical School
Boston, Massachusetts

Vasilios Chrisostomidis, DO
Associate Professor of Family Medicine
    and Community Medicine
Department of Family Medicine
University of Massachusetts Medical
    School
Worcester, Massachusetts

Dean A. Christian, MD[†]
Danville, Pennsylvania

Marissa T. Christian, PharmD
Clinical Pharmacy Specialist
Solid Organ Transplant
Penn State Health Milton S. Hershey
    Medical Center
Hershey, Pennsylvania

Justin Chu, DO
Emergency Medicine Physician
Vineland, New Jersey

Vivian Nnenna Chukwuma, MD
Resident
Department of Internal Medicine
Advocate Christ Medical Center
Oak Lawn, Illinois

Gustavo Churrango, MD
Advanced Gastroenterology
Central Main Medical Center
Lewiston, Maine

Joseph H. Cioffi, BA, MD
Resident
Department of Internal Medicine
George Washington University Hospital
Washington, District of Columbia

Michael Scott Clark, MD
Department of Neuroscience and
    Psychiatry
Outpatient Psychiatry
Market Liaison Institute
Novant Health
Charlotte, North Carolina

S. Lindsey Clarke, MD, FAAFP[†]
Medical University of South Carolina
    Area Health Education Consortium
    Professor (Greenwood/Family
    Medicine)
Director of Resident Education and
    Associate Program Director
Self Regional Healthcare
Greenwood, South Carolina

Karl T. Clebak, MD, MHA, FAAFP[†]
Associate Professor, Program Director
Department of Family and Community
    Medicine
Penn State Health Milton S. Hershey
    Medical Center
Hershey, Pennsylvania

Timothy J. Coker, MD, FAAFP[†]
Peterson Air Force Base, Colorado

Chelsea Elyse Cole, MD
Assistant Professor
UT Southwestern Medical Center
Dallas, Texas

Irene Coletsos, MD
Community Psychiatrist
Department of Behavioral Health
VinFen, Department of Mental Health
Quincy, Massachusetts

Jennifer R. Collins, PharmD
Clinical Pharmacy Specialist–Ambulatory
    Care
Community Health Network
Indianapolis, Indiana

Giancarlo Colón Rosa, MD
Resident Physician
Department of Internal Medicine
George Washington University Hospital
Washington, District of Columbia

Christina Colosimo, DO, MS
Chief Resident
Department of Trauma Surgery
Cooper University Hospital
Camden, New Jersey

Patrick Sean Connell, MD, PhD
Fellow
Department of Pediatric Cardiology
Baylor College of Medicine
Houston, Texas

Christina Conrad, DO
Department of Pediatric Emergency
    Medicine
Phoenix Children's Hospital
Phoenix, Arizona

Stephanie L. Conway-Allen, PharmD, RPh
Associate Professor
Department of Pharmacy Practice
Massachusetts College of Pharmacy and
    Health Sciences University
Worcester, Massachusetts

Ronald L. Cook, DO, MBA
Professor
Department of Family and Community
    Medicine
Texas Tech University Health Sciences
    Center School of Medicine
Lubbock, Texas

Tonya M. Cook, PharmD
Faculty, Clinical Pharmacist
Department of Family Medicine
    Residency
St. Mary's Medical Center Family
    Medicine Residency
Grand Junction, Colorado

Chloe Sabine Courchesne, MD
Assistant Professor
Department of Family Medicine
University of California, Irvine
Irvine, California

John Coward, MD
Hospitalist
Prisma Health
Columbia, South Carolina

Mary E. Cox, DO
Resident Physician
Department of Family Medicine
Novant Health Family Medicine
    Residency Program
Cornelius, North Carolina

Julie A. Creech, DO[†]
Family Medicine Physician, Sports
　Medicine Physician, Primary Care
　Sports Medicine Fellow
United States Air Force

Jason Cross, PharmD, BCPS, BCACP
Associate Professor of Pharmacy Practice
Massachusetts College of Pharmacy and
　Health Sciences University
Worcester, Massachusetts

Hongyi Cui, MD, PhD
Associate Professor of Surgery,
　Associate Director, Acute Care Surgery
Department of Surgery
University of Massachusetts Memorial
　Medical Center
Worcester, Massachusetts

Yuhamy Curbelo-Peña, MD[†]
Department of General Surgery
Vic University Hospital
Vic, Barcelona, Spain

Yulibeth Curbelo Peña, MD
Rehabilitation Department
Vall D'Hebron Hospital
Barcelona, Spain

Cragin D. Currence, MD
General Surgery Resident
Spartanburg Regional Health System
Spartanburg, South Carolina

Tina D'Amato, DO
Attending Family Physician
Charlotte Family Medicine
Charlotte, Vermont

Apaar Dadlani, MBBS
Resident Physician
Department of Internal Medicine
University of Louisville
Louisville, Kentucky

Jennifer Daily, MD
Associate Professor
Department of Family and Geriatric
　Medicine
University of Louisville School of Medicine
Louisville, Kentucky

Heather Ann Dalton, MD, FAAFP[†]
Hospice and Palliative Medicine Fellow
Department of Internal Medicine
UT Southwestern Medical Center
Dallas, Texas

Paul E. Daniel Jr., MD[†]
University of Massachusetts Medical
　School
University of Massachusetts Memorial
　Medical Center
Worcester, Massachusetts

Hillary J. Darrow, MD
Family Medicine Resident
Department of Family Medicine
　Residency
Carl R. Darnall Army Medical Center
Fort Hood, Texas

Akhil Das, MD, FACS
Professor
Department of Urology
Thomas Jefferson University
Philadelphia, Pennsylvania

Shilpa Das, DO, MS
Resident Physician
Department of Family Medicine
University of Maryland Medical Center
Baltimore, Maryland

Adrian DaSilva-DeAbreu, MD
Fellow
John Ochsner Heart & Vascular Institute
New Orleans, Louisiana

James Evan Davidson, MD
Chief Resident
Department of Internal Medicine
Augusta University Medical Center
Augusta, Georgia

Sarah E. Davis, DO
Physician
Department of Obstetrics and
　Gynecology
Cleveland Clinic Akron General
Akron, Ohio

Christopher Davis, MD, MPH
Resident Physician
Department of Family and Community
　Medicine
Penn State Health Milton S. Hershey
　Medical Center
Hershey, Pennsylvania

Fehima C. Dawy, MD
Resident
Department of Family and Community
　Medicine
University of Texas Health Science
　Center at San Antonio
San Antonio, Texas

Ana De Diego, MD
Resident Physician
Department of Internal Medicine
University of Miami at Holy Cross
Miami, Florida

Niyomi De Silva, MD
Associate Program Director
Department of Family Medicine
HCA Medical City Arlington
Arlington, Texas

Iain W. Decker, DO
Resident Physician
Department of Ophthalmology
Kettering Health Network Grandview
　Medical Center
Dayton, Ohio

Edward M. Degerman, MD
Sports Medicine Fellow
Department of Sports Medicine
SUNY Downstate Health Sciences
　University
Brooklyn, New York

Henry Del Rosario, MD
Assistant Professor
Department of Family Medicine and
　Community Health
University of Massachusetts Memorial
　Medical School
Worcester, Massachusetts

Collen del Valle, DO
Doctor of Osteopathic Medicine
University of North Texas Health Science
　Center
Texas College of Osteopathic Medicine
Fort Worth, Texas

Emilee J. Delbridge, PhD, LMFT
Assistant Professor of Clinical Family
　Medicine
Indianapolis, Indiana

Konstantinos E. Deligiannidis, MD, MPH,
　FAAFP
Assistant Professor
Department of Family Medicine
Donald and Barbara Zucker School of
　Medicine at Hofstra/Northwell
Hempstead, New York

Melissa Dennis, MD, MHA
Associate Chairman
OB Hospitalist
Department of Obstetrics and Gynecology
Advocate Illinois Masonic Medical Center
Chicago, Illinois

Yatri Desai, BS
Fourth Year Medical Student
Chicago College of Osteopathic Medicine
Midwestern University
Downers Grove, Illinois

Henry DeYoung, MD[†]
Lieutenant, VFA-106 Flight Surgeon
Department of Aviation Medicine
Virginia Beach, Virginia

Shaoshan Ding, MD
Practicing Physician

Laith Rommel Dinkha, DO
General Cardiologist
Department of Cardiology
Brooke Army Medical Center
Fort Sam Houston, Texas

Rebecca Dix, MD[†]
Springfield, Illinois

Amanda D. Dobbins, MD
Medical Resident
Department of Family Medicine
    Residency
Advocate Christ
Chicago, Illinois

Charles Doerner, DO
Fellow
Department of Cardiovascular Medicine
Largo Medical Center
Largo, Florida

Frank J. Domino, MD
Professor and Director of Predoctoral
    Education
Department of Family Medicine and
    Community Health
University of Massachusetts Medical
    School
Worcester, Massachusetts

Audrey Dong, DO
Resident
Department of Family Medicine
Penn State Health
State College, Pennsylvania

Heather C. Doty, DO
Novant Health Family Medicine
    Residency Program
Cornelius, North Carolina

Kyler M. Douglas, DO
Resident Doctor
Department of Family Medicine
Saint Louis University
St. Louis, Missouri

Joanna Drowos, DO, MPH, MBA
Associate Dean for Faculty Affairs
Associate Professor of Family Medicine
Charles E. Schmidt College of Medicine
Florida Atlantic University
Boca Raton, Florida

Sakshi Duggal, MBBS
Department of Family Medicine
Creighton University
Omaha, Nebraska

Maurice Duggins, MD, FAAFP
Faculty
Clinical Associate Professor
Department of Family and Community
    Medicine
Ascension Via Christi Family Medicine
    Residency
Kansas University School of Medicine–
    Wichita
Wichita, Kansas

Noel Dunn, MD[†]
Staff Physician
Department of Family Medicine
Madigan Army Medical Center
Tacoma, Washington

Maegen Dupper, MD
Associate Dean of Clinical Curriculum
Associate Professor of Medical
    Education, Family Medicine
California University of Science and
    Medicine
Colton, California

Muhammad I. Durrani, DO, MS[†]
Assistant Research Director, Core Faculty
Department of Emergency Medicine
Inspira Medical Center
Vineland, New Jersey

Sudeshna Dutta, MD
Resident
Department of Family Medicine
Creighton University
Omaha, Nebraska

Stephany Giraldo Eierle, DO, MPH
UMass Memorial WFMR PGY-2
Worcester, Massachusetts

Safiya Elahi, DO
Resident Physician
Department of Internal Medicine
University of Illinois at Chicago/Advocate
    Christ Medical Center
Oak Lawn, Illinois

William G. Elder, PhD
Professor and Chair
Department of Behavioral and Social
    Sciences
University of Houston
Houston, Texas

Pamela Ellsworth, MD
Professor of Urology
University of Central Florida
Orlando, Florida

Sara Elsayed, MD
Clinical Assistant Professor
Department of Family Medicine
MSU/MidMichigan Medical Center-
    Gratiot Family Medicine Residency
    Program
Alma, Michigan

Mohamad Elzaim, MD
Resident
Department of Family Medicine
Medical City Arlington
Arlington, Texas

Deborah R. Erlich, MD, MMedEd,
    FAAFP
Associate Professor
Department of Family Medicine
Family Medicine Clerkship Director
Tufts University School of Medicine
Boston, Massachusetts

Brooke Ersland, MD
Faculty
Department of Family Medicine
Methodist Charlton Family Medicine
    Residency
Dallas, Texas

Justin T. Ertle, MD
Assistant Professor
Department of Internal Medicine
Medical College of Georgia at Augusta
    University
Augusta, Georgia

Emily J. Eshleman, DO, MS
Resident Physician
Department of Family Medicine
University of Massachusetts Medical
    School
Worcester, Massachusetts

Frank Estrella, DO[†]
Department of Family Medicine
Riverside Methodist Hospital
Columbus, Ohio

Tyler Evans, DO
Resident PGY3
UT Southwestern Medical Center
Dallas, Texas

Pang-Yen Fan, MD
Professor of Medicine
Division of Renal Medicine
University of Massachusetts Medical
    School
Worcester, Massachusetts

Veronica Farrell, MSN, NP-C
Worcester, Massachusetts

Omofolarin Fasuyi, MD, MPH, FAAFP
Assistant Professor
Department of Family Medicine
Morehouse School of Medicine
Atlanta, Georgia

Rhonda A. Faulkner, PhD[†]
Director of Behavioral Medicine
Department of Family Medicine
AMITA Health Saint Joseph Hospital
    Chicago
University of Illinois College of Medicine
    Master Affiliate
Chicago, Illinois

Jeffrey P. Feden, MD, FACEP
Associate Professor, Clinician Educator
Department of Emergency Medicine
The Warren Alpert Medical School of
    Brown University
Providence, Rhode Island

A. Susan Feeney, DNP, FNP-BC, NP-C
Assistant Professor
Director of Nurse Practitioner Specialties
Graduate School of Nursing
University of Massachusetts Medical
    School
Worcester, Massachusetts

Ryan B. Feeney, PharmD, BCPS, BCGP
Clinical Pharmacist
Philadelphia, Pennsylvania

Neil Feldman, DPM[†]
Central Massachusetts Podiatry, PC
Worcester, Massachusetts

Nolan P. Feola, MD[†]
Capt., Eglin Air Force Base Family
    Medicine Residency
Eglin Air Force Base, Florida

Scott A. Fields, MD, MHA
Adjunct Associate Professor of Family
    Medicine
Oregon Health & Science University
Portland, Oregon

Matthew J. Filippo, DO
Associate Professor, Teaching/Clinical
    Psychiatrist
Department of Psychiatry
Advocate Lutheran General Hospital
Park Ridge, Illinois

Stanley Fineman, MD
Adjunct Associate Professor
Department of Pediatrics
Emory University School of Medicine
Atlanta, Georgia

Jorge Finke, MD
Bowdoin Street Health Center
Boston, Massachusetts

Megan Finneran, DO, MS
Resident Physician
Department of Neurosurgery
Carle BroMenn Medical Center
Normal, Illinois

Stephen Firkins, MD
Resident Physician
Department of Internal Medicine
The Ohio State University Wexner
    Medical Center
Columbus, Ohio

Zedeena Fisher, MD
Bayfront Health
St. Petersburg, Florida

Dylan T. Flaherty, DO
Internal Medicine Resident - PGY2
University of Louisville Health
Louisville, Kentucky

Theodore B. Flaum, DO
Associate Professor
Department of Osteopathic Manipulative
    Medicine
NYIT College of Osteopathic Medicine
Old Westbury, New York

Kyle J. Fletke, MD
Assistant Professor
Department of Family and Community
    Medicine
University of Maryland School of
    Medicine
Baltimore, Maryland

Suzanne Florczyk, PharmD
Clinical Pharmacist
Novant Health
Cornelius, North Carolina

Joseph A. Florence, MD
Professor and Director of Rural Programs
Department of Family Medicine
East Tennessee State University James
    H. Quillen College of Medicine
Johnson City, Tennessee

Michael P. Flynn, MD, MHS
Staff Physician
Atrius Health
PMG Physician Associates
Bourne, Massachusetts

Jay Fong, MD[†]
Assistant Professor
Department of Pediatrics
Division of Gastroenterology, Nutrition,
    and Hepatology
University of Massachusetts Medical
    School
Worcester, Massachusetts

Jane M. Forbes, MD
Chief Resident
UVA Family Medicine
Charlottesville, Virginia

Jennifer G. Foster, MD, MBA, FACP
Associate Professor of Medicine
Charles E. Schmidt College of Medicine
Boca Raton, Florida

Zoe Foster, MD, FAAFP
Program Director
Department of Family and Preventive
    Medicine
Prisma Health
University of South Carolina
Columbia, South Carolina

Danita R. Fox, MD
Family Medicine
Philadelphia, Pennsylvania

Robert L. Frachtman, MD, FACG
Clinical Assistant Professor of Internal
    Medicine
Department of Internal Medicine/
    Gastroenterology
Dell Medical School, The University of
    Texas at Austin
Austin, Texas

Daniel Jason Frasca, DO
Assistant Professor
Department of Soldier Care
Eisenhower Army Medical Center
Fort Gordon, Georgia

Erin Fredrickson, DO, MPH
Department of Family Medicine
University of Washington
Seattle, Washington

Eva Fremaint, MPAS, DMSc
PA-C
Department of U.S. Army

Bruce Palmer Freshley Jr., MD
Prisma Health
University of South Carolina School of
    Medicine-Greenville
Greenville, South Carolina

Minjin Fromm, MD
Assistant Professor
Department of Orthopedics and Physical
    Rehabilitation
University of Massachusetts Medical
    School
Worcester, Massachusetts

Katherine Gagan, MD
PGY-3
Tidelands Health MUSC Family Medicine
    Residency
Myrtle Beach, South Carolina

Steven W. Gale, MD
MCW-Prevea Family Medicine Residency
    Program
Green Bay, Wisconsin

Kelsey Gallagher, DO
Family Medicine
Amita Health Saint Joseph Hospital
Chicago, Illinois

Moises Gallegos, MD, MPH
Clerkship Director
Clinical Assistant Professor
Department of Emergency Medicine
Stanford University School of Medicine
Stanford, California

William T. Garrison, PhD†
Professor of Pediatrics
Department of Pediatrics
University of Massachusetts Medical
    School
Worcester, Massachusetts

Tamara L. Gayle, MD, MEd
Department of Pediatric Hospital Medicine
Children's National Medical Center
Washington, District of Columbia

Mawuse K. Gbegnon, MD
Resident
Department of Family Medicine
Novant Health Family Medicine
    Residency Program
Cornelius, North Carolina

Kamini Geer, MD, MPH
Program Director
AdventHealth Family Medicine Residency
East Orlando, Florida

Joanne E. Genewick, DO, FAIHM
Assistant Professor of Family Medicine
Mayo Clinic Alix School of Medicine
Assistant Professor of Family Medicine
Department of Family Medicine and
    Community Health
University of Minnesota
Consultant
Mayo Clinic Health System-Eastridge
Mankato, Minnesota

Michelle A. Georgia, DO
Resident Physician
Department of Pediatrics
University of Massachusetts
Worcester, Massachusetts

Fereshteh Gerayli, MD, FAAFP
Professor of Family Medicine
Johnson City Family Medicine Residency
    Program
James H. Quillen College of Medicine
East Tennessee State University
Johnson City, Tennessee

M. Alex Germano, MD
Assistant Professor
Department of Family and Community
    Medicine
Penn State College of Medicine
Hershey, Pennsylvania

Evangelos Giakoumatos, MD, MSc
Department of Family Medicine
Creighton University
Omaha, Nebraska

Lawrence M. Gibbs, MD, MSEd
Core Faculty
Department of Family Medicine
Methodist Family Medicine Residency
    Program
Dallas, Texas

Megan Gibson, MD†
Huntsville, Alabama

Cameron S. Gilbert, MD, USAF, CSARME†
Flight Surgeon
Moody Air Force Base, Georgia

Stephanie A. Gill, MD, MPH
Assistant Professor
Department of Family and Community
    Medicine
Penn State Health Milton S. Hershey
    Medical Center
Hershey, Pennsylvania

Daniel V. Girzadas Jr., MD
Department of Emergency Medicine
University of Illinois
Chicago, Illinois
Department of Emergency Medicine
Advocate Christ Medical Center
Oak Lawn, Illinois

Brian C. Glaser, MD
Family Medicine Residency Clinic
David Grant Medical Center
Travis Air Force Base, California

Erin M. Glembocki, MD
Resident Physician
Department of Family Medicine
ProHealth Care
Waukesha, Wisconsin

Lawrence Go, MD
Resident
Department of Family and Community
    Medicine
Penn State College of Medicine
Hershey, Pennsylvania

Krystyna Guinevere Golden, MD†
Resident Physician
Eglin Family Medicine Residency
Eglin Air Force Base Hospital
Eglin Air Force Base, Florida

Jeremy Golding, MD, FAAFP
Professor of Family Medicine and
    Obstetrics & Gynecology
University of Massachusetts Medical
    School
Department of Family Medicine and
    Community Health
University of Massachusetts Memorial
    Health Care
Hahnemann Family Health Center
Worcester, Massachusetts

Naga Bharani Goparaju, MD
Johnston Memorial Hospital
Abingdon, Virginia

Fredric D. Gordon, MD, FAASLD, AGAF
Professor of Medicine
Department of Transplantation and
    Hepatobiliary Diseases
Lahey Hospital & Medical Center
Burlington, Massachusetts

Melanie Rose Gordon, MD
Associate Professor
Core Teaching Faculty
Department of Internal Medicine
    Residency Program
Advocate Christ Medical Center
Oak Lawn, Illinois

Emily Ann Gorman, DO
Assistant Program Director
Department of Family Medicine
OhioHealth Riverside Family Medicine
Columbus, Ohio

Kiyomi K. Goto, DO
Assistant Professor
Department of Family and Community
    Medicine
Penn State Health
State College, Pennsylvania

Ginny L. Gottschalk, MD
Associate Professor
Department of Family and Community
    Medicine
University of Kentucky College of
    Medicine
Lexington, Kentucky

Nivas Govindarajan, MD, BS
Resident Physician
Department of North Texas GME
HCA Medical City Arlington
Arlington, Texas

Stephen Graber, MD
Loma Linda, California

Kristina Gracey, MD, MPH
Assistant Professor
Department of Family Medicine and
  Community Health
University of Massachusetts
Worcester, Massachusetts

Jennifer Grana, DO
Department of Family and Community
  Medicine
Penn State Health Milton S. Hershey
  Medical Center
Hershey, Pennsylvania

Mary Joyce Green, MD
Assistant Professor
Department of Family and Community
  Medicine
Penn State College of Medicine
Penn State Health Milton S. Hershey
  Medical Center
Hershey, Pennsylvania

Michael Allen Greene, MD
Program Director
Department of Family Medicine
Creighton University
Omaha, Nebraska

Ramanpreet Grewal, MD
Family Medicine
Galesburg Cottage Hospital
Galesburg, Illinois

Simon B. Griesbach, MD[†]
Assistant Director
Department of Family Medicine
Waukesha Family Medicine Residency at
  ProHealth Care
Waukesha, Wisconsin
Clinical Adjunct Assistant Professor
Department of Family Medicine and
  Community Health
Madison, Wisconsin
Assistant Clinical Professor
Department of Family and Community
  Medicine
Medical College of Wisconsin
Milwaukee, Wisconsin

Andrew Grimes, MD
Affiliate Clinical Faculty
Department of Perioperative Medicine
Dell Medical School, The University of
  Texas at Austin
Austin, Texas

Rebecca Groch, MD
Resident
Novant Health Department of Family
  Medicine Residency Program
Cornelius, North Carolina

Jennifer Grumet, MD
Clinical Assistant Professor
PA Studies Program
Chapman University
Irvine, California

Ankur Sudhir Gupta, MD, MS
Ophthalmologist
Department of Ophthalmology
Geisinger
Danville, Pennsylvania

Neena R. Gupta, MD[†]
Associate Professor
Department of Pediatric Nephrology
UMass Memorial Medical Center
Worcester, Massachusetts

Smriti Gupta, MD
Resident Physician
Department of Family Medicine
Penn State Health
State College, Pennsylvania

Sonia Gupta, MD
Resident
Department of Internal Medicine
Creighton University
Omaha, Nebraska

Zelibeth Gutierrez, MD
Department of Family Medicine
Tallahassee Memorial HealthCare Family
  Medicine Residency Program
Tallahassee, Florida

Christina Gutta, MD
Clinical Assistant Professor for
  Emergency Medicine and Primary Care
  Sports Medicine
Prisma Health-Upstate
Greenville, South Carolina

Emmeline Ha, MD
Health Policy Research Fellow
George Washington University
Washington, District of Columbia

Michael Haddadin, MD
Fellow
Department of Hematology Oncology
University of Massachusetts
Worcester, Massachusetts

Reem Hadi, MD
Board-Certified Family Physician
San Antonio, Texas

Janelle K. Hadley, MD, MPH
Resident Physician
Department of Family Medicine
Advocate Christ Family Medicine
  Residency
Oak Lawn, Illinois

Uruj Kamal Haider, MD
Assistant Professor
Department of Psychiatry
UMass Memorial
Worcester, Massachusetts

Shadi Hamdeh, MD
Department of Internal Medicine
Creighton University School of Medicine
Omaha, Nebraska

Hayley Bryton Hamilton-Bevil, MD, MPH
Resident
Department of Family Medicine
University of Texas Health San Antonio
San Antonio, Texas

Chad Hamner, MD
Medical Director
Department of Pediatric Trauma
Cook Children's Medical Center
Fort Worth, Texas

Robin Kang Hans, MD, MPH
Department of Family Medicine
San Joaquin General Hospital
French Camp, California

Thomas J. Hansen, MD[†]
System Vice President Chief Academic
  Officer
Department of Academic Affairs
Advocate Aurora Health
Downers Grove, Illinois

Allison Hargreaves, MD
Assistant Professor
Family Medicine and Community Health
University of Massachusetts Medical School
Worcester, Massachusetts

Ghulam Abbas Harrie, MD[†]
Faculty
PGH Family Medicine
Pontiac, Michigan

Colleen M. Harrington, MD, FACC, FASE
Assistant Professor of Medicine
Division of Cardiology
University of Massachusetts Medical School
Worcester, Massachusetts

Alyssa Jeanne Vest Hart, DO
Program Director
Department of Family Medicine
AMITA Health Saint Joseph Hospital Chicago
Chicago, Illinois

Madie D. Hartman, DO
Assistant Professor
Department of Family and Community Medicine
Penn State Health Milton S. Hershey Medical Center
Hershey, Pennsylvania

Fern R. Hauck, MD, MS
Professor
Department of Public Health Sciences
Department of Family Medicine
University of Virginia School of Medicine
Charlottesville, Virginia

Leesha A. Helm, MD, MPH
Assistant Professor
Department of Family and Community Medicine
Penn State Health Milton S. Hershey Medical Center
Hershey, Pennsylvania

Kayla Hempel, MD
Department of Emergency Department
Inspira Medical Center
Vineland, New Jersey

Scott T. Henderson, MD
Director Medical Services
Department of Student Health Center
University of Missouri
Columbia, Missouri

Matthew E. Herberg, MD[†]
Assistant Professor
Department of Otolaryngology
William Beaumont Army Medical Center
El Paso, Texas

Pablo I. Hernandez Itriago, MD, MHCM, FAAFP
Assistant Professor
Department of Family Medicine
University of Massachusetts Medical School
Chief Medical Officer
Edward M. Kennedy Community Health Center
Worcester, Massachusetts

Christopher R. Heron, MD, BS
Associate Professor
Department of Family and Community Medicine
Penn State Health Milton S. Hershey Medical Center
Hershey, Pennsylvania

Brian Hertz, MD[†]
Internal Medicine
Kaiser Permanente
San Rafael, California

Lisa Hertz, MD
Comprehensive GI Care
Los Alamitos, California

Joseph L. Hesse, MD
Resident Physician
Family Medicine Residency Program
Dell Medical School, The University of Texas at Austin
Austin, Texas

Mark L. Higdon, DO, FAAFP
Program Director
Novant Health Family Medicine Residency Program
Cornelius, North Carolina

Marilyn Hines, DO
Program Director
Chickasaw Nation Family Medicine Residency
Ada, Oklahoma

Kevin Hoang, MD
Resident
Department of Medicine
St. Elizabeth's Medical Center
Boston, Massachusetts

Linh Hoang, DO[†]
Family Medicine Physician
Houston, Texas

Joseph D. Hogue, MD, MBA
Program Director, Family Medicine Residency
Program Director, Transitional Year Residency
Division Chief, Mississippi Family Medicine
Baptist Memorial Hospital Desoto
Southaven, Mississippi

N. Wilson Holland, MD, FACP
Master Clinician Clinical Distinction, Adjunct Associate Professor
Department of Internal Medicine
Emory University School of Medicine
Atlanta, Georgia

Allison Holley, MD
Assistant Professor of Family Medicine
Florida Atlantic University College of Medicine
Boca Raton, Florida

Thomas Holmes, MD
Attending Physician
Lutheran General Hospital
Park Ridge, Illinois

Steven B. Holsten Jr., MD, FACS
Professor of Surgery
Vice Chair of Surgical Operations
Augusta University
Augusta, Georgia

Stanton C. Honig, MD[†]
Clinical Professor of Urology
Department of Urology
Yale University School of Medicine
New Haven, Connecticut

Maeve K. Hopkins, MD, MA[†]
Fellow, Maternal–Fetal Medicine
Hospital of the University of Pennsylvania
Philadelphia, Pennsylvania

Michael P. Hopkins, MD, MEd[†]
Professor
Department of Obstetrics and Gynecology
Northeast Ohio Medical University
Aultman Hospital
Canton, Ohio

Laura C. Horton, MD[†]
Gastroenterology Fellow
Department of Gastroenterology and Hepatology
Beth Israel Deaconess Medical Center
Chief Medical Resident
Department of Medicine
Brigham and Women's Hospital
Boston, Massachusetts

Matthew Houle, BS
Department of Gastroenterology and Liver Diseases
George Washington University School of Medicine and Health Sciences
Washington, District of Columbia

Steven A. House, MD, FAAFP, FAAHPM, HMDC
Professor
Department of Family and Geriatric Medicine
University of Louisville
Louisville, Kentucky

Jordan Howard-Young, MD
Assistant Professor
Department of Family Medicine and
    Community Health
UMass Chan Medical School
Worcester, Massachusetts

Amoreena Ranck Howell, MD, MSPH
Assistant Professor
Department of Family and Community
    Medicine
University of Maryland School of Medicine
Baltimore, Maryland

Dennis E. Hughes, DO, FACEP
360 Degree Medicine
Branson, Missouri

Pamela R. Hughes, MD[†]
Military Program Director
Department of Family Medicine
St Louis University (Southwest Illinois)
    Family Medicine Residency
O'Fallon, Illinois

Sarah Hutchings, MD
Southern Illinois University Family
    Medicine Residency
Springfield, Illinois

Michael Ibrahem, MD
Department of Family Medicine
University of Pittsburgh Medical Center
Pittsburgh, Pennsylvania

Antony Y. Ibrahim, MD
Resident Physician
Department of Family Medicine
Medical City Arlington
Arlington, Texas

Adedapo Iluyomade, MD, MBA
Clinical Faculty
Division of Cardiology
University of Miami Hospital and Clinics
Miami, Florida

Nathaniel John Irvine, MD[†]
Naval Hospital Jacksonville
Jacksonville, Florida

Bashyam Iyengar, MD, MPH
Ascension St. Vincent Family Residency
    Program
Jacksonville, Florida

Adam Jacob, DO
Resident
Department of Internal Medicine
George Washington University Hospital
Washington, District of Columbia

Siddharth Jain, BA
Chicago College of Osteopathic Medicine
Midwestern University
Downers Grove, Illinois

Vasudha Jain, MD
Myrtle Beach, South Carolina

Akash Jani, MD
Resident Physician
Department of Obstetrics & Gynecology
Advocate Illinois Masonic Medical Center
Chicago, Illinois

Ecler Ercole Jaqua, MD, DipABLM,
    DipABOM, FAAFP
Assistant Professor
Loma Linda, California

Melissa Jefferis, MD, FAAFP
Associate Program Director
Family Medicine Residency Program
Riverside Methodist Hospital
Columbus, Ohio

Sandya Gul Jiandani, MD
Family Medicine Resident PGY-3
Tallahassee Memorial Hospital Family
    Medicine Residency Program
Tallahassee, Florida

Dongsheng Jiang, MD, MSc
Associate Professor
Penn State University
State College, Pennsylvania

Joanna Jiang, MD
Medical Resident
Ohio State University
Columbus, Ohio

Nasheena Jiwa, MD
Physician/Fellow
Department of Pulmonary and Critical Care
University of Connecticut Health Center
Farmington, Connecticut

Brett Johnson, MD
Program Director, Family Medicine
Methodist Health System
Dallas, Texas

Jessica Johnson, MD, MPH
Clinical Assistant Professor
Department of Family Medicine
Brown University
Providence, Rhode Island

Tisha K. Johnson, MD, MPH[†]
Assistant Professor
Department of Preventive Medicine and
    Environmental Health
University of Kentucky
Lexington, Kentucky

Rutendo Jokomo-Nyakabau, MD
Physician
Creighton University
Omaha, Nebraska

Caitlin E. Jones, MD
General Surgery Resident
Department of Surgery
Medical College of Georgia
Augusta, Georgia

Stacy L. Jones, MD, MHA, FASA
The University of Arkansas for Medical
    Sciences
Little Rock, Arkansas

Melody A. Jordahl-Iafrato, MD, FAAFP
Assistant Program Director
Community Hospital East Family
    Medicine Residency
Department of Family Medicine
Community Hospital East
Indianapolis, Indiana

Jillian Joseph, MPAS, PA-C
Assistant Professor
Department of PA Studies
MCPHS University
Clinical Instructor
Department of Family Medicine and
    Community Health
UMass Medical School
Worcester, Massachusetts

Nisarg Joshi, MD, BS
Junior Attending, Vitreoretinal Surgery
    Fellow
Department of Ophthalmology
University of South Florida
Tampa, Florida

Vaidehi Joshi, MD, MHA
Resident Physician
Department of Family Medicine
Mount Carmel Health System
Westerville, Ohio

Patrick Wakefield Joyner, MD, MS[†]
Assistant Professor
Department of Orthopaedic Surgery
OrthoCollier
Naples, Florida

Khadija Kabani, DO, FAAFP
Associate Program Director
Department of Family Medicine
Methodist Health System
Dallas, Texas

Natasha S. Kadakia, DO[†]
Resident
Department of Internal Medicine
Advocate Christ Medical Center
Oak Lawn, Illinois

Afsha Rais Kaisani, MD
Core Faculty
Medical City Arlington Family Medicine
    Residency Program - HCA Medical
    City Healthcare UNT-TCU Graduate
    Medical Education Consortium
Arlington, Texas

Mwangi Kamau, MD
University of Massachusetts Medical School
Worcester, Massachusetts

Elijah Kamermans, MD
Resident
Department of Family and Community
    Medicine
Penn State University
State College, Pennsylvania

Evan Kang, MD†
Clinical Faculty
Lutheran General Hospital
Park Ridge, Illinois

Lovella Kanu, MD, FAAFP, Dipl. ABOM
Assistant Program Director
Advocate Family Medicine Residency
    Program
Oak Lawn, Illinois

Rahul Kapur, MD
Assistant Professor
Department of Family Medicine and
    Community Health
University of Minnesota
Minneapolis, Minnesota

Nioti Karim, MD
Houston, Texas

Mansi Katkar, MD
Resident Physician
Department of Internal Medicine
Advocate Lutheran General Hospital
Park Ridge, Illinois

Ravneet Kaur, MD
Department of Family Medicine
Creighton University School of Medicine
Omaha, Nebraska

Roop Kiran Kaur, MD
Voluntary Faculty
UB Rural Family Medicine Program
Olean, New York

Clara M. Keegan, MD
Associate Professor
Department of Family Medicine
The Robert Larner, M.D. College of
    Medicine at The University of Vermont
Burlington, Vermont

Darin N. Kennedy, MD
Assistant Professor
Atrium Health Family Medicine
Atrium CMC Mercy
Charlotte, North Carolina

Anila Khaliq, MD
Faculty
Department of Family Medicine
Touro College of Osteopathic Medicine
Middletown, New York

Niti N. Khambhati, MD
Resident Physician
Department of Family Medicine
Methodist Health System
Dallas, Texas

Husna Khan, DO
Resident
Department of Internal Medicine
Advocate Christ Medical Center
Oak Lawn, Illinois

Umair Usman Khan, MD
Resident Physician
Department of Family Medicine
Creighton University Family Medicine
Omaha, Nebraska

Natasha S. Khokhar, DO, MPH
Department of Family Medicine
San Joaquin General Hospital
French Camp, California

Barbara M. Kiersz Muller, DO
Family and Osteopathic Medicine
    Physician
Austin Regional Clinic—Far West
Austin, Texas

Gemma Kim, MD
Associate Professor
Department of Family Medicine
Desert Regional Medical Center
Palm Springs, California

Hyunyoung G. Kim, MD, MPH
Department of Family and Community
    Medicine
UT Health San Antonio
San Antonio, Texas

Judy Lu Kim, MD
People's Community Clinic
Austin, Texas

Peter Kim, MD
Medical City Arlington
Arlington, Texas

Walter M. Kim, MD, PhD
Lecturer
Department of Medicine
Harvard Medical School
Associate Physician
Division of Gastroenterology, Hepatology
    and Endoscopy
Brigham and Women's Hospital
Chief
Department of Gastroenterology
Lemuel Shattuck Hospital
Boston, Massachusetts

Brian J. Kimbrell, MD, FACS
Assistant Professor of Surgery
University of Florida
Trauma Medical Director
Medical Director of Critical Care
    Medicine
Blake Medical Center
Bradenton, Florida

LaRaey King, DO
Orlando, Florida

Thomas Kingsley, MD, MPH, MS
Assistant Professor of Medicine
Mayo Clinic
Rochester, Minnesota

Cecilia M. Kipnis, MD, FAAFP†
Assistant Program Director
Department of Family Medicine
Naval Hospital Jacksonville
Jacksonville, Florida

Ryan Kipp, MD, BS
Resident Physician
Department of Family and Community
    Medicine
Penn State Health Milton S. Hershey
    Medical Center
Hershey, Pennsylvania

Robert Kirchoff, MD, FASAM
Assistant Professor of Medicine
Alix School of Science and Medicine
Division of Hospital Internal Medicine
Mayo Clinic
Rochester, Minnesota

Marni Klessman Gleiber, MD
Assistant Professor of Physical Medicine
    and Rehabilitation
Florida Atlantic University, Charles E.
    Schmidt College of Medicine
Boca Raton, Florida

Laura K. Klug, PharmD
Associate Professor
Department of Pharmacy Practice and
    Family and Community Medicine
Creighton University
Omaha, Nebraska

Egle Klugiene, MD
Faculty Physician
Department of Family Medicine
MidMichigan Medical Center
Gratiot, Michigan

Daniel Kniaz, MD
Associate Director
Division of Nephrology
Lutheran General Hospital
Park Ridge, Illinois

Phillip Knouse, MD
Fellow Physician
Department of Hematology Oncology
Advocate Lutheran General Hospital
Park Ridge, Illinois

Sharon L. Koehler, DO, FACS[†]
Assistant Professor, Breast Surgery
Department of Clinical Specialties
New York Institute of Technology College
    of Osteopathic Medicine
Old Westbury, New York

Sydney E. Koenig, MD
Resident
Department of Family Medicine
HCA Memorial Health University Medical
    Center
Savannah, Georgia

Michael D. Kolman, DO
Department of Internal Medicine
Advocate Lutheran General Hospital
Park Ridge, Illinois

Alhang Konyak, MD, FAAFP
Program Director
Department of Family Medicine
Mercyhealth Family Medicine Residency
    Program
Loves Park, Illinois

Ashley Nicole Koontz, DO
PGY-1
Department of Family and Community
    Medicine
Penn State Health Milton S. Hershey
    Medical Center
Hershey, Pennsylvania

Scott E. Kopec, MD, FCCP
Associate Professor of Medicine
Program Director, Internal Medicine
    Residency
University of Massachusetts Medical School
Worcester, Massachusetts

Matthew J. Kor, MD
Resident Physician
Department of Family and Community
    Medicine
Penn State Health Milton S. Hershey
    Medical Center
Hershey, Pennsylvania

Merrill Alan Krolick, DO, FACC, FACP,
    FSCAI[†]
Chronic Stable Angina Pectoris
Largo Medical Center
Largo, Florida

E. James Kruse, DO
Associate Professor of Surgery
Chief of Surgical Oncology Section
Department of Surgery
Augusta University
Augusta, Georgia

Keshav Kukreja, MD[†]
Department of Internal Medicine
University of Texas Health Sciences
    Center at Houston
Houston, Texas

Daniel B. Kurtz, PhD, BS[†]
Utica College
Utica, New York

Lauren Elizabeth Kwan, MD
Resident
Department of Psychiatry and Behavioral
    Sciences
Vanderbilt University Medical Center
Nashville, Tennessee

Melinda Kwan, DO, MPH
Urgent Care Physician
Department of Urgent Care
Southwest Medical Associates
Las Vegas, Nevada

Rita M. Lahlou, MD, MPH
Assistant Professor
Department of Family Medicine
University of North Carolina
Chapel Hill, North Carolina

Jason Edward Lambrecht, MD, FHM,
    FACP, PharmD[†]
Assistant Professor
Critical Care Fellow
Department of Internal Medicine
Creighton University
Omaha, Nebraska

Stephen K. Lane, MD
Scituate, Massachusetts

Anne Campbell Larkin, MD
Associate Professor
Department of Surgery
University of Massachusetts Medical School
Worcester, Massachusetts

Shane L. Larson, MD[†]
Assistant Professor of Family Medicine
Uniformed Services University of the
    Health Sciences
Womack Army Medical Center
Fort Bragg, North Carolina

Rebecca A. Lauters, MD[†]
Assistant Program Director
Eglin Family Medicine Residency
Eglin Air Force Base
Eglin Air Force Base, Florida

Justin P. Lavin Jr., MD, FACOG
Professor and Chairman Emeritus
Department of Obstetrics and
    Gynecology
Cleveland Clinic Akron General
Akron, Ohio

Kelley V. Lawrence, MD, IBCLC
Assistant Campus Director
Department of UNC School of Medicine
    Charlotte Campus
Novant Health
Charlotte, North Carolina

Rondy Michael Lazaro, MD
Senior Instructor
Department of Physical Medicine and
    Rehabilitation
University of Rochester
Rochester, New York

Bianca Lee, DO, MS
Department of Internal Medicine
Nassau University Medical Center
East Meadow, New York

Daniel T. Lee, MD, MA
Clinical Professor
Department of Family Medicine
University of California, Los Angeles
Los Angeles, California

David L. Lee, MD
Assistant Professor
Department of Family and Community
    Medicine
Penn State Health Milton S. Hershey
    Medical Center
Hershey, Pennsylvania

Hobart Lee, MD, FAAFP
Associate Professor
Department of Family Medicine
Loma Linda University School of
    Medicine
Loma Linda, California

Joo Hyun Lee, MD
Resident Physician
Department of Population Health
The University of Texas at Austin
Austin, Texas

Blake Leeds, DO
University of Louisville School of
    Medicine
Louisville, Kentucky

F. Stuart Leeds, MD, MS
Associate Professor
Department of Family Medicine
Wright State University Boonshoft School
    of Medicine
Dayton, Ohio

Connie Leeper, MD, MPH
Assistant Professor
Department of Family, Internal, and Rural
    Medicine
University of Alabama
Tuscaloosa, Alabama

Angelia Leipelt, BA, IBCLC, ICCE, CLE
Lactation Consultant
Dignity Health Methodist Hospital of
    Sacramento
Sacramento, California

Samuel Michael Leschisin, MD
Department of Family Medicine
AMITA Health Saint Joseph Hospital
    Chicago
Chicago, Illinois

Nikki A. Levin, MD, PhD
Associate Professor
Department of Dermatology
University of Massachusetts Medical
    School
Worcester, Massachusetts

Gary I. Levine, MD
Associate Professor
Department of Family Medicine
Brody School of Medicine
East Carolina University
Greenville, North Carolina

Anqi Li, DO
Family Medicine Resident
Mercyhealth Family Medicine Residency
    Program
Rockford, Illinois

Lorena Likaj, MD, MPH
Resident
Department of Family Medicine
St. Francis Hospital
Wilmington, Delaware

Viktor Limanskiy, MD
Resident Physician
Department of Family Medicine
San Joaquin General Hospital
French Camp, California

Yea Ping Lin, MD, PhD, MPH, MS, BS
Resident Physician
Department of Family Medicine
    Residency Program
Desert Regional Medical Center
Palm Springs, California

Christopher Lin-Brande, MD[†]
Staff Physician
Department of Family Health Clinic
31st Medical Group
Aviano Air Base, Italy

Briana Lindberg, MD[†]
Sports Medicine Fellow
NCC Primary Care Sports Medicine
    Sports Medicine
National Capital Consortium
Fort Belvoir Community Hospital
Fort Belvoir, Virginia

Katelin M. Lisenby, PharmD, BCPS
Associate Clinical Professor
Department of Pharmacy Practice
Auburn University
Auburn, Alabama

Derek Lodico, DO[†]
Associate Professor
F. Edward Hebert School of Medicine
Chief Cardiothoracic Anesthesia
Department of Anesthesia, Critical Care,
    and Pain Medicine
Walter Reed National Military Medical
    Center
Bethesda, Maryland

Jayson R. Loeffert, DO
Assistant Professor
Department of Family and Community
    Medicine and Orthopedics and
    Rehabilitation
Penn State Health Milton S. Hershey
    Medical Center
Hershey, Pennsylvania

Keith Ranney Love, MD, BA
Fellow
Department of Cardiovascular Medicine
UMass Memorial Medical Center
Worcester, Massachusetts

Lily T. Luc, MD
Resident Physician
Department of Family & Community
    Medicine
Baylor College of Medicine
Houston, Texas

Daniel Ludi, MD
George Washington University
Washington, District of Columbia

Thanh-Ha Luong, MD
Attending
Oncology & Hematology
BronxCare Health System
Bronx, New York

Nica E. Lurtsema, MD, MPH
Resident Physician
Department of Family and Community
    Medicine
Texas Tech University Health Sciences
    Center
Lubbock, Texas

Ryan D. Lurtsema, MD
Assistant Professor
Sports Medicine, Family and Community
    Medicine
Texas Tech University Health Sciences
    Center
Lubbock, Texas

Andrew Lutzkanin, MD
Assistant Professor
Department of Family and Community
    Medicine
Penn State College of Medicine
Hershey, Pennsylvania

Ann M. Lynch, PharmD, RPh, AE-C
Professor
Department of Pharmacy Practice
Massachusetts College of Pharmacy and
    Health Sciences University
Worcester, Massachusetts

Jonathan Edward MacClements, MD,
    FAAFP
Professor
Department of Medical Education and
    Population Health
Dell Medical School, The University of
    Texas at Austin
Austin, Texas

Nathan J. Macedo, MD, MPH
Assistant Professor
Department of Family Medicine
UMass Chan Medical School-Baystate
Springfield, Massachusetts

Theodore E. Macnow, MD
Assistant Professor of Pediatrics
Department of Pediatric Emergency
UMass Memorial Children's Medical
    Center
Worcester, Massachusetts

Douglas William MacPherson, MD, MSc(CTM), FRCPC[†]
Associate Professor
Department of Pathology and Molecular Medicine
Michael G. Schulich School of Medicine, McMaster University
Hamilton, Ontario, Canada

Michael J. Maddaleni, MD
Department of Family Medicine/Sports Medicine
University of Massachusetts Medical School
Worcester, Massachusetts

Michelle Magid, MD, MBA[†]
Associate Professor
Department of Psychiatry
Dell Medical School, The University of Texas at Austin
Austin, Texas

Manju Mahajan, MD, FAAFP
Faculty
Department of Family Medicine and Community Health
Hahnemann Family Health Center
UMass Medical School
Worcester, Massachusetts

Deepali Maheshwari, DO, MPH[†]
Fellow
Department of Obstetrics and Gynecology
University of Massachusetts Medical School
Worcester, Massachusetts

Tauhid Mahmud, MD, MPH
Resident
Department of Family Medicine
University of Maryland Medical Center
Baltimore, Maryland

Stefany J. K. Malanka, MD
Resident
Department of Family Medicine
Creighton University School of Medicine
Omaha, Nebraska

Jose O. Malave, MD
Fellow
Department of Primary Care Sports Medicine
University of South Carolina
Greenville, South Carolina

Shivani Malhotra, MD, FAAFP
UAB Huntsville Family Medicine Residency Program
Huntsville, Alabama

Zaiba Malik, MD
Medical Director
Medpace
Cincinnati, Ohio
Assistant Professor
Wright State University Boonshoft School of Medicine
Dayton, Ohio

Samir Malkani, MD, MRCP–UK
Professor
Department of Medicine
University of Massachusetts Medical School
Worcester, Massachusetts

Naila Manahil, MD
Springfield, Illinois

Lee A. Mancini, MD, CSCS*D, CSN
Associate Professor
Department of Family Medicine and Community Health
Chief, Division of Sports and Exercise Medicine
Director, Primary Care Sports and Exercise Medicine Fellowship
University of Massachusetts
Worcester, Massachusetts

Eric J. Mao, MD
Assistant Professor
Department of Medicine
Division of Gastroenterology and Hepatology
University of California, Davis
Sacramento, California

Wendy K. Marsh, MD, MSc
Associate Professor
Department of Psychiatry
University of Massachusetts Medical School
Worcester, Massachusetts

Nicholas R. Martin, MD
PGY-2
Department of Family Medicine and Community Health
University of Massachusetts Medical School
Worcester, Massachusetts

Stephen A. Martin, MD, EdM
Associate Professor
Department of Family Medicine and Community Health
University of Massachusetts Medical School
Worcester, Massachusetts

Marni L. Martinez, APRN
Austin Gastroenterology
Austin, Texas

Valeria A. Martinez-Lebron, MD
Resident Physician
Department of Internal Medicine
George Washington University Hospital
Washington, District of Columbia

Patricia Martinez Quinones, MD, PhD
General Surgery Resident
Department of General Surgery
Augusta University
Augusta, Georgia

George W. Matar, MD
Resident Physician
Department of Family and Community Health
University Hospital Cleveland Medical Center
Cleveland, Ohio

Nikita Mathew, DO
Resident
Department of Family Medicine
HonorHealth
Scottsdale, Arizona

Donnah Mathews, MD, FACP
Assistant Professor
Department of Internal Medicine
Alpert School of Medicine at Brown University
Providence, Rhode Island

Samuel E. Mathis, MD
Assistant Professor
Department of Family Medicine
University of Texas Medical Branch
Galveston, Texas

Daniel R. Matta, MD
Family Medicine Residency Faculty
Department of Family Medicine
Tallahassee Memorial Hospital Family Medicine Residency Program
Tallahassee, Florida

Lindsey Matthews, DO
Resident
Department of Family Medicine
Novant Health
Cornelius, North Carolina

Douglas M. Maurer, DO, MPH, FAAFP[†]
Director, Medical Education and
    Research Division
Designated Institutional Official
Madigan Army Medical Center
Joint Base Lewis–McChord, Washington
Associate Professor of Family Medicine
Uniformed Services University of the
    Health Sciences
Bethesda, Maryland
Associate Professor of Family Medicine
University of Washington School of
    Medicine
Seattle, Washington

George Maxted, MD
Associate Clinical Professor
Department of Family Medicine
Tufts University School of Medicine
Boston, Massachusetts

Beth K. Mazyck, MD
Associate Professor
Department of Family Medicine and
    Community Health
University of Massachusetts Medical School
Worcester, Massachusetts

Andrew McBride, MD
Family Medicine Liaison
Department of Family Medicine
University of Colorado
Aurora, Colorado
Department of Family Medicine and
    Sports Medicine
Boulder Community Health
Boulder, Colorado

Margaret J. McCormick, MS, RN, CNE
Clinical Assistant Professor
Department of Nursing
Towson University
Towson, Maryland

Paul McFarlane, MBBS
Resident Physician
Department of Family Medicine
    Residency Program
Tallahassee Memorial Healthcare
Tallahassee, Florida

Joshua McGuire, MD
Resident Physician
Department of Family Medicine
Texas Tech University Health Sciences
    Center
Lubbock, Texas

James McKee, DO, MS
Sports Medicine Fellow
Family Medicine and Community Health
UMass Medical School
Worcester, Massachusetts

Marc McKenna, MD, CAQSM
Program Director
Chestnut Hill Family Medicine Residency
Philadelphia, Pennsylvania

Donna Marie McMahon, DO, FAAP
Associate Professor
Department of Clinical Specialties
NYIT College of Osteopathic Medicine
Old Westbury, New York

Brock McMillen, MD, FFAFP
Program Director, Indiana University-
    Methodist Family Medicine Residency
Assistant Professor of Clinical Family
    Medicine
Department of Family Medicine
Indiana University School of Medicine
Indiana University Health
Indianapolis, Indiana

Michael McShane, MD EdM
Assistant Professor
Department of Internal Medicine
Penn State College of Medicine
Hershey, Pennsylvania

Toussaint L. Mears-Clarke, MD
Faculty Physician
Department of Family Medicine
Family Medicine Residency Program
Dignity Health Methodist Hospital of
    Sacramento
Sacramento, California

Nolberto Adrián Medina-Gallardo, MD,
    PhD[†]
Digestive and General Surgeon Specialist
Attending, Department of General
    Surgery
Hospital Universitari de Vic
Consorci Hospitalari de Vic
Vic, Barcelona, Spain

Donna I. Meltzer, MD
Clinical Associate Professor
Department of Family, Population &
    Preventive Medicine
Stony Brook Medicine
Stony Brook, New York

Caleb J. Mentzer, DO
Assistant Professor
Department of Surgery
Division of Trauma, Critical Care, & Acute
    Care Surgery
Spartanburg Regional Medical Center
Spartanburg, South Carolina

Laura Mercurio, MD
Assistant Professor of Pediatrics and
    Emergency Medicine
Alpert Medical School of Brown University
Providence, Rhode Island

Marcelle Meseeha, MD
Assistant Professor
Department of Internal Medicine
Guthrie
Sayre, Pennsylvania

Eric Robert Messner, PhD, FNP-BC
Associate Medical Director
Department of Family and Community
    Medicine Inpatient Service
Assistant Professor
Department of Family and Community
    Medicine
Penn State Health Milton S. Hershey
    Medical Center
Hershey, Pennsylvania

Lemaat Michael, MD
Children's National Hospital
Washington, District of Columbia

Mark Micolucci, MD
Resident Physician
Department of Family Medicine
Prisma Health-Upstate
Greenville, South Carolina

Mariya Milko, DO, MS
Largo, Florida

Jan Estes Miller, MD
Associate Program Director
SSM Health St. Anthony Family Medicine
    Residency
Oklahoma City, Oklahoma

Jesse Miller, MD
Assistant Program Director
Primary Care Sports Medicine Fellowship
Department of Family and Preventive
    Medicine
Assistant Professor
Department of Family and Preventive
    Medicine
University of South Carolina
Columbia, South Carolina

Paul G. Millner, MD
Assistant Professor
Department of Internal Medicine
Creighton University Internal Medicine
    Department
Omaha, Nebraska

Hilary Mislan, MD
Director of Addiction Medicine and
    Chronic Pain
Family Health Center of Worcester
Worcester, Massachusetts

Abdul Salman Mohammed, MBBS, MD, RhMSUS
Attending Physician
Department of Rheumatology
Advocate Lutheran General Hospital
Park Ridge, Illinois

Linha Mazin Mohammed, MD
Resident Physician
Department of Family Medicine
Adventist Health Hanford Family Medicine Residency
Hanford, California

Hammad Mohsin, MD
Assistant Professor
Department of Psychiatry
Mather at Northwell Health
Port Jefferson, New York

Saadia Mohsin, MD
Ross Medical School
Miramar, Florida

Nicole Monk, DO
Resident Physician
Department of Family Medicine
Methodist Health System
Dallas, Texas

Katherine Montag Schafer, PharmD, BCACP
Assistant Professor
Department of Family Medicine and Community Health
University of Minnesota
Minneapolis, Minnesota

Robert A. Monteleone, MD
Program Director
Saint Francis Family Medicine Residency Program
Saint Francis Hospital
Wilmington, Delaware

Jon Daniel Montemayor, MD
Assistant Program Director
Family Medicine Program
Riverside Methodist Hospital
Columbus, Ohio

Rogerio Montes, MD
Family Medicine, PGY-2
Medical City Arlington
Arlington, Texas

Brandon J. Moore, PA-C, MPAS
US Department of Defense
Fort Bragg, North Carolina

Nicholas Moore, MD, FAAFP, CAQSM
Medical Director
Motor City Orthopedics & Sports Medicine
Associate Director
Providence Sports Medicine Fellowship Program
Assistant Professor
Michigan State University College of Human Medicine
Novi, Michigan

Wynne Morgan, MD
Assistant Professor
Department of Psychiatry
University of Massachusetts Medical School
Worcester, Massachusetts

Torb Morkeberg, DO
PGY-1
Department of Family Medicine and Community Health
University of Minnesota
Maplewood, Minnesota

Christopher Morrow, PA-C[†]
United States Army

Lindsay N. Moy, DO
Resident Physician
Department of Internal Medicine
Advocate Lutheran General Hospital
Park Ridge, Illinois

James Thomas Muller, DO
Physician
Department of Family Medicine
Novant Health Family Medicine Residency Program
Cornelius, North Carolina

Sahil Mullick, MD
Associate Program Director, Director of Inpatient Service, Assistant Clinical Professor, Hospitalist, Core Faculty
Department of Family and Community Medicine
Creighton University School of Medicine
Omaha, Nebraska

Pratha Muthiah, MD, MPH
Resident Physician
Department of Family Medicine
University Hospital Cleveland Medical Center
Cleveland, Ohio

Mark T. Nadeau, MD, MBA[†]
Professor and Program Director
Department of Family and Community Medicine
University of Texas Health Science Center at San Antonio
San Antonio, Texas

Vandana Nagpal, MD, FACP
Assistant Professor
Department of Medicine
University of Massachusetts
Worcester, Massachusetts

Rajasree Nair, MD
Clinic Medical Director
Methodist Charlton Family Medicine Residency
Methodist Health System
Dallas, Texas

Emilio Nardone, MD
Neurosurgery
Central Illinois NeuroHealth Sciences
Bloomington, Illinois

Munima Nasir, MD
Associate Professor
Department of Family and Community Medicine
Penn State Health Milton S. Hershey Medical Center
Hershey, Pennsylvania

Ashwin Nayak, MD
Clinical Assistant Professor
Stanford University School of Medicine
Stanford, California

Kristen Nayak, MD
Clinical Assistant Professor
Department of Medicine
Division of Primary Care and Population Health
Stanford University School of Medicine
Stanford, California

Jessica C. Nazzaro, DO
Obstetrics and Gynecology Resident
Aultman Hospital
Canton, Ohio

Michelle Nelson, MD
Core Faculty
Department of Family Medicine
MidMichigan Medical Center—Gratiot
Alma, Michigan

Vicki R. Nelson, MD, PhD
Associate Professor
Department of Family Medicine
Prisma Health-Upstate
University of South Carolina School of Medicine Greenville
Greenville, South Carolina

David Nesheim, MD
Pulmonary Critical Care Physician
Department of Internal Medicine
Advocate Lutheran General Hospital
Park Ridge, Illinois

Sandra N. New, DNP
Retired
Knoxville, Tennessee

Jacob Thomas Newman, DO
Resident Physician
Department of Internal Medicine
George Washington University Hospital
Washington, District of Columbia

Roland W. Newman II, DO
Assistant Professor
Associate Program Director - Family and
    Community Medicine Residency Program
Department of Family and Community
    Medicine
Penn State Health Milton S. Hershey
    Medical Center
Hershey, Pennsylvania

Nancy Nguyen, DO
Faculty Attending
Department of Family Medicine
Dignity Health Methodist Hospital
    of Sacramento Family Medicine
    Residency Program
Sacramento, California

Tam T. Nguyen, MD
Washington Township Medical Group
Union City, California

Tu Dan H. Nguyen, MD
Clinical Assistant Professor
Director of Sports Medicine
Department of UTHSC Family Medicine
Department of Memorial Family Medicine
    Residency Program
Memorial Hermann
Houston, Texas

Sarah E. Nickolich, MD
Assistant Professor
Department of Family and Community
    Medicine
Penn State Health Milton S. Hershey
    Medical Center
Hershey, Pennsylvania

Frederick W. Nielson, MD[†]
MAJ, USAF, MC
Department of Family Medicine
US Air Force
Eielson Air Force Base, Alaska

Bryan R. Norkus, MD
Associate Program Director
Arnett Family Medicine Residency
Adjunct Professor of Clinical Family
    Medicine
Department of Family Medicine
Indiana University School of Medicine
Lafayette, Indiana

Edward N. Northrup, MD
Resident Physician
Department of Emergency Medicine
Advocate Christ Medical Center
Oak Lawn, Illinois

Jonathan M. Novotney, DO[†]
Staff Family Physician
Fort Carson
Colorado Springs, Colorado

Crystal Nwagwu, MD
Assistant Professor
Baylor College of Medicine
Houston, Texas

Davis M. O'Brien, MD
Resident Physician
Department of Surgery
Medical College of Georgia
Augusta, Georgia

Jennifer Oberstar, MD
Assistant Professor
Department of Family Medicine and
    Community Health
University of Minnesota
Minneapolis, Minnesota

Adedotun Anthony Ogunsua, MD, MPH
Associate Professor
Idaho College of Osteopathic Medicine
Benefis Hospital
Great Falls, Montana

Arthur Ohannessian, MD
Assistant Professor
Department of Family Medicine
University of California, Los Angeles
Los Angeles, California

Cynthia Y. Ohata, MD
Associate Program Director
Department of Family Medicine
Advocate Christ Medical Center
Oak Lawn, Illinois

Smriti Ohri, MD
Assistant Professor
Department of Family Medicine
University of Connecticut
Hartford, Connecticut

Jacqueline L. Olin, CDCES, PharmD,
    FASHP, MS, FCCP, BCPS
Professor
Department of Pharmacy
Wingate University School of Pharmacy
Wingate, North Carolina

Kyle D. Olsen, DO[†]
Eglin Air Force Base Family Medicine
    Residency Program
Eglin Air Force Base, Florida

Adedamola Ayo Omole, MD
Adventist Health Hanford
Hanford, California

Cherry Onaiwu, MD, MS
Faculty
Department of Internal Medicine
CHI Baylor St. Luke's Health
Houston, Texas

Brooke Organ, DO[†]
Sports Medicine Physician
Department of Family Medicine
Scott Air Force Base, Illinois

Seniha Ozudogru, MD
Assistant Professor
Department of Neurology
University of Utah
Salt Lake City, Utah

Kelly Pagidas, MDCM, FACOG,
    FRCSC[†]
Providence, Rhode Island

Miguel A. Palacios, MD
Assistant Professor
Department of Family and Community
    Medicine
University of Texas Health San Antonio
San Antonio, Texas

Sally-Ann L. Pantin, MD, FAAFP
Associate Program Director
Mayo Clinic Florida Family Medicine
    Residency
Department of Family Medicine
Mayo Clinic School of Graduate Medical
    Education
Jacksonville, Florida

Afreen N. Papa, MD
Resident Physician
Department of Internal Medicine
Advocate Lutheran General Hospital
Park Ridge, Illinois

Jon S. Parham, DO, MPH, FAAFP
Associate Professor
Department of Family Medicine
University of Tennessee Graduate School
    of Medicine
Knoxville, Tennessee

Greer Park, DO
Resident
Department of Psychiatry
Advocate Lutheran General Hospital
Chicago, Illinois

Morgan J. Parker, DO
PGY-1 Resident
Department of Family Medicine
Novant Health
Cornelius, North Carolina

Douglas S. Parks, MD
Associate Professor
Department of Family Medicine
    Residency at Cheyenne
University of Wyoming
Laramie, Wyoming

Naomi Parrella, MD, FAAFP, Dipl. ABOM
Associate Professor and Medical Director
Department of Family Medicine
Department of Surgery
Rush University Medical Center
Chicago, Illinois

Elyas Parsa, DO
Program Director
Department of Family Medicine
San Joaquin General Hospital
French Camp, California

Michael T. Partin, MD
Assistant Professor
Department of Family and Community
    Medicine
Penn State Health Milton S. Hershey
    Medical Center
Hershey, Pennsylvania

Bindusri Paruchuri, MD
Chief Resident
Saint Francis Family Medicine
University of Tennessee Health Science
    Center
Memphis, Tennessee

Sandra Pasiah, MD
Resident Physician
Department of Internal Medicine
Advocate Christ Medical Center
Oak Lawn, Illinois

Avignat S. Patel, MD
Senior Physician
Department of Pulmonary Critical Care
    Medicine
Lahey Hospital and Medical Center
Burlington, Massachusetts
Assistant Professor
Department of Medicine
Tufts University School of Medicine
Boston, Massachusetts

Birju B. Patel, MD, FACP[†]
Adjunct Assistant Professor of Medicine
Emory University School of Medicine
Atlanta, Georgia

Krunal Patel, MD
Associate Professor of Medicine
University of Massachusetts Medical
    School
Worcester, Massachusetts

Mahesh C. Patel, MD
Associate Professor
Department of Internal Medicine-
    Infectious Diseases
University of Illinois at Chicago
Chicago, Illinois

Nihal K. Patel, MD
Assistant Clinical Professor
Department of Medicine
University of Connecticut School of
    Medicine
Harford, Connecticut

Preeya Patel, DO
Resident Physician
Department of Family Medicine
    Residency
Novant Health
Cornelius, North Carolina

Ruchita Patel, DO
Endocrinologist
Department of Internal Medicine
Advocate Christ Medical Center
Oak Lawn, Illinois

Jyothi R. Patri, MD, MHA, FAAFP,
    HMDC
Program Director
Adventist Health Hanford Family
    Medicine Residency Program
Adventist Health Hanford Central Valley
    Network
Hanford, California

Leila N. Patterson, MD
PGY2
Department of Family Medicine
Advocate Christ Medical Center
Oak Lawn, Illinois

Jared M. Patton, MD, MS[†]
Senior Medical Officer
Camp Kinser Branch Medical Clinic
United States Navy
Okinawa, Japan

Destiny D. Pegram, MD
Resident Physician
Department of Psychiatry
University of Massachusetts Medical
    School
Worcester, Massachusetts

Tristan Michael Alexander Pennella, DO
Family Medicine Resident
Mankato, Minnesota

Lauren Penwell-Waines, PhD
Associate Program Director
Novant Health Department of Family
    Medicine Residency Program
Cornelius, North Carolina

Jose Luis Perez-Lara, MD
Chief Pulmonary Fellow
Department of Pulmonary
BronxCare Health System
Bronx, New York

Christine S. Persaud, MD, MBA
Assistant Professor, Program Director-
    Sports Medicine Fellowship
Department of Orthopedic Surgery &
    Rehabilitation Medicine
SUNY Downstate Health Sciences
    University
Brooklyn, New York

Ian Paul Persits, DO, MS
Resident
Department of Internal Medicine
Cleveland Clinic Foundation
Cleveland, Ohio

Parvathi Perumareddi, DO
Associate Professor
Florida Atlantic University
Charles E. Schmidt College of Medicine
Boca Raton, Florida

Anna R. Peyton, DO
Resident Physician
Department of Family and Community
    Medicine Residency
Mercy Health Anderson Hospital
Cincinnati, Ohio

Kelsey E. Phelps, MD[†]
Assistant Professor of Family Medicine
Louisiana State University Rural Family
    Medicine Residency
Bogalusa Louisiana State University
Bogalusa, Louisiana

Teny Philip Thomas, MD
Clinical Educator
Pritzker School of Medicine
Northbrook Primary Care
NorthShore University Health System
Evanston, Illinois

Jason Philippe, MD
PGY-III Resident
Bayfront Health St. Petersburg
St. Petersburg, Florida

Jonathan A. Phillips, DO
Resident
Department of Internal Medicine/
    Pediatrics
University of Louisville
Louisville, Kentucky

Shawn Phillips, MD
Associate Professor
Department of Family and Community
    Medicine and Orthopedics and
    Rehabilitation
Penn State College of Medicine
Hershey, Pennsylvania

Grant Pierre, MD, CAQSM
Faculty Umass Sports Medicine
    Fellowship
Department of Family Medicine
University of Massachusetts
Worcester, Massachusetts

Anush S. Pillai, DO, FAAFP
Program Director
Family Medicine Residency Program
HCA Houston Healthcare West
Clinical Associate Professor
University of Houston, College of Medicine
Houston, Texas

Karly Pippitt, MD
Associate Professor, Clinic
Department of Family and Preventive
    Medicine
University of Utah
Salt Lake City, Utah

Yevgeniy Popov, DO, MPH
Fellow
Department of Rheumatology
University of Massachusetts Medical
    School
Worcester, Massachusetts

Stacy E. Potts, MD, Med
Vice Chair of Education
Health Department of Family Medicine
    and Community
University of Massachusetts
Worcester, Massachusetts

James E. Powers, DO, FACEP, FAAEM
Professor of Emergency Medicine
Campbell University School of
    Osteopathic Medicine
Lillington, North Carolina

Faruq Pradhan, MD
Gastroenterology Fellow
Banner University Medical Center
    Phoenix
Phoenix, Arizona

Timothy D. Prajka, DO
Resident Physician
Department of Family Medicine
Advocate Christ Medical Center
Oak Lawn, Illinois

Bethany Price, DO
Residency Faculty
Department of Family Medicine
Saint Mary's Family Medicine Residency
Grand Junction, Colorado

Simone Prioli, PA-C
Emergency Medicine
Boston, Massachusetts

Fabiola Puga Dueñas, MD
Department of Family Medicine
Tallahassee Memorial Hospital
Tallahassee, Florida

George G.A. Pujalte, MD, FACSM,
    FAMSSM, FAAFP[†]
Associate Professor
Department of Family Medicine, and
    Orthopedics and Sports Medicine
Mayo Clinic
Jacksonville, Florida

Vinay Krishna Pulusu, MD, MHA
Hospitalist
Clovis Community Medical Center
Fresno, California

Mantavya Punj, MD
Resident Physician
Department of Family Medicine
Mayo Clinic
Jacksonville, Florida

Natasha J. Pyzocha, DO, FAWM, FAAFP
Mont Vernon, New Hampshire

Jana W. Qiao, MD
Resident Physician
Department of Family Medicine
Penn State University
Hershey, Pennsylvania

Juan Qiu, MD, PhD
Professor
Department of Family and Community
    Medicine
Pennsylvania State University College of
    Medicine
State College, Pennsylvania

Christine A. Quartuccio-Carran, DO,
    FAAFP
Associate Program Director
Valley Health System Family Medicine
    Residency Program
Las Vegas, Nevada

Jeffrey D. Quinlan, MD, FAAFP[†]
Professor, Chair, and DEO
Department of Family Medicine
Roy J. and Lucille A. Carver College of
    Medicine, University of Iowa
Iowa City, Iowa

Raymundo A. Quintana, MD
Cardiovascular Diseases Fellow
Emory University School of Medicine
Atlanta, Georgia

Hannan Qureshi, MD
Resident Surgeon and Postdoctoral
    Research Fellow
Department of Otolaryngology—Head
    and Neck Surgery
University of Washington
Seattle, Washington

Radhika Ragam, MD
Department of Urology
Thomas Jefferson University
Philadelphia, Pennsylvania

Naureen Bashir Rafiq, MD[†]
Associate Professor
Department of Family Medicine
Creighton University School of Medicine
Omaha, Nebraska

Kalyanakrishnan Ramakrishnan, MD
Professor
Department of Family and Preventive
    Medicine
University of Oklahoma Health Sciences
    Center
Oklahoma City, Oklahoma

Muthalagu Ramanathan, MD
Professor of Internal Medicine
Department of Medicine
UMass Memorial Medical Center
Worcester, Massachusetts

Jason R. Ramos, MD, FAAFP
Family Medicine Program Director
Family Physician
Department of Family Medicine
Honor Community Health
Pontiac, Michigan

Ravishankar E. Rao, MD
Assistant Professor
Department of Family and Community
    Medicine
Penn State College of Medicine
Hershey, Pennsylvania

Umer Rashid, MD
Resident Physician
Department of Family Medicine
Adventist Health
Hanford, California

Tharani Ravi, MD
Assistant Professor
Department of Family and Community
    Medicine
University of Texas Health San Antonio
San Antonio, Texas

Akash Ray, DO
Department of Emergency Medicine
Inspira Medical Center
Vineland, New Jersey

Narothama Reddy Aeddula, MD, FACP,
   FASN, FNKF
Clinical Assistant Professor
Department of Medicine
Indiana University School of Medicine
Consultant Nephrologist
Department of Medicine
Deaconess Health System
Evansville, Indiana

Grant M. Reed, DO
Family Practice Physician
St. Margaret's Health
Peru, Illinois

Alexis Benavides Reedy-Cooper, MD,
   MPH
Assistant Professor
Department of Family and Community
   Medicine
Pennsylvania State University College of
   Medicine
Hershey, Pennsylvania

Robyn Lee Reese, DO
Resident Physician
Department of Family Medicine
Mayo Clinic
Jacksonville, Florida

Meghan E. Reeves, MD
Resident
Department of Family and Community
   Medicine
Penn State Health Milton S. Hershey
   Medical Center
Hershey, Pennsylvania

Brittany M. Reid, MBBS
Resident Physician
University of Massachusetts Medical
   School
Worcester, Massachusetts

Jennifer Reidy, MD, MS, FAAHPM
Chief
Department of Division of Palliative Care
UMass Memorial Medical Center
Associate Professor
Department of Family Medicine and
   Community Health
University of Massachusetts Medical School
Worcester, Massachusetts

Samuel Renier, MD
Department of Family Medicine
University of Minnesota
Minneapolis, Minnesota

Kimberly Resnick, MD
MetroHealth Medical Center
Associate Professor
Obstetrics and Gynecology
Case Western Reserve University
Cleveland, Ohio

Andrew J. Richardson, MD
Department of Family Medicine
Baylor Scott & White Health
College Station, Texas

Christopher J. Rider, MD
PGY-1
Florida State University Family Medicine
   Residency Program-BayCare Health
   System
Winter Haven, Florida

Maegan M. Riggin, MD
Resident Physician
Department of Family Medicine
Novant Health Family Medicine
   Residency Program
Cornelius, North Carolina

Bryce Ringwald, MD
Family Medicine Resident
OhioHealth Riverside Methodist Hospital
Columbus, Ohio

Sonia Rivera-Martinez, DO, FACOFP
Associate Professor
Department of Family Medicine
New York Institute of Technology College
   of Osteopathic Medicine
Old Westbury, New York

Daniel Rivlin, MD
Program Director, Mohs Micrographic
   Surgery
Department of Dermatology
Larkin Community Hospital
South Miami, Florida

Tazeen Rizvi, DO
Resident Physician
Department of Internal Medicine
Advocate Christ Medical Center
Oak lawn, Illinois

Jared M. Roberts
PGY-2
Penn State Health Milton S. Hershey
   Medical Center
Hershey, Pennsylvania

Sean C. Robinson, MD, CAQSM
Assistant Professor
Department of Family Medicine and
   Sports Medicine
Oregon Health & Science University
Portland, Oregon

Michelle Rodriguez, MD
Department of Family and Community
   Medicine
University of Texas Health Science
   Center at San Antonio
San Antonio, Texas

Benjamin Dale Rogers, MD[†]
Assistant Professor of Medicine
Division of Gastroenterology, Hepatology,
   and Nutrition
University of Louisville
Louisville, Kentucky

Hayley K. Rogers, MD
Department of Internal Medicine
George Washington University
Washington, District of Columbia

Tyler S. Rogers, MD
Assistant Professor
Department of Family Medicine
Martin Army Community Hospital
Fort Benning, Georgia
Fellow
Department of Family Medicine
Madigan Army Medical Center
Joint Base Lewis McChord, Washington

Cristhiam Rojas-Hernandez, MD
Assistant Professor
Department of Benign Hematology
The University of Texas MD Anderson
   Cancer Center
Houston, Texas

Leigh A. Romero, MD, CAQSM
Assistant Professor
Department of Population Health—Family
   Medicine
Dell Medical School, The University of
   Texas at Austin
Austin, Texas

Laura Ross, MD
Department of Internal Medicine
Novant Medical Center
Huntersville, North Carolina

Maria Rossi, MD, MS
Resident Physician
Department of Family Medicine
Southern Illinois University
Springfield, Illinois

Katherine L. Rotker, MD
Assistant Professor
Department of Urology
University of Massachusetts Medical
   Center
Worcester, Massachusetts

Lloyd A. Runser, MD, MPH, FAAFP[†]
Assistant Professor
Department of Family Medicine
Campbell University School of Medicine
Lillington, North Carolina
Associate Program Director
Novant Health Department of Family
    Medicine Residency Program
Charlotte, North Carolina
Assistant Professor
Department of Family Medicine
Virginia College of Medicine
Blacksburg, Virginia

Veronica J. Ruston, DO
General Medicine Physician
Phoenix, Arizona

Anup Sabharwal, MD, MBA, FACE,
    FASPC, FNLA
Professor
Department of Endocrinology, Diabetes,
    and Metabolism
Florida International University
Miami Beach, Florida

Afza Safeer, MD
PGY 1
University at Buffalo Family Medicine
    Residency Rural 1-2 Track
Olean, New York

Aashna Saini, MD
Resident Physician
Department of Obstetrics & Gynecology
University of Massachusetts Chan
    Medical School/UMass Memorial
    Medical Center
Worcester, Massachusetts

Yu Sakai, MD
Lemuel Shattuck Hospital
Boston, Massachusetts

Jeffrey T. Sakamoto, MD
Attending Physician
The Emergency Group
Honolulu, Hawaii

Kathryn Samai, PharmD, BCPS
Clinical Pharmacist of Emergency
    Medicine
Department of Pharmaceutical Care
    Services
Sarasota Memorial Healthcare System
Sarasota, Florida

Kyle M. Samyn, DO, MS
Resident Physician
Department of Family Medicine
Oakland Primary Care
Warren, Michigan

Vicente T. San Martin, MD
Medical Director
Department of Endocrinology
Macromedica Dominicana
Santo Domingo, Dominican Republic

Carolina Sanchez, MD
Department of Family and Community
    Medicine
University of Texas Health Science
    Center at San Antonio
San Antonio, Texas

Melanie Houston Sanders, MD
Clinical Assistant Professor
Medical Director of the Office of Clinical
    Skills
Greenville, North Carolina

Alejandro Folch Sandoval, MD
Clinical Fellow
Department of Division of Cardiovascular
    Medicine
University of Massachusetts Medical
    School
Worcester, Massachusetts

Adam K. Saperstein, MD[†]
Associate Professor
Department of Family Medicine
F. Edward Hebert School of Medicine
Uniformed Services University of the
    Health Sciences
Bethesda, Maryland

Luay Sarsam, MD
Department of Cardiovascular Disease
Arnot Ogden Medical Center
Elmira, New York

Durr-e-Shahwaar Sayed, DO
Attending Physician
Department of Family Medicine
Inspira Medical Group
Woodbury, New Jersey

Payam Sazegar, MD[†]
Kaiser Permanente San Diego Family
    Medicine Residency
San Diego, California

Christina Scartozzi, DO
Assistant Professor
Department of Family and Community
    Medicine
Penn State Health St. Joseph Medical
    Center
Reading, Pennsylvania

Richard Scharf, DO
Faculty attending
Rutgers Otolaryngology Residency Program
Cooperman Barnabas Medical Center
Livingston, New Jersey

Matthew J. Schear, DO, MS[†]
Cornea, External Diseases and Refractive
    Surgery
Department of Ophthalmology
Hudson Valley Eye Surgeons
Fishkill, New York

Daniel J. Schlegel, MD, MHA
Program Director
Penn State Hershey Family Medicine
    Residency Program
Assistant Professor
Department of Family and Community
    Medicine
Penn State Health Milton S. Hershey
    Medical Center
Hershey, Pennsylvania

Jennifer Schwartz, MD[†]
Newton Wellesley Hospital
Newton, Massachusetts

Ingrid U. Scott, MD, MPH[†]
Jack and Nancy Turner Professor of
    Ophthalmology
Professor of Public Health Sciences
Penn State College of Medicine
Hershey, Pennsylvania

Stephen Robert Scott, MD
Wellstar Atlanta Medical Center
Atlanta, Georgia

Timothy A. Scully, DO
Chief Resident
Department of Internal Medicine
Augusta University Medical Center
Augusta, Georgia

David P. Sealy, MD, CAQSM, FAAFP,
    FAMSSM
Professor
Department of Family Medicine/Sports
    Medicine
Medical University of South Carolina
Area Health Education Consortium
    Greenwood
Self Regional Healthcare, Primary Care
    Sports Medicine Fellowship
Greenwood, South Carolina

Stephen C. Sears, DO[†]
LT, MC (Flight Surgeon), USN
Aviation Medicine Department
United States Naval Hospital Yokosuka
Branch Health Clinic Iwakuni
Marine Corps Air Station
Iwakuni, Japan

Nighat Seema Ahmed, MD[†]
Diplomate American Board of Family
    Medicine
Diplomate American Board of Obesity
    Medicine
Assistant Professor
Florida State University College of
    Medicine
Tallahassee, Florida

Terry SeeToe, MD
Resident Physician
Department of Family Medicine
SUNY Downstate Health Sciences
    University
Brooklyn, New York

Jarrett Keller Sell, MD, FAAFP, AAHIVS
Associate Professor
Department of Family and Community
    Medicine
Penn State Health Milton S. Hershey
    Medical Center
Hershey, Pennsylvania

Anthony Shadiack, DO, CAQSM
Associate Program Director, Family
    Medicine
Grand Strand Medical Center
Myrtle Beach, South Carolina

Blake R. Shaffer, MD, MBS
Resident Physician
Department of Eglin Family Medicine
    Residency
Eglin Air Force Base Hospital
Eglin Air Force Base, Florida

Chirag N. Shah, MD
Associate Professor
Department of Emergency Medicine
Rutgers Robert Wood Johnson Medical
    School
New Brunswick, New Jersey

Hiral Shah, MD, FASGE, FAGA, FACG[†]
Program Director
Gastroenterology Fellowship
Lehigh Valley Health Network
Eastern Pennsylvania Gastroenterology
    and Liver Specialists
Allentown, Pennsylvania

Jay B. Shah, DO
Resident Physician
Department of Family Medicine
Advocate Christ Medical Center
Oak Lawn, Illinois

Nehal R. Shah, MD[†]
Assistant Professor of Medicine
Department of Internal Medicine
Virginia Commonwealth University
Richmond, Virginia

Samir A. Shah, AGAF, FACG,
    FASGE, MD
Clinical Professor of Medicine
Department of Medicine/Gastroenterology
Alpert Medical School of Brown University
Chief of Gastroenterology
Department of Gastroenterology
The Miriam Hospital
Providence, Rhode Island

Ammar Shahid, MD[†]
Department of Sports Medicine
Tower Health and Drexel University
Philadelphia, Pennsylvania

Esha Rajiv Sharma, MD, MPH
Resident Physician
Department of Family Medicine
Baptist Memorial Medical Education
    Program
Memphis, Tennessee

Denise Sharon, MD, PhD, FAASM[†]
Independent Contractor
PVHMC Adult and Children Sleep
    Disorders Center
Pomona Valley Hospital and Medical
    Center
Claremont, California

Erik C. Shaw, DO, MBMS
Resident Physician
Department of Family Medicine
Memorial Health University Medical
    Center/Mercer University College of
    Medicine
Savannah, Georgia

Vincent L. Shaw Jr., MD, CAQ-SM
Program Director
Department of Family Medicine
    Residency/Sports Medicine Fellowship
Baton Rouge General Medical Center
Baton Rouge, Louisiana

Karen Sheflin, DO
Assistant Professor
Department of Family Medicine
College of Osteopathic Medicine
New York Institute of Technology
Old Westbury, New York

Shelby L. Sheider, DO
Resident Physician
Department of Family Medicine
Martin Army Community Hospital
Fort Benning, Georgia

Zahra Sardar Sheikh, MD, MPH, CMD
Assistant Professor of Medicine
Department of Geriatric Medicine
University of Massachusetts
Worcester, Massachusetts

Jennifer M. Shoemaker, MD, MPH
Site Director, Amador Track
Sutter Family Medicine Residency
    Program
Jackson, California

Irfan H. Siddiqui, MD
Attending Physician, Faculty
Department of Internal Medicine
Advocate Christ Medical Center
Oak Lawn, Illinois

Kartik Sidhar, MD
Family Medicine Faculty
Department of Family Medicine
Department of Shadyside Family
    Medicine Residency
University of Pittsburgh Medical Center
Pittsburgh, Pennsylvania

Beshoy Sidhom, MD
Department of Family Medicine
University of Massachusetts
Worcester, Massachusetts

Karlynn Sievers, MD
Associate Program Director
Department of Family Medicine
St. Mary's Family Medicine Residency
    Program
Grand Junction, Colorado

Matthew A. Silva, PharmD, RPh, BCPS
Professor
Department of Pharmacy Practice
Massachusetts College of Pharmacy and
    Health Sciences
Worcester, Massachusetts

Sabrina L. Silver, DO, CAQSM[†]
Eglin Air Force Base, Florida

Algimantas Simpson, MD
Department of Family Medicine
Memorial Health University Hospital
Savannah, Georgia

Marvin H. Sineath Jr., MD, FAAFP,
    CAQSM
HCA-Memorial Health
Savannah, Georgia

Madhavi Singh, MD[†]
Assistant Professor
Department of Family and Community
    Medicine
Penn State College of Medicine
Hershey, Pennsylvania

Sareena Singh, MD, FACOG
Assistant Professor
Department of Obstetrics and
    Gynecology, Gynecologic Oncology
Northeast Ohio Medical University
Rootstown, Ohio

Brian G. Skotko, MD, MPP
Emma Campbell Endowed Chair on
    Down Syndrome
Department of Pediatrics
Massachusetts General Hospital
Associate Professor
Department of Pediatrics
Harvard Medical School
Boston, Massachusetts

Paul J. Sliskovich, MD
Department of Family Medicine
Creighton University
Omaha, Nebraska

Melissa L. Smith, MD
Lee's Summit, Missouri

Daniel S. Smoots, MD
HonorHealth Family Medicine
Phoenix, Arizona

Faraz A. Sohail, MD
Resident
Department of Internal Medicine
George Washington University
Washington, District of Columbia

D'Ann Wilson Somerall, FAANP,
    FNP-BC, DNP, CRNP, MAEd
Nurse Practitioner
Adjunct Assistant Professor
University of Alabama at Birmingham
    School of Nursing
Birmingham, Alabama

William E. Somerall Jr., MD, MAEd
Associate Professor
Department of School of Nursing
University of Alabama at Birmingham
Birmingham, Alabama

Ryan M. Song, MD
Resident Physician
Department of Internal Medicine
Advocate Lutheran General Hospital
Park Ridge, Illinois

Johan W. Sosa, MD
LaSalle, Illinois

Mikayla L. Spangler, PharmD
Associate Professor
Department of Pharmacy Practice and
    Family Medicine
Creighton University
Omaha, Nebraska

Dana Sprute, MD, MPH, FAAFP
Associate Professor, Division of Family
    Medicine
Department of Population Health
Dell Medical School, The University of
    Texas at Austin
Austin, Texas

Brianna Stadsvold, MD
Resident
Department of Surgery
Medical College of Georgia at Augusta
    University
Augusta, Georgia

Diana V. Steau, MD
Department of Family Medicine
Creighton University
Omaha, Nebraska

Ahja D. Steele, MD
Resident Physician
Department of Family Medicine
Advocate Health Care, Advocate Christ
    Medical Center
Oak Lawn, Illinnois

Daniel J. Stein, MD, MPH
Instructor/Associate Physician
Harvard Medical School
Department of Internal Medicine
    (Gastroenterology)
Brigham and Women's Hospital
Boston, Massachusetts

J. Herbert Stevenson, MD[†]
Sports Medicine, Department of Family
    Medicine and Community of Health
University of Massachusetts Medical
    School
Worcester, Massachusetts

Jenell Stewart, DO, MPH
Acting Assistant Professor
Department of Global Health and
    Medicine
University of Washington
Seattle, Washington

Sheila O. Stille, DMD, MAGD
Associate Professor
General Practice Program Director
University of Colorado School of Dental
    Medicine
Aurora, Colorado

Arvey Stone, MD
Morton Grove, Illinnois

Samantha Storti, MD
Resident
Department of Internal Medicine
Advocate Christ Medical Center
Oak Lawn, Illinois

Jeffrey Stovall, MD
Professor
Department of Psychiatry and Behavioral
    Sciences
Vanderbilt University School of Medicine
Nashville, Tennessee

Sibley Strader, MD
Department of Family Medicine and
    Community Health
University Hospitals Cleveland Medical
    Center
Cleveland, Ohio

Adam Strosberg, DNP, ARNP-BC
Adjunct Faculty
Department of Nursing
Christine E. Lynn College of Nursing,
    Florida Atlantic University
Boca Raton, Florida

Moiz A. Suhail, MD
Loyola University Medical Center
Maywood, Illinois

Sally Suliman, MD
Assistant Professor
Department of Pulmonary Critical Care
Banner University Medical Center
Phoenix, Arizona

Elizabeth Ashley Suniega, MD
Faculty Professor of Family Medicine
Department of Family Medicine
HCA Houston Healthcare West Family
    Medicine Residency Program
Houston, Texas

Jennifer E. Svarverud, DO[†]
Family Medicine Resident
Nellis Family Medicine Residency
Nellis Air Force Base, Nevada

Sasha Svendsen, MD
Child Abuse Pediatrician
UMass Memorial Children's Assistant
    Professor of Pediatrics
University of Massachusetts Chan
    Medical School
Worcester, Massachusetts

Adeem Tahira, DO
Novant Health Family Medicine
    Residency Program
Cornelius, North Carolina

Benjamin T. Tan, DO
Resident Physician
Department of Family Medicine
Mayo Clinic—Jacksonville
Jacksonville, Florida

Irene J. Tan, MD, FACR[†]
Clinical Professor of Medicine
Department of Medicine
Sidney Kimmel Medical College
Thomas Jefferson University
Department of Medicine, Division of
    Rheumatology
Einstein Medical Center Philadelphia
Philadelphia, Pennsylvania

Kathrine R. Tan, MD, MPH[†]
Team Lead, Domestic Response Team
Malaria Branch
Centers for Disease Control and
    Prevention
Atlanta, Georgia

Ying Tang, DO
Chief Resident
Department of Family Medicine Residency
Chickasaw Nation Medical Center
Ada, Oklahoma

Brice T. Taylor, MD, MSc[†]
Associate Professor
Department of Pulmonary and
    Critical Care
Atrium Health
Charlotte, North Carolina

Reggie Taylor, DO, MA
PGY-1
Family Medicine Residency Program
Carl R. Darnall Army Medical Center
Fort Hood, Texas

Jairo J. Tejada-Tejada, MD[†]
Resident
Department of Internal Medicine
BronxCare Health System
Bronx, New York

Yutthapong Temtanakitpaisan, MD,
    FACC, FSCAI
Interventional Cardiologist
Department of Cardiology
Bangkok Hospital Khon Kaen
Muang, Khon Kaen, Thailand

Jason Teng, MD[†]
Chief Resident
Stanford Emergency Medicine
    Department
Palo Alto, California

Allegra Tenkman, MD
Core Faculty
Department of Family Medicine
Mercy Health-Anderson Hospital Family
    and Community Medicine Residency
    Program
Cincinnati, Ohio

Erin Thomas, MD, BS
Medical Resident
Department of Internal Medicine
University of Massachusetts Medical
    School
Worcester, Massachusetts

Bradly J. Thrasher, DO
Assistant Professor
Department of Pediatrics
University of Louisville
Louisville, Kentucky

Rebecca Thrower, MD
Assistant Professor
Division of Family Medicine
Austin, Texas

Sarah Marie Tiggelaar, MD, FAAFP
Associate Program Director
UT Family Medicine Residency
Memphis, Tennessee

Robert J. Tiller, MD, FAAFP
Program Director
Department of Family Medicine
    Residency Program
Self Regional Healthcare
Greenwood, South Carolina

Jill N. Tirabassi, MD, MPH
Clinical Assistant Professor
Department of Family Medicine
Jacobs School of Medicine and
    Biomedical Sciences
Buffalo, New York

Andres A. Tirado Navales, MD[†]
Family and Community Medicine
    Resident
Penn State Health
State College, Pennsylvania

Rachelle Toman, MD, PhD
Family Medicine Residency Program
    Director and Medical Director
Georgetown University School of
    Medicine
Washington, District of Columbia

Veronica A. Torres, MD
Assistant Professor
Department of Family and Community
    Medicine
Baylor College of Medicine
Houston, Texas

Theresa A. Townley, MD, MPH[†]
Associate Professor
Department of Internal Medicines
Creighton University
Omaha, Nebraska

Anna Marie Tran, DO
Resident Physician - Family Medicine
Ascension St. Vincent's Hospital
Jacksonville, Florida

Huy T. Tran, MD[†]
Cerritos, California

Thomas Triantafillou, MD
Assistant Professor
Department of Medicine
Advocate Christ Medical Center
Oak Lawn, Illinois

Jonathan Triantafyllou, MD
Assistant Professor
Department of Family and Community
    Medicine
Penn State College of Medicine
Hershey, Pennsylvania

Alec L. Tributino, DO
Resident
Department of Family Medicine
University of Massachusetts
Worcester, Massachusetts

Zoltan Trizna, MD, PhD
Director
Dermatology and Dermatological Surgery
Austin, Texas

Pamela R. Tsinteris, MD, MPH
Family Physician, Program Director
    for Chronic Pain and Office Based
    Addiction Treatment Programs
Department of Family Medicine
Family Health Center of Worcester
Worcester, Massachusetts

Edison Tsui, MD
Hematology and Oncology
Springfield, Massachusetts

Jonathan Tsui, MD
Resident Physician
Department of Ophthalmology
Geisinger Eye Institute
Danville, Pennsylvania

Terrence Tsui, DO
Primary Care Sports Medicine Fellow
Department of Orthopaedics
Bayhealth Medical Center
Dover, Delaware

Matthew A. Tunzi, DO
Resident Physician
Department of Internal Medicine
San Antonio Uniformed Services Health
    Education Consortium
San Antonio, Texas

Alethea Y. Turner, DO, FAAFP
Associate Director
Department of Family Medicine
    Residency Program
HonorHealth
Scottsdale, Arizona

Bradley M. Turner, MD, MPH, MHA[†]
Associate Professor
Department of Pathology and Laboratory
    Medicine
University of Rochester
Rochester, New York

Rod J. Turner Jr., MD, MS
Primary Care Sports Medicine Fellow
UT Health Science Center at Houston
Houston, Texas

Sahel Uddin, DO
Resident
Department of Family and Community
    Medicine
Penn State Health Milton S. Hershey
    Medical Center
Hershey, Pennsylvania

Victoria Udezi, MD, MPH
Assistant Professor
Department of Family and Community
    Medicine
UT Southwestern Medical Center
Dallas, Texas

Lyncean Ung, DO
Nassau University Medical Center
East Meadow, New York

Joseph Francis Urbanik, DO
Chief Resident
Department of Internal Medicine
Advocate Aurora Lutheran General
    Hospital
Park Ridge, Illinois

Onameyore Utuama, MD, MPH
Hospitalist
Emory Healthcare
Atlanta, Georgia

Haris Vakil, MD
2nd Year Resident
Department of Family Medicine
UTMB
Galveston, Texas

Santiago O. Valdes, MD, FAAP
Associate Professor
Department of Pediatric Cardiology
Baylor College of Medicine/Texas
    Children's Hospital
Houston, Texas

Carrie Valenta, MD, FACP, FHM
Associate Professor
Department of Internal Medicine
University of Nebraska Medical Center
Omaha, Nebraska

Virginia J. Van Duyne, MD
Assistant Professor and Associate
    Residency Director
Department of Family Medicine and
    Community Health
University of Massachusetts Medical
    School
Worcester, Massachusetts

Christine M. Van Horn, MD, MS
Resident Physician
Department of Urology
University of Massachusetts Medical
    School
Worcester, Massachusetts

Staci Lynn Vanderjack, MD, MPH
Residency Faculty
Department of Family Medicine
Advocate Christ Family Medicine
    Residency
Oak Lawn, Illinois

Kathleen M. Vazzana, DO, MSc
Pediatric Rheumatologist
Department of Pediatric Rheumatology
Arnold Palmer Hospital for Children
Orlando, Florida

Benjamin J. Velky, MD
Faculty Physician
Department of Family Medicine
Montgomery Center for Family Medicine
Greenwood, South Carolina

Juan Carlos Venis, MD, MPH
Assistant Professor of Clinical Family
    Medicine
Department of Family Medicine
Indiana University School of Medicine
Indianapolis, Indiana

Ashley L. Vertente, MD, MBA
Resident Physician PGY2
Saint Francis Hospital
Wilmington, Delaware

Brian P. Vickery, MD
Associate Professor of Pediatrics
Emory University School of Medicine
Children's Healthcare of Atlanta
Atlanta, Georgia

Astrud S. A. Villareal, MD
Assistant Professor
Associate Program Director
Medical Director
Parkland Family Medicine Clinic
Department of Family and Community
    Medicine
UT Southwestern Medical Center
Dallas, Texas

Kirsten Vitrikas, MD[†]
Program Director
Department of Family Medicine
    Residency
David Grant USAF Medical Center
Travis Air Force Base, California

Dana Vlachos, DO
Faculty Attending
Department of Family Medicine
    Residency
Advocate Christ Medical Center
Oak Lawn, Illinois

Yongkasem Vorasettakarnkij, MD, MSc[†]
Assistant Professor
Department of Medicine
Chulalongkorn University
Cardiac Center
King Chulalongkorn Memorial Hospital
Thai Red Cross Society
Bangkok, Thailand

Rebecca Wadlinger, DO, MS, ATC
Assistant Professor, Team Physician
Primary Care Sports Medicine
Department of Orthopaedics
Pennsylvania State University/Penn
    State Health
State College, Pennsylvania

Christopher M. Wagner, MD
Resident Physician
Department of Internal Medicine
Advocate Lutheran General Hospital
Park Ridge, Illinois

Joseph R. Wagner, MD
Chair
Department of Urology
Hartford Healthcare
Hartford Hospital

Rachel P. Walker, BA, MD
Department of Family and Community
    Medicine
The University of Texas Health Science
    Center
San Antonio, Texas

Thomas A. Waller, MD
Assistant Professor of Family Medicine
Residency Director
Department of Family Medicine
Mayo Clinic Florida
Jacksonville, Florida

Anne Walsh, MMSc, PA-C, DFAAPA
Clinical Associate Professor
Department of PA Studies
Chapman University
Irvine, California

Grace Walter, MD
PGY-3
MedStar Health
Georgetown-Washington Hospital Center
Family Medicine Residency Program
Washington, District of Columbia

Thandi Walters, MD
Department of Family Medicine
Tallahassee Memorial Hospital
Tallahassee, Florida

Judy Wang, MD
Resident Physician
Family Medicine
University of Massachusetts
Worcester, Massachusetts

Samuel C. Wang, MD
Program Director
Memorial Family Medicine Residency
    Program
Houston, Texas

Sicong Wang, MD[†]
Department of Family Medicine
Madigan Army Medical Center
Joint Base Lewis–McChord, Washington

Daniel L. Warden, MD
Primary Care Sports Medicine Fellow
Department of Sports Medicine
Ascension Providence
Novi, Michigan

Waiz Wasey, MD
Assistant Professor Family Medicine,
    Sleep Medicine
Department of Family Medicine
Southern Illinois University
Springfield, Illinois

Lynn K. Weaver, MD
Resident
Department of Family and Community
    Medicine
Penn State College of Medicine
Hershey, Pennsylvania

Marianna G. Weaver, MA, DO
Resident Physician
Department of Medicine
University of Louisville Hospital
Louisville, Kentucky

Grant Wei, MD, FACEP
Associate Professor and Program
    Director
Department of Emergency Medicine
Rutgers Robert Wood Johnson Medical
    School
New Brunswick, New Jersey

Jill T. Wei Doherty, MD
Department of Family Medicine
Santa Monica Family Physicians
Santa Monica, California

Maggie C. Wertz, MD[†]
Faculty Physician
Eglin Family Medicine Residency
Eglin Air Force Base, Florida

Tyler Martin West, MD
PGY-1
Department of Family Medicine
Novant Health Family Medicine
    Residency Program
Cornelius, North Carolina

Daniel Jordan Whitaker, MD
Physician
Department of Family Medicine
Womack Family Medicine Residency
    Clinic
Fort Bragg, North Carolina

Cassandra Q. White, MD, FACS
Associate Professor
Department of Surgery
Augusta University
Augusta, Georgia

John J. Whitney, BS
Midwestern University
Downers Grove, Illinois

Todd A. Wical, DO[†]
Squadron Flight Surgeon
Department of Primary Care
Blanchfield Army Community Hospital
Fort Campbell, Kentucky

Joseph P. Wiedemer, MD, FAAFP
Associate Professor
Department of Family and Community
    Medicine
Penn State Health
State College, Pennsylvania

Marcy R. Wiemers, MD
Associate Professor
Department of Family and Community
    Medicine
University of Texas Health Science
    Center at San Antonio
San Antonio, Texas

Susanne Wild, MD
Clinical Associate Professor
Department of Family Medicine
Family Medicine Residency
University of Arizona College of
    Medicine—Phoenix
Phoenix, Arizona

Brittany L. Wiles, MD[†]
Naval Hospital Jacksonville
Jacksonville, Florida

Alec M. Wilhelmi, MD
Resident Physician
Department of Family Medicine and
    Population Health
Dell Medical School, The University of
    Texas at Austin
Austin, Texas

Ashley Rose Wilk, DO
Associate Program Director and Clinical
    Assistant Professor
Florida State University College of
    Medicine Residency at BayCare Health
    System
Winter Haven, Florida

Antonio A. Williams, MD
Associate Program Director and
    Department Chair
Morrow, Georgia

Faren H. Williams, MD, MS[†]
Clinical Professor
Department of Orthopedics and Physical
    Rehabilitation
University of Massachusetts Medical
    School
Worcester, Massachusetts

Katherine Williams, MD
Attending Physician
Department of Family Medicine
Summa Health Medical Group
Rootstown, Ohio

Nathaniel R. Wilson, MD
Resident Physician
Department of Internal Medicine
The University of Texas Health Science
    Center at Houston
Houston, Texas

Norton Winer, MD[†]
Assistant Clinical Professor of Neurology
Department of Neurology
University Hospitals Cleveland
Cleveland, Ohio

Robyn Wing, MD, MPH
Assistant Professor of Emergency
    Medicine & Pediatrics
Warren Medical School of Brown
    University
Providence, Rhode Island

Fawn J. Winkelman, DO
Affiliate Professor
Department of Osteopathic Family
    Medicine
Nova Southeastern University College of
    Osteopathic
Fort Lauderdale, Florida

Jay Winner, MD, FAAFP
Family Physician and Director Stress
    Reduction Program
Department of Family Medicine
Sansum Clinic
Santa Barbara, California

Christopher M. Wise, MD
Professor of Internal Medicine
Department of Internal Medicine/
    Rheumatology, Allergy, and
    Immunology
Virginia Commonwealth University Health
    System
Richmond, Virginia

Amy L. Wiser, MD
Assistant Professor Department of
    Family Medicine
Oregon Health & Science University
Portland, Oregon

Anita Wong, MD
Assistant Clinical Professor
Department of Family Medicine
University of California, Los Angeles
Los Angeles, California

William W. Wong, DO[†]
University of Massachusetts Medical
    School
Worcester, Massachusetts

J. Andrew Woods, PharmD, BCPS
Associate Professor of Pharmacy
Wingate University School of Pharmacy
Wingate, North Carolina

Jocelyn Worley, DO[†]
The University of Texas at Austin
Austin, Texas

Alexandra Wright, MBBS, Hons
Medical Resident
TMH Family Medicine Residency
Tallahassee, Florida

Frances Yung-tao Wu, MD
Clinical Assistant Professor
Department of Family Medicine
Rutgers Robert Wood Johnson Medical
    School
New Brunswick, New Jersey
Assistant Director
Department of Family Medicine
    Residency
Robert Wood Johnson University Hospital
    Somerset
Somerville, New Jersey

Sujitha Yadlapati, MD
Resident Physician
Department of Dermatology
HCA Corpus Christi Medical Center-Bay
    Area Program
McAllen, Texas

Pratiksha Yalakkishettar, MD[†]
Worcester, Massachusetts

Alice Yang, MD
Resident Physician
Department of Family Medicine
Family Medicine Residency Program
Dell Medical School, The University of
    Texas at Austin
Austin, Texas

Michael Y. Yang, MD, CAQ-SM[†]
Section Chief of Sports Medicine
Mercy Orthopedics and Sports Medicine
Mercy Catholic Medical Center
Darby, Pennsylvania

Wail Yar, MD, MPH
Resident Physician
Department of Family Medicine
Cleveland Clinic
Fellow
Department of Preventive Medicine
Case Western Reserve University
Cleveland, Ohio

Dinesh Yogaratnam, PharmD
Associate Professor
Department of Pharmacy Practice
Massachusetts College of Pharmacy and
    Health Sciences University
Worcester, Massachusetts

James R. Yon, MD
Department of Trauma and Acute Care
    Surgery
New Hanover Regional Medical Center
Wilmington, North Carolina

Kyung In Yoon, MD
Emergency Medicine Physician
Department of Emergency
Piedmont Fayette Hospital
Fayetteville, Georgia

Christine Young, MD
Associate Program Director
Department of Family Medicine
Mount Carmel Family Medicine
    Residency
Westerville, Ohio

Jocelyn C. Young, DO, MSc
Clinical Assistant Professor
Department of Family Medicine
SUNY Upstate Medical University
Assistant Clinical Professor
Department of Family Medicine
United Health Services/Wilson Family
    Medicine Residency Program
Faculty Physician
Department of Family Medicine
United Health Services Hospitals
Johnson City, New York

Faraz Yousefian, DO
Department of Internal Medicine
Texas Institute for Graduate Medical
    Education and Research
San Antonio, Texas

David H. Yun, MD[†]
Family Physician
Okubo Family Health Clinic
Joint Base Lewis–McChord, Washington

Christopher A. Zagar, MD, FAAFP
Assistant Program Director
Novant Health Family Medicine
    Residency Program
Cornelius, North Carolina
Chair, Department of Family Medicine
Novant Health Huntersville Medical
    Center
Huntersville, North Carolina
Adjunct Assistant Professor
Department of Family Medicine
Campbell University Jerry M. Wallace
    School of Osteopathic Medicine
Buies Creek, North Carolina

Mallory Zaino, MD
Resident Physician
Department of Internal Medicine
University of Louisville
Louisville, Kentucky

Rochelle Zak, MD
Associate Professor
Department of Medicine/Sleep Disorders
    Center
University of California at San Francisco
San Francisco, California

Abdel-Rahman Zakieh, MD, BS
Resident Physician
Department of Internal Medicine
Advocate Lutheran General Hospital
Park Ridge, Illinois

Brittany E. Zeller, DO
Resident Physician
Department of Family Medicine
Mount Carmel Family Medicine
    Residency
Westerville, Ohio

Jaimei Zhang, MD, MPH
Resident
Department of Family Medicine
University of North Carolina
Chapel Hill, North Carolina

Anna K. Zheng, MD
OB Lead
Department of Family Medicine
Edward M. Kennedy Community Health
  Center
Assistant Professor
Department of Family Medicine and
  Community Health
University of Massachusetts Medical
  Center
Worcester, Massachusetts

Erika Zimmons, DO, MS
Assistant Professor
Department of Family Medicine and
  Community Health
University of Massachusetts Medical
  School
Worcester, Massachusetts

Patrick M. Zito, DO, PharmD
Voluntary Assistant Professor
Department of Dermatology & Cutaneous
  Surgery
University of Miami Miller School of
  Medicine
Miami, Florida

Susan Zweizig, MD
Professor
Department of Obstetrics and
  Gynecology
University of Massachusetts
Worcester, Massachusetts

†*The views expressed are those of the authors and do not reflect the official policy of the Department of the Army, Department of the Navy, Department of the Air Force, the Department of Defense, or the United States Government.*

CONTENTS

Topics

Contents

Diagnosis and Treatment: An Algorithmic Approach

This section contains flowcharts (or algorithms) to help the reader in the diagnosis of clinical signs and symptoms and treatment of a variety of clinical problems. They are organized by the presenting sign, symptom, or diagnosis.

These algorithms were designed to be used as a quick reference and adjunct to the reader's clinical knowledge and impression. They are not an exhaustive review of the management of a problem, nor are they meant to be a complete list of diseases.

ABDOMINAL PAIN, CHRONIC

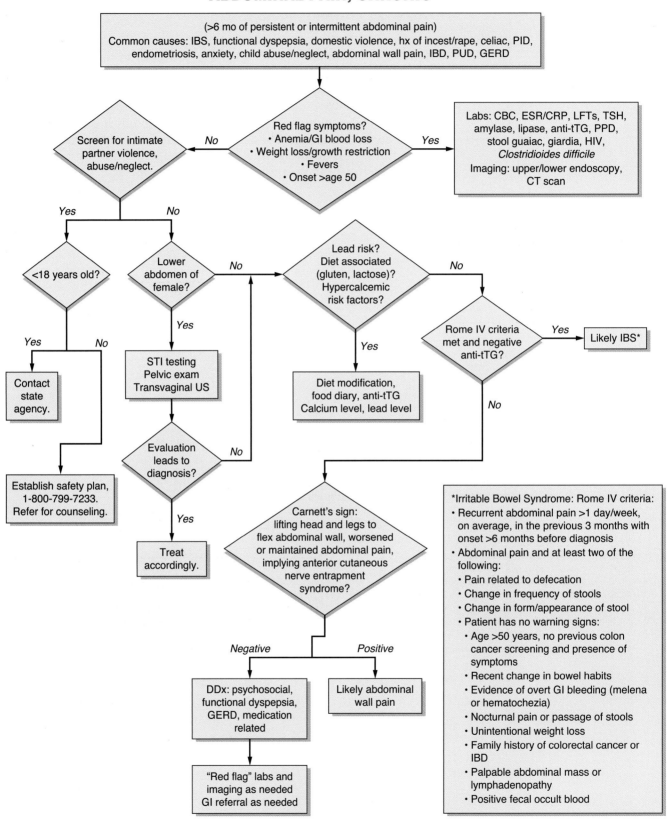

(>6 mo of persistent or intermittent abdominal pain)
Common causes: IBS, functional dyspepsia, domestic violence, hx of incest/rape, celiac, PID, endometriosis, anxiety, child abuse/neglect, abdominal wall pain, IBD, PUD, GERD

Red flag symptoms?
• Anemia/GI blood loss
• Weight loss/growth restriction
• Fevers
• Onset >age 50

No → Screen for intimate partner violence, abuse/neglect.

Yes → Labs: CBC, ESR/CRP, LFTs, TSH, amylase, lipase, anti-tTG, PPD, stool guaiac, giardia, HIV, *Clostridioides difficile*
Imaging: upper/lower endoscopy, CT scan

Yes → <18 years old?
No → Lower abdomen of female?

<18 years old?
Yes → Contact state agency.
No → Establish safety plan, 1-800-799-7233. Refer for counseling.

Lower abdomen of female?
No → Lead risk? Diet associated (gluten, lactose)? Hypercalcemic risk factors?
Yes → STI testing, Pelvic exam, Transvaginal US

STI testing → Evaluation leads to diagnosis?
No → (back to Lead risk?)
Yes → Treat accordingly.

Lead risk? Diet associated (gluten, lactose)? Hypercalcemic risk factors?
No → Rome IV criteria met and negative anti-tTG?
Yes → Diet modification, food diary, anti-tTG, Calcium level, lead level

Rome IV criteria met and negative anti-tTG?
Yes → Likely IBS*
No → (down to Carnett's sign)

Carnett's sign: lifting head and legs to flex abdominal wall, worsened or maintained abdominal pain, implying anterior cutaneous nerve entrapment syndrome?
Negative → DDx: psychosocial, functional dyspepsia, GERD, medication related → "Red flag" labs and imaging as needed, GI referral as needed
Positive → Likely abdominal wall pain

*Irritable Bowel Syndrome: Rome IV criteria:
• Recurrent abdominal pain >1 day/week, on average, in the previous 3 months with onset >6 months before diagnosis
• Abdominal pain and at least two of the following:
  • Pain related to defecation
  • Change in frequency of stools
  • Change in form/appearance of stool
• Patient has no warning signs:
  • Age >50 years, no previous colon cancer screening and presence of symptoms
  • Recent change in bowel habits
  • Evidence of overt GI bleeding (melena or hematochezia)
  • Nocturnal pain or passage of stools
  • Unintentional weight loss
  • Family history of colorectal cancer or IBD
  • Palpable abdominal mass or lymphadenopathy
  • Positive fecal occult blood

Kamini Geer, MD, MPH and LaRaey King, DO

Charles G, Chery M, Channell MK. Chronic abdominal pain: tips for the primary care provider. *Osteopath Fam Physician.* 2019;11(1):20–26.

ABDOMINAL PAIN, LOWER

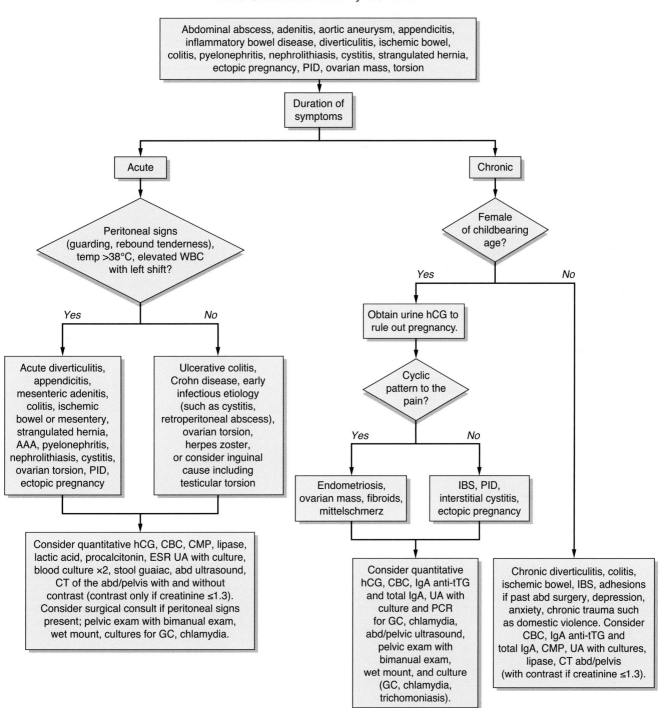

Kenneth A. Ballou, MD and Maegen Dupper, MD

Cartwright SL, Knudson MP. Diagnostic imaging of acute abdominal pain in adults. *Am Fam Physician* . 2015;91(7):452–459.

ABDOMINAL PAIN, UPPER

Right upper quadrant abdominal differential diagnosis:
- Biliary: cholecystitis, cholelithiasis, cholangitis
- Cardiac: myocardial infarction, pericarditis, angina
- Hepatic: abscess, hepatitis, mass
- Bowel: colitis, diverticulitis
- Pulmonary: pneumonia, emboli
- Renal: nephrolithiasis, pyelonephritis

Epigastric abdominal differential diagnosis:
- Biliary: cholecystitis, cholelithiasis, cholangitis
- Cardiac: myocardial infarction, pericarditis, angina
- Gastric: esophagitis, gastritis, GERD, functional dyspepsia, peptic ulcer disease
- Bowel: irritable bowel syndrome
- Pancreatic: mass, pancreatitis
- Vascular: aortic dissection, mesenteric ischemia

Left upper quadrant abdominal differential diagnosis:
- Cardiac: myocardial infarction, pericarditis, angina
- Gastric: esophagitis, gastritis, GERD, functional dyspepsia, peptic ulcer disease
- Pancreatic: mass, pancreatitis
- Renal: nephrolithiasis, pyelonephritis
- Pulmonary: pneumonia, emboli
- Vascular: aortic dissection, mesenteric ischemia
- Splenic: abscess, infection

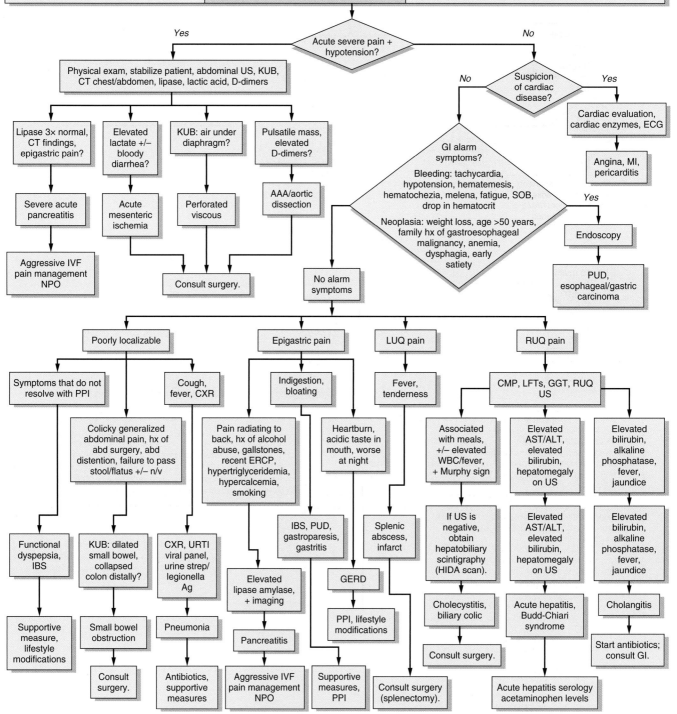

Brock McMillen, MD, FFAFP and Emilee J. Delbridge, PhD, LMFT

Vaghef-Davari F, Ahmadi-Amoli H, Sharifi A, et al. Approach to acute abdominal pain: practical algorithms. *Adv J Emerg Med.* 2019;4(2):e29.

ACETAMINOPHEN POISONING, TREATMENT

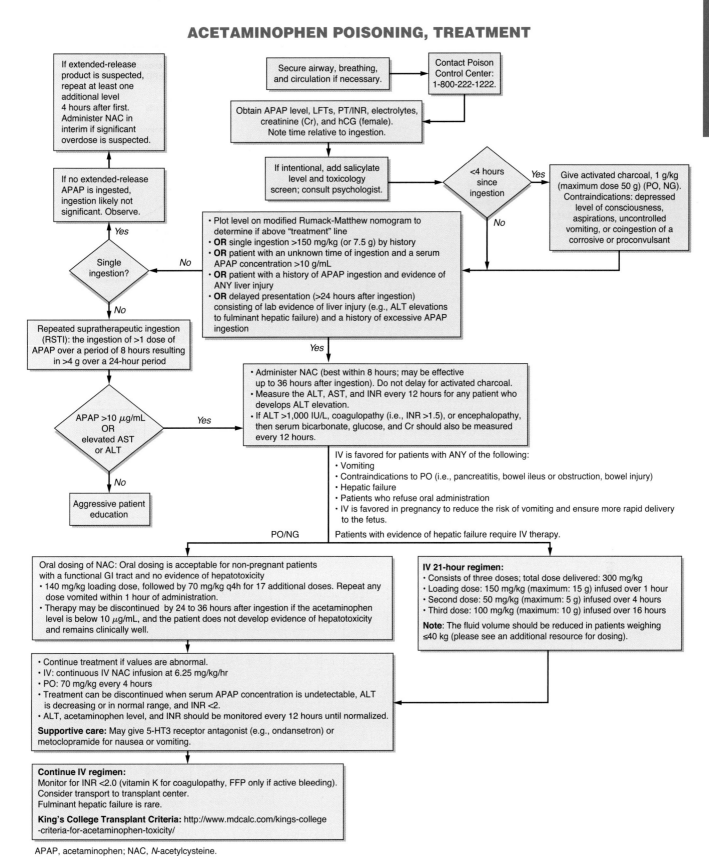

If extended-release product is suspected, repeat at least one additional level 4 hours after first. Administer NAC in interim if significant overdose is suspected.

Secure airway, breathing, and circulation if necessary.

Contact Poison Control Center: 1-800-222-1222.

Obtain APAP level, LFTs, PT/INR, electrolytes, creatinine (Cr), and hCG (female). Note time relative to ingestion.

If no extended-release APAP is ingested, ingestion likely not significant. Observe.

If intentional, add salicylate level and toxicology screen; consult psychologist.

<4 hours since ingestion — Yes → Give activated charcoal, 1 g/kg (maximum dose 50 g) (PO, NG). Contraindications: depressed level of consciousness, aspirations, uncontrolled vomiting, or coingestion of a corrosive or proconvulsant

No

Single ingestion? — Yes

No

- Plot level on modified Rumack-Matthew nomogram to determine if above "treatment" line
- **OR** single ingestion >150 mg/kg (or 7.5 g) by history
- **OR** patient with an unknown time of ingestion and a serum APAP concentration >10 g/mL
- **OR** patient with a history of APAP ingestion and evidence of ANY liver injury
- **OR** delayed presentation (>24 hours after ingestion) consisting of lab evidence of liver injury (e.g., ALT elevations to fulminant hepatic failure) and a history of excessive APAP ingestion

Yes

Repeated supratherapeutic ingestion (RSTI): the ingestion of >1 dose of APAP over a period of 8 hours resulting in >4 g over a 24-hour period

APAP >10 μg/mL OR elevated AST or ALT — Yes →

- Administer NAC (best within 8 hours; may be effective up to 36 hours after ingestion). Do not delay for activated charcoal.
- Measure the ALT, AST, and INR every 12 hours for any patient who develops ALT elevation.
- If ALT >1,000 IU/L, coagulopathy (i.e., INR >1.5), or encephalopathy, then serum bicarbonate, glucose, and Cr should also be measured every 12 hours.

No

Aggressive patient education

IV is favored for patients with ANY of the following:
- Vomiting
- Contraindications to PO (i.e., pancreatitis, bowel ileus or obstruction, bowel injury)
- Hepatic failure
- Patients who refuse oral administration
- IV is favored in pregnancy to reduce the risk of vomiting and ensure more rapid delivery to the fetus.

Patients with evidence of hepatic failure require IV therapy.

PO/NG

Oral dosing of NAC: Oral dosing is acceptable for non-pregnant patients with a functional GI tract and no evidence of hepatotoxicity
- 140 mg/kg loading dose, followed by 70 mg/kg q4h for 17 additional doses. Repeat any dose vomited within 1 hour of administration.
- Therapy may be discontinued by 24 to 36 hours after ingestion if the acetaminophen level is below 10 μg/mL, and the patient does not develop evidence of hepatotoxicity and remains clinically well.

IV 21-hour regimen:
- Consists of three doses; total dose delivered: 300 mg/kg
- Loading dose: 150 mg/kg (maximum: 15 g) infused over 1 hour
- Second dose: 50 mg/kg (maximum: 5 g) infused over 4 hours
- Third dose: 100 mg/kg (maximum: 10 g) infused over 16 hours

Note: The fluid volume should be reduced in patients weighing ≤40 kg (please see an additional resource for dosing).

- Continue treatment if values are abnormal.
- IV: continuous IV NAC infusion at 6.25 mg/kg/hr
- PO: 70 mg/kg every 4 hours
- Treatment can be discontinued when serum APAP concentration is undetectable, ALT is decreasing or in normal range, and INR <2.
- ALT, acetaminophen level, and INR should be monitored every 12 hours until normalized.

Supportive care: May give 5-HT3 receptor antagonist (e.g., ondansetron) or metoclopramide for nausea or vomiting.

Continue IV regimen:
Monitor for INR <2.0 (vitamin K for coagulopathy, FFP only if active bleeding).
Consider transport to transplant center.
Fulminant hepatic failure is rare.

King's College Transplant Criteria: http://www.mdcalc.com/kings-college-criteria-for-acetaminophen-toxicity/

APAP, acetaminophen; NAC, N-acetylcysteine.

Marissa T. Christian, PharmD, Ryan B. Feeney, PharmD, BCPS, BCGP, and Dean A. Christian, MD

Hodgman MJ, Garrard AR. A review of acetaminophen poisoning. *Crit Care Clin.* 2012;28(4):499–516.

ACIDOSIS

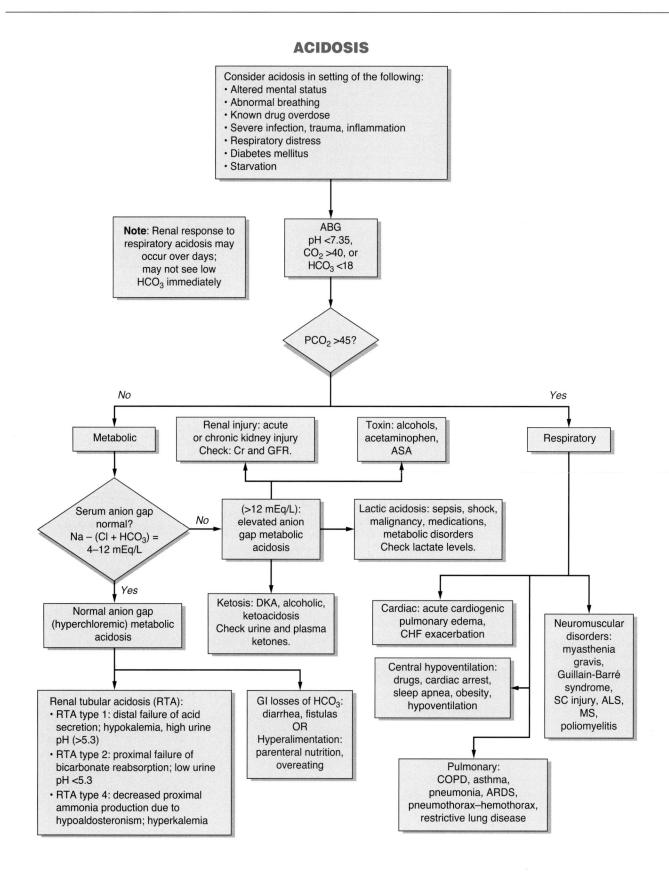

Consider acidosis in setting of the following:
- Altered mental status
- Abnormal breathing
- Known drug overdose
- Severe infection, trauma, inflammation
- Respiratory distress
- Diabetes mellitus
- Starvation

Note: Renal response to respiratory acidosis may occur over days; may not see low HCO_3 immediately

ABG
pH <7.35,
CO_2 >40, or
HCO_3 <18

PCO_2 >45?

No

Yes

Metabolic

Renal injury: acute or chronic kidney injury
Check: Cr and GFR.

Toxin: alcohols, acetaminophen, ASA

Respiratory

Serum anion gap normal?
$Na - (Cl + HCO_3) = 4–12$ mEq/L

No

(>12 mEq/L): elevated anion gap metabolic acidosis

Lactic acidosis: sepsis, shock, malignancy, medications, metabolic disorders
Check lactate levels.

Yes

Normal anion gap (hyperchloremic) metabolic acidosis

Ketosis: DKA, alcoholic, ketoacidosis
Check urine and plasma ketones.

Cardiac: acute cardiogenic pulmonary edema, CHF exacerbation

Neuromuscular disorders: myasthenia gravis, Guillain-Barré syndrome, SC injury, ALS, MS, poliomyelitis

Renal tubular acidosis (RTA):
- RTA type 1: distal failure of acid secretion; hypokalemia, high urine pH (>5.3)
- RTA type 2: proximal failure of bicarbonate reabsorption; low urine pH <5.3
- RTA type 4: decreased proximal ammonia production due to hypoaldosteronism; hyperkalemia

GI losses of HCO_3: diarrhea, fistulas
OR
Hyperalimentation: parenteral nutrition, overeating

Central hypoventilation: drugs, cardiac arrest, sleep apnea, obesity, hypoventilation

Pulmonary: COPD, asthma, pneumonia, ARDS, pneumothorax–hemothorax, restrictive lung disease

Shivani Malhotra, MD, FAAFP

Kraut JA, Madias NE. Serum anion gap: its uses and limitations in clinical medicine. *Clin J Am Soc Nephrol.* 2007;2(1):162–174.

ACNE

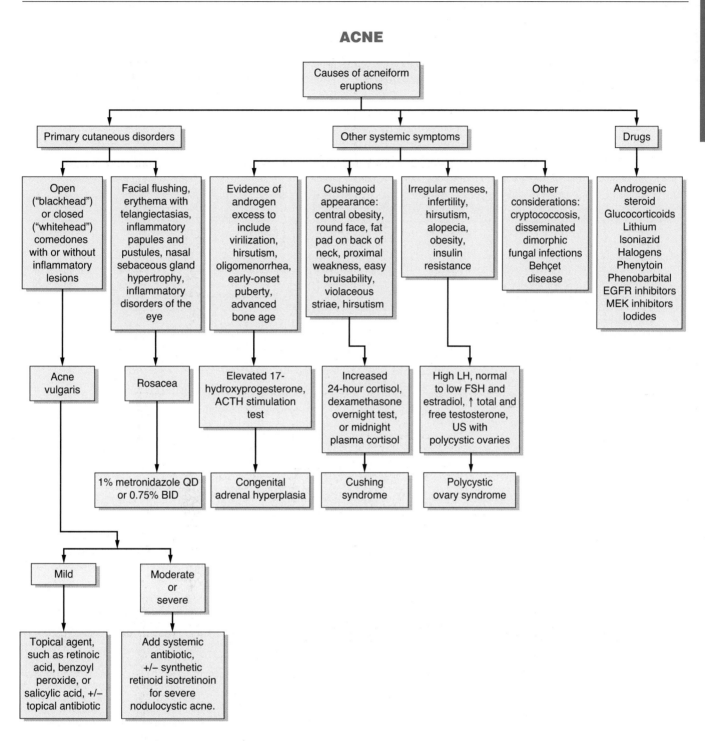

Christine A. Quartuccio-Carran, DO, FAAFP

Ogé LK, Broussard A, Marshall MD. Acne vulgaris: diagnosis and treatment. *Am Fam Physician*. 2019;100(8):475–484.

ALCOHOL WITHDRAWAL, TREATMENT

History: duration and quantity of alcohol intake for 2 weeks prior to presentation, time since last drink, previous episodes of alcohol withdrawal, concurrent substance use, preexisting medical and psychiatric conditions, prior detoxification admissions, prior seizure activity, living situation, social supports, stressors, triggers

Physical: VS (fever, tachycardia, tachypnea, hypertension), **CIWA** (see below), MSE (arousal, orientation, hallucinations), HEENT (diaphoresis, scleral icterus), CV (arrhythmias), evaluate s/sx of liver failure (ascites, varices, caput medusae, asterixis, palmar erythema), neuro (nystagmus, tremor, seizure activity)

Include assessment of conditions likely to *complicate*, *exacerbate*, or *precipitate* alcohol withdrawal: arrhythmias, CHF, CAD, dehydration, GI bleeding, infections, liver disease, pancreatitis, neurologic deficits.

Clinical Institute Withdrawal Assessment (CIWA) of Alcohol Scale (For patients in the ICU who cannot respond to questions, the MINDS protocol should be used.)
- Nausea and vomiting 0–7 (0, none; 4, intermittent; 7, constant nausea; frequent dry heaves/vomiting)
- Tremor 0–7 (0, none; 4, moderate; 7, severe; even with arms not extended)
- Paroxysmal sweats 0–7 (0, none; 4, beads of sweat; 7, drenching sweats)
- Anxiety 0–7 (0, none; 4, moderate; 7, acute panic state)
- Agitation 0–7 (0, none; 4, moderately restless; 7, constantly thrashing about or pacing)
- Tactile disturbances 0–7 (0, none; 1–3, for pruritus or paresthesias; 4–7, for hallucinations)
- Auditory disturbances 0–7 (0, none; 1–3, for increased sensitivity; 4–7, for hallucinations)
- Visual disturbances 0–7 (0, none; 1–3, for increased sensitivity; 4–7, for hallucinations)
- Headache 0–7 (0, no headache; 4, moderate; 7, extremely severe)
- Orientation 0–4 (0, fully oriented; 1, cannot do serial additions or is uncertain about date; 2, disoriented to date but within 2 calendar days; 3, disoriented to date by >2 days; 4, disoriented to place or person)

Mild withdrawal—CIWA 0–7 onset 5–8 hours after cessation or significant decrease in consumption: anxiety, restlessness, agitation, mild nausea, decreased appetite, sleep disturbance, facial sweating, mild tremulousness, fluctuating tachycardia and hypertension, possible mild cognitive impairment

Moderate withdrawal—CIWA 8–14 onset 24–48 hours after cessation: marked restlessness and agitation, moderate tremulousness with constant eye movement, diaphoresis, nausea, vomiting, anorexia, diarrhea

Severe withdrawal/delirium tremens—CIWA 15–30 onset 48–96 hours after alcohol cessation: marked tremulousness, fever, drenching sweats, severe hypertension and tachycardia, delirium

Good candidate for outpatient therapy:
- Not pregnant
- No comorbid illnesses requiring hospitalization
- No history of seizures
- Not a suicide risk
- Low risk of delirium tremens
- No history of unsuccessful outpatient detoxification
- Good access to follow-up medical care
- Tolerating oral medication
- Adequate social support available

Outpatient therapy contraindicated: pregnant, history of seizures or withdrawal seizures, chronic or acute comorbid illness requiring inpatient observation, lack of ability to follow-up

High risk of delirium tremens:
- Age >30 years
- Heavy drinking >8 years
- Drinking >100 g ethanol per day (>8 drinks per day)
- Random BAC >200 mg/dL
- Elevated MCV
- Cirrhosis

Admit to inpatient detoxification program:
- Replete thiamine IV as below before giving glucose and/or fluids containing dextrose to prevent Wernicke encephalopathy.
- VS q4h
- CIWA q4h
- Institute seizure precautions.
- IV fluids

Admit to ICU for inpatient detoxification:
- VS q15min
- CIWA q1h
- NPO, IV fluids
- Lateral decubitus position, restrain if necessary
- Glucose, sodium, potassium, phosphate, and magnesium replacement as needed

Treat as outpatient:
- Thiamine 100 mg once daily for 5 days
- Folic acid 1 g once daily for 5 days
- Evaluate daily until symptoms decrease.
- Assess blood pressure, heart rate, and CIWA-Ar score at each follow-up visit.
- Perform alcohol breath analysis randomly.
- Facilitate entry into a long-term outpatient therapy program (Alcoholics Anonymous).
- **If patient misses an appointment or resumes drinking, refer to addiction specialist or inpatient treatment facility.**
- Evaluate daily until symptoms decrease—usually for about 5 days. Face to face preferred but can alternate with telemedicine visits if necessary.
- Discuss any additional postwithdrawal treatment options through primary care or a specialized alcohol treatment program.

Labs:
- Toxicology screen/EtOH level to assess need for and timing of withdrawal regimen
- CBC, electrolytes, phosphate, magnesium; vitamin B_{12} and folate to be repleted regardless of blood levels
- Amylase/lipase if suspected pancreatitis
- PT, PTT if suspected liver failure
- LFTs, GGT
- UPT if premenopausal

Imaging:
- Head CT if history of trauma, mental status changes greater than expected, or focal neurologic changes
- Consider addition of EEG if focal neurologic signs or prolonged postictal state seizure.
- Consider addition of ECG if there is a history of cardiac problems.

Medications:
- Diazepam 5–20 mg IV q10min until calm and then q1h to maintain light somnolence for duration of delirium

If severe liver disease, severe asthma or respiratory failure, elderly, debilitated, or low serum albumin:
- Lorazepam 1–4 mg IV q10min until calm and then q1h to maintain light somnolence for duration of delirium

Example outpatient regimen:
Fixed diazepam schedule
Day 1: 10 mg q6h
Day 2: 10 mg q8h
Day 3: 10 mg q12h
Day 4/5: 10 mg at bedtime

Symptom-triggered diazepam schedule:
Give dose if CIWA >8.
Day 1: 10 mg q4h PRN
Day 2: 10 mg q6h PRN
Day 3: 10 mg q6h PRN
Days 4/5: 10 mg twice a day PRN
Pt with transaminitis, LFT >3 times normal USE Ativan in tapering doses over 5 days. May start with 2 mg q4h PRN

Fixed chlordiazepoxide (Librium) schedule:
Day 1: 50 mg PO q6h
Day 2: 25 mg q6h
Day 3: 25 mg q6h
Avoid in renal disease, liver disease, or elderly.

Discharge planning:
- CIWA scores <8–10 for 24 hours
- Begin 1:1 or group therapy.
- Discharge to treatment center, day program, home.
- Facilitate entry into Alcoholics Anonymous.
- Evaluate for outpatient treatment with benzodiazepine.
- Nutrition/social work consultation
- Close follow-up with primary care physician

Medications:
Nutritional replacement
- Thiamine 100 mg IV/IM or PO once daily for 5 days
- Folic acid 1 g PO once daily for 5 days

Sympatholytic adjunctive therapy (no effect on prevention of withdrawal seizure and should be used with benzodiazepine therapy)
- Atenolol 50–100 mg once daily
- Clonidine 0.2 mg 3 times daily

For hallucinations associated with withdrawal:
- Haloperidol 2–5 mg IM/PO q1–4h max 5 mg/day
- Use only in conjunction with benzodiazepines and with extreme caution because haloperidol may lower seizure threshold.
- Frequent reassurance, re-orientation to time and place, and nursing care are recommended nonpharmacologic interventions.

Supportive care
- Frequent reorientation to time and place may be needed for patient.
- Decrease stimulation.
- Encourage PO fluid intake of noncaffeinated beverages.

Medications:
Long-acting benzodiazepines (diazepam or chlordiazepoxide) provide lower chance of recurrent withdrawal or seizures. Symptom-triggered regimen is preferred over fixed dose regimen. If patient is at greater risk of complications, can consider front-loading approach (CIWA score of 19 or greater)

Symptom triggered (Assess using CIWA q1h. Once moderate symptoms controlled, can reduce assessment to q4–6h)
- Diazepam 10–20 mg (until CIWA-Ar <10)
  OR
- Chlordiazepoxide 50–100 (until CIWA-Ar <10)

Front loading
- Diazepam 10 mg PO q1h until CI WA-Ar <10

Fixed schedule
- Diazepam 20 mg PO q2–3h for three doses
  OR
- Chlordiazepoxide, 50 mg q6h for four doses, then 25 mg q6h for eight doses

Short-acting benzodiazepines (lorazepam) may have lower risk when there is concern about prolonged sedation, for example, h/o liver disease, LFT >3 times normal limit, elderly patients, or those with severe hepatic insufficiency.
- Lorazepam 1–2 mg PO q2–4h until CIWA <8

Astrud S. A. Villareal, MD, Tyler Evans, DO, and Victoria Udezi, MD, MPH

The ASAM clinical practice guideline on alcohol withdrawal management. *J Addict Med.* 2020;14(3S Suppl 1):1–72.

ALKALINE PHOSPHATASE ELEVATION

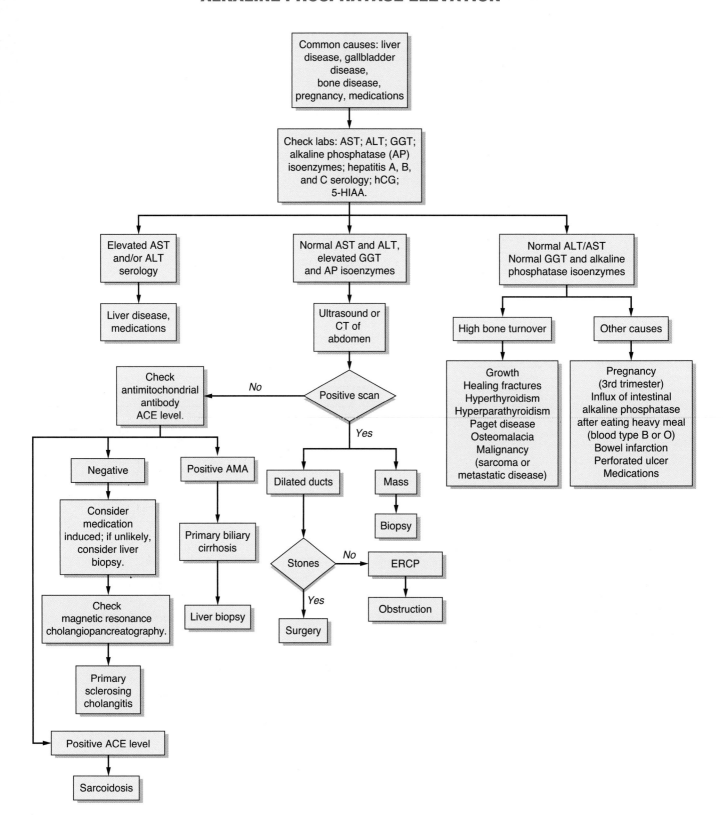

Reem Hadi, MD and Fozia Akhtar Ali, MD, FAAFP

Siddique A, Kowdley KV. Approach to a patient with elevated serum alkaline phosphatase. *Clin Liver Dis*. 2012;16(2):199–229.

AMENORRHEA, SECONDARY

Absence of menses >3 months in women with regular periods
OR
Absence of menses >6 months in women with irregular periods

↓

Common causes: pregnancy, ectopic pregnancy, anorexia/starvation, infection, PCOS, ovarian failure (menopause), pituitary adenoma, hypothyroidism, uterine causes (e.g., Asherman syndrome)

↓

Urine or serum hCG

(+)
Intrauterine pregnancy, ectopic pregnancy

(−)
Physical exam including vaginal and bimanual. Draw FSH; TSH; prolactin (PRL); and, if clinical hyperandrogenism present (hirsute, acne, oily skin), testosterone, DHEAS, +/− 17-hydroxyprogesterone.

↓

Is there a specific lab abnormality?

No

Perform progestational challenge (medroxy-progesterone) 10 mg daily × 10 days.

↓

Withdrawal bleeding?

Yes
Estrogen is present and endometrium functional; likely dx PCOS and other intermittent anovulatory states

No
Measure serum estrogen (E2).

Normal
Evaluate uterus and outflow tract (ultrasound, hysteroscopy) and also consider eating disorder, weight loss, and postcontraceptive amenorrhea.

Low
Primary and secondary hypothalamic amenorrhea—workup for celiac disease, diabetes, and consider MRI of sella

Yes

↑ ESH
Check E2.
Low
Menopause, primary ovarian insufficiency

↑ FSH
Check E2.
Low

Normal
Functional causes and PCOS

↑ TSH hypothyroidism (may also cause ↑ PRL)

↑ PRL
Rule out hypothyroidism with normal TSH.
↓
Repeat PRL.
↓
Stop medications potentially causing; e.g., phenothiazines.
↓
PRL >50–100 MRI of pituitary/sella (r/o prolactinoma)

↑ Testosterone and/or ↑ DHEAS
Androgen-secreting tumor (ovarian, adrenal) Consider Cushing disease.

Jeremy Golding, MD, FAAFP

Klein DA, Poth MA. Amenorrhea: an approach to diagnosis and management. *Am Fam Physician.* 2013;87(11):781–788.

ANEMIA

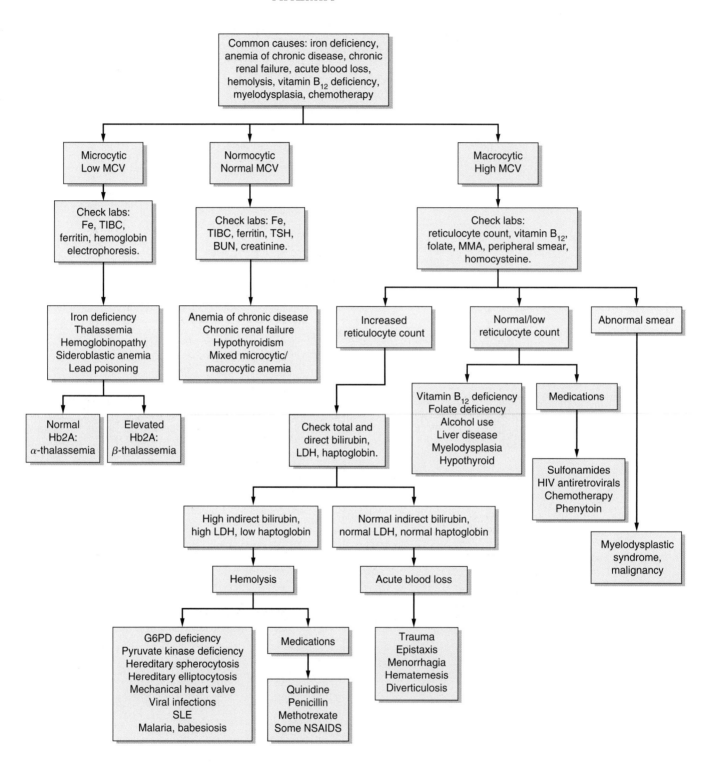

Brittany M. Reid, MBBS and Sandra S. Augusto, MD, MPH

Lanier JB, Park JJ, Callahan RC. Anemia in older adults. *Am Fam Physician.* 2018;98(7):437–442.

AST ELEVATION

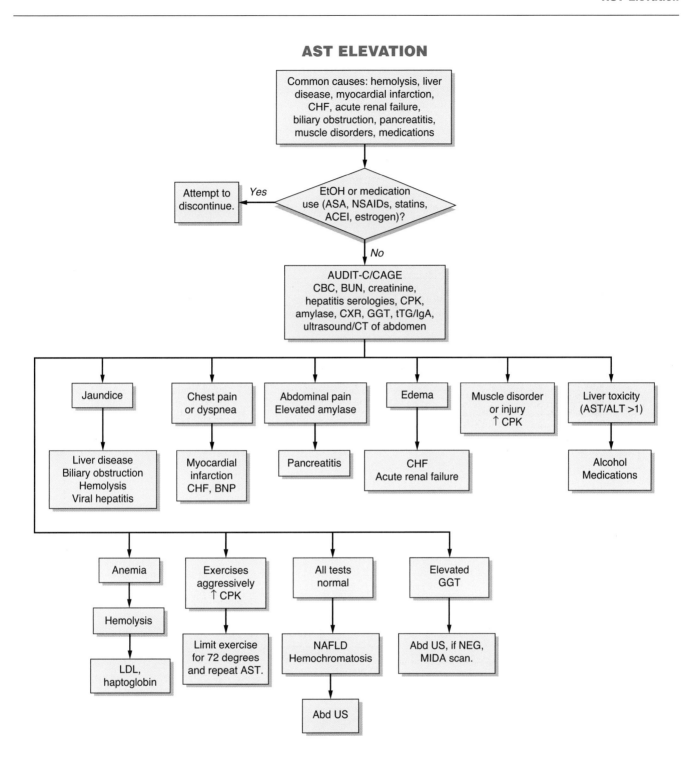

Bryce Ringwald, MD and Emily Ann Gorman, DO

Giboney PT. Mildly elevated liver transaminase levels in the asymptomatic patient. *Am Fam Physician*. 2005;71(6):1105–1110.

ASTHMA EXACERBATION, PEDIATRIC ACUTE

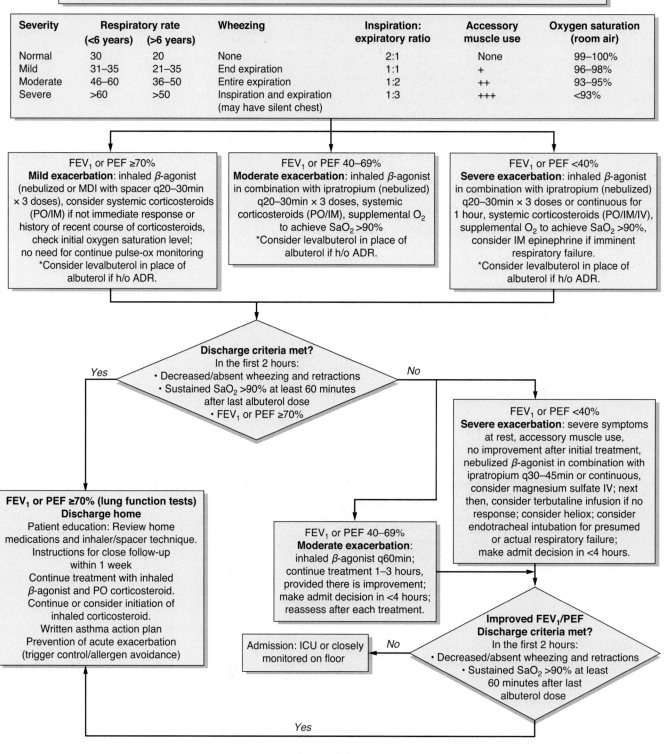

Jan Estes Miller, MD

National Asthma Education and Prevention Program. Expert Panel Report 3 (EPR-3): guidelines for the diagnosis and management of asthma—summary report 2007. *J Allergy Clin Immunol.* 2007;120(5 Suppl):S94–S138.

ASTHMA TREATMENT AND MAINTENANCE

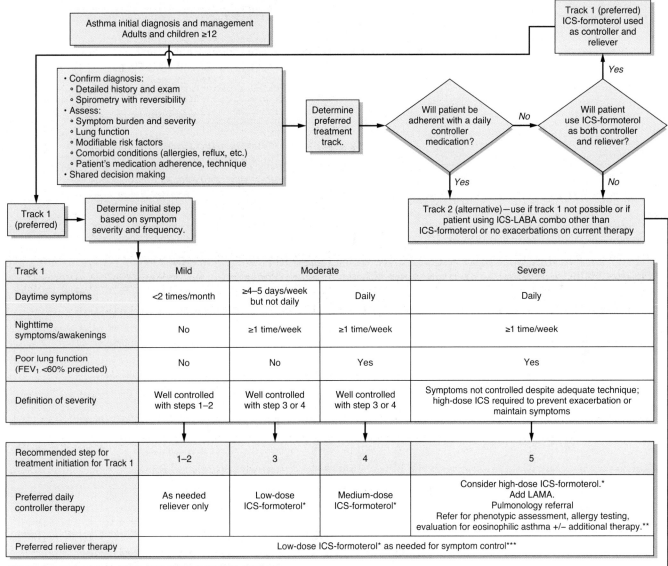

Asthma initial diagnosis and management
Adults and children ≥12

- Confirm diagnosis:
  - Detailed history and exam
  - Spirometry with reversibility
- Assess:
  - Symptom burden and severity
  - Lung function
  - Modifiable risk factors
  - Comorbid conditions (allergies, reflux, etc.)
  - Patient's medication adherence, technique
- Shared decision making

Determine preferred treatment track.

Will patient be adherent with a daily controller medication? —No→ Will patient use ICS-formoterol as both controller and reliever?

Yes ↓ (to Track 2) Yes ↑ → Track 1 (preferred) ICS-formoterol used as controller and reliever

No → Track 2 (alternative)—use if track 1 not possible or if patient using ICS-LABA combo other than ICS-formoterol or no exacerbations on current therapy

Track 1 (preferred) → Determine initial step based on symptom severity and frequency.

Track 1	Mild	Moderate		Severe
Daytime symptoms	<2 times/month	≥4–5 days/week but not daily	Daily	Daily
Nighttime symptoms/awakenings	No	≥1 time/week	≥1 time/week	≥1 time/week
Poor lung function (FEV$_1$ <60% predicted)	No	No	Yes	Yes
Definition of severity	Well controlled with steps 1–2	Well controlled with step 3 or 4	Well controlled with step 3 or 4	Symptoms not controlled despite adequate technique; high-dose ICS required to prevent exacerbation or maintain symptoms

Recommended step for treatment initiation for Track 1	1–2	3	4	5
Preferred daily controller therapy	As needed reliever only	Low-dose ICS-formoterol*	Medium-dose ICS-formoterol*	Consider high-dose ICS-formoterol.* Add LAMA. Pulmonology referral Refer for phenotypic assessment, allergy testing, evaluation for eosinophilic asthma +/– additional therapy.**
Preferred reliever therapy	Low-dose ICS-formoterol* as needed for symptom control***			

ICS, inhaled corticosteroid; LAMA, long-acting muscarinic antagonist.
*See Table 1 for low-, medium-, and high-dose ICS formulations.
***Maximum recommended dose of as needed ICS-formoterol is 72 μg/day of formoterol (54 μg metered dose).

Track 2 (alternative) → Determine initial step based on symptom severity and frequency.

Track 2	Mild		Moderate	Severe
Daytime symptoms	<2 times/month	≥2 times/month but <4–5 days/week	≥4–5 days/week but not daily	Daily
Nighttime symptoms/ awakenings	No	No	≥1 time/week	≥1 time/week
Poor lung function (FEV$_1$ <60% predicted)	No	No	Yes	Yes
Definition of severity	N/A	N/A	N/A	Symptoms not controlled despite adequate technique; high-dose ICS required to prevent exacerbation or maintain symptoms

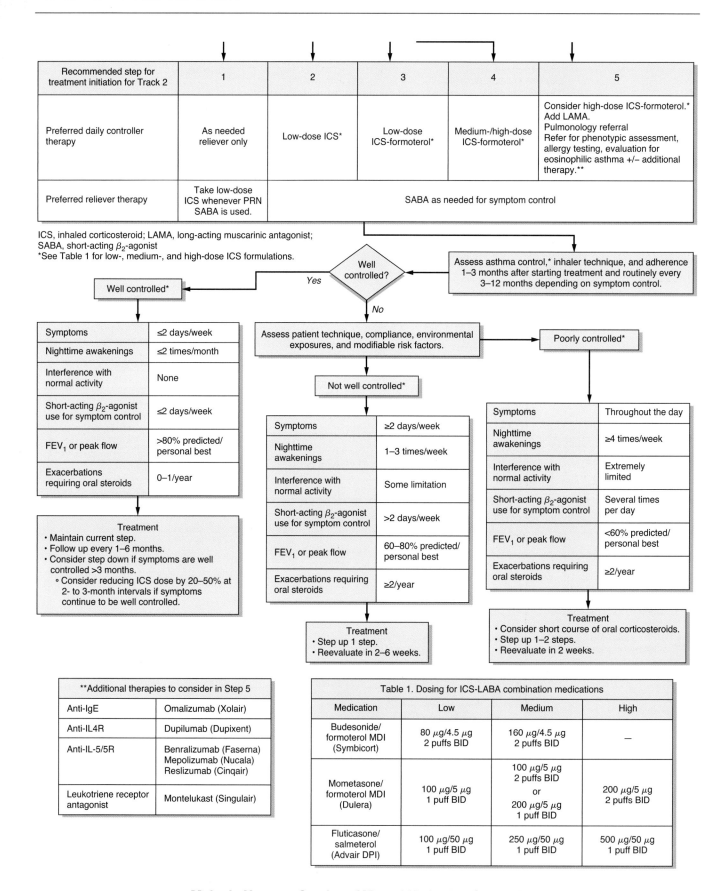

Recommended step for treatment initiation for Track 2	1	2	3	4	5
Preferred daily controller therapy	As needed reliever only	Low-dose ICS*	Low-dose ICS-formoterol*	Medium-/high-dose ICS-formoterol*	Consider high-dose ICS-formoterol.* Add LAMA. Pulmonology referral Refer for phenotypic assessment, allergy testing, evaluation for eosinophilic asthma +/– additional therapy.**
Preferred reliever therapy	Take low-dose ICS whenever PRN SABA is used.	SABA as needed for symptom control			

ICS, inhaled corticosteroid; LAMA, long-acting muscarinic antagonist; SABA, short-acting β_2-agonist
*See Table 1 for low-, medium-, and high-dose ICS formulations.

Assess asthma control,* inhaler technique, and adherence 1–3 months after starting treatment and routinely every 3–12 months depending on symptom control.

Well controlled?

Yes

Well controlled*

No

Assess patient technique, compliance, environmental exposures, and modifiable risk factors.

Poorly controlled*

Not well controlled*

Symptoms	≤2 days/week
Nighttime awakenings	≤2 times/month
Interference with normal activity	None
Short-acting β_2-agonist use for symptom control	≤2 days/week
FEV$_1$ or peak flow	>80% predicted/ personal best
Exacerbations requiring oral steroids	0–1/year

Treatment
• Maintain current step.
• Follow up every 1–6 months.
• Consider step down if symptoms are well controlled >3 months.
   ◦ Consider reducing ICS dose by 20–50% at 2- to 3-month intervals if symptoms continue to be well controlled.

Symptoms	≥2 days/week
Nighttime awakenings	1–3 times/week
Interference with normal activity	Some limitation
Short-acting β_2-agonist use for symptom control	>2 days/week
FEV$_1$ or peak flow	60–80% predicted/ personal best
Exacerbations requiring oral steroids	≥2/year

Treatment
• Step up 1 step.
• Reevaluate in 2–6 weeks.

Symptoms	Throughout the day
Nighttime awakenings	≥4 times/week
Interference with normal activity	Extremely limited
Short-acting β_2-agonist use for symptom control	Several times per day
FEV$_1$ or peak flow	<60% predicted/ personal best
Exacerbations requiring oral steroids	≥2/year

Treatment
• Consider short course of oral corticosteroids.
• Step up 1–2 steps.
• Reevaluate in 2 weeks.

**Additional therapies to consider in Step 5	
Anti-IgE	Omalizumab (Xolair)
Anti-IL4R	Dupilumab (Dupixent)
Anti-IL-5/5R	Benralizumab (Faserna) Mepolizumab (Nucala) Reslizumab (Cinqair)
Leukotriene receptor antagonist	Montelukast (Singulair)

Table 1. Dosing for ICS-LABA combination medications			
Medication	Low	Medium	High
Budesonide/ formoterol MDI (Symbicort)	80 μg/4.5 μg 2 puffs BID	160 μg/4.5 μg 2 puffs BID	–
Mometasone/ formoterol MDI (Dulera)	100 μg/5 μg 1 puff BID	100 μg/5 μg 2 puffs BID or 200 μg/5 μg 1 puff BID	200 μg/5 μg 2 puffs BID
Fluticasone/ salmeterol (Advair DPI)	100 μg/50 μg 1 puff BID	250 μg/50 μg 1 puff BID	500 μg/50 μg 1 puff BID

Melanie Houston Sanders, MD and Katherine Gagan, MD

Global Initiative for Asthma. Global strategy for asthma management and prevention, 2021. http://www.ginasthma.org/wp-content/uploads/2021/05/GINA-Main-Report-2021-V2-WMS.pdf. Accessed November 9, 2021.

ATAXIA

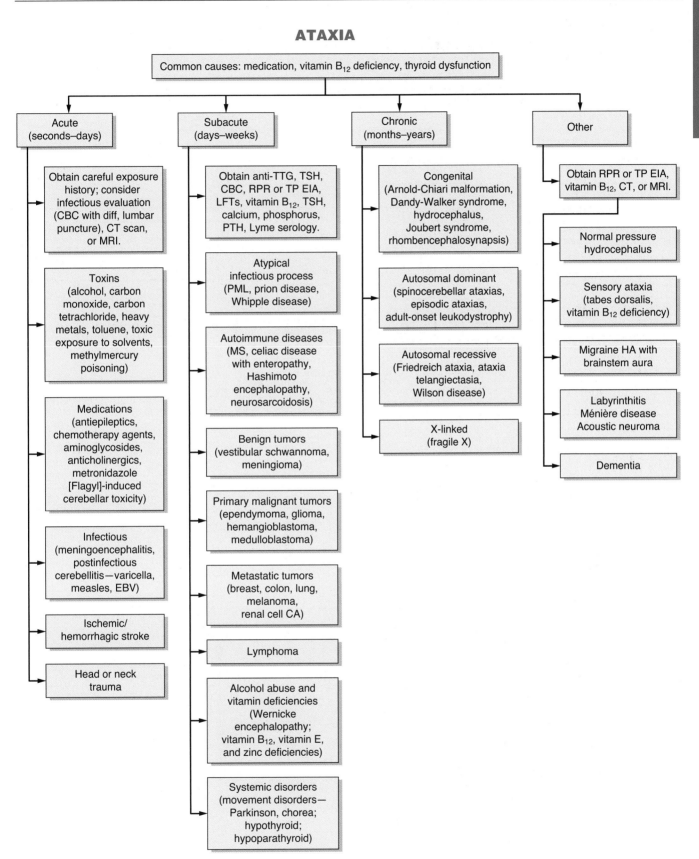

Common causes: medication, vitamin B$_{12}$ deficiency, thyroid dysfunction

Acute (seconds–days)

- Obtain careful exposure history; consider infectious evaluation (CBC with diff, lumbar puncture), CT scan, or MRI.
- Toxins (alcohol, carbon monoxide, carbon tetrachloride, heavy metals, toluene, toxic exposure to solvents, methylmercury poisoning)
- Medications (antiepileptics, chemotherapy agents, aminoglycosides, anticholinergics, metronidazole [Flagyl]-induced cerebellar toxicity)
- Infectious (meningoencephalitis, postinfectious cerebellitis—varicella, measles, EBV)
- Ischemic/hemorrhagic stroke
- Head or neck trauma

Subacute (days–weeks)

- Obtain anti-TTG, TSH, CBC, RPR or TP EIA, LFTs, vitamin B$_{12}$, TSH, calcium, phosphorus, PTH, Lyme serology.
- Atypical infectious process (PML, prion disease, Whipple disease)
- Autoimmune diseases (MS, celiac disease with enteropathy, Hashimoto encephalopathy, neurosarcoidosis)
- Benign tumors (vestibular schwannoma, meningioma)
- Primary malignant tumors (ependymoma, glioma, hemangioblastoma, medulloblastoma)
- Metastatic tumors (breast, colon, lung, melanoma, renal cell CA)
- Lymphoma
- Alcohol abuse and vitamin deficiencies (Wernicke encephalopathy; vitamin B$_{12}$, vitamin E, and zinc deficiencies)
- Systemic disorders (movement disorders—Parkinson, chorea; hypothyroid; hypoparathyroid)

Chronic (months–years)

- Congenital (Arnold-Chiari malformation, Dandy-Walker syndrome, hydrocephalus, Joubert syndrome, rhombencephalosynapsis)
- Autosomal dominant (spinocerebellar ataxias, episodic ataxias, adult-onset leukodystrophy)
- Autosomal recessive (Friedreich ataxia, ataxia telangiectasia, Wilson disease)
- X-linked (fragile X)

Other

- Obtain RPR or TP EIA, vitamin B$_{12}$, CT, or MRI.
- Normal pressure hydrocephalus
- Sensory ataxia (tabes dorsalis, vitamin B$_{12}$ deficiency)
- Migraine HA with brainstem aura
- Labyrinthitis Ménière disease Acoustic neuroma
- Dementia

Fozia Akhtar Ali, MD, FAAFP, Teny Philip Thomas, MD, and Maryse Emmerencia Bakouetila, MD

Brunberg JA; for Expert Panel on Neurologic Imaging. Ataxia. *AJNR Am J Neuroradiol.* 2008;29(7):1420–1422.

AZOTEMIA AND UREMIA

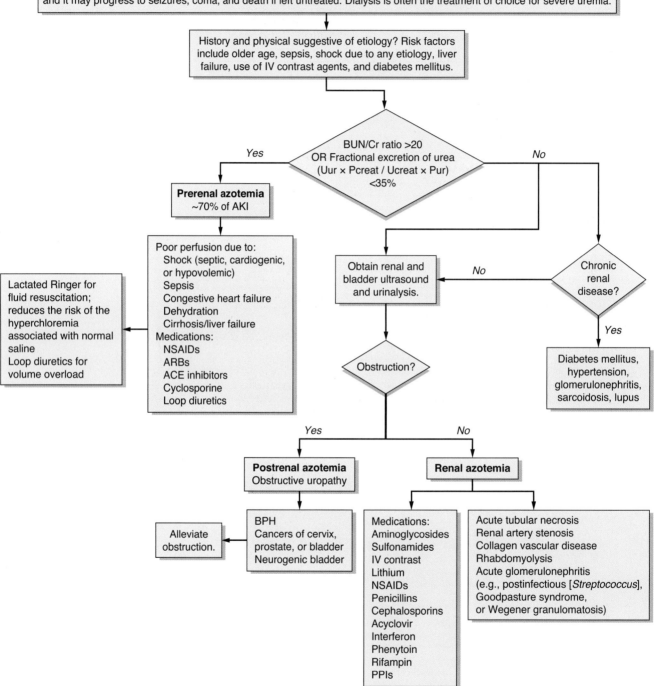

Azotemia is the elevation of blood urea nitrogen (BUN). It can be divided into prerenal, intrinsic renal, and postrenal azotemia based on the cause. This is important because treatments differ. Azotemia is called uremia if signs and symptoms, for example, nausea, vomiting, severe metabolic acidosis, hyperkalemia, and fluid overload, among others, develop. Uremia is mostly due to the accumulation of BUN and other toxins or waste products normally filtered by the kidney, and it may progress to seizures, coma, and death if left untreated. Dialysis is often the treatment of choice for severe uremia.

History and physical suggestive of etiology? Risk factors include older age, sepsis, shock due to any etiology, liver failure, use of IV contrast agents, and diabetes mellitus.

BUN/Cr ratio >20 OR Fractional excretion of urea $(U_{ur} \times P_{creat} / U_{creat} \times P_{ur})$ <35%

Yes

Prerenal azotemia
~70% of AKI

Poor perfusion due to:
  Shock (septic, cardiogenic, or hypovolemic)
  Sepsis
  Congestive heart failure
  Dehydration
  Cirrhosis/liver failure
Medications:
  NSAIDs
  ARBs
  ACE inhibitors
  Cyclosporine
  Loop diuretics

Lactated Ringer for fluid resuscitation; reduces the risk of the hyperchloremia associated with normal saline
Loop diuretics for volume overload

No

Obtain renal and bladder ultrasound and urinalysis.

Chronic renal disease?

No

Yes

Diabetes mellitus, hypertension, glomerulonephritis, sarcoidosis, lupus

Obstruction?

Yes

Postrenal azotemia
Obstructive uropathy

BPH
Cancers of cervix, prostate, or bladder
Neurogenic bladder

Alleviate obstruction.

No

Renal azotemia

Medications:
  Aminoglycosides
  Sulfonamides
  IV contrast
  Lithium
  NSAIDs
  Penicillins
  Cephalosporins
  Acyclovir
  Interferon
  Phenytoin
  Rifampin
  PPIs

Acute tubular necrosis
Renal artery stenosis
Collagen vascular disease
Rhabdomyolysis
Acute glomerulonephritis
(e.g., postinfectious [*Streptococcus*], Goodpasture syndrome, or Wegener granulomatosis)

Steven A. House, MD, FAAFP, FAAHPM, HMDC

Mercado MG, Smith DK, Guard EL. Acute kidney injury: diagnosis and management. *Am Fam Physician*. 2019;100(11):687–694.

CARDIAC ARRHYTHMIAS

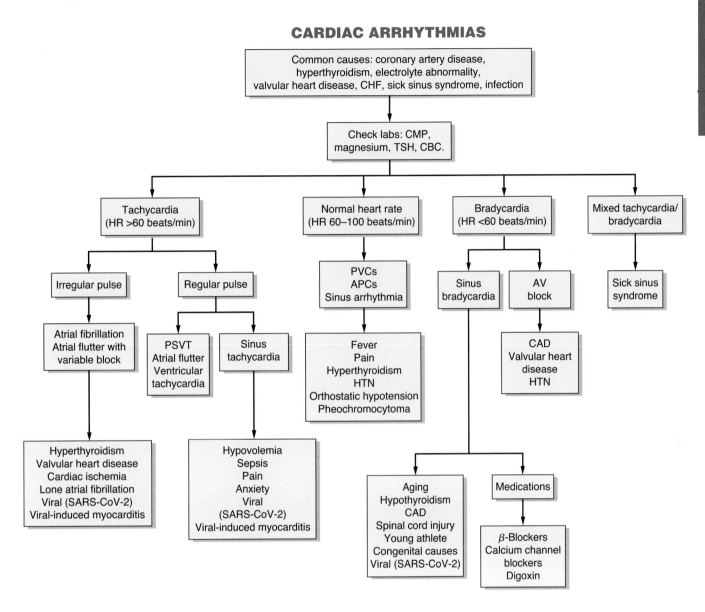

Frank Estrella, DO and Jon Daniel Montemayor, MD

Babapoor-Farrokhran S, Rasekhi RT, Gill D, et al. Arrhythmia in COVID-19 [published online ahead of print August 14, 2020]. *SN Compr Clin Med*. doi:10.1007/s42399-020-00454-2.

CERVICAL HYPEREXTENSION INJURY

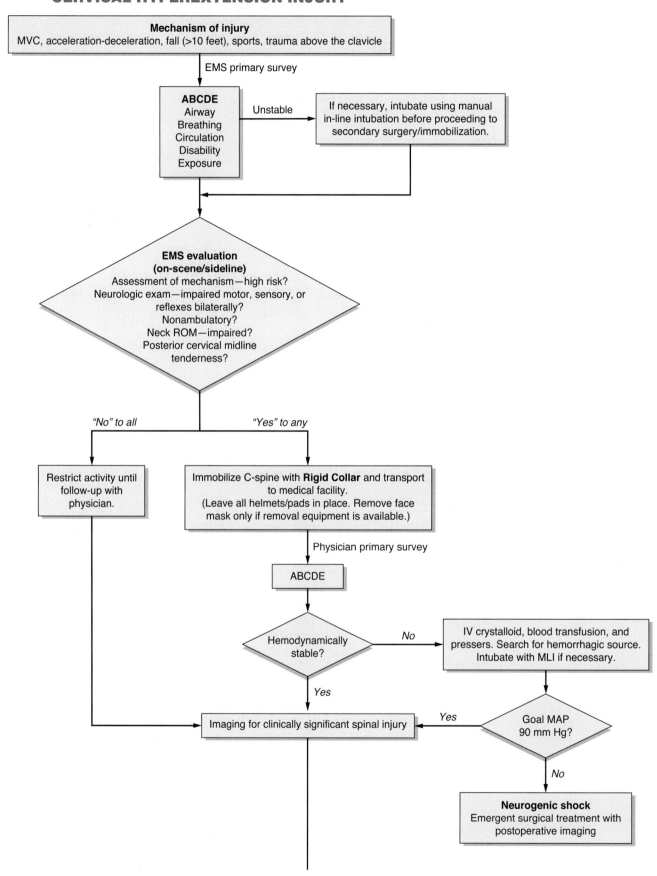

Mechanism of injury
MVC, acceleration-deceleration, fall (>10 feet), sports, trauma above the clavicle

EMS primary survey

ABCDE
Airway
Breathing
Circulation
Disability
Exposure

Unstable → If necessary, intubate using manual in-line intubation before proceeding to secondary surgery/immobilization.

**EMS evaluation
(on-scene/sideline)**
Assessment of mechanism—high risk?
Neurologic exam—impaired motor, sensory, or reflexes bilaterally?
Nonambulatory?
Neck ROM—impaired?
Posterior cervical midline tenderness?

"No" to all

"Yes" to any

Restrict activity until follow-up with physician.

Immobilize C-spine with **Rigid Collar** and transport to medical facility.
(Leave all helmets/pads in place. Remove face mask only if removal equipment is available.)

Physician primary survey

ABCDE

Hemodynamically stable?

No → IV crystalloid, blood transfusion, and pressers. Search for hemorrhagic source. Intubate with MLI if necessary.

Yes

Imaging for clinically significant spinal injury

Goal MAP 90 mm Hg?

Yes

No

Neurogenic shock
Emergent surgical treatment with postoperative imaging

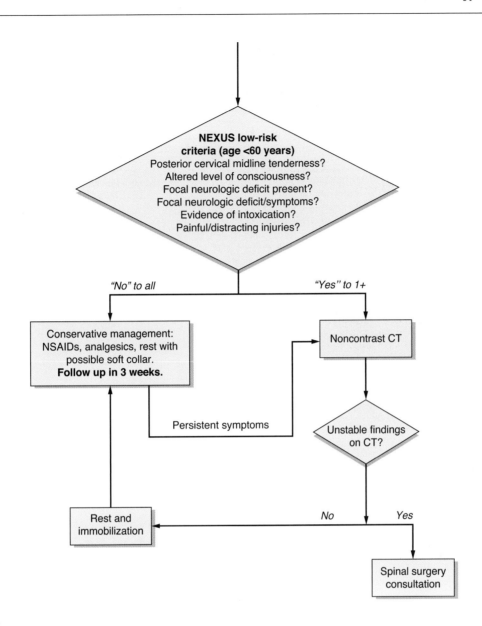

**NEXUS low-risk
criteria (age <60 years)**
Posterior cervical midline tenderness?
Altered level of consciousness?
Focal neurologic deficit present?
Focal neurologic deficit/symptoms?
Evidence of intoxication?
Painful/distracting injuries?

"No" to all

"Yes" to 1+

Conservative management:
NSAIDs, analgesics, rest with
possible soft collar.
Follow up in 3 weeks.

Noncontrast CT

Persistent symptoms

Unstable findings
on CT?

Rest and
immobilization

No

Yes

Spinal surgery
consultation

Ashley L. Vertente, MD, MBA and Michael Y. Yang, MD, CAQ-SM

Schleicher P, Pingel A, Kandziora F. Safe management of acute cervical spine injuries. *EFORT Open Rev.* 2018;3(5):347–357.

CHEST PAIN/ACUTE CORONARY SYNDROME

Common DDx: STEMI, NSTEMI/unstable angina, PE, aortic dissection, PTX, pericarditis, Boerhaave, anxiety, costochondritis, GI-related, domestic violence

ECG

STEMI criteria or STEMI equivalent

Alert cardiology

No STEMI criteria or STEMI equivalent

STEMI criteria

Any of the following

- 1 mm ST elevation in any two contiguous leads except V_2 and V_3
  - In women: 1.5 mm elevation in V_2 or V_3
  - In men <40 years: 2.5 mm elevation in V_2 or V_3
  - In men ≥40 years: 2 mm in V_2 or V_3

STEMI equivalents

- ST elevation in aVR with ST depression in six leads
- de Winter T waves
- ST depression in V_2 and V_3 and concerning posterior ECG

162–325 mg ASA
O_2 if SpO_2 <90%
SL NTG q5min × 3 PRN for pain (avoid in inferior STEMI)
Load with dual antiplatelet agent
  - Clopidogrel 300 mg ~OR~
  - Ticagrelor 180 mg ~OR~
  - Prasugrel 60 mg
Heparin bolus
Avoid morphine if possible (may interfere with antiplatelet agent).
Troponin, CXR

ASA 162–325 mg, serial troponin, serial ECG if continuing chest pain, CXR

Serial troponin positive

Yes — *No*

- Admit
- Heparin bolus
- ASA daily
- Consider nitrates, clopidogrel, β-blocker, ACEi, statin.

Risk stratify for CAD

High risk — Medium risk — Low risk

PCI available within 120 minutes

Yes — *No*

PCI

Administer thrombolytic within 30 minutes if unable to PCI within 120 minutes.

Cardiology evaluation for consideration of cardiac catheterization

Positive

Stress test

Negative

Discharge home with PCP follow-up.

Successful treatment

No — *Yes*

Consider CABG.

Medical therapy
- ASA 81 mg
- Clopidogrel 75 mg daily
- High-intensity statin
- β-blocker unless CHF or shock
- Cardiac rehabilitation
- ACE inhibitor for patients with reduced EF
- Consider aldosterone antagonist if EF <40%.

Review DDx: anxiety, GERD, PE, biliary dysfunction, MSK pain, domestic violence.

Jason Teng, MD and Moises Gallegos, MD, MPH

Thygesen K, Alpert JS, Jaffe AS, et al. Fourth universal definition of myocardial infarction (2018). *J Am Coll Cardiol.* 2018;72(18):2231–2264.

CHILD ABUSE: NONACCIDENTAL TRAUMA

When should you consider NAT in young children?

Skin Injury	**Age <6 months** • Any bruise or oral injury **Age 6 months–4 years** • Unexplained bruises in noncruising children • Bruises on the trunk, ear, neck, jaw line, cheek • Patterned bruising • Subconjunctival hemorrhage • Frenular tears
Burns	**Any age** • Unexplained burns • Burns in the shape of a heated object • Immersion burns • Burns on both the perineum and lower extremities
Fractures	**Age <6 months** • Any fracture **Age 6–11 months** • Linear parietal skull fractures without history • Any nonlinear parietal skull fracture • Any fracture of the ribs, femur, or humera • Nonskull fractures in nonambulatory children • Any other fracture without history **Age 12–23 months** • Any rib or femur fracture • Nonsupracondylar humerus fracture • Any other fracture without history **Age 24 months–4 years** • Any rib fracture • Any other fracture without history
Intracranial	**Age <12 months** • Any subdural hemorrhage or hygroma **Age 12 months–4 years** • Acute subdural hematoma without history of high energy trauma (e.g., MVC, long-distance fall)
Visceral	**Age <12 months** • Any visceral injury **Age 12 months–4 years** • Unexplained traumatic visceral injury • Trauma to pancreas • Proximal hollow viscus injury

When should you consider NAT in older children?

• When a child makes a disclosure
• When there is no or inconsistent history to explain an injury
• When a prepubertal child displays sexualized behaviors
• When a prepubertal child has genital injury or infection
• Any pregnancy in a child under 16 years old

Medical History

• If possible, interview the child separate from their guardian.
• Ask open-ended questions that do not introduce concepts of intentional injury or inappropriate behavior.
• When a child makes a disclosure, listen attentively, believe them, and thank them for telling you.

1. Obtain a focused injury history, especially a clear timeline.
2. PMH, that is, prior traumas, injuries, surgeries, hospitalizations
3. Family bleeding, bruising, bone, metabolic, or genetic history
4. Developmental and behavioral history
5. Social history, including living situation, other children in household, substance use, psychosocial stressors

Physical Examination

1. General assessment (alertness, demeanor, growth, evidence of neglect like severe caries, neglected wound care, etc.)
2. Skin exam, noting bruises, lacerations, burns, bites, etc.
3. Complete neurologic exam.
4. Consider secure photographs or sketches of physical signs.
5. If suspecting sexual violence, a specialized provider like a SANE nurse should perform the genital exam, if available.

Diagnostic Testing for Suspected NAT

1. Skeletal survey for those under 24 months
2. Head CT or MRI if <6 months or concerned for head trauma
3. Consider basic lab evaluation: AST/ALT, urine toxicology
4. If bruising: CBC, PT, aPTT, von Willebrand, factor VIII + IX
5. If fractures: Ca, Mg, phos, alk phos, PTH, vitamin D
6. If focal neuro findings or IC bleeding: Consult ophthalmology.

Management of Suspected NAT

1. Consult social work and child protection team.
2. Refer to child protection agencies when appropriate.
3. Document as objectively as possible.
4. Refer for mental health support early.

Cultural and Social Considerations

• Take the time to look into practices that differ from your own with a sense of curiosity and cultural humility, recognizing that parenting practices differ between cultures.
• NAT should never be the only thing on your differential.

• In many states, medical providers are mandated reporters when NAT is suspected, but we also have a responsibility to obtain a complete and accurate history to inform our degree of suspicion.
• The professional opinion of a medical providers is taken very seriously by child protective agencies and can have significant impact on the agencies' determinations.
• While investigating cases of suspected NAT is intended to protect children, many forms of agency involvement, particularly family separation, are inherently trauma inducing.

• Recognize that structural racism and other forms of oppression drive disparities in which families are suspected, referred, investigated, surveilled, and separated.
• Despite NAT being less likely to occur in families of color when controlling for other risk factors, children of color and Latinx children are overrepresented in child protective agencies, whereas cases of NAT among white, non-Latinx children are potentially missed.
• These structures of oppression, and the long history of medicine's involvement in their creation and perpetuation, create an understandable level of mistrust in some families.
• This mistrust can result in guarded responses, declining to volunteering information, or skepticism of medical recommendations, all of which may be misinterpreted by medical providers as suspicious.

Jordan Howard-Young, MD and Stephany Giraldo Eierle, DO, MPH

Child Welfare Information Gateway. *Child Welfare Practice to Address Racial Disproportionality and Disparity.* Washington, DC: Children's Bureau; 2021. https://www.childwelfare.gov/pubPDFs/racial_disproportionality.pdf. Accessed October 18, 2021.

CHRONIC JOINT PAIN AND STIFFNESS

Common causes: osteoarthritis, rheumatoid arthritis, septic arthritis, gout, pseudogout, fibromyalgia

→ Joint pain lasting >6 weeks

Yes / **No**

Yes branch

No systemic s/sx
Morning stiffness <1 hour

← <2,000 WBCs

Worse w/ weight-bearing ± Swelling
→ Osteoarthritis
→ Acetaminophen, NSAIDs, topical NSAIDs
→ Low-impact exercise, PT Staging with MRI Complementary therapies

Diffuse arthralgia, myalgia
→ Fibromyalgia
→ Graduated exercise program Pregabalin Amitriptyline Duloxetine

No branch

Warm, swollen joints
Morning stiffness >1 hour
± Systemic s/sx

→ Check ESR, Lyme serology, joint aspiration for cell count, cultures, crystals.

>3,000–50,000 WBCs >50% PMNs

Crystals present
- Urate, negative birefringence → Gout → NSAIDs colchicine, steroids
- Calcium phosphate dihydrate Positive birefringence → Pseudogout → NSAIDs intra-articular steroid

↑ESR
No crystals
Negative culture

→ Check autoimmune markers, systemic symptoms.

Variable cell counts Negative culture Symmetric joint involvement

Viral
→ Check for hep B, hep C, HIV, parvovirus B19, or other suspected viruses.
→ Joint treatment is largely supportive.

>50,000 WBCs >75% PMNs
→ Septic arthritis
→ Emergent empirical IV Abx. Consult orthopedics for irrigation, biopsy. Narrow Abx to clinical response, microbiology sensitivities.

Autoimmune / systemic branch

↑RF, anti-CCP
→ Rheumatoid arthritis
→ NSAIDs Methotrexate Biologics
→ NSAIDs, hydroxychloroquine

Malar rash Oral ulcers ↑ANA, anti-dsDNA, anti-Smith Ab
→ SLE
→ HLA-B27
→ Ankylosing spondylitis
→ NSAIDs PT

Asymmetric joints affected Involvement of SI joint, spine Negative RF
→ Spondyloarthropathy
- Urethritis Conjunctivitis → Reactive arthritis → Treat primary etiology. NSAIDs Sulfasalazine
- Scaly rash Dactylitis → Psoriatic arthritis → NSAIDs Methotrexate Biologics

Bilateral shoulder and hip involvement
→ Polymyalgia rheumatica
→ Oral steroids

Xerophthalmia Xerostomia
→ Sjögren syndrome
→ Hydroxychloroquine Steroids Methotrexate

IBD
→ IBD arthritis
→ Immunomodulators Anticytokines

Tristan Michael Alexander Pennella, DO and Joanne E. Genewick, DO, FAIHM

Pujalte GG, Albano-Aluquin SA. Differential diagnosis of polyarticular arthritis. *Am Fam Physician.* 2015;92(1):35–41.

CHRONIC OBSTRUCTIVE PULMONARY DISEASE (COPD), DIAGNOSIS AND TREATMENT

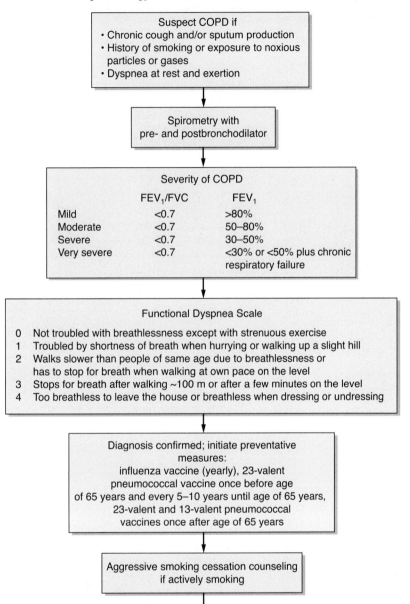

Suspect COPD if
- Chronic cough and/or sputum production
- History of smoking or exposure to noxious particles or gases
- Dyspnea at rest and exertion

Spirometry with pre- and postbronchodilator

Severity of COPD

	FEV$_1$/FVC	FEV$_1$
Mild	<0.7	>80%
Moderate	<0.7	50–80%
Severe	<0.7	30–50%
Very severe	<0.7	<30% or <50% plus chronic respiratory failure

Functional Dyspnea Scale

0 Not troubled with breathlessness except with strenuous exercise
1 Troubled by shortness of breath when hurrying or walking up a slight hill
2 Walks slower than people of same age due to breathlessness or has to stop for breath when walking at own pace on the level
3 Stops for breath after walking ~100 m or after a few minutes on the level
4 Too breathless to leave the house or breathless when dressing or undressing

Diagnosis confirmed; initiate preventative measures:
influenza vaccine (yearly), 23-valent pneumococcal vaccine once before age of 65 years and every 5–10 years until age of 65 years, 23-valent and 13-valent pneumococcal vaccines once after age of 65 years

Aggressive smoking cessation counseling if actively smoking

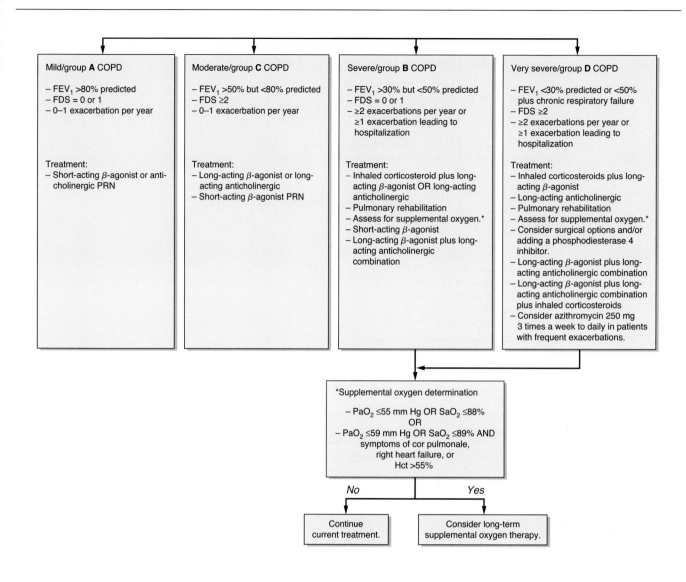

Mild/group A COPD

- FEV_1 >80% predicted
- FDS = 0 or 1
- 0–1 exacerbation per year

Treatment:
- Short-acting β-agonist or anti-cholinergic PRN

Moderate/group C COPD

- FEV_1 >50% but <80% predicted
- FDS ≥2
- 0–1 exacerbation per year

Treatment:
- Long-acting β-agonist or long-acting anticholinergic
- Short-acting β-agonist PRN

Severe/group B COPD

- FEV_1 >30% but <50% predicted
- FDS = 0 or 1
- ≥2 exacerbations per year or ≥1 exacerbation leading to hospitalization

Treatment:
- Inhaled corticosteroid plus long-acting β-agonist OR long-acting anticholinergic
- Pulmonary rehabilitation
- Assess for supplemental oxygen.*
- Short-acting β-agonist
- Long-acting β-agonist plus long-acting anticholinergic combination

Very severe/group D COPD

- FEV_1 <30% predicted or <50% plus chronic respiratory failure
- FDS ≥2
- ≥2 exacerbations per year or ≥1 exacerbation leading to hospitalization

Treatment:
- Inhaled corticosteroids plus long-acting β-agonist
- Long-acting anticholinergic
- Pulmonary rehabilitation
- Assess for supplemental oxygen.*
- Consider surgical options and/or adding a phosphodiesterase 4 inhibitor.
- Long-acting β-agonist plus long-acting anticholinergic combination
- Long-acting β-agonist plus long-acting anticholinergic combination plus inhaled corticosteroids
- Consider azithromycin 250 mg 3 times a week to daily in patients with frequent exacerbations.

*Supplemental oxygen determination

- PaO_2 ≤55 mm Hg OR SaO_2 ≤88%
OR
- PaO_2 ≤59 mm Hg OR SaO_2 ≤89% AND symptoms of cor pulmonale, right heart failure, or Hct >55%

No

Yes

Continue current treatment.

Consider long-term supplemental oxygen therapy.

William W. Wong, DO and Scott E. Kopec, MD, FCCP

Global Initiative for Chronic Obstructive Lung Disease. Global strategy for the diagnosis, management, and prevention of chronic obstructive pulmonary disease (2021 report). http://www.goldcopd.org/. Accessed July 23, 2021.

CIRRHOSIS

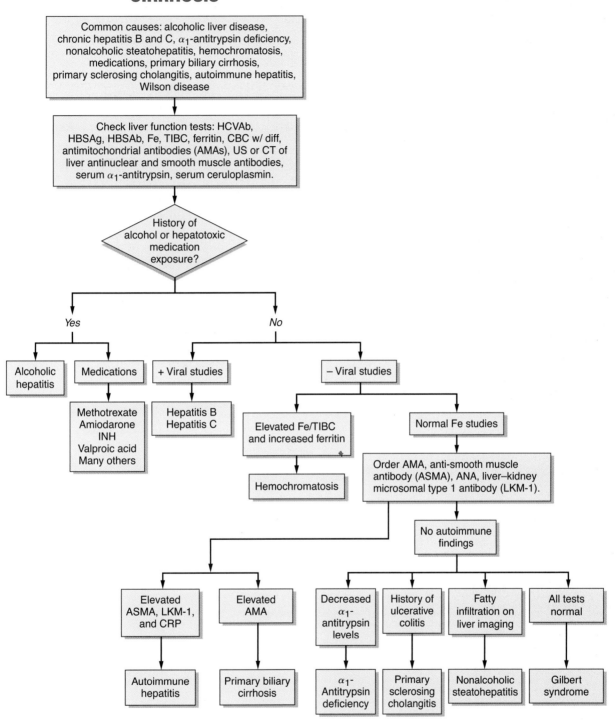

Common causes: alcoholic liver disease, chronic hepatitis B and C, α_1-antitrypsin deficiency, nonalcoholic steatohepatitis, hemochromatosis, medications, primary biliary cirrhosis, primary sclerosing cholangitis, autoimmune hepatitis, Wilson disease

Check liver function tests: HCVAb, HBSAg, HBSAb, Fe, TIBC, ferritin, CBC w/ diff, antimitochondrial antibodies (AMAs), US or CT of liver antinuclear and smooth muscle antibodies, serum α_1-antitrypsin, serum ceruloplasmin.

History of alcohol or hepatotoxic medication exposure?

Yes

Alcoholic hepatitis

Medications

Methotrexate
Amiodarone
INH
Valproic acid
Many others

No

+ Viral studies

Hepatitis B
Hepatitis C

− Viral studies

Elevated Fe/TIBC and increased ferritin

Hemochromatosis

Normal Fe studies

Order AMA, anti-smooth muscle antibody (ASMA), ANA, liver–kidney microsomal type 1 antibody (LKM-1).

No autoimmune findings

Elevated ASMA, LKM-1, and CRP

Autoimmune hepatitis

Elevated AMA

Primary biliary cirrhosis

Decreased α_1-antitrypsin levels

α_1-Antitrypsin deficiency

History of ulcerative colitis

Primary sclerosing cholangitis

Fatty infiltration on liver imaging

Nonalcoholic steatohepatitis

All tests normal

Gilbert syndrome

Shivani Malhotra, MD, FAAFP

Heidelbaugh JJ, Bruderly M. Cirrhosis and chronic liver failure: part I. Diagnosis and evaluation. *Am Fam Physician.* 2006;74(5):756–762.

CONCUSSION, SIDELINE EVALUATION
Stable, No C-Spine Injury

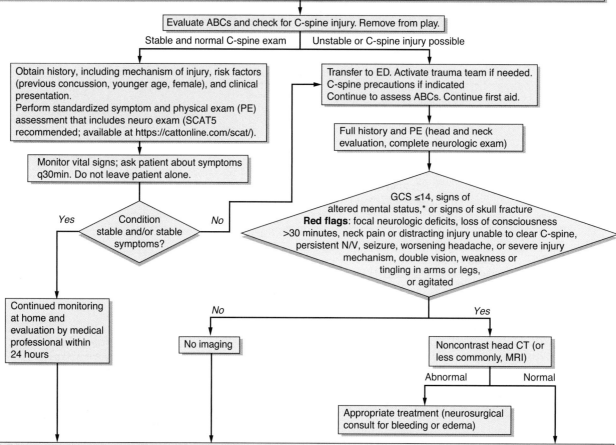

Concussion: traumatic event AND change in neurologic function OR one of the following signs/symptoms: **somatic** (HA, nausea/vomiting [N/V], dizziness, vertigo, visual problems, sensitivity to light or sound, numbness/tingling), **cognitive** (LOC, memory problems, feeling "foggy," slower reaction times, confusion), **emotional/behavioral** (i.e., irritability, sadness), **sleep** (i.e., drowsiness)

Evaluate ABCs and check for C-spine injury. Remove from play.

Stable and normal C-spine exam — Unstable or C-spine injury possible

Obtain history, including mechanism of injury, risk factors (previous concussion, younger age, female), and clinical presentation.
Perform standardized symptom and physical exam (PE) assessment that includes neuro exam (SCAT5 recommended; available at https://cattonline.com/scat/).

Transfer to ED. Activate trauma team if needed.
C-spine precautions if indicated
Continue to assess ABCs. Continue first aid.

Full history and PE (head and neck evaluation, complete neurologic exam)

Monitor vital signs; ask patient about symptoms q30min. Do not leave patient alone.

Yes — Condition stable and/or stable symptoms? — *No*

GCS ≤14, signs of altered mental status,* or signs of skull fracture **Red flags**: focal neurologic deficits, loss of consciousness >30 minutes, neck pain or distracting injury unable to clear C-spine, persistent N/V, seizure, worsening headache, or severe injury mechanism, double vision, weakness or tingling in arms or legs, or agitated

Continued monitoring at home and evaluation by medical professional within 24 hours

No — No imaging

Yes — Noncontrast head CT (or less commonly, MRI)

Abnormal — Normal

Appropriate treatment (neurosurgical consult for bleeding or edema)

A. Follow up with medical professional in next 24 hours.
- History and PE (including complete neurologic exam and symptom checklist)
- Patient should undergo physical and cognitive rest while symptoms persist.
- If at neurologic baseline, review Return to Play protocol and Return to Learn protocol.
- If not at neurologic baseline, consider ED evaluation or neuroimaging, close follow-up, and symptomatic treatment.
B. Consider neuropsych testing (paper-and-pencil, ImPACT, CogState, HeadMinder, ANAM, etc.).
- The ideal timing, frequency, and type of neuropsych testing have not been determined.
- Most concussions can be managed appropriately without the use of neuropsych testing.
- Neuropsych testing may be most helpful for high-risk athletes, those with prior concussions, and those who may downplay symptoms in an effort to return to play sooner.
C. Return to Learn protocol
- Once the patient can tolerate visual and auditory stimuli for 30–45 minutes, he or she may return to school.
- Academic adjustments such as a limited course load, reduced testing, or shortened classes may be necessary while recovering. Notify appropriate school personnel.
D. Return to Play protocol
- No athlete may return to play the same day. All school-aged athletes must return to school fully before they can return to play. Patient should not be on any medications to treat concussion symptoms before returning to play.
- Once asymptomatic at a stage for 24 hours, may move on to next stage; if symptoms arise, must take a 24-hour period of complete rest before dropping back one stage and starting from there
- Most athletes should return no sooner than 6 days after concussion. A minimum of 24 hours should occur between each stage.
    o Stage 1: no activity (complete physical AND cognitive rest; cognitive rest includes no driving)
    o Stage 2: light aerobic exercise (walking, swimming, or stationary cycling at <70% max HR)
    o Stage 3: sport-specific exercise (sport-specific drills such as skating or running; no head impact activities)
    o Stage 4: noncontact training drills (progression to more complex training drills such as passing; may start progressive resistance training)
    o Stage 5: full-contact practice
    o Stage 6: return to game play
E. Symptom management: If concussive symptoms (typically HA, sleep, cognitive, and mood disturbances) are persistent and interfering with function, consider symptomatic treatment.
- In the acute setting, ASA and NSAIDs should be used with caution due to increased risk of intracranial bleeding. Acetaminophen and physical modalities are OK.
- If HA persists for a few days, consider typical abortive treatment. There is no established role for pharmacotherapy in the acute treatment of concussion-induced sleep, cognitive, or mood disturbances.
- If symptoms persist beyond 4 weeks, consider referral to specialist (neurology, sports medicine, etc.). Multidisciplinary approach is often needed.

Signs of altered mental status: agitation, somnolence, repetitive questioning, or slow response to verbal communication.

Anthony Shadiack, DO, CAQSM

Harmon KG, Clugston JR, Dec K, et al. American Medical Society for Sports Medicine position statement on concussion in sport. *Br J Sports Med.* 2019;53(4):213–225.

CONGESTIVE HEART FAILURE: DIFFERENTIAL DIAGNOSIS

Common causes: CAD, MI, valvular disease, arrhythmia, idiopathic cardiomyopathy, pulmonary HTN, renal disease, medication noncompliance

Diagnosis made clinically.

History: exercise intolerance, dyspnea on exertion or at rest, cough, orthopnea, paroxysmal nocturnal dyspnea, chest discomfort, fatigue, weight gain

Exam: elevated jugular venous pressure, rales, S_3/S_4 gallop, hepatojugular reflux, increased abdominal distention, pallor, lower extremity edema

Testing: chest x-ray, ECG, troponin, echo, BNP, BMP, LFTs, TSH, UA, uric acid

Diagnosis of CHF: Framingham Diagnostic Criteria
Requires 2 major criteria or 1 major and 2 minor criteria

Major criteria
- Acute pulmonary edema
- Cardiomegaly
- Hepatojugular reflux
- Elevated jugular venous pressure
- Paroxysmal nocturnal dyspnea
- Rales
- S_3

Minor criteria
- Ankle edema
- Dyspnea on exertion
- Hepatomegaly
- Nocturnal cough
- Pleural effusion
- Tachycardia to >120 beats/min

97% and 89% sensitive for systolic and diastolic heart failure (HF), respectively

BNP <80

BNP 80–500

Indeterminate. Consider CHF AND alternative diagnoses:
- COPD
- Asthma
- Lung disease
- Pulmonary embolus

LVEF <50% (systolic HF)

LVEF >50% (diastolic HF)

BNP >500

Likely CHF

CHF essentially ruled out

Ischemic
- History of CAD/MI
- Positive stress test
- CAD on cardiac catheterization
- Troponin elevation

Evaluate for causes of CHF.
- Ischemic: CAD/MI
- Nonischemic: HTN, idiopathic CM, valvular disease, HOCM, arrhythmia, myocarditis/pericarditis, collagen vascular disease
- Due to volume: medication noncompliance, renal failure

Cardiac catheterization unless contraindicated

Nonischemic cardiomyopathy

Idiopathic cardiomyopathy

Other: HTN, thyrotoxicosis, alcoholism, chemotherapy induced, cocaine, autoimmune, collagen vascular disease, infiltrative (amyloid, hemochromatosis), obstructive sleep apnea

Tachycardia mediated (atrial fibrillation/flutter, SVT, frequent PVCs)

Valvular disease cardiomyopathy

Viral mediated (coxsackievirus, adenovirus, HIV, EBV)

Jeremy Golding, MD, FAAFP

King M, Kingery J, Casey B. Diagnosis and evaluation of heart failure. *Am Fam Physician.* 2012;85(12):1161–1168.

CONSTIPATION, DIAGNOSIS AND TREATMENT (ADULT)

Functional constipation
(Rome IV criteria)
- 2 of the following for 12 weeks in past 6 months:
  - <3 stools per week
  - For 25% of time, any of the following:
    - Hard stools
    - Straining
    - Manual assist
    - Sense of incomplete evacuation
    - Sense of anorectal blockade
- Rare loose stools without laxative use
- Does NOT meet criteria for IBS

Common causes: primary—functional, slow transit, pelvic floor dysfunction; secondary—IBS, diabetes mellitus, hypothyroidism, hypercalcemia, pregnancy, obstruction, medication side effect

History and physical:
Diet, fluid intake, exercise, Rome IV criteria, digital rectal exam, abdominal exam, neurologic exam

Red flags:
Unintentional weight loss, hematochezia, family Hx IBD or colon cancer, positive fecal occult, anemia, new onset in age >50 years, change in stool size, neurologic findings

Yes → Colonoscopy

No

Medication Hx: anticholinergics, opiates, calcium channel blockers, antidepressants, antacids

Yes → Consider medication effect: Adjust and/or begin with empiric treatment.

No → Diagnostic testing: CBC, glucose, creatinine, calcium, TSH

Positive →
Anemia
Hypothyroidism
Hypercalcemia
Diabetes mellitus

Negative

Empiric treatment:
Increase exercise and water intake; trial of 25–35 g/day of fiber (inulin up to 6 g/day or psyllium up to 35 g/day); increase exercise and water intake (2 L/day). All patients should be given bowel retraining (https://www.med.unc.edu/ibs/files/2017/10/BowelRetrain.pdf).

Symptoms improved?

No → Add polyethylene glycol and/or stimulant laxative.

Yes

Continue therapy.

Symptoms improved?

Yes → Continue therapy.

No →

Partial →

Treatment failure → Anorectal manometry with balloon expulsion

Normal ARM → Consider colonic transit time.

Abnormal ARM → Pelvic floor dysfunction

Add adjunctive agents such as lubiprostone and linaclotide.

Biofeedback; consider MRI/defecography and surgical referral.

Daniel J. Stein, MD, MPH and Stephen K. Lane, MD

Lacy BE, Mearin F, Chang L, et al. Bowel disorders. *Gastroenterology*. 2016;150(6):1393–1407.e5.

CONSTIPATION, TREATMENT (PEDIATRIC)

*Red flags:
No meconium passed >48 hours in a
  term newborn
Constipation <1 month of age
Family history of Hirschsprung disease
Ribbon stools
Blood in the stools in the absence of
  anal fissures
Failure to thrive
Fever
Bilious vomiting
Severe abdominal distension
Abnormal thyroid gland
Abnormal position of the anus
Perianal fistula
Absent anal or cremasteric reflex
Decreased lower extremity strength/
  tone/reflex
Sacral dimple
Tuft of hair on spine
Gluteal cleft deviation
Anal scars
Extreme fear during anal inspection

Rome Criteria
Rome IV infants and children <4 years
  ° ≥1 month with two or more of following
  • ≤2 BMs per week
  • History of excessive stool retention
  • History of painful or hard bowel movements
  • History of large-diameter stools
  • Presence of large fecal mass in rectum
  ° If child toilet-trained children include
  • ≥1 episode per week of incontinence
  • History of large stools that may block toilet
  ° Potential accompanying symptoms
  • Irritability, decreased appetite, early satiety which
    resolve immediately after passing of a large stool

Rome IV diagnostic children and adolescents aged
4–18 years (developmental age ≥4 years)
  ° ≥1 month with two or more of following, at least
    once a week
  • ≤2 bowel movements per week
  • ≥1 episode per week of incontinence after toilet
    training
  • History of retentive behavior or excessive volitional
    stool retention
  • History of painful or hard bowel movements
  • Presence of large fecal mass in rectum
  • History of large stools that may block toilet
  ° After appropriate evaluation, symptoms cannot be
    attributed to another medical condition.

Careful history and
physical exam;
digital rectal exam
is not required for
diagnosis.

Are red flags
present?

Yes

Obtain based on symptoms: CBC,
TSH, calcium, glucose, creatinine,
tissue transglutaminase (tTG), and
endomysium antibody (EMA).

Differential diagnosis:
Celiac disease
Hypothyroidism
Hypercalcemia
Hypokalemia
Diabetes mellitus
Drugs/toxins—opiates, anticholinergics,
antidepressants, chemotherapy, heavy
metals
Vitamin D intoxication
Botulism
Cystic fibrosis
Hirschsprung disease
Anal achalasia
Colonic inertia
Anal malformations
Pelvic mass
Spinal cord abnormalities
Abnormal abdominal musculature
Pseudoobstruction
Multiple endocrine neoplasia type 2B

No

Functional constipation

Fecal
impaction?

Yes

First line: polyethylene
glycol (PEG) 3350
1.0–1.5 g/kg/day orally
(as effective as enemas)

Second line: enemas
daily for 3–6 days

No

Initial therapy: PEG 0.4 g/kg/day orally
Maintenance therapy: PEG 0.2–0.8 g/kg/day
orally titrated to response; continue for
2 months until symptoms resolved for
1 month then D/C gradually.

PEG is superior to lactulose.

Education: recognition of withholding
behaviors; use of behavioral interventions:
regular toileting routines, diaries, reward
systems
Dietary/lifestyle recommendations:
– Normal fiber, fluid intake, physical activity
– No defined role for pre or probiotic

Refer for specialty evaluation.

A. Susan Feeney, DNP, FNP-BC, NP-C

Rasquin A, Di Lorenzo C, Forbes D, et al. Childhood functional gastrointestinal disorders: child/adolescent. *Gastroenterology.* 2006;130(5):1527–1537.

CONTRACEPTION

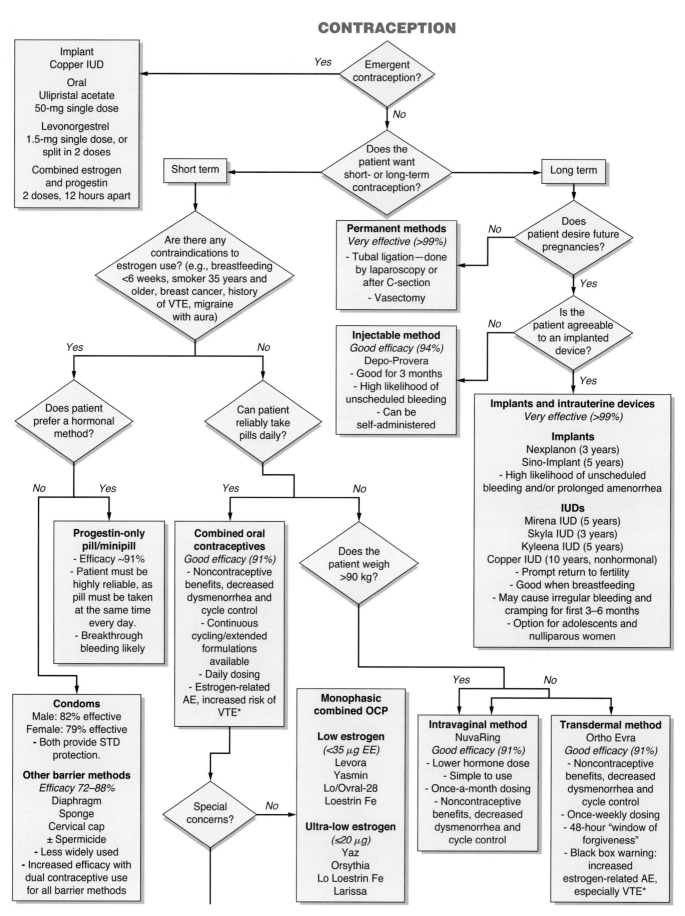

Emergent contraception? — Yes →

Implant
Copper IUD

Oral
Ulipristal acetate
50-mg single dose

Levonorgestrel
1.5-mg single dose, or
split in 2 doses

Combined estrogen
and progestin
2 doses, 12 hours apart

No ↓

Does the patient want short- or long-term contraception?

Short term ← | → Long term

Are there any contraindications to estrogen use? (e.g., breastfeeding <6 weeks, smoker 35 years and older, breast cancer, history of VTE, migraine with aura)

Yes | No

Does patient prefer a hormonal method?

No | Yes

Can patient reliably take pills daily?

Yes | No

Progestin-only pill/minipill
- Efficacy ~91%
- Patient must be highly reliable, as pill must be taken at the same time every day.
- Breakthrough bleeding likely

Combined oral contraceptives
Good efficacy (91%)
- Noncontraceptive benefits, decreased dysmenorrhea and cycle control
- Continuous cycling/extended formulations available
- Daily dosing
- Estrogen-related AE, increased risk of VTE*

Does the patient weigh >90 kg?

Condoms
Male: 82% effective
Female: 79% effective
- Both provide STD protection.

Other barrier methods
Efficacy 72–88%
Diaphragm
Sponge
Cervical cap
± Spermicide
- Less widely used
- Increased efficacy with dual contraceptive use for all barrier methods

Special concerns? — No →

Monophasic combined OCP

Low estrogen
(<35 μg EE)
Levora
Yasmin
Lo/Ovral-28
Loestrin Fe

Ultra-low estrogen
(≤20 μg)
Yaz
Orsythia
Lo Loestrin Fe
Larissa

Permanent methods
Very effective (>99%)
- Tubal ligation—done by laparoscopy or after C-section
- Vasectomy

← No — **Does patient desire future pregnancies?**

Yes ↓

Injectable method
Good efficacy (94%)
Depo-Provera
- Good for 3 months
- High likelihood of unscheduled bleeding
- Can be self-administered

← No — **Is the patient agreeable to an implanted device?**

Yes ↓

Implants and intrauterine devices
Very effective (>99%)

Implants
Nexplanon (3 years)
Sino-Implant (5 years)
- High likelihood of unscheduled bleeding and/or prolonged amenorrhea

IUDs
Mirena IUD (5 years)
Skyla IUD (3 years)
Kyleena IUD (5 years)
Copper IUD (10 years, nonhormonal)
- Prompt return to fertility
- Good when breastfeeding
- May cause irregular bleeding and cramping for first 3–6 months
- Option for adolescents and nulliparous women

Yes | No

Intravaginal method
NuvaRing
Good efficacy (91%)
- Lower hormone dose
- Simple to use
- Once-a-month dosing
- Noncontraceptive benefits, decreased dysmenorrhea and cycle control

Transdermal method
Ortho Evra
Good efficacy (91%)
- Noncontraceptive benefits, decreased dysmenorrhea and cycle control
- Once-weekly dosing
- 48-hour "window of forgiveness"
- Black box warning: increased estrogen-related AE, especially VTE*

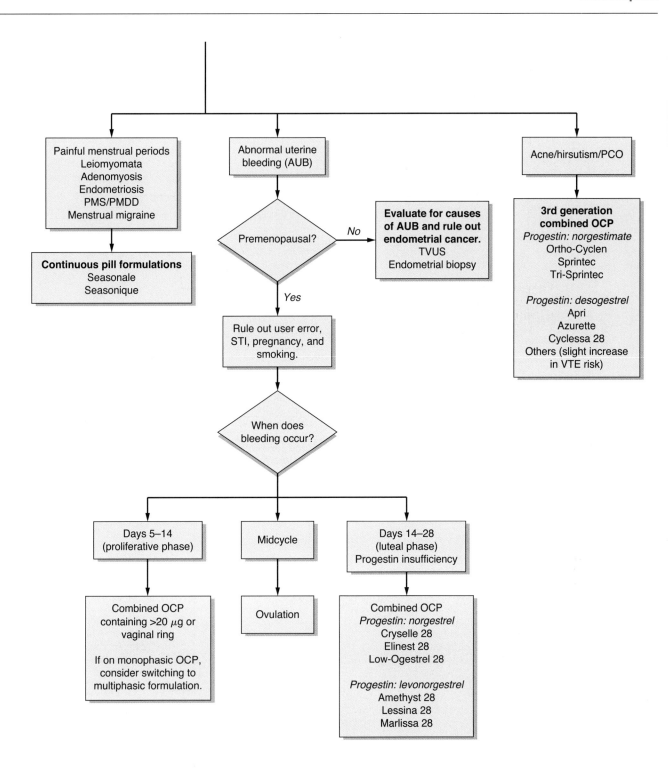

*Consult CDC MEC guidelines for contraindications to use.

Katherine Gagan, MD and Melanie Houston Sanders, MD

Curtis KM, Jatlaoui TC, Tepper NK, et al. U.S. selected practice recommendations for contraceptive use, 2016. *MMWR Recomm Rep.* 2016;65(4):1–66. doi:10.15585/mmwr.rr6504a1.

DEEP VENOUS THROMBOSIS, DIAGNOSIS AND TREATMENT

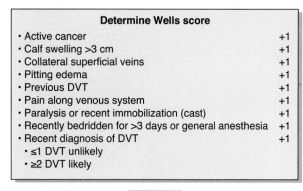

Determine Wells score

• Active cancer	+1
• Calf swelling >3 cm	+1
• Collateral superficial veins	+1
• Pitting edema	+1
• Previous DVT	+1
• Pain along venous system	+1
• Paralysis or recent immobilization (cast)	+1
• Recently bedridden for >3 days or general anesthesia	+1
• Recent diagnosis of DVT	+1

    • ≤1 DVT unlikely
    • ≥2 DVT likely

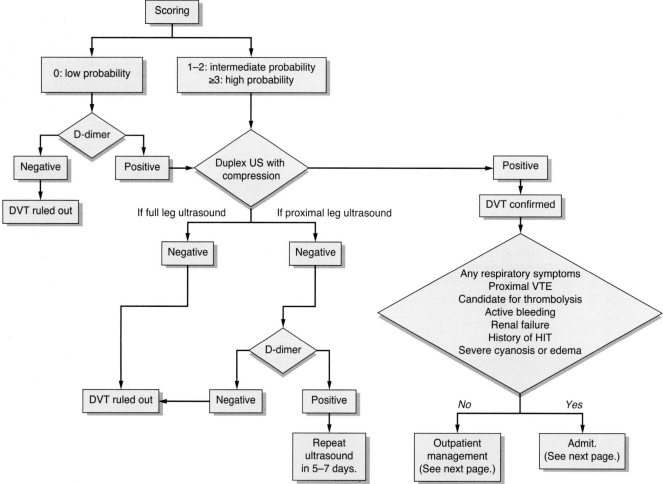

Scoring

0: low probability

1–2: intermediate probability
≥3: high probability

D-dimer

Negative → DVT ruled out

Positive →

Duplex US with compression → Positive → DVT confirmed

If full leg ultrasound → Negative → DVT ruled out

If proximal leg ultrasound → Negative → D-dimer

D-dimer → Negative → DVT ruled out

D-dimer → Positive → Repeat ultrasound in 5–7 days.

Any respiratory symptoms
Proximal VTE
Candidate for thrombolysis
Active bleeding
Renal failure
History of HIT
Severe cyanosis or edema

No → Outpatient management (See next page.)

Yes → Admit. (See next page.)

Treatment

```
     ┌─────────────┐                          ┌─────────────┐
     │  Outpatient │                          │  Inpatient  │
     │ management  │                          │ management  │
     │             │                          │ indications │
     └──────┬──────┘                          └──────┬──────┘
            │                                        │
            ▼                                        ▼
```

Outpatient management

Therapy options:

Low-molecular-weight heparin (LMWH), unfractionated heparin (UF), or fondaparinux with warfarin bridging

- Treatment with LMWH, UFH, or fondaparinux is recommended for at least 5 days AND until INR ≥2 for 2 consecutive days.
  - Enoxaparin 1 mg/kg SC BID OR
  - UFH preferred in patients with renal impairment
- Start warfarin on same days as LMWH, UFH, and fondaparinux.
  - Goal INR 2–3
  - Continue for 3–6 months after first DVT.
  - Warfarin is contraindicated in pregnancy.

LMWH, UF, or fondaparinux followed by dabigatran
- Dabigatran 150 mg BID after 7–10 days of LMWH and continue for at least 6 months
- Adjust dose for CrCl <50 mL/min.
- Do not use in CrCl <15 mL/min.

Direct oral anticoagulants (rivaroxaban or apixaban) does not need bridge.

- Rivaroxaban
  - 15 mg BID with food for 21 days followed by 20 mg daily for at least 3 months
  - Avoid in patients with CrCl < 30 mL/min.

- Apixaban
  - 10 mg BID for 7 days followed by 5 mg BID for at least 3 months

Inpatient management indications

- Massive DVT
- Symptomatic PE
- High-risk bleeding with anticoagulation therapy
- Comorbid condition
- Phlegmasia cerulea dolens
- History of HIT

- IV UFH : 80 U/kg bolus or to a max 5,000 units → continuous infusion with initial dose 18 U/kg/hr → titrate to goal PTT 60–85 seconds ~OR~
- UFH 250 U/kg SC BID ~OR~
- Enoxaparin 1.5 kg/mg SC daily ~OR~
- Fondaparinux 5–10 mg SC daily depending on weight

Jason Teng, MD and Moises Gallegos, MD, MPH

Lim W, Le Gal G, Bates SM, et al. American Society of Hematology 2018 guidelines for management of venous thromboembolism: diagnosis of venous thromboembolism. *Blood Adv.* 2018;2(22):3226–3256.

DEHYDRATION, PEDIATRIC

Causes of dehydration in pediatric patients include gastrointestinal losses (vomiting, diarrhea), losses from skin (sweat, fever, burns), and urinary loses (glycosuria, diuretics).

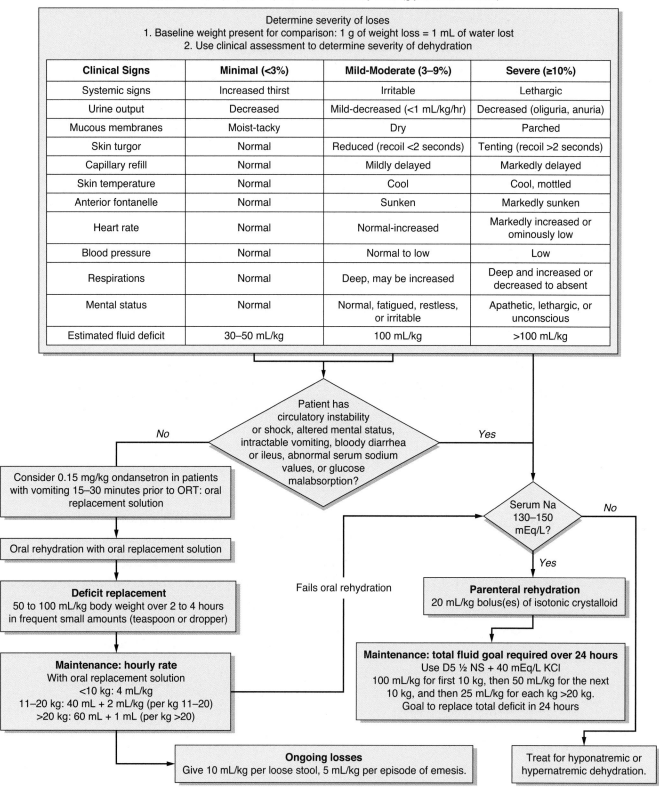

Determine severity of loses
1. Baseline weight present for comparison: 1 g of weight loss = 1 mL of water lost
2. Use clinical assessment to determine severity of dehydration

Clinical Signs	Minimal (<3%)	Mild-Moderate (3–9%)	Severe (≥10%)
Systemic signs	Increased thirst	Irritable	Lethargic
Urine output	Decreased	Mild-decreased (<1 mL/kg/hr)	Decreased (oliguria, anuria)
Mucous membranes	Moist-tacky	Dry	Parched
Skin turgor	Normal	Reduced (recoil <2 seconds)	Tenting (recoil >2 seconds)
Capillary refill	Normal	Mildly delayed	Markedly delayed
Skin temperature	Normal	Cool	Cool, mottled
Anterior fontanelle	Normal	Sunken	Markedly sunken
Heart rate	Normal	Normal-increased	Markedly increased or ominously low
Blood pressure	Normal	Normal to low	Low
Respirations	Normal	Deep, may be increased	Deep and increased or decreased to absent
Mental status	Normal	Normal, fatigued, restless, or irritable	Apathetic, lethargic, or unconscious
Estimated fluid deficit	30–50 mL/kg	100 mL/kg	>100 mL/kg

Patient has circulatory instability or shock, altered mental status, intractable vomiting, bloody diarrhea or ileus, abnormal serum sodium values, or glucose malabsorption?

No

Consider 0.15 mg/kg ondansetron in patients with vomiting 15–30 minutes prior to ORT: oral replacement solution

Oral rehydration with oral replacement solution

Deficit replacement
50 to 100 mL/kg body weight over 2 to 4 hours in frequent small amounts (teaspoon or dropper)

Maintenance: hourly rate
With oral replacement solution
<10 kg: 4 mL/kg
11–20 kg: 40 mL + 2 mL/kg (per kg 11–20)
>20 kg: 60 mL + 1 mL (per kg >20)

Yes

Serum Na 130–150 mEq/L?

No

Fails oral rehydration

Yes

Parenteral rehydration
20 mL/kg bolus(es) of isotonic crystalloid

Maintenance: total fluid goal required over 24 hours
Use D5 ½ NS + 40 mEq/L KCl
100 mL/kg for first 10 kg, then 50 mL/kg for the next 10 kg, and then 25 mL/kg for each kg >20 kg.
Goal to replace total deficit in 24 hours

Ongoing losses
Give 10 mL/kg per loose stool, 5 mL/kg per episode of emesis.

Treat for hyponatremic or hypernatremic dehydration.

Bindusri Paruchuri, MD and Sarah Marie Tiggelaar, MD, FAAFP

Santillanes G, Rose E. Evaluation and management of dehydration in children. *Emerg Med Clin North Am*. 2018;36(2):259–273. doi:10.1016/j.emc.2017.12.004.

DELIRIUM

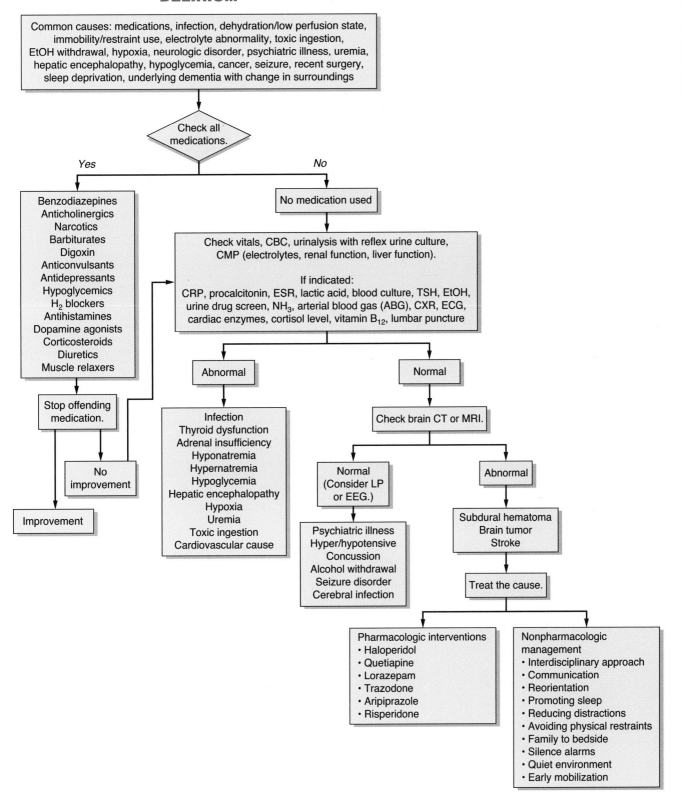

Common causes: medications, infection, dehydration/low perfusion state, immobility/restraint use, electrolyte abnormality, toxic ingestion, EtOH withdrawal, hypoxia, neurologic disorder, psychiatric illness, uremia, hepatic encephalopathy, hypoglycemia, cancer, seizure, recent surgery, sleep deprivation, underlying dementia with change in surroundings

Check all medications.

Yes — *No*

No medication used

Benzodiazepines
Anticholinergics
Narcotics
Barbiturates
Digoxin
Anticonvulsants
Antidepressants
Hypoglycemics
H_2 blockers
Antihistamines
Dopamine agonists
Corticosteroids
Diuretics
Muscle relaxers

Stop offending medication.

No improvement

Improvement

Check vitals, CBC, urinalysis with reflex urine culture, CMP (electrolytes, renal function, liver function).

If indicated:
CRP, procalcitonin, ESR, lactic acid, blood culture, TSH, EtOH, urine drug screen, NH_3, arterial blood gas (ABG), CXR, ECG, cardiac enzymes, cortisol level, vitamin B_{12}, lumbar puncture

Abnormal

Normal

Infection
Thyroid dysfunction
Adrenal insufficiency
Hyponatremia
Hypernatremia
Hypoglycemia
Hepatic encephalopathy
Hypoxia
Uremia
Toxic ingestion
Cardiovascular cause

Check brain CT or MRI.

Normal (Consider LP or EEG.)

Abnormal

Psychiatric illness
Hyper/hypotensive
Concussion
Alcohol withdrawal
Seizure disorder
Cerebral infection

Subdural hematoma
Brain tumor
Stroke

Treat the cause.

Pharmacologic interventions
• Haloperidol
• Quetiapine
• Lorazepam
• Trazodone
• Aripiprazole
• Risperidone

Nonpharmacologic management
• Interdisciplinary approach
• Communication
• Reorientation
• Promoting sleep
• Reducing distractions
• Avoiding physical restraints
• Family to bedside
• Silence alarms
• Quiet environment
• Early mobilization

Jason Philippe, MD and Holly L. Baab, MD

Oh ES, Fong TG, Hshieh TT, et al. Delirium in older persons: advances in diagnosis and treatment. *JAMA.* 2017;318(12):1161–1174. doi:10.1001/jama.2017.12067.

DEMENTIA

Common causes:
Alzheimer disease, Lewy body dementia, vascular dementia, frontotemporal dementia, neurosyphilis, NPH, HIV, depression

Concern for cognitive impairment:
Perform a cognitive screen with a validated tool (the Mini-Cog [mini-cog.com/], Mini-Mental State Examination [MMSE], Montreal Cognitive Assessment [MoCA]).

Failed screen?

Yes → / *No* →

No: Consider medication side effects: analgesics, anticholinergics, psychotropics, sedatives, benzodiazepines, etc.

Geriatric Depression Scale

- **Positive**
- **Negative**

Positive: Treat depression and reevaluate in 3 months.

Symptoms persist?

Laboratory studies
Routinely recommended:
TSH, vitamin B_{12}, CMP, CBC
High clinical suspicion:
syphilis, HIV, UA, heavy metals, LP

Abnormal labs

Thyroid disorder
Vitamin B_{12} deficiency
Electrolyte abnormalities
Uremia
Anemia
Infectious causes
Syphilis
HIV

Normal labs

Consider imaging:
CT or MRI (preferred) if abrupt or rapid decline, age <60 years, focal deficits, predisposing conditions (malignancy, anticoagulation)

Consider:
Neuropsychological testing or specialist evaluation

Abnormal
Vascular dementia (stepwise decline), normal-pressure hydrocephalus (gait disturbance, incontinence), frontotemporal disease (personality change), subdural hematoma

Normal
Alzheimer disease, Parkinson disease (shuffling gait, tremor), Lewy body dementia, chronic alcohol use

Treatment:
Alzheimer disease
Lewy body dementia
Vascular dementia

- **Mild:** Aducanumab
- **Mild to moderate:** Cholinesterase inhibitors (donepezil, galantamine, rivastigmine)
- **Moderate to severe:** Memantine

Stephen Graber, MD and Ecler Ercole Jaqua, MD, DipABLM, DipABOM, FAAFP

Oh ES, Rabins PV. Dementia. *Ann Intern Med*. 2019;171(5):ITC33–ITC48.

DEPRESSIVE EPISODE, MAJOR

Diagnostic criteria:

1. Depressed mood
2. Loss of interests/pleasure
3. Change in sleep
4. Change in appetite or weight
5. Change in psychomotor activity
6. Loss of energy
7. Trouble concentrating
8. Thoughts of worthlessness or guilt
9. Thoughts about death or suicide

Diagnosis requires at least 5 of the above symptoms and must include symptom 1 and/or 2.

Depression screen
Depressed mood and/or loss of interests/pleasure most days; most of the day >2 weeks

Imminent risk of serious self-harm or suicide?
— *Yes* → Refer to emergency mental health for treatment and stabilization.
— *No* →

Meets criteria →

Are medications, comorbid medical conditions, or substance use causing depression?
— *Yes* → Treat the underlying condition or change medications as indicated.
— *No* →

History of treatment-resistant depression, mania, hypomania, psychosis?
— *Yes* → Refer to mental health specialty care.
— *No* →

Consider if an anxiety disorder, substance use disorder, or posttraumatic stress disorder is also present.

Determine severity of the current depressive episode.

Severity is based on number of symptoms, intensity of those symptoms, and degree of functional disability.

Mild: ~5–6 symptoms that are distressing but manageable and result in minor functional impairment

Moderate: ~6–8 symptoms of intensity and degree of impairment that falls between that described as mild or severe

Severe: ~8–9 symptoms that are very distressing, unmanageable, and markedly interfere with social and/or occupational functioning

Mild
Offer monotherapy with antidepressant medication or psychotherapy, based on patient preference.

Moderate
Consider a combination of both antidepressant medication and psychotherapy.

Severe
Recommend a combination of both antidepressant medication and psychotherapy; consider psychiatry referral or inpatient stabilization.

Choosing an Antidepressant
First-line medications include SSRIs, SNRIs, bupropion, and mirtazapine.

Escitalopram: may be more effective, better tolerated, treats anxiety, safe in pregnancy and adolescents
Sertraline: most safety data in pregnancy
Fluoxetine: useful when doses may be missed
Duloxetine: useful in chronic pain and fibromyalgia
Bupropion: treats TUD, promotes weight loss, libido
Mirtazapine: sedating, promotes weight gain

If the patient has previously responded well to a specific medication, it is usually the best option.

Improving in 2–3 weeks?
— *No* → If partially responding and tolerating well, increase dose.
If not responding or tolerating poorly, change to a different antidepressant in the same or a different class.
If 2 or 3 antidepressant trials ineffective or patient status is worsening, refer to psychiatry.
— *Yes* → Maintain effective treatment; follow up in 1–3 months.

Jordan Howard-Young, MD and Stephany Giraldo Eierle, DO, MPH

U.S. Department of Veterans Affairs, U.S. Department of Defense. *VA/DoD Clinical Practice Guideline for Management of Major Depressive Disorder.* Washington, DC: U.S. Department of Veterans Affairs, U.S. Department of Defense; 2016.

DIABETIC KETOACIDOSIS (DKA), TREATMENT

DKA diagnostic criteria: serum glucose >250 mg/dL, arterial pH <7.3, serum bicarbonate <18 mEq/L, and elevated serum ketone level.
Complete initial evaluation. Check capillary glucose and serum/urine ketones to confirm hyperglycemia and ketonemia/ketonuria.

IV fluids

Start 1.0 L of 0.9% NaCl/hr.

Severe/shock

Administer 9% NaCl at 1.0–1.5 L over the 1st hour and then, if serum-corrected Na is high or normal, give 0.45% NaCl at 250–500 mL/hr depending on hydration state.

Hemodynamic monitoring and pressors

Mild dehydration

Evaluate corrected serum. Corrected Na = measured Na + 0.016 × (glucose − 100)

Corrected serum Na ≥135 mEq/L → 0.45% NaCl (250–500 mL/hr)

Corrected serum Na <135 mEq/L → 0.9% NaCl (250–500 mL/hr)

Insulin

Regular insulin 0.1 U/kg IV bolus 1–2 hours after starting IV fluids

. . . then 0.1 U/kg/hr IV

Uncomplicated DKA

Initiate rapid-acting insulin bolus 0.3 U/kg SC and then 0.2 U/kg SC 1 hour later.

Continue rapid-acting insulin 0.2 U/kg SC q2h.

If serum glucose does not fall by 50–70 mg/dL in 1st hour, double IV dose or double SC bolus dose.

Serum glucose <200 mg/dL

- 5% dextrose with 0.45% NaCl at 150–250 mL/hr
- Decrease insulin to 0.05–0.10 U/kg/hr IV.
- If using SC insulin instead of IV, decrease rapid-acting SC bolus to 0.1 U/kg SC q2h.

Keep serum glucose between 150 and 200 mg/dL until resolution of DKA.

Potassium

Urine output >50 mL/hr

K⁺ <3.3 mEq/L

Hold insulin until K⁺ >3.3 mEq/L. Give 20–30 mEq K⁺/hr.

K⁺ ≥5.3 mEq/L

Recheck every 2 hours.

K⁺ ≥3.3 and <5.3 mEq/L

Add 20–30 mEq K⁺ to each liter of IV fluid. Goal is K⁺ between 4 and 5 mEq/L.

Assess need for bicarbonate.

pH <6.9

Give 100 mEq of sodium bicarbonate in 400 mL sterile water. Give at rate of 200 mL/hr.

Repeat IV NaHCO₃ dose q2h until pH ≥6.9 and check serum K⁺.

Laboratory evaluation

Initial: CBC, CMP, ABG, serum ketones, Mg, phosphate, UA, ECG, HbA1c; if indicated, CXR, BCx, UCx, amylase, lipase

Serial: in addition to clinical monitoring, glucose, electrolytes, venous blood gas, urine output

Calculated: effective osmolality, anion gap, corrected Na⁺, urine output

Frequency: q1h initially and then q2–4h once stable until DKA resolution

Resolution of DKA*

Feed and change from IV to SC insulin regimen (0.5–0.8 U/kg/day for insulin-naive patients). Keep IV insulin running for 1–2 hours after SC doses. Look for causes of DKA.

*Resolution of DKA Criteria:
- Glucose level <200 mg/dL
- pH >7.3
- Serum bicarbonate level is 18 mEq/L or greater.

Astrud S. A. Villareal, MD, Collen Del Valle, DO, and Chelsea Elyse Cole, MD

Westerberg DP. Diabetic ketoacidosis: evaluation and treatment. *Am Fam Physician.* 2013;87(5):337–346.

DIARRHEA, CHRONIC

Common causes: infectious (bacterial, viral, parasitic), inflammatory bowel disease (IBD), irritable bowel syndrome (IBS), medications, endocrine diarrhea (tumors, systemic), malignancy, radiation, food additives, malabsorption syndromes (celiac disease, pancreatic insufficiency, bile acid malabsorption [BAM])

↓

History: characteristics of stool, associated symptoms, iatrogenic risk factors (medications, radiotherapy), antibiotics, recent hospitalization, medical and surgical history, dietary history (carbohydrates, sugar, alcohol, coffee, fatty food), recent travel, family history, sexual history, immunosuppression

↓

Alarm signs? GI bleeding, fever, significant weight loss?

Yes ←→ *No*

Labs: stool studies (multiplex PCR, culture, *Clostridium difficile*, ova + parasites, fat, electrolytes, calprotectin, blood), blood tests (TSH, glucose, celiac serology [TTG IgA], HIV Ab, GI peptide assays, C4/FGF19), hydrogen breath test

Medication induced?
Acid-reducing agents (PPIs, H$_2$ blockers), antacids (containing Mg), antibiotics, β-blockers, NSAIDs, colchicine, digoxin, SSRIs, metformin, olmesartan, mycophenolate mofetil, herbal medications, vitamin and mineral supplements, antineoplastic agents, sorbitol, fructose abuse, chronic laxative abuse

Abnormal / *Normal*

Stool positive for ova and parasites, *C. difficile* toxin, pathogenic bacteria, or PCR → infectious diarrhea

Positive fecal blood, leukocytes, calprotectin → inflammatory diarrhea → colonoscopy

Positive celiac serology → upper endoscopy

Positive fecal fat → see "Malabsorption Syndrome" algorithm

Positive hydrogen breath test → small intestinal bacterial overgrowth

Colonoscopy

Abnormal exam and/or biopsies / *Normal*

No / *Yes*

IBD, malignancy, ischemic colitis, infectious colitis, microscopic colitis

Evaluate for IBS/Rome criteria: recurrent abdominal pain, on average, at least 1 day/week in the last 3 months, associated with two or more of the following criteria:

- Related to defecation
- Associated with a change in frequency of stool
- Associated with a change in form (appearance) of stool

Consider alternative medications.

If no improvement with IBS treatment, consider empiric trial of bile acid sequestrants to determine if BAM is present.

Hayley K. Rogers, MD and Marie L. Borum, MD, EdD, MPH

Schiller LR. Evaluation of chronic diarrhea and irritable bowel syndrome with diarrhea in adults in the era of precision medicine. *Am J Gastroenterol.* 2018;113(5):660–669.

DIZZINESS

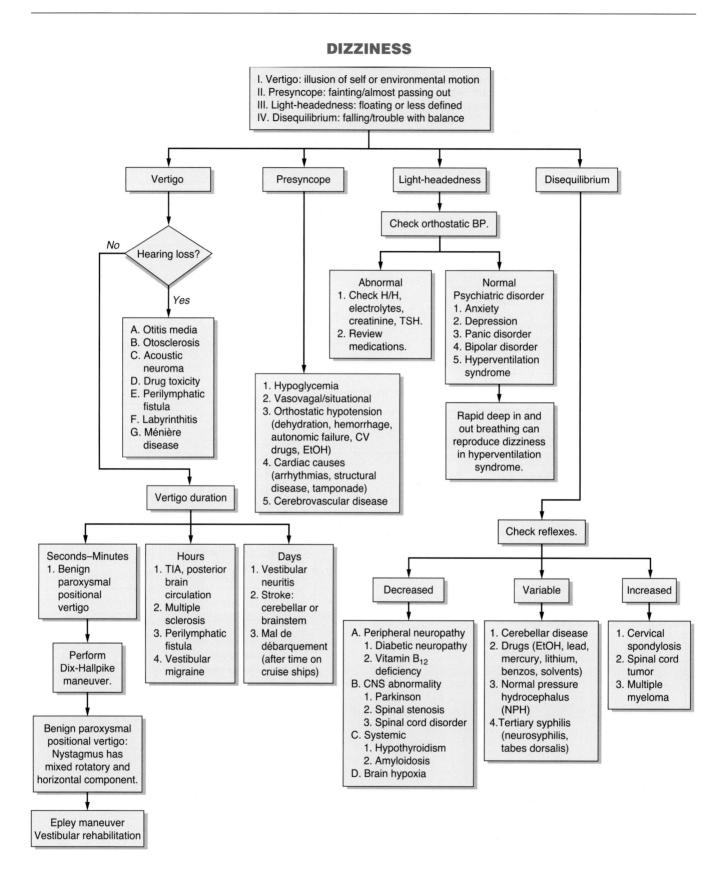

Jennifer G. Foster, MD, MBA, FACP

Stern SC, Cifu AS, Altkorn D, eds. *Symptom to Diagnosis: An Evidence-Based Guide*. 3rd ed. New York, NY: McGraw-Hill; 2014.

DYSPEPSIA

Dyspepsia: predominant symptom of epigastric pain for at least 1 month, associated with other symptoms, such as nausea, vomiting, or heartburn; common causes: GERD, peptic ulcer (<10%), gastroesophageal cancer (<1%), gastroparesis, functional dyspepsia (>70%)

Functional dyspepsia: dyspepsia with normal endoscopy. Main forms of functional dyspepsia: epigastric pain syndrome (intermittent pain/burning in epigastrium at least weekly) and postprandial distress syndrome (at least several episodes weekly of bothersome fullness after meals or early satiety). The two syndromes may both be present in the same patient.

Alarm features of dyspepsia: areas where gastric cancer is common (e.g., Southeast Asia), overt GI bleeding, progressive dysphagia and odynophagia, persistent vomiting, unintentional weight loss, family history upper GI cancer, palpable abdominal mass or lymphadenopathy, unexplained iron deficiency anemia

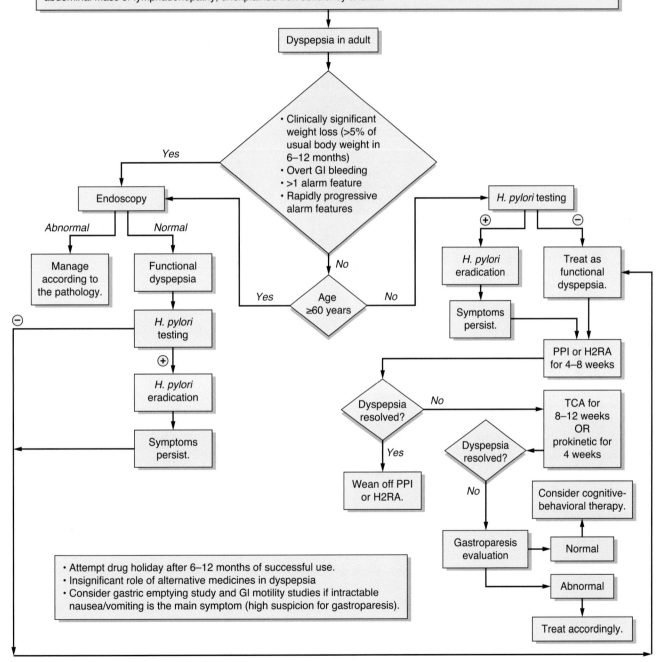

Kimberly Bibb, MD

Moayyedi P, Lacy BE, Andrews CN, et al. ACG and CAG clinical guideline: management of dyspepsia. *Am J Gastroenterol.* 2017;112(7):988–1013.

DYSPHAGIA

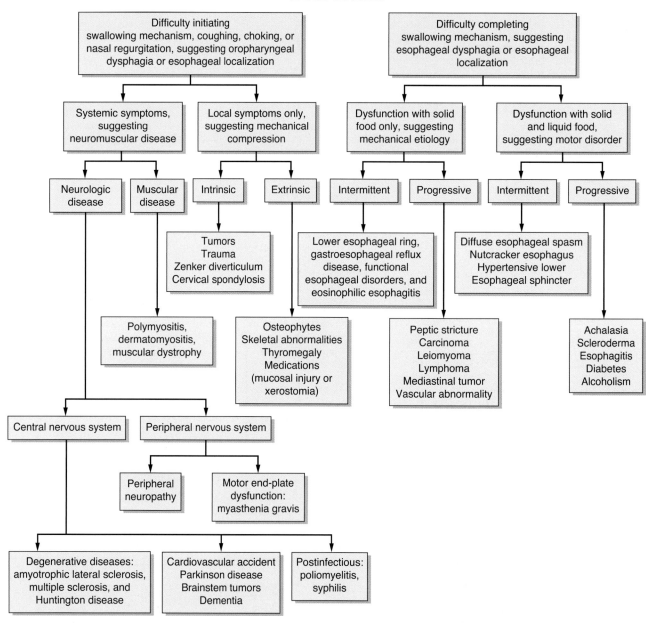

Joanna Drowos, DO, MPH, MBA

Wilkinson JM, Codipilly DC, Wilfahrt RP. Dysphagia: evaluation and collaborative management. *Am Fam Physician*. 2021;103(2):97–106.

ERYTHROCYTOSIS

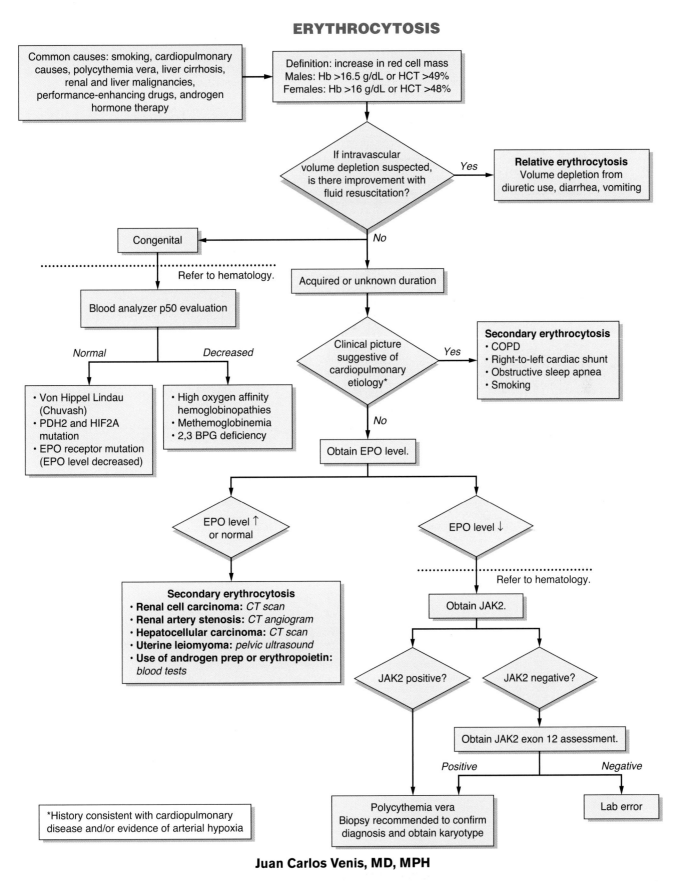

Common causes: smoking, cardiopulmonary causes, polycythemia vera, liver cirrhosis, renal and liver malignancies, performance-enhancing drugs, androgen hormone therapy

Definition: increase in red cell mass
Males: Hb >16.5 g/dL or HCT >49%
Females: Hb >16 g/dL or HCT >48%

If intravascular volume depletion suspected, is there improvement with fluid resuscitation? — **Yes** → **Relative erythrocytosis** Volume depletion from diuretic use, diarrhea, vomiting

No

Congenital
Refer to hematology.

Acquired or unknown duration

Blood analyzer p50 evaluation

Normal / *Decreased*

Clinical picture suggestive of cardiopulmonary etiology* — **Yes** → **Secondary erythrocytosis**
• COPD
• Right-to-left cardiac shunt
• Obstructive sleep apnea
• Smoking

No

• Von Hippel Lindau (Chuvash)
• PDH2 and HIF2A mutation
• EPO receptor mutation (EPO level decreased)

• High oxygen affinity hemoglobinopathies
• Methemoglobinemia
• 2,3 BPG deficiency

Obtain EPO level.

EPO level ↑ or normal

EPO level ↓
Refer to hematology.

Secondary erythrocytosis
• **Renal cell carcinoma:** *CT scan*
• **Renal artery stenosis:** *CT angiogram*
• **Hepatocellular carcinoma:** *CT scan*
• **Uterine leiomyoma:** *pelvic ultrasound*
• **Use of androgen prep or erythropoietin:** *blood tests*

Obtain JAK2.

JAK2 positive? / JAK2 negative?

Obtain JAK2 exon 12 assessment.

Positive / *Negative*

Polycythemia vera
Biopsy recommended to confirm diagnosis and obtain karyotype

Lab error

*History consistent with cardiopulmonary disease and/or evidence of arterial hypoxia

Juan Carlos Venis, MD, MPH

Tefferi A, Barbui T. Polycythemia vera and essential thrombocythemia: 2021 update on diagnosis, risk-stratification and management. *Am J Hematol.* 2020;95(12):1599–1613.

FATIGUE

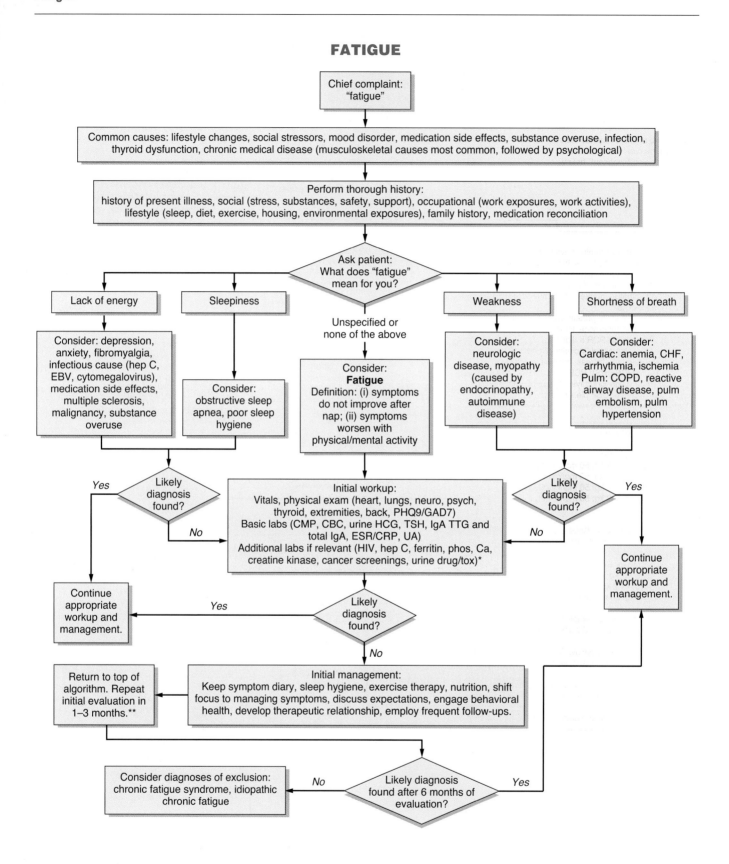

Judy Wang, MD and Stacy E. Potts, MD, Med

Wright J, O'Connor KM. Fatigue. *Med Clin North Am*. 2014;98(3):597–608.

FEVER IN FIRST 60 DAYS OF LIFE

Algorithm for:
- Well-appearing
- Full term (≤37 weeks)
- Previously healthy
- No focal source of infection

Ill-appearing or altered mental status? Initiate sepsis care with antibiotics listed in "Empiric Treatment" below.

Rectal temperature ≥38°C or 100.4°F

**HSV Risk Factors
- Ill-appearing, seizures, abnormal neurologic exam
- Maternal primary HSV or active lesions with vaginal delivery
- Vesicular rash, mucous membrane lesions
- Hepatosplenomegaly or ALT >40
- Household contact with active HSV lesions

Age <28 days?

Yes

1. Admit.
   CRP and/or procalcitonin, if available
2. CBC w/ diff, ALT, AST, UA, blood culture, straight catheterization urine culture
   If <21 days, obtain LP. If 22+ days and reassuring CBC/inflammatory markers (IM), may consider watching patient off of antibiotics
3. LP CSF: Gram stain, protein, glucose, culture. CSF HSV and enterovirus PCR.
4. Stool analysis and PCR if diarrhea
5. Respiratory viral panel (including COVID-19)
6. CXR if respiratory distress, hypoxia, crackles
7. HSV testing (CSF HSV PCR, serum HSV PCR, skin/eye/mouth swab PCR) if age <21 days OR age >21 days AND elevated transaminases or CSF pleocytosis.

Empiric treatment

Ampicillin (IM/IV)
<7 days and <2 kg: 50 mg/kg q12h
<7 days and >2 kg: 50 mg/kg q8h
≥7 days and <2 kg: 50 mg/kg q8h
≥7 days and >2 kg: 50 mg/kg q6h
AND
Gentamicin
<8 days: 2.5 mg/kg IV/IM q12h
8–90 days: 2.5 mg/kg IV/IM q8h

If concern for CNS disease, add cefotaxime (IM/IV)
≤7 days: <2 kg: 50 mg/kg q12h; >2 kg: 50 mg/kg q12h
>7 days: <1.2 kg: 50 mg/kg q12h; 1.2–2.0 kg: 50 mg/kg q8h; >2 kg: 50 mg/kg q6h

If <21 days, initiate empiric acyclovir therapy 20 mg/kg q8h if infant has **HSV risk factors.

If >21 days, add acyclovir if mucocutaneous vesicles, elevated transaminases, seizures, or CSF pleocytosis.

Add acyclovir 20 mg/kg q8h if mucocutaneous vesicles, elevated transaminases, seizures, or CSF pleocytosis.

Add vancomycin 15 mg/kg q8h if MRSA is suspected.

No

1. CBC w/ diff, UA, blood culture, straight catheterization urine culture
2. Respiratory viral panel (including COVID-19)
3. Stool analysis and culture if diarrhea
4. Consider HSV testing if risk criteria** are met in infants <42 days.
5. CXR if respiratory distress, hypoxia, crackles

Low-Risk Criteria
- WBC 5–15,000/μL
- Absolute band count ≤1,500/μL
- Inflammatory markers (IMs): procalcitonin (PCT) ≤0.5 ng/dL and/or C-reactive protein (CRP) <20 mg/dL
- UA <10 WBC/HPF and no bacteria
- Stool <5 WBC/HPF
- Stool culture
- Nontoxic appearance
- No focus of infection (i.e., bone, skin, etc.)
- Reliable PCP follow-up
- PCT <0.5 ng/dL

Yes

Outpatient management if patient able to be reevaluated in 24 hours
1. Consider empiric therapy with daily follow-up: ONLY if LP done; ceftriaxone IV/IM 50–100 mg/kg/day.
2. Await blood, urine cultures.

No

Admission recommended
1. Perform LP CSF: Gram stain, protein, glucose, culture.
2. Initiate empiric therapy: ceftriaxone IV/IM 50–100 mg/kg/day.
3. Await blood, urine cultures.
4. If MRSA is suspected, or ill-appearance, add vancomycin.
5. If mucocutaneous vesicles, seizures, or CSF pleocytosis, add acyclovir 20 mg/kg q8h.

Cultures at 24 hours?

Negative

Positive

Immediately reevaluate patient. LP recommended (if not already performed) and/or admission for IV antibiotics

Febrile?

No

Observe.

Yes

Febrile but low risk:
Clinical reexamination + repeat follow-up within 24 hours
Consider repeat ceftriaxone on case-specific basis.

Laura Mercurio, MD and Robyn Wing, MD, MPH

Pantell RH, Roberts KB, Adams WG, et al. Evaluation and management of well-appearing febrile infants 8 to 60 days old. *Pediatrics.* 2021;148(2):e2021052228.

FEVER OF UNKNOWN ORIGIN

Rachelle Toman, MD, PhD and Grace Walter, MD

Hersch EC, Oh RC. Prolonged febrile illness and fever of unknown origin in adults. *Am Fam Physician*. 2014;90(2):91–96.

GAIT DISTURBANCE

Common causes: infection, tumor, neuromuscular conditions, inflammation, musculoskeletal

↓

Typically multifactorial: Assess intrinsic and extrinsic factors.
History: sudden or insidious onset, associated falls, ADLs, physical limitations, diet
Exam: Consider standing, posture, stance (wide/narrow), walking, arm swing, turning, tandem, Romberg.

→ Extrinsic factors: footwear, eyewear, hearing aids, medications, drug use, substance use, diet, environmental hazards

↓

Associated pain or antalgic gait? (limp due to avoidance of pain)

Yes

Articular or nonarticular?

Articular

Mono or poly?

Mono → Check x-rays; consider arthrocentesis, ESR, or CRP. → Fracture, osteoarthritis, gout, transient synovitis, septic joint, Lyme disease, slipped epiphysis leg length discrepancy

Poly → Check ESR or CRP; consider ANA, RF or CCP, RPR. → Rheumatologic (osteoarthritis, reactive arthritis, SLE) Viral infection Fibromyalgia Malignancy

Nonarticular

Occult fracture
Neoplasm
Pes planus/cavus
Bursitis
Tendonitis

Vascular or neurogenic claudication

No

Neurologic symptoms or findings?

No

Cardiac disorders, depression, fear of falling, psychogenic

Yes

Confusion → Consider head CT. → Dementia Subdural NPH Stroke Neoplasm

Weakness → Cerebral palsy Myositis Muscular dystrophy Multiple sclerosis Myelopathy Stroke Decondition Spinal muscular atrophy Electrolyte imbalances

Numbness → Diabetes Vitamin B_{12} deficiency HIV Hyper- and hypothyroidism Heavy metal poisoning Neuropathy

Tremor → Parkinson disease Supranuclear palsy

Coordination deficit → Vertebrobasilar insufficiency Cerebellar dysfunction Vestibular disorders Neoplasm

Bryan R. Norkus, MD

Attaullah AHM, De Jesus O. *Gait Disturbances*. Treasure Island, FL: StatPearls Publishing; 2021. https://www-ncbi-nlm-nih-gov/books/NBK560610/. Accessed September 8, 2021.

GASTROESOPHAGEAL REFLUX DISEASE (GERD), DIAGNOSIS AND TREATMENT

Symptoms: burning sensation, acid reflux, chest pain, nocturnal/positional pain, antacid relief
Risk factors: obesity, recent weight gain, family history
Diagnosis: clinical symptoms of burning sensation, acid reflux, chest pain, nocturnal/positional pain, antacid relief +/– endoscopy testing

Encourage lifestyle modification, for example, weight loss (for BMI >30 or recent weight gain with normal BMI), tobacco cessation, diet changes, smaller meals, avoidance of late-night meals or immediate supine position postprandially, raising the head of the bed, and stress reduction. Avoid chocolate, caffeine, and alcohol.

Presence of "alarm features" (weight loss, dysphagia, epigastric mass, age >50 years at onset, regurgitation, odynophagia, N/V, choking)?

Yes

Endoscopy with biopsy

EGD with no evidence of GERD; consider ambulatory 24 pH monitoring while off PPI therapy.

EGD with proven evidence of GERD (LA grade C or D esophagitis, Barrett esophagus, or peptic stricture)

Acid exposure time (AET) <4% or <40 episodes of reflux in 24 hours—normal

4–6% AET inconclusive

>6% AET abnormal or >80 episodes of reflux in 24 hours

Consider additional testing/evaluate symptom association.

Nonerosive reflux disease (NERD)

No

Atypical symptoms (chronic cough, globus sensation, epigastric pain, nausea)?

Yes

Atypical GERD

Trial PPI × 8 weeks

Step-down OR on-demand therapy

Adequate response?

Yes

No

Consider other etiologies (H. pylori testing) OR endoscopy/ manometry/ pH monitoring.

No

Trial PPI or H2RA for 8 weeks

Adequate response?

Yes

Step-down OR on-demand therapy 8–12 weeks

Reevaluate.

Endoscopy if Tx needed for >10 years

No

Step-up therapy

Adequate response?

Yes

No

Consider other etiologies such as functional dyspepsia, NERD. Refer to GI.

Dylan T. Flaherty, DO and Benjamin Dale Rogers, MD

Gyawali CP, Kahrilas PJ, Savarino E, et al. Modern diagnosis of GERD: the Lyon Consensus. *Gut*. 2018;67(7):1351–1362.

GENITAL ULCERS

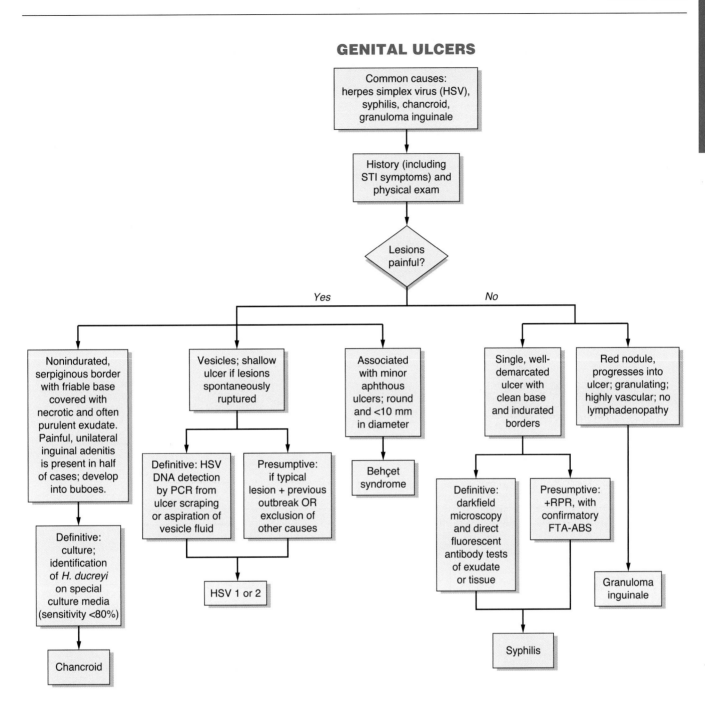

Frank J. Domino, MD

Roett MA. Genital ulcers: differential diagnosis and management. *Am Fam Physician*. 2020;101(6):355–361.

GRANULOCYTOSIS (LEUKOCYTOSIS)

WBC >11.0 × 10⁹/L

Common causes: infection, inflammation, drugs (steroid/lithium/β-agonists, G-CSF, GM-CSF, etc.), stress, smoking, asplenia/hyposplenism, pregnancy, myeloproliferative disorder, leukemia/lymphoma

Repeat CBC.
Order manual smear.

Leukocytosis confirmed? — *No* → No further workup necessary

Yes

Leukocytosis explained by additional pertinent history and/or physical examination? — *Yes* →

No

Patient presents with weight loss, fatigue, fevers, night sweats, splenomegaly, lymphadenopathy, bruising? Abnormal red blood cell (RBC) and platelet count? Risk or history of prior malignancy? — *Yes* →

Consider malignancy.
Review peripheral blood smear.
Hematology/oncology consultation
Bone marrow biopsy and flow cytometry, cytogenetics, or molecular testing on bone marrow or peripheral blood

No

Determine affected cell line.

LYMPHOCYTOSIS
(>4,500/mm³
[4.5 × 10⁹/L])

PLEOMORPHIC
(REACTIVE)

MONOMORPHIC
Suspect lymphoproliferative disorder.

Look for:
Infections
(viral, pertussis)
Hypersensitivity
Consider:
Immunization
Contact history
Chest x-ray
Viral panels

MONOCYTOSIS
(>880/mm³
[0.88 × 10⁹/L])
Look for:
Chronic infection
(EBV, fungal, protozoal, rickettsial)
Autoimmune
Splenectomy
Myelodysplastic syndrome
Consider:
Contact, travel, medical history, monospot test, PPD, ESR, CRP, ANA

If persistent

INCREASED BLASTS

BASOPHILIA
(>100/mm³
[0.1 × 10⁹/L])
Rare: Suspect MPN or CML.
Consider:
Karyotyping
BCR-ABL1
JAK2 V617F

Hematology/oncology consult
Bone marrow biopsy
Flow cytometry, cytogenetics, and molecular analysis of bone marrow or peripheral blood

EOSINOPHILIA
(>500/mm³ [0.5 × 10⁹])
Look for reactive etiology:
Allergic conditions
Eosinophilic esophagitis
Drug reaction
Dermatologic conditions
Parasitic infections
Consider:
Drug, travel history
Full skin exam and biopsy if indicated
Allergy/immunology testing
Stool for ova and parasites
Upper GI endoscopy

If negative, rule out myeloproliferative neoplasm, Hodgkin lymphoma.
Consider:
FISH/PCR for PDGFRA mutation

NEUTROPHILIA
(>7,000/mm³ [7 × 10⁹/L])

WBC >50,000: malignant

WBC <50,000: leukemoid reaction

Look for:
Infection
Chronic inflammation
Medications (including GM-CSF)
Splenectomy
Reactive (stressors, exercise, seizure, etc.)
Consider:
Medical, surgical drug, contact, social history
ESR, CRP, ANA
Blood smear review for nucleated RBCs
Blood culture, lumbar puncture
Additional system-specific studies

Edison Tsui, MD

George TI. Malignant or benign leukocytosis. *Hematology Am Soc Hematol Educ Program.* 2012;2012:475–484.

HEADACHE, CHRONIC

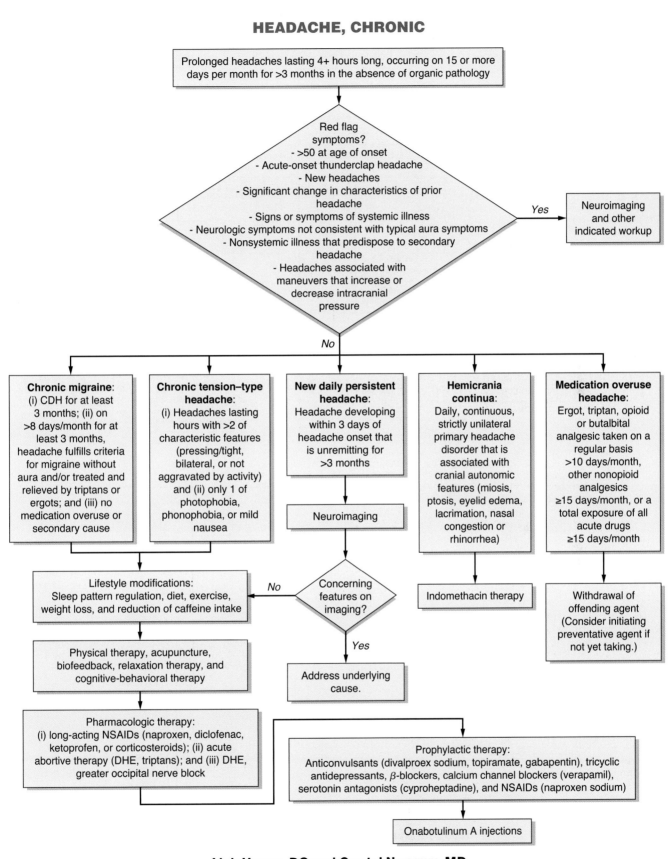

Linh Hoang, DO and Crystal Nwagwu, MD

Dodick D, Dilli E. *Chronic Daily Headache*. Mt. Royal, NJ: American Headache Society; 2018. https://americanheadachesociety.org/wp-content/uploads/2018/05/David_Dodick_and_Esma_Dilli_-_Chronic_Daily_Headache.pdf. Accessed November 23, 2021.

HEART MURMUR

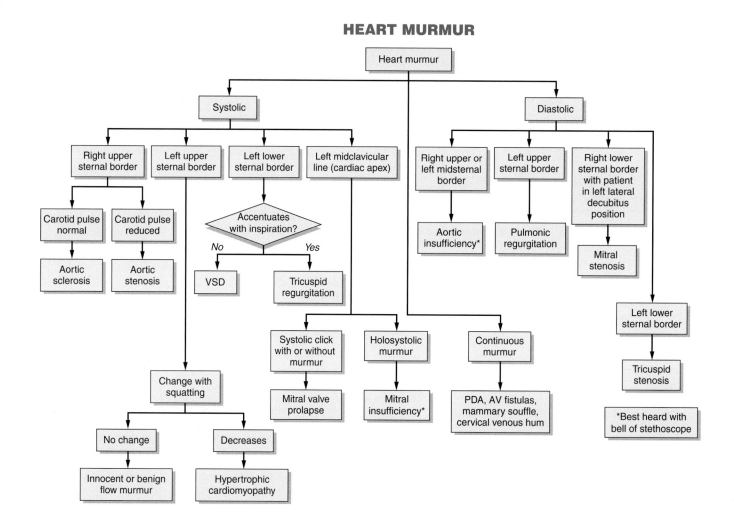

Roop Kiran Kaur, MD and Afza Safeer, MD

Bonow RO, Carabello BA, Chatterjee K, et al. 2008 Focused update incorporated into the ACC/AHA 2006 guidelines for the management of patients with valvular heart disease: a report of the American College of Cardiology/American Heart Association Task Force on Practice Guidelines (writing committee to revise the 1998 Guidelines for the Management of Patients With Valvular Heart Disease): endorsed by the Society of Cardiovascular Anesthesiologists, Society for Cardiovascular Angiography and Interventions, and Society of Thoracic Surgeons. *Circulation*. 2008;118(15):e523–e661.

HEMATEMESIS (BLEEDING, UPPER GASTROINTESTINAL)

Common causes:
PUD, Mallory-Weiss tear, esophagitis, gastritis, varices, epistaxis

Maintain two large-bore cannulas.
Transfuse pRBC to maintain Hb >7 mg/dL.

CBC, PT/INR, type and screen

Stable? — *No* →
ABC
Fluid resuscitation
Make patient NPO.
Consult gastroenterology.

Yes

Recent nose bleed? — *Yes* → Epistaxis
No

Start IV proton pump inhibitor.

Suspect variceal hemorrhage. ↔ Suspect nonvariceal hemorrhage.

Perform upper endoscopy.

Start IV octreotide drip (3–5 days) and broad-spectrum antibiotics (5–7 days).

Perform upper endoscopy with variceal ligation banding within 6–24 hours.

Has the bleeding stopped?

Yes — Start prophylactic nonselective β-blocker after octreotide complete.

Repeat endoscopy in 1–2 weeks and reband as needed.

No — Sengstaken-Blakemore tube

Consider emergent transjugular intrahepatic portosystemic shunt or surgery depending on local expertise.

No source identified
Consider repeat endoscopy and push enteroscopy.

Arteriovenous malformation, Dieulafoy ulcer
Endoscopic therapy with epinephrine, thermocoagulation, or clipping

Erosive esophagitis
Continue proton pump inhibitor therapy.

Peptic ulcer bleeding
Endoscopic therapy with epinephrine, thermocoagulation, and/or clips

Has the bleeding stopped?

Yes — Continue proton pump inhibitor therapy; eradicate *Helicobacter pylori* infection if present and consider discontinuing NSAIDs/blood thinners if possible.

No — Reattempt upper endoscopy; otherwise, consider arteriography with embolization or surgery.

Mallory-Weiss tear
Antiemetic and proton pump inhibitor; endoscopic treatment only if active bleeding

Frank J. Domino, MD

Kamboj AK, Hoversten P, Leggett CL. Upper gastrointestinal bleeding: etiologies and management. *Mayo Clin Proc.* 2019;94(4):697–703.

HEMATURIA

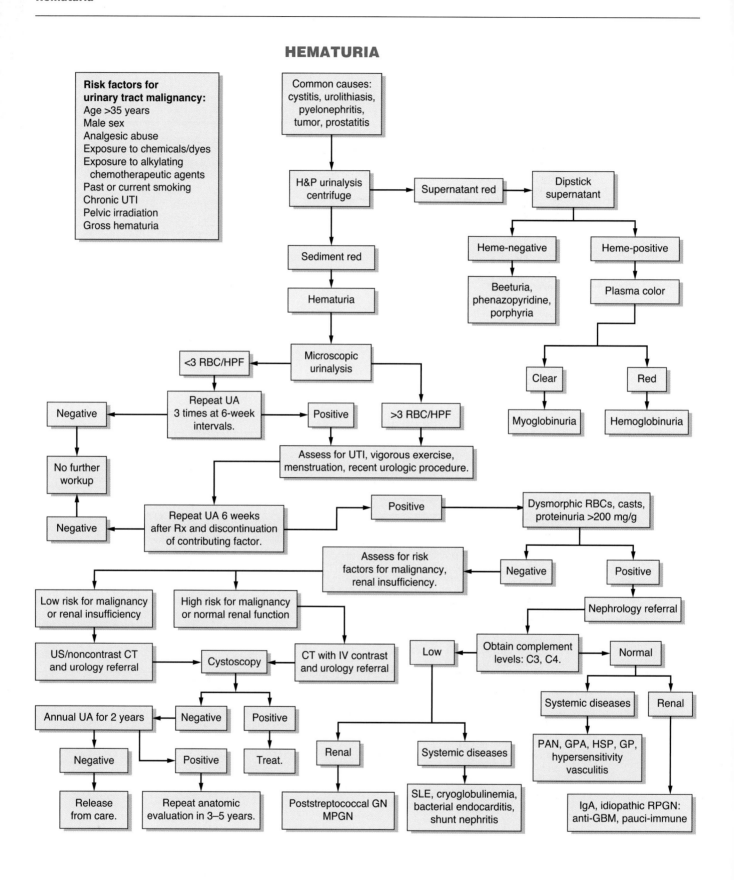

Risk factors for urinary tract malignancy:
Age >35 years
Male sex
Analgesic abuse
Exposure to chemicals/dyes
Exposure to alkylating chemotherapeutic agents
Past or current smoking
Chronic UTI
Pelvic irradiation
Gross hematuria

Common causes: cystitis, urolithiasis, pyelonephritis, tumor, prostatitis

H&P urinalysis centrifuge

Supernatant red

Dipstick supernatant

Heme-negative → Beeturia, phenazopyridine, porphyria

Heme-positive → Plasma color

Clear → Myoglobinuria

Red → Hemoglobinuria

Sediment red

Hematuria

Microscopic urinalysis

<3 RBC/HPF

Repeat UA 3 times at 6-week intervals.

Negative → No further workup

Positive

>3 RBC/HPF

Assess for UTI, vigorous exercise, menstruation, recent urologic procedure.

Repeat UA 6 weeks after Rx and discontinuation of contributing factor.

Negative

Positive → Dysmorphic RBCs, casts, proteinuria >200 mg/g

Negative

Positive → Nephrology referral

Assess for risk factors for malignancy, renal insufficiency.

Low risk for malignancy or renal insufficiency → US/noncontrast CT and urology referral

High risk for malignancy or normal renal function → CT with IV contrast and urology referral

Cystoscopy

Obtain complement levels: C3, C4.

Low

Normal → Systemic diseases, Renal

Annual UA for 2 years

Negative

Positive

Treat.

Renal

Systemic diseases

Negative → Release from care.

Positive → Repeat anatomic evaluation in 3–5 years.

Poststreptococcal GN MPGN

SLE, cryoglobulinemia, bacterial endocarditis, shunt nephritis

PAN, GPA, HSP, GP, hypersensitivity vasculitis

IgA, idiopathic RPGN: anti-GBM, pauci-immune

Michael T. Partin, MD and Karl T. Clebak, MD, MHA, FAAFP

Sharp VJ, Barnes KT, Erickson BA. Assessment of asymptomatic microscopic hematuria in adults. *Am Fam Physician*. 2013;88(11):747–754.

HEPATOMEGALY

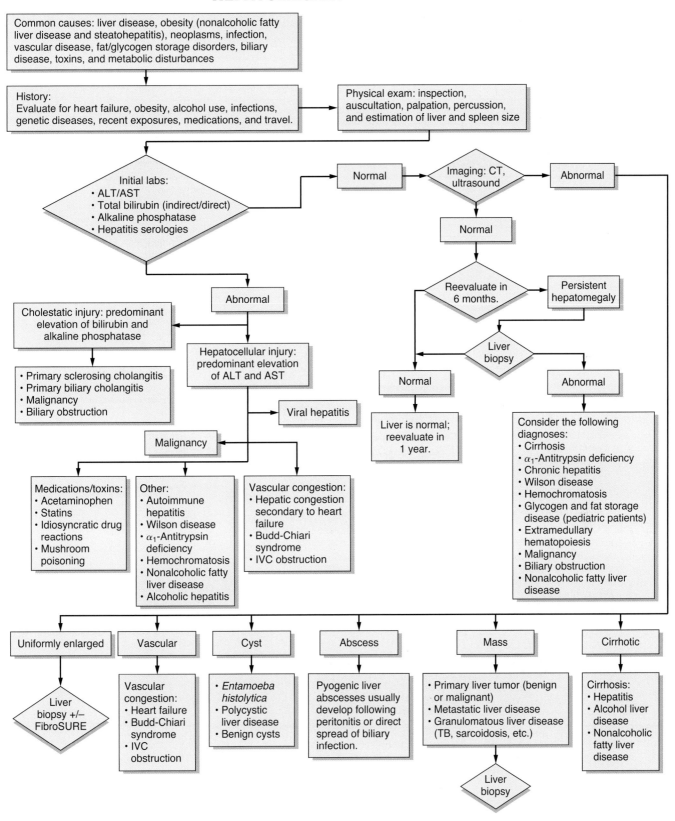

Nighat Seema Ahmed, MD

Kwo PY, Cohen SM, Lim JK. ACG clinical guideline: evaluation of abnormal liver chemistries. *Am J Gastroenterol.* 2017;112(1):18–35.

HYPERBILIRUBINEMIA AND JAUNDICE

Jaundice: a yellow discoloration of the skin, sclera and mucous membranes by bilirubin, a bile pigment formed by the breakdown of heme ring; detected when the serum bilirubin level >3 mg/dL

Bilirubin: a product of hemoglobin breakdown in the spleen; heme is converted to unconjugated bilirubin, bound to albumin, and transported to the liver where it is then conjugated.

Common causes of hyperbilirubinemia: Gilbert syndrome, hemolysis, hepatitis, and choledocholithiasis

Evaluation: CBC w/ diff; LFTs: AST, ALT, serum alkaline phosphatase (AP), total bilirubin (TB), and direct bilirubin (DB); haptoglobin, LDH; viral and autoimmune hepatitis serologies; amylase, lipase; hCG; US, CT, or MRI

DB >0.3 mg/dL? OR >50% of TB?

No → **Unconjugated hyperbilirubinemia**

Yes → **Conjugated hyperbilirubinemia**

Elevated AP?

Yes → **Intrahepatic**

No → **Prehepatic**

Obstruction on imaging?

No → **Intrahepatic**

Yes → **Extrahepatic**

Prehepatic

- Gilbert syndrome (mild defect in UDP glucuronosyltransferase [UGT] responsible for conjugation)
- Hemolytic anemic
- Reabsorption of large hematoma

Labs: anemia, possible reticulocytosis, mild TB elevation, increased indirect bilirubin (normal DB), normal AST/ALT

Intrahepatic

Unconjugated Hyperbilirubinemia

- Crigler-Najjar syndrome: more severe defect in UGT, usually presents during infancy

Conjugated Hyperbilirubinemia

- Dubin Johnson syndrome: defective secretion of conjugated bilirubin
- Rotor syndrome

Conjugated or Unconjugated Hyperbilirubinemia

- Hepatitis: viral, autoimmune, alcohol-related insult leading to inflammation that impedes or prevents transportation/secretion of conjugated bilirubin
- Medication or drug: acetaminophen
- Cirrhosis
- Congestive heart failure: hypoxic injury of hepatocytes leading to cellular injury

Intrahepatic Cholestasis (primary abnormality is elevated AP)

Other

- TPN
- Sepsis
- Sarcoidosis
- Pregnancy

Extrahepatic

Extrahepatic cholestasis (labs: elevated TB and DB, elevated AP/imaging: dilated bile ducts[s])

- Choledocholithiasis
- Chronic pancreatitis
- Cholangitis
- Biliary stricture
- Primary biliary cholangitis
- Primary sclerosing cholangitis
- Cholangiocarcinoma
- Pancreatic head tumor

Krunal Patel, MD and Gustavo Churrango, MD

Roche SP, Kobos R. Jaundice in the adult patient. *Am Fam Physician.* 2004;69(2):299–304.

HYPERCALCEMIA

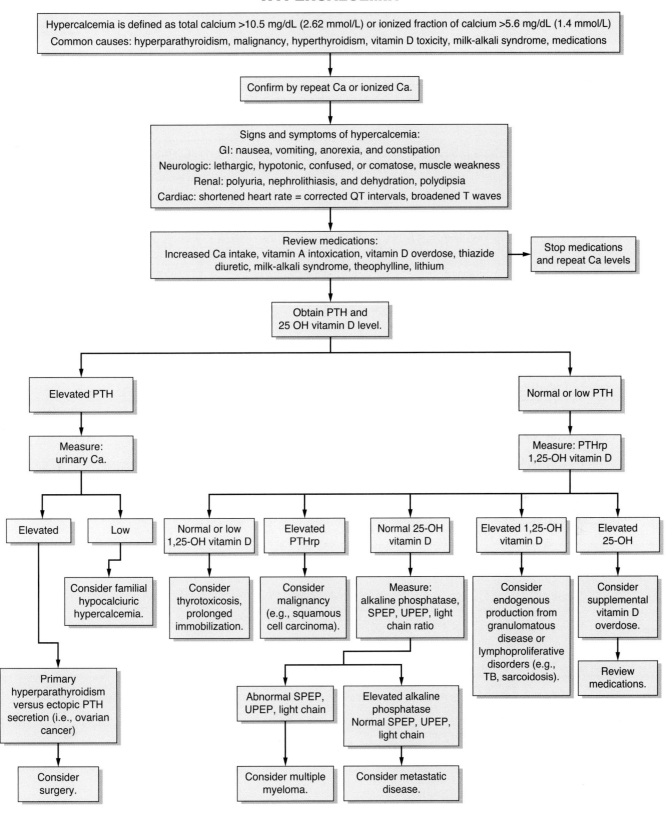

Hypercalcemia is defined as total calcium >10.5 mg/dL (2.62 mmol/L) or ionized fraction of calcium >5.6 mg/dL (1.4 mmol/L)
Common causes: hyperparathyroidism, malignancy, hyperthyroidism, vitamin D toxicity, milk-alkali syndrome, medications

Confirm by repeat Ca or ionized Ca.

Signs and symptoms of hypercalcemia:
GI: nausea, vomiting, anorexia, and constipation
Neurologic: lethargic, hypotonic, confused, or comatose, muscle weakness
Renal: polyuria, nephrolithiasis, and dehydration, polydipsia
Cardiac: shortened heart rate = corrected QT intervals, broadened T waves

Review medications:
Increased Ca intake, vitamin A intoxication, vitamin D overdose, thiazide diuretic, milk-alkali syndrome, theophylline, lithium

Stop medications and repeat Ca levels

Obtain PTH and 25 OH vitamin D level.

Elevated PTH

Normal or low PTH

Measure: urinary Ca.

Measure: PTHrp 1,25-OH vitamin D

Elevated

Low

Normal or low 1,25-OH vitamin D

Elevated PTHrp

Normal 25-OH vitamin D

Elevated 1,25-OH vitamin D

Elevated 25-OH

Consider familial hypocalciuric hypercalcemia.

Consider thyrotoxicosis, prolonged immobilization.

Consider malignancy (e.g., squamous cell carcinoma).

Measure: alkaline phosphatase, SPEP, UPEP, light chain ratio

Consider endogenous production from granulomatous disease or lymphoproliferative disorders (e.g., TB, sarcoidosis).

Consider supplemental vitamin D overdose.

Primary hyperparathyroidism versus ectopic PTH secretion (i.e., ovarian cancer)

Abnormal SPEP, UPEP, light chain

Elevated alkaline phosphatase Normal SPEP, UPEP, light chain

Review medications.

Consider surgery.

Consider multiple myeloma.

Consider metastatic disease.

Vasudha Jain, MD and John Coward, MD

Caroll MF, Schade DS. A practical approach to hypercalcemia. *Am Fam Physician*. 2003;67(9):1959–1966.
https://www.aafp.org/afp/2003/0501/p1959.html.

HYPERKALEMIA

K >5.5 mEq/L

Common causes: renal failure,
hyperglycemia, specimen delay and hemolysis, renal insufficiency, acidosis, rhabdomyolysis, insulin
deficiency, adrenal insufficiency, medications, massive blood transfusions, tumor lysis, ischemic bowel,
CHF, DMII, MI, burns, excessive exercise, anemia, RAASi usage

Repeat test—by serum,
not POC test

No ←

Symptoms present?
• Weakness, nausea, paresthesias,
palpitations, ileus, flaccid paralysis,
fasciculation
ECG changes present?
• Peaked T waves, ↑ PR interval,
↑ QRS width, sine wave pattern, PEA.
K >6.5 mEq/L

Yes → Treat as acute hyperkalemia.

No → See chronic hyperkalemia management.

Normal

Abnormal

Assess for pseudohyperkalemia:
ICV with K, hemolyzed sample,
mechanical trauma, clotting,
leukocytosis, thrombocytosis, fist
clench >1 minute

Check medications:
ACEI, ARBs, β-blockers, NSAIDs, penicillin K, TMP-SMX,
digitalis, K-sparing diuretics, heparin, cyclosporine, tacrolimus,
pentamidine, succinylcholine, direct renin agents, octreotide,
mannitol

Check herbal and natural product use:
Fruits, alfalfa, amino acids, dandelion, dried toad skin,
hawthorn berry, horsetail, lily of the valley, mildewed, nettle,
noni, juice, Siberian ginseng, OTC K salts, OTC K supplement

Suspicious medications
or herbs/supplements
found?

No → Check:
ABG, BMP, digoxin
level (if applicable),
CPK, urine K, BP,
ECG, O$_2$ saturation.

Yes → Discontinue use
or modify under
physician
guidance.

Urine K >30 mEq/L
or spot urine K/Cr
>200 mEq/g:
transcellular shift

Urine K <30 mEq/L
or spot urine K/Cr
<20 mEq/g: impaired
renal excretion

Acidosis
Rhabdomyolysis
Hyperglycemia
Burns

Renal insufficiency
Adrenal insufficiency
Hyporeninemic
Hypoaldosteronism

Acute hyperkalemia management: if ECG changes, moderate/severe symptoms, or
K >6.5 mEq/L
Membrane stabilizers
• Calcium chloride (CaCl)—higher bioavailability (3 times higher than calcium
gluconate): 10 mL of 10% CaCl over 2–5 minutes IV; may repeat in 5–10 minutes
• Calcium gluconate—less tissue toxicity: 30 mL of 10% Ca gluconate IV over
2–5 minutes; may repeat in 5–10 minutes
• Careful in potential dig toxicity as hypercalcemia can increase toxic effect of the drug
• Ca salts don't lower K.
• Action limited to 30–60 minutes
ICF shift
• Short-acting insulin: 10 units IV with glucose 50 g; works in 30–60 minutes
• β-Agonist: albuterol nebulizer; action in 30–60 minutes
K elimination
• K binding agents
• Sodium polystyrene sulfonate: works in several hours; 15–60 mg in 20% sorbitol
(60–240 mL) orally or rectal = 0.5–1 mEq/g reduction
• Patiromer sorbitex calcium: works in 7 hours; 4.2–16.8 g QD–BID; lowers K by
0.75 mEq/L
• Sodium zirconium cyclosilicate: works in 1 hour; 10 g TID; lowers K by 0.7 mEq/L
per 10-g dose
• Diuretics: loop diuretic in hypervolemic patients: furosemide 40 mg; works in
0.5–2 hours
• Dialysis: takes 1–8 hours; lowers K by 25–50 mEq/hr. Peritoneal dialysis works in
1–4 hours and lowers K by 50–70 mEq/24 hr.
• NaHCO$_3$: only use in patient with metabolic acidosis. Unsure of efficacy

Chronic hyperkalemia management: if K <6.5 and no ECG changes and no moderate/severe symptoms
• Dietary potassium counseling: Avoid salt substitutes.
• Manage RAASi therapy: Reduce or change medication if possible.
• Diuretic therapy
• Oral NaHCO$_3$ (if appropriate)
• Fludrocortisone: can increase fluid retention, HTN, vascular injury
• Consider potassium binders—see acute management (elimination section).
• Monitor potassium 2 times per year.
• Review medications, herbs, supplements.
• Multidisciplinary approach: patient education, physician education, dietitian, pharmacist

Anush S. Pillai, DO, FAAFP and Elizabeth Ashley Suniega, MD

Palmer BF, Carrero JJ, Clegg DJ, et al. Clinical management of hyperkalemia. *Mayo Clin Proc.* 2021;96(3):744–762.

HYPERLIPIDEMIA

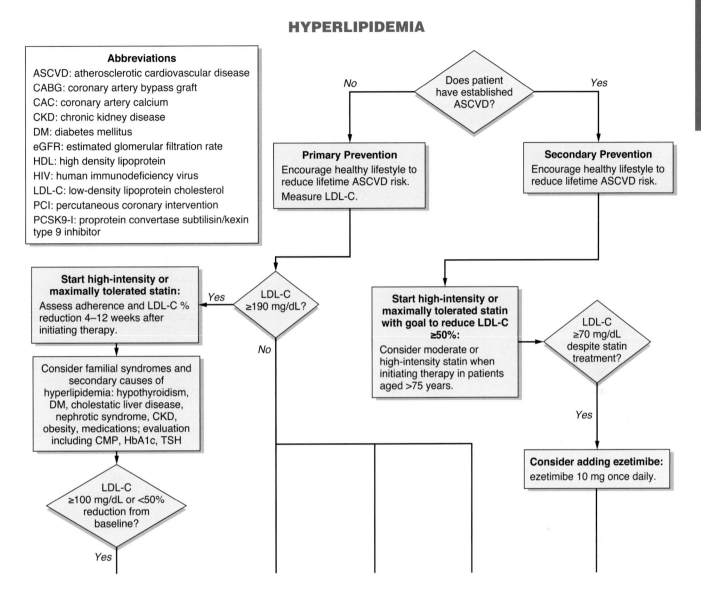

Abbreviations
ASCVD: atherosclerotic cardiovascular disease
CABG: coronary artery bypass graft
CAC: coronary artery calcium
CKD: chronic kidney disease
DM: diabetes mellitus
eGFR: estimated glomerular filtration rate
HDL: high density lipoprotein
HIV: human immunodeficiency virus
LDL-C: low-density lipoprotein cholesterol
PCI: percutaneous coronary intervention
PCSK9-I: proprotein convertase subtilisin/kexin type 9 inhibitor

Does patient have established ASCVD?

No → **Primary Prevention**
Encourage healthy lifestyle to reduce lifetime ASCVD risk.
Measure LDL-C.

Yes → **Secondary Prevention**
Encourage healthy lifestyle to reduce lifetime ASCVD risk.

LDL-C ≥190 mg/dL?

Yes → **Start high-intensity or maximally tolerated statin:**
Assess adherence and LDL-C % reduction 4–12 weeks after initiating therapy.

Consider familial syndromes and secondary causes of hyperlipidemia: hypothyroidism, DM, cholestatic liver disease, nephrotic syndrome, CKD, obesity, medications; evaluation including CMP, HbA1c, TSH

LDL-C ≥100 mg/dL or <50% reduction from baseline?

Yes

No

Start high-intensity or maximally tolerated statin with goal to reduce LDL-C ≥50%:
Consider moderate or high-intensity statin when initiating therapy in patients aged >75 years.

LDL-C ≥70 mg/dL despite statin treatment?

Yes → **Consider adding ezetimibe:** ezetimibe 10 mg once daily.

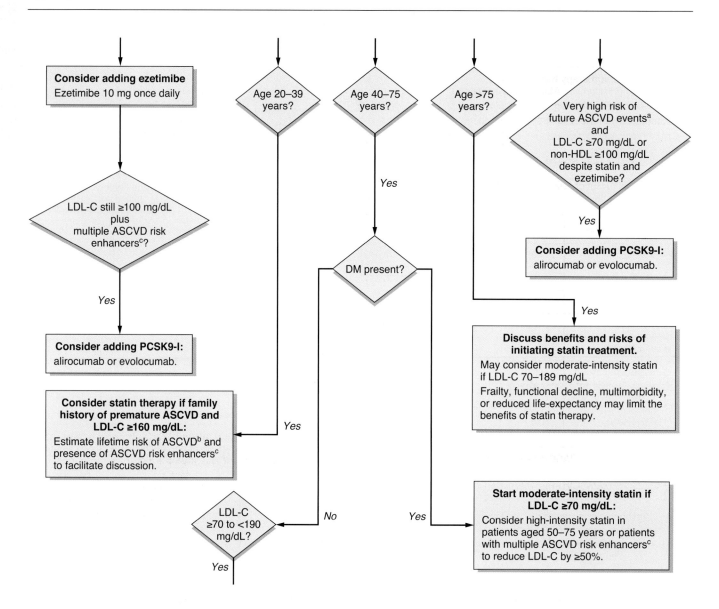

Consider statin therapy based on 10-year ASCVD risk[b] and presence of ASCVD risk enhancers[c]:

High Risk (≥20%): Start high-intensity statin to reduce LDL-C by ≥50%.

Intermediate Risk (≥7.5 to <20%): Start moderate-intensity statin to reduce LDL-C by ≥30%.
Consider measuring CAC to guide therapy.

Borderline Risk (5 to <7.5%): Consider moderate-intensity statin if ASCVD risk enhancers are present.

Low Risk (<5%): Emphasize healthy lifestyle to reduce ASCVD risk.

Reassess 4–12 weeks after start of treatment or after change in medication dose:
Assess for medication and lifestyle adherence.
Measure LDL-C and determine % reduction from baseline.
Reassess every 3–12 months.

LDL-C reduction	0%	30%–49%
Atorvastatin	40–□0 mg/day	10–20 mg/day
Rosuvastatin	20–40 mg/day	5–10 mg/day
Simvastatin		20–40 mg/day
Pravastatin		40–□0 mg/day
Lovastatin		40–□0 mg/day
Fluvastatin		40 mg twice daily
Fluvastatin □L		□0 mg/day
Pitavastatin		1–4 mg/day

[b]ASCVD Risk Predictor Plus
Available at:
http://tools.acc.org/ASCVD-Risk-Estimator-Plus/#!/calculate/estimate/

[c]ASCVD Risk Enhancers
Family history of premature ASCVD
Persistently elevated LDL-C ≥160 mg/dL
CKD
Metabolic syndrome
Conditions specific to women (e.g., history of preeclampsia or premature menopause before the age of 40 years)
Inflammatory diseases (e.g., rheumatoid arthritis, psoriasis, or chronic HIV infection)
Ethnicity (e.g., South Asian ancestry)
Persistently elevated triglycerides ≥175 mg/dL
High-sensitivity C-reactive protein ≥2.0 mg/dL
Lipoprotein (a) levels ≥50 mg/dL
Apolipoprotein B ≥130 mg/dL
Ankle-brachial index <0.9

[a]Very high risk of future ASCVD events is defined as a history of multiple major ASCVD events or 1 major ASCVD event plus multiple high-risk conditions.

Major ASCVD events include the following:
- Acute coronary syndrome within the past 12 months
- History of myocardial infarction beyond 12 months ago
- History of ischemic stroke
- Symptomatic peripheral arterial disease

High-risk conditions include the following:
- Age ≥65 years
- Heterozygous familial hypercholesterolemia
- History of prior CABG surgery or PCI outside of the major ASCVD event(s)
- Diabetes mellitus
- Hypertension
- CKD (eGFR 15–59 mL/min/1.73 m^2)
- Current smoking
- Persistently elevated LDL-C (≥100 mg/dL) despite maximally tolerated statin therapy plus ezetimibe
- History of congestive heart failure

Jason Cross, PharmD, BCPS, BCACP, Dinesh Yogaratnam, PharmD, and Sudeep K. Aulakh, MD, FACP, FRCPC

Grundy SM, Stone NJ, Bailey AL, et al. 2018 AHA/ACC/AACVPR/AAPA/ABC/ACPM/ADA/AGS/APhA/ASPC/NLA/PCNA guideline on the management of blood cholesterol: executive summary: a report of the American College of Cardiology/American Heart Association Task Force on Clinical Practice Guidelines. *J Am Coll Cardiol.* 2019;73(24):3168–3209.

HYPERNATREMIA

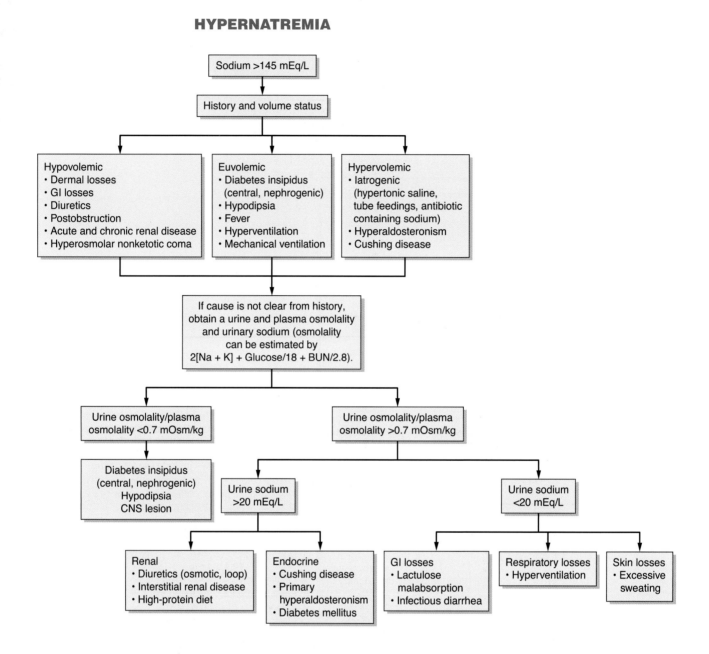

Sodium >145 mEq/L

History and volume status

Hypovolemic
• Dermal losses
• GI losses
• Diuretics
• Postobstruction
• Acute and chronic renal disease
• Hyperosmolar nonketotic coma

Euvolemic
• Diabetes insipidus (central, nephrogenic)
• Hypodipsia
• Fever
• Hyperventilation
• Mechanical ventilation

Hypervolemic
• Iatrogenic (hypertonic saline, tube feedings, antibiotic containing sodium)
• Hyperaldosteronism
• Cushing disease

If cause is not clear from history, obtain a urine and plasma osmolality and urinary sodium (osmolality can be estimated by 2[Na + K] + Glucose/18 + BUN/2.8).

Urine osmolality/plasma osmolality <0.7 mOsm/kg

Urine osmolality/plasma osmolality >0.7 mOsm/kg

Diabetes insipidus (central, nephrogenic) Hypodipsia CNS lesion

Urine sodium >20 mEq/L

Urine sodium <20 mEq/L

Renal
• Diuretics (osmotic, loop)
• Interstitial renal disease
• High-protein diet

Endocrine
• Cushing disease
• Primary hyperaldosteronism
• Diabetes mellitus

GI losses
• Lactulose malabsorption
• Infectious diarrhea

Respiratory losses
• Hyperventilation

Skin losses
• Excessive sweating

Timothy J. Coker, MD, FAAFP

Braun MM, Barstow CH, Pyzocha NJ. Diagnosis and management of sodium disorders: hyponatremia and hypernatremia. *Am Fam Physician.* 2015;91(5):299–307.

HYPERTRIGLYCERIDEMIA

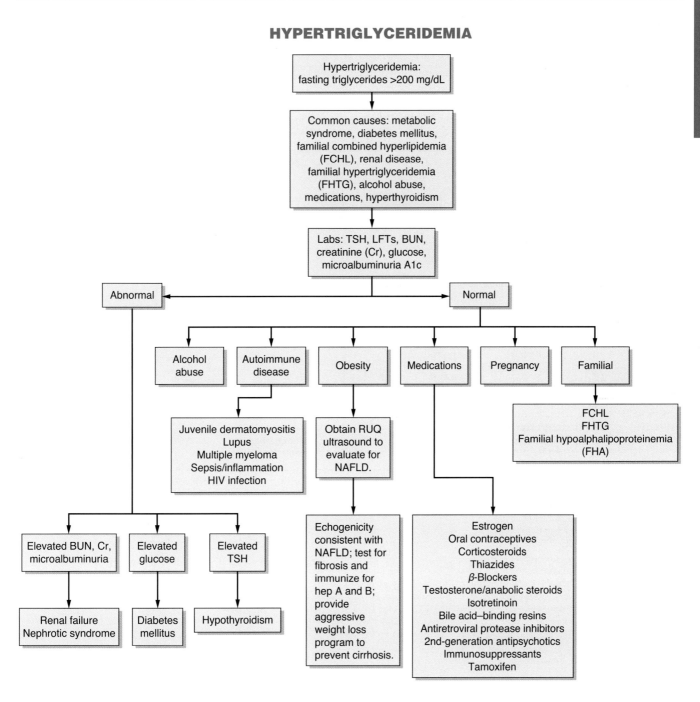

Steven W. Gale, MD and Timothy J. Coker, MD, FAAFP

Berglund L, Brunzell JD, Goldberg AC, et al; for Endocrine Society. Evaluation and treatment of hypertriglyceridemia: an Endocrine Society clinical practice guideline. *J Clin Endocrinol Metab.* 2012;97(9):2969–2989.

HYPOALBUMINEMIA

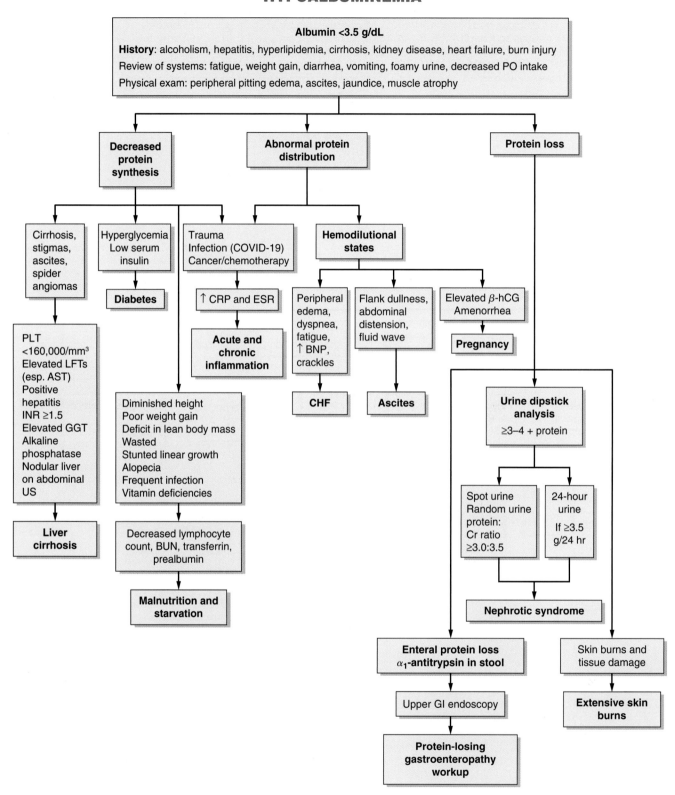

Anna Marie Tran, DO and Bashyam Iyengar, MD, MPH

Soeters PB, Wolfe RR, Shenkin A. Hypoalbuminemia: pathogenesis and clinical significance. *J Parenter Enteral Nutr.* 2019;43(2):181–193. doi:10.1002/jpen.1451.

HYPOCALCEMIA

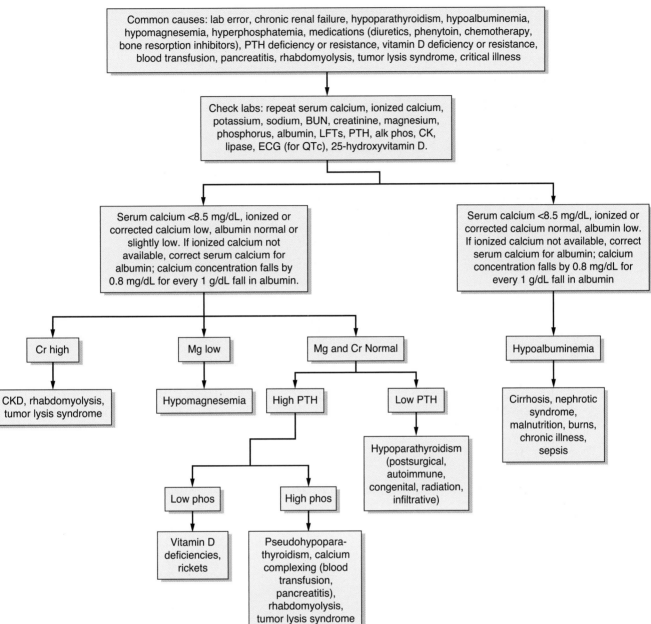

Common causes: lab error, chronic renal failure, hypoparathyroidism, hypoalbuminemia, hypomagnesemia, hyperphosphatemia, medications (diuretics, phenytoin, chemotherapy, bone resorption inhibitors), PTH deficiency or resistance, vitamin D deficiency or resistance, blood transfusion, pancreatitis, rhabdomyolysis, tumor lysis syndrome, critical illness

Check labs: repeat serum calcium, ionized calcium, potassium, sodium, BUN, creatinine, magnesium, phosphorus, albumin, LFTs, PTH, alk phos, CK, lipase, ECG (for QTc), 25-hydroxyvitamin D.

Serum calcium <8.5 mg/dL, ionized or corrected calcium low, albumin normal or slightly low. If ionized calcium not available, correct serum calcium for albumin; calcium concentration falls by 0.8 mg/dL for every 1 g/dL fall in albumin.

Serum calcium <8.5 mg/dL, ionized or corrected calcium normal, albumin low. If ionized calcium not available, correct serum calcium for albumin; calcium concentration falls by 0.8 mg/dL for every 1 g/dL fall in albumin

Cr high → CKD, rhabdomyolysis, tumor lysis syndrome

Mg low → Hypomagnesemia

Mg and Cr Normal → High PTH / Low PTH

Low PTH → Hypoparathyroidism (postsurgical, autoimmune, congenital, radiation, infiltrative)

High PTH → Low phos / High phos

Low phos → Vitamin D deficiencies, rickets

High phos → Pseudohypoparathyroidism, calcium complexing (blood transfusion, pancreatitis), rhabdomyolysis, tumor lysis syndrome

Hypoalbuminemia → Cirrhosis, nephrotic syndrome, malnutrition, burns, chronic illness, sepsis

Jeffrey T. Sakamoto, MD

Pepe J, Colangelo L, Biamonte F, et al. Diagnosis and management of hypocalcemia. *Endocrine*. 2020;69(3):485–495.

HYPOGLYCEMIA

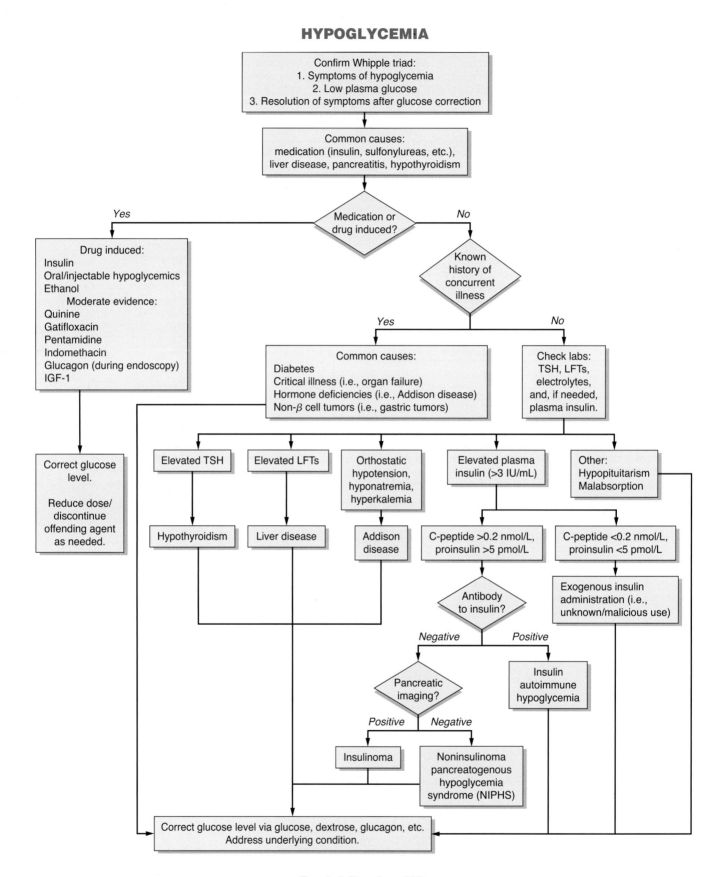

Frank J. Domino, MD

Kandaswamy L, Raghavan R, Pappachan JM. Spontaneous hypoglycemia: diagnostic evaluation and management. *Endocrine*. 2016;53(1):47–57.

HYPOKALEMIA

(K <3.5 mEq/L or 3.5 mmol/L)
- Basics: severe <2.5 mEq/L
- ECF = 2%; ICF = 98% (muscle 70%, liver, RBC, interstitial space)

Differential diagnosis

GI loss
Vomiting, diarrhea, nasogastric tube, laxative abuse, fistulas, villous adenoma, ureterosigmoidostomy, malabsorption, radiation enteropathy, clay

Renal loss:
Medications:
- Diuretics (thiazide and loop), amphotericin B, aminoglycosides, penicillin, antipseudomonal penicillins, foscarnet, cisplatin

Mineralocorticoid excess (HTN):
- Primary hypoaldosteronism, secondary hyperaldosteronism (CHF, cirrhosis, nephritic syndrome, renin-producing tumors), Bartter syndrome, Gitelman syndrome, exogenous mineralocorticoids, Liddle syndrome, vasculitis, hypomagnesemia, Fanconi syndrome, ingestion of glycyrrhizin

Osmotic diuresis (i.e., poorly controlled diabetes)
Renal tubular acidosis (type I and II)
COVID-19

Intracellular shift
Metabolic acidosis, insulin excess, β-adrenergic catecholamine excess (acute stress, β_2 agonists), hypokalemic periodic paralysis, intoxications (theophylline, caffeine, barium, toluene), hypothermia

Sweating

Poor intake
Alcoholism, tea and toast diet, anorexia nervosa, TPN, enteral nutrition

**Dialysis
Plasmapheresis**

Diagnosis and workup
- Start with history, physical. Check BMP, Mg, urine K, urine Cr, ECG.
- Urine Cl, UDS, TSH, CPK, or other studies based on H&P

Treatment and management
- Replete stores
- Stop loss—stop diuretics and address underlying cause. Change diuretic to RAASi (ACEi/ARB) or spironolactone.

Normal Mg
- Check urine K

Low Mg
- Replace Mg.
- Check for culprits like PPI use.

Outpatient management

Inpatient management

Urine K <15 mmol/day (UrK/Ucr <1.5)

Urine K >15 mmol/day (UrK/Ucr >1.5)

GI loss (diarrhea, vomiting, NG suction, IC shift)

Renal loss
- Check BP

Oral KCl (10 mEq to raise by 0.1 mEq/L)
- KCl preferred as most effective
- KHCO3 or KPhos if concomitant loss

Dietary K sources
- Banana (1 cm = 0.1 mEq)
- Grapefruit (14 mEq)
- Dried fruits, kiwi, broccoli, avocado

Repeat BMP in 3–4 days.

Check ECG.

If K <2.5 and moderate/severe symptoms
- KCl IV 10 mEq/hr
- 20–40 mEq/hr or higher via central line.
- Monitor BMP, ECG, telemetry.
- May combine PO/IV treatment as needed

If K >2.5 and mild symptoms—same as outpatient management and check BMP

BP low/normal
- Check HCO3.

BP high = hyperaldosteronism
- High renin and aldosterone = renal artery stenosis, renin secreting tumor
- Low renin, high aldosterone = primary aldosteronism → adrenal adenoma, adrenal hyperplasia
- Low renin, low aldosterone = Liddle syndrome, Cushing syndrome, mineralocorticoid excess, CAH, licorice use

Low HCO3 (metabolic acidosis, RTA1, RTA2, DKA)

High HCO3
- Check Ur Cl (metabolic alkalosis).

Ur Cl <10 mmol/day remote diuretic use or vomiting

Ur Cl >20 mmol/L diuretic use, low Mg, Bartter syndrome, Gitelman syndrome

Anush S. Pillai, DO, FAAFP and Nioti Karim, MD

Kardalas E, Paschou SA, Anagnostis P, et al. Hypokalemia: a clinical update. *Endocr Connect.* 2018;7(4):R135–R146.

HYPONATREMIA

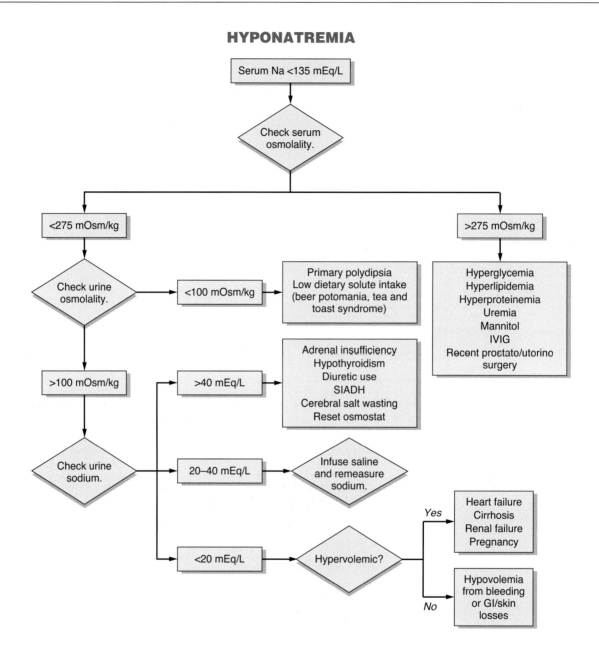

Serum Na <135 mEq/L

Check serum osmolality.

<275 mOsm/kg

>275 mOsm/kg

Check urine osmolality.

<100 mOsm/kg

Primary polydipsia
Low dietary solute intake
(beer potomania, tea and
toast syndrome)

Hyperglycemia
Hyperlipidemia
Hyperproteinemia
Uremia
Mannitol
IVIG
Recent prostate/uterine
surgery

>100 mOsm/kg

Check urine sodium.

>40 mEq/L

Adrenal insufficiency
Hypothyroidism
Diuretic use
SIADH
Cerebral salt wasting
Reset osmostat

20–40 mEq/L

Infuse saline
and remeasure
sodium.

<20 mEq/L

Hypervolemic?

Yes

Heart failure
Cirrhosis
Renal failure
Pregnancy

No

Hypovolemia
from bleeding
or GI/skin
losses

Ashwin Nayak, MD

Adrogué HJ, Madias NE. Hyponatremia. *N Engl J Med.* 2000;342(21):1581–1589.

HYPOTENSION

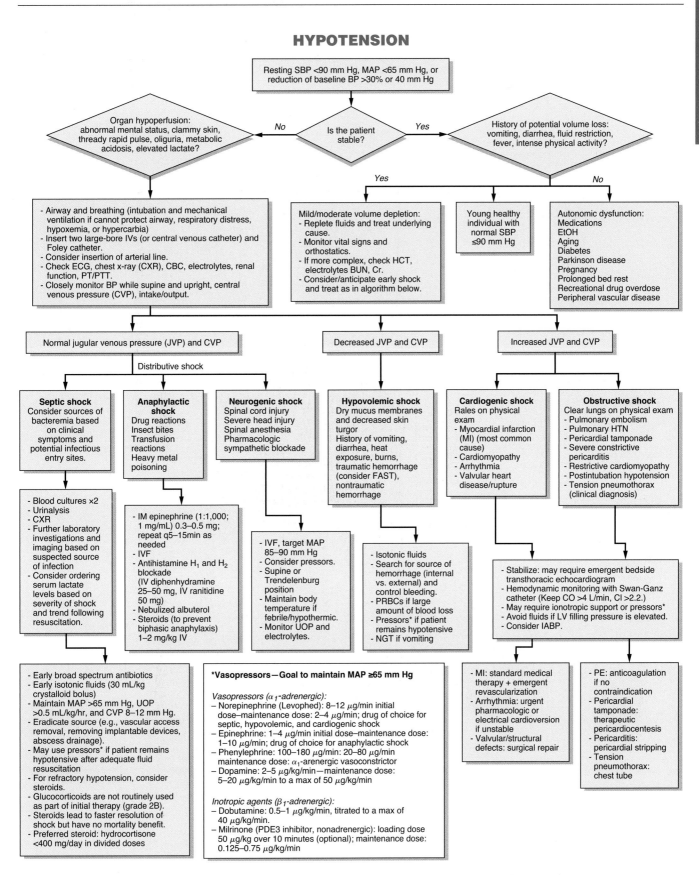

Sarah Bounader, MD and Sandra S. Augusto, MD, MPH

Thompson K, Venkatesh B, Finfer S. Sepsis and septic shock: current approaches to management. *Intern Med J.* 2019;49(2):160–170.

INFERTILITY

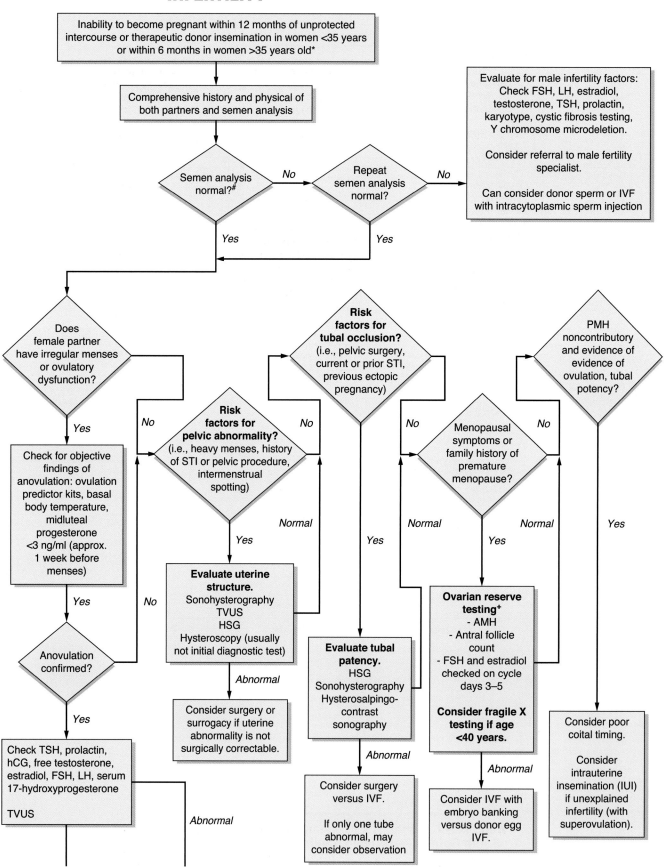

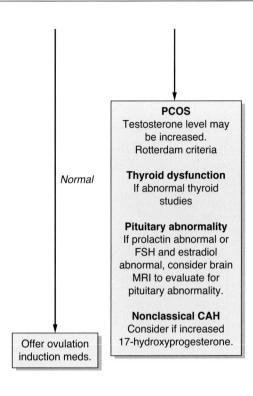

Normal

PCOS
Testosterone level may be increased.
Rotterdam criteria

Thyroid dysfunction
If abnormal thyroid studies

Pituitary abnormality
If prolactin abnormal or FSH and estradiol abnormal, consider brain MRI to evaluate for pituitary abnormality.

Nonclassical CAH
Consider if increased 17-hydroxyprogesterone.

Offer ovulation induction meds.

*Common causes of infertility
- Male factor (40–50%)
- Diminished ovarian reserve (premature menopause or advanced age)
- Tubal or uterine abnormality
- Ovulatory dysfunction (PCOS, thyroid abnormality, obesity/low BMI, eating disorder, hyperprolactinemia)
- Unknown (30%)

⁺Lab values consistent with reduced ovarian reserve
AMH <1 ng/mL
Antral follicle count <5–7
FSH >10 IU/L
Elevated estradiol (normal is <60–80 pg/mL)
History of poor response to IVF stimulation (<4 oocytes at egg retrieval)

#Lower limit cutoffs for normal semen analysis from WHO
Ejaculate volume 1.5 mL
pH ≥7.2.
Sperm concentration at least 15×10^6/mL
Minimum total sperm 39×10^6/ejaculate
Total motility 40%
No sperm agglutination

TVUS = transvaginal ultrasound
HSG = hysterosalpingogram
AMH = Anti-müllerian hormone
Nonclassical CAH: congenital adrenal hyperplasia

Katherine Gagan, MD and Melanie Houston Sanders, MD

American College of Obstetricians and Gynecologists. Infertility workup for the women's health specialist: ACOG Committee Opinion, Number 781. *Obstet Gynecol.* 2019;133(6):e377–e384.

KNEE PAIN

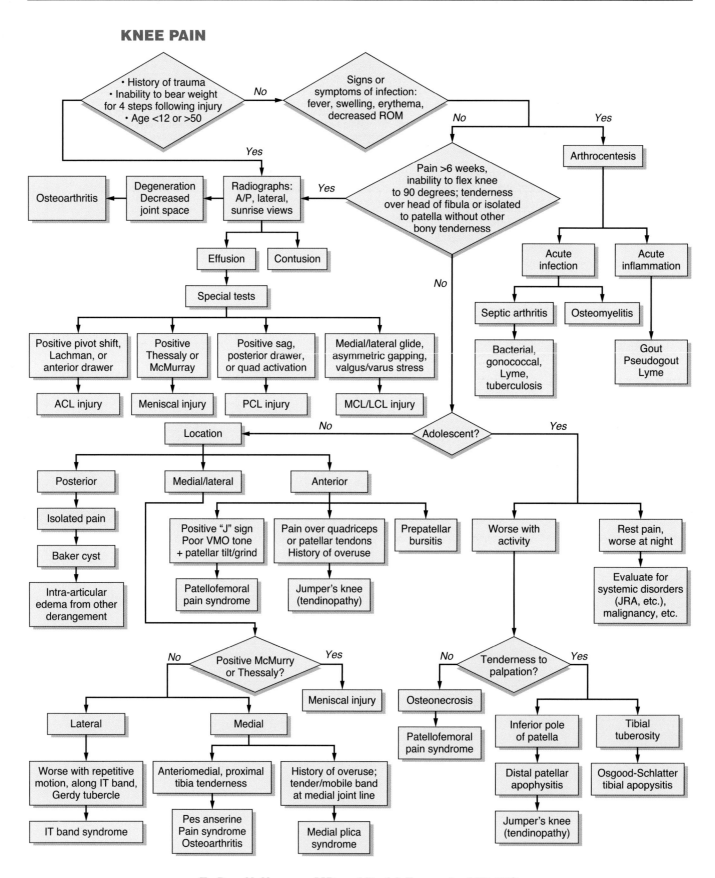

Tu Dan H. Nguyen, MD and Rod J. Turner Jr., MD, MS

Bunt CW, Jonas CE, Chang JG. Knee pain in adults and adolescents: the initial evaluation. *Am Fam Physician.* 2018;98(9):576–585.

LACTATE DEHYDROGENASE ELEVATION

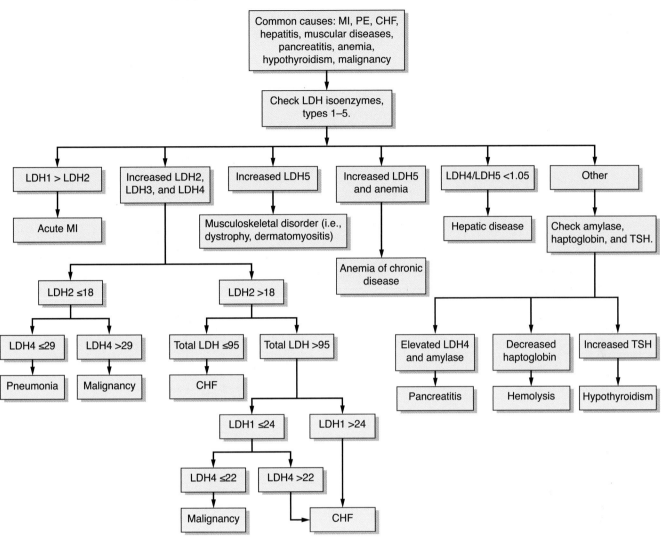

Naga Bharani Goparaju, MD and Pavan Annamaraju, MD

Lossos IS, Breuer R, Intrator O, et al. Differential diagnosis of pleural effusion by lactate dehydrogenase isoenzyme analysis. *Chest.* 1997;111(3):648–651.

LOW BACK PAIN, CHRONIC

Common causes: radiculitis, SI joint dysfunction, trauma, trochanteric bursitis, piriformis syndrome, osteoporosis, osteoarthritis, pars interarticularis fracture, ankylosing spondylitis, epidural abscess, malignancy, varicella zoster virus (postherpetic neuralgia), abdominal aortic aneurysm

↓

Pain >3 months

↓

Abnormal gait, bowel/bladder incontinence, acute urinary retention, bilateral sciatica, IV drug abuse, history of malignancy, pain worse when supine, saddle anesthesia, progressive neurologic symptoms, recent infection?

Yes → Urgent imaging (CT or MRI) and neurosurgical referral

No ↓

Fever or concern of infection?

No → Hx of trauma, osteoporosis, chronic steroid use?

Fever or concern of infection? **Yes** ↓

MRI or CT, CBC with diff, CRP/ESR, CMP, TB testing

Negative → Nonpharmacotherapy (left box)

Positive → Neurosurgical referral

Hx of trauma, osteoporosis, chronic steroid use? **No** → No need for imaging

Yes ↓ Plain x-rays

Plain x-rays *Positive* → Neurosurgical referral

Plain x-rays *Negative* → Nonpharmacotherapy (left box)

Nonpharmacotherapy: structured exercise, multidisciplinary rehab, weight loss, acupuncture, massage, spinal manipulation therapy, progressive relaxation, cognitive-behavioral therapy, stress management

Pharmacotherapy: topical or oral NSAIDs, skeletal muscle relaxants (i.e., tizanidine, cyclobenzaprine), antidepressants (i.e., duloxetine), anticonvulsants (i.e., topiramate), Botox, tramadol,* other opioids*

*Use with caution

↓

No improvement: Consider surgical or psychiatry referral or pain management.

No need for imaging ↓

Nonpharmacotherapy: structured exercise, multidisciplinary rehab, weight loss, acupuncture, massage, spinal manipulation therapy, progressive relaxation, cognitive-behavioral therapy, stress management

Pharmacotherapy: topical or oral NSAIDs, skeletal muscle relaxants (i.e., tizanidine, cyclobenzaprine), antidepressants (i.e., duloxetine), anticonvulsants (i.e., topiramate), Botox, tramadol,* other opioids*

*Use with caution

Zedeena Fisher, MD and Holly L. Baab, MD

Herndon CM, Zoberi KS, Gardner BJ. Common questions about chronic low back pain. *Am Fam Physician.* 2015;91(10):708–714.

LYMPHADENOPATHY

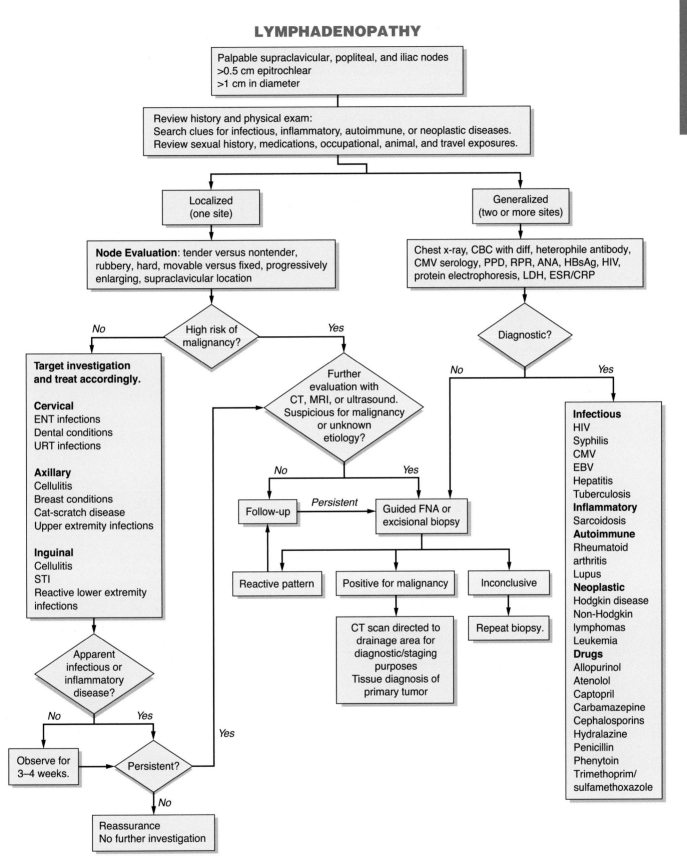

Palpable supraclavicular, popliteal, and iliac nodes
>0.5 cm epitrochlear
>1 cm in diameter

Review history and physical exam:
Search clues for infectious, inflammatory, autoimmune, or neoplastic diseases.
Review sexual history, medications, occupational, animal, and travel exposures.

Localized (one site)

Generalized (two or more sites)

Node Evaluation: tender versus nontender, rubbery, hard, movable versus fixed, progressively enlarging, supraclavicular location

Chest x-ray, CBC with diff, heterophile antibody, CMV serology, PPD, RPR, ANA, HBsAg, HIV, protein electrophoresis, LDH, ESR/CRP

High risk of malignancy?

Diagnostic?

No

Yes

No

Yes

Target investigation and treat accordingly.

Cervical
ENT infections
Dental conditions
URT infections

Axillary
Cellulitis
Breast conditions
Cat-scratch disease
Upper extremity infections

Inguinal
Cellulitis
STI
Reactive lower extremity infections

Further evaluation with CT, MRI, or ultrasound. Suspicious for malignancy or unknown etiology?

No

Yes

Follow-up

Persistent

Guided FNA or excisional biopsy

Reactive pattern

Positive for malignancy

Inconclusive

CT scan directed to drainage area for diagnostic/staging purposes
Tissue diagnosis of primary tumor

Repeat biopsy.

Apparent infectious or inflammatory disease?

No

Yes

Observe for 3–4 weeks.

Persistent?

Yes

No

Reassurance
No further investigation

Infectious
HIV
Syphilis
CMV
EBV
Hepatitis
Tuberculosis
Inflammatory
Sarcoidosis
Autoimmune
Rheumatoid arthritis
Lupus
Neoplastic
Hodgkin disease
Non-Hodgkin lymphomas
Leukemia
Drugs
Allopurinol
Atenolol
Captopril
Carbamazepine
Cephalosporins
Hydralazine
Penicillin
Phenytoin
Trimethoprim/sulfamethoxazole

Sarah Burroughs, DO and Evan Kang, MD

Gaddey HL, Riegel AM. Unexplained lymphadenopathy: evaluation and differential diagnosis. *Am Fam Physician*. 2016;94(11):896–903.

LYMPHOPENIA OR LYMPHOCYTOPENIA

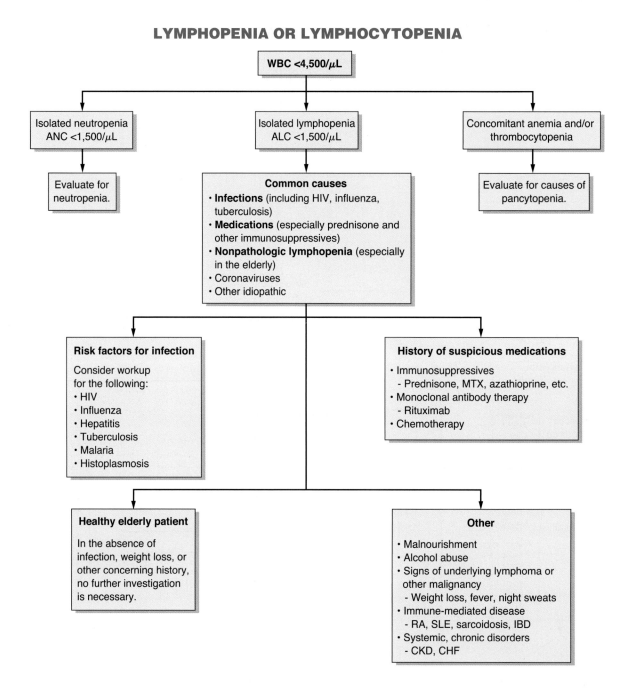

Jillian Joseph, MPAS, PA-C and Allison Hargreaves, MD

Warny M, Helby J, Nordestgaard BG, et al. Lymphopenia and risk of infection and infection-related death in 98,344 individuals from a prospective Danish population-based study. *PLoS Med.* 2018;15(11):e1002685. doi:10.1371/journal.pmed.1002685.

MENOPAUSE, EVALUATION AND MANAGEMENT PART I

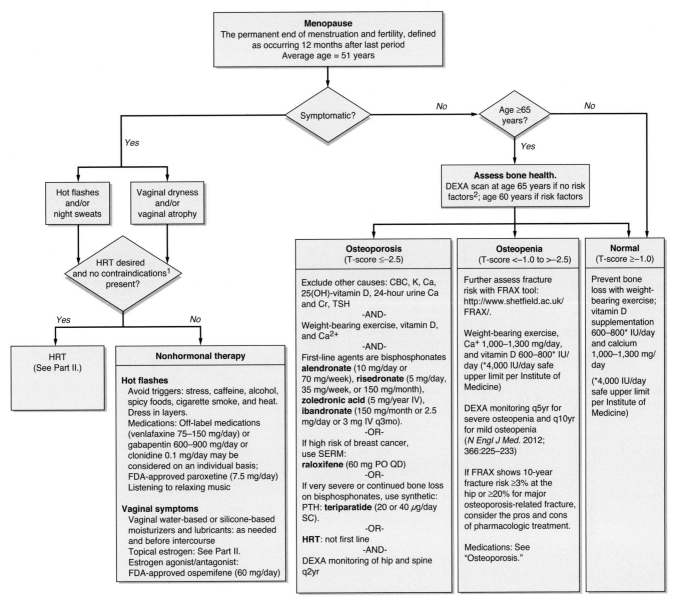

Menopause
The permanent end of menstruation and fertility, defined as occurring 12 months after last period
Average age = 51 years

Symptomatic?

No → **Age ≥65 years?** → No

Yes

- Hot flashes and/or night sweats
- Vaginal dryness and/or vaginal atrophy

HRT desired and no contraindications[1] present?

Yes → **HRT** (See Part II.)

No → **Nonhormonal therapy**

Hot flashes
Avoid triggers: stress, caffeine, alcohol, spicy foods, cigarette smoke, and heat. Dress in layers.
Medications: Off-label medications (venlafaxine 75–150 mg/day) or gabapentin 600–900 mg/day or clonidine 0.1 mg/day may be considered on an individual basis; FDA-approved paroxetine (7.5 mg/day)
Listening to relaxing music

Vaginal symptoms
Vaginal water-based or silicone-based moisturizers and lubricants: as needed and before intercourse
Topical estrogen: See Part II.
Estrogen agonist/antagonist: FDA-approved ospemifene (60 mg/day)

Yes → **Assess bone health.**
DEXA scan at age 65 years if no risk factors[2]; age 60 years if risk factors

Osteoporosis
(T-score ≤–2.5)

Exclude other causes: CBC, K, Ca, 25(OH)-vitamin D, 24-hour urine Ca and Cr, TSH
-AND-
Weight-bearing exercise, vitamin D, and Ca^{2+}
-AND-
First-line agents are bisphosphonates **alendronate** (10 mg/day or 70 mg/week), **risedronate** (5 mg/day, 35 mg/week, or 150 mg/month), **zoledronic acid** (5 mg/year IV), **ibandronate** (150 mg/month or 2.5 mg/day or 3 mg IV q3mo).
-OR-
If high risk of breast cancer, use SERM: **raloxifene** (60 mg PO QD)
-OR-
If very severe or continued bone loss on bisphosphonates, use synthetic: PTH: **teriparatide** (20 or 40 μg/day SC).
-OR-
HRT: not first line
-AND-
DEXA monitoring of hip and spine q2yr

Osteopenia
(T-score <–1.0 to >–2.5)

Further assess fracture risk with FRAX tool: http://www.shetfield.ac.uk/FRAX/.

Weight-bearing exercise, Ca$^+$ 1,000–1,300 mg/day, and vitamin D 600–800* IU/day (*4,000 IU/day safe upper limit per Institute of Medicine)

DEXA monitoring q5yr for severe osteopenia and q10yr for mild osteopenia (*N Engl J Med.* 2012; 366:225–233)

If FRAX shows 10-year fracture risk ≥3% at the hip or ≥20% for major osteoporosis-related fracture, consider the pros and cons of pharmacologic treatment.

Medications: See "Osteoporosis."

Normal
(T-score ≥–1.0)

Prevent bone loss with weight-bearing exercise; vitamin D supplementation 600–800* IU/day and calcium 1,000–1,300 mg/day

(*4,000 IU/day safe upper limit per Institute of Medicine)

PART II

HRT
(Use lowest effective dose for shortest duration possible.
Short-term use = 2–3 years; generally does not exceed 5 years)

Intact uterus?

Yes

No

Transdermal, oral, spray, gel, vaginal, or injectable estrogen + progesterone

Transdermal estrogen: Start 0.025 mg/day; max 0.10 mg/day

-OR-

Oral estrogen: 0.3 mg, 0.45 mg, max 0.625 mg/day conjugated estrogens; 0.5–1.0 mg/day micronized estradiol

-OR-

Spray or gel: estradiol spray 0.021 mg delivered per spray; max 3 sprays per day; 0.75 mg/day estradiol gel applied to large skin area

-OR-

Vaginal estrogen: 1 ring PV q3mo releases 50 or 100 μg/day estradiol.

-OR-

Injectable estrogen: 10–20 mg estradiol valerate IM q4wk

PLUS

Concomitant administration of one of the following:
1. **Medroxyprogesterone acetate (MPA)** 2.5 mg/day PO

-OR-

2. **Natural progesterone** 100–200 mg/day PO

Combined estrogen progesterone HRT

Combined estrogen and progesterone transdermal patches

Estradiol/levonorgestrel (delivers 0.045 mg/0.015 mg/day)

Estradiol/norethindrone acetate (delivers 0.05 mg/0.14 mg/day or = 0.05 mg/0.25 mg/day)

-OR-

Combined estrogen and progesterone pills

Estradiol 1 mg and drospirenone 0.5 mg

Ethinyl estradiol 2.5 or 5 μg and norethindrone acetate 0.5 or 1 mg

Conjugated estrogen 0.3, 0.45, or 0.625 mg and MPA 1.5, 2.5, or 5 mg

Estradiol 1 mg/norgestimate 0.9 mg

Topical estrogen therapy

Little or no estrogen is absorbed in bloodstream. Lower risk of side effects but no effect on vasomotor symptoms; for use in patients with vaginal symptoms only

Vaginal creams:
0.01% estradiol cream PV daily equivalent to 0.1 mg

0.625 mg conjugated estrogen/g: 0.5 g PV daily × 21 days, then off for 7 days

Vaginal tablet:
vaginal estradiol tablets 10–25 μg PV QD × 2 weeks and then vaginal estradiol tablets 10–25 μg PV twice weekly

Vaginal ring:
vaginal estradiol that delivers 7.5 μg/day estradiol; insert 1 ring PV q3mo.

Estrogen-only therapy
Transdermal
Oral
Spray/gel
Vaginal
Injectable

Do not use progesterone in women without a uterus.

Kelly Pagidas, MDCM, FACOG, FRCSC

ACOG Practice Bulletin No. 141: management of menopausal symptoms (Reaffirmed 2021). *Obstet Gynecol.* 2018;131(3):604.

MIGRAINE, TREATMENT

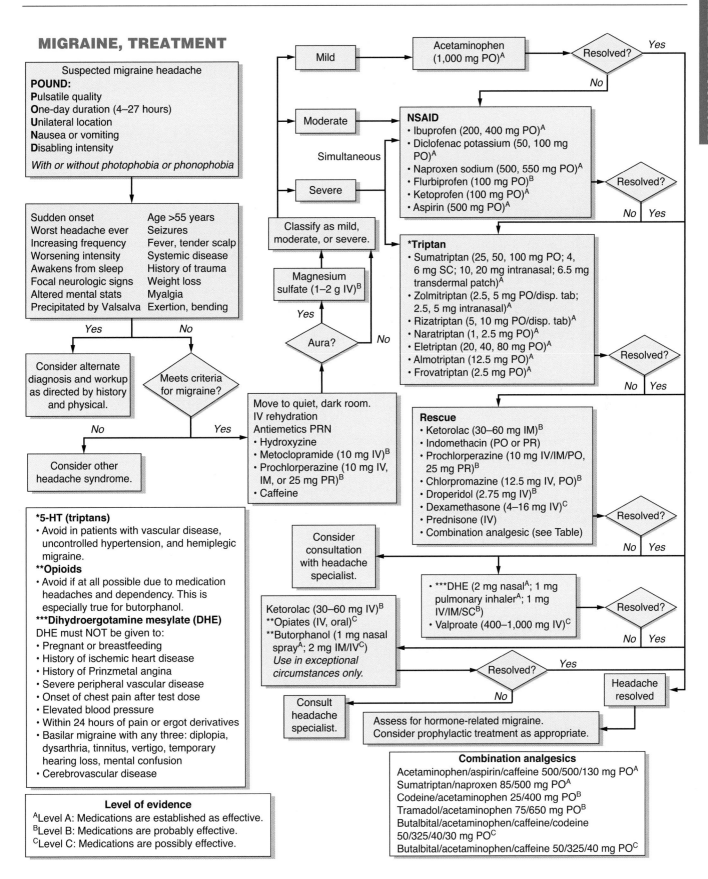

Suspected migraine headache
POUND:
Pulsatile quality
One-day duration (4–27 hours)
Unilateral location
Nausea or vomiting
Disabling intensity

With or without photophobia or phonophobia

Sudden onset — Age >55 years
Worst headache ever — Seizures
Increasing frequency — Fever, tender scalp
Worsening intensity — Systemic disease
Awakens from sleep — History of trauma
Focal neurologic signs — Weight loss
Altered mental stats — Myalgia
Precipitated by Valsalva — Exertion, bending

Yes / **No**

Consider alternate diagnosis and workup as directed by history and physical.

Meets criteria for migraine?

No / **Yes**

Consider other headache syndrome.

*5-HT (triptans)
• Avoid in patients with vascular disease, uncontrolled hypertension, and hemiplegic migraine.
**Opioids
• Avoid if at all possible due to medication headaches and dependency. This is especially true for butorphanol.
***Dihydroergotamine mesylate (DHE)
DHE must NOT be given to:
• Pregnant or breastfeeding
• History of ischemic heart disease
• History of Prinzmetal angina
• Severe peripheral vascular disease
• Onset of chest pain after test dose
• Elevated blood pressure
• Within 24 hours of pain or ergot derivatives
• Basilar migraine with any three: diplopia, dysarthria, tinnitus, vertigo, temporary hearing loss, mental confusion
• Cerebrovascular disease

Level of evidence
[A]Level A: Medications are established as effective.
[B]Level B: Medications are probably effective.
[C]Level C: Medications are possibly effective.

Mild → Acetaminophen (1,000 mg PO)[A] → Resolved? **Yes** / **No**

Moderate

Simultaneous

Severe

Classify as mild, moderate, or severe.

Magnesium sulfate (1–2 g IV)[B]

Yes

Aura? **No**

Move to quiet, dark room.
IV rehydration
Antiemetics PRN
• Hydroxyzine
• Metoclopramide (10 mg IV)[B]
• Prochlorperazine (10 mg IV, IM, or 25 mg PR)[B]
• Caffeine

NSAID
• Ibuprofen (200, 400 mg PO)[A]
• Diclofenac potassium (50, 100 mg PO)[A]
• Naproxen sodium (500, 550 mg PO)[A]
• Flurbiprofen (100 mg PO)[B]
• Ketoprofen (100 mg PO)[A]
• Aspirin (500 mg PO)[A]

Resolved? **No** / **Yes**

*Triptan
• Sumatriptan (25, 50, 100 mg PO; 4, 6 mg SC; 10, 20 mg intranasal; 6.5 mg transdermal patch)[A]
• Zolmitriptan (2.5, 5 mg PO/disp. tab; 2.5, 5 mg intranasal)[A]
• Rizatriptan (5, 10 mg PO/disp. tab)[A]
• Naratriptan (1, 2.5 mg PO)[A]
• Eletriptan (20, 40, 80 mg PO)[A]
• Almotriptan (12.5 mg PO)[A]
• Frovatriptan (2.5 mg PO)[A]

Resolved? **No** / **Yes**

Rescue
• Ketorolac (30–60 mg IM)[B]
• Indomethacin (PO or PR)
• Prochlorperazine (10 mg IV/IM/PO, 25 mg PR)[B]
• Chlorpromazine (12.5 mg IV, PO)[B]
• Droperidol (2.75 mg IV)[B]
• Dexamethasone (4–16 mg IV)[C]
• Prednisone (IV)
• Combination analgesic (see Table)

Consider consultation with headache specialist.

Resolved? **No** / **Yes**

• ***DHE (2 mg nasal[A]; 1 mg pulmonary inhaler[A]; 1 mg IV/IM/SC[B])
• Valproate (400–1,000 mg IV)[C]

Resolved? **No** / **Yes**

Ketorolac (30–60 mg IV)[B]
**Opiates (IV, oral)[C]
**Butorphanol (1 mg nasal spray[A]; 2 mg IM/IV[C])
Use in exceptional circumstances only.

Resolved? **Yes** / **No**

Consult headache specialist.

Headache resolved

Assess for hormone-related migraine.
Consider prophylactic treatment as appropriate.

Combination analgesics
Acetaminophen/aspirin/caffeine 500/500/130 mg PO[A]
Sumatriptan/naproxen 85/500 mg PO[A]
Codeine/acetaminophen 25/400 mg PO[B]
Tramadol/acetaminophen 75/650 mg PO[B]
Butalbital/acetaminophen/caffeine/codeine 50/325/40/30 mg PO[C]
Butalbital/acetaminophen/caffeine 50/325/40 mg PO[C]

Ekaterina Brodski-Quigley, MD, EdM

Marmura MJ, Silberstein SD, Schwedt TJ. The acute treatment of migraine in adults: the American Headache Society evidence assessment of migraine pharmacotherapies. *Headache*. 2015;55(1):3–20.

NAIL ABNORMALITIES

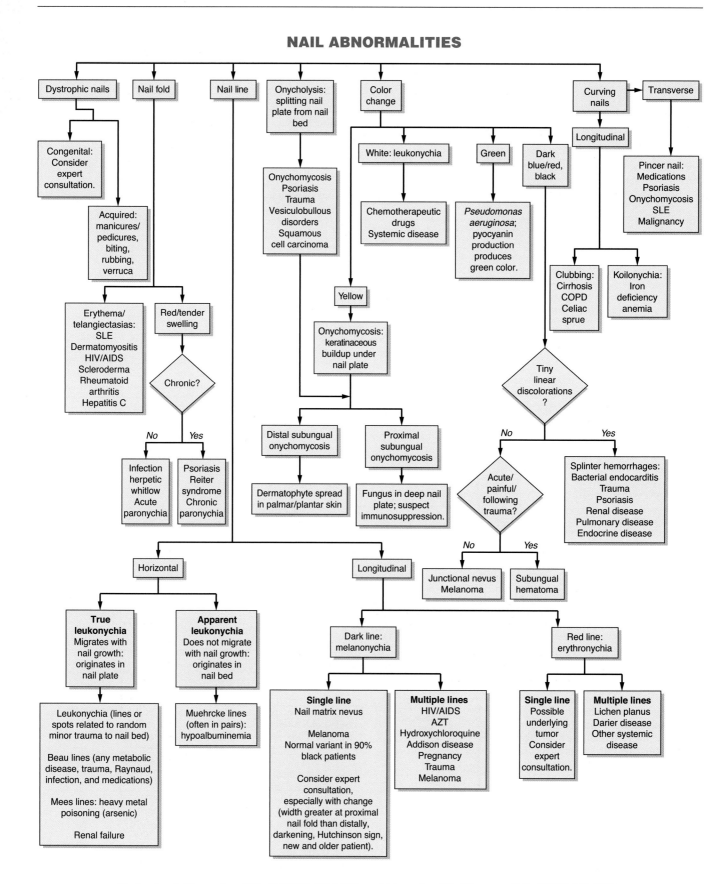

Natasha J. Pyzocha, DO, FAWM, FAAFP and Douglas M. Maurer, DO, MPH, FAAFP

Tully AS, Trayes KP, Studdiford JS. Evaluation of nail abnormalities. *Am Fam Physician*. 2012;85(8):779–787.

NEUTROPENIA

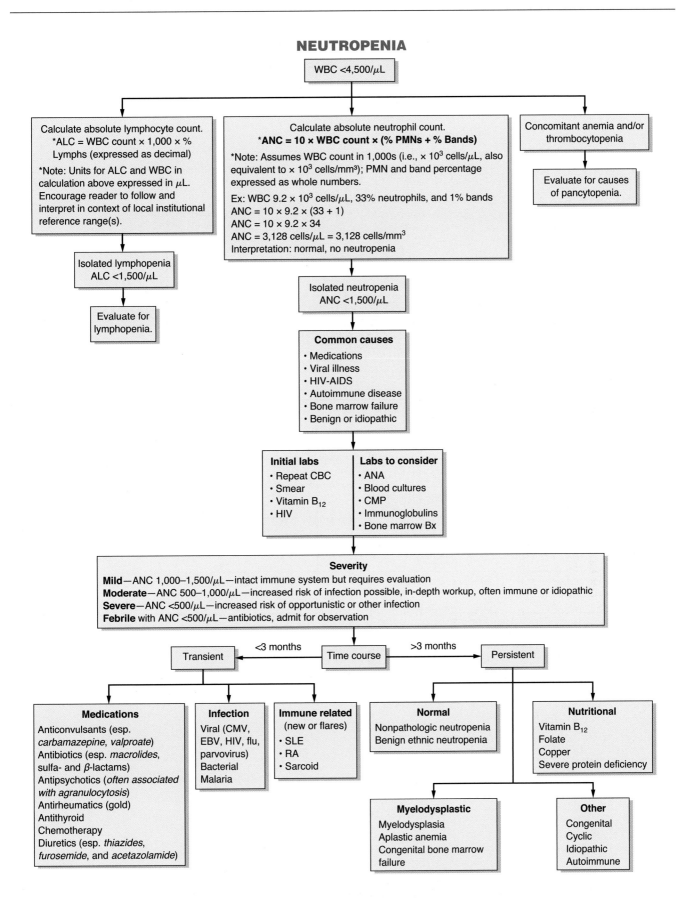

Ben Ayotte, MD, Robert Kirchoff, MD, FASAM, and Thomas Kingsley, MD, MPH, MS

Gibson C, Berliner N. How we evaluate and treat neutropenia in adults. *Blood.* 2014;124(8):1251–1258.

PAIN, CHRONIC, DIAGNOSIS

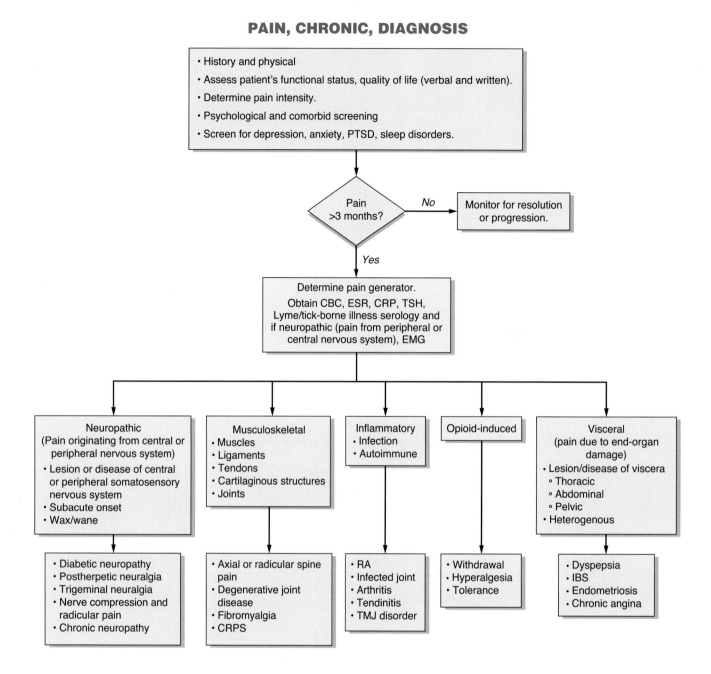

- History and physical
- Assess patient's functional status, quality of life (verbal and written).
- Determine pain intensity.
- Psychological and comorbid screening
- Screen for depression, anxiety, PTSD, sleep disorders.

Pain >3 months?

No → Monitor for resolution or progression.

Yes

Determine pain generator.
Obtain CBC, ESR, CRP, TSH, Lyme/tick-borne illness serology and if neuropathic (pain from peripheral or central nervous system), EMG

Neuropathic
(Pain originating from central or peripheral nervous system)
- Lesion or disease of central or peripheral somatosensory nervous system
- Subacute onset
- Wax/wane

Musculoskeletal
- Muscles
- Ligaments
- Tendons
- Cartilaginous structures
- Joints

Inflammatory
- Infection
- Autoimmune

Opioid-induced

Visceral
(pain due to end-organ damage)
- Lesion/disease of viscera
  - Thoracic
  - Abdominal
  - Pelvic
- Heterogenous

- Diabetic neuropathy
- Postherpetic neuralgia
- Trigeminal neuralgia
- Nerve compression and radicular pain
- Chronic neuropathy

- Axial or radicular spine pain
- Degenerative joint disease
- Fibromyalgia
- CRPS

- RA
- Infected joint
- Arthritis
- Tendinitis
- TMJ disorder

- Withdrawal
- Hyperalgesia
- Tolerance

- Dyspepsia
- IBS
- Endometriosis
- Chronic angina

Bruce Palmer Freshley Jr., MD and Christina Gutta, MD

Hooten M, Thorson D, Bianco J, et al. *Pain: Assessment, Non-Opioid Treatment Approaches and Opioid Management.* Bloomington, MN: Institute for Clinical Systems Improvement; 2017.

PALPABLE BREAST MASS

Obtain a detailed history and perform a clinical breast exam (CBE).

Order breast imaging:
- If <30 years old (yo), order a directed sonogram.
  - *If <30 yo and high clinical suspicion for malignancy or mass not visualized on ultrasound, also order a diagnostic mammogram.*
- If ≥30 yo, order a directed sonogram and diagnostic mammogram.

BI-RADS 1 or 3   BI-RADS 4 or 5   BI-RADS 2

Is clinical suspicion high or low?

Benign finding (i.e., cyst, lipoma, lymph node)   *Low*   *High*

Monitor

- If <30 yo, w/ CBE and/or sonogram every 6–12 months for 1–2 years
- If ≥30 yo, w/ CBE and sonogram/mammogram every 6 months for 1–2 years
- *CBE ideally performed on days 10–12 of menstrual cycle*

- Core needle biopsy by radiologist or surgeon
- If needle biopsy is not possible, refer to surgeon.

Is lesion unchanged?   *No*

Yes   Resume routine screening.

Stephen Robert Scott, MD and Antonio A. Williams, MD

Salzman B, Collins E, Hersh L. Common breast problems. *Am Fam Physician.* 2019;99(8):505–514.

PALPITATIONS, ADULT

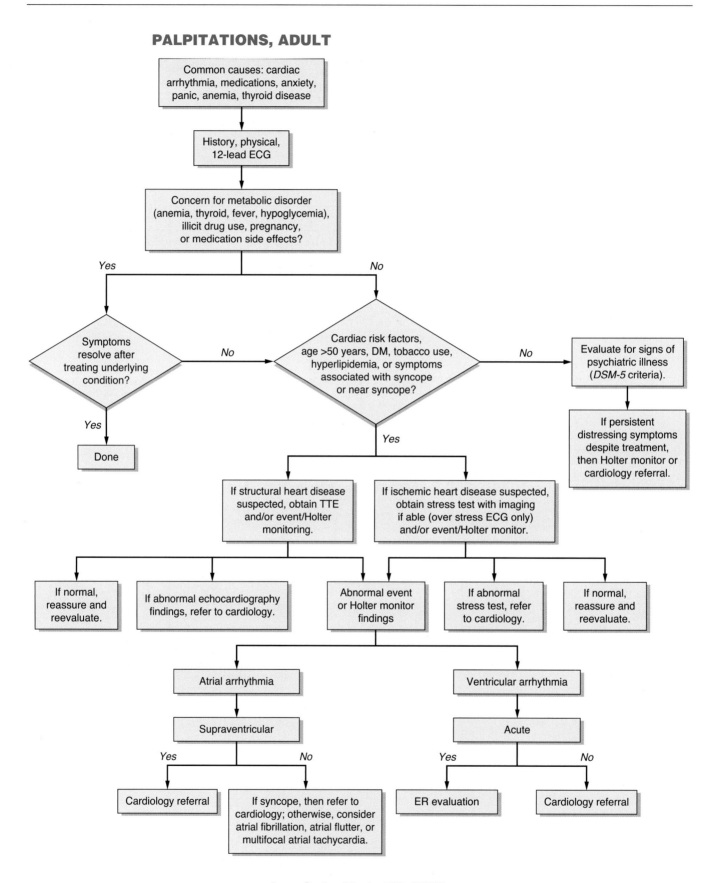

Juan Carlos Venis, MD, MPH

Wexler RK, Pleister A, Raman SV. Palpitations: evaluation in the primary care setting. *Am Fam Physician.* 2017;96(12):784–789.

PAP, NORMAL AND ABNORMAL IN NONPREGNANT WOMEN AGES 25 YEARS AND OLDER

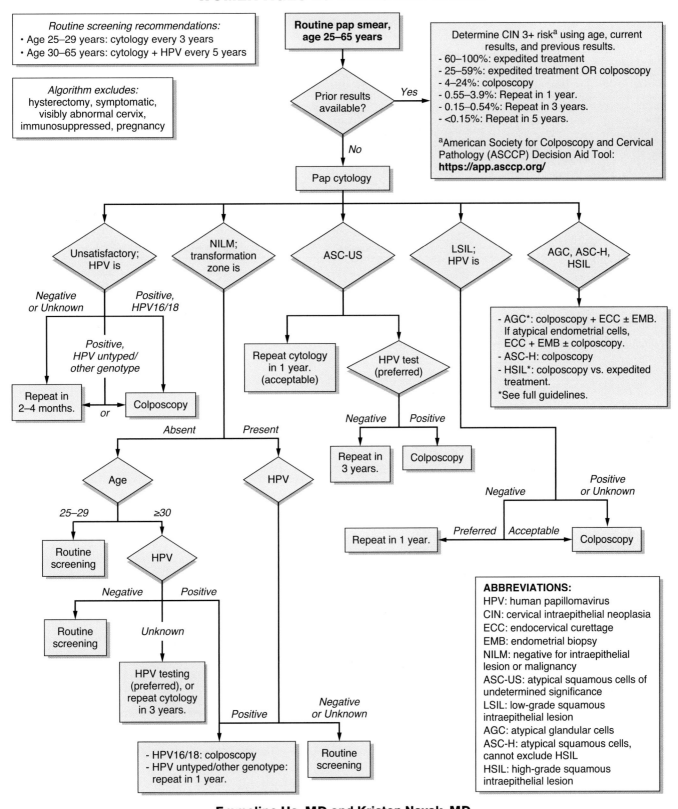

Emmeline Ha, MD and Kristen Nayak, MD

Perkins RB, Guido RS, Castle PE, et al; for 2019 ASCCP Risk-Based Management Consensus Guidelines Committee. 2019 ASCCP Risk-Based Management Consensus Guidelines for abnormal cervical cancer screening tests and cancer precursors. *J Low Genit Tract Dis.* 2020;24(2):102–131.

PAP, NORMAL AND ABNORMAL IN WOMEN AGES 21–24 YEARS

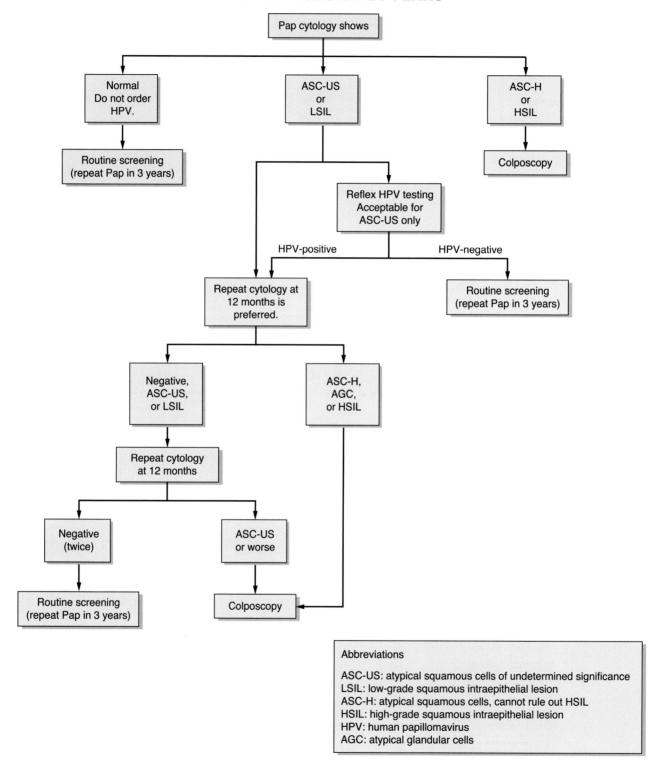

Pratiksha Yalakkishettar, MD and Manju Mahajan, MD, FAAFP

Perkins RB, Guido RS, Castle PE, et al. 2019 ASCCP risk-based management guidelines for abnormal cervical cancer screening tests and cancer precursors. *J Low Genit Tract Dis.* 2020;24(2):102–131.

PARKINSON DISEASE, TREATMENT

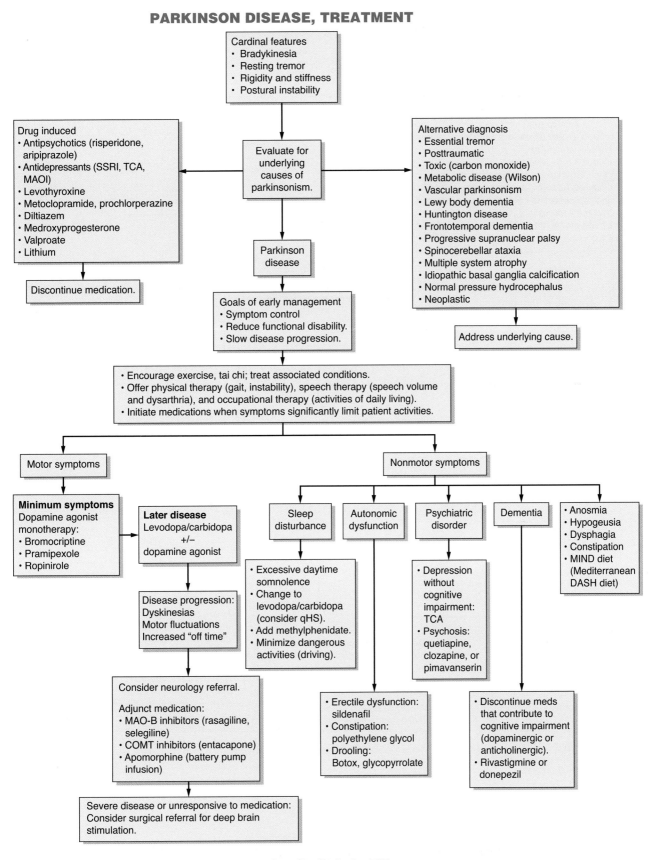

Cardinal features
- Bradykinesia
- Resting tremor
- Rigidity and stiffness
- Postural instability

Evaluate for underlying causes of parkinsonism.

Drug induced
- Antipsychotics (risperidone, aripiprazole)
- Antidepressants (SSRI, TCA, MAOI)
- Levothyroxine
- Metoclopramide, prochlorperazine
- Diltiazem
- Medroxyprogesterone
- Valproate
- Lithium

Discontinue medication.

Parkinson disease

Alternative diagnosis
- Essential tremor
- Posttraumatic
- Toxic (carbon monoxide)
- Metabolic disease (Wilson)
- Vascular parkinsonism
- Lewy body dementia
- Huntington disease
- Frontotemporal dementia
- Progressive supranuclear palsy
- Spinocerebellar ataxia
- Multiple system atrophy
- Idiopathic basal ganglia calcification
- Normal pressure hydrocephalus
- Neoplastic

Address underlying cause.

Goals of early management
- Symptom control
- Reduce functional disability.
- Slow disease progression.

- Encourage exercise, tai chi; treat associated conditions.
- Offer physical therapy (gait, instability), speech therapy (speech volume and dysarthria), and occupational therapy (activities of daily living).
- Initiate medications when symptoms significantly limit patient activities.

Motor symptoms

Nonmotor symptoms

Minimum symptoms
Dopamine agonist monotherapy:
- Bromocriptine
- Pramipexole
- Ropinirole

Later disease
Levodopa/carbidopa +/– dopamine agonist

Disease progression:
Dyskinesias
Motor fluctuations
Increased "off time"

Sleep disturbance
- Excessive daytime somnolence
- Change to levodopa/carbidopa (consider qHS).
- Add methylphenidate.
- Minimize dangerous activities (driving).

Autonomic dysfunction

Psychiatric disorder
- Depression without cognitive impairment: TCA
- Psychosis: quetiapine, clozapine, or pimavanserin

Dementia

- Anosmia
- Hypogeusia
- Dysphagia
- Constipation
- MIND diet (Mediterranean DASH diet)

Consider neurology referral.

Adjunct medication:
- MAO-B inhibitors (rasagiline, selegiline)
- COMT inhibitors (entacapone)
- Apomorphine (battery pump infusion)

- Erectile dysfunction: sildenafil
- Constipation: polyethylene glycol
- Drooling: Botox, glycopyrrolate

- Discontinue meds that contribute to cognitive impairment (dopaminergic or anticholinergic).
- Rivastigmine or donepezil

Severe disease or unresponsive to medication: Consider surgical referral for deep brain stimulation.

Saadia Mohsin, MD

Connolly BS, Lang AE. Pharmacological treatment of Parkinson disease: a review. *JAMA.* 2014;311(16):1670–1683.

PEDIATRIC EXANTHEMS, DIAGNOSTIC

URI symptoms present?

No →

Roseola (sixth disease, exanthem subitum)
- Herpes virus 6 and 7
- Incubation 5–15 days
- Rash: Erythematous maculopapular rash develops as fever resolves; starts on trunk and progresses to neck, extremities (rarely), face
- Prodrome: fever
- Enanthem: erythematous macules on soft palate
- Peak prevalence: 7–13 months

Yes →

Enanthem (involvement of mucous membranes)?

No → Vesicular?

No →

Erythema infectiosum (fifth disease)
- Human parvovirus B19
- Incubation 4–14 days
- Rash: intensely red malar rash "slapped cheek" followed in 1–2 days by reticular erythematous maculopapular rash on trunk, extremities, and buttocks; recrudescence can last up to months.
- Prodrome: generally mild; may have 1–4 days of headache, chills, URI symptoms
- Enanthem: none

Yes →

Varicella (chickenpox)
- Varicella zoster virus
- Incubation 14–16 days
- Rash: Macules form on trunk and spread to face and extremities; progress quickly in clusters to papules then teardrop-shaped vesicles ("dew drops on a rose petal") that crust over or umbilicate
- Prodrome: 1–2 days of fever, malaise, anorexia, headache
- Enanthem: Rarely, vesicles can lead to erosions of hard palate.

Yes → Vesicular?

No →

Yes →

Coxsackie virus (hand-foot-mouth disease)
- Coxsackie virus A16 (most common), A6, A10, and enterovirus 71
- Incubation 3–6 days
- Rash: ~2–3 mm erythematous macules and papules on palmar surface of hand, plantar surface of feet, buttocks, genitals, oral mucosa; progresses quickly through vesicular phase to form central gray ulcer
- Prodrome: 12–36 hours of cough, fever, malaise, anorexia, abdominal pain
- Enanthem: Occurs with exanthem as painful ulcerative lesions commonly found on tongue, hard palate, and buccal mucosa

Koplik spots (white papules on buccal mucosa)?

No →

Fast-spreading rash?

No →

Rubella (third disease, German measles)
- Rubella virus
- Incubation 14–17 days
- Rash: erythematous maculopapular rash with downward progression from face
- Prodrome: 1–7 days of malaise, painful lymphadenopathy
- Enanthem: Forchheimer spots (petechiae on soft palate)

Yes →

Scarlet fever (second disease)
- Group A streptococcus
- Incubation 1–5 days
- Rash: rapidly progressing erythematous macules and pinpoint, blanchable papules ("goose pimples") with sandpaper texture, greatest intensity at skin folds occurring almost simultaneously with fever
- Prodrome: 1–2 days of fever, sore throat, vomiting, abdominal pain
- Enanthem: progression from white to red strawberry tongue
- Perform rapid strep testing, a throat culture, and initiate treatment.

Yes →

Measles (first disease, rubeola)
- Measles virus
- Incubation 10–12 days
- Rash: erythematous maculopapular rash (developing as fever progresses) with downward progression from face and brownish hue during resolution
- Prodrome: 3–4 days of conjunctivitis, coryza, fever, cough
- Enanthem: Koplik spots

Jane M. Forbes, MD and Fern R. Hauck, MD, MS

Dyer JA. Childhood viral exanthems. *Pediatr Ann.* 2007;36(1):21–29.

PELVIC PAIN

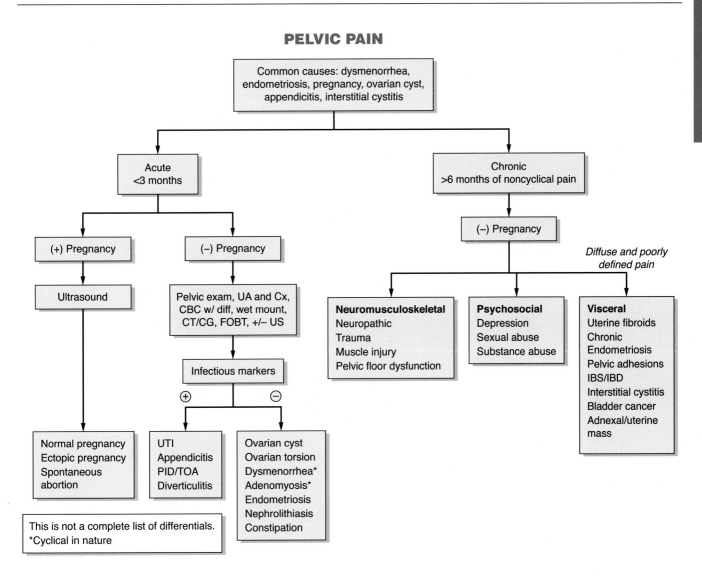

Rebecca Thrower, MD and Jocelyn Worley, DO

Learman LA, McHugh KW. ACOG Practice Bulletin Number 218: chronic pelvic pain. *Obstet Gynecol.* 2020;135(3):98–109.

POISON EXPOSURE AND TREATMENT
POISON EXPOSURE

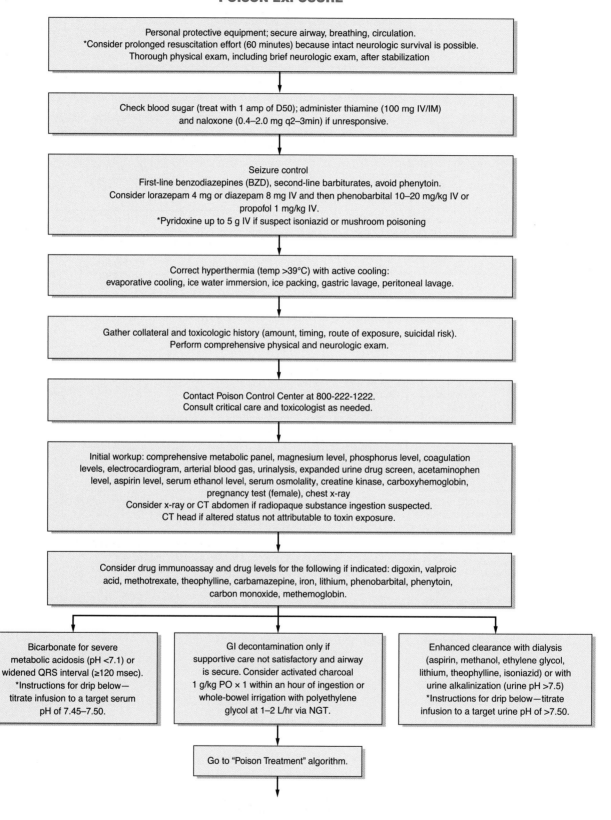

Personal protective equipment; secure airway, breathing, circulation.
*Consider prolonged resuscitation effort (60 minutes) because intact neurologic survival is possible.
Thorough physical exam, including brief neurologic exam, after stabilization

Check blood sugar (treat with 1 amp of D50); administer thiamine (100 mg IV/IM)
and naloxone (0.4–2.0 mg q2–3min) if unresponsive.

Seizure control
First-line benzodiazepines (BZD), second-line barbiturates, avoid phenytoin.
Consider lorazepam 4 mg or diazepam 8 mg IV and then phenobarbital 10–20 mg/kg IV or
propofol 1 mg/kg IV.
*Pyridoxine up to 5 g IV if suspect isoniazid or mushroom poisoning

Correct hyperthermia (temp >39°C) with active cooling:
evaporative cooling, ice water immersion, ice packing, gastric lavage, peritoneal lavage.

Gather collateral and toxicologic history (amount, timing, route of exposure, suicidal risk).
Perform comprehensive physical and neurologic exam.

Contact Poison Control Center at 800-222-1222.
Consult critical care and toxicologist as needed.

Initial workup: comprehensive metabolic panel, magnesium level, phosphorus level, coagulation
levels, electrocardiogram, arterial blood gas, urinalysis, expanded urine drug screen, acetaminophen
level, aspirin level, serum ethanol level, serum osmolality, creatine kinase, carboxyhemoglobin,
pregnancy test (female), chest x-ray
Consider x-ray or CT abdomen if radiopaque substance ingestion suspected.
CT head if altered status not attributable to toxin exposure.

Consider drug immunoassay and drug levels for the following if indicated: digoxin, valproic
acid, methotrexate, theophylline, carbamazepine, iron, lithium, phenobarbital, phenytoin,
carbon monoxide, methemoglobin.

Bicarbonate for severe
metabolic acidosis (pH <7.1) or
widened QRS interval (≥120 msec).
*Instructions for drip below—
titrate infusion to a target serum
pH of 7.45–7.50.

GI decontamination only if
supportive care not satisfactory and airway
is secure. Consider activated charcoal
1 g/kg PO × 1 within an hour of ingestion or
whole-bowel irrigation with polyethylene
glycol at 1–2 L/hr via NGT.

Enhanced clearance with dialysis
(aspirin, methanol, ethylene glycol,
lithium, theophylline, isoniazid) or with
urine alkalinization (urine pH >7.5)
*Instructions for drip below—titrate
infusion to a target urine pH of >7.50.

Go to "Poison Treatment" algorithm.

POISON TREATMENT

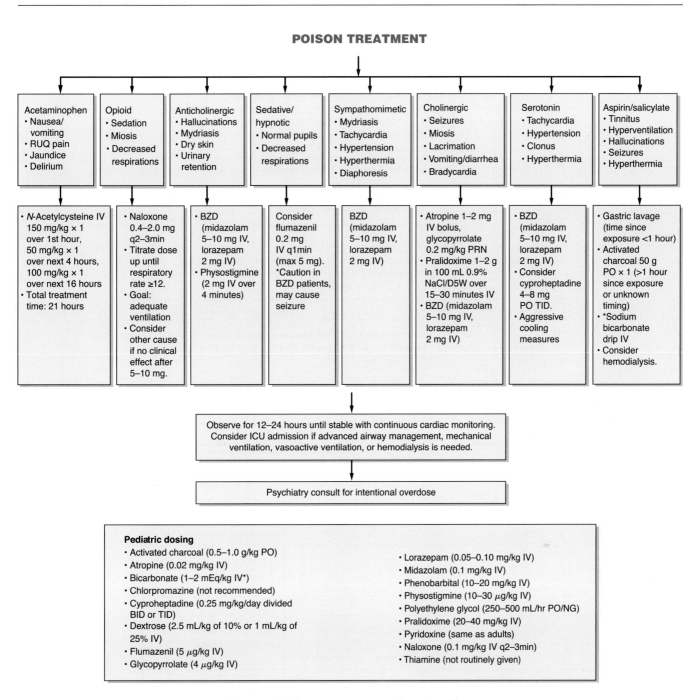

Acetaminophen
- Nausea/vomiting
- RUQ pain
- Jaundice
- Delirium

- *N*-Acetylcysteine IV 150 mg/kg × 1 over 1st hour, 50 mg/kg × 1 over next 4 hours, 100 mg/kg × 1 over next 16 hours
- Total treatment time: 21 hours

Opioid
- Sedation
- Miosis
- Decreased respirations

- Naloxone 0.4–2.0 mg q2–3min
- Titrate dose up until respiratory rate ≥12.
- Goal: adequate ventilation
- Consider other cause if no clinical effect after 5–10 mg.

Anticholinergic
- Hallucinations
- Mydriasis
- Dry skin
- Urinary retention

- BZD (midazolam 5–10 mg IV, lorazepam 2 mg IV)
- Physostigmine (2 mg IV over 4 minutes)

Sedative/hypnotic
- Normal pupils
- Decreased respirations

- Consider flumazenil 0.2 mg IV q1min (max 5 mg). *Caution in BZD patients, may cause seizure

Sympathomimetic
- Mydriasis
- Tachycardia
- Hypertension
- Hyperthermia
- Diaphoresis

BZD (midazolam 5–10 mg IV, lorazepam 2 mg IV)

Cholinergic
- Seizures
- Miosis
- Lacrimation
- Vomiting/diarrhea
- Bradycardia

- Atropine 1–2 mg IV bolus, glycopyrrolate 0.2 mg/kg PRN
- Pralidoxime 1–2 g in 100 mL 0.9% NaCl/D5W over 15–30 minutes IV
- BZD (midazolam 5–10 mg IV, lorazepam 2 mg IV)

Serotonin
- Tachycardia
- Hypertension
- Clonus
- Hyperthermia

- BZD (midazolam 5–10 mg IV, lorazepam 2 mg IV)
- Consider cyproheptadine 4–8 mg PO TID.
- Aggressive cooling measures

Aspirin/salicylate
- Tinnitus
- Hyperventilation
- Hallucinations
- Seizures
- Hyperthermia

- Gastric lavage (time since exposure <1 hour)
- Activated charcoal 50 g PO × 1 (>1 hour since exposure or unknown timing)
- *Sodium bicarbonate drip IV
- Consider hemodialysis.

Observe for 12–24 hours until stable with continuous cardiac monitoring. Consider ICU admission if advanced airway management, mechanical ventilation, vasoactive ventilation, or hemodialysis is needed.

Psychiatry consult for intentional overdose

Pediatric dosing
- Activated charcoal (0.5–1.0 g/kg PO)
- Atropine (0.02 mg/kg IV)
- Bicarbonate (1–2 mEq/kg IV*)
- Chlorpromazine (not recommended)
- Cyproheptadine (0.25 mg/kg/day divided BID or TID)
- Dextrose (2.5 mL/kg of 10% or 1 mL/kg of 25% IV)
- Flumazenil (5 μg/kg IV)
- Glycopyrrolate (4 μg/kg IV)

- Lorazepam (0.05–0.10 mg/kg IV)
- Midazolam (0.1 mg/kg IV)
- Phenobarbital (10–20 mg/kg IV)
- Physostigmine (10–30 μg/kg IV)
- Polyethylene glycol (250–500 mL/hr PO/NG)
- Pralidoxime (20–40 mg/kg IV)
- Pyridoxine (same as adults)
- Naloxone (0.1 mg/kg IV q2–3min)
- Thiamine (not routinely given)

*To mix a bicarbonate drip: 150 mEq (3 amps) NaHCO$_3$ in 1 L of D5W and then start at a rate of 150–200 mL/hr.

Christopher J. Rider, MD and Ashley Rose Wilk, DO

Thompson TM, Theobald J, Lu J, et al. The general approach to the poisoned patient. *Dis Mon.* 2014;60(11):509–524. doi:10.1016/j.disamonth.2014.10.002.

PRECOCIOUS PUBERTY

Signs of secondary sexual development in boys >9 years and girls >8 years

↓

Common causes:
medication, pituitary tumor, congenital adrenal hyperplasia, adrenal tumor, ovarian tumor, pseudoprecocious puberty

↓

X-ray to determine bone age

Bone age > chronologic age

Bone age = chronologic age

↓

Incomplete precocious puberty (premature adrenarche or thelarche)

Basal LH levels

>5 mIU/mL

<5 mIU/mL

GnRH stimulation test, LH, FSH

Gonadotropin-independent (peripheral) precocious puberty

Testosterone, estradiol, LH, FSH, cortisol, DHEA, DHEA-S, 17-hydroxyprogesterone, hCG (males), abdominal and pelvic US

In ♀, US + for ovarian cyst(s) or tumor

LH, FSH increased

Absent LH response

Gonadotropin-dependent (central) precocious puberty

Elevated hCG in ♂

Very high levels of testosterone in ♂

Pubertal values of testosterone in ♂ and estradiol in ♀, with bone and skin findings

Elevated testosterone in ♂ and estradiol in ♀

Estradiol, testosterone, TSH, MRI, of brain

Germ cell tumor

Leydig cell tumor

McCune-Albright syndrome

Exogenous sex steroids

CNS lesion

Abnormal TSH

Negative

Chronic primary hypothyroidism

Idiopathic precocious puberty

Elevated 17-hydroxyprogesterone

Congenital adrenal hyperplasia

Elevated DHEA, DHEA-S, findings on imaging

Adrenal tumor or cancer

Frank J. Domino, MD

Berberoğlu M. Precocious puberty and normal variant puberty: definition, etiology, diagnosis and current management. *J Clin Res Pediatr Endocrinol.* 2009;1(4):164–174.

PREOPERATIVE EVALUATION OF NONCARDIAC SURGICAL PATIENT

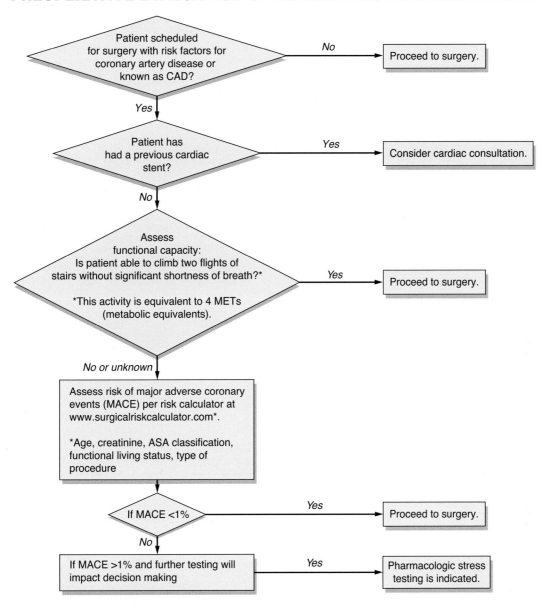

Patient scheduled for surgery with risk factors for coronary artery disease or known as CAD?
— No → Proceed to surgery.
— Yes ↓

Patient has had a previous cardiac stent?
— Yes → Consider cardiac consultation.
— No ↓

Assess functional capacity: Is patient able to climb two flights of stairs without significant shortness of breath?*
*This activity is equivalent to 4 METs (metabolic equivalents).
— Yes → Proceed to surgery.
— No or unknown ↓

Assess risk of major adverse coronary events (MACE) per risk calculator at www.surgicalriskcalculator.com*.
*Age, creatinine, ASA classification, functional living status, type of procedure
↓

If MACE <1%
— Yes → Proceed to surgery.
— No ↓

If MACE >1% and further testing will impact decision making
— Yes → Pharmacologic stress testing is indicated.

Andrew Grimes, MD and Stacy L. Jones, MD, MHA, FASA

Smilowitz NR, Berger JS. Perioperative cardiovascular risk assessment and management for noncardiac surgery: a review. *JAMA*. 2020;324(3):279–290.

PROTEINURIA

Defined as >150 mg/24 hr urine
Common causes and reasons to screen: hypertension, diabetes, glomerular disease, cardiovascular disease, congestive heart disease, multiple myeloma, nephrotic syndrome, fever, urinary tract infection, orthostatic hypertension, lupus. Perform history and physical.

If at any point in the workup there is high clinical suspicion for disease, if the patient is symptomatic, GFR <30, or if renal disease is discovered, then consult nephrology.

Underlying cause of proteinuria identified through history and physical exam?

Yes → Treat underlying cause.

No

Obtain urinalysis.

Normal GFR range for healthy adults: greater than 90 mL/min/1.73 m^2

Semiquantitative urinalysis ranges (albumin)
Negative: 0 mg/dL
Trace: 15–30 mg/dL
1+: 30–100 mg/dL
2+: 100–300 mg/dL
3+: 300–1,000 mg/dL
4+: >1,000 mg/dL

Albuminuria and GFR are independent risk factors for the progression of chronic kidney disease.

Trace to 2+.

2+ or greater

Obtain repeat urinalysis in 1–2 weeks.

2+ or greater → Obtain serum creatinine to determine GFR and urine albumin creatinine ratio (ACR) or instead evaluate with 24-hour urine.

<2+

ACR <300 mg/g without decreased GFR or 24-hour urine <2 g

ACR >30 mg/g + reduced GFR or ACR >300 mg/g or 24-hour urine > 2g

Transient (Consider fever, heavy physical activity, UTI, CHF, urologic hemorrhage, orthostatic proteinuria.)
Reassurance and f/u as needed

Evaluate for orthostatic proteinuria with first morning void and random void. If normal first morning void and elevated random sample, diagnose orthostatic proteinuria.

Obtain renal ultrasound and UPEP. Consult nephrology.

If UPEP abnormal, consult heme/onc; may be concern for multiple myeloma

Continue to monitor blood pressure, urinalysis, and renal function yearly.

Consider additional labs and evaluate for the following as clinically indicated:
• ANA (lupus)
• Antistreptolysin O titer (streptococcal glomerulonephritis)
• C3/C4 (glomerulonephritis)
• ESR (rule out inflammation/infection)
• Fasting glucose (diabetes)
• H/H (will be low in chronic renal failure)
• HIV, VDRL, hepatitis serologies
• Serum albumin and lipid levels (Consider nephrotic syndrome.)
• Serum electrolytes
• Serum urate (Elevation can cause tubulointerstitial disease.)
• Chest radiograph (systemic disease such as sarcoidosis, etc.)

Kyler M. Douglas, DO and Pamela R. Hughes, MD

Waheed S. Evaluation of proteinuria. https://bestpractice.bmj.com/topics/en-us/875. Updated September 9, 2021. Accessed September 24, 2021.

PULMONARY EMBOLISM, DIAGNOSIS

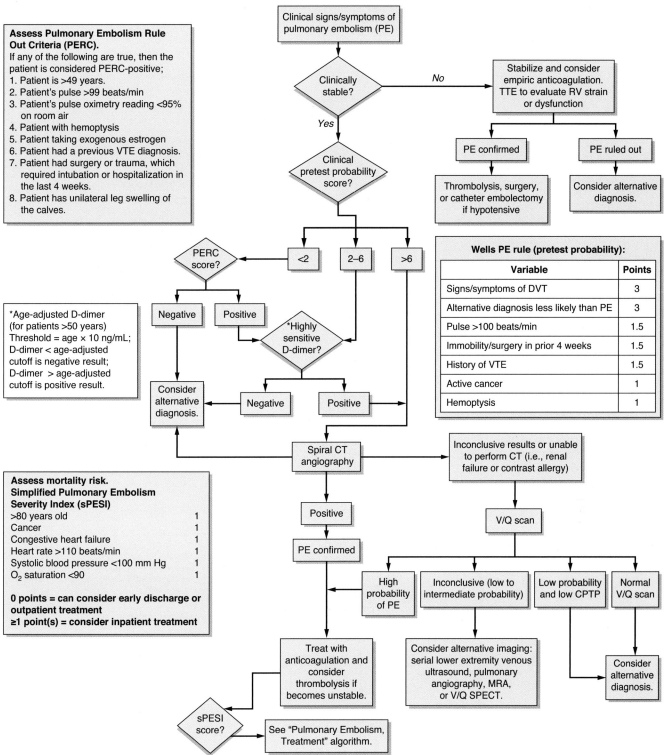

Assess Pulmonary Embolism Rule Out Criteria (PERC).
If any of the following are true, then the patient is considered PERC-positive;
1. Patient is >49 years.
2. Patient's pulse >99 beats/min
3. Patient's pulse oximetry reading <95% on room air
4. Patient with hemoptysis
5. Patient taking exogenous estrogen
6. Patient had a previous VTE diagnosis.
7. Patient had surgery or trauma, which required intubation or hospitalization in the last 4 weeks.
8. Patient has unilateral leg swelling of the calves.

*Age-adjusted D-dimer (for patients >50 years) Threshold = age × 10 ng/mL; D-dimer < age-adjusted cutoff is negative result; D-dimer > age-adjusted cutoff is positive result.

Assess mortality risk.
Simplified Pulmonary Embolism Severity Index (sPESI)

>80 years old	1
Cancer	1
Congestive heart failure	1
Heart rate >110 beats/min	1
Systolic blood pressure <100 mm Hg	1
O_2 saturation <90	1

0 points = can consider early discharge or outpatient treatment
≥1 point(s) = consider inpatient treatment

Clinical signs/symptoms of pulmonary embolism (PE)

Clinically stable? — No → Stabilize and consider empiric anticoagulation. TTE to evaluate RV strain or dysfunction
- PE confirmed → Thrombolysis, surgery, or catheter embolectomy if hypotensive
- PE ruled out → Consider alternative diagnosis.

Yes ↓

Clinical pretest probability score?
- <2 → PERC score?
- 2–6
- >6

PERC score?
- Negative → Consider alternative diagnosis.
- Positive → *Highly sensitive D-dimer?
  - Negative → Consider alternative diagnosis.
  - Positive → Spiral CT angiography

Wells PE rule (pretest probability):

Variable	Points
Signs/symptoms of DVT	3
Alternative diagnosis less likely than PE	3
Pulse >100 beats/min	1.5
Immobility/surgery in prior 4 weeks	1.5
History of VTE	1.5
Active cancer	1
Hemoptysis	1

Spiral CT angiography → Inconclusive results or unable to perform CT (i.e., renal failure or contrast allergy)
- Positive → PE confirmed → Treat with anticoagulation and consider thrombolysis if becomes unstable. → sPESI score? → See "Pulmonary Embolism, Treatment" algorithm.

Inconclusive results or unable to perform CT → V/Q scan
- High probability of PE → PE confirmed
- Inconclusive (low to intermediate probability) → Consider alternative imaging: serial lower extremity venous ultrasound, pulmonary angiography, MRA, or V/Q SPECT.
- Low probability and low CPTP → Consider alternative diagnosis.
- Normal V/Q scan → Consider alternative diagnosis.

Lawrence M. Gibbs, MD, MSEd and Melissa L. Smith, MD

Konstantinides SV, Meyer G, Becattini C, et al. 2019 ESC guidelines for the diagnosis and management of acute pulmonary embolism developed in collaboration with the European Respiratory Society (ERS). *Eur Heart J.* 2020;41(4):543–603.

PULMONARY EMBOLISM, TREATMENT

Probability of pulmonary embolism above treatment threshold

Anticoagulation contraindicated?
— Yes → **IVC filter**

No ↓

Massive pulmonary embolism?
(SBP <90 mm Hg for >15 minutes)
— Yes → **Thrombolysis contraindicated?**
- Prior intracranial bleed
- Ischemic stroke <3 months
- Suspected aortic dissection
- Active bleeding diathesis
- Recent brain or spinal surgery
- Closed head or facial trauma

No ↓

Benefits of thrombolysis may outweigh risks IF: hemodynamic instability, worsening oxygenation, severe RV, or major myocardial necrosis. Thrombolysis indicated?
— Yes → (to Thrombolysis contraindicated?)

Thrombolysis contraindicated? — Yes → **Embolectomy, per local expertise**

Thrombolysis contraindicated? — No → **Thrombolysis using tPA (can be given systemically or catheter directed based on bleeding risk)**

No ↓

History of heparin-induced thrombocytopenia?
— Yes (left) →
— Yes (from Clinical improvement?) →

Clinical improvement?
— No → **Embolectomy, per local expertise**
— Yes → **History of heparin-induced thrombocytopenia?**

No ↓

(left box) **History of heparin-induced thrombocytopenia? — Yes**

- Consider fondaparinux or argatroban (caution use of argatroban in liver disease) and vitamin K antagonist (warfarin) with at least 5 days of concomitant therapy. When used in combination, goal INR prior to discontinuation of the parenteral product is as follows: INR >2 (fondaparinux) or >4 (argatroban) × 24 hours. Of note, argatroban falsely elevates the INR, which could be misleading when given in combination with vitamin K antagonist. Once the INR is >4, discontinue the argatroban and recheck the INR in 4–6 hours with a goal INR of 2–3.
- Alternatively, consider using a new oral anticoagulant such as apixaban or rivaroxaban without need for parenteral bridging (of note, dabigatran and edoxaban require 5–10 days of parenteral therapy).
- Prior to using vitamin K antagonist (warfarin) for new-onset heparin-induced thrombocytopenia, be sure platelets are >150,000.

(lower left box) **History of heparin-induced thrombocytopenia? — No**

Begin either:
- Heparin infusion to therapeutic aPTT or therapeutic dose low-molecular-weight heparin (LMWH) and warfarin, discontinuing LMWH when INR >2 for at least 24 hours and minimum 5 days of concomitant therapy; goal INR 2–3

OR

- New oral anticoagulant such as apixaban or rivaroxaban without need for parenteral bridging (of note, dabigatran and edoxaban require 5–10 days of parenteral therapy). Stable, low-risk patients may be treated as outpatients with an appropriate regimen above.

Ryan B. Feeney, PharmD, BCPS, BCGP and Danita R. Fox, MD

Guyatt GH, Akl EA, Crowther M, et al; for American College of Chest Physicians Antithrombotic Therapy and Prevention of Thrombosis Panel. Executive summary: Antithrombotic Therapy and Prevention of Thrombosis, 9th ed: American College of Chest Physicians evidence-based clinical practice guidelines. *Chest.* 2012;141(2 Suppl):7S–47S.

RASH

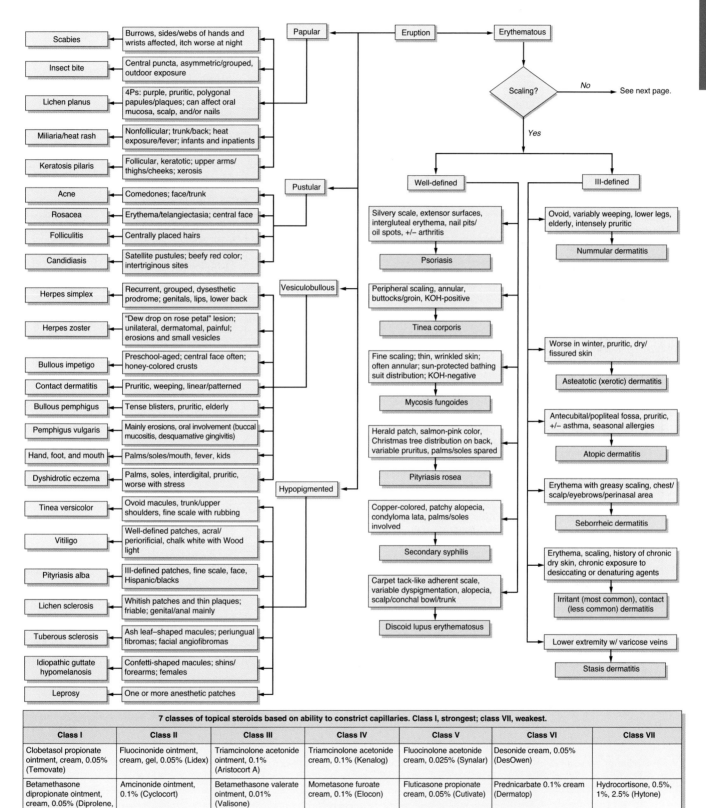

Scabies	Burrows, sides/webs of hands and wrists affected, itch worse at night
Insect bite	Central puncta, asymmetric/grouped, outdoor exposure
Lichen planus	4Ps: purple, pruritic, polygonal papules/plaques; can affect oral mucosa, scalp, and/or nails
Miliaria/heat rash	Nonfollicular; trunk/back; heat exposure/fever; infants and inpatients
Keratosis pilaris	Follicular, keratotic; upper arms/thighs/cheeks; xerosis

Papular

Acne	Comedones; face/trunk
Rosacea	Erythema/telangiectasia; central face
Folliculitis	Centrally placed hairs
Candidiasis	Satellite pustules; beefy red color; intertriginous sites

Pustular

Herpes simplex	Recurrent, grouped, dysesthetic prodrome; genitals, lips, lower back
Herpes zoster	"Dew drop on rose petal" lesion; unilateral, dermatomal, painful; erosions and small vesicles
Bullous impetigo	Preschool-aged; central face often; honey-colored crusts
Contact dermatitis	Pruritic, weeping, linear/patterned
Bullous pemphigus	Tense blisters, pruritic, elderly
Pemphigus vulgaris	Mainly erosions, oral involvement (buccal mucositis, desquamative gingivitis)
Hand, foot, and mouth	Palms/soles/mouth, fever, kids
Dyshidrotic eczema	Palms, soles, interdigital, pruritic, worse with stress

Vesiculobullous

Tinea versicolor	Ovoid macules, trunk/upper shoulders, fine scale with rubbing
Vitiligo	Well-defined patches, acral/periorificial, chalk white with Wood light
Pityriasis alba	Ill-defined patches, fine scale, face, Hispanic/blacks
Lichen sclerosis	Whitish patches and thin plaques; friable; genital/anal mainly
Tuberous sclerosis	Ash leaf–shaped macules; periungual fibromas; facial angiofibromas
Idiopathic guttate hypomelanosis	Confetti-shaped macules; shins/forearms; females
Leprosy	One or more anesthetic patches

Hypopigmented

Eruption → Papular / Erythematous

Erythematous → Scaling?
- No → See next page.
- Yes → Well-defined / Ill-defined

Well-defined:

Silvery scale, extensor surfaces, intergluteal erythema, nail pits/oil spots, +/– arthritis	→ **Psoriasis**
Peripheral scaling, annular, buttocks/groin, KOH-positive	→ **Tinea corporis**
Fine scaling; thin, wrinkled skin; often annular; sun-protected bathing suit distribution; KOH-negative	→ **Mycosis fungoides**
Herald patch, salmon-pink color, Christmas tree distribution on back, variable pruritus, palms/soles spared	→ **Pityriasis rosea**
Copper-colored, patchy alopecia, condyloma lata, palms/soles involved	→ **Secondary syphilis**
Carpet tack-like adherent scale, variable dyspigmentation, alopecia, scalp/conchal bowl/trunk	→ **Discoid lupus erythematosus**

Ill-defined:

Ovoid, variably weeping, lower legs, elderly, intensely pruritic	→ **Nummular dermatitis**
Worse in winter, pruritic, dry/fissured skin	→ **Asteatotic (xerotic) dermatitis**
Antecubital/popliteal fossa, pruritic, +/– asthma, seasonal allergies	→ **Atopic dermatitis**
Erythema with greasy scaling, chest/scalp/eyebrows/perinasal area	→ **Seborrheic dermatitis**
Erythema, scaling, history of chronic dry skin, chronic exposure to desiccating or denaturing agents	Irritant (most common), contact (less common) dermatitis
Lower extremity w/ varicose veins	→ **Stasis dermatitis**

7 classes of topical steroids based on ability to constrict capillaries. Class I, strongest; class VII, weakest.

Class I	Class II	Class III	Class IV	Class V	Class VI	Class VII
Clobetasol propionate ointment, cream, 0.05% (Temovate)	Fluocinonide ointment, cream, gel, 0.05% (Lidex)	Triamcinolone acetonide ointment, 0.1% (Aristocort A)	Triamcinolone acetonide cream, 0.1% (Kenalog)	Fluocinolone acetonide cream, 0.025% (Synalar)	Desonide cream, 0.05% (DesOwen)	
Betamethasone dipropionate ointment, cream, 0.05% (Diprolene, Diprosone)	Amcinonide ointment, 0.1% (Cyclocort)	Betamethasone valerate ointment, 0.01% (Valisone)	Mometasone furoate cream, 0.1% (Elocon)	Fluticasone propionate cream, 0.05% (Cutivate)	Prednicarbate 0.1% cream (Dermatop)	Hydrocortisone, 0.5%, 1%, 2.5% (Hytone)
Halobetasol propionate ointment, cream, 0.05% (Ultravate)	Desoximetasone ointment, cream, 0.25%; gel, 0.05% (Topicort)	Fluticasone propionate ointment, 0.05% (Cutivate)	Hydrocortisone valerate ointment, 0.2% (Westcort)	Hydrocortisone valerate cream, 0.2% (Westcort)	Alclometasone dipropionate ointment, cream, 0.05% (Aclovate)	

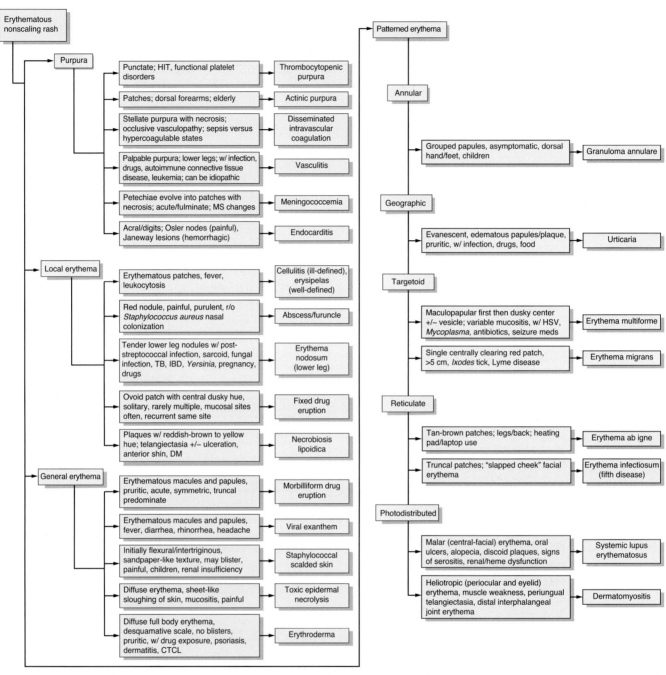

Erythematous nonscaling rash

Purpura
- Punctate; HIT, functional platelet disorders → Thrombocytopenic purpura
- Patches; dorsal forearms; elderly → Actinic purpura
- Stellate purpura with necrosis; occlusive vasculopathy; sepsis versus hypercoagulable states → Disseminated intravascular coagulation
- Palpable purpura; lower legs; w/ infection, drugs, autoimmune connective tissue disease, leukemia; can be idiopathic → Vasculitis
- Petechiae evolve into patches with necrosis; acute/fulminate; MS changes → Meningococcemia
- Acral/digits; Osler nodes (painful), Janeway lesions (hemorrhagic) → Endocarditis

Local erythema
- Erythematous patches, fever, leukocytosis → Cellulitis (ill-defined), erysipelas (well-defined)
- Red nodule, painful, purulent, r/o *Staphylococcus aureus* nasal colonization → Abscess/furuncle
- Tender lower leg nodules w/ post-streptococcal infection, sarcoid, fungal infection, TB, IBD, *Yersinia*, pregnancy, drugs → Erythema nodosum (lower leg)
- Ovoid patch with central dusky hue, solitary, rarely multiple, mucosal sites often, recurrent same site → Fixed drug eruption
- Plaques w/ reddish-brown to yellow hue; telangiectasia +/− ulceration, anterior shin, DM → Necrobiosis lipoidica

General erythema
- Erythematous macules and papules, pruritic, acute, symmetric, truncal predominate → Morbilliform drug eruption
- Erythematous macules and papules, fever, diarrhea, rhinorrhea, headache → Viral exanthem
- Initially flexural/intertriginous, sandpaper-like texture, may blister, painful, children, renal insufficiency → Staphylococcal scalded skin
- Diffuse erythema, sheet-like sloughing of skin, mucositis, painful → Toxic epidermal necrolysis
- Diffuse full body erythema, desquamative scale, no blisters, pruritic, w/ drug exposure, psoriasis, dermatitis, CTCL → Erythroderma

Patterned erythema

Annular
- Grouped papules, asymptomatic, dorsal hand/feet, children → Granuloma annulare

Geographic
- Evanescent, edematous papules/plaque, pruritic, w/ infection, drugs, food → Urticaria

Targetoid
- Maculopapular first then dusky center +/− vesicle; variable mucositis, w/ HSV, *Mycoplasma*, antibiotics, seizure meds → Erythema multiforme
- Single centrally clearing red patch, >5 cm, *Ixodes* tick, Lyme disease → Erythema migrans

Reticulate
- Tan-brown patches; legs/back; heating pad/laptop use → Erythema ab igne
- Truncal patches; "slapped cheek" facial erythema → Erythema infectiosum (fifth disease)

Photodistributed
- Malar (central-facial) erythema, oral ulcers, alopecia, discoid plaques, signs of serositis, renal/heme dysfunction → Systemic lupus erythematosus
- Heliotropic (periocular and eyelid) erythema, muscle weakness, periungual telangiectasia, distal interphalangeal joint erythema → Dermatomyositis

7 classes of topical steroids based on ability to constrict capillaries. Class I, strongest; class VII, weakest.						
Class I	**Class II**	**Class III**	**Class IV**	**Class V**	**Class VI**	**Class VII**
Clobetasol propionate ointment, cream, 0.05% (Temovate)	Fluocinonide ointment, cream, gel 0.05% (Lidex)	Triamcinolone acetonide ointment, 0.1% (Aristocort A)	Triamcinolone acetonide cream, 0.1% (Kenalog)	Fluocinolone acetonide cream, 0.025% (Synalar)	Desonide cream, 0.05% (DesOwen)	Hydrocortisone, 0.5%, 1%, 2.5% (Hytone)
Betamethasone dipropionate ointment, cream, 0.05% (Diprolene, Diprosone)	Amcinonide ointment, 0.1% (Cyclocort)	Betamethasone valerate ointment, 0.01% (Valisone)	Mometasone furoate cream, 0.1% (Elocon)	Fluticasone propionate cream, 0.05% (Cutivate)	Prednicarbate 0.1% cream (Dermatop)	
Halobetasol propionate ointment, cream, 0.05% (Ultravate)	Desoximetasone ointment, cream, 0.25%; gel, 0.05% (Topicort)	Fluticasone propionate ointment, 0.05% (Cutivate)	Hydrocortisone valerate ointment, 0.2% (Westcort)	Hydrocortisone valerate cream, 0.2% (Westcort)	Alclometasone dipropionate ointment, cream, 0.05% (Aclovate)	

Jennifer G. Foster, MD, MBA, FACP

Stern SC, Cifu AS, Altkorn D, eds. *Symptom to Diagnosis: An Evidence-Based Guide.* 3rd ed. New York, NY: McGraw-Hill; 2014.

RECTAL BLEEDING AND HEMATOCHEZIA

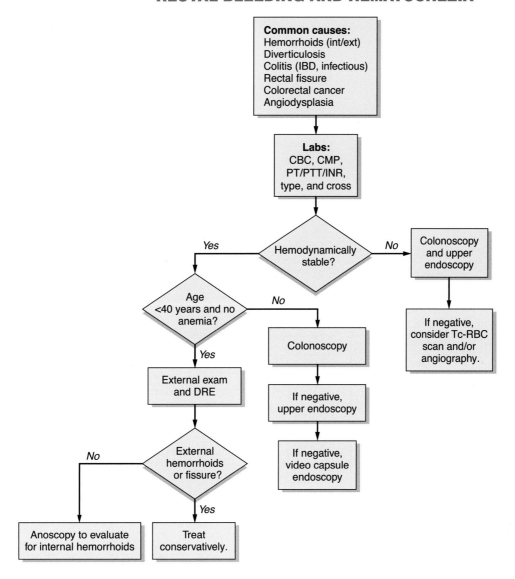

Common causes:
Hemorrhoids (int/ext)
Diverticulosis
Colitis (IBD, infectious)
Rectal fissure
Colorectal cancer
Angiodysplasia

Labs:
CBC, CMP,
PT/PTT/INR,
type, and cross

Hemodynamically stable?

Yes

No → Colonoscopy and upper endoscopy

If negative, consider Tc-RBC scan and/or angiography.

Age <40 years and no anemia?

No → Colonoscopy

If negative, upper endoscopy

If negative, video capsule endoscopy

Yes

External exam and DRE

External hemorrhoids or fissure?

No → Anoscopy to evaluate for internal hemorrhoids

Yes → Treat conservatively.

Allison Holley, MD

Almadi MA, Barkun AN. Patient presentation, risk stratification, and initial management in acute lower gastrointestinal bleeding. *Gastrointest Endosc Clin N Am.* 2018;28(3):363–377.

RED EYE

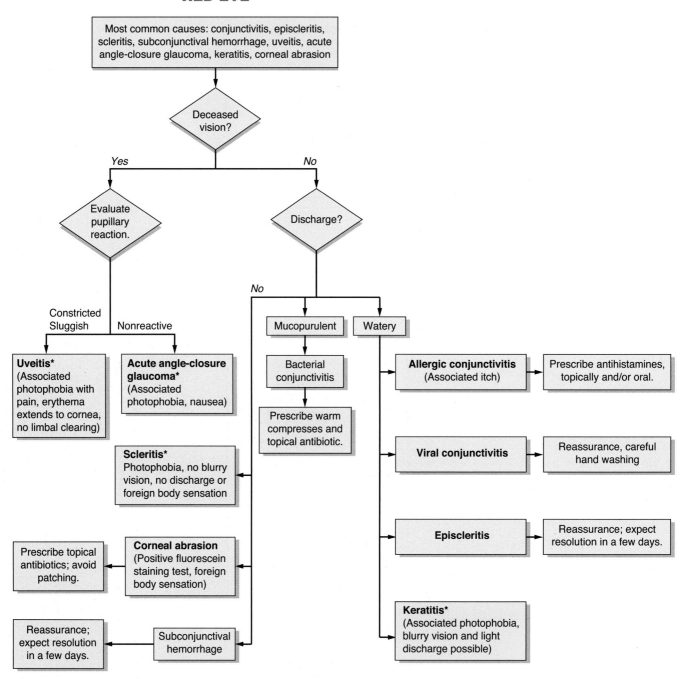

Most common causes: conjunctivitis, episcleritis, scleritis, subconjunctival hemorrhage, uveitis, acute angle-closure glaucoma, keratitis, corneal abrasion

Deceased vision?

Yes — Evaluate pupillary reaction.

No — Discharge?

Constricted Sluggish — **Uveitis*** (Associated photophobia with pain, erythema extends to cornea, no limbal clearing)

Nonreactive — **Acute angle-closure glaucoma*** (Associated photophobia, nausea)

No — Mucopurulent — Bacterial conjunctivitis — Prescribe warm compresses and topical antibiotic.

Watery

Allergic conjunctivitis (Associated itch) — Prescribe antihistamines, topically and/or oral.

Viral conjunctivitis — Reassurance, careful hand washing

Episcleritis — Reassurance; expect resolution in a few days.

Keratitis* (Associated photophobia, blurry vision and light discharge possible)

Scleritis* Photophobia, no blurry vision, no discharge or foreign body sensation

Corneal abrasion (Positive fluorescein staining test, foreign body sensation) — Prescribe topical antibiotics; avoid patching.

Subconjunctival hemorrhage — Reassurance; expect resolution in a few days.

*Urgent ophthalmology consultation.

Robert A. Baldor, MD, FAAFP

Cronau H, Kankanala RR, Mauger T. Diagnosis and management of red eye in primary care. *Am Fam Physician.* 2010;81(2):137–144.

SALICYLATE POISONING, ACUTE, TREATMENT

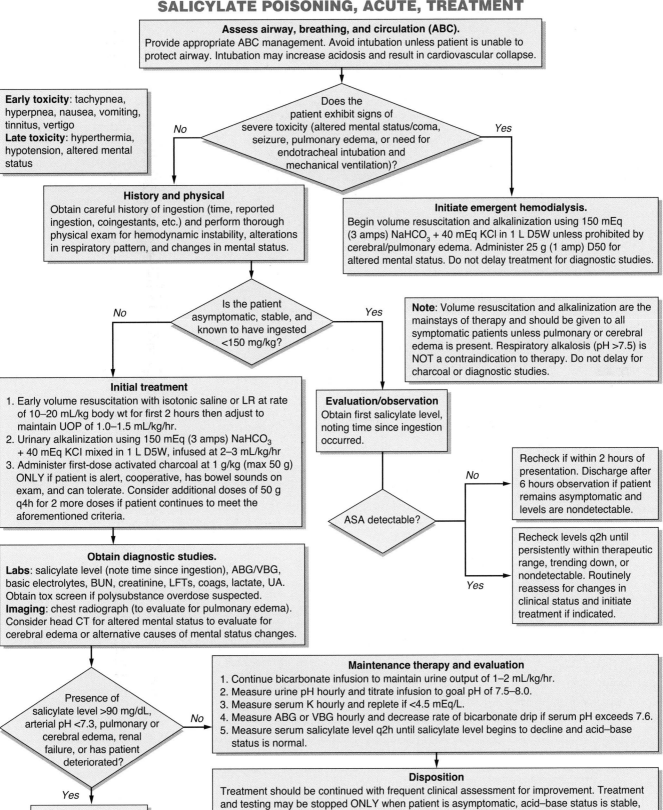

Assess airway, breathing, and circulation (ABC).
Provide appropriate ABC management. Avoid intubation unless patient is unable to protect airway. Intubation may increase acidosis and result in cardiovascular collapse.

Early toxicity: tachypnea, hyperpnea, nausea, vomiting, tinnitus, vertigo
Late toxicity: hyperthermia, hypotension, altered mental status

Does the patient exhibit signs of severe toxicity (altered mental status/coma, seizure, pulmonary edema, or need for endotracheal intubation and mechanical ventilation)?

No / *Yes*

History and physical
Obtain careful history of ingestion (time, reported ingestion, coingestants, etc.) and perform thorough physical exam for hemodynamic instability, alterations in respiratory pattern, and changes in mental status.

Initiate emergent hemodialysis.
Begin volume resuscitation and alkalinization using 150 mEq (3 amps) $NaHCO_3$ + 40 mEq KCl in 1 L D5W unless prohibited by cerebral/pulmonary edema. Administer 25 g (1 amp) D50 for altered mental status. Do not delay treatment for diagnostic studies.

Is the patient asymptomatic, stable, and known to have ingested <150 mg/kg?

No / *Yes*

Note: Volume resuscitation and alkalinization are the mainstays of therapy and should be given to all symptomatic patients unless pulmonary or cerebral edema is present. Respiratory alkalosis (pH >7.5) is NOT a contraindication to therapy. Do not delay for charcoal or diagnostic studies.

Initial treatment
1. Early volume resuscitation with isotonic saline or LR at rate of 10–20 mL/kg body wt for first 2 hours then adjust to maintain UOP of 1.0–1.5 mL/kg/hr.
2. Urinary alkalinization using 150 mEq (3 amps) $NaHCO_3$ + 40 mEq KCl mixed in 1 L D5W, infused at 2–3 mL/kg/hr
3. Administer first-dose activated charcoal at 1 g/kg (max 50 g) ONLY if patient is alert, cooperative, has bowel sounds on exam, and can tolerate. Consider additional doses of 50 g q4h for 2 more doses if patient continues to meet the aforementioned criteria.

Evaluation/observation
Obtain first salicylate level, noting time since ingestion occurred.

ASA detectable?

No

Recheck if within 2 hours of presentation. Discharge after 6 hours observation if patient remains asymptomatic and levels are nondetectable.

Yes

Recheck levels q2h until persistently within therapeutic range, trending down, or nondetectable. Routinely reassess for changes in clinical status and initiate treatment if indicated.

Obtain diagnostic studies.
Labs: salicylate level (note time since ingestion), ABG/VBG, basic electrolytes, BUN, creatinine, LFTs, coags, lactate, UA. Obtain tox screen if polysubstance overdose suspected.
Imaging: chest radiograph (to evaluate for pulmonary edema). Consider head CT for altered mental status to evaluate for cerebral edema or alternative causes of mental status changes.

Maintenance therapy and evaluation
1. Continue bicarbonate infusion to maintain urine output of 1–2 mL/kg/hr.
2. Measure urine pH hourly and titrate infusion to goal pH of 7.5–8.0.
3. Measure serum K hourly and replete if <4.5 mEq/L.
4. Measure ABG or VBG hourly and decrease rate of bicarbonate drip if serum pH exceeds 7.6.
5. Measure serum salicylate level q2h until salicylate level begins to decline and acid–base status is normal.

Presence of salicylate level >90 mg/dL, arterial pH <7.3, pulmonary or cerebral edema, renal failure, or has patient deteriorated?

No / *Yes*

Disposition
Treatment should be continued with frequent clinical assessment for improvement. Treatment and testing may be stopped ONLY when patient is asymptomatic, acid–base status is stable, AND salicylate level has fallen into therapeutic range (10–30 mg/dL).

Initiate hemodialysis.

Parvathi Perumareddi, DO

Juurlink DN, Gosselin S, Kielstein JT, et al; for EXTRIP Workgroup. Extracorporeal treatment for salicylate poisoning: systematic review and recommendations from the EXTRIP Workgroup. *Ann Emerg Med.* 2015;66(2):165–181.

SEIZURE, NEW ONSET

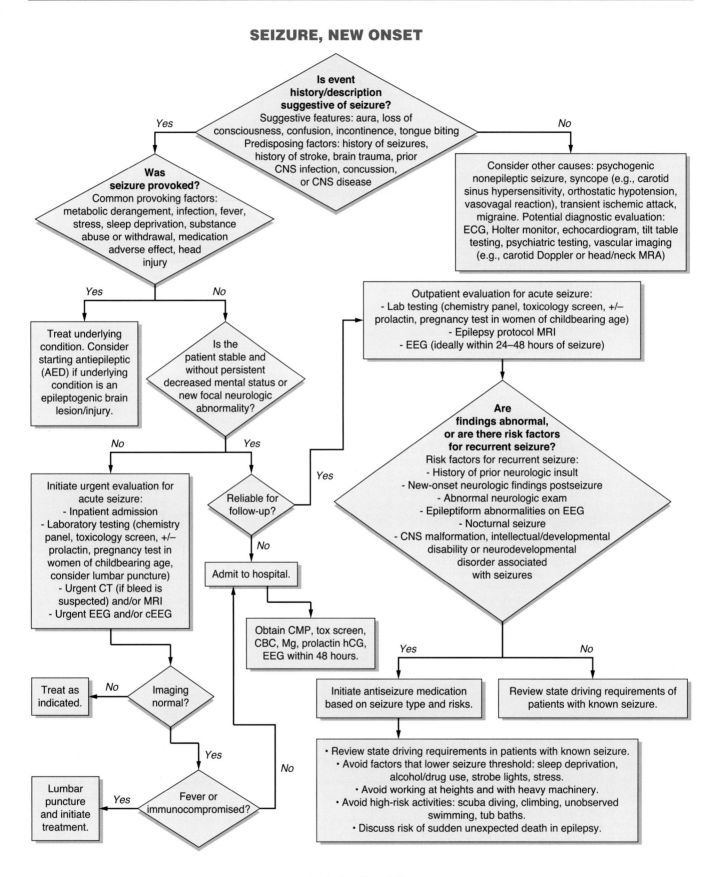

Is event history/description suggestive of seizure?
Suggestive features: aura, loss of consciousness, confusion, incontinence, tongue biting
Predisposing factors: history of seizures, history of stroke, brain trauma, prior CNS infection, concussion, or CNS disease

Yes → **Was seizure provoked?**
Common provoking factors: metabolic derangement, infection, fever, stress, sleep deprivation, substance abuse or withdrawal, medication adverse effect, head injury

No → Consider other causes: psychogenic nonepileptic seizure, syncope (e.g., carotid sinus hypersensitivity, orthostatic hypotension, vasovagal reaction), transient ischemic attack, migraine. Potential diagnostic evaluation: ECG, Holter monitor, echocardiogram, tilt table testing, psychiatric testing, vascular imaging (e.g., carotid Doppler or head/neck MRA)

Yes → Treat underlying condition. Consider starting antiepileptic (AED) if underlying condition is an epileptogenic brain lesion/injury.

No → **Is the patient stable and without persistent decreased mental status or new focal neurologic abnormality?**

Outpatient evaluation for acute seizure:
- Lab testing (chemistry panel, toxicology screen, +/– prolactin, pregnancy test in women of childbearing age)
- Epilepsy protocol MRI
- EEG (ideally within 24–48 hours of seizure)

No → Initiate urgent evaluation for acute seizure:
- Inpatient admission
- Laboratory testing (chemistry panel, toxicology screen, +/– prolactin, pregnancy test in women of childbearing age, consider lumbar puncture)
- Urgent CT (if bleed is suspected) and/or MRI
- Urgent EEG and/or cEEG

Yes → Reliable for follow-up?
Yes →
No → Admit to hospital.

Obtain CMP, tox screen, CBC, Mg, prolactin hCG, EEG within 48 hours.

Are findings abnormal, or are there risk factors for recurrent seizure?
Risk factors for recurrent seizure:
- History of prior neurologic insult
- New-onset neurologic findings postseizure
- Abnormal neurologic exam
- Epileptiform abnormalities on EEG
- Nocturnal seizure
- CNS malformation, intellectual/developmental disability or neurodevelopmental disorder associated with seizures

Yes → Initiate antiseizure medication based on seizure type and risks.

No → Review state driving requirements of patients with known seizure.

Treat as indicated. ← *No* — Imaging normal?
Yes →
Fever or immunocompromised? — *Yes* → Lumbar puncture and initiate treatment.
No →

- Review state driving requirements in patients with known seizure.
- Avoid factors that lower seizure threshold: sleep deprivation, alcohol/drug use, strobe lights, stress.
- Avoid working at heights and with heavy machinery.
- Avoid high-risk activities: scuba diving, climbing, unobserved swimming, tub baths.
- Discuss risk of sudden unexpected death in epilepsy.

Judy Lu Kim, MD

Gavvla JR, Schuele SU. New-onset seizure in adults and adolescents: a new review. *JAMA.* 2016;316(24):2657–2668.

SHOULDER PAIN, TREATMENT

Analgesics, NSAIDs, ice, activity modification

Positive apprehension testing—glenohumeral instability

OA

PT

IACS

Surgical evaluation if refractory

Anterior dislocation

X-ray if first time and available

Reduce if negative fracture.

Pain with shoulder active and passive ROM—adhesive capsulitis

Refer to PT. Consider IA CS injection.

Symptoms may take up to 1.5 years to resolve.

If not improving, consider:
– Repeat GH CS injection
– Distention
– Manipulation under anesthesia
– Surgical release
– ESWT

Acromioclavicular

OA

PT

IA CS

Surgical evaluation if refractory

Sprain/separation

Immobilization for comfort

I   II   III   IV–VI

2–3 days   4–6 weeks

Conservative treatment

Surgical repair

Pain with empty can and/or Hawkins testing—impingement syndrome

PT
CS
OMT
acupuncture

Surgery evaluation after 3 months if refractory

Rotator cuff

Myofascial or TrP

PT

Dry needling
TrP injection
OMT
Massage
Myofascial release
Acupuncture

Humeral Clavicle Scapula Fracture

Pain management Fracture management

Tendinopathy

PT
Consider PRP in first 3 months.
Acupuncture
TENS

SA or SD bursitis; CS

Surgical evaluation if refractory

Labral tear

PT

Tear

Partial   Complete

Consider early surgery if young and acute.

PT, NSAIDs, SA , CS, DPT, PRP

Surgical consult if:
– Not improving
– Disabling

Abbreviations:
NSAIDs, nonsteroidal anti-inflammatory drugs; TrP, trigger point; GH, glenohumeral; PT, physical therapy plus home exercise plan; OA, osteoarthritis; IA, intra-articular; CS, corticosteroid; OMT, osteopathic manipulative therapy; SA, subacromial; SD, subdeltoid; DPT, dextrose prolotherapy; PRP, platelet-rich plasma; TENS, transcutaneous electrical nerve stimulation; ESWT, extracorporeal shock wave therapy

Justin J. Chin, DO, Krystyna Guinevere Golden, MD, and Nolan P. Feola, MD

Greenberg DL. Evaluation and treatment of shoulder pain. *Med Clin N Am*. 2014;98(3):487–504.

SICKLE CELL ANEMIA, ACUTE, EVALUATION AND MANAGEMENT

This algorithm is meant to assist clinicians in the workup and management of common complications of sickle cell disease. It should not replace a physician's clinical judgment or be considered a standardized protocol for all patients.

Known Sickle Cell Patient (Part I of II)

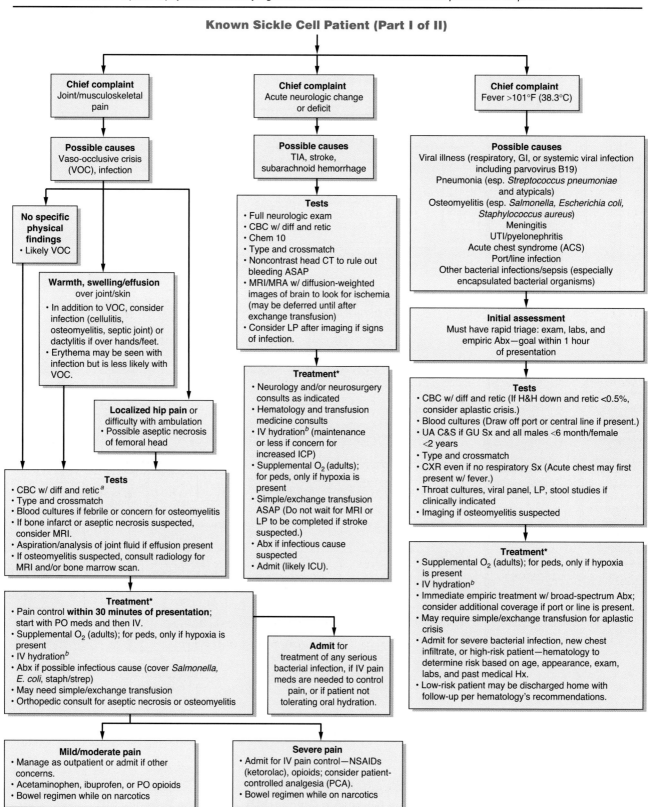

Chief complaint
Joint/musculoskeletal pain

Possible causes
Vaso-occlusive crisis (VOC), infection

No specific physical findings
• Likely VOC

Warmth, swelling/effusion over joint/skin
• In addition to VOC, consider infection (cellulitis, osteomyelitis, septic joint) or dactylitis if over hands/feet.
• Erythema may be seen with infection but is less likely with VOC.

Localized hip pain or difficulty with ambulation
• Possible aseptic necrosis of femoral head

Tests
• CBC w/ diff and retic [a]
• Type and crossmatch
• Blood cultures if febrile or concern for osteomyelitis
• If bone infarct or aseptic necrosis suspected, consider MRI.
• Aspiration/analysis of joint fluid if effusion present
• If osteomyelitis suspected, consult radiology for MRI and/or bone marrow scan.

Treatment*
• Pain control **within 30 minutes of presentation**; start with PO meds and then IV.
• Supplemental O_2 (adults); for peds, only if hypoxia is present
• IV hydration [b]
• Abx if possible infectious cause (cover *Salmonella, E. coli*, staph/strep)
• May need simple/exchange transfusion
• Orthopedic consult for aseptic necrosis or osteomyelitis

Mild/moderate pain
• Manage as outpatient or admit if other concerns.
• Acetaminophen, ibuprofen, or PO opioids
• Bowel regimen while on narcotics

Severe pain
• Admit for IV pain control—NSAIDs (ketorolac), opioids; consider patient-controlled analgesia (PCA).
• Bowel regimen while on narcotics

Chief complaint
Acute neurologic change or deficit

Possible causes
TIA, stroke, subarachnoid hemorrhage

Tests
• Full neurologic exam
• CBC w/ diff and retic
• Chem 10
• Type and crossmatch
• Noncontrast head CT to rule out bleeding ASAP
• MRI/MRA w/ diffusion-weighted images of brain to look for ischemia (may be deferred until after exchange transfusion)
• Consider LP after imaging if signs of infection.

Treatment*
• Neurology and/or neurosurgery consults as indicated
• Hematology and transfusion medicine consults
• IV hydration [b] (maintenance or less if concern for increased ICP)
• Supplemental O_2 (adults); for peds, only if hypoxia is present
• Simple/exchange transfusion ASAP (Do not wait for MRI or LP to be completed if stroke suspected.)
• Abx if infectious cause suspected
• Admit (likely ICU).

Admit for treatment of any serious bacterial infection, if IV pain meds are needed to control pain, or if patient not tolerating oral hydration.

Chief complaint
Fever >101°F (38.3°C)

Possible causes
Viral illness (respiratory, GI, or systemic viral infection including parvovirus B19)
Pneumonia (esp. *Streptococcus pneumoniae* and atypicals)
Osteomyelitis (esp. *Salmonella, Escherichia coli, Staphylococcus aureus*)
Meningitis
UTI/pyelonephritis
Acute chest syndrome (ACS)
Port/line infection
Other bacterial infections/sepsis (especially encapsulated bacterial organisms)

Initial assessment
Must have rapid triage: exam, labs, and empiric Abx—goal within 1 hour of presentation

Tests
• CBC w/ diff and retic (If H&H down and retic <0.5%, consider aplastic crisis.)
• Blood cultures (Draw off port or central line if present.)
• UA C&S if GU Sx and all males <6 month/female <2 years
• Type and crossmatch
• CXR even if no respiratory Sx (Acute chest may first present w/ fever.)
• Throat cultures, viral panel, LP, stool studies if clinically indicated
• Imaging if osteomyelitis suspected

Treatment*
• Supplemental O_2 (adults); for peds, only if hypoxia is present
• IV hydration [b]
• Immediate empiric treatment w/ broad-spectrum Abx; consider additional coverage if port or line is present.
• May require simple/exchange transfusion for aplastic crisis
• Admit for severe bacterial infection, new chest infiltrate, or high-risk patient—hematology to determine risk based on age, appearance, exam, labs, and past medical Hx.
• Low-risk patient may be discharged home with follow-up per hematology's recommendations.

Known Sickle Cell Patient (Part II of II)

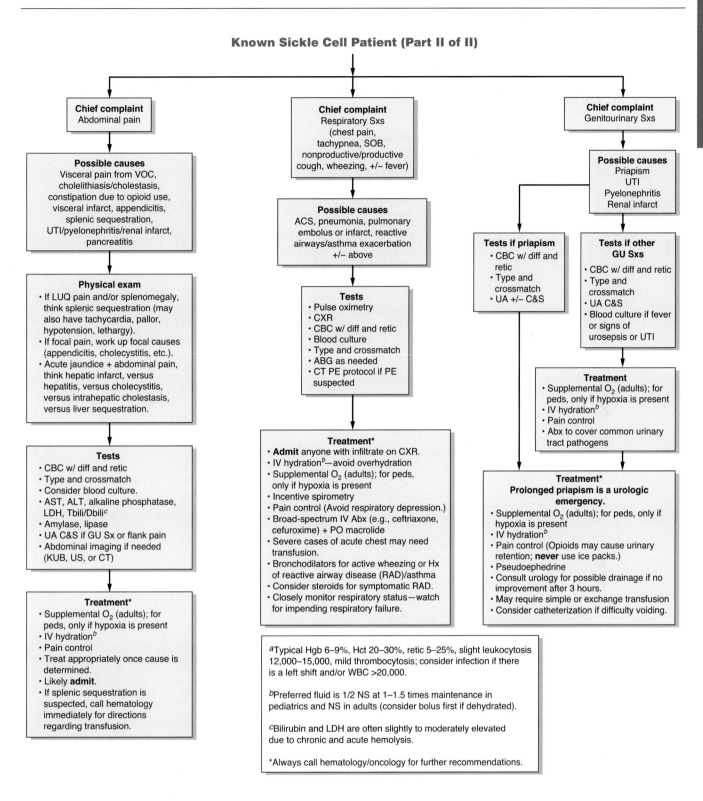

Chief complaint
Abdominal pain

Possible causes
Visceral pain from VOC, cholelithiasis/cholestasis, constipation due to opioid use, visceral infarct, appendicitis, splenic sequestration, UTI/pyelonephritis/renal infarct, pancreatitis

Physical exam
- If LUQ pain and/or splenomegaly, think splenic sequestration (may also have tachycardia, pallor, hypotension, lethargy).
- If focal pain, work up focal causes (appendicitis, cholecystitis, etc.).
- Acute jaundice + abdominal pain, think hepatic infarct, versus hepatitis, versus cholecystitis, versus intrahepatic cholestasis, versus liver sequestration.

Tests
- CBC w/ diff and retic
- Type and crossmatch
- Consider blood culture.
- AST, ALT, alkaline phosphatase, LDH, Tbili/Dbili[c]
- Amylase, lipase
- UA C&S if GU Sx or flank pain
- Abdominal imaging if needed (KUB, US, or CT)

Treatment*
- Supplemental O_2 (adults); for peds, only if hypoxia is present
- IV hydration[b]
- Pain control
- Treat appropriately once cause is determined.
- Likely **admit**.
- If splenic sequestration is suspected, call hematology immediately for directions regarding transfusion.

Chief complaint
Respiratory Sxs (chest pain, tachypnea, SOB, nonproductive/productive cough, wheezing, +/– fever)

Possible causes
ACS, pneumonia, pulmonary embolus or infarct, reactive airways/asthma exacerbation +/– above

Tests
- Pulse oximetry
- CXR
- CBC w/ diff and retic
- Blood culture
- Type and crossmatch
- ABG as needed
- CT PE protocol if PE suspected

Treatment*
- **Admit** anyone with infiltrate on CXR.
- IV hydration[b]—avoid overhydration
- Supplemental O_2 (adults); for peds, only if hypoxia is present
- Incentive spirometry
- Pain control (Avoid respiratory depression.)
- Broad-spectrum IV Abx (e.g., ceftriaxone, cefuroxime) + PO macrolide
- Severe cases of acute chest may need transfusion.
- Bronchodilators for active wheezing or Hx of reactive airway disease (RAD)/asthma
- Consider steroids for symptomatic RAD.
- Closely monitor respiratory status—watch for impending respiratory failure.

Chief complaint
Genitourinary Sxs

Possible causes
Priapism
UTI
Pyelonephritis
Renal infarct

Tests if priapism
- CBC w/ diff and retic
- Type and crossmatch
- UA +/– C&S

Tests if other GU Sxs
- CBC w/ diff and retic
- Type and crossmatch
- UA C&S
- Blood culture if fever or signs of urosepsis or UTI

Treatment
- Supplemental O_2 (adults); for peds, only if hypoxia is present
- IV hydration[b]
- Pain control
- Abx to cover common urinary tract pathogens

Treatment*
Prolonged priapism is a urologic emergency.
- Supplemental O_2 (adults); for peds, only if hypoxia is present
- IV hydration[b]
- Pain control (Opioids may cause urinary retention; **never** use ice packs.)
- Pseudoephedrine
- Consult urology for possible drainage if no improvement after 3 hours.
- May require simple or exchange transfusion.
- Consider catheterization if difficulty voiding.

[a]Typical Hgb 6–9%, Hct 20–30%, retic 5–25%, slight leukocytosis 12,000–15,000, mild thrombocytosis; consider infection if there is a left shift and/or WBC >20,000.

[b]Preferred fluid is 1/2 NS at 1–1.5 times maintenance in pediatrics and NS in adults (consider bolus first if dehydrated).

[c]Bilirubin and LDH are often slightly to moderately elevated due to chronic and acute hemolysis.

*Always call hematology/oncology for further recommendations.

Paul E. Daniel Jr., MD

National Heart, Lung, and Blood Institute. Evidence-based management of sickle cell disease: expert panel report, 2014. https://www.nhlbi.nih.gov/health-topics/evidence-based-management-sickle-cell-disease. Published September 2014. Accessed January 31, 2021.

SUICIDE, EVALUATING RISK FOR

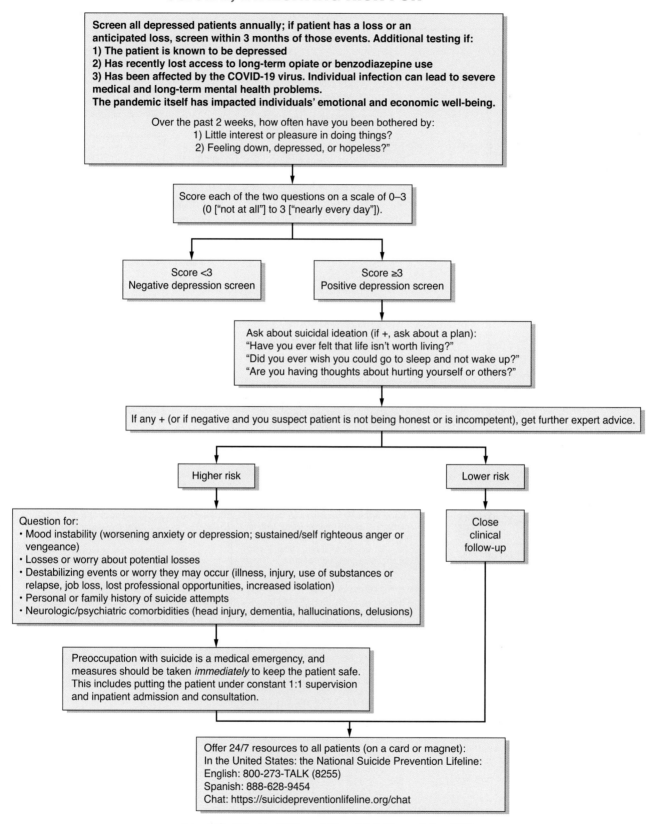

Screen all depressed patients annually; if patient has a loss or an anticipated loss, screen within 3 months of those events. Additional testing if:
1) The patient is known to be depressed
2) Has recently lost access to long-term opiate or benzodiazepine use
3) Has been affected by the COVID-19 virus. Individual infection can lead to severe medical and long-term mental health problems.
The pandemic itself has impacted individuals' emotional and economic well-being.

Over the past 2 weeks, how often have you been bothered by:
1) Little interest or pleasure in doing things?
2) Feeling down, depressed, or hopeless?"

Score each of the two questions on a scale of 0–3
(0 ["not at all"] to 3 ["nearly every day"]).

Score <3
Negative depression screen

Score ≥3
Positive depression screen

Ask about suicidal ideation (if +, ask about a plan):
"Have you ever felt that life isn't worth living?"
"Did you ever wish you could go to sleep and not wake up?"
"Are you having thoughts about hurting yourself or others?"

If any + (or if negative and you suspect patient is not being honest or is incompetent), get further expert advice.

Higher risk

Lower risk

Question for:
• Mood instability (worsening anxiety or depression; sustained/self righteous anger or vengeance)
• Losses or worry about potential losses
• Destabilizing events or worry they may occur (illness, injury, use of substances or relapse, job loss, lost professional opportunities, increased isolation)
• Personal or family history of suicide attempts
• Neurologic/psychiatric comorbidities (head injury, dementia, hallucinations, delusions)

Close clinical follow-up

Preoccupation with suicide is a medical emergency, and measures should be taken *immediately* to keep the patient safe. This includes putting the patient under constant 1:1 supervision and inpatient admission and consultation.

Offer 24/7 resources to all patients (on a card or magnet):
In the United States: the National Suicide Prevention Lifeline:
English: 800-273-TALK (8255)
Spanish: 888-628-9454
Chat: https://suicidepreventionlifeline.org/chat

Irene Coletsos, MD and Harold J. Bursztajn, MD

Posner K, Oquendo MA, Gould M, et al. Columbia Classification Algorithm of Suicide Assessment (C-CASA): classification of suicidal events in the FDA's pediatric suicidal risk analysis of antidepressants. *Am J Psychiatry.* 2007;164(7):1035–1043.

SYNCOPE

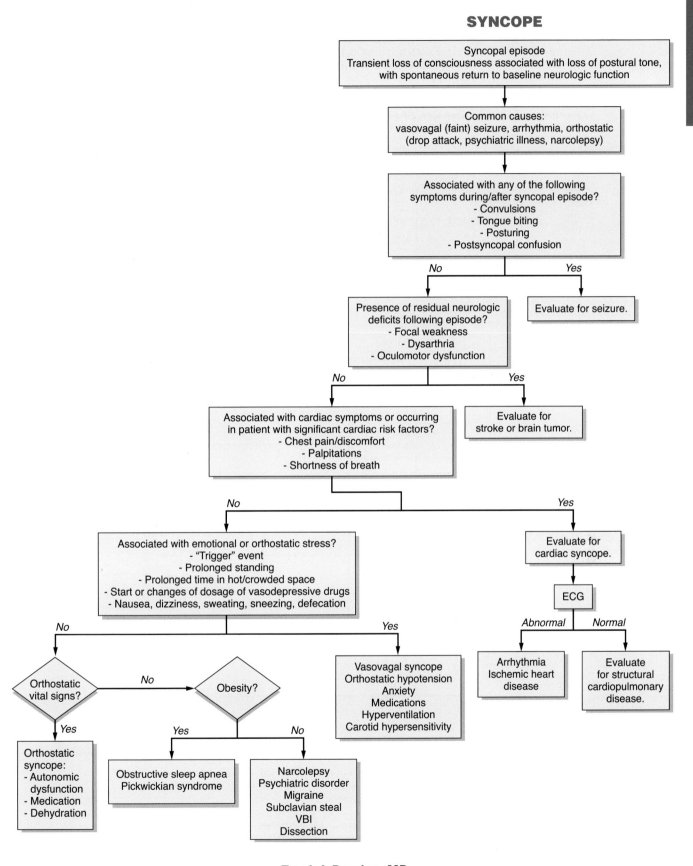

Syncopal episode
Transient loss of consciousness associated with loss of postural tone, with spontaneous return to baseline neurologic function

Common causes:
vasovagal (faint) seizure, arrhythmia, orthostatic (drop attack, psychiatric illness, narcolepsy)

Associated with any of the following symptoms during/after syncopal episode?
- Convulsions
- Tongue biting
- Posturing
- Postsyncopal confusion

No → Presence of residual neurologic deficits following episode?
- Focal weakness
- Dysarthria
- Oculomotor dysfunction

Yes → Evaluate for seizure.

Presence of residual neurologic deficits following episode?
No → Associated with cardiac symptoms or occurring in patient with significant cardiac risk factors?
- Chest pain/discomfort
- Palpitations
- Shortness of breath

Yes → Evaluate for stroke or brain tumor.

Associated with cardiac symptoms...
No → Associated with emotional or orthostatic stress?
- "Trigger" event
- Prolonged standing
- Prolonged time in hot/crowded space
- Start or changes of dosage of vasodepressive drugs
- Nausea, dizziness, sweating, sneezing, defecation

Yes → Evaluate for cardiac syncope.
→ ECG
Abnormal → Arrhythmia Ischemic heart disease
Normal → Evaluate for structural cardiopulmonary disease.

Associated with emotional or orthostatic stress?
No → Orthostatic vital signs?
Yes → Vasovagal syncope
Orthostatic hypotension
Anxiety
Medications
Hyperventilation
Carotid hypersensitivity

Orthostatic vital signs?
No → Obesity?
Yes → Orthostatic syncope:
- Autonomic dysfunction
- Medication
- Dehydration

Obesity?
Yes → Obstructive sleep apnea
Pickwickian syndrome
No → Narcolepsy
Psychiatric disorder
Migraine
Subclavian steal
VBI
Dissection

Frank J. Domino, MD

Runser LA, Gauer RL, Houser A. Syncope: evaluation and differential diagnosis. *Am Fam Physician.* 2017;95(5):303–312.

THROMBOCYTOPENIA

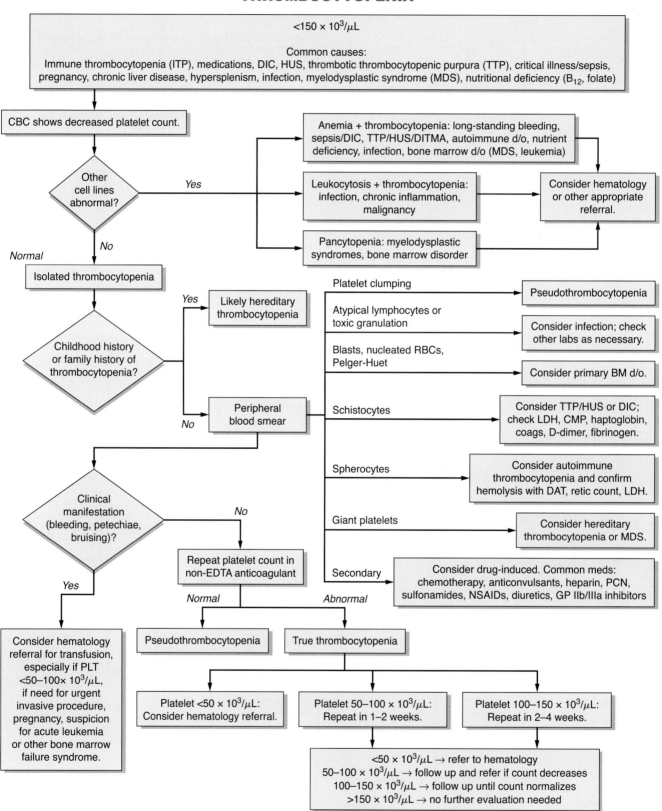

$<150 \times 10^3/\mu L$

Common causes:
Immune thrombocytopenia (ITP), medications, DIC, HUS, thrombotic thrombocytopenic purpura (TTP), critical illness/sepsis, pregnancy, chronic liver disease, hypersplenism, infection, myelodysplastic syndrome (MDS), nutritional deficiency (B_{12}, folate)

CBC shows decreased platelet count.

Other cell lines abnormal?

Yes

Anemia + thrombocytopenia: long-standing bleeding, sepsis/DIC, TTP/HUS/DITMA, autoimmune d/o, nutrient deficiency, infection, bone marrow d/o (MDS, leukemia)

Leukocytosis + thrombocytopenia: infection, chronic inflammation, malignancy

Pancytopenia: myelodysplastic syndromes, bone marrow disorder

Consider hematology or other appropriate referral.

Normal

No

Isolated thrombocytopenia

Childhood history or family history of thrombocytopenia?

Yes

Likely hereditary thrombocytopenia

No

Peripheral blood smear

Platelet clumping → Pseudothrombocytopenia

Atypical lymphocytes or toxic granulation → Consider infection; check other labs as necessary.

Blasts, nucleated RBCs, Pelger-Huet → Consider primary BM d/o.

Schistocytes → Consider TTP/HUS or DIC; check LDH, CMP, haptoglobin, coags, D-dimer, fibrinogen.

Spherocytes → Consider autoimmune thrombocytopenia and confirm hemolysis with DAT, retic count, LDH.

Giant platelets → Consider hereditary thrombocytopenia or MDS.

Secondary → Consider drug-induced. Common meds: chemotherapy, anticonvulsants, heparin, PCN, sulfonamides, NSAIDs, diuretics, GP IIb/IIIa inhibitors

Clinical manifestation (bleeding, petechiae, bruising)?

No

Repeat platelet count in non-EDTA anticoagulant

Yes

Consider hematology referral for transfusion, especially if PLT <50–$100 \times 10^3/\mu L$, if need for urgent invasive procedure, pregnancy, suspicion for acute leukemia or other bone marrow failure syndrome.

Normal

Pseudothrombocytopenia

Abnormal

True thrombocytopenia

Platelet $<50 \times 10^3/\mu L$: Consider hematology referral.

Platelet 50–$100 \times 10^3/\mu L$: Repeat in 1–2 weeks.

Platelet 100–$150 \times 10^3/\mu L$: Repeat in 2–4 weeks.

$<50 \times 10^3/\mu L \rightarrow$ refer to hematology
50–$100 \times 10^3/\mu L \rightarrow$ follow up and refer if count decreases
100–$150 \times 10^3/\mu L \rightarrow$ follow up until count normalizes
$>150 \times 10^3/\mu L \rightarrow$ no further evaluation needed

Jillian Joseph, MPAS, PA-C and Allison Hargreaves, MD

Gauer RL, Braun MM. Thrombocytopenia. *Am Fam Physician*. 2012;85(6):612–666.

TINNITUS

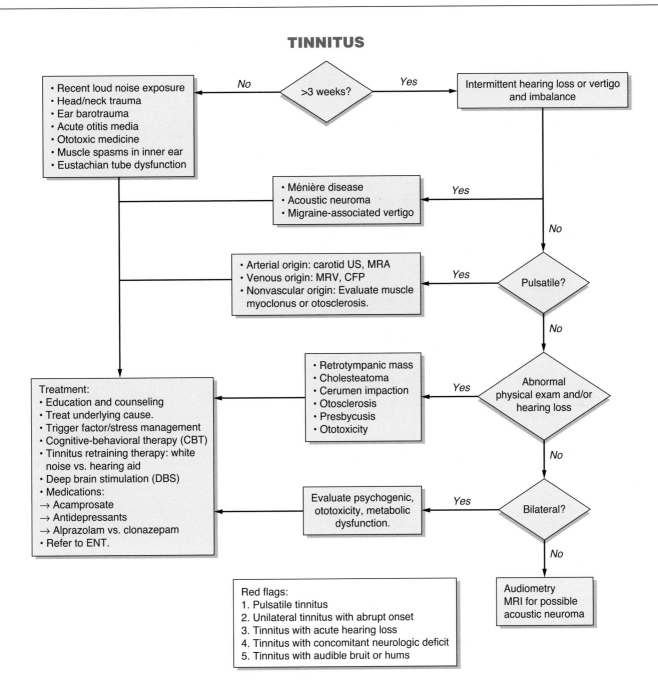

Red flags:
1. Pulsatile tinnitus
2. Unilateral tinnitus with abrupt onset
3. Tinnitus with acute hearing loss
4. Tinnitus with concomitant neurologic deficit
5. Tinnitus with audible bruit or hums

Dongsheng Jiang, MD, MSc and Juan Qiu, MD, PhD

Han BI, Lee HW, Ryu S, et al. Tinnitus update. *J Clin Neurol.* 2021;17(1):1–10.

TRANSIENT ISCHEMIC ATTACK AND TRANSIENT NEUROLOGIC DEFECTS

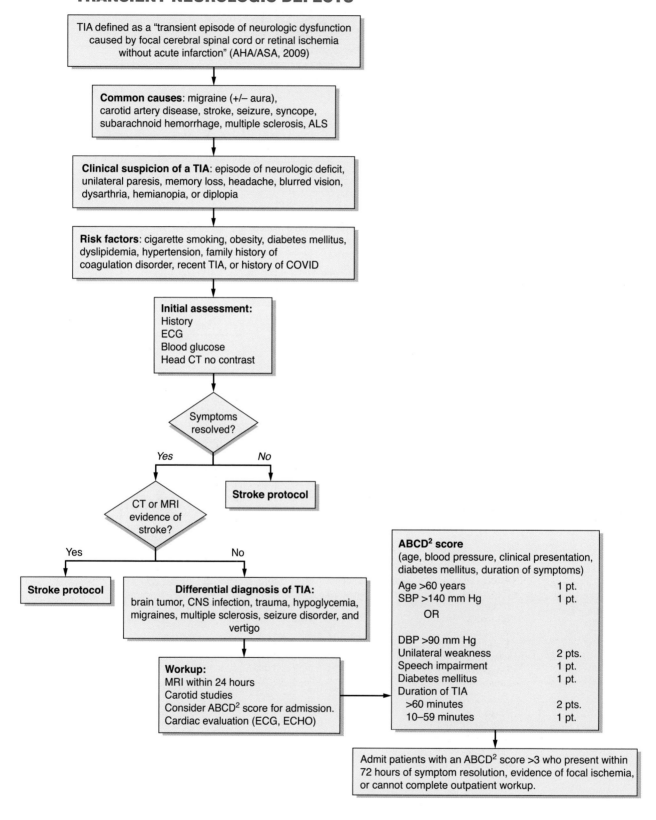

Saadia Mohsin, MD

Simmons BB, Cirignano B, Gadegbeku AB. Transient ischemic attack: part I. Diagnosis and evaluation. *Am Fam Physician*. 2012;86(6):521–526.

TREMOR

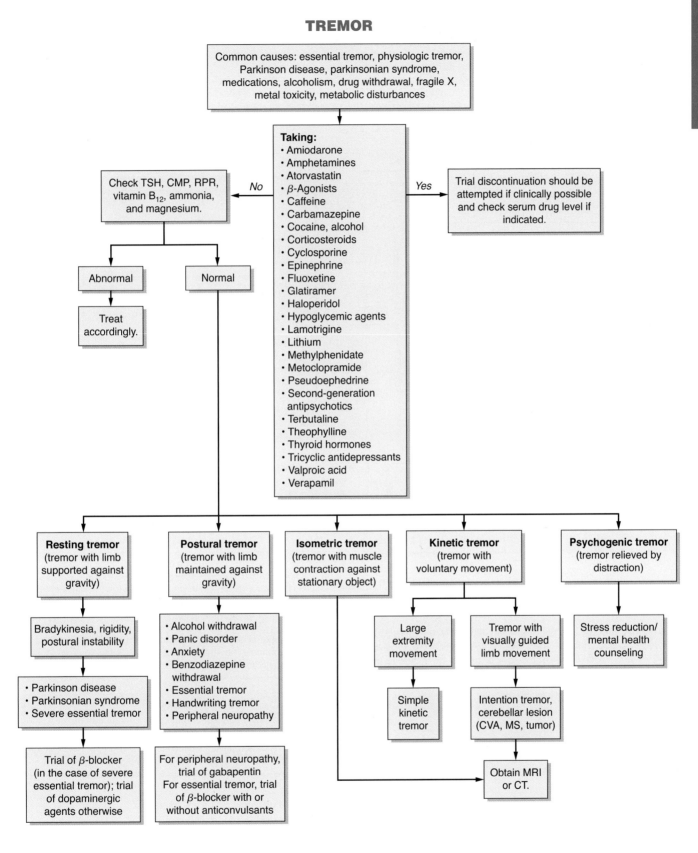

Marni Klessman Gleiber, MD

Crawford P, Zimmerman EE. Tremor: sorting through the differential diagnosis. *Am Fam Physician*. 2018;97(3):180–186.

TYPE 2 DIABETES, TREATMENT

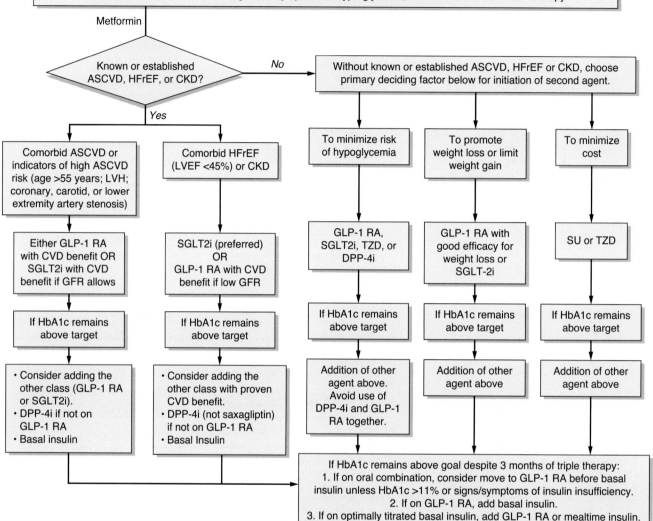

First-line therapy comprehensive lifestyle changes (including weight management and physical activity)
If HbA1c remains above goal, proceed below.
If initial HbA1c ≥8.5% or 1.5% above HbA1c target, can consider initiation of dual therapy (metformin + second agent)
If initial HbA1c ≥10%, BG >300 mg/dL, or symptoms of hyperglycemia, can consider basal insulin therapy

Metformin

Known or established ASCVD, HFrEF, or CKD?

No → Without known or established ASCVD, HFrEF or CKD, choose primary deciding factor below for initiation of second agent.

Yes

Comorbid ASCVD or indicators of high ASCVD risk (age >55 years; LVH; coronary, carotid, or lower extremity artery stenosis)

Comorbid HFrEF (LVEF <45%) or CKD

To minimize risk of hypoglycemia

To promote weight loss or limit weight gain

To minimize cost

Either GLP-1 RA with CVD benefit OR SGLT2i with CVD benefit if GFR allows

SGLT2i (preferred) OR GLP-1 RA with CVD benefit if low GFR

GLP-1 RA, SGLT2i, TZD, or DPP-4i

GLP-1 RA with good efficacy for weight loss or SGLT-2i

SU or TZD

If HbA1c remains above target

If HbA1c remains above target

If HbA1c remains above target

If HbA1c remains above target

If HbA1c remains above target

- Consider adding the other class (GLP-1 RA or SGLT2i).
- DPP-4i if not on GLP-1 RA
- Basal insulin

- Consider adding the other class with proven CVD benefit.
- DPP-4i (not saxagliptin) if not on GLP-1 RA
- Basal Insulin

Addition of other agent above. Avoid use of DPP-4i and GLP-1 RA together.

Addition of other agent above

Addition of other agent above

If HbA1c remains above goal despite 3 months of triple therapy:
1. If on oral combination, consider move to GLP-1 RA before basal insulin unless HbA1c >11% or signs/symptoms of insulin insufficiency.
2. If on GLP-1 RA, add basal insulin.
3. If on optimally titrated basal insulin, add GLP-1 RA or mealtime insulin.

Metformin therapy should be maintained, if indicated, whereas other oral agents may be discontinued on an individual basis to avoid unnecessarily complex or costly regimens, side effects, and hypoglycemia.

GLP-1 RA: with CVD benefit: liraglutide, semaglutide, dulaglutide; with greatest weight loss benefit: semaglutide, liraglutide, and dulaglutide
SGLT2i with CVD benefit: empaglifozin, canagliflozin, and dapagliflozin; requires renal dose adjustment
DPP-4i: linagliptin, saxagliptin, or sitagliptin; saxagliptin associated with increased risk of heart failure admissions
TZD: pioglitazone
SU: glimepiride, glyburide or glipizide
Basal (long-acting) insulin: insulin glargine, insulin detemir, insulin degludec. Start at 10 U or 0.1–0.2 U/kg/day SQ.

Glycemic Goals
- An HbA1c goal for newly diagnosed, nonpregnant adults with no comorbidities is <7%.
- If older age, multiple comorbidities, limited life expectancy, or high risk for hypoglycemia, higher HbA1c goals (such as <8%) may be appropriate.

Christine Chan, MD

American Diabetes Association. 12. Older adults: *Standards of Medical Care in Diabetes—2021. Diabetes Care.* 2021;44(Suppl 1):S168–S179.

VAGINAL BLEEDING, ABNORMAL

Common causes:
PCOS, hypothyroid, uterine
hyperplasia, pituitary adenoma
PALM-COEIN

PALM-COEIN
Structural: polyp, adenomyosis,
leiomyoma, malignancy, and
hyperplasia
Nonstructural: coagulopathy,
ovulatory dysfunction,
endometrial, iatrogenic, not
otherwise classified

History and physical exam,
including pelvic exam

Prepubescent

Consider CBC, pelvic US,
genital cultures, tumor markers,
and child abuse referral.

Reproductive age

Pap, hCG; consider genital cultures,
CBC, PT/INR, von Willebrand (vWF) antigen,
ristocetin cofactor, iatrogenic causes.

Postmenopausal

Pap, TVUS, endometrial
biopsy, TSH, prolactin,
genital cultures

GYN referral

Not pregnant; tests normal

Ovulatory dysfunction for >3 months

Adult

Age ≥45
years?

Yes

TVUS, prolactin,
endometrial biopsy

Normal results

Refer GYN

Abnormal results

Treat or refer.

No

Low BMI?

Yes

Refer/treat for
anorexia nervosa.

No

TSH, prolactin;
testosterone if hirsute

Adolescent

<3 years from menarche

Yes

Reassurance/
combination
contraceptive

Results normal, age
<45 years and without
risk for hyperplasia

Reassurance, treat
with hormones

Persistent
abnormal bleeding
despite treatment

US or EMB

Normal results,
age >45 years or high
risk for hyperplasia

Endometrial biopsy
and/or pelvic US

Normal results

Regulate with
hormones.

Abnormal results

Treat underlying condition or refer.

Abnormal results

Veronica Farrell, MSN, NP-C and Frank J. Domino, MD

Wouk N, Helton M. Abnormal uterine bleeding in premenopausal women. *Am Fam Physician.* 2019;99(7):435–443.

VITAMIN D DEFICIENCY

Risk factors/common causes:

- Age >65 years
- Insufficient sunlight exposure (homebound, veiled)
- Renal disease
- Liver disease
- Depression

- Dark skin
- Insufficient dietary intake
- GI malabsorption
- Obesity (BMI >30)
- Immigrants to colder climates
- Chronic use of glucocorticoids
- Periosteal bone pain (e.g., sternum, tibia)

- GI malabsorption (celiac, cystic fibrosis, inflammatory bowel disease)
- Pregnancy
- Medications: anticonvulsants, antiretroviral, and glucocorticoids
- Gastrectomy or extensive bowel surgery

Significant risk factors?

No → Low suspicion for vitamin D deficiency

Yes

Requirements:
<1 year old: 400 IU/day
>1 year old: 600 IU/day
To reach levels >30 ng/mL, may require 1,000 IU/day
Obese children: 2–3 times more vitamin D for their age group
Maintenance dose:
0–6 months: 1,000–2,000 IU/day
6 months–1 year: 1,500–2,000 IU/day
1–3 years: 2,500–3,000 IU/day
4–8 years: 3,000 IU/day
>8 years: 2,000 IU/day
Vitamin D deficiency:
0–1 year: 2,000 IU/day for 6 weeks or 50,000 IU weekly for 6 weeks followed by maintenance 400–1,000 IU/day
1–18 years: 2,000 IU/day for 6 weeks or 50,000 IU weekly for 6 weeks followed by maintenance 600–1,000 IU/day

Yes ← **Age <18 years?** → No

Lab: serum 25-hydroxyvitamin D concentration

Level <20 ng/mL (vitamin D deficiency)

Level <21–29 ng/mL (vitamin D insufficiency)

Level >30 ng/mL normal

Treatment

Treatment

Maintenance

Start 50,000 IU vitamin D_2 once a week for 8–12 weeks and then begin 2,000–3,000 IU vitamin D per day.

2,000–4,000 IU vitamin D per day

Supplement with 600–2,000 IU of vitamin D per day.

After 6 months, consider repeating serum 25-hydroxyvitamin D level.

Recheck serum 25-hydroxyvitamin D concentration.

Level <20 ng/mL? → No

Yes

Consult endocrinology if no malabsorptive disease.

Nighat Seema Ahmed, MD

Holick MF, Binkley NC, Bischoff-Ferrari HA, et al. Evaluation, treatment, and prevention of vitamin D deficiency: an Endocrine Society clinical practice guideline. *J Clin Endocrinol Metab*. 2011;96(7):1911–1930.

WEIGHT LOSS, UNINTENTIONAL

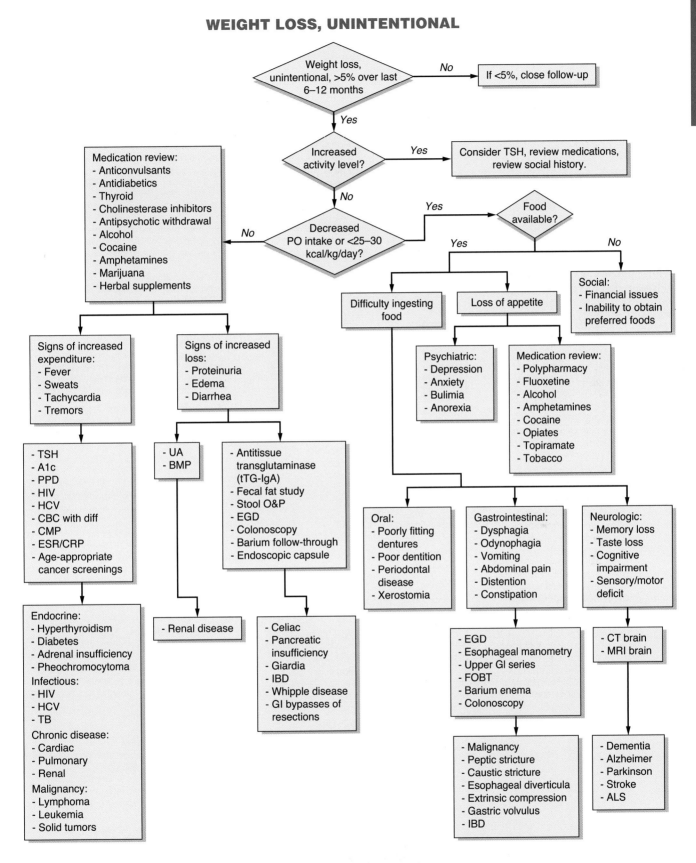

Megan Gibson, MD and Shivani Malhotra, MD, FAAFP

Gaddey HL, Holder K. Unintentional weight loss in older adults. *Am Fam Physician*. 2014;89(9):718–722.

ABNORMAL (DYSFUNCTIONAL) UTERINE BLEEDING

Rebecca A. Lauters, MD • Kyle D. Olsen, DO

BASICS

DESCRIPTION
- Abnormal uterine bleeding (AUB) is irregular uterine bleeding (heavy, prolonged, or frequent menstrual-like bleeding).
- May be acute or chronic (occurring >6 months)
- The International Federation of Gynecology and Obstetrics (FIGO) now uses AUB rather than dysfunctional uterine bleeding (DUB).

EPIDEMIOLOGY
Adolescent and perimenopausal women are affected most often.

Incidence
5% of reproductive-aged women will see a doctor in any given year for AUB.

Prevalence
3–30% of reproductive-aged women have AUB.

ETIOLOGY AND PATHOPHYSIOLOGY
- Anovulation accounts for 90% of AUB.
- Adolescent AUB is usually due to an immature hypothalamic-pituitary-ovarian (HPO) axis that leads to anovulatory cycles.
- The mnemonic PALM-COEIN was developed to describe AUB in reproductive aged women.
- PALM (structural causes): Polyp, Adenomyosis, Leiomyoma, and Malignancy and/or hyperplasia
- COEIN (nonstructural causes): Coagulopathy, Ovulatory disorders, Endometrial, Iatrogenic and Not yet classified
  - Coagulopathy
    ○ 20% of patients with heavy menstrual bleeding have a bleeding disorder.
    ○ Two most common: von Willebrand disease and thrombocytopenia
  - Diseases causing ovulatory dysfunction
    ○ Hyperparathyroidism, hypothyroidism, adrenal disorders, pituitary disease (prolactinoma), PCOS, eating disorders
  - Medications (iatrogenic causes)
    ○ Anticoagulants, steroids, tamoxifen (estrogen receptor antagonists), hormonal contraception, copper IUD, antipsychotic medications (mostly first generation), postmenopausal hormone replacement therapy, antiemetics (metoclopramide and domperidone specifically)
  - Other causes of AUB not defined in PALM-COEIN
    ○ Ectopic pregnancy, threatened or incomplete abortion or hydatidiform mole, upper genital tract infections, advanced or fulminant liver disease, chronic renal disease, nutritional deficiencies, inflammatory bowel disease, excessive weight gain, increased exercise

Genetics
Unclear but can include inherited disorders of hemostasis

RISK FACTORS
- Unopposed estrogen therapy (no. 1 risk factor for endometrial cancer)
- Increasing age, typically >40 years old; obesity; PCOS; diabetes mellitus; nulliparity; early menarche or late menopause (>55 years of age); chronic anovulation or infertility; history of breast cancer or endometrial hyperplasia; tamoxifen use; family history: gynecologic, breast, or colon cancer; thyroid disease

GENERAL PREVENTION
No direct preventive measure for AUB

COMMONLY ASSOCIATED CONDITIONS
Endometrial polyps, adenomyosis, leiomyoma, endometrial cancer, coagulopathy, PCOS, thyroid disorders, starvation (eating disorders), hyperprolactinemia, ovarian follicle decline (perimenopause), pregnancy, endometriosis

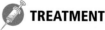
DIAGNOSIS

HISTORY
- Menstrual history
  - Onset, severity (quantified by pad/tampon use, presence and size of clots), timing of bleeding (unpredictable or episodic) over the last 6 months; also assess menopausal status.
- Association with other factors (e.g., coitus, contraception, weight loss/gain)
- Gynecologic history: gravidity and parity, STI history, previous Pap smear results
- Review of systems (Exclude symptoms of pregnancy, bleeding disorders, stress, exercise, recent weight change, visual changes, headaches, galactorrhea.)

ALERT
Postmenopausal bleeding is any bleeding that occurs >1 year after the last menstrual period; cancer must always be ruled out (1)[C].

PHYSICAL EXAM
Evaluate for:
- Body mass index, pallor, vital signs, visual field defects (pituitary lesion), vaginal discharge, hirsutism or acne, goiter, galactorrhea, purpura, ecchymosis
- Pelvic exam
  - Uterine irregularities and Tanner stage, foreign bodies, rule out rectal or urinary tract bleeding, include Pap smear and tests for STIs (1)[C]

Pediatric Considerations
Premenarchal children with vaginal bleeding should be evaluated for foreign bodies, physical/sexual abuse, possible infections, and signs of precocious puberty.

DIFFERENTIAL DIAGNOSIS
See "Etiology and Pathophysiology."

DIAGNOSTIC TESTS & INTERPRETATION
Initial Tests (lab, imaging)
- All patients: urine hCG and CBC
  - For acute heavy/hemorrhagic bleeding, a type and cross should be obtained.
- If disorder of hemostasis suspected, a partial thromboplastin time (PTT), prothrombin time (PT), activated partial thromboplastin time (aPTT), and fibrinogen level; if abnormal, get von Willebrand factor, ristocetin cofactor assay, and factor VIII.

- Consider other tests based on differential diagnosis.
  - TSH, prolactin level, follicle-stimulating hormone (FSH), STI screening, KOH prep, vaginitis panel
  - 17-Hydroxyprogesterone if congenital adrenal hyperplasia is suspected
  - Testosterone and/or dehydroepiandrosterone sulfate (DHEA-S) if PCOS
- TVUS in postmenopausal AUB
  - Postmenopausal endometrial thickness (ET) <4 mm does not require endometrial sampling unless bleeding is persistent or recurrent, whereas ET >4 mm should prompt further evaluation.
  - ET <5 mm: 99.6% negative predictive value (NPV) for ruling out endometrial cancer (2)
  - Incidentally found endometrial measurement >4 mm without associated bleeding in postmenopausal women should not trigger evaluation; however, assessment based on individual risk factors is appropriate.
- TVUS, sonohysterography, and hysteroscopy may be similarly effective in detection of intrauterine pathology in premenopausal women with AUB.

Follow-Up Tests & Special Considerations
It is appropriate to initiate medical therapy in females <35 years of age if low risk of uterine anatomic/histologic abnormality or adenomyosis prior to performing an endometrial biopsy (EMB).

Diagnostic Procedures/Other
- Pap smear to screen for cervical cancer if age >21 years (1)[C]
- EMB
  - Women age >45 years with AUB to rule out cancer or premalignancy
  - Postmenopausal women with ET ≥4 mm
  - Women aged 18 to 45 years with AUB, a history of unopposed estrogen, and failed medical management
  - Women any age without risk factors if they have abnormal findings following imaging (1)
  - Perform on or after day 18 of cycle, if known; secretory endometrium confirms ovulation occurred.
- Hysteroscopy with targeted biopsy if suspected intrauterine lesion with negative EMB
  - NPV for endometrial cancer with negative hysteroscopy at any age is 99.5%.

Test Interpretation
Pap smear could reveal carcinoma or inflammation indicative of cervicitis. Most EMBs show proliferative or dyssynchronous endometrium (suggesting anovulation) but can show simple or complex hyperplasia without atypia, hyperplasia with atypia, or endometrial adenocarcinoma.

TREATMENT

GENERAL MEASURES
NSAIDs (naproxen sodium 500 mg BID, mefenamic acid 500 mg TID, ibuprofen 600 to 1,200 mg/day)
- Decreases amount of blood loss and pain compared with placebo
- "Surgical" approaches (including LNG-IUD) generally superior to medical approaches for long-term control (3)[A]

MEDICATION

First Line

- Acute, emergent, nonovulatory bleeding (4)
  - Conjugated equine estrogen (Premarin): 25 mg IV q4h (max 6 doses) stops bleeding within 8 hours in 72% of individuals or 2.5 mg Premarin PO q6h should control bleeding in 12 to 24 hours (2)[A].
  - TXA 1.3 g PO or 10 mg/kg IV (max 600 mg/dose) TID
  - Intrauterine tamponade by filling 26F foley bulb with 30 mL saline
  - D&C if no response after 2 to 4 doses of Premarin or sooner if bleeding >1 pad per hour (1)[C]
  - Then change to oral contraceptive pill (OCP) or progestin for cycle regulation
- Acute, nonemergent, nonovulatory bleeding
  - Monophasic combined OCPs with 35 μg of estrogen TID for 7 days shown to stop bleeding in 88% of women
  - Medroxyprogesterone acetate 20 mg PO TID for 7 days shown to stop bleeding in 76% of women in 3 days
- Nonacute, nonovulatory bleeding
  - Levonorgestrel IUD (Mirena) is the most effective (71–95% decrease in blood loss) form of progesterone delivery and not inferior to surgical management (3)[A].
  - Progestins: medroxyprogesterone acetate (Provera) 10 mg/day for 5 to 10 days each month. Daily progesterone for 21 days per cycle results in significantly less blood loss (5)[A].
  - OCPs: 20 to 35 μg daily estrogen plus progesterone (Consider especially for anovulatory females <18 years old who are not yet sexually active.)
  - TXA 1.0–1.5 g PO 3 times a day; avoid in patients with hypercoagulable states.
- Do not use estrogen if contraindications (suspicion for endometrial hyperplasia or carcinoma, history of DVT, migraine with aura, or smoking in women >35 years of age [relative contraindication]).
- Precautions
  - Failed medical treatment requires further workup and consideration of surgical management.
  - Consider DVT prophylaxis when treating with high-dose estrogens (1)[C].

Second Line

- Gonadotropin-releasing hormone (GnRH) agonists
  - Leuprolide (varying doses and duration of action)
  - Elagolix 300 mg BID (6)
    - FDA approved for heavy menstrual bleeding due to uterine fibroids in premenopausal women combined with add-back therapy (1 mg estradiol/0.5 mg norethindrone acetate once a day)
- Danazol (200 to 400 mg/day for a maximum of 9 months) more effective than NSAIDs but limited by androgenic side effects and cost; now replaced by GnRH agonists
- Metformin or clomifene (Clomid) alone or in combination in women with PCOS who desire ovulation and pregnancy

ISSUES FOR REFERRAL

If an obvious cause for vaginal bleeding is not found in a pediatric patient, refer to a pediatric endocrinologist or gynecologist.

ADDITIONAL THERAPIES

- Antiemetics if treating with high-dose estrogen or progesterone (1)[C]
- Iron supplementation if anemia (usually iron deficiency) is identified
- Ulipristal acetate 5 mg or 10 mg (selective progesterone receptor modulator)
  - Found to be effective but currently suspended while undergoing evaluation of possible severe liver injury

SURGERY/OTHER PROCEDURES

- Hysterectomy in cases of endometrial cancer, if medical therapy fails, or if other uterine pathology is found
- Endometrial ablation, less expensive than hysterectomy and associated with high patient satisfaction; this is a permanent procedure and should be avoided in patients who desire continued fertility.
- Uterine artery embolization if bleeding is refractory to medications or confirmed fibroids

ADMISSION, INPATIENT, AND NURSING CONSIDERATIONS

- Significant hemorrhage causing acute anemia with signs of hemodynamic instability; with acute bleeding, replace volume with crystalloid and blood, as necessary.
- Pad counts and clot size can be helpful to determine and monitor amount of bleeding.
- Discharge criteria: hemodynamic stability and control of vaginal bleeding

 ONGOING CARE

FOLLOW-UP RECOMMENDATIONS

Once stable from acute management, recommend follow-up evaluation in 4 to 6 months for further evaluation.

Patient Monitoring

Women treated with estrogen or OCPs should keep a menstrual diary to document bleeding patterns and their relation to therapy.

DIET

No restrictions, although a 5% reduction in weight can induce ovulation in anovulation caused by PCOS

PATIENT EDUCATION

- https://www.acog.org/Patients
- https://www.uptodate.com (patient education)

PROGNOSIS

- Varies with pathophysiologic process
- Most anovulatory cycles can be treated with medical therapy and do not require surgical intervention.

COMPLICATIONS

Iron deficiency anemia, mood disorders

REFERENCES

1. Committee on Practice Bulletins—Gynecology. Practice Bulletin No. 128: diagnosis of abnormal uterine bleeding in reproductive-aged women. *Obstet Gynecol.* 2012;120(1):197–206.
2. Wong AS, Lao TT, Cheung CW, et al. Reappraisal of endometrial thickness for the detection of endometrial cancer in postmenopausal bleeding: a retrospective cohort study. *BJOG.* 2016;123(3):439–446.
3. Marjoribanks J, Lethaby A, Farquhar C. Surgery versus medical therapy for heavy menstrual bleeding. *Cochrane Database Syst Rev.* 2016;(1):CD003855.
4. ACOG Committee Opinion No. 557: management of acute abnormal uterine bleeding in nonpregnant reproductive-aged women. *Obstet Gynecol.* 2013;121(4):891–896.
5. Lethaby A, Irvine G, Cameron I. Cyclical progestogens for heavy menstrual bleeding. *Cochrane Database Syst Rev.* 2008;(1):CD001016.
6. Ali M, R SA, Al Hendy A. Elagolix in the treatment of heavy menstrual bleeding associated with uterine fibroids in premenopausal women. *Expert Rev Clin Pharmacol.* 2021;14(4):427–437.

ADDITIONAL READING

- Goldstein SR, Lumsden MA. Abnormal uterine bleeding in perimenopause. *Climacteric.* 2017;20(5):414–420.
- Lethaby A, Cooke I, Rees M. Progesterone or progestogen-releasing intrauterine systems for heavy menstrual bleeding. *Cochrane Database Syst Rev.* 2005;(4):CD002126.
- Practice Bulletin No. 136: management of abnormal uterine bleeding associated with ovulatory dysfunction. *Obstet Gynecol.* 2013;122(1):176–185.

 SEE ALSO

- Dysmenorrhea; Menorrhagia (Heavy Menstrual Bleeding)
- Algorithm: Abnormal Uterine Bleeding

 CODES

ICD10

- N93.9 Abnormal uterine and vaginal bleeding, unspecified
- N93.8 Other specified abnormal uterine and vaginal bleeding

CLINICAL PEARLS

- AUB is irregular uterine bleeding that occurs in the absence of pregnancy or pathology, making it a diagnosis of exclusion.
- Anovulation accounts for 90% of AUB.
- EMB should be performed in
  - Women age >45 years with AUB
  - Women aged 18 to 45 with AUB and a history of unopposed estrogen and failed medical management

ABNORMAL PAP AND CERVICAL DYSPLASIA

Anna K. Zheng, MD • Henry Del Rosario, MD

BASICS

DESCRIPTION

- Cervical dysplasia: premalignant cervical disease that is also called cervical intraepithelial neoplasia (CIN); precancerous epithelial changes in the transformation zone of the uterine cervix almost always associated with human papillomavirus (HPV) infections
- CIN encompasses a range of histologic diagnoses.
  - CIN I: mild dysplasia; low-grade lesion; cellular changes are limited to the lower 1/3 of the squamous epithelium.
  - CIN II: moderate dysplasia; high-grade lesion; cellular changes are limited to the lower 2/3 of the squamous epithelium.
  - CIN III or carcinoma in situ: severe dysplasia; high-grade lesion; cellular changes involve the full thickness of the squamous epithelium.
- System(s) affected: reproductive

Pediatric Considerations
Only 0.1% of cervical cancers occur before age 20 years. Screening any individual with a cervix age <21 years (regardless of sexual debut and history) does not reduce cervical cancer incidence and mortality compared with beginning screening at age 21 years.

Geriatric Considerations
- Any individual with a cervix and age >65 years who has had adequate prior screening and no history of CIN II+ in the last 20 years should not be screened for cervical cancer. Adequate prior screening is defined as three consecutive, negative cytology-only results or two consecutive, negative HPV testing alone or negative cytology "cotesting" with negative HPV results within 10 years before cessation of screening (with the most recent test within the last 5 years).
- Routine screening should continue for at least 25 years at 3-year intervals with HPV testing or cotesting after spontaneous regression or appropriate management of a high-grade precancerous lesion, even if this extends screening past the age 65 years (1)[C].

Pregnancy Considerations
- Squamous intraepithelial lesions can progress during pregnancy but often regress postpartum.
- Colposcopy only to exclude the presence of invasive cancer in high-risk individuals
- Unless cancer is identified or suspected, treatment of CIN is contraindicated during pregnancy.

EPIDEMIOLOGY
Cervical cancer is the fourth most common type of cancer in women worldwide. In the United States, cervical cancer has dropped to 20th place in causes of cancer death in 2021. Incidence of CIN III peaks between ages 25 and 29 years; invasive disease peaks 15 years later. Cervical cancer most commonly occurs in those aged 35 to 44 years. >15% of cervical cancer cases occur in those >65 years of age (occurs in those who did not get regular screening).

Incidence
In 2021, it was projected that there would be 14,480 new cases of cervical cancer diagnosed and 4,290 women will die from the disease. The incidence of cervical cancer in the United States has decreased by >50% in the past 40 years because of widespread cervical cancer screening tests.

Prevalence
Multiple studies in populations around the world have found that prevalence of high-grade dysplasia has fallen significantly in HPV-immunized populations (2).

ETIOLOGY AND PATHOPHYSIOLOGY
HPV is so common that most sexually active men and women will get at least one type of HPV at some point in their lives.

- High-risk HPV types: 16, 18, 31, 33, 35, 45, 52, and 58 are common oncogenic virus types for cervical cancer. HPV 16 and 18 are associated with ~70% of all cervical cancers.
- Most HPV infections are transient, becoming undetectable within 1 to 2 years. Persistent infections are what place women at significant risk for developing precancerous lesions. Compared to younger women, women age >30 years are less likely to clear a new HPV infection.
- Low-risk types: HPV viral types 6, 11, 42, 43, and 44 are considered common low-risk types and may cause genital warts. HPV 6 and 11 (cause 90% of benign anogenital warts) can lead to low-grade squamous intraepithelial lesion (LSIL) and CIN I.

RISK FACTORS
- HIV infection and other immunosuppressive conditions
- In utero exposure to diethylstilbestrol
- Cigarette smoking
- Multiple sexual partners
- Some correlation with low socioeconomic status, high parity, oral contraceptive use, and poor nutrition

GENERAL PREVENTION
Immunization: Immunization decreases high-risk HPV infections and CIN II/III cervical pathology for at least 5 to 7 years but has not yet been shown to decrease cervical cancer. It is likely that prevention of invasive cancer will be demonstrated within a few years. Ideally, HPV immunization of girls, boys, and any individual with a cervix should be initiated prior to first intercourse. Per the Advisory Committee on Immunization Practices (ACIP), offer HPV vaccine to adolescents 11 to 12 years of age and can start vaccination as early as 9 years old. Gardasil 9: The FDA approved in October 2018 for use in females and males ages 9 to 26 years and via shared clinical decision for ages 27 to 45 years; 88% effective preventing dysplasia due to HPV types 16 and 18 (75% of cervical cancer), types 6 and 11 (anogenital warts), and protection against five additional HPV types, which cause approximately 25% of CIN II+ lesions

- Vaccine schedule: If the first vaccine dose was given before the 15th birthday, only 2 doses are required to complete the series; 6 to 12 months apart. If vaccine began on or after the 15th birthday: 3 doses at 0, 2, and 6 months
- Immunocompromising conditions: 3 doses needed.
- Safe sex practices: condom use. Advise smoking cessation.

- Screening
  - Pap smear has been the main screening test for cervical cellular pathology, with or without cotesting for HPV. The U.S. Preventive Services Task Force recommends either cytology-only testing at 3-year intervals or primary HPV testing using an approved assay versus cotesting at 5-year intervals for women 30 to 65 years of age. Clinicians will choose to adopt the most feasible screening and testing approach depending on assay availability.
  - Screening recommendations by age and source (see algorithm "Pap, Normal and Abnormal in Nonpregnant Women Ages 25 Years and Older" and separate algorithm "Pap, Normal and Abnormal in Women Ages 21–24 Years").
  - <21 years: Do not screen (USPSTF/ASCCP/ACS/ASCP/ACOG) (3)[A].
  - Frequency of screening recommendation: USPSTF/ASCCP/ACS/ASCP generally agree by age and screen.
    ○ 21 to 29 years: Screen with cytology every 3 years. For patients ≥25 years, screen every 5 years with primary HPV testing using an assay method explicitly approved for primary HPV testing (preferred) or every 3 years with cytology (acceptable) (1).
    ○ 30 to 65 years: Screen with either primary HPV testing or cotesting every 5 years (1)[C]. Cytology every 3 years, if cotesting or HPV-only testing not available, is also acceptable (1),(3).
    ○ >65 years (who have had adequate prior screening and are not high risk): Do not screen (3)[A].
- Special circumstances: patients after hysterectomy with removal of the cervix and with no history of CIN II+: Do not screen (3)[A]. Patients with history of CIN II+ or status treatment should continue screening until at least 25 years following their diagnosis of CIN II+ (1)[C].
- HIV-positive patients: Screen individuals every 3 years in those who have had three consecutive normal annual Pap tests and every 3 years cotesting in ages ≥30 years.

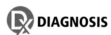DIAGNOSIS

HISTORY
Usually asymptomatic until there is invasive disease

PHYSICAL EXAM
Pelvic exam occasionally reveals external HPV lesions. Examine for exophytic or ulcerative cervical lesions, with or without bleeding.

DIFFERENTIAL DIAGNOSIS
Acute or chronic cervicitis; cervical glandular hyperplasia; uterine malignancy

DIAGNOSTIC TESTS & INTERPRETATION
- Current evidence indicates no clinically important differences between conventional cytology and liquid-based cytology in detecting cervical cancer precursors. Conventional Pap smear involves a cervical sample plated on a microscope slide with fixative. ThinPrep is a liquid-based collection and thin-layer preparation.
- To ensure an adequate sample of both the ecto- and endocervix, use a cytobrush and an extended tip spatula.

- The sensitivity and specificity of using HPV and cytology testing together (cotesting) for dysplasia is near 100% and 92.5%, respectively. Cotesting leads to earlier diagnosis of CIN III+ and cancer than does cytology alone. Testing for high-risk HPV using an assay specifically approved for primary screening without cytology is preferred for individuals with a cervix age ≥25 years, particularly for poorly screened or unscreened populations. Per updated 2019 ASCCP guidelines, cytology screening alone is also acceptable when HPV or cotesting is not feasible.
- Cytology report component: specimen type (conventional Pap smear or liquid based), adequacy (presence of endocervical cells), and categorization (negative for intraepithelial lesion or malignancy or epithelial cell abnormality; i.e., squamous/glandular)
- Bethesda 2014 system (cytologic grading) epithelial cell abnormalities
  – Squamous cell: atypical squamous cells (ASC) (of undetermined significance [ASC-US], cannot exclude high-grade squamous intraepithelial lesion or HSIL [ASC-H]). HPV, mild dysplasia, CIN I. Moderate/severe dysplasia CIS, CIN II, and CIN III
  – Glandular cell: atypical glandular cells (AGCs) favor neoplasia, not otherwise specified; AGCs: favor neoplasia. Adenocarcinoma in situ (AIS), adenocarcinoma

Diagnostic Procedures/Other
Clinical action depends on immediate risk of CIN III+ for cases age ≥25 years (1)[C]. Algorithms from 2012 ASCCP guidelines differ for women age 21 to 24 years, provided below (4)[C].

- ASC-US: (<25 years of age)
  – Option 1: HPV testing (preferred)
    ○ If HPV positive, proceed to clinical action depending on immediate CIN III+ risk (1),(4)[C].
    ○ If HPV negative, repeat cotesting at 3 years (4)[C].
  – Option 2: Repeat cytology at 1 year (acceptable) (4)[C].
    ○ If repeat cytology ASC or greater, proceed to colposcopy or other clinical action if immediate CIN III+ risk is known.
    ○ If repeat cytology is negative, proceed to routine screening.
- ASC-H (<25 years of age): colposcopy required
- LSIL (<25 years of age):
  – LSIL with negative HPV test: Repeat cotesting at 1 year (preferred).
    ○ If repeat cotesting is negative, repeat cotesting in 3 years.
    ○ If cotesting is positive, proceed to colposcopy or repeat cotesting in 1 year.
  – LSIL with no HPV test or positive HPV test: Proceed to colposcopy.
  – LSIL in pregnancy: colposcopy preferred, but it is acceptable to defer colposcopy to postpartum (4)[B]
- HSIL/CIN II or III+/AGCs/atypical endometrial cells (≥21 years): likely colposcopy but clinical action ultimately depends on immediate CIN III+ risk (1)[C]
- Age ≥25 years/special populations/rarely screened/status posttreatment/history of CIN II, CIN III, AIS or invasive cancer: clinical action only when immediate CIN III+ risk is ≥4% with stress on shared decision-making; can proceed to treatment if immediate CIN III+ risk is >60% and bypass colposcopy biopsy (1)

Test Interpretation
ASCs or columnar cells, coarse nuclear material, increased nuclear diameter, koilocytosis (HPV hallmark)

 ## TREATMENT

ASCCP smart-phone application includes 2019 guidelines: Evidence-based management phone application includes algorithms to guide Pap smear and postcolposcopic diagnostics and therapeutics are available online at https://www.asccp.org/mobile-app and https://www.asccp.org/management-guidelines (1),(4).

GENERAL MEASURES
Office evaluation and observation; promote smoking cessation; promote safe sex practices; promote immunization.

MEDICATION
Infective/reactive Pap smear: Treat organism/condition found on Pap smear results. Condyloma acuminatum treatment options: See chapter "Condylomata Acuminata."

SURGERY/OTHER PROCEDURES
- Expedited treatment that bypasses colposcopy biopsy is recommended for nonpregnant patients ≥25 years with immediate CIN III+ risk of >60% and is acceptable for immediate CIN III+ risk between 25% and 60% while stressing the importance of shared decision-making (1).
- Observation is preferred to treatment for CIN I (1). Colposcopy can be deferred for certain patients and repeat HPV testing or cotesting in 1 year is recommended if immediate CIN III+ risk is low risk (<4%).
- Excisional treatment is preferred to ablative treatment for histologic HSIL (CIN II or CIN III). For AIS, excision is recommended (1).
- If cervical malignancy, see "Cervical Malignancy."

 ## ONGOING CARE

FOLLOW-UP RECOMMENDATIONS
After treatment (excision or ablation) of HSIL, CIN II or III, or AIS and initial posttreatment management, women should reenter screening with HPV testing or cotesting at 3-year intervals for at least 25 years (1).

PATIENT EDUCATION
HPV vaccination, smoking cessation, protected intercourse, regular screening with Pap smear per guidelines

PROGNOSIS
- Progression of CIN to invasive cervical cancer is slow, and the likelihood of regression is high: Up to 43% of CIN II and 32% of CIN III lesions may regress. CIN III has a 30% probability of becoming invasive cancer over a 30-year period, although only about 1% if treated.
- CIN III becomes invasive: Lesions discovered early are amenable to treatment with excellent results and few recurrences.
- The 5-year survival rate for cervical cancer patients is 66.3%. The 5-year relative survival rate for patients diagnosed with localized disease is 91.9%.

COMPLICATIONS
Aggressive cervical surgery may be associated with cervical stenosis, cervical incompetence (leading to pre-term labor), and scarring affecting cervical dilatation in labor.

REFERENCES
1. Perkins RB, Guido RS, Castle PE, et al. 2019 ASCCP risk-based management consensus guidelines for abnormal cervical cancer screening tests and cancer precursors. *J Low Genit Tract Dis*. 2020;24(2):102–131.
2. Drolet M, Bénard É, Pérez N, et al. Population-level impact and herd effects following the introduction of human papillomavirus vaccination programmes: updated systematic review and meta-analysis. *Lancet*. 2019;394(10197):497–509.
3. Curry SJ, Krist AH, Owens DK, et al. Screening for cervical cancer: US Preventive Services Task Force recommendation statement. *JAMA*. 2018;320(7):674–686.
4. Massad LS, Einstein MH, Huh WK, et al. 2012 updated consensus guidelines for the management of abnormal cervical cancer screening tests and cancer precursors. *J Low Genit Tract Dis*. 2013;17(5 Suppl 1):S1–S27.

ADDITIONAL READING
American Society for Colposcopy and Cervical Pathology. Management guidelines. https://www.asccp.org/management-guidelines. Accessed November 25, 2021.

 ## SEE ALSO

- Cervical Malignancy; Condylomata Acuminata; Trichomoniasis; Vulvovaginitis, Prepubescent
- Algorithms: Pap, Normal and Abnormal in Nonpregnant Women Ages 25 Years and Older; Pap, Normal and Abnormal in Women Ages 21–24 Years

 ## CODES

ICD10
- R87.619 Unspecified abnormal cytological findings in specimens from cervix uteri
- N87.9 Dysplasia of cervix uteri, unspecified
- N87.1 Moderate cervical dysplasia

CLINICAL PEARLS
- Vaccine should be offered prior to onset of any sexual activity for maximum effectiveness.
- Know and adhere to recognized screening guidelines to avoid the harms of overscreening.
- Optimal screening strategy is in evolution. HPV-only screening is now preferred due to test being more sensitive than cytology alone (1), but the approved assay is not yet widely available in 2021.

ACETAMINOPHEN POISONING
Grant M. Reed, DO • Yatri Desai, BS

 BASICS

DESCRIPTION
- A disorder characterized by hepatic necrosis following large acetaminophen ingestions. Clinical manifestations of acetaminophen toxicity vary with time since ingestion and are accordingly classified into 4 stages.
- Single, large ingestions of acetaminophen account for a majority of poisoning, but it can also occur with ingestions of lesser amounts in individuals who regularly abuse alcohol, are chronically malnourished, or take medications impacting hepatic metabolism.
- Ingestions >12 g in adults and >250 mg/kg in children are likely to cause toxicity.
- The hepatic system is primarily impacted. Rare instances of cardiotoxicity and nephrotoxicity may occur, but evidence of direct injury to these systems is weak and not well-defined.
- Synonym(s): paracetamol poisoning

EPIDEMIOLOGY
- Hospitalizations due to acetaminophen toxicity from 1998 to 2011 were 67% due to intentional ingestion, 16% from unintentional ingestion, and 17% unspecified (1).
- Of the hospitalizations related to acetaminophen toxicity from 1998 to 2011, 83% were primarily adults and 69% were female (95% CI: 68–69%) (1).
- From 2008 to 2012, about 49% of unintentional acetaminophen related poison control calls were regarding children ≤5 years (1).

Incidence
Rates of acetaminophen related hospitalizations slowly increased prior to 2009. Discharges following toxicity decreased from 119.8 per 100,000 in 2009 to 108.6 per 100,000 in 2011 (1).

Prevalence
- According to 2008 to 2012 data from the American Association of Poison Control, there were an average 111,632 nationwide acetaminophen-related events per year (1).
- An estimated average of 10% of these events resulted in liver toxicity and 1% resulted in death (1).

ETIOLOGY AND PATHOPHYSIOLOGY
Pharmacokinetics (2)
- With oral therapeutic ingestion, acetaminophen is entirely absorbed from the duodenum and reaches peak serum concentrations of 10 to 20 μg/mL after up to 2 hours. This peak may be delayed with toxic ingestions.
- Therapeutic adult doses of acetaminophen are 325 to 1,000 mg q4–6h to a maximum dose of 4 g/day.
- Therapeutic pediatric doses are 10 to 15 mg/kg q4–6h, not to exceed 5 doses in 24 hours or 75 g/kg/day.
- The elimination half-life of acetaminophen ranges from 2 to 4 hours but may be delayed in extended-release formulation.

Pathophysiology (2)
- Ingestion of supratherapeutic doses of acetaminophen or subtherapeutic ingestions in individuals with compromised liver function causes acetaminophen poisoning and resulting hepatocellular damage.
- The liver metabolizes 96% of ingested acetaminophen and 2–4% is excreted unchanged in urine. Therapeutic doses break down into 90–95% benign metabolites and 5–10% of the toxic metabolite, *N*-acetyl-*p*-benzoquinone imine (NAPQI).

- NAPQI is rapidly conjugated with hepatic stores of glutathione to form a nontoxic metabolite to be excreted in the urine.
- Toxic ingestions of acetaminophen saturate the glucuronidation and sulfation pathways, depleting glutathione stores and result in accumulations of NAPQI that cause hepatocellular damage.

RISK FACTORS
- Concurrent poisoning with other substances impacting hepatic metabolism
- A psychiatric illness or history of suicide attempts
- Regular ingestion of large amounts of alcohol
- Chronic malnutrition and possible risk related to previous weight loss surgery

GENERAL PREVENTION
- Poison Control: (800) 222-1222 for consultations and management guidance
- FDA labeling guidance: http://www.fda.gov/Drugs/GuidanceComplianceRegulatoryInformation/Guidances/default.htm

Geriatric Considerations
There is an increased risk of hepatic damage in frail, elderly patients due to decreased hepatic metabolism and coingestion of other hepatotoxic medications. Keep dose of acetaminophen ≤3,000 mg/day in seniors and in patients with liver disease and/or alcohol abuse disorders (3).

Pediatric Considerations
Hepatic damage after ingestion of toxic acetaminophen doses can be less severe in young children, potentially because they have more stores of glutathione (3).

Pregnancy Considerations
There is an increased incidence of spontaneous abortion in pregnant patients with acetaminophen poisoning, especially with overdose at an early gestational age. Abortion incidence and possible fetal death is increased if *N*-acetylcysteine (NAC) treatment is delayed. IV NAC is generally preferred in pregnancy due to greater bioavailability (3).

DIAGNOSIS
Signs and symptoms of poisoning develop over the first 24 hours following large ingestions. Symptoms may develop gradually in those with a history of long-term ingestion near supratherapeutic doses. Presentation of symptoms varies and is divided into 4 stages (3):
- Stage 1—first 24 hours after ingestion
  - Patient may be asymptomatic in first 8 hours following ingestion. Symptoms may include nausea, emesis, anorexia, and diaphoresis.
  - Laboratory results are usually unremarkable at this time.
- Stage 2—days 2 to 3 following ingestion
  - Typically less nausea, vomiting, diaphoresis, and malaise than in stage 1
  - Right upper quadrant pain and hepatomegaly may become evident.
  - Elevated aminotransferases are usually seen.
- Stage 3—days 3 to 4 following ingestion
  - Stage I symptoms such as nausea, vomiting, and malaise reappear.
  - Severe poisonings may result in jaundice, confusion, somnolence, and coma.

  - Marked liver enzyme elevations which usually peak at this point; prolonged PT/INR; typically negative acetaminophen levels
  - Multiorgan failure and death most commonly occur in this stage
- Stage 4—days 5+ after ingestion
  - Possible recovery stage in patients with resolving stage 3 symptoms
  - Recovery may be prolonged, but is typically complete and without long-term sequelae. Laboratory abnormalities typically resolve.
  - Fulminant hepatic failure occurs in <1% of adults and is very rare in children <6 years of age.

HISTORY
Primary questions should focus on what was ingested (extended release, hydrocodone-acetaminophen, coingestants, etc.), how much was ingested, and time of ingestion. Was the ingestion intentional or accidental? Also ask regarding current or history of alcohol abuse, hepatitis, and previous surgeries.

PHYSICAL EXAM
Physical exam findings will likely vary depending on stage of toxicity. In general, a full physical examination is warranted with vitals assessment.
- Assess individual's general appearance for somnolence, fatigue, pallor, diaphoresis, and signs of dehydration.
- Look for signs of hepatotoxicity: hepatomegaly and RUQ pain.

DIFFERENTIAL DIAGNOSIS
- Consider presence of coingestants, especially alcohol, opiates, and aspirin.
- Other ingested toxins that produce severe acute hepatic injury, including the mushroom *Amanita phalloides* and products containing yellow phosphorus or carbon tetrachloride.
- Consider other causes of hepatitis: alcoholic, viral, ischemic.

DIAGNOSTIC TESTS & INTERPRETATION
Initial Tests (lab, imaging)
- Draw plasma acetaminophen levels on all patients ≥4 hours after ingestion (levels peak at 4 hours). Draw additional levels at 6 and 8 hours if extended-release form was ingested. Poison Control may help guide the frequency of exams, vitals, or any other ancillary testing that may be warranted (3).
  - If a sustained-released product has been ingested, obtain two serum acetaminophen levels 4 to 6 hours apart. Treat if either level is above the possible toxicity line.
  - For chronic toxicity or patients who present 24 hours postingestion, treat based on clinical effects, LFTs, and the acetaminophen level.
- Liver function tests: alanine transaminase (ALT), aspartate transaminase (AST), prothrombin time (PT)/international normalized ratio (INR), bilirubin, lactate dehydrogenase (LDH)
  - With severe poisonings, PT/INR rise in parallel with LFT changes.
  - With toxic ingestions, AST, ALT, and bilirubin levels begin to rise in stage 2 and peak in stage 3.
  - Improvement in ALT with therapy is an encouraging clinical sign.

- Additional labs: electrolytes, glucose, BUN, creatinine, urinalysis, urine drug screen (UDS), serum alcohol, and salicylate
  - Screen for coingestants with the above labs and consider searching for other medications/substances depending on the clinical history.
  - Obtain a pregnancy screen in females (urine or serum) as it can influence management.
  - Consider an arterial blood gas (ABG): Anion-gap metabolic acidosis due to accumulation of 5-oxoproline may rarely be seen.
- Imaging: No specific imaging is required.

Follow-Up Tests & Special Considerations
During recovery, liver tests should normalize and complete restoration of liver function without long-term sequelae is expected.

Diagnostic Procedures/Other
Advanced imaging of the liver and/or kidney with ultrasound or CT can be considered when acute hepatitis or kidney injury is present to rule out alternative causes. Otherwise, imaging is not required and any abnormal findings, if present, may be nonspecific.

 TREATMENT

- Immediately contact a local Poison Control Center for recommendations. Call (800) 222-1222 in the United States.
- NAC is a benign prodrug that provides cysteine as a substrate to detoxify acetaminophen metabolites and replenish glutathione stores in the liver. NAC administration may reduce mortality from 5% to 0.7%.
- The Rumack-Matthew nomogram (3):
  - A plot used to determine if acetaminophen levels are high enough to warrant treatment with NAC during acute toxic ingestions.
  - The nomogram is not intended for sustained-release products or chronic ingestions.
  - Give NAC when acetaminophen plasma levels measured ≥4 hours after ingestion are at the "treatment line" or higher on the Rumack-Matthew nomogram.
  - Treatment line acetaminophen plasma levels on the nomogram correspond to >150 μg/mL (993 μmol/L), >75 μg/mL (497 μmol/L), and >37 μg/mL (244 μmol/L) at 4, 8, and 12 hours after ingestion, respectively.
- Initiate NAC (Mucomyst) within 8 hours of ingestion whenever possible; single-dose activated charcoal (1 g/kg PO) may be effective if given within 1 to 4 hours of ingestion. *Never* delay oral NAC for activated charcoal.
- Ipecac and gastric lavage are no longer recommended for routine use at home or in health care facilities (4).

MEDICATION
First Line
- Empirically start NAC within 8 hours even while awaiting lab results. It may be effective up to ≥36 hours after ingestion.
  - NAC may be given PO or IV, depending on situation and availability. IV NAC has been shown to decrease the length of hospitalization compared to PO NAC (4).
  - A 2-bag regimen should be used to administer a total of 300 mg/kg IV NAC (Acetadote, Cetylev) over a 20-hour period to reduce adverse effects of NAC administration. Begin with a 200 mg/kg IV dose over 4 hours followed by a 100 mg/kg IV dose over 16 hours (5).

  - Use an oral loading dose of 140 mg/kg, then 70 mg/kg q4h for 17 additional doses (72-hour regimen).
- NAC precautions:
  - PO NAC may cause significant nausea and vomiting due to its sulfur content and is often poorly tolerated; consider a nasogastric tube.
  - IV NAC (Acetadote) may cause anaphylactoid reactions, (3–6%) including: rash, bronchospasm, pruritus, angioedema, tachycardia, or hypotension (higher rates seen in asthmatics and those with atopy). Reactions usually occur with the loading dose. To prevent this, slow or temporarily stop the infusion; may concurrently treat with antihistamines (5)
  - Nausea can be treated with metoclopramide, 1 to 2 mg/kg IV, or ondansetron, 0.15 mg/kg IV.
  - NAC failure rates range from 3% to 7% (4).
- Give single-dose activated charcoal within 1 to 4 hours of ingestion (especially in cases of coingestants). Do not delay NAC administration for use of activated charcoal.

Second Line
In massive ingestions (levels >1,000 mg/L, severe acidosis, coma/hypotension) or when severe renal failure is present, hemodialysis may improve survival (4).

ISSUES FOR REFERRAL
- Behavioral health evaluation for intentional ingestions
- Child abuse reporting if neglect led to overdose

ADMISSION, INPATIENT, AND NURSING CONSIDERATIONS
- Consider hospitalization for toxic ingestions with vital instability and/or laboratory abnormalities. Consider transfer to a psychiatric facility for intentional ingestions when medically stable.
- IV fluids are generally provided for hydration purposes.

 ONGOING CARE

FOLLOW-UP RECOMMENDATIONS
- Evaluate all patients at an accredited health care facility.
- Evaluate patients with evidence of organ failure, increased LFTs, or coagulopathy for emergency liver transplant (ELT) at a transplant center.
- Restrict activity if hepatic damage is significant.
- Outpatient management is adequate for nontoxic accidental ingestions.

DIET
No special diet, except with severe hepatic damage

PATIENT EDUCATION
- Counsel patients to avoid acetaminophen (Tylenol, others) or other forms of acetaminophen, particularly if using combination product(s) containing acetaminophen.
- Educate parents/caregivers during well-child visits regarding appropriate OTC dosing and medication storage.
- Provide anticipatory guidance for caregivers, family, and cohabitants of potentially suicidal patients.
- Educate patients on long-term acetaminophen therapy.

PROGNOSIS
- Complete recovery with early therapy is possible and more likely in stage 4 of toxicity (3).
- 10% of adult patients with severe liver complications develop necrosis, hepatic encephalopathy, or require transplant (1).
- Hepatic failure is rare in children <6 years of age (1).

COMPLICATIONS
Recovery after acute poisoning is complete and sequelae are rare.

REFERENCES
1. Major JM, Zhou EH, Wong H-L, et al. Trends in rates of acetaminophen-related adverse events in the United States. *Pharmacoepidemiol Drug Saf*. 2016;25(5):590–598.
2. McGill MR, Jaeschke H. Metabolism and disposition of acetaminophen: recent advances in relation to hepatotoxicity and diagnosis. *Pharm Res*. 2013;30(9):2174–2187.
3. Chiew AL, Buckley NA. Acetaminophen poisoning. *Crit Care Clin*. 2021;37(3):543–561.
4. Chiew AL, Gluud C, Brok J, et al. Interventions for paracetamol (acetaminophen) overdose. *Cochrane Database Syst Rev*. 2018;(2):CD003328.
5. O'Callaghan C, Graudins A, Wong A. A two-bag acetylcysteine regimen is associated with shorter delays and interruptions in the treatment of paracetamol overdose. *Clin Toxicol (Phila)*. 2021;17:1–5.

ADDITIONAL READING
- Burnham K, Yang T, Smith H, et al. A review of alternative intravenous acetylcysteine regimens for acetaminophen overdose. *Expert Rev Clin Pharmacol*. 2021;14(10):1267–1278.
- Mund ME, Quarcoo D, Gyo C, et al. Paracetamol as a toxic substance for children: aspects of legislation in selected countries. *J Occup Med Toxicol*. 2015;10:43.
- Serper M, Wolf MS, Parikh NA, et al. Risk factors, clinical presentation, and outcomes in overdose with acetaminophen alone or with combination products: results from the Acute Liver Failure Study Group. *J Clin Gastroenterol*. 2016;50(1):85–91.

 CODES

ICD10
- T39.1X4A Poisoning by 4-Aminophenol derivatives, undetermined, init
- K71.10 Toxic liver disease with hepatic necrosis, without coma
- T39.1X1A Poisoning by 4-Aminophenol derivatives, accidental, init

CLINICAL PEARLS
- Immediately consult Poison Control Center for management recommendations by calling (800) 222-1222 (United States).
- Give NAC when plasma acetaminophen concentrations (measured ≥4 hours after ingestion) are in the "possible risk" or higher levels. This corresponds to acetaminophen levels >150 μg/mL (993 μmol/L), >75 μg/mL (497 μmol/L), and >37 μg/mL (265 μmol/L) at 4, 8, and 12 hours after ingestion, respectively.
- Start NAC within 8 hours of ingestion for best chance of hepatic protection. Empirically give NAC in patients presenting near 8 hours while waiting for labs. A 2-bag IV dosing regimen over 20 hours is preferred.
- All patients with acetaminophen liver injury (even after 8 hours) should receive NAC.
- If using oral NAC, dilute with a beverage to increase palatability. Serve in a cup with lid and straw.
- For extended-release acetaminophen, follow plasma levels at 4, 6, and 8 hours after ingestion. Start NAC if any level is elevated.

ACNE ROSACEA
Shane L. Larson, MD

BASICS

DESCRIPTION
- Rosacea is a chronic condition characterized by recurrent episodes of facial flushing, erythema (due to dilatation of small blood vessels in the face), papules, pustules, and telangiectasia (due to increased reactivity of capillaries) in a symmetric, central facial distribution; sometimes associated with ocular symptoms (ocular rosacea)
- Four subtypes:
  - Erythematotelangiectatic rosacea (ETR)
  - Papulopustular rosacea (PPR)
  - Phymatous rosacea
  - Ocular rosacea
- System(s) affected: skin/exocrine
- Synonym(s): rosacea

Geriatric Considerations
- Chronic inflammatory dermatosis with middle-age onset
- Effects of aging might increase the side effects associated with oral isotretinoin used for treatment (at present, data are insufficient due to lack of clinical studies in elderly patients ≥65 years).

EPIDEMIOLOGY
Prevalence
- Predominant age of onset: 30 to 50 years
- Predominant sex: female > male. However, males are at greater risk for progression to later stages.
- More common in Fitzpatrick skin types I and II

ETIOLOGY AND PATHOPHYSIOLOGY
- No proven cause
- Possibilities include the following:
  - Thyroid and sex hormone disturbance
  - Alcohol, coffee, tea, spiced food overindulgence (unproven)
  - Demodex follicular parasite (suspected)
  - Exposure to cold, heat
  - Emotional stress
  - Dysfunction of the GI tract (possible association with *Helicobacter pylori*)

Genetics
- People of Northern European and Celtic background commonly afflicted
- Associated with three human leukocyte antigen (HLA) alleles: HLA-DRB1, HLA-DQB1, and HLA-DQA1 (MHC class II)

RISK FACTORS
- Exposure to spicy foods, hot drinks
- Environmental factors: sun, wind, cold, heat

GENERAL PREVENTION
No preventive measures known

COMMONLY ASSOCIATED CONDITIONS
- Seborrheic dermatitis of scalp and eyelids
- Keratitis with photophobia, lacrimation, visual disturbance
- Corneal lesions
- Blepharitis
- Uveitis

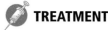

DIAGNOSIS

HISTORY
- Usually have a history of episodic flushing with increases in skin temperature in response to heat stimulus in mouth (hot liquids), spicy foods, alcohol, sun exposure
- Acne may have preceded onset of rosacea by years; nevertheless, rosacea usually arises de novo without preceding history of acne or seborrhea.
- Excessive facial warmth and redness are the predominant presenting complaints. Itching is generally absent.

PHYSICAL EXAM
- Rosacea has four subtypes:
  - The rosacea diathesis: episodic erythema, "flushing and blushing"
  - ETR: persistent erythema with telangiectases
  - PPR: persistent erythema, telangiectases, papules, pustules
  - Phymatous: persistent deep erythema, dense telangiectases, papules, pustules, nodules; rarely persistent "solid" edema of the central part of the face (phymatous)
- Progression from one subtype to another is hypothetical.
- Facial erythema, particularly on cheeks, nose, and chin. At times, entire face may be involved.
- Inflammatory papules are prominent; pustules and telangiectasia may be present.
- Comedones are absent (unlike acne vulgaris).
- Women usually have lesions on the chin and cheeks, whereas the nose is commonly involved in men.
- Ocular findings (mild dryness and irritation with blepharitis, conjunctival injection, burning, stinging, tearing, eyelid inflammation, swelling, and redness) are present in 50% of patients.

DIFFERENTIAL DIAGNOSIS
- Drug eruptions (iodides and bromides)
- Granulomas of the skin
- Cutaneous lupus erythematosus
- Carcinoid syndrome
- Acne vulgaris
- Seborrheic dermatitis
- Steroid rosacea (abuse)
- Systemic lupus erythematosus
- Lupus pernio (sarcoidosis)

DIAGNOSTIC TESTS & INTERPRETATION
- Diagnosis is based on physical exam findings.
- A recent change in classification has been proposed based on the phenotype that reflects the clinical presentation and to better focus treatment options, which are targeted to address the main clinical presentation (1).

Test Interpretation
Histology of affected skin may reveal:
- Inflammation around hypertrophied sebaceous glands, producing papules, pustules, and cysts
- Absence of comedones and blocked ducts
- Vascular dilatation and dermal lymphocytic infiltrate
- Granulomatous inflammation

TREATMENT

GENERAL MEASURES
- Proper skin care and photoprotection are important components of management plan (1)[B]. Use of mild, nondrying soap is recommended; local skin irritants should be avoided.
- Avoidance of triggers
- Reassurance that rosacea is completely unrelated to poor hygiene
- Treat psychological stress if present.
- Topical steroids should not be used because they may aggravate rosacea.
- Avoid oil-based cosmetics:
  - Others are acceptable and may help women tolerate symptoms.
- Electrodesiccation or chemical sclerosis of permanently dilated blood vessels
- Possible evolving laser therapy
- Support physical fitness.

MEDICATION
First Line
- Topical metronidazole preparations once (1% formulation) or twice (0.75% formulations) daily for 7 to 12 weeks was significantly more effective than placebo in patients with moderate to severe rosacea. A rosacea treatment system (cleanser, metronidazole 0.75% gel, hydrating complexion corrector, and sunscreen SPF 30) may offer superior efficacy and tolerability to metronidazole (2)[A].

- Azelaic acid (Finacea) is very effective as initial therapy; azelaic acid topical alone is effective for maintenance (3)[B].
- Topical ivermectin 1% cream (2)[A]
  - Recently found to be more effective than metronidazole for treatment of PPR
- Topical brimonidine tartrate 0.5% gel is effective in reducing erythema associated with ETR (4)[A].
  - α_2-Adrenergic receptor agonist; potent vasoconstrictor
- Oxymetazoline 1% cream, an α_{1A}-adrenergic receptor agonist, recently approved for the treatment of persistent erythema associated with rosacea in adults (5)[B]
- Doxycycline 40-mg dose is at least as effective as 100-mg dose and has a correspondingly lower risk of adverse effects but is much more expensive (6)[A].
- Precautions: Tetracyclines may cause photosensitivity; sunscreen is recommended.
- Significant possible interactions:
  - Tetracyclines: Avoid concurrent administration with antacids, dairy products, or iron.
  - Broad-spectrum antibiotics: may reduce the effectiveness of oral contraceptives; however, this finding has only been confirmed with rifampin; consider adding barrier method.

Second Line
- Topical erythromycin
- Topical timolol maleate 0.5%
- Topical clindamycin (lotion preferred)
  - Can be used in combination with benzoyl peroxide; commercial topical combinations are available.
- Possible use of calcineurin inhibitors (tacrolimus 0.1%; pimecrolimus 1%). Pimecrolimus 1% is effective to treat mild to moderate inflammatory rosacea.
- Permethrin 5% cream; similar efficacy compared to metronidazole for severe cases, oral isotretinoin at 0.3 mg/kg for a minimum of 3 months

Pediatric Considerations
Tetracyclines: not for use in children <8 years

Pregnancy Considerations
- Tetracyclines: not for use during pregnancy
- Isotretinoin: teratogenic; not for use during pregnancy or in women of reproductive age who are not using reliable contraception; requires registration with iPLEDGE program

ADDITIONAL THERAPIES
Cyclosporine 0.05% ophthalmic emulsion may be more effective than artificial tears for ocular rosacea.

SURGERY/OTHER PROCEDURES
Laser treatment is an option for progressive telangiectasias or rhinophyma.
- Pulsed dye laser (585 nm or 595 nm) is effective in treating telangiectases and erythema.
- CO_2 fractional ablative laser can be used to treat rhinophyma.

ONGOING CARE

FOLLOW-UP RECOMMENDATIONS
Outpatient treatment

Patient Monitoring
- Occasional and as needed
- Close follow-up and laboratory assessment for patients using isotretinoin per prescribing instructions and iPLEDGE program guidance
- Consider ophthalmology evaluation in patients with ocular symptoms.

DIET
Avoid alcohol and hot drinks of any type.

PROGNOSIS
- Slowly progressive
- Subsides spontaneously (sometimes)

COMPLICATIONS
- Rhinophyma (dilated follicles and thickened bulbous skin on nose), especially in men
- Conjunctivitis
- Blepharitis
- Keratitis
- Visual deterioration

REFERENCES

1. Schaller M, Almeida LM, Bewley A, et al. Rosacea treatment update: recommendations from the global ROSacea COnsensus (ROSCO) panel. *Br J Dermatol*. 2017;176(2):465–471.
2. van Zuuren EJ, Fedorowicz Z, Carter B, et al. Interventions for rosacea. *Cochrane Database Syst Rev*. 2015;(4):CD003262.
3. Thiboutot DM, Fleischer AB, Del Rosso JQ, et al. A multicenter study of topical azelaic acid 15% gel in combination with oral doxycycline as initial therapy and azelaic acid 15% gel as maintenance monotherapy. *J Drugs Dermatol*. 2009;8(7):639–648.
4. Fowler J Jr, Jackson M, Moore A, et al. Efficacy and safety of once-daily topical brimonidine tartrate gel 0.5% for the treatment of moderate to severe facial erythema of rosacea: results of two randomized, double-blind, and vehicle-controlled pivotal studies. *J Drugs Dermatol*. 2013;12(6):650–656.
5. Oxymetazoline cream (Rhofade) for rosacea. *Med Lett Drugs Ther*. 2017;59(1521):84–86.
6. Del Rosso JQ, Webster GF, Jackson M, et al. Two randomized phase III clinical trials evaluating anti-inflammatory dose doxycycline (40-mg doxycycline, USP capsules) administered once daily for treatment of rosacea. *J Am Acad Dermatol*. 2007;56(5):791–802.

ADDITIONAL READING

- Al Mokadem SM, Ibrahim AM, El Sayed AM. Efficacy of topical timolol 0.5% in the treatment of acne and rosacea: a multicentric study. *J Clin Aesthet Dermatol*. 2020;13(3):22–27.
- Del Rosso JQ, Tanghetti E, Webster G, et al. Update on the management of rosacea from the American Acne and Rosacea Society (AARS). *J Clin Aesthet Dermatol*. 2020;13(6 Suppl):17–24.
- Leyden JJ. Efficacy of a novel rosacea treatment system: an investigator-blind, randomized, parallel-group study. *J Drugs Dermatol*. 2011;10(10):1179–1185.
- Liu RH, Smith MK, Basta SA, et al. Azelaic acid in the treatment of papulopustular rosacea: a systematic review of randomized controlled trials. *Arch Dermatol*. 2006;142(8):1047–1052.
- Mikkelsen CS, Holmgren HR, Kjellman P, et al. Rosacea: a clinical review. *Dermatol Reports*. 2016;8(1):6387.

SEE ALSO

- Acne Vulgaris; Blepharitis; Dermatitis, Seborrheic; Lupus Erythematosus, Discoid; Uveitis
- Algorithm: Acne

CODES

ICD10
- L71.9 Rosacea, unspecified
- L71.8 Other rosacea

CLINICAL PEARLS

- Rosacea usually arises de novo without any preceding history of acne or seborrhea.
- Rosacea may cause chronic eye symptoms, including blepharitis.
- Avoid alcohol, sun exposure, and hot drinks.
- Medication treatment resembles that of acne vulgaris, with oral and topical antibiotics.

ACNE VULGARIS

Gary I. Levine, MD

BASICS

DESCRIPTION
Acne vulgaris is a disorder of the pilosebaceous units and a chronic inflammatory dermatosis notable for open/closed comedones, papules, pustules, nodules.

Geriatric Considerations
Favre-Racouchot syndrome: comedones on face/head due to sun exposure

Pregnancy Considerations
- May result in a flare or remission of acne
- Typically improves in 1st, may worsen in 3rd trimester
- Can use topical benzoyl peroxide, azelaic acid, erythromycin or clindamycin; oral erythromycin, azithromycin or cephalexin
- Avoid topical tretinoin and adapalene—may cause retinoid embryopathy; class C
- Contraindicated: isotretinoin (Category X), tazarotene, tetracycline, doxycycline, minocycline, sarecycline

Pediatric Considerations
- Neonatal acne (neonatal cephalic pustulosis)— newborn to 8 weeks; lesions limited to face; usually self-limited, Rx topical ketoconazole 2% cream
- Infantile acne—newborn to 1 year; lesions on face, neck, back, chest; topical/systemic Rx
- Early to middle childhood acne—1 to 7 years; rare; consider hyperandrogenism.
- Preadolescent acne—7 to 12 years; common, 47% of children, usually due to adrenal awakening, comedonal lesions
- Do not use tetracyclines in those <8 years old; other therapies similar to adolescent

EPIDEMIOLOGY
- Predominant age: early to late puberty, may persist in 20–40% of affected individuals into 4th decade
- Male > female (teen), female > male (adult)

Prevalence
- 80–95% of adolescents affected; 8% of adults aged 25 to 34 years; 3% at 35 to 44 years
- African Americans 37%, Caucasians 24%

ETIOLOGY AND PATHOPHYSIOLOGY
- Androgens (testosterone and dehydroepian-drosterone sulfate [DHEA-S]) stimulate sebum production/qualitative sebum changes and prolifera-tion of keratinocytes in follicles (1).
- Keratin plug obstructs follicle os, causing sebum accumulation and follicular distention.
- *Cutibacterium acnes* phylotype Ia, an anaerobe, colonizes and proliferates within a biofilm in the plugged follicle.
- *C. acnes* promote proinflammatory mediators, causing inflammation of follicle/dermis.

Genetics
Familial association in 50%

RISK FACTORS
- Increased endogenous androgenic effect
- Oily cosmetics, cocoa butter, polyvinyl chloride, chlorinated hydrocarbons, cutting oil

- Occluding skin surface (e.g., sports equipment such as helmets and shoulder pads), cell phones, hands against the skin, or pandemic masks ("maskne"— subset of acne mechanica)
- Numerous drugs, including androgenic steroids (e.g., steroid abuse, some birth control pills), lithium, phenytoin
- Endocrine disorders: PCOS, Cushing syndrome, congenital adrenal hyperplasia, androgen-secreting tumors, acromegaly
- Stress
- High-glycemic load, possibly high-dairy diets (skim milk), and whey protein supplements may exacerbate acne (1).
- Severe acne may worsen with smoking.

GENERAL PREVENTION
Avoidance of risk factors

COMMONLY ASSOCIATED CONDITIONS
- Acne conglobata, hidradenitis suppurativa
- Pomade acne
- SAPHO syndrome (synovitis, acne, pustulosis, hyperostosis, and osteitis)
- Pyogenic arthritis, pyoderma gangrenosum, and acne (PAPA) and seborrhea, acne, hirsutism, and alopecia (SAHA)
- Dark-skinned patients: 50% keloidal scarring and 50% acne hyperpigmented macules

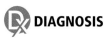

DIAGNOSIS

HISTORY
Ask about duration, relation to menses, medications, cleansing products, stress, smoking, exposures, diet, family history.

PHYSICAL EXAM
- Closed comedones (whiteheads), open comedones (blackheads)
- Nodules or papules, pustules, cysts
- Scars: ice pick, rolling, boxcar, atrophic macules, hypertrophic, depressed, sinus tracts
- Consistent grading is useful; no specific universal grading system is recommended per guidelines (2).
- Grading system (American Academy of Dermatology, 1990) (1)
  - Mild: few papules/pustules; no nodules
  - Moderate: some papules/pustules; few nodules
  - Severe: many papules/pustules/nodules
  - Very severe: acne conglobata, acne fulminans, acne inversa
- Most common areas affected are face, chest, back, and upper arms (greatest concentration of seba-ceous glands) (1).
- Adult female—facial lesion distribution not limited to mandibular and perioral lesion location, similar to adolescents

DIFFERENTIAL DIAGNOSIS
Folliculitis: gram-negative and gram-positive, acne (rosacea, cosmetica, steroid induced), perioral dermati-tis, pseudofolliculitis barbae, drug eruption, keratosis pilaris, sarcoidosis, seborrheic dermatitis, lupus erythematosus

DIAGNOSTIC TESTS & INTERPRETATION
Initial Tests (lab, imaging)
Only indicated if additional signs of androgen excess; if so, test for free and total testosterone and DHEA-S and consider LH and FSH (PCOS).

TREATMENT

- Comedonal (grade 1): keratolytic agent
- Mild inflammatory acne (grade 2): benzoyl peroxide +/− topical retinoid or benzoyl peroxide +/− topical antibiotic +/− topical retinoid
- Moderate inflammatory acne (grade 3): Add time-limited systemic antibiotic to grade 2 regimen.
- Severe inflammatory acne (grade 4): as in grade 3, or isotretinoin
- Topical retinoid plus a topical antimicrobial agent (such as BP) is first-line treatment for more than mild disease (3)[A].
- Topical retinoid + antibiotic (topical or PO) is better than either alone for mild/moderate.
- Topical retinoids are first-line agents for mainte-nance therapy (3)[A]. Avoid long-term antibiotics for maintenance.
- Avoid oral or topical antibiotics as monotherapy. Use with topical BP +/− topical retinoid (2)[C].
- Recommended vehicle type
  - Dry or sensitive skin: cream, lotion, or ointment
  - Oily skin, humid weather: gel, solution, wash
  - Hair-bearing areas: lotion, hydrogel, or foam
- Apply topical agents to entire affected area, not just visible lesions.
- Mild soap daily to control oiliness; avoid abrasives.
- Avoid drying agents; use gentle cleanser/noncomedogenic moisturizer to decrease irritation with keratolytic agents.

MEDICATION

> **ALERT**
> Most prescription branded topical medications are very expensive.

- Keratolytic agents (α-hydroxy acids, salicylic acid, topical retinoids, azelaic acid) (Side effects include dryness, erythema, and scaling; start with lower strength or alternate day Rx; increase as tolerated.)
- Tretinoin (Retin-A, Retin-A Micro, Avita, Atralin) varying strengths and formulations: wash skin; let skin dry 30 minutes before application to reduce irritation. Apply pea-sized dose at bedtime.
  - Retin-A Micro, Atralin, and Avita are less irritating and stable with BP.
  - May cause an initial flare of lesions; may be eased by every other day application for first 2 to 4 weeks
  - Avoid in pregnant and lactating women.
  - Cost varies based on formulation—$50 to $150 per tube for generic.
- Adapalene (Differin): 0.1%, apply topically HS
  - Effective; less irritation than tretinoin or tazarotene (3)[A]
  - May be combined with benzoyl peroxide (Epiduo) 0.1 or 0.3%/2.5%—very effective in skin of color
  - Available over-the-counter (OTC); *much* less expensive than other Rx retinoids ($10–$15)

- Tazarotene (Tazorac): Apply at bedtime. Most effective and most irritating; teratogenic, $400 per tube
- Azelaic acid (Azelex, Finevin): 20% topical BID
  - Keratinolytic, antibacterial, anti-inflammatory
  - Reduces postinflammatory hyperpigmentation in dark-skinned individuals
  - Side effects: erythema, dryness, scaling, hypopigmentation
  - Effective in postadolescent acne
  - Safe in pregnancy-risk Category B
  - 20% Rx >$400 per tube; OTC 10% and 15% formulations cost $10 to $40 per tube.
- Salicylic acid: 2%, less effective and less irritating than tretinoin. α-Hydroxy acids: available OTC
- Topical benzoyl peroxide: no resistance in *C. acnes*
  - 2.5% as effective as stronger preparations, gel penetrates better into follicles
  - When used with tretinoin, apply benzoyl peroxide in morning/tretinoin at night.
  - Side effects: concentration dependent irritation; may bleach clothes; photosensitivity
- Topical antibiotics (other than benzoyl peroxide): Do not use as monotherapy due to antibiotic resistance (2)[A].
  - Erythromycin 2%, clindamycin 1%, metronidazole gel or cream: once daily.
  - Benzoyl peroxide–erythromycin (Benzamycin): especially effective with azelaic acid
  - Benzoyl peroxide–clindamycin (BenzaClin, DUAC, Clindoxyl)
  - Benzoyl peroxide–salicylic acid (Cleanse & Treat, Inova): similar in effectiveness to benzoyl peroxide–clindamycin
  - Sodium sulfacetamide (Sulfacet-R, Novacet, Klaron): useful in acne with seborrheic dermatitis or rosacea
  - Dapsone (Aczone) 5% gel: useful in adult females with inflammatory acne; may cause yellow/orange skin discoloration when mixed with BP; very rare methemoglobinemia, expensive—$350 per tube
- Oral antibiotics: Use for shortest possible period, generally 6 to 12 weeks of therapy, limit to 3 months, max 6 months if necessary (2); use when acne is more severe, trunk involvement, unresponsive to topical agents, or at greater risk for scarring; do not use as monotherapy.
  - Tetracycline: 500 to 1,000 mg/day divided BID; high dose initially, taper in 6 months, less effective than doxycycline or minocycline (2), take fasting or without dairy, side effects: photosensitivity, esophagitis
  - Minocycline: 100 to 200 mg/day, divided daily—BID; side effects include photosensitivity, urticaria, gray-blue skin, vertigo, autoimmune hepatitis, lupus; extended release preparation better tolerated
  - Doxycycline: 20 to 200 mg/day, divided daily—BID; photosensitivity
  - Sarecycline (Seysara): 60 to 150 mg (1.5 mg/kg) given once daily, narrow spectrum, $1,000/month
  - Erythromycin: 500 to 1,000 mg/day; divided BID–QID; decreasing effectiveness due to *C. acnes* resistance
  - Trimethoprim-sulfamethoxazole (Bactrim DS, Septra DS): QD or BID
  - Azithromycin (Zithromax): 500 mg 3 days/week × 1 month, then 250 mg every other day × 2 months

- Oral retinoids
  - Isotretinoin: 0.5 to 1.0 mg/kg/day divided BID to maximum 2 mg/kg/day divided BID for very severe disease; 60–90% cure rate; usually given for 12 to 20 weeks; maximum cumulative dose = 120 to 150 mg/kg; 20% of patients relapse and require retreatment (1), 0.25 to 0.40 mg/kg/day in moderately severe acne
    - Side effects: teratogenic, pancreatitis, excessive drying of skin, hypertriglyceridemia, hepatitis, blood dyscrasias, hyperostosis, premature epiphyseal closure, night blindness, erythema multiforme, Stevens-Johnson syndrome, possible suicidal ideation, psychosis
    - Avoid tetracyclines or vitamin A during isotretinoin.
    - Monitor for pregnancy, psychiatric/mood changes, CBC, lipids, glucose, and LFTs at baseline and every month.
    - Patient and provider must register with iPLEDGE program (www.ipledgeprogram.com), two forms of effective contraception required
- Medications for women only
  - FDA-approved oral contraceptives (in order of possible effectiveness) (4)[B]
    - Drospirenone/ethinyl estradiol (Yaz), or drospirenone/ethinyl estradiol/levomefolate (Beyaz) > norgestimate/ethinyl estradiol (Ortho Tri-Cyclen) > norethindrone acetate/ethinyl estradiol (Estrostep)
    - Most combined contraceptives are also effective; may take 3 to 6 months
- Spironolactone (Aldactone); 25 to 200 mg/day; antiandrogen; reduces sebum production, not FDA-approved for acne Rx

ISSUES FOR REFERRAL
Management of acne scars

ADDITIONAL THERAPIES
- Acne hyperpigmented macules
  - Topical hydroquinone (1.5–10%), azelaic acid (20%) topically, topical retinoids, corticosteroids: low dose, dapsone 5% gel (Aczone): topical, anti-inflammatory; use in patients >12 years, sunscreen
- Light-based treatment—ultraviolet A/ultraviolet B (UVA/UVB), blue or blue/red light; pulse dye, infrared laser; photodynamic therapy with 5-aminolevulinic acid has best evidence.

SURGERY/OTHER PROCEDURES
- Comedo extraction after incising the layer of epithelium over closed comedo
- Inject large cystic lesions with 0.05 to 0.30 mL triamcinolone (Kenalog 2 to 5 mg/mL); 30-gauge needle, inject through pore, slightly distend cyst.
- Acne scar treatment: retinoids, steroid injections, cryosurgery, electrodesiccation, micro-/dermabrasion, chemical peels, laser resurfacing, pulsed dye laser, microneedling, fillers, punch elevation

COMPLEMENTARY & ALTERNATIVE MEDICINE
- Evidence suggests tea tree oil, seaweed extract, Kampo formulations, Ayurvedic formulations, rose extract, basil extract, epigallocatechin gallate, barberry extract, gluconolactone solution, and green tea extract may be useful (2).
- Dermocosmetics—limited data for acne Rx

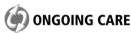
ONGOING CARE

FOLLOW-UP RECOMMENDATIONS
Limit use of oral antibiotics to 3 months; taper topical antibiotic (5),(6) as lesions resolve.

DIET
High-glycemic index foods and skim milk may worsen acne (2)[B].

PATIENT EDUCATION
Lesions may worsen during first 2 weeks of treatment; improvement typically seen after a minimum of 4 weeks of treatment.

PROGNOSIS
Gradual improvement over time (usually within 8 to 12 weeks after beginning therapy)

COMPLICATIONS
- Acne conglobata: severe confluent inflammatory acne with systemic symptoms. Facial scarring, psychological distress, including anxiety, depression, and suicidal ideation (1)
- Postinflammatory hyperpigmentation, keloids, scars—more common in skin of color

REFERENCES
1. Dawson AL, Dellavalle RP. Acne vulgaris. *BMJ*. 2013;346:f2634.
2. Zaenglein AL, Pathy AL, Schlosser BJ, et al. Guidelines of care for the management of acne vulgaris. *J Am Acad Dermatol*. 2016;74(5):945.e33–973.e33.
3. Kolli SS, Pecone D, Pona A, et al. Topical retinoids in acne vulgaris: a systematic review. *Am J Clin Dermatol*. 2019;20(3):345–365.
4. Lortscher D, Admani S, Satur N, et al. Hormonal contraceptives and acne: a retrospective analysis of 2147 patients. *J Drugs Dermatol*. 2016;15(6):670–674.
5. Marson JW, Baldwin HE. An overview of acne therapy, part 1: topical therapy, oral antibiotics, laser and light therapy, and dietary interventions. *Dermatol Clin*. 2019;37(2):183–193.
6. Marson JW, Baldwin HE. An overview of acne therapy, part 2: hormonal therapy and isotretinoin. *Dermatol Clin*. 2019;37(2):195–203.

SEE ALSO

Acne Rosacea, Algorithm: Acne

CODES

ICD10
L70.0 Acne vulgaris

CLINICAL PEARLS
- May need 8 to 12 weeks to see the effect of therapy
- Decrease topical frequency to every day or to every other day to lessen irritation.
- Use benzoyl peroxide every time a topical or oral antibiotic is used to reduce emergence of bacterial resistance.

ACUTE CORONARY SYNDROMES: NSTE-ACS (UNSTABLE ANGINA AND NSTEMI)

Keith Ranney Love, MD, BA • Alejandro Folch Sandoval, MD • Colleen M. Harrington, MD, FACC, FASE

BASICS

DESCRIPTION
- Unstable angina (UA) and non–ST-segment elevation myocardial infarction (NSTEMI) are acute coronary syndromes without ST-segment elevation (NSTE-ACS).
- NSTEMI is defined by the rise and fall of cardiac biomarkers (preferably troponin I or T) with at least one value above the 99th percentile upper reference limit and accompanied by one of the following: symptoms of ischemia, new ST-segment/T-wave changes (such as ST depression or T-wave inversions), development of pathologic Q waves on 12-lead ECG, or noninvasive imaging with evidence of myocardium at risk for ischemia or a new regional wall motion abnormality.
- UA is defined by the presence of clinical symptoms of cardiac ischemia (new-onset anginal chest pain, change in typical anginal pattern, development of angina at rest, or change in typical anginal equivalent), without evidence of myocardial necrosis as evidenced by normal cardiac biomarkers of injury (troponin). ECG changes, such as ST-segment depression or T-wave inversions, may be present.

EPIDEMIOLOGY
Incidence
Estimated annual incidence of new and recurrent MI is 605,000 and 200,000, respectively. In United States, average age at first MI is 65.6 years for males and 72.0 years for females (1).

Prevalence
An estimated 16.5 million Americans ≥20 years have coronary artery disease (CAD). Mortality: CAD is the leading cause of death in adults in the United States with overall age-adjusted mortality of 98.8/100,000. Death rate is higher in men.

ETIOLOGY AND PATHOPHYSIOLOGY
- NSTE-ACS primarily due to a sudden decrease in myocardial blood flow due to acute plaque rupture or plaque erosion leading to partially occluding thrombus
- Other mechanisms include (i) Dynamic obstruction triggered by intense spasm of an epicardial coronary artery (prinzmetal angina or coronary vasospasm induced by tobacco use, hyperventilation, magnesium deficiency, cocaine, or methamphetamine); (ii) increased myocardial oxygen demand resulting in supply-demand mismatch (type 2 NSTEMI) due to underlying causes such as pulmonary embolism, sepsis, shock, arrhythmias/tachycardia; (iii) coronary microvascular dysfunction or endothelial dysfunction without epicardial coronary obstruction; and (iv) less common causes include coronary arterial aneurysm, spontaneous coronary artery dissection, thromboembolism.

Genetics
CAD is generally a complex, polygenic disorder.

RISK FACTORS
- Traditional/classic: age (strongest risk factor), male sex, prior MI, hypertension (HTN), tobacco use, diabetes mellitus (DM), dyslipidemia, and family history of premature CAD (defined as age of onset prior to 55 years in males and 65 years in females)
- Novel/emerging risk factors: sedentary lifestyle, overweight/obesity (metabolic syndrome), inflammation (psoriasis, rheumatoid arthritis), psychosocial factors (anxiety/depression), chronic kidney disease (CKD), obstructive sleep apnea, environmental pollutants

GENERAL PREVENTION
Smoking cessation, a diet low in saturated fat, maintaining a normal body mass index, regular physical activity combined with risk factor control: glycemic control for patient with diabetes and blood pressure (BP) control in patients with HTN, risk-based statins; aspirin in those with documented CAD

COMMONLY ASSOCIATED CONDITIONS
Vascular disease, chronic kidney disease

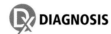

DIAGNOSIS

HISTORY
- Chest heaviness/tightness lasting ≥10 minutes; occurs with or without exertion. Pain or discomfort is typically retrosternal and can radiate to the neck, jaw, interscapular area, upper extremities, or epigastrium. Pain is typically described as a pressure, tightness, heaviness, squeezing, or fullness.
- Associated symptoms of palpitations, dyspnea, nausea, diaphoresis, light-headedness, syncope, or dysphoria can occur.
- Patients, especially elderly, diabetics, and women, can present without chest pain and with symptoms of dyspnea, diaphoresis, and extreme fatigue which represent "anginal equivalents."
- Risk factors for CAD; use of cocaine or amphetamines

PHYSICAL EXAM
General: Note vital signs (especially tachycardia or bradycardia, HTN or hypotension), widened pulse pressure, tachypnea, fever, poor dental hygiene. Cardiovascular: dysrhythmia, jugular venous distention (JVD), new murmur, rub or gallop, diminished peripheral pulses, carotid bruits. Respiratory: tachypnea, ↑ work of breathing, crackles. Musculoskeletal: Sharp pain reproducible with movement or palpation is unlikely to be cardiac. Skin: cool skin, pallor, diaphoresis, signs of dyslipidemia (xanthomas, xanthelasma)

DIFFERENTIAL DIAGNOSIS
- Cardiac: aortic dissection, myocarditis, pericarditis, pericardial effusion/cardiac tamponade, heart failure with preserved and reduced ejection fraction, hypertensive emergency, stress cardiomyopathy (Takotsubo), dysrhythmia, and mitral valve disease
- Pulmonary: pulmonary embolism, pneumothorax, pneumonia, pleuritis, bronchitis
- Psychiatric: panic attacks, anxiety
- Musculoskeletal: costochondritis, rib fracture
- Gastroenterology: gastroesophageal reflux disease, esophageal spasm, esophagitis, esophageal rupture or perforation, hiatal hernia, penetrating or perforating peptic ulcer, biliary or pancreatic pain

DIAGNOSTIC TESTS & INTERPRETATION
Initial Tests (lab, imaging)
- 12-lead ECG: should be obtained within 10 minutes of presentation; applies to both UA and NSTEMI
  - New ST-segment depression ≥0.5 mm in two or more contiguous leads and/or T-wave inversions ≥1 mm in two or more contiguous leads with prominent R wave or R/S ratio >1
  - ST depression and/or tall R wave in V_1/V_2 with upright T waves may indicate transmural STEMI of posterior wall. ECG with posterior leads ($V_7–V_9$) should be performed.
  - If initial ECG is nondiagnostic but symptoms persist with suspicion for ACS, perform serial ECGs at 15- to 30-minute intervals.
- Completed blood count and serum biomarkers (negative by definition in UA)
  - Troponin concentration rises 3 to 6 hours after onset of ischemic symptoms but can be delayed up to 8 to 12 hours (troponin T is not specific in patients with renal dysfunction).
  - Ultra-high sensitive troponins have a higher sensitivity than standard assays, but further validation is required.
  - CK-MB has been shown to have better specificity than troponins in post-PCI MI. Troponin elevation will resolve in 3 to 10 days; CK-MB will return to normal within 3 to 4 days.
  - Repeat biomarkers 8 to 12 hours from onset of symptoms.
- Chest x-ray, computed tomography with contrast to exclude other etiologies if applicable. Transthoracic echocardiography is recommended.

Follow-Up Tests & Special Considerations
- Fasting lipid profile, preferably within 24 hours. Activated partial thromboplastin time (aPTT); TSH, HgbA1c
- Urine drug screen in selected patients

Diagnostic Procedures/Other
- For low- to intermediate-risk patients with resolution of symptoms and nondiagnostic ECG with negative biomarkers, consider noninvasive cardiac testing with standard exercise treadmill test, exercise stress echocardiography, or myocardial perfusion imaging using single-photon emission computed tomography.
- Alternatively, coronary computed tomography angiography can be performed as well in the same population at low to intermediate risk.

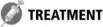

TREATMENT

GENERAL MEASURES
- Risk stratify (TIMI or GRACE score) to select use of early invasive approach (coronary angiography within 24 hours of admission) versus ischemia-guided therapy; urgent invasive management for very high-risk patients, such as those with hemodynamic instability or cardiogenic shock, recurrent or ongoing chest pain refractory to medical therapy, life-threatening arrhythmias or cardiac arrest, mechanical complications, acute heart failure, and recurrent dynamic ST-T wave changes
- Bed/chair rest with continuous ECG monitoring, maintain O_2 saturation >90%, and tight BP control. Discontinue NSAIDs if possible. Support smoking cessation. Correct electrolyte abnormalities (K+ and Mg++).

MEDICATION

First Line

- Antiplatelet therapy: Dual antiplatelet therapy is recommended for all patients with NSTE-ACS.
- Aspirin, nonenteric coated, initial dose of 162 to 325 mg chewed or crushed for all patients; decreases mortality and morbidity; maintenance dose of 75 to 100 mg/day indefinitely
- P2Y12 inhibitors:
  - Should be given at the time of diagnosis unless invasive approach is planned in a very high bleeding-risk patient
  - Ticagrelor, loading dose 180 mg PO, followed by 90 mg PO twice daily; avoid in patients with 2nd- and 3rd-degree heart block. Can cause dyspnea in some patients. Contraindicated in patients with severe liver dysfunction. PB2452, a monoclonal antibody fragment that binds ticagrelor, can be used as a reversal agent OR
  - Prasugrel 60 mg PO, followed by 10 mg PO daily. Often reserved for post-PCI patients treated with coronary stents; contraindicated in patients ≥75 years or those with history of CVA/TIA OR
  - Clopidogrel, loading dose 300 to 600 mg PO, followed by 75 mg PO daily. Use with caution in patients with thrombocytopenia and CKD. An estimated 15% of the general population clopidogrel "nonresponders." Resistance can be tested with P2Y12 assay, although routine screening is not currently recommended (1).
  - Patients unable to take aspirin should receive loading and maintenance dose of a P2Y12 inhibitor.
  - GP IIb/IIIa inhibitors: Add eptifibatide or tirofiban in select high-risk patients (persistent chest pain, large thrombus burden on angiography) after PCI.
- Supplemental oxygen may be given if oxygen saturations are <90% or in patients with heart failure symptoms.
- Nitroglycerin sublingual 0.4 mg every 5 minutes for total of 3 doses and then assess need for IV nitroglycerin. Avoid if hypotension or if used phosphodiesterase inhibitors within the past 24 to 48 hours. Nitroglycerin-induced hypotension may be attenuated with right ventricular infarction.
- Morphine sulfate 1 to 5 mg IV in patients with continuous ischemic chest pain, with increments of 2 to 8 mg repeated at 5- to 30-minute intervals
- Oral β-blocker therapy should be initiated within 24 hours in patients without signs of heart failure, cardiogenic shock, or other contraindications to β-blockade (2nd- or 3rd-degree heart block without a pacemaker, active asthma). Recommended dose is metoprolol tartrate 25 to 50 mg every 6 to 12 hours. IV therapy may be considered in patients with severe ischemia.
- In patients with concomitant ACS, stabilized heart failure, and reduced systolic function (LVEF <40%), the recommended β-blockers are metoprolol succinate, carvedilol, and bisoprolol.
- Lipid-lowering therapy: Initiate or continue high-intensity statin therapy (preferred due to nonlipid benefit on vascular function) with atorvastatin 80 mg daily or rosuvastatin 20 to 40 mg daily regardless of the patient's baseline LDL level. Ezetimibe, omega-3 fatty acids, PCSK9 inhibitors (evolocumab, alirocumab), and/or fibrates can be considered in statin-intolerant patients or as complimentary therapy.

- ACE inhibitor (ACEi) is recommended in all patients with ACS particularly in the presence of diabetes, LV dysfunction, or heart failure.
- Aldosterone antagonist (spironolactone or eplerenone) is recommended in NSTEMI for patients without significant renal dysfunction or hyperkalemia who are on a therapeutic dose of ACEi/ARB and β-blocker and have LVEF ≤40%, DM, or heart failure.
- Antithrombotic therapy: Initiate anticoagulant: enoxaparin or unfractionated heparin (UFH), fondaparinux, or bivalirudin. Bivalirudin has been associated with a lower bleeding risk.

Second Line

- Nondihydropyridine calcium channel blocker (CCB) (verapamil or diltiazem) to reduce myocardial oxygen demand when β-blockers are contraindicated if left ventricular ejection fraction is normal. Use oral long-acting CCB only after β-blockers and nitrates have been fully used. Long-acting CCBs are recommended in treatment of patients with epicardial or microvascular coronary artery spasm. Avoid in patients with heart block.
- Sublingual nitroglycerin as needed for angina; long-term nitrate therapy for recurrent angina
- Ranolazine indicated in treatment of chronic angina not responsive to other medications at 500 to 1,000 mg, twice a day. Benzodiazepines in patients with cocaine/methamphetamine intoxication. Avoid β-blockers in patients who use cocaine or methamphetamine.

ISSUES FOR REFERRAL

- Cardiology consultation is indicated for NSTE-ACS. Patients will need close follow-up with a cardiologist.
- Referral to exercise-based cardiac rehabilitation program prior to hospital discharge is associated with decreased morbidity and mortality. Referral to a dietitian should be considered.

SURGERY/OTHER PROCEDURES

- Coronary reperfusion strategies include PCI with stenting and CABG surgery.
- Mechanical circulatory support for patients with refractory shock

ADMISSION, INPATIENT, AND NURSING CONSIDERATIONS

- Admit patients with suspected NSTE-ACS.
- Considerations in special populations
  - Older population (≥75 years)
    ○ Benefit of early invasive management in elderly ≥ young population
    ○ Pharmacotherapy should be individualized based on weight, baseline characteristics, and comorbidities.
  - Pregnancy: Specific risk factors for ACS in pregnancy include advanced maternal age, gestational diabetes, and preeclampsia/eclampsia. Spontaneous coronary artery dissection and thromboembolism should be considered in evaluation of pregnant women with ACS. ACEi, ARBs, and statins are contraindicated.

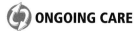 ONGOING CARE

FOLLOW-UP RECOMMENDATIONS

- Patients with low-risk suspected ACS who have normal serial ECGs and cardiac troponins may have a treadmill ECG, stress myocardial perfusion imaging, or stress echocardiography within 72 hours after discharge. Follow up 2 to 6 weeks (low risk) and 14 days (high risk).
- Patients with LVEF <40% are at increased risk of ventricular arrhythmias. Repeat LVEF evaluation 1 to 3 months postdischarge to reassess function and determine the need for ICD implantation.

DIET

Diet relationship to CAD is complex; patients should maintain a diet low in saturated and trans fats, low in sodium, and high in fiber.

PATIENT EDUCATION

Education on diet, exercise, smoking cessation, and lifestyle modification. It is safe to resume exercise; sexual activity within 2 weeks in asymptomatic patients after outpatient reevaluation. Recommend pneumococcal and influenza vaccination.

PROGNOSIS

UA/NSTEMI patients have lower in-hospital mortality than those with STEMI but a similar or worse long-term outcome.

COMPLICATIONS

Cardiogenic shock, heart failure, dysrhythmia (2), acute thromboembolic stroke, pericarditis/Dressler syndrome, depression (increases mortality risk)

REFERENCES

1. Collet JP, Cuisset T, Rangé G, et al. Bedside monitoring to adjust antiplatelet therapy for coronary stenting. *N Engl J Med.* 2012;367(22):2100–2109.
2. Benjamin EJ, Virani SS, Callaway CW, et al; American Heart Association Council on Epidemiology and Prevention Statistics Committee and Stroke Statistics Subcommittee. Heart disease and stroke statistics-2018 update: a report from the American Heart Association. *Circulation.* 2018;137(12):e67–e492.

 CODES

ICD10

- I24.9 Acute ischemic heart disease, unspecified
- I20.0 Unstable angina
- I21.4 Non-ST elevation (NSTEMI) myocardial infarction

CLINICAL PEARLS

- Dual antiplatelet therapy, antithrombotic therapy, β-blocker, high-dose statin therapy, and nitrates are the cornerstones of initial therapy and should be initiated promptly.
- Duration of antithrombotic therapy after NSTEMI depends on type of stent received and medications administered.

ACUTE CORONARY SYNDROMES: STEMI

Yutthapong Temtanakitpaisan, MD, FACC, FSCAI • Adedotun Anthony Ogunsua, MD, MPH

 BASICS

DESCRIPTION
Acute myocardial infarction (AMI) is the rapid development of myocardial necrosis resulting from a sustained and complete absence of blood flow to a portion of the myocardium. ST-segment elevation myocardial infarction (STEMI) occurs when coronary blood flow ceases, usually following complete atherothrombotic occlusion of a large coronary artery, resulting in transmural ischemia. This is accompanied by release of serum cardiac biomarkers and ST-segment elevation on an electrocardiogram (ECG).

EPIDEMIOLOGY
Incidence
There are >650,000 cases of AMI reported annually in the United States. Early revascularization and AMI management has improved mortality, with a 30-day survival of 95%.

Prevalence
- Atherosclerotic heart disease is the leading cause of morbidity and mortality in the United States.
- ~7.5 million people in the United States are affected by AMI.
- Prevalence increases with age and is higher in men (5.5%) compared to women (2.9%).

ETIOLOGY AND PATHOPHYSIOLOGY
- Atherosclerotic coronary artery disease (CAD): Atherosclerotic lesions can be fibrotic, calcified, or lipid laden. Thin-capped atheromas are more likely to rupture, causing atherothrombotic occlusion.
- Nonatherosclerotic causes:
  - Embolism from either infective vegetations, or thrombi originating within the right atrium across the foramen ovale ("paradoxical"), from the left atrium or from within the left ventricle
  - Spontaneous coronary artery dissection: prevalent in fibromuscular dysplasia (FMD) and in young women
  - Mechanical or iatrogenic obstruction: chest trauma, dissection of the aorta and/or coronary arteries
  - Coronary artery spasm from increased vasomotor tone; anginal variant
  - Arteritis and other etiologies: hematologic causes (disseminated intravascular coagulation [DIC], severe anemia), aortic stenosis, cocaine, IV drug use, severe burns, prolonged hypotension

RISK FACTORS
Advancing age, hypertension, tobacco use, diabetes mellitus, dyslipidemia, family history of premature onset of CAD, sedentary lifestyle

GENERAL PREVENTION
Smoking cessation/abstinence; healthy diet; weight loss/control; regular physical activity and exercise; control of hypertension, hyperlipidemia, and diabetes mellitus

COMMONLY ASSOCIATED CONDITIONS
Abdominal aortic aneurysm, cerebrovascular disease, atherosclerotic peripheral vascular disease

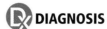 **DIAGNOSIS**

HISTORY
- Symptoms:
  - Classically, sudden onset of chest heaviness/tightness, with or without exertion, lasting minutes to hours
  - Pain/discomfort radiating to neck, jaw, interscapular area, upper extremities, and/or epigastrium
  - Patients with inferior MI may present primarily with abdominal discomfort.
- Previous history of myocardial ischemia (stable or unstable angina, AMI, coronary bypass surgery, or percutaneous coronary intervention [PCI])
- Assess risk factors for CAD, history of bleeding, noncardiac surgery, family history of premature CAD.
- Medications: Ask if recent use of phosphodiesterase type 5 inhibitors (if recent use, avoid concomitant nitrates).
- Tobacco, alcohol, and/or drug abuse (especially cocaine)

PHYSICAL EXAM
- General: restlessness, agitation, hypothermia, fever
- Neurologic: dizziness, syncope, fatigue, asthenia, disorientation (especially in the elderly)
- Cardiovascular (CV): dysrhythmia, hypotension, widened pulse pressure, S3 and S4, jugular venous distention (JVD)
- Respiratory: dyspnea, tachypnea, crackles, rales
- GI: abdominal pain, nausea, vomiting, hiccups
- Skin: cool skin, pallor, diaphoresis

Geriatric and Gender Considerations
- Elderly patients may have an atypical presentation, including silent or unrecognized MI. They may often present with syncope, weakness, shortness of breath, unexplained nausea, epigastric pain, altered mental status, or delirium.
- Women or patients with diabetes mellitus may present with typical and/or "atypical" symptoms such as fatigue, dyspnea, and malaise.

DIFFERENTIAL DIAGNOSIS
Unstable angina, aortic dissection, pulmonary embolism (PE), perforating gastric ulcer, pericarditis, dysrhythmias, gastroesophageal reflux disease (GERD), esophageal spasm, biliary/pancreatic pain, hyperventilation syndrome, anxiety/panic

DIAGNOSTIC TESTS & INTERPRETATION
Initial Tests (lab, imaging)
- 12-lead ECG:
  - ≥1 mm ST elevation in a regional pattern, involving at least two contiguous leads, with or without abnormal Q waves
  - STEMI of posterior wall: ST depression ± tall R waves in V_1–V_2
  - Absence of Q waves represents partial or transient occlusion or early infarction.
  - Consider right-sided and posterior chest leads if inferior MI pattern (examine V_3R, V_4R, V_7–V_9).
  - In the setting of ventricular pacing or a prior left bundle branch block (LBBB), the Sgarbossa criteria or BARCELONA algorithm (1) may be helpful.

- 2-Dimensional transthoracic echocardiography is useful in evaluating regional wall motion in MI, left ventricular function, mechanical complications, and mural thrombus.
- Once diagnosis is suspected, emergent coronary angiography with PCI is preferred.

Follow-Up Tests & Special Considerations
Serum biomarkers
- Troponin I and T (cTnI, cTnT) rise 3 to 6 hours after onset of ischemic symptoms.
- Elevations in cTnI persist for 7 to 10 days, whereas cTnT elevations persist for 10 to 14 days after MI.
- Myoglobin fraction of creatine kinase-MB (CK-MB) adds little diagnostic value in assessment of possible AMI to troponin testing.

Pregnancy Considerations
Pregnant patients presenting with STEMI will need discussion of risks and benefits of invasive coronary angiography with radiation exposure to fetus. Management should otherwise be the same as in nonpregnant patients.

Diagnostic Procedures/Other
- Portable chest x-ray; transthoracic echocardiography; chest computed tomography angiography (CTA) scan may occasionally be of value acutely in equivocal presentations to evaluate for alternative diagnoses (aortic dissection, PE, ventricular aneurysm).
- Coronary angiography is the definitive test.

ALERT
Patients with chronic kidney disease need special attention to amount of contrast media used.

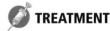 **TREATMENT**

GENERAL MEASURES
- See "Medication" for ED management.
- Following emergent revascularization, admit the patient to the coronary care unit (CCU) or a telemetry unit with continuous ECG monitoring and bed rest and use:
  - Antiarrhythmics as needed for unstable dysrhythmia
  - Dual antiplatelet therapy (DAPT) with continuation of aspirin 81 mg/day with clopidogrel 75 mg/day or prasugrel 10 mg/day or ticagrelor 90 mg twice daily

MEDICATION
Medication recommendations are based on the 2013 American College of Cardiology (ACC)/American Heart Association (AHA) guideline (2)[C] and 2017 European Society of Cardiology (ESC) guideline (3)[C].

First Line
- Supplemental oxygen 2 to 4 L/min for patients with oxygen saturation <90% or respiratory distress
- Nitroglycerin (NTG) sublingual 0.4 mg q5min for a total of 3 doses, followed by NTG IV if ongoing pain and/or hypertension and/or management of pulmonary congestion if no contraindications exist such as systolic <90 mm Hg or >30 mm Hg below baseline, right ventricle (RV) infarct, use of sildenafil or vardenafil within 24 hours or within 48 hours of tadalafil

- Morphine sulfate 4 to 8 mg IV with 2 to 8 mg IV repeated at 5- to 15-minute intervals to relieve pain, anxiety, or pulmonary congestion
- Antiplatelet agents:
  - Aspirin (ASA), non–enteric-coated, initial dose 162 to 325 mg chewed
  - A loading dose of a P2Y12 inhibitor is recommended for patients with STEMI for whom PCI is planned. Prasugrel or ticagrelor is preferred.
    - Prasugrel 60 mg loading dose. Prasugrel is contraindicated in patients with previous stroke/transient ischemic attack. Do not recommend in patients aged >75 years or lower body weight (<60 kg).
    - Ticagrelor 180 mg loading dose. Ticagrelor may cause transient dyspnea.
    - Clopidogrel 600 mg loading dose should be given if neither prasugrel nor ticagrelor is available.
    - Cangrelor may be considered in patients not pretreated with oral P2Y12 receptor inhibitors at the time of PCI or in those who are unable to take oral agents.
    - Standard recommendation for duration of DAPT is 6 to 12 months after PCI, depending on bleeding and ischemia risks.
- Anticoagulation therapy:
  - Unfractionated heparin (UFH) 70- to 100-U/kg IV bolus OR
  - Enoxaparin 0.5-mg/kg IV bolus OR
  - Bivalirudin 0.75-mg/kg IV bolus and then 1.75-mg/kg/hr infusion for up to 4 hours after procedure
- PCI versus fibrinolysis: Goal is to keep total ischemic time within 120 minutes. Door to needle time should be within 30 minutes or door to balloon time within 90 minutes.
  - Coronary reperfusion therapy
    - Primary PCI (balloon angioplasty, coronary stents) in the following:
      - Symptom onset of ≤12 hours
      - Symptom onset of ≤12 hours and contraindication to fibrinolytic therapy irrespective of time delay
      - Cardiogenic shock or acute severe heart failure (HF) irrespective of time delay from onset of MI
      - Evidence of ongoing ischemia 12 to 24 hours after symptom onset
  - Procedural considerations
    - Radial access is recommended over femoral access.
    - PCI of infarct-related artery (IRA) is indicated.
  - Fibrinolysis
    - If presenting to a hospital without PCI capability and cannot be transferred to a PCI-capable facility to undergo PCI within 120 minutes of first medical contact
    - If no contraindications, administer within 12 to 24 hours of symptom onset, if there is evidence of ongoing ischemia.
      - Alteplase (tPA): 15-mg IV bolus, followed by 0.75 mg/kg (up to 50 mg) IV over 30 minutes and then 0.5 mg/kg (up to 35 mg) over 60 minutes; maximum 100 mg over 90 minutes
      - Reteplase (rPA): 10 units IV bolus; give second bolus 30 minutes apart.
      - Tenecteplase (TNK-tPA): 30- to 50-mg (based on weight) IV bolus. Recommend to reduce to half dose in patients ≥75 years of age.

- Adjunctive antiplatelet therapy with fibrinolysis
  - Aspirin: 162- to 325-mg loading dose followed by 81 mg daily indefinitely
  - Clopidogrel (300-mg loading dose for patients <75 years of age, 75-mg dose for patients >75 years of age). Clopidogrel 75 mg daily should be continued for at least 14 days and up to 1 year.
- Adjunctive anticoagulation therapy with fibrinolysis
  - Use anticoagulants (UFH, enoxaparin, or fondaparinux) as ancillary therapy to reperfusion therapy for minimum of 48 hours and preferably duration of admission (up to 8 days) or until revascularization, if performed.
- Glycoprotein IIb/IIIa receptor antagonists at time of primary PCI in selected patients if there is no reflow or thrombotic complications (abciximab, eptifibatide, or tirofiban)
- ACE inhibitors should be initiated orally within 24 hours of STEMI in patients with anterior infarction, HF, diabetes, or ejection fraction (EF) ≤0.40 unless contraindicated.
- High-intensity statin therapy should be started as early as possible.
- Mineralocorticoid receptor antagonist (spironolactone, eplerenone) is recommended in patients with EF <40% and HF or diabetes, who are already receiving an ACE inhibitor and a β-blocker (BB), if there is no renal failure or hyperkalemia.

Second Line
Long-acting nondihydropyridine calcium channel blocker (CCB) when BB is ineffective or contraindicated and EF is normal; do not use immediate-release nifedipine.

ISSUES FOR REFERRAL
Transfer high-risk patients who receive fibrinolytic therapy as primary reperfusion therapy at a non–PCI-capable facility to a PCI-capable facility as soon as possible.

SURGERY/OTHER PROCEDURES
Urgent coronary artery bypass graft (CABG) surgery is indicated in patients with STEMI and coronary anatomy not amenable to PCI who have ongoing or recurrent ischemia, cardiogenic shock, severe HF, or other high-risk features.

ADMISSION, INPATIENT, AND NURSING CONSIDERATIONS
All STEMI patients should be admitted to a CCU or an intensive cardiac care unit for evaluation and treatment.

ONGOING CARE

FOLLOW-UP RECOMMENDATIONS
- STEMI patients should follow up with a cardiologist 1 to 2 weeks postdischarge, every 3 months for the first year, and then yearly.
- Emphasize medication adherence and encourage smoking cessation.
- Consider an exercise-based cardiac rehabilitation program.

DIET
Low-fat/healthy-fat diet: reduced intake of saturated fats (to <7% of total calories), eliminate *trans*-fatty acids (to <1% of total calories). Mediterranean diet is healthy.

PATIENT EDUCATION
May resume sexual activity 1 or more weeks after uncomplicated MI or 6 to 8 weeks after CABG; smoking cessation and low-fat diet

COMPLICATIONS
- Poor prognosis is associated with advanced age, diabetes, delayed or unsuccessful revascularization, reduced left ventricular systolic function, and evidence of congestive HF.
- HF, myocardial wall rupture, left ventricular aneurysm, pericarditis, dysrhythmias, acute mitral regurgitation, and depression (common)

REFERENCES
1. Di Marco A, Rodriguez M, Cinca J, et al. New electrocardiographic algorithm for the diagnosis of acute myocardial infarction in patients with left bundle branch block. *J Am Heart Assoc*. 2020;9(14):e015573.
2. O'Gara PT, Kushner FG, Ascheim DD, et al. 2013 ACCF/AHA guideline for the management of ST-elevation myocardial infarction: a report of the American College of Cardiology Foundation/American Heart Association Task Force on Practice Guidelines. *J Am Coll Cardiol*. 2013;61(4):e78–e140.
3. Ibanez B, James S, Agewall S, et al. 2017 ESC Guidelines for the management of acute myocardial infarction in patients presenting with ST-segment elevation: the Task Force for the management of acute myocardial infarction in patients presenting with ST-segment elevation of the European Society of Cardiology (ESC). *Eur Heart J*. 2018;39(2):119–177.

CODES

ICD10
- I24.9 Acute ischemic heart disease, unspecified
- I21.3 ST elevation (STEMI) myocardial infarction of unspecified site
- I25.10 Athscl heart disease of native coronary artery w/o ang pctrs

CLINICAL PEARLS
- STEMI occurs from occlusion of one or more coronary arteries resulting in transmural myocardial ischemia.
- Early revascularization with PCI within 90 minutes of presentation at a PCI-capable hospital is required, or within 120 minutes if transfer to a PCI-capable hospital is required.
- Fibrinolytic therapy should be initiated within 30 minutes if presenting to a hospital without PCI capability and the patient cannot be transferred to a PCI-capable facility to undergo PCI within 120 minutes of first medical contact.

ACUTE KIDNEY INJURY
Pratha Muthiah, MD, MPH

BASICS

DESCRIPTION
- An abrupt loss of kidney function, defined as one of the following (1):
  - Increase in serum creatinine (SCr) of ≥0.3 mg/dL within 48 hours
  - A 50% increase in SCr within 7 days
  - Urine output of <0.5 mL/kg/hr for >6 hours
- The result is retention of nitrogenous waste as well as electrolyte, acid–base, and volume homeostasis abnormalities (1).

EPIDEMIOLOGY
Incidence
- 5% of hospital and 30% of ICU admissions have acute kidney injury (AKI). 25% of patients develop AKI while in the hospital; 50% of these cases are iatrogenic.
- Developing AKI as an inpatient is associated with >4-fold increased risk of death (2).

ETIOLOGY AND PATHOPHYSIOLOGY
Three categories: prerenal, intrarenal, and postrenal
- Prerenal (reduced renal perfusion, typically reversible):
  - Decreased renal perfusion (often due to hypovolemia) leads to a decrease in glomerular filtration rate (GFR).
  - Caused by hypotension, volume depletion (GI losses, excessive sweating, diuretics, hemorrhage); renal artery stenosis/embolism; burns; heart/liver failure
  - If decreased perfusion is prolonged or severe, can progress to ischemic acute tubular necrosis (ATN).
- Intrarenal (intrinsic kidney injury, often from prolonged or severe renal hypoperfusion)
  - Acute tubular necrosis (ATN)—from prolonged prerenal azotemia, radiographic contrast material, aminoglycosides, nonsteroidal anti-inflammatory drugs (NSAIDs), or other nephrotoxic substances
  - Glomerulonephritis (GN)
  - Acute interstitial nephritis (AIN; drug induced), arteriolar insults, vasculitis, accelerated hypertension, cholesterol embolization (following an intra-arterial procedure), intrarenal deposition/sludging (uric acid nephropathy and multiple myeloma [Bence Jones proteins])
- Postrenal (obstruction of the collecting system)
  - Extrinsic compression (e.g., benign prostatic hypertrophy [BPH], carcinoma, pregnancy); intrinsic obstruction (e.g., calculus, tumor, clot, stricture, sloughed papillae); decreased function (e.g., neurogenic bladder), leading to obstruction of the urinary collection system

Genetics
No known genetic pattern

RISK FACTORS
- Chronic kidney disease (CKD)
- Comorbid conditions (e.g., diabetes mellitus, hypertension, heart failure, liver failure)
- Advanced age
- Radiocontrast material exposure (intravascular)
- Medications that impair autoregulation of GFR (NSAIDs, angiotensin converting enzyme inhibitors [ACEI], angiotensin II receptor blockers [ARB], cyclosporine/tacrolimus)
- Nephrotoxic medications (e.g., aminoglycoside antibiotics, platinum-based chemotherapy)
- Hypovolemia (e.g., diuretics, hemorrhage, GI losses)
- Sepsis, surgery, rhabdomyolysis
- Solitary kidney (risk in nephrolithiasis)
- BPH; malignancy (e.g., multiple myeloma)

GENERAL PREVENTION
- Maintain adequate renal perfusion with isotonic fluids, vasopressor support if necessary.
- Avoid nephrotoxic agents including (but not limited to) known nephrotoxic medications, herbal supplements, IV contrast.

COMMONLY ASSOCIATED CONDITIONS
Hyperkalemia, hyperphosphatemia, hypercalcemia, hyperuricemia, hydronephrosis, BPH, nephrolithiasis, congestive heart failure (CHF), uremic pericarditis, cirrhosis, CKD, malignant hypertension, vasculitis, drug reactions, sepsis, severe trauma, burns, transfusion reactions, recent chemotherapy, rhabdomyolysis, internal bleeding, dehydration

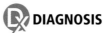

DIAGNOSIS

AKI is usually asymptomatic until the patient has experienced extreme loss of function. Oliguria can be present, but it is neither specific nor sensitive (3).

HISTORY
- Ascertain changes in oral intake, urine output, and body weight.
- Thorough medication history
- Prerenal: thirst, orthostatic symptoms
- Intrarenal: nephrotoxic medications, radiocontrast material, other toxins
- Postrenal: colicky flank pain that radiates to the groin suggests ureteric obstruction such as a stone; nocturia, frequency, and hesitancy suggest prostatic disease; suprapubic and flank pain are usually secondary to distension of the bladder and collecting system; anticholinergic drugs inhibit bladder emptying.
- Uremic symptoms: lethargy, nausea/vomiting, anorexia, pruritus, restless legs, sleep disturbance, hiccups
- Livedo reticularis, SC nodules, and ischemic digits despite good pulses suggest atheroembolization.
- Flank pain may suggest renal artery or vein occlusion.

PHYSICAL EXAM
- Uremic signs: altered sensorium, seizures, asterixis, myoclonus, pericardial friction rub, peripheral neuropathies
- Prerenal signs: tachycardia, decreased jugular venous pressure (JVP), orthostatic hypotension, dry mucous membranes, decreased skin turgor; comorbid stigmata of sepsis, liver disease, or heart failure
- Intrinsic renal signs: pruritic rash, livedo reticularis, SC nodules, ischemic digits despite good pulses
- Postrenal signs: suprapubic distension, flank pain, enlarged prostate

DIAGNOSTIC TESTS & INTERPRETATION
Initial Tests (lab, imaging)
- Compare to baseline renal function (creatinine [Cr]/GFR) (1)[A]
- Urinalysis: dipstick for blood and protein; microscopy for cells, casts, and crystals (1)[A]
- Sterile pyuria (especially WBC casts) suggests AIN; triad of fever, rash, and eosinophilia present in 10% of cases.
- Proteinuria, hematuria, and edema, often with nephritic urine sediment (RBCs and RBC casts), suggest GN or vasculitis.
- Casts: transparent hyaline casts—prerenal etiology; pigmented granular/muddy brown casts—ATN; WBC casts—AIN; RBC casts—GN
- Urine eosinophils: ≥1% eosinophils suggest AIN (poor sensitivity).
- Urine electrolytes in an oliguric state
  - $FENa = [(U_{Na} \times P_{Cr}) / (P_{Na} \times U_{Cr})] \times 100$
  - FENa <1%, likely prerenal; >2%, likely intrarenal
  - If patient on diuretics, use FE_{urea} instead of FE_{Na}: $FE_{urea} = [(U_{urea} \times P_{Cr}) / (P_{BUN} \times U_{Cr})] \times 100$; FE_{urea} <35% suggests prerenal etiology.
- CBC, BUN, SCr, electrolytes (including Ca/Mg/P); consider arterial or venous blood gas (ABG/VBG).
- BUN/Cr ratio not reliable in distinguishing prerenal azotemia from AKI (3)[B]
- Common lab abnormalities in AKI
  - Increased: potassium, phosphate, magnesium, uric acid
  - Decreased: hemoglobin, sodium calcium
- Calculate creatinine clearance (CrCl) to ensure appropriate medication dosing.
- Imaging:
  - Renal ultrasound (US): first line; excludes postrenal causes; identifies kidney size, hydronephrosis, and nephrolithiasis
  - Doppler-flow renal US: evaluates for renal artery stenosis/thrombosis; operator dependent
  - Abdominal x-ray (kidney, ureter, bladder [KUB]): identifies calcification, renal calculi, kidney size
- Novel biomarkers such as urinary IL-18, neutrophil gelatinase-associated lipocalin (NGAL), kidney injury molecule-1 (KIM-1), plasma cystatin C, TIMP-2, and *IGFBP7* under investigation (4)[C]

Follow-Up Tests & Special Considerations
- Consider CK (rhabdomyolysis) and immunologic testing (if GN or vasculitis suspected).
- Advanced imaging if initial tests unrevealing
  - Prerenal: US as effective as CT for obstruction
  - Noncontrast helical CT: most sensitive test for nephrolithiasis
  - Radionuclide renal scan: evaluates renal perfusion, function (GFR), and presence of obstructive uropathy and extravasation
  - MRI: acute tubulointerstitial nephritis with increased T2-weighted signal. Gadolinium contrast is contraindicated if GFR <30 mL/min due to risk of nephrogenic systemic fibrosis.

Diagnostic Procedures/Other
Cystoscopy with retrograde pyelogram evaluates for bladder tumor, hydronephrosis, obstruction, and upper tract abnormalities without risk of contrast nephropathy.

Test Interpretation
Kidney biopsy: last resort if patient does not respond to therapy or if diagnosis remains unclear; most useful to evaluate intrinsic AKI of unclear cause (AIN, GN, vasculitis, or renal transplant rejection)

TREATMENT

Fluid resuscitation is the mainstay of treatment of AKI, both in prerenal and intrinsic kidney injury. In severe cases of kidney injury, dialysis may be required, especially in cases where the patient is oliguric. The most important aspect of treating AKI is determining the underlying cause.

GENERAL MEASURES
- Identify and correct prerenal and postrenal causes.
- Stop nephrotoxic drugs and renally dose others.
- Strictly monitor intake/output and daily weight.
- Optimize cardiac output to maintain renal perfusion.
- Optimize nutrition and treat any infections.
- Indications for renal replacement therapy (RRT): volume overload, severe or progressive hyperkalemia, or severe metabolic acidosis refractory to medical management; advanced uremic complications (pericarditis, encephalopathy, bleeding diathesis); pulmonary edema

MEDICATION
First Line
- Find and treat the underlying cause.
- Prevent fluid overload, and correct electrolyte imbalances—particularly hyperkalemia.
  - If patient is oliguric and not volume overloaded, a monitored fluid challenge may help.
- Furosemide is ineffective in preventing and treating AKI but can (judiciously) be used to manage volume overload and/or hyperkalemia. Furosemide stress test may predict the likelihood of progressive AKI, need for RRT, and mortality (4)[B].
- Dopamine, natriuretic peptides, insulin-like growth factor, and thyroxine have no benefit in the treatment of AKI.
- Fenoldopam, a dopamine agonist, has been equivocal in decreasing risk of RRT and mortality in AKI; not currently recommended (1)[C]
- Hyperkalemia with ECG changes: Give IV calcium gluconate, isotonic sodium bicarbonate (only if acidemic, and avoid use of hypertonic "amps" of $NaHCO_3$), glucose with insulin, and/or high-dose nebulized albuterol (to drive K^+ into cells); Kayexalate and/or furosemide (to increase K^+ excretion); hemodialysis if severe/refractory
- Fluid restriction may be required for oliguric patients to prevent worsening hyponatremia.
- Metabolic acidosis (particularly pH <7.2): Sodium bicarbonate can be given (judiciously); be aware of volume overload, hypocalcemia, and hypokalemia.
- Effective strategies for AKI prevention: isotonic IVF, once-daily dosing of aminoglycosides; use of lipid formulations of amphotericin B, use of iso-osmolar nonionic contrast media
- Risk of contrast-induced AKI is reduced by avoidance of hypovolemia: isotonic saline 1 mL/kg/hr morning of procedure and continued until next morning or isotonic $NaHCO_3$ 3 mL/kg/hr × 1 hour before and 1 mL/kg/hr × 6 hours after contrast administration; N-acetylcysteine not of benefit

Second Line
- Tamsulosin or other selective α-blockers for bladder outlet obstruction secondary to BPH
- Dihydropyridine calcium channel blockers may have a protective effect in posttransplant ATN.

ISSUES FOR REFERRAL
- Consider nephrology consultation for the following:
  - Potential initiation of renal replacement therapy (RRT)
  - Persistent and prolonged anuria or oliguria
  - Refractory elevation in BUN and/or creatinine despite appropriate fluid and/or electrolyte replacement
  - Underlying structural or functional renal disease (e.g., glomerulonephropathies, SLE nephritis, cryoglobulinemia)
  - Renal transplant patients
- Consider urology consult for obstructive nephropathy.

SURGERY/OTHER PROCEDURES
- Relieve obstruction by retrograde ureteral catheters/percutaneous nephrostomy.
- Hemodialysis catheter placement

COMPLEMENTARY & ALTERNATIVE MEDICINE
Many herbal and dietary supplements are potentially nephrotoxic (aristolochic acid, ochratoxin A, Djenkol bean, impila, orellanine, cat's claw). Obtain a thorough medication history from the patient.

ADMISSION, INPATIENT, AND NURSING CONSIDERATIONS
- Treat life-threatening complications: hyperkalemia, metabolic acidosis, volume overload, and advanced uremia
- If hypovolemic, give isotonic IV fluids.
- Monitor fluid balance and daily weights.
- Consider urinary catheter placement to quantify urine output, weighing risks of catheter associated urinary tract infection (CAUTI). Remove as soon as possible.
- Stabilize renal function and ensure treatment plan prior to discharge.
- Dialysis if necessary

 ONGOING CARE

FOLLOW-UP RECOMMENDATIONS
Nephrology follow-up if persistent renal impairment and/or proteinuria

DIET
- Total caloric intake of 20 to 30 kcal/kg/day (1)
- Restrict Na^+ to 2 g/day (unless hypovolemic).
- Consider K^+ restriction (2 to 3 g/day) if hyperkalemic.
- If hyperphosphatemic, consider use of phosphate binders, although no evidence of benefit in AKI.
- Avoid magnesium- and aluminum-containing compounds.

PATIENT EDUCATION
- Keep well-hydrated. Avoid nephrotoxic drugs, such as NSAIDs and aminoglycosides.
- National Kidney Foundation. Acute kidney injury (AKI). https://www.kidney.org/atoz/content/AcuteKidneyInjury

PROGNOSIS
- Depending on the cause, comorbid conditions, and age of patient, mortality ranges from 5% to 80%.
- In cases of prerenal and postrenal AKI, short duration of AKI correlates with good rates of recovery. Intrarenal etiologies take longer to recover.
- Even with complete recovery from AKI, affected patients are at higher subsequent risk of developing CKD and ESRD.
- Among patients who require RRT for AKI, recovery more likely with higher baseline eGFR, AKI from ATN due to sepsis or surgery; recovery less likely with preexisting heart failure (5)

COMPLICATIONS
Death, sepsis, infection, seizures, paralysis, peripheral edema, CHF, arrhythmias, uremic pericarditis, bleeding, hypotension, anemia, hyperkalemia, uremia

REFERENCES
1. Kidney Disease: Improving Global Outcomes Acute Kidney Injury Work Group. KDIGO clinical practice guideline for acute kidney injury. *Kidney Inter Suppl*. 2012;2(Suppl 1):1–138.
2. Gonsalez SR, Cortês AL, da Silva AL, et al. Acute kidney injury overview: from basic findings to new prevention and therapy strategies. *Pharmacol Ther*. 2019;200:1–12.
3. Manoeuvrier G, Bach-Ngohou K, Batard E, et al. Diagnostic performance of serum blood urea nitrogen to creatinine ratio for distinguishing prerenal from intrinsic acute kidney injury in the emergency department. *BMC Nephrol*. 2017;18(1):173.
4. Koyner JL, Davison DL, Brasha-Mitchell E, et al. Furosemide stress test and biomarkers for the prediction of AKI severity. *J Am Soc Nephrol*. 2015;26(8):2023–2031.
5. Hickson LJ, Chaudhary S, Williams AW, et al. Predictors of outpatient kidney function recovery among patients who initiate hemodialysis in the hospital. *Am J Kidney Dis*. 2015;65(4):592–602.

ADDITIONAL READING
- Coca SG, Singanamala S, Parikh CR. Chronic kidney disease after acute kidney injury: a systematic review and meta-analysis. *Kidney Int*. 2012;81(5):442–448.
- Ergin B, Akin S, Ince C. Kidney microcirculation as a target for innovative therapies in AKI. *J Clin Med*. 2021;10(18):4041.
- Kidney Disease: Improving Global Outcomes. Guidelines. https://kdigo.org/guidelines/. Accessed November 12, 2021.

 SEE ALSO

- Chronic Kidney Disease; Glomerulonephritis, Acute; Hepatorenal Syndrome; Hyperkalemia; Prostatic Hyperplasia, Benign (BPH); Reye Syndrome; Rhabdomyolysis; Sepsis
- Algorithm: Anuria or Oliguria

 CODES

ICD10
- N17.0 Acute kidney failure with tubular necrosis
- N17.1 Acute kidney failure with acute cortical necrosis
- N17.8 Other acute kidney failure

CLINICAL PEARLS
- Three categories of AKI:
  - Prerenal: decreased renal perfusion (often from hypovolemia) leading to a decrease in GFR; reversible
  - Intrarenal: intrinsic kidney damage; ATN most common due to ischemic/nephrotoxic injury
  - Postrenal: extrinsic/intrinsic obstruction of the urinary collection system
- Indications for emergent hemodialysis: severe hyperkalemia, metabolic acidosis, or volume overload refractory to conservative therapy; uremic pericarditis, encephalopathy, or neuropathy; and selected alcohol and drug intoxications
- Management of ATN is supportive; no specific treatments are proven to effectively hasten recovery.
- Fluid management remains a mainstay of treatment in prerenal and intrinsic kidney injury.

ADENOMYOSIS

Bradley M. Turner, MD, MPH, MHA

 BASICS

DESCRIPTION

- Benign invasion of the endometrium into the myometrium, producing a diffusely enlarged uterus
- Considered a specific entity in the PALM-COEIN FIGO (polyp; adenomyosis; leiomyoma; malignancy and hyperplasia; coagulopathy; ovulatory dysfunction; endometrial; iatrogenic; and not yet classified—International Federation of Gynecology and Obstetrics) classification of causes of abnormal uterine bleeding
- Microscopically, there are ectopic, nonneoplastic endometrial glands and stroma surrounded by hypertrophic and hyperplastic myometrium.
- Can be either diffuse or focal, depending on the extent of myometrial invasion
- In some cases, it may manifest as a circumscribed myometrial mass referred to as an adenomyoma.
- Most commonly affects the posterior wall of the uterus
- Typically associated with the uterus; however, the term "adenomyosis" can also be applied to benign hyperplastic changes in the bile ducts, gallbladder, and ampulla of Vater.

EPIDEMIOLOGY

- Historically, adenomyosis had been found to present more frequently in the 4th and 5th decades; however, it is increasingly being identified in younger women with pain, abnormal uterine bleeding, infertility, or no symptoms at all, by using imaging techniques such as transvaginal ultrasound (TVUS) and magnetic resonance imaging (MRI) (1),(2).
- Wide variation among racial and ethnic groups and among different geographic regions (3)

Incidence

- Typically considered a uterine condition of women who are multiparous, have had prior cesarean section, or have had prior uterine surgery; however, an increasing amount of evidence suggests that there is also an association with infertility and reproductive failure.
- Variability in the criteria used for diagnosis makes an accurate determination of true incidence difficult.
- Depending on the criteria used for diagnosis, the incidence has been estimated as between 10% and 80%.
- The incidence has been reported to be higher in women presenting with endometriosis.

Prevalence

- As with incidence, an accurate determination of prevalence is difficult due to the variability in the criteria used for diagnosis.
- Depending on the criteria used for diagnosis, the prevalence has been reported to vary from 5% to 70%, with the mean frequency of adenomyosis at hysterectomy given as approximately 20–30%.

ETIOLOGY AND PATHOPHYSIOLOGY

- Adenomyosis has been described as an abnormal ingrowth and invagination of the basal endometrium into the inner layer of the myometrium (junctional zone [JZ]).
- The exact mechanism regarding how this occurs and is maintained is not clear and likely to be multifactorial.
- Two main theories predominate to explain the origin and pathogenesis of adenomyosis:
  - Dysregulated tissue injury and repair promoting cell migration and invagination of the endometrial basalis into the myometrium (1)
  - **De novo epithelial-mesenchymal transition** among displaced embryonic müllerian remnants or adult stem cells (1)
- Molecular alterations in eutopic endometrium seem to contribute to migration and survival of ectopic endometrial implants beyond the myometrial interface.
- Sex steroid hormone aberrations, inflammation, altered cell proliferation, and neuroangiogenesis are likely key pathogenic mechanisms of pain, bleeding, and infertility in adenomyosis.
- In women with adenomyosis, the JZ may represent a region of morphologic dysfunction and structural weakness, with varying susceptibility to invagination of endometrial stromal cells.
- Increased uterine pressure associated with pregnancy, leiomyomas, or other pathology may modulate the JZ environment, making it more susceptible to invagination of endometrial stromal cells.

Genetics

- DNA microarray and proteomics analysis have identified specific genes that are differentially expressed in adenomyosis and matched eutopic endometrium.
- Data suggest that genetic and epigenetic abnormalities contribute to the pathogenesis of adenomyosis.

RISK FACTORS

- Age >40 years; however, the disease has been increasing, identified in women of younger age, including adolescents. Reports suggest that early-stage adenomyosis might present a different clinical phenotype compared to late-stage disease.
- Multiparity
- Tamoxifen treatment
- Other possible risk factors:
  - Infertility and reproductive failure (growing body of literature)
  - Previous uterine surgery (studies have been inconsistent)
  - Smoking (studies have been inconsistent)

COMMONLY ASSOCIATED CONDITIONS

- Leiomyomas (uterine fibroids)
- Endometriosis
- Endometrial polyps
- Urinary tract dysfunction

DIAGNOSIS

- The diagnosis is made through physical examination, radiographic imaging, biopsy, and subsequent histopathologic evaluation.
- Pelvic pain, dysmenorrhea, and an enlarged uterus are the usual cues that prompt imaging by ultrasound or MRI; endometrial or uterine biopsies may be indicated in some cases.

HISTORY

- Presenting symptoms are nonspecific and one-third of patients with adenomyosis are asymptomatic (2).
- Symptoms often include the following:
  - Menorrhagia
  - Dysmenorrhea
  - Chronic pelvic pain
  - Abnormal uterine bleeding
- Urinary tract symptoms (e.g., stress urinary incontinence, urgency, daytime frequency, and urge urinary incontinence) have been associated with an increased incidence of adenomyosis; however, data are limited.

PHYSICAL EXAM

Uterus may be enlarged and tender.

DIFFERENTIAL DIAGNOSIS

- Pregnancy
- Benign uterine tumors
- Malignant uterine tumors
- Metastatic disease

DIAGNOSTIC TESTS & INTERPRETATION

Initial Tests (lab, imaging)

- A shared histologic and radiologic classification system defining the type and severity of adenomyosis has not been developed.
- A standard radiologic classification system defining the type and severity of adenomyosis has also not been developed.
- Recently, a uniform standardized reporting system of ultrasound findings of adenomyosis was developed by using the Morphological Uterus Sonographic Assessment (MUSA) criteria.
- TVUS is the imaging method of choice for initial evaluation of suspected adenomyosis (2)[C].
- TVUS can be either two- or three-dimensional (2)[C].
- Three-dimensional TVUS can provide JZ thickness.
- TVUS has a sensitivity of 65–81% and a specificity of 65–100%, with two-dimensional TVUS being slightly less sensitive and slightly more specific (1),(2)[B].
- TVUS is less sensitive with more interobserver variability than MRI in differentiating adenomyosis from leiomyoma.
- MRI has a pooled sensitivity of 77%, specificity of 89%, positive likelihood ratio of 6.5, and negative likelihood ratio of 0.2 for all subtypes, showing better results compared with those of TVUS.

- Leiomyomas are associated with adenomyosis in 36–50% of cases, making MRI an ideal imaging method (1)[C].
- MRI may be the preferred imaging method when available if cost is not a concern (4)[C].
- MRI should definitely be considered when TVUS cannot provide a definitive diagnosis.

Diagnostic Procedures/Other
- Uterine biopsy with histologic interpretation
- Uterine-sparing operative treatment (USOT) with histologic interpretation
- Hysterectomy with histologic interpretation

Test Interpretation
- The two-dimensional sonographic markers of adenomyosis include the following (1)[C]:
  - Uterine enlargement (with no visualized leiomyoma)
  - Cysts
  - Hyperechoic islands
  - Asymmetrical uterine wall thickening
  - Subendometrial echogenic linear striations
  - Translesional vascularity
  - Fan-shaped shadowing
  - Irregular and/or thickened JZ
  - Interrupted JZ
- Although several criteria have been proposed, a JZ thickness exceeding 12 mm seems to be highly predictive of adenomyosis (2)[B].
- Features of adenomyosis on MRI include low-intensity widening of the JZ on T2-weighted images, which corresponds to smooth muscle hyperplasia and thickening of the JZ (2)[C].
- Three objective parameters have been identified for an MRI diagnosis of adenomyosis:
  - Thickening of the JZ to at least 8 to 12 mm (2)[B]
  - JZ max/total myometrium >40% (2)[B]
  - JZ max–JZ min >5 mm (2)[B]
- Histologic interpretation has traditionally been considered the most practicable way to establish a definitive diagnosis of adenomyosis (1),(2)[C].
- Pathologic interpretation of uterine biopsy:
  - Presence of endometrial glands and stromal elements within the myometrium
  - Often difficult to definitively on smaller samples to diagnose adenomyosis due to sampling bias and/or biopsy artifact
- Pathologic interpretation of USOT and hysterectomy:
  - In morcellated specimens, diagnostic difficulty arises due to modification of the spatial arrangement of the tissue, leading to difficulty in referencing the surface. Sampling bias can also be an issue (1)[C].
  - Even in cases where the surface is accurately referenced, criteria vary among pathologists regarding the depth of invasion, which "definitively" defines adenomyosis (2)[C].

 TREATMENT

- There are no international guidelines to follow for medical or surgical treatment of adenomyosis.
- The mainstay of treatment has been surgical therapy.
- Medical therapy shows promise in certain patients.

MEDICATION
- Continuous use of oral contraceptive pills, high-dose progestins, and selective progesterone receptor modulators can temporarily improve the symptoms.
- Use of a levonorgestrel-releasing intrauterine device is also an effective, reversible, and long-term treatment used successfully to treat adenomyosis (1),(2)[C] and is the most effective first-line treatment (5)[C].
- Gonadotropin-releasing hormone (GnRH) agonists—used for management of menstrual bleeding and pain—and GnRH antagonists—used for treatment of leiomyomas and endometriosis—are both second-line options (5)[C].

ADDITIONAL THERAPIES
Selective progesterone receptor modulators, aromatase inhibitors, valproic acid, and anti-platelet therapy are under development for the treatment of adenomyosis (1),(2)[C].

SURGERY/OTHER PROCEDURES
- Hysterectomy is curative.
- USOT might be considered for women who wish to preserve fertility or do not wish to have a hysterectomy.
- USOT **excisional** techniques (1)[C]:
  - Complete excision (adenomyomectomy)
  - Cytoreduction (partial adenomyomectomy)
  - Uterine wedge resection
- USOT **nonexcisional** techniques (1)[C]:
  - Laparoscopic techniques including electrocoagulation and uterine artery ligation
  - Hysteroscopic techniques including endometrial ablation, endomyometrial resection
  - MRI or ultrasound-guided high-frequency ultrasound ablation (high-intensity focused ultrasound [HIFU])
  - Uterine artery embolization (UAE)
  - Other reported techniques include the following:
    - Alcohol instillation (cystic adenomyosis)
    - Radiofrequency ablation (focal adenomyosis)
    - Microwave ablation
    - Thermoablation (diffuse adenomyosis)
- Of the nonexcisional techniques, HIFU and UAE seem to offer the most encouraging results (1)[C].
- A systemic review of USOT for adenomyosis in reproductive-aged women suggests that excisional USOT—including uterine wedge resection, adenomyomectomy, and hysteroscopic excision—may possibly improve fertility, although the best method of surgery is yet to be seen (6)[C]. Nonexcisional USOT that may improve fertility include HIFU and radiofrequency ablation (6)[C].
- Hysterectomy, UAE, and endometrial ablation are only options if future fertility is not desired.

 ONGOING CARE

PATIENT EDUCATION
https://www.mayoclinic.org/diseases-conditions/adenomyosis/symptoms-causes/syc-20369138

PROGNOSIS
- Adenomyosis is a benign proliferation of endometrial tissue.
- Symptoms usually resolve after menopause.
- Hysterectomy is curative.
- Additional studies are still needed to determine the impact of untreated adenomyosis and USOT on fertility and reproductive outcomes.
- Additional studies are still needed to clarify the role of medical treatment in women with adenomyosis.
- A consensus on the criterion for diagnosing adenomyosis needs to be reached.

COMPLICATIONS
- Anemia from blood loss associated with heavy periods
- Patients with adenomyosis have been reported to be at increased risk for malignant disease; however, to date, there has not been sufficient morphologic, genetic, or epigenetic evidence to substantiate the malignant transformation of adenomyosis.

REFERENCES

1. Tan J, Yong P, Bedaiwy MA. A critical review of recent advances in the diagnosis, classification, and management of uterine adenomyosis. *Curr Opin Obstet Gynecol*. 2019;31(4):212–221.
2. Vannuccini S, Petraglia F. Recent advances in understanding and managing adenomyosis. *F1000Res*. 2019;8:F1000 Faculty Rev–283.
3. Upson K, Missmer SA. Epidemiology of adenomyosis. *Semin Reprod Med*. 2020;38(2-03):89–107.
4. Tellum T, Nygaard S, Lieng M. Noninvasive diagnosis of adenomyosis: a structured review and meta-analysis of diagnostic accuracy in imaging. *J Minim Invasive Gynecol*. 2020;27(2):408–418.e3.
5. Cope AG, Ainsworth AJ, Stewart EA. Current and future medical therapies for adenomyosis. *Semin Reprod Med*. 2020;38(2-03):151–156.
6. Kho KA, Chen JS, Halvorson LM. Diagnosis, evaluation, and treatment of adenomyosis. *JAMA*. 2021;326(2):177–178.

 CODES

ICD10
N80.0 Endometriosis of uterus

CLINICAL PEARLS
- Adenomyosis is often asymptomatic.
- MRI is more sensitive than TVUS, particularly in differentiating adenomyosis from leiomyoma.
- Histologic diagnosis is the gold standard.
- Various medical options exist; however, only hysterectomy is curative.

ADHESIVE CAPSULITIS (FROZEN SHOULDER)

Edwin Y. Choi, MD, MS, FAAFP, DFPHM • Daniel Jordan Whitaker, MD • Lea S. Choi, DO

 BASICS

DESCRIPTION
- Adhesive capsulitis (AC) or frozen shoulder:
  - Presents as progressive painful restriction in range of movement of the glenohumeral (GH) joint (1)
  - Course usually involves diminishment of pain but can have residual pain and limits of active and passive range of motion (ROM) (1).
- Subtypes:
  - Primary AC:
    - Idiopathic
    - Usually associated with diabetes mellitus (DM) (1)
    - Typically resolves in 9 to 18 months (2)
  - Secondary AC:
    - Typically due to prolonged immobilization
    - Most commonly due to a complication of rotator cuff impingement syndrome (rotator cuff tendonitis) that remains incompletely treated
    - Sometimes called "shoulder-hand-syndrome," which is a complex regional pain syndrome (or reflex sympathetic dystrophy), if it is characterized by shoulder pain, diffuse swelling, and decreased ROM (2)
- Clinical course:
  - Phase 1 (2 to 9 months): painful phase. Pain is constant. Diagnosis may be difficult if restricted movement is not present in early disease.
  - Phase 2 (4 to 12 months): stiffening or freezing phase. Movement becomes restricted, especially with external rotation.
  - Phase 3 (12 to 42 months): resolution or thawing phase; gradual return to normal shoulder mobility (2)

EPIDEMIOLOGY
Incidence
2.4/1,000 people per year (2)
Prevalence
2–5% in the general population, 10–20% among diabetes (2),(3)

ETIOLOGY AND PATHOPHYSIOLOGY
Underlying fundamental processes:
- Idiopathic
- Inflammation: Mast cells, T cells, B cells, and macrophages have been identified histologically, suggesting an inflammatory process. Studies confirm presence of elevated inflammatory cytokines such as IL-1, IL-6, TNF-α, COX-1, and COX-2 (3).
- Elevated markers for neoangiogenesis (CD34) and neoinnervation (GAP43, PGP9.5, NGFRp75) have been associated with AC which helps explain the acute painful phase. Additionally, one study showed that over expression of TGF-β led to the development of AC in rats (3).
- Scarring: Fibroblasts and myofibroblasts have been identified histologically. Capsular contracture reduces the joint volume to 3 to 4 mL compared to the normal 10 to 15 mL. Intracellular adhesion molecule-1 (ICAM-1) facilitates leukocyte endothelial transmigration. It is elevated in both AC and DM.

- This scarring primarily effects the rotator interval (coracohumeral ligament [CHL], biceps tendon, and GH capsule). A contracted CHL is an essential finding in AC (3).
- Contracture of the GH capsule from loss of synovial layer, capsular adhesions, and loss of capsular volume are seen in AC.

RISK FACTORS
- Shoulder immobilization; often due to impingement syndrome (most significant risk factor)
- Increasing age (1)
- Female gender (1)
- Diabetes (1)
- Thyroid disease (1)
- Atherosclerotic cardiovascular disease (ASCVD): cerebrovascular accident (CVA)/myocardial infarction (MI)/hyperlipidemia (2)
- Antiretroviral medication use
- Parkinson disease
- Trauma/surgery (1)
- Prior history of AC in contralateral shoulder

GENERAL PREVENTION
- Active lifestyle, while avoiding shoulder injury
- Control of diabetes, atherosclerotic disease, thyroid, and autoimmune conditions

COMMONLY ASSOCIATED CONDITIONS
DM, autoimmune disorders, Parkinson disease, highly active antiretroviral therapy (HAART) use, CVA/MI, cervical disc disease, thyroid disorders (1)

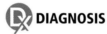 **DIAGNOSIS**

HISTORY
- Identify possible risk factors.
- Progressive and worsening stiffness of the GH joint
- Majority will have diffuse shoulder pain, especially at the beginning of the disease.
- On the late phase of the disease, stiffness becomes predominant.
- Rule out other pain invoking conditions such as fractures, osteoarthritis (OA), subacromial pathologies such as bursitis and rotator cuff tendinopathy, cervical radiculopathy, and GH arthrosis (3).

PHYSICAL EXAM
- Limitation in both active and passive ROM due to true mechanical restriction
- Capsular pattern of ROM restriction is demonstrated, with external rotation most affected, followed by abduction, and then flexion (1).
- Pain with rotator cuff impingement tests
- Inability to reach overhead or back pocket
- Scapular substitution frequently accompanies active shoulder movement.
- Loss of arm swing with gait

DIFFERENTIAL DIAGNOSIS
- Rotator cuff strain/tear/impingement syndrome
- GH or acromioclavicular joint OA
- Cervical strain/radiculopathy/OA

- Subacromial bursitis
- Parsonage-Turner syndrome: brachial plexus inflammation secondary to a trigger, such as an infection, trauma, or autoimmune condition
- Myofascial pain syndrome
- Calcific tendonitis
- Fracture
- Shoulder subluxation/dislocation
- Bony neoplasm/metastasis

DIAGNOSTIC TESTS & INTERPRETATION
AC is a clinical diagnosis that can further be guided by labs and images if needed. No single lab or imaging alone can make the diagnosis.

Initial Tests (lab, imaging)
- No labs are required for idiopathic AC. Blood tests can be used to check for associated/related conditions, such as diabetes, thyroid disease, a stroke, autoimmune diseases, and, in rare cases, Parkinson disease (e.g., thyroid-stimulating hormone, hemoglobin A1C, erythrocyte sedimentation rate).
- Imaging
  - Plain radiographs of the affected shoulder (posteroanterior, external rotation, axillary, and supraspinatus outlet views)
    - Preferred initial tests
    - In most cases, will be negative
    - Used primarily to rule out other pathologies such as GH OA, fractures, dislocation, or tumors (2)
  - Magnetic resonance imaging (MRI)
    - Not indicated unless there is a concomitant pathology in the shoulder or neurologic deficit
    - May show thickening of the joint capsule and the coracohumeral ligament along with edema and increased joint fluid (2)
    - Rotator interval/axillary joint capsule enhancement and inferior GH and/or coracohumeral ligament hyperintensity are the most diagnostic signs with sensitivity and specificity >80% (4).
  - Ultrasound (US)
    - Indications similar to those for MRI
    - Selection depends on individual cases and clinician's preference.
    - Can also reveal thickening of the coracohumeral ligament and soft tissues of the joint capsule and increased joint fluid
    - Doppler can show increased vascularity around the intra-articular portion of the biceps tendon and coracohumeral ligament.

Follow-Up Tests & Special Considerations
- Shared decision-making regarding treatment
- Pain referral for CRPS

Diagnostic Procedures/Other
Injection test can be helpful in differentiating AC from subacromial pathologies such as rotator cuff tendinopathy (which should improve with injection of local anesthetics, in contrast to AC). This should only be done if the diagnosis is still uncertain after a thorough history and physical.

TREATMENT

- In most cases, self-limited
- Physical therapy with exercises within the limits of pain
- Manage patient expectations; resolution often takes 18 months of medication and rehabilitation (2).
- Treat any underlying medical conditions associated with AC such as DM and thyroid disorders.

MEDICATION

- Medication should be used in conjunction with physical therapy to provide symptomatic relief.
- Acetaminophen or nonsteroidal anti-inflammatory drugs (NSAIDs) are first line of treatment.
- Glucocorticoid injections:
  - Single intra-articular corticosteroid injections and multisite injections showed great statistical and clinical outcomes for pain when used in the beginning of the disease (5). Intra-articular corticosteroid injections in patients with frozen shoulder for <1 duration showed greater benefits compared to other interventions and such benefits were shown to last as long as 6 months (5).
  - A course of physical therapy after an injection, for 4 to 6 weeks, with or without intra-articular corticosteroid appeared to be associated with short-term benefits of improving pain and ROM.
  - Injection may be diluted with a local anesthetic such as lidocaine. Triamcinolone 20 to 40 mg or methylprednisolone 20 to 40 mg can be used.
  - Hydrodilatation with normal saline combined with intra-articular corticosteroid injection may expedite ROM recovery compared to corticosteroid injection alone (3).
- Although a short course of oral glucocorticoid can temporarily provide pain relief and improved mobility, the benefits were not greater than a few weeks. Studies have shown that intra-articular corticosteroid injections are more effective than oral steroid treatment (3).

ISSUES FOR REFERRAL

Surgical referral can be considered if patients fail to make progress with conservative management for one year.

ADDITIONAL THERAPIES

- Exercise and physical therapy:
  - Gentle ROM exercises should be offered to every patient.
  - Exercises should be performed daily and as tolerated. A structured plan should be given to the patient (6).
  - Physical therapy has been found to be beneficial especially in phases 2 and 3 of AC. Best data supports its use in conjunction with other treatment such as corticosteroid injections.
- Laser has been suggested as a possible treatment, particularly for pain relief; not enough evidence for support

- Suprascapular nerve block can provide temporary pain relief and may be a therapeutic option for AC refractory to intra-articular corticosteroid injections; however, there is a lack of high-quality evidence for support (3).
- Other therapies that have been studied include whole-body cryotherapy and intra-articular injection of botulinum toxin type A, both of which have demonstrated to improve pain and ROM but with limited evidence (3).

SURGERY/OTHER PROCEDURES

- Should be reserved for patients who do not respond to conservative measures for at least 1 year or is not showing any improvement conservatively
- Some of the most common procedures include manipulation under anesthesia (MUA), arthroscopic capsular release (ARC), distension arthrogram, among others (2). One study comparing ARC, MUA, and physiotherapy showed that although all three treatments led to substantial improvements in pain and function, none of the treatments were clinically superior to another (7).

 ONGOING CARE

FOLLOW-UP RECOMMENDATIONS

- After establishing a diagnosis, assess the need for pain control and start the patient on NSAIDs, in combination with a gentle exercise program with guidance with physical therapy.
- Follow up in 3 to 4 weeks: if no significant improvement, may consider intra-articular corticosteroid injections (5)
- Physical therapy should be concurrently used because it can hasten the rate of recovery and increase ROM (5).
- For secondary AC, consider evaluation by a multidisciplinary team.
- If no improvement, consider surgical intervention (2).

PATIENT EDUCATION

- Patient education is important; explain prognosis and ensure compliance with treatment.
- Climbing the wall: Face a wall and place the hand from the affected shoulder flat on the surface of the wall; use the fingers to "climb" the wall; pause 30 seconds every few inches. Repeat the exercise after turning the torso 90 degrees to wall (abduction).
- In case of secondary AC, address the importance of treating underlying causes.

PROGNOSIS

- Recovery is dependent on onset of treatment, symptoms, and comorbidities in patient.
- Variable duration, lasting 1 to 3 years without intervention (1)
- Patients with idiopathic frozen shoulder have a good rate of recovery (5).

REFERENCES

1. Zreik NH, Malik RA, Charalambous CP. Adhesive capsulitis of the shoulder and diabetes: a meta-analysis of prevalence. *Muscles Ligaments Tendons J.* 2016;6(1):26–34.
2. Rangan A, Goodchild L, Gibson J, et al. Frozen shoulder. *Shoulder Elbow.* 2015;7(4):299–307.
3. Le HV, Lee SJ, Nazarian A, et al. Adhesive capsulitis of the shoulder: review of pathophysiology and current clinical treatments. *Shoulder Elbow.* 2017;9(2):75–84.
4. Suh CH, Yun SJ, Jin W, et al. Systematic review and meta-analysis of magnetic resonance imaging features for diagnosis of adhesive capsulitis of the shoulder. *Eur Radiol.* 2019;29(2):566–577.
5. Challoumas D, Biddle M, McLean M, et al. Comparison of treatments for frozen shoulder: a systematic review and meta-analysis. *JAMA Netw Open.* 2020;3(12):e2029581.
6. Jain TK, Sharma NK. The effectiveness of physiotherapeutic interventions in treatment of frozen shoulder/adhesive capsulitis: a systematic review. *J Back Musculoskelet Rehabil.* 2014;27(3):247–273.
7. Rangan A, Brealey SD, Keding A, et al. Management of adults with primary frozen shoulder in secondary care (UK FROST): a multicentre, pragmatic, three-arm, superiority randomised clinical trial. *Lancet.* 2020;396(10256):977–989.

 CODES

ICD10
- M75.00 Adhesive capsulitis of unspecified shoulder
- M75.01 Adhesive capsulitis of right shoulder
- M75.02 Adhesive capsulitis of left shoulder

CLINICAL PEARLS

- Frozen shoulder or AC is generally a self-limiting global restriction in ROM of the shoulder joint. Up to 15% will have disability long-term.
- Natural course consists of a painful phase, freezing phase, and thawing phase. It occurs mostly in older women; total prevalence is 2–5% of the general population and roughly 10–20% of the diabetic population.
- An active and passive ROM restriction will be present. Most common is an inability to externally rotate the shoulder. Other signs include pain on provocation of subacromial space and inability to reach overhead or for back pocket.
- Plain x-rays are the preferred initial imaging modality. MRI and US are done only if there is concomitant pathology or neurologic deficit.
- Treatment includes pain control and physical therapy; can progress to glucocorticoid therapy with a consideration for surgery
- Resolution of symptoms often takes ≥18 months.

ADOPTION, INTERNATIONAL
Heather C. Doty, DO • Carley Borrelli, MD

BASICS

DESCRIPTION
- Although international adoptions have decreased in the past 15 years, they still represent a significant portion of ~135,000 yearly U.S. adoptions.
- Diverse birth countries, disease exposures, and unknown health histories make international adoption particularly complex.
- Multidisciplinary teams are often necessary for appropriate care. Many parents planning to adopt seek advice from their primary care provider.

EPIDEMIOLOGY
Incidence
- 1,622 children were adopted internationally in 2020. This number has decreased every year since 2004 when international adoption numbers peaked at 22,986.
- 15% of current U.S. adoptions are international.
- In 2020, the most common countries of origin for internationally adopted children were China (~40%), India, Ukraine, Colombia, South Korea, Nigeria, and Ethiopia.
- In 2018, 52% of internationally adopted children were <5 years, 33% were ages 5 to 12 years, and 15% were 13 to 17 years. More females than males were adopted internationally (52% vs 48%) (1).

RISK FACTORS
- Unknown birth, medical, and vaccination histories
- Possible in utero or postnatal toxin exposure
- Inadequate nutrition (before or after birth)
- Exposures to infectious diseases not commonly seen in the United States
- Overcrowded or institutionalized living situations (e.g., orphanages)
- History of neglect, deprivation, or abuse

GENERAL PREVENTION
- Prospective adoptive parents are required to have a medical exam, typically performed by a primary care physician, in order to verify sufficient medical and psychological capacity to adopt a child from a foreign country. Exam requirements vary by country.
- A State Department-approved physician must examine the child in their native country before immigration to the United States. This is a limited examination targeted at identifying diseases that would exclude qualifying for a visa.
- Children should optimally be examined by a physician within 2 weeks of arrival in the United States.
- A follow-up visit 4 to 6 weeks after their postadoption appointment is also recommended.
- Screen for hearing, vision, growth, and developmental delay.
- Review immunization records (if available).
- A travel medicine visit is encouraged for family members who are traveling to the adopted child's country of origin.
- A preadoption visit can help clarify medical diagnoses and review available medical records (including photos and/or video) to confirm/refute specific diagnoses.

COMMONLY ASSOCIATED CONDITIONS
- 80% of international adoptees have medical or developmental issues; 20% of these are severe (2).
- Infectious diseases:
  - Hepatitis A/B/C
  - Intestinal parasites
  - Tuberculosis (TB), primarily latent
  - Syphilis, including inadequately treated
  - HIV
  - *Helicobacter pylori*
- Emotional or behavioral problems
- Developmental delay
- Fetal alcohol spectrum disorder
- Feeding difficulties, malnutrition, rickets
- Anemia
- Congenital anomalies (e.g., cleft lip/palate, orthopedic deformities)
- Prematurity or low birth weight
- Inadequate immunizations
- Lead poisoning
- Sensorineural and conductive hearing loss
- Strabismus, blindness

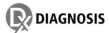**DIAGNOSIS**

HISTORY
- Medical records are often limited or difficult to access.
- Review chronic medical conditions, allergies, and medications.
- Review immunization records carefully. Records that are "too perfect" should raise suspicion.
  - Some vaccinations (e.g., *Haemophilus influenzae* type B [Hib], pneumococcal, varicella) are not routine in other countries.
- Review family history and birth/prenatal history, including exposures.
- Review documented history of emotional or nutritional deprivation and physical, emotional, or sexual abuse.
- Review time (if any) spent in orphanage or other institution.
- Growth charts are critical—review carefully. The first sign of malnutrition is failure to gain weight, followed by slowed linear growth, and a lag in head circumference.
- Review or observe (as able) data regarding developmental milestones, behavior, attachment, parent stress, and parent–child interactions.
- Review laboratory results and screening test results.
- Review testing and treatment of tuberculosis.

PHYSICAL EXAM
- This may be the child's first comprehensive exam; be sensitive to cues the child is providing and use a translator as necessary.
- Comprehensive physical exam. Highlight:
  - Growth parameters
  - General appearance; presence of features suggestive of genetic disorder, syndromes, or congenital defects
  - Skin—congenital skin abnormalities, rash, infection, bruises, scars, or signs of prior abuse (2)
  - Genitalia—signs of abuse or ritual cutting

- Ocular—assess red reflex, extraocular movements, and funduscopic exam
- Neurologic—sensorimotor skills, coordination, reflexes, strength, and spinal exam
- Oral exam—tooth development and signs of decay
- Abdomen—hepatosplenomegaly
- Assess development using a validated instrument, the date of birth may be unknown. Assess development at each visit to identify delay and potential need for additional services. About 50–90% of internationally adopted children are delayed on adoption; most have normal cognition at long-term follow-up.

DIAGNOSTIC TESTS & INTERPRETATION
- Developmental screening
- Hearing and vision screening
  - Formal audiologic exam is recommended for all internationally adopted children.
  - Funduscopic exam is recommended for children with a birth weight <1500 g.

Initial Tests (lab, imaging)
- Based on history and physical exam (3)[A]:
  - Hepatitis A (Hep A IgM, Hep A IgG); hepatitis B (HBsAg, HBsAb, HBcAb); hepatitis C (enzyme immunoassay [EIA])
  - HIV 1 and 2 antibody testing/ELISA
  - Syphilis: nontreponemal (RPR, VDRL, or ART) and treponemal (MHA-TP, FTA-ABS, or TPPA)
  - Tuberculin skin test (TST) in all ages or interferon-γ release assay ages ≥5 years
    - Consider interferon γ release assay in children who have received the BCG vaccine.
    - Consider repeat test after 6 months to rule out exposure prior to leaving country of birth.
  - Three stool specimens from three separate days for ova and parasites, specific request for *Giardia intestinalis* and *Cryptosporidium* species testing of one sample
  - CBC with indices and differential; blood lead concentration for ages ≤6 years
  - Thyroid-stimulating hormone (TSH)
  - Urinalysis
  - Hemoglobinopathy/blood disorder screen: sickle cell, thalassemia, glucose-6-phosphate dehydrogenase (G6PD) deficiency
  - Newborn screening panel
  - Ricket screen if growth delay, institutionalized, or history of limited sunlight or poor vitamin D intake
  - Repeat all testing performed before adoption even if results are normal, as results may be unreliable.
- Consider:
  - Antibody titers depending on veracity of immunization records (4)[C]
  - Stool cultures for bacterial pathogens (diarrhea)
  - *H. pylori* testing (dyspepsia, abdominal pain, or anemia)
  - Ca^{++}, PO_4, alkaline phosphate, and 25-hydroxyvitamin D level (rickets)
  - >12 months of age: for Chagas disease via *Trypanosoma cruzi*, serologic testing in adoptees from endemic countries (Mexico, Central, and South America)
  - Testing for malaria, typhoid fever, leprosy, and melioidosis if child with unexplained fever, splenomegaly, anemia, or eosinophilia from a country where the disease is endemic

Follow-Up Tests & Special Considerations

- HIV: Confirm antibody positive in children <18 months with DNA PCR (may represent maternal antibody).
- Hep C: Confirm positive tests with recombinant immunoblot assay (RIBA) and/or HCV RNA PCR; an initial positive in children <18 months may be due to maternal antibody, repeat after 18 months of age.
- Positive TST (TB): Do *not* attribute to bacillus Calmette-Guérin (BCG) vaccine. Evaluate for active disease; treat latent TB infection (LTBI).
- Test for intestinal parasites if GI symptoms persist.
- Eosinophilia >450 cells/mm³ with negative stool ova and parasites: serologic testing for *Schistosoma*, *Toxocara canis*, lymphatic filariasisfor children >2 years old from sub-Saharan Africa, Egypt, Southern Asia, Western Pacific Islands, the NE coast of Brazil, Guyana, Haiti, and the Dominican Republic (4)[A]
  – Add *Strongyloides* for adoptees from sub-Saharan African, Latin American, and Southeast Asian countries.
- Behavioral concerns may first present during adolescence, even for children adopted in infancy.
- For children with history of treated congenital syphilis, follow with ophthalmologic, audiologic, neurologic, and developmental screening.

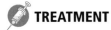 TREATMENT

GENERAL MEASURES
- Regular diet for children who arrive malnourished
- Monitor linear growth.
- Consider early intervention for children with suspected delays.
- Involve parents in local and online support groups.
- Postadoption depression may occur in parents.

MEDICATION
- Immunizations: Catch up vaccines per CDC schedule (http://www.cdc.gov/vaccines/schedules/).
  – No further Hep B vaccine if HBsAg positive, HBsAb and HBcAb positive, or HBsAb positive and HBV vaccine given appropriately
  – MMR for vaccination for mumps and rubella, even if measles antibodies present (4)[C]
- Possible approaches (3)[A]:
  – Repeating questionable vaccinations negates the need to obtain serologic tests.
  – To minimize/avoid vaccine administration, check antibody titers—infants 6 to 12 months: polio; diphtheria; children, >1 year: Hep A; MMR; varicella (4)[C]
- Ensure adoptive parents, caretakers, and household members are up-to-date with Tdap, Hep A/B, and measles vaccines (2)[C].

ISSUES FOR REFERRAL
- Time referrals and elective procedures to allow adjustment to new home
- Individual and/or family counseling does help adjustment.
- Internationally adopted children may exhibit self-stimulating behaviors (e.g., rocking, head banging) related to prior sensory deprivation. These behaviors typically decrease with time, and no treatment is necessary if the child is otherwise developing normally. If in doubt, refer to developmental pediatrics or occupational therapy.
  – If a child continues to have disruptive behaviors, or would rather self-soothe than seek nurturing human interaction, consider intervention.
- Refer to pediatric ophthalmology for strabismus (seen in 10–25% of previously institutionalized adoptees).
- Refer to audiology and/or ENT for concerns, questionable screening results, or if slow to acquire language skills.
- No longer hearing one's native language slows speech development. Speech therapy helps children from non–English-speaking countries.

ONGOING CARE

FOLLOW-UP RECOMMENDATIONS
Patient Monitoring
- Regular well-child visits, particularly within first months of entry into the United States
- Close monitoring of developmental milestones, behavior, and attachment

DIET
- Regular diet, with specific attention to known nutritional deficiencies within country of origin (http://adoptionnutrition.org)
- Up to 68% of international adoptees fall >2 standard deviations below the mean for one or more growth parameters; most begin to follow an appropriate growth curve (<2 deviations from the mean) within 9 to 12 months of arrival.

PATIENT EDUCATION
- Allow ad lib access to healthy foods to promote self-regulatory eating behaviors.
- Toileting: Some children may not be trained yet; others may regress in their new home. Time, positive reinforcement, and avoiding punishment often resolve this issue as the child adjusts to new surroundings.
- Sleeping: Children must learn to trust their new home and parents. Avoid aggressive sleep rules. Parents should be present physically and emotionally to establish safety and promote bedtime ritual.
- Language: Adoptive family should learn key phrases in the child's native language prior to adoption. When using translator services, be careful to avoid perception of translator use equating to potential return to native country.
- Adopted children may grieve lost family, relationships, and culture; encourage parents to acknowledge this and openly work through it. Provide counseling if needed.
- Encourage families to learn about the child's culture and ethnicity of origin (2).

PROGNOSIS
- Recovery from developmental delay correlates with time spent in institutional setting.
  – Risk of long-term developmental, behavioral, or academic problems increases with adoption age.
  – Rate of recovery exceeds rate of normal development.
- Children may regress in previously acquired skills.
- A desire to search for biologic family is common in adolescence (2).
- American Academy of Pediatrics' Council on Foster Care, Adoption, and Kinship Care (https://www.aap.org/en/community/aap-councils/council-on-foster-care-adoption-and-kinship-care/)

REFERENCES

1. U.S. Department of State, Bureau of Consular Affairs. Intercountry adoption. https://travel.state.gov/content/travel/en/Intercountry-Adoption.html. Accessed October 20, 2021.
2. Barratt MS. International adoption. *Pediatr Rev*. 2013;34(3):145–146.
3. American Academy of Pediatrics. Medical evaluation of internationally adopted children for infectious diseases. In: Pickering LK, ed. *Red Book: 2012 Report of the Committee on Infectious Diseases*. 29th ed. Elk Grove Village, IL: American Academy of Pediatrics; 2012:239–240.
4. Feja KN, Tolan RW Jr. Infections related to international travel and adoption. *Adv Pediatr*. 2013;60(1):107–139.

ADDITIONAL READING

- Centers for Disease Control and Prevention. ACIP vaccine recommendations and guidelines. https://www.cdc.gov/vaccines/hcp/acip-recs/index.html. Accessed November 12, 2021.

CODES

ICD10
- Z02.82 Encounter for adoption services
- Z62.821 Parent-adopted child conflict

CLINICAL PEARLS

- Internationally adopted children may exhibit self-stimulating behaviors (e.g., rocking, head banging) that usually decrease over time. Refer to developmental or occupational specialist when concerns persist.
- A preadoption visit can identify medical concerns, ensure travel safety for prospective parents, and prepare resources prior to a child's arrival.
- Initial labs for internationally adopted children include Hep A/B/C, HIV 1/2, CBC, TSH, lead, G6PD deficiency, hemoglobin electrophoresis, PPD/TST (or IGRA ages ≥5 years), ova and parasites (three stool specimens, including single specimen for *Giardia* and *Cryptosporidium* antigens), and urinalysis.
- If initially negative, repeat HIV, Hep B/C, and TST at 6 months.
- Catch up immunizations according to recommended schedules (https://www.cdc.gov/vaccines/hcp/acip-recs/index.html).
- Ensure that appropriate immunizations are up-to-date for adoptive family and caretakers.

ADVANCE CARE PLANNING

Heather Ann Dalton, MD, FAAFP • Christopher Lin-Brande, MD

BASICS

DESCRIPTION

- Advance care planning (ACP) allows patients to have a voice in the decisions that affect their care after they lose the ability to do so for themselves.
- There are several methods of addressing goals of care as patients age:
  - Advance directives, including living wills (LWs) and heath care durable powers of attorney (DPOAs)
  - Physician/medical orders for life-sustaining treatment (POLST/MOLST) and directives to physicians
  - Facilitated conversations with family and significant others
- ACP is an important aspect of patient-centered care as the population ages and individuals lose decision-making capacity, when new chronic medical conditions are diagnosed, or in the setting of severe acute illnesses like COVID-19.
- ACP helps to interpret patient wishes in the context of individual illness circumstances, negotiate conflicts in decisions, and allow patients determine what is in their best interest based on personal values.
- Definitions
  - Advance directives (1): written instructions to guide decision-making in the event a patient is unable to provide informed consent
    - LWs and DPOAs usually only take effect if the patient has been determined to lack capacity to decide care for himself or herself; otherwise, patient preference takes precedence (even if contradictory to an LW).
    - Done appropriately, these help patients avoid languishing in poor quality of life states, often with associated complex ethical dilemmas.
  - LW: a patient's explicit written instructions of his or her wishes regarding medical care
    - Each state has specific legal requirements. Certain states do not recognize LWs but have other "medical directive" forms. LWs and medical directives can take effect immediately (e.g., when a patient is diagnosed with a terminal illness) or when a patient can no longer make decisions for himself or herself.
    - LWs have direct treatment instructions.
    - Challenges of LWs include lack of standardization, potential completion too far in advance of use, and narrow scope.
    - LWs do not expire, but they can be revised.
    - The LW is NOT a medical directive, so it cannot prevent life-sustaining treatment in an emergent situation (as a POLST can [see next]).

- DPOA: a written document designating a surrogate decision maker in the event a patient cannot speak for himself or herself
  - A health care proxy (HCP) speaks on behalf of the patient to make decisions aligned as closely as possible to the patient's wishes. Ideally, this is someone the patient knows and trusts. It is also helpful if this individual has had discussions with the patient about his or her values and desires.
  - If multiple HCP are named, disagreements about who speaks for the patient must be resolved before a decision can be made.
  - If there is a conflict between an LW provision and an HCP decision, different states have varying rules regarding precedence. In some states, the DPOA supersedes the LW; in other states, the most recently executed document is legally binding.
  - If a patient has had goals of care discussions with friends or family but does not have a legally named HCP, those discussions can still help inform the decision-making process.
- POLST/MOLST: a medical directive which, unlike an LW, directs point of care decision-making by EMS for patients at the end of life
  - Designed to minimize confusion in emergent situations, these are adjunctive documents to LWs and DPOAs that provide clear instruction regarding resuscitation, intubation, and other life-saving treatments.
  - They are portable and follow a patient across different care settings. Given their simplicity, a POLST/MOLST is more likely to be followed than an LW, which can be difficult to locate.
  - Although EMS may be concerned about the legal implications of withholding life-sustaining treatment, POLST forms provide legal protection if patient wishes are followed.
  - Patients with POLST documents have fewer unwanted interventions.
- Nursing home residents and patients with dementia often do not have capacity to complete legal documents related to LW and DPOA.
- ACP should be completed while patients are able to make decisions about their future care.
- There are no guidelines for when to initiate discussions about ACP; age 65 years may be an appropriate time for a realistic conversation prior to the onset of dementia or other incapacitating illness. Each conversation must be individualized.

Pediatric Considerations
- Pediatric ACP (pACP) is less common.
- For children with serious acute or terminal illness, it is a difficult (but important) part of treatment.
  - Provider fears about increasing parental distress when discussing pACP are unfounded.
  - pACP may unburden parents from difficult decisions and is associated with increased positive emotions, understanding of the patient's illness, and provider rapport.

TREATMENT

- Suggested discussion points:
  - All adult patients:
    - Discuss basic medical decision-making.
    - Assess willingness to engage in ACP. Do not force patients if they are not ready to have this potentially emotionally charged conversation.
    - Ask patients to identify who they would like to make decisions for them if they were unable to do so.
    - Encourage patients to inform trusted family or friends about new diagnoses or changes in health.
    - Discuss what values are most important to patients.
    - Document decisions concisely and clearly.
  - Any patient with a chronic or terminal illness:
    - Discuss the natural course of disease progression, including time course and end-of-life expectations.
      - For example:
        - Chronic obstructive lung disease: exacerbations, decreased ability to perform activities of daily living, supplemental oxygen, mechanical ventilation
        - Diabetes: macrovascular and microvascular complications (heart attack, stroke, dementia, dialysis, amputations)
        - Malignancy: possibility of chronic pain, inability to swallow/poor appetite necessitating alternative feeding options, ascites and therapeutic procedures, treatment side effects
  - "Elderly patients":
    - Consider routine discussions of ACP around age 65 years. It is crucial to speak with patients while they still have decision-making capacity. Discussions should be repeated regularly to ensure patient preferences have not changed.
    - Refer patients to legal services for advance directive/DPOA.
    - Complete POLST forms in clinic, if applicable in your state.

– Any change in clinical status (including frequent ER visits or hospitalizations):
  ○ Changes in functional status should prompt a discussion about prognosis and future wishes. Hospitalizations are important milestones to discuss recovery or decline.
  ○ Consider palliative care services.
  ○ Consider support services to prevent caregiver burnout.
• At the end of life, if it is the patient's desire, it is important to engage hospice services in a timely manner.
  – ACP discussions are often complicated by social, familial, cultural, and medical factors. It is important to be sensitive to each patient's individual context.
  – Do not force the conversation if a patient is resistant or unprepared to discuss ACP.
    ○ Motivational interviewing can be used to gauge interest and readiness to discuss ACP.
    ○ Addressing implications for friends and family who may be burdened with decision-making may help promote ACP conversations.
  – The first time ACP is brought up often serves as an introduction to the topic and an opportunity for the patient to consider options. Subsequent visits can address specific scenarios and choices.
  – Avoid medical jargon (i.e., CPR, mechanical ventilation, parenteral nutrition, etc.) when addressing options. Patients may not understand the severity of illness or the implications of advanced life-saving interventions.

ONGOING CARE

Reimbursement: The Centers for Medicare & Medicaid Services reimburses physicians for ACP discussions.

• Current CPT codes are 99497 for the first 30 minutes of discussion and completion of forms and 99498 for each additional 30 minutes (2).
• There are no limits to the number of times ACP can be reported in a given period of time.
• An advance directive does not have to be completed in order to bill for services.
• No specific diagnosis is required for the ACP codes (3).

FOLLOW-UP RECOMMENDATIONS
Patient Monitoring
• There are no specific guidelines for how often an LW or DPOA discussion should be revisited after completion.
• When there is a new diagnosis or a significant change in clinical status, have the patient consider how it would affect his or her ACP decision-making.
• Have patients display POLST/MOLST forms prominently for ease of visibility to EMS.

PATIENT EDUCATION
• See references for links: The National Hospice and Palliative Care Organization, National Institute on Aging, Aging with Dignity, National Healthcare Decisions Day, and the American Bar Association have resources to help patients.
• Online platforms such as MyDirectives allow patients to specify their wishes electronically.
• DeathWise is a nonprofit organization with worksheets patients can use for the health, financial, care of body, and service components of ACP.

COMPLICATIONS
• Often LWs, DPOAs, and POLSTs are completed, but physicians do not have access to them. Electronic health records are a convenient place to store documents, but they may be difficult to retrieve.
  – Any ACP form should be part of the medical record with open access (if possible) to facilitate appropriate decision-making.
  – Medical bracelets or other devices are often used to notify EMS of patient directives.
• Emergency rooms are vulnerable to uncertainty about what interventions patients want if they cannot communicate for themselves and guiding documents are not readily available.
  – POLST forms can help avoid confusion.
• There is often misunderstanding on the part of both doctors and patients regarding do not resuscitate (DNR) and do not intubate (DNI) orders.
  – DNR/DNI orders can be reversed or should not be honored in certain situations.
  – DNR/DNI in a person with a chronic progressive illness does not necessarily mean DNR/DNI for an acute reversible process.
  – The prognosis for successful resuscitation on a hospital ward is approximately 14%; it is 50–80% for patients undergoing surgery.

REFERENCES

1. American Association of Retired Persons. Advance directive forms by state. http://www.aarp.org/home-family/caregiving/free-printable-advance-directives/. Accessed July 19, 2021.
2. Centers for Medicare and Medicaid Services. Medicare Learning Network: advance care planning. https://www.cms.gov/outreach-and-education/medicare-learning-network-mln/mlnproducts/downloads/advancecareplanning.pdf. Accessed July 19, 2021.
3. Bosisio F, Barazzetti G. Advanced care planning: promoting autonomy in caring for people with dementia. *Am J Bioeth*. 2020;20(8):93–95.

ADDITIONAL READING

• Aging with Dignity. Five wishes. https://www.agingwithdignity.org. Accessed October 3, 2021.
• American Bar Association. Tool kit for health care advance planning. https://www.americanbar.org/groups/law_aging/resources/health_care_decision_making/consumer_s_toolkit_for_health_care_advance_planning.html. Accessed October 3, 2021.
• DeathWise: http://deathwise.wpengine.com/
• Heyland DK. Engaging seriously ill older patients in advance care planning. https://psnet.ahrq.gov/webmm/case/404/engaging-seriously-ill-older-patients-in-advance-care-planning. Accessed October 3, 2021.
• MyDirectives: https://www.mydirectives.com/
• National Healthcare Decisions Day: https://theconversationproject.org/nhdd/
• National Hospice and Palliative Care Organization, CaringInfo: http://www.caringinfo.org/i4a/pages/index.cfm?pageid=1.

 CODES

ICD10
• Z71.89 Other specified counseling
• Z51.5 Encounter for palliative care
• Z66 Do not resuscitate

CLINICAL PEARLS
• ACP is an important and underutilized element of compassionate and comprehensive patient-centered care.
• The primary barriers to discussing advance directives from the patient perspective include lack of knowledge, fear of burdening family, and a desire for physicians to initiate the discussion.
• The primary barriers to discussing advance directives from the physician perspective include discomfort with the topic, lack of emotional support, lack of reimbursement, and lack of time to fully address the topic.
• Fewer unwanted interventions occur in the emergency room and inpatient setting when ACP is actively reviewed and wishes are documented and conveyed appropriately.

AIR TRAVEL EMERGENCIES
Theodore E. Macnow, MD • Michelle A. Georgia, DO

BASICS

DESCRIPTION
Physicians commonly help with in-flight medical events (IME). Many IME fall outside a practitioner's normal scope of practice. The aircraft environment is cramped with limited medical resources. Despite these obstacles, health care workers should be prepared to render assistance in these situations.

EPIDEMIOLOGY
Incidence
- 4 billion passengers travel annually worldwide (1).
- Exact incidence of IMEs is unknown.
- Airlines estimate an IME occurs on 1 in 40 flights, most are minor and handled by the flight crew.
- Other databases, which include only more serious IMEs, estimate incidence at 1 in 600 flights (2).
- Airline estimates are that there is an IME in 1 per 7,500 to 40,000 airline passengers 250 to 1,500 events/day worldwide (3).
- The likelihood of encountering an IME is increasing because of larger aircrafts, longer flights, and an aging population.
- The most common IMEs involve syncope/near syncope (32.7%), gastrointestinal (14.8%), respiratory (10.1%), and cardiovascular symptoms (7%) (3).
- In otherwise healthy passengers, vasovagal syncope represents up to 90% of IMEs.
- 5% of passengers suffer from a chronic illness and account for two-thirds of IMEs.
- 15% of ground-based physician calls are for pediatric passengers (1).
- 3% of IMEs are fatal; however, death may be underreported as it is often not declared in-flight.

ETIOLOGY AND PATHOPHYSIOLOGY
Hypobaric hypoxia: Atmospheric pressure of oxygen drops from 160 mm Hg at sea level to 120 mm Hg at cruising altitude in a pressurized cabin.

- In healthy people, the arterial oxygen tension drops from 100 to about 60 mm Hg with associated mean inflight oxygen saturations of 93% (range: 85 to 98) (4).

ALERT
Passengers with chronic obstructive pulmonary disease (COPD) or other pulmonary disorders have a lower baseline PaO$_2$, so the drop in oxygen tension may occur on the steep part of the hemoglobin dissociation curve and result in more significant hypoxemia.

ALERT
Passengers with unstable angina or heart failure may not be able to compensate for hypoxia.

- Gas expansion: Gases expand about 30% in flight. This can lead to a pneumothorax, wound dehiscence or perforation from bowel gas expansion, sinus pressure, and tympanic membrane rupture in children with ear infections.
- Venous thromboembolism: There is an increased risk for clotting because of prolonged sitting, hypoxic conditions, and dehydration. There is an increased risk of deep vein thromboses (DVTs) on longer flights and in passengers with underlying medical conditions.
- Stress: Travelling is mentally and physically stressful, which may lead to psychiatric emergencies or acute coronary syndrome (ACS).

- Insomnia: Passengers have disrupted circadian rhythms, which may trigger seizures and contribute to medication nonadherence.
- Turbulence: Motion sickness is common and traumatic injury can result from falling luggage.
- Medication nonadherence: Forgotten or checked medications may lead to glycemic control problems, seizures, blood pressure instability, and inaccessible as needed medications.
- Decreased access to food and drink: Vasovagal syncope may result from dehydration. Diabetics may suffer hypoglycemia.
- Low air humidity: Cabin air is less than 20% relative humidity which contributes to dehydration, epistaxis, and asthma or COPD exacerbations.
- Viral infections: Parainfluenza and influenza are the most common viruses communicated by proximity. The cabin air is filtered and not infectious.

ALERT
Transmission of SARS-CoV2 virus can occur on air travel. Like other viruses, the risk is mostly from proximity to infected, possibly asymptomatic passengers rather than cabin air flow. Risk may be mitigated by following applicable guidelines for mask-wearing, social distancing, and quarantining.

RISK FACTORS
- Recent surgery: Passengers are at risk for wound dehiscence, bowel perforation, and compartment syndrome from gas expansion.
- COPD, asthma, CHF, or coronary artery disease: Passengers may suffer from hypoxemia and not be able to compensate appropriately.
- Recent cast placement: Passengers are at risk for compartment syndrome due to tissue edema.
- Hypercoagulability: Passengers with inherited or acquired hypercoagulable conditions, pregnancy, medications, heart disease, or recent surgery are at increased risk for DVTs.
- Recent scuba diving: Passengers are at risk for decompression syndromes.
- Long flights: The effects of hypoxia are cumulative and time-dependent.

GENERAL PREVENTION
General guidelines:
- Travelers should discuss medications with their doctor and bring necessary medications and equipment onboard.
- Supplemental inflight oxygen is required for patients with a baseline PaO$_2$ < 70 mm Hg or who are unable to walk a flight of stairs or 150 feet without becoming short of breath or experiencing angina.

Pregnancy Considerations
Women are generally safe to fly until 36 weeks' gestation.

Pediatric Considerations
Travelers with children should bring liquid formulations of medication in allowed quantities on the plane. Children with asthma should have a rescue inhaler with spacer and facemask.
- Specific guidelines:
  - Avoid flying 10 to 14 days after surgery (varies by type of surgery).
  - Casts may need to be bivalved if applied 24 to 48 hours before a flight.
  - Avoid scuba diving 24 hours before flying.

- DVT prevention (5)[C]:
  - Adequately hydrate.
  - Avoid venous stasis by standing, stretching, and exercising legs in flight.
  - Passengers with risk factors may need compression stockings, aspirin, or anticoagulation.

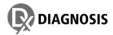

DIAGNOSIS

HISTORY
- Symptoms vary based on emergency; if patient is alert, gather as much history as possible.
- Ask about past medical and surgical history, medications and compliance, and allergies.
- Inquire about illicit drug or alcohol use.
- Document findings and recommendations and save a secure copy for your records.

PHYSICAL EXAM
- Wear all available PPE. There are protective gloves available on board.
- May need to obtain blood pressure by palpitation due to noise.
- Assess vital signs. Signs of dehydration including skin perfusion
- General appearance and mental status
- If stethoscope available on in-flight kit—auscultation as best as possible

ALERT
Assess for tension pneumothorax by listening for decreased lung sounds and contralateral tracheal deviation. A tension pneumothorax requires needle decompression.

DIFFERENTIAL DIAGNOSIS
- **Syncope or near-syncope:** vasovagal syncope, dehydration, hypoglycemia, intoxication, medication reaction or toxicity, ACS, arrhythmia, cerebrovascular accident, pulmonary thrombosis/air embolism, and hypoxia
- **Chest pain:** ACS, pulmonary embolism, pneumothorax, bronchospasm, aortic dissection, gastroesophageal reflux, musculoskeletal etiology, and anxiety
- **Shortness of breath:** COPD or asthma exacerbation, pneumonia, pulmonary thrombosis/air embolism, toxic exposure
- **Stroke-like symptoms:** cerebrovascular accident, transient ischemic attack, hypoglycemia, seizure, syncope, intracranial mass, and complex migraine
- **Seizure:** seizure, syncope, hypoglycemia, eclampsia, cardiac arrest
- **Gastrointestinal illness:** motion sickness, foodborne illness, gastritis, enteritis, gastroesophageal reflux, pancreatitis, medication or substance withdrawal
- **Obstetric emergency:** preterm labor, miscarriage, eclampsia, placenta previa
- **Allergic reaction:** urticaria, anaphylaxis, dermatitis
- **Cardiac arrest:** arrhythmia, pulmonary embolism, respiratory arrest, ACS, intoxication, syncope
- **Altered mental status:** use or withdrawal from drugs or alcohol (consider GI absorption from smuggling), hypoglycemia, panic attack, DKA, hypoxia, psychiatric emergency
- **Trauma:** may result from turbulence or falling luggage

DIAGNOSTIC TESTS & INTERPRETATION
- The automated external defibrillator (AED) can be used as a cardiac monitor.
- Ask other passengers for equipment (i.e., glucometer, MDI spacer, or pulse oximeter).

TREATMENT

GENERAL MEASURES

- **First aid and CPR:** If there is no pulse or not breathing, start CPR, BLS, ALS, and PALS as appropriate. Airline crew members are trained in first aid and CPR.
- **Ask for help:** Ask the flight crew and other passengers for equipment, medications, expertise, and lifting assistance.
- **Oxygen:** All flights have oxygen at 2 to 5 L per minute by facemask. This oxygen delivery at cruising altitude mimics conditions at sea level. Oxygen should be applied in all cases of respiratory distress, chest pain, seizures, and altered mental status.
- **Ground-based physician support:** Many airlines contract with companies that offer inflight medical advice, interpreter services, recommendations for diversion, and sometimes telemedicine technology.
- **Request to fly at lower attitude:** Flying below 22,500 feet with cabin pressurization mimics sea level oxygen pressure. Flying lower uses more fuel and is slower so may not be optimal to reach a hospital quickly.
- **Request a diversion:** The pilot can request an expedited landing, medical services on arrival, or a closer destination. Medical emergencies that involve resuscitation, persistent abnormal vital signs, chest pain, stroke symptoms, respiratory distress, unconsciousness, obstetrics, or psychiatric emergencies should be considered for diversion.

Table 1. FAA-Mandated Contents of Emergency Medical Kit

Equipment	Oropharyngeal airways (3 sizes)
	Cardiopulmonary resuscitation mask
	Manual resuscitation devices, 3 masks
	Adhesive tape, 1-inch
	Alcohol sponges
	Intravenous administration set
	Needles
	Protective gloves
	Sphygmomanometer
	Stethoscope
	Tape scissors
	Tourniquet
	Instructions on kit use
Medications	Analgesic, nonnarcotic
	Antihistamine, 50 mg, injectable
	Antihistamine tablets, 25 mg
	Aspirin tablets, 325 mg
	Atropine, 0.5 mg, 5 mL
	Bronchodilator, inhaled (i.e., albuterol)
	Dextrose, 50%/50 mL, injectable
	Epinephrine 1:1,000, 1 mL, injectable
	Epinephrine 1:10,000, 2 mL, injectable
	Lidocaine, 5 mL, 20 mg/mL, injectable
	Nitroglycerine tablets
	Saline solution (minimum 500 mL)

MEDICATION

- All U.S. commercial aircrafts have an emergency medical kit (EMK) as well as basic first aid kits on the aircraft. The contents vary among countries, airlines, and aircrafts. Many airlines have adopted a more extensive EMK.
- The minimal contents in the EMK required by the Federal Aviation Administration are described in Table 1.
- All aircraft are equipped with an AED.

ALERT

- Not usually found in the EMK are glucometers, intubation equipment, ACLS drugs, narcotics, insulin, or antibiotics. Consider asking other passengers for needed medications or equipment.
- In a 2019 survey, only 35% of EMKs contain naloxone.

Pediatric Considerations

EMKs do not include liquid or suppository medications. Consider crushing tablets or asking other passengers for medication or equipment. A toilet paper roll or cut soda bottle can be taped to an albuterol pump to make a spacer.

ADDITIONAL THERAPIES

- **Cardiac arrest:** CPR; early defibrillation; epinephrine 1:10,000 q3–5min (adults: 1 mg IV, pediatric: 0.01 mg/kg IV); lidocaine or atropine when indicated. Recommend diversion.
- **Acute coronary syndrome:** oxygen by facemask, aspirin 325 mg PO, nitroglycerin (0.4 mg sublingually q5–10min if systolic blood pressure > 100 mm Hg). Apply AED. Recommend diversion.
- **Asthma/COPD exacerbation:** oxygen, albuterol 2.5 mg inhaled (repeat as needed), steroid (if available), epinephrine 1:1,000 (autoinjector: adult: 0.3 mg, pediatric [<25 kg]: 0.15 mg IM; ampule: adult: 0.3 mg, pediatric: 0.01 mg/kg) if significant respiratory distress. Consider diversion.
- **Allergic reaction:** diphenhydramine (PO or IV, adult: 25 to 50 mg, pediatric: 1 mg/kg); if anaphylaxis, epinephrine 1:1,000 (autoinjector: adult: 0.3 mg, pediatric [<25 kg]: 0.15 mg IM; ampule: adult: 0.3 mg, pediatric: 0.01 mg/kg); NS (IV, adults: 1 L, pediatric: 20 mL/kg) steroid (if available); divert if anaphylaxis.
- **Vasovagal syncope:** Elevate legs. If alert and oriented, offer oral liquids. Consider IV fluid bolus. Consider hypoglycemia and offer oral glucose. Monitor blood pressure. Consider diversion if remains symptomatic or has persistent abnormal vital signs.
- **Gastrointestinal:** Oral antiemetic and antacid may be available from the EMK or other passengers. If there is abdominal pain, consider diversion.
- **Tension pneumothorax:** needle thoracostomy 4th or 5th intercostal space anterior axillary line
- **Psychiatric emergency:** Consider intoxication, hypo/hyperglycemia, and hypoxia. Attempt verbal de-escalation. If aggression, established airline protocol should be implemented prior to chemical restraint. Ask patient and other passengers if they have oral anxiolytics. If restraint is necessary, it should be by four passengers, one on each limb. Monitor the patient for signs of respiratory distress or ACS if restrained. Consider diversion.
- **Opioid Ingestion:** Rescue breathing as needed. Naloxone if available in EMK or from other passengers 0.4 to 0.8 mg IV or 2 mg intranasal or IM.

 ONGOING CARE

PROGNOSIS

- The Aviation Medical Assistance Act of 1998 protects volunteer in-flight physicians from malpractice. No physician has been successfully sued in the United States for volunteering care in an IME.
- When overhead paged for assistance, health care workers responded 76% of the time, physicians in 48% of cases (2).
- The correlation of the inflight and hospital diagnosis is about 80%. 60% of IMEs improve with help from a health care provider (6).

REFERENCES

1. Rotta AT, Alves PM, Nerwich N, et al. Characterization of in-flight medical events involving children on commercial airline flights. *Ann Emerg Med*. 2020;75(1):66–74.
2. Peterson DC, Martin-Gill C, Guyette FX, et al. Outcomes of medical emergencies on commercial airline flight. *N Engl J Med*. 2013;368(22): 2075–2083.
3. Martin-Gill C, Doyle TJ, Yealy DM. In-flight medical emergencies: a review. *JAMA*. 2018;320:2580–2590.
4. Humphreys S, Deyermond R, Bali I, et al. The effect of high altitude commercial air travel on oxygen saturation. *Anaestesia*. 2005;60:458–460.
5. Aerospace Medical Association Medical Guidelines Task Force. Medical Guidelines for Airline Travel, 2nd ed. *Aviat Space Environ Med*. 2003; 74(5 Suppl):A1–19.
6. Nable JV, Tupe CL, Gehle BD, et al. In-flight medical emergencies during commercial travel. *N Engl J Med*. 2015;373:939–945.

ADDITIONAL READING

Khatib AN, Carvalho AM, Primavesi R, et al. Navigating the risks of flying during COVID-19: a review for safe air travel. *J Travel Med*. 2020;27(8):taaa12.

 SEE ALSO

- AirRx: downloadable smartphone app with information on protocols, diagnoses, and treatments for managing IMEs
- Printable cards for management of common IMEs (3)

CLINICAL PEARLS

- Medical emergencies on airplanes are common. Most are minor.
- Equipment and drugs on board airplanes vary widely.
- All flights are equipped with AEDs and oxygen.
- Many airlines partner with ground-based physician support to help the flight crew and volunteers in IMEs.
- Utilize passengers as a resource for help, information, and supplies.

ALCOHOL USE DISORDER (AUD)

Eric Robert Messner, PhD, FNP-BC • Curtis W. Bone, MD, MHS

 BASICS

DESCRIPTION
- Any pattern of alcohol use causing significant physical, mental, or social dysfunction. Key features are tolerance, withdrawal, and persistent use despite problems.
- The severity of AUD exists on a spectrum but is classified as mild, moderate, or severe based on the number of symptoms. 2 to 3 of the *DSM-5* criteria for substance use disorders (see below) is considered mild disease. 6 or more is classified as severe AUD.
  - Continued use despite related social or interpersonal problems or physical or psychological problems
  - Recurrent use in hazardous situations
  - Failure to fulfill obligations at work, school, or home
  - Cravings, tolerance, withdrawal
  - Using more than intended or for longer periods of time than intended
  - Persistent desire or attempts to cut down/stop
  - Social, occupational, or recreational activities sacrificed for alcohol use
- "Risky drinking" or "unhealthy use" refers to individuals who do not meet formal criteria for AUD or have not been identified as experiencing AUD yet drink at levels that place them at increased risk of negative outcomes.
  - Women: >3 drinks per day, >7 drinks per week
  - Men: >4 drinks per day, >14 drinks per week
- Binge drinking
  - Drinking that brings blood alcohol levels to 0.08 g/dL
  - Usually 4 drinks for women and 5 drinks for men in 2 hours
- National Institute on Alcohol Abuse and Alcoholism criteria for "at-risk" drinking: men: >14 drinks a week or >4 per occasion; women: >7 drinks a week or >3 per occasion
- The 2015–2020 Dietary Guidelines for Americans defines moderate drinking as up to 1 drink per day for women and up to 2 drinks per day for men.

Geriatric Considerations
- Multiple drug interactions
- Signs and symptoms may be different or attributed to chronic medical problem or dementia.
- Accelerated aging from frequent alcohol use together with increased consumption in middle-age and older adults increases risk of cognitive decline and dementia (1).

Pediatric Considerations
- Children of alcoholics are at increased risk; 2.5% of adolescents have AUD; 13.4% of youth age 12 to 20 years report binge drinking in the past month; negative effect on maturation and normal brain development
- Early-onset drinkers (those who start drinking before age 21 years) are 4 times more likely to develop a problem than those who begin after age 21 years.

EPIDEMIOLOGY
- Predominant age 18 to 25 years, but all ages affected; male > female (3:1)
- Young drinkers through college age commonly engage in heavy to binge drinking (4 drinks for women and 5 drinks for men in 2 hours) to extreme binge drinking (>15 drinks in one session) on weekends.
- New data reflects increased drinking in middle-age to older adults and binge drinking, especially in women, increasing risk of cognitive decline and dementia (2).
- Global increase in AUD over the past 20 years. The COVID-19 pandemic has been associated with increases in alcohol consumption on a global scale.
- In the United States, recent increases in AUD come from a dramatic rise in AUD in women (84%) as compared to men (35%).
  - Stems from increases in heavy and binge drinking in adolescent girls as well as women
  - Women also tend to experience more alcohol-related health issues than men (3).

Prevalence
- 27% of Americans age ≥18 years reported binge drinking in the past month; 7% reported heavy alcohol use in the past month; 15 million adults (6%) age >18 years has AUD.
- Excess drinking cost $249 billion in 2010 in the United States, and kills 88,000 Americans per year: approximately 1 in 10 working-age adults
- In the United States, harmful alcohol use is the third leading cause of preventable death and has become a major public health crisis (4).

ETIOLOGY AND PATHOPHYSIOLOGY
- Multifactorial: genetic, environment, psychosocial
- Alcohol is a CNS depressant, facilitating γ-aminobutyric acid (GABA) inhibition and blocking *N*-methyl-D-aspartate receptors.

Genetics
50–60% of risk is genetic.

RISK FACTORS
- Family history; depression; anxiety disorders; bipolar disorder; eating disorders
- Tobacco use; other substance abuse
- Male gender; lower socioeconomic status; unemployment; poor self-esteem
- Posttraumatic stress disorder; antisocial personality disorder; criminal behavior

GENERAL PREVENTION
- Counsel patients with family history and risk factors.
- USPSTF recommended in 2018 to screen adults for alcohol use and provide brief counseling to those with risky drinking habits.
- Screening and brief intervention (SBI) (1)

COMMONLY ASSOCIATED CONDITIONS
- Cardiomyopathy; atrial fibrillation; hypertension
- Peptic ulcer disease; cirrhosis; fatty liver; cholelithiasis; hepatitis; pancreatitis
- Diabetes mellitus; malnutrition; upper GI malignancies
- Peripheral neuropathy, seizures
- Abuse and violence
- Behavioral disorders (depression, bipolar, schizophrenia): >50% of patients have a comorbid substance abuse problem.

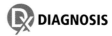 **DIAGNOSIS**

HISTORY
- Thorough behavioral history
- Anxiety, depression, insomnia, psychological and social dysfunction, marital, or relationship problems, domestic violence
- Repeated attempts to stop/reduce drinking, blackouts; loss of interest in nondrinking activities
- Employment problems (tardiness, absenteeism, decreased productivity, interpersonal problems, frequent job loss)
- Complaints about alcohol-related behavior; frequent trauma, MVAs, ED visits
- Physical symptoms: anorexia, nausea, vomiting, abdominal pain, palpitations, headache

PHYSICAL EXAM
- Physical exam may be completely normal.
- General: fever, agitation, diaphoresis
- Cardiovascular: hypertension, dilated cardiomyopathy, tachycardia, arrhythmias
- Respiratory: aspiration pneumonia
- GI: stigmata of chronic liver disease, peptic ulcer disease, pancreatitis, esophageal malignancies, esophageal varices
- Musculoskeletal: poorly healed fractures, myopathy, osteopenia, osteoporosis, bone marrow suppression
- Neurologic: tremors, cognitive deficits (e.g., memory impairment), peripheral neuropathy, Wernicke-Korsakoff syndrome (from severe acute deficiency of thiamine: Korsakoff psychosis is a chronic neurologic sequela of Wernicke encephalopathy. Wernicke encephalopathy has the traditional triad of ophthalmoplegia, ataxia, and confusion.
- Dermatologic: burns (e.g., cigarettes), bruises, poor hygiene, palmar erythema, spider telangiectasias

DIFFERENTIAL DIAGNOSIS
- Other substance use disorders
- Depression, dementia; cerebellar ataxia; cerebrovascular accident (CVA); benign essential tremor; seizure disorder
- Hypoglycemia; diabetic ketoacidosis; viral hepatitis

DIAGNOSTIC TESTS & INTERPRETATION
Screening
- CAGE questionnaire: (**C**ut down, **A**nnoyed, **G**uilty, and **E**ye opener): >2 "yes" answers is 74–89% sensitive, 79–95% specific for AUD; less sensitive for white women, college students, elderly; not an appropriate tool for less severe forms of alcohol abuse
- Single question for unhealthy use: "How many times in the last year have you had X or more drinks in 1 day?" (X = 5 for men, 4 for women); 81.8% sensitive, 79% specific for AUDs (1)[C]

- Alcohol Use Disorders Identification Test (AUDIT): 10 items, if >4: 70–92% sensitive, better in populations with low incidence of alcoholism: https://www.nams.sg/helpseekers/alcohol/self-assessment-tool/Pages/default.aspx
- AUDIT-C is a three-item screening tool. Scores >4 for men and >3 for women are concerning for alcohol misuse.
  - Q#1: How often did you have a drink containing alcohol in the past year?
  - Q#2: How many drinks containing alcohol did you have on a typical day when you were drinking in the past year?
  - Q#3: How often did you have six or more drinks on one occasion in the past year?

Initial Tests (lab, imaging)
- CBC; liver function tests (LFTs); electrolytes; BUN/creatinine; lipid panel; thiamine; folate; hepatitis A, B, and C serology
- Amylase, lipase (if GI symptoms present)
- Serum levels increased in chronic abuse:
  - AST/ALT ratio >2.0; γ-glutamyl transferase (GGT); carbohydrate-deficient transferrin; uric acid
  - Elevated mean corpuscular volume (MCV); ↑ prothrombin time, triglycerides and cholesterol (total)
- Often decreased
  - Calcium, magnesium, potassium, phosphorus; BUN; hemoglobin, hematocrit, platelet count
  - Serum protein, albumin; thiamine; folate
- CT scan or MRI of brain: cortical atrophy, lesions in thalamic nucleus, and basal forebrain
- Abdominal ultrasound (US): ascites, periportal fibrosis, fatty infiltration, inflammation

Test Interpretation
Sequelae of chronic AUD: liver: inflammation or fatty infiltration (alcoholic hepatitis), periportal fibrosis (alcoholic cirrhosis occurs in only 10–20% of alcoholics); gastric mucosa: inflammation, ulceration; pancreas: inflammation, liquefaction necrosis; heart: dilated cardiomyopathy; immune system: decreased granulocytes; endocrine organs: elevated cortisol levels, testicular atrophy, decreased female hormones; brain: cortical atrophy, enlarged ventricles

 TREATMENT

For management of acute withdrawal, see "Alcohol Withdrawal."

GENERAL MEASURES
- Brief interventions and counseling by clinicians have proven effective for problem drinking.
- Treat comorbid problems (sleep, anxiety, etc.), but use extreme caution in prescribing medications with cross tolerance to alcohol (benzodiazepines).
- Group programs and/or 12-step programs help patients accept treatment and develop insight.

MEDICATION
First Line
Long-term treatment of AUD is initiated after resolution of acute withdrawal:
- FDA approved
  - Naltrexone: 50 to 100 mg/day PO or 380 mg IM once every 4 weeks; most evidence-based FDA-approved medication for AUD. Opiate antagonist reduces craving and likelihood of relapse and decreases number of heavy drinking days among people with AUD (IM route may enhance compliance and efficacy) (3)[B]; will precipitate withdrawal if patient is on opioids

  - Acamprosate (Campral): 666 mg PO TID after withdrawal completed; consider if contraindication to naltrexone. Reduces relapse risk. If helpful, use for 1 year; caution if creatinine clearance is low
- Supplements for all
  - Thiamine: 100 mg/day (first dose IV prior to glucose to avoid Wernicke encephalopathy)
  - Folic acid: 1 mg/day
  - Multivitamin: daily
- Contraindications
  - Naltrexone: pregnancy, acute hepatitis, hepatic failure
  - Acamprosate: GFR <30 (5)[C]

ALERT
Treat acute symptoms if in alcohol withdrawal; give thiamine 100 mg/day with first dose prior to glucose.

Second Line
Non–FDA-approved medications for long-term treatment of AUD (Initiate after resolution of acute withdrawal.)

- Topiramate (Topamax): 25 to 300 mg/day PO or divided BID; may enhance abstinence (off-label FDA use)
- Baclofen: initial dose 5 mg TID; initial dose may be titrated to 10 mg TID with max dose 60 mg/day in 3 divided doses. Well tolerated in patients with cirrhosis. Doses beyond 60 mg/day provide no identifiable benefit.
- Gabapentin: initial dose 300 to 600 mg QHS for insomnia and/or cravings related to alcohol use; can titrate to 600 mg TID
- Disulfiram: 250 to 500 mg/day PO; FDA approved but not considered first line given unproven efficacy and severe risks; may provide psychological deterrent; most effective if used with close supervision; extreme caution with use given potential for severe emesis in population at risk of esophageal varices. Severe reactions may involve myocardial infarction, upper GI bleed, seizure, and death.
- Selective serotonin reuptake inhibitors may be beneficial if comorbid depression exists.
- Varenicline may provide benefit to patients with AUD who also smoke (5)[C].

ISSUES FOR REFERRAL
Addiction specialist, 12-step or long-term program, behavioral health professional

 ONGOING CARE

FOLLOW-UP RECOMMENDATIONS
Patient Monitoring
- Outpatient detoxification: daily visits (not recommended for patients with heavy alcohol abuse)
- Early outpatient rehabilitation: weekly visits; detoxification alone is not sufficient.

PATIENT EDUCATION
- Center for Substance Abuse Treatment: (800) 662-HELP or https://www.samhsa.gov/find-help
- Alcoholics Anonymous: http://www.aa.org/
- Secular Organizations for Sobriety: http://www.sossobriety.org/

PROGNOSIS
- Chronic relapsing disease; mortality rate more than twice general population, death 10 to 15 years earlier
- Abstinence benefits: survival, mental health, family, employment
- 12-step programs, cognitive behavior, and motivational therapies are often effective during 1st year following treatment.

REFERENCES
1. Huffstetler AN, Kuzel AJ, Sabo TR, et al. Practice facilitation to promote evidence-based screening and management of unhealthy alcohol use in primary care: a practice-level randomized controlled trial. BMC Fam Pract. 2020;21(1):93.
2. Sullivan EV, Pfefferbaum A. Brain-behavior relations and effects of aging and common comorbidities in alcohol use disorder: a review. Neuropsychology. 2019;33(6):760–780.
3. Guinle MIB, Sinha R. The role of stress, trauma, and negative affect in alcohol misuse and alcohol use disorder in women. Alcohol Res. 2020;40(2):5.
4. Abraham AJ, Andrews CM, Harris SJ, et al. Availability of medications for the treatment of alcohol and opioid use disorder in the USA. Neurotherapeutics. 2020;17(1):55–69.
5. Litten RZ, Wilford BB, Falk DE, et al. Potential medications for the treatment of alcohol use disorder: an evaluation of clinical efficacy and safety. Subst Abus. 2016;37(2):286–298.

ADDITIONAL READING
- National Institute on Alcohol Abuse and Alcoholism. Helping patients who drink too much: a clinician's guide. http://www.niaaa.nih.gov/guide. Accessed September 20, 2020.
- National Institute on Alcohol Abuse and Alcoholism. Rethinking Drinking: alcohol & your health. http://www.rethinkingdrinking.niaaa.nih.gov. Accessed September 20, 2020.
- Tucker JA, Chandler SD, Witkiewitz K. Epidemiology of recovery from alcohol use disorder. Alcohol Res. 2020;40(3):2.

 CODES

ICD10
- F10.10 Alcohol abuse, uncomplicated
- F10.20 Alcohol dependence, uncomplicated
- F10.239 Alcohol dependence with withdrawal, unspecified

CLINICAL PEARLS
- CAGE questionnaire: >2 "yes" answers is 74–89% sensitive, 79–95% specific for AUD; less sensitive for white women, college students, elderly; not an appropriate tool for less severe forms of alcohol abuse
- Single question for unhealthy use screening: "How many times in the last year have you had X or more drinks in 1 day?" (X = 5 for men, 4 for women); 81.8% sensitive, 79% specific for AUDs
- National Institute on Alcohol Abuse and Alcoholism criteria for "at-risk" drinking: men >14 drinks a week or >4 per occasion; women: >7 drinks a week or >3 per occasion

ALCOHOL WITHDRAWAL

Melanie Rose Gordon, MD

 BASICS

DESCRIPTION
Alcohol withdrawal syndrome (AWS) is a spectrum of symptoms resulting from abrupt cessation or reduction in alcohol intake, after a period of prolonged use. It ranges from minor symptoms such as tremors, and insomnia, to major complications such as seizures, and delirium tremors. Symptoms generally start within a few hours of the last drink and peak at 24 to 48 hours.

EPIDEMIOLOGY
Incidence
- According to National Survey Drug Use and Health, in 2019, 14.5 million Americans met diagnostic criteria for alcohol use disorder (AUD). Approximately 50% of those with AUD have experienced AWS in their lifetime. <4% were offered FDA-approved medications to treat AUD.
- 2–7% of patients admitted to hospital with heavy alcohol use are at increased risk of AWS.
- 32% of emergency room visits are alcohol related.

Prevalence
- AUD are among the most prevalent mental disorders with 12-month and lifetime prevalence of 13.9% and 29.1%, respectively.
- Higher prevalence among men, younger and unmarried adults, and those with lower socioeconomic status

ETIOLOGY AND PATHOPHYSIOLOGY
- Consumption of alcohol stimulates the neurotransmitter γ-aminobutyric acid (GABA), resulting in decreased excitability, with chronic alcohol ingestion, this repeated stimulation downregulates GABA inhibitory effects.
- Concurrently, alcohol ingestion inhibits glutamate on the central nervous system (CNS), with chronic alcohol use upregulation of excitatory *N*-methyl-D-aspartate glutamate receptors.
- When alcohol is abruptly stopped, the joint effect of a downregulated inhibitory system (GABA modulated) and upregulated excitatory system (glutamate modulated) results in brain hyperexcitability no longer suppressed by alcohol; clinically seen as AWS

Genetics
Etiology of AUD is multifactorial; evidence suggests genetic predisposition is present in half of individuals with AUD.

RISK FACTORS
- Long duration of heavy alcohol consumption
- Prior history of alcohol withdrawal episodes, alcohol withdrawal seizures, and delirium tremens (DTs)
- Elevated blood pressure on presentation, comorbid medical conditions or surgical illness
- Physiologic dependence on benzodiazepines (BZDs) or barbiturates

Geriatric Considerations
Elderly with AUD are more susceptible to withdrawal, and chronic comorbid conditions place them at higher risk of complications from withdrawal.

Pregnancy Considerations
Inpatient hospitalization for acute alcohol withdrawal management is recommended in pregnancy.

GENERAL PREVENTION
- The U.S. Preventive Services Task Force recommends universal screening for all adults to reduce unhealthy alcohol use.
- The single screening question, "How many times in the past year have you had 5 or more (men) 4 or more (women) drinks in 1 day" is the most sensitive and specific question for detecting unhealthy alcohol use.
- Brief, standard assessment screening tools include CAGE, AUDIT, or AUDIT-C to detect unhealthy alcohol use.

COMMONLY ASSOCIATED CONDITIONS
- General: weight loss and poor nutrition, dehydration
- Renal: electrolyte abnormalities (hyponatremia, hypokalemia, hypomagnesemia, hypophosphatemia)
- GI: hepatitis, cirrhosis, esophageal varices, GI bleed, pancreatitis, portal hypertension
- Heme: thrombocytopenia, macrocytic anemia
- Cardiovascular: hypertension, atrial fibrillation, other arrhythmias, hyperlipidemia
- CNS: seizures, hallucinations, memory deficits, atrophy, Wernicke-Korsakoff syndrome
- Peripheral nervous system: neuropathy
- Pulmonary: aspiration pneumonitis or pneumonia; increased risk of anaerobic infections
- Psychiatric: depression, posttraumatic stress disorder, bipolar disease, polysubstance use disorder
- Reproductive: sexual dysfunction and amenorrhea

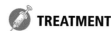 **DIAGNOSIS**

- *Diagnostic and Statistical Manual of Mental Disorders,* 5th edition diagnostic criteria for AWS:
  - Two (or more) of the following present within a few hours after the cessation or reduction of heavy and prolonged alcohol ingestion:
    ○ Autonomic hyperactivity
    ○ Hand tremor
    ○ Insomnia
    ○ Psychomotor agitation
    ○ Anxiety
    ○ Nausea or vomiting
    ○ Generalized seizures
    ○ Transient visual, auditory, or tactile hallucinations or illusions
  - Signs or symptoms cause significant impairment in social, occupation, or occupation areas.
  - Signs and symptoms are not secondary to an underlying medical or mental condition.
- Clinical manifestations
  - AWS can be divided into three cluster of symptoms
  - Autonomic hyperactivity: onset a few hours of cessation and peak 24 to 48 hours
  - Neural excitation: Alcohol withdrawal–associated seizures are often brief and typically occur 12 to to 48 hours after last drink.
  - Alcohol withdrawal delirium: onset 48 to 72 hours after cessation

HISTORY
Essential historical information should be as follows:
- Duration and quantity of alcohol intake, time since last drink
- Prior symptoms of alcohol withdrawal, or hx of prior admissions for AUD
- Concurrent substance use
- Preexisting medical and psychiatric conditions, prior seizure activity
- Social history: living situation, social support, stressors, and triggers

PHYSICAL EXAM
Should include assessment of conditions that are exacerbated by AWS
- Cardiovascular: arrhythmias, heart failure, coronary artery disease
- GI: GI bleed, liver disease, pancreatitis
- Neuro: oculomotor dysfunction, gait ataxia, neuropathy
- Psych: orientation, memory (may be complicated by hepatic encephalopathy)
- General: hand tremor (six to eight cycles per second), infections

DIFFERENTIAL DIAGNOSIS
- Cocaine and amphetamines intoxication
- Opioid, marijuana, and other sedating substances withdrawal
- Anticholinergic drug toxicity
- Neuroleptic malignant syndrome
- ICU delirium
- Sepsis, CNS infection, or hemorrhage
- Mania, psychosis, anxiety, or panic disorder
- Thyroid crisis

DIAGNOSTIC TESTS & INTERPRETATION
Initial Tests (lab, imaging)
- Blood alcohol level, urine drug screen
- Complete blood count; comprehensive metabolic panel
- Lipase; amylase, GGT
- Head CT for patients whose presentations differ from their typical withdrawal symptoms or mental status atypical for withdrawal
- If first seizure, full neurologic workup, including EEG, brain imaging, and lumbar puncture

Follow-Up Tests & Special Considerations
- For patients reporting abnormal pain, elevate amylase or lipase, consider abdominal ultrasound or CT.
- Electrocardiogram is suggested for patients >50 years or for patients with history of cardiac problems.

Test Interpretation
Rate of metabolism of alcohol varies but is generally 10 to 15 mg/dL/hr, patients with prolonged alcohol use metabolize at a faster rate of 20 to 30 mg/dL/hr. Using these calculations can approximate when withdrawal symptoms may increase.
- Blood alcohol concentration (BAC): <100% may see loss of coordination and mood changes.
- BAC: 80 is considered legal intoxication in United States.
- BAC: 100 to 199 neurologic impairment, slower reaction time or ataxia
- BAC: 200 to 299 obvious intoxication is present, unless person has marked tolerance.
- BAC: >300 can be associated with slurred speech, amnesia, coma, and death.

TREATMENT

GENERAL MEASURES
- Goals of therapy:
  - "Provide a safe withdrawal from the drug(s) of dependence."
  - "Provide humane withdrawal and protect patient's dignity."
  - "Prepare patient for ongoing treatment of his or her dependence on alcohol."

- The Clinical Institute Withdrawal Assessment of Alcohol Scale, Revised (CIWA-Ar) is useful for deciding medication dosing and frequency for AWS. Severity of symptoms are rated on a scale from 0 to 7, with 0 being without symptoms and 7 being the maximum score (except orientation and clouding of sensorium, scale 0 to 4).
  - Nausea and vomiting
  - Tactile disturbances
  - Tremor
  - Auditory disturbances
  - Paroxysmal sweats
  - Visual disturbances
  - Anxiety
  - Headache or fullness in head
  - Agitation
  - Orientation and clouding of sensorium
- The maximum CIWA-Ar score achievable is 67.
  - Mild withdrawal = score <8: likely resolve without medication
  - Moderate withdrawal = 8 to 14: often require management with medication
  - Severe withdrawal = >15 are associated with the highest risk of seizures and development of DTs.
- Frequent reevaluation with CIWA-Ar score is crucial.

MEDICATION

First Line

- BZD monotherapy remains the treatment of choice for CIWA scores >10.
- BZD should be based on the following considerations:
  - Agents with rapid onset control agitation more quickly (e.g., IV diazepam).
  - Long-acting BZDs (diazepam, chlordiazepoxide) are more effective at preventing breakthrough seizures and contribute to reduction in breakthrough or rebound symptoms.
  - Short-acting BZDs (lorazepam, oxazepam) are preferable when prolonged sedation is a concern (e.g., elderly patients or other serious concomitant medical illness) and preferable with severe hepatic impairment.
- BZD dosages will vary by patient.
- Can use symptom-triggered or fixed-schedule regimens
  - Symptom-triggered regimens are preferred and associated with lower BZD amounts and reduce hospitalization length of stay.
  - Fixed-schedule regimens are appropriate if nursing staff do not have training for symptom triggered regime, in patient with severe coronary artery disease, or if history of past withdrawal seizures.
- Symptom-triggered regimen: Administer one of the following medications every 4 to 6 hours, with added doses PRN when CIWA-Ar ≥8. Assess need for further medications 1 hour after each dose.
  - Chlordiazepoxide: 50 to 100 mg PO
  - Diazepam: 10 to 20 mg PO
  - Oxazepam: 30 to 60 mg PO
  - Lorazepam: 2 to 4 mg PO
- Fixed-schedule regimen: Administer one of the following medications every 6 hours:
  - Chlordiazepoxide: 50 mg PO for 4 doses and then 25 mg PO for 8 doses
  - Diazepam: 10 mg PO for 4 doses and then 5 mg PO for 8 doses
  - Lorazepam: 2 mg PO for 4 doses and then 1 mg PO for 8 doses
  - Important to monitor closely and provide additional BZDs if CIWA-Ar ≥8

- Folic acid: 1 mg daily
- Thiamine: 50 to 100 mg daily
  - Do not administer IV glucose before giving thiamine because this may precipitate Wernicke encephalopathy and Korsakoff psychosis.
- Correct electrolyte abnormalities/imbalance as they occur.

Second Line

- Gabapentin: reduces alcohol consumption, cravings, and may be effective for mild withdrawal.
- β-Blockers (e.g., atenolol or propranolol) and α_2-agonists (e.g., clonidine) help to control hypertension and tachycardia but do not prevent severe symptoms such as DT or seizures; not used as monotherapy
- Carbamazepine: associated with reduced seizures and effective at mild withdrawal; should not be used as a monotherapy
- If the patient exhibits significant agitation and alcoholic hallucinosis, an antipsychotic (haloperidol) can be used, but requires close observation because of lower seizure threshold.

ADDITIONAL THERAPIES

Peripheral neuropathy and cerebellar dysfunction merit physical therapy evaluation.

ADMISSION, INPATIENT, AND NURSING CONSIDERATIONS

Criteria for inpatient admission:

- CIWA-Ar score >15 or severe withdrawal
- Presence of ataxia, nystagmus, confusion which may indicate Werniecke encephalopathy
- Severe nausea or vomiting that prevents ingestion of medications
- Poor ability to follow up or no reliable social support
- Pregnancy
- History of severe withdrawal symptoms
- History of seizure disorder, withdrawal seizures, or DTs
- Presence of cardiovascular disease
- Concurrent psychiatric illness, associated medical or surgical illness that requires treatment

 ONGOING CARE

FOLLOW-UP RECOMMENDATIONS

- Managing alcohol withdrawal is only first step toward treating patient's underlying AUD.
- Discharge arrangements should include:
  - Development of plan to engage patient in further treatment
  - Transition to outpatient substance use counseling, peer support groups, and/or residential treatment facility
  - Prescription of available FDA-approved medication-assisted treatment
- Acamprosate (666 mg PO TID): glutamate and GABA modulator indicated to reduce cravings
  - Contraindications: renal impairment (CrCl <30 mL/min)
  - Compliance may be issue due to multidosing each day; recent studies question benefits.
- Naltrexone (50 mg/day PO; 380 mg IM every 4 weeks): opiate receptor antagonist, reduce craving. Initiate therapy after patient is opioid free for at least 7 days.
  - Contraindications: acute hepatitis/liver failure, concomitant opioid therapy
  - Effective in short term (3 to 6 months)

- Disulfiram (250 mg/day PO): creates adverse reaction to alcohol by interfering with aldehyde dehydrogenase, blocking alcohol metabolism, leading to an accumulation of acetaldehyde
  - Second-line option due to limited evidence of efficacy for relapse prevention
  - Contraindications: concomitant use of ethanol-containing products, foods, or medications; psychosis, severe myocardial disease, diabetes, seizures, emphysema, severe liver and renal disease, pregnancy, and coronary occlusion

Patient Monitoring

Frequent follow-up to monitor for relapse

DIET

Advance as tolerated

PATIENT EDUCATION

- Alcoholics Anonymous: http://www.aa.org/
- SMART Recovery (Self-Management and Recovery Training): http://www.smartrecovery.org/ (not spiritually based)
- National Institute on Alcohol Abuse and Alcoholism: http://www.niaaa.nih.gov/guide/
- FamilyDoctor.Org: alcohol withdrawal syndrome (Spanish resources available)

PROGNOSIS

Mortality from severe withdrawal (DTs) is 1–5%.

COMPLICATIONS

Occurs more frequently in individuals who have prior episodes of withdrawal or concomitant illnesses

ADDITIONAL READING

- Muncie HL Jr, Yasinian Y, Oge' L. Outpatient management of alcohol withdrawal syndrome. *Am Fam Physician*. 2013;88(9):589–595.
- Rastegar DA, Fingerhood MI. *The American Society of Addiction Medicine Handbook of Addiction Medicine*, 2nd edition. Oxford, United Kingdom: Oxford University Press; 2020.

 SEE ALSO

Substance Use Disorders

CODES

ICD10

- F10.239 Alcohol dependence with withdrawal, unspecified
- F10.230 Alcohol dependence with withdrawal, uncomplicated
- F10.231 Alcohol dependence with withdrawal delirium

CLINICAL PEARLS

- Any BZD dose should be patient specific, sufficient to achieve and maintain a "light somnolence" (e.g., sleeping but easily arousable), and should be tapered off carefully to prevent BZD withdrawal.
- Administer thiamine before patient receives glucose so to not precipitate Wernicke encephalopathy.
- Avoid administering diazepam and lorazepam intramuscularly because of erratic absorption.
- Managing AWS is the first step toward treating AUD. Ensure patient has outpatient follow-up to continue treatment.

ALOPECIA
Mallory Zaino, MD

BASICS

DESCRIPTION
- Alopecia: absence of hair from areas where it normally grows
  - Anagen phase: growing hairs, 90% scalp hair follicles at any time, lasts 2 to 6 years
  - Catagen phase: regression of follicle, <1% follicles, lasts 3 weeks
  - Telogen phase: Resting phase lasts 2 to 3 months, 50 to 150 telogen hairs shed per day.
- Classified as scarring (cicatricial), nonscarring (noncicatricial), or structural
- Scarring (cicatricial) alopecia
  - Inflammatory disorders leading to permanent hair loss and follicle destruction
  - Includes lichen planopilaris, frontal fibrosing alopecia, and discoid lupus erythematosus
- Nonscarring (noncicatricial) alopecia
  - Lack of inflammation, no destruction of follicle
  - Includes androgenic alopecia, alopecia areata (AA), telogen effluvium, anagen effluvium
- Structural hair disorders
  - Brittle or fragile hair from abnormal hair formation or external insult

EPIDEMIOLOGY
Prevalence
- Androgenic alopecia:
  - In males, 30% Caucasian by 30 years of age, 50% by 50 years of age, and 80% by 70 years of age
  - In females, 70% of women >65 years of age
- AA: 1/1,000 with lifetime risk of 1–2%, men and women affected equally
- Scarring alopecia: rare, 3–7% of all hair disorder patients

ETIOLOGY AND PATHOPHYSIOLOGY
- Scarring (cicatricial) alopecia
  - Inflammatory disorders leading to permanent destruction of the follicle
  - Slick smooth scalp without follicles evident
  - Three major subtypes based on type of inflammation: lymphocytic, neutrophilic, and mixed
  - Primary scarring includes discoid lupus, lichen planopilaris, dissecting cellulitis of scalp, primary fibrosing, among others.
  - Secondary scarring from infection, neoplasm, radiation, surgery, and other physical trauma, including tinea capitis
  - Central centrifugal cicatricial alopecia most common form of scarring hair loss in African American women; etiology unknown but likely secondary to hair care practices
- Nonscarring (noncicatricial) alopecia
  - Focal alopecia
  - AA
    - Patchy hair loss, usually autoimmune in etiology, T cell–mediated inflammation resulting in premature transition to catagen then telogen phases
    - May occur with hair loss in other areas of the body (alopecia totalis [entire scalp]), alopecia universalis (rapid loss of all body hair)
    - Nail disease frequently seen
    - High psychiatric comorbidity (1)
  - Alopecia syphilitica: "moth-eaten" appearance, secondary syphilis
  - Postoperative, pressure-induced alopecia: from long periods of pressure on one area of scalp

- Temporal triangular alopecia: congenital patch of hair loss in temporal area, unilateral or bilateral
- Traction alopecia: patchy, due to physical stressor of braids, ponytails, hair weaves
- Pattern hair loss
  - Androgenic alopecia: hair transitions from terminal to vellus hairs
  - Male pattern hair loss: androgen-mediated hair loss in specific distribution; bitemporal, vertex occurs where androgen sensitive hairs are located on scalp. This is a predominantly hereditary condition (2).
    - Increased androgen receptors, increased 5-α reductase leads to increased testosterone conversion in follicle to dihydrotestosterone (DHT). This leads to decreased follicle size and vellus hair (2).
    - Norwood Hamilton classification type I to VII
    - Female pattern hair loss: thinning on frontal and vertex areas (Ludwig classification, grade I to III). Females with low levels of aromatase have more testosterone available for conversion to DHT (3). This carries an unclear inheritance pattern (2).
    - Polycystic ovarian syndrome, adrenal hyperplasia, and pituitary hyperplasia all lead to androgen changes and can result in alopecia.
  - Medications (hormone replacement therapy, oral contraceptive pills)
  - Drugs (testosterone, progesterone, danazol, adrenocorticosteroids, anabolic steroids)
- Trichotillomania: intentional pulling of hair from scalp; may present in variety of patterns
- Diffuse alopecia
  - Telogen effluvium: sudden shift of many follicles from anagen to telogen phase resulting in decreased hair density but not bald areas
    - May follow major stressors, including childbirth, injury, illness; occurs 2 to 3 months after event
    - Can be chronic with ongoing illness, including SLE, renal failure, IBS, HIV, thyroid disease, pituitary dysfunction
    - Adding or changing medications (oral contraceptives, anticoagulants, anticonvulsants, SSRIs, retinoids, β-blockers, ACE inhibitors, colchicine, cholesterol-lowering medications, etc.)
    - Malnutrition from malabsorption, eating disorders; poor diet can contribute.
  - Anagen effluvium
    - Interruption of the anagen phase without transition to telogen phase; days to weeks after inciting event
    - Chemotherapy is most common trigger.
    - Radiation, poisoning, and medications can also trigger.
- Structural hair disorders
  - Multiple inherited hair disorders including Menkes disease, monilethrix, and so forth. These result in the formation of abnormal hairs that are weakened.
  - May also result from chemical or heat damaging from hair processing treatments

Genetics
Family history of early patterned hair loss is common in androgenic alopecia, also in AA.

RISK FACTORS
- Genetic predisposition
- Chronic illness including autoimmune disease, infections, cancer
- Physiologic stress including pregnancy and childbirth
- Poor nutrition

- Medication, chemotherapy, radiation
- Hair chemical treatments, braids, weaves/extensions

GENERAL PREVENTION
Minimize risk factors where possible.

COMMONLY ASSOCIATED CONDITIONS
- See "Etiology and Pathophysiology."
- Vitiligo—4.1% patients with AA, may be the result of similar autoimmune pathways (4)

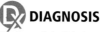

DIAGNOSIS

The diagnosis is clinical, made by history and examination.

HISTORY
- Description of hair loss problem: rate of loss, duration, location, degree of hair loss, other symptoms including pruritus, infection, hair care, and treatments
- Associated symptoms: pruritus, pain, or burning
- Hair styling practices: use of prolonged heat, coloring, bleaching, chemical relaxers, and hair styling (braids and ponytails)
- Medications
- Medical illness including chronic disease, recent illness, surgeries, pregnancy, thyroid disorder, iron deficiency, poisonings, exposures
- Psychological stress
- Dietary history and weight changes
- Family history of hair loss or autoimmune disorders

PHYSICAL EXAM
- Pattern of hair loss
  - Generalized, patterned, focal
  - Assess hair density, vellus versus terminal hairs, broken hair.
- Scalp scaling, inflammation, papules, pustules
- Presence of follicular ostia to determine class of alopecia
- Hair pull test
  - Pinch 25 to 50 hairs between thumb and forefinger and exert slow, gentle traction while sliding fingers up.
    - Normal: 1 to 2 dislodge
    - Abnormal: ≥6 hairs dislodged
    - Broken hairs (structural disorder)
    - Broken-off hair at the borders patch that are easily removable (in AA)
- Hair loss at other sites, nail disorders, skin changes
- Clinical signs of thyroid disease, lupus, or other diseases
- Clinical signs of virilization: acne, hirsutism, acanthosis nigricans, truncal obesity

DIFFERENTIAL DIAGNOSIS
Search for type of alopecia and then for reversible causes.

DIAGNOSTIC TESTS & INTERPRETATION
Initial Tests (lab, imaging)
- No testing may be indicated depending on clinical appearance.
- Nonandrogenic alopecia
  - TSH, CBC, ferritin
  - Consider: LFT, BMP, zinc, VDRL, ANA, prolactin all depending on clinical history and exam
- Androgenic alopecia: especially in females
  - Consider free testosterone and dehydroepiandrosterone sulfate.

Diagnostic Procedures/Other

- Light hair-pull test: Pull on 25 to 50 hairs; ≥6 hairs dislodged is consistent with shedding (effluvium, AA).
- Direct microscopic exam of the hair shaft
  - Anagen hairs: elongated, distorted bulb with root sheath attached
  - Telogen hairs: rounded bulb, no root sheath
  - Exclamation point hairs: club-shaped root with thinner proximal shaft (AA)
  - Broken and distorted hairs may be associated with multiple hair dystrophies
- Biopsy: scarring (cicatricial) alopecia or if diagnosis remains unknown
  - Recommend two 4-mm punch biopsies.
  - In scarring alopecia, take the biopsy at the edge of inflammation.
    - Lymphocytic inflammation with perifollicular fibrosis
  - In nonscarring alopecia, take the biopsy at an area with thinning hair but not complete hair loss.
    - Androgenic alopecia: ratio of terminal: vellus hair follicle <2:1, variable size of hair shafts, follicular miniaturization
    - Telogen effluvium: increased ratio of catagen: telogen, no change in number of hair follicles, no miniaturization of follicle
    - AA: increased ratio of catagen: telogen, no change in number of hair follicles, follicular miniaturization
- Ultraviolet light fluorescence and potassium hydroxide prep (to rule out tinea capitis)

 TREATMENT

GENERAL MEASURES

- Consider potential harms and benefits to the patient prior to treatment. Many will gain an improved quality of life that is of benefit (2)[A].
- Stop any possible medication causes if possible; this will often resolve telogen effluvium (5)[C].
- Treat underlying medical causes (e.g., thyroid disorder, syphilis).
- Traction alopecia: Change hair care practices; education
- Trichotillomania: often requires psychological intervention to induce behavior change

MEDICATION

- Nonscarring
- **Androgenic alopecia**: Treatment must be continued indefinitely; can use in combination
  - Minoxidil (Rogaine) (6)[A]: 2% topical solution (1 mL BID) for women, 5% topical solution (1 mL BID) or foam (daily) for men; works in 60% of cases (3)[C]
    - Unclear mechanism of action; appears to prolong anagen phase
    - Adverse effects: skin irritation, hypertrichosis of face/hands, tachycardia; Category C in pregnancy (3)[C]
  - Finasteride (Propecia) (6)[A]: 1 mg/day for men and women (off-label) (7)[C]; 30–50% improvement in males, poor data in females (2)[C]
    - 5-α reductase inhibitor, reduces DHT in system, increases total and anagen hairs, slows transition of terminal to vellus hairs
    - Adverse effects: loss of libido, gynecomastia, depression. Caution in liver disease; absolutely no use or contact during pregnancy, Category X, reliable contraception required in female use (7)[C]

- Spironolactone (Aldactone): 100 to 200 mg/day (off-label) (3)[C]
  - Aldosterone antagonist, antiandrogen; blocks the effect of androgens, decreasing testosterone production
  - Adverse effects: dose-dependent, hyperkalemia, menstrual irregularity, fatigue; Category D in pregnancy
- Ketoconazole: decreases DHT levels at follicle, works best with minoxidil in female androgenic alopecia (7)[C]
- Combination: Finasteride + minoxidil has superior efficacy to monotherapy (2)[C].
- **AA**: no FDA-approved treatment; high rate of spontaneous remission in patchy AA
- Intralesional steroids
  - Triamcinolone: 2.5 to 5.0 mg/mL (3)[C]
    - Inject 0.1 mL into deep dermal layer at 0.5 to 1.0 cm intervals with 1/2 inch 30-gauge needle, every 4 to 6 weeks; maximum 20 mg/session (1)[C]
    - Adverse effects: local burning, pruritus, skin atrophy
  - Systemic glucocorticoids: Use in extensive, multifocal AA; may induce regrowth but requires long-term monthly treatment to maintain growth (1)[C]
    - Adverse effects: hyperglycemia, adrenal insufficiency, osteoporosis, cataracts, obesity
  - PUVA light therapy + prednisone: moderate effectiveness in diffuse AA
  - Tinea capitis: See "Tinea (Capitis, Corporis, Cruris)."

SURGERY/OTHER PROCEDURES

- Wigs, hairpieces, extensions
- Surgical: graft transplantation, flap transplantation, or excision of the scarred area; used primarily in scarring alopecia
- Platelet-rich plasma: has been shown to restore dormant hair follicles and stimulate new hair growth

COMPLEMENTARY & ALTERNATIVE MEDICINE

- Many herbal medications are available; no clear evidence at this time
- Volumizing shampoos can help remaining hair look fuller.

 ONGOING CARE

DIET

If nutritional deficit noted, supplementation may be necessary.

PATIENT EDUCATION

National Alopecia Areata Foundation: www.naaf.org

PROGNOSIS

- *Androgenic alopecia*: Prognosis depends on response to treatment.
- *AA*: often regrows within 1 year even without treatment. Recurrence common. 10% have severe, chronic form; poor prognosis more likely with long duration, extensive hair loss, autoimmune disease, nail involvement, and young age
- *Telogen effluvium*: maximum shedding 3 months after the inciting event and recovery following correction of the cause. Usually subsides in 3 to 6 months but takes 12 to 18 months for cosmetically significant regrowth; rarely, permanent hair loss, usually with long-term illness

- *Anagen effluvium*: Shedding begins days to a few weeks after the inciting event, with recovery following correction of the cause; rarely, permanent hair loss
- *Traction alopecia*: excellent prognosis with behavior modification
- *Cicatricial alopecia*: hair follicles permanently damaged; prognosis depends on type of alopecia and available treatments.
- *Tinea capitis*: excellent prognosis with treatment

REFERENCES

1. Alkhalifah A. Alopecia areata update. *Dermatol Clin*. 2013;31(1):93–108.
2. Blumeyer A, Tosti A, Messenger A, et al; for European Dermatology Forum. Evidence-based (S3) guideline for the treatment of androgenetic alopecia in women and in men. *J Dtsch Dermatol Ges*. 2011;9(Suppl 6):S1–S57.
3. Rathnayake D, Sinclair R. Innovative use of spironolactone as an antiandrogen in the treatment of female pattern hair loss. *Dermatol Clin*. 2010;28(3):611–618.
4. Kumar S, Mittal J, Mahajan B. Colocalization of vitiligo and alopecia areata: coincidence or consequence? *Int J Trichology*. 2013;5(1):50–52.
5. Harrison S, Bergfeld W. Diffuse hair loss: its triggers and management. *Cleve Clin J Med*. 2009;76(6):361–367.
6. Adil A, Godwin M. The effectiveness of treatments for androgenetic alopecia: a systematic review and meta-analysis. *J Am Acad Dermatol*. 2017;77(1):136–141.e5.
7. Atanaskova Mesinkovska N, Bergfeld WF. Hair: what is new in diagnosis and management? Female pattern hair loss update: diagnosis and treatment. *Dermatol Clin*. 2013;31(1):119–127.

 SEE ALSO

- Hyperthyroidism; Lichen Planus; Lupus Erythematosus, Systemic (SLE); Polycystic Ovarian Syndrome (PCOS); Syphilis; Tinea (Capitis, Corporis, Cruris)
- Algorithm: Alopecia

 CODES

ICD10

- L65.9 Nonscarring hair loss, unspecified
- L64.9 Androgenic alopecia, unspecified
- L63.9 Alopecia areata, unspecified

CLINICAL PEARLS

- History and physical are necessary in determining type of alopecia for appropriate treatment.
- Treatment of underlying medical condition or removal of triggering medication will often resolve hair loss.
- Educating the patient about the nature of the condition and expectations is key to care.
- Alopecia can affect the psychological condition of the patient, and it may be necessary to address this in any type of hair loss.

ALTITUDE ILLNESS
Andrew McBride, MD

BASICS

DESCRIPTION

- A spectrum of cerebral and pulmonary syndromes ranging from mild discomfort to fatal illness that occur on ascent to higher altitudes as a direct result of inadequate acclimatization
- Categories of altitude: intermediate, 1,520 to 2,440 m; high, 2,440 to 4,270 m; very high, 4,270 to 5,490 m; and extreme, >5,490 m
- Altitude illness can affect anyone, including experienced and fit individuals. For most, it is an unpleasant (self-limited) syndrome that does not require medical intervention (1).
- Acute mountain sickness (AMS): symptoms associated with a physiologic response to a hypobaric, hypoxic environment. Onset usually occurs within 6 to 12 hours after ascending >2,500 m. Neurologic symptoms predominate, ranging from mild/moderate headache and malaise to severe impairment.
- High-altitude pulmonary edema (HAPE): noncardiogenic pulmonary edema; typically after 2 or more days at altitudes >3,000 m, rare between 2,500 and 3,000 m
- High-altitude cerebral edema (HACE): a potentially fatal neurologic syndrome considered to be the end stage of AMS; onset after at least 2 days at altitudes >4,000 m
- System(s) affected: nervous/pulmonary (2)
- Synonym(s): mountain sickness

Geriatric Considerations
- Risk does not increase with age.
- Age alone should not preclude travel to high altitude; allow extra time to acclimate.
- Worsening of preexisting medical problems referred to as altitude-exacerbated conditions

Pediatric Considerations
- Altitude illness seems to have the same incidence in children as in adults; diagnosis may be delayed in younger children.
- Any child who experiences behavioral symptoms after recent ascent should be presumed to have an altitude-related illness.

Pregnancy Considerations
- The risk during pregnancy is unknown.
- No evidence suggests that exposure to high altitudes (1,500 to 3,500 m) poses a risk to a pregnancy.

EPIDEMIOLOGY
Most epidemiologic studies are limited to relatively homogeneous male populations.

Incidence
- AMS: 10–25% of unacclimatized persons who ascend to 2,500 m; 50–85% at altitudes of 4,500 to 5,500 m
- HAPE/HACE: 0.5–1.0% of unacclimatized persons with 2 or more days of exposure at altitudes exceeding 3,000 m. Risk increases with rate of ascent.
- Above 2,500 m (8,200 feet), for every 1,000-m increase in altitude, there is a 13% increase in the AMS (3).

ETIOLOGY AND PATHOPHYSIOLOGY
- Individuals with a prior history of AMS, HACE, or HAPE are at a higher risk for recurrent AMS.
- Hypobaric hypoxia and hypoxemia are the pathophysiologic precursors to altitude illness.
- Symptoms of AMS may be the result of cerebral swelling, either through vasodilatation induced by hypoxia or through cerebral edema.
- Other mechanisms include impaired cerebral autoregulation, release of vasogenic mediators, and alteration of the blood–brain barrier.
- HAPE is a noncardiogenic pulmonary edema characterized by exaggerated pulmonary hypertension leading to vascular leakage through overperfusion, stress failure, or both.

Genetics
Genetic factors involved in predisposition to developing AMS are poorly understood.

RISK FACTORS
- Failure to properly acclimatize at a lower altitude
- Ascent rate >300 to 500 m/day
- Extreme altitude
- Increased duration at high altitude
- Higher altitude during sleep cycle
- Prior history of altitude illness
- Cardiac congenital abnormalities
- Female gender
- History of migraines (4)
- Younger age (<46 years)
- History of anxiety (5)

GENERAL PREVENTION
- General guidelines
  - Preacclimatization (exposure of hypoxia prior to ascent) protects against altitude illness.
  - Staged ascent (spending 6 to 7 days) at 2,200 to 3,000 m can also prevent altitude illness (6).
  - >2,500 m, do not ascend faster than 500 m/day; rest every 3 to 4 days (2).
  - Lower sleeping elevation: "Climb high and sleep low" for anyone going >3,500 m.
  - Avoid heavy exertion for the first 1 to 3 days at altitude.
  - Avoid respiratory depressants (alcohol and sedatives).
  - Preascent physical conditioning is not preventive.
- Pharmacologic prophylaxis
  - Acetazolamide, dexamethasone, and ibuprofen (see "Treatment")
  - For prevention of HAPE only (if at risk):
    - Consider nifedipine, β-agonists, and tadalafil (see "Treatment").

DIAGNOSIS

HISTORY
- AMS:
  - Symptoms include headache, anorexia, irritability, marked fatigue, nausea, vomiting, dizziness, light-headedness, dyspnea with exertion, or insomnia.

- Severity has been studied using the Lake Louise diagnostic criteria, which ranks from 0 (none) to 3 (severe) (7).
  - Headache, gastrointestinal symptoms, fatigue and/or weakness, dizziness/light-headedness, and AMS Clinical Functional Score (symptom affect on activities)
  - AMS is considered diagnostic with a headache score of at least 1 point and a total score of at least 3 points.
- HAPE symptoms: reduced exercise tolerance, exertional dyspnea, and cough followed by dyspnea at rest, cyanosis, and productive cough that may contain pink frothy sputum (6)
- HACE symptoms: altered mental status (irrational behavior, lethargy, obtundation, coma)
  - May progress to ataxia and confusion (2)

PHYSICAL EXAM
- HAPE
  - Lung crackles or wheezing
  - Central cyanosis
  - Tachycardia
  - Tachypnea
- HACE
  - Abnormal mental status exam (behavioral change, lethargy, obtundation, coma)
  - Truncal ataxia
  - Papilledema, retinal hemorrhage, cranial nerve palsies
  - Focal neurologic deficits (rare)

DIFFERENTIAL DIAGNOSIS
- AMS/HACE
  - Dehydration
  - Ingestion of toxins, drugs, or alcohol
  - Subarachnoid hemorrhage, CNS mass, cerebrovascular accident
  - Migraine headache
  - Carbon monoxide exposure
  - CNS infection
  - Acute psychosis
- HAPE
  - Pneumonia
  - Cardiogenic pulmonary edema
  - Spontaneous pneumothorax
  - Pulmonary embolism
  - Asthma
  - Bronchitis
  - Myocardial infarction
  - Hyperventilation syndrome
- Onset of symptoms >3 days at a given altitude, the absence of headache, or the lack of rapid response to oxygen or descent suggests an alternative diagnosis.

DIAGNOSTIC TESTS & INTERPRETATION
Initial Tests (lab, imaging)
- AMS: Laboratory studies are nonspecific and rarely required for diagnosis.
- HAPE: Severe hypoxemia demonstrated with oximetry or blood gas analysis.
- Chest radiographs usually show patchy infiltrates. Clear lung fields suggest an alternate diagnosis.
- ECG may show sinus tachycardia or right-sided heart strain (1).

TREATMENT

GENERAL MEASURES
- Individuals without previous altitude exposure should adhere to acclimatization guidelines.
- Stop ascent, acclimatize at the same altitude, and/or descend if symptoms do not abate over 24 hours. Definitive treatment is to descend to a lower altitude. Dramatic improvement accompanies even modest reductions in altitude.
- Oxygen helps relieve symptoms. Give continuously by cannula or mask and titrate to SaO_2 >90% (1).
- AMS
  - Acetazolamide reduces mild to moderate symptoms of AMS (see "Medication").
  - Dexamethasone may also be effective in treating moderate AMS (see "Medication").
- HAPE
  - Oxygen therapy
  - Minimize exertion and keep patient warm.
  - Immediate descent or evacuation to a lower altitude
  - Portable hyperbaric therapy (2 to 15 psi using Gamow bag or Chamberlite) is an effective and practical alternative when descent is not possible.
  - Nifedipine (see "Medication")
- HACE
  - Immediate descent
  - Supplemental oxygen (highest flow available; maintain SaO_2 >90%)
  - Dexamethasone (see "Medication")
  - Portable hyperbaric therapy if available and unable to descend

MEDICATION
First Line
- Oxygen: 2 to 15 L/min to maintain SaO_2 >90% until symptoms improve
- Acetazolamide: If patient has a history of problems at altitude and/or plans to ascend >500 m/day above 2,500 m, consider therapy for primary prevention. Avoid in patients with a sulfonamide allergy.
  - Primary prevention of AMS: Adult dosing 125 mg PO BID starting 24 hours before ascent and continued for 2 to 4 days at a stable altitude; pediatric dosing 2.5 mg/kg (maximum 125 mg) every 12 hours (6).
  - Treatment of AMS: 250 mg PO BID until symptoms resolve; pediatric dose: 2.5 mg/kg q12h (6)
- Dexamethasone: may significantly reduce the incidence and severity of AMS. Adverse side effects are rare.
  - Prevention of AMS: 2 mg PO q6h or 4 mg PO q12h, starting 1 day before ascent and discontinued cautiously after 2 days at maximum altitude. Do not use for pediatric prevention (6).
  - Treatment of AMS: 4 mg PO/IV/IM q6h; pediatric dose: 0.15 mg/kg dose q6h (6)
  - Treatment of HACE: 8 mg PO/IV/IM initially and then 4 mg q6h; pediatric dose: 0.15 mg/kg dose q6h (6)

- Nifedipine (reduces pulmonary arterial pressure) (1)
  - Prevention of HAPE: 30 mg extended-release PO BID starting 1 day prior to ascent and continued for 2 days at maximum altitude (6)
  - Treatment of HAPE: 30 mg extended-release PO q12h (likely unnecessary if oxygen is available)
- Tadalafil: Consider for the prevention of HAPE (1).
  - Prevention HAPE: 10 mg PO BID 1 day prior to ascent in HAPE-susceptible individual (6).
- Adjunct therapy
  - Salmeterol
    - Possible treatment of HAPE (not well studied): 125 μg inhaled BID starting 1 day before ascent and continued for 2 days at maximum altitude
  - NSAIDs: possible benefit in AMS prevention and treatment of associated headache
    - Aspirin: 325 mg PO q4h for total 3 doses
    - Ibuprofen: 400 to 600 mg PO q8h
  - Antiemetics
    - Prochlorperazine: 10 mg PO/IM q6–8h
    - Promethazine: 25 to 50 mg PO/IM/PR q6h
- Other trialed therapies
  - Gingko balboa: no benefit over placebo in reducing the risk of AMs (8)
  - Coca-containing products have been used in the Andes but have not been well studied (6).
  - Simulated altitude or remote ischemic preconditioning (RIPC), as well as supplementation of antioxidants, medroxyprogesterone, iron, or *Rhodiola crenulata* lack quality evidence supporting their use (8).
  - Furosemide: previously studied for treatment of AMS or HACE, 20 to 80 mg PO/IV q12h for a total of 2 doses. Currently out of favor; not recommended for prophylaxis; not established for use in HAPE (6)

ADMISSION, INPATIENT, AND NURSING CONSIDERATIONS
Outpatient treatment for mild cases

ONGOING CARE

FOLLOW-UP RECOMMENDATIONS
Patient Monitoring
- For mild cases, no follow-up is needed.
- For more severe cases, follow closely until symptoms subside.

PATIENT EDUCATION
Counsel patients about the risks of high-altitude travel and how to recognize symptoms of high-altitude illness.

PROGNOSIS
Most cases of mild to moderate AMS are self-limiting and do not require medical intervention. Patients may resume ascent once the symptoms subside. HAPE and HACE respond well to descent, evacuation, and/or pharmacologic treatment if identified early.

COMPLICATIONS
High-altitude retinal hemorrhage can cause visual changes but is usually asymptomatic.

REFERENCES
1. Davis C, Hackett P. Advances in the prevention and treatment of high altitude illness. *Emerg Med Clin North Am*. 2017;35(2):241–260.
2. Bärtsch P, Swenson ER. Clinical practice: acute high-altitude illnesses. *N Engl J Med*. 2013;368(24):2294–2302.
3. Meier D, Collet T, Locatelli I, et al. Does this patient have acute mountain sickness? The rational clinical examination systematic review. *JAMA*. 2017;318(18):1810–1819.
4. Richalet JP, Larmignat P, Poitrine E, et al. Physiological risk factors for severe high-altitude illness: a prospective cohort study. *Am J Respir Crit Care Med*. 2012;185(2):192–198.
5. Boos CJ, Bass M, O'Hara JP, et al. The relationship between anxiety and acute mountain sickness. *PLoS One*. 2018;13(6):e0197147.
6. Armstrong C. Acute altitude illness: updated prevention and treatment guidelines from the Wilderness Medical Society. *Am Fam Physician*. 2020;101(8):505–507.
7. Roach RC, Hackett PH, Oelz O, et al. The 2018 Lake Louise Acute Mountain Sickness Score. *High Alt Med Biol*. 2018;19(1):4–6.
8. Gonzalez G, Molano Franco D, Nieto Estrada VH, et al. Interventions for preventing high altitude illness: part 2. Less commonly-used drugs. *Cochrane Database Syst Rev*. 2018;(3):CD012983.

 CODES

ICD10
- T70.20XA Unspecified effects of high altitude, initial encounter
- T70.20XD Unspecified effects of high altitude, subsequent encounter
- T70.20XS Unspecified effects of high altitude, sequela

CLINICAL PEARLS
- Slow ascent and timely descent are important to prevent and treat of high-altitude illnesses.
- Lack of symptom resolution with appropriate descent suggests an alternative diagnosis.
- High-flow oxygen, followed by oxygen titrated to maintain SaO_2 >90%, is the first-line treatment for all patients with more than mild altitude illness.

ALZHEIMER DISEASE

John P. Barrett, MD, MPH, MS

 BASICS

DESCRIPTION
- Alzheimer disease (AD) is a progressive, irreversible, degenerative neurologic disease that results in neuron death.
- AD represents 60–80% of dementia.
- AD is the sixth leading cause of death in the United States (1).
- People ≥65 years with new AD live 4 to 8 years on average.
- AD is underdiagnosed (~50%) and >50% with AD unaware of diagnosis
- Economic burden in 2018: ~$305 billion, projected $1.1 trillion by 2050 (1)
- Dementia should be distinguished from:
  - Age-related cognitive decline: lifelong changes in mental ability and memory; part of normal aging
  - Mild cognitive impairment (MCI): greater impairment than cognitive decline
    - MCI: People are generally able to live independently from a cognitive perspective.
    - MCI: affects 15–20% of those ≥65 years, with 32–38% developing dementia within 5 years
- AD diagnostic classification:
  - Preclinical AD: no cognitive symptoms, AD biomarkers present
  - MCI due to AD: often only memory symptoms
  - Dementia due to AD:
    - Early stage: memory impairment >MCI
    - Middle stage: impairment in communication and response to environment
    - Late stage: lose ability to appropriately recognize and respond to environment
- System(s) affected: nervous
- Synonym(s): presenile dementia; senile dementia of the Alzheimer type

EPIDEMIOLOGY
- Predominant age: >65 years
- Incidence: females = males
- Prevalence: females > males

Incidence
New cases of AD in the United States: 484,000/year (1)
- 65 to 75 years: 2 new cases per 1,000 people
- 75 to 84 years: 11 new cases per 1,000 people
- ≥85 years: 37 new cases per 1,000 people

Prevalence
~5.8 million in United States; ~44 million worldwide
- 13.8 million in United States by 2050
- 1 in 10 of those ≥65 years have AD dementia.
- 32% of those ≥85 years have AD dementia.
- ~200,000 in United States with early-onset AD (<65 years)

ETIOLOGY AND PATHOPHYSIOLOGY
- Progressive, irreversible disease where cognitive impairment worsens over time
- β-amyloid plaques outside of neurons and τ protein tangles inside of neurons, resulting in loss of connections and neuron death
- Age, genetics, systemic diseases, lifestyle behaviors may influence AD progression.

Genetics
- Autosomal dominant: <5% of AD, usually early onset (<65 years)
- Familial inheritance AD (nonautosomal dominant): 15–25% of AD

RISK FACTORS
- Nonmodifiable risk factors: (1),(2),(3)
  - Age, gender (due to longer lifespan in women)
  - Family history, genetic mutations
  - APOE-e4 gene variant: e4 heterozygous 2- to 3-fold risk; e4 homozygous 8-fold risk
  - Racial and ethnic differences in AD exist.
- Cardiovascular disease–related risk factors:
  - Hypertension (HTN) (especially in midlife years); hyperlipidemia
  - Obesity, diabetes, and impaired glucose processing
  - Tobacco use, unhealthy diet, lack of physical activity
  - Cerebrovascular (stroke) risks and injury
- Other potentially modifiable risk factors:
  - Less years of formal education (<8th grade)
  - Lack of continuous brain activity—learning
  - Traumatic brain injuries: repetitive mild and moderate/severe
  - Lack of social engagement
  - Late-life depression
  - Poor quality and inadequate sleep
  - Hearing and vision deficits
  - High alcohol consumption
  - Possible environmental factors (e.g., pollution)

GENERAL PREVENTION
- Cognitive decline and impairment are top concerns of people ≥50 years.
- HTN management, increased physical activity, and cognitive training may delay/prevent cognitive decline, MCI, and AD (3)[B].
- NSAIDs, estrogen, and vitamin E do not delay AD onset; insufficient evidence for statins and proton pump inhibitors (3)[B].
- Healthy lifestyles may prevent or delay AD (3)[B].
- Treat psychiatric conditions and avert delirium during hospitalizations.

COMMONLY ASSOCIATED CONDITIONS
- Down syndrome
- Depression

DIAGNOSIS

- "Welcome to Medicare" preventive visit and Medicare Annual Wellness Visit both require assessment of cognitive function.
- Diagnosis of dementia requires exclusion of delirium. Delineating specific dementia type requires a thorough H&P, cognitive, and other diagnostic tests.
  - 2000 *DSM-IV-TR* criteria: progressive impairment in ≥2 areas of memory, executive function, attention, language, or visuospatial skills and significant interference in ability to function in work, home, or social interactions
  - 2013 *DSM-5* uses term "neurocognitive disorder" instead of dementia; impairment in one or more cognitive areas sufficient to disrupt independent living: complex attention, executive function, learning and memory, language, perceptual motor, social cognition

HISTORY
- Include informant: family member, caregiver, or friend.
- Alzheimer's Association 10 signs (1):
  - Memory loss that disrupts daily life
  - Difficulty completing familiar tasks
  - Challenges in planning and problem solving
  - New problems with words in speaking or writing
  - Trouble with visual images or spatial relationships
  - Changes in mood or personality
  - Misplacing things, losing ability to retrace steps
  - Decreased or poor judgment
  - Withdrawal from work or social activities
  - Confusion with time and place

PHYSICAL EXAM
- Exam to rule out other causes of dementia or delirium
- Noncognitive portions of physical exam often normal for age except in late stage AD (2),(3)
- Neuro: speech, language, vision, hearing, gait, balance, reflexes, muscle strength and tone, tremor, abnormal movements (akathisia, bradykinesia/dyskinesia)
- Late stage: skin lesions, nutrition-hydration status
- Brief cognitive testing, such as: Mini-Cog, Montreal Cognitive Assessment (MoCA), Mini-Mental State Examination (MMSE, under copyright, fee for use)
- Assess depression: Patient Health Questionnaire-9, Geriatric Depression Scale (GDS).
- Functional assessment: instrumental activities of daily living (IADLs), Functional Activities Questionnaire (FAQ)

DIFFERENTIAL DIAGNOSIS
- Other dementias (most common):
  - Vascular (large and microvessel, mixed); mixed type (with AD)
  - Frontotemporal lobar degeneration; dementia with Lewy bodies
  - Parkinson; normal pressure hydrocephalus
  - Creutzfeldt-Jakob; Huntington; Wernicke-Korsakoff
- Metabolic: hyper-/hypothyroid, vitamin-nutrient deficiency, uremia/renal, hepatic, hyponatremia
- Autoimmune: vasculitis, end-stage multiple sclerosis
- Infectious: HIV, syphilis, Lyme disease, varicella-zoster virus, prion
- Depression; brain tumor: primary or metastatic; subdural hematoma (usually acute presentation)
- Medications, drug-alcohol reactions/addiction

DIAGNOSTIC TESTS & INTERPRETATION
Neuropsychological testing for atypical symptoms, young age, unclear presentation, or need to determine independent decision making

Initial Tests (lab, imaging)
- To help rule out other causes of dementia (2)
  - Complete blood count with differential; homocysteine level
  - Chemistry panel; thyroid function, syphilis testing, lipid panel, vitamin B$_{12}$
  - Special considerations: ESR, HIV, folate, C-reactive protein, HbA1c

- Imaging (biomarkers): Different professional standards exist; may help determine cause of dementia
  – Consider MRI (preferred) or computed tomography (CT) scan if MRI contraindicated.
    ○ Initial AD evaluation; recent or rapid decline, age <65 years, history of stroke, atypical presentation, concern for cancer, high bleeding risk
  – Single-photon emission CT (SPECT) and positron emission tomography (PET): rarely indicated; *insufficient evidence to use alone*

Follow-Up Tests & Special Considerations
- Consider genetic testing with concern for autosomal dominant and familial AD.
- Cerebrospinal fluid biomarker testing not currently indicated

 ## TREATMENT

GENERAL MEASURES
- Optimize treatment of risk factors and associated comorbid conditions (e.g., hearing).
- Advanced care planning before individual loses ability for independent decisions
- Assess caregiver support and burnout.

ALERT
American Geriatrics Society recommends "Don't prescribe cholinesterase inhibitors (ChEIs) for dementia without periodic assessment for perceived cognitive benefits and adverse gastrointestinal effects" in its Choosing Wisely statement.

MEDICATION
First Line
- Acetylcholinesterase inhibitors (ChEIs) (2)[A]
  – Best in mild to moderate disease; *may* be effective in Lewy body dementia
  – ChEIs equally effective; GI and other side effects, such as bradycardia/syncope
  – When used for at least 6 months, may provide mild benefit in cognition and behavior
  – Try different ChEI if no benefit.
  – Donepezil (Aricept): Start at 5 mg/day PO; may increase to 10 mg/day after 1 month, may increase to 23 mg/day after 3 months if needed
  – Orally disintegrating tablets; generic available
  – Caution with digoxin or β-blockers (Donepezil may prolong PR interval.)
  – Rivastigmine (Exelon): Start at 1.5 mg PO BID, increase by 1.5 mg BID every 2 weeks; maintenance 6 to 12 mg/day total
  – Capsule, solution, or patch (reduced side effects)
  – Galantamine (Razadyne): Start at 4 mg BID for 4 weeks, increase by 4 mg BID every month: goal of 16 to 24 mg/day dose
  – Tablets, solution, extended-release (ER) capsule, and transdermal formulations
- Vitamin E—2,000 IU/day, mixed results, side effects exist (2)[B]

- Memantine, a *N*-methyl-ᴅ-aspartate (NMDA) receptor antagonist for moderate to severe AD
  – Monotherapy or in combination with acetylcholinesterase inhibitors (2)[A]
  – Memantine immediate release: 5 mg/day; titrate up to 10 mg BID, adding 5 mg/day qwk PRN
  – Memantine ER: 7 mg/day up to 28 mg/day, adding 7 mg/day qwk PRN
- Aducanumab (Aduhelm): monoclonal antibody therapy targeting β-amyloid. Limited benefit with side-effect concerns. Recommend against routine use; aducanumab evaluation by physicians who specialize in AD (4)[C]
- Neuropsychiatric symptoms: assessment for delirium and reversible causes (sleep hygiene, hearing, environment changes); for moderate to severe symptoms, consider second-line care.

Second Line
- For moderate to severe depression: selective serotonin reuptake inhibitors (SSRIs) preferred
- Insomnia: Medications have little efficacy for sleep in AD (2)[A],(3)[A].
  – Avoid antihistamines in elderly.
  – Caution and use lowest dose possible: risperidone, trazodone, sleep aid (e.g., zolpidem)
- Moderate agitation, anxiety/restlessness: may consider low-dose risperidone or SSRIs (citalopram) (2)[B].
- Cautious use of low-dose risperidone for severe psychosis
- Precautions
  – Avoid anticholinergic drugs when possible.
  – Benzodiazepines may produce paradoxical excitation or daytime drowsiness.
  – Triazolam (Halcion) can produce confusion, memory loss, and psychotic behavior.
  – Donepezil: caution with anticholinergics, sick sinus syndrome, and history of peptic ulcers

ISSUES FOR REFERRAL
Consider geriatric psychiatry referral for AD patients with behavioral symptoms requiring psychotropic medications.

ADDITIONAL THERAPIES
- Exercise to reduce restlessness; cognitive stimulation therapy
- Consider occupational, music, aroma, and pet therapy.

 ## ONGOING CARE

FOLLOW-UP RECOMMENDATIONS
Patient Monitoring
- Medication reconciliation each visit, including OTCs
- Recommend healthy lifestyle: exercise, nutrition, sleep, being socially and cognitive activity stimulation.
- Inform about unproven products advertised to improve brain health: some medications, nutritional supplements, and brain games.
- Frequently assess medication side effects and effectiveness (ChEIs/memantine).
- Late AD may require skilled care placement.

- Advanced care planning is Medicare reimbursable.
- National Highway Traffic Safety Administration's safe driving assessment: https://www.nhtsa.gov/older -drivers/driving-safely-while-aging-gracefully

PATIENT EDUCATION
- Alzheimer's Association: https://www.alz.org/
- Early advanced care planning, such as advanced directives, financial planning, caregiver support

PROGNOSIS
Average survival from diagnosis is 4 to 8 years, and initial diagnosis is often delayed.

COMPLICATIONS
- Hostility, agitation, wandering, falls, "sundowning," depression, suicide
- Infections, inadequate nutrition/hydration, drug toxicity

REFERENCES
1. Alzheimer's Association. 2021 Alzheimer's disease facts and figures. *Alzheimers Dement*. 2021;17(3):327–406.
2. Atri A. The Alzheimer's disease clinical spectrum: diagnosis and management. *Med Clin North Am*. 2019;103(2):263–293.
3. Livingston G, Huntley J, Sommerlad A, et al. Dementia prevention, intervention, and care: 2020 report of the Lancet Commission. *Lancet*. 2020;396(10248):413–446.
4. Cummings J, Aisen P, Apostolova LG, et al. Aducanumab: appropriate use recommendations. *J Prev Alzheimers Dis*. 2021;8(4):398–410.

ADDITIONAL READING
The Gerontological Society of America. *The GSA KAER Toolkit for Primary Care Teams*. Washington, DC: The Gerontological Society of America; 2020. https://www.geron.org/images/gsa/Marketing/KAER /GSA_KAER-Toolkit_2020_Final.pdf.

 ## SEE ALSO

Delirium; Depression; Hypothyroidism, Adult; Substance Use Disorders

CODES

ICD10
- G30 Alzheimer's disease
- G30.1 Alzheimer's disease with late onset
- G30.9 Alzheimer's disease, unspecified

CLINICAL PEARLS
- AD is very common, >32% in those >85 years, and greatly underdiagnosed.
- Imaging not needed for diagnosis for typical AD
- Early diagnosis allows advance care planning (e.g., advanced directives) and caregiver support.
- Atypical antipsychotic medications increase mortality.

AMENORRHEA

Rachel Ceccarelli, DO, MPH • Jeremy Golding, MD, FAAFP

 BASICS

DESCRIPTION
- Primary amenorrhea
  - No menses by age 13 years with absence of secondary sexual characteristics OR
  - No menses by age 15 years with normal secondary characteristics
- Secondary amenorrhea: cessation of menses for 3 months if previously normal menstrual cycles or 6 months if a history of irregular cycles
- System(s) affected: endocrine/metabolic; reproductive

Pregnancy Considerations
Pregnancy is by far the most common cause of secondary amenorrhea.

EPIDEMIOLOGY
Prevalence
- Primary amenorrhea: <1% of female population
- Secondary amenorrhea: 3–4% of female population
- No evidence for race and ethnicity affecting prevalence

ETIOLOGY AND PATHOPHYSIOLOGY
Absence of menses that can be temporary, intermittent, or permanent due to dysfunction of the hypothalamus, pituitary, uterus, ovaries, or vagina
- Primary amenorrhea
  - Gonadal dysgenesis (e.g., Turner syndrome [45,X]) or failure (e.g., autoimmune, idiopathic)
  - Anatomic abnormalities (e.g., müllerian agenesis, imperforate hymen, transverse vaginal septum)
  - Hypothalamic-pituitary abnormalities
    - Functional hypothalamic amenorrhea (reduced GnRH secretion, e.g., weight loss/anorexia nervosa)
    - Physiologic delay of puberty
    - Central lesions (tumors, hypophysitis, granulomas)
    - Pituitary dysfunction (hyperprolactinemia, abnormal follicle-stimulating hormone [FSH], luteinizing hormone [LH], or GnRH)
    - Thyroid dysfunction
  - Polycystic ovarian syndrome (PCOS)
  - Androgen insensitivity syndrome
- Secondary amenorrhea
  - Pregnancy
  - Hypothalamic dysfunction (reduced GnRH secretion)
    - Functional hypothalamic amenorrhea (stress, anorexia nervosa, and/or excessive exercise)
    - Hypothalamic tumors
    - Severe systemic illness (e.g., diabetes mellitus type 1 or celiac disease)
  - Pituitary disease (e.g., hyperprolactinemia, Sheehan syndrome, Cushing syndrome)
  - Thyroid disease
  - PCOS
  - Ovarian disorders (e.g., primary ovarian insufficiency [due to chemotherapy, radiation, fragile X syndrome] or ovarian tumors)
  - Anatomic abnormalities (e.g., intrauterine adhesions [Asherman syndrome], obstructive fibroids, polyps, iatrogenic cervical stenosis)
- Pathophysiology varies, depending on etiology.

Genetics
May occur with Turner syndrome or testicular feminization

RISK FACTORS
- Obesity
- Excessive exercise (commonly associated "female athlete triad")
- Eating disorders
- Malnutrition
- Stress (emotional or illness-induced [e.g., myocardial infarct, severe burns])
- Family history of amenorrhea or early menopause
- Treatment with antipsychotic medications

GENERAL PREVENTION
Maintenance of proper body mass index (BMI) and healthy lifestyle with respect to food and exercise

COMMONLY ASSOCIATED CONDITIONS
- Primary ovarian insufficiency may be associated with autoimmune abnormalities (autoimmune thyroiditis, type 1 diabetes).
- PCOS is associated with insulin resistance and obesity.
- Decreased exposure to estrogen may increase risk for osteopenia or osteoporosis.

 DIAGNOSIS

HISTORY
- Review of systems, including weight change, symptoms of pregnancy or menopause, virilizing changes, cyclic pelvic pain, galactorrhea, headaches, vision changes, fatigue, palpitations, polyuria/polydipsia
- Growth and pubertal development history, including age of breast development, pubertal growth spurt, and adrenarche (early sexual maturation)
- History of chronic illness, trauma, surgery, medications (including contraceptives), prior chemotherapy or radiation
- Obstetric history
- Psychiatric history
- Social history, including diet and exercise history, drug abuse, sexual history, and stress
- Family history of delayed or absent puberty

PHYSICAL EXAM
- General appearance
- Vital signs, height, weight, growth percentile and BMI, hypotension, bradycardia, hypothermia (anorexia nervosa)
- HEENT exam: evidence of dental erosions, trauma to palate (bulimia), visual field defect, funduscopic changes, cranial nerve findings (prolactinoma), webbed neck (Turner syndrome), thyromegaly
- Skin exam: evidence of androgen excess (acne, hirsutism), acanthosis nigricans (PCOS), fine downy hair on body (anorexia nervosa), striae, vitiligo, easy bruisability
- Breast: state of development, evidence of galactorrhea (prolactinoma), shield chest (Turner syndrome)
- Pelvic exam: presence or absence of pubic hair (if sparse: androgen insensitivity or deficiency); clitoromegaly (androgen excess); distention or bulging of external vagina (imperforate hymen); thin, pale

vaginal mucosa without rugae (estrogen deficiency and ovarian failure); presence of cervical mucus (evidence for estrogen production); blind vaginal pouch (müllerian agenesis, androgen insensitivity syndrome); ovarian enlargement (tumors, PCOS, autoimmune oophoritis)

DIAGNOSTIC TESTS & INTERPRETATION
Initial Tests (lab, imaging)
- Primary amenorrhea
  - Serum human chorionic gonadotropin (hCG), prolactin (PRL), thyroid-stimulating hormone (TSH), and FSH
  - If no or minor breast development:
    - Low FSH suggests primary hypothalamic-pituitary etiology or constitutional delay of puberty.
    - High FSH suggests gonadal failure, and karyotype analysis should be performed.
  - If normal breast development:
    - If low FSH, evaluate for anatomic abnormalities. If uterus is absent or abnormal, perform karyotype analysis, testosterone level, and dehydroepiandrosterone sulfate (DHEA-S).
- Secondary amenorrhea
  - Serum hCG, PRL, TSH, and FSH
    - PRL >100 ng/mL: suggests empty sella syndrome or pituitary adenoma; however, levels can transiently increase with stress. Repeat level and if elevated, perform MRI for evaluation.
    - PRL elevated but <100 ng/mL: Evaluate for other etiologies, of which medications are most common.
    - If FSH high: Consider primary ovarian insufficiency or natural menopause.
  - To determine endogenous estrogen production, perform a progestin challenge (see "Treatment"): if withdrawal bleed, likely chronic anovulation (most commonly PCOS). If no withdrawal bleed, perform estrogen and progestin challenge (see "Treatment"):
    - If no bleed: Consider outflow tract obstruction or hypoestrogenism.
    - If bleed occurs: Check FSH/LH: elevated in premature ovarian failure; decreased in pituitary tumors, eating disorders, chronic illness.
- If there is evidence for hyperandrogenism, measure total testosterone, DHEA-S, and 17-OH progesterone levels. Initiate evaluation for androgen-secreting tumor if testosterone >200 ng/dL.
- Imaging is not generally indicated as a first approach.
- US may show ovarian cysts (PCOS), presence or absence of uterus, and endometrial thickness (consider MRI if unable to tolerate US probe).

Follow-Up Tests & Special Considerations
- Women <30 years with ovarian failure (see below) should have karyotype analysis and be investigated for premutations of *FMR1* gene (fragile X syndrome) and for adrenal antibodies.
- If absence of uterus or foreshortened vagina, karyotype analysis should also be performed.
- Laparoscopy: diagnosis of streak ovaries (Turner syndrome) or polycystic ovaries
- Hysterosalpingogram: Rule out Asherman syndrome and other etiologies of outflow obstruction.

Diagnostic Procedures/Other
- If constitutional delay is suspected, obtain bone age.
- If hypothalamic amenorrhea from functional suppression is suspected, consider dual energy x-ray absorptiometry (DEXA) scan to assess bone loss (1).

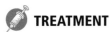

TREATMENT

GENERAL MEASURES
Identify and correct underlying pathology if possible.

MEDICATION
- Progesterone challenge and replacement: medroxyprogesterone (Provera): 10 mg/day for 10 days will result in withdrawal bleed within 7 days of last dose if hypothalamic-pituitary-gonadal axis is intact (i.e., amenorrhea is a consequence of anovulation and lack of progesterone), although experts disagree (2).
- Estrogen replacement: Cycling with a combination oral contraceptive (containing 35 or 50 μg of estrogen) or conjugated estrogen (Premarin) 0.625 mg for 25 days with progesterone added as above for the last 10 days will result in a withdrawal bleed if the uterus and lower genital tract are normal (hypothalamic-pituitary axis pathologic).
- Use of hormonal therapies will not correct the underlying problem. Other drugs might be required to treat specific conditions (e.g., bromocriptine for hyperprolactinemia).
- Use of hormonal replacement therapy is not recommended for long-term management of amenorrhea in older women.
  - May be safe for symptom management in young women
  - Give to maintain secondary sex characteristics and to prevent osteoporosis in adolescents and young women (3)[A].
- Combination estrogen/progesterone contraceptives (oral contraceptive pills [OCPs], patch, ring) replace estrogen and prevent pregnancy.
  - Have a positive effect on bone mineral density in oligo-/amenorrheic women but not in functional hypothalamic amenorrhea (4)[A]
  - Can decrease hirsutism in PCOS
- Calcium supplementation: 1,500 mg/day if cause is hypoestrogenism
- Because PCOS is related to insulin resistance, metformin (Glucophage) has been used (start at 500 mg BID) to correct metabolic abnormalities, improve ovulation, and restore normal menstrual patterns. Of note, treatment with metformin has shown an increase in clinical pregnancy rates but not in live birth rates (5)[A].
- Functional hypothalamic amenorrhea appears to improve with administration of exogenous leptin (still under investigation) (6)[C].
- Contraindications to estrogen administration
  - Pregnancy, thromboembolic disease, previous myocardial infarction or cerebrovascular accident, estrogen-dependent malignancy, severe hepatic impairment or disease

- Precautions
  - Patients with amenorrhea who desire pregnancy should not be given hormone replacement therapy but should receive treatment for infertility based on the specific cause.

ISSUES FOR REFERRAL
Many causes of amenorrhea require referral to specialists in ob/gyn, endocrine, surgery, and/or psychiatry.

SURGERY/OTHER PROCEDURES
- Hymenectomy for primary amenorrhea if due to imperforate hymen
- Lysis of adhesions in Asherman syndrome is often effective in restoring regular menses and fertility.
- If karyotype is XY, gonads must be removed due to increased risk of tumors.
- Patients with congenital short vagina can undergo surgery to create a functioning vagina.
- Treatment of prolactinomas may include surgical resection.

 ONGOING CARE

FOLLOW-UP RECOMMENDATIONS
If excessive exercise is suspected, activity level should be reduced by 25–50%.

Patient Monitoring
- Depends on the cause and treatment chosen
- If hormonal replacement is used, discontinue after 6 months to assess spontaneous resumption of menses.

DIET
- Correct overweight or underweight by dietary management and behavior modification.
- If PCOS is the etiology, a weight-loss diet will help restore ovulation.

PATIENT EDUCATION
- Educate on the circumstances and complications of her condition and its underlying etiology.
- Specific educational resources are helpful (e.g., prenatal classes and menopause support groups).
- Discuss the expected duration of amenorrhea (temporary or permanent), effect on fertility, and the long-term sequelae of untreated amenorrhea (e.g., osteoporosis, vaginal dryness).
- Appropriate contraceptive advice should be given because fertility returns before menses.
- Additional support may be needed if the amenorrhea is associated with a reduction in, or loss of, fertility.

PROGNOSIS
Reflects the underlying cause. In functional hypothalamic amenorrhea, one study demonstrated 83% reversal rate in presence of obvious contributing factor.

COMPLICATIONS
- Estrogen-deficiency symptoms (e.g., hot flashes, vaginal dryness) and osteoporosis in prolonged hypoestrogenic amenorrhea
- Increased risk of endometrial cancer in patients whose amenorrhea is secondary to anovulation with estrogen excess (obesity, PCOS)
- Premature ovarian failure may increase cardiovascular risk.

REFERENCES
1. Gordon CM. Clinical practice. Functional hypothalamic amenorrhea. *N Engl J Med.* 2010;363(4):365–371.
2. Klein DA, Poth MA. Amenorrhea: an approach to diagnosis and management. *Am Fam Physician.* 2013;87(11):781–788.
3. Marjoribanks J, Farquhar C, Roberts H, et al. Long term hormone therapy for perimenopausal and postmenopausal women. *Cochrane Database Syst Rev.* 2012;(7):CD004143.
4. Liu SL, Lebrun CM. Effect of oral contraceptives and hormone replacement therapy on bone mineral density in premenopausal and perimenopausal women: a systematic review. *Br J Sports Med.* 2006;40(1):11–24.
5. Tang T, Lord JM, Norman RJ, et al. Insulin-sensitising drugs (metformin, rosiglitazone, pioglitazone, D-chiro-inositol) for women with polycystic ovary syndrome, oligo amenorrhoea and subfertility. *Cochrane Database Syst Rev.* 2012;(5):CD003053.
6. Chou SH, Chamberland JP, Liu X, et al. Leptin is an effective treatment for hypothalamic amenorrhea. *Proc Natl Acad Sci U S A.* 2011;108(16):6585–6590.

ADDITIONAL READING
- Practice Committee of American Society for Reproductive Medicine. Current evaluation of amenorrhea. *Fertil Steril.* 2008;90(Suppl 5):S219–S225.
- Santoro N. Update in hyper- and hypogonadotropic amenorrhea. *J Clin Endocrinol Metab.* 2011;96(11):3281–3288.

 SEE ALSO

- Hyperthyroidism; Hypothyroidism, Adult; Osteoporosis and Osteopenia
- Algorithms: Amenorrhea, Primary (Absence of Menarche by Age 16 Years); Amenorrhea, Secondary; Delayed Puberty

 CODES

ICD10
- N91.1 Secondary amenorrhea
- N91.2 Amenorrhea, unspecified
- N91.0 Primary amenorrhea

CLINICAL PEARLS
- First evaluate whether amenorrhea is primary or secondary and exclude pregnancy. TSH and PRL are usual first blood tests.
- Progestin challenge may cause withdrawal bleed in women with intact hypothalamic-pituitary-gonadal axis.

ANAL FISSURE

Anne Walsh, MMSc, PA-C, DFAAPA • Jennifer Grumet, MD • Lisa Hertz, MD

BASICS

DESCRIPTION
Anal fissure (fissure in ano): longitudinal tear in the lining of the anal canal distal to the dentate line, most commonly at the posterior midline; characterized by a knifelike tearing sensation on defecation, often associated with bright red blood per rectum. This common benign anorectal condition is often confused with hemorrhoids; may be acute or chronic (>4 to 8 weeks in duration and may be associated with the presence of hypertrophic papilla and sentinel pile (skin tag).

EPIDEMIOLOGY
- Affects all ages. Common in infants 6 to 24 months; not common in older children, suspect abuse, or trauma; elderly less common due to lower resting pressure in the anal canal
- Sex: male = female; women more likely to get anterior midline fissures (25%) versus men (8%)

Incidence
Exact incidence is unknown (1). Patients often treat with home remedies and do not seek medical care.

Prevalence
- 80% of infants, usually self-limited
- 10–20% of adults, most of whom do not seek medical advice

ALERT
Secondary fissures:

- Lateral fissure: Rule out infectious disease.
- Atypical fissure: Rule out Crohn disease.

ETIOLOGY AND PATHOPHYSIOLOGY
High-resting pressure within the anal canal (usually as a result of constipation/straining) coupled with decreased perfusion of the posterior canal leads to ischemia of the anoderm, resulting in splitting of the anal mucosa during defecation and spasm of the exposed internal sphincter.

Genetics
None known

RISK FACTORS
- Constipation (25% of patients)
- Diarrhea (6% of patients)
- Passage of hard or large-caliber stool
- Low fiber diet
- High-resting pressure of internal anal sphincter (prolonged sitting, obesity)
- Trauma (sexual activity or abuse, foreign body, childbirth, mountain biking)
- Prior anal surgery with scarring/stenosis
- Inflammatory bowel disease (Crohn disease)
- Infection (chlamydia, syphilis, herpes, tuberculosis)

GENERAL PREVENTION
All measures to prevent constipation; avoid straining and prolonged sitting on toilet.

COMMONLY ASSOCIATED CONDITIONS
Posterior midline location: constipation, irritable bowel syndrome; other/multiple locations: Crohn disease, tuberculosis, leukemia, and HIV

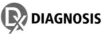

DIAGNOSIS

HISTORY
- Severe, sharp rectal pain, often with and following defecation but can be continuous; bright red blood on the stool or when wiping
- Occasionally, anal pruritus or perianal irritation

PHYSICAL EXAM
- Gentle spreading of the buttocks with close inspection of the anal verge will reveal a tender, smooth-edged tear in the anodermal tissue, typically posterior midline, occasionally anterior midline, rarely eccentric to midline. Digital rectal exam and anoscopy are painful and can be deferred if inspection confirms the diagnosis.
- Minimal edema, erythema, or bleeding may be seen.
- Chronic fissures may demonstrate rolled edges, exposed muscle fibers, hypertrophic papillae at proximal end, and a sentinel pile (tag) at distal end.

DIFFERENTIAL DIAGNOSIS
- Thrombosed external hemorrhoid: swollen, painful mass at anal verge
- Perirectal abscess: tender, warm erythematous induration or fluctuance
- Perianal fistula: abnormal communication between rectum and perianal epithelium with feculent or purulent drainage
- Pruritus ani: shallow excoriations and erythema rather than true fissure

DIAGNOSTIC TESTS & INTERPRETATION
Diagnostic Procedures/Other
- Avoid anoscopy/sigmoidoscopy initially unless necessary for other diagnoses or chronic fissures.
- Due to pain, some patients may require exam under anesthesia in order to confirm the diagnosis.

TREATMENT

The goal of treatment is to avoid repeated tearing of the anal mucosa with resultant spasm of the internal anal sphincter by decreasing the patient's high sphincter tone and addressing its underlying cause.

GENERAL MEASURES
- Wash area gently with warm water; consume high-fiber diet; increase fluids; add daily fiber supplement; avoid constipation; maintain healthy weight.
- Medical therapy for chronic fissures usually initiated in a stepwise manner when needed: topical nitrates, topical calcium channel blockers, botulinum toxin injections

MEDICATION
First Line
Acute fissures—50% will heal spontaneously with supportive measures (1)[B].
- Stool softeners (docusate) orally daily
- Osmotic laxatives (polyethylene glycol) orally daily as needed
- Fiber supplements (psyllium, methylcellulose, inulin) orally daily and increase fluid intake
- Topical analgesics (2% lidocaine gel or 3% cream) 2 to 3 times daily for pain control
- Topical lubricants/emollients (Balneol lotion, glycerin ointment, petroleum jelly) for comfort with defecation
- Topical hydrocortisone 1% cream short-term for inflammation/pruritus
- Sitz baths (plain, warm-hot water soak of perineum for 10 to 20 minutes) 2 to 3 times daily after bowel movements

Second Line
Chronic fissures—will not heal without treatment, due to persistent internal sphincter spasm and ischemia (2):
- Chemical sphincterotomy—first-line treatment
  - Topical nitroglycerin 0.2–0.4% ointment applied BID; nitroglycerin 0.4% ointment available commercially (Rectiv) marginally but significantly better than placebo in healing (48.6% vs. 37%); late recurrence common (50%) (2); reduces resting anal pressure through the release of nitric oxide and vasodilation. Headache, hypotension, dizziness are major side effects (20–30%).
  - Topical calcium channel blockers (nifedipine 0.2–0.3% gel, diltiazem 2% ointment), applied 2 to 4 times per day, relax the internal sphincter muscle, thereby reducing the resting anal pressure; no better than nitrates for healing but fewer side effects (1)[C]. Oral calcium channel blockers confer lower healing rates, more side effects, and equal rates of recurrence (3)[A].
  - Botulinum toxin (Botox) 4 mL (20 units) injected into the internal sphincter muscle: no better than topical nitrates for healing but fewer side effects; inhibits the release of acetylcholine from nerve endings to inhibit muscle spasm (4)[C]
  - Minoxidil 5% gel topically achieved better and more rapid healing of chronic fissures compared to topical glyceryl trinitrate in one small randomized controlled trial (5).

ISSUES FOR REFERRAL
- Persistent symptoms despite medical therapy, usually tried for 90 to 120 days prior to colorectal surgery referral. Select patients with chronic fissure may be referred directly for surgical therapy due to proven superior healing rates (1)[C].
- Late recurrence, which is common (50%) particularly if the underlying issue remains untreated (constipation, irritable bowel)
- Secondary fissures (suspected infectious or inflammatory bowel disease)

ADDITIONAL THERAPIES

Anococcygeal support (modified toilet seat) may offer some advantage in chronic fissures to avoid surgery.

SURGERY/OTHER PROCEDURES

- Surgery typically reserved for failure of medical therapy
- Lateral internal sphincterectomy (LIS) involves division of the internal sphincter muscle and is the surgical procedure of choice (95% healing) (1)[C].
  - Risk for fecal or flatus incontinence: up to 47% short term, up to 15% long term (6)
  - Open and closed techniques have similar results and are equally acceptable (1)[C].
  - May be repeated for recurrent fissures with similar outcomes (1)[C]
  - Not typically performed on women of childbearing potential due to increased risk of fecal incontinence with or without subsequent obstetrical injury (1)
- Anocutaneous flap safe alternative to LIS in patients without anal hypertonia with less incontinence but lower healing rates (1)[B]
- Botulinum toxin injections also first-line treatment; less effective (60–80% healing) than surgery but fewer complications (4)[C]
  - Risk for fecal or flatus incontinence: 18% short term, no long term
  - May be repeated as needed with same efficacy; lower doses as effective as higher doses with lower rates of complications including incontinence and recurrence (7)[A]
  - Higher doses combined with fissurectomy may be as effective as surgical sphincterotomy (8)[C].
- Controlled pneumatic balloon dilation may be used by gastroenterologists if surgical referral not available; should not be used first line as benefits are not well documented. Uncontrolled manual dilation is no longer recommended.

COMPLEMENTARY & ALTERNATIVE MEDICINE

Alternative therapies (hibiscus and other herbal extracts, clove and coconut oil, essential oils, homeopathic and ayurvedic medications, anal self-massage) need further study before they can be recommended as first-line treatment.

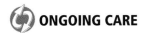 ONGOING CARE

DIET

High fiber (>25 g/day; augment with daily fiber supplements); increase fluid intake, decrease caffeine.

PATIENT EDUCATION

- Avoid prolonged sitting or straining during bowel movements; drink plenty of fluids; avoid constipation; lose weight if obese.
- Avoid use of triple antibiotic ointment and long-term use of steroid creams to anal area.
- Use a finger cot or glove when applying nitroglycerin ointment and apply first dose before bedtime to minimize side effects.
- Topical medications should be applied directly to anal verge; no need to insert rectally.

PROGNOSIS

Most acute fissures heal within 6 weeks with conservative therapy. Medical therapy is less likely to be successful for chronic anal fissures (40% failure rate) but should remain first-line treatment.

COMPLICATIONS

- Chronic fissure is a complication of nonhealing acute fissure.
- Recurrence is a common complication especially when underlying cause is not addressed.
- Abscess and fistula formation are less common complications.
- Fecal and flatus incontinence are primarily associated with surgery (5–47% postop), which may become permanent (up to 8% long term, primarily to flatus).

REFERENCES

1. Stewart DB Sr, Gaertner W, Glasgow S, et al. Clinical practice guideline for the management of anal fissures. *Dis Colon Rectum*. 2017;60(1):7–14.
2. Altomare DF, Binda GA, Canuti S, et al. The management of patients with primary chronic anal fissure: a position paper. *Tech Coloproctol*. 2011;15(2):135–141.
3. Sahebally SM, Ahmed K, Cerneveciute R, et al. Oral versus topical calcium channel blockers for chronic anal fissure—a systematic review and meta-analysis of randomized controlled trials. *Int J Surg*. 2017;44:87–93.
4. Wald A, Bharucha AE, Cosman BC, et al. ACG clinical guideline: management of benign anorectal disorders. *Am J Gastroenterol*. 2014;109(8):1141–1157.
5. Emile SH, Abdel-Razik MA, Elshobaky A, et al. Topical 5% minoxidil versus topical 0.2% glyceryl trinitrate in treatment of chronic anal fissure: a randomized clinical trial. *Int J Surgery*. 2020;75:152–158.
6. Acar T, Acar N, Güngör F, et al. Comparative efficacy of medical treatment versus surgical sphincterotomy in the treatment of chronic anal fissure. *Nig J Clin Prac*. 2020;23(4):539–544.
7. Lin JX, Krishna S, Su'a B, et al. Optimal dosing of botulinum toxin for treatment of chronic anal fissure: a systematic review and meta-analysis. *Dis Colon Rectum*. 2016;59(9):886–894.
8. Barnes TG, Zafrani Z, Abdelrazeq AS. Fissurectomy combined with high-dose botulinum toxin is a safe and effective treatment for chronic anal fissure and a promising alternative to surgical sphincterotomy. *Dis Colon Rectum*. 2015;58(10):967–973.

ADDITIONAL READING

- Fargo MV, Latimer KM. Evaluation and management of common anorectal conditions. *Am Fam Physician*. 2012;85(6):624–630.
- Gee T, Hisham RB, Jabar MF, et al. Ano-coccygeal support in the treatment of idiopathic chronic posterior anal fissure: a prospective non-randomised controlled pilot trial. *Tech Coloproctol*. 2013;17(2):181–186.
- Sinha R, Kaiser AM. Efficacy of management algorithm for reducing need for sphincterotomy in chronic anal fissures. *Colorectal Dis*. 2012;14(6):760–764.
- Sobrado Júnior CW, Hora JAB, Sobrado LF, et al. Anoplasty with skin tag flap for the treatment of chronic anal fissure. *Rev Col Bras Cir*. 2019;46(3):e20192181.
- Sugerman DT. JAMA patient page. Anal fissure. *JAMA*. 2014;311(11):1171.
- Yiannakopoulou E. Botulinum toxin and anal fissure: efficacy and safety systematic review. *Int J Colorectal Dis*. 2012;27(1):1–9.

 CODES

ICD10

- K60.2 Anal fissure, unspecified
- K60.0 Acute anal fissure
- K60.1 Chronic anal fissure

CLINICAL PEARLS

- Avoid anoscopy or sigmoidoscopy initially unless necessary for other diagnoses.
- Best chance to prevent recurrence is to treat the underlying cause (e.g., chronic constipation).
- No medical therapy approaches the cure rate of surgery for chronic fissure.

ANEMIA, APLASTIC

Muthalagu Ramanathan, MD

BASICS

DESCRIPTION

- Pancytopenia due to hypocellular bone marrow without the presence of infiltrates or fibrosis; classified as acquired (much more common) and congenital
- Acquired aplastic anemia: insidious onset; due to exogenous insult triggering an autoimmune reaction; often responsive to immunosuppression
- Congenital forms: rare, mostly present in childhood (exception is atypical presentation of Fanconi syndrome in adults; 30s for males and 40s for females)
- The occurrence of specific mutations in genes of the telomere complex in acquired aplastic anemia has blurred the distinction between the congenital and acquired forms.
- System(s) affected: heme/lymphatic/immunologic
- Synonym(s): hypoplastic anemia; panmyelophthisis; refractory anemia; aleukia hemorrhagica; toxic paralytic anemia

ALERT
- Early intervention for aplastic anemia greatly improves the chances of treatment success.
- Hematopoietic growth factors require close monitoring in newly diagnosed patients.

Geriatric Considerations
The elderly are often exposed to large numbers of drugs and therefore may be more susceptible to acquired aplastic anemia.

Pediatric Considerations
- Congenital forms of aplastic anemia require different treatment regimens than acquired forms.
- Acquired aplastic anemia is seen in children exposed to ionizing radiation or treated with cytotoxic chemotherapeutic agents.

Pregnancy Considerations
- Pregnancy is a real but rare cause of aplastic anemia. Symptoms may resolve after delivery and with termination.
- Complications in pregnancy can occur from low platelet counts and paroxysmal nocturnal hemoglobinuria–associated aplastic anemia.

EPIDEMIOLOGY
- Predominant age: biphasic 15 to 25 years (more common) and >60 years
- Predominant sex: male = female

Incidence
- 2 to 3 new cases per million per year in Europe and North America
- The incidence is 3-fold higher in Thailand and China versus the Western world.

ETIOLOGY AND PATHOPHYSIOLOGY
- Idiopathic (~70% of the cases)
- Drugs: phenylbutazone, chloramphenicol, sulfonamides, gold, cytotoxic drugs, antiepileptics (felbamate, carbamazepine, valproic acid, phenytoin)
- Viral: HIV, Epstein-Barr virus (EBV), nontypeable postinfectious hepatitis (not A, B, or C), parvovirus B19 (mostly in the immunocompromised), atypical mycobacterium
- Toxic exposure (benzene, pesticides, arsenic)

- Radiation exposure
- Immune disorders (systemic lupus erythematosus, eosinophilic fasciitis, graft versus host disease)
- Pregnancy (rare)
- Congenital (Fanconi anemia, dyskeratosis congenita, Shwachman-Diamond syndrome, amegakaryocytic thrombocytopenia)
- The immune hypothesis: activation of T cells with associated cytokine production leading to destruction or injury of hematopoietic stem cells. This leads to a hypocellular bone marrow without marrow fibrosis.
- The activation of T cells likely occurs because of both genetic and environmental factors. Exposure to specific environmental precipitants, diverse host, genetic risk factors, and individual differences in characteristics of immune response likely account for variations in its clinical manifestations and patterns of responsiveness to treatment.
- Telomerase deficiency leads to short telomeres. This leads to impaired regenerative capacity and hence a reduction in marrow progenitors and qualitative deficiency in the repair capacity of hematopoietic tissue.
- Reduction of natural killer cells in the bone marrow
- A somatic mutation of the PIGA gene underlies the clonal disease paroxysmal nocturnal hemoglobinuria: There is direct evidence that the expansion of the PIGA mutant clone results from Darwinian selection exerted by a glycosylphosphatidylinositol (GPI)-specific autoimmune attack (1).

Genetics
- Telomerase mutations found in a small number of patients with acquired and congenital forms. These mutations render carriers more susceptible to environmental insults.
- Mutations in genes called *TERC* and *TERT* were found in pedigrees of adults with acquired aplastic anemia who lacked the physical abnormalities or a family history typical of inherited forms of bone marrow failure. These genes encode for the RNA component of telomerase.
- HLA-DR2 incidence in aplastic anemia is twice that in the normal population.

RISK FACTORS
- Treatment with high-dose radiation or chemotherapy
- Exposure to toxic chemicals
- Use of certain medications
- Certain blood diseases, autoimmune disorders, and serious infections
- Tumors of thymus (red cell aplasia)
- Pregnancy, rarely

GENERAL PREVENTION
- Avoid possible toxic industrial agents.
- Use safety measures when working with radiation.

DIAGNOSIS

HISTORY
- Solvent and radiation history; family, environmental, travel, and infectious disease history
- Patients are often asymptomatic but may have frequent infections, fatigue, shortness of breath, headache, or bleeding/bruising.

PHYSICAL EXAM
- Mucosal hemorrhage, petechiae
- Pallor
- Fever
- Hemorrhage, menorrhagia, occult stool blood, melena, epistaxis
- Dyspnea
- Palpitations
- Progressive weakness
- Retinal flame hemorrhages
- Systolic ejection murmur
- Weight loss
- Signs of congenital aplastic anemia
  – Short stature
  – Microcephaly
  – Nail dystrophy
  – Abnormal thumbs
  – Oral leukoplakia
  – Hyperpigmentation (café au lait spots) or hypopigmentation

DIFFERENTIAL DIAGNOSIS
Includes other causes of bone marrow failure and pancytopenia

- Hypoplastic myelodysplastic syndrome (MDS)
- Marrow replacement
  – Acute lymphoblastic leukemia
  – Lymphoma
  – Hairy cell leukemia (increased reticulin and infiltration of hairy cells)
  – Large granular lymphocyte leukemia
  – Fibrosis
- Megaloblastic hematopoiesis
  – Folate deficiency
  – Vitamin B_{12} deficiency
- Paroxysmal nocturnal hemoglobinuria, hemolytic anemia (dark urine), pancytopenia, and venous thrombosis (classically hepatic veins)
- Systemic lupus erythematosus
- Prolonged starvation or anorexia nervosa (Bone marrow is gelatinous with loss of fat cells and increased ground substance.)
- Transient erythroblastopenia of childhood
- Drug-induced agranulocytosis that may be reversible on withdrawal of drug
- Overwhelming infection
  – HIV with myelodysplasia
  – Viral hemophagocytic syndrome

DIAGNOSTIC TESTS & INTERPRETATION
Antinuclear antibody (ANA) and anti-DNA

Initial Tests (lab, imaging)
- CBC: pancytopenia, anemia (usually normocytic), leukopenia, neutropenia, thrombocytopenia
- Decreased absolute number of reticulocytes
- Viral serology: hepatitis A, B, C; EBV; cytomegalovirus (CMV); HIV
- Vitamin B_{12} and folate levels
- Increased serum iron secondary to transfusion
- Normal total iron-binding capacity (TIBC)
- High mean corpuscular volume (MCV) >104
- CD34+ cells decreased in blood and marrow
- Urinalysis: hematuria
- Abnormal liver function tests (hepatitis)

- Increased fetal hemoglobin (Fanconi)
- Increased chromosomal breaks under specialized conditions (Fanconi)
- Molecular determination of abnormal gene (Fanconi)
- Human leukocyte antigen (HLA) testing on patients and immediate families
- CT of thymus region if thymoma-associated RBC aplasia suspected
- Radiographs of radius and thumbs (if congenital anemia suspected)
- Renal ultrasound (to rule out congenital anemia or malignant hematologic disorder)
- Chest x-ray to exclude infections such as mycobacterial infection

Diagnostic Procedures/Other
Bone marrow aspiration and biopsy

Test Interpretation
- Normochromic RBC
- Bone marrow
  - Decreased cellularity (<10%): no fibrosis, no malignant cells or dysplastic cells seen
  - Decreased megakaryocytes
  - Decreased myeloid precursors
  - Decreased erythroid precursors
  - Prominent fat spaces and marrow stroma, polyclonal plasma cells

TREATMENT

Two major options: immunosuppressive therapy plus growth factor therapy and hematopoietic stem cell transplantation. Treatment decisions are based on age of the patient, severity of disease, and availability of a HLA-matched sibling donor for transplantation.

GENERAL MEASURES
- Supportive measures: RBC and platelet transfusions. Use only irradiated leukocyte-reduced or CMV-negative blood especially if patient is a candidate for hematopoietic stem cell transplantation.
- Antibiotics, antifungals, antivirals when appropriate, especially if absolute neutrophil count (ANC) <100 cells/μL
- Oxygen therapy for severe anemia
- Good oral hygiene
- Control menorrhagia with norethisterone or oral contraceptive pills.
- Transfusion support (judiciously prescribed RBCs for severe anemia; platelets for severe thrombocytopenia)
  - Transfuse when
    ○ Hb <7 g/dL or if Hb <8 g/dL and symptomatic ± congestive heart failure (CHF)
    ○ Platelet count is <10 × 10⁹ or if <20 × 10⁹ with fever/bleeding

MEDICATION
First Line
- Corticosteroids (methylprednisolone) are often given with immunosuppressive regimens.
- Immunosuppressive therapy
  - A combination of antithymocyte globulin (ATG) plus cyclosporine. ATG eliminates lymphocytes, and cyclosporine blocks T-cell function.

- ATG
  - Horse serum containing polyclonal antibodies against human T cells
  - First-choice treatment for patients >40 years of age and for younger patients without a compatible donor. Consider in patients 30 to 40 years of age.
  - May be used as a single agent but has better response in combination with cyclosporine
- Cyclosporine following initial ATG therapy for minimum of 6 months
  - Monitor through blood levels. Normal values for assays vary.
  - Note: Relapses may occur after the initial response to the immunosuppressive therapy if cyclosporine is discontinued too early. Restarting cyclosporine can lead to a response in up to 25% of patients.
- Eltrombopag day 1 to 6 months along with immunosuppression with ATG + cyclosporine
- Granulocyte-colony stimulating factor (G-CSF)
  - May be used in conjunction with ATG and cyclosporine
  - Shows faster neutrophil recovery, but survival is not improved
  - Treatment is costly and is disputed in two randomized trials.
- Stem cell transplant: matched sibling allogeneic stem cell transplant for age <20 years and ANC <500 or age 20 to 40 years and ANC <200

Second Line
- Rabbit ATG + cyclosporine
- Campath
- Androgen such as danazol can be used in a subset of patients who have anemia as a predominant feature.
- Matched unrelated donor stem cell transplant
- Eltrombopag as monotherapy in relapsed refractory AA
- Cytoxan 50 mg/kg daily for 4 days can be used for refractory disease.

SURGERY/OTHER PROCEDURES
- First-line hematopoietic stem cell transplantation is recommended for patients with an HLA-identical donor and severe aplastic anemia when age <20 years and ANC <500 or age 20 to 40 years and ANC <200. Consider in patients 40 to 50 years of age in good general medical condition.
- Patients >40 years of age have higher rates of graft versus host disease and graft rejection. Individuals with potentially poor-prognosis mutations such as mutations in ASXL1 or DNMT3A tend to have worse outcomes from IST, and we may be more likely to suggest HCT for these individuals.
- Unrelated donor transplants should be considered for patients age <40 years without HLA-matched sibling donor who fail first-line immunosuppressive therapy.
- Thymectomy for thymoma

ADMISSION, INPATIENT, AND NURSING CONSIDERATIONS
If neutropenic, use antiseptic mouthwash such as chlorhexidine and avoid foods that can expose patient to bacteria, such as uncooked foods.

ONGOING CARE

PATIENT EDUCATION
- Avoid people who are ill and large crowds.
- Wash your hands often, brush and floss your teeth; regular dental care
- Pneumonia vaccine and annual flu shot
- Aplastic Anemia and MDS International Foundation, Inc., 800-747-2828. Website: http://www.aamds.org

PROGNOSIS
- Hematopoietic stem cell transplantation with HLA-matched sibling
  - Age <16 years, 91% at 5 years
  - Age >16 years, 70–80% at 5 years
- Immunosuppressive therapy using ATG and cyclosporine: overall survival of 75%; 90% among responders at 5 years

COMPLICATIONS
- Infection (fungal, sepsis)
- Graft versus host disease in bone marrow transplant recipients (acute 18%; chronic 26%)
- Hemorrhage
- Transfusion hemosiderosis, transfusion hepatitis
- Heart failure
- Development of secondary cancer: leukemia or myelodysplasia (15–19% risk at 6 to 10 years)

REFERENCE
1. Luzatto L, Risitano AM. Advances in understanding the pathogenesis of acquired aplastic anaemia. *Br J Haematol*. 2018;182(6):758–776.

SEE ALSO

- Lupus Erythematosus, Systemic (SLE); Myelodysplastic Syndromes (MDS)
- Algorithm: Anemia

CODES

ICD10
- D61 Other aplastic anemias and other bone marrow failure syndromes
- D61.0 Constitutional aplastic anemia
- D61.01 Constitutional (pure) red blood cell aplasia

CLINICAL PEARLS
- Acquired aplastic anemia has an insidious onset and is caused by an exogenous insult triggering an autoimmune reaction. This form is usually responsive to immunosuppressive therapy.
- Immunosuppressive therapy using ATG and cyclosporine + eltrombopag: ORR of 94% and overall survival of 90% among responders at 5 years

ANEMIA, CHRONIC DISEASE

Andrew McBride, MD

BASICS

DESCRIPTION
- Otherwise known as anemia of chronic inflammation
- During chronic systemic infection, inflammation, or malignancy, the production of proinflammatory mediators causes inhibition of erythropoiesis as well as the imbalance in iron homeostasis (1).
- Anemia of chronic disease (ACD) is characterized as a normocytic, normochromic, hypoproliferative anemia and classically has low serum iron levels, elevated ferritin levels, and elevated total iron-binding capacity (TIBC) (1),(2).
- Anemia is typically mild to moderate with hemoglobin (Hgb) rarely <8 g/dL.

EPIDEMIOLOGY
Incidence
There is limited data on the incidence of ACD.

Prevalence
ACD is the second most common anemia after iron deficiency anemia (IDA) due to the aging population and the high prevalence of chronic infections and inflammatory disorders in the United States. Overall, the estimated worldwide prevalence of undifferentiated anemia is 24.8% (3).

ETIOLOGY AND PATHOPHYSIOLOGY
- Production of red blood cells is decreased as a result of functional iron deficiency.
- In general, the severity of the anemia will correspond with the severity of the underlying disease (1).
- Proinflammatory cytokines such as interleukins (IL), tumor necrosis factor (TNF), bone morphogenic proteins (BMP), and interferons (IFN) create changes in iron homeostasis in several ways (1):
  - Dysregulating iron homeostasis
  - Diminishing proliferation as well as differentiation of red blood cell progenitor cells
  - Blunting the erythropoietic response
  - Increasing erythrocyte phagocytosis and apoptosis
- Iron overload and the proinflammatory cytokines IL-1, IL-6, and BMP6 increase the production of the iron-regulating hormone hepcidin in hepatocytes, macrophages, and enterocytes (1).
  - Hepcidin binds to ferroportin causing internalization and degradation, preventing efflux of iron from stores in macrophages and hepatocytes, stopping iron absorption by duodenal enterocytes.
    - This results in low serum iron levels and inhibited erythropoiesis known as iron-restricted erythropoiesis.
  - As a result, iron delivery to erythroid progenitor cells within bone marrow is reduced and erythropoiesis is diminished, causing anemia.
- Erythropoietin (EPO) production and the response to EPO by erythroid bone marrow is suppressed by proinflammatory cytokines such as IL-1, TNF-α, and IFN-γ (1).
- Inflammatory cytokines may also cause erythrophagocytosis and oxidative damage, reducing RBC survival.

RISK FACTORS
Risk factors for anemia of chronic disease include hepatic disease, renal disease, and other infections or autoimmune causes of the commonly associated conditions below.

GENERAL PREVENTION
Prevention of anemia of chronic disease involves timely and undergoing treatment of the associated conditions below.

COMMONLY ASSOCIATED CONDITIONS
- Chronic systemic diseases
  - Rheumatoid arthritis (RA), systemic lupus erythematosus (SLE), sarcoidosis, temporal arteritis, inflammatory bowel disease (IBD), systemic inflammatory response syndrome (SIRS)
- Hepatic disease or failure
- Congestive heart failure or coronary artery disease
- Chronic kidney disease (CKD)
- Acute or chronic infections
  - Viral
    - HIV, HCV
  - Bacterial
    - Abscess, subacute bacterial endocarditis, tuberculosis, osteomyelitis
  - Fungal
  - Parasitic
- Malignancies
- Cytokine dysregulation (anemia of aging)
- Hypometabolic states
  - Protein malnutrition, thyroid disease, panhypopituitarism, diabetes mellitus, Addison disease

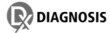**DIAGNOSIS**

HISTORY
- ACD is often discovered incidentally on routine CBC with differential.
- ACD presents with the underlying causative infectious, inflammatory, or malignant process without any source of occult bleeding; often, patients will have mild and vague anemia symptoms, such as fatigue, light-headedness, and palpitations (1).
- Those with a cardiovascular condition may experience symptoms of angina, shortness of breath, and reduced exercise capacity with even a moderately low Hgb level (10 to 11 g/dL).

PHYSICAL EXAM
Physical exam findings are associated with the underlying condition.

DIFFERENTIAL DIAGNOSIS
- IDA
- Anemia of CKD
- Drug-induced marrow suppression or hemolysis
- Endocrine disorders
- Thalassemia
- Sideroblastic anemia
- Dilutional anemia

DIAGNOSTIC TESTS & INTERPRETATION
Initial Tests (lab, imaging)
- Hgb/Hct, mean corpuscular volume (MCV), reticulocyte count, ferritin, B$_{12}$/folate, serum iron, TIBC
- Hgb (1)
  - Typically, <13 g/dL in males or <12 g/dL in females
  - An Hgb of <8 g/dL suggests a concurrent secondary cause for the anemia.
- MCV
  - Usually normal (80 to 100 fL), but microcytosis may be present with concurrent iron deficiency or long-standing disease (<25% of cases)
- RBC morphology
  - Normocytic and normochromic
  - Increased protoporphyrin levels

- Serum ferritin
  - Nonspecific acute phase reactant
  - Normal or slightly elevated (30 to 200 μg/L)
  - In CKD, ferritin can reach 800 μg/L.
  - Serum ferritin levels <30 μg/L suggests coexisting iron deficiency.
- Serum iron levels
  - Low due to increased retention and decreased release from stores
  - <50
- TIBC
  - Extremely low
  - <300
- Absolute reticulocyte count
  - Inappropriately low (reticulocyte index, 20,000 to 25,000/mL) due to reduced erythropoiesis
- Serum B$_{12}$ and folate
  - Diminished due to decreased absorption or lacking in diet

	IDA	ACD	IDA + ACD
Iron	Low	Low	Low
Reticulocyte count	Low	Low	Low
Transferrin, TIBC	High	Low	Normal/high
Transferrin saturation	Low	Normal	Low
Ferritin	Low	Normal/high	Normal
sTfR index	High	Low/normal	High
Hepcidin	Low	High	Normal
EPO	High	Normal/high	High
Inflammatory markers	Normal	High	High

Diagnostic Procedures/Other
- Traditional gold standard: bone marrow biopsy with Prussian blue stainable iron combined with anemia, hypoferremia, and low TSAT (1)
  - Staining is qualitative and may not be accurate.
- Reticulocyte Hgb concentration <28 pg (2)
- Measuring the hepcidin level via enzyme-linked immunosorbent essay can help differentiate iron deficiency anemia from anemia of chronic disease (2),(4).
- Soluble transferrin receptor (sTfR) and the sTfR/log ferritin index
  - Ratio reflects erythropoiesis within bone marrow and differentiates among ACD, IDA, and ACD + IDA.
    - However, sTfR alone may have greater clinical value than the sTfR index because transferrin is not affected by chronic disease/inflammation, unlike ferritin. Elevated sTfR indicates IDA, whereas normal values are more consistent with ACD
- Functional test: supplemental iron increase H/H in IDA and little effect on ACD
- Although a known cause of anemia may be present, iron, B$_{12}$, and folate deficiencies should be ruled out.

TREATMENT

GENERAL MEASURES

- Primary management should focus on the underlying cause of ACD (1).
  - Treatment of the primary disease will generally restore Hgb back to baseline.
- In cases where primary treatment is not possible (e.g., terminal cancer, end-stage renal disease), additional treatment can be considered.
  - The two main forms of treatment are erythropoietin-stimulating agents (ESAs) and transfusions.
  - ACD is frequently responsive to ESAs (epoetin-α, darbepoetin) in pharmacologic doses (5).
  - Replete iron to maximize ESA effectiveness.
  - Transfusion should only be initiated in severe anemia or acute symptoms.
- Currently, no target Hgb exists, but treatment to Hgb >13 g/dL is associated with adverse outcomes (1).
- Coexisting B_{12} or folate deficiency should be considered and corrected in severe cases of anemia.
  - Reduced dietary intake of nutrients is common among patients who are chronically ill.
  - Patients who regularly undergo hemodialysis will often lose these during treatment.

MEDICATION

- ESAs
  - Specifically approved for CKD, but there is evidence that they may also have applications in RA, IBD, HIV, and cancer
  - Indication for ESA therapy is an Hgb <10 g/dL (5)[C].
  - ESAs do not improve symptoms or outcomes in mild anemia of CHF.
  - Do not use in certain cancers: breast, cervical, head and neck, lymphoid, and non–small cell lung cancers. Do not administer to patients with active malignancy not receiving curative therapy.
- Epoetin-α (1),(5),(6)
  - Indications
    - Hgb <10 g/dL
    - Fatigue or exertional intolerance
    - CKD (eGFR <60 mL/min)
    - Anemia due to IBD, RA, hepatitis C
    - Chemotherapy in patients with specific malignancies (palliative therapy)
  - Dosing and schedule
    - Lowest effective dose to maintain an Hgb level generally between 10 and 12 g/dL (1),(5),(6)
    - CKD associated: Start 50 to 100 U/kg SC/IV 3 times per week.
  - Patients with cancer who are undergoing chemotherapy: 150 U/kg SC 3 times per week or 40,000 U once a week
  - Adverse effects:
    - Increased risk of cardiovascular complications, mortality, and thromboembolism
    - Pure red cell aplasia (decrease in Hgb, low reticulocyte count, normal WBC and platelets)
    - Risk of tumor progression in certain cancer patients
- Darbepoetin-α
  - Long-acting, molecularly modified EPO preparation with a half-life 3 to 4 times longer than recombinant human EPO, reducing the frequency of injections to weekly or biweekly
  - Dosing and schedule
    - Administer SC/IV q1–2wk; hold if Hgb >12 g/dL; IV route is preferred in hemodialysis patients.
  - Adverse effects
    - Similar to EPO
- Epoetin-α or darbepoetin-α dose adjustments
  - Follow FDA-approved labeling.
  - Treatment beyond 6 to 8 weeks without appropriate rise of Hgb (>1 to 2 g/dL) is not recommended.

First Line

Either epoetin-α or darbepoetin-α may be chosen as first-line treatment. These should be started along with treatment of the underlying chronic disease.

ADDITIONAL THERAPIES

- Iron (5)
  - Indications
    - Coexisting iron deficiency
    - Resistance to EPO
  - Forms
    - Oral: ferrous sulfate. Poorly tolerated (GI side effects); incomplete absorption (due to hepcidin).
    - Intravenous: ferric gluconate, iron sucrose, iron dextran (potential allergic and anaphylactoid reactions), ferumoxytol
  - Adverse effects
    - May stimulate hepcidin production and exacerbate iron restriction
  - Benefits
    - Relatively safe
    - Inexpensive
    - May decrease ESA requirements (DRIVE study)
- Transfusions
  - 1 to 2 U packed red blood cells (1)
  - Indications
    - Life-threatening/severe anemia: A "restrictive threshold" of Hgb 7 to 8 g/dL to guide transfusion in asymptomatic patients should be used (7)[A].
    - Patients with underlying cardiac or pulmonary disease, active ACS, elderly patients, or patients with acute bleeding or hemorrhagic shock may require transfusion at Hgb of higher threshold (>10 g/dL).
    - Symptomatic anemia (chest pain, SOB, reduced exercise capacity) and/or ECG changes
    - Lack of response to medical therapy
  - Possible adverse effects
    - Infection (HIV, hepatitis)
    - Volume overload
    - Transfusion reaction
  - Specific benefits
    - Rapid correction of anemia
  - When an infection occurs during EPO therapy, it is best to cease EPO therapy and rely on transfusion therapy instead until the infection is properly treated.
- Future directions (1)
  - Antihepcidin antibodies, hepcidin-production inhibitors
  - Anti-BMP, anti–IL-6 antibodies
  - Ferroportin stabilizers
  - Vitamin D (lowers hepcidin)
  - Heparin (impairs hepcidin transcription)

 ONGOING CARE

FOLLOW-UP RECOMMENDATIONS

In situations where anemia is refractory to treatment of the underlying disease and the above agents, referral to a hematologist should be considered.

Patient Monitoring

- Hgb should not be increased >11 to 12 g/dL because normalization of Hgb has been associated with higher mortality (6).
- Baseline and periodic monitoring of transferrin saturation and ferritin levels every 3 months may be of value (5).

DIET

Many chronic conditions associated with ACD are impacted by diet. A well-balanced diet rich in fruits and vegetables including iron-rich foods may be beneficial in treatment.

PATIENT EDUCATION

Patients receiving medical therapy should be advised about the following possible risks:

- Mortality, cardiovascular complications, thromboembolism, progression of cancer

PROGNOSIS

ACD does not typically progress.

COMPLICATIONS

- Adverse effects of ACD:
  - Mortality
  - Cardiovascular complications
  - Symptoms affecting daily life
- Adverse effects of ESAs:
  - Heightened risk of mortality and/or cardiovascular complications in CKD patients
  - Heightened risk of mortality and/or tumor progression in cancer patients
  - Elevated risk of thromboembolism

REFERENCES

1. Gangat N, Wolanskyj AP. Anemia of chronic disease. *Semin Hematol*. 2013;50(3):232–238.
2. Thomas DW, Hinchliffe RF, Briggs C, et al; for British Committee for Standards in Haematology. Guidelines for the laboratory diagnosis of functional iron deficiency. *Br J Haematol*. 2013;161(5):639–648.
3. McLean E, Cogswell M, Egli I, et al. Worldwide prevalence of anaemia, WHO Vitamin and Mineral Nutrition Information System, 1993–2005. *Public Health Nutr*. 2009;12(4):444–454. doi:10.1017/S1368980008002401.
4. Karlsson T. Evaluation of a competitive hepcidin ELISA assay in the differential diagnosis of iron deficiency anaemia with concurrent inflammation and anaemia of inflammation in elderly patients. *J Inflamm (Lond)*. 2017;14(1):21.
5. Kidney Disease: Improving Global Outcomes Anemia Work Group. KDIGO clinical practice guideline for anemia in chronic kidney disease. *Kidney Inter Suppl*. 2012;2(4):279–335.
6. Babitt JL, Lin HY. Mechanisms of anemia in CKD. *J Am Soc Nephrol*. 2012;23(10):1631–1634.
7. Carson JL, Carless PA, Hebert PC. Transfusion thresholds and other strategies for guiding allogeneic red blood cell transfusion. *Cochrane Database Syst Rev*. 2012;(4):CD002042.

 SEE ALSO

Anemia, Iron Deficiency; Iron Studies; Microcytic Anemia

CODES

ICD10

- D63.1 Anemia in chronic kidney disease
- D63.8 Anemia in other chronic diseases classified elsewhere

CLINICAL PEARLS

- ACD is the second most common anemia seen clinically.
- One of the most common diagnostic problems is making the distinction between ACD, IDA, and combined ACD + IDA.
  - Iron level is usually nondiagnostic.
  - Use markers such as transferrin/TIBC, TSAT, sTfR, sTfR index, hepcidin, and ferritin to distinguish.
- IV iron should be given to all patients treated with ESAs.
- Hgb should be kept in low to normal range.

ANEMIA, IRON DEFICIENCY
Deborah R. Erlich, MD, MMedEd, FAAFP

BASICS

DESCRIPTION
- Low serum iron associated with low hemoglobin (Hgb) or microcytic, hypochromic red blood cells (RBCs)
- Because normal Hgb varies with age and sex, anemia is defined as Hgb level 2 standard deviations below normal for age and sex (1).
- Onset acute (rapid blood loss) or chronic (slow blood loss, deficient iron intake, or poor absorption)
- Both low Hgb per RBC and fewer RBC in total lead to blood oxygen deficiency, which can have serious systemic consequences.
- System(s) affected: hematologic, lymphatic, immunologic, cardiac, and gastrointestinal (GI) systems

Geriatric Considerations
- Iron deficiency anemia (IDA) is associated with increased hospitalization, morbidity, and mortality in older adults (2).
- Older patients with suspected IDA should undergo endoscopy to evaluate for occult GI malignancy (3)[C].

Pediatric Considerations
- Risks for IDA in children include low birth weight, history of prematurity, lead exposure, low income status, and immigrant status. Additionally, infants who drink cow's milk before 12 months of age have a higher risk for IDA.
- The U.S. Preventive Services Task Force (USPSTF) did not find sufficient evidence for screening low-risk infants; the Centers for Disease Control and Prevention (CDC) recommends screening high-risk infants at 6 to 12 months, and the AAP recommends universal screening at 12 months (1).
- Should screening be done, include both Hgb and ferritin.

Pregnancy Considerations
- The USPSTF did not find sufficient evidence for screening pregnant women for IDA; the CDC recommends screening women for anemia at the first prenatal visit and giving low-dose iron to all pregnant women, whereas the American College of Obstetricians and Gynecologists (ACOG) recommends screening all pregnant women for IDA and treating those with IDA.
- Iron supplements are recommended during pregnancy to improve maternal hematologic indexes, although significant clinical outcomes have not been proven (4)[A].

EPIDEMIOLOGY
- Iron deficiency is the most common nutritional deficiency in the world (5),(6), and IDA is the most common cause of anemia (50%) (5).
- Predominant age: all ages but especially toddlers and menstruating and pregnant women
- Predominant sex: female
- Predominant race: Mexican American and black females (5)
- Common in both developing and developed countries

Incidence
- Adults: men 2%, women 15–20% annually
- Infants and toddlers: 3–5% annually
- Pregnant patients: may be as high as 20% (1)

Prevalence
2 billion people worldwide (6)
- Infants and children age <12 years: 4–7%
- Men: 2–5%
- Menstruating women: 30% (6)

ETIOLOGY AND PATHOPHYSIOLOGY
Depletion of iron stores leads to decrease in both reticulocyte count and production of Hgb. Causes:
- Blood loss (menses, GI bleeding, trauma)
- Poor iron intake
- Poor iron absorption (e.g., atrophic gastritis, postgastrectomy, celiac disease)
- Increased demand for iron (e.g., infancy, adolescence, pregnancy, breastfeeding)

RISK FACTORS
- Premenopausal woman
- Frequent blood donor
- Pregnancy/lactation, young maternal age
- Strict vegan diet
- Use of NSAIDs
- Hospitalized with frequent blood draws
- Living in or visiting countries with endemic hookworm infection

GENERAL PREVENTION
- Consider screening asymptomatic pregnant women and high-risk children at 1 year of age (guidelines vary) (1)[C].
- Supplementation in asymptomatic children aged 6 to 12 months if at risk for IDA (e.g., malnutrition, abuse, cow's milk <12 months) (1),(4)
- Iron- and vitamin C–rich diet for menstruating women
- Iron 30 mg/day for asymptomatic pregnant women (4)

COMMONLY ASSOCIATED CONDITIONS
- GI tract malignancy, peptic ulcer disease (PUD), *Helicobacter pylori* infection, irritable bowel disease
- Hookworm or other parasitic infestations
- Menometorrhagia
- Pregnancy
- Obesity treated with gastric bypass surgery
- Malnutrition
- Medications such as NSAIDs or antacids

DIAGNOSIS

HISTORY
- Asymptomatic in most cases; symptoms may occur in severe anemia:
  - Weakness, fatigue, and/or malaise
  - Exertional dyspnea
  - Angina with coronary artery disease
  - Headaches or inability to concentrate
  - Melena
  - Pica (ice chewing)

PHYSICAL EXAM
- Pallor (skin, conjunctivae, sublingual)
- Tachycardia, tachypnea
- Cool extremities
- Brittle nails/hair
- Signs of heart failure

DIFFERENTIAL DIAGNOSIS
- GI bleeding (e.g., gastritis, PUD, carcinoma, varices, celiac disease)
- Chronic intravascular hemolysis (e.g., paroxysmal nocturnal hemoglobinuria, malfunctioning prosthetic valve)
- Defective iron usage (e.g., thalassemia trait, sideroblastosis, G6PD deficiency)
- Defective iron reutilization (e.g., infection, inflammation, cancer, hypothyroid, chronic diseases)
- Hypoproliferation (e.g., decreased erythropoietin from hypothyroidism, renal failure)

- Other anemias such as anemia of chronic disease, thalassemia, lead poisoning

DIAGNOSTIC TESTS & INTERPRETATION
Initial Tests (lab, imaging)
- Test with signs and symptoms of anemia, and fully evaluate if iron deficiency is confirmed (1),(6).
- Obtain: Hgb, HCT, ferritin, serum iron, total iron-binding capacity (TIBC)
- Hgb (to define anemia):
  - <13 g in men and <12 g in women (6)
  - Hgb 2 standard deviations below normal for age and sex (1)
  - Patients with comorbidities (e.g., chronic hypoxemia, smokers, high altitudes) may be anemic at higher Hgb levels.
- Mean corpuscular volume (MCV): <80 Fl
  - MCV may be low normal in mild anemia or hidden by large cells (reticulocytes, macrocytes).
- Ferritin is most sensitive and specific for diagnosing iron deficiency as cause of anemia (6):
  - <15 μg/L diagnoses IDA (<30 μg/L likely) (1).
  - >100 μg/L rules out iron deficiency.
- Iron studies:
  - Decreased: ferritin, serum iron, transferrin saturation (TF = (serum iron) $\times$ 100 / total iron-binding capacity)
  - Increased: TIBC, transferrin
- Red cell distribution width (RDW) increases with a mixed population of cells (e.g., mixed IDA and vitamin B_{12} deficiency)
- CBC with differential, peripheral smear, reticulocyte count, and index
  - Peripheral smear usually shows hypochromia and microcytosis but may be normal, and reticulocyte production index is low (1).
- When clinical suspicion is high for a comorbidity
  - Consider testing for G6PD deficiency.
  - Evaluate for thalassemia.
    - Very low MCV <80, elevated Hgb A2 or Hgb F, family history, and especially high or high normal RBC count
    - Microcytosis with ovalocytosis and unresponsive to iron suggests the thalassemia trait.
- Celiac disease: IgA antiendomysial antibodies (IgA anti-EmA) and/or IgA antitissue transglutaminase (IgA anti-TTG)
- TSH for hypothyroidism
- An empiric trial of iron at 3 mg/kg/day may help diagnose decreased iron stores in children; reticulocytes become elevated in 7 to 10 days or Hgb increases >1 g/dL weekly, indicating iron deficiency.
- Drugs that may alter lab results:
  - Iron supplements or multivitamin–mineral preparations that contain iron
- Disorders that may alter lab results:
  - Elevated ferritin: acute inflammation, acute or chronic liver disease, Hodgkin disease, acute leukemia, solid tumors, fever, renal dialysis
  - Elevated Hgb: smoking, chronic hypoxemia, high altitude

Diagnostic Procedures/Other
- Stool guaiac (low sensitivity, so if negative, consider further evaluation)
- Stool for ova and parasites if at risk
- Colonoscopy and endoscopy to evaluate for bleeding sites and colorectal and gastric carcinoma for:
  - Premenopausal women with negative GYN workup and/or lack of response to iron
  - Men and postmenopausal women (1)[C]
- Bone marrow aspiration rarely performed

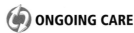

TREATMENT

GENERAL MEASURES
- Search for underlying cause and correct.
- Avoid transfusions, except in rare cases.

MEDICATION
- Elemental iron 100 to 200 mg/day for adults (whether pregnant or not) (4),(6)[C]
- Elemental iron 3 to 6 mg/kg/day for children (6)
- Ferrous sulfate 325 mg TID, ferrous gluconate 300 mg 1 to 3 tablets BID–TID or ferrous fumarate 324 mg 1 tablet BID on an empty stomach 1 hour before meals (1)[C]
- Constipation will occur in ~1/4 of patients. Consider a stool softener along with iron.
  - Medications that reduce gastric acid secretion such as proton pump inhibitors and H_2 antagonists reduce iron absorption (1).
  - Special oral iron formulations (e.g., enteric-coated iron) are expensive and reduce symptoms only to the degree that they reduce the delivery of iron.
- IV iron is indicated for patients who cannot tolerate the side effects of oral replacement (e.g., pregnant women or patients with GI disorders) or for patients who do not sufficiently respond to oral replacement. Other indications for IV iron: bariatric surgery status, heavy uterine bleeding, malabsorption, inflammatory bowel disease, ongoing/severe losses
- Outside of the United States, IV iron is becoming first line ahead of oral iron for its superiority in efficacy and toxicity.
- IV iron formulations available in the United States:
  - Low-molecular-weight iron dextran 1,000 mg over 1 hour
  - Ferumoxytol 510 mg over 3 minutes
  - Ferric carboxymaltose 750 mg over 15 minutes
- Liquid iron preparations (used for children) can also be used in adults when tablets are not absorbed or low tolerance requires a dose reduction.
  - Continued bleeding and untreated hypothyroidism are causes for "failure to respond" to iron.
  - Formula to determine elemental iron needed: elemental iron (mg) = dose (mL) = 0.0442 (desired Hgb − observed Hgb) × LBW + (0.26 × LBW)
    - Desired Hgb = target Hgb in g/dL
    - Observed Hgb = current Hgb in g/dL
    - LBW = lean body weight in kg
    - For males: LBW = 50 kg + 2.3 kg for each inch of height >5 feet
    - For females: LBW = 45.5 kg + 2.3 kg for each inch of height >5 feet
    - Normal Hgb (males and females)
      - >15 kg (33 lb) . . . 14.8 g/dL
      - <15 kg (33 lb) . . . 12.0 g/dL
- Relative contraindications for oral iron:
  - Tetracycline
  - Allopurinol
  - Antacids
  - Penicillamine
  - Fluoroquinolones
  - Vitamin E
- Consider parenteral iron for patients with an Hgb level <6 g/dL, malabsorption, chronic kidney disease, or failure to respond to higher oral doses with concomitant vitamin C (6).
- Issues for parenteral iron formulations:
  - Give test dose for iron dextran prior to first dose to avoid anaphylaxis; ferric gluconate or iron sucrose may be safer alternative. Dimercaprol increases risk of nephrotoxicity.

- Dosing is product dependent; refer to individual product for suggested dosing.
- Precautions
  - Iron may cause dark stools and constipation.
  - Iron overdose is highly toxic; absorption is limited to 1 to 2 mg daily (6); keep tablets and liquids out of reach of small children.
- Blood transfusion for severe acute blood loss or severely symptomatic patients (e.g., demand ischemia due to anemia). Hgb threshold varies by risk factors and clinical scenario. Pregnant women with Hgb <6 should be transfused (1)[C].

ISSUES FOR REFERRAL
- Men and postmenopausal women with IDA (Test for colon cancer.)
- Pregnant women with Hgb level <9 g/dL
- Men or nonpregnant women with an Hgb level <6 g/dL
- Failure to respond to a 4- to 6-week trial of oral iron

ADDITIONAL THERAPIES
Nutrition plays a large role in iron deficiency. Patients should be educated on food sources of iron.

ONGOING CARE

FOLLOW-UP RECOMMENDATIONS
Patient Monitoring
- Monitor patients every 3 months after Hgb normalizes for a year and then yearly (1)[C].
- Hgb increases 1 g/dL every 3 to 4 weeks.
- Iron stores may take up to 4 weeks to correct after Hgb normalizes.

DIET
- Iron-rich foods include red meat, poultry, fish and eggs (all heme iron sources, best absorbed); and lentils, beans, dark green vegetables, raisins, tofu, and iron-fortified breads/cereals (all non-heme iron sources, less well absorbed) (7).
- Foods and beverages containing ascorbic acid (vitamin C) enhance iron absorption when taken simultaneously, such as citrus, tomatoes, dark green leafy vegetables, and berries (6).
- Avoid milk or dairy products within 2 hours of iron tablet ingestion.
- Limit milk to 16 oz/day (adults).
- Limit tea, coffee, and caffeinated beverages.
- Increase fluid and dietary fiber to decrease likelihood of constipation.
- Limit foods with high levels of chemicals (phytates and polyphenols).

PATIENT EDUCATION
- http://familydoctor.org/familydoctor/en/diseases-conditions/anemia.html
- http://patient.info/pdf/4392.pdf

PROGNOSIS
- IDA can be resolved with iron therapy if the underlying cause is discovered and appropriately treated.
- Treat coexisting subclinical hypothyroidism and IDA together. Failure to treat hypothyroidism results in poor response to iron therapy.

COMPLICATIONS
- Hidden bleeding, particularly a bleeding malignancy (3)
- Ischemic events or heart failure, especially in elderly
- Poor growth, failure to thrive, motor and cognitive developmental delay in children (5)

REFERENCES
1. Short MW, Domagalski JE. Iron deficiency anemia: evaluation and management. *Am Fam Physician*. 2013;87(2):98–104.
2. Goodnough LT, Schrier SL. Evaluation and management of anemia in the elderly. *Am J Hematol*. 2014;89(1):88–96.
3. Lanier JB, Park JJ, Callahan RC. Anemia in older adults. *Am Fam Physician*. 2018;98(7):437–442.
4. McDonagh M, Cantor A, Bougatsos C, et al. *Routine Iron Supplementation and Screening for Iron Deficiency Anemia in Pregnant Women: A Systematic Review to Update the U.S. Preventive Services Task Force Recommendation. Evidence Syntheses No. 123*. Rockville, MD: Agency for Healthcare Research and Quality; 2015.
5. Centers for Disease Control and Prevention. Iron deficiency—United States, 1999–2000. *MMWR Morb Mortal Wkly Rep*. 2002;51(40):897–899.
6. Camaschella C. Iron-deficiency anemia. *N Engl J Med*. 2015;372(19):1832–1843.
7. National Institutes of Health Office of Dietary Supplements. Iron: fact sheet for health professionals. https://ods.od.nih.gov/factsheets/Iron-HealthProfessional/. Accessed September 18, 2020.

ADDITIONAL READING
- Auerbach M, Deloughery T. Single-dose intravenous iron for iron deficiency: a new paradigm. *Hematology Am Soc Hematol Educ Program*. 2016;2016(1):57–66.
- Chertow GM, Mason PD, Vaage-Nilsen O, et al. On the relative safety of parenteral iron formulations. *Nephrol Dial Transplant*. 2004;19(6):1571–1575.
- Johnson-Wimbley TD, Graham DY. Diagnosis and management of iron deficiency anemia in the 21st century. *Therap Adv Gastroenterol*. 2011;4(3):177–184.
- USPSTF Recommendations. Iron Deficiency Anemia in Pregnant Women: Screening and Supplementation. Released September 2015. Accessed June 29, 2018.

 SEE ALSO

Algorithm: Anemia

CODES

ICD10
- D50.9 Iron deficiency anemia, unspecified
- D62 Acute posthemorrhagic anemia
- D50.0 Iron deficiency anemia secondary to blood loss (chronic)

CLINICAL PEARLS
- Risk factors for IDA include pre-menopausal women, pregnancy/lactation, vegan diet,
- Initial testing includes Hbg/Hct, ferritin, serum iron, TIBC; with clinical suspicion, consider TSH, IgA anti-TTG
- Empiric treatment: FeSO4 325 mg TID on empty stomach 1 hour before meals
- IV iron formulations in US: Low-molecular-weight iron dextran 1,000 mg over 1 hour
- Ferumoxytol 510 mg over 3 minutes, Ferric carboxymaltose 750 mg over 15 minutes

ANEMIA, SICKLE CELL
Joseph P. Wiedemer, MD, FAAFP • Smriti Gupta, MD

 BASICS

DESCRIPTION
- Hereditary, hemoglobinopathy marked by chronic hemolytic anemia, acute episodes of painful crises, and increased susceptibility to infections
- The heterozygous condition (Hb AS), sickle cell trait, is usually asymptomatic without anemia.
- Synonym(s): sickle cell disease (SCD); Hb SS disease

Pediatric Considerations
- Sequestration crises and hand–foot syndrome seen typically in infants/young children.
- Strokes occur mainly in childhood.
- Adolescence/young adulthood:
  - Frequency of complications and organ/tissue damage increases with age.
  - Psychological complications: body image, interrupted schooling, restriction of activities; stigma of disease; low self-esteem

Pregnancy Considerations
- Complicated, especially during 3rd trimester and delivery
  - Fetal mortality 35–40%. Fetal survival is >90% if the fetus reaches the 3rd trimester.
  - High prevalence of small for gestational age (SGA) babies
  - 6 times higher maternal mortality compared to control (1)
- Increased risk of thrombosis, preterm delivery, pain, toxemia, infection, pulmonary infarction, and phlebitis
- Partial exchange transfusion in 3rd trimester may reduce maternal morbidity and fetal mortality but is controversial.
- Chronic transfusions have been effective in diminishing pain episodes in pregnant women. However, this method should be used with caution due to risk of alloimmunization.

EPIDEMIOLOGY
Prevalence
- ~100,000 Americans have sickle cell anemia (SCA), and ~3 million people in the United States have sickle cell trait.
- The condition affects mainly people of African descent. Hispanic, Middle Eastern, Asian Indian, and Mediterranean ancestry may also be affected.

ETIOLOGY AND PATHOPHYSIOLOGY
- Hemoglobin S (HbS) results from the substitution of the amino acid valine for glutamic acid at the sixth position of the β-globin chain. Hydrophobic valine residues interact with other hydrophobic residues, contributing to HbS polymerization.
- HbS polymerization occurs in the RBC with increased concentrations of HbS and in deoxygenated states, resulting in RBC sickling.
- Sickle RBCs exhibit increased adhesion, are inflexible and have decreased ability to maneuver through small vessels leading to increased blood viscosity, stasis, and vaso-occlusion of small arterioles and capillaries, resulting in ischemia.
- Chronic anemia; crises:
  - Vaso-occlusive crisis: tissue ischemia and necrosis; progressive organ failure/tissue damage from repeated episodes
  - Hand–foot syndrome: Vessel occlusion/ischemia affects small blood vessels in hands or feet.

- Aplastic crisis: suppression of RBC production by severe infection (e.g., parvovirus and other viral infections)
  - Suppression of RBC production
  - Hyperhemolytic crisis: accelerated hemolysis with reticulocytosis; increased RBC fragility/shortened lifespan
  - Sequestration crisis: splenic sequestration of blood (only in young children as spleen is later lost to autoinfarction)
- Susceptibility to infection: impaired/absent splenic function leading to decreased ability to clear infection; defect in alternate pathway of complement activation
- Increased red cell destruction causes decreased hemoglobin levels and results in anemia and fatigue.

Genetics
- Autosomal recessive. Homozygous condition, Hb SS; heterozygous condition, Hb AS
- The heterozygote condition can also be combined with other hemoglobinopathies: Sickle cell hemoglobin C (HbSC) disease and Sβ + thalassemia are clinically similar to the heterozygous condition, whereas Sβ thalassemia is clinically similar to the homozygous condition.

RISK FACTORS
- Vaso-occlusive crisis ("painful crisis"): hypoxia, dehydration, high altitudes, stress, fever, infection, acidosis, cold, anesthesia, strenuous physical exercise, alcohol, smoking
- Aplastic crisis (suppression of RBC production): severe infections, human parvovirus B19 infection, folic acid deficiency
- Hyperhemolytic crisis (accelerated hemolysis with reticulocytosis): acute bacterial infections, exposure to oxidant

GENERAL PREVENTION
- Prevention of crises
  - Avoid hypoxia, dehydration, cold, infection, fever, acidosis, and anesthesia.
  - Prompt management of fever, infections, pain
  - Avoid alcohol and smoking. Avoid high-altitude areas.
- Minimizing trauma: Aseptic technique is imperative.

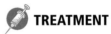 **DIAGNOSIS**

HISTORY
- Often asymptomatic in early months of life due to presence of fetal hemoglobin
- In those >6 months of age, earliest symptoms are irritability and painful swelling of the hands and feet (hand–foot syndrome). May also see pneumococcal sepsis or meningitis, severe anemia and acute splenic enlargement (splenic sequestration), acute chest syndrome, pallor, jaundice, or splenomegaly
- Manifestations in older children include anemia, severe or recurrent musculoskeletal or abdominal pain, aplastic crisis, acute chest syndrome, splenomegaly or splenic sequestration, and cholelithiasis.
- Painful crises in bones, joints, abdomen, back, and viscera account for 90% of all hospital admissions.
- Acute chest syndrome: tachycardia, fever, bilateral infiltrates caused by pulmonary infarctions

DIAGNOSTIC TESTS & INTERPRETATION
Initial Tests (lab, imaging)
- Screening test: Sickledex test/hemoglobin electrophoresis (diagnostic test of choice); SCA (FS pattern)
  - 80–100% HbS, variable amounts of HbF, and no HbA1
  - Sickle cell trait (FS pattern): 30–45% HbS, 50–70% HbA1, minimal HbF
- Hemoglobin ~5 to 10 g/dL; RBC indices: mean corpuscular volume (MCV) normal to increased; mean corpuscular hemoglobin concentration (MCHC) increased; reticulocytes 3–15%
- Leukocytosis; bands in absence of infection, platelets elevated; peripheral smear: sickled RBCs, nucleated RBCs, Howell-Jolly bodies
- Serum bilirubin mildly elevated (2 to 4 mg/dL); ferritin very elevated in patients with multiple previous transfusions; serum lactate dehydrogenase (LDH) elevated, fecal/urinary urobilinogen high
- Haptoglobin absent or very low
- Urine analysis: hemoglobinuria, hematuria (sickle cell trait may have painless hematuria), increased albuminuria (Monitor for progressive kidney disease.)
- Imaging depends on clinical circumstances.
  - Bone scan to rule out osteomyelitis
  - CT/MRI to rule out CVA; high index of suspicion required for any acute neurologic symptoms other than mild headache
  - Chest x-ray: may show enlarged heart; diffuse alveolar infiltrates in acute chest syndrome
  - Transcranial Doppler: Start at age 2 years; repeat yearly. Transcranial Doppler ultrasound identifies children age 2 to 16 years at higher risk of stroke; may be normal in clinically silent strokes
  - ECG to detect pulmonary hypertension and echocardiogram every other year from age 15 years and older

TREATMENT

GENERAL MEASURES
- Painful crises: hydration, analgesics; oxygen regardless of whether the patient is hypoxic
- Retinal evaluation starting at school age to detect proliferative sickle retinopathy
- Occupational therapy, cognitive and behavioral therapies, support groups
- All standard childhood vaccinations should be administered accordingly.
- Special immunizations
  - Influenza vaccine yearly
  - Conjugated pneumococcal vaccine (PCV13) at ages 2, 4, and 6 months; booster at 12 to 15 months
  - Patients <5 years of age with incomplete vaccination history should receive catch-up doses accordingly.
  - Adults age ≥19 years who have functional asplenia and have not received pneumococcal vaccination should receive 1 dose PCV13, followed by administration of PPSV23 at least 8 weeks later. A second PPSV23 dose is recommended 5 years after the first PPSV23 dose for persons aged 19 to 64 years old with functional or anatomic asplenia (1)[C].

- Meningococcal vaccine:
  - 6 weeks old: Hib-MenCY at ages 2, 4, 6, and 12 months
  - 9 months old: 2 doses of MCV4 separated by 3 months
  - ≥2 years of age: 2 doses of MCV4-D-CRM separated by 2 months; boosters recommended every 5 years

MEDICATION
First Line
- Prophylactic penicillins indicated in infants and children starting at 2 months: A dose of 125 mg BID is recommended for children <3 years. A dose of 250 mg BID is recommended for children 3 to 5 years. Amoxicillin 20 mg/kg/day is an alternative to penicillin. Penicillin can be discontinued at age 5 unless they have had a splenectomy or invasive pneumococcal infection.
- Supplemental oxygen
- Painful crises (mild, outpatient)
  - Nonopioid analgesics (ibuprofen)
- Painful crises (severe, hospitalized)
  - Parenteral opioids (e.g., morphine on fixed schedule); patient-controlled analgesia (PCA) pump may be useful. Patients given strong opioids in the acute care setting should be safely monitored.
- Hydroxyurea for prevention of painful acute chest syndrome, vaso-occlusive episodes, and very severe anemia. Increases fetal hemoglobin concentration. Infants and children >9 months of age with SCA should be started on hydroxyurea to prevent complications. Adults: Start 15 mg/kg/day single daily dose; children: 20 mg/kg/day; titrate upward every 8 weeks (max dose of 35 mg/kg/day). Monitor blood counts (avoid severe neutropenia, thrombocytopenia).
- Acute chest syndrome: Patients may deteriorate quickly; monitor patients with vaso-occlusive crisis with incentive spirometry. Treat with aggressive management with oxygen, analgesics, antibiotics, and simple or exchange transfusion.
- Empiric antibiotics to cover *Mycoplasma pneumoniae* and *Chlamydia pneumoniae* (cephalosporins or azithromycin). If osteomyelitis, cover for *Staphylococcus aureus* and *Salmonella* (e.g., ciprofloxacin).
- Precautions: Avoid high-dose estrogen oral contraceptives; consider Depo-Provera. G-CSF use is contraindicated as it may lead to vaso-occlusive episodes and multiorgan failure.

Second Line
Folic acid: 0 to 6 months: 0.1 mg/day; 6 to 12 months: 0.25 mg/day; 1 to 2 years: 0.5 mg/day; >2 years of age: 1 mg/day

ADDITIONAL THERAPIES
Transfusions and additional therapies
- Transfusion for aplastic crises, severe complications (i.e., CVA), prophylactically before surgery, and treatment for acute chest syndrome; prophylactic transfusions for primary or secondary stroke prevention in children
- Preoperative transfusions have been shown to reduce the risk of perioperative complications with goal hemoglobin >10 g/dL.
- Chelation with oral deferasirox if the patient is multiply transfused (after age 2 years).
- Red cell exchange is indicated to minimize the level of HbS (<30%) as well as prevent iron overload.

SURGERY/OTHER PROCEDURES
- Hematopoietic stem cell transplant (HSCT): curative. Matched sibling allogeneic stem cell transplant has 90% overall survival and event-free survival. Alternative sources of allogeneic stem cells (cord blood and haploidentical donors) are also being considered.
- Endothelin-1 has therapeutic potential for prevention of renal and pulmonary complications of sickle cell disease.
- Oral therapy with L-glutamine has been shown to reduce oxidative stress and fewer episodes of sickle cell-related pain in patients ages >5.
- Monoclonal antibodies that bind P-selectin show promise to be immunologic treatments to reduce the frequency of and time to pain crisis in conjunction with hydroxyurea therapies.

ADMISSION, INPATIENT, AND NURSING CONSIDERATIONS
Admission criteria/initial stabilization: severe pain, suspected infection or sepsis, evidence of acute chest syndrome

 ONGOING CARE

FOLLOW-UP RECOMMENDATIONS
Patient Monitoring
- Treat infections early. Parents/patients: Any temperature of ≥101°F (38.3°C) requires immediate medical attention.
- Monitor for hepatitis C and hemosiderosis in patients who receive chronic transfusions.
- Periodic eye evaluations: starting at age 10 years for proliferative sickle retinopathy; rescreen 1- to 2-year intervals.
- Biannual examination for hepatic, renal, and pulmonary dysfunction
- Neuroimaging screening for risk of stroke: transcranial Doppler beginning at age 2 years and continuing up to age 16 years
- Baseline pulmonary evaluation at each visit to assess for wheezing, shortness of breath, or cough (indicators of disease severity and pulmonary hypertension). Echocardiography for symptomatic patients; right heart catheterization for diagnosis
- Screening for albuminuria should be performed annually starting at age 10, with introduction of ACE/ARB therapy for management of confirmed albuminuria.
- SCD may be considered a provoking factor for VTE, but decisions on anticoagulation duration and prophylaxis should be a shared decision-making process.

DIET
- Avoid alcohol (leads to dehydration); maintain hydration.
- Multivitamin without iron is recommended; vitamin D deficiency and decreased bone marrow density in SCD patients

PATIENT EDUCATION
- SickleCellKids.org—education website for children with SCA: http://www.sicklecelldisease.org
- American Sickle Cell Anemia Association: http://www.ascaa.org

PROGNOSIS
- Anemia occurs in infancy; sickle cell crises at 1 to 2 years of age; some children die in their 1st year.
- In adulthood, fewer crises but more complications. Median age of death is 42 years for men and 48 years for women.

COMPLICATIONS
- Alloimmunization, bone infarct and osteomyelitis, aseptic necrosis of femoral head
- Cerebral strokes (peak age 6 to 7 years), impaired mental development, even without history of stroke
- Cholelithiasis/abnormal liver function
- Chronic leg ulcers, poor wound healing
- Impotence, priapism, hematuria/hyposthenuria, renal complications (proteinuria)
- Retinopathy, splenic infarction (by age 10 years)
- Acute chest syndrome (infection/infarction) leading to chronic pulmonary disease
- Infections (pneumonia, osteomyelitis, meningitis, pyelonephritis); sepsis (leading cause of morbidity and mortality)
- Hemosiderosis (secondary to multiple transfusions)
- Risk of opioid tolerance and substance abuse in chronic, uncontrolled patients

REFERENCE
1. Onimoe G, Rotz S. Sickle cell disease: a primary care update. *Cleve Clin J Med*. 2020;87(1):19–27.

 SEE ALSO

Algorithm: Anemia

CODES

ICD10
- D57.212 Sickle-cell/Hb-C disease with splenic sequestration
- D57.211 Sickle-cell/Hb-C disease with acute chest syndrome
- D57.21 Sickle-cell/Hb-C disease with crisis

CLINICAL PEARLS
- >100,000 Americans have SCA (~1 in 365 African Americans). The majority of newborns with SCD are born in Nigeria, the Republic of Congo, and India.
- The preferred maintenance IV fluid is 1/2 NS because NS may theoretically increase the risk of sickling.
- Painful crises in bones, joints, abdomen, back, and viscera account for 90% of all hospital admissions. Management of pain should follow individualized pain plans or hospital protocol for SCD crises without discrimination.
- Acute chest syndrome: tachycardia, fever, bilateral infiltrates caused by pulmonary infarctions

ANEURYSM OF THE ABDOMINAL AORTA

Katyayini Aribindi, MD • Jeffrey Chen, MD

 BASICS

DESCRIPTION
- There are two types of aneurysms: true and false. A true aneurysm involves all three vessel wall layers. False aneurysms or pseudoaneurysms occur when the intimal and medial layers are disrupted, and the dilated segment is surrounded by the adventitia only, and possibly a perivascular clot. Ruptures are usually higher with false aneurysms due to poor support of the aneurysmal wall.
- Abdominal aortic aneurysm (AAA) is the most common true arterial aneurysm. False aneurysms of the abdominal aorta are usually due to trauma or infection.
- The average diameter of the infrarenal aorta is 2.0 cm; an aortic diameter of ≥3.0 cm is considered aneurysmal.
- In men, AAA diameters are predictive of clinical events. In women, aneurysms are still defined as >3.0 cm, but the aortic scaling index (ASI; diameter [cm]/body surface area [m²]) is more predictive of clinical events.
- System(s) affected: cardiovascular; neurologic; heme/lymphatic/immunologic
- Synonym(s): aortic aneurysms; AAA

Geriatric Considerations
Incidence of AAA, risk of rupture, and operative morbidity and mortality all rise with age.

Pediatric Considerations
Rare in children; may be associated with umbilical artery catheters, connective tissue diseases, arteritides, or congenital abnormalities

EPIDEMIOLOGY
- Estimated prevalence of AAA in developed countries is 2–8%. Age-related increase is seen more with men than women.
- Ultrasound studies show that 4–8% of older men have an occult AAA.
- 90% of all AAA >4 cm are related to atherosclerotic disease, with the vast majority located infrarenally.
- Predominant sex: male > female

Incidence
- Roughly 15,000 deaths per year and the 15th leading cause of death in United States
- 0.4–0.67% in Western populations or 2.5 to 6.5 aneurysms per 1,000 patient-years
- If stratified into years, the incidence of AAA is increased in the older populations. For example, the incidence increases from 55 to 298 per 100,000 patient-years if comparing men aged 65 to 74 years versus men >85 years of age.

Prevalence
- The prevalence of AAA-associated mortality has decreased by 50% since the 1990s, likely due to the decline in cigarette smoking, increased screening for AAA detection, and early interventions.
- With the increasing life expectancy in developed countries, the prevalence of AAA is expected to increase, but the decreased prevalence of smoking will have the opposite effect.

ETIOLOGY AND PATHOPHYSIOLOGY
- AAAs are caused by degradations of abnormal production of elastin and collagen, the structural components of the aortic wall.

- There are many causes of aortic aneurysms: inflammation, degenerative disorders, vasculitis, infections, and trauma. However, the vast majority of AAA are caused by inflammation with atherosclerosis as the inciting factor.
- B-cell and T-cell lymphocytes, macrophages, inflammatory cytokines, and matrix metalloproteinases degrade elastin and collagen, thus decreasing the aortic wall strength, leading to a decreased ability to accommodate the pulsatile flow.
- Histopathology shows elastin and collagen destruction, decreased vascular smooth muscle, ingrowth of new blood vessels, and subsequent inflammation.
- Although most aortic aneurysms are caused by inflammatory or degenerative destruction of elastin and collagen, infections, trauma, and connective tissues disorders can also degrade elastin and collagen, leading to similar presentations.
- The natural course of a AAA is progressive expansion, based on a variety of factors, the most important being on going smoking.

Genetics
- Familial aggregations exist with aneurysms developing at an earlier age.
- Familial abdominal aortic aneurysms have a variable polygenetic inheritance pattern.
- Monogenetic inheritance patterns such as: Marfan syndrome (fibrillin-1 defect), Ehlers-Danlos syndrome (type IV collagen defect), or Loeys-Dietz syndrome are more commonly associated with thoracoabdominal aortic aneurysms.

RISK FACTORS
Older age, male sex, Caucasian race, family history, smoking, hypertension (HTN), hyperlipidemia, atherosclerosis, peripheral aneurysms, obesity

GENERAL PREVENTION
- Address cardiovascular disease risk factors.
- Follow screening guidelines: U.S. screening for detection of AAA in male patients, 65 to 75 years, who have ever smoked.

COMMONLY ASSOCIATED CONDITIONS
- HTN, myocardial infarction (MI), heart failure, carotid artery atherosclerosis, and/or lower extremity peripheral arterial disease, tobacco abuse
- Screening for thoracic aneurysm should also be considered.
- 20% of patients with AAA have concurrent thoracic aneurysm (1).

DIAGNOSIS
- Asymptomatic AAA (majority)
  - USPSTF recommends a one-time screen for an AAA by abdominal ultrasound for men aged 65 to 75 years with a smoking history (2)[A].
  - Selective screening for AAAs in nonsmoker men aged 65 to 75 years can be offered based on personal or family history and patient's preferences (2)[A].
  - Women with a first-degree relative with an AAA can be offered screening via abdominal ultrasound (1)[C].

ALERT
- Symptomatic: The triad of shock, pulsatile mass, and abdominal pain always suggest rupture of AAA, and immediate surgical evaluation is recommended (1)[A].

- Hemodynamically stable patients (shock is absent as the rupture is contained) may undergo a CT abdomen with IV contrast for evaluation of an AAA.
- Unstable patients (rupture is uncontained) undergo a focused bedside ultrasound and surgical repair if AAA is present.
- Unusual presentations:
  - Primary aortoenteric fistula: erosion/rupture of AAA into duodenum
  - Aortocaval fistula: erosion/rupture of AAA into vena cava or left renal vein: 3–6%
  - Inflammatory aneurysm: encasement by thick inflammatory rind; can cause chronic abdominal pain, weight loss, and elevated ESR. Surrounding viscera may be densely adherent.

HISTORY
- Abdominal, back, or flank pain; AAA risk factors, hypotension if presenting in an emergency situation
- Found on routine screening if presenting in an outpatient setting

PHYSICAL EXAM
- Pulsatile supraumbilical mass
- In one study, sensitivity varied based on abdominal girth and size of aneurysm. However, the sensitivity was 100% of aneurysms >5.0 cm when the girth was <100 cm. The sensitivity and specificity varied from 23% to 68% and 75% to 91%, respectively (3).
- Encroachment by aneurysm
  - Vertebral body erosion, gastric outlet obstruction, ureteral obstruction
  - Lower extremity ischemia secondary to embolization of mural thrombus
- Rupture leads to tachycardia, hypotension, evidence of shock and anemia, and possible flank contusion (Grey Turner sign).

DIFFERENTIAL DIAGNOSIS
- Other abdominal masses
- Other causes of abdominal or back pain (e.g., peptic ulcer disease, renal colic, diverticulitis, appendicitis, incarcerated hernia, bowel obstruction, GI hemorrhage, arthritis, metastatic disease, MI)

DIAGNOSTIC TESTS & INTERPRETATION
Initial Tests (lab, imaging)
- If rupturing AAA is considered: complete blood chemistry (chemistries, PT/INR, PTT, type and cross), ECG
- Ultrasound: simplest and least expensive diagnostic procedure with a high sensitivity (94–100%) and specificity (98–100%); test of choice for an asymptomatic AAA (1)[A]
- Surveillance of asymptomatic aneurysm
  - 2.6 to 2.9 cm: Screen at 5-year intervals.
  - 3.0 to 3.9 cm: Screen at 3-year intervals.
  - 4.0 to 5.4 cm: Screen every 6 to 12 months.
- CT scans are preferred preoperative study (caution with IV contrast in renal failure) if a symptomatic AAA is suspected (1).
- MRI/MRA can visualize AAA but is often not possible in emergent situations.
- Aortography does not define outer dimensions of aneurysm.
- Abdominal x-rays can be diagnostic if calcifications exist; not a diagnostic tool of choice

Follow-Up Tests & Special Considerations
- Evaluation for coronary artery disease is appropriate prior to elective AAA repair, including stress test, echocardiography, and ECG if appropriate.

- If AAA was discovered at any location, then full assessment of entire aorta, including thoracic aorta and aortic valve, is recommended (1)[C].

Diagnostic Procedures/Other

ALERT
Use clinical judgment: Patients with known AAA having abdominal or back pain symptoms may be rupturing despite a negative CT scan.

 TREATMENT

GENERAL MEASURES
- Treat atherosclerotic risk factors: HTN, dyslipidemia, diabetes mellitus, and smoking (2)[A].
- Smoking was associated with a 0.35 mm/year AAA growth, twice as fast as AAA growth in nonsmokers, and is the most important AAA outcome predictor (1).
- Emergent treatment in unstable or symptomatic patients requires immediate vascular surgery consultation, adequate IV access and resuscitation, type and cross for multiple units, and rapid bedside ultrasound (1).
- Less acute treatment of AAA/prevention of rupture is elective repair and risk factor modification.

MEDICATION
- β-Blockers, aspirin, and statins theoretically reduce the rate of growth of AAAs by decreasing shear wall stress, inflammation, and prevention of an intraluminal mural thrombus. However, there are conflicting RCT and meta-analysis trials. Because concomitant atherosclerosis is often a precipitating factor in AAAs, their use is recommended for reduced mortality in patients with coronary artery disease or its equivalents (4)[A].
- The use of ACE inhibitors has shown to be inconclusive with regard to growth of AAA; however, studies do indicate a decreased rate of AAA rupture (4)[A].
- Doxycycline and roxithromycin, previously theorized to decreased wall inflammation, have not been shown to have any effect on AAA (5).

SURGERY/OTHER PROCEDURES
Current recommendations are the following:
- Elective
  - 5.5-cm diameter is threshold for repair in "average" patient (1)[C].
  - Younger, low-risk patients with long-life expectancy may prefer early repair.
  - Saccular aneurysms should be considered for elective repair (1)[C].
  - Women or AAA with high risk of rupture: Consider elective repair at 4.5 to 5.0 cm.
    - Consider delayed repair in high-risk patients.
    - 5% perioperative mortality for open elective repair (1)
- High risk of rupture
  - Expansion >0.5 cm/year
  - Smoking/COPD severe/steroids
  - Family history; multiple relatives
  - HTN if poorly controlled
  - Shape nonfusiform
- High-risk patients for elective repair
  - Risk factors for open repair include age >75 years, COPD, chronic kidney disease with Cr >1.75, and suprarenal clamp site.
  - The leading cause of early mortality after AAA repair is coronary artery disease, with open AAA repair being much higher risk than endovascular AAA repair (1)[C].
- The RCT IMPROVE trial showed a similar 30-day mortality for patients with ruptured AAA who under-

went endovascular repair versus open repair (35.4% vs. 37.4%); 1-year follow-up all-cause mortality between the two groups (41.1% vs. 45.1%) (5)[A]
- Although difficult to quantify, perioperative morbidity rates are lower for EVAR, suggesting that an EVAR is preferable in patients with a ruptured AAA with poor prognostic factors for an open repair, such as SBP <80 mm Hg, age >80 years, Cr >1.3 on admission, ischemic heart disease, female sex, and hemoglobin <9.0 on admission (2),(5)[A].
- Contraindications for AAA endovascular repair are an aortic neck >32 mm and a ruptured AAA with aortic neck length <7 mm. In these patients, an open AAA repair is performed due to anatomic constrictions.

ADMISSION, INPATIENT, AND NURSING CONSIDERATIONS
Risk of abdominal compartment syndrome after repair, 4–12%; usually associated with large fluid resuscitation

 ONGOING CARE

FOLLOW-UP RECOMMENDATIONS
Patient Monitoring
- May do a CT scan 5 years after an open repair for possible late aortic dilatation or pseudoaneurysm (2)[C]
- Follow-up imaging should be tailored to patient. Once renal function stabilizes postoperatively, a CT can be performed to evaluate the endograft (2)[C].
- Aggressive risk factor modification always recommended postoperatively (2)[A]

DIET
Low-fat, low-salt, and low-caffeine diet; nutrition optimized prior to elective repair

PATIENT EDUCATION
Smoking cessation, aerobic exercise, aggressive control of atherosclerotic risk factors such as HTN

PROGNOSIS
- Naturally progressive disorder, expands at an average rate of 0.3 to 0.4 cm/year. A fast expansion is considered >0.6 cm/year and should be evaluated for operative management.
- Possibility of rupture increases with an aneurysm diameter of >5.5 cm or a fast rate of expansion (>0.5 cm over a 6-month period), continued cigarette use, female sex, recent surgery, uncontrolled HTN, and aneurysm couture.

COMPLICATIONS
- Emergent AAA repair and elective AAA repair have similar complications, with a higher incidence in emergent AAA repair.
- Complications include MI, respiratory failure, and acute kidney injury in the early period.
- Late complications such as aortic graft infection, aortoenteric fistula, and graft occlusion have similar rates between emergent and elective repair.
- Ischemic bowel and abdominal compartment syndrome are complications usually after a ruptured open AAA repair given the massive blood loss, increased operative time, and magnitude of fluid resuscitation.

REFERENCES

1. Chaikof EL, Dalman RL, Eskandari MK, et al. The Society for Vascular Surgery practice guidelines on the care of patients with an abdominal aortic aneurysm. *J Vasc Surg.* 2018;67(1):2.e2–77.e2.
2. LeFevre ML; for U.S. Preventive Services Task Force. Screening for abdominal aortic aneurysm: U.S. Preventive Services Task Force recommendation statement. *Ann Intern Med.* 2014;161(4):281–290.
3. Fink HA, Lederle FA, Roth CS, et al. The accuracy of physical examination to detect abdominal aortic aneurysm. *Arch Intern Med.* 2000;160(6):833–836.
4. Guessous I, Periard D, Lorenzetti D, et al. The efficacy of pharmacotherapy for decreasing the expansion rate of abdominal aortic aneurysms: a systematic review and meta-analysis. *PLoS One.* 2008;3(3):e1895.
5. Braithwaite B, Cheshire NJ, Greenhalgh RM, et al; for IMPROVE Trial Investigators. Endovascular strategy or open repair for ruptured abdominal aortic aneurysm: one-year outcomes from the IMPROVE randomized trial. *Eur Heart J.* 2015;36(31):2061–2069.

ADDITIONAL READING

- Aggarwal S, Qamar A, Sharma V, et al. Abdominal aortic aneurysm: a comprehensive review. *Exp Clin Cardiol.* 2011;16(1):11–15.
- Kuivaniemi H, Ryer EJ, Elmore JR, et al. Understanding the pathogenesis of abdominal aortic aneurysms. *Expert Rev Cardiovasc Ther.* 2015;13(9):975–987.
- Mussa FF. Screening for abdominal aortic aneurysm. *J Vasc Surg.* 2015;62(3):774–778.
- Sweeting MJ, Thompson SG, Brown LC, et al; for RESCAN Collaborators. Meta-analysis of individual patient data to examine factors affecting growth and rupture of small abdominal aortic aneurysms. *Br J Surg.* 2012;99(5):655–665.

 SEE ALSO

Aortic Dissection; Arteritis, Temporal; Ehlers-Danlos Syndrome; Marfan Syndrome; Polyarteritis Nodosa; Turner Syndrome

CODES

ICD10
- I71.4 Abdominal aortic aneurysm, without rupture
- I71.3 Abdominal aortic aneurysm, ruptured

CLINICAL PEARLS

- Men with a smoking history aged 65 to 75 years should undergo a one-time screening abdominal ultrasound to evaluate for an AAA. Men and women with a first-degree relative with an AAA should be considered for a screening abdominal ultrasound.
- Larger AAAs should be screened more often, with elective repair with AAA >5.5 cm or an expansion of >0.5 cm every 6 months.
- Patients with a ruptured AAA present in shock, with abdominal pain and a pulsatile mass. A bedside ultrasound should be done quickly to evaluate for an AAA, or an emergent CT scan can be performed if the patient is hemodynamically stable.
- AAAs are treated either open or endovascularly as an elective or emergent procedure. 30-day and 1-year mortality between the two methods remain the same; however, there is increased mortality with an emergent AAA repair.
- Patients require aggressive risk factor modification, especially smoking cessation.

ANGIOEDEMA

Kathryn M. Brown, MD, MS • Katherine Montag Schafer, PharmD, BCACP

BASICS

- All patients presenting with angioedema (AE) should be treated with antihistamine, corticosteroids, and, if needed, epinephrine.
- If AE thought to be related to allergen exposure, to prevent recurrence, need to attempt to identify the causative agent and patient should be educated to avoid exposure.
- Recurrent AE not related to allergen exposure requires referral to specialist to clarify diagnosis and determine if alternative treatments are available.

DESCRIPTION

- AE is acute, localized swelling of skin, mucosa, and submucosa caused by extravasation of fluid into the affected tissues.
- AE commonly occurs as a part of the presentation of urticaria, but when it presents without wheals, it should be diagnosed as a distinct disease.
- AE develops in minutes to hours and resolves in hours to days but can be life-threatening if the upper airway is involved.
- Two major classifications of AE exist, both with unique subtypes (1),(2):
  - Acquired AE (AAE): involves all cases that are not considered to be hereditary AE (HAE)
    ○ Idiopathic histaminergic AAE (IH-AAE): no cause identified, response to antihistamine treatment
    ○ Idiopathic nonhistaminergic AAE (InH-AAE): no cause identified, no response to antihistamine treatment
    ○ Angiotensin-converting enzyme inhibitor (ACEI)-related AAE (ACEI-AAE)
    ○ C1-inhibitor (C1-INH) deficiency–related AAE (C1-INH-AAE)
  - HAE: mediated by changes in the genes that regulate the compliment cascade also known as bradykinin mediated AE
    ○ C1-INH HAE: caused by C1-INH deficiency
    ○ FXII-HAE: Patients have a normal C1-inhibitor but an FXII mutation.
    ○ U-HAE: Patients have a normal C1-inhibitor, unknown cause.
- Synonym(s): angioneurotic edema; Quincke edema

EPIDEMIOLOGY

- Predominant age of onset
  - AAE:
    ○ IH-AAE, InH-AAE, ACEI-AAE: any age
    ○ C1-INH-AAE: >40 years
  - HAE: infancy to 2nd decade of life
- Predominant gender: male = female, except FXII-HAE which predominantly affects females

Prevalence

- AAE:
  - IH-AAE: most common form of AE
  - ACEI-AAE: 0.1–2.2% of patients receiving ACEI
    ○ When compared to whites, the incidence of AE related to ACEI use are as high as 4 times that of whites. Note: Race is now recognized as a social, not biologic, construct and decisions about initiation of ACEI should not be influenced by self identified race.
  - C1-INH-AAE: 1:500,000
- HAE
  - C1-INH-HAE: 1:10,000 to 100,000

ETIOLOGY AND PATHOPHYSIOLOGY

- AAE:
  - IH-AAE: due to release of vasoactive substances
  - ACEI-AAE: thought to be due to elevated plasma levels of bradykinin
  - C1-INH-AAE: nongenetic changes to C1-INH function, can be due to autoantibodies
    ○ Can be associated with other lymphoproliferative conditions like systemic lupus erythematosus
- HAE:
  - Attacks are triggered by prolonged mechanical pressure, cold, heat, trauma, emotional stress, menses, illness, and inflammation.
  - C1-INH-HAE
    ○ Type I: decreased production of C1-INH
    ○ Type II: Normal or high levels of C1-INH; however, is dysfunctional
  - FXII-HAE
    ○ Normal C1-INH with presence of mutation in coagulation factor XII gene
    ○ Formerly type III HAE
    ○ Symptoms often estrogen dependent, provoked with estrogen administration (hormone replacement therapy or oral contraceptives) or with pregnancy
  - U-HAE
    ○ Normal C1-INH, without presence of factor XII gene mutation

Genetics

- HAE types I and II are autosomal dominant, whereas HAE with normal C1-INH is dominant X-linked.
- Spontaneous genetic mutations responsible for 25% of HAE cases

RISK FACTORS

- Consuming medications and foods that can cause allergic reactions
- Preexisting diagnosis of HAE or AAE
- Positive family history

GENERAL PREVENTION

- Avoid known triggers.
- Do not use ACE inhibitors in type I or II HAE.

COMMONLY ASSOCIATED CONDITIONS

- Quincke disease (AE of the uvula)
- Urticaria

DIAGNOSIS

- AAE:
  - Lack of positive family history of AE
  - Assess for:
    ○ Exposure to common allergens: foods, (shellfish, nuts, eggs, milk, wheat soy), latex, insect bites/stings, medication (antibiotics, aspirin, narcotics, NSAIDs, and OCPs)
      ▪ Allergy can be confirmed with positive skin prick test.
    ○ Exposure to ACE
    ○ Exposure to physical stimuli (cold or vibration)
  - If ACEI, allergy or other causes have been ruled out, then deemed idiopathic (IH-AAE).
    ○ If AE recurs despite prophylactic antihistamine use, then deemed InH-AAE.
- HAE:
  - Positive family history of AE in second-degree relative
  - C1-INH-HAE, FXII-HAE, and U-HAE require laboratory confirmation.

HISTORY

- Acute, typically asymmetric, swelling with onset in minutes to hours (3)
- In comparison with urticaria, AE presents without wheals, typically is nonpruritic but can cause a painful, burning sensation (3).
- Recent exposure to food allergens or medications (3)
- Identify potential triggers such as environmental exposure or trauma (3).
- Family history of AE (3)
- Recent infection, history of autoimmune disease, or malignancy (4)

PHYSICAL EXAM

- Vitals: Symptoms of hypotension, tachycardia, and tachypnea indicate systemic involvement and increased severity (4).
- Tense, nonpitting skin swelling that is skin colored or slightly erythematous (3)
- Commonly affects the mucous membranes of the face including periorbital, lips, tongue, or larynx but can involve any part of the body (3)
- Evaluate for involvement of oropharynx or symptoms such as stridor (4).
- GI tract involvement is more common in forms of HAE and may manifest as intermittent, unexplained abdominal pain (3).

ALERT

- Select history and exam findings increase the likelihood for early intubation and tracheostomy, including involvement of the anterior tongue, base of the tongue or larynx, stridor within 4 hours of onset of symptoms, and drooling (5)[C].
- Patients with HAE are at higher risk for intubation, tracheostomy, and death, although these complications can occur with any subtype (4)[C].

DIFFERENTIAL DIAGNOSIS

Urticaria; anaphylaxis; contact dermatitis; food/drug allergy; erysipelas; connective tissue disease: systemic lupus erythematosus, dermatomyositis; lymphedema; insect bite reaction; diffuse subcutaneous infiltrative process (6)[C]

DIAGNOSTIC TESTS & INTERPRETATION

Initial Tests (lab, imaging)

- Initial diagnosis should be based on history and clinical assessment alone (4)[C].
- Laboratory testing includes CBC, ESR, complement testing (C4, C1-INH, C1-INH function), allergy testing, and screening for paraproteinemia (SPEP, UPEP) (3)[C],(5).
- Complement testing assists in distinguishing between various types of AE; this assessment should be done in collaboration with an allergy specialist (5)[C]:
  - Low serum C4 is a sensitive but nonspecific screening test for hereditary and acquired C1-INH deficiency.
  - If C4 is normal, determine C1-INH level and function and recheck C4 during an acute attack.
  - If C4 level and C1-INH level and function are still normal, consider other causes and/or requires genetic assessment (i.e., FXII gene).
  - If C4 level, C1-INH level, and C1-INH function are low, these indicate C1-INH-HAE type I.
  - C1-INH-HAE, type II is characterized by low C4 and low C1-INH function, but C1-INH level can be normal or elevated.

- For recurrent AE with urticaria, complement levels should be obtained in addition to allergy testing for potential triggers (5)[C].
- Abdominal radiographs and CT scan can demonstrate GI AE or ileus (5)[C].
- C1-INH deficiency may occur in association with internal malignancy. In rare cases, AE can be a paraneoplastic disease. Imaging (CT scan, radiography, etc.) would be done as part of a neoplastic workup for patients with AAE (5)[C].

Follow-Up Tests & Special Considerations

If C4 and C1q antigen are low (as in AAE), neoplastic and autoimmune workup is warranted. CBC, a peripheral smear, protein electrophoresis, immunophenotyping of lymphocytes, and imaging studies are often undertaken to rule out hematologic malignancies or cancer (3)[C].

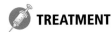 TREATMENT

GENERAL MEASURES

- Intubation if airway is threatened (4)[C]
- Eliminate suspected trigger (3)[C].
- Volume replacement is essential for patients who are unstable or refractory to initial therapy (4)[C].

MEDICATION

First Line

- If AE presenting with signs of anaphylaxis (hypotension, respiratory compromise): epinephrine 1:1,000; 0.1 mg/kg (maximum 0.3 mg for children, 0.5 mg for adults) intramuscularly q5–15min (4),(7)[C]
- If cause of AE is unknown, use first-line therapy:
  - Epinephrine, if airway involvement
  - H_1 antagonist (IV diphenhydramine, adult: 25 to 50 mg, children: 1 mg/kg, maximum 50 mg). In older adults, side effects can include delirium, urinary retention, constipation, and increased ocular pressure (4),(7)[C].
  - H_2 antagonists (IV ranitidine, adult: 50 mg, children: 1 mg/kg, maximum 50 mg) (4),(7)[C]
  - Corticosteroids (IV hydrocortisone, adult: 200 mg, children: maximum 100 mg; or IV methylprednisolone, adult: 50 to 100 mg, children: 1 mg/kg, maximum 50 mg) (4),(7)[C]
- IH-AAE (1),(5)
  - Acute treatment: first-line therapy, as above (4)
  - Prevention: second-generation antihistamines (cetirizine, fexofenadine, loratadine, etc.), administered daily; may need to escalate to higher than standard doses, up to 4 times labeled dosing, before considering treatment failure or alternative diagnosis, that is, InH-AAE (1)
- InH-AAE
  - Acute treatment: Antihistamines are ineffective; corticosteroids, epinephrine, if upper airway involvement
  - Prevention: Consider tranexamic acid: adult up to 3 g/day or specialty referral for immunosuppressive agents (1).
- ACEI-AAE
  - Acute treatment:
    - Remove causative agent.
    - May be ineffective: first-line therapy, as above
    - Off-label: bradykinin receptor antagonist (icatibant), C1-INH replacement (Berinert, Ruconest), kallikrein inhibitor (ecallantide)
  - Prevention: Remove causative agent; angiotensin receptor blockers (ARBs) are an appropriate substitute as the it has a low incidence of cross-reactivity.

- C1-INH-AAE
  - Acute treatment:
    - Off label: bradykinin receptor antagonist (icatibant), C1-INH replacement (Berinert, Ruconest), kallikrein inhibitor (ecallantide)
    - H1/H2 antagonists, corticosteroids, and epinephrine are ineffective and not recommended (8)[C].
    - Associated improvement through treatment of underlying disease (8)[C]
  - Prevention: possible remission through treatment of underlying disease
- FXII-HAE/U-HAE:
  - Patients with U-HAE/HXII-HAE do not respond to corticosteroids and antihistamine.
  - Treatment choice should be driven by allergy/immunology specialist and may include C1-INH agents, icatibant, ecallantide, progesterone, danazol, and tranexamic acid (1).
  - Prevention: in women, symptoms may be provoked by hormone therapy or pregnancy. Avoidance of these conditions may prevent clinical attacks (1).

Second Line

HAE acute treatment: FFP can be considered if first-line treatments unavailable; however, can potentially worsen attack, so caution is required (8)[C]

ISSUES FOR REFERRAL

Patients presenting with first episode of AE with a positive family history or recurrent AE will benefit from management from allergy/immunology specialist for diagnosis, treatment selection, education, and formation of emergency and procedural action plans (4)[C].

SURGERY/OTHER PROCEDURES

Tracheostomy if progressive laryngeal edema prevents endotracheal intubation

ADMISSION, INPATIENT, AND NURSING CONSIDERATIONS

Need for admission is based on severity of airway involvement. Ishoo criteria can be used for risk stratification. All patients with respiratory distress or in need of airway support will benefit from treatment in an intensive care unit (4)[C].

 ONGOING CARE

FOLLOW-UP RECOMMENDATIONS

Patient Monitoring

- Diagnostic workup if symptoms are severe, persistent, or recurrent
- For those with recurrent AE, specialty management is recommended.

DIET

Avoid identified food allergens.

PATIENT EDUCATION

Educate on avoidance of identified triggers, types of treatment, when to seek emergency care, and wearing medical alert bracelet.

PROGNOSIS

- AE symptoms often resolve in hours to 2 to 4 days. If airway is compromised, AE can be life-threatening.
- Patients with HAE have an average of 20 attacks per year; each may last 3 to 5 days. Prophylaxis can decrease the frequency of events and number of missed days of school or work.

COMPLICATIONS

Anaphylaxis

REFERENCES

1. Cicardi M, Aberer W, Baneri A, et al. Classification, diagnosis, and approach to treatment for angioedema: consensus report from the Hereditary Angioedema International Working Group. Allergy. 2014;69(5):602–616.
2. Reichman ME, Wernecke M, Graham DJ, et al. Antihypertensive drug associated angioedema: effect modification by race/ethnicity. Pharmacoepidemiol Drug Saf. 2017;26(10):1190–1196.
3. Temiño VM, Peebles RS Jr. The spectrum and treatment of angioedema. Am J Med. 2008;121(4):282–286.
4. Bernstein JA, Cremonesi P, Hoffmann TK, et al. Angioedema in the emergency department: a practical guide to differential diagnosis and management. Int J Emerg Med. 2017;10(1):15.
5. LoVerde D, Files DC, Krishnaswamy G. Angioedema. Crit Care Med. 2017;45(4):725–735.
6. Radonjic-Hoesli S, Hofmeier KS, Micaletto S, et al. Urticaria and angioedema: an update on classification and pathogenesis. Clin Rev Allergy Immunol. 2018;54(1):88–101.
7. Simons FE, Ardusso LR, Bilò MB, et al; for World Allergy Organization. World Allergy Organization anaphylaxis guidelines: summary. J Allergy Clin Immunol. 2011;127(3):587–593.
8. Zuraw BL, Bernstein JA, Lang DM, et al; for American Academy of Allergy, Asthma and Immunology, American College of Allergy, Asthma and Immunology. A focused parameter update: hereditary angioedema, acquired C1 inhibitor deficiency, and angiotensin-converting enzyme inhibitor-associated angioedema. J Allergy Clin Immunol. 2013;131(6):1491–1493.

 SEE ALSO

Anaphylaxis; Urticaria

CODES

ICD10

- T78.3XXA Angioneurotic edema, initial encounter
- D84.1 Defects in the complement system

CLINICAL PEARLS

- AE is an acute, localized swelling of skin, mucosa, and submucosa caused by extravasation of fluid into the affected tissues.
- If AE occurs in the presence of wheals, the patients should be diagnosed with urticaria and not AE.
- Onset is in minutes to hours and often resolves in hours to days, but it can be life-threatening if the upper airway is involved.
- There are two major classifications of AE: AAE and HAE.
- Any recurrent AE requires referral for specialist management.

ANKLE FRACTURES
Jeffrey P. Feden, MD, FACEP

BASICS

- Bones: tibia, fibula, talus
- Mortise: tibial plafond, medial and lateral malleolus
- Ligaments: syndesmotic, lateral collateral, and medial collateral (deltoid) ligament

DESCRIPTION

- Two common classification systems help describe fractures (but do not always predict fracture stability).
  - Danis-Weber system: based on level of the fibular fracture in relationship to the ankle joint
    - Type A (30%): below ankle joint; usually stable
    - Type B (63%): at the level of the ankle joint; may be stable or unstable
    - Type C (7%): above ankle joint; usually unstable
  - Lauge-Hansen (LH): based on foot position and direction of applied force relative to the tibia
    - Supination-adduction (SA)
    - Supination-external rotation (SER): most common (40–75% of fractures)
    - Pronation-abduction (PA)
    - Pronation-external rotation (PER)
- Stability-based classification
  - Stable
    - Isolated lateral malleolar fractures (Weber A/B) without talar shift and with negative stress test
    - Isolated nondisplaced medial malleolar fractures
  - Unstable
    - Bi- or trimalleolar fractures
    - High fibular fractures (Weber C) or lateral malleolar fracture with medial injury and positive stress test
    - Lateral malleolar fracture with talar shift/tilt (bimalleolar equivalent)
    - Displaced medial malleolar fractures
- Pilon fracture: tibial plafond fracture due to axial loading (unstable)
- Maisonneuve: fracture of proximal 1/3 of fibula associated with ankle fracture (unstable); high risk of peroneal nerve injury

Pediatric Considerations

- Ankle fractures are more common than sprains in children compared to adults because ligaments are stronger than physis.
- Talar dome: osteochondral fracture of talar dome; suspect in child with nonhealing ankle "sprain" or recurrent effusions
- Tillaux: isolated Salter-Harris III of distal tibia with growth plate involvement
- Triplane fracture: Salter-Harris IV with fracture lines oriented in multiple planes: 2-, 3-, and 4-part variants

EPIDEMIOLOGY

- Ankle fractures are responsible for 9% of all adult and 5% of all pediatric fractures.
- Peak incidence: females 45 to 64 years; males 8 to 15 years (Average is 46 years).

Incidence

107 to 184 per 100,000 people per year

ETIOLOGY AND PATHOPHYSIOLOGY

- Most common: falls (38%), inversion injury (32%), sports related (10%)
- Plantar flexion (joint less stable in this position)
- Axial loading: tibial plafond or pilon fracture

RISK FACTORS

- Age, fall, fracture history, polypharmacy, intoxication
- Obesity, sedentary lifestyle
- Sports, physical activity
- History of smoking or diabetes
- Alcohol or slippery surfaces

GENERAL PREVENTION

- Nonslip, flat, protective shoes
- Fall precautions in elderly

COMMONLY ASSOCIATED CONDITIONS

- Most ankle fractures are isolated injuries, but 5% have associated fractures, usually in ipsilateral lower limb.
- Ligamentous or cartilage injury (sprains)
- Ankle or subtalar dislocation
- Other axial loading or shearing injuries (i.e., vertebral compression or contralateral pelvic fractures)

DIAGNOSIS

HISTORY

- Location of pain, timing, and mechanism of injury (Key historical element is exact mechanism.)
- Weight-bearing status after injury
- History of ankle injury or surgery
- Tetanus status
- Assess for safety and fall risk (especially in elderly).

PHYSICAL EXAM

- Examine skin integrity (open vs. closed fracture).
- Assess point of maximal tenderness.
- Assess neurovascular status and ability to bear weight.
- Consider associated injuries.
- Assess ankle stability: anterior drawer test for the anterior talofibular ligament (ATFL), talar tilt test for lateral and medial ligaments, squeeze test and external rotation stress test for the tibiofibular syndesmosis.

DIFFERENTIAL DIAGNOSIS

- Ankle sprain
- Other fractures: talus, 5th metatarsal, calcaneus

DIAGNOSTIC TESTS & INTERPRETATION

- Plain radiographs: first line for suspected fractures based on pretest probability (Ottawa Rules)
- Ottawa Ankle Rules (OAR): Overall sensitivity of 98% in adults increases to 99.6% if applied within the first 48 hours after trauma (1)[A].
- OAR: obtain films in patients aged 18 to 55 years if:
  - Tenderness at the posterior edge of distal 6 cm of tibia or tip of the medial malleolus, or
  - Tenderness at the posterior edge or distal 6 cm of fibula or tip of the lateral malleolus, or
  - Inability to bear weight both immediately and in the ED for four steps, or
  - Tenderness at navicular or 5th metatarsal (Ottawa Foot Rules)

- If initial x-ray is normal, but severe symptoms persist past 48 to 72 hours, obtain repeat x-rays.
- In children >1 year old, OAR sensitivity is 98.5%.
- OAR not valid for intoxicated patients, those with multiple injuries, or sensory deficits (neuropathy)
- Three standard views
  - Anteroposterior (AP)
  - Lateral: Talar dome/distal tibia incongruity indicates instability.
  - Mortise (15- to 25-degree internal rotation view): symmetry of mortise; space between the medial malleolus and talus should be ≤4 mm.
  - Additional stress view may demonstrate instability (e.g., increased medial clear space with manual external rotation).

Pediatric Considerations

- Consider tenderness over distal fibula with normal films as Salter-Harris I.
- Stress views unnecessary in children and may cause physeal damage.
- Salter-Harris V often missed, diagnosed when leg length discrepancy or angular deformity after Salter-Harris I; rare, 1% of fractures

Follow-Up Tests & Special Considerations

- CT recommended for operative planning in trimalleolar, Tillaux, triplane, pilon fractures, or fractures with intra-articular involvement
- MRI not routinely indicated; does not increase sensitivity for detecting complex ankle fractures
  - MRI useful for chronic instability, osteochondral lesions, occult fractures, and unexpected stiffness in children

Diagnostic Procedures/Other

- Ultrasound for soft tissue injury associated with displaced fractures
- Bone scan or MRI for stress fracture

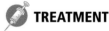

TREATMENT

GENERAL MEASURES

- Immobilize in temporary cast/splint and protect with crutches/non–weight-bearing.
  - 1 to 2 weeks to allow decreased swelling, if not open or irreducible fracture (2)[C]
- Ice and elevate the extremity; pain due to swelling best controlled with elevation
  - Compression stockings offer no benefit for swelling (3)[A].
- Closed ankle fractures—must determine stability
  - Stable = nonoperative
  - Unstable = surgery
  - Lateral shift of talus ≥2 mm or displacement of either malleolus by 2 to 3 mm = surgery (2)[C]
  - In adults with displaced fractures: insufficient evidence if surgery or nonoperative management produces superior long-term outcomes (4)[A]
- Stable syndesmosis injury = nonoperative
- Fracture dislocations: urgent reduction
  - Do not wait for imaging if neurovascular compromise or obvious deformity.
  - Flex hip and knee 90 degrees for easier reduction.
  - Postreduction: neurovascular exam and x-rays

MEDICATION

First Line
- NSAIDs and/or acetaminophen for pain
- Initial IM pain injection (i.e., ketorolac, ≥50-kg adult: 60 mg or 30 mg q6h, max 120 mg daily; children 2 to 16 years old, <50 kg or age of ≥65 years: 1 mg/kg, 30 mg, or 15 mg q6h, max 60 mg daily)
- For suspected open fractures: tetanus booster, broad-spectrum cephalosporin and aminoglycoside within 3 hours postinjury (2)[C]
- Intra-articular or hematoma block

Second Line
Opioid analgesics as adjunctive therapy

ISSUES FOR REFERRAL
- Consultation for neurovascular compromise, tenting of skin or open fracture, displaced or unstable fracture, compartment syndrome
- All other fractures: Follow up within 1 week and remain non–weight-bearing. Consult orthopedics if uncomfortable with routine fracture management.

ADDITIONAL THERAPIES
- Nonoperative = cast immobilization
  - No difference in type of immobilization (Air-Stirrup, cast, orthosis) (3)[A]
  - Initially non–weight-bearing with crutches and then advance to 50% with crutches; full weight-bearing after 6 weeks postinjury
  - If removable cast, gentle range of motion exercises at 4 weeks
- Open ankle fractures (2%)
  - Remove gross debris/contamination in ED.
  - Duration of optimal antibiotic therapy controversial
  - Surgical emergency; best if repaired within 24 hours

SURGERY/OTHER PROCEDURES
- Surgical options
  - Open reduction and internal fixation (ORIF); preferred in athletes and unstable fractures
  - External fixation may be preferred in extreme tissue injury or comminuted fractures; may have more malunion compared to ORIF but no difference in wound complications
- Timing of surgery
  - Immediately if neurovascular compromise, open fracture, unsuccessful reduction, tissue necrosis (2)[C]
  - Otherwise delay >5 days postinjury because inflammation can affect wound healing (2)[C].
- Length of recovery is usually 6 to 8 weeks.

Pediatric Considerations
- Salter-Harris I and II = nonoperative
  - Distal tibia: long leg cast for 4 to 6 weeks and then short leg cast for 2 to 3 weeks (5)[C]
  - Distal fibula: posterior splint or ankle brace 3 to 4 weeks, weight-bearing; if displaced, then short leg cast 4 to 6 weeks, non–weight-bearing (5)[C]
  - Limit reduction attempts because of potential injury to growth plate (5),(6)[C].
  - Reduction not recommended if presenting ≥1 week postinjury (5)[C]
  - Intra-articular displacement of ≥2 mm in child with >2 years growth remaining = ORIF (6)[C]

- Salter-Harris III and IV:
  - Distal tibia: if >2 mm displacement = ORIF (6)[C]
  - Distal fibula: rare, usually stable after tibial reduction (6)[C]
  - Tillaux and triplane: ORIF if displaced ≥2 mm (5),(6)[C]

Geriatric Considerations
- Higher surgical risk due to age/comorbidities
- Osteoporosis increases risk of implant/fixation failure (4)[A].
- Risks from surgery/anesthesia: wound healing problems, pulmonary embolism, mortality, amputation, reoperation

ADMISSION, INPATIENT, AND NURSING CONSIDERATIONS
- Admit if:
  - Emergency surgery required
  - Patient nonadherent, lacks social support, unable to maintain non–weight-bearing status, or has significant associated injuries
  - Concerning mechanism of injury (i.e., syncope, myocardial infarction, head injury)
- Nursing: non–weight-bearing; maintain splint/cast; apply ice; keep leg elevated; pain control; assist ADLs.
- Discharge criteria:
  - Ambulates with walker or crutches
  - Medical workup (if needed) completed
  - Orthopedic follow-up arranged

 ONGOING CARE

FOLLOW-UP RECOMMENDATIONS
Patient Monitoring
- Orthopedic follow-up: serial x-rays
  - In children, sclerotic lines on x-ray (Parker-Harris growth arrest lines) indicate growth disturbance (5)[C].
- Immobilize for 4 to 6 weeks and then progressive activity, weight-bearing, with removable splint or boot (3)[A].
- Physical therapy referral: no difference in outcomes between stretching, manual therapy, exercise program (3)[A].

DIET
NPO if surgery is being considered

PATIENT EDUCATION
- Ice and elevate for 2 to 3 weeks; use crutches/cane as instructed; splint/cast care (avoid getting wet, etc.)
- Notify physician if swelling increases, paresthesias, pain, or change in color of extremity.

PROGNOSIS
- Good results can be achieved without surgery if fracture is stable.
  - Most return to activity within 3 to 4 months.
- Most athletes return to preinjury activity levels.
- Increasing age, not injury severity, is associated with worsening mobility after fracture.

COMPLICATIONS
- Displaced fracture or instability
- Delayed union, malunion, or nonunion (0.9–1.9%)
- Postsurgical wound problems: loss of fixation, further surgery, amputation
- Deep venous thrombosis
- Complex regional pain syndrome, extensor retinaculum syndrome in children (5)[C]
- Infection (osteomyelitis)
- Posttraumatic arthritis, degenerative joint disease, growth arrest in children

REFERENCES
1. Polzer H, Kanz KG, Prall WC, et al. Diagnosis and treatment of acute ankle injuries: development of an evidence-based algorithm. Orthop Rev (Pavia). 2012;4(1):e5.
2. Mandi DM. Ankle fractures. Clin Podiatr Med Surg. 2012;29(2):155–186.
3. Lin CW, Donkers NA, Refshauge KM, et al. Rehabilitation for ankle fractures in adults. Cochrane Database Syst Rev. 2012;(11):CD005595.
4. Donken CC, Al-Khateeb H, Verhofstad MH, et al. Surgical versus conservative interventions for treating ankle fractures in adults. Cochrane Database Syst Rev. 2012;(8):CD008470.
5. Parrino A, Lee MC. Ankle fractures in children. Curr Orthop Pract. 2013;24:617–624.
6. Kay RM, Matthys GA. Pediatric ankle fractures: evaluation and treatment. J Am Acad Orthop Surg. 2001;9(4):268–278.

 CODES

ICD10
- S82.899A Oth fracture of unsp lower leg, init for clos fx
- S82.899B Oth fracture of unsp lower leg, init for opn fx type I/2
- S82.56XA Nondisp fx of medial malleolus of unsp tibia, init

CLINICAL PEARLS
- OAR are nearly 100% sensitive in determining the need for x-rays.
- Assess neurovascular status, ability to bear weight, and associated injuries.
- Assess joint above/below to avoid overlooking extent of injury (i.e., Maisonneuve).
- Normal x-rays with point tenderness suggest Salter-Harris type I fractures in children.
- Assessment of fracture stability (using classification systems) often dictates conservative versus operative management.

ANKYLOSING SPONDYLITIS

Lindsay N. Moy, DO • Abdul Salman Mohammed, MBBS, MD, RhMSUS

BASICS

DESCRIPTION
- Ankylosing spondylitis (AS) is an axial inflammatory spondyloarthropathy (axSpA) characterized by chronic low back pain (>3 months duration) and evidence of sacroiliitis (sclerosis, erosions, and changes in joint width) on plain radiography.
- Systems affected: musculoskeletal; ophthalmic; cardiovascular; neurologic; pulmonary
- Synonyms: Marie–Strümpell disease; "bamboo spine"

EPIDEMIOLOGY
- Peak age of onset 20 to 30; rarely occurs after age 40 years
- Male > female (approximately 2 to 3:1)

Incidence
Age- and gender-adjusted rate of 6.3 to 7.3/100,000 person-years

Prevalence
~0.55% for AS and ~1.4% for all axSpA in the United States (1)

ETIOLOGY AND PATHOPHYSIOLOGY
- Autoinflammation at sites of bacterial exposure (e.g., intestines) or mechanical stress in genetically susceptible individuals (2)
- Inflammation at the insertion of tendons, ligaments, and fasciae to bone (enthesopathy) causes erosion, remodeling, and new bone formation.

Genetics
- 85–95% of patients with AS are *HLA-B27*–positive.
- Other genetic associations include endoplasmic reticulum aminopeptidase 1 (*ERAP1*), interleukin-23 receptor (*IL23R*), and gene deserts on chromosome *2p15* and *21q22* (2).

RISK FACTORS
Positive family history
- HLA-B27–positive child of a parent with AS has a 10–30% risk of developing the disease.

COMMONLY ASSOCIATED CONDITIONS
- Peripheral arthritis (30%)
- Enthesopathy (29%): Achilles tendonitis, plantar fasciitis
- Uveitis (25–35%)
- Psoriasis (10%)
- Dactylitis "sausage digit" (6%)
- Inflammatory bowel disease "IBD" (4%) (3)[A]
- Peripheral spondyloarthritis (SpA): psoriatic arthritis, reactive arthritis, IBD-related arthritis, juvenile idiopathic arthritis
- Aortitis, aortic regurgitation, and cardiac conduction defects

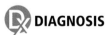

DIAGNOSIS

HISTORY
- Inflammatory back pain
  - Insidious onset typically at age <40; duration >3 months; morning stiffness in spine lasting >1 hour; nighttime awakenings secondary to back pain; pain and stiffness increase at rest and improve with activity.

- Alternating buttock/hip pain and constitutional symptoms (fatigue, poor sleep, weight loss, low-grade fever) are common.
- Other symptoms associated with enthesopathy (Achilles tendon pain, plantar fascia pain), dactylitis (sausage digits), iritis (unilateral pain, red eye, photophobia, vision changes/blurring)

PHYSICAL EXAM
- Sacroiliac joint tenderness, loss of lumbar lordosis, and cervical spine rotation
- Diminished range of motion in the lumbar spine in all three planes of motion
- Modified Wright-Schober test for lumbar spine flexion:
  - Mark patient's back over the L5 spinous process (or at the dimples of Venus) and measure 10 cm above and 5 cm below this point. Instruct the patient to flex forward at the hip. Normal is at least 5 cm of expansion between these two marks on maximal flexion.
- Thoracocervical kyphosis (usually after at least 10 years of symptoms)
  - Occiput–wall distance increased (distance between occiput and wall when standing with back flat against a vertical surface; zero is normal)
- Respiratory excursion of chest wall decreased
  - Measure circumference of chest wall at the 4th intercostal space. Normal is an increase >5 cm during maximal respiratory excursion; <2.5 cm is consistent with AS.
- Tenderness of tendon insertional sites—Achilles, plantar fascia
- Peripheral oligoarthritis/dactylitis seen mostly with peripheral SpA
- Extra-articular manifestations: uveitis, psoriasis, IBD
- Aortic regurgitation murmur (1%)

DIFFERENTIAL DIAGNOSIS
- Mechanical low back pain
- Nonradiographic axSpA (features of AS with evidence of sacroiliitis on MRI but not on plain radiographs—can progress to AS)
- Other inflammatory arthritis
- Osteoarthritis or erosive osteochondritis of the axial spine
- Diffuse idiopathic skeletal hyperostosis (DISH)
- Osteitis condensans ilii: benign sclerotic changes in the iliac portion of the SI joint after pregnancy
- Infectious arthritis or discitis, unilateral sacroiliitis: tuberculosis, brucellosis, bacterial infection (particularly in IV drug users)
- Vertebral compression fracture
- Familial Mediterranean fever
- Fibromyalgia—tender points can mimic enthesitis findings

DIAGNOSTIC TESTS & INTERPRETATION
- ESR and C-reactive protein (CRP) may be mildly elevated or normal; if high, correlates with disease activity and prognosis
- Absence of rheumatoid factor
- Mild normochromic anemia (15%)
- Mild elevation of alkaline phosphatase may be present in severe disease.
- Synovial fluid: mild leukocytosis

- SI joints: Oblique projection is preferred.
  - Joint abnormalities are graded as detailed below:
    - Grade 0: normal; grade 1: suspected joint changes; grade 2: mild erosions or sclerosis without joint width changes; grade 3: moderate or severe sacroiliitis with erosions, sclerosis, increased joint space, or partial ankylosis; grade 4: complete ankylosis
- Spine: lateral view preferred
  - Early plain radiograph changes: "shiny corners" due to osteitis and sclerosis at site of annulus fibrosus attachments to the corners of vertebral bodies with "squaring" due to erosion and remodeling of vertebral body; contrast-enhanced MRI is more sensitive for detecting early changes.
  - Late changes: ossification of annulus fibrosis resulting in bony bridging between vertebral bodies (syndesmophytes) giving classic "bamboo spine" appearance; ankylosis of apophyseal joints, ossification of spinal ligaments, and/or spondylodiscitis also occurs.
- Peripheral joints
  - Asymmetric pericapsular ossification, sclerosis, loss of joint space, and erosions may occur.
  - Ultrasound can be used to identify enthesitis.

Initial Tests (lab, imaging)
Diagnosis is based off of the Assessment of SpondyloArthritis international Society (ASAS) modified Berlin algorithm:
- If a patient has low back pain for at least 3 months and there is concern for AS based off of history and physical, obtain an anterior-posterior x-ray of the sacroiliac joints.
  - If sacroiliitis is noted to be grade 2 bilaterally or grade 3 unilaterally and the patient has at least one other typical SpA symptom (as listed below), this is sufficient for diagnosis of AS.
  - If the plain AP x-ray is negative for sacroiliitis, but the patient has at least 4 of the following 11 symptoms, this is considered sufficient for diagnosis of AS: inflammatory back pain; heel pain (enthesopathy); dactylitis; uveitis; positive family history for SpA; inflammatory bowel disease; alternating buttock pain; psoriasis; asymmetric arthritis; positive response to NSAIDs; elevated ESR or CRP.
  - If the plain AP x-ray is negative for sacroiliitis and the patient has 2 to 3 of the above symptoms, a positive HLA-B27 is enough for diagnosis.
  - If the plain AP x-ray is negative for sacroiliitis and the patient only has 0 to 1 of the above symptoms, as well as a positive HLA-B27, further workup is recommended with MRI sacrum to assess for sacroiliitis.

Test Interpretation
Erosive changes and new bone formation at bony attachment of the tendons and ligaments result in ossification of periarticular soft tissues.

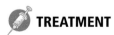

TREATMENT

GENERAL MEASURES
- Symptom control, maintaining spinal flexibility and normal posture, reducing functional limitations, maintaining work ability, and decreasing disease complications are primary treatment goals.
- Aggressive physical therapy is the most important nonpharmacologic management.

MEDICATION

First Line

- Nonsteroidal anti-inflammatory drugs (NSAIDs) are first-line pharmacologic agent for pain and stiffness in AS (4)[A].
  - Naproxen, up to 500 mg BID; celecoxib, up to 200 mg BID; ibuprofen, up to 800 mg TID
- Precautions
  - Consider CVD, GI, and renal risks of NSAIDs. Use with caution in patients with a bleeding diathesis or on anticoagulants.
- Injection of intra-articular corticosteroids into SI joints and prostheses can provide transient relief, but systemic corticosteroids are not recommended (5)[C].
- Surgery may be an option for those with atlantoaxial subluxation complicated by neurologic impairment.

Pregnancy Considerations

Infants exposed to NSAIDs in 1st trimester may have a higher incidence of cardiac malformations.

Second Line

- Biologic agents: tumor necrosis factor (TNF)-α antagonists
  - Recommended for active disease after lack of response to at least two different NSAIDs over 1 month (5)[C]
  - FDA-approved agents for AS include etanercept (recombinant TNF receptor fusion protein), infliximab (chimeric monoclonal IgG1 antibody to TNF-α), adalimumab (fully humanized IgG1 monoclonal antibody to TNF-α), golimumab (human IgG1 kappa monoclonal antibody to TNF-α), and certolizumab pegol (pegylated humanized monoclonal antibody to TNF-α).
- Precautions with TNF-α blockers
  - Anti-TNFs increase the risk of serious bacterial, mycobacterial, fungal, opportunistic, and viral infections. Screen for tuberculosis and hepatitis B.
  - Lymphomas, nonmelanoma skin cancers, and other malignancies have been reported in patients receiving anti-TNFs.
  - Immunizations (especially live vaccines) should be updated before initiating anti-TNFs; live vaccines are contraindicated once patients receive anti-TNFs.
- Disease-modifying antirheumatic drugs (DMARDs), such as methotrexate and sulfasalazine, are ineffective for axial disease; sulfasalazine may be effective for peripheral arthritis; this class may be considered in patients with contraindications to TNF agents (5)[C].

ISSUES FOR REFERRAL

- Coordinate care with a rheumatologist for diagnosis, monitoring, and management (anti-TNF therapy).
- Management of aortic regurgitation, uveitis, spinal fractures, pulmonary fibrosis, hip joint involvement, renal amyloidosis, and cauda equina syndrome may require referral to appropriate specialty.

ADDITIONAL THERAPIES

Bisphosphonate medications if osteopenia or osteoporosis is present

SURGERY/OTHER PROCEDURES

- Evaluate for C-spine ankylosis/instability before intubation in patients with AS undergoing surgery.
- Vertebral osteotomy can improve posture for patients with severe cervical or thoracolumbar flexion.

ONGOING CARE

FOLLOW-UP RECOMMENDATIONS

Patient Monitoring

- Monitor posture and range of motion with 6- to 12-month visits; increase frequency if higher disease activity.
- Bath Ankylosing Spondylitis Disease Activity Index (BASDAI) or Ankylosing Spondylitis Disease Activity Score (ASDAS) can be used to measure disease activity.
- Fall prevention/evaluation
- Regular-interval monitoring of CRP or ESR
- Screening for osteopenia/osteoporosis with dual energy x-ray absorptiometry scan

PATIENT EDUCATION

- Maintain physical activity and posture.
- Swimming, water aerobics, tai chi, and walking are excellent activities.
- Avoid trauma/contact sports.
- Arthritis Foundation: http://www.arthritis.org
- Spondylitis Association of America: http://www.spondylitis.org

PROGNOSIS

Extent and rapidity of progression of ankylosis are highly variable.

COMPLICATIONS

- MSK/spine: osteoporosis, spinal fusion causing kyphosis, c-spine fracture or subluxation, cauda equina syndrome (rare)
- Pulmonary: restrictive lung disease, upper lobe fibrosis (rare)
- Cardiac: conduction defects at atrioventricular (AV) node, aortic insufficiency, aortitis, pericarditis (extremely rare)
- Eye: uveitis, cataracts
- Renal: IgA nephropathy, amyloidosis ($<1\%$)
- GI: microscopic, subclinical ileal, and colonic mucosal ulcerations in up to 50% of patients, mostly asymptomatic

REFERENCES

1. Reveille JD, Weisman MH. The epidemiology of back pain, axial spondyloarthritis and HLA-B27 in the United States. *Am J Med Sci*. 2013;345(6): 431–436.
2. Dougados M, Baeten D. Spondyloarthritis. *Lancet*. 2011;377(9783):2127–2137.
3. de Winter JJ, van Mens LJ, van der Heijde D, et al. Prevalence of peripheral and extra-articular disease in ankylosing spondylitis versus non-radiographic axial spondyloarthritis: a meta-analysis. *Arthritis Res Ther*. 2016;18(1):196.
4. Kroon FP, van der Burg LR, Ramiro S, et al. Nonsteroidal anti-inflammatory drugs (NSAIDs) for axial spondyloarthritis (ankylosing spondylitis and non-radiographic axial spondyloarthritis). *Cochrane Database Syst Rev*. 2015;(7):CD010952.
5. Ward MM, Deodhar A, Akl EA, et al. American College of Rheumatology/Spondylitis Association of America/Spondyloarthritis Research and Treatment Network 2015 recommendations for the treatment of ankylosing spondylitis and nonradiographic axial spondyloarthritis. *Arthritis Rheumatol*. 2016;68(2):282–298.

ADDITIONAL READING

- Adams K, Bombardier C, van der Heijde DM. Safety of pain therapy during pregnancy and lactation in patients with inflammatory arthritis: a systematic literature review. *J Rheumatol Suppl*. 2012;90:59–61.
- Garg N, van den Bosch F, Deodhar A. The concept of spondyloarthritis: where are we now? *Best Pract Res Clin Rheumatol*. 2014;28(5):663–672.
- Gensler L, Inman R, Deodhar A. The "knowns" and "unknowns" of biologic therapy in ankylosing spondylitis. *Am J Med Sci*. 2012;343(5):360–363.
- Jo S, Han J, Lee YL, et al. Regulation of osteoblasts by alkaline phosphatase in ankylosing spondylitis. *Ann Rheum Dis*. 2019;22(2):252–261.
- Mease PJ. Fibromyalgia, a missed comorbidity in spondyloarthritis: prevalence and impact on assessment and treatment. *Curr Opin Rheumatol*. 2017;29(4):304–310.
- Rudwaleit M, van der Heijde D, Khan MA, et al. How to diagnose axial spondyloarthritis early. *Ann Rheum Dis*. 2004;53(5):535–543.
- Sieper J. Treatment challenges in axial spondylarthritis and future directions. *Curr Rheumatol Rep*. 2013;15(9):356. doi:10.1007/s11926-013-0356-9.
- Sieper J, Rudwaleit M, Baraliakos X, et al. The Assessment of Spondyloarthritis International Society (ASAS) handbook: a guide to assess spondyloarthritis. *Ann Rheum Dis*. 2009;68(Suppl 2):ii1–ii44.
- van der Heijde D, Ramiro S, Landewé R, et al. 2016 Update of the ASAS-EULAR management recommendations for axial spondyloarthritis. *Ann Rheum Dis*. 2017;76(6):978–991.

SEE ALSO

Arthritis, Psoriatic; Arthritis, Rheumatoid (RA); Crohn Disease; Reactive Arthritis (Reiter Syndrome); Ulcerative Colitis

CODES

ICD10

- M45.0 Ankylosing spondylitis of multiple sites in spine
- M45.6 Ankylosing spondylitis lumbar region
- M45.7 Ankylosing spondylitis of lumbosacral region

CLINICAL PEARLS

- Diagnosis of AS is suggested by a history of inflammatory back pain, evidence of limited chest wall expansion, restricted spinal motion in all planes, radiographic evidence of sacroiliitis, and a therapeutic response to NSAIDs.
- HLA-B27 testing supports the diagnosis if clinical features are not definitive.
- MRI is more sensitive at detecting SI joint inflammation than plain radiography.
- Physical therapy is important in helping to maintain posture and mobility.
- NSAIDs and TNF-α blockers are the mainstays of pharmacologic treatment of AS.

ANOREXIA NERVOSA

Anqi Li, DO • Alhang Konyak, MD, FAAFP

BASICS

DESCRIPTION
- An eating disorder characterized by the restriction of food intake leading to significantly low weight with intense fear of weight gain
- *Diagnostic and Statistical Manual of Mental Disorders*, 5th edition (*DSM-5*), divides anorexia into two types:
  - Restricting type: not engaged in binge eating or purging behaviors (last 3 months)
  - Binge eating/purging type: regularly engaged in binge eating or purging behaviors (last 3 months)
- System(s) affected: nervous, cardiovascular, endocrine, metabolic, pulmonary, gastrointestinal, reproductive, ophthalmic, taste, and dermatologic
- Severity of anorexia nervosa (AN) is based on BMI (per *DSM-5*):
  - Mild: BMI $\geq$17 kg/m^2
  - Moderate: BMI 16.00 to 16.99 kg/m^2
  - Severe: BMI 15.00 to 15.99 kg/m^2
  - Extreme: BMI <15 kg/m^2

EPIDEMIOLOGY
- Predominant age: 15 to 24 years
- Predominant sex: female > male (10:1 to 20:1 female-to-male ratio)

Prevalence
- 0.9–2.0% in women (1.1–3.0% in young females)
- 0.1–0.3% in men (higher in gay and bisexual men)

ETIOLOGY AND PATHOPHYSIOLOGY
- Complex relationships among genetic, biologic, environmental, psychological, and social factors that result in the development of this disorder
- Parenting style that leads to high expectation may result in children struggle for control.
- Serotonin, norepinephrine, and dopamine neuronal systems are implicated.

Genetics
- Evidence of higher concordance rates in monozygotic than in dizygotic twins
- First-degree female relative with eating disorder increases risk 6- to 10-fold.
- One genome-wide significant locus identified for AN on chromosome 12

RISK FACTORS
- Female gender
- Adolescence
- Body dissatisfaction, negative self-evaluation
- Perfectionism, high parental demands, academic pressure, severe life stressors
- History of sexual or physical abuse
- Participation in sports or activities that emphasize leanness: ballet, figure skating, gymnastics, cheerleading
- Type 1 diabetes mellitus
- Family history of substance abuse, affective disorders, or eating disorders

GENERAL PREVENTION
Prevention programs can reduce risk factors and future onset of eating disorders.
- Target adolescents and young women $\geq$15 years of age.
- Encourage realistic and healthy weight management strategies and attitudes.

- Promote self-esteem.
- Reduce focus on thin as ideal.
- Decrease co-occurring anxiety/depressive symptoms and improve stress management.

COMMONLY ASSOCIATED CONDITIONS
- Suicide, mood and anxiety disorders
- Substance use disorder
- Cluster C personality disorder

DIAGNOSIS

HISTORY
- Onset may be insidious or stress related.
- Patient unlikely to self-identify problem
- Restriction of required energy intake, leading to significantly low body weight
- Fear of weight gain and/or distorted body image
- Report feeling fat even when emaciated
- Preoccupation with body size, weight control
- Elaborate food preparation and eating rituals
- Other possible signs and symptoms:
  - Extensive exercise
  - Amenorrhea
  - Weakness, fatigue, cognitive impairment
  - Cold intolerance
  - Constipation, bloating, early satiety
  - Growth arrest, delayed puberty
  - Fractures
- Screening
  - Clinician-administered eating disorder screen for primary care to identify patients with eating disorders
    - Are you satisfied with your eating patterns? (No is abnormal.)
    - Do you ever eat in secret? (Yes is abnormal.)
    - Does your weight affect the way you feel about yourself? (Yes is abnormal.)
    - Have any members of your family suffered with an eating disorder? (Yes is abnormal.)
    - Do you currently suffer with or have you ever suffered in the past with an eating disorder? (Yes is abnormal.)

PHYSICAL EXAM
- May be normal
- Abnormal vital signs: hypothermia, bradycardia, orthostatic hypotension
- Body weight <85% of expected (may wear extra clothes or hide heavy objects to increase weight on scale)
- Cardiac: dysrhythmias, midsystolic click from mitral valve prolapse
- Skin/extremities: dry skin; lanugo hair on extremities, face, and trunk; hair loss; peripheral edema
- Neurologic and abdominal exams: to rule out other causes of weight loss and vomiting
- Gynecologic: amenorrhea

DIFFERENTIAL DIAGNOSIS
- Hyperthyroidism, adrenal insufficiency
- IBS, malabsorption
- Immunodeficiency, chronic infections
- Uncontrolled diabetes
- Bulimia, body dysmorphic disorder
- Depressive, anxiety, or conversion disorders

DIAGNOSTIC TESTS & INTERPRETATION
Screening tools:
- SCOFF questionnaire (1)[B]
- Eating Disorder Screen for Primary Care

Initial Tests (lab, imaging)
- Vitals: hypotension, bradycardia, hypothermia
- UA: low specific gravity, ketone, low urine creatinine excretion
- CBC: anemia, leukopenia, thrombocytopenia
- Low-serum LH, FSH; low-serum testosterone in men
- Thyroid function tests: low thyroid-stimulating hormone with normal T_3/T_4
- LFT: abnormal liver enzymes
- Chem 7: altered BUN, creatinine clearance; electrolyte disturbances including hyponatremia, hypokalemia
- Hypoglycemia, hypercholesterolemia, hypercortisolemia, hypophosphatemia, hypomagnesemia
- Low vitamin D and hypocalcemia
- 12-Lead ECG to assess for prolonged QT interval
- If underweight for >6 months: DEXA scan to assess for diminished bone density

Follow-Up Tests & Special Considerations
Weighting is an anxiety-provoking test but an important marker to assess progress. Ask staff to be nonjudgmental. Try to weight patients in a gown, as many may intend to exaggerate their weight by hiding heavy objects or wearing baggy clothes.

Test Interpretation
- Osteoporosis/osteopenia, pathologic fractures
- Sick euthyroid syndrome, dehydration
- Cardiac impairment
- Renal impairment
- AN may exist concurrently with chronic medical disorders.

TREATMENT

GENERAL MEASURES
- OP treatment:
  - Interdisciplinary team (primary care physician, mental health provider, dietitian)
  - Average weekly weight gain goal: 0.5 to 1.0 kg, with stepwise increase in calories
  - CBT
  - Focus on health, not weight gain alone.
  - Build trust and a treatment alliance.
  - Involve the patient in establishing diet and exercise goals.
  - Help the patient to recognize feelings that lead to disordered eating.
  - In chronic cases, goal may be to achieve a safe weight rather than a healthy weight.
- Inpatient treatment:
  - If possible, admit to a specialized eating disorders unit.
  - Monitor vital signs, electrolytes, cardiac function, edema, and weight.
  - Assess risk for refeeding syndrome.
  - Initial supervised meals may be necessary.
  - Stepwise increase in activity
  - Tube feeding or TPN is used only as a last resort.

- Psychotherapy (e.g., CBT or family therapy) should be offered (2),(3)[A].
- CBT has demonstrated effectiveness as a means of improving treatment adherence and minimizing dropout among patients with AN (4)[A].

MEDICATION

First Line

- No medications are available that effectively treat patients with AN, but pharmacotherapy may be used as an adjuvant to CBTs (5)[A].
- If medications are used, start with low doses due to increased risk for adverse effects.
- SSRIs may:
  - Help to prevent relapse after weight gain
  - Treat comorbid depression or OCD
  - Use of atypical antipsychotics is being studied with mixed findings to date. Olanzapine is potentially beneficial as an adjuvant treatment of underweight individuals in the inpatient settings.
- Attend to black box warnings.
- Bupropion should be avoided because it is associated with a higher incidence of seizures.

Second Line

- Management of osteopenia:
  - Primary treatment is weight gain.
  - Elemental calcium 1,200 to 1,500 mg/day plus vitamin D 800 IU/day
  - No indication for bisphosphonates in AN
  - Weak evidence for use of hormone-replacement therapy
- Psyllium to prevent constipation

ISSUES FOR REFERRAL

Patients with AN require an interdisciplinary team (primary care physician, mental health provider, nutritionist).

COMPLEMENTARY & ALTERNATIVE MEDICINE

- Acupuncture
- Relaxation therapy

ADMISSION, INPATIENT, AND NURSING CONSIDERATIONS

- Suggested physiologic values to admit: heart rate <40 beats/min, BP <90/60 mm Hg, symptomatic hypoglycemia, temperature <97.0°F (36.1°C), dehydration, other cardiovascular abnormalities, weight <75% of expected, rapid weight loss, lack of improvement while in OP therapy
- Suggested psychological indications: poor motivation/insight, lack of cooperation with OP treatment, inability to eat, need for nasogastric feeding, suicidal intent or plan, severe coexisting psychiatric disease, problematic family environment
- Suggested lab indications: potassium <3 mmol/L, prolonged QTC (>0.499 ms), urine specific gravity >1.03 or <1.01

Pediatric Considerations

- Children often present with nausea, abdominal pain, fullness, and inability to swallow.
- Additional indications for hospitalization: heart rate <50 beats/min, orthostatic BP, hypokalemia or hypophosphatemia, rapid weight loss even if weight not <75% below normal
- Children and adolescents should be offered family-based therapy and treatment.

Geriatric Considerations

- Late-onset AN (>50 years of age) may be a long-term disease or triggered by death of loved one, marital discord, divorce, or depression.
- Always consider other organic causes of weight loss.
- Discharge when medically stable. Arrange OP appointment with mental health provider and primary care provider.

 ONGOING CARE

FOLLOW-UP RECOMMENDATIONS

- Close follow-up until patient demonstrates forward progress in care plan
- Family and individual therapy is extremely important for long-term outcomes.
- CBT is helpful for the treatment of AN and may aid in the prevention of relapse.
- Emphasize importance of moderate activity for health.

Patient Monitoring

- Level of exercise activity
- Weigh weekly until stable, then monthly.
- Depression, suicidal ideation

DIET

- Dietary consultation while patient is hospitalized
- Nutritional education programs

PATIENT EDUCATION

- http://www.mayoclinic.org/diseases-conditions /anorexia/home/ovc-20179508
- National Alliance on Mental Illness: https://www .nami.org/About-Mental-Illness/Mental-Health -Conditions/Eating-Disorders

PROGNOSIS

- Prognosis: ~50% recover, 30% improve, 20% are chronically ill.
- Mortality: 5–18% (annual mortality rate of 5 per 1,000 person-years)

ALERT

High risk of suicide (approximately 1 in 5 individuals with AN who died had committed suicide) (6)[A]

COMPLICATIONS

- Refeeding syndrome
- Cardiac arrhythmia, cardiac arrest, cardiomyopathy, congestive heart failure
- Delayed gastric emptying, necrotizing colitis
- Seizures, Wernicke encephalopathy, peripheral neuropathy, cognitive deficits
- Osteopenia, osteoporosis

Pregnancy Considerations

- Fertility may be affected.
- Behaviors may persist, decrease, or recur during pregnancy and the postpartum interval.
- Increased risk for preterm labor, operative delivery, and infants with low birth weight; anemia, genitourinary infections, and labor induction should be managed as high risk.

REFERENCES

1. Cotton MA, Ball C, Robinson P. Four simple questions can help screen for eating disorders. *J Gen Intern Med*. 2003;18(1):53–56.
2. Hay PJ, Claudino AM, Touyz S, et al. Individual psychological therapy in the outpatient treatment of adults with anorexia nervosa. *Cochrane Database Syst Rev*. 2015;(7):CD003909.
3. Bulik CM, Berkman ND, Brownley KA, et al. Anorexia nervosa treatment: a systematic review of randomized controlled trials. *Int J Eat Disord*. 2007;40(4):310–320.
4. Galsworthy-Francis L, Allan S. Cognitive behavioural therapy for anorexia nervosa: a systematic review. *Clin Psychol Rev*. 2014;34(1):54–72.
5. Claudino AM, Hay P, Lima MS, et al. Antidepressants for anorexia nervosa. *Cochrane Database Syst Rev*. 2006;(1):CD004365.
6. Arcelus J, Mitchell AJ, Wales J, et al. Mortality rates in patients with anorexia nervosa and other eating disorders. A meta-analysis of 36 studies. *Arch Gen Psychiatry*. 2011;68(7):724–731.

ADDITIONAL READING

American Psychiatric Association. *Practice Guideline for the Treatment of Patients with Eating Disorders*. 3rd ed. Arlington, VA: American Psychiatric Association; 2006.

 SEE ALSO

- Amenorrhea; Bulimia Nervosa; Osteoporosis and Osteopenia
- Algorithm: Weight Loss, Unintentional

CODES

ICD10

- F50.01 Anorexia nervosa, restricting type
- F50.02 Anorexia nervosa, binge eating/purging type
- F50.00 Anorexia nervosa, unspecified

CLINICAL PEARLS

- "Are you satisfied with your eating patterns?" or "Do you worry that you have lost control over how you eat?" may help to screen those with an eating problem.
- Assess for suicide risk.
- Studies have shown patients with AN will not accept medications unless combined with psychotherapy.
- To care for a patient with AN, an interdisciplinary team that includes a medical provider, a dietitian, and a behavioral health professional is the most accepted approach.

ANTIPHOSPHOLIPID ANTIBODY SYNDROME

Narothama Reddy Aeddula, MD, FACP, FASN, FNKF • Krishna Baradhi, MD

 BASICS

DESCRIPTION

Antiphospholipid antibody syndrome (APS) is a systemic autoantibody-mediated thrombophilic disorder characterized by recurrent arterial or venous thrombosis and/or recurrent fetal loss in the presence of persistent antiphospholipid antibodies (APAs) as evidenced by lupus anticoagulant (LAC), anticardiolipin antibodies (aCL), and/or anti–β_2 glycoprotein-I (GPI) antibody. The APAs enhance clot formation by interacting with phospholipid-binding plasma proteins. The resulting APS can cause morbidity and mortality in both pregnant and nonpregnant individuals:

- Types of APS (based on clinical presentation)
  - Primary: no underlying condition evident
  - Secondary: most commonly associated with autoimmune diseases like systemic lupus erythematosus (SLE); transient APAs have been linked to certain infections, drugs, and malignancies.
  - Catastrophic APS (CAPS) a.k.a. Asherson syndrome (<1%)
    - Most severe form of disease; characterized by thrombotic microangiopathy and associated with multiorgan failure
    - High mortality if treatment is delayed

Pregnancy Considerations

- Complications include maternal venous thromboembolism, stroke, fetal demise, preeclampsia and placental insufficiency, fetal growth retardation, miscarriage, and preterm birth.
- Triple antibody positivity is considered the most noteworthy risk factor.
- Low-dose aspirin and low-molecular-weight heparin (LMWH) or unfractionated heparin are the drugs of choice in pregnancy.
- Prophylactic-dose heparin is recommended in the postpartum period (unless patient is on therapeutic anticoagulation) given high risk of thrombosis during this time. With adequate treatment, >70% of patients with APS deliver viable infants.

EPIDEMIOLOGY

- The prevalence of APAs increases with age but is not necessarily associated with a higher risk of thrombosis.
- For APS, female > male

Incidence

- Incidence of APS is around 5 new cases per 100,000 persons per year.
- In patients with positive APAs without prior risk of thrombosis, the annual incident risk of thrombosis is 0–3.8%. This risk is increased to 5.3% in those with triple positivity. 10–15% of recurrent abortions are attributable to APS.

Prevalence

Prevalence around 40 to 50 cases per 100,000 persons per year. APAs are present in 1–5% of the general population and in ~40% of those with SLE. A higher prevalence of 10–15 % is seen in those with venous thromboembolism, fetal loss, and stroke. Estimates in United States suggest that APS are associated with approximately 50,000 pregnancy losses.

ETIOLOGY AND PATHOPHYSIOLOGY

- Anti–β_2-GP1 antibodies play a central role in the pathogenesis of APS. The procoagulant effect is mediated by various possible mechanisms:
  - Endothelial effects: inhibition of prostacyclin production and loss of annexin V cellular shield

- Platelet activation resulting in adhesion and aggregation
- Interference of innate anticoagulant pathways (such as inhibition of protein C)
- Complement activation
- Pregnancy-related complications are also a result of autoantibody-mediated effects:
  - Interference with expression of trophoblastic adhesion molecules resulting in abnormal placentation and placental thrombosis
- Proposed mechanisms: excess production of natural antibodies, molecular mimicry due to infections, exposure of phospholipid antigens during platelet activation, cardiolipin peroxidation, and genetic predisposition
- A "second hit" by environmental factors is often required to manifest APS.

Genetics

Most cases of APS are acquired. There are a few studies of familial occurrence of aCL and LAC. A valine 247/leucine polymorphism in β_2-GP1 could be a genetic risk for the presence of anti–β_2-GP1 antibodies and APS.

RISK FACTORS

- Age >55 years in males, >65 years in females
- Cardiovascular risk factors (hypertension [HTN], hyperlipidemia, diabetes, obesity, smoking, combined oral contraceptive use)
- Underlying autoimmune disease (SLE, rheumatoid arthritis, collagen vascular disease, Sjögren syndrome, idiopathic thrombocytopenic purpura, Behçet syndrome)
- Positive APAs
- Surgery, immobilization, pregnancy

GENERAL PREVENTION

Risk factor modification: Control HTN and diabetes; smoking cessation; avoidance of oral contraceptives in high-risk patients; start thromboprophylaxis in established cases; preconception assessment

COMMONLY ASSOCIATED CONDITIONS

- Autoimmune diseases: SLE (most common), scleroderma, Sjögren syndrome, dermatomyositis, and rheumatoid arthritis
- SLE is the most common autoimmune disease associated with APS.
- Malignancy
- Infections: viral, bacterial, parasitic, and rickettsial
- Certain drugs associated with APA production without increased risk of thrombosis: phenothiazines, hydralazine, procainamide, and phenytoin
- Hemolysis, elevated liver enzymes, and low platelet count in association with pregnancy (HELLP) syndrome
- Sneddon syndrome (APS variant syndrome with livedo reticularis, HTN, and stroke)

DIAGNOSIS

Sapporo criteria (also called Sydney criteria), revised 2006:

- At least one of the following clinical criteria:
  - Vascular thrombosis
    - ≥1 clinical episodes of arterial, venous, or small vessel thrombosis, occurring within any tissue or organ and confirmed by unequivocal imaging studies or histopathology without associated inflammation in the vessel wall
    - Superficial venous thrombosis does not meet the criteria for APS.

- Complications of pregnancy (any one of the following):
  - ≥3 consecutive spontaneous abortions before the 10th week of pregnancy, unexplained by maternal/paternal chromosomal abnormalities or maternal anatomic/hormonal causes
  - ≥1 unexplained deaths of morphologically normal fetuses (documented by ultrasonography or by direct examination) at ≥10th week of gestation
  - ≥1 premature births of morphologically normal newborn babies at ≤34th week of pregnancy due to severe preeclampsia, eclampsia, or placental insufficiency
- AND the presence of at least one of three laboratory findings (confirmed on ≥2 occasions at least 12 weeks apart):
  - LAC detected in blood
  - Anticardiolipin IgG and/or IgM antibodies present at moderate or high levels in the blood (>40 GPL or MPL or >99th percentile) via a standardized ELISA
  - Anti–β_2-GP1 IgG and/or IgM antibodies in blood at a titer >99th percentile by standardized ELISA

HISTORY

- History of venous thromboembolism or arterial thrombosis (stroke, MI)
- History of recurrent fetal loss or other obstetric complications
- Bleeding from thrombocytopenia if severe or acquired factor II deficiency
- Personal or family history of autoimmune disease

PHYSICAL EXAM

- Signs of venous thrombosis in extremities
- Skin manifestations, including a vasculitic rash in the form of palpable purpura or livedo reticularis, superficial thrombophlebitis, or lower extremity ulcers
- Livedo reticularis
- Cardiac murmurs
- Focal neurologic or cognitive deficits

DIFFERENTIAL DIAGNOSIS

- Thrombophilic conditions
  - Inherited: deficiency of protein C, protein S, antithrombin III; mutation of factor V Leiden, prothrombin gene mutation
  - Acquired: neoplastic and myeloproliferative disorders, hyperviscosity syndromes, nephrotic syndrome
- Embolic disease secondary to atrial fibrillation, LV dysfunction, endocarditis, cholesterol emboli
- Disseminated intravascular coagulation
- Paroxysmal nocturnal hemoglobinuria
- Heparin-induced thrombocytopenia
- Behçet syndrome
- CAPS: hemolytic-uremic syndrome, TTP, or malignant HTN

DIAGNOSTIC TESTS & INTERPRETATION

- LAC assay and IgG and IGM aCL by ELISA and anti–β_2-GP1 IgG and IgM antibodies are diagnostic tests of choice.
- The LAC assay combines at least two out of three screening tests (prolongation of aPTT, dilute Russell viper venom time [dRVVT], and kaolin clotting) with two confirmatory tests.
- A weakly positive LAC result should be considered clinically important (1).
- Anti–β_2-GP1 antibodies are important in the pathogenesis of thrombosis. A positive LAC assay recognizes antibodies against β_2-GP1 and prothrombin.

- Although testing for antibodies to phosphatidyl-serine and prothrombin can help to assess the risk of thrombosis, routine evaluation for prothrombin antibodies is not recommended.
- The clinical significance of other autoantibodies (annexin V, phosphatidic acid, and phosphatidylinositol) remains unclear.
- The utility of β_2-GP1 anti-domain I antibodies is being evaluated thoroughly for its diagnostic and risk stratification value.

Initial Tests (lab, imaging)
- CBC, PT/INR, aPTT, LAC, aCL, anti-β_2-GP1 antibodies (2)[B]
- Prevalence of APAs in SLE ranges from 11% to 87%; hence, it is important to screen for SLE.
- Imaging is based on clinical picture, suspected sites of thrombosis, and organ involvement.

Follow-Up Tests & Special Considerations
- The results of LAC are difficult to interpret in patients treated with warfarin. Unfractionated heparin or LMWH and fondaparinux do not affect the LAC assay.
- Repeat testing at 12 weeks for persistence of APA.

Diagnostic Procedures/Other
Biopsy of the affected organ system may be necessary to distinguish from vasculitis.

Test Interpretation
Usual finding is thrombosis and minimal vascular or perivascular inflammation:
- Acute changes: capillary congestion and noninflammatory fibrin thrombi
- Chronic changes: ischemic hypoperfusion, atrophy, and fibrosis

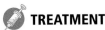
TREATMENT

MEDICATION
First Line
- Primary thromboprophylaxis: is controversial in patients with APS and no clinical symptoms (3)[B]. A 2018 Cochrane review involving nine studies and 1,044 randomized participants failed to show conclusive benefit of aspirin in patients without a thrombotic event. Low-dose aspirin or heparin is indicated only in patients with a high risk of thrombosis because the overall risk of thrombosis is <4%.
- Secondary thromboprophylaxis: All symptomatic, nonpregnant patients with APS need indefinite anticoagulation. The target INR depends on the severity and type of thrombosis:
  - Venous thrombosis (first episode): warfarin with target INR of 2.0 to 3.0 (3)[B]
  - Arterial thrombosis or recurrent venous thrombosis despite anticoagulation: warfarin with target INR 3.0 to 4.0
  - LMWH and fondaparinux are alternatives.
- Direct oral anticoagulants (DOACs) such as rivaroxaban, apixaban, and dabigatran; all have been approved for treatment of DVT/PE; however, studies in APS are lacking; a prospective randomized trial in 2016 of warfarin versus rivaroxaban in patients with thrombotic APS showed increase in endogenous thrombin potential in patients who switched to rivaroxaban. The 15th International Congress on Antiphospholipid Antibodies Task Force published in 2017 concluded that there is insufficient evidence

to recommend DOACs in APS. DOACs may be alternatives to warfarin in patients intolerant to warfarin. A 3-year, open-label, randomized noninferiority trial in 2019 did not show noninferiority of rivaroxaban to dose-adjusted VKAs for thrombotic APS and moreover showed a non-statistically significant near doubling of the risk for recurrent thrombosis.
  - Rituximab may be an option in severe cases, possibly in those with thrombotic microangiopathy (4).
- Danaparoid, fondaparinux, and argatroban can be considered in heparin-induced thrombocytopenia.
- Statins can decrease proinflammatory and prothrombotic state in APS but not recommended in the absence of hyperlipidemia.
- Hydroxychloroquine can be added in recalcitrant APS.
- Eculizumab may be useful in refractory cases.
- Vitamin D deficiency/insufficiency should be corrected in all APA-positive patients, but its role in APS needs further study.
- Low-dose aspirin is superior to low-dose aspirin with low-dose warfarin due to decreased bleeding risk with no differences in number of thrombosis.
- CAPS: Anticoagulants and high-dose steroids may suffice in less severe cases. Aggressive treatment with either IVIG or plasma exchange is often required in severe cases. These measures have improved survival up to 66%.
- Treatment in pregnancy:
  - Patients with APS and no prior thrombotic events may be offered low-dose aspirin during pregnancy; treatment decisions should be individualized though.
  - For women with no prior history of thrombosis and ≥2 early miscarriages, treat with either 81 mg aspirin alone or in combination with unfractionated heparin (5,000 to 10,000 U SC q12h) or LMWH (prophylactic dose). In those with a previous late pregnancy loss (>10 weeks' gestation) or preterm (<34 weeks) delivery due to severe preeclampsia, a combination of aspirin and heparin is recommended.
  - Preconception assessment and treatment with low-dose aspirin, vitamin D, and folate should be offered in selected patients.
  - In those with a history of thrombosis, low-dose aspirin plus either therapeutic low-dose heparin (dosed every 8 to 12 hours to maintain mid-interval aPTT or factor Xa levels) or LMWH (therapeutic dose)
  - Refractory cases: Up to 30% of patients have recurrent pregnancy loss despite the use of aspirin and heparin. There is no role for warfarin due to risk of teratogenicity. Such cases are best managed in consultation with a maternal–fetal medicine specialist.

SURGERY/OTHER PROCEDURES
Patients with thrombosis may require thrombectomy or an IVC filter, when anticoagulation is contraindicated.

ONGOING CARE

FOLLOW-UP RECOMMENDATIONS
Patient Monitoring
- Standard guidelines for monitoring to maintain INR at therapeutic goal on warfarin therapy
- Close monitoring is required during pregnancy.

DIET
Heart-healthy diet. Patients on warfarin should avoid foods rich in vitamin K (kale, spinach, sprouts, greens).

PATIENT EDUCATION
- Compliance with warfarin therapy to keep INR at goal
- Awareness of drug and diet interactions with warfarin
- Avoid oral hormonal contraceptives.

PROGNOSIS
- Pulmonary HTN, neurologic involvement, myocardial ischemia, nephropathy, gangrene of extremities, and CAPS are associated with a worse prognosis.
- 30% risk of recurrent thrombosis in the absence of adequate anticoagulation

COMPLICATIONS
- Pregnancy complications and pulmonary HTN are associated with higher morbidity and mortality.
- Thrombotic complications are the common cause of death.

REFERENCES

1. Bertolaccini ML, Amengual O, Andreoli L, et al. 14th International Congress on Antiphospholipid Antibodies Task Force. Report on antiphospholipid syndrome laboratory diagnostics and trends. *Autoimmun Rev.* 2014;13(9):917–930.
2. Giannakopoulos B, Passam F, Ioannou Y, et al. How we diagnose the antiphospholipid syndrome. *Blood.* 2009;113(5):985–994.
3. Lim W, Crowther MA, Eikelboom JW. Management of antiphospholipid antibody syndrome: a systematic review. *JAMA.* 2006;295(9):1050–1057.
4. Arachchillage DJ, Cohen H. Use of new oral anticoagulants in antiphospholipid syndrome. *Curr Rheumatol Rep.* 2013;15(6):331.

ADDITIONAL READING

de Jesús GR, Benson AE, Chighizola CB, et al. 16th International Congress on Antiphospholipid Antibodies Task Force Report on Obstetric Antiphospholipid Syndrome. *Lupus.* 2020;29(12):1601–1615.

CODES

ICD10
- D68.61 Antiphospholipid syndrome
- D68.69 Other thrombophilia
- D68.62 Lupus anticoagulant syndrome

CLINICAL PEARLS
- APS is a multisystem autoimmune disorder with recurrent arterial/venous thrombosis and fetal loss and positive APAs.
- Both clinical and laboratory criteria are required for diagnosis. The latter must be confirmed on two separate occasions at least 12 weeks apart.
- Thrombotic manifestations of APS require lifelong anticoagulation.

ANXIETY (GENERALIZED ANXIETY DISORDER)

Rhonda A. Faulkner, PhD • Daniella Davida Brutman, MD

BASICS

DESCRIPTION
- Persistent, excessive, and difficult-to-control worry associated with significant symptoms of motor tension, autonomic hyperactivity, and/or disturbances of sleep or concentration
- System(s) affected: nervous (increased sympathetic tone and catecholamine release), cardiac (tachycardia), pulmonary (dyspnea), and GI (nausea, irregular bowels)

EPIDEMIOLOGY
Prevalence
- Lifetime prevalence in United States 5.1–11.9%
- Onset at any age but typically during adulthood; median age of onset in the United States is 31 years.
- Female > male (2:1)
- Generally recurrent and chronic in nature; fluctuates in severity
- COVID-19 survivors have increased incidence of anxiety, depression, and posttraumatic stress disorder (PTSD) (1).

ETIOLOGY AND PATHOPHYSIOLOGY
- May be mediated by abnormalities of neurotransmitter systems (i.e., serotonin, norepinephrine, and γ-aminobutyric acid [GABA])
- Associated with altered regional brain function (increased activity in the amygdala and prefrontal cortex)

Genetics
A serotonin transporter gene (5HT1A) may contribute to GAD.

RISK FACTORS
- Adverse life events (illness, poverty, etc.)
- Family history
- Comorbid psychiatric disorders (2)

GENERAL PREVENTION
- Physical activity and cardiorespiratory fitness are associated with decreased generalized anxiety and depression.
- Cognitive-behavioral therapy (CBT) and parental intervention in children with early anxiety may protect against GAD (2).

COMMONLY ASSOCIATED CONDITIONS
- Major depressive disorder (>60%), dysthymia, bipolar disorder, schizophrenia
- Alcohol/drug abuse; cigarette smoking in adolescence
- Panic disorder, agoraphobia, phobia, social anxiety disorder, anorexia nervosa, PTSD, obsessive-compulsive disorder (OCD), ADHD
- Somatoform and pain disorders

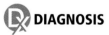

DIAGNOSIS

HISTORY
- Diagnosis is primarily through history. Pathologic anxiety must be distinguished from normal anxiety reactions.
- DSM-5 criteria are as follows:
  - Symptoms of excessive anxiety and worry occur more often than not for at least 6 months.
  - Difficult to control the worry

- At least three additional criteria for diagnosis of GAD in adults; only one in children
  - Restlessness or feeling keyed up or on edge
  - Easily fatigued
  - Difficulty concentrating or mind going blank
  - Irritability
  - Muscle tension
  - Sleep disturbances (difficulty falling or staying asleep)
- Persistent worry must cause significant distress or impairment in social, occupational, or other areas of functioning.
- Focus of anxiety and worry is not consistent with or limited to the occurrence of other types of psychiatric disorders and is not directly related to PTSD.
- Symptoms are not the result of a substance, another medical condition, or other DSM-5 diagnosis.

PHYSICAL EXAM
Useful for identifying other differential diagnoses. No specific physical findings in GAD; patients may exhibit irritability, bitten nails, tremor, or clammy hands.

DIFFERENTIAL DIAGNOSIS
- Cardiovascular: ischemic heart disease, mitral valve prolapse, cardiomyopathies, arrhythmias, congestive heart failure
- Respiratory: asthma, chronic obstructive pulmonary disease, pulmonary embolism
- CNS: stroke, seizures, dementia, migraine, vestibular dysfunction, neoplasms
- Metabolic and hormonal: hyper- or hypothyroidism, pheochromocytoma, adrenal insufficiency, Cushing syndrome, hypokalemia, hypoglycemia, hyperparathyroidism
- Drug-induced anxiety: alcohol, sympathomimetics (cocaine, amphetamine, caffeine), corticosteroids, herbals (ginseng)
- Withdrawal: alcohol, sedative-hypnotics
- Psychiatric: panic disorder, OCD, PTSD, social phobia, adjustment disorder, and somatization disorder

DIAGNOSTIC TESTS & INTERPRETATION
Initial Tests (lab, imaging)
- Laboratory tests are normal. Initial tests may include thyroid-stimulating hormone, CBC, BMP, urine drug screen, and ECG.
- GAD-2: two-question self-reporting scale (22% positive predictive value [PPV]/78% negative predictive value [NPV])
- PHQ-4 provides a very brief screen for both anxiety and depression (2).

Diagnostic Procedures/Other
Psychological testing
- GAD-7: provides more detailed information for treatment (29% PPV/71% NPV); also may be indicative of panic disorder (GAD-7: 29% PPV/71% NPV)
- Hamilton Anxiety Scale (HAM-A), Anxiety Disorders Interview Schedule (ADIS-IV)
- Children: ADIS-IV Parent and Child Version, Multidimensional Anxiety Scale for Children (MASC), Screen for Child Anxiety Related Emotional Disorders (SCARED)

TREATMENT

GENERAL MEASURES
- Assess for suicidality.
- Identify and treat coexisting substance abuse and other psychiatric conditions.
- Delayed treatment may result in poorer clinical outcomes compared with patients treated within 1 year of symptom onset.
- Remission may not occur until 4 to 6 months of treatment. Treat for ≥12 months.
- Psychotherapeutic approaches
  - Psychological treatments are effective in treating GAD: number needed to treat (NNT) = 2 (3)[A].
  - CBT: most well-studied psychological treatment; may improve comorbid conditions; treatment of choice when available (2)[A]
  - Relaxation/mindfulness training (2)[A]
  - Psychodynamic psychotherapy: patient discovering and verbalizing unconscious conflicts (2)[C]

MEDICATION
First Line
- SSRIs and SNRIs have demonstrated efficacy, are well tolerated, do not cause abuse/dependence, and treat comorbid depression. Data to compare between agents are limited (4)[A].
- Medication selection based on side effect profile, drug–drug interactions, and/or patient treatment history/preference.
- For SSRIs/SNRIs, start at lowest available dose, uptitrate every 2 to 4 weeks, use highest tolerated FDA-approved dose for at least 4 to 6 weeks before deeming ineffective or switching to a different SSRI/SNRI. Taper gradually to discontinue.
- Switching between medications without adequate dose or duration of therapy can lead to ineffective treatment.
- Common side effects of SSRIs: nausea, diarrhea, insomnia, agitation or sedation, drug interactions, weight gain, and sexual side effects (decreased libido, delayed orgasm)
- Common side effects of SNRIs: nausea, dizziness, insomnia, sedation, constipation, sweating, and blood pressure elevation
- SSRI: escitalopram (Lexapro): initially 10 mg/day; may titrate to a max of 20 mg/day (5)[A]
- SNRIs:
  - Duloxetine (Cymbalta): initially 30 mg/day; may titrate by 30 mg/day qwk to a max of 120 mg/day; doses >60 mg/day rarely more effective (5)[A]
  - Venlafaxine XR (Effexor XR): initially 37.5 to 75.0 mg; may titrate up by 75 mg every 4 days to a max of 225 mg/day (5)[A]
- Pregabalin (Lyrica): decreases anxiety scores and reduces relapse at 75 to 300 mg BID; less sexual dysfunction and sleep disruption than SSRIs. Taper to discontinue; rapid onset of action (off-label) (5)[A]

Second Line
- Sertraline (Zoloft): initially 25 mg/day; may titrate by 25 to 50 mg/day qwk to a max of 200 mg/day (5)[B]
- Azapirones: buspirone (BuSpar): less dependence risk; 15 mg/day divided BID–TID initially; max of 60 mg/day divided BID–TID (5)[B]
- Fluoxetine (Prozac): 10 to 20 mg/day; may titrate up to 60 mg/day (off-label) (5)[B]

- Mirtazapine (Remeron): 15 mg nightly; titrate in increments of 15 mg qwk; max dose 45 mg daily; use as monotherapy or adjunct to SSRI; most common side effect is drowsiness (off-label) (5)[B].
- Paroxetine (Paxil): initially 10 to 20 mg/day; may titrate by 10 mg/day qwk to a max of 50 mg/day (no added benefit >20 mg/day); efficacious but poorly tolerated (5)[A]
- Quetiapine (Seroquel): optimal dose 150 mg/day. Efficacious but less well tolerated than SSRIs. Consider as augmentation (5)[A].
- Citalopram (Celexa) likely has efficacy for GAD but does not have FDA indication.
- Benzodiazepines: efficacious in the short term, less effective long term, risk for dependence/abuse (4),(5)[A]
  – Clonazepam (Klonopin): 0.25 mg BID; may increase to 4 mg/day divided BID
  – Diazepam (Valium): 2 to 5 mg BID–QID; may increase to max of 40 mg/day
  – Lorazepam (Ativan): 0.5 mg BID–TID; may increase to 6 mg/day divided TID
  – Alprazolam (Xanax): 0.25 mg TID; may increase to 4 mg/day
- Hydroxyzine (Vistaril, Atarax): CNS depressant, antihistamine, anticholinergic; decreased risk of dependence; usual dose: 50 to 100 mg PO QID; limit use in the elderly (3)[B].

Geriatric Considerations
- Avoid TCAs and long-acting benzodiazepines; benzodiazepines may cause delirium.
- Pregabalin may cause dizziness and somnolence.

Pediatric Considerations
- CBT is first-line treatment for pediatric patients with mild to moderate GAD.
- CBT with SSRI is first-line treatment with severe GAD
- Black box warning (SSRIs): Antidepressants increase the risk of suicidal thinking and behavior in children, adolescents, and young adults.
- Studies have also shown increase in suicide attempts in adolescents after SSRI discontinuation.
- SSRIs and SNRIs have all been shown to be effective.
- SSRIs are first-line choice among medications.
- Anxiety and ADHD often co-occur. Treat the more debilitating first and consider using nonstimulating medications.

Pregnancy Considerations
- Buspirone: Category B: secreted in breast milk; inadequate studies to assess risk
- Benzodiazepines: Category D: may cause lethargy and weight loss in nursing infants; avoid breastfeeding if the mother is taking chronically or in high doses.
- SSRIs: If possible, taper and discontinue. After 20 weeks' gestation, there is increased risk of pulmonary hypertension; mild transient neonatal syndrome of CNS; and motor, respiratory, and GI signs. Studies regarding risk of autism show mixed results. Most are Category C, with the exception of:
  – Paroxetine: Category D: conflicting evidence regarding risk of congenital cardiac defects and other congenital anomalies in 1st trimester
  – Hydroxyzine: Category C: case reports of neonatal withdrawal

- Benzodiazepines: age >65 years, respiratory disease/sleep apnea, contraindicated with narrow-angle glaucoma, precaution with open-angle glaucoma; sudden discontinuation increases seizure risk. Long-term use has potential for tolerance and dependence; use with caution in patients with history of substance abuse.
- Buspirone: hepatic and/or renal dysfunction; monoamine oxidase inhibitor (MAOI) treatment
- SSRIs: Use caution in those with comorbid bipolar disorder; may increase risk of serotonin syndrome, especially in combination with other serotonergic drugs

COMPLEMENTARY & ALTERNATIVE MEDICINE
- Probable benefit but more study needed for acupuncture, yoga, massage, tai chi, and aromatherapy (6)[B]
- Kava: some evidence for benefit over placebo in mild to moderate anxiety but concern regarding potential hepatotoxicity. Safety is affected by manufacturing quality, plant part used, dose, and interactions with other substances (6)[B].
- Strong evidence to support regular physical activity to significantly relieve anxiety (6)[A],(7)
- Possible benefit from repetitive transcranial magnetic stimulation to the right dorsal lateral prefrontal cortex for pharmacotherapy treatment refractory patients
- Cannabidiol may have beneficial role in the treatment of anxiety-related disorders and COVID-19–related anxiety; more longitudinal studies are needed.
- Psilocybin with behavioral intervention may have a substantial additive benefit, but more research is needed (8).

 ## ONGOING CARE

FOLLOW-UP RECOMMENDATIONS
Patient Monitoring
- Clinical follow-up with patient every 6 months is recommended.
- Follow up within 2 to 4 weeks from starting new medications.
- Medications should be continued past the initial period of response and recommend continued treatment for 12 months.
- Monitor mental status on benzodiazepines and avoid drug dependence or abrupt discontinuation.
- Monitor all patients for suicidal ideation, especially those on SSRIs and SNRIs.

DIET
- Limit caffeine intake.
- Avoid alcohol (drug interactions, high rate of abuse, increased anxiety) and nicotine.

PATIENT EDUCATION
- Regular exercise may be beneficial for anxiety and comorbid conditions.
- Psychoeducation regarding normal versus pathologic anxiety and the physiology of anxiety can be helpful.

PROGNOSIS
- Probability of recovery is 40–60%, but relapse is common.
- Comorbid psychiatric disorders and poor relationships with spouse or family make relapse more likely.

REFERENCES
1. Mazza MG, De Lorenzo R, Conte C, et al. Anxiety and depression in COVID-19 survivors: role of inflammatory and clinical predictors. *Brain Behav Immun*. 2020;89:594–600.
2. Patel G, Fancher TL. In the clinic. Generalized anxiety disorder. *Ann Intern Med*. 2013;159(11):ITC6-1–ITC6-12.
3. Cuijpers P, Sijbrandij M, Koole S, et al. Psychological treatment of generalized anxiety disorder: a meta-analysis. *Clin Psychol Rev*. 2014;34(2):130–140.
4. Huh J, Goebert D, Takeshita J, et al. Treatment of generalized anxiety disorder: a comprehensive review of the literature for psychopharmacologic alternatives to newer antidepressants and benzodiazepines. *Prim Care Companion CNS Disord*. 2011;13(2):PCC.08r00709.
5. Slee A, Nazareth I, Bondarpnek P, et al. Pharmacological treatments for generalised anxiety disorder: a systematic review and network meta-analysis. *Lancet*. 2019;393(10173):768–777.
6. Sarris J, Moylan S, Camfield DA, et al. Complementary medicine, exercise, meditation, diet, and lifestyle modification for anxiety disorders: a review of current evidence. *Evid Based Complement Alternat Med*. 2012;2012:809653.
7. Kandola A, Stubbs B. Exercise and anxiety. *Adv Exp Med Biol*. 2020;1228:345–352.
8. Goldberg SB, Pace BT, Nicholas CR, et al. The experimental effects of psilocybin on symptoms of anxiety and depression: a meta-analysis. *Psychiatry Res*. 2020;284:112749.

 ## SEE ALSO

Algorithms: Anxiety; Depressive Episode, Major

CODES

ICD10
F41.1 Generalized anxiety disorder

CLINICAL PEARLS
- Psychiatric comorbidities, especially depression, are common with GAD; patients are at increased risk for suicidality.
- CBT and SSRIs/SNRIs are the treatments of choice.
- Start medication at low doses, with careful titration to full therapeutic dosing, to minimize side effects and maximize efficacy.
- Benzodiazepines may be used initially but should be tapered and withdrawn if possible.

AORTIC VALVULAR STENOSIS

Jeremy Golding, MD, FAAFP

 BASICS

DESCRIPTION

Aortic stenosis (AS) is a narrowing of the aortic valve area causing obstruction to left ventricular (LV) outflow. The disease has a long asymptomatic latency period, but development of severe obstruction or onset of symptoms such as syncope, angina, and congestive heart failure (CHF) are associated with a high mortality rate without surgical intervention.

EPIDEMIOLOGY

AS is the most common primary valve disease leading to surgery or catheter intervention in Europe and North America, with a growing prevalence due to the aging population (1). Cause by age at presentation:
- <30 years: congenital
- 30 to 65 years: congenital or rheumatic fever (RF)
- >65 years: degenerative calcification of aortic valve

Prevalence
- Affects 1.3% of population 65 to 74 years old, 2.4% 75 to 84 years old, 4% >84 years old
- Bicuspid aortic valve: 1–2% of population. Bicuspid aortic valve predisposes to development of AS at an earlier age.

ETIOLOGY AND PATHOPHYSIOLOGY
- Progressive aortic leaflet thickening and calcification results in LV outflow obstruction. Obstruction causes increased afterload and, over time, decreased cardiac output.
- Increase in LV systolic pressure is required to preserve cardiac output; this leads to development of concentric LV hypertrophy (LVH). The compensatory LVH preserves ejection fraction but adversely affects heart functioning.
  - LVH impairs coronary blood flow during diastole by compression of coronary arteries and reduced capillary ingrowth into hypertrophied muscle.
  - LVH results in diastolic dysfunction by reducing ventricular compliance.
- Diastolic dysfunction necessitates stronger left atrial (LA) contraction to augment preload and maintain stroke volume. Loss of LA contraction by atrial fibrillation can induce acute deterioration.
- Diastolic dysfunction may persist after relief of AS due to the presence of interstitial fibrosis.
- Angina: increased myocardial demand due to higher LV pressure. Myocardial supply is compromised due to LVH.
- Syncope (exertional): can be multifactorial from inability to augment cardiac output due to the fixed obstruction to LV outflow; arrhythmias; or most commonly, abnormal baroreceptor response resulting in failure to appropriately augment blood pressure.
- Heart failure: Eventually, LVH cannot compensate for increasing afterload resulting in high LV pressure and volume, which are accompanied by an increase in LA and pulmonary pressures.
- Degenerative calcific changes to aortic valve (2)
  - Mechanism involves mechanical stress to valve leaflets as well as atherosclerotic changes to the valve tissue. Bicuspid valves are at higher risk for mechanical stress.
  - Early lesions: subendothelial accumulation of oxidized LDL and macrophages and T lymphocytes (inflammatory response)

- Disease progression: Fibroblasts undergo transformation into osteoblasts; protein production of osteopontin, osteocalcin, and bone morphogenic protein-2 (BMP-2), which modulates calcification of leaflets
- Congenital: unicuspid valve, bicuspid valve, tricuspid valve with fusion of commissures, hypoplastic annulus
- RF: chronic scarring with fusion of commissures

RISK FACTORS
- Congenital unicommissural valve or bicuspid valve
  - Unicommissural valve: Most cases were detected during childhood.
  - Bicuspid valve: predisposes to the development of AS earlier in adulthood (4th to 5th decade) compared to tricuspid valve (6th to 8th decade)
- RF
  - Prevalence of chronic rheumatic valvular disease has declined significantly in the United States.
  - Most cases are associated with mitral valve disease.
- Degenerative calcific changes
  - Most common cause of acquired AS in the United States
  - Risk factors are similar to that of coronary artery disease (CAD) and include the following: hypercholesterolemia, hypertension, smoking, male gender, age, and diabetes mellitus.

COMMONLY ASSOCIATED CONDITIONS
- CAD (50% of patients)
- Hypertension (40% of patients): results in "double-loaded" left ventricle (dual source of increased afterload as a result of obstruction from AS and hypertension)
- Aortic insufficiency (common in calcified bicuspid valves and rheumatic disease)
- Mitral valve disease: 95% of patients with AS from RF also have mitral valve disease.
- LV dysfunction and CHF
- Acquired von Willebrand disease: Impaired platelet function and decreased vWF results in bleeding (ecchymosis and epistaxis) in 20% of AS patients. Severity of coagulopathy is directly related to severity of AS.
- Gastrointestinal arteriovenous malformations (AVMs)
- Cerebral or systemic embolic events due to calcium emboli

DIAGNOSIS

HISTORY
- Primary symptoms: angina, syncope, and heart failure. Angina is the most frequent symptom. Syncope is often exertional. Heart failure symptoms include fatigue, exertional dyspnea, orthopnea, paroxysmal nocturnal dyspnea, and shortness of breath.
- Palpitations
- Neurologic events (transient ischemic attack or cerebrovascular accident) secondary to embolization
- Geriatric patients may have subtle symptoms such as fatigue and exertional dyspnea.
- Note: Symptoms do not always correlate with valve area (severity of AS) but most commonly occur when aortic valve area is <1 cm², jet velocity is >4.0 m/s, or the mean transvalvular gradient is ≥40 mm Hg.

PHYSICAL EXAM
- Auscultation
  - Harsh, systolic crescendo–decrescendo murmur is best heard at 2nd right sternal border and radiates into the carotid arteries. Peak of murmur correlates with severity of stenosis; later peaking murmur suggests greater severity.
  - High-pitched blowing diastolic murmur suggests associated aortic insufficiency.
  - Paradoxically split S_2 or absent A_2. Note: Normally split S_2 reliably excludes severe AS.
  - S_4 due to stiffening of the left ventricle
- Other associated signs include *pulsus parvus et tardus*: decreased and delayed carotid upstroke. LV heave; findings of CHF: pulmonary and/or lower extremity edema

DIFFERENTIAL DIAGNOSIS
- Mitral regurgitation: High-frequency, pansystolic murmur, best heard at the apex, often radiates to the axilla.
- Hypertrophic obstructive cardiomyopathy: also systolic crescendo–decrescendo murmur but best heard at left sternal border and may radiate into axilla. Murmur intensity increases by changing from squatting to standing and/or by Valsalva maneuver.
- Discrete fixed subaortic stenosis: 50–65% has associated cardiac deformity (patent ductus arteriosus [PDA], ventricular septal defect [VSD], aortic coarctation).
- Aortic supravalvular stenosis: Williams syndrome, homozygous familial hypercholesterolemia

DIAGNOSTIC TESTS & INTERPRETATION
Initial Tests (lab, imaging)
- Chest x-ray (CXR)
  - May be normal in compensated, isolated valvular AS
  - Boot-shaped heart reflective of concentric hypertrophy
  - Poststenotic dilatation of ascending aorta and calcification of aortic valve (seen on lateral PA CXR)
- ECG: often normal ECG (ECG is nondiagnostic), or may show LVH, LA enlargement, and nonspecific ST- and T-wave abnormalities
- Echo indications
  - Initial workup
    - Doppler echocardiogram: primary test in the diagnosis and evaluation of AS (1)[A]
    - Assesses valve anatomy and severity of disease
    - Assesses LV wall thickness, size, and function, and pulmonary artery pressure
  - In known AS and changing signs/symptoms
  - In known AS and pregnancy due to hemodynamic changes of pregnancy
- Echo findings
  - Aortic valve thickening, calcification
  - Decreased aortic valve excursion
  - Reduced aortic valve area
  - Transvalvular gradient across aortic valve
  - LVH and diastolic dysfunction
  - LV ejection fraction
  - Wall-motion abnormalities suggesting CAD
  - Evaluate for concomitant aortic insufficiency or mitral valve disease.
- AS severity based on echo values (2)
  - Stage A (at risk): bicuspid aortic valve, sclerosis, or other congenital abnormality; mean pressure gradient: 0 mm Hg; jet vel. <2 m/s
  - Stage B (progressive): bicuspid or trileaflet valve
    - Mild: mean pressure gradient: <20 mm Hg; jet vel. 2.0 to 2.9 m/s
    - Moderate: mean pressure gradient: 20 to 40 mm Hg; jet vel. 3.0 to 3.9 m/s

- Stage C (asymptomatic severe AS):
  - C1 (without LV dysfunction): AVA ≤1.0 or AVAi ≤0.6 cm²/m²; mean pressure gradient: 40 to 60 mm Hg; jet vel. ≥4 to 5 m/s
  - C2 (with LV dysfunction): AVA ≤1.0 or AVAi ≤0.6 cm²/m²; mean pressure gradient: ≥40 mm Hg; jet vel. ≥4 m/s
- Stage D (symptomatic severe AS):
  - D1 (high gradient): AVA ≤1.0 cm²; mean pressure gradient: >40 mm Hg; jet vel. >4 m/s
  - D2 (low flow/low gradient with reduced EF <50%): AVA ≤1.0 cm²; mean pressure gradient: <40 mm Hg; jet vel. <4 m/s
  - D3 (low gradient, normal EF ≥50% or paradoxical low-flow severe AS): AVA ≤1.0 cm²; AVAi ≤0.6 cm²/m² and stroke volume index <35 mL/m²; mean pressure gradient: <40 mm Hg; jet vel. <4 m/s

Diagnostic Procedures/Other
- Exercise stress testing
  - Asymptomatic patients with severe AS: helpful to uncover subtle symptoms or changes, abnormal BP (increase <20 mm Hg), and ECG changes (ST depressions). 1/3 of patients develop symptoms with exercise testing; STOP testing at this point.
  - Symptomatic patients: DO NOT perform exercise stress testing because it may induce hypotension or ventricular tachycardia.
  - CHF patients: Dobutamine stress echocardiography is reasonable to evaluate patients with low-flow/low-gradient AS and LV dysfunction.
- Cardiac catheterization
  - Perform prior to aortic valve replacement (AVR) in patients with suspected CAD. Determines need for coronary artery bypass graft (CABG). If unambiguous diagnosis of AS, perform only coronary angiography.
  - Can also use if noninvasive testing is inconclusive or if there is discrepancy between severity of symptoms and findings on echo
  - Measures transvalvular flow and transvalvular pressure gradient, which facilitates calculation of effective valve area
  - Hemodynamic measurements with infusion of dobutamine can be useful for evaluation of patients with low-flow/low-gradient AS and LV dysfunction.

Test Interpretation
- Aortic valve: nodular calcification on valve cusps (initially at bases), cusp rigidity, cusp thickening, and fibrosis
- LVH, myocardial interstitial fibrosis
- 50% incidence of concomitant CAD

TREATMENT

MEDICATION
- No effective medical therapy for severe or symptomatic AS
- Prevention: currently no recommended medical therapy. Statins have been thought to slow progression if initiated during mild disease. However, this has not been supported by large, randomized controlled trials.
- Antibiotic prophylaxis against recurrent RF is indicated for patients with rheumatic AS (penicillin G 1,200,000 U IM q4wk; duration varies with age and history of carditis).
- Antibiotic prophylaxis is no longer indicated for prevention of infective endocarditis.
- Comorbidities: hypertension: angiotensin-converting enzyme (ACE) inhibitors, start with low dose and increase cautiously. Be cautious of vasodilators, which may cause hypotension.

SURGERY/OTHER PROCEDURES
- AVR is recommended for most symptomatic patients with evidence of significant AS on echocardiography (3).
- Indications for AVR surgery:
  - Symptomatic and severe high-gradient AS by history or exercise testing (2)[B] when surgical risk is low or intermediate
  - Asymptomatic, severe AS and LVEF <50% (2)[B]
  - Severe AS (stage C or D) when undergoing other cardiac surgery (2)[B]
- AVR surgery is reasonable in patients who are:
  - Asymptomatic with severe AS (C1) with jet vel. ≥5 m/s and low surgical risk, decreased exercise tolerance, or have an exercise fall in blood pressure (2)[B]
  - Symptomatic stage D2, with a low-dose dobutamine stress with jet vel. ≥4.0 m/s or mean pressure gradient ≥40 mm Hg with ≤1.0 cm² at any dobutamine dose (2)[B]
  - Symptomatic stage D3 with LVEF >50% if clinical and hemodynamic data support valve obstruction as likely cause of symptoms (2)[C]
  - Stage B who are undergoing other cardiac surgery, or asymptomatic stage C1 with rapid disease progression and low surgical risk (2)[C]

ALERT
Note: If the aortic valve area is >1.5 cm² and the gradient is <15 mm Hg, there is no benefit from AVR.

- Transcatheter AVR (TAVR) offers a less invasive option for some patients (1).
  - For those who are high at surgical risk and considered inoperable, TAVR has demonstrated superiority to medical therapy.
  - For those who are high at surgical risk, TAVR has demonstrated noninferiority to surgical AVR (1).
  - For those who are intermediate at surgical risk, TAVR may emerge as a reasonable alternative to surgical risk, although this indication has not yet been approved in the United States.
  - Valve-in-valve TAVR can be considered in high-risk patients with failed surgically implanted bioprosthetic valves.
- Percutaneous balloon valvuloplasty may have role in palliation or as a bridge to valve replacement in hemodynamically unstable or high-risk patients but is not recommended as an alternative to valve replacement.

ONGOING CARE

FOLLOW-UP RECOMMENDATIONS
- Advise patients to immediately report symptoms referable to AS.
- Asymptomatic patients: yearly history and physical
- Serial ECHO: yearly for severe AS, every 1 to 2 years for moderate AS, every 3 to 5 years for mild AS

PATIENT EDUCATION
Physical activity limitations
- Asymptomatic mild AS: no restrictions
- Asymptomatic moderate to severe AS: Avoid strenuous exercise. Consider exercise stress test prior to starting exercise program.

PROGNOSIS
- Although survival in asymptomatic patients is comparable to that in age- and sex-matched control patients, it decreases rapidly after symptoms appear (3).
- 25% mortality per year in symptomatic patients who do not undergo valve replacement; average survival is 2 to 3 years without AVR surgery.
- Median survival in symptomatic AS: heart failure: 2 years; syncope: 3 years; angina: 5 years
- Perisurgical mortality: AVR surgery has 4% mortality rate; AVR + CABG has 6.8% mortality rate.
- Adverse postoperative prognostic factors: age, heart failure New York Heart Association (NYHA) class III/IV, cerebrovascular disease, renal dysfunction, CAD

REFERENCES

1. Baumgartner H, Falk V, Bax JJ, et al; for ESC Scientific Document Group. 2017 ESC/EACTS guidelines for the management of valvular heart disease. Eur Heart J. 2017;38(36):2739–2791.
2. Nishimura RA, Otto CM, Bonow RO, et al. 2017 AHA/ACC focused update of the 2014 AHA/ACC guideline for the management of patients with valvular heart disease: a report of the American College of Cardiology/American Heart Association Task Force on Clinical Practice Guidelines. Circulation. 2017;135(25):e1159–e1195.
3. Grimard BH, Safford RE, Burns EL. Aortic stenosis: diagnosis and treatment. Am Fam Physician. 2016;93(5):371–378.

 CODES

ICD10
- I35.0 Nonrheumatic aortic (valve) stenosis
- I06.0 Rheumatic aortic stenosis
- Q23.0 Congenital stenosis of aortic valve

CLINICAL PEARLS
- AS is diagnosed on physical exam by a systolic crescendo–decrescendo murmur and delayed and diminished pulses.
- Symptomatic AS most commonly presents as angina, syncope, and heart failure.
- Symptomatic AS has a very poor prognosis, unless treated with surgical intervention.

APPENDICITIS, ACUTE

Elijah Kamermans, MD • M. Alex Germano, MD

BASICS

DESCRIPTION
- Acute inflammation of the appendix
- Simple or uncomplicated appendicitis occurs when there is no clinical or radiologic sign of perforation. Complicated or perforated appendicitis is defined by a palpable mass and phlegmon or abscess on imaging.
- Arising from the base of the cecum in right lower quadrant (RLQ), the appendix can be anterior, posterior, medial, or lateral to the cecum as well as in the pelvis. Vascular supply provided by appendicular artery, a branch of the ileocolic artery; nerve supply derived from the superior mesenteric plexus
- Most common cause of acute surgical abdomen

EPIDEMIOLOGY
- Predominant age: 10 to 30 years; rare in infancy
- Predominant sex: slight male predominance
  - Ages 10 to 30 years: male > female (3:2)
  - Age >30 years: male = female

Incidence
- 1 case per 1,000 people per year
- Lifetime incidence 1 in every 15 people (7%)

Pregnancy Considerations
- Most common extrauterine surgical emergency
- Incidence similar in pregnancy
- Higher rate of perforation; more likely to present with peritonitis

ETIOLOGY AND PATHOPHYSIOLOGY
Obstruction of the appendiceal lumen is thought to lead to distention, ischemia, and bacterial overgrowth. Without intervention, appendicitis can lead to perforation and subsequent abscess formation or generalized peritonitis. Causes of obstruction:
- Fecaliths (most common)
- Lymphoid tissue hyperplasia (in children)
- Vegetable, fruit seeds, and other foreign bodies
- Intestinal worms (ascarids)
- Strictures, fibrosis, neoplasms

Genetics
First-degree relative with history of appendicitis increases risk; no direct genetic link has been found.

RISK FACTORS
Adolescent males, familial tendency, intra-abdominal tumors

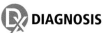 DIAGNOSIS

- Diagnosis relies on history and physical examination with supporting laboratory studies and imaging.
- Scoring systems
  - Modified Alvarado Scoring System (MASS): The use of MASS in the diagnosis of acute appendicitis improves diagnostic accuracy and reduces negative appendectomy and complication rates.
  - Supplement MASS in female patients with additional investigations (e.g., abdominal ultrasound or laparoscopy).
  - Migratory right iliac fossa pain (1 point)
  - Nausea/vomiting (1 point)
  - Anorexia (1 point)
  - Tenderness in right iliac fossa (2 points)
  - Rebound tenderness in right iliac fossa (1 point)
  - Elevated temperature (1 point)
  - Leukocytosis (2 points)
  - A MASS score >7 suggests appendicitis without the need for further imaging.
- A MASS score of 3 or lower does not warrant a CT as appendicitis is seen as less likely. A MASS score of 4 to 6 would require a CT scan for diagnosis of appendicitis (1). A cutoff point of 6 for the MASS score yields higher sensitivity but is also associated with a higher negative appendectomy rate (normal appendix).
- Pediatric Appendicitis Score—helps predict the likelihood of acute appendicitis (diagnosis is still clinical)

HISTORY
- Classic history is vague periumbilical pain, followed by anorexia, nausea, and vomiting. Over the next 4 to 48 hours, pain migrates to the RLQ.
- Only 50% of patients present with a classic history.
- Pain before vomiting (~100% sensitive), abdominal pain (~100%), pain migration (50%)
- Anorexia (~100%), nausea (90%), vomiting (75%), obstipation
- Atypical symptoms and pain suggest a retrocecal or pelvic appendix.

PHYSICAL EXAM
- Fever; temperature >100.4°F (may be absent); tachycardia
- RLQ tenderness; maximal tenderness at McBurney point (1/3 the distance from the anterior superior iliac spine to the umbilicus)
- Voluntary and involuntary guarding
- Rovsing sign: RLQ pain with palpation of left lower quadrant
- Psoas sign: pain with right thigh extension (retrocecal appendix)
- Obturator sign: pain with internal rotation of flexed right thigh (pelvic appendix); local and suprapubic pain on rectal exam (pelvic appendix)
- Pelvic and rectal exams are helpful to assess other causes of lower abdominal pain (e.g., pelvic inflammatory disease, prostatitis).
- Serial exams can be useful in indeterminate cases.

DIFFERENTIAL DIAGNOSIS
- GI
  - Gastroenteritis, inflammatory bowel disease
  - Diverticulitis, ileitis
  - Cholecystitis, pancreatitis
  - Intussusception, volvulus
- Gynecologic
  - Pelvic inflammatory disease, ectopic pregnancy
  - Ovarian cyst, ovarian torsion, tubo-ovarian abscess
  - Endometriosis
  - Ruptured graafian follicle
- Urologic
  - Testicular torsion, epididymitis
  - Kidney stones, prostatitis, cystitis, pyelonephritis
- Systemic
  - Diabetic ketoacidosis
  - Henoch-Schönlein purpura
  - Sickle cell crisis
  - Porphyria
- Other
  - Acute mesenteric lymphadenitis
  - No organic pathologic condition
  - Hernias
  - Psoas abscess
  - Rectus sheath hematoma
  - Epiploic appendagitis
  - Pneumonia (basilar)

Pediatric Considerations
- Decreased diagnostic accuracy of history and physical exam
- Higher fever; more vomiting and diarrhea

Pregnancy Considerations
- Appendicitis is more difficult to diagnose in pregnancy.
- Normal inflammatory response is suppressed.
- Appendix displaced out of pelvis by gravid uterus

Geriatric Considerations
Decreased diagnostic accuracy, more likely to be atypical presentation

DIAGNOSTIC TESTS & INTERPRETATION

Initial Tests (lab, imaging)
- Leukocytosis: WBC >10,000/mm³ (70%)
- Polymorphonuclear predominance—"left shift" (>90%)
- Urinalysis: hematuria, pyuria (30%)
- Human chorionic gonadotropin (hCG) (If positive, rule out ectopic pregnancy.)
- C-reactive protein: nonspecific inflammatory marker; when paired with an elevated WBC, increases predictive value for appendicitis
- Drugs may alter lab results: antibiotics, steroids.
- Imaging if the diagnosis is not clear; helps to detect complications (abscess, perforation)
- Plain films: minimal utility, nonspecific findings, may visualize fecalith
- CT with contrast: sensitivity 91–98%; specificity 95–99%; imaging modality of choice. Consider radiation dose, particularly in young patients.
- Ultrasound: alternative in pregnancy, children, and women with suspected gynecologic pathology. Sensitivity and specificity vary in the skill of the ultrasonographer. Increasing use adult populations, with positive predictive value approaching 100% in some studies (2)[B]. Can rule in appendicitis but cannot reliably exclude the diagnosis. An effective strategy is to start with ultrasound and, if negative, obtain a CT scan if suspicion warrants.
- MRI: increasing use in pregnant patients. May help in patients with contrast allergies renal failure. Limitations include cost, availability, and time required to complete study.
- Radioisotope-labeled WBC scans: may be used in patients with indeterminate CT scans and suspected appendicitis as an alternative to observation or surgery. Limitations include availability and time required to complete study.

Diagnostic Procedures/Other
Exploratory laparotomy/laparoscopy. Acceptable appendectomy rates vary based on age and gender and may be higher for females of childbearing age than males.

Test Interpretation
- Acute appendiceal inflammation, local vascular congestion, obstruction
- Gangrene, perforation with abscess (15–30%)
- Fecalith

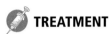

TREATMENT

GENERAL MEASURES
- Surgery (appendectomy) has been the standard of care for acute, uncomplicated appendicitis. There is growing evidence for medical management in select cases—antibiotic therapy, with appendectomy reserved for those who do not respond to treatment (3).
- Delay in surgery for complicated appendicitis is associated with increased complications and cost (4).
- Surgery is indicated for complicated or perforated appendicitis with abscess formation <3 cm. For a drainable abscess >3 cm, percutaneous drainage and antibiotics are the recommendation (5).
- Treatment of pain does not affect the Alvarado score or increase the chance of delayed or unnecessary interventions significantly (6).

MEDICATION
First Line
- Uncomplicated acute appendicitis: perioperative dose of antibiotic: single dose of cefoxitin or ampicillin/sulbactam (Unasyn) or cefazolin plus metronidazole
- Nonoperative antibiotic of choice: ertapenem for 3 days followed by 7 days PO levofloxacin and metronidazole (7)[B]
- Gangrenous or perforating appendicitis
  – Broadened antibiotic coverage for aerobic and anaerobic enteric pathogens
  – Piperacillin and tazobactam (Zosyn) or ticarcillin and clavulanate (Timentin) or a 3rd-generation cephalosporin plus metronidazole are initial options.
  – Adjust dosage and choice of antibiotic based on intraoperative cultures.
  – Continue antibiotics for at least 7 days postoperatively or until patient becomes afebrile with normal WBC count.

Second Line
- Uncomplicated acute appendicitis: clindamycin plus one of the following: ciprofloxacin, levofloxacin, gentamicin, or aztreonam
- In the case of acute appendicitis complicated by abscess formation or phlegmon in pediatric patients, some studies show initial conservative management with antibiotics alone to carry fewer risks and complications than emergent appendectomy.
- Gangrenous or perforated appendicitis: ciprofloxacin or levofloxacin plus metronidazole or monotherapy with a carbapenem (imipenem and cilastatin, meropenem, ertapenem)

ISSUES FOR REFERRAL
All cases of appendicitis require emergent surgical consultation.

SURGERY/OTHER PROCEDURES
- The American College of Surgeons, Society for Surgery of the Alimentary Tract, and others recommend surgery as the treatment of choice.
- Antibiotic treatment might be used as an alternative in specific patients or if surgery is contraindicated.
- Nonoperative management with antibiotics with up to a reported 39% recurrence rate at 5 years for uncomplicated acute appendicitis (7)[B]

ADMISSION, INPATIENT, AND NURSING CONSIDERATIONS
- Admit all patients with appendicitis.
- Fluid resuscitation with normal saline (NS) or lactated Ringer (LR) solution
- Correct fluid and electrolyte deficits.
- Discharge when tolerating oral intake, return of bowel function, afebrile, normal WBC.

ONGOING CARE

FOLLOW-UP RECOMMENDATIONS
- Return to work in 1 to 2 weeks is typically following most cases of uncomplicated appendicitis.
- Restrict activity for 4 to 6 weeks after surgery: no heavy lifting (>10 lb) or strenuous physical activity.
- If managed nonoperatively and patient is >40 years, consider colonoscopy to rule out malignancy.

PATIENT EDUCATION
Postoperative warning signs:
- Anorexia, nausea, vomiting
- Abdominal pain, fever, chills
- Signs/symptoms of wound infection

PROGNOSIS
- Generally uncomplicated course in young adults with unruptured appendicitis
- Extremes of age and appendiceal rupture increase morbidity and mortality.
- Morbidity rates
  – Nonperforated appendicitis: 3%
  – Perforated appendicitis: 47%
- Mortality rates
  – Unruptured appendicitis: 0.1%
  – Ruptured appendicitis: 3%
  – Patients >60 years of age make up 50% of total deaths from appendicitis.
  – Older patients with ruptured appendix: 15%

Pediatric Considerations
- Rupture earlier
- Rupture rate: 15–60%

Pregnancy Considerations
- Rupture rate: 40%
- Fetal mortality rate: 2–8.5%

Geriatric Considerations
Rupture rate: 67–90%

COMPLICATIONS
- Intestinal fistulas
- Intestinal obstruction, paralytic ileus, incisional hernia
- Liver abscess (rare), pyelophlebitis
- Stump appendicitis: recurrence of appendicitis at appendiceal stump after appendectomy; incidence 0.15% (8)[B]

REFERENCES

1. McKay R, Shepherd J. The use of the clinical scoring system by Alvarado in the decision to perform computed tomography for acute appendicitis in the ED. *Am J Emerg Med*. 2007;25(5):489–493.
2. Benedetto G, Ferrer Puchol MD, Llavata Solaz A. Suspicion of acute appendicitis in adults. The value of ultrasound in our hospital. *Radiologia*. 2019;61(1):51–59.
3. Flum DR, Davidson GH, Monsell SE, et al; for CODA Collaborative. A randomized trial comparing antibiotics with appendectomy for appendicitis. *N Engl J Med*. 2020;383(20):1907–1919.
4. Symer MM, Abelson JS, Sedrakyan A, et al. Early operative management of complicated appendicitis is associated with improved surgical outcomes in adults. *Am J Surg*. 2018;216(3):431–443.
5. Miftaroski A, Kessler U, Monnard E, et al. Two-step procedure for complicated appendicitis with perityphlitic abscess formation. *Swiss Med Wkly*. 2017;147:w14422.
6. Snyder MJ, Guthrie M, Cagle S. Acute appendicitis: efficient diagnosis and management. *Am Fam Physician*. 2018;98(1):25–33.
7. Salminen P, Tuominen R, Paajanen H, et al. Five-year follow-up of antibiotic therapy for uncomplicated acute appendicitis in the APPAC randomized clinical trial. *JAMA*. 2018;320(12):1259–1265.
8. Dikicier E, Altintoprak F, Ozdemir K, et al. Stump appendicitis: a retrospective review of 3130 consecutive appendectomy cases. *World J Emerg Surg*. 2018;13:22.

ADDITIONAL READING
Bhangu A, Søreide K, Di Saverio S, et al. Acute appendicitis: modern understanding of pathogenesis, diagnosis, and management. *Lancet*. 2015;386(10000):1278–1287.

 SEE ALSO

Algorithm: Abdominal Rigidity

 CODES

ICD10
- K35.80 Unspecified acute appendicitis
- K35.2 Acute appendicitis with generalized peritonitis
- K35.3 Acute appendicitis with localized peritonitis

CLINICAL PEARLS
- Anorexia with periumbilical pain localizing to RLQ is the classic history for acute appendicitis.
- Diagnosis is more challenging in children, pregnant patients, and the elderly due to varying symptoms and signs.
- In equivocal cases, CT is the diagnostic test of choice. Ultrasound and MRI are alternatives.
- Acute appendicitis is the most common surgical emergency during pregnancy.

APPROACH TO TRAVEL MEDICINE COUNSELING

Melissa Jefferis, MD, FAAFP

 BASICS

DESCRIPTION

Pretravel consultations are an important way to assess trip plans, determine potential health hazards, discuss risks and methods of prevention.

EPIDEMIOLOGY

Incidence

There were 1.33 billion international tourist travel arrivals in 2017 (CDC). Illness and injury are common during travel.

RISK FACTORS

Risks vary by destination, length of the trip, planned activities, age, and health status of the traveler.

- Traveler details
  - Past medical history (age, gender, medical conditions, allergies, medications)
    - Flying is contraindicated within 3 weeks of a myocardial infarction and within 10 days of a thoracic or abdominal surgery.
    - If preexisting eustachian tube dysfunction, use of a vasoconstricting nasal spray immediately before air travel may lessen the occurrence of otitis or barotrauma (1).
    - See *CDC Yellow Book* for list of special considerations for travelers with chronic medical illnesses including cardiovascular diseases, pulmonary diseases, diabetes, and severe allergic reactions.
  - Special conditions (pregnancy, breastfeeding, disability or handicap, immunocompromised state, older age)
    - Flying is generally discouraged after the 36th week of pregnancy. Many airlines require a provider letter if flying after this time.
  - Immunization history
  - Prior travel experience (previous malaria prophylaxis, experience with altitude, illnesses related to prior travel)
- Trip details
  - Itinerary (countries/specific regions, rural or urban; side trips)
  - Timing (length, season, time until departure)
  - Reason for travel
  - Special activities (disaster relief, medical care, high altitude or climbing, diving, cruise ship, rafting, cycling, extreme sports)

GENERAL PREVENTION

- Routine vaccinations
  - *Haemophilus influenzae* type b
  - Hepatitis B—for last minute travelers, can offer accelerated vaccine schedule for hepatitis A and hepatitis B with Twinrix or accelerated schedule for hepatitis B alone with Heplisav-B
  - Influenza
  - Measles, mumps, rubella—more common in countries without routine childhood immunization, including Europe
  - Meningococcal—outbreaks common in sub-Saharan Africa especially during the dry season (December through June). Saudi Arabia requires the quadrivalent vaccine for Hajj pilgrims. Hajj visas require vaccine to be administered ≥10 days and ≤3 years (≤5 years for conjugate vaccine) before arriving in Saudi Arabia (2).
  - Pneumococcal
  - Polio—wild poliovirus type 1 circulates currently in Afghanistan and Pakistan (2).

- Rotavirus—common in developing countries; does not usually cause travelers' diarrhea in adults, so vaccination is only recommended for children
  - Tetanus, diphtheria, pertussis
  - Varicella—more common in countries without routine childhood immunization
  - Zoster—stress may trigger reactivation.
  - Human papillomavirus (HPV)—sexual activity during travel may lead to HPV infection.
- Travel-specific vaccinations (destination dependent)
  - Cholera (not available in the United States)—observing safe food, water, sanitation, and hand washing recommendations while in affected countries will have virtually no risk of acquiring cholera.
  - Hepatitis A
  - Japanese encephalitis
  - Rabies—if immunoglobulin would be difficult to obtain, consider vaccination to simplify postexposure prophylaxis.
  - Tick-borne encephalitis (not available in U.S.)
  - Typhoid—highest risk in India, Pakistan, and Bangladesh. Do not give live oral vaccine to pregnant women, immunocompromised patients, or if antibiotics taken in the previous 72 hours (2).
  - Yellow fever—highest risk in sub-Saharan Africa and the Amazon regions of South America. Vaccination is not considered valid until 10 days after administration (2).
- Malaria prophylaxis
  - Based on destination, types of planned activities, and patient preferences. CDC has up-to-date recommendations.
  - Chloroquine-sensitive malaria (2),(3)
    - Chloroquine—begin 1 to 2 weeks prior to travel, continue 4 weeks after leaving malaria-endemic area; may increase QTc interval (particularly if given with other QTc-prolonging drugs)
      - Adult dose: 300-mg base (500-mg salt) orally once weekly
      - Pediatric dose: 5 mg/kg base (8.3 mg/kg salt) orally once weekly (up to 300-mg base per dose)
    - Hydroxychloroquine—begin 1 to 2 weeks prior to travel, continue for 4 weeks after leaving malaria-endemic area; dosed weekly
      - Adult dose: 310-mg base (400-mg salt) orally once weekly
      - Pediatric dose: 5 mg/kg base (6.5 mg/kg salt) orally once weekly (up to 310 mg base per dose)
  - Chloroquine-resistant malaria (2),(3)
    - Atovaquone/proguanil—begin 1 to 2 days before travel and continue for 1 week after leaving malaria-endemic area.
      - Adult dose: 250 mg/100 mg atovaquone/proguanil PO daily
      - Pediatric dose: Tablets contain 62.5 mg/25 mg atovaquone/proguanil hydrochloride.
        - 5 to 10 kg: 1/2 pediatric tablet daily
        - 10 to 20 kg: 1 pediatric tablet daily
        - 20 to 30 kg: 2 pediatric tablets daily
        - 30 to 40 kg: 3 pediatric tablets daily
        - >40 kg: 1 adult tablet daily
    - Doxycycline—begin 1 to 2 days before travel and continue for 4 weeks after leaving malaria-endemic area.
      - Adult dose: 100 mg orally daily
      - Pediatric dose: ≥8 years old 2.2 mg/kg up to adult dose of 100 mg daily

- Mefloquine—begin 1 to 2 weeks before travel and continue for 4 weeks after leaving malaria-endemic area; has a number of drug interactions; not recommended for people with cardiac conduction abnormalities (especially ventricular arrhythmias), major psychiatric disorders, or seizures
    - Adult dose: 228-mg base (250-mg salt) orally once weekly
    - Pediatric dose
      - ≤9 kg: 4.6 mg/kg base (5 mg/kg salt) orally once weekly
      - 10 to 19 kg: 1/4 tablet once weekly
      - 20 to 30 kg: 1/2 tablet once weekly
      - 31 to 45 kg: 3/4 tablet once weekly
      - >45 kg: 1 tablet once weekly
- Protection against mosquitoes and ticks
  - Avoid areas of known outbreaks of communicable disease. Refer to the CDC travelers' health Web site for updates.
  - Avoid peak exposure times and places.
    - Mosquitoes may bite at any time of the day.
    - Peak biting activity for vectors of some diseases (such as dengue, Zika, and chikungunya) is during daylight hours (1).
    - Peak biting activity for vectors of other diseases (such as malaria, West Nile, and Japanese encephalitis) are most active in twilight periods (dawn and dusk) or after dark.
  - Wear appropriate clothing: Minimize exposed skin.
  - Check for ticks.
  - Bed nets
  - Insecticides and repellants—reapply regularly.
    - DEET, Picaridin
    - Oil of lemon eucalyptus, IR3535, 2-Undecanone
- Zika virus
  - Single-stranded RNA virus of the Flaviviridae family, genus *Flavivirus*
  - Most infections are asymptomatic.
  - Pregnant women should avoid travel to any area with risk of Zika virus transmission. Vertical transmission can lead to congenital Zika. Congenital Zika sequelae can include microcephaly with brain anomalies and fetal loss.
- SARS-Coronavirus-2
  - Consider delaying or cancelling trips planned if case numbers are high in originating location or destination.
  - Check travel restrictions, including testing requirements, before you go.
  - Do not travel if you have any symptoms. Avoid contact with anyone who is sick.
  - Bring extra supplies, such as masks and hand sanitizer.
  - Wear a mask.
  - Respect physical distancing recommendations by staying at least 6 feet apart from others.
  - Wash your hands often or use hand sanitizer (with at least 60% alcohol).
- Traveler's diarrhea
  - Symptoms range from mild abdominal cramping and urgent loose stools to severe abdominal pain, fever, vomiting, and bloody diarrhea.
  - Differs from food poisoning in which preformed toxins are ingested in food. Nausea and vomiting may both be present, although usually resolve within 12 hours.
  - Approximately 80–90% bacterial, 5–8% viral, 10% protozoal (1)
  - Most common bacteria is enterotoxigenic *Escherichia coli*. Common viruses include norovirus, rotavirus, and astrovirus. Most common protozoa is *Giardia* (2).

- Length—bacterial causes last 3 to 7 days if untreated. Viral lasts 2 to 3 days. Protozoal can last weeks to months if not treated.
- High-risk areas include Asia, Middle East, Africa, Mexico, and Central and South America (2).
- Intermediate-risk areas include countries in Eastern Europe, South Africa, and some of the Caribbean islands (2).
- Strategies to minimize diarrhea (2)
  - Wash hands or use sanitizer prior to eating.
  - Avoid raw or undercooked meat, fish, or shellfish, salads, uncooked vegetables, unpasteurized fruit juices, or unpasteurized milk or milk products.
  - Avoid unpeeled raw fruit. Peel it yourself if possible.
  - Tap water may be unsafe for drinking, making ice, preparing food, washing dishes, or brushing teeth; use sealed bottled water if possible.
- For high-risk patients—bismuth subsalicylate reduces incidence of travelers' diarrhea by 50%; 2 oz of liquid or two chewable tablets QID (not recommended for children <3 years or pregnant women) (2)
- Treatment based on severity of disease (2)
  - Mild—diarrhea is tolerable, not distressing, and does not interfere with activities; does not require antibiotics
  - Moderate—diarrhea is distressing and interferes with planned activities. Antibiotics such as fluoroquinolones, azithromycin, or rifaximin. Loperamide can be used as a monotherapy.
  - Severe—incapacitating diarrhea. Azithromycin is preferred agent, although fluoroquinolones and rifaximin can also be used.
- Antibiotic options for travelers' diarrhea treatment
  - Azithromycin 1,000 mg one-time dose, if symptoms not resolved in 24 hours, then continue daily dosing for 3 days. Alternate dosing is 500 mg daily for 3 days.
  - Ciprofloxacin 750 mg one-time dose, if symptoms not resolved in 24 hours, then continue daily dosing for 3 days. Alternate dosing is 500 mg BID × 3 days.
  - Rifaximin 200 mg TID × 3 days
- Adjunct medications
  - Loperamide
    - 4 mg initially followed by 2 mg after each loose stool (max 16 mg/day)
    - Pediatric dose
    - Not recommended for children <6 years
    - 6 to 8 years—2 mg initial dose, followed by 1 mg after each loose stool (max 4 mg/day)
    - 9 to 11 years—2 mg after initial dose, followed by 1 mg after each loose stool (max 6 mg/day)
    - ≥12 years: Refer to adult dosing.
  - Diphenoxylate
    - 5 mg (2 tablets) TID or QID until control achieved (max 20 mg/day)
    - Pediatric dose: not recommended for children <2 years; 0.3 to 0.4 mg/kg/day in 4 divided doses
- Altitude illness
  - More likely at an altitude of 8,000 feet (2,500 m) or higher, although can occur at lower altitudes. Children and adults are equally susceptible. Factors that increase risk are elevation at destination, rate of ascent, and exertion (2).
  - Acute mountain sickness (AMS)—most common. Typically presents with headache starting 2 to 12 hours after arrival. Other symptoms include fatigue, loss of appetite, nausea, and vomiting; usually resolves within 24 to 48 hours of acclimatization (2)
  - High-altitude cerebral edema (HACE)—severe progression of AMS. Rare, although most often associated with high-altitude pulmonary edema (HAPE). Lethargy, drowsiness, confusion, ataxia; requires immediate descent (2)
  - HAPE—can occur by itself or with AMS and HACE. Symptoms begin with shortness of breath on exertion and progress to shortness of breath at rest, weakness, and cough. Supplemental oxygen and immediate descent. HACE and HAPE can be fatal, although HAPE is more rapidly fatal (2).
  - Preventive measures
    - Ascend gradually—from low altitude to <9,000 feet in 1 day. >9,000 feet, don't climb >1,600 feet per day. Plan an extra day for acclimatization every 3,300 feet (2).
    - In first 48 hours, avoid alcohol and only perform mild exercise.
  - Preventive medications
    - Recommended for those at high risk for AMS (based on rate of ascent or history of HACE or HAPE): Consider for those at moderate risk.
    - Acetazolamide—AMS/HACE prevention dose: 125 mg BID (250 mg BID if >100 kg); pediatric dose: 2.5 mg/kg q12h (2)
      - AMS treatment dose: 250 mg BID; pediatric dose: 2.5 mg/kg q12h; used as an adjunct to dexamethasone
    - Dexamethasone—usually reserved for treatment; prevention dose: 2 mg q6h or 4 mg q12h; should not be used for prophylaxis in pediatric patients (2)
      - AMS treatment dose: 4 mg q6h PO, IV, or IM (2)
      - HACE treatment dose: 8 mg once, then 4 mg q6h PO, IV, or IM; pediatric dose: 0.15 mg/kg/dose q6h up to 4 mg (2)
    - Nifedipine—for prevention and treatment of HAPE; dose: 30 mg SR q12h (2)
    - Tadalafil—for prevention of HAPE only; dose: 10 mg BID (2)
    - Sildenafil—for HAPE prevention; dose: 50 mg q8h (2)
- Jet lag
  - Before travel, adjust sleep cycle (and possibly meal times) 1 to 2 hours earlier or later (depending on direction of travel) for several days prior to departure.
  - Drink plenty of water to remain hydrated.
  - Optimize sunlight exposure to destination.
  - Sedative hypnotics (nonbenzodiazepine), such as zolpidem, can be useful.
  - If using benzodiazepines, use short-acting agents, such as temazepam.
- Motion sickness
  - High-risk individuals
    - Children ages 2 to 12 years
    - Women, especially when pregnant, menstruating, or on hormones
    - People who get migraines
  - Prevention strategies
    - Avoidance of known triggers
    - Strategic positioning (front of car, overwing of aircraft)
  - Treatment
    - Dimenhydrinate: pediatric dose: 1.0 to 1.5 mg/kg 1 hour before travel and every 6 hours during the trip
    - Diphenhydramine: pediatric dose: 0.5 to 1.0 mg/kg/dose up to 25 mg 1 hour before travel and every 6 hours during the trip
    - Scopolamine: transdermal patch to hairless area behind ear at least 4 hours prior to exposure and every 3 days as needed; should not be used in children
- Environmental hazards
  - Avoid walking barefoot (parasites can enter skin).
  - Avoid swimming in freshwater where there is a risk for schistosomiasis or leptospirosis.

- Use sunscreen.
- If scuba diving, avoid flying or altitude exposure >2,000 feet (2).
  - ≥12 hours after surfacing from nondecompression dive
  - ≥18 hours after repetitive dives or multiple days of diving
  - 24 to 28 hours after a dive that required decompression stops
- Other information
  - Avoid contact with animals because bites and scratches may transmit rabies.
  - Discuss risks such as traffic accidents, alcohol misuse, personal assault, robbery, and water safety.
  - Check hotels or other sleeping locations for bed bugs on bedding and furniture.
  - Consider travel insurance (including coverage for evacuation).
  - Hand carry medications and supplies.
  - Include medications to manage exacerbations or complications of existing chronic diseases.
  - Avoid areas with known outbreaks of communicable disease. Reference the CDC Travelers' Health Web site before travel.
  - The Department of State's Smart Traveler Enrollment Program provides destination-specific travel alerts.

REFERENCES

1. Bagshaw M, DeVoll J, Jennings R, et al. *Medical Guidelines for Airline Passengers*. Alexandria, VA: Aerospace Medical Association; 2002. https://www.asma.org/asma/media/asma/Travel-Publications/paxguidelines.pdf. Accessed December 8, 2019.
2. Brunette GW, Nemhauser JB, Kozarsky PE, et al. *CDC Yellow Book 2020: Health Information for International Travel*. New York, NY: Oxford University Press; 2019.
3. Sanford C, McConnell A, Osborn J. The pretravel consultation. *Am Fam Physician*. 2016;94(8):620–627.

ADDITIONAL READING

- Centers for Disease Control and Prevention. Travelers' health. https://wwwnc.cdc.gov/travel. Accessed January 3, 2021.
- Sanford CA, Pottinger PS, Jong EC. *The Travel and Tropical Medicine Manual*. 5th ed. St. Louis, MO: Elsevier; 2017.
- U.S. Department of State—Bureau of Consular Affairs. Travel.State.Gov. https://travel.state.gov/content/travel.html. Accessed January 15, 2021.
- World Travel & Tourism Council: https://wttc.org/

 CODES

ICD10
- Z71.9 Counseling, unspecified
- Z71.89 Other specified counseling

CLINICAL PEARLS

- The COVID-19 pandemic has drastically altered the landscape of domestic and international travel.
- The CDC Travelers' Health Web site is a useful point-of-care tool for destination-specific travel advice (https://wwwnc.cdc.gov/travel/).
- To allow adequate time for vaccine response and delivery of necessary pretrip medications, patients should seek advice several weeks prior to anticipated travel.

ARTERITIS, TEMPORAL

Irfan H. Siddiqui, MD • Sandra Pasiah, MD

BASICS

DESCRIPTION
- Technically termed giant cell arteritis (GCA)
- A chronic, generalized, cellular, and humoral immune-mediated vasculitis of large- and medium-sized vessels, predominantly affecting the cranial arteries originating from the aortic arch, although vascular involvement may be widespread. Inflammation of the aorta is observed in 50% of cases.
- Frequent features include fatigue, headaches, jaw claudication, visual symptoms, scalp tenderness, constitutional symptoms, polymyalgia rheumatica (PMR) symptoms, and aortic arch syndrome (decreased or absent peripheral pulses, discrepancies of blood pressure, arterial bruits).
- Considered medical emergency due to risk of irreversible vision loss if not treated due to ophthalmic artery occlusion

EPIDEMIOLOGY
- Most common form of systemic vasculitis affecting persons ≥50 years old
- 80% of cases occur ages 70 to 80.
- Women are affected about 2 to 3 times more than men in persons of Northern European descent.
- Most common vasculitis in individuals of Northern European descent
- Rare in persons of Asian or African descent
- Lower BMI associated with increased risk

Incidence
- Incidence varies by ethnicity.
- Prevalence in Northern Europeans is 2 per 1,000 persons.
- Peaks in patients 70 to 80 years old

ETIOLOGY AND PATHOPHYSIOLOGY
- The exact etiology of GCA remains unknown, although current theory suggests that advanced age, ethnicity, and specific genetic predisposition lead to a maladaptive response to endothelial injury, intimal hyperplasia, and ultimately vascular stenosis.
- GCA is a chronic, systemic vasculitis primarily affecting the elastic lamina of medium- and large-sized arteries. Histopathology of affected arteries is marked by transmural inflammation of the intima, media, and adventitia, as well as patchy infiltration by lymphocytes, macrophages, and multinucleated giant cells. Mural hyperplasia can result in arterial luminal narrowing, resulting in subsequent distal ischemia.
- Current theory regarding the etiology of GCA is that a maladaptive response to endothelial injury leads to an inappropriate activation of T-cell–mediated immunity via immature antigen-presenting cells. The subsequent release of cytokines within the arterial vessel wall can attract macrophages and multinucleated giant cells, which form granulomatous infiltrates and give diseased vessels their characteristic histology. This also leads to an oligoclonal expansion of T-cells directed against antigens in or near the elastic lamina. Ultimately, this cascade results in vessel wall damage, intimal hyperplasia, and eventual stenotic occlusion.

- In recent years, GCA and PMR have increasingly been considered to be closely related conditions.
- Varicella zoster virus has been proposed as possible immune trigger for GCA; however, this has not been substantiated, and adjunctive treatment with antivirals remains controversial.

Genetics
The gene for *HLA-DRB1*04* has been identified as a risk factor for GCA, and polymorphisms of *ICAM-1* and *PTPN-22* have also been implicated.

RISK FACTORS
- Increasing age (>70 years) is the greatest risk factor.
- Females
- Genetic predisposition—occasional family clustering has been reported.
- Environmental factors influence susceptibility
- History of smoking
- Early menopause (<43 years) and lower BMI at menopause in women 50 to 69 years old

COMMONLY ASSOCIATED CONDITIONS
Population studies have shown 40–60% of patients diagnosed with GCA also have PMR symptoms, and 16–21% of patient with PMR have GCA.

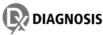

DIAGNOSIS

HISTORY
- Most common presenting symptom is headache (2/3 of patients).
- Constitutional symptoms (fever, fatigue, weight loss)
- Any visual disturbances (amaurosis fugax, diplopia)
- Vision loss (20% of patients); unilateral is most common, often proceeds to bilateral if untreated.
- Jaw claudication (presence of symptom significantly increases likelihood of a positive biopsy)
- Scalp tenderness or sensitivity
- Claudication of upper extremities or tongue
- Symptoms of PMR (shoulder and hip girdle pain and stiffness)
- Distal extremity swelling/edema
- Upper respiratory symptoms

PHYSICAL EXAM
- Temporal artery abnormalities (beading, prominence, tenderness)
- Typically appear "ill"
- Decreased peripheral pulses in the presence of large vessel diseases
- Funduscopic exam shows pale and edema of the optic disc, scattered cotton wool patches, and small hemorrhages.
- Unlike other forms of vasculitis, GCA rarely involves the skin, kidneys, and lungs.
- Supraclavicular, axillary, and supraorbital bruits

DIFFERENTIAL DIAGNOSIS
- Migraines
- Herpes zoster
- Other vasculitis (Takayasu arteritis, Wegener, PAN)
- Other rheumatologic condition (RA, PMR, MCTD)

DIAGNOSTIC TESTS & INTERPRETATION
- American College of Rheumatology 1990 classification criteria are as follows:
  - Age >50 years
  - New localized headache
  - Temporal artery abnormality (tenderness to palpation, decreased or absent pulses)
  - ESR >50 mm/hr
  - Abnormal temporal artery biopsy showing vasculitis with predominance of mononuclear cell infiltration or granulomatous inflammation
- 3 or more of the ACR criteria demonstrate a sensitivity of 94.5% and a specificity of 91.2%.

Initial Tests (lab, imaging)
- ESR >50 mm/hr (86% sensitivity), although nonspecific (27%); infrequently, may be normal
- C-reactive protein (CRP) >2.45 mg/dL is a more sensitive marker of inflammation (97% sensitivity) and is associated with increased odds of a positive biopsy result.
- A normal ESR and/or CRP renders the diagnosis of GCA unlikely.
- Acute-phase reactants (fibrinogen, interleukin-6) are frequently elevated but very nonspecific and reserved for diagnostically difficult cases.
- Mild anemia: very nonspecific but may be associated with a lower rate of ischemic complications
- Color Doppler US of the temporal artery may identify vascular occlusion, stenosis, or edema ("halo sign"); it is low cost and noninvasive but also very operator dependent and does not significantly improve on the clinical exam. It may aid in the diagnosis of larger vessel involvement.
- Atherosclerotic disease with carotid intima-media thickness >0.9 mm may mimic halo sign.
- MRI and MRA may be beneficial in diagnosis (78% sensitive, 90% specific) if performed within 5 days of steroids.
- Positron emission tomography (PET), like MRI/MRA and color Doppler, may be useful in diagnostically difficult cases to quantify the inflammatory burden and early in the course of disease, as the metabolic changes occur prior to structural vascular damage, but it also lacks studies to support its use.

Follow-Up Tests & Special Considerations
- Development of aortic aneurysms (late and potentially serious complication of GCA) can lead to aortic dissection.
- Due to the risk of irreversible vision loss, treatment with high-dose steroids should be started on strong clinical suspicion of GCA, prior to the temporal biopsy being done.

Diagnostic Procedures/Other

- Gold standard diagnostic study: histopathologic examination of the temporal artery biopsy specimen (Do not delay starting medication if suspicion as pathology remains up to 14 days after starting steroids.)
- Overall sensitivity is 87%.
- The temporal artery is chosen because of its accessibility in the systemic disease; alternatively, facial artery or other cranial arteries may be used.
- Length of biopsy specimen should be at least 2 cm to avoid false-negative results because skip lesions may occur.
- Diagnostic yield of biopsy may be increased if procedure is coupled with imaging (high-resolution MRI or color Doppler US).
- Bilateral temporal artery biopsy should not be performed, unless the initial histopathology is negative and the suspicion for GCA remains high.
- May be negative in up to 42% of patients with GCA, especially in large vessel disease, and a negative biopsy alone should not dictate treatment
- Biopsy results are not affected by prior glucocorticoids, so treatment should not be delayed.

Test Interpretation

- Inflammation of the arterial wall, with fragmentation and disruption of the internal elastic lamina
- Multinucleated giant cells are found in <50% of cases and are not specific for the disease.
- GCA occurs in three histologic patterns: classic, atypical, and healed.

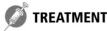 TREATMENT

MEDICATION

First Line

Glucocorticoids:

- The typical dose of prednisone is between 60 and 80 mg/day (or 1 mg/kg/day), and the dose may be titrated up to relieve symptoms. Steroids should not be in the form of alternate day therapy because this is more likely to lead to a relapse of vasculitis (1)[A].
- IV steroids indicated if vision loss has been noted, otherwise PO steroids are equally as effective (1)[C].
- Given risk of irreversible vision loss, immediate steroid therapy should be initiated prior to confirmation by biopsy.
- The initial dose of steroids is continued for 2 to 4 weeks and slowly tapered over 9 to 12 months. Tapering may require ≥2 years (1)[A]. Assess for relapse during taper by monitoring symptoms, ESR, CRP.
- Tocilizumab (an IL-6 receptor antagonist) 162 mg SQ weekly or biweekly in addition to prednisone may be superior to prednisone alone although it does carry a black box warning regarding increased risk of opportunistic infections.
- It has been suggested that low-dose aspirin might be effective for patients with GCA.

Second Line

- Methotrexate as an adjunct to glucocorticoid therapy may have a modest effect in decreasing the relapse rate of GCA.
- Cyclophosphamide have shown some benefit in patients who have not adequately responded to glucocorticoids.
- Azathioprine and abatacept can also be used as adjuncts to glucocorticoids.
- Therapies directed at TNF as adjunct to steroids have not shown significant benefit (1)[B].

 ONGOING CARE

FOLLOW-UP RECOMMENDATIONS

Sun avoidance and protection of the head and the face from photodamage may eventually prove to be important preventive measures for GCA.

Patient Monitoring

- GCA is typically self-limited and lasts several months or years.
- Overall, GCA does not seem to decrease longevity. Nevertheless, it may lead to serious complications such as visual loss, which occurs in about 15–20% of patients.
- Another complication of GCA is the development of aortic aneurysms, usually affecting the ascending aorta. Yearly, chest x-rays may be useful to identify this problem.
- About 50% of the patients with GCA will eventually develop PMR (stiffness of shoulder and hip girdle).
- Low-dose aspirin should be given as indicated by atherosclerosis guidelines.

DIET

Calcium and vitamin D supplementation should be administered for osteoporosis prevention associated with prolonged corticosteroid therapy.

PATIENT EDUCATION

- Consequences of discontinuing steroids abruptly (adrenal insufficiency, disease relapse)
- Risks of long-term steroid use (infection, hyperglycemia, weight gain, impaired wound healing, osteoporosis, hypertension)
- Possibility of relapse and importance of reporting new headaches and vision changes to provider immediately

PROGNOSIS

- Variable duration of disease, from 1 year to chronic course
- Life expectancy is not affected by the disease unless severe aortitis is present.
- Once vision loss has occurred, it is unlikely to be recovered, but treatment resolves the other symptoms and prevents future vision loss and stroke.

- In most patients, glucocorticoid therapy can eventually be discontinued without complications. In patients with chronic disease, however, prednisone may need to be continued for years.
- Disease relapse is possible.

COMPLICATIONS

- Vision loss with delayed diagnosis
- Glucocorticoid-related toxicity

REFERENCE

1. Borchers AT, Gershwin ME. Giant cell arteritis: a review of classification, pathophysiology, geoepidemiology and treatment. *Autoimmun Rev.* 2012;11(6–7):A544–A554.

ADDITIONAL READING

De Miguel E, Beltran LM, Monjo I, et al. Atherosclerosis as a potential pitfall in the diagnosis of giant cell arteritis. *Rheumatology (Oxford).* 2018;57(2):318–321.

 SEE ALSO

Depression; Fibromyalgia; Headache, Cluster; Headache, Tension; Polymyalgia Rheumatica; Polymyositis/Dermatomyositis

 CODES

ICD10

- M31.6 Other giant cell arteritis
- M31.5 Giant cell arteritis with polymyalgia rheumatica

CLINICAL PEARLS

- Due to the risk of irreversible vision loss, treatment with high-dose steroids (prednisone 60 mg/day) should be started immediately in patients suspected of GCA.
- Temporal artery biopsy is the gold standard for diagnosis. Temporal artery biopsy is not likely to be affected by a few weeks of treatment.
- Treatment consists of a very slow steroid taper. Bone protection therapy and low-dose aspirin should be considered.
- Normal ESR level = value of age / 2 for men and age + 10 / 2 for women
- Patients on corticosteroids should be placed on therapy to minimize osteoporosis, unless there are contraindications.

ARTHRITIS, JUVENILE IDIOPATHIC

Donna Marie McMahon, DO, FAAP • Kathleen M. Vazzana, MSc, DO

 BASICS

DESCRIPTION

- Juvenile idiopathic arthritis (JIA) is the most common chronic pediatric rheumatologic disease.
- JIA can be associated with significant disability.
  - Age of onset: <16 years of age
  - Common symptoms: joint swelling, restricted range of motion, warmth, redness, pain
  - ≥6 weeks of symptoms prior to diagnosis
- Seven (International League of Associations for Rheumatology [ILAR]) subtypes determined by clinical characteristics in first 6 months of illness (1):
  - Systemic: 10%; preceded by febrile onset of ≥2 weeks with rash, serositis, hepatospleno-megaly, or lymphadenopathy (1)
  - Polyarticular rheumatoid factor (RF) (+): 2–7%; ≥5 joints involvement (1); large and small joints; RF positive on two tests ≥3 months apart (2)
  - Polyarticular RF (−): 10–30%; ≥5 (large and small) joints involved (1); RF (−) (2)
  - Oligoarticular: 30–60%; involvement of 1 to 4 joints; risk for chronic uveitis in antinuclear antibodies (ANA) (+) females (1) and axial skeletal involvement in older boys (2). Types: (i) persistent (40%): knee, ankle, elbow; (ii) extended type (20%): >4 joints after first 6 months
  - Psoriatic arthritis: 5%; arthritis with psoriasis or arthritis with >2 of the following: dactylitis, nail changes (pitting), psoriasis in first-degree relative (1)
  - Enthesitis-related arthritis: 1–11%; arthritis and enthesitis or one of them plus at least two of the following: sacroiliac or lumbosacral pain, Reiter syndrome or acute anterior uveitis in first-degree relative, acute symptomatic anterior uveitis, human leukocyte antigen (HLA)-B27 (+), history of ankylosing spondylitis, sacroiliitis with inflammatory bowel disease, onset of arthritis in male >6 years old (1)[C]
  - Undifferentiated arthritis (11–21%): presents with overlapping symptoms in ≥2 categories above or arthritis that does not fulfill above categories (2)
- Systems affected: musculoskeletal, hematologic, lymphatic, immunologic, dermatologic, ophthalmologic, gastrointestinal (GI)
- Synonyms: juvenile chronic arthritis; juvenile arthritis; juvenile rheumatoid arthritis (JRA); Still disease (2)

EPIDEMIOLOGY

Male = female (1); onset: throughout childhood; 54% of cases occur in children 0 to 5 years.

Incidence

2 to 20/100,000 children <16 years in developed nations

Prevalence

16 to 150/100,000 children <16 years in developed nations (1)

ETIOLOGY AND PATHOPHYSIOLOGY

- Humoral and cellular immunodysregulation. T lymphocytes play a key role.
- Genetic predisposition; IL2RA/CD25 and VTCN1 implicated as genetic loci
- Environmental triggers, possibly infectious
  - Rubella or parvovirus B19 (3)
  - Heat shock proteins (3)
- Immunoglobulin or complement deficiency

RISK FACTORS

Female gender 3:1

COMMONLY ASSOCIATED CONDITIONS

Other autoimmune disorders, chronic anterior uveitis (iridocyclitis), nutritional impairment, growth issues (3)[C]

 DIAGNOSIS

Clinical criteria: age of onset <16 years and >6 weeks duration of objective arthritis (swelling or restricted range of motion of a joint with heat, pain, or tenderness and no other form of childhood arthritis) in ≥1 joints

HISTORY

- Arthralgias, fever, fatigue, malaise, myalgias, weight loss, morning stiffness, rash
- Limp if lower extremity involvement
- Arthritis for ≥6 weeks

PHYSICAL EXAM

- Arthritis: swelling, effusion, loss of musculoskeletal landmarks, limited range of motion, tenderness, pain with motion, warmth
- Rash, rheumatoid nodules (uncommon), lymph-adenopathy, hepato- or splenomegaly, enthesitis, dactylitis (mainly in psoriatic type)

DIFFERENTIAL DIAGNOSIS

- Legg-Calvé-Perthes, toxic synovitis, growing pains, Perthes disease
- Septic arthritis, osteomyelitis, viral infection, myco-plasmal infection, Lyme disease
- Reactive arthritis: postinfectious, rheumatic fever, Reiter syndrome
- Inflammatory bowel disease
- Hemoglobinopathies, hemarthrosis, rickets
- Leukemia (particularly acute lymphocytic leukemia), bone tumors (osteoid osteoma), neuroblastoma
- Vasculitis, Henoch-Schönlein purpura, Kawasaki disease
- Systemic lupus erythematosus, dermatomyositis, mixed connective tissue disease, sarcoidosis, systemic sclerosis, collagen disorders
- Farber disease
- Accidental or nonaccidental trauma

DIAGNOSTIC TESTS & INTERPRETATION

Initial Tests (lab, imaging)

- CBC: Leukocyte count is normal or elevated (systemic); lymphopenia, reactive thrombocytosis, anemia; liver function test (LFT; hepatic involvement) and renal function studies (prior to therapy with nephrotoxic drugs)
- Joint-fluid aspiration/analysis to exclude infection
- ESR and C-reactive protein typically elevated; C-reactive protein often disproportionately high
- Myeloid-related proteins (MRP 8/14) associated with flares
- ANA-positive patients have increased risk of uveitis; ANA positive in up to 70% with oligoarticular JIA

- RF (+): 2–10% (usually polyarticular); poor prognosis
- HLA-B27 positive: enthesitis-related arthritis
- Diagnostic radiography, MRI, ultrasound, and CT; no one modality has superior diagnostic value (4)[A]
- Radiograph of affected joint(s): *early* radiographic changes: soft tissue swelling, periosteal reaction, juxta-articular demineralization; *later* changes: joint space loss, articular surface erosions, subchondral cyst formation, sclerosis, joint fusion
- If orthopnea, obtain ECG to rule out pericarditis.
- Radionuclide scans: for infection/malignancy
- CT is best for bony abnormalities. MRI can assess synovial hypertrophy and cartilage degeneration; MRI more sensitive to monitor disease activity and clinical responsiveness to treatment in peripheral joints

Follow-Up Tests & Special Considerations

Use pediatric (not adult) controls when interpreting results of dual energy x-ray absorptiometry

Diagnostic Procedures/Other

- **Ultrasound**: Assess for inflammation (4)[A].
- **Synovial biopsy**: if synovial fluid cannot be aspirated or if infection is suspected in spite of negative synovial fluid culture

Test Interpretation

Synovial biopsy → synovial cell hyperplasia, hyperemia, infiltration of small lymphocytes and mononuclear cells

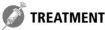 **TREATMENT**

GENERAL MEASURES

- Goal is to control active disease, minimize extra-articular manifestations, and achieve clinical remission.
- All patients require regular (every 3 to 4 months for oligoarticular JIA and in ANA-positive patients) ophthalmic exams to uncover asymptomatic eye disease, particularly for the first 3 years following diagnosis.
- Moist heat or electric blanket for morning stiffness
- Splints for contractures
- Aerobic exercise: weight-bearing or aquatic therapy to improve functional capacity

MEDICATION

First Line

- ≤4 joints
  - NSAIDs (ibuprofen, naproxen, celecoxib): adequate in ~50%; symptoms often improve within days; full efficacy 2 to 3 months
    - Precautions: may worsen bleeding diatheses; use caution in renal insufficiency and hypovolemic states; take with food.
    - Significant drug interactions: may lower serum levels of anticonvulsants and blunt the effect of loop diuretics; NSAIDs may increase serum methotrexate levels.

- Intra-articular long-acting corticosteroids: immediately effective; improve synovitis, joint damage, contractures, prevent leg length discrepancy (4)[B]
  - Indication: patients with oligoarthritis who fail a 2-month NSAID trial or with poor prognosis (2)
- ≥5 joints
  - If high disease activity or a failed 1 to 2 months NSAID trial → methotrexate (5)[C]

Second Line
- 30–40% of patients require addition of disease-modifying antirheumatic drugs (DMARDs): methotrexate, sulfasalazine, leflunomide, and tumor necrosis factor (TNF) antagonists (etanercept, infliximab, adalimumab); newer biologic therapies, including IL-1 and IL-6 receptor antagonists, are currently under investigation.
- Methotrexate: 10 mg/m²/week PO or SC
- Sulfasalazine: oligoarticular and HLA-B27 spondylarthritis
- Etanercept: 0.8 mg/kg (max of 50 mg/dose) given SC q1wk or 0.4 mg/kg SC twice a week (max of 25 mg/dose)
- Infliximab: 5 mg/kg q6–8wk
- Adalimumab: if weight 15 kg to <30 kg, 20 mg SC q2wk; if weight ≥30 kg, 40 mg SC q2wk
- Rituximab: for polyarticular RF+ who have failed two TNF-α inhibitors (4)
- Tocilizumab: for RF-pJIA who have failed two TNF-α inhibitors (4)
- Begin treatment with TNF-α inhibitors in children with a history of arthritis in ≤4 joints and significant active arthritis despite treatment with methotrexate or arthritis in ≥5 joints and any active arthritis following an adequate trial of methotrexate (6)[C].
- Anakinra: IL-1 receptor antagonist. Begin treatment with anakinra in children with systemic arthritis and active fever whose treatment requires a second medication, in addition to systemic glucocorticoids (6).

ISSUES FOR REFERRAL
- Consult pediatric rheumatologist for assistance with management of JIA.
- Orthopedics as needed for articular complications
- Ophthalmology to evaluate for uveitis and continued screening
- Physical therapy to maintain range of motion, improve muscle strength, and prevent deformities
- Occupational therapy to maintain and improve appropriate age-related functional activities
- Behavioral health if difficulty coping with disease

SURGERY/OTHER PROCEDURES
- Total hip and/or knee replacement for severe disease
- Soft tissue release if splinting/traction unsuccessful
- Correct limb length or angular deformities
- Synovectomy is rarely performed.

ADMISSION, INPATIENT, AND NURSING CONSIDERATIONS
- Hospitalize if:
  - Patient unable to ambulate
  - Signs/symptoms of pericarditis
  - Persistent fever or diagnostic confusion to facilitate evaluation and workup
  - Need for surgery
- Discharge when fever and serositis resolved.

ONGOING CARE

FOLLOW-UP RECOMMENDATIONS
Patient Monitoring
Determined by medication and disease activity
- NSAIDs: periodic CBC, urinalysis, LFTs, renal function tests
- Aspirin and/or other salicylates: transaminase and salicylate levels weekly for 1 month and then every 3 to 4 months
- Methotrexate: monthly LFTs, CBC, BUN, creatinine

PATIENT EDUCATION
- Psychosocial needs; school issues; behavioral strategies for dealing with pain and noncompliance; available health care resources; support groups
- http://www.rheumatology.org/I-Am-A/Patient-Caregiver

PROGNOSIS
- 50–60% of patients will ultimately achieve remission.
- Functional ability depends on adequacy of therapy (disease control, maintaining muscle and joint function).
- Poor prognosis: patients with active disease at 6 months; polyarticular disease; extended pauciarticular disease course; female gender; RF (+); ANA (+); persistent morning stiffness; rapid appearance of erosions; hip involvement

COMPLICATIONS
- Blindness, band keratopathy, glaucoma, short stature, micrognathia if temporomandibular joint involvement, debilitating joint disease, disseminated intravascular coagulation, hemolytic anemia
- NSAIDs: peptic ulcer, GI hemorrhage, CNS reactions, renal disease, leukopenia
- DMARDs: bone marrow suppression, hepatitis, renal disease, dermatitis, mouth ulcers, retinal toxicity (antimalarials; rare)
- TNF antagonists: higher risk of infection
- Osteoporosis, avascular necrosis
- Methotrexate: Folate supplementation decreases hepatic/GI symptoms; may reduce stomatitis
- Macrophage activation syndrome: decreased blood cell precursors secondary to histiocyte degradation of marrow

REFERENCES

1. Giancane G, Alongi A, Ravelli A. Update on the pathogenesis and treatment of juvenile idiopathic arthritis. *Curr Opin Rheumatol.* 2017;29(5):523–529.
2. Saad N, Onel K. Overview of juvenile idiopathic arthritis. *Open Orthop J.* 2020;14:101–109.
3. Collado P, Vojinovic J, Nieto JC, et al; for Omeract Ultrasound Pediatric Group. Toward standardized musculoskeletal ultrasound in pediatric rheumatology: normal age-related ultrasound findings. *Arthritis Care Res (Hoboken).* 2016;68(3):348–356.
4. Webb K, Wedderburn LR. Advances in the treatment of polyarticular juvenile idiopathic arthritis. *Curr Opin Rheumatol.* 2015;27(5):505–510.
5. Beukelman T, Patkar NM, Saag KG, et al. 2011 American College of Rheumatology recommendations for the treatment of juvenile idiopathic arthritis: initiation and safety monitoring of therapeutic agents for the treatment of arthritis and systemic features. *Arthritis Care Res (Hoboken).* 2011;63(4):465–482.
6. Grevich S, Shenoi S. Update on the management of systemic juvenile idiopathic arthritis and role of IL-1 and IL-6 inhibition. *Adolesc Health Med Ther.* 2017;8:125–135.

ADDITIONAL READING

- Chausset A, Pereira B, Echaubard S, et al. Access to paediatric rheumatology care in juvenile idiopathic arthritis: what do we know? A systematic review. *Rheumatology (Oxford).* 2020;59(12):3633–3644.
- Ringold S, Angeles-Han ST, Beukelman T, et al. 2019 American College of Rheumatology/Arthritis Foundation guideline for the treatment of juvenile idiopathic arthritis: therapeutic approaches for non-systemic polyarthritis, sacroiliitis, and enthesitis. *Arthritis Rheumatol.* 2019;71(6):846–863.
- Shenoi S. Juvenile idiopathic arthritis—changing times, changing terms, changing treatments. *Pediatr Rev.* 2017;38(5):221–232.
- Shoop-Worrall SJW, Wu Q, Davies R, et al. Predicting disease outcomes in juvenile idiopathic arthritis: challenges, evidence and new directions. *Lancet Child Adolesc Health.* 2019;3(10):725–733.

CODES

ICD10
- M08.90 Juvenile arthritis, unspecified, unspecified site
- M08.80 Other juvenile arthritis, unspecified site
- M08.00 Unsp juvenile rheumatoid arthritis of unspecified site

CLINICAL PEARLS
- JIA is the most common form of arthritis in children.
- Consider JIA in any child presenting with a limp.
- High-titer RF correlates with disease severity; prognosis worse if positive RF titers
- DMARDs improve JIA-associated symptoms.
- NSAIDs are typically first-line choice of medication.

ARTHRITIS, PSORIATIC

Nikki A. Levin, MD, PhD • Zainab Abbas, MD

 BASICS

A chronic, destructive, seronegative arthropathy most common in patients with long-standing psoriasis

DESCRIPTION

- Psoriatic arthritis (PsA) is a seronegative spondyloarthropathy characterized by inflammatory arthritis and enthesitis.
- Five patterns of arthritis in PsA:
  - Asymmetric oligoarthritis: <5 joints
  - Distal interphalangeal (DIP) joint predominant: osteoarthritis-like, associated with nail psoriasis
  - Symmetric polyarthritis: may be indistinguishable from rheumatoid arthritis (RA)—typically milder
  - Spondyloarthritis: asymmetric and discontinuous, unlike ankylosing spondylitis (AS)
  - Arthritis mutilans: destructive, resorptive arthritis; produces "opera-glass" or "telescoping" digit
- Psoriasis may be limited in extent.
  - Course of arthritis and extent of psoriasis do not correlate.
  - Other extra-articular features, such as iritis, are less common.
  - Damaging joint disease may occur in 40–60%. Characteristic radiologic changes include "pencil-in-cup" deformity and periostitis.
- Rheumatoid factor (RF) and anti–cyclic citrullinated peptide (anti-CCP) antibody are usually negative. HLA-B27 may be positive.

EPIDEMIOLOGY

- Peak onset age: 30 to 50 years
- Predominant gender: female = male
- Polyarthritis is more common in women.
- Spondylitis in up to 25%, more common in males
- Psoriasis precedes arthritis in most patients by an average of 12 years. Arthritis preceding psoriasis occurs in up to 15% of patients, usually children. Arthritis and psoriasis may present simultaneously.
- Psoriasis occurs in 2–3% of the U.S. population; 6–42% will develop PsA (1).

Prevalence

Prevalence: 1 to 2/1,000 population (1)

ETIOLOGY AND PATHOPHYSIOLOGY

- CD4+/CD8+ T cells; tumor necrosis factor α (TNF-α); interleukins 1 (IL-1), 6, 8, and 10; and matrix metalloproteases present in synovial fluid
- Osteoclast precursor cell upregulation
- Unknown. Probably multifactorial: immunologic, genetic, environmental factors

Genetics

- 30–40% concordance in identical twins
- HLA-B27 in 15–50% with PsA (spondylitis pattern) versus 90% in AS
- Other HLA associations in PsA: HLA-B7, HLA-B38, HLA-B39, HLA-Cw6

RISK FACTORS

- Psoriasis
- Family history of PsA
- Obesity

GENERAL PREVENTION

No known prevention strategies; unknown whether early treatment of psoriasis prevents onset of PsA

COMMONLY ASSOCIATED CONDITIONS

Psoriasis

 DIAGNOSIS

- A history of inflammatory arthritis, dactylitis, or enthesitis in patients with existing psoriasis helps establish the diagnosis. It can be difficult to differentiate PsA from other inflammatory arthropathies.
- Use Classification of Psoriatic Arthritis (CASPAR) criteria (91% sensitivity; 99% specificity) to screen patients for PsA. Inflammatory articular disease (joint, spine, or entheseal) with ≥3 points from the following five categories:
  - Evidence of current psoriasis, a personal or family history of psoriasis (2 points)
  - Typical psoriatic nail dystrophy, including onycholysis, pitting, and hyperkeratosis (1 point)
  - Negative RF (ELISA preferred) (1 point)
  - Current or prior history of dactylitis (1 point)
  - Radiologic evidence of new bone formation (excluding osteophyte formation) on plain radiographs of the hand or foot (1 point)

HISTORY

History and physical exam help establish the diagnosis of PsA.

- (Generally) long-standing history of psoriasis
- Morning stiffness of hands, feet, or low back for >30 minutes
- Pain of involved joints
- Swelling or redness of peripheral joints
- Low back or buttock pain
- Ankle or heel pain
- Dactylitis or uniform swelling of an entire digit

PHYSICAL EXAM

- Affected peripheral joints may have overlying erythema, warmth, and swelling.
  - Synovitis
  - Dactylitis
  - Swelling of tendons (e.g., Achilles tendon) and tenderness at insertion sites (e.g., calcaneus)
  - Limited range of motion of axial skeleton
  - Pain with stress of the sacroiliac joint
- Well-demarcated pink-to-red erythematous plaques with a white silvery scale; common locations include scalp, ears, trunk, buttocks, gluteal cleft, elbows and forearms, knees and legs, and palms and soles.
- Nails may be dystrophic with pits, oil spots, crumbling, leukonychia, and red lunulae.

DIFFERENTIAL DIAGNOSIS

- Reactive arthritis
- Psoriasis and RA
- Psoriasis and osteoarthritis
- Psoriasis and polyarticular gout
- Psoriasis and AS

DIAGNOSTIC TESTS & INTERPRETATION

Initial Tests (lab, imaging)

- Serum RF (usually negative)
- Anti-CCP (usually negative)
- Antinuclear antibodies (usually negative)
- Acute-phase reactants (ESR and C-reactive protein) may be elevated.
- HLA-B27 is noted in 50–70% with axial disease and <15% with peripheral disease.
- Baseline radiographs of affected joints
- Plain radiographs may aid diagnosis, assess joint damage, disease progression, and response to therapy.
- Juxta-articular new bone formation (periostitis) and marginal joint erosions that progress centrally ("pencil-in-cup" erosions) are characteristic radiographic features.

Follow-Up Tests & Special Considerations

Follow-up radiographs; interval based on severity

Diagnostic Procedures/Other

Diagnosis is typically clinical.

Test Interpretation

Biopsy of skin or synovium is not usually required.

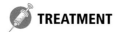 **TREATMENT**

GENERAL MEASURES

Physical therapy and/or occupational therapy benefit all stages of disease.

- Treatment algorithms for PsA are based on severity of joint symptoms, extent of structural damage, and severity of psoriasis. Patients with moderate to severe arthritis should be started on disease-modifying antirheumatic drugs (DMARDs) to reduce or prevent joint damage and preserve joint integrity and function.
- In addition to pharmacotherapy, patients should be educated on lifestyle modifications such as smoking cessation, weight reduction, joint protection, physical activity, exercise, and stress coping mechanisms (2).

MEDICATION

First Line

- NSAIDs to control symptoms of mild disease. Intermittent intra-articular glucocorticoid injections may help.
- There are no systematic trials of NSAIDs for PsA. Dose NSAID to suppress mild inflammation. NSAID selection is based on patient preference and dosing convenience. Sample NSAIDs include ibuprofen 400 to 800 mg PO TID–QID, naproxen 250 to 500 mg PO BID–TID, diclofenac 100 to 150 mg QD, indomethacin 100 to 150 mg QD.
- Monotherapy is as effective as combination therapy (≥2 drugs from the following: analgesics, NSAIDs, opioids, opioid-like drugs, and neuromodulators [antidepressants, anticonvulsants, and muscle relaxants]) (3)[A].

Second Line

- Recommended DMARDs include sulfasalazine, leflunomide, methotrexate. There is no evidence to support the use of combination DMARD therapy.
- Initial dosing regimens for DMARDs: sulfasalazine (2 to 3 g/day PO divided in BID dosing), leflunomide (loading dose of 100 mg/day PO for 3 days and then 20 mg/day PO), methotrexate (1 test dose of 2.5 to 5.0 mg PO to assess for significant bone marrow suppression and then 15 to 25 mg once weekly), azathioprine (0.5 mg/kg/day, with a max dose of 2.5 mg/kg/day if no signs of cytopenia at lower doses)
- Avoid systemic corticosteroids if possible (may help in short term for severe flares while initiating a biologic agent).
- Biologic therapies, particularly anti–TNF-α agents are indicated for patients who do not respond to at least one standard DMARD or in patients with poor prognosis, even if they have not failed a standard DMARD (4)[A],(5).
- Dosing regimens for anti–TNF-α agents:
  – Adalimumab 40 mg SC q2wk
  – Certolizumab pegol 200 mg every 2 week; for maintenance dosing or 400 mg every 4 weeks
  – Etanercept 50 mg SC weekly
  – Golimumab 50 mg SC monthly
  – Infliximab 5 mg/kg at 0, 2, and 6 weeks, q8wk afterward)
- Anti–IL-17 agents include:
  – Ixekizumab 80 mg q2wk (6)
  – Secukinumab 150 mg weekly from 0 to 4 weeks and then monthly (6)
  – Brodalumab 210 mg SC × 1 weekly from 0 to 2 and then q2wk (7)
- Anti–IL-12/IL-23 agents include:
  – Ustekinumab is currently dosed at 45 or 90 mg (depending on weight) at 0, 4, and 12 weeks and then q12wk thereafter (3).
- IL-23 selective inhibitor include:
  – Guselkumab 100 mg SC × 1 at 0 and 4 week and then Q8wk (8)
- PDE4 inhibitors include:
  – Apremilast 30 mg PO BID (6)
- JAK1 and JAK3 inhibitors include:
  – Tofacitinib citrate dosed at 5 mg PO BID immediate release or 11 mg once daily extended release (1)
- Selective T-cell costimulation blocker:
  – Abatacept dosed at 125 mg once weekly SC or according to body weight. Following the initial IV infusion (using the weight-based dosing), repeat IV infusion (using the same weight-based dosing) q2wk and q4wk after the initial infusion, and q4wk thereafter (1).
- Above medications are FDA-approved for PsA.
- Do not use anti-TNF agents in the setting of active infection (including TB and hepatitis B). Do not use anti-TNF agents with concurrent live vaccinations, with New York Heart Association classes III to IV congestive heart failure, with malignancy, or in patients with a history of demyelinating disease.
- Do not use ustekinumab in patients with active infection, mycobacterial or *Salmonella* infection, with concurrent live vaccinations, including bacillus Calmette-Guérin vaccination or with history of malignancy.

Pregnancy Considerations

- Avoid teratogenic medications (e.g., methotrexate, leflunomide) during pregnancy.
- Adalimumab, etanercept, golimumab, infliximab, ustekinumab, and certolizumab pegol, secukinumab, are currently listed as Category B medications. Apremilast, abatacept, tofacitinib citrate, ixekizumab, guselkumab are listed as pregnancy Category C medication.

ISSUES FOR REFERRAL

- Rheumatology
- Dermatology

SURGERY/OTHER PROCEDURES

Joint fusion or replacement for advanced destruction

 ONGOING CARE

FOLLOW-UP RECOMMENDATIONS

Epidemiologic data suggest a relationship between psoriasis, metabolic syndrome, myocardial infarction, and stroke. Control of weight, blood pressure, lipids, and glucose is recommended (2).

PATIENT EDUCATION

- National Psoriasis Foundation: https://www.psoriasis.org/about-psoriatic-arthritis/
- Arthritis Foundation: http://www.arthritis.org/about-arthritis/types/psoriatic-arthritis/
- American College of Rheumatology: https://www.rheumatology.org

PROGNOSIS

- Course is typically insidious with chronic joint disease and recurring/remitting skin disease.
- Prognosis is more favorable than for RA (except for patients who develop arthritis mutilans).

COMPLICATIONS

- Disability
- Psychosocial impact of PsA: anxiety and depression (9)

REFERENCES

1. Ritchlin CT, Colbert RA, Gladman DD. Psoriatic arthritis. *N Engl J Med*. 2017;376(10):957–970.
2. Ahmed N, Prior JA, Chen Y, et al. Prevalence of cardiovascular-related comorbidity in ankylosing spondylitis, psoriatic arthritis and psoriasis in primary care: a matched retrospective cohort study. *Clin Rheumatol*. 2016;35(12):3069–3073.
3. Gossec L, Smolen JS, Ramiro S, et al. European League Against Rheumatism (EULAR) recommendations for the management of psoriatic arthritis with pharmacological therapies: 2015 update. *Ann Rheum Dis*. 2016;75(3):499–510.
4. Coates LC, Kavanaugh A, Mease PJ, et al. Group for Research and Assessment of Psoriasis and Psoriatic Arthritis 2015 treatment recommendations for psoriatic arthritis. *Arthritis Rheumatol*. 2016;68(5):1060–1071.
5. Qiu M, Xu Z, Gao W, et al. Fourteen small molecule and biological agents for psoriatic arthritis: a network meta-analysis of randomized control trials. *Medicine (Baltimore)*. 2020;99(31):e21447.
6. Ash Z, Gaujoux-Viala C, Gossec L, et al. A systematic literature review of drug therapies for the treatment of psoriatic arthritis: current evidence and meta-analysis informing the EULAR recommendations for the management of psoriatic arthritis. *Ann Rheum Dis*. 2012;71(3):319–326.
7. Singh JA, Guyatt F, Ogdie A, et al. Special article: 2018 American College of Rheumatology/National Psoriasis Foundation Guideline for the Treatment of Psoriatic Arthritis. *Arthritis Rheumatol*. 2019;71(1):5–32.
8. Mease PJ, Rahman P, Gottlieb AB, et al. Guselkumab in biologic-naïve patients with active psoriatic arthritis (DISCOVER-2): a double-blind, randomized, placebo-controlled phase 3 trial. *Lancet*. 2020;395(10230):1126–1136.
9. Zhao SS, Miller N, Harrison N, et al. Systematic review of mental health comorbidities in psoriatic arthritis. *Clin Rheumatol*. 2020;39(1):217–225.

ADDITIONAL READING

- Iragorri N, Hazlewood G, Manns B, et al. Psoriatic arthritis screening: a systematic review and meta-analysis. *Rheumatology (Oxford)*. 2019;58(4):692–707.
- Perez-Chada LM, Merola JF. Comorbidities associated with psoriatic arthritis: review and update. *Clin Immunol*. 2020;214:108397.
- Ruyssen-Witrand A, Perry R, Watkins C, et al. Efficacy and safety of biologics in psoriatic arthritis: a systematic literature review and network meta-analysis. *RMD Open*. 2020;6(1):e001117.

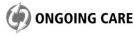 CODES

ICD10

- L40.50 Arthropathic psoriasis, unspecified
- L40.51 Distal interphalangeal psoriatic arthropathy
- L40.53 Psoriatic spondylitis

CLINICAL PEARLS

- One in 4 patients with psoriasis develops PsA.
- The severity of psoriasis correlates with the likelihood of developing arthritis, not the severity of arthritis.
- Commonly overlooked locations of psoriasis include scalp, ears, umbilicus, and gluteal cleft.
- Osteoarthritis and polyarticular gout may mimic or coexist with PsA.
- The polyarticular pattern of PsA mimics RA. The presence of both enthesitis and psoriasis helps differentiate PsA from RA.
- Therapies for PsA are rapidly expanding and include NSAIDS, DMARDS, immunosuppressants, and biologics.

ARTHRITIS, RHEUMATOID (RA)

Theresa A. Townley, MD, MPH • Sonia Gupta, MD

BASICS

DESCRIPTION
- Rheumatoid arthritis (RA) is a chronic inflammatory disease primarily causing synovial inflammation leading to the destruction of bone and cartilage (1).
- Classification: based on the duration of disease (1)
  - Early: ≤6 months
  - Established: ≥6 months
  - Based on the disease activity: low, moderate, high, or remission

EPIDEMIOLOGY
Incidence
Annual incidence: United States is approximately 40/100,000 persons.

Prevalence
- Prevalence: 0.5–1% of the general population worldwide
- Female:male, 2:1

ETIOLOGY AND PATHOPHYSIOLOGY
The cause remains uncertain; often precipitated by stress or insult (e.g., infection, smoking, trauma)

Genetics
HLA-DRB1

RISK FACTORS
Females at a younger age (5th to 6th decade), first- and second-degree relative), North American regions, Native Americans, smoking, obesity, lower socioeconomic status infections

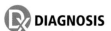**DIAGNOSIS**

HISTORY
Arthritis is insidious in onset, symmetrically involving small joints, morning stiffness ≥1 hour, low-grade fever, and weight loss.

PHYSICAL EXAM
- Swelling and tenderness of metacarpophalangeal (MCP), proximal interphalangeal (PIP), metatarsophalangeal (MTP), and spare distal interphalangeal (DIP) joints
- Ulnar deviation, boutonnière deformity, MCP joint subluxation, radial deviation at the wrist
- Subcutaneous nodules
- Keratoconjunctivitis, rales, and decrease breath sound; pericardial friction rubs; splinter hemorrhage, palpable purpura, skin ulceration, and nail fold infarcts; sensory and/or motor deficit

DIFFERENTIAL DIAGNOSIS
Systemic lupus erythematosus, osteoarthritis, viral hepatitis, tophaceous gout, calcium pyrophosphate dihydrate deposition (CPPD), arthropathy, polymyalgia rheumatica (PMR), postinfectious reactive arthritis, Lyme arthritis

DIAGNOSTIC TESTS & INTERPRETATION
- Elevated ESR and CRP
- Serology: rheumatoid factor and anti–cyclic citrullinated peptide (anti-CCP) antibodies
- X-ray to follow the progression and identify destruction of disease. MRI of hands and wrists (erosions, pannus, synovitis). Ultrasound can assess synovial thickening/erosions.
- Diagnostic criteria
  - American College of Rheumatology criteria (1)
    - At least one joint with clinical synovitis that cannot be explained by another condition
    - The score of ≥6 to classify as RA joint involvement
      - 1 large joint (0 points), 2 to 10 large joints (1 points), 1 to 3 small joints (2 points), 4 to 10 small joints (3 points), >10 joints (5 points)
  - Serology
    - Negative RF or low-positive anti-CCP antibodies (0 points)
    - Low-positive RF or low-positive anti-CCP antibodies (2 points)
    - High-positive RF or high-positive anti-CCP antibodies (3 points)
  - Acute phase reactants
    - Normal CRP or ESR (0 points)
    - Abnormal CRP or ESR (1 point)
  - Duration of symptoms
    - <6 weeks (0 points)
    - ≥6 weeks (1 point)

Follow-Up Tests & Special Considerations
Laboratory monitoring for DMARD (2): CBC, liver transaminases, serum creatinine

Diagnostic Procedures/Other
- Joint aspiration to exclude crystal arthropathy and septic arthritis
- Synovial fluid analysis in RA: yellowish-white, turbid, white blood cell increased (3,500 to 50,000 cells/mm), protein: ~4.2 g/dL (42 g/L), serum-synovial glucose difference >30 mg/dL

Test Interpretation
- Anti-CCP antibodies are present in 60–70% of patients with RA but are 90–98% specific for RA. They are often present years before clinical arthritis. It correlates with erosive disease.
- Rheumatoid factor is positive in 50% of patients at the time of diagnosis and an additional 20–35% becomes positive in 6 months.
- Imaging: x-ray to follow the progression and identify destruction of disease. MRI of hands and wrists (erosions, pannus, synovitis); ultrasound can assess synovial thickening/erosions.

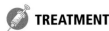 **TREATMENT**

GENERAL MEASURES
Smoking cessation, well-balanced diet, regular physical activity, good dental hygiene

MEDICATION
- DMARDs: azathioprine, cyclosporine, glucocorticoids, gold, intramuscular and oral, hydroxychloroquine, leflunomide, methotrexate (MTX), minocycline, penicillamine, sulfasalazine
- Biologic agent: abatacept, adalimumab, anakinra, certolizumab, etanercept, golimumab, infliximab, rituximab, tocilizumab, tofacitinib
- Strong recommendations (2)
  - If the disease activity is low, use DMARD monotherapy (MTX preferred) over double or triple therapy.
  - If the disease activity remains moderate or high despite DMARD monotherapy, use combination traditional DMARDs or TNF inhibitor or non-TNF biologic rather than continuing traditional DMARD monotherapy.
  - If the patient's disease is in remission, do not discontinue all RA therapies.
  - If disease flares in patient on traditional DMARD, TNF inhibitor, or non-TNF biologics therapy, add a short-term glucocorticoid at the lowest possible dose and for the shortest possible duration.
  - If the patient is in remission, taper medication off.
- Before starting medication
  - Screening for hepatitis B and hepatitis C infection
  - Tuberculin skin test (TST) or interferon-γ release assay (IGRA) before biologic
  - Baseline ophthalmologic examination for patients receiving hydroxychloroquine use

ISSUES FOR REFERRAL
Orthopedics for surgery

SURGERY/OTHER PROCEDURES
Synovectomy, tendon alignment, arthrodesis

COMPLEMENTARY & ALTERNATIVE MEDICINE
Psychosocial interventions, physical, and occupational therapy

ADMISSION, INPATIENT, AND NURSING CONSIDERATIONS
For serious infection, diverticulitis, and gastrointestinal perforation

 ONGOING CARE

DIET
Avoid fatty foods and eat lots of fruits and vegetables.

PROGNOSIS
Poor prognosis with autoantibody and longer disease duration, HLA, erosive disease

COMPLICATIONS
Anemia, lymphoproliferative disease, leukemia, focal glomerulonephritis, depression, carpal tunnel syndrome

REFERENCES
1. Aletaha D, Neogi T, Silman AJ, et al. 2010 Rheumatoid arthritis classification criteria: an American College of Rheumatology/European League Against Rheumatism collaborative initiative. *Arthritis Rheum*. 2010;62(9):2569–2581.
2. Singh JA, Saag KG, Bridges SL Jr, et al. 2015 American College of Rheumatology guideline for the treatment of rheumatoid arthritis. *Arthritis Rheumatol*. 2016;68(1):1–26.

ADDITIONAL READING
- Cush JJ. Rheumatoid arthritis: early diagnosis and treatment. *Med Clin North Am*. 2021;105(2):355–365.
- Sánchez-Flórez JC, Seija-Butnaru D, Valero EG, et al. Pain management strategies in rheumatoid arthritis: a narrative review [published online ahead of print October 8, 2021]. *J Pain Palliat Care Pharmacother*. doi:10.1080/15360288.2021.1973647.

 CODES

ICD10
- M06.9 Rheumatoid arthritis, unspecified
- M05.60 Rheu arthritis of unsp site w involv of organs and systems
- M05.30 Rheumatoid heart disease w rheumatoid arthritis of unsp site

CLINICAL PEARLS
- Early treatment with DMARDs is essential.
- MTX is the first-line treatment for active disease and glucocorticoids are used for flares if patients are already on DMARD therapy.

ARTHRITIS, SEPTIC
Ravishankar E. Rao, MD

BASICS

DESCRIPTION
- Infection due to bacterial invasion of the joint space
- Systems affect: musculoskeletal
- Synonyms: suppurative arthritis; infections arthritis; pyarthrosis; pyogenic arthritis; bacterial arthritis

EPIDEMIOLOGY
Gender differences:
- Gonococcal: female > male
- Nongonococcal: male > female

Incidence
- May occur at any age, bimodal incidence with peaks in childhood and age 55+
- 40 to 60 cases per 100,000 population/year overall (1)
- 70 cases per 100,000 population/year in immuno-compromised and patients with prosthetic joints
- Disseminated gonococcal infection is 3 cases per 100,000 population/year

Prevalence
- 27% of patients presenting with monoarticular arthritis have nongonococcal septic arthritis (1).
- Given rising prevalence of prosthetic joints, infected hardware is now most common form of septic arthritis (~2–10% of all joint recipients).

ETIOLOGY AND PATHOPHYSIOLOGY
- Multiple pathogens
- Nongonococcal:
  - *Staphylococcus aureus* (most common in adults)
    - MRSA risk increased in elderly, intravenous drug users (IVDU), postsurgical
  - *Streptococcus* spp. (second most common in adults)
  - Gram-negative rods (GNR): IVDU, trauma, extremes of age, immunosuppressed
- *Neisseria gonorrhoeae* (most common in young, sexually active adults)
- Polymicrobial infections: *Pantoea agglomerans*, *Nocardia asteroides*; typically occur after penetrating trauma such as bite wounds or organic foreign body penetration
- Other: rickettsial (e.g., Lyme), fungal, mycobacterial
- Risk by specific age:
  - <1 month: *S. aureus*, group B streptococcus (GBS), GNR
  - 1 month to 4 years: *S. aureus*, *Streptococcus pneumoniae*, *Neisseria meningitidis*
  - 16 to 40 years: *N. meningitidis*, *S. aureus*
  - >40 years: *S. aureus*
- Patients with native joint infection are at increased risk for infection of prosthesis (of same joint should it require replacement).
- Specific high-risk groups:
  - Rheumatoid arthritis (RA): *S. aureus*
  - IVDU: *S. aureus*, GNR, opportunistic pathogens
  - Neonates: GBS
  - Immunocompromised: gram-negative bacilli, fungi
  - Trauma patients with open injuries: mixed flora
- Pathogenesis:
  - Hematogenous spread (most common)
  - Direct inoculation by microorganisms secondary to trauma or iatrogenesis (e.g., joint surgery)
  - Adjacent spread (e.g., osteomyelitis)

- Pathophysiology:
  - Microorganisms initially enter through synovial membrane and spread to the synovial fluid.
  - Resulting inflammatory response releases cytokines and destructive proteases leading to systemic symptoms and joint damage.

RISK FACTORS
- Age >80 years
- Low socioeconomic status, alcoholism
- Cellulitis and skin ulcers
- Violation of joint capsule
  - Prior orthopedic surgery
  - Intra-articular injection
  - Trauma
- History of previous joint disease
  - Inflammatory arthritis (RA: 10-fold increased risk)
  - Osteoarthritis
  - Crystal arthritides
- Systemic illness
  - Diabetes mellitus, liver disease, HIV, malignancy, end-stage renal disease/hemodialysis, immuno-suppression, sickle cell anemia
- Risks for hematogenous spread
  - IVDU, severe sepsis/systemic infection

GENERAL PREVENTION
- Prompt treatment of skin and soft tissue infections
- Control risk factors.
- Immunizations (*S. pneumoniae*, *N. meningitidis*)

COMMONLY ASSOCIATED CONDITIONS
Preexisting joint conditions, previous joint trauma or surgery, prosthetic joint

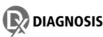

DIAGNOSIS

HISTORY
- Typically presents with a combination of joint pain, swelling, warmth, and decreased range of motion
- Nongonococcal arthritis: mostly monoarticular (80%)
  - Typically large joints: knee (50%), hip (20%), shoulder (8%), ankle (7%)
  - Most patients report fever.
  - IV drug users may develop infection in axial joints (e.g., sternoclavicular joint).
  - Prosthetic joints may be minimally symptomatic and present with draining sinus over joint.
  - Patients on chronic immunosuppressive drugs and those receiving articular corticosteroid injections may have atypical presentations (absent fever or joint pain).
- Pediatric considerations:
  - Infants may avoid moving limb (often mistaken for neurologic problem).
  - Hip pain may commonly refer to knee and/or thigh.
- Gonococcal arthritis
  - Bacteremic phase
    - Migratory polyarthritis, tenosynovitis, high fever, chills, pustules (dermatitis–arthritis syndrome)
  - Localized phase
    - Less symptomatic—often monoarticular, low-grade fever
- Approximately 22% of all patients with culture-proven septic arthritis had no associated risk factors or underlying joint disease.

PHYSICAL EXAM
- Physical exam has poor sensitive and specificity for septic arthritis; however, common findings include:
  - Fever
  - Limited range of motion
  - Joint effusion and tenderness
  - Erythema and warmth over affected joint
  - Pain with passive range of motion
- Hip and shoulder involvement may reveal severe pain with range of motion and less obvious swelling.
- Infants with septic hip arthritis maintain the joint in flexion and external rotation as position of comfort.
- Purpura associated with disseminated gonococcal infection

DIFFERENTIAL DIAGNOSIS
- Crystal arthritis: gout, pseudogout, calcium oxalate, cholesterol
- Infectious arthritis: fungi, spirochetes, rheumatic fever, HIV, viral
- Inflammatory arthritis: RA, spondyloarthropathy, systemic lupus erythematosus, sarcoidosis
- Osteoarthritis
- Trauma: meniscal tear, fracture, hemarthrosis
- Other: bursitis, cellulitis, tendinitis

DIAGNOSTIC TESTS & INTERPRETATION
Initial Tests (lab, imaging)
- Synovial fluid analysis is the gold standard of diagnosis.
  - Obtain prior to antibiotic therapy when possible.
  - Include Gram stain, culture, cell count/differential, and crystal analysis.
  - Use blood culture bottles to increase yield.
  - Gram stain (sensitivity 29–65%); culture (positive in 80%) (1)
  - >50,000 WBCs/HPF with >90% polymorpho-nuclear leukocytes is suggestive.
    - Synovial WBC (sWBC) *count alone is insufficient to rule in or rule out septic arthritis* (1).
    - Likelihood of septic arthritis increases as sWBC rises >100,000/HPF (1).
  - Analysis of synovial fluid leukocyte esterase is associated with a high negative predictive value (NPV) (2)
  - Crystals (e.g., urate or calcium pyrophosphate) *do not exclude concurrent infectious arthritis.*
  - Prosthetic joint: WBC count is unreliable; a lower number of sWBCs may indicate infection.
- Serum tests:
  - WBC count alone is neither sensitive nor specific.
  - ESR >15 mm/hr has sensitivity up to 94% but poor specificity (3)[B].
  - CRP >20 mg/L has sensitivity of 92% (3)[B].
  - Synovial lactate is a potential biomarker to rule out septic arthritis when <250 U/L; however, more study is needed (1),(4).
  - Blood cultures positive in ~50% of cases
- Other tests:
  - Disseminated gonococcus: culture blood, cervix, urine, urethra, pharynx in addition to joint fluid
  - Suspect Lyme arthritis: PCR and serum titers for *Borrelia* IgM and IgG indicate exposure.
- Pediatrics: No single lab test distinguishes septic arthritis from transient synovitis.
  - The combination of fever, non–weight-bearing, and elevated ESR/CRP is suspicious; obtain synovial fluid for analysis when possible.

- Imaging:
  - Can help identify effusion but does not further differentiate causes of arthritis
  - Plain films
    - Nondiagnostic for septic arthritis; useful for trauma, soft tissue swelling, osteoarthritis, or osteopenia
    - May show nonspecific inflammatory arthritic changes (i.e., erosions, joint destruction, or joint space loss)
  - Ultrasound
    - Useful for guiding arthrocentesis
    - Recommended for aspiration of deep joints such as the hip
  - MRI
    - Highly sensitive for effusion, may help differentiate between transient synovitis and septic arthritis in children
  - Other imaging
    - CT is not routinely indicated.
    - Bone scans are not performed unless there is concurrent suspicion for osteomyelitis.

Diagnostic Procedures/Other
Arthrocentesis in all suspected cases (prior to starting antibiotics)
- Avoid contaminated tissue (e.g., overlying cellulitis) when performing arthrocentesis.

Test Interpretation
Synovial biopsy shows polymorphonuclear leukocytes and (possibly) the causative organism.

 TREATMENT

GENERAL MEASURES
- Admit for parenteral antibiotics and monitoring.
  - Begin antibiotics immediately after arthrocentesis.
- Drainage of purulent material is *required* if:
  - Pediatric: Surgical drainage and irrigation is recommended if hip involvement due to high risk of avascular necrosis.
  - Prosthetic joint: antibiotics and consult with orthopedics for consideration of revision arthroplasty, resection arthroplasty, or débridement
- Antibiotic therapy for a total of 4 to 6 weeks in most cases
  - Native joint infections require at least 2 weeks; prosthetics longer.
  - Each case should be evaluated individually and contextually, consulting infectious disease specialists when appropriate.
  - Exception: gonococcal arthritis; treated for 2 to 3 weeks
- Intra-articular antibiotics are not typically recommended or used.

MEDICATION
First Line
- Initial antibiotic choice is guided by Gram stain or most likely organism based on age, clinical history, and risk factors (1)[C].
- Nongonococcal (1),(2)[C]:
  - Gram-positive cocci:
    - Vancomycin 15 to 20 mg/kg 2 to 3 times daily or linezolid 600 mg twice daily

- Gram-negative bacilli:
  - Cefepime 2 g twice daily or ceftriaxone 2 g daily or ceftazidime 2 g 3 times daily or cefotaxime 2 g 3 times daily
  - For cephalosporin allergy: Consider treatment with ciprofloxacin 400 mg 3 times daily.
- Negative Gram stain:
  - Vancomycin 15 to 20 mg/kg 2 to 3 times daily plus 3rd-generation cephalosporin until cultures and susceptibilities return
- Duration of therapy: typically 2 weeks of IV and additional 2 to 4 weeks PO while monitoring therapeutic response closely
- Gonococcal:
  - Ceftriaxone 1 g IV/IM daily for 7 to 14 days
    - Continue at least 24 to 48 hours after symptom resolution.
    - May require concurrent drainage of affected joint
    - Concomitant treatment for *Chlamydia* (doxycycline 100 mg twice daily or azithromycin 1 g once)
- Other considerations:
  - Narrow antibiotic therapy based on culture results
  - Consider *Salmonella* in pediatric patients with history of sickle cell disease.
    - 3rd-generation cephalosporins in this instance
  - Lyme arthritis
    - Doxycycline 100 mg PO twice daily -or- amoxicillin 500 mg PO 3 times daily for 28 days if no neurologic involvement, otherwise ceftriaxone 2 g IV daily

ISSUES FOR REFERRAL
Infectious disease and orthopedic consultations
- ID specialist consult for IVDU and immunosuppressed patients
- Orthopedic consultation for prosthetic joint infections (1)[C]

SURGERY/OTHER PROCEDURES
- Consider drainage in all cases—particularly shoulder, hip, and prosthetic joints (1)[C].
- Other treatment options include repeat needle aspiration, arthroscopy, or arthrotomy.

ADMISSION, INPATIENT, AND NURSING CONSIDERATIONS
Mean duration of hospitalization is 12 days.

 ONGOING CARE

FOLLOW-UP RECOMMENDATIONS
Patient Monitoring
- Can monitor synovial fluid to verify decreasing WBC and sterile fluid after initial treatment
- If no improvement in 24 hours, reevaluate and consider arthroscopy.
- Follow up at 1 week and 1 month after stopping antibiotics to exclude relapse.

PROGNOSIS
- Early treatment improves functional outcome.
- Delayed recognition/treatment is associated with higher morbidity and mortality.
- Elderly, concurrent RA, *S. aureus* infections, and infection of hip and shoulder also increase risk of poor outcome.

COMPLICATIONS
- Mortality rates between 3% and 25% (1)
- Limited joint range of motion, ankylosis, osteomyelitis, postinfectious synovitis
- Secondary osteoarthritis; flail, fused, or dislocated joint; sepsis, septic necrosis
- Sinus formation
- Osteomyelitis, postinfectious synovitis
- Limb length discrepancy (primarily in cases prior to skeletal maturity)

REFERENCES
1. Long B, Koyfman A, Goggleib M. Evaluation and management of septic arthritis and its mimics in the emergency department. *West J Emerg Med.* 2019;20(2):331–341.
2. Carpenter CR, Schuur JD, Everett WW, et al. Evidence-based diagnostics: adult septic arthritis. *Acad Emerg Med.* 2011;18(8):781–796.
3. Hariharan P, Kabrhel C. Sensitivity of erythrocyte sedimentation rate and C-reactive protein for the exclusion of septic arthritis in emergency department patients. *J Emerg Med.* 2011;40(4):428–431.
4. Shu E, Fashidpour L, Young M, et al. Utility of point-of-care synovial lactate to identify septic arthritis in the emergency department. *Am J Emerg Med.* 2019;37(3):502–505.

ADDITIONAL READING
- Hassan AS, Rao A, Manadan AM, et al. Peripheral bacterial septic arthritis: review of diagnosis and management. *J Clin Rheumatol.* 2017;23(8):435–442.
- Ritchie B, Porritt K, Marin T, et al. Diagnostic test accuracy of serum procalcitonin compared with C-reactive protein for bone and joint infection in children and adolescents: a systematic review and meta-analysis [published online ahead of print August 20, 2021]. *JBI Evid Synth.* doi:10.11124/JBIES-20-00357.
- Ross JJ. Septic arthritis of native joints. *Infect Dis Clin North Am.* 2017;31(2):203–218.

CODES

ICD10
- M00.079 Staphylococcal arthritis, unspecified ankle and foot
- M00.829 Arthritis due to other bacteria, unspecified elbow
- M00.011 Staphylococcal arthritis, right shoulder

CLINICAL PEARLS
- Arthrocentesis and synovial fluid analysis are mandatory in cases of suspected septic arthritis.
- Gram stain has variable sensitivity in septic arthritis. sWBC count is generally >50,000/HPV but is unreliable as a sole diagnostic feature and should be interpreted in context.
- Early IV antibiotics and (if necessary) drainage of infected joints are critical to successful management.
- Crystalline disease may coexist with septic arthritis.
- Initial antibiotic therapy is guided by arthrocentesis results (Gram stain), age, and patient-specific risk factors.

ARTHROPOD BITES AND STINGS

James E. Powers, DO, FACEP, FAAEM

 BASICS

DESCRIPTION

- Arthropods are the largest division of the animal kingdom. Two classes, insects and arachnids, have the greatest impact on human health.
- Arthropods affect humans by inoculating poison, microorganisms, or irritative substances through a bite or sting; by invading tissue; or by contact allergy to their skin, hairs, or secretions.
- Transmission of infectious microorganisms during feeding is of the greatest concern.
- Sequelae of bites, stings, or contact include
  – Local redness with itch, pain, and swelling: common, usually immediate and transient
  – Large local reactions that increase over 24 to 48 hours
  – Systemic reactions with anaphylaxis, neurotoxicity, organ damage, or other systemic toxin effects
  – Tissue necrosis or secondary infection
  – Infectious disease transmission: Presentation may be delayed weeks to years.

EPIDEMIOLOGY

Incidence

- 33,671 cases of arthropod exposures were reported in 2016. This is a small fraction of arthropod encounters.
- Systemic reactions to *Hymenoptera* venom occur in 0.5–3.3% of population and most fatalities involve those with no prior allergic reaction.

Prevalence

Widespread, with regional and seasonal variations

ETIOLOGY AND PATHOPHYSIOLOGY

- Arthropods: four medically important classes
  – Insects: *Hymenoptera* (bees, wasps, hornets, fire ants), mosquitoes, bed bugs, flies, lice, fleas, beetles, caterpillars, and moths
  – Arachnids: spiders, scorpions, mites, and ticks
  – Chilopods: centipedes
  – Diplopods: millipedes
- Four general categories of pathophysiologic effects: toxic, allergic, infectious, and traumatic
  – Toxic effects of venom: local (tissue inflammation or destruction) versus systemic (neurotoxic or organ damage)
  – Allergic: Antigens in saliva or venom may cause local inflammation. Exaggerated immune responses may result in anaphylaxis or serum sickness.
  – Trauma: Mechanical injury from biting or stinging causes pain, swelling, and portal of entry for bacteria and secondary infection. Retention of arthropod parts can cause a granulomatous reaction.
  – Infection: Arthropods may transmit bacterial, viral, and protozoal diseases.

Genetics

Family history of atopy may be a factor in the development of more severe allergic reactions.

RISK FACTORS

- Previous sensitization
- Certain outdoor activities, occupations, and travel exposures increase risk.
- Greater risk for adverse outcome in young, elderly, immunocompromised, and those with chronic or poorly controlled cardiac or respiratory disease
- Increased risk of anaphylaxis in patients with mastocytosis

GENERAL PREVENTION

- Avoid common arthropod habitats.
- Insect repellents (not effective for bees, spiders, scorpions, caterpillars, bed bugs, fleas, ants)
  – N,N-diethyl-meta-toluamide (DEET)
    o Most effective broad-spectrum repellent against biting arthropods (1),(2)[A]
    o Formulations with higher concentrations (20–50%) are first-line choice in areas of endemic arthropod-borne diseases (2)[A].
    o Concentrations >30% have longer duration of action. No significant protection benefits with DEET concentrations >50%.
    o Safe for children >6 months of age; pregnant and lactating women (2)[B]
  – Picaridin (icaridin)
    o 20% spray comparable to 20% DEET for mosquito protection (2)[A]
  – P-menthane-3,8-diol (PMD; lemon eucalyptus extract)
    o 30% concentrations give 4 to 5 hours of protection against mosquitoes and ticks (1)[A].
    o Not recommended for children <3 years old
  – IR3535: less effective in most studies; not appropriate for malaria-endemic regions (1)[B]
- Barrier methods: clothing, bed nets
  – Wear long pants, long-sleeved shirts, and hats.
  – Permethrin: synthetic insecticide derived from chrysanthemum plant. Do not apply directly to skin. Permethrin-impregnated clothing provides good protection against arthropods and is safe for children of all ages and for pregnant women.
  – Mosquito nets: advised for all travelers to disease-endemic areas at risk from biting arthropods. Permethrin-treated nets may offer additional protection (2)[B].
- Desensitization 75–95% effective for *Hymenoptera*-specific venom
  – Skin tests to determine sensitivity
  – Refer to allergist/immunologist.
- Fire ant control (but not elimination) possible
  – Baits; sprays; dusts; aerosols; biologic agents
- Risk of tick-borne diseases may be decreased by prompt removal of ticks within 24 hours of attachment.

DIAGNOSIS

HISTORY

- Sudden onset of pain or itching with visualization of arthropod
- Many cases unknown to patient or asymptomatic initially (bed bugs, lice, scabies, ticks). Consider in patients presenting with localized erythema, urticaria, wheals, papules, pruritus, or bullae.
- Identify insect by its habitat or remnants brought by patient.
- History of prior exposure useful but not always available or reliable
- Travel, occupational, social, and recreational history

PHYSICAL EXAM

- If stinger is still present in skin, remove by flicking or scraping away from skin.
- Anaphylaxis is a clinical diagnosis. Signs and symptoms include (3)[A]
  – Erythema, urticaria, angioedema
  – Itching/edema of lips, tongue, uvula; drooling
  – Respiratory distress, wheeze, repetitive cough, stridor, dysphonia
  – Hypotension, dysrhythmia, syncope, chest pain

- If anaphylaxis not present, exam focuses on the sting or bite itself. Common findings include local erythema, swelling, wheals, urticaria, papules, or bullae; excoriations from scratching
- Look for arthropod infestation (lice, scabies) or attached ticks. Body lice usually found in seams of clothing; skin scraping to identify scabies
- Signs of secondary bacterial infection after 24 to 48 hours: increasing erythema, pain, fever, lymphangitis, or abscess

DIFFERENTIAL DIAGNOSIS

- Urticaria and localized dermatologic reactions:
  – Contact dermatitis, drug eruption, mastocytosis, bullous diseases, dermatitis herpetiformis, tinea, eczema, vasculitis, pityriasis, erythema multiforme, viral exanthem, cellulitis, abscess, impetigo, folliculitis, erysipelas, necrotizing fasciitis
- Anaphylactic-type reactions
  – Cardiac, hemorrhagic, or septic shock; acute respiratory failure, asthma; angioedema, urticarial vasculitis; flushing syndromes (catecholamines, vasoactive peptides); syncope
  – Differential diagnosis of the acute abdomen should include black widow spider bite.

DIAGNOSTIC TESTS & INTERPRETATION

Initial Tests (lab, imaging)

Seldom needed; basic lab parameters usually normal

Follow-Up Tests & Special Considerations

- Severe envenomations may affect organ function and require lab monitoring (CBC, comprehensive metabolic panel, prothrombin time/international normalized ratio).
- Potential arthropod-borne diseases:
  – Ticks: Lyme disease, Rocky Mountain spotted fever (RMSF), relapsing fever, anaplasmosis, babesiosis, tularemia; ehrlichiosis, Powassan disease; Heartland virus (HRTV); Bourbon virus
  – Flies: tularemia, leishmaniasis, African trypanosomiasis, bartonellosis, loiasis
  – Fleas: plague, tularemia, murine typhus
  – Chigger mites: scrub typhus
  – Body lice: epidemic typhus, relapsing fever
  – Kissing bugs: Chagas disease
  – Mosquitoes: malaria, yellow fever, dengue fever, West Nile virus, equine encephalitis, chikungunya, Zika virus
- With history of anaphylaxis, significant systemic symptoms, progressively severe reactions, refer to allergist for formal testing (3)[B].

Diagnostic Procedures/Other

Skin and immunologic tests available to identify specific allergens

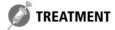 **TREATMENT**

ALERT

- Rapid anaphylaxis is severe and potentially life-threatening. Most deaths due to anaphylaxis occur within 30 to 60 minutes of sting.
- Give epinephrine as soon as diagnosis of anaphylaxis is suspected. Delay is associated with increased fatality (3),(4)[A].
- Antihistamines and steroids do not replace epinephrine and are never initial therapy in anaphylaxis; no direct outcome data regarding their effectiveness in anaphylaxis available (3)[A]
- Airway management critical for angioedema

GENERAL MEASURES
Relieve itching, pain, and swelling; local wound care, ice compress, analgesics

MEDICATION

First Line
- For arthropod bites/stings with anaphylaxis
  - Expert opinion consensus (3)[C]
  - Epinephrine: most important: IM injection in midanterolateral thigh
    - IM injection: epinephrine 1:1,000 (1 mg/mL): adult: 0.3 to 0.5 mg per dose; pediatric: Give 0.01 mg/kg to a maximum dose of 0.3 mg per dose, can repeat every 5 to 15 minutes to total of three injections (3),(4)[A].
  - Oxygen up to 100%, as needed
  - IV fluids: Establish 1 to 2 large-bore IV lines. Normal saline bolus 1 to 2 L IV; repeat as needed (pediatrics 20 to 30 mL/kg) (4)[A].
  - H_1 antagonists: diphenhydramine 25 to 50 mg IV (pediatrics 1 to 2 mg/kg) (3)[A]
  - H_2 antihistamines: ranitidine 50 mg IV (4)[A]
  - β_2 Agonists: albuterol for bronchospasm nebulized 2.5 to 5.0 mg in 3 mL (4)[A]
  - *Corticosteroids: although frequently used, there is no benefit in acute anaphylaxis;* questionable benefit in preventing biphasic allergic reactions
- Arthropod bites/stings without anaphylaxis
  - Tetanus booster, as indicated
  - Oral antihistamines
    - Diphenhydramine adults: 25 to 50 mg PO/IV/IM every 4 to 6 hours. Pediatrics: 1 to 2 mg/kg to a max dose of 50 mg PO/IV/IM; daily maximum dose of 300 mg for adults and pediatrics
    - Cetirizine adults: 5 to 10 mg PO daily; pediatrics: 6 to 23 months—2.5 mg PO daily; 2 to 5 years—5 mg PO daily; 6 years and older—5 to 10 mg PO daily
    - H_2 blockers: ranitidine adults: 150 mg PO 1 to 2 times daily as needed; pediatrics: 2 to 4 mg PO 1 to 2 times daily as needed
  - Oral steroids: Consider short course for severe pruritus or local reactions; prednisone or prednisolone 1 to 2 mg/kg once daily
  - Consider topical steroid cream or ointment for 3 to 5 days.
    - OTC 1% hydrocortisone
    - May consider higher potency such as triamcinolone 0.1%, fluocinolone 0.025%
  - Wound care: antibiotics only if infection
  - Other specific therapies:
    - Scorpion stings: Treat excess catecholamine release (nitroprusside, prazosin, β-blockers). Atropine for hypersalivation (4). Only one FDA-approved scorpion antivenom. Use only in consultation with toxicologist.
    - Black widow bites: Treat muscle spasms with benzodiazepines and opioid analgesics (4). Antivenom: for severe symptoms only (5)[B]; available but should be administered in conjunction with toxicologist
    - Consult poison control hotline for questions regarding management: 1-800-222-1222.
  - Fire ants: characteristically cause sterile pustules; leave intact—do not open or drain.
  - Brown recluse spider: pain control, supportive treatment; surgical consult if débridement needed
  - Ticks: early removal. Associated with Lyme disease, RMSF, ehrlichiosis, babesiosis.
  - Pediculosis: head, pubic, and body lice
    - First line: permethrin 1% topical lotion
    - Alternatives: Pyrethrins, ivermectin orally shown to be effective but not FDA-approved for pediculosis
    - Repeat treatment in 7 to 10 days.
  - *Sarcoptes scabiei* scabies
    - Permethrin 5% cream is drug of choice: Apply to entire body. Wash off after 8 to 14 hours. Repeat in 1 week.
    - Ivermectin: 200 μg/kg PO once; repeat in 2 weeks shown to be effective but not FDA-approved for scabies
    - 2018 Cochrane review found no difference in efficacy of permethrin compared to systemic or topical ivermectin (6).

ISSUES FOR REFERRAL
Patients with history of anaphylaxis, severe systemic symptoms, or progressively severe reactions benefit from consultation with allergy/immunology.

SURGERY/OTHER PROCEDURES
Débridement and delayed skin grafting may be needed for severe brown recluse spider and other bites.

COMPLEMENTARY & ALTERNATIVE MEDICINE
- Cool compresses
- Calamine lotion not shown to have benefit.
- A paste of 3 tsp of baking soda and 1 tsp water may help salve bites.

ADMISSION, INPATIENT, AND NURSING CONSIDERATIONS
- Anaphylaxis, vascular instability, neuromuscular events, pain, GI symptoms, renal damage/failure
- All patients with anaphylaxis should be observed for 1 hour after symptoms resolve. Those with severe anaphylaxis or who require more than one dose of epinephrine should undergo extended observation (7)[C].

 ONGOING CARE

FOLLOW-UP RECOMMENDATIONS
- Venom immunotherapy is the cornerstone of treatment for *Hymenoptera*; 80–98% effective (3)[A]
- Provide epinephrine for patient self-administration if history of anaphylaxis (3)[A]. Consider "med-alert" identifiers.

Patient Monitoring
- Monitor for delayed effects, including infectious diseases from arthropod bites.
- Serum sickness reactions, vasculitis (rare)

PATIENT EDUCATION
Arthropod avoidance and preventive measures

PROGNOSIS
- Excellent for local reactions
- For systemic reactions, best prognosis with early intervention to prevent cardiorespiratory collapse

COMPLICATIONS
- Scarring; secondary bacterial infections; arthropod-associated infectious diseases
- Psychological effects, phobias

REFERENCES

1. Alpern JD, Dunlop SJ, Dolan BJ, et al. Personal protection measures against mosquitoes, ticks, and other arthropods. *Med Clin North Am.* 2016;100(2):303–316.
2. Moore SJ, Mordue Luntz AJ, Logan JG. Insect bite prevention. *Infect Dis Clin North Am.* 2012;26(3):655–673.
3. Lieberman P, Nicklas RA, Randolph C, et al. Anaphylaxis—a practice parameter update 2015. *Ann Allergy Asthma Immunol.* 2015;115(5):341–384.
4. Singer E, Zodda D. Allergy and anaphylaxis: principles of acute emergency management. *Emerg Med Pract.* 2015;17(8):1–19; quiz 20.
5. Erickson TB, Cheema N. Arthropod envenomation in North America. *Emerg Med Clin North Am.* 2017;35(2):355–375.
6. Rosumeck S, Nast A, Dressler C. Ivermectin and permethrin for treating scabies. *Cochrane Database Syst Rev.* 2018;4(4):CD012994.
7. Shaker MS, Wallace DV, Golden DBK, et al. Anaphylaxis-a 2020 practice parameter update, systematic review, and Grading of Recommendations, Assessment, Development and Evaluation (GRADE) analysis. *J Allergy Clin Immunol.* 2020;145(4):1082–1123.

ADDITIONAL READING

- Centers for Disease Control and Prevention. Parasites—scabies. Medication. https://www.cdc.gov/parasites/scabies/health_professionals/meds.html. Accessed August 15, 2020.
- Centers for Disease Control and Prevention. Parasites. Treatment. https://www.cdc.gov/parasites/lice/head/treatment.html. Accessed August 22, 2020.
- Centers for Disease Control and Prevention. West Nile virus. Prevention. http://www.cdc.gov/westnile/faq/repellent.html. Accessed August 20, 2020.
- Juckett G. Arthropod bites. *Am Fam Physician.* 2013;88(12):841–847.
- Mutebi JP, Gimnig JE. Environmental hazards & other noninfectious health risk. In: Centers for Disease Control and Prevention. *CDC Yellow Book 2020: Health Information for International Travel.* https://wwwnc.cdc.gov/travel/yellowbook/2020/noninfectious-health-risks/mosquitoes-ticks-and-other-arthropods
- Warrell DA. Venomous bites, stings, and poisoning: an update. *Infect Dis Clin North Am.* 2019;33:17–38.

CODES

ICD10
- T63.481A Toxic effect of venom of arthropod, accidental, init
- T63.301A Toxic effect of unsp spider venom, accidental, init
- T63.484A Toxic effect of venom of oth arthropod, undetermined, init

CLINICAL PEARLS
- Urgent administration of epinephrine is the key to successful treatment of anaphylaxis.
- Local treatment and symptom management are sufficient in most insect bites and stings.
- Tick-borne illness is on the rise in the United States.

ASCITES
Sara Elsayed, MD • Ahmed Aldabdob, MD

 BASICS

DESCRIPTION
- Accumulation of fluid in the peritoneal cavity; may occur in conditions that cause generalized edema
- Refractory ascites: ascitic fluid that recurs after paracentesis or cannot be prevented by treatment
- Men generally have no fluid in peritoneal cavity; women may have up to 20 mL depending on menstrual phase.

EPIDEMIOLOGY
- Children: most commonly associated with nephrotic syndrome and malignancy
- Adults: cirrhosis (81%), cancer (10%), heart failure (3%), other (6%)

Incidence
~50–60% of cirrhotic patients develop ascites within 10 years (1). The presence of ascites in cirrhotic patients is a poor prognostic indicator with a survival rate of 50% at 2 years.

Prevalence
10% of patients with cirrhosis have ascites.

ETIOLOGY AND PATHOPHYSIOLOGY
- Portal hypertension versus nonportal hypertension
  - Cannot reliably establish/confirm etiology without paracentesis
  - Serum-ascites albumin gradient (SAAG): (serum albumin level: ascites albumin level) helps to differentiate
- High portal pressure (SAAG ≥1.1)
  - Cirrhosis is the most common cause of ascites in the United States.
  - Hepatitis (alcoholic, viral, autoimmune, medications)
  - Acute liver failure
  - Liver malignancy (primary or metastatic)
  - Elevated right-sided filling pressures from heart failure or constrictive pericarditis
  - Hepatic venous thrombosis (Budd-Chiari syndrome)
  - Portal vein thrombosis
- Normal portal pressure (SAAG <1.1)
  - Peritoneal carcinomatosis
  - Tuberculosis (TB)
  - Severe hypoalbuminemia (nephrotic syndrome; severe enteropathy with protein loss)
  - Meigs syndrome (ovarian cancer)
  - Lymphatic leak (chylous ascites)
  - Pancreatitis
  - Inflammatory (vasculitis, lupus serositis, sarcoidosis)
  - Other infections (parasitic, fungal)
  - Hemoperitoneum (trauma or ectopic pregnancy)
- Pathogenesis of ascites in the setting of portal hypertension (cirrhotic ascites)
  - Most ascites is due to portal hypertension leading to backward transmission of increased pressure to the visceral capillary bed with subsequent dilation and shift of fluid to the peritoneal cavity. This dilation further increases portal pressure and decreases systemic blood volume with resultant hypotension. Systemic hypovolemia stimulates neurohormonal mechanisms (renin angiotensin system and antidiuretic hormone) for sodium retention as an attempt to compensate for decreased systemic volume and pressure.

RISK FACTORS
- Cirrhosis—hepatitis B and C; alcohol abuse
- Congestive heart failure (CHF); advanced kidney disease; malignancy
- TB

GENERAL PREVENTION
Lifestyle—appropriate diet; physical activity; safe sexual practices; avoid alcohol misuse and hepatotoxic medications.

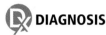 **DIAGNOSIS**

HISTORY
- Address risk factors (e.g., EtOH use, TB exposure, prior malignancies, sexual partners, transfusion history, metabolic syndrome, increased risk of nonalcoholic steatohepatitis progressing to cirrhosis, previous history of cardiac illness).
- Assess for symptoms of underlying disease (chest pain, dyspnea, orthopnea, peripheral edema, asterixis, weight loss, night sweats, chronic cough).
- Assess for complications (fever/abdominal pain might indicate spontaneous bacterial peritonitis [SBP], progressive dyspnea due to increased abdominal girth).
- Progressive abdominal distention may be painful.

PHYSICAL EXAM
- Abdominal distention with flank/shifting dullness is the most sensitive (83%) and specific (56%) exam finding; requires >1,500 mL of fluid to detect
- Signs of right-sided heart failure suggesting cardiac cirrhosis
- Edema (penile/scrotal, pedal), increased jugular venous pressure
- Stigmata of chronic liver cirrhosis (palmar erythema, spider angiomata, dilated abdominal wall collateral veins)
- Other signs of advanced liver disease: jaundice, muscle wasting, gynecomastia, leukonychia, asterixis
- Signs of underlying malignancy: cachexia; supraclavicular (Virchow) node suggests upper abdominal malignancy.

DIFFERENTIAL DIAGNOSIS
- Obesity
- Large ovarian tumors
- Bowel obstruction
- Massive splenomegaly

DIAGNOSTIC TESTS & INTERPRETATION
Initial Tests (lab, imaging)
- Ultrasound (can detect small volumes of ascitic fluid ~100 mL)
- Diagnostic paracentesis for fluid analysis to determine etiology and rule out infection in all inpatients and outpatients with clinically new-onset ascites
  - Paracentesis complication rate is 1%. The presence of coagulation abnormalities does not preclude paracentesis, unless there is evidence of disseminated intravascular coagulopathy or primary fibrinolysis (1).
  - Routine attempts to correct platelet or coagulation defects not needed prior to paracentesis
  - Ascitic fluid analysis (1)[C]:
    - Cell count and differential:
      - Polymorphonuclear (PMN) leukocytes ≥250 cells/mm³ is diagnostic of SBP.
    - Albumin to calculate SAAG (obtained by subtracting ascitic fluid albumin from serum albumin obtained on the SAME day):
      - <1.1 g indicates a low portal pressure exudative process (i.e., inflammatory, biliary/pancreatic, carcinomatosis, TB).
      - ≥1.1 g indicates portal hypertensive/transudative process (cirrhosis, CHF, constrictive pericarditis, thrombosis).
    - Total protein (low in cirrhosis, nephrotic disease and high in cardiac ascites) levels <10 g/dL in

cirrhotic patients without SBP indicate increased risk and warrant antibiotic prophylaxis .
  - Other tests (based on clinical scenario to rule out etiologies other than cirrhosis) (1)[C]:
    - Bacterial Gram stain/culture if infection suspected (Cirrhotic patients with ascites can fail to mount fever or leukocytosis.)
      - Fluid cultures are traditionally positive in 50–90% of cases of SBP.
      - Yield is improved if inoculated to blood culture bottles at bedside and if fluid is obtained before first dose of antibiotics.
    - Amylase (suspicion for bowel perforation, choledocholithiasis, or pancreatitis)
    - Triglyceride if fluid appears milky
    - Cytology if concern for malignancy (less sensitive in the absence of carcinomatosis)
    - Lactate dehydrogenase (LDH): An ascitic fluid-to-serum LDH ratio >1.0 can indicate infection, perforation, or tumor.
    - Carcinoembryonic antigen and alkaline phosphatase (elevated in viscous perforation)
- Mycobacterial culture/polymerase chain reaction for suspicion of TB
- Blood urea nitrogen/creatinine, electrolytes (renal function)
  - Brain natriuretic peptide (heart failure)
  - Liver function tests and hepatitis serologies (hepatitis)
- Abdominal ultrasound (US) can confirm ascites; highly sensitive, cost-effective, involves no radiation
- Portal US Doppler can detect thrombosis or cirrhosis.
- CT scan for intra-abdominal pathology (malignancy)
- MRI preferred for evaluation of liver disease or confirmation of portal vein thrombosis

Diagnostic Procedures/Other
Laparoscopy: if imaging and paracentesis are nondiagnostic
- Allows for direct visualization and biopsy of peritoneum, liver, and intra-abdominal lymph nodes
- Preferred for evaluating suspected peritoneal TB or malignancies

Test Interpretation
Cytology may reveal malignant cells: adenocarcinoma (ovary, breast, GI tract) or primary peritoneal carcinoma (most commonly associated with ascites).

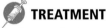 **TREATMENT**

For all patients, first-line treatment consists of:
- Daily weight
- Restrict dietary sodium to ≤2 g/day if the cause is due to portal hypertension (high SAAG).
- Water restriction (1.0 to 1.5 L/day) only necessary if serum sodium <120 to 125 mEq/L
- Avoid alcohol and ensure adequate nutrition if liver disease.
- Baclofen may be used to reduce alcohol craving/consumption in EtOH cirrhosis.

MEDICATION
ALERT
- Care with diuresis; aggressive diuresis can induce prerenal acute kidney injury (AKI), encephalopathy, and hyponatremia. Monitor creatinine and electrolytes closely. Serum creatinine >2 mg/dL or serum sodium <120 mmol/L warrants withdrawal of diuretics.
- Avoid nonsteroidal anti-inflammatory drugs (can exacerbate oliguria/azotemia).

- Angiotensin-converting enzyme (ACE) inhibitors and angiotensin receptor blockers (ARBs) may be harmful in patients with cirrhosis/ascites due to an increased risk of hypotension and renal failure. Avoid in refractory ascites.
- Consider discontinuing β-blockers in patients with refractory ascites, SBP, worsening hypotension (SBP <90 mm Hg), AKI, hyponatremia <130 mEq/L, or azotemia.

First Line
- Sodium restriction and diuretics are the mainstay of treatment for patients with elevated portal pressures; other causes (e.g., carcinomatosis) are less likely to respond to medical therapy.
  - Spironolactone 100 to 400 mg daily PO; typical initial dose is 100 to 200 mg given in AM.
    - Diuretic of choice due to antialdosterone effects; can be used as single agent in minimal ascites. Monitor for hyperkalemia.
  - Furosemide 40 to 160 mg daily PO; typical initial dose is 40 mg given in AM.
    - Antinatriuretic effect helps achieve negative sodium balance.
    - Preferred in combination with spironolactone rather than as monotherapy
  - Most common (and preferred) regimen is spironolactone and furosemide together (maintaining a 100:40 ratio) for maximum efficacy and to maintain potassium homeostasis.
    - Titrate dose to desired result ([i] daily weight loss no more than 0.5 kg/day in patients without peripheral edema and 1 kg/day in patients with peripheral edema; [ii] Urinary sodium output more than the sodium intake) and monitor renal function regularly.
    - Follow daily weight.
    - Adjust ratio to maintain normal potassium.
- Diuretic-intractable/refractory ascites (10% of patients—50% mortality in 6 months) defined as:
  - i) Persistent or worsening ascites despite maximum doses of spironolactone (400 mg/day) and furosemide (160 mg/day) for at least 1 week
  - ii) Recurrence of grade 2 or 3 ascites within 4 weeks of achieving minimal ascites
  - iii) Diuretic-induced complications like hepatic encephalopathy, hyponatremia to <125 mEq/L, renal impairment with creatinine rise of 100% to >2.0
- Treatment:
  - *Ensure compliance with dietary sodium restriction using* 24-hour urine sodium excretion.
  - Discontinue diuretics if urinary sodium excretion under diuretic therapy is <30 mmol/day.
  - Therapeutic paracentesis or serial large-volume paracentesis (LVP) (see "Surgery/Other Procedures")
  - IV furosemide reduces eGFR dramatically in ascitic patients and is best avoided.

Second Line
- Midodrine 7.5 mg TID can be used for refractory ascites or hypotensive patients, it was found to improve response to diuretics, improve hyponatremia, mean arterial pressure, and may improve survival (1)[B]. Titrate to blood pressure response.
- Alternatives to spironolactone: amiloride up to 40 mg/day; triamterene up to 200 mg/day in divided doses (1)[C]
- Alternatives to furosemide: torsemide up to 100 mg/day; bumetanide up to 4 mg/day (1)[C]
- Vaptans may have a beneficial effect on hyponatremia and ascites, but routine use in ascites is not yet supported. FDA has recommended to avoid use in chronic liver disease due to potential to induce serious liver injury (2)[A].

ISSUES FOR REFERRAL
Liver transplant is the definitive treatment for portal hypertension. Consider referral for transplant in patients with decompensated liver disease, whether or not ascites is present/controlled (1)[B].

SURGERY/OTHER PROCEDURES
- Therapeutic paracentesis
  - Initial therapy if tense ascites is present (1)[C]
  - Serial (generally every 2 weeks) paracenteses can be used as second line after diuretics in patients with elevated portal pressures.
  - Complications: infection, hemodynamic collapse, acute renal failure
  - Similar complication rate as diuretics
  - Replace albumin when removing >5 L of ascites: 5.5 to 8.0 g albumin for each liter removed. Albumin replacement decreases renal dysfunction, postparacentesis hyponatremia, and overall morbidity; likely not needed for malignant ascites
  - Continue diuretics at 50% of the previous dose if transitioning to serial paracentesis in patients failing diuretic monotherapy.
- Transjugular intrahepatic portosystemic shunt (TIPS)
  - Only for patients with elevated portal pressures with refractory ascites
  - Fluoroscopically placed conduit from portal to hepatic vein for intractable ascites
    - At time of placement, portal pressure should drop ≥20 mm Hg (or to <12 mm Hg), and ascites should be controllable with diuretics.
    - Yearly US to confirm shunt function
    - 4 weeks after TIPS, urinary sodium and serum creatinine improve significantly and can normalize after 6 to 12 months in combination with diuretics. Shunt dilation and/or replacement may be required after 2 years.
    - TIPS is superior to paracentesis for controlling ascites; no difference in mortality
- Automated low-flow ascites pump drains ascitic fluid from peritoneal cavity to urinary bladder for elimination; mainly used in patients with contraindication to TIPS placement or liver transplant
- Cell free and concentrated ascites reinfusion:
  - Used for management of malignant ascites. Protein collected from filtration and concentration of ascitic fluid is reinfused intravenously.
- Peritoneovenous shunt (LeVeen or Denver shunt): drains ascites directly into the inferior vena cava
  - Trials show poor long-term shunt patency, no survival advantage over medical therapy.
  - Complications include bacteremia, bowel obstruction, and variceal bleed.
  - Reserved for patients with refractory ascites who are not candidates for TIPS or liver transplant and who can't tolerate repeat paracentesis (1)[C]
- Indwelling catheters with external drainage
  - Most useful in malignant ascites as a palliative measure (can be drained at home)
  - Overall low rate of infection
- Avoid percutaneous endoscopic gastrostomy (PEG) tube placement in patients with ascites due to high postprocedure mortality rate (1)[B].

 ## ONGOING CARE

PROGNOSIS
- Prognosis varies depending on underlying cause.
- Ascites in itself is rarely life-threatening but can signify life-threatening underlying disease (e.g., cancer, end-stage liver disease).

COMPLICATIONS
- SBP
  - Ascitic fluid PMN leukocyte count ≥250 cells/mm³ or positive culture
    - Broad-spectrum antibiotics are as follows: Cefotaxime 2 g q8h or similar 3rd-generation cephalosporin is the treatment of choice for suspected SBP; covers 95% of flora (including *Escherichia coli*, *Klebsiella*, pneumococci); broader coverage often required for hospital-acquired infections
    - Levofloxacin is an alternative for patients who are not on long-term fluoroquinolones or who are allergic to penicillins or β-lactams.
    - Consider SBP prophylaxis in GI bleeding, previous SBP episode, or ascitic fluid protein <10 g hospitalized for reasons other than SBP.
    - Suspect primary bacterial peritonitis (PBP) due to bowel perforations when ascitic fluid >250 cells/mm³ (often >5,000 cells/mm³) and any two of the following:
      - Ascitic fluid total protein >1 g/dL (often >3 g/dL)
      - Ascitic fluid glucose <50 mg/dL (or 2.8 mmol/L)
      - Ascitic fluid LDH that is 3-fold greater than serum LDH
- Hepatorenal syndrome: Type 1 is rapid acute worsening of renal function evolving in the setting of a known precipitating factor. Type 2 is more slowly progressive in the setting of refractory ascites.
- Cellulitis is common in obese patients with brawny edema. Treat with diuretics and antibiotics (1)[B].

REFERENCES
1. Gallo A, Dedionigi C, Civitelli C, et al. Optimal management of cirrhotic ascites: a review for internal medicine physicians. *J Transl Int Med*. 2020;8(4):220–236.
2. Kockerling D, Nathwani R, Forlano R, et al. Current and future pharmacological therapies for managing cirrhosis and its complications. *World J Gastroenterol*. 2019;25(8):888–908.

ADDITIONAL READING
Long B, Koyfman A. The emergency medicine evaluation and management of the patient with cirrhosis. *Am J Emerg Med*. 2018;36(4):689–698.

 SEE ALSO

- Cirrhosis of the Liver; Hepatorenal Syndrome
- Algorithms: Congestive Heart Failure: Differential Diagnosis; Nephrotic Syndrome

CODES

ICD10
- R18.8 Other ascites
- R18.0 Malignant ascites
- K70.31 Alcoholic cirrhosis of liver with ascites

CLINICAL PEARLS
- Cirrhosis is the most common cause of ascites.
- Patients with new-onset ascites or hospitalized patients with ascites should undergo diagnostic paracentesis.
- Avoid ACE inhibitors, ARBs, and β-blockers in patients with ascites.
- Most common cause of "diuretic-intractable ascites" is nonadherence with dietary sodium restriction.
- Diuretics are first-line agents in the treatment of ascites. Serial paracentesis or TIPS is second line.

ASTHMA
Stacy E. Potts, MD, MEd

BASICS

DESCRIPTION
- A heterogeneous disease characterized as chronic inflammation of the airway (1)
- Common triggers: exercise, allergen-irritant exposure, change in weather, laughter, or viral respiratory infections
- Patient may experience symptom-free periods alternating with sporadic flare-up (exacerbations).
- Most common asthma phenotypes:
  - Allergic asthma: usually present since childhood and has strong family history of allergic diseases
  - Nonallergic asthma
  - Late-onset asthma: more common in females
  - Asthma with fixed airflow limitation: due to airway remodeling
  - Asthma with obesity
- Asthma severity is assessed retrospectively from treatment required to control symptoms.
  - Mild asthma: well controlled with Step 1 or 2 treatment (i.e., with as-needed ICS-formoterol alone or with low-intensity maintenance controller treatment)
  - Moderate asthma: well controlled with Step 3 or 4 treatment (i.e., low- or medium-dose ICS-LABA
  - Severe asthma: remains "uncontrolled" with optimized treatment with high-dose ICS-LABA or that requires high-dose ICS-LABA to prevent it from becoming "uncontrolled"

EPIDEMIOLOGY
Incidence
Traffic-related air pollution may be attributable to 13% of global asthma incidence.

Prevalence
Asthma affects 235 million individuals worldwide.
- 490,000 deaths worldwide reported in 2017
- Asthma affects about 10% of children ages 5 to 18 years in the United States.
- Asthma prevalence is greater in boys than girls; however, in adults, women are more affected.
- Obesity is associated with increased prevalence and incidence of asthma.
- Rate of asthma deaths largest among those aged >65

ETIOLOGY AND PATHOPHYSIOLOGY
Airway hyperreaction begins with inflammatory cell infiltration and degranulation, subbasement fibrosis, mucus hypersecretion, epithelial injury, significant smooth muscle hypertrophy and hyperreactivity, angiogenesis that then leads to intermittent airflow obstruction due to reversible bronchospasm.

Genetics
Genetic association with increased interleukin (IL) or IgE production and airway hyperresponsiveness leading to asthma

RISK FACTORS
- Host factors: genetic predisposition, sex, race, obesity, preterm, or small for gestational age (SGA)
- Environmental: viral infections, animal and airborne allergens, tobacco smoke exposure, pollution, stress
- Aspirin or NSAIDs hypersensitivity
- Persons with food allergies and asthma are at increased risk for fatal anaphylaxis from those foods.

COMMONLY ASSOCIATED CONDITIONS
- Atopy: eczema, allergic conjunctivitis, allergic rhinitis
- Obesity (associated with higher asthma rates)
- Gastroesophageal reflux disease (GERD)
- Obstructive sleep apnea (OSA)

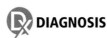

DIAGNOSIS

HISTORY
History of variable respiratory symptoms:
- More than one symptom such as wheeze, SOB, cough, chest tightness
- Symptoms worse at night, vary in time and intensity, worse with common triggers

PHYSICAL EXAM
- May be normal
- Focus on
  - Use of accessory muscles
  - Rhinitis, nasal polyps, swollen nasal turbinates
  - Expiratory wheezing, prolonged expiratory phase. Note: Wheezing may be absent in severe exacerbation due to severely reduced airflow.
  - Skin: eczema

DIFFERENTIAL DIAGNOSIS
- In children
  - Upper airway diseases (allergic rhinitis or sinusitis)
  - Large airway obstruction (foreign body aspiration, vocal cord dysfunction, vascular ring or laryngeal web, laryngotracheomalacia, enlarged lymph nodes, or tumor)
  - Small airway obstruction (viral bronchiolitis, cystic fibrosis, bronchopulmonary dysplasia, heart disease, primary ciliary dyskinesia, bronchiectasis)
  - Other causes (recurrent cough, chronic upper airway cough syndrome, aspiration/GERD)
- In adults
  - Chronic obstructive pulmonary disease, bronchiectasis, heart failure, pulmonary embolism, tumor, pulmonary infiltration with eosinophilia, Churg-Strauss syndrome, medication-induced cough (ACE inhibitors), vocal cord dysfunction

DIAGNOSTIC TESTS & INTERPRETATION
Initial Tests (lab, imaging)
- Blood tests are not required but may find eosinophilia or elevated serum IgE levels (allergic asthma).
- Documented variable expiratory airflow limitation:
  - Spirometry with methacholine challenge: Normal test does not rule out asthma; measures the FVC and the FEV_1; a reduced predicted ratio of FEV_1/FVC with reversibility (increase of 200 mL and 12% of FEV_1/FVC from baseline) after using a short-acting bronchodilator (SABA)
  - Excessive variability in twice-daily peak expiratory flow (PEF) in 2 weeks (daily PEF variability >10%)
  - Bronchial challenge test: used mainly in adults, positive when there is a fall in FEV_1 >20% with methacholine or histamine; or >15% with hypertonic saline or mannitol challenge
  - Exercise challenge test: fall in FEV_1 >10% and 200 mL from baseline
  - Significant increase in lung function after 4 weeks of anti-inflammatory treatment
- Chest x-ray is used to exclude alternative diagnoses.

Follow-Up Tests & Special Considerations
- Asthma action plan: Patients monitor their own symptoms and/or peak flow measurements. Reassess action plan every 3 to 6 months.
- Assess asthma symptoms control with simple screening tools, such as consensus-based Global Initiative for Asthma (GINA) symptom control tool or Primary Care Asthma Control Screening Tool (PACS).

Diagnostic Procedures/Other
- Allergy skin testing is not useful for diagnosis of asthma but may be to evaluate atopic triggers.
- Measurement of fractional concentration of exhaled nitric oxide (FENO) suggests eosinophilic airway inflammation.

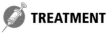

TREATMENT

GENERAL MEASURES
- Focus on symptom control and prevention of exacerbations.
- Use of holding chambers ("spacers") with inhaled agents improves clinical outcomes.
- Written asthma self-management action plan
- Encourage physical activity, weight loss, smoking cessation, avoidance of irritants, emotional stress.
- Avoidance of occupational exposure
- Annual influenza vaccine
- Pneumococcal vaccine recommended for high-risk patients
- Patients at risk for anaphylaxis carry EpiPen.
- Controller medications: used for regular maintenance, reduce airway inflammation, control symptoms, and reduce risk of exacerbations:
  - Inhaled corticosteroids (ICS)
  - Long-acting β-agonist (LABA) (formoterol, salmeterol)
- The ICS can be delivered by regular daily treatment or, in mild asthma, by as-needed low-dose ICS-formoterol.
- Treatment of asthma with SABAs alone is no longer recommended by the GINA guidelines for adults and adolescents.
  - ICS therapy is essential to reduce risk of death and severe exacerbations.
- Reliever (rescue medication) provided to all patients for as-needed relief of breakthrough symptoms
  - SABA–albuterol/levalbuterol
- Add-on therapies for patients with severe asthma, when patients persist with symptoms despite optimized treatment with high-dose controller medications (ICS + LABA)

Pediatric Considerations
- Tiotropium is not indicated in children <12 years.
- Reliever for all management steps in children 6 to 11 years is as-needed SABA.
- School-based programs including asthma self-management reduce emergency department visits, hospitalizations, and days of reduced activity.

Pregnancy Considerations
- Do not use bronchial provocation test nor step down controller treatment until after delivery.
- Asthma symptoms tend to worsen in 1/3 of patients, 1/3 improves, and 1/3 remains unchanged.
- Exacerbations are common in 2nd trimester.
- Poorly controlled asthma results in low birth weight, increased prematurity, and perinatal mortality.
- All short-acting agents (SABA) are pregnancy Category C as well as ICS.
- Cessation of ICS during pregnancy is a significant risk factor for exacerbation.
- Montelukast and zafirlukast are Category B but are not studied extensively in pregnancy.

Geriatric Considerations
- Underdiagnosed due to comorbidities
- Management challenges due to comorbidities (like arthritis) and due to polypharmacy

MEDICATION
First Line
- Initial recommended controllers by patient's presenting symptoms
- Stepwise approach for asthma treatment for adolescents (>12 years) and adults:
  - Step 1: symptom-driven treatment:
    ○ First: symptom-driven as-needed low-dose ICS-formoterol; controller alternatives: low-dose ICS whenever SABA taken; preferred reliever: ICS-formoterol
  - Step 2: low-dose controller + as-needed reliever:
    ○ First: low-dose ICS + SABA; controller alternatives: LTRA or low-dose ICS whenever SABA taken (separate or combined)
  - Step 3: one or two controllers + as-needed reliever:
    ○ First (adults/adolescents): low-dose ICS-LABA; controller alternatives: medium-dose ICS or low-dose ICS with LRTA. Preferred reliever: as-needed low-dose ICS/formoterol as both controller + reliever for those on maintenance therapy; first (ages 6 to 11 years) and second alternative (adults/adolescents): medium-dose ICS + SABA; third: low-dose ICS + LTRA
  - Step 4: two or more controllers + as-needed reliever:
    ○ First (adults/adolescents): medium-dose ICS-LABA as controller; controller alternatives: high-dose ICS, add-on tiotropium, or LTRA. Consider house dust mite SLIT for sensitized patient with normal spirometry and allergic rhinitis; preferred reliever low-dose ICS-formoterol for those prescribed bud-form/BDP-form maintenance and reliever therapy, otherwise SABA reliever when on other ICS-LABA
  - Step 5: high-dose ICS-LABA, referral for phenotype assessment and consider add-on therapy (i.e., LAMA, anti-IgE, anti-IL5/5R, anti-IL4, tiotropium) or add low-dose OCS while considering risks versus benefits

- Combination therapy with an LABA + ICS resulted in fewer asthma exacerbations than treatment with ICS alone.
- COVID-19 special considerations
  - Patients with asthma should continue taking their prescribed asthma medications, particularly ICS-containing medication and oral corticosteroids if prescribed.
  - Where possible, avoid use of nebulizers due to the risk of transmitting infection to other patients and to health care workers and avoid spirometry in patients with suspected or confirmed COVID-19.
  - COVID-19 vaccination is recommended for people with asthma.

ISSUES FOR REFERRAL
- Specialized testing (e.g., bronchoprovocation)
- Specialized treatments (e.g., immunotherapy)
- Poorly controlled asthma, frequent exacerbation, or multiple emergency department visits
- Occupational asthma due to legal implications

ADDITIONAL THERAPIES
- Exercise-induced bronchoconstriction (EIB): pharmacotherapy show to reduce symptoms, SABA prior exercise, or LTRA/chromones
- Allergen immunotherapy when clear relationship between symptoms and exposure
- Management of acute exacerbation of asthma
  - Outpatient:
    ○ Mild: speak in full sentence, HR <120 beats/minute, oxygen saturation 90–95%, and peak flow >50% of predicted can be managed as outpatient in clinic; should start SABA with ICS or formoterol/ICS and prednisolone; if symptoms resolve within 1 hour, could be discharged home with close follow-up
    ○ Severe symptoms: not able to speak in full sentence, HR >120 beats/minute, oxygen saturation <90%, peak flow <50% predicted, drowsy, confused, or silent chest; transfer to inpatient facility.
  - Treatment for severe:
    ○ Oxygen: to maintain saturation 93–95%
    ○ SABA: within 1 hour of arrival, initially around the clock followed by on demand
    ○ Systemic steroids: Oral is as effective as IV. 50 mg prednisolone (morning dose) or 200 mg hydrocortisone divided in doses. Duration should be 5 to 7 days.
    ○ Epinephrine: only when asthma is associated with angioedema or anaphylaxis
    ○ Avoid sedative.
    ○ Vital signs, pulse oximetry, response and duration of response to SABA, a lung function such as PEF or FEV_1
    ○ Asthma education
  - Discharge criteria
    ○ Minimal or absent asthma symptoms
    ○ Hypoxia has resolved.
    ○ FEV_1 or PEF ≥70% predicted or personal best
    ○ Bronchodilator response sustained ≥60 minutes

 ## ONGOING CARE
Smoking cessation if indicated

FOLLOW-UP RECOMMENDATIONS
- Identify triggers and control exposures.
- Consider stepping down treatment once symptoms are controlled for 3 months.

PATIENT EDUCATION
- American Academy of Allergy, Asthma & Immunology: 800-822-2762 or http://www.aaaai.org/
- Asthma and Allergy Foundation of America: 800-727-8462 or http://www.aafa.org/

PROGNOSIS
Prognosis is good for male patients, nonsmokers, and children with mild disease.

COMPLICATIONS
- Atelectasis, pneumonia, medication-specific side effects/adverse effects/interactions
- Respiratory failure; death: ~50% of asthma deaths occur in the elderly (age >65 years)

REFERENCE
1. Global Initiative for Asthma. Global strategy for asthma management and prevention, 2021. https://ginaastma.org/wp-content/uploads/2021/05/GINA-Main-Report-2021-V2-WMS.pdf. Accessed October 20, 2021.

ADDITIONAL READING
Cloutier MM, Baptist AP, Blake KV, et al.; and National Asthma Education and Prevention Program Coordinating Committee Expert Panel Working Group. 2020 Focused updates to the asthma management guidelines: a report from the National Asthma Education and Prevention Program Coordinating Committee Expert Panel Working Group. *J Allergy Clin Immunol*. 2020;146(6):1217–1270.

 ## CODES

ICD10
- J45.20 Mild intermittent asthma, uncomplicated
- J45.52 Severe persistent asthma with status asthmaticus
- J45.51 Severe persistent asthma with (acute) exacerbation

CLINICAL PEARLS
- SABA plus ICS or formoterol/ICS is the most effective rescue therapy for acute asthma symptoms.
- Holding chambers should be used by all.
- ICSs are the preferred long-term control therapy for patients of all ages.

ATELECTASIS

Keshav Kukreja, MD • Adrian DaSilva-DeAbreu, MD • Raymundo A. Quintana, MD

BASICS

DESCRIPTION
- Atelectasis is defined as the incomplete expansion of lung tissue due to collapse or closure. The loss of lung volume and function leads to impaired airway mucus clearance.
- Broadly categorized as:
  - Obstructive: airway blockage
  - Nonobstructive: loss of contact between the parietal and visceral pleurae, replacement of lung tissue by scarring or infiltrative disease, surfactant dysfunction, and parenchymal compression
- Symptoms depend on the rate of collapse, the amount of lung involved, and whether the patient has underlying lung disease and/or comorbidities.
- Reduced respiratory gas exchange can cause hypoxemia.

EPIDEMIOLOGY
- Mean age is 60 years, but all ages are susceptible.
- Male = female; no racial or socioeconomic predilection

Incidence
- Rounded atelectasis can be seen in up to 65–70% of asbestos workers.
- Lobar atelectasis is variable based on the collateral ventilation and number of lobes involved.

Prevalence
Postoperative atelectasis, especially after major cardiovascular or gastrointestinal (GI) procedures; can be seen in up to 90% of patients

ETIOLOGY AND PATHOPHYSIOLOGY
- Obstructive (resorptive) atelectasis is caused by intrinsic airway blockage and is the most common variety. It can be caused by luminal blockage (i.e., foreign body, mucus plug, asthma, cystic fibrosis, trauma, mass lesion) or airway wall abnormality (i.e., congenital malformation and emphysema).
  - Distal to the obstruction, alveolar air is rapidly reabsorbed into the deoxygenated venous system, causing complete collapse of the alveolar tissue.
  - Fraction of inspired oxygen (FiO_2): Compared to the rapid dissociation of O_2 distal to the obstruction, the 79% atmospheric nitrogen in atmosphere dissociates more slowly from the alveoli. This prevents collapse by maintaining positive pressure inside the alveoli. However, with increased FiO_2, the concentration of nitrogen is decreased, allowing rapid development of atelectasis at the onset of obstruction.
  - The patency and function of the collateral ventilatory systems in each lobe (pores of Kohn, canals of Lambert, and fenestrations of Boren) depends on multiple patient factors including age, underlying lung disease, and FiO_2.
  - In patients with emphysema, the fenestra of Boren become enlarged, which acts as a compensatory mechanism and can lead to a delay in atelectasis despite an obstructing lesion or mass.
- Nonobstructive atelectasis
  - Passive atelectasis (i.e., during a pleural effusion or pneumothorax) is due to pleural membrane separation of the visceral and parietal layers.
  - Compression atelectasis occurs with space-occupying lesions, cardiomegaly, abscess, or significant lymphadenopathy.
    - Increased chest wall pressure compresses the alveoli, leading to diminished functional residual capacity (FRC) or resting lung volume.
  - Adhesive atelectasis in the setting of acute respiratory distress syndrome (ARDS), radiation, smoke inhalation, or uremia. The underlying surfactant dysfunction causes increased surface tension and alveoli collapse.
  - Cicatrization represents pleural or parenchymal scarring and is common in granulomatous disease (i.e., sarcoidosis), toxic or radiation exposure, and drug-induced fibrosis (i.e., amiodarone, cyclophosphamide).
  - Replacement atelectasis: diffuse tumor (i.e., bronchioalveolar cell carcinoma) manifestation resulting in complete lobar collapse
- Rounded atelectasis is a distinct form of atelectasis seen in patients with asbestos exposure as a result of their significant pleural disease.
- Others
  - Hypoxemia from a pulmonary embolus
  - Muscular weakness: due to anesthesia side-effect, or in neuromuscular diseases with respiratory muscle involvement

Pediatric Considerations
Children are at a higher risk of developing atelectasis due to their less developed collateral ventilation and compensatory mechanisms.

RISK FACTORS
- Critical care and prolonged immobilization
- General anesthesia (including long-acting muscle relaxants, postoperative epidural anesthesia)
- Positive fluid balance
- Massive blood transfusion (≥4 units)
- Nasogastric tube placement
- Hypothermia
- Mechanical ventilation with high tidal volume (Vt >10 mL/kg) and plateau pressure (>30 cm H_2O)
- Patient risk factors for postoperative atelectasis:
  - Age >60 years and <6 years
  - Chronic obstructive pulmonary disease (COPD)
  - Obstructive sleep apnea
  - Congestive heart failure (CHF)
  - Alcohol abuse, smoking
  - Pulmonary hypertension
  - Albumin <3.5 g/dL
  - Hemoglobin <10 g/dL
  - BMI >27 kg/m^2 (weak evidence)
  - ASA class II+ functional dependence in activities of daily living (ADLs)
  - Surgical procedures: cardiothoracic, vascular, upper GI, neurosurgical, oromaxillofacial, and ENT
  - Often a precursor to more serious pulmonary complications (1)
- Right middle lobe syndrome (Brock syndrome): wedge-shaped density extending inferiorly and anteriorly from the hilum. Best seen on lateral chest radiography; no consistent clinical definition

GENERAL PREVENTION
- Early mobilization, deep breathing exercises, coughing, and frequent changes in body position
- Preoperative physical therapy lowered rates of atelectasis, pneumonia, and length of stay (LOS) in patients undergoing elective cardiac surgery. However, there was no change in other postoperative pulmonary complications or mortality (2)[A]. Furthermore, large RCTs are needed before conclusions can be drawn regarding the efficacy of chest physiotherapy and incentive spirometry (IS).

- Mechanical ventilation settings with high Vt (Vt >10 mL/kg) and plateau pressures (>30 cm H_2O) and without positive end-expiratory pressure (PEEP) are associated with postoperative pulmonary complications (i.e., pneumonia, respiratory failure):
  - Minimize ventilator-induced injury by employing low Vt and plateau pressures at sufficient PEEP.
  - Ensure lower FiO_2 during anesthetic induction and intraoperatively to prevent nitrogen washout.
- Continuous positive airway pressure (CPAP) during anesthesia induction and reversal of anesthesia-induced atelectasis after intubation by a recruitment maneuver may decrease postoperative pulmonary complications (3)[C].

COMMONLY ASSOCIATED CONDITIONS
- Obstructive lung diseases (COPD and asthma)
- Trauma
- ARDS, neonatal RDS, pulmonary edema, pulmonary embolism, pneumonia, pleural effusion, pneumothorax
- Respiratory syncytial virus (RSV), bronchiolitis
- Bronchial stenosis, pulmonic valve disease, and pulmonary hypertension
- Neuromuscular disorders (muscular dystrophy, spinal muscular atrophy, spinal cord injury, and Guillain-Barré syndrome) and cystic fibrosis

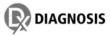
DIAGNOSIS

HISTORY
- Frequently asymptomatic
- Tachypnea and sudden-onset dyspnea
- Nonproductive cough
- Pleuritic pain on affected side
- History of smoking, COPD, pulmonary insufficiency, exposure to radiation, asbestos, or other air pollutants

PHYSICAL EXAM
- Signs of hypoxia or cyanosis
- Tracheal or precordial impulse displacement toward the affected side; dullness to percussion
- Bronchial breathing in patent airway
- Wheezing or absent breath sounds in occluded airway
- Diminished chest expansion

DIFFERENTIAL DIAGNOSIS
See "Etiology and Pathophysiology."

DIAGNOSTIC TESTS & INTERPRETATION
Initial Tests (lab, imaging)
- CBC and respiratory Gram stain, culture, and viral panel if infection suspected
- ABG: Despite hypoxemia, $PaCO_2$ level is usually normal or low.
- Chest x-ray (CXR), PA, and lateral
  - Displaced hilum, mediastinal shift toward the side of atelectatic lung, volume loss in ipsilateral hemithorax, raised diaphragm
  - Crowding of the ribs and silhouetting of the diaphragm or heart border
  - Compensatory hyperlucency of remaining lobes of affected lung and compensatory hyperinflation in unaffected lung
  - Lobar collapse
  - Wedge-shaped densities: obstructive atelectasis

- Small, linear bands (Fleischner lines) often at lung bases: discoid (subsegmental or plate) atelectasis
- Direct signs: displacement of fissures and opacification of the collapsed lobe. Right upper lobe collapse may display the inverted "S sign of Golden," representing neoplastic shift of the minor fissure.
- Air bronchograms: Pleural fluid or air may indicate compressive atelectasis.
- Adhesive atelectasis may present as a diffuse reticular granular pattern, which can progress to a pulmonary edema pattern and to bilateral opacification in severe cases.
- Pleural-based round density: round atelectasis
- Complete atelectasis of entire lung: opacification of the entire hemithorax and a shift of the mediastinum to atelectatic lung

Follow-Up Tests & Special Considerations
- Chest CT or MRI may be indicated to visualize airway and mediastinal structures and identify cause of atelectasis in unclear cases.
- Pulmonary function tests (PFTs) can help identify obstructive or restrictive disease and decreased respiratory muscle pressures.
- Hypoalbuminemia (albumin <3.5 g/L) is a powerful marker of increased risk for postoperative pulmonary complications, including atelectasis.

Diagnostic Procedures/Other
Flexible fiber-optic bronchoscopy can be considered in unexplained or refractory cases.

TREATMENT

GENERAL MEASURES
- Identify and treat the underlying etiology.
- PEEP for prevention following surgery or general anesthesia (3)[C]
- Lay on unaffected side, encourage frequent coughing, deep breathing exercises, and early mobility.
- IS every hour while awake
  - Frequently used despite lack of evidence for IS preventing postoperative pulmonary complications after coronary artery bypass grafting (CABG) (4)[A]
- Mechanical ventilate with PEEP in severe respiratory distress or hypoxemia:
  - Lower Vt (6 mL/kg) and lower plateau pressures (<30 mm Hg) associated with reduced mortality
  - PEEP 15 to 20 mL may be necessary to maintain arterial O_2 saturation in surfactant-impaired lung regions.

MEDICATION
First Line
Pharmacotherapy should address underlying etiology:
- Antibiotics for infection
- Chemotherapy or radiation for malignancy
- Inhalers and steroids for asthma
- Effective analgesia to permit deep inspiration and coughing
- Mucolytics can be considered to promote airway clearance (i.e., N-acetylcysteine and saline).

Pediatric Considerations
- Dornase alfa may be effective clearing mucinous secretions in refractory mucous plugging in children (used in cystic fibrosis).
- Chest physiotherapy (i.e., percussion, drainage, deep insufflation, and saline lavage) is the most commonly utilized therapy in the inpatient setting.

- Other physically stimulating modalities (mechanical insufflation-exsufflation, intrapulmonary percussive ventilation, intermittent positive pressure breathing) may have utility in patients with neuromuscular disease and cystic fibrosis to enhance mucus clearance.
- Applying continuous distending pressure has shown some benefit in the treatment of preterm infants with RDS and has the potential to reduce lung damage particularly if used early (5)[A].
- In obstructive atelectasis, bronchoscopy remains controversial. However, in the presence of a mucus plug or cast, bronchoscopy may be beneficial.

Second Line
Fiber-optic bronchoscopy to improve airway clearance has been efficacious in several studies; however, there is debate regarding its efficacy in the treatment of atelectasis. It may be beneficial in those with unsuccessful attempts or contraindications to chest physiotherapy (i.e., chest wall trauma).

SURGERY/OTHER PROCEDURES
Appropriate surgical resection for underlying disease (i.e., tumor, severe lymphadenopathy)

> **ALERT**
> The association between postoperative atelectasis and fever is likely coincidental rather than causal.

ADMISSION, INPATIENT, AND NURSING CONSIDERATIONS
Ensure adequate oxygenation (may start with 100% FiO_2 then taper) and humidification. Note: if obstructive atelectasis is suspected, then judiciously increase FiO_2 to prevent nitrogen washout, which can hasten atelectasis.

ONGOING CARE

FOLLOW-UP RECOMMENDATIONS
Patient Monitoring
- Frequency/adequacy of monitoring will vary by underlying cause and concurrent comorbidities.
- For uncomplicated cases of atelectasis associated (i.e., those associated with asthma or infection), outpatient monitoring may be appropriate.

PATIENT EDUCATION
Maximize mobility as tolerated and encourage frequent coughing and deep breathing exercises. Seek further treatment or return to ED for worsening symptoms or shortness of breath.

PROGNOSIS
- Postoperative atelectasis usually spontaneous resolves within 24 hours but can persist for days.
- Resolution of lobar atelectasis due to endobronchial obstruction depends on treatment of underlying disease or malignancy.
- Surgical intervention is indicated only for resectable etiologies (i.e., tumor) or if atelectasis is severe and causes chronic infections and bronchiectasis.

COMPLICATIONS
- Pneumonia or other pulmonary infections
- Acute atelectasis: hypoxemia, respiratory failure, postobstructive drowning of the lung
- Chronic atelectasis: bronchiectasis, pleural effusion, empyema

REFERENCES
1. Restrepo RD, Braverman J. Current challenges in the recognition, prevention and treatment of perioperative pulmonary atelectasis. *Expert Rev Respir Med*. 2015;9(1):97–107.
2. Hulzebos EH, Smit Y, Helders PP, et al. Preoperative physical therapy for elective cardiac surgery patients. *Cochrane Database Syst Rev*. 2012;(11):CD010118.
3. Baltieri L, Santos LA, Rasera I Jr, et al. Use of positive pressure in the bariatric surgery and effects on pulmonary function and prevalence of atelectasis: randomized and blinded clinical trial. *Arq Bras Cir Dig*. 2014;27(Suppl 1):26–30.
4. Freitas ER, Soares BG, Cardoso JR, et al. Incentive spirometry for preventing pulmonary complications after coronary artery bypass graft. *Cochrane Database Syst Rev*. 2012;(9):CD004466.
5. Ho JJ, Henderson-Smart DJ, Davis PG. Early versus delayed initiation of continuous distending pressure for respiratory distress syndrome in preterm infants. *Cochrane Database Syst Rev*. 2002;(2):CD002975.

ADDITIONAL READING
- Brower RG. Consequences of bed rest. *Crit Care Med*. 2009;37(Suppl 10):S422–S428.
- Guimarães MM, El Dib R, Smith AF, et al. Incentive spirometry for prevention of postoperative pulmonary complications in upper abdominal surgery. *Cochrane Database Syst Rev*. 2009;(3):CD006058.
- Mavros MN, Velmahos GC, Falagas ME. Atelectasis as a cause of postoperative fever: where is the clinical evidence? *Chest*. 2011;140(2):418–424.
- Tusman G, Böhm SH, Warner DO, et al. Atelectasis and perioperative pulmonary complications in high-risk patients. *Curr Opin Anaesthesiol*. 2012;25(1):1–10.
- Wu KH, Lin CF, Huang CJ, et al. Rigid ventilation bronchoscopy under general anesthesia for treatment of pediatric pulmonary atelectasis caused by pneumonia: a review of 33 cases. *Int Surg*. 2006;91(5):291–294.

 ## CODES

ICD10
J98.11 Atelectasis

CLINICAL PEARLS
- Low serum albumin (<3.5 g/L) is a strong predictor of postoperative pulmonary complications, including atelectasis.
- Anesthesia-induced atelectasis occurs in almost all anesthetized patients but can be reduced by employing PEEP intraoperatively or when reversing anesthesia.
- Early mobilization, coughing, deep breathing exercises, and treating the underlying cause are the mainstays of therapy.
- Bronchogenic carcinoma can present as atelectasis and must be excluded in all patients >35 years.
- In complete atelectasis of an entire lung, the mediastinal ipsilateral shift separates atelectasis from massive pleural effusion.
- No strong clinical evidence supports atelectasis as an early cause of postoperative fever.

ATRIAL FIBRILLATION AND ATRIAL FLUTTER

Bianca Lee, DO, MS • Lyncean Ung, DO

 BASICS

This topic covers both atrial fibrillation (AFib) and atrial flutter (AFlut).

DESCRIPTION

- AFib: paroxysmal or continuous supraventricular tachyarrhythmia characterized by rapid, uncoordinated atrial electrical activity and an irregularly irregular ventricular response. In most patients, the ventricular rate is rapid because the atrioventricular (AV) node is bombarded with very frequent atrial electrical impulses (400 to 600 beats/minute).
- AFlut: paroxysmal or continuous supraventricular tachyarrhythmia with rapid but organized atrial electrical activity. The atrial rate is typically between 250 and 350 beats/minute and is often manifested as "saw-tooth" flutter (F) waves on the ECG, particularly in the inferior leads and V_1. AFlut commonly occurs with 2:1 or 3:1 AV block, so the ventricular response may be regular and typically at a rate of 150 beats/minute.
- AFib and AFlut are related arrhythmias, sometimes seen in the same patient. Distinguishing the two is important because there may be implications for management.
- Clinical classifications:
  - Paroxysmal: self-terminating episodes, usually <7 days
  - Persistent: sustained >7 days, usually requiring pharmacologic or electrical cardioversion to restore sinus rhythm
  - Permanent: Sinus rhythm cannot be restored or maintained.
  - Nonvalvular AFib: absence of moderate-to-severe mitral stenosis or a mechanical heart valve
- Lone AFib occurs in patients <60 years (with possible genetic predisposition) who have no clinical or echocardiographic evidence of cardiovascular disease, including hypertension (HTN).

EPIDEMIOLOGY

- Incidence/prevalence increases significantly with age.
- Young patients with AFib, particularly lone AFib, are most commonly males.

Incidence

- AFib: from <0.1%/year <40 years to >1.5%/year >80 years
- Lifetime risk: 25% for those ≥40 years
- AFlut is less common.

Prevalence

- Estimated at 0.4–1% in general population, with 2.7 million patients in America
- Increases with age, up to 8% in those ≥80 years

ETIOLOGY AND PATHOPHYSIOLOGY

- Cardiac: HTN, acute coronary syndrome (ACS), congestive heart failure (CHF), valvular heart disease, cardiomyopathy, pericarditis, and infiltrative heart disease
- Pulmonary: pulmonary embolism (PE), chronic obstructive pulmonary disease (COPD), obstructive sleep apnea, pneumonia
- Ingestion: ethanol, caffeine, nicotine
- Endocrine: hyperthyroidism, diabetes mellitus (DM)

- Obesity
- Postoperative: cardiac, pulmonary, or esophageal
- Idiopathic: lone AFib
- Iatrogenic: amiodarone
- Patients with paroxysmal episodes are usually associated with premature atrial beats and/or bursts of tachycardia, originating in pulmonary vein ostia or other sites.
- Many patients with AFib are thought to have some degree of atrial fibrosis or scarring.
- Autonomic (vagal and sympathetic) tone may play a role in triggering the arrhythmia.
- The presence of AFib is associated with electrical and structural remodeling processes that promote arrhythmia maintenance in the atria, termed "AFib begets AFib."

Genetics

Familial forms are rare but do exist. There are ongoing efforts to identify the genetic underpinnings of such cases.

RISK FACTORS

Age, HTN, and obesity are the most important risk factors for both AFib and AFlut.

GENERAL PREVENTION

Adequate control of HTN may prevent development of AFib due to hypertensive heart disease and is the most significant modifiable risk factor for AFib. Weight reduction may decrease the risk of AFib in obese patients. Ethanol consumption may trigger AFib.

COMMONLY ASSOCIATED CONDITIONS

HTN, stroke, and other cardiac diseases

 DIAGNOSIS

HISTORY

Symptoms vary from none to mild (palpitations, lightheadedness, fatigue, poor exercise capacity) to severe (angina, dyspnea, syncope).

PHYSICAL EXAM

- AFib: irregularly irregular heart rate and pulse, pulse deficit
- AFlut: similar to AFib but may have regular pulse

DIFFERENTIAL DIAGNOSIS

- Multifocal atrial tachycardia
- Sinus tachycardia with frequent atrial premature beats
- Paroxysmal supraventricular tachycardia (Wolff-Parkinson-White [WPW], atrioventricular nodal reentry tachycardia [AVNRT])

DIAGNOSTIC TESTS & INTERPRETATION

- Screening with ECG to detect asymptomatic cases of AFib has not been shown to detect more cases than screening focused on pulse palpation (1)[A].
- AFib: The ECG is diagnostic, with findings of low-amplitude fibrillatory waves without discrete P waves and an irregularly irregular pattern of QRS complexes. There is often tachycardia in the absence of heart rate–controlling medications (2).

- AFlut: The ECG is diagnostic. Saw-tooth F waves are the classic sign, generally best seen in the inferior leads, although ventricular rate may need to be slowed to see the waves. QRS complexes may be regular or irregular; there is usually tachycardia (2).
- Ambulatory rhythm monitoring (e.g., telemetry, Holter monitoring, event recorders) is helpful in confirming suspected paroxysmal AFib or AFlut and monitoring for recurrence (2).

Initial Tests (lab, imaging)

Thyroid-stimulating hormone, electrolytes, complete blood count, complete metabolic panel, 2D transthoracic echocardiogram, prothrombin time/international normalized ratio (INR) (if anticoagulation is contemplated); digoxin level (if appropriate)

Follow-Up Tests & Special Considerations

- Occasional Holter monitoring and/or exercise stress testing to assess for adequacy of rate and/or rhythm control
- Chest x-ray (CXR) for cardiopulmonary disease
- ECG for signs of cardiac hypertrophy, ischemia, and/or other arrhythmias
- Transesophageal echocardiogram to detect left atrial appendage thrombus if cardioversion is planned
- Sleep study may be useful if sleep apnea is suspected.

Test Interpretation

Evaluate for presence of atrial dilatation and fibrosis, atrial thrombus (especially in atrial appendage), valvular heart disease, cardiomyopathy.

🩺 TREATMENT

- Two primary issues in the management of AFib and/or AFlut: decisions on heart rate control (control ventricular rate while allowing AFib to continue) or rhythm control (terminate AFib and restore normal sinus rhythm) and decision to anticoagulate or not.
- Anticoagulation therapy to prevent thromboembolism (primarily stroke) reduces risk of stroke by about 2/3. Several calculators exist for estimating yearly risk of thromboembolic event (ATRIA, CHA_2DS_2VASc). If risk is sufficiently low, or risk of bleeding is high (HAS-BLED tool may assist in evaluation), no anticoagulation may be indicated. Clinical judgment and patient preference remain important.

MEDICATION

- American Heart Association/American College of Cardiology anticoagulation guidelines (the same for AFib and AFlut) (3)[C]:
  - CHA_2DS_2VASc scoring (**C**HF [1 point], **H**TN [1 point], **A**ge ≥75 years [2 points], **D**M [1 point], prior **S**troke or transient ischemic attack [TIA] or thromboembolism [2 points], **V**ascular disease [1 point], **A**ge 65 to 74 years [1 point], female **S**ex **c**ategory [1 point]). CHA_2DS_2VASc is the recommended stroke risk assessment for patients with nonvalvular AFib (3)[C].
    - In patients with nonvalvular AFib and a CHA_2DS_2VASc score of 0 in males or 1 in females, anticoagulant therapy may be omitted (3)[C].

○ In patients with nonvalvular AFib and a CHA_2DS_2VASc score of 1 in males and 2 in females (with one non–sex-related risk factor), oral anticoagulant therapy may be considered (3)[C].

○ In patients with nonvalvular AFib with any high-risk factors for stroke (prior TIA/cerebrovascular accident [CVA]/thromboembolism) or a CHA_2DS_2VASc score ≥2 in men or ≥3 in women should receive oral anticoagulants unless contraindicated (3)[C].

– DOAC (direct-acting oral anticoagulant)/NOAC (non–vitamin K oral anticoagulant) agents are recommended over warfarin for most patients with nonvalvular atrial fibrillation who should receive anticoagulant therapy (3)[C]. Oral anticoagulants include warfarin (3)[C] with maintenance of an INR of 2.0 to 3.0, dabigatran (Pradaxa), rivaroxaban (Xarelto), apixaban (Eliquis), or edoxaban (Savaysa) (3)[C]. Patients with mechanical valves should be treated with warfarin to maintain an INR of 2.0 to 3.0 or 2.5 to 3.5 dependent on the type and location of the prosthesis (2)[B].

– The selection of an anticoagulant should be individualized; consider the risks of each agent, cost, patient preference, and tolerability.

ALERT
Renal and hepatic functions should be evaluated prior to initiation of direct thrombin or factor Xa inhibitors (3)[C]. Limited information is available about safety in patients on renal dialysis. Additional dosing considerations of age ≥80 years or weight ≤60 kg are recommended with apixaban (3)[C]. Dosing of such agents may need individualized adjustment. Specific reversal agents for life-threatening bleeding or urgent procedure are available:

- Idarucizumab (Praxbind) for dabigatran (3)[C]
- Coagulation factor Xa (recombinant), inactivated-zhzo (Andexxa) for apixaban and rivaroxaban (3)[C].

- In addition to anticoagulation, initial rate control must be achieved followed by a decision regarding long-term strategy: rate-control alone or rhythm control. Four classes of medications are available to achieve ventricular rate control: β-blockers (i.e., metoprolol), nondihydropyridine calcium channel blockers (i.e., verapamil, diltiazem), digoxin, and amiodarone. Optimal target for ventricular rate has not been firmly established, but there is evidence that aggressive control of the ventricular rate (<80 beats/minute) offers no benefit beyond more modest rate control (i.e., resting heart rate <110 beats/minute) (2)[C].
- Patients in whom rate control cannot be achieved or who continue to have persistent symptoms despite reasonable heart rate control may require attempts at restoration of sinus rhythm.
- Restoration of sinus rhythm using electrical or pharmacologic cardioversion may significantly reduce the symptom burden of AFib or AFlut in many patients and may also be useful for controlling ventricular rate.
- Randomized clinical trials (AFFIRM and RACE) comparing the outcomes of rate versus rhythm control found no difference in morbidity, mortality, and stroke rates in patients assigned to one therapy or the other (2).

ISSUES FOR REFERRAL
Management of AFib or AFlut refractory to standard medical therapy (i.e., unable to achieve adequate rate control with medication or development of significant bradycardia with treatment) may require the use of more aggressive treatments.

SURGERY/OTHER PROCEDURES
- Electrophysiologic study and ablation may be considered for patients with either AFib or AFlut. In the case of AFlut, ablation is a procedure viewed as a first-line therapy. Ablation of AFib may be reasonable in symptomatic patients with heart failure with reduced ejection fraction (HFrEF) to lower mortality and reduce hospitalization (3)[B].
- Cardiac surgery (e.g., the maze procedure, occlusion of the left atrial appendage) may be considered in patients planning to undergo cardiac surgery for other reasons.
- Percutaneous left atrial appendage (LAA) occlusion with WATCHMAN device may be considered in those at increased risk of stroke and systemic embolism with contraindications to long-term anticoagulation (3)[B].

COMPLEMENTARY & ALTERNATIVE MEDICINE
The use of herbal remedies, dietary supplements, and vitamins should be thoroughly assessed to avoid medication interactions.

ADMISSION, INPATIENT, AND NURSING CONSIDERATIONS
- Patients with significant symptoms, RVR, AFib/AFlut triggered by an acute process (e.g., ACS, CHF, PE), or in whom antiarrhythmic therapy is being started likely require admission to the hospital for a period of stabilization.
- Acute therapy for symptomatic patients with AFib or AFlut:
  – IV β-blockers or nondihydropyridine calcium channel blockers (e.g., diltiazem, verapamil) for control of ventricular rate in patients without preexcitation (3)[C].
  – IV amiodarone or digoxin may be considered in patients with severe left ventricular dysfunction or hemodynamic instability (3)[C].
- Urgent direct-current cardioversion is recommended in patients with hemodynamic instability or inadequate rate control (3)[C].
- Consider the initiation of anticoagulation therapy.

 ## ONGOING CARE

Consider elective expert consultation.

FOLLOW-UP RECOMMENDATIONS
Patient Monitoring
- Adequate anticoagulation levels with warfarin should be determined weekly during initiation and at least monthly when stable (3)[A].
- If NOACs are employed, hepatic and renal functions should be reevaluated at least annually (3)[B].

DIET
Patients on warfarin should attempt to consume a stable amount of vitamin K.

PATIENT EDUCATION
For overweight and obese patients, weight loss combined with risk factor modification have demonstrated beneficial effects on controlling AFib (3)[C].

PROGNOSIS
AFib and AFlut may increase morbidity and mortality, but the overall prognosis is a function of underlying heart disease and adherence with therapy.

COMPLICATIONS
- Embolic stroke
- Peripheral arterial embolization
- Bleeding with anticoagulation
- Tachycardia-induced cardiomyopathy with prolonged periods of inadequate rate control

REFERENCES

1. Jonas DE, Kahwati LC, Yun JDY, et al. Screening for atrial fibrillation with electrocardiography: evidence report and systematic review for the US Preventive Services Task Force. *JAMA.* 2018;320(5):485–498.
2. January CT, Wann LS, Alpert JS, et al. 2014 AHA/ACC/HRS guideline for the management of patients with atrial fibrillation: executive summary: a report of the American College of Cardiology/American Heart Association Task Force on Practice Guidelines and the Heart Rhythm Society. *Circulation.* 2014;130(23):2071–2104.
3. January CT, Wann LS, Calkins H, et al. 2019 AHA/ACC/HRS focused update of the 2014 AHA/ACC/HRS guideline for the management of patients with atrial fibrillation: a report of the American College of Cardiology/American Heart Association Task Force on Clinical Practice Guidelines and the Heart Rhythm Society. *Circulation.* 2019;140(2):e125–e151.

CODES

ICD10
- I48.91 Unspecified atrial fibrillation
- I48.92 Unspecified atrial flutter
- I48.0 Paroxysmal atrial fibrillation

CLINICAL PEARLS
Reevaluation of the need for and choice of anticoagulation therapy at periodic intervals is recommended to reassess stroke and bleeding risks.

ATRIAL SEPTAL DEFECT

Marvin H. Sineath Jr., MD, FAAFP, CAQSM • Sydney E. Koenig, MD

 BASICS

DESCRIPTION

- Anatomy
  - Opening in the atrial septum allowing flow of blood between the two atria
  - Patent foramen ovale is not considered an atrial septal defect (ASD) because no septal tissue is missing.
- Types classified by location and abnormal embryogenesis (1)
  - 75%: ostium secundum defect, located in the mid-septum
  - 15–20%: ostium primum defect, located in the inferior septum, associated with cleft mitral valve and failure of endocardial cushion development
  - 5–10%: sinus venosus defect, located in the superior-posterior septum near the orifice of the superior vena cava, associated with partial defect in right upper pulmonary venous return
  - <1%: coronary sinus defect, absence of the entire common wall between the coronary sinus and the left atrium
- Hemodynamic effects
  - Left-to-right shunting in late ventricular systole and early diastole
  - Degree depends on size of the defect and relative pressures of the two ventricles.
  - Causes excessive blood flow through the right-sided circulation, ultimately leading to reactive pulmonary hypertension and heart failure
- Systems affected: cardiovascular; pulmonary

Pediatric Considerations
- Most cases of ASD are detected and corrected in the pediatric population.
- The smaller the defect and the younger the child, the greater the chance of spontaneous closure.

EPIDEMIOLOGY
Incidence
- Predominant age: present from birth, may be diagnosed at any age
- Female-to-male ratio 2–4:1 (2)
- No race predilection
- 1/1,500 live births (2)
- Ostium secundum alone accounts for >90% of all congenital heart lesions in the adult population (3)

Prevalence
ASDs account for 13% of congenital heart disorders.

ETIOLOGY AND PATHOPHYSIOLOGY
- Flow across ASD usually left-to-right shunt because of higher left-sided pressures:
  - Minimal right-to-left shunting in early ventricular systole, especially during inspiration
  - Increased right-sided pressure/pulmonary arterial hypertension can cause reversal of shunt flow (Eisenmenger syndrome) with resulting cyanosis and clubbing.
- Symptoms typically occur due to right ventricular and pulmonary vascular volume overload and right-sided heart failure.

Genetics
- Majority of cases are spontaneous, although rare familial cases exist (2).
- 25% prevalence in Down syndrome
- 5% with chromosomal abnormalities

RISK FACTORS
- Family history, other congenital heart defects
- Maternal age >35 years
- Gestational exposures: thalidomide, alcohol, tobacco, elevated blood glucose (4).

COMMONLY ASSOCIATED CONDITIONS
- 70% ASDs are isolated but may occur as a component of other complex cardiac structural defects, including anomalous pulmonary venous return.
- May be associated with rare underlying genetic syndromes, including Holt-Oram (ASD present in 66%), Ellis-van Creveld, VACTERL syndrome, Down syndrome, or Noonan syndrome (4)

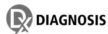 **DIAGNOSIS**

HISTORY
- Most ASDs are small, asymptomatic in throughout childhood, and only found as an incidental cardiac murmur on routine physical examination.
- Infants with large ASDs may present with right-sided heart failure (more advanced, only 10% at diagnosis), tachypnea, recurrent respiratory infections, or failure to thrive.
- Uncorrected defects usually become symptomatic by 40 years of age and may present with palpitations (most frequently), exercise intolerance, dyspnea, syncope, peripheral edema, cyanosis, or fatigue (4).
- Children and young adults are rarely symptomatic but may present with exercise intolerance or atrial arrhythmias (4).

PHYSICAL EXAM
- Children and young adults are mostly asymptomatic, although they can rarely exhibit cyanosis and hyperdynamic precordium.
- Signs vary according to extent of shunting.
- Cardiac palpation
  - Hyperdynamic precordium over the right ventricle (4)
  - Palpable pulmonary artery pulse at the left upper sternal border
- Cardiac auscultation
  - *Fixed, widely split S_2 (key physical finding)*
  - May also have
    - Systolic ejection murmur (pulmonic flow murmur)
    - Low-pitched diastolic rumble (tricuspid flow murmur)
    - Diastolic murmur (pulmonic regurgitation)
    - Systolic murmur (mitral regurgitation)
    - Fourth heart sound in the setting of right-sided heart failure
- Signs of Eisenmenger syndrome:
  - Cyanosis and clubbing
  - Jugular venous distention and edema

DIFFERENTIAL DIAGNOSIS
- Other congenital heart disease
- Right bundle branch block (for widely split S_2)

DIAGNOSTIC TESTS & INTERPRETATION
Initial Tests (lab, imaging)
- Best initial test is transthoracic echocardiogram (TTE) with Doppler imaging of the entire atrial septum: sensitive for secundum (89%), primum (100%), and sinus venosus (44%) defects.

- If TTE is nondiagnostic or shows evidence of right ventricular overload, progression to transesophageal echocardiography (TEE) is warranted.
- Oximetry at rest and with activity: Cyanosis or SpO_2 <90% may suggest Eisenmenger syndrome (right-to-left shunting). In certain subsets of patients, these signs may only appear with activity (5).
- ECG is not typically diagnostic but may show various signs of right- or left-sided heart strain, inverted P wave in lead III (in sinus venosus), or leftward axis (ostium primum or sinus venosus) (4).

Follow-Up Tests & Special Considerations
- Bubble contrast enhancement may be helpful.
- TEE may be required to define ASD morphology and to locate the pulmonary veins; often used prior to percutaneous closure. TEE has excellent sensitivity and specificity.

Diagnostic Procedures/Other
- Echocardiography is first line as noted above.
- Cardiac catheterization: used to characterize ASDs and concomitant heart disease and to assess presence of pulmonary vascular resistance or hypertension (particularly if considering surgery) (1). This procedure is not indicated in young patients unless part of a planned closure, evaluating another disease simultaneously, or other visualization methods are insufficient (5).
- Cardiac magnetic resonance: noninvasive follow-up to echocardiography, used to evaluate sinus venosus defects/pulmonary veins, shunt fraction, and right ventricular function (4),(5)
- Exercise testing: may be used to document change over time (1)
- Chest x-ray: may be used to identify right ventricular or pulmonary artery enlargement
- Cardiac CT: may further define ASD but with significant radiation exposure

 TREATMENT

GENERAL MEASURES
- 75% of small secundum ASDs (<8 mm) will close spontaneously by 18 months of age; however, close follow-up is warranted (4).
- Surgical closure usually required for primum and sinus venosus defects (4).

MEDICATION
First Line
- Treatment of secondary cardiac or pulmonary vascular disease
  - Atrial fibrillation/supraventricular tachycardia (SVT) with anticoagulation and cardioversion/sinus rhythm or rate control (1)
  - Heart failure with diuretics, oxygen, digoxin, etc.
  - Remodeling therapy with prostaglandins, endothelin blockers, and PDE-5 inhibitors for patients with severe pulmonary arterial hypertension (5)
- Consider pulmonary vasodilator therapy for adults with progressive/severe pulmonary vascular disease (1).

Second Line
- Antibiotic prophylaxis is NOT recommended for unrepaired/isolated ASDs or as prophylaxis against infective endocarditis during dental procedures.
- To prevent thrombus formation after device deployment, aspirin alone or a combination of aspirin and clopidogrel 75 mg for at least 6 months is recommended.

SURGERY/OTHER PROCEDURES
- The majority of small secundum defects, <6 mm, close spontaneously by 2 years of age. Closure is generally indicated in children with defects > 8 mm, defects of any size in children >5 years with related symptoms.
- Closure for secundum defects is not recommended in asymptomatic patients before 2 years of age given the possibility of spontaneous closure. It is also contraindicated in patients with irreversible, severe pulmonary hypertension without continued shunting (1).
- In adults, secundum closure via percutaneous transcatheter device or surgery to reduce subsequent morbidity and mortality indicated in patients with right heart enlargement with or without symptoms, pulmonary systemic flow ratio of 2:1 (or >1.5:1 and <21 years old per the AHA), or symptoms including documented orthodeoxia/platypnea or paradoxical embolism (1). Treatment with a closure device does not significantly affect aortic/mitral valve function.
- Surgical repair is standard for a sinus venosus, coronary sinus, or primum ASD (1),(4).
- Percutaneous closure with a closure device is considered the treatment of choice of secundum ASD in adults (5),(6). It is safe and effective with satisfactory long-term clinical follow-up. In addition, the use of closure device does not significantly affect aortic or mitral valve function (6).
- Maze procedure may be considered before or after closure for patients with intermittent or chronic atrial tachyarrhythmias (1).

 ONGOING CARE

FOLLOW-UP RECOMMENDATIONS
- Outpatient cardiologist visits: every 3 months to 5 years depending on physiologic stage of the defect (5)
- ECG: every 1 to 5 years depending on physiologic stage of the defect
- TTE: every 1 to 5 years depending on physiologic stage of the defect
- Exercise stress test: every 6 to 24 months for advanced disease

Patient Monitoring
- In otherwise asymptomatic healthy children, follow up until defect has closed or become negligible in size.
- ASDs repaired in adulthood may require periodic long-term follow-up (1).
- ASDs repaired in childhood generally do not have late complications.
- Pregnancy is well tolerated in cases with repaired/small unrepaired ASDs but is not recommended in cases of unrepaired ASD/Eisenmenger syndrome due to increased risk of maternal and fetal mortality (1).

- Recommend consultation in patients with unrepaired ASDs prior to scuba diving or high-altitude travel.

PATIENT EDUCATION
For patient education materials on this topic, consult the American Heart Association or Mayo Clinic ASD webpages.

PROGNOSIS
- ASD closure in asymptomatic, minimally symptomatic, and symptomatic adults reduces morbidity especially if performed before 25 years of age (3),(5).
- ASD repair deferred until after adolescence may not decrease long-term risk of future atrial arrhythmias.
- In one study, prognosis after ASD closure saw a >20% reduction in pulmonary resistance by pretreatment with PAH therapies and pulmonary remodeling treatments (5)
- Unoperated ASDs: up to 25% mortality by 27 years, up to 90% mortality by 60 years, increased rates of atrial arrhythmias, reduced functional capacity, greater degrees of pulmonary arterial hypertension (3),(5)

COMPLICATIONS
- Unrepaired: congestive heart failure, stroke, atrial arrhythmias, increased infection risk (pulmonary, cerebral abscess, infective endocarditis). Rarer complications include pulmonary arterial hypertension/Eisenmenger syndrome, paradoxical embolism (5).
- Surgically repaired: late-onset arrhythmias 10 to 20 years after surgery (5%), perioperative atrial tachyarrhythmias (10–13% of patients, increased risk of arrhythmia-associated embolic events (3)
- Device closure: device embolization (1%), cardiac perforation, thrombus formation, endocarditis, supraventricular arrhythmias, and device erosions

REFERENCES

1. Warnes CA, Williams RG, Bashore TM, et al. ACC/AHA 2008 guidelines for the management of adults with congenital heart disease: a report of the American College of Cardiology/American Heart Association Task Force on Practice Guidelines (writing committee to develop guidelines on the management of adults with congenital heart disease). Developed in collaboration with the American Society of Echocardiography, Heart Rhythm Society, International Society for Adult Congenital Heart Disease, Society for Cardiovascular Angiography and Interventions, and Society of Thoracic Surgeons. *J Am Coll Cardiol.* 2008;52(23):e143–e263.
2. Baglivo M, Dassati S, Krasi G, et al. Atrial septal defects, supravalvular aortic stenosis and syndromes predisposing to aneurysm of large vessels. *Acta Biomed.* 2019;90(10-S):53–57.
3. Oster M, Bhatt AB, Zaragoza-Macias E, et al. Interventional therapy versus medical therapy for secundum atrial septal defect: a systematic review (part 2) for the 2018 AHA/ACC Guideline for the Management of Adults With Congenital Heart Disease: a report of the American College of Cardiology/American Heart Association Task Force on Clinical Practice Guidelines. *J Am Coll Cardiol.* 2019;73(12):1579–1595.
4. Geva T, Martins JD, Wald RM. Atrial septal defects. *Lancet.* 2014;383(9932):1921–1932.
5. Stout KK, Daniels CJ, Aboulhosn JA, et al. 2018 AHA/ACC guideline for the management of adults with congenital heart disease: executive summary. *J Am Coll Cardiol.* 2019;73(12):1494–1563.
6. Scacciatella P, Marra S, Pullara A, et al. Percutaneous closure of atrial septal defect in adults: very long-term clinical outcome and effects on aortic and mitral valve function. *J Invasive Cardiol.* 2015;27(1):65–69.

ADDITIONAL READING

Nishimura RA, Carabello BA, Faxon DP, et al. ACC/AHA 2008 guideline update on valvular heart disease: focused update on infective endocarditis: a report of the American College of Cardiology/American Heart Association Task Force on Practice Guidelines: endorsed by the Society of Cardiovascular Anesthesiologists, Society for Cardiovascular Angiography and Interventions, and Society of Thoracic Surgeons. *Circulation.* 2008;118(8):887–896.

 SEE ALSO

Aortic Valvular Stenosis; Coarctation of the Aorta; Patent Ductus Arteriosus; Pulmonary Valve Stenosis; Tetralogy of Fallot; Ventricular Septal Defect

CODES

ICD10
- Q21.2 Atrioventricular septal defect
- Q21.1 Atrial septal defect
- I23.1 Atrial septal defect as current complication following acute myocardial infarction

CLINICAL PEARLS
- ASD is often missed due to subtle clinical presentation.
- Ideally, hemodynamically significant ASDs should be closed in early childhood, although some benefit from closure is present in older patients.
- Many ASDs can be treated by catheter-directed percutaneous closure rather than open-heart surgery.
- Routine endocarditis prophylaxis is not recommended for unrepaired ASDs.
- Generally, symptomatic and hemodynamically significant ASDs are repaired; management of asymptomatic small ASDs is debated.
- Patent foramina ovalia, unlike large ASDs, are very common and generally require no treatment in asymptomatic individuals.

ATTENTION DEFICIT/HYPERACTIVITY DISORDER, ADULT

Alexis Benavides Reedy-Cooper, MD, MPH

BASICS

- Adult attention deficit hyperactivity disorder (adult ADHD) is a pattern of behaviors that include inattention and/or hyperactivity or impulsivity. It is present in multiple settings that impair social, academic, or work performance.
- Complications of adult ADHD include employment, financial, and interpersonal difficulties as well as increased risk for driving accidents and suicide.
- Adult ADHD typically begins in childhood; 30–60% of patients diagnosed with ADHD as a child will continue to meet criteria as adults.

DESCRIPTION

- Symptoms include difficulty concentrating, impulsivity, and hyperactivity/overactivity. Impairment in executive functioning and emotional dysregulation are common features.
- The three main types of ADHD are (i) hyperactivity-impulsivity predominant, (ii) inattentive predominant, and (iii) combined. The combined type is the most common, followed by the inattentive and hyperactive types.

EPIDEMIOLOGY
Prevalence
ADHD affects approximately 4.4–5.2% of adults between 18 and 44 years of age (1). ADHD is more common in men than women. This could be due to underrecognition in women. Women are less likely to be referred for assessment and more likely to be undiagnosed or misdiagnosed (2).

ETIOLOGY AND PATHOPHYSIOLOGY
Genetics
- ADHD appears to have a genetic component, with heritability of approximately 0.8, suggesting that genetic factors would account for about 65% of phenotypic variance.
- First-degree relatives of persons with ADHD reported to have 4 to 5 times greater risk than general population.

RISK FACTORS
- Studies have shown that the risk of ADHD is increased among offsprings of mothers who smoked or had obesity and diabetes during pregnancy. Risk is also increased in those who had lead exposure in childhood. It is unknown whether these associations are causal (3).
- Premature birth; very low birth weight; and extreme neglect, abuse, or social deprivation also increase the risk as do certain infections during pregnancy, at birth, and in early childhood.
- Other factors associated with increased risk for ADHD include high blood pressure (BP) or maternal stress in pregnancy, obesity and diabetes in pregnancy, seizures or brain injury in childhood, and other neurodevelopmental disorders including autism spectrum disorder and learning disabilities.

COMMONLY ASSOCIATED CONDITIONS
- Substance use and substance abuse disorders
- Mood and anxiety disorders
- Intellectual disabilities
- Obsessive-compulsive disorder (OCD)
- Tic disorders
- Delayed sleep-wake phase disorder

DIAGNOSIS

- Diagnosis is made from patient's history and detailing patient's current level of functioning in at least two different settings (e.g., work and home).
- It is important to gather history of patient's childhood and school performance.

HISTORY
- Commonly reported symptoms of ADHD include poor concentration, disorganization, failure to complete projects, poor performance at work, and difficulty controlling temper
- *DSM-5* criteria include (1):
  - At least five symptoms of inattention or hyperactivity/impulsivity
  - Several symptoms must be present before age 12 (if not diagnosed in childhood, this is established by a historical assessment of childhood symptoms).
  - Symptoms must be present in two or more settings (home, work, etc.).
  - There must be clear evidence that symptoms interfere with or reduce quality of social, academic, or work functioning.
  - Symptoms must be present for more than 6 months.
- History of medication or substances including anticonvulsants, steroids, antihistamines, nicotine, and caffeine that have side effects that impact attentiveness and mimic ADHD symptoms
- History of thyroid disorders, head injury or trauma, liver disease, seizure disorders
- Ask about cardiovascular disease, neurodevelopmental disorders including autism spectrum disorder, tic disorders, learning disabilities.
- Ask about family history of ADHD as well as other psychiatric and neurologic problems.

PHYSICAL EXAM
- Physical exam is key to ruling out other medical conditions.
- Focus on thyroid and neurologic examinations; look for findings suggestive of substance abuse.
- Record BP and baseline weight; monitor if starting medical treatment.

DIFFERENTIAL DIAGNOSIS
Hearing impairment, hyperthyroid/hypothyroid, sleep deprivation, sleep apnea, phenylketonuria, OCD, lead toxicity, substance abuse (4)

DIAGNOSTIC TESTS & INTERPRETATION
- Adult ADHD screening tools:
  - Retrospective scales include the Childhood Symptom Scale and the Wender Utah Rating Scale
  - Current symptom scales include the Adult ADHD Rating Scale IV, Adult ADHD Self-Report Scale Symptom Checklist, and the Conners Adult ADHD Rating Scale (1). These scales can take 5 to 20 minutes to complete.
- Provider/patient screening checklist
  - https://add.org/wp-content/uploads/2015/03/adhd-questionnaire-ASRS111.pdf
  - https://nyulangone.org/files/psych_adhd_screener_0.pdf
- Developments in imaging techniques have revealed structural and functional brain differences between individuals with and without ADHD, but there is no evidence for clinical utility (1).

Initial Tests (lab, imaging)
- Thyroid-stimulating hormone (TSH)
- ECG with concerns for cardiac disease in patient or family history
- Urine toxicology screen to rule out concomitant substance abuse disorder

Follow-Up Tests & Special Considerations
- Liver function test monitoring (with atomoxetine)
- Consider polysomnography in patients with sleep disorder symptoms to rule out sleep apnea
- A history of childhood behaviors is helpful, but adult patients often don't accurately recall childhood symptomology.
- Inquire about family history of ADHD, family and personal substance abuse, and tic disorders to facilitate formulation of an accurate diagnosis and recognition of high-risk behaviors.
- Caution against stimulant use in pregnancy because of high risk of low fetal birth weight and preterm birth. Risks and benefits of treatment must be discussed in detail with patient and preferably with her spouse (5)[B].
- Caution against use of stimulants in adult patients with cardiac history.

ALERT
Mood disorders, generalized anxiety disorders, and substance abuse can also coexist with adult ADHD; treating both the ADHD and comorbid conditions will improve the patient's prognosis.

TREATMENT

- Most of the research and medication trials have been performed in children.
- There is increasing evidence that stimulants and nonstimulants used in children are also effective in adults (4)[A].

ALERT
Because stimulant medication may induce dependency, substance abuse, and diversion, it is recommended to do pill counts, screen urine for drugs, monitor behavior, and query prescription databases. Misuse of amphetamines may cause sudden death and serious cardiovascular adverse events.

GENERAL MEASURES
When substance abuse is not present, stimulants are first-line treatment for ADHD and highly efficacious. There are multiple formulations of stimulants, and patients may require trials of different dosages, formulations, and medications before an optimal response in symptoms and functions is achieved. Nonstimulants are useful when there is abuse potential, comorbid conditions, or poor response to stimulants.

MEDICATION
- Medications should be titrated slowly to effective dose to avoid side effects.
- Stimulants are more effective than antidepressants or nonstimulants, but up to 30% discontinue medications because of side effects.

- Stimulants can be grouped into those related to methylphenidate and those related to amphetamine. Both groups include both short- and long-acting preparations. Recent evidence suggests that adherence and persistence rates improve in those using long-acting agents (1).
- Antidepressants studied for ADHD include bupropion, which has been shown to have a medium effect compared with stimulants (4)[A].

First Line

- Stimulants: methylphenidate (Concerta, Ritalin), dexmethylphenidate (Focalin), dextroamphetamine/amphetamine (Adderall), dextroamphetamine (Dexedrine), lisdexamfetamine (Vyvanse)
  - Methylphenidate preparations are available in short-acting, intermediate-acting, long-acting, and patch formulations.
  - Ritalin LA may be used for patients naive to stimulants. It can be started at 20 mg daily and dose titrated by 10-mg increments weekly to symptoms response; max dose of 60 mg/day
  - Concerta ER is another option in adults up to 65 years of age. Starting dose of 18 mg/day; adjust in increments of 18 mg weekly until symptoms improve. Max dose 72 mg/day; also has an oral osmotic release to decrease abuse potential
  - Dextroamphetamine is commonly used (half-life of 4 to 6 hours) with an initial dose of 5 mg BID; titrate up by 5 mg weekly to maximum of 20 mg BID.
  - Dextroamphetamine/amphetamine (Adderall) is a 75%/25% mix that also comes in an extended-release form. Initial dosing can be started at 5 mg BID for short acting or 20 mg daily for long acting and increased by 5 mg/week for short acting and 10 mg/week long acting to a maximum of 40 to 60 mg total daily.
  - Lisdexamfetamine (Vyvanse) is an extended-release stimulant that is a prodrug requiring metabolization to active component, dextroamphetamine.
  - Common side effects of stimulants include hypertension (HTN), tachycardia, insomnia, weight loss, stomach upset, increased anxiety/irritability, or worsening of tics (4)[A].
- Nonstimulants:
  - Atomoxetine (Strattera) has been shown effective in adults with ADHD when compared to placebo (6)[B]. It may be given as a single dose or split dose and has low abuse potential, making it a better choice over a stimulant medication for patients with substance abuse history. Onset of effect may take up to 4 weeks. Atomoxetine may be particularly useful when anxiety, mood or tics co-occur with ADHD. There are rare cases of liver damage associated with these medications. Monitor for increased suicidal thinking.
  - Antidepressants: best used for those at high risk or with history of substance abuse disorder. Bupropion (Wellbutrin) is effective in adults with ADHD symptoms, especially if they have comorbid depression (5)[A].
  - Tricyclic antidepressants (desipramine and nortriptyline) have also shown to be effective in ADHD (1).
  - α_2-Agonists (guanfacine, clonidine) have been found to be effective in children and adolescents; however, their efficacy, safety, and tolerability have not been studied extensively in adults (7)[C]. These may be used with comorbid tics and/or disruptive behavior disorders.
  - Combining stimulants with a nonstimulant medication such as atomoxetine, guanfacine, or clonidine has shown positive effects among patients who are resistant to stimulants alone.

ISSUES FOR REFERRAL

Patients with comorbid conditions may need referral for diagnosis and treatment. Consider referral to obstetrician experienced in high-risk pregnancies when treating pregnant women with ADHD.

ADDITIONAL THERAPIES

- Cognitive-behavioral therapy (CBT) can be useful in conjunction with medication to help patient modify and cope with symptoms. CBT helps reduce impairments resulting from executive dysfunction (EDF) that is not optimally ameliorated with medication (1).
- Among adults with ADHD and EDFs, addition of memantine as an adjunct to extended-release methylphenidate was associated with improved executive functioning, supporting the need for further research.

COMPLEMENTARY & ALTERNATIVE MEDICINE

- There is mixed evidence that fatty acid supplementation in addition to medication may be beneficial in the treatment of ADHD (8)
- Eliminating artificial food coloration only shows a mild benefit in decreasing ADHD symptoms (9)
- Behavioral therapy
  - Providing rewards can motivate desired behaviors in this population
  - Multiple trials show improved behaviors in parents who learn methods encouraging appropriate behaviors (10).
  - Classroom performance also shows significant improvement in schools emphasizing learning, minimizing punishment, and increasing a positive learning environment (10).

 ONGOING CARE

Transfer from pediatric to adult care must be closely coordinated to avoid hiatus in treatment.

FOLLOW-UP RECOMMENDATIONS

- Close follow-up of medication as dose is titrated and to monitor for side effects.
- Repeat screening checklists to quantify benefit of interventions as needed.
- Reinforce behavioral change (e.g., self-initiated through CBT), which is essential goal of long-term management.

PATIENT EDUCATION

Support groups (e.g., http://www.chadd.org and http://www.add.org) assist the newly diagnosed adult by providing education, treatment options, available resources, and peer support.

REFERENCES

1. Young JL, Goodman DW. Adult attention-deficit/hyperactivity disorder diagnosis, management, and treatment in the DSM-5 era. *Prim Care Companion CNS Disord*. 2016;18(6). doi:10.4088/PCC.
2. National Institute for Health and Care Excellence. *NICE Guideline, No. 87. Attention Deficit Hyperactivity Disorder: Diagnosis and Management*. London, United Kingdom: National Institute of Health and Care Excellence; 2018.
3. Volkow ND, Swanson JM. Clinical practice: adult attention deficit–hyperactivity disorder. *N Engl J Med*. 2013;369(20):1935–1944.
4. Castells X, Ramos-Quiroga JA, Bosch R, et al. Amphetamines for attention deficit hyperactivity disorder (ADHD) in adults. *Cochrane Database Syst Rev*. 2011;(6):CD007813.
5. Verbeeck W, Tuinier S, Bekkering GE. Antidepressants in the treatment of adult attention-deficit hyperactivity disorder: a systematic review. *Adv Ther*. 2009;26(2):170–184.
6. Asherson P, Bushe C, Saylor K, et al. Efficacy of atomoxetine in adults with attention deficit hyperactivity disorder: an integrated analysis of the complete database of multicenter placebo-controlled trials. *J Psychopharmacol*. 2014;28(9):837–846.
7. Hirota T, Schwartz S, Correll CU. Alpha-2 agonists for attention-deficit/hyperactivity disorder in youth: a systematic review and meta-analysis of monotherapy and add-on trials to stimulant therapy. *J Am Acad Child Adolesc Psychiatry*. 2014;53(2):153–173.
8. Millichap JG, Yee MM. The diet factor in attention–deficit/hyperactivity disorder. *Pediatrics*. 2012;129(2):330–337.
9. Sonuga-Barke EJS, Brandeis D, Cortese S, et al. Nonpharmacological interventions for ADHD: systematic review and meta-analyses of randomized controlled trials of dietary and psychological treatments. *Am J Psychiatry*. 2013;170(3):275–289.
10. Feldman HM, Reiff MI. Attention deficit-hyperactivity disorder in children and adolescents. *N Eng J Med*. 2014;370(9):838–846.

ADDITIONAL READING

American Psychiatric Association. *Diagnostic and Statistical Manual of Mental Disorders*. 5th ed. Arlington, VA: American Psychiatric Association; 2013.

CODES

ICD10

- F90.9 Attention-deficit hyperactivity disorder, unspecified type
- F90.1 Attn-defct hyperactivity disorder, predom hyperactive type
- F90.0 Attn-defct hyperactivity disorder, predom inattentive type

CLINICAL PEARLS

- Adult ADHD results in inattention, easy distractibility, hyperactivity, and impulsive behavior; it is associated with low self-esteem, problematic interpersonal relationships, and difficulty meeting academic and job expectations.
- Psychotropic medications plus cognitive behavioral treatments are the cornerstone of management.
- Substance abuse is a common comorbidity; recommend use of nonstimulant medication in those at high risk.

ATTENTION DEFICIT/HYPERACTIVITY DISORDER, PEDIATRIC

Katherine Williams, MD

 BASICS

DESCRIPTION

- Attention deficit hyperactivity disorder (ADHD) is a neurodevelopmental disorder that manifests in early childhood characterized by distractibility, impulsivity, hyperactivity, and/or inattention.
- Three subsets: predominantly hyperactivity (ADHD-H), predominantly inattentive (ADHD-I), or combined (ADHD-C)
- System(s) affected: nervous
- Synonym(s): attention deficit disorder; hyperactivity

EPIDEMIOLOGY

- Predominant age: onset <12 years; lasts into adolescence and adulthood
- Predominant sex: male > female (2:1); ADHD-I is more common in girls.

Prevalence
9–15% of children 4 to 17 years

ETIOLOGY AND PATHOPHYSIOLOGY
Not definitive—suggested pathogenesis includes imbalance of catecholamine metabolism and structural brain differences. Environmental influences are controversial.

Genetics
Familial pattern

RISK FACTORS

- Family history
- Medical causes (affecting brain development)—including prenatal tobacco exposure and prematurity

COMMONLY ASSOCIATED CONDITIONS

- Mood disorders—depression, anxiety
- Behavior disorders—oppositional defiant disorder, conduct disorder
- Austism spectrum disorder
- Physiologic disorders—sleep disorders, tics
- Learning disabilities, developmental coordination syndrome, language disorder
- Substance use disorders

DIAGNOSIS

- American Academy of Pediatrics (AAP) guidelines recommend *DSM-5* criteria to establish diagnosis (1)[C].
- *DSM-5* criteria for children <17 years: ≥6 inattention criteria and/or ≥6 hyperactivity/impulsivity criteria. Symptoms must occur often, be present before age of 12 years, for >6 months, be noticed in ≥2 settings (e.g., home, school), reduced quality of social or scholastic functioning, be excessive for development level of child, and are not better explained by or occur with another mental disorder (e.g., depression, anxiety, or personality disorder) (2)[C].
- Inattention
  - Careless mistakes in tasks; difficulty sustaining attention or in organizing
  - Does not seem to listen
  - Does not follow through or finish tasks
  - Avoids tasks that require sustained mental effort
  - Loses things
  - Forgetful in daily activities
  - Distracted by external stimuli
  - Forgetful

- Hyperactivity/impulsivity
  - Fidgets
  - Difficulty remaining seated
  - Runs/climbs excessively or inappropriately; difficulty playing quietly
  - Acts as if "driven by a motor" or seeming to always be "on the go"
  - Talks excessively
  - Blurts out answers before question is complete
  - Has difficulty waiting turn
  - Interrupts others
- Children undergoing extreme stress (divorce, illness, homelessness, abuse) may demonstrate ADHD behaviors secondary to stress (1)[C]. This can be assessed using the American Academy of Child and Adolescent Psychiatry (AACAP) screening tool.
- If diagnostic behaviors are noted in only one setting, explore the stressors in that setting.
- The diagnostic behaviors are more noticeable in tasks that require concentration or boredom tolerance.

HISTORY

- Birth and development history
- Psychosocial evaluation of home environment
- School performance and school absences
- Psychiatric history or history of comorbid disorder(s)
- Cardiac history

PHYSICAL EXAM

- Baseline weight, heart rate, blood pressure for future monitoring
- Note any soft neurologic signs, such as tics, clumsiness, mixed handedness.
- Assess hearing and vision.

DIFFERENTIAL DIAGNOSIS

- Activity level appropriate for age
- Dysfunctional family situation or abuse
- Learning disability (e.g., dyslexia)
- Hearing/vision/language disorder
- Autism spectrum disorders
- Oppositional/defiant disorder or conduct disorder
- Seizure disorder
- Neurodevelopmental syndromes (e.g., fragile X)
- Lead poisoning
- Sequelae of central nervous system infection/trauma
- Medication effect
- Any of the comorbid conditions that could mimic primary ADHD (learning disorders, mood disorders, etc.)

DIAGNOSTIC TESTS & INTERPRETATION

- Behavior rating scales completed by parents, caregivers, and teachers prior to initiation of therapy and then repeated after therapy
- National Institute for Children's Health Quality. Caring for Children with ADHD: A Resource Toolkit for Clinicians. https://www.nichq.org/resource/caring-children-adhd-resource-toolkit-clinicians.
- Testing for learning disability through the school

Initial Tests (lab, imaging)
Rarely needed; consider lead

Diagnostic Procedures/Other
ECG prior to stating stimulant medication if positive family history of premature CV disease

 TREATMENT

GENERAL MEASURES

- Identify treatment goals based on behaviors which are most harmful to the child's development.
- Coordinate school and home behavioral plan.
- Children age 4 to 5 should begin with behavioral interventions (2)[C].
- Age 6 to 17 begin with behavioral interventions (2)[C] and consider medication if behavioral goals are not being met over time.
- Behavioral counseling can be beneficial for both parents and child, including parent training, academic training, and social training.
- Behavioral modifications should involve repeated positive reinforcement with limiting negative comments, reward systems (i.e., star charts for younger children, privileges for older children), environmental changes at both home and school (time out, quiet time), token economy (reward for positive, loss of reward for negative behavior).

MEDICATION

- Stimulant medications are often considered first line as they have highest efficacy but also carry greater risks.
- Atomoxetine may be used first line, especially if there is risk of diversion in the home, growth concerns (poor weight gain, sleep issues, etc.), or if parents wish to try nonstimulant medication.
- Stimulant choice should be based on cost, formulary, convenience, and duration. A second type of stimulant should be tried if the first treatment fails (2)[C].
- All stimulant capsules can be opened and sprinkled (Note: Concerta is a pill).

First Line
Stimulant:

- Methylphenidate
  - Short acting
    - Ritalin, Methylin
    - Effects seen within 30 minutes; duration 3 to 5 hours
  - Intermediate acting
    - Metadate ER: onset within 20 to 60 minutes and lasts for 8 hours
  - Long acting
    - Methylphenidate CD: 30% immediate release and 70% delayed release for duration over 8 to 12 hours (bimodal)
    - Cotempla XR-ODT: 25% immediate release and 75% extended release for duration up to 12 hours
    - Quillivant XR: 20% immediate release and 80% extended release with duration up to 12 hours
    - Quillichew ER: continuous release over 6 to 8 hours with duration up to 13 hours
    - Ritalin LA: 50% immediate release and 50% delayed release over 8 to 12 hours
    - Concerta: 20% immediate release and 80% continuous release for duration over 10 to 12 hours
    - Aptensio XR: 40% immediate release and 60% controlled release for duration of 12 hours
    - Adhansia XR: 20% immediate release and 80% controlled release for duration of 16 hours
    - Jornay PM: Nighttime dosing where <5% of drug available within the first 10 hours of administration with a peak concentration at 14 hours and steady decline after
    - Daytrana transdermal patch: onset 2 hours after application with duration of 9 to 12 hours

- Dexmethylphenidate
  - Focalin: duration 5 to 6 hours
  - Focalin XR: 50% immediate release and 50% delayed release over 10 to 12 hours
- Serdexmethylphenidate-dexmethylphenidate
  - Azstarys: 70% prodrug delayed and 30% immediate release drug; onset within 1 hour and duration of 13 hours
- Amphetamine
  - Immediate release
    - Evekeo/Evekeo ODT: onset within 20 to 60 minutes with duration 4 to 6 hours
  - Extended release
    - Dyanavel XR: combination of immediate and extended release for duration of 13 hours
    - Adzenys ER/ODT: combination of 50% immediate release and 50% extended release; duration over 10 to 12 hours
- Dextroamphetamine
  - Immediate release
    - Dexedrine, ProCentra: onset within 20 to 60 minutes for duration of 4 to 6 hours
  - Extended release
    - Dextroamphetamine SR: combination of immediate release and continuous release for duration over 8 to 12 hours
- Dextroamphetamine/amphetamine mixed salts
  - Short acting
    - Adderall: onset within 20 to 60 minutes with duration of 4 to 6 hours
  - Long acting
    - Adderall XR: combination of immediate and continuous release for duration of 10 to 12 hours
    - Mydayis: combination of immediate and 2 different delayed-release beads for duration up to 16 hours
- Lisdexamfetamine
  - Vyvanse: prodrug converted to dextroamphetamine with effect over 10 hours
- Precautions:
  - If not responding, check compliance and consider another diagnosis.
  - Some children experience withdrawal (tearfulness, agitation) after a missed dose or when medication wears off. A small, short-acting dose at 4 PM may help to prevent this.
  - Stimulants are drugs of abuse and should be monitored carefully.
  - Drug holidays are not recommended but may be tried in weight loss or ADHD-I.
- Common adverse effects:
  - Anorexia, insomnia, growth delay, GI effects, CV effects, and headache
  - Rare: priapism, psychosis, tics, suicidal thinking
- Significant possible interactions: may increase levels of anticonvulsants, SSRIs, tricyclics, and warfarin
- High-caffeine energy drinks, albuterol inhalers, and decongestants may increase side effects.
- The FDA reports permanent skin discoloration with Daytrana patches.

Pregnancy Considerations
Medications are Category C: caution in pregnancy.

Second Line
Nonstimulant:
- SNRI
  - Atomoxetine (Strattera): Effects last at least 10 to 12 hours but must be taken daily without drug holidays.
  - Viloxazine (Qelbree): lasts throughout the day, must be taken daily without drug holidays

- α_2-Agonist
  - Modest efficacy, high side effects. Consider consultation before use.
    - Clonidine XR (Kapvay): duration at least 10 to 12 hours
    - Guanfacine XR (Intuniv): duration at least 10 to 12 hours

ALERT
- SNRIs carry a "black box" warning regarding potential exacerbation of suicidality (similar to SSRIs). Close follow-up is recommended.
- Side effects similar to stimulants including CV/GI effects, and the rare side effects of tics and priapism
- Associated with hepatic injury in a small number of cases; check liver enzymes if symptoms develop.

ISSUES FOR REFERRAL
Refer for children if there are additional mental health issues developmental issues, or poor response to treatment.

COMPLEMENTARY & ALTERNATIVE MEDICINE
Surveys have shown that parents of children with ADHD use herbals and complementary treatments frequently (20–60%) but very limited evidence to support any intervention.

 ONGOING CARE

FOLLOW-UP RECOMMENDATIONS
Patient Monitoring
- Office visits to monitor side effects and efficacy: End points are improved grades, rating scales, family interactions, and peer interactions.
- Monitor growth (especially weight), HR, and BP.

DIET
- There is "insufficient evidence to suggest that dietary interventions reduce the symptoms of ADHD" (2)[C].
- The AAP recommends that a trial of a preservative-free food coloring–free diet is a reasonable intervention.

PATIENT EDUCATION
- Excellent reference: http://www.parentsmedguide.org
- Teacher's reference: ADDitude toolkit for parents and teachers
- CHADD's National Resource Center for teachers
- Key points for parents:
  - Find things the child is good at and emphasize these; reinforce good behavior; give one task at a time; stop behavior with quiet discipline; coordinate homework with teachers; and have external organization tools—charts, schedules, token systems.
  - Develop an individualized education plan (IEP) with the school.
- Support groups:
  - Children and Adults with Attention Deficit Disorder (CHADD): http://www.chadd.org
  - Attention Deficit Disorder WareHouse: http://www.addwarehouse.com
  - Center for Parent Information and Resources (CPIR): https://www.parentcenterhub.org

PROGNOSIS
- May last into adulthood; plan for a transition at age 17 years.
- Relative deficits in academic and social functioning may persist into late adolescence/adulthood.
- Encourage career choices that allow autonomy and mobility.

COMPLICATIONS
- Untreated ADHD can lead to failing in school, parental abuse, social isolation, and poor self-esteem.
- Possible withdrawal when medication wears off
- Decreased rate of growth
- Increased risk of substance abuse, which may decrease with treatment of ADHD
- Increased incidence of automobile accidents and injuries, which decreases with medication

REFERENCES
1. American Psychiatric Association. *Diagnostic and Statistical Manual of Mental Disorders*. 5th ed. Arlington, VA: American Psychiatric Association; 2013.
2. Wolraich M, Brown L, Brown RT, et al; for Subcommittee on Attention-Deficit/Hyperactivity Disorder, Steering Committee on Quality Improvement and Management. ADHD: clinical practice guideline for the diagnosis, evaluation, and treatment of attention-deficit/hyperactivity disorder in children and adolescents. *Pediatrics*. 2011;128(5):1007–1022.

ADDITIONAL READING
- Felt BT, Biermann B, Christner JG, et al. Diagnosis and management of ADHD in children. *Am Fam Physician*. 2014;90(7):456–464.
- Laforett DR, Murray DW, Kollins SH. Psychosocial treatments for preschool-aged children with attention-deficit hyperactivity disorder. *Dev Disabil Res Rev*. 2008;14(4):300–310.
- National Institute for Children's Health Quality. Caring for children with ADHD: a resource toolkit for clinicians. https://www.nichq.org/resource/caring-children-adhd-resource-toolkit-clinicians. Published 2002. Accessed September 8, 2019.
- See "Patient Education."

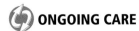 CODES

ICD10
- F90.2 Attention-deficit hyperactivity disorder, combined type
- F90.0 Attention-deficit hyperactivity disorder, predominantly inattentive type
- F90 Attention-deficit hyperactivity disorders

CLINICAL PEARLS
- Identify treatment goals before initiating any intervention and make treatment plan based on these goals.
- Behavioral therapy for child and parents and coordination with teachers and behavioral specialists in schools are critical for both short- and long-term success.
- Due to heavy genetic component, parents may also have ADHD and may have difficulty helping the child with organization.
- AAP recommends behavioral interventions for age 4 to 5 years and behavioral interventions plus stimulant medications as first-line treatment for age 6 to 17 years.
- Multiple medications—stimulants first line; titrate to patient response with close monitoring of response and side effects

ATYPICAL MOLE (DYSPLASTIC NEVUS) SYNDROME

Sahil Mullick, MD • Stefany J. K. Malanka, MD

BASICS

Atypical mole syndrome (AMS), also known as dysplastic nevi syndrome (DNS), B-K mole syndrome, Clark nevi syndrome, or familial atypical multiple mole melanoma (FAMMM) syndrome, is a condition characterized by a large number of pigmented nevi with architectural disorder, which arise sporadically or by inheritance and are associated with an increased risk of melanoma.

DESCRIPTION
There is no consensus on criteria for AMS.
- Elevated total body nevi count, including clinically atypical nevi, is usually >50 and often >100.
  - Larger number in hereditary AMS versus sporadic atypical nevi (as few as <10)
- Increased risk of melanoma
  - Up to 90% occurrence by age 80 years in certain high-risk individuals
  - Earlier onset than in sporadic melanoma
  - More arise de novo than from an existing nevus
  - Higher risk for appearance at unusual sites (e.g., scalp, eyes, and sun-protected areas)
- Median age of diagnosis for melanoma in AMS is 10 to 20 years earlier than the general population, with documented cases of melanoma as early as in the 2nd and 3rd decades of life.

EPIDEMIOLOGY
Incidence
Uncertain due to phenotype variability, limited data

Prevalence
Affects between 2% and 8% of fair-skinned adults as well as those with high exposure to ultraviolet radiation

ETIOLOGY AND PATHOPHYSIOLOGY
- Cyclin-dependent kinase inhibitor 2A (CDKN2A) mutations have been observed in familial DNS and multiple melanomas. The CDKN2A gene on 9p21 encodes for the proteins p16 and p14. p16 binds to CDK4/6 and is a negative cell-cycle regulator via inhibition of the CDK-cyclin D interaction needed for cell cycle progression from G1 to S. p14 functions by stabilizing the tumor-suppressor protein p53 in the G1 phase of the cell cycle.
- Familial cases of germline CDKN2A mutations are transmitted in an autosomal dominant fashion.
- No clear somatic mutation patterns in sporadic cases

Genetics
CDKN2A gene mutation is observed in 25–40% of hereditary cases, with autosomal dominant inheritance but variable expressivity and incomplete penetrance.

RISK FACTORS
Family history of melanoma or multiple nevi, sun exposure, neonatal blue-light phototherapy, history of painful sunburns

GENERAL PREVENTION
- Primary prevention with sun avoidance, sun protection
- Secondary prevention of melanoma with routine skin exams, biopsy of suspect lesions, and environmental risk mitigation as above

COMMONLY ASSOCIATED CONDITIONS
- Malignant melanoma, including ocular melanoma
- Ocular nevi
- Pancreatic cancer in CDKN2A mutation

DIAGNOSIS

AMS is a clinical diagnosis with various classification schemes proposed. Although not widely accepted, diagnostic criteria, as defined by the NIH, require the three features of (i) malignant melanoma in ≥1 first- or second-degree relatives; (ii) numerous melanocytic nevi (frequently >50), some of which are clinically atypical; and (iii) nevi that have certain histologic features (1).

HISTORY
- Changing lesions: bleeding, scaling, size, texture, nonhealing, hyper- or hypopigmentation
- Large number of nevi
- Congenital nevi
- Sun exposure
- Prior skin biopsies
- Prior melanoma
- Immunosuppression (e.g., AIDS, chemotherapy, pancreatic cancer)
- First- or second-degree relatives with:
  - AMS
  - Melanoma
  - Pancreatic cancer

PHYSICAL EXAM
- Full-body skin exams, with photography to track new and changing nevi
- Goal to distinguish melanoma from atypical mole (AM)
- ABCDE mnemonic for skin lesions concerning for melanoma: Asymmetry, Border irregularity, Color variegation, Diameter >6 mm, and Evolving lesion
  - AM is often defined as ≥5 mm and at least two other features.
  - Melanoma typically has several characteristics of ABCDEs, with increased specificity for melanoma if lesion diameter is >6 mm.
- "Ugly duckling sign" (2)[B]:
  - Melanoma screening strategy for increasing accuracy of diagnosis of melanoma by identifying malignant nevi straying from the predominant nevus pattern when numerous atypical nevi are present
- Most common features of AM on dermoscopy include (3)[C]:
  - Reticular pattern most common
  - Uniform pigmentation most common followed by multifocal hypo/hyperpigmentation
  - Homogenous brown globules
  - Pigmentation with central heterogeneity and abrupt termination
- Dermatoscopic features more suggestive of melanoma include (4)[C]:
  - Depigmented areas
  - Whitish veil
  - Homogenous areas distributed irregularly, in multiple areas, or >25% of total lesion
  - ≥4 colors

DIFFERENTIAL DIAGNOSIS
- Common nevus: acquired or congenital
- Melanoma
- Seborrheic keratosis
- Dermatofibroma
- Lentigo
- Pigmented actinic keratosis
- Pigmented basal cell carcinoma
- Blue rubber bleb nevus syndrome

DIAGNOSTIC TESTS & INTERPRETATION
Diagnosis is first suspected with history and physical exam and then confirmed by biopsy and histopathology.

Initial Tests (lab, imaging)
- Dermoscopy can be used for a more detailed exam of nevus to aid in distinguishing between benign and malignant lesions as well as for further classification to any of the 11 subtypes; however, the degree of success is dependent on the skill of the examiner.
- Reflectance confocal microscopy (RCM) may provide more specificity than dermoscopy in distinguishing AM from melanoma.
- When the total nevus count is high and following each nevus is impractical, total body photography may aid in the evaluation of evolving nevi as well as documenting new nevi.

Follow-Up Tests & Special Considerations
Genetic testing is available for CDKN2A mutations, but it is not recommended outside of research studies because results cannot be adequately used for management or surveillance.

Diagnostic Procedures/Other
- Biopsy is recommended for any lesion where melanoma cannot be excluded.
- Biopsy entails full-thickness biopsy of the entire lesion with a narrow 1- to 3-mm margin of normal skin down to fat for adequate depth assessment (5)[C].
  - Excisional biopsy, elliptical or punch excision, provides the most accurate diagnosis and should be performed when possible.
  - Scoop shave biopsy can also be used, but care must be taken to not transect the lesion.
- Reexcision of mild to moderately dysplastic nevi with positive margins may not change pathologic diagnosis or outcomes (studies inconclusive) (6)[A], but for severely dysplastic nevi, consider reexcision, with surgical margins of 2 to 5 mm (7)[C].

Test Interpretation
"Dysplastic nevus" is a term more accurately reserved as a histologic diagnosis. Features may include melanocyte proliferation in the dermoepidermal junction extending through at least three rete ridges in a specific pattern, fusing of rete ridges, dermal fibrosis, neovascularization, and interstitial lymphocytic inflammation (7)[C].

TREATMENT

MEDICATION
No medications have been shown to treat AMS (7)[C].

ISSUES FOR REFERRAL
- Dermatologist for routine skin exam for those patients at high risk for melanoma
- Ophthalmologic exams for ocular nevi/melanoma screening/papilledema
- Oncology or specialized genetics study group involvement if strong family predisposition to pancreatic cancer

ADDITIONAL THERAPIES
- Topical chemo- and immunotherapies have been unsuccessfully attempted to treat AMs (7)[C].
- Laser treatment should be avoided because it is both unsafe and ineffective for melanocytic nevi (7)[C].

SURGERY/OTHER PROCEDURES
Surgical excision of all atypical nevi is not recommended because most melanomas in AMS appear de novo on healthy skin and therefore has low clinical value and is not cost-effective. Excision of all atypical nevi also leads to both poor cosmetic outcomes and a false sense of security. Lesions suspicious for melanoma should be biopsied or removed surgically.

 ONGOING CARE

FOLLOW-UP RECOMMENDATIONS
Close follow-up with a dermatologist or other physician experienced with assessment of atypical nevi:
- Total body skin exam (including nails, scalp, genital area, and oral mucosa) every 6 months initially, starting at puberty; may be reduced to annually once nevi are stable
- Total body photography at baseline and intervals to track new and changing nevi
- Dermoscopic evaluation of suspicious lesions
- Excision of suspicious lesions
- Ocular exam for those with familial AMS

Patient Monitoring
Monthly self-exams of skin

PATIENT EDUCATION
For young adults with fair skin, counsel to minimize exposure to ultraviolet radiation to reduce risk of skin cancer (USPSTF grade B).
- Fair skin: light eye, hair, or skin color, freckles
- Educate on sun avoidance, proper application of sunscreen, use of protective clothing (e.g., hats), avoidance of tanning booths and sunburns.
- Teach "ABCDE" mnemonic + "ugly duckling sign" to assess nevi and identify potential melanomas.
- Provide instruction on skin self-exam techniques.
- A sample listing of patient-centric review sources on this topic are as follows:
  - American Academy of Dermatology (https://www.verywellhealth.com/the-abcdes-of-skin-cancer-514388)
  - Skin Cancer Foundation (https://www.skincancer.org/risk-factors/atypical-moles/)
  - Melanoma Research Foundation (https://melanoma.org/melanoma-education/what-melanoma-looks-like/)

PROGNOSIS
- Most AM either regress or do not change.
- Multiple classification schemes have been developed over the years to delineate risk of melanoma in patients with AMS. Individuals with a family history of melanoma are at greatest risk. The Rigel classification system can be applied in the clinical setting. Points are assigned based on incidence of melanoma, with 1 point given for a personal history with melanoma and 2 points for each family member with melanoma (modified nuclear family consisting of first-degree relatives plus grandparents and uncles/aunts) and stratified as follows:
  - Score = 0, Rigel group 0, 6% 25-year accumulated risk for melanoma
  - Score = 1, Rigel group 1, 10% risk
  - Score = 2, Rigel group 2, 15% risk
  - Score ≥3, Rigel group 3, 50% risk
- The *CDKN2A* mutation has also been associated with a 60–90% risk of melanoma by age 80 years and a 17% risk for pancreatic cancer by age 75 years.

COMPLICATIONS
- Malignant melanoma
- Poor cosmetic outcomes from biopsy

REFERENCES
1. Goldsmith LA, Askin FB, Chang AE, et al. Diagnosis and treatment of early melanoma: NIH consensus development panel on early melanoma. *JAMA.* 1992;268(10):1314–1319.
2. Gaudy-Marqueste C, Wazaefi Y, Bruneu Y, et al. Ugly duckling sign as a major factor of efficiency in melanoma detection. *JAMA Dermatol.* 2017;153(4):279–284.
3. Hofmann-Wellenhof R, Blum A, Wolf IH, et al. Dermoscopic classification of atypical melanocytic nevi (Clark nevi). *Arch Dermatol.* 2001;137(12):1575–1580.
4. Salopek TG, Kopf AW, Stefanato CM, et al. Differentiation of atypical moles (dysplastic nevi) from early melanomas by dermoscopy. *Dermatol Clin.* 2001;19(2):337–345.
5. Strazzula L, Vedak P, Hoang MP, et al. The utility of re-excising mildly and moderately dysplastic nevi: a retrospective analysis. *J Am Acad Dermatol.* 2014;71(6):1071–1076.
6. Vuong KT, Walker J, Powell HB, et al. Surgical re-excision vs. observation for histologically dysplastic naevi: a systematic review of associated clinical outcomes. *Br J Dermatol.* 2018;179(3):590–598.
7. Duffy K, Grossman D. The dysplastic nevus: from historical perspective to management in the modern era: part I. Historical, histologic, and clinical aspects. *J Am Acad Dermatol.* 2012;67(1):1.e1–1.e18.

ADDITIONAL READING
- Czajkowski R, Placek W, Drewa G, et al. FAMMM syndrome: pathogenesis and management. *Dermatol Surg.* 2004;30(2, Pt 2):291–296.
- Duffy K, Grossman D. The dysplastic nevus: from historical perspective to management in the modern era: part II. Molecular aspects and clinical management. *J Am Acad Dermatol.* 2012;67(1):19.e1–19.e12, quiz 31–32.

- Farber MJ, Heilman ER, Friedman RJ. Dysplastic nevi. *Dermatol Clin.* 2012;30(3):389–404.
- Friedman RJ, Farber MJ, Warycha MA, et al. The "dysplastic" nevus. *Clin Dermatol.* 2009;27(1):103–115.
- Goldstein AM, Tucker MA. Dysplastic nevi and melanoma. *Cancer Epidemiol Biomarkers Prev.* 2013;22(4):528–532. doi:10.1158/1055-9965.EPI-12-134.
- Matichard E, Le Hénanff A, Sanders A, et al. Effect of neonatal phototherapy on melanocytic nevus count in children. *Arch Dermatol.* 2006;142(12):1599–1604.
- Moloney FJ, Guitera P, Coates E, et al. Detection of primary melanoma in individuals at extreme high risk: a prospective 5-year follow-up study. *JAMA Dermatol.* 2014;150(8):819–827.
- Naeyaert JM, Brochez L. Clinical practice. Dysplastic nevi. *N Engl J Med.* 2003;349(23):2233–2240.
- Newton JA, Bataille V, Griffiths K, et al. How common is the atypical mole syndrome phenotype in apparently sporadic melanoma? *J Am Acad Dermatol.* 1993;29(6):989–996.
- Perkins A, Duffy RL. Atypical moles: diagnosis and management. *Am Fam Physician.* 2015;91(11):762–767.
- Robson ME, Storm CD, Weitzel J, et al. American Society of Clinical Oncology policy statement update: genetic and genomic testing for cancer susceptibility. *J Clin Oncol.* 2010;28(5):893–901.
- Silva JH, Sá BC, Avila AL, et al. Atypical mole syndrome and dysplastic nevi: identification of populations at risk for developing melanoma—review article. *Clinics (Sao Paulo).* 2011;66(3):493–499.

 CODES

ICD10
- D22.9 Melanocytic nevi, unspecified
- D22.4 Melanocytic nevi of scalp and neck
- D22.30 Melanocytic nevi of unspecified part of face

CLINICAL PEARLS
- In describing nevi, "atypical" is a clinical term, whereas "dysplastic" is a histologic term.
- AMS is a risk factor for melanoma while most atypical moles/dysplastic nevi are not precursors of melanoma. Melanoma in AMS tends to arise from healthy skin despite a large number of atypical nevi.
- ~20% of individuals with familial AMS will develop pancreatic cancer by age 75 years.
- Patients with AMS tend to produce neoplasms in unusual sites such as the scalp, eyes, and sun-protected areas (e.g., gluteal folds).

AUTISM SPECTRUM DISORDERS

Afsha Rais Kaisani, MD • Rogerio Montes, MD • Niyomi De Silva, MD

 BASICS

DESCRIPTION

- Group of neurodevelopmental disorders of early childhood characterized by (i) persistent deficits in social communication and interaction and (ii) restricted, repetitive patterns of behavior, interests, or activities
- *Diagnostic and Statistical Manual of Mental Disorders*, 5th edition: umbrella term autism spectrum disorder (ASD), which encompasses a group of pervasive developmental disorders with designations for varying severities and associated symptoms
- ASD combines former diagnoses, including autistic disorder, childhood disintegrative disorder, Asperger disorder, pervasive developmental disorder not otherwise specified (PDD-NOS), early infantile autism, childhood autism, Kanner autism, high-functioning autism, and atypical autism, many of which are still used by ICD-10 coding.
- Although symptoms must be present in early development period, they may not be apparent until social demands exceed capacity.
- Symptoms must cause functional impairment. Severity levels:
  – Level 1: requiring support
  – Level 2: requiring substantial support
  – Level 3: requiring very substantial support
- Specifiers for associated symptoms include with catatonia; intellectual impairment; language impairment; known medical or genetic condition; and neurodevelopmental, mental, or behavioral disorders.
- Important to distinguish ASD from symptoms that could be better explained by intellectual disability or global developmental delay

EPIDEMIOLOGY
Predominant age: onset in early childhood; predominant sex: male > female (4:1)

Pediatric Considerations
Symptom onset can often be seen in children <3 years of age but may not become apparent until social demands exceed capacity.

Incidence
Estimated 1 in every 110 children in the United States diagnosed per year

Prevalence
- According to the Centers for Disease Control and Prevention (CDC) in 2016, an estimated prevalence of 1 in every 54 children between the ages of 3 and 17 years carried a diagnosis of ASD.
- This has been a steady increase since 2000 when the CDC reported the prevalence to be 1 in 150, likely due to changes in definition and increased awareness.
- In 2016, there was no difference in prevalence of non-Hispanic white children diagnosed with ASD compared to non-Hispanic black children. However, the number of Hispanics diagnosed with ASD is lower.

ETIOLOGY AND PATHOPHYSIOLOGY
- No single cause has been identified.
- General consensus: A genetic abnormality leads to altered neurologic development.
- Epidemiologic evidence does not support association between immunizations and ASD.

Genetics
- Genetic concordance: A 2009 Swedish population-based cohort study of 2 million subjects showed a cumulative risk of 59% for monozygotic twins.
- The American College of Medical Genetics and Genomics practice guidelines list the risk of siblings of children diagnosed with ASD without an identifiable cause to be:
  – 7% if the affected child is female
  – 4% if the affected child is male
  – >30% if there are two or more affected children

RISK FACTORS
- Male sex, advanced paternal age, family history, very low birth weight
- Perinatal insults including toxic exposures, teratogens, prenatal infections, use of selective serotonin reuptake inhibitors (SSRI) or valproate during pregnancy

GENERAL PREVENTION
- Screening for early intervention is associated with improved prognosis, yet the median age of diagnosis in the United States is >4 years.
- Routine screening for ASD with a validated tool is recommended at 18- and 24-month well-child visits to assist with early detection.
- Screening is indicated after 24 months if parents or clinician have concerns about ASD as less severe presentations may pass earlier routine screening.
- Children with false positives for ASD frequently have some form of developmental disorder which also benefits from early intervention.
- Screening can be difficult due to variability of signs and symptoms of ASD along with the lack of unanimous consensus of social developmental milestones, thus leading to delayed diagnosis.

COMMONLY ASSOCIATED CONDITIONS
- Intellectual disability (seizure in severe cases)
- Attention deficit hyperactivity disorder (ADHD), anxiety, depression, or obsessive behavior
- Motor impairments including hypotonia, apraxia, toe walking, or gross motor delays
- Phenylketonuria (PKU), tuberous sclerosis, fragile X syndrome, Angelman syndrome, Rett syndrome, CHARGE syndrome, Joubert syndrome, Smith-Lemli-Opitz syndrome, Timothy syndrome, and fetal alcohol syndrome (rare)
- Sleep issues: insomnia, circadian rhythm sleep–wake disorder, sleep-related movement disorder
- Change in bowel habits, abdominal pain

 DIAGNOSIS

HISTORY
- Listen to parents' concerns and test early for suspicion of a neurodevelopmental disorder.
- Impairment in social-emotional reciprocity:
  – Failure of normal back-and-forth conversations; reduced sharing of interests, emotions, or affect; failure to initiate or respond to social interaction
- Deficits in nonverbal communication:
  – Abnormal eye contact or body language; deficits in understanding and use of gestures; lack of facial expression and nonverbal communication

- Deficits in developing, maintaining, and understanding relationships:
  – Difficulties adjusting behavior to suit various social contexts
  – Difficulties in sharing imaginative play or in making friends
  – Absence of interest and developing peer relationships
- Repetitive and stereotyped behavior patterns
  – Stereotyped or repetitive motor movements, use of objects, or speech
  – Insistence on sameness, inflexible adherence to routines, or ritualized patterns of behavior with intolerance to change
  – Highly restricted, fixated interests that are abnormal in intensity or focus
  – Hyper- or hyporeactivity to sensory input or unusual interest in sensory aspects of the environment
- Prenatal, neonatal, and developmental history; seizure disorder
- Family history of autism, genetic disorders, learning disabilities, psychiatric illness, or neurologic disorders

PHYSICAL EXAM
- Measurement of growth parameters including height, weight, and head circumference, as macrocephaly is present in 25% of ASD
- Vision, hearing, speech/language, and communication assessments
- Developmental and sensorimotor testing
- Complete neurologic exam
- Examination for dysmorphic features consistent with genetic disorders
- Wood lamp skin exam to rule out skin manifestations of neurocutaneous disorders

DIFFERENTIAL DIAGNOSIS
- Behavioral disorder: anxiety, obsessive-compulsive, reactive attachment
- Development disorders: elective mutism, Rett syndrome, language disorder, hearing impairment, intellectual disability/global developmental delay, social communication disorder
- Others: fetal alcohol disorder, tic disorder, fragile X syndrome, acquired epileptic aphasia

DIAGNOSTIC TESTS & INTERPRETATION
- The Modified Checklist for Autism in Toddlers (M-CHAT): commonly used test to screen for ASDs in children 12 to 30 months of age. Additional information is needed for children <12 months (https://mchatscreen.com) (1)[B].
- The Modified Checklist for Autism in Toddlers Revised with Follow-up (M-CHAT-R/F) shows improved PPV and lower false-positive rate in children aged 16 to 30 months, especially those with cultural barriers (https://mchatscreen.com/mchat-rf/) (1)[B].
- Infant-Toddler Checklist (parent questionnaire) can identify language delay in low-risk patients between 12 to 18 months of age; also useful in identifying infant siblings of children with ASD at increased risk for ASD (1)[B]
- Screening Tool for Autism in Toddlers & Young Children (STAT) shows promising evidence as level 2 screening to detect 2-year-olds with autism with other developmental disorders (1)[B].

- Social Communication Questionnaire (SCQ) (formerly Autism Screening Questionnaire)—used for children age 4+ years. Use carefully, as it may identify overlapping symptoms with other conditions (1)[B].
- ASD screening tools for older children: Autism Spectrum Quotient-Child and Childhood Autism Spectrum Test (ages 4 to 11), Autism Spectrum Screening Questionnaire (ages 7 to 16), and the Developmental Behaviour Checklist (ages 4 to 18 with intellectual disabilities)

Initial Tests (lab, imaging)
- Chromosomal microarray (CMA), DNA analysis (fragile X), and karyotype testing
- Complete blood count, serum lead, thyroid-stimulating hormone, and PKU screening
- Metabolic testing if signs of lethargy, limited endurance, hypotonia, recurrent vomiting and dehydration, developmental regression, or specific food intolerance
- Consider TORCH (toxoplasmosis, others [syphilis, varicella-zoster, parvovirus B19], rubella, cytomegalovirus, and herpes) infection workup if microcephaly present.
- SCQ
- Consider MRI if focal neurologic symptoms.

Follow-Up Tests & Special Considerations
- Children with ASD have the same general health care needs as other children and should receive the same preventative care.
- Follow-up appointments and testing recommended as indicated for comorbidities
- Consider additional hearing tests with audiometry and brainstem auditory evoked response (BAER) or consultation to audiology.
- Speech and language evaluation
- Evaluation by multidisciplinary team; includes a psychiatrist, genetic counselor, neurologist, psychologist, and other autism specialists
- Intellectual level needs to be established and monitored
- Tests used to follow autism are the following:
  – Gilliam Autism Rating Scale (GARS)
  – Childhood Autism Rating Scale (CARS)
  – Autism Diagnostic Interview-Revised (ADI-R)
  – Autism Diagnostic Observation Schedule-Generic (ADOS-G)

Diagnostic Procedures/Other
Electroencephalogram if displaying signs or symptoms suggestive of seizures

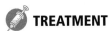

TREATMENT

GENERAL MEASURES
- Early intensive behavioral intervention with applied behavior analysis, focused on learning and reinforcing acceptable behaviors. Treatment addresses social communication, language, play skills, and maladaptive behavior to improve cognitive, language, and adaptive skills.
- Cognitive-behavioral therapy has been shown to reduce anxiety in older children with ASD with average to above-average IQ.
- Targeted play therapy has led to improvements in early social communication skills.

- Programs for training and educating parents to improve language skills and decrease disruptive behavior
- Core features of education program:
  – Individualized program with high staff-student ratio 1:2
  – Specialized teacher training with ongoing evaluation of teachers and programs
  – 25 hr/week of specialized services
  – A structured routine environment
  – Ongoing program evaluation and adjustment with routine functional analysis of individual child behavioral problems

MEDICATION
First Line
- Currently, the only FDA-approved psychotropic medications for ASD are risperidone and aripiprazole. Risperidone (approved age >5 years; oral; 0.25 mg/day in <20 kg; 0.5 mg/day in >20 kg with effective dose range 0.5 to 3.0 mg/day PO divided doses) has shown short-term efficacy for treatment for irritability, repetitive behaviors, and social withdrawal. Aripiprazole (approved ages 6 to 17 years; oral; initial dose 2 mg daily for 2 days, increase up to 5 mg daily; max 15 mg/day) has shown efficacy for treating short-term irritability, and repetitive movements.
- Stimulants (such as methylphenidate) have been efficacious in treating concomitant symptoms of ADHD (impulsiveness, hyperactivity, and inattention); however, the magnitude of response is less than in typically developing children, and adverse effects are frequent.
- SSRIs have limited evidence for autism. It has shown help in reducing ritualistic behavior, improving mood and language skills; initial choice for anxiety and depressive mood
- Melatonin used for patients with concomitant sleep disorders has shown mixed efficacy.

ISSUES FOR REFERRAL
Refer early for evaluation of behavior and language, genetic counseling, and audiology. Consider referrals to psychiatry, ophthalmology, otolaryngology, neurology, nutrition. Refer family members to support groups.

COMPLEMENTARY & ALTERNATIVE MEDICINE
- Medications such as secretin, intravenous immunoglobulin, and vitamins and minerals have shown no benefit and may carry significant risks.
- Therapies such as auditory integration therapy and hyperbaric oxygen have shown no benefit.
- Music, massage, therapeutic horseback riding, and other pet therapies would merit further review.

ONGOING CARE

FOLLOW-UP RECOMMENDATIONS
Patient Monitoring
- Constant monitoring by caregivers; evaluation every 6 to 12 months by physician for symptom and medical management
- Intellectual and language testing every 2 years in childhood

DIET
Insufficient evidence for recommendations of any certain dietary modifications for ASD; gluten- and casein-free diets without benefit across several randomized clinical trials

PATIENT EDUCATION
- Refer parents to the Partners in Policymaking course (https://partnersonlinecourses.com/) for advocacy.
- Economic costs: Due to caretaker burden, family earnings are less among families with ASD children.

PROGNOSIS
- Prognosis influenced by IQ, early intervention, strength of early language skills, and psychiatric comorbidities
- General expected course is for a lifelong need for supervised structured care; some patients will develop gainful employment, independent living, and social relationships.

COMPLICATIONS
- Increased risk for physical and sexual abuse
- With pica, increased risk of lead poisoning
- Gastrointestinal issues: weight abnormalities and abnormal stool patterns

REFERENCE
1. Hyman SL, Levy SE, Myers SM; Council on Children with Disabilities, Section on Developmental and Behavioral Pediatrics. Identification, evaluation, and management of children with autism spectrum disorder. Pediatrics. 2020;145(1):e20193447.

ADDITIONAL READING
Sanchack K, Thomas C. Autism spectrum disorder: primary care principles. Am Fam Physician. 2016;94(12):972–979.

 SEE ALSO

Algorithm: Intellectual Disability

CODES

ICD10
- F84.5 Asperger's syndrome
- F84 Pervasive developmental disorders
- F84.2 Rett's syndrome

CLINICAL PEARLS

American Academy of Pediatrics ALARM mnemonic:
- **A**SD is prevalent (screen all children between 18 and 24 months).
- **L**isten to parents when they feel something is wrong.
- **A**ct early: Screen children with delayed language and social developmental milestones.
- **R**efer to multidisciplinary teams.
- **M**onitor support for patient and families.

BABESIOSIS

Frederick W. Nielson, MD

BASICS

DESCRIPTION
- Rare tick-borne hemolytic disease caused by intraerythrocytic protozoan parasites of the genus *Babesia*
- Infrequently reported outside the United States
  - Sporadic cases have been reported from:
    - France, Italy, the United Kingdom, Ireland, the former Soviet Union, Mexico (1)
    - China, Italy, and Turkey have reported a reemergence of cases.
  - In the United States, infections have been reported in many states. The most endemic areas are:
    - Islands off the coast of Massachusetts (including Nantucket and Martha's Vineyard)
    - New York (including Long Island, Shelter Island, and Fire Island), Connecticut
    - Asymptomatic infection common in these areas (1)
- Incubation period varies from 5 to 33 days:
  - Most patients do not recall specific tick exposure.
  - After transfusion of infected blood, the incubation period can be up to 9 weeks (1).
- System(s) affected: cardiovascular, gastrointestinal, hemic/lymphatic/immunologic, musculoskeletal, nervous, pulmonary, renal/urologic

Pediatric Considerations
Transplacental and perinatal transmission rarely reported (1),(2)

Geriatric Considerations
- Morbidity and mortality higher in patients >60 years
- Cases more common in patients >70 years who have medical comorbidities.

EPIDEMIOLOGY
- Babesiosis affects patients of all ages. Most patients present in their 40s or 50s (1).
- Coinfection with other tick-borne illness is increasingly recognized.

Incidence
- Cases reported to the Centers for Disease Control and Prevention appear to be on the rise from 911 in 2012 peaking at 2,368 in 2017 before falling slightly to 2,101 in 2018.
- Prevalence is difficult to estimate due to lack of surveillance and asymptomatic infections.
- Transfusion-associated babesiosis and transplacental/perinatal transmission have been reported (1).
- In patients at high risk for tick-borne diseases, seroconversion data show antibodies to *Babesia microti* in 7 of 671 individuals (1%) (1).

ETIOLOGY AND PATHOPHYSIOLOGY
- *B. microti* (in the United States) and *Babesia divergens* and *Babesia bovis* (in Europe) cause most human infections (1). *B. divergens* and a new strain *Babesia duncani* appear to be more virulent. Other species identified in case reports. All share morphologic, antigenic, and genetic characteristics (1).
- Ixodid (hard-bodied) ticks, particularly *Ixodes dammini* (*Ixodes scapularis*: deer tick) and *Ixodes ricinus*, are the primary vectors.
- The white-footed deer mouse is the primary reservoir.
- Infection is passed to humans through the saliva of a nymphal-stage tick during a blood meal. Sporozoites introduced at the time of the bite enter red blood cells and form merozoites through binary fission (classic morphology on blood smear). Humans are a dead-end host for *B. microti*.

RISK FACTORS
- Residing in endemic areas
- Asplenia
- Immunocompromised state

GENERAL PREVENTION
- Avoid endemic regions during the peak transmission months of May to September (1).
- Appropriate insect repellent is advised during outdoor activities, especially in wooded or grassy areas:
  - 10–35% N,N-diethyl-meta-toluamide (DEET) provides adequate skin protection (1).
  - Acaricides, such as permethrin, provide impregnated clothing with even further protection.
- Early removal of ticks—daily skin checks
- Examine pets for ticks; flea/tick control for pets

COMMONLY ASSOCIATED CONDITIONS
- Coinfection with *Borrelia burgdorferi* and *B. microti*, particularly in endemic areas. Coinfection rates may be as high as ~27%.
- Coinfection with *Ehrlichia* (1)

DIAGNOSIS

HISTORY
- The tick must remain attached for at least 24 hours before the transmission of *B. microti* occurs (1).
- Travel/exposure history
- Comorbidities (immunosuppression, chronic disease)
- Fever (68–89%), fatigue (78–79%), chills (39–68%), sweats (41–56%), headache (32–75%), myalgia (32–37%), anorexia (24–25%), cough (17–23%), arthralgias (17–32%), nausea (9–22%). Other symptoms reported by case reports include abdominal pain, vomiting, diarrhea, and emotional lability.

PHYSICAL EXAM
- High fever (up to 40°C [104°F])
- Hemodynamic instability (shock in extremely ill)
- Hepatomegaly and splenomegaly (mild if noted)
- Rash (uncommon; if rash is present, consider concurrent Lyme disease)
- Central nervous system involvement includes headache, photophobia, neck and back stiffness, altered sensorium, and emotional lability
- Jaundice and dark urine may develop later in course of illness.

DIFFERENTIAL DIAGNOSIS
- Bacterial sepsis
- Hepatitis
- Lyme disease, ehrlichiosis, Rocky Mountain spotted fever
- Leishmaniasis
- Malaria
- HIV, Epstein-Barr virus
- Hemolysis, elevated liver enzymes, and low platelet syndrome (in pregnancy)

DIAGNOSTIC TESTS & INTERPRETATION
Initial Tests (lab, imaging)
- Diagnosis requires a high index of clinical suspicion. Nonspecific laboratory clues include evidence of mild to severe hemolytic anemia, normal to slightly depressed leukocyte count, elevated lactate dehydrogenase or transaminase level, elevated blood urea nitrogen and creatinine, proteinuria and hemoglobinuria (1),(2).
- Definitive diagnosis is made by blood smear.
  - Wright- or Giemsa-stained peripheral blood smear demonstrates intraerythrocytic parasites (2)[B].
  - Dividing "cross-like" tetrads of merozoites (Maltese cross) are pathognomonic (2).
  - Serial blood smears may be required (low parasite load early in the illness) (2).
  - Can be confused with *Plasmodium falciparum* on peripheral smear
- If blood smears are negative but suspicion remains, IgM serologies through indirect immunofluorescent antibody testing (IFAT) for *B. microti* antigen:
  - Positive titer results vary by lab. Titers of >1:64 or a 4-fold increase from baseline are consistent with *B. microti* infection. Titers may be >1:1,024 in acute infection (2)[B]. Titers often elevated 8 to 12 months and can persist for years.
  - In New England, seroprevalence is 0.5–16%
- Detection of *B. microti* by polymerase chain reaction (PCR) is more sensitive and equally specific in acute cases. PCR can also be used to monitor disease progression (2)[B]. Newer real-time PCR tests have a sensitivity and specificity approaching 100%.
- If lab tests are inconclusive and infection is strongly suspected, inoculation of laboratory animals with patient blood can reveal *B. microti* organisms in the blood of the animal within 2 to 4 weeks (2).

Follow-Up Tests & Special Considerations

Monitoring intraerythrocytic parasitemia helps guide treatment.

Diagnostic Procedures/Other

Based on blood smear, history, and epidemiologic information (2)

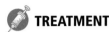 **TREATMENT**

GENERAL MEASURES

- In areas endemic for Lyme disease and ehrlichiosis, consider adding doxycycline 100 mg BID PO to empirically treat coinfection until serologic testing is complete (1)[C].
- Drug resistance has emerged in severely immuno-compromised patients (2).
- Consider treating asymptomatic patients if parasitemia persists for >3 months; otherwise, do not treat in absence of symptoms (1).

MEDICATION

First Line

- Mild to moderate infection with *B. microti*: 7 to 10 days of atovaquone 750 mg PO (with a fatty meal) BID plus azithromycin 500 mg/day PO BID on day 1, followed by 250 mg/day . Pediatrics: atovaquone 20 mg/kg (max 750 mg) BID and azithromycin 10 mg/kg (max 500 mg) on day 1 and then 5 mg/kg (max 250 mg) (3)[C]. For severe *B. microti* infection the same dosing is recommended but azithromycin can be given IV. Alternative treatment option includes oral quinine 650 mg TID or QID plus IV clindamycin 300 to 600 mg QID for 7 to 10 days. Pediatrics: clindamycin 7 to 10 mg/kg (max 600 mg) TID or QID and quinine 8 mg/kg (max 650 mg) TID (3).
- Persistent or relapsing babesiosis: Treat for 6 weeks, including 2 weeks after *Babesia* is no longer detected on blood smear.

Second Line

- Combination of quinine sulfate 650 mg PO TID and clindamycin 600 mg PO TID or 1.2 g parenterally BID for 7 to 10 days is the most commonly used treatment. Pediatric: quinine 8 mg/kg (max 650 mg) every 6 to 8 hours for 7 to 10 days and clindamycin 7 to 10 mg/kg (max 600 mg) PO q6–8h for 7 to 10 days. Some experts prefer this regimen for severe infections (3)[C].
- Other drugs including tetracycline, primaquine, sulfadiazine (Microsulfon), and sulfadoxine/pyrimethamine (Fansidar) have been evaluated. Results vary. Pentamidine (Pentam) is moderately effective in diminishing symptoms and decreasing parasitemia (1)[C].

> **ALERT**
> Clindamycin can lead to *Clostridium difficile*–associated diarrhea.

ISSUES FOR REFERRAL

Severe disease: Consider consultation with hematology and infectious disease for exchange transfusion in extremely ill patients (blood parasitemia >10%, massive hemolysis, and asplenia) (2)[C].

ADMISSION, INPATIENT, AND NURSING CONSIDERATIONS

Select patients with severe babesiosis and organ compromise may be considered for exchange transfusion.

 ONGOING CARE

FOLLOW-UP RECOMMENDATIONS

- If left untreated, silent babesiosis may persist for months or years (2).
- Alkaline phosphatase levels >125 U/L, white blood cell counts >5 × 10⁹/L, history of cardiac abnormality, history of splenectomy, presence of heart murmur, and parasitemia of 4% or higher are associated with disease severity.

Patient Monitoring

The need for monitoring depends on disease severity. Severe infections: Follow hematocrit and parasitemia levels until clinical improvement, and parasitemia is <5%. Mild to moderate: Expect clinical improvement within 48 hours and complete resolution within 3 months.

COMPLICATIONS

- Many remain asymptomatic.
- Complications in hospitalized patients: congestive heart failure (12%), disseminated intravascular coagulation (18%), acute respiratory distress syndrome (21%), renal failure (6%), coma/lethargy (9%), death (9%)
- Other reported complications include neutropenia and myocardial infarction.
- In asplenic patients, warm autoimmune hemolytic anemia has been reported.

REFERENCES

1. Ortiz JF, Millhouse PW, Morillo Cox Á, et al. Babesiosis: appreciating the pathophysiology and diverse sequela of the infection. *Cureus*. 2020;12(10):e11085. doi:10.7759/cureus.11085.
2. Vannier E, Krause PJ. Human babesiosis. *N Engl J Med*. 2012;366(25):2397–2407.
3. Krause PJ, Auwaerter PG, Bannuru EE, et al. Clinical practice guidelines by the Infectious Diseases Society of America (IDSA): 2020 Guidelines on the diagnosis and management of babesiosis. *Clin Infect Dis*. 2021;72(2):e49–e64. doi:10.1093/cid/ciaa1216.

ADDITIONAL READING

- Curcio SR, Tria LP, Gucwa AL. Seroprevalence of *Babesia microti* in individuals with lyme disease. *Vector Borne Zoonotic Dis*. 2016;16(12):737–743.
- Saetre K, Godhwani N, Maria M, et al. Congenital babesiosis after maternal infection with *Borrelia burgdorferi* and *Babesia microti*. *J Pediatric Infect Dis Soc*. 2018;7(1):e1–e5.
- Sanchez E, Vannier E, Wormser GP, et al. Diagnosis, treatment, and prevention of Lyme disease, human granulocytic anaplasmosis, and babesiosis: a review. *JAMA*. 2016;315(16):1767–1777.
- Woolley AE, Montgomery MW, Savage WJ, et al. Post-babesiosis warm autoimmune hemolytic anemia. *N Engl J Med*. 2017;376(10):939–946.

 CODES

ICD10

B60.0 Babesiosis

CLINICAL PEARLS

- Ticks must remain in place for 24 hours to transmit infection. Encourage daily "tick checks" if people are exposed in high-risk areas.
- Most patients do not recall tick exposure, and incubation can last up to a month.
- Left untreated, silent babesial infection may persist for months or years.
- First-line treatment for mild or moderate disease is atovaquone plus azithromycin.
- Patients with mild-to-moderate disease should show clinical improvement within 48 hours after starting therapy. Symptoms should fully resolve in 3 months.
- Coinfection with *B. burgdorferi* and *Ehrlichia* species is common in endemic areas. In areas endemic for Lyme disease and ehrlichiosis, consider adding doxycycline until serologic testing is completed.

BACK PAIN, LOW
Vasilios Chrisostomidis, DO

 BASICS

DESCRIPTION
- Low back pain (LBP) is extremely common and includes a wide range of symptoms involving the lumbosacral spine and pelvic girdle.
- Characterized by duration or associated symptoms
- Duration (1)[A]
  - Acute (<6 weeks)
  - Subacute (>6 weeks but <3 months)
  - Chronic (>3 months)
- Associated symptoms (1)[A]
  - Localized/nonspecific "mechanical" LBP
  - Back pain with lower extremity symptoms
  - Systemic and visceral symptoms
- A specific cause is not found for most patients with LBP. Most cases resolve in 4 to 6 weeks.
- Rule out "red" flag symptoms indicating the need for immediate intervention.
- System(s) affected: musculoskeletal, neurologic
- Synonym(s): lumbago, lumbar sprain/strain, low back syndrome

EPIDEMIOLOGY
Incidence
- 1-year incidence for first episode: 6.3–15.3% (2)
- 1-year incidence for *any* episode: 1.5–3.6% (2)
- A very common primary care complaint (1)

Prevalence
- Lifetime prevalence: 84% (1)
- Global point prevalence: 9% (1)
- Chronic point prevalence in United States: 13.1%
- Predominant sex: male = female
- Age: The highest incidence is in the 3rd decade (20 to 29 years); overall prevalence increases with age until 65 years and then declines (1).

ETIOLOGY AND PATHOPHYSIOLOGY
LBP can be commonly due to muscle spasm/tension. Estimated 39% of chronic LBP due to disk degeneration. 30% estimated to be from facet joint syndrome. Other possibilities include sacroiliac injuries/degeneration and spinal stenosis. Age-related degenerative changes of the lumbosacral spine and atrophy of supporting musculature may contribute as well (2)[A].

RISK FACTORS
- Age (1)[A]
- Activity (lifting, sudden twisting, bending) (1)[A]
- Obesity (1)[A]
- Sedentary lifestyle (1)[A]
- Physically strenuous work (1)[A]
- Psychosocial factors—anxiety, depression, stress (1)[A]
- Genetic factors (2)
- Heavy operating equipment (2)
- Poor flexibility (2)
- Smoking (1)[A]

GENERAL PREVENTION
- Maintain normal weight (1)[A].
- Adequate physical fitness and activity (1)[A]
- Stress reduction (1)[A]
- Proper lifting technique and good posture
- Smoking cessation
- There is insufficient evidence to recommend for or against routine preventive measures in adults.

 DIAGNOSIS

HISTORY
- Onset of pain (sudden or gradual) (1)
- Pain from spinal structures (musculature, ligaments, facet joints and disks) can refer to the thigh region but rarely below the knee. However, facet pain most commonly radiates to sacroiliac joint/PSIS region (1).
- Sacroiliac pain often refers to the thigh and can radiate below the knee (1).
- Irritation, impingement, or compression of lumbar nerve roots often results in more leg pain than back pain (1).
- Pain from the L1–L3 nerve roots radiates to the hip and/or thigh, whereas pain from the L4–S1 nerve roots radiates below the knee.
- Red flags
  - Recent trauma
  - Neurologic deficits
    - Bowel/bladder incontinence or urinary retention
    - Saddle anesthesia
    - Weakness, falls
  - Night pain, sweats, fever, weight loss
  - Age >70 years with or without trauma
  - Age >50 years with minor trauma
  - History of cancer
  - Osteoporosis
  - Immunosuppression, prolonged glucocorticoid use
  - IV drug use/fever (3)
- Yellow flags (predicting poor long-term prognosis):
  - Lack of social support
  - Unsupportive work environment
  - Depression and/or anxiety
  - Abuse of alcohol or other substances
  - History of physical or sexual abuse
  - Excessive mobility in spine or other joints (2)
  - Fear of reinjury, movement, or pain (2)
  - Low expectation of recovery (2)
  - Passive coping style (2)
- Pain can be provoked with motion: flexion–extension, side-bending rotation, sitting, standing, and lifting. Pain often relieved with rest.
- Radicular pain may radiate to buttocks, thighs, and lower legs.

Pediatric Considerations
Back pain is not normal in children and must be carefully evaluated. Trauma from high impact or hyperextension sports would be the leading cause requiring further evaluation.

PHYSICAL EXAM
- Observe gait, positioning, and facial expressions.
- Test lumbar spine range of motion.
- Evaluate for point tenderness or muscle spasm.
- Evaluate for signs of muscle atrophy.
- Complete thorough physical exam to assess for wide differential (full differential listed in subsequent section).
  - Completely evaluate reflexes, strength, pulses, sensation.
  - Slump test: Have patient sit on table and slump shoulders forward. Then, have patient touch chin to chest and attempt to have them extend one leg at a time. Do this while continually reassessing for symptom reproduction; can be indicative of disk herniation
  - Straight leg test: Raise the patient's leg straight while the patient is lying down. Keep the knee straight. For more specificity, dorsiflex ankle while lifting leg. This can also evaluate for herniated disk.
  - Evaluate for saddle anesthesia, anal wink reflex.
  - FABER and FADIR test of hips bilaterally
  - Evaluate for psychological distress that may be contributing.
  - Stork test: Stand on one leg with opposite hip held in flexion. Extend back. Pain in lumbosacral area is a positive test—consider spondylolisthesis versus facet OA.
  - Waddell sign—overreaction to physical exam, widespread tenderness—may indicate psychological component/underlying depression

DIFFERENTIAL DIAGNOSIS
- Localized/nonspecific "mechanical" LBP (87%) (1)[A]
  - Lumbar strain/sprain (70%)
  - Disk/facet degeneration (10%)
  - Osteoporotic compression fracture (4%)
  - Spondylolisthesis (2%)
  - Severe scoliosis, kyphosis
  - Asymmetric transitional vertebrae (<1%)
  - Traumatic fracture (<1%)
- Back pain with lower extremity symptoms (7%) (1)[A]
  - Disk herniation (4%)
  - Spinal stenosis (3%)
- Systemic and visceral symptoms (1)[A]
  - Neoplasia (0.7%)
    - Multiple myeloma; metastatic carcinoma
    - Lymphoma/leukemia
    - Spinal cord tumors, retroperitoneal tumors
  - Infection (0.01%)
    - Osteomyelitis
    - Septic discitis
    - Paraspinous abscess; epidural abscess
    - Shingles
  - Inflammatory disease (0.03%)
    - Ankylosing spondylitis, psoriatic spondylitis
    - Reactive arthritis
    - Inflammatory bowel disease
  - Visceral disease (0.05%)
    - Prostatitis
    - Endometriosis
    - Chronic pelvic inflammatory disease
    - Nephrolithiasis, pyelonephritis
    - Perinephric abscess
    - Aortic aneurysm
    - Pancreatitis; cholecystitis
    - Penetrating ulcer
  - Other
    - Osteochondrosis
    - Paget disease
    - Cauda equina syndrome

DIAGNOSTIC TESTS & INTERPRETATION
Initial Tests (lab, imaging)
- No clinical benefit of routine imaging (2)
  - Imaging only recommended for progressive, severe neurologic deficits or in the setting of "red flags" (2)
  - Significant amount of false positives; evidence of possible herniated disk material seen in 20–76% of asymptomatic patients on computed tomography (CT), magnetic resonance imaging (MRI), myelography (2)
- X-ray of the lumbar spine (1),(4)[A]
  - Not recommended for initial presentation without red flags. Defer films for 6 weeks, unless there is a history of acute trauma (fall, etc.) or high risk of disease.
  - Useful to evaluate bony etiology (e.g., fracture)
- MRI of the lumbar spine (1),(4)[A] for patients presenting with neurologic deficits, failure to improve with 6 weeks of conservative treatment, or if there is a strong suspicion of cancer or cauda equina syndrome
  - Useful for suspected herniated disk, nerve root compression, or metastatic disease

- CT scan of the lumbar spine (1),(4)[A]
  - Appropriate alternative to MRI for patient with pacemaker, metallic hardware, or other contraindication to MRI
- Labs are unnecessary with initial presentation if no related red flags, signs, or symptoms (1),(4)[A].
- If infection or bone marrow neoplasm is suspected, consider (1),(4)[A]
  - Complete blood count (CBC) with differential
  - Erythrocyte sedimentation rate (ESR)
  - C-reactive protein (CRP) level
  - 3-phase bone scan

Diagnostic Procedures/Other
Neurosurgical consult for acute neurologic deficits or suspected cauda equina syndrome (1)[A]

 TREATMENT

The primary goal is to provide supportive care and allow return to functional activity. Patients should be aware of alarm symptoms to prompt a return visit.

MEDICATION
First Line
- Physical therapy
  - For patients with sciatica, early referral to physical therapy improves short- and long-term outcomes.
  - McKenzie method is a reasonable approach for those patients who feel better with low back extension (standing up straight) (3).
  - Manual medicine, osteopathic manipulative treatments (OMTs): myofascial release, counterstrain, bilateral ligamentous techniques as well as muscle energy techniques as tolerated
- Patient education
  - Reassure patients that pain is usually self-limited; treatment should relieve pain and improve function.
  - Limit bed rest to <48 hours.
  - Encouraging activity as tolerated leads to quicker recovery; walk as much as possible.
  - Early intervention with formal physical therapy (2),(5)
  - Sit on straight backed chair (not sofa or soft cushioned chair) to maintain lumbar lordosis.
  - Strong evidence that intensive patient education is effective for long-term pain control and ability to return to work (3)
- Medications (1),(4)[A]
  - Acetaminophen 325 to 650 mg PO q4–6h PRN pain (max 4 g/day)
  - Nonsteroidal anti-inflammatory drugs (NSAIDs)
    - Ibuprofen 400 to 600 mg PO 3 to 4 times daily (max 3,200 mg/day)
    - Naproxen 250 to 500 mg PO q12h (max 1,500 mg/day)
  - Adding B vitamins (at least 50 mg of vitamin B_1 [thiamine], 50 mg of vitamin B_6 [pyridoxine], and 2,000 μg of B_{12} [cyanocobalamin]) to NSAIDs reduced medication needs and pain scores compared to NSAIDs alone (5)[A].
- Obstetric considerations
  - Use medications cautiously in pregnancy—benefit must clearly outweigh risk.
- OMT and chiropractic care may be used in a multidisciplinary approach; may be used in the general population as well as the obstetric patient

Second Line
- Second-line therapy for moderate to severe pain (1),(4)[A]
  - Cyclobenzaprine 5 to 10 mg PO up to TID PRN (max 30 mg/day)
  - Tizanidine 2 mg PO up to TID PRN

- Avoid opioid use (If so, ≤4 days, maximum) for LBP; opioids in the setting of LBP do *not* have a significantly better effect than NSAIDs plus placebo or placebo alone and may cause chronic opioid dependence and/or chronic LBP.
  - Single, small trial with topiramate has showed that it is better than placebo at improving pain/function (3).
  - Topical lidocaine likely no better than placebo (3)
  - Use of diazepam (Valium) with naproxen regimen *does not* improve disability or pain scores.
- Other treatments (1),(4)[A]
  - Antidepressants (1),(4)[A]
    - Tricyclic antidepressants (amitriptyline, nortriptyline, desipramine) have been shown in randomized trials to provide a small pain reduction in patients. No clear evidence that selective serotonin reuptake inhibitors are more effective than placebo in cases of chronic LBP. Treatment of concurrent depression may have positive effect on LBP.
    - Cymbalta has shown superiority to other antidepressants in decreasing pain for chronic LBP. Typically uptitrate to 60 mg daily (3).
- Injections
  - Facet: Therapeutic facet joint nerve blocks in the lumbar spine and lumbar intra-articular injections have all shown benefit.
  - Epidural: provide short-term relief of persistent pain associated with documented radicular symptoms caused by herniated disk (1),(4)
  - Lumbar radiofrequency: Recent RCT showed no clinically significant improvement of LBP when radiofrequency was done with exercise program versus exercise program alone.

Geriatric Considerations
- Older persons taking nonselective NSAIDs should use a proton pump inhibitor or misoprostol for gastrointestinal protection.
- Patients taking a COX-2 selective inhibitor with aspirin should use a proton pump inhibitor or misoprostol for gastrointestinal protection.
- Age-related decline in cytochrome P450 function and polypharmacy (common in elderly patients) increases risk for adverse medication reactions.

COMPLEMENTARY & ALTERNATIVE MEDICINE
- Recent guideline updates suggest *not* recommending acupuncture.
- Yoga can help with chronic LBP (1),(4)[A]. Recent data suggest yoga as effective for chronic LBP as physical therapy and that yoga can improve long-term function and reduce pain overall.
- Spinal manipulative therapy (including osteopathic treatment) is as effective as NSAIDs and exercise for pain and functional status.

 ONGOING CARE

FOLLOW-UP RECOMMENDATIONS
- Regular exercise to manage weight and control symptoms (4)[A]
- Strongly encourage patients to remain active.
- Educate patients regarding chronicity, recurrence, and red flags (4)[A].

Patient Monitoring
- Reassurance is important. Follow up within 2 to 4 weeks of initial presentation to monitor progress. Most patients spontaneously improve.
  - Assess severity and quality of pain, range of motion, and other historical features (red flags).
- Reevaluate for organic causes if no adequate improvement.

COMPLICATIONS
- Regular NSAID use can increase risk of gastrointestinal toxicity and nephrotoxicity (1)[A].
- Acetaminophen has potential hepatotoxicity in high doses. Recommendations indicate 4 g should be the highest daily dose (1)[A].
- Centrally acting skeletal muscle relaxants and opioid agonists carry the risk for sedation, confusion, dependence, and abuse (1)[A]. Proceed with extreme caution if patients are requiring pain medications long term.

REFERENCES
1. Golob AL, Wipf JE. Low back pain. *Med Clin North Am*. 2014;98(3):405–428.
2. Delitto A, George SZ, Van Dillen LR, et al; for Orthopaedic Section of the American Physical Therapy Association. Low back pain. *J Orthop Sports Phys Ther*. 2012;42(4):A1–A57.
3. Will JS, Bury DC, Miller JA. Mechanical low back pain. *Am Fam Physician*. 2018;98(7):421–428.
4. Chaparro LE, Furlan AD, Deshpande A, et al. Opioids compared with placebo or other treatments for chronic low back pain: an update of the Cochrane Review. *Spine (Phila Pa 1976)*. 2014;39(7):556–563.
5. Calderon-Ospina CA, Nava-Mesa MO, Arbeláez Ariza CE. Effect of combined diclofenac and B vitamins (thiamine, pyridoxine, and cyanocobalamin) for low back pain management: systematic review and meta-analysis. *Pain Med*. 2020;21(4):766–781.

ADDITIONAL READING

Andronis L, Kinghorn P, Qiao S, et al. Cost-effectiveness of non-invasive and non-pharmacological interventions for low back pain: a systematic literature review. *Appl Health Econ Health Policy*. 2017;15(2):173–201.

 SEE ALSO

Algorithm: Low Back Pain, Acute

CODES

ICD10
- M54.5 Low back pain
- G89.29 Other chronic pain
- M53.3 Sacrococcygeal disorders, not elsewhere classified

CLINICAL PEARLS
- Most cases resolve spontaneously within 4 to 12 weeks of onset.
- Assess for red flag symptoms, such as bowel/bladder incontinence, history of cancer, or recent trauma.
- Labs and imaging studies are unnecessary for most cases of back pain if no red flag symptoms are present. Symptoms typically will resolve in ≤6 weeks.
- With no red flags, physical activity as tolerated speeds recovery.
- Early intervention with formal physical therapy and spinal manipulative therapy can reduce symptoms, strengthen musculature, and speed up recovery.

BACTERIURIA, ASYMPTOMATIC

Onameyore Utuama, MD, MPH • Kitty Brigitta Carter-Wicker, MD • Omofolarin Fasuyi, MD, MPH, FAAFP

BASICS

DESCRIPTION
Asymptomatic bacteriuria (ASB) is specific bacterial growth $\geq 10^5$ CFU/mL in one and two consecutive midstream urine samples for men and women, respectively >18 years. This definition applies to individuals with no clinical symptoms (1).

EPIDEMIOLOGY
Incidence
- Premenopausal females: 1–5%
- Pregnancy: 2–10%
- Older females and males: 4–19%
- Institutionalized older population: 15–50%

Prevalence
- Variable, increased with age, female gender, sexual activity, and presence of genitourinary (GU) abnormalities
- Pregnancy: 2–10%
- Short- and long-term indwelling catheter 9–23% and 100%, respectively
- Long-term care residents in women 25–50% and men 15–40%

ETIOLOGY AND PATHOPHYSIOLOGY
- Microbiology is similar to that of other UTI, with bacteria originating from periurethral area, vagina, or gut.
- Organisms are less virulent in ASB than those causing UTI.
- The most common organism is *Escherichia coli*. Other common organisms are *Klebsiella pneumoniae*, *Enterobacter*, *Proteus mirabilis*, *Staphylococcus aureus*, group B *Streptococcus* (GBS), and *Enterococcus*.

Genetics
Genetic variations that reduce toll-like receptor 4 (*TLR4*) function have been associated with ASB by lowering innate immune response and delaying bacterial clearance.

RISK FACTORS
- Pregnancy
- Older age
- Female gender
- Sexual activity, use of diaphragm with spermicide
- GU abnormalities: neurogenic bladder, urinary retention, urinary catheter use (indwelling, intermittent, or condom catheter)

- Institutionalized elderly population
- Diabetes mellitus
- Immunocompromised status
- Spinal cord injuries or functional impairment
- Hemodialysis

COMMONLY ASSOCIATED CONDITIONS
Depends on the risk factors

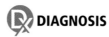

DIAGNOSIS

HISTORY
- Asymptomatic
- Lack of symptoms attributable to UTI such as fever, acute dysuria (<1 week), new or worsening urinary urgency/frequency/incontinence, or acute gross hematuria

PHYSICAL EXAM
- Afebrile
- No suprapubic and costovertebral angle tenderness

DIFFERENTIAL DIAGNOSIS
- UTI
- Uncomplicated cystitis
- Contaminated urine specimen

DIAGNOSTIC TESTS & INTERPRETATION
Initial Tests (lab, imaging)
- Urinalysis (UA):
  - The presence of pyuria, leukocyte esterase, and nitrite in ASB is common.
- Urine culture
- Screening urine culture in asymptomatic patients is indicated in only two conditions:
  - Pregnancy: screening between 12 and 16 weeks' gestation or at first prenatal visit if later (1)[A]
  - Prior to transurethral resection of prostate (TURP) (1)[A] or any urologic interventions when mucosal bleeding is anticipated (1)[C]
- Screening for ASB in men and nonpregnant women is not recommended.

Follow-Up Tests & Special Considerations
- Noncontaminated urine specimen should be used for urine culture.
- In pregnancy, periodic screening urine culture should be done after ASB treatment (1)[A] but not required in GBS bacteriuria (2).

Test Interpretation
- Patient with significant bacteriuria with or without pyuria and without symptoms referable to UTI should be diagnosed as ASB per Infectious Diseases Society of America.
  - Significant bacteriuria is defined based on type of urine specimen, sex, and the amount of bacteria.
  - By midstream, clean catch specimen
    - Male: >100,000 CFU/mL of single bacteria species
    - Female: the same criteria as male but needs two positive consecutive specimens
    - By catheterized specimen male and female: >100 CFU/mL of one bacterial species; required one-time collection only
- The presence of pyuria or leukocyte esterase is common but not a marker of infection.
- Positive nitrite is an indicator of the presence of bacteriuria but cannot differentiate UTI from ASB or poor collection technique.

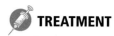

TREATMENT

GENERAL MEASURES

ALERT
- Antibiotic treatment of ASB is indicated in only two conditions:
  - Pregnancy (1)[A]
    - Rationale: Treatment prevents up to 70% of pregnant women from developing acute pyelonephritis, which reduces the risk of low birth weight and preterm delivery that are perinatal complications (1).
  - Prior to TURP (1)[A]
    - Rationale: Antibiotic treatment can effectively prevent postprocedure bacteremia and sepsis.
- Treatment of ASB in other conditions (nonpregnant women, diabetic women, indwelling catheter, patients with spinal cord injury, or the elderly living in the community) does not provide any known clinical benefit, does not reduce the risk of symptomatic infection, nor improve morbidity or mortality. It increases health care cost, adverse drug side effects, development of resistant organisms, and reinfection rate (1).
- Recommendation against screening all nonrenal solid organ transplant or after 1 month following renal transplant; inadequate evidence to guide management in nonurologic procedure (3)[A]

MEDICATION

- Pregnancy
  - Intrapartum antibiotic prophylaxis with IV penicillin or clindamycin (penicillin allergy) is recommended for women with GBS bacteriuria occurring at any stage of pregnancy and of any colony count to prevent GBS disease in the newborn.
  - No consensus on choice of antibiotics and duration of treatment in pregnancy; however, the cure rate is higher for the 4 to 7 days of treatment than 1-day treatment (1)[A].
  - Choice of antibiotics should be guided by bacterial pathogen, local resistance rate, adverse effects, and comorbidities of patients (1).
  - Common oral antibiotics (FDA-B) that have been used
    - Nitrofurantoin 100 mg BID for 5 days (low level of resistance, may cause hemolysis in glucose-6-phosphate dehydrogenase deficiency)
    - Amoxicillin/clavulanate 500/125 mg BID for 5 to 7 days
    - Cefuroxime 250 mg BID for 5 days
    - Cephalexin 500 mg BID for 5 days
    - Fosfomycin 3 g for 1 single dose (not effective when glomerular filtration rate is <30 mL/min, may be used in highly resistant bacteria such as methicillin-resistant *S. aureus* [MRSA], vancomycin-resistant enterococci [VRE], and extended-spectrum β-lactamase [ESBL]-producing organism bacteria) (4)
  - Avoid trimethoprim in 1st trimester and near term. Avoid sulfa after 32 weeks' gestation.
  - Contraindicated: fluoroquinolones (FDA-C), tetracyclines (FDA-D)
- Prior to invasive urologic interventions
  - Initiate antibiotic the night before or immediately before the procedure (1)[A].
  - Antibiotic should be continued until the indwelling catheter is removed postprocedure (1)[B].

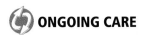 **ONGOING CARE**

FOLLOW-UP RECOMMENDATIONS

No consensus on screening frequency of ASB in pregnancy, but monthly screening of urine culture after ASB treatment is recommended except GBS (1).

Patient Monitoring

Development of any signs/symptoms of UTI should warrant antibiotic treatment.

DIET

Daily cranberry juice or cranberry capsules twice daily may reduce the frequency of ASB during pregnancy, but it has not been confirmed in large study (5) (see "Additional Reading").

PATIENT EDUCATION

Patient should seek medical attention when UTI symptoms develop.

COMPLICATIONS

- Late pregnancy pyelonephritis occurs in 20–35% of women with untreated bacteriuria (20- to 30-fold higher than women with negative initial screening urine cultures or in whom bacteriuria was treated). Pyelonephritis is associated with premature delivery and worse fetal outcomes (infant with group B streptococcal infections, low-birth-weight infant). Antimicrobial treatment will decrease the risk of subsequent pyelonephritis from 20–35% to 1–4% and the risk of having a low-birth-weight baby from 15% to 5%.
- If bacteriuria remains untreated in patients who undergo traumatic urologic procedures, up to 60% develop bacteremia after the procedure and 5–10% progress to severe sepsis/septic shock.

REFERENCES

1. Nicolle LE, Bradley S, Colgan R, et al. Infectious Diseases Society of America guidelines for the diagnosis and treatment of asymptomatic bacteriuria in adults. *Clin Infect Dis*. 2005;40(5):643–654.
2. Zolotor AJ, Carlough MC. Update on prenatal care. *Am Fam Physician*. 2014;89(3):199–208.
3. Nicolle LE, Gupta K, Bradley SF, et al. Clinical practice guideline for the management of asymptomatic bacteriuria: 2019 update by the Infectious Diseases Society of America. *Clin Infect Dis*. 2019;68(10):e83–e110. https://doi.org/10.1093/cid/ciy1121.
4. Kalinderi K, Delkos D, Kalinderis M, et al. Urinary tract infection during pregnancy: current concepts on a common multifaceted problem. *J Obstet Gynaecol*. 2018;38(4):448–453.
5. Wing DA, Rumney PJ, Hindra S, et al. Pilot study to evaluate compliance and tolerability of cranberry capsules in pregnancy for the prevention of asymptomatic bacteriuria. *J Altern Complement Med*. 2015;21(11):700–706.

ADDITIONAL READING

- Köves B, Cai T, Veeratterapillay R, et al. Benefits and harms of treatment of asymptomatic bacteriuria: a systematic review and meta-analysis by the European Association of Urology Urological Infection Guidelines Panel. *Eur Urol*. 2017;72(6):865–868.
- Wing DA, Rumney PJ, Preslicka CW, et al. Daily cranberry juice for the prevention of asymptomatic bacteriuria in pregnancy: a randomized, controlled pilot study. *J Urol*. 2008;180(4):1367–1372.

 CODES

ICD10

- N39.0 Urinary tract infection, site not specified
- B96.20 Unsp Escherichia coli as the cause of diseases classd elswhr
- B96.1 Klebsiella pneumoniae as the cause of diseases classd elswhr

CLINICAL PEARLS

- ASB is a common and benign disorder for which treatment is not indicated in most patients.
- The presence of pyuria, leukocyte esterase, and nitrite is common in ASB and not an indication for antimicrobial treatment.
- Antibiotic treatment is indicated for ASB in pregnancy, patients who require TURP, or any urologic interventions with mucosal bleeding.
- Treatment of ASB in other conditions does not decrease the frequency of UTI or improve outcome.
- Overtreatment of ASB may result in negative consequences such as antimicrobial resistance, adverse drug reaction, and unnecessary cost.

BALANITIS, PHIMOSIS, AND PARAPHIMOSIS
Nathan J. Macedo, MD, MPH

BASICS

DESCRIPTION
- Balanitis:
  - Balanitis is an inflammation of the glans penis.
  - Posthitis is an inflammation of the foreskin or prepuce.
  - Balanoposthitis is inflammation of both the glans penis and the foreskin.
  - Balanitis xerotica obliterans (BXO) is lichen sclerosus of the glans penis (uncommon).
- Phimosis and paraphimosis:
  - Phimosis: tightness of the distal penile foreskin that prevents it from being drawn back from over the glans
  - Paraphimosis: constriction by foreskin of an uncircumcised penis, preventing the foreskin from returning to its position over the glans; occurs after the retracted foreskin becomes swollen and engorged; a urologic emergency
- System(s) affected: renal/urologic; reproductive; skin/exocrine

ALERT
- Recurrent infection and irritations (condom catheters) can lead to phimosis.
- Recurrent balanitis, either chemical or infectious, can lead to an acquired phimosis.
- Inappropriate forced reduction of a physiologic foreskin can lead to chronic scarring and acquired phimosis; unfortunately, many times done due to instructions from health care providers
- Paraphimosis is a pediatric emergency; if left untreated, can lead to necrosis and autoamputation

EPIDEMIOLOGY
- Balanitis: predominant age: adult; predominant gender: male only
- Phimosis/paraphimosis: predominant age: infancy and adolescence; unusual in adults; risk returns in geriatrics; predominant sex: male only

Incidence
Balanitis: will affect 3–11% of males

Prevalence
Phimosis: in the United States: 8% of boys age 6 years and 1% of men >16 years of age (1)

ETIOLOGY AND PATHOPHYSIOLOGY
- Balanitis:
  - Allergic reaction (condom latex, contraceptive jelly, soaps)
  - Infections (*Candida albicans*, *Borrelia vincentii*, streptococci, *Trichomonas*, HPV)
  - Fixed-drug eruption (sulfa, tetracycline)
  - Plasma cell infiltration (Zoon balanitis)
  - Autodigestion by activated pancreatic transplant exocrine enzymes

- Phimosis:
  - Physiologic: present at birth; resolves spontaneously during the first 2 to 3 years of life through nocturnal erections, which slowly dilate the phimotic ring
  - Acquired: recurrent inflammation, trauma, or infections of the foreskin
- Paraphimosis:
  - Often iatrogenically or inadvertently induced by the foreskin not being pulled back over the glans after voiding, cleaning, cystoscopy, or catheter insertion

Geriatric Considerations
Condom catheters can predispose to balanitis.

Pediatric Considerations
Oral antibiotics predispose male infants to *Candida balanitis*. Most phimosis referrals seen in pediatric urology clinics are normal physiologically phimotic foreskins (2). Inappropriate care of physiologic phimosis can lead to acquired phimosis by repeated forced reduction of the foreskin. Uncircumcised penises require no special care and with normal hygiene, most foreskins will become retractile over time.

RISK FACTORS
- Balanitis:
  - Presence of foreskin
  - Morbid obesity
  - Poor hygiene
  - Diabetes; probably most common
  - Nursing home environment
  - Condom catheters
  - Chemical irritants
  - Edematous conditions: CHF, nephrosis
- Phimosis:
  - Poor hygiene
  - Diabetes by repeated balanitis
  - Frequent diaper rash in infants
  - Recurrent posthitis
- Paraphimosis:
  - Presence of foreskin
  - Inexperienced health care provider (leaving foreskin retracted after catheter placement)
  - Poor education about care of the foreskin

GENERAL PREVENTION
- Balanitis:
  - Proper hygiene and avoidance of allergens
  - Circumcision
- Phimosis/paraphimosis:
  - If the patient is uncircumcised, appropriate hygiene and care of the foreskin are necessary to prevent phimosis and paraphimosis.

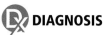

DIAGNOSIS

HISTORY
- Balanitis:
  - Pain
  - Drainage
  - Dysuria
  - Odor
  - Ballooning of foreskin with voiding
  - Redness
- Phimosis:
  - Painful erections
  - Recurrent balanitis
  - Foreskin balloons when voiding.
  - Inability to retract foreskin at appropriate age
- Paraphimosis:
  - Uncircumcised
  - Pain
  - Drainage
  - Voiding difficulty

PHYSICAL EXAM
- Balanitis:
  - Erythema
  - Tenderness
  - Edema
  - Discharge
  - Ulceration
  - Plaque
- Phimosis:
  - Foreskin will not retract.
  - Secondary balanitis
  - Physiologic phimosis—preputial orifice appears normal and healthy.
  - Pathologic phimosis—preputial orifice has fine white fibrous ring of scar.
- Paraphimosis:
  - Edema of prepuce and glans
  - Drainage
  - Ulceration

DIFFERENTIAL DIAGNOSIS
- Balanitis:
  - Leukoplakia
  - Lichen planus
  - Psoriasis
  - Reactive arthritis (formerly known as Reiter syndrome)
  - Lichen sclerosus et atrophicus
  - Erythroplasia of Queyrat
  - BXO: atrophic changes at end of foreskin; can form band that prevents retraction
- Phimosis/paraphimosis:
  - Penile lymphedema, which can be related to insect bites, trauma, or allergic reactions
  - Penile tourniquet syndrome: foreign body around penis, most commonly hair
  - Anasarca

DIAGNOSTIC TESTS & INTERPRETATION

Initial Tests (lab, imaging)
- Microbiology culture
- Wet mount
- Serology for syphilis
- Serum glucose; ESR (if concerns about reactive arthritis)
- STI testing
- HIV testing
- Gram stain

Diagnostic Procedures/Other
Biopsy, if persistent

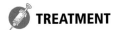 # TREATMENT

GENERAL MEASURES
- Consider circumcision for recurrent balanitis and paraphimosis.
- Warm compresses or sitz baths
- Local hygiene

MEDICATION
- Balanitis:
  - Allergic/irritant:
    ◦ Hydrocortisone 1% BID
  - Antifungal:
    ◦ Clotrimazole (Lotrimin) 1% BID
    ◦ Nystatin (Mycostatin) BID–QID
    ◦ Fluconazole: 150 mg PO single dose
  - Antibacterial:
    ◦ Bacitracin QID
    ◦ Neomycin–polymyxin B–bacitracin (Neosporin) QID
    ◦ If cellulitis, cephalosporin or sulfa drug PO or parenteral:
      ▪ Dermatitis: topical steroids QID
      ▪ Zoon balanitis: topical steroids QID
- Phimosis:
  - 0.05% fluticasone propionate daily for 4 to 8 weeks with gradual traction placed on foreskin
  - 1% pimecrolimus BID for 4 to 6 weeks; not for use in children <2 years
- Paraphimosis:
  - Manual reduction, if possible (should be done with the patient sedated). Place the middle and index fingers of both hands on the engorged skin proximal to the glans. Place both thumbs on glans and, with gentle pressure, push on the glans and pull on the foreskin to attempt reduction. If unsuccessful, a dorsal slit will be necessary, with eventual circumcision after the edema resolves.

- Osmotic agents: granulated sugar placed on edematous tissue for several hours to reduce edema
- Puncture technique: Multiple punctures of foreskin with a 21-gauge needle will allow edematous fluid to escape and thus allow reduction.
- Dorsal slit; done by surgeon or urologist
- BXO:
  - 0.05% betamethasone BID
  - 0.1% tacrolimus BID

ISSUES FOR REFERRAL
Recurrent infections or development of meatal stenosis

SURGERY/OTHER PROCEDURES
- Balanitis and phimosis: Consider circumcision as preventive measure.
- For paraphimosis:
  - Represents a true surgical emergency to avoid necrosis of glans
  - Dorsal slit with delayed circumcision, if reduction is not possible
  - Operative exploration if the possibility of penile tourniquet syndrome cannot be eliminated. Hair removal cream can be applied if a hair is thought to be the cause of the tourniquet.

ADMISSION, INPATIENT, AND NURSING CONSIDERATIONS
- Admission criteria/initial stabilization
  - Uncontrolled diabetes
  - Sepsis
- Appropriate hygiene if condom catheters are used
- Discharge upon resolution of problem

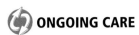 # ONGOING CARE

FOLLOW-UP RECOMMENDATIONS
Patient Monitoring
Balanitis:
- Every 1 to 2 weeks until etiology has been established
- Persistent balanitis may require biopsy to rule out malignancy or BXO.
- Evaluation for resolution of phimosis

DIET
Weight reduction, if obese

PATIENT EDUCATION
- Need for appropriate hygiene
- Appropriate foreskin care
- Avoidance of known allergens such as soaps
- No sexual activity for 2 to 3 weeks after circumcision

PROGNOSIS
Should resolve with appropriate treatment

COMPLICATIONS
- Meatal stenosis
- Premalignant changes from chronic irritation
- UTIs
- Acquired phimosis
- Unreducible paraphimosis can lead to gangrene.
- Posthitis (inflammation of the prepuce)

REFERENCES

1. Oster J. Further fate of the foreskin. Incidence of preputial adhesions, phimosis, and smegma among Danish schoolboys. *Arch Dis Child*. 1968;43(228):200–203.
2. Mcgregor TB, Pike JG, Leonard MP. Pathologic and physiologic phimosis: approach to the phimotic foreskin. *Can Fam Physician*. 2007;53(3):445–448.

 ## SEE ALSO

Reactive Arthritis (Reiter Syndrome)

 ## CODES

ICD10
- N48.1 Balanitis
- N47.1 Phimosis
- N48.0 Leukoplakia of penis

CLINICAL PEARLS
- Balanitis is an inflammation of the glans penis. Posthitis is an inflammation of the foreskin. BXO is lichen sclerosus of the glans penis.
- With recurrent infections and a plaque, a biopsy should be done to rule out BXO or malignancy.
- If there is a true phimosis that interferes with appropriate hygiene, treat the phimosis with steroids or circumcision.

BARRETT ESOPHAGUS

Daniel J. Stein, MD, MPH

BASICS

DESCRIPTION
- Metaplasia of the distal esophageal mucosa from native stratified squamous epithelium to abnormal columnar (intestinalized) epithelium; likely a consequence of chronic GERD
- Predisposes to the development of adenocarcinoma of the esophagus

EPIDEMIOLOGY
- Predominant age >50 years, more common in men
- Estimated to be present in 1–2% of adult population
- Very rare in pediatric population

Incidence
- 10–15% of patients undergoing endoscopy for evaluation of reflux symptoms
- Incidence of esophageal adenocarcinoma (EAC) is rising in the United States (1); 6-fold increase (to 2.5 cases per 100,000) since 1970s
- Annual incidence of adenocarcinoma in all Barrett patients estimated at 0.5% per year
- Attributed to changes in smoking and obesity rather than reclassification or overdiagnosis

Prevalence
Difficult to ascertain, may be as many as 1.5 to 2 million adults in the United States (extrapolated from a 1.6% prevalence in Swedish general population)

ETIOLOGY AND PATHOPHYSIOLOGY
- Chronic gastric reflux injures the esophageal mucosa, triggering columnar metaplasia. Refluxed bile acids likely induce differentiation in gastroesophageal junction (GEJ) cells.
- Columnar cells in the esophagus have higher malignant potential than squamous cells. Activation of *CDX2* gene and overexpression of HER2/neu (ERBB2) oncogene promotes carcinogenesis.
- Elevated levels of COX-2, a mediator of inflammation and regulator of epithelial cell growth, are associated with Barrett esophagus (BE) (1).
- Classic progression: normal epithelium → esophagitis/reflux exposure → metaplasia (BE) → dysplasia (low → high-grade) → adenocarcinoma

Genetics
- Familial predisposition to GERD and BE with multiple genetic markers have been identified.
- Acquired genetic changes lead to adenocarcinoma and are being investigated as biomarkers for risk stratification and early detection.

RISK FACTORS
- Chronic reflux (>5 years)
- Hiatal hernia
- Age >50 years
- Male gender
- White ethnicity—incidence in white males is much higher than white women and African American men
- Smoking history
- Intra-abdominal obesity
- Family history—at least one first-degree relative with BE or EAC

GENERAL PREVENTION
Weight loss, smoking cessation, robust intake of fruits and vegetables, and moderate wine consumption may decrease risk of BE and lower progression to esophageal cancer (1)[C].

COMMONLY ASSOCIATED CONDITIONS
GERD, obesity, hiatal hernia

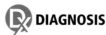

DIAGNOSIS

HISTORY
- Assess underlying risk factors.
- Common GERD symptoms: heartburn, regurgitation
- Atypical symptoms include chest pain, odynophagia, chronic cough, water brash, globus sensation, laryngitis, or wheezing.
- Symptoms suggestive of complicated GERD or cancer include weight loss, anorexia, dysphagia, odynophagia, hematemesis, or melena.

ALERT
BE is not by itself symptomatic; up to 50% of EAC and BE patients do not report GERD.

PHYSICAL EXAM
- No findings on physical exam are specific for BE.
- Findings similar to GERD

DIFFERENTIAL DIAGNOSIS
- Erosive esophagitis
- Uncomplicated GERD
- Hiatal hernia

DIAGNOSTIC TESTS & INTERPRETATION
Endoscopy with multiple biopsies demonstrating intestinal metaplasia extending ≥1 cm proximal to the GEJ is required to diagnose BE.
- Gastric cardia–type epithelium on pathology does not have clear malignant significance and may reflect sampling error.
- Specialized intestinal metaplasia at the GEJ: unclear significance, cancer risk difficult to assess with varying definitions of GEJ landmarks

ALERT
- Endoscopic screening is controversial and has not been prospectively studied. Consider screening men with chronic GERD (>5 years) and/or frequent GERD symptoms with two or more risk factors: age >50 years, white ethnicity, central obesity, smoking history, family history of BE or EAC (ACG), or patients with multiple risk factors (1),(2)[B].
- Screening for BE in the general population with GERD is *not* routinely recommended (1),(2)[C].

Initial Tests (lab, imaging)
None
- *Helicobacter pylori* testing is *not* indicated. Meta-analyses show an inverse relationship between *H. pylori* infections and BE, which may be related to decreased acid production.
- No current biomarkers are effective for diagnosis; some under investigation for risk stratification (1)[B]

Diagnostic Procedures/Other
- Endoscopy: Visual identification of columnar epithelium (reddish, velvety appearance) replacing squamous epithelium (pale, glossy appearance) of the distal esophagus is standard for diagnosis/monitoring.
- Biopsies are needed to confirm the diagnosis.
- Classify disease extent: long segment (≥3 cm) versus short segment (<3 cm).

- The Prague grading system used to describe BE using the squamocolumnar junction and GEJ. "C" represents circumferential extent of the columnar changes. "M" indicates the maximal proximal extent of columnar mucosa.
- Advanced imaging techniques, such as narrow band imaging (NBI) and confocal laser endomicroscopy (not in routine use), may help identify dysplasia.
- Consider brush cytology with wide-area transepithelial sampling increases detection of dysplasia (3)[A].
- Systematic endoscopic biopsies confirm diagnosis:
  - Seattle protocol: four-quadrant biopsies at regular intervals with biopsies of visible mucosal irregularities; more time-consuming but higher diagnostic yield than random biopsies (1)[A]
  - Capsule endoscopy has lower sensitivity than conventional endoscopy.

Test Interpretation
- Specialized intestinal metaplasia (also called specialized columnar epithelium) is diagnostic (4)[C].
- Diagnosis of dysplasia (and grade) should be confirmed by two gastrointestinal pathologists before treatment. Benign BE is established by a single pathologist report (4)[C].
- Cardia-type columnar epithelium may predispose to malignancy (unclear risk); International Consensus Group recommends defining BE by the presence of columnar mucosa in the esophagus (noting if intestinal metaplasia is present) (4)[C].
- If screening endoscopy reveals erosive esophagitis, repeat endoscopy after 8 to 12 weeks of proton pump inhibitor (PPI) therapy to exclude underlying BE; defer biopsies until healing occurs (2)[C].

TREATMENT

MEDICATION
- The goal of medical therapy is to control GERD and reduce esophagitis.
- Neither suppression of gastric acid production via high-dose PPIs nor reduction in esophageal acid exposure via antireflux surgery induces regression of BE. These therapies may, however, decrease progression/cancer risk (1)[A],(5)[B].

First Line
- Unlike the stepwise management of GERD without evidence of BE, all patients with BE should be treated with a daily PPI.
- Dose PPIs 30 to 60 minutes before a meal (ideally, the first meal of the day).
- Patients should remain on lifetime PPI therapy. If GERD symptoms were initially present, PPI should be increased until symptoms are controlled (2)[A].

ALERT
Titrate PPI therapy to symptoms; routine pH monitoring is *not* recommended (1)[C]. In patients with symptoms uncontrolled on PPI, manage according to current standards for treatment of uncontrolled GERD.

ISSUES FOR REFERRAL
- Most patients with low-grade dysplasia (except those who do not desire intervention) and all those with high-grade dysplasia or intramucosal carcinoma should be referred for endoscopic eradication of their Barrett.

- Initiate PPI therapy prior to endoscopy to reduce reactive esophagitis/atypia (2)[C].
- Refer patients considering esophagectomy (rare) to a high-volume institution.

ADDITIONAL THERAPIES

- Aspirin combined with high-dose twice-daily PPI may reduce progression to dysplasia (not yet routinely recommended).
  - COX-2 selective inhibitor celecoxib use not shown to affect progression of Barrett dysplasia to adenocarcinoma (1)[A]
  - Consider low-dose aspirin in patients with BE and risk factors for cardiovascular disease (1)[C].
- Statins, alone or in combination with aspirin or NSAIDs, may be effective in chemoprevention but are not yet routinely recommended (1)[B].
- No dysplasia: No other therapy is generally indicated; continue regular surveillance assuming good overall patient health (3)[C],(4).
- Treatment of dysplasia:
  - Low-grade dysplasia: Refer for consideration of endoscopic therapy (usually radiofrequency ablation or cryotherapy) to reduce the risk of progression to adenocarcinoma (3)[C],(4).
  - High grade dysplasia: Refer for endoscopic mucosal resection and/or endoscopic therapy to prevent progression to adenocarcinoma unless unable to tolerate the procedure (3)[C],(4).
  - Intramucosal carcinoma: endoscopic resection if possible, followed by ablation of remaining Barrett, with surgery as a backup (6)[C]
  - More advanced carcinoma: Refer to oncology and surgery to discuss resection.
  - Indeterminate grade dysplasia should have a re-evaluation with biopsies on increased PPI dosage.
  - Endoscopic eradication is successful in >90% of patients but often requires multiple sessions and can be associated with complications (3).
  - Patients with prior ablation need ongoing surveillance for recurrence.

ALERT

Endoscopic eradication not recommended for most BE without dysplasia; therapy should be individualized. Continue surveillance in these patients.

SURGERY/OTHER PROCEDURES

Antireflux surgery such as fundoplication may control GERD symptoms but have not been shown to reverse BE, decrease risk of cancer, or be superior to medical therapy (1)[A].

ALERT

Antireflux surgery does not appear to decrease risk of esophageal cancer.

- Esophagectomy is definitive but should only be considered after failure of minimally invasive endoscopic eradication therapy for high-grade dysplasia (1)[B]. Morbidity and mortality are higher than with endoscopic treatment.
  - Preferred for patients with evidence of submucosal invasion (stage T1SM2 or higher) or T1a patients with poor differentiation, lymphovascular invasion, or incomplete endoscopic mucosal resection
  - Added benefit of lymph node removal
  - Mortality rate: <5% in patients with high-grade dysplasia who are otherwise healthy
  - Serious postoperative complications: 30–50%
  - Should ideally be performed by an experienced surgeon in a high-volume center (1)[A]

COMPLEMENTARY & ALTERNATIVE MEDICINE

A prospective study of 339 men and women with BE found those taking either a multivitamin, vitamin C, or vitamin E once a day were less likely to develop EAC.

Geriatric Considerations

Surveillance or no treatment may be preferable to endoscopic eradication therapy or esophagectomy in patients who are poor operative candidates. Discontinue surveillance in patients who are not candidates for treatment.

 ONGOING CARE

FOLLOW-UP RECOMMENDATIONS

- Surveillance (to detect high-grade dysplasia or early carcinoma), although controversial, is recommended in patients with histologically confirmed BE, especially for those in high-risk groups.
- Surveillance intervals depend on grade of dysplasia (1)[C].
- Patients diagnosed with BE on initial exam do not require endoscopy in 1 year (2)[C].
- No dysplasia: Survey every 3 to 5 years.
  - Discontinue surveillance if life expectancy is ≤5 years (4)[C].
- Low-grade dysplasia not planning for ablation: Survey every 6 to 12 months (2),(3)[C],(4).
  - Routine surveillance if patients have confirmed absence of low-grade dysplasia after two consecutive endoscopies (4)[C]
- Indefinite for dysplasia: Repeat after 3 to 6 months of increased acid suppression, and if unchanged, survey every 12 months (4)[C].
- High-grade dysplasia without eradication therapy: Survey every 3 months. With eradication therapy: Survey every 3 months for 4, then every 6 months twice, and then every 12 months (1),(2)[C].

ALERT

Adherence to recommended surveillance protocols may improve rates of dysplasia and cancer detection.

- Continue surveillance even if the patient has had endoscopic ablation therapy, antireflux surgery, or esophagectomy.

DIET

Avoid foods that trigger reflux: caffeine, alcohol, chocolate, peppermint, carbonated drinks, garlic, onions, spicy foods, fatty foods, citrus, and tomato-based products.

PATIENT EDUCATION

- Lifestyle modifications: smoking cessation, weight loss, avoid supine position after meals, avoid tight-fitting clothes, elevate head of bed
- No evidence that treating GERD reverses BE or necessarily prevents esophageal cancer

PROGNOSIS

Annual incidence of esophageal cancer in patients with BE is estimated 0.12–0.6% per year:

- Low-grade dysplasia: may be transient; cancer risk 0.7–0.8% per year (3)
- High-grade dysplasia: cancer risk 5–9% per year (2),(3)
- Promising areas for research include the use of biomarkers for risk stratification, chemoprevention of neoplastic progression, capsule endoscopy for screening, and the use of vitamins and antioxidants for prevention and treatment.

COMPLICATIONS

Same as GERD: stricture, bleeding, ulceration

REFERENCES

1. Spechler SJ, Sharma P, Souza RF, et al; for American Gastroenterological Association. American Gastroenterological Association medical position statement on the management of Barrett's esophagus. *Gastroenterology*. 2011;140(3):1084–1091.
2. Shaheen NJ, Falk GW, Iyer PG, et al. ACG clinical guideline: diagnosis and management of Barrett's esophagus. *Am J Gastroenterol*. 2016;111(1): 30–50.
3. Qumseya B, Sultan S, Bain P, et al; for Standards of Practice Committee of the American Society for Gastrointestinal Endoscopy. ASGE Guideline on screening and surveillance of Barrett's esophagus. *Gastrointest Endosc*. 2019;90(3):335–359.
4. Bennett C, Moayyedi P, Corley DA, et al; for BOB CAT Consortium. BOB CAT: a large-scale review and Delphi consensus for management of Barrett's esophagus with no dysplasia, indefinite for, or low-grade dysplasia. *Am J Gastroenterol*. 2015;110(5):662–682.
5. Singh S, Garg SK, Singh PP, et al. Acid-suppressive medications and risk of oesophageal adenocarcinoma in patients with Barrett's oesophagus: a systematic review and meta-analysis. *Gut*. 2014;63(8):1229–1237.
6. Wani S, Qumseya B, Sultan S, et al; for Standards of Practice Committee. Endoscopic eradication therapy for patients with Barrett's esophagus–associated dysplasia and intramucosal cancer. *Gastrointest Endosc*. 2018;87(4):907–931.e9.

ADDITIONAL READING

- Dunbar KB, Spechler SJ. Controversies in Barrett esophagus. *Mayo Clin Proc*. 2014;89(7):973–984.
- Zimmerman TG. Common questions about Barrett esophagus. *Am Fam Physician*. 2014;89(2):92–98.

CODES

ICD10

- K22.70 Barrett's esophagus without dysplasia
- K22.719 Barrett's esophagus with dysplasia, unspecified
- K22.710 Barrett's esophagus with low grade dysplasia

CLINICAL PEARLS

- The incidence of esophageal cancer is rising faster than any other major malignancy. BE is a precursor to esophageal carcinoma.
- The highest incidence of BE is in white males >50 years of age.
- Patients with BE should be on PPI therapy.
- Endoscopic eradication therapy is preferred for dysplasia with or without submucosal invasion.
- Esophagectomy is generally limited to patients with invasive carcinoma or those failing to respond to endoscopic therapy.

BASAL CELL CARCINOMA
Karl T. Clebak, MD, MHA, FAAFP • Jana W. Qiao, MD

BASICS

DESCRIPTION
Basal cell carcinoma (BCC) is the most common type of skin cancer, originating from the basal cell layer of the skin appendages.
- Rarely metastasizes but is locally invasive and capable of local tissue destruction and disfigurement

EPIDEMIOLOGY
Most common cancer in Europe, Australia, and the United States. The most common type of skin cancer.

Incidence
- Over 2 million new cases each year in the United States; 2.5 times more common than squamous cell carcinoma (SCC)
- Highest incidence in the world is in Australia.
- White individuals have a 1 in 5 chance of developing BCC during their lifetime.
- Most common skin cancer in Asian and Hispanic individuals; second most common skin cancer in African American/black individuals (1)
- Predominant age: generally >60 years
- Predominant sex: male > female (2:1 ratio)

Prevalence
Not well established

ETIOLOGY AND PATHOPHYSIOLOGY
UV radiation induces inflammation and cyclooxygenase activation in the skin.

Genetics
Several genetic conditions increase the risk of developing BCC:
- Albinism (recessive alleles)
- Xeroderma pigmentosum (autosomal recessive)
- Bazex-Dupré-Christol syndrome (rare, X-linked dominant)
- Nevoid BCC syndrome/Gorlin syndrome (rare, autosomal dominant)
- Cytochrome P450 CYP2D6 and glutathione S-transferase detoxifying enzyme gene mutations (especially in truncal BCC, marked by clusters of BCCs and a younger age of onset)
- Mutations in the tumor suppressor gene patched, or activated mutations in smoothened, resulting in upregulation of hedgehog pathway signaling

RISK FACTORS
- Chronic sun exposure (UV radiation); increased susceptibility in the following phenotypes:
  - Light complexion: skin type I (burns but does not tan) and skin type II (usually burns sometimes tans)
  - Red or blond hair
  - Blue or green eyes
- Tendency to sunburn
- Male sex, although increasing risk in women due to lifestyle changes, such as tanning beds
- Previous history of nonmelanoma skin cancer
- Family history of skin cancer
- Chronic immunosuppression: transplant recipients (5 to 10 times higher incidence), patients with HIV (2 times higher incidence), or lymphomas
- Arsenic exposure
- Immunosuppression
- UV radiation and/or use of tanning devices
- Xeroderma pigmentosum

GENERAL PREVENTION
- Use broad-spectrum sunscreens of at least SPF 30 daily and reapply after swimming or sweating.
- Avoid overexposure to the sun. Avoid tanning beds.
- The USPSTF concludes that the current evidence is insufficient to assess the balance of benefits and harms of visual skin examination by a clinician to screen for skin cancer in adults. The American Cancer Society recommends cancer-related checkups every 3 years in patients 20 to 39 years old and yearly in patients ≥40 years.

COMMONLY ASSOCIATED CONDITIONS
- Cosmetic disfigurement (head and neck most often affected)
- Loss of vision with orbital involvement
- Loss of nerve function due to perineural spread or extensive and deep invasion
- Ulcerating neoplasms are prone to infections.

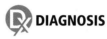

DIAGNOSIS

HISTORY
- Exposure to risk factors, family history of skin cancer
- History of a growing, ulcerating, or bleeding skin lesion often in a sun-exposed area

PHYSICAL EXAM
- 80% on face and neck, 20% on trunk and lower limbs
- Nodular: most common (50–80%); presents as pinkish, pearly papule, plaque, or nodule, often with telangiectatic vessels, ulceration, and a rolled periphery, usually on the head or neck
- Pigmented: presents as a translucent papule with "floating pigment"; more commonly seen in darker skin types; may give a blue, brown, or black appearance and be confused with melanoma (2)
- Superficial: 10–30%; light red, scaly plaque resembling eczema or psoriasis but with thin, rolled borders and central clearing, usually on trunk or extremities; least invasive of BCC subtypes (2)
- Morpheaform (sclerosing): 5–10%; resembles scar-like waxy plaque with poorly defined borders, occasionally with ulceration; most common on head or neck (2)

DIFFERENTIAL DIAGNOSIS
- SCC
- Sebaceous hyperplasia
- Epidermal inclusion cyst
- Intradermal nevi (pigmented and nonpigmented)
- Molluscum contagiosum
- Actinic keratosis
- Nummular dermatitis
- Psoriasis
- Melanoma (pigmented lesions)
- Atypical fibroxanthoma
- Fibrous papule
- Keratoacanthoma

DIAGNOSTIC TESTS & INTERPRETATION
Initial Tests (lab, imaging)
- Biopsy is necessary to confirm the diagnosis.
- Dermoscopy may improve diagnostic accuracy of BCCs.

Diagnostic Procedures/Other
- Clinical diagnosis and histologic subtype are confirmed through skin biopsy and pathologic examination.
- Shave biopsy is typically sufficient and used for nodular lesions. For flat lesions, punch biopsy or a shave biopsy with a scoop technique allows for the assessment of depth of tumor and perineural invasion.

Test Interpretation
- Nodular BCC
  - Extending from the epidermis are nodular aggregates of basaloid cells.
  - Tumor cells are uniform; rarely have mitotic figures; large, oval, hyperchromatic nuclei with little cytoplasm, surrounded by a peripheral palisade
  - Increased mucin in dermal stroma
- Superficial BCC
  - Appear as buds of basaloid cells attached to undersurface of epidermis
  - Peripheral palisading
- Morpheaform BCC
  - Thin cords and strands of basaloid cells; embedded in dense, fibrous, scar-like stroma
  - Less peripheral palisading and retraction, greater subclinical involvement
- Infiltrating BCC
  - Like morpheaform BCC but no scar-like stroma and thicker, spiky, irregular strands
  - Less peripheral palisading and retraction, greater subclinical involvement
- Micronodular BCC
  - Small, nodular aggregates of tumor cells
  - Less retraction artifact and higher subclinical involvement than nodular BCC

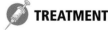

TREATMENT

GENERAL MEASURES
The National Comprehensive Cancer Network (NCCN) recommendations outline the following approaches:
- Low-risk BCC: curettage and electrodesiccation, standard excision, radiation therapy
- High-risk BCC: standard excision, Mohs surgery, radiation therapy

MEDICATION
- May be especially useful in those who cannot tolerate surgical procedures, who refuse to have surgery, and who have low-risk superficial and/or nodular BCC
  - 5-Fluorouracil (5-FU) cream inhibits thymidylate synthetase, interrupting DNA synthesis for superficial lesions in low-risk areas; primary treatment only; 5% applied BID for 3 to 10 weeks
  - Imiquimod (Aldara) cream approved for treatment of low-risk superficial BCC; daily dosing for 6 to 12 weeks; 80% clearance rate (3)[A]

- Emerging therapies:
  - Vismodegib, a sonic hedgehog pathway inhibitor; for patients with advanced BCC failing other options; also beneficial for multiple BCC and BCC nevus syndrome
  - Intralesional injection: Efficacy for small (<1 cm) nodular and superficial BCCs varies from 67% to 94% based on the type of agent used (3)[C]. Ingenol mebutate: from the plant *Euphorbia peplus*; in one trial, 63% of lesions, significant histologic cure rates were seen 85 days after treatment.
  - Laser therapy: Evidence for monotherapy is currently lacking in randomized controlled trials, but anecdotal evidence supports treatment for superficial BCC; one retrospective study with superpulsed carbon dioxide therapy for superficial and nodular BCC showed no recurrence in 3-year follow-up (3)[B].

First Line
Typically surgical excision (see "Surgery/Other Procedures")

ADDITIONAL THERAPIES
- Radiation therapy
  - Useful for patients, typically older (>60 years), who cannot not undergo surgery and for unresectable tumors
  - Used following surgery as adjuvant therapy, particularly if margins of tumor were not cleared
  - Cure rate is ~90%.
  - Recurrence rates are 4–16%.
- Photodynamic therapy (PDT)
  - PDT uses photosensitizing agents (injected or topical) which becomes accumulated in the target cells.
  - Methyl aminolevulinate and 5-aminolevulinic acid, photosensitizers, are activated by specific wavelengths of light that destroy local tissue.
  - Currently approved in Canada, Europe, Australia, and New Zealand; off-label treatment for BCC in the United States

SURGERY/OTHER PROCEDURES
- Surgical excision is first-line treatment; specific treatment selection varies with extent and location of lesion as well as tumor border demarcation.
- High-risk areas
  - Inner canthus, nasolabial sulcus, philtrum, preauricular area, retroauricular sulcus, lip, temple, "mask areas" of the face
- Curettage and electrodesiccation
  - If nodular lesion <1 cm, in low-risk area, not deeply invasive
  - Avoid in the hair-bearing areas due to risk of the tumor extending down follicular structures.
  - 5-year cure rate of 91–97%; recurrence as high as 27% for high-risk lesions (3)
  - Pathology sample sent at time of curettage and electrodesiccation to ensure absence of high-risk pathology
- Excision with postoperative margin assessment
  - Treatment of choice for low-risk lesions <2 cm in diameter
  - Goal is 4-mm margin.

- 5-year cure rate of 98%
- Cryosurgery
  - Reserved for nodular and superficial BCC, not indicated for tumors with depth exceeding 3 mm
  - Contraindicated in hair-bearing areas and over the lower extremities (3)
  - Typically for tumors with low risk of recurrence
  - Mean recurrence rates range from 0% to 39% across different studies.
- Mohs surgery
  - Surgical procedure where thin layers of the tumor are progressively removed and examined to determine tumor boarder, allowing only cancer-free tissue to remain
  - Preferred microsurgically controlled surgical treatment for lesions in high-risk areas, recurrent lesions, and lesions exhibiting an aggressive growth pattern
  - 5-year recurrence rates up to 10.1% in primary BCC, 17.4% in recurrent BCC
  - Requires referral to appropriately trained dermatologic surgeon

COMPLEMENTARY & ALTERNATIVE MEDICINE
In patients with a previous nonmelanoma skin cancer, β-carotene has not been shown to reduce the incidence of new skin cancers.

ADMISSION, INPATIENT, AND NURSING CONSIDERATIONS
Outpatient, unless extensive lesion

 ONGOING CARE

FOLLOW-UP RECOMMENDATIONS
- Seek shade, especially between 10 AM and 4 PM.
- Oral retinoids may prevent the development of new BCCs in patients with Gorlin syndrome, renal transplant recipients, and patients with severe actinic damage.

Patient Monitoring
- Every 6 to 12 months for first 2 to 5 years and then annually for life. If no recurrence within the first 2 years, decreased frequency of monitoring can be considered.
- Increased risk of other skin cancers
- Recurrence:
  - Local: Follow NCCN 2021 guidelines for primary treatment.
  - Regional: surgery and/or radiation therapy
  - Metastatic: multidisciplinary tumor board consultation

PATIENT EDUCATION
- Monthly skin self-exam
- Educate patients concerning adequate vitamin D intake. Use broad-spectrum UVA/UVB sunscreen SPF ≥15.
- Keep newborns out of the sun. Apply sunscreen to babies ≥6.

PROGNOSIS
- Proper treatment yields 90–95% cure.
- Most recurrences happen within 5 years. BCCs that develop in the head or neck area have a higher risk of recurring.
- Development of new BCCs: Many patients (30–50%) will develop a new lesion within 5 year.

COMPLICATIONS
- Recurrence rates > 5 years postoperatively are up to 56% in primary BCC, 14% in recurrent BCC; long-term follow-up in high-risk tumors is indicated.
- Usually, recurrences will appear within 5 years.
- Metastasis: rare (<0.1%) but metastatic disease usually fatal within 8 months
  - Head and neck location, depth, tumor diameter > 4cm are risk factors for metastasis and death.

REFERENCES
1. Hogue L, Harvey VM. Basal cell carcinoma, squamous cell carcinoma, and cutaneous melanoma in skin of color patients. *Dermatol Clin*. 2019;37(4):519–526.
2. Cameron MC, Lee E, Hibler BP, et al. Basal cell carcinoma: epidemiology; pathophysiology; clinical and histological subtypes; and disease associations. *J Am Acad Dermatol*. 2019;80(2):303–317.
3. Cameron MC, Lee E, Hibler BP, et al. Basal cell carcinoma: contemporary approaches to diagnosis, treatment, and prevention. *J Am Acad Dermatol*. 2019;80(2):321–339.

ADDITIONAL READING
Dzubow L, Goldberg LH, Lebwohl M, et al. *Basal Cell Carcinoma Prevention Guidelines*. New York, NY: The Skin Cancer Foundation; 2021. http://www.skincancer.org/skin-cancer-information/basal-cell-carcinoma/bcc-prevention-guidelines. Accessed October 13, 2021.

CODES

ICD10
- C44.711 Basal cell carcinoma of skin of unspecified lower limb, including hip
- C44.51 Basal cell carcinoma of skin of trunk
- C44.61 Basal cell carcinoma of skin of upper limb, including shoulder

CLINICAL PEARLS
- BCC is the most common cancer and skin malignancy, originating from the basal cell layer of the skin appendages.
- Chronic sun exposure and fair skin type increase risk with 80% on face and neck.
- Nodular type most common; telangiectasia seen at the borders

BED BUGS
Fawn J. Winkelman, DO • Adam Strosberg, DNP, ARNP-BC

BASICS

DESCRIPTION
- Nocturnal obligate blood parasites residing in furniture and bedding
- 5 to 7 mm oval, reddish brown, flat, wingless morphology
- Microscopic evidence suggests a mature bed bug *Cimex lectularius* is approximately the size of an apple seed (1).

EPIDEMIOLOGY
Incidence
- Bed bug infestations are increasing in incidence and becoming more difficult to treat (2).
- Resurgence due to changes in pesticide, increased travel, use of secondhand furniture, and high turnover rates of hotel guests

Prevalence
- Infestations have increased by 10–30% across the United States (1) in public places (schools, hospitals, hotels/motels, aircraft) over the past decade (3).
- The global population of bed bugs (*C. lectularius* and *Cimex hemipterus*, family Cimicidae) has undergone a significant resurgence since the late 1990s. This is likely due to an increase in global travel, trade, and the number of insecticide-resistant bed bugs. The global bed bug population is estimated to be increasing by 100–500% annually (4). It will be interesting to see what (if any) impact the COVID-19 travel restrictions have on the incidence of infestation.
- There are over 75 species of Insecta: Hemiptera: Cimicidae ("bed bugs") with the two genera and species implicated in human infestations being *C. lectularius* and *C. hemipterus* (1).
- *C. lectularius* lives in urban environments and *C. hemipterus* lives in tropical climates.

ETIOLOGY AND PATHOPHYSIOLOGY
- Insect family Cimicidae
- Three species bite humans: *C. lectularius*, *C. hemipterus*, and *Leptocimex boueti* (3)[B].
- Most prevalent species is *C. lectularius* (3)[B]
- Found in tropical and temperate climates
- Hide in crevices of mattresses, box springs, headboards, and baseboards
- Infestations occur in hotels/motels, hospitals, cinemas, vehicles, aircraft, and homes.
- Unlike other infestations, they are not associated with hygienic deficiencies.
- Reactions range from an absent or minimal response to the typical pruritic, erythematous maculopapular rash. Less commonly, there is an urticarial or anaphylactoid response.
- Skin reactions are due to host immunologic response to parasite salivary proteins.
- Urticarial reactions are mediated via immunoglobulin (Ig) G antibody response to salivary proteins (5)[B].
- Bullous reactions caused by an IgE-mediated hypersensitivity to nitrophorin in bug saliva (5)[B].
- Bugs are attracted to body warmth and exhaled carbon dioxide (6).
- Bites do not transmit other known pathogens.

RISK FACTORS
- Immunocompromised
- High hotel turnover
- Secondhand furniture in home

GENERAL PREVENTION
- Traps typically use carbon dioxide and heat to attract and trap bugs but can be cost prohibitive (7)[B].
- Vector control: Vacuum regularly; reduce clutter; seal cracks in walls; inspect luggage and clothing.
- Launder all bedding and clothing in >130°F (50°C) for 2 hours or place in 20°F (−5°C) or cooler environment for at least 5 days.
- If present in the home, eradicate using professional extermination services. Some pest control companies use canines to detect live bed bugs and eggs based on pheromones from the bed bugs (7)[B].

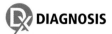

DIAGNOSIS

HISTORY
- Recent travel
- Bed bug sighting; blood specks on sheets
- New skin lesions in the morning
- Intense pruritus, pain, or burning

PHYSICAL EXAM
- Characteristic lesions are erythematous pruritic papules in an irregular linear pattern (1).
- Found on body surfaces exposed during sleeping such as face, neck, arms, legs, and shoulders
- May appear hours to days after being bitten
- Patients are usually asymptomatic but may present with papular urticaria, diffuse urticaria, bullous lesions, and/or anaphylactoid symptoms.

DIFFERENTIAL DIAGNOSIS
- Urticaria; insect or spider bite; scabies
- Dermatitis herpetiformis

DIAGNOSTIC TESTS & INTERPRETATION
Initial Tests (lab, imaging)
- Skin scraping with mineral oil preparation
- Skin biopsy

Test Interpretation
- Skin scraping is negative with mineral oil, which helps to exclude scabies.
- Skin biopsy shows nonspecific perivascular eosinophilic infiltrate consistent with arthropod bite reaction.

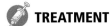 **TREATMENT**

GENERAL MEASURES

- Treatment should address three areas: treatment of the skin, eradication of the infestation, and assessment for potential behavioral health consequences (1).
- Most patients present for the treatment of skin irritation and lesions.
- Disease is self-limited and resolves within 1 to 2 weeks.
- Treat symptomatically.

MEDICATION

First Line

- Oral antihistamines (i.e., diphenhydramine, hydroxyzine)
- Topical antipruritics (i.e., pramoxine/calamine ointment or doxepin cream)
- Topical low-potency to mid-potency corticosteroids for 2 weeks (i.e., hydrocortisone, triamcinolone)
- Systemic corticosteroids (severe cases)

ADDITIONAL THERAPIES

- If secondarily infected, use topical or oral antibiotics against *Staphylococcus* and *Streptococcus* spp. (i.e., cephalexin, tetracycline, doxycycline, clindamycin, topical mupirocin).
- Epinephrine for anaphylaxis
- Professional extermination may be necessary.
- The CDC recommends a comprehensive integrated pest management program—remove clutter, seal cracks, heat treatment, vacuum, and nonchemical pesticides.
- New approaches (more research necessary) include xenointoxication (oral arthropodicidal agent) toxic to the bed bugs.

 ONGOING CARE

FOLLOW-UP RECOMMENDATIONS

- Not necessary as disease is self-limited
- May need specific care in extreme cases or if anaphylactoid reactions
- Consider behavioral health consultation depending on the severity of the patient's emotional reaction to the infestation.

PATIENT EDUCATION

- Avoid scratching to prevent superinfection.
- Inspect bedding, furniture, and luggage regularly.
- CDC: www.cdc.gov/parasites/bedbugs/
- EPA: http://www.epa.gov/bedbugs
- Myth 1: *Bed bugs are invisible.* They are nocturnal and hide during the daytime. Adult bugs are ~1/4-inch long, and eggs are the size of a pin head.
- Myth 2: *Bed bugs reproduce rapidly.* Their life cycle is 4 to 5 weeks, longer than the house fly.
- Myth 3: *Bed bugs can live without feeding.* Bugs can live 3 to 5 months without a blood meal.
- Tips to prevent and control bed bugs
  - Ensure infestation is bed bugs (not fleas, other insects, and/or ticks).
  - Regularly wash and heat dry your clothing and bedding, especially if it touches the floor.
  - EPA tips: https://www.epa.gov/bedbugs/top-ten-tips-prevent-or-control-bed-bugs

COMPLICATIONS

- Bed bug dermatitis, allergic reactions, asthma exacerbations, anaphylaxis
- Significant psychological distress (insomnia, depression, anxiety, delusional parasitosis) (5)
- Secondary bacterial infections
- Transmission of blood-borne diseases (rare)

REFERENCES

1. McNeil C, Jarrett A, Shreve M. Bed bugs: current treatment guidelines. *J Nurs Pract.* 2017;13(6):381–388.
2. Woloski JR, Burman D, Adebona O. Mite and bed bug infections. *Prim Care.* 2018;45(3):409–421.
3. Studdiford JS, Conniff KM, Trayes KP, et al. Bedbug infestation. *Am Fam Physician.* 2012;86(7):653–658.
4. Lai O, Ho D, Glick S, et al. Bed bugs and possible transmission of human pathogens: a systematic review. *Arch Dermatol Res.* 2016;308(8):531–538.
5. Williams K, Willis MS. Bedbugs in the 21st century: the reemergence of an old foe. *Lab Med.* 2012;43(5):141–148.
6. Vaidyanathan R, Feldlaufer MF. Bed bug detection: current technologies and future directions. *Am J Trop Med Hyg.* 2013;88(4):619–625.
7. Ogg B. Bed bug myths—rely on research for facts. *The Nebline.* 2012;347–348.

ADDITIONAL READING

- Lancaster Extension Education Center: http://lancaster.unl.edu/pest/bugs.shtml
- National Pesticide Information Center: http://npic.orst.edu/

 CODES

ICD10

- S00.96XA Insect bite (nonvenomous) of unspecified part of head, initial encounter
- S10.96XA Insect bite of unspecified part of neck, initial encounter
- S40.269A Insect bite (nonvenomous) of unspecified shoulder, initial encounter

CLINICAL PEARLS

- 90% of infestations occur within 3 feet of bedding.
- Wash bedding/clothing regularly in hot water and vacuum carpet daily or steam clean daily.
- Inspect furniture, bedding, and luggage regularly.
- Bed bugs are largely resistant to over-the-counter (OTC) products (permethrin, cyfluthrin, bifenthrin, and deltamethrin or fluvalinate and esfenvalerate).

BEHAVIORAL PROBLEMS, PEDIATRIC

Ginny L. Gottschalk, MD • William G. Elder, PhD

 BASICS

DESCRIPTION

Behavior that disrupts at least one area of psycho-social functioning. Commonly reported behavioral problems are as follows:

- Noncompliance: active or passive refusal to do as requested by parent or other authority figure
- Temper tantrums: loss of internal control that leads to crying, whining, breath holding, or aggressive behavior
- Sleep problems: difficulty going to sleep or staying asleep at night, nightmares, and night terrors
- Nocturnal enuresis: bed wetting that occurs in children >5 years of age for >3 months with no medical problems
  - Primary: children who have never been dry at night
  - Secondary: children dry at night for at least 6 months
  - Monosymptomatic enuresis: only have bedwetting
  - Nonmonosymptomatic enuresis: bedwetting in addition to daytime incontinence, urgency, voiding difficulties or voiding <4 or >7 times per day
- Functional encopresis: repeated involuntary fecal soiling that is not caused by organic defect or illness
- Problem eating: "picky eating," difficult mealtime behaviors
- Thumb-sucking: can be problematic if persists past eruption of primary teeth as teeth alignment may be impacted

EPIDEMIOLOGY

- Noncompliance issues: manifest as children develop autonomy; slightly more common in males; decreases with age
- Temper tantrums: 5–7% of children between 1 and 3 years of age have temper tantrums lasting at least 15 minutes three or more times per week; 20% of 2-year-olds, 18% of 3-year-olds, and 10% of 4-year-olds have at least one temper tantrum every day (1).
- Sleep problems
  - Night waking in 25–50% of infants 6 to 12 months
  - Bedtime refusal in 10–30% of toddlers
  - Nightmares in 10–50% of preschoolers; peaks between ages 6 and 10 years
  - Night terrors in 1–6.5% early childhood; peaks between ages 4 and 12 years
  - Sleepwalking frequently in 3–5%; peaks between ages 4 and 8 years (2)
- Nocturnal enuresis
  - Common, 5–10% of 7 year olds and 3% of teenagers (3) wet the bed.
- Functional encopresis: rare before age 3 years, most common in 5- to 10-year-olds; more common in boys (4)
- Problem eating: Prevalence peaks at 50% at 24 months of age; no relation to sex/ethnicity/income (5)
- Thumb-sucking: decreases with age; most children spontaneously stop between 2 and 4 years (5).

COMMONLY ASSOCIATED CONDITIONS

- Noncompliance: If excessive or aggressive, rule out depression, compulsive patterns, adjustment disorder, inappropriate discipline.
- Temper tantrums: difficult child temperament, stress, normal development
- Sleep problems: inconsistent bedtime routine or sleep schedule, stimulating bedtime environment; can be associated with hyperactive behavior, poor impulse control, and poor attention in young children. Acute or chronic anxiety is associated with insomnia. Long-acting stimulant medications may disturb sleep quality.
- Enuresis: associated with constipation, heavy snoring, sleep apnea, and psychiatric conditions such as ADHD
- Functional encopresis: enuresis, UTIs, ADHD

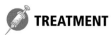 **DIAGNOSIS**

HISTORY

- Noncompliance: history from caregivers and teachers, if possible; direct observation of child or child–caregiver interaction
  - Criteria: problematic for at least some adults, leading to difficult interactions for at least 6 months
  - Reduces child's ability to take part in structured activities
  - Creates stressful relationships with compliant children
  - Disrupts academic progress; places child at risk for physical injury
- Temper tantrums: focus on development, family functioning, or violence; may consist of stiffening limbs and arching back, dropping to floor, shouting, screaming, crying, pushing/pulling, stomping, hitting, kicking, throwing, or running away (1)[C]
- Sleep disorders: Ask about sleep and bedtime routine, bedtime problems, excessive daytime sleepiness, awakenings during the night, regularity and duration of sleep, and snoring (BEARS) screen (2)[C].
- Nocturnal enuresis: onset and duration; dry overnight previously; daytime wetting or any associated genitourinary symptoms; family history of enuresis; medical and psychosocial history; constipation; sleep problems; child and caregiver's motivation for treatment; voiding diary (3)[C]
- Encopresis: fecal continence ever attained; triggering event; how often and where does child stool; pain or blood with defecation; how much stool passed accidentally; history of trauma or abuse; rectal prolapse; prior surgery (4)[C]
- Problem eating: review of child's diet, growth curves, nutritional needs, and caregiver's response to behavior (5)

PHYSICAL EXAM

- Nocturnal enuresis
- Generally normal and may not be required for treatment

- If there is concern, focus on signs of occult spinal dysraphism (3)[C].
- Functional encopresis
  - Abdominal exam for masses or tenderness; rectal exam for tone, size of rectal vault, fecal impaction, masses, fissures, hemorrhoids; back for dimpling or hair tufts (4)[C]

DIFFERENTIAL DIAGNOSIS

- Temper tantrums: language deficits or autism disruptive mood dysregulation disorder (DMDD)—distinguishable because of baseline irritable mood between outbursts and older age (6 to 18 years)
- Normal development, including

DIAGNOSTIC TESTS & INTERPRETATION

Initial Tests (lab, imaging)

- For enuresis: urinalysis to rule out UTI and glycosuria; ultrasound of the pelvis if constipation is a concern (3)[C]
- For functional encopresis: TSH for hypothyroidism or celiac disease if poor growth or family history; urinalysis and culture if enuresis or features of UTI
  - Spine imaging if evidence of spinal dysraphism or if both encopresis and daytime enuresis; barium enema if suspect Hirschsprung disease (4)[C]

Follow-Up Tests & Special Considerations

Sleep disorders: Sleep studies may be performed in children if there is a history of snoring and/or observed apnea spells to rule out obstructive sleep apnea (OSA); daytime ADHD-type symptoms may be present (2)[C].

Diagnostic Procedures/Other

- Pediatric Symptom Checklist: https://brightfutures.org/mentalhealth/pdf/professionals/ped_sympton_chklst.pdf
- National Initiative for Children's Healthcare Quality (NICHQ) Vanderbilt Assessment (ADHD screen): http://www.myadhd.com/vanderbiltparent6175.html
- Child Sexual Behavior Inventory: completed by female caregiver to assist with differentiation of normative versus abnormal behaviors particularly those related to sexual abuse: https://www.nctsn.org/measures/child-sexual-behavior-inventory

TREATMENT

GENERAL MEASURES

- Educate caregiver about specific behavioral problem.
- Parent management training programs and techniques are effective for many child behavior problems.
- Noncompliance: For extreme disobedience, consider parent training programs; may need formal screening for ADHD, obsessive-compulsive disorder (OCD), oppositional defiant disorder (ODD), or conduct disorder (CD)

- Temper tantrums: Remind caregiver this is a normal development.
  - Child is experiencing fatigue, anger, or frustration but does not have another means to cope.
  - Usually occur so child can get what they want, to avoid or escape doing something they do not want to do, or to seek parental attention
  - Identify triggers such as hunger, over tiredness, or changing activities and try to prevent tantrums.
  - Other methods for dealing with a tantrum include one of the following:
    - Ignore the tantrum; place child in time-out (1 minute for each year of age); hold/restrain child until calm; provide child with clear, firm, and consistent instructions as well as enough time to obey (1)[C].
- Sleep problems: Educate caregiver at well child checks about importance of bed routine and consistency and consistency in response to sleep disruptions. Specific recommendations may also include:
  - Graduated extinction: ignore cries for specified period; check in at increasing intervals.
  - Fading: gradual decrease in direct contact with the child as they fall asleep; goal is for the child to fall asleep independently.
  - If fearful, special routines or aromatherapy sprays may help the child feel more secure (2)[C].
- Nocturnal enuresis
- Ensure family and child know this is not caused by poor parenting skills or psychological factors.
- Regularly waking the child to void and limiting fluids are not supported by evidence.
- Nonmonosymptomatic: aggressive treatment of constipation when accompanying enuresis; generally, treat daytime symptoms first.
- Monosymptomatic: first line: enuresis alarm and desmopressin
  - Alarm: motivated family and child; used nightly; discontinue after 6 weeks if no progress; if helpful, use until 14 consecutive dry nights achieved (3)[C].
- Functional encopresis
  - First disimpaction: manually, with enemas or polyethylene glycol solution
  - Maintenance therapy: No quick fix, results take months to achieve, and relapses are common.
    - Medical: polyethylene glycol, fiber, lactulose, sorbitol, magnesium citrate
    - Behavior modification: toileting after meals for 10 minutes 2 to 3 times a day, star charts, and rewards (4)[C]
- Problem eating
  - Avoid punishment, prodding, or rewards. Offer a variety of healthy foods at every meal; limit milk to 24 oz/day and decrease juice (5)[C].
- Normative sexual behavior: no treatment needed; caregivers should not punish or admonish; gently redirect behavior when in public setting.
  - Curiosity about sex characteristics is common in children as young as 2 to 5 years old, including interest in looking at others, intruding on physical boundaries, and touching their mother's breasts. Sexual play such as "doctor" is common; 60–80% of children engage in sexual play before age 13 (6)
- Thumb-sucking: Praise children when not sucking their thumb, offer alternatives that are soothing (e.g., stuffed toys), negative reinforcement such as a bandage around or bitters on the thumb (5)

MEDICATION

Most pediatric behavioral issues respond well to nonpharmacologic therapy:

- Sleep disorders
  - Cognitive-behavioral therapy and sleep hygiene are first-line treatment; no recommended pharmacotherapy
  - After behavioral methods are exhausted, melatonin 0.5 to 10.0 mg PO can be tried in concert with behavior modification. However, this is not approved by the FDA for children (2)[C].
- Nocturnal enuresis
  - First line: Desmopressin decreases urine production. One-third are dry with med, one-third have no benefit, and one-third have intermediate response. Safe for long-term use and few side effects. Chronic polydipsia can lead to hyponatremia and is only contraindication. Give 1- to 2-week trial. Dosing: 0.2 to 0.4 mg 1 hour before bedtime
  - Second line: Anticholinergic agent (e.g., oxybutynin) works as control, not cure; oxybutynin 2.5 to 5.0 mg before bedtime
  - Third line: tricyclic antidepressants (e.g., imipramine) used by specialists (3)[C]

ISSUES FOR REFERRAL

- Tantrums that are more severe, occur after the age of 5 years, or those who exhibit self-injurious behaviors, slow recovery time from tantrums, more tantrums in the home than outside the home, or more aggressive behaviors toward others may require referral to a psychologist or psychiatrist (1)[C].
- Children with chronic insomnia or anxiety that interferes with sleep should be referred to a psychologist or psychiatrist (2)[C].
- With enuresis and OSA symptoms, refer for sleep studies because surgical correction of airway obstruction often improves or cures enuresis and daytime wetting (3)[C].
- Must distinguish sexual behavior problems: Developmentally inappropriate behaviors—greater frequency or earlier age than expected—becomes a preoccupation, recurs after adult intervention/corrective efforts. If abuse is not suspected, consider referral to a child psychologist. If abuse is suspected, must report to child protective services.
- If disimpaction by either manual or medical methods is unsuccessful, consult gastroenterology or general surgery. Patients who show no improvement after 6 months of maintenance medical therapy should be referred to gastroenterology (4)[C].
- Thumb-sucking resistant to behavioral intervention and threatening permanent dentition and bite may be evaluated by a pediatric dentist for use of habit-breaking dental appliances (5)[C].

 ONGOING CARE

DIET

Nutrition is very important in behavioral issues. Avoiding high-sugar foods and caffeine and providing balanced meals have been shown to decrease aggressive and noncompliant behaviors in children.

PATIENT EDUCATION

- See *Parent Training Programs: Insight for Practitioners* at: http://www.cdc.gov/violenceprevention/pdf/Parent_Training_Brief-a.pdf
- *The Happiest Baby Guide to Great Sleep: Simple Solutions for Kids from Birth to 5 Years.* Harvey Karp, MD. New York, HarperCollins Publishers 2012, 384 pp.

REFERENCES

1. Daniels E, Mandleco B, Luthy KE. Assessment, management, and prevention of childhood temper tantrums. *J Am Acad Nurse Pract*. 2012;24(10):569–573.
2. Bhargava S. Diagnosis and management of common sleep problems in children. *Pediatr Rev*. 2011;32(3):91–99.
3. Névéus T, Fonseca E, Franco I, et al. Management and treatment of nocturnal enuresis—an updated standardization document from the International Children's Continence Society. *J Pediatr Urol*. 2020;16(1):10–19.
4. Har AF, Croffie JM. Encopresis. *Pediatr Rev*. 2010;31(9):368–374.
5. Nasir A, Nasir L. Counseling on early childhood concerns: sleep issues, thumb-sucking, picky eating, school readiness, and oral health. *Am Fam Physician*. 2015;92(4):274–278.
6. Mesman GR, Harper SL, Edge NA, et al. Problematic sexual behavior in children. *J Pediatr Health Care*. 2019;33(3):323–331.

CODES

ICD10
- F91.9 Conduct disorder, unspecified
- F91.1 Conduct disorder, childhood-onset type
- F91.2 Conduct disorder, adolescent-onset type

CLINICAL PEARLS

- Well-child visits provide opportunities for screening for these common conditions.
- Noncompliance: In extreme disobedience, child may need to be screened for ADHD, OCD, ODD, or CD.
- Self-injurious behaviors, slow recovery time, more tantrums in the home than outside the home, or more aggressive behaviors toward others may require referral to a psychologist or psychiatrist.
- Parental education, including a review of age-appropriate discipline, is a key component of treatment.
- Temper tantrums in toddlers are common, often occurring at least one per day.

BELL PALSY

Daniel R. Matta, MD • Paul McFarlane, MBBS

BASICS

DESCRIPTION
An acute, usually unilateral peripheral facial nerve palsy. The etiology is largely idiopathic; however, many cases have been attributable to herpes simplex virus (HSV) type 1. An ischemic process involving the facial nerve has also been posited as a likely cause for Bell palsy.

EPIDEMIOLOGY
- Affects 0.002% of the population annually
- No geographic or gender predominance
- Affects all ages with a median age of onset of 40 years but with highest incidence in persons over 70 years
- Occurs with equal frequency on the left and right sides of the face

Incidence
Most population studies have shown an annual incidence of 15–30 per 100,000.

ETIOLOGY AND PATHOPHYSIOLOGY
- Inflammation of cranial nerve VII causes edema of perineurium and subsequent compression and possibly degeneration of both the nerve and the associated vasa nervorum.
- Infectious, immune, and ischemic mechanisms suggested, with activation of latent herpes virus (HSV type 1 and herpes zoster virus) in cranial nerve ganglia as the most likely infectious etiology.

RISK FACTORS
- Pregnancy, with increased risk seen in patients with chronic hypertension, maternal obesity, and severe preeclampsia
- Immunocompromised status
- Diabetes mellitus
- Age >30 years
- Upper respiratory infection
- Chronic hypertension
- Obesity

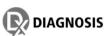

DIAGNOSIS

The diagnosis of Bell palsy is based on a thorough history and examination. Labs and diagnostic images may be considered when other differentials are probable based on history and exam.

HISTORY
- Onset: typically rapid (over 24–48 hours)
- Key features: unilateral lower motor neuron-type facial weakness, with no other neurologic or systemic signs. A patient may present for medical attention as they may complain of inability to close the eyelid or find liquids leaking from the affected side of the mouth.
- Course is progressive with peak weakness occurring at up to 3 weeks after first day of noted weakness. Symptoms may take up to several months to improve.
- Although strokes may present with facial weakness, it is not usually the presenting symptom. Furthermore, stoke lesions (affecting the ipsilateral facial nerve nucleus or facial nerve tract in the pons) that can mimic Bell palsy is rare.

- Associated symptoms:
  - Mastoid or postauricular pain
  - Hyperacusis: increased sensitivity to sounds (nerve to the stapedius muscle)
  - Dysgeusia: alteration of taste on the ipsilateral anterior 2/3 of the tongue (chorda tympani branch of the facial nerve)
  - Numbness on the ipsilateral side of the face
  - Decreased lacrimation or salivation (parasympathetic effects)
- Asking the patient about a travel history (or if they live in a Lyme endemic area) or presence of skin rashes may help to elicit a more likely cause for the patient's facial nerve weakness (such as herpes zoster, Lyme disease, or sarcoidosis).

PHYSICAL EXAM
- Neurologic
  - Flaccid paralysis of muscles on the affected side, including the forehead
    - Impaired ability to raise the ipsilateral eyebrow
    - Impaired closure of the ipsilateral eye
    - Impaired ability to smile, grin, or purse the lips
    - Bell phenomenon: upward diversion of the eye with attempted closure of the lid
- Determine if the weakness is caused by either a central (upper motor neuron) or peripheral (lower motor neuron) lesion
  - In contrast to low motor neuron lesions, the forehead muscles are usually spared in upper motor neuron lesions.
  - Patients may complain of numbness, but no deficit is present on sensory testing.
  - Subtle deficits in other cranial nerves, especially trigeminal, glossopharyngeal, and hypoglossal, may be present, but if these signs are prominent, the diagnosis of Bell palsy is doubtful.
- Head, ears, eyes, nose, and throat (HEENT)
  - Carefully examine to exclude a space-occupying lesion.
  - Perform pneumatic otoscopic exam.
- Skin: Examine for erythema migrans (Lyme disease) and vesicular rash (herpes zoster virus).

DIFFERENTIAL DIAGNOSIS
- Up to 50% of cases of peripheral facial nerve palsy may not be due to Bell palsy.
- Consider other differentials for peripheral facial nerve palsy if "red flags" below exist:
  - Gradual onset over weeks to months
  - Concomitant vertigo or hearing loss
  - Constitutional symptoms and/or cervical lymphadenopathy
  - Evidence of Lyme disease
  - Failure of improvement within 3 months or worsening of weakness over several months.
- Facial cranial nerve palsy etiologies include:
  - Congenital causes: genetic syndromes, birth-related trauma, developmental hypoplasia of facial muscles
  - Acquired causes: infective (Ramsay Hunt syndrome, Lyme, TB, HIV), inflammatory (vasculitis, sarcoidosis, autoimmune), neoplastic (benign, malignant), cerebrovascular (stroke, aneurysm), and traumatic

- Clinical approach based on facial palsy pattern (1)[B]:
  - Recurrent, ipsilateral palsy: neoplasm of the nerve (schwannoma) or adjacent structures (parotid, temporal bone, or cerebellopontine angle [CPA])
  - Bilateral palsy: neurologic (Guillain-Barré syndrome) or associated with neoplasm (lymphoma, disseminated carcinomatosis, malignant pachymeningitis); rare: cryptococcal meningitis associated with HIV, autoimmune (MS, myasthenia gravis, Sjögren), sarcoidosis, granulomatosis with polyangiitis
  - Palsy at birth: segmental developmental palsy (associated with synkinesis, recovers spontaneously)
  - Facial palsy syndromes: Ramsay-Hunt (rash in the ear [zoster oticus] and/or mouth caused by VZV); Melkersson-Rosenthal (orofacial edema, recurrent facial palsy, and fissured tongue); Heerfordt-Waldenström (parotid enlargement, anterior uveitis, facial palsy, and fever)

DIAGNOSTIC TESTS & INTERPRETATION
Bell palsy is a clinical diagnosis. It is not necessary to obtain routine lab testing or diagnostic imaging in new-onset Bell palsy (2)[C]. However, further testing may be considered in:
- Atypical presentation of facial palsy
- Recurrent facial palsy
- Slowly progressive disease >3 weeks
- Lack of improvement after 4 months

Initial Tests (lab, imaging)
- Blood glucose level
- CBC, CRP/ESR to rule out inflammatory process
- Consider rapid plasma reagin (RPR), Lyme serology, and/or HIV test if indicated.
- Consider titers for VZV, rubella, cytomegalovirus, hepatitis A, hepatitis B, and hepatitis C.
- Salivary polymerase chain reaction (PCR) for HSV-1 or herpes zoster virus (mostly for research purposes)

Follow-Up Tests & Special Considerations
- Trauma: facial radiographs to evaluate for fractures
- Contrast-enhanced CT: to evaluate for stroke or temporal bone fracture
- Gadolinium-enhanced MRI: to evaluate for brain or parotid neoplasms
- Invasive diagnostic procedures are not indicated because biopsy could further damage the nerve.

Diagnostic Procedures/Other
- Electrodiagnostic studies may be offered to patients with complete paralysis for prognostic purposes, but it does not change the management.
- Parotid gland biopsy: considered if no recovery with negative imaging at 7 months

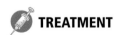

TREATMENT

GENERAL MEASURES
- Artificial tears should be used frequently to lubricate the cornea.
- The ipsilateral eye should be patched or taped shut at night to avoid drying and infection.

MEDICATION

- Recovery from Bell's palsy is possible without treatment, particularly in patients who do not have a complete palsy.
- Corticosteroids decrease inflammation and limit nerve damage, thereby increase the number of patients who make full recovery and reduce disabling sequelae (NNT = 10) (3)[A].
- Antiviral alone has no benefit over placebo (4); hence, the use of antivirals as a monotherapy in new-onset Bell palsy is not recommended (2).
- According to a 2012 Guideline from the American Academy of Neurology (AAN), for patients with new-onset Bell palsy, antivirals (in addition to steroids) might be offered to increase the probability of recovery of facial function (Level C evidence). Patients offered antivirals should be counseled that a benefit from antivirals has not been established, and, if there is a benefit, it is likely to be modest at best (4)[B].
- Corticosteroids:
  - Recommended in all Bell palsy cases (2),(5)[A]
  - Should be started within 72 hours of symptoms onset (2)[A]
  - A 10-day course of oral steroids is recommended. This may be either:
    ○ Prednisolone 50 mg PO daily for 10 days or
    ○ Prednisone 60 mg daily for 5 days and then tapering dose (by 10 mg/day) the next 5 days (3)[A].
  - Precautions: Use with discretion in patients with peptic ulcer disease and diabetes.
  - Contraindications: documented hypersensitivity, preexisting infections (TB, systemic mycosis)
- If antiviral is being used, consider valacyclovir 1,000 mg PO TID for 7 days. Acyclovir is another option, though with reduced bioavailability.
  - Precautions: Use with discretion in patients with chronic kidney disease.

Pregnancy Considerations
Steroids should be used cautiously during pregnancy; consult with an obstetrician. Acyclovir and valacyclovir are considered Category B drugs in pregnancy by the U.S. FDA.

ISSUES FOR REFERRAL
Refer to a facial nerve specialist when they experience worsening neurologic findings at any point, ocular symptoms developing at any point, or incomplete recovery at 3 months after onset of initial symptoms (2)[C].

ADDITIONAL THERAPIES
- Insufficient evidence that physical therapy combined with drug treatment has a positive effect on recovery compared with drug treatment only (2),(6)[C]
- Electrostimulation and mirror biofeedback rehabilitation have limited evidence of effect.
- Acupuncture with strong stimulation has shown some therapeutic promise but no clear recommendation.

SURGERY/OTHER PROCEDURES
- Surgical treatment of Bell palsy remains controversial and is reserved for intractable cases.
- There is insufficient evidence to decide whether surgical intervention is beneficial or harmful in the management of Bell palsy (2)[B].
- In those cases where surgical intervention is performed, cranial nerve XII is surgically decompressed at the entrance to the meatal foramen where the labyrinthine segment and geniculate ganglion reside.
- Decompression surgery should not be performed >14 days after the onset of paralysis because severe degeneration of the facial nerve is likely irreversible after 2 to 3 weeks.

 ONGOING CARE

FOLLOW-UP RECOMMENDATIONS
Patient Monitoring
- Start steroid treatment immediately and followed for 12 months.
- Patients who do not recover complete facial nerve function should be referred to ENT and/or ophthalmology specialist(s) for further management.

PATIENT EDUCATION
FamilyDoctor.org from AAFP: https://familydoctor.org/condition/bells-palsy

PROGNOSIS
- Most patients achieve complete spontaneous recovery within 2 weeks. >80% recover within 3 months.
- 85% of untreated patients will experience the first signs of recovery within 3 weeks of onset.
- 16% are left with a partial palsy, motor synkinesis, and autonomic synkinesis.
- 7% may have recurrence, which may be on the affected or opposite side.
- 5% experience severe sequelae, and a small number of patients experience permanent facial weakness and dysfunction.
- The Sunnybrook and House-Brackmann (H-B) facial grading systems are clinical prognostic models that identify Bell palsy patients at risk for nonrecovery at 12 months (7)[B].
- Poor prognostic factors include the following:
  - Age >60 years
  - History of recurrence
  - Complete facial weakness
  - Diabetes mellitus; HTN
  - House-Brackmann (H-B) grade ≤II
- Treatment with corticosteroids and the Sunnybrook score are significant factors for predicting nonrecovery at 1 month.
- Patients with no improvement or progression of symptoms should be referred to ENT (5)[A] and may require neuroimaging to rule out neoplasms (5)[A].

COMPLICATIONS
- Corneal abrasion or ulceration
- Steroid-induced hyperglycemia, psychological disturbances; avascular necrosis of the hips, knees, and/or shoulders

REFERENCES

1. Hohman MH, Hadlock TA. Etiology, diagnosis, and management of facial palsy: 2000 patients at a facial nerve center. *Laryngoscope*. 2014;124(7):E283–E293.
2. Baugh RF, Basura GJ, Ishii LE, et al. Clinical practice guideline: Bell's palsy. *Otolaryngol Head Neck Surg*. 2013;149(3 Suppl):S1–S27.
3. Madhok VB, Gagyor I, Daly F, et al. Corticosteroids for Bell's palsy (idiopathic facial paralysis). *Cochrane Database Syst Rev*. 2016;7(7):CD001942.
4. Gagyor I, Madhok VB, Daly F, et al. Antiviral treatment for Bell's palsy (idiopathic facial paralysis). *Cochrane Database Syst Rev*. 2019;9(9):CD001869
5. de Almeida JR, Guyatt GH, Sud S, et al; and Bell Palsy Working Group, Canadian Society of Otolaryngology—Head and Neck Surgery, Canadian Neurological Sciences Federation. Management of Bell palsy: clinical practice guideline. *CMAJ*. 2014;186(12):917–922.
6. Ferreira M, Marques EE, Duarte JA, et al. Physical therapy with drug treatment in Bell palsy: a focused review. *Am J Phys Med Rehabil*. 2015;94(4):331–340.
7. Kanerva M, Jonsson L, Berg T, et al. Sunnybrook and House-Brackmann systems in 5397 facial gradings. *Otolaryngol Head Neck Surg*. 2011;144(4):570–574.

ADDITIONAL READING
Reich SG. Bell's palsy. *Continuum (Minneap Minn)*. 2017;23(2, Selected Topics in Outpatient Neurology):447–466.

 SEE ALSO

Amyloidosis; Diabetes Mellitus, Type 1; Diabetes Mellitus, Type 2; Herpes Simplex; Herpes Zoster (Shingles); Lyme Disease; Sarcoidosis; Sjögren Syndrome

 CODES

ICD10
G51.0 Bell's palsy

CLINICAL PEARLS
- Look closely at the voluntary movement on the upper part of the face on the affected side; in Bell palsy, all of the muscles are involved (weak or paralyzed), whereas in a stroke, the upper muscles (forehead) are spared (because of bilateral innervation).
- No need to obtain routine labs or diagnostic imaging in a typical new-onset Bell palsy
- Initiate steroids immediately following the onset of symptoms.
- Protect the affected eye with lubrication and taping.
- In areas with endemic Lyme disease, consider Lyme until proven otherwise.

BILE ACID MALABSORPTION

Sanjiv Chopra, MBBS, MACP • Laura C. Horton, MD

BASICS

DESCRIPTION
- Bile acid malabsorption occurs when increased primary bile acids in the colon lead to chronic diarrhea and abdominal symptoms such as discomfort and bloating.
- Definitions (1)
  - Type 1: Secondary to ileal dysfunction (e.g., Crohn disease, ileal resection, or radiation injury)
  - Type 2: Idiopathic
  - Type 3: Secondary to GI disorders other than ileal dysfunction (e.g., chronic pancreatitis, postcholecystectomy, celiac disease, bacterial overgrowth, and others)
  - Type 4: Increased bile acid synthesis induced by metformin *(does not cause malabsorption but can cause similar symptoms to bile acid malabsorption due to effects of increased bile acid levels in colon)*

EPIDEMIOLOGY
Prevalence
- Overall prevalence is estimated to be approximately 1% in Western countries (1).
- Among patients with Crohn disease, with ileal resection, prevalence may be as high as 90% (1).
- Among patients with functional diarrhea or diarrhea-predominant irritable bowel syndrome (IBS-D), ~30–40% shown to have dysregulation bile acid synthesis (1)
- Bile acid malabsorption has been observed in up to 43% of patients with microscopic colitis, although data is conflicting and this was not replicated in other studies (1).
- Prevalence of type 3 and type 4 bile acid malabsorption unknown (1)

ETIOLOGY AND PATHOPHYSIOLOGY
- Primary bile acids are synthesized from cholesterol in the liver and secreted in bile after storage in the gallbladder, where they emulsify fats and play a role in micelle formation (1),(2),(3).
- ~95% of bile acids are actively absorbed in the terminal ileum via the apical sodium bile acid transporter (2).
- In the colon, secondary bile acids are formed by modification of primary bile acids by intestinal bacteria; these modifications increase passive absorption of secondary bile acids in the colon. Ultimately, a small amount of bile acids is passively reabsorbed in the colon (3).
- After reabsorption in the ileum or colon, primary and secondary bile acids return to the liver via the portal vein for reuse (2).
- Bile acid malabsorption in the ileum leads to increased levels of bile acids in the colon. There, the bile acids cause diarrhea via multiple mechanisms: stimulation of water, electrolyte, and mucus secretion; stimulation of colonic motility; alterations to microbiome (1).

Genetics
Genetic variants in proteins involved in enterohepatic circulation of bile acids may contribute to bile acid malabsorption in murine models

RISK FACTORS
- Inflammatory bowel disease (IBD), primarily Crohn disease (ileal resection or ileal disease)
- Radiation therapy associated ileitis (e.g., pelvic radiation therapy)
- Cholecystectomy
- Microscopic colitis

GENERAL PREVENTION
No specific measures for prevention

COMMONLY ASSOCIATED CONDITIONS
- Crohn disease
- Celiac disease
- IBS-D
- Functional diarrhea

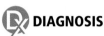

DIAGNOSIS

HISTORY
Diarrhea is the hallmark of bile acid malabsorption. Other associated symptoms include abdominal discomfort, bloating, and fecal urgency (1),(2),(3).

PHYSICAL EXAM
No specific findings on physical examination

DIFFERENTIAL DIAGNOSIS
Other causes of chronic diarrhea including IBD, celiac disease, lactase deficiency, small intestinal bacterial overgrowth, parasitic infection, lymphoma, microscopic colitis, endocrine dysfunction, and others

DIAGNOSTIC TESTS & INTERPRETATION
Diagnostic tests may detect reduced ileal bile acid absorption, reduced hepatic feedback inhibition, and/or increased hepatic bile acid synthesis.

Initial Tests (lab, imaging)
Evaluate initially for other causes of chronic watery diarrhea; nonexhaustive list below
- Upper endoscopy and colonoscopy with biopsies (Evaluate for celiac disease, IBD, microscopic colitis.)
- Stool ova and parasites, *Giardia* antigen (parasitic diseases)
- Thyroid function testing (hyperthyroidism)
- Breath test (small intestinal bacterial overgrowth)
- Complete medication reconciliation (medication-induced diarrhea)
- Hemoglobin A1c (diabetes mellitus)
- Dietary history (osmotic diarrhea, e.g., sorbitol)

Follow-Up Tests & Special Considerations

- An empiric trial of bile acid sequestrant (cholestyramine, colesevelam, or colestipol) may be considered in lieu of diagnostic testing, as many of the below tests have limited availability or are still investigational. Reported response rates to a trial of first-line cholestyramine vary; response rate up to 96% in severe bile acid malabsorption (3)
- 75SeHCAT (75-selenium homocholic acid taurine) (3)
  - Quantifies ileal reabsorption of a radiolabeled bile acid at 7 days; reduced retention may indicate type 1 bile acid malabsorption
  - Cutoffs for disease are <15% retention (mild), <10% (moderate), or <5% (severe)
  - Limited availability
- Fasting serum 7α-hydroxy-4-cholesten-3-one (C4) (1),(2),(3)
  - Serum C4 is a direct measurement of bile acid synthesis; high fasting serum C4 levels (cutoff value >48 ng/mL) may indicate reduced ileal reabsorption.
  - Commercially available through Mayo Clinic; preferred over fecal testing
- 48-hour fecal bile acid test (1)
  - Patients consume high-fat diet for 4 days, and collect stool for the last 48 hours; total and primary bile acids and fecal fat levels quantified
  - Criteria diagnostic for bile acid malabsorption: total fecal bile acids ≥2,337 μmol/48 hr, primary bile acids >10%, or total fecal bile acids ≥1,000 μmol/48 hr plus primary bile acids >4%
- Serum fasting fibroblast growth factor 19 (FGF-19) (1)
  - Inversely correlated with serum fasting C4; measures bile acid synthesis. Poor test characteristics and not widely used.

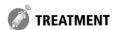 ## TREATMENT

MEDICATION

- Bile acid sequestrants are the mainstay of treatment and may improve abdominal symptoms and stooling.
- 70–96% patients with chronic diarrhea from bile acid malabsorption respond to short course of cholestyramine (3); initiate at 4 g once daily and increase frequency up to 4 times daily.

First Line

- 70–96% patients with chronic diarrhea from bile acid malabsorption respond to short course of cholestyramine; initiate at 4 g once daily and increase frequency up to 4 times daily. The other available bile acid sequestrants are colesevelam and colestipol.
- Increase dose of bile acid sequestrant gradually to avoid side effects (e.g., constipation, nausea, abdominal discomfort).
- Bile acid sequestrants may interfere with the absorption of other medications; other medications should be taken 1 hour before or 4 to 6 hours after bile acid sequestrant.

Second Line

Farnesoid X receptor (FXR agonists) reduce electrolyte secretion in the colon which is upregulated by primary bile acids. These are still under investigation.

ADMISSION, INPATIENT, AND NURSING CONSIDERATIONS

Bile acid malabsorption rarely requires inpatient management.

 ## ONGOING CARE

In patients with bile acid malabsorption due to IBD, treatment of IBD may improve malabsorption symptoms.

FOLLOW-UP RECOMMENDATIONS

No specific follow-up recommendations

Patient Monitoring

Monitor for fat-soluble vitamin malabsorption in patients on long-term bile acid sequestrants (e.g., follow vitamin A and E levels and prothrombin time) (1).

DIET

Low-fat diet may complement pharmacologic treatment and improve symptoms.

PROGNOSIS

Prognosis is excellent with appropriate diagnosis and treatment.

COMPLICATIONS

- Rarely, volume depletion due to watery diarrhea may occur but is unlikely.
- Fat-soluble vitamin malabsorption may occur in patients on chronic treatment bile acid sequestrants (1).

REFERENCES

1. Camilleri M, Vijayvargiya P. The role of bile acids in chronic diarrhea. *Am J Gastroenterol.* 2020;115(10):1596–1603.
2. Johnston I, Nolan J, Pattni SS, et al. New insights into bile acid malabsorption. *Curr Gastroenterol Rep.* 2011;13(5):418–425.
3. Barkun AN, Love J, Gould M, et al. Bile acid malabsorption in chronic diarrhea: pathophysiology and treatment. *Can J Gastroenterol.* 2013;27(11): 653–659.

 ## CODES

ICD10

E78.70 Disorder of bile acid and cholesterol metabolism, unspecified

CLINICAL PEARLS

- Suspect bile acid malabsorption in patients with diarrhea who also complain of abdominal discomfort, bloating, and fecal urgency.
- Consider empiric treatment with a short course of bile acid sequestrant (cholestyramine as first line) in patients with chronic diarrhea as an empiric treatment for bile acid malabsorption.

BIPOLAR I DISORDER
Wendy K. Marsh, MD, MSc

BASICS

DESCRIPTION
- An episodic mood disorder of at least one manic or mixed (mania and depression) episode that causes marked impairment, psychosis, and/or hospitalization; major depressive episodes are not required but usually occur.
- Symptoms are not caused by a substance or general medical condition.

Geriatric Considerations
In new onset in older patients (>50 years of age), a workup for organic or chemically induced pathology is strongly recommended.

Pediatric Considerations
Diagnosis is based on the same set of symptoms applied to adults. Need for clarity of symptoms is critical to differentiate between attention deficit hyperactivity disorder (ADHD), oppositional defiant disorder (ODD), disruptive mood dysregulation, and other diagnoses with overlapping symptoms that are common in childhood.

Pregnancy Considerations
- Pregnancy does not reduce risk of mood episodes.
- Need to weigh risk of fetal and maternal exposure to mood episode to that of medication
- Avoid divalproex (Depakote) due to high teratogenicity risk.
- Postpartum carries high risk of severe acute episode with psychosis and/or infanticidal ideation.

EPIDEMIOLOGY
Onset usually between 15 and 30 years of age, average age of 25 years

Prevalence
- 1.0–1.6% lifetime prevalence
- Manic episodes more common in men; depressive episodes more common in women

ETIOLOGY AND PATHOPHYSIOLOGY
- Dysregulation of biogenic amines or neurotransmitters (particularly serotonin, norepinephrine, and dopamine)
- MRI findings suggest abnormalities in prefrontal cortical areas, striatum, and amygdala that predate illness onset (1)[C].

Genetics
- Monozygotic twin concordance 40–70%; dizygotic 5–25%
- 50% have at least one parent with a mood disorder.
- First-degree relatives are 7 times more likely to develop BP-I than the general population.

RISK FACTORS
Genetics, major life stressors, or substance abuse

GENERAL PREVENTION
Treatment adherence and education help to prevent relapses.

COMMONLY ASSOCIATED CONDITIONS
Substance abuse (60%), ADHD, anxiety disorders (~50%), and eating disorders

DIAGNOSIS

- The diagnosis of BP-I requires at least one manic or mixed episode (simultaneous mania and depression). Although a depressive episode is not necessary for the diagnosis, 80–90% of people with BP-I also experience depression.
- Manic episode, *DSM-5* criteria (2)
  – Distinct period of abnormally and persistently elevated, expansive, or irritable mood plus increased activity or energy for at least 1 week (or any duration if hospitalization is necessary)
  – During the period of mood disturbance, three or more of the "DIG FAST" symptoms must persist (four if the mood is only irritable) and must be present to a significant degree.
    ○ Distractibility
    ○ Insomnia, decreased need for sleep
    ○ Grandiosity or inflated self-esteem
    ○ Flight of ideas or racing thoughts
    ○ Agitation or increase in goal-directed activity
    ○ Speech pressured/more talkative than usual
    ○ Taking risks: excessive involvement in pleasurable activities that have a high potential for painful consequences (e.g., financial or sexual)
  – Mixed specifier: when three or more symptoms of opposite mood pole are present during primary mood episode, for example, mania with mixed features (of depression, like sad mood, low self-esteem and thoughts of death)

HISTORY
- Collateral information makes diagnostics more complete and is often necessary for a clear history.
- History: safety concerns (e.g., Suicidal/homicidal ideation? Safety plan? Psychosis present?), physical well-being (e.g., Number of hours of sleep? Weight change? Substance abuse?), personal history (e.g., Talkative? Risky driving? Excessive spending? Credit card debt? Promiscuity? Other risk-taking behavior? Legal trouble?), substance use (e.g., Did the mood change precede or occur subsequent to substance use?)

PHYSICAL EXAM
- Mental status exam in acute mania
  – General appearance: disorganized or discombobulated, psychomotor agitation, bright clothing, excessive makeup
  – Speech: pressured, difficult to interrupt
  – Mood/affect: euphoria, irritability, expansive, labile
  – Thought process: flight of ideas (streams of thought occur to patient at rapid rate), easily distracted
  – Thought content: grandiosity, paranoia, hyperreligiosity
  – Perceptual abnormalities: 3/4 of manic patients experience delusions, grandiose, or paranoia.
  – Suicidal/homicidal ideation: aggression toward self or others; suicidal ideation is common with mixed episode.
  – Insight/judgment: poor/impaired
- See "Bipolar II Disorder" for an example of a mental status exam in depression.
- With mixed episodes, patients may exhibit a combination of manic and depressive mental states.

DIFFERENTIAL DIAGNOSIS
- Other psychiatric considerations: unipolar depression ± psychotic features, schizophrenia, schizoaffective disorder, personality disorders (particularly antisocial, borderline, histrionic, and narcissistic), ADD ± hyperactivity, substance-induced mood disorder
- Medical considerations: epilepsy (e.g., temporal lobe), brain tumor, infection (e.g., AIDS, syphilis), stroke, endocrine (e.g., thyroid) disease, multiple sclerosis
- In children, consider ADHD and ODD.

DIAGNOSTIC TESTS & INTERPRETATION
- BP-I is a clinical diagnosis.
- The Mood Disorder Questionnaire is a self-assessment screen for history of mood elevation (thus presumed bipolar diagnosis) (sensitivity 73%, specificity 90%).
- Patient Health Questionnaire-9 helps to determine the presence and severity of a depressive episode.

Initial Tests (lab, imaging)
- TSH, CBC, BMP, LFTs, RPR, HIV, ESR
- Drug/alcohol screen with each presentation
- Dementia workup if new onset in elderly
- Consider brain imaging (CT, MRI) with initial onset of mania to rule out organic cause (e.g., tumor, infection, or stroke), especially with onset in elderly and if psychosis is present.

Diagnostic Procedures/Other
Consider EEG if presentation suggests temporal lobe epilepsy (hyperreligiosity, hypergraphia).

TREATMENT

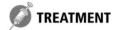

GENERAL MEASURES
- Ensure safety.
- Psychotherapy for depression (e.g., cognitive-behavioral therapy, social rhythm, interpersonal) in conjunction with medications
- Regular daily schedule especially sleep, clean from substances, avoid blue light (screens) in evening, exercise, a healthy diet

MEDICATION
- Acute mania (3),(4)[B]
  – First line
    ○ Lithium monotherapy
    ○ Atypical antipsychotic: quetiapine, risperidone/paliperidone, aripiprazole, asenapine, orcariprazine monotherapy
    ○ Divalproex
    ○ Lithium or divalproex plus atypical antipsychotic
  – Second line
    ○ Olanzapine; carbamazepine; lithium plus divalproex; lithium or divalproex plus olanzapine; ziprasidone; haloperidol
    ○ Electroconvulsive therapy (ECT)
- Acute bipolar I depression (4)
  – First line
    ○ Quetiapine
    ○ Lithium; lamotrigine; lurasidone
  – Second line
    ○ Divalproex; cariprazine
    ○ SSRI/bupropion adjunctive
    ○ Olanzapine* + fluoxetine
    ○ ECT
- *Side effects concerns: Weight gain, metabolic syndrome, and extrapyramidal symptoms (EPS) warrant vigilance and monitoring by the clinician.

- Treatment mood stabilizer(s) or other psychotropic medications. When combining, use different classes (e.g., an atypical antipsychotic and/or an antiseizure medication and/or lithium).
  - Lithium (Lithobid, Eskalith, generic): dosing: 600 to 1,200 mg/day divided BID–QID; start 600 to 900 mg/day divided BID–TID, titrate based on blood levels. *Warning*: caution in kidney and heart disease; use can lead to diabetes insipidus or thyroid disease over time. Caution with diuretics or ACE inhibitors; dehydration can lead to toxicity (seizures, encephalopathy, arrhythmias). Pregnancy requires close monitoring and risks to fetus (Ebstein anomaly). *Monitor*: Check ECG >40 years, TSH, BUN, creatinine, electrolytes at baseline and every 6 months; check level 5 to 7 days after initiation or dose change, then every 2 weeks × 3, and then every 3 months (plasma range: 0.8 to 1.2 mmol/L).
- Anti-convulsants
  - Divalproex sodium, valproic acid (Depakote, Depakene, generic): dosing: Start 250 to 500 mg BID–TID; maximum 60 mg/kg/day. Black box warnings: hepatotoxicity, pancreatitis, thrombocytopenia, pregnancy Category D (high risk for multiple major malformations) Rec. avoiding in reproductive age women. Monitor CBC and LFTs at baseline and every 6 months; check level 5 days after initiation and dose changes (plasma range: 50 to 125 μg/mL).
  - Carbamazepine (Equetro, Tegretol, generic): dosing: 800 to 1,200 mg/day PO divided BID–QID; start 100 to 200 mg PO BID and titrate up to lowest effective dose. *Warning*: Do not use with tricyclic antidepressant (TCA) or within 14 days of an MAOI. Caution in kidney/heart disease; risk of aplastic anemia/agranulocytosis, enzyme inducer; pregnancy Category D. Monitor CBC and LFTs at baseline and every 3 to 6 months; check level 4 to 5 days after initiation and dose changes (plasma range: 4 to 12 μg/mL)
  - Lamotrigine (Lamictal, generic): dosing: 200 to 400 mg/day; start 25 mg/day for 2 weeks, then 50 mg/day for 2 weeks, then 100 mg/day for 1 week, and then 150 mg/day. (Note: Use different dosing if adjunct to valproate.) *Warning*: Titrate slowly (risk of Stevens-Johnson syndrome); caution with kidney/liver/heart disease; pregnancy relative safety but needs close
  - Oxcarbazepine (Trileptal) dosing: 300 mg PO QD. Titrate to 1,800 to 2,400/day max.
- Atypical antipsychotics
  - Side effects: orthostatic hypotension, metabolic side effects (glucose and lipid dysregulation, weight gain), tardive dyskinesia, neuroleptic malignant syndrome (NMS), prolactinemia (except aripiprazole [Abilify]), increased risk of death in elderly with dementia-related psychosis, pregnancy growing data on relative safety, watch for metabolic AE above
  - Monitor LFTs, lipids, glucose at baseline, 3 months and annually; check for EPS with Abnormal Involuntary Movement Scale (AIMS) and assess weight (with abdominal circumference) at baseline; at 4, 8, and 12 weeks; and then every 3 to 6 months; monitor for orthostatic hypotension 3 to 5 days after starting or changing dose.

  - Aripiprazole: dosing: 15 to 30 mg/day; less likely to cause metabolic side effects
  - Asenapine: dosing: 5 to 10 mg sublingual BID
  - Cariprazine (Vraylar) dosing: 1.5 to 3.0 mg/day only for depression; 3 to 6 mg/day mood elevation
  - Lurasidone (Latuda) dosing: 20 to 60 mg/day;
  - Olanzapine (Zyprexa, Zydis, generic): dosing: 5 to 20 mg/day; most likely to cause metabolic side effects (weight gain, diabetes)
  - Paliperidone (Invega) dosing: 6 mg every morning; may cause agranulocytosis, cardiac arrhythmias. IM preparation available
  - Quetiapine (Seroquel, Seroquel XR, generic): dosing: in mania, 200 to 400 mg BID; in bipolar depression, 50 to 300 mg QHS; XR dosing 50 to 400 mg QHS
  - Risperidone (Risperdal, Risperdal Consta, generic): dosing: 1 to 6 mg/day divided QD–QID; IM preparation available (q2wk)
  - Ziprasidone (Geodon): dosing: 40 to 80 mg BID; less likely to cause metabolic side effects. Caution: QTc prolongation (>500 ms) has been associated. Consider ECG at baseline.
- Avoid TCAs and serotonin norepinephrine reuptake inhibitor (SNRI); due to increased risk of mood cycling risk

ISSUES FOR REFERRAL
- Refer to psychiatry, depends on knowledge level of the doctor, stability of patient.
- Patients benefit from a multidisciplinary team, including a primary care physician, psychiatrist, and therapist.

ADDITIONAL THERAPIES
- Modest evidence supports transcranial magnetic stimulation, ketamine infusion, ar/modafinil, sleep deprivation, and levothyroxine bipolar depression.
- Blue-blocking glasses or dark therapy for mania. Full spectrum 10,000 lux midmorning light for depression

ADMISSION, INPATIENT, AND NURSING CONSIDERATIONS
- Admit if dangerous to self or others.
- To admit involuntarily, the patient must have a psychiatric diagnosis (e.g., BP-I) and present a danger to self or others, or the mental disease must be inhibiting the person from obtaining basic needs (e.g., food, clothing, shelter).
- Nursing: Alert staff to potentially dangerous or agitated patients. Acute suicidal threats need continuous observation.

 ## ONGOING CARE

FOLLOW-UP RECOMMENDATIONS
- Regularly scheduled visits support adherence with treatment.
- Frequent communication among primary care doctor, psychiatrist, and therapist

Patient Monitoring
Mood charts are helpful to monitor symptoms.

PATIENT EDUCATION
- National Alliance on Mental Illness (NAMI): http://www.nami.org/
- National Institute of Mental Health (NIMH): http://www.nimh.nih.gov/index.shtml

PROGNOSIS
- Frequency and severity of episodes are related to medication adherence, consistency with therapy, quality of sleep, and support systems.
- 40–50% of patients experience another manic episode within 2 years of first episode.
- 25–50% attempt suicide, and 15% die by suicide.
- Substance abuse, unemployment, psychosis, depression, and male gender are associated with a worse prognosis.

REFERENCES
1. American Psychiatric Association. *Diagnostic and Statistical Manual of Mental Disorders*. 5th ed. Arlington, VA: American Psychiatric Association; 2013.
2. Ostacher MJ, Tandon R, Suppes T. Florida Best Practice Psychotherapeutic Medication Guidelines for Adults with Bipolar Disorder: a novel, practical, patient-centered guide for clinicians. *J Clin Psychiatry*. 2016;77(7):920–926.
3. Parikh SV, LeBlanc SR, Ovanessian MM. Advancing bipolar disorder: key lessons from the Systematic Treatment Enhancement Program for Bipolar Disorder (STEP-BD). *Can J Psychiatry*. 2010;55(3):136–143.
4. Yatham LN, Kennedy SH, Parikh SV, et al. Canadian Network for Mood and Anxiety Treatments (CANMAT) and International Society for Bipolar Disorders (ISBD) collaborative update of CANMAT guidelines for the management of patients with bipolar disorder: update 2018. *Bipolar Disord*. 2018;20(2):97–170.

ADDITIONAL READING
Salcedo S, Gold AK, Sheikh S, et al. Empirically supported psychosocial interventions for bipolar disorder: current state of the research. *J Affect Disord*. 2016;201:203–214.

 ## SEE ALSO

Algorithm: Depressive Episode, Major

CODES

ICD10
- F31.9 Bipolar disorder, unspecified
- F31.10 Bipolar disorder, current episode manic without psychotic features, unspecified
- F31.30 Bipolar disord, crnt epsd depress, mild or mod severt, unsp

CLINICAL PEARLS
- BP-I is characterized by at least one manic or mixed episode that causes marked impairment; major depressive episodes usually occur but are not necessary.
- 25–50% of BP-I patients attempt suicide, and 15% die by suicide.
- There is no known way to prevent BP-I, but treatment adherence and education helps reduce further episodes.
- Goal of treatment is to decrease the intensity, length, and frequency of episodes as well as greater duration of euthymia (healthy mood) between episodes.

BIPOLAR II DISORDER
Wendy K. Marsh, MD, MSc

 BASICS

DESCRIPTION
A mood disorder characterized by at least one episode of major depression (with or without psychosis) and at least one episode of hypomania, a nonsevere mood elevation

Geriatric Considerations
In new onset in older patients (>50 years of age), a workup for organic or chemically induced pathology is strongly recommended.

Pediatric Considerations
Diagnosis is based on the same set of symptoms applied to adults. Need for clarity of symptoms is critical to differentiate between attention deficit hyperactivity disorder (ADHD), oppositional defiant disorder (ODD), disruptive mood dysregulation, and other diagnoses with overlapping symptoms that are common in childhood.

Pregnancy Considerations
- Pregnancy does not reduce risk of mood episodes.
- Need to weigh risk of exposure to mood episode to that of medication
- Avoid divalproex (Depakote) due to high teratogenicity risk.
- Postpartum caries high risk of severe acute episode with psychosis and/or infanticidal ideation.

EPIDEMIOLOGY
Onset usually between 15 and 30 years of age

Prevalence
- 0.5–1.0% lifetime prevalence
- More common in women

ETIOLOGY AND PATHOPHYSIOLOGY
Dysregulation of biogenic amines or neurotransmitters (particularly serotonin, norepinephrine, and dopamine)

Genetics
Heritability estimate: >77%

RISK FACTORS
Genetics, major life stressors, or substance misuse

GENERAL PREVENTION
Treatment adherence and education can help to prevent further episodes.

COMMONLY ASSOCIATED CONDITIONS
Substance misuse, ADHD, anxiety disorders, and eating disorders

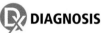 **DIAGNOSIS**

- *DSM-5* criteria: one hypomanic episode and at least one major depressive episode. Mood elevation symptoms cause unequivocal change in functioning noticed by others but not severe enough to cause marked impairment (1)[C].
- Hypomania is a distinct period of persistently elevated, expansive, or irritable mood, different from usual euthymic mood, including increase in activity or energy lasting at least 4 days:
  - The episode must include at least three of the "DIG FAST" symptoms *plus increased energy* below (four if the mood is only irritable):
    ○ Distractibility
    ○ Insomnia, decreased need for sleep
    ○ Grandiosity or inflated self-esteem

○ Flight of ideas or racing thoughts
○ Agitation or increase in goal-directed activity (socially, at work or school, or sexually)
○ Speech pressured/more talkative than usual
○ Taking risks: excessive involvement in pleasurable activities that have high potential for painful consequences (e.g., sexual or financial)
- Major depression: Depressed mood or diminished interest and four or more of the "SIG E CAPS" symptoms are present during the same 2-week period:
  - Sleep disturbance (e.g., trouble falling asleep, early-morning awakening)
  - Interest: loss or anhedonia
  - Guilt (or feelings of worthlessness)
  - Energy, loss of
  - Concentration, loss of
  - Appetite changes, increase or decrease
  - Psychomotor changes (retardation or agitation)
  - Suicidal/homicidal thoughts
  - Rapid cycling is ≥4 mood episodes in 12 months (major depression or hypomania).
  - Mixed specifier: when three or more symptoms of opposite mood pole are present during primary mood episode, for example, hypomania with mixed features (of depression)
- Note: If symptoms have *ever* met criteria for a full manic episode, for example, hospitalization was necessary secondary to manic/mixed symptoms or psychosis was present, then the diagnosis is BP-I.

HISTORY
- Collateral information makes diagnostics more complete and is often necessary for a clear history.
- History: safety concerns (e.g., Suicidal/homicidal ideation? Safety plan? Psychosis present?), physical well-being (e.g., Number of hours of sleep? Substance abuse?), personal history (e.g., Risky driving? Excessive spending? Credit card debt? Promiscuity? Other risk-taking behavior? Legal trouble?), substance use (e.g., did the mood change precede or occur subsequent to substance use)

PHYSICAL EXAM
- Mental status exam in hypomania
  - General appearance: usually appropriately dressed may be bright colors or eye-catching style, often with psychomotor agitation
  - Speech: may be pressured, talkative, difficult to interrupt
  - Mood/affect: euphoria, irritability, congruent, or expansive
  - Thought process: may be easily distracted, difficulty concentrating on one task
  - Thought content: usually positive, with "big" plans
  - Perceptual abnormalities: none
  - Suicidal/homicidal ideation: low incidence of homicidal or suicidal ideation
  - Insight/judgment: usually stable/may be impaired by distractibility or grandiosity
- Mental status exam in depression
  - General appearance: unkempt, psychomotor retardation, poor eye contact
  - Speech: low, soft, monotone
  - Mood/affect: sad, depressed/congruent, flat
  - Thought process: ruminating thoughts, generalized slowing
  - Thought content: preoccupied with negative or nihilistic ideas

- Perceptual abnormalities: 15% of depressed patients experience hallucinations or delusions.
- Suicidal/homicidal ideation: Suicidal ideation is very common.
- Insight/judgment: often impaired

DIFFERENTIAL DIAGNOSIS
- Other psychiatric considerations: BP-I disorder, unipolar depression, personality disorders (particularly borderline, antisocial, and narcissistic), ADHD, substance-induced mood disorder
- Medical considerations: epilepsy (e.g., temporal lobe), brain tumor, infection (e.g., AIDS, syphilis), stroke, endocrine (e.g., thyroid disease), multiple sclerosis, autoimmune

DIAGNOSTIC TESTS & INTERPRETATION
- BP-II is a clinical diagnosis.
- Mood Disorder Questionnaire, self-assessment screen for history of mood elevation (thus presumed bipolar diagnosis)
- Hypomania Checklist-32 distinguishes between BP-II and unipolar depression (sensitivity 80%, specificity 51%) (2)[B].
- Patient Health Questionnaire-9 helps to determine the presence and severity of depression.

Initial Tests (lab, imaging)
- Rule out organic causes of mood disorder during initial episode.
- Drug/alcohol screen is prudent with each presentation.
- Dementia workup if new onset in elderly
- With initial presentation: Consider CBC, chem 7, TSH, LFTs, ANA, RPR, HIV, and ESR.
- Consider brain imaging (CT, MRI) with initial onset of hypomania to rule out organic cause, especially with onset in the elderly.

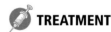 **TREATMENT**

GENERAL MEASURES
- Ensure safety.
- Psychotherapy for depression (e.g., CBT, social rhythm, interpersonal, family focused) in conjunction with medications
- Regular circadian rhythm/daily sleep and activity schedule, exercise, a healthy diet
- Sobriety, substance free
- Stress reduction

MEDICATION
- Acute mood elevation (3),(4)[C]
  - First line
    ○ Quetiapine, lithium
    ○ Atypical, other: cariprazine, risperidone, aripiprazole, ziprasidone, asenapine
    ○ Divalproex (avoid in reproductive age women)
  - Second line
    ○ Haloperidol, paliperidone
    ○ Lithium plus divalproex
    ○ Lithium or divalproex plus atypical
- Acute bipolar II depression (4)
  - First line
    ○ Quetiapine
  - Second line
    ○ Lithium, lamotrigine, lurasidone, cariprazine
    ○ Bupropion adjunct
    ○ ECT

- When combining, use different classes (e.g., an atypical antipsychotic and/or an antiseizure medication and/or lithium) (2)[A].
  - Lithium (Lithobid, Eskalith, generic): dosing: 600 to 1,200 mg/day divided BID–QID; start 600 to 900 mg/day divided BID–TID, titrate based on blood levels. *Warning*: Caution in kidney and heart disease; use can lead to diabetes insipidus or thyroid disease. Caution with diuretics or ACE inhibitors; dehydration can lead to toxicity (seizures, encephalopathy, arrhythmias). Pregnancy requires close monitoring. *Monitor*: Check ECG >40 years, TSH, BUN, creatine, electrolytes at baseline and every 6 months. Check level 5 to 7 days after initiation or dose change, then every 2 weeks × 3, and then every 3 months (goal: 0.8 to 1.2 mmol/L).
  - Anti-convulsants
    - Divalproex sodium, valproic acid (Depakote, Depakene, generic): dosing: Start 250 to 500 mg BID–TID; maximum 60 mg/kg/day. Black box warnings: hepatotoxicity, pancreatitis, thrombocytopenia, pregnancy Category D. Monitor CBC and LFTs at baseline and every 6 months; check level 5 days after initiation and dose changes (goal: 50 to 125 μg/mL).
    - Lamotrigine (Lamictal, generic): dosing: 200 to 400 mg/day; start 25 mg/day for 2 weeks, then 50 mg/day for 2 weeks, then 100 mg/day for 1 week, and then 150 mg/day. (Note: Use half dosing if adjunct to valproate.) *Warning*: Titrate slowly (risk of Stevens-Johnson syndrome); caution with kidney/liver/heart disease; pregnancy Category C
  - Atypical antipsychotics
    - Side effects: orthostatic hypotension, metabolic side effects (glucose and lipid dysregulation, weight gain), tardive dyskinesia, neuroleptic malignant syndrome (NMS), prolactinemia (except aripiprazole), increased risk of death in elderly with dementia-related psychosis, pregnancy Category C
    - Monitor LFTs, lipids, glucose at baseline, 3 months and annually; check for EPS with Abnormal Involuntary Movement Scale (AIMS), and assess weight (with abdominal circumference) at baseline; at 4, 8, and 12 weeks; and then every 3 to 6 months; monitor for orthostatic hypotension 3 to 5 days after starting or changing dose.
    - Aripiprazole (Abilify): dosing: 10 to 30 mg/day; less likely to cause metabolic side effects than other AAP
    - Asenapine: dosing: 5 to 10 mg sublingual BID
    - cariprazine (Vraylar): dosing: 1.5 to 3 mg for depression, up to 6 mg for mood elevation
    - Lurasidone (Latuda): dosing: 20 to 60 mg/day; less likely to cause metabolic side effects
    - Paliperidone (Invega): dosing: 6 mg every morning; may cause agranulocytosis, cardiac arrhythmias

- Quetiapine (Seroquel, Seroquel XR, generic): dosing: in mania, 200 to 400 mg BID; in bipolar depression, 50 to 600 mg QHS; XR dosing 50 to 400 mg QHS
- Risperidone (Risperdal, Risperdal Consta, generic): dosing: 1 to 6 mg/day divided QD–QID; IM preparation available (q2wk)
- Ziprasidone (Geodon): dosing: 40 to 80 mg BID; less likely to cause metabolic side effects. Caution: QTc prolongation (>500 ms) has been associated with use (0.06%). Consider ECG at baseline.
- Unipolar antidepressants
  - Bupropion (Wellbutrin): dosing: 150 to 300 mg PO every day. Use only with antimanic agent.
  - Avoid TCAs and serotonin-norepinephrine reuptake inhibitors—increases mood cycling risk.

ISSUES FOR REFERRAL
- Refer to psychiatry recommended, depends on knowledge level of the doctor, stability of patient.
- Patients benefit from a multidisciplinary team, including a primary care physician, psychiatrist, and therapist.

ADDITIONAL THERAPIES
- Modest evidence supports transcranial magnetic stimulation, vagus nerve stimulation, ketamine infusion, sleep deprivation, and hormone therapy (e.g., thyroid) in bipolar depression.
- Blue-blocking glasses or dark therapy for mood elevation

ADMISSION, INPATIENT, AND NURSING CONSIDERATIONS
- Admit if dangerous to self or others.
- To admit involuntarily, the patient must have a psychiatric diagnosis (e.g., BP-I) and present a danger to self or others, or the mental disease must be inhibiting the person from obtaining basic needs (e.g., food, clothing).
- Nursing: Alert staff to potentially dangerous or agitated patients. Acute suicidal threats need continuous observation.

ONGOING CARE

FOLLOW-UP RECOMMENDATIONS
Regularly scheduled visits support adherence with treatment.

Patient Monitoring
Mood charts are helpful to monitor symptoms.

PATIENT EDUCATION
- National Alliance on Mental Illness (NAMI): http://www.nami.org/
- National Institute of Mental Health (NIMH): http://www.nimh.nih.gov/index.shtml

PROGNOSIS
- Frequency and severity of episodes are related to medication adherence, consistency with therapy, quality of sleep, and support systems.

- 25–50% attempt suicide and 15% die by suicide.
- Substance abuse, unemployment, psychosis, depression, and male gender are associated with a worse prognosis.

REFERENCES
1. American Psychiatric Association. *Diagnostic and Statistical Manual of Mental Disorders*. 5th ed. Arlington, VA: American Psychiatric Association; 2013.
2. Ostacher MJ, Tandon R, Suppes T. Florida best practice psychotherapeutic medication guidelines for adults with bipolar disorder: a novel, practical, patient-centered guide for clinicians. *J Clin Psychiatry*. 2016;77(7):920–926.
3. Parikh SV, LeBlanc SR, Ovanessian MM. Advancing bipolar disorder: key lessons from the Systematic Treatment Enhancement Program for Bipolar Disorder (STEP-BD). *Can J Psychiatry*. 2010;55(3):136–143.
4. Yatham LN, Kennedy SH, Parikh SV, et al. Canadian Network for Mood and Anxiety Treatments (CANMAT) and International Society for Bipolar Disorders (ISBD) collaborative update of CANMAT guidelines for the management of patients with bipolar disorder: update 2018. *Bipolar Disord*. 2018;20(2):97–170.

ADDITIONAL READING
Salcedo S, Gold AK, Sheikh S, et al. Empirically supported psychosocial interventions for bipolar disorder: current state of the research. *J Affect Disord*. 2016;201:203–214.

 SEE ALSO

Algorithm: Depressive Episode, Major

 CODES

ICD10
F31.81 Bipolar II disorder

CLINICAL PEARLS
- BP-II is characterized by at least one episode of major depression and one episode of hypomania.
- Patients may not recognize symptoms and or decline treatment during a hypomanic episode; they may enjoy the elevated mood and productivity.
- Patients with BP-II are at great risk of both attempting and completing suicide.

BITES, ANIMAL AND HUMAN
Kathryn Samai, PharmD, BCPS • Brian J. Kimbrell, MD, FACS

BASICS

DESCRIPTION
- Animal bite rates vary by species: dogs (60–90%), cats (5–20%), rodents (2–3%), humans (2–3%), and (rarely) other animals, including snakes.
- System(s) affected: potentially any

Pediatric Considerations
Young children are more likely to sustain bites and have bites that include the face, upper extremity, or trunk.

EPIDEMIOLOGY
- All ages, but children > adults
- Dog bites: male > female patients; cat bites: female > male patients

Incidence
- 3 to 6 million animal bites per year in the United States (1)
- Account for 1% of all injury-related ED visits
- 1–2% will require hospital admission, and 20 to 35 victims die from dog bite complications, annually.

ETIOLOGY AND PATHOPHYSIOLOGY
- Dog bites are far more common than cat bites; most dog bites are from a domestic pet known to the victim.
- Most (~90%) cat bites are provoked.
- Human bite wounds are typically incurred by striking another in the mouth with a clenched fist.
- Human bites also occur incidentally (e.g., paronychia due to nail biting; thumb sucking; or nonmalicious bites to the face, breasts, or genital areas).
- Animal bites can cause tears, punctures, scratches, avulsions, or crush injuries.
- Contamination by oral flora leads to infection.
- Cat bites are more often puncture-type wound.

RISK FACTORS
- Older and/or male dogs are more likely to bite.
- Clenched-fist human bites are frequently associated with the use of alcohol or drugs.
- Patients presenting >8 hours following the bite are at greater risk of infection.

GENERAL PREVENTION
- Instruct children and adults about animal hazards.
- Enforce animal control laws.
- Educate pet owners.

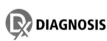
DIAGNOSIS

HISTORY
- Detailed history of the incident (provoked or unprovoked), type/breed of animal, vaccine status, whereabouts of animal
- Site of the bite
- Geographic setting
- Underlying medical history—particularly comorbid diseases and immunocompromise
- Ascertain immunization history (tetanus and rabies, in particular).

PHYSICAL EXAM
- Dog bites
  - Hands and face most common site of injury in adults and children, respectively
  - More likely to have associated crush injury

- Cat bites
  - Predominantly involve the hands, followed by lower extremities, face, and trunk
- Human bites
  - Intentional bite: semicircular or oval area of erythema and bruising, with/without break in skin
  - Clenched-fist injury: small wounds over the metacarpophalangeal joints from striking the fist against another's teeth
  - Signs of wound infection include fever, erythema, swelling, tenderness, purulent drainage, and lymphangitis.
- Document neurovascular status.
- Signs of tenosynovitis (hand/finger bites): finger held in flexion, fusiform swelling, pain along tendon sheath, pain with active/passive extension of the affected digit

> **ALERT**
> Cat bites are twice as likely to become infected as are dog bites and have higher risks of osteomyelitis, tenosynovitis, and septic arthritis.

Pediatric Considerations
Human bite marks on a child with an intercanine distance >3 cm are likely from an adult and should raise concerns about child abuse.

DIFFERENTIAL DIAGNOSIS
Evaluate for other possible causes of trauma.

DIAGNOSTIC TESTS & INTERPRETATION
Initial Tests (lab, imaging)
- Gram stain and culture wound drainage
  - If wound fails to heal, culture for atypical pathogens (fungi, *Nocardia*, and mycobacteria); keep bacterial cultures for 7 to 10 days (some pathogens are slow-growing).
- 85% of bite wounds will yield a positive culture; most are polymicrobial.
- Obtain aerobic and anaerobic blood cultures before starting antibiotics if bacteremia is suspected.
- Recent antibiotic therapy may alter culture results.
- Obtain radiograph to check for fractures in clenched-fist injuries.

> **ALERT**
> If bite wound is near a bone or joint, obtain a plain radiograph to check for bone injury (baseline imaging is also helpful for later comparison if osteomyelitis is suspected) (2).

Follow-Up Tests & Special Considerations
- Plain radiograph and/or MRI for suspected osteomyelitis
- CT scan for severe skull bites. Ultrasound can detect abscess formation.

Diagnostic Procedures/Other
Surgical exploration may be needed to determine the extent of injuries or to drain deep infections (e.g., tendon sheath), especially in serious hand wounds.

Test Interpretation
Most common microorganisms include:
- Dog bites (3),(4)
  - *Pasteurella* spp. present in 50% of bites
  - Streptococci spp., *Staphylococcus aureus*, *Staphylococcus intermedius*, *Neisseria* spp., *Capnocytophaga canimorsus*, *Bacteroides* spp., *Fusobacterium* spp.

- Cat bites (4)
  - *Pasteurella* spp. in 75% of bites
  - Streptococcus spp. (including *Streptococcus pyogenes*), Staphylococcus spp. (including methicillin-resistant *S. aureus* [MRSA]), *Neisseria* spp., Moraxella spp., *Porphyromonas* spp., *Fusobacterium* spp., *Bacteroides* spp.
- Human bites
  - *Eikenella corrodens* (15–29%), *Streptococcus* spp., *S. aureus* (including MRSA), and various anaerobic bacteria (e.g., *Fusobacterium*, *Peptostreptococcus*, *Prevotella*, and *Porphyromonas* spp.)
  - Although rare, case reports suggest transmission of viruses (hepatitis B/C, HIV, and herpes simplex).
- Aquatic bites
  - *S. aureus*, *Streptococcus* spp., *Vibrio* spp. (saltwater, brackish water), *Aeromonas* spp. (freshwater), *Mycobacterium* spp., *Pseudomonas* spp.
- Reptile bites
  - *Pseudomonas aeruginosa*, *Proteus* spp., *Salmonella*, *Bacteroides fragilis*, and *Clostridium* spp.
- Rodent bites
  - *Streptobacillus moniliformis* or *Spirillum minus*, which causes rat-bite fever
- Monkey bites
  - All monkey bites can transmit rabies, and bites of a macaque monkey may transmit herpes B virus, which is potentially fatal.
- Ungulate (hooved animals) bites
  - Pigs are the most likely to bite; commonly polymicrobial infections (*Staphylococcus* and *Streptococcus* spp., *Haemophilus influenzae*, *Pasteurella*, *Actinobacillus* and *Flavobacterium* spp.)

> **ALERT**
> Asplenic patients and those with underlying hepatic disease are at risk for bacteremia and fatal sepsis after dog bites infected with *C. canimorsus*.

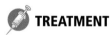
TREATMENT

GENERAL MEASURES
- Complete and submit bite report per local policy.
- Elevate the injured extremity to prevent swelling.
- Contact local health department to determine rabies prevalence in biting species.
- Snake bite: If venomous, transport for appropriate evaluation and antivenom; be sure patient is stable for transport; assess coagulation and renal status.

MEDICATION
- Determine need for antirabies therapy: rabies immunoglobulin and human diploid cell rabies vaccine for those bitten by wild animals (primary vector in the United States is bat or raccoon), rabid pets, unvaccinated pets, or in situations where the animal cannot be quarantined for 10 days.
- Refer to most common microbial organisms to determine antibiotic coverage for unusual animals.

> **ALERT**
> Refer to state and local health authorities for rabies consultation (https://www.cdc.gov/rabies/resources/contacts.html).

- Tetanus toxoid (Td) for previously immunized with >10 years since their last dose (2)[C]; tetanus, diphtheria, and pertussis (Tdap) formulation is generally preferred to Td (2)[C].
- Anti-HBs negative patients bitten by HBsAg-positive individuals should receive both hepatitis B immunoglobulin (HBIG) and hepatitis B vaccine.
- HIV postexposure prophylaxis is generally not recommended for human bites, unless there is significant blood exposure to broken skin.
- Monkey bite: Contact CDC; consider an antiviral, such as valacyclovir, active against herpes B virus.
- Preemptive antibiotics recommended only for human bites and high-risk wounds (deep puncture, crush injury, venous or lymphatic compromise, hands or near joint, face or genital area, immunocompromised hosts, requiring surgical repair, asplenic, advanced liver, edema)
- Duration of antibiotic therapy: preemptive, 3 to 5 days; treatment of cellulitis/skin abscess, 5 to 10 days

ALERT
Consider community-acquired MRSA as possible pathogen (from human skin or colonized pet). If high suspicion, doxycycline or TMP-SMX provide good coverage.

First Line
- For preemptive and empiric treatment, amoxicillin and clavulanate is first-line antibiotic (2)[B].
  - Adults: amoxicillin and clavulanate 875/125 mg PO BID
  - Children: amoxicillin and clavulanate <3 months: 30 mg/kg/day PO q12h; ≥3 months and <40 kg: 25 to 45 mg/kg/day q12h; >40 kg: use adult dosing.
- Patients with deep or severe wound infections, systemic infections requiring IV therapy, and the immunocompromised:
  - Adults: ampicillin and sulbactam 3.0 g IV q6h or piperacillin and tazobactam 3.375 g IV q6h (2)
  - Children: ampicillin and sulbactam 200 mg/kg/day (dosed on ampicillin component) IV given in 4 divided doses to maximum of 3 g per dose

Second Line
- Alternative oral regimens
  - Adults: clindamycin (300 mg PO TID) plus either trimethoprim-sulfamethoxazole (TMP-SMX; 1 DS tablet PO BID) or ciprofloxacin (500 to 750 mg PO BID)
  - Children: clindamycin 25 to 30 mg/kg/day PO in 3 divided doses to a maximum of 400 mg per dose plus TMP-SMX (8 to 10 mg/kg/day of trimethoprim) PO in 2 divided doses to a maximum of 160 mg TMP per dose
  - Avoid 1st-generation cephalosporins (e.g., cephalexin), penicillinase-resistant penicillins (e.g., dicloxacillin), macrolides (e.g., erythromycin), and clindamycin (when not administered with another agent) because they lack activity against *Pasteurella multocida* (dog/cat bites) and *Eikenella corrodens* (human bites).
- Alternative intravenous regimens
  - Adults: ciprofloxacin 400 mg IV q12h or levofloxacin 750 mg IV every day with metronidazole 500 mg IV q8h

Pregnancy Considerations
Pregnant women who cannot take penicillins or cephalosporin due to severe allergy
- Azithromycin
- Observe closely and note potential increased risk of treatment failure.

ISSUES FOR REFERRAL
- Deep wounds to the hand and face should be referred to a hand surgeon or plastic surgeon.
- Bites from primates or unusual species of animals should be referred to infectious disease specialist.

SURGERY/OTHER PROCEDURES
- Copious irrigation of the wound with normal saline via a catheter tip to reduce risk of infection
- Débride devitalized tissue.
- Débridement of puncture wounds is not advised.
- Consider primary closure if the wound is clean after irrigation, the bite is <12 hours old, and in bites to the face (cosmesis).
- Infected wounds and those at high risk for infection (cat bites, human bites, bites to the hand, crush injuries, presentation >12 hours from injury) should be left open.
- Delayed primary closure in 3 to 5 days is an option for infected wounds.
- Splint injured hand.
- Large, gaping wounds should be reapproximated with widely spaced sutures or adhesive strips.
- Consider surgical consultation for deep, severe, or complex bite wounds; bites to vital structures should be treated as possible penetrating traumatic injuries.

ADMISSION, INPATIENT, AND NURSING CONSIDERATIONS
Patients with deep or severe wound infections, systemic infections requiring IV therapy, and the immunocompromised generally require inpatient admission.

 ONGOING CARE

FOLLOW-UP RECOMMENDATIONS
Patient Monitoring
- Recheck for infection in 24 to 48 hours.
- Daily follow-up for infections to ensure resolution
- Base revisions of antibiotic therapy on culture results and clinical response.

PATIENT EDUCATION
Educate patients about how to be safe around animals and avoid animal bites.

PROGNOSIS
Wounds should improve and close over 7 to 10 days.

COMPLICATIONS
- Septic arthritis
- Osteomyelitis
- Extensive soft tissue injuries with scarring
- Hemorrhage
- Gas gangrene
- Sepsis
- Meningitis
- Endocarditis
- Posttraumatic stress disorder
- Death

REFERENCES
1. Murphy J, Qaisi M. Management of human and animal bites. *Oral Maxillofac Surg Clin North Am*. 2021;33(3):373–380.
2. Stevens DL, Bisno AL, Chambers HF, et al. Practice guidelines for the diagnosis and management of skin and soft tissue infections: 2014 update by the Infectious Disease Society of America. *Clin Infect Dis*. 2014;59(2):e10–e52.
3. Baxter M, Denny KJ, Keijzers G. Antibiotic prescribing in patients who presented to the emergency department with dog bites: a descriptive review of current practice. *Emerg Med Australas*. 2020;32(4):578–585.
4. Greene SE, Fritz SA. Infectious complications of bite injuries. *Infect Dis Clin North Am*. 2021;35(1):219–236.

ADDITIONAL READING
- Bula-Rudas FJ, Olcott JL. Human and animal bites. *Pediatr Rev*. 2018;39(10):490–500.
- Jakeman M, Oxley JA, Owczarczak-Garstecka SC, et al. Pet dog bites in children: management and prevention. *BMJ Paediatr Open*. 2020;4(1):e000726.
- World Health Organization. Animal bites. http://www.who.int/news-room/fact-sheets/detail/animal-bites. Accessed September 16, 2020.

 SEE ALSO

Bartonella Infections; Cellulitis; Rabies; Snake Envenomation

CODES

ICD10
- S61.459A Open bite of unspecified hand, initial encounter
- S01.85XA Open bite of other part of head, initial encounter
- S20.97XA Other superficial bite of unspecified parts of thorax, initial encounter

CLINICAL PEARLS
- Dog bites are the most common form of animal bite.
- Cleanse, débride, and culture if any signs of infection.
- Antibiotic prophylaxis is recommended for human bites and high-risk wounds.
- Consider rabies and tetanus vaccination.
- Adjust antibiotic choice and duration of therapy based on culture results and clinical improvement.
- Animal and human bites require close follow-up, looking for signs of infection or other complications.

BLADDER CANCER

Veronica A. Torres, MD • Lily T. Luc, MD

BASICS

DESCRIPTION
- Primary malignant neoplasms arising in the urinary bladder
- There are three types that begin in cells in the lining of the bladder: transitional cell carcinoma, squamous cell carcinoma, and adenocarcinoma.
- Most common type is transitional cell carcinoma (90%) (1).
- The spectrum of bladder cancer includes nonmuscle invasive, muscle invasive, and metastatic disease.
- Rhabdomyosarcoma of the bladder may occur in children.

EPIDEMIOLOGY
Incidence
- Increases with age (median age at diagnosis is 73 years) (2)
- More common in Caucasians than in Asians or African Americans
- Male > female (4:1); but in smokers, risk is 1:1.
- 34.2/100,000 men per year (2)
- 8.5/100,000 women per year
- 19.7/100,000 men and women per year (2)

Prevalence
In 2018, 723,745 cases in the United States (2)

ETIOLOGY AND PATHOPHYSIOLOGY
Unknown, other than related to risk factors:
- 75% is nonmuscle invasive (in lamina propria or mucosa) (3):
  - Usually highly differentiated with long survival
  - Initial event seems to be the activation of an oncogene on chromosome 9 in superficial cancers (1).
- 25% of tumors are muscle invasive (deeper than lamina propria) at presentation (3):
  - Tend to be high grade with worse prognosis
  - Associated with other chromosome deletions

Genetics
Genetic effects may play a direct role in the initiation and progression of bladder cancer. Most studies showed a small increase in risk in relatives of those with bladder cancer. Patients with Lynch syndrome has up to 20% lifetime risk of developing bladder cancer.

RISK FACTORS
- Smoking is the single greatest risk factor (increases risk 4-fold) and increases risk equally for men and women (4).
- There is a slight but significant increased risk with the use of pioglitazone, possibly in a dose- and time-dependent manner; may also be present with other thiazolidinediones (5)
- Other risk factors (4):
  - Positive family history, especially in relatives diagnosed before age 60 years
  - Occupational carcinogens in dye, rubber, paint, plastics, metal, carbon black dust, petroleum, and automotive exhaust

- Schistosomiasis in Mediterranean (squamous cell) cancer
- Arsenic in well water
- History of bladder radiation, pelvic irradiation, or certain anticancer drugs like cyclophosphamide or ifosfamide
- Chronic lower UTI
- Chronic indwelling urinary catheter
- Cyclophosphamide exposure

ALERT
Any smoker who presents with microscopic or gross hematuria or irritative voiding symptoms such as urgency and frequency not clearly due to UTI should be evaluated by cystoscopy for the presence of a bladder neoplasm.

GENERAL PREVENTION
- Avoid smoking and other risk factors.
- Counseling of individuals with occupational exposure
- The U.S. Preventive Services Task Force has concluded that there is insufficient evidence to determine the balance between risk and harm of screening for bladder cancer.

COMMONLY ASSOCIATED CONDITIONS
Smoking

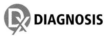DIAGNOSIS

HISTORY
- Painless hematuria is the most common symptom.
- Urinary symptoms (frequency, urgency, dysuria)
- Abdominal or pelvic pain in advanced disease
- Exposures (see "Risk Factors")

PHYSICAL EXAM
Normal in early cases, pelvic or abdominal mass in advanced disease, wasting in systemic disease

DIFFERENTIAL DIAGNOSIS
- UTI
- Nephrolithiasis
- Interstitial cystitis/nephritis
- Papillary urothelial hyperplasia
- Renal cell carcinoma
- Other urinary tract neoplasms

DIAGNOSTIC TESTS & INTERPRETATION
Initial Tests (lab, imaging)
- Urinalysis is the initial test in patients presenting with gross hematuria or urinary symptoms such as frequency, urgency, and dysuria.
- Urine cytology (Consult your local lab for volume needed and proper fixative/handling.)
- Cystoscopy with biopsy is the gold standard for at-risk patients with painless hematuria.
- Transurethral resection of bladder tumor (TURBT) is required to determine the histologic grade and depth of invasion (3).

- CT or MRI performed at the time of TURBT is indicated to rule out secondary primary lesion and is helpful in staging.

Follow-Up Tests & Special Considerations
- Urine cytology: 34–55% sensitive, >90% specific (3)
- Urine-based tumor markers: sensitivity ranges from 50% to 80%, and specificity ranges from 70% to 90%. However, none of the urine markers is sensitive enough to rule out bladder cancer on its own and thus are not recommended as part of routine testing.
  - Fluorescence in situ hybridization (FISH) assay: can be used to predict and assess response to intravesical bacillus Calmette-Guérin (BCG) therapy
- Liver function tests, alkaline phosphatase if metastasis suspected
- Done for staging and to evaluate extent of disease but not for diagnosis itself:
  - CT urogram replacing IVP to image upper tracts if there is a suspicion of disease there
  - Diffusion-weighted MRI and multidimensional CT scan are undergoing studies for use in diagnosis and staging of bladder tumors.
  - For invasive disease, metastatic workup should include chest x-ray and PET scan.
  - Bone scan should be performed if the patient has bone pain or if alkaline phosphatase is elevated.
- Urologic CT scan (abdomen, pelvis, with and without contrast) or MRI (40–98% accurate), with MRI slightly more accurate, is recommended if metastasis is suspected
- Regular cystoscopy (initiated at 3 months postprocedure) is indicated after TURBT and intravesical chemotherapy for superficial bladder cancers. Urinary biomarkers should not be routinely used for follow-up.

Test Interpretation
- Characterized as superficial (nonmuscle invasive) or invasive (muscle invasive)
- Superficial lesions (70–80%)
  - Ta: noninvasive papillary carcinoma, tend to recur.
  - Tis: carcinoma in situ; flat lesion, high grade
  - T1: extends into submucosa, lamina propria. Usually high grade
- Invasive cancer
  - T2: invasion into muscle
    - pT2a: invasion into superficial muscle
    - pT2b: invasion into deep muscle
  - T3: invasion into perivesical fat
    - pT3a: microscopic
    - pT3b: macroscopic
  - T4: invasion into adjacent organs
    - T4a: invades prostate, uterus, vagina, or bowel
    - T4b: invades abdominal wall, pelvic wall, or other organs
- N1 to N3: invades lymph nodes
- M: metastasis to bone or soft tissue

TREATMENT

For nonmuscle-invasive bladder cancer, the treatment includes a complete TURBT and a single dose of intravesical chemotherapy; additional intravesical chemotherapy depends on risk of recurrence and progression. For muscle-invasive cancer, a radical cystectomy with pelvic lymphadenectomy is preferred. A recent Cochrane review compared open radical cystectomy with robotic radical cystectomy and did not find significant differences in time to recurrence, rates of major complications, quality of life, or positive margin rates.

MEDICATION

First Line
- Single immediate installation of intravesical chemotherapy (e.g., mitomycin, epirubicin, or gemcitabine) after TURBT is recommended for low-risk superficial lesions (3).
- Six-week induction course of intravesical BCG or Mitomycin C after TURBT in high-risk superficial lesions has been shown to decrease recurrence and delay disease progression (3),(6).
- Chemotherapy is the first-line treatment for metastatic bladder cancer:
  - Methotrexate, vinblastine, doxorubicin, cisplatin (MVAC) is the preferred regimen.

Second Line
- A recent review showed that gemcitabine plus cisplatin may be better tolerated and result in equivalent survival to MVAC.
- Checkpoint inhibition immunotherapy is preferred for patients who progressed after platinum-based therapy.

ISSUES FOR REFERRAL

Patients with microscopic or gross hematuria not otherwise explained or resolving should be referred to a urologist for cystoscopy.

ADDITIONAL THERAPIES

Radiotherapy:
- In the United States, used for patients with muscle-invasive cancer who are not surgical candidates or who want to preserve their native bladder (3)
- Preoperative (radical cystectomy) radiotherapy also an option

SURGERY/OTHER PROCEDURES

Surgery is definitive therapy for superficial and invasive cancer:
- Superficial cancer: TURBT
- Invasive cancer:
  - Radical cystectomy and bilateral pelvic lymphadenectomy is the gold standard (3).
  - Partial cystectomy may be an option in select cases.
  - May require prostatectomy in men or complete hysterectomy and bilateral salpingo-oophorectomy in women (7)

ADMISSION, INPATIENT, AND NURSING CONSIDERATIONS

Need for surgery or intensive therapy

 ONGOING CARE

FOLLOW-UP RECOMMENDATIONS
- Superficial cancers
  - Urine cytology alone has not been shown to be sufficient for follow-up.
  - Cystoscopy every 3 months for 18 to 24 months, every 6 months for the next 2 years and then annually (6)
- Follow-up for invasive cancers depends on the approach to treatment.
- Patients treated with BCG require lifelong follow-up.

DIET
Continue adequate fluid intake.

PATIENT EDUCATION
Smoking cessation

PROGNOSIS
- Prognosis depends on the stage of the cancer, grade (how the cells look under the microscope), presence of carcinoma in situ in other parts of the bladder, patient's age, and general health.
- 5-year relative survival rates (2)
  - Overall survival: 77.1%
    - In situ: 96.0%
    - Localized: 69.6%
    - Regional metastasis: 37.5%
    - Distant metastasis: 6.4%
- Superficial bladder cancer
  - Prognosis depends on how many tumors there are, size of the tumors, and whether it recurred after treatment.
  - Single immediate installation of intravesical chemotherapy after TURBT decreases tumor recurrence 10–15% versus TURBT alone (6)
  - BCG treatment decreases risk of recurrence and progression in high-risk superficial lesions.
- Invasive cancer
  - T2 disease: Radical cystectomy results in 60–75% 5-year survival.
  - T3 or T4 disease: Radical cystectomy results in 20–40% 5-year survival.
  - Neoadjuvant chemotherapy with cystectomy has led to varying degrees of increased survival.
  - Radiation with chemotherapy has led to varying degrees of increased survival.
- Metastatic cancer
  - MVAC resulted in mean survival of 12.5 months.

COMPLICATIONS
- Superficial bladder cancer
  - Local symptoms
    - Dysuria, frequency, nocturia, pain, passing debris in urine
    - Bacterial cystitis
    - Perforation
  - General symptoms
    - Flulike symptoms
    - Systemic infection
- Invasive cancer
  - Symptoms related to definitive treatment, including incontinence, bleeding
  - Patients with neobladder at risk for azotemia and metabolic acidosis

REFERENCES

1. Li HT, Duymich CE, Weisenberger DJ, et al. Genetic and epigenetic alterations in bladder cancer. *Int Neurourol J*. 2016;20(Suppl 2):S84–S94.
2. National Cancer Institute Surveillance, Epidemiology, and End Results Program. *Cancer stat facts: bladder cancer*. https://seer.cancer.gov /statfacts/html/urinb.html. Accessed August 9, 2021.
3. Kamat AM, Hahn NM, Efstathiou JA, et al. Bladder cancer. *Lancet*. 2016;388(10061):2796–2810.
4. Saginala K, Barsouk A, Aluru JS, et al. Epidemiology of bladder cancer. *Med Sci (Basel)*. 2020;8(1):15.
5. Tang H, Shi W, Fu S, et al. Pioglitazone and bladder cancer risk: a systematic review and meta-analysis. *Cancer Med*. 2018;7(4):1070–1080.
6. Chang SS, Boorjian SA, Chou R, et al. Diagnosis and treatment of non-muscle invasive bladder cancer: AUA/SUO guideline. *J Urol*. 2016;196(4):1021.
7. Spiess PE, Agarwal N, Bangs R, et al. Bladder Cancer, Version 5.2017, NCCN Clinical Practice Guidelines in Oncology. *J Natl Compr Canc Netw*. 2017;15(10):1240–1267.

ADDITIONAL READING

DeGeorge KC, Holt HR, Hodges SC. Bladder cancer: diagnosis and treatment. *Am Fam Physician*. 2017;96(8):507–514.

 SEE ALSO

- Hematuria
- Algorithm: Hematuria

CODES

ICD10
- C67.8 Malignant neoplasm of overlapping sites of bladder
- C67 Malignant neoplasm of bladder
- C67.6 Malignant neoplasm of ureteric orifice

CLINICAL PEARLS
- Painless hematuria should be evaluated with cystoscopy.
  - Do not perform cystoscopy or imaging in asymptomatic, never-smoking women <50 years with microscopic hematuria with <25 RBC/HPF.
- Be aware of potential link between pioglitazone treatment and risk for bladder cancer.
- Worst outcomes for patient who continues to smoke
- The U.S. Preventive Services Task Force recommends against routine screening for bladder cancer.

BORDERLINE PERSONALITY DISORDER

Rebecca Groch, MD • Lauren Penwell-Waines, PhD • Michael Scott Clark, MD

BASICS

DESCRIPTION

A psychiatric disorder that begins no later than adolescence or early adulthood, borderline personality disorder (BPD) is a consistent and pervasive pattern of unstable and reactive moods and sense of self, impulsivity, and volatile interpersonal relationships (1):

- Common behaviors and variations:
  - Unstable self-image
  - Unstable goals, aspirations, values, and plans
  - Self-mutilation: pinching, scratching, cutting
  - Suicide: ideation, history of attempts, plans
  - Splitting: idealizing then devaluing others
  - Presentation of helplessness or victimization
  - High utilization of emergency department and resultant inpatient hospitalizations for psychiatric treatment
- High rate of associated mental disorders
- Typically display little insight into behavior

Geriatric Considerations
Symptoms generally improve with age. Illness (both acute and chronic) may exacerbate feelings of fear and helplessness.

Pediatric Considerations
Diagnosis is rarely made in children. Axis I disorders and general medical conditions (GMCs) are more probable.

Pregnancy Considerations
Pregnancy may exacerbate stress or increased fears, resulting in escalation of borderline behaviors.

EPIDEMIOLOGY
Onset no later than adolescence or early adulthood (may go undiagnosed for years)

Prevalence
- 0.5–5.9% of U.S. population
- 10% of all psychiatric outpatients and between 15% and 25% of patients in psychiatry inpatient settings have BPD (2).

ETIOLOGY AND PATHOPHYSIOLOGY
Undetermined but generally accepted that BPD is due to a combination of the following:
- Hereditary temperamental traits
- Environment (i.e., history of childhood sexual and/or physical abuse, history of childhood neglect, ongoing conflict in home, maladaptive parenting styles)
- Insufficient modulation by prefrontal region over limbic structures

Genetics
First-degree relatives are at greater risk for this disorder (undetermined if due to genetic or psychosocial factors).

RISK FACTORS
- Childhood sexual and/or physical abuse and neglect
- Disrupted family life
- Physical illness and external social factors may exacerbate BPD.

GENERAL PREVENTION
Tends to be a multigenerational problem. Children, caregivers, and significant others should have some time and activities away from the borderline individual, which may protect them.

COMMONLY ASSOCIATED CONDITIONS
Other psychiatric disorders

DIAGNOSIS

- The comprehensive evaluation should identify
  - Comorbid conditions
  - Functional impairments
  - Adaptive/maladaptive coping styles
  - Psychosocial stressors
  - Patient strengths; needs/goals
- Initial assessment should focus on risk factors:
  - Establish treatment agreement with patient and outline treatment goals.
  - Assess suicide ideation, self-harm behavior, psychosis.

HISTORY
- Clinic visits for problems that do not have biologic findings
- Conflicts with medical staff members
- Idealizing or unexplained anger at physician
- History of unrealistic expectations of physician (e.g., "I know you can take care of me." "You're the best, unlike my last provider.")
- Obtain collateral information (i.e., from family, partner) about patient behaviors.
- History of interpersonal difficulties, affective instability, and impulsivity
- History of self-injurious behavior, possibly with suicidal threats or attempts

PHYSICAL EXAM
- Thorough physical examination to help lower suspicion of organic disease (especially thyroid disease) (1),(2)
- Often no gross abnormalities found other than related to scarring from self-mutilation.

DIFFERENTIAL DIAGNOSIS
- Mood disorders:
  - In particular, disruptive mood dysregulation disorder, a pediatric diagnosis characterized by severe recurrent temper outbursts manifesting verbally or behaviorally and grossly out of proportion to the situation, may appear quite similar to the acting out and intense emotions seen in BPD. Look for other symptoms characteristic of BPD to differentiate (1).
- Psychotic disorder
  - Although auditory and visual hallucinations may be present, they typically are in the context of situational crises and are not accompanied by disordered thoughts, bizarre delusions, flat affect, or other negative symptoms.
- Attention deficit hyperactivity disorder (ADHD)— BPD has more severe emotional dysregulation and less severe impulsivity.
- GMC
- Substance use disorder (SUD)

DIAGNOSTIC TESTS & INTERPRETATION
- Consider age of onset. To meet criteria for BPD, borderline pattern of behaviors will be present from adolescence or early adulthood.
- Formal psychological testing
- Rule out personality change due to a GMC (1)[C].

Initial Tests (lab, imaging)
Thyroid stimulating hormone (TSH) and urine drug screen to rule out GMC and SUD

Diagnostic Procedures/Other
According to *Diagnostic and Statistical Manual of Mental Disorders, 5th edition (DSM-5)* criteria, patient must meet at least five of the following criteria (1)[C]:
- Attempt to avoid abandonment
- Volatile interpersonal relationships
- Identity disturbance
- Impulsive behavior:
  - In ≥2 areas
  - Impulsive behavior is self-damaging.
- Suicidal or self-mutilating behavior
- Mood instability
- Feeling empty
- Is unable to control anger or finds it difficult
- Paranoid or dissociative when under stress

TREATMENT

- Outpatient psychotherapy for BPD is the preferred treatment (3),(4)[C]:
  - Dialectical behavior therapy (DBT) combines cognitive behavioral techniques for emotional regulation and reality testing with concepts of distress tolerance, acceptance, and self-awareness.
    - Following a dialectal process, therapists are tough-minded allies who validate feelings and are unconditionally accepting while also reminding patients to accept their dire level of emotional dysfunction and to apply better alternative behaviors.
- Other empirically supported treatments to consider include transference-focused (psychodynamic) psychotherapy, cognitive-behavioral therapy (CBT), mentalization, schema-focused therapy, and mindfulness-based therapies.

GENERAL MEASURES

- Patients with BPD require more medical care and increased "intentionality" by the provider.
- Focus on patient management rather than on "fixing" behaviors:
  - Schedule consistent follow-up appointments to relieve patient anxiety.
  - Meet with and rely on treatment team to avoid splitting of team by patient and to provide opportunity to discuss patient issues.
  - Set appropriate boundaries for communication.
  - Treatment is usually most effective when both medications and psychotherapy are used simultaneously.

MEDICATION

- Although no specific medications are approved by the FDA to treat BPD, pharmacotherapy can be used for symptom management for comorbid Axis I disorders (2)[A].
  - Affective dysregulation: mood stabilizers, selective serotonin reuptake inhibitors (SSRIs), and monoamine oxidase inhibitors (MAOIs)
  - Impulsive-behavioral control: SSRIs and mood stabilizers
  - Cognitive-perceptual symptoms: antipsychotics on a short-term basis
- Consider high rate of self-harm and suicidal behavior when prescribing (2)[A].
- Anxiolytics are typically contraindicated due to reduced inhibition that may lead to increased impulsivity.
- SSRIs are having a less prominent role with more emphasis on mood stabilizers and atypical antipsychotics, but research is uncertain and inconclusive.

ISSUES FOR REFERRAL

- Urgency for scheduled follow-up depends on community resources (e.g., outpatient day programs for suicidal patients; substance abuse programs)
- With increased risk for self-harm or self-defeating behaviors and low community resources, the patient can/will have increased need for frequent visits.

SURGERY/OTHER PROCEDURES

There is emerging but inconclusive evidence for the use of transcranial stimulation to improve executive functioning (5).

COMPLEMENTARY & ALTERNATIVE MEDICINE

Omega-3 fatty acid dietary supplementation has shown beneficial effects for decreasing emotional reactivity (2)[B].

ADMISSION, INPATIENT, AND NURSING CONSIDERATIONS

- Hospitalizations should be limited and of short duration to adjust medications, implement psychotherapy for crisis intervention, and stabilize patients from psychosocial stressors.
- Extended inpatient hospitalization should be considered for the following reasons:
  - Persistent/severe suicidal ideation or risk to others
  - Comorbid substance use and/or nonadherence to outpatient or partial hospitalization treatments
  - Comorbid Axis I disorders that may increase threat to life for the patient (i.e., eating disorders, mood disorders)

 ## ONGOING CARE

FOLLOW-UP RECOMMENDATIONS

- Schedule visits that are short, more frequent, and focused to relieve patients' anxiety about relationships with their physician/provider and to help reduce risk of provider burnout.
- Emphasize importance of healthy lifestyle modifications (i.e., exercise, rest, diet).

Patient Monitoring

Monitor for suicidal ideation/behaviors or other self-harm behaviors.

PATIENT EDUCATION

Include patients in the diagnosis so they can make sense of their disease process and participate in the treatment strategy.

PROGNOSIS

Borderline behaviors may decrease with age and over time.

REFERENCES

1. American Psychiatric Association. *Diagnostic and Statistical Manual of Mental Disorders*. 5th ed. Arlington, VA: American Psychiatric Association; 2013.
2. Leichsenring F, Leibing E, Kruse J, et al. Borderline personality disorder. *Lancet*. 2011;377(9759):74–84.
3. Doering S. Borderline personality disorder in patients with medical illness: a review of assessment, prevalence, and treatment options. *Psychosom Med*. 2019;81(7):584–594. doi:10.1097/PSY.0000000000000724.
4. Rao S, Heidari P, Broadbear JH. Developments in diagnosis and treatment of people with borderline personality disorder. *Curr Opin Psychiatry*. 2020;33(5):441–446. doi:10.1097/YCO.0000000000000625.
5. Lisoni J, Miotto P, Barlati S, et al. Change in core symptoms of borderline personality disorder by tDCS: a pilot study. *Psychiatry Res*. 2020;291:113261.

 ## CODES

ICD10

F60.3 Borderline personality disorder

CLINICAL PEARLS

- BPD may be discerned by the impropriety of reactions to situations others find or minor.
- View BPD as a chronic condition with waxing and waning features. It is important to adjust medications/treatments as clinically appropriate when symptoms change.
- If there are problems with the patient disrespecting the physician or support staff, clear guidelines should be established with the treatment team and then with the patient.
- When considering terminating care, the patient may improve if empathetically confronted about certain behaviors and is given clear guidelines on how to behave in the clinic. It is the patient's job to follow the guidelines, and it is you and your team's job to enforce the guidelines. Designate a well-trained support staff to be the primary contact person for the patient.
- Have an agenda when you visit with BPD patients. Be cordial and identify one to two issues to be discussed per clinic visit. Frequently scheduled visits can help with this.
- Regularly scheduled psychotherapy improves medical care by becoming the "home" for mental health treatment, leaving the physician to focus on the patient's immediate medical issues.

BRAIN INJURY, TRAUMATIC

James R. Yon, MD • Christina Colosimo, DO, MS

 BASICS

DESCRIPTION
- Traumatic brain injury (TBI) is defined as an alteration in brain function or other evidence of brain pathology, caused by an external force.
- System(s) affected: neurologic; psychiatric; cardiovascular; endocrine/metabolic; gastrointestinal; pulmonary
- Synonym(s): head injury, concussion

EPIDEMIOLOGY
Incidence
- Sixty-nine million individuals worldwide are estimated to sustain a TBI each year.
- 801,700 ED visits and 326,600 hospitalizations per year in the United States
- 61,000 deaths per year; ~30% of all injury-related deaths
- Incidence in males twice that of females

Prevalence
- Predominant age: 0 to 4 years, 15 to 19 years, and >65 years
- Predominant gender: male > female (2:1)

ETIOLOGY AND PATHOPHYSIOLOGY
- Centers for Disease Control and Prevention (CDC) TBI data in 2017, mechanism of injury of hospitalized patients (male vs. female percentage)
  – Unintentional falls (35.6 vs. 23.9)
  – Motor vehicle crashes (22.5 vs. 10.8)
  – Unintentionally being struck by or against an object (2.3 vs. 0.9)
  – Intentional self-harm (0.8 vs. 0.3)
  – Assault (7.5 vs. 1.7)
  – Children 0 to 17 years
    ○ Falls (7.7)
    ○ Motor vehicle crashes (6.8)
- Contact sports account for 45% of TBI emergency room visits for children related to sports and recreation.
- Primary insult: direct mechanical damage
- Secondary insult: actuation of complex cellular and molecular cascades that promote cerebral edema, ischemia, and apoptotic cell death

RISK FACTORS
Alcohol and drug use, prior/recurrent head injury, contact sports, seizure disorder, ADHD, male sex

Geriatric Considerations
Subdural hematomas are common after a fall or blow in elderly; symptoms may be subtle and not present until days after trauma. Many elderly patients are on antiplatelet or anticoagulation therapy.

GENERAL PREVENTION
- Safety education and fall prevention
- Seat belts; bicycle and motorcycle helmets
- Protective headgear for contact sports

Pediatric Considerations
Child abuse: Consider if dropped or fell <4 feet (e.g., off bed, couch), suspicious history, significant injury present, or any retinal hemorrhages.

DIAGNOSIS

HISTORY
- Loss of consciousness (LOC), headache, vomiting, amnesia, confusion, dizziness, sensitivity to light
- Epidural hemorrhage from blunt trauma: 30% with a "lucid interval" (initial LOC followed by recovery of consciousness and then LOC recurs and persists)

PHYSICAL EXAM
- Neurologic and cognitive testing is important.
- Repeat neurologic exams every 30 minutes until 2 hours after Glasgow Coma Scale (GCS) reaches 15, then hourly for 4 hours, and then every 2 hours.
- Evidence of increased intracranial pressure (ICP) (elevated BP, decreased pulse rate, or slow/irregular breathing [Cushing triad]—only 30% have all three)
- Signs of basilar skull fracture: raccoon eyes, Battle sign, hemotympanum, CSF rhinorrhea or otorrhea

DIFFERENTIAL DIAGNOSIS
Other causes of altered mental status (e.g., toxicologic, infectious, metabolic, vascular)

DIAGNOSTIC TESTS & INTERPRETATION
Initial Tests (lab, imaging)
- Mild TBI and concussions cognitive screening tests
- Evaluate for coagulopathy.
- Type and screen for possible surgical intervention.
- Perform drug and alcohol screening.
- Noncontrasted CT head is the study of choice to review bone windows, tissue windows, and subdural space.

Pediatric Considerations
Skull radiographs are not indicated unless abuse is suspected, in which case they can detect fractures not seen under CT; no return to activity until they are asymptomatic and return to school should precede return to sport/physical activity (1)[A].

TREATMENT

GENERAL MEASURES
Acute management depends on injury severity. Most patients need no interventions.
- Immediate goal: Determine who needs further therapy, imaging studies (CT), and hospitalization to prevent further injury.
- For the mildly injured patient
  – Early education is beneficial for recovery (1)[A].
  – Graduated return to cognitive and physical activity when there are no evident signs or symptoms (physical, cognitive, emotional, or behavioral) on neuropsychological and clinical evaluation (2)[A]
- For the moderate to severely injured patient
  – Avoid hypotension or hypoxia. Head injury causes increased ICP secondary to edema, and cerebral perfusion pressure (CPP) should be maintained between 60 and 70 mm Hg (3)[A].
  – 30-degree head elevation decreases ICP and improves CPP.

– Hyperventilation (hypocapnia)
  ○ Use should be limited to patients with impending herniation while preparing for definitive treatment or intraoperatively; risk of worsening cerebral ischemia and organ damage (3)
– Mild systematic hypothermia lowers ICP but leads to increased rates of pneumonia. Selective brain cooling may also decrease ICP with improved outcomes at 2 years postinjury. A meta-analysis showed that when hypothermia was maintained for more than 48 hours, reduction in mortality was the greatest and neurologic outcome were the best (4).
– 3% hypertonic saline and mannitol effectively reduce ICP; however, 3% hypertonic saline effectively increases CPP, whereas mannitol has a more sustained effect on ICP (5). In regard to refractory intracranial hypertension, hypertonic saline is preferred (6).
- Seizure prophylaxis
  – Does not change morbidity or mortality. Consider phenytoin or levetiracetam for 1 week postinjury or longer for patients with early seizures, dural-penetrating injuries, multiple contusions, and/or subdural hematomas requiring evacuation (7)[A].

MEDICATION
First Line
- Pain control is important in patients with a TBI. In individuals with severe brain injuries who can't communicate, there are scales such as the Nociception Coma Scale (NCS) that can be used (8).
- Increased ICP
- Hypertonic saline: 2 mL/kg IV decreases ICP without adverse hemodynamic status; preferred agent (3),(9)[A]
- Mannitol: 0.25 to 2.00 g/kg (0.25 to 1.00 g/kg in children) given over 30 to 60 minutes in patients with adequate renal function. Prophylactic use is associated with worse outcomes (9)[A].
- Sedation
  – Propofol: preferred due to short duration of action. Avoid high doses to prevent propofol infusion syndrome. When combined with morphine, it can also effectively decrease ICP and decrease use of other meds (9)[A].
  – Midazolam: similar sedating effect to propofol but may cause hypotension (9)[A]
  – A systematic review that no one sedative agent is more efficacious than the other for improvement of patient-centered outcomes, ICP, or CPP in critically ill adults with severe TBI (10).
- Seizures
  – Phenytoin (Dilantin): 15 mg/kg IV (1 mg/kg/min IV, not to exceed 50 mg/min). Stop infusion if QT interval increases by >50%.

ALERT
Avoid corticosteroid use because it increases mortality rates and risk of developing late seizures (9)[A].

ISSUES FOR REFERRAL
Consult neurosurgery for:
- All penetrating head trauma
- All abnormal head CTs

ADDITIONAL THERAPIES

- Emerging therapies with limited but promising evidence: coma arousal therapy: amantadine, zolpidem, and levodopa/carbidopa; post-coma therapy: bromocriptine
- Mixed results for therapeutic hypothermia with defined physiologic parameters (11)[A]
- In a systematic review and meta-analysis, TXA was found to have no significant difference in incidence of thromboembolic complications (1.7% in TXA vs. 1.4% in placebo group) (12)[A]. In the TBI population, it demonstrated a reduction in deaths.

SURGERY/OTHER PROCEDURES

- Early evacuation of trauma-related intracranial hematoma decreases mortality especially with GCS <6 and CT evidence of hematoma, cerebral swelling, or herniation.
- CSF drainage reduces ICP but has not been demonstrated to have long-term benefit.
- CSF leakage often resolves in 24 hours with bed rest but if not may require surgical repair (3)[A].

COMPLEMENTARY & ALTERNATIVE MEDICINE

Music therapy in conjunction with multimodal stimulation improves awareness in comatose TBI patients (11)[B].

ADMISSION, INPATIENT, AND NURSING CONSIDERATIONS

- Abnormal GCS or CT
- Persistent neurologic deficits (e.g., confusion, somnolence)
- Patient with no competent adult at home for observation
- Possibly admit: LOC, amnesia, patients on anticoagulants with negative CT
- C-spine immobilization should be considered in all head trauma.
- Use normal saline for resuscitation fluid.
- Discharge criteria: normal CT with return to normal mental status and responsible adult to observe patient at home (see "Patient Monitoring")

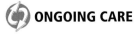 ONGOING CARE

FOLLOW-UP RECOMMENDATIONS

- Schedule regular follow-up within a week to determine return to activities.
- Rehabilitation indicated following a significant acute injury. Set realistic goals.
- For patients on anticoagulants, net benefit to restarting therapy after discharge despite increased bleeding risk

Patient Monitoring

Patient should be discharged to the care of a competent adult with clear instructions on signs and symptoms that warrant immediate evaluation (e.g., changing mental status, worsening headache, focal findings, or any signs of distress). Patients should be monitored but not awakened from sleep.

DIET

As tolerated, monitor for signs of nausea.

PATIENT EDUCATION

Proper counseling, symptomatic management, and gradual return to normal activities are essential.

PROGNOSIS

- Gradual improvement may continue for years
- Mortality rate for TBI is 30 per 100,000 annually in the United States.
- Poor prognostic factors: low GCS on admission, nonreactive pupils, old age, comorbidity, midline shift, nonambulatory
- 50% of patients with mild TBI will returned to work by 1 month after injury and more than 80% by 6 months.

COMPLICATIONS

- Chronic subdural hematoma, which may follow even "mild" head injury, especially in the elderly; often presents with headache and decreased mentation
- Seizures: incidence of late seizures after TBI, over 30 years is 2% for mild injuries, 4% for moderate injuries, and over 15% for severe injuries (13); 5% in hospitalized patients
- Postconcussion syndrome can follow mild head injury without LOC and includes headaches, dizziness, fatigue, and subtle cognitive or affective changes.
- Second-impact syndrome occurs when the CNS loses autoregulation. An individual with a minor head injury is returned to a contact sport, and, following even minor trauma (e.g., whiplash), the patient loses consciousness and may quickly herniate, with a 50% mortality. A similar syndrome of malignant edema can occur in children with even a single injury.

REFERENCES

1. Nygren-de Boussard C, Holm LW, Cancelliere C, et al. Nonsurgical interventions after mild traumatic brain injury: a systematic review. Results of the International Collaboration on Mild Traumatic Brain Injury Prognosis. *Arch Phys Med Rehabil*. 2014;95(Suppl 3):S257–S264.
2. McCrory P, Meeuwisse WH, Aubry M, et al. Consensus statement on concussion in sport: the 4th International Conference on Concussion in Sport held in Zurich, November 2012. *Br J Sports Med*. 2013;47(5):250–258.
3. Tsang KK, Whitfield PC. Traumatic brain injury: review of current management strategies. *Br J Oral Maxillofac Surg*. 2012;50(4):298–308.
4. Peterson K, Carson S, Carney N. Hypothermia treatment for traumatic brain injury: a systematic review and meta-analysis. *J Neurotrauma*. 2008;25(1):62–71. doi:10.1089/neu.2007.0424.
5. Shi J, Tan L, Ye J, et al. Hypertonic saline and mannitol in patients with traumatic brain injury: a systemic and meta-analysis. *Medicine (Baltimore)*. 2020;99(35):e21655. doi:10.1097/D.0000000000021655.
6. Gu J, Huang H, Huang Y, et al. Hypertonic saline or mannitol for treating elevated intracranial pressure in traumatic brain injury: a meta-analysis of randomized controlled trials. *Neurosurg Rev*. 2019;42(2):499–509. doi.org/10.1007/s10143-018-0991-8.
7. Agrawal A, Timothy J, Pandit L, et al. Posttraumatic epilepsy: an overview. *Clin Neurol Neurosurg*. 2006;108(5):433–439.
8. Schnakers C, Chatelle C, Vanhaudenhuyse A, et al. The Nociception Coma Scale: a new tool to assess nociception in disorders of consciousness. *Pain*. 2010;148(2):215–219.
9. Meyer MJ, Megyesi J, Meythaler J, et al. Acute management of acquired brain injury part II: an evidence-based review of pharmacological interventions. *Brain Inj*. 2010;24(5):706–721.
10. Roberts DJ, Hall RI, Kramer AH, et al. Sedation for critically ill adults with severe traumatic brain injury: a systematic review of randomized controlled trials. *Crit Care Med*. 2011;39(12):2743–2751.
11. Crossley S, Reid J, McLatchie R, et al. A systematic review of therapeutic hypothermia for adult patients following traumatic brain injury. *Crit Care*. 2014;18(2):R75.
12. Yokobori S, Yatabe T, Kondo Y, et al. Efficacy and safety of tranexamic acid administration in traumatic brain injury patients: a systematic review and meta-analysis. *J Intensive Care*. 2020;8:46. doi:10.1186/s40560-020-00460-5.
13. Ding K, Gupta PK, Diaz-Arrastia R. Epilepsy after traumatic brain injury. In: Laskowitz D, Grant G, eds. *Translational Research in Traumatic Brain Injury*. Boca Raton, FL: CRC Press/Taylor and Francis Group; 2016: chap 14. https://www.ncbi.nlm.nih.gov/books/NBK326716/. Accessed October 25, 2021.

 CODES

ICD10

- S06.9X0A Unsp intracranial injury w/o loss of consciousness, init
- S06.5X0A Traum subdr hem w/o loss of consciousness, init
- S06.6X0A Traum subrac hem w/o loss of consciousness, init

CLINICAL PEARLS

- TBI involves two distinct phases: the primary mechanical insult and secondary dysregulation of the cerebrovascular system with cerebral edema, ischemia, and cell-mediated death.
- Indications for imaging include evidence of skull fracture, altered consciousness, neurologic deficit, persistent vomiting, scalp hematoma, abnormal behavior, coagulopathy, age >65 years.

BREAST ABSCESS

Kelley V. Lawrence, MD, IBCLC • Lindsey Matthews, DO • Mawuse K. Gbegnon, MD

BASICS

DESCRIPTION
- Breast abscess: localized accumulation of infected fluid within the breast parenchyma
- Mastitis: breast inflammation with or without infection. This can be associated with lactation (puerperal) or nonlactational.
- Associated with lactation or fistulous tracts secondary to squamous epithelial neoplasm or duct occlusion
- System(s) affected: skin/exocrine, immune
- Synonym(s): mammary abscess; peripheral breast abscess; subareolar abscess; puerperal abscess

Pregnancy Considerations
Most commonly associated with postpartum lactation

EPIDEMIOLOGY
- Most common benign breast problem during pregnancy and puerperal period (1)
- Predominantly reproductive age and perimenopausal (between ages 18 and 50)
  - Puerperal abscess: lactational
  - Subareolar abscess: reproductive age through postmenopause (2)
    - 90% of nonlactational breast abscesses are subareolar (1).
    - Nipple piercing associated in increased risk of subareolar abscess (3)
    - Smoking linked to recurrences (3)
- Predominant sex: female
- Higher incidence in African American, diabetic, smoking, or obese women (3)

Incidence
- Ranges estimate up to 11% of breastfeeding women; the Academy of Breastfeeding Medicine cites 3% (2),(4).
- Puerperal abscess has highest incidence within 12 weeks postpartum (3) and while weaning from breastfeeding (4).

Prevalence
Transient condition; recurrences are most strongly associated with smoking, surgical treatment, and increased age (3).

ETIOLOGY AND PATHOPHYSIOLOGY
- Puerperal abscesses:
  - Likely that bacteria (often from infants oral flora) gain entry through cracks/fissures in the nipple (1)
  - Insufficient treatment of mastitis
  - Unattended postpartum engorgement and other situations leading to breast milk stasis (4)
  - Lactose-rich milk and plugged lactiferous duct causing stasis, leading to microbial growth and subsequent abscess formation
- Subareolar abscess:
  - Associated with squamous metaplasia of the lactiferous duct epithelium, keratin plugs, ductal ectasia, fistula formation (2)
  - Higher incidence in patients with nipple piercings (3)
- Microbiology
  - Staphylococcus aureus is most common cause for lactational abscesses (3),(4).
  - Methicillin-resistant S. aureus (MRSA) is a significant cause (4).
  - Less common causes (3)
    - Streptococcus pyogenes, Escherichia coli, Bacteroides, Corynebacterium, Pseudomonas, Proteus

- Anaerobes and mixed flora are more common in subareolar abscesses.
- In patients with breast implants, coagulase negative S. aureus is more common.
- In nonlactational abscesses, lack of growth is a common result.

Genetics
No current evidence to support a genetic predisposition to breast abscess formation (lifestyle/environment have been implicated more often)

RISK FACTORS
- Maternal age >30 (5)
- Primiparous (5)
- Pregnancy ≥41 weeks' gestation (5)
- Puerperal mastitis
  - Up to 11% progression to abscess (3)
  - Most often due to inadequate antibiotic and anti-inflammatory treatment of mastitis (4)
  - Risk factors (stasis) (4):
    - Infrequent or missed feeds
    - Poor latch, weak or uncoordinated suckling
    - Damage or irritation of the nipple
    - Nipple inversion or retraction
    - Inefficient removal of milk (by baby or pump)
    - Oversupply of milk
    - Illness in mother or baby
    - Rapid weaning
    - Plugged duct
    - Pressure on the breast (i.e., tight bra, car seatbelt)
    - Maternal stress and fatigue
- General risk factors (3)
  - Smoking; diabetes; obesity
  - African American
  - Nipple piercing
- Medically related risk factors
  - Steroids
  - Breast implants
  - Lumpectomy with radiation
  - Inadequate antibiotics to treat mastitis
  - Topical antifungal medication used for mastitis

GENERAL PREVENTION
- Frequent breast emptying with on-demand feeding and/or pumping to prevent mastitis
- Early treatment of mastitis with milk expression, antibiotics, and compresses
- Smoking cessation to minimize occurrence/recurrence

COMMONLY ASSOCIATED CONDITIONS
Lactation, mastitis, weaning

DIAGNOSIS

HISTORY
- Tender breast lump, usually unilateral
- Breastfeeding, weaning, or returning to work
- Decreased breast milk supply on affected breast
- Perimenopausal/postmenopausal
- Systemic malaise (usually less than with mastitis)
- Localized erythema, edema, pain
- Fever, nausea, vomiting
- Spontaneous nipple drainage
- Prior breast infection
- Diabetes

PHYSICAL EXAM
- Fever, tachycardia (not always present)
- Erythema of overlying skin

- Palpable mass, sometimes fluctuant
- Tenderness on palpation
- Induration
- Local edema
- Draining pus or skin ulceration
- Nipple and/or skin retraction
- Regional lymphadenopathy
- Puerperal abscesses are generally peripheral; nonlactational abscesses are more commonly found in periareolar/subareolar region.

DIFFERENTIAL DIAGNOSIS
- Engorgement
- Plugged milk duct
- Mastitis
- Galactocele (sometimes referred to as a milk lake)
- Fibrocystic breasts
- Fat necrosis
- Tuberculosis (may be associated with HIV infection)
- Sarcoid; granulomatous mastitis
- Syphilis
- Foreign body reactions (e.g., to silicone and paraffin)
- Mammary duct ectasia
- Carcinoma (inflammatory or primary squamous cell)

DIAGNOSTIC TESTS & INTERPRETATION
Initial Tests (lab, imaging)
- Ultrasound helps identify fluid collection (6).
  - The preferred imaging modality for abscesses (1)[C]
- CBC (leukocytosis), elevated ESR
- Culture and sensitivity of expressed breast milk or infected aspirate to identify pathogen
  - The presence of pathogenic bacteria or high bacteria count (e.g., $> 10^3$/mL) indicates mastitis; low predictive value, clinical context is needed (1)[C]

Follow-Up Tests & Special Considerations
Mammogram to rule out malignancy (generally not done during acute phase)

Diagnostic Procedures/Other
- Aspiration (+/− ultrasound guided) for culture
  - Can be diagnostic and therapeutic
  - Does not exclude malignancy
  - Cytology (particularly in nonlactating patient)
- Mammography has limited value in the acute assessment of breast abscesses or mastitis (1)[C].

Test Interpretation
- Abscesses on ultrasound can be hypoechoic, well-circumscribed, and/or macro-lobulated.
  - If ultrasound negative for pocket of fluid, consider alternative diagnoses.
  - If multiloculated on imaging, refer to breast surgical/interventional specialist.
- Utilize culture sensitivities to guide antibiotic therapy when possible.

TREATMENT

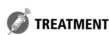

GENERAL MEASURES
- Cold and/or warm compresses for pain control (4)[C]
- Continue to breastfeed or express milk to drain the affected breast (4)[A].
- Antibiotic treatment without puerperal abscess drainage is ineffective (5)[A].
  - Acceptable to start antibiotics while working to get patient to drainage/aspiration

MEDICATION
Combination of antibiotics plus drainage for cure

First Line
- Optimal antibiotic first-line treatment for mastitis or methicillin-sensitive *S. Aureus* breast abscess includes dicloxacillin 500 mg q6h, flucloxacillin 500 mg q6h, or 1st-generation cephalosporin (but may be less preferred due to broader spectrum of coverage); clindamycin if severely penicillin-allergic (1),(4)[C]
- Breast abscess first-line treatment includes empiric antibiotics to cover community-acquired MRSA.
  - Nonsevere infection:
    - Clindamycin 300 to 450 mg PO QID as alternative for penicillin-allergic and if concern for anaerobes (2)[C]
    - TMP-SMZ DS 1 to 2 PO BID for 10 to 14 days (4)[C]
      - Mothers should discontinue breastfeeding if infant is <2 months of age.
    - Dicloxacillin plus metronidazole if non-lactational (3)[B]
      - *Contraindications*: antibiotic allergy
    - Doxycycline 100 mg BID for 7 to 10 days (1)[C]
  - In severe infections, may consider daptomycin or inpatient admission for IV vancomycin

Second Line
Consult infectious disease specialist if inadequate response to antibiotic treatment plus drainage.

ISSUES FOR REFERRAL
- Patient must be stable for outpatient referral.
- If showing signs of hemodynamic instability, patient should be referred for inpatient stabilization and care (rare).

ADDITIONAL THERAPIES
- NSAIDs for analgesia, anti-inflammatory effect, and/or antipyresis (4)[B]
- Rest, adequate fluid intake, good nutrition (4)[B]
- Application of heat to the breast just prior to feeding/milk-expression may help with adequate milk flow (4)[C].
- Cold packs applied after a feeding/milk-expression can reduce pain and edema (4)[C].

SURGERY/OTHER PROCEDURES
- Drain all abscesses and treat with antibiotics (2)[A].
- Current best practice recommendation suggest
  - Aspiration (using 18–21-gauge needle) with or without US guidance for abscesses <3 cm (1),(2) [B] (Serial aspirations may be necessary.)
  - Consider US-guided percutaneous catheter placement if abscess >3 cm (2)[B].
  - Consider incision and drainage (I&D) using 15 blade scalpel if abscess is >5 cm, recurrent, or chronic (2)[B].
- Ongoing research indicates that an algorithmic approach may provide more consistent outcomes (7)[C].
  - Consider needle aspiration for abscesses <5 cm on US, no skin changes (defined as ulceration, desquamation, or frank extrusion of purulence), and fewer than 5 days of symptoms.
  - US-guided aspiration of breast abscess is preferred to I&D in most cases due to better cosmesis and faster recovery (7)[B].

- Ongoing research also investigating use of pigtail catheter insertion and/or vacuum-assisted biopsy/aspiration (6)[B]
- Biopsy nonpuerperal abscesses to rule out malignancy; remove all fistulous tracts in nonlactating patients as well (2)[C].

COMPLEMENTARY & ALTERNATIVE MEDICINE
- Lecithin supplementation
- Acupuncture may help with breast engorgement and prevention of breast abscess.
- Breast lymphatic massage may ease engorgement.
- Judicious use of cabbage leaves applied over affected area (to decrease inflammation and milk production)

ADMISSION, INPATIENT, AND NURSING CONSIDERATIONS
- Outpatient, unless systemically immunocompromised, septic, or requiring inpatient antibiotic treatment
- Hospital-grade breast pump should be made available to patient from time of admission.

 ## ONGOING CARE
- If lactational, continue effective milk removal to prevent recurrence.
- If planning to wean from breastfeeding, avoid abrupt discontinuation of feeding.
- Consider smoking cessation to decrease risk of nonlactational abscess recurrence.

FOLLOW-UP RECOMMENDATIONS
Patient Monitoring
- Ensure complete resolution to exclude malignancy.
- Close outpatient follow-up until resolution as abscesses may require serial aspirations or drainage

DIET
No dietary patterns have been associated with breast abscess formation.

PATIENT EDUCATION
- Wound care, rest, breast milk emptying
- Continue with breastfeeding or pumping (if breast-feeding is not possible due to location of abscess; infant mouth not to come in contact with affected tissue) to prevent engorgement.

PROGNOSIS
- Drained abscess heals from inside out (in 8 to 10 days).
- Subareolar abscesses frequently recur, even after I&D and antibiotics; may require surgical removal of ducts

COMPLICATIONS
- Fistula: mammary duct or milk fistula
- Poor cosmetic outcome
- Early cessation of breastfeeding (4)

REFERENCES
1. Boakes E, Woods A, Johnson N, et al. Breast infection: a review of diagnosis and management practices. *Eur J Breast Health*. 2018;14(3):136–143.
2. Lam E, Chan T, Wiseman SM. Breast abscess: evidence based management recommendations. *Expert Rev Anti Infect Ther*. 2014;12(7):753–762.
3. David M, Handa P, Castaldi M. Predictors of outcomes in managing breast abscesses—a large retrospective single-center analysis. *Breast J*. 2018;24(5):755–763.
4. Amir L; for Academy of Breastfeeding Medicine Protocol Committee. ABM Clinical Protocol #4: mastitis, revised March 2014. *Breastfeed Med*. 2014;9(5):239–243.
5. Irusen H, Rohwer AC, Steyn DW, et al. Treatments for breast abscesses in breastfeeding women. *Cochrane Database Syst Rev*. 2015;(8):CD010490.
6. Colin C, Delov AG, Peyron-Faure N, et al. Breast abscesses in lactating women: evidences for ultrasound-guided percutaneous drainage to avoid surgery. *Emerg Radiol*. 2019;26(5):507–514.
7. Barron AU, Luk S, Phelan HA, et al. Do acute-care surgeons follow best practices for breast abscess management? A single-institution analysis of 325 consecutive cases. *J Surg Res*. 2017;216:169–171.

ADDITIONAL READING
Hale TW, Rowe HE. *Medications and Mothers' Milk. A Manual of Lactation Pharmacology*. New York, NY: Springer; 2017.

 ## CODES

ICD10
- N61 Inflammatory disorders of breast
- O91.13 Abscess of breast associated with lactation
- O91.12 Abscess of breast associated with the puerperium

CLINICAL PEARLS
- Up to 11% of cases of puerperal mastitis progress to abscess formation (most often due to inadequate therapy).
- Risk factors for mastitis result from milk stasis (poor milk transfer, infrequent feeds, missing feeds, weaning) (2),(4).
- Treat abscesses not associated with lactation with antibiotics that cover anaerobic bacteria and work up for malignancy. Doxycycline is also an option for lactating women (if needed) for treatment duration <3 weeks.
- The treatment of choice for most breast abscesses is the combination of antibiotics plus aspiration.
- US-guided aspiration of breast abscess is preferred to I&D in most cases due to better cosmesis and faster recovery (7)[B].
- If lactational, continue to empty the breast (feeding, pumping, or expression of breast milk) (4).

BREAST CANCER

Anne Campbell Larkin, MD

BASICS

Most commonly diagnosed cancer (CA) in women and the second most common cause of CA death for U.S. women. Females have a ~2.6% or 1 in 39 chance of dying from breast cancer in the United States.

DESCRIPTION
- Malignant neoplasm of cells native to the breast—epithelial, glandular, or stroma
- Types: ductal carcinoma in situ (DCIS), infiltrating ductal carcinoma, infiltrating lobular carcinoma, Paget disease, phyllodes tumor, inflammatory breast cancer (BC), angiosarcoma

EPIDEMIOLOGY
Incidence
- Estimated new female DCIS: 49,290; invasive BC: 281,550 in 2021
- Estimated deaths in 2021: females 43,600
- Incidence rates of BC have increased by 0.5% per year in recent years.

Prevalence
There are >3.8 million breast cancer survivors in US.

ETIOLOGY AND PATHOPHYSIOLOGY
- Genes such as *BRCA1* and *BRCA2* function as tumor suppressor genes, and mutation leads to cell cycle progression and limitations in DNA repair.
- Mutations in estrogen/progesterone induce cyclin D1 and *c-Myc* expression, leading to cell cycle progression.
- Additional tumors (33%) may cross talk with estrogen receptors and epidermal growth factors receptors (EGFR), leading to similar abnormal cellular replication.

Genetics
- Criteria for additional risk evaluation/gene testing in affected BC individual
  - BC at age ≤50 years
  - BC at any age and
    - ≥1 family member with BC ≤50 years of age or ovarian/fallopian tube/primary peritoneal CA
    - ≥2 family members with BC or pancreatic CA
    - Population at increased risk (e.g., Ashkenazi Jew with BC or ovarian CA at any age)
  - Triple-negative BC (ER−, PR−, HER2−)
  - Two BC primaries
  - Ovarian/fallopian tube/primary peritoneal CA
  - ≥1 family member with BC and CA of thyroid, adrenal cortex, endometrium, pancreas, central nervous system, diffuse gastric, aggressive prostate (Gleason >7), leukemia, lymphoma, sarcoma, dermatologic manifestations, and/or macrocephaly, gastrointestinal (GI) hamartomas
  - Male BC
- Criteria for additional risk evaluation/gene testing in unaffected BC individual
  - First- or second-degree relative with BC ≤45 years of age
  - ≥2 breast primaries in one individual
  - ≥1 ovarian/fallopian tube/primary peritoneal CA from same side of family
  - ≥2 w/ breast primaries on same side of family
  - ≥1 family member with BC and CA of thyroid, adrenal cortex, endometrium, pancreas, CNS, diffuse gastric, aggressive prostate, leukemia, lymphoma, sarcoma, dermatologic manifestations, and/or macrocephaly, GI hamartomas
  - Ashkenazi Jew with BC/ovarian CA at any age
  - Male BC
  - Known BC *susceptibility gene* mutation in a family member

- *BRCA1* and *BRCA2* are inherited in an autosomal fashion and account for 5–10% of female and 5–20% of male CAs; 15–20% familial BCs
  - Mutations higher in Ashkenazi Jewish descent
  - Mutation in *BRCA* raises risk to 45–65% from 7% at age 70 years.

RISK FACTORS
- National Cancer Institute BC Risk calculator: https://bcrisktool.cancer.gov
- Hormone replacement therapy (combination estrogen-progesterone and estrogen only agents [but not vaginal estrogen]) during perimenopause increases breast cancer risk for 10 years after medication is discontinued.
- Relative risk (RR) >4.0:
  - Age >65 years
  - Biopsy confirmed atypical hyperplasia
  - *BRCA* mutation
  - DCIS
  - Lobular carcinoma in situ (LCIS)
  - Personal history of early-onset BC (<40 years)
  - ≥2 first-degree relatives diagnosed at an early age
- RR 2.1 to 4.0:
  - Personal history of BC (40+ years)
  - Postmenopausal
  - History of radiation
  - First-degree relative of BC
- RR 1.1 to 2.0:
  - Alcohol use
  - Ashkenazi Jewish descent
  - Diethylstilbestrol exposure
  - Early menarche (<12 years old)
  - Late menopause (>55 years old)
  - High socioeconomic status
  - First pregnancy at >30 years
  - Proliferative breast disease without atypia (fibroadenoma or ductal hyperplasia)
  - Dense breasts (>50%)
  - Nulliparous/no history of full-term pregnancy
  - No history of breastfeeding
  - History of obesity
  - History of endometrial or ovarian CA
  - Hormone replacement therapy
  - Recent oral contraceptive pill use
  - Tall height
- Patients with 20–25% lifetime risk should receive an annual MRI beginning at age 30 years:
  - *BRCA* mutation
  - First-degree relative with *BRCA* mutation
  - History of radiation age 10 to 30 years
  - Li-Fraumeni or Cowden syndrome or first-degree relative with the same
- Patients with 15–20% lifetime risk:
  - Personal history of BC, DCIS, LCIS, atypical ductal hyperplasia, atypical lobular hyperplasia
  - History of dense or unevenly dense breasts

GENERAL PREVENTION
- Maintain healthy weight—obesity increases BC risk; physical activity and healthy diet are key.
- Limit alcohol use—≥1 serving of alcohol per day is recommended.
- High serum 25-OH vitamin D levels correlate with lower breast cancer risk; consider vitamin D supplementation.
- Medication: The U.S. Preventative Services Task Force (USPSTF) recommends that clinicians offer to prescribe risk-reducing medications, such as tamoxifen, raloxifene, or aromatase inhibitors, to women who are at increased risk for breast cancer

and at low risk for adverse medication effects (B recommendation).
  - The National Cancer Institute Risk Assessment Tool can be used to determine risk.
  - Greater risk was defined as >3% where the risk of medication harms are low.
- Breast self-exams (BSE): American Cancer Society no longer recommend routine monthly BSE.
- Clinical breast exam (CBE):
  - USPSTF: insufficient evidence to assess clinical benefits and harms
  - American Cancer Society (ACS): no clear benefit or structured guidelines in average-risk women (1)
- Mammography:
  - USPSTF: women should undergo biennial mammogram starting at age 50 until age 74
  - American Cancer Society: Women should have annual mammograms starting at age 45 to 54, then women 55 and over should have biennial mammograms or can continue yearly screening if desired (1).
    - Women ages 40 to 44 have the choice to begin annual screening mammograms if desired.

COMMONLY ASSOCIATED CONDITIONS
- Genetic syndromes and mutations such as BRCA1, BRCA2, Li-Fraumeni, and Cowden disease
- History of high-risk breast lesions such as atypical ductal hyperplasia (ADH), atypical lobular hyperplasia (ALH), and LCIS
- Obesity

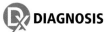

DIAGNOSIS

HISTORY
- Painless lump in breast or axilla
- Swelling, thickening, redness, or dimpling of the skin
- Nipple discharge (bloody), erosion, or retraction
- Abnormal findings or calcifications on screening mammography

PHYSICAL EXAM
- Visualize breasts with patient sitting and supine looking for skin dimpling, peau d'orange, and asymmetry.
- Palpation of all four breast quadrants and regional lymph node exam: cervical, supraclavicular, infraclavicular, axillary

DIFFERENTIAL DIAGNOSIS
- Benign breast disease:
  - Fibrocystic disease
  - Fibroadenoma
  - Intraductal papilloma (bloody nipple discharge)
  - Duct ectasia
  - Simple cyst
  - Sclerosing adenosis
  - Fat necrosis (history of serial/parallel breast trauma)
- Infection (abscess, cellulitis, mastitis)

DIAGNOSTIC TESTS & INTERPRETATION
Initial Tests (lab, imaging)
- Mammography (MMG) BI-RADS: Breast Imaging–Reporting and Data System is a quality assurance (QA) method published by the American Radiology Society.
  - BI-RADS has been extended to breast US and MRI interpretation as well.
  - Components of BI-RADS report:
    - Indication for study and type of examination
    - Overall breast composition, including breast density
      - A—breasts are almost entirely fatty tissue
      - B—scattered areas of fibroglandular density

- C—heterogenously dense
- D—extremely dense
  - Description of abnormalities and important findings
    - Uses standard BI-RADS descriptors
  - Comparison to prior images and summary report, including final BI-RADS assessment category
- Final BI-RADS assessment category:
  - BI-RADS 0: incomplete; additional imaging evaluation needed
    - Commonly occurs on screening studies
  - BI-RADS 1: negative
    - Continue with current screening guidelines
  - BI-RADS 2: benign
    - No further action needed
  - BI-RADS 3: probably benign, possibility of malignancy is <2%
    - Follow-up imaging should occur in 6 months for 1 year; consider imaging every 6 to 12 months for 2 to 3 years.
    - Can consider biopsy if patients is anxious or follow-up is uncertain
  - BI-RADS 4: suspicious
    - Patient and clinician should discuss possible management plans and likely a biopsy.
  - BI-RADS 5: highly suggestive of malignancy
    - Diagnostic imaging needed with follow-up and biopsy
  - BI-RADS 6: known biopsy—proven malignancy
    - Includes patients with biopsy-proven cancers that have yet to be surgically removed
- Calcifications on screening mammography need to be evaluated with diagnostic mammogram (Dx MMG) and stereotactic guided biopsy.
- Palpable masses on exam
  - Palpable mass ≥30 years:
    - Obtain Dx MMG and US to determine cystic versus solid.
      - If BI-RADS 1 to 3, then get US ± biopsy.
      - If BI-RADS 4 to 6, then get core needle biopsy ± surgical excision.
  - Palpable mass <30 years:
    - Obtain US ± Dx MMG ± biopsy.
      - If low clinical suspicion, may observe for 1 to 2 menstrual cycles for resolution
  - Spontaneous, reproducible nipple discharge:
    - Obtain Dx MMG ± US.
      - If negative, then consider ductogram or MRI ± surgical excision.
  - Asymmetric thickening/nodularity <30 years:
    - Obtain US ± Dx MMG ± biopsy.
  - Asymmetric thickening/nodularity ≥30 years:
    - Obtain Dx MMG+ US ± biopsy.
  - Skin changes, peau d'orange:
    - Obtain Dx MMG ± US ± biopsy for underlying mass.
      - If no mass, then perform punch biopsy of skin change.
- Palpable lymph nodes: Obtain CT chest, abdomen/pelvis, and bone scan.

Follow-Up Tests & Special Considerations
- Advanced disease (stage IIIA or higher):
  - Chest CT, abdominal ± pelvis CT, FDG positron emission tomography (PET)/CT scan, bone scan or sodium fluoride PET/CT if FDG-PET/CT indeterminate
- Most common metastasis:
  - Lungs, liver, bone, brain
- Bone scan if:
  - Localized bone pain or elevated alkaline phosphate
- Abdominal ± pelvis CT if:
  - Abdominal symptoms, elevated alkaline phosphate, abnormal LFTs

- Chest CT if:
  - Pulmonary symptoms present
- Brain/spine MRI if:
  - CNS/spinal cord symptoms

Diagnostic Procedures/Other
- Axillary lymph nodes should have US of axilla during workup and core needle biopsy or FNA if suspicious nodes are identified.
  - Otherwise sentinel lymph node biopsy should occur during index operation.
- Hematoma, bruising, and/or reactive lymph nodes

Test Interpretation
- Surgical pathology results should note:
  - Ductal/lobular/other
  - Invasive/noninvasive
  - Margins
  - Nodal involvement
- Tumor receptor status: ER, PR, HER2 assay

 ## TREATMENT

MEDICATION
- Neoadjuvant chemotherapy:
  - Locally advanced (large tumor and/or positive lymph nodes)
  - Early operable BC to facilitate breast conservation surgery
  - Triple negative BC and tumor size >0.5 cm
  - HER2 (+) tumors ≥2 cm with positive lymph nodes
- Consider 21-gene PT-PCR assay in ER/PR(+) tumors with (−) nodes
- Dose-dense chemotherapy demonstrates overall survival advantage in early BC.
  - Doxorubicin/cyclophosphamide (AC) weekly or every 2 weeks paclitaxel for HER2 negative BC
- Anti-HER2/neu antibody (e.g., trastuzumab with or without pertuzumab) in HER2/neu-positive patients

ISSUES FOR REFERRAL
Premenopausal women should be referred to fertility expert prior to chemotherapy initiation.

ADDITIONAL THERAPIES
- Radiation therapy (RT)
  - Upon completion of surgery ± chemotherapy, whole breast radiation should be offered for patients undergoing breast conservation therapy (BCT) prior to starting endocrine therapy.
  - Mastectomy versus lumpectomy + RT overall survival is similar.
  - Postmastectomy RT is offered if tumor >5 cm, ≥1 lymph nodes are involved, chest wall/skin involvement, unable to obtain clear margins.
- Hormone therapy for ER+ tumors
  - DCIS:
    - Tamoxifen 200 mg QD for 5 years
    - Age <60 and postmenopausal: may consider use of aromatase inhibitors (AI)
    - Age >60: selective estrogen receptor modulator (SERM) or AI equally effective
  - Invasive cancer:
    - SERM (tamoxifen 20 mg QD): premenopausal at diagnosis: 5-year treatment and consider for additional 5 years
    - Aromatase inhibitors (anastrozole 1 mg QD, letrozole 2.5 mg QD, and exemestane 25 mg QD): postmenopausal women, 5-year treatment following endocrine therapy for 4.5 to 6 years, or endocrine therapy for up to 10 years
- Advanced disease
  - Hormone therapy and cytotoxic therapy
  - Bisphosphonates skeletal complications

- Anti–vascular endothelial growth factor (anti-VEGF) antibody
- Anti-HER2/neu antibody in select HER2/neu-positive patients

Pregnancy Considerations
- Treatment varies on trimester.
- Surgical options:
  - Mastectomy or breast conservation
    - BCT can be offered at any point in pregnancy but may require delay in adjuvant RT.

SURGERY/OTHER PROCEDURES
- Breast-conserving therapy (lumpectomy) offered if negative margins can be achieved and the patient will also receive adjuvant RT.
- Mastectomy indicated for multicentric disease, large tumor to breast size ratio, inflammatory BC, T_4 disease, contraindication to RT, patient preference.
- Evaluation of axillary nodes: preoperative US and biopsy for all patients with clinically suspicious axillary nodes. If biopsy is positive, an axillary node dissection should be performed.

 ## ONGOING CARE

FOLLOW-UP RECOMMENDATIONS
- Every 4 to 6 months for 5 years and then annually
- No evidence to support the use of routine complete blood count, LFTs, "tumor markers," bone scan, chest x-ray, liver US, CT scans, MRI, PET
- Mammogram 6 months postradiation then annually
- Annual gynecologic exam on endocrine therapy; bone mineral density at baseline and follow-up when on aromatase inhibitors or with ovarian failure secondary to treatment

DIET
Active lifestyle, healthy diet, limited alcohol intake

PROGNOSIS
5-year survival (SEER 18, all races, females)
- Localized 98.8%
- Regional 85.5%
- Distant 27.4%
- Unknown 54.5%
- All stages 89.9%

REFERENCE
1. American Cancer Society. *About Breast Cancer*. Atlanta, GA: American Cancer Society; 2021. http://www.cancer.org. Accessed August 11, 2021.

 ## CODES

ICD10
- C50.52 Malignant neoplasm of lower-outer quadrant of breast, male
- C50.929 Malignant neoplasm of unspecified site of unspecified male breast
- C50.812 Malignant neoplasm of overlapping sites of left female breast

CLINICAL PEARLS
- U.S. women; lifetime risk of 1 in 8
- Excessive alcohol use, high body mass index (BMI), and physical inactivity are modifiable risk factors.
- Normal mammography does not exclude the possibility of CA with a palpable mass.

BREASTFEEDING

Angelia Leipelt, BA, IBCLC, ICCE, CLE • Ronald G. Chambers Jr., MD, FAAFP

BASICS

- Breastfeeding is the natural process of feeding human milk directly from the breast.
- Breast milk is the preferred nutritional source and the normal and physiologic way to feed all new-borns and infants.
- Breast milk contains over 200 active components which provide nutrition, fight pathogens, promote healthy gut microbiome, and aid in maturity of immune system.
- The American Academy of Pediatrics (AAP), the American Academy of Family Physicians (AAFP), and the American Congress of Obstetricians and Gynecologists (ACOG) recommend exclusive breastfeeding for 6 months, with continuation of breastfeeding for ≥1 year as desired by mother and infant (1)[A].

DESCRIPTION

- Maternal benefits (as compared with mothers who do not breastfeed) include:
  - Rapid involution/decreased postpartum bleeding
  - Decreased risk of postpartum depression and increased bonding
  - Postpartum weight loss
  - Decreased risk of breast cancer and association of decreased risk of premenopausal and postmeno-pausal ovarian cancer (2), decreased risk of type 2 diabetes, hypertension, hyperlipidemia, rheuma-toid arthritis, and cardiovascular disease
  - Decreased risk of prematurity
  - Increased bone density
- Infant benefits include the following (1):
  - Ideal food: easily digestible, nutrients well ab-sorbed, less constipation
  - Lower rates of virtually all infections via maternal antibody protection
    - Fewer respiratory and GI infections
    - Decreased risk of ear infections, bacterial meningitis, pneumonia, and sepsis
    - Decreased incidence of otitis media and necro-tizing enterocolitis
  - Decreased incidence of obesity and type 1 and 2 diabetes
  - Decreased incidence of allergies, clinical asthma, and atopic dermatitis in childhood
  - Decreased risk of developing celiac disease and inflammatory bowel disease
  - Decreased risk of childhood leukemia
  - Decreased risk of sudden infant death syndrome (SIDS)
  - Enhanced neurodevelopmental performance including intelligence (3)
  - Increased attachment between mother and baby

EPIDEMIOLOGY

Incidence

- According to CDC Breastfeeding Scorecard, U.S. breastfeeding rates are on the rise in 2018: any breastfeeding: 83.2%. (however, differs among dif-ferent sociodemographic and culture) (4)
- Breastfeeding at 6 months: 57.6%
- Breastfeeding at 12 months: 35.9%
- Exclusive breastfeeding at 3 months: 46.9%
- Exclusive breastfeeding at 6 months: 24.9%

ETIOLOGY AND PATHOPHYSIOLOGY

- The mechanism of milk production is based on several hormones: Prolactin triggers milk production and oxytocin releases milk based on supply and demand. Endocrine control system triggers making of colostrum at 5 months' gestation.
- Alveoli make milk in response to hormone prolactin. Sucking stimulates secretion of prolactin, which triggers milk production.
- Stimulation of areola causes secretion of oxytocin. Oxytocin is responsible for let-down reflex when myoepithelial cells contract and milk is ejected into milk ducts.
- Endocrine/metabolic: Cystic fibrosis, diabetes, galac-tosemia, phenylketonuria, and thyroid dysfunction may cause delayed lactation or decreased milk.

GENERAL PREVENTION

Most vaccinations can be given to breastfeeding mothers, including COVID-19 immunization. The CDC recommends that the diphtheria-tetanus-acellular pertussis, hepatitis B, inactivated influenza virus (as opposed to live attenuated), measles-mumps-rubella (MMR), and inactivated polio and varicella vaccines can be given. The CDC recommends avoiding the yellow fever or smallpox vaccine in breastfeeding mothers (5).

DIAGNOSIS

PHYSICAL EXAM

Breast examination during pregnancy, assess for scars, lumps, or flat/inverted nipples. Confirm history of infertility, endocrine disorders, breast and hormonal pathology, overall health and psychosocial concerns, perinatal complications, and previous breastfeeding problems.

ALERT

A breast lump should be followed to complete resolu-tion or worked up if present and not just attributed to changes from lactation.

TREATMENT

GENERAL MEASURES

Breastfeeding initiation

- Initiate breastfeeding immediately after birth, ideally placing the infant naked on mother's chest uninter-rupted skin-to-skin *in first hour* (1),(6).
- As baby opens wide, bring baby close, tucking baby in "belly to belly." Line baby's nose to nipple, baby tilts its head back with wide open mouth, bring baby close as baby latches to ensure baby's gum takes in more of the areola.
- Baby's lips are flanged, rounded cheeks, no clicking or popping sounds, and absence of nipple pain when latched.
- Feed baby 2 to 8 times for first 24 hours and 8 or more times per 24 hours, feeding 10 or more minutes.
- Observation of a nursing session by an experienced physician, nurse, or IBCLC

- Avoid supplementation with formula or water and/or artificial nipples unless medically indicated.
- Contraindications to breastfeeding are few (WHO) (1).
  - Maternal HIV (in industrialized world) or human T-cell leukemia virus (HTLV) infection
  - Active untreated tuberculosis
  - Active herpes simplex virus (HSV) lesions on the breast
  - Substances of abuse without evaluation
  - Review medications that will pass into human milk.
  - Infants with galactosemia or maple syrup urine disease should not be fed with breast milk. Infants with phenylketonuria may be fed breast milk under close observation.
  - Mothers who develop varicella 5 days before through 2 days after delivery
  - Maternal hepatitis is *not* a contraindication.

ISSUES FOR REFERRAL

- Refer to trained physician, nurse, or IBCLC for inpatient and/or outpatient teaching.
- Frequent follow-up if having problems with latching, sore nipples, breast pain, overactive letdown, over supply inadequate milk production

COMPLEMENTARY & ALTERNATIVE MEDICINE

Galactagogues

- Metoclopramide, domperidone, oxytocin, fenugreek, goat's rue, and milk thistle have mixed results in improving milk production, but efficacy and safety data are lacking in literature.

ONGOING CARE

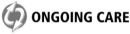

FOLLOW-UP RECOMMENDATIONS

See mother and baby within a few days of hospital discharge, especially if first time breastfeeding.

- Risk factors for suboptimal initiation
  - Breast surgery or reduction surgery prior to preg-nancy may disrupt breast milk production.
  - Severe postpartum hemorrhage may lead to Sheehan syndrome, associated with difficulty breastfeeding due to poor milk production.
  - Other factors: delivery mode, duration of labor, gestational age, maternal infection, parity, culture, mother–baby separation, maternal anxiety, use of artificial nipple, and non–breast milk fluids

Patient Monitoring

- Monitor maternal breast milk supply concerns.
- Monitor infant's weight, behavior, and output closely.
- Supplementation with pumped milk and/or infant formula if infant has lost ≥10% of birth weight.
- Supplementation without persistent breast stimula-tion with frequent feedings or breast pump use will decrease milk production and decrease breastfeed-ing success.

DIET

- For mothers:
  - Drink plenty of fluids to satisfy thirst and optimal hydration.
  - Breastfeeding mothers may require ~500 more calories per day.
  - Limit caffeine to <300 mg/day.
  - Alcohol should be avoided. Possible long-term effects of alcohol in maternal milk remain unknown.
- For infants:
  - In 2008, the AAP increased its recommended daily intake of vitamin D for infants from 200 to 400 IU. For exclusively breastfed babies, this will require taking a vitamin supplement, such as Poly-Vi-Sol or Vi-Daylin vitamin drops, 0.5 mL/day, beginning in the first few days of life (1).
  - In 2010, the AAP recommended adding supplementation for breastfed infants with oral iron 1 mg/kg/day beginning at age 4 months.
    - Preterm infants fed by human milk should receive an iron supplement of 2 mg/kg/day by 1 month of age, and this should be continued until the infant is weaned to iron-fortified formula or begins eating complementary foods that supply the 2 mg/kg of iron.

PATIENT EDUCATION

- Support measures to normalize breastfeeding have been shown to be successful with respect to child and maternal health outcomes.
  - Emphasize importance of exclusive breastfeeding for first 6 weeks of life to allow adequate buildup of sufficient milk supply.
  - Regular promotion of the advantages of breastfeeding/risks of not breastfeeding (6)[A]
- Milk usually transitions to mature milk about day 3 to 5 postpartum.
- Signs of adequate nursing
  - Baby feeding on demand (8 to 12 feedings per 24 hours by day 2)
  - Baby should have 6 to 8 wet diapers per day and 3 to 4 bowel movements per day by day 6 to 8.
  - Proper latching and positioning
  - Baby satisfied; appropriate weight gain (average 1 oz/day in first few months)
- Weaning
  - Solid food may be introduced at 4 months with continuation of breastfeeding.
  - Mothers returning to work/school should be introduced to alternative feeding methods 1 to 2 weeks prior. Initiate breast pumping plan.
- Family planning
  - Options include lactational amenorrhea method (LAM), barrier methods, implants, Depo-Provera, PO contraception, and intrauterine devices (IUDs). ACOG recommends that progesterone-only pills be used 2 to 3 weeks postpartum, and that Depo-Provera, IUDs, combined OCPs, and Implanon can be used 6 weeks postpartum.
  - Monitor for changes in milk supply after starting a contraceptive.

COMPLICATIONS

- Breast milk jaundice should be considered if jaundice persists for >1 week in an otherwise healthy, well-hydrated newborn. It peaks at 10 to 14 days.
- Plugged duct
  - Mother is well except for sore lump in one or both breasts and is without fever. Use moist, hot packs on lump prior to, and during, nursing; more frequent nursing on affected side
- Mastitis (see "Mastitis")
  - Sore lump in one or both breasts plus maternal fever and/or redness on skin overlying lump
  - Use moist, hot packs on lump prior to, and during, nursing.
  - Antibiotics covering for *Staphylococcus aureus* (most common organism)
  - Other possible sources of fever should be ruled out, that is, endometritis and pyelonephritis.
  - Mother should get increased rest; use acetaminophen (Tylenol) PRN.
  - Fever should resolve within 48 hours or consider changing antibiotics. Lump should resolve. If it continues, an abscess may be present, requiring surgical drainage.
- Milk supply inadequate
  - Review health concerns, weight gain, signs of adequate supply; technique, frequency, and duration of nursing and any use of supplementation.
- Sore nipples
  - Check technique and improve latch-on.
  - Baby should be taken off the breast by breaking the suction with a finger in the mouth.
  - Check for signs of thrush in baby and on mother's nipple. If affected, treat both.
  - Check for evidence of ankyloglossia (tongue tie) in the infant. Correction of ankyloglossia may lead to decreased nipple soreness and improved breastfeeding.
  - Nipple bleb (a blister on the nipple that can be filled with serous fluid or another fluid) due to improper positioning. Moist heat and improve latching techniques.
- Flat or inverted nipples
  - When stimulated, inverted nipples will retract inward, flat nipples remain flat; check for this on initial prenatal physical.
- Engorgement
  - Develops after milk transitions day 3 or 4, resolves within a day or 2
  - Signs are warm, hard, sore breasts.
    - Frequent nursing; breastfeed long enough to empty breasts.
    - Pump to relieve discomfort.
    - Explore reasons for ongoing problems.

REFERENCES

1. Johnston M, Landers S, Noble L, et al. Breastfeeding and the use of human milk. *Pediatrics*. 2012;129(3):e827–e841.
2. Westerfield KL, Koenig K, Oh R. Breastfeeding: common questions and answers. *Am Fam Physician*. 2018;98(6):368–373.
3. Horta BL, Loret de Mola C, Victora CG. Breastfeeding and intelligence: a systematic review and meta-analysis. *Acta Paediatr*. 2015;104(467):14–19.
4. Centers for Disease Control and Prevention. *Breastfeeding Report Card—United States, 2018*. Atlanta, GA: Centers for Disease Control and Prevention; 2018. http://www.cdc.gov/breastfeeding/pdf/2018breastfeedingreportcard.pdf. Accessed October 18, 2021.
5. Centers for Disease Control and Prevention. *Breastfeeding Vaccinations*. Atlanta, GA: Centers for Disease Control and Prevention; 2010. http://www.cdc.gov/breastfeeding/recommendations/vaccinations.htm. Accessed October 18, 2021.
6. American College of Obstetricians and Gynecologists Women's Health Care Physicians; Committee on Health Care for Underserved Women. Committee Opinion No. 570: breastfeeding in underserved women: increasing initiation and continuation of breastfeeding. *Obstet Gynecol*. 2013;122(2, pt 1):423–427.

ADDITIONAL READING

- American Academy of Pediatrics, American College of Obstetricians and Gynecologists. *Breastfeeding Handbook for Physicians*. 2nd ed. Elk Grove Village, IL: American Academy of Pediatrics; 2014.
- National Library of Medicine. Drugs and lactation database: COVID-19 vaccine. https://www.ncbi.nlm.nih.gov/books/NBK565969/?report=reader. Published 2006. Updated September 20, 2021. Accessed October 18, 2021.

 CODES

ICD10

Z39.1 Encounter for care and examination of lactating mother

CLINICAL PEARLS

- Women who do not receive support are at risk for shorter durations of breastfeeding.
- Virtually all mothers can breastfeed with accurate information, support from family, the health care system, and society at large.
- Breast milk is the optimal food for infants, with myriad health benefits for mothers and children.

BRONCHIECTASIS

Mary Joyce Green, MD • Jared M. Roberts

BASICS

DESCRIPTION
- Bronchiectasis is an irreversible dilatation of ≥1 airways accompanied by recurrent transmural bronchial infection/inflammation and chronic mucopurulent sputum production.
- It may be focal or diffused.

EPIDEMIOLOGY
- Predominant age: most commonly presents in 6th decade of life
- Predominant sex: female > male (1)

Incidence
- Incidence has decreased in the United States for two reasons:
  - Widespread childhood vaccination against pertussis
  - Effective treatment of childhood respiratory infections with antibiotics
- Among children, incidence may be higher in indigenous or socioeconomically disadvantaged group (2).

Prevalence
- In the United States, prevalence estimated to be 139/100,000 (3)
- Higher among women versus men (180 vs. 95/100,000) and to increase substantially with age (from 7/100,000 to 812/100,000 aged 34 and ≥75 years (3)

ETIOLOGY AND PATHOPHYSIOLOGY
- Frequently idiopathic
- Chronic infections (PTB), autoimmune disease, genetic causes (cystic fibrosis (CF)), chronic obstructive pulmonary disease (COPD), connective tissue disease, allergic bronchopulmonary aspergillosis (ABPA) (4)
- Vicious circle hypothesis: Transmural infection, generally by bacterial organisms, causes inflammation and obstruction of airways. Damaged airways and dysfunctional cilia foster bacterial colonization, which leads to further inflammation and obstruction.

RISK FACTORS
- Nontuberculous mycobacterial infection is both a cause and a complication of non-CF bronchiectasis.
- Severe respiratory infection in childhood (measles, adenovirus, influenza, pertussis, or bronchiolitis)
- Systemic diseases (e.g., rheumatoid arthritis and inflammatory bowel disease)
- Chronic rhinosinusitis
- Recurrent pneumonia
- Aspirated foreign body
- Immunodeficiency
- Congenital abnormalities

GENERAL PREVENTION
- Routine immunizations against pertussis, measles, *Haemophilus influenzae* type B, influenza, and pneumococcal pneumonia
- Genetic counseling if congenital condition is etiology
- Smoking cessation

COMMONLY ASSOCIATED CONDITIONS
- Mucociliary clearance defects
  - Primary ciliary dyskinesia
  - Young syndrome (secondary ciliary dyskinesia)
  - Kartagener syndrome
- Other congenital conditions
  - α_1-Antitrypsin deficiency
  - Marfan syndrome
  - Cartilage deficiency (Williams-Campbell syndrome)
- COPD

- Pulmonary fibrosis, causing traction bronchiectasis
- Postinfectious conditions
  - Bacteria (*H. influenzae* and *Pseudomonas aeruginosa*)
  - Mycobacterial infections (tuberculosis [TB] and *Mycobacterium avium* complex [MAC])
  - Whooping cough
  - *Aspergillus* species
  - Viral (HIV, adenovirus, measles, influenza virus)
- Immunodeficient conditions
  - Primary: hypogammaglobulinemia
  - Secondary: ABPA, posttransplantation
  - Sequelae of toxic inhalation or aspiration (e.g., chlorine, luminal foreign body)
- Rheumatic/chronic inflammatory conditions
  - Rheumatoid arthritis
  - Sjögren syndrome
  - Systemic lupus erythematosus
  - Inflammatory bowel disease
- Miscellaneous
  - Yellow nail syndrome

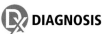

DIAGNOSIS

- Typical symptoms include chronic productive cough, wheezing, and dyspnea.
- Symptoms are often accompanied by repeated respiratory infections.
- Once diagnosed, investigate etiology.

HISTORY
- Any predisposing factors (congenital, infectious, and/or exposure related)
- Immunization history
- Symptoms are commonly present for many years and include the following:
  - Chronic cough (90%)
  - Sputum: may be copious and purulent (90%)
  - Rhinosinusitis (60–70%)
  - Fatigue: may be a dominant symptom (70%)
  - Dyspnea (75%)
  - Chest pain: may be pleuritic (20–30%)
  - Hemoptysis (20–30%)

PHYSICAL EXAM
- Fever may indicate exacerbation.
- Wheezing (20%)
- Bibasilar crackles (60%)
- Rhonchi (44%)
- Digital clubbing (3%)
- Chest deformities may be present.

DIFFERENTIAL DIAGNOSIS
- CF
- COPD
- Asthma
- Chronic bronchitis
- Pulmonary TB
- ABPA

DIAGNOSTIC TESTS & INTERPRETATION
- Spirometry
  - Moderate airflow obstruction and hyperresponsive airways
  - Forced expiratory volume in the 1st second of expiration (FEV_1): <80% predicted and FEV_1/FVC <0.7
  - Special tests
  - Ciliary biopsy by electron microscopy
- Sputum culture
  - *H. influenzae*, nontypeable form (42%)
  - *P. aeruginosa* (18%)

- Cultures may also be positive for *Streptococcus pneumoniae, Moraxella catarrhalis*, MAC, and *Aspergillus*.
  - Screen for TB and non-TB in selected individuals.
  - Of all isolates, 30–40% will show no growth.
- Special tests
  - Sweat test for CF
  - CBC with differential to determine possible underlying primary versus secondary immune etiology
  - Purified protein derivative (PPD) test for TB
  - Skin test for *Aspergillus;* can alternatively test for antibodies against *Aspergillus* (total IgE, IgG specific antibodies, IgE specific antibodies)
  - HIV
  - Serum Igs to test for humoral immunodeficiency
  - Protein electrophoresis to test for α_1-antitrypsin deficiency
  - Barium swallow to look for abnormalities of deglutition, achalasia, esophageal hypomotility
  - pH probe to characterize reflux
  - Screening tests for rheumatologic diseases
  - Testing for primary biliary dyskinesia
- Chest radiograph
  - Nonspecific; increased lung markings or may appear normal
- Chest computed tomography (CT)
  - Noncontrast high-resolution chest CT is the most important diagnostic tool.
  - Bronchi are dilated and do not taper, resulting in "tram track sign"; parallel opacities seen on scan
  - Varicose constrictions and balloon cysts may be seen.
  - For focal bronchiectasis, rule out endobronchial obstruction.
  - For exclusively upper lobe bronchiectasis, consider CF and ABPA.

Diagnostic Procedures/Other
- Bronchoscopy may be used to obtain cultures and evacuate sputum.
- Bronchoscopy for hemoptysis
- Bronchoscopy may be useful to rule out airway-obstructing lesions with focal bronchiectasis.

Test Interpretation
Bronchoscopy findings include the following:
- Dilatation of airways and purulent secretions
- Thickened bronchial walls with necrosis of bronchial mucosa
- Peribronchial scarring

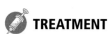

TREATMENT

- Treat underlying conditions.
- Recognize an acute exacerbation with four out of nine criteria.
  - Change in sputum production
  - Increased dyspnea
  - Increased cough
  - Fever
  - Increased wheezing
  - Malaise, fatigue, lethargy
  - Reduced pulmonary function
  - Radiographic changes
  - Changes in chest sounds
- Non-CF bronchiectasis: Determine cause of exacerbations; promote good bronchopulmonary hygiene via daily airway clearance.
- Consider surgical resection of damaged lung for focal disease that is refractory to medical management.
- Medical management: Reduce morbidity by controlling symptoms and preventing disease progression.

- Patients with non-CF bronchiectasis may not respond to CF treatment regimens in the same way as patients with CF do.

MEDICATION

First Line
- Antibiotics
  - Potentially useful in acute exacerbations
  - Sputum culture and sensitivity should direct therapy; antibiotic selection is complicated by a wide range of pathogens and resistant organisms.
  - May start empiric antibiotics while awaiting culture results. Consider covering *Pseudomonas* infection until results are back.
  - Patients may require twice the usual dose and longer treatment for 14 days (10 to 21 days) for an acute exacerbation.
- Ciprofloxacin: 750 mg PO q12h for adults
- Amoxicillin clavulanate (Augmentin): 500 mg PO q8–12h; pediatric: base dosing on amoxicillin content
- Trimethoprim sulfamethoxazole /(SMX): 160 mg trimethoprim /800 mg SMX PO q12h; pediatric: ≥2 months, 8 mg/kg trimethoprim and 40 mg/kg SMX PO/24 hours, administered in 2 divided doses q12h
- Doxycycline and cefaclor given PO are also effective.
- Macrolides: appear to have immunomodulatory benefits
- Although chronic therapy decreases sputum production, number of exacerbations, and hospitalizations, there is a risk of emergence of resistance to antibiotics (5),(6).
- Long-term antibiotic therapy is indicated in adults with ≥3 exacerbations per year or who have persistent significant symptoms:
  - *P aeruginosa* colonized: Treat with inhaled antibiotic (colistin: first line; gentamicin: second line); consider long-term oral macrolide (azithromycin or erythromycin) in patients who cannot tolerate inhaled antibiotics or as an adjunct to inhaled antibiotics in severe cases (ERS) (7).
  - Non–*P. aeruginosa* colonized: long-term macrolide, doxycycline as second line; inhaled gentamicin if long-term oral therapy is contraindicated
  - With macrolide treatment, use caution in patients susceptible to QTc prolongation.
- Should be administered IV in cases of severe infection (8)
- All patients considered for chronic therapy with azithromycin should be screened for non-TB mycobacterial infection prior (8).
- Bronchodilators
  - There is limited evidence for use of bronchodilators in patients without breathlessness.
  - Use bronchodilators before physiotherapy, mucoactive drugs, and before inhaled antibiotics.
- Inhaled corticosteroids
  - Do not routinely recommend inhaled corticosteroids to patients, unless they have concomitant asthma/COPD (BTS/ERS) (4),(7)
- Mucoactive agents:
  - Whereas nebulized dornase and high-dose anti-inflammatory agents such as ibuprofen have some benefit in CF-related bronchiectasis, there is no role of such agents in non–CF-related bronchiectasis. In fact, nebulized dornase in adults can be harmful with more frequent exacerbations and decline in lung function.
  - Nebulized saline or hypertonic saline (7% saline) use prior to airway clearance techniques can help augment sputum production (9)[B].
  - Mannitol may improve quality of life and reduce sputum plugging (BTS) (4).

ADDITIONAL THERAPIES
Sputum clearance techniques, including chest physiotherapy (percussion and postural drainage) and pulmonary rehabilitation (improves exercise tolerance)

SURGERY/OTHER PROCEDURES
- Surgery if area of bronchiectasis is localized and symptoms remain intolerable despite medical therapy or if disease is life-threatening (9)
- Surgery effectively improves symptoms in 80% of these cases.

ADMISSION, INPATIENT, AND NURSING CONSIDERATIONS
Bronchiectasis can present as life-threatening massive hemoptysis. In this situation, in addition to airway protection and resuscitation, bronchial artery embolization or surgical intervention is necessary to control bleeding (10).

ONGOING CARE

Long-term outpatient treatment recommendations for bronchiectasis in children and adults (9):

- Children and adults with CF and non–CF-related bronchiectasis should be treated by comprehensive interdisciplinary chronic disease management programs.
- In children, aim to achieve normal growth and development.
- Patients with primary and secondary immune deficiencies should be under joint care with a clinical immunologist.
- Patient with CF should be referred to a CF center.
- Patient should be informed of the various techniques for airway clearance.
- Pulmonary rehabilitation should be offered to patients with symptoms of breathlessness affecting activities of daily living (9)[B].
- In situation of an acute exacerbation, use and modify antibiotics as per sputum microbiology.
- Consider suitability of long-term antibiotics for patients with recurrent exacerbations.
- Noninvasive ventilation can improve quality of life in patients with chronic respiratory failure and can reduce hospitalizations.
- Consider lung transplant evaluation in patients with declining respiratory status and FEV_1 <30%. However, because non-CF bronchiectasis has significantly lower mortality hazard compared to CF-related bronchiectasis, separate referral and listing criteria should be considered.

FOLLOW-UP RECOMMENDATIONS
Regular exercise is recommended.

Patient Monitoring
- Serial spirometry at least annually (9)
- Chest CTs to monitor progression of disease may be indicated with some conditions such as bronchiectasis with MAC infections.
- Routine microbiologic sputum analysis

PATIENT EDUCATION
http://www.lung.org/

PROGNOSIS
- Mortality rate (death due directly to bronchiectasis) is 10.6–29.7%.
- *Pseudomonas* infection, low body mass index, and advanced age are associated with poorer prognosis (5).

COMPLICATIONS
- Hemoptysis
- Recurrent pulmonary infections
- Pulmonary hypertension
- Cor pulmonale
- Lung abscess

REFERENCES

1. Weycker D, Edelsberg J, Oster G, et al. Prevalence and economic burden of bronchiectasis. *Clin Pulm Med*. 2005;12(4):205–209.
2. El Boustany P, Gachelin E, Colomban C, et al. A review of non-cystic fibrosis bronchiectasis in children with a focus on the role of long-term treatment with macrolides. *Pediatr Pulmonol*. 2019;54(4):487–496. doi:10.1002/ppul.24252.
3. Weycker D, Hansen GL, Seifer FD. Prevalence and incidence of noncystic fibrosis bronchiectasis among US adults in 2013. *Chron Respir Dis*. 2017;14(4):377–384. doi:10.1177/1479972317709649.
4. Hill AT, Sullivan AL, Chalmers JD, et al. British Thoracic Society guideline for bronchiectasis in adults. *Thorax*. 2019;74(Suppl 1):1–69. doi:10.1136/thoraxjnl-2018-212463.
5. Hnin K, Nguyen C, Carson KV, et al. Prolonged antibiotics for non-cystic fibrosis bronchiectasis in children and adults. *Cochrane Database Syst Rev*. 2015;(8):CD001392.
6. Welsh EJ, Evans DJ, Fowler SJ, et al. Interventions for bronchiectasis: an overview of Cochrane systematic reviews. *Cochrane Database Syst Rev*. 2015;(7):CD010337.
7. Polverino E, Goeminne PC, McDonnell MJ, et al. European Respiratory Society guidelines for the management of adult bronchiectasis. *Eur Respir J*. 2017;50(3):1700629. doi:10.1183/13993003.00629-2017.
8. O'Donnell AE. Bronchiectasis: which antibiotics to use and when? *Curr Opin Pulm Med*. 2015;21(3):272–277.
9. Pasteur MC, Bilton D, Hill AT; for British Thoracic Society Non-CF Bronchiectasis Guideline Group. British Thoracic Society guideline for non-CF bronchiectasis. *Thorax*. 2010;65(Suppl 1):i1–i58.
10. Wurzel D, Marchant JM, Yerkovich ST, et al. Short courses of antibiotics for children and adults with bronchiectasis. *Cochrane Database Syst Rev*. 2011;(6):CD008695.

ADDITIONAL READING

Kaehne A, Milan SJ, Felix LM, et al. Head-to-head trials of antibiotics for bronchiectasis. *Cochrane Database Syst Rev*. 2018;(9):CD012590.

CODES

ICD10
- Q33.4 Congenital bronchiectasis
- A15.0 Tuberculosis of lung
- J47.0 Bronchiectasis with acute lower respiratory infection

CLINICAL PEARLS
- Symptoms of bronchiectasis include chronic productive cough, wheezing, and dyspnea often accompanied by repeated respiratory infections.
- A chest x-ray has poor sensitivity and specificity for the diagnosis; a noncontrast high-resolution chest CT is the most important diagnostic tool.
- Current practice guidelines recommend treating acute exacerbations with a 14-day course of antibiotics. Frequent exacerbations may be treated with prolonged and aerosolized antibiotics.

BRONCHIOLITIS
Dennis E. Hughes, DO, FACEP

 BASICS

DESCRIPTION
- Inflammation and obstruction of small airways and reactive airways generally affecting infants and young children—upper respiratory infection (URI) prodrome followed by increased respiratory effort, crackles, and wheezing
- Usual course: insidious, acute, progressive
- Leading cause of hospitalizations in infants and children in most Western countries. It is the most common cause of lower respiratory infections (LRTI) in children <24 months of age.
- Predominant age: newborn—2 years (peak age <6 months). Neonates are not protected despite transfer of maternal antibody.
- Predominant sex: male > female

EPIDEMIOLOGY
Incidence
- Accounts for ~$1.7B in health care cost in United States. Incidence is estimated at 3.2/1,000. Almost 100% of children experience RSV infection by two seasons.
- Usually seasonal (October to May in the Northern Hemisphere) and often occurs in epidemics—in subtropical regions, RSV is endemic year-round
- Responsible for 18.8% (90,000 annually) of all pediatric hospitalizations (excluding live births) in children <2 years
- Incidence increasing since 1980 (with concomitant increase in relative rate of hospitalization from 2002 to 2007); of those <12 months with condition, the hospitalization rate ~2–3%

Prevalence
There is a 21–25% prevalence of bronchiolitis in children <12 months of age; decreasing to 13% from 12 to 24 months of age in the United States.

ETIOLOGY AND PATHOPHYSIOLOGY
RSV accounts for 70–85% of all cases (children <12 months of age), but rhinovirus, parainfluenza virus, adenovirus, influenza virus, *Mycoplasma pneumoniae*, and *Chlamydophila pneumoniae* have all been implicated:
- Infection results in necrosis and lysis of epithelial cells and subsequent release of inflammatory mediators.
- Edema and mucus secretion, which combined with accumulating necrotic debris and loss of cilia clearance, result in airflow obstruction.
- Ventilation/perfusion mismatching resulting in hypoxia
- Air trapping is caused by dynamic airways narrowing during expiration, which increases work of breathing.
- Bronchospasm appears to play little or no role.

RISK FACTORS
- Secondhand cigarette smoke
- Low birth weight, premature birth
- Immunodeficiency
- Formula feeding (little or no breastfeeding)

- Contact with infected person (primary mode of spread)
- Children in daycare environment
- Congenital cardiopulmonary disease
- <12 weeks of age

GENERAL PREVENTION
- Hand washing or use of alcohol-based hand rubs (preferred)—this simple exercise has been estimated to have the largest impact on prevention of transmission.
- Contact isolation of infected babies
- Persons with colds should keep contact with infants to a minimum.
- Breastfeeding of infants for at least 6 months has been associated with reduced morbidity of disease.
- Palivizumab (Synagis), a monoclonal product, administered monthly, October to May, 15 mg/kg IM; used for RSV prevention ONLY in high-risk patients (see American Academy of Pediatrics [AAP] recommendations) (1)

Pediatric Considerations
Prior infection does not seem to confer subsequent immunity.

COMMONLY ASSOCIATED CONDITIONS
- Upper respiratory congestion
- Conjunctivitis
- Pharyngitis
- Otitis media
- Diarrhea

 DIAGNOSIS

History and physical examination should be the basis for the diagnosis of bronchiolitis; ancillary testing only indicated if clinical picture is unclear (no single of group of tests confirmatory for bronchiolitis)

HISTORY
- Irritability
- Anorexia
- Fever
- Noisy breathing (due to rhinorrhea)
- Cough
- Grunting
- Cyanosis
- Apnea
- Vomiting

PHYSICAL EXAM
- Tachypnea
- Retractions (increased work of breathing)
- Rhinorrhea
- Wheezing
- Upper respiratory findings: pharyngitis, conjunctivitis, otitis

DIFFERENTIAL DIAGNOSIS
- Other pulmonary infections such as pertussis, croup, or bacterial pneumonia
- Aspiration

- Vascular ring
- Foreign body
- Asthma
- Heart failure
- Gastroesophageal reflux
- Cystic fibrosis

DIAGNOSTIC TESTS & INTERPRETATION
Laboratory and other ancillary testing (including chest x-ray) are not required if clinical diagnosis is bronchiolitis. Recent meta-analysis found no single history or physical factor that predicted airspace disease on chest radiograph.

Initial Tests (lab, imaging)
- Arterial oxygen saturation by pulse oximetry. Results need to be interpreted in clinical context. Transient hypoxemia is a common phenomenon in healthy infants (1); capnography not found to aid in prediction of disease severity or need for hospitalization. AAP guidelines suggest intermittent versus continuous pulse oximetry be considered.
- Rapid respiratory viral antigen testing is not necessary during RSV season because the disease is managed symptomatically but may be useful for epidemiologic, hospital cohorting, or in the very young to reduce unnecessary other workup; also indicated in infants admitted while receiving palivizumab prophylaxis (If positive, prophylaxis may be discontinued as recent data suggests no benefit in using palivizumab.)
- The AAP does not recommend routine RSV testing in infants and children with bronchiolitis.
- Chest x-ray findings are variable and may include atelectasis, peribronchial cuffing, hyperinflation, and perihilar infiltrates (AAP, others do not recommend routine chest radiographs in clinical picture of acute bronchiolitis) (1).

Diagnostic Procedures/Other
Point of care ultrasound (POCUS) is being utilized to assist with diagnosis of pneumonia in bronchiolitis with accuracy comparable to radiographs. Also, use of a POCUS-derived scoring system may prognosticate patients who need escalation of therapy (2).

 TREATMENT

The cornerstone of therapy is supportive to include upper airway suctioning, prevention of significant and prolonged hypoxia, and dehydration. The other interventions noted have historically varying effect on the course of the illness despite numerous studies. Recent clinical practice guidelines do not support the routine use of corticosteroids, bronchodilators, or epinephrine. Despite the recommendations against such treatments, some estimated 50% of patients receive some combination of medication during their course (3). Parental education and support is vital (1)[A].

GENERAL MEASURES

To prevent the transmission of RSV (most common infectious etiology of bronchiolitis), it is recommended that caregivers disinfect hands with alcohol-based skin cleaners both before and after contact with patients. Family should also be instructed on similar measures to reduce transmission.

MEDICATION

First Line

- Humidified oxygen for hypoxia of <90% (many feel that transient pulse oximetry in 85–90% range during sleeping in clinically well-appearing infant may be observed) (1)[C]
- Nebulized hypertonic saline (3%) can be effective in reducing LOS in hospitalized patients but not recommended use in the ED (more recent literature review shows some signal of benefit) (1),(4).
- Antibiotics only if secondary bacterial infection present (rare); not indicated for routine use (1)[B]
- Positive-pressure ventilation (PPV) in the form of continuous positive airway pressure (CPAP) can be used in cases of respiratory failure. There is limited clinical evidence other than observational studies.
- High-flow nasal cannula oxygen widely used in various settings to improve oxygen saturation with resultant reduction in end-tidal CO_2 ($ETCO_2$) and respiratory rate, but overall effectiveness remains unproven to date. Recent RCT indicates that high-flow oxygen therapy is effective in treating those potentially needing escalated therapy (5).

ADDITIONAL THERAPIES

- Ribavirin and palivizumab for patients at high risk (for prophylaxis per CDC/AAP guidelines)
- Heliox therapy (70% helium and 30% oxygen) may be of benefit early in moderate to severe bronchiolitis to reduce degree of respiratory distress due to air flow restriction, but Cochrane Review found little evidence of sustained benefit at 24 hours.
- Although not routinely recommended, inhaled β-agonists (albuterol) can be effective in selected cases (particularly in patients with a history of bronchospasm). Many clinicians will attempt an empiric trial of bronchodilators in a primary presentation to judge the clinical response (some argue that this condition maybe asthma equivalent).

ADMISSION, INPATIENT, AND NURSING CONSIDERATIONS

- Bronchiolitis can be associated with apnea in children <6 weeks of age.
- Respiratory rate >45 breaths/min with respiratory distress or apnea
- Hypoxia is common, so clinical criteria are more helpful (pulse oximetry <94% used by many as cutoff).
- Ill or toxic appearance
- Underlying heart condition, respiratory condition, or immune suppression
- High risk for apnea (age <30 days, preterm birth [<37 weeks])
- Dehydrated or unable to feed (<50% of normal intake suggested as threshold for hospitalization consideration)

- Uncertain home care
- Use of respiratory distress assessment instrument may aid in determining admission. The five best predictors of admission, age, respiratory rate, heart rate, oxygen saturation, and duration of symptoms, were recently incorporated into a scoring instrument.
- Supplemental oxygen for pulse oximetry <94% on room air if clinically indicated (i.e., retractions, increased WOB, etc.). AAP recommends O_2 saturation >90% if infant otherwise well.
- IV fluids indicated only if tachypnea precludes oral feeding; weight-based maintenance rate plus insensible losses
- Discharge criteria
  – Normal respiratory rate and no oxygen requirement: Recent small studies suggest that after a period of observation, children can be safely discharged on home oxygen with home health follow-up. Despite reassuring appearance, the clinical course is unpredictable, so follow-up and parental education is important.

ONGOING CARE

FOLLOW-UP RECOMMENDATIONS

Patient Monitoring

- Hospitalization is usually required only if oxygen is a requirement or unable to feed/drink.
- For a hospitalized patient, monitor as needed depending on the severity of the infection.
- If the patient is receiving home care, follow daily by telephone call for 2 to 4 days; the patient may need frequent office visits.

PATIENT EDUCATION

- American Academy of Pediatrics: http://www.aap.org
- American Academy of Family Physicians: http://www.familydoctor.org

PROGNOSIS

- Recovery time is variable. 40% can have symptoms at 14 days and 10% at 4 weeks.
- Mortality statistics differ but probably <1%.
- High-risk infants (bronchopulmonary dysplasia, congenital heart disease) may have a prolonged course.

COMPLICATIONS

- Bacterial superinfection
- Bronchiolitis obliterans
- Apnea
- Respiratory failure
- Death
- Increased incidence of development of reactive airway disease (asthma)

REFERENCES

1. Ralston SL, Lieberthal AS, Meissner HC, et al. Clinical practice guideline: the diagnosis, management, and prevention of bronchiolitis. Pediatrics. 2014;134(5):e1474–e1502. Pediatrics. 2015;136(4):782.
2. Biagi C, Pierantoni L, Baldazzi M, et al. Lung ultrasound for the diagnosis of pneumonia in children with acute bronchiolitis. BMC Pulm Med. 2018;18(1):191.
3. George S. Bronchiolitis: translating evidence into practice. Emerg Med Australas. 2018;30:292.
4. Hsieh CW, Chen C, Su HC, et al. Exploring the efficacy of using hypertonic saline for nebulizing treatment in children with bronchiolitis: a meta-analysis of randomized controlled trials. BMC Pediatr. 2020;20(1):434.
5. Franklin D, Babl FE, Schlapbach LJ, et al. A randomized trial of high flow nasal oxygen therapy in infants with bronchiolitis. N Engl J Med. 2018;378(12):1121–1131.

ADDITIONAL READING

- Chandelia S, Kumar D, Chadha N, et al. Magnesium sulfate for treating bronchiolits for children up to two years of age. Cochrane Database Syst Rev. 2020;12(12):CD012965.
- Joseph MM, Edwards A. Acute bronchiolitis: assessment and management in the emergency department. Pediatr Emerg Med Pract. 2019;16(10):1–24.
- Kyler KE, McCulloh RJ. Current concepts in the evaluation and management of bronchiolitis. Infect Dis Clin North Am. 2018;32(1):35–45.
- Oakley E, Brys T, Borland M, et al. Medication use in infants admitted with bronchiolitis. Emerg Med Australas. 2018;30(3):389–397.
- Rivera-Sepulveda AV, Rebman T, Gerard J, et al. Physician compliance with bronchiolitis guidelines in pediatric emergency departments. Clinical Pediatrics (Phil). 2019;58(9):1008–1018.

CODES

ICD10

- J21.9 Acute bronchiolitis, unspecified
- J21.0 Acute bronchiolitis due to respiratory syncytial virus
- J21.8 Acute bronchiolitis due to other specified organisms

CLINICAL PEARLS

- Bronchiolitis is the leading cause of hospitalizations in infants and children—especially <3 months of age.
- Diagnosis is a clinical one of children in the first 2 years of life, associated with rhinorrhea, cough, labored breathing, and irritability.
- RSV causes the majority of bronchiolitis. Chest x-ray is not indicated.
- Parental education and support is essential.
- Treatment: nasal and upper airway suctioning mainstay of treatment

BRONCHITIS, ACUTE

Ghazaleh Bigdeli, MD, FCCP

 BASICS

- Acute bronchitis is a common clinical condition characterized by an acute onset but persistent cough, with or without sputum production. It is typically self-limited, resolving within 1 to 3 weeks. Symptoms result from inflammation of the lower respiratory tract and are most frequently due to viral infection.
- Treatment is focused on patient education and supportive care. Antibiotics are not needed for the great majority of patients with acute bronchitis but are greatly overused for this condition. Reducing antibiotic use for acute bronchitis is a national and international health care priority.

DESCRIPTION

- Acute bronchitis is a lower respiratory tract infection that causes reversible bronchial inflammation, involving the large airways, without evidence of pneumonia.
- Cough, the predominant symptom, may last as long as 3 weeks (1).
- Generally self-limited, with complete healing and full return of function (1)
- Most infections are viral if no underlying cardiopulmonary disease is present (1).
- Synonym(s): tracheobronchitis

Geriatric Considerations
Can be serious, particularly if part of influenza, with underlying COPD or CHF

Pediatric Considerations
- Usually occurs in association with other conditions of upper and lower respiratory tract (trachea usually involved)
- If repeated attacks occur, child should be evaluated for anomalies of the respiratory tract, immune deficiencies, or for asthma.
- Acute bronchitis caused by RSV may be fatal.
- Antitussive medication not indicated in patients age <6 years (1)

EPIDEMIOLOGY

- Predominant age: all ages
- Predominant gender: male = female

Incidence
It accounts for approximately 10% of ambulatory care visits in the United States, or 100 million visits per year. The incidence of acute bronchitis is highest in late fall and winter when transmission of respiratory viruses peaks (1),(2).

ETIOLOGY AND PATHOPHYSIOLOGY

- Viruses are the most commonly identified pathogens in patients with acute bronchitis (about 60%). The most common viral causes of acute bronchitis include (1):
  - Influenza A and B
  - Parainfluenza
  - Coronavirus types 1 to 3
  - Rhinoviruses
  - Respiratory syncytial virus
  - Human metapneumovirus
- Bacteria are detected in 1–10% of cases of acute bronchitis.
- Atypical bacteria, such as *Mycoplasma pneumoniae*, *Chlamydophila pneumoniae*, and *Bordetella pertussis*, are rare causes of acute bronchitis.

- Approximately 10% of patients presenting with a cough lasting at least 2 weeks have evidence of B. pertussis infection.
- Possible fungal infections
- Chemical irritants
- Acute bronchitis causes an injury to the epithelial surfaces, resulting in an increase in mucus production and thickening of the bronchiole wall.

Genetics
No known genetic pattern

RISK FACTORS

- Infants
- Elderly
- Air pollutants
- Smoking
- Secondhand smoke
- Environmental changes
- Chronic bronchopulmonary diseases
- Chronic sinusitis
- Tracheostomy or endobronchial intubation
- Bronchopulmonary allergy
- Hypertrophied tonsils and adenoids in children
- Immunosuppression
  - Immunoglobulin deficiency
  - HIV infection
  - Alcoholism
- Gastroesophageal reflux disease (GERD)

GENERAL PREVENTION

- Avoid smoking and secondhand smoke.
- Control underlying risk factors (i.e., asthma, sinusitis, and reflux).
- Avoid exposure, especially daycare.
- Pneumovax, influenza immunization

COMMONLY ASSOCIATED CONDITIONS

- Allergic rhinitis
- Sinusitis
- Pharyngitis
- Epiglottitis (rare but can be rapidly fatal)
- Coryza
- Croup
- Influenza
- Pneumonia
- Asthma
- COPD/emphysema
- GERD

DIAGNOSIS

- Acute bronchitis should be suspected in patients with an acute onset but persistent cough (often lasting 1 to 3 weeks) who do not have clinical findings suggestive of pneumonia (e.g., fever, tachypnea, rales, signs of parenchymal consolidation) and do not have chronic obstructive pulmonary disease.
- In most cases, the diagnosis can be made based on the history and physical examination.
- Testing is generally reserved for cases in which pneumonia is suspected, clinical diagnosis is uncertain, or when results would change management.

HISTORY

- Cough for >5 days and no evidence of pneumonia, asthma, exacerbation of COPD
- Cough is initially dry and nonproductive, then productive; later, mucopurulent sputum, which may indicate secondary infection
- Cough lasts >5 days.
- Dyspnea, wheeze, and fatigue may occur.
- Possible contact with others who have respiratory infections
- Fever may suggest pneumonia or influenza infection.

PHYSICAL EXAM

- Fever
- Tachypnea
- Pharynx injected
- Rhonchi, wheezing
- No evidence of pulmonary consolidation, rales, etc.

DIFFERENTIAL DIAGNOSIS

- Pneumonia
- COVID-19
- Postnasal drip syndrome
- Common cold
- Acute sinusitis
- Bronchopneumonia
- Influenza
- Bacterial tracheitis
- Bronchiectasis
- Asthma
- Reactive airways dysfunction syndrome (RADS)
- Allergy
- Eosinophilic pneumonitis
- Aspiration
- Retained foreign body
- Inhalation injury
- Cystic fibrosis
- Bronchogenic carcinoma
- Heart failure
- GERD
- Chronic cough
- ACE inhibitor use

DIAGNOSTIC TESTS & INTERPRETATION

Initial Tests (lab, imaging)
- None normally needed; diagnosis is based on history and physical exam showing no postnasal drip or rales.
- For a complicated picture, consider the following:
  - CBC with differential
  - Influenza titers (if appropriate for time of year)
  - Viral panel/testing for SARS-CoV-2 (COVID-19) is recommended for all patients during the COVID-19 pandemic.
- No testing needed unless concerned about pneumonia
- Pulse oximetry if underlying pulmonary disease is present
- CXR are only indicated if:
  - Dyspnea, bloody sputum, or rusty sputum color
  - Pulse >100 beats/min
  - Respiratory rate >24 breaths/min
  - Oral body temperature >100°F (37.8°C)
  - Focal consolidation, egophony, or fremitus on chest examination

Follow-Up Tests and Special Considerations
- Arterial blood gases: hypoxemia (rarely)
- Pulmonary function tests (seldom needed during acute stages): increased residual volume, decreased maximal expiratory rate (1)
- Sputum culture in those patients intubated or with tracheostomy
- Procalcitonin

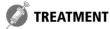 **TREATMENT**

GENERAL MEASURES
- Outpatient treatment unless elderly or complicated by severe underlying disease
- Rest
- Stop smoking and avoid secondhand smoke.
- Steam inhalations
- Vaporizers
- Adequate hydration
- Antitussives (honey 1 tbsp every 2 to 3 hours PRN)
- Antibiotics are not recommended (2)[A].
- Treat associated illnesses (e.g., GERD).

MEDICATION

ALERT
Antibiotics are not recommended unless a treatable pathogen has been identified or significant comorbidities are present. This should be explained to patients who likely expect an antibiotic to be prescribed.

First Line
- Supportive; increased fluids (Cough results in increased fluid loss.)
- Antipyretic analgesic such as aspirin, acetaminophen, or ibuprofen
- Decongestants if accompanied by sinus condition
- Cough suppressant for troublesome cough (not with COPD); nonpharmacologic therapy: honey (1 tbsp every 2 to 4 hours PRN), throat lozenges, hot tea; smoking cessation and avoidance of secondhand smoke is a reasonable first step.
- Pharmacologic therapy: benzonatate (Tessalon), guaifenesin with dextromethorphan; not indicated in children age <6 years (1)[C]
- Mucolytic agents are not recommended.
- Inhaled β-agonist (e.g., albuterol) or in combination with high-dose inhaled corticosteroids for cough with bronchospasm in those with known airflow obstruction (1),(3)[B]
- If influenza is highly suspected and symptom onset is <48 hours: oseltamivir (Tamiflu), zanamivir (Relenza) (1)[B], IV peramivir (Rapivab), or baloxavir marboxil (Xofluza)
- Antibiotics ONLY if a treatable cause (i.e., pertussis) is identified (1)[A].
  - Clarithromycin (Biaxin): 500 mg q12h or azithromycin (Zithromax) Z-Pak for atypical or pertussis infection
  - In patients with acute bronchitis of a suspected bacterial cause, azithromycin tends to be more effective in terms of lower incidence of treatment failure and adverse events than amoxicillin or amoxicillin-clavulanic acid but not more effective than doxycycline.
    - Doxycycline: 100 mg/day × 10 days if *Moraxella*, *Chlamydia*, or *Mycoplasma* suspected
    - Quinolone for more serious infections or other antibiotic failure or in elderly or patients with multiple comorbidities

- Contraindication(s): Doxycycline and quinolones should not be used during pregnancy or in children.
- Precautions:
  - Multiple antibiotics have the potential to interfere with the effectiveness of oral contraceptives.
  - Antibiotic use can be associated with *Clostridium difficile* infections.
  - Cough and cold preparations should not be used in children <6 years (1)[B].

Second Line
Other antibiotics if indicated by sputum culture

ISSUES FOR REFERRAL
- Complications such as pneumonia or respiratory failure
- Comorbidities such as COPD
- Cough lasting >3 months

ADDITIONAL THERAPIES
- Antipyretic for fever (e.g., acetaminophen, or ibuprofen)
- Inhaled β-agonist (e.g., albuterol) or in combination with high-dose inhaled corticosteroids for cough with bronchospasm (1)[B]
- Oral corticosteroids probably not indicated with exception in COVID-19 infection (1)

COMPLEMENTARY & ALTERNATIVE MEDICINE
Throat lozenges for pharyngitis

ADMISSION, INPATIENT, AND NURSING CONSIDERATIONS
- Hypoxia—may require supplemental oxygen
- Respiratory failure that may require CPAP/bilevel ventilation
- Severe bronchospasm
- Exacerbation of underlying disease
- Bronchodilators if patient is bronchospastic
- IV fluids may be helpful if patient is dehydrated.
- Ensure patient comfort and monitor for signs of deterioration, especially if underlying lung disease exists.
- May need to follow oxygen saturation in patients with underlying lung disease
- Discharge criteria: improvement in symptoms and comorbidities

 ONGOING CARE

FOLLOW-UP RECOMMENDATIONS
- Usually a self-limited disease not requiring follow-up
- Cough may linger for several weeks.
- In children, if recurrent, need to consider other diagnoses, such as asthma (2)

Patient Monitoring
- Oximetry until no longer hypoxemic
- Recheck for chronicity.

DIET
Increased fluids (3 to 4 L/day) while febrile

PATIENT EDUCATION
- For patient education materials favorably reviewed on this topic, contact the American Lung Association: 1740 Broadway, New York, NY 10019 (212) 315-8700; www.lung.org.
- American Academy of Family Physicians: www.familydoctor.org

PROGNOSIS
- Usual: complete resolution
- Can be serious in the elderly or debilitated
- Cough may persist for several weeks after an initial improvement.
- Postbronchitic reactive airways disease (rare)
- Bronchiolitis obliterans and organizing pneumonia (rare)

COMPLICATIONS
- Superinfection such as bronchopneumonia
- Bronchiectasis
- Hemoptysis
- Acute respiratory failure
- Chronic cough

REFERENCES
1. Albert RH. Diagnosis and treatment of acute bronchitis. *Am Fam Physician*. 2010;82(11):1345–1350.
2. Gonzales R, Anderer T, McCulloch CE, et al. A cluster randomized trial of decision support strategies for reducing antibiotic use in acute bronchitis. *JAMA Intern Med*. 2013;173(4):267–273.
3. Becker LA, Hom J, Villasis-Keever M, et al. Beta2-agonists for acute cough or a clinical diagnosis of acute bronchitis. *Cochrane Database Syst Rev*. 2015;(9):CD001726.

 SEE ALSO

- Asthma; Chronic Obstructive Pulmonary Disease and Emphysema
- Algorithm: Cough, Chronic

CODES

ICD10
- J20.9 Acute bronchitis, unspecified
- J68.0 Bronchitis and pneumonitis due to chemicals, gases, fumes and vapors
- B97.0 Adenovirus as the cause of diseases classified elsewhere

CLINICAL PEARLS
- Acute bronchitis is a common and generally self-limited disease.
- Treat cough with honey (1 tbsp every 2 to 4 hours PRN), benzonatate (Tessalon), guaifenesin with dextromethorphan.
- It does not require treatment with antibiotics. This needs to be explained to patients who expect antibiotics to be prescribed.
- Cough may linger for several weeks after the resolution of other symptoms.
- Recurrent or seasonal episodes may suggest another disease process, such as asthma.
- Fever is uncommon and should prompt investigation for pneumonia or influenza.

BULIMIA NERVOSA
Amanda D. Dobbins, MD • Dana Vlachos, DO

BASICS

DESCRIPTION
An eating disorder which includes binge eating and inappropriate compensatory behaviors

- Binge eating is characterized by eating, in a discrete period of time (usually within 2-hour period), an amount of food that is definitely larger than most people would eat during a similar period of time and a sense of lack of control over eating during the episode, followed by recurrent inappropriate compensatory behavior to prevent weight gain, such as self-induced vomiting, misuse of laxatives or diuretics (or other medications), excessive exercise, and fasting after the binge.
- Binge eating and inappropriate compensatory behaviors both occur on average, at least once a week for 3 months.
- DSM-5 classifies bulimia nervosa severity as the following:
  - Mild: 1 to 3 episodes of inappropriate compensatory behaviors per week
  - Moderate: 4 to 7 episodes of inappropriate compensatory behaviors per week
  - Severe: 8 to 13 episodes of inappropriate compensatory behaviors per week
  - Extreme: 14 or more episodes of inappropriate compensatory behaviors per week
- System(s) affected: oropharyngeal, endocrine/metabolic, gastrointestinal, dermatologic, cardiovascular, pulmonary, psychiatric

EPIDEMIOLOGY
- Predominant age: adolescents and young adults but can occur in all age groups and ethnicities worldwide
- Mean age of onset: 18 to 21 years
- Predominant sex: female > male (13:1)

Incidence
18.5% to 26.9%, declining in incidence over time in recent studies (1)

Prevalence
Up to 3% of females and ~1% of males in their lifetime

ETIOLOGY AND PATHOPHYSIOLOGY
- Combination of biologic, psychological, environmental, and social factors.
- Strong evidence of serotonergic dysregulation
- Multiple studies demonstrate altered brain function and structure in bulimia nervosa.

Genetics
Heritability estimated to be up to 41% in recent studies (2)

RISK FACTORS
- Female gender
- History of obesity and dieting
- Body dissatisfaction: critical comments about weight, body shape, or eating: low self-esteem
- Depression, social anxiety, severe life stressor
- Poor impulse control, substance abuse
- Perfectionist or obsessive thinking; environment stressing high achievement, physical fitness, (e.g., armed forces, ballet, cheerleading, gymnastics, or modeling)
- Family history of substance abuse, affective disorders, eating disorder, or obesity
- Diabetes: type 1 > type 2
- Childhood trauma (sexual or physical abuse, neglect)

GENERAL PREVENTION
- Realistic and healthy weight management strategies and attitudes
- Decrease body dissatisfaction and promote self-esteem.
- Reduce focus on thin as ideal.

COMMONLY ASSOCIATED CONDITIONS
- Major depression, dysthymia, anxiety, obsessive-compulsive, bipolar disorders
- Substance use disorder
- Personality disorders: borderline, schizotypal, antisocial (3)

DIAGNOSIS

HISTORY
- Patients unlikely to self-identify binge eating or purging behaviors; corroborate with parent/relative
- Unhappiness and/or preoccupation with weight and diet attempts
- Pattern of binge eating and compensatory behaviors
  - Binging
  - Vomiting (often with little effort)
  - Vigorous aerobic exercise
  - Distress/shame related to loss of control
- Depressed mood and self-depreciation following the binges
- Other possible signs and symptoms
  - Requesting weight loss help and mildly underweight to overweight
  - Diet pill, diuretic, laxative, ipecac, and thyroid medication use/abuse, frequent fluctuations in weight
  - Menstrual disturbances or amenorrhea
  - Fatigue and lethargy
  - Abdominal pain, bloating, constipation, diarrhea, rectal prolapse
  - Sore throat and thermal tooth sensitivity
  - Omission/underdosing insulin in diabetes patients
- Screening
  - Do you currently suffer with or have you ever suffered in the past with an eating disorder? (Yes is abnormal.)
  - Have any members of your family suffered with an eating disorder? (Yes is abnormal.)
  - Does your weight affect the way you feel about yourself? (Yes is abnormal.)
  - Do you ever eat in secret? (Yes is abnormal.)
  - Are you satisfied with your eating patterns? (No is abnormal.)

PHYSICAL EXAM
- Often normal with normal weight or overweight range
- Tachycardia
- Erosion of dental enamel
- Perimylolysis, cheilosis, gingivitis
- Sialadenosis (parotid gland swelling and/or asymptomatic, noninflammatory parotid gland enlargement)
- Epigastric tenderness to palpation
- Calluses, abrasions, bruising on hand, thumb (Russell sign)
- Peripheral edema

DIFFERENTIAL DIAGNOSIS
- Anorexia, binge eating/purging type; distinguished by BMI <18.5 kg/m^2
- Major depressive disorder

- Other metabolic disorders: Addison disease, celiac disease, diabetes mellitus, hyperthyroidism, hypothyroidism, hyperpituitarism
- Genetic syndromes: Kleine-Levin syndrome, Prader-Willi syndrome
- Body dysmorphic or borderline personality disorder

DIAGNOSTIC TESTS & INTERPRETATION
- All lab results may be within normal limits and are not necessary for diagnosis.
- Psychological self-report screening tests may be helpful, but diagnosis is based on meeting the *DSM-5* criteria:
  - SCOFF Questionnaire (4)[B]
  - Primary Care Evaluation of Mental Disorders Patient Health Questionnaire

Initial Tests (lab, imaging)
- Complete blood count, comprehensive metabolic panel, and liver function tests
  - Hypokalemia, hypochloremia, hypomagnesemia, hyponatremia, hypocalcemia, hypophosphatemia, hypoglycemia
  - Serum amylase levels and pH derangements
  - Elevated blood urea nitrogen
- Urinalysis: increased urine specific gravity

Diagnostic Procedures/Other
- Pregnancy test
- Electrocardiogram: bradycardia or arrhythmias, conduction defects, depressed ST segment due to hypokalemia

TREATMENT
Cognitive-behavioral therapy (CBT) and nutritional rehabilitation should be considered as first-line treatment (5),(6),(7)[A].

GENERAL MEASURES
- Multidisciplinary team
  - Primary care physician, behavioral health provider, nutritionist
- Build trust; increase motivation for change.
- Assess psychological and nutritional status.
- Consider evidence-based self-help program.
- CBT for bulimia nervosa (6),(7)[A]
  - Twenty 45- to 50-minute appointments for 16 weeks
  - Involve patient in establishing goals.
  - Self-monitoring of food intake, frequency of binges/purges, related antecedents, consequences, thoughts, and emotions
  - Self-monitoring of weight once per week
  - Educate about ineffectiveness of purging for weight control and adverse outcomes.
  - Establish prescribed eating plan to develop regular eating habits and realistic weight goal.
  - Gradually introduce feared foods into diet and challenge fear of loss of control.
  - Problem-solve how to cope with triggers.
  - Decrease ruminations about calories, weight, and purging.
  - Establish relapse prevention plan.
  - Gradual laxative withdrawal
- Interpersonal therapy (may act more slowly than CBT)
- Transdiagnostic CBT
- Dialectical behavior therapy
- Family therapy for adolescents
- Nutritional education, relaxation techniques
- Educate patient to brush teeth and use baking soda to rinse mouth after vomiting.

MEDICATION

First Line

- Selective serotonin reuptake inhibitors (SSRIs) (8)[A], particularly fluoxetine (Prozac) titrated to 60 mg/day, are effective in reducing symptoms with relatively few side effects. Higher doses than standard doses for depression are often needed.
  - Combination of medication and CBT has been shown to have added benefit over medication or therapy alone.
  - Maintain full therapeutic dose for at least 6 to 12 months (9).
  - Avoid bupropion: contraindicated due to its association with seizures in patients who purge
- If no response to treatment, consider patients may vomit medications.

Second Line

- Select different SSRI (citalopram, fluvoxamine, and sertraline).
- Ondansetron (Zofran) 4 to 8 mg TID between meals can help prevent vomiting.
- Third-line therapies are available for those who fail first- and second-line therapies but are rarely used due to side effect profiles.
- The anticonvulsant topiramate may have some usefulness in helping to diminish binge–purge episodes in bulimic patients (10).

ISSUES FOR REFERRAL

Patients with bulimia require a multidisciplinary team, including a primary care physician, behavioral health provider, and a nutritionist. Important part of treatment is to arrange mental health therapist for psychotherapy.

COMPLEMENTARY & ALTERNATIVE MEDICINE

Bright light therapy is potentially acutely effective at improving disordered eating and mood (11).

ADMISSION, INPATIENT, AND NURSING CONSIDERATIONS

- Admission (to a specialized eating disorders unit if available) is indicated for one or more of the following:
  - ≤75% median body mass index for age and sex
  - Dehydration; electrolyte disturbance (hypokalemia, hyponatremia, hypophosphatemia)
  - ECG abnormalities (e.g., prolonged QTc or severe bradycardia)
- Severe bradycardia (<50 beats/min daytime; <45 beats/min at night)
  - Hypotension (<90/45 mm Hg)
  - Hypothermia (body temperature <96°F, 35.6°C)
  - Orthostatic increase in pulse (>20 beats/min) or decrease in blood pressure (>20 mm Hg systolic or >10 mm Hg diastolic)
  - Failure of outpatient treatment
  - Acute food refusal, uncontrollable bingeing and purging
  - Acute medical complications of malnutrition (e.g., syncope, seizures, cardiac failure, pancreatitis)
  - Comorbid psychiatric or medical condition that prohibits or limits appropriate outpatient treatment (e.g., severe depression, suicidal ideation, obsessive compulsive disorder, type 1 diabetes mellitus) (12)
- During admission:
  - Supervised meals and bathroom privileges
  - Monitor weight, physical activity, electrolytes, and cardiac activity.
  - Gradually shift control to patients as they demonstrate improvement.

ONGOING CARE

FOLLOW-UP RECOMMENDATIONS

Patient Monitoring

- Binge–purge activity, including antecedents and consequences, level of exercise activity
- Self-esteem, comfort with body and self, ruminations and depressive symptoms
- Repeat any abnormal lab values weekly until stable.

DIET

- Balanced diet, normal eating pattern
- Nutritional rehabilitation aims to restore a structured and consistent meal pattern: three meals and two snacks per day

PATIENT EDUCATION

https://www.nami.org/Learn-More/Mental-Health -Conditions/Eating-Disorders/Overview

PROGNOSIS

- An estimated 45–70% will have a full recovery or improvement of symptoms, and 20–30% may experience relapse (13),(14).
- Positive prognostic factors: younger age at presentation, shorter duration of illness, less frequent symptoms, absence of laxative use, close social relationships, and a good therapeutic response within the first month of treatment
- Negative prognostic factors: overemphasis on body shape and weight, history of physical abuse, disturbed family relationships, poor motivation, self-injurious behaviors, and presence of a personality disorder (13)

COMPLICATIONS

- Substance use disorder
- Osteopenia/osteoporosis/stress fracture
- Gastric dilatation/Boerhaave syndrome/Mallory-Weiss tears
- Spontaneous pneumomediastinum
- Potassium depletion, cardiac arrhythmia, cardiac arrest
- Suicide

Pregnancy Considerations

- Binging/purging behaviors may persist, increase, or decrease with pregnancy.
- Increased risk for miscarriage, preterm delivery, operative delivery, and infants with low birth weight should be managed as high risk (10).

REFERENCES

1. van Eeden A, van Hoeken D, Hoek HW. Incidence, prevalence and mortality of anorexia nervosa and bulimia nervosa. *Curr Opin Psychiatry*. 2021;34(6):515–524.
2. Yao S, Larsson H, Norring C, et al. Genetic and environmental contributions to diagnostic fluctuation in anorexia nervosa and bulimia nervosa. *Psychol Med*. 2021;51(1):62–69. doi:10.1017/S0033291719002976.
3. Udo T, Grilo CM. Psychiatric and medical correlates of DSM-5 eating disorders in a nationally representative sample of adults in the United States. *Int J Eat Disord*. 2019;52(1):42–50. doi:10.1002/eat.23004.
4. Cotton MA, Ball C, Robinson P. Four simple questions can help screen for eating disorders. *J Gen Intern Med*. 2003;18(1):53–56.
5. Linardon Jake, Wade TD, de la Piedad GX, et al. The efficacy of cognitive-behavioral therapy for eating disorders: a systematic review and meta-analysis. *J Consult Clin Psychol*. 2017;85(11):1080–1094.
6. Hay PP, Bacaltchuk J, Stefano S, et al. Psychological treatments for bulimia nervosa and binging. *Cochrane Database Syst Rev*. 2009;(4):CD000562.
7. Shapiro JR, Berkman ND, Brownley KA, et al. Bulimia nervosa treatment: a systematic review of randomized controlled trials. *Int J Eat Disord*. 2007;40(4):321–336.
8. Bacaltchuk J, Hay P, Trefiglio R. Antidepressants versus psychological treatments and their combination for bulimia nervosa. *Cochrane Database Syst Rev*. 2001;(4):CD003385.
9. Yager J, Devlin M, Halmi K, et al. 2014. Guideline watch: *Practice Guideline for the Treatment of Patients with Eating Disorders*, 3rd edition. *Focus (Am Psychiatr Publ)*. 2012;12(4):416–431.
10. Mazzeo SE, Slof-Op't Landt MC, Jones I, et al. Associations among postpartum depression, eating disorders, and perfectionism in a population-based sample of adult women. *Int J Eat Disord*. 2006;39:202–211. https://doi.org/10.1002/eat.20243.
11. Beauchamp MT, Lundgren JD. A systematic review of bright light therapy for eating disorders. *Prim Care Companion CNS Disord*. 2016;18(5). doi:10.4088/PCC.16r02008.
12. Golden NH, Katzman DK, Sawyer SM, et al; for the Society for Adolescent Health and Medicine. Position paper of the Society for Adolescent Health and Medicine: medical management of restrictive eating disorders in adolescents and young adults. *J Adolesc Health*. 2015;56(1):121–125. doi:10.1016/j.jadohealth.2014.10.259.
13. Castillo M, Weiselberg W. Bulimia nervosa/purging disorder. *Curr Prob Pediatr Adolesc Health Care*. 2017;47(4):85–94. doi:10.1016/j.cppeds.2017.02.004.
14. Olmsted MP, MacDonald DE, McFarlane T, et al. Predictors of rapid relapse in bulimia nervosa. *Int J Eat Disord*. 2015;48(3):337–340. doi:10.1002/eat.22380.

CODES

ICD10

F50.2 Bulimia nervosa

CLINICAL PEARLS

- Asking "Are you satisfied with your eating patterns?" and/or "Do you worry that you have lost control over how much you eat?" may help to screen for an eating problem.
- Consider multidisciplinary team approach with PCP, behavioral health provider, and nutritionist.
- SSRIs, particularly fluoxetine (60 mg daily), may be helpful as a first step or as an adjunctive treatment with CBT.
- Pharmacotherapy alone is reasonable if specialized nutritional rehabilitation and psychotherapy are not available.

BUNION (HALLUX VALGUS)

Jennifer G. Chang, MD

BASICS

DESCRIPTION
- Lateral deviation of the great toe ("Hallux abducto valgus" derives from the Latin for "big toe askew.")
- Associated medial deviation of the 1st metatarsal, leading to a medial prominence of the 1st metatar-sophalangeal (MTP) joint (also known as "bunion")
- Progressive subluxation of the 1st MTP joint in later stages
- System(s) affected: musculoskeletal/skin

EPIDEMIOLOGY
- Predominant age: more common in adults
- Gender difference: female > male by ~2:1
- More common in shoe-wearing populations
- Commonly bilateral

Incidence
Unknown and difficult to assess

Prevalence
- Prevalence increases with age, particularly in females.
- Adults (age 18 to 65 years): estimated prevalence of 23%
- Elderly (>65 years) adults: estimated prevalence of 35.7%
- Juvenile hallux valgus: more common in girls (>80% of cases)

ETIOLOGY AND PATHOPHYSIOLOGY
Multifactorial and controversial. Contributing factors may include underlying anatomy and repetitive external forces:
- Absence of muscles that directly stabilize the 1st MTP allows relatively unopposed forces to influence lateral deviation of the proximal phalanx and medial deviation of the 1st metatarsal head.
- Medial MTP joint capsule and medial collateral ligament are chronically stretched and may eventually rupture, decreasing stability and causing progressive subluxation of the 1st MTP joint.
- Lateral joint capsule and collateral ligaments also contract.
- Lateral and plantar migration of abductor hallucis muscle moves the great toe into plantar flexion and lateral pronation.

Genetics
- Cohort and twin studies suggest heritability
- Genome wide association studies suggest sex-specific differences in genetic mechanisms

RISK FACTORS
- Genetic predisposition
- Abnormal biomechanics (i.e., flexible flat feet)
- Foot deformities: joint laxity, hindfoot pronation, Achilles tendon tightness, pes planus (fallen arches), metatarsus primus varus

- Amputation of 2nd toe
- Inflammatory joint disease
- Neuromuscular disorders (cerebral palsy, stroke)
- Improper footwear (high heels; narrow toe box)

GENERAL PREVENTION
Proper footwear may decrease the progression of the disease.

COMMONLY ASSOCIATED CONDITIONS
- Medial bursitis of the 1st MTP joint (most common)
- Hammertoe deformity of the 2nd phalanx
- Plantar callus
- Metatarsalgia
- Degeneration of 1st metatarsal head cartilage (hallux rigidus)
- Pronated feet; ankle equinus
- Onychocryptosis (ingrown toenail)
- Entrapment of the medial dorsal cutaneous nerve
- Synovitis of the MTP joint

DIAGNOSIS
- Based on clinical exam
- Radiographs are used for staging.

HISTORY
- Painful MTP joint (most common symptom in adults)
- Abnormal position of great toe
- Enlargement of the MTP joint medially (patients complain of a "bump")
- Shoes do not fit properly.
- Pain with ambulation
- Skin irritation, blister, or callus at the 1st MTP

PHYSICAL EXAM
- Observe gait; may be antalgic due to pain
- Medial prominence at the MTP joint
- Skin changes: erythema, blistering, callus or ulceration at the MTP joint
- Great toe over- or underriding the 2nd toe
- Examine the entire 1st metatarsal and toe for:
  - 1st MTP range of motion
  - 1st tarsometatarsal (TMT) mobility
  - Neurovascular integrity
  - Degenerative osteoarthritis

DIFFERENTIAL DIAGNOSIS
- Trauma: turf toe; sesamoiditis; stress fracture
- Infection: osteomyelitis; septic arthritis
- Joint disorder: osteoarthritis; rheumatoid arthritis; pseudogout; gout
- Tendon disorder: tendinosis; tenosynovitis; tendon rupture
- Other: bursitis; ganglion cyst; foreign body granuloma

DIAGNOSTIC TESTS & INTERPRETATION
Initial Tests (lab, imaging)
- Weight-bearing AP and lateral radiographs (sesamoid view optional) to assess:
  - Joint congruency and degenerative changes
  - Lateral sesamoid bone displacement
  - Rounded 1st metatarsal head
  - Longer 1st metatarsal
- Radiographic parameters:
  - Hallux valgus angle (HVA): Long axis of the 1st MT and proximal phalanx is normally <15 degrees.
  - Intermetatarsal angle (IMA): Between long axis of 1st and 2nd metatarsal is normally <9 degrees.
  - Distal metatarsal articular angle (DMAA): Between 1st metatarsal long axis and line through base of distal articular cap is normally <15 degrees.
  - Hallux valgus interphalangeus: Between long axis of distal phalanx and proximal phalanx is normally <10 degrees.

TREATMENT
- Primary indication for treatment is pain.
- There are conservative (nonoperative) and surgical approaches.
- Only surgical approaches can correct the hallux valgus deformity.
- Surgical treatment is generally more effective in improving pain but has attendant risks.

GENERAL MEASURES
Nonoperative treatment options may improve symptoms and delay the progression of hallux valgus deformity, although high-quality evidence is limited:
- Proper fitting footwear: low-heeled, wide-toe shoes to decrease stress on MTP joint
- Orthotics: correct foot alignment (pes planus and overpronation). Improving gait may prevent bunion formation and reduce pressure on the MTP.
- Splinting: in theory, stabilizes and balances soft tissue structures around the MTP. Limited evidence shows improvement in degree of angulation in mild hallux valgus. Dynamic splint use may reduce pain.
- Foot mobilization and exercise, combined with a toe separator, may improve pain scores, strength and range of motion in moderate hallux valgus (1)[B].
- Pads/spacers: Pads decrease friction on the MTP joint. A toe spacer in the 1st interdigital space may reduce pain (2)[C].

MEDICATION
- Topical (NSAIDs) and oral medications (NSAIDs, acetaminophen) can be used to relieve pain. Other topical options include capsaicin cream.
- Corticosteroid injections may improve pain (rarely used outside of postoperative setting).

ISSUES FOR REFERRAL
Surgery is indicated for patients with severe pain, dysfunction, or persistent symptoms that do not abate with conservative therapy.

ADDITIONAL THERAPIES
Custom orthoses are a safe intervention that may decrease pain at 6 and 12 months compared with no treatment; however, this improvement is less than that seen with surgical intervention (3)[B].

SURGERY/OTHER PROCEDURES
- >100 different surgical techniques exist to treat hallux valgus.
- No single technique is proven superior; no universally accepted standard exists for procedure selection.
- Minimally invasive techniques are gaining popularity.
- Choice of technique depends on disease severity, radiographic findings, and patient/surgeon-specific factors:
  - Arthrodesis: fusion of the 1st MTP joint; used for severe and/or recurrent hallux valgus; fusion of the 1st TMT joint (modified Lapidus) is considered for TMT joint hypermobility.
  - Arthroplasty: removing the joint or replacing it with a prosthesis; high revision rates
  - Exostectomy/bunionectomy: removing the medial bony prominence of the MTP joint (less common now)
  - Soft tissue realignment: alters the function of surrounding ligaments and tendons; used for minor deformities or as an adjunct to bony correction techniques
  - Osteotomy and realignment: various techniques; can correct large deformities, but evidence of long-term outcome is lacking (4)[C]
  - Mini-tight rope procedure: use of a FiberWire to correct the misalignment of the deformity
- Some patients may have little to no improvement in symptoms despite interventions. Providers should establish realistic expectations prior to surgery.
- In pediatric patients, surgery should generally be delayed until skeletal maturity (5)[C].

COMPLEMENTARY & ALTERNATIVE MEDICINE
Marigold ointment may reduce pain and soft tissue swelling related to bunion.

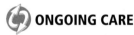 ONGOING CARE

FOLLOW-UP RECOMMENDATIONS
- Postoperative treatment includes physical therapy, physiotherapy, supportive footwear, continuous passive motion, or manual manipulation.
- Time until full weight-bearing depends on the surgical procedure.

PROGNOSIS
Patient outcome varies depending on biomechanical factors, severity of the deformity, and treatment modality used. The radiologic HA angle predicts surgical outcomes. Patients with an HA angle <37 degrees have a higher chance of having the deformity successfully corrected with surgery compared with patients with an HA angle >37 degrees (6)[B].

COMPLICATIONS
- Risks associated with surgery include infection, persistent pain, and poor cosmetic result.
- Additional risks vary with the surgical procedure.
- Other complications may include the following:
  - Early swelling
  - Hallux varus
  - Recurrence of bunion
  - Metatarsal fracture
  - Decreased sensation over the 1st metatarsal or phalanx

REFERENCES
1. Abdalbary SA. Foot mobilization and exercise program combined with toe separator improves outcomes in women with moderate hallux valgus at 1-year follow-up a randomized clinical trial. *J Am Podiatr Med Assoc.* 2018;108(6):478–486.
2. Tehraninasr A, Saeedi H, Forogh B, et al. Effects of insole with toe-separator and night splint on patients with painful hallux valgus: a comparative study. *Prosthet Orthot Int.* 2008;32(1):79–83.
3. Torkki M, Malmivaara A, Seitsalo S, et al. Surgery vs orthosis vs watchful waiting for hallux valgus: a randomized controlled trial. *JAMA.* 2001;285(19):2474–2480.
4. Choi JH, Zide JR, Coleman SC, et al. Prospective study of treatment of adult primary hallux valgus with scarf osteotomy and soft tissue realignment. *Foot Ankle Int.* 2013;34(5):684–690.
5. Chell J, Dhar S. Pediatric hallux valgus. *Foot Ankle Clin.* 2014;19(2):235–243.
6. Deenik AR, de Visser E, Louwerens JW, et al. Hallux valgus angle as main predictor for correction of hallux valgus. *BMC Musculoskelet Disord.* 2008;9:70.

ADDITIONAL READING
- Barnish MS, Barnish J. High-heeled shoes and musculoskeletal injuries: a narrative systematic review. *BMJ Open.* 2016;6(1):e010053.
- Dayton P, Sedberry S, Feilmeier M. Complications of metatarsal suture techniques for bunion correction: a systematic review of the literature. *J Foot Ankle Surg.* 2015;54(2):230–232.
- Dux K, Smith N, Rottier FJ. Outcome after metatarsal osteotomy for hallux valgus: a study of postoperative foot function using revised foot function index short form. *J Foot Ankle Surg.* 2013;52(4):422–425.
- Fraissler L, Konrads C, Hoberg M, et al. Treatment of hallux valgus deformity. *EFFORT Open Rev.* 2016;1(8):295–302.
- Hsu YH, Liu Y, Hannan MT, et al. Genome-wide association meta-analyses to identify common genetic variants associated with hallux valgus in Caucasian and African Americans. *J Med Genet.* 2015;52(11):762–769.
- Kaufmann G, Dammerer D, Heyenbrock F, et al. Minimally invasive versus open chevron osteotomy for hallux valgus correction: a randomized controlled trial. *Int Orthop.* 2019;43(2):343–350.
- Khan MT. The podiatric treatment of hallux abducto valgus and its associated condition, bunion, with Tagetes patula. *J Pharm Pharmacol.* 1996;48(7):768–770.
- Nix S, Smith M, Vicenzino B. Prevalence of hallux valgus in the general population: a systematic review and meta-analysis. *J Foot Ankle Res.* 2010;3:21.
- Nix SE, Vicenzino BT, Collins NJ, et al. Characteristics of foot structure and footwear associated with hallux valgus: a systematic review. *Osteoarthritis Cartilage.* 2012;20(10):1059–1074.
- Plaass C, Karch A, Koch A, et al. Short term results of dynamic splinting for hallux valgus—a prospective randomized study. *Foot Ankle Surg.* 2020;26(2):146–150.
- Sanhudo JAV, Pereira TAP. Current trends in fixation techniques. *Foot Ankle Clin.* 2020;25(1):97–108.
- Smyth NA, Aiyer AA. Introduction: why are there so many different surgeries for hallux valgus? *Foot Ankle Clin.* 2018;23(2):171–182.
- Trnka HJ, Krenn S, Schuh R. Minimally invasive hallux valgus surgery: a critical review of the evidence. *Int Orthop.* 2013;37(9):1731–1735.

 CODES

ICD10
- M20.10 Hallux valgus (acquired), unspecified foot
- M20.11 Hallux valgus (acquired), right foot
- M20.12 Hallux valgus (acquired), left foot

CLINICAL PEARLS
- Avoid footwear with high heels, pointed toe boxes, or inadequate toe space to reduce development or progression of bunions.
- Surgery generally results in superior outcomes for pain relief in appropriately selected patients.
- No single surgical method has shown to be superior for long-term pain relief.
- Establish realistic expectations prior to surgery to improve patient satisfaction with surgical outcomes.

BURNS

Caleb J. Mentzer, DO • Cragin D. Currence, MD • James R. Yon, MD

BASICS

DESCRIPTION
- Tissue injuries caused by application of heat, chemicals, electricity, or irradiation
- Extent of injury (depth of burn) is a result of intensity and duration of exposure.
  - 1st degree involves superficial layers of epidermis.
  - 2nd degree involves varying amounts of epidermis (with blister formation) and part of the dermis.
  - 3rd degree involves destruction of all skin elements (full thickness) with coagulation of subdermal plexus.
- System(s) affected: endocrine/metabolic, pulmonary, skin/exocrine

Geriatric Considerations
- Prognosis is worse for severe burns.
- Patients >60 years of age account for 11% of all burns.

Pediatric Considerations
Consider child abuse or neglect when dealing with hot water burns in children; abuse accounts for 15% of pediatric burns. Special concerns are sharply demarcated wounds, immersion injuries, and suspect stories. Involve child welfare services early.

EPIDEMIOLOGY
- Predominant age: 30 years; 13% infants; 11% >60 years of age
- Predominant gender: Males account for 70%.

Incidence
Per year in the United States
- 1.2 to 2.0 million burns; 700,000 emergency room visits; 45,000 to 50,000 hospitalizations; 3,900 deaths owing to burn-related complications
- In children: 250,000 burns; 15,000 hospitalizations; 1,100 deaths
- Estimated total cost of $2 billion annually for burn care
- House fires cause 75% of deaths.
- Burn deaths decreasing nationally due to improved prevention and treatment
- Increase in burns from the illegal production of methamphetamines. Patients can present with a combination of chemical burn, thermal burn, and explosion injury.

ETIOLOGY AND PATHOPHYSIOLOGY
- Open flame and hot liquid are the most common causes of burns (heat usually ≥45°C): flame burns more common in adults; scald burns are more common in children.
- Caustic chemicals or acids (may show little signs or symptoms for the first few days)
- Electricity (may have significant injury with very little damage to overlying skin)
- Excess sun exposure

RISK FACTORS
- Water heaters set too high
- Workplace exposure to chemicals, electricity, or irradiation
- Young children and older adults with thin skin are more susceptible to injury.

- Carelessness with burning cigarettes: related to 18% of fatal fires in 2006
- Inadequate or faulty electrical wiring
- Lack of smoke detectors: Lacking or nonfunctioning smoke alarms are implicated in 63% of residential fires.
- Arson: cause of 12.4% of fires that resulted in fatalities in 2012

GENERAL PREVENTION
Home safety education should be a key mechanism for injury prevention.
- Families educated on home safety were more likely to have safe hot water temperatures.
- Safety education results in more families having functioning smoke alarms and increased use of fireguards.

COMMONLY ASSOCIATED CONDITIONS
Smoke inhalation syndrome
- May involve thermal burn to respiratory mucosa (e.g., trachea, bronchi) as well as carbon monoxide inhalation
- Occurs within 72 hours of burn
- Should be suspected in all burns occurring in an enclosed space or exposure to explosions

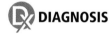

DIAGNOSIS

HISTORY
- History of source of burn
- In children or elderly: Check for consistency between the history and the burn's physical characteristics.

PHYSICAL EXAM
- 1st degree: erythema of involved tissue, skin blanches with pressure; skin may be tender.
- 2nd degree: Skin is red and blistered; skin is very tender.
- 3rd degree: Burned skin is tough and leathery; skin is nontender.
- Rule of 9s
  - Each upper extremity: adult and child 9%
  - Each lower extremity: adult 18%; child 14%
  - Anterior trunk: adult and child 18%
  - Posterior trunk: adult and child 18%
  - Head and neck: adult 10%; child 18%
- Quick estimate: The surface area of the patient's hand (palmar surface plus fingers) is 1% of the body surface area (BSA).
- Careful documentation of extent of burn and the estimated depth of burn
- Check for any signs suggestive of potential airway involvement: singed nasal hair, facial burns, carbonaceous sputum, progressive hoarseness, inflamed oropharynx, circumferential burns around the neck, tachypnea.

DIAGNOSTIC TESTS & INTERPRETATION
- Children: glucose (hypoglycemia may occur in children because of limited glycogen storage)
- Smoke inhalation: arterial blood gas, carboxyhemoglobin
- Electrical burns: ECG, urine myoglobin, creatine kinase isoenzymes

Initial Tests (lab, imaging)
- Labs: hematocrit; type and crossmatching; electrolytes, including BUN and creatinine; urinalysis
- Imaging: chest radiograph; xenon scan is useful in suspected smoke inhalation.

Diagnostic Procedures/Other
Bronchoscopy may be necessary in smoke inhalation to evaluate lower respiratory tract (1)[A].

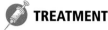

TREATMENT

- Prehospital care
  - Remove the patient from the source of burn.
  - Extinguish and remove all burning clothing.
  - Room-temperature water may be poured onto burn but only in the first 15 minutes following burn exposure.
  - Wrap patient to prevent hypothermia.
  - All patients to receive 100% oxygen via face mask
- Hospitalization for all serious burns
  - 2nd-degree burns >10% of BSA
  - Any 3rd-degree burn
  - Burns of hands, feet, face, or perineum
  - Electrical or lightning burns
  - Inhalation injury
  - Chemical burns
  - Circumferential burn
- Transfer to burn center for (2)[C]
  - 2nd- and 3rd-degree burns >10% of BSA in patients <10 years and >50 years of age
  - 2nd-degree burns >20% of BSA and full-thickness burns >5% BSA in any age range
  - 3rd-degree burns in any age group
  - Burns of hands, feet, face, or perineum
  - Electrical or lightning burns
  - Inhalation injury
  - Chemical burns
  - Circumferential burn
  - Burns in patients with additional trauma (fractures, etc.) in which the burn is the more severe injury; otherwise, send to trauma center for stabilization
  - Burn injuries in patients with preexisting medical conditions that could affect management, mortality, or recovery

GENERAL MEASURES
- Based on depth of burns and accurate estimate of total BSA involved (rule of 9s)
- Tetanus prophylaxis (if not current)
- Remove all rings, watches, and other items from injured extremities to avoid tourniquet effect.
- Remove clothing and cover all burned areas with dry sheets.
- Flush area of chemical burn (for ~2 hours).
- For all major burns, use 100% oxygen administration; consider early intubation.
- Do not apply ice to burn site.
- Nasogastric tube (high risk of paralytic ileus)
- Foley catheter
- Analgesia
- ECG monitoring in first 24 hours following electrical burn

- Whirlpool hydrotherapy followed by silver sulfadiazine (Silvadene) occlusive dressings in severe burns
- Daily or BID cleansing with dressing changes
- Burn fluid resuscitation
  - Calculate fluid resuscitation from time of burn, not from time treatment begins.
  - 2 to 4 mL lactated Ringer × body weight (kg) × % BSA burn (1/2 given in first 8 hours, in second 8 hours, and in third 8 hours); in children, this is given in addition to maintenance fluids and is adjusted according to urine output and vital signs. Protocol-based resuscitation leads to superior outcomes.
  - Colloid solutions are not recommended during the first 12 to 24 hours of resuscitation (3)[A].
  - Other: Use of biologic membranes or skin substitutes may be indicated for burn coverage.
- Inhalation injury
  - Intubation, ventilation with positive end-expiratory pressure assistance. Employ lung protective ventilation strategies.
  - Hyperbaric oxygen treatment may be useful in patients with carbon monoxide levels >25%; patients with coma, focal neurologic deficit, ischemic ECG changes; and pregnant patients.
  - Prophylactic antibiotics and steroids are not indicated (4)[C].

MEDICATION

First Line
- IV morphine or hydromorphone (Dilaudid) for severe pain
- Oral analgesics, such as acetaminophen (Tylenol) with codeine, acetaminophen with oxycodone (Percocet), or acetaminophen with hydrocodone (Lortab) for moderate pain
- Silver sulfadiazine (Silvadene): Apply topically to burn site (can cause leukopenia). Do not use in sulfa-allergic patients, women who are pregnant/ breastfeeding, or infants (<2 months).
- Neosporin or bacitracin ointment: Apply to facial burns.
- Mupirocin: has potent inhibitory activity against methicillin-resistant *Staphylococcus aureus* (MRSA)
- Acticoat A.B. (a dressing consisting of two sheets of high-density polyethylene mesh coated with nano-crystalline silver) has a more controlled, prolonged release of silver, allowing less frequent dressing changes.
- Electrical burn with myoglobinuria will require alkalinization of urine and mannitol.
- Consider H_2 blockers (e.g., famotidine) or proton pump inhibitors (e.g., lansoprazole, pantoprazole) for stress ulcer prophylaxis in severely burned patients.
- Tetanus toxoid/tetanus immunoglobulin
- There is no clear indication for prophylactic systemic antibiotics.
- Use of negative pressure wound therapy may result in a low-protease environment with higher levels of angiogenic factor (vascular endothelial growth factor [VEGF]) during wound healing, leading to more chaotic, hyperkeratinized, thickened epidermis when compared with a standard hydrocolloid dressing.

Second Line
- Mafenide (Sulfamylon) for full-thickness burn, best against *Pseudomonas* (*caution*: metabolic acidosis, painful)
- Silver nitrate 0.5% (messy, leeches electrolytes from burn, causes water toxicity)

- Povidone-iodine (Betadine) may result in iodine absorption from burn and "tan eschar," makes débridement more difficult.
- Travase (enzymatic débridement)

SURGERY/OTHER PROCEDURES
- Escharotomy may be necessary in constricting circumferential burns of extremities or chest due to compartment syndrome.
- Tangential excision with split-thickness skin grafts: Early excision of burns results in a significant reduction in mortality (excluding patients with inhalational injury) and a significant decrease in hospital length of stay (5)[B].
- Various dressings (e.g., biosynthetic, biologic) are available to help reduce the number of dressing changes and promote healing.

ONGOING CARE

FOLLOW-UP RECOMMENDATIONS
Early mobilization is the goal.

DIET
- High-protein, high-calorie diet when bowel function resumes
- Nasogastric tube feedings may be required in early postburn period.
- Total parenteral nutrition if NPO is expected for >5 days
- Early initiation of enteral nutrition in the first 24 hours of admission results in shorter intensive care unit (ICU) stay and lower wound infection rates.

PATIENT EDUCATION
- Use of sunscreen: Skin grafts or newly epithelialized skin is highly sensitive to sun exposure and thermal extremes.
- Prevent access to electrical cords/outlets.
- Isolate household chemicals.
- Use low-temperature setting for water heater (<54°C).
- Household smoke detectors with special emphasis on maintenance
- Family/household evacuation plan
- Proper storage and use of flammable substances
- Burn management: http://www.aafp.org/afp/2000/1101/p2029.html
- Burn prevention: http://www.aafp.org/afp/2000/1101/p2032.html

PROGNOSIS
- 1st-degree burn: complete resolution
- 2nd-degree burn: epithelialization in 10 to 14 days (deep 2nd-degree burns probably will require skin graft)
- 3rd-degree burn: no potential for reepithelialization; skin graft is required.
- Baux score (sum of age and TBSA burned) and Denver 2 score (pulmonary score ranging 0 to 3, using PaO_2/FiO_2 cutoffs of 100, 175, and 250), renal score (0 to 3, using creatinine cutoffs of 1.8, 2.5, and 5.0 mg/dL), hepatic score (0 to 3, using bilirubin cutoffs of 2, 4, and 8 mg/dL), and cardiac score (0 to 3, based on number and dosage of inotropes) can be used to estimate mortality (6)[B].
- Length of hospital stay and need for ICU care depend on extent of burn, smoke inhalation, comorbidities, and age.

- Burn size is correlated to complications; >60% TBSA burned in children and >40% in adults are at increased risk for mortality and morbidity (6)[B].
- A 50% survival rate can be expected with a 62% burn in patients aged 0 to 14 years, 63% burn in patients aged 15 to 40 years, 38% burn in patients aged 40 to 65 years, and 25% burn in patients >65 years of age.
- 90% of survivors can be expected to return to an occupation comparable to their preburn employment.

COMPLICATIONS
- Gastroduodenal ulceration (Curling ulcer)
- Marjolin ulcer: malignant squamous cell carcinoma developing in old burn site
- Signs of infection: discoloration, green fat, edema, eschar separation, and conversion of 2nd-degree to 3rd-degree wound
- Biopsy is the best way to diagnose wound infection.
- Burn wound sepsis: most commonly *S. aureus* (including MRSA), vancomycin-resistant enterococci, and gram-negative organisms
- Pneumonia
- Decreased mobility with possibility of future flexion contractures
- Hypertrophic scarring common with burns

REFERENCES
1. Dries DJ, Endorf FW. Inhalation injury: epidemiology, pathology, treatment strategies. *Scand J Trauma Resusc Emerg Med*. 2013;21:31.
2. Bezuhly M, Fish JS. Acute burn care. *Plast Reconstr Surg*. 2012;130(2):349e–358e.
3. Perel P, Roberts I, Ker K. Colloids versus crystalloids for fluid resuscitation in critically ill patients. *Cochrane Database Syst Rev*. 2013;(2):CD000567.
4. ISBI Practice Guidelines Committee, Steering Subcommittee, Advisory Subcommittee. ISBI practice guidelines for burn care. *Burns*. 2016;42(5): 953–1021.
5. Ong YS, Samuel M, Song C. Meta-analysis of early excision of burns. *Burns*. 2006;32(2):145–150.
6. Jeschke MG, Pinto R, Kraft R, et al; and Inflammation and the Host Response to Injury Collaborative Research Program. Morbidity and survival probability in burn patients in modern burn care. *Crit Care Med*. 2015;43(4):808–815.

CODES

ICD10
- T30.0 Burn of unspecified body region, unspecified degree
- T30.4 Corrosion of unspecified body region, unspecified degree

CLINICAL PEARLS
- 1st degree: erythema of involved tissue; skin blanches with pressure. Skin may be tender.
- 2nd degree: Skin is red and blistered. Skin is very tender.
- 3rd degree: Burned skin is tough and leathery. Skin is not tender.

BURSITIS, PES ANSERINE (PES ANSERINE SYNDROME)

Jennifer Schwartz, MD

 BASICS

DESCRIPTION

- The pes anserinus ("goosefoot") is the combined insertion of the sartorius, gracilis, and semitendinosus tendons on the anteromedial tibia.
- There is a bursa that lies under the pes anserinus (between the semitendinosus tendon and the tibial attachment of the medical collateral ligament).
- *Pes anserine tendino-bursitis (PATB)* is due to irritation of the bursa and/or tendons in this area.

EPIDEMIOLOGY

Prevalence

One of the most frequent soft tissue pain syndromes in the knee

ETIOLOGY AND PATHOPHYSIOLOGY

PATB is thought to occur due to:

- Overuse injury
- Excessive valgus and rotary stresses
- Mechanical forces and degenerative changes
- Direct trauma

RISK FACTORS

- More common in middle-aged, overweight females
- Other risk factors include:
  - Pes planus; genu valgum
  - Long-distance/hill running, cycling, swimming ("breaststroker's knee")
  - Sports with side-to-side/cutting activity (soccer, basketball, racquet sports)

COMMONLY ASSOCIATED CONDITIONS

- Osteoarthritis (OA)
  - Increased incidence of PATB in patients with symptomatic OA (1)[C]
  - Prevalence of OA and PATB reported as high as 75% (2)[C]
  - Higher grades of OA associated with a thicker pes anserine bursa and larger area of bursitis (3)[C]
- Medial meniscal tear
- Type II diabetes

 DIAGNOSIS

Largely a clinical diagnosis

HISTORY

- Medial knee pain at the pes anserine insertion is the most common complaint.
  - Pain is located 4 to 6 cm below the medial joint line on the anteromedial aspect of the tibia.
- Pain is exacerbated by knee flexion:
  - Going up or down stairs
  - Getting up out of a chair or from a sitting position
  - Sitting cross-legged

PHYSICAL EXAM

- Common findings include:
  - Tenderness to palpation or localized swelling at the pes anserine insertion
    - Caution: 30% of asymptomatic patients will have tenderness to deep palpation in this area. Be sure to examine both sides and correlate physical exam with history.
  - Pain worsens with flexion of the knee against resistance.
- Findings that suggest an alternative diagnosis: joint effusion, tenderness directly over the joint line, locking of the knee, systemic signs such as fever

DIFFERENTIAL DIAGNOSIS

- Medial collateral ligament injury
- Medial meniscal injury
- Medial compartment OA
- Medial plica syndrome
- Tibial stress fracture
- Septic arthritis

DIAGNOSTIC TESTS & INTERPRETATION

Initial Tests (lab, imaging)

- Primarily a clinical diagnosis
- Lab work not indicated
- Imaging is not indicated unless there is concern for underlying bony injury/fracture, ligamentous injury, or meniscal tear.

Follow-Up Tests & Special Considerations

- X-ray
  - Can demonstrate underlying osteoarthritis
- Ultrasound (US)
  - Can demonstrate focal edema within the pes anserine bursa but has poor correlation with clinical findings
  - Many patients with the clinical diagnosis of pes anserine bursitis have no morphologic changes of the pes anserine complex on US.
- MRI: T2-weighted axial images are best to see inflammation of the bursa.
  - No large studies have evaluated the correlation between a clinical diagnosis of pes anserine bursitis and radiographic evidence of pes anserine pathology on MRI.
  - May see fluid in the pes bursa on MRI in 5% of asymptomatic patients

 TREATMENT

Pes anserine bursitis is often self-limited. Conservative therapy is most common:

- Relative rest and activity modification to avoid offending movements (especially knee flexion)
- Ice to the affected area
- NSAIDs for pain control
- Physical therapy (PT) for knee strengthening and treatment of other underlying pathology
- Kinesio taping
  - One study showed Kinesio taping to be more effective than PT + naproxen (Naprosyn) to decrease pain in patients with PATB (4)[C].
- Corticosteroid injection
  - Steroid injections and PT found to be equally as effective for acute pain in PATB (2)[C]. Steroid injections may be preferred in some cases due to the immediate results and risk of low PT compliance.

– When considering steroid injection for symptomatic OA, also consider performing an injection at the pes anserine bursa—PATB pain can affect function in patients with both diagnoses (1)[C].
- Weight loss to improve biomechanical forces at the knee

MEDICATION

First Line
- NSAIDs: i.e., ibuprofen (800 mg PO TID) or naproxen (500 mg PO BID)
- Corticosteroid injection combined with local anesthetic:
  – Inject at the point of maximal tenderness using standard aseptic technique.
  – ∼2 mL of anesthetic (i.e., 1% lidocaine) and 1 mL of steroid (i.e., 40 mg of methylprednisolone) is injected into the bursa using a small (e.g., 25-gauge, 1-inch) needle.
  – Insert needle perpendicular to the skin until bone is felt and then withdraw slightly before injecting.
  – Avoid injecting directly into the tendon.
- US-guided injection is superior to blind injection (5)[C].

Second Line
Platelet-rich plasma injections can also provide pain relief (6)[C].

ADDITIONAL THERAPIES
- Hamstring and Achilles stretching
- Quadriceps and adductor strengthening
- Extra corporeal shock wave therapy (ESWT) can decrease pain in PATB (7)[C].

SURGERY/OTHER PROCEDURES
- No role for surgery in routine isolated cases
- Drainage or removal of bursa may be used in severe/refractory cases.

 ONGOING CARE

Home exercise program focusing on flexibility and strengthening

DIET
Consider dietary changes as part of a comprehensive weight-loss program if obesity is a contributing factor.

PROGNOSIS
Most cases of pes anserine syndrome respond to conservative therapy. Recurrence is common, and multiple treatments may be required.

REFERENCES

1. Glenn SH, Daniel CH. Pay attention to the pes anserine in knee osteoarthritis. *Current Sports Medicine Reports*. 2018;17(2):41.
2. Sarifakioglu B, Afsar SI, Yalbuzdag SA, et al. Comparison of the efficacy of physical therapy and corticosteroid injection in the treatment of pes anserine tendino-bursitis. *J Phys Ther Sci*. 2016;28(7):1993–1997.
3. Uysal F, Akbal A, Gökmen F, et al. Prevalence of pes anserine bursitis in symptomatic osteoarthritis patients: an ultrasonographic prospective study. *Clin Rheumatol*. 2015;34(3):529–533.
4. Homayouni K, Foruzi S, Kolhori F. Effect of kinesiotaping versus non-steroidal anti-inflammatory drugs and physical therapy for treatment of pes anserinus tendino-bursitis: a randomized comparative clinical trial. *Phys Sportsmed*. 2016;44(3):252–256.
5. Finnoff JT, Nutz DJ, Henning PT, et al. Accuracy of ultrasound-guided versus unguided pes anserinus bursa injections. *PM R*. 2010;2(8):732–739.
6. Rowicki K, Płomiński J, Bachta A. Evaluation of the effectiveness of platelet rich plasma in treatment of chronic pes anserinus pain syndrome. *Ortop Traumatol Rehabil*. 2014;16(3):307–318.
7. Khosrawi S, Taneri P, Ketabi M. Investigating the effect of extracorporeal shock wave therapy on reducing chronic pain in patients with pes anserine bursitis: a randomized, clinical-controlled trial. *Adv Biomed Res*. 2017;6:70.

ADDITIONAL READING

- Alvarez-Nemegyei J. Risk factors for pes anserinus tendinitis/bursitis syndrome: a case control study. *J Clin Rheumatol*. 2007;13(2):63–65.
- Chatra PS. Bursae around the knee joints. *Indian J Radiol Imaging*. 2012;22(1):27–30.
- Mohseni M, Graham C. Pes anserine bursitis. In: StatPearls [Internet]. Treasure Island, FL: StatPearls Publishing; 2019. https://pubmed.ncbi.nlm.nih.gov/30422536/. Accessed October 4, 2021.
- Rennie WJ, Saifuddin A. Pes anserine bursitis: incidence in symptomatic knees and clinical presentation. *Skeletal Radiol*. 2005;34(7):395–398.
- Wittich CM, Ficalora RD, Mason TG, et al. Musculoskeletal injection. *Mayo Clin Proc*. 2009;84(9):831–836; quiz 837.

 CODES

ICD10
M70.50 Other bursitis of knee, unspecified knee

CLINICAL PEARLS
- Consider pes anserine syndrome in patients presenting with medial knee pain.
- Pes anserine syndrome is relatively common in athletes and in older, obese patients with OA.
- Tenderness over the insertion of the pes anserine tendon on the medial aspect of the tibia 4 to 6 cm distal to the joint line is common in asymptomatic patients as well—correlation of the entire clinical picture is necessary for accurate diagnosis.
- Consider pes anserine syndrome in patients who have persistent symptoms associated with medial-sided OA.
- Treatment is typically conservative. A local steroid/anesthetic injection may provide pain relief and enhance rehabilitation.

CANDIDIASIS, MUCOCUTANEOUS

Karlynn Sievers, MD • Tonya M. Cook, PharmD

BASICS

DESCRIPTION
- Heterogeneous group of mucocutaneous infections with commensal *Candida* species
- Characterized by superficial infection of the skin, mucous membranes, and nails
- >20 *Candida* species cause infection in humans. *Candida albicans* is responsible for 70% of fungal infections worldwide.
  - *Candida auris* is an emerging global pathogen with a high propensity to develop drug resistance (1).
- Candidiasis affects:
  - Aerodigestive system
    - Oropharyngeal candidiasis (thrush): mouth, pharynx
    - Angular cheilitis: corner of the mouth
    - Esophageal candidiasis
    - Gastritis and/or ulcers, associated with thrush; alimental or perianal
  - Other systems
    - Candida vulvovaginitis: vaginal mucosa and/or vulvar skin
    - Candidal balanitis: glans of the penis
    - Candidal paronychia: nail bed or nail folds
    - Folliculitis
    - Interdigital candidiasis: webs of the digits
    - Candidal diaper dermatitis and intertrigo (within skin folds)
- Synonym(s): monilia; thrush; yeast; intertrigo

ALERT
Vaginal antifungal creams and suppositories can weaken condoms and diaphragms.

Pregnancy Considerations
- Vaginal candidiasis is common during pregnancy—extend treatment (typically a full 7-day course).
- Vaginal yeast infection at birth increases the risk of newborn thrush but is of no overall harm to baby.

EPIDEMIOLOGY
- Common in the United States; particularly with immunodeficiency and/or uncontrolled diabetes
- Age considerations
  - Infants and seniors: thrush and cutaneous infections (infant diaper rash)
  - Women (prepubertal through postmenopausal): yeast vaginitis

Incidence
Unknown—mucocutaneous candidiasis is common in immunocompetent patients. Complication rates are low.

Prevalence
Candida species are normal flora of oral cavity and GI tract that are present in >70% of the U.S. population.

ETIOLOGY AND PATHOPHYSIOLOGY
C. albicans (responsible for 80–92% vulvovaginal and >80% of oral isolates). Altered cell–mediated immunity against *Candida* species (either transient or chronic) increases susceptibility to infection.

Genetics
Chronic mucocutaneous candidiasis is a heterogeneous, genetic syndrome that typically presents in infancy.

RISK FACTORS
- Immune suppression (antineoplastic treatments, transplant patients, cellular immune defects, HIV/AIDS)
- Malignant diseases
- Corticosteroid use
- Smoking and alcoholism
- Hyposalivation (Sjögren disease, drug-induced xerostomia, radiotherapy) (2)
- Broad-spectrum antibiotic therapy
- Douches, chemical irritants, birth control pills, intrauterine devices, and concurrent vaginitides
- Denture wear, poor oral hygiene (2)
- Endocrine alterations (diabetes mellitus, pregnancy, renal failure, hypothyroidism)
- Uncircumcised men at higher risk for balanitis

GENERAL PREVENTION
- Use antibiotics and steroids judiciously; rinse mouth after using inhaled steroids.
- Avoid douching.
- Minimize perineal moisture (wear cotton underwear; frequent diaper changes).
- Clean dentures often; use well-fitting dentures and remove during sleep.
- Optimize glycemic control in diabetics.
- Preventive regimens during cancer treatments, especially in patients with hematologic malignancies
- Treat with HAART in HIV-infected patients; antifungal prophylaxis not recommended unless HIV-infected adults have frequent or severe recurrences

COMMONLY ASSOCIATED CONDITIONS
- HIV
- Diabetes mellitus
- Cancer and other immunosuppressive conditions that cause leukopenia

DIAGNOSIS

HISTORY
- Infants/children
  - Oral: adherent white patches on oral mucosae or on the tongue that do not wipe away easily
  - Perineal: erythematous rash with characteristic satellite lesions; painful if skin layer eroded
  - Angular cheilitis: painful fissures at mouth corners
- Adults
  - Vulvovaginal lesions; whitish "curd-like" discharge; pruritus; burning
  - Balanitis: erythema, erosions, scaling; dysuria
- Immunocompromised hosts
  - Oral: white, raised, painless, distinct patches; red, slightly raised patches/petechiae
  - Esophagitis: dysphagia, odynophagia, retrosternal pain; usually concomitant thrush
  - GI symptoms: abdominal pain
  - Folliculitis: follicular pustules

PHYSICAL EXAM
- Infants/children
  - Oral: white, raised, distinct patches within the mouth; when wiped off, reveals red base
  - Perineal: erythematous maculopapular rash with satellite pustules or papules
  - Angular cheilitis: tender fissures in mouth corners, often cracked and bleeding
- Adults
  - Vulvovaginal: thick, whitish, cottage cheese–like discharge; vagina or perineum erythema
  - Balanitis: erythema, linear erosions, scaling
  - Interdigital: redness, excoriation at base and web spaces of fingers and/or toes, possible maceration
- Immunocompromised hosts
  - Oral: white, raised, nontender, distinct patches; red, slightly raised patches; thick, dark-brownish coating; deep fissures (2)
  - Esophagitis: Often, oral thrush is visible.
  - Folliculitis: follicular pustules

DIFFERENTIAL DIAGNOSIS
- For oral candidiasis, consider leukoplakia; lichen planus; geographic tongue; herpes simplex; erythema multiforme; pemphigus, burning mouth syndrome
- Baby formula or breast milk can mimic thrush—easier to remove than thrush.
- Hairy leukoplakia: does not rub off; dorsum and lateral margins of tongue
- Angular cheilitis from vitamin B or iron deficiency, staphylococcal infection, or edentulous overclosure
- Bacterial vaginosis and *Trichomonas vaginalis* tend to have more odor, itch, and a different discharge.

DIAGNOSTIC TESTS & INTERPRETATION
Initial Tests (lab, imaging)
- 10% KOH slide preparation: mycelia (hyphae) or pseudomycelia (pseudohyphae) yeast forms
- Associated with normal vaginal pH (<4.5)

Diagnostic Procedures/Other
- If first-line treatment fails, obtain samples for culture.
- Esophagitis or hyperplastic candidiasis may require endoscopy with biopsy (if suspicious for cancer).

Test Interpretation
Biopsy: epithelial parakeratosis with polymorphonuclear leukocytes in superficial layers; periodic acid–Schiff staining reveals candidal hyphae.

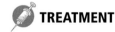

TREATMENT

GENERAL MEASURES
Screen for immunodeficiency (diabetes, HIV, autoimmune disease).

MEDICATION

First Line

- Vaginal (choose 1)
  - Miconazole (Monistat) 2% cream: one applicator or 200 mg (one suppository), intravaginally QHS for 7 days
  - Clotrimazole (Gyne-Lotrimin, Mycelex): intravaginal suppository (100 mg QHS for 7 days; 200 mg QHS for 3 days; 500 mg daily for 1 day) or 2% cream (one applicator QHS for 3 days)
  - Fluconazole 150 mg PO single dose
- Oropharyngeal
  - Mild disease
    ○ Clotrimazole (Mycelex): oral 10-mg troche; 20 minutes 5 times daily for 7 to 14 days
    ○ Nystatin suspension: 100,000 U/mL swish and swallow 400,000 to 600,000 U QID
    ○ Nystatin pastilles: 200,000 U each, QID daily for 7 to 14 days (3)
    ○ Denture wearers
      ■ Nystatin ointment: 100,000 U/g under denture and corners of mouth for 3 weeks
  - Moderate to severe disease
    ○ Fluconazole: 200 mg load and then 100 to 200 mg (>14 days of age: 6 mg/kg × 1 dose and then 3 mg/kg q24h × 7 to 14 days [max 100 mg/day])
- Esophagitis
  - Fluconazole: PO 400 mg load and then 200 to 400 mg/day for 14 to 21 days or IV 400 mg (6 mg/kg) daily
  - Alternative options are available if fluconazole is not tolerated; systemic antifungal therapy is always required (4).

Pregnancy Considerations

2% miconazole cream, intravaginally, for 7 days in uncomplicated candidiasis; systemic amphotericin B for invasive candidiasis

Second Line

- Vaginal
  - Topical antifungals, with no one preferred agent recommended (4)
  - Alternatively, fluconazole 150 mg in a single dose (4)
  - For recurrent cases (≥4 symptomatic episodes in 1 year): induction therapy with 10 to 14 days of topical or oral azole and then fluconazole 150 mg once per week for 6 months (4)
    ○ In HIV patients: Concerns with this regimen include emergence of drug resistance (5)[A].
- Oropharyngeal
  - Miconazole oral gel (20 mg/mL): QID, swish and swallow.
  - Itraconazole (Sporanox) suspension: 200 mg (20 mL) daily; swish and swallow for 7 to 14 days.
  - Posaconazole (Noxafil) oral suspension: 400 mg BID for 3 days and then 400 mg daily for up to 28 days
  - Amphotericin B (Fungizone) oral suspension (100 mg/mL): 1 mL QID daily, swish and swallow; use between meals.

- Esophagitis
  - Amphotericin B (variable dosing) IV dose of 0.3 to 0.7 mg/kg daily or an echinocandin should be used for patients who cannot tolerate oral therapy.
  - For refractory disease:
    ○ Could consider amphotericin B, itraconazole, posaconazole, voriconazole, isavuconazole (3)
    ○ Echinocandins (may be first choice in severe disease in patients with immunodeficiency) (3)
    ○ Several new agents are under investigation (3).
- Continue treatments for 2 days after infection gone:
  - Contraindications
    ○ Ketoconazole, itraconazole, or nystatin (if swallowed): severe hepatotoxicity
    ○ Amphotericin B: can cause nephrotoxicity
  - Precautions
    ○ Miconazole: can potentiate the effect of warfarin but drug of choice in pregnancy
    ○ Fluconazole: renal excretion; rare, hepatotoxicity; resistance frequent
    ○ Posaconazole: can cause GI discomfort or QT prolongation (3)
    ○ Voriconazole: transient visual disturbances; clinical hepatitis, cholestasis, and fulminant liver failure (rare) (3)
- Possible interactions (rarely seen with topical treatment)
  - Fluconazole
    ○ Rifampin and tolbutamide: decreased fluconazole concentrations
    ○ Warfarin, phenytoin, cyclosporine: altered metabolism; check levels.
  - Itraconazole: potent CYP3A4 inhibitor. Carefully assess all coadministered medications.

ISSUES FOR REFERRAL

- Evaluate patients with recurrent superficial candidal infections for immunodeficiency (5)[A].
- GI candidiasis

ADDITIONAL THERAPIES

- For infants with thrush: Boil pacifiers and bottle nipples; assess mother's breasts/nipples for *Candida* infection.
- For denture-related candidiasis: Remove dentures at night. Disinfect dentures (using soak solution of white vinegar, 2% chlorhexidine gluconate solution, or 0.1% hypochlorite solution) and treat orally (2).

COMPLEMENTARY & ALTERNATIVE MEDICINE

Probiotics: *Lactobacillus* and *Bifidobacterium* may inhibit *Candida* spp.

ADMISSION, INPATIENT, AND NURSING CONSIDERATIONS

Proper oral hygiene. Protocols for brushing, denture care, and oral cavity moistening reduce oral candidiasis.

 ONGOING CARE

FOLLOW-UP RECOMMENDATIONS

Patient Monitoring

Immunocompromised persons benefit from regular evaluation and screening.

DIET

Active culture yogurt or other live lactobacillus may decrease colonization; indeterminate evidence

PATIENT EDUCATION

- Advise patients at risk for recurrence about potential for overgrowth with antibacterial therapy.
- Oral "azole" medications should be avoided in the first trimester. Thereafter, only give orally when benefits outweigh risks.

PROGNOSIS

Benign prognosis in immunocompetent patients; may have significant morbidity in immunosuppressed persons

COMPLICATIONS

In HIV patients, moderate immunosuppression (e.g., CD4 200 to 500 cells/mm^3) may be associated with chronic candidiasis (5)[A]. With more severe immunosuppression (e.g., CD4 <100 cells/mm^3), esophagitis or systemic fungal infections are possible.

REFERENCES

1. Hendrickson JA, Hu C, Aitken SL, et al. Antifungal resistance: a concerning trend for the present and future. *Curr Infect Dis Resp.* 2019;21(12):47.
2. Millsop J, Fazel N. Oral candidiasis. *Clin Dermatol.* 2016;34(4):487–494.
3. Quindós G, Gil-Alonso S, Marcos-Arias C, et al. Therapeutic tools for oral candidiasis: current and new antifungal drugs. *Med Oral Patol Oral Cir Bucal.* 2019;24(2):e172–e180.
4. Pappas P, Kauffman C, Andes D, et al. Clinical practice guideline for the management of candidiasis: 2016 update by the Infectious Diseases Society of America. *Clin Infect Dis.* 2016;62(4):e1–e50.
5. Wang X, van de Veerdonk FL, Netea MG. Basic genetics and immunology of *Candida* infections. *Infect Dis Clin North Am.* 2016;30(1):85–102.

ADDITIONAL READING

Nambiar M, Varma SR, Jaber M, et al. Mycotic infections—mucormycosis and oral candidiasis associated with Covid-19: a significant and challenging association. *J Oral Microbiol.* 2021;13(1):1967699.

 SEE ALSO

Candidiasis, Invasive; HIV/AIDS

CODES

ICD10

- B37.9 Candidiasis, unspecified
- B37.2 Candidiasis of skin and nail
- B37.89 Other sites of candidiasis

CLINICAL PEARLS

- Candidiasis is typically a clinical diagnosis. KOH preparations are a simple confirmatory office test. Culture and biopsy are rarely needed.
- Person-to-person transmission is rare.
- Obtain a biopsy if there is concern for oral cancer.
- Oral antifungal medications are hepatically metabolized and may have serious side effects.

CAPACITY (COMPETENCE) DETERMINATION AND INFORMED CONSENT

Jon S. Parham, DO, MPH, FAAFP • Sandra N. New, DNP

BASICS

- Personal autonomy in decision-making is a fundamental personal freedom.
- Capacity determination is an inherent element of the informed consent process.
- It is universally presumed that patients ≥18 years (or an emancipated minor under individual state laws) have legal and clinical capacity to give informed consent for health care testing, interventions, and treatment or to refuse same no matter the harm or benefit until proven otherwise.

DESCRIPTION

- Capacity:
  - Involves a clinical evaluation by an authorized health care provider
  - Focuses on perceived ability of patient to participate with understanding in the process of informed consent
- Competence:
  - A legal determination of abilities, performed by a court judge
  - Involves medical information but not limited to medical issues
- Capacity is the currently preferred term to competence: legal and medical capacity.
- A capacity determination is needed when arriving at a health care decision for testing, treatment or an intervention involving risk of harm or no improvement.
  - Any treating health care provider can evaluate capacity, including the provider also obtaining informed consent (although a psychiatrist or neuropsychiatric consultant is often asked to weigh in, other health care providers can determine capacity).
- Medical capacity is determined by:
  - Clinical observation and response to questions
  - Capacity assessment tool(s)
  - Cognitive assessment tool(s)
  - Interviews with a guardian or designated health care power of attorney (if indicated)

- The four "C"s of capacity are:
  - Context: comprehension of their health status
  - Choices: able to describe options
  - Consequences: able to explain possible outcomes
  - Consistency: continuity of choice selection
- Adequate cognition is a fundamental component but not the sole determinant of capacity (1).

EPIDEMIOLOGY

Most U.S. adults do not have an advanced directive—population studies show approximately 1/3 have completed an advanced directive (2).

Incidence

Need for capacity determination has been increased due to:

- Increasing patient longevity
- Prolonged chronic disease states
- Better patient rehabilitation opportunities
- Safer anesthetics and advanced postsurgery care

Prevalence

Prevalence varies based on the patient risk factors (pretest probability) and physician experience:

- ~3% of healthy outpatient seniors lack capacity (3).
- Highest rate of incapacity (68%) is in learning disabled patients.

ETIOLOGY AND PATHOPHYSIOLOGY

- Dementia is the most likely cause for individuals to be found incapable of making health care decisions in the outpatient setting.
- Capacity is a dynamic state; reassessment is necessary with each significant health care decision and informed consent.

RISK FACTORS

- For incapacity:
  - Longevity, multiple comorbidities, hospitalized for medical reasons
  - Never married, never worked outside home
- Insufficient informed consent:
  - Patient factors:
    - Health illiteracy
    - Excessive information
  - Provider factors:
    - Inexperience with process (e.g., house staff)
    - Insufficient discussion time

GENERAL PREVENTION

Early assessment and periodic reassessment of capacity in:

- Dynamic patient conditions, like electrolyte imbalance, closed head injuries, delirium states
- After procedures with anesthesia or analgesics
- Enhancement and dissipation of mind altering substances

COMMONLY ASSOCIATED CONDITIONS

- Dementia/Alzheimer disease, Parkinson disease, and traumatic brain injury
- Schizophrenia, depression, and substance abuse
- Acute illness, metabolic derangement

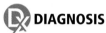

DIAGNOSIS

In patients without capacity, physicians are unable or unwilling to recognize the incapacity 42% of the cases (1)[C].

HISTORY

Family or frequent observers are resources regarding behavior patterns and reasoning displayed by patients.

- Engage in a deliberate approach, initially assessing for:
  - Communication barriers: physical impairments, lack of language fluency, medical jargon
  - Reversible causes of incapacity: metabolic derangements, medication side effects, serious illness, delirium
  - Health belief system; cultural differences; religious, political viewpoints, or adverse historical events

PHYSICAL EXAM

Verbal patient responses, facial expression, and body language often confirm capacity or suggest "warning signs" to obtain more formal evaluation.

DIAGNOSTIC TESTS & INTERPRETATION

Initial Tests (lab, imaging)

Screening for capacity occurs with:

- Informal patient conversations
- Discussions inherent to medical history taking
- Informed consent discussions

Follow-Up Tests & Special Considerations

- Four common tools for the formal evaluation of capacity
  - MacArthur Competence Assessment Tool for Treatment (MacCAT-T)—gold standard
    - Assesses: understanding, reasoning, appreciation, expression of choice
    - Semi-structured interview, 20 minutes
  - Aid to Capacity Evaluation (ACE)
    - Semi-structured interview, 7 questions
    - Found predictive for medical and psychiatric patients, except for schizophrenic patients (4)[A]
  - Assessment of Capacity for Everyday Decision-Making (ACED)
    - Semi-structured interview
    - Used with cognitively impaired seniors to measure capacity to perform independent activities of daily living
  - Capacity Assessment Tool (CAT)
    - Structured interview
    - Assesses capacity to discern between two intervention choices
- Special situation/considerations for assessment of capacity for informed consent
  - Communication impairments
    - Translators of all languages, including for deaf/mute and blind combined with deafness
    - Health literacy level accommodation
  - Patient participation in research or experimental intervention protocols
  - Patient refusal to participate in informed consent
  - Child or adolescent as patient

Diagnostic Procedures/Other

Cognitive screening (e.g., Mini-Mental State Examination) can contribute to (but not substitute for) capacity determination.

Test Interpretation

Capacity definition is state specific. Capacity determination in the informed consent process is determined by the treating provider (1)[C].

TREATMENT

GENERAL MEASURES

Steps to take if a patient fails to have capacity or fails to display ability to participate in informed consent:

- Determine the acuity of the need for decision-making: (e.g., decisions regarding emergency care—"loss of life or limb"—are made by treating provider).
- Correct any reversible causes of impaired capacity (e.g., electrolyte rebalance or language translation).

- Reframe questions that help determine capacity or simplify explanation in informed consent.
- Seek out next of kin to become a proxy decision maker with understanding of patient's values.
- Court appointed guardian process is lengthy and usually is not necessary.

ISSUES FOR REFERRAL

Specialist consultation is not usually necessary to determine capacity for medical decision-making. As indicated, consider consulting with the following expert services:

- Psychiatry; neuropsychiatry; medical ethics; health care attorney

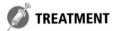 ## ONGOING CARE

The following in rank order have responsibility for medical decision-making/informed consent if patient lacks capacity:

- Spouse (unless legally separated)
- Adult child
- A parent
- An adult sibling
- An adult who has provided unique care and has a special knowledge of the patient values and is accessible (5)[C]

FOLLOW-UP RECOMMENDATIONS

Reassessment of patients is a provider responsibility:

- At each significant medical decision point
- If the patient shows signs of change in capacity

REFERENCES

1. Barstow C, Shahan B, Roberts M. Evaluating medical decision-making capacity in practice. *Am Fam Physician*. 2018;98(1):40–46.
2. Yadav KN, Gabler NB, Cooney E, et al. Approximately one in three US adults completes any type of advanced directive for end-of-life care. *Health Aff (Millwood)*. 2017;36(7):1244–1251.
3. Sessums LL, Zembrzuska H, Jackson JL. Does this patient have medical decision-making capacity? *JAMA*. 2011;306(4):420–427.
4. Downey LVA, Zun L. Who has the ability to consent? *Prim Care Companion CNS Disord*. 2020;22(4):20m02619.
5. Weiss BD, Berman EA, Howe CL, et al. Medical decision-making for older adults without family. *J Am Geriatr Soc*. 2012;60(11):2144–2150.

ADDITIONAL READING

- Baón-Pérez BS, Álvarez-Marrodán I, Navío-Acosta M, et al. Spanish validation of the MacArthur Competence Assessment Tool for clinical research interview for assessing patients' mental capacity to consent to clinical research. *J Empir Res Hum Res Ethics*. 2017;12(5):343–351.
- Klein CC, Jolson MB, Lazarus M, et al. Capacity to provide informed consent among adults with bipolar disorder. *J Affect Disord*. 2019;242:1–4.
- Mandarelli G, Sabatello U, Lapponi E, et al. Treatment decision-making capacity in children and adolescents hospitalized for an acute mental disorder: the role of cognitive functioning and psychiatric symptoms. *J Child Adolesc Psychopharmacol*. 2017;27(5):462–465.

CLINICAL PEARLS

- Use a structured approach to assessing decision-making capacity, including an assessment of language barriers, identification and remediation of reversible causes of incapacity and a comprehensive interview to assess the ability to consent. Include appropriate formal assessment tools.
- Capacity is dynamic. Reassess at new (or changing) significant health care decision/informed consent points.
- The order of succession for decision-making is: spouse, adult child, parent, adult sibling, adult with close relationship.
- Integrate formal assessment with individual patient context to determine capacity.

C

CARBON MONOXIDE POISONING

Beshoy Sidhom, MD • Sandra S. Augusto, MD, MPH

 BASICS

DESCRIPTION

- Carbon monoxide (CO) is an odorless, tasteless, colorless gas produced during the incomplete combustion of carbon-based compounds. If inhaled, CO may cause nonspecific symptoms and is potentially fatal.
  - CO inhalation leads to displacement of oxygen from binding sites on hemoglobin to form carboxyhemoglobin (COHb).
  - The formation of COHb leads to tissue hypoxia from decreased oxygen carrying capacity and a left shift of the oxyhemoglobin dissociation curve.
  - CO binds to mitochondrial cytochrome oxidase, impairing adenosine triphosphate (ATP) production. It also binds to myoglobin, affecting muscle function.
- System(s) affected: cardiovascular, pulmonary, musculoskeletal, nervous

Pregnancy Considerations
Tissue hypoxia due to CO poisoning may cause significant fetal abnormalities because CO has a stronger affinity and a longer half-life when bound to fetal hemoglobin. The fetus is therefore susceptible to adverse outcomes even if the mother is unaffected.

EPIDEMIOLOGY

Incidence
- CO poisoning is the third leading cause of poisoning death in the United States.
- Accounts for 50,000 ER visits annually (16 cases per 100,000 population); 1–3% are fatal.
- Approximately 15,000 intentional poisoning occur per year, accounting for 2/3 reported deaths (10-fold higher than unintentional poisonings).
- Results in approximately 1,200 to 1,600 deaths a year in the United States due to fire- and non–fire-related poisoning.
- Vague symptoms may cause patients to not seek care, leading to underdiagnosis.

Prevalence
- More prevalent during the winter months in areas with colder climate
- Occupational exposure to methylene chloride, an industrial solvent that is a component of paint remover, can also lead to CO poisoning.

ETIOLOGY AND PATHOPHYSIOLOGY

- CO is rapidly absorbed through the lungs, binding hemoglobin with 210 to 240 times the affinity of oxygen. This stabilizes hemoglobin in the relaxed high affinity state (R state), reducing oxygen-carrying capacity and delivery, leading to left shift of the oxyhemoglobin dissociation curve.
- CO inactivates cytochrome oxidase. This leads to decreased ATP production, especially in tissues with high metabolic demands (brain, heart). The electron transport chain continues, generating superoxide radicals, leading to further damage.
- Increased peroxynitrite production contributes to impaired mitochondrial function and hypoxia.
- CO displaces NO from platelets, leading to platelet activation and aggregation. Oxidative stress, lipid peroxidation, and apoptosis are additional effects.
- Mitochondrial dysfunction and hypoxia leads to myocardial stunning and injury.
- Proteases released from neutrophil degranulation interact with xanthine hydrogenase forming xanthine oxidase. This inhibits endogenous defense against oxidative stress.

- Brain hypoxia leads to excitatory amino acid production and increased nitrite levels, resulting in further ischemia.
- CO also initiates an inflammatory cascade that can lead to oxidative degradation of nervous system lipids and delayed neurologic damage.
- CO also promotes the release of NO which can lead to profound hypotension.

RISK FACTORS
- Alcohol and tobacco use
- Patients with severe COPD regardless of current tobacco smoke exposure
- Closed or improperly ventilated spaces
- Fires and fire-related injuries
- High-risk vocations: coal miners, auto mechanics, paint stripping, work in the solvent industry
- Exposure to exhaust from motor vehicles, faulty furnaces, stoves, generator use (power outages and storms), and other fuel burning devices
- If exposed, infants, elderly patients, and patients with comorbid conditions such as cardiovascular disease, anemia, and chronic respiratory conditions have increased risk for poor outcomes.
- Increased endogenous CO production occurs in patients with hemolytic anemia.

GENERAL PREVENTION
- Appropriate ventilation around fuel-burning devices
- Installation of in-home CO monitors or alarms
- Postexposure determination of CO source to limit future exposures, eliminate source, and initiate treatment
- Public policy to ensure building code safety
- Limiting occupational exposures for those who work with automobiles, paint, solvents, or mines

COMMONLY ASSOCIATED CONDITIONS
- CO and cyanide poisoning often occur simultaneously after smoke inhalation and have synergistic effects.
- Intentional poisoning often occurs in the context of coingestion of other substances (~40%).
- Up to 50–75% of fire-related injuries have a component of CO poisoning.

DIAGNOSIS

- Clinical triad of (i) relevant symptoms, (ii) history of CO exposure, (iii) and elevated COHb levels (1)
- An elevated COHb level of >3% in a nonsmoker and >10% in smokers confirms exposure. The COHb level does not correlate with the severity of the illness or long-term prognosis but is necessary for the diagnosis (1),(2),(3),(4).
- Older pulse oximeters do not differentiate COHb from oxyhemoglobin, with normal oximeter readings in a hypoxic patient (3). Eight-wavelength CO oximeters can detect CO exposure but cannot reliably make a definitive diagnosis of CO poisoning (1),(2).

HISTORY
- The diagnosis of CO poisoning is dependent on duration and mechanism of exposure. No single symptom is sensitive or specific. A high index of suspicion is necessary.
- Common symptoms include the following:
  - Headache (84% of patients)
  - Confusions/impaired judgment
  - Dizziness
  - Nausea/vomiting
  - Fatigue
  - Chest pain and shortness of breath

- Patients may also present with visual disturbances, seizures, syncope, arrhythmias, and loss of consciousness.
- Some patients may present with cardiopulmonary symptoms such as chest pain, palpitations, or shortness of breath.
- Long-term (subacute) exposure is defined as >24 hours and occurs with repeated exposure to low concentrations of CO. Symptoms include chronic fatigue, emotional distress, memory deficits, difficulty working, sleep disturbances, vertigo, neuropathy, recurrent infections, polycythemia, paresthesia, abdominal pain, and diarrhea.
- Exclude pregnancy in all female patients.

PHYSICAL EXAM
- Pulse oximetry does not distinguish between oxygenated hemoglobin, deoxygenated hemoglobin, COHb, and methemoglobin. Therefore, patients exposed to CO must have COHb levels measured with a co-oximeter (blood gas analysis).
- Findings vary. Patients often report confusion or have altered mental status.
- Classically described "cherry red" skin coloring of lips and skin is rare (<1% of cases)
- Examine for signs of burns of the skin and oropharynx (enclosed space fires) or other secondary injuries.
- Full neurologic and mental status examinations; confusion/CNS depression, ataxia, visual field defects, papilledema, and nystagmus
- Respiratory depression or tachypnea, and cyanosis
- Tachycardia, hypotension, cardiac dysrhythmias
- As noted above, pulse oximetry is often misleading.

DIFFERENTIAL DIAGNOSIS
- Cyanide toxicity (also co-existent)
- Methylene chloride (dichloromethane) inhalation or ingestion
- Viral syndromes
- Behavioral disorders (major depressive disorder)
- Infections (meningitis or encephalitis)
- Metabolic causes (hypoglycemia, electrolyte impairment)
- Alcohol intoxication, opiates, acetylsalicylic acid (ASA) overdose
- Trauma
- CNS lesions
- Coingestion of other substance

DIAGNOSTIC TESTS & INTERPRETATION
Initial Tests (lab, imaging)
- Diagnosis requires a recent history of CO exposure, consistent symptoms, and demonstration of an elevated COHb level.
- Chronic CO intoxication is more difficult to diagnose due to a lack of a clear eliciting event.
- Noninvasive COHb measurement should not be used to diagnose CO poisoning (2)[A].
- Arterial or venous blood gas is recommended:
  - COHb levels of >3% in nonsmokers, >10% in smokers. COHb may be low despite significant poisoning (e.g., treatment with O_2 or significant time elapses before the level is drawn).
  - Significant metabolic acidosis; anion gap >16
  - Elevated lactate confers worse prognosis.
  - PaO_2 tends to be normal because O_2 dissolved in blood is not affected by CO.
- Basic labs: serum chemistries, CBC

- ECG in all patients
  - Cardiac enzymes in patients with moderate or severe poisoning. If elevated, there is an increased risk of mortality in all patients (~24%) and is even higher in the following populations (2)[B]:
    - Patients ≥65 years
    - Patients with cardiac risk factors or anemia
    - Symptoms suggestive of cardiac ischemia
- Pregnancy test in all women of childbearing age
- Toxicology screen (particularly important in intentional poisoning)
- CK to evaluate for rhabdomyolysis
- Head CT/MRI scan can help to rule out other neurologic causes; may also show infarction due to hypoxia/ischemia. Long-term white matter hyperintensities and hippocampal atrophy also occur.

Follow-Up Tests & Special Considerations
- Consider CO poisoning in younger patients with chest pain or symptoms suggestive of ischemia.
- Consider the diagnosis in afebrile patients with vague or "flulike" symptoms. CO poisoning and the flu are both common during the winter time.
- Patients may present as a group (coworkers, family members, school children) with similar symptoms.
- Patients with intentional poisoning should undergo behavioral evaluation when stable.
- Implement suicide precautions if appropriate.

 TREATMENT

GENERAL MEASURES
- Prompt removal from the CO source and initiation of oxygen therapy to displace CO
- Supportive care as necessary
- Intubation and mechanical ventilation may be necessary for severe intoxication, particularly if the patient is unable to protect their airway or if there are signs of respiratory failure.
- Poison Control: 800-222-1222 (United States)

MEDICATION
- 100% oxygen via nonrebreathing reservoir facemask until COHb is normal (<3%) and patient is asymptomatic, regardless of oxygen saturation or PO_2 (1)[C],(2),(4)[A]
- CO has a half-life of 250 to 320 minutes in room air, and this half-life is reduced to 90 minutes with oxygen therapy via a nonrebreather mask.

Second Line
Hyperbaric oxygen therapy (not always readily available)

ADDITIONAL THERAPIES
- Hyperbaric oxygen (HBO_2) is associated with lower long and short-term mortality rates and long-term neuropsychiatric symptoms, although criteria for starting therapy remains unclear (5).
- NBO_2 and HBO_2 reduce the elimination half-life of COHb to ~85 minutes and 20 minutes, respectively (1).
- If HBO_2 is unavailable, administer NBO_2 until CO has normalized and symptoms have resolved (2),(4).
- HBO_2 therapy may reduce permanent neurologic deficit by reversing inflammatory response and mitochondrial dysfunction (1)[C].
- Optimal HBO_2 protocols are unclear (4)[C].
- HBO_2 currently recommended for:
  - Exposure >24 hours (4)[C]
  - Levels >25% (1),(4)[C]
  - CO level >20% in pregnant patient
  - Loss of consciousness (1),(4)[C]
  - Abnormal neurologic or psychiatric signs (1)[C]

- Cardiovascular dysfunction or end organ ischemia (1)[C]
  - Severe acidosis (1),(4)[C]
- Empirically treat patients for cyanide poisoning who present with CO poisoning from a house fire, if the pH is <7.20 or plasma lactate is >10 mmol/L (1),(4)[C].
- HBO_2 not as likely to be helpful if >24 hours has elapsed since exposure. Greatest benefit occurs if initiated as early as possible, within 6 hours of exposure being the goal.
- Expert consensus favors HBO_2 therapy for pregnant women (4)[C].
- In the United States, locating a hyperbaric oxygen chamber location can be found via the Undersea and Hyperbaric Medical Society website (www.uhms.org) or via the Divers Alert Network Emergency hotline (1-919-684-8111).

ADMISSION, INPATIENT, AND NURSING CONSIDERATIONS
- Patients whose symptoms do not improve after 4 to 5 hours of 100% O_2 should be transported to the nearest HBO_2 facility. Hospitalize patients with severe poisoning, ECG or laboratory evidence of end-organ damage, and those with concerning medical or social factors.
- Admit unconscious patients with CO poisoning to ICU following intubation.
- Patients with accidental poisoning and mild symptoms that resolve in the ED can be safely discharged.

 ONGOING CARE

FOLLOW-UP RECOMMENDATIONS
- All patients treated for acute CO poisoning should follow up in 1 to 2 months after discharge (1),(4).
- If there are behavioral or cognitive concerns, pursue neuropsychological evaluation, particularly following intentional CO poisoning.
- Long-term cognitive, psychiatric, speech, occupational, and physical rehab may be necessary.

Patient Monitoring
Repeat measurement of COHb levels with arterial blood gases.

PATIENT EDUCATION
- Professional installation and maintenance of combustion devices
- Consumer Product Safety Commission hotline 1-800-638-2772
- CO detector in bedrooms and by potential CO sources
- Annual furnace inspections (6)[B]
- Avoid use of combustion engines indoors; periodic furnace inspection
- www.cdc.gov/co/default.htm

PROGNOSIS
Although most patients completely recover, chronic neuropsychiatric impairment is described in 12–68% of patients.

COMPLICATIONS
- High-activity metabolic tissues are at higher risk.
- Cardiac:
  - Myocardial infarction (acute and long term)
  - Demand ischemia
  - Reduced left ventricular function
  - Dysrhythmia (prolonged QT)
- Pulmonary:
  - Inhalation injury
  - Pulmonary edema
  - Pneumonia (aspiration)
  - Acute respiratory failure
- Neurologic:
  - Anoxic encephalopathy
  - Vestibular and motor deficits

- Hippocampal atrophy
- Cognitive dysfunction
- Delayed posthypoxic leukoencephalopathy
- Diffuse brain atrophy
- Parkinsonism
- Behavioral:
  - Depression, anxiety
  - Irritability, moodiness, and violence

Geriatric Considerations
Increased number of comorbid leading to possibility of complications and worse outcomes

REFERENCES

1. Rose JJ, Wang L, Xu Q, et al. Carbon monoxide poisoning: pathogenesis, management, and future directions of therapy. *Am J Respir Crit Care Med*. 2017;195(5):596–606.
2. Wolf SJ, Maloney GE, Shih RD, et al; for American College of Emergency Physicians Clinical Policies Subcommittee (Writing Committee) on Carbon Monoxide Poisoning. Clinical policy: critical issues in the evaluation and management of adult patients presenting to the emergency department with acute carbon monoxide poisoning. *Ann Emerg Med*. 2017;69(1):98–107.e6.
3. Weaver LK. Clinical practice. Carbon monoxide poisoning. *N Engl J Med*. 2009;360(12):1217–1225.
4. Hampson NB, Piantadosi CA, Thom SR, et al. Practice recommendations in the diagnosis, management, and prevention of carbon monoxide poisoning. *Am J Respir Crit Care Med*. 2012;186(11):1095–1101.
5. Huang CC, Ho CH, Chen YC, et al. Hyperbaric oxygen therapy is associated with lower short- and long-term mortality in patients with carbon monoxide poisoning. *Chest*. 2017;152(5):943–953.
6. Rupert DJ, Poehlman JA, Damon SA, et al. Risk and protective behaviours for residential carbon monoxide poisoning. *Inj Prev*. 2013;19(2):119–123.

ADDITIONAL READING
- Centers for Disease Control and Prevention: http://www.cdc.gov/co
- Jung JW, Lee JH. Serum lactate as a predictor of neurologic outcome in ED patients with acute carbon monoxide poisoning. *Am J Emerg Med*. 2019;37(5):823–827. doi:10.1016/j.ajem.2018.07.046.

CODES

ICD10
- T58.0 Toxic effect of carbon monoxide from motor vehicle exhaust
- T58.2 Toxic effect of carbon monoxide from incomplete combustion of other domestic fuels
- T58.9 Toxic effect of carbon monoxide from unspecified source

CLINICAL PEARLS
- CO poisoning warrants a high index of suspicion. Consider in patients exposed to fire; during the winter months, in young patients with chest pain; and when patients present as a group.
- Noninvasive pulse oximeters are not reliable for the diagnosis of CO poisoning.
- If CO poisoning is suspected, remove individuals from the source and immediately administer 100% oxygen.
- Although not required in all cases, consider HBO_2 for the treatment of CO poisoning if it is available.

CARDIOMYOPATHY

Yousef Ahmed, MD • Henry DeYoung, MD • Derek Lodico, DO

BASICS

DESCRIPTION
- Cardiomyopathies are myocardial diseases which result in structural and functional heart abnormalities in the absence of coronary artery disease, congenital heart disease, valvular disease, or hypertension which could sufficiently explain the clinical myocardial dysfunction (1).
- Current classification scheme attempt to differentiate between myocardial diseases confined to the myocardium (primary) and those due to systemic disorders (secondary). Specific causes of myocardial dysfunction due to other cardiovascular disorders are considered a third, separate category (1).
- Classification of cardiomyopathies
  - Primary (mainly involves the myocardium)
    - Genetic
      - Hypertrophic cardiomyopathy (HCM)
      - Arrhythmogenic right ventricular cardiomyopathy/dysplasia (ARVC/D)
      - Left ventricular (LV) noncompaction (LVNC)
      - Glycogen storage (Danon type, PRKAG2)
      - Conduction defects
      - Mitochondrial myopathies
      - Ion channel disorders: long QT syndrome (LQTS), Brugada syndrome, short QT syndrome, and catecholaminergic polymorphic ventricular tachycardia (CPVT)
    - Mixed (genetic and nongenetic)
      - Dilated cardiomyopathy (DCM)
      - Restrictive (nonhypertrophied and nondilated)
    - Acquired
      - Myocarditis, stress cardiomyopathy, peripartum, tachycardia induced, infants of type 1 diabetic mothers
  - Secondary (multiorgan involvement; see list below)
    - Specific: ischemic, valvular, hypertensive, and congenital heart disease
- Patients with end-stage cardiomyopathy have stage D heart failure or severe symptoms at rest refractory to standard medical therapy.
- Systems affected: cardiovascular, renal, hepatic, and pulmonary

Pediatric Considerations
Progressive course and early diagnosis may alter disease course. Causes: DCM, HCM, RCM, LVNC in childhood, endocrine, uremic, nutritional

Pregnancy Considerations
Peripartum cardiomyopathy (PPCM) may occur in peripartum women well before and up to months after delivery.

EPIDEMIOLOGY
Predominant age: Ischemic cardiomyopathy is the most common etiology; predominantly in patients aged >50 years. Consider uncommon causes in young. In the young, HCM is the most common cause of sudden cardiac death and important underlying cause of heart failure disability.

Incidence
DCM: 5 to 8 new cases per 100,000 population annually

Prevalence
- DCM: roughly 1:2,500; third most common cause of heart failure and most common reason for heart transplantation

- HCM: at least 1:500 of the adult population
- RCM: more commonly seen in the tropics

ETIOLOGY AND PATHOPHYSIOLOGY
- HCM: hypertrophied, nondilated left ventricle without other systemic or cardiac disease which could produce wall thickening
- ARVC/D: involves the right ventricle with progressive loss of myocytes and fatty/fibrofatty tissue replacement; can be associated with myocarditis (adenovirus or enterovirus)
- LVNC: congenital cardiomyopathies with "spongy" appearance of the LV myocardium
- LQTS: most common ion channelopathy with prolonged ventricular repolarization and QTc
- DCM: Ventricular chamber enlargement and systolic dysfunction with normal LV wall thickness result in progressive heart failure and further complications; strong genetic component with infectious and toxic etiologies
- RCM: normal/decreased ventricular volume with restrictive physiology, biatrial enlargement, and impaired ventricular filling
- Myocarditis: acute or chronic inflammation of the myocardium produced by toxins, drugs, or infectious causes
- PPCM: a form of DCM with LV systolic dysfunction and heart failure of unknown etiology
- Stress cardiomyopathies: triggered by profound psychological stress resulting in acute but rapidly reversible LV systolic dysfunction
- Endocrine: diabetes mellitus, hyperthyroidism, hypothyroidism, hyperparathyroidism, pheochromocytoma, acromegaly
- Nutritional deficiencies: beriberi, pellagra, scurvy, selenium, carnitine, kwashiorkor
- Autoimmune/collagen: systemic lupus erythematosus, dermatomyositis, rheumatoid arthritis, scleroderma, polyarteritis nodosa
- Infectious causes
  - Viral (e.g., HIV, coxsackievirus, adenovirus)
  - Bacterial and mycobacterial (e.g., diphtheria, rheumatic fever)
  - Parasitic (e.g., toxoplasmosis, *Trypanosoma cruzi*)
- Infiltrative (2): amyloidosis, Gaucher disease, Hurler disease, Hunter disease, Fabry disease
- Storage: hemochromatosis, glycogen storage disease (type II, Pompe), Niemann-Pick disease
- Neuromuscular/neurologic: Duchenne and Emery-Dreifuss muscular dystrophies, Friedreich ataxia, myotonic dystrophy, neurofibromatosis, tuberous sclerosis
- Toxic: alcohol, drugs and chemotherapy (anthracyclines, cyclophosphamide, trastuzumab [Herceptin]), radiation, heavy metal, chemical agents
- Inflammatory (granulomatous): sarcoidosis
- Idiopathic
- Endomyocardial: endomyocardial fibrosis, hypereosinophilic syndrome (Loeffler endocarditis)

Genetics
Autosomal dominant HCM is the most common form of primary genetic cardiomyopathy, which is commonly caused by many mutations that encode contractile proteins of the cardiac sarcomere. Genetic causes of DCM are less common, accounting for 1/3 cases, with mostly autosomal dominant inheritance. LVNC and ARVC are also inherited in an autosomal dominant fashion in addition to LQTS and other ion-channel disorders.

RISK FACTORS
- Hypertension
- Hyperlipidemia
- Obesity
- Coronary artery disease
- Diabetes mellitus
- Smoking
- Physical inactivity
- Excessive alcohol intake
- Dietary sodium
- Obstructive sleep apnea
- Chemotherapy

GENERAL PREVENTION
Reduce salt and water intake, and perform home blood pressure (BP) and daily weight measurements.

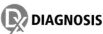

DIAGNOSIS

HISTORY
- Dyspnea at rest or with exertion
- Paroxysmal nocturnal dyspnea
- Orthopnea
- Postprandial dyspnea
- Right upper quadrant pain or bloating
- Fatigue
- Syncope
- Edema

PHYSICAL EXAM
- Tachypnea
- Cheyne-Stokes breathing
- Low pulse pressure
- Cool extremities
- Jugular venous distinction
- Bibasilar rales
- Tachycardia
- Displaced point of maximal impulse (PMI)
- S_3 gallop
- Blowing systolic murmur
- Hepatosplenomegaly
- Ascites
- Edema

DIFFERENTIAL DIAGNOSIS
- Severe pulmonary disease
- Primary pulmonary hypertension
- Recurrent pulmonary embolism
- Constrictive pericarditis
- Some advanced forms of malignancy
- Anemia

DIAGNOSTIC TESTS & INTERPRETATION
- ECG: LV hypertrophy, interventricular conduction delay, atrial fibrillation, evidence of prior Q-wave infarction
- Hyponatremia
- Prerenal azotemia
- Anemia
- Mild elevation in troponin
- Elevated B-type natriuretic peptide (BNP) or pro-BNP
- Mild hyperbilirubinemia
- Elevated liver function tests
- Elevated uric acid

Initial Tests (lab, imaging)
- ECG
- Chest radiograph
  - Cardiomegaly
  - Increased vascular markings to the upper lobes
  - Pleural effusions may or may not be present.
- Echocardiography
  - In DCM, four-chamber enlargement and global hypokinesis are present.
  - In HCM, severe LV hypertrophy is present.
  - Segmental contraction abnormalities of the LV are indicative of previous localized myocardial infarction.
- Cardiac MRI
  - May be useful to characterize certain nonischemic cardiomyopathies
- Stress myocardial perfusion imaging (MPI)
  - Recommended in those with new-onset LV dysfunction or when ischemia is suspected

Diagnostic Procedures/Other
Cardiac catheterization
- Helpful to rule out ischemic heart disease
- Characterize hemodynamic severity
- Pulmonary artery catheters may be reasonable in patients with refractory heart failure to help guide management.

TREATMENT

See "Heart Failure, Chronic" for detailed treatment protocols.

GENERAL MEASURES
- Reduction of filling pressures
- Treatment of electrolyte disturbances

MEDICATION
First Line
- Systolic failure syndromes
  - Either an ACE inhibitor or an ARB is equally effective and should be considered in all patients; initiate at low doses and titrate as tolerated to target doses (3)[A].
  - Sacubitril/valsartan (Entresto), a combination drug containing a neprilysin inhibitor and valsartan (ARNI), was approved in 2015 for the treatment of systolic heart failure (ejection fraction [EF] <40%) as an alternative to an ACE/ARB (4)[A].
  - In patients who have been stable on an ACE or ARB, morbidity and mortality may be further reduced (all-cause mortality reduction approximately NNT 33 over 2 years treatment) by replacement with an ARNI (4)[A], with careful monitoring needed for hypotension and angioedema.
  - Loop diuretics
    ○ May need to be given IV initially and then orally as patient stabilizes
  - Furosemide, 40 to 120 mg/day or TID (3)[A]
  - β-Blockers
    ○ Use with caution in acutely decompensated or low-cardiac output states.
    ○ Initiate with low doses and titrate as tolerated.
  - Metoprolol succinate, 12.5 to 200 mg/day; carvedilol, 3.125 to 25 mg BID; or bisoprolol, 1.25 to 10 mg/day (3)[A]
  - Patients with New York Heart Association (NYHA) II to IV heart failure, EF <35%, on standard therapy: aldosterone antagonists: spironolactone or eplerenone (3)[A]
  - Digoxin, 0.125 to 0.250 mg/day for symptomatic patients on standard therapy (3)[B]
  - Combination hydralazine/isosorbide dinitrate is first-line treatment in African American patients with classes III and IV symptoms already on standard therapy and for all patients with reduced EF and symptoms incompletely responsive to ACE inhibitor and β-blocker (3)[A].
    ○ Contraindications
      ▪ β-Blockers: low cardiac output, 2nd- or 3rd-degree heart block
      ▪ Avoid use of diltiazem and verapamil in patients with systolic dysfunction.
      ▪ Aldosterone antagonists: oliguria, anuria, renal dysfunction
      ▪ Loop diuretics: hypokalemia, hypomagnesemia
      ▪ ACE inhibitors: pregnancy, angioedema
      ▪ ARNIs: patients currently on an ACE inhibitor or who have taken one in the past 36 hours, patients with a history of angioedema
- Precautions
  - In patients with chronic kidney disease, digoxin dosage should be ≤0.125 mg/day and drug levels followed carefully to avoid toxicity.
  - Closely monitor electrolytes.
  - ACE inhibitors and ARNIs: Initiate with care if BP is low.
  - β-Blockers: Avoid in patients with evidence of poor tissue perfusion; they may further depress systolic function.
  - Milrinone, dobutamine: long-term use associated with increased mortality
- Medications to avoid
  - NSAIDs
  - Glitazones
  - Cilostazol

Second Line
- Inotropic therapy (e.g., dobutamine or milrinone) for cardiogenic shock and support prior to surgery or cardiac transplantation (3)[B]
- Continuous inotrope infusion may be considered in stage D outpatients for symptom control in those who are not eligible for transplantation or mechanical circulatory support (3)[B].

ISSUES FOR REFERRAL
Management by a heart failure team improves outcomes and facilitates early transplant referral.

ADDITIONAL THERAPIES
- Prophylactic implantable cardioverter-defibrillator (ICD) should be considered for patients with a left ventricular ejection fraction (LVEF) <35% and mild to moderate symptoms (3)[A].
- Cardiac resynchronization therapy (CRT) is recommended and should be considered for patients in sinus rhythm with a QRS >150 ms, LVEF <35%, in functional class (FC) I to III, and ambulatory FC IV patients (3)[A].
- Patients with severe, refractory heart failure with no reasonable expectation of improvement should not be considered for an ICD. Palliative care is a reasonable option in such patients.
- Consideration of an LV assist device as "permanent" or destination therapy or cardiac transplantation is reasonable in selected stage D patients.

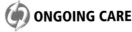

ONGOING CARE

DIET
Low fat, low salt, fluid restriction

PROGNOSIS
~20–40% of patients in NYHA FC IV die within 1 year. With a transplant, 1-year survival is as high as 94%.

COMPLICATIONS
Worsening congestive heart failure syncope, renal failure, arrhythmias, or sudden death

REFERENCES
1. Maron BJ, Towbin JA, Thiene G, et al. Contemporary definitions and classification of the cardiomyopathies: an American Heart Association Scientific Statement from the Council on Clinical Cardiology, Heart Failure and Transplantation Committee; Quality of Care and Outcomes Research and Functional Genomics and Translational Biology Interdisciplinary Working Groups; and Council on Epidemiology and Prevention. *Circulation*. 2006;113(14):1807–1816.
2. Seward JB, Casaclang-Verzosa G. Infiltrative cardiovascular diseases: cardiomyopathies that look alike. *J Am Coll Cardiol*. 2010;55(17):1769–1779.
3. Yancy CW, Jessup M, Bozkurt B, et al. 2017 ACC/AHA/HFSA focused update of the 2013 ACCF/AHA guideline for the management of heart failure: a report of the American College of Cardiology/American Heart Association Task Force on Clinical Practice Guidelines and the Heart Failure Society of America. *Circulation*. 2017;136(6):e137–e161.
4. McMurray JJ, Packer M, Desai AS, et al; for PARADIGM-HF Investigators and Committees. Angiotensin-neprilysin inhibition versus enalapril in heart failure. *N Engl J Med*. 2014;371(11):993–1004.

 SEE ALSO

- Alcohol Use Disorder (AUD); Alcohol Withdrawal; Amyloidosis; Diabetes Mellitus, Type 1; Diabetes Mellitus, Type 2; Hypertension, Essential; Hypertrophic Cardiomyopathy; Hypothyroidism, Adult; Protein–Energy Malnutrition; Rheumatic Fever; Sarcoidosis
- Algorithm: Congestive Heart Failure: Differential Diagnosis

 CODES

ICD10
- I42.9 Cardiomyopathy, unspecified
- I42.0 Dilated cardiomyopathy
- I42.5 Other restrictive cardiomyopathy

CLINICAL PEARLS
- Cardiomyopathy represents the end-stage of a large number of disease processes involving the heart muscle.
- Ischemic, hypertensive, postviral, familial, alcoholic, and incessant tachycardia-induced are the most common cardiomyopathy varieties seen in the United States.
- Core therapy for heart failure applies salt restriction, diuretics, ACE inhibitors, β-blockers, digoxin, and electrical treatments, such as cardiac resynchronization and implantable defibrillators, as appropriate.

CAROTID SINUS HYPERSENSITIVITY

Afsha Rais Kaisani, MD • Nicholas Broughton, DO • Niyomi De Silva, MD

 BASICS

DESCRIPTION
- The carotid sinus is located near the bifurcation of the internal and external carotid arteries and contains baroreceptors that are responsive to increases or decreases in arterial pressure.
- The carotid sinuses play a central role in blood pressure (BP) homeostasis.
- An endogenous increase in BP or external pressure applied to a carotid sinus causes an increase in the baroreceptor firing rate and activates vagal efferents and/or inhibits the sympathetic discharge to the heart and blood vessels, resulting in a slowing of the heart rate and drop in BP.
- In carotid sinus hypersensitivity (CSH), stimulation of one or both carotid sinuses, such as mechanical forces with turning neck) causes an exaggerated baroreceptor response that can result in dizziness or syncope.
- There are three definitions for CSH (1):
  - Standard criteria: a pause in heart rate of ≥3 seconds in response to carotid sinus massage (CSM) and/or vasodepression of ≥50 mm Hg drop in systolic BP or both of the above
  - Krediet criteria: a pause in heart rate of ≥6 seconds in response to CSM and/or a fall in MAP to a value <60 mm Hg for ≥6 seconds
  - Kerr criteria: a pause in heart rate in response to CSM >95th percentile of the population response (7.3 seconds asystole), and/or vasodepression in response to CSM >95th percentile of the population response (>77 mm Hg fall in systolic BP), or both
- CSH is generally divided into three subtypes, based on response to CSM:
  - Cardioinhibitory (70–75%): asystole for at least 3 seconds
  - Vasodepressive (5–10%): fall in systolic BP of at least 50 mm Hg
  - Mixed (20–25%): combination of the first 2 subtypes
- Carotid sinus syndrome (CSS) typically (but not consistently) refers to CSH *with syncope and may be classified as:*
  - Spontaneous CSS: syncope after accidental mechanical manipulation (trigger) of the carotid sinuses (e.g., shaving, tight collars, or tumors)
  - Induced CSS: syncope diagnosed by CSM although no mechanical trigger is found

EPIDEMIOLOGY
- Disease of elderly; most often occurs in male patients >65 years.
- Associated with a history of coronary artery disease (CAD) and hypertension (HTN), with right CSH > left CSH

Prevalence
- In 2006, CSH was found in 39% of unselected adults >65 years of age using standard diagnostic criteria, and found to be comparable with 2019 review of prevalence data (2).
- CSH may be a cause of the symptoms in 30% of elderly patients with unexplained syncope.

ETIOLOGY AND PATHOPHYSIOLOGY
- The exact site of the abnormality that causes hypersensitivity response in patients with CSH remains unknown. Changes in any part of the reflex arc or the target organs may give rise to this condition, or it may be a part of a generalized autonomic disorder associated with autonomic dysregulation.
- Associated with resting sympathetic overactivity and increased baroreflex sensitivity
- Bradycardia and asystole seen in cardioinhibitory and mixed CSH subtypes appear to be mediated by vagal efferents, whereas vasodilatation and arterial hypotension in the vasodepressor and mixed subtypes are attributed to decrease sympathetic tone.
- Symptomatic CSH has been shown to be associated with impaired cerebral autoregulation, and in asymptomatic CSH, it was found to be normal.
- Atherosclerosis may diminish carotid sinus compliance, resulting in a reduction in afferent impulse traffic in the baroreflex pathway (3).
- CSH is often idiopathic but can be caused by:
  - Carotid body tumors
  - Inflammatory and malignant lymph nodes in the neck
  - Extensive scarring from prior neck surgery in the area of the carotid sinus
  - Metastatic cancer

RISK FACTORS
- Advanced age, male gender
- CAD
- HTN
- DM

COMMONLY ASSOCIATED CONDITIONS
- Carotid sinus syncope, sick sinus syndrome
- Atrioventricular block
- CAD
- HTN
- Orthostatic hypotension
- Vasovagal syncope
- Alzheimer disease
- Parkinson disease

DIAGNOSIS

HISTORY
- Recurrent syncope: usually sudden, unexplained, of short duration, seemingly spontaneous, and with complete recovery, although fractures and other injuries may occur
- Unexplained falls: Evidence of a causal relationship is suggested between falls and the cardioinhibitory subgroup.
- Dizziness: manifests as transient light-headedness or presyncope but not usually as true vertigo; associated more with vasodepressor and mixed subtypes
- Syncope may be associated with prodrome or retrograde amnesia.
- Causative or exacerbating factors
  - Any CSM-like maneuver such as shaving, wearing tight collars, or turning one's head sharply
  - Neck tumors, extensive neck scarring secondary to radical dissection or radiation fibrosis, and neck trauma

- Certain medications can potentiate symptoms associated with CSH:
  - Digoxin or β-blockers (especially with cardioinhibitory subtype)
  - Physostigmine, morphine, methacholine increase vagal sensitivity and may predispose to cardioinhibitory subtype of CSH.

PHYSICAL EXAM
Normal unless carotid baroreceptor is stimulated, then
- Bradycardia
- Hypotension
- Pallor
- Diaphoresis

DIFFERENTIAL DIAGNOSIS
- Neurocardiogenic syncope
- Postural hypotension
- Situational syncope
- Postural tachycardia syndrome (POTS)
- Primary autonomic insufficiency
- Hypovolemia
- Dysrhythmias
- Sick sinus syndrome
- Cerebrovascular insufficiency
- Other causes of syncope (e.g., metabolic, psychogenic)
- ECG may demonstrate sinus pause(s) or atrial-ventricular block.
- Carotid duplex scan to rule out carotid stenosis in presence of a bruit (see the following section)

DIAGNOSTIC TESTS & INTERPRETATION
Diagnostic Procedures/Other
- CSM is indicated in patients >40 years of age with syncope of unknown etiology after a negative initial evaluation (4)[B].
- Commonly accepted technique for accurate diagnosis involves the following steps:
  - Patient in supine position for 5 minutes with continuous BP monitoring and ECG (on footplate-type tilt table for increased diagnostic accuracy); baseline BP and ECG are recorded.
  - For 5 to 10 seconds, apply firm longitudinal massage over the right carotid sinus (between the superior border of the thyroid and the angle of the mandible) at the site of maximal pulsation:
    - Note that light pressure over the carotid sinus will not reliably produce a hypersensitivity response.
    - Record symptoms, BP, and note ECG changes.
    - Discontinue if asystole ≥3 seconds.
  - If initial test nondiagnostic, apply pressure to the left carotid sinus while the patient remains supine; if still nondiagnostic, repeat in 70-degree head-up tilt (first on the right then, if necessary, the left), allowing time for hemodynamic adjustment to the head-up position.
  - Evidence behind the testing strategy
  - Right side first: Up to 66% with CSH have positive response on the right; if a positive right response, no need to repeat test on the left side
  - 30% of CSM exams are found to be nondiagnostic in the supine position; positive predictive value increases from 77% to 96% with a specificity of 93% by performing CSM in the 70-degree position.

- Absolute contraindications for CSM testing
- Carotid bruit present: must examine via carotid ultrasound with Doppler first:
  ○ No testing if >70% stenosis
  ○ Supine only testing if 50–70% stenosis
- Myocardial infarction, transient ischemic attack, or stroke within the past 3 months
- Relative contraindications to CSM testing
- History of ventricular tachycardia or ventricular fibrillation
- False-positive results with CSM are relatively common in the elderly. Care should be taken to exclude other causes of syncope.
- Neurologic and cardiovascular complications have been reported during CSM. Cardiovascular complications (primarily arrhythmia) are extremely rare. Transient neurologic symptoms and signs occur in up to 0.9% of patients. Persistent neurologic deficits are extremely rare following CSM. Correctly performed CSM should be considered a safe, low-risk procedure (3)[C].

Test Interpretation
Standard positive response criteria (asystole ≥3 seconds and/or drop in systolic BP ≥50 mm Hg) is based on historical observations, although expert review of more recent data suggest these criteria may be too sensitive (5)[C].

- Specificity of the CSM technique increases if reproduction of a patient's syncope is demonstrated during a test (4)[B].

TREATMENT

GENERAL MEASURES
- No treatment is required for isolated CSH in asymptomatic individuals.
- High-dietary salt intake and increased fluid intake may be helpful to maintain intravascular volume in patients with vasodepressor subtype and absence of other cardiovascular disease.
- Evaluation for driving restrictions

MEDICATION
First Line
No single agent has demonstrated long-term effectiveness for treatment of recurrent and symptomatic CSH.

Second Line
- Fludrocortisone or midodrine may be used to improve orthostatic symptoms in patients with vasodepressor subtype (not approved by FDA for this indication). However, fludrocortisone causes sodium and water retention and should be used with caution in elderly patients with heart disease. An adverse effect with midodrine is that it increases mean ambulatory BP (3)[C].
- Atropine may be used in the acute setting in patients with cardioinhibitory subtype with bradycardia.
- Some evidence of benefit from sertraline and fluoxetine in patients unresponsive to pacemakers (3)[C]

SURGERY/OTHER PROCEDURES
- 2017 ACC/AHA/HRS (6)[A] Guideline for the Evaluation and Management of Patients With Syncope notes that evidence is very limited and thus recommendation strength not high. Available evidence does not support the use of pacing for reflex-mediated syncope beyond patients with recurrent vasovagal syncope and asystole documented by implantable loop recorder.
- Permanent pacing may reduce the frequency of symptoms but may not completely eliminate them.
- Surgery for patients with CSH secondary to mass effect from tumor burden
- Carotid sinus denervation by surgery or radiation therapy is no longer recommended because of the high rate of complications.

 ## ONGOING CARE

PATIENT EDUCATION
- Avoid precipitating maneuvers (as described above) that place pressure on the neck, such as tight collars and neckties.
- With syncope, restrict driving or other potentially hazardous activities until the patient is cleared by the physician (4).
- Avoid precipitating medications like vasodilators and those temporally related to symptoms.
- Teach patient to assume supine position if prodromal symptoms or presyncope occurs.
- Explain diagnosis, provide reassurance, and explain risk of recurrence.

PROGNOSIS
- The presence of CSH has not been demonstrated to confer an independent mortality risk.
- Untreated CSS patients have a syncope recurrence rate as high as 62% within 4 years.
- Patients with cardioinhibitory CSH who received a pacemaker had a significant reduction in their mean number of falls, from 9.3 to 4.1 falls in a 1-year follow-up period (3).

COMPLICATIONS
CSH, according to Kerr criteria, is associated with increased mortality. Further evaluation is needed to predict future falls, syncope, and ability of criteria to identify patients who would benefit from pacing (1)[B].

REFERENCES
1. McDonald C, Pearce MS, Newton JL, et al. Modified criteria for carotid sinus hypersensitivity are associated with increased mortality in a population-based study. *Europace*. 2016;18(7):1101–1107.
2. Kadermuneer P, Sandeep R, Haridasan V, et al. Prevalence and one-year outcome of carotid sinus hypersensitivity in unexplained syncope: a prospective cohort study from South India. *Indian Heart J*. 2019;71(1):1–6.
3. Seifer C. Carotid sinus syndrome. *Cardiol Clin*. 2013;31(1):111–121.
4. Moya A, Sutton R, Ammirati F, et al; for Task Force for the Diagnosis and Management of Syncope of the European Society of Cardiology (ESC). Guidelines for the diagnosis and management of syncope (version 2009). *Eur Heart J*. 2009;30(21):2631–2671.
5. Krediet CT, Parry SW, Jardine DL, et al. The history of diagnosing carotid sinus hypersensitivity: why are the current criteria too sensitive? *Europace*. 2011;13(1):14–22.
6. Varosy PD, Chen LY, Miller AL, et al. Pacing as a treatment for reflex-mediated (vasovagal, situational, or carotid sinus hypersensitivity) syncope: a systematic review for the 2017 ACC/AHA/HRS guideline for the evaluation and management of patients with syncope: a report of the American College of Cardiology/American Heart Association Task Force on Clinical Practice Guidelines and the Heart Rhythm Society. *Circulation*. 2017;136(5):e123–e135.

ADDITIONAL READING
- Amin V, Pavri BB. Carotid sinus syndrome. *Cardiol Rev*. 2015;23(3):130–134.
- Kapoor JR. Carotid sinus hypersensitivity: a diagnostic pearl. *J Am Coll Cardiol*. 2009;4(17):1633.
- Kerr SRJ, Pearce MS, Brayne C, et al. Carotid sinus hypersensitivity in asymptomatic older persons: implications for diagnosis of syncope and falls. *Arch Intern Med*. 2006;166(5):515–520.
- Parry SW, Richardson DA, O'Shea D, et al. Diagnosis of carotid sinus hypersensitivity in older adults: carotid sinus massage in the upright position is essential. *Heart*. 2000;83(1):22–23.

 ## SEE ALSO

Syncope

CODES

ICD10
G90.01 Carotid sinus syncope

CLINICAL PEARLS
- Consider CSH as a potential cause for syncope, dizziness, or unexplained falls, especially in the elderly.
- Diagnose CSH via CSM (using firm pressure for 5 to 10 seconds), producing asystole of at least 3 seconds and/or a drop in systolic BP of at least 50 mm Hg.
- Remember to auscultate for carotid artery bruit prior to considering CSM.
- Consider dual-chamber pacemaker in patients with recurrent syncope and cardioinhibitory or mixed CSH subtypes.
- The finding of CSH does not exclude other causes of syncope.

CAROTID STENOSIS

Evangelos Giakoumatos, MD, MSc • Naureen Bashir Rafiq, MD

 BASICS

Carotid stenosis may be caused by atherosclerosis, intimal fibroplasia, vasculitis, adventitial cysts, or vascular tumors; atherosclerosis is the most common etiology.

DESCRIPTION
- Narrowing of the carotid artery lumen is typically due to atherosclerotic changes in the vessel wall. Atherosclerotic plaques are responsible for 90% of extracranial carotid lesions and up to 30% of all ischemic strokes.
- A "hemodynamically significant" carotid stenosis produces a drop in pressure or a reduction in flow. It corresponds approximately to a 60–99% diameter-reducing stenosis.
- Carotid lesions are classified by the following:
  - Symptom status
    - Asymptomatic: tend to be homogenous and stable
    - Symptomatic: tend to be heterogeneous and unstable; present with stroke or transient cerebral ischemic attack
  - Degree of stenosis
    - High grade: 80–99% stenosis
    - Moderate grade: 50–79% stenosis
    - Low grade: <50% stenosis

EPIDEMIOLOGY
More common in men and with increasing age (see "Risk Factors")

Incidence
Unclear (Asymptomatic patients often go undiagnosed.)

Prevalence
- Moderate stenosis
  - Age <50 years: men 0.2%, women 0%
  - Age >80 years: men 7.5%, women 5%
- Severe stenosis
  - Age <50 years: men 0.1%, women 0%
  - Age >80 years: men 3.1%, women 0.9%

ETIOLOGY AND PATHOPHYSIOLOGY
- Atherosclerosis begins during adolescence, consistently at the carotid bifurcation. The carotid bulb has unique blood flow dynamics. Hemodynamic disturbances cause endothelial injury and dysfunction. Plaque formation in vessel wall results and stenosis then ensues.
- Initial cause is not well understood, but certain risk factors are frequently present (see "Risk Factors"). Tensile stress on the vessel wall, turbulence, and arterial wall shear stress seem to be involved.

Genetics
- Increased incidence among family members
- Genetically linked factors
  - Diabetes mellitus (DM), race, hypertension (HTN), family history, obesity
  - In a recent single nucleotide polymorphism study, the following genes were strongly associated with worse carotid plaque: *TNFSF4*, *PPARA*, *TLR4*, *ITGA2*, and *HABP2*.

RISK FACTORS
- Nonmodifiable factors: advanced age (>65 years old), male sex, family history, coronary artery disease (CAD), peripheral artery disease, aortic aneurysmal disease, congenital arteriopathies
- Modifiable factors: smoking, diet, dyslipidemia, physical inactivity, obesity, HTN, DM
- Possible factors: *Chlamydia pneumoniae* and *Cytomegalovirus*

GENERAL PREVENTION
- Antihypertensive treatment to maintain BP <140/90 mm Hg (systolic BP of 150 mm Hg is target in elderly). See "Hypertension, Essential."
- Smoking cessation to reduce the risk of atherosclerosis progression and stroke
- Lipid control: regression of carotid atherosclerotic lesions seen with statin therapy

COMMONLY ASSOCIATED CONDITIONS
- Transient ischemic attack (TIA)/stroke
- CAD/myocardial infarction (MI)
- Peripheral vascular disease (PVD)
- HTN
- DM
- Hyperlipidemia

 DIAGNOSIS

Screening for carotid stenosis is not recommended. However, in the setting of symptoms suggestive of stroke or TIA, workup for this condition may be indicated.

HISTORY
- Identification of modifiable and nonmodifiable comorbidities (see "Risk Factors")
- History of cerebral ischemic event
- Stroke, TIA, amaurosis fugax (monocular blindness), aphasia
- CAD/MI
- Peripheral arterial disease
- Review of systems, with focus on risk factors for
  - Cardiovascular disease
  - Stroke (HTN and arrhythmias)

PHYSICAL EXAM
- Lateralizing neurologic deficits: contralateral motor and/or sensory deficit
- Amaurosis fugax: ipsilateral transient visual obscuration from retinal ischemia
- Visual field defect
- Dysarthria, aphasia (in the case of dominant hemisphere involvement, usually left)
- Carotid bruit (low sensitivity and specificity)

DIFFERENTIAL DIAGNOSIS
- Aortic valve stenosis
- Aortic arch atherosclerosis
- Arrhythmia with cardiogenic embolization
- Migraine
- Brain tumor
- Metabolic disturbances
- Functional/psychological deficit
- Seizure

DIAGNOSTIC TESTS & INTERPRETATION
Initial Tests (lab, imaging)
Workup for suspected TIA/stroke may include the following:
- CBC with differential
- Basic metabolic panel
- ESR (if temporal arteritis a consideration)
- Glucose/hemoglobin A1c
- Fasting lipid profile
- Duplex ultrasonography is the recommended initial diagnostic test in asymptomatic patients with known or suspected carotid stenosis.
- Duplex ultrasound (US) identifies ≥50% stenosis, with 98% sensitivity and 88% specificity.

Follow-Up Tests & Special Considerations
- Proceed to imaging if there is suggestion of stenosis from history or physical exam.
- Other noninvasive imaging techniques can add detail to duplex results:
  - CT angiography
    - 88% sensitivity and 100% specificity
    - Requires IV contrast with risk for subsequent renal morbidity
  - MR angiography
    - 95% sensitivity and 90% specificity
    - Evaluates cerebral circulation (extracranial and intracranial) as well as aortic arch and common carotid artery
    - The presence of unstable plaque can be determined if the following characteristics are seen:
      - Presence of thin/ruptured fibrous cap
      - Presence of lipid-rich necrotic core
      - Tends to overestimate degree of stenosis

Diagnostic Procedures/Other
Cerebral angiography is the traditional gold standard for diagnosis:
- Delineates the anatomy pertaining to aortic arch and proximal vessels
- The procedure is invasive and has multiple risks:
  - Contrast-induced renal dysfunction (1–5% complication rate)
  - Thromboembolic-related complications (1–2.6% complication rate) and neurologic complications
  - Should be used only when other tests are not conclusive

Test Interpretation
- Stenosis consistently occurs at the carotid bifurcation, with plaque formation most often at the level of the proximal internal carotid artery:
  - Plaque is thickest at the carotid bifurcation.
  - Plaque occupies the intima and inner media and avoids outer media and adventitia.
- Plaque histology
  - Homogenous (stable) plaques seldom hemorrhage or ulcerate:
    - Fatty streak and fibrous tissue deposition
    - Diffuse intimal thickening
  - Heterogenous (unstable) plaques may hemorrhage or ulcerate:
    - Presence of lipid-laden macrophages, necrotic debris, cholesterol crystals
    - Ulcerated plaques
  - Soft and gelatinous clots with platelets, fibrin, and red and white blood cells

 TREATMENT

Smoking cessation, BP control, antiplatelet medication, and statin medication are the primary treatments for both asymptomatic and symptomatic carotid stenosis.

GENERAL MEASURES
- Lifestyle modifications: dietary control and weight loss, exercise of 30 min/day at least 5 days/week
- Patients should be advised to quit smoking and offered smoking cessation intervention to reduce the risk of atherosclerotic progression and stroke.
- Control of HTN with antihypertensive agents to maintain BP <140/90 mm Hg; <150/90 mm Hg in the elderly. In carefully selected individuals, tighter blood pressure control might reduce cerebrovascular events, but this remains uncertain.

MEDICATION
- Antihypertensive treatment (<140/90 mm Hg), <150/90 mm Hg in the elderly
- Diet, smoking cessation, and exercise are useful adjuncts to therapy.
- Statin initiation is recommended; choose moderate-to high-intensity statin therapy for anti-inflammatory benefit.
- A comprehensive program that includes tight control of HTN with ACEI or ARB treatment reduces the risk in individuals with diabetes. Stroke prevention benefit of intensive glucose-lowering therapy has not been established (1)[A].
- Aspirin: 75 to 325 mg/day
- If patient has sustained TIA or ischemic stroke, antiplatelet therapy with
  – Aspirin alone (75 to 325 mg/day), or
  – Clopidogrel alone (75 mg/day), or
  – Aspirin plus extended-release dipyridamole (25 and 200 mg BID, respectively)
  – A combination of clopidogrel plus aspirin is NOT recommended within 3 months post-TIA or CVA.

ISSUES FOR REFERRAL
- For acute symptomatic stroke, order imaging and contact neurology.
- For known carotid stenosis, some suggest duplex imaging every 6 months if stenosis is >50% and patient is a surgical candidate.

SURGERY/OTHER PROCEDURES
- Symptomatic carotid stenosis (history of ischemia ipsilateral to stenosis)
  – Carotid endarterectomy (CEA) is of some benefit in 50–69% symptomatic stenosis, highly beneficial for those with 70–99% stenosis without near-occlusion and has no benefit in people with carotid near-occlusion (2)[A].
  – CEA is recommended for patients with a life expectancy of at least 5 years. The anticipated rate of perioperative stroke or mortality must be <6% (3)[B].
  – Treatment with aspirin (81 to 325 mg/day) is recommended for all patients who are having CEA. Aspirin should be started prior to surgery and continued for at least 3 months postsurgery but may be continued indefinitely (3)[B].
  – Carotid artery stenting (CAS) provides similar long-term outcomes as CEA (4)[A]. Age should be considered when planning a carotid intervention.
    ○ CAS has an increased risk of adverse cerebrovascular events in the elderly compared to the young but similar mortality risk. CEA is associated with similar neurologic outcomes in the elderly and young, at the expense of increased mortality (5)[A].
    ○ CAS is suggested in selected patients with neck anatomy unfavorable for arterial surgery and those with comorbid conditions that greatly increase the risk of anesthesia and surgery.
    ○ Dual antiplatelet therapy with aspirin (81 to 325 mg/day) plus clopidogrel (75 mg/day) is recommended for 30 days post-CAS.
- Asymptomatic patients
  – As compared with CAS, CEA is the preferred option for the management of asymptomatic carotid stenosis if a surgical option is chosen. CAS has the potential for increased risks of periprocedural stroke and periprocedural death (6)[A].
  – The advantage of surgical compared with medical therapy has decreased with contemporary medical management. It is not possible to make an evidence-based recommendation for or against surgical therapy with current literature (1)[A].

ADMISSION, INPATIENT, AND NURSING CONSIDERATIONS
- Any patient with presentation of acute symptomatic carotid stenosis should be hospitalized for further diagnostic workup and appropriate therapy.
- Rapid evaluation for symptoms compatible with TIA should be obtained in the emergency department (ED) or inpatient setting.
- Discharge criteria: 24 to 48 hours post-CEA, if ambulating, taking adequate PO intake, and neurologically intact

 ONGOING CARE

FOLLOW-UP RECOMMENDATIONS
Patient Monitoring
- Duplex at 2 to 6 weeks postoperatively
- Duplex every 6 to 12 months
- Reoperative CEA or CAS is reasonable, if there is rapidly progressive restenosis.
- Patients with any of the following: renal failure, heart failure, diabetes, and age >80 years have a high readmission rate following CEA; thus, intensive medical therapy and rigorous follow-up is recommended.

DIET
Heart-healthy diet low in saturated fat, no trans fat

PATIENT EDUCATION
For patient education materials on this topic, consult the following:
- American Heart Association: http://www.heart.org
- Mayo Clinic information: http://www.mayoclinic.org/diseases-conditions/carotid-artery-disease/basics/definition/con-20030206

COMPLICATIONS
- Untreated: TIA/stroke (risk of ipsilateral stroke approximately 1.68% per year)
- Postoperative (status post CEA)
  – Perioperative (within 30 days)
    ○ Stroke/death, cranial nerve injury, hemorrhage, hemodynamic instability, MI
  – Late (>30 days postop)
    ○ Recurrent stenosis, false aneurysm at surgical site

REFERENCES

1. Meschia JF, Bushnell C, Boden-Albala B, et al; and American Heart Association Stroke Council, Council on Cardiovascular and Stroke Nursing, Council on Clinical Cardiology, Council on Functional Genomics and Translational Biology, Council on Hypertension. Guidelines for the primary prevention of stroke: a statement for healthcare professionals from the American Heart Association/American Stroke Association. *Stroke.* 2014;45(12):3754–3832.
2. Orrapin S, Rerkasem K. Carotid endarterectomy for symptomatic carotid stenosis. *Cochrane Database Syst Rev.* 2017;(6):CD001081.
3. Chaturvedi S, Bruno A, Feasby T, et al. Carotid endarterectomy—an evidence-based review: report of the Therapeutics and Technology Assessment Subcommittee of the American Academy of Neurology. *Neurology.* 2005;65(6):794–801.
4. Bonati LH, Lyrer P, Ederle J, et al. Percutaneous transluminal balloon angioplasty and stenting for carotid artery stenosis. *Cochrane Database Syst Rev.* 2012;(9):CD000515.
5. Antoniou GA, Georgiadis GS, Georgakarakos EI, et al. Meta-analysis and meta-regression analysis of outcomes of carotid endarterectomy and stenting in the elderly. *JAMA Surg.* 2013;148(12):1140–1152.
6. Moresoli P, Habib B, Reynier P, et al. Carotid stenting versus endarterectomy for asymptomatic carotid artery stenosis: a systematic review and meta-analysis. *Stroke.* 2017;48(8):2150–2157.

ADDITIONAL READING
- Go C, Avgerinos ED, Chaer RA, et al. Long-term clinical outcomes and cardiovascular events after carotid endarterectomy. *Ann Vasc Surg.* 2015;29(6):1265–1271.
- Jonas DE, Feltner C, Amick HR, et al. Screening for asymptomatic carotid artery stenosis: a systematic review and meta-analysis for the U.S. Preventive Services Task Force. *Ann Intern Med.* 2014;161(5):336–346.
- Paraskevas KI, Mikhailidis DP, Veith FJ. Comparison of the five 2011 guidelines for the treatment of carotid stenosis. *J Vasc Surg.* 2012;55(5):1504–1508.
- Rundek T, Sacco R. Risk factor management to prevent first stroke. *Neurol Clin.* 2008;26(4):1007–1045, ix.

 SEE ALSO

Algorithms: Stroke; Transient Ischemic Attack and Transient Neurologic Defects

CODES

ICD10
- I65.29 Occlusion and stenosis of unspecified carotid artery
- I65.21 Occlusion and stenosis of right carotid artery
- I65.22 Occlusion and stenosis of left carotid artery

CLINICAL PEARLS
- Atherosclerosis is responsible for 90% of all cases of carotid artery stenosis.
- Duplex US is the best initial imaging modality.
- Antiplatelet therapy and aggressive treatment of vascular risk factors are the mainstays of medical therapy.
- Compared with CEA, CAS increases the risk of any stroke and decreases the risk of MI. For every 1,000 patients opting for stenting rather than endarterectomy, 19 more patients would have strokes and 10 fewer would have MIs.

C

CARPAL TUNNEL SYNDROME
Rahul Kapur, MD • Samuel Renier, MD

 BASICS

DESCRIPTION
- Symptomatic compression neuropathy of the median nerve
- Increased pressure within the carpal tunnel leads to compression of the median nerve and characteristic motor–sensory findings.
- The dorsal aspect of the carpal tunnel is composed of the carpal bones. The transverse carpal ligament defines the palmar boundary.
  - The carpal tunnel contains nine flexor tendons and the median nerve.
- Symptoms most commonly affect the dominant hand; >50% of patients will experience bilateral symptoms.
- System(s) affected: musculoskeletal, nervous

ALERT
- Increased incidence during pregnancy (up to 20–45%)
- Increased incidence with chronic hemodialysis (2–31%)

EPIDEMIOLOGY
- Predominant age: 40 to 60 years
- Predominant sex: female > male (3:1 to 10:1)

Incidence
- Two peaks: late 50s (women), late 70s (both genders)
- Incidence up to 276/100,000 has been reported.
- Incidence increases with age.

Prevalence
- 4% in women and 2% in men; 50 cases per 1,000 individuals per year in United States
- 14% in patients with diabetes without neuropathy and 30% in patients with diabetic neuropathy
- Rising prevalence may be the result of increasing lifespan and increasing prevalence of diabetes.
- Most expensive upper extremity musculoskeletal disorder; >$2 billion per year
- Carpal tunnel release (CTR) is one of the most frequently performed hand/wrist procedures, with approximately 600,000 CTR procedures per year.
- Median time lost by U.S. workers with carpal tunnel syndrome (CTS) = 28 days

ETIOLOGY AND PATHOPHYSIOLOGY
- Combination of mechanical trauma, inflammation, increased pressure, and ischemic injury to the median nerve within the carpal tunnel
- Acute CTS caused by rapid and sustained pressure in carpal tunnel, usually secondary to trauma, may require urgent surgical decompression.
- Distal radius fractures and volar lunate dislocations increase risk.
- Chronic CTS divided into four categories:
  - Idiopathic: combination of edema and fibrous hypertrophy without inflammation
  - Anatomic: persistent median artery, ganglion cyst, infection, space-occupying lesion in carpal tunnel
  - Systemic: associated with conditions such as obesity, diabetes, hypothyroidism, rheumatoid arthritis, amyloidosis, scleroderma, renal failure, and drug toxicity
  - Exertional: repetitive use of hands and wrists, repeated palmar impact, use of vibratory tools

Genetics
- Unknown; however, a familial type has been reported.
- More likely to experience CTS if there is a first-degree relative with CTS.

RISK FACTORS
- Prolonged postures in extremes of wrist flexion and extension including activities such as gardening, cycling, or tennis; repetitive exposure to vibration (motorcycle riding)
  - There is insufficient evidence to implicate computer use in the development of CTS.
  - Jobs most at risk for CTS: use of vibratory tools, food processing and packing, dairy and poultry workers, and assembly workers
- Alterations of fluid balance: pregnancy, rheumatoid arthritis, obesity, renal failure, hypothyroidism, congestive heart failure, hemodialysis
  - CTS is the most common neuropathy in patients with rheumatoid arthritis.
- Neuropathic factors: diabetes, alcoholism, vitamin deficiency, or exposure to toxins
- More common in patients with concomitant migraine headaches

GENERAL PREVENTION
There is no known prevention for CTS. It is recommended to take occasional (e.g., hourly) breaks when doing repetitive work involving hands or if prolonged occupational exposure to vibratory tools. It is suspected that weight loss may help prevent CTS.

COMMONLY ASSOCIATED CONDITIONS
- Diabetes, obesity; pregnancy; hypothyroidism
- Osteoarthritis of small joints of hand and wrist
- Hyperparathyroidism, hypocalcemia
- Hemodialysis

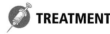 **DIAGNOSIS**

HISTORY
- Nocturnal pain, numbness, and tingling of the thumb, index, long, and radial portion of the ring fingers; patients may not localize or alternatively describe the entire hand as being affected.
- Hand weakness during tasks such as opening jars is often noted early in the disorder.
- Atypical presentation involves paresthesias in radial digits, with pain radiating proximally along median nerve to elbow and sometimes the shoulder.
- Symptoms characteristically are relieved by shaking or rubbing the hands ("Flick sign").
- During waking hours, symptoms occur when driving, talking on the phone, and occasionally when using the hands for repetitive maneuvers.
- Presence of predisposing factors, such as diabetes, rheumatoid arthritis, chronic hemodialysis, obesity, acromegaly, pregnancy, or occupational exposure

PHYSICAL EXAM
- Durkan compression test: Direct compression of median nerve at carpal tunnel for 30 seconds elicits symptoms (87% sensitivity, 90% specificity).
- Positive Phalen sign: Holding the wrist in fully flexed position for 60 seconds precipitates paresthesias, numbness, or pain (68% sensitivity, 73% specificity).
- Positive Tinel sign: Tapping over the palmar surface of the wrist proximal to the carpal tunnel may produce an electric sensation along the distribution of the median nerve (50% sensitivity, 77% specificity).

- Square-sign test: Positive if measurement of wrist width/height >0.7 (53% sensitivity, 80% specificity)
- Loss of two-point discrimination
- Decreased sensation to pain
- Wasting of thenar musculature is a late sign and should not be used to rule out CTS (16% sensitivity, 94% specificity).

DIFFERENTIAL DIAGNOSIS
- Cervical spondylosis (carpal tunnel may also occur with cervical spine disease; "double crush")
- Generalized peripheral neuropathy
- Brachial plexopathy, in particular upper trunk
- CNS disorders (multiple sclerosis, cerebral infarction)
- Thoracic outlet syndrome
- Pronator syndrome (median nerve compression at the elbow)
- Anterior interosseous syndrome
- Ulnar nerve compression
- Musculoskeletal disorders of the wrist:
  - Trauma or distal radius fracture
  - Degenerative joint disease
  - Rheumatoid arthritis
  - Ganglion cyst
  - de Quervain tenosynovitis
- Scleroderma

DIAGNOSTIC TESTS & INTERPRETATION
- The most accurate screening forms are the CTS-6, Kamath and Stothard questionnaire, and Katz and Stirrat hand symptom diagram.
- No laboratory test is diagnostic.
  - Normal serum thyrotropin (thyroid-stimulating hormone [TSH]), HbA1c, ESR, and normal serum chemistries help exclude secondary conditions associated with CTS.
- Special tests
  - Electrodiagnostic studies
    - Sensitivity 85%; specificity 95%
    - Most useful with low pretest probability and suspicion of alternate peripheral neuropathy, radiculopathy, or "double-crush" phenomenon with compression at multiple locations
    - Nerve conduction studies compare latency and amplitude of median nerve signals across the carpal tunnel
- The most sensitive indicator is median sensory distal latency, which is prolonged in CTS.
- Standard radiographs of the wrist evaluate bony anatomy and degenerative joint disease but are not necessary to diagnose CTS.
- Ultrasound—rapid, noninvasive, painless modality; sensitivity 87%; specificity 83%; hypoechoic median nerve cross-sectional area >9 mm
- Magnetic resonance imaging is of limited benefit.

TREATMENT

GENERAL MEASURES
- Strong evidence supports immobilization (brace/splint/orthosis) and the use of local steroid (methylprednisolone) injection in improving patient-reported outcomes.
- Strong evidence indicates that surgical treatment of CTS results in better functional improvements at 1 year compared with nonoperative treatment.
- A trial of nonoperative management is generally recommended for patients with mild to moderate CTS symptoms.

MEDICATION

First Line

Mainstay treatments for mild to moderate CTS include night splinting (12 weeks) and local corticosteroid injection.

- Recent research has shown significantly improved outcomes in pain, function, and remission of nocturnal paresthesia with a single local corticosteroid injection compared to night splints at 1-, 3-, and 6-month follow-up (1)[A].
- A positive response to injection may signal a higher likelihood of benefit of surgery.
- Side effects of injection include reducing collagen and proteoglycan synthesis, limiting tenocytes, and reducing mechanical strength of tendon, leading to further degeneration and risk for rupture.
- No evidence supports multiple trials of injection; thus, surgery should be considered for those with refractory or recurrent symptoms.
- Those with moderate to severe disease benefit from early surgery.

Second Line

- Oral corticosteroids are less effective than local corticosteroid injection but more effective than placebo in the short term; long-term benefits of oral corticosteroid use have not been shown (2)[A].
  - The long-term risks of even a short course of steroids should be balanced with the limited potential benefit of symptom improvement.
- Gabapentin shown to be effective in managing CTS symptoms.
  - 300 mg daily been shown to be more effective than 100 mg daily while maintaining minimal to no side effects (3)[A].
- Although commonly used, nonsteroidal anti-inflammatory medications provide no significant improvement in symptoms compared to placebo.
  - Contraindications: GI intolerance
  - Precautions: GI side effects of NSAIDs may preclude their use in selected patients.
- Hand therapy has been shown to improve patient function (4)[B].

ISSUES FOR REFERRAL

Preoperative electrodiagnostic studies are generally obtained prior to any surgical intervention.

SURGERY/OTHER PROCEDURES

- Completely dividing the transverse carpal ligament provides symptom relief in >95% of patients.
- Surgical decompression is an outpatient procedure performed under local or regional anesthesia.
- Incisional healing generally takes 2 weeks; an additional 2 weeks may be required before using the affected hand for tasks requiring strength.
- Complete resolution of numbness in 93.8% of patients with severe CTS by EMG at follow-up of 9.3 years (5)[B].
- The approach should be based on surgeon and patient preference.
  - Endoscopic surgery results in higher patient satisfaction rates, greater key pinch strength, earlier return to work times, and lower incidence of scar-related complications (6)[A].
  - Patients undergoing endoscopic release are at greater risk of transient nerve injury, but this effect is not permanent (6)[A].

COMPLEMENTARY & ALTERNATIVE MEDICINE

- No trial data support the use of vitamin B_6 in the prevention or treatment of CTS.

- Acupuncture shown to be as effective as short-term oral prednisolone therapy and may be used as an alternative therapy or as an adjuvant.
- No data to support chiropractic therapy as a treatment for CTS.

ADMISSION, INPATIENT, AND NURSING CONSIDERATIONS

Outpatient

 ONGOING CARE

FOLLOW-UP RECOMMENDATIONS

Patient Monitoring

- Patients treated nonoperatively (splinting, injections) require follow-up over 4 to 12 weeks to ensure adequate progress.
- There is only limited, low-quality evidence to suggest that rehabilitation exercises such as wrist immobilization, ice therapy, and multimodal hand rehabilitation are beneficial.
- 7–20% of patients treated surgically may experience recurrence.

DIET

Insufficient evidence to suggest a specific diet helps reduce risk or alleviate symptoms of CTS.

PROGNOSIS

- Approximately 85% of patients who initially respond to conservative therapy will experience reemergence of symptoms within 4 years.
- A positive Phalen test and thenar wasting are factors that have been associated with poorer outcomes with conservative management.
- Patients with severe CTS may not recover completely after surgical release. Paresthesias and weakness may persist, but nighttime symptoms generally resolve.
- If untreated, more severe cases of CTS can lead to numbness and weakness in the hand, atrophy of the thenar muscles, and permanent loss of median nerve function.

COMPLICATIONS

- Postoperative infection (rare)
- Injury to the median nerve or its recurrent (motor) branch
- Pillar pain (tenderness adjacent to the actual ligament release sites of the trapezial ridge and hook of hamate) in the months following CTR (prevalence of 6–36%)

REFERENCES

1. de Moraes VY, Queiroz Jr J, Raduan-Neto J. Nonsurgical treatment for symptomatic carpal tunnel syndrome: a randomized clinical trial comparing local corticosteroid injection versus night orthosis. *J Hand Surg Am*. 2021;46(4):295.e1–300.e1.
2. Huisstede BM, Randsdorp MS, van den Brink J, et al. Effectiveness of oral pain medication and corticosteroid injections for carpal tunnel syndrome: a systematic review. *Arch Phys Med Rehabil*. 2018;99(8):1609.e10–1622.e10.
3. Eftekharsadat B, Babaei-Ghazani A, Habibzadeh A. The efficacy of 100 and 300 mg gabapentin in the treatment of carpal tunnel syndrome. *Iran J Pharm Res*. 2015;14(4):1275–1280.
4. Ostergaard PJ, Meyer MA, Earp BE. Non-operative treatment of carpal tunnel syndrome. *Curr Rev Musculoskelet Med*. 2020;13(2):141–147.
5. Tang CQY, Lai SWH, Tay SC. Long-term outcome of carpal tunnel release surgery in patients with severe carpal tunnel syndrome. *Bone Joint J*. 2017;99-B(10):1348–1353.
6. Li Y, Luo W, Wu G, et al. Open versus endoscopic carpal tunnel release: a systematic review and meta-analysis of randomized controlled trials. *BMC Musculoskelet Disord*. 2020;21(1):272.

ADDITIONAL READING

- Calandruccio JH, Thompson NB. Carpal tunnel syndrome: making evidence-based treatment decisions. *Orthop Clin North Am*. 2018;49(2):223–229.
- Dabbagh A, MacDermid JC, Yong J, et al. Diagnosing carpal tunnel syndrome: diagnostic test accuracy of scales, questionnaires, and hand symptom diagrams—a systematic review. *J Orthop Sports Phys Ther*. 2020;50(11):622–631.
- Graham B, Peljovich AE, Afra R, et al. The American Academy of Orthopaedic Surgeons evidence-based clinical practice guideline on: management of carpal tunnel syndrome. *J Bone Joint Surg Am*. 2016;98(20):1750–1754.
- Hermiz SJ, Kalliainen LK. Evidence-based medicine: current evidence in the diagnosis and management of carpal tunnel syndrome. *Plast Reconstr Surg*. 2017;140(1):120e–129e.
- Ingram J, Mauck BM, Thompson NB, et al. Cost, value, and patient satisfaction in carpal tunnel surgery. *Orthop Clin North Am*. 2018;49(4):503–507.
- Kronlage SC, Menendez ME. The benefit of carpal tunnel release in patients with electrophysiologically moderate to severe disease. *J Hand Surg Am*. 2015;40(3):438.e1–444.e1.
- Paryavi E, Zimmerman RM, Means KR Jr. Endoscopic compared with open operative treatment of carpal tunnel syndrome. *JBJS Rev*. 2016;4(6):e2. doi:10.2106/JBJS.RVW.15.00071.

 SEE ALSO

- Arthritis, Rheumatoid (RA); Hypoparathyroidism; Lupus Erythematosus, Systemic (SLE); Scleroderma
- Algorithms: Carpal Tunnel Syndrome; Pain in Upper Extremity

 CODES

ICD10

- G56.0 Carpal tunnel syndrome
- G56.01 Carpal tunnel syndrome, right upper limb
- G56.02 Carpal tunnel syndrome, left upper limb

CLINICAL PEARLS

- Paresthesias associated with CTS are characteristically confined to the thumb, index, long, and radial half of the ring fingers of the affected hand.
- Thenar atrophy is a late finding, indicating severe nerve damage, and is associated with a higher likelihood of failure with conservative management.
- The Durkan (carpal compression) test is superior to Tinel sign (tapping on median nerve over carpal tunnel) and Phalen maneuver (holding wrists in flexion) for the clinical diagnosis of CTS.
- Often, the diagnosis is clinical; electrodiagnostic studies provide objective evidence of nerve compression and are sensitive and specific for diagnosis.
- Steroid injection and night splinting are mainstays of treatment for mild to moderate CTS.
- Surgical release of the carpal tunnel is >90% effective long term.

CATARACT
Yasir Ahmed, MD • Ingrid U. Scott, MD, MPH

BASICS

DESCRIPTION
- A cataract is any opacity or discoloration of the lens, localized or generalized; the term is usually reserved for changes that affect visual acuity (1).
- Etymology: from Latin *catarractes*, for "waterfall"; named after foamy appearance of opacity
- Leading cause of blindness worldwide, estimated 20 million people (1)
- Types include the following:
  - Age related: approximately 90% of cases
  - Metabolic (diabetes via accelerated sorbitol pathway, hypocalcemia, Wilson disease)
  - Congenital (1/250 newborns; 10–38% of childhood blindness)
  - Systemic disease associated (myotonic dystrophy, atopic dermatitis [AD])
  - Secondary to associated eye disease, so-called complicated (e.g., uveitis associated with juvenile rheumatoid arthritis or sarcoid, tumor such as melanoma or retinoblastoma)
  - Traumatic (e.g., heat, electric shock, radiation, concussion, perforating eye injuries, intraocular foreign body)
  - Toxic/nutritional (e.g., corticosteroids)
- Morphologic classification:
  - Nuclear: exaggeration of normal aging changes of *central* lens nucleus, often associated with myopia due to increased refractive index of lens (Some elderly patients consequently may be able to read again *without spectacles*, so-called "second sight.")
  - Cortical: outer portion of lens; may involve anterior, posterior, or equatorial cortex; radial, spoke-like opacities
  - Subcapsular: Posterior subcapsular cataract has more profound effect on vision than nuclear or cortical cataract; patients particularly troubled under conditions of miosis; near vision frequently impaired more than distance vision
- System(s) affected: nervous

Geriatric Considerations
Some degree of cataract formation is expected in all people >70 years of age.

Pediatric Considerations
See "Congenital cataract"; may present as leukokoria

Pregnancy Considerations
See "Congenital cataract" (i.e., medications, metabolic dysfunction, intrauterine infection, and malnutrition)

EPIDEMIOLOGY
Incidence
- ~48% of the 37 million cases of blindness worldwide result from cataracts (1).
- Leading cause of treatable blindness and vision loss in developing countries (1)
- Predominant age: depends on type of cataract

Prevalence
- Cataract type and prevalence are highly variable based on population demographics.
- An estimated 50% of people 65 to 74 years of age and 70% of people >75 years of age have age-related cataract.

ETIOLOGY AND PATHOPHYSIOLOGY
- Age-related cataract:
  - Continual addition of layers of lens fibers throughout life creates hard, dehydrated lens nucleus that impairs vision (nuclear cataract).
  - Aging alters biochemical and osmotic balance required for lens clarity; outer lens layers hydrate and become opaque, adversely affecting vision.
- Congenital:
  - Usually unknown etiology
  - Drugs (corticosteroids in 1st trimester, sulfonamides)
  - Metabolic (diabetes in mother, galactosemia in fetus)
  - Intrauterine infection during 1st trimester (e.g., rubella, herpes, mumps)
  - Maternal malnutrition
- Other cataract types:
  - Common feature is a biochemical/osmotic imbalance that disrupts lens clarity.
  - Local changes in lens protein distribution lead to light scattering (lens opacity).

Genetics
- Congenital (e.g., chromosomal disorders [Down syndrome])
- Genetics of age-related cataracts is not yet established but likely multifactorial contribution.

RISK FACTORS
- Aging
- Cigarette smoking
- Ultraviolet (UV) sunlight exposure
- Diabetes
- Prolonged high-dose steroids
- Positive family history
- Alcohol

GENERAL PREVENTION
- Use of UV protective glasses
- Avoidance of tobacco products
- Effective control of diabetes
- Care with high-dose, long-term steroid use (systemic therapy > inhaled treatment)
- Protective methods using pharmaceutical intervention (e.g., antioxidants, acetylsalicylic acid [ASA], hormone replacement therapy [HRT]) show no proven benefit to date.

COMMONLY ASSOCIATED CONDITIONS
- Diabetes (especially with poor glucose control)
- Myotonic dystrophy (90% of patients develop a visually innocuous change in 3rd decade; becomes disabling in 5th decade)
- AD (10% of patients with severe AD develop cataracts in 2nd to 4th decades; often bilateral)
- Neurofibromatosis type 2

- Associated ocular disease or "secondary cataract" (e.g., chronic anterior uveitis, acute [or repetitive] angle-closure glaucoma or high myopia)
- Drug induced (e.g., steroids, chlorpromazine)
- Trauma

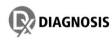

DIAGNOSIS

HISTORY
- Age-related cataract:
  - Decreased visual acuity, blurred vision, distortion, or "ghosting" of images (1)
  - Problems with visual acuity in any lighting condition
  - Falls or accidents; injuries (e.g., hip fracture)
- Congenital: often asymptomatic; leukokoria; parents notice child's visual inattention or strabismus.
- Other types of cataract:
  - May also present with decreased visual acuity
  - Appropriate clinical history or signs to help with diagnosis

PHYSICAL EXAM
- Visual acuity assessment for all cataracts
  - Glare testing allows further assessment of visual dysfunction.
- Age-related cataract: lens opacity on eye examination
- Congenital:
  - Lens opacity present at birth or within 3 months of birth
  - Leukocoria (white pupil), strabismus, nystagmus, signs of an associated syndrome (as with Down or rubella syndrome)
  - *Note*: must always rule out ocular tumor; early diagnosis and treatment of retinoblastoma may be lifesaving.
- Other types of cataract: may present with decreased visual acuity associated with characteristic physical findings (e.g., metabolic, trauma)

DIFFERENTIAL DIAGNOSIS
- An opaque-appearing eye may be due to opacities of the cornea (e.g., scarring, edema, calcification), lens opacities, tumor, or retinal detachment. Biomicroscopic examination (slit lamp) or careful ophthalmoscopic exam should provide a diagnosis.
- In the elderly, visual impairment is often due to multiple factors such as cataract and macular degeneration, both contributing to visual loss.
- Age-related cataract is significant if symptoms and ophthalmic exam support cataract as a major cause of vision impairment.
- Congenital lens opacity in the absence of other ocular pathology may cause severe amblyopia.
- *Note*: Cataract *does not* produce a relative afferent pupillary reaction defect. Abnormal pupillary reactions mandate further evaluation for other pathology.

DIAGNOSTIC TESTS & INTERPRETATION
- Visual quality assessment: Glare testing, contrast sensitivity is sometimes indicated.
- Retinal/macular function assessment: potential acuity meter testing
- Workup of the underlying process

Test Interpretation

Consistent with lens changes found in the type of cataract; however, diagnosis is made by clinical examination

TREATMENT

- Outpatient (usually)
- ~1.64 million cataract extractions in the United States yearly (2)

GENERAL MEASURES

Eye protection from UV light

MEDICATION

There are currently no medications to prevent or slow the progression of cataracts.

ISSUES FOR REFERRAL

If the patient has cataracts and symptoms do not seem to support recommendation for surgery, a second opinion by another ophthalmologist may be indicated.

SURGERY/OTHER PROCEDURES

- Age-related cataract:
  - Surgical removal is indicated if visual impairment producing symptoms are distressing to the patient, interfering with lifestyle or occupation, or posing a risk for fall or injury (2)[A].
  - Because significant cataracts may develop gradually, the patient may not be aware of how it has changed their lifestyle. The physician may note a significant cataract, and the patient reports "no problems." Thus, evaluation requires an effective physician-patient relationship.
  - Preoperative evaluation: by the primary care physician:
    - Patients on anticoagulants may need to be temporarily discontinued 1 to 2 weeks before surgery if possible (but usually not necessary, thus need to discuss with ophthalmologist).
    - Patients who have ever taken an α-blocker such as tamsulosin (Flomax) should alert their ophthalmologist due to increased risk of intraoperative floppy iris syndrome [IFIS] even in patients who no longer use these drugs.
  - Anesthesia: usually topical with sedation and monitoring of vital signs, sometimes local injection as well
  - Surgical technique: cataract extraction via phacoemulsification through small incisions created by blade or laser, followed by implantation of a prosthetic intraocular lens; lenses have power calculated based on the size of the eye and curvature of the cornea usually to correct for distance vision; surgery performed on one (usually worse) eye, with contralateral surgery after recovery and if deemed necessary
    - Laser-assisted cataract surgery: Laser allows automated completion of certain steps of cataract surgery such as incisions, opening the lens capsule, and breaking up

the cataract before surgical removal with phacoemulsification (3).
  - Postoperative care: usually protective eye shield as directed, topical antibiotic, NSAIDs, and steroid ophthalmic medications; avoid lifting or bending for at least a week. Keeping eye protected in general.
- Congenital cataract:
  - Treatment is surgical removal of cataract. Newborns may require surgery within days to reduce the risk of severe amblyopia. The use of lens implants is controversial because the eyes are growing.
  - Postoperative care: long-term patching program for the good eye to combat amblyopia; refractive correction of operative eye, with multiple repeat examinations; challenging for physician and parents

ONGOING CARE

FOLLOW-UP RECOMMENDATIONS

Patient Monitoring

- As the cataract progresses, the glasses or contact lens prescription may change to maintain vision. When this is no longer successful and interferes with patient's activities of daily living, surgery is indicated.
- Following surgery, spectacle correction may still be required to maximize near and/or far visual acuity. Refraction is usually prescribed several weeks after surgery.

PATIENT EDUCATION

Medline Plus on cataracts at: https://www.nlm.nih.gov/medlineplus/cataract.html

PROGNOSIS

- Ocular prognosis is good after cataract removal if no prior or coexisting ocular disease: 94.3% of otherwise healthy eyes achieve best-corrected visual acuity of 20/40 or better. Success rates are lower with comorbidities such as diabetes and glaucoma (4).
- Posterior capsular opacification can occur after cataract surgery and can cause a decrease in vision (14.7–42.7% of eyes, usually treated with Nd:YAG laser capsulotomy in the office with a rate of 4–25.3%).
- In congenital cataracts, prognosis often is poorer because of the high risk of amblyopia.

COMPLICATIONS

- Vary widely from delay in visual recovery or protracted visual discomfort to blindness and loss of the eye
- Complications are uncommon in general (<2% of eyes). Among the complications, a posterior capsular rupture is significant as it may require additional steps during surgery (5)[B].
- Poor preoperative visual acuity is related to surgical complications.

REFERENCES

1. Asbell PA, Dualan I, Mindel J, et al. Age-related cataract. *Lancet*. 2005;365(9459):599–609.
2. Riaz Y, Mehta JS, Wormald R, et al. Surgical interventions for age-related cataract. *Cochrane Database Syst Rev*. 2006;(4):CD001323.
3. Kolb CM, Shajari M, Mathys L, et al. Comparison of femtosecond laser-assisted cataract surgery and conventional cataract surgery: a meta-analysis and systematic review. *J Cataract Refract Surg*. 2020;46(8):1075–1085.
4. Biber JM, Sandoval HP, Trivedi RH, et al. Comparison of the incidence and visual significance of posterior capsule opacification between multifocal spherical, monofocal spherical, and monofocal aspheric intraocular lenses. *J Cataract Refract Surg*. 2009;35(7):1234–1238.
5. Lundström M, Barry P, Henry Y, et al. Visual outcome of cataract surgery; study from the European Registry of Quality Outcomes for Cataract and Refractive Surgery. *J Cataract Refract Surg*. 2013;39(5):673–679.

 SEE ALSO

- Floppy Iris Syndrome
- Algorithm: Cataracts

CODES

ICD10

- H26.049 Anterior subcapsular polar infantile and juvenile cataract, unspecified eye
- H26.069 Combined forms of infantile and juvenile cataract, unspecified eye
- H26.231 Glaucomatous flecks (subcapsular), right eye

CLINICAL PEARLS

- Cataracts are the leading cause of blindness worldwide; most cataracts are age-related.
- The primary indication for cataract surgery is visual impairment leading to significant lifestyle changes for the patient.
- For congenital cataracts, always consider ocular tumor because early diagnosis and treatment of retinoblastoma may be lifesaving.

CELIAC DISEASE
Lloyd A. Runser, MD, MPH, FAAFP • Maegan M. Riggin, MD

BASICS

DESCRIPTION
- An immune-mediated reaction to dietary gluten (found in wheat, barley, rye) primarily affecting the small intestine in genetically predisposed individuals. Affected individuals cannot tolerate gliadin (a component of gluten found in rye, barley, and wheat).
- Presentations
  - Typical
    - Diarrheal illness characterized by villous atrophy with symptoms of malabsorption (steatorrhea, weight loss, vitamin deficiencies, anemia); resolves with a gluten-free diet (GFD)
    - <50% of adults present with gastrointestinal (GI) symptoms.
  - Atypical
    - Minor GI symptoms, with a myriad of extraintestinal manifestations (e.g., anemia, LFTs, dental enamel defects, neurologic symptoms, infertility)
  - Asymptomatic (silent) disease
    - Found when screening first-degree relatives
    - Positive laboratory tests and genetics, without signs/symptoms; normal histology on biopsy
- System(s) affected: GI
- Synonym(s): celiac sprue; gluten-sensitive enteropathy

EPIDEMIOLOGY
Incidence
- 1 to 13/100,000 worldwide (1)
- 6.5/100,000 in United States (2)
- Primarily affects those of Northern European ancestry
- Predominant sex: female > male (3:2)

Prevalence
- 0.7% in the United States; an estimated 3 million Americans have celiac disease (3).
- 1% worldwide (1)

ETIOLOGY AND PATHOPHYSIOLOGY
Sensitivity to gluten, specifically gliadin protein fraction. Tissue transglutaminase (tTG) modification of the gliadin protein leads to immunologic cross-reactivity, inflammation, and tissue damage (villous atrophy) with subsequent GI symptoms and malabsorption.

Genetics
Homogenicity for *HLA-DQ2/DQ8* increases risk of celiac disease and enteropathy-associated T-cell lymphoma.

RISK FACTORS
- First-degree relatives: 5–20% incidence (1)
- Second-degree relatives

Pediatric Considerations
No other risk factors (e.g., grain processing, genetically modified organisms, hygiene and illness during childhood, breastfeeding, time of introduction of solid foods, pollution, tobacco use, and medication) explain why some susceptible individuals develop celiac, whereas others do not (4).

COMMONLY ASSOCIATED CONDITIONS
- *Dermatitis herpetiformis (DH)*: 85% of patients with DH have celiac disease. All patients should follow GFD (1).
- Secondary lactase deficiency
- Osteopenia and osteoporosis
- Thyroid disease: Hashimoto thyroiditis
- Type 1 diabetes: 3–10% of patients with type 1 diabetes also have celiac disease (1).

- Symptomatic iron deficiency: 10–15% have celiac disease.
- Elevated AST and ALT (with no direct cause)
- Hyposplenism
- Oral apthous ulcers
- Irritable bowel syndrome (IBS)
- Restless leg syndrome
- Celiac disease is associated with increased risk for adenocarcinoma and lymphoma of the small bowel.
  - The risk of lymphoproliferative malignancies depends on small intestinal histopathology.
  - Little to no increased risk in latent celiac disease (seropositive but normal biopsy)
- Associated autoimmune conditions (type 1 diabetes, autoimmune thyroiditis, primary biliary cirrhosis, autoimmune hepatitis, psoriasis, Sjögren disease)
- Associated genetic conditions (Down syndrome, IgA deficiency, Turner syndrome, Williams syndrome)

Pregnancy Considerations
- Prevalence of celiac disease: 2.5 to 3.5 times higher in women with unexplained infertility
- Up to 19% of men with celiac disease have androgen resistance. Semen quality and likelihood of pregnancy increase with GFD.
- Higher rates of low birth weight, prematurity, spontaneous abortions, intrauterine growth restriction, and stillbirths

Pediatric Considerations
Children with celiac disease at higher risk for type 1 diabetes, Down syndrome, Turner syndrome, Williams syndrome, IgA deficiency, and autoimmune thyroid disease (5)[C].

DIAGNOSIS

HISTORY
- Diarrhea and cramping are the most common GI symptoms.
- Other symptoms include: Steatorrhea (fatty stools); abdominal pain or distension; nausea, vomiting, flatulence; weight loss, weakness, fatigue; muscle cramps; bone and joint pain; paresthesias in hands and feet; constipation
- Clinical signs include: delayed puberty; iron deficiency anemia; recurrent aphthous stomatitis; dental enamel hyperplasia; anxiety, depression; migraines; anorexia; encopresis
- In children, malabsorption may manifest as failure to thrive, short stature, or chronic fatigue (5).

PHYSICAL EXAM
Physical examination is often normal. Findings include:
- Orthostatic hypotension
- Peripheral edema
- Oropharynx: aphthous stomatitis, glossitis, cheilosis
- Skin: dermatitis herpetiformis (symmetric erythematous papules and blisters on elbows, knees, buttocks, and back), signs of anemia
- Abdomen: distention

DIFFERENTIAL DIAGNOSIS
- Gluten allergy—type II allergic reaction with signs of anaphylaxis
- Nonceliac gluten sensitivity—GI symptoms and/or systemic symptoms improved by GFD but without biomarkers characteristic of celiac disease
- Short bowel syndrome, small intestinal bacterial overgrowth

- Lactose intolerance; dyspepsia
- Gastroesophageal reflux disease (GERD)
- Pancreatic exocrine insufficiency
- Crohn disease; Whipple disease
- Tropical sprue; hypogammaglobulinemia
- Intestinal lymphoma; microscopic colitis
- Autoimmune enteropathy; HIV enteropathy
- Acute enteritis; radiation enteritis
- Eosinophilic gastroenteritis; giardiasis
- Irritable bowel syndrome (IBS)

DIAGNOSTIC TESTS & INTERPRETATION
Tissue biopsy is the gold standard for diagnosis.

Initial Tests (lab, imaging)
- Do not base diagnosis solely on serology in adults. Patients with symptoms highly suggestive of celiac disease or those with positive serologies should undergo endoscopy for small bowel biopsy while on a gluten-containing diet.
- Biopsy and histologic examination of duodenal bulb during routine upper endoscopy increases the diagnostic yield of celiac disease. Sampling of the duodenal bulb and the distal duodenum is recommended to improve histologic confirmation of celiac disease.
- IgA anti-tTG is the preferred serologic test in patients >2 years (1)[C].
- Total serum IgA to screen for IgA deficiency

> **ALERT**
> Positive IgA tTG has high sensitivity and specificity (sensitivity, 95–98%; specificity, 95%) if on normal (non–gluten-free) diet for at least 4 weeks.

- IgA-deficient patients have false-negative IgA anti-tTG antibodies.
- IgA deficiency is 10 to 15 times more prevalent in patients with celiac disease.
- The tTG antibody test is the preferred test (over the deamidated gliadin peptide [DGP] antibody).

Follow-Up Tests & Special Considerations
- If patient is IgA deficient OR if IgA anti-tTG are negative, follow up with anti-DGP IgA and IgG.
  - Sensitivity, 94%; specificity, 99% (~anti-tTG)
- Do not use HLA DQ serotyping for initial diagnosis. Consider if discrepant serology–histology results in patients unable to test on GFD and children with Down syndrome (1)[C].
- Consider bone mineral density testing at the time of diagnosis and after 1 year (if osteopenia/osteoporosis on initial testing) or 2 years (if normal initially and patient still symptomatic or nonadherent to diet).
- Younger age on diagnosis, less severe initial histologic damage, and male gender increase likelihood for achieving mucosal recovery.
- Members of a family who have more than one individual with CD are at higher risk. Screen family members including second-degree relatives (1)[C].

Pediatric Considerations
- Test symptomatic pediatric patients with IgA and IgA anti-tTG antibodies.
- Periodic monitoring with IgA anti-tTG Ab can assess dietary adherence.
- Negative serology cannot rule out CD.
- Consider HLA for high-risk children with negative serology.
- Limit IgA antiendomysial antibodies to patients with illnesses that increase false-positive tTG Ab, such as type I diabetes or autoimmune liver disease.

Diagnostic Procedures/Other
- Endoscopy with a minimum of four biopsies of distal duodenum and two of duodenal bulb at time of initial evaluation correctly diagnose 95% of children (1)[C].
- Video capsule endoscopy is a promising alternative with a sensitivity and specificity of 80% and 95%; particularly helpful if antibody screening and clinical picture are consistent with celiac disease despite nondiagnostic duodenal biopsies

Test Interpretation
Small-bowel biopsy
- Villous atrophy, hyperplasia and lengthening of crypts, infiltration of plasma cells, and intraepithelial lymphocytosis in lamina propria
- Villous atrophy also caused by Crohn disease, radiation enteritis, Giardia, and other food intolerances

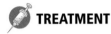

TREATMENT

GENERAL MEASURES
- Gluten-free diet (GFD)—avoid wheat, barley, and rye.
  - Rice, corn, and nut flour are safe and palatable substitutes (1)[C].
  - Grains: uncontaminated oats, rice, corn, tapioca, quinoa, amaranth, sorghum
- Levels of IgA antigliadin normalize with gluten abstinence.
- *Lifelong* abstinence is required; immune response to gluten will recur with resumption of gluten intake.

MEDICATION
First Line
Usually no medications. GFD is primary treatment.

Second Line
- In refractory disease, consult with GI for consideration of choice, dosing, and duration of second-line agents:
  - Steroids (prednisone (1)[C] or budesonide (1)[B])
  - Azathioprine (used with caution; use may lead to lymphoma) (1)[C]
  - Cyclosporine
  - Infliximab
  - Cladribine
- Depending on disease severity, patients may develop nutritional deficiencies that require appropriate supplementation.

ISSUES FOR REFERRAL
- Additional nutritional support with qualified dietitian
- Refractory celiac disease
- Child with positive celiac serology

COMPLEMENTARY & ALTERNATIVE MEDICINE
- Many alternative therapies are under development. Future treatment may include predigestion of gluten with peptidase, tight junction blockade, transglutaminase 2 or HLA DQ2/DQ8 blockers, and induction of immune tolerance (4).
- Patients with celiac disease are at increased risk for pneumococcal infection. Pneumococcal vaccination should be considered, especially for those between the ages of 15 and 64 years who may not have received vaccination.

ONGOING CARE

FOLLOW-UP RECOMMENDATIONS
- Consultation with registered dietitian
- Screen for osteoporosis and treat accordingly.
- Follow-up with GI at 3 to 6 months for serology and 12 months for repeat biopsy if indicated

Patient Monitoring
- Repeat EGD if no clinical response to GFD or relapse in symptoms (1)[C].
- Follow anti-tTG IgA or deaminated antigliadin antibodies as a measure of response/compliance with diet (vs. antigliadin IgA or IgG).

DIET
- Remove gluten: wheat, rye, barley, and products with gluten additives (processed food/meat, medications, hygiene products).
- Dietary change is challenging (especially identifying sources of "hidden" gluten) and should be coordinated with a skilled registered dietitian.

PATIENT EDUCATION
- Discuss how to recognize gluten in various products; highlight potential complications and outcomes of failing to follow a GFD.
- Support groups and self-education
- Celiac Disease Foundation: https://www.celiac.org/; Quick Start Gluten-Free Diet Guide for Celiac Disease & Non-Celiac Gluten Sensitivity: http://celiac.org/wp-content/uploads/2013/12/quick-start-guide.pdf
- National Celiac Association: https://nationalceliac.org/; Beyond Celiac: https://www.beyondceliac.org/

PROGNOSIS
- Good prognosis if adherent to GFD
- Patients should see improvement within 7 days of dietary modification.
- Symptoms usually resolve in 4 to 6 weeks.
- It is unknown whether strict dietary adherence decreases cancer risk.

COMPLICATIONS
- Malignancy: Untreated and refractory patients have increased cancer risk, but successful treatment decreases risk to population baseline (1)[C].
- Refractory disease (rare ~1–2% of all patients)
  - May respond to prednisone
  - May need total parenteral nutrition
- Osteoporosis
- Dehydration; electrolyte depletion
- Vitamin deficiency

REFERENCES

1. Rubio-Tapia A, Hill ID, Kelly CP, et al; for American College of Gastroenterology. ACG clinical guidelines: diagnosis and management of celiac disease. *Am J Gastroenterol*. 2013;108(5):656–677.
2. Riddle MS, Murray JA, Porter CK. The incidence and risk of celiac disease in a healthy US adult population. *Am J Gastroenterol*. 2012;107(8):1248–1255.
3. Rubio-Tapia A, Ludvigsson JF, Brantner TL, et al. The prevalence of celiac disease in the United States. *Am J Gastroenterol*. 2012;107(10):1538–1544.
4. King JA, Jeong J, Underwood FE. Incidence of celiac disease is increasing over time: a systematic review and meta-analysis. *Am J Gastroenterology*. 2020;115(4):507–525. doi:10.14309/ajg.0000000000000523.
5. Bingham SM, Bates MD. Pediatric celiac disease: a review for non-gastroenterologists. *Curr Probl Pediatr Adolesc Health Care*. 2020;50(5):100786.

ADDITIONAL READING
- Husby S, Koletzko S, Korponay-Szabo I, et al. European Society of Paediatric Gastroenterology, Hepatology, and Nutrition guidelines for diagnosing celiac disease 2020. *J Pediatr Gastroenterol Nutr*. 2020;70(1):141–156.
- Husby S, Murray JA, Katzka DA. AGA clinical practice update on diagnosis and monitoring of celiac diease—changing utility of serology and histologic measures: expert review. *Gastroenterology*. 2019;156(4):885–889. doi:10.1053/j.gastro.2018.12.010.
- Lebwohl B, Sanders DS, Green PHR. Coeliac disease. *Lancet*. 2019;391(10115):70–81.
- Vaquero L, Rodriguez-Martin L, Leon F, et al. New coeliac disease treatments and their complications. *Gastroenterol Hepatol*. 2018;41(3):191–204.

 SEE ALSO

Algorithms: Diarrhea, Chronic; Malabsorption Syndrome

 CODES

ICD10
K90.0 Celiac disease

CLINICAL PEARLS
- Screen for celiac disease in patients with nonspecific GI symptoms, presumed IBS, dermatitis herpetiformis, unexplained transaminitis, or unexplained iron deficiency anemia.
- Test total IgA levels along with IgA anti-tTG antibodies in patients >2 years of age. Positive serology is not definitive.
- Diagnostic testing must be completed while on a gluten-containing diet.
- Endoscopic biopsy with histologic examination of the intestinal mucosa is the gold standard for diagnosis.
- Standard of treatment is a gluten-free diet. Patient symptoms should improve in 7 days if fully compliant.

CELLULITIS

Karl T. Clebak, MD, MHA, FAAFP • Jarrett Keller Sell, MD, FAAFP, AAHIVS • Lynn K. Weaver, MD

 BASICS

Skin infections are a common health burden with >650,000 admissions per year in the United States (1).

DESCRIPTION

- An acute bacterial infection of the dermis and subcutaneous tissue
- Types and locations:
  - Periorbital cellulitis: bacterial infection of the eyelid and surrounding tissues
  - Orbital cellulitis: infection of the eye posterior to the septum; sinusitis is most common risk factor.
  - Facial cellulitis: preceded by upper respiratory infection or otitis media
  - Buccal cellulitis: infection of cheek in children associated with bacteremia (common before *Haemophilus influenzae* type B vaccine)
  - Peritonsillar cellulitis: common in children; associated with fever, sore throat, and "hot potato" speech
  - Perianal cellulitis: sharply demarcated, bright, perianal erythema
  - Necrotizing cellulitis: gas-producing bacteria in the lower extremities; more common in diabetics

EPIDEMIOLOGY

- Predominant sex: male = female
- Seasonality increased hospitalizations for cellulitis in the summer with fewer in the winter months (2)

Incidence

27 annual visit rates per 1,000 people for purulent SSTI in 2015 (1); 0.2 to 24.6 per 1000 person years 200/100,000 patient/years

Prevalence

Visits to U.S. ambulatory practices for purulent skin and soft tissue infection (SSTI) range from 5.4 to 11.35 million visits annually (1); 3.3 million new cases in the United States in 2012 costing $15 billion

ETIOLOGY AND PATHOPHYSIOLOGY

Cellulitis is caused by bacterial penetration through a compromise in the epidermis, the protective barrier of the skin.

- Microbiology
  - β-Hemolytic streptococci (groups A, B, C, G, and F), *Staphylococcus aureus*, including MRSA, and gram-negative aerobic bacilli are most common.
  - *S. aureus* seen in periorbital and orbital cellulitis and IV drug users
  - *Pseudomonas aeruginosa* seen in diabetics and other immunocompromised patients
  - *H. influenza* causes buccal cellulitis.
  - Clostridia and non–spore-forming anaerobes: necrotizing cellulitis (crepitant/gangrenous)
  - *Streptococcus agalactiae*: cellulitis following lymph node dissection
  - *Pasteurella multocida* and *Capnocytophaga canimorsus*: cellulitis preceded by bites
  - *Streptococcus iniae*: immunocompromised hosts
  - Rare causes: *Mycobacterium*, fungal (mucormycosis, aspergillosis, syphilis)

Genetics
No genetic pattern

RISK FACTORS

- Disruption of skin barrier: trauma, infection, insect bites, injection drug use, body piercing, maceration
- Inflammation: excoriating skin disorders or radiation therapy
- Edema due to venous insufficiency; lymphatic obstruction due to surgery or congestive heart failure (CHF)
- Elderly, diabetes, hypertension, obesity
- Tinea pedis
- Previous episode of cellulitis
- Recurrent cellulitis:
  - Cellulitis recurrence score (predicts recurrence of lower extremity cellulitis based on presence of lymphedema, chronic venous insufficiency, peripheral vascular disease, and deep venous thrombosis) (3)[A]
  - Recurrent cellulitis is seen in immunocompromised patients (HIV/AIDS), steroids and TNF-α inhibitor therapy, diabetes, hypertension, cancer, peripheral arterial or venous diseases, chronic kidney disease, dialysis, IV or SC drug use (3).

GENERAL PREVENTION

- Good skin hygiene keeping skin well hydrated to avoid dryness and cracking
- Elevation of the extremity, compression stockings, pneumatic pressure pumps to decrease edema
- Maintain glycemic control and proper foot care in diabetic patients.

COMMONLY ASSOCIATED CONDITIONS
Abscess, lymphedema, venous insufficiency, obesity

 DIAGNOSIS

Clinical diagnosis presenting as an area of rapidly spreading unilateral erythema, warmth, swelling, and/or tenderness.

HISTORY

- Previous trauma, surgery, animal/human bites, dermatitis, and fungal infection are portals of entry.
- Pain, itching, and/or burning
- Fever, chills, and malaise

PHYSICAL EXAM

- Assess vital signs for hemodynamic stability.
- Localized pain and tenderness with erythema, induration, swelling, and warmth
- Regional lymphadenopathy
- Purulent drainage
- Orbital cellulitis: proptosis, globe displacement, limitation of ocular movements, vision loss, diplopia
- Facial cellulitis: malaise, anorexia, vomiting, pruritus, burning, anterior neck swelling

DIFFERENTIAL DIAGNOSIS
Toxic shock syndrome, venous stasis dermatitis, deep vein thrombosis, thrombophlebitis, bursitis, dermatitis, herpes zoster, osteomyelitis, malignancy, drug reaction, sunburn, insect stings, erythema nodosum

DIAGNOSTIC TESTS & INTERPRETATION
Initial Tests (lab, imaging)

- If there are signs of systemic disease (fever, heart rate >100 bpm, or systolic blood pressure <90 mm Hg): blood cultures, CPK, CRP. Consider serum lactate levels.
- Swab open wounds for culture.
- Plain radiographs, CT, and MRI are useful if osteomyelitis, fracture, necrotizing fasciitis, retained foreign body.
- MRI and ultrasound are most useful for evaluation of potential underlying abscesses.
- Gallium-67 scintigraphy helps detect cellulitis superimposed on chronic limb lymphedema.
- Procalcitonin is not useful in diagnosing early cellulitis (4).

Diagnostic Procedures/Other
Consider lumbar puncture in children with *H. influenzae* type B or if meningeal signs and facial cellulitis.

TREATMENT

GENERAL MEASURES

- Immobilize/elevate involved limb to reduce swelling.
- Sterile saline dressings or cool aluminum acetate compresses for pain relief
- Edema: compression stockings, pneumatic pumps; diuretic therapy for CHF patients
- Mark the borders of erythema to monitor progression and response to therapy.
- Tetanus immunization if needed

MEDICATION
First Line

- Target treatment if known pathogen and/or with certain exposures (animal bites)
- Empiric antibiotic selection:
  - Nonpurulent cellulitis
    - With nonpurulent drainage, target treatment toward β-hemolytic streptococci and MSSA.
    - Outpatient: treatment duration of 5 to 10 days (5)[C]; shorter courses of 5 days have been shown to be as effective as longer courses.
      - Oral: for mild cellulitis
        - Cephalexin 500 mg PO q6h; children: 25 to 50 mg/kg/day in 3 to 4 doses
        - Dicloxacillin 500 mg PO q6h; children: 25 to 50 mg/kg/day in 4 doses
        - Clindamycin 300 to 450 mg PO q6–8h; children: 20 to 30 mg/kg/day in 4 doses
      - IV: for rapidly progressing cellulitis
        - Cefazolin 1 to 2 g IV q8h; children: 100 mg/kg/day IV in 2 to 4 divided doses
        - Oxacillin 2 g IV q4h; children: 150 to 200 mg/kg/day IV in 4 to 6 doses
        - Nafcillin 2 g IV q4h; children: 150 to 200 mg/kg/day IV in 4 to 6 doses
        - Clindamycin 600 to 900 mg IV q8h; children: 25 to 40 mg/kg/day IV in 3 to 4 doses

- Purulent cellulitis (probable CA-MRSA)
  - Culture purulent wounds and follow up in 48 hours.
  - Incise and drain abscesses and start empiric antibiotic therapy. Modify based on culture results; tailor duration based on clinical response (6)[C]:
    - Oral
      - Clindamycin 300 to 450 mg PO; children: 40 mg/kg/day in 3 to 4 doses
      - Trimethoprim-sulfamethoxazole (TMP-SMX) 1 DS tab PO BID; children: dose based on TMP at 8 to 12 mg/kg/day divided in 2 doses
      - Doxycycline 100 mg PO BID; children >8 years of age: ≤45 kg: 4 mg/kg/day divided in 2 doses; >45 kg: 100 mg PO BID
      - Minocycline 200 mg PO once and then 100 mg PO BID; children >8 years old: 4 mg/kg PO once and then 4 mg/kg PO BID
      - Linezolid 600 mg PO BID; children <12 years: 10 mg/kg/dose (max 600 mg/dose) PO TID; ≥12 years: 600 mg PO BID
      - Tedizolid 200 mg PO once daily; children: Dosing is not established.
    - IV
      - Vancomycin 15 to 20 mg/kg/dose IV every 8 to 12 hours
      - Daptomycin 4 mg/kg/dose IV once daily; if bacteremia is present or suspected: 6 mg/kg IV once daily
      - Linezolid 600 mg IV BID
      - Tedizolid 200 mg IV once daily
      - Ceftaroline 600 mg IV q12h
      - Tigecycline 100 mg IV once, thereafter 50 mg IV q12h
- Necrotizing cellulitis: requires broad-spectrum coverage to cover clostridial and anaerobic species: ampicillin-sulbactam 1.5 to 3.0 g q6–8h IV or piperacillin-tazobactam 3.37 g q6–8h IV plus ciprofloxacin 400 mg q12h IV plus clindamycin 600 to 900 mg q8h IV; consider intensive care and emergent surgical consultation.
- Freshwater exposure: penicillinase-resistant: penicillin plus gentamicin or fluoroquinolone; salt water exposure: doxycycline 200 mg IV in 2 divided doses
- Bites: The combination of amoxicillin and clavulanic acid is recommended for human and dog bites. Ticarcillin and clavulanic acid or the combination of a 3rd-generation cephalosporin (i.e., ceftriaxone) plus metronidazole provides adequate parenteral therapy for animal or human bites. If allergic to penicillin, use fluoroquinolone plus metronidazole.
- Facial cellulitis in adults: ceftriaxone IV
- Diabetic foot infection:
  - Mild/moderate: cephalexin or cephalexin plus doxycycline or TMP-SMX plus amoxicillin clavulanate
  - Severe: ampicillin-sulbactam or imipenem-cilastatin or meropenem; alternative: combinations of targeting anaerobes as well as gram-positive and gram-negative aerobes
- If severe infection, toxicity, immunocompromised patients, or worsening infection despite empirical therapy, admit for empiric antibiotic therapy covering MRSA.

- Recurrent streptococcal cellulitis: penicillin 250 mg BID, or if penicillin-allergic, use erythromycin 250 mg BID
- Dalbavancin, a 2nd-generation lipoglycopeptide antibiotic with MRSA coverage, can be used to treat cellulitis and be administered rarely as once a week (6)[C].

Pediatric Considerations
- Avoid doxycycline in children ≤8 years old and during pregnancy.
- The Melbourne ASSET tool is helpful in determining the need for IV antibiotics in pediatric populations (sensitivity 60%, specificity 93%) (7).

Second Line
Mild infection
- Penicillin allergy: erythromycin 500 mg PO q6h

SURGERY/OTHER PROCEDURES
- Débridement for gas and purulent matter
- Intubation or tracheotomy may be needed for cellulitis of the head or neck.

ADMISSION, INPATIENT, AND NURSING CONSIDERATIONS
- Severe infection, suspicion of deeper or rapidly spreading infection, tissue necrosis, or severe pain
- Marked systemic toxicity or worsening symptoms that do not resolve after 24 to 48 hours of therapy
- Patients with underlying risk factors or severe comorbidities

 ONGOING CARE

FOLLOW-UP RECOMMENDATIONS
Patient Monitoring
- Repeat relevant labs if patient is toxic or not improving.
- Symptomatic improvement usually occurs in 24 to 48 hours, but visible improvement may take 72 hours.

DIET
Glucose control in diabetics

PATIENT EDUCATION
Good skin hygiene

PROGNOSIS
- Low-dose penicillin prophylaxis in patients with recurrent cellulitis decreases recurrence.
- Older age, higher BMI, and diabetes mellitus have been shown to lower early response to antibiotics.

COMPLICATIONS
- Local abscess
- Bacteremia, sepsis
- Superinfection with gram-negative organisms
- Lymphangitis
- Thrombophlebitis or venous thrombosis
- Bacterial meningitis
- Gangrene

REFERENCES
1. Fritz SA, Shapiro DJ, Hersh AL. National trends in incidence of purulent skin and soft tissue infections in patients presenting to ambulatory and emergency department settings, 2000-2015. *Clin Infect Dis.* 2020;70(12):2715–2718. doi:10.1093/cid/ciz977.
2. Peterson RA, Polgreen LA, Cavanaugh JE, et al. Increasing incidence, cost, and seasonality in patients hospitalized for cellulitis. *Open Forum Infect Dis.* 2017;4(1):ofx008.
3. Tay EY, Fook-Chong S, Oh CC, et al. Cellulitis recurrence score: a tool for predicting recurrence of lower limb cellulitis. *J Am Acad Dermatol.* 2015;72(1):140–145.
4. Brindle RJ, Ijaz A, Davies P. Procalcitonin and cellulitis: correlation of procalcitonin blood levels with measurements of severity and outcome in patients with limb cellulitis. *Biomarkers.* 2019;24(2):127–130.
5. Stevens DL, Bisno AL, Chambers HF, et al. Practice guidelines for the diagnosis and management of skin and soft tissue infections: 2014 update by the Infectious Diseases Society of America. *Clin Infect Dis.* 2014;59(2):e10–e52.
6. Bender S, Oakden K. New developments and treatment options of cellulitis in the hospital. In: Conrad K, ed. *Clinical Approaches to Hospital Medicine: Advances, Updates and Controversies.* Cham, Switzerland: Springer; 2018:77–87.
7. Ibrahim LF, Hopper SM, Donath S, et al. Development and validation of a cellulitis risk score: the Melbourne ASSET Score. *Pediatrics.* 2019;143(2):e20181420.

ADDITIONAL READING
- Kaye KS, Petty LA, Shorr AF, et al. Current epidemiology, etiology, and burden of acute skin infections in the United States. *Clin Infect Dis.* 2019;68(Suppl 3): S193–S199. doi:10.1093/cid/ciz002.
- Webb E, Neeman T, Bowden FJ, et al. Compression therapy to prevent recurrent cellulitis of the leg. *N Engl J Med.* 2020;383(7):630–639.

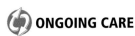 CODES

ICD10
- L03.312 Cellulitis of back [any part except buttock]
- L03.032 Cellulitis of left toe
- L03.211 Cellulitis of face

CLINICAL PEARLS
- *S. aureus* and group A *Streptococcus* are the most common organisms causing cellulitis.
- Consider MRSA if cellulitis does not respond to antibiotics within 48 hours or if purulence present.
- Rapid expansion of infected area with discoloration and severe pain may suggest necrotizing fasciitis, requiring urgent surgical evaluation.
- Venous stasis dermatitis often mimics cellulitis leading to improper use of antibiotics.

CELLULITIS, ORBITAL

Frances J. Boly, DO • Tazeen Rizvi, DO

 BASICS

DESCRIPTION
- Acute, severe, vision-threatening infection of orbital contents posterior to the orbital septum also referred to as postseptal cellulitis
- Preseptal (previously referred to as periorbital) cellulitis is anterior to the septum. Location determines the appropriate workup and treatment.
- Synonym(s): postseptal cellulitis

EPIDEMIOLOGY
- No difference in frequency between genders in adults; higher incidence in boys in childhood
- More common in children
- Orbital cellulitis is much less common than preseptal cellulitis (1).

Incidence
The incidence of orbital cellulitis has declined since introduction of routine *Haemophilus influenzae* type b (Hib) vaccination.

ETIOLOGY AND PATHOPHYSIOLOGY
- Sinusitis is classically associated with orbital cellulitis. Local skin conditions surrounding the eyelids and lashes are typically associated with preseptal cellulitis.
- The ethmoid sinus is separated from the orbit by the lamina papyracea ("layer of paper"), a thin bony separation, and is often the source of contiguous spread of infection to the orbit. The ethmoid sinus is present at birth.
- The orbital septum is a connective tissue barrier that extends from the skull into the lid and separates the preseptal from the orbital space.
- Cellulitis in the closed bony orbit causes proptosis, globe displacement, orbital apex syndrome (mass effect on the cranial nerves), optic nerve compression, and vision loss.
- Cultures of surgical specimens in adults often grow multiple organisms. In over 1/3 of cases, no pathogen is recovered. Blood cultures typically do not grow an organism.
- Most common organisms (2):
  – *Staphylococcus aureus, Streptococcus pneumoniae, Streptococcus anginosus*
- Less common organisms:
  – Rare cases of orbital cellulitis caused by non–spore-forming anaerobes, *Eikenella corrodens, Aeromonas hydrophila, Pseudomonas aeruginosa,* and *Mycobacterium tuberculosis* (3)
  – In immunocompromised patients, mucormycosis and aspergillosis should be considered as a cause of orbital cellulitis (4).
- *Haemophilus* is no longer the leading cause of orbital cellulitis. MRSA is increasingly a consideration.

Genetics
No known genetic predisposition

RISK FACTORS
- Sinusitis present in 80–100% of cases. Pansinusitis is often observed in adults (1).
- Orbital trauma, retained orbital foreign body (FB), ophthalmic surgery, and/or history of sinus surgery (1)

- Dental, periorbital, skin, or intracranial infection; acute dacryocystitis (inflammation of the lacrimal sac) and acute dacryoadenitis (inflammation of the lacrimal gland)
- Immunosuppressed patients are at increased risk of adverse outcomes.

GENERAL PREVENTION
- Routine Hib vaccination
- Appropriate treatment of bacterial sinusitis
- Proper wound care and perioperative monitoring of orbital surgery and trauma
- Avoid trauma to the sinus and orbital regions.

COMMONLY ASSOCIATED CONDITIONS
- Sinusitis, especially pansinusitis in adults
- Trauma and intraorbital FB
- Preseptal cellulitis
- Adverse outcomes include neurotrophic keratitis, secondary glaucoma, septic uveitis or retinitis, exudative retinal detachment, meningitis, cranial nerve palsies, panophthalmitis, inflammatory or infectious neuritis, retinal vein occlusion, central retinal artery occlusion, orbital abscess, subperiosteal abscess, orbital apex syndrome, subdural or brain abscess, and death.

 DIAGNOSIS

HISTORY
- Complaints of acute onset red, swollen, tender eye or eyelid, and pain with eye movements
- History of surgery, trauma, sinus or upper respiratory infection, dental infection
- Malaise, fever, stiff neck, mental status changes
- Specific signs of orbital cellulitis include:
  – Proptosis, double vision, ophthalmoplegia, vision loss (or decreased field of vision), pain with eye movement, decreased color vision (differentiating green and red)

ALERT
- Differentiating orbital from preseptal cellulitis is the critical diagnostic step. Preseptal cellulitis can be identified by exam or following CT scan.
- Both preseptal and orbital cellulitis present with a red, swollen painful eye or eyelid.
- Diplopia, ophthalmoplegia, painful extraocular movements, proptosis, vision loss, and fever suggest orbital involvement.
- Contrast CT is the imaging method of choice and must be done for suspicion of orbital cellulitis (5).
- Treat with immediate IV antibiotics, hospital admission, and ophthalmology referral.
- Monitor frequently for vision loss, cavernous sinus thrombosis, abscess, and meningitis.

PHYSICAL EXAM
Vital signs
- Assess visual acuity (with glasses if required).
- Lid exam and palpation of the orbit
- Pupillary reflex for afferent pupillary defect
- Extraocular movements; assess for pain with eye movement—if present, then concerning for orbital cellulitis.

- Red desaturation: Patient views red object with one eye and compares to the other; reduced red color may indicate optic nerve involvement.
- Proptosis; pain with palpation
- Confrontation visual field testing

DIFFERENTIAL DIAGNOSIS
- Preseptal cellulitis
  – Eyelid erythema with or without conjunctival erythema, afebrile, no pain on eye movement, no diplopia, normal eye exam, vision intact
- Metastatic tumors and autoimmune inflammation may masquerade as orbital cellulitis in rare cases; usually present with painless slow onset of symptoms
- Idiopathic orbital inflammatory disease (orbital pseudotumor)
  – Afebrile, normal WBCs; usually subacute, may have pain, responds to steroids after ruling out orbital cellulitis
- Orbital FB
- Arteriovenous fistula (carotid-cavernous fistula)
  – Spontaneous or due to trauma; bruit may be present; insidious, subacute onset
- Cavernous sinus thrombosis
  – Signs of orbital cellulitis with cranial nerves III, IV, V, and VI findings; often bilateral and acute
  – Severely ill
- Acute thyroid orbitopathy
  – Afebrile; possible signs of thyroid disease
  – Bilateral orbital involvement
- Orbital tumor
  – Rhabdomyosarcoma, acute lymphoblastic leukemia, or metastatic tumors
  – Unilateral
  – Slow onset
- Trauma, insect bite, ruptured dermoid cyst
- Clinical signs help distinguish preseptal from orbital cellulitis. Preseptal infection causes erythema, induration, and tenderness of the eyelid and/or periorbital tissues, and patients rarely show signs of systemic illness. Local skin trauma, lacerations, or bug bites can be seen. Extraocular movements and visual acuity are intact.
- Orbital cellulitis also presents with red, swollen, painful eye or eyelid. More specific symptoms include proptosis, conjunctival edema, ophthalmoplegia, painful eye movements, and decreased visual acuity.

DIAGNOSTIC TESTS & INTERPRETATION
- CBC with differential, C-reactive protein, ESR. Inflammatory markers can be higher with orbital cellulitis versus preseptal.
- Swab cultures of eye secretions or nasopharyngeal aspirates are often contaminated by normal flora but may identify causative organism(s).
- Cultures from orbital and sinus abscesses at the time of surgery more often yield positive results but should be limited to cases where invasive procedures are indicated. Cultures from sinus aspirates and abscesses may grow multiple organisms (6).
- Blood cultures (usually negative) should be obtained prior to initiation of antibiotic therapy in ill-appearing or febrile patients.

Initial Tests (lab, imaging)
- CT scan of orbits and sinuses with axial and coronal views, with and without contrast, is imaging modality of choice (7)[C]. US and MRI are alternatives.
  - Thin section (2 mm) CT, coronal and axial views with bone windows to differentiate preseptal from orbital cellulitis, confirm extension into orbit, detect coexisting sinus disease, and identify orbital or subperiosteal abscesses that may require surgery
  - Deviation of medial rectus indicates intraorbital involvement.
- MRI offers superior soft tissue resolution for identification of cavernous sinus thrombosis but is less effective for bone imaging.
- US is used to rule out orbital myositis, locate FBs or abscesses, and follow progression of drained abscess (8).

Follow-Up Tests & Special Considerations
- Frequent eye exam and vital signs (q4h)
- Identify associated conditions, such as meningitis or orbital abscess.

Diagnostic Procedures/Other
Consult ophthalmology for slit lamp and dilated funduscopic exam; to evaluate proptosis, color vision, automated visual field; and need for surgery.

TREATMENT
Admit patients with orbital cellulitis for monitoring and treatment with broad-spectrum IV antibiotics.

MEDICATION
- Empiric antibiotic therapy to cover pathogens associated with acute sinusitis (*S. pneumoniae*, *H. influenzae*, *Moraxella catarrhalis*, *Streptococcus pyogenes*), as well as for *S. aureus*, *S. anginosus*, and anaerobes
- Modify IV antibiotic treatment when culture and sensitivity results are available. Duration of IV therapy is usually a week. Additional PO therapy depends on response.
- Consider treatment of MRSA for severe infection or based on local resistance patterns.
- PO antibiotic therapy for 2 to 3 weeks or longer (3 to 6 weeks) is recommended for patients with severe sinusitis and bony destruction.

First Line
- Ampicillin/sulbactam (Unasyn) or ceftriaxone plus metronidazole or clindamycin if anaerobic infection is suspected
  - Ampicillin/sulbactam: 3 g IV q6h for adult; 200 to 300 mg/kg/day divided q6h for children
  - Ceftriaxone: 1 to 2 g IV q12h for adults or 100 mg/kg/day divided BID in children with maximum 4 g/day
  - Clindamycin: 600 mg IV q8h for adults; 20 to 40 mg/kg/day IV q6–8h for children (6)
  - Metronidazole: 500 mg IV q8h for adult; 30 to 35 mg/kg/day divided q8h for children

ALERT
In severe orbital cellulitis, in suspected or proven MRSA infection, vancomycin remains the parenteral drug of choice. Use in conjunction with agents to cover gram-negative bacteria.

- Vancomycin: 1 g IV q12h for adults; 40 mg/kg/day IV divided q8–12h, max daily dose 2 g for children

Second Line
Any number of antibiotic regimens have been reported as successful. There is no definitive consensus for best choice (1).

ISSUES FOR REFERRAL
Always admit to the hospital and consult with ophthalmology. Consider consultation with ID and ENT for orbital cellulitis; neurology/neurosurgery if intracranial spread is suspected

ADDITIONAL THERAPIES
- Steroid use is controversial.
- PO steroids as an adjunct to IV antibiotics for orbital cellulitis may speed resolution of inflammation.
- Nasal decongestants are often recommended.
- Topical erythromycin or nonmedicated ophthalmic ointment protects the cornea from exposure in cases with severe proptosis.
- Children may be treated with amoxicillin/clavulanate 20 to 40 mg/kg/day divided TID or in adults 250 to 500 mg TID (9).

SURGERY/OTHER PROCEDURES
- IV antibiotic therapy is the initial therapy. 80–90% of cases respond to medical therapy without surgery.
- Surgical intervention warranted for visual loss, complete ophthalmoplegia, well-defined large abscess (>10 mm) on presentation or no clinical improvement after 24 to 48 hours of antibiotic therapy
- Trauma cases may need débridement or FB removal.
- Orbital abscess may need surgical drainage.
- Surgical drainage with 4 to 8 weeks of antibiotics is the treatment of choice for brain abscess.
- Surgical interventions may include external ethmoidectomy, endoscopic ethmoidectomy, uncinectomy, antrostomy, and subperiosteal drainage.

ADMISSION, INPATIENT, AND NURSING CONSIDERATIONS
Patients with orbital cellulitis should be admitted for IV antibiotics and serial eye exams to evaluate progression of infection or involvement of optic nerve.
- Follow temperature, WBC, visual acuity, pupillary reflex, ocular motility, and proptosis.
- Repeat CT scan or surgical intervention may be required for worsening orbital cellulitis cases

 ## ONGOING CARE

FOLLOW-UP RECOMMENDATIONS
Patient Monitoring
Serial visual acuity testing and slit lamp exams

ALERT
Bedside exam q4h is indicated, as complications can develop rapidly.

PATIENT EDUCATION
- Maintain proper hand washing and good skin hygiene.
- Avoid skin or lid trauma.

PROGNOSIS
Historically, blindness occurred in 20% and death in 17% of cases before antibiotics. Vision loss occurs in 3–11% of cases (1).

COMPLICATIONS
- Vision loss, CNS involvement, and death
- Permanent vision loss
  - Corneal exposure
  - Optic neuritis
  - Endophthalmitis
  - Septic uveitis or retinitis
  - Exudative retinal detachment
  - Retinal artery or vein occlusions
  - Globe rupture
  - Orbital compartment syndrome
- CNS complications
  - Intracranial abscess, meningitis, cavernous sinus thrombosis

REFERENCES
1. El Mograbi A, Ritter A, Najjar E, et al. Orbital complications of rhinosinusitis in the adult population: analysis of cases presenting to a tertiary medical center over a 13-year period. *Ann Otol Rhinol Laryngol*. 2019;128(6):563–568.
2. Danishyar A, Sergent SR. *Orbital Cellulitis*. In: StatPearls [Internet]. Treasure Island, FL: StatPearls Publishing; 2021. Updated August 12, 2021. https://www.ncbi.nlm.nih.gov/books/NBK507901/.
3. Hamed-Azzam S, AlHashash I, Briscoe D, et al. Common orbital infections~state of the art~part 1. *J Opthalmic Vis Res*. 2018;13(2):175–182.
4. Sagiv O, Thakar SD, Kandl TJ, et al. Clinical course of preseptal and orbital cellulitis in 50 immunocompromised patients with cancer. *Ophthalmology*. 2018;125(2):318–320.
5. Khan SA, Hussain A, Phelps PO. Current clinical diagnosis and management of orbital cellulitis. *Expert Rev Ophthalmol*. 2021;16(5):387–399.
6. Bedwell J, Bauman NM. Management of pediatric orbital cellulitis and abscess. *Curr Opin Otolaryngol Head Neck Surg*. 2011;19(6):467–473.
7. Mahalingam-Dhingra A, Lander L, Preciado DA, et al. Orbital and periorbital infections: a national perspective. *Arch Otolaryngol Head Neck Surg*. 2011;137(8):769–773.
8. Schramm VL, Myers EN, Kennerdell JS. Orbital complications of acute sinusitis: evaluation, management, and outcome. *Otolaryngology*. 1978;86(2):ORL221–30.
9. Daoudi A, Ajdakar S, Rada N, et al. Orbital and periorbital cellulitis in children. Epidemiological, clinical, therapeutic aspects and course. *J Fr Ophtalmol*. 2016;39(7):609–614.

CODES

ICD10
- H05.019 Cellulitis of unspecified orbit
- H05.011 Cellulitis of right orbit
- H05.012 Cellulitis of left orbit

CLINICAL PEARLS
- Most cases of orbital cellulitis arise from sinusitis.
- CT of orbits and sinuses with axial and coronal views with and without contrast is diagnostic modality of choice.
- Patients with orbital cellulitis must be admitted for visual monitoring and IV antibiotic therapy.
- Older age (>10 years) and diplopia predict need for surgical intervention in children.
- Ophthalmoplegia, mental status changes, contralateral cranial nerve palsy, or bilateral orbital cellulitis raise suspicion for intracranial involvement.

CELLULITIS, PERIORBITAL

Fozia Akhtar Ali, MD, FAAFP • Hayley Bryton Hamilton-Bevil, MD, MPH

 BASICS

DESCRIPTION
- An acute bacterial infection of the skin and subcutaneous tissue anterior to the orbital septum; does not involve the orbital structures (globe, fat, and ocular muscles)
- Synonym(s): preseptal cellulitis

ALERT
It is essential to distinguish periorbital cellulitis from orbital cellulitis. Orbital cellulitis is a potentially life-threatening condition. *Orbital cellulitis is posterior to the orbital septum; symptoms include restricted eye movement, pain with eye movement, proptosis, and vision changes.*

EPIDEMIOLOGY
- Occurs more commonly in children; mean age 21 months
- 3 times more common than orbital cellulitis (1)[C]

Incidence
Increased incidence in the winter months (due to increased cases of sinusitis) (1)[C]

ETIOLOGY AND PATHOPHYSIOLOGY
- The anatomy of the eyelid distinguishes periorbital (preseptal) from orbital cellulitis:
  - A connective tissue sheet (orbital septum) extends from the orbital bones to the margins of the upper and lower eyelids; it acts as a barrier to infection of deeper orbital structures.
  - Infection of tissues anterior to the orbital septum is periorbital (preseptal) cellulitis.
  - Infection deep to the orbital septum is orbital (postseptal) cellulitis.
- Periorbital cellulitis typically arises from a contiguous infection of soft tissues of the face.
  - Sinusitis (via lamina papyracea) extension
  - Local trauma; insect or animal bites
  - Foreign bodies
  - Dental abscess extension
  - Hematogenous seeding
- Common organisms (1)[C]
  - *Staphylococcus aureus*, typically MSSA (MRSA is increasing.)
  - *Staphylococcus epidermidis*
  - *Streptococcus pyogenes*
- Atypical organisms
  - *Acinetobacter* sp.; *Nocardia brasiliensis*
  - *Bacillus anthracis*; *Pseudomonas aeruginosa*
  - *Neisseria gonorrhoeae*; *Proteus* sp.
  - *Pasteurella multocida*; *Mycobacterium tuberculosis*; *Trichophyton* sp. (ringworm)

- Since vaccine introduction, the incidence of *Haemophilus influenzae* disease has decrease (should still be suspected in unimmunized or partially immunized patients).

Genetics
No known genetic predisposition

RISK FACTORS
- Contiguous spread from upper respiratory infection
- Acute sinusitis
- Conjunctivitis
- Blepharitis
- Dental infection
- Local skin trauma/puncture wound
- Insect bite
- Bacteremia

GENERAL PREVENTION
- Avoid trauma around the eyes.
- Avoid swimming in fresh or salt water with facial skin abrasions.
- Routine vaccination: particularly *H. influenzae* type B and *Streptococcus pneumoniae*

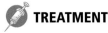 **DIAGNOSIS**

HISTORY
- Induration, erythema, warmth, and/or tenderness of periorbital soft tissue, usually with normal vision and normal eye movements
- Chemosis (conjunctival swelling), proptosis; pain with extraocular eye movements can occur in severe cases of periorbital cellulitis and are concerning for orbital cellulitis.
- Fever (not always present)

ALERT
Pain with eye movement, fever, and conjunctival swelling raise the suspicion for orbital cellulitis.

PHYSICAL EXAM
- Vital signs and general appearance (Patients with orbital cellulitis often appear systemically ill.)
- Inspect eyes and surrounding structures—lids, lashes, conjunctiva, and skin.
- Erythema, swelling, and tenderness of lids without orbital congestion
  - Violaceous discoloration of eyelid is more commonly associated with *H. influenzae.*
- Evaluate for skin break down.
- Look for vesicles to rule out herpetic infection.
- Inspect nasal vaults and palpate sinuses for signs of acute sinusitis.

- Examine oral cavity for dental abscesses.
- Test ocular motility and visual acuity.

DIFFERENTIAL DIAGNOSIS
- Orbital cellulitis
  - Orbital cellulitis may have the same signs and symptoms as periorbital cellulitis, with fever, proptosis, chemosis, ophthalmoplegia, decreased visual acuity, pain with ocular movement.
- Abscess
- Dacryocystitis
- Hordeolum (stye)
- Allergic inflammation
- Orbital or periorbital trauma
- Idiopathic inflammation from orbital pseudotumor
- Orbital myositis
- Rapidly progressive tumors
  - Rhabdomyosarcoma
  - Retinoblastoma
  - Lymphoma
- Leukemia

DIAGNOSTIC TESTS & INTERPRETATION
Initial Tests (lab, imaging)
- CBC with differential
- Blood cultures (low yield) (2)[C]
- Wound culture of purulent drainage (if present)
- Imaging is indicated if there is suspicion for orbital cellulitis (marked eyelid swelling, fever, and leukocytosis or failure to improve on appropriate antibiotics within 24 to 48 hours).
- CT to evaluate the extent of infection and detect orbital inflammation or abscess:
  - CT with contrast, thin sections (2 mm); coronal and axial views with bone windows
  - The classic sign of orbital cellulitis on CT scan is bulging of the medial rectus.

Follow-Up Tests & Special Considerations
- Children with periorbital or orbital cellulitis often have underlying sinusitis.
- If a child is febrile, <15 months old, and appears toxic, admit for blood cultures, antibiotic therapy, and consider lumbar puncture.

 TREATMENT

MEDICATION
- Treat periorbital cellulitis with oral antibiotics and ensure close follow-up.
- Empiric antibiotic treatment should cover the most likely organisms (*Staphylococcus* and *Streptococcus*).

- Observe local prevalence of MRSA to determine need for coverage.
- No evidence that IV antibiotics are more effective than PO in reducing recovery time or preventing secondary complications in simple periorbital cellulitis (1)[C]
- No evidence for benefit of steroid use

First Line
- Uncomplicated posttraumatic periorbital cellulitis
  - Usually due to skin flora, including *Staphylococcus* and *Streptococcus*
  - Cephalexin 500 mg PO q6h or dicloxacillin 500 mg PO q6h
  - Clindamycin 300 mg PO TID, doxycycline 100 mg PO BID, or trimethoprim-sulfamethoxazole (TMP-SMX) 1 to 2 DS tablets PO q12h if MRSA is suspected
- Extension from sinusitis
  - Amoxicillin-clavulanate 875 mg PO BID
  - 3rd-generation cephalosporin (e.g., cefdinir 300 mg PO BID)
- Dental abscess
  - Amoxicillin-clavulanate 875 mg PO BID or clindamycin 300 mg PO TID
- Bacteremic cellulitis
  - May be associated with meningitis
  - Ceftriaxone 1 g IV q24h plus vancomycin 15 mg/kg/dose IV q8–12h or clindamycin 600 to 900 mg IV q8h to cover MRSA
  - Duration of therapy: A 10- to 14-day course is usually sufficient. Follow patients treated with oral antibiotics for presumed periorbital cellulitis closely (daily follow-up until improvement occurs) for response to antibiotics and possible progression to orbital cellulitis. If symptoms do not improve within 24 hours, reevaluate for IV antibiotic therapy.

ISSUES FOR REFERRAL
Consult ENT and ophthalmology if there is concern for orbital cellulitis or if patients do not respond quickly to first-line treatment (3).

SURGERY/OTHER PROCEDURES
- Usually not indicated in uncomplicated cases
- If there is an abscess or potential compromise of critical structures, orbital surgery is indicated.
- Diplopia is the strongest clinical predictor for surgery.

ADMISSION, INPATIENT, AND NURSING CONSIDERATIONS
- If the patient is stable and there are no systemic signs of toxicity, mild cases in adults and children >1 year of age can be safely managed on an outpatient basis.
- Consider hospitalization and IV antibiotics:
  - If patient appears systemically ill
  - Children <1 year of age (3),(4)[C]
  - Patients not immunized against *S. pneumoniae* or *H. influenzae*
  - If patients do not improve or deteriorate within 24 hours of oral antibiotics
  - High suspicion for orbital cellulitis (eyelid swelling with reduced vision, diplopia, abnormal light reflexes, or proptosis)
- No strict guidelines indicate when to switch from parenteral to PO therapy. In general, a switch from IV to PO antibiotics is reasonable once eyelid edema and erythema have significantly improved.
- A 10- to 14-day course of antibiotics is indicated.

 ONGOING CARE

FOLLOW-UP RECOMMENDATIONS
Patient Monitoring
Follow for signs of orbital involvement, including decreased visual acuity or painful/limited ocular motility.

PATIENT EDUCATION
- Maintain good skin hygiene.
- Avoid skin trauma.
- Report early skin changes (swelling, redness, and pain) if recurrent after a course of therapy.

PROGNOSIS
- With timely treatment, patients do well.
- Recurrent periorbital cellulitis occurs with ≥3 periorbital infections in 1 year with at least 1 month of in between episodes; must be differentiated from treatment failure due to antibiotic resistance (1)[C]

COMPLICATIONS
- Orbital cellulitis; orbital abscess formation
- Scarring

- Vision loss
- Cavernous sinus thrombosis
- Osteomyelitis

REFERENCES
1. Hauser A, Fogarasi S. Periorbital and orbital cellulitis. *Pediatr Rev*. 2010;31(6):242–249.
2. Baring DE, Hilmi OJ. An evidence based review of periorbital cellulitis. *Clin Otolaryngol*. 2011;36(1):57–64.
3. Upile NS, Munir N, Leong SC, et al. Who should manage acute periorbital cellulitis in children? *Int J Pediatr Otorhinolaryngol*. 2012;76(8):1073–1077.
4. Williams KJ, Allen RC. Paediatric orbital and periorbital infections. *Curr Opin Ophthalmol*. 2019;30(5):349–355.

ADDITIONAL READING
- Baiu I, Melendez E. Periorbital and orbital cellulitis. *JAMA*. 2020;323(2):196.
- Ekhlassi T, Becker N. Preseptal and orbital cellulitis. *Dis Mon*. 2017;63(2):30–32.

 CODES

ICD10
L03.211 Cellulitis of face

CLINICAL PEARLS
- Periorbital (preseptal) and orbital (postseptal) cellulitis occur most commonly in children.
- CT scan of sinuses and orbits can differentiate periorbital cellulitis from orbital cellulitis.
- Orbital cellulitis typically has fever, pain with eye movement, diplopia, and/or proptosis.
- Prompt imaging and consultation is necessary if there is a concern for orbital cellulitis.

C

CEREBRAL PALSY
Elyas Parsa, DO • Robin Kang Hans, MD, MPH

 BASICS

DESCRIPTION
Cerebral palsy (CP) is a group of clinical syndromes characterized by motor and postural dysfunction due to permanent and nonprogressive disruptions in the developing brain. Motor impairment resulting in activity limitation is necessary for this diagnosis. CP is classified by the nature of the movement disorder and its functional severity.

EPIDEMIOLOGY
Incidence
- Overall, 1.5 to 3.0/1,000 live births
- Incidence increases as gestational age (GA) at birth decreases:
  - 146/1,000 for GA of 22 to 27 weeks
  - 62/1,000 for GA of 28 to 31 weeks
  - 7/1,000 for GA of 32 to 36 weeks
  - 1/1,000 for GA of 37+ weeks
- Incidence increases as birth weight decreases (1).

ETIOLOGY AND PATHOPHYSIOLOGY
- Multifactorial; CP results from static injury or lesions in the developing brain, occurring prenatally, perinatally, or postnatally.
- Cytokines, free radicals, and inflammatory response are likely contributing factors.
- Spastic CP is most common, usually related to premature birth, with either periventricular leukomalacia or germinal matrix hemorrhage.

Genetics
There are reports of associations between CP and polymorphisms of certain genes: thrombophilic, cytokines, and apolipoprotein E.

RISK FACTORS
- Prenatal: congenital anomalies, multiple gestation, in utero stroke, intrauterine infection (cytomegalovirus [CMV], varicella), intrauterine growth retardation (IUGR), clinical and histologic chorioamnionitis, antepartum bleeding, maternal factors (cognitive impairment, seizure disorders, hyperthyroidism), abnormal fetal position (e.g., breech)
- Perinatal: preterm birth, low-birth weight, periventricular leukomalacia, perinatal hypoxia/asphyxia, intracranial hemorrhage/intraventricular hemorrhage, neonatal seizure or stroke, hyperbilirubinemia
- Postnatal: traumatic brain injury or stroke, sepsis, meningitis, encephalitis, asphyxia, and progressive hydrocephalus

GENERAL PREVENTION
- Effective prevention strategies include antenatal corticosteroids, magnesium sulfate, and neonatal hypothermia (2).
- Treating mothers with magnesium sulfate during preterm delivery is neuroprotective for fetus and may reduce the risk of CP. Effect on term fetus is unknown (3)[B].
- Term born infants who experience intrapartum hypoxia have benefit from therapeutic hypothermia (4).

COMMONLY ASSOCIATED CONDITIONS
- Seizure disorder
- Intellectual and speech and language impairments
- Behavioral problems
- Hearing and visual impairments
- Feeding impairment, swallowing dysfunction, and aspiration: when severe, may require gastrostomy feedings
- Poor dentition, excessive drooling
- GI conditions: constipation (59%), vomiting (22%), gastroesophageal reflux
- Decreased linear growth and weight abnormalities (under- and overweight)
- Osteopenia
- Bowel and bladder incontinence
- Orthopedic: contractures, hip subluxation/dislocation, scoliosis (60%)

DIAGNOSIS
- Guidelines for early and accurate diagnosis (5):
  - International guidelines for early diagnosis of CP before 12 months of age: Tools for detection include neuroimaging and Prechtl General Movements Assessment (GMA) (6) before 5 months and use of the Hammersmith Infant Neurologic Examination (HINE) (7) in a longitudinal fashion between 3 and 12 months.
- A clinical diagnosis including
  - Delayed motor milestones
  - Abnormal tone
  - Abnormal neurologic exam suggesting a cerebral etiology for motor dysfunction
  - Absence of regression (not losing function)
  - Absence of underlying syndromes or alternative explanation for etiology
- Although the pathologic lesion is static, clinical presentation may change as the infant grows and develops.

HISTORY
Ask about prenatal, perinatal, and postnatal risk factors.
- Neurobehavioral signs (poor feeding/frequent vomiting/irritability)
- Timing of motor milestones
- Abnormal spontaneous general movements
- Asymmetry of movements such as early hand preference
- Regression of motor skills does not occur with CP.

PHYSICAL EXAM
- Spasticity: increased tone/reflexes/clonus
- Dyskinesia: abnormal movements
- Hypotonia: decreased tone
- Ataxia: abnormal balance/coordination
- Tone: may be increased or decreased
- Trunk and head control: often poor but may be advanced due to high tone

- Reduced strength and motor control
- Persistence of primitive reflexes
- Asymmetry of movement or reflexes
- Decreased joint range of motion and contractures
- Brisk deep tendon reflexes, clonus
- Delayed motor milestones: serial exams most effective
- Gait abnormalities: scissoring, toe-walking
- CP is classified by the following:
  - Spasticity
    - Unilateral: hemiplegic
    - Bilateral: diplegic (lower extremity [LE] > upper extremity [UE] involvement) or quadriplegic (UE ≥ LE involvement)
  - Dystonia: hypertonia and reduced movement
  - Choreoathetosis: irregular spasmodic involuntary movements of the limbs or facial muscles
  - Ataxia: loss of orderly muscular coordination
  - The Manual Ability Classification System (MACS) can be used to assess UE and fine motor function.

DIFFERENTIAL DIAGNOSIS
Benign congenital hypotonia, brachial plexus injury, familial spastic paraplegia, dopa-responsive dystonia, transient toe-walking, muscular dystrophy, metabolic disorders (e.g., glutaric aciduria type 1), mitochondrial disorders, genetic disorders (e.g., Rett syndrome)

DIAGNOSTIC TESTS & INTERPRETATION
Laboratory testing is not needed to make diagnosis but can help exclude other etiologies.
- Testing for metabolic and genetic syndromes (8)[C]
  - Considered if no specific etiology is identified by neuroimaging or there are atypical features in clinical presentation
  - Detection of certain brain malformations may warrant genetic or metabolic testing to identify syndromes.
- Diagnostic testing for coagulopathies should be considered in children with hemiplegic CP with cerebral infarction identified on neuroimaging (8)[C].

Initial Tests (lab, imaging)
- Neuroimaging is not essential, but it is recommended in children with CP for whom the etiology has not been established (8)[C].
- MRI is preferred to CT (8)[C].
- Abnormalities found in 80–90% of patients: brain malformation, cerebral infarction, intraventricular or other intracranial hemorrhage, periventricular leukomalacia, ventricular enlargement, or other CSF space abnormalities

Diagnostic Procedures/Other
- Screening for comorbid conditions: developmental delay/intellectual impairment, vision/hearing impairments, speech and language disorders, feeding/swallowing dysfunction, or seizures
- Electroencephalograms (EEGs) should only be obtained if there is a history of suspected seizures.

TREATMENT

Focuses on control of symptoms; treatments reduce spasticity to prevent painful contractures, manage comorbid conditions, and optimize functionality and quality of life.

GENERAL MEASURES
- Early intervention for children 0 to 3 years (6)[A]
- Various therapies enhance function:
  - Physical therapy to improve posture stability and gait, motor strength and control, and prevent contractures
  - Occupational therapy to increase functional activities of daily living
  - Speech therapy for verbal and nonverbal speech and to aid in feeding
- Equipment optimizes participation in activities:
  - Orthotic splinting (ankle–foot orthosis)
  - Spinal bracing (body jacket) may slow down scoliosis.
  - Augmentative communication with pictures, switches, or computer systems for nonverbal individuals
  - Crutches, walkers, gait trainers, and wheelchairs for mobility and standers for weight bearing

MEDICATION

First Line
- Diazepam (7)[A]
  - A γ-aminobutyric acid-A (GABA$_A$) agonist that facilitates CNS inhibition at spinal and supraspinal levels to reduce spasticity
  - Used for short-term treatment for generalized spasticity; insufficient evidence on motor function
  - Adverse effects: ataxia and drowsiness
  - Adult dose: 2 to 12 mg/dose PO q6–12h
  - Pediatric dose (<12 years and <15 kg): <8.5 kg: 0.5 to 1.0 mg HS; 8.5 to 15.0 kg: 1 to 2 mg HS; children 5 to 16 years of age and ≥15 kg: 1.25 mg TID
- Botulinum toxin type A (7)[A]
  - Acts at neuromuscular junction to inhibit the release of acetylcholine to reduce tone
  - Injected directly into muscles of interest for localized spasticity; insufficient evidence on motor function
  - Higher functional benefit when combined with occupational therapy
  - Lasts for 12 to 16 weeks following injection

Second Line
- Baclofen (7)[A]
  - A GABA$_B$ agonist, facilitates presynaptic inhibition of mono- and polysynaptic reflexes
  - Adverse effects: drowsiness and sedation
  - Abrupt withdrawal symptoms: spasticity, hallucinations, seizures, confusion, hyperthermia

  - Adults: Initial dose is 5 mg TID; increase dosage every 3 days to an average maintenance dose of 20 mg TID, 80 mg/day maximum.
  - Pediatric dose (>2 years): initial 10 to 15 mg/day. Titrate to effective dose (maximum 40 mg/day). <8 years old: 60 mg/day maximum; >8 years old: 60 mg/day maximum
- Intrathecal baclofen (baclofen pump) (9)[A]
  - Continuous intrathecal route allows greater maximal response with smaller dosage to reduce spasticity.
  - May help ambulatory individuals with gait but no improvement seen in nonambulatory patients
  - Adverse effects: infection, catheter malfunction, CSF leakage

ADDITIONAL THERAPIES
Multidisciplinary care including ophthalmology; neurology; orthopedics; physiatry along with physical, occupational, and speech therapists

SURGERY/OTHER PROCEDURES
- Dorsal root rhizotomy selectively cuts dorsal rootlets from L1–S2. Decreases spasticity in lower limbs when done in conjunction with physiotherapy but associated with adverse effects. Evidence is lacking as to long-term outcomes.
- Surgical treatment of joint dislocations/subluxation, scoliosis management, tendon lengthening, gastrostomy

COMPLEMENTARY & ALTERNATIVE MEDICINE
- Therapeutic horse riding or hippotherapy improves postural control and balance.
- Aquatherapy improves gross motor function in patients with various motor severities.

ONGOING CARE

PROGNOSIS
Reduced lifespan strongly associated with level of functional impairment and intellectual disability

REFERENCES

1. Sadowska M, Sarecka-Hujar B, Kopyta I. Cerebral palsy: current opinions on definition, epidemiology, risk factors, classification and treatment options. *Neuropsychiatr Dis Treat.* 2020;16:1505–1518.
2. Novak I, Morgan C, Fahey M, et al. State of the evidence traffic lights 2019: systematic review of interventions for preventing and treating children with cerebral palsy. *Curr Neurol Neurosci Rep.* 2020;20(2):3.
3. Nguyen TM, Crowther CA, Wilkinson D, et al. Magnesium sulphate for women at term for neuroprotection of the fetus. *Cochrane Database Syst Rev.* 2013;(2):CD009395.
4. Badawi N, Mcintyre S, Hunt RW. Perinatal care with a view to preventing cerebral palsy. *Dev Med Child Neurol.* 2021;63(2):156–161.
5. Maitre NL, Burton VJ, Duncan AF, et al. Network implementation of guideline for early detection decreases age at cerebral palsy diagnosis. *Pediatrics.* 2020;145(5):e20192126.
6. Spittle A, Orton J, Anderson P, et al. Early developmental intervention programmes post-hospital discharge to prevent motor and cognitive impairments in preterm infants. *Cochrane Database Syst Rev.* 2012;(12):CD005495.
7. Delgado MR, Hirtz D, Aisen M, et al; and the Quality Standards Subcommittee of the American Academy of Neurology, Practice Committee of the Child Neurology Society. Practice parameter: pharmacologic treatment of spasticity in children and adolescents with cerebral palsy (an evidence-based review): report of the Quality Standards Subcommittee of the American Academy of Neurology and the Practice Committee of the Child Neurology Society. *Neurology.* 2010;74(4):336–343.
8. Ashwal S, Russman BS, Blasco PA, et al; for the Quality Standards Subcommittee of the American Academy of Neurology, Practice Committee of the Child Neurology Society. Practice parameter: diagnostic assessment of the child with cerebral palsy: report of the Quality Standards Subcommittee of the American Academy of Neurology and the Practice Committee of the Child Neurology Society. *Neurology.* 2004;62(6):851–863.
9. Pin TW, McCartney L, Lewis J, et al. Use of intrathecal baclofen therapy in ambulant children and adolescents with spasticity and dystonia of cerebral origin: a systematic review. *Dev Med Child Neurol.* 2011;53(10):885–895.

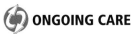 CODES

ICD10
- G80.9 Cerebral palsy, unspecified
- G80.1 Spastic diplegic cerebral palsy
- G80.2 Spastic hemiplegic cerebral palsy

CLINICAL PEARLS
- Management should focus on maximizing functioning and quality of life using multidisciplinary team approach.
- Regression of motor skills does not occur with CP.

CERVICAL HYPEREXTENSION INJURIES

Shane L. Larson, MD • Brock A. Benedict, DO

BASICS

DESCRIPTION

- Class of neck injuries typically seen in rapid, forceful extension of the cervical spine
- Flexion–extension injuries ("whiplash") are usually from motor vehicle accidents (MVAs).
- Other causes include falls, violence, or sports-related injuries (1).
- May involve:
  - Injury to vertebral and paravertebral structures: fractures, dislocations, ligamentous tears, and disc disruption/subluxation
  - Spinal cord injury (SCI): traumatic central cord syndrome (CCS) secondary to cord compression or vascular insult, SCI without radiologic abnormality (SCIWORA)
  - Blunt cerebrovascular injury (BCVI): vertebral artery or carotid artery dissection
  - Soft tissue injury: cervical strain/sprain (i.e., whiplash), cervical stingers (see "Brachial Plexopathy")

EPIDEMIOLOGY

- Predominant age: SCI average age of injury 43 years, CCS average age 53 years
- Trauma and sports injuries are more common in young adults (average age 29 years).
- Most (~80%) new SCI cases are male (1).

Incidence

In the United States

- Cervical fractures: 2 to 5/100 blunt trauma patients
- CCS: 4/100,000 people/year
- BCVI: estimated 1/1,000 of hospitalized trauma patients; incidence increased with cervical spine or thoracic injury.
- Cervical strain: 3 to 4/1,000 people/year
- Whiplash is the most common injury in MVAs and accounts for 28% of all ED visits for MVAs.
- Incidence of whiplash is 70 to 328/100,000 with rates highest in 20- to 24-year-old females.
- 2–6% of patients with blunt trauma have SCI. 80% are below the C2 level (2).
- The incidence of traumatic SCI is approximately 54 cases per million population per year (1).

ETIOLOGY AND PATHOPHYSIOLOGY

Blunt trauma due to MVAs, falls, sports injuries, and violence (primarily gunshot wounds)

RISK FACTORS

- Whiplash: initial injury, no seat belt use, female gender
- Chronic pain and/or disability: litigation, previous neck pain or injury, female gender, report of headache/low back pain at onset, low education level (3)[C]
- Fractures: osteoporosis, conditions predisposing to spinal rigidity, such as ankylosing spondylitis or other spondyloarthropathies
- CCS: preexisting spinal stenosis present in >50%
  - Acquired: prior trauma, spondylosis
  - Congenital: Klippel-Feil syndrome (congenital fusion of any two cervical vertebrae)

GENERAL PREVENTION

Seat belts, rule changes, proper technique, and proper use of protective equipment for sports activities can prevent or minimize injury.

COMMONLY ASSOCIATED CONDITIONS

Closed head injuries, whiplash-associated disorders (WADs), SCI, soft tissue trauma

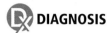

DIAGNOSIS

HISTORY

Usually acute presentation with mechanism of cervical hyperextension and complaints of neck pain, stiffness, or headaches ± neurologic symptoms; include Glasgow Coma Scale (GCS)

PHYSICAL EXAM

- External signs of trauma on the head and neck such as abrasions, lacerations, or contusions provide clues to mechanism and associated injuries.
- Presence, severity, and location of neck tenderness help localize involved structure(s):
  - Posterior, midline bony tenderness raises concern for underlying fracture.
  - Paraspinal or lateral soft tissue tenderness suggests muscular/ligamentous injury.
  - Anterior tenderness concerning for vascular injury
- Carotid bruit suggests carotid dissection
- Neurologic exam: Paresthesias, weakness suggests SCI or stroke secondary to BCVI:
  - CCS often presents as
    - Distal > proximal symptom distribution, upper extremity > lower extremity
    - Extremity weakness/paralysis predominates
    - Variable sensory changes below level of lesion (including paresthesias and dysesthesia)
    - Bladder/bowel incontinence may occur.

DIFFERENTIAL DIAGNOSIS

- Acute or chronic disc pathology (herniation or internal disruption)
- Osteoarthritis
- Cervical radiculopathy
- For CCS
  - Bell cruciate palsy
  - Bilateral brachial plexus injuries
  - Carotid or vertebral artery dissection

DIAGNOSTIC TESTS & INTERPRETATION

Initial Tests (lab, imaging)

- Low-risk patients can be cleared clinically (without imaging) using either the Canadian C-Spine Rule (CCR) or the National Emergency X-Ray Utilization Study (NEXUS) criteria (4)[B]:
  - CCR: Stable, ≥16-year-old patient with acute head and neck trauma and no history of cervical spine disease/surgery can be cleared if all of the following conditions are met:
    - GCS ≥15
    - No dangerous mechanism or extremity paresthesias
    - Age <65 years
    - At least one "low-risk factor" (i.e., simple rear-end MVA, ambulation at the accident scene, no midline cervical tenderness, delayed onset of neck pain, or sitting at the time of exam)
  - NEXUS: clinically clear if all of the following:
    - No posterior, midline C-spine tenderness
    - No evidence of intoxication
    - Normal level of alertness
    - No focal/neurologic deficits
    - No distracting injury
  - Reported sensitivity/specificity: CCR (90–100%/1–77%), NEXUS (83–100%/13–46%) (5)[B]

- In patients with high-risk mechanism or concerning historical/physical exam, recommend imaging based on the suspected injury and level of clinical suspicion:
  - Plain radiographs: in some patients who cannot be cleared clinically but are still in low-suspicion category: sensitivity for C-spine injury 39%:
    - Dynamic: flexion–extension; only if asymptomatic and no neurologic deficits or mental impairment, poor identification of ligamentous injury, limited diagnostic value
  - Axial CT from occiput to T1 with coronal and sagittal reconstructions has replaced plain radiography as the test of choice for cases with moderate to high clinical suspicion of C-spine injury, given high sensitivity (90–100%).
  - MRI: test of choice in CCS with direct visualization of traumatic cord lesions (edema or hematomyelia), soft tissue compressing cord, and/or stenosis of canal; detects ligamentous injury and abnormalities of intervertebral discs and soft tissues; MRI is less helpful for fractures.
  - CT angiography: visualization of cervical and cerebral vascular structures to detect BCVI, sensitivity approaches 100% when a ≥16-slice CT scanner is used. MR angiography is an alternative, although sensitivity of 47–50% limits utility.

Test Interpretation

- CCS: thought to be due to white matter axonal disruption of the lateral column, particularly the corticospinal tracts
- BCVI: intimal disruption, leading to thrombosis and embolization
- Acute cervical strain/sprain: Models suggest myofascial tearing, edema, and inflammation.

Geriatric Considerations

- Degenerative changes of the C-spine may be confused with acute traumatic change; osteopenia may limit fracture visualization on x-ray—CT is more accurate.
- Degenerative disease and osteopenia increase risk of upper cervical spine injuries (even with low-velocity trauma).

Pediatric Considerations

SCIWORA: high incidence at <9 years accounting for up to 50% of pediatric cervical spine injuries. MRI helps detect injury.

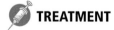

TREATMENT

GENERAL MEASURES

- Whiplash/WAD
  - Limited or no benefit to cervical collar. If provided, use for <72 hours.
  - No advantage to engaging early multiprofessional intervention (e.g., pain management and psychology) (5)[C]
  - No outcome differences with physical therapy (PT) versus passive (immobilization, rest) treatment; advance activity levels as tolerated
  - No preferred approach to treatment in absence of fracture
- Fractures
  - Stability determined by imaging
  - Decompression and stabilization are indicated for:
    - Incomplete SCIs with spinal canal compromise
    - Clinical deterioration or failure to improve despite conservative management

– Hangman fracture: traumatic spondylolisthesis of C2 with bilateral fractures through C2 pedicles, often with anterior subluxation of C2 over C3; can be unstable:
  ○ Managed with halo vest immobilization for 12 weeks until flexion–extension films normal
– Odontoid fractures: Treat according to type:
  ○ I: through apex; usually stable; external immobilization with a cervical collar (less often halo vest) for up to 12 weeks
  ○ II: most common, at base of dens, usually unstable; nonunion rates of up to 67% with halo immobilization alone, especially with dens displacement >6 mm or age >50 years
  ○ III: through C2 body, usually stable; immobilization in halo or cervical collar for 12 to 20 weeks
– Hyperextension teardrop fractures
  ○ If stable, rigid collar or cervicothoracic brace for 8 to 14 weeks
  ○ If unstable, halo brace for up to 3 months
• CCS: neck immobilization with cervical collar, PT/occupational therapy (OT)
• Cervical strain: no difference in outcomes with active (PT) versus passive (immobilization, rest) treatment; may use soft cervical collar for 10 days for symptomatic relief and then mobilize and increase activity as tolerated; no clear EBM guidelines

MEDICATION
• Fractures: pain control with analgesics
• CCS: Within 8 hours of injury, consider methylprednisolone 30 mg/kg IV over 15 minutes and then continuous infusion 5.4 mg/kg/hr IV for 23 hours. Further improvement in motor function recovery may be seen if infusion is continued for 48 hours, especially if initial bolus administration is delayed after injury (6),(7)[A].
• BCVI: Anticoagulation with IV heparin, followed by warfarin therapy for 3 to 6 months and then long-term antiplatelet therapy; antiplatelet agent as sole initial therapy in patients with contraindications to anticoagulation
• Cervical strain: NSAIDs or acetaminophen. There is little benefit to adding cyclobenzaprine for acute cervical strain.

ISSUES FOR REFERRAL
• If cervical spine injury is suspected, immobilize patient and send to ED for evaluation and clearance.
• Emergent consultation from a spine surgeon for any concern for unstable fracture or SCI

SURGERY/OTHER PROCEDURES
• Fractures
  – Hangman fracture: surgical fixation for excessive angulation or subluxation, disruption of intervertebral disc space, or failure to obtain alignment with external orthosis
  – Odontoid fractures
    ○ Type II: Early surgical stabilization is recommended in setting of age >50 years, dens displacement >5 mm, and specific fracture patterns.
    ○ Type III: Surgical intervention is often reserved for cases of nonunion/malunion after trial of external immobilization.

• CCS: Surgical decompression/fixation is indicated in setting of unstable injury, herniated disc, or when neurologic function deteriorates.
• BCVI: Surgical and/or angiographic intervention may be required if there is evidence of pseudoaneurysm, total occlusion, or transection of the vessel.

ADMISSION, INPATIENT, AND NURSING CONSIDERATIONS
• Varies by injury; clinical judgment, imaging findings, concomitant injuries, and need for operative intervention
• Advanced Trauma Life Support protocol with backboard and collar

 ONGOING CARE

FOLLOW-UP RECOMMENDATIONS
Patient Monitoring
Follow patients with known injuries using serial imaging under the care of a specialist.

PATIENT EDUCATION
ThinkFirst Foundation: http://www.thinkfirst.org

PROGNOSIS
• Presenting neurologic status is the most important factor in determining prognosis.
• Fractures
  – Hangman fracture: 93–100% fusion rate after 8 to 14 weeks external immobilization
  – Odontoid fracture, fusion rate by type: type I, ~100% with external immobilization alone; type II, nonunion rates of up to 67% with halo immobilization alone, especially with dens displacement >6 mm or age >50 years; type III, 85% with external immobilization, 100% with surgical fixation
• BCVI: Patients have fewer neurologic sequelae with early diagnosis and antithrombotic therapy.
• CCS
  – Spontaneous recovery of motor function in >50% over several weeks. Younger patients are more likely to regain function.
  – Leg, bowel, and bladder functions return first, followed by upper extremities.
• WAD: Prognostic factors for development of late whiplash syndrome (>6 months of symptoms affecting normal activity) include increased initial pain intensity, pain-related disability, and cold hyperalgesia.

COMPLICATIONS
• Fractures: instability or malunion/nonunion necessitating second operation, reactions, and infection related to orthosis
• BCVI: embolic ischemic events and pseudoaneurysm formation

REFERENCES
1. Jara-Almonte G, Pawar C. Emergency department management of cervical spine injuries. *Emerg Med Pract*. 2021;23(10):1–28.
2. Masson de Almeida Prado R, Masson de Almeida Prado JL, Ueta RHS, Guimarães JB, Yamada AF. Subaxial spine trauma: radiological approach and practical implications [published online ahead of print September 25, 2021]. *Clin Radiol*. doi:10.1016/j.crad.2021.09.006.
3. Walton DM, Macdermid JC, Giorgianni AA, et al. Risk factors for persistent problems following acute whiplash injury: update of a systematic review and meta-analysis. *J Orthop Sports Phys Ther*. 2013;43(2):31–43.
4. Stiell IG, Clement CM, McKnight RD, et al. The Canadian C-spine rule versus the NEXUS low-risk criteria in patients with trauma. *N Engl J Med*. 2003;349(26):2510–2518.
5. Michaleff ZA, Maher CG, Verhagen AP, et al. Accuracy of the Canadian C-spine rule and NEXUS to screen for clinically important cervical spine injury in patients following blunt trauma: a systematic review. *CMAJ*. 2012;184(16):E867–E876.
6. Jull G, Kenardy J, Hendrikz J, et al. Management of acute whiplash: a randomized controlled trial of multidisciplinary stratified treatments. *Pain*. 2013;154(9):1798–1806.
7. Bracken MB. Steroids for acute spinal cord injury. *Cochrane Database Syst Rev*. 2012;(1):CD001046.

ADDITIONAL READING
• Puvanesarajah V, Qureshi R, Cancienne JM, et al. Traumatic sports-related cervical spine injuries. *Clin Spine Surg*. 2017;30(2):50–56.
• Siasios I, Fountas K, Dimopoulos V, et al. The role of steroid administration in the management of dysphagia in anterior cervical procedures. *Neurosurg Rev*. 2018;41(1):47–53.

 CODES

ICD10
• S13.4XXA Sprain of ligaments of cervical spine, initial encounter
• S13.101A Dislocation of unspecified cervical vertebrae, init encntr
• S14.109A Unsp injury at unsp level of cervical spinal cord, init

CLINICAL PEARLS
• Use NEXUS or CCR to determine need for imaging in every patient with a potential neck injury.
• Always perform imaging if clinical judgment suggests the need to do so.
• Inquire about preexisting cervical spine conditions, especially in the elderly, because this may increase risk of injury or change radiographic interpretation.
• Suspect SCI until fully cleared through exam and imaging.
• Consider BCVI when neurologic deficits are inconsistent with level of known injury or in the setting of a significant mechanism of injury.

CERVICAL MALIGNANCY

Linha Mazin Mohammed, MD

BASICS

DESCRIPTION
- Cervical cancer is a malignant neoplasm arising from the uterine cervix.
- Most cervical cancers begin in the transformation zone.
- 60–75% are from squamous epithelium, and 25–40% are glandular.

EPIDEMIOLOGY
Incidence
- Cervical cancer is the fourth most common cancer in women worldwide and the most common gynecologic cancer.
- Eighty-four percent of cervical cancer cases are from resource-limited regions.
- The disease has a bimodal distribution, with the highest risk among women aged 40 to 59 years and >70 years. However, in recent years, there has been an increase in incidence in women aged 30 to 35 years.

Prevalence
- In 2018, the American Cancer Society (ACS) estimates 13,240 new cases of invasive cancer and 4,170 deaths in the United States.
- In the United States, Hispanic women are at highest risk followed by African Americans, Asians, and whites. American Indians and Alaskan natives have the lowest risk, perhaps attributed to low screening rates.

ETIOLOGY AND PATHOPHYSIOLOGY
- Human papillomavirus (HPV) infection with high-risk (HR) serotypes is the most important etiologic factor.
- HPV infection has high prevalence with nearly 80 million people infected in the United States and 14 million new cases each year worldwide.
- HR serotypes 16 and 18 account for 70% of all cervical cancer.
- Persistent HR-HPV infection promotes coding errors in the cell cycle, resulting in dysplastic changes to the endocervical cellular lining. In addition, HPV activates E6 and E7 oncogenic proteins, which in turn inactivate p53 and Rb tumor suppressor genes.
- Tumor growth is via lymphatic and hematogenous spread (Halstedian growth).

Genetics
There is a broad separation of HPV types based on their associated risk of cervical cancer:
- High risk—This includes HPV 16, 18, 31, 33, 35, 39, 45, 51, 52, 56, 58, 59, and 68.
- Low risk—6, 11, 40, 42, 43, 44, 53, 54, 61, 72, 73, and 81

RISK FACTORS
- Persistent HPV infection is the primary risk factor for developing cervical cancer.
- Other risk factors include: lack of or decreased access to health care and ability to obtain regular Pap tests, early coitarche, multiple sexual partners, unprotected sex, a history of sexually transmitted infections (STIs), low socioeconomic status, obesity (increases the risk for adenocarcinoma type), nonwhite race, first birth prior to age of 20, high parity (>3 full-term deliveries), cigarette smoking (doubles the risk), immunosuppression (HIV/AIDS, chemotherapy), diethylstilbestrol (DES) exposure in utero, oral contraceptive use of >5 years (risk back to baseline after >10 years of nonuse), family history of cervical cancer

GENERAL PREVENTION
- The cornerstone of prevention not only includes routine screening with a Pap test (or HPV test) but also vaccination against HR-HPV. Also important is education on safe sex practices and smoking cessation.
- HPV vaccines protect against HPV serotypes most commonly associated with cervical cancer development, 16 and 18, as well the serotypes responsible for warts (6 and 11).
- The three FDA-approved vaccines are four-serotype Gardasil 4, nine-serotype Gardasil 9, and two-serotype (HPV 16 and 18) Cervarix.
- Vaccination is recommended for:
  – Everyone through the age of 26
  – Girls and boys ages 11 or 12 years in 2 doses, 6 to 12 months apart. It can also be given as early as 9 years of age.
  – Children ≥15 years should receive 3 doses over the course of 6 months.
  – Immunocompromised patients aged 9 to 26 years, men who have sex with men, and the LGBTQ community
- Routine screening with a Pap test (or HPV test) is essential for identifying precursors and early-stage disease. Screening has the potential to prevent up to 80% of cervical cancer worldwide.
- Current guidelines from the U.S. Preventive Services Task Force (USPSTF), as endorsed by The Society of Gynecologic Oncology (SGO), American College of Obstetricians and Gynecologists (ACOG), and the American Society for Colposcopy and Cervical Pathology (ASCCP), recommend screening as follows:
  – Women aged 21 to 29 years: cytology alone every 3 years (1)[C]
  – Women aged 30 to 65 years: cytology alone every 3 years or HR-HPV testing (using an assay specifically approved by the FDA for HPV-screening-only testing) alone every 5 or cytology plus HR-HPV every 5 years (1)[C]
- An alternative screening algorithm using a risk-based strategy and specific FDA-approved high-risk HPV tests followed by cytology for positive screens is a recommended alternative.
- The International Federation of Gynecology and Obstetrics (FIGO) recommends visual inspection with acetic acid (VIA) or Lugol iodine (VILI) as alternatives to Pap smears in resource-poor settings.
- Despite HPV vaccination, cervical cancer screening remains the main preventive measure for both vaccinated and unvaccinated women.

COMMONLY ASSOCIATED CONDITIONS
- Condyloma acuminata
- Preinvasive/invasive lesions of the vulva, vagina, oral, anal, and oropharyngeal cancers

DIAGNOSIS

HISTORY
- Patients with HPV infection may be asymptomatic. Early stages can be discovered incidentally as a result of cervical cancer screening.
- The most common symptoms of cervical cancer are irregular or heavy bleeding and postcoital vaginal bleeding. Other symptoms include vaginal discharge.
- Less common symptoms include low back pain with radiation down posterior leg, lower extremity edema, vesicovaginal and rectovaginal fistula, and urinary symptoms.

PHYSICAL EXAM
- Thorough pelvic exam is essential:
  – Many patients have a normal exam, especially with microinvasive disease.
  – Lesions may be exophytic, endophytic, polypoid, papillary, ulcerative, or necrotic.
  – May have watery, purulent, or bloody discharge.
- In women with symptoms of cervical cancer, bimanual and rectovaginal examination should be performed to evaluate uterine size; vaginal wall; rectovaginal septum; and parametrial, uterosacral, and pelvic sidewall involvement.
- Enlarged supraclavicular or inguinal lymphadenopathy, lower extremity edema, ascites, or decreased breath sounds with lung auscultation may indicate metastases or advanced stage disease.

DIFFERENTIAL DIAGNOSIS
- Marked cervicitis and erosion
- Glandular hyperplasia
- Sexually transmitted infections
- Cervical condyloma, leiomyoma, or polyp
- Metastasis from endometrial carcinoma or gestational trophoblastic neoplasia

DIAGNOSTIC TESTS & INTERPRETATION
Initial Tests (lab, imaging)
- Colposcopy with directed biopsies and/or biopsy of gross lesions are the definitive means of diagnosis.
- CBC may show anemia.
- Urinalysis may show hematuria.
- In advanced disease, BUN, creatinine, and liver function tests (LFTs) may be helpful.
- CT scan of the chest, abdomen, and pelvis and/or a positron emission tomography (PET) scan for metastatic workup
- Apart from chest x-ray (CXR) and intravenous pyelogram (IVP), imaging does not alter tumor stage.
- MRI of the abdomen may be helpful in evaluating parametrial involvement in patients who are surgical candidates or for planning radiation therapy.

Follow-Up Tests & Special Considerations
- Exam under anesthesia may be helpful in determining clinical stage, disease extent, and suitability for surgery.
- Endocervical curettage and cervical conization as indicated to determine depth of invasion and presence of lymphovascular involvement
- Cystoscopy to evaluate bladder invasion
- Proctoscopy for invasion into rectum

Test Interpretation
- Majority of cases are invasive squamous cell types arise from the ectocervix.
- Adenocarcinomas arise from endocervical mucus-producing glandular cells. Often, a "bulky," "barrel-shaped" cervix is present on exam.
- Other cell types include rare mixed cell types, neuroendocrine tumors, sarcomas, lymphomas, and melanomas.

TREATMENT

GENERAL MEASURES
- Improve nutritional state, correct anemia (Hb <12 g/dL), and treat pelvic infections.
- Lymph node evaluation is key to staging and treatment

C

- Correction of urinary tract obstruction is important prior to beginning chemoradiation.
- Pretreatment evaluation should be done prior to chemotherapy for lymph nodes involvement using PET/CT scan.

MEDICATION

- Chemoradiation with a cisplatin-containing regimen has superior survival over pelvic and extended-field radiation alone.
- Neoadjuvant chemotherapy may improve survival for early and locally advanced tumors, but more data are needed.
- Adjuvant chemotherapy after chemoradiation may improve progression-free survival in patients who receive primary chemoradiation for stages IIB to IVA tumors. The OUTBACK trial will further investigate these findings (http://www.clinicaltrials.gov).
- The addition of the antiangiogenesis drug bevacizumab to standard combination chemotherapy (cisplatin/topotecan or cisplatin/paclitaxel) for recurrent, persistent, or metastatic disease has been shown to improve overall survival.

First Line

- Chemoradiation is the primary treatment of choice for stages IB2 to IVA.
- The preferred regimen is weekly cisplatin + radiation therapy or carboplatin (if intolerant to cisplatin).
- The preferred first-line therapy for recurrent or metastatic disease is a combination of cisplatin/paclitaxel/bevacizumab.

Second Line

Other recommended regimen include cisplatin and fluorouracil.

ISSUES FOR REFERRAL

Multidisciplinary management of patients as needed and in a timely fashion

ADDITIONAL THERAPIES

- Chemoradiation (without surgery) is the first-line therapy for tumors stage IIB and higher (gross lesions with obvious parametrial involvement) and for most bulky stage IB2 tumors.
- Combination of external beam pelvic radiation and brachytherapy is usually employed.
- If para-aortic lymph node metastases are suspected, extended-field radiation or lymph node dissection prior to radiation therapy may be performed.

SURGERY/OTHER PROCEDURES

- Surgical management is an option for patients with early-stage tumors.
- Removal of precursor lesions (cervical intraepithelial neoplasia [CIN]) by loop electrosurgical excision procedure (LEEP), cold knife conization, laser ablation, or cryotherapy
- Stage IA1 (lesions with <3-mm invasion from basement membrane) without lymphovascular space invasion: option of conization or simple extrafascial hysterectomy
- Stage IA2 (lesions with >3-mm but <5-mm invasion from basement membrane): option of radical hysterectomy with lymph node dissection or radiation depending on clinical setting. Robotic radical hysterectomy (RRH) has demonstrated to be superior to laparoscopic radical hysterectomy and open radical hysterectomy in intraoperative blood loss, length of hospital stay, and intraoperative and postoperative complications; RRH can be regarded as a safe and effective therapeutic procedure for the management of cervical cancer.
- Stages IA2 to IB1: Fertility-sparing radical trachelectomy may be considered in selected patients.

- Stages IB1 to IIA (gross lesions without obvious parametrial involvement): option of radical hysterectomy with lymph node sampling or primary chemoradiation with brachytherapy and teletherapy, depending on clinical setting. In stage IB, when comparing adjuvant radiotherapy with no adjuvant radiotherapy, there is no significant difference in survival at 5 years between women who received radiation and those who received no further treatment (risk ratio [RR] = 0.8, 95% confidence interval [CI] 0.3–2.4). However, women who received radiation had a significantly lower risk of disease progression at 5 years (RR 0.6, 95% CI 0.4–0.9).
- Stage IVA (lesions limited to central metastasis to the bladder and/or rectum): Primary pelvic exenteration may be feasible.
- Stage IVB (lesions spread to distant organs): Treatment goal is palliation; therefore, early referral to palliative care should be made.

Pregnancy Considerations

- Management is guided by consideration of stage of lesion, gestational age, and maternal assessment of risks and benefits from treatment.
- Abnormal cytology is best followed up by colposcopy with directed biopsies.
- In pregnant women diagnosed with cervical cancer before 16 weeks of gestation, treatment should be started immediately.
- In pregnant women with early stages (IA1, IA2, IB) diagnosed after 16 weeks of gestation, treatment may be delayed to allow for fetal maturity.
- In pregnant women with advance disease (stage IB2) diagnosed after 16 weeks, treatment may be based on gestational age at the time of diagnosis. Microinvasive carcinoma: conization or trachelectomy. If depth of invasion ≤3 mm, follow up at the 6-week postpartum visit.
- Invasive carcinoma requires definitive therapy, with timing determined by maternal preference, stage of disease, and gestational age at the time of diagnosis.

ADMISSION, INPATIENT, AND NURSING CONSIDERATIONS

- Signs of active bleeding
- Urinary symptoms
- Dehydration
- Complications from surgery, chemotherapy, or radiation
- Active vaginal bleeding can be controlled with timely vaginal packing and radiation therapy.
- Recognition of ureteral blockage, hydronephrosis, urosepsis, and timely intervention
- Discharge criteria based on multidisciplinary assessment

 ONGOING CARE

FOLLOW-UP RECOMMENDATIONS

Patient Monitoring

- With completion of definitive therapy and based on individual risk factors, patients are evaluated with physical/pelvic examinations:
  – Every 3 to 6 months for 2 years
  – Every 6 to 12 months until the 5th year
  – Yearly thereafter
- Pap smears may be performed yearly but have a low sensitivity for detecting recurrence.
- CT and PET scan are useful in locating metastases when recurrence is suspected. Preferably 3 to 4 months posttreatment
- Signs of recurrence include vaginal bleeding, unexplained weight loss, leg edema, and pelvic or thigh pain.

PATIENT EDUCATION

- ACOG: http://www.acog.org
- SGO: http://www.sgo.org; the Foundation for Women's Cancer: http://www.foundationfor womenscancer.org
- ACS: http://www.cancer.org; the National Cancer Institute: http://www.cancer.gov

PROGNOSIS

- If detected early, invasive cervical cancer can be treated successfully.
- The 5-year survival rate for early-stage (stage 1A, in which the cancer has minimal spread to the inside of the cervix) is estimated at 92%.
- The 5-year survival rate by stage (2012 ACS): Stage IB—80%; stage IIA—63%; stage IIB—58%; stage III—30%; stage IVA—16%
- An elevated squamous cell carcinoma antigen (SCC-Ag) serum levels estimated by ELISA technique can be used to predict the clinical response to neoadjuvant chemotherapy and residual disease. Persistently elevated SCC-Ag level at 2 to 3 months after RT had a significantly higher incidence of treatment failure.
- Serum SCC-Ag levels are also useful for monitoring treatment efficacy, disease progression, recurrence, and poor prognosis in SCCs. The combination of clinical pelvic examination and SCC-Ag levels provides useful information for the further need of treatment.

COMPLICATIONS

- Loss of ovarian function from radiotherapy or indication for bilateral oophorectomy
- Hemorrhage
- Pelvic infection
- Genitourinary fistula
- Bladder dysfunction, sexual dysfunction
- Ureteral obstruction with renal failure
- Bowel obstruction
- Pulmonary embolism
- Lower extremity lymphedema

REFERENCE

1. Curry SJ, Krist AH, Owens DK, et al; for U.S. Preventive Services Task Force. Screening for cervical cancer: US Preventive Services Task Force recommendation statement. *JAMA.* 2018;320(7):674–686.

 SEE ALSO

Abnormal Pap and Cervical Dysplasia

CODES

ICD10

- C53.9 Malignant neoplasm of cervix uteri, unspecified
- C53.0 Malignant neoplasm of endocervix
- C53.1 Malignant neoplasm of exocervix

CLINICAL PEARLS

- Cervical cancer is the second most common malignancy in women worldwide. Improving access to screening is likely to have the greatest impact in the reduction of the burden of disease.
- Women with cervical cancer may be asymptomatic and have a normal physical exam.
- Surgical management is an option for patients with early-stage tumors.
- Chemoradiation is the first-line therapy for higher stage tumors.

CHICKENPOX (VARICELLA ZOSTER)

Daniel R. Matta, MD • Joseph A. Chen, MD

 BASICS

DESCRIPTION

- Highly contagious, generalized exanthem characterized by crops of pruritic vesicles on the skin and mucous membranes following exposure to varicella-zoster virus (VZV)
- VZV is acquired through inhalation of respiratory droplets from an infected host and through direct contact with vesicles.
- VZV establishes latency in the dorsal root ganglia; reactivation results in herpes zoster (shingles).
- Outbreaks tend to occur late winter through early spring in temperate climates.
- Usual incubation period is 14 to 16 days (range 10 to 21 days) after exposure to varicella OR shingles rash. Patients are infectious from ~48 hours before appearance of vesicles until the final lesions have crusted.
- Historically, most acquire chickenpox during childhood and developed lifelong immunity. The varicella vaccine became available in 1995 (1). Varicella is currently part of recommended primary vaccination schedule for children.
- System(s) affected: nervous, skin/exocrine

EPIDEMIOLOGY

- Peak incidence 3 to 9 years but may occur at any age
- Predominant gender: male = female

Incidence

- Decreasing incidence since routine vaccination; estimated 3.5 million cases annually prior to vaccine, with an incidence of 8–9% in children aged 1 to 9 years
- Reported U.S. varicella cases: 1991: 147,076; 2017: 8,775 cases (1)
- Prior to vaccine, ~100 deaths per year were reported in the United States; in 2015, only 6 reported deaths (1)
- U.S. rates: 1994, prior to vaccine: 136/100,000 persons; 2013 to 2014: <0.001/100,000 persons
- In developing countries, varicella is still associated with a severe disease burden.
- Susceptible (nonimmune) individuals exposed to varicella are at risk to develop disease and are also potentially infectious for 21 days.

ETIOLOGY AND PATHOPHYSIOLOGY

- Viral particles are inhaled via respiratory droplets where they invade respiratory epithelium. Replication in regional respiratory tract lymph nodes is followed by primary viremia (4 to 6 days after exposure). A second phase of viral replication and a secondary viremia (14 to 16 days after exposure) contributes to epidermal invasion and the characteristic skin lesions.
- Skin lesions are histologically identical to herpes simplex virus.
- In fatal cases, intranuclear inclusions are found in vascular endothelium and most organs.
- VZV is a double-stranded DNA virus of the α-Herpesviridae subfamily.
- Humans are primary disease reservoir.

RISK FACTORS

Nonimmune, immunocompromised (especially children with leukemia/lymphoma in remission or receiving high-dose corticosteroids), pregnancy

Geriatric Considerations

- Infection is more severe in adults; reactivation of latent infection causes shingles.
- The CDC recommends vaccinating all immunocompetent adults ≥50 years old with recombinant varicella vaccine (Shingrix). The live attenuated vaccine (Zostavax) is no longer available for use in the United States as of 2020.
- The recombinant zoster vaccine (Shingrix) is administered as a 2-dose series separated by 2 to 6 months. This vaccine can be given to patients with a history of shingles or who have already had a dose of the live attenuated zoster vaccine.
- Primary viral pneumonia is the most common cause of death from varicella.

Pediatric Considerations

- Neonates born to mothers who develop chickenpox from 5 days before to 2 days after delivery are at risk for serious disease and should receive varicella-zoster immune globulin (VZIG).
- Newborns are at highest risk for severe disease during the 1st month of life, especially if mother is seronegative.
- Delivery prior to 28 weeks increases risk.
- Varicella bullosa is seen mainly in children <2 years. Lesions appear as bullae instead of vesicles. The clinical course is otherwise similar.
- Septic complications and encephalitis are the most common causes of death from zoster in children.
- Avoid aspirin/acetylsalicylic acid in children because of link to Reye syndrome.

Pregnancy Considerations

- 25% risk of transplacental infection
- Congenital malformations are seen in 2% of patients when the fetus is infected during the 1st or 2nd trimester, characterized by limb hypoplasia, localized muscle atrophy, encephalitis, low birth weight, cutaneous scarring, cortical atrophy, chorioretinitis, and microcephaly.
- Morbidity (e.g., pneumonia) is increased in women infected during pregnancy.
- Women who contract chickenpox can breastfeed as normal. However, open vesicles on the breast should be covered to minimize transmission.

GENERAL PREVENTION

- Isolate hospitalized patients.
- When indicated, administer passive immunization using VZIG within 96 hours after exposure. VZIG recommended for:
  - Patients exposed to chickenpox or shingles who are immunocompromised, newborns of mothers with onset of chickenpox <5 days before delivery or <2 days after delivery, premature infants (<28 weeks) exposed in neonatal period either whose mothers are not immune, or babies who weigh <1,000 g regardless of maternal immunity
- Active immunization prevents or reduces the severity of varicella if given within 72 hours of exposure.

- Active immunization: varicella virus vaccine (Varivax): live attenuated vaccine recommended by ACIP for immunization of healthy patients ≥12 months who have not had chickenpox
  - 12 months to 12 years: initial dose 0.5 mL SC at age 12 to 15 months; second dose at age 4 to 6 years. Single dose is 85–94% effective in preventing severe disease. The 2-dose regimen is 96–98% effective. Breakthrough disease has shorter duration and lower fever incidence (2)[A].
  - ≥13 years: two 0.5 mL SC doses 4 to 8 weeks apart, seroconversion rates 78–82% after 1 dose, 99% after 2 doses; adult efficacy in lower end of this range
  - 2014 U.S. estimate: 91% one or more dose vaccine coverage for children 19 to 35 months (3)
  - Vaccine side effects include pain and redness at the vaccine site (19% of children; 24% of teens and adults). 1 in 10 develops fever. 1 in 25 will develop a mild varicella-like rash up to 1 month after vaccination.
  - Vaccine contraindications
    - Severe allergic reaction (e.g., anaphylaxis) to a previous dose or vaccine component
    - Severe immunodeficiency (e.g., HIV patients with low CD4 counts, chemotherapy, congenital immunodeficiency, long-term immunosuppressive therapy)
    - Pregnancy
- MMRV vaccine, combines the measles, mumps, and rubella vaccine with varicella, is equally effective. There are rare reports of an increased risk of febrile seizures 5 to 12 days after vaccination in 1/2,300 to 2,600 patients.
- May be considered for a subset of HIV-positive children in CDC class I with CD4 >25%
  - Vaccine recipients who develop a rash should avoid contact with immunocompromised people, pregnant women who have never had chickenpox, and their newborns.
  - Allow at least 3 months between doses 1 and 2 in children needing catch-up vaccination.

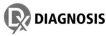 **DIAGNOSIS**

HISTORY

- Prodromal symptoms: fever, malaise, anorexia, headache
- Malaise, muscle aches, arthralgias, and headache are more common in adults.
- Subclinical in ~4% of cases
- Characteristic rash

PHYSICAL EXAM

- Characteristic rash: crops of vesicles on erythematous base
- Lesions erupt in successive crops.
- Fever (usually <102°F)
- Progress from macule to papule to vesicle and then begin to crust
- Pruritic rash is present in various stages of development and healing.

DIFFERENTIAL DIAGNOSIS
- Herpes zoster: shingles
- Insect bites
- Smallpox
- Impetigo
- Coxsackievirus infection
- Scabies
- Dermatitis herpetiformis
- Drug rash

DIAGNOSTIC TESTS & INTERPRETATION
The diagnosis of chickenpox is primarily clinical. Testing is generally reserved for complicated cases or epidemiologic studies.

Initial Tests (lab, imaging)
- VZV polymerase chain reaction (PCR) is the current method of choice (best is fluid from intact vesicle).
- Marked leukocytosis suggests secondary infection.
- Multinucleated giant cells on Tzanck smear from vesicle scrapings
- Isolate virus from human tissue culture technically difficult (positive in <40% of cases)
- Direct immunofluorescence is more sensitive and quicker to perform.

Follow-Up Tests & Special Considerations
- Serologies show acute (IgM) or prior (IgG) infection.
- Visualization by electron microscopy, tissue culture (costly), and various methods of acute and convalescent sera collection: latex agglutination (most available), enzyme immunoassay, indirect immunofluorescence antibody, fluorescent antibody to membrane assay, or PCR assay, which can detect wild from vaccine viral strains
- Vaccine-modified cases difficult to diagnose; PCR testing of skin lesions is most sensitive and specific for diagnosing varicella, especially in vaccinated persons.

 ## TREATMENT
Generally outpatient, except for complicated cases

GENERAL MEASURES
- Supportive/symptomatic treatment
- Oral antihistamines and/or oatmeal baths for itch
- Calamine lotion for itch
- Acetaminophen and/or ibuprofen for pain and fever
- Clipping fingernails closely can help prevent scarring or excoriations leading to secondary infections.

MEDICATION
First Line
- Supportive: antipyretics for fever; avoid aspirin in children.
- Local and/or systemic antipruritic agents for itching
- VZIG available for passive immunization for:
  – Immunocompromised patients, newborn infants to mothers with signs and symptoms of varicella at the time of delivery; premature infants born at 28 weeks or more whose mothers do not have evidence of immunity to varicella; premature infants <28 weeks' gestation or who weigh <1,000 g regardless of maternal immunity
  – Give VZIG within 96 hours after exposure (4).

- Acyclovir: decreases duration of fever and shortens time of viral shedding; recommended for unvaccinated adolescents >12, children treated with inhaled steroids or intermittent oral steroids (5), adults, and high-risk patients (immunocompromised); most beneficial if initiated early in the disease (≤24 hours)
  – 2- to 16-year-old patients: 20 mg/kg/dose (max 800 mg/dose) QID for 5 days
  – Immunocompetent adults: 800 mg 5 times daily for 5 days
  – Immunocompromised adults: 10 mg/kg/dose IV q8h for 7 days. Use IBW in obese patients.
  – For more complicated disease, IV acyclovir has better bioavailability than oral agents.
- Contraindication
  – Hypersensitivity to the drug
- Precautions
  – Renal insufficiency with acyclovir
  – Concurrent administration of probenecid increases half-life; increased effects with zidovudine (e.g., drowsiness, lethargy)

Second Line
Valacyclovir: ≥2 years: 20 mg/kg/dose (max 1,000 mg/dose) TID for 5 days

ADMISSION, INPATIENT, AND NURSING CONSIDERATIONS
Severe complications including septicemia, necrotizing fasciitis, and osteomyelitis may require inpatient care. Newborns and immunocompromised individuals are at higher risk of severe varicella and may need hospital monitoring.

 ## ONGOING CARE

FOLLOW-UP RECOMMENDATIONS
Patient Monitoring
- Not needed in mild cases. Intensive supportive care may be required in the setting of complications.
- Activity as tolerated. Children may return to school when lesions have completely scabbed.

DIET
No special diet

PATIENT EDUCATION
- In otherwise healthy children, chickenpox is rarely serious and the recovery is almost always complete.
- Native chickenpox typically confers lifelong immunity.
- A second attack is rare, but subclinical infection can occur; occasionally, after vaccination in children
- Latent infection may recur years later as shingles in adults.
- Fatalities are rare.

COMPLICATIONS
- Although only 2% of cases are reported after 2nd decade, 35% of deaths occur in this age group.
- Secondary bacterial infection: cellulitis, abscess, erysipelas, sepsis, septic arthritis/osteomyelitis, or staphylococcal pyomyositis

- Pneumonia: 20–30% of adults with chickenpox have lung involvement; 1/400 is hospitalized.
- Encephalitis
- Meningitis; Reye syndrome
- Purpura, thrombocytopenia
- Glomerulonephritis; arthritis; hepatitis

REFERENCES
1. Centers for Disease Control and Prevention. Nationally notifiable infectious diseases and conditions, United States: annual tables. https://wonder.cdc.gov/nndss/nndss_annual_tables_menu.asp. Accessed August 18, 2021.
2. Ayoade F, Kumar S. *Varicella Zoster*. In: StatPearls [Internet]. Treasure Island, FL: StatPearls Publishing; 2021. https://pubmed.ncbi.nlm.nih.gov/28846365/.
3. Berger S. *Varicella-Zoster: Global Status*. Los Angeles, CA: GIDEON Informatics; 2021.
4. Hill HA, Elam-Evans LD, Yankey D, et al. National, state, and selected local area vaccination coverage among children aged 19-35 months—United States, 2014. *MMWR Morb Mortal Wkly Rep*. 2015;64(33):889–896.
5. Centers for Disease Control and Prevention. Updated recommendations for use of VariZIG—United States, 2013. *MMWR Morb Mortal Wkly Rep*. 2013;62(28):574–576.

ADDITIONAL READING
Centers for Disease Control and Prevention. Recommended child and adolecent immunization schedule for ages 18 years or younger, United States, 2021. https://www.cdc.gov/vaccines/schedules/downloads/child/0-18yrs-child-combined-schedule.pdf.

 ## SEE ALSO

Herpes Zoster (Shingles)

CODES

ICD10
- B01.9 Varicella without complication
- B02.9 Zoster without complications
- P35.8 Other congenital viral diseases

CLINICAL PEARLS
- Varicella zoster infection is more likely to produce serious illness in adults than in children.
- Introduction of the varicella vaccine has significantly reduced morbidity and mortality. Currently, 2 doses of vaccine are recommended during childhood.
- Recombinant zoster vaccine is recommended for immunocompetent persons ≥50 years of age to decrease chance of shingles.

CHILD ABUSE
Wynne Morgan, MD • Sasha Svendsen, MD

BASICS

DESCRIPTION
- Types of abuse: neglect (most common and highest mortality), physical abuse, emotional/psychological abuse, sexual abuse, and sexual exploitation
- Neglect includes physical (e.g., failure to provide necessary food or shelter or lack of appropriate supervision), medical (e.g., failure to provide necessary medical or mental health treatment), educational (e.g., failure to educate a child or attend to special education needs), and emotional (e.g., inattention to a child's emotional needs, failure to provide psychological care, or permitting the child to use alcohol or other drugs).
- System(s) affected: gastrointestinal (GI), endocrine/metabolic, musculoskeletal, nervous, renal, reproductive, skin/exocrine, pulmonary, cardiac, immune, and psychiatric
- Synonym(s): nonaccidental trauma; child maltreatment; inflicted injury

EPIDEMIOLOGY
Prevalence
Children's Bureau report for federal fiscal year (FFY) 2019 (1):
- Child Protective Services agencies received an estimated 4.4 million referrals alleging maltreatment, with a national screened-in referral rate of 32.2 referrals per 1,000 children).
- Approximately 3.5 million children received either an investigation or alternative response. Of those investigated, just >650,000 children (8.9 per 1,000) were found to be victims of abuse or neglect.
- Neglect is the most common type of reported maltreatment at 74.9%, followed by physical abuse at 17.5%, and sexual abuse at 9.3%.
- The overall rate of child fatalities was 2.5 deaths per 100,000 children in the national population. The rate of child fatalities is slightly higher in boys compared to girls.
- The majority of perpetrators are the parents of their victims (77.5%).

RISK FACTORS
- American Indian or Alaska Native children had the highest rates of victimization, followed by African-American children.
- Children in the age group of birth to 1 year had the highest rate of victimization at 25.3 per 1,000 infants and the highest rate of mortality from maltreatment.
- Girls have a slightly higher rate of victimization when compared to boys.
- Military families are a risk of abuse, especially around times of deployment.
- Child risk factors include chronic illness, physical/congenital disability, developmental delay, preterm, unintended pregnancy
- Caregiver risk factors include poverty, substance misuse, lower educational status, parental history of abuse, parental mental health issues, young and/or unmarried mother, poor support network, and domestic violence (2).

GENERAL PREVENTION
- Know your patients and ask about their family situations; screen for risk factors at prenatal, postnatal, and pediatric visits.
- Physicians can educate parents on a range of normal behaviors to expect in infants and children:
  – E.g., anticipatory guidance on ways to handle crying infants; methods of discipline for toddlers

- Train first responders, teachers, and childcare workers to look for signs of abuse and know methods for reporting.
- Some studies suggest developing screening tools to identify high-risk families early and offer interventions such as early childhood home visitation programs.

COMMONLY ASSOCIATED CONDITIONS
- Failure to thrive
- Prematurity
- Developmental delays
- Poor school performance
- Poor social skills
- Low self-esteem
- Anxiety or depression

DIAGNOSIS

- Relatively minor skin injuries, frenulum tears, or bruising in precruising infants may be the first indications of child physical abuse; these relatively minor, unexplained injuries have been termed "sentinel injuries."
- In a retrospective study of infants who were diagnosed with abuse, 27.5% had a sentinel injury (80% had a bruise), and in 41.9% of those cases, the parent reported that a medical provider was aware of the injury (3).
- Patients may present with seemingly unrelated complaints; multiple studies have documented repeated visits (to the primary care physician or to the emergency department [ED]) before child abuse is suspected.
- Infants with injuries caused by child abuse often present with vague complaints; thus, it is important to have high index of suspicion when evaluating infants for fussiness.
- Documentation
  – The medical record is a legal document.
  – Critical elements include the following:
    ○ Brief statement of child's disclosure or caregiver's explanation, including any alternate explanations offered (Use direct quotations when possible.)
    ○ Time the incident occurred and date/time of disclosure
    ○ Whether witnesses were present
    ○ Developmental abilities of child
    ○ Objective medical findings
- DO NOT use terms such as "rule out," "R/O," and "alleged." They may cause ambiguity; clearly state objective findings and medical provider's opinion.
- The history from the caregiver should be obtained separately from the child. Consideration should be given to obtain the history from the child separate to the caregiver when indicated.
- Any description of abuse given by the child should be recorded word for word using quotation marks in the child's own language and attributed to the child whenever possible.
- The child should not be rewarded after a disclosure (e.g., "Tell me what happened and you can go back to your mom . . .").
- Remember this is a medical history and the medical provider is obtaining information needed for diagnostic and treatment decisions.
- Documentation should include disposition of patient and record any report made to child welfare.

HISTORY
- Use nonjudgmental, open-ended questions (ask: who, what, when, and where; NEVER why).
- Use quotes whenever possible.
- Do not obtain history from the caregiver in front of the child.
- Document past medical history, developmental history, child's temperament, and thorough social history including objective documentation of family interactions.
- History of a sentinel injury should prompt consideration of abuse; it may be the first and only abusive injury; there may be escalating and repeated violence.
- The following historical elements may suggest abusive injury:
  – No explanation or vague explanation of injury
  – Important detail of explanation changes dramatically
  – Explanation is inconsistent with pattern, age, or severity of injury.
  – Explanation is inconsistent with child's physical or developmental abilities.
  – Different witnesses provide different history.
  – There is considerable delay in seeking treatment.
  – Denial of trauma in a child with injury
- Nonspecific symptoms of abuse:
  – Behavior changes; self-destructive behavior
  – Anxiety and/or depression
  – Sleep disturbances, night terrors
  – School problems

PHYSICAL EXAM
- Examine child in a comfortable setting:
  – Explain what the exam will involve and why procedures are needed.
  – Allow child to choose who will be in the room.
  – Completely undress the child and have them wear a gown to perform a complete physical examination, including thorough skin exam.
- Complete a general assessment for signs of physical abuse, neglect, and self-injurious behaviors:
  – Measurements, photographs, and careful objective descriptions are critical for accurate diagnosis.
  – Encourage communication and collaboration with specialist and child abuse assessment team.
- A thorough physical exam may include:
  – Skin (completely undress, including diaper)
  – Head (including fontanels), eyes, ears, nose, and mouth
  – Chest/abdomen
  – Anogenital area
  – Extremities
  – Review growth charts
- Physical abuse findings
  – Skin markings (e.g., lacerations, burns, bruises, patterned injuries, bites)
  – Immersion injuries with clearly demarcated borders
  – Oral trauma (e.g., torn frenulum, loose teeth)
  – Ear bruising
  – Eye trauma (e.g., hyphema, subconjunctival hemorrhage)
  – Head/abdominal blunt trauma
  – Fractures
- Sexual abuse findings
  – Unexplained penile, vaginal, hymenal, perianal, or anal injuries/bleeding/discharge
  – Pregnancy or sexually transmitted infections (STIs)
  – The majority of anogenital exams of children who have been sexually abused are completely normal.
- Neglect findings
  – Low-growth parameter trends, unclean, unkempt
  – Rashes
  – Fearful or overly trusting

– Clinging to or avoiding caregiver
– Abnormal development or growth parameters

DIFFERENTIAL DIAGNOSIS

- Physical trauma mimics
  – Accidental injury; toxic ingestion
  – Bleeding disorders (e.g., classic hemophilia)
  – Metabolic or congenital conditions
  – Conditions with skin manifestations (e.g., congenital dermal melanocytosis, Henoch-Schönlein purpura, meningococcemia, erythema multiforme, hypersensitivity, staphylococcal scalded skin syndrome, chickenpox, impetigo)
  – Cultural practices (e.g., cupping, coining)
- Neglect mimics
  – Endocrinopathies (e.g., diabetes mellitus)
  – Constitutional growth delay
  – GI (clefts, malabsorption, irritable bowel)
  – Seizure disorder
- Skeletal trauma mimics
  – Obstetrical trauma
  – Nutritional (scurvy, rickets)
  – Infection (congenital syphilis, osteomyelitis)
  – Osteogenesis imperfecta

DIAGNOSTIC TESTS & INTERPRETATION
Initial Tests (lab, imaging)

- Directed by history and physical exam findings:
  – Urinalysis (abdominal/flank/back/genital trauma), urine DNA probe for STIs
  – Complete blood count, coagulation studies
  – Electrolytes, creatinine, blood urea nitrogen, glucose
  – Liver and pancreatic function tests (abdominal trauma)
  – Guaiac stool (abdominal trauma)
- In cases of suspected neglect:
  – Stool exam, calorie count, purified protein derivative and anergy panel, sweat test, lead and zinc levels
- In cases of suspected sexual abuse:
  – STI testing: gonorrhea, chlamydia, *Trichomonas*; also consider HIV, hepatitis B and C serologies, syphilis.
  – The American Academy of Pediatrics (AAP) recommends the use of NAATs when evaluating children and adolescents for *Chlamydia trachomatis* and *Neisseria gonorrhoeae*.
  – Serum pregnancy test
- Skeletal survey is a mainstay of child abuse evaluation; 22 radiographs
  – It is recommended for:
    ○ Infants <6 months with bruising, regardless of pattern (given rarity of accidental bruising in young nonmobile infants)
    ○ Children with bruising attributed to abuse or domestic violence
    ○ Children <12 months with bruising on the cheek, eye area, ear, neck, upper arm, upper leg, hand, foot, torso, buttocks, or genital area
    ○ All children <2 years old with fractures and poorly explained injuries
  – Suspected intracranial and extracranial injury:
    ○ Computed tomography (CT) scan of head
    ○ Consider magnetic resonance imaging of head/neck, looking at subtle findings, brain parenchyma, intracerebral edema, or hemorrhage.
  – Intra-abdominal injuries: CT scan of abdomen with IV contrast
- High-risk imaging findings:
  – Fractures in nonambulatory patients (Children who are not walking or cruising rarely have bruising or fractures from short "falls.")
  – Corner or bucket-handle fractures
  – Posterior rib fractures in infants
  – Rupture of liver/spleen in abdominal blunt trauma

Follow-Up Tests & Special Considerations

- Red flags
  – History that is inconsistent with the injury
  – No explanation offered for the injury or injury blamed on sibling or another child
  – History that is inconsistent with the child's developmental level
- Maintain a high level of suspicion when exam findings indicate multiple types of injury.
- Patterns suggestive of abuse
  – Bruises seen away from bony prominences
  – Bruises to face, back, abdomen, arms, buttocks, ears, hands
  – Multiple bruises in clusters or uniform shape
  – Patterned injuries (such as bite marks or the imprint of an object like a belt or cord) should be considered highly concerning for inflicted injury.
- TEN-4 method to identify bruises suggestive of child abuse:
  – T: torso
  – E: ear
  – N: neck
  – 4: any bruise on a child <4 months old
- In cases of sexual abuse where there is concern for exposure to body fluids, forensic evidence kit collection may be indicated up to 120 hours postassault.

 TREATMENT

GENERAL MEASURES
All cases of suspected child abuse or neglect require a mandatory report to state child welfare agencies.

MEDICATION
First Line

- Consider antibiotics postexposure prophylaxis in postpubertal children as indicated for STIs. Of note, do not prophylactically treat prepubertal children with antibiotics for STIs.
- If exposure to body fluids is of concern, consider HIV postexposure prophylaxis.

ALERT
Emergency contraception reduces rate of pregnancy after sexual assault:

- Levonorgestrel (Plan B): single dose of 1.5 mg or two 0.75-mg doses taken together or 12 hours apart; effective up to 72 hours OR
- Ulipristal (Ella): 30-mg single dose as soon as possible; effective up to 120 hours

ISSUES FOR REFERRAL
When responding to possible abuse, consider:

- The child's safety. Is the child at imminent risk for additional harm if sent back to the environment where the possible perpetrator has access to the child?
- Work with child welfare to ensure family is complying with a plan of safe care that may include the following:
  – Mental health referrals for the victim and other family members, including siblings
  – Any follow-up with medical subspecialties, as needed
  – Continue to support the caregivers through the process when possible.

ADMISSION, INPATIENT, AND NURSING CONSIDERATIONS
Admission if:

- Moderate to severe injuries or unstable
- Acute psychological trauma
- Unable to coordinate a safe discharge plan

 ONGOING CARE

PATIENT EDUCATION

- National Child Abuse Hotline: 1-800.4.A.CHILD (800.422.4453)
- National Toll-Free Crisis Hotline Numbers—Child Welfare Information Gateway: https://www.childwelfare.gov/pubs/reslist/tollfree/
- Trauma resources: National Child Traumatic Stress Network (NCTSN), www.NCTSN.org

PROGNOSIS
Without intervention, child abuse is often a chronic and escalating phenomenon.

COMPLICATIONS
Sexual, physical, and emotional abuse in childhood are risk factors for poorer adult mental and physical health. This includes maltreatment, depression, substance misuse, suicide attempts, and risky sexual behaviors.

REFERENCES

1. U.S. Department of Health & Human Services, Administration for Children and Families. Administration on Children, Youth and Families, Children's Bureau. Child maltreatment 2017. https://www.acf.hhs.gov/cb/research-data-technology/statistics-research/child-maltreatment. Accessed December 20, 2021.
2. Christian CW, Crawford-Jakubiak JE, Flaherty EG, et al; for Committee on Child Abuse and Neglect, American Academy of Pediatrics. The evaluation of suspected child physical abuse. *Pediatrics*. 2015;135(5):e1337–e1354.
3. Sheets LK, Leach ME, Koszewski IJ, et al. Sentinel injuries in infants evaluated for child physical abuse. *Pediatrics*. 2013;131(4):701–707.

 CODES

ICD10

- T74.12XA Child physical abuse, confirmed, initial encounter
- T74.32XA Child psychological abuse, confirmed, initial encounter
- T74.22XA Child sexual abuse, confirmed, initial encounter

CLINICAL PEARLS

- Mandated reporting is required for suspected child abuse and neglect; the medical provider does not have to prove abuse before reporting.
- When a bruise is present, it should be considered as potentially sentinel for physical abuse if no plausible explanation is given.
- High index of suspicion is important for prevention and recognition of abuse. Vague complaints and repeated visits to the office and/or ED should prompt further consideration.
- Neglect is the most common and lethal form of abuse.
- Detailed and comprehensive physical exam with documentation is key.

C

CHLAMYDIA INFECTION (SEXUALLY TRANSMITTED)

Casandra Cashman, MD, FAAFP

 BASICS

DESCRIPTION

- *Chlamydia trachomatis* is an intracellular membrane-bound prokaryotic organism. Chlamydia derives from the Greek word for "cloak."
- Chlamydia is the most common bacterial sexually transmitted infection (STI) in the United States.
- Transmitted through vaginal, anal, or oral sex; transmitted vertically during vaginal delivery
- Most cases are asymptomatic, especially in females. Untreated disease can lead to pelvic inflammatory disease (PID), ectopic pregnancy, and infertility.
- System(s) affected: reproductive

Pregnancy Considerations

Perinatal acquisition may result in neonatal pneumonia and/or conjunctivitis.

EPIDEMIOLOGY

Incidence

- Mandatory reporting started in 1985; there has generally been a steady increase in incidence since.
- ~1.8 million *reported* cases in 2019 (most recent CDC data). Increasing incidence reflects broader screening, improved testing, and better reporting (rather than a large increase in disease burden).
- Swedish new variant of *C. trachomatis* (nvCT) first reported in 2006; often produces false-negative tests; largely confined to Nordic countries

Prevalence

- 553/100,000 people in the United States
- Young females, ethnic minorities most affected
- Highest prevalence ages 20 to 24 years, followed by ages 15 to 19 years
- Predominant sex: females > males. Females have 2 times higher reported incidence and prevalence than males. This likely reflects increased testing in females. Increasing use of highly sensitive nucleic acid amplification test (NAAT) urine screening may increase identification in males.
- Infection rates ~6 times higher in blacks than whites. Rates are higher in larger urban areas.
- Highest male prevalence in heterosexual adolescents
- Estimated to affect ~2% of young sexually active individuals in the United States

ETIOLOGY AND PATHOPHYSIOLOGY

C. trachomatis serotypes D to K associated with genital tract infections. Chlamydia is an obligate intracellular organism. Chlamydia has biphasic life cycle. Exists extracellularly as elementary body (EB) that is metabolically inactive and infectious. Once taken up by host cell (typically columnar epithelium of the genital tract), the EB prevents lysosomal phagocytosis and transforms to reticulate body (RB) which requires energy from host cell to synthesize RNA, DNA, and proteins. After taking up host cell residence, EB are released and are capable of infecting neighboring cells or spreading the infection through sexual contact.

RISK FACTORS

Risk correlates with:

- Number of lifetime sexual partners and number of concurrent sexual partners
- No use of barrier contraception during intercourse
- Black/Hispanic/Native American and Alaskan Native ethnicity

- Men who have sex with men (MSM) may be at higher risk for rectal and pharyngeal chlamydia than other groups; consider testing with NAAT when appropriate (1).

GENERAL PREVENTION

- Screen populations with prevalence >5% at least annually.
- Screening recommended if new or >1 sex partner in past 6 months; attending an adolescent clinic, family planning clinic, STD or abortion clinic, or attending a jail or other detention center clinic. Screen if rectal pain, discharge or tenesmus, testicular pain; test all individuals with urethral or cervical discharge.
- All sexually active women ≤25 years of age should be screened at least yearly. Repeat testing in ~3 months is recommended for those who screen positive because reinfection rate is high regardless of whether the sexual partner is treated (2)[A].
- Consider screening sexually active men ≤25 years of age particularly in high-risk populations.
- Screen high-risk MSM annually with genital and extragenital screening (3)[A].
- NAAT is the preferred screening test in all circumstances except child sexual abuse involving boys or rectal/oropharyngeal testing in prepubescent girls. For these situations, culture and susceptibility testing is preferred (3)[A].
- Acceptable to screen women for chlamydia on same day as intrauterine device (IUD) insertion—treat if positive (no need to remove IUD in this circumstance) (4)[B]

COMMONLY ASSOCIATED CONDITIONS

- Females
  - PID: ~10% develop PID within 12 months if untreated.
  - Infertility, ectopic pregnancy
  - Chronic pelvic pain
  - Urethral syndrome (dysuria, frequency, and pyuria in the absence of infection)
  - Arthritis (less common)
  - Spontaneous abortion
- Males
  - Epididymitis and nongonococcal urethritis
  - Reiter syndrome (HLA-B27)
  - Proctitis
- Neonates
  - Inclusion conjunctivitis (occurs in ~40% of exposed neonates)
  - Otitis media
  - Pneumonia
  - Pharyngitis
- Diseases caused by other chlamydial species
  - Lymphogranuloma venereum (LGV): *C. trachomatis* serotypes L1 to L3
  - Trachoma: *C. trachomatis* serotypes A to C

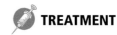 **DIAGNOSIS**

Many patients are asymptomatic.

Pregnancy Considerations

- Test all patients at first prenatal visit.
- Obtain repeat testing 3 to 4 weeks after treatment for all pregnant patients with confirmed chlamydial infection. Test again 3 months after.
- Repeat screening in 3rd trimester in high-risk patients (2)[A].

HISTORY

- Complete sexual history, including number of sex partners (lifetime and past year), prior history of STIs, use of barrier protection, commercial sex work, oral or anal receptive intercourse, and partner fidelity
- In females, the most common symptoms are:
  - Mucopurulent vaginal discharge, dysuria (urethral syndrome), bartholinitis, abdominopelvic pain (endometritis, salpingitis/PID), right upper quadrant pain (Fitz-Hugh–Curtis syndrome)
- In males, the most common symptoms are:
  - Dysuria, urethral discharge (urethritis), scrotal pain (epididymitis), rectal pain or discharge (proctitis), acute arthritis (Reiter syndrome)

PHYSICAL EXAM

- Men and women: external genitalia (rash, lesions), urethral discharge, inguinal lymphadenopathy, pharyngeal exudate, and perianal lesions
- Women: cervix (discharge, motion tenderness), bimanual examination for cervical motion tenderness, uterine, ovarian/adnexal tenderness or mass
- LGV (*C. trachomatis* serovars L1, L2, or L3): Primary lesion is a small papule that may ulcerate at the site of transmission after an incubation period of 3 to 30 days. Unilateral tender lymphadenopathy. With rectal transmission, LGV causes an invasive proctocolitis.

DIFFERENTIAL DIAGNOSIS

- *Neisseria gonorrhoeae*: urethritis, proctitis, epididymitis, cervicitis, PID, Bartholin abscess
- *Mycoplasma* or *Ureaplasma urealyticum*: urethritis, epididymitis, Reiter disease, PID
- *C. trachomatis* (serotypes L1 to L3): LGV, proctitis
- Trichomoniasis

DIAGNOSTIC TESTS & INTERPRETATION

Initial Tests (lab, imaging)

- NAAT: sensitivity >95%; specificity >99%
- Urine test is similarly sensitive to cervical swabs but preferably is collected on first catch urine. Self-collected vaginal swabs are most sensitive (3)[A].
- Lab result may remain positive for 3 weeks after successful treatment.
- Test for concurrent STIs, including gonorrhea, HIV, and syphilis; perform cervical cancer (Pap smear) screening according to recommended guidelines.

Follow-Up Tests & Special Considerations

See "Patient Monitoring."

TREATMENT

GENERAL MEASURES

- Offer patients concurrent testing for gonorrhea, HIV (after counseling and consent), and possibly syphilis. Ensure women are up-to-date with recommended cervical cancer screening.
- Consider treating gonorrhea empirically.
- Test and treat all partners (most recent partner and all partners within the past 60 days).

MEDICATION

First Line

- https://www.cdc.gov/std/treatment-guidelines/chlamydia.htm
- Treatment of chlamydial urethritis, cervicitis (including sexual partners of infected persons)
- Azithromycin 1 g PO single dose *or*
- Doxycycline 100 mg PO BID for 7 days
- First-line PID treatment (outpatient)
  – Ceftriaxone 250 mg IM × 1 *plus* doxycycline 100 mg PO for 14 days with or without metronidazole 500 mg PO BID for 14 days *or (Please note updated uncomplicated gonorrhea treatment guidelines published December 2020, which recommend 500 mg of ceftriaxone IM for patients under 150 kg, and 1 g for patients over 150 kg.)*
  – Cefoxitin 2 g IM × 1 with probenecid 1 g PO × 1 *plus* doxycycline 100 mg PO for 14 days with or without metronidazole 500 mg PO BID for 14 days
- Azithromycin and ceftriaxone may be given simultaneously in the office to treat both chlamydia and gonorrhea. This reduces nonadherence.
- Asymptomatic rectal chlamydia is most effectively treated with doxycycline 100 mg BID × 7 days. Azithromycin 1 g for 1 day is slightly less effective but can also be used, especially if compliance or medication availability is an issue (5)[A].

ALERT
Use azithromycin with caution in patients with known QT prolongation, hypokalemia, hypomagnesemia, bradycardia, or who are currently treated with antiarrhythmics.

Pregnancy Considerations
- Tetracyclines (doxycycline) and quinolones (ofloxacin, levofloxacin) are contraindicated in pregnant women.
- Consider the following:
  – Azithromycin 1 g PO *or*
  – Amoxicillin 500 mg PO TID for 7 days *or*
  – Erythromycin base 500 mg PO QID for 7 days

ALERT
Tetracyclines and quinolones are contraindicated in young children:

- <45 kg: erythromycin base or ethinyl succinate 500 mg/kg/day PO QID for 14 days
- >45 kg but <8 years: azithromycin 1 g PO once
- >8 years: adult regimen
- Rule out sexual abuse in children with chlamydial infections.

Second Line
For chlamydial urethritis/cervicitis
- Erythromycin base 500 mg PO QID for 7 days OR erythromycin ethylsuccinate 800 mg PO QID for 7 days
- Levofloxacin 500 mg PO daily for 7 days OR ofloxacin 300 mg PO BID for 7 days

ADDITIONAL THERAPIES
Patient-delivered partner therapy (PDPT) or expedited partner therapy (EPT): Provide medications or prescriptions to take to sexual partners of persons infected with STIs without clinical assessment.

- EPT reduces recurrence more effectively than traditional partner referral.
- http://www.cdc.gov/std/ept/legal/

ADMISSION, INPATIENT, AND NURSING CONSIDERATIONS
- Inpatient treatment of PID: pregnancy, lack of response or intolerance to oral medicines, suspicion of poor compliance, severe clinical illness, pelvic abscess, and possible need for surgical intervention
- Otherwise, treat PID as outpatient unless moderately or severely ill.

 ONGOING CARE

FOLLOW-UP RECOMMENDATIONS
Abstain from sexual contact for at least 7 days after treatment (single-dose treatment) or until completion of the full course of other antibiotics.

Patient Monitoring
- Test of cure not routinely recommended except in pregnancy. Do not repeat NAAT <3 weeks after testing; may be falsely positive due to nonviable organisms
- Test of cure in 3 to 4 weeks in pregnancy as well as test for reinfection in 3 months
- Consider rescreening higher risk pregnant women in 3rd trimester even if initial screening negative.
- Test for reinfection (not cure) 3 months after treatment or, if not possible, then at next presentation to medical care if within 12 months.
- Sexual partners should be treated. Some states allow for EPT.

PATIENT EDUCATION
- Counsel regarding safe sexual practices, barrier protection, and abstinence.
- Complete antibiotic course (patient and partners)

PROGNOSIS
Prognosis is good following therapy.

COMPLICATIONS
- Both sexes: Chlamydial infection enhances transmission of and susceptibility to HIV.
- Females: tubal infertility (most common cause of acquired infertility), tubal (ectopic) pregnancy, chronic pelvic pain
  – Annual screening of sexually active women would prevent 61% of chlamydia-related PID.
- Males: transient oligospermia and postepididymitis urethral stricture (rare)

REFERENCES

1. Centers for Disease Control and Prevention. Sexually transmitted disease surveillance 2019: chlamydia. https://www.cdc.gov/std/stats19/chlamydia.htm. Accessed August 16, 2021.
2. Centers for Disease Control and Prevention. Sexually transmitted infections treatment guidelines, 2021: chlamydial infection. https://www.cdc.gov/std/treatment-guidelines/chlamydia.htm. Accessed August 16, 2021.
3. Centers for Disease Control and Prevention. Recommendations for the laboratory-based detection of *Chlamydia trachomatis* and *Neisseria gonorrhoeae*—2014. http://www.cdc.gov/mmwr/preview/mmwrhtml/rr6302a1.htm. Accessed Sept. 21, 2020.
4. Sufrin CB, Postlethwaite D, Armstrong MA, et al. *Neisseria gonorrhea* and *Chlamydia trachomatis* screening at intrauterine device insertion and pelvic inflammatory disease. *Obstet Gynecol.* 2012;120(6):1314–1321.
5. Elgalib A, Alexander S, Tong CY, et al. Seven days of doxycycline is an effective treatment for asymptomatic rectal *Chlamydia trachomatis* infection. *Int J STD AIDS.* 2011;22(8):474–477.

ADDITIONAL READING

- Elwell C, Mirrashidi K, Engel J. Chlamydia cell biology and pathogenesis. *Nat Rev Microbiol.* 2016;14(6):385–400.
- He W, Jin Y, Zhu H, et al. Effect of *Chlamydia trachomatis* on adverse pregnancy outcomes: a meta-analysis. *Arch Gynecol Obstet.* 2020;302(3):553–567.

 SEE ALSO

Cervicitis, Ectropion, and True Erosion; Epididymitis; Gonococcal Infections; HIV/AIDS; Pelvic Inflammatory Disease; Syphilis; Urethritis

 CODES

ICD10
- A56.8 Sexually transmitted chlamydial infection of other sites
- A56.01 Chlamydial cystitis and urethritis
- A56.02 Chlamydial vulvovaginitis

CLINICAL PEARLS

- *C. trachomatis* is common in young sexually active individuals. Annual screening is recommended in sexually active women 25 years of age and younger and in other individuals with known risk factors.
- To prevent recurrence, treat patients and their partners concurrently.
- Doxycycline is the most effective treatment for rectal chlamydia.
- Test of cure is only recommended for pregnant patients 3 to 4 weeks after treatment for an identified chlamydia infection. Test for reinfection 3 months afterward. Repeat screens in 3rd trimester for high-risk patients regardless of initial test results.

CHOLELITHIASIS

Hongyi Cui, MD, PhD

 BASICS

DESCRIPTION
- The presence of cholesterol, pigment, or mixed stones (calculi) within the gallbladder
- Synonym(s): gallstones

Pediatric Considerations
- Uncommon in children <10 years
- Most gallstones in children are pigment stones associated with blood dyscrasias.

EPIDEMIOLOGY
Incidence
- Increased in Native Americans and Hispanics
- Increases with age ~1–3% per year; peaks at 7th decade
- 2% of the U.S. population develops gallstones annually.

Prevalence
- 8–10% of the U.S. population with gallstones
- 20% >65 years of age
- Female > male (2 to 3:1)

ETIOLOGY AND PATHOPHYSIOLOGY
- Gallstone formation is a complex process mediated by genetic, metabolic, immune, and environmental factors. Gallbladder sludge (a mixture of cholesterol crystals, calcium bilirubinate granules, and mucin gel matrix) serves as the nidus for gallstone formation.
- Bile supersaturated with cholesterol (cholesterol stones) precipitates as microcrystals that aggregate and expand. Stone formation is enhanced by biliary stasis or impaired gallbladder motility.
- Decrease in bile phospholipid (lecithin) or decreased bile salt secretion
- Excess unconjugated bilirubin in patients with hemolytic diseases; passage of excess bile salt into the colon with subsequent absorption of excess unconjugated bilirubin in patients with inflammatory bowel disease (IBD) or after distal ileal resection (black or pigment stones)
- Hydrolysis of conjugated bilirubin or phospholipid by bacteria in patients with biliary tract infection or stricture (brown stones or primary bile duct stones; rare in the Western world and common in Asia)

RISK FACTORS
- Age peaks in patients 60 to 80 years of age.
- Female gender, pregnancy, multiparity, obesity, and metabolic syndrome
- Caucasian, Hispanic, or Native American descent
- High-fat diet rich in cholesterol
- Cholestasis or impaired gallbladder motility in association with prolonged fasting, long-term total parenteral nutrition (TPN), following vagotomy, long-term somatostatin therapy, and rapid weight loss
- Hereditary (p.D19H variant for the hepatic canalicular cholesterol transporter ABCG5/ABG8)
- Short gut syndrome, terminal ileal resection, IBD
- Hemolytic disorders (hereditary spherocytosis, sickle cell anemia, etc.), cirrhosis (black/pigment stones)
- Medications (birth control pills, estrogen replacement therapy at high doses, and long-term corticosteroid or cytostatic therapy)
- Viral hepatitis, biliary tract infection, and stricture (promotes intraductal formation of pigment stones)

GENERAL PREVENTION
- Regular exercise and dietary modification may reduce the incidence of gallstone formation.
- Lipid-lowering drugs (statins) may prevent cholesterol stone formation by reducing bile cholesterol saturation.
- Ursodiol (Actigall) taken during rapid weight loss helps prevent gallstone formation.

COMMONLY ASSOCIATED CONDITIONS
90% of people with gallbladder carcinoma have gallstones and chronic cholecystitis.

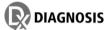 **DIAGNOSIS**

HISTORY
- Most patients are asymptomatic (80%): 2% become symptomatic each year. Over their lifetime, <50% of patients with gallstones develop symptoms.
- Episodic right upper quadrant or epigastric pain lasting >15 minutes and sometimes radiating to the back (biliary colic—due to transient cystic duct obstruction)
- Pain is usually postprandial, particularly following a fatty meal but sometimes awakens patients from sleep.
- Most patients develop recurrent symptoms after a first episode of biliary colic.
- Other symptoms include nausea, vomiting, indigestion or bloating sensation, and fatty food intolerance.
- Gallstone-related complications (such as gallstone pancreatitis) may be first manifestation of gallstone disease.

PHYSICAL EXAM
- Physical exam is *usually normal* in patients with cholelithiasis in the absence of an acute attack.
- Epigastric and/or right upper quadrant tenderness (Murphy sign) is a traditional physical finding associated with acute cholecystitis. Murphy sign has limited sensitivity and specificity.
- Charcot triad: fever, jaundice, right upper quadrant pain historically associated with cholangitis
- Reynolds pentad: fever, jaundice, right upper quadrant pain, hemodynamic instability, mental status changes; also classically associated with ascending cholangitis
- Flank and periumbilical ecchymoses (Cullen sign and Grey Turner sign) in patients with acute hemorrhagic pancreatitis
- Courvoisier sign: palpable mass in the right upper quadrant in patient with obstructive jaundice most commonly due to malignant tumors within the biliary tree or pancreas

DIFFERENTIAL DIAGNOSIS
- Peptic ulcer diseases and gastritis
- Hepatitis
- Pancreatitis
- Cholangitis
- Gallbladder cancer
- Gallbladder polyps
- Acalculous cholecystitis
- Biliary dyskinesia
- Choledocholithiasis

DIAGNOSTIC TESTS & INTERPRETATION
Ultrasound is the preferred diagnostic modality for cholelithiasis.

Initial Tests (lab, imaging)
- Leukocytosis and elevated C-reactive protein level are common in acute calculus cholecystitis.
- Ultrasound (US) is the preferred imaging modality. US detects gallstones in 97–98% of patients.
- Thickening of the gallbladder wall (≥5 mm), pericholecystic fluid, and direct tenderness when the probe is pushed against the gallbladder (sonographic Murphy sign) are associated with acute cholecystitis.
- CT scan has no advantage over US except for detecting distal common bile duct (CBD) stones.
- MR cholangiopancreatography (MRCP) is reserved for cases of suspected CBD stones. However, MRCP has no therapeutic value, and preoperative MRCP is not more cost-effective than initial cholecystectomy with cholangiography in the diagnosis of patients with suspected CBD stones and patients with mild to moderate gallstone pancreatitis (GP).
- Endoscopic US is as sensitive as endoscopic retrograde cholangiopancreatography (ERCP) for detection of CBD stones in patients with GP.
- Hepatobiliary iminodiacetic acid (HIDA) scan is useful in diagnosing acute cholecystitis secondary to cystic duct obstruction. It is also useful in differentiating acalculous cholecystitis from other causes of abdominal pain. False-positive tests can result from a fasting state, insufficient resistance of the sphincter of Oddi, and gallbladder agenesis.
- Cholecystokinin (CCK)-HIDA is specifically used to diagnose gallbladder dysmotility (biliary dyskinesia).
- 10–30% of gallstones are radiopaque calcium or pigment-containing gallstones (visible on plain x-ray). A "porcelain gallbladder" is a calcified gallbladder (also visible by x-ray) that is associated with chronic cholecystitis and gallbladder cancer.

Test Interpretation
- Pure cholesterol stones are white or slightly yellow.
- Pigment stones may be black or brown. Black stones contain polymerized calcium bilirubinate, most often secondary to cirrhosis or hemolysis; these almost always form within the gallbladder.
- Brown stones are associated with biliary tract infection, caused by bile stasis, and as such primarily form in the bile ducts.

 TREATMENT

GENERAL MEASURES
- Treat symptomatic cholelithiasis.
- Conservative therapy is preferred during pregnancy; surgery in the 2nd trimester if necessary.
- Prophylactic cholecystectomy for patients with calcified (porcelain) gallbladder (risk for gallbladder cancer), patients with large stones (≥3 cm), patients with sickle cell disease, pediatric gallstones, patients planning an organ transplant, and patients with recurrent pancreatitis due to microlithiasis
- In morbidly obese patients, cholecystectomy may be performed in combination with bariatric procedures to reduce subsequent stone-related comorbidities.
- Prophylactic cholecystectomy is recommended for gallstones discovered incidentally during open abdominal surgery.

C

Geriatric Considerations
Gallstones are more common in the elderly. Age alone should not alter the therapeutic plan.

MEDICATION
First Line
- Analgesics for pain relief
  - NSAIDs are the first-choice treatment for pain control, which is equivalent to opioid therapy.
  - Opioids are an option for patients who cannot tolerate or fail to respond to NSAIDs.
- Antibiotics for patients with acute cholecystitis
- Prophylactic antibiotics in low-risk patients do not prevent infections during laparoscopic cholecystectomy (LC).

ISSUES FOR REFERRAL
Patients with retained or recurrent bile duct stones following cholecystectomy should be referred for ERCP.

SURGERY/OTHER PROCEDURES
- Surgery should be considered for patients who have symptomatic cholelithiasis or gallstone-related complications (e.g., cholecystitis) or in asymptomatic patients with immune suppression, calcified gallbladder, giant gallstones (≥3 cm), or family history of gallbladder cancer.
- Open and LC have similar mortality and complication rates. LC offers less pain and quicker recovery and is the current gold-standard treatment.
- In well-selected patients, robotic cholecystectomy (RC) is an alternative to LC. RC is associated with higher cost and has not been shown to be superior to LC in terms of pain and risk of complication. Surgery-related complications include CBD injury (0.4–0.6%), right hepatic duct/artery injury, retained stones, bile leak, biloma formation, and bile duct stricture. Bile spillage during LC has been shown to be a risk factor for surgical site infection.
  - Conversion to open procedure is based on clinical judgment. This should not be viewed as a surgical complication but rather a decision to carry out the operation in the safest manner. Male gender, previous upper abdominal surgery, thickened gallbladder wall, and acute cholecystitis increase the likelihood of need to convert to an open procedure.
  - In 10–15% of patients with symptomatic cholelithiasis, CBD stones are detected by intraoperative cholangiogram (IOC). CBD stone(s) can be removed by laparoscopic CBD exploration or postoperative ERCP.
  - IOC helps delineate bile duct anatomy when dissection is difficult. Routine use of IOC is controversial and may be associated with decreased incidence and severity of bile duct injury.
- Early LC (<24 hours after diagnosis of biliary colic) decreases hospital stay and operating time.
- For patients with acute cholecystitis, early LC (<7 days of clinical presentation) is safe and may shorten the total hospital stay versus delayed LC (>6 weeks after index admission with acute cholecystitis) (1)[A].
- Laparoscopic fundus-first cholecystectomy and partial/subtotal cholecystectomy are viable options in difficult operative conditions (such as severe cholecystitis).

- Percutaneous cholecystostomy (PC) is used for high-risk patients with cholecystitis or gallbladder empyema. Interval cholecystectomy is recommended.
- Symptomatic patients who are not candidates for surgery or those who have small gallstones (5 mm or smaller) in a functioning gallbladder with a patent cystic duct are candidates for oral dissolution therapy (ursodiol [Actigall]). The recurrence rate is >50% once medication is discontinued.
- Cystic duct stenting via ERCP is a viable option for managing severe acute cholecystitis, gallbladder hydrops, or empyema in patients unfit for surgery. It can be used as a bridge to laparoscopic cholecystectomy.
- Extracorporeal shock wave lithotripsy is a non-invasive therapeutic alternative for symptomatic patients who are not candidates for surgery. It helps break down large bile duct stones before ERCP. Complications include biliary pancreatitis, hepatic hematoma, incomplete ductal stone clearance, and recurrence.

ADMISSION, INPATIENT, AND NURSING CONSIDERATIONS
For patients with symptomatic cholelithiasis, LC is typically an outpatient procedure. For patients with complications (i.e., cholecystitis, cholangitis, pancreatitis), inpatient care is necessary.
- Acute phase: NPO, IV fluids, and antibiotics
- Adequate pain control with narcotics and/or NSAIDs

 ONGOING CARE

FOLLOW-UP RECOMMENDATIONS
Patient Monitoring
- Follow for signs of symptomatic cholelithiasis.
- Follow patients on oral dissolution agents with serial liver enzymes, serum cholesterol, and imaging.

DIET
A low-fat diet may help.

PATIENT EDUCATION
- Change in lifestyle (e.g., regular exercise) and dietary modification (low-fat diet and reduction of total caloric intake) may reduce gallstone-related hospitalizations.
- Patients with asymptomatic gallstones should be educated about the typical symptoms of biliary colic and gallstone-related complications.

PROGNOSIS
- <50% of patients with gallstones become symptomatic.
- Cholecystectomy-related mortality is <0.5% in elective cases and 3–5% in emergency cases; morbidity is <10% in elective cases and 30–40% in emergency cases.
- ~10–15% of patients have associated choledocholithiasis.
- After cholecystectomy, stones may recur within the biliary tree in patients with associated risk factors.

COMPLICATIONS
- Acute cholecystitis (90–95% secondary to gallstones)
- GP; ERCP ± sphincterotomy offers no clear benefit in patients with mild GP but reduces complications in those with severe GP (2)[A].
- CBD stones with obstructive jaundice and acute cholangitis. In patients undergoing ERCP for CBD stones, early LC reduces the risk of recurrent biliary events (3)[B].
- Biliary-enteric fistula and gallstone ileus
- Bouveret syndrome is a variant of gallstone ileus where the gallstone lodges in the duodenum or pylorus causing a gastric outlet obstruction.
- Gallbladder cancer
- Mirizzi syndrome (extrinsic bile duct obstruction caused by gallstones lodged in gallbladder or cystic duct)

REFERENCES
1. Chung AY, Duke MC. Acute biliary disease. *Surg Clin North Am*. 2018;98(5):877–894.
2. Burstow MJ, Yunus RM, Hossain MB, et al. Meta-analysis of early endoscopic retrograde cholangiopancreatography (ERCP) ± endoscopic sphincterotomy (ES) versus conservative management for gallstone pancreatitis (GSP). *Surg Laparosc Endosc Percutan Tech*. 2015;25(3):185–203.
3. Huang RJ, Barakat MT, Girotra M, et al. Practice patterns for cholecystectomy after endoscopic retrograde cholangiopancreatography for patients with choledocholithiasis. *Gastroenterology*. 2017;153(3):762.e2–771.e2.

ADDITIONAL READING
Peponis T, Eskesen TG, Mesar T, et al. Bile spillage as a risk factor for surgical site infection after laparoscopic cholecystectomy: a prospective study of 1,001 patients. *J Am Coll Surg*. 2018;226(6):1030–1035.

 SEE ALSO

Cholangitis, Acute; Choledocholithiasis

 CODES

ICD10
- K80.20 Calculus of gallbladder w/o cholecystitis w/o obstruction
- K80.21 Calculus of gallbladder w/o cholecystitis with obstruction
- K80.01 Calculus of gallbladder w acute cholecystitis w obstruction

CLINICAL PEARLS
- Most gallstones are asymptomatic.
- Transabdominal US is the imaging modality of choice for cholelithiasis (sensitivity, 97%; specificity, 95%).
- Laparoscopic cholecystectomy is the preferred surgical procedure for symptomatic cholelithiasis and gallstone-related complications.
- Acute acalculous cholecystitis is associated with bile stasis and gallbladder ischemia.
- Prophylactic cholecystectomy is not indicated in patients with asymptomatic gallstones.

CHRONIC COUGH

Jacqueline L. Olin, CDCES, PharmD, FASHP, MS, FCCP, BCPS • Brian Hertz, MD •
J. Andrew Woods, PharmD, BCPS

BASICS

DESCRIPTION
- Chronic cough is defined as a cough that persists for >8 weeks in adults.
- In children, chronic cough is often defined as a cough of >4 weeks in duration.
- Subacute cough describes a cough lasting 3 to 8 weeks.
- Patients present because of fear of the causative illness (e.g., cancer), annoyance, self-consciousness, and hoarseness.
- System(s) affected: gastrointestinal (GI), pulmonary

EPIDEMIOLOGY
- Predominant age: all age groups
- Predominant sex: male = female, with females more likely to seek out medical attention

Incidence
Persistent unexplained cough occurs in up to 10% of patients presenting with chronic cough and up to 46% referred to specialty cough clinics (1).

Prevalence
Chronic cough is one of the most common reasons for primary care visits.

ETIOLOGY AND PATHOPHYSIOLOGY
Varies with findings and disorders implicated
- Often multiple etiologies, but most are related to bronchial irritation. Frequent etiologies (account for >90% of cases) in nonsmokers include the following:
  - Upper airway cough syndrome (UACS) and other upper airway abnormalities, including allergic and vasomotor rhinitis syndromes
  - Chronic rhinitis with postnasal drip (allergic, nonallergic, chronic sinusitis, etc.)
  - Postviral cough
  - Asthma
  - Gastroesophageal reflux disease (GERD)
- Other causes:
  - ACE inhibitors
  - Chronic smoking or exposure to smoke or pollutants
  - Aspiration
  - Bronchiectasis
  - Infections (e.g., pertussis, tuberculosis)
  - Nonasthmatic eosinophilic bronchitis (NAEB)
  - Cystic fibrosis
  - Sleep apnea
  - Restrictive lung diseases
  - Neoplasms: bronchogenic or laryngeal
  - Psychogenic (habit cough)
- Cough hypersensitivity syndrome defines a syndrome of cough with characteristic trigger symptoms not adequately explained by other medical conditions.

- Etiologies of chronic cough in young children differ from those in older children and adults with asthma, protracted bacterial bronchitis, and UACS as most common causes (2),(3).

RISK FACTORS
Although various conditions may contribute to chronic cough, the main causes include smoking and pulmonary diseases.

COMMONLY ASSOCIATED CONDITIONS
Patients with UACS, asthma, and GERD may present with chronic cough as the only symptom and not the usual symptoms associated with the diagnoses.

DIAGNOSIS

HISTORY
- Patient's age, associated signs/symptoms, medical history, medication history (i.e., ACE inhibitors), environmental and occupational exposures, potential for aspiration, and smoking history may make some causes more likely.
- The character of cough or description of sputum quality is rarely helpful in predicting the underlying cause.
- Cough diaries have not correlated well with objective measures.
- Hemoptysis or signs of systemic illness preclude empiric therapy.

PHYSICAL EXAM
- Signs and symptoms are variable and related to the underlying cause; usually, a nonproductive cough with no other signs or symptoms
- Possible signs and symptoms of UACS, sinusitis, GERD, congestive heart failure, chronic stressors
- Absence of additional signs/symptoms of a particular condition not necessarily helpful
  - For example, 5% of patients with GERD have no other signs or symptoms and sometimes have poor response to empiric proton pump inhibitor (PPI) trials.

DIAGNOSTIC TESTS & INTERPRETATION
- Evaluation often starts with empiric therapy directed at likely underlying etiology and/or simple testing such as a chest x-ray (CXR).
- Extensive testing only if indicated by the history and physical

Pediatric Considerations
Children with chronic cough not responsive to an inhaled β-agonist and without overt stressors should undergo spirometry (if age-appropriate) and foreign body evaluation (CXR).

Initial Tests (lab, imaging)
- Evaluation will be dictated by findings in the comprehensive history and physical.
- Evaluation of peak flow may be indicated.
- If considering neoplasm, heart failure, or infectious etiologies, CXR or B-type natriuretic peptide (BNP) may be indicated.
- In cases of failure to respond to initial trial of empiric therapy, CXR may also be beneficial.

Follow-Up Tests & Special Considerations
- Examples:
  - If considering chronic obstructive pulmonary disease (COPD), asthma, or restrictive lung disease: spirometry
  - If suspicious of cystic fibrosis: sweat chloride testing
  - If suspicious of hypereosinophilic syndrome, tuberculosis, or malignancy: sputum for eosinophils and cytology
- If abnormal CXR, suspected neoplasm, or underlying pulmonary disorder, consider a chest CT.
- Consider pulmonary consultation.
- Consider specialist cough clinic.
- Refer to gastroenterologist for endoscopy.

Diagnostic Procedures/Other
If diagnosis suggested and inadequate response to initial measures, other procedures can be considered:
- Pulmonary function testing
- Purified protein derivative (PPD) skin testing
- Allergen testing
- 24-hour esophageal pH monitor
- Bronchoscopy, if history of hemoptysis or smoking with normal CXR
- Endoscopic or video fluoroscopic swallow evaluation or barium esophagram
- Sinus CT
- Ambulatory cough monitoring and cough challenge with citric acid, capsaicin, or other bronchodilator (at specialized cough clinic)
- Echocardiogram

Test Interpretation
Specific to underlying cause

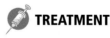

TREATMENT

GENERAL MEASURES
- With chronic cough, empiric treatment should be directed at the most common causes as clinically indicated (UACS, asthma, GERD) (1),(3)[C].
- Empiric trial of nasal steroids and/or antihistamines should be considered if allergic symptoms or postnasal drip is present.

- With concomitant complaints of heartburn and regurgitation, GERD should be considered as a potential etiology (3)[C].
- In patients with cough associated with the common cold, nonsedating antihistamines were not found to be effective in reducing cough (1),(3)[C].
- Many patients will have resolution of cough after smoking cessation.
- When indicated, ACE inhibitor therapy should be switched in patients in whom intolerable cough occurs. It may take several days or weeks for cough to resolve after stopping ACE inhibitor therapy.
- Empirically treat postnasal drip and GERD.
- Empiric PPIs are not recommended in children or adults in the absence of a GERD diagnosis (3)[C].
- Multimodality speech pathology therapy had a positive benefit on cough severity in some adults (1)[C].
- Attempt maximal therapy for single most likely cause for several weeks and then search for coexistent etiologies.

MEDICATION
- Treatments (nasal steroids, classic antihistamines, antacids, bronchodilators, inhaled corticosteroids, PPIs, antibiotics) should be directed at the specific cause of cough.
- If history and physical exam suggest GERD, may want to trial empiric PPI therapy prior to further diagnostic testing
- The FDA issued a public health advisory stating that OTC cough and cold medicines, including antitussives, expectorants, nasal decongestants, antihistamines, or combinations, should not be given to children <2 years. Subsequently, manufacturers have changed labeling to state "do not use" in children <4 years. In 2017, the FDA issued a contraindication to codeine for cough treatment in children <12 years.
- Routine empiric treatment of children with chronic cough with leukotriene receptor antagonists lacks evidence and cannot be recommended.

First Line
In adults:
- Nasal steroids: fluticasone, budesonide, others, 1 spray BID for those with allergic rhinitis symptoms or postnasal drip or an empiric trial of PPI (omeprazole, others) once a day

Second Line
- A peripherally acting antitussive agent has been used:
  – In patients >10 years, benzonatate (Tessalon Perles) 100 to 200 mg PO TID as needed (maximum 600 mg/day)
- Gabapentin was evaluated in a randomized, double-blind, placebo-controlled trial of patients with refractory chronic cough. Gabapentin demonstrated improved cough-specific quality of life compared

to placebo. Nausea and fatigue occurred in 31%. A therapeutic trial with a risk-benefit assessment at 6 months is suggested (1)[C].
- A comparative effectiveness review of 49 studies with common opioid and nonanesthetic antitussives stated there is some efficiency for treating cough in adults, but evidence is limited (4)[C].
- Studies evaluating inhaled corticosteroid use in chronic cough for patients without additional indication such as asthma did not show consistent benefits (1)[C].

ISSUES FOR REFERRAL
Patients with chronic cough may benefit from evaluation by pulmonary, gastroenterology, ear/nose/throat (ENT), and/or allergy specialists. Consider specialist cough clinic.

SURGERY/OTHER PROCEDURES
Fundoplication may be effective for cough secondary to refractory GERD.

 ONGOING CARE

FOLLOW-UP RECOMMENDATIONS
Consider stepwise withdrawal of medications after resolution of cough.

Patient Monitoring
Frequent follow-up is necessary to assess the effectiveness of treatment.

DIET
Dietary modification: Patients with GERD may benefit by avoiding ethanol, caffeine, nicotine, citrus, tomatoes, chocolate, and fatty foods.

PATIENT EDUCATION
- Reassure patient that most cases of chronic cough are not life-threatening and that the condition can usually be managed effectively.
- Counsel that several weeks to a month may be needed for significant reduction or elimination of cough.
- Prepare the patient for the possibility of multiple diagnostic tests and therapeutic regimens because the treatment is very often empiric.

PROGNOSIS
- >80% of patients can be effectively diagnosed and treated using a systematic approach.
- Cough from any cause may take weeks to months until resolution, and resolution depends greatly on efficacy of treatment directed at underlying etiology.

COMPLICATIONS
- Cardiovascular: arrhythmias, syncope
- Stress urinary incontinence
- Abdominal and intercostal muscle strain
- GI: emesis, hemorrhage, herniation

- Neurologic: dizziness, headache, seizures
- Respiratory: pneumothorax, laryngeal, or tracheo-bronchial trauma
- Skin: petechiae, purpura, disruption of surgical wounds
- Medication side effects
- Other: negative impact on quality of life

REFERENCES
1. Gibson P, Wang G, McGarvey L, et al; and CHEST Expert Cough Panel. Treatment of unexplained chronic cough: CHEST guideline and expert panel report. *Chest*. 2016;149(1):27–44.
2. Chang AB, Oppenheimer JJ, Weinberger M, et al; and CHEST Expert Cough Panel. Etiologies of chronic cough in pediatric cohorts: CHEST guideline and expert panel report. *Chest*. 2017;152(3):607–617.
3. Michaudet C, Malaty J. Chronic cough: evaluation and management. *Am Fam Physician*. 2017;96(9):575–580.
4. Yancy WS Jr, McCrory DC, Coeytaux RR, et al. Efficacy and tolerability of treatments for chronic cough: a systematic review and meta-analysis. *Chest*. 2013;144(6):1827–1838.

 SEE ALSO

- Asthma; Bronchiectasis; Eosinophilic Pneumonias; Gastroesophageal Reflux Disease; Laryngeal Cancer; Lung, Primary Malignancies; Pertussis; Pulmonary Edema; Rhinitis, Allergic; Sinusitis; Tuberculosis
- Algorithm: Cough, Chronic

 CODES

ICD10
- R05 Cough
- J44.9 Chronic obstructive pulmonary disease, unspecified
- J41.0 Simple chronic bronchitis

CLINICAL PEARLS
- Chronic cough is defined as a cough that persists for >8 weeks in adults.
- In patients with chronic cough, most frequent etiologies include a history of smoking, asthma, UACS, and GERD.
- The FDA issued a public health advisory stating that OTC cough and cold medicines should not be given to children <2 years. OTC cough expectorant and suppressant product labels state "do not use" in children <4 years. Codeine is contraindicated for cough treatment in children <12 years.

CHRONIC KIDNEY DISEASE

Tyler Martin West, MD • Mark L. Higdon, DO, FAAFP

 BASICS

Chronic kidney disease (CKD) is defined as structural or functional abnormalities of the kidney, as determined by either pathologic abnormalities or markers of damage (abnormalities in blood or urine tests, histology, imaging studies) or a glomerular filtration rate (GFR) <60 mL/min/1.73 m². Findings present for ≥3 months. CKD is classified based on the cause, GFR category (G1 to G5), and albuminuria category (A1 to A3).

DESCRIPTION
- Kidney Disease: Improving Global Outcomes (KDIGO) categories by GFR estimation (in mL/min/1.73 m²): G1: kidney damage with normal or increased GFR ≥90; G2: mild ↓ GFR 60 to 89; G3a: mild to moderate ↓ GFR 45 to 59; G3b: moderate to severe ↓ GFR 30 to 44; G4: severe ↓ GFR 15 to 29; G5: kidney failure: GFR <15 or dialysis
- CKD per albumin-to-creatinine ratio (ACR) category: A1: normal to mildly increased: <30 mg/g or <3 mg/mmol; A2: moderately increased: 30 to 300 mg/g or 3 to 30 mg/mmol; A3: severely increased: >300 mg/g or >30 mg/mm

EPIDEMIOLOGY
- African Americans are 3.6 times more likely to develop CKD than Caucasians.
- Similar in both sexes; however, rate of end-stage renal disease (ESRD) is 1.6 times higher in males than females.

Incidence
Estimated annual incidence of 1,700/1 million population

Prevalence
Overall prevalence of CKD (stages 1 to 5) is 14.8%. Unadjusted prevalence and incidence rates of ESRD (stage 5) are 1,752 and 362.4/1 million, respectively. Numbers do not reflect the burden of earlier stages of CKD (stages 1 to 4), which are estimated to affect 13.1% of the population in the United States. Prevalence increases with age and peaks after 70.

ETIOLOGY AND PATHOPHYSIOLOGY
Progressive destruction of kidney nephrons; GFR will drop gradually, and plasma Cr values will approximately double, with 50% reduction in GFR and 75% loss of functioning nephrons mass. Hyperkalemia usually develops when GFR falls to <20 to 25 mL/min. Anemia develops from decreased renal synthesis of erythropoietin.
- Renal parenchymal/glomerular
  - Nephritic: hematuria, red blood cell (RBC) casts, hypertension (HTN), variable proteinuria
    ○ Focal proliferative: IgA nephropathy, systemic lupus erythematosus (SLE), Henoch-Schönlein purpura, Alport syndrome, proliferative glomerulonephritis, crescentic glomerulonephritis
    ○ Diffuse proliferative: membranoproliferative glomerulonephritis, SLE, cryoglobulinemia, rapidly progressive glomerulonephritis (RPGN), Goodpasture syndrome
  - Nephrotic: proteinuria (>3.5 g/day), hypoalbuminemia, hyperlipidemia, and edema
    ○ Minimal change disease, membranous nephropathy, focal segmental glomerulosclerosis
    ○ Amyloidosis, diabetic nephropathy

- Vascular: HTN, thrombotic microangiopathies, vasculitis (Wegener), scleroderma, crush injury
- Interstitial tubular: infections, obstruction, toxins, allergic interstitial nephritis, multiple myeloma, connective tissue disease, cystic disease, nephrolithiasis
- Postrenal: obstruction (benign prostatic hyperplasia [BPH]), neoplasm, neurogenic bladder

Genetics
- Alport syndrome, Fabry disease, sickle cell anemia, SLE, and autosomal dominant polycystic kidney disease can lead to CKD.
- Polymorphisms in gene that encodes for podocyte nonmuscle myosin IIA are more common in African Americans than Caucasians and appear to increase risk for nondiabetic ESRD.

RISK FACTORS
Type 1 or 2 diabetes mellitus (DM) (most common), age > 60 years, low socioeconomic status, obesity, smoking, drug use, chronic infection (hepatitis B/C, HIV), CVD (HTN, renal artery stenosis, atherosclerosis), prior kidney transplant, BPH, autoimmune disease, vasculitis, connective tissue disease, nephrotoxic drugs (nonsteroidal anti-inflammatory drugs [NSAIDs], lithium, sulfonamide, aminoglycosides, vancomycin, PPIs, allopurinol, loop diuretics, chemotherapeutic agents), congenital anomalies, obstructive uropathy, renal aplasia/hypoplasia/dysplasia/reflux nephropathy)

GENERAL PREVENTION
The U.S. Preventive Services Task Force has concluded the evidence is insufficient to recommend screening asymptomatic adults for CKD (1)[C].

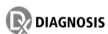 **DIAGNOSIS**

HISTORY
Patients with CKD stages 1 to 3 are usually asymptomatic; can present with oliguria, nocturia, polyuria, change in urinary frequency, bone disease, edema, HTN, dyspnea, fatigue, depression, weakness, pruritus, ecchymosis, anorexia, nausea, vomiting, hyperlipidemia, claudication, erectile dysfunction, decreased libido, amenorrhea

PHYSICAL EXAM
Check for volume status (pallor, BP/orthostatic; edema; jugular venous distention; weight), skin for sallow complexion or uremic frost, ammonia-like odor, murmurs, bruits, pericarditis, pleural effusions, enlarged prostate, central nervous system changes such as asterixis, confusion, seizures, coma, and peripheral neuropathy.

DIAGNOSTIC TESTS & INTERPRETATION
Initial Tests (lab, imaging)
GFR can be estimated using the Modification of Diet in Renal Disease (MDRD) and Chronic Kidney Disease-Epidemiology Collaboration (CKD-EPI) equations, Cr clearance using the Cockcroft-Gault formula to determine medication dosage, UA to assess for evidence of damage (WBC casts in pyelonephritis, RBC casts in glomerulonephritis/vasculitis, Na, Cr, urea, albuminuria), US (initial imaging test of choice to assess for cysts, masses, hydronephrosis, kidney size).

Follow-Up Tests & Special Considerations
- Hematology: normochromic, normocytic anemia; increased bleeding time
- Chemistry: elevated BUN, Cr, hyperkalemia, metabolic acidosis, increased parathyroid hormone (PTH), hyperlipidemia, hyperphosphatemia, decreased 25-(OH) vitamin D, hypocalcemia, decreased albumin
- Serology: antinuclear antibody (ANA); double-stranded DNA, antineutrophil cytoplasmic antibody; complements (C3, C4, CH50); antiglomerular basement membrane (anti-GBM) antibodies; hepatitis B, C; and HIV screening
- Serum and urine immunoelectrophoresis

ALERT
Drugs that may alter lab result:
- Cimetidine: inhibits Cr tubular secretion
- Trimethoprim: inhibits Cr and K⁺ secretion and may cause/worsen hyperkalemia
- Cefoxitin and flucytosine: increases serum Cr
- Diltiazem and verapamil (like angiotensin-converting-enzyme inhibitors [ACE-Is]/angiotensin receptor blockers [ARBs]) have significant antiproteinuric effects in patients with CKD.

Diagnostic Procedures/Other
- Biopsy: hematuria, proteinuria, acute/progressive renal failure, nephritic or nephrotic syndrome
- In patients with an estimated GFR(eGFR) <60 mL/min/1.73 m², there is some evidence for a one-time cystatin-C GFR estimation.
- ECG: Assess for abnormal heart rhythms due to electrolyte imbalances.

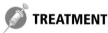 **TREATMENT**

MEDICATION
- HTN: Adults with elevated blood pressure and CKD G1 to G3 should be treated to a target systolic blood pressure of 120 using standardized office measurements. Renal transplant patients should have a target blood pressure of <130/80 mm Hg (2)[C].
  - ACE-I or ARB recommended for diabetic and nondiabetic adults with albumin excretion >30 mg/24 hr based on evidence of benefits.
    ○ An ACE-I or ARB can still be considered in patients with no albuminuria. Those patients, however, are at less risk of CKD progression.
    ○ Avoid combining ACE-I, ARB, and DRI therapy in diabetic and non-diabetic patients with CKD.
    ○ Advise contraception in women who are receiving ACE-I or ARB therapy and discontinue in women who are considering pregnancy or have become pregnant (3)[C].
  - CCB or ARB is first line in adult kidney transplant patients for prevention of allograft failure and minimization of possible drug-induced side effects.
  - In children with CKD, 24-hour mean arterial pressure by ambulatory blood pressure monitoring (ABPM) should be lowed to <50th percentile for age, sex, and height. In this population, and ACE-I or ARB is first line.
  - A combination between a low-sodium diet plus the use of an ACE-I or ARB leads to significant reduction in proteinuria (4)[C].

- Secondary hyperparathyroidism
- For GFR <45, monitor for hyperphosphatemia, hypocalcemia, and vitamin D deficiency if intact PTH is elevated.
- Calcimimetic agents (oral cinacalcet or IV etelcalcetide) are not U.S. Food and Drug Administration-approved for use in patients with CKD not on dialysis. These should be reserved for ESRD patients (4)[C].
- Hyperphosphatemia: Maintain normal serum phosphate levels using the following:
  - Stages 3 to 5 CKD (not on dialysis): Restrict dietary phosphate to 800 to 1,000 mg/day.
  - Noncalcium phosphate binders (with meals): sevelamer, lanthanum
  - Calcium binders have not been associated with improvement in mortality or cardiovascular outcomes (4)[C].
  - Vitamin D: inactive vitamin D 25 (ergocalciferol or cholecalciferol), calcitriol (active vitamin D 1,25 [OH]): Vitamin D may increase absorption of phosphate by intestines and should not be started until serum phosphate concentration is controlled.
- Anemia: Treat with iron replacement therapy with or without erythropoietin-stimulating agents (ESAs). Consider ESA if Hb >9 g/dL and <10 g/dL. ESA initiation not recommended for Hb >10 g/dL. If using ESA, goal Hb range 10 to 11 g/dL, not to exceed 11.5 g/dL.
- Hyperlipidemia: statins with low-density lipoprotein (LDL) goal <70
- Glycemic control: Goal HbA1c range 6.5–8.0%. HbA1c may be falsely low in patients with decreased RBC; glucose logs may be more accurate reflection of glycemic control. Metformin use should be reviewed for GFR between 30 and 44 and discontinued if GFR <30 mL/min/1.73 m². Use sodium-glucose cotransporter-2 (SGLT2) inhibitors along with metformin in patients with type 2 DM and GFR >30 mL/min/1.73 m² (3)[C]. SGLT2 inhibitors can be used for patients with and without DM to control disease progression.
- Metabolic acidosis: Start treatment when bicarbonate <22 mEq/L with goal to maintain in normal range.

ISSUES FOR REFERRAL
- Nephrology consult:
  - GFR <15: immediate, GFR 15 to 29: urgent, GFR 30 to 59: nonurgent referral, GFR 60 to 89: not required unless with comorbidities
  - Rapid decline of eGFR (>5 mL/min/1.73 m² per year), patients without diabetes with heavy proteinuria (24-hour urine protein >500 mg, urine PCR >.5, urine ACR >300), patients with diabetes with >3 g proteinuria or hematuria, management of complications (metabolic management, electrolyte abnormalities, acidosis, etc.)
- Urology consult for hematuria, renal masses, complex renal cysts, symptomatic nephrolithiasis, hydronephrosis
- Registered Dietitian/psychology/social work/physical therapy/occupational therapy consultation to assist with dietary options, behavioral modification, access to food resources, and mobility
- Renal replacement: Prepare for dialysis or transplant when GFR <30 mL/min/1.73 m².

ADDITIONAL THERAPIES
- Aspirin for secondary prevention for patients with established cardiovascular disease
- For mild pain associated with CKD, acetaminophen is considered first-line therapy. Oral, parental, and even topical NSAIDs are generally not recommended.
- For moderate to severe pain, opioids may be indicated, but the risk of overdose or toxicity is increased because many are renally excreted. Oxycodone, fentanyl, and methadone are preferred, but dose adjustment is still recommended. Meperidine is contraindicated in CKD. Codeine and morphine should be used with caution.
- Chronic pain syndromes may be treated with anticonvulsants and gabapentinoids, which should be renally dosed.

ADMISSION, INPATIENT, AND NURSING CONSIDERATIONS
- For use of contrast in imaging, patients should have eGFR > 30 mL/min/1.73 m². Volume expansion with IV isotonic saline prior to and following iodinated contrast is recommended.
- Metformin should be held prior to iodinated contrast imaging and resumed 48 hours.

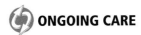 ONGOING CARE

FOLLOW-UP RECOMMENDATIONS
Patient Monitoring
- Monitor for changes in blood pressure, serum creatinine, and serum potassium within 2 to 4 weeks of initiation of ACE-I or ARB. If >30% increase in creatinine, correct acute kidney injury, reassess medications, reduce/stop the current ACE-I or ARB dose Discontinue therapy in the setting of symptomatic hypotension or uncontrolled hyperkalemia.
- For patients taking metformin, monitor eGFR annually and vitamin B$_{12}$ levels after taking metformin >4 years.
- Monitor creatinine levels in pregnant patients with CKD closely.
- Monitor Hgb annually for GFR 30 to 59 and biannually for GFR <30, calcidiol levels, HbA1c 2 to 4 times a year, volume status, electrolytes, kidney function (urine albumin, GFR, serum creatinine).
- Calcium, phosphate, PTH, alkaline phosphate beginning at CKD stage G3

DIET
- <2 g sodium per day. Limit processed foods, refined carbohydrates, sweetened beverages. Restrict potassium and phosphorus. Restrict protein to 0.8 g/kg/day. Restrict fluids depending on volume status.
- Nutritional consult for CKD diet

PROGNOSIS
Progression is defined as 25% decrease in GFR from baseline. Rapid progression is decrease in GFR by >5 mL/min/1.73 m²/year. Patients with CKD gradually progress to ESRD. 5-year survival rate for U.S. patients on dialysis is ~35%.

COMPLICATIONS
HTN, anemia, secondary hyperparathyroidism, renal osteodystrophy, sleep disturbances, infections, malnutrition, electrolyte imbalances, platelet dysfunction/bleeding, pseudogout, gout, metabolic calcification, sexual dysfunction

REFERENCES

1. Moyer VA. Screening for chronic kidney disease: U.S. Preventive Services Task Force recommendation statement. *Ann Intern Med*. 2012;157(8):567–570.
2. Kidney Disease: Improving Global Outcomes (KDIGO) Blood Pressure Work Group. KDIGO 2021 Clinical Practice Guideline for the Management of Blood Pressure in Chronic Kidney Disease. *Kidney Int*. 2021;99(3S):S1–S87.
3. Kidney Disease: Improving Global Outcomes (KDIGO) Diabetes Work Group. KDIGO 2020 Clinical Practice Guideline for Diabetes Management in Chronic Kidney Disease. *Kidney Int*. 2020;98(4S):S1–S115.
4. U.S. Department of Veterans Affaris. VA/DoD Clinical Practice Guideline: management of chronic kidney disease (CKD) (2019). https://www.healthquality.va.gov/guidelines/CD/ckd/. Accessed October 18, 2021.

 CODES

ICD10
- N18.9 Chronic kidney disease, unspecified
- Q63.9 Congenital malformation of kidney, unspecified
- N18.3 Chronic kidney disease, stage 3 (moderate)

CLINICAL PEARLS
- CKD is defined based on >3 months of kidney functional or structural abnormalities and classified based on GFR and albuminuria.
- ACE-I and ARB are first line for HTN treatment in CKD with albuminuria.
- Care should be taken in prescribing medication in CKD due to reduced renal clearance of certain medications.
- Consider nonurgent nephrologist referral for GFR ≥59 and urgent nephrologist referral for GFR ≥29.
- CKD progression should be monitored closely and managed by a multidisciplinary team to ensure proper nutrition, pain control, mobility, and access to care.

CHRONIC OBSTRUCTIVE PULMONARY DISEASE AND EMPHYSEMA

Christopher M. Wagner, MD • David Nesheim, MD

 BASICS

DESCRIPTION

- The Global Initiative for Chronic Obstructive Lung Disease (GOLD) defines COPD as follows:
  - "COPD is a common, preventable, and treatable disease that is characterized by persistent respiratory symptoms and airflow limitation that is due to airway and/or alveolar abnormalities usually caused by significant exposure to noxious particles or gases and influenced by host factors including abnormal lung development" (1).
- This new definition no longer includes the terms "emphysema" and "chronic bronchitis."
- COPD is now the third leading cause of death worldwide, with 90% of these deaths occurring in low- and middle-income countries. COPD was responsible for 3.2 million deaths globally in 2019 (2).

EPIDEMIOLOGY

Incidence
The incidence of COPD is 8.9/1,000 person-years.

ETIOLOGY AND PATHOPHYSIOLOGY
Exposure to noxious gases or particles (see "Risk Factors") leading to the following pathologic processes in the lung:
- Impaired gas (carbon dioxide and oxygen) exchange
- Persistent airway obstruction
- Destruction of lung parenchyma

Genetics
- Genetics may contribute to host response to noxious gases or particles.
- Antiprotease deficiency (due to α_1-antitrypsin deficiency) is an inherited, rare disorder due to two autosomal codominant alleles.

RISK FACTORS
- Smoking tobacco or marijuana: including passive smoking and water pipe
- History of severe childhood respiratory infections
- Aging—including healthy aging as well as the cumulative summation of lung exposure over time
- Lower level of education and lower socioeconomic status
- Asthma and airway hyperreactivity
- Indoor air pollution (especially indoor biomass cooking worldwide)
- Occupational organic or inorganic dusts

GENERAL PREVENTION
Smoking cessation—and general avoidance of noxious material—is the most important preventative measure.

COMMONLY ASSOCIATED CONDITIONS
- Pulmonary: lung cancer, chronic respiratory failure, acute bronchitis, sleep apnea, pulmonary hypertension (HTN), asthma
- Cardiac: coronary artery disease, arrhythmia
- Ear/nose/throat (ENT): chronic sinusitis, laryngeal carcinoma
- Miscellaneous: malnutrition, osteoporosis, muscle dysfunction, depression

DIAGNOSIS
The diagnosis of COPD requires three features:
- A postbronchodilator forced expiratory volume in 1 second (FEV_1)/forced vital capacity (FVC) ratio of <0.7, which confirms the presence of persistent airflow limitation.
- Appropriate symptoms including dyspnea, chronic cough, sputum production, and/or wheezing
- Significant exposure to noxious stimuli, such as history of smoking cigarettes or environmental exposures

HISTORY
- Discuss patient's use of tobacco and/or cannabis.
- Consider indoor pollution and occupational exposures.
- Review possible causes of exacerbation (e.g., cold weather, recent upper respiratory infection, pneumonia, noncompliance with medications).
- Exacerbation: increased frequency of sputum production; change in sputum color, frequency and/or amount; fevers; wheezing; chest tightness/pain

PHYSICAL EXAM
- Prolonged expiration, wheezing
- Barrel chest, diminished breath sounds, distant heart sounds
- Accessory muscle use, pursed lip breathing, cyanosis
- Clubbing not typical for COPD, however, may indicate another process (e.g., lung cancer)

DIFFERENTIAL DIAGNOSIS
- Asthma (including occupational), reactive airways dysfunction syndrome (RADS)
- Interstitial lung disease, bronchiectasis, primary alveolar hypoventilation, bronchiolitis obliterans
- Lung cancer
- Chronic pulmonary embolism
- Sleep apnea, congestive heart failure (CHF), gastroesophageal reflux disease
- Cystic fibrosis

DIAGNOSTIC TESTS & INTERPRETATION
Initial Tests (lab, imaging)
- Spirometry (see "Diagnostic Procedures/Other")
- Arterial blood gases (ABGs) may show hypercapnia and hypoxia.
- CBC may reveal polycythemia, reflecting chronic hypoxia.
- BMP may reveal elevated CO_2, indicative of chronic CO_2 retention.
- Imaging (CXR, CT chest) important to rule out other conditions; CXR: hyperinflation, flat diaphragms, and possibly bullous changes

Follow-Up Tests & Special Considerations
- Pulse oximetry to assess need for oxygen, both at rest and with exertion
- α_1-Antitrypsin screening for those with COPD age <45 years, have a blood relative with this disease, or spirometry out of proportion to tobacco use
- Chest CT may show parenchymal destruction and bullae.

Diagnostic Procedures/Other
Pulmonary function testing without/with bronchodilator
- Decreased postbronchodilator FEV_1:FVC ratio <0.7. This is the diagnostic criteria for airway obstruction; repeat spirometry recommended if between 0.6 and 0.8
- Reduced FEV_1
- Normal or increased FVC
- Normal or increased total lung capacity
- Increased residual volume and functional residual capacity
- Diffusing capacity is normal or reduced.
- Typically not bronchodilator responsive (change in FEV_1 or FVC of ≥12% and change in volume of ≥200 mL)

Test Interpretation
- Staging: GOLD criteria for airflow limitation (1)
  - Grade 1: FEV_1 ≥80% predicted
  - Grade 2: FEV_1 50–80% predicted
  - Grade 3: FEV_1 30–50% predicted
  - Grade 4: FEV_1 <30% predicted or FEV_1 <50% predicted plus chronic respiratory failure
  - FEV_1 was previously used to grade severity; however, it was found to correlate poorly with patients' functional capacity and risk for exacerbation.
- Symptom severity assessments:
  - COPD Assessment Tool (CAT), which is an 8-item questionnaire worth 5 points each (overall score range 0 to 40) that determine disease-specific, health-related quality of life
  - Modified Medical Research Council (mMRC) questionnaire, which evaluates breathlessness based on scale of 0 (breathless with strenuous exercise) to 4 (too breathless to leave the house or breathless when dressing or undressing)
  - GOLD severity assessment based on symptom burden and risk of exacerbation
- The ABCD assessment tool incorporates severity of patient's symptoms and exacerbation history.
  - Group A: low risk, less symptoms: 0 to 1 exacerbation per year and no prior hospitalization for exacerbation; and CAT score <10 or mMRC grade 0 to 1
  - Group B: low risk, more symptoms: 0 to 1 exacerbation per year and no prior hospitalization for exacerbation; and CAT score ≥10 or mMRC grade ≥2
  - Group C: high risk, less symptoms: ≥2 exacerbations per year or ≥1 hospitalization for exacerbation; and CAT score <10 or mMRC grade 0 to 1
  - Group D: high risk, more symptoms: ≥2 exacerbations per year or ≥1 hospitalization for exacerbation; and CAT score ≥10 or mMRC grade ≥2

TREATMENT

GENERAL MEASURES
- Smoking cessation: This is the most important intervention to decrease risk of disease progression.
- Home oxygen: should be initiated at partial pressure of arterial oxygen (PaO$_2$) ≤55 mm Hg or pulse oximetry trends ≤88%, or if PaO$_2$ between 55 and 60 mm Hg and evidence of erythrocytosis or cor pulmonale
- Influenza and pneumococcal immunizations
- Pulmonary rehabilitation
- NPPV may improve hospitalization-free survival in hypercapnic patients after recent hospitalization.

MEDICATION
First Line
- Minimally symptomatic, low risk of exacerbation (category A):
  – First line: a short-acting bronchodilator to use as a rescue drug
  – Short-acting β-agonists: albuterol, levalbuterol
  – Short-acting muscarinic antagonists: ipratropium, oxitropium
- More symptomatic, low risk of exacerbation (category B)
  – First line: regular use of long-acting bronchodilator in addition to as needed short-acting bronchodilator
  – Second line: If uncontrolled symptoms with a single long-acting agent, then use combined long-acting β-agonists (LABA)–long-acting muscarinic antagonists (LAMA) rather than steroids.
  – LABA: formoterol, arformoterol, salmeterol
  – LAMA: tiotropium, aclidinium, umeclidinium, glycopyrrolate
- Minimally symptomatic, high risk of exacerbation (category C)
  – First line: LAMA
  – Second line:
    ○ LAMA-LABA combination
    ○ LABA and inhaled corticosteroid (ICS)
- More symptomatic, high risk of exacerbation (category D)
  – First line: LAMA-LABA combination
  – Second line: can add triple therapy with LAMA-LABA and ICS therapy
    ○ PD4 inhibitor (roflumilast) if FEV$_1$ <50% and chronic bronchitis. Chronic macrolide therapy if former smoker and frequent exacerbations; theophylline not preferred due to side effects

Second Line

ALERT
Precautions

- β-Agonists: sinus tachycardia, arrhythmias in susceptible patients; can consider levalbuterol
- Anticholinergics: minimal systemic absorption in inhaled form; urinary retention possible
- ICS: increased risk of pneumonia; oral candidiasis
- Corticosteroids: weight gain, diabetes, adrenal suppression, osteoporosis, infection (pneumonia)

- Macrolides: Long-term use can possibly lead to bacterial resistance and hearing impairment.
- Theophylline: arrhythmia, CNS symptoms, nausea, vomiting

ISSUES FOR REFERRAL
Severe exacerbation, frequent hospitalizations, rapid progression, weight loss, severe disease, or surgical evaluation

ADDITIONAL THERAPIES
- Pulmonary rehabilitation program for patients with high symptom burden and risk of exacerbations
- Acute COPD exacerbations: Mild to moderate exacerbations can be treated with short-acting bronchodilators and possibly short courses of steroids and/or antibiotics (5 to 7 days). Severe exacerbations require inpatient admission (see below).

SURGERY/OTHER PROCEDURES
Lung reduction surgery, bronchoscopic lung reduction, surgical bullectomy, lung transplantation

ADMISSION, INPATIENT, AND NURSING CONSIDERATIONS
- Severe acute exacerbation: Maintain oxygenation, short-acting inhaled β-agonists/inhaled anticholinergic agents, and oral or IV corticosteroids prednisone (up to 1 mg/kg/day commonly 40 mg/day for 5 days). Antibiotics for moderate/severe exacerbations with increased sputum volume or sputum purulence; optimal antibiotic therapy has not been determined; noninvasive positive pressure ventilation if necessary
- May lead to acute or acute on chronic respiratory failure requiring ICU admission and intubation
- Prior to discharge: Assess proper inhaler use, prescribe proper maintenance inhalers, and ensure understanding; assess need for home oxygen.

ALERT
If not already in place, have patient delineate an advance directive.

ONGOING CARE

FOLLOW-UP RECOMMENDATIONS
- May taper or stop oral steroids as outpatient
- Pulmonary rehabilitation program for patients with high symptom burden and risk of exacerbations

Patient Monitoring
Follow-up should be initially within 4-week period and a 12-week period after an exacerbation; paying attention to symptoms, medication compliance, and the need for oxygen in 4 weeks. Additionally, spirometry should be repeated in 12 weeks.

DIET
Referral for nutritional support indicated in malnourished patients

PATIENT EDUCATION
American Lung Association: www.lung.org/lung-disease/copd/

PROGNOSIS
- Supplemental oxygen, when indicated, is shown to increase survival (may only require at night).
- Smoking cessation improves prognosis.
- For severe upper lobe disease and poor control or poor postrehabilitation exercise capacity, lung volume reduction surgery may be considered.
- For very severe disease unresponsive to all interventions, patient may be candidate for lung transplant.
- 4-year mortality estimates range from 28% for mild to moderate COPD to 62% for moderate to severe COPD.

COMPLICATIONS
- Malnutrition, poor sleep quality, infections, secondary polycythemia
- Acute or chronic respiratory failure, bullous lung disease, pneumothorax
- Arrhythmias, cor pulmonale, pulmonary HTN

REFERENCES
1. Global Initiative for Chronic Obstructive Lung Disease. Global strategy for the diagnosis, management, and prevention of chronic obstructive pulmonary disease: 2020 report. www.goldcopd.org. Accessed August 9, 2020.
2. Halpin DMG, Celli BR, Criner GJ, et al. The GOLD Summit on chronic obstructive pulmonary disease in low- and middle-income countries. *Int J Tuberc Lung Dis.* 2019;23(11):1131–1141.

 SEE ALSO

Bronchitis, Acute

 CODES

ICD10
- J44.9 Chronic obstructive pulmonary disease, unspecified
- J43.9 Emphysema, unspecified
- J42 Unspecified chronic bronchitis

CLINICAL PEARLS
- Smoking cessation remains the most important intervention to prevent disease or delay disease progression.
- Consider screening PFTs on any high-risk patient.
- Home oxygen evaluation is important because supplemental oxygen improves mortality.
- Regularly reevaluate disease burden to titrate short and long acting medication regimen.
- Influenza/pneumococcal vaccines should be current.
- Discuss advance directives before patient is seriously ill.

CHRONIC PAIN MANAGEMENT: AN EVIDENCE-BASED APPROACH

Jennifer Reidy, MD, MS, FAAHPM • Vandana Nagpal, MD, FACP

 BASICS

- Chronic pain is defined as pain persisting beyond the time anticipated for normal tissue healing, usually >3 months.
- Over time, neuroplastic changes in the CNS transform pain into a chronic experience with emotional, psychological, and cognitive dimensions.
- An epidemic of undertreated pain coexists with an epidemic of prescription drug abuse in the United States.
- People of color, especially African Americans, are often undertreated.
- Opioid medications should be prescribed using an evidence/systems-based approach and only when indicated for chronic, nonmalignant pain.

EPIDEMIOLOGY

Incidence
- Chronic pain has been reported by as many as 20–40% of patients in primary care.
- The annual economic cost of chronic pain in the United States is estimated at $560 to $635 billion (1).

Prevalence
In the United States, an estimated 20% (50 million) adults reported some level of chronic pain on cross-sectional household surveys in 2016. The prevalence was higher among women and those with lower socioeconomic status (https://www.cdc.gov/mmwr/volumes/67/wr/mm6736a2.htm).

ALERT
Opioid-related overdoses are at an all-time high. Deaths have surged during the COVID-19 pandemic (https://www.cdc.gov/drugoverdose/resources/covid-drugs-QA.html?CDC_AA_refVal=https%3A%2F%2Fwww.cdc.gov%2Fcoronavirus%2F2019-ncov%2Fneed-extra-precautions%2Fother-at-risk-populations%2Fpeople-who-use-drugs%2FQA.html#increased-use).

ETIOLOGY AND PATHOPHYSIOLOGY
- With intense, repeated, or prolonged stimulation of damaged or inflamed tissues, the threshold for activating primary afferent pain fibers is lowered, the frequency of firing is higher, and there is increased response to noxious and/or normal stimuli (peripheral and central sensitization). The amygdala, prefrontal cortex, and cortex relay emotions related to the pain experience, and these areas undergo structural and functional changes over time.
- Patients often have an identifiable etiology, but pain levels can be worse than observable tissue injury. Many patients have no obvious source of chronic pain.

Genetics
A genetic polymorphism in opioid receptors may affect patient's response to individual opioids.

RISK FACTORS
- Traumatic: motor vehicle accidents, repetitive motion injuries, falls
- Postsurgical: back surgeries, amputations, thoracotomies
- Psychiatric comorbidities: substance abuse, depression, posttraumatic stress disorder (PTSD)

GENERAL PREVENTION
- Prevent work-related injuries through ergonomic workplace design.
- Varicella vaccine and rapid treatment of shingles to lower risk of postherpetic neuralgia
- Tight glycemic control for diabetic patients, prevention of alcohol abuse, smoking cessation

COMMONLY ASSOCIATED CONDITIONS
Any chronic disease and/or its treatment can cause chronic pain.

 DIAGNOSIS

Two general categories of pain:
- Nociceptive pain (response to tissue damage):
  - *Somatic*: skin, bone, soft tissue disease; described as well localized, sharp, stabbing, aching
  - *Visceral*: visceral inflammation/injury; described as poorly localized, dull, aching; may refer to sites remote from lesion; can wax and wane
- Neuropathic pain: damaged peripheral or central nerves; described as burning, tingling, and/or numbness
  - Sympathetically mediated pain: Peripheral nerve injury can cause severe burning pain, swelling of the affected limb, and focal changes in sweat production and skin appearance (e.g., complex regional pain syndrome).

HISTORY
- Pain history: location, onset, intensity, duration, quality, temporal pattern, exacerbating agents, alleviators, prior treatments
- Assess and document how pain affects patient's functioning and quality of life.
- Screen for personal or family history of substance abuse (including tobacco addiction), mental health conditions, and/or sexual abuse.
- Standardized tools: pain severity—Brief Pain Inventory (Short Form); mood—Patient Health Questionnaire-9 (PHQ-9); substance abuse—Screener and Opioid Assessment for Patients with Pain (SOAPP)
- Stratify patients according to risk of chronic opioid therapy and need for increased monitoring; a positive screen does not automatically exclude patients from opioid therapy.

PHYSICAL EXAM
Exam is guided by history and includes functional and behavioral assessments.

DIFFERENTIAL DIAGNOSIS
Aberrant drug-taking behaviors could be related to:
- Inadequate analgesia ("pseudoaddiction"), disease progression, opioid-resistant pain, opioid-induced hyperalgesia, opioid tolerance, substance use disorder, self-medication of nonpain symptoms, criminal intent (diversion), and poor health literacy

DIAGNOSTIC TESTS & INTERPRETATION
Base testing on history, exam, and differential diagnosis.

Initial Tests (lab, imaging)
- Urine drug screen: qualitative analysis for drugs of abuse and quantitative analysis for individual drugs
- Most tests are immunoassays, which detect morphine and heroin but often not other opioids.

Follow-Up Tests & Special Considerations
For chronic opioid therapy, consider random urine drug screens.

Diagnostic Procedures/Other
Consider interventional pain clinic for complex injections and nerve blocks.

Test Interpretation
There is a possibility of false-positive urine drug screen due to commonly prescribed medications. Laboratory-based chromatography/spectrometry can identify specific drugs.

 TREATMENT

- Goals of treatment are to restore function and decrease pain.
- Treatment should always include exercise, cognitive-behavioral therapy (CBT), patient and family education, yoga, massage, relaxation techniques, support groups, mindfulness, meditation, and acupuncture.
- For complex regional pain syndrome, sympathetic block may decrease risk of chronic pain.
- Evidence on use of cannabis for chronic pain is low quality and controversial (2)[A].

GENERAL MEASURES
- Keep a pain and function diary; record medication use.
- CDC: https://www.cdc.gov/drugoverdose/prescribing/guideline.html
- AAPM: https://academic.oup.com/painmedicine/article/21/7/1331/5817092
- VA: https://www.healthquality.va.gov/guidelines/Pain/cot/

MEDICATION
- Management varies depending on type of pain (neuropathic vs nociceptive).
- Use sequential time-limited trials of medications; start at low doses and gradually increase until effect or dose-limiting side effects are reached.
- Combination acetaminophen/NSAID products with opioids can lead to serious acetaminophen/NSAID toxicities if patients exceed recommended doses.
- Note: Be aware of implicit bias. A meta-analysis and systematic review found that blacks/African Americans were at greatest risk for undertreatment regardless of pain type (traumatic or not) or type of analgesia (opioids or not) (3)[A].
- For mild to moderate chronic noncancer pain
  - Acetaminophen: daily dose not to exceed total 4 g in healthy adults and 2 g in elderly patients with hepatic disease or current/past alcohol use
  - NSAIDs: Use COX-2 selective inhibitors with caution because of cardiac risks (may have less gastric risk). If high cardiac risk, consider nonselective COX inhibitor (naproxen) with or without gastric prophylaxis.

- Topical agents: NSAIDs (diclofenac gel 1–3% BID), lidocaine (4% gel OTC is less effective but more affordable than 5% patch), ketamine 0.5–10% BID–QID, capsaicin 0.035–0.1% QD–QID
- Tramadol: an opioid analgesic with weak serotonin-norepinephrine reuptake inhibitor (SNRI), may be helpful in neuropathic pain but has ceiling dose, risk of seizures and requires dose adjustment for renal and hepatic failure (initial dose 50 mg q6h PRN, ceiling dose 400 mg/day or 300 mg/day for older adults).
- For neuropathic pain
  - Classes of medications include (i) tricyclic antidepressants (desipramine [25 to 100 mg QD but start with 10 mg QD in frail elderly] and nortriptyline [25 to 100 mg QD but start with 10 mg QD in frail elderly]); (ii) SNRI antidepressants (duloxetine 30–60 mg BID); (iii) anticonvulsants (α2-δ ligands, gabapentin [initial dose 300 mg/day and titrate to max of 3,600 mg/day in 3 divided doses] and pregabalin [100 to 300 mg/day in 2 to 3 divided doses]); and (iv) last line is opioids, including tramadol.
- For moderate to severe chronic pain
  - Morphine, oxycodone, hydromorphone, oxymorphone, fentanyl. Check opioid equianalgesic table vetted by your institution.
    - Avoid morphine in patients with renal insufficiency.
    - Methadone should only be prescribed by experienced providers due to many drug interactions and risk of potentially fatal cardiac arrhythmias.
  - No evidence supports any of these opioids as superior to other or having improved side effect profile.
  - Once stable dose of opioids is established, change to sustained-release formulations if pain is constant or frequent; short-acting formulations for breakthrough/episodic pain only.
  - Common side effects: constipation: Senna should be coprescribed with opioids; also nausea, sedation, mental status changes, and pruritus.
  - Coprescribe nasal naloxone for patients on chronic opioids (see "Ongoing Care") (4)[C].

ALERT
Patients on chronic opioid therapy must agree to monitoring. Use universal precautions (see "Ongoing Care").

SURGERY/OTHER PROCEDURES
Consider interventional procedures, including joint injections, nerve blocks, spinal cord stimulation, and intrathecal medication among others, as needed.

COMPLEMENTARY & ALTERNATIVE MEDICINE
- For adults with chronic low back pain, consider mindfulness-based stress reduction (MBSR) or CBT (5)[A].
- Yoga as effective as standard physical therapy for moderate to severe chronic low back pain (4)[A]

 ONGOING CARE

FOLLOW-UP RECOMMENDATIONS
Patient Monitoring
- Maintain a nonjudgmental approach.
- Assess and document benefits, risks, pain levels, functioning, and quality of life.
- *Universal precautions*:
  - Informed consent for opioid therapy
  - Written agreement between patient and clinician
  - One prescriber and one pharmacy
  - No after-hours prescriptions or early refills
  - Mandatory police reporting for medication thefts
  - Random urine drug tests, pill/patch counts
  - Continue with physical therapy, counseling, and psychiatric medications.
  - Participate in state's prescription drug monitoring program: http://www.cdc.gov/drugoverdose/pdmp/.
  - Taper and discontinue medications (5% dose reduction per week) if patient does not benefit, if side effects outweigh benefits. If medications are abused or diverted, more rapid taper is appropriate. If addiction is suspected, always offer treatment for substance abuse.
  - Patients on long-term opioid therapy may see improvement in pain, function, and quality of life with voluntary dose reductions (6)[A].
- Nasal naloxone
  - Naloxone kit: two 1 mg/mL prefilled syringes with intranasal mucosal atomization device; takes effect in 2 to 5 minutes, lasts 30 to 90 minutes

PATIENT EDUCATION
American Chronic Pain Association: https://theacpa.org

COMPLICATIONS
- Rate of addiction in chronic pain patients ~3–19%; aberrant medication-taking behaviors ~5–24%
- Definitions
  - Addiction: chronic biopsychological disease characterized by impaired control over drug use, compulsive use, and continued use despite harm
  - Physical dependence: withdrawal syndrome produced by abrupt cessation or rapid dose reduction
  - Tolerance: state of adaptation when a drug induces changes that diminish its effects over time
  - Diversion: selling drugs or giving them to persons other than for whom they are prescribed

REFERENCES
1. Institute of Medicine, Committee on Advancing Pain Research, Care, and Education. *Relieving Pain in America: A Blueprint for Transforming Prevention, Care, Education, and Research*. Washington, DC: National Academies Press; 2011.
2. Fisher E, Moore RA, Fogarty AE, et al. Cannabinoids, cannabis, and cannabis-based medicine for pain management: a systematic review of randomised controlled trials. *Pain*. 2021;162(Suppl 1):S45–S66. doi:10.1097/j.pain.0000000000001929.
3. Meghani SH, Byun E, Gallagher RM. Time to take stock: a meta-analysis and systematic review of analgesic treatment disparities for pain in the United States. *Pain Med*. 2012;13(2):150–174.
4. Saper RB, Lemaster C, Delitto A, et al. Yoga, physical therapy, or education for chronic low back pain: a randomized noninferiority trial. *Ann Intern Med*. 2017;167(2):85–94.
5. Cherkin DC, Sherman KJ, Balderson BH, et al. Effect of mindfulness-based stress reduction vs cognitive behavioral therapy or usual care on back pain and functional limitations in adults with chronic low back pain: a randomized clinical trial. *JAMA*. 2016;315(12):1240–1249.
6. Frank JW, Lovejoy TI, Becker WC, et al. Patient outcomes in dose reduction or discontinuation of long-term opioid therapy: a systematic review. *Ann Intern Med*. 2017;167(3):181–191.
7. Puntillo F, Giglio M, Brienza N, et al. Impact of COVID-19 pandemic on chronic pain management: looking for the best way to deliver care. *Best Pract Res Clin Anaesthesiol*. 2020;34(3):529–537. doi:10.1016/j.bpa.2020.07.00.

ADDITIONAL READING
- Bohnert ASB, Guy GP Jr, Losby JL. Opioid prescribing in the United States before and after the Centers for Disease Control and Prevention's 2016 opioid guideline. *Ann Intern Med*. 2018;169(6):367–375.
- Boston University School of Medicine. SCOPE of Pain (Safer/Competent Opioid Prescribing Education). https://www.scopeofpain.org. Accessed November 13, 2021.

 SEE ALSO

The SARS-CoV-2 pandemic led to a significant decrease in access to clinics and procedures for chronic pain management (7).

 CODES

ICD10
- G89.29 Other chronic pain
- G89.21 Chronic pain due to trauma
- G89.28 Other chronic postprocedural pain

CLINICAL PEARLS
- Start with the presumption that a patient's pain is *real*.
- Emphasize that a pain-free life may not be possible—better function and quality of life are shared goals.
- Use a multidisciplinary approach with nonpharmacologic therapies and thoughtful medication use with clear goals, expectations, and documentation of care plan.
- Universal precautions are a systems-based approach for opioid prescription in cases of chronic pain.

CIRRHOSIS OF THE LIVER

Liam P. Burke, MD

 BASICS

DESCRIPTION
A chronic disease with inflammation, necrosis, fibrosis, hepatocellular dysfunction, and vascular remodeling potentially leading to liver failure and/or cancer

EPIDEMIOLOGY
- Predominant age at diagnosis: 40 to 60 years old
- Predominant sex: male > female; more women with cirrhosis from alcohol abuse
- Liver disease and cirrhosis are the 9th leading cause of death among U.S. adult males; 12th overall leading cause of death in United States
- Nonalcoholic steatohepatitis (NASH) is an increasingly common cause of cirrhosis (projected to become the leading cause in the next decade).

Incidence
Roughly 30,000 cases of cirrhosis diagnosed each year and very likely an underestimate as many patients are unaware that they have cirrhosis.

Prevalence
- 0.3% of Americans are diagnosed with cirrhosis (~630,000) and 2% with chronic liver disease.
- Highest prevalence of cirrhosis in non-Hispanic blacks, Mexican Americans, and people living below the federal poverty level

ETIOLOGY AND PATHOPHYSIOLOGY
- Chronic hepatitis C virus (HCV) (26%)
- Alcohol abuse (21%), NASH/obesity (~10%)
- Hepatitis B virus (HBV) plus hepatitis D infection (15%)
- Other: hemochromatosis, autoimmune hepatitis, primary biliary cirrhosis, secondary biliary cirrhosis, biliary atresia, idiopathic biliary fibrosis, primary sclerosing cholangitis, Wilson disease, α_1-antitrypsin deficiency, granulomatous disease (e.g., sarcoidosis); drug-induced liver disease (e.g., methotrexate, α-methyldopa, amiodarone); venous outflow obstruction (e.g., Budd-Chiari syndrome, veno-occlusive disease); chronic right-sided heart failure; tricuspid regurgitation; and rare genetic, metabolic, and infectious causes
- Hepatocellular injury results in cellular hyperplasia (regenerating nodules), fibrous changes, and angiogenesis. Distortions in blood flow result in portal hypertension.

Genetics
Hemochromatosis, Wilson disease, and α_1-antitrypsin deficiency in adults are associated with cirrhosis.

RISK FACTORS
Alcohol abuse, intravenous drug abuse, obesity

GENERAL PREVENTION
- Mitigate risk factors (e.g., alcohol abuse; screen for hepatitis C); >80% of chronic liver disease is preventable.
- Limit alcohol consumption and advise weight loss in overweight or obese patients.

COMMONLY ASSOCIATED CONDITIONS
HCV, alcohol and drug abuse, diabetes, depression, obesity

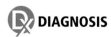 **DIAGNOSIS**

HISTORY
- Review risk factors (alcohol abuse, viral hepatitis, family history of primary liver cancer, other liver disease, or autoimmune disease).

- Symptoms
  - Fatigue, malaise, weakness
  - Anorexia, weight loss (weight gain if ascites/edema)
  - Right upper abdominal pain
  - Tea-colored urine, clay-colored stools
  - Edema, abdominal swelling/bloating, pruritus
  - Bruising, bleeding, hematemesis, hematochezia, melena
  - Absent/irregular menses, chronic anovulation
  - Diminished libido, erectile dysfunction
  - Night blindness

PHYSICAL EXAM
Physical exam may be normal until end-stage disease—many relate to manifestations of portal hypertension and/or hyperestrinism.
- Skin changes: spider angiomas, palmar erythema, jaundice, scleral icterus, ecchymoses, caput medusa, hyperpigmentation, decreased body hair, facial telangiectasias
- Hepatomegaly; splenomegaly (if portal hypertension)
- Abdominal fluid wave, shifting dullness (ascites)
- Gynecomastia, Dupuytren contractures
- Pretibial, presacral pitting edema, and clubbing (especially in hepatopulmonary syndrome)
- Asterixis, mental status changes (hepatic encephalopathy)
- Muscle wasting, weakness
- Fetor hepaticus (in severe portosystemic shunting)

DIFFERENTIAL DIAGNOSIS
Steatohepatitis, other causes of portal hypertension (e.g., portal vein thrombosis, lymphoma); metastatic or multifocal cancer in the liver; vascular congestion (e.g., cardiac cirrhosis); acute alcoholic hepatitis

DIAGNOSTIC TESTS & INTERPRETATION
Fibrosis-4 (FIB-4) index: age; aspartate aminotransferase (AST); alanine aminotransferase (ALT); platelet count (1)

Initial Tests (lab, imaging)
- AST/ALT: mildly elevated, typically AST > ALT; enzymes may normalize as cirrhosis progresses.
- Elevated alkaline phosphatase (ALP), γ-glutamyl transpeptidase (GGT), and total/direct bilirubin
- Anemia from hemolysis, folate deficiency, and/or splenomegaly
- Thrombocytopenia (<110; 95% specific for cirrhosis); FIB-4 <1.45 or AST to platelet ratio index (APRI) <0.7 unlikely to have cirrhosis
- Impaired synthetic liver function denoted by hypoalbuminemia, low cholesterol, prolonged prothrombin time (PT), international normalized ratio (INR), and partial thromboplastin time (PTT); coagulopathy of vitamin K–dependent clotting factors (II, VII, IX, X)
- Progressive cirrhosis indicated by hyperammonemia, elevated BUN, hyperkalemia, and hyponatremia
- Hepatorenal syndrome: creatinine clearance <40 mL/min (or serum creatinine >1.5) with urine volume <500 mL/day and urine sodium <10 mEq/L
- Abdominal ultrasound q6–12mo to screen for hepatocellular carcinoma (HCC)
- Doppler ultrasound or elastography to assess liver parenchyma and Doppler for hepatic/portal vein

Follow-Up Tests & Special Considerations
Consider:
- Hepatitis serologies
- Serum ethanol and GGT if alcohol abuse suspected
- Antimitochondrial antibody to screen for primary biliary cirrhosis

- Anti–smooth muscle and antinuclear antibodies to screen for chronic active (autoimmune) hepatitis
- Transferrin saturation (>50%) and ferritin (markedly increased) to screen for hemochromatosis; if abnormal, check hemochromatosis (HFE) genetics/mutation analysis.
- α_1-Antitrypsin phenotype screen
- Ceruloplasmin to screen for Wilson disease; if low, check copper excretion (serum copper plus 24-hour urine copper).
- α-Fetoprotein level to screen for HCC

Diagnostic Procedures/Other
- Liver biopsy: required for definitive diagnosis, percutaneous if INR <1.5 and no ascites; otherwise, transjugular; biopsy recommended if noninvasive markers incongruent with imaging
- Ultrasound-based elastography: noninvasive alternative to liver biopsy, increasing availability; evaluates fibrosis
- Endoscopy (EGD) if esophageal varices/portal hypertensive gastropathy are a concern
- Magnetic resonance elastography: best imaging in obese or nonalcoholic fatty liver disease (NAFLD)

Test Interpretation
Fibrous bands and regenerative nodules are classic biopsy features of cirrhosis. Other histologic patterns:
- Alcoholic liver disease: steatosis, polymorphonuclear (PMN) leukocyte infiltrate, ballooning degeneration of hepatocytes, Mallory bodies, giant mitochondria
- HBV/HCV: periportal lymphocytic inflammation
- NASH: same as alcoholic liver disease; steatosis may "burn-out" in advanced disease.
- Biliary cirrhosis: PMN infiltrate in wall of bile ducts, inflammation increased in portal spaces, progressive loss of bile ducts in portal spaces
- Hemochromatosis: intrahepatic iron stores increased via iron stain or weighted biopsy tissue
- α_1-Antitrypsin deficiency: positive periodic acid–Schiff bodies in hepatocytes

 TREATMENT

Outpatient care except for major GI bleeding, altered mental status, sepsis/infection, rapid hepatic decompensation, or renal failure

GENERAL MEASURES
- Abstain from alcohol, drugs, and hepatotoxic medications and herbs.
- Pneumococcal-23, hepatitis A/B, and influenza vaccinations
- Weight loss, exercise, and control of lipids/glucose
- Key initial step is determining compensated versus uncompensated disease (ascites; spontaneous bacterial peritonitis [SBP]; hepatic encephalopathy, coagulopathy, variceal hemorrhage)

MEDICATION
First Line
Treat the underlying cause first (note prescribing precautions in decompensated cirrhosis) to delay progression of disease.
- HCV: Goal is to eradicate viral RNA in serum. Simplified treatment with direct acting antivirals (DAAs) recommended if without cirrhosis (e.g., FIB-4 < 3.25, FibroScan <12.5 kPa, normal biopsy, or platelet count >150,000) with glecaprevir-pibrentasvir for 8 weeks in genotypes 1 to 6, or sofosbuvir-velpatasvir for 12 weeks duration in genotypes 1, 2, 4, 5, and 6; if

cirrhosis, past treatment failure, eGFR <30 mL/min/m², hepatitis B, HIV, suspected HCC then specialty referral

- HBV: In compensated cirrhosis with viremia, goal of treatment is to reduce HCC risk and decompensation with 48-week therapy. If decompensated, indefinite therapy recommended. Entecavir 0.5 to 1.0 mg PO daily, tenofovir 300 mg PO daily, and telbivudine 600 mg PO daily are first line.
- NAFLD: weight loss of 7–10% to improve histopathologic features. Improved fitness and/or >150 min/week of physical activity improves metabolic and hepatic indices.
- Alcoholic hepatitis: Treat alcohol withdrawal; Maddrey Discriminant Function score for risk stratification; >32 indicates poor prognosis, patients may benefit from prednisolone 40 mg/day for 28 days with 2 to 4 week; taper to reduce short-term mortality; pentoxifylline for patients who cannot tolerate steroids
- Hereditary hemochromatosis: phlebotomy every 1 to 2 weeks as tolerated to goal serum ferritin of 50 to 100 μg/L (often to <40 μg/L) and then 2 to 6 times per year as needed; deferoxamine 40 mg/kg/day over 8 to 12 hours for 5 to 7 days in dyserythropoietic syndrome and chronic hemolytic anemia to reduce iron overload quickly
- Primary biliary cirrhosis: ursodeoxycholic acid (ursodiol) 13 to 15 mg/kg PO divided BID–QID with food; bile acid sequestrants are first-line therapy for pruritus: cholestyramine 4 to 8 g PO BID; antihistamines; rifampicin 150 to 300 mg PO BID or naltrexone 50 mg/day can be used for pruritus if ursodiol is ineffective. Evaluate and treat for malabsorption, fat-soluble vitamin deficiencies, metabolic bone disease, hypercholesterolemia, hypothyroidism, and anemia.
- Wilson disease: initial treatment with penicillamine 1,000 to 1,500 mg/day PO BID–QID or trientine 750 to 1,500 mg/day PO BID–TID on empty stomach. Trientine 750 to 1,500 mg/day PO BID–TID is better tolerated. After 1 year, zinc acetate 150 mg/day PO BID–TID for maintenance; zinc for presymptomatic, pregnant, and pediatric populations
- Autoimmune hepatitis: Treat if AST or ALT >10 times ULN, or if either >5 times ULN and γ globulins >2 times ULN with prednisone 30 mg/day × 1 week, then 20 mg/day for 1 week, then 10 mg/day for 2 weeks with, maintenance of 5 mg/day with azathioprine 50 mg/day throughout; after induction, treat to normal transaminases. Discontinue maintenance after at least 24 months of treatment if AST and ALT are normal.
- Esophageal varices: for primary prophylaxis of variceal bleed, propranolol >40 mg, carvedilol 6.25 mg, or nadolol 40 mg PO daily, to lower portal pressure by 20 mm Hg, systolic pressure from 90 to 100 mm Hg, and pulse rate by 25%; PPI indicated when varices require banding, and also for portal hypertensive gastropathy
- Ascites/edema: low-sodium (<2 g/day) diet and spironolactone 100 to 400 mg/day with or without furosemide 40 to 160 mg/day PO; torsemide may substitute for furosemide. If serum sodium <120 mmol/L, then 1.0 to 1.5 L/day water restriction. If new onset, rule out SBP. If history of SBP, consider SBP prophylaxis (TMP-SMX DS daily, norfloxacin 400 mg PO daily).
- Encephalopathy: lactulose 15 to 45 mL BID; titrate to induce 2 to 3 loose bowel movements daily. Combination therapy with rifaximin (550 mg PO BID) is recommended regimen to prevent recurrent hepatic encephalopathy.
- Pruritus: ursodiol, cholestyramine, or antihistamines (e.g., hydroxyzine)

- Renal insufficiency: Stop NSAIDs, diuretics, and nephrotoxic drugs; normalize electrolytes; and hospitalize for plasma expansion or dialysis.
- Prophylactic antibiotics for invasive procedures, GI bleeding, or history of SBP

Second Line
HBV: adefovir 10 mg PO daily second line; PEG-IFN α2a 180 μg SC weekly for 48 weeks in compensated cirrhosis if not contraindicated; lamivudine not recommended as first-line agent due to resistance

ISSUES FOR REFERRAL
Evaluate for liver transplant at onset of complications (ascites, variceal bleeding, encephalopathy), jaundice, or liver lesion suggestive of HCC and/or when evidence of hepatic dysfunction develops (Child-Turcotte-Pugh [CTP] >7 and Model for End-Stage Liver Disease [MELD] >10).

SURGERY/OTHER PROCEDURES
- Varices: endoscopic ligation, 4 to 6 treatments (if acute bleed, use pre-esophagogastroduodenoscopy [EGD] octreotide as vasoconstrictor); transjugular intrahepatic shunt (TIPS) second-line or salvage therapy for acute bleed
- Ascites: if tense, therapeutic paracentesis every 2 weeks PRN; caution if pedal edema absent
- Fulminant hepatic failure: liver transplantation
- HCC: curable if small with radiofrequency ablation or resection and transplant

COMPLEMENTARY & ALTERNATIVE MEDICINE
- Zinc sulfate 220 mg BID may improve dysgeusia and appetite; adjunct for hepatic encephalopathy
- Milk thistle may lower transaminases and improve symptoms

ADMISSION, INPATIENT, AND NURSING CONSIDERATIONS
Major GI bleeding, altered mental status, sepsis/infection, rapidly progressing hepatic decompensation, renal failure

ONGOING CARE
- Monitor liver enzymes, sodium, creatinine, platelets, and PT q6–12mo; calculate MELD score.
- Serial α-fetoprotein and liver ultrasound screening q6–12mo in patients with cirrhosis. Patients >55 years with chronic HBV or HCV, elevated INR, or low platelets are at highest risk for HCC.
- MRI with contrast best follow-up test for HCC if α-fetoprotein elevated and/or liver mass found on ultrasound
- EGD at cirrhosis diagnosis and every 3 years (compensated) and every 1 year (decompensated) to screen for varices

FOLLOW-UP RECOMMENDATIONS
Regular physical conditioning may help with fatigue.

Patient Monitoring
- Monitor for nonspecific symptoms such as fatigue, weakness, reduced appetite, itchy skin at each visit.
- Change in mental status, jaundice, or abdominal pain are major concerns.

DIET
Protein (1.2 to 1.5 g/kg body weight daily), high fiber, multivitamin (without iron), sodium restriction (<2 g/day), combined with fluid restriction, essential if ascites/edema

PATIENT EDUCATION
- Educate about when to seek emergency care (e.g., hematemesis, altered mental status).
- Drug, alcohol, and smoking cessation (no cannabis)
- Update required immunizations; HCV transmission precautions

PROGNOSIS
- 5 to 20 years of asymptomatic disease from time of initial diagnosis
- MELD score and CTP score historically used to provide prognostic information. These scores lack contribution of nutritional assessment; sarcopenia (muscle wasting) suggested as an important predictor of mortality in patients with cirrhosis
- After onset of complications, death typically within 5 years without transplant
  – 5% per year develop HCC
  – 50% of cirrhotics develop ascites over 10 years; 50% 5-year survival after ascites develop
  – Acute variceal bleeding is the most common fatal complication; 30% mortality
  – Median survival after complications (ascites, variceal bleeding, encephalopathy) is 1.5 years.
  – With transplant, 85% survive 1 year; after transplant, ~5% annual mortality
- <25% of eligible patients receive a transplant because of donor organ shortage

COMPLICATIONS
Ascites, edema, infections, hepatic encephalopathy, GI bleeding, esophageal varices, gastropathy, colopathy, hepatorenal syndrome, hepatopulmonary syndrome, HCC, fulminant hepatic failure, complications after transplant (e.g., surgical, rejection, infections)

REFERENCE
1. Vallet-Pichard A, Mallet V, Nalpas B, et al. FIB-4: an inexpensive and accurate marker of fibrosis in HCV infection. comparison with liver biopsy and fibrotest. *Hepatology*. 2007;46(1):32–36.

ADDITIONAL READING
Chalasani N, Younossi Z, Lavine JE, et al. The diagnosis and management of nonalcoholic fatty liver disease: practice guidance from the American Association for the Study of Liver Diseases. *Hepatology*. 2018;67(1):328–357.

 ## SEE ALSO

Algorithm: Cirrhosis

 ## CODES

ICD10
- K74.60 Unspecified cirrhosis of liver
- K70.30 Alcoholic cirrhosis of liver without ascites
- K74.69 Other cirrhosis of liver

CLINICAL PEARLS
- 80% of chronic liver disease that leads to cirrhosis is preventable (primarily alcohol abuse).
- After diagnosis of cirrhosis, abdominal ultrasound every 6 months for early detection of HCC
- Update necessary immunizations and treat underlying cause (HCV, alcohol abuse, etc.).
- Rule out SBP in patients presenting with ascites.

CLOSTRIDIUM DIFFICILE INFECTION

Alexis Benavides Reedy-Cooper, MD, MPH

BASICS

DESCRIPTION
- A gram-positive, spore-forming anaerobic bacillus that releases toxins to produce clinical disease
- Infection caused by *Clostridioides difficile* is frequently associated with antibiotic use, hospitalization, residence at long-term care facilities, and age.
- Severity of infection ranges from asymptomatic carrier to diarrhea, colitis, sepsis, perforation, and death.
- Transmission of spores is typically person-to-person via the fecal-oral route but may also occur through exposure to contaminated surfaces or equipment. *C. difficile* spores can survive on dry surfaces for up to 5 months.
- System(s) affected: gastrointestinal
- Synonym(s): *Clostridioides difficile* infection, *C. difficile*–associated disease or diarrhea (CDAD); *C. difficile* infection; *C. difficile* colitis; *C. diff*

EPIDEMIOLOGY
Incidence
- Colonization with *C. difficile* found in:
  - 2–10% of community, 3–18% of inpatients, 4–20% of long-term residents (1)
- Global estimated incidence of *C. difficile* infection 50/100,000/year; hospitalization rates are increasing (2).
- National incidence of health care–associated *C. difficile* infection 73/100,000 persons (3)
- National incidence of community-acquired *C. difficile* infection 52/100,000 persons

Prevalence
- Prevalence increasing in the United States in both health care settings and the community
- *C. difficile* accounted for 12% of health care–associated infections in 2010.
- >2 million cases of *C. difficile*–associated disease in U.S. hospitals from 1993 to 2005

ETIOLOGY AND PATHOPHYSIOLOGY
- *C. difficile* is an anaerobic toxin-producing, gram-positive bacillus bacteria existing in vegetative and spore forms. Spores can survive for months in harsh conditions and outside of the body.
- Spread by fecal-oral contact. Acid-resistant spores pass through stomach to reside mostly in the colon.
- Colonic colonization causes disruptions in barrier functions of the normal microbiome (4).
- *C. difficile* is noninvasive. Toxins mediate disease:
  - Toxins A (enterotoxin) and B (cytotoxin) attract neutrophils and monocytes, degrading colonic epithelial cells and causing clinical disease.
- The hypervirulent strain BI/NAP1/027 of *C. difficile* is associated with higher rates of colectomy and death.

Genetics
No known genetic factors

RISK FACTORS
- Host risk factors
  - Age >65 years
  - Hospitalization or long-term health care facility
  - Comorbidities, including inflammatory bowel disease, immunosuppression, chronic liver disease, and end-stage renal disease
  - Enteral feeding
  - Previous *C. difficile* infection

- Factors that disrupt normal colonic microbiota:
  - Exposure to antibiotics (including perioperative prophylaxis)
  - Commonly implicated antibiotics: ampicillin, amoxicillin, clindamycin (most common), cephalosporins, and fluoroquinolones
  - Chronic acid suppression (4).
- Recurrence from prior infection
  - Recurrence rates are ~20%; recurrence more likely with each additional episode (4)
- Community-acquired *C. difficile* infections (no overnight admission in >12 weeks) are more frequent in patients without other risk factors (younger, no recent antibiotic exposure).
- Risk increases with length of hospital stay, duration of antibiotics exposure and number of antibiotics used (5).

Geriatric Considerations
C. difficile is the most common cause of acute diarrheal illness in long-term care facilities.

Pediatric Considerations
- Neonates have a higher rate of *C. difficile* colonization (25–80%) but are generally less symptomatic than adults.
- Frequently serve as carrier for infection in adults

GENERAL PREVENTION
- Antibiotic stewardship programs decrease the incidence of *C. difficile* infection.
- Society for Healthcare Epidemiology of America (SHEA)/Infectious Diseases Society of America (IDSA) guidelines for prevention (6):
  - For health care workers, patients, and visitors:
    - Contact precautions, including gloves and gowns, on entry to room
    - Alcohol-based hand sanitizers are not effective. Hand washing with soap and water before and after patient interaction is recommended.
    - Accommodate patients with *C. difficile* infection in private rooms, if possible.
  - Environmental cleaning and disinfection
    - Disinfect with hypochlorite or other spore-killing solution.
    - Identify and reduce environmental sources.
  - Antimicrobial restrictions
    - Minimize the frequency and duration of antibiotic therapy. Use particular care when prescribing commonly implicated antibiotics.

COMMONLY ASSOCIATED CONDITIONS
Pseudomembranous colitis, toxic megacolon, sepsis, colonic perforation

DIAGNOSIS

HISTORY
- Common presenting symptoms include diarrhea and abdominal cramping or pain.
- Age and underlying comorbidities
- Recent antibiotic use (Risk of *C. difficile* infection may persist for 3 months after antibiotic is discontinued.)
- Proton pump inhibitor or H$_2$-receptor blocker use
- Diarrhea (defined as >3 stools in 24 hours) that is watery, foul-smelling, and sometimes bloody (1)
- Fever (<10%), anorexia, nausea
- Recent hospitalization or stay at nursing facility
- Gastrointestinal manipulations like tube feeding, enemas, surgery

PHYSICAL EXAM
- Abdominal exam: look for tenderness, increasing distension, diminished bowel sounds, peritoneal signs.
- Initial presentation can be fulminant and rapidly fatal; assessment of severity is key to management.
- Look for signs of systemic illness including fever, tachycardia, hypotension, dehydration.

DIFFERENTIAL DIAGNOSIS
- Infectious causes
  - *Salmonella*
  - *Shigella*
  - *Campylobacter*
  - Shiga toxin–producing *Escherichia coli* infection
- Noninfectious causes
  - Intestinal obstruction
  - Ischemic bowel disease
  - Inflammatory bowel disease: ulcerative colitis, Crohn disease
  - Gastrointestinal cancer
  - Drug-associated diarrhea
  - Foodborne illness
  - Other antibiotic associated diarrhea (75% of antibiotic diarrhea not associated with *C. difficile*)

DIAGNOSTIC TESTS & INTERPRETATION
Initial Tests (lab, imaging)
- CBC, BMP, lactate to evaluate leukocytosis and serum creatinine, aids in assessment of severity of disease
- Several stool tests are available for diagnosis.
  - Glutamate dehydrogenase (GDH) assay (sensitivity, 85–95%; specificity, 89–99%)
  - Enzyme immunoassays which detect toxin A or toxin B (sensitivity 63–94%)
  - Nucleic acid amplification tests (NAATs)
  - Cell culture cytotoxicity assays (gold standard)
- Stepwise approach to testing often used by may vary by facility
  - For example, GED plus toxin assay with NAAT testing for discrepant results
- Repeat testing during the same episode of diarrhea is not recommended. Stool carriage persists for 3 to 6 weeks after successful treatment.
- Routine radiologic examination is not recommended in the absence of signs of systemic disease or clinical suspicion for complicated/severe disease.
  - Plain films may show thumbprinting and colonic distension.
  - CT may show mucosal thickening, colonic wall thickening, pericolonic inflammation, or signs of complicated infection in severe cases (i.e., extraluminal air).

Diagnostic Procedures/Other
Endoscopy can evaluate for presence of pseudomembranes and exclude other conditions.
- Although not all patients with *C. difficile* infection have pseudomembranes, their presence is pathognomonic.
- Flexible sigmoidoscopy may miss 15–20% of pseudomembranes (from the proximal colon).

Test Interpretation
SHEA/IDSA guidelines (6)
- Mild or moderate disease: leukocytosis with white blood cell (WBC) count <15,000 cells/μL and a serum creatinine level <1.5 times the premorbid level
- Severe, uncomplicated disease: leukocytosis with WBC count >15,000 cells/μL or a serum creatinine level >1.5 times the premorbid level
- Severe, complicated disease: hypotension, sepsis, markedly elevated WBC count, and imaging findings of complicated disease

TREATMENT

GENERAL MEASURES
- Antimotility agents are contraindicated.
- Avoid indiscriminate use of antibiotics.
- Proton pump inhibitors are associated with recurrent infection but have not been shown to be causal.
- Discontinue offending antibiotic, whenever possible.

MEDICATION

First Line
- Mild or moderate infection (nonfulminant), first episode
  - Vancomycin 125 mg given QID for 10 days
  - Fidaxomicin 200 mg given BID for 10 days
    - Associated with fewer relapses
  - Only if above agents are unavailable, then reasonable to use metronidazole, 500 mg TID PO for 10 days
  - If patient is unable to take oral medications, then intravenous (IV) metronidazole or intraluminal (PO) vancomycin can be used.
- First recurrence
  - If a standard regimen was used for the initial episode, use vancomycin taper: 125 mg QID for 10 to 14 days, BID for a week, QD for a week, and then every 2 or 3 days for 2 to 8 weeks.
  - Fidaxomicin 200 mg given BID for 10 days if VAN was used for the initial episode
- Second recurrence
  - Vancomycin taper and/or pulse: vancomycin 125 mg PO QID for 10 to 14 days, then 125 mg PO BID for 7 days, then 125 mg PO once daily for 7 days, and then 125 mg PO every 2 to 3 days for 2 to 8 weeks:
    - Pulse dosing every 2 to 3 days allows spores to germinate and then be killed.
  - Vancomycin 125 mg PO QID for 10 days followed by rifaximin 400 mg TID for 20 days, OR
  - Fidaxomicin 200 mg given BID for 10 days, OR
  - Fecal microbiota transplantation should be considered with recurrence after ≥3 treatment courses.
- Severe infection
  - Enteral vancomycin is first-line therapy in patients with severe C. difficile infection:
    - 125 mg PO QID for 10 to 14 days
    - Fidaxomicin 200 mg given BID for 10 days
    - Vancomycin retention enema if unable to take PO or if there is evidence of poor gastrointestinal motility
- Fulminant infection: Consider surgical and critical care consultation.
  - Vancomycin 500 mg PO QID or by nasogastric tube. If ileus or PO is not an option, consider vancomycin 500 mg rectally.
  - Intravenously administered metronidazole (500 mg every 8 hours)

> **ALERT**
> When using vancomycin to treat C. difficile infection, use oral or rectal formulations. IV formulations (not excreted into the colonic lumen) are ineffective.

Second Line
- Oral metronidazole
- 500 mg PO TID for 10 to 14 days
- Vancomycin: for patients who cannot tolerate or have failed metronidazole therapy and for pregnancy
- Fecal transplant: stool from healthy, screened donor. Administered via either rectal or oral route. Highly effective for recurrent infections (80–90% cure rate) after offending antibiotic stopped; recipient gut flora transformed in as few as 3 days following fecal transplantation (7)[A].

SURGERY/OTHER PROCEDURES
- Severe abdominal pain or signs of hemodynamic instability in the setting of known infection should prompt surgical and critical care consultation.
- Perforation of the colon (8)[A]

> **ALERT**
> BI/NAP1/027 strain is commonly associated with fulminant colitis, often requiring surgical intervention in younger patients with severe disease.

COMPLEMENTARY & ALTERNATIVE MEDICINE
- Adjunctive IV immunoglobulin (IVIG) has shown promise; more data needed before routine use
- Probiotics Lactobacillus acidophilus and Saccharomyces boulardii have inhibitory effects on C. difficile and can help prevent C. difficile infection.
- Other investigational treatments:
  - Newer antibiotics (rifalazil, tolevamer, and ramoplanin)
  - Monoclonal antibodies to modulate toxin effects
  - Vaccine form of C. difficile antitoxin antibody

ADMISSION, INPATIENT, AND NURSING CONSIDERATIONS
- Admission criteria/initial stabilization
  - Hypovolemia
  - Inability to keep up with enteric losses
  - Hematochezia
  - Electrolyte disturbances
- IV fluids to maintain volume status
- Discharge criteria
  - Decreased diarrhea severity and frequency
  - Tolerating oral diet and medications

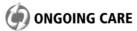 ONGOING CARE

FOLLOW-UP RECOMMENDATIONS
Do not repeat testing for toxins because patients may shed for weeks following an acute infection.

Patient Monitoring
- Relapses of colitis occur in 15–30%.
- Relapses typically occur 2 to 10 days after discontinuing antibiotics.

DIET
- Regular diet
- NPO if severe colitis and surgical evaluation pending

PATIENT EDUCATION
Educate patients about C. difficile transmission, the importance of appropriate hand washing with soap and water and not relying on alcohol-based sanitizers as well as avoidance of unnecessary use of antibiotics to prevent unnecessary risk of C. difficile infection.

PROGNOSIS
- Most patients improve with conservative management and oral antibiotics.
- 1–3% of patients develop severe/fulminant colitis requiring emergency colectomy.

REFERENCES
1. Guh AY, Kutty PK. Clostridioides difficile infection. Ann Intern Med. 2018;169(7):ITC49–ITC64.
2. Balsells E, Shi T, Leese C, et al. Global burden of Clostridium difficile infections: a systematic review and meta-analysis. J Glob Health. 2019;9(1): 010407. doi: 10.7189/jogh.09.010407.
3. Guh AY, Mu Y, Winston LG, et al; for Emerging Infections Program Clostridioides difficile Infection Working Group. Trends in U.S. burden of Clostridioides difficile infection and outcomes. N Engl J Med. 2020;382(14):1320–1330. doi:10.1056/NEJMoa1910215.
4. Leffler DA, Lamont JT. Clostridium difficile infection. N Engl J Med. 2015;372(16):1539–1548.
5. McDonald LC, Gerding DN, Johnson S, et al. Clinical practice guidelines for Clostridium difficile infection in adults and children: 2017 update by the Infectious Diseases Society of America (IDSA) and Society for Healthcare Epidemiology of America (SHEA). Clin Infect Dis. 2018;66(7):e1–e48.
6. Cohen SH, Gerding DN, Johnson S, et al; for Society for Healthcare Epidemiology of America, Infectious Diseases Society of America. Clinical practice guidelines for Clostridium difficile infection in adults: 2010 update by the Society for Healthcare Epidemiology of America (SHEA) and the Infectious Diseases Society of America (IDSA). Infect Control Hosp Epidemiol. 2010;31(5):431–455.
7. Shankar V, Hamilton MJ, Khoruts A, et al. Species and genus level resolution analysis of gut microbiota in Clostridium difficile patients following fecal microbiota transplantation. Microbiome. 2014;2:13.
8. Debast SB, Bauer MP, Kuijper EJ; and European Society of Clinical Microbiology and Infectious Diseases. European Society of Clinical Microbiology and Infectious Diseases: update of the treatment guidance document for Clostridium difficile infection. Clin Microbiol Infect. 2014;20(Suppl 2):1–26.

CODES

ICD10
- A04.7 Enterocolitis due to Clostridium difficile
- A04.71 Enterocolitis due to Clostridium difficile, recurrent
- A04.72 Enterocolitis due to Clostridium difficile, not specified as recurrent

CLINICAL PEARLS
- C. difficile is spread by fecal-oral contact.
- Alcohol-based hand sanitizers are ineffective against C. difficile. Wash hands with soap and water.
- Testing and treatment of asymptomatic patients is not recommended.
- C. difficile and organismal by-products (e.g., toxin) are identifiable from stool samples.
- Patients may shed organism or toxin for weeks after treatment. Repeat toxin assays following treatment are not helpful.
- Vancomycin or fidaxomicin is now considered first line.
- Consider probiotic use when prescribing antibiotics to potentially decrease risk of development of C. difficile infection.
- Metronidazole is no longer recommended as first-line treatment (in combination with vancomycin or as monotherapy), unless vancomycin and fidaxomicin are not viable options.

COLIC, INFANTILE
Daniel T. Lee, MD, MA • Phillip Charles Brown, MD • Arthur Ohannessian, MD

 BASICS

DESCRIPTION
- Colic is defined as excessive crying in an otherwise healthy baby.
- A commonly used criteria is the Wessel criteria or the Rule of Three, when crying lasts for:
  - >3 hr/day
  - >3 days/week
  - Persists >3 weeks
- Many clinicians do not strictly adhere to the criterion of persistence for >3 weeks because few parents or clinicians will wait that long before evaluation or intervention.
- Colic usually peaks at 6 weeks of life.
- Some clinicians feel that colic represents the extreme end of the spectrum of normal crying, whereas most feel that colic is a distinct clinical entity.

EPIDEMIOLOGY
Incidence
- Predominant age group is between 2 weeks and 4 months of age.
- Equal predominance among males and females, breastfed versus formula-fed, and full term versus preterm

Prevalence
- Wide range from 8% to 40% of infants; however, more likely affects 10–25% of infants
- Causes 10–20% of pediatric visits during the early weeks of an infant's life

Pediatric Considerations
This is a problem during infancy.

ETIOLOGY AND PATHOPHYSIOLOGY
The cause is unknown. Factors that may play a role include the following:
- Infant gastroesophageal reflux disease
- Fruit juice intolerance
- Swallowing air during the process of crying, feeding, or sucking
- Overfeeding or feeding too quickly; underfeeding has also been proposed
- Inadequate burping after feeding
- Family tension and/or stress
- Parental anxiety, depression, and/or fatigue
- Parent–infant interaction mismatch
- Infant's inability to console him or herself when dealing with stimuli
- Hypersensitivity after exposure to prolonged environmental stimuli
- Possible early manifestation of childhood migraine
- Intolerance to cow's milk, soy milk, or breast milk protein
- Increases in the gut hormone motilin, causing hyperperistalsis
- Functional lactose overload (i.e., breast milk that has a lower lipid content can have faster transit time in the intestine, leading to more lactose fermentation in the gut and hence gas and distension)
- Intestinal immaturity leading to incomplete absorption of carbohydrates in the small intestine resulting in excessive gas when the unabsorbed carbohydrate is fermented by colonic bacteria
- Alterations in fecal microflora
- Tobacco smoke exposure
- Prenatal exposure to maternal smoking or nicotine replacement therapy
- Immature motor regulation
- Increased serotonin concentration

RISK FACTORS
- Physiologic predispositions in an infant may play a role, but no definitive risk factors have been established.
- Emerging data suggest maternal smoking or exposure to nicotine replacement therapy during pregnancy is associated with higher incidence of infantile colic.
- Infants with a maternal history of migraine headaches are twice as likely to have colic.

GENERAL PREVENTION
Colic is generally not preventable.

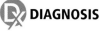 **DIAGNOSIS**

HISTORY
- Evaluation for Wessel criteria: Crying lasts for >3 hr/day, >3 days/week, and persists >3 weeks.
- Episodes usually have a clear beginning and end.
- The crying is generally spontaneous, without preceding events triggering the episodes.
- The crying is typically different from normal crying. Colicky crying may be louder, more turbulent, variable in pitch, and appears more like screaming.
- Episodes of colic may be associated with hypertonia, which may include facial flushing, circumoral pallor, tense abdomen, arching of the back, tightening of the arms, clenching of the fingers, or drawing up of the legs.
- The infant may be difficult to soothe or console despite all of the parents' efforts.
- The infant acts normally when not colicky.
- Assess the support system of caregivers and families, including coping skills.

PHYSICAL EXAM
- A comprehensive physical exam is normal.
- Because excessive crying may be a risk factor for abuse, be sure to examine the child carefully for signs of shaken baby syndrome or other types of child abuse.

DIFFERENTIAL DIAGNOSIS
Any organic cause for excessive or qualitatively different crying in infants such as:
- Infectious causes such as meningitis, sepsis, otitis media, or UTI
- Gastrointestinal causes such as gastroesophageal reflux disease, intussusception, lactose intolerance, constipation, anal fissure, or strangulated hernia
- Trauma, which includes foreign bodies, corneal abrasion, occult fracture, digit or penile hair tourniquet syndrome, or child abuse

DIAGNOSTIC TESTS & INTERPRETATION
Initial Tests (lab, imaging)
Infantile colic is a clinical diagnosis. No testing is typically performed unless clinical symptoms imply other causes (UTI, weight loss, etc.).

Diagnostic Procedures/Other
A thorough history and physical exam should be performed to rule out other causes. Otherwise, no diagnostic procedures or imaging are indicated.

 TREATMENT

GENERAL MEASURES
- Soothe by holding and rocking the baby (1)[B].
- Use a pacifier (1)[B].
- Use of gentle rhythmic motion (e.g., strollers, infant swings, car rides) (1)[B]
- White noise (e.g., vacuum cleaner, clothes dryer, white noise machine) (1)[B]
- Crib vibrators or car ride simulators have not proven to be helpful (1)[B].
- Providing a warm bath (1)[B]
- Increased carrying or use of infant carrier has not been shown to improve colic (1)[B].
- Frequent burping does not significantly lower colic events (and may increase rate of regurgitation) (2).
- Employ the 5 Ss (need to be done concurrently):
  - Swaddling: tight wrapping with blanket; may be especially beneficial in infants <8 weeks old (3)[B]
  - Side: laying baby on side
  - Shushing: loud white noise
  - Swinging: rhythmic, jiggle motion
  - Sucking: on a nipple, finger, or pacifier
  - (Bonus "S"): "Stay calm." The baby may not understand what is said but rather how it is said (e.g., "Everything will be fine; I am here now.").

MEDICATION
- No medication has been found to be universally beneficial in treating infantile colic. Probiotics are safe and effective. Their use is discussed in the "Complementary & Alternative Medicine" section.
- Dicyclomine (Bentyl) may have some benefit, but the potential serious adverse effects, such as apnea, seizures, and syncope, have precluded its use. Furthermore, the manufacturer has made the medication contraindicated for infants <6 months (4)[B].
- Simethicone has not been shown to be beneficial (4)[B].
- Omeprazole has not been shown to be beneficial.

ISSUES FOR REFERRAL
Excessive vomiting, poor weight gain, recurrent respiratory diseases, or bloody stools should prompt referral to a specialist.

COMPLEMENTARY & ALTERNATIVE MEDICINE

- There is no clear evidence that probiotics are more effective than placebo at preventing infantile colic; however, daily crying time may reduce with probiotics (specifically *Lactobacillus reuteri*) (5).
- *Lactobacillus reuteri* DSM 17938 was found to shorten duration of crying in a 2020 systematic review, but acupuncture was not found to be effective in treatment (6).
- A recent study indicates that *Bifidobacterium animalis* subsp. *lactis* may be the most efficacious probiotic. However, more data is needed (7).
- Anecdotal evidence that car rides, both real and simulated, can be effective. You can find a 10-hour recording of a simulated car ride at the following link: https://www.youtube.com/watch?v=8KAXmle-T_4.
- Providing "white noise," such as running a vacuum cleaner, clothes dryer, white noise generator, or infant sound machine. Avoid excessively loud and/or prolonged noise to minimize potential adverse effects on hearing or auditory development.
- Herbal teas and supplements may help but are not recommended because of limited, inconclusive evidence.
  – Herbal teas containing mixtures of chamomile, vervain, licorice, and balm-mint used up to TID may be beneficial. However, the study used high dosages, raising clinical concerns that this therapy may impair needed milk consumption in infants and be impractical to administer. In addition, preparations used in the study may not be commercially available in the United States.
  – There is evidence supporting the effectiveness of different preparations of fennel, such as oils, teas, and herbal compounds, in treating infantile colic (7)[A].
- A home-based intervention focusing on reducing infant stimulation and synchronizing infant sleep-wake cycles with the environment, as well as parental support, has been shown to be effective.
- Use of music may help.
- Chiropractic treatment has shown no benefit over placebo (8).
- Infant massage has not been shown to be helpful.

ONGOING CARE

FOLLOW-UP RECOMMENDATIONS
Frequent outpatient visits as needed for parental reassurance, education, and monitoring and to ensure the health of the infant and parents

Patient Monitoring
Follow for proper feeding, growth, and development.

DIET
- If breastfeeding:
  – Continue breastfeeding; switching to formula unlikely to help
  – Low likelihood of therapeutic benefit from eliminating milk products, eggs, wheat, nuts, soy, and/or fish from the maternal diet of breastfeeding mothers but may be beneficial if the mother is atopic or the infant has symptoms of cow's milk allergy (1)[B].

- If formula feeding:
  – Feeding the infant in a vertical position using a curved bottle or bottle with collapsible bag may help to reduce air swallowing.
  – If no intervention or dietary change has been effective, consider a 1-week trial of hypoallergenic formulas such as whey hydrolysate (e.g., Good Start) or casein hydrolysate (e.g., Alimentum, Nutramigen, Pregestimil) (1)[B],(4)[C].
  – Adding fiber to formula also has not been shown to be helpful (1)[B].
- Supplementing with sucrose solution may be helpful, but the effect may be short-lived (<1 hour) (1),(4)[B].
- Switching to soy protein formula is unlikely to be helpful.
- Despite the proposed mechanism of functional lactose overload, use of lactase enzymes in formula or breast milk or given directly to the infant has no therapeutic benefit (1)[B].

PATIENT EDUCATION
- Reassure parents that colic is not the result of bad parenting and advise parents about having proper rest breaks, adequate sleep, and help in caring for the infant.
- Parents need to develop their own personal coping strategies to deal with colic episodes to avoid risk of harm to infant.
- Explain the spectrum of crying behavior.
- Avoid over- or underfeeding.
- Instruct parents regarding beneficial feeding techniques such as improved bottles (low air, curved) and sufficient burping after feeding.
- Information for parents of colicky infants can be found at the following link from the American Academy of Family Physician: https://www.aafp.org/afp/2004/0815/p741.html.

PROGNOSIS
- Usually subsides by 3 to 6 months of age, often on its own
- Despite apparent abdominal pain, colicky infants eat well and gain weight normally.
- A few studies indicate temper tantrums may be more common among formerly colicky infants as studied in toddlers up to 4 years old.
- Colic has no bearing on the baby's intelligence or future development.

COMPLICATIONS
- Colic is self-limiting, and there is no proven untoward lasting effects to the infant.
- Possible associations with increased risk/incidence of postpartum depression among either or both parents, child abuse, caregiver burnout, and early cessation of breastfeeding

REFERENCES
1. Johnson JD, Cocker K, Chang E. Infantile colic: recognition and treatment. *Am Fam Physician*. 2015;92(7):577–582.
2. Kaur R, Bharti B, Saini SK. A randomized controlled trial of burping for the prevention of colic and regurgitation in healthy infants. *Child Care Health Dev*. 2015;41(1):52–56.
3. van Sleuwen BE, L'hoir MP, Engelberts AC, et al. Comparison of behavior modification with and without swaddling as interventions for excessive crying. *J Pediatr*. 2006;149(4):512–517.
4. Wade S, Kilgour T. Extracts from "clinical evidence": infantile colic. *BMJ*. 2001;323(7310):437–440.
5. Ong TG, Gordon M, Banks SS, et al. Probiotics to prevent infantile colic. *Cochrane Database Syst Rev*. 2019;(3):CD012473.
6. Hjern A, Lindblom K, Reuter A, et al. A systematic review of prevention and treatment of infantile colic. *Acta Paediatr*. 2020;109(9):1733–1744.
7. Anheyer D, Frawley J, Koch AK, et al. Herbal medicines for gastrointestinal disorders in children and adolescents: a systematic review. *Pediatrics*. 2017;139(6):e20170062.
8. Dobson D, Lucassen PL, Miller JJ, et al. Manipulative therapies for infantile colic. *Cochrane Database Syst Rev*. 2012;(12):CD004796.

ADDITIONAL READING
- Gelfand AA, Thomas KC, Goadsby PJ. Before the headache: infant colic as an early life expression of migraine. *Neurology*. 2012;79(13):1392–1396.
- Johnson JD, Cocker K, Chang E. Infantile colic: recognition and treatment. *Am Fam Physician*. 2015;92(7):577–582.
- Savino F, Pelle E, Palumeri E, et al. *Lactobacillus reuteri* (American Type Culture Collection Strain 55730) versus simethicone in the treatment of infantile colic: a prospective randomized study. *Pediatrics*. 2007;119(1):e124–e130.

 ## CODES

ICD10
R10.83 Colic

CLINICAL PEARLS
- Colic is defined as excessive crying in an otherwise healthy baby (3 hr/day, 3 day/week, persists >3 weeks).
- Excessive crying may be a risk factor for shaken baby syndrome or other forms of child abuse.
- Usually subsides spontaneously by 3 to 6 months of age
- Provide advice, support, and reassurance to parents.
- Prevent caregiver burnout by advising parents to get proper rest breaks, sleep, and help in caring for the infant.
- Employ the 5 Ss (need to be done concurrently):
  – Swaddling: tight wrapping with blanket
  – Side: laying baby on side
  – Shushing: loud white noise
  – Swinging: rhythmic, jiggle motion
  – Sucking: on a nipple, finger, or pacifier
  – (Bonus "S"): "Stay calm." The baby may not understand what is said but rather how it is said (e.g., "Everything will be fine; I'm here now.").

COLITIS, ISCHEMIC

Marie L. Borum, MD, EdD, MPH • Joseph H. Cioffi, BA, MD

 BASICS

Ischemic colitis (IC) results from decreased blood flow to the colon with resultant inflammation and tissue damage.

DESCRIPTION

- More common in the elderly; can affect patients of all ages
- IC is self-limited and reversible in 80% of patients:
  – 20% of patients progress to full-thickness necrosis requiring surgical intervention.
- Most commonly, ischemia is related to a nonocclusive reduction in blood flow.
- Presentation varies, but patients with acute IC typically present with localized abdominal pain and tenderness. Frequent loose, bloody stools may be seen within 12 to 24 hours of onset.
- Laboratory and radiographic findings are nonspecific and must be correlated with clinical presentation.
- Colonoscopy is the gold standard for diagnosis of IC.
- Most patients recover with supportive care (IV fluids, bowel rest, and clinical monitoring).

EPIDEMIOLOGY

- More common in women (57–76%—particularly after age 69) (1)
- Evidence of IC is seen in 1 of every 100 endoscopies.

Geriatric Considerations

Rare in patients <60 years old. Average age at diagnosis is 70.

Incidence

4.5 to 44 cases per 100,000 in the general population (may be underestimated due to nonspecific clinical manifestations)

Prevalence

19 cases per 100,000 in the general population

ETIOLOGY AND PATHOPHYSIOLOGY

- Local hypoperfusion in the colon compromises the ability to meet metabolic demands. Reperfusion injury may also play a role.
- The colon is perfused by both the superior and inferior mesenteric arteries (SMAs and IMAs) and branches of the internal iliac arteries. Occlusion of branches of the SMA or IMA rarely leads to ischemic consequences due to extensive collateral circulation.
- Watershed areas of the colon (splenic flexure and rectosigmoid junction) are supplied by narrow terminal branches of the SMA and IMA respectively and are most susceptible to ischemic damage.
- The left colon is more commonly affected than the right; isolated right-sided disease has the worst prognosis.
- The rectum is often spared because of additional blood supply from the internal iliac arteries.
- Type I: unidentified etiology
  – Likely small vessel disease; treat supportively.
- Type II: etiology identified
  – Treat the underlying cause (1).
    o Hypoperfusion from shock, trauma
    o Embolic occlusion of mesenteric vessels
    o Hypercoagulable states, vasculitis

- o Sickle cell disease
- o Arterial thrombosis; venous thrombosis
- o Mechanical obstruction of the colon (e.g., tumor, adhesions, hernia, volvulus, prolapse, diverticulitis)
- o Surgical complications
- o Medications (intestinally active vasoconstrictive substances, medications that induce hypotension and thus hypoperfusion)
- o Cocaine abuse
- o Aortic dissection
- o Strenuous physical activity (e.g., long-distance running)
- Repeated episodes of ischemia and inflammation may result in chronic colonic ischemia, possible stricture formation, recurrent bacteremia, and sepsis. These patients may have unresolving areas of colitis and require segmental colonic resection.

Genetics

- Various coagulopathies have been related to IC including deficiencies of protein C, protein S, antithrombin III, and factor V Leiden mutation.
- Routine coagulation testing not justified except in younger patients and patients with recurrent IC (1)

RISK FACTORS

- Age >60 years (90% of patients)
- Smoking (most common cause of recurrent IC) (1)
- Hypertension, diabetes mellitus (1)
- Rheumatologic disorders/vasculitis
- Cerebrovascular disease, ischemic heart disease (1)
- Recent abdominal surgery, i.e., ileostomy
- Constipation, constipation-inducing medications (1)
- History of vascular surgery (1)
- Chronic obstructive pulmonary disease (COPD)
- Hypoalbuminemia; hemodialysis
- Hypercoagulability, oral contraceptive (1)
- Immunosuppression (via medication-related affects or CMV-induced IC) (2)
- IBS (1)

Dx DIAGNOSIS

- Diagnosis is based on history, risk factors, and physical examination (3)[A].
- Laboratory values and radiographic findings are usually nonspecific (3)[A].
- Colonoscopy is diagnostic (3)[A].

HISTORY

- Abdominal pain is the most common symptom (4)[A]. Pain may be out of proportion to physical examination findings.
- Sudden-onset, mild to moderate abdominal pain with tenderness over the affected segment of bowel (5)[A]
- Sudden urge to defecate followed by passage of either bright red or maroon stool typically within 12 to 24 hours of abdominal pain onset (5)[A]
- Lower GI bleeding is rarely heavy (3)[A].

PHYSICAL EXAM

- Individual signs and symptoms are poorly predictive of IC (6)[C].
- Vital signs: hypotension; tachycardia
- Tenderness over the involved segment of bowel (5)[A]
- Abdominal distention with vomiting (due to possible associated ileus) (3)[A]
- In the uncommon setting of transmural ischemia, patients may develop peritoneal signs such as rebound and guarding (7)[A].

DIFFERENTIAL DIAGNOSIS

- Infectious colitis (7)[A]
- Inflammatory bowel disease (ulcerative colitis, Crohn disease) (7)[A]
- Colon cancer, diverticulitis (7)[A]
- Pseudomembranous colitis (6)[A]

DIAGNOSTIC TESTS & INTERPRETATION

- Depends on clinical presentation, extent of colonic involvement, transmural involvement, acuity (3)[A]
- CT scan is the initial diagnostic test for patients with nonspecific abdominal pain (6)[A].
- Colonoscopy for definitive diagnosis (3)[A]
- Radiographic tests and laboratory values are otherwise nonspecific (6)[A].

Initial Tests (lab, imaging)

- The following lab markers of ischemia are not specific to IC but can help determine disease severity (6)[A]:
  – CBC (leukocytosis) (6)[A]
  – BMP, ABG (signs of metabolic acidosis) (6)[A]
  – Lactate, LDH, CPK, amylase (6)[A]
  – Alkaline phosphatase (6)[A]
  – Albumin (5)[B]
- Abdominal plain film:
  – 20% of patients show thumbprinting and mural thickening; may predict worse prognosis (7)[A]
- Abdominal CT scan with contrast (3)[A]:
  – Thickening of the colonic wall and pericolonic fat stranding (5)
  – Other findings include hyperdense mucosa, submucosal edema, and mesenteric inflammation (3)[A].
  – Pneumatosis, pneumoperitoneum, and free peritoneal fluid suggest advanced ischemia (3)[A].
- Multiphasic CTA should be performed for suspected right-sided IC or if acute mesenteric ischemia cannot be excluded (5)[B].

Follow-Up Tests & Special Considerations

- Stool cultures, fecal leukocytes, stool ova, and parasites to rule out infection (6)[A]
- Patients undergoing aortic surgery may benefit from postoperative colonoscopy within 2 to 3 days to look for signs of IC (5)[A].
- If indicated, cardiac workup including electrocardiogram, Holter monitoring, or transthoracic echocardiogram to exclude cardiogenic embolism (6)[A]
- Drug and toxicology screening (5)[A]
- If colon cancer screening is indicated, perform several weeks following recovery from the ischemic insult (1).

Diagnostic Procedures/Other
- Colonoscopy is gold standard; sigmoidoscopy used to evaluate postoperative left-sided ischemia (3)[A]
- Cyanotic hemorrhagic tissue and edematous mucosa suggest ischemia (5)[A].
  - Segmental distribution (watershed), hemorrhagic nodules, and rectal sparing (5)[A]
  - "Colon single-stripe sign" is a single line of erythema, with a 75% histopathologic yield (5)[A].
  - Routine biopsy no longer advised, as results are typically nonspecific (3)[A]
- In cases of isolated right IC, noninvasive vascular imaging studies are recommended to evaluate acute SMA occlusion (5)[A].

Test Interpretation
Biopsied specimens reveal mucosal infarction and ghost cells, which show normal cellular outlines but lack intracellular contents (3)[A].

 TREATMENT
- Treatment depends on disease severity (3)[A].
- Continuous clinical monitoring, including vital signs and serial abdominal exams (7)[A]
- In the absence of colonic necrosis or perforation, most patients respond to supportive care (1)[A]:
  - Bowel rest (5)[A]
  - IV fluids to maintain hemodynamic stability (5)[A]
  - Avoid intestinally active vasoconstrictive medications (5)[A].
  - Avoid systemic corticosteroids—may worsen ischemia and increase risk of perforation (3)[A].
- If ileus is present, place nasogastric tube (3)[A].
- If radiographic abnormalities present, serial abdominal x-rays help follow improvement (5)[A].
- If signs of clinical deterioration are present despite supportive care (increased abdominal pain, peritoneal signs, persistent diarrhea, bleeding, or sepsis), consider surgery (3)[A].

MEDICATION
Specific medications have been associated with IC, including (1)[B]:
- Constipation-inducing medications (i.e., opioids)
- Immunomodulators (anti-TNFα inhibitors, type 1 interferon-α/β)
- Illicit drugs (cocaine, amphetamines)

First Line
Consider broad-spectrum antibiotics covering aerobic and anaerobic bacteria to avoid bacterial translocation secondary to colonic mucosal damage (5)[A].
- Ciprofloxacin 400 mg IV BID or 500 mg PO BID
- Metronidazole 500 mg PO/IV TID

ISSUES FOR REFERRAL
- If cardiac workup reveals CHF or cardiac arrhythmias, initiate appropriate treatment (5)[A].
- If signs of clinical deterioration are present despite supportive care (increased abdominal pain, peritoneal signs, persistent diarrhea, bleeding, or sepsis), consider surgery (3)[A].

SURGERY/OTHER PROCEDURES
- 20% of patients require surgical intervention (4)[A].
- Surgery may be indicated for:
  - Peritoneal signs, increased abdominal tenderness, new-onset shock, lactic acidosis, or acute renal failure (3)[A]
  - Pneumatosis intestinalis, portal vein air, or free peritoneal air (3)[A]
  - Diarrhea, lower GI bleeding, or exudative colitis persisting past 14 days (3)[A]
- Most common surgical intervention is colectomy with end ileostomy (6)[A].
  - Cholecystectomy may prevent resuscitation-related acute acalculous cholecystitis (3)[A].

COMPLEMENTARY & ALTERNATIVE MEDICINE
- Ginko biloba extract has been studied as an adjunct to general treatment.
- Weight loss supplements/herbal supplements (Ephedra, ma huang, bitter orange, white willow bark) have been implicated in cases of IC.

ADMISSION, INPATIENT, AND NURSING CONSIDERATIONS
- ICU patients represent a difficult population to diagnose IC given the concurrent comorbidities and clinical care (sedation/ventilation) that can mask the characteristic signs and symptoms.
- Consider bedside colonoscopy in critically ill patients.

 ONGOING CARE

DIET
- Bowel rest until symptoms resolve
- Parenteral nutrition for patients needing prolonged bowel rest who have contraindications to surgery

PATIENT EDUCATION
Risks of IC with the use of weight loss medications/herbal supplements

PROGNOSIS
- In most patients, IC symptoms resolve in 24 to 48 hours.
- Radiographic or endoscopic resolution within 2 weeks
- Right-sided IC is the most significant predictor of outcome. Right-sided IC has a 2-fold increase in mortality and a 4-fold increase in morbidity (5).
- Secondary cardiovascular prevention minimizes recurrence.
- Male gender, low hemoglobin, low serum albumin, high BUN, and presence of metabolic acidosis are poor prognostic factors (1).
- Chronic kidney disease, COPD, long-term care facilities increase mortality in IC (1).

COMPLICATIONS
20–30% of patients develop chronic IC with persistent diarrhea or stricture formation requiring surgery.

REFERENCES
1. Brandt LJ, Feuerstadt P, Longstreth GF, et al. ACG clinical guideline: epidemiology, risk factors, patterns of presentation, diagnosis, and management of colon ischemia (CI). *Am J Gastroenterol.* 2015;110(1):18–45.
2. Doulberis M, Panagopoulos P, Scherz S, et al. Update on ischemic colitis: from etiopathology to treatment including patients of intensive care unit. *Scand J Gastroenterol.* 2016;51(8):893–902.
3. Moszkowicz D, Mariani A, Trésallet C, et al. Ischemic colitis: the ABCs of diagnosis and surgical management. *J Visc Surg.* 2013;150(1):19–28.
4. Yadav S, Dave M, Edakkanambeth Varayil J, et al. A population-based study of incidence, risk factors, clinical spectrum, and outcomes of ischemic colitis. *Clin Gastroenterol Hepatol.* 2015;13(4):731–738.e6.
5. Feuerstadt P, Brandt LJ. Update on colon ischemia: recent insights and advances. *Curr Gastroenterol Rep.* 2015;17(12):45.
6. Ahmed M. Ischemic bowel disease in 2021. *World J Gastroenterol.* 2021;27(29):4746–4762.
7. Sardar P, White CJ. Chronic mesenteric ischemia: diagnosis and management. *Prog Cardiovasc Dis.* 2021;65:71–75.

ADDITIONAL READING
- Cosse C, Sabbagh C, Browet F, et al. Serum value of procalcitonin as a marker of intestinal damages: type, extension, and prognosis. *Surg Endosc.* 2015;29(11):3132–3139.
- Giannetti A, Matergi M, Biscontri M, et al. Multiparametric ultrasound in the diagnosis and monitoring of ischemic colitis: description of a case of ischemic colitis of the right colon and revision of the literature. *J Ultrasound.* 2019;22(4):477–484.
- Huber TS, Björck M, Chandra A, et al. Chronic mesenteric ischemia: clinical practice guidelines from the Society for Vascular Surgery. *J Vasc Surg.* 2021;73(1S):87S–115S.
- Puga AM, Lopez-Oliva S, Trives C, et al. Effects of drugs and excipients on hydration status. *Nutrients.* 2019;11(3):669.

 CODES

ICD10
- K55.9 Vascular disorder of intestine, unspecified
- K55.0 Acute vascular disorders of intestine
- K55.1 Chronic vascular disorders of intestine

CLINICAL PEARLS
- Suspect IC in patients with multiple risk factors who present with abdominal pain and loose bloody stools.
- Colonoscopy is the diagnostic gold standard.
- Most often, IC is self-limited and responds well to conservative management with IV fluids, bowel rest, and empiric broad-spectrum antibiotics.
- Peritoneal signs or lack of clinical improvement suggests more extensive ischemia and need for surgical intervention.

COLON CANCER
Laura B. Bishop, MD

BASICS

DESCRIPTION
- Colon and rectal cancers (CRC) are often grouped together but are two distinct clinical entities that differ in their prognosis, presentation, staging and management.
- CRC is the second leading cause of cancer deaths and the third most common cancer in men and women in the United States.
- Screening for colon cancer reduces the incidence of and mortality from colon cancer.

EPIDEMIOLOGY
Incidence
- Estimated that in 2019 in the United States, there are 101,420 new cases of colon cancer and 44,180 new cases of rectal cancer per the American Cancer Society.
- Colorectal cancer is expected to cause about 51,020 deaths during 2019.
- Incidence is relatively equal between men and women. Internationally, CRC is the third most common cancer in men and the second most common in women.
- Recent databases suggest a trend toward increased incidence in the age >50 population.

Prevalence
- The lifetime risk for developing colon cancer in the United States is about 1 in 22 (4.49%) for men and 1 in 24 (4.15%) for women.
- Incidence and death rates have been declining due to improved screening, prevention, and treatment.

ETIOLOGY AND PATHOPHYSIOLOGY
- Progression from the first abnormal cells to the appearance of colon cancer usually occurs over 10 to 15 years, a disease characteristic that contributes to the effectiveness of screening and prevention.
- High-risk polyp findings include multiple polyps, villous or dysplastic polyps, and larger polyps. Hyperplastic polyps are less likely to evolve into CRC.
- Multiple genetic and environmental factors have been linked to the development of CRC.

Genetics
- <10% of CRC cases are linked to an inherited gene. Patients with early-onset CRC have a higher percentage of genetic causes, suggesting that genetic counseling and perhaps a colorectal cancer–specific multigene panel could be recommended for patients with early-onset CRC or their first-degree family members.
  - Many of these are inherited in an autosomal dominant fashion:
    - APC, a tumor suppressor gene, is altered in familial adenomatous polyposis (FAP).
    - Genes encoding DNA mismatch repair (MMR) enzymes are implicated in hereditary nonpolyposis colon cancer (HNPCC), formerly Lynch syndrome, including hMLH1, hMSH2, hMSH6, hPMS1, hPMS2, and others.
    - STK11, a tumor suppressor gene, is altered in Peutz-Jeghers syndrome.
  - A smaller portion of patients with familial CRC may have a recessive gene.
    - MUTYH defects lead to issues with the base excision repair gene. This MUTYH-associated polyposis (MAP) may present as a variant form of FAP.
- Sporadic cases of CRC have been linked to oncogenes: KRAS, C-MYC, C-SRC, HER-2/neu, BRCA1, BRCA2, TP53 and others.

RISK FACTORS
- Age
  - >90% of people diagnosed with sporadic colon cancer are >50 years of age.
  - However, younger patients are more likely to have advanced disease at the time of diagnosis due to low suspicion of cancer and decreased access to care.
- Personal history of colorectal polyps
  - Risk increases with multiple polyps, villous polyps, larger polyps (>1 cm), and presence of dysplasia.
- Personal history of cancer
  - 30% increase in risk of developing metachronous (new primary tumors unrelated to the patients' previous cancers) colon cancer
  - 2–4% incidence of local recurrence with colon cancer, 3–5% incidence of synchronous colon cancer
  - History of radiation therapy to the abdomen/pelvis
- Personal history of inflammatory bowel disease (IBD)
  - Prevalence of CRC in ulcerative colitis and Crohn disease is ~3%, with a cumulative risk of CRC of 2% at 10 years, 8% at 20 years, and 18% at 30 years.
  - Ulcerative colitis with pancolitis up to 10-fold risk of CRC, 8 to 10 years after initial diagnosis.
- Family history of CRC
  - Having a single first-degree relative with a history of CRC increases risk ~1.7-fold.
  - Risk is more than double for those who have a history of CRC or polyps in:
    - Any first-degree relative <50 years of age
    - ≥2 first-degree relatives, regardless of age
    - One first-degree and one second-degree relative
- Inherited syndromes
  - HNPCC
    - Often develops at young age (Average age at diagnosis of CRC is 48 years.)
    - Often presents with right-sided lesions and cancer often recurs
    - Lifetime risk of CRC is 52–69%; also associated with endometrial and other cancers
    - Accounts for ~3% of all CRC
  - FAP
    - Affected individuals develop hundreds to thousands of polyps in colon and rectum, typically presenting during childhood.
    - CRC usually present by age 40 years in untreated patients; however most have prophylactic colectomies.
    - Accounts for <1% of CRC
    - Variants include Gardner and Turcot syndromes as well as attenuated FAP (AFAP).
  - Peutz-Jeghers syndrome
    - Individuals may have hyperpigmented mucocutaneous lesions (mouth, hands, feet) and large polyps in GI tract discovered as an adolescent.
    - 81–93% risk for CRC and other cancers
  - BRCA1 and BRCA2 syndromes
    - Some data suggests that carriers of BRCA1 may have increased risk for early CRC; however, more evidence is needed to recommend early screening.
- Race and ethnicity
  - African Americans have the highest CRC incidence and mortality rates in the United States. These disparities require more research but may be associated with diet, stressors, decreased insurance coverage, perceptions surrounding colorectal screening, provider bias/systemic racism, issues following up polyps, mistrust in clinical trials, and decreased provider referral opportunities.
- Lifestyle factors
  - Smoking, obesity, sedentary activity, insulin resistance, high-fat and low-fiber diet, and potentially microbiota

GENERAL PREVENTION
- Several options exist for colon cancer screening. Stool-based testing such as guaiac fecal occult blood test (gFOBT) and fecal immunochemical test (FIT) or FIT-DNA tests are less invasive, but endoscopic testing (flexible sigmoidoscopy or colonoscopy) offers ability to provide intervention if polyp discovered.
- Lifestyle factors that may reduce risk:
  - No study has evidence strong enough to modify risk stratification/screening based on protective factors.
  - Regular physical activity, diet high in fiber and fruits/vegetables
  - There is conflicting evidence on folic acid, calcium, vitamin D, magnesium, NSAIDs, fish oil, and statins.

ALERT
The U.S. Preventive Services Task Force (USPSTF) strongly recommends screening for colorectal cancer from 50 to 75 years (A) and states there is a moderate certainty of moderate benefit from screening between 45 and 50 years (B). American Cancer Society and others also recommend initiating screening at 45 years. For persons ages 76 to 85 years old, screening should be based on overall health status and life expectancy and should involve shared decision-making between the patient and health care provider.

- Screening methods:
  - Visualization-based tests:
    - Colonoscopy every 10 years
    - Flexible sigmoidoscopy every 5 years
    - Flexible sigmoidoscopy every 10 years + FIT yearly
  - Stool-based tests:
    - FIT annually
    - High-sensitivity fecal occult blood testing annually
    - FIT-DNA (sDNA) test every 1 to 3 years
  - Imaging-based tests:
    - CT colonography every 5 years
  - For patients who have a positive FIT, FOBT, or stool DNA test, a colonoscopy is recommended.
- Screening in high-risk groups:
  - The American College of Gastroenterology recommends screening black patients starting at age 45 years.
  - People with a history of polyps need frequent colonoscopy screening, with the interval depending on polyp number, size, and histology (1).
  - People who have a first-degree relative or two second-degree relatives with CRC or adenomatous polyps before age 60 years should begin colonoscopy at age 40 or 10 years younger than the youngest age of relative at cancer diagnosis, whichever is earlier.
  - IBD patients should have surveillance colonoscopies every 1 to 2 years 8 to 10 years after diagnosis.
  - People with prior abdominal/pelvic radiation should be screened; however, recommendations vary typically starting between 30 and 40 years and occurring every 5 to 10 years thereafter.
  - Genetic testing may be appropriate for individuals with a strong family history of CRC or polyps:
    - Family members of a person with HNPCC should start colonoscopy at 25 years.
    - Individuals with suspected FAP should have yearly flexible sigmoidoscopy beginning at age 10 to 12 years; if polyps are seen, a colonoscopy is recommended.

- Frequency of follow-up of polyps:
  - <1 year:
    - Following piecemeal (unable to remove with single loop) removal of a large polyp >15 mm
    - Serrated polyposis syndrome; meets one of the following criteria:
      - At least 5 serrated polyps proximal to sigmoid, with 2 or more 10 mm
      - Any serrated polyps proximal to sigmoid with family history of serrated polyposis syndrome
      - 20 serrated polyps of any size throughout the colon
  - 1 year:
    - Known FAP or at risk based on family history
  - 1 to 2 years:
    - IBD (Crohn or ulcerative colitis)
  - <3 years:
    - >10 adenomatous polyps
  - 3 years:
    - 3 to 10 tubular adenomas
    - Tubular adenoma 10 mm or larger
    - Sessile serrated polyp 10 mm or larger
    - Villous adenomatous polyp
    - High-grade dysplastic adenoma or serrated polyp on pathology
    - Sessile serrated polyp with dysplasia
    - Serrated adenoma
  - 5 years:
    - 1 sessile serrated polyp <10 mm without dysplasia;
    - History of colon cancer s/p surgery if initial 1 year follow-up is normal
    - One first-degree relative with CRC or advanced adenoma diagnosed before 60 years of age
    - Two first-degree relatives diagnosed at any age
  - 10 years:
    - Normal screening colonoscopy with no polyps
    - Hyperplastic polyps in rectum or sigmoid colon, <10 mm
    - <3 tubular adenomatous polyps on pathology, all <10 mm in size (can repeat in 5 years with risk factors)
    - One first-degree relative with CRC or advanced adenoma diagnosed at ≥60 years
    - Two second-degree relatives with CRC

COMMONLY ASSOCIATED CONDITIONS

- Polyposis syndromes that have increased association with colorectal cancer including HNPCC, Gardner, Crail (Turcot), FAP, Peutz-Jeghers, and juvenile polyposis syndromes
- IBDs including Crohn disease and particularly ulcerative colitis with pancolitis

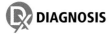 DIAGNOSIS

HISTORY

- Most patients with colon cancer are asymptomatic.
- Microcytic, iron-deficiency anemia in men of any age and postmenopausal women is CRC until proven otherwise; diagnostic colonoscopy.
- Symptoms may indicate advanced disease.
  - Abdominal pain or cramping
  - Change in bowel habits or in the caliber of stool (tenesmus, constipation, diarrhea)
  - Rectal bleeding, dark stools, or blood in stool
  - Weakness or fatigue
  - Unintentional weight loss

PHYSICAL EXAM

- Signs of anemia (pallor, systolic flow murmurs, etc.)
- Weight loss
- Palpable abdominal mass (late presentation)
- Must include digital rectal exam

DIFFERENTIAL DIAGNOSIS

>95% of colon cancers are adenocarcinomas. Other colonic tumors include carcinoid tumors, lymphomas, and Kaposi sarcoma in HIV.

DIAGNOSTIC TESTS & INTERPRETATION

Initial Tests (lab, imaging)

- Should any screening method identify an increased risk, colonoscopy must be performed because it can be both diagnostic and therapeutic.
- For biopsy-confirmed colorectal cancer, obtain:
  - CBC, ferritin with iron panel
  - CEA—primarily used for detection of persistent or recurrent disease in the future

Follow-Up Tests & Special Considerations

- Contrasted CT chest, abdomen, and pelvis to evaluate for metastatic disease; if found, brain MRI
- Intraoperative ultrasound may be used to evaluate solid organs (e.g., the liver) after tumor resection.
- In selected cases, positron emission tomography (PET) may be used to detect metastatic disease, particularly if contrast cannot be used.
- Staging of colon cancer
  - The American Joint Committee on Cancer (AJCC) tumor-node metastasis staging is preferred.
    - Stage 0: limited to the mucosa (carcinoma in situ or intramucosal carcinoma) (Tis, N0, M0)
    - Stage I: invades mucosa (T1) or muscularis propria (T2); no invasion of lymph nodes or distant sites (T1, N0, M0 or T2, N0, M0)
    - Stage IIA: invades pericolorectal tissues; no lymph nodes or distant sites (T3, N0, M0)
    - Stage IIB: penetrates to surface of visceral peritoneum; no lymph nodes or distant sites (T4a, N0, M0)
    - Stage IIC: directly invades or adherent to other organs or structures (T4b, N0, M0)
    - Stage IIIA: invades submucosa or muscularis propria with spread to 1 to 3 lymph nodes; no distant sites (T1, N1, M0 or T2, N1, M0)
    - Stage IIIB: invades pericolorectal tissues or surface of visceral peritoneum + spread to 1 to 3 lymph nodes; no distant sites (T3, N1, M0 or T4a, N1, M0)
    - Stage IIIC: invades pericolorectal tissues or peritoneum or other organs and to ≥4 nearby lymph nodes; no distant sites (any T3 or T4, N2, M0)
    - Stage IVA: any level of invasion with spread to one organ or site (any T, any N, M1a)
    - Stage IVB: any level of invasion with spread to more than one organ or site or peritoneum (any T, any N, M1b)

 TREATMENT

ADDITIONAL THERAPIES

Adjuvant chemotherapy is most clearly beneficial for stage III (node-positive) disease, in which improvements of 30% can be achieved in both disease recurrence and overall survival, compared with untreated controls. Chemotherapeutic regimens for metastatic disease may extend overall survival from 6 months to 2 years. Often used therapies are FOLFOX (folinic acid, 5-fluorouracil, oxaliplatin), FOLFIRI (folinic acid, leucovorin, 5-fluorouracil, irinotecan) or CAPEOX (capecitabine, oxaliplatin). Additional agents may be added depending on tumor genetics including bevacizumab, encorafenib, pembrolizumab, panitumumab, entrectinib, regorafenib, ramucirumab, cetuximab, nivolumab, and ziv-aflibercept.

SURGERY/OTHER PROCEDURES

- Localized cancer
  - Surgery is the primary treatment and often requires regional lymph node removal as well.
  - Without significant complications, primary anastomosis can be possible for local cancers.
    - Obstructing lesions tend to require resections with diversion followed by colectomy with regional lymphadenectomy
  - Minimally invasive (i.e., laparoscopic) surgery has fewer complications, less blood loss, shorter hospital stay, less time to bowel movement, and lower 30-day mortality when compared to open surgery with equivalent oncologic outcomes.
- Locally advanced cancers
  - Often require multiorgan resection
- Metastatic cancer
  - Depending on patient comorbidities and goals of care, it can be reasonable to aggressively resect metastatic lesions isolated to the liver/lungs in addition to the primary tumors.

 ONGOING CARE

FOLLOW-UP RECOMMENDATIONS

Patient Monitoring

- Risk of recurrence is greatest in first 4 years; 80% in first 2.5
- H&P and CEA every 3 to 6 months for 5 years
- Annual CT of chest, abdomen, pelvis for 3 years
- Surveillance colonoscopy 1 year after initial surgery and then every 5 years if normal
- CEA is used to detect recurrences after resection of primary colon cancer. CEA levels decrease and normalize within 4 to 6 weeks after surgery.

PATIENT EDUCATION

American Cancer Society: Colorectal Cancer Screening Decision Aid

PROGNOSIS

5-year relative survival rate after surgical:

- Stage I: 85–95%
- Stage II: 60–80%
- Stage III: 30–60%
- Stage IV: 25–40% following resection of hepatic metastases with clear margins

COMPLICATIONS

- Chemotherapy: hair loss, nausea, vomiting, bruising, fatigue, increased risk for infections
- Radiation therapy: skin irritation, nausea, rectal pain, incontinence, bladder irritation, fatigue, and sexual problems

REFERENCE

1. Gupta S, Lieberman D, Anderson JC, et al. Recommendations for follow-up after colonoscopy and polypectomy: a consensus update by the US Multi-Society Task Force on Colorectal Cancer. *Gastrointest Endosc.* 2020;91(3):463–485.e5.

 CODES

ICD10

- C18.9 Malignant neoplasm of colon, unspecified
- C18.2 Malignant neoplasm of ascending colon
- C18.8 Malignant neoplasm of overlapping sites of colon

CLINICAL PEARLS

Microcytic, iron deficiency anemia in men and postmenopausal women is CRC until proven otherwise and colonoscopy should be performed.

COLONIC POLYPS

Maximos Attia, MD, FAAFP • Marcelle Meseeha, MD

 BASICS

DESCRIPTION
- Intraluminal colonic tissue growth; most commonly sporadic or part of polyposis syndromes
- Generally slow growing with low malignant potential; due to high prevalence in population, however, resection is generally recommended to eliminate risk.
- Size classification:
  - Diminutive ≤5 mm, small 6 to 9 mm, large ≥10 mm
- Morphologic classification:
  - Depressed, flat, sessile, or pedunculated
- Clinical significance:
  - >95% of colonic adenocarcinomas arise from polyps.

EPIDEMIOLOGY
Colorectal polyps are more common in non-Caucasian men in Western countries.

Incidence
Incidence increases with age.

Prevalence
- 15–20% of all adults
- 30% of U.S. population >50 years
- 6% of children
- 12% of children with lower GI bleed

ETIOLOGY AND PATHOPHYSIOLOGY
- Mucosal
  - Neoplastic
    - Adenomatous polyps (tubular >80%, villous 5–15%, tubulovillous 5–15%)
    - Serrated polyps
    - Sessile serrated polyps (SSPs) are common, more in proximal colon, with low malignant potential if no dysplasia and significant malignant potential if dysplastic.
    - Traditional serrated adenoma is uncommon, more often noted in distal colon, with significant malignant potential.
  - Nonneoplastic polyps (hyperplastic, juvenile polyps, hamartomas, inflammatory pseudopolyps)
    - Hyperplastic polyps are very common, more in distal colon, with very low malignant potential.
    - Juvenile polyps are common in childhood, benign hamartomas, more in rectosigmoid, and not premalignant.
- Submucosal (lipomas, lymphoid aggregates, carcinoids)

Genetics
- Inactivation of tumor suppressor genes as adenomatous polyposis coli (APC) or mismatch repair genes (*MLH1*) causes polyps to grow into cancer.
- Familial adenomatous polyposis (FAP) is autosomal dominant. By age 40 years, almost all patients develop colorectal cancer (CRC).
- MUTYH-associated polyposis (MAP) is autosomal recessive caused by biallelic mutations in MUTYH gene.
- Juvenile polyposis syndrome (JPS) is autosomal dominant. 50–60% of patients have a mutation in the SMAD4 or BMPR1A gene. By age 35 years, 20% of patients develop CRC.

RISK FACTORS
- Family history of intestinal polyposis, polyps, or CRC
- Advancing age; male
- High-fat, low-fiber diet; tobacco use
- Excessive alcohol intake: >8 drinks a week
- Inflammatory bowel disease is associated with a decreased prevalence of colon polyps (but with higher risk of colon cancer).

GENERAL PREVENTION
- Low-fat, high-fiber diet
- Avoid smoking.
- Decrease alcohol intake.
- Use of NSAIDs and calcium is associated with decreased incidence and recurrence of polyps.
- No lower rates of CRC with azathioprine, 6-mercaptopurine, folate, calcium, multivitamins, or statins

COMMONLY ASSOCIATED CONDITIONS
Hereditary polyposis syndromes:
- Adenomatous
  - FAP
    - Classic (CFAP)
    - Attenuated (AFAP)
  - MAP
  - FAP variants:
    - Gardner syndrome
    - Turcot syndrome
- Hamartomatous
  - Peutz-Jeghers syndrome (PJS)
  - JPS
  - Familial juvenile polyposis
  - Cowden syndrome

ALERT
JPS imposes a higher risk of CRC, although juvenile polyps are not premalignant.

DIAGNOSIS

HISTORY
- Generally asymptomatic
- Painless rectal bleeding, bright or dark red, mixed with stools, dripping, or on wiping
- Diarrhea or mucous stool
- Abdominal pain
- Constipation
- Chronic bleeding, resulting in iron deficiency anemia

- McKittrick-Wheelock syndrome; large hypersecretory rectosigmoid villous adenoma, resulting in persistent severe diarrhea, electrolyte disorder, dehydration, and prerenal acute renal failure
- Social and family history

PHYSICAL EXAM
- Usually normal
- Rectal polyps noted as prolapsed or palpated on digital rectal examination (DRE)
- Fecal occult blood test (FOBT) by DRE is less effective than FOBT by stool passed spontaneously.

DIAGNOSTIC TESTS & INTERPRETATION
Initial Tests (lab, imaging)
- CBC; anemia with chronic bleeding
- Basic metabolic panel; electrolyte disorder with hypersecretory adenomas
- FOBT, insensitive screening test, because small polyps don't usually bleed:
  - Guaiac (gFOBT)—uses a chemical indicator with color change in presence of blood
  - Immunochemical (iFOBT or fecal immunochemical test [FIT])—uses antibodies against human hemoglobin
- Stool DNA test is more sensitive and less specific than FIT.

Diagnostic Procedures/Other
- Colonoscopy is the gold standard test for detection of polyps and allows for concurrent polypectomy; not a perfect screening test, with increased miss rate with right-sided colon polyps, smaller polyp size, low quality of colon prep, less endoscopist experience
- Computed tomographic colonography (CTC) is less sensitive with flat polyps and requires excellent bowel preparation.
- Double-contrast barium enema
- Colon capsule endoscopy
- Enhanced optical technologies can potentially differentiate between neoplastic and nonneoplastic colonic lesions (1)[A].
- Enhanced optical technologies include:
  - Narrowed spectrum endoscopy (narrow-band imaging [NBI])
  - Image-enhanced endoscopy (i-scan)
  - Fujinon intelligent chromoendoscopy (FICE)
  - Confocal laser endomicroscopy (CLE)
- Patients with >10 colorectal adenomas should undergo genetic testing for APC and MUTYH (2)[C].

Test Interpretation
- Tubular adenoma
  - Gross: tends to be polypoid
  - Micro: dysplastic epithelium, tubular architecture
- Villous adenoma:
  - Gross: tends to be sessile
  - Micro: dysplastic epithelium, fingerlike projections

- Tubulovillous adenomas have a combination of tubular and villous architecture.
- Hyperplastic polyps are composed of hyperplastic colonic mucosa.
- Hamartomatous polyps include muscularis mucosa.
- Juvenile polyp
  – Gross: pedunculated, smooth red mass, 1 to 3 cm (3)

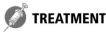 TREATMENT

SURGERY/OTHER PROCEDURES
- Colonic polypectomy; diagnostic, therapeutic:
  – Snare polypectomy with electrocautery for pedunculated polyps
  – Endoscopic mucosal resection for sessile polyps
  – Endoscopic submucosal dissection
- Colorectal surgery; prophylactic in FAP and MAP and when there are numerous polyps or persistent bleeding (2),(3)[C]:
  – Total colectomy ileorectal anastomosis
  – Proctocolectomy ileal pouch anal anastomosis
- Chemoprevention: NSAIDs and calcium may reduce incidence and recurrence of polyps in patients with FAP and MAP (4).

 ONGOING CARE

FOLLOW-UP RECOMMENDATIONS
Follow-up colonoscopy in (5):
- 10 years if no polyps or distal small hyperplastic polyps (<10 mm) (5)[B]
- 3 to 5 years in hyperplastic polyps ≥10 mm (5)[C]
- 7 to 10 years if 1 to 2 small tubular adenomas (<10 mm) (5)[B]
- 3 to 5 years if 3 to 4 small tubular adenomas (<10 mm) (5)[C]
- 3 years if 5 to 10 small tubular adenomas (<10 mm) (5)[B]
- 1 year if >10 adenomas (5)[C]
- 3 years if one or more adenomas ≥10 mm (5)[A]
- 3 years if one or more adenomas with tubulovillous or villous features of any size or with high-grade dysplasia (HGD) (5)[B]
- 6 months if adenoma ≥20 mm or SSP ≥20 mm, with piecemeal resection (5)[B]
- 5 to 10 years if 1 to 2 small SSPs (<10 mm) (5)[C]
- 3 to 5 years if 3 to 4 small SSPs (<10 mm) (5)[C]
- 3 years if 5 to 10 small SSPs (<10 mm) (5)[C]
- 3 years if SSP ≥10 mm or with dysplasia or traditional serrated adenoma (5)[C]
- Different consideration is given for polyps that meet criteria for serrated polyposis syndrome (5)[B]

Patient Monitoring
- Colonoscopy for CRC screening starts at age 45 years and earlier for at-risk patients. The U.S. Preventive Services Task Force, American College of Gastroenterology (ACG), and American Cancer Society (ACS) recommend that people at average risk for CRC start screening at age 45 years through age of 75 years, may extend to 85 years, based on life expectancy and overall health.
- Stop screening if life expectancy is <10 years.
- In CFAP and AFAP, screen for extracolonic manifestations: thyroid cancer, desmoid tumors, and gastroduodenal polyposis (every 6 months to 5 years) (2)[C].
- In families, lifetime screening for mutation carriers (2)[C]:
  – In CFAP: with sigmoidoscopy or colonoscopy, every 1 to 2 years starting at age of 10 to 11 years
  – In AFAP and MAP: with colonoscopy, every 1 to 2 years starting at age of 18 to 20 years
- After colorectal surgery, surveillance of the rectum (every 6 to 12 months) or pouch (every 6 months to 5 years) is indicated (2)[C].
- First-degree relatives of patients with JPS require screening by colonoscopy and upper endoscopy after age 12 years (3)[C].
- Genetic evaluation is recommended for any patient with >10 adenomas cumulatively over lifespan (5).

DIET
Low-fat, high-fiber diet (insufficient evidence)

PATIENT EDUCATION
Importance of colonoscopy as a screening tool

PROGNOSIS
- Regression or no change in size, more with small hyperplastic polyps and with patients on NSAIDs
- Recurrence: Juvenile polyps recur in 45% of children with multiple polyps and 17% with solitary polyps (3).
- Risk factors for colon cancer:
  – Polyp pathology
    ○ Adenomatous
    ○ Serrated
    ○ With HGD
    ○ With >25% villous histology
    ○ Polyp size >1 cm in diameter
    ○ Polyps located in proximal colon
    ○ More than three polyps
- Recurrence rates <10% postpolypectomy
- Ineffective endoscopic resection of precancerous lesions results in lingering cancer.

COMPLICATIONS
- Polyps: progression to cancer
- Polypectomy: bleeding 2–11%, perforation 0–1%, higher with endoscopic submucosal dissection
- Colonoscopy: complications related to anesthesia and procedure itself

REFERENCES
1. Shaukat A, Kahi CJ, Burke CA, et al. ACG clinical guidelines: colorectal cancer screening 2021. *Am J Gastroenterol*. 2021;116(3):458–479.
2. Stoffel EM, Mangu PB, Limburg PJ; for American Society of Clinical Oncology. Hereditary colorectal cancer syndromes: American Society of Clinical Oncology clinical practice guideline endorsement of the familial risk-colorectal cancer: European Society for Medical Oncology clinical practice guidelines. *J Oncol Pract*. 2015;11(3):e437–e441.
3. Thakkar K, Fishman DS, Gilger MA. Colorectal polyps in childhood. *Curr Opin Pediatr*. 2012;24(5):632–637.
4. Ichkhanian Y, Zuchelli T, Watson A, et al. Evolving management of colorectal polyps. *Ther Adv Gastrointest Endosc*. 2021;14:26317745211047010.
5. Gupta S, Lieberman D, Anderson JC, et al. Recommendations for follow-up after colonoscopy and polypectomy: a consensus update by the US Multi-Society Task Force on Colorectal Cancer. *Gastrointest Endosc*. 2020;91(3):463–485.e5.

ADDITIONAL READING
- Kaltenbach T, Anderson JC, Burke CA, et al. Endoscopic removal of colorectal lesions—recommendations by the US Multi-Society Task Force on Colorectal Cancer. *Gastrointest Endosc*. 2020;9(3):486.
- Rex DK, Boland CR, Dominitz JA, et al. Colorectal cancer screening: recommendations for physicians and patients from the U.S. Multi-Society Task Force on Colorectal Cancer. *Gastroenterology*. 2017;153(1):307–323.
- Wolf AMD, Fontham ETH, Church TR, et al. Colorectal cancer screening for average-risk adults: 2018 guideline update from the American Cancer Society. *CA Cancer J Clin*. 2018;68(4):250–281.

 SEE ALSO

Colon Cancer; Rectal Cancer

 CODES

ICD10
- K63.5 Polyp of colon
- D12.6 Benign neoplasm of colon, unspecified
- K51.40 Inflammatory polyps of colon without complications

CLINICAL PEARLS
- Colonoscopy is the gold standard for diagnosing polyps.
- Biopsy small hyperplastic polyps to differentiate adenomatous and serrated polyps.
- Use of NSAIDs and calcium is associated with decreased incidence and recurrence of polyps.
- The progression from normal mucosa to polyp to carcinoma takes years to develop.

COMMUNITY ACQUIRED METHICILLIN-RESISTANT *STAPHYLOCOCCUS AUREUS* (CA-MRSA) SKIN INFECTIONS

Stephen A. Martin, MD, EdM • Paul P. Belliveau, PharmD

 BASICS

DESCRIPTION

- Community-acquired methicillin-resistant *Staphylococcus aureus* (CA-MRSA) has unique properties that allow the organism to cause skin and soft tissue infections (SSTIs) in healthy hosts:
  - CA-MRSA has a different virulence and disease pattern than hospital-acquired MRSA (HA-MRSA).
- CA-MRSA infections generally impact patients who have not been recently (<1 year) hospitalized or had a medical procedure (e.g., dialysis, surgery, catheters).
- Incidence of CA-MRSA increased in the United States from 2000 until 2010–2013 when it plateaued for adults and decreased for children.
- CA-MRSA typically causes mild to moderate SSTIs (abscesses, furuncles, and carbuncles).
- Severe or invasive CA-MRSA disease is less frequent but can include the following:
  - Osteomyelitis
  - Sepsis
  - Septic thrombophlebitis
  - Necrotizing fasciitis
  - Necrotizing pneumonia with abscesses
- Although less frequent, HA-MRSA can still cause SSTIs in the community.
- System(s) affected: skin, soft tissue

EPIDEMIOLOGY
- Predominant age: all ages, generally younger
- Predominant sex: female > male

Incidence
- SSTI incidence for adult ambulatory care peaked in 2010 at 35 per 1,000 population and has since plateaued.
- SSTI incidence for pediatric ambulatory care visits peaked in 2011 at 26 per 1,000 population, decreasing to 13 per 1,000 in 2015.
- The incidence of MRSA-related hospitalizations decreased from 2010 to 2014.
- Among people who inject drugs, the incidence of MRSA-related skin abscesses is increasing. Patients should care for substance misuse and linked with syringe exchange programs.

Prevalence
- Local epidemiology patterns vary.
- 25–30% of U.S. population colonized with *S. aureus*; up to 7% are colonized with MRSA.
- CA-MRSA isolated in ~60% of SSTIs presenting to emergency departments (range 15–74%).
- CA-MRSA accounts for up to 75% of all community staphylococcal infections in children.

ETIOLOGY AND PATHOPHYSIOLOGY
- First noted in 1980. Current epidemic began in 1999. The USA300 clone is predominant.
- CA-MRSA is distinguished from HA-MRSA by:
  - Lack of a multidrug-resistant phenotype
  - Presence of exotoxin virulence factors
  - Type IV *Staphylococcus* cassette cartridge (contains the methicillin-resistant gene *mecA*)

RISK FACTORS
~50% of patients have no obvious risk factor. Recognized risk factors include the following:
- Antibiotic use in the past month, particularly cephalosporins and fluoroquinolones
- Abscess
- Reported "spider bite"
- Intravenous (IV) or intradermal drug use
- HIV infection
- Hemodialysis catheter presence
- History of MRSA infection
- Close contact with a similar infection
- Children, particularly in daycare centers
- Resident in long-term care facility
- Competitive athletes
- Incarceration

GENERAL PREVENTION
- Colonization (particularly of the anterior nares) is a risk factor for subsequent *S. aureus* infection. It is unclear whether this is similar for CA-MRSA. Oropharyngeal and inguinal colonization are equally prevalent.
- CA-MRSA is transmitted easily through environmental and household contact.
- CDC guidance for prevention of MRSA in athletes: http://www.cdc.gov/mrsa/community/team-hc -providers/advice-for-athletes.html

COMMONLY ASSOCIATED CONDITIONS
Many patients are otherwise healthy.

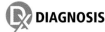 **DIAGNOSIS**

HISTORY
- Review risk factors.
- "Spider bite" is commonly confused with MRSA— patients often report a history of spider bite.
- Prior CA-MRSA skin infection
- Risk factors alone cannot rule in or rule out a CA-MRSA infection.

PHYSICAL EXAM
- Abscess, sometimes with surrounding cellulitis. Nonsuppurative cellulitis is a much less common presentation of CA-MRSA.
- Erythema, warmth, tenderness, swelling
- Fluctuance
- Folliculitis, pustular lesions
- Tissue necrosis

DIFFERENTIAL DIAGNOSIS
SSTIs due to other organisms

DIAGNOSTIC TESTS & INTERPRETATION
Initial Tests (lab, imaging)
- Wound cultures establish definitive diagnosis. Culture a purulent lesion if there are systemic signs of illness or if the patient is immunocompromised (1)[B].
- Susceptibility testing; many labs use oxacillin instead of methicillin.
- "D-zone disk-diffusion test" evaluates for inducible clindamycin resistance if CA-MRSA is resistant to erythromycin.

- Ultrasound may help identify abscesses versus a non-drainable phlegmon; evidence suggests abscesses shallower than 0.4 cm may not need incision and drainage (I&D) (2),(3)[A].
- Look for fascial plane edema on CT or MRI if necrotizing fasciitis is suspected. DO NOT DELAY surgical intervention to obtain imaging in such cases.

Diagnostic Procedures/Other
I&D for purulent lesions; needle aspiration not recommended (1). An effective alternative to I&D is the loop drainage technique.

 TREATMENT

- For purulent infections, surgical drainage for abscesses, wound culture, and narrow-spectrum antimicrobials.
- See "Alert" section regarding use of antibiotics in uncomplicated cases.
- Use antibiotics active against HA-MRSA for patients with abscesses if patients do not respond to initial antibiotic treatment, have markedly impaired host defenses, or present with systemic inflammatory response syndrome (SIRS) and hypotension (1).
- Packing may not improve outcomes (3)[A].
- Moist heat may work for small abscesses.
- Extended antibiotic coverage for CA-MRSA is not warranted for nonsuppurative cellulitis (4)[A].
- Routine elimination of MRSA colonization is not recommended in patients with active infection or for their close contacts.
- Most CA-MRSA infections are localized SSTIs and do not require hospitalization or vancomycin.
- Base initial antibiotic coverage on local CA-MRSA prevalence and individual risk factors.
- CDC guidance: http://www.cdc.gov/mrsa/pdf /Flowchart_pstr.pdf

GENERAL MEASURES
- Modify therapy based on culture and susceptibility.
- Treat underlying conditions that may predispose susceptibility to bacterial infection (e.g., tinea pedis).
- Restrict contact (e.g., sports competition) if wound cannot be covered.
- Elevate affected area.

MEDICATION

ALERT
Studies have shown a role for narrow-spectrum antibiotics in addition to surgical drainage. Clindamycin or trimethoprim/sulfamethoxazole (TMP/SMX) for abscesses <5 cm results in improved cure rates at 7 to 14 days (number needed to treat is 7 to 14) (5)[A].

First Line
Antibiotics for CA-MRSA SSTIs: 7- to 14-day course (depends on severity and clinical response):
- TMP/SMX: DS (160 mg TMP and 800 mg of SMX) 1 to 2 tablet(s) PO q12h; children, 8 to 12 mg/kg/day PO of trimethoprim component in 2 divided doses.
- Doxycycline or minocycline: 100 mg PO q12h. Children, >8 years and <45 kg, 2 to 5 mg/kg/day PO in 1 to 2 divided doses, not to exceed 200 mg/day; >8 years and >45 kg, use adult dosing; taken with a full glass of water

- Clindamycin: 300 to 450 mg PO q6h. Children, 30 to 40 mg/kg/day PO in 3 divided doses. Taken with full glass of water. Check D-zone test in erythromycin-resistant, clindamycin-susceptible *S. aureus* isolates (a positive test indicates induced resistance—choose a different antibiotic).
- CA-MRSA is resistant to β-lactams (including oral cephalosporins and antistaphylococcal penicillins) and often macrolides, azalides, and quinolones.
- Although most CA-MRSA isolates are susceptible to rifampin, this drug should *never* be used as a single agent because of concerns regarding resistance. The role of combination therapy with rifampin in CA-MRSA SSTIs is not clearly defined.
- There has been increasing resistance to clindamycin, both initial (~33%) and induced.
- Although CA-MRSA isolates are susceptible to vancomycin, oral vancomycin cannot be used for CA-MRSA SSTIs due to limited absorption.

Second Line
Treat severe CA-MRSA SSTIs requiring hospitalization and HA-MRSA SSTIs using the following:

- Vancomycin: generally, 1 g IV q12h (30 mg/kg/day IV in 2 divided doses). Children: 40 mg/kg/day IV in 4 divided doses. Vancomycin-like antibiotics that require only 1 or 2 doses are also available (6)[A].
- Linezolid: 600 mg IV/PO q12h. Children, uncomplicated: <5 years of age, 30 mg/kg/day IV/PO in 3 divided doses; 5 to 11 years of age, 20 mg/kg/day IV/PO in 2 divided doses; >11 years, use adult dosing. Children, complicated: birth to 11 years, 30 mg/kg/day IV/PO in 3 divided doses; older, use adult dosing
  - Linezolid seems to be more effective than vancomycin for treating people with SSTIs, but current studies have high risk of bias.
- Clindamycin: 600 mg IV q8h; children, 10 to 13 mg/kg/dose IV q6–8h up to 40 mg/kg/day.
- Daptomycin: 4 mg/kg/day IV; children, 1 to <2 years, 10 mg/kg IV once daily; 2 to 6 years, 9 mg/kg IV once daily; 7 to 11 years, 7 mg/kg IV once daily; 12 to 17 years, 5 mg/kg IV once daily; ≥18 years, adult dosing.
  - Do not use if pulmonary involvement.
- Ceftaroline: 600 mg IV q12h; children, 0* to <2 months, 6 mg/kg IV q8h; 2 months to <2 years, 8 mg/kg IV q8h; ≥2 years to <18 years and ≤33 kg, 12 mg/kg IV q8h; ≥2 years to <18 years and >33 kg, 400 mg IV q8h OR 600 mg IV q12h; ≥18 years, adult dosing. *Gestational age 34 weeks and older and postnatal age 12 days and older.

Pediatric Considerations
- Tetracyclines not recommended for patients age <8 years for CA-MRSA (in contrast with their position as treatment of choice in tickborne rickettsial diseases).
- TMP/SMX not recommended for patients <2 months.
- Daptomycin is not recommended in pediatric patients <1 year of age (risk of potential muscular, neuromuscular, and/or nervous system side effects).
- Daptomycin dosage adjustment for pediatric patients with renal impairment has not been established.
- Ceftaroline dosage adjustment for pediatric patients with CrCl ≤50 mL/min/1.73 m^2 has not been established.

Pregnancy Considerations
- Tetracyclines are contraindicated.
- TMP/SMX not recommended in 1st or 3rd trimester

Geriatric Considerations
A recent review notes no prospective trials in this age group and recommends use of general adult guidelines.

ISSUES FOR REFERRAL
Consider consultation with infectious disease specialist if:
- Refractory CA-MRSA infection
- Plan to attempt decolonization

SURGERY/OTHER PROCEDURES
Concern for serious SSTIs (including necrotizing fasciitis) mandates prompt surgical evaluation.

ADMISSION, INPATIENT, AND NURSING CONSIDERATIONS
- Consider admission if:
  - Systemically ill. Extensive soft tissue involvement
  - Comorbidities that may delay or complicate resolution of SSTI; immunocompromised status
  - Failure to improve despite appropriate oral antibiotic therapy
  - Presence of SSTI complications (sepsis, necrotizing fasciitis) and comorbidities
- Alternatives to inpatient admission include observation units and outpatient parenteral antimicrobial therapy (OPAT) in carefully selected cases
- Nursing: contact precautions
- If admitted for IV therapy, assess the following before discharge:
  - Afebrile for 24 hours
  - Clinically improved
  - Able to take oral medication
  - Has adequate social support and is available for outpatient follow-up

 ## ONGOING CARE

Patients who present with IV drug use should be effectively connected to ongoing substance use disorder care.

FOLLOW-UP RECOMMENDATIONS
Patient Monitoring
For outpatients: Promptly return for care with systemic symptoms, worsening local symptoms, or failure to improve within 48 hours. Consider a follow-up within 48 hours of initial visit to assess response and review culture.

PATIENT EDUCATION
- Cover draining wounds with clean, dry bandages.
- Clean hands regularly with soap and water or alcohol-based gel; hot soapy shower daily.
- Do not share items that may be contaminated (including razors or towels).
- Clean clothes, towels, and bed linens.
- CDC MRSA education: https://www.cdc.gov/mrsa/
- A mixture of 1/4 cup household bleach diluted in 1 gallon of water can be used to clean potentially contaminated surfaces.

PROGNOSIS
In outpatients, improvement should occur within 48 hours.

COMPLICATIONS
- Necrotizing pneumonia or empyema (after an influenza-like illness); necrotizing fasciitis
- Sepsis syndrome; pyomyositis and osteomyelitis
- Purpura fulminans
- Disseminated septic emboli; endocarditis

REFERENCES

1. Stevens DL, Bisno AL, Chambers HF, et al; for Infectious Diseases Society of America. Practice guidelines for the diagnosis and management of skin and soft tissue infections: 2014 update by the Infectious Diseases Society of America. *Clin Infect Dis.* 2014;59(2):e10–e52.
2. Breyre A, Frazee BW. Skin and soft tissue infections in the emergency department. *Emerg Med Clin North Am.* 2018;36(4):723–750.
3. Loewen K, Schreiber Y, Kirlew M, et al. Community-associated methicillin-resistant *Staphylococcus aureus* infection: literature review and clinical update [published correction appears in *Can Fam Physician.* 2017;63(8):596. *Can Fam Physician.* 2017;63(7):512–520.
4. Shuman EK, Malani PN. Empirical MRSA coverage for nonpurulent cellulitis: swinging the pendulum away from routine use. *JAMA.* 2017;317(20):2070–2071.
5. Frazee B. Antibiotics for simple skin abscesses: the new evidence in perspective. *Emerg Med J.* 2018;35(4):277–278.
6. Chambers HF. Pharmacology and the treatment of complicated skin and skin-structure infections. *N Engl J Med.* 2014;370(23):2238–2239.

ADDITIONAL READING
- Bystritsky R, Chambers H. Cellulitis and soft tissue infections. *Ann Intern Med.* 2018;168(3):ITC17–ITC32.
- Lee AS, de Lencastre H, Garau J, et al. Methicillin-resistant *Staphylococcus aureus*. *Nat Rev Dis Primers.* 2018;4:18033.
- Russell FM, Rutz M, Rood LK, et al. Abscess size and depth on ultrasound and association with treatment failure without drainage. *West J Emerg Med.* 2020;21(2):336–342.

 ## CODES

ICD10
- A49.02 Methicillin resis staph infection, unsp site
- A41.02 Sepsis due to Methicillin resistant Staphylococcus aureus
- J15.212 Pneumonia due to Methicillin resistant Staphylococcus aureus

CLINICAL PEARLS
- Incise and drain abscesses and send purulent material for culture and sensitivity.
- Local susceptibility patterns of CA-MRSA should guide empiric antibiotic treatment.
- Expect clinical improvement within 48 hours.

COMPLEMENTARY AND ALTERNATIVE MEDICINE

James Thomas Muller, DO • Kelley V. Lawrence, MD, IBCLC • Kimberly M. Chekan, DO, MPH

BASICS

DESCRIPTION

- Complementary and alternative medicine (CAM) are medical and health care systems, practices, and products that are not currently considered as part of conventional Western medicine and can be used in conjunction with conventional medicine.
- *Alternative medicine* is used in place of conventional medicine to promote healing of conditions not fully explained by the conventional biomedical model or for which the effectiveness of therapy is not yet established by clinical research.
- *Integrative medicine* is the combination of allopathic and/or osteopathic medicine with CAM and may be provided to the patient by a single licensed medical professional trained in CAM or by a group of diverse health care providers.
- *Holistic* is a descriptive term for a practitioner's approach to patient care that assesses the emotional, spiritual, mental, and physical state of wellness of the patient and works to provide comprehensive care.
- Manipulative and body-based methods include:
  - Massage therapy is manipulation of soft tissues using knowledge of anatomy and physiology to restore function, promote relaxation, and relieve pain.
  - Tenets of osteopathic manipulative treatment (OMT) from American Osteopathic Association:
    ○ Rational treatment is based on an understanding of the basic principles of body unity, self-regulation, and the interrelationship of structure and function; structure and function are reciprocally interrelated; the body is capable of self-regulation, self-healing, and health maintenance; the body is a unit; the person is a unit of body, mind, and spirit.
  - Chiropractic therapy focuses on imbalances in the musculoskeletal and nervous system to treat back, neck, and joint pain.
  - Cupping uses pressure suction to help improve blood flow to skin, decrease pain, and reduce inflammation.
- Mind–body medicine include:
  - Meditation is a practice of detachment in which a person sits quietly, generally focusing on the breath, while releasing thoughts from the mind with the intention to center self, restore balance, and enhance well-being.
  - Yoga is an exercise of mindfulness, meditation, strength, and balance, composed of *asanas* (postures) and *pranayamas* (focused breathing).
  - Aromatherapy uses highly concentrated plant extracts to stimulate healing.
- Alternative medical systems include:
  - Traditional Chinese medicine (TCM) incorporates Chinese herbs and acupuncture. Acupuncture is the practice of regulating *chi* by inserting thin needles at specific points along meridian pathways of the body.
  - Ayurvedic medicine originated in India and uses healing modalities and herbs to integrate and balance the body, mind, and spirit.
  - Homeopathy proposes that dilute quantities of an offending agent can stimulate innate immunity.
  - Naturopathy includes herbs, vitamins, supplements, dietary counseling, homeopathic remedies, manipulative therapies, acupuncture, and hydrotherapy.
- Energy therapies
  - *Reiki*, "source energy," involves laying hands lightly on patient or holding the hands just above the body and facilitates spiritual and physical healing by stimulating life force energy.
- Common reasons patients choose CAM
  - Additive therapy to address issues not covered by conventional medical treatment
  - Conventional medicine has been unsuccessful in fully addressing ailment.
  - Preventative health care and/or a desire for a more holistic/natural/noninvasive approach to well-being
  - Concern about medication side effects
  - Cultural or familial belief system more aligned with "natural" solutions

EPIDEMIOLOGY
All ages use CAM; most common use is among 30 to 69 year old females. More prevalent use of CAM among adults with higher levels of education, high socioeconomic status, living in West, former tobacco use disorder, and/or recently hospitalized. Cancer survivors are more likely to use CAM (1).

Prevalence
CAM is most frequently used to treat musculoskeletal issues; 59–90% of patients claim that use of alternative therapy helped their chronic pain (1).

GENERAL PREVENTION
Many core principles of CAM therapy are used for general prevention of chronic disease.

COMMONLY ASSOCIATED CONDITIONS
Acute/chronic pain; osteoarthritis; fibromyalgia; poor quality sleep; fatigue; symptoms from cancer diagnosis and side effects from treatment; headache/migraine; irritable bowel syndrome (IBS); depression/anxiety; low libido; weight loss; asthma; eczema; tinnitus; autoimmune disease

DIAGNOSIS

HISTORY
- What has you interested in pursuing CAM and what prior knowledge do you have about CAM?
- What is your biggest concern today and why?
- Past medical history, surgical history, family history, social history
- Prescription medications; vitamins; herbals; supplements; over-the-counter medications
- Nutritional habits; exercise regimen; sleep
- Social interactions; support system; mood; spirituality
- What treatments have you tried in the past? What has worked and not worked?
- What are your goals for your health and how do I (your provider) fit into your goals?
- What are your beliefs about your body and your health?

PHYSICAL EXAM
- Vital signs. General appearance including body mass index/body composition
- General physical examination—targeted by history to focus on particular system
- Osteopathic scan and screen physical exam for somatic dysfunction

DIAGNOSTIC TESTS & INTERPRETATION
Initial Tests (lab, imaging)
In addition to routine annual testing: vitamin testing, inflammatory markers, endocrine abnormality testing

Follow-Up Tests & Special Considerations
Special CAM considerations without evidence supporting safety or efficacy: food intolerance testing, *Candida* testing, postchelator challenge, adrenal stress profile (2)[C]

Diagnostic Procedures/Other
OMT (3)[A]
- Diagnosing somatic dysfunctions: "Impaired or altered function of related components of the body framework system: skeletal, arthrodial, and myofascial structures, and their related vascular, lymphatic, and neural elements" (4).
  - Tissue texture changes; asymmetry; restricted range of motion; tenderness

TREATMENT

- OMT
  - Used to relieve somatic dysfunctions in following regions: head, cervical, thoracic, lumbar, sacrum, innominates, upper extremities, lower extremities, abdomen, rib cage by applying manually guided forces to improve function and help restore homeostasis (4)
  - Techniques: soft tissue, myofascial release, balanced ligamentous tension, muscle energy, direct articulatory, Still technique, facilitated positional release, high velocity, low amplitude
  - Evidence for use in chronic low back pain (4)[A]
- Acupuncture
  - For chronic low back pain, recurrent headache/migraine (1)[A], chemotherapy-induced nausea and vomiting (5)[A]
- Cupping
  - Cupping reduces chronic low back pain (6)[A].
- Massage therapy
  - Most studies discuss the effect of massage therapy on neck pain, low back pain, cancer pain (7)[A].

MEDICATION
- Evidence supports safety and efficacy of:
  - Enteric-coated peppermint oil for abdominal pain associated with IBS
  - Ashwagandha effective in helping reduce stress and anxiety
- Variable evidence supports safety and efficacy of:
  - Ginger for nausea, including that associated with chemotherapy
  - Saffron (*Crocus sativus L.*) reduces depressive symptoms in mothers with mild postpartum depression.

- Riboflavin for migraine prophylaxis 400 mg daily for 3 months before seeing effects
- Arnica and turmeric for knee osteoarthritis
- Oral probiotics to decrease necrotizing enterocolitis in preterm infants, to prevent URIs in children, to shorten duration of acute and antibiotic-associated diarrhea and as prophylaxis for traveler's diarrhea
- Vitamin D3 800 IU or more per day may reduce falls and fractures in the elderly.
- *Ginkgo biloba* improves cognition in patients with dementia.

ISSUES FOR REFERRAL
Minimal provider education and training in CAM. Seeking more expertise if patient interested in CAM; confirming certification and training of CAM providers when referring a patient

ADDITIONAL THERAPIES
Variable evidence supports safety and efficacy of:
- Massage (30 minutes × 3) during labor shortens the second stage and reduces pain.
- Yoga throughout pregnancy shortens labor by 140 to 190 minutes.
- Exercise in both preconception and early pregnancy reduces chance of gestational diabetes mellitus.
- Exercise has a small to moderate effect in reducing symptoms in persons with diagnosed anxiety disorders.

ADMISSION, INPATIENT, AND NURSING CONSIDERATIONS
Many hospitals provide CAM services including TCM, hypnosis, reflexology, aromatherapy, homeopathy, yoga, herbal medicine, OMT, and chaplain services.

 ONGOING CARE

FOLLOW-UP RECOMMENDATIONS
Maintain contact between primary care provider and CAM providers; make sure records are shared between both providers.

Patient Monitoring
Dietary supplements are the most commonly used CAM therapy. Many health care providers report they lack the resources and training to respond to patient questions regarding supplements and herbal medicines; important to include all supplements on medication list

DIET
Nutrition plans to consider with weight loss and inflammation reduction: ketogenic; intermittent fasting; Mediterranean; paleo

PATIENT EDUCATION
The National Center for Complementary and Integrative Health (https://nccih.nih.gov/)

COMPLICATIONS

ALERT
Be aware, patients may delay seeking medical care or may consider replacement of curative conventional treatment. Ginkgo, goldenseal, and St. John's wort account for most reported herb–drug interactions

Herbs with possible adverse effects
- Black cohosh (*Actaea racemosa*) reduces effectiveness of statins.
- California poppy (*Eschscholzia californica*): may cause respiratory depression, drowsiness; contains opioids
- Ephedra (*Ephedra spp.*): sympathomimetic; insomnia, gastric distress
- Ginkgo (*Ginkgo biloba*): increased bleeding time
- Goldenseal (*Hydrastis canadensis*) interferes with nearly all prescription medications.
- Guarana (*Paullinia cupana*): tachycardia, hypertension; contains caffeine
- Kava (*Piper methysticum*): decreases use of niacin; possibly hepatotoxic
- Licorice (*Glycyrrhiza spp.*): Long-term use depletes serum potassium
- Senna (*Cassia senna*): depletes serum potassium
- St. John's wort (*Hypericum perforatum*): numerous drug interactions; induces CYP3A4 pathway, increasing metabolism: cyclosporine, tacrolimus, warfarin, protease inhibitors, theophylline, venlafaxine, digoxin, oral contraceptives
- Wormwood (*Artemisia absinthium*): elevates serotonin level, may raise blood pressure
- Yohimbe (*Pausinystalia yohimbe*): elevates blood pressure

Geriatric Considerations
- *Ginkgo biloba* commonly interacts with warfarin (Coumadin).
- Incorporating integrative medicine into palliative care may be beneficial.
- Tai chi and yoga may reduce risk/fear of falls and improve mobility in elderly. Gentle chair yoga, as well as massage, acupuncture, and Reiki may be beneficial for fatigue in elderly cancer patients.

Pediatric Considerations
- Carob bean juice and preparation including *Matricaria chamomilla* and apple pectin were shown to significantly reduce the duration of diarrhea.
- Peppermint oil can decrease duration, frequency, and severity of pain in children suffering from undifferentiated functional abdominal pain.
- Different fennel preparations were found to be useful in treating infantile colic.
- Psyllium fiber may be a useful adjunct for constipation and decreasing pain episodes in patients with IBS.
- Iron is a leading cause of accidental poisoning in children <6 years of age.
- Vitamin A is the most common cause of hypervitaminosis.

REFERENCES
1. Urits I, Schwartz RH, Orhurhu V, et al. A comprehensive review of alternative therapies for the management of chronic pain patients: acupuncture, tai chi, osteopathic manipulative medicine, and chiropractic care. *Adv Ther*. 2021;38(1):76–89.
2. Jones SL, Campbell B, Hart T. Laboratory tests commonly used in complementary and alternative medicine: a review of the evidence. *Ann Clin Biochem*. 2019;56(3):310–325.
3. Task Force on the Low Back Pain Clinical Practice Guidelines. American Osteopathic Association guidelines for osteopathic manipulative treatment (OMT) for patients with low back pain. *J Am Osteopath Assoc*. 2016;116(8):536–549.
4. Licciardone JC, Schultz MJ, Amen B. Osteopathic manipulation in the management of chronic pain: current perspectives. *J Pain Res*. 2020;13:1839–1847.
5. Li QW, Yu MW, Wang XM, et al. Efficacy of acupuncture in the prevention and treatment of chemotherapy-induced nausea and vomiting in patients with advanced cancer: a multi-center, single-blind, randomized, sham-controlled clinical research. *Chin Med*. 2020;15:57.
6. Moura CC, Chaves ÉCL, Cardoso ACLR, et al. Cupping therapy and chronic back pain: systematic review and meta-analysis. *Rev Lat Am Enfermagem*. 2018;26:e3094.
7. Miake-Lye IM, Mak S, Lee J, et al. Massage for pain: an evidence map. *J Altern Complement Med*. 2019;25(5):475–502.

ADDITIONAL READING
American Osteopathic Association. Tenets of osteopathic medicine. https://osteopathic.org/about/leadership/aoa-governance-documents/tenets-of-osteopathic-medicine. Accessed December 6, 2021.

 CODES

ICD10
Z76.89 Persons encountering health services in other specified circumstances

CLINICAL PEARLS
- Enteric-coated peppermint oil may help IB-associated abdominal pain.
- Ashwagandha may help to reduce stress and anxiety.
- Riboflavin is helpful for migraine prophylaxis 400 mg daily—may take 3 months to see effects.
- OMT is helpful for chronic low back pain.
- Ginkgo, goldenseal, and St. John's wort account for most herb–drug interactions.
- Tai chi can help with balance and reduce risk of falls in the elderly.

COMPLEX REGIONAL PAIN SYNDROME

Dennis E. Hughes, DO, FACEP

 BASICS

DESCRIPTION

- Complex regional pain syndrome (CRPS) is a pain syndrome that can be chronic and debilitating. It is divided into two subtypes and can result in significant physical and psychosocial short and long-term disability. Most cases are a result of a physical insult to an extremity such as trauma or surgery. The lack of a dermatomal distribution distinguishes CRPS from other pain syndromes.
  - Type I: no nerve injury (reflex sympathetic dystrophy [RSD])
  - Type II: associated with a demonstrable nerve injury (causalgia)
- Synonym(s): traumatic erythromelalgia; Weir Mitchell causalgia; causalgia; RSD; posttraumatic neuralgia; sympathetically maintained pain

EPIDEMIOLOGY

- Peak age 50 to 70 years
- Predominant gender: female > male (3:1, 60–81%), favoring postmenopausal
- Rarely seen in pediatrics—cases in this age group predominantly involve lower extremities in females.
- Recent studies found 3.8% occurrence after wrist fracture and 7% occurrence after intra-articular ankle fracture—both independent strong risk for CRPS. Fractures and sprains are associated ~60% of cases, the remaining 40% have less precise or no recognized inciting event. Upper extremities are more commonly involved.
- More prevalent in patients that report higher than usual expected pain in early phases of trauma. Latency depends on normal injury recovery time—prolonged pain (greater than 2 months) after injury hints at diagnosis.

Incidence

Incidence of 5.46 to 26.2/100,000 for type I and 0.82/100,000 for type II in United States

ETIOLOGY AND PATHOPHYSIOLOGY

- Poorly understood activation of abnormal sympathetic reflex that lowers pain threshold. It is agreed that the process is multifactorial and involves both central and peripheral nervous systems.
  - Increased excitability of nociceptive neurons in the spinal cord; "central sensitization"
  - Exaggerated responses to normally nonpainful stimuli (hyperalgesia, allodynia)
  - The exaggerated inflammatory response results in afferent neurons releasing increased amounts of neuropeptides (1).
- Type II is associated with physical injury to nerve. This represents a minority of cases.
- Emerging information reveals CNS changes (functional, anatomic, biochemical) in addition to spinal level changes. Increased levels of immunomodulators suggest autoimmune component. The lack of a definitive pathophysiologic mechanism has led to suggest that CRPS is a "functional neurologic syndrome" (2).

Genetics

No known genetic pattern

RISK FACTORS

- Minor or severe trauma (upper extremity fracture-particularly distal radius noted in a significant number of those with CRPS)
- Surgery (particularly carpal tunnel release)
- Lacerations, burns, frostbite
- Casting/immobilization after extremity injury
- Penetrating injury (case reports of CRPS developing after snakebites)
- Polymyalgia rheumatica
- Myocardial infarction, cerebral vascular accident
- Reports of CRPS development after "innocuous" events such as IV catheters, IM injections

GENERAL PREVENTION

- Early mobilization and avoiding prolonged immobilization has proven benefit in reducing incidence of CRPS.
- One study of wrist fractures found that addition of 500 mg/day of vitamin C lowered rates of CRPS.
- There is evidence that limiting use of tourniquets, liberal regional anesthetic use, and ensuring adequate perioperative analgesia can reduce the incidence of CRPS-I.

COMMONLY ASSOCIATED CONDITIONS

- Serious injury to bone and soft tissue
- Herpes zoster
- Postherpetic neuralgia results from partial or complete damage to afferent nerve pathways.
- Pain occurs in dermatomes as a sequela of herpes zoster.
- Signal exists for patients having comorbid painful conditions or psychiatric diagnosis at increased risk of developing CRPS.

DIAGNOSIS

Unprovoked pain is the hallmark of the condition, and the diagnosis of CRPS is excluded by the existence of conditions that would otherwise account for the degree of symptoms. Budapest clinical diagnostic criteria (3),(4) can aid in establishing diagnosis:

- Continuing pain which is disproportionate to any inciting event
- At least one symptom in three of the four following categories:
  - Sensory: hyperalgesia and/or allodynia
  - Vasomotor: skin, temperature, color asymmetry
  - Sudomotor/edema: edema, sweating changes, or sweating asymmetry
  - Motor/trophic: decreased range of motion or motor dysfunction and/or trophic changes (hair, nail, skin)
- Must display one sign at the time of the evaluation in two or more of the following:
  - Sensory: hyperalgesia (to pinprick) or allodynia (to light touch, pressure, or joint movement)
  - Vasomotor: evidence of temperature, skin, color asymmetry

  - Sudomotor/edema: evidence of edema or sweating changes or asymmetry
  - Motor/trophic: decreased range of motion; motor dysfunction; or trophic changes in hair, nails, skin
- There is no other diagnosis that explains the signs and symptoms.

HISTORY

The patient commonly complains of persistent burning pain, swelling, and poor function after extremity injury. The severity of the preceding injury may vary from fracture to relatively minor trauma (4).

PHYSICAL EXAM

The affected extremity appears swollen with erythematous, shiny skin with brittle nails, and reduced hair. There will be limited range of motion—both active and passive.

DIFFERENTIAL DIAGNOSIS

- Infection
- Hypertrophic scar
- Neuroma
- CNS tumor or syrinx
- Deep vein thrombosis or thrombophlebitis
- Thoracic outlet syndrome
- Connective tissue disorder
- Factitious

DIAGNOSTIC TESTS & INTERPRETATION

The diagnosis of CRPS does not require any specific testing—it is a clinical diagnosis. It is a symptom-based diagnosis of exclusion. Testing is performed to rule out other potential etiologies of clinical symptoms (5).

Initial Tests (lab, imaging)

- CBC, erythrocyte sedimentation rate (ESR)
- Plain radiographs may show patchy demineralization within 3 to 6 weeks of onset of CRPS that are more pronounced than would be seen from disuse alone.
- Three-phase bone scanning has varying sensitivity but is most accurate for support of the diagnosis when there is diffuse activity (especially on phase 3).
- Bone density

Diagnostic Procedures/Other

- Electromyelography (EMG) shows nerve injury with type II CRPS.
- Sudomotor function testing (resting sweat testing, resting skin temperature, quantitative sudomotor axon reflex testing; all related to increased autonomic activity of the affected limb)

Test Interpretation

- Partial or complete damage to afferent nerve pathways and probably reorganized central pain pathways
- Nerves most commonly involved are median and sciatic.
- Atrophy in affected muscles
- Incomplete nerve plexus lesion

TREATMENT

GENERAL MEASURES
Discourage maladaptive behaviors (pain medication seeking, secondary gain). Principle of functional restoration is a stepwise and multidisciplinary approach. Early and aggressive mobilization seems to lessen the duration. Avoidance of opiates cannot be overemphasized.

MEDICATION
First Line
- NSAIDs recommended early in course but mixed support in literature
- The following have literature support of either limited or suggestive benefit in treatment of CRPS-I:
  - Corticosteroids (prednisone 30 mg/day × 2 to 12 weeks with taper) are the only class of drugs that have direct clinical trial support early in the course. A recent retrospective case review found that patients showed significant improvement with various measurable physical parameters after treatment with prednisolone (30 mg starting dose tapering by 5 mg every 3 days for a total of 3 weeks treatment) (6)[C].
  - Gabapentin 600 to 1,800 mg/day for 8 weeks following diagnosis (3)[C]
  - 50% DMSO cream applied to affected extremity up to 5 times daily
  - N-Acetylcysteine 600 mg TID
  - Bisphosphonates (alendronate) at 40 mg/day (however, optimal dose uncertain) (3)[C]
  - Nifedipine 20 mg/day showed benefit early in the course of the condition.
- Although many have advocated the use of tricyclic antidepressants in the treatment of CRPS, there is no credible evidence of improvement of pain. They may be helpful in controlling depressive symptoms that develop with disease progression.

ISSUES FOR REFERRAL
- After 2 months of the illness, psychological evaluation generally is indicated to identify and treat any comorbid conditions. Depressive symptoms frequently develop.
- Physical therapy and occupational therapy early for guided motor and mirror therapy

ADDITIONAL THERAPIES
Type I
- Physical and occupational therapy (beneficial to the overall prognosis for recovery) should be initiated early in the course of treatment
  - "Mirror therapy" has shown good results.
  - Case reports of patients responding favorably to passive ROM treatment under sedation followed by multiple physical therapy sessions
- Transcutaneous nerve stimulation
- Psychotherapy
- Use of subdissociative (0.2 to 0.5 mg/kg) infusions of ketamine has shown some promise, but effects seem to be time limited; systemic literature review failed to find a high-quality support for ketamine treatment.

SURGERY/OTHER PROCEDURES
- Type II responds more favorably to nerve-directed treatment.
  - Sympathetic blocks
  - Cervicothoracic or lumbar sympathectomies have little data to support their use and should be used judiciously and after all other therapies have failed.
- Anesthetic blockade (chemical or surgical) of sympathetic nerve function
  - Transient relief suggests that chemical or surgical sympathectomy will be helpful.
  - Little in the way of quality, clinical trials exist to support local sympathetic blockage as the gold standard of therapy.
- IV regional sympathetic block with guanethidine or reserpine by pain specialist or anesthetist
- Transcutaneous electric nerve stimulation (controversial)
- Inject myofascial painful trigger points.
- Dorsal root ganglion (DRG) stimulation higher rate of success than spinal cord stimulation in recent comparative study; more specific target as DRG home of soma of sensory neurons
- Intrathecal analgesia
- Amputation as a last resort in severe cases, with patients reporting improved quality of life
- Single case study of topical 5% lidocaine revealed significant pain reduction and improved range of motion and function.
- Osteopathic manipulation (case report literature)

COMPLEMENTARY & ALTERNATIVE MEDICINE
- Vitamin C (500 mg/day) may help to prevent CRPS in those with wrist fracture (3).
- Briskly rub the affected part several times per day.
- Acupuncture
- Hypnosis can be suggested.
- Relaxation training (alternate muscle relaxing and contracting)
- Biofeedback
- Whirlpool baths

ADMISSION, INPATIENT, AND NURSING CONSIDERATIONS
Only for proposed surgical therapy

 ONGOING CARE

FOLLOW-UP RECOMMENDATIONS
Weekly, to monitor progress and initiate additional modalities as needed

PATIENT EDUCATION
- Counsel to remain active physically.
- Reflex Sympathetic Dystrophy Syndrome Association: http://rsds.org/; 203-877-3790

PROGNOSIS
Most improve with early treatment, but symptoms may be lifelong if there is limited response to initial treatments.

COMPLICATIONS
- Depression
- Disability
- Opioid dependence

REFERENCES
1. Prasad Md A, Chakravarthy Md K. Review of complex regional pain syndrome and the role of the neuroimmune axis. *Mol Pain*. 2021;17:17448069211006617.
2. Chang C, McDonnell P, Gershwin ME. Complex regional pain syndrome—autoimmune or functional neurologic syndrome. *J Transl Autoimmun*. 2020;4:100080.
3. Shim H, Rose J, Halle S, et al. Complex regional pain syndrome: a narrative review for the practising physician. *Br J Anaesth*. 2019;123(2): e424–e433.
4. Goebel A, Barker C, Birklein F, et al. Standards for diagnosis and management of complex regional pain syndrome: results of a European Pain Federation task force. *Eur J Pain*.2019;23(4): 641–651.
5. Mesaroli G, Hundert A, Birnie KA, et al. Screening and diagnostic tools for complex regional pain syndrome: a systematic review. *Pain*. 2021;162(5):1295–1304.
6. Birklein F, Dimova V. Complex regional pain syndrome up-to-date. *Pain Rep*. 2017;2(26):e624.

ADDITIONAL READING
Eldufani J, Elahmer N, Blaise G. A medical mystery of complex regional pain syndrome. *Heliyon*. 2020;6(2):e03329. Published 2020 Feb 19.

 CODES

ICD10
- G90.52 Complex regional pain syndrome I of lower limb
- G90.523 Complex regional pain syndrome I of lower limb, bilateral
- G56.4 Causalgia of upper limb

CLINICAL PEARLS
- A pain syndrome disproportioned to injury
- Pain control and early mobility are the key to recovery.
- Avoid use of opiate analgesics.
- Use a multidisciplinary approach.

CONDYLOMATA ACUMINATA

Caroline R. Campbell, MD • M. Ashleigh Brown, DO • E. James Kruse, DO

BASICS

DESCRIPTION
- Condylomata acuminata are soft, skin-colored, fleshy lesions (commonly called genital warts) that are caused by human papillomavirus (HPV):
  - Warts appear singly or in groups (a single wart is a "condyloma"; multiple warts are "condylomas" or "condylomata"); small or large; typically appear on the anogenital skin (penis, scrotum, introitus, vulva, perianal area); and may occur in the anogenital tract (vagina, cervix, rectum, urethra, anus); also conjunctival, nasal, oral, and laryngeal warts
- System(s) affected: skin/exocrine, reproductive, occasionally respiratory
- HIV considerations:
  - Treatment of external genital warts should not be different for HIV-infected persons (1).
  - Lesions may be larger or more numerous (1).
  - May not respond as well to therapy as immunocompetent persons (1)

Pediatric Considerations
- Consider sexual abuse if seen in children, although children can be infected by other means (e.g., transfer from wart on another child's hand or prolonged latency period) (2).
- American Academy of Pediatrics recommends all school-aged children who present with lesions be evaluated for abuse and screened for other STDs (2).

Pregnancy Considerations
- Warts often grow larger during pregnancy and regress spontaneously after delivery.
- Neonatal infection is thought to occur through vertical transmission. Incidence remains controversial. Cesarean section is not absolutely indicated for maternal condylomata (3).
- Cervical infection has been found to be a risk factor for preterm birth (3).
- Few documented cases of laryngeal papillomas due to HPV transmission at the time of delivery. Although rare, the condition is life-threatening.
- HPV vaccination is contraindicated in pregnancy.
- Treatment during pregnancy is somewhat controversial but may include topical trichloroacetic acid (TCA), cryotherapy, electrocautery, or surgical excision.
- The safety of imiquimod, sinecatechins, podophyllin, and podofilox during pregnancy has not been established (3).

EPIDEMIOLOGY
- HPV types 6 and 11 associated with 90% of condylomata acuminata. Types 16, 18, 31, 33, and 35 may be found in warts and may be associated with high-grade intraepithelial dysplasia in immunocompromised states such as HIV.
- Highly contagious; incubation period may be from 1 to 8 months. Initial infections may very well go unrecognized, so a "new" outbreak may be a relapse of an infection acquired years prior.
- Predominant age: 15 to 30 years
- Predominant sex: 1:1 male to female
- Most infections are transient and clear spontaneously within 2 years.

Incidence
One study population demonstrated that from 2007 to 2010, with the introduction of HPV vaccines, the incidence of genital warts decreased 35% (from 0.94% per year to 0.61% per year) in females <21 years and decreased 19% in males <21 years.

Prevalence
- Most common viral sexually transmitted infection (STI) in the United States. Most sexually active men and women will have acquired a genital HPV infection, usually asymptomatic, at some time.
- Estimated 6.2 million Americans become infected with genital HPV each year.
- Peak prevalence in ages 17 to 33 years
- 10–20% of sexually active women may be actively infected with HPV. Studies in men suggest a similar prevalence.
- Pregnancy and immunosuppression favor recurrence and increased growth of lesions.

ETIOLOGY AND PATHOPHYSIOLOGY
HPV is a circular, double-stranded DNA molecule. There are >120 HPV subtypes. HPV types that cause genital warts do not cause anogenital cancers.

RISK FACTORS
- Usually acquired by unprotected sexual activity
  - Young adults and adolescents
  - Multiple sexual partners; short interval between meeting new sex partner and first intercourse
  - Not using protective barriers
  - Young age of commencing sexual activity
  - History of other STI
- Immunosuppression (particularly HIV)
- Cigarette smoking
- Use of oral contraceptives
- Radiation therapy

GENERAL PREVENTION
- Sexual abstinence or monogamy
- HPV vaccination is for prevention of HPV infections and HPV-associated cancers. This vaccine is targeted to adolescents before the period of their greatest risk for exposure to HPV. The vaccine does not treat previous infections:
  - A 2-dose schedule (0, 6 to 12 months) will have efficacy equivalent to a 3-dose schedule (0, 1 to 2, 6 months) if the HPV vaccination series is initiated before the 15th birthday (4).
  - The 9-valent HPV (9vHPV; Gardasil 9) vaccine protects against the two most common HPV serotypes (types 6 and 11, which cause most anogenital warts) and the two most cancer-promoting types (16 and 18) as well as 31, 33, 45, 52, and 58 (4).
  - Quadrivalent HPV (4vHPV) and 9vHPV vaccines (Gardasil and Gardasil 9) are licensed for use in females and males aged 9 through 45 years (5).
  - The Advisory Committee on Immunization Practices (ACIP) has recommended routine vaccination at age 11 or 12 years for females since 2006 and since 2011 for males (4).
- Use of condoms is partially effective, although warts may be easily spread by lesions not covered by a condom (e.g., 40% of infected men have scrotal warts).
- Abstinence until treatment completed

COMMONLY ASSOCIATED CONDITIONS
- >90% of cervical cancer associated with HPV types 16, 18, 31, 33, and 35
- 60% of oropharyngeal and anogenital squamous cell carcinomas are associated with HPV.
- STIs (e.g., gonorrhea, syphilis, chlamydia), AIDS

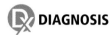

DIAGNOSIS

HISTORY
- Explore sexual history, contraception use, and other lifestyle topics.
- Most warts are asymptomatic but symptoms include
  - Pruritus, burning, redness, pain, bleeding
  - Vaginal discharge
  - Large warts may cause obstructive symptoms in the anus (with defecation) or vaginal canal (with intercourse or childbirth).

PHYSICAL EXAM
- Lesions often have a typical rough, warty appearance with multiple fingerlike projections but may be soft, sessile, and smooth.
- Large lesions are cauliflower-like and may grow to >10 cm.
- Most common sites: penis, vaginal introitus, and perianal region
- May be seen anywhere on the anogenital epithelium or in the anogenital tract
- Warts often occur in clusters.
- Bleeding or irritation of the lesions may be noted.

DIFFERENTIAL DIAGNOSIS
- Condylomata lata (flat warts of syphilis)
- Lichen planus
- Normal sebaceous glands
- Seborrheic keratosis
- Molluscum contagiosum
- Keratomas, micropapillomatosis
- Scabies
- Crohn disease
- Skin tags
- Melanocytic nevi
- Vulvar intraepithelial neoplasia
- Squamous cell carcinoma

DIAGNOSTIC TESTS & INTERPRETATION
- Diagnosis is usually clinical, made by unaided visual examination of the lesions.
- Biopsy
- Acetowhitening test: Subclinical lesions can be visualized by applying moistened gauze soaked with 5% acetic acid (vinegar) to the affected area for 5 minutes. Using a 10× hand lens or colposcope, warts appear as tiny white papules. A shiny white appearance of the skin represents foci of epithelial hyperplasia (subclinical infection), but because of low specificity, the CDC recommends against routine use of this test to screen for HPV mucosal infection.

Initial Tests (lab, imaging)
- Usually not required for diagnosis
- Serologic tests for syphilis may be helpful to rule out condylomata lata.
- Other testing for STIs
- Pap smear may be indicated.

Follow-Up Tests & Special Considerations
Because squamous cell carcinoma may resemble or coexist with condylomata, biopsy may be considered for lesions refractory to therapy.

Diagnostic Procedures/Other
- Biopsy with highly specialized identification techniques, such as HPV DNA detected through polymerase chain reaction, is rarely useful.
- Colposcopy, antroscopy, anoscopy, and urethroscopy may be required to detect anogenital tract lesions.
- Screening men who have sex with men (MSM) with anal Pap smears is controversial.

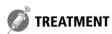 **TREATMENT**

GENERAL MEASURES
- Approximately, 30% resolve spontaneously in 4 months.
- Change therapy if no improvement after three treatments, clearance not complete after six treatments, or therapy's duration or dosage exceeds manufacturer's recommendations.
- Appropriate screening/counseling of partners

MEDICATION
First Line
- No single therapy for genital warts is ideal for all patients or clearly superior to other therapies.
- Recommendations for external genital warts, patient applied:
  - Podofilox (Condylox) (3)[A]: antimitotic action; apply 0.5% solution or gel to warts twice daily (allowing to dry) for 3 consecutive days at home followed by 4 days of no therapy; may repeat up to 4 total cycles; maximum of 0.5 mL/day or area <10 cm^2
  - Imiquimod (Aldara) (3)[A]: immune enhancer; self-treatment with a 5% cream applied once daily at bedtime 3 times weekly until warts resolve for up to 16 weeks. Wash off with soap and water 6 to 10 hours after application. Imiquimod has been noted to weaken condoms and diaphragms; therefore, patients should refrain from sexual contact while the cream is on the skin.
  - Sinecatechins (Veregen): immune enhancer and antioxidant, extract from green tea; apply a 0.5-cm strand of ointment 3 times daily for up to 16 weeks. Do not wash off after.
- Recommendations for external genital warts, provider applied:
  - Cryotherapy: liquid nitrogen applied to warts for two bursts of approximately 10 seconds (or whatever time is needed to freeze the wart without extension significantly deep or lateral to the wart) with thawing in between; usually requires 2 to 3 weekly sessions (3)[A]
  - Podophyllin 10–25% in tincture of benzoin. Apply directly to warts, air-dry in office before coming into contact with clothes. Wash off in 1 to 4 hours. Repeat every 7 days in office until gone (3)[A].
  - TCA: 80% solution. Apply only to warts; powder/talc to remove unreacted acid. Repeat in office at weekly intervals; ideal for isolated lesions in pregnancy (3)[A]
- Recommendations for exophytic cervical warts: biopsy to exclude high-grade squamous intraepithelial lesion (SIL) (3)[A]
- Recommendations for vaginal warts: cryotherapy or TCA or bichloroacetic acid (BCA) 80–90% (3)[A]

- Recommendations for urethral meatus warts: cryotherapy or podophyllin 10–25% in compound tincture of benzoin (3)[A]
- Recommendations for anal warts: cryotherapy, TCA or BCA 80–90%, or surgery; specialty consultation for intra-anal warts (3)[A]

Pregnancy Considerations
Cryotherapy, surgery, or TCA; medications contraindicated in pregnancy: podophyllin, podophyllotoxin, sinecatechins, interferon, and imiquimod (3)[C]

Second Line
Intralesional interferon, photodynamic therapy, topical cidofovir (3)[A]

SURGERY/OTHER PROCEDURES
- Larger warts may require surgical excision, laser treatment, or electrocoagulation (including infrared therapy):
  - Precaution: Laser treatment may create smoke plumes that contain HPV. CDC recommendation is for the use of a smoke evacuator no <2 inches from the surgical site. Masks are recommended; N95 the most efficacious (6)
- Intraurethral, external (penile and perianal), anal, and oral lesions can be treated with fulgurating CO_2 laser. Oral or external penile/perianal lesions can also be treated with electrocautery or surgery.

 ONGOING CARE

FOLLOW-UP RECOMMENDATIONS
No restrictions, except for sexual contact

Patient Monitoring
- Patients should be seen every 1 to 2 weeks until lesions resolve.
- Patients should follow up 3 months after completion of treatment.
- Persistent warts require biopsy.
- Sexual partners require monitoring.

PATIENT EDUCATION
- Provide information on HPV, STI prevention, and condom use.
- Explain to patients that it is difficult to know how or when a person acquired an HPV infection; a diagnosis in one partner does not prove sexual infidelity in the other partner.
- Emphasize the need for women to follow recommendations for regular Pap smears.

PROGNOSIS
- Asymptomatic infection persists indefinitely.
- Treatment has not clearly been shown to decrease transmissible infectivity.
- Warts may clear with treatment or resolve spontaneously. However, recurrences are frequent, particularly in the first 3 months, and may necessitate repeated treatments.

COMPLICATIONS
- Cervical dysplasia (probably does not occur with type 6 or 11, which cause most warts)
- Malignant change: Progression of condylomata to cancer rarely, if ever, occurs, although squamous cell carcinoma may coexist in larger warts.
- Urethral, vaginal, or anal obstruction from treatment
- The prevalence of high-grade dysplasia and cancer in anal canal is higher in HIV-positive than in HIV-negative patients, probably because of increased HPV activity.

REFERENCES
1. Gormley RH, Kovarik CL. Human papillomavirus-related genital disease in the immunocompromised host: part II. *J Am Acad Dermatol*. 2012;66(6):883.e1–883.e17, quiz 899–900.
2. Unger ER, Fajman NN, Maloney EM, et al. Anogenital human papillomavirus in sexually abused and nonabused children: a multicenter study. *Pediatrics*. 2011;128(3):e658–e665.
3. Workowski KA, Bolan GA; for Centers for Disease Control and Prevention. Sexually transmitted diseases treatment guidelines, 2015. *MMWR Recomm Rep*. 2015;64(RR-03):1–137.
4. Meites E, Kempe A, Markowitz LE. Use of a 2-dose schedule for human papillomavirus vaccination—updated recommendations of the Advisory Committee on Immunization Practices. *MMWR Morb Mortal Wkly Rep*. 2016;65(49):1405–1408.
5. U.S. Food and Drug Administration. FDA approves expanded use of Gardasil 9 to include individuals 27 through 45 years old. https://www.fda.gov/NewsEvents/Newsroom/PressAnnouncements/ucm622715.htm. Accessed December 12, 2018.
6. Bryant C, Gorman R, Stewart J, et al. *NIOSH Health Hazard Evaluation Report*. Bryn Mawr, PA: National Institute for Occupational Safety and Health; 1988. HETA 85-126-1932.

ADDITIONAL READING
- Bauer HM, Wright G, Chow J. Evidence of human papillomavirus vaccine effectiveness in reducing genital warts: an analysis of California public family planning administrative claims data, 2007–2010. *Am J Public Health*. 2012;102(5):833–835.
- Giuliano AR, Palefsky JM, Goldstone S, et al. Efficacy of quadrivalent HPV vaccine against HPV infection and disease in males. *N Engl J Med*. 2011;364(5):401–411.
- Gormley RH, Kovarik CL. Human papillomavirus-related genital disease in the immunocompromised host: part I. *J Am Acad Dermatol*. 2012;66(6):867.e1–867.e14, quiz 881–882.
- Yanofsky V, Patel R, Goldenberg G. Genital warts: a comprehensive review. *J Clin Aesthet Dermatol*. 2012;5(6):25–36.

 CODES

ICD10
A63.0 Anogenital (venereal) warts

CLINICAL PEARLS
- Condylomata acuminata are soft, skin-colored, fleshy lesions caused by HPV subtypes 6, 11, 16, 18, 31, 33, and 35.
- The majority of sexually active men and women will have acquired a genital HPV infection, usually asymptomatic, at some time.
- No single therapy for genital warts is ideal for all patients or clearly superior to other therapies.
- 9vHPV vaccine is effective in preventing HPV infection, particularly if administered prior to the onset of engaging in sexual activity. Gardasil is approved and recommended for use in males and females aged 9 to 45 years.

CONJUNCTIVITIS, ACUTE
Frances Yung-tao Wu, MD

BASICS

DESCRIPTION
- Inflammation of the bulbar and/or palpebral conjunctiva of <4 weeks' duration
- System(s) affected: nervous, skin/exocrine
- Synonym(s): pink eye

Geriatric Considerations
- Suspect bacterial, autoimmune, or irritative process.
- If purulent, risk of bacterial cause increases with age and long-term care facility residence, with age >65 years and bilateral lid adherence. Risk for bacterial infection is >70%.

Pediatric Considerations
- Neonatal conjunctivitis may be gonococcal, chlamydial, irritative, or related to dacryocystitis.
- Pediatric ER study; 78% positive bacterial culture, mostly *Haemophilus influenzae*; 13% no growth; other studies showed >50% adenovirus.
- Children <5 years of age 7× more likely have bacterial involvement than older patients.
- Despite lack of evidence, daycare regulations may require a child with presumed conjunctivitis to be treated with a topical antibiotic before returning (1)[A].

EPIDEMIOLOGY
- Predominant age
  - Pediatric: viral, bacterial
  - Adult: viral, bacterial, allergic
- Predominant sex: male = female

Incidence
1–2% of ambulatory office visits, up to 3% of ER visits

ETIOLOGY AND PATHOPHYSIOLOGY
- Viral
  - Adenovirus (common cold), coxsackievirus (implicated in recent hemorrhagic conjunctivitis epidemics in Asia and Middle East)
  - Enterovirus (acute hemorrhagic conjunctivitis)
  - Herpes simplex; herpes zoster or varicella
  - Measles, mumps, or influenza
  - COVID-19
- Bacterial
  - *Staphylococcus aureus*, MRSA, or *Staphylococcus epidermidis*
  - *Streptococcus pneumoniae*
  - *H. influenzae* (children)
  - *Pseudomonas* spp. or anaerobes (contact lens users)
  - *Acanthamoeba*-contaminated contact lens solution (rare; ~30 cases/year in US).
  - *Neisseria gonorrhoeae*
  - *Chlamydia trachomatis*: gradual onset 1 to 4 weeks
- Allergic
  - Hay fever, seasonal allergies, atopy
- Nonspecific
  - Irritative: topical medications, wind, dry eye, UV light exposure, smoke, chlorine
  - Autoimmune: Sjögren syndrome, pemphigoid, Wegener granulomatosis, Reiter syndrome, sarcoid
  - Rare: *Rickettsia*, fungal, parasitic, tuberculosis, syphilis, Kawasaki disease, chikungunya, Graves disease, gout, carcinoid, psoriasis, Stevens-Johnson syndrome, molluscum contagiosum, rosacea, squamous neoplasia

RISK FACTORS
- History of contact with infected persons
- Sexually transmitted disease (STD) contact: gonococcal, chlamydial, syphilis, or herpes

- Contact lenses: pseudomonal or acanthamoeba keratitis
- Epidemic bacterial (streptococcal) conjunctivitis reported in school settings, epidemic adenoviral transmission in crowded settings

GENERAL PREVENTION
- Wash hands frequently.
- Eyedropper technique: while eye is closed and head back, several drops over nasal canthus and then open eyes to allow liquid to enter. Never touch tip of dropper to skin or eye.
- Prevention of zoster (shingles) by vaccination is recommended in 50- to 70-year-old adults.

COMMONLY ASSOCIATED CONDITIONS
- Viral infection (e.g., common cold)
- Possible sexually transmitted infection

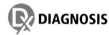**DIAGNOSIS**

HISTORY

ALERT
Red flag: Any decrease in visual acuity is not consistent with conjunctivitis alone; must document normal vision for diagnosis of true isolated conjunctivitis

- Viral: contact or travel
  - May start with one eye and then both
  - If herpetic, recurrences or vesicles on skin
- Bacterial: difficult to distinguish from viral. Assume bacterial in contact lens wearer, unless cultures are negative. If recent STD, suspect chlamydia or gonococcal infection. Nursing home residents may have MRSA conjunctivitis and should be cultured.
- Allergic: itching, atopy, seasonal, dander
- Irritative: feels dry, exposure to wind, tear-film deficit may persist 30 days after acute conjunctivitis, chemicals such as chlorine from pools or drug: atropine, aminoglycosides, iodide, phenylephrine, antivirals, bisphosphonates, retinoids, topiramate, chamomile, COX-2 inhibitors, immune modulators
- Foreign body: Redness may persist 24 hours after removal.

PHYSICAL EXAM
- General: common to all types of conjunctivitis
  - Red eye, conjunctival injection
  - Foreign body sensation
  - Eyelid sticking or crusting, discharge
  - Normal visual acuity and pupillary reactivity
- Viral
  - Upper respiratory "cold" symptoms and preauricular lymphadenopathy may be present.
  - Hemorrhagic coxsackievirus, adenoviral epidemics seen in health care facilities and community
  - Severe viral: herpes simplex or zoster:
    ○ Burning sensation, rarely itching
    ○ Unilateral, dermatomal distribution herpetic skin vesicles in zoster
    ○ Palpable preauricular node
  - Bacterial (non-STD): may be epidemic
  - Mild pruritus, discharge mild to heavy
  - Conjunctival chemosis/edema
  - If contact lens user, must rule out pseudomonal (or other bacterial) keratitis. If long-term care resident, culture to rule out MRSA.
- Bacterial: gonococcal (or meningococcal) hyperacute infection
  - Rapid onset 12 to 24 hours

- Severe purulent discharge
- Chemosis/conjunctival/eyelid edema
- Rapid growth of superior corneal ulceration
- Preauricular adenopathy
- Signs of STDs (chlamydia, GC, HIV, etc.)
- Allergic
  - Itching predominant, chemosis, edema
  - Seasonal or animal dander allergies
- Nonspecific irritative
  - Dry eyes, intermittent redness, chemical/drug exposure
  - Foreign body: may have redness and discharge 24 hours after removal
- Must document normal visual acuity
- Cornea should be clear and without fluorescein uptake. Cloudy or ulcerated cornea signifies keratitis; consult ophthalmologist.
- Fluorescein stain exam is recommended. Evert lid to inspect for foreign bodies.
- Skin: Look for herpetic vesicles, nits on lashes (lice), scaliness (seborrhea), lid inflammation (blepharitis, rosacea, or styes).
- Limbal flush at corneal margin if uveitis
- If pupil is irregular (i.e., penetrating foreign body), emergent referral is warranted.
- Discharge on lid margin but no conjunctival injection: blepharitis

DIFFERENTIAL DIAGNOSIS
- Punctate keratitis due to prolonged contact lens wear
- Phlyctenular conjunctivitis: localized nodules with hyperemia from immune response to *Staphylococcus* and TB
- Uveitis (iritis, iridocyclitis, choroiditis): limbal flush (red band at corneal margin), hazy anterior chamber, and decreased visual acuity
- Acute glaucoma (emergency): headache, corneal clouding, poor visual acuity
- Corneal ulcer, keratitis, or foreign body: lesions or tear-film deficits on fluorescein exam
- Dacryocystitis: tenderness and swelling over tear sac (below medial canthus)
- Scleritis and episcleritis: red injected vessels radially oriented, sectoral (pie wedge), nodularity of sclera
- Pingueculitis: inflammation of a yellow nodular or wedge-like area of chronic conjunctival degeneration (pinguecula)
- Ophthalmia neonatorum: neonates in the first 2 days of life (gonococcal; 5 to 12 days of life): chlamydial, herpes simplex virus (HSV)
- Blepharitis: Lid margins are inflamed producing itching, scale, or discharge but no conjunctival injection.

DIAGNOSTIC TESTS & INTERPRETATION
- Usually not needed initially for most common causes, if COVID-19 epidemic related, consider viral PCR or antigen.
- Culture swab if STD suspected severe symptoms, contact lens user, or failed prior treatment.
- Viral swab (10-minute test) for adenovirus is costly, and may not be tolerated by children.

Diagnostic Procedures/Other
- Fluorescein exam to rule out corneal ulcer, herpes zoster, or abrasion.
- Remove small, superficial foreign bodies with irrigation or moistened swab.
- Refer cases of prolonged symptoms (>7 days) to confirm diagnosis and exclude need for biopsy.

💉 TREATMENT

GENERAL MEASURES
- Viral conjunctivitis does not require antibiotics, most resolve spontaneously.
- Clean external eyelid with wet cloth up to 4×/day.
- Stop use of contact lenses as long as eye is red.
- Eye patching is not beneficial.

MEDICATION

First Line
- Viral (nonherpetic)
  - Artificial tears for symptomatic relief
  - Vasoconstrictor/antihistamine (e.g., naphazoline/pheniramine) QID for severe itching
  - May consider topical antibiotic (see bacterial below) if return to daycare requires treatment
  - If very severe or prolonged, refer to ophthalmologist for possible steroid
- Viral (herpetic) (ophthalmology consultation)
  - Ganciclovir gel: 0.15%, 5 times per day for 7 days (2)[B]
  - Acyclovir: PO 400 mg 5 times per day for HSV; 800 mg for zoster for 7 days
- Bacterial (nonsexually transmitted): 3 days of cool compresses before starting antibiotic reduces unnecessary antibiotic use.
  - If preferred may use topical antibiotics (NNT 7 by day 6) (immediate topical antibiotics may allow for earlier return to school for some children):
  - Bacitracin ophthalmic ointment (over the counter [OTC]): Apply 3 to 4 times per day for 5 to 7 days.
  - Povidone-iodine 1.25% ophthalmic solution (antimicrobial lubricant OTC) 1 gtt 4 times per day for 5 to 7 days (1)[A]
  - Polymyxin B-trimethoprim solution 1 gtt 6 times per day for 5 to 7 days
  - Erythromycin ophthalmic ointment: 1/2 inch 2 to 4 times per day for 5 days
  - Sodium sulfacetamide (Bleph-10) (10% solution): 2 drops q4h (while awake) for 5 days
  - Tobramycin or gentamicin: 0.3% ophthalmic drops/ointment q4h (drops) to q8h (ointment) for 7 days
- Bacterial (gonococcal)
  - Neonates: Hospitalize for IV ceftriaxone or cefotaxime.
  - Adults: ceftriaxone: 1 g IM as single dose and topical bacitracin ophthalmic ointment 1/2 inch QID. Neonates 25 to 50 mg/kg IV or IM, not to exceed 125 mg, as a single dose. Chlamydia in neonates requires oral erythromycin: 50 mg/kg/day divided q6h PO for 14 days, max 3 g/day.
- Allergic and atopic: OTC medications are efficacious, no definitive evidence favoring one over another, cost varies widely (3)[A].
  - Ketotifen (Zaditor, Alaway, and other generics OTC): 0.25% 1 drop 2 times per day
  - Ketorolac (Acular): 0.1% 1 drop 4 times per day
  - Cetirizine (Zerviate): 24% 1 drop 2 times per day
  - Olopatadine (Pataday, Patanol): 0.1% 1 drop 2 times per day or 0.2% 1 drop daily
  - Cromolyn (Opticrom): 4% 1 drop 4 times per day
  - Naphazoline (Vasocon-A, Naphcon-A, Opcon-A, Visine-A: OTC) 1 drop 4 times a day
  - Azelastine (Astelin): 0.05% 1 drop 2 times per day
  - Nedocromil (Alocril): 2% 1 drop 2 times per day
  - Alcaftadine (Lastacaft): 0.25% 1 drop daily
  - Emedastine (Emadine): 0.05% 1 drop 2 times/day
  - Oral nonsedating antihistamines (cetirizine [Zyrtec] 10 mg/day, fexofenadine [Allegra] 60 mg BID, etc.) may treat nasal symptoms but cause ocular drying; oral antihistamine (e.g., diphenhydramine 25 mg TID) in severe cases of itching

- Contraindications: steroids not beneficial in treatment of bacterial keratitis (4)[A]. Any topical steroid requires baseline and periodic specialist's exam for corneal ulcers, glaucoma, and cataracts, especially in children <10 years. Topical immune modulators (tacrolimus, cyclosporine) should be reserved for specialist use only in the most difficult cases.
- Precautions
  - Do not allow dropper to touch the eye.
  - Case reports of eye irritation from gentamicin in infants, moxifloxacin in adults, sulfacetamide in allergic individuals
  - Vasoconstrictor/antihistamine: rebound vasodilation after prolonged use

Second Line
- Viral and allergic: numerous OTC products, oral montelukast 10 mg daily
- Bacterial: second line (quinolones used as postoperative or for known resistant organisms)
  - Ofloxacin: 0.3% 1 gtt QID for 7 days
  - Ciprofloxacin: 0.3% 1 gtt QID for 7 days
  - Levofloxacin: 0.3% 1 gtt QID for 7 days
  - Azithromycin: 1.5% BID for 3 days

ISSUES FOR REFERRAL
- Refer to ophthalmology for decreased visual acuity, suspected herpetic keratitis/contact lens–related conjunctivitis or immunocompromised (HIV).
- Refer for prolonged symptoms or worsening over 7 days (concern for severe adenoviral keratitis) .

COMPLEMENTARY & ALTERNATIVE MEDICINE
- Usually benign and self-limited; saline flushes, cool compresses, and similar treatments help.
- Mandarin orange yogurt oral showed improvement over 2 weeks for allergic pollen conjunctivitis in a small study.

ADMISSION, INPATIENT, AND NURSING CONSIDERATIONS
- Acute gonococcal conjunctivitis (or very rare case of meningococcal conjunctivitis) requires inpatient treatment with ceftriaxone 50 mg/kg IV everyday (pediatric), 1 g IM for one (adult) along with ophthalmologic consultation.
- Admission criteria/initial stabilization
  - Penetrating ocular trauma, gonococcal conjunctivitis

ONGOING CARE

FOLLOW-UP RECOMMENDATIONS
- If not resolved within 5 to 7 days, reconsider diagnosis or consult specialist; some epidemic keratoconjunctivitis and other adenoviral conjunctivitis typically last 1 to 2 weeks.
- Children may be excluded from school until eye is no longer red, depending on school policy. Allergic conjunctivitis (noncontagious) should return to school with doctor's note.

Patient Monitoring
Patient should follow up in 1 day if any worsening.

PATIENT EDUCATION
- No contact lenses until eyes are fully healed (~1 week). Discard current contact lenses.
- Adenovirus may persist on surfaces up to 28 days, instruct to practice soap hand-washing and hypochlorite wipe use for surfaces.
- Discard old eye makeup, especially mascara.
- Cool, moist compresses can ease irritation and itch.

PROGNOSIS
- Viral: 5 to 10 days of symptoms for pharyngitis with conjunctivitis, 2 weeks with adenovirus
- Herpes simplex: 2 to 3 weeks of symptoms
- Most common bacterial—H. influenzae, Staphylococcus, Streptococcus: self-limited; 74–80% resolution within 7 days, whether treated or not

COMPLICATIONS
- Corneal scars with herpes simplex
- Lid scars, conjunctival scars, symblepharon, or entropion may occur with varicella zoster and chlamydia or any severe inflammation.
- Corneal ulcers or perforation
- Hypopyon: pus in anterior chamber
- Chlamydial neonatal (ophthalmic): could have concomitant pneumonia
- Otitis media may follow H. influenzae conjunctivitis.
- Very rarely N. meningitidis conjunctivitis may be followed by meningitis.

REFERENCES

1. Steeples L, Mercieca K. Acute conjunctivitis in primary care: antibiotics and placebo associated with small increase in the proportion cured by 7 days compared with no treatment. Evid Based Med. 2012;17(6):177–178.
2. Wilhelmus KR. Antiviral treatment and other therapeutic interventions for herpes simplex virus epithelial keratitis. Cochrane Database Syst Rev. 2015;(1):CD002898.
3. Castillo M, Scott NW, Mustafa MZ, et al. Topical antihistamines and mast cell stabilisers for treating seasonal and perennial allergic conjunctivitis. Cochrane Database Syst Rev. 2015;(6):CD009566.
4. Herretes S, Wang X, Reyes JM. Topical corticosteroids as adjunctive therapy for bacterial keratitis. Cochrane Database Syst Rev. 2014;(10):CD005430.

🔁 SEE ALSO

- Rhinitis, Allergic
- Algorithm: Eye Pain

CODES

ICD10
- H10.30 Unspecified acute conjunctivitis, unspecified eye
- H10.33 Unspecified acute conjunctivitis, bilateral
- H10.32 Unspecified acute conjunctivitis, left eye

CLINICAL PEARLS
- Conjunctivitis does not cause decreased acuity or photophobia. If visual acuity is decreased, consider more serious ophthalmic disorders.
- Culture discharge in all contact lens wearers and nursing home residents. Consider referral, discard current lenses, and use spectacles for visual correction until eyes are fully healed.
- Antibiotics are of no value in viral conjunctivitis (most cases of infectious conjunctivitis).
- Cool compresses for 3 days before using any antibiotic is appropriate for treating conjunctivitis in healthy adults and children >1 month.

CONSTIPATION
Daniel R. Matta, MD • Alexandra Wright, MBBS, Hons

BASICS

- Unsatisfactory defecation characterized by infrequent stools, difficult stool passage, or both
- Characteristics include <3 bowel movements a week, hard stools, excessive straining, prolonged time spent on the toilet, a sense of incomplete evacuation, and abdominal discomfort/bloating.

DESCRIPTION

Geriatric Considerations
Colorectal neoplasms may be associated with constipation. Consider new-onset constipation after age 50 years a "red flag." Use warm water enemas (instead of sodium phosphate enemas) for impaction in geriatric patients. Sodium phosphate enemas have been associated with fatalities and severe electrolyte disturbances.

Pediatric Considerations
Consider Hirschsprung disease (absence of colonic ganglion cells) in cases of pediatric constipation. Hirschsprung disease accounts for 25% of all newborn intestinal obstructions and can present as milder cases diagnosed in older children with chronic constipation, abdominal distension, and decreased growth. Hirschsprung has a 5:1 male-to-female ratio and is associated with inherited conditions (e.g., Down syndrome).

Pregnancy Considerations
Avoid misoprostol.

EPIDEMIOLOGY
- More pronounced in children and elderly
- Predominant sex: female > male (2:1)
- Nonwhites > whites

Incidence
- 5 million office visits annually
- 100,000 hospitalizations

Prevalence
- 16% of adults >18 years, rising to 33% of adults >60 years of age
- 3% of pediatric visits relate to constipation.

ETIOLOGY AND PATHOPHYSIOLOGY
Defecation reflex is a reflex that can be inhibited by voluntarily contracting the external sphincter or facilitated by straining to contract the abdominal muscles while voluntarily relaxing the anal sphincter. Rectal distention initiates the defecation reflex. The urge to defecate occurs with an increase in rectal pressure. Distention of the stomach also initiates rectal contractions and a desire to defecate (gastrocolic reflex).

RISK FACTORS
- Extremes of age
- Polypharmacy
- Sedentary lifestyle or condition
- Low-fiber diet and inadequate fluid intake

GENERAL PREVENTION
High-fiber diet, adequate fluids, exercise, and training to "obey the urge" to defecate

COMMONLY ASSOCIATED CONDITIONS
- General debilitation (disease or aging)
- Dehydration
- Hypothyroidism
- Hypokalemia
- Hypercalcemia
- Nursing home resident

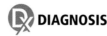

DIAGNOSIS

ALERT
Red flags:

- New onset after age of 50 years
- Hematochezia/melena
- Unintentional weight loss
- Family history of colon cancer
- Anemia
- Neurologic defects

HISTORY
- Assess onset of symptoms, number of bowel movements per week, straining, completeness of evacuation, and use of manual manipulation.
- Identify red flags; evaluate diet, lifestyle, prescription, and OTC medication use; identify reversible causes; ask about history of sexual abuse, opioid use.
- Bristol Stool Form Scale—seven categories of consistency (1)
- A diary of dietary intake and bowel patterns helps to measure treatment response.
- Rome III criteria:
  - At least two of the following for 12 weeks in the previous 6 months:
    - <3 stools per week
    - Straining at least 1/4 of the time
    - Hard stools at least 1/4 of time
    - Need for manual assist at least 1/4 of time
    - Sense of incomplete evacuation at least 1/4 of time
    - Sense of anorectal blockade at least 1/4 of time
  - Loose stools rarely seen without use of laxatives
  - Frequent constipation but does not meet irritable bowel syndrome (IBS) criteria
  - Although there can be overlap, the history of primary constipation differs from constipation-predominant IBS.
    - In primary constipation, pain and bloating are relieved by adequate defecation. In IBS, pain and bloating predominate and are not readily relieved by defecation.
- Bowel Function Index—for opioid-induced constipation (OIC) score of 0 to 100, mean of three variables; ease of defecation, completeness of emptying, patient's rating of constipation severity

PHYSICAL EXAM
- Vital signs
- Abdominal exam, previous surgical scars, hypoactive bowel sounds, tenderness, and masses
- Gynecologic exam: Evaluate for masses and rectocele.
- Digital rectal exam: Evaluate for structural lesions: masses, stool, fissures, and hemorrhoids; assess for pelvic floor dyssynergia and sphincter tone
- Neurologic exam

DIFFERENTIAL DIAGNOSIS
- Primary constipation (primary problem is within the GI tract) has four subtypes.
  - Normal colonic transit time most common subtype; can be difficult to differentiate from constipation-predominant IBS
  - Slow colonic transit time
  - Pelvic floor/anal sphincter dysfunction (defecatory disorders)
  - Combination pelvic floor/anal sphincter dysfunction and slow transit
- Secondary constipation (outside the GI tract)
  - Endocrine dysfunction (diabetes mellitus, hypothyroid)
  - Metabolic disorder (increased calcium, decreased potassium)
  - Mechanical (obstruction, rectocele)
  - Pregnancy
  - Neurologic disorders (Hirschsprung, multiple sclerosis, spinal cord injuries, Parkinson disease)
- Congenital
  - Hirschsprung disease/syndrome
  - Hypoganglionosis
  - Congenital dilation of the colon
  - Small left colon syndrome
- Medication effect
  - Opioids
  - Antidepressants
  - Antipsychotics
  - Antacids (calcium, aluminum)
  - Nondihydropyridine calcium channel blockers, especially verapamil
  - Iron and multivitamins with iron
  - Diuretics
  - Overuse of antidiarrheal medications

DIAGNOSTIC TESTS & INTERPRETATION
Identify red flags, secondary causes, and reversible conditions. If none present, go to first-line treatment.

Initial Tests (lab, imaging)
- CBC to screen for iron deficiency anemia
- Consider toxicology screen if illicit opioid use is suspected.
- Calcium, glucose, and thyroid function testing (TSH) based on history and exam. If red flags are present, refer for sigmoid/colonoscopy.

Follow-Up Tests & Special Considerations
For patients with pelvic floor dysfunction, suspected defecatory disorders or exam abnormalities (e.g., rectocele), and/or patients who are refractory to initial treatment, refer to an experienced subspecialist. A physical therapist experienced in biofeedback can also be very helpful.

Diagnostic Procedures/Other
- Anorectal manometry (ARM)
- Balloon expulsion testing (BET)
- Surface electromyelography
- Barium or magnetic resonance defecography
- Radiopaque markers and scintigraphy

Test Interpretation
- ARM and BET recommended for all refractory cases
- If ARM and BET are negative, barium or magnetic resonance defecography to evaluate transit time
- Consider biofeedback.

 TREATMENT

Address immediate concerns:
- Bloating/discomfort/straining: osmotic agents
- Postoperative, after childbirth, hemorrhoids, fissures: stool softener to aid defecation
- If impacted, manual disimpaction and then treat any underlying conditions

GENERAL MEASURES
In patients with no known secondary causes, conservative nonpharmacologic treatment is recommended.
- Eliminate medications that cause constipation.
- Increase fluid intake.
- Increase soluble fiber in diet.
- Encourage regular defecation attempts after eating.
- Regular exercise
- Enemas if other methods fail (Avoid sodium phosphate enemas in geriatric patients.)

MEDICATION
Nonprescription medications are first line. If patient goals are not reached, advance to prescription medications.

First Line
Bulking agents (accompanied by adequate fluids)
- Osmotic laxatives
  - Polyethylene glycol (PEG) (MiraLAX) 17 g/day PO dissolved in 4 to 8 oz of beverage (current evidence shows PEG to be superior to lactulose) (2)[B]
  - Lactulose (Chronulac, Enulose) 15 to 60 mL PO QHS (flatulence, bloating, cramping)
  - Sorbitol: 15 to 60 mL PO QHS (as effective as lactulose)
  - Magnesium salts (milk of magnesia): 15 to 30 mL PO once daily; avoid in renal insufficiency.
- Hydrophilic colloids (bulk-forming agents)
  - Psyllium (Konsyl, Metamucil, Perdiem Fiber): 1 tbsp in 8-oz liquid PO daily up to TID
  - Methylcellulose (Citrucel): 1 tbsp in 8-oz liquid PO daily up to TID
  - Polycarbophil (Mitrolan, FiberCon): 2 caplets with 8-oz liquid PO up to QID
- Stool softeners
  - Docusate sodium (Colace): 50 to 100 mg PO TID

Second Line
- Stimulants (irritate bowel, causing muscle contraction; usually combined with a softener; work in 8 to 12 hours)
  - Senna/docusate (Senokot-S, Ex-Lax, Peri-Colace): 1 to 2 tablets or 15 to 30 mL PO at bedtime
  - Bisacodyl (Dulcolax, Correctol): 1 to 3 tablets PO daily
- Lubricants (soften stool and facilitate passage of the feces by its lubricating oily effects)
  - Mineral oil (15 to 45 mL/day)
  - Short-term use only; can bind fat-soluble vitamins, with the potential for deficiencies; may similarly decrease absorption of some drugs
  - Avoid in those at risk for aspiration (lipoid pneumonia).

- Suppositories
  - Osmotic: sodium phosphate
  - Lubricant: glycerin
  - Stimulatory: bisacodyl
  - Enemas: saline (Fleet enema)
- Long-term prescription agents
  - Lubiprostone (Amitiza): a selective chloride channel activator; 24 μg PO BID
  - Prucalopride (Motegrity): a serotonin-4 receptor antagonist; adult dose: 2 mg PO once daily, for CrCl <30 use 1 mg once daily; increased incidence of suicidal ideation reported in clinical trials
- Guanylate cyclase-C agonists (adult use only)
  - Plecanatide (Trulance): dose: 3 mg PO once daily
  - Linaclotide (Linzess): dose: 145 μg PO once daily; can use lower dose 72 μg once daily
- OIC
- Trial of laxatives first, followed by peripherally acting μ-opioid receptor antagonists
  - Methylnaltrexone (Relistor): dose: 38 to <62 kg: 8 mg; 62 to 114 kg: 12 mg SC every other day PRN
  - Naloxegol (Movantik): dose: 12.5 to 25.0 mg PO daily; discontinue other laxatives for 3 days when initiating naloxegol; avoid in patients on strong CYP3A4 inhibitors due to increased naloxegol levels and risk of opioid withdrawal.
  - Naldemedine (Symproic): dose: 0.2 mg PO daily; monitor for opioid withdrawal in patients on strong CYP3A4 inhibitors or P-gp inhibitors.
- Linaclotide (Linzess): dose 145 μg PO once daily; can use lower dose 72 μg once daily
- Prokinetic agents (partial 5-HT4 agonists): cisapride (Propulsid) has been withdrawn due to cardiac side effects; only available via IND protocols; tegaserod (Zelnorm) available for IBS-C; side effects include cardiac events, ischemic colitis, and suicidal ideation.

ADDITIONAL THERAPIES
- Other nonpharmacologic therapies include biofeedback, a first-line recommendation for patients with refractory constipation due to functional conditions involving dyssynergic defecation or inadequate propulsive force.
- Behavior therapy
- Acupuncture: initial randomized trial effective at 20 weeks; longer term trials needed (3)[B]

SURGERY/OTHER PROCEDURES
Surgery rarely indicated; sometimes required for anatomic findings (rectocele or enterocoele)

ADMISSION, INPATIENT, AND NURSING CONSIDERATIONS
- Toxic megacolon
- Manual disimpaction occasionally required in chronic refractory cases

 ONGOING CARE

DIET
Increase soluble fiber (bloating and gas can be problematic with insoluble fiber):
- Gradually increase intake to 25 g/day over a 6-week period.
- Oat bran (hard outer layer of cereal grains)
- Peas; onions; lentils; beans; seeds; nuts; and fruits, including bananas, apples, and strawberries
- Encourage liberal intake of fluids.

PATIENT EDUCATION
- Occasional mild constipation is normal.
- Bowel training: The best time to move bowels is in the morning, after eating breakfast, when the normal bowel transit and defecation reflexes are functioning.

PROGNOSIS
- Occasional constipation responds well to simple measures.
- Habitual constipation can be a lifelong nuisance.
- Patients with neurologic compromise can suffer from obstipation, impaction, and toxic megacolon.
- No evidence for laxative dependence or harm from stimulant use; melanosis coli may develop but is a benign condition.

COMPLICATIONS
- Volvulus
- Toxic megacolon
- Acquired megacolon in severe, long-standing cases
- Fluid and electrolyte depletion: laxative abuse
- Rectal ulceration (stercoral ulcer) related to recurrent fecal impaction
- Anal fissures

REFERENCES
1. Lewis SJ, Heaton KW. Stool form scale as a useful guide to intestinal transit time. *Scand J Gastroenterol*. 1997;32(9):920–924.
2. Lee-Robichaud H, Thomas K, Morgan J, et al. Lactulose versus polyethylene glycol for chronic constipation. *Cochrane Database Syst Rev*. 2010;(7):CD007570.
3. Liu Z, Yan S, Wu J, et al. Acupuncture for chronic severe functional constipation: a randomized trial. *Ann Intern Med*. 2016;165(11):761–769.

ADDITIONAL READING
Bharucha AE, Lacy BE. Mechanisms, evaluation and management of chronic constipation. *Gastroenterology*. 2020;158(5):1232–1249.e3.

 CODES

ICD10
- K59.00 Constipation, unspecified
- K59.01 Slow transit constipation
- K59.09 Other constipation

CLINICAL PEARLS
- Constipation (especially with normal transit time) is common. Reversible risk factors include inadequate hydration, sedentary lifestyle, poor dietary habits, and medication side effects.
- Red flags: onset >50 years, hematochezia/melena, unintentional weight loss, anemia, neurologic defects
- Osmotic agents (PEG) are the most clinically effective."

CONTRACEPTION

Chloe Sabine Courchesne, MD

BASICS

DESCRIPTION
- Medications or procedures that control timing of pregnancies and prevent unintended pregnancies
- Options are divided into two major categories: hormonal and nonhormonal.

EPIDEMIOLOGY
Incidence
- The estimated prevalence of contraception use in the United States among women 15 to 49 years is 65%.
- 45% of pregnancies in the United States are unintended. Half occur in women using reversible contraception. Unintended pregnancies are associated with increased risk of adverse maternal and infant outcomes.

RISK FACTORS
Unintended pregnancy: higher rates among women ages 18 to 24 and >40, unmarried women, women with less than a college education, and minority women

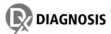

DIAGNOSIS

HISTORY
- Review past medical, family, social, obstetric, and gynecologic histories including menstrual history, prior contraceptive use, and prior sexually transmitted infections (STIs).
- Screen for hypertension.
- In family history of thrombophilia, consider testing before initiation of estrogen-containing contraception.
- Contraindications: See CDC medical eligibility criteria (MEC) (1).
  - Estrogen-progestin contraceptives
    - Common absolute: age ≥35 years and smoking ≥15 cigarettes per day, <21 days postpartum, SBP ≥160 mm Hg or DBP ≥100 mm Hg, current/prior venous thromboembolism (VTE), thrombophilia, long-standing/complicated diabetes, ischemic heart disease, systemic lupus, migraine with aura, breast cancer
    - Common relative: age ≥35 years and smoking <15 cigarettes per day, breastfeeding <42 days postpartum, SBP 140 to 159 mm Hg or DBP 90 to 99 mm Hg (or well-controlled on medications), bariatric surgery, migraines without aura but ≥35 years, breast cancer history
  - Progestin-only (pill/Depo/implant)
    - Absolute: current breast cancer
    - Common relative: bariatric surgery, heart disease, stroke, lupus, migraine with aura
  - Levonorgestrel—intrauterine device (IUD)
    - Common absolute: postseptic abortion, postpartum sepsis, current breast cancer, distorted uterine cavity
    - Absolute contraindications for initiation but do not require discontinuation: cervical/endometrial cancer, PID, known untreated chlamydia, or gonorrhea infection
    - Common relative: heart disease, lupus

- Copper IUD ("ParaGard")
  - Absolute: same as levonorgestrel IUD, okay to use in breast cancer
  - Absolute contraindications for initiation but not continuation: same as levonorgestrel IUD
  - Relative: thrombocytopenia, solid organ transplant

DIAGNOSTIC TESTS & INTERPRETATION
Initial Tests (lab, imaging)
- A pregnancy test
- Consider testing for gonorrhea and chlamydia prior to IUD insertion.
- Pap smear if indicated

TREATMENT

GENERAL MEASURES
Method(s) should be selected based on patient preference, effectiveness, need for STI prevention, side effects, and contraindications.

MEDICATION
- Estrogen-progestin contraceptives
  - Mechanism of action: suppression of ovulation, thickening of cervical mucus, and endometrial changes
  - Efficacy: failure rate of 9% with typical use and 0.3% with perfect use at 1 year (2)
  - Side effects: irregular bleeding, nausea, headaches, mastalgia, depression
  - Combined oral contraceptives (COCs)
    - COCs all contain ethinyl estradiol but differ in the amount (10 to 50 μg) and type of progestin.
    - Dosing
      - Most have 21 active days and 7 placebo days.
      - Alternatively, active pills can be taken continuously with scheduled withdrawal bleeds.
    - Initiation
      - Recommended: "quick start" (Begin pill on the day medication is obtained.)
      - Alternative: Begin the pill on the 1st day of menses or first Sunday.
        - Note: If not starting pill within 5 days of start of menses, backup contraception is recommended for 7 days.
  - Weekly hormonal patch
    - Applied transdermally and changed weekly for 3 weeks. No patch worn during week 4 for withdrawal bleeding, unless user prefers fewer yearly periods (continuous cycling).
    - Ortho Evra, Xulane:
      - 20 μg/day ethinyl estradiol and 150 μg/day norelgestromin
      - Produces higher serum estrogen levels than oral 20-μg pill (slightly increased risk of VTE)
      - Application site irritation; reduced efficacy in women >90 kg
    - Twirla:
      - 30 μg/day of ethinyl estradiol and 120 μg/day of levonorgestrel
      - Common adverse reactions: application site disorders, nausea, headache, weight gain
      - Contraindicated in women with a BMI ≥30kg/m². Reduced effectiveness in women with a BMI ≥25 to <30 kg/m²

- Vaginal contraceptive ring
  - Ring is inserted in the vagina and remains in place for 3 weeks followed by 1 week of ring-free interval; may also use continuous cycling for 4 weeks, then immediately replaced with a new ring (off-label). Common adverse reactions: headaches, nausea and vomiting, vulvovaginal mycotic infection, vaginal discharge, UTI
  - NuvaRing:
    - 15 μg/day of ethinyl estradiol and 120 μg/day of etonogestrel absorbed via vaginal wall
    - Although systemic exposure to estrogen is about 50% of exposure with COCs, the risk of VTE is similar.
  - Annovera:
    - Single ring is cleaned and used for up to one year.
    - Not adequately evaluated in females with a BMI >29 kg/m².
- Progestin-only birth control
  - Mechanism of action: Primary mechanism is ovulation inhibition with possible secondary benefit from thickening of cervical mucus and thinning of endometrial lining.
  - Progestin-only pill (Micronor)
    - Efficacy: failure rate of about 0.3% with perfect use, 9% with typical use at 1 year (2)
    - Can be used in some women with contraindications to estrogen, including, e.g., breastfeeding women
    - Dosing: 1 pill at the same time daily, no placebo days
    - Side effects: irregular bleeding
  - Injectable contraceptive (medroxyprogesterone acetate) (Depo-Provera)
    - Efficacy: failure rate of 0.2% with perfect use, 6% with typical use at 1 year (2)
    - Dosing: one injection every 3 months. Contraceptive levels of hormone persist for up to 4 months.
    - Side effects: irregular bleeding, weight gain (average of 5 lb/year of use), amenorrhea, depression
- LARCs: IUDs and implantable devices
  - Mirena (52-mg levonorgestrel-releasing IUD):
    - Primary mechanism of action: produces sterile inflammatory reaction due to foreign body that is toxic to sperm and ova, thickens cervical mucus
    - Efficacy: failure rate of 0.2% with both perfect and typical use at 1 year (2)
    - Dosing: 20 μg/day initially; reduces to 10 μg/day (approved for 6 years; used off-label for 7 years)
    - Safe and recommended in nulliparous women/teenagers
    - Can be inserted immediately postpartum or immediately following D&C for miscarriage or abortion; associated with higher rates of expulsion compared to delayed placement (6 to 10 weeks)
    - Side effects: irregular bleeding for first 3 to 6 months that usually resolves; may see amenorrhea after 1 year
    - Side effect management: Consider NSAIDs, COCs, or progestin-only pills for spotting and cramps.

- Liletta (52-mg levonorgestrel-releasing IUD):
  - Dosing: 18.6 μg/day initially; reduces to 12.6 μg/day (approved for 5 years)
- Kyleena (19.5-mg levonorgestrel-releasing IUD):
  - Dosing: 17.5 μg/day initially; reduced to 7.5 μg/day (approved for 5 years)
- Skyla (13.5-mg levonorgestrel-releasing IUD):
  - Dosing:14 μg/day initially; reduces to 5 μg/day (approved for 3 years)
  - Smaller insertion tube; more bleeding days than Mirena
- ParaGard (copper IUD):
  - Primary mechanism of action: produces sterile inflammatory reaction
  - Efficacy: failure rate of 0.6% with perfect use, 0.8% with typical use at 1 year (2)
  - Approved for 10 years
  - Same insertion timing as levonorgestrel-IUD
  - Side effects: increased menstrual bleeding and cramping
- Nexplanon (etonogestrel implant):
  - Mechanism of action: inhibits ovulation
  - Efficacy: failure rate of 0.05% with perfect use, 0.3% with typical use at 1 year
  - Dosing: semirigid plastic rod containing 68 mg of etonogestrel; initially 60 to 70 μg/day; subsequently 25 to 30 μg/day
  - Up to 3 years
  - Inserted only by certified providers, but technique is simple to learn
  - Side effects: menstrual irregularities (common for 6 to 12 months, may persist for 3 years)
- Emergency contraception: initiated as soon as possible after unprotected intercourse. Copper IUD is the most effective, followed by ulipristal, levonorgestrel, and Yuzpe method.
  - Copper IUD (ParaGard): up to 5 days after intercourse; 0.04 to 0.19% failure rate
  - Ulipristal acetate (Ella): 30 mg once; selective progesterone modulator, up to 5 days after intercourse 2% failure rate
  - Levonorgestrel: 1.5 mg taken as two 0.75-mg tablets (Plan B) or one 1.5-mg tablet (Plan B One-Step); most effective within 72 hours. 1.1–2.4% failure rate. Less nausea than "Yuzpe regimen." Available over the counter; likely ineffective for women with BMI >30
  - "Yuzpe regimen" 50 μg/0.25 mg, 2 tablets q12h (4 tablets total). Any OCP may be used as long as the dose of estrogen component ≥100 μg/dose. 3.2% failure rate. *Note*: Antiemetic should be given 1 to 2 hours.

ADDITIONAL THERAPIES
- Male condoms: failure rate of 2% with perfect use, 18% with typical use at 1 year (2)
- Spermicides: All contain nonoxynol-9; may alter vaginal flora and mucosal barrier. Failure rate: 28% with typical use at 1 year (2)

- Sponge (Today Sponge): Soft foam disk contains nonoxynol-9. Moisten with water before use; effective for 24 hours; must leave in for 6 hours after use. Failure rate: 12–24% with typical use (2)
- Diaphragm: latex or silicone dome-shaped device with flexible spring-activated rim, prevents sperm from entering cervix; used with spermicides. Failure rate: 12% with typical use, 6% with perfect use at 1 year (2)
- Phexxi: nonhormonal spermicidal prescription contraceptive approved by the FDA in 2020. It is a combination of lactic acid, citric acid, and potassium bitartrate indicated as an on demand method of contraception. Administer single-dose applicator vaginally immediately before or up to 1 hour prior to each episode of intercourse. May be used with other methods except vaginal ring. Avoid use in women with a history of recurrent UTIs or urinary tract abnormalities. Common side effects: discomfort, mycotic infection, UTI, and bacterial vaginosis. Failure rate: 13.7%

SURGERY/OTHER PROCEDURES
Permanent sterilization
- Female: tubal ligation. Failure rate: 0.5% at 1 year (2)
- Male: vasectomy. Failure rate: 0.15% at 1 year (2)

COMPLEMENTARY & ALTERNATIVE MEDICINE
- Fertility awareness methods. Failure rate: 24% at 1 year typical use (2)
- Withdrawal method: failure rate: 22% at 1 year (2)
- Lactational amenorrhea method: effective only if the infant is <6 months old and exclusively breastfeeding, and mother has not resumed regular menses. Failure rate: 7% at 1 year typical use

Pediatric Considerations
AAP and ACOG recommend LARCs as first-line agents.

 ONGOING CARE

FOLLOW-UP RECOMMENDATIONS
Patient Monitoring
- 2 to 3 months postinitiation to assess tolerance
- Check for IUD strings 1 month after insertion; spontaneous expulsion rate highest in the 1st month
- BP check within 3 months of initiating on estrogen-containing methods

DIET
St. John's wort may alter estrogen levels.

PATIENT EDUCATION
- Diaphragm: Insert before intercourse using spermicide per manufacturer's recommendations.
- Male condom: Describe proper use.
- IUD: Patient should monitor presence of the string monthly.

- Backup birth control is needed for the first 7 days with quick start.
- STI prevention
- Timing of various methods
- Useful patient education materials: https://www.reproductiveaccess.org/contraception/ and https://www.cdc.gov/reproductivehealth/contraception/

COMPLICATIONS
- Estrogen-progestin contraceptives:
  - Serious (requires discontinuation): stroke, thromboembolism, hypertension, myocardial infarction, and cholestatic jaundice
- Injectable contraceptive:
  - Decreased bone mineral density (BMD) if used for ≥2 years. Mostly recovers after discontinuation. Consider calcium/vitamin D supplementation if prolonged use.
- Nexplanon: insertion site reaction including pain, bleeding, paresthesias, and infection
- IUDs:
  - Uterine perforation
  - Absolute risk of ectopic pregnancy is reduced with IUD, but if pregnancy does occur, there is a higher risk that it will be ectopic.
- Sponge and diaphragm: toxic shock syndrome

REFERENCES
1. Centers for Disease Control and Prevention. US Medical Eligibility Criteria (US MEC) for contraceptive use, 2016. https://www.cdc.gov/reproductivehealth/contraception/mmwr/mec/summary.html. Accessed October 15, 2021.
2. Trussell J. Contraceptive failure in the United States. *Contraception*. 2011;83(5):397–404.

 SEE ALSO

https://www.reproductiveaccess.org/contraception/: information for providers and patients, updated regularly

CODES

ICD10
- Z30.9 Encounter for contraceptive management, unspecified
- Z30.41 Encounter for surveillance of contraceptive pills
- Z30.431 Encounter for routine checking of intrauterine contracep dev

CLINICAL PEARLS
LARC methods provide high efficacy and convenience for patients.

COR PULMONALE

Andres A. Tirado-Navales, MD • Madhavi Singh, MD

 BASICS

DESCRIPTION

- The term "cor pulmonale" derives from the Latin *cor* (heart) and *pulmonale* (lungs). Hence, cor pulmonale is a cardiac complication of primary pulmonary disease.
- Acute or chronic pulmonary processes can lead to increased right-sided cardiac pressures. Resultant pulmonary hypertension (PH) subsequently induces structural alterations and/or impairs right ventricle (RV) function.
- PH is defined by a mean pulmonary artery pressure (mPAP) ≥25 mm Hg at rest measured by right heart catheterization.
- PH may be secondary to abnormalities of the pulmonary system, including disorders of the lung parenchyma, pulmonary circulation, chest wall, and/or ventilatory mechanisms. The pathophysiologic mechanisms of pulmonary arterial hypertension (WHO Group I) and PH secondary to pulmonary processes are biologically and clinically distinct. Therefore, for the purposes of this review, pulmonary arterial hypertension (WHO Group I) will not be considered as a cause of cor pulmonale.
- Cor pulmonale may occur in acute or chronic setting.
  - Acute: rapid increase of pulmonary arterial pressure resulting in RV overload, dysfunction, and potential cardiovascular collapse
  - Chronic: progressive hypertrophy and dilation of the RV over months to years, leading to dysfunction and potential failure

EPIDEMIOLOGY

- ~6–7% of all types of adult heart disease in United States. Globally, the incidence of cor pulmonale is widely variable due to air pollution, tobacco use, and toxic exposure.
- An estimated 10–30% of heart failure admissions in the United States are the result of cor pulmonale, most commonly related to chronic obstructive pulmonary disease (COPD).

Incidence
Difficult to assess: Best estimate is 1/10,000 to 3/10,000 per year.

Prevalence
Difficult to assess: Best estimate is 2/1,000 to 6/1,000.

ETIOLOGY AND PATHOPHYSIOLOGY

- Acute: A sudden event, such as large pulmonary embolism (PE), increases resistance to blood flow in the pulmonary vasculature, causing a quick and significant increase of pressure proximal to the right ventricular outflow tract. The RV may not be able to generate adequate force to overcome this pressure, leading to low RV cardiac output, which ultimately leads to a decreased left ventricle (LV) cardiac output. Increased RV pressures in conjunction with a low cardiac output may cause coronary ischemia, further impairing cardiac output and potentially causing complete cardiovascular collapse.
- Chronic: a disorder of the pulmonary system leading to chronic hypoxia, which results in progressive vasoconstriction of the pulmonary vasculature. Over time, the pulmonary arterial system hypertrophies and intrinsic vasoactive mechanisms (mediated by nitric oxide, cyclooxygenase, and endothelin) become dysregulated, leading to an increase in pulmonary vasculature resistance. Evidence also supports the involvement of capillary and postcapillary pulmonary vasculature to varying degrees in all PH groups.

- Increased pulmonary vascular resistance yields PH. PH transmits increased pressures and volumes to the thin-walled, low-pressure RV causing maladaptive remodeling (concentric hypertrophy, followed by eccentric dilation), which is frequently associated with tricuspid regurgitation and subsequent impairment in RV systolic and diastolic function.
- Indicators for the presence of PH in these patients may include a disproportionally low diffusing capacity of the lungs for carbon monoxide (DLCO) and an elevated pCO$_2$.
- Pulmonary disorders
  - Lung parenchymal disease: COPD (most common), interstitial lung disease (ILD), and pulmonary fibrosis
  - Pulmonary circulation: thromboembolic disease (associated with WHO Group IV PH)
  - Chest wall: severe obesity, kyphoscoliosis
  - Ventilation: obstructive sleep apnea (OSA) and obesity hypoventilatory syndrome; neuromuscular diseases such as Guillain-Barré syndrome, muscular dystrophy, myasthenia gravis, spinal cord injuries
  - Left ventricular failure is not considered a cause of cor pulmonale.

RISK FACTORS

- Acute cor pulmonale (most commonly caused by PE)
- Chronic cor pulmonale (most commonly caused by underlying pulmonary disorder)
  - Risk factors associated with pulmonary disorders
    - Tobacco use (COPD)
    - Occupational exposures (ILD)
    - Hypercoagulable state (chronic thromboembolic disease)
    - Obesity, age (chest wall/ventilatory abnormalities)

GENERAL PREVENTION
Management of underlying pulmonary disorders, including aggressive correction of hypoxia and acidosis, which may contribute to worsening PH

COMMONLY ASSOCIATED CONDITIONS
PH, defined as the presence of a resting mPAP >25 mm Hg

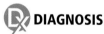 **DIAGNOSIS**

HISTORY

- Dyspnea is the most common symptom. Although nonspecific, dyspnea may be present at rest, with exertion, or manifests as paroxysmal nocturnal dyspnea.
- Other pulmonary symptoms: pleuritic chest pain, cough, hemoptysis
- General heart failure symptoms: fatigue, lethargy, syncope; exertional angina less likely
- Right-sided heart failure symptoms: anorexia, early satiety, digital cyanosis, clubbing, right upper quadrant discomfort (hepatic congestion), lower extremity edema
- Hoarseness secondary to compression of the left recurrent laryngeal nerve by enlarged pulmonary vessels
- Cardiovascular collapse, shock, and/or cardiac arrest may occur in acute or advanced chronic setting.

PHYSICAL EXAM

- Peripheral edema is the most common sign of right-sided heart failure, although it is nonspecific.
- General: pallor, diaphoresis, clubbing, cyanosis, tachypnea
- Neck: jugular venous distention, with prominent *a*-wave

- Lungs: tachypnea, wheezing
- Heart
  - Increased intensity of pulmonic component of second heart sound (P$_2$)
  - Splitting of S$_2$ over the cardiac apex with inspiration
  - Audible right-sided S$_3$ or S$_4$
  - RV heave
  - Pansystolic murmur heard best at right midsternal border increasing with inspiration, consistent with tricuspid regurgitation (typically a late sign)
- Abdomen: hepatomegaly
- Extremities: clubbing, cyanosis, bilateral lower extremity edema, may also show signs of deep vein thrombosis (DVT) such as tenderness or unilateral swelling

DIFFERENTIAL DIAGNOSIS
Other causes of right-sided failure:

- Left-sided heart failure
- WHO Groups I, II, and V PH
- Right-sided intrinsic cardiomyopathy

DIAGNOSTIC TESTS & INTERPRETATION

- 2D echocardiogram (1)[C]
  - Initial diagnostic test of choice
  - Elevated pulmonary arterial pressures
  - Right ventricular hypertrophy
  - Bulging of the interventricular septum into the LV with systole
  - Flattening of the interventricular or interatrial septum
  - Dilation and hypokinesis of the RV
  - Tricuspid regurgitation
  - Dilation of the right atrium
  - Main pulmonary artery to ascending aorta diameter ratio >1
  - Acute thromboembolic pulmonary disease as evidenced by right ventricular hypokinesis with sparing of the apex (McConnell sign)
  - Echocardiography can over- or underestimate the pulmonary arterial pressures depending on image quality or operator. Pulmonary arterial pressures should therefore be verified by right heart catheterization.
- MRI
  - If echocardiography is inconclusive or as a substitute
  - Most accurate modality for diagnosing emphysema and ILD
  - Can assess cardiac pressures, size, function, myocardial mass, and viability
- Right heart catheterization
  - Gold standard for diagnosis of PH and therefore critical for diagnosis of cor pulmonale
  - Elevated central venous pressure (CVP)
  - Mean PAP ≥25 mm Hg at rest

Initial Tests (lab, imaging)

- CBC may show signs of polycythemia due to chronic hypoxia.
- Basic metabolic panel (BMP) may demonstrate elevated creatinine secondary to poor cardiac output.
- Liver function tests (LFTs) may be abnormal due to proximal hepatic congestion or poor distal cardiac output secondary to RV failure.
- Brain natriuretic peptide (BNP) and cardiac troponin can be elevated secondary to right ventricular strain.
- D-dimer may be positive as evidence of underlying thromboembolic pulmonary disease.
- Arterial blood gas may show hypercapnia due to COPD or hypoxemia due to ILD.
- Arterial blood gases of COPD patients show a decreased PaO$_2$ with normal or increased PaCO$_2$.

- ECG often shows signs of right-sided enlargement.
  – Right axis deviation
  – An R/S wave ratio >1 in V_1
  – Right ventricular hypertrophy (R wave in V_1 and V_2 with S waves in V_5 and V_6)
  – Right atrial enlargement as evidenced by P pulmonale (increased amplitude of P wave in leads II, III, and avF with a "tent-like" appearance)
  – Incomplete or complete right bundle branch block
  – $S_1S_2S_3$ pattern or $S_1Q_3T_3$ inverted pattern
- Chest x-ray
  – Cardiomegaly
  – Enlargement of the central pulmonary arteries and reduced size of peripheral vessels (oligemia)
  – Reduced retrosternal space due to right ventricular enlargement on lateral views
  – Enlargement of the right atrium resulting in prominence of the right heart border
  – Evidence of COPD, ILD, and structural disease (i.e., kyphosis)
  – Evidence of PE (Westermark sign, Fleischner sign, and Hampton hump)
- Spiral computed tomography (CT) scan of chest
  – Diagnosis of acute PE
  – Diagnosis of COPD and ILD
- Ventilation/perfusion (V/Q) scan
  – High specificity and sensitivity for acute and chronic thromboembolic disease
  – Screening method of choice for chronic thromboembolic PH because of its higher sensitivity compared with CT pulmonary angiogram
  – May be used for diagnosis of acute thromboembolic disease if contraindication to chest spiral CT
  – Diagnosis of chronic thromboembolic disease (WHO Group IV PH) may warrant confirmation by pulmonary angiography.
- Pulmonary angiography
  – Gold standard in diagnosis of chronic thromboembolic pulmonary disease
- Polysomnography
  – Gold standard for diagnosis of OSA
- Pulmonary function tests (PFTs)
  – DLCO: A decrease in lung volume combined with decreased diffusion capacity for carbon monoxide may indicate ILD. COPD is associated with a decreased DLCO.
  – Obstructive or restrictive ventilatory defects (ILD, chest wall abnormalities, and COPD)
  – Decreased exercise capacity on cardiopulmonary exercise testing
  – Larger than expected impairment in gas exchange both at rest or during exercise

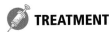 TREATMENT

Reduce symptoms, improve quality of life, and increase survival. Reduce disease burden via oxygenation, preservation of cardiac function, and attenuation of PH.

GENERAL MEASURES
- Treat underlying disease (2)[C]
  – For underlying pulmonary disease, long-acting bronchodilators, long-acting antimuscarinic agents, and/or inhaled corticosteroids may be beneficial for long-term disease management.
  – For underlying chronic thromboembolic disease, anticoagulation may be indicated.
- Supportive therapy as necessary
  – Continuous positive airway pressure/bilevel positive airway pressure may be used for hypoxia/sleep disorders.

  – Ventilation using positive-pressure masks, negative-pressure body suits, or mechanical ventilation is suggested for patients with neuromuscular disease.
  – Phlebotomy may be indicated for severe polycythemia or signs and symptoms of hyperviscosity (hematocrit >55%).

MEDICATION
- Oxygen (3)[A]
  – Long-term continuous oxygen therapy improves the survival of hypoxemic patients with COPD and cor pulmonale.
  – All patients with PH whose PaO_2 is consistently <55 mm Hg or saturation ≤88% at rest, during sleep, or with ambulation should be prescribed oxygen to keep O_2 >92 mm Hg.
  – Exposure to high altitude should be avoided. Supplemental oxygen should be used during altitude exposure or air travel as needed to maintain oxygen saturations >91%.
- Preservation of cardiac function
  – Inotropes: Dobutamine and milrinone may improve cardiac output.
  – Diuretics: decrease RV filling pressures and reduce peripheral edema secondary to RHF
    ○ Excessive volume depletion should be avoided.
    ○ Monitor closely for metabolic alkalosis because this may suppress ventilatory drive and contribute to hypoxia.
- Ameliorate PH
  – Treatment of underlying disease is hallmark of management (2)[C].
  – When refractory to traditional medical treatment, advanced therapies may be beneficial, although evidence is lacking.
  – For chronic thromboembolic–associated PH (WHO Group IV), riociguat may be used (4)[C].

ISSUES FOR REFERRAL
Patients with cor pulmonale should be referred to a specialized center for expert consultation.

SURGERY/OTHER PROCEDURES
- Endarterectomy for chronic thromboembolic disease (WHO Group IV) is the gold standard. However, about on third of patients in this group are found to be inoperable.
  – Balloon pulmonary angioplasty is an option that may provide improvement in hemodynamic measurements, with low mortality rate in inoperable patients (4)[C].
- Lung volume reduction surgery (LVRS) is a surgical option that may be beneficial for patients with advanced upper-lobe predominant emphysema who have poor disease control despite maximal medical therapy (5).
- Moderate to severe disease refractory to medication may require lung and/or heart transplantation.

 ONGOING CARE

DIET
Salt and fluid restriction

PATIENT EDUCATION
- Smoking cessation and avoidance of exposure to secondary smoke is strongly recommended.
- Level of physical activity should be discussed with physician.
- Pregnancy should be avoided.

PROGNOSIS
Patients with cor pulmonale resulting from COPD have a greater likelihood of dying than do similar patients with COPD alone. In patients with COPD and mild disease (PAP 20 to 35 mm Hg), 5-year survival is 50%.

REFERENCES
1. Simonneau G, Gatzoulis MA, Adatia I, et al. Updated clinical classification of pulmonary hypertension. *J Am Coll Cardiol.* 2013;62(Suppl 25):D34–D41.
2. Nathan SD, Barbera JA, Gaine SP, et al. Pulmonary hypertension in chronic lung disease and hypoxia. *Eur Respir J.* 2019;53(1):1801914. doi:10.1183/13993003.01914-2018.
3. Galiè N, Humbert M, Vachiery JL, et al. 2015 ESC/ERS guidelines for the diagnosis and treatment of pulmonary hypertension: the Joint Task Force for the Diagnosis and Treatment of Pulmonary Hypertension of the European Society of Cardiology (ESC) and the European Respiratory Society (ERS): endorsed by: Association for European Paediatric and Congenital Cardiology (AEPC), International Society for Heart and Lung Transplantation (ISHLT). *Eur Heart J.* 2016;37(1):67–119.
4. Kim NH, Delcroix M, Jais X, et al. Chronic thromboembolic pulmonary hypertension. *Eur Respir J.* 2019;53(1):1801915. doi:10.1183/13993003.01915-2018.
5. DeCamp M, Lipson D, Krasna M, et al. The evaluation and preparation of the patient for lung volume reduction surgery. *Proc Am Thorac Soc.* 2008;5(4):427–431.

ADDITIONAL READING
Galiè N, McLaughlin VV, Rubin LJ, et al. An overview of the 6th World Symposium on Pulmonary Hypertension. *Eur Respir J.* 2019;53(1):1802148. doi:10.1183/13993003.02148-2018.

 SEE ALSO

- Chronic Obstructive Pulmonary Disease and Emphysema; Pulmonary Arterial Hypertension; Pulmonary Embolism
- Algorithm: Congestive Heart Failure: Differential Diagnosis

 CODES

ICD10
- I27.81 Cor pulmonale (chronic)
- I26.09 Other pulmonary embolism with acute cor pulmonale

CLINICAL PEARLS
- Treatment of cor pulmonale requires treatment of the underlying disease. Therefore, accurate diagnosis of primary pulmonary disease is critical to clinical management and treatment therapy.
- Continuous, long-term oxygen therapy improves life expectancy and quality of life in cor pulmonale.
- Referral of patients with cor pulmonale to a specialized center is strongly recommended.

CORNEAL ABRASION AND ULCERATION

Christine S. Persaud, MD, MBA • Edward M. Degerman, MD

 BASICS

DESCRIPTION
- Corneal abrasions: result from cutting, scratching, or abrading the thin, protective, clear coat of the exposed anterior portion of the ocular epithelium. These injuries cause pain, tearing, photophobia, foreign body sensation, and a gritty feeling (1).
- Corneal ulceration: break in the epithelial layer of the cornea leading to exposure of the underlying corneal stroma, which results in a corneal ulcer. Superficial ulcers, limited to loss of the corneal epithelium, are the most common form of ulceration (2).
- Corneal abrasion and ulceration can both lead to impaired vision from scarring.

EPIDEMIOLOGY
Incidence
Eye-related diagnoses make up 8% of total ER visits and are commonly caused by direct/minor trauma. Of those eye-related visits caused by injury, 64% are corneal abrasions (3). Abrasions are the third leading cause of red eye, following conjunctivitis and subconjunctival hemorrhage (4).

ETIOLOGY AND PATHOPHYSIOLOGY
- Most often caused by mechanical trauma but may also result from foreign bodies: sand and dust, contact lenses wear, or chemical and flash burns
- Corneal ulceration seen with contact lenses use, HIV, trauma, ocular surface disease. Edema plays a major role in epithelial defect. Edema can lead to trauma, ischemia, and increased intraocular pressure. Excessive fluid disrupts the normal architecture of the epithelial layer (1).
- Causes of ulcerations include:
  - Gram-positive organisms ~29–53% (*Staphylococcus aureus* and coagulase-negative *Streptococcus* are common.)
  - Gram-negative organisms ~47–50% (*Pseudomonas* most common, followed by *Serratia marcescens*, *Proteus mirabilis*, and gram-negative enteric bacilli)
  - Herpes simplex with bacterial superinfection
  - Varicella virus
  - Autoimmune disorder: Sjögren, rheumatoid arthritis, inflammatory bowel disease
- Increased risk of corneal ulceration in HIV, diabetes mellitus (DM), and immunocompromise
- Eyelid abnormalities (chronic blepharitis, entropion)
- Nutritional deficiencies (vitamin A and protein undernutrition)
- Dry eyes/bullous keratopathy/mucous membrane pemphigoid

RISK FACTORS
- History of trauma (direct blunt trauma, chemical burn, radiation exposure, etc.)
- Contact lenses wear
- Male gender
- Age: 20 to 34 years old
- Job (construction, manufacturing); lack of eye protection

GENERAL PREVENTION
- Protective eyewear during work (auto mechanics, metal workers, miners, etc.) and during sports
- With the increasing use of face masks during the COVID-19 pandemic, a case has even been reported of corneal abrasion from removal of face mask with the edge of the mask causing a corneal abrasion (5).

COMMONLY ASSOCIATED CONDITIONS
- Vitamin A deficiency is associated with corneal ulcers.
- Neuropathy of cranial nerve (CN) V
- DM, thyroid dysfunction, immunocompromised states, connective tissue disease
- Critically ill patients who lack blinking reflex or inability to close their eyes and those on intermittent positive pressure from ventilation (6)

 DIAGNOSIS

HISTORY
Check for recent ocular trauma and acute pain. Other symptoms include photophobia, pain with extraocular muscle movement, eye twitching, excessive tearing, blepharospasm, foreign body sensation, gritty feeling, blurred or decreased vision, nausea, and headache.

PHYSICAL EXAM
- Gross examination of the anatomy: eyelids, surface of the eye, pupils, and extraocular muscles
- Snellen chart for visual acuity
- Tonometry for pressure measurements
- Penlight
- Fluorescein stain
- Wood's lamp (7)

DIFFERENTIAL DIAGNOSIS
- Corneal abrasion
  - Acute angle-closure glaucoma
  - Conjunctivitis
  - Infective keratitis
    - Uveitis and Iritis
    - Keratoconjunctivitis (4),(7)
- Corneal ulceration
  - Herpes zoster
    - Herpes zoster ophthalmicus

DIAGNOSTIC TESTS & INTERPRETATION
Initial Tests (lab, imaging)
- Ulcer culture
- Pretreatment with topical antibiotics may alter culture results.

Diagnostic Procedures/Other
- Slit lamp and fluorescein dye to identify and evaluate corneal abrasions
- Trauma/foreign body has geographic shape; if due to contact lenses, several punctate lesions (7)
- Document visual acuity.
- If ocular penetration with presence or suspicion of retained foreign body, ocular CT scan for metallic objects or MRI for nonmetalic objects should be considered.

Test Interpretation
Scraping culture/staining identifies bacteria, yeast, or intranuclear inclusions to help narrow diagnosis

 TREATMENT

GENERAL MEASURES
- Most uncomplicated corneal abrasions heal in 24 to 48 hours.
- May not require follow-up if lesion is <4 mm, uncomplicated abrasion, normal vision, and resolving symptoms
- But untreated abrasions can lead to corneal ulceration
- Do not rinse with tap or bottled water because it may contain microorganisms such as acanthamoeba instead rinse with a saline solution or multipurpose contact lenses solutions.
- Patching not recommended
  - Does not reduce pain
  - Delays healing and can increase risk of infection (1)[A]

MEDICATION

- Treatment guidelines: pain control, infection prevention, and daily symptom monitoring
- Oral analgesic: narcotics, acetaminophen, NSAIDs
- Topical anesthetics include proparacaine hydrochloride 0.1–0.5%, tetracaine hydrochloride 1%.
  - Proparacaine may be less cytotoxic than tetracaine (1)[B].
  - Topical anesthetics should be avoided after initial examination because they can delay healing and cause corneal damage.
- Topical cycloplegic agents like 1% atropine one drop every 8 hours has been recommended (8).
- Frequent use of artificial tears (8)

First Line
- Ophthalmic NSAIDs: Diclofenac 0.1% one drop QID helps relieve moderate pain:
  - Alternatives include ketorolac 0.5% one drop QID and bromfenac 0.09%.
  - Caution: Ophthalmic NSAIDs may rarely cause corneal melting and perforation.
  - Caution in patients with bleeding tendency
  - Topical NSAIDs should be discontinued once pain decreases as it delays corneal wound healing.
- Ophthalmic antibiotics may help prevent further infection and ulceration (9)[C].
- Some ophthalmic antibiotics include bacitracin 500 IU BID or QID, ofloxacin/ciprofloxacin 0.3%, gentamicin 0.3%, erythromycin 0.5%, polymyxin B/trimethoprim (Polytrim), and tobramycin 0.3%.
  - Broad spectrum antibiotics such as Polytrim are used for large dirty abrasions to prevent ulcerations.
  - Abrasions caused by contact lenses are typically treated with antibiotics with gram-negative coverage/antipseudomonals such as gentamicin, tobramycin, norfloxacin, or ciprofloxacin.
- Large corneal abrasions (>4 mm) or very painful abrasions should be treated with a combination of topical antibiotic and topical NSAID.
- Fungal keratitis is treated with a protracted course of topical antifungal agents (by ophthalmologist).
- Herpetic keratitis should be referred promptly to ophthalmologist and treated initially with trifluridine:
  - Vidarabine and acyclovir are alternatives.

ISSUES FOR REFERRAL
- Chemical burn
- Evidence of corneal ulcer or infiltrate

- Failure to heal after 3 to 4 days
- Inability to remove a foreign body
- Increase size of abrasion after 24 hours
- Penetrating injury
- Presence of hyphema (blood) or hypopyon (pus)
- Rust ring
- Vision loss of >20/40
- Worsening symptoms or no improvement after 24 hours (7)

ADDITIONAL THERAPIES
Novel approaches are being studied including the use of nanofibers loaded with antibiotic moxifloxacin HCl and antiscarring agent pirfenidone, used as an ocular insert (10).

ONGOING CARE

FOLLOW-UP RECOMMENDATIONS
Patient Monitoring
- Follow-up not necessary for small (<4 mm), uncomplicated abrasions, normal vision, and resolving symptoms
- Lesions >4 mm, decreased vision, and abrasions due to contact lenses need follow-up within 24 hours (4)[C].

PATIENT EDUCATION
Prevention of abrasions and proper handling of contact lenses can prevent recurrence of corneal ulcers.

PROGNOSIS
- Corneal abrasions heal within 24 to 72 hours.
- Ophthalmology consult with penetrating eye injury

COMPLICATIONS
- Recurrence
- Scarring of the cornea
- Loss of vision

REFERENCES
1. Malafa MM, Coleman JE, Bowman RW, et al. Perioperative corneal abrasion: updated guidelines for prevention and management. *Plast Reconstr Surg*. 2016;137(5):790e–798e.
2. Belknap EB. Corneal emergencies. *Top Companion Anim Med*. 2015;30(3):74–80.
3. Fusco N, Stead TG, Lebowitz D, et al. Traumatic corneal abrasion. *Cureus*. 2019;11(4):e4396.
4. Wipperman JL, Dorsch JN. Evaluation and management of corneal abrasions. *Am Fam Physician*. 2013;87(2):114–120.
5. Au SCL, Ko CKL. Corneal abrasion from removing face mask during the COVID-19 pandemic. *Vis J Emerg Med*. 2021;22:100958.
6. Ting DSJ, Deshmukh R, Said DG, et al. Care for critically Ill patients with COVID-19: don't forget the eyes. *Eye (Lond)*. 2020;34(7):1253–1254.
7. Pflipsen M, Massaquoi M, Wolf S. Evaluation of the painful eye. *Am Fam Physician*. 2016;93(12):991–998.
8. Davids A, White T. What is the best treatment of corneal abrasion? *Evid Based Pract*. 2020;23(5):16–17.
9. Fraser S. Corneal abrasion. *Clin Ophthalmol*. 2010;4:387–390.
10. Tawfik EA, Alshamsan A, Abul Kalam M, et al. In vitro and in vivo biological assessment of dual drug-loaded coaxial nanofibers for the treatment of corneal abrasion. *Int J Pharm*. 2021;604:120732.

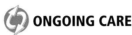 CODES

ICD10
- S05.00XA Inj conjunctiva and corneal abrasion w/o fb, unsp eye, init
- H16.009 Unspecified corneal ulcer, unspecified eye
- H16.049 Marginal corneal ulcer, unspecified eye

CLINICAL PEARLS
- Contact lenses use should be discontinued until corneal abrasion or ulcer is healed and pain is fully resolved.
- Eye patching is not recommended.
- Prescribe topical and/or oral analgesic medication for symptom relief and consider ophthalmic antibiotics.
- Healing can take 2 to 3 days for small abrasion (4 mm) for larger one may take 4 to 5 days.
- Treatment usually involves frequent topical antimicrobials application (e.g., every 1 to 2 hours).
- Prompt referral to an ophthalmologist should be made with suspicion of an ulcer, recurrence of abrasion, retained foreign body, viral keratitis, significant visual loss, or lack of improvement despite therapy.

CORNS AND CALLUSES
Tu Dan H. Nguyen, MD

BASICS

DESCRIPTION
- A callus (tyloma) is a diffuse area of hyperkeratosis, usually without a distinct border.
  - Typically, the result of exposure to repetitive forces, including friction and mechanical pressure; tend to occur on the palms of hands and soles of feet (1)
- A corn (heloma) is a circumscribed hyperkeratotic lesion with a central conical core of keratin that causes pain and inflammation. The conical core in a corn is a thickening of the stratum corneum.
  - Typically occur at pressure points, poor fitting shoes, an underlying bone lesion/spur (1)
- Hard corn or heloma durum (more common): often on toe surfaces, especially 5th toe (proximal interphalangeal [PIP]) joint
- Soft corn or heloma molle: commonly in the interdigital space
- Digital corns are also known as clavi or heloma durum.
- Intractable plantar keratosis is usually located under a metatarsal head (1st and 5th most common), is typically more difficult to resolve, and often is resistant to usual conservative treatments.

EPIDEMIOLOGY
Corns and calluses have the largest prevalence of all foot disorders.

Incidence
- Incidence of corns and calluses increases with age.
- Less common in pediatric patients
- Women affected more often than men
- Blacks report corns and calluses 30% more often than whites.

Prevalence
- 9.2 million Americans
- ~38/1,000 people affected

ETIOLOGY AND PATHOPHYSIOLOGY
Increased activity of keratinocytes in superficial layer of skin leads to hyperkeratosis. This is a normal response to excess friction, pressure, or stress.
- Calluses typically arise from repetitive friction, motion, or pressure to skin. The increased pressure is often secondary to a metatarsal deformity (long metatarsal or plantarflexed metatarsal) or another bone spur or deformity.

- Hard corns are an extreme form of callus with a keratin-based core. Often found on the digital surfaces and commonly linked to bony protrusions, causing skin to rub against shoe surfaces.
- Soft corns arise from increased moisture from perspiration leading to skin maceration, along with mechanical irritation, especially between toes.

Genetics
No true genetic basis was identified because most corns and calluses are due to mechanical stressors on the foot/hands.

RISK FACTORS
- Extrinsic factors producing pressure, friction, and local stress
  - Ill-fitting shoes or walking barefoot
  - Not using socks/gloves
  - Activities that increase stress applied to skin of hands or feet (manual labor, running, walking, sports)
- Intrinsic factors
  - Bony prominences: bunions, hammertoes, mallet deformities, deformed metatarsals
  - Motor or sensory neuropathy such as secondary to diabetes
  - Abnormal gait

GENERAL PREVENTION
External irritation and pressure are by far the most common cause of calluses and corns. General measures to reduce friction or pressure on the skin are recommended to reduce incidence of callus formation. Examples include wearing shoes that fit well and using socks and gloves.

Geriatric Considerations
In elderly patients, especially those with neurologic or vascular compromise, skin breakdown from calluses/corns may lead to increased risk of infection/ulceration. 30% of foot ulcers in the elderly arise from eroded hyperkeratosis. Regular foot exams are emphasized for these patients as well as diabetic patients (2).

COMMONLY ASSOCIATED CONDITIONS
- Foot ulcers: especially noted in diabetic patients or patients with neuropathy or vascular compromise
- Infection: look for warning signs including
  - Increasing size, redness, pain, or swelling
  - Purulent drainage
  - Fever
  - Change in color of fingers or toes
- Signs of gangrene (color change, coolness)

DIAGNOSIS
- Most commonly a clinical diagnosis based on visualization of the lesion
- Examination of footwear may also provide clues.

HISTORY
- Careful history can usually pinpoint cause.
- Ask about neurologic, vascular history, and diabetes. These may be risk factors for progression of corns/calluses to frank ulcerations and infection.

PHYSICAL EXAM
- Calluses
  - Thickening of skin without distinct borders
  - Often on feet, hands; especially over palms of hands, soles of feet
  - Colors range from white to gray-yellow, brown, red.
  - May be painless or tender
  - May throb or burn
- Corns
  - Hard corns
    ○ Commonly on feet: dorsum of toes or 5th PIP joint
    ○ Varied texture: dry, waxy, and transparent to a hornlike mass
    ○ Distinct borders
    ○ Often painful
  - Soft corns
    ○ Commonly between toes, especially between 4th and 5th digits at the base of the web space
    ○ Often yellowed, macerated appearance
    ○ Often extremely painful

DIFFERENTIAL DIAGNOSIS
- Plantar warts (typically a loss of skin lines within the wart), which are viral in nature
- Porokeratoses (blocked sweat gland)
- Underlying ulceration of skin, with or without infection (important to rule out especially with diabetic patients)

DIAGNOSTIC TESTS & INTERPRETATION
Initial Tests (lab, imaging)
- Radiographs may be warranted if no external cause is found. Look for abnormalities in foot structure and bone spurs.
- Use of metallic radiographic marker and weight-bearing films often highlight the relationship between the callus and bony prominence.

Follow-Up Tests & Special Considerations

Evaluate chronic conditions (diabetes) and recurrent infections (tinea pedis) that could worsen symptoms.

Diagnostic Procedures/Other

Biopsy with microscopic evaluation in rare cases

Test Interpretation

Abnormal accumulation of keratin in epidermis, stratum corneum

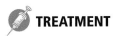 TREATMENT

GENERAL MEASURES
- Most therapy for corns and calluses can be done as self-care in the home.
- In office débridement of affected tissue and use of protective padding
- Use sandpaper discs or pumice stones over hard, thickened areas of skin; can be done safely at home.
- Use bandages, soft foam padding, or silicone sleeve over the affected area to decrease friction on the skin and promote healing with digital clavi.
- Use socks or gloves regularly.
- Padding to offload bony prominences
- Low-heeled shoes; soft upper with deep and wide toe box
- Avoidance of activities that contribute to painful lesions
- Prefabricated or custom orthotics

MEDICATION
- Keratolytic agents, such as urea, ammonium lactate, or salicylic acid plaster/ointment can be applied safely (3).
- Intralesional bleomycin injections have shown improvement in size and pain of warts.

Geriatric Considerations

Use of salicylic acid corn plasters can cause skin breakdown and ulceration in patients with thin, atrophic skin; diabetes; and those with vascular compromise. The skin surrounding the callus will often turn white and can become quite painful. Sometimes the acids are weak enough to not penetrate the thick skin but they can burn the adjacent skin, making the condition worse. Aggressive use of pumice stones can also lead to skin breakdown, especially surrounding the callus.

ISSUES FOR REFERRAL
- May benefit from referral to podiatrist if use of topical agents and shoe changes are ineffective
- Abnormalities in foot structure may require surgical treatment.
- Diabetic, vascular, and neuropathic patients may benefit from referral to podiatrist for regular foot exams to prevent infection or ulceration.

SURGERY/OTHER PROCEDURES
- Surgical treatment to areas of protruding bone where corns and calluses form
- Rebalancing of foot pressure through functional foot orthotics
- Shaving or cutting off hardened area of skin using a chisel or 15-blade scalpel. For corns, remove keratin core and place pad over area during healing.

COMPLEMENTARY & ALTERNATIVE MEDICINE
- May benefit from urea-based lotions, creams, or ointments
- Warm water/Epsom salt soaks

ADMISSION, INPATIENT, AND NURSING CONSIDERATIONS
- Admission usually not necessary, unless progression to ulcerated lesion with signs of severe infection, gangrene
- May require aggressive débridement in operating room if an abscess or deep-space infection is suspected. Deep-space infections can develop where an abscess can penetrate into tendon sheaths and/or deep compartments within the foot or hand, potentially leading to rapid sepsis. Vascular status must be assessed and vascular referral considered.
- Nursing
  – Wound care, dressing changes for infected lesions
  – Shoe wear modification

 ONGOING CARE

PATIENT EDUCATION
- General information: http://www.mayoclinic.org/diseases-conditions/corns-and-calluses/basics/definition/con-20014462
- American Podiatric Medical Association: http://www.apma.org

PROGNOSIS

High recurrence rate. Complete cure is possible once factors causing pressure or injury are eliminated.

COMPLICATIONS

Ulceration, infection

REFERENCES

1. Becker BA, Childress MA. Common foot problems: over-the-counter treatments and home care. *Am Fam Physician*. 2018;98(5):298–303.
2. Pinzur MS, Slovenkai MP, Trepman E, et al; for Diabetes Committee of American Orthopaedic Foot and Ankle Society. Guidelines for diabetic foot care: recommendations endorsed by the Diabetes Committee of the American Orthopaedic Foot and Ankle Society. *Foot Ankle Int*. 2005;26(1):113–119.
3. Phillips S, Seiverling E, Silvis M. Pressure and Friction Injuries in Primary Care. *Prim Care*. 2015;42(4):631–644.

ADDITIONAL READING
- American College of Foot and Ankle Surgeons: http://www.acfas.org/
- Theodosat A. Skin diseases of the lower extremities in the elderly. *Dermatol Clin*. 2004;22(1):13–21.

CODES

ICD10

L84 Corns and callosities

CLINICAL PEARLS

Most therapy for corns and calluses can be done as self-care in the home using padding over the affected area to decrease friction or pressure. However, if simple home care is not helpful, then removal of the lesions is often immediately curative. Cryotherapy may worsen discomfort and is not warranted for treatment.

CORONARY ARTERY DISEASE AND STABLE ANGINA

Merrill Alan Krolick, DO, FACC, FACP, FSCAI • Charles Doerner, DO

 BASICS

DESCRIPTION

- Coronary artery disease (CAD) refers to the atherosclerotic narrowing of the epicardial coronary arteries. It may manifest insidiously as angina pectoris or as an acute coronary syndrome (ACS).
- Stable angina is a chest discomfort due to myocardial ischemia that is predictably reproducible at a certain level of exertion or emotional stress.
- The spectrum of ACS includes unstable angina (UA), non–ST elevation myocardial infarction (NSTEMI), and ST elevation myocardial infarction (STEMI). See chapters on ACS for further information.
- Definitions
  - Typical angina: exhibits three classical characteristics: (i) substernal chest pressure, pressure or heaviness that may radiate to the jaw, back, or arms and generally lasts from 2 to 15 minutes; (ii) occurs at a certain level of myocardial oxygen demand from exertion, emotional stress, or increased sympathetic tone; and (iii) relieved with rest or sublingual nitroglycerin
  - Atypical angina: exhibits two of the above typical characteristics
  - Noncardiac chest pain: exhibits ≤1 of the above typical characteristics
  - Anginal equivalent: Patients may present without chest discomfort but with nonspecific symptoms such as dyspnea, diaphoresis, fatigue, belching, nausea, light-headedness, or indigestion that occur with exertion or stress. Patients with diabetes mellitus, women, and the elderly may present with more atypical features as compared to the general population.
  - UA: anginal symptoms that are new or more frequent, more severe, or occurring with lessening degrees of myocardial demand; it is considered ACS but does not present with cardiac biomarker elevation. (See "Acute Coronary Syndromes: NSTE-ACS (Unstable Angina and NSTEMI).")
  - NSTEMI: elevation of cardiac biomarker (troponin) with either anginal symptoms, ischemic ECG changes other than ST elevation, or both. (See "Acute Coronary Syndromes: NSTEACS (Unstable Angina and NSTEMI).")
  - STEMI: presents with typical symptoms as mentioned above with ST elevations noted on ECG; generally caused by acute plaque rupture and complete obstruction of culprit vessel and may present prior to laboratory detection of troponin. (See "Acute Coronary Syndromes: STEMI.")
- Canadian Cardiovascular Society grading scale:
  - Class I: Angina does not limit ordinary physical activity, occurring only with strenuous or prolonged exertion (7 to 8 metabolic equivalents [METs]).
  - Class II: Angina causes slight limitation of ordinary activity. It occurs when walking rapidly, uphill, or >2 blocks; climbing >1 flight of stairs; or with emotional stress (5 to 6 METs).
  - Class III: Angina causes marked limitation of ordinary physical activity. It occurs when walking 1 to 2 blocks or climbing one flight of stairs (3 to 4 METs).
  - Class IV: Angina occurs with any physical activity and may occur at rest (1 to 2 METs).

Geriatric Considerations

- The elderly may present with atypical symptoms.
- Physical limitations may delay recognition of angina until it occurs with minimal exertion or at rest.
- Maintain a high degree of suspicion during evaluation of dyspnea and other nonspecific complaints.
- Geriatric patients may be very sensitive to the side effects of medications used to treat angina.

EPIDEMIOLOGY

- CAD is the leading cause of death for adults both in the United States and worldwide.
- The cost of CAD in the United States was $555 billion in 2016 and is expected to rise to $1.1 trillion by 2035.
- ~80% of CAD is preventable with a healthy lifestyle.

Incidence

In the United States, the lifetime risk of a 40-year-old developing CAD is 49% for men and 32% for women.

Prevalence

In the United States, 28.4 million people carry a diagnosis of CAD, whereas 7.12 million have angina pectoris.

ETIOLOGY AND PATHOPHYSIOLOGY

- Anginal symptoms occur during times of myocardial ischemia caused by a mismatch between coronary perfusion and myocardial oxygen demand.
- Atherosclerotic narrowing of the coronary arteries is the most common etiology of angina, but it may also occur in those with significant aortic stenosis, pulmonary hypertension, hypertrophic cardiomyopathy, coronary spasm, or volume overload.
- Sensory nerves from the heart enter the spinal cord at levels C7–T4, causing diffuse referred pain/discomfort in the associated dermatomes.

RISK FACTORS

- Traditional risk factors: hypertension, ↓ HDL, ↑ LDL, smoking, diabetes, premature CAD in first-degree relatives (men <55 years old; women <65 years old), age (>45 years for men; >55 years for women)
- Nontraditional risk factors: obesity, sedentary lifestyle, chronic inflammation, abnormal ankle-brachial indices, renal disease

GENERAL PREVENTION

- Smoking cessation
- Regular aerobic exercise program
- Weight loss for obese patients (goal body mass index [BMI] <25 kg/m^2). A plant-based or Mediterranean-like diet is recommended.
- Blood pressure (BP) control (goal <140/90 mm Hg; consider <130/80 mm Hg for those with 10-year ASCVD risk ≥10%) (1)[C].
- Type 2 diabetes management: Consider more aggressive hemoglobin A1c (HbA1c) goal of 6.5–7% in younger, recently diagnosed individuals.
- At least moderate-intensity statin therapy for those with diabetes age 40 to 75 years and those with 10-year ASCVD risk ≥7.5–20% (Recommendations of advisory organizations vary, and the American College of Cardiology/American Heart Association risk calculator overestimates risk in many by as much as 50%–100%.)
- Low-dose aspirin should no longer be recommended for routine primary prevention of myocardial infraction (MI) without objective evidence of CAD. Benefits and harms are closely balanced, with no strong evidence for reduction in all-cause mortality, but with evidence for a reduction in cardiovascular events at the cost of increased major GI bleeding. A shared decision-making approach may consider aspirin for primary prevention in patients aged 40 to 59 years at highest risk for CAD and at low risk for GI bleeding. Likelihood of benefit is low. Aspirin should not be recommended for those over age 60 (USPSTF 2021 "D" level recommendation). It may be used for those with high clinical suspicion in the interim prior to stress testing/catheterization.

COMMONLY ASSOCIATED CONDITIONS

Hyperlipidemia, peripheral vascular disease, cerebrovascular disease, hypertension, obesity, diabetes

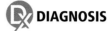 **DIAGNOSIS**

HISTORY

- Careful history is important to elicit symptoms.
- Pain may be described with a clenched fist over the center of the chest (Levine sign).
- Discomfort is usually not affected by position or deep inspiration.
- Episodes of angina are generally of the same character and in the same location as previous episodes.
- Recent decrease in level of physical activity may be due to worsening anginal symptoms.
- Dyspnea on exertion may present as the only symptom. Atypical symptoms are more likely in women, the elderly, and diabetic patients.
- May present with symptoms similar to gastric reflux or GI upset (indigestion, nausea, diaphoresis)

PHYSICAL EXAM

- Normal cardiac exam does not exclude the diagnosis of angina or CAD.
- Cardiac exam may reveal dysrhythmias, heart murmurs indicative of valvular disease, gallops, or signs of congestive heart failure.
- Evidence of peripheral vascular disease (diminished pulses, bruits, abdominal aortic aneurysm [AAA]) may or may not be noted.

DIFFERENTIAL DIAGNOSIS

- Vascular: aortic dissection, pericarditis, myocarditis, MI, vasospasm
- Pulmonary: pleuritis, pulmonary embolism, pneumothorax
- Gastroesophageal: gastric reflux, esophageal spasm, peptic ulcer
- Musculoskeletal: costochondritis, arthritis, muscle strain, rib fracture
- Other: anxiety, psychosomatic, cocaine abuse

DIAGNOSTIC TESTS & INTERPRETATION

Initial Tests (lab, imaging)

- Serial cardiac troponins for those presenting acutely with symptoms
- Complete blood count, lipid profile, HbA1c for risk stratification
- Basic metabolic panel to rule out electrolyte abnormalities and assess renal function
- ECG
  - Should be obtained unless there is a noncardiac cause of the chest pain
  - Frequently unremarkable between anginal episodes; may show signs of myocardial ischemia during symptomatic episodes, evidence of old MI
  - Left bundle branch block or ventricular pacing makes interpretation for ischemia unreliable.
- Chest x-ray may exclude other causes of pain.

Follow-Up Tests & Special Considerations

- Goal is to detect high-risk coronary lesions where intervention would improve long-term mortality or alleviate anginal symptoms.
- Stress testing is most helpful for patients at intermediate risk of CAD.
  - Exercise testing for those who can physically exercise (≥5 METs)
    - Standard exercise ECG for those with normal baseline ECG (i.e., without left bundle branch block or ventricular pacing)
    - Exercise stress testing with echo or perfusion imaging for those with abnormal baseline ECG or in premenopausal women

– In patients who cannot tolerate exercise, consider pharmacologic stress testing.

• Echocardiogram should be obtained in patients with a new or loud (≥III/VI) murmur, evidence of MI, symptoms of heart failure, concern for hypertrophic cardiomyopathy or pericardial effusion, and in those with new arrhythmias. A normal echocardiogram does not rule out CAD.

• Echocardiogram can be considered in patients with hypertension or diabetes and abnormal ECG.

• CT coronary angiography or cardiac MRI can be considered as a supplement/alternative to stress testing in patients with continued symptoms despite negative stress testing, inconclusive stress testing, or need for better anatomic definition of disease.

Diagnostic Procedures/Other

• Cardiac catheterization with coronary angiography is the gold standard for confirmation and delineation of coronary disease and direction of interventional therapy or surgery. It is indicated if noninvasive testing suggests a high-risk lesion or if patient fails to respond to appropriate medical management.

• Significant CAD is defined as ≥50% stenosis of the left main coronary artery or ≥70% stenosis of other major coronary arteries by angiography.

TREATMENT

GENERAL MEASURES

• AHA/ACC -recommended BP control goal for most patients with significant CAD: <130/80 mm Hg (1) [C]. Individualize goal based on patient preferences.

• Smoking cessation goal: complete cessation, no exposure to secondhand smoke or e-cigarettes

• Physical activity goal: 30 to 60 minutes of moderate aerobic activity, at least 5 (preferably 7) days/week

• Weight management goal: BMI 18.5 to 24.9 kg/m^2; waist circumference <35 inches (women) or <40 inches (men)

• Individualize glycemic control goals in diabetics: Avoid hypoglycemic episodes.

MEDICATION

First Line

• β-Blockers: decrease myocardial oxygen demand by lowering heart rate, BP, and contractility
  – Improve mortality in patients with MI or heart failure and should be used as initial therapy
  – Can improve symptoms of angina
  – Metoprolol (25 to 400 mg daily [succinate] or divided BID [tartrate]) or carvedilol (3.125 to 25.000 mg BID). Adjust doses according to clinical response. Maintain resting heart rate 50 to 60 beats/min.
  – Side effects: bradycardia, fatigue, and sexual dysfunction predominantly in men

• Calcium channel blockers (CCBs): cause arterial vasodilation, decreased myocardial oxygen demand, and improved coronary blood flow. Similar effectiveness to β-blockers; may be used instead of, or in addition to β-blockers. Only long-acting CCBs should be used:
  – Dihydropyridine CCBs: Nifedipine (30 to 90 mg/day), amlodipine (5 to 10 mg/day), or felodipine (2.5 to 10 mg/day) work predominantly on arterial vasodilation and can improve coronary blood flow.
  – Nondihydropyridine CCBs: Diltiazem (120 to 480 mg/day) or verapamil (120 to 480 mg/day) also have negative inotropic effects and should not be used in those with ejection fracture <40% because they may precipitate heart failure. Side effects include constipation and peripheral edema.

• Nitrates: dilate systemic veins and arteries (including coronary vessels) and cause decreased preload. At higher doses, they decrease BP.
  – Sublingual nitroglycerin (0.4 mg every 5 minutes for up to 3 doses) used for acute anginal episodes
  – Long-acting nitrates such as isosorbide mononitrate (30 to 240 mg daily [extended release]) can be used for angina prophylaxis.
  – Side effects include headache and hypotension but tend to improve with continued usage.
  – Contraindicated with concomitant phosphodiesterase type 5 inhibitor use (e.g., sildenafil)

• Lipid-lowering agents:
  – High-intensity statin therapy is indicated for all patients with CAD regardless of lipid levels.
  – Statin therapy should also be strongly considered for those with high CAD risk. (Lifetime ASCVD risk ≥7.5–10%, <75 to 80 years. Evidence for benefit is sparse for statins in primary prevention after 75 years, and many recommend DE-prescribing statins in this age group if not used for treatment.)
  – Atorvastatin (40 to 80 mg/day) and rosuvastatin (20 to 40 mg/day) are high-intensity statins.
  – Statins reduce risk of MI and revascularization need. Side effects include myalgias, transaminitis, rhabdomyolysis (rare), and impaired glucose tolerance.
  – Ezetimibe may be added to statin therapy if LDL is not at goal after maximally tolerated dose of statin, especially in secondary prevention.
  – Proprotein convertase subtilisin/kexin type 9 inhibitors further reduce LDL levels when used in combination with statins for high-risk patients and reduce cardiovascular events in highly selected patients but are very expensive.

• Antiplatelets: decrease risk of thrombosis
  – Aspirin (75 to 162 mg/day) decreases risk of first MI and reduces adverse cardiovascular events in those with stable angina.
  – Clopidogrel (75 mg/day) may be used in patients with contraindications to aspirin.
  – Dual antiplatelet therapy with aspirin + clopidogrel, prasugrel, or ticagrelor is indicated after MI or percutaneous coronary intervention (PCI) (use prasugrel only after PCI. Do not use in patient with CVA history).

• Angiotensin-converting enzyme inhibitors (ACEIs): act on the renin-angiotensin-aldosterone system to reduce BP and afterload. They also have effects on cardiac remodeling after MI.
  – ACEIs such as lisinopril (5 to 40 mg/day) and enalapril (2.5 to 20.0 mg BID) have been shown to reduce both cardiovascular death and MI in patients with CAD and left ventricular systolic dysfunction.
  – Angiotensin receptor blockers such as candesartan (4 to 32 mg daily) may be used in patients intolerant to ACEIs.
  – Side effects include cough (ACEIs predominantly), hyperkalemia, and angioedema.

Second Line

Ranolazine (500 to 1,000 mg BID) decreases calcium overload in myocytes, acting as an antianginal/anti-ischemic agent.

• It does not affect HR or BP and may be used as an adjunctive therapy when symptoms persist despite optimal dose of other antianginals. Side effects: nausea, constipation, dizziness, QT prolongation, headache

SURGERY/OTHER PROCEDURES

• Revascularization should be considered if optimal medical therapy is inadequate to control symptoms.

• PCI with balloon angioplasty and/or stent placement (with drug-eluting or bare-metal stent) is performed for significant lesions. Additional techniques include laser therapy and atherectomy.

• PCI does not appear to decrease mortality or risk of MI versus aggressive medical management in those with stable angina.

• Coronary artery bypass graft (CABG) is preferred over PCI for those with severe left main coronary stenosis, significant lesions in ≥3 major coronary arteries, and for lesions not amenable to PCI.

COMPLEMENTARY & ALTERNATIVE MEDICINE

Relaxation/stress reduction therapy for angina

ONGOING CARE

FOLLOW-UP RECOMMENDATIONS

Lifestyle modifications should be aggressively stressed at every visit.

Patient Monitoring

Frequent follow-up after initial event: every 4 to 6 months in first year and then 1 to 2 times per year

DIET

• Plant-based or Mediterranean-like diet is recommended and shown to lower all-cause mortality compared to standard diet. Eating fatty fish like salmon recommended (but not omega-3 supplements)

• Adherence to dietary modification for comorbid conditions (diabetes, heart failure, hypertension)

PROGNOSIS

Variable; depends on severity of symptoms, extent of CAD, and left ventricular function

COMPLICATIONS

ACS, arrhythmia, cardiac arrest, heart failure

REFERENCE

1. Whelton PK, Carey RM, Aronow WS, et al. 2017 ACC/AHA/AAPA/ABC/ACPM/AGS/APhA/ASH/ASPC/NMA/PCNA guideline for the prevention, detection, evaluation, and management of high blood pressure in adults: a report of the American College of Cardiology/American Heart Association Task Force on Clinical Practice Guidelines. *J Am Coll Cardiol.* 2018;71(19):e127–e248.

SEE ALSO

Algorithm: Chest Pain/Acute Coronary Syndrome

CODES

ICD10

• I25.119 Athscl heart disease of native cor art w unsp ang pctrs
• I25.118 Athscl heart disease of native cor art w oth ang pctrs
• I20.9 Angina pectoris, unspecified

CLINICAL PEARLS

• Maximize antianginal therapy: Combine β-blockers, CCBs, and nitrates as tolerated, along with high-intensity statin therapy. PCI may be considered for those with stable ischemic heart disease who continue to have angina on maximally tolerated medical therapy. PCI is first-line treatment for those with UA/NSTEMI/STEMI.

• Lifestyle changes and optimal medical therapy must be emphasized to prevent progression of atherosclerosis and to control contributing risk factors.

COSTOCHONDRITIS

Smriti Ohri, MD • Scott A. Fields, MD, MHA

 BASICS

DESCRIPTION
- Anterior chest wall pain and tenderness of the costochondral and costosternal regions, most often affecting the 2nd to 5th costal cartilages
- System(s) affected: musculoskeletal
- Synonym(s): costosternal syndrome; parasternal chondrodynia; anterior chest wall syndrome

EPIDEMIOLOGY
- Predominant age: 20 to 40 years
- Predominant gender: female

Incidence
- 30% emergency room visits for chest pain
- 13% primary care visits for chest pain

ETIOLOGY AND PATHOPHYSIOLOGY
Although not fully understood, inflammation can be caused by pulling from adjoining muscles at costochondral or costosternal regions.

RISK FACTORS
- Unusual physical activity or upper extremity overuse
- Recent trauma (including motor vehicle accident, domestic violence) or new-onset physical activity
- Recent upper respiratory infection (URI) with coughing

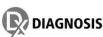 **DIAGNOSIS**

- Pain is usually sharp, achy, or pressure-like, involving multiple (and mostly unilateral 2nd to 5th) costal cartilages.
- Exacerbated by upper body movements and exertional activities
- Reproduced by palpation of the affected cartilage segments
- Chest tightness is often associated with the pain.

HISTORY
- A complete and thorough history (including a cardiac risk factor evaluation) is mandatory for an accurate diagnosis.
- Social history: careful screening and evaluation for domestic violence and substance abuse

PHYSICAL EXAM
- A thorough cardiopulmonary exam to exclude other conditions presenting with chest pain
  - Cardiac rhythm; murmurs; gallops, rubs
  - Adventitious lung sounds—rales, rhonchi, wheezes, rubs
- Tenderness over the costochondral junctions is necessary to establish the diagnosis but does not completely exclude other causes of chest pain.
- If swelling or redness of costal cartilage is present, the presentation is often termed Tietze syndrome (also an inflammatory condition generally involving single costal cartilage of rib 2).
- Movement of upper extremity of the same side may reproduce the pain.

Pediatric Considerations
- Consider psychogenic chest pain in children who perceive family discord.
- Consider slipping rib syndrome in children with chronic chest and abdominal pain (1).

Geriatric Considerations
Consider herpes zoster in elderly patients.

DIFFERENTIAL DIAGNOSIS
- Consider alternate diagnosis if presence of other signs and symptoms, like shortness of breath, dyspnea on exertion, cough, fever, tachycardia, and hypotension.
- Cardiac
  - Coronary artery disease (CAD); acute coronary syndrome (ACS)
  - Cardiac contusion from trauma
  - Aortic aneurysm
  - Pericarditis
  - Myocarditis
- Gastrointestinal
  - Gastroesophageal reflux
  - Peptic esophagitis
  - Esophageal spasm
  - Cholecystitis
- Musculoskeletal (1)
  - Fibromyalgia
  - Slipping rib syndrome
  - Costovertebral arthritis
  - Painful xiphoid syndrome
  - Rib trauma
- Psychogenic
  - Panic attacks
- Respiratory
  - Pulmonary embolism
  - Pneumonia
  - Chronic cough
  - Pneumothorax
- Other
  - Domestic violence and abuse
  - Herpes zoster
  - Spinal tumor
  - Metastatic cancer
  - Substance abuse (cocaine)

DIAGNOSTIC TESTS & INTERPRETATION
- Primarily a clinical diagnosis
- Laboratory exams and imaging to rule out other diagnoses
- ESR is inconsistently elevated.

Initial Tests (lab, imaging)
Imaging is not indicated for the diagnosis of costochondritis.

Diagnostic Procedures/Other

- None indicated for the diagnosis of costochondritis
- Consider ECG in patients age >35 years and for patients with history of or at risk for CAD (2)[C].
- Consider chest x-ray in patients with appropriate cardiopulmonary symptoms (2)[C].
- Consider CT imaging if high suspicion of aortic dissection, infectious or neoplastic process (2)[C].
- Consider spiral CT for pulmonary embolism and D-dimer if history or risk factors are present.

Test Interpretation

Costochondral joint inflammation

 ## TREATMENT

Reassurance of benign nature of condition and potential for long, slow recovery from pain

GENERAL MEASURES

- Rest and heat (or ice) massage
- Stretching exercises
- Minimize symptom-provoking activities (e.g., reduce frequency or intensity of exercise/work activity).

MEDICATION

- Pain relief with NSAIDs (ibuprofen, naproxen, or diclofenac), acetaminophen or other analgesics
- Use of skeletal muscle relaxants may be beneficial if associated with muscle spasm.

ISSUES FOR REFERRAL

- Consider referral to physical therapy for pain reduction and improvement in function (3)[B].
- Refractory cases of costochondritis can be treated with local injections of combined lidocaine/corticosteroid into costochondral areas; rarely necessary (2)[C]

- Consider referral to gastroenterology or cardiology if an alternate diagnosis meriting special input is suspected.

COMPLEMENTARY & ALTERNATIVE MEDICINE

Limited data but may be safely tried if patient interested

- Chiropractic manipulation; exercise prescription
- Dry needling by properly trained providers (4)[C]
- Acupuncture (5)[C]
- Massage

ADMISSION, INPATIENT, AND NURSING CONSIDERATIONS

Only if cardiac or other serious etiology of chest pain is being considered

 ## ONGOING CARE

FOLLOW-UP RECOMMENDATIONS

Follow-up within 1 week if diagnosis is unclear or symptoms do not abate with conservative treatment

PATIENT EDUCATION

- Educate regarding the self-limited (although potentially recurrent) nature of the illness.
- Instruct patient on proper physical activity regimens to avoid overuse syndromes.
- Avoid sudden, significant changes in activity.

PROGNOSIS

- Self-limited illness lasts for weeks to months and usually abates by 1 year: sometimes chronic particularly in adolescents
- Often recurs

COMPLICATIONS

May be refractory or recurrent

REFERENCES

1. Ayloo A, Cvengros T, Marella S. Evaluation and treatment of musculoskeletal chest pain. *Prim Care.* 2013;40(4):863–887, viii.
2. Proulx AM, Zryd TW. Costochondritis: diagnosis and treatment. *Am Fam Physician.* 2009;80(6):617–620.
3. Zaruba RA, Wilson E. Impairment based examination and treatment of costochondritis: a case series. *Int J Sports Phys Ther.* 2017;12(3):458–467.
4. Westrick RB, Zylstra E, Issa T, et al. Evaluation and treatment of musculoskeletal chest wall pain in a military athlete. *Int J Sports Phys Ther.* 2012;7(3):323–332.
5. Lin K, Tung C. Integrating acupuncture for the management of costochondritis in adolescents. *Med Acupunct.* 2017;29(5):327–330.

 ## CODES

ICD10

M94.0 Chondrocostal junction syndrome [Tietze]

CLINICAL PEARLS

- A common disorder, accounting for up to 30% of all cases of chest pain
- Diagnosis is primarily clinical. Lab and other testing is done to exclude other conditions based on patient risk.
- Self-limited (potentially recurrent) condition. Activity modification helps prevent recurrence.

COUNSELING TYPES
William T. Garrison, PhD

BASICS

DESCRIPTION

- Psychotherapeutic and counseling interventions play an important role in the management of chronic and acute-onset diseases and disorders. They are typically the primary initial mode of evaluation and/or treatment for most mild to moderate psychiatric disorders that reach criteria using the *DSM-5* (1) or *ICD-11* diagnostic classification systems.
- Treatment and successful control of either medical or psychological conditions typically benefit from some form of professional counseling. Best outcomes occur when they are employed by a skilled practitioner. However, psychotherapy differs from generic counseling, which can take many forms and is delivered commonly in nonmedical settings. In recent years, attempts to integrate counseling and psychotherapy within primary care practices have increased.
- Counseling approaches are usually tailored to the specific presenting problem or issue and serve educational and emotional support functions. Typically, counseling in medical settings will be time-limited and problem-focused and often not intended to lead to major medical symptom relief or major behavioral changes but to improve patient coping.
- The goals of psychotherapy range from increasing individual psychological insight and motivation for change to reduction of interpersonal conflict in the marriage or family, reduction of chronic or acute emotional suffering, or reversal of dysfunctional or habitual behaviors. There are several general classes of psychotherapy, starting with individual, marital, or family approaches. In addition, a number of psychological theories guide various methods and treatment philosophies. The following is a brief overview of commonly used psychotherapeutic and counseling methods.
  - Psychodynamic therapy: Unconscious conflict manifests as patient's symptoms/problem behaviors:
    - Short-term (4 to 6 months) and long-term (≥1 year)
    - Focus is on increasing insight of underlying conflict or processes to initiate symptomatic change.
    - Therapist actively helps patient identify patterns of behavior stemming from existence of an unconscious conflict or beliefs and motivations that may not be accurately perceived by the individual.
  - Cognitive-behavioral therapy (CBT): Patterns of thoughts and behaviors can lead to development and/or maintenance of symptoms. Thought patterns may not accurately reflect reality and may lead to psychological distress:
    - CBT aims at modifying thought patterns by increasing cognitive flexibility and changing dysfunctional behavioral patterns.
    - CBT encourages patient self-monitoring of symptoms and the precursors or results of maladaptive behavior.
    - Uses therapist-assisted challenges to patient's basic beliefs/assumptions

    - May use *exposure*, a procedure derived from basic learning theories, which encourages gradual steps toward change, at a speed that is tolerated by the patient
    - CBT can be offered in group or individual formats, for adults or children.
    - A CBT practitioner attempts to combine practical interventions with emotional supports.
  - Dialectical behavior therapy (DBT): Techniques such as social skills training, mindfulness, and problem solving are used to modulate impulse control and affect management:
    - DBT is a therapy approach that derives from CBT but emphasizes emotional control in relationships.
    - Originally used in treatment of patients with self-destructive behaviors (e.g., cutting, suicide attempts)
    - Seeks to change rigid patterns of cognitions and behaviors that have been maladaptive
    - Uses both individual and group treatment modalities
    - The DBT therapist takes an active role in interpretation and support.
  - Interpersonal psychotherapy: Interpersonal relationships in a patient's life are linked to symptoms. Therapy seeks to alleviate symptoms and improve social adjustment through exploration of patient's relationships and experiences. Focus is on one of four potential problem areas:
    - Grief or loss
    - Interpersonal role disputes
    - Role transitions
    - Interpersonal deficits: Therapist works with the patient in resolving the problematic interpersonal issues to facilitate change in symptoms.
  - Family therapy: focuses on the family as a unit of intervention
    - Uses psychoeducation to increase patient's and family's insight
    - Teaches communication and problem-solving skills
  - Motivational interviewing (MI): focuses on motivation as a key to successful change process
    - Short-term and problem-focused. Many therapists use MI prior to initiating other therapies.
    - Focuses on identifying discrepancies between goals and behavior and the patient's desire to change
    - "5 As" model is a brief counseling framework developed specifically for physicians to effect behavioral change in patients:
      - Assess for a problem.
      - Advise making a change.
      - Agree on action to be taken.
      - Assist with self-care support to make the change.
      - Arrange follow-up to support the change.
  - Supportive and informational counseling (heterogeneous treatment)
    - Often focuses on situational factors maintaining symptoms
    - Often encourages the use of community resources

    - Behavioral therapy: relatively nontheoretical approach to behavioral change or symptom reduction/eradication through application of principles of stimulus and response. Motivational interviewing is often performed at the onset of behavioral and parenting counseling or therapy.

Pediatric Considerations

- Important distinctions are made between psychotherapy and counseling for children/teens compared to adults/couples.
- The focus of evaluation must include attention to parent and family processes and factors. Interventions typically include interactions and sessions with parents as well as collateral work with teachers and other school personnel.
- Younger children will often be evaluated and diagnosed through behavioral descriptions provided by parents and other adults who know them well as well as through direct observation and/or play techniques. Children of all ages should be screened using behavioral checklists that are standardized and norm-referenced for age and gender.
- Any child or teenager who requests counseling should be interviewed initially by the primary care provider and referred appropriately. Most referrals will be in response to parental request, however.
- Psychotherapeutic interventions with the strongest empirical basis with children include behavior therapy/modification, CBT, and family/parenting therapy. Play therapy has the least empirical support but has been found to be useful for developing rapport and for treating trauma in younger children. Insight-oriented therapies appear to be more effective with older children (10 years or older).
- There is controversy regarding the efficacy of psychopharmacologic treatment in preadolescents, although clear benefits have been demonstrated in some studies as well as clinical practice. Treatment guidelines for mild to moderate depressed mood and/or anxiety disorders typically recommend pediatric CBT initially, and studies have typically supported this approach in preteen and milder cases. Medications should be considered in more severe presentations.

EPIDEMIOLOGY

- 19 million adults suffer from clinical depression, and over 20 million adults have a diagnosable anxiety disorder in the U.S.
- One in four Americans report seeking some form of mental health treatment in their adult life. This includes generic counseling in nonmedical settings such as work, clergy, or school settings and also includes visits to primary care providers. It is estimated that between 3.5% and 5% of adults in the United States participate in formal mental health psychotherapy annually. Recent estimates emerging from the COVID-19 pandemic suggest these rates have increased since spring 2020.
- Public health experts report that the majority of those adults with diagnosable psychiatric disorders do not receive professional mental health services. This is due to multiple factors, including failure to identify, noncompliance with psychiatric referral, regional shortages of providers, economic or insurance barriers, and excessive time duration from referral to an available service.

RISK FACTORS

The need for psychotherapy or counseling services is associated with a host of socioeconomic and biogenetic factors, including the general effects of poverty, family or marital dysfunction, life stressors, medical diseases or conditions, and individual biologic predisposition to mental health disorders.

GENERAL PREVENTION

It is generally assumed that early identification and intervention of child and adolescent psychopathology increases the likelihood of reducing the risk for adult psychopathology, but this has not been sufficiently validated in all categories of psychological disorders. Data support such claims in disorders such as childhood ADHD, anxiety disorders, and habit disorders of childhood, however. A range of evidence-based therapies now exist that are designed for children and adults.

 TREATMENT

GENERAL MEASURES

There is evidence of a "dose effect" in psychotherapy outcomes research, with some investigators suggesting that 6 to 8 sessions are necessary to yield positive initial effects in adults, and upward of 15 to 20 sessions for longer term, sustainable therapeutic effects. This dose effect may not be applicable to counseling services with primarily informational or emotional/supportive functions. Also, long-term therapy should be evaluated at 3- to 6-month intervals to determine efficacy.

MEDICATION

- Psychotherapy is most likely to be accompanied by use of pharmaceutical adjuncts in moderate to severe cases of psychological dysfunction that do not respond to other therapies or in cases of extremely poor quality of life or high risk. The most common examples are in cases of clinical depression or anxiety that clearly incapacitates the patient or significantly reduces his or her quality of life. Patients at risk for suicide or who represent a danger to others are also candidates for acute psychopharmacotherapy. Studies suggest that verbal and behaviorally oriented therapies can add efficacy to medication treatment in both depression and anxiety and reduce the risk of relapse.
- There is controversy in the research field regarding the efficacy of medication alone versus psychotherapy alone versus combined treatments. The most recent consensus has been that combined treatments in moderate to severe psychological dysfunction are most likely to render positive short-term results and increase the likelihood that such effects can be sustained over time. Many patients in mental health settings do not require psychotropic medications.

ADDITIONAL THERAPIES

- Anxiety disorders
  - Panic disorder with and without agoraphobia: CBT, psychodynamic therapy
  - Generalized anxiety disorder: CBT

- Obsessive-compulsive disorder: CBT
- Posttraumatic stress disorder: CBT, play therapy with children
- Specific phobia: CBT
- Social phobia: CBT
- Mood disorders
  - Unipolar depression: CBT, interpersonal therapy, psychodynamic therapy
  - Bipolar disorder: family therapy, interpersonal therapy, CBT/DBT
  - Schizophrenia: psychodynamic therapy, family therapy, CBT/DBT
- Eating disorders
  - Binge eating disorder: CBT/DBT, interpersonal therapy, behavior modification
  - Bulimia nervosa: CBT/DBT, interpersonal therapy, behavior modification
- Personality disorders
  - Borderline: DBT, CBT
- Substance use disorders
  - Alcohol: counseling, CBT, motivational interviewing
  - Cocaine, heroin, opioids, cannabis: CBT, counseling
  - Smoking: motivational interviewing, behavioral modification with evidence-based medications

COMPLEMENTARY & ALTERNATIVE MEDICINE

A host of nonempirically based psychological and nutritional therapies can be found outside of mainstream medicine and psychological science. Very little or no evidence exists to support many experimental therapies, but all have the considerable power of the placebo effect fueling their anecdotal supports or claims. Placebo effects are also thought to be powerfully enhanced by the use of ingested or applied substances that create real physiologic, although not therapeutic, changes in the patient. If it makes them feel different, they are more likely to believe it helps. Placebo alone accounts for moderate amounts of perceived symptom improvement in a range of psychiatric medications as well as nonregulated supplements.

 ONGOING CARE

FOLLOW-UP RECOMMENDATIONS

Patient Monitoring

There is evidence of a "dose effect" in psychotherapy outcomes research, with investigators suggesting upward of 20 sessions for sustainable therapeutic effects. This dose effect may not be applicable to counseling services with primarily informational or emotional/supportive functions. Because many patients cease attendance to psychotherapy sessions after one or a few sessions, most interventions of this type cannot be accurately evaluated by the referring provider. Long-term therapy should also be evaluated for effectiveness at regular periods. Patients at suicidal risk need to be monitored more often and in-person.

REFERENCE

1. American Psychiatric Association. *Diagnostic and Statistical Manual of Mental Disorders*. 5th ed. Arlington, VA: American Psychiatric Association; 2013.

ADDITIONAL READING

- Bortolotti B, Menchetti M, Bellini F, et al. Psychological interventions for major depression in primary care: a meta-analytic review of randomized controlled trials. *Gen Hosp Psychiatry*. 2008;30(4):293–302.
- Eddy KT, Dutra L, Bradley R, et al. A multidimensional meta-analysis of psychotherapy and pharmacotherapy for obsessive-compulsive disorder. *Clin Psychol Rev*. 2004;24(8):1011–1030.
- Furukawa TA, Watanabe N, Churchill R. Combined psychotherapy plus antidepressants for panic disorder with or without agoraphobia. *Cochrane Database Syst Rev*. 2007;(1):CD004364.
- Hunot V, Churchill R, Silva de Lima M, et al. Psychological therapies for generalised anxiety disorder. *Cochrane Database Syst Rev*. 2007;(1):CD001848.

CODES

ICD10

- Z71.9 Counseling, unspecified
- Z71.89 Other specified counseling
- Z63.9 Problem related to primary support group, unspecified

CLINICAL PEARLS

- Combined medication and psychotherapeutic treatments in moderate to severe psychological dysfunction are most likely to render positive short-term results and increase the likelihood such effects can be sustained over time.
- Relapse is common over time and/or as treatments are discontinued or not reevaluated.
- Children <10 years may benefit significantly from counseling or behavior therapy alone for symptom relief.
- Older children and those with more severe symptoms typically require psychopharmacologic options in concert with counseling and/or cognitive-behavioral therapy approaches.

C

CROHN DISEASE

Eric J. Mao, MD • Samir A. Shah, AGAF, FACG, FASGE, MD

 BASICS

DESCRIPTION
- A chronic, progressive inflammatory GI tract disorder, most commonly involving the terminal ileum (80%)
- Hallmark features of Crohn disease (CD)
  - Transmural inflammation that can result in fibrotic strictures, fistulas, fissures, or abscesses
  - Noncaseating granulomas (30%)
  - Skip lesions: diseased mucosa interspersed with normal mucosa; can be continuous, mimicking ulcerative colitis (UC)
  - Diverse presentations: ileitis (1/3), ileocolitis (1/3); isolated colitis (1/3)

EPIDEMIOLOGY
Incidence
- 3 to 20 cases per 100,000 person-years in North America; incidence rising globally
- Bimodal age distribution: Predominant age is 15 to 30 years, with a second smaller peak at 50 to 80 years.
- Women slightly more affected than men; increased incidence in northern climates
- Increased risk in whites versus nonwhites: 2- to 5-fold
Prevalence
247 cases per 100,000 persons

ETIOLOGY AND PATHOPHYSIOLOGY
- General: Clinical manifestations result from activation of inflammatory cells and subsequent tissue injury.
- Multifactorial: Genetics, environmental triggers, commensal microbial antigens, and immunologic abnormalities result in inflammation and tissue injury.
Genetics
- 15% of CD patients have a first-degree relative with inflammatory bowel disease (IBD); first-degree relative of an IBD patient has 3- to 30-fold increased risk of developing IBD by age 28 years.
- Associated genetic syndromes: Turner and Hermansky-Pudlak syndromes, glycogen storage disease type 1b

RISK FACTORS
Environmental factors
- Cigarette smoking doubles the risk of CD; tobacco cessation reduces flares and relapses.
- Dietary factors: higher incidence if diet high in refined sugars, animal fat or protein, processed or ultraprocessed foods

COMMONLY ASSOCIATED CONDITIONS
- Extraintestinal manifestations
  - Arthritis (20%): seronegative, small and large joints (ankylosing spondylitis [AS] or sacroiliitis [SI], associated with HLA-B27)
  - Skin disorders (10%): erythema nodosum, pyoderma gangrenosum, psoriasis
  - Ocular disease (5%): uveitis (associated with HLA-B27), iritis, episcleritis

  - Kidney stones: calcium oxalate stones (from steatorrhea and diarrhea) or uric acid stones (from dehydration and metabolic acidosis)
  - Osteopenia and osteoporosis; hypocalcemia
  - Hypercoagulability: venous thromboembolism prophylaxis essential in hospitalized patients
  - Gallstones: cholesterol stones resulting from impaired bile acid reabsorption
  - Primary sclerosing cholangitis (PSC) (5%)
- Conditions associated with increased disease activity
  - Peripheral arthropathy (not SI and AS)
  - Episcleritis (not uveitis)
  - Oral aphthous ulcers and erythema nodosum
- Complications: GI bleed, toxic megacolon, bowel obstruction, bowel perforation, peritonitis, malignancy, intra-abdominal fistula, perianal disease

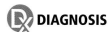 **DIAGNOSIS**

HISTORY
Hallmarks: crampy abdominal pain (+/− bleeding), prolonged diarrhea, fatigue, weight loss, fever, perianal disease. Children may present with failure to thrive.
- Factors exacerbating CD: concurrent infection, smoking, NSAIDs, antibiotics, stress

PHYSICAL EXAM
Presentation varies with location of disease.
- General: signs of sepsis/disease activity (fever, tachycardia, hypotension) or wasting/malnutrition
- Abdominal: focal or diffuse tenderness, distension, rebound/guarding, rectal bleeding, palpable mass
- Perianal: fistulae, fissures, abscess
- Skin: erythema nodosum, pyoderma gangrenosum; psoriasis

DIFFERENTIAL DIAGNOSIS
- Acute, severe abdominal pain: perforated viscus, pancreatitis, appendicitis, diverticulitis, bowel obstruction, kidney stones, ovarian torsion
- Chronic diarrhea with crampy pain (colitis-like): UC, radiation colitis, infection, drugs, ischemia, microscopic colitis, IBD, celiac disease, malignancy (lymphoma, carcinoma), carcinoid, segmental colitis associated with diverticulosis
- Wasting illness: malabsorption, malignancy

DIAGNOSTIC TESTS & INTERPRETATION
Initial Tests (lab, imaging)
- CBC, serum chemistries, LFTs, erythrocyte sedimentation rate (ESR), C-reactive protein (CRP), serum iron, vitamin B_{12}, vitamin D-25 OH, stool calprotectin
- If diarrhea, stool specimen for routine culture, *Clostridium difficile*, and ova and parasites in at-risk populations
- With severe flares, KUB to rule out toxic megacolon
- Ileocolonoscopy provides the greatest diagnostic sensitivity and specificity; biopsy normal and abnormal mucosa (1)[C]
- Upper endoscopy for patients with upper GI signs or symptoms (1)[C]
  - Signs of upper GI CD: antral narrowing, segmental stricturing, inflammatory mucosa

- Small bowel: sensitivity of CT or magnetic resonance enterography (MRE) better than small bowel follow through. MRE has no radiation exposure (important in younger patients). Capsule endoscopy allows small bowel visualization but no biopsy.
  - Signs of small bowel disease: narrowed lumen with nodularity (string sign); bowel loop separation (transmural inflammation); increased bowel wall enhancement or thickening suggests inflammation.
- Perianal disease: endoscopic ultrasound (EUS) or MRI pelvis, exam under anesthesia
- Contraindications to endoscopy: perforated viscus, recent myocardial infarction, severe diverticulitis, toxic megacolon
- In some cases, unprepared limited sigmoidoscopy allows adequate visualization to assess severity, extent, aspirate stool for *C. difficile*, obtain biopsies to assess histologic severity, and exclude other disorders (e.g., cytomegalovirus) in CD.

Follow-Up Tests & Special Considerations
- Evidence of complications
  - Stricture: obstructive signs—nausea, vomiting, pain, weight loss, diarrhea, or inability to pass gas/feces
  - Abscess/inflammatory mass: localized abdominal peritonitis with fever and abdominal pain; diffuse peritonitis suggests perforation or abscess rupture (may be masked by steroids, opiates).
  - Fistula:
    - Enteroenteric: asymptomatic or a palpable, commonly indolent, abdominal mass
    - Enterovesicular: pneumaturia, recurrent UTI
    - Retroperitoneal: psoas abscess, ureteral obstruction
    - Enterovaginal: vaginal passage of gas or feces; clear, nonfeculent drainage from ileal fistula (may be misdiagnosed as primary vaginal infection)
- Treatment goals
  - Steroid-free clinical remission
  - Biochemical (CRP and ESR) and biologic (calprotectin) remission
  - Radiologic response by cross-sectional or ultrasound imaging
  - Endoscopic response and remission (2)
  - Symptoms may not correlate with disease activity, so objective testing (biomarkers, imaging, endoscopy) is crucial.

Diagnostic Procedures/Other
How to distinguish CD from UC:
- CD: small bowel or colonic disease, rectal sparing; skip lesions; granulomas, perianal fistula or abscess; RLQ pain; rectal bleeding is uncommon.
- UC: continuous colonic involvement including the rectum; LLQ pain; rectal bleeding common

ALERT
CD can mimic UC with continuous bowel involvement; 10–15% of cases are difficult to differentiate.

TREATMENT

- Disease activity: Harvey Bradshaw Index or Crohn Disease Activity Index (CDAI)
- Disease severity: risk stratification for rapidly progressive disease
  - Risk factors for high-risk disease: age at diagnosis <30, extensive anatomic involvement, perianal or severe rectal disease, deep ulcers/severe endoscopic disease, prior surgical resection, stricturing/penetrating behavior, extraintestinal manifestation
- Disease severity considers longitudinal factors and prognosis, whereas disease activity is a one-time assessment of symptoms; disease severity/risk assessment should drive therapy decisions.
- Low-risk disease: budesonide or prednisone taper with or without immunomodulator
- Moderate-/high-risk disease: biologic monotherapy or biologic combination therapy with immunomodulator

MEDICATION

- Mild to moderate CD
  - Asymptomatic with mild endoscopic disease: observation alone
  - No role for mesalamine in CD (1)[A]
  - Antibiotics not recommended (1)[C]
  - Induction:
    - Controlled ileal release budesonide (9 mg/day for 8 weeks and then discontinued over 2-week taper) for distal ileum and/or right colon involvement OR prednisone taper
  - Maintenance:
    - Stop therapy and observe or consider immunomodulator/biologic therapy.
- Moderate to severe CD
  - Induction:
    - Biologic as initial induction agent to avoid corticosteroids
    - May need budesonide or prednisone 40 to 60 mg/day for short-term to alleviate symptoms (1)[C]
  - Maintenance:
    - No role for mesalamine
    - If steroids required for induction, consider biologic and/or immunomodulator.
- Immunomodulators:
  - Thiopurines: azathioprine or 6-mercaptopurine for maintenance but not induction (1)[C]
  - Methotrexate (SC or IM): effective for induction and maintenance of steroid-dependent CD (1)[C]; take with folic acid 1 mg/day.
- Anti–tumor necrosis factor (anti-TNF): infliximab, adalimumab, certolizumab pegol for induction and maintenance (1)[A],(3)[A]
  - Test for TB and HBV infection prior to anti-TNF initiation.
- Combination therapy: anti-TNF and immunomodulator
  - Combination therapy with standard dose immunomodulator is more effective than either alone.
  - Combining anti-TNF with low-dose immunomodulator reduces immunogenicity against anti-TNF.
  - Rare complication: hepatosplenic T-cell lymphoma (fatal, seen in young males) on anti-TNF and thiopurine

- Antileukocyte trafficking: vedolizumab for induction and maintenance (1)[A],(3)[B]
  - Gut-selective; no risk of progressive multifocal leukoencephalopathy (PML)
- Anti–IL-12/IL-23: ustekinumab for induction and maintenance (1)[A],(3)[B]

First Line
For moderate to severe CD patients naive to biologic drugs:

- Infliximab, adalimumab, or ustekinumab recommended over certolizumab to induce remission (3)[A]
- Vedolizumab recommended over certolizumab to induce remission (3)[C]

Second Line
- For moderate to severe CD patients who never responded to anti-TNFα (primary nonresponse):
  - Ustekinumab is recommended to induce remission (3)[A].
  - Vedolizumab is recommended over no therapy to induce remission (3)[C].
- For moderate to severe CD patients who previously responded to anti-TNFα (secondary nonresponse):
  - Adalimumab or ustekinumab is recommended to induce remission (3)[A].
  - Vedolizumab is recommended over no therapy to induce remission (3)[C].

ADDITIONAL THERAPIES
- Oral lesions: triamcinolone acetonide in benzocaine and carboxymethyl cellulose or topical sucralfate for aphthous ulcers, cheilitis
- Gastroduodenal CD: Case reports show success of anti-TNF therapy; symptomatic relief possible from proton pump inhibitors, H_2 receptor blockers, and/or sucralfate

 ONGOING CARE

FOLLOW-UP RECOMMENDATIONS
- Monitor CBC, BMP, LFTs every 3 to 4 months.
- Actively monitor disease with CRP and/or calprotectin every 6 months.
- With azathioprine or 6-mercaptopurine therapy, check TPMT/NUDT15 genotype/activity prior to initiation and thiopurine metabolites 1 month afterward.

Patient Monitoring
- Vaccinations
  - Check titers; avoid live vaccines (MMR, varicella, Zostavax) in patients on immunosuppressive therapy.
  - Regardless of immunosuppression: HPV, influenza, pneumococcal, meningococcal, hepatitis A and B, Tdap, and varicella zoster for those ≥18 years
  - COVID-19 vaccine is recommended for all IBD patients.

- Cancer prevention
  - Colonoscopy with targeted biopsies every 1 to 5 years after 8 to 10 years of CD with colonic involvement; consider chromoendoscopy if available (4)[C]; in PSC patients, annual screening colonoscopy recommended
  - Annual PAP smears if immunocompromised
  - Annual skin exam
- Bone health
  - Calcium and vitamin D supplementation with each course of corticosteroids or if vitamin D deficient
  - Bone density assessment if previous steroid use, maternal history of osteoporosis, malnourished, amenorrheic, postmenopausal

REFERENCES

1. Lichtenstein GR, Loftus EV, Isaacs KL, et al. ACG clinical guideline: management of Crohn's disease in adults. *Am J Gastroenterol*. 2018;113(4):481–517.
2. Colombel JF, D'haens G, Lee WJ, et al. Outcomes and strategies to support a treat-to-target approach in inflammatory bowel disease: a systematic review. *J Crohns Colitis*. 2020;14(2):254–266.
3. Feuerstein JD, Ho EY, Shmidt E, et al. AGA clinical practice guidelines on the medical management of moderate to severe luminal and perianal fistulizing Crohn's disease. *Gastroenterology*. 2021;160(7):2496–2508.
4. Murthy SK, Feuerstein JC, Nguyen GC, et al. AGA clinical practice update on endoscopic surveillance and management of colorectal dysplasia in inflammatory bowel diseases: expert review. *Gastroenterology*. 2021;161(3):1043–1051.e4.

 CODES

ICD10
- K50.0 Crohn's disease of small intestine
- K50.113 Crohn's disease of large intestine with fistula
- K50.011 Crohn's disease of small intestine with rectal bleeding

CLINICAL PEARLS
- Cigarette smoking doubles the risk of CD; tobacco cessation reduces flares and need for surgery.
- MRE allows assessment of luminal and extraluminal CD without radiation exposure.
- Assess for TB and HBV infection prior to initiating biologic therapy.
- Test for *C. difficile* infection when evaluating diarrhea in all CD patients.
- Hospitalized CD patients require deep vein thrombosis prophylaxis.
- Anti-TNF therapy effective in delaying or preventing postoperative recurrence in CD
- Disease severity rather than disease activity should drive therapy decisions.

CROUP (LARYNGOTRACHEOBRONCHITIS)

Afsha Rais Kaisani, MD • Antony Y. Ibrahim, MD • Niyomi De Silva, MD

 BASICS

Croup is a self-limited upper respiratory infection causing inflammation of the larynx and subglottic airway that presents with barking cough and inspiratory stridor. Although usually mild, croup can cause significant respiratory distress and even death.

DESCRIPTION
- Croup is referred to as viral laryngotracheitis (LT) or laryngotracheobronchitis (LTB). It is a common viral illness presenting with nonspecific upper respiratory symptoms.
- Croup causes upper airway inflammation and obstruction leading to pathognomonic barking cough and inspiratory stridor; symptoms start abruptly and are worse at nighttime.

EPIDEMIOLOGY
- Most commonly affects children aged 6 months to 3 years of age, with average affected age around 2.5 years old. Although rare, croup can affect children as young as 3 months and as old as 7 years.
- Predominant sex: male > female (1.5:1)
- Most often occurs in the last fall and early winter, but may present year-round

Incidence
- Accounts for 1.3% of emergency department cases
- The vast majority are considered mild cases, but 3–7% of cases require hospitalization.
- <3% require laryngoscopic or airway procedures.
- 4.4% of children returned to the emergency department within 48 hours (1).

Prevalence
60% of barking cough resolved within 48 hours and only 2% have symptoms persisting for longer than 5 nights (1).

ETIOLOGY AND PATHOPHYSIOLOGY
- Infection of the larynx and subglottic region, causing narrowing of the airway secondary to inflammation and edema
- Small children have narrow airway enabling greater ease of edema collection. Negative-pressure inspiration pulls airway walls closer together creating inspiratory stridor.
- Typically caused by viruses that initially infect oropharyngeal mucosa and migrates inferiorly, most common pathogen being parainfluenza virus (types 1 to 4), responsible for >80% of cases
  – Type 1 is the most common.
  – Type 3 is affiliated with bronchiolitis and pneumonia in young infants and children.
  – Type 4, further categorized into subtypes 4A and 4B, is not well understood but is associated with a milder illness.
- Other viruses: RSV, paramyxovirus, influenza virus type A or B, adenovirus, rhinovirus, enteroviruses (coxsackie and echo), reovirus, measles virus where vaccination not common, and metapneumovirus
- *Mycoplasma pneumoniae* and *Corynebacterium diphtheriae* have been reported but are rare.

Genetics
Congenital subglottic stenosis, which is a narrowing of the lumen of the cricoid region, can present as recurrent croup.

RISK FACTORS
Prior intubations, prematurity, and age <3 years increase the risks for recurrent croup (more than two episodes per year) (2).

GENERAL PREVENTION
Croup spreads through droplets. Children should be considered contagious up to 3 days after the start of illness and/or until afebrile. There is not a specific vaccine for croup, but seasonal influenza vaccine may contribute to decreased risk.

COMMONLY ASSOCIATED CONDITIONS
- Some evidence suggests croup hospitalization may be associated with future development of asthma.
- If recurrent (>2 episodes in a year) or during first 90 days of life, consider host factors or allergic factors.
- Underlying anatomic abnormality (e.g., subglottic stenosis, paradoxical vocal cord dysfunction)
- Consider gastroesophageal reflux disease diagnostic consideration for patients with recurrent croup symptoms.

DIAGNOSIS

- Croup is a clinical diagnosis; most children present with acute onset of classic "seal-like" barking cough, inspiratory stridor, hoarseness, and chest wall indrawing.
- Low-to-moderate grade fever, but absence of fever should not reduce suspicion for croup.
- Severity is determined by clinical inspection for signs of respiratory distress: nasal flaring, retractions, tripoding, sniffing position, abdominal breathing, and tachypnea. Although uncommon, hypoxia, cyanosis, and fatigue are late signs of severity.
- For cases presenting with more severe symptoms or not improving as rapidly as expected, SARS-CoV-2 testing should be considered (3).
- Westley Croup Severity Score is the commonly used scoring system. It looks at five clinical features and scores are as follows: ≤2 mild; 3 to 7 moderate; 8 to 11 severe; ≥12 impending respiratory failure.
  – Level of consciousness: normal, including sleep = 0; disoriented = 5
  – Cyanosis: none = 0; with agitation = 4; at rest = 5
  – Stridor: none = 0; with agitation = 1; at rest = 2
  – Air entry: normal = 0; decreased = 1; markedly decreased = 2
  – Retractions: none = 0; mild = 1; moderate = 2; severe = 3

HISTORY
Croup is primarily a clinical diagnosis, characterized by abrupt onset of barking cough, inspiratory stridor, and hoarseness (2).

PHYSICAL EXAM
- Vital signs can demonstrate tachypnea and tachycardia.
- Pulse oximetry often is normal as there is no disturbance of alveolar gas exchange; however, oxygen saturation might be decreased in severe cases.
- Breathing sounds and voice are important for diagnosis; typically, the patient will present with hoarseness, stridor, and/or inspiratory wheezing to auscultation.
  – Substantial wheezing, rhonchi, and rales should prompt alternative diagnosis.
- Decreased breath sounds and respiratory effort may indicate the child is progressing into respiratory failure and less able to mount an effort to move air (2).

DIFFERENTIAL DIAGNOSIS
- Upper respiratory infection
- Foreign body aspiration requires high index of suspicion.
- Bacterial tracheitis: high fever, barking cough, respiratory distress, and rapid deterioration
- Retropharyngeal or peritonsillar abscess: similar septic appearance with dysphonia
- Allergic reaction (acute angioneurotic edema) includes spasmodic croup with classic nocturnal exacerbations.
- Epiglottitis: rapid onset, high fever, dysphonia, drooling, and prototypical posture of extended chin and leaning forward. The incidence of epiglottitis has significantly decreased with widespread vaccination against *Haemophilus influenzae* being replaced by strep and staph organisms.
- Others: subglottic stenosis, thermal injury/smoke inhalation, hemangioma, airway anomalies (e.g., tracheo-/laryngomalacia), other anatomic obstructions including subglottic cyst (2)
- SARS-CoV-2 presents with more severe symptoms and response to treatment is not as rapid as expected (3).

DIAGNOSTIC TESTS & INTERPRETATION
- LTB is a clinical diagnosis and does not require confirmatory testing.
- Blood work not required; if done, WBC counts may be mildly elevated with a predominance of lymphocytes.
  – An elevated WBC shift to the left (bandemia) would suggest bacterial etiology (epiglottitis, bacterial tracheitis, peritonsillar, and/or retropharyngeal abscess).
- Rapid antigen or viral culture tests should be reserved for patients in whom initial treatment is ineffective.
- If imaging were to be done, posteroanterior and lateral neck films will show funnel-shaped subglottic region with normal epiglottis: "steeple" or "pencil point" sign (present in 40–60% of children with LTB).
  – A steeple sign can be seen in patients without croup warranting other considerations.
  – All patients should be monitored during imaging; airway obstruction may occur rapidly.

- When suspecting an alternative diagnosis, the following findings can be appreciated:
  - Retropharyngeal abscess: bulging of posterior pharyngeal wall
  - Epiglottitis: thumb sign, which is a thickened epiglottis
- Polymerase chain reaction testing from nasopharyngeal mucosa is used when SARS-CoV-2 is suspected as the cause of croup (3).

Initial Tests (lab, imaging)

Radiographic imaging is not routinely indicated. CT of the neck can be considered for patients with suspected abscess, tumor, or foreign body aspiration (2).

Diagnostic Procedures/Other

Laryngoscopy should be reserved for atypical presentations or when alternate diagnosis are suspected (2). Specifically, those that are hospitalized but not intubated or those with a history of intubation and under 36 months of age.

 ## TREATMENT

- Treatment is supportive; severity of illness may dictate additional measurements.
- The limited experience with COVID-19 croup suggests cases can present with severe pathology and may not improve as rapidly as with typical croup. In a recent case study, patients required >1 dose of glucocorticosteroids before clinical improvement was noted (3).

GENERAL MEASURES

- Symptomatic treatment
- Minimize lab tests, imaging, and procedures that upset the child; agitation worsens tachypnea and can be more detrimental than accepting a clinical diagnosis.
- Pulse oximetry and oxygen should be administered for hypoxemia or severe respiratory distress.
- Frequent clinical checks may be more sensitive in identifying worsening disease.
- Heliox is a helium and oxygen mixture used for respiratory conditions and it seems to improve airflow resistance by decreasing gas density. However, data is limited on its benefits (2)[B].

MEDICATION

First Line

- Nebulized epinephrine and corticosteroid
- Corticosteroids: Oral corticosteroids should be used in patients with any severity. They provide faster resolution and decrease hospital admission by decreasing laryngeal mucosa edema.
  - Dexamethasone is the preferred corticosteroid due to its easy single dosing and ability to be given orally, intramuscular, and intravenous. It is also the least expensive steroids. Optimal dosage is unclear, but 0.60 mg/kg is the most commonly used range.
  - Other steroids (betamethasone, budesonide, prednisolone) are beneficial. In randomized trials comparing prednisolone to dexamethasone, the latter is more commonly used in the emergency department, but they have no difference in efficacy in the community.

- Racemic or L-epinephrine (equal efficacy and side effect profiles). It is reserved for moderate-to-severe cases with stridor at rest.
  - Racemic epinephrine is dosed at 0.05 mL/kg of 2.25% (max 0.5 mL) solution nebulized in normal saline to total volume of 3 mL. L-epinephrine is dosed at 0.5 mL/kg (max 5 mL) of a 1:1,000 via nebulizer. Onset of action is within 1 to 5 minutes, and duration is of approximately 2 hours. Repeat as necessary as long as side effects are tolerated. Observe child for 2 hours to ensure no recurrence after epinephrine wears off.
- Antibiotic is not indicated because this is a viral illness.
- Oxygen as needed
- Humidified air has shown no clinical benefit in moderate-to-severe croup (2).

SURGERY/OTHER PROCEDURES

- Intubation rarely is required; tube 0.5 to 1.0 mm smaller than normal
- Intubation may be required for fatigue due to work of breathing or obstruction.

ADMISSION, INPATIENT, AND NURSING CONSIDERATIONS

- Outpatient care for mild cases
- In most cases, observation in the emergency department after medical management is sufficient.
- Admission criteria: poor response to therapy or recurrent stridor at rest after epinephrine wears off, increased oxygen requirement, pneumonia, or other serious conditions
- Discharge criteria
  - At least 2 hours since last epinephrine
  - Received dose of steroids
  - No stridor at rest, no difficulty breathing
  - Normal air entry, color, and consciousness

 ## ONGOING CARE

FOLLOW-UP RECOMMENDATIONS

Patient Monitoring

Most with croup do not require specific follow-up.

DIET

- Cool, liquid diet is better tolerated.
- Frequent small feedings

PATIENT EDUCATION

- Croup is usually a self-limited and mild disease, but some will need more intense hospital care.
- Avoid agitation, which may worsen symptoms; dressed lightly; use antipyretics as needed. Keep hydrated with liquids, ice pops, etc.
- Emergency ambulance for cyanosis, lethargy, struggling to breathe, drooling and unable to swallow
- Croup is contagious in the first few days, and good hand hygiene is very important.

- The cough may linger for a few weeks.
- Parents of patients with COVID-19–related croup should be counseled on quarantine guidelines.

PROGNOSIS

- Prognosis is good. The few cases that are severe respond to intensive respiratory management.
- Recurrence is rare in viral-mediated disease. If croup recurs, consider an anatomic, allergic, or obstructive etiology.

COMPLICATIONS

- Subglottic stenosis in intubated patients
- Bacterial tracheitis
- Cardiopulmonary arrest
- Pneumonia (2)

REFERENCES

1. Hanna J, Brauer PR, Morse E, et al. Epidemiological analysis of croup in the emergency department using two national datasets. *Int J Pediatr Otorhinolaryngol*. 2019;126:109641.
2. Smith DK, McDermott AJ, Sullivan JF. Croup: diagnosis and management. *Am Fam Physician*. 2018;97(9):575–580.
3. Venn AMR, Schmidt JM, Mullan PC. Pediatric croup with COVID-19. *Am J Emerg Med*. 2021;43:287.e1–287.e3.

CODES

ICD10

- J05.0 Acute obstructive laryngitis [croup]
- J20.9 Acute bronchitis, unspecified
- J38.5 Laryngeal spasm

CLINICAL PEARLS

- LT and LTB outbreaks are most common in fall and winter time for population aged 6 months to 3 years. Symptoms often occur at night.
- It is a clinical diagnosis, thus medical management and stabilization of the patient take priority over lab testing or radiographic images.
- Recurrent episodes should be followed up with a search for anatomic or allergic etiology.
- Consider other diagnoses in acute presentations with toxic appearance: epiglottitis, abscess, bacterial tracheitis.
- Be aware of severity should the child become less noisy; less air movement can be sign of respiratory failure.
- Foundation of treatment is oxygen, oral/IM steroids, and nebulized epinephrine.

C

CRYPTORCHIDISM

Pamela Ellsworth, MD

BASICS

DESCRIPTION
- Incomplete or improper descent of one or both testicles; also called *undescended testes* (1)
- Normally descent is in month 7 to 8 of gestation. The cryptorchid testis may be palpable or nonpalpable.
- Can be congenital or acquired
- Types of cryptorchidism
  - Pre-scrotal: at or above scrotal inlet
  - Abdominal: testis located inside the internal inguinal ring
  - Canalicular: testis located between the internal and external inguinal rings
  - Ectopic: located outside the normal path of testicular descent; may be ectopic to perineum, femoral canal, superficial inguinal pouch (most common), suprapubic area, or opposite hemiscrotum
  - Retractile: fully descended testis that moves freely between the scrotum and the groin
  - Iatrogenic: Previously descended testis becomes undescended due to scar tissue after inguinal surgery.
  - Also may be referred to as palpable versus nonpalpable (1)
- System(s) affected: reproductive
- Synonym(s): undescended testes (UDT)

EPIDEMIOLOGY
Incidence
- Predominant age: newborn, more common in premature newborns
- Predominant sex: male only

Prevalence
- In the United States, cryptorchidism occurs in 1–3% of full-term and 15–30% of premature newborn males (2).
- Spontaneous testicular descent occurs by age 1 to 3 months in 50–70% of full-term males.
- Descent at 6 to 9 months of age is rare (1).

ETIOLOGY AND PATHOPHYSIOLOGY
- Not fully understood, may involve alterations in
  - Mechanical factors (gubernaculum, length of vas deferens and testicular vessels, groin anatomy, epididymis, cremasteric muscles, and abdominal pressure), hormonal factors (gonadotropin, testosterone, dihydrotestosterone, and müllerian-inhibiting substance), and neural factors (ilioinguinal nerve and genitofemoral nerve)
  - Insulin-like growth factor 3 (IGF-3) or androgen receptor gene (1)
  - Environmental factors acting as endocrine disruptors
- Major regulators of testicular descent are the Leydig cell–derived hormones, testosterone, and IGF-3.
- Risk of ascent as high as 32% in retractile testis

Genetics
Increased risk of UDT in first-degree relatives suggests a genetic etiology.

RISK FACTORS
- Family history: highest risk if brother had UDT, followed by uncle and then father
- Low birth weight, prematurity, and small for gestational age (1)
- Retractile testes are at increased risk for ascent.
- Maternal smoking and diabetes during gestation (3)

COMMONLY ASSOCIATED CONDITIONS
- Anatomic anomalies: inguinal hernia/hydrocele, abnormalities of vas deferens and epididymis, hypospadias, meningomyelocele
- Endocrine disorders: intersex abnormalities, hypogonadotropic hypogonadism, germinal cell aplasia
- Genetic disorders: prune-belly syndrome, Prader-Willi syndrome, Kallmann syndrome, cystic fibrosis
- Wilms tumor

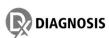

DIAGNOSIS

HISTORY
≥1 testicles in a site other than the scrotum

PHYSICAL EXAM
- Performed with warm hands, with child in sitting, standing, and squatting position
- A Valsalva maneuver and applied pressure to lower abdomen may help to identify the testes, especially a gliding testis.

- Failure to palpate a testis after repeated exams suggests an intra-abdominal or atrophic testis.
- An enlarged contralateral testis in the presence of a nonpalpable testis suggests testicular atrophy/absence.
- Testes should be palpated for quality and position at each recommended well-child visit (1)[B].

DIFFERENTIAL DIAGNOSIS
- Retractile testis (hypermobile testis): a normally descended testis that ascends into the inguinal canal because of an active cremasteric reflex (more common in males 4 to 6 years of age)
- Atrophic testis: may occur as a result of neonatal torsion
- Vanished testis may be the result of a lack of development or in utero torsion.

DIAGNOSTIC TESTS & INTERPRETATION
Initial Tests (lab, imaging)
- If only single testis not palpable in an otherwise normal male, no need for lab tests or imaging.
- In phenotypic male newborn with bilateral, nonpalpable UDTs, hormone levels help determine whether the testes are ectopic or absent (1)[A].
  - Luteinizing hormone (LH), follicle-stimulating hormone (FSH), müllerian-inhibiting substance (MIS), testosterone, serum electrolytes, karyotype
- If bilateral nonpalpable testes presents at >3 months of age, evaluate for disorders of sexual development (4) and evaluate for congenital adrenal hyperplasia.
- Ultrasound or other imaging should not delay referral to a specialist, as they are rarely needed in decision making (1)[B].

Follow-Up Tests & Special Considerations
In infants <6 months of age, periodic examination to determine if testis becomes palpable a prior to further intervention (1)

Pediatric Considerations
Without spontaneous testicular descent by 6 months (gestational age adjusted), infant should be referred to urology, and surgery should be performed within 1 year (1)[B].
- In children with retractile testes, yearly examinations to rule out subsequent ascent (1)[B]

Diagnostic Procedures/Other
Laparoscopy can confirm presence or absence of testis when nonpalpable and determine the feasibility of performing a standard orchidopexy.

Test Interpretation

Higher incidence of carcinoma in UDT and alterations in spermatogenesis. Histologic changes occur by 1.5 years of age (5).

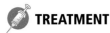

TREATMENT

GENERAL MEASURES
- Rule out retractile testis.
- Appropriate health care: outpatient until surgery is performed
- American Urological Association (AUA) guidelines on cryptorchidism do not recommend use of hormonal therapy to induce testicular descent due to low response rate and lack of evidence for long-term efficacy (1).

MEDICATION
Medical therapy is not indicated in the United States per the AUA guidelines on cryptorchidism 2014 (1).

ISSUES FOR REFERRAL
- ≥1 testes not descended by 6 months age (1)[B]
- Bilateral nonpalpable UDTs (1)
- Newly diagnosed cryptorchidism after 6 months of age (1)[B]

SURGERY/OTHER PROCEDURES
- Benefits: avoids torsion, averts trauma, decreases but does not eliminate risk of malignancy, and prevents further alterations in spermatogenesis
- If no spontaneous testicular descent by 6 months of age (gestational age adjusted), surgery should be performed within 1 year (1)[B].
- Prepubertal orchidopexy decreases risk of testicular cancer (1).
- Laparoscopy/abdominal exploration is performed first if testis is nonpalpable.
- If palpable, an inguinal approach is usually performed. If low-lying, a single-incision scrotal approach can also be considered but may increase the risk of hernia.

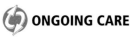

ONGOING CARE

FOLLOW-UP RECOMMENDATIONS
- Initial follow-up within 1 month of surgery and periodically thereafter to assess testicular size/growth
- Patients with retractile testes should be examined at least annually to monitor for secondary ascent until testis is no longer retractile (1)[B].

Patient Monitoring
- Patients should be followed after surgery to evaluate testicular growth.
- Testicular tumors occur mainly during or after puberty; thus, these children should be taught self-examination.

DIET
No restrictions

PATIENT EDUCATION
Discuss with parents about causes, treatments, patient's reproductive potential, and increased risk for testicular cancer.

PROGNOSIS
- Disorder is usually corrected with surgical therapy; however, there are possible lifelong consequences.
- If testicle is absent or orchiectomy is required, may consider placement of testicular prosthesis.
- Early orchidopexy may decrease risk of testicular damage and risk of malignancy.

COMPLICATIONS
- Paternity rates are similar to the general population for men with a unilateral UDT, although lower (33–65%) for men with bilateral UDT.
- Abnormalities also have been identified in the contralateral descended testis, suggesting that unilateral cryptorchidism is a bilateral disease.

REFERENCES

1. Kolon TF, Herndon CDA, Baker LA, et al. Evaluation and treatment of cryptorchidism. https://www.auanet.org/guidelines/guidelines/cryptorchidism-guideline. Accessed October 26, 2021.
2. Sijstermans K, Hack WW, Meijer RW, et al. The frequency of undescended testis from birth to adulthood: a review. *Int J Androl*. 2008;31(1):1–11.
3. Zhang L, Wang XH, Zheng XM, et al. Maternal gestational smoking, diabetes, alcohol drinking, pre-pregnancy obesity and the risk of cryptorchidism: a systematic review and meta-analysis of observational studies. *PLoS One*. 2015;10(3):e0119006.
4. Docimo SG, Silver RI, Cromie W. The undescended testicle: diagnosis and management. *Am Fam Physician*. 2000;62(9):2037–2044, 2047–2048.
5. Park KH, Lee JH, Han JJ, et al. Histological evidences suggest recommending orchiopexy within the first year of life for children with unilateral inguinal cryptorchid testis. *Int J Urol*. 2007;14(7):616–621.

ADDITIONAL READING

- Braga LH, Lorenzo AJ. Cryptorchidism: a practical review for all community healthcare providers. *Can Urol Assoc J*. 2017;11(1–2 Suppl 1):S26–S32.
- Fantasia J, Aidlen J, Lathrop W, et al. Undescended testes: a clinical and surgical review. *Urol Nurs*. 2015;35(3):117–126.
- Foresta C, Zuccarello D, Garolla A, et al. Role of hormones, genes, and environment in human cryptorchidism. *Endocr Rev*. 2008;29(5):560–580.
- Smith S, Nguyen HT. Barriers to implementation of guidelines for the diagnosis and management of undescended testis. *F1000Res*. 2019;8:F1000 Faculty Rev-326.
- Wood HM, Elder JS. Cryptorchidism and testicular cancer: separating fact from fiction. *J Urol*. 2009;181(2):452–461.

 ## CODES

ICD10
- Q53.9 Undescended testicle, unspecified
- Q53.10 Unspecified undescended testicle, unilateral
- Q53.20 Undescended testicle, unspecified, bilateral

CLINICAL PEARLS
- If testicular descent does not occur by 6 months of age, it is unlikely to occur. Refer to urologist at 6 months.
- Children with bilateral, nonpalpable UDTs require laboratory evaluation to determine if viable testicular tissue is present and to rule out disorder of sexual differentiation.
- Radiologic imaging has no role in the initial evaluation of cryptorchidism.
- The risk of infertility is increased with bilateral UDTs.

CUSHING DISEASE AND CUSHING SYNDROME

Joumana Chaiban, MD, MBA, FACE • Safiya Elahi, DO • Husna Khan, DO

 BASICS

DESCRIPTION

- Cushing syndrome is defined as excessive glucocorticoid exposure from exogenous (steroid medications) or less commonly from endogenous sources (pituitary, adrenal, pulmonary, etc.).
- Cushing disease is glucocorticoid excess due to excessive adrenocorticotropic hormone (ACTH) secretion from a pituitary tumor.
- System(s) affected: endocrine/metabolic, musculoskeletal, skin/exocrine, cardiovascular; neuropsychiatric

Pediatric Considerations
- Rare in infancy and childhood
- Cushing disease accounts for approximately 75% of all cases of Cushing syndrome in children >7 years.
  - Rarely, Cushing disease (ACTH-producing pituitary adenoma) can be the initial manifestation of multiple endocrine neoplasia (MEN) type 1 in pediatric patients.
- In children <7 years, adrenal causes of Cushing syndrome (adenoma, carcinoma, or bilateral hyperplasia) are more common.
- The most common presenting symptom is lack of growth and weight gain.

Pregnancy Considerations
- Pregnancy may exacerbate the disease.
- Cortisol levels increase in normal pregnancy.

EPIDEMIOLOGY

Incidence
U.S. endogenous causes of Cushing syndrome are rare—around 8 cases per million population.

Prevalence
2–5% prevalence reported in difficult-to-control diabetics with obesity and hypertension (HTN)

ETIOLOGY AND PATHOPHYSIOLOGY
- Exogenous
  - Prolonged glucocorticoid use (most commonly in chronic disorders like asthma, chronic obstructive pulmonary disease, etc.)
- Endogenous glucocorticoid secretion
  - Endogenous ACTH–dependent hypercortisolism: 80–85%
    ○ ACTH-secreting pituitary tumor (Cushing disease): ~75%
    ○ Ectopic ACTH production (e.g., small cell carcinoma of lung, neuroendocrine tumors of the lung, or rarely thyroid, thymus, and pancreas)
  - Endogenous ACTH–independent hypercortisolism: ~15–20%
    ○ Adrenal adenoma
    ○ Adrenal carcinoma
- Pediatric/adolescent
  - Adrenal hyperplasia secondary to McCune-Albright syndrome: mean age 1.2 years
  - Adrenocortical tumors: mean age 4.5 years
  - Ectopic ACTH syndrome: mean age 10.1 years
  - Primary pigmented nodular adrenocortical disease: mean age 13.0 years
  - Cushing disease: mean age 14.1 years
- Pregnancy
  - Pituitary-dependent Cushing syndrome
  - Adrenal causes
  - ACTH-independent adrenal hyperplasia

Genetics
- MEN
- Carney complex (an inherited multiple neoplasia syndrome)
- McCune-Albright syndrome (mutation of GNAS1 gene)
- Familial isolated pituitary adenomas (mutations in the aryl hydrocarbon receptor–interacting protein gene)
- Activating somatic mutations of the USP8 (ubiquitin-specific protease 8) gene are found in a large proportion of Cushing disease cases. Presence of USP8 mutation in pituitary tumors is linked to higher incidence of tumor recurrence after transsphenoidal surgery.

RISK FACTORS
Prolonged use of corticosteroids

GENERAL PREVENTION
Avoid corticosteroid exposure, when possible.

COMMONLY ASSOCIATED CONDITIONS
Psychiatric disorders, diabetes, HTN, hypokalemia, infections, dyslipidemia, osteoporosis, and poor physical fitness

DIAGNOSIS

HISTORY
- Weight gain: 95%
- Decreased libido: 90%
- Menstrual irregularity: 80%
- Depression/emotional lability: 50–80%
- Easy bruising: 95%
- Diabetes or glucose intolerance: 90%
- Classical features may be absent in ectopic ACTH syndrome, especially in paraneoplastic syndrome. Hypokalemia is common in addition to catabolic effects of cortisol.

PHYSICAL EXAM
- Obesity (usually central): 95%
- Facial plethora: 90%
- Moon face (facial adiposity): 90%
- Thin skin: 85%
- HTN: 75%
- Hirsutism: 75%
- Proximal muscle weakness: 90%
- Purple striae on the skin
- Increased adipose tissue in neck and trunk, supraclavicular fat pads, buffalo hump
- Acne
- Skeletal growth retardation in children (epiphyseal plates remain open): 70–80%

DIFFERENTIAL DIAGNOSIS
- Obesity
- Type 2 diabetes mellitus (T2DM)
- HTN
- Metabolic syndrome X
- Polycystic ovarian disease
- Pseudo-Cushing (e.g., alcoholism, physical stress, severe major depression)

DIAGNOSTIC TESTS & INTERPRETATION

Initial Tests (lab, imaging)
- Endocrine Society guidelines (1)[C] recommend testing for Cushing syndrome with the following:
  - Adrenal incidentaloma
  - Multiple progressive features suggestive of Cushing syndrome
  - Unusual features for age such as early osteoporosis and HTN
  - Abnormal growth and increased weight in children

- Labs
  - Screening tests
    ○ It is important to differentiate Cushing from pseudo-Cushing (e.g., obesity, alcoholism, depression).
    ○ Most widely used are the late-night salivary cortisol, 24-hour urinary free cortisol (UFC), or low-dose dexamethasone suppression testing.
    ○ Cortisol levels may vary day-to-day and a single urine free cortisol or late night salivary cortisol may not reflect the extent of cortisol exposure.
    ■ Endocrine Society Guidelines recommend biochemical diagnosis based on three different approaches:
      □ Assessing daily cortisol excretion: measuring 24-hour UFC level:
        • Obtain at least two measurements to rule out intermittent hypercortisolism.
        • Measure concomitant 24-hour urinary creatinine excretion to verify adequacy of collection as results may be falsely low if renal impairment (GFR <60 mL/min).
        • Overall sensitivity and specificity: 90–97% and 85–99%, respectively
        • Avoid drinking excessive amounts of water due to risk of false-positive values.
      □ Documenting loss of diurnal variation: late-night salivary cortisol:
        • Obtain at least two measurements.
        • Cortisol secretion is highest in the morning and lowest between 11 PM and midnight.
        • Licorice, chewing tobacco, and steroid-containing oral gels may lead to false-positive results. Nocturnal shift-workers, or those with oral diseases with insufficient saliva quantity may have false-negative results.
        • The nadir of serum cortisol is maintained in Pseudo-Cushing but not in Cushing syndrome. Sensitivity and specificity are >90–95%.
      □ Documenting loss of feedback inhibition of cortisol on hypothalamic-pituitary-adrenal (HPA) axis: low-dose dexamethasone suppression testing:
        • Dexamethasone 1 mg given between 11 PM and midnight, and fasting plasma cortisol is measured between 8 and 9 AM the following morning.
        • A serum cortisol level <1.8 μg/dL excludes Cushing syndrome, but specificity is limited.
        • Test of choice in subclinical Cushing syndrome (those with subtle increase in cortisol without signs of overt hormonal excess; follow such patients for possible progression)
        • The presence of pseudo-Cushing states (depression, obesity, etc.), hepatic or renal disease, or any drug that induces cytochrome P450 enzymes may cause a false result. Measuring a concomitant dexamethasone level may be helpful.
  - Other available screening tests
    ○ Awake midnight plasma cortisol samples on three consecutive nights. A late-evening serum cortisol >7.5 μg/dL has a sensitivity of 99% and specificity of 100%. Persistently elevated serum cortisol implies Cushing syndrome; nadir of serum cortisol is maintained in obese patients but not in Cushing.
    ○ Corticotropin-releasing hormone (CRH) after dexamethasone: although not a reliable method to distinguish pseudo-Cushing from Cushing

- After excluding pseudo-Cushing and physiologic hypercortisolism, a referral to an endocrinologist is helpful for further testing to establish the cause of Cushing.
- Localization tests: Once the diagnosis of Cushing syndrome is confirmed:
  – Morning ACTH levels:
    ○ Less than 10 pg/mL: ACTH-independent Cushing
    ○ More than 20 pg/mL: ACTH-dependent Cushing
    ○ 10 to 20 pg/mL: CRH stimulation test is recommended to differentiate between the two forms.
- High-dose suppression test: 8 mg of oral dexamethasone is given at 11 PM, with measurement of an 8-AM cortisol level the next day.
  – A baseline 8-AM cortisol measurement is also obtained the morning prior to ingesting dexamethasone. Suppression of serum cortisol level to <50% of baseline is suggestive of a pituitary source of ACTH rather than ectopic ACTH or primary adrenal disease. Sensitivity and specificity are 95% and 100%.
  – Another approach is to measure 8-AM cortisol after 8-mg dexamethasone given the night before: Cushing disease: cortisol suppressed to <5 μg/dL.
- Factitious Cushing syndrome is rare. Consider if incongruous hormonal lab results with normal adrenal findings on imaging.
- Imaging
  – Confirm Cushing diagnosis before imaging studies due to the possibility of both pituitary and adrenal incidentalomas.
    ○ Dotatate PET/CT, a high-resolution diagnostic tool is quite useful in identifying tumors missed by other forms of imaging (2), with a sensitivity of around 90–91%.
    ○ Up to 19% of ectopic ACTH-secreting tumors can remain occult despite conventional body imaging and modalities of nuclear imaging such as scintigraphy/SPECT.
    ○ Octreotide scintigraphy to look for occult ACTH-secreting tumor
    ○ Chest CT scan if ectopic ACTH secretion is suspected
    ○ Abdominal CT scan if adrenal disease is suspected
    ○ Pituitary MRI scan if pituitary tumor is suspected (all patients with ACTH-dependent hypercortisolism)

ALERT
- Antiepileptic drugs, progesterone, oral contraceptives, rifampin, and spironolactone may cause a false-positive dexamethasone suppression test.
- Pregnancy: UFC is recommended instead of dexamethasone in the initial evaluation of pregnant women (or on birth control pills). Only UFC in the 2nd or 3rd trimester >3 times the upper limit of normal is suggestive of Cushing syndrome.

Diagnostic Procedures/Other
Testing for associated findings can be useful, including:
- Thyroid function, T2DM, osteoporosis
- Polycystic ovarian syndrome/hyperandrogenism
- Oligomenorrhea/hypogonadism
- Hypercoagulable state/venous thromboembolism
- Metastases from malignant tumors
- Atrial fibrillation
- Hypokalemia
- Growth hormone reduction

 ## TREATMENT
Surgical resection once the cause has been established is the most effective treatment.

MEDICATION
- Medical therapy is usually ineffective for long-term treatment; used in preparation for surgery or as adjunctive after surgery, pituitary radiotherapy
- Metyrapone, ketoconazole, and mitotane lower cortisol by direct inhibiting synthesis and secretion in the adrenal gland. Replacement glucocorticoid therapy is often required (3).
- Metyrapone is notable for rapid onset of action as nadir of cortisol levels after a single dose is 2 hours. Mitotane inhibits steroidogenic enzymes in the adrenal gland inducing a chemical adrenalectomy. Long ½-life due to accumulation in adipose tissue. Ketoconazole inhibits adrenal enzymes leading to nadir of cortisol in 2 to 3 days.
- Etomidate (IV) inhibits the adrenal corticosteroid synthesis and is effective in rapidly lowering cortisol levels in severe Cushing syndrome.
- Mifepristone, a potent glucocorticoid receptor antagonist, is FDA approved to control hyperglycemia in adults with endogenous Cushing syndrome who have type 2 diabetes or glucose intolerance secondary to hypercortisolism that has not responded to (or who are not candidates for) surgery.
- Pasireotide, a somatostatin receptor ligand, is approved for the treatment of Cushing disease when surgery is not successful or cannot be performed (4). Hyperglycemia is a common and significant adverse side effect.
- Osilodrostat (a CYP11B1 and CYP11B2 inhibitor) inhibits steroidogenesis. Comparable to metyrapone, and superior to ketoconazole, in inhibition of cortisol production (5)[B].
- Pituitary tumor–directed agents such as retinoic acid, silibinin (inhibitor of heat shock protein overexpressed in Cushing disease tumors), and roscovitine (cyclin-dependent kinase inhibitor) may be effective in managing Cushing disease.

SURGERY/OTHER PROCEDURES
- Transsphenoidal surgery:
  – Primary treatment for Cushing disease: remission range of 95–90%
  – Resection of the ACTH-producing ectopic tumor
- Adrenal surgery
  – For hormonally active, unilateral adrenal adenomas, surgery is the treatment of choice. Decision for surgery is individualized for cortisol-secreting tumors with mild symptoms.
  – For nodular hyperplasia, bilateral adrenalectomy is usually recommended.
  – For patients with Cushing disease, bilateral laparoscopic adrenalectomy can be considered if persistent disease after pituitary surgery and radiotherapy. It requires lifelong glucocorticoid and mineralocorticoid replacement. Preferred in women of child-bearing age, due to teratogenicity of available medications
    ○ Synchronous bilateral adrenalectomy is effective and safe for patients with unmanageable ACTH-dependent hypercortisolism.
    ○ If malignancy is suspected further diagnostic procedures and/or adrenalectomy are indicated.

- Radiotherapy and stereotactic radiosurgery (SRS) second-line treatment for persistent hypercortisolism after surgery and has become the modality of choice for small adenoma tumors in sellar and parasellar regions.
  – Conventional radiation therapy for large tumors, or close proximity to optic nerve.
- Risk of hypopituitarism with radiation therapy.

 ## ONGOING CARE

PATIENT EDUCATION
Education about diet and monitoring daily weight, early treatment of infections and emotional lability

PROGNOSIS
- Generally chronic course with cyclic exacerbations and rare remissions
- Recurrence rate is 20% for adrenal tumors.
- Poor with small cell carcinoma of the lung producing ectopic hormone.
- After surgery, a drop in cortisol level is a predictor.
- Some patients may need supraphysiologic steroid replacement postsurgery, tapered over months.

REFERENCES
1. Nieman LK, Biller BMK, Findling JW, et al. Treatment of Cushing's syndrome: an Endocrine Society clinical practice guideline. *J Clin Endocrinol Metab*. 2015;100:2807–2831.
2. Wannachalee T, Turcu AF, Bancos I, et al. The clinical impact of [68 Ga]-DOTATATE PET/CT for the diagnosis and management of ectopic adrenocorticotropic hormone-secreting tumours. *Clin Endocrinol (Oxf)*. 2019;91(2):288–294.
3. Nieman LK, Ilias I. Evaluation and treatment of Cushing's syndrome. *Am J Med*. 2005;118(12):1340–1346.
4. Ferriere A, Tabarin A. Cushing's syndrome: treatment and new therapeutic approaches. *Best Pract Res Clin Endocrinol Metab*. 2020;34(2):101381.
5. Creemers SG, Feelders RA, De Jong FH, et al. Osilodrostat is a potential novel steroidogenesis inhibitor for the treatment of Cushing syndrome: an in vitro study. *J Clin Endocrinol Metab*. 2019;104(8):3437–3449.

 ## SEE ALSO

Algorithm: Cushing Syndrome

 ## CODES

ICD10
- E24.9 Cushing's syndrome, unspecified
- E24.0 Pituitary-dependent Cushing's disease
- E24.2 Drug-induced Cushing's syndrome

CLINICAL PEARLS
- Cushing disease is due to excessive ACTH secretion from a pituitary tumor.
- Cushing syndrome is due to excessive corticosteroid exposure from exogenous sources (medications) or endogenous sources (pituitary, adrenal, pulmonary, etc.) or tumor.
- Depression, alcoholism, medications, eating disorders, and other conditions can cause mild clinical and laboratory findings similar to those in Cushing syndrome (pseudo-Cushing syndrome).

C

CUTANEOUS DRUG REACTIONS

David H. Yun, MD • Jonathan M. Novotney, DO • Sicong Wang, MD

BASICS

DESCRIPTION
- An adverse cutaneous reaction in response to administration of a drug. Rashes are the most common form of adverse drug reaction (ADR).
- Severity can range from mild eruptions that resolve within 24 hours after the removal of the inciting agent, to severe skin damage with multiorgan involvement.
- Morbilliform and urticarial eruptions are the most common, accounting for approximately 94% of cutaneous drug reactions.
- Approximately 2% are severe and life-threatening.

EPIDEMIOLOGY
- All ages affected
- Immunosuppressed individuals at increased risk
- Patients with AIDS are 8.7 times more likely to develop cutaneous drug reactions compared to general population.
- Increased likelihood of severe cutaneous and systemic reactions in geriatric population; unclear if due to polypharmacy or change in drug metabolism
- Difficult to distinguish from viral exanthems in pediatric patients

Incidence
In the United States, incidence of 1–3% in hospitalized patients; estimated 1/1,000 hospitalized patients has had a severe cutaneous reaction.

ETIOLOGY AND PATHOPHYSIOLOGY
Two classifications of ADR:
- Predictable (type A): dose dependent, known pharmacologic effect of drug, and drug–drug interaction
- Unpredictable (type B): drug intolerance, drug idiosyncrasy secondary to abnormality in metabolism, drug allergy, and drug pseudoallergy
- Immunologically mediated reaction: immunoglobulin (Ig) E–mediated reaction (type I hypersensitivity), cytotoxic/IgG/IgM induced (type II), immune complex reactions (type III), and delayed-type hypersensitivity (type IV) with T cells, eosinophils, neutrophils, and monocytes
- >700 drugs are known to cause cutaneous drug reactions.
  - Morbilliform/urticarial/exfoliative erythroderma: penicillins, cephalosporins, sulfonamides, tetracyclines, ibuprofen, naproxen, allopurinol, acetylsalicylic acid, radiocontrast media (1)
  - Acneiform: OCPs, corticosteroids, iodinated compounds, hydantoins, lithium
  - Fixed drug eruptions: NSAIDs, sulfonamides, tetracycline, barbiturates, salicylates, OCPs
  - Acute generalized exanthematous pustulosis (AGEP): penicillins, cephalosporins, macrolides, calcium channel blockers, antimalarials, carbamazepine, acetaminophen, terbinafine, nystatin, vancomycin
  - Drug rash with eosinophilia and systemic symptoms (DRESS) syndrome: anticonvulsants, sulfonamides, dapsone, minocycline, allopurinol
  - Erythema multiforme/Stevens-Johnson syndrome (SJS)/toxic epidermal necrolysis (TEN): >100 drugs reported. Most common include sulfonamides, cephalosporins, NSAIDs, barbiturates, hydantoins, anticonvulsants tetracycline, terbinafine, allopurinol.
  - Lichenoid: thiazides, NSAIDs, gold, ACE inhibitors, proton pump inhibitors, antimalarials, sildenafil
  - Photosensitivity: doxycycline, thiazides, sulfonylureas, quinolones, sulfonamides, NSAIDs
  - Hypersensitivity vasculitis: hydralazine, penicillins, cephalosporins, thiazides, gold, sulfonamides, NSAIDs, propylthiouracil
  - Sweet syndrome (acute febrile neutrophilic dermatosis): sulfa drugs, granulocyte colony-stimulating factor (G-CSF), granulocyte-macrophage colony-stimulating factor (GM-CSF), diazepam, minocycline, nitrofurantoin, captopril, penicillamine

Genetics
Genetics may play a role because certain HLA antigens have been associated with increased predisposition to specific drug eruptions:
- *HLA-B*5801*, *HLA-B*5701*, and *HLA-B*1502* have been linked to allopurinol-induced and carbamazepine-induced SJS/TEN, respectively.
- HLA-DQB1*0301 allele found in 66% of patients of erythema multiforme compared with 31% of control subjects
- HLA class I antigens, such as *HLA-A2*, *HLA-B12*, and *HLA-B22*, have been linked to TEN and fixed drug eruptions, respectively.
- CYP2C9*3 variants linked to phenytoin-induced SJS/TEN

RISK FACTORS
Previous drug reaction, polypharmacy, concurrent infection, immunocompromised, disorders of metabolism, and certain genetic HLA haplotypes

GENERAL PREVENTION
Always ask patients about prior adverse drug events. Be aware of medications with higher incidence of reactions as well as drug–drug reaction.

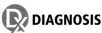**DIAGNOSIS**

HISTORY
- Any new medication within the preceding 6 weeks (oral, parenteral, and topical agents, including over-the-counter drugs, vitamins, and herbal remedies)
- Consider other etiologies: unrelated acute or chronic urticaria, bacterial infections, viral exanthems, or underlying skin disease including cutaneous lymphoma.

PHYSICAL EXAM
May present as a number of different eruption types, including, but not limited to the following:
- Morbilliform eruptions (exanthems)
  - Most frequent cutaneous reaction (75–95%); difficult to distinguish from viral exanthem; often secondary to an antibiotic
  - Starts on trunk as pruritic red macules and papules, then extends symmetrically to extremities in confluent fashion, sparing face, palms, soles, and mucous membranes
  - Onset usually 7 to 21 days after drug initiation (2)
- Urticaria
  - Pruritic erythematous wheals distributed anywhere on the body, including mucous membranes
  - Lesions can vary in size and shape (e.g., round oval, rhomboid) and may change over time.
  - Angioedema, a related manifestation, may appear as asymmetric soft tissue swelling which can compromise airway and be life-threatening.
  - Individual lesions usually fade within 24 hours, but new lesions may develop.

- Acneiform eruptions
  - Folliculocentric, monomorphous pustules typically involving the face, trunk, and proximal extremities, can also present in areas atypical of acne vulgaris such as forearms and legs.
  - Distinguished from acne vulgaris by absence of comedones
- Fixed drug eruptions
  - Solitary/few, sharply demarcated, round and/or oval erythematous plaques with dusky center that may leave postinflammatory hyperpigmentation; occur on skin or on mucous membrane
  - Appear shortly after drug exposure and recur in identical location after reexposure; some patients have a refractory period during which the drug fails to activate lesions.
  - Onset usually 30 minutes to 8 hours after administration of drug
- AGEP
  - Rapidly appearing multiple nonfollicular sterile pustules on erythematous background typically involving intertriginous areas
  - Usually resolves within 1 to 3 days after removal of offending drug leaving a desquamation pattern
  - AGEP often causes fever and marked leukocytosis with neutrophilia and/or eosinophilia.
- DRESS syndrome
  - Drug-induced, multiorgan inflammatory response which may be life-threatening
  - Presentation can involve cutaneous eruptions (typically pruritic erythematous papules and patchy erythematous macules), fever, eosinophilia (most cases but not all), hepatic dysfunction, renal dysfunction, and lymphadenopathy.
  - Onset usually 2 to 8 weeks after drug exposure
  - Symptoms and organ involvement may worsen after discontinuation of offending agent and persist for months.
  - Mucosal involvement rare (3)
- Erythema multiforme
  - Acute, immune-mediated, mucocutaneous condition
  - Most commonly associated with herpes simplex virus (HSV) and other viral/bacterial etiologies (i.e., *Mycoplasma*); less likely secondary to drug exposure (<10% of cases)
  - Palpable classic target lesions and/or two-zone atypical target lesions with localized erythema
  - Most commonly distributed symmetrically on extensor surfaces of acral extremities; may involve mucus membrane (25–60%)
- SJS/TEN
  - Classification and distinction between SJS and TEN determined by affected body surface area (BSA)
    ○ SJS: <10% BSA; SJS–TEN overlap: 10–30% BSA; TEN: >30% BSA
  - TEN strongly associated with drug intake (>95%); SJS less strongly associated (~50%)
  - Onset is usually 4 to 28 days but as delayed as 8 weeks after starting offending drug: flat atypical two-zone target lesions and erythematous macules that are truncal and generalized with mucosal involvement
  - May develop confluent areas of bullae, erosions, and necrosis; significant risk for infection and sepsis
  - SJS: 1–5% mortality; TEN: 25–35% mortality
- Lichenoid eruptions
  - Eruption of violaceous, pruritic polygonal papules symmetrically distributed favoring extensor surfaces/sun-exposed areas

- Time frame of onset varies depending on causative medication.
- Chronic lesions persist for weeks/months after the drug discontinued.
- Photosensitivity reaction
  - Phototoxic reactions: usually occur within minutes to hours after sunlight exposure with exaggerated sunburn reaction
  - Photoallergic reactions: more pruritic than painful; photodistributed sparing scalp, submental, and periorbital areas
- Hypersensitivity vasculitis
  - Nonblanching petechiae/palpable purpura which commonly present on lower extremities
  - Onset usually 7 to 21 days after drug exposure
  - Biopsy shows inflammation and necrosis of vessel walls.
  - Renal, hepatic, pulmonary, GI, and CNS involvement possible but uncommon
- Sweet syndrome
  - Fever; neutrophilia; tender, edematous violaceous papules; plaques; or nodules, with or without pustules/vesicles that spontaneously resolve
  - Classically seen in young women after a mild respiratory illness or GI infection
- Exfoliative dermatitis/erythroderma
  - Severe end-stage dermatosis that develops from other drug reactions; commonly associated with systemic manifestations such as fever and chills
  - Generalized erythema with exfoliation and/or fine desquamation of large confluent areas
  - Increased risk of secondary infection and insensible fluid and temperature loss with hemodynamic instability

DIFFERENTIAL DIAGNOSIS

- Viral exanthem: Presence of fever, lymphocytosis, and other systemic findings may help in narrowing differential.
- Primary dermatosis (e.g., pustular psoriasis): Correlation of drug withdrawal to rash resolution may clarify diagnosis; skin biopsy is helpful.
- Bacterial infection: Cultures of pustules may distinguish primary infection from AGEP and acneiform eruptions.

DIAGNOSTIC TESTS & INTERPRETATION

Initial Tests (lab, imaging)
Selection of initial tests should be guided by clinical history and physical exam findings. CBC with differential; significant eosinophilia may be seen in DRESS and other drug-induced allergic reactions. LFT, urinalysis, and serum creatinine to assess for internal organ involvement; chest x-ray if suspected vasculitis

Diagnostic Procedures/Other
- Special tests depend on suspected mechanism:
  - Type I: skin/intradermal testing, radioallergosorbent test (RAST)
  - Type II: direct/indirect Coombs test
  - Type III: ESR, C-reactive protein, ANA, complement components, cryoglobulin assays
  - Type IV: patch testing, lymphocyte proliferation assay (investigational)
  - Anaphylaxis/nonimmunologic mast and basophil cell reaction: plasma histamine, serum tryptase levels, 24-hour urine N-methylhistamine
- Cultures useful in excluding infectious etiology; skin biopsy is nonspecific but useful in characterizing an eruption and excluding primary skin pathologies.
- Develop a timeline documenting the onset and duration of all drugs, dosages, and onset of cutaneous eruption (1)[A].

Test Interpretation
- Nonspecific histologic findings are superficial epidermal and dermal infiltrates composed variably of lymphocytes, neutrophils, and eosinophils.
- SJS/TEN: partial or full-thickness necrosis of the epidermis necrotic keratinocytes, vacuolization leading to subepidermal blister at basal membrane zone

TREATMENT

GENERAL MEASURES
- Monitor for signs of impending cardiovascular collapse: Anaphylactic reactions, DRESS, SJS/TEN, extensive bullous reactions, and generalized erythroderma may require inpatient treatment.
- Do not rechallenge with drugs causing urticaria, bullae, angioedema, DRESS, anaphylaxis, or erythema multiforme.

MEDICATION
- Immediate withdrawal of offending drug. Depending on the type of eruption, symptomatic treatment may be useful, but most require no additional therapy except cessation of offending agent.
- Anaphylaxis or widespread urticaria: epinephrine 0.1 to 0.5 mg (1:1,000 [1 mg/mL] solution) IM in the mid-outer thigh every 5 to 15 min; prednisone PO 1 mg/kg in tapering doses may be given for severe refractory cases.
- Acute urticaria (<6 weeks) and chronic urticaria (>6 weeks): 2nd-generation antihistamines (preferred, less sedating): cetirizine 10 to 20 mg daily, loratadine 10 to 20 mg daily, fexofenadine 180 mg daily. H$_2$ antagonists: ranitidine 150 mg BID
- Erythema multiforme
  - Treatment is generally supportive with management of suspected underlying infection.
  - Recurrent, HSV associated: prophylaxis with acyclovir 400 mg BID, valacyclovir 500 mg BID, or famciclovir 250 mg BID (4)[C]
  - "Magic mouthwash" and oral antiseptic helpful for mucosal erosions. Consider ophthalmology consult for severe ocular involvement (4)[C].
- SJS/TEN: Treatment is supportive. Consult with a dermatologist, ophthalmologist, and gynecologist as applicable. Systemic corticosteroid use remains controversial. Consider IVIG 2 to 3 g/kg for severe disease, although limited studies have not shown survival benefits in adults. In pediatric SJS/TEN patients, IVIG and systemic glucocorticoids appear to improve outcome; varied success rates reported with use of antitumor necrosis factor-α agents, cyclosporine, cyclophosphamide, and plasmapheresis. Avoid débridement and consider using detached epidermis as natural biologic dressing to minimize risk for hypertrophic scars (5)[C].
- DRESS: prompt removal of offending drug and supportive measures; high-potency topical steroids for rash; systemic steroids with severe organ involvement; appropriate supportive multidisciplinary care guided by organ involvement (6)[C]

ONGOING CARE

FOLLOW-UP RECOMMENDATIONS
Patient Monitoring
- For urticarial, bullous, DRESS, or erythema multiforme spectrum lesions, close follow-up is needed; may even require hospitalization if suspicious for life-threatening type including SJS/TEN and DRESS
- Patients with anaphylaxis/angioedema should be given EpiPens to be kept at home, work, and in the car for secondary prevention and a Med-Alert bracelet; label the patient's medical record with the agent and reaction.
- If the patient needs to take the inciting drug (e.g., antibiotic) in the future, induction of drug tolerance or graded challenge procedures may be necessary.

PROGNOSIS
- Majority of cases are self-limiting upon removal of offending drug.
- Eruptions generally begin fading within days after removing offending agent. With morbilliform eruptions, eruption may spread distally even when agent is removed, resolving over time.
- Anaphylaxis, angioedema, DRESS, SJS/TEN, and bullous reactions are potentially fatal.
- Severity-of-illness score for toxic epidermal necrolysis (SCORTEN), a prognostic scoring system, can be used to guide management of hospitalized patients of SJS/TEN; also, may be helpful when discussing prognosis

COMPLICATIONS
Anaphylaxis, bone marrow suppression, hepatitis (dapsone, hydantoin), renal failure, psychological trauma, sepsis, and pulmonary and thyroid toxicity

REFERENCES

1. Joint Task Force on Practice Parameters, American Academy of Allergy, Asthma and Immunology, American College of Allergy, Asthma and Immunology, et al. Drug allergy: an updated practice parameter. Ann Allergy Asthma Immunol. 2010;105(4):259–273.
2. Ahmed AM, Pritchard S, Reichenberg J. A review of cutaneous drug eruptions. Clin Geriatr Med. 2013;29(2):527–545.
3. Cacoub P, Musette P, Descamps V, et al. The DRESS syndrome: a literature review. Am J Med. 2011;124(7):588–597.
4. Sokumbi O, Wetter DA. Clinical features, diagnosis, and treatment of erythema multiforme: a review for the practicing dermatologist. Int J Dermatol. 2012;51(8):889–902.
5. Dodiuk-Gad RP, Chung WH, Valeyrie-Allanore L, et al. Stevens-Johnson syndrome and toxic epidermal necrolysis: an update. Am J Clin Dermatol. 2015;16(6):475–493.
6. Hoetzenecker W, Nägeli M, Mehra ET, et al. Adverse cutaneous drug eruptions: current understanding. Semin Immunopathol. 2016;38(1):75–86.

 CODES

ICD10
- L27.1 Loc skin eruption due to drugs and meds taken internally
- L50.0 Allergic urticaria
- R21 Rash and other nonspecific skin eruption

CLINICAL PEARLS
- Virtually, any drug can cause a rash; antibiotics are the most common culprits that cause cutaneous drug reactions.
- Focus on drug history with new suspicious skin eruptions.
- Usually self-limited after withdrawal of offending agent
- Symptoms such as tongue swelling/angioedema, skin necrosis, blisters, high fever, dyspnea, and mucous membrane erosions signify more severe drug reactions.
- Useful resources: Drug Eruption Reference Manual by Jerome Litt; www.drugeruptiondata.com

CYCLIC VOMITING SYNDROME
Joanna Jiang, MD • Stephen Firkins, MD

BASICS

DESCRIPTION
- An idiopathic chronic functional GI disorder characterized by discrete, recurrent, stereotypical paroxysmal episodes of high-intensity nausea and vomiting lasting hours to days
- Subsets
  - Cyclic vomiting syndrome (CVS) plus two or more neuromuscular disorders in association
  - Catamenial CVS: associated with menstrual cycle
  - Note: Cannabis hyperemesis syndrome (CHS) is distinct from CVS.
- CVS has four distinct phases:
  - Interepisodic: symptom-free period
  - Prodromal: minutes to hours of nausea with or without abdominal pain
  - Vomiting: hours to days
  - Recovery: Nausea remits and patient recovers appetite, strength, and energy (1)[B].

EPIDEMIOLOGY
Incidence
- 3 per 100,000 annually in children
- Limited data in adults

Prevalence
- 0.04–2% in general population
- 1–2% in children (2)
- Female > male (55:45)
- More common in children; mean age of diagnosis is 35 years in adults and ages 3 to 7 in children.
- Average of 3 years from symptom onset to diagnosis

ETIOLOGY AND PATHOPHYSIOLOGY
- Strong link between CVS and migraine: similar symptoms, frequent family history of migraines, and effectiveness of antimigraine therapy
- One proposed mechanism:
  - Heightened neuronal excitability owing to enhanced ion permeability, mitochondrial deficits, or hormonal state → increased susceptibility to physical or psychological trigger → release of corticotropin-releasing factor (CRF) → vomiting
  - Vomiting perpetuated by altered brainstem regulation → sustained vomiting
- Possible maternal inheritance, based on family history of migraines and link to mitochondrial DNA (mtDNA) mutations
- Multiple theories:
  - GI motility dysfunction
  - Autonomic dysfunction: sympathetic (1)[B]
  - Food allergy or intolerance

Genetics
- Likely matrilineal inheritance, especially with childhood onset
- A3243G or other mtDNA mutations including mitochondrial dysfunction
- Ion channel mutations
- Several polymorphisms have been identified. 165119T more common in children with CVS

RISK FACTORS
- Family history of migraine headaches
- Depression and/or anxiety
- Chronic cannabis use
- Possibly food allergies
- Hypothalamic-pituitary-adrenal axis dysfunction

GENERAL PREVENTION
- No primary prevention measures exist.
- Secondary prevention of attacks relies on multidisciplinary approach to trigger avoidance, comorbidity treatment, and prophylactic medication use.

COMMONLY ASSOCIATED CONDITIONS
- Irritable bowel syndrome (67%)
- Headaches (52%)
- Motion sickness (46%)
- Migraines (11–40%)
- Seizure disorder (5.6%)
- Cannabis use

DIAGNOSIS

HISTORY
- Children often present with bilious emesis (83%), severe abdominal pain (80%), and/or hematemesis.
- Episodes are often triggered by stressors or concurrent illness.
- The North American Society for Pediatric Gastroenterology, Hepatology, and Nutrition consensus criteria for diagnosing CVS
  - At least five attacks in any interval or >2 attacks during a 6-month period
  - Episodes intense nausea and vomiting lasting 1 hour to 10 days, at least 1 week apart
  - Stereotypical symptoms and pattern in each patient
  - Vomiting at least 4 times per hour for at least 1 hour during episode
  - Return to baseline between episodes
  - Not attributable to another disorder
  - All six criteria must be met.
- Rome IV criteria for adults
  - Stereotypical onset (acute) and duration (<1 week) of vomiting episodes
  - ≥3 discrete episodes in the prior year and 2 episodes in the past 6 months at least 1 week apart
  - Absence of nausea and vomiting between episodes
  - All three criteria should be fulfilled for at least 3 months.
- Adult hallmarks
  - Prominence of epigastric or diffuse abdominal pain
  - Increased prevalence of anxiety and depression
  - Normal or rapid gastric emptying
  - Successful suppression of attacks by chronic amitriptyline therapy (1)[B]

PHYSICAL EXAM
Evaluate for dehydration (seen in 30%).
- Orthostatic hypotension, tachycardia, dry mucous membranes
- General physical exam often otherwise normal

DIFFERENTIAL DIAGNOSIS
- GI disorders: GERD, *Helicobacter pylori*, peptic ulcer disease, cholelithiasis, pancreatitis, appendicitis, obstruction, gastroparesis
- Neurologic disorders: migraine headaches, Chiari malformation, intracranial mass
- Renal disorders: nephrolithiasis, obstruction
- Metabolic and endocrine disorders: porphyria, Addison disease, diabetic ketoacidosis, hyperemesis gravidarum, pheochromocytoma
- Behavioral disorders: Münchausen by proxy, anxiety, bulimia nervosa, depression, panic disorder

- Pregnancy
- Cannabinoid abuse—CHS: Symptoms include episodic nausea, vomiting, abdominal pain, and compulsive bathing with hot water; associated with high-dose (nearly daily) cannabis use
- Any child with suspected CVS should be evaluated for a possible metabolic or neurologic etiology if:
  - Child is <2 years of age.
  - Vomiting episodes are associated with prior fasting or increased protein intake.
  - Any focal findings on neurologic exam
  - Hypoglycemia, anion gap metabolic acidosis, hyperammonemia, or other findings suggestive of metabolic disorders

DIAGNOSTIC TESTS & INTERPRETATION
CVS is a diagnosis of exclusion. Labs and imaging are needed to identify and exclude other diagnoses and complications.

Initial Tests (lab, imaging)
- Electrolytes: hypokalemia
- CBC: hemoconcentration and leukocytosis
- Amylase and lipase
- ESR
- Hepatic transaminases: hepatitis or biliary disease
- Urinalysis: granular casts, ketones
- Urine drug screen: THC (false positives can occur, especially after IV PPI administration)
- Pregnancy test
- Lactate, ammonia, amino acids, urine organic acids, adrenocorticotropic hormone—particularly for acute episodes in children to exclude metabolic disease
- Upper GI series to exclude malrotation
- Abdominal US to exclude transient hydronephrosis, ureteropelvic junction obstruction, and biliary disease
- GI referral and esophagogastroduodenoscopy (EGD) in adults and patients with alarm symptoms (hematemesis, dysphagia, etc.)

Follow-Up Tests & Special Considerations
- Counseling—behavioral health for management of anxiety, depression, eating disorders, or cannabis abuse (if applicable)
- CT or MRI of head—assess for structural lesions of the brain or causes of increased ICP
- CT of the abdomen and pelvis—evaluate biliary and urinary tracts to exclude structural causes

Diagnostic Procedures/Other
- EGD: to evaluate for clinical suspicion of peptic ulcer disease or signs of hematemesis
- Electroencephalogram: seizure disorder evaluation
- Gastric emptying studies: Exclude gastroparesis (1)[B].
- Autonomic testing
- Neuropsychiatric testing

TREATMENT

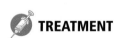

GENERAL MEASURES
- Patient reassurance
- Avoid triggers (stress, sleep deprivation, chocolate, cheese, monosodium glutamate, red wine).
- Nonstimulating environment
- Relaxation techniques and psychological testing
- Avoid recreational drugs (marijuana).

MEDICATION

First Line

- For patients who present to the ED, early treatment with antiemetics may decrease hospitalization.
- Abortive medications (should be administered in the prodrome or shortly after vomiting begins):
  - Sumatriptan: selective serotonin agonist (5-HT_{1B}, 5-HT_{1D}); >40 kg = 20 mg intranasal route or 3 to 6 mg subcutaneous route
  - Aprepitant: neurokinin 1 antagonist; 30 min before vomiting, days 2 and 3—if <15 kg = 80 mg/40 mg/40 mg; if 15 to 20 kg = 80 mg/80 mg/80 mg; if >20 kg = 125 mg/80 mg/80 mg
- Prophylactic medications (decrease frequency or severity by >50%):
  - Many prophylactic medications for CVS are pregnancy risk Category C or greater risk. Therefore, discussion of risk versus benefit of treatment during pregnancy is necessary.
    - Amitriptyline (67–82%): first-line in adults and children >5 years: 0.2 to 2.0 mg/kg/day; not recommended for children <5 years; slow titration over 2 to 3 weeks to avoid side effects
    - Cyproheptadine (39–66%): children 2 to 5 years: 0.25 to 0.50 mg/kg/day divided BID–TID; appetite stimulant; usually first-line treatment for children <5 years; especially if associated with migraines
    - Propranolol (57%): children: 0.5 mg/kg/day divided BID–TID; adults: 10 to 20 mg/day BID to TID especially if associated with migraines
  - Supportive medications:
    - Anticonvulsants, mitochondrial supplements (coenzyme Q10, riboflavin), calcium channel blockers (1)
    - Topiramate: adults with CVS and chronic headaches; 20 to 100 mg daily; 2 mg/kg/day divided BID
    - Ondansetron: children: 0.3 to 0.4 mg/kg/dose (<16 mg) q6h; adults: 4 mg IV/PO q6–8h
    - Lorazepam: children: 0.05 to 0.10 mg/kg/dose IV (not to exceed 4 mg/dose); adults: 1 mg PO QID to reduce anxiety

Second Line

- Abortive
  - Seek to use IV, rectal, or dermal medications to decrease repeated vomiting.
  - Diphenhydramine: children: 1.25 mg/kg/dose q6h, not to exceed 300 mg/day; adults: 25 to 50 mg q4–6h PRN
  - Metoclopramide: 0.1 mg/kg/dose q6h
  - Chlorpromazine + diphenhydramine: 0.5 to 1.0 mg/kg q8h
  - Ketorolac: 0.5 to 1.0 mg/kg/dose <10 mg q8h
  - Hydromorphone: children: 0.015 mg/kg/dose IV for 1 dose; adults: 2 to 4 mg PO PRN or 0.5 to 2.0 mg IM/SC for 1 dose
- Prophylactic
  - Phenobarbital (79%): 2 to 3 mg/kg/day
  - Erythromycin (75%): 20 mg/kg/day divided BID–TID
  - Valproic acid: 10 to 40 mg/kg/day (avoid if possible and substitute adjunctive mitochondrial supplements)
  - Levetiracetam: 500 to 3,000 mg daily adults
  - Zonisamide: 100 to 700 mg daily adults
  - Pizotifen: 0.25 mg BID–TID
  - Flunarizine: 5 mg once a day
  - Mirtazapine: 7.5 to 15 mg once at night

- Aprepitant: twice weekly—<40 kg = 40 mg; 40 to 60 kg = 80 mg; >60 kg = 125 mg
- Erythromycin: 20 mg/kg/day divided 4 times in a day
- Rescue therapy
  - Sedative medications
  - Most episodes (72%) end with premonitory sleep, and therefore, induced sleep can cause symptomatic relief and may shorten an episode.

ISSUES FOR REFERRAL

- Regular behavioral health appointments and consultation with a gastroenterologist can decrease episodes of CVS and reduce inappropriate pharmacotherapy. An initial referral to a gastroenterologist is needed for patients with suspected CVS.
- Referral to appropriate allied health specialist (psychologist, psychiatrist, neurologist, sleep, or substance use specialist) as indicated (1)

ADDITIONAL THERAPIES

Relaxation techniques:

- Deep breathing
- Biofeedback
- Guided imagery

COMPLEMENTARY & ALTERNATIVE MEDICINE

- Coenzyme Q10 10 mg/kg/day divided BID for prevention up to 300 mg daily
- L-carnitine 50 to 100 mg/kg/day divided BID for prevention up to 3 g daily
- Riboflavin 10 mg/kg/day divided BID for prevention
- While marijuana is a potential treatment for intractable vomiting, regular use may cause cannabinoid hyperemesis syndrome (CHS).

ADMISSION, INPATIENT, AND NURSING CONSIDERATIONS

- Admission criteria/initial stabilization
  - Severe dehydration
  - Failure of outpatient management
  - Increased anion gap that reflects severe dehydration or metabolic decompensation
  - IV fluids or IV medications
  - Lorazepam 1 to 2 mg IV q3h main approach to induce sleep most effective in acute crisis
- IV fluids: replacement of ongoing losses; 5–10% dextrose-containing fluids or normal saline with added potassium to attenuate any metabolic crisis
- Nursing
  - Decrease stimulation; avoid noise and bright light.
  - Encourage relaxation techniques.
  - Avoid unnecessary interruptions during sleep.
- Discharge criteria
  - Vomiting and electrolyte imbalances resolved
  - Pain managed with oral analgesia
  - Euvolemia
  - Appropriate oral intake

 ONGOING CARE

FOLLOW-UP RECOMMENDATIONS

Patient Monitoring

- Weekly appointments for severe cases
- Monitor for hypokalemia, acid–base disturbances, and ketosis if ongoing emesis.
- Regular outpatient visits for support

DIET

- Foods rich in carbohydrates, vitamins, and minerals
- A low-amine diet may help in children.
- Limit fats and spicy foods
- Avoid trigger foods: chocolate, cheese, and monosodium glutamate.
- Consistent meal schedules

PATIENT EDUCATION

- A vomiting diary identifies potential triggers in 75% of children
- Stress management
- Sleep hygiene
- Regular, moderate exercise
- Cyclic Vomiting Syndrome Association website: http://www.cvsaonline.org

PROGNOSIS

- Usually lasts 2.5 to 5.5 years
- Vomiting resolves in 70% of children. Many continue to have somatic symptoms (headache; abdominal pain).
- 35% develop recurrent/migraine headaches.
- 50–75% of patients treated prophylactically are asymptomatic at 1 year.
- 13% are nonresponsive to therapy. Risk factors for nonresponse include poorly controlled migraines, psychiatric conditions, chronic narcotic use, and marijuana use.

COMPLICATIONS

Occur during vomiting phase:

- Esophagitis
- Mallory-Weiss tear
- Weight loss

REFERENCES

1. Venkatesan T, Levinthal DJ, Tarbell SE, et al. Guidelines on management of cyclic vomiting syndrome in adults by the American Neurogastroenterology and Motility Society and the Cyclic Vomiting Syndrome Association. *Neruogastroenterol Motil.* 2019;31(Suppl 2):e13604.
2. Kovacic K, Li BUK. Cyclic vomiting syndrome: a narrative review and guide to management. *Headache.* 2021;61(2):231–243.

CODES

ICD10
- G43.A0 Cyclical vomiting, not intractable
- G43.A1 Cyclical vomiting, intractable

CLINICAL PEARLS

- CVS is more common in children than adults. The average age of diagnosis is 5 years.
- A food diary helps identify patterns and triggers for vomiting cycles.
- Proper sleep hygiene, stress management, and appropriate diet help mitigate symptoms.
- Treatment in the vomiting phase often requires a combination of pharmacologic and psychosocial interventions, with sumatriptan or aprepitant being the preferred abortive treatments.
- Long-term prophylaxis can help reduce frequency and duration of recurrent vomiting cycles. Amitriptyline is the drug of choice in patients age >5 years.

CYSTIC FIBROSIS

Ryan D. Lurtsema, MD • Nica E. Lurtsema, MD, MPH

BASICS

DESCRIPTION
- Cystic fibrosis (CF) is an autosomal recessive mutation that most prominently affects the pulmonary and pancreatic systems but may involve any organ system.
- Due to improvements in medical care leading to a dramatic increase in survival, adults living with CF now outnumber children (1).

EPIDEMIOLOGY
Although CF is the most common lethal inherited disease in Caucasians, it is found in every racial group.

Incidence
Number of infants born with CF in relation to the total number of live births in the United States
- 1 in 3,200 Caucasians
- 1 in 10,000 Latin Americans
- 1 in 10,500 Native Americans
- 1 in 15,000 African Americans
- 1 in 30,000 Asian Americans

Prevalence
There are >30,000 patients with CF living in the United States and 70,000 worldwide. The median predicted survival for CF patients in the United States was 46.2 years (95% CI, 45.2–47.6).

ETIOLOGY AND PATHOPHYSIOLOGY
- Primary defect is abnormal function of an epithelial chloride channel protein encoded by the *CFTR* (CF transmembrane conductance regulator) gene on chromosome band 7q31.2. *CFTR* is a regulated chloride channel that affects the activity of chloride and sodium channels on the cell surface, with mutations leading to abnormally viscous secretions that alter organ functions.
- Obstruction, infection, and inflammation negatively affect lung growth, structure, and function, leading to decreased mucociliary clearance, intense neutrophilic response with infection, and eventual degradation of supporting tissues leading to bronchiectasis and eventual failure.

Genetics
- CF is an autosomal recessive, single-gene disorder. There exist >1,500 mutations in the *CFTR* gene that can cause varying severity of phenotypic CF. Most common is the deltaF508 mutation, which accounts for 85.3% of cases in the United States, followed by the G542X (4.5%) and G551D (4.3%) mutations.
- The severity of disease can also be affected by modifier genes (*CFTM1* for meconium ileus), GERD, severe respiratory infection, or environmental factors such as smoke exposure.

GENERAL PREVENTION
Preconception counseling
- American Congress of Obstetricians and Gynecologists recommends preconception or 1st/2nd trimester genetic analysis for all North American couples.
- Newborn screening has been integral in early diagnosis, with 62.4% of new CF cases in 2019 identified with this method.
- Patients diagnosed prior to onset of symptoms have better lung function and nutritional outcomes.

COMMONLY ASSOCIATED CONDITIONS
- CF-related diabetes (CFRD)
  - May present as steady decline in weight, lung function, or increased frequency of exacerbation
  - Leading comorbid complication (20.7%)
  - Result of progressive insulin deficiency
  - Early screening and treatment may improve survival.
- Upper respiratory
  - Rhinosinusitis is seen in up to 100% of patients with CF.
  - Nasal polyps are seen in up to 86% of patients.
- The GI tract
  - Pancreatic exocrine insufficiency (85–90%)
  - Malabsorption of fat, protein, and fat-soluble vitamins (A, D, E, and K)
  - Hepatobiliary disease (12.6%) including focal biliary cirrhosis and cholelithiasis
  - Meconium ileus at birth (10–15%)
  - Distal intestinal obstruction syndrome (DIOS): (5.3%)
  - GERD (32.7%)
- Endocrine
  - Bone mineral disease (16.6%)
  - Joint disease (3.0%)
  - Hypogonadism
  - Frequent low testosterone levels in men
  - Menstrual irregularities
- Reproductive organs
  - Congenital bilateral absence of the vas deferens with obstructive azoospermia in 98% of males
- Depression (12.8%)

Pregnancy Considerations
- Pulmonary disease may worsen during pregnancy.
- CF may cause increased incidence of preterm delivery, IUGR, and cesarean section.
- Advances in fertility treatments now allow men with CF to father children.

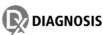

DIAGNOSIS

Criteria for diagnosis of CF
- At least one of the following:
  - One or more typical phenotypic features of CF:
    - Chronic pulmonary disease
    - Chronic sinusitis
    - Characteristic GI and nutritional abnormalities
    - Salt loss syndromes
    - Obstructive azoospermia
  - History of CF in a sibling
  - Positive newborn screening test
- PLUS at least one:
  - Elevated sweat chloride concentration on two or more occasions
  - Two mutations known to cause CF on separate alleles
  - Abnormalities in nasal potential difference (NPD) testing that are typical of CF

HISTORY
- History during prenatal period:
  - Routine prenatal ultrasonography indicates hyperechogenic bowel.
    - The risk is highest if there is evidence of meconium peritonitis, bowel dilatation, or absent gallbladder. Parents should be offered CF carrier screening if these findings are present.
- History during neonatal period:
  - Meconium ileus (20%) (generally considered pathognomonic for CF)
  - Prolonged jaundice
- History during infancy:
  - Failure to thrive
  - Chronic diarrhea
  - Anasarca/hypoproteinemia
  - Pseudotumor cerebri (vitamin A deficiency)
  - Hemolytic anemia (vitamin E deficiency)
- History during childhood:
  - Recurrent endobronchial infection
  - Bronchiectasis
  - Chronic pansinusitis
  - Steatorrhea
  - Poor growth
  - DIOS
  - Allergic bronchopulmonary aspergillosis (ABPA)
- History during adolescence and adulthood (7% diagnosed >18 years old):
  - Recurrent endobronchial infection
  - Bronchiectasis
  - ABPA
  - Chronic sinusitis
  - Hemoptysis
  - Pancreatitis
  - Portal hypertension
  - Azoospermia
  - Delayed puberty
- Suspect with failure to thrive, steatorrhea, and recurrent respiratory problems
  - Chronic/recurrent respiratory symptoms, including airway obstruction and infections
  - Persistent infiltrates on chest x-rays (CXRs)
  - Hypochloremic metabolic acidosis

PHYSICAL EXAM
- Respiratory: rhonchi or crackles, hyperresonance on percussion, and nasal polyps
- GI: hepatosplenomegaly when cirrhosis present
- Other: digital clubbing, growth retardation, and pubertal delay

DIFFERENTIAL DIAGNOSIS
- Immunologic
  - Severe combined immunodeficiency
- Pulmonary
  - Difficult-to-manage asthma
  - Chronic obstructive pulmonary disease
  - Recurrent pneumonia
  - Chronic/recurrent sinusitis
  - Primary ciliary dyskinesia
- GI
  - Celiac disease
  - Protein-losing enteropathy
  - Pancreatitis of unknown etiology
  - Shwachman-Diamond syndrome

DIAGNOSTIC TESTS & INTERPRETATION

Initial Tests (lab, imaging)
- Newborn screening tests blood levels of immunoreactive trypsin (IRT).
- Sweat test (gold standard)
  - Sweat chloride (<40 mmol/L is normal.)
    - ○ >60 mmol/L on two occasions is positive for CF.
- CFTR mutation analysis
  - Allele-specific PCR identifies >90% of mutations; finite chance of false-negative
  - Full-sequence testing is more costly and time consuming.
- NPD (when sweat test and DNA testing inconclusive)
- CXR

Follow-Up Tests & Special Considerations
To further investigate the presence of CF-related complications, these tests are generally ordered:
- Sputum culture (common CF organisms)
- Pulmonary function tests (PFTs)
- 72-hour fecal fat, stool elastase
- Oral glucose tolerance test annually after age 10 years
- Head CT: Abnormal sinus CT findings are nearly universal in CF.
- Chest CT: after abnormal CXR
- Referral to CF facility within first 24 to 72 hours of diagnosis recommended (2)[C]

Diagnostic Procedures/Other
Flexible bronchoscopy with bronchoalveolar lavage

 TREATMENT

GENERAL MEASURES
- Cystic Fibrosis Foundation guidelines call for:
  - Four office visits, four respiratory cultures, PFTs q6mo, and at least one evaluation by a multidisciplinary team, including dietitian, GI, and social worker per year
  - PFT goals: >75% predicted for adults, >100% predicted for children <18 years old
  - Annual screening for ABPA for patients >6 years with total serum IgE concentration
  - Annual influenza vaccination for all CF patients age >6 months
  - Screen all adults and children >8 years with risk factors for osteoporosis with a DEXA scan.
  - Annual measurement of fat-soluble vitamins to rule out vitamin deficiencies
  - Annual LFTs
  - Decrease exposure to tobacco smoke.
  - COVID-19 vaccination for all eligible age groups
  - Telehealth with home-based spirometry is a viable option for disease monitoring.
- All patients should be followed in a CF center (accredited sites listed at https://www.cff.org/).
- Infant care:
  - Monthly visits for first 6 months of life and then every 2 months until 1 year of life
  - Fecal elastase testing and salt supplementation
  - Consider palivizumab for RSV prophylaxis in infants with CF <2 years.

MEDICATION
- Pathogens for pulmonary infections: MRSA and MSSA, *Stenotrophomonas maltophilia*, *Pseudomonas aeruginosa*, *Burkholderia cepacia*, nontuberculous mycobacteria
  - Antibiotics should be targeted to most likely pathogen with most courses lasting 2 weeks.
- Pulmonary infections:
  - Antibiotics, oral
    - ○ *Staphylococcus aureus*: Bactrim (MRSA), doxycycline (MRSA), or cephalexin
    - ○ *P. aeruginosa*: fluoroquinolones
  - Antibiotics, inhaled
    - ○ Tobi (tobramycin): For *P. aeruginosa*, nebulize twice daily for 28 days; stop for 28 days and then resume use.
    - ○ Colistin (more commonly used in Europe)
    - ○ Cayston (aerosolized aztreonam)
  - Antibiotics, IV
    - ○ *S. aureus*: cefazolin or nafcillin
    - ○ MRSA: vancomycin or linezolid
    - ○ *P. aeruginosa*: piperacillin/tazobactam (Zosyn) or ceftazidime plus aminoglycoside (tobramycin)
- Medications recommended for chronic use in pulmonary disease:
  - Recombinant human DNAse (dornase alfa)
  - Hypertonic saline (7%)
  - High-dose ibuprofen in patients 6 to 17 years old with $FEV_1 \geq 60$ PPV
  - Inhaled tobramycin or aztreonam in *P. aeruginosa*–positive patients
  - Azithromycin in *P. aeruginosa*–positive patients
  - Ivacaftor and lumacaftor: CFTR potentiators approved in 2015 for patients with two copies of the F508del mutation
- Inhaled steroids are not recommended for chronic use in the absence of asthma or ABPA.
- Insufficient evidence for chronic use of inhaled β-agonist, inhaled anticholinergics, leukotriene modifiers, inhaled colistin
- Pancreatic enzymes, often combined with H_2 blockers or PPI to increase effectiveness
- Fat-soluble vitamin supplementation (A, D, E, and K)
- Ursodeoxycholic acid has not been proven effective for cholestasis.

ADDITIONAL THERAPIES
- High-frequency chest wall oscillation vest is the most widely used airway clearance technique, with aerobic exercise being a useful adjunct.
- CF-related bone disease: Consider bisphosphonate therapy.

SURGERY/OTHER PROCEDURES
- Timing for lung transplantation (bilateral) is polyfactorial. Key indications for referral are:
  - FEV_1 <50% predicted for those with a rapidly declining FEV_1 (>20% relative decline within 12 months)
  - FEV_1 <40% predicted with additional markers of shortened survival
  - FEV_1 <30% predicted for all others
- 5-year posttransplant survival is up to 62%.
- Liver transplantation is reserved for progressive liver failure ± portal hypertension with GI bleeding.
- Nasal polypectomy in 4.5% of CF patients

ADMISSION, INPATIENT, AND NURSING CONSIDERATIONS
- Pulmonary exacerbation (most common reason for admission)
- Bowel obstruction
- Pancreatitis in pancreatic-sufficient patients
- Always admit on contact precautions and to private rooms.
- Increased salt loss increases risk of hyponatremic hypochloremic dehydration.
- Cautious use of IV fluids with worsening lung disease

 ONGOING CARE

FOLLOW-UP RECOMMENDATIONS
- Upon discharge for a pulmonary exacerbation, follow up with CF specialist within 2 to 4 weeks.
- Routine clinic visits every 3 months with airway cultures and PFTs as indicated
- Annual comprehensive nutritional evaluation

DIET
High-calorie, high-fat diet titrated to specific BMI goals established by the Cystic Fibrosis Foundation. If not meeting nutritional goals, consider referral to dietitian, pancreatic enzymes, or supplemental tube feeds.

PATIENT EDUCATION
Cystic Fibrosis Foundation: https://www.cff.org

PROGNOSIS
- Median survival is 39.3 years.
- Progression of lung disease usually determines length of survival.

REFERENCES

1. Cystic Fibrosis Foundation. Understanding changes in life expectancy. https://www.cff.org/Research/Researcher-Resources/Patient-Registry/Understanding-Changes-in-Life-Expectancy/. Accessed November 20, 2021.
2. Borowitz D, Robinson KA, Rosenfeld M, et al. Cystic Fibrosis Foundation evidence-based guidelines for management of infants with cystic fibrosis. *J Pediatr*. 2009;155(6 Suppl):S73–S93.

 CODES

ICD10
- E84.9 Cystic fibrosis, unspecified
- E84.11 Meconium ileus in cystic fibrosis
- E84.0 Cystic fibrosis with pulmonary manifestations

CLINICAL PEARLS
- Meconium ileus is virtually pathognomonic for CF.
- When sweat test is equivocal, CFTR genetic testing is diagnostic.
- Consider CF in any child with chronic diarrhea, especially with poor growth or failure to thrive.
- All children with nasal polyps, digital clubbing, or bronchiectasis should be evaluated.
- A rapid decline in pulmonary function suggests resistant organisms (e.g., *B. cepacia*), CFRD, ABPA, or GERD.

DE QUERVAIN TENOSYNOVITIS

Lee A. Mancini, MD, CSCS*D, CSN • Nicholas R. Martin, MD • Jessica Z. Andrade, DO

BASICS

DESCRIPTION
- First identified in 1895 by Fritz De Quervain, de Quervain tenosynovitis is a painful condition due to stenosis of the tendon sheath in the 1st dorsal compartment of the radial aspect of the wrist.
- Caused by repetitive motion of the extensor pollicis brevis (EPB) and abductor pollicis longus (APL) over the radial styloid with resultant metaplastic changes of the surrounding tendon sheath

EPIDEMIOLOGY
- The predominant age range is 30 to 50 years.
- Women are affected more commonly than men (1).
- With new occupational and professional demands, the prevalence of this condition is increasing gradually.

Incidence
- The overall incidence of de Quervain tenosynovitis is 0.9/1,000 person-years.
- For patients age >40 years, the incidence is 1.4/1,000 person-years compared with 0.6/1,000 person-years for those <20 years.
- Women have an incidence rate ratio of 2.8/1,000 person-years compared with 0.6/1,000 person-years in men.
- The incidence ratio rate of de Quervain tenosynovitis is 1.3/1,000 person-years in blacks and 0.8/1,000 person-years in whites (1).

Prevalence
Currently estimated at 1.3% in females and 0.5% in males

ETIOLOGY AND PATHOPHYSIOLOGY
- Repetitive motions of the wrist and/or thumb result in microtrauma, metaplastic thickening of the tendons (EPB, APL), and narrowing of the surrounding tendon sheath.
- EPB and APL movement is resisted as they glide over the radial styloid causing pain with movements of the thumb and wrist.
- Among individual undergoing release of the 1st dorsal compartment, histopathology of the tendon sheaths was characterized by myxoid degeneration with dense fibrous tissue and mucopolysaccharide accumulation.
- Cadaveric analyses have identified an additional septum within the 1st dorsal compartment in 34–44% of individuals and subcompartmentalization has been reported in 86–94% of patients with de Quervain tenosynovitis (2).

RISK FACTORS
- Women age 30 to 50 years
- Pregnancy (primarily 3rd trimester and postpartum)
- African American

- Systemic diseases (e.g., rheumatoid arthritis)
- Participation in activities that include repetitive motion or forceful grasping with thumb and wrist deviation such as golf, fly fishing, racquet sports, rowing, or bicycling, video gaming, and more recently text messaging
- Repetitive movements with the hand/thumb requiring forceful grasping with wrist involving ulnar/radial deviation; dental hygienists, musicians, carpenters, assembly workers, and machine operators
- Recent analyses suggest anatomic variability including tendon insertion variation and subcompartmentalization of the 1st dorsal compartment may be the greatest risk factors.

GENERAL PREVENTION
Avoid overuse or repetitive movements of the wrist and/or thumb associated with forceful grasping and ulnar/radial deviation.

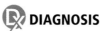

DIAGNOSIS

HISTORY
- Repetitive motion activity; overuse of wrist or thumb
- Gradually worsening pain along the radial aspect of the thumb and wrist with certain movements, particularly ulnar deviation of the wrist
- Pregnancy
- Sports, leisure, and occupational history
- Trauma (rare)

PHYSICAL EXAM
- Pain over the radial styloid exacerbated when patients move the thumb or make a fist
- Crepitus with movement of the thumb
- Swelling over the radial styloid and base of the thumb
- Decreased range of motion of the thumb
- Pain over the 1st dorsal compartment on resisted thumb abduction or extension
- Tenderness may extend proximally or distally along the tendons with palpation or stress.
- Finkelstein test: Ask the patient to actively ulnar deviate off the edge of a table and the examiner grasps the affected thumb and passively continues to deviate the hand in the ulnar direction. A positive test occurs when there is pain along the distal radius.
- Eichhoff test: Patient grasps a flexed thumb, and the examiner deviates the wrist in an ulnar direction.
- Finkelstein test is more sensitive for determining tenosynovitis of the APL and EPB tendons (3)[A].

DIFFERENTIAL DIAGNOSIS
- Scaphoid fracture
- Scapholunate ligament tear

- Dorsal wrist ganglion
- Osteoarthritis of the 1st carpometacarpal (CMC) joint
- Flexor carpi radialis tendonitis
- Infectious tenosynovitis
- Tendonitis of the wrist extensors
- Intersection syndrome
- Trigger thumb

DIAGNOSTIC TESTS & INTERPRETATION
Initial Tests (lab, imaging)
- Primarily a clinical diagnosis
- Radiographs of the wrist to rule out other pathology, such as CMC arthritis, if the diagnosis is in question
- MRI is the imaging test of choice to rule out coexisting soft tissue injury or wrist joint pathology.

Follow-Up Tests & Special Considerations
- Ultrasound can help to detect anatomic variations in the 1st dorsal extensor compartment of the wrist and target corticosteroid injections (4),(5).
- Ultrasound imaging has been reported as 100% sensitive for detection of pathology (2).

Test Interpretation
Inflamed and thickened retinacular sheath of the tendon

TREATMENT

- Most cases of de Quervain tenosynovitis are self-limited.
- Rest and NSAIDs (3)[A]
- Ice (15 to 20 minutes 5 to 6 times a day)
- Immobilization with a thumb spica splint (3)[A]
- Occupational therapy
- Acupuncture
- Corticosteroid injection (preferably ultrasound guided)
- Consider surgery if conservative measures fail >6 months.

GENERAL MEASURES
- If full relief is not achieved, a corticosteroid injection of the tendon sheath can improve symptoms.
- Anatomic variation, including subcompartmentalization of the 1st dorsal compartment or the EPB tendon traveling in a separate compartment, may complicate treatment. Ultrasound can distinguish these variants and improve anatomic accuracy of injections (4).
- Surgical release may be indicated after 3 to 6 months of conservative treatment if symptoms persist. Surgery is highly effective and has a relatively low rate of complications.

MEDICATION

First Line
Splinting, rest, and NSAIDs

Second Line
- Corticosteroid injection of the tendon sheath has shown significant cure rates. Additional injections are sometimes required.
- Corticosteroid injection plus immobilization is more effective than immobilization alone (6)[B].
- Ultrasound-guided percutaneous tenotomy, retinaculum release, and/or injection of platelet-rich plasma are newer techniques that show promise for treatment of de Quervain tenosynovitis.

ISSUES FOR REFERRAL
Referral to a hand surgeon is indicated if there is no improvement with conservative therapy.

ADDITIONAL THERAPIES
- Hand therapy, along with iontophoresis/phonophoresis, may help improve outcomes in persistent cases.
- Patients may use thumb-stretching exercises as part of their rehabilitation.

SURGERY/OTHER PROCEDURES
- Indicated for patients who have failed conservative treatment
- Endoscopic release may provide earlier relief, fewer superficial radial nerve complications, and greater patient satisfaction with resultant scar compared to open release (6)[B].

ADMISSION, INPATIENT, AND NURSING CONSIDERATIONS
Hospitalization for care associated with surgical treatment

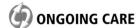 ONGOING CARE

FOLLOW-UP RECOMMENDATIONS
- Additional corticosteroid injection may be performed at 4 to 6 weeks if symptoms persist. Caution with repeat steroid injections.
- Avoid repetitive motions and activities that cause pain.

DIET
As tolerated

PATIENT EDUCATION
Activity modification: Avoid repetitive movement of the wrist/thumb and forceful grasping.

PROGNOSIS
- Extremely good with conservative treatment
- Complete resolution can take up to 1 year.
- 95% success rates have been shown with conservative therapy >1 year.
- Up to 1/3 of patients will have persistent symptoms.

COMPLICATIONS
- Most complications are secondary to treatment. These include GI, renal, and hepatic injury secondary to NSAID use.
- Nerve damage may occur during surgery.
- Hypopigmentation, fat atrophy, bleeding, infection, and tendon rupture have been reported as potential adverse events from corticosteroid injection. Ultrasound guidance reduces the rate of complications.
- If not appropriately treated, thumb flexibility may be lost due to fibrosis.

REFERENCES

1. Wolf JM, Sturdivant RX, Owens BD. Incidence of de Quervain's tenosynovitis in a young, active population. *J Hand Surg Am.* 2009;34(1):112–115.
2. Dunn CL, Polmear MM, Nesti LK. Dispelling the myth of work-related de Quervain's tenosynovitis. *J Wrist Surg.* 2019;8:90–92.
3. Huisstede BM, Coert JH, Fridén J, et al; for European HANDGUIDE Group. Consensus on a multidisciplinary treatment guideline for de Quervain disease: results from the European HANDGUIDE study. *Phys Ther.* 2014;94(8):1095–1110.
4. Lee KH, Kang CN, Lee BG, et al. Ultrasonographic evaluation of the first extensor compartment of the wrist in de Quervain's disease. *J Orthop Sci.* 2014;19(1):49–54.
5. Di Sante L, Martino M, Manganiello I, et al. Ultrasound-guided corticosteroid injection for the treatment of de Quervain's tenosynovitis. *Am J Phys Med Rehabil.* 2013;92(7):637–638.
6. Kang HJ, Koh IH, Jang JW, et al. Endoscopic versus open release in patients with de Quervain's tenosynovitis: a randomised trial. *Bone Joint J.* 2013;95-B(7):947–951.

ADDITIONAL READING

- Ali M, Asim M, Danish SH, et al. Frequency of de Quervain's tenosynovitis and its association with SMS texting. *Muscles Ligaments Tendons J.* 2014;4(1):74–78.
- Ashraf MO, Devadoss VG. Systematic review and meta-analysis on steroid injection therapy for de Quervain's tenosynovitis in adults. *Eur J Orthop Surg Traumatol.* 2014;24(2):149–157.
- Cavaleri R, Schabrun SM, Te M, et al. Hand therapy versus corticosteroid injections in the treatment of de Quervain's disease: a systematic review and meta-analysis. *J Hand Ther.* 2016;29(1):3–11.
- Goel R, Abzug JM. de Quervain's tenosynovitis: a review of the rehabilitative options. *Hand (N Y).* 2015;10(1):1–5.
- Kume K, Amano K, Yamada S, et al. In de Quervain's with a separate EPB compartment, ultrasound-guided steroid injection is more effective than a clinical injection technique: a prospective open-label study. *J Hand Surg Eur Vol.* 2012;37(6):523–527.
- Kwon BC, Choi SJ, Koh SH, et al. Sonographic identification of the intracompartmental septum in de Quervain's disease. *Clin Orthop Relat Res.* 2010;468(8):2129–2134.
- Orlandi D, Corazza A, Fabbro E, et al. Ultrasound-guided percutaneous injection to treat de Quervain's disease using three different techniques: a randomized controlled trial. *Eur Radiol.* 2015;25(5):1512–1519.
- Pagonis T, Ditsios K, Toli P, et al. Improved corticosteroid treatment of recalcitrant de Quervain tenosynovitis with a novel 4-point injection technique. *Am J Sports Med.* 2011;39(2):398–403.
- Peters-Veluthamaningal C, van der Windt DA, Winters JC, et al. Corticosteroid injection for de Quervain's tenosynovitis. *Cochrane Database Syst Rev.* 2009;(3):CD005616.
- Rousset P, Vuillemin-Bodaghi V, Laredo JD, et al. Anatomic variations in the first extensor compartment of the wrist: accuracy of US. *Radiology.* 2010;257(2):427–433.
- Scheller A, Schuh R, Hönle W, et al. Long-term results of surgical release of de Quervain's stenosing tenosynovitis. *Int Orthop.* 2009;33(5):1301–1303.
- Walker-Bone K, Palmer KT, Reading I, et al. Prevalence and impact of musculoskeletal disorders of the upper limb in the general population. *Arthritis Rheum.* 2004;51(4):642–51.

 SEE ALSO

Algorithm: Pain in Upper Extremity

 CODES

ICD10
M65.4 Radial styloid tenosynovitis [de Quervain]

CLINICAL PEARLS

- Repetitive movements of the wrist and thumb, and activities that require forceful grasping, are the most common causes of de Quervain tenosynovitis.
- Anatomic variations of the 1st dorsal compartment and metaplastic changes are identified in a majority of cases.
- Initial treatment is typically conservative.
- Corticosteroid injections are helpful and have lower complication rates if done under ultrasound guidance.
- Combined orthosis/corticosteroid injection approaches are more effective than either intervention alone.
- Ultrasound-guided percutaneous retinacular release and endoscopic surgery are helpful for recalcitrant cases.

D

DEEP VEIN THROMBOPHLEBITIS

Umer Rashid, MD • Jyothi R. Patri, MD, MHA, FAAFP, HMDC

 BASICS

DESCRIPTION
- Development of blood clot within the deep veins, usually accompanied by inflammation of the vessel wall
- Major clinical consequences are embolization (usually to the lung), recurrent thrombosis, and postphlebitic syndrome.

EPIDEMIOLOGY
- Age- and gender-adjusted incidence of venous thromboembolism (VTE) is 100 times higher in the hospital than in the community. Almost half of all VTEs occur either during or soon after discharge from a hospital stay or surgery.
- 10–30% of patients diagnosed with deep venous thrombosis (DVT) and/or pulmonary embolism (PE) will die within 1 month of diagnosis.
- One-third (about 33%) of people with DVT/PE will have a recurrence within 10 years.
- Of patients with VTE, 20% are complicated with PE. The 28-day DVT fatality rate is 5.4%; at 1 year, 20%; at 3 years, 29%.

Incidence
- In the United States, VTE incidence is 50.4/100,000 person per year.
- Increased incidence in Caucasian and African American populations and with aging
- Most common site: lower extremity DVT
- Incidence in pregnancy: ~0.5 to 3/1,000
- 1–5% of central venous catheters are complicated by thrombosis.

Prevalence
- Variable; depends on medical condition or procedure
- At the time of DVT diagnosis, as many as 40% of patients also have asymptomatic PE; conversely, 30% of patients diagnosed with PE do not have a demonstrable source.
- Present in 11% of patients with acquired brain injury entering neurorehabilitation

ETIOLOGY AND PATHOPHYSIOLOGY
Factors involved may include venous stasis, endothelial injury, and hypercoagulability (Virchow triad).

Genetics
- Factor V Leiden, the most common thrombophilia, is found in 5% of the population and in 10–65% of all VTE events and increases VTE risk 3- to 6-fold.
- Prothrombin G20210A is found in 3% of Caucasians; increases the risk of thrombosis ~3-fold

RISK FACTORS
- Acquired: previous DVT, cancer, immobilization, trauma, traumatic brain injury, recent major surgery, medications (oral/transdermal contraceptives, estrogens, tamoxifen, glucocorticoids), obesity, smoking, antiphospholipid syndrome, acute infectious process, thrombocytosis, pregnancy/puerperium, central venous catheters, inflammatory bowel disease
- Hereditary: deficiencies of protein C, protein S, or antithrombin III; factor V Leiden R506Q, prothrombin G20210A mutation, dysfibrinogenemia, elevated factor VIII activity, hyperhomocysteinemia

GENERAL PREVENTION
- Mechanical thromboprophylaxis for patients with high bleeding risk
- For acutely ill and for critically ill hospitalized patients at increased risk of thrombosis, low-molecular-weight heparin (LMWH), low-dose unfractionated heparin, or fondaparinux are recommended (1)[C].

 DIAGNOSIS

HISTORY
- Higher clinical suspicion in patient with risk factors (see "Risk Factors" section)
- DVT is classified as provoked or idiopathic based on underlying risk factors.
- Clinical assessment of bleeding risk (bleeding with the previous history of anticoagulation, history of liver disease, recent surgeries, history of GI bleed) is important prior to initiating treatment.
- Modified Wells criteria, a validated clinical prediction rule, is useful to determine the pretest probability of having a DVT.
  - Active cancer (treatment ongoing or within last 6 months) (+1 point)
  - Calf swelling >3 cm when compared to the asymptomatic leg (+1 point)
  - Collateral superficial veins (nonvaricose) (+1 point)
  - Pitting edema in the symptomatic leg (+1 point)
  - Previous documented DVT (+1 point)
  - Swelling of the entire leg (+1 point)
  - Localized tenderness along deep venous system (+1 point)
  - Paralysis, paresis, or recent cast immobilization of lower extremities (+1 point)
  - Recently bedridden >3 days or major surgery in past 4 weeks (+1 point)
  - Alternative diagnosis at least as likely (−2 points)
- Interpretation: score of 0, DVT unlikely; score of 1 to 2, moderate risk; score of ≥3, DVT likely. D-dimer testing and/or ultrasound should follow based on Wells criteria score.

PHYSICAL EXAM
- Symptoms may present as pain, swelling, or discoloration but may be nonspecific or absent.
- Edema, due to swelling of collateral veins, is the most specific symptom.
- Resistance to dorsiflexion of the foot (Homan sign) is unreliable and nonspecific.

DIFFERENTIAL DIAGNOSIS
Cellulitis, fracture, ruptured synovial cyst (Baker cyst), lymphedema, calf muscle strain/tear/hematoma, Achilles tendon tear, extrinsic compression of vein (e.g., by tumor/enlarged lymph nodes), compartment syndrome, and localized allergic reaction

DIAGNOSTIC TESTS & INTERPRETATION
Initial Tests (lab, imaging)
- Routine laboratory testing (CBC, metabolic panel, coagulation studies) is not useful for diagnosis.
- D-dimer (sensitive but not specific; has high negative predictive value [NPV]), indicated in patients with a low and moderate pretest probability of DVT or PE but not indicated in high pretest probability patients; false positives in liver disease, inflammation, malignancy, trauma, pregnancy, and recent surgery

- Patients with a prior DVT and those with malignancy have higher rates of VTE, which decreases the NPV of Wells criteria.
- Compression ultrasound (CUS): first-line imaging for DVT due to its noninvasive nature and ease of use
- In patients with suspected DVT, the diagnosis process should be guided by the assessment of the pretest probability.
  - Low pretest probability: high-sensitivity D-dimer assay sufficient to exclude DVT if negative. If positive, follow with CUS.
  - Moderate pretest probability: high-sensitivity D-dimer assay preferred as an initial test; if positive, follow with CUS.
  - High pretest probability: CUS initial test; if positive CUS, then treat DVT. If negative, no further testing is necessary; if continued concern, may repeat CUS in 24 hours
- Other imaging modalities, such as CT venography and magnetic resonance venography, are rarely used but maybe better than CUS for demonstrating new from old thrombosis.
- Contrast venography and impedance plethysmography are now rarely used.

Follow-Up Tests & Special Considerations
- In young patients and/or those of concern or with idiopathic/recurrent VTE, consider thrombophilia testing (factor V Leiden mutation, prothrombin G20210A genetic assay, ATIII functional assay, protein C functional assay, protein S antigen, and functional assay and free S, phospholipid-dependent tests and anticardiolipin antibodies, lupus anticoagulant [drawn before initiation of heparin]).
- Risk of an underlying malignancy is more likely if recurrent VTE, risk 3.2 (95% CI 2.0–4.8). Unprovoked VTE, 4.6 times higher (vs. secondary); upper extremity DVT, not catheter associated, odds ratio (OR) 1.8; abdominal DVT, OR 2.2 (2); bilateral lower extremity DVT, OR 2.1 (2)

TREATMENT

MEDICATION
Consider starting therapy before diagnosis confirmation in patients with high pretest probability and acceptable risk of bleeding.
- Anticoagulation is the mainstay of therapy. For patients with PE or proximal DVT, long-term therapy (at least 3 months) is recommended. Duration of therapy after 3 months is case-by-case basis.
- Indefinite anticoagulation is considered if there is a low risk of bleeding if index event is unprovoked PE and/or if D-dimer is positive 1 month after stopping anticoagulation.
- Direct oral anticoagulants (dabigatran, rivaroxaban, apixaban, or edoxaban) recommended instead of vitamin K antagonists for the first 3 months of treatment in patients with lower extremity DVT or PE and no cancer (2)[B]
- Use and choice of anticoagulation should be considered based on the patient's history, bleeding risk, cost, and ease of compliance.

First Line

- Unfractionated heparin
  - IV drip: initial dose of 80 U/kg followed by continuous infusion of 18 U/kg/hr. Target aPTT ratio >1.5 times control. Monitor aPTT every 6 hours and adjust infusion rate accordingly until two successive values are within the therapeutic range.
- LMWH
  - Enoxaparin (Lovenox): 1 mg/kg/dose SC q12h or 1.5 mg/kg daily
  - Dalteparin (Fragmin): 200 U/kg SC q24h or 100 U/kg SC q12h
- Direct and indirect factor Xa inhibitors
  - Fondaparinux (Arixtra): 5 mg (body weight <50 kg), 7.5 mg (body weight = 50 to 100 kg), or 10 mg (body weight >100 kg) SC once daily
  - Rivaroxaban (Xarelto): 15 mg PO twice daily with food for the first 3 weeks then 20 mg PO every day with food
  - Apixaban (Eliquis): 10 mg PO twice daily for 1 week followed by 2.5 to 5.0 mg PO twice daily
  - Edoxaban (Savaysa): Initially give parenteral anticoagulants for 5 to 10 days and then transition to 60 mg PO daily (>60 kg), 30 mg PO daily (≤60 kg).
- Thrombin inhibitors
  - Dabigatran (Pradaxa): Initially give parenteral anticoagulants for 5 to 10 days and then transition to 150 mg PO twice daily for creatinine clearance >30 mL/min.
- Vitamin K antagonists
  - Warfarin (Coumadin): Start with 2 to 5 mg/day. Adjust to a target INR of 2 to 3; overlap with a parenteral anticoagulant for a minimum of 5 days until therapeutic INR is sustained ≥24 hours.
- Adverse effects
  - All anticoagulants increase the risk of bleeding.
  - Heparin and LMWH can also cause heparin-induced thrombocytopenia (HIT) (LMWH has a lower risk) and injection site irritation.
  - Warfarin is teratogenic.
  - Dosage adjustments may be required for patients with decreased creatinine clearance.

Second Line

Heparin can be given by intermittent SC self-injection.

Pregnancy Considerations

- Warfarin (Coumadin) is a teratogen. It is contraindicated in pregnancy but is safe during breastfeeding.
- LMWH is recommended over unfractionated heparin for treatment of acute DVT and PE in pregnancy.
- Enoxaparin, dalteparin, fondaparinux, and apixaban are pregnancy Category B.
- Dabigatran, rivaroxaban, edoxaban are pregnancy Category C.

SURGERY/OTHER PROCEDURES

- In selected patients with proximal DVT (acute iliofemoral DVT <14 days, good functional status, >1 year of life expectancy), may consider catheter-directed thrombolysis/open thrombectomy
- Thrombolysis (systemic or catheter-directed) reduces the incidence of a postthrombotic syndrome (PTS) after a proximal (iliofemoral or femoral) DVT by one third.

- Thrombectomy is recommended in patients with limb-threatening ischemia due to iliofemoral venous outflow obstruction.
- IVC filter
  - Not routinely inserted in patients with acute DVT
  - It may be considered in patients with DVT or PE with absolute contraindication to anticoagulation or recurrent embolism despite adequate anticoagulation.
  - Special considerations can be given to patients who are chronically immobile, such as spinal cord injury patients.

ADMISSION, INPATIENT, AND NURSING CONSIDERATIONS

- In patients with acute PE, if the following criteria are met, then hospital admission is not necessary. Patients who meet these criteria but are admitted may be discharged early (<5 days of inpatient treatment) (2):
  - The patient is clinically stable with good cardiopulmonary reserve.
  - No recent bleeding, severe renal or liver disease, or severe thrombocytopenia <70,000
  - Expected to be compliant
  - The patient feels well enough to be treated at home.
- Admission for respiratory distress, elevated cardiac biomarkers, right ventricular dysfunction, candidate for thrombolysis, active bleeding, renal failure, phlegmasia alba dolens, phlegmasia cerulea dolens, history of HIT
- In medically stable and properly anticoagulated patients, an overlap of anticoagulation and warfarin monitoring may be done as an outpatient.
- Limb elevation and graduated compression stockings for symptomatic relief

 ONGOING CARE

FOLLOW-UP RECOMMENDATIONS

- Resumption of normal activity with avoidance of prolonged immobility
- Compression stockings are not routinely recommended for the prevention of PTS after acute DVT (2)[B] but can be used for patients who already present with symptoms of PTS.

Patient Monitoring

- Monitor platelet counts while on heparin, LMWH, and fondaparinux for HIT.
- An anti-Xa activity level may help guide LMWH titration of therapy.
- Investigate significant bleeding (e.g., hematuria or GI hemorrhage) because anticoagulant therapy may unmask a preexisting lesion (e.g., cancer, peptic ulcer disease, or arteriovenous [AV] malformation).

PATIENT EDUCATION

Dietary habits should be discussed when warfarin is initiated to ensure that intake of vitamin K–rich foods are monitored.

PROGNOSIS

- 20% of untreated proximal (iliofemoral, femoral, or popliteal) lower extremity DVTs progress to PE, and 10–20% of those are fatal. However, with anticoagulant therapy, mortality is decreased 5- to 10-fold.
- DVT confined to the infrapopliteal veins has a small risk of embolization but can propagate proximally.
- Up to 75% of patients with symptomatic DVT present with PTS after 5 to 10 years.

COMPLICATIONS

PE (fatal in 10–20%), arterial embolism (paradoxical embolization) with AV shunting, chronic venous insufficiency, PTS, treatment-induced hemorrhage, soft tissue ischemia associated with massive clot and high venous pressures; phlegmasia cerulea dolens (rare but a surgical emergency)

REFERENCES

1. Holbrook A, Schulman S, Witt DM, et al. Evidence-based management of anticoagulant therapy: antithrombotic therapy and prevention of thrombosis, 9th ed: American College of Chest Physicians evidence-based clinical practice guidelines. *Chest.* 2012;141(Suppl 2):e152S–e184S.
2. Kearon C, Akl EA, Ornelas J, et al. Antithrombotic therapy for VTE disease: CHEST guideline and expert panel report. *Chest.* 2016;149(2):315–352.

 SEE ALSO

Antithrombin Deficiency; Factor V Leiden; Protein C Deficiency; Protein S Deficiency; Prothrombin 20210 (Mutation); Pulmonary Embolism

CODES

ICD10

- I80.209 Phlbts and thombophlb of unsp deep vessels of unsp low extrm
- I80.299 Phlebitis and thombophlb of deep vessels of unsp low extrm
- I80.10 Phlebitis and thrombophlebitis of unspecified femoral vein

CLINICAL PEARLS

- Many cases of VTE are asymptomatic.
- At the time of DVT diagnosis, as many as 40% of patients also have asymptomatic PE.
- Wells criteria is useful to determine the pretest probability of a DVT, but follow-up testing and/or imaging should be done if moderate to high probability.
- Choice of anticoagulant therapy should be individualized based on patient's history and compliance.

DEHYDRATION

Tu Dan H. Nguyen, MD

BASICS

DESCRIPTION
- A state of negative fluid balance; strictly defined as free water deficiency
- The two types of dehydration:
  - Water loss
  - Salt and water loss (combination of dehydration and hypovolemia)

EPIDEMIOLOGY
- Responsible for 10% of all pediatric hospitalizations in the United States
- Gastroenteritis, one of its leading causes, accounts to 13/1,000 children <5 years of age annually in the United States.

Incidence
- More than half a million hospital admissions annually in the United States for dehydration
- Of hospitalized older persons, 8% are dehydrated (1).
- Worldwide, ~3 to 5 billion cases of acute gastroenteritis occur each year in children <5 years of age, resulting in nearly 2 million deaths.

ETIOLOGY AND PATHOPHYSIOLOGY
- Negative fluid balance occurs when ongoing fluid losses exceed fluid intake.
- Fluid losses can be insensible (sweat, respiration), obligate (urine, stool), or abnormal (diarrhea, vomiting, osmotic diuresis in diabetic ketoacidosis).
- Negative fluid balance can lead to severe intravascular volume depletion (hypovolemia) and end-organ damage from inadequate perfusion.
- The elderly are at increased risk as kidney function, urine concentration, thirst sensation, aldosterone secretion, release of vasopressin, and renin activity are all significantly lowered with age.
- Decreased intake
- Increased output: vomiting, diarrheal illnesses, sweating, frequent urination
- "Third spacing" of fluids: effusions, ascites, capillary leaks from burns, or sepsis

Genetics
Some causes of dehydration have a genetic component (diabetes), whereas others do not (gastroenteritis).

RISK FACTORS
- Children <5 years of age at highest risk
- Elderly
- Decreased cognition
- Lack of access to water such as in critically sick intubated patients
- Increased exertion in high temperature

GENERAL PREVENTION
- Patient/parent education on early signs of dehydration
- Universal precautions (including hand hygiene)

Geriatric Considerations
Systematically assessing risk factors helps with early prevention and management of dehydration in the elderly, especially those in long-term care facilities.

Clinical Finding	Mild	Moderate	Severe
Dehydration: children	5–10%	10–15%	>15%
Dehydration: adults	3–5%	5–10%	>10%
General condition: infants	Thirsty, alert, restless	Lethargic/drowsy	Limp, cold, cyanotic extremities, may be comatose
General condition: older children	Thirsty, alert, restless	Alert, postural dizziness	Apprehensive, cold, cyanotic extremities, muscle cramps
Quality of radial pulse	Normal	Thready/weak	Feeble or impalpable
Quality of respiration	Normal	Deep	Deep and rapid/tachypnea
BP	Normal	Normal to low	Low (shock)
Skin turgor	Normal skin turgor	Reduced skin turgor, cool skin	Skin tenting, cool, mottled, acrocyanotic skin
Eyes	Normal	Sunken	Very sunken
Tears	Present	Absent	Absent
Mucous membranes	Moist	Dry	Very dry
Urine output	Normal	Reduced	None passed in many hours
Anterior fontanelle	Normal	Sunken	Markedly sunken

COMMONLY ASSOCIATED CONDITIONS
- Hypo-/hypernatremia
- Hypokalemia
- Hypovolemic shock
- Renal failure
- Rhabdomyolysis
- Heat illness

DIAGNOSIS

Calculate percent dehydration = (preillness weight − illness weight)/preillness weight × 100. Supplement this along with the ongoing fluid loss.

HISTORY
- Fever
- Intake (including description and amount)
- Diarrhea (including duration, frequency, consistency, ± mucus/blood)
- Vomiting (including duration, frequency, consistency, ± bilious/nonbilious)
- Urination pattern
- Sick contacts
- Medication history (e.g., diuretics, laxatives)

PHYSICAL EXAM
- The most useful signs for identifying dehydration in children are prolonged capillary refill time, abnormal skin turgor, and abnormal respiratory pattern.
- Vitals: pulse, BP, temperature
- Orthostatic vital signs: Take BP and heart rate (HR) while supine, sitting, and standing.
  - Systolic BP decrease of 20 mm Hg, diastolic BP decrease by 10 mm Hg, or HR increase by 20 bpm suggests hypovolemia (2).
- Weight loss: <5%, 10%, or >15%
- Mental status
- Head: sunken anterior fontanelle (for infants)
- Eyes: sunken, ± tear production
- Mucous membranes: tacky, dry, or parched
- Capillary refill: ranges from brisk to >3 seconds
- Darker urine color

DIFFERENTIAL DIAGNOSIS
- Decreased intake: ineffective breastfeeding, inadequate thirst response, anorexia, malabsorption, metabolic disorder, obtunded state
- Excessive losses: gastroenteritis, diarrhea, febrile illness, diabetic ketoacidosis, hyperglycemia, hyperosmolar hyperglycemic state, diabetes insipidus, intestinal obstruction, sepsis

DIAGNOSTIC TESTS & INTERPRETATION
Initial Tests (lab, imaging)
- For mild dehydration: generally not necessary (Urine specific gravity can be helpful if obtained.)
- For moderate to severe dehydration
  - Electrolytes, BUN, creatinine, and glucose
  - Urinalysis (specific gravity, hematuria, glucosuria)
- Imaging does not play a role in the diagnosis of dehydration, unless the specific condition causing the dehydration requires imaging.
- In adults, inferior vena cava collapsibility is a surrogate marker for volume status.

Pediatric Considerations
Infants and the elderly may not concentrate urine maximally, making urine specific gravity less helpful.

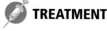

TREATMENT

MEDICATION
First Line
- Oral rehydration is the first-line treatment in dehydrated children. If this is unsuccessful, use IV rehydration. If IV unobtainable, nasogastric (NG) or intraosseous (IO) rehydration can be considered (3).
- Oral rehydration is the first-line treatment in dehydrated adults as long as they can tolerate fluids. Have a lower threshold for IV rehydration if needed.
- If the patient is experiencing excessive vomiting, consider using an antiemetic.

- Ondansetron (PO or SL, IV if needed) may be effective in decreasing the rate of vomiting, improving the success rate of oral hydration, preventing the need for IV hydration, and preventing the need for hospital admission (4),(5).
- Other antiemetics can be used.

Second Line
- Loperamide may reduce the duration of diarrhea compared with placebo in children with mild to moderate dehydration (two randomized controlled trials [RCTs] yes, one RCT no).
- In children ages 3 to 12 years with mild diarrhea and minimal dehydration, loperamide decreases diarrhea duration and frequency when used with oral rehydration.

Pediatric Considerations
Given a higher risk for serious adverse events, loperamide is not indicated for children <3 years of age with acute diarrhea.

ISSUES FOR REFERRAL
- For severe dehydration, critical care referral and ICU-level care may be warranted.
- Surgical consultation for acute abdominal issues if needed

SURGERY/OTHER PROCEDURES
For specific underlying causes of dehydration, such as intestinal obstruction or appendicitis

ADMISSION, INPATIENT, AND NURSING CONSIDERATIONS
- Intractable vomiting/diarrhea
- Electrolyte abnormalities
- Hemodynamic instability
- Inability to tolerate oral rehydration therapy (ORT)
- Stabilize airway, breathing, circulation.
- If mild dehydration, try ORT.
- If excessive vomiting/severe dehydration with shock, start IV access and IV fluids immediately.
- IV fluids
  - Stage I
    - For moderate to severe dehydration in children: isotonic saline or Ringer lactate solution bolus of 10 to 20 mL/kg; may repeat up to 60 mL/kg; if still hemodynamically unstable, consider colloid replacement (blood, albumin, fresh frozen plasma) and address other causes for shock.
    - For moderate to severe hypovolemia in adults: isotonic saline or Ringer lactate 20 mL/kg/hr until normal state of consciousness returns/vital signs stabilize. Also consider colloid replacement if continued fluids required beyond 3 L.
  - Stage II: Replace fluid deficit along with maintenance over 48 hours; fluid deficit = preillness weight − illness weight
  - An alternative IV treatment option for moderate (10%) dehydration in children
    - Bolus with NS/LR at 20 mL/kg for 1 hour

  - Replete fluid deficit with D5 1/2 NS + 20 mEq KCl/L at 10 mL/kg for 8 hours (hours 2 to 9).
  - Replete 1.5 for maintenance fluids with D5 1/4 NS + 20 mEq/L of KCl for 16 hours (hours 10 to 24).
- An alternative to IV fluids is hypodermoclysis, the subcutaneous infusion of fluids into the body (adults).
  - Indications: hydration of patients with mild to moderate dehydration who do not tolerate oral intake because of cognitive impairment, severe dysphagia, advanced terminal illness, or intractable vomiting. It is also indicated to prevent dehydration, especially in frail elderly residents living in long-term care settings who reject the oral route for any reason; useful technique for patients with difficult IV access
  - Contraindications: severe dehydration or shock, patients with coagulopathy or receiving full anticoagulation, patients with severe generalized edema (anasarca) or congestive heart failure, and those with fluid overload (6)
- Strict inputs and outputs: oral and IV input and output of urine and stool, which may include weighing wet diapers
- Discharge criteria
  - Input > output
  - Underlying etiology treated and improving

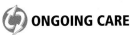 ## ONGOING CARE

FOLLOW-UP RECOMMENDATIONS
Activity as tolerated
- If mild to moderate dehydration, the patient may be mobile without restrictions, although watch for orthostasis/falls.
- If moderate to severe dehydration, bed rest

Patient Monitoring
Ongoing surveillance for recurrence

DIET
- Bland food bananas, rice, applesauce, toast (BRAT) diet
- If diarrhea, lactose-free feeds may reduce the duration of diarrhea in children with mild to severe dehydration, compared with lactose-containing feeds.
- Small frequent sips of room temperature liquids
- Oral rehydration solutions are available commercially.
- Continue breastfeeding ad lib.

PATIENT EDUCATION
- Patients should seek medical care if they (or their child) feel faint or dizzy when rising from a sitting or lying position, becomes lethargic and/or confused, or complains of a rapid HR.

- Patients should call their physician if they are unable to keep down any fluids, vomiting has been going on >24 hours in an adult or >12 hours in a child, diarrhea has lasted >2 days in an adult/child, or an infant/child is much less active than usual or is very irritable.
- http://www.mayoclinic.org/diseases-conditions/dehydration/basics/definition/con-20030056

PROGNOSIS
Self-limited if treated early; potentially fatal if untreated and persistent

COMPLICATIONS
- Seizures
- Renal failure
- Cardiovascular arrest

REFERENCES
1. Thomas DR, Cote TR, Lawhorne L, et al; for Dehydration Council. Understanding clinical dehydration and its treatment. *J Am Med Dir Assoc.* 2008;9(5):292–301.
2. Lanier JB, Mote MB, Clay EC. Evaluation and management of orthostatic hypotension. *Am Fam Physician.* 2011;84(5):527–536.
3. Rouhani S, Meloney L, Ahn R, et al. Alternative rehydration methods: a systematic review and lessons for resource-limited care. *Pediatrics.* 2011;127(3):e748–e757.
4. Colletti JE, Brown KM, Sharieff GQ, et al. The management of children with gastroenteritis and dehydration in the emergency department. *J Emerg Med.* 2010;38(5):686–698.
5. Carter B, Fedorowicz Z. Antiemetic treatment for acute gastroenteritis in children: an updated Cochrane systematic review with meta-analysis and mixed treatment comparison in a Bayesian framework. *BMJ Open.* 2012;2(4):e000622.
6. Lopez JH, Reyes-Ortiz CA. Subcutaneous hydration by hypodermoclysis. *Rev Clin Gerontol.* 2010;20(2):105–113.
7. Canavan A, Arant BS Jr. Diagnosis and management of dehydration in children. *Am Fam Physician.* 2009;80(7):692–6.

 ### SEE ALSO

Oral Rehydration

 ### CODES

ICD10
- E86.0 Dehydration
- E87.1 Hypo-osmolality and hyponatremia
- E86.1 Hypovolemia

CLINICAL PEARLS
- Dehydration is the result of a negative fluid balance and is a common cause of hospitalization in both children and the elderly.
- Begin by assessing the level of dehydration, determining the underlying cause, and calculating necessary replacement.
- Treatment is directed at restoring fluid balance via oral rehydration (first-line) therapy or IV fluids and treating underlying causes.

Holliday-Segar Method for Determining Maintenance ORT in Children (7)

Body Weight	Daily Water Requirement	Hourly Water Requirement
≤23 lb (10 kg)	100 mL/kg	4 mL/kg
24–44 lb (11–20 kg)	1,000 mL, plus 50 mL/kg for each kg between 11 and 20 kg	40 mL, plus 2 mL/kg for each kg between 11 and 20 kg
>44 lb (20 kg)	1,500 mL, plus 20 mL/kg for each kg >20 kg	60 mL, plus 1 mL/kg for each kg >20 kg

DELIRIUM

Dongsheng Jiang, MD, MSc • Shaoshan Ding, MD

BASICS

DESCRIPTION
- A temporary neurocognitive complication of illness and/or medication(s) manifested by new confusion and impaired attention
- Requires evaluation to decrease morbidity and mortality

EPIDEMIOLOGY
- Predominant age: older persons
- Predominant sex: male = female

Incidence
- >50% in older ICU patients
- 11–51% in postoperative patients
- 19% after intracranial surgery and 42% after neurovascular surgery (1)
- 10–40% in hospitalized older patients
- 20–22% in nursing home/post–acute-care patients

Prevalence
- 1–2% in outpatients
- 8–17% in older ED patients
- 14% in older postacute care patients
- 18–35% in hospitalized general medicine patients

ETIOLOGY AND PATHOPHYSIOLOGY
- Multifactorial: believed to result from a decline in physiologic reserves with aging, resulting in a vulnerability to new stressors
- Often interaction between predisposing and precipitating risk factors

RISK FACTORS
- Predisposing risk factors
  - Advanced age, >70 years
  - Preexisting cognitive impairment
  - Functional impairment
  - Dehydration
  - History of alcohol abuse
  - Malnutrition
  - Hearing or vision impairment
  - Multiple comorbidities
- Precipitating risk factors
  - Severe illness in any organ system(s)
  - Medical devices (urinary catheter, restraints)
  - Polypharmacy (≥5 medications)
  - Specific medications, especially benzodiazepines, opioids, and anticholinergics diphenhydramine, high-dose neuroleptics
  - Pain
  - Any iatrogenic event
  - Surgery
  - Sleep deprivation

COMMONLY ASSOCIATED CONDITIONS
Multiple but most common are the following:
- New medicine or medicine changes
- Infections (especially lung, urine, and blood stream, but consider meningitis as well)
- Toxic metabolic (especially low sodium, elevated calcium, renal failure, and hepatic failure)

- Heart attack or stroke
- Alcohol or drug withdrawal
- Preexisting cognitive impairment increases risk.

DIAGNOSIS

- Delirium is a diagnosis of exclusion.
- Diagnosis is made using a careful history, behavioral observation, and cognitive assessment.
  - *Diagnostic and Statistical Manual of Mental Disorders*, 5th edition, diagnostic criteria include (2):
    - Disturbance in attention and awareness
    - Change in cognition not due to dementia or coma
    - Presence of an additional disturbance in cognition (e.g., memory deficit, language, visuospatial ability, disorientation or perception)
    - Onset over short period (hours to days) and fluctuates during course of day
    - Evidence from history, exam, or lab that disturbance is caused by physiologic consequence of medical condition, intoxicating substance, medication use, or more than one cause.
  - The Confusion Assessment Method (CAM) is the most well validated and tested clinical tool (sensitivity 94–100% and specificity 90–95% (3)[B]) and has been adapted for ICU setting in adults (CAM-ICU) and children (pediatric CAM-ICU [pCAM-ICU]).

ALERT
- Four key diagnostic features of the CAM:
  - Acute change in mental status
  - Fluctuating course
  - Inattention
  - Disorganized thinking or altered level of consciousness
- Several nondiagnostic symptoms may be present:
  - Short- and long-term memory problems
  - Sleep–wake cycle disturbances
  - Hallucinations and/or delusions
  - Emotional lability
  - Tremors and asterixis
- Subtypes based on level of consciousness
  - Hyperactive delirium (15%): Patients are loud, agitated, restless, and disruptive.
  - Hypoactive delirium (20%): quietly confused; sleepy; may sit and not eat, drink, or move
  - Mixed delirium (50%): features of both hyperactive and hypoactive delirium
  - Normal consciousness delirium (15%): still displays disorganized thinking, along with acute onset, inattention, and fluctuating mental status
  - Subsyndromal delirium (23%): some delirium symptoms but does not progress to full delirium

HISTORY
- Time course of mental status changes
- Recent medication changes
- Symptoms of infection

- New neurologic signs
- Abrupt change in functional ability

PHYSICAL EXAM
- Comprehensive cardiorespiratory exam is essential.
- Focal neurologic signs are usually absent.
- Mini-Mental State Examination (MMSE) is the most well-known and studied cognitive screen, but it may not be the most appropriate in an acute care setting; shorter cognitive screens have been studied in delirious patients (i.e., Short Blessed Test [SBT], Brief Alzheimer Screen [BAS], and Ottawa 3DY) and may be helpful if performed serially over time.
- Gastrointestinal/genitourinary exam for constipation/urinary retention

DIFFERENTIAL DIAGNOSIS
- Depression (disturbance of mood, normal level of consciousness, fluctuates weeks to months)
- Acute stress disorder (disturbance of mood, normal level of consciousness, precipitated by traumatic event)
- Bipolar disorder, manic episode (pressured speech, impulsivity, fluctuates weeks to months, rarely sudden onset in older adults)
- Dementia (insidious onset, memory problems, normal level of consciousness, fluctuates days to weeks)
- Psychosis (rarely sudden onset in older adults)
- Seizure disorders (i.e., nonconvulsive status epilepticus)

DIAGNOSTIC TESTS & INTERPRETATION
Initial Tests (lab, imaging)
- Labs: guided by history and physical exam
  - Complete blood count (CBC), comprehensive metabolic panel (CMP), urinalysis (UA), urine culture, blood culture
  - Medication levels (digoxin, theophylline, antiepileptics) where applicable
- Chest radiograph
- Electrocardiogram as necessary

Follow-Up Tests & Special Considerations
- If preliminary lab tests do not indicate a precipitator of delirium, consider:
  - Arterial blood gases
  - Troponin
  - Toxicology screen
  - Ammonia
  - Thyroid stimulating hormone (TSH)
  - Thiamine
- Noncontrast-enhanced head CT scan if
  - Recent fall
  - Receiving anticoagulants
  - New focal neurologic signs
  - Ruling out mass before lumbar puncture

Diagnostic Procedures/Other
- Lumbar puncture (rarely necessary)
- Electroencephalogram (rarely necessary)

TREATMENT

- The best treatment is prevention:
  - There is strong evidence for multicomponent non-pharmacologic interventions.
  - The Hospital Elder Life Program (HELP) is a widely used approach (3),(4),(5):
    - Address acute medical issues (e.g., treat underlying disorder, stabilize vitals, maintain hydration).
    - Reorientation strategies:
      - Use orientation boards, clocks, calendars.
      - Provide eyeglasses, hearing aids, interpreters; encourage family involvement.
    - Optimize hydration and nutrition.
    - Early mobilization
    - Avoid restraints.
    - Encourage self-care.
    - Normalize sleep–wake cycle (discourage napping, open curtains during day, prioritize uninterrupted sleep).
    - Pain control with nonopioids
    - Drug adjustments (avoid or reduce psychoactive drugs and anticholinergic medications, prioritize nonpharmacologic approaches)
    - Pharmacologic management of symptoms (reserve for severe circumstances)
  - Addressing six risk factors (i.e., cognitive impairment, sleep deprivation, dehydration, immobility, vision impairment, and hearing impairment) in at-risk hospitalized patients can reduce the incidence of delirium by 33%.

GENERAL MEASURES

- De-escalation skill training for staff
- Look for underlying causes: hypotension, hypoxia, hypoglycemia, drug overdose or withdrawal, and others.
- Remove unnecessary tubes/catheters.
- Actively involve family members in care.
- Postoperative patients should be monitored for
  - Myocardial infarction/ischemia
  - Infection (i.e., pneumonia, urinary tract infection)
  - Pulmonary embolism
  - Urinary or stool retention (attempt catheter removal by postoperative day 2)
  - Anemia/bleeding
- Anesthesia route (general vs. epidural) may affect the risk of delirium. Depth of anesthesia likely affects risk of delirium.
- ICU sedation and avoidance of benzodiazepines may reduce risk.
- Multifactorial treatment: Identify contributing factors and provide preemptive care to avoid iatrogenic problems, with special attention to
  - CNS oxygen delivery (attempt to attain):
    - SaO_2 >90% with goal of SaO_2 >95%
    - Systolic BP <2/3 of baseline or >90 mm Hg
    - Hematocrit >30%
  - Fluid/electrolyte balance
    - Sodium, potassium, and glucose normal (glucose <300 mg/dL in diabetics)
    - Treat fluid overload or dehydration.
  - Treat pain
    - Scheduled acetaminophen with PRN morphine for breakthrough pain for example

- Avoid meperidine (Demerol).
- Eliminate unnecessary medications.
  - Investigate new symptoms as potential medication side effects (i.e., Beers medications).
- Constipation and urinary retention can cause delirium, so monitor and regulate bowel/bladder function.
  - Bowel movement at least every 48 hours
  - Screen for urinary retention.
- Prevent major hospital-acquired problems.
  - Use a pressure-reducing mattress.
  - Avoid urinary catheters.
  - Encourage incentive spirometry.
  - Venous thromboembolism (VTE) prophylaxis if bedfast
  - Early mobilization
  - Environmental stimulation
    - Glasses and hearing aids
    - Clock and calendar
    - Soft lighting with curtains open during the day
    - Music and television, if desired
  - Sleep
    - Quiet and dark environment
    - Soft music
    - Therapeutic massage
- Restraints increase risk of delirium and falls/injury.
  - Use as a last resort for patients at risk for self-injury or risk for injuring caregivers. Remove as soon as possible.

MEDICATION

- Nonpharmacologic approaches are preferred for initial treatment, but medication may be needed for severe agitation and injurious behaviors, especially in the ICU setting.
- No FDA-approved medication for delirium
- No evidence to support the use of medicine for prophylaxis

First Line

- For symptomatic management of intolerable agitation or hallucinations:
  - Antipsychotics (in alphabetical order)
    - Aripiprazole (Abilify) 2 to 5 mg PO daily to BID
    - Haloperidol (Haldol): initially, 0.25 to 0.50 mg PO/IM; reevaluate and potentially redose hourly until symptoms controlled and then use effective dose up to QID PRN. Critical care guidelines do not support use of antipsychotics for prevention of ICU delirium.
    - Olanzapine (Zyprexa) 2.5 to 5.0 mg PO daily to BID
    - Quetiapine (Seroquel) 12.5 to 25.0 mg PO BID–TID
    - Risperidone (Risperdal) 0.25 to 0.50 mg PO daily
- Contraindications: Avoid haloperidol in patients with parkinsonism or Parkinson disease.
- Precautions: Antipsychotics may cause extrapyramidal effects and increase fall risk.
- Antipsychotics may prolong the QT interval. Aripiprazole (Abilify) has minimal or no QT prolonging effect.

- For management of sedation in ICU patient
  - Alpha 2-agonist dexmedetomidine is preferred for sedation in ICU patients and is the only medication that has been found to possibly shorten delirium duration. The primary adverse effects of this medication include hypotension and bradycardia. Some studies have also found use of clonidine as an oral bridge off of dexmedetomidine.
- Melatonin and melatonin agonists are gaining interest as sleep aids in ICU patients.

Second Line

- Benzodiazepines should generally be avoided except in alcohol withdrawal, or if patient takes regularly at baseline, or when antipsychotic is contraindicated. Benzodiazepines can cause delirium. Lorazepam (Ativan): initially, 0.25 to 0.50 mg PO/IM/IV TID–QID PRN; may need to adjust to effect
- Cholinesterase inhibitors should be avoided.

REFERENCES

1. Kappen PR, Kakar E, Dirven CMF, et al. Delirium in neurosurgery: a systematic review and meta-analysis [published online ahead of print August 16, 2021]. *Neurosurg Rev.* doi:10.1007/s10143-021-01619-w.
2. American Psychiatric Association. *Diagnostic and Statistical Manual of Mental Disorders.* 5th ed. Arlington, VA: American Psychiatric Association; 2013.
3. Hshieh TT, Inouye SK, OH ES. Delirium in the elderly. *Psychiatr Clin North Am.* 2018;41(1):1–7.
4. Bellelli G, Brathwaite JS, Mazzola P. Delirium: A Marker of Vulnerability in Older People. *Front Aging Neurosci.* 2021;13:626127.
5. Duning T, Ilting-Reuke K, Beckhuis M, et al. Postoperative delirium—treatment and prevention. *Curr Opin Anaesthesiol.* 2021;34(1):27–32.

 SEE ALSO

- Dementia; Depression; Substance Use Disorders
- Algorithm: Delirium

 CODES

ICD10

- R41.0 Disorientation, unspecified
- F19.931 Oth psychoactive substance use, unsp w withdrawal delirium
- F10.231 Alcohol dependence with withdrawal delirium

CLINICAL PEARLS

- The criteria for delirium include an acute onset of fluctuating mental status, inattention, and either disorganized thinking or altered level of consciousness.
- Primary treatment for delirium is to identify and treat the underlying causes.
- Nonpharmacologic measures are preferable.
- Delirium may not resolve as soon as the treatable contributors resolve; may take weeks or months

DEMENTIA
Hammad Mohsin, MD • Swagato Bhattacharyya, DO

 BASICS

DESCRIPTION
Dementia refers to cognitive decline from previous level of performance in various cognitive domains (attention, executive function perceptual-motor, social cognition, language, and memory) interfere significantly with ADLs in the absence of delirium or any other mental disorder.

- *DSM-5* classifies dementias under neurocognitive disorders (major and mild) and specifies the cause of neurocognitive decline secondary to the following:
  - Alzheimer dementia (AD)
  - Vascular dementia (VaD)
  - Lewy body dementia
  - Parkinson disease dementia
  - Frontotemporal dementia
  - Creutzfeldt-Jakob disease (CJD)
  - HIV dementia
  - Substance-/medication-induced neurocognitive disorder

EPIDEMIOLOGY
Incidence
- In 2011, average annual incidence for AD was 0.4% in ages 65 to 74, 3.2% in ages 75 to 84, and 7.6% in ages ≥85.
- Annual incidence of Alzheimer and other dementias expected to double by 2050

Prevalence
- In patients age ≥65 years
  - AD: 11.3% (5.3% in ages 65 to 74, 13.8% in ages 75 to 84, 34.6% in ages >85)
  - VaD: 1.6%
  - Other: 13%
- Estimated 5 to 6 million Americans living with dementia
- Expected to increase to 14 million by 2050

ETIOLOGY AND PATHOPHYSIOLOGY
- AD: involves β-amyloid protein accumulation and/or neurofibrillary tangles (NFTs), synaptic dysfunction, neurodegeneration, and eventual neuronal loss
- Age, genetics, systemic disease, smoking, and other host factors may influence the β-amyloid accumulation and/or the pace of progression toward the clinical manifestations of AD.
- VaD: cerebral atherosclerosis/emboli with clinical/subclinical infarcts

Genetics
- AD: positive family history in 50%, but 90% AD is sporadic: *APOE4* increases risk but full role unclear.
- Familial/autosomal dominant AD accounts for <5% AD: amyloid precursor protein (APP), presenilin-1 (PSEN-1), and presenilin-2 (PSEN-2).

RISK FACTORS
- Age is the strongest factor.
- Sex: female > male
- Genetic predisposition
- Hypertension: AD; VaD
- Hypercholesterolemia: AD; VaD
- Diabetes: VaD
- Obesity: VaD
- Cigarette smoking: VaD
- Endocrine/metabolic abnormalities: hypothyroidism, Cushing syndrome; thiamine and vitamin B_{12} deficiency
- Chronic alcoholism, other drugs
- Lower educational status
- Head injury early in life
- Sedentary lifestyle

GENERAL PREVENTION
- Treat reversible causes of dementia, such as drug-induced, alcohol-induced, and vitamin deficiencies.
- Treat hypertension, hypercholesterolemia, and diabetes.
- No evidence for statins (or any other specific medication) to prevent onset of dementia (1)[A]
- BP control and low-dose aspirin may prevent or lessen cognitive decline in VaD.
- Maintain or increase physical activity and exercise.
- Continue cognitively stimulating activities and social interactions.

COMMONLY ASSOCIATED CONDITIONS
- Anxiety and major depression
- Psychosis (delusions; delusions of persecution are common)
- Delirium
- Behavioral disturbances (agitation, aggression)
- Sleep disturbances

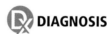 **DIAGNOSIS**

Clinical diagnosis

HISTORY
Requires a family member or someone who knows the patient well to describe changes in the patient's cognition and behavior.

- Probable diagnosis AD (2):
  - Age between 40 and 90 years (usually >65 years)
  - Progressive cognitive decline of insidious onset
  - No disturbances of consciousness
  - Deficits in areas of cognition
  - No other explainable cause of symptoms
  - Specifically rule out thyroid disease, vitamin deficiency (B_{12}), grief reaction, and depression.
  - Supportive factors: family history of dementia

PHYSICAL EXAM
Clinical Assessment
- Physical exam to assess for neurologic deficits, motor and gait abnormalities, tremors, etc.
- No disturbances of consciousness
- Can start with brief initial screening tests for cognitive impairment
  - Mini-Cog test
  - General Practitioner Assessment of Cognition
  - Ascertain Dementia 8-item Informant Questionnaire
- If screening is positive, should be screened for depression (such as with PHQ-2 and PHQ-9, and geriatric depression scale), and can be assessed by other cognitive assessment tools.
- Cognitive decline demonstrated by standardized instruments, including the following:
  - Mini-Mental State Examination (MMSE)
  - Montreal Cognitive Assessment (MoCA) test
  - ADAS-Cog
  - Use caution in relying solely on cognition scores, especially in those with learning difficulty, language barriers, or similar limitations.
- Neuropsychological testing extensively evaluates multiple cognitive domains and can help discriminate between normal aging and dementia. This may be useful in difficult situations when history and mental status examination do not agree, most useful when repeated over time.

DIFFERENTIAL DIAGNOSIS
- Major depression
- Medication side effect
- Chronic alcohol use
- Delirium
- Subdural hematoma
- Normal pressure hydrocephalus
- Brain tumor
- Thyroid disease
- Parkinson disease
- Vitamin B_{12} deficiency
- Toxins (aromatic hydrocarbons, solvents, heavy metals, marijuana, opiates, sedative-hypnotics)

Initial Tests (lab, imaging)
- Used to rule out causes
  - CBC, CMP
  - Thyroid-stimulating hormone
  - Vitamin B_{12} level
- Select patients based on clinical suspicion
  - HIV, rapid plasma reagin (RPR)
  - Erythrocyte sedimentation rate (ESR)
  - Folate
  - Heavy metal and toxicology screen
- Research studies with cerebrospinal fluid (CSF) biomarkers in patient with confirmed AD have shown decreased β-amyloid (1 to 42) and increased τ and p-τ levels, which are specific features of AD, and CSF τ proteins are increased in CJD (3)[A].
- Neuroimaging (CT/MRI of brain):
  - Routine neuroimaging generally recommended to evaluate for dementia, can help to distinguish specific types of dementia with structural imaging finding
  - Early age of onset (<65 years), rapid progression, focal neurologic deficits, cerebrovascular disease risk, or atypical symptoms: neuroimaging (MRI/CT) to rule out other causes
- Important findings
  - AD: diffuse cerebral atrophy starting in association areas, hippocampus (hippocampal atrophy may be the earliest sign), amygdala
  - VaD: old infarcts, including lacunar

Follow-Up Tests & Special Considerations
- Genetic testing for dementia not recommended, such as testing for *APOE4* for Alzheimer, unless there are multiple family members diagnosed with AD at a young age.
- LP and CSF analysis can be considered in atypical presentations to identify infectious, inflammatory, or neoplastic etiologies.

Diagnostic Procedures/Other
PET scan not routinely recommended; has been approved to differentiate between Alzheimer disease and frontotemporal dementia

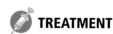 **TREATMENT**

GENERAL MEASURES
- Daily schedules and written directions
- Emphasis on nutrition, personal hygiene, accident-proofing the home, safety issues, sleep hygiene, and supervision
- Socialization (adult daycare)
- Sensory stimulation (display of clocks and calendars) in the early to middle stages
- Occupational training and structured physical exercise program
- Discussion with the family concerning support and advance directives

MEDICATION

- Cognitive dysfunction
- Medications for AD (4)[A] show a small improvement in some cognitive measures, but it remains unclear if the improvement is clinically significant and associated with side effects.
- Cognitive dysfunction, mild
  - Cholinesterase inhibitors: donepezil (Aricept), 5 to 10 mg/day; rivastigmine (Exelon), 1.5 to 6.0 mg BID, transdermal system 4.6 mg/24 hr and 9.5 mg/24 hr; galantamine (Razadyne), 4 to 12 mg BID, extended release 8 to 24 mg/day
    - Adverse events: nausea, vomiting, diarrhea, anorexia, nightmares, bradycardia/syncope
    - Galantamine warning: associated with mortality in patients with mild cognitive impairment in clinical trial
    - It is suggested to consider cholinesterase inhibitor for patients with mild to moderate dementia (MMSE 10 to 26). Responses may be quite variable.
    - Start drug with lowest acquisition cost; also consider adverse event profile, adherence, medical comorbidity, drug interactions, and dosing profiles.
- Cognitive dysfunction, moderate to severe
  - Cholinesterase inhibitors
  - Memantine (Namenda), NMDA receptor antagonist, 5 to 20 mg/day
    - Adverse events: dizziness, confusion, headache, constipation
    - Generally well tolerated with fewer side effects compared to cholinesterase inhibitors
    - Not shown to be beneficial in milder forms of AD
  - Combination cholinesterase inhibitor and memantine
    - The patients with moderate to advanced dementia (MMSE <17), recommendations are to add memantine (10 mg BID) to a cholinesterase inhibitor, or using memantine alone in patients who do not tolerate or benefit from a cholinesterase inhibitor.
    - In patients with severe dementia (MMSE <10), it is suggested continuing memantine. However, in advanced dementia, medications can be discontinued to maximize quality of life and patient comfort.
  - Other medications
    - Aducanumab (Aduhelm)—recombinant monoclonal antibody against β-amyloid, FDA approved for treatment of mild AD, administered in research settings
      - Clinical benefits from trials have been inconsistent.
- Commonly associated conditions
  - Psychosis and agitation/aggressive behavior:
    - Look for precipitating factors (infection, pain, depression, medications).
    - Nonpharmacologic therapies (behavioral interventions, music therapy, etc.) are preferred as first-line treatment.
    - Mood stabilizers (valproic acid, carbamazepine) have been used, although evidence is lacking.
    - For moderate/severe symptoms; antipsychotics: Initiate low doses; risperidone 0.25 to 1.00 mg/day; olanzapine 1.25 to 5.00 mg/day; quetiapine 12.5 to 50.0 mg/day; aripiprazole 5 mg/day; ziprasidone 20 mg/day
    - Atypical antipsychotic, quetiapine, is often first line due to decreased extrapyramidal side effect.
    - Novel antipsychotic, pimavanserin (selective 5-HT2A receptor inverse agonist) has shown to effectively treat Parkinson disease psychosis with minimal risk of worsening motor function associated with other treatment (5)[B].

ALERT

Black box warning on antipsychotics due to increased mortality in elderly with dementia

Geriatric Considerations

- Initiate pharmacotherapy at low doses and titrate slowly up if necessary.
- Benzodiazepines are potentially inappropriate for older adults, yet their use persists.

ALERT

Benzodiazepine use is associated with increased fall risk (6)[A].

- Watch decreased renal function and hepatic metabolism.

First Line

Nonpharmacologic management: environmental modifications, caregiver training, music therapy, exercise, pet therapy

Second Line

- Cholinesterase inhibitors, memantine, atypical antipsychotics, antidepressants, mood stabilizers, methylphenidate, benzodiazepines, melatonin
- Antidepressants not clearly superior to placebo in treating depression (HTA-SADD)

ISSUES FOR REFERRAL

Neuropsychiatric evaluation helpful in early stages or mild cognitive impairment

ADDITIONAL THERAPIES

Behavioral modification

- Socialization, such as adult daycare, to prevent isolation and depression
- Sleep hygiene program as alternative to pharmaceuticals for sleep disturbance
- Scheduled toileting to prevent incontinence

ADMISSION, INPATIENT, AND NURSING CONSIDERATIONS

Psychiatry admission may be required because of safety concerns (self-harm/harm to others), self-neglect, aggressive behaviors, or other behavioral issues.

 ONGOING CARE

FOLLOW-UP RECOMMENDATIONS

Patient Monitoring

- Progression of cognitive impairment by use of standardized tool (e.g., MMSE, ADAS-Cog)
- Development of behavioral problems: sleep, depression, psychosis, aggression
- Adverse events of pharmacotherapy
- Nutritional status
- Caregiver evaluation of stress

PATIENT EDUCATION

- Advance care planning: Discuss safety, management of finances, medical decision making, possible skilled facility placement; legal guardianship, if necessary
- Advance directives, health care proxy should be established early on if possible.
- National Institute on Aging: https://www.nia.nih.gov/health/topics/dementia

PROGNOSIS

- AD: usually steady progression leading to profound cognitive impairment:
  - Average survival of AD is about 10 years.
- VaD: incrementally worsening dementia but cognitive improvement is unlikely
- Secondary dementias: Treatment of the underlying condition may lead to improvement; commonly seen with normal pressure hydrocephalus, hypothyroidism, and brain tumors
- For patients with late-stage dementia, palliative and hospice care can be beneficial.

COMPLICATIONS

- Wandering
- Sundowner syndrome is common in older people (who are sedated) and also in people who have dementia (can have adverse reaction to even small dose of psychoactive substances).
- Falls with injury
  - Hip fracture; head trauma/hematomas
- Neglect and abuse
- Caregiver burnout—can refer to respite care and support groups

REFERENCES

1. McGuinness B, Craig D, Bullock R, et al. Statins for the prevention of dementia. *Cochrane Database Syst Rev.* 2009;(2):CD003160.
2. Blass DM, Rabins PV. In the clinic. Dementia. *Ann Intern Med.* 2008;148(7):ITC4-1–ITC4-16.
3. van Harten AC, Kester MI, Visser PJ, et al. Tau and p-tau as CSF biomarkers in dementia: a meta-analysis. *Clin Chem Lab Med.* 2011;49(3):353–366.
4. Birks J. Cholinesterase inhibitors for Alzheimer's disease. *Cochrane Database Syst Rev.* 2006;(1):CD005593.
5. Cummings J, Isaacson S, Mills R, et al. Pimavanserin for patients with Parkinson's disease psychosis: a randomised, placebo-controlled phase 3 trial. *Lancet.* 2014;383(9916):533–540.
6. Seppala LJ, Wermelink AMAT, de Vries M, et al; for EUGMS Task and Finish Group on Fall-Risk-Increasing Drugs. Fall-risk-increasing drugs: a systematic review and meta-analysis: II. Psychotropics. *J Am Med Dir Assoc.* 2018;19(4):371.e11–371.e17.

ADDITIONAL READING

Lyketsos CG, Colenda CC, Beck C, et al; for Task Force of American Association for Geriatric Psychiatry. Position statement of the American Association for Geriatric Psychiatry regarding principles of care for patients with dementia resulting from Alzheimer disease. *Am J Geriatr Psychiatry.* 2006;14(7):561–572.

 SEE ALSO

Algorithm: Dementia

CODES

ICD10

- F03 Unspecified dementia
- G30.9 Alzheimer's disease, unspecified
- F01.50 Vascular dementia without behavioral disturbance

CLINICAL PEARLS

- Medications for AD show a small, statistically significant improvement in some cognitive measures, but it remains unclear if the improvement is clinically significant.
- Do not forget the role of adult protective services in case of elderly abuse—elder abuse hotline: 800-922-2275.
- A particular concern in nursing homes relates to finding alternatives to the use of physical restraints and antipsychotic medications.

DEMENTIA, VASCULAR
Birju B. Patel, MD, FACP • N. Wilson Holland, MD, FACP

BASICS

Vascular dementia is a heterogeneous disorder caused by the sequelae of cerebrovascular disease that manifests in cognitive impairment affecting memory, thinking, language, behavior, judgment, and executive dysfunction.

DESCRIPTION
- Vascular dementia (previously known as multi-infarct dementia) was first mentioned by Thomas Willis in 1672. Later, it was further described in the late 19th century by Binswanger and Alzheimer as a separate entity from dementia paralytica caused by neurosyphilis. This concept has evolved tremendously since the advent of neuroimaging modalities.
- Synonym(s): vascular cognitive impairment (VCI); vascular cognitive disorder (VCD); poststroke dementia; Binswanger disease. *Diagnostic and Statistical Manual of Mental Disorders* (Fifth Edition) (*DSM-5*) categorizes vascular dementia as mild or major VCD.

EPIDEMIOLOGY
Common cause of dementia in the elderly and it frequently overlaps with Alzheimer dementia

Incidence
About 6 to 12 cases per 1,000/person age >70 years

Prevalence
- ~1.2–4.2% in those age >65 years
- 14–32% prevalence of dementia after a stroke

ETIOLOGY AND PATHOPHYSIOLOGY
No set pathologic criteria exist for the diagnosis of vascular dementia such as those that exist for Alzheimer dementia. Pathology includes the following:
- Large vessel disease: cognitive impairment that follows a stroke
- Small vessel disease (subcortical) includes white matter changes (leukoaraiosis), subcortical infarcts, and incomplete infarction. This is usually the most common cause of multi-infarct dementia. Lacunar infarcts and deep white matter changes are typically included in this category.
- Transient ischemic attack (TIA)/stroke
- Vascular, demographic, genetic factors
  – Vascular disease (i.e., hypertension [HTN], peripheral vascular disease [PVD], atrial fibrillation, hyperlipidemia, diabetes) (1)[B],(2)[C]

Genetics
- Cerebral autosomal dominant arteriopathy with subcortical infarcts and leukoencephalopathy (CADASIL) is caused by a mutation in the *NOTCH3* gene on chromosome 19 that results in leukoencephalopathy and subcortical infarcts. This is clinically manifested in recurrent strokes, migraine with aura, and vascular dementia.
- *Apolipoprotein E* gene type: Those with ApoE4 subtypes are at higher risk of developing both vascular and Alzheimer dementia.
- Amyloid precursor protein (APP) gene: leads to a form of vascular dementia called heritable cerebral hemorrhage with amyloidosis

RISK FACTORS
- Age (risk doubles every 5 years)
- Previous stroke
- Tobacco use
- Diabetes (especially with frequent hypoglycemia)
- Atherosclerotic heart disease; HTN; atrial fibrillation; PVD
- Hyperlipidemia
- Metabolic syndrome
- Low socioeconomic status (3)[C]

GENERAL PREVENTION
- Optimization and aggressive treatment of vascular risk factors, such as HTN, diabetes, and hyperlipidemia
- HTN is the single most modifiable risk factor and treatment for it must be optimized.
- Smoking is associated with white matter changes on imaging, which may be associated with small vessel disease and vascular dementia progression.
- Lifestyle modification: weight loss, physical activity, smoking cessation
- Hearing loss should be corrected.
- Depression and social isolation should be evaluated.
- Cognitively stimulating activity can be beneficial.
- Medication management for vascular risk reduction: aspirin usage, statin therapy for hyperlipidemia, antihypertensive therapy (4)[B]

COMMONLY ASSOCIATED CONDITIONS
- CADASIL
- Cerebral amyloid angiopathy (CAA) causes ischemic white matter damage due to amyloid deposition in penetrating cortical vessels.

DIAGNOSIS

Differentiation between Alzheimer dementia and vascular dementia can be difficult, and significant overlap is seen in the clinical presentation of these two dementias. The diagnosis of vascular dementia is a clinical diagnosis. Memory impairment is less prominent in vascular dementia versus Alzheimer dementia. The neuropsychological pattern observed in vascular dementia is impaired recall, relatively intact recognition, less severe forgetfulness with greater benefit from cues, and more executive dysfunction.

HISTORY
- Gradual, stepwise progression is typical with multi-infarct dementia.
- Ask about onset and progression of cognitive impairment and the specific cognitive domains involved.
- Ask about vascular risk factors and previous attempts to control these risk factors.
- Ask about medication compliance.
- Ask about urinary incontinence and gait disturbances. Abnormal gait and falls are strong predictors of development of vascular dementia, particularly unsteady, frontal, and hemiparetic types of gait.

- Look for early symptoms, including difficulty performing cognitive tasks, memory, mood, and assessment of instrumental activities of daily living (IADLs).
- History may include TIAs, cerebrovascular accidents (CVAs), coronary atherosclerotic heart disease, atrial fibrillation, hyperlipidemia, and/or PVD. Small vessel disease usually presents with executive dysfunction. Large vessel disease usually presents with gait, visuospatial, and language dysfunction.

PHYSICAL EXAM
- Screen for HTN. Average daily home blood pressure (BP) is associated with progression of cerebrovascular disease and cognitive decline in the elderly.
- Focal neurologic deficits may be present.
- Gait assessment is important, especially looking at gait initiation, gait speed, and balance (5).
- Check for carotid bruits as well as abdominal bruits and assess for presence of PVD.
- Check body mass index and waist circumference.
- Do a thorough cardiac evaluation that includes looking for arrhythmias (i.e., atrial fibrillation).

DIFFERENTIAL DIAGNOSIS
- Alzheimer dementia
- Depression
- Delirium
- CNS tumors
- Hypothyroidism/hyperthyroidism
- Vitamin B$_{12}$ deficiency

DIAGNOSTIC TESTS & INTERPRETATION
- Cognitive testing, such as Saint Louis University Mental Status (SLUMS) and Montreal Cognitive Assessment (MoCA), provides more definitive information in terms of cognitive deficits, especially executive function, which may be lost earlier in vascular dementia. The Mini-Mental State Examination is not sensitive in distinguishing Alzheimer dementia from vascular dementia because it does not have good measures of executive function.
- Neuropsychological testing may also be beneficial, especially in evaluating multiple cognitive domains and their specific involvements and deficits.

Initial Tests (lab, imaging)
As appropriate, consider complete blood count, comprehensive metabolic profile, lipid panel, thyroid function, hemoglobin A1C, and vitamin B$_{12}$.
- Cognitive deficits observed clinically do not always have to correlate with findings found on neuroimaging studies.
- MRI is the gold standard of imaging (6).
- White matter changes and specific location of these changes can be associated with executive dysfunction and episodic memory impairment.

Follow-Up Tests & Special Considerations
Consider referral to a cognitive specialist for complex cases.

TREATMENT

Prevention is the real key to treatment:
- Control of risk factors, including HTN, hyperlipidemia, and diabetes
- Avoidance of tobacco and smoking cessation
- Healthy, low-cholesterol diet

MEDICATION
- Clinical evidence for use of acetylcholinesterase inhibitors and memantine reveals limited benefit in vascular dementia but may slow cognitive decline in patients with mixed Alzheimer and vascular dementia.
- Controlling BP with any antihypertensive medications, treatment of dyslipidemia (e.g., statins), and treatment of diabetes are very important.
- Selective serotonin reuptake inhibitors (SSRIs) may be of benefit for agitation and psychosis in vascular dementia.

ADDITIONAL THERAPIES
- Limit alcohol drink intake to ≤1/day in women and 2/day in men.
- Preventing new CVAs is key in managing vascular dementia; aspirin and other anti-platelet agents may be useful if no contraindications.

SURGERY/OTHER PROCEDURES
Patients with symptomatic carotid artery stenosis should be referred to a vascular surgeon to be evaluated for carotid endarterectomy. Carotid endarterectomy is recommended over carotid artery stenting in patients >70 years of age if perioperative morbidity/mortality are <6%.

COMPLEMENTARY & ALTERNATIVE MEDICINE
Ginkgo biloba should be avoided due to increased risk of bleeding, especially in CAA.

ADMISSION, INPATIENT, AND NURSING CONSIDERATIONS
- Remain sensitive to functional assessment and avoidance of pressure ulcers after CVAs.
- Avoid Foley catheter usage unless necessary due to increased risk of infection.
- Nonpharmacologic approaches to behavior management should be attempted prior to medication usage.
- Providing optimal sensory input to patients with cognitive impairment is important during hospitalizations to avoid delirium and confusion. Patients should be given frequent cues to keep them oriented to place and time. They should be informed of any changes in the daily schedule of activities and evaluations. Family and caregivers should be encouraged to be with patients with dementia as much as possible to further help them from becoming confused during hospitalization. Recreational, physical, occupational, and music therapy can be beneficial during hospitalization in avoiding delirium and preventing functional decline.
- Depression can present as "pseudodementia" with worsening confusion during hospitalization and is a treatable condition.

 ONGOING CARE

Vascular dementia is a condition that should be followed with multiple visits in the office setting with goals of optimizing cardiovascular risk profiles for patients. Future planning and advanced directives should be addressed early. Family and caregiver evaluation and burden should also be evaluated.

FOLLOW-UP RECOMMENDATIONS
Perform regular follow-up with a primary care provider or geriatrician for risk factor modification and education on importance of regular physical and mental exercises as tolerated.

Patient Monitoring
Appropriate evaluation and diagnosis of this condition, need for future planning, optimizing vascular risk factors, lifestyle modification counseling, therapeutic interventions

DIET
- The American Heart Association diet and Dietary Approaches to Stop Hypertension (DASH) diet is recommended for optimal BP and cardiovascular risk factor control.
- Low-fat, decreased concentrated sweets and carbohydrates, especially in those with metabolic syndrome

PATIENT EDUCATION
- Lifestyle modification is important in vascular risk reduction (smoking cessation, exercise counseling, dietary counseling, weight-loss counseling).
- Optimizing vascular risk factors via medications (i.e., HTN, diabetes, atrial fibrillation, PVD, heart disease)
- Avoiding smoking, including secondhand smoke
- Home BP monitoring and glucometer testing of blood sugars if HTN, impaired glucose tolerance, and/or diabetes is present

PROGNOSIS
- Vascular dementia with previous CVA results in a worse prognosis.
- Lost cognitive abilities that persist after initial recovery of deficits from stroke do not usually return. Some individuals can have intermittent periods of self-reported improvement in cognitive function.
- Risk factors for progression of cognitive and functional impairment poststroke include age, prestroke cognitive abilities, depression, polypharmacy, and decreased cerebral perfusion during acute stroke.
- Unsteady or frontal gait can be a predictor for risk of development of vascular dementia.

COMPLICATIONS
- Physical disability from stroke
- Severe cognitive impairment

REFERENCES
1. Kalaria RN. The pathology and pathophysiology of vascular dementia. *Neuropharmacology.* 2018;134(pt B):226–239.
2. Dichgans M, Leys D. Vascular cognitive impairment. *Circ Res.* 2017;120(3):573–591.
3. Sundbøll J, Horváth-Puhó E, Adelborg K, et al. Higher risk of vascular dementia in myocardial infarction survivors. *Circulation.* 2018;137(6): 567–577.
4. White WB, Wolfson L, Wakefield DB, et al. Average daily blood pressure, not office blood pressure, is associated with progression of cerebrovascular disease and cognitive decline in older people. *Circulation.* 2011;124(21):2312–2319.
5. Montero-Odasso M, Verghese J, Beauchet O, et al. Gait and cognition: a complementary approach to understanding brain function and the risk of falling. *J Am Geriatr Soc.* 2012;60(11):2127–2136.
6. Iadecola C, Duering M, Hachinski V, et al. Vascular cognitive impairment and dementia: JACC Scientific Expert Panel. *J Am Coll Cardiol.* 2019;73(25):3326–3344.

 SEE ALSO

Alzheimer Disease; Depression; Mild Cognitive Impairment

 CODES

ICD10
- F01.50 Vascular dementia without behavioral disturbance
- F01.51 Vascular dementia with behavioral disturbance

CLINICAL PEARLS
- Executive dysfunction and gait abnormalities are often seen early and are more pronounced in vascular dementia as opposed to Alzheimer dementia.
- Memory is relatively preserved in vascular dementia when compared with Alzheimer dementia in the early stages of this disease.
- Stepwise progression, as opposed to progressive decline in Alzheimer dementia, is typical.
- Considerable overlap exists between vascular dementia and Alzheimer dementia in clinical practice, and classification into one of these categories is often difficult. Patients can have mixed etiologies as well.

D

DENTAL INFECTION

Stephanie A. Gill, MD, MPH

BASICS

DESCRIPTION
- Pain ± swelling in the head and neck region with odontogenic (teeth and supporting structures) origin of infection; if left untreated, can lead to serious and potentially life-threatening illnesses
- Assume any head and neck infection or swelling to be odontogenic in origin until proven otherwise.
- System(s) affected: oropharynx, throat, dental, gastrointestinal
- Synonym(s): odontogenic infections, dental abscess

EPIDEMIOLOGY
- More than 90% of all head and neck infections have an odontogenic origin.
- 17% of 5- to 19-year-olds have untreated dental caries.
- 26% of individuals age >20 years have untreated dental caries (1).
- Rates of untreated dental caries are higher in Latino (18%) and non-Latino black (21%) children/teens (1)[A].
- 92% of adults 20 to 64 years have had dental caries in their permanent teeth.
- 17% of adults age >64 years are edentulous (1).

ETIOLOGY AND PATHOPHYSIOLOGY
- Dental caries represent the most common chronic disease worldwide.
- Caries or trauma can lead to death of the tooth pulp, which can lead to infection and/or abscess of adjacent tissues via direct or hematogenous bacterial colonization.
- Caries (tooth decay; "cavity") represent a contagious bacterial infection causing demineralization and destruction of the tooth tissue (enamel, dentin, and cementum).
- *Streptococcus mutans* is easily transmitted to newly dentate infants by caregivers.
- Acidic secretions from *S. mutans* are implicated in early caries.
- Often there is polymicrobial mix of anaerobes in dental abscess (viridans streptococci and *Streptococcus anginosus*).
- Anaerobes, including peptostreptococci, *Bacteroides*, *Prevotella*, and *Fusobacterium*, have also been implicated; lactobacilli not seen in healthy subjects but common in patients with extensive caries (2)
- Caries (and subsequent other infections) are preventable with good oral hygiene, low-cariogenic diet, access to fluoride, and professional dental care.
- Fluoride supplementation has dramatically decreased dental caries.

RISK FACTORS
- Low socioeconomic status
- Parent and/or sibling with history of caries or existing untreated dental caries (especially in past 12 months)

- Previous dental caries
- Poor access to dental/health care; lack of dental insurance; fear of dentist
- Poor oral hygiene; poor nutrition, including diet containing high level of sugary foods and drinks
- Trauma to the teeth or jaw
- Inadequate access to and use of fluoride
- Gingival recession (increased risk of root caries)
- Physical and mental disabilities
- Poorly controlled systemic diseases (e.g., diabetes)
- Decreased salivary flow (e.g., use of anticholinergic medications, immunologic diseases, radiation therapy to head and neck)

GENERAL PREVENTION
- Most dental problems can be avoided through flossing/use of interdental brushes; brushing with fluoride toothpaste, systemic fluoride (fluoridated bottled water; fluoride supplements for high-risk patients and in non-fluoridated areas); fluoride varnish for all children age <6 years and moderate- to high-risk patients; regular dental cleanings (1),(3).
- Prevent transmission of *S. mutans* from mother/caregiver to infant by improving maternal dentition, chlorhexidine gluconate rinses, and use of xylitol products for mother especially during first 2 years of a child's life. Avoid smoking, which is linked to severe periodontal disease (2).
- Good control of systemic diseases (e.g., diabetes)
- Fluoride varnish provided by dental or medical primary care providers twice per year (2),(3)

COMMONLY ASSOCIATED CONDITIONS
- Extensive caries, crowding, multiple missing teeth
- Periapical and periodontal abscess
- Soft tissue cellulitis
- Periodontitis (deep inflammation ± infection of gingiva, alveolar bone support, and ligaments)

DIAGNOSIS

HISTORY
- Pain of involved tooth; can be referred to ears, jaw, cheek, neck, or sinuses; unexplained headaches
- Hot/cold sensitivity
- Pain can be unprovoked, intermittent, and/or constant.
- Pain with biting or chewing
- Trismus (inability to open mouth)
- Bleeding or purulent drainage from gingival tissues
- When severe infection (systemic)
  - Fever
  - Difficulty breathing or swallowing
  - Raspy voice
  - Mental status changes
- Evaluate children <4 years with stiff neck, sore throat, and dysphagia for retropharyngeal abscess.

PHYSICAL EXAM
- Gingival edema and erythema
- Cheek (extraoral) or vestibular (intraoral) swelling
- Fluctuant mass at involved site
- Suppuration of gingival margin
- Submandibular or cervical lymphadenopathy
- Severe (systemic) infection may present with dysphagia, fever, and signs of airway compromise.

DIFFERENTIAL DIAGNOSIS
- Bacterial or viral pharyngitis
- Pericoronitis (inflammation ± infection of gum flap over mandibular last molar, typically 3rd molars)
- Otitis media or externa; sinusitis
- Headache/migraine
- Viral (HSV1, herpangina, hand-foot-mouth disease) or aphthous stomatitis
- Temporomandibular joint (TMJ) dysfunction (myofascial pain, ± internal derangement of TMJ)
- Parotitis
- Jaw pain can be anginal equivalent, especially in women and especially lower left side of the jaw.

DIAGNOSTIC TESTS & INTERPRETATION
Initial Tests (lab, imaging)
- No initial labs needed, unless patient looks acutely ill
- If acutely ill
  - Consider CBC with differential.
  - If abscess present, drain/aspirate pus and culture for aerobes and anaerobes (4).
  - Typically polymicrobial infections with anaerobic gram-negative rods and anaerobic gram-positive cocci (4)
- Individual films of suspected teeth, including root apices; test with palpation, percussion, and cold sensitivity.
- Panoramic film or CT scan of the teeth and jaw to evaluate the extent of infection

Follow-Up Tests & Special Considerations
- Panoramic radiograph, particularly if trismus present
- CT scan can be helpful if facial swelling extends below inferior border of mandible or into infraorbital space. This helps to locate for potential incision and drainage by oral and maxillofacial surgeon or ENT.

TREATMENT

- Isolated pain (no swelling or systemic signs of infection) does not warrant antibiotic use.
- If localized, consider incision and drainage.
- Appropriate pain control: anti-inflammatory agents are first line; short-course opioids in some cases (5)[A]

- Refer to oral health provider for definitive treatment: root canal, extraction, gum therapy (4).
- If infection is severe (systemic symptoms), consider hospitalization with IV antibiotics until stable; may need intraoral or extraoral incision and drainage; definitive treatment (extraction or root canal therapy) necessary to prevent progression or recurrence

GENERAL MEASURES
- Ibuprofen 600 to 800 mg (pediatrics: 10 mg/kg) q6h or acetaminophen 650 to 1,000 mg (pediatrics: 10 to 15 mg/kg) q4–6h PRN for pain
- For more severe pain, consider acetaminophen with ibuprofen (synergistic effect) + short course of opioids.
- Local nerve block with long-acting anesthetic (bupivacaine); avoid penetrating infection to avoid tracking infection.

MEDICATION
First Line
- Amoxicillin: 500 mg TID for 7 to 10 days; in children, 40 to 60 mg/kg/day divided TID
- If penicillin allergic, use clindamycin 300 mg PO TID for 7 days.

Second Line
If long-standing infection or no response to first-line treatment
- Clindamycin: 300 mg PO TID for 7 to 10 days
- Amoxicillin/clavulanic acid (500 mg/125 mg), 1 tablet PO TID for 7 days
- If severe infection, consider IV antibiotics (ampicillin-sulbactam, cefoxitin, cefotetan).
- Consider double coverage with metronidazole 500 mg PO TID for 7 days for better bone penetration and good anaerobic coverage. Do not use metronidazole alone; will increase development of resistant strains; can be used with amoxicillin or clindamycin.

ISSUES FOR REFERRAL
Consult an oral health provider and ensure definitive follow-up.

SURGERY/OTHER PROCEDURES
- Incise and drain large, fluctuant abscesses.
- Root canal or extraction is definitive treatment.

ADMISSION, INPATIENT, AND NURSING CONSIDERATIONS
Criteria for hospital admission: swelling involving deep spaces of the neck, floor of the mouth, or infraorbital region; deviation of the airway; unstable vital signs; fever (>101°F); chills; raspy voice; confusion or delirium; or evidence of invasive infection or cellulitis

- Ensure secure airway.
- IV fluid resuscitation if necessary
- Ensure good oral hygiene.
- Rinse or swab mouth with chlorhexidine gluconate BID.
- Use warm saltwater rinses several times per day, especially after incision and drainage; ice packs to decrease swelling and encourage drainage
- Discharge patient when
  - Airway not compromised
  - Abscess and sepsis eliminated
  - Able to take PO intake and ambulate

 ONGOING CARE
Educate regarding proper oral hygiene, need for follow-up dental care, and potential medical complications that arise due to lack of dental care.

FOLLOW-UP RECOMMENDATIONS
- Follow up with oral health provider within 24 hours.
- Ensure adequate PO intake, including protein.

DIET
- Maintain a healthy diet; bacteria thrive on refined sugar and starch.
- Avoid sugary foods that stick between the teeth.
- Avoid the use of sugary/carbonated drinks throughout day; water as beverage of choice between meals

Pediatric Considerations
In children, limit the frequency of sugary drinks and advise against sleeping with a bottle; fluoride varnish twice a year (more for higher risk children) for children age <6 years (3)

PATIENT EDUCATION
- Control caries and periodontal disease.
- Biannual dental visits at a minimum
  - Limit the frequency of sugar/carbonated drinks and sugary or sticky foods.
- In young children, avoid sleeping with a bottle to decrease the chance of dental caries.
- Brush twice daily and use floss/interdental brush daily.

PROGNOSIS
Prognosis is excellent with proper treatment.

COMPLICATIONS
- Ludwig angina
- Retropharyngeal and mediastinal infection
- Osteomyelitis
- Endocarditis/cardiac tamponade
- Submental infection
- Submandibular infection
- Can cause unstable diabetes in diabetics/worsen preexisting heart disease
- Brain abscess/death

REFERENCES
1. National Center for Health Statistics. *Health, United States, 2018: With Chartbook on Long-term Trends in Health.* Hyattsville, MD: 2021. https://www.cdc .gov/nchs/data/hus/hus19-508.pdf. Accessed August 21, 2021.
2. Chaffee BW, Gansky SA, Weintraub JA, et al. Maternal oral bacterial levels predict early childhood caries development. *J Dent Res.* 2014;93(3):238–244.
3. Chou R, Cantor A, Zakher B, et al. Preventing dental caries in children <5 years: systematic review updating USPSTF recommendation. *Pediatrics.* 2013;132(2):332–350.
4. Robertson D, Smith AJ. The microbiology of the acute dental abscess. *J Med Microbiol.* 2009;58(pt 2):155–162.
5. Bali RK, Sharma P, Gaba S, et al. A review of complications of odontogenic infections. *Natl J Maxillofac Surg.* 2015;6(2):136–143.

ADDITIONAL READING
- Clark MB, Douglass AB, Maier R, et al. *Smiles for Life: A National Oral Health Curriculum.* 3rd ed. Leawood, KS: Society of Teachers of Family Medicine; 2010. http://www.smilesforlifeoralhealth .com/buildcontent.aspx?tut=555&pagekey=62948& cbreceipt=0. Accessed October 18, 2021.
- Flynn TR. What are the antibiotics of choice for odontogenic infections, and how long should the treatment course last? *Oral Maxillofac Surg Clin North Am.* 2011;23(4):519–536.
- Stephens MB, Wiedemer JP, Kushner GM. Dental problems in primary care. *Am Fam Physician.* 2018;98(11):654–660.
- Tadakamadla J, Boccalari E, Rathore V, et al. In vitro studies evaluating the efficacy of mouth rinses on Sars-Cov-2: A systematic review. *J Infect Public Health.* 2021;14(9):1179–1185.
- U.S. Preventive Services Task Force. Dental caries in children from birth through age 5 years: screening. http://www.uspreventiveservicestaskforce.org/Page /Topic/recommendation-summary/dental-caries-in -children-from-birth-through-age-5-years-screening. Accessed August 21, 2021.

 CODES

ICD10
- K02.9 Dental caries, unspecified
- K04.7 Periapical abscess without sinus
- K12.2 Cellulitis and abscess of mouth

CLINICAL PEARLS
- Do not ignore tooth pain.
- Treat patients with facial swelling aggressively because infections can spread quickly, leading to significant morbidity or even death.
- Prevention (oral hygiene, fluoride, dental visits) is the key to avoiding odontogenic infections.
- When indicated, amoxicillin and clindamycin are generally the antibiotics of choice for odontogenic infections.

D

DEPRESSION

Grant M. Reed, DO • Johan W. Sosa, MD

 BASICS

DESCRIPTION

A primary mood disorder characterized by a sustained feeling of sadness and/or decreased interest in all or most activities once enjoyed (anhedonia), which represents a change from previous functioning

EPIDEMIOLOGY

Incidence
- In the United States, 8.1% of adults age ≥20 years experienced depression in a given 2-week period between 2013 and 2016.
- 19.2% lifetime risk of having major depressive disorder (MDD)

Prevalence
- Non-Hispanic Asian adults had the lowest prevalence of depression (3.1%) compared with Hispanic (8.2%), non-Hispanic white (7.9%), and non-Hispanic black (9.2%) adults. This pattern was observed among both men and women.
- Among all race and Hispanic-origin groups (except non-Hispanic Asian), men had a significantly lower prevalence of depression compared with women.
- Prevalence decreases with increasing levels of family income for both men and women.
- Predominant age: low risk before early teens but highest prevalence in teens and young adults

ETIOLOGY AND PATHOPHYSIOLOGY

There are diverse theories regarding the pathophysiology; none proven

Genetics
Multiple gene loci place a person at increased risk when faced with environmental stressor; twin studies suggest 37% concordance.

RISK FACTORS
- Female > male (2:1)
- Severity of first episode
- Persistent sleep disturbances
- Presence of chronic disease(s), recent myocardial infarction (MI), cardiovascular accident (CVA)
- Strong family history (depression, bipolar, suicide, substance abuse), spouse with depression
- Childhood trauma/maltreatment
- Substance abuse and dependence, domestic abuse/violence
- Losses, stressors, unemployment
- Single, divorced, or unhappily married

COMMONLY ASSOCIATED CONDITIONS
- Bipolar disorder, cyclothymic disorder, grief reaction, anxiety disorders, somatoform disorders, schizophrenia/schizoaffective disorders
- Medical comorbidity
- Substance abuse

 DIAGNOSIS

DSM-5 requires the following criteria for MDD:
- Criterion A: ≥5 of the following symptoms present nearly every day during the same 2-week period, with at least 1 of the 5 being either depressed mood or loss of interest or pleasure:
  - Depressed mood most of the day by subjective report or observation from other people
  - Markedly diminished interest or pleasure in all activities most of the day by subjective report or observation from other people
  - Decreased or increased appetite or significant weight loss without dieting or weight gain
  - Insomnia or hypersomnia
  - Fatigue or energy loss
  - Agitation, restlessness, or slowed speech or body movements observable by others
  - Worthlessness, excessive/inappropriate guilty feelings
  - Diminished thinking/concentration, poor memory, indecisiveness
  - Recurrent thoughts of death, suicidal ideations, or suicide attempt or a specific plan for committing suicide
- Criterion B: Symptoms cause significant social, occupational, or functional distress or impairment.
- Criterion C: symptoms not attributable to substance effects or other medical conditions

HISTORY

The mnemonic "SIGECAPS" is helpful.
- Sleep: changes in sleep habits from baseline, including excessive sleep, early waking, or inability to fall asleep
- Interest: loss of interest in previously enjoyable activities (anhedonia)
- Guilt: excessive or inappropriate guilt that may or may not be related to a specific problem or circumstance
- Energy: perceived lack of energy
- Concentration: inability to concentrate on specific tasks
- Appetite: an increase or decrease in appetite
- Psychomotor: restlessness and agitation or the perception that everyday activities are too strenuous to manage
- Suicidality: the desire to end one's life or hurt oneself, harmful thoughts directed internally, or recurrent thoughts of death or homicidality

Geriatric Considerations
- Often difficult to diagnose due to medical comorbidities
- Can present as memory difficulties
- Geriatric Depression Scale (GDS 15) improves rate of diagnosis in primary care setting.

Pediatric Considerations
Can present with somatic symptoms (headaches, GI upset), irritability or anger, concentration difficulties in school, frequent absences from school, or a sudden change in grades

PHYSICAL EXAM

A comprehensive physical and mental status examination
- Level of consciousness and orientation
- Appearance: hygiene, posture, clothing
- Attitude: hostility, apathy
- Behavior: eye contact, psychomotor agitation or retardation
- Mood: depressed, anxious, angry, elated, tearful, etc.
- Affect: mood-congruent, flat, labile, manic, etc.
- Memory: intact immediate, recent, and remote
- Speech: fluency, repetition, comprehension
- Thought processes/content: presence of delusions, hallucinations, suicidal/homicidal thoughts, flight of ideas or tangentiality, grandiosity, obsessions/compulsions
- Insight: understanding of own illness
- Judgment: capacity to make rational decisions

DIFFERENTIAL DIAGNOSIS
- Mental health conditions:
  - Depressed phase of bipolar disorder—inquire if prior mania, family or personal history of bipolar disorder, prior agitation, or excitement with antidepressant medication
  - Adjustment disorder with depressed mood
  - Substance abuse–related mood disorders

- Medical comorbidity: adrenal diseases, hypothyroidism, diabetes, hypercalcemia, liver or renal failure, malignancy, sleep disorders, chronic fatigue syndrome, fibromyalgia, lupus
- Neurologic or cognitive disorders such as neurodegenerative CNS disease, dementia, or delirium
- Deficiencies: vitamin B_3, vitamin B_{12}, or folate

DIAGNOSTIC TESTS & INTERPRETATION
- The Patient Health Questionnaire-9 (PHQ-9) is a brief screening test valid for diagnosis of MDD in primary care settings. A score of 10 or higher indicates that depression is likely present.
- Other validated scales include Beck Depression Inventory, Zung Self-Rating Depression Scale, or GDS 15.

Initial Tests (lab, imaging)
To rule out medical causes
- CMP to evaluate kidney and liver function

Follow-Up Tests & Special Considerations
- TSH
- CBC
- Consider urine drug screen if symptoms suggest intoxication or concerning historical.

TREATMENT

American Psychiatric Association (APA) 2010 treatment guideline recommend the following (1)[C]:
- Acute phase (first 3 months of treatment)
  - Full evaluation, including risk to self and others, with selection of appropriate treatment setting. Goal should be symptom remission.
    - For mild to moderate depression, either psychotherapy and/or medication is appropriate.
    - For refractory or severe depression, both medication and psychotherapy are preferred.
    - Hospitalization is indicated for those at risk of harm to self or others, if the patient is incapacitated so as to be unable to take care of themselves, or if there is no support system to assist with treatment.
  - See within 2 to 4 weeks of starting medication and q2wk until improvement, then monthly.
  - Continue to increase dosage q3–4wk until remission. Full medication effect is achieved in 4 to 6 weeks. Augmentation with a second medication may be necessary.
  - ≥6 visits recommended for monitoring (younger patients, those at high suicide risk, see within 1st week, and follow frequently).
- Continuation phase (4 to 9 months of treatment)/maintenance phase (9+ months of treatment)
  - Monitor for relapse; q3–6mo if stable
  - Use depression rating scales and patient reports to monitor response.
  - For patients not responding to medication alone, psychotherapy should be added.
  - Once remission achieved, dosage should be continued for at least 6 to 9 months to reduce relapse; cognitive-behavioral therapy (CBT) is also effective in reducing relapse (visits typically q2wk).
  - Medications should be tapered gradually (weeks to months) to allow for the detection of recurring symptoms and to minimize discontinuation syndromes.

GENERAL MEASURES
Psychotherapy
- CBT: combines cognitive psychotherapy with behavioral therapy; proven effective (NNT = 2.75)

- Interpersonal psychotherapy (IPT): identifies a trigger of the depressive episode, facilitates mourning, promotes recognition of affects, resolves role disputes and role transitions, and builds social skills
- Psychodynamic psychotherapy: used to identify unconscious thoughts leading to current behavior
- Family and marital therapy: addresses family or relationship-oriented problems
- Problem-solving therapy: combines elements of CBT and IPT into a brief treatment lasting 6 to 12 sessions; may have a role in those with mild symptoms of depression
- Supportive psychotherapy: improves self-esteem, psychological functioning, and adaptive skills by focusing on current, problematic relationships or maladaptive patterns of behavior and/or emotional responses
- For the initial treatment of unipolar major depression, consider either psychotherapy alone or in combination with medications.

MEDICATION

Start at the lowest available dose and maintain highest effectively tolerated FDA-approved dose for at least 4 to 6 weeks before deeming ineffective. Effectiveness is comparable between and within drug classes, selection should be based on provider familiarity and patient characteristics/preferences such as:

- Safety and side effect profile
- Comorbid illnesses and concurrent medications
- Specific depressive symptoms
- Ease of use (frequency of dosing) or cost
- Patient preference

First Line

Selective serotonin reuptake inhibitors (SSRIs) (brand name): starting dose; usual dose [special notes]

- Citalopram (Celexa): 20 mg/day; 20 to 40 mg/day (FDA warning: doses >40 mg/day risk of QTc prolongation)
- Escitalopram (Lexapro): 10 mg/day; 10 to 20 mg/day (causes dose-dependent QTc prolongation)
- Fluoxetine (Prozac): 20 mg/day; 20 to 40 mg/day (FDA approved for teens)
- Fluvoxamine (Luvox): 50 mg QHS; 50 to 200 mg/day (off label for depression; primarily used for OCD)
- Paroxetine (Paxil): 20 mg/day or Paxil CR 25 mg/day; 20 to 40 mg/day or Paxil CR 50.0 to 62.5 mg/day
- Sertraline (Zoloft): 50 mg/day; 50 to 200 mg/day
- Common adverse effects: sexual dysfunction (20%), nausea, GI upset, dizziness, insomnia, headache, weight gain. Adverse effects typically resolve within the 1st week.
- Abrupt discontinuation may cause withdrawal symptoms (i.e., dizziness, nausea, headache, paresthesia).

Pregnancy Considerations

- SSRIs (most are pregnancy Category C): Fluoxetine, sertraline, and bupropion are widely used and considered safe. After 20 weeks' gestation, there is an increased risk of pulmonary HTN; mild transient neonatal syndrome of CNS; and motor, respiratory, and GI signs.
- Paroxetine (pregnancy Category D): There is conflicting evidence regarding the risk of congenital cardiac defects and other congenital anomalies in the 1st trimester.
- Newborns of mothers on antidepressants may exhibit a brief period of withdrawal symptoms.

Pediatric Considerations

See "Depression, Pediatric" topic.

Second Line

- Tricyclic (TCAs) and tetracyclic antidepressants
  - Amitriptyline** (Elavil): 25 to 50 mg QHS; 100 to 300 mg/day (serotonin > norepinephrine reuptake inhibitor)
  - Amoxapine (Asendin): 25 mg QHS or TID; 200 to 300 mg/day (norepinephrine > serotonin reuptake inhibitor)
  - Clomipramine** (Anafranil): 25 mg QHS or TID; 100 to 250 mg/day (serotonin > norepinephrine reuptake inhibitor)
  - Desipramine** (Norpramin): 25 mg/day; 150 to 300 mg/day (may be sedating for some, activating for others)
  - Doxepin** (Sinequan): 25 mg QHS up to 150 mg/day; 150 to 300 mg/day (highly sedating and causes weight gain)
  - Imipramine** (Tofranil): 25 mg QHS or 150 mg/day; 150 to 300 mg/day (serotonin > norepinephrine reuptake inhibitor)
  - Maprotiline** (Ludiomil): 25 mg QHS; 100 to 225 mg QHS (potent norepinephrine reuptake inhibitor)
  - Nortriptyline (Pamelor): 25 mg QHS; 50 to 150 mg/day (norepinephrine > serotonin reuptake inhibitor)
  - Protriptyline (Vivactil): 10 mg QHS up to 10 mg TID; 15 to 60 mg QHS(better tolerated due to low affinity for H1/M1 receptors)
  - Trimipramine** (Surmontil): 25 mg QHS; 150 to 300 mg/day (serotonin reuptake inhibitor)
  - **Drugs are highly sedating and associated with weight gain.
  - Similar efficacy to SSRIs; however, therapy is limited by adverse effects (1)[C].
  - Avoid use when these comorbidities are present: arrhythmias and other significant cardiac disease, seizure disorders, osteoporosis, glaucoma.
  - Common adverse effects: orthostatic hypotension, dry mouth, blurred vision, constipation, urinary retention, tachycardia, confusion/delirium
- Serotonin modulators
  - Nefazodone (Serzone): 100 mg BID; 300 to 600 mg/day (not commonly used because of risk of liver failure)
  - Trazodone (Desyrel/Trialodine): 50 mg BID; 200 to 400
  - Vilazodone (Viibryd): 10 mg QHS titrated to 20 mg QHS in week 2; 20 to 40 mg/day (Take with food.)
  - Vortioxetine (Trintellix): 5 to 10 mg/day; 20 mg/day
  - Common adverse effects: somnolence, dizziness, constipation or diarrhea, sexual dysfunction
- Monoamine oxidase inhibitors (MAOIs)
  - Phenelzine (Nardil): 15 mg/day titrated to 15 mg TID over 2 to 3 days; 60 to 90 mg/day
  - Selegiline (Eldepryl): 6 mg/24 hr; 6 to 12 mg/24 hr
  - Tranylcypromine (Parnate): 10 mg/day; 30 to 60 mg/day
  - Common adverse effects: hypotension, sexual dysfunction, sleep disturbance

ALERT

- Black box warning: increased risk of suicidality in children, adolescents, and young adults up to age 25 years who are treated with antidepressants. Although this has not been extended to adults, suicide risk assessments are warranted for all patients.
- Serotonin syndrome: a rare but potentially lethal complication from rapid increase in dose or new addition of medication with serotonergic effects.
- Antidepressants can precipitate manic episodes in those with bipolar disorder. Use with caution if a personal or family history.
- TCAs can be fatal in overdose.
- Allow 14-day period off of all antidepressants before starting MAOIs.

ISSUES FOR REFERRAL

Refer immediately if presence of active suicidal plan or intent, severe self-neglect, or significant risk of self-harm.

ADDITIONAL THERAPIES

- Electroconvulsive therapy (ECT) is indicated for severe refractory depression or severe depression with psychotic features or catatonia and those with an urgent need for response (suicidal or nutritionally compromised).
- Repetitive transcranial magnetic stimulation (rTMS) may be helpful for treatment-resistant depression.

SURGERY/OTHER PROCEDURES

Deep Brain Stimulation and Deep Cortical Stimulation are investigational treatments for resistant depression.

COMPLEMENTARY & ALTERNATIVE MEDICINE

Not regulated by FDA

- Hypericum perforatum (St. John's wort): 300 to 1,800 mg/day
- Light therapy: effective for seasonal affective disorder

ADMISSION, INPATIENT, AND NURSING CONSIDERATIONS

Patients at risk for suicide should be treated as inpatients.

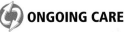 ONGOING CARE

PATIENT EDUCATION

- Depression is a common, treatable medical illness and not a character defect.
- Medications may need to be taken for at least 2 to 4 weeks before any beneficial effect is noted. It may take 6 to 8 weeks to reach maximal efficacy.
- Recommend exercise, good sleep hygiene, nutrition, and decreased use of tobacco and alcohol.
- The National Suicide Prevention Lifeline, 800-273-TALK (8255), is a free 24-hour hotline.

PROGNOSIS

- 70% show significant improvement.
- 50% will relapse over their lifetime.

REFERENCE

1. American Psychiatric Association. Practice guideline for the treatment of patients with major depressive disorder. 2010. https://psychiatryonline.org/pb/assets/raw/sitewide/practice_guidelines/guidelines/mdd.pdf. Accessed January 18, 2021.

 SEE ALSO

Depression, Geriatric; Depression, Pediatric; Depression, Postpartum; Depression, Treatment Resistant; Suicide; Suicide, Pediatric

 CODES

ICD10

- F32.9 Major depressive disorder, single episode, unspecified
- F33.9 Major depressive disorder, recurrent, unspecified
- F34.1 Dysthymic disorder

CLINICAL PEARLS

- Therapeutic alliance is important to treatment success.
- Given the high recurrence rates, long-term treatment is often necessary.

DEPRESSION, ADOLESCENT
Margo L. Bailey-Leatherwood, MD, MS • Lovella Kanu, MD, FAAFP, Dipl. ABOM

BASICS

DESCRIPTION
- *DSM-5* depressive disorders include major depressive disorder (MDD), disruptive mood dysregulation disorder (DMDD), persistent depressive disorder (PDD), premenstrual dysphoric disorder, substance/medication-induced depressive disorder, and other nonspecific depression. This chapter focuses on MDD as it relates to the adolescent patient.
- MDD is a primary mood disorder characterized by sadness and/or irritable mood with impairment of functioning; abnormal psychological development; and a loss of self-worth, energy, and interest in typically pleasurable activities.
- DMDD is characterized by having severe, recurrent outbursts along with persistent irritability and anger.
- PDD is characterized by a depressed mood for most days lasting at least 1 year in a child/adolescent.
- Adolescents with depression are likely to suffer broad functional impairment across social, academic, family, and occupational domains, along with a high incidence of relapse and a high risk for substance abuse and other psychiatric comorbidity.

EPIDEMIOLOGY
Incidence
During adolescence, the cumulative probability of depression ranges from 5% to 20% (1).

Prevalence
- MDD: 6–12% of adolescents; twice as common in females
- DMDD: 2–5%; more prominent in males (2)

ETIOLOGY AND PATHOPHYSIOLOGY
- Unclear; low levels of neurotransmitters (serotonin, norepinephrine); decreased functioning of the dopamine system also contributes.
- External factors may affect neurotransmitters independently.
- Hormonal changes during puberty

Genetics
- Offspring of parents with depression have 3 to 4 times increased rates of depression compared with offspring of parents without mood disorder (1).
- Family studies indicate that anxiety in childhood tends to precede adolescent depression (1).

RISK FACTORS
- Prior depressive episodes
- History of insomnia, anxiety disorders, attention deficit hyperactivity disorder (ADHD), body dysmorphic disorder, chronic childhood illness, and/or learning disabilities
- Increased screen time (3)
- Female gender
- General stressors: adverse life events, difficulties with peers, loss of a loved one, academic difficulties, abuse, chronic illness, tobacco abuse, and low socioeconomic status
- LGBTQ identified

GENERAL PREVENTION
- Some evidence indicates that child and adolescent mental health can be improved by successfully treating maternal depression (1)[A].
- The United States Preventive Services Task Force (USPSTF) recommends the screening of adolescents (12 to 18 years of age) for MDD when systems are in place to ensure accurate diagnosis, appropriate treatment, and follow-up.

COMMONLY ASSOCIATED CONDITIONS
- 20% meet the criteria for generalized anxiety disorder.
- Also associated with behavioral disorders, substance abuse, eating disorders

DIAGNOSIS

HISTORY
- Adolescents may present with medically unexplained somatic complaints (fatigue, irritability, headache).
- Based on *DSM-5* criteria, ≥5 of the following symptoms have been present during the same 2-week period and represent a change from previous functioning: At least one of the symptoms is either depressed mood or loss of interest or pleasure (2):
  - Criterion A
    - Depressed mood most of the day, nearly every day, either subjective report or observation by others (feelings of sadness, emptiness, hopelessness; in children, can be irritability)
    - Markedly diminished interest or pleasure in all activities most of the day, nearly every day
    - Significant weight loss when not dieting or weight gain (>5% body weight in 1 month)
    - Insomnia or hypersomnia
    - Psychomotor agitation or retardation nearly every day
    - Fatigue or loss of energy
    - Feelings of worthlessness or excessive or inappropriate feelings of guilt nearly every day
    - Diminished ability to think or concentrate, or indecisiveness, nearly every day
    - Recurrent thoughts of death, recurrent suicidal ideation, or attempt
  - Criterion B. Symptoms cause clinically significant distress or impairment in social, occupational, or other important areas of functioning.
  - Criterion C. Episode is not attributable to substances' effects or other medical conditions.
  - Criterion D. Episode is not better explained by a schizoaffective, schizophreniform, or delusional disorder.
  - Criterion E. There has never been a manic or hypomanic episode.

PHYSICAL EXAM
- Psychomotor retardation/agitation may be present.
- Clinicians should carefully assess patients for signs of self-injury (such as wrist lacerations) or abuse.

DIFFERENTIAL DIAGNOSIS
- Normal bereavement
- Substance-induced mood disorder

- Bipolar disorder
- Adjustment disorder with depressed mood
- Mood disorder secondary to a medical condition (thyroid, anemia, vitamin deficiency, diabetes)
- Organic CNS diseases
- Malignancy
- Infectious mononucleosis or other viral diseases
- ADHD, posttraumatic stress disorder (PTSD), eating disorders, and anxiety disorders
- Sleep disorder
- Sadness

DIAGNOSTIC TESTS & INTERPRETATION
Initial Tests (lab, imaging)
May be used to rule out other diagnoses (i.e., CBC, TSH, glucose, vitamin B_{12}, folate, monospot, and urine drug)

Follow-Up Tests & Special Considerations
None with sufficient sensitivity/specificity for diagnosis

Diagnostic Procedures/Other
- Depression is primarily diagnosed after a formal interview, with supporting information from caregivers and teachers.
- Standardized tests are useful as screening tools and to monitor response to treatment but should not be used as the sole basis for diagnosis:
  - Beck Depression Inventory II (BDI-II): ages 13 to 18 years (1)[A]
  - Children's Depression Inventory 2 (CDI 2): ages 7 to 17 years
  - Center for Epidemiological Studies Depression Scale for Children (CES-DC): ages 6 to 17 years
  - Patient Health Questionnaire-9 (PHQ-9): ages 13 to 17 years with ideal cut point of 11 or higher (instead of 10 used for adults)
- The USPSTF recommends screening for MDD in adolescents ages 12 to 18 years but states that current evidence is insufficient to assess benefits and harms for screening children aged 11 years or younger (4)[B].
- The evaluation of adolescents who screen positive for depression should include assessment of potential for harm to self and others using structured screening and interview tools (5).

TREATMENT

GENERAL MEASURES
- Active support and monitoring with short validated scales should be used in mild cases for 6 to 8 weeks.
- Psychotherapy and/or medication should be considered if active support and monitoring do not improve symptoms (6)[A].
- Treatment should include psychoeducation, supportive management, and family and school involvement (7)[C].
- Initial management should include treatment planning and ensuring that the patient and family are comfortable with the plan (7)[C].

- A Cochrane review showed that there was no significant difference between remission rates for adolescents treated with cognitive-behavioral therapy (CBT) versus medication or combination therapy immediately postintervention (6)[A].
- A multitreatment meta-analysis showed that combined fluoxetine/CBT had higher efficacy than monotherapies, but other selective serotonin reuptake inhibitors (SSRIs), such as sertraline and escitalopram, were better tolerated (7)[A].

MEDICATION

First Line

- Fluoxetine: for depression in age >8 years. Starting dose 10 mg/day; effective dose 10 to 60 mg/day. The most studied SSRI and with the most favorable effectiveness and safety data has the longest half-life of the SSRIs and is not generally associated with withdrawal symptoms between doses or on discontinuation (6)[A].
- Escitalopram: for depression in age >12 years. Starting dose of 5 mg/day; effective dose of 10 to 20 mg/day (6)[A].
- Citalopram: for depression in age >12 years. Starting dose of 10 mg/day; effective dose of 10 to 40 mg/day (6)[A].
- Sertraline: for depression in age >12 years. Starting dose of 25 mg/day; effective dose of 50 to 200 mg/day (6)[A].
- Can titrate dose every 1 to 2 weeks if no significant adverse effects emerge (headaches, GI upset, insomnia, agitation, behavior activation, suicidal thoughts) (6)[A].

ALERT

SSRI black box warning to monitor for worsening condition, behavior changes, and suicidal thoughts (6)[A]

- Because of this increased risk for suicidality, it is important to closely monitor for suicidality and other adverse effects after initiating pharmacotherapy in an adolescent child. Follow-up in 2 weeks is recommended.
- Given their rates of increased drug metabolism, adolescents may be at higher risk for withdrawal symptoms from SSRIs than adults; if these are present, twice-daily dosing may be considered (7)[A].
- All other SSRIs except fluoxetine should be slowly tapered when discontinued (6)[A].

Pediatric Considerations

- Tricyclic antidepressants (TCAs) have not been proven to be effective in adolescents and should not be used (6)[A].
- Paroxetine (SSRI): Avoid use due to short half-life, associated withdrawal symptoms, and higher association with suicidal ideation.

ISSUES FOR REFERRAL

- Collaborative care interventions between mental health and primary care have a greater improvement in depressive symptoms after 12 months (6)[B].
- Refer to a child psychiatrist for severe, recurrent, or treatment-resistant depression or if the patient has comorbidities.

COMPLEMENTARY & ALTERNATIVE MEDICINE

- Physical exercise and light therapy may have a mild to moderate effect (8)[B].
- St. John's wort, acupuncture, S-adenosylmethionine, and 5-hydroxytryptophan have not been shown to have an effect or have inadequate studies to support use in adolescent depression.

ADMISSION, INPATIENT, AND NURSING CONSIDERATIONS

If severely depressed, psychotic, suicidal, or homicidal, one-on-one supervision may be needed.

ONGOING CARE

- Antidepressant treatment should be continued for 6 to 12 months at full therapeutic dose after the resolution of symptoms at the same dosage.
- After resolution of symptoms, monitor monthly for 6 months, then regularly for the next 18 months (6).

FOLLOW-UP RECOMMENDATIONS

Patient Monitoring

- SSRI medications include black box warning to monitor for worsening condition, behavior changes, and suicidal thoughts (6)[A].
- Systematic and regular tracking of goals and outcomes from treatment should be performed, including assessment of depressive symptoms and functioning in home, school, and peer settings (6)[A].
- Diagnosis and initial treatment should be reassessed if no improvement is noted after 6 to 8 weeks of treatment (6)[A].
- The goal of treatment should be sustained symptom remission and restoration of full function.
- Educate patients and family members about the causes, symptoms, course and treatments of depression, risks of treatments, and risk of no treatment.

PROGNOSIS

- 60–90% of episodes remit within 1 year.
- 50–70% of remissions develop subsequent depressive episodes within 5 years.
- Depression in adolescence predicts mental health disorders in adult life, psychosocial difficulties, and ill health (2)[A].

COMPLICATIONS

- Treatment-induced mania, aggression, or lack of improvement in symptoms
- School failure/refusal
- 1/3 of adolescents with suicidal ideation go on to make an attempt (7).

REFERENCES

1. Thapar A, Collishaw S, Pine DS, et al. Depression in adolescence. *Lancet*. 2012;379(9820):1056–1067.
2. American Psychiatric Association. *Diagnostic and Statistical Manual of Mental Disorders*. 5th ed. Arlington, VA: American Psychiatric Association; 2013.
3. Liu M, Wu L, Yao S. Dose-response association of screen time-based sedentary behaviour in children and adolescents and depression: a meta-analysis of observational studies. *Br J Sports Med*. 2016;50(20):1252–1258.
4. Siu AL; for U.S. Preventive Services Task Force. Screening for depression in children and adolescents: US Preventive Services Task Force recommendation statement. *Ann Intern Med*. 2016;164(5):360–366.
5. Lewandowski RE, Acri MC, Hoagwood KE, et al. Evidence for the management of adolescent depression. *Pediatrics*. 2013;132(4):e996–e1009.
6. Cheung AH, Zuckerbrot RA, Jensen PS, et al. Guidelines for Adolescent Depression in Primary Care (GLAD-PC): part II. Treatment and ongoing management. *Pediatrics*. 2018;141(3):e20174082.
7. Nock MK, Green JG, Hwang I, et al. Prevalence, correlates, and treatment of lifetime suicidal behavior among adolescents: results from the National Comorbidity Survey Replication Adolescent Supplement. *JAMA Psychiatry*. 2013;70(3):300–310.
8. Larun L, Nordheim LV, Ekeland E, et al. Exercise in prevention and treatment of anxiety and depression among children and young people. *Cochrane Database Syst Rev*. 2006;(3):CD004691.

CODES

ICD10

- F32.9 Major depressive disorder, single episode, unspecified
- F33.9 Major depressive disorder, recurrent, unspecified
- F32.8 Other recurrent depressive disorders

CLINICAL PEARLS

- Adolescent depression is underdiagnosed and often presents with irritability and anhedonia.
- Fluoxetine is the most studied FDA-approved for treatment of adolescent depression.
- Escitalopram, citalopram, and sertraline are also FDA-approved antidepressants.
- CBT combined with fluoxetine is efficacious for adolescents with major depression.
- Paroxetine and TCAs should not be used to treat adolescent depression.
- Referral to a child psychiatrist is appropriate for complex cases or treatment-resistant depression.
- Monitor all adolescents with depression for suicidality, especially during the 1st month of treatment with an antidepressant.

D

DEPRESSION, GERIATRIC

Assim M. AlAbdulKader, MD, MPH, FAAFP

 BASICS

DESCRIPTION

A primary mood disorder characterized by a depressed mood and/or a markedly decreased interest or pleasure in normally enjoyable activities most of the day, almost every day for at least 2 weeks, and causing significant distress or impairment in daily functioning. The geriatric population can have variable presentations and comorbid conditions that present different challenges than treating depression in the younger population.

EPIDEMIOLOGY

Incidence
- 2–10% of community-dwelling elderly
- 5–10% seen in primary care clinics
- 10–37% of hospitalized elderly patients
- 12–27% of nursing home residents

Prevalence
- The Global Burden of Disease Study (2015) estimated the prevalence of depressive disorders among older adults (>60 years old) of 4–6% among males and 5–8% among females.
- Suicide is the 11th leading cause of death in the United States for all ages. The elderly account for 24% of all completed suicides with the highest rates for males aged >85 years.

ETIOLOGY AND PATHOPHYSIOLOGY
- A complex interaction between heritable, biologic, psychological, and environmental factors
- Abnormalities in neurotrophins, neurogenesis, neuroimmune systems, and neuroendocrine systems

Genetics
Possible mechanisms, including genetic influences on monoamine transmission and associated transcriptional and translational activity and dysregulation in biologic processes and proteostasis involving C-peptide, FABP-liver, and ApoA-IV proteins

RISK FACTORS
- Female sex
- Lower socioeconomic status
- Widowed, divorced, or separated marital status
- Chronic physical health/chronic pain
- Family history of depression
- Death of a loved one
- Caregiving
- Functional/cognitive impairment
- Lack/loss of social support/social isolation
- Significant loss of independence
- Insomnia/sleep disturbance

GENERAL PREVENTION
Limited, but growing body of evidence suggest these interventions to prevent depression in the elderly:
- Following traditional dietary patterns (e.g., Mediterranean, Japanese, or Norwegian)
- Increasing the consumption of foods rich in omega-3 polyunsaturated fatty acids (e.g., salmon, tuna, sardine, mackerel)
- Engaging in regular physical activity and exercise

COMMONLY ASSOCIATED CONDITIONS
Chronic disease (e.g., coronary artery diseases [CAD], cerebrovascular diseases [CVD], cancer, Parkinson disease)

 DIAGNOSIS

Diagnostic and Statistical Manual of Mental Disorders, 5th edition *(DSM-5)* criteria

HISTORY
- Depressed mood most of the day, nearly every day, and/or loss of interest/pleasure in life for at least 2 weeks
- Other common symptoms include the following:
  – Feeling hopeless, helpless, or worthless
  – Insomnia and loss of appetite/weight (alternatively, hypersomnia with increased appetite/weight in atypical depression)
  – Fatigue and loss of energy
  – Somatic symptoms (headaches, chronic pain)
  – Neglect of personal responsibility or care
  – Psychomotor retardation or agitation
  – Diminished concentration, indecisiveness
  – Thoughts of death or suicide
- Screening with "SIGECAPS"
  – **S**leep: changes in sleep habits from baseline, including excessive sleep, early waking, or inability to fall asleep
  – **I**nterest: loss of interest in previously enjoyable activities (anhedonia)
  – **G**uilt: excessive or inappropriate guilt that may or may not focus on a specific problem or circumstance
  – **E**nergy: perceived lack of energy
  – **C**oncentration: inability to concentrate on specific tasks
  – **A**ppetite: increase/decrease in appetite
  – **P**sychomotor: restlessness and agitation or the perception that everyday activities are too strenuous to manage
  – **S**uicidality: desire to end life or hurt oneself, harmful thoughts directed internally, recurrent thoughts of death or thoughts of homicidality

PHYSICAL EXAM
Mental status examination, focused neurologic and physical examination to rule out other underlying conditions

DIFFERENTIAL DIAGNOSIS
Concurrent medical conditions, cognitive disorders, and medications may cause symptoms that mimic depression:
- Medical conditions: hypothyroidism, vitamin B_{12} or folate deficiency, liver or renal failure, cancers, stroke, sleep disorders, electrolyte imbalances, Cushing disease, chronic fatigue syndrome
- Cognitive disorders: delirium, dementia and other neurodegenerative disorders

- Medications: interferon-α, β_2-blockers, isotretinoin, benzodiazepines, glucocorticoids, GnRH agonists, levodopa, clonidine, H_2 blockers, baclofen, phenobarbital, topiramate, triptans, varenicline, metoclopramide, reserpine
- Other psychiatric disorders

DIAGNOSTIC TESTS & INTERPRETATION
Initial Tests (lab, imaging)
Initial laboratory evaluation to rule out potential medical factors that could be causing symptoms
- Thyroid-stimulating hormone (hypothyroidism)
- CBC (anemia, infection)
- Vitamin B_{12}, folic acid (deficiencies)
- Urinalysis (urinary tract infection, glucosuria)
- Comprehensive metabolic panel
- Urine toxicology screen
- 24-hour urine free cortisol (Cushing disease)

Follow-Up Tests & Special Considerations
Additional testing for possible confounding medical disorders, as warranted (e.g., sleep study)

Diagnostic Procedures/Other
Validated screening tools and rating scales (1)[A]:
- Geriatric Depression Scale (GDS): 15- or 30-point scales
- Patient Health Questionnaire (PHQ-2 and PHQ-9)
- Hamilton Depression Rating Scale (HDRS): 17- or 21-item, clinician-administered scale
- Beck Depression Inventory (BDI): 21- or 13-item, self-report rating
- Cornell Scale for Depression in Dementia

Test Interpretation
Refer to appropriate scoring and interpretation instructions.

 TREATMENT

Although 50% reduction in symptoms alone is considered clinically meaningful, the goal is to treat the patient to the point of remission (i.e., essentially the absence of depressive symptoms).

GENERAL MEASURES
- Lifestyle modifications:
  – Improve nutrition.
  – Encourage social interactions.
  – Exercise and physical activity may be beneficial for depression in the elderly (2)[A].
- Psychotherapy: Studies do show some benefit in depressed elderly (3)[B]:
  – Cognitive-behavioral therapy (CBT)
  – Psychodynamic psychotherapy

MEDICATION
Conservative initial dosing of antidepressants in the elderly, starting with 1/2 of the usual initiation dose and titrating dose every 2 to 4 weeks, as tolerated, to reach an adequate treatment dose

First Line

- Selective serotonin reuptake inhibitors (SSRIs) have been found to be effective in treating depression in the elderly and are considered first-line for pharmacotherapy (3)[A].
- No single SSRI clearly outperforms others in the class; choice of medication often reflects side effect profile or practitioner familiarity (4)[A]:
  - Citalopram: Start at 10 mg/day; treatment range 10 to 20 mg/day
  - Sertraline: Start at 25 mg/day; treatment range 50 to 200 mg/day
  - Escitalopram: Start at 5 to 10 mg/day; treatment range 10 to 20 mg/day
  - Fluoxetine: Start at 10 mg/day; treatment range 20 to 60 mg/day
  - Paroxetine: Start at 10 mg/day; treatment range 20 to 40 mg/day
- SSRIs should not be used concomitantly with monoamine oxidase inhibitors (MAOIs).
- Common side effects: increased risk of falls, nausea, diarrhea, sexual dysfunction

Second Line

Atypical antidepressants: more effective than placebo in the treatment of depression in the elderly, although additional studies are needed to better delineate patient factors that determine response:

- Bupropion: Start at 150 mg/day. Increase dose in 3 to 4 days. Treatment range from 300 to 450 mg/day. Avoid in patients with elevated seizure risk, tremors, or anxiety (5)[A].
- Venlafaxine: Start at 37.5 mg/day extended-release and titrate weekly. Treatment range 150 to 225 mg/day; monitor BP at higher doses (5)[C].
- Duloxetine: Start at 20 to 30 mg/day. Treatment range from 60 to 120 mg/day. May also be associated with elevated BP (5)[A]
- Mirtazapine: Start at 7.5 to 15.0 mg nightly. Treatment range 30 to 45 mg/day; problems with dry mouth, weight gain, sedation, and cognitive dysfunction (5)[A]
- Desvenlafaxine: 50 mg/day in the AM; higher doses do not confer additional benefit; 50 mg every other day if CrCl <30 mL/min (5)[A]

ISSUES FOR REFERRAL

Depression with suicidal ideation, psychotic depression, bipolar disorder, comorbid substance abuse issues, polypharmacy, severe or refractory illness

ADDITIONAL THERAPIES

For patients who have not responded to initial SSRI trial:

- Try a different SSRI medication, switch to an atypical antidepressant, or augment initial antidepressant with bupropion.
- 2nd-generation antipsychotic agents (5)[C]:
  - Aripiprazole: 2 to 5 mg/day. Treatment range 5 to 15 mg/day; can produce sedation, weight gain
  - Used for augmentation in conjunction with other antidepressant medications

- Tricyclic antidepressants (TCAs):
  - Nortriptyline: 25 to 50 mg nightly. Treatment range 75 to 150 mg nightly; anticholinergic effects, weight gain, increase risk of falls (5)[C]
  - TCAs have been shown to be effective in treating depression. However, difficult for elderly patients to tolerate due to side effect profile and are potentially lethal in overdose, limiting their use as initial agents (1)[A]
- MAOIs effective in the treatment of depression in the elderly. They are not used frequently in clinical practice due to potential side effects and necessary dietary restrictions (1)[A].
- Although not FDA-approved, buspirone, lithium, or triiodothyronine used off-label to augment a primary antidepressant
- Evidence for benefit of antidepressants in the treatment of depression in patients with dementia is equivocal. Consideration should be made for a limited trial with close monitoring for symptom improvement or side effects and used only in patients with severe symptoms.
- Electroconvulsive therapy (ECT) has been shown to produce remission of depressive symptoms in the elderly. However, due to lack of consistent evidence, it should only be considered as an option for patients with severe or psychotic depression.

COMPLEMENTARY & ALTERNATIVE MEDICINE

- St. John's wort may have minimal benefit but has drug interactions.
- Tryptophan and hydroxytryptophan: 150 to 300 mg/day; possible efficacy

ADMISSION, INPATIENT, AND NURSING CONSIDERATIONS

Inpatient care is indicated if imminent safety risk is present (e.g., acutely suicidal) or if unable to adequately care for themselves due to depression.

 ONGOING CARE

FOLLOW-UP RECOMMENDATIONS

Due to the delay of benefit following the initiation of antidepressant therapy, it is necessary to ensure open communication with the patient to prevent premature discontinuation of therapy. An adequate explanation of potential side effects with instructions to call the office before discontinuing therapy is imperative.

Patient Monitoring

- A patient with severe depression who exhibits suicidality will require admission.
- Monitor for worsening anxiety symptoms or increase in suicidality especially in the week following initiation or switching of antidepressants.

DIET

Patients taking MAOIs need to avoid foods high in tyramine (i.e., certain cheeses and wines).

PATIENT EDUCATION

- Depression is a treatable illness.
- Medications need to be taken for 2 to 4 weeks before any beneficial effect is noted and may take 6 to 8 weeks to reach maximum efficacy.

- Depression is often a recurring illness.
- National Suicide Prevention Lifeline at 1-800-273-TALK (8255) is a free, 24-hour hotline available.

PROGNOSIS

Estimates vary for initial clinical response and remission (between 30% and 70%).

COMPLICATIONS

- Impairment in social, occupational, or interpersonal functioning
- Difficulty performing activities of daily living and self-care
- Increase in medical services utilization and increased costs of care
- Increased risk of suicide

REFERENCES

1. Taylor WD. Clinical practice. Depression in the elderly. *N Engl J Med.* 2014;371(13):1228–1236.
2. Blake H, Mo P, Malik S, et al. How effective are physical activity interventions for alleviating depressive symptoms in older people? A systematic review. *Clin Rehabil.* 2009;23(10):873–887.
3. Wilson KC, Mottram PG, Vassilas CA. Psychotherapeutic treatments for older depressed people. *Cochrane Database Syst Rev.* 2008;(1):CD004853.
4. Ruhé HG, Huyser J, Swinkels JA, et al. Switching antidepressants after a first selective serotonin reuptake inhibitor in major depressive disorder: a systematic review. *J Clin Psychiatry.* 2006;67(12):1836–1855.
5. Nelson JC, Delucchi K, Schneider LS. Efficacy of second generation antidepressants in late-life depression: a meta-analysis of the evidence. *Am J Geriatr Psychiatry.* 2008;16(7):558–567.

 SEE ALSO

Algorithms: Depressed Mood Associated with Medical Illness; Depressive Episode, Major

 CODES

ICD10

- F32.9 Major depressive disorder, single episode, unspecified
- F03 Unspecified dementia
- F43.21 Adjustment disorder with depressed mood

CLINICAL PEARLS

- Late-life depression (LLD) is not a normal part of aging.
- Depression in the elderly may be difficult to diagnose due to medical and cognitive comorbidities.
- Depression may present primarily with cognitive dysfunction, and this may improve with treatment of the depression.
- SSRIs are considered first-line therapy. A full remission may take upward of 12 weeks of treatment.
- A multidisciplinary approach to the treatment of depression is often the most efficacious.

DEPRESSION, POSTPARTUM

Uruj Kamal Haider, MD • Destiny D. Pegram, MD

BASICS

DESCRIPTION
- Major depressive disorder (MDD) that recurs or has its onset in the postpartum period
- May also occur in mothers adopting a baby or in fathers
- Postpartum depression (PPD) is similar to nonpregnancy depression (sleep disorders, anhedonia, psychomotor changes, etc.); it most often has its onset within the first 12 weeks postpartum yet can occur within 1 year after delivery.
- Different from postpartum "blues" (sadness and emotional lability), which is experienced by 30–70% of women and has an onset and resolution within first 10 days postpartum

EPIDEMIOLOGY

Incidence
10–20% of women have a new episode of major or minor depression during postpartum period (1).

Prevalence
- >50% of women with PPD enter pregnancy depressed or have an onset during pregnancy (2).
- As many as 19.2% women suffer from depression within 3 months postpartum period.

ETIOLOGY AND PATHOPHYSIOLOGY
- May be related to sensitivity in hormonal fluctuations, including estrogen; progesterone; and other gonadal hormones as well as neuroactive steroids; cytokines; hypothalamic–pituitary–adrenal (HPA) axis hormones; altered fatty acid, oxytocin, and arginine vasopressin levels; and genetic and epigenetic factors
- Multifactorial including biologic–genetic predisposition in terms of neurobiologic deficit, destabilizing effects of hormone withdrawal at birth, inflammation, and psychosocial stressors

RISK FACTORS
- Previous episodes of PPD, history of MDD, or anxiety and depression during pregnancy
- History of premenstrual dysphoria, family history of depression
- Poor pregnancy outcomes (preterm birth, stillbirth, neonatal death, major malformations)
- Substance use, unwanted or unplanned pregnancy, multiple psychosocial stressors, lack of social support, intimate partner violence
- Young maternal age, multiple births; African Americans and Hispanics may have higher rates of PPD.
- Postpartum pain, sleep disturbance, and fatigue
- Recent immigrant status, history of adverse childhood experiences
- Decision to decrease antidepressants during pregnancy
- Gestational diabetes

GENERAL PREVENTION
- Universal screening, using validated rating scales, during pregnancy and postpartum year for better detection. Evidence suggests that screening pregnant and postpartum women for depression reduces depressive symptoms in women with depression and reduces the prevalence of depression in a given population. Evidence for pregnant women was less robust but is also consistent with the evidence for postpartum women regarding the benefits of screening, the benefits of treatment, and screening instrument accuracy (3)[A].
- Psychotherapy/counseling, particularly using cognitive behavioral therapy (CBT) and interpersonal therapy (IPT) based interventions, has been shown to be effective in small randomized trials in the prevention of PPD in at-risk individuals, but the USPSTF concludes that further research is needed (4)[A].
- Use of selective serotonin reuptake inhibitors (SSRIs), specifically sertraline, may be effective in preventing PPD in women at high risk for PPD (4)[A].

COMMONLY ASSOCIATED CONDITIONS
- Bipolar mood disorder, depressive disorder not otherwise specified, dysthymic disorder, cyclothymic disorder, MDD
- Postpartum blues

DIAGNOSIS

HISTORY
- Decreased interest in formerly compelling or pleasurable activities, depressed/low mood, guilt, low self-esteem
- Increased/decreased sleep, decreased energy, decreased concentration, increased/decreased appetite
- Psychomotor agitation or retardation, suicidal ideation

DIFFERENTIAL DIAGNOSIS
- Baby blues: not a psychiatric disorder; mood lability resolves within days.
- Postpartum psychosis: a psychiatric emergency
- Postpartum anxiety/panic disorder
- Postpartum obsessive-compulsive disorder
- Hypothyroidism
- Postpartum thyroiditis: can occur in up to 5.7% of patients in the United States and can present as depression
- Bipolar disorder, depressive episode

DIAGNOSTIC TESTS & INTERPRETATION

Initial Tests (lab, imaging)
No blood testing is necessary, but selective tests based on history and symptoms might include complete blood count (CBC), thyroid-stimulating hormone (TSH), vitamin B_{12} level

Follow-Up Tests & Special Considerations
Urine analysis, urine drug screen, β-hCG

Diagnostic Procedures/Other
- Edinburgh Postnatal Depression Scale is a validated screening tool.
- The Patient Health Questionnaire-9 (PHQ-9) is a validated commonly used screening tool.
- Edinburgh Postnatal Depression Scale (partner version): to be completed by mother's partner to obtain his/her view of mother's depression

TREATMENT

GENERAL MEASURES
- Assess for the presence of suicidal ideation.
- Assess for the presence of homicidal ideation and thoughts of harming the baby (infanticide).
- Assess for symptoms of psychosis including delusions and hallucinations.
- Suicidal ideation, homicidal ideation, or infanticide ideation may require immediate hospitalization.
- Psychotherapy is considered first-line treatment for mild depressive episodes.
- Strongly consider pharmacotherapy when symptoms of depression are moderate to severe.
- Outpatient individual psychotherapy in combination with pharmacotherapy may be beneficial.

MEDICATION

First Line
- For nonbreastfeeding women, selection of antidepressants is similar to nonpostpartum patients.
- SSRIs are generally effective and safe. Paroxetine has been associated with fetal cardiac defects when used during pregnancy:
  - Sertraline (Zoloft): 50 to 200 mg/day PO, fluoxetine (Prozac): 20 to 60 mg/day PO
  - Paroxetine (Paxil): 20 to 50 mg/day; PO given at bedtime; (associated with very small increase in risk of cardiovascular defects with first trimester use), citalopram (Celexa): 20 to 40 mg/day PO, escitalopram (Lexapro): 10 to 20 mg/day PO
- Serotonin-norepinephrine reuptake inhibitors (SNRIs):
  - Venlafaxine (Effexor XR): 75 to 225 mg/day PO, desvenlafaxine (Pristiq): 50 to 100 mg/day PO
  - Duloxetine (Cymbalta): 60 to 120 mg/day PO
- Atypical antidepressants:
  - Bupropion (Wellbutrin): 150 to 450 mg/day PO (no sexual dysfunction, activating)
  - Mirtazapine (Remeron): 15 to 45 mg/day PO at bedtime; (increases appetite and is sedating at lower doses, no sexual dysfunction)
- Tricyclic antidepressants (TCAs), particularly nortriptyline, have been shown to be as effective as SSRIs, yet are more lethal in overdose and have increased rates of unfavorable side effects. Nortriptyline: 75 to 150 mg/day PO given at bedtime
- Bipolar disorder requires treatment with mood stabilizer.

- Among breastfeeding mothers: Breastfeeding should generally not preclude treatment with antidepressants.
  - SSRIs and some other antidepressants are considered a reasonable option during breastfeeding.
  - All antidepressants are excreted in breast milk but are generally compatible with lactation.
  - Sertraline and paroxetine have the lowest translactal passage and are considered most compatible with breastfeeding.
  - Translactal passage is greater with fluoxetine, citalopram (5)[B], and venlafaxine.
  - Start with low doses and increase slowly. Minimize polypharmacy. Attempt to maximize use of only one psychotropic medication at a time. Monitor infant for adverse side effects.
  - Continuing an efficacious medication is preferred over switching antidepressants to avoid exposing the mother and infant to the risks of untreated PPD (5)[B].
  - Breastfeeding women need additional education and support regarding the risks and benefits of use of antidepressants during breastfeeding.
  - Consider negative effects of untreated PPD on infant and child development.
  - Discussions of the treatment options with the patient and her partner when possible. Take into account the patient's personal psychiatric history and previous response to treatment, the risks of no treatment or undertreatment, available data about the safety of medications during breastfeeding, and her individual expectations and treatment preferences.
  - For further information: https://www.ncbi.nlm.nih.gov/books/NBK501922/?report=classic

Second Line
Consider switching to a different antidepressant if patient has a lack of response. Augmentation may be necessary in the setting of treatment resistant PPD. Electroconvulsive therapy (ECT) is an option for depressed postpartum women who do not respond to antidepressant medications, have severe or psychotic symptoms, cannot tolerate antidepressant medications, are actively engaged in suicidal self-destructive behaviors, or have a previous history of response to ECT.

ISSUES FOR REFERRAL
- Obtain psychiatric consultation for patients with psychotic symptoms.
- Strongly consider immediate hospitalization if delusions or hallucinations are present.
- Hospitalization is indicated if mother's ability to care for self and/or infant is significantly compromised.

ADDITIONAL THERAPIES
- CBT and IPT are evidence-based treatments shown to effectively treat PPD.
- Psychoeducation, listening visits (nondirective counseling), and psychodynamic psychotherapy may also improve symptoms of PPD.

SURGERY/OTHER PROCEDURES
Brexanolone was approved by the FDA in March 2019 for PPD. It is a rapidly acting antidepressant that is administered as a continuous IV infusion over a period of 60 hours. There is restricted access to this medication. It is only administered at sites enrolled in the Risk Evaluation and Mitigation Strategy Program, and it is very expensive. Consider in women with severe PPD who refuse or do not respond to ECT (6).
- Requires constant monitoring with pulse oximetry
- FDA recommends that providers monitor patient at least every 2 hours for excessive sedation and loss of consciousness.
- Side effects include dry mouth, hot flashes/flushing, diarrhea, dyspepsia, excessive sedation, loss of consciousness, and dizziness.

COMPLEMENTARY & ALTERNATIVE MEDICINE
- Breastfeeding has been associated with reduced stress and improved maternal mood.
- Infant massage, infant sleep intervention, exercise, and bright light therapy may be beneficial.

ADMISSION, INPATIENT, AND NURSING CONSIDERATIONS

ALERT
Obtain psychiatric consultation for patients with refractory depression or psychotic symptoms. If delusions or hallucinations are present, strongly consider immediate hospitalization. The psychotic mother should *not* be left alone with the baby.

- Admission criteria/initial stabilization: presence of suicidal or homicidal ideation and/or psychotic symptoms and/or thoughts of harming baby and/or inability to care for self or infant, severe weight loss
- Discharge criteria: absence of suicidal or homicidal ideation and/or psychotic symptoms and/or thoughts of harming the baby; mother must be able to care for self and infant.

 ONGOING CARE

FOLLOW-UP RECOMMENDATIONS
Patient Monitoring
- Collaborative care approach, including primary care visits and case manager follow-ups
- Consultation with the infant's doctor, particularly if the mother is breastfeeding while taking psychotropic medications

DIET
- Good nutrition and hydration, especially when breastfeeding
- Mixed evidence to support the addition of multivitamin with minerals and omega-3 fatty acids

PATIENT EDUCATION
- *This Isn't What I Expected: Overcoming Postpartum Depression*, by Karen R. Kleiman and Valerie Davis Raskin
- Web resources: Postpartum Support International: http://www.postpartum.net/, La Leche League: http://www.llli.org/, http://www.womensmentalhealth.org/

PROGNOSIS
- Treatment of maternal depression to remission has been shown to have a positive impact on children's mental health.
- Some patients, particularly those with undertreated or undiagnosed depression, may develop chronic depression requiring long-term treatment.
- Untreated maternal depression is linked to impaired mother–infant bonding and cognitive and language development delay in infants and children.
- Postpartum psychosis is associated with tragic outcomes such as maternal suicide and infanticide.

COMPLICATIONS
- Suicide, self-injurious behavior, psychosis
- Neglect of baby, harm to the baby
- Preterm and low-birth-weight baby

REFERENCES

1. Stuart-Parrigon K, Stuart S. Perinatal depression: an update and overview. *Curr Psychiatry Rep.* 2014;16(9):468.
2. Wisner KL, Sit DK, McShea MC, et al. Onset timing, thoughts of self-harm, and diagnoses in postpartum women with screen-positive depression findings. *JAMA Psychiatry.* 2013;70(5):490–498.
3. O'Connor E, Rossom RC, Henninger M, et al. Primary care screening for and treatment of depression in pregnant and postpartum women: evidence report and systematic review for the US Preventive Services Task Force. *JAMA.* 2016;315(4):388–406.
4. O'Connor E, Senger CA, Henninger ML, et al. Interventions to prevent perinatal depression: evidence report and systematic review for the US Preventive Services Task Force. *JAMA.* 2019;321(6):588–601.
5. Gavin NI, Gaynes BN, Lohr KN, et al. Perinatal depression: a systematic review of prevalence and incidence. *Obstet Gynecol.* 2005;106(5 Pt 1): 1071–1083.
6. Leader LD, O'Connell M, VandenBerg A. Brexanolone for postpartum depression and practical considerations. *Pharmacotherapy.* 2019;39(11):1105–1112.

CODES

ICD10
- F53 Puerperal psychosis
- O90.6 Postpartum mood disturbance

CLINICAL PEARLS
- Universal screening for depression is recommended during the 1st and 3rd trimester and at regular intervals during the postpartum period.
- Early diagnosis and treatment are vital, as untreated PPD can lead to developmental difficulties for the infant and prolonged disability and suffering for the mother.
- Psychotherapy may be an effective monotherapy for mild to moderate depressive systems. In severe PPD, use of medications is strongly urged.
- Antidepressant treatment is safe during pregnancy and breastfeeding and treatment should be individualized for each mom (5)[B].

DEPRESSION, TREATMENT RESISTANT

Michelle Magid, MD, MBA

BASICS

DESCRIPTION
- Major depressive disorder (MDD) that has failed to respond to ≥2 adequate trials of antidepressant therapy in ≥2 different classes is considered to be "treatment resistant."
- Individual antidepressants must be given for 6 weeks at standard doses before being considered a failure.

EPIDEMIOLOGY
- Depression affects >16 million people in the United States and >350 million people worldwide.
- The average adult has a 16% lifetime risk of MDD, with majority experiencing onset before the age of 30.
- Approximately 1/3 of patients with MDD will develop treatment-resistant depression.

ETIOLOGY AND PATHOPHYSIOLOGY
- Unclear. Low levels of neurotransmitters (serotonin, norepinephrine, dopamine, and γ-aminobutyric acid [GABA]) have been indicated.
- Serotonin has been linked to irritability, hostility, and suicidal ideation.
- Norepinephrine has been linked to low energy.
- Dopamine may play a role in low motivation and depression with psychotic features.
- GABA can help with feelings of anxiety, stress, and fear.
- Environmental stressors, such as abuse and neglect, may affect both the function and levels of neurotransmitters.
- Inflammation and oxidative stress in the brain can contribute to treatment-resistant depression.

Genetics
A genetic abnormality in the serotonin transporter gene (5-HTTLPR) may increase risk for treatment-resistant depression.

RISK FACTORS
- Severity of disease
- Mislabeling bipolar patients as depressed
- Comorbid medical disease (including chronic pain)
- Comorbid personality disorder
- Comorbid anxiety disorder
- Comorbid substance use disorder
- Genetic familial predisposition to poor response to antidepressants

GENERAL PREVENTION
- Medication adherence in combination with psychotherapy
- Maintenance electroconvulsive therapy (ECT) may prevent relapse.

COMMONLY ASSOCIATED CONDITIONS
- Suicide
- Bipolar disorder
- Substance use disorders
- Anxiety disorders
- Dysthymia
- Eating disorders
- Somatic symptom disorders

DIAGNOSIS

HISTORY
- Symptoms are the same as in MDD. However, patients do not respond to standard form of treatment.
- Important to screen for suicidality in treatment-resistant depression
- Screening with SIGECAPS
  – Sleep: too much or too little
  – Interest: inability to enjoy activities
  – Guilt: excessive and uncontrollable
  – Energy: poor
  – Concentration: inability to focus on tasks
  – Appetite: too much or too little
  – Psychomotor changes: restlessness/agitation or slowing/lethargy noted by others
  – Suicidality: desire to end life or feeling hopeless

PHYSICAL EXAM
Mental status exam may reveal poor hygiene, limited eye contact, poor relatedness, restricted affect, tearfulness, weight loss or gain, psychomotor retardation or agitation.

DIFFERENTIAL DIAGNOSIS
- Bipolar disorder
- Persistent depressive disorder
- Posttraumatic stress disorder
- Dementia
- Early-stage Parkinson disease
- Personality disorder
- Medical illness such as malignancy, thyroid disease, HIV, anemia
- Substance use disorders

DIAGNOSTIC TESTS & INTERPRETATION
Initial Tests (lab, imaging)
Used to rule out medical factors that could be causing/contributing to treatment resistance
- CBC, complete metabolic profile
- Urine drug screen
- Thyroid-stimulating hormone (TSH)
- 25-OH vitamin D, vitamin B_{12}, folate
- Urinalysis
- FSH, LH if applicable
- HCG, if applicable

- Testosterone, if applicable
- CT or MRI of the brain if neurologic disease, tumor, or dementia is suspected

Follow-Up Tests & Special Considerations
Delirium and dementia often look like depression.

Diagnostic Procedures/Other
Depression is a clinical diagnosis. Use validated depression rating scales to assist:
- Beck Depression Inventory
- Hamilton Depression Rating Scale
- Patient Health Questionnaire 9 (PHQ-9)
- Edinburgh Postnatal Depression Scale if pregnant or postpartum

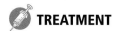

TREATMENT

MEDICATION
First Line
Please see "Depression" topic. When those fail, augmentation and combination strategies are as follows:
- Antidepressants in combination
  – Citalopram (start 20 mg/day; max dose 40 mg/day) + bupropion (start 100 mg BID; max dose 450 mg total) (1),(2)[B]
  – Tricyclic antidepressants (TCAs) and selective serotonin reuptake inhibitors (SSRIs) may be used in combination. Proceed with caution due to risk of serotonin syndrome; citalopram (start 20 mg/day; max dose 40 mg/day) + nortriptyline (start 50 mg at bedtime; max dose 150 mg at bedtime)
  – Serotonin and norepinephrine reuptake inhibitors (SNRI) and noradrenergic and specific serotonergic antidepressant (NaSSA) may also be used in combination, such as venlafaxine extended release (start 75 mg/day; max dose 225 mg/day) and mirtazapine (start 15 mg/day; max dose 45 mg/day).
- Antidepressants + antipsychotics
  – Citalopram (start 20 mg/day; max dose 40 mg/day) + aripiprazole (start 2 mg/day; up to 20 mg/day, different mechanism of action at higher doses) OR + risperidone (start 0.5 to 1.0 mg at bedtime; max dose 6 mg/day) OR + quetiapine (start 25 mg at bedtime; titrate to 100 to 300 mg at bedtime; max dose 600 mg/day) (1)[A],(2)
  – Olanzapine/fluoxetine combination (start 3 mg/25 mg to 12 mg/50 mg at bedtime) (1)[A],(2)
- Antidepressant + lithium
  – TCA: nortriptyline (start 50 mg at bedtime; max dose 150 mg at bedtime) + lithium (start 300 mg at bedtime; max dose 900 mg BID)
  – SSRI: citalopram (start 20 mg/day; max dose 40 mg QD) + lithium (start 300 mg at bedtime; max dose 900 mg BID) (1)[A],(2)

- In all combinations, citalopram (Celexa) can be replaced with other SSRIs such as fluoxetine (Prozac) 20 to 80 mg/day, sertraline (Zoloft) 50 to 200 mg/day, and escitalopram (Lexapro) 10 to 20 mg/day, vortioxetine (Trintellix) 5 to 20 mg/day or with SNRIs duloxetine (Cymbalta) 30 to 120 mg/day, venlafaxine XR (Effexor XR) 75 to 225 mg/day, or desvenlafaxine (Pristiq) 50 to 100 mg/day, or with a NaSSA mirtazapine (Remeron) 15 to 45 mg at bedtime.
- Maximum doses for medication in treatment-resistant cases may be higher than in treatment-responsive cases.

Second Line
- Citalopram (start 20 mg/day; max dose 40 mg/day) + triiodothyronine (T3) (12.5 to 50.0 μg/day) (1),(2)[B]
- Citalopram (start 20 mg/day; max dose 40 mg/day) + buspirone (start 7.5 mg twice a day; max dose 30 mg twice a day) (1)[B],(2)
- Citalopram (start 20 mg/day; max dose 40 mg/day) + lisdexamfetamine (Vyvanse) (20 to 50 mg every morning) (1)[B],(2)
- Antidepressant in combination with therapy, particularly, cognitive-behavioral therapy (CBT) (3)[A]
- Monoamine oxidase inhibitor (MAOI)
  - Tranylcypromine (Parnate): Start 10 mg BID and increase 10 mg/day every 1 to 3 weeks; max dose 60 mg/day
  - Selegiline transdermal (Emsam patch): Apply 6-mg patch daily and increase 3 mg/day; max dose 12 mg/day
  - Side-effect profile (e.g., hypertensive crisis), drug–drug interactions, and dietary restrictions make MAOIs less appealing. Patch version does not require dietary restrictions at lower doses.
  - High risk of serotonin syndrome if combined with another antidepressant. 2-week washout period is advised.

ISSUES FOR REFERRAL
Treatment-resistant depression should be managed in consultation with a psychiatrist.

ADDITIONAL THERAPIES
- First line
  - ECT: brief administration of electrical stimulation to the brain via superficial electrode placement
    ○ Safe and cost-effective option for treatment-resistant and life-threatening depression, with a 66.6% response rate (4)[A]
    ○ Known to rapidly relieve suicidality, psychotic depression, and catatonia
    ○ Cognitive side effects during treatment can occur but are more likely with bilateral lead placement.
    ○ Three types of lead placements
      ■ Right unilateral
      ■ Bitemporal
      ■ Bifrontal

- Second line
  - Deep brain stimulation (DBS): surgical implantation of intracranial electrodes, connected to an impulse generator implanted in the chest wall:
    ○ Reserved for those who have failed medications, psychotherapy, and ECT
    ○ Preliminary data is promising, showing 40–70% response rate and 35% remission rate. Further trials are being done.
  - Transcranial magnetic stimulation (TMS): noninvasive brain stimulation technique that is generally safe
    ○ Currently, only FDA-approved for less severe forms of the illness
  - Vagus nerve stimulation (VNS): surgical implantation of electrodes onto left vagus nerve
    ○ Its use in treatment-resistant depression has become limited in recent years.
  - Ketamine (0.5 mg/kg single-dose infusion over 40 minutes): Studies show evidence of rapid improvement in mood and suicidal thinking. Currently used off-label for treatment-resistant depression (2)[B],(4). Esketamine, an intranasal spray, in conjunction with an oral antidepressant, has been FDA approved for treatment-resistant depression. Dosing is 28 mg, 56 mg, or 84 mg twice a week for 1 to 4 weeks, followed by taper and/or maintenance treatment.
    ○ The effects of ketamine and esketamine appear temporary, usually lasting days to weeks (5). Continued studies are focusing on dosing and frequency of administration to maintain longer lasting response and remission.

ADMISSION, INPATIENT, AND NURSING CONSIDERATIONS
- Inpatient care is indicated for severely depressed, psychotic, catatonic, or suicidal patients.
- Discharge criteria: symptoms improving, no longer suicidal, psychosocial stressors addressed

 ONGOING CARE

FOLLOW-UP RECOMMENDATIONS
- Frequent visits (i.e., every month)
- During follow-up, evaluate side effects, dosage, and effectiveness of medication as well as need for referral to ECT or ketamine/esketamine treatment.
- Patients who have responded to ECT or ketamine/esketamine treatment may need maintenance treatments (q2–12 wk) to prevent relapse.
- Combination of lithium/nortriptyline after ECT appears to be as effective as maintenance ECT in reducing relapse.

DIET
Patients on MAOIs need dietary restriction of foods rich in tyramine.

PATIENT EDUCATION
- Educate patients that depression is a medical illness, not a character defect.
- Review signs and symptoms of worsening depression and when patient needs to come in for further evaluation.
- Discuss safety plan to address suicidal thoughts.

PROGNOSIS
With medication adherence, close follow-up, improved social support, and psychotherapy, prognosis improves.

COMPLICATIONS
- Suicide
- Disability
- Poor quality of life

REFERENCES
1. McIntyre RS, Filteau MJ, Martin L, et al. Treatment-resistant depression: definitions, review of the evidence, and algorithmic approach. *J Affect Disord*. 2014;156:1–7.
2. Taylor RW, Marwood L, Oprea E, et al. Pharmacological Augmentation in Unipolar Depression: A Guide to the Guidelines. *Int J Neuropsychopharmacol*. 2020;23(9):587–625.
3. Wiles NJ, Thomas L, Turner N, et al. Long-term effectiveness and cost-effectiveness of cognitive behavioural therapy as an adjunct to pharmacotherapy for treatment-resistant depression in primary care: follow-up of the CoBalT randomised controlled trial. *Lancet Psychiatry*. 2016;3(2):137–144.
4. Ross EL, Zivin K, Maixner DF. Cost-effectiveness of electroconvulsive therapy vs pharmacotherapy/psychotherapy for treatment-resistant depression in the United States. *JAMA Psychiatry*. 2018;75(7):713–722.
5. Sanacora G, Frye MA, McDonald W, et al. A consensus statement on the use of ketamine in the treatment of mood disorders. *JAMA Psychiatry*. 2017;74(4):399–405.

CODES

ICD10
- F32.9 Major depressive disorder, single episode, unspecified
- F33.9 Major depressive disorder, recurrent, unspecified

CLINICAL PEARLS
- Treatment-resistant depression is common, affecting 1/3 of those with MDD.
- Combination and augmentation strategies with antidepressants, antipsychotics, therapy, and mood stabilizers can be helpful.
- ECT and ketamine/esketamine should be considered in severe and life-threatening cases. DBS is still experimental but showing excellent promise.

DERMATITIS HERPETIFORMIS

Abdul Aleem, MD • Hiral Shah, MD, FASGE, FAGA, FACG

BASICS

DESCRIPTION
- Dermatitis herpetiformis (DH) presents as a chronic, relapsing, polymorphous, intensely pruritic, erythematous papulovesicular eruption with symmetrical distribution primarily involving extensor skin surfaces of the elbows, knees, buttocks, back, and scalp.
- DH is an autoimmune disease associated with gluten sensitivity with genetic, environmental, and immunologic influences.
- DH is distinguished from other bullous diseases by characteristic histologic and immunologic findings as well as associated gluten-sensitive enteropathy (GSE).
- System(s) affected: skin
- Synonym(s): Duhring disease, Duhring-Brocq disease

EPIDEMIOLOGY
- Occurs most frequently in those of Northern European origin
- Rare in persons of Asian or African American origin
- Predominant age: most common in 4th and 5th decades but may present at any age
- Childhood DH is rare in most countries, although an Italian study showed 27% of patients were age of <10 years and 36% age of <20 years.
- Predominant gender: adults: male > female (1.5:1 in the United States, 2:1 worldwide); children: female > male

Incidence
1/100,000 persons per year in the United States

Prevalence
11/100,000 persons in the U.S. population; as high as 39/100,000 persons worldwide

ETIOLOGY AND PATHOPHYSIOLOGY
- Evidence suggests that epidermal transglutaminase (eTG) 3, a keratinocyte enzyme involved in cell envelope formation and maintenance, is the autoantigen in DH.
- eTG is highly homologous with tissue transglutaminase (tTG), which is the antigenic target in celiac disease and GSE.
- The initiating event for DH is presumed to be the interaction of wheat peptides with tTGs, which results in the formation of an autoantigen with high affinity for particular class II major histocompatibility complex (MHC) molecules.
- Presentation of the autoantigen leads to activation of T cells and the humoral immune system.
- IgA antibodies against tTG cross-react with eTG and result in IgA-eTG immune complexes that are deposited in the papillary dermis. Subsequent activation of complement and recruitment of neutrophils to the area result in inflammation and microabscesses.
- Skin eruption may be delayed up to 5 to 6 weeks after exposure to gluten.
- Gluten applied directly to the skin does not result in the eruption, whereas gluten taken by mouth or rectum does. This implies necessary processing by the GI system.
- Thought to be immune complex–mediated disease

Genetics
- High association with human leukocyte antigen (HLA)-DQ2 (95%), with remaining patients being positive for DQ8, DR4, or DR3
- Strong association with combination of alleles DQA1*0501 and DQB1*0201/0202, DRB1*03 and DRB1*05/07, or DQA1*0301 and DQB1*0302

RISK FACTORS
- GSE: >90% of those with DH will have GSE, which may be asymptomatic.
- Family history of DH or celiac disease

GENERAL PREVENTION
Gluten-free diet (GFD) results in improvement of DH and reduces dependence on medical therapy. GFD also may reduce the risk of lymphomas associated with DH.

COMMONLY ASSOCIATED CONDITIONS
- Hypothyroidism is the most common condition associated with DH.
- GSE, gluten ataxia
- Gastric atrophy, hypochlorhydria, pernicious anemia
- GI lymphoma, non-Hodgkin lymphoma
- Hyperthyroidism, thyroid nodules, thyroid cancer
- IgA nephropathy
- Autoimmune disorders, including systemic lupus erythematosus, dermatomyositis, Sjögren syndrome, rheumatoid arthritis, sarcoidosis, Raynaud phenomenon, insulin-dependent diabetes mellitus, myasthenia gravis, Addison disease, vitiligo, alopecia areata, primary biliary cirrhosis, and psoriasis

DIAGNOSIS

Diagnosis of DH involves a clinicopathologic correlation among clinical presentation, histologic and direct immunofluorescence (DIF) evaluation, serology, and response to therapy or dietary restriction.

HISTORY
- Waxing and waning, intensely pruritic eruption with papules and tiny vesicles .
- Eruption may worsen with gluten intake.
- GI symptoms may be absent or may not be reported until prompted.

PHYSICAL EXAM
- The classic lesions of DH are described as symmetric, grouped, erythematous papules and vesicles.
- More commonly presents with erosions, excoriations, lichenification, hypopigmentation, and/or hyperpigmentation secondary to scratching and healing of old lesions
- Areas involved include extensor surfaces of elbows (90%), knees (30%), shoulders, buttocks, and sacrum. The scalp is also frequently affected. Oral lesions are rare.
- In children, purpura may be visible on digits and palmoplantar surfaces.
- Adults with associated enteropathy are most often asymptomatic, with about 20% experiencing steatorrhea and <10% with findings of bloating, diarrhea, or malabsorption.
- Children with associated enteropathy may present with abdominal pain, diarrhea, iron deficiency, and reduced growth rate.

DIFFERENTIAL DIAGNOSIS
- In adults
  - Bullous pemphigoid: linear deposition of C3 and IgG at the basement membrane zone
  - Linear IgA disease: homogeneous and linear deposition of IgA at the basement membrane zone, absence of GSE
  - Prurigo nodularis
  - Urticaria: wheals, angioedema, dermal edema
  - Erythema multiforme

- In children
  - Atopic dermatitis: face and flexural areas
  - Scabies: interdigital areas, axillae, genital region
  - Papular urticaria: dermal edema
  - Impetigo

DIAGNOSTIC TESTS & INTERPRETATION
Initial Tests (lab, imaging)
- Serum IgA tTG antibodies: Detection of tTG antibodies was noted to be up to 95% sensitive and >90% specific for DH in patients on unrestricted diets (1),(2)[A].
- Serum IgA eTG antibodies: Antibodies to eTG, the primary autoantigen in DH, were shown to be more sensitive than antibodies to tTG in the diagnosis of patients with DH on unrestricted diets (95% vs. 79%) but is not widely available in all labs (1),(2)[A].
- Serum IgA endomysial antibodies (EMA): Antibodies to EMA have a sensitivity between 50% and 100% and a specificity close to 100% in patients on unrestricted diets but is more expensive, time-consuming, and operator-dependent than tTG (2).

Follow-Up Tests & Special Considerations
- Serologic assessment of anti-tTG and anti-eTG correlate with intestinal involvement of disease and in conjunction with anti-EMA may be useful in monitoring major deviations from GFD (1),(2).
- Genetic testing for haplotypes HLA-DQ2 and HLA-DQ8 can also be offered to patients to determine genetic susceptibility, to screen patients with high risk of CD, or if the diagnosis is not clear (1).

Diagnostic Procedures/Other
- The gold standard test to establish a diagnosis of DH is DIF of the perilesional skin that demonstrate characteristic granular IgA deposits in dermal papillae and/or basement membrane (1),(2)[A]. It is this key diagnostic feature that differentiates this blistering skin condition from all other dermatologic diseases (3).
- DIF has a sensitivity and specificity of close to 100% (1).
- In patients with high suspicion for DH with a negative DIF, another perilesional skin biopsy should be obtained from a different site (1).
- Histopathology of these lesions with routine staining reveals neutrophilic microabscesses in the tips of the dermal papillae and may show subepidermal blistering (1),(2).

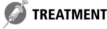
TREATMENT

GENERAL MEASURES
- GFD is the mainstay of treatment in DH and can lead to complete resolution of symptoms (1),(2)[A].
- Typically requires 18 to 24 months of strict adherence to GFD prior to resolution of skin lesions without any additional treatment
- Lesions can recur within 12 weeks of reintroduction of gluten.

MEDICATION
- Despite being on GFD, the lesions of DH take several months to clear, and active lesions warrant additional treatment (3).
- Medications are useful for immediate symptom management but should only be used as an adjunct to dietary modification (2).

First Line
- Dapsone is approved by the FDA for use in DH and is the most widely used medication (2),(4)[A].

- Initial dosing of 25 to 50 mg/day on a strict GFD typically results in improvement of symptoms within 24 to 48 hours (1),(3)[C].
- It is recommended to use minimum effective dose with slow titration based on patient's response and tolerability. Average maintenance dose is 1 mg/kg/day (50 to 150 mg/day) and can be increased up to 200 mg to obtain better symptom control.
- Minor outbreaks on the face and scalp are common even with treatment; not ideal for long-term use in DH
- Dapsone works by inhibiting neutrophil recruitment and IL-8 release, inhibiting the respiratory burst of neutrophils, and protecting cells from neutrophil-mediated injury, thereby suppressing the skin reaction. It has no role in preventing IgA deposition or mitigating the immune reaction in the gut (2),(4).
- Precautions
  - Common side effects include nausea, vomiting, headache, dizziness, weakness, and hemolysis.
  - A drop in hemoglobin of 1 to 2 g is characteristic with dapsone 100 mg/day.
  - G6PD deficiency increases severity of hemolytic stress. Dapsone should be avoided, if possible, in those who are G6PD-deficient.
  - Dose-related methemoglobinemia may occur with doses >100 mg/day. Cimetidine may reduce the severity of this side effect.
  - Risk of distal motor neuropathy

ALERT
- Monitor for potentially fatal dapsone-induced sulfone syndrome: fever, jaundice and hepatic necrosis, exfoliative dermatitis, lymphadenopathy, methemoglobinemia, and hemolytic anemia.
- Can occur 48 hours or 6 months after treatment, most often 5 weeks after initiation

Pediatric Considerations
- <2 years: Dosing is not established.
- >2 years: 0.5 to 1.0 mg/kg/day

Pregnancy Considerations
- Category C: Safety during pregnancy is not established.
- Secreted in breast milk and will produce hemolytic anemia in infants
- Adherence to a strict GFD 6 to 12 months before conception should be considered with the hope of eliminating need for dapsone during pregnancy.

Second Line
- High-potency topical steroids can be used acutely to control symptoms until dapsone becomes effective (1)[C].
- Sulfapyridine (1 to 2 g/day) is FDA-approved for use in DH and is thought to be the active metabolite in sulfasalazine (2 to 4 g/day) (2),(5)[B]. Common side effects include nausea, vomiting, and anorexia. Enteric-coated form may reduce side effects. Other side effects include agranulocytosis, hypersensitivity reactions, hemolytic anemia, proteinuria, and crystalluria (2),(5).
- Topical steroids and 3rd-generation antihistamines can be used to provide relief from symptoms of pruritus and itching.

ISSUES FOR REFERRAL
Over time, the management of DH warrants an interdisciplinary treatment that includes providing a referral to dermatologist, gastroenterologist, and registered dietitian (1),(2).

ADDITIONAL THERAPIES
A single case report described topical dapsone therapy as potential alternative treatment or as an adjunct to oral dapsone to decrease systemic exposure and risk of severe side effects. However, it has not been studied extensively (6)[C].

 ## ONGOING CARE

FOLLOW-UP RECOMMENDATIONS
Patient Monitoring
- Every 6 to 12 months by physician and dietitian to evaluate GFD adherence and recurrence of symptoms
- Adherence to GFD can be monitored with serologic levels of anti-tTG, anti-eTG, and EMA levels (1).
- Patients on dapsone require lab monitoring weekly for the 1st month, biweekly for 2 months, and then every 3 months for the duration of medication use (1),(5).

DIET
- Grains that should be avoided: wheat (includes spelt, kamut, semolina, and triticale), rye, and barley (including malt)
- Safe grains (gluten-free): rice, amaranth, buckwheat, corn, millet, quinoa, sorghum, teff (an Ethiopian cereal grain), and oats
- Care should be taken to avoid gluten-free grains that are contaminated with sources of gluten during processing such as oats.
- Sources of gluten-free starches that can be used as flour alternatives
  - Cereal grains: amaranth, buckwheat, corn, millet, quinoa, sorghum, teff, rice (white, brown, wild, basmati, jasmine), and Montina
  - Tubers: arrowroot, jicama, taro, potato, and tapioca
  - Legumes: chickpeas, lentils, kidney beans, navy beans, pea beans, peanuts, and soybeans
  - Nuts: almonds, walnuts, pistachios, chestnuts, hazelnuts, and cashews
  - Seeds: sunflower, flax, and pumpkin

PATIENT EDUCATION
- Patients started on dapsone should be made aware of potential hemolytic anemia and the signs associated with methemoglobinemia.
- American Academy of Dermatology, 930 N. Meacham Road, P.O. Box 4014, Schaumburg, IL 60168-4014; (708) 330-0230
- The University of Chicago Celiac Disease Center, 5841 S. Maryland Ave., Mail Code 4069, Chicago, IL 60637; (773) 702-7593; www.celiacdisease.net or http://www.cureceliacdisease.org/
- Gluten Intolerance Group of North America, 31214-124 Ave. SE, Auburn, WA 98092; (206) 246-6652; fax (206) 246-6531; https://www.gluten.org/
- The Celiac Disease Foundation, 13251 Ventura Blvd., #1, Studio City, CA 9160; (818) 990-2354; fax (818) 990-2379

PROGNOSIS
- DH is a chronic disease with excellent prognosis, provided strict adherence to a GFD is maintained.
- 10- to 15-year survival rates do not seem to differ from general population.
- Remission in 10–15%
- Skin disease responds readily to dapsone. Occasional new lesions (2 to 3 per week) are to be expected and are not an indication for altering daily dosage.
- Strict adherence to a GFD improves clinical symptoms and decreases dapsone requirement. GFD is the only sustainable method of eliminating cutaneous and GI disease.
- Risk of lymphoma may be decreased in those who maintain a GFD.

COMPLICATIONS
- Majority of complications are associated with GSE.
- Malnutrition, weight loss, nutritional deficiencies (folate, vitamin B_{12}, iron)
- Abdominal pain, dyspepsia
- Osteoporosis, dental abnormalities
- Autoimmune diseases
- Lymphomas

REFERENCES
1. Antiga E, Caproni M. The diagnosis and treatment of dermatitis herpetiformis. *Clin Cosmet Investig Dermatol.* 2015;8:257–265.
2. Bolotin D, Petronic-Rosic V. Dermatitis herpetiformis. Part II. Diagnosis, management, and prognosis. *J Am Acad Dermatol.* 2011;64(6):1027–1034.
3. Reunala T, Salmi TT, Hervonen K. Dermatitis herpetiformis: pathognomonic transglutaminase IgA deposits in the skin and excellent prognosis on a gluten-free diet. *Acta Derm Venereol.* 2015;95(8):917–922.
4. Wozel G, Blasum C. Dapsone in dermatology and beyond. *Arch Dermatol Res.* 2014;306(2):103–124.
5. Willsteed E, Lee M, Wong LC, et al. Sulfasalazine and dermatitis herpetiformis. *Australas J Dermatol.* 2005;46(2):101–103.
6. Handler MZ, Chacon AH, Shiman MI, et al. Letter to the editor: application of dapsone 5% gel in a patient with dermatitis herpetiformis. *J Dermatol Case Rep.* 2012;6(4):132–133.

ADDITIONAL READING
- Bolotin D, Petronic-Rosic V. Dermatitis herpetiformis. Part I. Epidemiology, pathogenesis, and clinical presentation. *J Am Acad Dermatol.* 2011;64(6):1017–1026.
- Cardones AR, Hall RP III. Management of dermatitis herpetiformis. *Immunol Allergy Clin North Am.* 2012;32(2):275–281.
- Cardones AR, Hall RP III. Pathophysiology of dermatitis herpetiformis: a model for cutaneous manifestations of gastrointestinal inflammation. *Immunol Allergy Clin North Am.* 2012;32(2):263–274.
- Kárpáti S. An exception within the group of autoimmune blistering diseases: dermatitis herpetiformis, the gluten-sensitive dermopathy. *Immunol Allergy Clin North Am.* 2012;32(2):255–262.
- Paek SY, Steinberg SM, Katz SI. Remission in dermatitis herpetiformis: a cohort study. *Arch Dermatol.* 2011;147(3):301–305.

 ## SEE ALSO

- Celiac Disease
- Algorithm: Rash

CODES

ICD10
L13.0 Dermatitis herpetiformis

CLINICAL PEARLS

- DH is a chronic, relapsing, intensely pruritic rash that often presents with erosions, excoriations, lichenification, and pigmentary changes secondary to scratching and healing of old papulovesicular lesions.
- Strong association with GSE
- Diagnosis established with perilesional skin biopsy showing DIF demonstrating granular IgA deposits in the dermal papillae
- Serologic levels of IgA transglutaminase aid in diagnosis and monitoring of deviations from GFD.
- Mainstay of treatment is a GFD with dapsone used primarily for short-term symptom relief.

DERMATITIS, ATOPIC
Dennis E. Hughes, DO, FACEP

 BASICS

DESCRIPTION
- A chronic, relapsing, inflammatory, intensely pruritic skin diease
- Early-onset cases have coexisting allergen sensitization more often than late onset.
- Clinical phenotypical presentation is highly variable, suggesting multifactorial pathophysiology.
- May have significant effect on quality of life for patient and family—recurrent symptoms affect lifestyle and mental health.

EPIDEMIOLOGY
- 45% of all cases begin in the first 6 months of life with 80–95% onset prior to age 5 years.
- 50–66% of affected children will have a spontaneous remission before adolescence.
- Also, may have late-onset dermatitis in adults or relapse of childhood condition—primarily hand eczema
- Darker pigmented individuals are affected more often than whites.
- 60% incidence if one parent previously affected; rises to 80% if both parents previously affected. Monozygotic twins have 80% concordance for the disorder.

Incidence
Varies worldwide, but all countries' populations are affected. The only consistent signal favored lower incidence in rural versus urban locations (exceptions are Canada, Mexico) (1).

Prevalence
Approaching 20% prevalence in children and 10% in young adults; still present in later adulthood 2%

ETIOLOGY AND PATHOPHYSIOLOGY
- Current understanding is atopic dermatitis is a systemic T-helper cell driven disorder.
- Alteration in stratum corneum results in transepidermal water loss and defect in barrier function.
- Epidermal adhesion is reduced either as a result of (i) genetic mutation resulting in altered epidermal proteins or (ii) defect in immune regulation causing an altered inflammatory response.
- Interleukin-31 (IL-31) upregulation is thought to be a major factor in pruritus mediated by cytokines and neuropeptides rather than histamine excess.

Genetics
- Recent discovery of association between atopic dermatitis (AD) and mutation in the filaggrin gene (*FLG*), which codes for a skin barrier protein
- Both epidermal and immune coding likely involved

RISK FACTORS
- "Itch–scratch cycle" (stimulates histamine release)
- Skin infections
- Emotional stress
- Irritating clothes and chemicals
- Excessively hot or cold climate
- Food allergy in children (in some cases). Studies of breastfeeding conveying decreased risk versus increased risk are mixed in conclusion (2).
- Exposure to tobacco smoke
- Some evidence suggests that repeated exposure to "hard" water may exacerbate condition.
- Family history of atopy
  - Asthma
  - Allergic rhinitis

COMMONLY ASSOCIATED CONDITIONS
- Food sensitivity/allergy in many cases; strong association with asthma and allergic rhinitis
- Association with both cutaneous and extracutaneous infections: URI, OM, UTI, cellulitis, erysipelas, zoster, endocarditis, MRSA, MSSA, pharyngitis, and rarely sepsis
- Hyper-IgE syndrome (Job syndrome)
  - AD
  - Elevated IgE
  - Recurrent pyodermas
  - Decreased chemotaxis of mononuclear cells

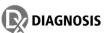 **DIAGNOSIS**

Clinical diagnosis

HISTORY
- Presence of major symptoms, including relapsing of condition, family history, typical distribution, and morphology necessary to make diagnosis of AD
- Most prevalent symptoms: itch (54%), dryness and scaling (19.6%), inflamed skin (7.2%), skin pain (8.2%), sleep disturbance (11.4%) (3)

PHYSICAL EXAM
Primarily skin manifestations
- Distribution of lesions
  - Infants: trunk, face, and flexural surfaces; diaper-sparing
  - Children: antecubital and popliteal fossae
  - Adults: hands, feet, face, neck, upper chest, and genital areas
- Morphology of lesions
  - Infants: erythema and papules; may develop oozing, crusting vesicles
  - Children and adults: Lichenification and scaling are typical with chronic eczema as a result of persistent scratching and rubbing (lichenification rare in infants).
- Associated signs
  - Facial erythema, mild to moderate
  - Perioral pallor
  - Infraorbital fold (Dennie sign/Morgan line)—atopic pleat
  - Dry skin progressing to ichthyosis
  - Increased palmar linear markings
  - Pityriasis alba (hypopigmented asymptomatic areas on face and shoulders)
  - Keratosis pilaris

DIFFERENTIAL DIAGNOSIS
- Photosensitivity rashes
- Contact dermatitis (especially if only the face is involved)
- Scabies
- Seborrheic dermatitis (especially in infants)
- Psoriasis or lichen simplex chronicus if only localized disease is present in adults
- Rare conditions of infancy
  - Histiocytosis X
  - Wiskott-Aldrich syndrome
  - Ataxia-telangiectasia syndrome
- Ichthyosis vulgaris

DIAGNOSTIC TESTS & INTERPRETATION
Initial Tests (lab, imaging)
- No test is diagnostic.
- Serum IgE levels are elevated in as many as 80% of affected individuals, but test is not routinely ordered.
- Eosinophilia tends to correlate with disease severity.
- Scoring atopic dermatitis (SCORAD) is scoring system for AD comprising scores for area, intensity, and subjective symptoms.

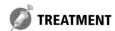 **TREATMENT**

GENERAL MEASURES
- Minimize flare-ups and control the duration and intensity of flare-up.
- Avoid agents that may cause irritation (e.g., wool, perfumes).
- Minimize sweating.
- Lukewarm (not hot) bathing. No evidence significantly guides frequency of bathing, but a minimum of twice weekly and when hygiene dictates for with post bath skin care supported (1).
- Avoid alkaline soaps. Hypoallergenic cleansers with a slightly acidic (pH 5–6) with gentle mechanical removal of crusts, scale, and bacterial skin contaminants.
- Sun exposure may be helpful.
- Humidify the house.
- Avoid excessive contact with water.
- Avoid lotions that contain alcohol.
- If very resistant to treatment, search for a coexisting contact dermatitis.

Pediatric Considerations
Chronic potent fluorinated corticosteroid use may cause striae, hypopigmentation, or atrophy, especially in children.

MEDICATION

First Line

- Frequent systemic lubrication with thick emollient creams (e.g., Eucerin, Vaseline) over moist skin is the mainstay of treatment before any other intervention is considered. The "soak and seal" method is recommended.
- Infants and children: 0.5–1% topical hydrocortisone creams or ointments (Use the "fingertip unit [FTU]" dosing.)
- Adults: higher potency topical corticosteroids in areas other than face and skin folds
- Short-course, higher potency corticosteroids for flares; then, return to the lowest potency (creams preferred) that will control dermatitis.
- Antihistamines for pruritus (e.g., hydroxyzine 10 to 25 mg at bedtime and as needed)

Second Line

- Topical immunomodulators (tacrolimus or pimecrolimus) for episodic use for children >2 years. There is a black box warning from the FDA regarding potential cancer risk (no increased incidence noted over last 15 years of clinical use) (4).
- Plastic occlusion in combination with topical medication to promote absorption
- For severe AD, consider systemic steroids for 1 to 2 weeks (e.g., prednisone 2 mg/kg/day PO [max 80 mg/day] initially, tapered over 7 to 14 days)—should be used very infrequently, and most reserve oral steroids only in cases where immunotherapy is being considered (5).
- Topical tricyclic doxepin, as a 5% cream, may decrease pruritus.
- Modified Goeckerman regimen (tar and ultraviolet light)
- Topical antibiotics promptly at the first sign of secondary skin infection
- Dupilumab, a biologic that targets mediators of inflammation (IL-22, IL-17, IFN-γ), is FDA approved for moderate to severe atopic dermatitis in adults, adolescents 12–17 years of age. It has just recently completed Phase 3 trials for children 6–11 of age with significant reduction in symptoms and improved QOL. It is used in combination with topical corticosteroids (6).

ISSUES FOR REFERRAL

- Ophthalmology evaluation for persistent vernal conjunctivitis
- If using topical steroids around eyes for extended periods, ophthalmology follow-up for cataract evaluation
- For consideration of systemic immunotherapy (cyclosporine, azathioprine, methotrexate) in the most severe cases and when associated mental health affects QOL (5)

ADDITIONAL THERAPIES

- Methods to reduce house mite allergens (micropore filters on heating, ventilation, and air-conditioning systems; impermeable mattress covers)
- Behavioral relaxation therapy to reduce scratching

- Bleach baths may reduce staph colonization, but definitive evidence for benefit in the condition is lacking. Recommend 1/2 cup of standard 6% household bleach for a full tub of water and soak for 5 to 10 minutes, blotting skin dry upon leaving the bath.

COMPLEMENTARY & ALTERNATIVE MEDICINE

- Evening primrose oil (includes high content of fatty acids)
  - May decrease prostaglandin synthesis
  - May promote conversion of linoleic acid to omega-6 fatty acid
- Probiotics may reduce the severity of the condition, thus reducing medication use.

 ONGOING CARE

FOLLOW-UP RECOMMENDATIONS

Patient Monitoring

Evaluate to ensure that secondary bacterial or fungal infection does not develop as a result of disruption of the skin barrier. Most patients with AD are colonized by *Staphylococcus*. There is a little evidence for the routine use of antimicrobial interventions to reduce skin bacteria, but treatment of clinical infection with coverage for *Staphylococcus* is recommended.

DIET

- Trials of elimination may find certain "triggers" in some patients.
- Breastfeeding in conjunction with maternal hypoallergenic diets may decrease the severity in some infants (varying opinions).

PATIENT EDUCATION

- http://www.aad.org/skin-conditions/dermatology-a-to-z/atopic-dermatitis
- National Eczema Association: www.nationaleczema.org

PROGNOSIS

- Chronic disease
- Declines with increasing age
- 90% of pediatric patients have spontaneous resolution by puberty.
- Localized eczema (e.g., chronic hand or foot dermatitis, eyelid dermatitis, or lichen simplex chronicus) may continue in some adults.

COMPLICATIONS

- Cataracts are more common in patients with AD.
- Skin infections (usually *Staphylococcus aureus*); sometimes subclinical
- Eczema herpeticum
  - Generalized vesiculopustular eruption caused by infection with herpes simplex or vaccinia virus
  - Causes acute illness requiring hospitalization
- Atrophy and/or striae if fluorinated corticosteroids are used on face or skin folds
- Systemic absorption may occur if large areas of skin are treated, particularly if high-potency medications and occlusion are combined.

REFERENCES

1. Silverberg JI, Barbarot S, Gadkari A, et al. Atopic dermatitis in the pediatric population: a cross-sectional, international epidemiologic study. *Ann Allergy Asthma Immunol*. 2021;126(4):417–428.e2.
2. Lin HP, Chiang BL, Yu HH, et al. The influence of breastfeeding in breast-fed infants with atopic dermatitis. *J Microbiol Immunol Infect*. 2019;52(1):132–140.
3. Silverberg JL, Gelfand JM, Margolis DJ, et al. Patient burden and quality of life in atopic dermatitis in US adults: a population-based cross-sectional study. *Ann Allergy Asthma Immunol*. 2018;121(3):340–347.
4. Ohssuki M, Morimoto H, Nakagawa H. Tacrolimus ointment for the treatment of adult and pediatric atopic dermatitis: review on safety and benefits. *J Dermatol*. 2018;45(8):936–942.
5. Wollenberg A, Christen-Zäch S, Taieb A, et al. ETFAD/EADV Eczema Task Force 2020 position paper on diagnosis and treatment of atopic dermatitis in adults and children. *J Eur Acad Dermatol Venereol*. 2020;34(12):2717–2744.
6. Paller AS, Siegfried EC, Thaçi D, et al. Efficacy and safety of dupilumab with concomitant topical corticosteroids in children 6 to 11 years old with severe atopic dermatitis: a randomized, double-blinded, placebo-controlled phase 3 trial. *J Am Acad Dermatol*. 2020;83(5):1282–1293.

ADDITIONAL READING

Wei W, Anderson P, Gadkari A, et al. Extent and consequences of inadequate disease control among adults with a history of moderate to severe atopic dermatitis. *J Dermatol*. 2018;45(2):150–157.

 SEE ALSO

Algorithm: Rash

CODES

ICD10

- L20.9 Atopic dermatitis, unspecified
- L20.89 Other atopic dermatitis
- L20.83 Infantile (acute) (chronic) eczema

CLINICAL PEARLS

- Institute early and proactive treatment to reduce inflammation. Use the lowest potency topical steroid that controls symptoms.
- Monitor for secondary bacterial infection.
- Frequent systemic lubrication with thick emollient creams (e.g., Eucerin, Vaseline) over moist skin is the mainstay of treatment before any other intervention is considered.

DERMATITIS, CONTACT
Konstantinos E. Deligiannidis, MD, MPH, FAAFP

 BASICS

DESCRIPTION
- A cutaneous reaction to an external substance
- Each type has a different mechanism, whereas the clinical presentation is the same (1).
- Primary irritant dermatitis (ID) is a result of direct damage to the stratum corneum by chemicals or physical agents that occurs faster than the skin is able to repair itself, which results in an inflammatory nonimmunologic cutaneous reaction. Prior sensitization is not required (2). ID occurs immediately or within 48 hours of exposure.
- Allergic contact dermatitis (ACD) affects only individuals previously sensitized to a substance. It represents a delayed hypersensitivity reaction, requiring several hours or days for the cascade of cellular immunity to manifest itself (2).
- System(s) affected: skin/exocrine
- Synonym(s): dermatitis venenata

EPIDEMIOLOGY
Common

Incidence
Occupational contact dermatitis accounts for up to 70% of occupational skin disease occurrences and affects 20.5/100,000 workers per year in one Australian study.

Prevalence
- Florists, hairdressers, cooks, beauticians, and metal-working machine operators have the highest incidence.
- Predominant sex: male = female
  - Variations due to differences in exposure to offending agents as well as normal cutaneous variations between males and females (eccrine and sebaceous gland function and hair distribution)

Geriatric Considerations
Increased incidence of ID secondary to skin dryness

Pediatric Considerations
Increased incidence of positive patch testing due to better delayed hypersensitivity reactions (3)

ETIOLOGY AND PATHOPHYSIOLOGY
Hypersensitivity reaction to a substance generating cellular immunity response
- Plants
  - Urushiol (allergen): poison ivy, poison oak, poison sumac
  - Primary contact: plant (roots/stems/leaves)
  - Secondary contact: clothes/fingernails (not blister fluid—the established eruption is not itself contagious or transmissible)

- Chemicals
  - Nickel: jewelry, zippers, hooks, and watches (4)
  - Potassium dichromate: tanning agent in leather
  - Paraphenylenediamine: hair dyes, fur dyes, and industrial chemicals
  - Turpentine: cleaning agents, polishes, and waxes
  - Soaps and detergents
- Topical medicines
  - Neomycin: topical antibiotics
  - Thimerosal (Merthiolate): preservative in topical medications
  - Anesthetics: benzocaine
  - Parabens: preservative in topical medications
  - Formalin: cosmetics, shampoos, and nail enamel

Genetics
Increased frequency of ACD in families with allergies

RISK FACTORS
- Occupation
- Hobbies
- Travel
- Cosmetics
- Jewelry

GENERAL PREVENTION
- Avoid causative agents.
- Use of protective gloves (with cotton lining) may be helpful.

 DIAGNOSIS

HISTORY
- Itchy rash
- Assess for prior exposure to irritating substance.

PHYSICAL EXAM
- Acute
  - Papules, vesicles, bullae with surrounding erythema
  - Crusting and oozing
  - Pruritus
- Chronic
  - Erythematous base
  - Thickening with lichenification
  - Scaling
  - Fissuring
- Distribution
  - Where epidermis is thinner (eyelids, genitalia)
  - Areas of contact with offending agent (e.g., nail polish)
  - Palms and soles relatively more resistant, although hand dermatitis is common
  - Deeper skin folds spared
  - Linear arrays of lesions
  - Lesions with sharp borders and sharp angles are pathognomonic.
  - Well-demarcated area with a papulovesicular rash

DIFFERENTIAL DIAGNOSIS
- Based on clinical impression
  - Appearance, periodicity, and localization
- Groups of vesicles
  - Herpes simplex
- Diffuse bullous or vesicular lesions
  - Bullous pemphigoid
- Photodistribution
  - Phototoxic/allergic reaction to systemic allergen
- Eyelids
  - Seborrheic dermatitis
- Scaly eczematous lesions
  - Atopic dermatitis
  - Nummular eczema
  - Lichen simplex chronicus
  - Stasis dermatitis
  - Xerosis
- Id reaction (see separate chapter)

DIAGNOSTIC TESTS & INTERPRETATION
Diagnostic Procedures/Other
Consider patch tests for suspected allergic trigger (systemic corticosteroids or recent, aggressive use of topical steroids may alter results).

Test Interpretation
- Intercellular edema
- Bullae

 TREATMENT

GENERAL MEASURES
- Identify and remove offending agent (5)[C]:
  - Avoidance
  - Work modification
  - Protective clothing
  - Barrier creams, especially high-lipid content moisturizing creams (e.g., Keri lotion, petrolatum, coconut oil)
- Topical soaks with cool tap water, Burow solution (1:40 dilution), saline (1 tsp/pt water), or silver nitrate solution
- Lukewarm water baths
- Aveeno oatmeal baths
- Emollients (white petrolatum, Eucerin)

MEDICATION
First Line
- Topical medications (4)[A]
  - Lotion of zinc oxide, talc, menthol 0.15% (Gold Bond), phenol 0.5%
  - Corticosteroids for ACD as well as ID
    - High-potency steroids: fluocinonide (Lidex) 0.05% gel, cream, or ointment TID–QID
    - Use high-potency steroids only for a short time and then switch to low- or medium-potency steroid cream or ointment. Avoid long-term daily use (6)[C].
    - Caution regarding face/skin folds: Use lower potency steroids (4)[C] and avoid prolonged usage. Switch to lower potency topical steroid once the acute phase is resolved.

- Calamine lotion for symptomatic relief
- Topical antibiotics for secondary infection (bacitracin, erythromycin)
- Systemic
  - Antihistamine
    - Hydroxyzine: 25 to 50 mg PO QID, especially useful for itching
    - Diphenhydramine: 25 to 50 mg PO QID
    - Cetirizine: 10 mg PO BID–TID
- Corticosteroids
  - Prednisone: Taper starting at 60 to 80 mg/day PO, over 10 to 14 days, occasionally 21 days.
  - Used for moderate to severe cases, particularly involving face or genitals
  - Little published evidence to compare appropriate length of treatment, but clinical experience suggests that short courses of therapy (i.e., 5 to 7 days) are not adequate to prevent rebound dermatitis.
  - Treatment for up to 21 days for severe/extensive rash resulting from exposure to potent allergens like urushiol (e.g., poison ivy) is commonly recommended to prevent reemergence of dermatitis upon taper (rebound), although 14 days is usually adequate.
  - May use burst dose of steroids for up to 5 days for less persistent immunogens or less severe dermatitis
- Antibiotics for secondary skin infections
  - Dicloxacillin: 250 to 500 mg PO QID for 7 to 10 days
  - Amoxicillin-clavulanate (Augmentin): 500 mg PO BID for 7 to 10 days
  - Erythromycin: 250 mg PO QID in penicillin-allergic patients
  - Trimethoprim-sulfamethoxazole (Bactrim DS): 160 mg/800 mg (1 tablet) PO BID for 7 to 10 days (suspected resistant *Staphylococcus aureus*)
- Precautions
  - Antihistamines may cause drowsiness.
  - Prolonged use of potent topical steroids may cause local skin effects (atrophy, stria, telangiectasia).
  - Use tapering dose of oral steroids if using >5 days.

Second Line
Other topical or systemic antibiotics, depending on organisms and sensitivity

Pregnancy Considerations
Usual caution with medications

ISSUES FOR REFERRAL
May need referral to a dermatologist or allergist if refractory to conventional treatment

COMPLEMENTARY & ALTERNATIVE MEDICINE
The use of complementary and alternative treatment is a supplement and not an alternative to conventional treatment.

ADMISSION, INPATIENT, AND NURSING CONSIDERATIONS
Rarely needs hospital admission

 ONGOING CARE

FOLLOW-UP RECOMMENDATIONS
Stay active, but avoid overheating.

Patient Monitoring
- As necessary for recurrence
- Patch testing for etiology after resolved

DIET
No special diet

PATIENT EDUCATION
- Avoidance of irritating substance
- Cleaning of secondary sources (nails, clothes)
- Fallacy of blister fluid spreading disease

PROGNOSIS
- Self-limited
- Benign
- 55% of patients still had contact dermatitis at 2 years after diagnosis.
- Improvement in rash less likely for those who remain in the same or similar profession
- Increased length of exposure and atopy are poor prognostic indicators.

COMPLICATIONS
- Generalized eruption secondary to autosensitization
- Secondary bacterial infection

REFERENCES
1. Sultan TA, Hatem AMA. Management of contact dermatitis. *J Dermatol Dermatol Surg.* 2015;19(2):86–91.
2. Tan CH, Rasool S, Johnston GA. Contact dermatitis: allergic and irritant. *Clin Dermatol.* 2014;32(1):116–124.
3. Admani S, Jacob SE. Allergic contact dermatitis in children: review of the past decade. *Curr Allergy Asthma Rep.* 2014;14(4):421.
4. Usatine RP, Riojas M. Diagnosis and management of contact dermatitis. *Am Fam Physician.* 2010;82(3):249–255.
5. Fonacier L, Bernstein DI, Pacheco K, et al. Contact dermatitis: a practice parameter—update 2015. *J Allergy Clin Immunol Pract.* 2015;3(3 Suppl): S1–S39. doi:10.1016/j.jaip.2015.02.009.
6. Nassau S, Fonacier L. Allergic contact dermatitis. *Med Clin North Am.* 2020;104(1):61–76.

ADDITIONAL READING
- Martin SF. Contact dermatitis: from pathomechanisms to immunotoxicology. *Exp Dermatol.* 2012;21(5):382–389.
- Pelletier JL, Perez C, Jacob SE. Contact dermatitis in pediatrics. *Pediatr Ann.* 2016;45(8):e287–e292.
- Rashid RS, Shim TN. Contact dermatitis. *BMJ.* 2016;353:i3299.

 SEE ALSO

Algorithm: Rash

 CODES

ICD10
- L25.9 Unspecified contact dermatitis, unspecified cause
- L23.9 Allergic contact dermatitis, unspecified cause
- L25.5 Unspecified contact dermatitis due to plants, except food

CLINICAL PEARLS
- Commonly occurs on hands and face
- Anyone exposed to irritants or allergic substances is predisposed to contact dermatitis, especially in occupations that have high exposure to chemicals.
- The most common allergens causing contact dermatitis are plants of the *Toxicodendron* genus (poison ivy, poison oak, poison sumac).
- Poison-ivy dermatitis typically requires 10 to 14 days (occasionally more) of topical or oral steroid therapy to prevent recurrent eruption.
- Worldwide, nickel is the number one patch-tested allergen causing ACD.
- The usual treatment for contact dermatitis is avoidance of the allergen or irritating substance and temporary use of topical steroids.
- A contact dermatitis eruption presents in a nondermatomal geographic fashion due to the skin being in contact with an external source.

D

DERMATITIS, DIAPER
Dennis E. Hughes, DO, FACEP

 BASICS

DESCRIPTION
- Diaper dermatitis is a rash occurring under the covered area of a diaper (named for typical location, not etiology). It is usually initially a contact irritant dermatitis but can be caused by or contributed to by systemic conditions.
- System(s) affected: skin/exocrine
- Synonym(s): diaper rash; nappy rash; napkin dermatitis

Geriatric Considerations
Incontinence is a significant cofactor in the elderly population.

EPIDEMIOLOGY
Incidence
- The most common dermatitis found in infancy
- Peak incidence: 7 to 12 months of age, then decreases
- Lower incidence reported in breastfed babies due to lower pH, urease, protease, and lipase activity

Prevalence
Prevalence has been variably reported from 4% to 35% in the first 2 years of life. Upward of 75% of infants will have episodes of varying duration and severity in United States. Severity varies: 58% slight symptoms; 34% moderate; 8% severe. Underreporting contributes to difficulty in determining impact of condition (1).

ETIOLOGY AND PATHOPHYSIOLOGY
- Immature infant skin with histologic, biochemical, functional differences compared to mature skin (2)
- Wet skin is central in the development of diaper dermatitis, as prolonged contact with urine or feces results in susceptibility to chemical, enzymatic, and physical injury; wet skin is also penetrated more easily.
- Fecal proteases and lipases are irritants.
- Superhydrase urease enzyme found in the stratum corneum liberates ammonia from cutaneous bacteria.
- Fecal lipase and protease activity is increased by acceleration of GI transit; thus, a higher incidence of irritant diaper dermatitis is observed in babies who have had diarrhea in the previous 48 hours.

- Once the skin is compromised, secondary infection by *Candida albicans* is common. 40–75% of diaper rashes that last >3 days are colonized with *C. albicans*.
- Bacteria may play a role in diaper dermatitis through reduction of fecal pH and resulting activation of enzymes.
- Allergy is exceedingly rare as a cause in infants.

RISK FACTORS
- Infrequent diaper changes
- Improper laundering (cloth diapers)
- Family history of dermatitis
- Hot, humid weather
- Recent treatment with oral antibiotics
- Diarrhea (>3 stools per day increases risk)
- Dye allergy
- Eczema may increase risk.

GENERAL PREVENTION
Most effectively managed by prevention including rigorous attention to hygiene

COMMONLY ASSOCIATED CONDITIONS
- Contact (allergic or irritant) dermatitis
- Seborrheic dermatitis
- Psoriasis
- Candidiasis
- Atopic dermatitis

 DIAGNOSIS

Correct diagnosis is key. Ensure that no stigmata of systemic conditions exist. The initial presentation of diseases other than contact irritant dermatitis may be in the diaper area. Avoid assuming that all diaper-area dermatitis is simple contact/irritant dermatitis by performing an appropriate general skin examination (3).

HISTORY
- Onset, duration, and change in the nature of the rash
- Presence of rashes outside the diaper area
- Associated scratching or crying
- Contact with infants with a similar rash
- Recent illness, diarrhea, or antibiotic use
- Fever
- Pustular drainage
- Lymphangitis

PHYSICAL EXAM
- Mild forms consist of shiny erythema ± scale.
- Margins are not always evident.
- Moderate cases have areas of papules, vesicles, and small superficial erosions.
- It can progress to well-demarcated ulcerated nodules that measure ≥1 cm in diameter.
- It is found on the prominent parts of the buttocks, medial thighs, mons pubis, and scrotum.
- Skin folds are spared or involved last.
- *Tidemark dermatitis* refers to the bandlike form of erythema of irritated diaper margins.
- Diaper dermatitis can cause an id reaction (autoeczematous) outside the diaper area.

DIFFERENTIAL DIAGNOSIS
- Contact dermatitis
- Seborrheic dermatitis
- Candidiasis
- Atopic dermatitis
- Scabies
- Acrodermatitis enteropathica (deficiency in zinc)
- Letterer-Siwe disease
- Congenital syphilis
- Child abuse
- Streptococcal/staphylococcal infection
- Kawasaki disease
- Biotin deficiency
- Psoriasis
- HIV infection

DIAGNOSTIC TESTS & INTERPRETATION
Initial Tests (lab, imaging)
Rarely needed

Follow-Up Tests & Special Considerations
- Consider a culture of lesions or a potassium hydroxide (KOH) preparation.
- The finding of anemia in association with hepatosplenomegaly and the appropriate rash may suggest a diagnosis of Langerhans cell histiocytosis or congenital syphilis.
- Finding mites, ova, or feces on a mineral oil preparation of a burrow scraping can confirm the diagnosis of scabies.

Test Interpretation
- Biopsy is rare.
- Histology may reveal acute, subacute, or chronic spongiotic dermatitis.

TREATMENT

Prevention is the key to treatment of this condition.

GENERAL MEASURES

- Expose the buttocks to air as much as possible.
- Use mild, slightly acidic or neutral pH cleanser with water; no rubbing and pat dry.
- Avoid impermeable waterproof pants during treatment (day or night); they keep the skin wet and subject to rash or infection.
- Change diapers frequently, even at night, if the rash is extensive.
- Super-absorbable diapers are beneficial, as they wick urine away from skin and still allow air to permeate. Manufacturer-associated data indicates diapers with a mesh-like top sheet construction may be superior in allowing stool to separate from skin.
- Discontinue using baby lotion, powder, ointment, or baby oil (except zinc oxide).
- Use of appropriately formulated baby wipes (alcohol free and fragrance free) is safe and as effective as water. Those baby wipes commercially marketed as safe for sensitive skin appear to be generally equally effective (4).
- Apply zinc oxide ointment or other barrier cream to the rash at the earliest sign and BID or TID (e.g., Desitin or Balmex). Thereafter, apply to clean, thoroughly dried skin.
- Cornstarch can reduce friction. Avoid talcum-containing products.

MEDICATION

First Line

- For a pure contact dermatitis, a low-potency topical steroid (hydrocortisone 0.5–1% TID for 3 to 5 days) and removal of the offending agent (urine, feces) should suffice.
- If candidiasis is suspected or diaper rash persists, use an antifungal such as miconazole nitrate 2% cream, miconazole powder, econazole (Spectazole), clotrimazole (Lotrimin), or ketoconazole (Nizoral) cream at each diaper change. Candida superinfection is common in persistent dermatitis in the moist diaper area.
- If inflammation is prominent, consider a very low-potency steroid cream such as hydrocortisone 0.5–1% TID along with an antifungal cream ± a combination product such as clioquinol–hydrocortisone (Vioform–Hydrocortisone) cream.
- If a secondary bacterial infection is suspected, use an antistaphylococcal oral antibiotic or mupirocin (Bactroban) ointment topically.

- Precautions: Avoid high- or moderate-potency steroids often found in combination of steroid antifungal mixtures—these should never be used in the diaper area.

Second Line

- Sucralfate paste for resistant cases
- Recent study suggests that use of hydrocolloid dressings can speed healing of rash.
- Case reports support the use of immune modulators such as topical tacrolimus (0.03%) in refractory cases; however, it is not approved for children <2 year of age. Recent literature review by American Academy of Allergy and American College of Allergy found no findings to suggest harm (5).

ISSUES FOR REFERRAL

Consider if a systemic disease such as Langerhans cell histiocytosis, acrodermatitis enteropathica, or HIV infection is suspected.

ADMISSION, INPATIENT, AND NURSING CONSIDERATIONS

- Admission criteria/initial stabilization
  - Febrile neonates
  - Recalcitrant rash suggestive of immunodeficiency
  - Toxic-appearing infants
- Assist first-time parents with hygiene education.

 ONGOING CARE

FOLLOW-UP RECOMMENDATIONS

Patient Monitoring

Recheck weekly until clear, then at times of recurrence.

PATIENT EDUCATION

Patient education is vital to the treatment and prevention of recurrent cases.

PROGNOSIS

- Quick, complete clearing with appropriate treatment
- Secondary candidal infections may last a few weeks after treatment has begun.

COMPLICATIONS

- Secondary bacterial infection (Consider community-acquired methicillin-resistant *Staphylococcus aureus* [MRSA] in pustular dermatitis that does not respond to normal therapy.)
- Rare complication is inoculation with group A β-hemolytic *Streptococcus* resulting in necrotizing fasciitis.
- Secondary yeast infection

REFERENCES

1. Blume-Peytavi U, Kanti V. Prevention and treatment of diaper dermatitis. *Pediatr Dermatol*. 2018;35 Suppl 1:s19–s23.
2. Burdall O, Willgress L, Goad N. Neonatal skin care: Developments in care to maintain neonatal barrier function and prevention of irritant diaper dermatitis. *Pediatr Dermatol*. 2019;36(1):31–35.
3. Lebsing S, Chaiyarit J, Techasatian L. Diaper rashes can indicate systemic conditions other than diaper dermatitis. *BMC Dermatol*. 2020;20(1):7.
4. Price AD, Lythgoe J, Ackers-Johnson J, et al. The BaSICS (Baby Skin Integrity Comparison Survey) study: a prospective experimental study using maternal observations to report the effect of baby wipes on the incidence of diaper dermatitis in infants, from birth to eight weeks of age. *Pediatr Neonatol*. 2021;62(2):138–145.
5. Leung AKC, Leong KF, Lam JM. Successful treatment of recalcitrant granuloma gluteale infantum with topical tacrolimus 0.03% ointment. *Case Rep Pediatr*. 2021;2021:9994067.

ADDITIONAL READING

Madhu R, Vijayabhaskar C, Anandan V, et al. Indian Academy of Pediatrics Guidelines for Pediatric Skin Care. *Indian Pediatr*. 2021;58(2):153–161.

 SEE ALSO

Algorithm: Rash

 CODES

ICD10

- L22 Diaper dermatitis
- B37.2 Candidiasis of skin and nail

CLINICAL PEARLS

- Hygiene is the main preventative measure.
- Look for secondary infection in persistent cases (*Candida*, *Staphylococcus* spp).

DERMATITIS, SEBORRHEIC

Dellyse Bright, MD • Darin N. Kennedy, MD

BASICS

DESCRIPTION
Chronic, superficial, recurrent inflammatory skin disorder affecting sebum-rich, hairy regions of the body, especially the scalp, eyebrows, and face and to lesser extent, chest, and back

EPIDEMIOLOGY
Incidence
- Predominant age: infancy (1), adolescence (2), and adulthood
- Predominant sex: male > female

Prevalence
- Seborrheic dermatitis: 1–3%; in immunosuppressed individuals up to 83% (2)
- Infantile seborrheic dermatitis: up to 71% in the first 3 months of life, all ethnicities, all climates (1)

ETIOLOGY AND PATHOPHYSIOLOGY
- Skin surface yeast such as *Malassezia* may be a contributing factor (3).
- Genetic and environmental factors: Flares are common with stress/illness.
- Parallels increased sebaceous gland activity in infancy and adolescence or as a result of some acnegenic drugs.
- Seborrheic dermatitis is more common in immunosuppressed patients, suggesting that immune mechanisms are implicated in the pathogenesis of the disease, although the mechanisms are not well defined (3).

Genetics
Positive family history; no genetic markers have been identified to date.

RISK FACTORS
- Immunosuppressed conditions such as AIDS, lymphoma, organ transplantation (2),(4)
- Parkinson disease, epilepsy, traumatic brain, and spinal cord injury (4)
- Emotional stress (2)
- Obesity (2)
- Oily skin (2)
- Acne (2)
- Medications may cause flares/induce seborrheic dermatitis: buspirone, chlorpromazine, cimetidine, ethionamide, griseofulvin, haloperidol, interferon-α, methyldopa, psoralen, IL-2 (2)

GENERAL PREVENTION
Seborrheic skin should be washed more often than usual to soften the affected areas.

COMMONLY ASSOCIATED CONDITIONS
- Parkinson disease
- AIDS

DIAGNOSIS

Diagnosis of seborrheic dermatitis is usually made by history and physical exam. If unclear, a punch biopsy of the skin will confirm the diagnosis.

HISTORY
- Intermittent active phases manifest with burning, scaling, and itching, alternating with inactive periods; activity is increased in winter and early spring, with remissions commonly occurring in summer.
- Infants (1)
  - Cradle cap: greasy scaling of the scalp with occasional erythema
  - Diaper and/or axillary rash
  - Age of onset: ~1 month
  - Usually self-resolves by 8 to 12 months
- Adults
  - Red, greasy, scaling rash consisting of macules and plaques with indistinct margins
  - Red, smooth, glazed appearance in skin folds
  - Hypopigmented, scaling macules on skin of color (5)
  - Minimal pruritus
  - Chronic waxing and waning course
  - Bilateral and symmetric
  - Most commonly located in hairy skin areas: scalp and scalp margins, eyebrows and eyelid margins, nasolabial folds, ears and retroauricular folds, presternal area, middle to upper back, buttock crease, inguinal area, genitals, and armpits

PHYSICAL EXAM
- Scalp appearance varies from mild, patchy scaling to widespread, thick, adherent crusts. Plaques are rare.
- Seborrheic dermatitis can spread onto the forehead, the posterior part of the neck, and the postauricular skin, as in psoriasis.
- Skin lesions manifest as brawny or yellow greasy scaling over red, inflamed skin.
- Hypopigmentation can be seen in skin tones of color.
- Infectious eczematoid dermatitis, with oozing and crusting, suggests secondary infection.
- Seborrheic blepharitis may occur independently.

DIFFERENTIAL DIAGNOSIS
- Atopic dermatitis: Distinction may be difficult in infants.
- Psoriasis
  - More common on the extensor surfaces of the knees, elbows, and the nail beds are usually involved.
  - Scalp psoriasis will be more sharply demarcated than seborrheic dermatitis with crusted, infiltrated plaques rather than mild scaling and erythema.
- Candida
- Tinea cruris/capitis: Suspect these when usual medications fail or hair loss occurs.

- Eczema of auricle/otitis externa
- Rosacea
- Discoid lupus erythematosus: Skin biopsy will be beneficial.
- Histiocytosis X: may appear as seborrheic-like eruption
- Dandruff: scalp only, noninflammatory
- Drug eruption

DIAGNOSTIC TESTS & INTERPRETATION
Diagnostic Procedures/Other
- Consider biopsy if:
  - Usual therapies fail.
  - Petechiae are noted.
  - Histiocytosis X is suspected.
- Consider fungal cultures if:
  - Refractory to treatment
  - Pustules and alopecia are present.

Test Interpretation
Nonspecific changes

- Hyperkeratosis, acanthosis, accentuated rete ridges, focal spongiosis, and parakeratosis are characteristic.
- Parakeratotic scale around hair follicles and mild superficial inflammatory lymphocytic infiltrate

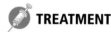

TREATMENT

GENERAL MEASURES
- Increase frequency of shampooing.
- Sunlight in moderate doses may be helpful.
- Infants (cradle cap)
  - As above, increasing frequency of shampooing with a mild, nonmedicated shampoo may help.
  - Remove thick scale by applying warm mineral oil and then wash off 1 hour later with a mild soap and a soft-bristle toothbrush or terrycloth washcloth.
- Adults
  - Wash all affected areas with antiseborrheic shampoos. Start with over-the-counter products (i.e., selenium sulfide), allowing shampoo/lotion to remain on the skin for several minutes before washing off, and increase to more potent preparations (those containing coal tar, sulfur, or salicylic acid) if no improvement is noted.
  - For dense scalp scaling, 10% liquor carbonic detergents in Nivea oil may be used at bedtime, covering the head with a shower cap. This should be done nightly for 1 to 3 weeks.

MEDICATION

First Line

- Cradle cap: Use a coal tar shampoo or ketoconazole shampoo if the nonmedicated shampoo is ineffective. Massage in and allow to remain on for several minutes before removing.
- Adults
  - Topical antifungal agents
    - Ketoconazole 2% or miconazole 2% shampoo twice a week (allow to remain on scalp for several minutes before washing off) for clearance and then once a week or every other week for maintenance (2),(3)
    - Ketoconazole 2% or sertaconazole 2% cream may be used to clear scales in other areas (2).
    - Ciclopirox 1% shampoo twice weekly (2),(3)
    - Facial hair can also be treated with ketoconazole 2% shampoo (3).
  - Topical corticosteroids
    - Begin with 1% hydrocortisone and advance to more potent (fluorinated) steroid preparations daily for 2 to 4 weeks (3).
      - Avoid continuous use of potent steroids to reduce the risk of skin atrophy, hypopigmentation, and/or systemic absorption (especially in infants, children and elderly).
      - Precautions: Fluorinated corticosteroids and higher concentrations of hydrocortisone (e.g., 2.5%) may cause atrophy or striae if used on the face or on skin folds.
  - Other topical agents
    - Coal tar 1% shampoo twice a week
    - Selenium sulfide 2.5% shampoo twice a week
    - Zinc pyrithione 1% shampoo twice a week
    - Lithium gluconate/succinate 8% ointment/gel twice a week (6)
- Once controlled, washing with zinc soaps or selenium lotion with periodic use of steroid cream may help to maintain remission.

Second Line

- Calcineurin inhibitors (3),(6)[A] (Not linked to skin atrophy and hypopigmentation. Just as effective as topical steroids; potentially more side effects)
  - Pimecrolimus 1% cream BID (6)
  - Tacrolimus 0.1% ointment (6)
- Systemic antifungal therapy
  - For severe or recalcitrant seborrheic dermatitis (3),(4)
    - Itraconazole: 200 mg/day, effective with good safety profile (3),(4)
    - Ketoconazole: 200 mg/day, associated with more relapses (4)
    - Terbinafine: 250 mg/day × 4 to 6 weeks or pulse therapy 250 mg/day × 12 days/month for 3 months (4)
    - Daily regimen for 1 to 2 months followed by twice-weekly dosing for chronic maintenance treatment
    - Monitor potential hepatotoxic effects.
- Low-molecular-weight hyaluronic acid
  - Hyaluronic acid sodium salt gel 0.2% BID

ISSUES FOR REFERRAL

- No response to first-line therapy and concerns regarding systemic illness (e.g., HIV)
- Resistant SD in adults should prompt testing for HIV.

COMPLEMENTARY & ALTERNATIVE MEDICINE

- Honey, antifungal, antioxidant, and antibacterial: effective in remission of and prevention of relapses of SD (3)
- Aloe vera, anti-inflammatory and antifungal: reduction in pruritus and scaling associated with SD (3)
- Borage oil containing essential amino acid gamma-lineolic acid (GLA): may be effective in infantile SD (3)
- Tea-tree essential oil, antifungal, anti-inflammatory, and antioxidant: effective in mild to moderate cases (3)
- Quassia Amara extract, anti-inflammatory and antifungal, especially against *Malassezia* yeast: outperformed topical 2% ketoconazole and 1% ciclopiroxolamine (3)

 ONGOING CARE

Individuals with coiled hair or hair that is heat and/or chemically treated will need less drying agents to prevent hair breakage compared to those with straighter hair who may prefer drying agents. Applying shampoos and other topical treatments directly to scalp instead of hair shaft can decrease risk of hair damage (5).

FOLLOW-UP RECOMMENDATIONS

Patient Monitoring

Every 2 to 12 weeks depending on the disease severity and the patient's response to therapy

PATIENT EDUCATION

http://familydoctor.org/familydoctor/en/diseases-conditions/seborrheic-dermatitis.html

PROGNOSIS

- In infants, seborrheic dermatitis usually remits after 6 to 8 months.
- In adults, seborrheic dermatitis is usually chronic and relapsing, with exacerbations and remissions. Disease is usually controlled with shampoos and topical steroids.
- Erythema or hypopigmentation typically resolves with treatment (5).

COMPLICATIONS

- Skin atrophy/striae are possible from fluorinated corticosteroids, especially if used on the face.
- Glaucoma and/or cataracts can result from use of fluorinated steroids around the eyes.
- Photosensitivity is caused occasionally by tar-containing products.
- Herpes keratitis is a rare complication of herpes simplex: Instruct patient to stop eyelid steroids if herpes simplex develops.

REFERENCES

1. Victoire A, Magin P, Coughlan J, et al. Interventions for infantile seborrhoeic dermatitis (including cradle cap). *Cochrane Database Syst Rev.* 2019;3(3):CD011380.
2. Okokon EO, Verbeek JH, Ruotsalainen JH, et al. Topical antifungals for seborrhoeic dermatitis. *Cochrane Database Syst Rev.* 2015;(5):CD008138.
3. Borda L, Perper M, Keri JE. Treatment of seborrheic dermatitis: a comprehensive review. *J Dermatolog Treat.* 2019;30(2):158–169.
4. Gupta AK, Richardson M, Paquet M. Systematic review of oral treatments for seborrheic dermatitis. *J Eur Acad Dermatol Venereol.* 2014;28(1):16–26.
5. Elgash M, Dlova N, Ogunleye T, et al. Seborrheic dermatitis in skin of color: clinical considerations. *J Drugs Dermatol.* 2019;18(1):24–27.
6. Kastarinen H, Oksanen T, Okokon EO, et al. Topical anti-inflammatory agents for seborrhoeic dermatitis of the face or scalp. *Cochrane Database Syst Rev.* 2014;2014(5):CD009446.

ADDITIONAL READING

- Borda LJ, Wikramanayake TC. Seborrheic dermatitis and dandruff: a comprehensive review. *J Clin Investig Dermatol.* 2015;3(2):10.13188/2373-1044.1000019.
- Clark GW, Pope SM, Jaboori KA. Diagnosis and treatment of seborrheic dermatitis. *Am Fam Physician.* 2015;91(3):185–190.
- Dessinioti C, Katsambas A. Seborrheic dermatitis: etiology, risk factors, and treatments: facts and controversies. *Clin Dermatol.* 2013;31(4):343–351.
- Hay RJ. *Malassezia*, dandruff and seborrhoeic dermatitis: an overview. *Br J Dermatol.* 2011;165(Suppl 2):2–8.
- Kim GK, Del Rosso J. Topical pimecrolimus 1% cream in the treatment of seborrheic dermatitis. *J Clin Aesthet Dermatol.* 2013;6(2):29–35.

 SEE ALSO

Algorithm: Rash

 CODES

ICD10

- L21.9 Seborrheic dermatitis, unspecified
- L21.1 Seborrheic infantile dermatitis
- L21.0 Seborrhea capitis

CLINICAL PEARLS

- Search for an underlying systemic disease in a patient who is unresponsive to usual therapy.
- In infants, seborrheic dermatitis is usually self-limited.
- In adults, seborrheic dermatitis is usually chronic, with exacerbations and remissions. Disease is usually easily controlled with shampoos and topical steroids.

DERMATITIS, STASIS

Joseph A. Florence, MD • Fereshteh Gerayli, MD, FAAFP

BASICS

DESCRIPTION
- Chronic, eczematous, erythema, scaling, and noninflammatory edema of the lower extremities accompanied by cycle of scratching, excoriations, weeping, crusting, and inflammation in patients with chronic venous insufficiency (CVI), due to impaired circulation and other factors (nutritional edema)
- Clinical skin manifestation of CVI usually appears late in the disease.
- May present as a solitary lesion; can be associated with venous leg ulcer, which is located on the medial or lateral side of the ankle
- System(s) affected: skin/exocrine
- Synonym(s): gravitational eczema; varicose eczema; venous dermatitis

EPIDEMIOLOGY
Incidence
- In the United States: common in patients age >50 years (6–7%)
- Predominant age: adult, geriatric
- Predominant sex: female > male

Geriatric Considerations
Common in this age group:
- Estimated to affect 15 to 20 million patients age >50 years in the United States

ETIOLOGY AND PATHOPHYSIOLOGY
- Incompetence of perforating veins, superficial venous thrombosis from varicose veins, and deep vein thrombosis (DVT) can each contribute to CVI leading to venous hypertension (HTN) and cutaneous inflammation. This can be a pathway to venous leg ulcer.
- Deposition of fibrin around capillaries
- Microvascular abnormalities
- Ischemia
- Continuous presence of edema in ankles, usually present because of venous valve incompetency (varicose veins)
- Weakness of venous walls in lower extremities
- Trauma to edematous, eczematized skin
- Itch may be caused by inflammatory mediators (from mast cells, monocytes, macrophages, or neutrophils) liberated in the microcirculation and endothelium.
- Abnormal leukocyte–endothelium interaction is proposed to be a major factor.
- A cascade of biochemical events leads to ulceration.

Genetics
Familial link probable

RISK FACTORS
- Atopy
- Chronic edema
- Old age
- Obesity
- Previous DVT
- Previous pregnancy
- Prolonged standing
- Secondary infection
- Superimposition of itch–scratch cycle
- Trauma
- Low-protein diet

- Genetic propensity
- Tight garments that constrict the thigh
- Vein stripping
- Vein harvesting for coronary artery bypass graft surgery
- Previous cellulitis

GENERAL PREVENTION
- Use compression stockings to avoid recurrence of edema and to mobilize the interstitial lymphatic fluid from the region of stasis dermatitis and also following DVT.
- Topical lubricants twice a day to prevent fissuring and itching

COMMONLY ASSOCIATED CONDITIONS
- Varicose veins
- Venous insufficiency
- Other eczematous disease
- Hyperhomocysteinemia
- Venous HTN

DIAGNOSIS

HISTORY
- Itching, pain, and burning may precede skin signs, which are aggravated during evening hours.
- Insidious onset
- Usually bilateral
- Description may include aching/heavy legs.
- Erythema, scaling, edema of lower extremities
- Noninflammatory edema preceded the skin eruption and ulceration.
- Edema initially develops around the ankle.

PHYSICAL EXAM
- Evaluation of the lower extremities characteristically reveals:
  - Bilateral scaly, eczematous patches, papules, and/or plaques
  - Violaceous (sometimes brown), erythematous lesions due to deoxygenation of venous blood (postinflammatory hyperpigmentation and hemosiderin deposition within the cutaneous tissue)
- Distribution: medial aspect of ankle, with frequent extension onto the foot and lower leg, occasionally lateral side of ankle
- Brawny induration
- Stasis ulcers (frequently accompany stasis dermatitis) secondary to minor trauma
- Excoriations
- Weeping, crusting, inflammation of the skin
- Varicosities are often associated with ulcers.
- Clinical inspection reveals swelling and warmth.
- Skin changes are more common in the lower 1/3 of the extremity and medially.
- Early signs include prominent superficial veins and pitting ankle edema.
- May present as a solitary lesion mimicking a neoplasm

DIFFERENTIAL DIAGNOSIS
- Other eczematous diseases:
  - Atopic dermatitis
  - Uremic dermatitis
  - Contact dermatitis (due to topical agents used to self-treat)

- Neurodermatitis
- Arterial insufficiency
- Sickle cell disease causing skin ulceration
- Cellulitis
- Erysipelas
- Tinea dermatophyte infection
- Pretibial myxedema
- Nummular eczema
- Lichen simplex chronicus
- Xerosis
- Asteatotic eczema
- Amyopathic dermatomyositis

DIAGNOSTIC TESTS & INTERPRETATION
Initial Tests (lab, imaging)
Duplex ultrasound imaging is helpful in diagnosis.

Diagnostic Procedures/Other
- Rule out arterial insufficiency. Check peripheral pulses; ankle brachial pressure index (ABPI or ABI)
- Check for diabetes.

Test Interpretation
- ABPI <0.8 is suggestive of arterial insufficiency.
- ABPI can be elevated, >1.2 in diabetic patients and others with distal small vessel calcifications.
- Arterial duplex ultrasound and angiography are the gold standards.

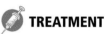TREATMENT

GENERAL MEASURES
Primary role of treatment is to reverse effects of venous HTN. Appropriate health care:
- Outpatient:
  - Reduce edema:
    ○ Leg elevation: legs above the level of heart for 30 minutes, 3 to 4 times daily. Avoid prolonged dependent position.
    ○ Compression therapy: This is the mainstay of treatment of venous stasis ± ulcers. Compression bandages can be safely applied in patients with ABI of 0.8 to 1.2.
    ○ Elastic bandage wraps: Ace bandages or Unna paste boot (zinc gelatin) or compression stockings
    ○ Graduated elastic compression of 30 to 40 mm Hg at the ankle improves ulcer healing rate and may prevent ulcer recurrence (1)[A].
    ○ Compression bandages containing both elastic and inelastic components (mixed component systems) are as effective as four-layer bandages, are easier to apply, and have less slippage and associated with favorable quality of life outcomes.
    ○ High compression is contraindicated in arterial insufficiency.
    ○ Pneumatic compression devices are beneficial, especially in nonambulatory patients and those with a component of arterial insufficiency (2)[B].
- Improvement of lipodermatosclerosis:
  - Activity:
    ○ Avoid standing still.
    ○ Stay active and exercise regularly.
    ○ Elevate foot of bed unless contraindicated.

- Inpatient, for endovascular radiofrequency ablation, vein stripping, sclerotherapy, or skin grafts:
  - Venous ulcer treatment: Treat infection: Débride the ulcer base of necrotic tissue (surgical necrotomy if possible, or enzymatic débridement with collagenase).
    - Autolytic: Modern wound dressings (hydrogel, hydrocolloids, alginate, foam bandages, plain nonadherent dressing) are better than traditional wet to dry dressing because they maintain moist wound environment, with less tissue damage on removal, and less frequent changing requirement (2)[A]. However, there is no difference in healing rate of venous stasis ulcers by use of hydrocolloid dressing versus simple nonadherent dressing when used beneath compression.
    - Biologic: Topical application of granulocyte-macrophage colony-stimulating factor promotes healing of ulcers (insufficient evidence).
    - Mechanical: wet to dry dressings, hydrotherapy, and irrigation
    - Surgical: modifying cause of venous HTN (by venous ligation, valvuloplasty, and endoscopic perforator vein surgery); treat ulcer by graft.

MEDICATION

First Line
- Pentoxifylline 400 mg TID is effective in treating venous leg ulcer.
- The use of low-dose aspirin because adjuvant treatment for venous leg ulcers is not supported (3)[A].
- In light of increasing bacterial resistance to antibiotics, current guidelines recommend the use of antibacterial preparations only for clinical infection (cellulitis, increased pain, warmth, malodorous exudate), not for bacterial colonization (4)[A].
- If secondary infection, treat with PO antibiotics for *Staphylococcus* or *Streptococcus* organisms (e.g., dicloxacillin 250 mg QID, cephalexin 500 mg BID, or levofloxacin 500 mg daily).
- If MRSA suspected, clindamycin 300 mg QID, doxycycline 100 mg BID, TMP/SMX or IV vancomycin
- There is no reliable evidence in the effectiveness of topical antiseptics such as povidone-iodine, peroxide-based preparations, mupirocin, chlorhexidine (4)[A].
- Uncomplicated stasis dermatitis can be treated with short courses (about 2 weeks) of topical steroids (2)[B] (topical triamcinolone 0.1% cream/ointment BID).
- Topical antipruritic: pramoxine, camphor, menthol, and doxepin
- Topical anesthetic (lidocaine/prilocaine) may reduce pain during débridement.
- Systemic steroids for severe cases
- Silver sulfadiazine (SSD) has a positive effect in wound healing (2)[A].

Second Line
- Consider antibiotics on basis of culture results of exudate from infected ulcer craters.
- Lubricants when dermatitis is quiescent
- Chronic stasis dermatitis can be treated with topical emollients (e.g., white petroleum, lanolin).
- Antipruritic medications (e.g., diphenhydramine, cetirizine hydrochloride)
- Hydrocolloid or a foam dressing may reduce ulcer pain; no evidence that ibuprofen dressings offer pain relief

ISSUES FOR REFERRAL
Consider referral for:
- Nonhealing ulcer
- Arterial insufficiency
- Uncertain diagnosis
- Rheumatoid arthritis
- Patch testing to evaluate for contact dermatitis
- Associated disease (e.g., symptomatic varicose veins)

ADDITIONAL THERAPIES
If the patient is on amlodipine, consider discontinuing.

SURGERY/OTHER PROCEDURES
Sclerotherapy and surgery may be required for associated disease.

 ## ONGOING CARE

FOLLOW-UP RECOMMENDATIONS
Patient Monitoring
- If Unna boot compression is used: Cut off and reapply boot once a week. Unna boots reduce edema by compression and prevent scratching.
- Regular use of high-compression stockings reduces chance of recurrent venous ulcer (5)[A].

DIET
Lose weight, if overweight.

PATIENT EDUCATION
- Encourage staying active to keep circulation and leg muscles in good condition. Walking is ideal.
- Keep legs elevated while sitting or lying.
- Do not wear girdles, garters, or pantyhose with tight elastic tops.
- Do not scratch.
- Avoid leg injury.
- Elevate foot of bed with 2- to 4-inch blocks.
- Apply compression stockings prior to getting out of bed when less edema is present. Regular use of high-compression stockings may prevent recurrence of venous ulcers.

PROGNOSIS
- Chronic course with intermittent exacerbations and remissions
- The healing process for ulceration is often prolonged and may take months.

COMPLICATIONS
- Sensations of itching, pain, and burning have negative impact on the quality of life.
- Secondary bacterial infection
- DVT
- Bleeding at dermatitis sites
- Squamous cell carcinoma in edges of long-standing stasis ulcers
- Scarring, which in turn leads to further compromise to blood flow and increased likelihood of minor trauma

REFERENCES
1. O'Meara S, Cullum N, Nelson EA, et al. Compression for venous leg ulcers. *Cochrane Database Syst Rev.* 2012;(11):CD000265.
2. Evidence-based (S3) guidelines for diagnostics and treatment of venous leg ulcers. *J Eur Acad Dermatol Venereol.* 2016;30(11):1843–1875.
3. Jull A, Wadham A, Bullen C, et al. Low dose aspirin as adjuvant treatment for venous leg ulceration: pragmatic, randomised, double blind, placebo controlled trial (Aspirin4VLU). *BMJ.* 2017;359:j5157.
4. O'Meara S, Al-Kurdi D, Ologun Y, et al. Antibiotics and antiseptics for venous leg ulcers. *Cochrane Database Syst Rev.* 2014;(1):CD003557.
5. Nelson EA, Bell-Syer SE. Compression for preventing recurrence of venous ulcers. *Cochrane Database Syst Rev.* 2012;(8):CD002303.

ADDITIONAL READING
- Coleridge-Smith PD. Leg ulcer treatment. *J Vasc Surg.* 2009;49(3):804–808.
- Coleridge-Smith P, Labropoulos N, Partsch H, et al. Duplex ultrasound investigation of the veins in chronic venous disease of the lower limbs—UIP consensus document. Part I. Basic principles. *Eur J Vasc Endovasc Surg.* 2006;31(1):83–92.
- Collins L, Seraj S. Diagnosis and treatment of venous ulcers. *Am Fam Physician.* 2010;81(8):989–996.
- Partsch H, Flour M, Smith P; for International Compression Club. Indications for compression therapy in venous and lymphatic disease consensus based on experimental data and scientific evidence. Under the auspices of the IUP. *Int Angiol.* 2008;27(3):193–219.
- Sippel K, Mayer D, Ballmer B, et al. Evidence that venous hypertension causes stasis dermatitis. *Phlebology.* 2011;26(8):361–365.

 ## SEE ALSO
- Varicose Veins
- Algorithm: Rash

 ## CODES

ICD10
- I83.10 Varicose veins of unsp lower extremity with inflammation
- I83.11 Varicose veins of right lower extremity with inflammation
- I83.12 Varicose veins of left lower extremity with inflammation

CLINICAL PEARLS
- Treatment of edema associated with stasis dermatitis via elevation and/or compression stockings or bandages is essential for optimal results.
- Pentoxifylline may improve venous ulcer healing.
- No difference in healing rate of venous stasis ulcers by use of hydrocolloid dressing versus simple nonadherent dressing when used beneath compression. Decision about the dressing should be based on local cost and patient or physician's preferences.
- Mild topical corticosteroids reduce inflammation and itching; however, these may potentiate infection; high-potency topical corticosteroids should be avoided due to increased risk of atrophy and ulceration.

DIABETES MELLITUS, TYPE 1
Vicente T. San Martin, MD • David T. Broome, MD

 BASICS

DESCRIPTION
- Type 1 diabetes mellitus (T1DM) is a chronic disease caused by insulin deficiency following β-cell destruction.
- Results in hyperglycemia and potential end-organ complications
- Features include:
  - Usually rapid onset
  - Absolute insulin dependence
  - Polyphagia, polydipsia, polyuria, and nocturia
  - Ketosis or diabetic ketoacidosis (DKA)
  - Body habitus: usually normal or thin physique at diagnosis
- System(s) affected: endocrine, metabolism, cardio-vascular, neurologic, renal, ocular

Pregnancy Considerations
- T1DM confers maternal and fetal risk (spontane-ous abortion, fetal anomalies, preeclampsia, fetal demise, macrosomia, neonatal hypoglycemia, and neonatal hyperbilirubinemia).
- Preconception counseling should address the importance of glycemic control as close to normal as safely possible to reduce congenital anomalies.
- Glycemic targets during pregnancy: fasting <95 mg/dL, and 1-hour postprandial <140 mg/dL, or 2-hour postprandial <120 mg/dL
- Glycated hemoglobin (HbA1c) is slightly lower dur-ing pregnancy due to increased RBC turnover. The HbA1c target should ideally be <6% if achieved without hypoglycemia but can be relaxed to <7% if necessary to prevent hypoglycemia (1)[B].
- Dilated eye examinations should occur before preg-nancy or in the 1st trimester and monitored every trimester and 1-year postpartum (1)[B].
- Women with T1DM should be prescribed low-dose aspirin 60 to 150 mg/day (usual dose 81 mg/day) by the end of the first trimester in order to lower the risk of preeclampsia (if no contraindication) (1)[C].

EPIDEMIOLOGY
Age of presentation is bimodal: at 4 to 6 years of age and at 10 to 14 years of age (early puberty) (2).

Incidence
- In the United States, incidence is 23.6/100,000 in non-Hispanic white children and adolescents (3).
- Lower rates in other racial and ethnic groups

Pediatric Considerations
In infants and toddlers, symptoms of T1DM may be subtle or masquerade as an intercurrent illness.

Prevalence
The U.S. prevalence of type 1 diabetes ranges from 2.6/1000 to 3.7/1000 (4).

ETIOLOGY AND PATHOPHYSIOLOGY
There are two main categories of T1DM: immune-mediated and idiopathic diabetes (1):
- Immune-mediated diabetes: cellular-mediated autoimmune destruction of β cells of the pancreas (markers: autoantibodies to insulin, GAD65, tyrosine phosphatases IA-2 and IA-2β, including zinc transporter 8 autoantibody [ZnT8A]). Obtain 3 antibody tests (GAD65, IA-2A, ZnT8) to rule out MODY-monogenic diabetes.

- Idiopathic diabetes: no known etiology for perma-nent insulinopenia; prone to ketoacidosis but have no evidence of autoimmunity
- At least one autoantibody is present in 85–90% of individuals (1).

Genetics
- HLA associations, with linkage to the DQA and DQB genes, and it is influenced by the DRB genes (HLA-DQA1, HLA-DQB1, and DLA-DRB1). These antibodies can be predisposing or protective (1).
- The major susceptibility locus maps to the HLA class II genes at 6p21 (accounting for 30–50% of genetic T1DM), but there are >40 loci (5).

RISK FACTORS
- Risk factors: viral infections, vitamin D deficiency, perinatal factors (maternal age, history of pre-eclampsia, neonatal jaundice), high birth weight for gestational age, and lower gestational age at birth
- Increased susceptibility to T1DM is inheritable:
  - T1DM in monozygous twins with long-term follow-up is >50%.
  - Among first-degree relatives, siblings are at a higher risk (5–10% risk by age 20 years) than offspring.
  - Offsprings of fathers with diabetes are at a higher risk (~12%) than offsprings of mothers with diabetes (~6%) (5).

GENERAL PREVENTION
Although there is currently a lack of accepted screening programs, providers should consider referring relatives of those with type 1 diabetes for risk assessment in a clinical research study (http://www.diabetestrialnet.org) (1).

COMMONLY ASSOCIATED CONDITIONS
Autoimmune diseases, such as primary adrenal insuf-ficiency (Addison disease), celiac disease, autoimmune hepatitis, pernicious anemia, myasthenia gravis, vit-iligo, Graves disease, and Hashimoto hypothyroidism

 DIAGNOSIS

HISTORY
New-onset polyuria and polydipsia
- Polyuria may present as nocturia, bed-wetting, or incontinence in a previously continent child.
- Polyuria may be difficult to appreciate in diaper-clad children.
- Polyuria occurs when serum glucose concentration rises >180 mg/dL (10 mmol/L).

PHYSICAL EXAM
- Weight loss, increased fatigue, lethargy, muscle cramps
- Ketosis/DKA leads to abdominal discomfort, nausea.
- Vision changes, such as blurriness (5)

DIFFERENTIAL DIAGNOSIS
- Type 2 diabetes
- Monogenic diabetes considered when (1):
  - Diabetes diagnosed before 6 months of age should have immediate genetic testing.
  - Strong family history of diabetes without classic features of type 2 diabetes
  - Nonobese diabetic child with negative autoantibodies

- Secondary diabetes
  - Pancreatic disease (chronic pancreatitis, cystic fibrosis, hereditary hemochromatosis)
  - Endocrine-associated diabetes: acromegaly, Cushing syndrome, pheochromocytoma, glucagonoma, neuroendocrine tumors
  - Drug- or chemical-induced diabetes: glucocor-ticosteroids, HIV protease inhibitors, atypical antipsychotics, tacrolimus, cyclosporine, immune checkpoint inhibitors
- Acute poisonings (salicylate poisoning can mimic DKA)

DIAGNOSTIC TESTS & INTERPRETATION
Initial Tests (lab, imaging)
- Criteria for the diagnosis of diabetes:
  - Fasting (>8 hours) glucose ≥126 mg/dL (7.0 mmol/L) on more than one occasion
  - Random glucose of ≥200 mg/dL (11.1 mmol/L) in a patient with classic symptoms of hyperglycemia
  - Oral glucose tolerance test (OGTT): plasma glucose ≥200 mg/dL 2 hours after a glucose load of 1.75 g/kg (max dose 75 g)
  - HbA1c level ≥6.5%
- Other tests to consider:
  - Urinalysis for glucose, ketones, and albuminuria (urine albumin:creatinine ratio)
  - Pancreatic autoantibodies: islet cell, IAA, GAD, IA2A, and ZnT8A
  - Serum β-hydroxybutyrate (BHB) and urine ketones
  - Fructosamine
- C-peptide level if needed to differentiate from type 2 diabetes because low or no C-peptide indicates insulinopenia

Follow-Up Tests & Special Considerations
Patients should be screened for thyroid disease on diagnosis and periodically thereafter (1)[C].

Test Interpretation
In the absence of unequivocal hyperglycemia, results should be confirmed by repeat testing.

 TREATMENT

GENERAL MEASURES
Insulin is the mainstay of therapy with education regarding matching of mealtime insulin dose to carbohydrate intake, premeal blood glucose level, and anticipated activity.
- Premeal blood glucose goal: 90 to 130 mg/dL (5.0 to 7.2 mmol/L)
- Bedtime/overnight blood glucose levels goal: 90 to 150 mg/dL (5.0 to 8.3 mmol/L)
- Pediatric A1c goal: <7.5% (A1c <7.0% is reason-able if achieved without excessive hypoglycemia.)
- Adult A1c goal: <7.0% (A1c <6.5% reasonable in select individuals); less stringent A1c goals (such as <8%) may be appropriate for elderly patients and other special populations.

MEDICATION

- Most treated with multiple daily injections (MDIs) of prandial insulin and basal insulin, or continuous subcutaneous insulin infusion (CSII).
- Use rapid-acting insulin analogs to reduce hypoglycemia risk.
- Types of injectable insulin:
  – Long-acting insulin analogs: insulin glargine, insulin detemir, and insulin degludec. These should not be mixed with other insulins in the same syringe.
  – Intermediate-acting insulin (NPH) can be mixed with other insulins.
  – Short-acting (regular) insulin
  – Rapid-acting insulin analogs: insulin lispro, insulin aspart, and insulin glulisine

First Line

- Flexible intensive insulin therapy is the gold standard.
- MDI or CSII have equal efficacy (1).
- Total initial dose is 0.2 to 0.4 units/kg/day for insulin-naive patients (up to 1.0 unit/kg/day in puberty).
- ~50% of total dose given as basal insulin, with the rest as bolus insulin.
- MDI regimen (1):
  – Basal, long-acting insulin once or twice a day
  – Prandial, short-acting insulin based on number of carbohydrate portions (e.g., 1:10, meaning 1 U of insulin for every 10 g of carbohydrates)
  – Correctional short-acting mealtime insulin based on premeal blood glucose level and sensitivity factor (e.g., 1 U for every 50 mg/dL over 150 mg/dL, where 50 mg/dL is the sensitivity factor)
- CSII regimen:
  – CSII and continuous glucose monitoring (CGM) should be encouraged when there is active patient/family participation (1).

Second Line

- Twice-daily injections with NPH along with regular or rapid-acting insulin (not physiologic, but lower cost and fewer injections)
- Pramlintide: delays gastric emptying, blunts pancreatic secretion of glucagon, and enhances satiety
- Pancreatic and islet transplantation have been shown to normalize glucose levels but require lifelong immunosuppression; reserved for simultaneous renal transplantation, recurrent DKA, or severe hyperglycemia

ISSUES FOR REFERRAL

New and established diagnoses of type 1 diabetes would benefit from endocrinology referral.

ADDITIONAL THERAPIES

- Inhaled rapid-acting insulin (may be used for mealtime coverage)
- Investigational agents (not yet FDA-approved): insulin icodec (super-long-acting insulin), metformin, GLP-1 receptor agonists, DPP-4 inhibitors, SGLT-1/ SGLT-2 inhibitors (1)[C]

SURGERY/OTHER PROCEDURES

- All patients with T1DM should have basal insulin continued if not eating prior to a procedure.
- If patients are not eating on the morning prior to a procedure/surgery, prandial insulin should be held.

ADMISSION, INPATIENT, AND NURSING CONSIDERATIONS

Newly diagnosed patients with T1DM may require hospitalization during initiation of insulin therapy.

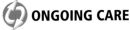 ## ONGOING CARE

FOLLOW-UP RECOMMENDATIONS

Regular aerobic exercise with care to avoid hypoglycemia:

- To reduce hypoglycemia, patients should lower basal requirements (temporary basal rate if using an insulin pump), or be advised to eat/drink 15 to 30 g of carbohydrates prior to vigorous exercise.
- Some patients may require both measures to reduce hypoglycemic events.

Patient Monitoring

- Blood pressure (BP) checks at every routine visit with a goal BP of <130/80 mm Hg
- Home blood glucose monitoring with home blood glucose meter or CGM: Glucose checks should be done at least 4 to 6 times/day.
- Comprehensive foot exam at least annually
- Quarterly measurement of HbA1c
- For patients of all ages with diabetes and atherosclerotic cardiovascular disease (ASCVD), high-intensity statin therapy should be added to lifestyle therapy.
- For patients with diabetes age 40 to 75 years and >75 years without ASCVD, use moderate-intensity statin in addition to lifestyle therapy.
- Annual screenings:
  – Albuminuria for earliest signs of possible nephropathy (urine albumin:creatinine ratio)
  – Initial dilated comprehensive eye exam within 5 years of diagnosis and then every 1 to 2 years
  – Monofilament testing with pinprick, temperature, and vibration sensation for screening of peripheral neuropathy 5 years after diagnosis and then annually
  – Annual influenza vaccine in patients ≥6 months of age
  – Pneumococcal pneumonia with 13-valent pneumococcal conjugate vaccine (PCV13) is recommended before age 2 years. People aged 2 to 64 years should also receive a 23-valent pneumococcal polysaccharide vaccine (PPSV23). At age >65 years, regardless of vaccine history, PPSV23 is recommended.
  – Hepatitis B vaccination to unvaccinated adults aged 19 to 59 years. Consider administering 3-dose series of hepatitis B vaccine to unvaccinated adults with diabetes ages ≥60 years.

DIET

- American Diabetes Association diet: http://www.diabetes.org/food-and-fitness/food/
- Carbohydrate counting using insulin-to-carbohydrate ratio with all meals and snacks allows patient flexibility in eating.

PATIENT EDUCATION

Patient education of their diagnosis, carbohydrate counting, nutritional recommendations is important.

PROGNOSIS

- Initial remission or 3 to 6 month "honeymoon phase" with decreased insulin needs and easier control
- Prognosis improves with careful blood glucose monitoring, improvement in insulin delivery regimens, and appropriate glycemic control.

COMPLICATIONS

- Microvascular disease (retinopathy, nephropathy, neuropathy)
- Macrovascular disease (coronary and cerebral artery disease)
- Chronic foot ulcers/amputations
- Hypoglycemia (recommend checking glucose before driving)
- DKA
- Excessive weight gain
- Increased risk of serious infection
- Increased risk of preeclampsia and preterm delivery

REFERENCES

1. American Diabetes Association. Standards of medical care in diabetes—2020. *Diabetes Care.* 2020;43(Suppl 1):S1–S2.
2. Felner EI, Klitz W, Ham M, et al. Genetic interaction among three genomic regions creates distinct contributions to early- and late-onset type 1 diabetes mellitus. *Pediatr Diabetes.* 2005;6(4):213–220.
3. Bell RA, Mayer-Davis EJ, Beyer JW, et al; for SEARCH for Diabetes in Youth Study. Diabetes in non-Hispanic white youth: prevalence, incidence, and clinical characteristics: the SEARCH for Diabetes in Youth Study. *Diabetes Care.* 2009;32(Suppl 2):S102–S111.
4. Menke A, Orchard TJ, Imperatore G, et al. The prevalence of type 1 diabetes in the United States. *Epidemiology.* 2013;24(5):773–774.
5. Steck AK, Rewers MJ. Genetics of type 1 diabetes. *Clin Chem.* 2011;57(2):176–185.

 ## CODES

ICD10

- E10.319 Type 1 diabetes mellitus with unspecified diabetic retinopathy without macular edema
- E10.321 Type 1 diabetes mellitus with mild nonproliferative diabetic retinopathy with macular edema
- E10.351 Type 1 diabetes mellitus with proliferative diabetic retinopathy with macular edema

CLINICAL PEARLS

- The age of presentation of T1DM is bimodal: one peak at 4 to 6 years of age and a second peak at 10 to 14 years of age.
- Therapy with MDI or CSII and the use of a multidisciplinary team care approach are associated with improved glycemic control, resulting in better long-term outcomes.
- Adult A1c goal is <7.0%; less stringent A1c goals may be appropriate for elderly patients and other special populations.

DIABETES MELLITUS, TYPE 2

Samir Malkani, MD, MRCP–UK • Sanaa Ayyoub, MD

BASICS

DESCRIPTION
Diabetes mellitus (DM) type 2 is due to a progressive insulin secretory defect in the setting of insulin resistance.

Geriatric Considerations
Monitor for hypoglycemia; adjust doses for renal/hepatic dysfunction and cognitive function; less aggressive glucose targets than younger patients

Pediatric Considerations
Incidence is increasing and parallels obesity epidemic.

Pregnancy Considerations
- Diet, metformin, glyburide, and insulin are all options for treatment of gestational diabetes.
- In gestational diabetes, screen for diabetes/prediabetes with oral glucose tolerance test (OGTT) 6 to 12 weeks postpartum and every 3 years.

EPIDEMIOLOGY
Incidence
1.5 million new cases in the United States each year

Prevalence
Estimated 30.3 million Americans (9.4% of the population); 90–95% are likely type 2.

ETIOLOGY AND PATHOPHYSIOLOGY
- Peripheral insulin resistance and defective insulin secretion with increased hepatic gluconeogenesis
- Genetic factors: usually polygenic; rarely monogenic (e.g., peroxisome proliferator–activated receptor [PPAR] γ and insulin gene mutations)
- Obesity (body mass index [BMI] $\geq$25 kg/m^2) and visceral adiposity
- Gut microbiome changes
- Drug or chemical induced (e.g., glucocorticoids, antiretroviral therapy, atypical antipsychotics, organ transplant immunosuppressants)

Genetics
- Small causal effect of common polymorphisms; 50% concordance in monozygotic twins
- Family history is strongly predictive of risk.

RISK FACTORS
- Parental history of type 2 diabetes
- Gestational diabetes or history of baby with birth weight $\geq$4 kg (9 lb)
- Polycystic ovarian syndrome (PCOS)
- Hypertriglyceridemia or low high-density lipoprotein (HDL)
- Ethnicity: African American, Latino, Native American, Asian, and Pacific Islander
- Sedentary lifestyle, visceral obesity

GENERAL PREVENTION
- Maintenance of normal weight, or weight loss of 7% body weight, decrease intake of carbohydrates and overall calories; moderate-intensity exercise (150 min/week)
- Metformin, α-glucosidase inhibitors, thiazolidinediones (TZDs), and glucagon-like peptide-1 receptor agonist (GLP-1 RA) in prediabetes

COMMONLY ASSOCIATED CONDITIONS
Hypertension, dyslipidemia, metabolic syndrome, fatty liver disease, PCOS, acanthosis nigricans, hemochromatosis

DIAGNOSIS

HISTORY
Polyuria, polydipsia, polyphagia, weight loss, fatigue, blurry vision, neuropathy, and frequent infections. Many individuals are asymptomatic.

PHYSICAL EXAM
BMI, waist circumference, funduscopic exam, oral exam, cardiopulmonary exam, abdominal exam for hepatomegaly, focused neurologic exam, and diabetic foot exam

DIFFERENTIAL DIAGNOSIS
- Type 1 DM—low or absent insulin, C-peptide, positive β-cell autoantibodies, ketosis
- DM is one of the features of Cushing syndrome, acromegaly, and glucagonoma.

DIAGNOSTIC TESTS & INTERPRETATION
Initial Tests (lab, imaging)
Criteria for diagnosis
- HbA1c $\geq$6.5% *or*
- Hyperglycemic symptoms and random plasma glucose $\geq$200 mg/dL (11.1 mmol/L) *or*
- Fasting plasma glucose (FPG) $\geq$126 mg/dL (7.0 mmol/L) *or*
- 2-hour plasma glucose $\geq$200 mg/dL (11.1 mmol/L) during OGTT with 75-g glucose load
- If equivocal, perform different test on same sample or a repeat test in a separate sample.

TREATMENT

Tight glucose control prevents long-term microvascular complications, but benefits on macrovascular outcomes are less apparent. Individuals likely to benefit from a more aggressive target are those without preexisting DM complications, with recent diagnoses of DM, and with long life expectancy.
- Use patient-centered approach.
- Dietary modification, regular exercise, control of cardiovascular (CV) risk factors (blood pressure [BP] and lipids)
- HbA1c targets—ADA recommendations (1) and ACP targets differ (2).
  - A1c <7.0: long life expectancy, no cardiovascular disease (CVD), short duration of DM, no history of hypoglycemia
  - A1c <8.0%: limited life expectancy, advanced micro- or macrovascular complications, extensive comorbidities, history of severe hypoglycemia or long-standing DM where lower goal is difficult to attain
  - The ACP recommends an HbA1c between 7% and 8% in most patients (2).
  - ADA recommends preprandial glucose 80 to 130 mg/dL; postprandial glucose <180 mg/dL

- Combine drugs from different classes for complementary action. Start monotherapy with metformin (if not contraindicated), but if A1c is $\geq$9%, start dual therapy; if A1c $\geq$10%, BG 300 mg/dL, and patient is symptomatic, consider adding insulin with/without GLP-1 analog.
- Always consider side effect profile, CV benefit, renal benefit, and cost.

GENERAL MEASURES
- Diabetic foot exam at every visit
- Nephropathy: annual urine microalbumin-to-creatinine ratio and plasma creatinine (eGFR)
- Retinopathy: annual diabetic eye exam
- If 40 to 75 years old, prescribe moderate- to high-intensity statin.
- If >50 years old, low-dose aspirin if one additional CV risk factor and low GI bleed risk
- Hypertension: goal BP <140/80 mm Hg
- Pneumococcal (PPSV23) for all adults; pneumococcal conjugate vaccine (PCV13) for patients >65 years (and some younger—see CDC) and annual influenza vaccine

MEDICATION
First Line
Metformin
- Reduces hepatic gluconeogenesis and multiple other mechanisms of action
- Preferred due to high efficacy in lowering glucose, good safety profile, low hypoglycemia risk, low cost, and weight loss
- Some studies suggest CV benefit; dosage: 500 to 2,000 mg in divided doses BID or extended release QD
- Avoid in severe acute illnesses (e.g., liver disease, cardiogenic shock, pancreatitis, hypoxia) due to risk of lactic acidosis.
- Caution with acute heart failure, alcohol abuse, elderly; associated with vitamin B$_{12}$ deficiency
- In CKD for eGFR 30 to 45, reduce dose to $\leq$1,000 mg; stop if eGFR <30.
- Severe diarrhea in 10% of patients requiring switch to another agent

Second and Third Line
- General principles
  - If HbA1c not at goal, add second/third agent.
  - If patient has CAD, heart failure, or CKD, consider drugs that improve outcomes with these conditions.
  - Consider drug-specific side effects such as weight gain, hypoglycemia.
  - Cost of drug is an important consideration.
  - Seek patient input to optimize adherence.
- GLP-1 RA (incretins)
  - Enhance glucose-dependent insulin release.
  - Promote weight loss, no risk of hypoglycemia; some improve CV outcomes.
  - Small risk of acute pancreatitis. Use cautiously in CKD $\geq$ stage 4. May exacerbate gastroparesis. Most are injectable, expensive.
  - Contraindicated in personal/family history of medullary thyroid cancer or multiple endocrine neoplasia (MEN) type 2

- Exenatide (Byetta): 5 to 10 μg SC BID or exenatide ER (Bydureon) 2 mg/week
- Liraglutide (Victoza): 0.6 to 1.8 mg/day; improved CV outcomes (3)
- Dulaglutide (Trulicity): 0.75 to 4.50 mg weekly; improved CV outcomes (3)
- Lixisenatide (Adlyxin): up to 20 μg SC QD
- Semaglutide injection (Ozempic): 0.25 to 1.00 mg weekly; improved CV outcomes (3); oral (Rybelsus) 3 to 14 mg daily neutral CV risk (4)
- SGLT2 inhibitors
  - Inhibit renal glucose reabsorption
  - Cause weight loss, no hypoglycemia risk
  - Canagliflozin, dapagliflozin, and empagliflozin reduced heart failure admissions and slowed progression of renal disease (3).
  - Empagliflozin and canagliflozin improved CV mortality (3).
  - Canagliflozin slowed progression of renal disease, death from renal causes in those with albuminuria and GFR of 30 to 90 (5).
  - Dapagliflozin slowed progression of renal disease, and reduced mortality from renal or CV causes, in patients with GFR 25 to 75 (6).
  - Increase in genital mycotic infections and UTI. Increased risk of euglycemic diabetic ketoacidosis (DKA); relatively expensive
  - Do not initiate therapy if eGFR <45.
  - Canagliflozin (Invokana): 100 to 300 mg/day
  - Dapagliflozin (Farxiga): 5 to 10 mg daily
  - Empagliflozin (Jardiance): 10 to 25 mg daily
  - Ertugliflozin (Steglatro): 5 to 15 mg daily
- Dipeptidyl peptidase-4 (DPP-4) inhibitors
  - Inhibit DPP-4 enzyme, which deactivates endogenous GLP-1 and GIP
  - Low risk for hypoglycemia; reduce dose in renal impairment except linagliptin.
  - Weight neutral
  - No evidence for CV risk reduction (7).
  - Sitagliptin (Januvia): 100 mg/day
  - Saxagliptin (Onglyza): 2.5 or 5.0 mg daily
  - Linagliptin (Tradjenta): 5 mg/day
  - Alogliptin (Nesina): 25 mg/day
- Sulfonylureas
  - Stimulate β-cell production of insulin
  - Caution with renal or liver disease, sulfa allergy, creatinine clearance <50 mL/min
  - May cause weight gain, hypoglycemia
  - Inexpensive
  - Glipizide (Glucotrol): 2.5 to 40.0 mg/day
  - Glipizide extended-release: 5 to 20 mg/day
  - Glyburide (DiaBeta, Micronase): 1.25–20.00 mg/day, Glynase: 0.75 to 12.00 mg/day
  - Glimepiride (Amaryl): 1 to 8 mg/day
- TZD
  - Increases insulin sensitivity; activates PPARs
  - Pioglitazone reduces triglycerides (7); low cost
  - Can worsen heart failure symptoms
  - Increased risk of fractures/low bone mass
  - Pioglitazone (Actos): 15 to 45 mg/day
  - Rosiglitazone (Avandia): 4 to 8 mg/day
- Insulin
  - Increases glucose disposal, inhibits hepatic glucose production
  - Potent glucose lowering; safe
  - Consider as initial therapy in those with A1c >10%, catabolic symptoms, ketosis.

- Use as additional therapy after dual/triple therapy has been tried.
- Weight gain; high hypoglycemia risk
- Analogs have lower hypoglycemia risk than NPH and regular insulin but more expensive.
- Neutral effects on CV outcomes
- Basal insulin start with 0.1 to 0.3 U/kg/day. Titrate up for desired result. Add mealtime (rapid-/short-acting) insulin if postmeal glucose is high. Mealtime starting dose can be 4 U or 10% of basal dose.
- Rapid-acting analogs—lispro (Humalog), aspart (Novolog), glulisine (Apidra): duration of action 3 to 5 hours; ultrarapid (Fiasp and lispro-aabc) quicker onset
- Inhaled insulin (Afrezza): rapid onset of action; duration of action 4.5 hours
- Short-acting insulin—human regular (Humulin R/Novolin R/ReliOn R): duration of action 6 to 8 hours
- Intermediate-acting insulin—human NPH (Humulin N/Novolin N/ReliOn N): duration 13 to 20 hours; human regular U-500 (Humulin R U-500): duration 6 to 10 hours
- Basal insulin analogs—glargine U-100 (Lantus, Basaglar): duration 22 to 24 hours; Glargine U-300 (Toujeo): duration 36 hours; detemir (Levemir): duration 21.5 hours; degludec U-100, U-200 (Tresiba): duration 42 hours
- Premixed insulin products—NPH/regular 70/30 (Novolin 70/30, Humulin 70/30), 70/30 and 50/50 aspart mix (Novolog mix), 75/25 and 50/50 lispro mix (Humalog mix)
- Amylinomimetic
  - Delays gastric emptying, blunts glucagon, enhances satiety
  - Causes weight loss
  - Reduce prandial insulin by 50%.
  - Pramlintide (Symlin): 60 to 120 μg SC premeal
- α-Glucosidase inhibitors
  - Slows intestinal carbohydrate digestion
  - Avoid in renal insufficiency and bowel diseases.
  - Decreases postprandial hyperglycemia
  - Acarbose (Precose): 25 to 100 mg TID
  - Miglitol (Glyset): 25 to 100 mg TID
- Meglitinides
  - Mechanism similar to SU but much shorter duration of action
  - Take at beginning of meals.
  - Repaglinide (Prandin): 0.5 to 4.0 mg TID
  - Nateglinide (Starlix): 60 to 120 mg TID
- Combination therapy
  - Drugs from different classes with complementary mechanisms of actions can be combined.

SURGERY/OTHER PROCEDURES
For patients with BMI >35 kg/m^2, consider bariatric surgery.

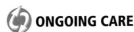 ONGOING CARE

PATIENT EDUCATION
Diabetes self-management education

PROGNOSIS
Normal lifespan with good management

COMPLICATIONS
- Emergencies: hyperosmolar coma, DKA
- ASCVD, peripheral vascular disease, stroke, foot ulcers, Charcot joints
- Microvascular: neuropathy, retinopathy, diabetic CKD
- Ophthalmic: blindness, cataracts, glaucoma
- GI: fatty liver disease, gastroparesis

REFERENCES
1. American Diabetes Association. Standards of Medical Care in Diabetes–2021. *Diabetes Care*. 2021;44(Suppl 1):S1–S232.
2. Qaseem A, Wilt TJ, Kansagara D, et al; for Clinical Guidelines Committee of the American College of Physicians. Hemoglobin A1c targets for glycemic control with pharmacologic therapy for nonpregnant adults with type 2 diabetes mellitus: a guidance statement update from the American College of Physicians. *Ann Intern Med*. 2018;168(8):569–576.
3. Acharya T, Deedwania P. Cardiovascular outcome trials of the newer anti-diabetic medications. *Prog Cardiovasc Dis*. 2019;62(4):342–348.
4. Husain M, Birkenfeld AL, Donsmark M, et al. Oral semaglutide and cardiovascular outcomes in patients with type 2 diabetes. *N Engl J Med*. 2019;381(9):841–851.
5. Perkovic V, Jardine MJ, Neal B, et al. Canagliflozin and renal outcomes in type 2 diabetes and nephropathy. *N Engl J Med*. 2019;380(24):2295–2306.
6. Heerspink HJL, Stefánsson BV, Correa-Rotter R, et al. Dapagliflozin in patients with chronic kidney disease. *N Engl J Med*. 2020;383(15):1436–1446.
7. Carbone S, Dixon DL, Buckley LF, et al. Glucose-lowering therapies for cardiovascular risk reduction in type 2 diabetes mellitus: state-of-the-art review. *Mayo Clin Proc*. 2018;93(11):1629–1647.

 SEE ALSO

- Diabetes Mellitus, Type 1; Diabetic Ketoacidosis; Hypertension, Essential
- Algorithm: Type 2 Diabetes, Treatment

 CODES

ICD10
- E11.329 Type 2 diabetes mellitus with mild non-proliferative diabetic retinopathy without macular edema
- E11.331 Type 2 diabetes mellitus with moderate nonproliferative diabetic retinopathy with macular edema
- E11.359 Type 2 diabetes mellitus with proliferative diabetic retinopathy without macular edema

CLINICAL PEARLS
Individualize A1c targets based on life expectancy and comorbidities. Hypoglycemia poses more short-term danger than hyperglycemia.

DIABETIC KETOACIDOSIS

Daniel R. Matta, MD • Zelibeth Gutierrez, MD

BASICS

DESCRIPTION
- A life-threatening medical emergency in diabetics, which most commonly occurs in patients with type 1 diabetes
- Characterized by a biochemical triad of hyperglycemia, ketosis, and high anion gap metabolic acidosis
- Rarely, it can occur in the absence of hyperglycemia (i.e., euglycemic DKA) during pregnancy and in individuals taking sodium-glucose cotransporter-2 inhibitors (1).
- System(s) affected: endocrine/metabolic, neurology

EPIDEMIOLOGY
Incidence
Incidence by age group: 1 to 17 (10.1%), 18 to 44 (53.3%), 45 to 64 (27.1 %), 65 to 84 (8.7%), and 85+ (0.8%) (2)

ETIOLOGY AND PATHOPHYSIOLOGY
- Impaired glucose utilization secondary to insulin deficiency leading to the activation of counterregulatory mechanisms (gluconeogenesis, glycogenolysis, proteolysis), which further increase blood glucose level and trigger ketone bodies production. Resulting ketonemia and hyperglycemia lead to osmotic diuresis, dehydration, electrolytes disturbances and acidosis.
- Leading causes include medication noncompliance and infection. Other precipitating factors are:
  - First presentation of DM
  - Myocardial infarction (MI); cerebrovascular accident (CVA)
  - Medications (corticosteroids, sympathomimetics, atypical antipsychotics, SGLT2 inhibitors)
  - Alcohol and Illicit drugs (cocaine)
  - Trauma; surgery
  - Emotional stress and psychiatric comorbidities
  - Pregnancy

RISK FACTORS
- Type 1 DM
- Ketosis-prone type 2 DM (Hispanic and African American ethnicity, G6PD deficiency)

GENERAL PREVENTION
- Close monitoring of glucose during periods of stress, illness, and trauma with "sick day" management instructions
- Careful insulin control and regular monitoring of blood glucose levels along with education on symptom recognition

COMMONLY ASSOCIATED CONDITIONS
>30% of patients have features of both DKA and hyperosmolar hyperglycemic syndrome (HHS).

DIAGNOSIS

- Diagnostic criteria (1)[C]
  - Hyperglycemia (usually 250–800 mg/dL) as rapidly assessed on fingerstick glucose testing and confirmed on serum chemistry
  - Low HCO_3 (usually ≤18 mEq/L)
  - Metabolic acidosis on arterial blood gases (ABGs) (pH <7.3)
  - Anion gap = serum sodium − (serum chloride + bicarbonate); >10 mmol
  - Positive B-hydroxybutyrate (B-OHB) in serum is highly sensitive and specific.
- Diagnosis can be stratified into three levels of severity.

DKA	Mild	Moderate	Severe
Plasma glucose (mg/dL)	>250	>250	>250
Arterial pH	7.25–7.30	7.00–7.24	<7.00
Serum bicarbonate (mEq/L)	15–18	10–15	<10
Urine ketone	+	+	+
Serum B-OHB	> 3 mmol/L	>3 mmol/L	>3 mmol/L
Effective serum osmolality	Variable	Variable	Variable
Anion gap	>10	>12	>12
Mental status	Alert	Alert/drowsy	Stupor/coma

- Note that there is considerable variability ranging from euglycemia to severe hyperglycemia with acidosis, dehydration, and coma. Individualization of treatment based on clinical and laboratory assessment is needed (1).

HISTORY
- Recent illness, injury, or surgery
- Changes in diet or medications. Missed insulin doses/noncompliance, insulin pump failure
- Polyuria, polydipsia, polyphagia, weight loss
- Generalized weakness, malaise, fatigue, lethargy, nausea, vomiting, abdominal pain
- Anorexia or increased appetite

PHYSICAL EXAM
- Vital signs: hypotension, tachycardia, fever, or hypothermia
- Tachypnea, hyperpnea, Kussmaul respirations
- Fruity odor of ketotic breath (acetone smell)
- Abdominal tenderness, decreased bowel sounds
- Dry mucous membranes, poor skin turgor, dehydration
- Decreased reflexes
- Altered mental status, coma

DIFFERENTIAL DIAGNOSIS
- Hyperosmolar hyperglycemic state
- Alcoholic ketoacidosis, starvation ketosis, lactic acidosis
- Toxic ingestions (e.g., salicylates, methanol, ethylene glycol)
- Uremia/chronic renal failure
- Sepsis
- Acute pancreatitis

DIAGNOSTIC TESTS & INTERPRETATION
Initial Tests (lab, imaging)

ALERT
- Important labs:
  - β-hydroxybutyrate (β-HOB) is the predominant ketone produced and is preferred over serum ketones. β-HB >3 mg/dL is abnormal and should be decreased to <1.5 mg/dL within 12 to 24 hours.
  - ABG or venous blood gases (VBG) for pH assessment: VBG pH correlates with 0.03 lower than ABG pH
  - Urinalysis: ketonuria, glycosuria.
  - Creatinine and BUN: Markedly increased serum ketones may cross-react and cause a falsely high serum creatinine.
  - Electrolytes derangements: hypomagnesemia, hypophosphatemia, base deficit with high anion gap
  - Decreased total body K^+: Severe acidosis causes an artificially elevated K^+ level.
  - Pseudohyponatremia secondary to hyperglycemia or hypertriglyceridemia: It is now accepted to correct Na^+ concentration by adding 2.4 mmol/L to measured Na^+ for every 100 mg/dL increase in serum glucose above 100 mg/dL.
  - Calculate serum osmolality: If calculated osmolality <320 mOsm/kg, consider etiologies other than diabetic ketoacidosis (DKA) especially in patients with altered mentation.
  - HbA1c (glycosylated hemoglobin) helps assess long-term history of diabetic control.
  - CBC: Consider DKA related leukocytosis versus infection.
- Other tests:
  - Blood and urine culture, chest x-ray, and lumbar puncture based on clinical suspicion for infection
  - ECG: frequently shows sinus tachycardia (nonspecific), changes consistent with electrolyte abnormalities, and/or ischemic changes with MI as a precipitation factor
  - Troponin
  - Head CT scan if CVA or cerebral edema suspected

Follow-Up Tests & Special Considerations
Elevated lipase and amylase might not be reliable for diagnosis of pancreatitis in DKA.

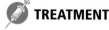

TREATMENT

Goals
- Fluid resuscitation
- Resolution of anion gap acidosis and ketosis
- Insulin therapy to normalize serum glucose
- Correction of electrolytes
- Identify and treat precipitating cause(s).

GENERAL MEASURES
- Severe DKA requires an ICU setting.
- Start isotonic crystalloid solution (e.g., 0.9% saline or lactated Ringer bolus).
- Check serum glucose every hour along with serum electrolytes, BUN, creatinine, venous pH, and glucose every 2 to 4 hours until stable.

MEDICATION
First Line
- Intravenous fluid (IVF) is a priority (1)[C],(2)[C].
  - ADA recommends administration of 1,000 to 1,500 mL of normal saline in the first hour.
  - After the first hour, IVF infusion rate should be adjusted based on hemodynamics and electrolytes (usually 250 to 500 mL/hr in patients without cardiac, renal, or hepatic compromise).
  - There is no data to refute or support use of 0.45% NaCl in patients with normal to high corrected Na$^+$ concentration after initial fluid resuscitation, but risk of hyperchloremic metabolic acidosis with continuous 0.9% NaCl should be considered.
  - When glucose is 200 mg/dL, change to 5% dextrose with 0.45% NaCl at same rate to prevent hypoglycemia.
    - The "two bag method" is an emerging fluid management strategy that consists in running two bags of 0.45% NaCl one with and another without dextrose 10%. Infusion rates are adjusted based on hourly glucose level to maintain a total infusion rate of 250 mL/hr. This method has been associated with earlier correction of acidosis compared to conventional fluid replacement (1),(3).
- Insulin: Start IV infusion after initial IVF resuscitation and correction of hypokalemia (<3.3 mg/dL) (1)[C],(3)[C].
  - Optional initial bolus 0.1 U/kg IV and then continuous infusion at 0.1 U/kg/hr (Do not use initial insulin bolus in children.)
  - If bolus not given, 0.14 U/kg/hr continuous infusion is recommended (1).
  - Aim for rate of serum glucose reduction of 50 to 75 mg/dL/hr in the first hour; adjust infusion rate every hour until steady decline is achieved.
  - ADA recommends reducing infusion rate to 0.02 to 0.05 U/kg/hr IV to maintain serum glucose between 150 to 200 mg/dL until correction of acidosis.
  - Use of basal insulin (glargine 0.25 U/kg SC) within 12 hours of starting treatment may result in reduction of time to gap closure, shorter hospital stay, and less rebound hyperglycemia (1).
  - Overlap and continue IV insulin infusion for 1 to 2 hours after SC insulin is initiated.
- Potassium: Start replacement with 20 to 30 mEq/L of K$^+$ in 1 L IVFs when serum K$^+$ ≤5.2 mg/dL and if urine output is adequate.
  - Hold insulin if K$^+$ ≤3.3 mg/dL; give IV potassium 20 to 30 mEq/hr with fluids until >3.3 mg/dL to prevent cardiac arrhythmia. For each 0.1 unit of pH, serum K$^+$ will change by ~0.6 mEq in opposite direction.
- Phosphorus: Routine replacement not recommended because it may lead to hypocalcemia; if very low (<1.0 mg/dL), give 20 to 30 mEq/L of K-Phos in fluids.

- Sodium bicarbonate: Available evidence does not support its use in patients with pH 6.9 or higher (1),(3). Patients with pH <6.9 or life-threatening hyperkalemia are at increased risk for poor outcome; therefore, ADA recommends slow administration of 100 mEq NaCHO over 2 hours in such cases. NaCHO$_3$ use may increase risk of cerebral edema, especially in children (3).
- Magnesium: If magnesium ≤1.2 mg/dL or <1.8 and patient is symptomatic, magnesium treatment should be considered.
- Precautions
  - Insulin pump should be stopped.
  - If glucose does not fall by 10% in first hour, give regular insulin 0.14 U/kg IV bolus and then continuous infusion at previous rate.
  - If using bicarbonate, add 100 mmol or 2 ampules of sodium bicarbonate to 400 mL isotonic solution with 20 mEq KCL >200 mL/hr for 2 hours until venous pH is >7.0 and then stop infusion (4).

Second Line
- Rapid-acting subcutaneous insulin can be considered for patients who are alert, tolerating oral intake, serum bicarbonate >10 mEq/L, and pH >7.0.
- Load with 0.3 U/kg SC, followed by 0.1 to 0.2 U/kg q1–2h. Once glucose <200 mg/dL, reduce dosing to 0.05 to 0.1 U/kg q1–2h till resolution of ketoacidosis.

Pediatric Considerations
- Initial insulin infusion rates of 0.05 to 0.1 U/kg/h are recommended (3)[C].
- Cerebral edema is a rare complication (~1%) but has a mortality of 20–50%:
  - Perform repeat neurologic examination. Treatment should be started as soon as suspected based on clinical assessment and not be delayed because of neuroimaging (3)[C].

Pregnancy Considerations
- DKA per se is not an indication for emergency delivery; imperative to stabilize mother first
- Euglycemic DKA
- β-Tocolytics and corticosteroids can trigger DKA (5).
- Perinatal death: 9–35% (5)

ISSUES FOR REFERRAL
ADA 2021 Diabetes Care Guidelines recommend outpatient follow-up within 1 month or 1 to 2 weeks for poorly controlled diabetics.

ADMISSION, INPATIENT, AND NURSING CONSIDERATIONS
ADA admission criteria: blood glucose >250 mg/dL; pH <7.3; HCO$_3$ ≤15 mEq/L; ketones in urine; ICU setting for severe DKA (6)

Pediatric Considerations
Discharge whe DKA has resolved anion gap <12, glucose <200 mg/dL; pH >7.3; bicarbonate >18 mEq/L. Patient must be tolerating PO intake and able to resume home medication regimen.

ONGOING CARE

DIET
- NPO initially, advance diet when nausea and vomiting are controlled.
- Avoid foods with high glycemic index (e.g., soft drinks, fruit juice, white bread, added sugar).

PATIENT EDUCATION
- Self-monitoring of glucose, glucose goals, and when to call PCP
- Recognition and prevention of hypoglycemia
- Healthy nutritional choices
- Sick day management
- Proper use of insulin syringes/needles

PROGNOSIS
- Worse in the extremes of age and in the setting of coma and hypotension
- Overall DKA mortality of 0.5–2%

COMPLICATIONS
- Cerebral edema (most common cause of death in children with DKA)
- Pulmonary edema, respiratory distress, myocardial infarction
- Vascular thrombosis
- Hypokalemia, hyperkalemia, hypophosphatemia
- Cardiac dysrhythmia (secondary to hypokalemia or acidosis)
- Acute renal failure
- Late hypoglycemia (secondary to treatment)
- Infection

REFERENCES
1. Karslioglu French E, Donihi AC, Korytkowski MT. Diabetic ketoacidosis and hyperosmolar hyperglycemic syndrome: review of acute decompensated diabetes in adult patients. *BMJ*. 2019;365:l1114.
2. Kamleshun R, Jyotsnav J. An update on the incidence and burden of diabetic ketoacidosis in the U.S. *Diabetes Care*. 2020;43(12):e96–e97.
3. Cashen K, Petersen T. Diabetic ketoacidosis. *Pediatric Rev*. 2019;40(8):412–420.
4. Kitabchi AE, Umpierrez GE, Miles JM, et al. Hyperglycemic crises in adult patients with diabetes. *Diabetes Care*. 2009;32(7):1335–1343.
5. Sibai BM, Viteri OA. Diabetes ketoacidosis in pregnancy. *Obstet Gynecol*. 2014;123(1):167–178.
6. American Diabetes Association Index. *Diabetes Care*. 2021;44(Suppl 1):S226–S232.

 CODES

ICD10
- E10.11 Type 1 diabetes mellitus with ketoacidosis with coma
- E10.10 Type 1 diabetes mellitus with ketoacidosis without coma
- E13.11 Other specified diabetes mellitus with ketoacidosis with coma

CLINICAL PEARLS
- DKA is defined by a classic clinical triad of hyperglycemia, ketosis, and high anion gap metabolic acidosis.
- Admit if blood glucose >250 mg/dL, pH <7.3, HCO$_3$ ≤15 mEq/L, and ketones in urine.
- Potassium is falsely elevated due to acidosis; start replacement when K$^+$ ≤5.2 mg/dL and urine output is adequate.

DIABETIC POLYNEUROPATHY

Samir Malkani, MD, MRCP–UK

BASICS

DESCRIPTION
Peripheral nerve dysfunction seen in diabetes; several patterns described:
- Symmetric polyneuropathy
  - Distal sensory or sensorimotor
- Mononeuropathy, radiculopathy, and polyradiculopathy
  - Cranial neuropathy
  - Focal limb or truncal neuropathy
  - Radiculoplexus neuropathy (diabetic amyotrophy)
- Acute painful small fiber neuropathy
- Autonomic neuropathies
- Chronic inflammatory demyelinating polyneuropathy (CIDP)

EPIDEMIOLOGY
Prevalence
- Generalized polyneuropathy
  - 10% at diabetes diagnosis
  - 50% at 10 years
  - Cross-sectional prevalence: 15% by symptoms; 50% by nerve conduction
- Autonomic neuropathy: 16.7% in a United Kingdom study

ETIOLOGY AND PATHOPHYSIOLOGY
- Metabolic derangement due to hyperglycemia
  - Aldose reductase converts excess glucose to sorbitol, which causes nerve damage.
  - Nonenzymatic glycation of neural proteins and lipids forms damaging advanced glycosylation end products.
  - Protein kinase C activation causes vascular endothelial changes.
  - Oxidative stress from excessive production of reactive oxygen species
  - Cyclooxygenase-2 and poly (ADP-ribose) polymerase activation
- Vasculopathy causing nerve ischemia: predominant factor in mononeuropathies

RISK FACTORS
- Poor glycemic control
- Duration of diabetes
- Hypertension
- Hyperlipidemia
- Tobacco and alcohol consumption

GENERAL PREVENTION
- Maintenance of normal blood sugar
- Exercise and appropriate diet

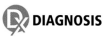

DIAGNOSIS

HISTORY
- Most common form (typical): symmetric distal sensory or sensorimotor polyneuropathy
  - Distressing numbness, tingling, pain of legs/feet, usually worse at night; allodynia; hyperalgesia
  - Often silent sensory loss, patient unaware
  - Ataxia and falls due to proprioceptive loss
  - Neuropathic foot ulcers due to analgesia and repetitive injury
  - Neuropathic degeneration of foot joints

- Hands involved late
- Distal muscle involvement, usually mild
- Symmetric proximal polyneuropathy
  - Proximal leg weakness and wasting
  - Muscles of shoulder girdle rarely involved
  - Pain and sensory changes less prominent
- Focal cranial or limb mononeuropathy
  - May involve 3rd, 4th, 6th, or 7th cranial nerve
  - Femoral, sciatic, or peroneal neuropathy: weakness or pain in nerve distribution
  - Any major peripheral nerve can be involved.
- Truncal neuropathies: painful radiculopathy over dermatomes
- Lumbar radiculoplexus neuropathy (diabetic amyotrophy)
  - Unilateral hip, thigh pain
  - Pelvic girdle and thigh weakness with atrophy
  - Recovery over months
- Diabetic autonomic neuropathy
  - GI: nocturnal diarrhea, sometimes alternating with constipation; gastroparesis with postprandial fullness; nausea and vomiting
  - Cardiovascular: postural dizziness, exercise intolerance
  - Urogenital: urinary hesitancy, overflow incontinence; erectile dysfunction; vaginal dryness; sexual dysfunction
  - Sudomotor: anhidrosis or hyperhidrosis; gustatory sweating of head and upper body
- CIDP: progressive, severe motor loss
- Diabetic cachexia: painful small fiber neuropathy with prominent weight loss and depression

PHYSICAL EXAM
- Symmetric distal polyneuropathy
  - "Stocking-and-glove" distal sensory loss
  - Large fiber neuropathy: loss of perception of vibration and light touch (10-g monofilament)
  - Small fiber involvement: loss of temperature and pinprick
  - Absent ankle reflexes
  - Wasting, weakness of small muscles in foot; changes to arch of foot or clawing of toes
  - With small fiber involvement, there may be lack of objective sensory deficit despite pain.
- Symmetric proximal polyneuropathy
  - Proximal leg, arm wasting, and weakness
  - Loss of patellar reflexes
- Focal cranial or limb mononeuropathy
  - 3rd cranial nerve palsy: painful ophthalmoplegia and ptosis; preserved pupillary reflexes (in contrast to compressive palsies)
  - 6th cranial nerve: lateral gaze palsy
  - Femoral neuropathy: weakness of lower leg extension, hip flexion, quadriceps wasting, absent patellar reflex, sensory loss in anterior thigh
  - Sciatic neuropathy: pain or sensory loss in back of thigh and leg; weakness of hamstrings, lower leg muscles
  - Peroneal neuropathy: foot drop
- Truncal neuropathies: sensory loss along dermatome
- Lumbar radiculoplexopathy (amyotrophy)
  - Weakness and wasting pelvic girdle and thigh
  - Sensory loss in L2–L3
  - Absent patellar reflex

- Autonomic neuropathy
  - Cardiovascular: resting tachycardia; orthostatic hypotension
  - Gastroparesis: postprandial distension; gastric splash
- CIDP: motor weakness

DIFFERENTIAL DIAGNOSIS
- Uremic polyneuropathy
- Drug induced
  - Antineoplastic drugs: cisplatin, vincristine
  - Isoniazid
  - Amiodarone
- Toxic
  - Chronic arsenic poisoning
  - n-Hexane, methyl-n-butyl ketone
- Nutritional deficiency
  - Usually associated with alcoholism
- Paraneoplastic polyneuropathy
- Hypothyroidism

DIAGNOSTIC TESTS & INTERPRETATION
Initial Tests (lab, imaging)
- Fasting plasma glucose, 2-hour glucose tolerance test, or hemoglobin A1c for diagnosis and to assess glycemic control; may occur in "prediabetes"
- Serum vitamin B_{12}
- Thyroid function
- Creatinine and BUN
- Syphilis testing
- Serum protein electrophoresis
- 25-OH vitamin D
- In mononeuropathy/mononeuritis multiplex, test for vasculitis, paraproteinemia, and sarcoid.
- In radiculopathy or mononeuropathy, imaging studies to exclude compressive lesions

Diagnostic Procedures/Other
- Bedside testing of vibration perception with 128-Hz tuning fork, monofilament perception of 10-g filament, pinprick and temperature testing
- Quantitative sensory testing for vibratory and thermal thresholds
  - Standardized measures for assessing severity and risk of foot ulceration
- Electromyogram nerve conduction velocity
  - Useful to confirm mononeuropathy and entrapment syndromes
  - Sensitive but nonspecific index of presence and severity of diabetic polyneuropathy
  - In small unmyelinated fiber painful neuropathy, test may be normal.
- Lumbar puncture
  - In CIDP, elevation of spinal fluid protein
- Skin biopsy with epidermal nerve fiber density
  - Enables direct study of small nerve fibers that are difficult to assess electrophysiologically
- Corneal confocal microscopy
  - Noninvasive approach. Loss of corneal innervation correlates with neuropathy

Test Interpretation
- In nerve biopsy of peripheral nerve, wallerian degeneration, focal axonal swellings containing neurofilaments, axonal atrophy, and demyelination are seen.
- Thick neural capillary basement membrane and endothelial proliferation
- Obliterative microvascular lesions and perivascular inflammation

TREATMENT

GENERAL MEASURES
- Maintain blood glucose control.
- Provide appropriate footwear to prevent pressure damage to insensate feet.

MEDICATION
Specific treatment to reverse nerve damage, other than improved glucose control, is not available. Current therapies target pain-relief.

First Line
Management of pain and sensory neuropathy
- Calcium channel modulators: gabapentin (off-label) (1),(2),(3)
  – Binds Ca^{2+} channel–associated protein α_2-δ; inhibits neurotransmitter release
  – Dose range 300 to 1,200 mg TID, NNT ~4 to 8
  – Reduce dose in renal insufficiency.
  – Adverse effects: dizziness, fatigue, edema
- Calcium channel modulators: pregabalin (1),(2),(3)
  – Binds same calcium channel as gabapentin
  – Linear pharmacokinetics and quicker onset of action compared to gabapentin
  – Usual dose: 150 to 600 mg/day, NNT ~4 to 10
  – Adverse effects are dizziness and edema.
- Duloxetine (1),(2),(4)
  – Selective serotonin and norepinephrine reuptake inhibitor
  – Usual dose is 30 to 60 mg/day; NNT ~4 to 9
  – Adverse effects are nausea and dizziness.
- Tricyclic antidepressants (TCA) (off-label) (1),(2),(4)
  – Analgesia may be related to effects on sodium channels; NNT ~2 to 5, NNH ~3 to 16
  – Amitriptyline 25 to 150 mg at bedtime
  – Nortriptyline (25 to 150 mg); desipramine (25 to 200 mg) less sedating than amitriptyline but limited trial data
    ○ Anticholinergic effects and cardiac arrhythmias may occur.
- Management of autonomic neuropathy
  – Orthostatic hypotension
    ○ Fludrocortisone (off-label) (1)
    ○ Midodrine (off-label) (1)
  – Gastroparesis
    ○ Metoclopramide (1) or domperidone
    ○ Erythromycin (off-label)
  – Diabetic diarrhea
    ○ Loperamide
    ○ Clonidine (off-label)
    ○ Octreotide (off-label)
    ○ Antibiotics for bacterial overgrowth
  – Hyperhidrosis
    ○ Propantheline (off-label)
    ○ Topical glycopyrrolate (1)

Geriatric Considerations
Anticholinergic effects of TCAs may cause urinary retention and cardiac arrhythmias.

Second Line
- Antidepressants
  – Venlafaxine (75 to 225 mg daily) (off-label) (1),(2),(4), NNT ~2 to 5
    ○ Serotonin-norepinephrine reuptake inhibitor
- Topical therapies
  – Capsaicin (2),(4),(5) 0.075% cream applied TID
    ○ Depletes C fibers in skin of substance P
    ○ Limited data on efficacy
  – Lidocaine (2),(4),(5) 5% (700 mg) patches applied daily to feet (off-label):
    ○ Causes sodium channel blockade
- Opiate analgesia
  – Tramadol (off-label) (1),(2),(4): 100 to 400 mg/day, NNT ~3 to 9
    ○ Binds opiate receptors; also inhibits reuptake of norepinephrine and serotonin; fewer opiate side effects
  – Tapentadol (1),(2),(4)
    ○ Binds to μ-opiate receptor and inhibits norepinephrine uptake

ISSUES FOR REFERRAL
If CIDP is suspected, refer to neurologist for investigation and treatment.

ADDITIONAL THERAPIES
- Transcutaneous electrical nerve stimulation
- Percutaneous nerve stimulation
- Electrical spinal cord stimulation
- Actovegin, dextromethorphan with quinidine

SURGERY/OTHER PROCEDURES
Electrical spinal cord stimulation

COMPLEMENTARY & ALTERNATIVE MEDICINE
Acupuncture, Reiki, electromagnetic field treatment: no convincing trial data

 ONGOING CARE

PROGNOSIS
- Generalized symmetric polyneuropathies
  – Usually slow, chronic progression
  – Insensitive but painless foot as pain lessens
- Focal neuropathies
  – Recovery over months to years

COMPLICATIONS
- Claw foot deformity
- Neurotropic ulceration
  – Painless ulcers on weight-bearing area
  – Callus formation is a precursor to ulceration.
- Neuropathic arthropathy
  – Results in complete disorganization of joint structure in foot, Charcot joint

REFERENCES
1. Pop-Busui R, Boulton AJ, Feldman EL, et al. Diabetic neuropathy: a position statement by the American Diabetes Association. *Diabetes Care*. 2017;40(1):136–154.
2. Liampas A, Rekatsina M, Vadalouka A, et al. Pharmacological management of painful peripheral neuropathies: a systematic review. *Pain Ther*. 2021;10(1):55–68.
3. Derry S, Bell RF, Straube S, et al. Pregabalin for neuropathic pain in adults. *Cochrane Database Syst Rev*. 2019;(1):CD007076.
4. Alam U, Sloan G, Tesfaye S. Treating pain in diabetic neuropathy: current and developmental drugs. *Drugs*. 2020;80(4):363–384.
5. Azmi S, Alam U, Burgess J, et al. State-of-the-art pharmacotherapy for diabetic neuropathy. *Expert Opin Pharmacother*. 2021;22(1):55–68.

ADDITIONAL READING
- Jensen TS, Karlsson P, Gylfadottir SS, et al. Painful and non-painful diabetic neuropathy, diagnostic challenges and implications for future management. *Brain*. 2021;144(6):1632–1645.
- Patel K, Horak H, Tiryaki E. Diabetic neuropathies. *Muscle Nerve*. 2021;63(1):22–30.
- Vinik AI. Clinical practice. Diabetic sensory and motor neuropathy. *N Engl J Med*. 2016;374(15):1455–1464.

 SEE ALSO

Diabetes Mellitus, Type 1; Diabetes Mellitus, Type 2

CODES

ICD10
- E10.42 Type 1 diabetes mellitus with diabetic polyneuropathy
- E11.42 Type 2 diabetes mellitus with diabetic polyneuropathy
- E13.42 Oth diabetes mellitus with diabetic polyneuropathy

CLINICAL PEARLS
- Occasionally, when glycemic control improves dramatically, as can occur when treatment for diabetes is initiated, there may be a worsening of neuropathy symptoms (described as treatment-induced neuropathy). Symptoms usually stabilize and gradually improve as glycemic control is maintained.
- It is common to combine agents with different mechanisms of action in the management of neuropathic pain. Topical therapies can be combined with systemic therapies. There is limited evidence-based data to support combination oral therapy, and maximizing the dose of a single agent may be more efficacious.

DIARRHEA, ACUTE
Marie L. Borum, MD, EdD, MPH • Daniel Ludi, MD

BASICS

DESCRIPTION
- An abnormal increase in stool water content, volume, or frequency (≥3 in 24 hours) for <14 days duration
- Most commonly secondary to infectious etiology; often self-limited
- Acute viral diarrhea (50–70%)
  - Most common cause of infectious diarrhea; noninflammatory (watery)
  - Frequently presents with associated nausea and/or vomiting
  - Symptoms usually develop after an incubation period of ~1 day and last for 1 to 3 days; typically self-limited
- Bacterial diarrhea (15–20%)
  - Most common infectious cause of inflammatory (bloody) diarrhea
  - Incubation period variable; diarrhea caused by preformed enterotoxin presents within 1 to 6 hours of contaminated food ingestion, whereas bacterial infection typically presents within 1 to 3 days.
  - Symptoms usually resolve in 1 to 7 days; antibiotic use attenuates length and/or severity of disease.
  - Suspect when concurrent illness in others who have shared potentially contaminated food.
- Protozoal infections (10–15%)
  - Typically cause noninflammatory (watery) diarrhea
  - Long incubation period and prolonged disease course, symptoms develop approximately 7 days after exposure and commonly last >7 days.
  - Suspect when outbreaks of watery diarrhea in areas with contaminated water or food supply
- Traveler's diarrhea (TD) typically begins 3 to 7 days after arrival in foreign location and resolves within 5 days; rapid onset, generally self-limited

EPIDEMIOLOGY
- In developing countries, acute diarrhea is more common in children; no age predilection in developed countries
- Acute diarrhea accounts for >128,000 U.S. hospital admissions and ~2.5 million annual deaths worldwide (1).

Prevalence
- Second leading cause of death in children <5 years and seventh leading cause of death among all ages worldwide
- Affects 11% of the general population
- In developing world, acute diarrhea is largely due to contaminated food and water.

ETIOLOGY AND PATHOPHYSIOLOGY
- Bacterial
  - *Escherichia coli*
  - *Salmonella, Shigella, Campylobacter jejuni*
  - *Vibrio parahaemolyticus, Vibrio cholerae*
  - *Yersinia enterocolitica*
  - *Clostridium difficile*
  - *Staphylococcus aureus*
  - *Bacillus cereus*
  - *Clostridium perfringens*
  - *Listeria monocytogenes*
- Viral
  - *Rotavirus* and *Norovirus* (most common)
  - Adenovirus
  - Astrovirus
  - Cytomegalovirus (in immunocompromised)
- Protozoal
  - *Giardia lamblia*
  - *Entamoeba histolytica*
  - *Cryptosporidium*
  - *Isospora belli*
  - *Cyclospora, Microspora*
- Pathophysiology (1)
  - Noninflammatory: most commonly viral. Increased intestinal secretions without disruption of intestinal mucosa; watery character
  - Inflammatory: generally invasive or toxin-producing bacteria; disrupts mucosal integrity with subsequent tissue invasion/damage; bloody character
- Viral diarrhea: changes in small intestine cell morphology, including villous shortening, increased number of crypt cells, and increased cellularity of the lamina propria
- Bacterial diarrhea: Bacterial invasion of colonic wall leads to mucosal hyperemia, edema, and leukocytic infiltration.

RISK FACTORS
- Travel to developing countries
- Failure to observe food/water precautions
- Immunocompromised host (HIV, malignancy, chemotherapy)
- Recent hospitalization
- Antibiotic use
- Proton pump inhibitor (PPI) use
- Daycare exposure
- Fecal-oral sexual contact
- Nursing home residence
- Pregnancy (12-fold increase for listeriosis) (1)

GENERAL PREVENTION
- Frequent hand washing reduces incidence of diarrhea by approximately 30%.
- Proper food and water precautions, particularly during foreign travel—"boil it, peel it, cook it, or forget it"
- Avoid undercooked meat, raw fish, unpasteurized milk.
- Rotavirus vaccine (for infants)
- Typhoid fever and cholera vaccine (for travel to endemic areas)
- TD prevention:
  - Pretravel counseling on high-risk food/beverage
  - Consider daily prophylaxis with bismuth subsalicylate (BSS) in all travelers (can reduce the risk of TD by up to 60%); usual dosing of 2 tablets (262 mg each) or 2 oz (60 mL) liquid formulation 4 times daily
  - Do not use routine antibiotic prophylaxis.
  - When indicated, the Infectious Disease Society of America recommends chemoprophylaxis with fluoroquinolones: norfloxacin 400 mg/day or ciprofloxacin 500 mg orally once or twice daily.
  - Probiotics, prebiotics, and synbiotics have unclear benefit as prophylaxis.

COMMONLY ASSOCIATED CONDITIONS
- Inflammatory bowel disease (IBD)
- Immunocompromised (HIV, malignancy, chemotherapy)

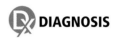

DIAGNOSIS

HISTORY
- Duration of symptoms <14 days
- Historical clues for dehydration: orthostatic hypotension, dizziness, increased thirst, decreased urine output, or altered mental status
- Description of stool—characteristics and output
  - Frequency; quantity; consistency; character: presence of mucus, blood, or fat; floating
  - *Giardia* associated with pale, greasy stools
- Weight loss
- Associated symptoms: change in appetite, abdominal pain or bloating, nausea/vomiting, or fever
- Risk factors of acute diarrhea (see "Risk Factors")
- Cirrhosis (associated with *Vibrio*)
- Hemochromatosis (associated with *Yersinia*)

PHYSICAL EXAM
- Assess degree of dehydration (1); ill-appearing, dry mucous membranes, tachycardia, orthostatic hypotension, decreased skin turgor, delayed capillary refill, altered mental status; can be absent in early dehydration
- Fever is more suggestive of inflammatory diarrhea.
- Thyroid: Assess for enlargement or nodules.
- Abdomen: Assess for distention, rigidity, rebound tenderness.
- Rectum: blood, tenderness, stool consistency

Geriatric Considerations
Fecal impaction or obstructing neoplasm can cause overflow diarrhea with chronic constipation.

DIFFERENTIAL DIAGNOSIS
- IBD
- Malabsorption
- Medications (cholinergic agents, magnesium-containing antacids, chemotherapy, antibiotics)
- Diverticulitis, ischemic colitis
- Spastic (irritable) colon
- Fecal impaction
- Endocrinopathies: thyroid disease
- Neoplasia

DIAGNOSTIC TESTS & INTERPRETATION
Initial Tests (lab, imaging)
- Reserve laboratory testing for patients with persistent fever, moderate-severe disease characterized by passage of ≥6 stools per day, duration of >72 hours, dysentery, profuse watery diarrhea, immunosuppression, or if suspected outbreak (2)[C].
- Complete blood count (CBC)
  - Leukocytosis, anemia (blood loss), eosinophilia (parasite infection), thrombocytopenia (hemolytic uremic syndrome [HUS])
- Basic metabolic panel (BMP)
  - Serum electrolytes, BUN and creatinine (may elevate with volume depletion), nonanion gap metabolic acidosis

- Stool sample
  - Occult blood (IBD, bowel ischemia, and certain bacterial infections)
  - Fecal leukocytes: useful to distinguish inflammatory diarrhea from noninflammatory but should not be used to determine the infectious cause of diarrhea
  - Stool ova and parasites
  - Stool culture
  - Multiplex stool testing (PCR testing for bacterial, viral, and parasitic causes of diarrhea)
  - *C. difficile* toxin (especially IBD, recently hospitalized, or recent antibiotic use) (3)[C]
  - *Giardia* ELISA >90% sensitive in at-risk population
- Abdominal radiographs (flat plate and upright) if severe abdominal pain or concern for obstruction
- Abdominal CT scan is preferred to evaluate intra-abdominal disease (4)[C].

Diagnostic Procedures/Other
- Consider sigmoidoscopy or colonoscopy in patients with persistent diarrhea, when there is no clear diagnosis after routine blood and stool tests, and if empiric or supportive therapy is ineffective.
- Consider colonoscopy in immunocompromised patients to evaluate for CMV colitis.

 ## TREATMENT

GENERAL MEASURES
- Oral rehydration and electrolyte management are key to successful treatment.
- Oral intake, as tolerated—"if the gut works, use it"
- Balanced electrolyte rehydration solutions recommended in elderly and profuse, watery TD (2)[C]
- IV fluids if patient cannot tolerate oral rehydration or presents with severe dehydration

MEDICATION

First Line
- Consider empiric antibiotics (fluoroquinolones or macrolides) in patients with signs and symptoms of systemic infection, severe disease, or clear cases of TD (2)[C].
  - Fever; bloody diarrhea; fecal leukocytes
  - Immunocompromised host
  - Signs of severe volume depletion
- Tailor antibiotics to stool culture results (2)[C].
  - *Giardia*: metronidazole 250 mg PO TID for 5 to 7 days, tinidazole 2 g PO once
  - *E. histolytica*: metronidazole 500 to 750 mg PO TID for 7 to 10 days, tinidazole 2 g PO daily for 3 to 5 days
  - *Shigella*: ciprofloxacin 500 mg PO BID for 3 to 5 days or ceftriaxone 1 to 2 g IM/IV daily for 5 days
  - *Campylobacter*: azithromycin 500 mg PO daily for 3 to 5 days or erythromycin 500 mg PO QID for 5 days
  - *C. difficile*: The Infectious Disease Society of America now recommends fidaxomicin 200 mg PO BID for 10 days as first-line therapy. Vancomycin 125 to 500 mg PO QID for 10 to 14 days can be used as alternative; consider fecal microbiota transplant in recurrent mild to moderate *C. difficile* infections.
  - TD: ciprofloxacin 500 mg PO BID for 1 to 3 days, azithromycin (if suspicion of quinolone-resistant pathogens) 500 mg PO daily or 1 g PO daily for 1 to 3 days, rifaximin 200 mg PO TID for 3 days; can combine with loperamide; loperamide or BSS may be used alone in cases of mild TD (5)[C].

- General considerations
  - Antibiotics are not recommended in *Salmonella* infections unless caused by *Salmonella typhosa* or if the patient is febrile or immunocompromised.
  - Avoid antibiotics in patients with *E. coli* 0157:H7 due to risk for HUS.
  - Antibiotics are not indicated for foodborne toxigenic diarrhea.
  - Avoid antimotility agents (e.g., loperamide) in patients with febrile or bloody diarrhea or antibiotic-associated colitis.
  - Antimotility agents used with antibiotics may speed recovery from TD.
  - Antibiotics are not recommended for the treatment of mild TD (5)[C].

COMPLEMENTARY & ALTERNATIVE MEDICINE
- Bismuth subsalicylate may help control rate of diarrhea stools (2),(6)[C].
- Probiotics are recommended for prevention of antibiotic-associated diarrhea and *C. difficile* infection recurrence and to treat acute infectious diarrhea in setting of symptomatic IBS (6)[C].
- Probiotic use >10^{10}/g may help in patients with antibiotic-associated diarrhea (2)[A].
- Avoid probiotics in immunocompromised patients (5)[A].

ADMISSION, INPATIENT, AND NURSING CONSIDERATIONS
Outpatient management, except for patients who are severely ill with signs of volume depletion

 ## ONGOING CARE

DIET
- Early oral refeeding is encouraged. Regular diets are as effective as restricted diets.
- The traditional bananas, rice, applesauce, toast (BRAT) diet has little evidence-based support (despite heavy clinical use) and may result in suboptimal nutrition.
- During periods of active diarrhea, coffee, alcohol, dairy products, fruits, vegetables, red meats, and heavily seasoned foods may exacerbate symptoms.

PATIENT EDUCATION
See "General Prevention."

PROGNOSIS
Acute diarrhea is rarely life-threatening if adequate hydration is maintained.

COMPLICATIONS
- Volume depletion, shock, sepsis
- HUS with *E. coli* 0157:H7
- Guillain-Barré syndrome with *C. jejuni*
- Reactive arthritis with *Salmonella*, *Shigella*, and *Yersinia*
- Functional bowel disorders (e.g., postinfectious irritable bowel syndrome [PI-IBS])

REFERENCES

1. Hamilton KW, Cifu AS. Diagnosis and management of infectious diarrhea. *JAMA*. 2019;321(9):891–892.
2. Riddle MS, DuPont HL, Connor BA. ACG clinical guideline: diagnosis, treatment, and prevention of acute diarrheal infections in adults. *Am J Gastroenterol*. 2016;111(5):602–622.
3. Khanna S, Shin A, Kelly CP. Management of *Clostridium difficile* infection in inflammatory bowel disease: expert review from the Clinical Practice Updates Committee of the AGA Institute. *Clin Gastroenterol Hepatol*. 2017;15(2):166–174.
4. DuPont HL. Acute infectious diarrhea in immunocompetent adults. *N Engl J Med*. 2014;370(16):1532–1540.
5. Riddle MS, Connor BA, Beeching NJ, et al. Guidelines for the prevention and treatment of travelers' diarrhea: a graded expert panel report. *J Travel Med*. 2017;24(Suppl 1):S57–S74.
6. Wilkins T, Sequoia J. Probiotics for gastrointestinal conditions: a summary of the evidence. *Am Fam Physician*. 2017;96(3):170–178.

ADDITIONAL READING

- da Cruz Gouveia MA, Lins MTC, da Silva GAP. Acute diarrhea with blood: diagnosis and drug treatment. *J Pediatr (Rio J)*. 2020;96(Suppl 1):20–28.
- Florez ID, Niño-Serna LF, Beltrán-Arroyave CP. Acute infectious diarrhea and gastroenteritis in children. *Curr Infect Dis Rep*. 2020;22(2):4.
- Islam S. Clinical uses of probiotics. *Medicine (Baltimore)*. 2016;95(5):e2658.

 ## SEE ALSO

Botulism; Cholera; Food Poisoning, Bacterial

CODES

ICD10
- R19.7 Diarrhea, unspecified
- A09 Infectious gastroenteritis and colitis, unspecified
- A08.4 Viral intestinal infection, unspecified

CLINICAL PEARLS
- Viruses are the most common causes of acute diarrheal illness in the United States.
- Oral rehydration is the most important and effective treatment for acute diarrhea.
- Routine stool culture is not recommended, unless patients present with bloody diarrhea, fever, severe dehydration, signs of inflammatory disease, persistent symptoms >7 days, or have a history of immunosuppression.
- Start empiric antibiotics in patients who are severely ill or immunocompromised.

DIARRHEA, CHRONIC

Marie L. Borum, MD, EdD, MPH • Jacob Thomas Newman, DO

BASICS

DESCRIPTION
- An increase in frequency of defecation, urgency, or decrease in stool consistency (typically >3 loose stools per day) for >4 weeks (1),(2)
  - Abnormal stool form is the most important defining factor; frequent defecation with normal consistency is termed pseudodiarrhea (1).
- Etiologies fall into the following categories: osmotic, secretory, malabsorptive, inflammatory, infectious, and hypermotility (2),(3).
- Infectious causes of chronic diarrhea are uncommon in immunocompetent patients.

EPIDEMIOLOGY
Incidence
Difficult to estimate as definitions vary.

Prevalence
Varies by etiology. Worldwide prevalence is ~20% (2). U.S. prevalence is ~6.6% (4).

ETIOLOGY AND PATHOPHYSIOLOGY
Disturbances in luminal water and electrolyte balance cause increased water volume in the stool.
- Osmotic (fecal osmotic gap >100 mOsm/kg) (3),(5). Resolves with a fasting trial (2)
  - Carbohydrate malabsorption
    - Disaccharides (e.g., lactose), monosaccharides (e.g., fructose), and polyols (common sugar substitutes)
  - Mg, phosphate, and sulfate ingestion
- Secretory (fecal osmotic gap <50 mOsm/kg) (1),(6). Does not resolve with a fasting trial (2)
  - Alcoholism, stimulant laxative ingestion
  - Bacterial enterotoxins (i.e., cholera)
  - Postcholecystectomy/ileal resection <100 cm
    - Excessive intestinal bile salts cause choleretic diarrhea; resolves in 6 to 12 months
  - Disordered motility
    - Postvagotomy, autonomic neuropathy
    - Hyperthyroidism
  - Neuroendocrine tumors
    - VIPoma
    - Carcinoid syndrome, gastrinoma, somatostatinoma
  - Metastatic medullary thyroid cancer
  - Adrenal insufficiency
  - Noninvasive infection: giardiasis, cryptosporidiosis
  - Microscopic colitis
  - Protein-losing enteropathy
- Malabsorptive (1),(6)
  - Celiac disease, Whipple disease
  - Tropical sprue, giardiasis
  - Chronic mesenteric ischemia, lymphatic obstruction
  - Short bowel syndrome: Ileal resection of >100 cm leads to insufficient small bowel bile salts.
  - Small intestinal bacterial overgrowth (SIBO)
  - Pancreatic exocrine insufficiency
- Inflammatory (1),(6)
  - IBD—ulcerative colitis; Crohn disease
  - Microscopic colitis
  - Diverticulitis; vasculitis; radiation enterocolitis
  - Infections: *Clostridium difficile, Entamoeba histolytica,* cytomegalovirus, tuberculosis
  - Neoplasms: colon cancer, lymphoma
- Hypermotility (normal fecal osmotic gap; 50 to 100 mOsm/kg) (1)
  - Irritable bowel syndrome (IBS)
  - Functional diarrhea
    - Pain differentiates IBS from functional diarrhea (2),(5)

- Drugs (1),(3),(6)
  - Adverse effect of >700 drugs, most commonly: NSAIDs, PPIs, colchicine, metformin, digoxin, ACE inhibitors, β-blockers, newer gliptins, theophyllines, antibiotics, SSRIs, antineoplastic agents
    - Drug-induced diarrhea is confirmed by the resolution of symptoms with medication discontinuation (3).
  - Factitious diarrhea: excessive laxative use
- Herbal products: St. John's wort, echinacea, garlic, saw palmetto, ginseng, etc.
- Infectious (1)
  - Bacterial: *C. difficile, M. avium intracellulare*
  - Viral: cytomegalovirus
  - Parasitic: *Giardia lamblia, Cryptosporidium, Isospora, E. histolytica*
  - Helminthic: *Strongyloides*
- Food allergies (1)

Genetics
- Celiac disease is associated with HLA-DQ2 and HLA-DQ8 haplotypes on major histocompatibility complex (MHC) class II (5).
- Inflammatory bowel disease (IBD) is polygenic. First-degree relative of IBD patients are at 10-fold increase of developing IBD (5).
- CF is caused by a mutation in the CF transmembrane conductance regulator (CFTR) anion channel, resulting in abnormal exocrine gland secretions of chloride.

RISK FACTORS
- Osmotic
  - Excess ingestion of nonabsorbable carbohydrates (i.e., artificial sweeteners)
  - Magnesium-containing antacids (3),(5)
  - Lactose intolerance, celiac disease
- Secretory (1)
  - Postsurgical: extensive small bowel resection/ileal surgery, vagotomy, bile acid malabsorption
  - History of neuroendocrine disease or stimulant laxative abuse
  - Dysmotility syndromes
  - Medications (i.e., NSAIDs, caffeine, metformin, colchicine, carbamazepine) (3),(5)
- Malabsorptive
  - CF; chronic alcohol abuse, celiac disease
  - Chronic pancreatitis/pancreatic insufficiency (fat malabsorption)
  - Medications (e.g., orlistat, acarbose)
- Inflammatory
  - IBD, NSAID use (3), radiation
  - HIV/AIDS
  - Antibiotic use (commonly clindamycin, amoxicillin, ampicillin, cephalosporins) (3)
  - Antineoplastic drugs (i.e., 5-fluorouracil, methotrexate, irinotecan) (3)
  - Immunosuppressant therapy
- Hypermotility
  - Psychosocial stress, preceding infection
  - Stimulant medications (i.e., macrolides, metoclopramide, senna) (3),(5)
- Genetic predisposition

ALERT
Diabetes mellitus and cholecystectomy can cause secretory and osmotic diarrhea.

GENERAL PREVENTION
Varies by etiology; treat the underlying cause.

COMMONLY ASSOCIATED CONDITIONS
- Extraintestinal manifestations of IBD include arthralgias, aphthous stomatitis, uveitis/episcleritis, erythema nodosum, pyoderma gangrenosum, perianal fistulas, rectal fissures, ankylosing spondylitis, and PSC.
- Celiac disease is associated with dermatitis herpetiformis, T1DM, and IgA deficiency.
- Many patients with IBS have behavioral comorbidities.
- Latex-food allergy syndrome: associated allergies to latex and banana, avocado, kiwi, and walnut (1)

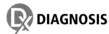

DIAGNOSIS

HISTORY
- Detailed history of symptoms (1),(2),(3):
  - Onset, pattern, and frequency of stooling, aggravating or alleviating factors
  - Stool volume and quality (including presence of blood or mucus)
  - Travel history, antibiotic use, diet patterns
  - Current medications and supplements
  - Family history (especially IBD, colorectal cancer, or CF)
- Alarm features such as rectal bleeding/melena, unintentional weight loss, fevers, or nocturnal symptoms
- Skin changes (rashes, hives), arthritis, ocular problems, heat intolerance, polyuria/polydipsia, headache, fever, flushing, alcohol intake
- Food allergies are rare, occurring in only 1–2% of adults. Consider in patients with hives (1).
- Flatus and bloating are predominant features of carbohydrate malabsorption (1).
- Prior surgery or radiation therapy (2),(6)
- Systemic illness: endocrine, immunologic
- IBS or functional diarrhea by Rome IV criteria (2),(5),(6):
  - IBS: recurrent abdominal pain at least 1 day/week in the preceding 3 months (symptoms >6 months); and ≥2 of:
    - Related to defecation
    - Change in frequency of stool
    - Change in form of stool
  - Functional diarrhea: ≥25% loose or watery stools without prominent abdominal pain or bloating for >3 months (symptoms >6 months)

PHYSICAL EXAM
- General: volume depletion, nutritional status, recent weight loss, anasarca (1),(2)
- Skin: flushing (carcinoid), erythema nodosum (IBD), pyoderma gangrenosum (IBD), ecchymoses (vitamin K deficiency), dermatitis herpetiformis (celiac disease), hyperpigmentation (Addison disease) (1),(2)
- HEENT: iritis/uveitis (IBD), lid lag (hyperthyroid)
- Neck: goiter (hyperthyroid), lymphadenopathy (Whipple disease)
- Cardiovascular: tachycardia (hyperthyroid), heart murmur (carcinoid syndrome) (2),(6)
- Pulmonary: wheezing (carcinoid)
- Abdomen: hyperactive bowel sounds (IBD), distension, and/or diffuse tenderness (IBD/IBS)
- Anorectal: anorectal fistulas or anal fissures (IBD), fecal impaction (overflow incontinence)
- Extremities: arthritis (IBD)
- Neurologic: tremor (hyperthyroid)

DIFFERENTIAL DIAGNOSIS
See "Etiology and Pathophysiology," "Commonly Associated Conditions," and "Risk Factors."

DIAGNOSTIC TESTS & INTERPRETATION

Initial Tests (lab, imaging)
Test patients with alarm symptoms or persistent symptoms and no identifiable cause.

- Blood: CBC, electrolytes (Mg, P, Ca), total protein, albumin, thyroid-stimulating hormone, free T_4, erythrocyte sedimentation rate, C-reactive protein (CRP), IgA anti–tissue transglutaminase (TTG), iron studies (1),(6)
  - Normal CRP (<10 mg/L) or fecal calprotectin (<50 μg/g) level effectively rules out IBD for patients who meet Rome IV diagnostic criteria for IBS without alarm features (5)[A].
- Stool: fecal WBC, lactoferrin/calprotectin (preferred), culture, ova and parasite, *Giardia* antigen, *C. difficile* toxin, electrolytes, occult blood, osmolality, qualitative fecal fat (Sudan stain) (1)
  - Fecal osmotic gap = 290 mOsm/kg − 2(Na[feces] + K[feces])
  - *C. difficile* testing only in diarrheal stools (5)[C]
- CT or MRI to evaluate the GI tract structure (i.e., IBD, malignancy, chronic pancreatitis) (1)

Follow-Up Tests & Special Considerations
- Celiac disease: antiendomysial antibody IgA, anti-TTG IgA (sensitivity and specificity >90%) in patients without IgA deficiency, antigliadin antibodies (AGA) IgA, serum IgA level (10% of celiac patients have IgA deficiency—may cause false-negative results)
  - IgA TTG positive result should be confirmed by duodenal biopsy (2).
- Chronic pancreatic insufficiency: fecal elastase and chymotrypsin (1)[C]
- Protein-losing enteropathy: fecal α_1-antitrypsin (1)[C]
- Microscopic colitis: normal-appearing mucosal biopsy from colon (5)[C],(6)[C]
- Carbohydrate malabsorption: fecal pH (<7.0) and hydrogen breath test
- SIBO: hydrogen breath test and proximal jejunal aspirate with >10^5 colony-forming units per milliliter coliform bacteria (5)
- Recent hospitalization or antibiotics: *C. difficile* toxin
- HIV ELISA, *Isospora/Cryptosporidium* stains (1)[C]
- Consider testing for protozoa, atypical infections, *Strongyloides*, and tropical sprue in travelers and migrants of endemic areas (1)[C].
- Allergy testing (1)[C]
- Laxative abuse: stool osmotic gap (6)[C]
- Neuroendocrine tumor (6)[C]
  - Serum: chromogranin A, VIP, gastrin, calcitonin
  - Urine: 5-HIAA, histamine
  - Imaging: CT or MRI abdomen (5)

Diagnostic Procedures/Other
- Ileocolonoscopy with biopsies: IBD, microscopic colitis, CMV colitis, and colorectal neoplasia
- Flexible sigmoidoscopy: if pregnant, with comorbidities, or if left-sided symptoms predominate (tenesmus and urgency)
- Esophagogastroduodenoscopy (EGD) with biopsies if malabsorption is suspected
- CT or magnetic resonance enterography (1)

Test Interpretation
- Celiac disease:
  - Marsh classification: intraepithelial lymphocytosis, crypt hyperplasia, villous atrophy
- Crohn disease: cobblestoning, linear ulcerations, skip lesions, noncaseating granulomas

- Ulcerative colitis: crypt abscesses, superficial inflammation, continuous rectal lesion
- Lymphocytic colitis: high intraepithelial lymphocytes, high inflammatory cells within the lamina propria, normal mucosal architecture
- Melanosis coli suggests laxative abuse (1),(3).

TREATMENT

GENERAL MEASURES
- Volume resuscitation, electrolyte repletion
- If stable, generally outpatient treatment (1)[C]

MEDICATION
First Line
- Based on underlying cause:
  - Lactose intolerance: lactose-free diet
  - Postcholecystectomy or ileal resection: cholestyramine or colestipol 2 to 16 g/day PO split BID
  - Diabetes: glucose control
  - Hyperthyroidism: methimazole 5 to 20 mg/day PO, propylthiouracil (PTU) 100 to 150 mg/day PO divided; thyroid ablation
  - *C. difficile*: 10 days of: vancomycin 125 mg PO q6h or metronidazole (Flagyl) 500 mg PO q8h or fidaxomicin 200 mg PO BID
  - *G. lamblia*: metronidazole 250 mg PO q8h ×5 to 7 days, nitazoxanide 500 mg PO q12h ×3 days (1)[A]
  - Whipple disease: ceftriaxone 2 g IV for 14 days then Bactrim DS 160/800 mg PO BID for 1 to 2 years
  - SIBO: rifaximin 550 mg PO BID, fluoroquinolones 250 to 750 mg PO BID, metronidazole 500 mg PO q6–8h
  - Pancreatic insufficiency: pancrelipase
  - HIV/AIDS: antiretroviral therapy (HAART)
  - Microscopic colitis: budesonide 9 mg/day PO, mesalamine 800 mg PO TID, bismuth subsalicylate (Pepto-Bismol) 786 mg PO TID
  - IBD: 5-ASA, short courses of corticosteroids and/or antibiotics, immunomodulators, anti-TNF therapy
  - Neuroendocrine tumor: octreotide 100 to 600 μg/day SC (1)[C]
  - Celiac disease: gluten-free diet
  - IBS diarrhea predominant: rifaximin 550 mg PO TID ×14 days, alosetron 0.5 to 1.0 mg PO BID, peppermint oil, eluxadoline 100 mg PO BID; TCAs may also be considered (1)[C].
- Symptom relief (1)[C]:
  - Loperamide 4 to 8 mg/day PO divided; only use if infectious etiology is ruled out
  - Diphenoxylate-atropine 1 to 2 tabs BID–QID
  - Fiber supplementation
  - Bismuth subsalicylate 525 to 1,050 mg every 0.5 to 1 hour; max dose 4.2 g/day (1)[C]

ISSUES FOR REFERRAL
Gastroenterology referral for suspected inflammatory diarrhea or suspected diagnoses requiring endoscopy/biopsy (e.g., celiac disease/microscopic colitis)

SURGERY/OTHER PROCEDURES
- Resection of neuroendocrine tumors
- Intestinal resection for refractory IBD
- Fecal transplant for recurrent *C. difficile*

ADMISSION, INPATIENT, AND NURSING CONSIDERATIONS
Consider inpatient hospitalization if patient is hemodynamically unstable, has severe electrolyte abnormalities, dehydration, malnutrition, AKI, or is unable to tolerate oral intake.

ONGOING CARE

DIET
- Elimination diet: Avoid gluten-containing foods, nonabsorbable carbohydrates, lactose-containing products, and food allergens.
- Low FODMAP diet helps symptoms in up to 75% of IBS patients (1),(2).
- High carbohydrate intake and obesity have been linked to chronic diarrhea (4).

PATIENT EDUCATION
- Chronic diarrhea is generally defined as three or more loose bowel movements per day for over 4 weeks.
- Wide variation in "normal" bowel habits
- Restrict colon stimulants.

PROGNOSIS
Varies according to etiology

COMPLICATIONS
- Fluid and electrolyte imbalances, AKI
- Malnutrition, anemia, weight loss
- Malignancy (colon cancer [IBD], lymphoma [IBD therapies], small bowel cancer [celiac, Crohn])
- Infection with immunosuppressive therapies for IBD

REFERENCES

1. Schiller LR, Pardi DS, Sellin JH. Chronic diarrhea: diagnosis and management. *Clin Gastroenterol Hepatol*. 2017;15(2):182–193.e3.
2. Chu C, Rotondo-Trivette S, Michail S. Chronic diarrhea. *Curr Probl Pediatr Adolesc Health Care*. 2020;50(8):100841.
3. Philip NA, Ahmed N, Pitchumoni CS. Spectrum of drug-induced chronic diarrhea. *J Clin Gastroenterol*. 2017;51(2):111–117.
4. Singh P, Mitsuhashi S, Ballou S, et al. Demographic and dietary associations of chronic diarrhea in a representative sample of adults in the United States. *Am J Gastroenterol*. 2018;113(4):593–600.
5. Burgers K, Lindberg B, Bevis ZJ. Chronic diarrhea in adults: evaluation and differential diagnosis. *Am Fam Physician*. 2020;101(8):472–480.
6. Schiller LR. Evaluation of chronic diarrhea and irritable bowel syndrome with diarrhea in adults in the era of precision medicine. *Am J Gastroenterol*. 2018;113(5):660–669.

 SEE ALSO

Algorithm: Diarrhea, Chronic

CODES

ICD10
K52.9 Noninfective gastroenteritis and colitis, unspecified

CLINICAL PEARLS
- A comprehensive medical history guides the appropriate workup and avoids unnecessary testing.
- Consider IBS, IBD, malabsorption syndromes, celiac disease, prescribed or OTC medication use, herbal product use, and chronic infections (immunocompromised) in the differential diagnosis.
- Treatment is based on the underlying cause.

D

DIFFUSE INTERSTITIAL LUNG DISEASE

J. Andrew Woods, PharmD, BCPS • Jacqueline L. Olin, CDCES, PharmD, FASHP, MS, FCCP, BCPS • Brice T. Taylor, MD, MSc

 BASICS

DESCRIPTION
- Interstitial lung diseases (ILDs) represent a diverse group of chronic progressive lung diseases associated with alveolar inflammation and/or potentially irreversible pulmonary fibrosis.
- >200 individual diseases may present with similar characteristics, making ILD difficult to classify.
- A classification scheme proposed by the American Thoracic Society and European Respiratory Society includes these subtypes:
  - Known causes (environmental, occupational, or drug-associated disease)
  - Systemic disorders (e.g., sarcoidosis, Wegener granulomatosis, collagen vascular disease)
  - Rare lung diseases (e.g., pulmonary histiocytosis, lymphangioleiomyomatosis)
  - Idiopathic interstitial pneumonias (IIPs)
- Based on clinical, radiologic, and histologic features, IIPs are further subclassified into the following diagnoses:
  - Major IIPs, including idiopathic pulmonary fibrosis (IPF), nonspecific interstitial pneumonia (NSIP), respiratory bronchiolitis-associated ILD (cryptogenic organizing pneumonia [COP], etc.)
  - Rare IIPs
  - Unclassifiable IIPs
- Classification of IIPs and relationships between the subtypes are difficult to classify due to mixed patterns of injury.

Pediatric Considerations
ILD in infants and children represents a heterogeneous group of respiratory disorders. Diseases result from a variety of processes involving genetic factors and inflammatory or fibrotic responses, and processes are distinct from those that cause ILD in adults. Some diseases result from developmental disorders and growth abnormalities in infancy.

EPIDEMIOLOGY
Incidence
Exact incidence and prevalence are difficult to determine because of differences in case definitions and procedures used in diagnosis. U.S. incidence: 16.3 to 17.4

Prevalence
Prevalence in United States: 42.7 to 63 cases/100,000 in the general population and pediatric ILD of 3.6/1 million

ETIOLOGY AND PATHOPHYSIOLOGY
- Alveolar inflammation may progress into irreversible fibrosis.
- Varying degrees of ventilatory dysfunction occur among the ILD subtypes.
- ILD associated with collagen vascular disease and systemic connective disorders can manifest involvement of skin, joints, muscular, and ocular systems.

- Some types of ILD are associated with specific exposures:
  - Medications (amiodarone, antibiotics [especially nitrofurantoin], chemotherapy agents, gold, illicit drugs)
  - Inorganic dusts (silicates, asbestos, talc, mica, coal dust, graphite)
  - Organic dusts (moldy hay, inhalation of fungi, bacteria, animal proteins)
  - Metals (tin, aluminum, cobalt, iron, barium)
  - Gases, fumes, vapors, aerosols

Genetics
Role of genetic factors is unknown.

RISK FACTORS
- Environmental or occupational exposure to inorganic or organic dusts
- 66–75% of patients with ILD have a history of smoking.
- Due to diversity of diseases, age is not a reliable predictor of pathology:
  - Most patients with connective tissue disease–related pathology and inherited subtypes present between ages 20 and 40 years
  - Median age of patients with IPF is 66 years. Studies of clinical predictors of survival including age, ethnicity, and smoking status have been inconsistent.

COMMONLY ASSOCIATED CONDITIONS
Many systemic disorders and primary diseases are associated with ILD. A partial list includes the following:
- Collagen vascular disease
- Sarcoidosis
- Amyloidosis
- Goodpasture syndrome
- Churg-Strauss syndrome
- Wegener granulomatosis

DIAGNOSIS

Diagnosis of IPF requires exclusion of other known ILD causes, the presence of a UIP pattern on high-resolution computed tomography (HRCT), and/or surgical lung biopsy pattern (1).

HISTORY
- Progressive exertional dyspnea and nonproductive cough; may also have hemoptysis or fatigue
- Obtaining a history of illness duration (acute vs. chronic), potential environmental/occupational exposures, travel, medical conditions (including systemic diseases), and medication reconciliation is important in assessing the cause of the ILD.
- Some cases of lung disease may occur weeks to years after discontinuation of an offending agent.

PHYSICAL EXAM
Physical findings are usually nonspecific. Some common features include the following:
- Fine crackles (typically present on auscultation of lung bases on posterior axillary line)
- Inspiratory "squeaks"
- Clubbing of the digits and cyanosis in advanced disease

DIFFERENTIAL DIAGNOSIS
- Acute pulmonary edema
- Diffuse hemorrhage
- Atypical pneumonia
- Diffuse bronchoalveolar cell carcinoma or lymphatic spread of tumor

DIAGNOSTIC TESTS & INTERPRETATION
Initial Tests (lab, imaging)
- O₂ saturation
- Peak expiratory flow rate
- CBC with differential, comprehensive metabolic profile, CRP, or erythrocyte sedimentation rate (ESR)
- Chest x-ray (CXR): most commonly reticular pattern, less commonly nodular or mixed patterns

Follow-Up Tests & Special Considerations
HRCT of the chest is the most useful tool for diagnosing then distinguishing among ILD subclasses, especially if normal CXRs:
- If indicated, arterial blood gas (ABG), hypersensitivity pneumonitis panel, plasma ACE inhibitor concentration (sarcoidosis)
- If a systemic disorder is suspected, consider antinuclear antibody (ANA), rheumatoid factor (RF), antineutrophil cytoplasmic antibodies (ANCA), anti-cyclic citrullinated peptide (anti-CCP), and a myositis panel.

Diagnostic Procedures/Other
- Pulmonary function test (PFT; spirometry, lung volumes, carbon monoxide diffusing capacity)
  - Commonly demonstrates a restrictive defect (decreased vital capacity and total lung capacity)
  - Forced vital capacity (FVC) has been shown to decline 100 to 200 mL/year in the placebo arm of IPF patients in clinical trials.
- Bronchoscopy
  - Bronchoalveolar lavage (BAL) cellular analysis studies may be useful in distinguishing subtypes (including sarcoidosis, hypersensitivity pneumonitis, cancer). If performed, the BAL target site should be chosen based on the HRCT finding.
  - Bronchoscopic transbronchial lung biopsy may help diagnose sarcoidosis and, on occasion, is sufficiently supportive of other ILD diagnoses.
- Thoracoscopic surgery for lung biopsy has the greatest diagnostic specificity for ILDs but is less frequently used; given improved specificity of HRCT, may be indicated if a diagnosis cannot be determined from transbronchial biopsy or HRCT

Test Interpretation

- Diagnostic classifications of IIPs are based on histo-pathologic patterns seen on lung biopsy.
- Characteristic changes on HRCT may help to distinguish between the following subtypes:
  - Reticulonodular, ground-glass opacities, and, in later stages, honeycombing may be seen.
  - Associated hilar and mediastinal adenopathy are characteristic of stage I and II sarcoidosis.
- No specific test is the gold standard, which emphasizes the importance of a multidisciplinary consensus for diagnosis with clinical, radiologic, and pathologic findings.

TREATMENT

- Evidence does not support the routine use of any specific therapy for ILD in general, especially IPF.
- No survival benefit of home oxygen use in ILD
- Corticosteroids have a role in some ILD subtypes.
- Current evidence does not clearly support routine use of noncorticosteroid anti-inflammatory agents for IPF, including cyclosporine, colchicine, cyclophosphamide, cytokines, sildenafil, dual endothelin receptor antagonists (bosentan, macitentan), etanercept, methotrexate, or interferon.
- Current evidence does not support the routine use of antimicrobials, specifically co-trimoxazole and doxycycline, for IPF.
- Clinical trials have indicated that anticoagulation (warfarin), ambrisentan, imatinib, and the combination of prednisone, azathioprine, and N-acetylcysteine are ineffective, potentially harmful, and therefore not recommended in the treatment of IPF.
- Thrombomodulin alfa was not effective in improving 3-month survival following acute exacerbation of IPF in an RCT despite early promise in a small historical control study.

GENERAL MEASURES

- Avoid/minimize offending environmental/occupational exposures/medications.
- Smoking cessation
- Supplemental oxygen, if indicated
- Annual influenza vaccination and pneumococcal vaccination, when indicated

MEDICATION

First Line

- Corticosteroids are most effective for certain ILDs, especially exacerbations of sarcoidosis, nonspecific interstitial pneumonia (NSIP), cryptogenic organizing pneumonia (COP), and hypersensitivity pneumonitis. However, response rates have been variable across and within subtypes. The optimal dose and duration of therapy are unknown.
  - Common starting dose of prednisone is 0.5 to 1.0 mg/kg/day for 4 to 12 weeks with potential up-titration based on patient response.
- In patients with ILD associated with systemic sclerosis, nintedanib (Ofev), a tyrosine kinase inhibitor, reduced the rate of FVC decline versus placebo at 52 weeks.
- Nintedanib has been shown to significantly decrease the annual rate of FVC decline in patients with progressive fibrosing ILDs in comparison to placebo.

- Two antifibrotic agents approved for IPF exhibited modest slowing of FVC decline over 52 weeks compared to placebo. Both decreased all-cause mortality rates. It is not clear if FVC is the most conclusive meaningful efficacy variable for IPF.
  - Pirfenidone (Esbriet) decreased the rate of decline in FVC compared to placebo with a significant improvement in progression-free survival, and pooled analysis reveals a significant reduction in all-cause death and death from IPF and reduce respiratory-related hospitalizations in IPF. Common adverse effects are GI related (nausea, vomiting, anorexia, weight loss, GERD, and dyspepsia), rash, insomnia, dizziness, fatigue, and aminotransferase elevation; most are mild to moderate and do not result in pirfenidone discontinuation. Pirfenidone is not recommended for patients with severe liver impairment or ESRD.
  - Pirfenidone is titrated over 2 weeks to 801 mg PO 3 times daily with food.
  - Nintedanib reduced the annual rate of decline in FVC, and fewer acute exacerbations occurred compared to placebo. The most common adverse effects are GI upset (nausea, vomiting, diarrhea, abdominal pain), anorexia, aminotransferase elevation, and hypertension. It is not recommended in moderate to severe liver impairment and can cause birth defects.
  - Nintedanib is given at 150 mg PO twice daily with food.
  - Adding pirfenidone to nintedanib may convey a synergistic effect but could be limited by GI upset. Further investigation is warranted.

Second Line

- The addition of tacrolimus to corticosteroids (with cyclosporine, cyclophosphamide, or no additional therapy) may improve event-free survival in patients with ILD complicated with polymyositis or dermatomyositis.
- Several second-line agents have been used in Wegener granulomatosis:
  - Cyclophosphamide is commonly used in treatment of Wegener granulomatosis. It is given 1.5 to 2.0 mg/kg/day PO for 3 to 6 months.
  - Methotrexate has been used in treatment of mild Wegener granulomatosis in combination with corticosteroids. A studied dosing regimen consisted of an initial dose of 0.3 mg/kg (max dose of 15 mg) once weekly, with 2.5 mg titration each week (max dose of 25 mg/week).
  - Other second-line agents that have been studied include mycophenolate mofetil and rituximab.

SURGERY/OTHER PROCEDURES

- Single- or double-lung transplantation may be a treatment of last resort. Lung transplant among selected IPF patients has demonstrated median survival of 4.5 years. Some ILDs associated with systemic disease may recur in the recipient lung.
- Alveolar type II cell intratracheal transplantation may benefit patients with moderate to progressive IPF.
- Clinical trials to assess the safety and efficacy of allogeneic human mesenchymal stem cell infusion in patients with mild to moderate IPF are ongoing.

ONGOING CARE

FOLLOW-UP RECOMMENDATIONS

Follow-up testing should include PFTs, 6-minute walk test, pulse oximetry, and CXR.

PATIENT EDUCATION

National Heart, Lung, and Blood Institute: http://www.nhlbi.nih.gov/health/health-topics/topics/ipf/

PROGNOSIS

Median survival of 2.5 to 3 years

COMPLICATIONS

- Cor pulmonale
- Pulmonary hypertension
- Pneumothorax
- Progressive respiratory failure

REFERENCE

1. Raghu G, Martine RJ, Myers JL, et al. Diagnosis of idiopathic pulmonary fibrosis: an official ATS/ERS/JRS/ALAT clinical practice guideline. *Am J Resp Crit Care Med*. 2018;198(5):e44–e68.

ADDITIONAL READING

- Glassberg MK, Minkiewicz J, Toonkel RL, et al. Allogeneic human mesenchymal stem cells in patients with idiopathic pulmonary fibrosis via intravenous delivery (AETHER): a phase I safety clinical trial. *Chest*. 2017;151(5):971–978.
- Kondoh Y, Azuma A, Inoue Y, et al. Thrombomodulin alfa for acute exacerbation of idiopathic pulmonary fibrosis. A randomized, double-blind placebo controlled trial. *Am J Respir Crit Care Med*. 2020;201(9):1110–1119.
- Serro-Mollar A, Gay-Jordi G, Guillamat-Prats R, et al. Safety and tolerability of alveolar type II cell transplantation in idiopathic pulmonary fibrosis. *Chest*. 2016;150(3):533–543.

CODES

ICD10

- J84.9 Interstitial pulmonary disease, unspecified
- J84.10 Pulmonary fibrosis, unspecified
- J84.111 Idiopathic interstitial pneumonia, not otherwise specified

CLINICAL PEARLS

- ILD differs from chronic obstructive pulmonary disease (COPD); anatomically, ILD involves the lung parenchyma (i.e., alveoli), and COPD involves both airways and alveoli.
- In some cases, avoiding or minimizing offending environmental/occupational exposures, medications, and smoking may alter disease severity.

D

DIVERTICULAR DISEASE
Brianna Stadsvold, MD • Davis M. O'Brien, MD • Steven B. Holsten Jr., MD, FACS

BASICS

DESCRIPTION
Diverticulum (single) or diverticula (multiple) are outpouchings of the colonic wall. Diverticular disease is a spectrum of diseases impacting the entire GI tract (except the rectum):

- Asymptomatic diverticulosis: common incidental finding on routine colonoscopy or imaging
- Symptomatic diverticulosis: also known as symptomatic uncomplicated diverticular disease (SUDD); recurrent abdominal pain attributed to diverticulosis without colitis or diverticulitis (1)
- Acute diverticulitis: diverticular disease with associated inflammation and/or infection
  - Uncomplicated diverticulitis: abdominal pain and leukocytosis without peritoneal signs or systemic toxicity
  - Complicated diverticulitis: secondary abscess formation, bowel obstruction, perforation, peritonitis, fistula, or stricture in the setting of diverticular inflammation
- Diverticular bleeding
  - Accounts for >40% of lower GI bleeds; often presents as painless hematochezia unless associated with active diverticulitis
  - Bleeding is more common with right-sided diverticula.

EPIDEMIOLOGY
Incidence
- Diverticular disease accounts for <300,000 hospitalizations per year in the United States.
- Diverticulitis occurs in 1–2% of the general population and in 4% of patients with diverticulosis over the course of their lifetime (1).
- Diverticular bleeding occurs in 3–5% of patients with diverticulosis.

Prevalence
- Prevalence of diverticulosis and the number of diverticula increase with age.
  - Diverticulosis occurs in 20% of those age 40 years, 60% of those age 60 years, and 70% by the age of 80 years.
  - Incidence of diverticulitis increased from 62 to 75/100,000 from 1998 to 2005; largest increase in patients <45 years of age—mostly due to changes in diet
- Male = female overall; more common in men <65 years of age and more common in women >65 years

ETIOLOGY AND PATHOPHYSIOLOGY
Diverticula form at points of weakness along the intestinal wall where small blood vessels (vasa recta) penetrate through the muscular layer of the colon.

- Age-related degeneration of the mucosal wall; increased intraluminal pressure from dense, fiber-depleted stools; and abnormal colonic motility contribute to diverticulosis
- Most right-sided diverticula are true diverticula (involves all layers of the colonic wall).
- Most left-sided diverticula are pseudodiverticula (outpouchings of the mucosa and submucosa only).

- Diverticulitis occurs when local inflammation and infection contribute to tissue necrosis with risk for mucosal micro- or macroperforation. Microscopy reveals inflammation with lymphocytic infiltrate, ulceration, mucin depletion, necrosis, Paneth cell metaplasia, and cryptitis.
- Alterations in intestinal microbiota contribute to chronic inflammation (1).
- Thinning of the vasa recta over the neck of the diverticula increases susceptibility to bleeding.
- Diverticular disease and irritable bowel syndrome may represent the same disease continuum.

Genetics
- Although genetics may play a role, there is no known genetic pattern.
- Asian and African populations have lower overall prevalence but develop diverticular disease with adoption of a Western lifestyle.

RISK FACTORS
- Age >40 years
- Low-fiber diet
- Sedentary lifestyle, obesity
- Previous diverticulitis. Risk rises with the number of diverticula.
- Smoking increases the risk of perforation (1).
- Risk of diverticular bleeding increases with NSAIDs, steroids, and opiate analgesics. Calcium channel blockers and statins protect against diverticular bleeding.

GENERAL PREVENTION
- High-fiber diet or nonabsorbable fiber (psyllium)
- Regular physical activity

COMMONLY ASSOCIATED CONDITIONS
Colon cancer, connective tissue diseases, obesity, irritable bowel syndrome, and inflammatory bowel disease

DIAGNOSIS

HISTORY
- Diverticulosis
  - 80–85% of patients are asymptomatic. Of the 15–20% with symptoms, 1–2% will require hospitalization, and 0.5% will undergo surgery.
  - The most common symptom is dull, colicky abdominal pain, typically in the LLQ. Pain can be exacerbated by eating and by passing bowel movement or flatus.
  - Diarrhea or constipation is common.
- Acute diverticulitis: uncomplicated (85%) and complicated (15%)
  - Abdominal pain: acute onset, typically in LLQ
  - Fever and/or chills
  - Anorexia, nausea (20–62%), or vomiting
  - Constipation (50%) or diarrhea (25–35%)
  - Dysuria and urinary frequency suggest bladder or ureteral irritation.
  - Pneumaturia and fecaluria if associated with a colovesical fistula
- Diverticular bleeding
  - Melena, hematochezia (0.5/1,000 person-years)
  - Painless rectal bleeding
- Immunocompromised patients may not present with fever or leukocytosis and are at higher risk for perforation and abscess formation.

PHYSICAL EXAM
- Diverticulosis
  - Exam is usually normal.
  - May have intermittent distension or tympany
  - May have heme + stools
- Acute diverticulitis
  - Abdominal tenderness (usually LLQ)
  - Abdominal distension and tympany
  - Rebound tenderness, involuntary guarding, or rigidity suggests perforation and/or peritonitis.
  - Palpable mass in LLQ (20%)
  - Bowel sounds hypoactive (could be high-pitched and intermittent if obstruction is present)
  - Rectal exam may reveal tenderness or a mass.
  - Colovaginal, colovesical, and perirectal fistulae are rarely the initial presentation.

DIFFERENTIAL DIAGNOSIS
Urinary tract infection, nephrolithiasis, irritable bowel syndrome, lactose intolerance, carcinoma, inflammatory bowel disease, fecal impaction, bowel obstruction, angiodysplasia, ischemic colitis, acute appendicitis, ectopic pregnancy

DIAGNOSTIC TESTS & INTERPRETATION
Initial Tests (lab, imaging)
- Diverticulosis: no labs or imaging needed
- Acute diverticulitis
  - WBC count is normal in up to 45% of cases. As diverticulitis worsens, WBC count becomes elevated with left shift.
  - Hemoglobin normal (unless bleeding)
  - ESR elevated
  - Urinalysis may show microscopic pyuria or hematuria.
  - Urine culture: usually normal; persistent infection is suspicious for colovesical fistula.
  - Blood cultures positive in systemic cases
  - Plain films of the abdomen (acute abdominal series—supine and upright) to assess for free air under the diaphragm (bowel perforation) and signs of bowel obstruction (dilated loops of bowel)
  - CT scan with IV, oral, and/or rectal contrast (sensitivity: 98%, specificity: 99%) to stage disease and determine treatment plan (2)[A]
  - Ultrasound and MRI (sensitivity: 94%, specificity: 92%) are useful alternatives.
  - Barium enema is not recommended due to risk of peritoneal extravasation.
- Diverticular bleeding
  - Anemia with bleeding
  - Obtain coagulation panel for coagulopathy.

Diagnostic Procedures/Other
Diverticular bleeding

- Endoscopy to evaluate GI bleeding
- NG lavage to exclude upper GI bleeding
- Angiography if bleeding obscures endoscopy or when endoscopy cannot visualize a source
- ^{99m}Tc-pertechnetate–labeled RBC scan (more sensitive) with follow-up angiography to localize bleeding (not studied in a comparison trial)

TREATMENT

GENERAL MEASURES
- Diverticulosis: outpatient therapy with fiber supplementation and/or bulking agents (psyllium) (>30 g/day) (2)[A]
- Uncomplicated diverticulitis: outpatient therapy (see exceptions below) with or without oral antibiotics. 1–2% of subjects require hospitalization for toxicity, septicemia, peritonitis, or failure of symptoms to resolve. Up to 30% of patients may require surgery at first episode of diverticulitis.
- Complicated diverticulitis: hospitalization, bowel rest, and IV antibiotics. Hinchey classification (severity):
  - Stage I: diverticulitis + confined paracolic abscess
  - Stage II: diverticulitis + distant abscess
  - Stage III: diverticulitis + purulent peritonitis
  - Stage IV: diverticulitis + fecal peritonitis
- Symptomatic improvement is expected within 2 to 3 days. Antibiotics should be continued for 7 to 10 days.
- Diverticular bleeding: 80% of cases resolve spontaneously.

MEDICATION
First Line
- Symptomatic diverticulosis: cyclical rifaximin 400 mg PO BID for 7 days every month or continuous mesalamine 800 mg PO BID (2)[C]
- Acute diverticulitis
  - The routine use of antibiotics in uncomplicated diverticulitis is controversial (2),(3)[C].
  - Outpatient oral antibiotics: Cover for anaerobes and gram-negative bacteria with:
    - A fluoroquinolone (ciprofloxacin 750 mg BID or levofloxacin 750 mg QD) *plus* metronidazole 500 mg TID (may use clindamycin if metronidazole intolerant) or
    - Trimethoprim/sulfamethoxazole DS BID *plus* metronidazole 500 mg TID
    - Treat for 7 to 10 days.
  - Inpatient: Use IV antibiotics.
    - Monotherapy with a β-lactam/β-lactamase inhibitor: piperacillin/tazobactam (3,375 g IV QID) or ampicillin/sulbactam 3 g IV q6h or ertapenem (1 g IV QD)
    - Penicillin-allergic patient: quinolone (levofloxacin 750 mg IV QD plus metronidazole 500 mg IV TID)
    - Unresponsive or severe disease: imipenem or meropenem
  - Recurrences of acute diverticulitis may be decreased by using mesalamine ± rifaximin or probiotics.
- Diverticular bleeding
  - Consider vasopressin 0.2 to 0.3 U/min through selective intra-arterial catheter.
- Precautions
  - Avoid morphine and other opiates that may increase intraluminal pressure or promote ileus.
  - Increased fiber intake is not recommended in the acute management of diverticulitis.

Second Line
- Outpatient: amoxicillin/clavulanate monotherapy (875/125 mg BID) (contraindicated in patients with clearance <30 mL/min) or moxifloxacin (400 mg PO QD) *plus* metronidazole (500 mg PO TID)
- Severely ill inpatients: ampicillin (500 mg IV q6h) + metronidazole (500 mg IV TID) + a quinolone *or* ampicillin + metronidazole + an aminoglycoside

ISSUES FOR REFERRAL
- Acute diverticulitis patients should follow up with a gastroenterologist or surgeon after resolution of diverticulitis (6 to 8 weeks) for colonoscopy to exclude malignancy, fistula, strictures, or inflammatory bowel disease (2).
- Acute complicated diverticulitis should have appropriate surgical and critical care/infectious disease consultations.

SURGERY/OTHER PROCEDURES
- Acute diverticulitis
  - Indications for emergent surgery: peritonitis, uncontrolled sepsis, perforation, obstruction
  - Hinchey I and II: consultation to interventional radiology to drain large abscesses (>4 cm)
  - Hinchey III or IV: frequently requires surgery during the same hospital admission
  - Elective colon resection in recurrent diverticulitis is a case-by-case decision and is typically performed during the quiescent phase following appropriate nonoperative treatment (2).
  - Immunocompromised patients are more likely to present with acute complicated diverticulitis, fail medical management, and have complications from elective surgery.
- Diverticular bleeding
  - Endoscopy and hemostasis via epinephrine injection, electrocautery, or clipping
  - Angiography is preferred over endoscopy in unstable patients to identify the bleeding source and embolize the feeding artery.
  - Massive or recurrent bleeding requires limited or subtotal colectomy to control hemorrhage.

COMPLEMENTARY & ALTERNATIVE MEDICINE
Probiotics have been used to prevent recurrence with mixed success.

ADMISSION, INPATIENT, AND NURSING CONSIDERATIONS
- Admit for systematic toxicity, sepsis, and/or peritonitis (complicated diverticulitis).
- Consider admitting patients with uncomplicated diverticulitis and the following: elderly, immunocompromised, evidence of microperforation, marked leukocytosis, temperature >39°C, intolerance of PO intake, severe abdominal pain, or unreliable follow-up.

ONGOING CARE

FOLLOW-UP RECOMMENDATIONS
Patient Monitoring
- Follow up outpatients 2 to 3 days after initiating antibiotic therapy and then weekly thereafter until symptom resolution.
  - Repeat imaging and/or inpatient therapy may be required if there is disease progression at follow-up.
- Colonoscopy should be performed in 6 to 8 weeks (unless done within the past year).

DIET
- Bowel rest with NPO during acute diverticulitis; advance diet as tolerated as bowel function returns
- Patients with known diverticulosis or a history of diverticulitis should consume a high-fiber diet to prevent recurrence (3).
- Avoiding nuts and popcorn is not necessary (3).

PROGNOSIS
- Good with early detection and prompt treatment
- After first episode of diverticulitis, there is a 33% chance of recurrence. After a second episode, there is a 66% chance of further recurrence.
- Most complications occur during first bout of diverticulitis.
- Younger patients are more likely to have recurrence.
- Rebleeding occurs in up to 6%.

COMPLICATIONS
Hemorrhage, perforation, peritonitis, obstruction, abscess, or colovesicular/colovaginal fistula

REFERENCES
1. Tursi A, Scarpignato C, Strate LL, et al. Colonic diverticular disease. *Nat Rev Dis Primers*. 2020;6(1):20.
2. Eckmann JD, Shaukat A. Updates in the understanding and management of diverticular disease. *Curr Opin Gastroenterol*. 2022;38(1):48–54.
3. Stollman N, Smalley W, Hirano I; for American Gastroenterological Association Institute Clinical Guidelines Committee. American Gastroenterological Association Institute guideline on the management of acute diverticulitis. *Gastroenterology*. 2015;149(7):1944–1949.

ADDITIONAL READING
- Böhm SK. Excessive body weight and diverticular disease. *Visc Med*. 2021;37(5):372–382.
- Katz LH, Guy DD, Lahat A, et al. Diverticulitis in the young is not more aggressive than in the elderly, but it tends to recur more often: systematic review and meta-analysis. *J Gastroenterol Hepatol*. 2013;28(8):1274–1281.
- Maguire LH. Genetic risk factors for diverticular disease-emerging evidence. *J Gastrointest Surg*. 2020;24(10):2314–2317.
- Nally DM, Kavanagh DO. Current controversies in the management of diverticulitis: a review. *Dig Surg*. 2019;36(3):195–205.

CODES

ICD10
- K57.92 Diverticulitis of intestine, part unspecified, without perforation or abscess without bleeding
- K57.13 Diverticulitis of small intestine without perforation or abscess with bleeding
- K57.21 Diverticulitis of large intestine with perforation and abscess with bleeding

CLINICAL PEARLS
- Diverticulosis is common in elderly patients with a sedentary lifestyle who consume a Western diet.
- Patients with diverticulosis benefit from a high-fiber diet.
- Antibiotics may not be necessary for low-risk patients with acute uncomplicated diverticulitis.
- Not all patients with recurrent diverticulitis require surgical intervention (colectomy).
- Dietary restrictions do not prevent recurrent diverticulitis.
- After an episode of diverticulitis, patients should undergo colonoscopy to rule out malignancy.
- Diverticular disease is a common cause of GI bleeding.

D

DOMESTIC VIOLENCE

Rhonda A. Faulkner, PhD • Alyssa Jeanne Vest Hart, DO • Radhika Agarwal, MD

BASICS

DESCRIPTION
- Domestic violence (DV) is the behavior in any relationship that is used to gain or maintain power and control over an intimate partner.
- May include physical, sexual, and/or emotional abuse; economic or psychological actions; or threats of actions that influence another person
- Although women are at greater risk of experiencing DV, it occurs among patients of any race, age, sexual orientation, religion, gender, socioeconomic background.
- Synonym(s): intimate partner violence (IPV); spousal abuse; family violence

EPIDEMIOLOGY
Prevalence
- DV occurs in 1 of 4 American families. In the United States, lifetime estimates of DV are 22–39% for women. DV affects both sexes, but women are more likely to be victims and report partner violence than men.
- Each year, nearly 5.3 million incidents of DV occur among U.S. women ≥18 years old and 3.2 million incidents among men.
- DV results in nearly 2 million injuries and up to 4,000 deaths annually in the United States.
- Costs of DV are estimated to exceed $5.8 billion annually.
- DV survivors have a 1.6- to 2.3-fold increase in health care use.
- DV incidents increased by 8.1% in during lockdown restrictions in the COVID-19 pandemic.

Geriatric Considerations
4–6% of elderly are abused, with ~2 million elderly persons experiencing abuse and/or neglect each year. In 90% of cases, the perpetrator is a family member.

Pediatric Considerations
- >3 million children aged 3 to 17 years are at risk for witnessing acts of DV.
- ~1 million abused children are identified in the United States each year.
- Children living in violent homes are at increased risk of physical, sexual, and/or emotional abuse; anxiety and depression; decreased self-esteem; emotional, behavioral, social, and/or physical disturbances; and lifelong poor health.

Pregnancy Considerations
- DV occurs during 7–20% of pregnancies. Women with unintended pregnancy are at 3 times greater risk of DV.
- 25% of abused women report exacerbation of abuse during pregnancy. There is a positive correlation between DV and postpartum depression.

RISK FACTORS
- Patient/victim risk factors
  - Substance abuse (drug or alcohol), high-risk sexual behavior
  - Poverty/financial stressors/unemployment/less education

- Recent loss of social support, family disruption and life cycle changes, social isolation
  - Prior history of abusive relationships or experiencing abuse as child
  - Mental or physical disability in family
  - Pregnancy
  - Attempting to leave the relationship
- Perpetrator risk factors
  - Substance abuse, depression, personality disorders
  - Young age
  - Unemployment, recent job loss or instability, low academic achievement
  - Witnessing/experiencing violence as child
  - Threatening to self or others, violence to children or outside the home
  - Owns weapons
- Relational risk factors
  - Marital conflict or instability, economic stress, traditional gender role norms, poor family functioning, obsessive/controlling relationship

Geriatric Considerations
Factors associated with geriatric abuse: increasing age, nonwhite race, low-income status, functional impairment, cognitive disability, substance use, poor emotional state, low self-esteem, cohabitation, and lack of social support

Pediatric Considerations
Factors associated with child abuse or neglect: low-income status, low maternal education, nonwhite race, large family size, young maternal age, single-parent household, parental psychiatric disturbances, and presence of a stepfather

DIAGNOSIS

- DV is often underdiagnosed, with only 10–12% of physicians conducting routine screening.
- The U.S. Preventive Services Task Force (USPSTF) in 2013 issued guidelines recommending that clinicians screen all women of reproductive age for DV and provide or refer women to intervention services when appropriate (1)[A].
- Other recommendations:
  - The World Health Organization (WHO) recommends against DV screening; however, they recommend asking about exposure to DV when assessing conditions that may be caused or complicated by abuse (2)[C].
  - There is no evidence of harm in screening for DV.

Pregnancy Considerations
American College of Obstetrics and Gynecologists (ACOG) and AMA guidelines on DV recommend that physicians routinely assess all pregnant women for DV. ACOG recommends periodic screening throughout obstetric care (at the first prenatal visit, at least once per trimester, at the postpartum checkup).

Pediatric Considerations
American Academy of Pediatrics (AAP) and AMA recommend that physicians remain alert for signs and symptoms of child physical and sexual abuse in the routine exam.

- Barriers to screening: time constraints, discomfort with the subject, fear of offending the patient, and lack of perceived skills and resources to manage DV
- Abused patients may refuse to disclose abuse for many reasons, which include the following:
  - Not feeling emotionally ready to admit the situation, shame and self-blame, fear of rejection by the physician, fear of retribution from abuse, belief that abuse will not happen again, belief that no alternatives or available resources exist

HISTORY
- Physicians should introduce the subject of DV in a general way (i.e., "I routinely ask all patients about domestic violence. Have you ever been in a relationship where you were afraid?").
- Screen patient alone, without partner or others present.
- Ask screening questions in patient's primary language; do not use children or other family members as interpreters.
- HITS questions: Each HITS question is scored on a 5-point scale (never, rarely, sometimes, fairly often and frequently, with a score of >10 indicating likely victimization; sensitivity 30–100% and specificity 86–96%). "How often does your partner:
  - **H**urt you physically? **I**nsult or talk down to you? **T**hreaten you with harm? **S**cream or curse at you?"
- Partner Violence Scale (sensitivity, 35–71%; specificity, 80–94%)
  - "Have you ever been hit, kicked, punched, or otherwise, hurt by someone within the past year? If so, by whom?"
  - "Do you feel safe in your current relationship?"
  - "Is there a partner from a previous relationship who is making you feel unsafe now?"
- SAFE questions
  - **S**tress/safety: "Do you feel safe in your relationship?"
  - **A**fraid/abused: "Have you ever been in a relationship where you were threatened, hurt, or afraid?"
  - **F**riends/family: "Are your friends or family aware that you have been hurt? Could you tell them, and would they be able to give you support?"
  - **E**mergency plan: "Do you have a safe place to go and the resources you need in an emergency?"
- Assess pregnancy difficulties such as poor/late prenatal care, low-birth-weight babies, and perinatal deaths as well as repeat abortions (unplanned pregnancy may be a result of sexual assault or reproductive coercion).
- Pelvic and abdominal pain, chronic without demonstrable pathology, gynecologic disorders
- Headaches, back pain
- Sexually transmitted infections (STIs)
- Depression, suicidal ideation, anxiety, fatigue, eating disorders, substance abuse

- Overuse of health services/frequent emergency room visits
- Nonadherence with medication/treatment plan and/or missed appointments

PHYSICAL EXAM

- Clinical presentation/psychological signs and symptoms
  - Delay in seeking treatment, inconsistent explanation of injuries, reluctance to undress
  - Signs of battered woman syndrome and/or posttraumatic stress disorder (PTSD) (flat affect/avoidance of eye contact, evasiveness, heightened startle response, sleep disturbance, traumatic flashbacks)
  - Suspicious partner accompaniment at appointment; overly solicitous partner and/or refusal to leave exam room
- Physical signs and symptoms
  - Tympanic membrane rupture
  - Rectal or genital injury (centrally located injuries with bathing-suit pattern of distribution—concealable by clothing)
  - Head and neck injuries (site of 50% of abusive injuries)
  - Scrapes, loose or broken tooth, bruises, cuts, or fractures to face or body
  - Knife wounds, cigarette burns, bite marks, welts with outline of weapon (such as belt buckle)
  - Defensive posture injuries
  - Injuries inconsistent with explanation or in various stages of healing
  - Malnutrition or pressure ulcers in the elderly

DIAGNOSTIC TESTS & INTERPRETATION

Initial Tests (lab, imaging)

Liver function tests (LFTs), amylase, lipase if abdominal trauma is suspected, BUN and creatinine if malnutrition/dehydration is suspected, pregnancy test and STD testing (HIV Ab/Ag, syphilis screen, gonorrhea and chlamydia NAAT, trichomonas) in cases of sexual abuse, x-ray if suspected fracture, radiographic skeletal survey for children <2 years old if physical abuse is suspected

 TREATMENT

- Treatment includes initial diagnosis; ongoing medical care; emotional support, counseling, and patient education regarding the DV cycle; referrals to community and supportive services as needed.
- On diagnosis, use the SOS-DoC intervention:
  - **S**: Offer *S*upport and assess *S*afety:
    - Support: "You are not to blame. I am sorry this is happening to you. There is no excuse for DV."
    - Remind patient of your commitment to confidential communication.
    - Safety: Listen and respond to safety issues for the patient: "Do you feel safe going home?"; "Are your children safe?"
  - **O**: Discuss *O*ptions, including safety planning and follow-up:

- Provide information about DV and help when needed. Make referrals to local resources.
  - "Do you need or want to access a safety shelter or DV service agency?"
  - "Do you want police intervention and if so, would you like me to call the police so they can make a report with you?"
  - Offer numbers to local resources and National DV Hotline: 1-800-799-SAFE (open 24/7; can provide physicians in every state with information on local resources).
  - **S**: Validate patient's *S*trengths:
    - "It took courage for you to talk with me today. You have shown great strength in very difficult circumstances."
  - **Do**: *Do*cument observations, assessment, and plans:
    - Use patient's own words regarding injury and abuse. Language should be chosen carefully; "patient reports" as opposed to "patient denies/claims," which may suggest the clinician does not believe the patient.
    - Legibly document injuries: Use a body map.
    - If possible, photograph patient's injuries if given consent. Photographs must include the patient's face or identifying features with the injury in order to be useful as legal evidence.
    - Make patient safety plan. Prepare patient to get away in an emergency:
      - Encourage patient to prepare an emergency kit to keep in a safe place: keys (house and car); important papers (Social Security card, birth certificates, photo ID/driver's license, passport, green card); cash, food stamps, credit cards; medication for self and children; children's immunization records; important phone numbers/addresses (friends, family, local shelters); personal care items (e.g., extra glasses).
    - Encourage patient to arrange a signal with someone to let that person know when she or he needs help.
  - **C**: Offer *C*ontinuity:
    - Offer a follow-up appointment and assess barriers to access.

GENERAL MEASURES

- Reporting child and elder abuse to protective services is mandatory in most states. Several states have laws requiring mandatory reporting of IPV.
- Contact the local DV program to find out about laws and community resources before they are needed.
- Display resource materials (National DV Hotline: 1-800-799-SAFE) in the office, all exam rooms, and restrooms.

ADDITIONAL THERAPIES

- National DV Hotline: 1-800-799-SAFE (7233)
- Post in all exam rooms posters in both English and Spanish; available at http://www.thehotline.org/resources/download-materials/

 ONGOING CARE

FOLLOW-UP RECOMMENDATIONS

- Schedule prompt follow-up appointment. Inquire about what occurred since last visit.
- DV often requires multiple interventions over time before it is resolved.

PATIENT EDUCATION

- Counsel patients about nonviolent ways to resolve conflict and about the cycle of violence.
- Counsel parents about developmentally appropriate ways to discipline their children and about the negative consequences of arguments on children and each other.
- National Coalition Against Domestic Violence: http://www.ncadv.org/
- CDC: http://www.cdc.gov/violenceprevention/

PROGNOSIS

Most DV perpetrators do not voluntarily seek therapy unless pressured by partners or on legal mandate. Current evidence is insufficient on effectiveness of therapy for perpetrators.

REFERENCES

1. U.S. Preventive Services Task Force. *Intimate Partner Violence and Abuse of Elderly and Vulnerable Adults: Screening.* Rockville, MD: Agency for Healthcare Research and Quality; 2013.
2. Sumner SA, Mercy JA, Dahlberg LL, et al. Violence in the United States: status, challenges, and opportunities. *JAMA.* 2015;314(5):478–488.

ADDITIONAL READING

Lee ASD, McDonald LR, Will S, et al. Improving provider readiness for intimate partner violence screening. *Worldviews Evid Based Nurs.* 2019;16(3):204–210.

CODES

ICD10

- T74.91XA Unspecified adult maltreatment, confirmed, initial encounter
- T74.11XA Adult physical abuse, confirmed, initial encounter
- T74.31XA Adult psychological abuse, confirmed, initial encounter

CLINICAL PEARLS

- Display resource materials in the office (e.g., posting abuse awareness posters/National DV Hotline, 1-800-799-SAFE, in both English and Spanish, in all exam rooms and restrooms).
- Given the high prevalence of DV and the lack of harm and potential benefits of screening, routine screening is recommended.
- For those who screened positive, offer resources, reassure confidentiality, and provide close follow-up.

D

DOWN SYNDROME
Brian G. Skotko, MD, MPP

BASICS

DESCRIPTION
- Down syndrome (DS) is a congenital condition associated with intellectual disability and an increased chance of multisystem medical problems.
- Synonym: trisomy 21

Pediatric Considerations
Murmur may not be present at birth.

Geriatric Considerations
Life expectancy has increased to ~60 years.

Pregnancy Considerations
- The American College of Obstetricians and Gynecologists (ACOG), the Society for Maternal-Fetal Medicine (SMFM) and the American College of Medical Genetics and Genomics (ACMG) recommends all women be offered traditional prenatal screening and diagnostic testing for DS.
- ACOG and the SMFM acknowledge that any women may choose noninvasive prenatal screening (NIPS). ACMG recommends all women be offered NIPS (1),(2).

EPIDEMIOLOGY
Incidence
In the United States, 1/792 live births, ~5,300 births per year

Prevalence
~212,000 persons in the United States (3)

ETIOLOGY AND PATHOPHYSIOLOGY
- Etiology: presence of all or part of an extra chromosome 21
- Trisomy 21: 95% of DS, an extra chromosome 21 is found in all cells due to nondisjunction, usually in maternal meiosis.
- Translocation DS: 3–4% of DS, extra chromosome 21q material is translocated to another chromosome (usually 13, 14, or 21); ~25% have parental origin.
- Mosaic trisomy 21: 1–2% of DS, manifestations may be milder.

Genetics
- Online Mendelian Inheritance in Man (OMIM) 190685
- Inheritance: most commonly sporadic nondisjunction resulting in trisomy 21
- Chance of having another child with DS is
  – 1% (or age risk, whichever is greater) after conceiving a pregnancy with nondisjunction trisomy 21
  – 10–15% for mothers/sisters and 3–5% for fathers/brothers who carry balanced translocation with chromosome 21
  – 100% if the parental balanced translocation is 21;21 (45,t[21;21])
  – Unclear after child with mosaic DS but ~1%

RISK FACTORS
- DS believed to occur in all races and ethnicities with equal frequency, although live birth prevalence may differ based on different elective termination rates
- Chance of having an infant with DS increases with mother's age.

GENERAL PREVENTION
Preimplantation diagnosis with in vitro fertilization (IVF), prenatal diagnosis followed by termination, and adoption are current options for expectant parents who do not wish to raise a child with DS.

COMMONLY ASSOCIATED CONDITIONS
- Cardiac
  – Congenital heart defects (40–50%)
- GI/growth
  – Feeding problems are common in infancy.
  – Structural defects (~12%)
  – Gastroesophageal reflux
  – Constipation
  – Celiac disease (~5%)
- Pulmonary
  – Tracheal stenosis/tracheoesophageal fistula
  – Pulmonary hypertension
  – Obstructive sleep apnea (50–75%)
- Genitourinary
  – Cryptorchidism, hypospadias
- Hematologic/neoplastic
  – Transient myeloproliferative disorder (~10%): generally resolves spontaneously; can be preleukemic (acute megakaryoblastic leukemia [AMKL]) in 20–30%
  – Leukemia (AMKL or acute lymphoblastic leukemia [ALL]) in 0.5–1%
  – Decreased risk of most solid tumors; increased risk of germ cell tumors/testicular cancer
- Endocrine
  – Hypothyroidism: congenital or acquired (13–63%)
  – Diabetes
- Skeletal
  – Atlantoaxial instability (15%): ~2% symptomatic
  – Short stature is common.
  – Scoliosis (Some cases have adult onset.)
  – Hip problems (1–4%)
- Immune/rheumatologic
  – Abnormal immune function with increased rate of respiratory infections
  – Increased risk of autoimmune disorders, including Hashimoto thyroiditis, celiac disease, and alopecia
- Neurologic
  – Intellectual ability ranging from mild to severe disability. Average is moderate intellectual disability.
  – Autism spectrum disorder (<18%)
  – Hypotonia
  – Seizures (8%); typically occurring <1 year of age (infantile spasms) or >30 years of age
  – Alzheimer disease: At least 40% at age 40 years develop signs of dementia; percentage increases with age.
- Psychiatric
  – Attention deficit hyperactivity disorder (ADHD), obsessive-compulsive disorder (OCD), and autism spectrum disorder increased frequency in children.
  – Generalized depression and anxiety with increased frequency in young adults/adults
  – Down syndrome disintegrative disorder is a very rare clinical regression syndrome that can occur in adolescents or young adults (4).

- Sensory
  – Hearing loss (75%): mostly conductive due to high frequency of asymptomatic middle ear effusion; otitis media (50–70%)
  – Visual impairment (60%): strabismus (refractive errors, 15%), myopia, hyperopia, nystagmus, cataracts (15%)
- Dermatologic
  – Xerosis, eczema, palmoplantar hyperkeratosis, atopic or seborrheic dermatitis, onychomycosis, syringomas, furunculosis/folliculitis, hidradenitis suppurativa

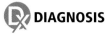

DIAGNOSIS

HISTORY
~85% of mothers of infants with DS learn of the diagnosis postnatally, although this is changing with the availability of prenatal screening such as NIPS.

PHYSICAL EXAM
- In November 2015, DS-specific growth charts were released. These charts do not represent "optimal" growth of children with DS; 50% BMI on the DS-specific growth curves corresponds to the 85% (overweight) on the standard NCHS growth curves (5).
- Infants and children
  – Brachycephaly (100%)
  – Hypotonia (80%)
  – Small ears, often low set and simplified
  – Upslanting palpebral fissure (90%)
  – Epicanthic folds (90%)
  – Brushfield spots
  – Depressed nasal bridge
  – Short neck, often with increased nuchal folds
  – Single palmar crease, single flexion crease on 5th finger
  – Increased space between toes 1 and 2, 5th finger clinodactyly, brachydactyly

DIAGNOSTIC TESTS & INTERPRETATION
Initial Tests (lab, imaging)
- Maternal prenatal screening includes the following:
  – 1st trimester: combined screen (maternal age, β-human chorionic gonadotropin [β-hCG], pregnancy-associated plasma protein A [PAPP-A], and nuchal translucency)
  – 2nd trimester: quad screen (α-fetoprotein, β-hCG, estriol, inhibin A)
  – Sequential screen (combined screen in 1st trimester, if abnormal, obtain amniocentesis *or* await 2nd trimester quad screening)
  – Integrated screen (combined screening in 1st trimester plus quad screen in 2nd trimester)
  – NIPS with cell-free DNA (beginning ~10 weeks' gestation) (1)
- Prenatal diagnosis includes the following:
  – Chorionic villus sampling: 1st trimester, ~99% accurate, ~1% miscarriage
  – Amniocentesis: 2nd trimester, ~99% accurate, ~0.25% miscarriage rate

- Postnatal diagnosis
  - Fluorescence in situ hybridization (FISH) can be performed at time of clinical suspicion, but karyotype should always be done to differentiate genetic type of DS.
  - Parental (and adult-aged sibling) karyotype is indicated only if translocation DS found in child.
- Work-up for newborns
  - Echo, with or without murmur
  - CBC with differential (to look for transient myelo-proliferative disorder)
  - Thyroid-stimulating hormone (TSH)
  - Audiogram
  - Ophthalmologic exam (look for red reflex)
  - Swallowing study for those with feeding difficulties
  - Car-seat test

Follow-Up Tests & Special Considerations
- After delivering a prenatal diagnosis, the clinician should offer "Understanding a Down Syndrome Diagnosis" (http://understandingdownsyndrome.org).
- If the diagnosis is postnatal, the mother and her partner should be informed of the diagnosis promptly by a physician (preferably the obstetrician and pediatrician or family physician), on the basis of clinical observations and before the karyotype is available, but with consideration of extenuating circumstances (e.g., mother's medical condition). The spouse/partner and infant should be present unless this would cause undue delay. The meeting should be private. Refer to the baby by name.
- In the postnatal setting, the clinician should be knowledgeable on the subject of DS and should conduct a discussion with content that is current, respectful, balanced, informative, and realistic but not overly pessimistic, concentrating on what is relevant to the 1st year of life.
- Cardiac follow-up, as indicated

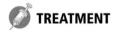 ## TREATMENT

ISSUES FOR REFERRAL
- Infant stimulation programs (early Intervention)
- Lactation consultant
- Physical/occupational/speech therapy
- Pediatric cardiologist, if indicated

SURGERY/OTHER PROCEDURES
Repair of congenital anomalies is appropriate.

COMPLEMENTARY & ALTERNATIVE MEDICINE
- There is no evidence to support the use of supplements in children with DS.
- Craniosacral manipulation is dangerous due to potential atlantoaxial instability.

ADMISSION, INPATIENT, AND NURSING CONSIDERATIONS
If the social situation indicates adoption, consider the National Down Syndrome Adoption Network (NDSAN) (http://www.ndsan.org/) national registry of families seeking to adopt a child with DS.

 ## ONGOING CARE

FOLLOW-UP RECOMMENDATIONS
Patient Monitoring
- The American Academy of Pediatrics recommends ongoing assessment and review, at least annually, the following surveillance:
  - Vision: Assess for strabismus, cataracts, and nystagmus by ophthalmologist by 6 months, annually between ages 1 and 5 years, every 2 years ages 5 to 13 years, every 3 years ages 13 to 21 years.
  - Hearing: neonatal screen with auditory brainstem response (ABR) or otoacoustic emissions (OAE), then audiogram every 6 months until age 3 years, and then annually
  - Thyroid: initial newborn screen. Repeat TSH at 6 months, 12 months, and then annually (5)[C].
  - Screening for celiac disease (total IgA and tissue transglutaminase [tTG]-IgA) annually, if symptomatic
  - Three-view cervical spine films if patient symptomatic, beginning at 3 to 5 years of age
  - Hemoglobin annually to screen for iron deficiency anemia
  - Repeat echocardiogram in teens if with murmur or fatigue
  - Integrating specific aspects of DS care into the electronic health record can improve adherence to guidelines that span the life of the child (6)[B].
- Adults with DS: A comprehensive approach to medical care is also necessary (7).

DIET
- No special diet, but caloric needs are lower in adolescents/adults with DS than their peers.
- Obesity is prevalent at all ages.

PATIENT EDUCATION
- Down Syndrome Clinic to You (DSC2U), an online health and wellness portal for patients with DS, their caregivers, and primary care providers; https://www.dsc2u.org
- National Down Syndrome Congress: 800-232-NDSC; https://www.ndsccenter.org/
- National Down Syndrome Society: 800-221-4602; https://www.ndss.org/
- The LuMind IDSC Down Syndrome Foundation provides information on the latest research for people with DS: www.lumindidsc.org.
- Lettercase provides peer-reviewed booklet for parents who have received a prenatal diagnosis of DS and have not yet made a decision about their pregnancy: https://www.lettercase.org/.
- Down Syndrome Pregnancy provides free downloadable books and articles for expectant mothers who have decided to continue their pregnancies after a prenatal diagnosis of DS: http://downsyndromepregnancy.org/.
- Understanding a Down Syndrome Diagnosis provides an overview of DS and select resources: http://understandingdownsyndrome.org/.

PROGNOSIS
- 99% of young adults/adults with DS report being happy with their lives.
- Life expectancy ~60 years

REFERENCES
1. Gregg AR, Skotko BG, Benkendorf JL, et al. Noninvasive prenatal screening for fetal aneuploidy, 2016 update: a position statement of the American College of Medical Genetics and Genomics. *Genet Med.* 2016;18(10):1056–1065.
2. Rose NC, Kaimal AJ, Dugoff L, et al. Screening for fetal chromosomal abnormalities: ACOG Practice Bulletin, Number 226. *Obstet Gynecol.* 2020;136(4):e48–e69.
3. De Graaf G, Buckley F, Skotko B. People living with Down syndrome in the USA: births and population. https://go.dselink.net/us-population-factsheet. Accessed December 27, 2021.
4. Santoro SL, Cannon S, Capone G, et al. Unexplained regression in Down syndrome: 35 cases from an international Down syndrome database. *Genet Med.* 2020;22(4):767–776.
5. Zemel BS, Pipan M, Stallings VA, et al. Growth charts for children with Down syndrome in the United States. *Pediatrics.* 2015;136(5):e1204–e1211.
6. Santoro SL, Bartman T, Cua CL, et al. Use of electronic health record integration for down syndrome guidelines. *Pediatrics.* 2018;142(3):e20174119.
7. Tsou AY, Bulova P, Capone G, et al. Medical care of adults with Down syndrome: a clinical guideline. *JAMA.* 2020;324(15):1543–1556.

ADDITIONAL READING
- Antonarakis SE, Skotko BG, Rafii MS, et al. Down syndrome. *Nat Rev Dis Primers.* 2020;6(1):9.
- Skotko B. Publications. http://brianskotko.com/publications/. Accessed December 27, 2021.
- Bull MJ; for Committee on Genetics. Health supervision for children with Down syndrome. *Pediatrics.* 2011;128(2):393–406.
- Bull MJ. Down syndrome. *N Engl J Med.* 2020;382(24):2344–2352.

 ## SEE ALSO

Algorithm: Intellectual Disability

 ## CODES

ICD10
- Q90.0 Trisomy 21, nonmosaicism (meiotic nondisjunction)
- Q90 Down syndrome
- Q90.1 Trisomy 21, mosaicism (mitotic nondisjunction)

CLINICAL PEARLS
- 99% of young adults/adults with DS report being happy with their lives.
- DS specialty clinics, including virtual ones like dsc2u.org, may improve medical outcomes.

D

DRUG ABUSE, PRESCRIPTION

Matthew A. Silva, PharmD, RPh, BCPS • Hilary Mislan, MD

BASICS

Controlled substances are prone to misuse and diversion. Universal precautions should be used for monitoring of all patients prescribed controlled substances to identify substance use disorder in affected patients. Patients with substance use disorder should be offered treatment (and/or referred as needed).

DESCRIPTION
- Prescription drug abuse behaviors exist on a continuum and may include the following:
  - Use of medication for medical reasons other than what the prescriber intended
  - Use of medication for nonmedical reasons such as to get high (dissociative effects) or to enhance performance
  - Use of medication for any reason by someone other than the person for whom the medication was originally prescribed
- Commonly abused prescription medications include opioid analgesics (morphine, oxycodone, hydrocodone, oxymorphone, hydromorphone, fentanyl, methadone, buprenorphine), stimulants (amphetamine, methylphenidate), benzodiazepines (alprazolam, clonazepam, lorazepam), and barbiturates (secobarbital, amobarbital).
- *Diversion* is a term used to describe the rerouting of medications from prescriptions or other legitimate supplies for recreational use or criminal activity, such as selling prescription medication for personal profit.

EPIDEMIOLOGY
- More than half of ED-related visits are related to abused or misused pharmaceuticals (opioid and nonopioid).
- In the United States in 2016, there were 17,087 overdose deaths involving prescription opioids, which account for 27% of all drug overdose deaths that year.

Incidence
- Predominant sex: males > females
- Predominant age: highest among adults 18 to 25 years (mean 22 years), then adolescents and teens 12 to 17 years, followed by adults ≥26 years

Prevalence
- Lifetime prevalence of prescription drug abuse is highest for opioids, benzodiazepines, and stimulants.
- In the United States in 2016, the CDC found that 4.3% reported misuse of prescription pain relievers, 2.1% for prescription stimulants, 2.2% for prescription tranquilizers, and 0.6% for prescription sedatives.

ETIOLOGY AND PATHOPHYSIOLOGY
Opioids, benzodiazepines, stimulants, and barbiturates produce euphoria, tolerance, and dependence leading to misuse and addiction.

Genetics
Variant alleles affect the expression and function of opioid, dopamine, acetylcholine, serotonin, and γ-aminobutyric acid, helping to explain susceptibility to different forms.

RISK FACTORS
- Sociodemographic, psychiatric, pain- and drug-related factors
- Genetics, environment, family history
- Ongoing opioid prescription (3+ months) greatly increases risk of opioid-related overdose at 1 (4-fold) and 5 years (30-fold).

GENERAL PREVENTION
- Limit or avoid prescribing controlled medications on the first visit (until the relationship is established). Limit initial quantity of opioid pain medication prescribed to a few days (1)[A].
- Screen by asking questions about unhealthy drug use (including prescription drugs, USPSTF-B recommendation).
- Take a thorough history, review records, and perform periodic urine drug screens (UDSs) before deciding if a controlled substance is indicated.
- Try all available nonopioid treatments for pain before prescribing opioids for chronic pain.
- Avoid prescribing benzodiazepines. Use other treatments for anxiety (cognitive-behavioral therapy, mindfulness, selective serotonin reuptake inhibitors, PRN H_1 blocker, buspirone).
- Avoid benzodiazepines and hypnotics in elderly.
- Patients should give good informed consent about risks of controlled medications before starting AND every 3 months while continuing treatment.
- Develop/adopt standard practice agreements for prescribing and monitoring controlled substances.
- Wean/stop prescription analgesics for chronic pain if ineffective for improving pain and function, if aberrant behaviors suggesting opioid use present, or if patient overdoses.
- Dose reduction of chronic opioids can decrease risk while improving pain, function, and quality of life.
- Prescription monitoring programs (PMPs) reduce doctor shopping but not ED visits for overdose and prescription drug abuse–related deaths (2)[A].
- Identify and treat underlying substance use disorder.
- Prescribe intranasal naloxone to all patients prescribed chronic opioids and provide education to patient and family members on proper use in case of overdose.

COMMONLY ASSOCIATED CONDITIONS
- Opioids: tolerance (loss of effectiveness over time), opioid-induced hyperalgesia, dependence (uncomfortable withdrawal symptoms), addiction (which can lead to loss of savings, job, close relationships and incarceration, hepatitis C virus or HIV infection, etc.), overdose/death, depression, constipation, low testosterone, and sexual dysfunction
- Benzodiazepines and barbiturates: dependence (withdrawal can cause seizures, delirium tremens, death), psychosis, anxiety, sleep driving, blackout states, cognitive impairment, impaired driving; increased fall risk and mortality in elderly patients
- Stimulants: dependence, hypertension, tachyarrhythmias, myocardial ischemia, seizures, hypothermia, psychosis, hallucinations, paranoia, anxiety

DIAGNOSIS

- Initial screening: "How many times in the past year have you used an illegal drug or used a prescription medication for nonmedical reasons?"; primary care setting sensitivity of 100% and specificity of ~75% (3)[C]
- Other screening tools: Drug Abuse Screening Test (DAST) helps determine involvement with drugs over the past year. Assess alcohol use with CAGE or Alcohol Use Disorders Identification Test (AUDIT). Consult the *DSM-5* criteria for substance use disorders.

HISTORY
Consider aberrant behaviors when taking a history. Patient may ask for dose escalations and early refills ("spilled the bottle . . . ," "pharmacist shorted me . . . ," etc.). Patients may have a strong preference for one drug, make appointments at end of day and after hours, and/or show hostile/threatening or flattering behavior.

PHYSICAL EXAM
- Monitor patients for signs of sedation, confusion, or intoxication (can include slurred speech and unsteady gait in case of benzodiazepines).
- Physical exam findings in opioid withdrawal include dilated pupils, frequent yawning, tachycardia, elevated blood pressure, and piloerection. Physical exam findings in benzodiazepine withdrawal include tachycardia, elevated blood pressure, and tremors.
- There are often no physical exam findings during a visit when a patient is misusing a prescription medication, other objective findings such as urine drug testing should be used in monitoring.

DIAGNOSTIC TESTS & INTERPRETATION
UDSs are recommended to ensure safe use of medication and prevent diversions (4)[C]. Random pill counts are useful for identifying misuse and abuse behaviors, or medication diversion.

Initial Tests (lab, imaging)
- UDSs: Ensure the panel includes semisynthetics (hydrocodone, hydromorphone, oxycodone) and synthetics (methadone, fentanyl, propoxyphene, meperidine) along with tramadol and buprenorphine. Test for other drugs of abuse such as benzodiazepines (clonazepam, alprazolam, lorazepam are ordered individually), cocaine, amphetamine, alcohol metabolites, and consider other drugs that may be highly prevalent in your area (such as gabapentin, PCP, barbiturates).
- Codeine will be positive for codeine plus morphine.
- Morphine will be positive for morphine.
- Oxycodone (OxyContin) will be positive for oxycodone and oxymorphone.
- Hydrocodone will be positive for hydrocodone and hydromorphone.
- Buprenorphine will be positive for buprenorphine and norbuprenorphine.
- Diazepam will be positive for nordiazepam, oxazepam, and temazepam.
- Chlordiazepoxide will be positive for nordiazepam and oxazepam.
- Alprazolam will be positive for α-hydroxyalprazolam.
- Clonazepam will be positive for 7-aminoclonazepam.
- Lorazepam will be positive for lorazepam-glucuronide.

Follow-Up Tests & Special Considerations
Random pill counts are useful for identifying patients taking more controlled substance than prescribed. Random urine drug testing can also be concurrently collected.

Test Interpretation
- Screening drug tests (by enzyme-linked immunosorbent assay method) may result in false positives from interactions with other commonly prescribed medications or substances people are frequently exposed to (such as energy drinks causing a false positive amphetamine screen), so treatment decisions should be based on highly specific confirmation testing (such as by gas chromatography/mass spectrometry).
- Full opioid metabolite

- Results are positive if drugs (or metabolites of drugs) that are not prescribed are present; positive in presence of illicit drugs (e.g., cocaine)
- Suspect diversion when negative for prescribed drug at a time when the patient reported taking it.
- Ingestion of poppy seeds can cause positive morphine and codeine on UDS confirmation testing. Advise patients prescribed controlled substances to avoid eating poppy seeds to avoid confusion from this.

TREATMENT

Addiction is a treatable chronic disease. The general approach to treatment includes inpatient, residential, or outpatient detoxification as required; counseling and intensive counseling as needed; and ongoing medication-assisted treatment (MAT) with buprenorphine or injectable naltrexone.

- Buprenorphine/naloxone: Begin taper to initiate discontinuation whenever there is evidence of prescription opioid abuse (4)[C]. Some situations indicate immediate discontinuation rather than taper (e.g., diversion or plan to switch to buprenorphine/naloxone treatment).
- Opioid discontinuation through interdisciplinary pain care programs, buprenorphine-assisted programs, and detoxification programs have achieved opioid discontinuation rates >85%.
- Benzodiazepines cannot be stopped abruptly for risk of seizures and death. Discontinue via slow taper or at a controlled detoxification program.
- Amphetamines can be stopped abruptly without risk of severe withdrawal or death.

GENERAL MEASURES
A variety of treatments are available including inpatient programs (detoxification and sometimes induction onto MAT), outpatient programs (MAT and behavioral health), and peer-led support services.

MEDICATION
Short-term opioid detoxification programs use clonidine, buprenorphine, or methadone under the direction of an addiction specialist. Long-term MAT with buprenorphine/naloxone, methadone, or naltrexone is more effective than short-term detoxification.

- Buprenorphine and naloxone MAT
  - Any provider (MD, DO, NP, or PA) may prescribe buprenorphine/naloxone after completing training and obtaining an X waiver. For details, see https://www.samhsa.gov/medication-assisted-treatment/become-buprenorphine-waivered-practitioner. An alternative pathway without formal training and certification is now available, allowing eligible providers to treat up to 30 patients.
  - Buprenorphine without naloxone is more prone to misuse. Naloxone-based formulations discourage misuse (such as by sniffing or IV) because naloxone displaces buprenorphine binding to opioid receptors when taken parenterally (naloxone is not well absorbed sublingually).
  - Buprenorphine is now also available as a monthly long-acting injectable into the subcutaneous tissue of the abdomen. This dosage form is administered by a nurse at clinic, eliminating the need for daily dosing and diversion-related issues while creating an opportunity to offer support. The injectable form is expensive.
  - Buprenorphine/naloxone doses should be titrated to the maximum of 24 mg/day for patients who continue to use other opioids. Methadone or detoxification followed by naltrexone should be offered for those unable to abstain from opioids on maximal buprenorphine/naloxone dosing.

  - Buprenorphine/naloxone should be continued as long as the patient takes prescribed doses and remains engaged in care; discontinue if there is evidence of buprenorphine/naloxone diversion.
  - Naltrexone (oral or long-acting injectable [very expensive]) (1) is another opioid antagonist that reduces cravings for opioids and blocks opioid-euphoria when ingested and does not require special training to prescribe. Naltrexone should not be started until a person has been off opioids for 7 days to avoid precipitating acute, severe withdrawal. This washout requirement for injectable naltrexone means fewer patients will be successful starting buprenorphine/naloxone, but once started, effectiveness of injectable naltrexone is similar.
  - Buprenorphine/naloxone and methadone are similarly effective when used in long-term opioid maintenance therapy, and both are effective in the treatment of chronic pain for people with opioid dependence.
- Methadone
  - Only an addiction specialist may dispense methadone for treatment of opioid use disorder at a certified opioid treatment program.

First Line
Treatment plans should be adjusted to fit specific patient needs. Some patients are able to achieve remission on their own, with peer support or with behavioral health support alone but many require MAT. The best medication is the medication that the patient will take.

ISSUES FOR REFERRAL
Enlist the help of chemical dependency groups/addiction specialists/pain management and psychiatry/psychology when patients have polysubstance abuse and to treat underlying mood and anxiety disorders, posttraumatic stress disorder, and ADHD.

ADDITIONAL THERAPIES
- Behavioral health support (individual counseling, group therapy which may include a variety of clinical approaches). This can also be available as intensive outpatient programs and partial hospitalization programs.
- SMART Recovery and 12-step programs such as AA and NA.
- Residential treatment programs (range in length from acute detoxification, short-term rehabilitation, transitional support programs, crisis stabilization units, to long-term residential programs including halfway houses and sober houses)
- Al-Anon/Alateen and Learn to Cope provide helpful free support groups for family members.

COMPLEMENTARY & ALTERNATIVE MEDICINE
Mindfulness and meditation, acupuncture, or yoga may help with stress reduction.

ADMISSION, INPATIENT, AND NURSING CONSIDERATIONS
Indications for detoxification programs include continued use of opioids despite outpatient treatment, concomitant alcohol and benzodiazepine dependence (increased risk of seizures), mental confusion/delirium, history of seizures, psychosis, suicidal ideation, serious, or absence of social support.

ONGOING CARE

Treatment with MAT should continue for as long as the patient benefits from it.

FOLLOW-UP RECOMMENDATIONS
Expert opinion suggests high-frequency visits (such as weekly) when a patient begins MAT.

Patient Monitoring
Monitor patients with in-person check-ins, drug testing, and review of the PMP.

PATIENT EDUCATION
- Controlled medication should be inaccessible to others (ideally in locked box/bag). Diverting medication may result in legal charges.
- Address "Red flags"; dose escalation when necessary; provide support and strategies for managing stress, cravings, and preoccupation about the next dose.

PROGNOSIS
The majority of patients with substance use disorder are able to achieve remission.

COMPLICATIONS
Misuse of opioids and benzodiazepines may lead to overdose and death. Misuse of stimulants may lead to psychosis and cardiac conditions such as myocardial infarction and arrhythmias.

REFERENCES

1. Onwuchekwa Uba R, Ankoma-Darko K, Park SK. International comparison of mitigation strategies for addressing opioid misuse: a systematic review. *J Am Pharm Assoc (2003)*. 2020;60(1):195–204.
2. Fink DS, Schleimer JP, Sarvet A, et al. Association between prescription drug monitoring programs and nonfatal and fatal drug overdoses: a systematic review. *Ann Intern Med*. 2018;168(11):783–790.
3. Smith PC, Schmidt SM, Allensworth-Davies D, et al. A single-question screening test for drug use in primary care. *Arch Intern Med*. 2010;170(13):1155–1160.
4. Manchikanti L, Abdi S, Atluri S, et al. American Society of Interventional Pain Physicians (ASIPP) guidelines for responsible opioid prescribing in chronic non-cancer pain: part I—evidence assessment. *Pain Physician*. 2012;15(Suppl 3):S1–S65.

 SEE ALSO

https://www.cdc.gov/drugoverdose/pdf/pdo_checklist-a.pdf

CODES

ICD10
- F19.10 Other psychoactive substance abuse, uncomplicated
- F11.10 Opioid abuse, uncomplicated
- F15.10 Other stimulant abuse, uncomplicated

CLINICAL PEARLS

- Most licensed physicians and nurse practitioners may now provide MAT with buprenorphine without the requirement of special certification.
- Conduct frequent UDSs (weekly to every 3 months) for all patients prescribed controlled substances.
- Discontinue prescription opioid analgesics if pain or functionality does not improve or if there is evidence of abuse or diversion (e.g., positive UDSs, driving while intoxicated [DWI], overdose, early refills).

DUCTAL CARCINOMA IN SITU

Anne Campbell Larkin, MD

 BASICS

DESCRIPTION

- Ductal carcinoma in situ (DCIS) is a heterogeneous group of lesions that have the presence of a clonal proliferation of neoplastic, *noninvasive* epithelial cells confined to ducts and lobules.
- Considered a premalignant lesion
- Can be classified as low, intermediate, or high grade
- Mortality from DCIS with subsequent progression to invasive breast carcinoma (IBC) is low, regardless of histologic type or type of treatment.

EPIDEMIOLOGY

Incidence

- Average annual percentage increase of 1%
- Estimated 62,738 new diagnoses of DCIS in 2019
- Estimated 49,290 new diagnoses of DCIS in 2021
- DCIS accounts for approximately 80–85% of in situ breast carcinomas (lobular carcinoma in situ [LCIS] accounts for approximately 15–20%).
- Represents ~26% of all new breast cancers
- Incidence rate comparable in different ethnicities
- More stable incidence in women 50 to 69 years old
- Increasing incidence in women <50 and >70 years old

ETIOLOGY AND PATHOPHYSIOLOGY

- A nonobligate precursor to IBC
- Poorly understood spectrum of polyclonal and clonal epithelial proliferative lesions—final step prior to IBC
  - The changes necessary for transition to IBC are poorly understood.
- Molecular evidence suggests that low- and high-grade DCIS are genetically distinct lesions.
  - High-grade DCIS associated with a higher likelihood of progression to invasive disease

Genetics

- Low-grade DCIS typically expresses estrogen receptor (ER) and progesterone receptor (PR), without HER2 protein overexpression or amplification.
- High-grade DCIS not consistently ER+ or PR+
  - Frequent HER2 protein overexpression and amplification (even more frequent compared to IBC)
  - Commonly associated with p53 gene mutations
- *BRCA1* and *BRCA2* associations observed
- Consider genetic counseling in high-risk DCIS patients.

RISK FACTORS

- Similar to IBC, although not as strongly associated
- Female gender, nulliparity, late age at first birth or menopause, first-degree relative with breast cancer, long-term use of postmenopausal combined estrogen and progestin therapy, history of atypical ductal hyperplasia (ADH), dense breast tissue are all risk factors.
- Association with age, body mass index, smoking, lactation, early menarche, alcohol consumption, and oral contraceptive use is less clear.

GENERAL PREVENTION

- Screening may result in overdiagnosis with little or no reduction in the incidence of advanced cancers.
- Women with increased risk should have more aggressive screening (risk assessment tool available at http://bcrisktool.cancer.gov).
- General screening guidelines—U.S. Preventive Services Task Force (USPSTF):
  - Biennial mammography for women aged 50 to 74 years (B recommendation)
  - The decision to start screening mammography in women <50 years should be an individual one.

- Insufficient evidence regarding benefits and harms of screening mammography if ≥75 years old
- Insufficient evidence to assess the benefits and harms of digital breast tomosynthesis (DBT) as a primary screening method (I statement)
- Insufficient evidence to assess the balance of benefits and harms of adjunctive screening using breast ultrasonography (US), magnetic resonance imaging (MRI), DBT, or other methods in women identified to have dense breasts on an otherwise negative screening mammogram (I statement)
- General screening guidelines—National Comprehensive Cancer Network (NCCN):
  - Women should be familiar with their breasts and promptly report changes; periodic consistent breast self-exam (BSE) may facilitate breast self-awareness.
  - Clinical breast exam (CBE):
    - USPSTF states evidence is insufficient to assess benefits and harms when added to mammography screening for women ≥40 years.
    - WHO states CBE may be beneficial in settings with weak health settings (mammography not accessible) for women 50 to 69 years old.
    - NCCE recommends annual CBE in women starting at age 40 years, and from age 25 to 39 years, perform BSE with CBE every 1 to 3 years.
- Risk reduction:
  - Assess familial/genetic history.
  - Lifestyle modifications: Limit alcohol intake to <1 drink per day, exercise, maintain a healthy diet, and weight control.
  - Hormonal risk reduction agent recommended in certain high-risk women ≥35 years old; tamoxifen for premenopausal women and raloxifene for postmenopausal women
  - Benefits of aromatase inhibitors are less clear.

 DIAGNOSIS

HISTORY

- Most DCIS is now diagnosed by screening mammography (presence of microcalcifications in approximately 72%); patients may be asymptomatic with nonpalpable mass (12%).
- More advanced lesions may present with a palpable mass, spontaneous nipple discharge, or Paget disease.

PHYSICAL EXAM

- CBE with patient in upright and supine position; evaluating for asymmetry, spontaneous discharge, skin changes (peau d'orange, erythema, scaling); nipple retraction/excoriation (Paget disease)
- Palpation of all breast quadrants, including lymph node examination (axillary, supraclavicular, and cervical)
- Positive clinical findings: Refer for consideration of diagnostic imaging and/or surgical evaluation unless <30 years old with a low clinical suspicion (observe 1 to 2 menstrual cycles; refer if clinical findings persist).

DIFFERENTIAL DIAGNOSIS

Usual ductal hyperplasia, flat epithelial atypia, ADH, LCIS, microinvasive carcinoma

DIAGNOSTIC TESTS & INTERPRETATION

Initial Tests (lab, imaging)

- Mammography BI-RADS: Breast Imaging–Reporting and Data System is a quality assurance (QA) method published by the American Radiology Society.
  - BI-RADS has been extended to breast US and MRI interpretation as well.

- Components of BI-RADS report:
  - Indication for study and type of examination
  - Overall breast composition, including breast density
    - A—breasts are almost entirely fatty tissue
    - B—scattered areas of fibroglandular density
    - C—heterogeneously dense
    - D—extremely dense
  - Description of abnormalities and important findings
    - Uses standard BI-RADS descriptors
  - Comparison to prior images and summary report, including final BI-RADS assessment category
  - Final BI-RADS assessment category and screening recommendations:
    - BI-RADS 0: incomplete; additional imaging evaluation needed
      - Commonly occurs on screening studies; consider diagnostic workup.
    - BI-RADS 1: negative
      - Continue with current screening guidelines.
    - BI-RADS 2: benign
      - No further action needed; continue current screening guidelines.
    - BI-RADS 3: probably benign, possibility of malignancy is <2%
      - Follow-up imaging should occur in 6 months for 1 year; consider imaging every 6 to 12 months for 2 to 3 years.
      - Can consider biopsy if patients is anxious or follow-up is uncertain
    - BI-RADS 4: suspicious
      - Patient and clinician should discuss possible management plans and likely a biopsy.
    - BI-RADS 5: highly suggestive of malignancy
      - Diagnostic imaging needed with follow-up and biopsy
    - BI-RADS 6: known biopsy—proven malignancy
      - Includes patients with biopsy-proven cancers that have yet to be surgically removed
- DCIS most often seen as clustered microcalcifications
- After *diagnostic* imaging, tissue biopsy should be considered.

Follow-Up Tests & Special Considerations

- US not typically recommended for *screening*
- Sensitivity of breast MRI screening > mammography; with decreased specificity resulting in increased number of false positives
- Screening MRI only recommended in certain women:
  - *BRCA* mutation—*commence at age 25 to 29 years*
  - First-degree relative of *BRCA* carrier—*commence at age 25 to 29 years*
  - ≥20% lifetime risk of breast cancer defined by models that are largely based on family history—*annual breast MRI to begin 10 years prior to the youngest family member but not prior to age 25 years*
  - Thoracic radiation between the ages of 10 and 30 years—*annual breast MRI to begin 10 years after radiation therapy but not prior to age 25 years*
  - Presence of Li-Fraumeni, *PTEN*, or Bannayan-Riley-Ruvalcaba syndrome in patient or first-degree relative
  - ≥20% risk of breast cancer based on gene and/or risk level: ATM, CDH1, CHEK2, PALB2, PTEN, STK11, TP53
- The NCCN Panel has included breast MRI as indicated during the initial workup of DCIS.

- Pathology
  - Tissue is necessary for diagnosis: typically core needle (CN) or vacuum-assisted (VA) biopsy (mammographic/stereotactic, US, or MRI guided).
    - Open surgical biopsy can be performed in patients not amenable to CN or VA biopsy, but this is rare.
  - Fine-needle aspiration (FNA) is not adequate for specific diagnosis of DCIS.
  - Histologic classification
    - Classified as either low, intermediate, or high grade based on architectural patterns (comedo, solid, cribriform, clinging, papillary, and micro-papillary), nuclear grade (I, II, or III), and the absence or presence of necrosis
    - Ductal intraepithelial neoplasia (DIN) is an alternative histologic classification incorporating size as a discriminating factor.
    - Grade is more important for prognosis, risk for progression, and local recurrence.
    - Comedo-type necrosis (necrosis filling central portion of involved duct) is typically seen in high-grade DCIS, with varying degrees of necrosis in other types of DCIS.
  - Determination of ER and PR status (1)[A]

 ## TREATMENT

MEDICATION
- Secondary chemoprevention following breast-conserving surgery for ER+ DCIS:
  - Tamoxifen for premenopausal patients or tamoxifen or an aromatase inhibitor for postmenopausal patients for 5 years
  - There may be some advantage for aromatase inhibitor therapy in patients <60 years old or patients with concerns for thromboembolism (1)[C].
  - Considered in lumpectomy patients with or without whole breast radiation (1)[A]
  - Adjuvant chemotherapy is not indicated.

SURGERY/OTHER PROCEDURES
- Surgery is the primary treatment option.
  - Options for surgery are based on risk of recurrence, anatomic location, extent of disease, and the ability to achieve "negative" margins (1)[A].
- Positive margins are considered "ink on tumor."
- Totality of evidence does not support the routine practice of obtaining negative margin widths wider than 2 mm (1)[C].
- Margins <1 mm considered inadequate (1)[A]
- Margins <1 mm at the breast fibroglandular boundary (chest wall or skin) do not mandate surgical excision but may be an indication for higher boost dose radiation in patients opting for breast conservation (1)[A].
- DCIS with microinvasion, defined as no invasive focus >1 mm in size, should be considered as DCIS when considering the optimal margin width (1)[C]. When there is only minimal or focal DCIS involvement near the margin, clinical judgment can be applied to determine if reexcision may be avoided in individual cases (1)[C].
- Surgical options include the following:
  - Breast conservation (lumpectomy) without lymph node procedure, without breast radiation therapy (1)[A]
  - Breast conservation (lumpectomy) without lymph node procedure, with whole breast radiation therapy, with or without boost to tumor bed (1)[A]
  - A sentinel lymph node biopsy may be considered if the lumpectomy is in an anatomic location compromising the performance of a future sentinel lymph node procedure (1)[C].

- Patients not amenable to margin-free lumpectomy should have total mastectomy (1)[C].
  - Mastectomy with or without sentinel node biopsy plus optional breast reconstruction (1)[A]
  - Mastectomy provides maximum local control.
  - A complete axillary lymph node dissection should not be performed in the absence of evidence of invasive cancer and proven axillary metastatic disease.
  - Long-term cause-specific survival seems to be equivalent to lumpectomy with whole breast radiation (1)[A].
  - A sentinel lymph node biopsy should be considered in patients with seemingly pure DCIS to be treated with mastectomy (1)[C].
- Radiation considerations:
  - Radiation decreases recurrence rates by about 50% but with no overall survival benefit.
  - Drawbacks to radiation therapy include:
    - The patient's burden of daily treatment for 6 weeks and short-term side effects, such as fatigue and skin toxicity
    - A slightly increased risk of secondary cancers
    - Inability to receive radiation therapy again in the ipsilateral breast should an invasive carcinoma develop.
- DCIS recurrence considerations:
  - Recurrence generally requires mastectomy.
  - Rates of recurrence for DCIS and IBC are similar:
    - ~50% of recurrences are pure DCIS; ~50% are IBC.
  - Recurrence should be treated with wide local excision, chest wall radiation, and consideration for systemic hormonal treatment (1)[A].
- Secondary chemoprevention following breast-conserving surgery for ER + DCIS:
  - Tamoxifen for premenopausal patients or tamoxifen or an aromatase inhibitor for postmenopausal patients for 5 years
  - There may be some advantage for aromatase inhibitor therapy in patients <60 years old or patients with concerns for thromboembolism (1)[C].
  - Considered in lumpectomy patients with or without whole breast radiation (1)[A]. Adjuvant chemotherapy is not indicated.

ADMISSION, INPATIENT, AND NURSING CONSIDERATIONS
Breast-conserving surgery is typically an outpatient procedure.

 ## ONGOING CARE

FOLLOW-UP RECOMMENDATIONS
- History and physical exam should occur every 6 to 12 months for the first 5 years and then annually after that.
- Mammography every 12 months (first mammogram 6 to 12 months after breast conservation therapy) (1)[C]
- If treated with tamoxifen or an aromatase inhibitor, monitor per NCCN guidelines for breast cancer risk reduction (1)[C].

PROGNOSIS
- Good prognosis: 10-year breast cancer–specific survival rates of >95%; overall mortality after diagnosis of treated pure DCIS generally >98%
- Risk of local recurrence after mastectomy generally reported as 1–2% (higher in some studies)

- Higher risk of local recurrences after breast-conserving therapy occurs in:
  - Younger age (particularly before age 40 years) patients
  - Larger tumor size
  - High nuclear grade
  - Comedo-type necrosis
  - Close/positive margin status (related to DCIS volume)
- ER+ tumors are associated with lower risk for recurrence.
- There is interest in identifying subsets of patients who have low rates of ipsilateral breast tumor recurrence such that they might safely forgo radiation.
  - The Oncotype DX DCIS test may help clinicians in selecting which patients with DCIS might safely forgo radiation therapy after breast-conserving surgery.
    - The test results in an Oncotype DX DCIS score, with the following risk categories:
      - DCIS score <39—low risk of recurrence
        - Radiation therapy benefits likely to be small and will not outweigh the risks of side effects.
      - DCIS score 39 to 54—intermediate risk of recurrence
        - Radiation therapy benefits unclear relative to the risks of side effects.
      - DCIS score 55 to 100—high risk of recurrence
        - Radiation therapy benefits are likely to be greater than the risks of side effects.

REFERENCE
1. National Comprehensive Cancer Network. NCCN clinical practice guidelines in oncology: breast cancer (Version 3.2018) 2018. http://www.nccn.org. Accessed November 8, 2018.

 ## SEE ALSO

Breast Cancer

 ## CODES

ICD10
- D05.10 Intraductal carcinoma in situ of unspecified breast
- D05.11 Intraductal carcinoma in situ of right breast
- D05.12 Intraductal carcinoma in situ of left breast

CLINICAL PEARLS
- DCIS is a heterogeneous group of *noninvasive* neoplastic breast ductal epithelial cell lesions.
- The incidence of DCIS has continued to increase in women <50 and >70 years of age, with a more stable incidence in women 50 to 69 years of age.
- The goal of DCIS treatment is to prevent recurrence and progression to IBC.
- The Oncotype DX DCIS score may help clinicians in selecting which patients with DCIS who may safely forgo radiation therapy after breast-conserving surgery.
- Current standard of care is breast-conserving therapy with consideration for postoperative whole breast radiation therapy and/or postsurgical tamoxifen or aromatase inhibitor therapy, unless otherwise contraindicated.
- With appropriate therapy, the overall prognosis of pure DCIS is excellent.

DUPUYTREN CONTRACTURE

Karl T. Clebak, MD, MHA, FAAFP • Shawn Phillips, MD • Ashley Nicole Koontz, DO

BASICS

DESCRIPTION
- Palmar fibromatosis; caused by progressive fibrous proliferation and tightening of the fascia of the palms, resulting in flexion deformities and loss of function
- Not the same as "trigger finger," which is caused by thickening of the distal flexor tendon
- Similar change rarely occurs in plantar fascia, usually appearing simultaneously.
- System(s) affected: musculoskeletal
- Dupuytren diathesis is an aggressive heritable form associated with age of onset <40, bilateral presentation to include radial digits, plantar fibromatosis (Ledderhose), and penile fibromatosis (Peyronie) (1).
- Synonyms: morbus Dupuytren; Dupuytren disease; "Celtic hand"; Viking's disease; palmar fascial fibromatosis, contracture of palmar fascia

EPIDEMIOLOGY
Prevalence
- Increases with age; mean prevalence in Western countries: 12%, 21%, and 29% at ages 55, 65, and 75 years, respectively. Norway: 30% of males >60 years; Spain: 19% of males >60 years
- More common in Caucasian men of Scandinavian or Northern European ancestry
- Mean age of onset is 60 years with typical age range of onset between 40 and 80 years.

ETIOLOGY AND PATHOPHYSIOLOGY
- Definitive etiology unknown; possibly oxidative stress, altered wound repair, and/or abnormal immune response
- Occurs in three stages (Luck classification) (1):
  - Proliferative phase: proliferation of myofibroblasts with nodule development on palmar surface
  - Involutional stage: myofibroblasts spread along palmar fascia to fingers with cord development via production of more type 3 collagen
  - Residual phase: fibroblasts are predominant with dense collagen leading to cord tightening and contracture formation

Genetics
- Autosomal dominant with incomplete penetrance:
  - Siblings with 3-fold risk
- 68% of male relatives of affected patients develop disease at some time.
- Possible association with HLA alleles

RISK FACTORS
- Smoking (mean 16 pack-years, odds ratio: 2.8)
- Increasing age
- Male/Caucasian; male > female (range 3.5:1 to 9:1)
- Vibration exposure and manual work—risk doubles if regular (weekly) exposure
- Diabetes mellitus (increases with duration of DM, usually mild; middle and ring finger involved)

- Excessive alcohol consumption
- Northern European ethnicity
- Family history
- Hand trauma
- Low body weight and BMI

GENERAL PREVENTION
Avoid risk factors, especially if a strong family history.

COMMONLY ASSOCIATED CONDITIONS
- Alcoholism
- Epilepsy (inconstant data)
- DM
- Chronic lung disease
- Occupational hand trauma (vibration)
- Hypercholesterolemia
- Carpal tunnel syndrome
- Peyronie disease
- HIV
- Cancer
- Adhesive capsulitis of shoulder

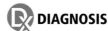

DIAGNOSIS

Diagnosis is largely clinical, based on history and physical exam.

HISTORY
- Caucasian male aged 40 to 80 years
- Family history and additional risk factors as listed above.
- Commonly report loss of ability to complete iADLs (1)
- Gradual onset of initially painless nodule of the palm
- Progression to include:
  - Pain of palpable nodule
  - Loss of function of affected finger
- Ring finger or middle finger most common, but any digit can be involved (1)
- Metacarpophalangeal joint is most commonly affected; proximal and distal interphalangeal joints are rarely affected (1).

PHYSICAL EXAM
- Visual inspection and palpation of the affected region of the palm to assess for nodule or cordlike band
- Assess for contracture of the affected finger.
  - More common in ulnar digits
  - Hueston tabletop test—ask patient to lay hands flat on table, positive if patient is unable to lie fingers flat (2)
  - Garrod nodes—callous over knuckles; associated with severe disease progression
- Tubiana staging (3)
  - 0: no extension deficit, no disease
  - N: no extension deficit, nodule present on exam
  - I: 1 to 45 degrees of extension deficit (surgical referral warranted)
  - II: 46 to 90 degrees of extension deficit

- III: 91 to 135 degrees of extension deficit
- IV: >135 degrees of extension deficit

DIFFERENTIAL DIAGNOSIS
- Camptodactyly: early teens; tight fascial bands on ulnar side of small finger
- Diabetic cheiroarthropathy: all four fingers
- Volkmann ischemic contracture
- Trigger finger (thickening of the distal flexor tendon)
- Ganglion cyst

DIAGNOSTIC TESTS & INTERPRETATION
Initial Tests (lab, imaging)
Diagnosis based on history and physical, testing is not routinely indicated. MRI can assess cellularity of lesions that correlate with recurrence after surgery.

TREATMENT

No definitive cure exists. Patients must be educated that risk for recurrence exists with all treatment, surgical and nonsurgical.

GENERAL MEASURES
- Observation for mild disease is reasonable
- Extension splinting
- Physical therapy for range of motion
- See indications for surgical referral below.

MEDICATION
- Steroid injection:
  - Can treat acute nodules or painful knuckle pads
  - Serial triamcinolone injections improved long-term outcomes when combined with needle aponeurotomy (4)[B].
  - Steroid alone associated with 50% recurrence in 1 to 3 years.
- Clostridial collagenase injections (FDA-approved 2010):
  - Degrades collagen to allow manual rupture of diseased cord
  - Best for isolated cord of MCP joint
  - 5-year recurrence rate of 47%; comparable with surgical recurrence rates (5)[B]
  - More rapid recovery of hand function compared to limited fasciectomy with fewer serious adverse events (6)[B]
  - Complications: injection site reaction, skin tear
  - Can do two cords concurrently
  - Can be effective for postsurgical recurrence

First Line
- Clostridial collagenase injections (FDA-approved 2010):
  - Degrades collagen to allow manual rupture of diseased cord
  - Best for isolated cord of MCP joint
  - 5-year recurrence rate of 47%; comparable with surgical recurrence rates (5)[B]
  - More rapid recovery of hand function compared to limited fasciectomy with fewer serious adverse events (6)[B]

– Complications: injection site reaction, skin tear
– Can do two cords concurrently
– Can be effective for postsurgical recurrence
• Steroid injection:
– Can treat acute nodules or painful knuckle pads
– Serial triamcinolone injections improved long-term outcomes when combined with needle aponeurotomy (4)[B].
– Steroid alone associated with 50% recurrence in 1 to 3 years

ISSUES FOR REFERRAL
Indications for orthopedic surgery referral:
• Any involvement of PIP joints
• MCP joints contracted >30 degrees
• Impaired function
• Disabling deformity

ADDITIONAL THERAPIES
Percutaneous and needle fasciotomy:
• Best for MCP joint; improvement of 93% versus 57% for PIP joint
• Recurrence common; 50%
• Shown to be effective for recurrent disease
• Better for MCP joints in patients with comorbid conditions; lower complication rate but higher recurrence
• At 3 months and 1 year, outcomes of needle fasciotomy and collagenase injections are the same (7)[B].

SURGERY/OTHER PROCEDURES
• Dermofasciectomy/limited fasciectomy/segmental aponeurectomy:
– Greater initial correction over nonincisional treatment; higher complication rates
– Percutaneous aponeurotomy and lipofilling (PALF) is a new, minimally invasive procedure that appears to have shorter convalescence, less long-term complications, similar operative contraction correction, and no significant difference at 1 year in results versus limited fasciectomy (8)[A].
• Indications:
– Any involvement of the PIP joints
– MCP joints contracted at least 30 degrees
– Positive Hueston tabletop test (Patient is unable to lay palm flat on a table.)
• May require skin grafts for wound closure with severe cutaneous shrinkage
• 80% have full range of movement with early surgery.
• Amputation of 5th digit if severe and deforming
• MCP joints respond better to surgery than PIP joints, especially if contracted >45 degrees.

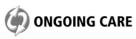 ONGOING CARE

FOLLOW-UP RECOMMENDATIONS
Patient Monitoring
Regular follow-up every 6 months to 1 year

PATIENT EDUCATION
• Avoid risk factors (alcohol, vibratory exposure, etc.), especially if strong family history.
• Mild disease: Passively stretch digits twice a day and avoid recurrent gripping of tools.

PROGNOSIS
• Unpredictable but usually slowly progressive
• 10% may regress spontaneously.
• Dupuytren diathesis predicts aggressive course. Features include ethnicity (Nordic), family history, bilateral lesions outside of palm, age <50 years—all factors with 71% risk of recurrence compared to baseline 23% without any risk factors.
• Prognosis better for MCP versus PIP joint after surgery and collagenase injection

COMPLICATIONS
• Complex regional pain syndrome
• Operative nerve injury
• Postoperative recurrence in 46–80%
• Postoperative hand edema and skin necrosis
• Digital infarction
• Limited hand function

REFERENCES
1. Dutta A, Jayasinghe G, Deore S, et al. Dupuytren's contracture—current concepts. *J Clin Orthop Trauma*. 2020;11(4):590–596.
2. Hueston JT. The table top test. *Hand*. 1982;14(1):100–103.
3. Mella JR, Guo L, Hung V. Dupuytren's contracture: an evidence based review. *Ann Plast Surg*. 2018;81(6S Suppl 1):S97–S101.
4. McMillan C, Binhammer P. Steroid injection and needle aponeurotomy for Dupuytren disease: long-term follow-up of a randomized controlled trial. *J Hand Surg Am*. 2014;39(10):1942–1947.
5. Peimer CA, Blazar P, Coleman S, et al. Dupuytren contracture recurrence following treatment with collagenase *Clostridium histolyticum* (CORDLESS [Collagenase Option for Reduction of Dupuytren Long-Term Evaluation of Safety Study]): 5-year data. *J Hand Surg Am*. 2015;40(8):1597–1605.
6. Zhou C, Hovius SE, Slijper HP, et al. Collagenase *Clostridium histolyticum* versus limited fasciectomy for Dupuytren's contracture: outcomes from a multicenter propensity score matched study. *Plast Reconstr Surg*. 2015;136(1):87–97.
7. Scherman P, Jenmalm P, Dahlin LB. One-year results of needle fasciotomy and collagenase injection in treatment of Dupuytren's contracture: a two-centre prospective randomized clinical trial. *J Hand Surg Eur Vol*. 2016;41(6):577–582.
8. Kan HJ, Selles RW, van Nieuwenhoven CA, et al. Percutaneous aponeurotomy and lipofilling (PALF) versus limited fasciectomy in patients with primary Dupuytren's contracture: a prospective, randomized, controlled trial. *Plast Reconstr Surg*. 2016;137(6):1800–1812.

ADDITIONAL READING
• Ball C, Pratt AL, Nanchahal J. Optimal functional outcome measures for assessing treatment for Dupuytren's disease: a systematic review and recommendations for future practice. *BMC Musculoskelet Disord*. 2013;14:131.
• Collis J, Collocott S, Hing W, et al. The effect of night extension orthoses following surgical release of Dupuytren contracture: a single-center, randomized, controlled trial. *J Hand Surg Am*. 2013;38(7):1285–1294.e2.
• Eaton C. Evidence-based medicine: Dupuytren contracture. *Plast Reconstr Surg*. 2014;133(5):1241–1251.
• Henry M. Dupuytren's disease: current state of the art. *Hand (N Y)*. 2014;9(1):1–8.
• Lanting R, Broekstra DC, Werker PM, et al. A systematic review and meta-analysis on the prevalence of Dupuytren disease in the general population of Western countries. *Plast Reconstr Surg*. 2014;133(3):593–603.
• Michou L, Lermusiaux JL, Teyssedou JP, et al. Genetics of Dupuytren's disease. *Joint Bone Spine*. 2012;79(1):7–12.
• Sweet S, Blackmore S. Surgical and therapy update on the management of Dupuytren's disease. *J Hand Ther*. 2014;27(2):77–83; quiz 84.
• van Rijssen AL, Werker PM. Percutaneous needle fasciotomy for recurrent Dupuytren disease. *J Hand Surg Am*. 2012;37(9):1820–1823.

 CODES

ICD10
M72.0 Palmar fascial fibromatosis [Dupuytren]

CLINICAL PEARLS
• Dupuytren contracture is a fixed flexion deformity of (most commonly) the 4th and 5th digits due to palmar fibrosis. 90% of cases are progressive; not trigger finger, which is due to thickening of the distal flexor tendon
• Refer patients with involvement of the PIP joints or MCP involvement with contractures of >30 degrees.
• Both surgical and enzymatic fasciotomy have high rate of recurrence.

DYSHIDROSIS

Benjamin T. Tan, DO • Robyn Lee Reese, DO

BASICS

DESCRIPTION

- A common chronic dermatitis often involving the palms and soles. The precise definition is frequently debated, with many terms being used interchangeably. Efforts are being made to more specifically define dyshidrosis, and literature supports the presence of several different classes within the family "dyshidrosis."
- Dyshidrotic eczema
  - Common, chronic, or recurrent; nonerythematous; symmetric vesicular eruption primarily of the palms, soles, and interdigital areas
  - Associated with burning, itching, and pain
- Pompholyx (from Greek "bubble")
  - Rare condition characterized by abrupt onset of large bullae
  - Often used interchangeably with dyshidrotic eczema (small vesicles); however, may be a distinct entity
- Lamellar dyshidrosis
  - Fine, spreading, exfoliation of the superficial epidermis in the same distribution as described above
- System(s) affected: dermatologic, exocrine, immunologic
- Synonym(s): cheiropompholyx, keratolysis exfoliativa, vesicular palmoplantar eczema, desquamation of interdigital spaces pompholyx, acute and recurrent vesicular hand dermatitis, recurrent vesicular palmoplantar dermatitis

EPIDEMIOLOGY

Incidence
- Mean age of onset is 40 years and younger.
- Male = female
- Comprises 5–20% of hand eczema cases

Prevalence
20 cases per 100,000 people

ETIOLOGY AND PATHOPHYSIOLOGY

- Exact mechanism unknown; thought to be multifactorial (allergies, genetics, and dermatophyte infection implicated)
- Dermatopathology: intraepidermal spongiosis without effect on eccrine sweat glands
- Vesicles remain intact due to thickness of stratum corneum of palmar/plantar skin (1).
- Immunologic reaction: theorized that rapid rise in immunoglobulin levels may precipitate vesicle formation
- Aggravating factors (debated)
  - Hyperhidrosis (in 40% of patients with the condition)
  - Detergents/solvents
  - Increased water exposure (e.g., florists, hair stylists, health care workers)
  - Climate: hot/cold weather; humidity
  - Contact sensitivity (in 30–67% of patients with the condition) (2)
  - Metals: nickel, cobalt, and chromate sensitivity (may include implanted orthopedic or orthodontic metals) (1)
  - Stress
  - Dermatophyte infection (present in 10% of patients with the condition) (2)
  - Prolonged wear of occlusive gloves
  - Cement workers
  - IV immunoglobulin therapy
  - Smoking
  - Sunlight/UVA radiation

Genetics
- Atopy: 50% of patients with dyshidrotic eczema have atopic dermatitis (1).
- Rare autosomal dominant form of pompholyx found in Chinese population maps to chromosome 18q22.1–18q22.3 (2)

RISK FACTORS
- Many risk factors are disputed in the literature, with none being consistently associated.
- Atopy
- Other dermatologic conditions
  - Atopic dermatitis (early in life)
  - Contact dermatitis (later in life)
  - Dermatophytosis
- Sensitivity to
  - Foods
  - Drugs: neomycin, quinolones, acetaminophen, and oral contraceptives
  - Contact and dietary: nickel (more common in young women), chromate (more common in men), and cobalt (1)
  - Smoking

GENERAL PREVENTION
- Control emotional stress.
- Avoid excessive sweating.
- Avoid exposure to irritants.
- Avoid diet high in metal salts (chromium, cobalt, nickel).
- Avoid smoking.

COMMONLY ASSOCIATED CONDITIONS
- Atopic dermatitis
- Allergic contact dermatitis
- Parkinson disease
- HIV (2)

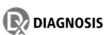

DIAGNOSIS

HISTORY
- Episodes of pruritic rash
- Recent emotional stress
- Familial or personal history of atopy
- Exposure to allergens or irritants
  - Occupational, dietary, or household
  - Cosmetic and personal hygiene products
  - Vesicular eruption typically occurs 24 hours after allergen challenge (1).
- Costume jewelry use
- IV immunoglobulin therapy
- HIV
- Smoking

PHYSICAL EXAM
- Transient, often recurrent, symmetrical vesicular eruptions located on volar and plantar surfaces and lateral fingers. Lesions may not heal completely between flares (1).
- Prodrome: Intense pruritus may occur prior to vesicular eruption.
- Early findings
  - 1 to 2 mm, clear, nonerythematous, deep-seated vesicles (lasting 2 to 3 weeks)
  - Has a "tapioca" appearance
- Late findings
  - Unroofed vesicles with inflamed bases
  - Desquamation (terminal phase)
  - Peeling, rings of scale, or lichenification common

DIFFERENTIAL DIAGNOSIS
- Vesicular tinea pedis/manuum
- Vesicular id reaction
- Contact dermatitis (allergic or irritant)
- Scabies
- Chronic vesicular hand dermatitis
- Drug reaction
- Dermatophytid
- Bullous disorders: dyshidrosiform bullous pemphigoid, pemphigus, bullous impetigo, epidermolysis bullosa
- Pustular psoriasis
- Acrodermatitis continua
- Erythema multiforme
- Herpes simplex infection
- Pityriasis rubra pilaris
- Vesicular mycosis fungoides
- Palmoplantar pustulosis (PPP)

DIAGNOSTIC TESTS & INTERPRETATION

Follow-Up Tests & Special Considerations
- Skin culture in suspected secondary infection (most commonly, *Staphylococcus aureus*) (3)
- Consider antibiotics based on culture results and severity of symptoms.

Diagnostic Procedures/Other
- Diagnosis is based on clinical exam.
- Potassium hydroxide (KOH) wet mount (if concerned about dermatophyte infection)
- Patch test (if suspecting allergic cause) (3)

Test Interpretation
- Fine, 1- to 2-mm spongiotic, intraepidermal vesicles with little to no inflammatory change
- No eccrine glandular involvement
- Thickened stratum corneum
- Pompholyx may be confused with PPP but will contain the following distinguishing histopathologic features that PPP will not: vesicles with spongiosis and neutrophils only on the top, without microabscesses on the edges of vesicles (4).

TREATMENT

GENERAL MEASURES
- Avoid possible causative factors: stress, direct skin contact with irritants, nickel, occlusive gloves, household cleaning products, smoking, sweating.
- Use moisturizers/emollients for symptomatic relief and to maintain effective skin barrier (3).
- Skin care
  - Avoid shoes with known irritants (e.g., leather, rubber soles).
  - Wear socks and gloves made of cotton and change frequently.
  - Wash infrequently in lukewarm water, carefully dry, and then apply emollient.
  - Avoid direct contact with fresh fruit (5)[C].

MEDICATION

First Line
- Mild cases: topical steroids (high potency) (2)[B]
  - Considered cornerstone of therapy but limited published evidence
  - Use limited to 2 weeks each episode due to risk of infection (3)[B]

- Moderate to severe cases
  - Ultra high-potency topical steroids with occlusion over treated area (3)[B]
  - Prednisone 40 to 100 mg/day tapered after blister formation ceases (2)[B]
    - Limited use due to significant side effects (3)[B]
  - Psoralens plus ultraviolet-A (PUVA) therapy, either systemic/topical or immersion in psoralens (2)[B]
- Recurrent cases (3)[B]
  - Systemic steroids at onset of itching prodrome
  - Prednisone 60 mg PO for 3 to 4 days

Second Line
- Topical calcineurin inhibitors (Mitigate the long-term risks of topical steroid use.)
  - Topical tacrolimus (6)[B]
  - Topical pimecrolimus (6)[B]
  - May not be as effective on plantar surface
- Other therapies (typically with dermatology consultation)
  - Oral cyclosporine (3)[B]; monitor for hypertension and renal injury.
  - Injections of botulinum toxin type A (BTXA) (6)[B]
    - Newer topical forms of BTXA currently being developed show promise.
    - Painful, requires nerve block
  - Systemic alitretinoin (teratogenic) (5)[B]
  - Topical bexarotene (a teratogenic retinoid X receptor agonist approved for use in cutaneous T-cell lymphoma) (6)[B]
  - Methotrexate (6)[C] (significant side effects including GI intolerance and hepatotoxicity) (3)[B]
  - Azathioprine (1)[C] (6- to 8-week onset of action; must monitor for GI side effects, liver toxicity, blood dyscrasia)
  - Disulfiram or sodium cromoglycate in nickel-allergic patients (1)[C]
  - Mycophenolate mofetil (2)[C] (GI side effects; benefit: no hepatotoxicity with long-term use) (3)[B]
  - Tap water iontophoresis (2)[C]

ISSUES FOR REFERRAL
- Allergist (if allergen testing required)
- Psychologist (if stress modification needed)

ADDITIONAL THERAPIES
- Other oral agents:
  - Thalidomide (do not use in pregnancy/no available studies on efficacy)
  - Dapsone 100 to 150 mg daily (also limited literature on efficacy; may be used in combination with steroids) both significant side effects; very limited use (3)[B]
- Radiation therapy (1)[C]
- UV-free phototherapy (5)[C]
- Treat underlying dermatophytosis (1).
- BTXA in those in which excessive sweating is an exacerbating factor (3)[B]

COMPLEMENTARY & ALTERNATIVE MEDICINE
- Conservative management:
  - Antihistamines: hydroxyzine, cetirizine, loratadine
  - Soaks/cold compresses of weak solutions of potassium permanganate, Burow solution (aluminum acetate), or vinegar 15 minutes, 4 times daily (3)[C]
- Exposure to sunlight as maintenance therapy, 12 minutes every other day, 10 to 15 exposures (5)[C]
- Dandelion juice (not for atopic patients) (6)[C]
- Cognitive relaxation techniques (3)[B]

 ONGOING CARE

FOLLOW-UP RECOMMENDATIONS
Patient Monitoring
- Dyshidrotic Eczema Area and Severity Index (DASI) (1)
- Parameters used in the DASI score
  - Number of vesicles per square centimeter
  - Erythema
  - Desquamation
  - Severity of itching
  - Surface area affected
- Grading: mild (0 to 15), moderate (16 to 30), severe (31 to 60)
- Monitor BP and glucose in patients receiving systemic corticosteroids.
- Monitor for adverse effects of medications.

DIET
- Consider diet low in metal salts if history of nickel sensitivity (3)[B].
- Updated recommendations for low-cobalt diet are available (1).

PATIENT EDUCATION
- Instructions on self-care, complications, and avoidance of triggers/aggravating factors
- American Academy of Dermatology: dyshidrotic eczema at: https://www.aad.org/public/diseases/eczema/dyshidrotic-eczema#overview

PROGNOSIS
- Condition is benign.
- Usually heals without scarring
- Lesions may spontaneously resolve.
- Recurrence is common.

COMPLICATIONS
- Quality of life impact: skin tightening, pain, and decreased dexterity
- Secondary bacterial infections with or without steroid use (*S. aureus* most common)
- Dystrophic nail changes
- Fissures and ulcerations
- Psychological distress
- Lymphedema

REFERENCES

1. Veien NK. Acute and recurrent vesicular hand dermatitis. *Dermatol Clin*. 2009;27(3):337–353.
2. Wollina U. Pompholyx: a review of clinical features, differential diagnosis, and management. *Am J Clin Dermatol*. 2010;11(5):305–314.
3. Lofgren SM, Warshaw EM. Dyshidrosis: epidemiology, clinical characteristics, and therapy. *Dermatitis*. 2006;17(4):165–181.
4. Masuda-Kuroki K, Murakami M, Kishibe M, et al. Diagnostic histopathological features distinguishing palmoplantar pustulosis from pompholyx. *J Dermatol*. 2019;46(5):399–408.
5. Letić M. Use of sunlight to treat dyshidrotic eczema. *JAMA Dermatol*. 2013;149(5):634–635.
6. Wollina U. Pompholyx: what's new? *Expert Opin Investig Drugs*. 2008;17(6):897–904.

ADDITIONAL READING

- Agner T, Aalto-Korte K, Andersen KE, et al; for European Environmental and Contact Dermatitis Research Group. Classification of hand eczema. *J Eur Acad Dermatol Venereol*. 2015;29(12):2417–2422.

- Chen JJ, Liang YH, Zhou FS, et al. The gene for a rare autosomal dominant form of pompholyx maps to chromosome 18q22.1–18q22.3. *J Invest Dermatol*. 2006;126(2):300–304.
- Gerstenblith MR, Antony AK, Junkins-Hopkins JM, et al. Pompholyx and eczematous reactions associated with intravenous immunoglobulin therapy. *J Am Acad Dermatol*. 2012;66(2):312–316.
- Guillet MH, Wierzbicka E, Guillet S, et al. A 3-year causative study of pompholyx in 120 patients. *Arch Dermatol*. 2007;143(12):1504–1508.
- Hsu CY, Wang YC, Kao CH, et al. Dyshidrosis is a risk factor for herpes zoster. *J Eur Acad Dermatol Venereol*. 2015;29(11):2177–2183.
- Molin S, Diepgen TL, Ruzicka T, et al. Diagnosing chronic hand eczema by an algorithm: a tool for classification in clinical practice. *Clin Exp Dermatol*. 2011;36(6):595–601.
- Nishizawa A. Dyshidrotic eczema and its relationship to metal allergy. *Curr Probl Dermatol*. 2016;51:80–85.
- Schuttelaar ML, Coenraads PJ, Huizinga J, et al. Increase in vesicular hand eczema after house dust mite inhalation provocation: a double-blind, placebo-controlled, cross-over study. *Contact Dermatitis*. 2013;68(2):76–85.
- Stuckert J, Nedorost S. Low-cobalt diet for dyshidrotic eczema patients. *Contact Dermatitis*. 2008;59(6):361–365.
- Sumila M, Notter M, Itin P, et al. Long-term results of radiotherapy in patients with chronic palmoplantar eczema or psoriasis. *Strahlenther Onkol*. 2008;184(4):218–223.
- Waldman RA, DeWane ME, Sloan B, et al. Dupilumab for the treatment of dyshidrotic eczema in 15 consecutive patients. *J Am Acad Dermatol*. 2020;82(5):1251–1252.

 SEE ALSO

Algorithm: Rash

 CODES

ICD10
L30.1 Dyshidrosis [pompholyx]

CLINICAL PEARLS

- Dyshidrosis is a transient, recurrent, vesicular eruption, most commonly of the palms, soles, and interdigital areas.
- Etiology and pathophysiology are unknown but are most likely related to a combination of genetic and environmental factors.
- Best prevention is effective skin care and limiting exposure to irritating agents.
- Treatments are based on disease severity; preferred treatments include topical steroids, oral steroids, and calcineurin inhibitors.
- Condition, although benign and self-healing, can be chronic and debilitating with major concern for superimposed bacterial infection that may be avoided by preventative measures, early treatment, and recognition.

DYSMENORRHEA

Maggie C. Wertz, MD

BASICS

DESCRIPTION
- Pelvic pain occurring at/around time of menses; a leading cause of absenteeism for women <30 years old
- Primary dysmenorrhea: pelvic pain without pathologic physical findings; diagnosis of exclusion
- Secondary dysmenorrhea: often more severe, results from specific pelvic pathology; often resistant to typical treatments for dysmenorrhea; severity based on activity impairment:
  – Mild: painful, rarely limits daily function, or requires analgesics
  – Moderate: daily activity affected, rare absenteeism, requires analgesics
  – Severe: daily activity affected, likelihood of absenteeism increased, limited benefit from analgesics
- System affected: reproductive
- Synonym(s): menstrual cramps

EPIDEMIOLOGY
- Predominant age
  – Primary: onset 6 to 12 months after the start of menarche, teens to early 20s
  – Secondary: 20s to 30s
- Predominant sex: women only

Prevalence
- Up to 90% of menstruating females have experienced primary dysmenorrhea (1).
- Up to 42% lose days of school/work monthly due to dysmenorrhea.
- Up to 20% reported impairment in daily activities and/or sleep.

ETIOLOGY AND PATHOPHYSIOLOGY
- Primary: Elevated prostaglandin (PGF2α) production through indirect hormonal control (decrease in progesterone at start of menses leads to increase in prostaglandins) causes nonrhythmic hypercontractility and increased uterine muscle tone with vasoconstriction and resultant uterine ischemia. Ischemia results in hypersensitization of type C pain nerve fibers; intensity of cramps directly proportional to amount of PGF2α released (1)
- Secondary:
  – Endometriosis (most common cause)
  – Adenomyosis
  – Congenital abnormalities of uterine/vaginal anatomy
  – Cervical stenosis
  – Pelvic inflammatory disease
  – Ovarian cysts
  – Pelvic tumors, especially leiomyomata (fibroids) and uterine polyps

Genetics
Not well studied

RISK FACTORS
- Primary (1),(2)
  – Cigarette smoking
  – Alcohol use
  – Early menarche (age <12 years)
  – Age <30 years
  – Family history of dysmenorrhea
  – Irregular/heavy menstrual flow
  – Nonuse of oral contraceptives
  – Sexual abuse/history of sexual assault
  – Psychological symptoms (depression, anxiety, increased stress, etc.)
  – Nulliparity

- Secondary
  – Pelvic infection
  – Use of intrauterine device (IUD) in the few months following insertion
  – Structural pelvic malformations
  – Family history of endometriosis in first-degree relative

GENERAL PREVENTION
- Primary: regular exercise; early childbirth and higher parity; use of hormonal contraceptives
- Secondary: Reduce risk of sexually transmitted infections (STIs).

Pediatric Considerations
Onset with first menses raises probability of genital tract anatomic abnormality (i.e., transverse vaginal septum, imperforate or minimally perforated hymen, uterine anomalies).

COMMONLY ASSOCIATED CONDITIONS
- Irregular/heavy menstrual periods
- Longer menstrual cycle length/duration of bleeding
- Anxiety/depression
- Decreased quality of life

DIAGNOSIS

Typically, a clinical diagnosis based on characteristic symptom history of suprapubic/low back cramping/pain occurring at or near menstrual flow onset lasting for 8 to 72 hours (2)

HISTORY
- Primary: onset once ovulatory cycles are established in adolescents; 6 to 12 months after menarche on average
- Patients may have associated nausea, vomiting, diarrhea, headache, fatigue, insomnia, pain radiating into the low back or inner thighs, and rarely syncope and fever. These are all considered to be secondary to prostaglandin release.
- Recurrence at or just before the onset of the menstrual flow
  – Pelvic pain occurring between menstrual periods is not likely to be dysmenorrhea.
  – Present with most menstrual periods (cyclic)
- Acute relief associated with the following:
  – Use of analgesics, especially NSAIDs
  – Local topical heat application
  – Orgasm
- Response to NSAIDs helps confirm diagnosis.
- Impact of symptoms on daily activities can help determine severity.
- Secondary: can be associated with chronic pelvic pain, midcycle pain, dyspareunia, abnormal uterine bleeding, typical onset after age 25 years, nonmidline pain, progression of severity, lack of response to NSAIDs/hormonal treatment and infertility.

PHYSICAL EXAM
- Primary: Physical exam is typically normal. Examine to rule out secondary dysmenorrhea only if the history is inconsistent with primary dysmenorrhea. Pelvic exam is recommended if patient is sexually active to rule out infection.
- Secondary: Evaluate for cervical discharge, uterine enlargement, tenderness, irregularity, or fixation.

DIFFERENTIAL DIAGNOSIS
- Primary: History is characteristic.
- Secondary
  – Endometriosis (most common)
  – Pelvic/genital infection
  – Complication of pregnancy
  – Missed/incomplete abortion
  – Ectopic pregnancy
  – Uterine/ovarian neoplasm
  – UTI
  – Complication with IUD use
  – Congenital uterine or cervical anomaly
  – Adenomyosis
  – Leiomyomata (fibroids)
  – Pelvic adhesions
  – Inflammatory bowel disease
  – Irritable bowel syndrome
  – Chronic pelvic pain (idiopathic)

DIAGNOSTIC TESTS & INTERPRETATION
Initial Tests (lab, imaging)
All tests should only be performed if indicated based on history or if patient has symptoms refractory to first-line therapies; most cases of primary dysmenorrhea can be diagnosed on history alone.
- Pregnancy test
- Urine testing for infection
- Gonorrhea/chlamydia cervical testing, especially in women age <25 years and in high-prevalence areas
- Primary: Consider pelvic ultrasound to rule out secondary abnormalities.
- Secondary: ultrasound and/or laparoscopy to define anatomy for severe/refractory cases. MRI may be useful as second-line noninvasive imaging if ultrasound is nondiagnostic and fibroids, ovarian torsion, deep endometriosis, or adenomyosis is suspected.

Follow-Up Tests & Special Considerations
Counsel regarding appropriate preventive measures for STI and pregnancy.

Diagnostic Procedures/Other
Laparoscopy is rarely needed and is usually only considered in cases of suspected endometriosis or pelvic adhesions not definitively identified on transvaginal ultrasound.

Test Interpretation
- Primary: none
- Secondary: Specific anatomic abnormalities may be noted (see "Differential Diagnosis").

Pregnancy Considerations
Consider ectopic pregnancy when pelvic pain occurs with vaginal bleeding in a patient with a positive pregnancy test.

TREATMENT
- Reassure the patient that treatment success is very likely with adherence to recommendations.
- Relief may require the use of several treatment modalities at the same time.

GENERAL MEASURES
- Regular exercise (1),(3)[A] and topical local heat (1)[C] are noninvasive general measures to relieve pain. Local heat in conjunction with the use of an NSAID is superior to an NSAID alone (1)[C].

- High-frequency transcutaneous electrical nerve stimulation (TENS) has been found to be beneficial (1),(4). Low-frequency TENS is not recommended because it is not superior to placebo.
- Secondary dysmenorrhea: treatment of suspected/confirmed underlying cause of pain

MEDICATION

First Line

- NSAIDs: inhibit the peripheral production of prostaglandins. No NSAID has been found to be superior to others. Medication should be taken on scheduled dosing starting 1 to 2 days prior to onset of menses and continued for 2 to 3 days (1),(2). If one NSAID preparation does not work, another NSAID preparation should be tried. Each preparation should be taken as prescribed for at least 3 menstrual cycles prior to determining effectiveness.
  - Ibuprofen 400 mg PO q8h
  - Naproxen sodium 500 mg PO q12h
  - Celecoxib 400 mg PO × 1 and then 200 mg PO q12h
  - Mefenamic acid 500 mg PO × 1 and then 250 mg PO q6h (not to exceed 3 days)
- Hormonal contraceptives: recommended for primary dysmenorrhea in women desiring contraception (2)[B]. Directly suppresses ovulation and limits endometrial growth resulting in reduced prostaglandin production, intrauterine pressure, and uterine contractions. Continuous rather than cyclic dosing has been found to be superior for pain control (4). Amenorrhea by any means can improve symptoms of dysmenorrhea. Estrogen-containing contraceptives are recommended first line for secondary dysmenorrhea due to endometriosis, although progestin-only methods have also been shown to be beneficial (2)[B].
  - Low- and high-dose combined oral contraceptives (COCs) along with transdermal and intravaginal combined contraceptives have all been found to be superior to placebo (1)[C].
  - Levonorgestrel IUDs are just as effective as COCs (4)[C].
  - Progestin-only contraceptions including subcutaneous and subdermal preparations appear to decrease primary dysmenorrhea but to a lesser extent than combined options and IUDs (1),(2)[B].
- Potential contraindications to NSAIDs and COCs
  - Platelet disorders
  - Gastric ulceration or gastritis
  - Personal and family history of thromboembolic disorders
  - Vascular disease
  - Migraines with aura
  - Active smoking
- Precautions for first-line options:
  - GI irritation
  - Lactation
  - Coagulation disorders
  - Impaired renal function
  - Heart failure
  - Liver dysfunction
  - Pregnancy
  - Hypertension

- Significant possible interactions
  - Coumadin-type anticoagulants
  - Aspirin with other NSAIDs

Second Line

- Acetaminophen and acetaminophen with caffeine are superior to placebo and have less potential side effects than NSAIDs (1)[B].
- Behavioral interventions, such as relaxation exercises including yoga, may help alleviate pain in primary dysmenorrhea.
- Nifedipine may be effective in some women and may be used in women trying to conceive (pregnancy Category C).

SURGERY/OTHER PROCEDURES

Laparoscopic uterosacral nerve ablation and presacral neurectomy have been shown to relieve pain at 6 and 12 months, respectively, but are still reserved for patients with pain resistant to all other first- and second-line treatments (1),(4)[B]. Hysterectomy is effective for dysmenorrhea but should only be considered in very rare occasions and when all desired childbearing is complete (1).

COMPLEMENTARY & ALTERNATIVE MEDICINE

- Chinese herbal medicine shows promising evidence of decreasing pain, but more evidence is needed.
- Acupuncture treatments have been shown to decrease pain in dysmenorrhea, but further randomized, well-designed studies are needed. Additionally, these treatments must be frequent and timely for effectiveness.
- Acupoint stimulation, particularly noninvasive stimulation (acupressure), has had inconclusive results for pain relief.
- Aromatherapy abdominal massage performed daily for 10 minutes, 7 days prior to onset of menses can decrease primary dysmenorrhea.
- Further research needed to determine benefit and safety for regular use of oral fennel, oral ginger, oral fenugreek, oral valerian, extracorporeal magnetic innervation, vitamin K_1 injection into the spleen-6 acupuncture point, use of high-frequency vibratory stimulation tampon, transdermal nitroglycerin, and vaginal sildenafil.

ADMISSION, INPATIENT, AND NURSING CONSIDERATIONS

Both primary and secondary dysmenorrhea are usually managed in the outpatient setting.

- Primary: outpatient care
- Secondary: usually outpatient care

 ONGOING CARE

FOLLOW-UP RECOMMENDATIONS
Normal

DIET
Insufficient evidence for any specific dietary changes

PATIENT EDUCATION
Reassure the patient that primary dysmenorrhea is treatable with the use of NSAIDs, COCs, IUD, exercise or local heat, and that it will usually abate with age and parity.

PROGNOSIS
- Primary: reduced with age and parity
- Secondary: likely to require therapy based on underlying cause

COMPLICATIONS
- Primary: anxiety and/or depression
- Secondary: infertility from underlying pathology

REFERENCES

1. Burnett M, Lemyre M. No. 345—primary dysmenorrhea consensus guideline. *J Obstet Gynaecol Can*. 2017;39(7):585–595.
2. Osayande AS, Mehulic S. Diagnosis and initial management of dysmenorrhea. *Am Fam Physician*. 2014;89(5):341–346.
3. Brown J, Brown S. Exercise for dysmenorrhoea. *Cochrane Database Syst Rev*. 2010;(2):CD004142.
4. Oladosu FA, Tu FF, Hellman KM. Nonsteroidal anti-inflammatory drug resistance in dysmenorrhea: epidemiology, causes, and treatment. *Am J Obstet Gynecol*. 2018;218(4):390–400.

ADDITIONAL READING

- Ryan SA. The treatment of dysmenorrhea. *Pediatr Clin North Am*. 2017;64(2):331–342.
- Woo HL, Ji HR, Pak YK, et al. The efficacy and safety of acupuncture in women with primary dysmenorrhea: a systematic review and meta-analysis. *Medicine (Baltimore)*. 2018;97(23):e11007.

 SEE ALSO

- Dyspareunia; Endometriosis; Menorrhagia (Heavy Menstrual Bleeding); Premenstrual Syndrome (PMS) and Premenstrual Dysphoric Disorder (PMDD)
- Algorithm: Pelvic Pain

CODES

ICD10
- N94.6 Dysmenorrhea, unspecified
- N94.4 Primary dysmenorrhea
- N94.5 Secondary dysmenorrhea

CLINICAL PEARLS

- Dysmenorrhea is a leading cause of absenteeism for women age <30 years.
- In women who desire contraception, hormonal contraceptives are the preferred treatment.
- All NSAIDs studied have been found to be equally effective in the relief of dysmenorrhea and should be initiated 1 to 2 days prior to onset of menses with scheduled dosing for at least 2 to 3 days with each menstrual cycle.

DYSPAREUNIA

Janelle K. Hadley, MD, MPH • Staci Lynn Vanderjack, MD, MPH

 BASICS

DESCRIPTION

- Recurrent and persistent genital or pelvic pain associated with sexual activity, which is not exclusively due to intensity of intercourse, lack of lubrication or vaginismus. It can be associated with distress and can negatively impact relationships, self-esteem, and sexual satisfaction.
- It is important to note that while dyspareunia and vaginismus have previously been viewed as separate conditions, they were combined into genito-pelvic pain and penetration disorder as described by the *DSM-5* (1).
  - Many individuals have sexual practices that do not include penetration; these individuals can also be impacted by these conditions (1).
- May be the result of organic, emotional, or psychogenic causes
  - Primary: present throughout one's sexual history
    ○ Potential relationship exists between primary dyspareunia and vaginismus, low libido, and arousal disorders.
  - Secondary: arising from a specific event or condition (e.g., menopause, endometriosis, pelvic inflammatory disease [PID], depression, drugs)
  - Superficial: pain at, or near, the introitus or vaginal barrel associated with penetration
  - Deep: pain after penetration located at the cervix or lower abdominal area
  - Complete: present under all circumstances
  - Situational: occurring selectively with specific situations
  - Idiopathic: no identifiable cause or presence despite treatment
- System(s) affected: reproductive

EPIDEMIOLOGY

- Predominant age: all ages
- Predominant sex: female > male

Incidence

>50% of all sexually active women will report dyspareunia at some time.

Geriatric Considerations

Incidence increases dramatically in postmenopausal women primarily because of vaginal atrophy.

Prevalence

Most sexually active women will experience dyspareunia at some time in their lives.

- ~15% (4–40%) of adult women will have dyspareunia on a few occasions during a year.
- ~1–2% of women will have painful intercourse on a more-than-occasional basis.
- Male prevalence is ~1%.

ETIOLOGY AND PATHOPHYSIOLOGY

- Disorders of vaginal outlet
  - Adhesions
  - Condyloma
  - Clitoral irritation
  - Episiotomy scars
  - Fissures
  - Hymenal ring abnormalities
  - Inadequate lubrication
  - Infections
  - Lichen planus
  - Lichen sclerosus
  - Postmenopausal atrophy
  - Psoriasis
  - Trauma
  - Vulvar papillomatosis
  - Vulvar vestibulitis/vulvodynia
- Disorders of vagina
  - Abnormality of vault owing to surgery or radiation
  - Congenital malformations
  - Inadequate lubrication
  - Infections
  - Inflammatory or allergic response to foreign substance
  - Masses or tumors
  - Pelvic relaxation resulting in rectocele, uterine prolapse, or cystocele
- Disorders of pelvic structures
  - Endometriosis
  - Levator ani myalgia/spasm
  - Malignant or benign tumors of the uterus
  - Ovarian pathology
  - Pelvic adhesions
  - PID
  - Pelvic venous congestion
  - Prior pelvic fracture
  - Uterine fibroids
- Disorders of the GI tract
  - Constipation
  - Diverticular disease
  - Fistulas
  - Hemorrhoids
  - Inflammatory bowel diseases
- Disorders of the urinary tract
  - Interstitial cystitis
  - Ureteral or vesical lesions
  - Urethritis
- Chronic disease
  - Behçet syndrome
  - Diabetes
  - Sjögren syndrome
  - Fibromyalgia
  - Multiple sclerosis
  - Neuropathies and chronic pain syndromes
- Male
  - Peyronie disease
  - Cancer of penis
  - Genital muscle spasm
  - Infection or irritation of penile skin
  - Infection of seminal vesicles
  - Lichen sclerosus
  - Musculoskeletal disorders of pelvis and lower back
  - Penile anatomy disorders
  - Phimosis
  - Prostate infections and enlargement (e.g., chronic prostatitis)
  - Testicular disease
  - Obstruction of ejaculatory duct (e.g., torsion of spermatic cord, calculus, cyst)
  - Urethritis
- Psychological disorders
  - Anxiety
  - Conversion reactions
  - Depression
  - Fear
  - Hostility toward partner
  - Phobic reactions
  - Psychological trauma/PTSD

RISK FACTORS

- Fatigue
- Stress
- Depression and anxiety
- Diabetes
- Estrogen deficiency
  - Menopause
  - Lactation
- Previous PID
- Vaginal surgery or trauma
- Alcohol/marijuana consumption
- Medication side effects (antihistamines, tamoxifen, bromocriptine, low-estrogen oral contraceptives, SSRIs, depo-medroxyprogesterone, desipramine)
- History of sexual abuse
- Black race

Pregnancy Considerations

- Pregnancy has a potent influence on sexuality; dyspareunia is common in late pregnancy and postpartum.
  - Breastfeeding, perineal pain, fatigue, and stress can be risk factors in postpartum period.
- Episiotomies do not have a protective effect.
  - Women who experience delivery interventions including episiotomy are at greater risk than women who deliver over an intact perineum or have an unsutured tear.

GENERAL PREVENTION

N/A

COMMONLY ASSOCIATED CONDITIONS

Vaginismus

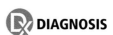 **DIAGNOSIS**

HISTORY

- Identify pain characteristics:
  - Onset
  - Duration
  - Location: entry versus deep, single versus multiple sites; positional
  - Intensity/quality: varying degrees of pelvic/genital pressure, aching, tearing, and/or burning
  - Pattern (precipitating or aggravating factors): when pain occurs (at entry, during, or after intercourse)
  - Relief measures: Avoid intercourse, change positions, and have intercourse only at certain times of the month.
- Include menstrual, anatomic, obstetric/gynecologic, sexual, domestic violence, and sexual assault histories with past medical, surgical, and psychosocial history
- Specifically, for male dyspareunia, symptoms must be present for 3 months or longer (2).

PHYSICAL EXAM

- A complete exam, including a focused pelvic exam, to identify pathology
  - Exam must include inspection and palpation of urethra, vulva, and vaginal areas; palpation of the uterine, bladder, and adnexal structures; rectovaginal exam; penis, scrotum, pelvic floor muscles and digital rectal exam.
  - Sensory mapping with a cotton-tipped applicator to identify sensitive and painful areas
- Because examination often reproduces the pain, examiner should be cautious and sensitive to patient's anxiety.

DIFFERENTIAL DIAGNOSIS

Vaginismus (genito-pelvic pain penetration disorder)

- If pain prevents penetration, severe vaginismus may be present.

DIAGNOSTIC TESTS & INTERPRETATION
Initial Tests (lab, imaging)
Based on history and exam findings
- Wet mount
- Gonorrhea and chlamydia cultures
- Herpes culture of lesions if present
- Urinalysis and urine culture
- Pap smear
- Glycohemoglobin
- GAD-7 and PHQ-9

Follow-Up Tests & Special Considerations
- Serum estradiol if vulvodynia or atrophic vaginitis
- Voiding cystourethrogram if urinary tract involvement
- GI contrast studies if GI symptoms
- Ultrasound and CT scan are of limited value; perform if clinically indicated.

Diagnostic Procedures/Other
Based on history and exam findings
- Colposcopy and biopsy if vaginal/vulvar lesions
- Laparoscopy if complex deep-penetration pain
- Cystoscopy if urinary tract involvement
- Colonoscopy if GI involvement

Test Interpretation
Depends on etiology

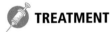 TREATMENT

GENERAL MEASURES
- Educate the patient and partner regarding the nature of the problem. Reassure both that there are solutions to the problem.
- Initiate specific treatment when initial evaluation identifies an organic cause.
- Once organic causes are ruled out, treatment is a multidimensional and multidisciplinary approach; medications alone don't resolve (3)[A].
  - Individual behavioral therapy
    ○ Indicated to help the patient deal with intrapersonal issues and assess the role of the partner
  - Couple behavioral therapy
    ○ Indicated to help resolve interpersonal problems
    ○ May involve short-term structured intervention or sexual counseling
    ○ Designed to desensitize systemically uncomfortable sexual responses and intercourse through a series of interventions over a period of weeks
    ○ Interventions range from muscle relaxation and mutual body massage to sexual fantasies and erotic massage.

MEDICATION
First Line
Depends on the etiology
- Antibiotics, antifungals, or antivirals, as indicated, for infection
- Vaginal moisturizers and lubricants for dryness
- Analgesics like NSAIDs and topical anesthetics for pain
- Topical/vaginal estrogen for vaginal and vulvar atrophy
  - Available data support the use of estrogen over other vaginal therapies for postmenopausal vaginal symptoms (4)[A], although vaginal lubricants have an important role in management of atrophy-associated symptoms and may be as effective so should be tried first.

- Neuropathic pain associated with vulvar vestibulitis/vulvodynia may respond to tricyclic antidepressants (amitriptyline or nortriptyline) or gabapentin.
- In observational studies, pain with ejaculation improved or resolved completely with tamsulosin (5).
- If no identifiable source is identified, can also consider imipramine or gabapentin given success in chronic pain

Second Line
- Ospemifene for moderate to severe symptoms due to menopause-related vulvovaginal atrophy (1)[C]
- Intravaginal DHEA (prasterone) for moderate to severe symptoms due to menopause-related vulvovaginal atrophy

ISSUES FOR REFERRAL
Referral for long-term therapy may be necessary.

ADDITIONAL THERAPIES
Physical therapy for pelvic floor muscle pain (This is first line if vaginismus is present.)

SURGERY/OTHER PROCEDURES
- Consideration of surgical interventions for dyspareunia due to altered anatomy, uterine position, fibroids, or prior pelvic surgery
  - Laparoscopic excision of endometriotic lesions or pelvic adhesions
  - Surgical vestibulectomy can be considered if medical measures fail with vulvar vestibulitis.
  - Fractional CO$_2$ laser treatments demonstrate improvement in symptoms of vulvovaginal atrophy (although this should only be used in a research setting) (1).
- FDA warns against the use of medical devices for unapproved uses including "vaginal rejuvenation" procedures.

COMPLEMENTARY & ALTERNATIVE MEDICINE
- Sitz baths may relieve painful inflammation.
- Perineal massage
- Antioxidants may improve symptoms associated with endometriosis.

 ONGOING CARE

FOLLOW-UP RECOMMENDATIONS
Patient Monitoring
- Outpatient follow-up depends on therapy.
- Every 6 to 12 months once resolved

DIET
A high-fiber diet may help if constipation is a contributing cause.

PATIENT EDUCATION
- Boston Women's Health Book Collective, Norsigian J. *Our Bodies, Ourselves*. New York, NY: Touchstone; 2011.
- Kegel exercise information
- Provide couples with information about sexual arousal techniques.

PROGNOSIS
Depends on underlying cause but most patients will respond to treatment

REFERENCES

1. ACOG Practice Bulletin No. 141: management of menopausal symptoms. *Obstet Gynecol*. 2014;123(1):202–216.
2. Luzzi G, Lamont L. A guide to sexual pain in men. *Practitioner*. 2005;249(1667):73, 75, 77 passim.
3. Weinberger JM, Houman J, Caron AT, et al. Female sexual dysfunction: a systematic review of outcomes across various treatment modalities. *Sex Med Rev*. 2019;7(2):223–250. doi:10.1016/j.sxmr.2017.12.004.
4. Pitsouni E, Grigoriadis T, Douskos A, et al. Efficacy of vaginal therapies alternative to vaginal estrogens on sexual function and orgasm of menopausal women: a systematic review and meta-analysis of randomized controlled trials. *Eur J Obstet Gynecol Reprod Biol*. 2018;229:45–56.
5. Demyttenaere K, Huygens R. Painful ejaculation and urinary hesitancy in association with antidepressant therapy: relief with tamsulosin. *Eur Neuropsychopharmacol*. 2002;12(4):337–341. doi:10.1016/s0924-977x(02)00040-8.

ADDITIONAL READING
- Seehusen DA, Baird DC, Bode DV. Dyspareunia in women. *Am Fam Physician*. 2014;90(7):465–470.
- Sorensen J, Bautista KE, Lamvu G, et al. Evaluation and treatment of female sexual pain: a clinical review. *Cureus*. 2018;10(3):e2379.

 SEE ALSO
- Balanitis, Phimosis, and Paraphimosis; Endometriosis; Genito-Pelvic Pain/Penetration Disorder (Vaginismus); Pelvic Inflammatory Disease; Sexual Dysfunction in Women; Vulvovaginitis, Estrogen Deficient; Vulvovaginitis, Prepubescent
- Algorithms: Dyspareunia; Vaginal Discharge

CODES

ICD10
- N94.1 Dyspareunia
- F52.6 Dyspareunia not due to a substance or known physiol cond

CLINICAL PEARLS
- Thorough history to determine if patient feels pain before, during, or after intercourse will help identify cause.
  - Pain before intercourse suggests a phobic association with penetration or the anticipated sexual activity and/or the presence of vestibulitis.
  - Pain during intercourse combined with the location of the pain is most predictive of the causes of pain.
  - Introital pain after intercourse suggests vestibulitis in women of childbearing age, hypertonic pelvic floor, or vulvovaginal dystrophia.
  - A sudden symptom onset can suggest a psychosexual etiology, whereas gradual onset of symptoms is more likely physical or anatomic.
- Potential relationship exists between primary dyspareunia and vaginismus, low libido, and arousal disorders.
- Episiotomy does not offer any benefit in the prevention of dyspareunia; an episiotomy in fact may cause more future discomfort.

DYSPEPSIA, FUNCTIONAL

Briana Lindberg, MD • Kristina Burgers, MD

 BASICS

DESCRIPTION
- The presence of bothersome postprandial fullness, early satiety, or epigastric pain/burning in the absence of causative structural disease (to include normal upper endoscopy) for at least 1 to 3 days per week for the preceding 3 months, with initial symptom onset at least 6 months prior to diagnosis (Rome IV criteria)
- Rome IV criteria divide patients into two subtypes:
  - Postprandial distress syndrome (PDS)
  - Epigastric pain syndrome (EPS)
- System(s) affected: GI
- Synonym(s): idiopathic dyspepsia, nonulcer dyspepsia, nonorganic dyspepsia, PDS, and EPS

EPIDEMIOLOGY
Incidence
Unknown; accounts for 70% of patients with dyspepsia and ~5% of primary care visits

Prevalence
- 10–20% prevalence worldwide (varies based on criteria)
- More common in Western cultures
- PDS may be more common in Eastern cultures.
- Predominant age: adults (can be seen in children)
- Predominant gender: female > male

ETIOLOGY AND PATHOPHYSIOLOGY
Unknown but proposed mechanisms or associations include gastric motility disorders, visceral pain hypersensitivity, *Helicobacter pylori* infection, alteration in upper GI microbiome, postinfectious complications, immune activation, inflammation, and gut-brain axis disorders

Genetics
Possible link to G-protein β_3 subunit 825 CC genotype, serotonin transport genes, and/or cholecystokinin-A-receptor gene polymorphisms

Geriatric Considerations
Patients age >60 years with new-onset dyspepsia should undergo endoscopy.

Pediatric Considerations
Be alert for family system dysfunction.

Pregnancy Considerations
Pregnancy may exacerbate symptoms.

RISK FACTORS
- Other functional disorders: fibromyalgia, temporomandibular joint pain, chronic fatigue syndrome
- Anxiety/depression, psychosocial stressors (e.g., divorce; unemployment; history of physical, sexual, or emotional trauma/abuse)
- Smoking
- Female gender

GENERAL PREVENTION
Avoid foods and habits known to exacerbate symptoms.

COMMONLY ASSOCIATED CONDITIONS
Other functional bowel disorders

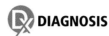 **DIAGNOSIS**

HISTORY
- Postprandial fullness (1)
- Early satiety (1)
- Epigastric pain (1)
- Epigastric burning (1)
- Symptoms for 3 months (1)
- Alarm features include (2),(3),(4):
  - Unintended weight loss
  - Progressive dysphagia
  - Odynophagia
  - Persistent vomiting
  - GI bleeding
  - Family history of upper GI cancer
  - Age ≥60 years

PHYSICAL EXAM
- Document weight status and vital signs.
- Examine for signs of systemic illness.
  - Murphy sign for cholecystitis
  - Rebound and guarding for ulcer perforation
  - Palpate during muscle contraction to assess for abdominal wall pain.
  - Jaundice
  - Thyromegaly

DIFFERENTIAL DIAGNOSIS
- Peptic ulcer disease; gastroesophageal reflux disease
- Cholecystitis; choledocholithiasis
- Gastric or esophageal cancer; esophageal spasm
- Malabsorption syndromes; celiac disease
- Pancreatic cancer; pancreatitis

- Inflammatory bowel disease; carbohydrate malabsorption; gastroparesis
- Ischemic bowel disease
- Intestinal parasites
- Irritable bowel syndrome
- Ischemic heart disease
- Diabetes mellitus; thyroid disease; connective tissue disorders
- Medication effects

DIAGNOSTIC TESTS & INTERPRETATION
Initial Tests (lab, imaging)
- Functional dyspepsia is a diagnosis of exclusion. Order labs based on clinical suspicion (2)[C].
- Test for *H. pylori* (stool antigen or urea breath test) in areas of high *H. pylori* prevalence (2),(4)[A].
- CBC (if anemia or infection are suspected)
- Liver-associated enzymes/right upper quadrant ultrasound (if hepatobiliary disease is suspected)
- Pancreatic enzymes (if pancreatic disease is suspected)
- Upper endoscopy for patients age >60 years to rule out malignancy (4)[C]
- Upper endoscopy is unlikely to change outcomes or management (2),(5)[C].
- Self-report questionnaires can track symptoms (3)[C].

Diagnostic Procedures/Other
- Esophageal manometry or gastric accommodation studies are rarely needed (3)[C].
- Motility studies are unnecessary, unless gastroparesis is strongly suspected (4)[C].

Test Interpretation
None (By definition, this a functional disorder.)

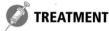 **TREATMENT**

GENERAL MEASURES
- Reassurance/physician support is helpful (2),(3)[C].
- Treatment is based on presumed etiologies.
- Discontinue offending medications (3)[C].
- Routine endoscopy not recommended in dyspeptic patients age <60 years even without alarm features (4)[B]

MEDICATION

First Line

- Treat *H. pylori* if confirmed on testing (3),(4)[A].
- Trial of once daily proton pump inhibitor (PPI) medication (e.g., omeprazole 20 mg PO QD) or H₂ receptor antagonist for up to 8 weeks in patients without alarm symptoms—most effective for patients with EPS (3),(4),(5)[A]
- Prokinetics have been proposed as first-line agents in PDS, although efficacy data for metoclopramide, 5 to 10 mg PO TID 30 minutes before meals (only agent approved in United States) are limited (5)[C]. Prokinetics should be prescribed at the lowest effective dose to avoid potential side effects (4)[C]. Use with caution in elderly patients due to side effects of tardive dyskinesia and parkinsonian symptoms.

Second Line

- Trial of tricyclic antidepressant (TCA) medication is more helpful for EPS than PDS (e.g., amitriptyline 25 mg PO QD, can uptitrate to 50 mg PO QD), with an NNT of 6 (2),(4)[A]. Caution in elderly. There is no benefit to SSRI/SNRI.
- Trazodone 25 mg at bedtime is an alternative (2),(5)[A]. Consider buspirone or mirtazapine if no response or if contraindications to TCA (2)[B].
- Gabapentin 300 mg twice daily can be a useful adjunct, particularly for treatment of gastrointestinal pain symptoms (6)[B].

ADDITIONAL THERAPIES

- Stress reduction (2),(5)[C]
- Psychotherapy and/or cognitive-behavioral therapy effective in some patients (2)[C],(3),(4)[B]
- Patients should be given a positive diagnosis and reassured of benign prognosis (2)[C].

COMPLEMENTARY & ALTERNATIVE MEDICINE

Alternative medicine approaches need further study and are not currently recommended (4)[C].

- STW 5 (Iberogast®) shown to be helpful in some studies (2)[C].
- Probiotics have theoretical benefit but lack consistent trial data to support routine use (2)[C].
- Hypnotherapy may help (3)[B].
- Transcutaneous electroacupuncture may help (3)[B].

ONGOING CARE

FOLLOW-UP RECOMMENDATIONS

Patient Monitoring

- Provide ongoing support and reassurance.
- Upper endoscopy if persistent symptoms
- Change medications if no difference in symptoms after 4 weeks (3)[C].
- Discontinue medications once symptoms resolve (3)[C].

DIET

- Limited data to support dietary modification
- Consider limiting fatty foods (2),(5)[C].
- Avoid foods that exacerbate symptoms: wheat and cow milk proteins, peppers or spices, coffee, tea, and alcohol (2),(5)[C].

PATIENT EDUCATION

Reassurance and stress reduction techniques

PROGNOSIS

Long-term/chronic symptoms with symptom-free periods

COMPLICATIONS

Iatrogenic, from evaluation to rule out serious pathology

REFERENCES

1. Stanghellini V, Chan FK, Hasler WL, et al. Gastroduodenal disorders. *Gastroenterology*. 2016;150(6):1380–1392.
2. Talley NJ, Ford AC. Functional dyspepsia. *N Engl J Med*. 2015;373(19):1853–1863.
3. Miwa H, Kusano M, Arisawa T, et al; for Japanese Society of Gastroenterology. Evidence-based clinical practice guidelines for functional dyspepsia. *J Gastroenterol*. 2015;50(2):125–139.
4. Moayyedi PM, Lacy BE, Andrews CN, et al. ACG and CAG clinical guideline: management of dyspepsia. *Am J Gastroenterol*. 2017;112(7):988–1013.
5. Talley NJ, Walker MM, Holtmann G. Functional dyspepsia. *Curr Opin Gastroenterol*. 2016;32(6):467–473.
6. Shafigh-Ardestani M, Karami-Horestani M, Emami B, et al. Evaluating the effect of oral gabapentin on the improvement of gastrointestinal symptoms in patients with functional dyspepsia resistant to conventional treatments. *Adv Biomed Res*. 2019;8:53.

ADDITIONAL READING

- Garcia-Etxebarria K, Carbone F, Teder-Laving M, et al. A survey of functional dyspepsia in 361,360 individuals: phenotypic and genetic cross-disease analyses [published online ahead of print August 11, 2021]. *Neurogastroenterol Motil*. 2021:e14236. doi:10.1111/nmo.14236.
- Grossman D, Tack J, Ford A, et al. Neuromodulators for functional gastrointestinal disorders (disorders of gut–brain interaction): a Rome Foundation working team report. *Gastroenterology*. 2018;154(4):1140–1171.
- Lu Y, Chen M, Huang Z, et al. Antidepressants in the treatment of functional dyspepsia: a systematic review and meta-analysis. *PLoS One*. 2016;11(6):e0157798.
- Masuy I, Van Oudenhove L, Tack J. Treatment options for functional dyspepsia. *Aliment Pharmacol Ther*. 2019;49(9):1134–1172.

SEE ALSO

- Irritable Bowel Syndrome
- Algorithm: Dyspepsia

CODES

ICD10

K30 Functional dyspepsia

CLINICAL PEARLS

- Dyspepsia without underlying organic disease is classified as being functional or idiopathic.
- Consider empiric acid suppression therapy as first line for functional dyspepsia.
- Extensive diagnostic testing is not recommended unless alarm symptoms are present.

D

DYSPHAGIA
Felix B. Chang, MD, DABMA, ABIHM, ABIM

BASICS

Impaired passage of the alimentary bolus from the mouth to stomach (1)[C]

DESCRIPTION
- Oropharyngeal: difficulty transferring food bolus from oropharynx to proximal esophagus
- Esophageal: difficulty moving food bolus through the body of the esophagus to the pylorus

EPIDEMIOLOGY
5–8% of the general population >50 years of age

Incidence
Esophageal food impaction 25 per 100,000 persons per year

Prevalence
- From 14% to 33% among community-dwelling individuals 65 years old or greater
- In hospital settings, can be as high as 40%
- Nursing home residents range from 29% to 32%.
- 30–40% in older people living independently
- 44% in patients in geriatrics acute care
- 60% in older patients that are institutionalized

ETIOLOGY AND PATHOPHYSIOLOGY
- Oropharyngeal (transfer dysphagia):
  - Functional due to disordered motor function in the oropharynx
  - Mechanical causes: pharyngeal and laryngeal cancer, acute epiglottitis, carotid body tumor, pharyngitis, tonsillitis, strep throat, lymphoid hyperplasia of lingual tonsil, lateral pharyngeal pouch, hypopharyngeal diverticulum
  - Neuromyogenic: stroke, head trauma, Parkinson and parkinsonism, amyotrophic lateral sclerosis, myasthenia, myopathies (polymyositis, dermatomyositis, muscular dystrophies), alcoholic, thyrotoxicosis, hypothyroidism, amyloidosis, Cushing syndrome
- Esophageal:
  - Mechanical: carcinomas, esophageal diverticula, esophageal webs, Schatzki ring, structures (peptic, chemical, trauma, radiation), foreign body
  - Extrinsic mechanical lesions: peritonsillar abscess, thyroid disorders, tumors, mediastinal compression, vascular compression (enlarged left atrium, aberrant subclavius, aortic aneurysm), osteoarthritis of the cervical spine, adenopathy, esophageal duplication cyst
- Neuromuscular: achalasia, diffuse esophageal spasm, hypertonic lower esophageal sphincter, scleroderma, nutcracker esophagus, CVA, Alzheimer disease, Huntington chorea, Parkinson disease, multiple sclerosis, skeletal muscle disease (polymyositis, dermatomyositis), neuromuscular junction disease (myasthenia gravis, Lambert-Eaton syndrome, botulism), hyper- and hypothyroidism, Guillain-Barré syndrome, systemic lupus erythematosus, acute lymphoblastic leukemia, amyloidosis, diabetic neuropathy, brainstem tumors, Chagas disease
- Infection: diphtheria, chronic meningitis, tertiary syphilis, Lyme disease, rabies, poliomyelitis, CMV, esophagitis (*Candida*, herpetic)

RISK FACTORS
- Children: hereditary and/or congenital malformations
- Adults: age >50 years; elderly: GERD, stroke, COPD, chronic pain
- Smoking, excess alcohol intake, obesity

- Medications: quinine, potassium chloride, vitamin C, tetracycline, Bactrim, clindamycin, NSAIDs, procainamide, anticholinergics, bisphosphates, anticonvulsants (phenobarbital, carbamazepine, and phenytoin); antihistaminics, antidepressants (amitriptyline, imipramine), antipsychotics (haloperidol, phenothiazine, butyrophenone, thioxanthene); drugs for overactive bladder oxybutynin; opiates; antimigraine drugs such as rizatriptan; antihypertensive (ACE, ARB, calcium channel blockers, β-blockers, α_2-agonist); diuretics (HCTZ and chlorothiazide); cytotoxic (antineoplastics; interferon-α, ribavirin); appetite suppressants sibutramine; β_2-agonist bronchodilators, muscle relaxants
- Xerostomia is reported with ACE inhibitors, antiarrhythmics, antiemetics, diuretics, SSRI.
- Mucositis by cytotoxic chemotherapy, and molecular target treatment as sunitinib, everolimus
- Neurologic events or diseases: CVA, myasthenia gravis, multiple sclerosis, Parkinson disease, amyotrophic lateral sclerosis (ALS), Huntington chorea, dementia
- HIV patients with CD4 cell count <100 cells/mm^3
- Trauma or irradiation of head, neck, and chest; mechanical lesions
- Extrinsic mechanical lesions: lung, thyroid tumors, lymphoma, metastasis
- Iron deficiency
- Anterior cervical spine surgery (up to 71% in the first 2 weeks postop; 12–14% at 1 year postop)
- Dysphagia lusoria (vascular abnormalities causing dysphagia): complete vascular ring, double aortic arch, right aortic arch with retroesophageal left subclavian artery and left ligamentum arteriosum, and right aortic arch with mirror-image branching and left ligamentum arteriosum

GENERAL PREVENTION
- Correct poorly fitting dentures.
- Educate patients to prolong chewing and drink adequate volumes of water at meals.
- Liquid and soft food diet as appropriate
- Avoid alcohol with meals.
- Prophylactic swallowing exercises in patients with head and neck cancer undergoing chemoradiation

COMMONLY ASSOCIATED CONDITIONS
Peptic structure, esophageal webs and rings, carcinoma, history of stroke, dementia, pneumonia

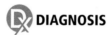

DIAGNOSIS

HISTORY
- Dysphagia to both solids and liquids from the onset of deglutition likely represents an esophageal motility disorder.
- Oropharyngeal dysphagia presents as difficulty initiating the swallowing process.
- Dysphagia for solids that progresses to involve liquids more likely reflects mechanical obstruction.
- Progressive dysphagia is usually caused by cancer or a peptic stricture. Intermittent dysphagia is most often related to a lower esophageal ring.
- Inquire about heartburn, weight loss, hematemesis, coffee ground emesis, anemia, regurgitation of undigested food particles, and respiratory symptoms.
- Inquire about regurgitation, aspiration, or drooling immediately after swallowing as this may represent oropharyngeal dysphagia.

- Does the food bolus feel stuck?
  - Upper sternum or back of throat may represent oropharyngeal dysphagia, whereas sensation over the lower sternum is typical of esophageal dysphagia.
- Is odynophagia (pain) present?
  - May represent inflammation, achalasia, diffuse esophageal spasm, esophagitis, pharyngitis, pill-induced esophagitis, cancer
- Have globus sensation ("lump in the throat")?
  - Potentially indicates cricopharyngeal or laryngeal disorders
- History of sour taste in the back of the throat or chronic heartburn suggests GERD.
- Inquire about alcohol and/or tobacco use.
- Are there associated symptoms such as weight loss or chest pain?
  - Double aortic arch, right aortic arch with retroesophageal left subclavian artery and left ligamentum arteriosum
  - Anticholinergics, antihistamines, and some antihypertensives can decrease salivary production.
- Halitosis: Rule out diverticulum. Prior history of a connective tissue disorder
- Changes in speech, hoarseness, weak cough, dysphonia? Rule out neuromuscular dysfunction.
- Dysphagia may be the first symptom of a neuromuscular disorder, such as amyotrophic lateral sclerosis or myasthenia gravis.

PHYSICAL EXAM
- Skin: telangiectasia, sclerodactyly, calcinosis (r/o autoimmune disease); Raynaud phenomenon, sclerodactyly may be found in CREST syndrome or systemic scleroderma; stigmata of alcohol abuse (palmar erythema; telangiectasia)
- Head, eye, ear, nose, throat (HEENT):
  - Oropharyngeal: pharyngeal erythema/edema, tonsillitis, pharyngeal ulcers or thrush, odynophagia (bacterial, viral, fungal infections); tongue fasciculations (ALS)
  - Neck: masses, lymphadenopathy, neck tenderness (thyroiditis), goiter
- Neurologic:
  - Cranial nerve exam: sensory: cranial nerves V, IX, and X; motor: cranial nerves V, VII, X, XI, and XII
  - CNS, mental status exam, strength testing, Horner syndrome, ataxia, cogwheel rigidity (CVA, dementia, Parkinson disease, Alzheimer disease)
    - Eye position, extraocular motility
- Informal bedside swallowing evaluation: Observe level of consciousness, postural control-upright position, oral hygiene, mobilization of oral secretions.

DIFFERENTIAL DIAGNOSIS
See "Etiology and Pathophysiology."

DIAGNOSTIC TESTS & INTERPRETATION
Adults (2)[C]:
- EGD is recommended for the initial assessment of patient with esophageal dysphagia; barium esophagography is recommended as an adjunct if EGD findings are negative (3)[C].
- Fiberoptic endoscopic examination of swallowing (FEES)
- Ambulatory 24-hour pH testing if reflux is suspected
- Esophageal manometry if history suggest dysmotility disorder achalasia, diffuse esophageal spasm, scleroderma esophagus, nutcracker esophagus, hypertensive LES, ineffective esophageal motility, collagen vascular disease (scleroderma, CREST).
- Videofluoroscopic swallowing study (VFSS): oropharyngeal dysphagia
- Do not order "formal" swallow evaluation in stroke patients unless they fail their initial swallow screen.

Initial Tests (lab, imaging)
- CBC (infection and inflammation)
- Antiacetylcholine antibodies (myasthenia)
- Thyroid function studies to detect dysphagia associated with hypothyroidism or hyperthyroidism, cobalamin levels serum protein, and albumin levels for nutritional assessment
- Barium swallow: detects strictures or stenosis; if endoscopy fails to identify an abnormality

Follow-Up Tests & Special Considerations
- CT scan of chest; MRI of brain and cervical spine
- VFSS (lips, tongue, palate, pharynx, larynx, proximal esophagus)
- Fiberoptic endoscopy and videofluoroscopy are similar in terms of diagnostic sensitivity.
- For accurate diagnosis of eosinophilic esophagitis; biopsies from normal-appearing mucosa in the midthoracic and distal esophagus should be requested for all patients with unexplained solid food dysphagia (3)[B].

Diagnostic Procedures/Other
- Endoscopy with biopsy; esophageal manometry; esophageal pH monitoring
- Patients with persistent oropharyngeal symptoms and a negative initial workup should be referred for EGD to rule out esophageal pathology (3)[C].

 ## TREATMENT

GENERAL MEASURES
Exclude cardiac disease. Ensure airway patency and adequate pulmonary function. Assess nutritional status. Speech therapy

MEDICATION
Modify medications taken by patient according to patient functional swallowing ability (3)[C].

First Line
- For esophageal spasms: calcium channel blockers: nifedipine 10 to 30 mg TID; imipramine 50 mg at bedtime; sildenafil 50 mg/day PRN
- For esophagitis: Patients <50 years who have esophageal dysphagia and no other worrisome symptoms should undergo a 4-week trial of acid suppression therapy prior to endoscopy (3)[B].
  - Antacids (calcium carbonate, magnesium hydroxide, aluminum hydroxide, sodium bicarbonate-based)
  - H$_2$ blockers:
    ○ Cimetidine: up to 1,600 mg orally per day in 2 or 4 divided doses for 12 weeks
    ○ Ranitidine: initial 150 mg orally 4 times daily and maintenance 150 mg orally twice daily
    ○ Nizatidine: 150 mg orally twice daily for 12 weeks
    ○ Famotidine: 20 to 40 mg orally twice daily for 12 weeks
- Proton pump inhibitors:
  - Omeprazole: 20 mg once daily for 4 to 8 weeks
  - Lansoprazole: 30 mg once daily for up to 8 weeks
  - Rabeprazole: 20 mg orally once daily for 4 to 8 weeks
  - Esomeprazole: 20 to 40 mg orally once daily for 4 to 8 weeks
  - Pantoprazole: 40 mg orally once daily for up to 8 weeks

ISSUES FOR REFERRAL
- Gastroenterology: endoscopy, refractory symptoms
- Surgery: dilation, esophageal myotomy, biopsy
- A speech-language pathologist should be part of multidisciplinary team for treating patients with head and neck cancers.

ADDITIONAL THERAPIES
Speech therapy to assess swallowing; nutritional evaluation and positioning, physical therapy for muscle-strengthening exercise bedtime, remaining upright after eating
- Self-expanded metal stent is safe, effective, and quicker in palliating dysphagia compared to other modalities.
- Do not recommend percutaneous feeding tubes in patient with advance dementia; instead, offer careful hand feeding.
- Enteral tube feedings using an NG or gastrostomy tube may be required for patients with high risk of aspiration or who require supplemental nutrition or hydration.

SURGERY/OTHER PROCEDURES
- Esophageal dilatation (pneumatic or bougie) for achalasia. Esophageal stent; laser for cancer palliation
- Treat underlying problem (e.g., thyroid goiter, vascular ring, esophageal atresia).
- Nd:YAG laser incision of lower esophageal rings refractory to dilation
- Photodynamic therapy (cancer). Cricopharyngeal myotomy (oropharyngeal dysphagia)
- Surgery for Zenker diverticulum, refractory strictures, or myotomy (for achalasia)
- Percutaneous endoscopic gastrostomy (PEG) decreases risk of dysphagia when compared with nasogastric tube.

COMPLEMENTARY & ALTERNATIVE MEDICINE
- Acupuncture may augment swallowing training to improve dysphagia following a stroke.
- Insufficient evidence for routine use of botulinum toxin

ADMISSION, INPATIENT, AND NURSING CONSIDERATIONS
- Complete or partial esophageal obstruction associated with malnutrition or dehydration
- Need for enteral feeding
- Hospitalization with total or near-total obstruction of esophageal lumen
- Hospitalization may be needed for endoscopy and/or esophageal dilatation and is generally indicated for diagnostic or therapeutic surgical procedures.
- IV fluids for dehydrated, hypovolemic patients, and patients with impaired consciousness
- Discharge when tolerating adequate diet without nausea/pain

 ## ONGOING CARE

Swallow therapy may reduce the incidence of chest infections or pneumonia after stroke (4)[A].

FOLLOW-UP RECOMMENDATIONS
Soft-pureed diet may be useful in mechanical esophageal narrowing. In severe or prolonged dysphagia, enteral feeding using nasogastric tube or gastrostomy may be required.

Patient Monitoring
Medications should be reviewed.

DIET
See "General Prevention."

PATIENT EDUCATION
Safe swallowing:
- Drink using small sips of liquids, without any gulping. Sit upright at 90 degrees and avoid drinking or eating when lying down or slouched.
- Eat slowly, small bites of food, chew food completely before swallowing, not swallow any drink or food before taking more. Not use drinks to wash down food. Refrain from talking when food is in their mouth.

PROGNOSIS
- 45% reported mortality within 12 months in nursing home residents with oropharyngeal dysphagia an aspiration
- Oropharyngeal dysphagia is generally associated with poorer prognosis.
- Swallowing treatment showed a reduced incidence of pneumonia but no difference in swallow quality of life scores (4)[A]

COMPLICATIONS
- Oropharyngeal: pneumonia, lung abscess, aspiration pneumonia, airway obstruction
- Malnutrition and dehydration, frailty
- Contribute to the development of sarcopenia, reduce immunity, impaired wound healing.
- Aspiration pneumonia in 50% of patients undergoing modified barium swallow studies.

REFERENCES
1. Pasha SF, Acosta RD, Chandrasekhara V, et al; for ASGE Standards of Practice Committee. The role of endoscopy in the evaluation and management of dysphagia. *Gastrointest Endosc*. 2014;79(2):191–201.
2. American College of Radiology. ACR appropriateness criteria for dysphagia. https://www.guidelinecentral.com/summaries/acr-appropriateness-criteria-dysphagia/. Accessed September 28, 2019.
3. Wirth R, Dziewas R. Dysphagia and pharmacotherapy in older adults. *Curr Opin Clin Nutr Metab Care*. 2019;22(1):25–29.
4. Bath PM, Lee HS, Eventon LF. Swallowing therapy for dysphagia in acute and subacute stroke. *Cochrane Database Syst Rev*. 2018;10(10):CD000323.

ADDITIONAL READING
- Christmas C, Rogus-Pulia N. Swallowing disorders in the older population. *J Am Geri Soc*. 2019;67(12):2643–2649
- Wilkinson JM, Halland M. Esophageal motility disorders. *Am Fam Physician*. 2020;102(5):291–296.
- Xin Li L, Deng K. Acupuncture combined with swallowing training for poststroke dysphagia: a meta-analysis of randomised controlled trials. *Acupunct Med*. 2019;37(2):81–90.

CODES

ICD10
- R13.10 Dysphagia, unspecified
- R13.12 Dysphagia, oropharyngeal phase
- R13.14 Dysphagia, pharyngoesophageal phase

CLINICAL PEARLS
- Esopahagogastroduodenoscopy is recommended for the initial evaluation of esophageal dysphagia, with barium esophagography as an adjunct.
- Palliative care goals are to minimize coughing, chocking, and drooling.

ECTOPIC PREGNANCY

Kristina Gracey, MD, MPH

 BASICS

DESCRIPTION

Ectopic: pregnancy implanted outside the uterine cavity. Subtypes include:

- Tubal: pregnancy implanted in any portion of the fallopian tube. Abdominal: pregnancy implanted intra-abdominally, most commonly after tubal abortion or rupture of tubal ectopic pregnancy. Heterotopic: pregnancy: implanted intrauterine with a separate pregnancy implanted outside the uterine cavity. Ovarian: implantation of pregnancy in ovarian tissue. Cervical: implantation of pregnancy in cervix. Intraligamentary: implantation of pregnancy within the broad ligament

EPIDEMIOLOGY

Incidence

- The true incidence is difficult to estimate. Incidence is likely between about 6 and 20 per 1,000 pregnancies in the United States. About 1 in 10 first-trimester pregnancies presenting to the emergency with pain and/or bleeding are due to ectopic pregnancy. In the United States, ectopic pregnancy is the leading cause of first-trimester maternal deaths.
- Heterotopic pregnancy, although rare (1:30,000), occurs with greater frequency (1/1,000) in women undergoing in vitro fertilization (IVF); increasing incidence of nontubal, and particularly cesarean scar ectopic pregnancies, due in part to more cesarean sections and more IVF
- ~33% recurrence rate if prior ectopic pregnancy

ETIOLOGY AND PATHOPHYSIOLOGY

95–97% of ectopic pregnancies occur in the fallopian tube, of which, 55–80% in the ampulla, 12–25% in the isthmus, and 5–17% in the fimbria. One risk factor for a tubal pregnancy is impaired movement of the fertilized ovum to the uterine cavity due to dysfunction of the tubal cilia, scarring, or narrowing of the tubal lumen.

RISK FACTORS

- History of pelvic inflammatory disease (PID), endometritis, or current gonorrhea/chlamydia infection, pelvic adhesive disease (infection or prior surgery)
- Previous ectopic pregnancy, history of tubal surgery (~33% of pregnancies after tubal ligation are ectopic.)
- Use of an intrauterine device (IUD): IUD reduces absolute risk of ectopic pregnancy, but there is an increased likelihood of ectopic location if pregnancy occurs.
- Use of assisted reproductive technologies
- Tobacco use; patients with disorders that affect ciliary motility may be at increased risk (e.g., endometriosis, Kartagener).

GENERAL PREVENTION

Reliable contraception or abstinence, and screening for and treatment of STIs (i.e., gonorrhea, chlamydia) that can cause PID and tubal scarring

 DIAGNOSIS

HISTORY

In >50% of presenting cases, patients have sudden-onset abdominal pain coupled with cessation of/or irregular menses and acute vaginal bleeding (the classic triad). Other common symptoms include nausea and/or vomiting, vaginal bleeding, and pain referred to the shoulder (from hemoperitoneum).

PHYSICAL EXAM

- Abdominal tenderness ± rebound tenderness associated with vaginal bleeding
- Palpable mass on pelvic exam (adnexal or cul-de-sac fullness), cervical motion tenderness
- In cases of rupture and significant intraperitoneal bleeding, signs of shock such as pallor, tachycardia, and hypotension may be present.

DIFFERENTIAL DIAGNOSIS

Missed, threatened, inevitable, or completed abortion (miscarriage), gestational trophoblastic neoplasia ("molar pregnancy"), appendicitis, salpingitis, PID, ruptured corpus luteum or hemorrhagic cyst, ovarian tumor, benign or malignant, ovarian torsion, cervical polyp, cancer, trauma, or cervicitis

DIAGNOSTIC TESTS & INTERPRETATION

Initial Tests (lab, imaging)

- CBC and ABO type and antibody screen
- Transvaginal US (TVUS) is the gold standard for diagnosis:
  - Failure to visualize a normal intrauterine gestational sac when serum human chorionic gonadotropin (hCG) is above the discriminatory level (>1,500 to 2,000 IU/L) suggests an abnormal pregnancy of unknown location (PUL).
  - An hCG level of 3,500 IU/L is associated with a 99% probability of detecting a normal intrauterine gestational sac in clinical practice.
  - These values are not validated for multiple gestations.
- If TVUS unavailable or inconclusive for intrauterine pregnancy (IUP), check hCG: Serial quantitative serum levels normally increase by at least 53% every 48 hours: Abnormal rise (<35%) should prompt workup for gestational abnormalities. Clinical impression of acute abdomen/intraperitoneal bleeding concurrent with a positive hCG level is indicative of ectopic pregnancy until proven otherwise.
- MRI may also be useful but costly and rarely used if TVUS is available; benefits particularly for abdominal or cesarean scar pregnancy

Follow-Up Tests & Special Considerations

Serum progesterone level: >20 mg/mL associated with lower risk of ectopic pregnancy. In women with pain and/or bleeding who have an inconclusive US, serum progesterone level <3.2 ng/mL ruled out a viable pregnancy in 99.2% of women; may provide additional data for PUL but does not predict ectopic pregnancy (1)[B]

Diagnostic Procedures/Other

In the setting of an undesired pregnancy, sampling of the uterine cavity with endometrial biopsy or D&C can identify the presence/absence of intrauterine chorionic villi. When an IUP has been evacuated by curettage, hCG levels should drop by 50% within 48 hours. Historically, culdocentesis was performed to confirm suspected hemoperitoneum prior to surgical management. Currently, TVUS quantification of pelvic fluid is sufficient.

Test Interpretation

Products of conception (POC; especially chorionic villi) outside the uterine cavity

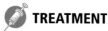 **TREATMENT**

MEDICATION

- Methotrexate: treatment for unruptured tubal pregnancy or for remaining POCs after laparoscopic salpingostomy. Methotrexate inhibits DNA synthesis via folic acid antagonism by inactivating dihydrofolate reductase.
- If TVUS is suggestive but not diagnostic, in the hemodynamically stable patient who qualifies for medical management, confirm suspected US findings with 2 hCG levels drawn 48 hours apart. Rise <35% is consistent with nonviable pregnancy.
- Most effective when pregnancy is <3 cm diameter, hCG <5,000 mIU/mL, and no fetal heart movement is seen. Success rate is 88% if hCG <1,000 mIU/mL, 71% if hCG 1,000 to 2,000 mIU/mL, 38% if 2,000 to 5,000 mIU/mL:
  - Three main dosage regimens exist (2), but single-dose regimen is preferred for simplicity, safety, and comparable effectiveness to multidose regimens (2),(3)[A]:
    ○ Single: IM methotrexate 50 mg/m^2 of body surface area (BSA); may repeat once if <15% decline in hCG between day 4 and 7. Follow hCG weekly.
    ○ Double dose: methotrexate 50 mg/m^2 of BSA once and then repeated on day 4; if <15% decline in hCG between day 4 and 7, may repeat third dose on day 7. Repeat hCG as needed on days 11 and 14 until decreases >15% in the interval and then weekly. If not dropping by day 14, refer for surgical management.
    ○ Multidose: methotrexate 1 mg/kg IM/IV every other day, with leucovorin 0.1 mg/kg IM in between. Maximum 4 doses until hCG drop below 15%; course may be repeated 7 days after last dose if necessary.
  - Contraindications: hemodynamic instability or any evidence of rupture, moderate to severe anemia, severe hepatic or renal dysfunction, immunodeficiency
  - Relative contraindications: fetal heart activity seen, large gestational sac (>3 cm, less effective), noncompliance or limited access to hospital or transportation, hCG >5,000 mIU/mL

- Precautions: immunologic, hematologic, renal, GI, hepatic, and pulmonary disease, or interacting medications
- Pretreatment testing: serum hCG, CBC, liver and renal function tests, blood type and screen
- Patient counseling: During therapy, refrain from use of alcohol, aspirin, NSAIDs, and folate supplements (decreases efficacy of methotrexate); avoid excessive sun exposure due to risk of sensitivity. Adherence to scheduled follow-up appointments is critical. Increased abdominal pain may occur during treatment; however, severe pain, nausea, vomiting, bleeding, dizziness, or light-headedness may indicate treatment failure and require urgent evaluation.
- Rupture of ectopic pregnancy during methotrexate treatment ranges from 7% to 14%.
- Side effects include stomatitis; conjunctivitis; abdominal cramping; and rarely neutropenia, pneumonitis, or alopecia (3).
- Systemic methotrexate may be offered in some kinds of nontubal ectopic pregnancies, but data is limited.

ISSUES FOR REFERRAL
Consider gynecologic consultation if not experienced in medical management and for surgical care.

ADDITIONAL THERAPIES
- Physician or patient may elect for surgical treatment as primary method and then postop hCG should guide need for supplemental methotrexate.
- After evidence of medical failure or tubal rupture, surgery is necessary.
- Treatment of cervical, ovarian, abdominal, or other ectopic pregnancy is complicated and requires immediate specialist referral.
- Follow all patients treated medically to an hCG of 0 to ensure that there is no need for surgical intervention.
- Offer anti-D Rh prophylaxis at a dose of 50 μg to all Rh-negative women who have a surgical procedure to manage an ectopic pregnancy or if there has been significant bleeding or abdominal pain.
- Expectant management of ectopic (confirmed on TVUS) may be offered to women who are clinically stable and have low and decreasing hCG level initially <1,500 mIU/mL (1)[B].
- Expectant management to allow for spontaneous resolution of PUL is acceptable in asymptomatic patients with no evidence of rupture or hemodynamic instability coupled with an appropriately low hCG and no extrauterine mass suggestive of ectopic. Ruptured tubal pregnancies may occur even with extremely low hCG levels (<100 mIU/mL) (4).
- With expectant management of PUL, repeat TVUS weekly (or when hCG above discriminatory zone) until location is confirmed or clinical picture is unstable.

SURGERY/OTHER PROCEDURES
- Indications include ruptured ectopic pregnancy, inability to comply with medical follow-up, previous tubal ligation, known tubal disease, current heterotopic pregnancy, desire for permanent sterilization at time of diagnosis.
- Laparoscopy is the first-line surgical management (1)[A].

- Salpingectomy (tubal removal) is preferred and is indicated for uncontrolled bleeding, recurrent ectopic pregnancy, severely damaged tube, large gestational sac, or patient's desire for sterilization (1)[B].
- Salpingostomy (preservation of tube) is considered in patients who wish to maintain fertility particularly if contralateral tube is damaged/absent (1)[C]. No difference in recurrence rate compared to salpingectomy. Persistent trophoblastic tissue with salpingostomy remains in the fallopian tube in 4–15% of cases; will need to follow weekly hCG
- Surgical treatment is first line for cesarean and cornual pregnancies.

ADMISSION, INPATIENT, AND NURSING CONSIDERATIONS
- Fails criteria for methotrexate management, suspicion of rupture, orthostatic, shock, and severe abdominal pain requiring IV narcotics
- Inpatient observation in the setting of an uncertain diagnosis, particularly with an unreliable patient, may be appropriate.
- Surgical emergency: Two IV access lines should be placed immediately if suspicion of rupture; aggressive resuscitation as needed. Blood product transfusion if necessary en route to OR. In cases of shock, pressors and cardiac support may be necessary.
- IV fluids are unnecessary for a stable ectopic pregnancy being medically treated but are critical for a surgical patient who is bleeding.
- Strict input/output, hourly vitals, orthostatics if mobile, frequent abdominal exams, serial hematocrit, pad counts if heavy vaginal bleeding
- Discharge criteria: afebrile, abdominal pain resolving or resolved, diagnosis established, surgical treatment, and recovery is complete

 ## ONGOING CARE

FOLLOW-UP RECOMMENDATIONS
Patient Monitoring
- Serial serum quantitative hCG until level drops to zero: After methotrexate administration, a strict monitoring protocol should be followed. Following salpingostomy, weekly levels are appropriate. Following salpingectomy, further follow-up may be unnecessary.
- Pelvic US for persistent or recurrent masses
- Pain control: brief course of narcotics usually necessary with medical or surgical management
- Liver and renal function tests weekly following methotrexate administration if repeat dosing is required
- Delay of subsequent pregnancy for at least 3 months after treatment with methotrexate due to teratogenicity (folate deficiency) (1)[C]

DIET
During treatment, avoid alcohol and foods and vitamins high in folate (leafy greens, liver, edamame) due to interaction with methotrexate efficacy.

PATIENT EDUCATION
- Signs and symptoms of ectopic pregnancy should be reviewed.
- Patients should be encouraged to plan subsequent pregnancies and seek early medical care on discovery of future pregnancies.

PROGNOSIS
- Chronic ectopic pregnancies are rare and treated with surgical removal of the fallopian tube.
- Future fertility depends on fertility prior to ectopic pregnancy and degree of tubal compromise. In women with normal fertility, treatment options have no differences in future fertility rates. In women with subfertility, expectant or medical treatments confer better future fertility (1)[C].
- ~66% of women with a history of ectopic pregnancy will have a future IUP if they are able to conceive.
- If infertility persists beyond 12 months, the fallopian tubes should be evaluated.

COMPLICATIONS
Hemorrhage and hypovolemic shock, persistent trophoblastic tissue after medical or surgical management, infection, infertility, blood transfusions with associated infections/transfusion reaction, disseminated intravascular coagulation in the setting of massive hemorrhage

REFERENCES

1. Diagnosis and management of ectopic pregnancy: Green-top Guideline No. 21. *BJOG*. 2016;123(13):e15–e55.
2. Mergenthal MC, Senapati S, Zee J, et al. Medical management of ectopic pregnancy with single-dose and 2-dose methotrexate protocols: human chorionic gonadotropin trends and patient outcomes. *Am J Obstet Gynecol*. 2016;215(5):590.e1–590.e5.
3. Yuk JS, Lee JH, Park WI, et al. Systematic review and meta-analysis of single-dose and non-single-dose methotrexate protocols in the treatment of ectopic pregnancy. *Int J Gynaecol Obstet*. 2018;141(3):295–303.
4. Committee on Practice Bulletins—Gynecology. ACOG Practice Bulletin No. 191 summary: tubal ectopic pregnancy. *Obstet Gynecol*. 2018;131(2):409–411.

 ## CODES

ICD10
- O00.9 Ectopic pregnancy, unspecified
- O00.1 Tubal pregnancy
- O00.0 Abdominal pregnancy

CLINICAL PEARLS
- 97% of ectopic pregnancies occur in the fallopian tube.
- Diagnosis requires high clinical suspicion in the setting of abdominal pain and a positive pregnancy test until IUP is confirmed.

EJACULATORY DISORDERS

Payam Sazegar, MD

BASICS

DESCRIPTION
- Group of dysfunctions involving altered time and control (premature ejaculation [PE], delayed ejaculation [DE]), presence (anejaculation [AE]), direction (retrograde ejaculation [RE]), volume (perceived ejaculate volume reduction [PEVR]), or force (decreased force of ejaculation [DFE]) of ejaculation
- PE is defined (*DSM-V*, 2013) as a persistent/recurrent pattern of ejaculation occurring during partnered sexual activity within 1 minute following vaginal penetration and before the individual wishes it + present for 6 months + causing significant distress for individual.
  - Natural biologic response is to ejaculate within 2 to 5 minutes after vaginal penetration.
  - Ejaculatory control is an acquired behavior that increases with experience.
  - Comorbidities common (diabetes, hypertension, sexual desire disorder, erectile dysfunction [ED])
- DE: prolonged time to ejaculate (>30 minutes) despite desire, stimulation, and erection; problematic for couples trying to conceive
- Aspermia (lack of sperm in the ejaculate):
  - AE: lack of emission or contractions of bulbospongiosus muscle
  - RE: partial or complete ejaculation of semen into the bladder
  - Obstruction: ejaculatory duct obstruction or urethral obstruction
- Also:
  - Painful ejaculation: genital or perineal pain during or after ejaculation
  - Ejaculatory anhedonia: normal ejaculation lacking orgasm or pleasure
  - Hematospermia: presence of blood in the ejaculate (often not a serious condition)

EPIDEMIOLOGY
Prevalence
- PE is common; reported prevalence in U.S. males in up to 20–30%.
- DE is reported in 5–8% of men age 18 to 59 years, but <3% have the problem for >6 months.
- Predominant age: all sexually mature age groups
- Predominant sex: male only

ETIOLOGY AND PATHOPHYSIOLOGY
Male sexual response:
- Erection mediated by parasympathetic nervous system
- Normal ejaculation consists of three phases:
  - Emission phase: Semen is deposited into urethra by contraction of prostate, seminal vesicles, vas deferens; under autonomic sympathetic control
  - Ejaculation phase: semen forcibly propelled out of urethra by rhythmic contractions of the bulbospongiosus and ischiocavernosus muscles. This is mediated by the somatic nervous system on the motor branches of the pudendal nerve. Bladder neck contracture by α-adrenergic receptors ensures anterograde ejaculation.
  - Orgasm: the pleasurable sensation associated with ejaculation (cerebral cortex); smooth muscle contraction of accessory sexual organs; release of pressure in posterior urethra

- PE:
  - Hypersensitivity/hyperexcitability of glans penis
  - 5-hydroxytryptamine (5-HT) receptor sensitivity
  - Psychogenic (inexperience, anxiety/guilt, low frequency of sex, relationship problems)
  - Urologic (ED, prostatitis, urethritis)
  - Endocrine (hyperthyroid, obesity, diabetes)
  - Lack of physical or sexual activity
  - Withdrawal/detox of prescription or illicit drugs
- DE:
  - Rarely due to underlying painful disorder (e.g., prostatitis, seminal vesiculitis)
  - Often has psychogenic component
  - No relation to testosterone levels
  - Sexual performance anxiety and other psychosocial factors
  - Medications may impair ejaculation (e.g., MAOIs, SSRIs, α- and β-blockers, thiazides, antipsychotics, tricyclic and quadricyclic antidepressants, NSAIDs, opiates, alcohol).
- Never any ejaculate:
  - Congenital structural disorder (müllerian duct cyst, wolffian abnormality)
  - Acquired (radical prostatectomy, postinfectious, posttraumatic, T10–T12 neuropathy)
- AE:
  - Retroperitoneal lymph node (LN) dissection
  - Spinal cord injury or other (traumatic) sympathetic nerve injury
  - Medications (α- and β-blockers, benzodiazepines, SSRIs, MAOIs, TCAs, antipsychotics, aminocaproic acid)
  - Diabetes mellitus (DM) (neuropathy)
  - Radical prostatectomy
- RE:
  - Transurethral resection of the prostate (25%) or other prostate resection procedures
  - Surgery on the neck of the bladder
  - Extensive pelvic surgery
  - Retroperitoneal LN dissection for testicular cancer (also may produce failure of emission)
  - Neurologic disorders (multiple sclerosis [MS], DM)
  - Medications (tamsulosin, other α-blockers, SSRIs, antipsychotics)
  - Urethral stricture (may be posttraumatic)
- Painful ejaculation:
  - Infection or inflammation (orchitis, epididymitis, prostatitis, urethritis)
  - Ejaculatory duct obstruction
  - Seminal vesicle calculi
  - Obstruction of the vas deferens
  - Psychological/functional
- Hematospermia (often unable to find cause):
  - Usually not a serious condition
  - Inflammation/infection
  - Calculi: bladder, seminal vesicle, prostate, urethra
  - Trauma to genital area (cycling, constipation, masturbation)
  - Obstruction
  - Cyst
  - Tumor (1–3% prostate cancers present with hematospermia)
  - Arteriovenous malformations
  - Iatrogenic
  - Hypertension

COMMONLY ASSOCIATED CONDITIONS
- Neurologic disorders (e.g., multiple sclerosis)
- Diabetes
- Prostatitis
- Ejaculatory duct obstruction
- Urethral stricture
- Psychological disorders
- Endocrinopathies
- Relationship/interpersonal difficulties

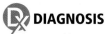 DIAGNOSIS

Based on a good history. Start by asking if ejaculation occurs before individual wishes OR does not occur following normal stimulation (including masturbation).

HISTORY
Detailed sexual history, including:
- Time frame of the problem
- Quality of patient's sexual response
- Sense of ejaculatory control and sexual distress
- Overall assessment of the relationship
- Ask specific questions because patients often reluctant to discuss openly.
- Detailed history of recent and current medications
- History of past trauma or recent infections
- Past surgical history with particular attention to genitourinary (GU) surgeries
- Supplements and alternative therapies tried
- Many men do not distinguish initially between problems related to erection and ejaculation.
- Some men have unrealistic expectations of ejaculatory response and frequency.
- Include the sexual partner in the interview, especially if the patient expresses a belief that he is not meeting his partner's needs.
- In review of systems, elicit any evidence of testosterone deficiency or prolactin excess, especially if anhedonia present.

PHYSICAL EXAM
- Check vitals. Look for focal neurologic signs (MS, spinal cord injury) and psychiatric disorders.
- Thorough GU exam, including:
  - Size and texture of testes and epididymis
  - Verification of the presence of the vas deferens
  - Location and patency of urethral meatus
  - Digital rectal examination to evaluate prostate consistency, size, and possible midline lesions

DIAGNOSTIC TESTS & INTERPRETATION
- Laboratory test results may be normal.
- Fasting glucose or HgbA1c to rule out diabetes
- Postorgasmic urinalysis will confirm RE. Semen fructose level, sperm count, and viscosity can be measured. Patient may complain of cloudy urine.
- AE will have fructose negative, sperm negative, and nonviscous postorgasmic urinalysis.
- In painful ejaculation, urinalysis and urine culture needed to rule out infection
- If prostate cancer is considered, check prostate-specific antigen (PSA).
- In anhedonia, consider checking testosterone, prolactin, glucose, and thyroid levels.

- In hematospermia, painful ejaculation, or if ejaculatory duct obstruction is considered, transrectal ultrasound (TRUS) may be helpful.
- TRUS-guided seminal vesicle aspiration if ejaculatory duct obstruction is present
- If suspicious of anatomic abnormality, can get scrotal US and/or MRI

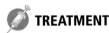 **TREATMENT**

GENERAL MEASURES
- Identifying any medical cause (even if not reversible) helps patient accept condition.
- Improve partner communication.
- Psychological counseling for patient and partner
- Reduce performance pressure through reassurance.
- Use of a variety of resources may be necessary (e.g., psychiatrist, psychologist, sex therapist, vascular surgeon, urologist, endocrinologist, neurologist).
- PE:
  – Use sensate focus therapy (gradual progression of nonsexual contact to sexual contact).
  – Quiet vagina: Female partner stops moving just prior to ejaculation.
  – Techniques to learn ejaculatory control (e.g., coronal squeeze technique [squeezing the glans penis until ejaculatory urge ceases] or start-and-stop technique [cessation of penile stimulation when ejaculation approaches and resumption of stimulation when ejaculatory feeling ends]) (1)[B]
- DE:
  – Change to antidepressant less likely to cause DE (citalopram, fluvoxamine, nefazodone) (2)[B]
- AE/RE:
  – Discontinue offending medications.
  – Diabetic control
  – If urethral obstruction present, refer to urology.
  – RE may be helped if intercourse occurs when bladder is full.
  – Consider penile vibratory stimulation (effective in spinal cord injuries >T10) or electroejaculation (place on monitor if lesions above T6 because autonomic dysreflexia may result) to collect sperm in AE cases.
- Painful ejaculation:
  – Counseling may be beneficial.
  – If seminal vesicle stones are possible, refer to urology.
- Hematospermia:
  – Often resolves spontaneously, without known cause. Reassure initially.
  – May try empiric antibiotic, but little evidence to support
  – If persistent or high degree of suspicion for abnormality, refer to urologist.

MEDICATION
- PE:
  – Treat underlying ED (a common comorbidity) with PDE5 inhibitors (3)[A].
- First line:
  – Dapoxetine, a short-acting SSRI, used "on-demand" 30 to 60 mg 1 to 2 hours prior to sex has good efficacy (2),(3),(4)[A]; best efficacy but higher cost
  – Other "on-demand" options include clomipramine 20 to 50 mg 4 to 24 hours before intercourse, sertraline 50 mg 4 to 8 hours before intercourse, and paroxetine 20 mg 3 to 4 hours before intercourse (2),(3),(4)[A].

  – Daily dosing of clomipramine 20 to 50 mg, sertraline 25 to 200 mg, fluoxetine 5 to 20 mg, or paroxetine 10 to 40 mg can delay ejaculation within 1 to 3 weeks of starting (2),(3)[A].
  – PDE5 inhibitor with or without SSRI (3)[A]
  – Topical anesthetic gel (e.g., 2.5% prilocaine ± 2.5% lidocaine [EMLA]) 2.5 g applied under a condom for 30 minutes prior to intercourse (5)[A]
  – Tramadol 5 to 50 mg used "on demand" 2 hours before sex; effective in many studies (6)[A]; now available in spray form
  – Second line: behavioral/sex therapy, pelvic floor muscle therapy (1),(2)[B]
- DE:
  – No "approved" drugs; many options
  – Consider switching antidepressants to bupropion, nefazodone, and mirtazapine.
  – Patients who must continue SSRIs may respond to bupropion and buspirone (2),(7)[B].
  – Sex therapy, self-stimulation therapies (1),(2)[B]
  – Some evidence that amantadine or cyproheptadine may be helpful (2),(7)[B]
- AE and RE:
  – First line: pseudoephedrine 60 mg PO daily to QID or imipramine 25 to 75 mg PO BID (8)[A]
  – α-Agonists and antihistamines can be helpful but are not approved by the FDA.
  – Second line: for RE, can try postejaculation bladder harvest of sperm (if fertility desired); for AE, can try midodrine, penile vibratory stimulation, or electroejaculation (2),(8)[B]
- Painful ejaculation:
  – Treat underlying infection/inflammatory process.
  – α-Blockers may have some benefit.

ISSUES FOR REFERRAL
The following conditions, when suspected, should be referred to a urologist:
- Ejaculatory duct obstruction
- Seminal vesicle or prostatic stones
- Urethral obstruction
- Vas deferens obstruction
- Calculi
- Persistent or severe hematospermia (2)[B]

SURGERY/OTHER PROCEDURES
Surgical treatment of ejaculatory duct obstruction:
- Transurethral resection of the ejaculatory ducts

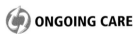 **ONGOING CARE**

PATIENT EDUCATION
See "General Measures."

PROGNOSIS
Often improves with therapy and counseling

COMPLICATIONS
Psychological impact on some males: signs of severe inadequacy, self-doubt, additional anxiety, and guilt

REFERENCES

1. Pastore A, Palleschi G, Fuschi A, et al. Pelvic muscle floor rehabilitation as a therapeutic option in lifelong premature ejaculation: long-term outcomes. *Asian J Androl.* 2018;20(6):572–575.
2. Althof SE, McMahon CG. Contemporary management of disorders of male orgasm and ejaculation. *Urology.* 2016;93:9–21.
3. Sun Y, Yang L, Bao Y, et al. Efficacy of PDE5Is and SSRIs in men with premature ejaculation: a new systematic review and five meta-analyses. *World J Urol.* 2017;35(12):1817–1831.
4. Sridharan K, Sivaramakrishnan G, Sequeira R, et al. Pharmacological interventions for premature ejaculation: a mixed-treatment comparison network meta-analysis of randomized clinical trials. *Int J Impot Res.* 2018;30(5):215–223.
5. Butcher MJ, Zubert T, Christiansen K, et al. Topical agents for premature ejaculation: a review. *Sex Med Rev.* 2020;8(1):92–99.
6. Kirby EW, Carson CC, Coward RM. Tramadol for the management of premature ejaculation: a timely systematic review. *Int J Impot Res.* 2015;27(4):121–127.
7. Abdel-Hamid I, Ali O. Delayed ejaculation: pathophysiology, diagnosis, and treatment. *World J Mens Health.* 2018;36(1):22–40.
8. Shoshany O, Abhyankar N, Elyaguov J, et al. Efficacy of treatment with pseudoephedrine in men with retrograde ejaculation. *Andrology.* 2017;5(4):744–748.

ADDITIONAL READING

- Jiann B. The office management of ejaculatory disorders. *Transl Androl Urol.* 2016;5(4):526–540.
- Mehta A, Sigman M. Management of the dry ejaculate: a systematic review of aspermia and retrograde ejaculation. *Fertil Steril.* 2015;104(5):1074–1081.
- Otani T. Clinical review of ejaculatory dysfunction. *Reprod Med Biol.* 2019;18(4):331–343.

 CODES

ICD10
- F52.4 Premature ejaculation
- N53.11 Retarded ejaculation
- N53.14 Retrograde ejaculation

CLINICAL PEARLS
- If ED is contributing to ejaculatory difficulty, management of ED should precede attempted management of ejaculatory disorders.
- Medications should always be thoroughly reviewed because they may be the primary cause of ejaculatory disorders.
- PE and DE generally have both psychogenic and physical causes, whereas AE and RE are due to organic neurogenic/autonomic dysfunction.
- A multidisciplinary approach, including the primary care physician, urologists, psychologists, and other appropriate health care professionals, is essential to the proper treatment of ejaculatory disorders.

ELDER ABUSE

Thomas Triantafillou, MD • Vivian Nnenna Chukwuma, MD

 BASICS

DESCRIPTION

Elder abuse (EA) is a public health concern (autonomy, wellbeing). Defined as: (i) intentional actions that cause harm or create a serious risk of harm to a vulnerable elder (financial, physical, emotional, impaired capacity for self-care or self-protection risk) by a caregiver or other person who stands in a trust relationship, or (ii) failure by a caregiver to satisfy the elder's basic needs or to protect the elder from harm (National Academy of Sciences, 2003). In 2009, the estimated cost was approximately $2.9 billion, a 12% increase from the preceding year (National Committee for the Prevention of Elder Abuse).

EPIDEMIOLOGY

Incidence

The global incidence of EA is around 16% (World Health Organization [WHO]). In the United States, it is estimated that 10% of the population are victims of EA and as many as 5 million elders are affected each year.

Prevalence

EA in both the community and in institutions has increased during the COVID-19 pandemic (WHO). The estimated annual prevalence per 1,000 people of key forms of violence is: 22 for physical and sexual abuse, 17 for intimate partner violence, fatal suicide 0.17, nonfatal self-harm 0.27, and 9.7 to 32.6 for violence by older adults with dementia against others (1).

ETIOLOGY AND PATHOPHYSIOLOGY

The etiology of EA involves biopsychosocial factors in combination with increased dependence on the caregiver by the victim in a suboptimal environment with poor behavioral coping methods, further compounded by increased stress.

RISK FACTORS

The victim: advanced age; female gender; low socioeconomic status; exploitable resources; social isolation; lack of purpose; PTSD in veterans; poor self-perceived health; loss of sense of control; health care insecurity; prior history of abuse in life; functional dependence; cognitive impairment; mental illness or substance use; polyvictimization (victim's perception of EA, protecting the offender, perpetrator influence on the victim). The abuser: early child abuse; history of violence; mental illness or substance use; high stress or poor coping; poor physical or cognitive health; inadequate training or supervision; poor prior relationship between the caregiver and the victim; financial dependency on the victim.

GENERAL PREVENTION

Complete annual wellness visits to discuss advanced care plan, power of attorney for health or finances, goals of care (GOC), degree of self-sufficiency, the role of the caregiver, the risk of caregiver burnout. Assess caregiver stress and burden (meet without patient). Screen for risk or presence of mood disorders (depression: PHQ-2 or PHQ-9; anxiety: General Anxiety Disorder-7 (GAD-7); loneliness: 3-item UCLA) or cognitive impairment (Folstein Mini-Mental State Examination [MMSE], Montreal Cognitive Assessment [MoCA], Saint Louis University Mental Status [SLUMS]). Encourage socialization. Refer to community programs: Department of Aging, Adult Protective Services (APS), Alzheimer's Association.

COMMONLY ASSOCIATED CONDITIONS

Conditions commonly associated with EA can be risk factors. They include social isolation, increased dependence for activities of daily living/instrumental activities of daily living (ADLs/IADLs), depression, cognitive impairment, and aggressive behavior.

 DIAGNOSIS

There is no golden standard for EA screen. The U.S. Preventive Services Task Force has not recommended screening for EA. However, when there is a high clinical suspicion, EA should be considered. Types of EA: physical or sexual, violation of personal rights, material exploitation, neglect (includes abandonment), financial, and psychological. The context can vary from self-neglect, institutional (nursing home, assisted living), or domestic (home). Most commonly, the abuser in a domestic environment is a family member. Screening tools (2),(3): (i) hospital: Elderly Indicators of Abuse (E-IOA); (ii) emergency department: Elder Abuse Instrument (EAI), ED Senior Abuse Identification (AID); (iii) nursing home: Elder Psychological Abuse Scale (EPAS); and (iv) general: Elder Abuse Suspicion Index (EASI); Hwalek-Sengstock Elder Abuse Screening Test (H-S/EAST); Vulnerability Abuse Screening Scale (VASS); Lichtenberg Financial Decision Screening Scale (LFDSS)

HISTORY

Use a culture-sensitive history with a focus on prior or current advance care plan. Do a review of living arrangements, degree of physical or cognitive function, who the caregivers are, and if there is evidence of caregiver burnout.

PHYSICAL EXAM

- It is important to document positive and negative findings in your physical exam and to be detailed because they can be admissible in court. Assess for unexplained fractures.
- General overall appearance: cachexia; hygiene and clothing; if bedbound, record integrity of mattress and sheets; evidence of falls, including broken eyeglasses
- Oral exam: dentition, oral ulcers
- Skin exam: large bruises (>5 cm) located at the face, lateral arm, back, or inner thighs
  - Patterned injury suggesting inappropriate restraint such as bite marks, ligature marks around wrists, ankles, or neck
  - Burn marks in patterns inconsistent with unintentional injury e.g., stocking and glove pattern suggesting forced immersion
  - Open wounds, cuts, punctures, untreated injuries in various stages of healing, traumatic alopecia, or scalp swelling
  - Check for pressure ulcers on the bony prominences of the patient.

DIFFERENTIAL DIAGNOSIS

- Dementia (FAST 6 or 7), or dementia in a withdrawn or malnourished patient
- Elderly with Alzheimer, mixed, or lewy body dementia (LBD) can present with delusions.

- Psychosis
- Substance use disorders
- Parkinson disease resulting in fractures or bruises
- Coagulopathy with advanced malignancy or other conditions
- Antiplatelet therapy associated with bruising
- Wasting from malignancy, infections, or chronic disease
- Delirium due to electrolyte, trauma, infection, heart disease, urine retention, constipation, end-of-life
- Thyroid disorder associated with altered mental status, delirium, depression, frailty, or anxiety
- Fixed drug reaction, fragile photo-aged skin, steroid purpura, allergic reaction
- Fracture from osteoporosis

DIAGNOSTIC TESTS & INTERPRETATION

Initial Tests (lab, imaging)

CBC, CMP, UA, vitamin B_{12}, folic acid, RPR, TSH, PT/INR (if bruising)

Follow-Up Tests & Special Considerations

- Anemia: iron, TIBC, ferritin
- Change in mental status: vitamin B_1, vitamin B_6; consider toxicology; consider encephalopathy panel.
- Trauma: image to assess for new or old fractures. Consider CT head imaging to look for hemorrhage (e.g., subdural).

Diagnostic Procedures/Other

- Use tools to assess for cognitive impairment such as MMSE (proprietary), MoCA (forgetfulness, MCI), SLUMS
- Depression screening tools such as the Geriatric Depression Scale, PHQ2 or PHQ9, and GAD-7
- Documentation
  - Can document "suspected mistreatment" but avoid making definitive diagnosis of EA (or dementia) in your initial assessment, unless it is obvious. Document the abuser's name, relationship, and contact information.
  - Pictures need to include the patient's name, medical number, date and time taken, a ruler (used for measurement), name of witnesses that took image. Take pictures of torn clothes.
- Include anatomical diagrams.
- In some states, reporting is only mandated when the patient cannot (i.e., for cognitive or physical reasons) do so. The law protects those who report in "good faith." The identity of the reporter shall not be disclosed except with the written permission of the reporter or by order of a court.

 TREATMENT

- Most states require all health care providers to report suspected EA to a local agency such as the APS (https://www.preventfamilyviolence.org/adult-protective-services-numbers) with limited evidence on effectiveness of other interventions (4).
- The treatment plan should be centered around action items related but not limited to: the vulnerable older adult, trusted other, or context (Abuse Intervention Model: domain I/II/III) (5).

- Domain I—vulnerable older adult (victim): Consider virtual education interventions (Elder Abuse Training Institute Island; Ejaz et al). Consider a Family-Based Cognitive Behavioral Social Work (FBCBSW) approach to reduce emotional and financial neglect.
  - Impaired physical function: Assess need for assist devices or physical therapy.
  - Impaired cognition: Make recommendations for a healthy diet, activity, and sleep habits customized to the patient's capabilities.
  - Emotional distress or mental illness: Assess presence of depression (PHQ-2 or PHQ-9), anxiety (GAD-7). When appropriate, use medications for mood or mental illness.
- Domain II—trusted others (perpetrator)
  - Dependence on the vulnerable elder: Share with the perpetrator resources to support financial planning to allow mitigation of dependence on the victim.
  - Mood or substance use or pathologic personality traits: Ask the perpetrator to follow with their clinical provider. Report to law enforcement entities if the patient's life is threatened.
- Domain III—context of abuse (circumstances)
  - Social isolation: Provide resources to expand a patient's social network. Can consider a trial of care at assisted living or a nursing home. Work closely with social work (clinic; home health).
  - Low-quality relationship between victim-perpetrator: Seek help from social work or psychologist.
  - Cultural norms: Address taboos related to diagnosis such as dementia in a culture-sensitive manner and customize the plan of care to the patient.

MEDICATION
None

ISSUES FOR REFERRAL
Mood or behavior concern: behavioral health services; cognitive assessment: neurocognitive specialist

ADDITIONAL THERAPIES
Physical and occupational therapy for ambulation, safety assessment, cognition assessment

COMPLEMENTARY & ALTERNATIVE MEDICINE
Relaxation or well-being techniques

ADMISSION, INPATIENT, AND NURSING CONSIDERATIONS
- Victims of abuse should not be transferred or discharged without reliable follow-up, including:
  - A home visit either by PCP or by APN, combined with home health services
  - Report to the state's APS or a designated alternative (e.g., if patient resides in nursing home, then report to that state's regulatory entity, public health department, and Ombudsman). With physical harm, report to local law enforcement.
  - Follow-up with appropriate mental health care
- Manage uncontrolled chronic conditions due to neglect (i.e., wound care from ulcers or infections).
- Hospital security may need to be notified if restricted visitor access to a patient is required.
- Locations for disposition: friend or family member, nursing home, assisted living facility

ONGOING CARE

FOLLOW-UP RECOMMENDATIONS
- Although evidence is unclear on a change in outcomes from any education intervention, information about responsibilities should be shared with the person responsible for the patient.
- Educate caregivers on signs and effects of caregiver burnout matched with resources for home aid services.
- Review your state requirements on reporting: http://www.napsa-now.org/wp-content/uploads/2014/11/Mandatory-Reporting-Chart-Updated-FINAL.pdf.
- Contact the APS. A helpful resource is http://www.napsa-now.org/get-help/help-in-your-area/.
- Contact the Department of Aging to request an assessment at home including a review of services that can support the patient to be independent in the community.
- ED providers should report to the Long-Term Care Ombudsman.

Patient Monitoring
The patient should have frequent home or clinic visits.

DIET
Mediterranean, or MIND diet

PATIENT EDUCATION
- For EA resources in your state, https://ncea.acl.gov, or call 800-677-1166
- Other useful resources for families
  - Eldercare locator, 800-677-1116, https://eldercare.acl.gov/Public/Index.aspx
  - Alzheimer's Association, 800-272-3900
  - National Organization for Victim Assistance, https://www.trynova.org/

PROGNOSIS
EA and self-neglect are associated with an overall increased risk in mortality.

COMPLICATIONS
Associated outcomes: mortality; hospitalizations; functional health decline; loneliness; depression

REFERENCES

1. Rosen T, Makaroun LK, Conwell Y, et al. Violence in older adults: scope, impact, challenges, and strategies for prevention. *Health Aff (Millwood)*. 2019;38(10):1630–1637.
2. Van Royen K, Van Royen P, De Donder L, et al. Elder abuse assessment tools and interventions for use in the home environment: a scoping review. *Clin Interv Aging*. 2020;15:1793–1807.
3. Ries NM, Mansfield E. Elder abuse: the role of general practitioners in community-based screening and multidisciplinary action. *Aust J Gen Pract*. 2018;47(4):235–238.
4. Baker PRA, Francis DP, Hairi NN, et al. Interventions for preventing abuse in the elderly. *Cochrane Database Syst Rev*. 2016;2016(8):CD010321.
5. Mosqueda L, Burnight K, Gironda MW, et al. The Abuse Intervention Model: a pragmatic approach to intervention for elder mistreatment. *J Am Geriatr Soc*. 2016;64(9):1879–1883.

ADDITIONAL READING
- American Bar Association Commission on Law and Aging. Adult protective services reporting chart (laws current as of December 2019). https://www.americanbar.org/content/dam/aba/administrative/law_aging/2020-elderabuse-reporting-chart.pdf. Published December 2019. Accessed January 3, 2022.
- Cooper C, Katona C, Finne-Soveri H, et al. Indicators of elder abuse: a crossnational comparison of psychiatric morbidity and other determinants in the Ad-HOC study. *Am J Geriatr Psychiatry*. 2006;14(6):489–497.
- Hoover RM, Polson M. Detecting elder abuse and neglect: assessment and intervention. *Am Fam Physician*. 2014;89(6):453–460.

SEE ALSO

- Tools on EA for clinicians from Weill Cornell Medicine: https://elderabuseemergency.org/ElderWP/
- National Council on Aging: https://www.ncoa.org

CODES

ICD10
- T74.11XA Adult physical abuse, confirmed, initial encounter
- T74.21XA Adult sexual abuse, confirmed, initial encounter
- T74.01XA Adult neglect or abandonment, confirmed, initial encounter

CLINICAL PEARLS
- To reduce the risk of EA, strengthen the patients' social support, address depression, provide the patient with assistive devices, screen for cognitive impairment with a trial of medication if possible, and identify caregiver burnout.
- Refer to the Department of Aging for services such as home aid when ADLs or IADLs are impaired.
- Patient with capacity: The APS cannot act if a patient has the capacity to make decisions and elects not to report the abuse. Patient with impaired capacity: A medicolegal process along with guidance from the APS can lead to guardianship.

ENCOPRESIS

Jay Fong, MD • William T. Garrison, PhD

 BASICS

DESCRIPTION

- Voluntary or involuntary fecal soilage in a (typically) previously toilet-trained individual
  - Age may be chronologic or developmental.
  - No underlying organic disease
  - At least one event per month for 3 months
  - Classified into functional constipation (retentive encopresis) and functional nonretentive fecal incontinence (FNRFI); both cause fecal incontinence. There is no constipation in FNRFI. *Functional constipation is more common.*
- Adult encopresis (fecal incontinence) is a separate topic.
- System(s) affected: GI; psychological
- Synonyms(s): fecal incontinence, soiling

EPIDEMIOLOGY

Incidence

Predominant sex: male > female (4 to 6:1). Constipation accounts for 3% of general pediatric referrals; up to 84% of constipated children have fecal incontinence at some point.

Prevalence

Occurs in 1–3% of children 4 years of age

ETIOLOGY AND PATHOPHYSIOLOGY

- In 90% of cases, encopresis develops as a consequence of chronic constipation, with resulting overflow incontinence (*retentive encopresis*). The other 10% are caused by specific organic etiologies.
- Chronic constipation with irregular and incomplete evacuation results in progressive rectal distension and stretching of the internal/external anal sphincters.
- Chronic rectal distension causes habituation, leading to the loss of sensing the normal urge to defecate. Eventually, soft or liquid stool leaks around the retained fecal mass.
- Many children voluntarily withhold stool in response to the urge to defecate for fear of pain or a preoccupation with not interrupting social activities.
- Psychological
  - Stool withholding, fear, anxiety
  - Difficulty with toilet training, including unusual anxiety or conflict with parent
  - Resistance to using public toilet facilities, such as school bathrooms or outdoor toilets
  - Known association with sexual abuse in boys; likely similar association in girls
  - Developmental delay
- Anatomic
  - Rectal distension and desensitization
  - Anal fissure or painful defecation
  - Muscle hypotonia
  - Slow intestinal motility
  - Hirschsprung disease
  - Cystic fibrosis
  - Spinal cord defects (e.g., spina bifida)
  - Congenital anorectal malformations
  - Anal stenosis
  - Anterior displacement of the anus

- Postoperative stricture of anus or rectum
  - Pelvic mass
  - Neurofibromatosis
- Dietary or metabolic
  - Inadequate dietary fiber; excessive protein or milk intake; inadequate water intake
  - Hypothyroidism; hypercalcemia; hypokalemia
  - Diabetes insipidus; diabetes mellitus
  - Food allergy
  - Gluten enteropathy
- Medication side effects

Genetics

None known; although incidence may be higher in children with family history of constipation

RISK FACTORS

- Male gender
- Constipation
- Very low birth weight
- Painful defecation
- Difficulty with bowel training, including social pressure related to early daycare placement
- Organic/anatomic causes
- Anxiety and depression
- Insufficient fluid or fiber intake
- Refusal to use public restrooms
- Attention deficit
- History of abuse

GENERAL PREVENTION

Family education: toilet training when ready; optimize fluid and fiber intake.

COMMONLY ASSOCIATED CONDITIONS

- Constipation, Hirschsprung disease
- Cerebral palsy, cystic fibrosis
- Developmental and behavioral diagnoses, urinary incontinence

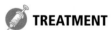 **DIAGNOSIS**

HISTORY

- Signs/symptoms of constipation:
  - Hard, large-caliber stools
  - <3 defecations per week
  - Pain or discomfort with stool passage
  - Withholding stool
  - Blood on stool or in diaper/toilet bowl
  - Decreased appetite
  - Abdominal pain that improves with stool passage
  - Hiding while defecating before child is toilet-trained; avoiding use of the toilet
  - Diet low in fiber or fluids, high in dairy products
  - No stool passage in the first 48 hours of life
  - Pasty stool on underclothes
  - Recurrent UTIs
- Abrupt onset after age 5 years more likely to be associated with psychological trauma
- Overlap with attention deficit disorder (ADD) common in children >5 years
- Medication use: opiates, phenobarbital, and tricyclic antidepressants (TCAs)
- Family history of constipation

PHYSICAL EXAM

- Neurologic exam of lower extremities and perineal area, with attention to S1–S4 distribution, perineal sensation, cremasteric reflex, and anal sphincter tone
- Genital examination and digital rectal exam: Assess for anal fissures, sphincter tone, rectal distension/impaction, occult or visible blood.
- Abdominal exam: bowel sounds, percussion note (tympany), abdominal distension; palpate for stool (most common in left lower quadrant).

DIAGNOSTIC TESTS & INTERPRETATION

Most cases diagnosed by history and physical

Initial Tests (lab, imaging)

Used only to rule out organic causes

- UA/urine culture: UTI/glucosuria
- Thyroid function tests: hypothyroidism
- Electrolyte panel, including calcium: hypokalemia, hypercalcemia, or hyperglycemia
- Abdominal plain films if impaction is suspected and not detected by abdominal or rectal exam

Follow-Up Tests & Special Considerations

- Failure to pass meconium within 48 hours of birth, failure to thrive, bloody diarrhea, or bilious vomiting in a neonate should be promptly evaluated to exclude aganglionic megacolon.
- Constipation and diarrhea, rash, failure to thrive, or recurrent pneumonia should prompt evaluation for cystic fibrosis. Patients with abdominal distension or ileus should be evaluated for possible obstruction.

Diagnostic Procedures/Other

Manometric studies may be useful in patients who have constipation that does not respond to treatment.

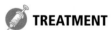 **TREATMENT**

GENERAL MEASURES

- Anticipatory toilet training advice about when children should reduce reliance on diapers or use pull-ups during the daytime hours (average age for toilet training in girls is 29 months; 31 months for boys)
- Eliminate impaction prior to maintenance therapy.
- Avoid frequent and repeated rectal exams, enemas, and suppositories, especially in infants.
- Once stools are regular in frequency, child should sit on toilet BID at the same time each day for 10 to 15 minutes and for 10 to 15 minutes after meals. Incorporate positive reinforcement for successful bowel movements.

MEDICATION

- Remove impaction and start maintenance treatment.
- No randomized controlled studies have compared methods of disimpaction: can use oral agents, enemas, and rectal suppositories; oral agents are least traumatic. Glycerin suppositories are best option for infants.

First Line

- Disimpaction with polyethylene glycol (PEG)
  - Give 17 g (240 mL) water or juice: 1.0 to 1.5 g/kg/day for 3 days for disimpaction.
  - 0.4 to 0.8 g/kg/day for maintenance
- Disimpaction with mineral oil for child >1 year; give 15 to 30 mL/year of age to max 240 mL.
  - Maintenance: 1 to 3 mL/kg/day or divided BID
  - May mix with orange juice to make palatable; avoid in infants to avoid aspiration pneumonia.
- Other maintenance regimens include the following:
  - Milk of magnesia (MOM) 400 mg (5 mL): 1 to 2 mL/kg/day BID
  - Lactulose 10 g (15 mL): 1 to 3 mL/kg/day divided BID
  - Senna syrup 8.8 g sennoside (5 mL): age 2 to 6 years: 2.5 to 7.5 mL/day divided BID; age 6 to 12 years: 5 to 15 mL/day divided BID
  - Bisacodyl suppository 10 mg: 0.5 to 1 suppository once or twice per day

ISSUES FOR REFERRAL

If symptoms do not improve after 6 months of compliance with a multifactorial treatment model, refer to pediatric gastroenterologist for further evaluation and guidance.

ADDITIONAL THERAPIES

Behavioral treatment and counseling

SURGERY/OTHER PROCEDURES

If ongoing constipation is refractory to a combination of medical and behavioral therapy, consider anorectal manometry to evaluate for internal anal sphincter achalasia (or ultrashort-segment Hirschsprung disease). If present, this condition can be treated successfully in most patients with an internal sphincter myectomy.

COMPLEMENTARY & ALTERNATIVE MEDICINE

- Children with volitional stool holding who receive behavioral treatment in addition to medications are more likely to have resolution of encopresis at 3 and 6 months than with medication alone (1)[A].
- No evidence that biofeedback training adds benefit to conventional treatment for functional fecal incontinence in children (2)[A]
- Behavioral interventions combined with laxative therapy (rather than laxative therapy alone) improve continence in children with functional fecal incontinence associated with constipation (1)[B].

ADMISSION, INPATIENT, AND NURSING CONSIDERATIONS

- Admission criteria/initial stabilization
  - Continued soiling and recurrent impaction on outpatient medical therapy, whether from lack of medication efficacy or patient nonadherence
  - Decreased intake leading to malnutrition or dehydration
  - Recalcitrant vomiting or concern for obstruction
  - Involve appropriate agencies if concern for abuse.
  - Hospital admission and abdominal films may be necessary to ensure complete removal of impaction. This may include direct gastric administration of balanced electrolyte–PEG solutions if the patient cannot tolerate by mouth. Serial abdominal films and observation of rectal effluent can help determine treatment adequacy.

- IV fluids if the patient is dehydrated and has difficulty tolerating oral intake
- Nursing to document stool output and character
- Discharge criteria
  - Stools that are looser in consistency and clearer in appearance are a successful inpatient end point.
  - Abdominal radiographs showing less fecal loading (compared with a pretreatment radiograph) with improving serial abdominal exams

 ONGOING CARE

The patient and family should be encouraged to keep records of bowel movements successfully passed as well as soiling episodes as well as incorporating a reward system to promote continued efforts at sitting on the toilet regularly. An open channel of communication between the patient and clinician care team will be vital to plan on close follow-up, especially after hospitalizations for rectal disimpaction and bowel preparations.

FOLLOW-UP RECOMMENDATIONS

Follow up monthly at first with clinician to review the patient's stooling regimen, conduct a physical exam, and readjust the home regimen as needed to ensure continued progress and remission of symptoms.

Patient Monitoring

- Continue maintenance treatment for 6 months to 2 years with visits every 4 to 10 weeks for support and to ensure compliance; more frequent visits with oppositional or anxious children
- Telephone or virtual visits can be used to adjust doses and to provide ongoing encouragement.
- Treat recurrences of impaction promptly.
- Emphasize compliance with medication and self-initiation of regular bathroom visits.
- Children who do not progress using a well-designed behavior plan should be referred for more in-depth mental health evaluation and counseling.

DIET

Adequate fluid and fiber intake (2)[A]. Reduce cow's milk products. Avoid excessive consumption of bananas, rice, apples, and gelatin.

PATIENT EDUCATION

- Demystify defecation.
- Carefully explain the treatment plan including medications and dietary changes.
- Avoid punishment for inadvertent soiling.
- In children >4 years of age, explain to parents how overreliance on diapers and pull-ups (while convenient) can prolong the problem.
- Always attempt to use positive reinforcement for successful toilet sits and medication compliance.
- If positive approach is unsuccessful, consider removing desired privileges (e.g., TV, video games) for noncompliance with behavioral plan. Some children respond well to a token economy (earned privileges) to promote desired behavior.
- Encourage regular physical activity.

PROGNOSIS

- Many children exhibit a good response and relapse due to parental noncompliance.
- From 30% to 50% of children may still have encopresis after 5 years of treatment.
- Children with psychosocial or emotional problems preceding the encopresis are more recalcitrant to treatment.

COMPLICATIONS

- Colitis due to excessive enema/suppository
- Perianal dermatitis
- Anal fissure

REFERENCES

1. Brazzelli M, Griffiths PV, Cody JD, et al. Behavioural and cognitive interventions with or without other treatments for the management of faecal incontinence in children. *Cochrane Database Syst Rev.* 2011;(12):CD002240.
2. Tabbers MM, DiLorenzo C, Berger MY, et al; for European Society for Pediatric Gastroenterology, Hepatology, and Nutrition, North American Society for Pediatric Gastroenterology. Evaluation and treatment of functional constipation in infants and children: evidence-based recommendations from ESPGHAN and NASPGHAN. *J Pediatr Gastroenterol Nutr.* 2014;58(2):258–274.

ADDITIONAL READING

- Baird DC, Bybel M, Kowalski AW. Toilet training: common questions and answers. *Am Fam Physician.* 2019;100(8):468–474.
- Constipation Guideline Committee of the North American Society for Pediatric Gastroenterology, Hepatology and Nutrition. Evaluation and treatment of constipation in infants and children: recommendations of the North American Society for Pediatric Gastroenterology, Hepatology and Nutrition. *J Pediatr Gastroenterol Nutr.* 2006;43(3):e1–e13.
- Lu PL, Mousa HM. Constipation: Beyond the old paradigms. *Gastroenterol Clin North Am.* 2018;47(4):845–862.

CODES

ICD10

- R15.9 Full incontinence of feces
- R15.1 Fecal smearing
- F98.1 Encopresis not due to a substance or known physiol condition

CLINICAL PEARLS

- 90% of encopresis results from chronic constipation.
- Address toddler constipation early by decreasing excessive milk intake, increasing fruits/vegetables intake, and ensuring adequate fluid and fiber intake.
- Eliminate fecal impaction before initiating maintenance therapy.

ENDOCARDITIS, INFECTIVE

Theodore B. Flaum, DO • Ian Paul Persits, DO, MS

BASICS

Infective endocarditis (IE) is an infection of the inner layer of the heart including the valves (native/prosthetic), interventricular septum, intracardiac devices, chordae tendineae, and mural endocardium. IE occurs worldwide and is generally fatal if left untreated.

DESCRIPTION
- An infection of the valvular (primarily) and/or mural (rarely) endocardium
- System(s) affected: cardiovascular, endocrine/metabolic, hematologic/lymphatic, immunologic, pulmonary, renal/urologic, skin/exocrine, neurologic
- Synonym(s): bacterial endocarditis; subacute bacterial endocarditis (SBE); acute bacterial endocarditis (ABE)

EPIDEMIOLOGY
More common in males (range is 3:2 to 9:1). >50% of cases in the United States occur in individuals >60 years of age.

Incidence
- Native valve endocarditis has variable rates of incidence due to changes in definition over the years.
- 1.5–3% incidence 1 year after prosthetic valve replacement; 3–6% 5 years postreplacement
- Increasing incidence of cardiovascular device–related infections due to higher frequency of implantable devices.
- Can be community- or hospital-acquired
- Most commonly affects the mitral valve and aortic valve (increased left-sided pressures and turbulent flow)

ETIOLOGY AND PATHOPHYSIOLOGY
IE is most commonly caused by a nonbacterial thrombus that adheres to an endocardial surface, coupled with a bacterial source sufficient to seed the thrombus. This can occur from direct bacterial invasion or valvular trauma:
- Native valve endocarditis
  - Acute: *Staphylococcus aureus*; *Streptococcus* groups A, B, C, G; *Streptococcus pneumoniae*; *Staphylococcus lugdunensis*; *Enterococcus* spp.; *Haemophilus influenzae* or *parainfluenzae*; *Neisseria gonorrhoeae*
  - Subacute: α-hemolytic streptococci, *Streptococcus bovis*, *Enterococcus* spp., *S. aureus*, *Staphylococcus epidermidis*; HACEK organisms
- Intravenous drug abuse endocarditis (IVDA) (most commonly tricuspid valve): *S. aureus*, *Enterococcus* spp.; *Pseudomonas aeruginosa*, *Burkholderia cepacia*, other bacilli (gram-negative); *Candida* spp.
- Prosthetic valve endocarditis
  - Early (≥12 months after valve implantation): *S. aureus*, *S. epidermidis*; gram-negative bacilli; *Candida* spp., *Aspergillus* spp.
  - Late (>12 months after valve implantation): α-hemolytic streptococci, *S. aureus*, *Enterococcus* spp., *S. epidermidis*, *Candida* spp., *Aspergillus* spp.

- Culture-negative endocarditis: 10% of cases; *Bartonella quintana* (homeless); *Brucella* spp., fungi, *Coxiella burnetii* (Q fever), *Chlamydia trachomatis*, *Chlamydophila psittaci*, HACEK organisms
- Device-related endocarditis: coagulase-negative staphylococci or *S. aureus*

RISK FACTORS
- Injection drug use, IV catheterization, certain malignancies (colon cancer), poor dentition/infection, chronic hemodialysis, age >60 years, male sex
- High risk with:
  - Structural heart disease, prosthetic cardiac valves, valvular disease, implantable devices, total parenteral nutrition
  - Previous IE
  - Congenital heart disease (CHD): unrepaired cyanotic CHD, including palliative shunts and conduits; repaired CHD with prosthetic device during the first 6 months; repaired CHD with residual defects at or near prosthetic site; cardiac transplant with valvulopathy (1)[B]

GENERAL PREVENTION
- Good oral hygiene
- Antibiotic prophylaxis is only recommended in patients with a high risk of adverse outcomes if IE were to occur (1)[B]—(see "Risk Factors"). Administer 30 to 60 minutes prior to the procedure (exception vancomycin which should be administered 120 minutes prior to the procedure).
- *Procedures requiring prophylaxis*
  - Oral/upper respiratory tract procedures/biopsies: Amoxicillin 2 g PO 30 to 60 minutes before procedure or ampicillin 2 g IV/IM are first-line prophylactic choices. Clindamycin no longer recommended for dental prophylaxis because it is associated with more frequent and severe adverse effects (i.e., *Clostridium difficile* infection)
  - GI/GU: Only consider coverage for *Enterococcus* (with penicillin, ampicillin, piperacillin, or vancomycin) for patients with an established infection undergoing procedures (1)[B].
  - Cardiac valvular surgery or placement of prosthetic intracardiac/intravascular materials: perioperative cefazolin 1 to 2 g IV 30 minutes preoperative or vancomycin 15 mg/kg (maximum 1 g) (penicillin-allergic patients) 60 minutes preoperative (1)[B]
  - Skin/soft tissue: incision and drainage of infected tissue; use agents active against skin pathogens (e.g., cefazolin 1 to 2 g IV q8h or vancomycin 15 mg/kg q12h; max 1 g) if penicillin-allergic or if methicillin-resistant *S. aureus* (MRSA) suspected.

COMMONLY ASSOCIATED CONDITIONS
Most patients with IE have preexisting conditions (see high-risk above).

DIAGNOSIS

- Modified Duke Criteria (1)[B] (definite: 2 major criteria, or 1 major and 3 minor criteria, or 5 minor criteria; possible: 1 major and 1 minor or 3 minor criteria)
- Major clinical criteria
  - Positive blood culture: isolation of typical microorganism for IE from two separate blood cultures or persistently positive blood culture
  - Single positive blood culture for *C. burnetii* or anti–phase-1 IgG antibody titer >1:800
  - Positive echocardiogram: presence of vegetation, abscess, or new partial dehiscence of prosthetic valve
  - New valvular regurgitation (change in preexisting murmur not sufficient)
- Minor criteria
  - Predisposing heart condition or IV drug use
  - Fever ≥38.0°C (100.4°F)
  - Vascular phenomena: arterial emboli, septic pulmonary infarcts, mycotic aneurysm, intracranial hemorrhage, conjunctival hemorrhage, Janeway lesions
  - Immunologic phenomena: glomerulonephritis, Osler nodes, Roth spots, rheumatoid factor (RF)
  - Microbiologic evidence

HISTORY
- Fever (>38°C), chills, cough, dyspnea, orthopnea; especially in subacute endocarditis: night sweats, weight loss, fatigue
- Review risk factors.
- Symptoms of transient ischemic attack, cerebrovascular accident (CVA), or myocardial infarction (MI) on presentation

PHYSICAL EXAM
- Most patients with IE have new murmur/change to an existing murmur. Signs of heart failure are common if valve function is compromised.
- Peripheral stigmata of IE: splinter hemorrhages in fingernail beds, Osler nodes, Roth spots, Janeway lesions, palatal/conjunctival petechiae, splenomegaly, hematuria
- Neurologic findings consistent with CVA

DIFFERENTIAL DIAGNOSIS
Vasculitis, temporal arteritis, fever of unknown origin, infected central venous catheter, marantic endocarditis, connective tissue diseases, intra-abdominal infections, rheumatic fever, salmonellosis, brucellosis, Lyme disease, malignancy, tuberculosis, atrial myxoma, septic thrombophlebitis

DIAGNOSTIC TESTS & INTERPRETATION
- If not critically ill; three sets of blood cultures drawn >2 hours apart from different sites *before administration* of *antibiotics* with repeat cultures in 48 to 72 hrs until bacterial clearance
- If acutely ill, draw three sets of blood cultures over 1 hour *prior to empiric therapy* (1)[A].
- Leukocytosis

- Anemia; decreased C3, C4, CH50; and RF in subacute endocarditis
- ESR, C-reactive protein (CRP)
- Hematuria
- Consider serologies for *Chlamydia*, Q fever, *Legionella*, and *Bartonella* in "culture-negative" endocarditis.
- Transthoracic (TTE) or transesophageal echocardiogram (TEE [preferred]) (1)[A]
- CT scan
- Emboli, abscesses, and/or infarction
- Immune-complex glomerulonephritis

Initial Tests (lab, imaging)
Routine laboratory findings are often nonspecific and often are a manifestation of secondary sequelae of IE.
- Laboratory findings:
  - Nonspecific
    ○ Elevated inflammatory markers
    ○ Leukocytosis, +RF
    ○ Normochromic normocytic anemia
  - Findings related to secondary system involvement
    ○ RBC casts
    ○ Microscopic hematuria, proteinuria, pyuria
- Imaging
  - ECG: New/evolving signs of conduction disease (atrioventricular blocks and/or bundle branch blocks) are often a sign of paravalvular and/or myocardial involvement.
  - TTE/TEE: new or worsening valvular regurgitation, new partial dehiscence of prosthetic valve, new intracardiac shunting, presence of vegetations

Follow-Up Tests & Special Considerations
If indicated, follow-up imaging to evaluate for secondary system involvement or to rule out other causes:
- Chest x-ray: may reveal evidence of septic pulmonary emboli or signs of congestive heart failure
- CT chest/abdomen/pelvis: Evaluate distal sites of infections and/or infarction.

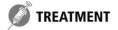 TREATMENT

MEDICATION
First Line
- Start empiric treatment after three sets of blood cultures have been drawn. Results guide treatment.
  - Native valves: ampicillin-sulbactam IV with gentamicin IV/IM. If penicillin-allergic, use vancomycin IV with gentamicin IV/IM and with ciprofloxacin PO/IV (2)[A].
  - Prosthetic valves: vancomycin IV with gentamicin IV/IM and rifampin PO, if <12 months postsurgery. If >12 months, use native valve regimen (2)[A].
- Penicillin-susceptible viridans streptococci or *S. bovis*
  - Native valve: penicillin G IV continuously or ceftriaxone IV/IM for 4 weeks (1)[B]
  - Prosthetic valve: penicillin G IV for 6 weeks or ceftriaxone IV/IM ± gentamicin IV/IM for 2 weeks (1)[B]

- Penicillin-resistant viridans streptococci or *S. bovis*
  - Native valve: penicillin G IV + gentamicin IV/IM (1)[B]
  - Prosthetic valve: penicillin G IV or ceftriaxone IV/IM for 6 weeks + gentamicin IV/IM for 2 weeks (1)[B]
- Penicillin-susceptible *Staphylococcus*
  - Native valve: oxacillin or nafcillin IV for 6 weeks. For oxacillin-resistant strains, use vancomycin IV for 6 weeks (1)[B].
  - Prosthetic valve: oxacillin or nafcillin IV + rifampin IV/PO for 6 weeks, + gentamicin IV for first 2 weeks. For oxacillin-resistant strains, use vancomycin IV, + rifampin IV/PO, both for 6 weeks, + gentamicin IV/IM for the first 2 weeks (1)[B].
- Penicillin-resistant *Staphylococcus*
  - Native valve: vancomycin for 6 weeks or daptomycin IV for 6 weeks
  - Prosthetic valve: vancomycin + rifampin IV/PO + gentamicin IV/IM for 2 weeks
- Penicillin-sensitive *Enterococcus*
  - Native or prosthetic valve: ampicillin IV or penicillin G IV + gentamicin IV for 4 to 6 weeks (1)[B].
- *HACEK* organisms: ceftriaxone IM or IV for 4 weeks (1)[B] *or* ampicillin-sulbactam IV for 4 weeks *or* ciprofloxacin PO or IV for 4 weeks (1)[B]

SURGERY/OTHER PROCEDURES
Surgery is required in 50% of IE cases. Indications (2)[A]:
- Heart failure due to aortic or mitral valve disease
  - Prevention of embolism: aortic or mitral valve vegetations >10 mm with prior embolic episodes; isolated very large vegetation >15 mm; in patients with major ischemic stroke, surgery is delayed for at least 4 weeks, if possible (3)[C].
- Uncontrolled infection: persistent fever and positive cultures >7 to 10 days; infection caused by fungi or resistant organism; presence of abscess, fistula, false aneurysm, or enlarging vegetations
- Early prosthetic valve IE

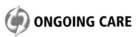 ONGOING CARE

FOLLOW-UP RECOMMENDATIONS
Patient Monitoring
- Baseline ECG; monitor ECG for conduction disturbances/MI in initial weeks of therapy.
- TTE at the conclusion of therapy
- Blood cultures q48h until negative

PROGNOSIS
The 1-year mortality of IE is 30%. Late complications contribute to poor prognosis. These include heart failure, reinfection, and cerebral emboli. The 10-year survival is 60–90% (4)[A].

COMPLICATIONS
- Cerebral complications are the most frequent and severe, occurring in 15–20% of patients (1)[A].
- Emboli: arterial, infectious (e.g., abscesses of heart, lung, brain, meninges, bone, pericardium)
  - Neurologic events are the most frequent complications in patients with IE requiring ICU admission. Ischemic stroke is the presenting symptom of IE in 20% of cases (4)[A].

- Inflammatory/immune disorders (e.g., arthritis, myositis, glomerulonephritis)
- Other complications: congestive heart failure, ruptured valve cusp, sinus of Valsalva aneurysm, arrhythmia, and mycotic aneurysms

REFERENCES
1. Baddour LM, Wilson WR, Bayer AS, et al; for American Heart Association Committee on Rheumatic Fever, Endocarditis, and Kawasaki Disease of the Council on Cardiovascular Disease in the Young, Council on Clinical Cardiology, Council on Cardiovascular Surgery and Anesthesia, and Stroke Council. Infective endocarditis in adults: diagnosis, antimicrobial therapy, and management of complications: a scientific statement for healthcare professionals from the American Heart Association. *Circulation*. 2015;132(15):1435–1486.
2. Habib G, Lancellotti P, Antunes MJ, et al. 2015 ESC guidelines for the management of infective endocarditis: The Task Force for the Management of Infective Endocarditis of the European Society of Cardiology (ESC). Endorsed by: European Association for Cardio-Thoracic Surgery (EACTS), the European Association of Nuclear Medicine (EANM). *Eur Heart J*. 2015;36(44):3075–3128.
3. Byrne JG, Rezai K, Sanchez JA, et al. Surgical management of endocarditis: the Society of Thoracic Surgeons clinical practice guideline. *Ann Thorac Surg*. 2011;91(6):2012–2019.
4. El-Dalati S, Cronin D, Shea M, et al. Clinical practice update on infectious endocarditis. *Am J Med*. 2020;133(1):44–49.

 CODES

ICD10
- I33.0 Acute and subacute infective endocarditis
- I39 Endocarditis and heart valve disord in dis classd elswhr
- A54.83 Gonococcal heart infection

CLINICAL PEARLS
- Preprocedural antibiotic prophylaxis is recommended for patients with artificial heart valves, a previous history of IE, CHD, and cardiac transplants with valvulopathy.
- TEE/TTE and blood cultures are the mainstays for diagnosing IE.
- The most commonly identified organisms are viridans *Streptococcus* spp./ and *Staphylococcus*.
- Valves most commonly involved: (i) mitral valve, (ii) aortic valve, (iii) combination of aortic and mitral valves, (iv) tricuspid valve, (v) pulmonic valve

ENDOMETRIAL CANCER AND UTERINE SARCOMA

Sareena Singh, MD, FACOG • Kimberly Resnick, MD

BASICS

DESCRIPTION
- Endometrial cancer: malignancy of the endometrial lining of the uterus
  - Two types
    - Type I: estrogen-dependent, grade 1 or grade 2, better prognosis, endometrioid histology
    - Type II: estrogen-independent, higher grade, more aggressive, includes grade 3 endometrioid and nonendometrioid: serous, clear cell, mucinous, poor prognosis (1)[A]
- Cell types: adenocarcinoma, adenosquamous (malignant squamous elements), clear cell, and papillary serous
- Sarcomas: malignancy of the uterine mesenchyme and mixed tumors
  - Mixed müllerian sarcoma (carcinosarcoma): Heterologous sarcoma elements are not native to the müllerian system (e.g., cartilage or bone); homologous sarcoma elements are native to the müllerian system (40–50% prevalence of all sarcomas).
  - Leiomyosarcoma develops in the myometrium, characterized by cellular atypic mitoses and coagulative necrosis (30% prevalence of all sarcomas).
  - Endometrial stromal sarcoma develops from the stromal component of the endometrium (15% prevalence of all sarcomas).
  - Poorer prognosis (2)[C]
- Predominant age
  - Endometrial cancer: Most patients are postmenopausal:
    - Average age of diagnosis: 63 years old
  - Sarcomas: occur in both pre- and postmenopausal:
    - Average age of diagnosis: 40 to 69 years old (2)[C]
- 70% of endometrial cancer is stage I at the time of diagnosis.
- System(s) affected: reproductive
- Synonym(s): uterine cancer; endometrial cancer; corpus cancer

Pregnancy Considerations
This malignancy is not associated with pregnancy.

EPIDEMIOLOGY
Incidence
- Endometrial cancer is the most common gynecologic malignancy, fourth most common cancer in women, and eighth leading cause of cancer-related death in women worldwide.
- In the United States, it is estimated that endometrial cancer will account for 61,380 new cases and 10,920 deaths in 2017 according to SEER database.
- Incidence higher in Caucasian than African American, but African Americans have stage matched higher mortality (3).

Prevalence
Approximately 500,000 women in the United States

ETIOLOGY AND PATHOPHYSIOLOGY
Continuous estrogen stimulation unopposed by progesterone
- Endometrial: unopposed estrogen
  - Estrogen replacement therapy without concomitant progesterone increases the risk. Addition of progesterone decreases risk to that of general population.
- Sarcomas: etiology unknown

Genetics
- Endometrial: Lynch syndrome (hereditary nonpolyposis colorectal cancer); lifetime risk up to 30% (3); Cowden syndrome
- Sarcoma: African American, higher incidence of leiomyosarcoma, childhood retinoblastoma survivors

RISK FACTORS
- Early menarche/late menopause
- Nulliparity
- Personal or family history of colon or reproductive system cancer
- Obesity
- Diabetes mellitus
- Hypertension
- Polycystic ovarian syndrome
- Increasing age
- Estrogen-secreting tumor
- Endometrial hyperplasia
- Unopposed estrogens
- Tamoxifen use

GENERAL PREVENTION
- In young women who are obese or anovulatory, the risk of endometrial cancer can be reduced by taking oral contraceptive pills, permanently losing weight, or taking cyclic progesterone to prevent unopposed estrogen's effects on the uterus.
- Estrogen replacement therapy should always include progesterone unless the woman has had a hysterectomy.
- Cigarette smoking has been associated with a lower risk of type I endometrial cancer; however, it is not recommended secondary to its many health risks and increase risk of type II endometrial cancer.

COMMONLY ASSOCIATED CONDITIONS
- Endometrial hyperplasia: 1–25% will progress to endometrial adenocarcinoma:
  - Simple without atypia
  - Complex without atypia
  - Simple with atypia
  - Complex with atypia
    - 43% with complex hyperplasia with atypia have concurrent endometrial cancer.
- Endometrial cancer patients should be screened regularly for breast and colon cancer per routine screening guidelines.
- Patients who have breast or colon cancer are at increased risk for endometrial cancer.
- Granulosa cell tumors of the ovary produce estrogen; these patients will have an increased risk of endometrial cancer.

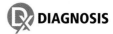

DIAGNOSIS

HISTORY
- Endometrial cancer
  - Postmenopausal bleeding is the most frequent sign. Any spotting or abnormal discharge mandates evaluation.
  - Premenopausal patients with history of anovulation and heavy, irregular, or prolonged periods that fail multiple medical managements mandate evaluation.
- Sarcoma
  - Mixed müllerian sarcoma: bleeding and prolapsing tissue, pain (2)[C]
  - Leiomyosarcoma: pelvic pain, pressure, uterine mass, abnormal bleeding

PHYSICAL EXAM
Pelvic exam: enlarged uterus, fixed

DIFFERENTIAL DIAGNOSIS
- Atypical complex hyperplasia: a premalignant lesion of the endometrium
- Cervical cancer
- Ovarian cancer invading the uterus
- Endometriosis
- Adenomyosis
- Leiomyoma

DIAGNOSTIC TESTS & INTERPRETATION
Initial Tests (lab, imaging)
- Liver and renal function tests
- Transvaginal ultrasound usually shows increased endometrial thickness (>4 mm in postmenopausal patients or in patients with irregular or heavy periods if >35 years of age, 100% NPV) (1)[A].
- Levels of cancer antigen 125 (CA-125) may be elevated when intra-abdominal disease is present (1)[A].
- Chest x-ray (CXR): Most common site of metastases is the lung.
- Mammogram and colonoscopy: Endometrial cancer is associated with breast and colon cancer.
- Routine preoperative MRI, CT, or PET scan: not recommended (3)

Follow-Up Tests & Special Considerations
- Endometrial cancer is mostly localized to the uterus; therefore, preoperative evaluation for metastasis is not needed unless metastasis is already suspected (2)[A].
- CT scan, PET/CT, MRI, CA-125: not part of the routine evaluation but may be needed if metastasis is suspected, patient is a poor operative candidate, or pathology returns high grade (G3 endometrioid, papillary serous, clear cell, carcinosarcoma) (2)
- MRI has been reported to show the depth of myometrial penetration accurately but is not always cost-effective.

Diagnostic Procedures/Other

- Office endometrial biopsy (90% accurate): If negative with high suspicion for cancer or patient continues to have bleeding, a dilation and curettage (D&C) is necessary (2)[B]. Endometrial stromal sarcoma and leiomyosarcoma rarely are diagnosed preoperatively. Any patient with history of irregular, heavy, or prolonged periods should undergo endometrial biopsy prior to endometrial ablation procedures.
- Fractional D&C is 99% accurate except in cases of sarcoma.
- If surgical approach is favored, D&C with hysteroscopic guidance is recommended over D&C alone, due to its ability to pick up discrete lesions (2)[A].
- Meta-analyses suggest hysteroscopic peritoneal dissemination of malignant cells; unknown significance of that dispersion

Test Interpretation

- International Federation of Gynecology and Obstetrics Staging System: revised 2009
  - Stage I (confined to corpus uteri)
    ○ A: no or <1/2 myometrial invasion
    ○ B: invasion ≥1/2 the myometrium
  - Stage II: Tumor invades cervical stroma but does not extend beyond the uterus.
  - Stage III: local and/or regional spread
    ○ A: uterine serosal and/or adnexal invasion
    ○ B: vaginal and/or parametrial involvement
    ○ C: metastases to pelvic and/or para-aortic lymph nodes
    ○ IIIC1: +pelvic nodes
    ○ IIIC2: +para-aortic lymph nodes positive pelvic lymph nodes
  - Stage IV: Tumor invades bladder and/or bowel mucosa and/or distant metastases:
    ○ A: Tumor invades bladder and/or bowel mucosa.
    ○ B: distant metastases, including intra-abdominal metastases and/or inguinal lymph nodes (1)[A]
- Uterine sarcoma criteria for diagnosis: mitotic index, cellular atypia, and areas of coagulative necrosis separated from tumor

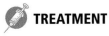 ## TREATMENT

GENERAL MEASURES

- Main treatment for uterine cancer is surgery.
- Radiation is used to prevent tumor recurrence at the vaginal cuff.

MEDICATION

First Line

- Endometrial
  - Chemotherapy for advanced or recurrent disease incurable with surgery and radiation
    ○ Paclitaxel + carboplatin (2)[B]
    ○ Doxorubicin + cisplatin + paclitaxel
- Hormonal therapy
  - Medroxyprogesterone acetate: for recurrence or metastases
  - Megestrol (Megace) 160 mg/day for at least 2 months for women with premalignant lesions, atypical complex hyperplasia, or well-differentiated endometrial cancer in patients desiring fertility. Follow with D&C to determine cancer resolution.
  - Levonorgestrel-containing intrauterine device: as mentioned earlier for patients who desire future fertility

- Sarcoma
  - Chemotherapy
    ○ Doxorubicin as single agent or in combination
- Hormonal
  - Tamoxifen or aromatase inhibitors; not fully studied, +/− progesterone
  - Progesterones

ADDITIONAL THERAPIES

Radiation therapy

- Nonoperative candidates: radiation therapy alone
- Low risk: no adjuvant radiation therapy
- Intermediate risk: Consider adjuvant vaginal brachytherapy; reduces local recurrences but has no effect on overall survival
- Vaginal brachytherapy is equivalent to whole pelvic radiation in regard to overall survival (3).
- High risk: chemotherapy and radiation therapy in some cases

SURGERY/OTHER PROCEDURES

Surgical staging

- Extrafascial hysterectomy and bilateral salpingo-oophorectomy
- Cytologic washings
- Pelvic and para-aortic lymph node dissection
- Omental sampling, as indicated, and for papillary serous (3)
- Optimal tumor debulking (1)[A], survival advantage
- LAP2 trial: minimally invasive and laparotomy similar 5-year survival (3)

Geriatric Considerations

Older (and obese) patients may be at high risk for surgery. Alternative radiation or progesterone therapy can be considered.

ADMISSION, INPATIENT, AND NURSING CONSIDERATIONS

- Admission criteria/initial stabilization
  - Excessive vaginal bleeding
  - Preoperative stabilization
- Nursing: routine; ensure postoperative pain is controlled.
- Postsurgical criteria: pain controlled, tolerating diet, ambulating, and voiding

 ## ONGOING CARE

FOLLOW-UP RECOMMENDATIONS

Follow-up visit with speculum and rectovaginal exam every 3 to 6 months for 2 years, then every 6 months for 3 years, and then annually for life (2)[C]

Patient Monitoring

- Annual CXR is no longer recommended.
- CT scan or PET/CT scan of the chest, abdomen, and pelvis should be used only to investigate suspicion of recurrent disease, not routinely.
- Control comorbid conditions.

DIET

As tolerated and according to comorbidities

PATIENT EDUCATION

After surgery:

- No intercourse for ~6 weeks
- No lifting >10 to 15 lb
- No driving until pain free
- Do not expect resumption of full activity for 6 weeks.

PROGNOSIS

5-year survival rates

- Uterine adenocarcinoma

Stage	Survival (%)
IA	88
IB	75
II	69
IIIA	58
IIIB	50
IIIC	47
IVA	17
IVB	15

- Uterine carcinosarcoma

Stage	Survival (%)
I	70
II	45
III	30
IV	15

COMPLICATIONS

- Surgical: excessive bleeding, wound infection, lymphedema, deep vein thrombosis (DVT), and damage to the urinary or intestinal systems
- Radiation: diarrhea, ileus, bowel obstruction or fistula, radiation cystitis, proctitis, vaginal stenosis, DVT
- Chemotherapy: per the drug given

REFERENCES

1. Creasman W. Revised FIGO staging for carcinoma of the endometrium. *Int J Gynaecol Obstet*. 2009;105(2):109.
2. Committee on Practice Bulletins—Gynecology and the Society of Gynecologic Oncology. Practice Bulletin No. 149: endometrial cancer. *Obstet Gynecol*. 2015;125(4):1006–1026.
3. Sorosky JI. Endometrial cancer. *Obstet Gynecol*. 2012;120(2, Pt 1):383–397.

 ## SEE ALSO

- Cervical Malignancy
- Algorithm: Pelvic Pain

 ## CODES

ICD10

- C54.1 Malignant neoplasm of endometrium
- C55 Malignant neoplasm of uterus, part unspecified
- C54.2 Malignant neoplasm of myometrium

CLINICAL PEARLS

- Most common presenting symptom is abnormal uterine bleeding.
- Any patient with history of irregular, heavy, or prolonged periods should undergo endometrial biopsy.
- Primary cause is unopposed estrogen.
- Endometrial thickness on transvaginal ultrasound of <5 mm makes endometrial cancer very unlikely.
- Primary treatment is with surgery, with possible chemotherapy ± radiation.

E

ENDOMETRIOSIS

Kenneth A. Ballou, MD

 BASICS

DESCRIPTION
- Endometriosis is a common but potentially painful and debilitating estrogen-dependent gynecologic condition affecting women of predominately reproductive age (1).
- Symptoms and signs generally consist of pelvic and/or abdominal pain, pelvic mass, and/or decreased fertility.
- Due to estrogen-dependent implants of endometrial tissue found outside the uterus. Although endometriomas have been recorded in liver, bowel, umbilicus, lung, and other tissue, the most common pathologic sites are:
  - Peritoneum (bladder, cul-de-sac, pelvic walls, ligaments, and fallopian tubes)
  - Ovaries
  - Rectovaginal septum
- Ectopic endometrial implants proliferate and slough with the menstrual cycle.
- Stage I (minimal) to IV (severe). Staging is useful in therapeutic planning but does not correlate with pain severity.

EPIDEMIOLOGY
Prevalence
- Female only
- Affects 6–10% of fertile women (1)
- Found in 20–50% of infertile women (1)
- Found in 71–87% of women with chronic pelvic pain (1)

Pediatric Considerations
Endometriosis may begin with puberty, as endometrial implants are dependent on ovarian hormones. This can lead to debilitating pelvic pain and severe dysmenorrhea associated with missed school and family/social activities.

Pregnancy Considerations
The presence of endometriosis decreases fecundability from 15–20% to 2–10% per month. 25–50% of infertile women have endometriosis. However, pelvic endometriosis generally improves during pregnancy.

Geriatric Considerations
Although menopause often results in a resolution of symptoms, pelvic endometriosis may extend into menopause and may be exacerbated by hormone replacement therapy (HRT).

ETIOLOGY AND PATHOPHYSIOLOGY
- Not fully understood; several factors are believed to play a role, including immunologic changes and genetic predisposition in the presence of abnormal proliferating endometrial tissue implants causing chronic peritoneal inflammation.
- Theories include:
  - Sampson theory: Retrograde menstruation results in peritoneal implantation and disease.
  - Halban theory: Distant disease is probably caused by hematogenous/lymphatic dissemination or metaplastic transformation.
  - Coelomic metaplasia: Coelomic epithelium remains undifferentiated in the peritoneal cavity and differentiates to form functioning endometrium.

- Endometrial-associated infertility is multifactorial:
  - Pelvic inflammation
  - Anatomic disruption of pelvic structures (Involvement of the fallopian tube may cause isthmic tubal obstruction.)
  - Proliferation and activation of peritoneal macrophages (may predispose to gamete phagocytosis)
  - Alteration in eutopic endometrium

Genetics
Odds ratio of symptomatic endometriosis with a first-degree affected relative is 7.2. Those with affected first-degree relatives have a 26% chance of severe manifestations versus 12% if no first-degree affected relatives.

RISK FACTORS
- Family history
- Menstruation and ovulation
- Delayed childbirth

GENERAL PREVENTION
- Suppression of heavy menstruation and ovulation with oral contraceptives during adolescence may delay sequelae.
- Some factors are considered protective:
  - Fruits, green vegetables, n-3 long-chain fatty acids
  - Aerobic exercise may decrease pelvic pain.
- Early diagnosis and treatment might help prevent sequelae.

COMMONLY ASSOCIATED CONDITIONS
Associated with increased risks for cancer of the ovary, breast, endometrium; increased risk for cutaneous melanoma, non-Hodgkin lymphoma, autoimmune diseases, asthma, and cardiovascular disease

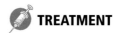 DIAGNOSIS

HISTORY
- Dysmenorrhea (50–90% of cases) due to deep infiltrating endometrial implants
- Dyspareunia due to lesions of the cul-de-sac, uterosacral ligaments, and posterior vaginal fornix
- Dyschezia due to involvement of the rectosigmoid colon and rectovaginal regions
- Chronic pelvic pain (≥6 months) that worsens with time and begins 1 to 2 days prior to menstrual cycles
- Hematochezia
- Cyclic nausea, abdominal distention
- Infertility (late finding)
- History of pelvic pain, infertility, and hysterectomy in first- or second-degree relative

PHYSICAL EXAM
- Focal pain/tenderness on pelvic exam is associated with endometriosis in 66% of patients.
- Pelvic mass may be present.
- Immobile pelvic organs (frozen pelvis)
- Rectovaginal exam revealing uterosacral nodules, beading, or tenderness
- An exquisitely tender "barb" stabbing pain in the region of the uterosacral ligament is found in severe cases.

DIFFERENTIAL DIAGNOSIS
Differential diagnosis of pelvic pain includes all causes of acute abdomen and
- Pelvic adhesions
- Nonspecific dysmenorrhea
- Acute salpingitis/pelvic inflammatory disease
- Ruptured ovarian cyst
- Uterine leiomyomas
- Adenomyosis
- Irritable bowel syndrome
- Inflammatory bowel disease
- Pelvic malignancy
- Complications of intrauterine/ectopic pregnancy
- Cystitis
- Depression
- History of sexual abuse
- Chronic pain syndrome

DIAGNOSTIC TESTS & INTERPRETATION
Initial Tests (lab, imaging)
- Labs are only useful to rule out other diagnoses; there are no useful labs to rule in endometriosis.
- CA-125 levels are not recommended (2)[C] due to low sensitivity.
- If history and physical exam reveal adnexal pain or tenderness with/without fullness on pelvic exam
  - Transvaginal ultrasound (US) and MRI are equally effective in detecting ovarian endometriomas: sensitivity, 80–90%; specificity, 60–98% for both.
  - US is preferred (less costly).
  - Both modalities are poor in detecting peritoneal implants and adhesions.

Diagnostic Procedures/Other
Definitive diagnosis is made only by microscopic characteristics of tissue biopsied during laparoscopy or laparotomy (1).

Test Interpretation
- Laparoscopically visualized red and blue-black lesions described as "powder-burns," adhesions, and "chocolate cysts" on the ovarian and peritoneal surfaces
- Histologically described endometrial glands and stroma on analysis of biopsied lesions

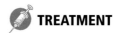 TREATMENT

GENERAL MEASURES
Management is dependent on multiple factors:
- Age and reproductive desires of the patient
- The certainty of the diagnosis
- The degree of degradation on quality of life due to pain and infertility
- The threat to other organ systems: GI tract, bladder

MEDICATION
Medications are used to improve the patient's quality of life through symptom relief and to prevent progression of the disease and its potential to cause organ dysfunction. Unfortunately, few studies of medical therapy report patient-relevant outcomes. Many women gain only limited or intermittent benefit from medical therapies (3)[A].

First Line

Women found to have endometriomas during incidental surgery or studies may not need any treatment. Others with minimal symptoms may find sufficient relief with NSAID medications. Increased exercise, especially aerobic, may help others.

- Cyclic combined oral contraceptive pills (OCPs) suppress ovulation.
- NSAIDs initiated at the beginning or just before menses. Evidence is inconclusive on effectiveness (4)[A].

Second Line

- Low-dose OCPs or low-dose progestins with recommendations to switch from cyclic to continuous combined contraception for 3 to 6 months if symptoms persist or if there is chronic, noncyclic pelvic pain (5)[A]. Evidence for combined hormonal contraception is of relatively low quality.
- Levonorgestrel intrauterine device (IUD) (Mirena) found to decrease recurrence of painful menstruation (although not FDA-approved for this indication)
- Medroxyprogesterone acetate 150 mg IM 3 months. Prolonged use may lead to loss of bone mineral density of uncertain clinical significance.
- Gonadotropin-releasing hormone (GnRH) agonists: inhibit pituitary gonadotropin synthesis and induce a hypoestrogenic state
- Norethindrone acetate 5 mg PO once daily plus conjugated equine estrogen 0.625 mg PO once daily

Third Line

If symptoms and signs continue, physicians should be experienced in the use and side effects of GnRH analogues prior to their use (symptoms return in as many as 70% of treated patients):

- Leuprolide acetate (Lupron Depot) 3.75 mg IM each month or 11.25 mg IM every 3 months (gluteal)
- Nafarelin (Synarel) intranasal one spray (200 μg) in one nostril each morning and the other nostril each evening (start between days 2 and 4 of menstrual cycle)
- Goserelin (Zoladex) implant 3.6 mg SC in upper abdominal wall every 28 days
- Danazol: also effective, with side effects similar to GnRH analogs
- Aromatase inhibitors (anastrozole and letrozole) prolong the remission induced by GnRH medications.

ALERT

Calcium (1,000 to 1,500 mg/day) with vitamin D 1,000 to 2,000 IU daily or low-dose estrogen with progestogen (1),(6)[C] is recommended when using GnRH agonists to prevent calcium loss.

ISSUES FOR REFERRAL

- Refer early to a physician with expertise in medical and surgical treatment of endometriosis, especially if the patient desires to conceive in the future.
- Indications for referral to a specialty gynecologist include the following:
  - Need for definitive diagnosis
  - Failure to respond to a conservative or first-line therapy
  - Chronic pelvic pain
  - Delayed fertility

ADDITIONAL THERAPIES

Regular exercise and counseling for pain-management strategies. Narcotics are contraindicated for chronic pain.

SURGERY/OTHER PROCEDURES

Surgery (laparoscopy or laparotomy) is both diagnostic and therapeutic (first line or when conservative measures fail):

- Peritoneal endometriosis: laser ablation/excision/fulguration
- Ovarian endometriosis (endometriomas) >3 to 4 cm: ablation, excision, drainage
- Lysis of adhesions (LOA)
- Hysterectomy with bilateral salpingo-oophorectomy for debilitating symptoms refractory to other medical or surgical treatments:
  - Relieves pain in 80–90%, but pain recurs in 10% within 1 to 2 years after surgery
  - Postoperative HRT should include estrogen and progestogen or progesterone.
- Interruption of nerve pathways: Laparoscopic ablations and presacral neurectomy improve dysmenorrhea.
- Fertility procedures: Ablation or excision of lesions with LOA is recommended to treat infertility in stages I and II disease:
  - Spontaneous conception should be attempted for 1 year prior to assisted reproduction techniques.
  - Disease does not endanger in vitro fertilization (IVF) pregnancies.

ALERT

Surgery for endometriomas may decrease ovarian reserve in advanced disease.

COMPLEMENTARY & ALTERNATIVE MEDICINE

- Osteopathic manipulative therapy found to improve quality of life (2)[C]
- Postsurgical use of Chinese herbal medicine has been found to be effective.
- Acupuncture may be more effective than danazol to decrease pain, irregular menstruation, and perineal swelling.
- Botulinum toxin injections have been used to control pain.

ONGOING CARE

FOLLOW-UP RECOMMENDATIONS

Routine gynecologic care

Patient Monitoring

Symptomatic and asymptomatic pelvic masses (http://www.acog.org/)

PROGNOSIS

- Excellent, especially if diagnosis and treatment plans are initiated early in disease course
- Poor for recovery of fertility if the disease has progressed to stage III/IV
- Symptoms and signs improve after bilateral oophorectomy.

COMPLICATIONS

Sequelae include chronic pelvic pain, reduced quality of life, repetitive surgical intervention, depression, medication side effects and costs, and infertility.

REFERENCES

1. Practice Bulletin No. 114: management of endometriosis. *Obstet Gynecol.* 2010;116(1):223–236.
2. Daraï C, Deboute O, Zacharopoulou C, et al. Impact of osteopathic manipulative therapy on quality of life of patients with deep infiltrating endometriosis with colorectal involvement: results of a pilot study. *Eur J Obstet Gynecol Reprod Biol.* 2015;188:70–73.
3. Becker CM, Gattrell WT, Gude K, et al. Reevaluating response and failure of medical treatment of endometriosis: a systematic review. *Fertil Steril.* 2017;108(1):125–136.
4. Allen C, Hopewell S, Prentice A, et al. Nonsteroidal anti-inflammatory drugs for pain in women with endometriosis. *Cochrane Database Syst Rev.* 2009;(2):CD004753.
5. Jensen JT, Schlaff W, Gordon K. Use of combined hormonal contraceptives for the treatment of endometriosis-related pain: a systematic review of the evidence. *Fertil Steril.* 2018;110(1):137–152.e1.
6. Giudice LC. Clinical practice. Endometriosis. *N Engl J Med.* 2010;362(25):2389–2398.

ADDITIONAL READING

- Brown J, Farquhar C. Endometriosis: an overview of Cochrane Reviews. *Cochrane Database Syst Rev.* 2014;(3):CD009590.
- Davis L, Kennedy SS, Moore J, et al. Oral contraceptives for pain associated with endometriosis. *Cochrane Database Syst Rev.* 2007;(3):CD001019.
- de Ziegler D, Borghese B, Chapron C. Endometriosis and infertility: pathophysiology and management. *Lancet.* 2010;376(9742):730–738.
- Fujii S. MR imaging of endometriosis. In: Harada T, ed. *Endometriosis: Pathogenesis and Treatment.* Tottori, Japan: Springer; 2014:311–320.
- Jacobson TZ, Duffy JM, Barlow D, et al. Laparoscopic surgery for pelvic pain associated with endometriosis. *Cochrane Database Syst Rev.* 2009;(4):CD001300.
- Koga K, Yoshino O, Hirota Y, et al. Infertility treatment of endometriosis patients. In: Harada T, ed. *Endometriosis: Pathogenesis and Treatment.* Tottori, Japan: Springer; 2014:431–444.
- Practice Committee of American Society for Reproductive Medicine. Treatment of pelvic pain associated with endometriosis. *Fertil Steril.* 2008;90(Suppl 5):S260–S269.
- Rubin R. Botulinum toxin to treat endometriosis pain. *JAMA.* 2019;322(8):716.
- Schrager S, Falleroni J, Edgoose J. Evaluation and treatment of endometriosis. *Am Fam Physician.* 2013;87(2):107–113.
- Zhu X, Hamilton KD, McNicol ED. Acupuncture for pain in endometriosis. *Cochrane Database Syst Rev.* 2011;(9):CD007864.
- Zondervan KT, Becker CM, Missmer SA. Endometriosis. *N Engl J Med.* 2020;382(13):1244–1256.

 ## CODES

ICD10

- N80.2 Endometriosis of fallopian tube
- N80.5 Endometriosis of intestine
- N80.0 Endometriosis of uterus

CLINICAL PEARLS

- Severe dysmenorrhea and dyspareunia are never normal. Failure to respond to NSAIDs and/or OCPs warrants further investigation.
- A rectovaginal exam can be useful in patients suspected of having endometriosis.

E

ENDOMETRITIS AND OTHER POSTPARTUM INFECTIONS

Justin P. Lavin Jr., MD, FACOG • Sarah E. Davis, DO

BASICS

DESCRIPTION
- Endometritis (infection of the endometrium) is the most common postpartum infection.
- Bacterial infection of genital tract, manifesting after delivery with a peak incidence at postpartum day 7 (most patients will have been discharged), can occur as late as 6 weeks postpartum.
- Postpartum infections of the myometrium and parametrial tissues are less common. Vaginal and cervical infections, perianal cellulitis, pelvic cellulitis, pelvic abscess, septic pelvic vein thrombophlebitis, and parametrial phlegmon are other (generally rare) postpartum infections of the pelvic region.
- System(s) affected: reproductive
- Synonym(s): postpartum infection; endometritis; endoparametritis; endomyometritis; myometritis; endomyoparametritis; metritis; metritis with pelvic cellulitis

EPIDEMIOLOGY
Incidence
Occurs in women of childbearing years

Prevalence
- Occurs after 1–3% of all births
- Infection 10 times more likely after cesarean section
  - 2–15% of infections begin prior to labor.
  - 30–35% occur after labor in absence of appropriate antibiotic prophylaxis; 2–15% occur after labor with appropriate prophylaxis.
  - Fifth leading cause of maternal mortality, accounting for 11% of maternal deaths

ETIOLOGY AND PATHOPHYSIOLOGY
- Endometritis is more common in labors complicated by chorioamnionitis.
- Other infections follow trauma to the perineum, vagina, cervix, and uterus.
- Postpartum infections are typically polymicrobial, involving organisms ascending from the lower genital tract:
  - Aerobic isolates (70%): *Streptococcus faecalis, Streptococcus agalactiae, Streptococcus viridans, Staphylococcus aureus, Escherichia coli*
  - Anaerobic isolates (80%): *Peptococcus* sp., *Peptostreptococcus* sp., *Clostridium* sp., *Bacteroides bivius, Bacteroides fragilis, Fusobacterium* sp.
- Other genital *Mycoplasma*
- Consider herpes simplex virus and cytomegalovirus, particularly in immunocompromised patients failing to improve on appropriate antibiotics.
- Thrombosis of any pelvic vein, including vena cava
- Phlegmon on leaves of the broad ligament

RISK FACTORS
- Cesarean delivery is the primary risk factor.
- Chorioamnionitis
- Bacterial vaginosis
- Group B streptococcal colonization of genital tract
- HIV infection
- Prolonged labor
- Prolonged rupture of membranes; heavily meconium-stained amniotic fluid
- Multiple vaginal examinations
- Internal fetal monitoring during labor
- Operative vaginal delivery; manual extraction of the placenta; care in a teaching hospital
- Low socioeconomic status
- Obesity
- Anemia

GENERAL PREVENTION
- Intrapartum prophylaxis for group B colonization of genital tract
- Vaginal delivery
  - Avoid unnecessary vaginal examinations.
  - Treat chorioamnionitis during labor.
  - Avoid manual placental extraction and retained placental products.
  - Consider antibiotic prophylaxis for third- and fourth-degree laceration.
  - Aseptic technique for operative vaginal delivery
  - A recent large multicenter trial suggests benefit from prophylaxis with amoxicillin and clavulanic acid for operative vaginal delivery (1)[B].
  - In contrast, antibiotic prophylaxis for manual removal of the placenta has not been demonstrated to be effective.
- Cesarean delivery
  - Preoperative paint and scrub with 10% povidone-iodine scrub or an alcohol-based solution decreases puerperal infection by up to 38%.
  - Prophylactic antibiotics before both emergency and scheduled cesarean deliveries prior to skin incision reduce postpartum infection (2)[A].
    - Administer antibiotics within 1 hour of the start of surgery (3).
    - Should be repeated for lengthy procedures or excessive blood loss (3)
    - Appropriate administration of antibiotics results in a 40% reduction in postpartum maternal infections without any increase in neonatal infections (2)[A],(3).
  - Extended coverage with cephalosporin and azithromycin further decreases infection risk and is cost-effective (3),(4)[A].
  - Vaginal preparation with povidone-iodine solution or chlorhexidine-alcohol solutions immediately before cesarean delivery reduces the risk of postoperative endometritis (5)[A].
  - Weight-based antibiotic dosage helps ensure appropriate tissue concentrations prior to skin incision.
  - Placental removal with gentle traction
  - Use of multiple interventions as a bundle are more effective than individual components.

COMMONLY ASSOCIATED CONDITIONS
- Chorioamnionitis
- Wound infection

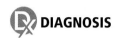

DIAGNOSIS

HISTORY
- History of cesarean delivery or chorioamnionitis
- Fever and chills
- Malaise
- Headache
- Anorexia
- Abdominal pain
- Heavy vaginal bleeding or foul smelling lochia

PHYSICAL EXAM
- Oral temperature >38°C (100.4°F)
- Tachycardia
- Uterine tenderness on exam (key finding)
- Other localized abdominopelvic tenderness on exam
- Purulent or malodorous lochia
- Heavy vaginal bleeding
- Ileus
- Group A or B streptococcal bacteremia may have no localizing signs.

DIFFERENTIAL DIAGNOSIS
- "5 Ws": Wind (pneumonia); Water (UTI); Wound infection; Wow (mastitis); Wonder drug (medication-related fever)
- Viral syndrome; dehydration
- Pelvic abscess
- Thrombophlebitis
- Thyroid storm
- Appendicitis

DIAGNOSTIC TESTS & INTERPRETATION
Initial Tests (lab, imaging)
- CBC: Interpret with care. (Physiologic leukocytosis may be as high as 20,000 WBCs.)
- CMP
- Diagnosis often made on clinical grounds. Potential testing includes:
  - Genital tract cultures and rapid test for group B streptococci (may be done during labor)
  - Amniotic fluid Gram stain: usually polymicrobial
  - Uterine tissue cultures: Prep the cervix with Betadine and use a shielded specimen collector or Pipelle; difficult to obtain without contamination
- If the patient meets criteria for SIRS and or suspected sepsis, follow institution guidelines for appropriate workup and identification (i.e., serum lactate, fluid resuscitation, two sets of blood cultures, and timely administration of broad spectrum antibiotics).

- If patient not responding to antibiotics in 24 to 48 hours:
  - Ultrasound for retained products of conception, pelvic abscess, or mass
  - CT or MRI looking for pelvic vein thrombophlebitis, abscess, or deep-seated wound infection

Diagnostic Procedures/Other
Paracentesis/culdocentesis with culture rarely necessary

Test Interpretation
- Superficial layer of infected necrotic tissue in microscopic sections of uterine lining
- >5 neutrophils per high-power field in superficial endometrium; ≥1 plasma cell in endometrial stroma

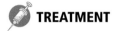

TREATMENT

MEDICATION

First Line
Clindamycin 900 mg IV q8h + gentamicin 5 mg/kg IV q24h (6)[A]
- Potential side effects include nephrotoxicity, ototoxicity, pseudomembranous colitis, or diarrhea (in up to 6%).

Second Line
- Ampicillin/sulbactam 3 g IV q6h
- Metronidazole 500 mg IV or PO q8–12h + penicillin 5,000,000 U IV q6h, or
- Ampicillin 2 g IV q6h + gentamicin 5 mg/kg IV q24h (6)[A]
- Cefoxitin 2 g IV q6h. Add ampicillin 2 g IV q6h, if clinical failure after 48 hours (6)[A].
- Cefotetan 2 g IV q12h. Add ampicillin 2 g IV q6h, if clinical failure after 48 hours (6)[A].
- Note: Base therapy on cultures, sensitivities, and clinical response.
- Contraindications
  - Drug allergy
  - Renal failure (aminoglycosides)
  - Avoid sulfa, tetracyclines, and fluoroquinolones before delivery and if breastfeeding. Metronidazole is relatively contraindicated if breastfeeding.
- Precautions
  - Clindamycin and other antibiotics occasionally cause pseudomembranous colitis.
  - Antibiotic-associated diarrhea (Clostridium difficile)
  - Gentamicin can cause renal injury.
- Note: Consider adding a macrolide antibiotic (for chlamydia coverage) for infections occurring after 48 hours.
- Note: Heparin typically indicated for septic pelvic vein thrombophlebitis; requires 10 days of full anticoagulation

SURGERY/OTHER PROCEDURES
- Ultrasound to look for retained products of conception if not responsive to initial therapy
- Curettage for retained products of conception
- Surgery or image-guided drainage to drain abscess
- Surgery to decompress the bowel
- Surgical drainage of a phlegmon is not advised unless it is suppurative. Surgical removal of other inflamed tissue is usually not required.

ADMISSION, INPATIENT, AND NURSING CONSIDERATIONS
- Inpatient care is recommended for postpartum infections.
- Many infections occur after hospital discharge. Therefore, education regarding the importance of fever, pain, heavy vaginal bleeding, foul smelling lochia, or other signs of infection should occur prior to discharge (1).
- IV antibiotics and close observation for severe infections
- Open and drain infected wounds.
- Optimize fluid status.

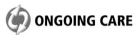

ONGOING CARE

FOLLOW-UP RECOMMENDATIONS

Patient Monitoring
- Individualize according to severity.
- IV antibiotics can be stopped when the patient is afebrile for 24 to 48 hours.
- Oral antibiotics on discharge are not necessary, unless patient was bacteremic; then continue oral antibiotics to complete a 7-day course.

DIET
As tolerated, although may be limited by ileus

PATIENT EDUCATION
- Advise patient to contact physician with fever >38°C (100.4°F) postpartum, heavy vaginal bleeding, foul-smelling lochia, or other symptoms of infection.
- Information available at http://www.healthline.com/health/pregnancy/complications-postpartum-endometritis

PROGNOSIS
With supportive therapy and appropriate antibiotics, most patients improve quickly and recover without complication.

COMPLICATIONS
- Resistant organisms; peritonitis; pelvic abscess
- Septic pelvic thrombophlebitis
- Ovarian vein thrombosis
- Sepsis; death

REFERENCES

1. Knight M, Chiocchia V, Partlett C, et al. Prophylactic antibiotics in the prevention of infection after operative vaginal delivery (ANODE): a multicentre randomised controlled trial. Lancet. 2019;393(10189):2395–2403.
2. Bollig C, Nothacker M, Lehane C, et al. Prophylactic antibiotics before cord clamping in cesarean delivery: a systematic review. Acta Obstet Gynecol Scand. 2018;97(5):521–535.
3. Committee on Practice Bulletins-Obstetrics. ACOG Practice Bulletin No. 199: use of prophylactic antibiotics in labor and delivery. Obstet Gynecol. 2018;132(3):e103–e119.
4. Tita AT, Szychowski JM, Boggess K, et al. Adjunctive azithromycin prophylaxis for cesarean delivery. N Engl J Med. 2016;375:1231–1241.
5. Haas DM, Morgan S, Contreras K, et al. Vaginal preparation with antiseptic solution before cesarean section for preventing postoperative infections. Cochrane Database Syst Rev. 2018;7(7):CD007892.
6. French LM, Smaill FM. Antibiotic regimens for endometritis after delivery. Cochrane Database Syst Rev. 2004;(4):CD001067.

 SEE ALSO

Algorithm: Pelvic Pain

 CODES

ICD10
- O86.12 Endometritis following delivery
- O86.4 Pyrexia of unknown origin following delivery
- O86.13 Vaginitis following delivery

CLINICAL PEARLS
- Postpartum endometritis follows 1–3% of all births.
- Infections are typically polymicrobial and involve organisms ascending from the lower genital tract.
- Evidence supports antibiotic prophylaxis prior to skin incision for all cesarean deliveries but not for operative vaginal deliveries.
- Clindamycin 900 mg IV q8h and gentamicin 5 mg/kg q24h are recommended as first-line therapy for endometritis. Treat until the patient is afebrile for 24 to 48 hours and stop antibiotics completely (unless there is documented bacteremia, which requires a 7-day course of therapy).
- If no improvement occurs on antibiotics, consider retained placental products, abscess, wound infection, hematoma, cellulitis, phlegmon, or septic pelvic vein thrombosis.

E

ENURESIS

Joseph L. Hesse, MD • Swati B. Avashia, MD, FAAP, FACP

BASICS

DESCRIPTION
- Classification
  - Primary nocturnal enuresis (NE): 80% of all cases; person who has never established urinary continence on consecutive nights for a period of ≥6 months
  - Secondary NE: 20% of cases; resumption of enuresis after at least 6 months of urinary continence
- NE: intermittent nocturnal incontinence after the anticipated age of bladder control (age 5 years)
  - Primary monosymptomatic NE (PMNE): bedwetting with no history of bladder dysfunction or other lower urinary tract (LUT) symptoms
  - Nonmonosymptomatic NE (NMNE): bed-wetting with LUT symptoms such as frequency, urgency, daytime wetting, hesitancy, straining, weak or intermittent stream, posturination dribbling, lower abdominal or genital discomfort, or sensation of incomplete emptying

ALERT
Adult-onset NE with absent daytime incontinence is a serious symptom; complete urologic evaluation and therapy are warranted.

- System(s) affected: nervous, renal/urologic
- Synonym(s): bed-wetting; sleep enuresis; nocturnal incontinence; primary NE

EPIDEMIOLOGY
Incidence
- Depends on family history
- Spontaneous resolution: 15% per year

Prevalence
- Very common; 5 to 7 million children in the United States (1)
- 10% of 7-year-olds; 3% of 11- to 12-year-olds; 0.5–1.7% at 16 to 17 years old (2)
- 1.5 to 2 times more common in males than females
- Nocturnal > day (3:1)

Geriatric Considerations
Infrequent; often associated with daytime incontinence (formerly referred to as diurnal enuresis)

ETIOLOGY AND PATHOPHYSIOLOGY
- A disorder of sleep arousal, a low nocturnal bladder capacity, and nocturnal polyuria are the three factors that interrelate to cause NE.
- Both functional and organic causes (below); many theories, none absolutely confirmed
- Detrusor instability
- Deficiency of arginine vasopressin (AVP); decreased nocturnal AVP or decreased AVP stimulation secondary to an empty bladder (Bladder distension stimulates AVP.)
- Maturational delay of CNS
- Severe NE with some evidence of interaction between bladder overactivity and brain arousability: association with children with severe NE and frequent cortical arousals in sleep
- Organic urologic causes in 1–4% of enuresis in children: urinary tract infection (UTI), occult spina bifida, ectopic ureter, lazy bladder syndrome, irritable bladder with wide bladder neck, posterior urethral valves, neurologic bladder dysfunction
- Organic nonurologic causes: epilepsy, diabetes mellitus, food allergies, obstructive sleep apnea, chronic renal failure, hyperthyroidism, pinworm infection, sickle cell disease
- NE occurs in all stages of sleep.

Genetics
Most commonly, NE is an autosomal-dominant inheritance pattern with high penetrance (90%).
- 1/3 of all cases are sporadic.
- 75% of children with enuresis have a first-degree relative with the condition.
- Higher rates in monozygotic versus dizygotic twins (68% vs. 36%)
- If both parents had NE, risk in child is 77%; 44% if one parent is affected. Parental age of resolution often predicts when child's enuresis should resolve.

RISK FACTORS
- Family history
- Stressors (emotional, environmental) common in secondary enuresis (e.g., divorce, death)
- Constipation and/or encopresis
- Organic disease: 1% of monosymptomatic NE (e.g., urologic and nonurologic causes)
- Psychological disorders
  - Comorbid disorders are highest with secondary NE: depression, anxiety, social phobias, conduct disorder, hyperkinetic syndrome, internalizing disorders.
  - Association with ADHD; more pronounced in ages 9 to 12 years
- Altered mental status or impaired mobility

GENERAL PREVENTION
No known measures

COMMONLY ASSOCIATED CONDITIONS
- Obstructive sleep apnea syndrome (10–54%) (1): Atrial natriuretic factor inhibits renin-angiotensin-aldosterone pathway leading to diuresis.
- Constipation (33–75%) (1)
- Behavioral problems (specifically ADHD in 12–17%) (1)
- Overactive bladder or dysfunctional voiding (up to 41%) (1)
- UTI (18–60%) (1)

DIAGNOSIS

HISTORY
- Age of onset, duration, severity
- LUT symptoms
- Daily intake patterns
- Voiding and stooling patterns (voiding diary); constipation issues
- Psychosocial history (patient, parental, school/bullying, etc.)
- Family history of enuresis
- Investigation and previous treatment history

PHYSICAL EXAM
- ENT: evaluation for adenotonsillar hypertrophy (associated with sleep apnea)
- Abdomen: enlarged bladder, kidneys, fecal masses, or impaction
- Back: Look for dimpling or tufts of hair on sacrum.
- Genital urinary exam
  - Males: meatal stenosis, hypospadias, epispadias, phimosis
  - Females: vulvitis, vaginitis, labial adhesions, ureterocele at introitus; evidence of abuse
- Rectal exam: tone, fecal soiling, fecal impaction
- Neurologic exam, especially lower extremities

DIFFERENTIAL DIAGNOSIS
- Primary NE
  - Delayed physiologic urinary control
  - UTI (both)
  - Spina bifida occulta
  - Obstructive sleep apnea (both)
  - Idiopathic detrusor instability
  - Previously unrecognized myelopathy or neuropathy (e.g., multiple sclerosis, tethered cord, epilepsy)
  - Anatomic urinary tract abnormality (e.g., ectopic ureter)
- Secondary NE
  - Acute situational stress (most common cause)
  - Bladder outlet obstruction
  - Neurologic disease, neurogenic bladder (e.g., spinal cord injury)

DIAGNOSTIC TESTS & INTERPRETATION
Initial Tests (lab, imaging)
- Only obligatory test in children is urinalysis.
- Urinalysis and urine culture: UTI, pyuria, hematuria, proteinuria, glycosuria, and poor concentrating ability (low specific gravity) may suggest organic etiology, especially in adults.
- Urinary tract imaging is usually not necessary.
- If abnormal clinical findings or adult onset: renal and bladder US
- IV pyelogram, voiding cystourethrogram (VCUG), or retrograde pyelogram is rarely indicated (1).
- MRI if spinal dysraphism is suspected

Follow-Up Tests & Special Considerations
- Secondary enuresis (if not psychosocial factors identified): serum glucose, BUN, creatinine, thyroid-stimulating hormone (TSH), urine culture
- In children, imaging and urodynamic studies are helpful for significant daytime symptoms, history of UTIs, suspected structural abnormalities, and in refractory cases.

Diagnostic Procedures/Other
Urodynamic studies may be beneficial in adults and NMNE.

Test Interpretation
- Dysfunctional voiding
- Detrusor instability and/or reduced bladder capacity most common findings

TREATMENT

GENERAL MEASURES
- Use nonpharmacologic approaches as first line before prescribing medications (1)[A].
- Simple behavioral interventions (e.g., scheduled wakening, positive reinforcement, bladder training, diet changes) are effective, although less so than alarms or medications (1)[B]; found to achieve dryness in 15–20% of cases (3)
  - Explain the three pathophysiologic factors (fragmented sleep, low nocturnal bladder capacity, and increased nocturnal urine production).
  - Encourage normal drinking patterns during daytime hours and reduction of intake 2 hours prior to sleep.
  - Emphasize regular bedtime with full night's sleep.
  - Scheduled voiding before bed
  - Scheduled waking for nighttime voiding
  - Nightlights to light the way to the bathroom

- – Reward system for dry nights
- – Use pull up over regular underwear or cloth underwear with built in waterproof barrier.
- – "Cleanliness training": child helps with changing wet bedding
- Do not shame or punish bed-wetting but have the child participate in removing and laundering soiled bedding and garments.
- Secondary enuresis:
  - – Referral for behavioral counseling if suspicion
  - – Stool softeners and cathartics if constipation present
- If behavioral interventions alone have no success, combined therapy (e.g., enuresis alarm, bladder training, motivational therapy, and pelvic floor muscle training) is more effective than each component alone or than pharmacotherapy (1)[A].
- Enuresis alarms (bells or buzzers)
  - – Considered first line; most effective treatment
  - – 66–70% success rate; must be used nightly for 2 to 4 months; offers cure; significant parental involvement; disruption of sleep for entire family
  - – If successful, it should be used until 14 consecutive dry nights achieved (2)[B].
- See "Patient Education" for options.

MEDICATION

First Line

Desmopressin (DDAVP): synthetic analogue of vasopressin that decreases nocturnal urine output (2)[A]

- Intranasal DDAVP: adults only, 20 mg (2 sprays) intranasally at bedtime
- FDA recommends against use in children due to reports of severe hyponatremia resulting in seizures and deaths in children using intranasal formulations of desmopressin.
- Oral DDAVP: safe in children. Begin at 0.2 mg tablet taken at bedtime on empty stomach; after 14 days of inefficient treatment, can titrate to 0.4 mg (2).
  - – Maximally effective in 1 hour; effect lasts 8 to 10 hours.
  - – If treatment is successful, can be continued for 3 months, then stop for 2 weeks for test of dryness.
  - – High relapse rate after discontinuation without a structured withdrawal program. If relapse occurs, oral desmopressin can continue to be prescribed in 3-month blocks.
  - – Suspend dose in children who experience acute condition affecting fluid/electrolyte balances (fever, vomiting, diarrhea, vigorous exercise).
  - – 60–70% success; 30% of children have full response and 40% have partial response.

Pediatric Considerations

FDA recommends against using intranasal formulations of desmopressin in children due to reports of severe hyponatremia resulting in seizures and deaths (3)[A].

Second Line

- Imipramine (Tofranil): tricyclic antidepressant, anticholinergic effects; increases bladder capacity, antispasmodic properties
  - – Primarily in adults; use in children is reserved for resistant cases and initiated by specialists.
  - – Dose: adults, 25 to 75 mg and children >6 years, 10 to 25 mg PO at bedtime; increase by 10 to 25 mg at 1- to 2-week intervals; treat for 2 to 3 months; then taper.
  - – 40% success rate, but relapses after discontinuation are high (2).
  - – Pretreatment ECG recommended identifying underlying rhythm disorders.

- Anticholinergics: Monotherapy is not recommended in children.
  - – Oxybutynin (Ditropan, Ditropan XL, Oxytrol patch): anticholinergic; smooth muscle relaxant, antispasmodic; may increase functional bladder capacity and aids in timed voiding (4)[B]
    - ○ 30–50% success; 50% relapse after stopped
    - ○ Ditropan: adults: 5 mg PO TID–QID; children >5 years old with overactive bladder who have failed alarm therapy and desmopressin can try 5 mg at bedtime.
    - ○ Ditropan XL: adults: 5 mg/day PO; increase to 30 mg/day PO (5- to 10-mg tablet).
    - ○ Oxytrol patch: 1 patch every 3 to 4 days (3.9 mg/patch) (Periodic trials of the medication, i.e., weekends or weeks at a time, will help determine efficacy and resolution of primary disturbance.)
  - – Tolterodine (Detrol, Detrol LA): anticholinergic; fewer side effects than Ditropan (4)[B]
    - ○ Detrol: 1 to 2 mg PO BID in adults, 2 mg at bedtime in children >5 years old
    - ○ Detrol LA: 2 to 4 mg/day
- Precautions
  - – Oxybutynin: glaucoma, myasthenia gravis, GI or genitourinary obstruction, ulcerative colitis, constipation, megacolon; use a decreased dose in the elderly.
  - – Tolterodine: urinary retention, gastric retention, constipation, uncontrolled narrow-angle glaucoma; significant drug interactions with CYP2D6, CYP3A3/4 substrates
  - – Desmopressin: Avoid in patients at risk for electrolyte changes or fluid retention (congestive heart failure [CHF], renal insufficiency). Stop during gastroenteritis or other acute illness with risk of dehydration.
  - – Imipramine: Do not use with monoamine oxidase inhibitors (MAOIs), hypotension, and arrhythmias; low-toxic therapeutic ratio
- Combination therapy with DDAVP and oxybutynin has better results than individual use (4)[B].

ALERT
Imipramine: cardiotoxicity and death with overdose

ISSUES FOR REFERRAL
- Primary NE: persistent enuresis despite nonpharmacologic and pharmacologic therapies
- Diurnal incontinence or nonmonosymptomatic enuresis with voiding dysfunction or underlying medical condition

ADDITIONAL THERAPIES
Individual and family psychotherapy, crisis intervention

SURGERY/OTHER PROCEDURES
Only for surgically correctable causes (e.g., tethered cord, ectopic ureter, benign prostatic hypertrophy, obstructive sleep apnea)

COMPLEMENTARY & ALTERNATIVE MEDICINE
Acupuncture has small amounts of supportive data (3)[B].

 ## ONGOING CARE

FOLLOW-UP RECOMMENDATIONS
Patient Monitoring
- When starting with nonpharmacologic treatment, patient should be seen in clinic every 1 to 3 months.
- If starting enuresis alarm, patient should return in 1 week to assess response.
- If starting DDAVP, patient should return in 1 to 2 weeks to assess response and then return at least every 3 months.

DIET
- Limit fluid and caffeine intake 2 hours before sleep.
- Limit dairy products and sweetened drinks for 4 hours before sleep (decrease osmotic diuresis) (5).

PATIENT EDUCATION
Web resources for hypnosis scripts, alarms, and supplies
- www.hypnoticworld.com/hypnosis-scripts/habits-disorders/enuresis
- http://wetstop.com
- https://bedwettingstore.com
- www.dri-sleeper.com
- www.nitetrain-r.com
- Parents can search their App Store for free bed-wetting diary apps (e.g., My Dryness Tracker).

PROGNOSIS
In children, NE is usually self-limiting; 1% will persist as adult; evaluate for organic causes.

COMPLICATIONS
UTI, perineal excoriation, psychological disturbance (especially in children)

REFERENCES

1. Baird DC, Seehusen DA, Bode DV. Enuresis in children: a case based approach. *Am Fam Physician*. 2014;90(8):560–568.
2. Kuwertz-Bröking E, von Gontard A. Clinical management of nocturnal enuresis. *Pediatr Nephrol*. 2018;33(7):1145–1154.
3. Jain S, Bhatt GC. Advances in the management of primary monosymptomatic nocturnal enuresis in children. *Paediatr Int Child Health*. 2016;36(1):7–14.
4. Bayne AP, Skoog SJ. Nocturnal enuresis: an approach to assessment and treatment. *Pediatr Rev*. 2014;35(8):327–335.
5. Traisman E. Enuresis: evaluation and treatment. *Pediatr Ann*. 2015;44(4):133–137.

 ## SEE ALSO

- Incontinence, Urinary Adult Female; Incontinence, Urinary Adult Male
- Algorithm: Enuresis, Secondary

CODES

ICD10
- N39.44 Nocturnal enuresis
- R32 Unspecified urinary incontinence
- F98.0 Enuresis not due to a substance or known physiol condition

CLINICAL PEARLS
- Initial evaluation is history, exam, and urinalysis.
- For PMNE in children, if the condition is not distressing to child and caretakers, treatment is unnecessary.
- Behavioral and lifestyle interventions are the first-line treatment for PMNE; alarms and desmopressin are the most effective treatments.
- Dryness is possible for most children.
- Secondary enuresis: most often due to psychosocial factors

EPICONDYLITIS

Julie A. Creech, DO • Brooke Organ, DO • Sabrina L. Silver, DO, CAQSM

BASICS

DESCRIPTION

- Tendinopathy of the elbow characterized by pain and tenderness at the myotendinous junctions or tendinous insertions of the wrist flexors/extensors at the humeral epicondyles
- Although commonly known as medial and lateral epicondylitis, without microscopic histologic examination, the more appropriate term is medial epicondyle tendinopathy (MET) and lateral epicondyle tendinopathy (LET).
- Most commonly secondary to chronic (overuse) pathology, although acute (traumatic) etiology can occur
- Two types
  - MET ("golfer's elbow")
    - Involves the wrist flexors and pronators, which originate at the medial epicondyle
  - LET ("tennis elbow")
    - Involves the wrist extensors and supinators, which originate at the lateral epicondyle
    - Most commonly involves the extensor carpi radialis brevis (ERCB) tendon
- May be caused by various different athletic or occupational activities
- Common in carpenters, plumbers, gardeners, and overhead athletes
- 75% of cases involve the dominant arm.

EPIDEMIOLOGY

- Predominant age: >40 years
- Predominant sex: male = female

Incidence

- Common overuse injury
- Lateral > medial
- Estimated between 1% and 3%

Prevalence

- LET: 1.3%
- MET: 0.4%

ETIOLOGY AND PATHOPHYSIOLOGY

- Acute (tendonitis)
  - Rare, uncommon pathology
  - Inflammatory response to injury or sudden, violent contraction
- Chronic (tendinosis)
  - Overuse injury
  - Repetitive wrist flexion or extension places strain across enthesis of flexor/extensor group.
  - Degeneration, calcium deposition, fibroblast proliferation, microvascular proliferation, hyaline cartilage destruction, diminished restorative inflammatory response
- Aggravating activities
  - Tool/racquet griping
  - Shaking hands
  - Occupational (painters, mechanics, cooks)
  - Sports (golf, tennis, archery, pitchers)

RISK FACTORS

- Repetitive wrist motions
  - Flexion/pronation: medial
  - Extension/supination: lateral
- Smoking
- Obesity
- Upper extremity forceful activities

GENERAL PREVENTION

- Limit overuse of the wrist flexors, extensors, pronators, and supinators.
- Use proper techniques when working with hand tools or playing racquet sports.
- Use lighter tools and smaller grips.

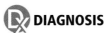 DIAGNOSIS

HISTORY

- Insidious onset
- Pain localized to lateral or medial elbow
- Aching pain, often radiates from epicondyle to forearm or wrist
- Pain with gripping
- Sensation of mild forearm weakness

PHYSICAL EXAM

- Localized pain just distal to the affected epicondyle
- MET
  - Tenderness at origin of wrist flexor tendons
  - Increased pain with resisted wrist flexion and pronation
  - Normal elbow range of motion
  - Increased pain with gripping
- LET
  - Tenderness at origin of wrist extensors
  - Increased pain with resisted wrist extension/supination
  - Normal elbow range of motion
  - Increased pain with gripping

DIFFERENTIAL DIAGNOSIS

- Arthritis, such as posterior osteophytes
- Epicondylar fractures
- Posterior interosseous nerve entrapment (lateral elbow pain)
- Ulnar neuropathy (medial elbow pain)
- Synovitis
- Thoracic outlet syndrome
- Medial collateral ligament injury
- Referred pain from shoulder or neck

DIAGNOSTIC TESTS & INTERPRETATION

Initial Tests (lab, imaging)

No imaging is required for initial evaluation and treatment of a classic overuse injury.

Follow-Up Tests & Special Considerations

- Anteroposterior/lateral radiographs if decreased range of motion, trauma, or no improvement with initial conservative therapy. Assess for fractures or signs of arthritis.
- For recalcitrant cases
  - Musculoskeletal ultrasound (US) reveals abnormal tendon appearance (e.g., hypoechoic, tendon thickening, partial tear at tendon origin, calcifications). US can also guide injections of steroid and/or anesthetic.
  - MRI can show intermediate or high T2 signal intensity within the common flexor or extensor tendon or the presence of peritendinous soft tissue edema.

Diagnostic Procedures/Other

Infiltration of local anesthetic with subsequent resolution of symptoms supports the diagnosis if clinically in doubt.

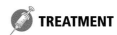 TREATMENT

GENERAL MEASURES

Initial treatment consists of activity modification, counterforce bracing, oral or topical NSAIDs, ice, and physical therapy.

- If left untreated, symptoms typically last between 6 months and 2 years. For patients with good function and minimal pain, consider conservative management using a "wait and see" approach based on patient preference.
- Modify activity, encourage relative rest, and correct faulty biomechanics.
- Bracing
  - Wrist extensor splints (WESs) inhibit contraction of extensor muscle and decreases tendon movement, thereby decreasing stress at the common extensor origin in LET (1)[B].
  - Counterforce bracing with a forearm strap is easy and inexpensive. Systematic reviews are inconclusive about overall efficacy, but initial bracing may improve the ability to perform daily activities in the first 6 weeks.
  - Consider cock-up wrist splinting for repetitive daily activities if counterforce bracing fails; can also use at nighttime to provide relative rest
- Ice frequently after activities
- Physical therapy
  - Infiltration of local anesthetic can reduce pain and may permit better participation in physical therapy.
  - Eccentric strength training and stretching program
  - US therapy
  - Corticosteroid iontophoresis
  - Dry needling

MEDICATION

First Line
- Topical NSAIDs: Low-quality evidence suggests topical NSAIDS are significantly more effective than placebo with respect to pain and number needed to treat (NNT = 7) to benefit in the short term (up to 4 weeks) with minimal adverse effects (2)[A].
- Oral NSAIDs: unclear efficacy with respect to pain and function, but may offer short-term pain relief; associated with adverse GI effects (2)[A]

Second Line
Corticosteroid injections: short-term (≤8 weeks) reduction in pain; no benefits found for intermediate or long-term outcomes (3)[A]

ISSUES FOR REFERRAL
Failure of conservative therapy

ADDITIONAL THERAPIES
Given the mechanism of injury, many new treatments are targeted at tendon regeneration.
- Glyceryl trinitrate (GTN) transdermal patch
  - Nitric oxide (NO) is a small free radical generated by NO synthesis. NO is expressed by fibroblasts and is postulated to aid in collagen synthesis. Topical application of GTN theoretically improves healing by this mechanism. 1/4 of a 5-mg/24-hr GTN transdermal patch is applied once daily for up to 24 weeks.
  - Significant decreases in pain are seen at 3 weeks and 6 months compared to placebo patch.
- Extracorporeal shock wave therapy (ESWT) is a noninvasive, nonelectrical therapy found to be 89% effective in treating LET in some studies and is noted to be as effective as WES (1)[B].
- Prolotherapy
  - Injection of a dextrose solution into and around the tendon attachment stimulates a localized inflammatory response, leading to increased blood flow to stimulate healing.
- Platelet-rich plasma (PRP) injections
  - Injection of supraphysiologic autologous PRP leads to a local inflammatory response. Platelets degranulate, release growth factors, and stimulate the physiologic healing cascade.
  - PRP treatment of chronic LET significantly reduces pain and increases function. The benefit exceeds that of corticosteroid injection even after a follow-up of 1 year (4)[A].
- US-guided percutaneous needle tenotomy
  - Injection of a local anesthetic followed by US-guided tendon fenestration, aspiration, and abrasion of the underlying bone; thought to break apart scar tissue and stimulate inflammation and healing
  - Usually requires referral to sports medicine or orthopedic physician with specific equipment and training

- Autologous tenocyte injection (ATI)
  - Two-step process
  - Small number of tenocytes are harvested, often from patellar tendon, and cultured.
  - Cultured tenocytes are then injected into tendon to help stimulate regeneration.
- Botulinum toxin A for chronic LET
  - Injections into the forearm extensor muscles (60 U) can be performed in the outpatient setting.

SURGERY/OTHER PROCEDURES
- Surgical intervention required in only 2.8% of patients
- Elbow surgery may be indicated in refractory cases:
  - Involves débridement and tendon release
  - Can be performed open or arthroscopically
  - Improvements in VAS, DASH scores, and grip strength seen in 5-year study (5)[B]
- Denervation of the lateral humeral epicondyle
  - Transection of the posterior cutaneous nerve of the forearm with implantation into the triceps may help with chronic symptoms and pain.

COMPLEMENTARY & ALTERNATIVE MEDICINE
Acupuncture: effective for short-term pain relief for lateral epicondyle pain

 ONGOING CARE

PROGNOSIS
Good: Majority resolve with conservative care.

REFERENCES
1. Aydın A, Atiç R. Comparison of extracorporeal shock-wave therapy and wrist-extensor splint application in the treatment of lateral epicondylitis: a prospective randomized controlled study. *J Pain Res.* 2018;11:1459–1467.
2. Pattanittum P, Turner T, Green S, et al. Non-steroidal anti-inflammatory drugs (NSAIDs) for treating lateral elbow pain in adults. *Cochrane Database Syst Rev.* 2013;(5):CD003686.
3. Krogh TP, Bartels EM, Ellingsen T, et al. Comparative effectiveness of injection therapies in lateral epicondylitis: a systematic review and network meta-analysis of randomized controlled trials. *Am J Sports Med.* 2013;41(6):1435–1446.
4. Mi B, Liu G, Zhou W, et al. Platelet rich plasma versus steroid on lateral epicondylitis: meta-analysis of randomized clinical trials. *Phys Sportsmed.* 2017;45(2):97–104.
5. Han SH, Lee JK, Kim HJ, et al. The result of surgical treatment of medial epicondylitis: analysis with more than a 5-year follow-up. *J Shoulder Elbow Surg.* 2016;25(10):1704–1709.

ADDITIONAL READING
- Cullinane FL, Boocock MG, Trevelyan FC. Is eccentric exercise an effective treatment for lateral epicondylitis? A systematic review. *Clin Rehabil.* 2014;28(1):3–19.
- Dingemanse R, Randsdorp M, Koes BW, et al. Evidence for the effectiveness of electrophysical modalities for treatment of medial and lateral epicondylitis: a systematic review. *Br J Sports Med.* 2014;48(12):957–965.
- Green S, Buchbinder R, Barnsley L, et al. Acupuncture for lateral elbow pain. *Cochrane Database Syst Rev.* 2002;(1):CD003527.
- Lin YC, Wu WT, Hsu YC, et al. Comparative effectiveness of botulinum toxin versus non-surgical treatments for treating lateral epicondylitis: a systematic review and meta-analysis. *Clin Rehabil.* 2018;32(2):131–145.
- Mattie R, Wong J, McCormick Z, et al. Percutaneous needle tenotomy for the treatment of lateral epicondylitis: a systematic review of the literature. *PM R.* 2017;9(6):603–611.
- Ozden R, Uruç V, Doğramaci Y, et al. Management of tennis elbow with topical glyceryl trinitrate. *Acta Orthop Traumatol Turc.* 2014;48(2):175–180.

 SEE ALSO

Algorithm: Pain in Upper Extremity

 CODES

ICD10
- M77.00 Medial epicondylitis, unspecified elbow
- M77.10 Lateral epicondylitis, unspecified elbow
- M77.01 Medial epicondylitis, right elbow

CLINICAL PEARLS
- MET (golfer's elbow) is characterized by pain and tenderness at the tendinous origins of the wrist flexors at the medial epicondyle.
- LET (tennis elbow) is characterized by pain and tenderness at the tendinous origins of the wrist extensors at the lateral epicondyle.
- Left untreated, symptoms typically last between 6 months and 2 years
- Most patients improve using conservative treatment with bracing, activity modification, and physical therapy.
- Newer therapies such as ATI, prolotherapy, and tenotomy are directed toward tendon regeneration.

E

EPIDIDYMITIS
Katherine L. Rotker, MD • Matthew Chabot, MD

BASICS

DESCRIPTION
- Inflammation (infectious or noninfectious) of epididymis resulting in scrotal pain and swelling, induration of the posterior epididymis, eventual scrotal wall edema, involvement of the adjacent testicle, and hydrocele formation
- Acute epididymitis: scrotal pain for <6 weeks
- Chronic epididymitis: scrotal pain for ≥6 weeks
- Epididymitis with involvement of testis is named epididymo-orchitis.
- Classification: infectious (bacterial, viral, fungal, parasitic) versus noninfectious (chemical, traumatic, autoimmune, idiopathic, industrial, noninfectious, vaso-epididymal reflux syndrome, vasal reflux syndrome); chronic versus acute
- System(s) affected: reproductive

EPIDEMIOLOGY
- Predominant age: usually younger, sexually active men or older men with UTIs; in older men, commonly secondary to bladder outlet obstruction (i.e., benign prostatic hyperplasia [BPH])
- Predominant sex: male only

Pediatric Considerations
In prepubertal boys: Epididymitis is found to be the most common cause of acute scrotum—more common than testicular torsion.

Incidence
- Common (600,000 cases annually in the United States) (1)
- 1 in 1,000 adult males per year
- 1.2 in 1,000 boys age 2 to 13 years per year (2),(3)

Prevalence
Common

ETIOLOGY AND PATHOPHYSIOLOGY
- Infectious epididymitis
  - Retrograde passage of urinary bacteria from the prostate or urethra to the epididymis via the ejaculatory ducts and the vas deferens; rarely, hematogenous spread
  - Causative organism is identified in 80% of patients and varies according to patient age.
- Noninfectious epididymitis
  - Often no etiology is found, however, can be instigated by trauma, autoimmune disease, or vasculitis
  - Likely secondary to reflux of sterile urine causing a chemical inflammation rather than infectious
  - Can develop as a sequelae of strenuous exercise with a full bladder when urine is pushed through internal urethral sphincter (located at proximal end of prostatic urethra) or prolonged periods of sitting
  - Reflux of urine through orifice of ejaculatory ducts at verumontanum may occur with history of urethritis/prostatitis because inflammation may produce rigidity in musculature surrounding orifice to ejaculatory ducts, holding them open.
  - Exposure of epididymis to foreign fluid may produce inflammatory reaction within 24 hours.
- <14 years of age
  - Cause largely unknown, although likely from anatomic abnormalities resulting in urine reflux such as vesicoureteral reflux, ectopic ureter, or anorectal malformation (rectourethral fistula)
  - May also be part of postinfectious syndrome from *Mycoplasma pneumoniae*, enterovirus, or adenovirus
  - Henoch-Schönlein purpura may present as acute scrotum.

- 14 to 35 years of age
  - Usually *Chlamydia trachomatis* (serous urethral discharge) or *Neisseria gonorrhoeae* (purulent discharge) in sexually active males
  - With anal intercourse, likely *Escherichia coli* or *Haemophilus influenzae*
- >35 years
  - Commonly enteric bacteria but occasionally *Staphylococcus aureus* or *Staphylococcus epidermidis*
  - In elderly men, often with distal urinary tract obstruction, BPH, UTI, or catheterization
  - Tuberculosis (TB), if sterile pyuria, nodularity of vas deferens (hematogenous spread), and recent infection. TB is the most common granulomatous disease affecting the epididymitis (4).
  - Sterile urine reflux after transurethral prostatectomy
  - Granulomatous reaction following BCG intravesical therapy for bladder cancer
- Amiodarone may cause noninfectious epididymitis; dose dependent and usually resolves with decreasing drug dosage (<200 mg/day)
- Syphilis, blastomycosis, coccidioidomycosis, and cryptococcosis are rare causes, but brucellosis can be a common cause in endemic areas.

RISK FACTORS
- UTI
- Prostatitis
- Indwelling urethral catheter
- Urethral instrumentation or transurethral surgery
- Urethral or meatal stricture
- Transrectal prostate biopsy
- Prostate brachytherapy (seeds) for prostate cancer
- Anal intercourse
- High-risk sexual activity
- Strenuous physical activity
- Prolonged sedentary periods
- Bladder obstruction (BPH, prostate cancer)
- HIV-immunosuppressed patient
- Severe Behçet disease
- Presence of foreskin
- Constipation
- Increased intra-abdominal pressure (due to frequent physical strain)
  - Military recruits, especially who begin physically unprepared
  - Laborers; restaurant kitchen workers
  - Full bladder during intense physical exertion

GENERAL PREVENTION
- Safer sexual practices
- Mumps vaccination
- Antibiotic prophylaxis for urethral manipulation
- Early treatment of prostatitis/BPH
- Vasectomy or vasoligation during transurethral surgery
- Avoid vigorous rectal exam with acute prostatitis.
- Emptying the bladder prior to physical exertion
- Physically conditioning the body prior to engaging in regular intense physical exertion
- Treat constipation.

COMMONLY ASSOCIATED CONDITIONS
- Prostatitis/urethritis/orchitis
- Hematospermia
- Constipation
- UTI

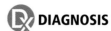

DIAGNOSIS

HISTORY
- Gradual onset of scrotal pain, sometimes radiating to the groin region over 1 to 2 days
- Urethral discharge or symptoms of UTI, such as frequency of urination, dysuria, cloudy urine, or hematuria
- Detailed sexual history, especially new exposures
- Fever only in 11–19% (3)
- Progresses from the posterior-lying epididymis to the body/head of epididymis
- Entire hemiscrotum may become swollen and red; the testis becomes indistinguishable from the epididymis; the scrotal wall becomes thick and indurated, and reactive hydrocele may occur.
- Noninfectious epididymitis
  - Unilateral scrotal pain/swelling preceded by prolonged intense physical exertion with full bladder
  - No symptoms of infection

Pediatric Considerations
- Bacteremia from *H. influenzae* infection may produce acute epididymitis.
- Must rule out testicular torsion (with scrotal ultrasound) in adolescent males particularly age >13 years
- History not helpful in distinguishing epididymitis from testicular torsion

Geriatric Considerations
Diabetics with sensory neuropathy may have no pain despite severe infection/abscess.

PHYSICAL EXAM
- Epididymis is markedly tender to palpation.
- The tail of the epididymis is larger in comparison with the contralateral side.
- Elevation of the testes/epididymis reduces the discomfort (Prehn sign).
- Absence of a cremasteric reflex should raise suspicion for testicular torsion.

DIFFERENTIAL DIAGNOSIS
- Testicular/testicular appendage torsion
- Urethritis/orchitis
- Testicular trauma
- Epididymal congestion following vasectomy
- Testicular malignancy
- Epididymal cyst
- Inguinal hernia
- Spermatocele
- Hydrocele
- Hematocele
- Varicocele
- Epididymal adenomatoid tumor
- Epididymal rhabdomyosarcoma
- Vasculitis (Henoch-Schönlein purpura)

DIAGNOSTIC TESTS & INTERPRETATION
Initial Tests (lab, imaging)
- All suspected cases should be evaluated for objective evidence of inflammation by one of the following:
  - Urinalysis/urine culture preferably on first-void urine to evaluate for positive leukocyte esterase and bacteriuria
  - Urine culture/Gram stain urethral discharge; ≥2 WBC per oil immersion field; evaluate for gonococcal infection.
  - Microscopic examination of sediment from a spun first-void urine with ≥10 WBC per high-power field
- Urine gonorrhea and chlamydia testing for all suspected cases (4)[A]

- CRP >24 mg/L suggestive of epididymitis (5)[C]
- A clear urinalysis and negative culture suggest noninfectious epididymitis.
- If testicular torsion/mass cannot be excluded (especially in children), Doppler ultrasound is test of choice (2),(3).
- In adult men, ultrasound: sensitivity and specificity of 100% in evaluation of acute scrotum (6) compared to sensitivity of 63.6–100% and specificity of 97–100% in children (3)

Pediatric Considerations
Further radiographic imaging in children should be done to rule out anatomic abnormalities.

Diagnostic Procedures/Other
This is a clinical diagnosis.

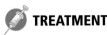 ## TREATMENT

GENERAL MEASURES
- Bed rest or restriction on activity
- Scrotal elevation, athletic scrotal supporter
- Ice pack wrapped in towel
- Avoid constipation.
- Spermatic cord block with local anesthesia in severe cases
- If noninfectious epididymitis:
  - No strenuous physical activity and avoidance of any Valsalva maneuvers for several weeks
  - Empty bladder prior to strenuous exercises.

MEDICATION
First Line
- Sexually active adults <35 years: doxycycline 100 mg PO BID for 10 days (*C. trachomatis* coverage) PLUS ceftriaxone 250 mg IM × 1 (*N. gonorrhoeae* coverage). Treat all sexual partners within last 60 days (2)[C],(4)[A].
- ≥35 years, not suspecting STD with enteric etiology (i.e., bacteriuria due to bladder outlet obstruction, prostate biopsy, urinary instrumentation, systemic disease, and/or immunosuppression)
  - Levofloxacin 500 mg/day PO for 10 days OR
  - Ofloxacin 300 mg PO BID for 10 days (2)[C],(4)[A]
  - Note: 2016 FDA black box warning on fluoroquinolones due to disabling and potentially permanent side effects. Consider trimethoprim-sulfamethoxazole for milder infections.
- Men who practice insertive anal intercourse: ceftriaxone 250 mg IM × 1 plus fluoroquinolone as above; if HIV positive, usually no difference in treatment (2)[C],(4)[A]
- Analgesia:
  - NSAIDs (e.g., naproxen or ibuprofen) for mild to moderate pain
  - Consider steroid if patient cannot tolerate NSAID.
  - Acetaminophen with codeine or oxycodone for moderate to severe pain
- Septic or toxic patient
  - 3rd-generation cephalosporin or aminoglycoside
- For Behçet, sarcoid, Henoch-Schönlein purpura
  - Steroids, such as methylprednisolone, 40 mg/day recommended
- Chronic epididymitis: 2-week course of NSAIDs, scrotal icing/elevation; if no improvement, may add TCA or neuroleptic (2)

Second Line
- Trimethoprim-sulfamethoxazole (Bactrim, Septra) double strength PO BID for 10 to 14 days; increasing bacterial resistance may limit effectiveness.
- Add rifampin (rifampicin) or vancomycin, as required.

Pediatric Considerations
- May be postinfectious inflammatory condition; treat with anti-inflammatories and analgesics.
- Antibiotic therapy can be reserved for young infants until positive urine cultures (2).

ISSUES FOR REFERRAL
- If suspicion is high for testicular torsion, then urgent ultrasound or referral to emergency department for possible surgery (1)[C]
- Epididymitis in ages <14 years requires a urology referral due to high incidence of associated urogenital abnormalities.
- If medical management fails, should be referred to urologist to rule out anatomic abnormality or chemical epididymitis
- If HIV positive, CMV, salmonella, toxoplasmosis, *Ureaplasma urealyticum*, *Corynebacterium* sp., *Mycoplasma* sp., and *Mima polymorpha* must also be considered.

SURGERY/OTHER PROCEDURES
- Vasostomy to drain infected material if severe or refractory case
- Scrotal exploration if unable clinically to distinguish between epididymitis and testicular torsion
- Drainage of abscesses, epididymectomy (acute suppurative), or epididymo-orchiectomy in severe cases refractory to antibiotics
- Surgery to correct underlying anatomic abnormality or obstruction

ADMISSION, INPATIENT, AND NURSING CONSIDERATIONS
- Intractable pain
- Sepsis
- Abscess
- Persistent vomiting
- Scheduled surgery
- Purulent drainage
- Most cases can be managed with outpatient care.

 ## ONGOING CARE

FOLLOW-UP RECOMMENDATIONS
Patient Monitoring
- Routine follow-up in 1 week. Follow up within 72 hours if symptoms fail to improve with treatment for reevaluation of diagnosis and therapy (4)[A].
- Swelling and tenderness after antibiotic course should be evaluated for abscess, tumor, infarction, cancer, TB, and fungal epididymitis (4)[A].
- In noninfectious epididymitis, follow up in 4 weeks to assess efficacy of NSAIDs and lifestyle changes.

DIET
If constipation is contributing to pain or chemical epididymitis, then consider constipation prevention (high-fiber diet) and/or treatment.

PATIENT EDUCATION
- Stress completing course of antibiotics, even when asymptomatic.
- Early recognition and treatment of UTI or prostatitis
- Safer sexual practices. Avoid sex until antibiotic course completed and partner treated if likely STD.
- If treated for STI, refer sexual partners for evaluation of *N. gonorrhoeae* or *C. trachomatis* if sexual contact within 60 days preceding onset of symptoms or most recent sexual partner if >60 days (4)[A].
- If noninfectious epididymitis, then educate on noninfectious etiology and proper lifestyle changes.

PROGNOSIS
- Pain improves within 1 to 3 days, but induration may take several weeks/months to completely resolve.
- If bilateral involvement, sterility may result.
- In noninfectious epididymitis, symptoms usually resolve in <1 week.

COMPLICATIONS
- Recurrent epididymitis
- Infertility
- Oligospermia
- Testicular necrosis or atrophy
- Secondary abscess formation
- Fournier gangrene (necrotizing synergistic infection)

REFERENCES
1. Trojian TH, Lishnak TS, Heiman D. Epididymitis and orchitis: an overview. *Am Fam Physician*. 2009;79(7):583–587.
2. McConaghy JR, Panchal B. Epididymitis: an overview. *Am Fam Physician*. 2016;94(9):723–726.
3. Tekgul S, Dogan HS, Kocvara R, et al; for European Society for Paediatric Urology and European Association of Urology. *EAU Guidelines on Paediatric Urology*. Arnhem, Netherlands: European Association of Urology; 2016.
4. Workowski KA, Bolan GA; for Centers for Disease Control and Prevention. Sexually transmitted diseases treatment guidelines, 2015. *MMWR Recomm Rep*. 2015;64(RR-03):1–137.
5. Crawford P, Crop JA. Evaluation of scrotal masses. *Am Fam Physician*. 2014;89(9):723–727.
6. Rizvi SA, Ahmad I, Siddiqui MA, et al. Role of color Doppler ultrasonography in evaluation of scrotal swellings: pattern of disease in 120 patients with review of literature. *Urol J*. 2011;8(1):60–65.

ADDITIONAL READING
- Somekh E, Gorenstein A, Serour F. Acute epididymitis in boys: evidence of a post-infectious etiology. *J Urol*. 2004;171(1):391–394.
- Tracy CR, Steers WD, Costabile R. Diagnosis and management of epididymitis. *Urol Clin North Am*. 2008;35(1):101–108.
- Wolin LH. On the etiology of epididymitis. *J Urol*. 1971;105(4):531–533.

 ## CODES

ICD10
- N45.1 Epididymitis
- N45.2 Orchitis
- N45.3 Epididymo-orchitis

CLINICAL PEARLS
- With epididymitis, pain is gradual in onset, and the tenderness is mostly posterior to the testis. With testicular torsion, the symptoms are quite rapid in onset, the testis will be higher in the scrotum and may have a transverse lie, and the cremasteric reflex will be absent. The absence of leukocytes on urine analysis and decreased blood flow on scrotal ultrasound with Doppler will suggest torsion.
- Prostatic massage is contraindicated in epididymitis because of the risk for worsening local infection. The potential for sepsis is increased with acute prostatitis.
- Noninfectious epididymitis is a clinical diagnosis of exclusion, and infectious causes are much more common but must be considered in certain occupations, such as soldiers and laborers.

EPISCLERITIS

Daniel J. Schlegel, MD, MHA

BASICS

- Episcleritis is irritation and inflammation of the episclera, a thin layer of tissue covering the sclera. It is not an infection.
- Episcleritis is the localized inflammation of the vascular connective tissue superficial to the sclera.
- Usually a self-limited condition, typically resolving without treatment within 3 weeks
- Topical lubricants and/or topical corticosteroid treatment may relieve symptoms while awaiting spontaneous resolution.

DESCRIPTION
- Edema and injection confined to the episcleral tissue
- Two types
  - Simple (diffuse scleral involvement—more common)
  - Nodular (focal area[s] of involvement—less common)

EPIDEMIOLOGY
Slight female predominance (~60–65%)

Incidence
- May occur at any age
- Peak incidence in 40s to 50s
- Community incidence not well-known (~20 to 50 cases per 100,000 person-years)

Prevalence
Not historically well-known; a recent community study found a prevalence of 53 cases per 100,000 persons.

ETIOLOGY AND PATHOPHYSIOLOGY
- Etiology: usually idiopathic, but other causes may be found (either nonimmune or immune)

- Pathophysiology:
  - Nonimmune (e.g., dry eye syndrome, with histology showing widespread vasodilation, edema, lymphocytic infiltration)
  - Immune (systemic vasculitis or rheumatologic disease)

COMMONLY ASSOCIATED CONDITIONS
- Usually not associated with another condition
- Less commonly associated conditions include the following:
  - Rheumatoid arthritis
  - Vasculitis
  - Inflammatory bowel disease
  - Ankylosing spondylitis
  - Systemic lupus erythematosus
  - Gout
  - Herpes zoster
  - Hypersensitivity disorders
    - Rosacea
    - Contact dermatitis
    - Penicillin sensitivity
    - Erythema multiforme

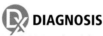

DIAGNOSIS

Episcleritis is a clinical diagnosis (1),(2)[C].

HISTORY
- History should elicit potential causative factors, recurrence, or associated systemic disease (2).
- Pain is often absent; when present, it is usually mild and localized to the eye (1),(2).
- Mild tearing may be present (2).

PHYSICAL EXAM
- Check visual acuity; decreased vision is very unusual with episcleritis, and its presence should raise suspicion for another condition such as scleritis (1),(2).
- The white sclera will have a pink or purplish hue.
- Focal hyperemia (2),(3)
- Pupils equal and reactive (2)
- Superficial episcleral vascular dilation (1),(2)
- Episcleral edema (1),(2)
  - Diffuse in simple episcleritis
  - Focal in nodular episcleritis
- Tenderness over involved area may be present (2) but is usually absent (3).
- Superficial episcleral vascular hyperemia blanches with topical phenylephrine (1),(3).

ALERT
Recurrent episodes, difficulty confirming the diagnosis, or worsening symptoms should prompt an ophthalmology referral.

DIFFERENTIAL DIAGNOSIS
- Scleritis
- Bacterial conjunctivitis
- Viral conjunctivitis
- Herpes (ulcerative) keratitis
- Superficial keratitis
- Increased intraocular pressure (ocular hypertension)

DIAGNOSTIC TESTS & INTERPRETATION
Most patients with episcleritis do not require any further lab work or diagnostic studies (4)[C].

TREATMENT

MEDICATION
Treatment for episcleritis typically consists of symptomatic relief. The goal is to suppress the inflammation, which will, in turn, relieve the discomfort or pain (5).

First Line
Topical lubricants such as artificial tears are typically used for initial management of symptomatic episcleritis (2)[C].

Second Line
- Topical corticosteroids are useful when discomfort is not sufficiently controlled by conservative measures (2),(4),(6)[C].
  - Fluorometholone 0.1% drops 4 times daily; if not effective, may increase frequency
  - Prednisolone 0.5–1% eye drops
- Refractory episcleritis may be treated with oral NSAIDs (4)[C].

ISSUES FOR REFERRAL
Ophthalmology referral advised:
- If prescribing corticosteroid eye drops
- Recurrent episodes, uncertain diagnosis, and/or worsening symptoms
- Rarely, episcleritis may progress to scleritis.

ADDITIONAL THERAPIES
- Topical NSAIDs have not been shown to have a significant benefit over artificial tears (7)[B].
- When episcleritis results from viral infection, appropriate antiviral therapy is indicated (6)[C].

ONGOING CARE

FOLLOW-UP RECOMMENDATIONS
Episcleritis is usually self-limited (up to 21 days) and does not typically require follow-up.

PROGNOSIS
Most patients have no ocular complications and make a full recovery.

COMPLICATIONS
Associated complications are rare.
- Anterior uveitis may occur in 4–16% of cases (1),(6)[C].
- Decreased vision may occur in 0–4% of cases (1),(6)[C].
- Ocular hypertension has been reported in 0–3.5% of cases (1),(6)[C].

REFERENCES

1. Sainz de la Maza M, Molina N, Gonzalez-Gonzalez LA, et al. Clinical characteristics of a large cohort of patients with scleritis and episcleritis. *Ophthalmology*. 2012;119(1):43–50.
2. Cronau H, Kankanala RR, Mauger T. Diagnosis and management of red eye in primary care. *Am Fam Physician*. 2010;81(2):137–144.
3. Galor A, Thorne JE. Scleritis and peripheral ulcerative keratitis. *Rheum Dis Clin North Am*. 2007;33(4):835–854.
4. Kirkwood BJ, Kirkwood RA. Episcleritis and scleritis. *Insight*. 2010;35(4):5–8.
5. Daniel Diaz J, Sobol EK, Gritz DC. Treatment and management of scleral disorders. *Surv Ophthalmol*. 2016;61(6):702–717.
6. Berchicci L, Miserocchi E, Di Nicola M, et al. Clinical features of patients with episcleritis and scleritis in an Italian tertiary care referral center. *Eur J Ophthalmol*. 2014;24(3):293–298.
7. Williams CP, Browning AC, Sleep TJ, et al. A randomised, double-blind trial of topical ketorolac vs artificial tears for the treatment of episcleritis. *Eye (Lond)*. 2005;19(7):739–742.

CODES

ICD10
- H15.109 Unspecified episcleritis, unspecified eye
- H15.129 Nodular episcleritis, unspecified eye
- H15.102 Unspecified episcleritis, left eye

CLINICAL PEARLS
- Episcleritis typically is a benign, self-limited disorder, usually resolving within 3 weeks of symptom onset.
- Often not painful and presents without decrease in visual acuity
- Although treatment is often not needed, when employed, the goal is symptomatic relief while awaiting spontaneous resolution.
- Topical lubricants and/or topical corticosteroid treatment may relieve symptoms.
- Associated complications are uncommon and not severe but may include anterior uveitis, decreased vision, and ocular hypertension.
- Episcleritis can be an early presentation of scleritis, which is more severe. Accurate diagnosis of episcleritis is important.

E

EPISTAXIS
Christopher R. Heron, MD, BS • Ryan Kipp, MD, BS

BASICS

DESCRIPTION
- Hemorrhage from the nose involving either the anterior or posterior mucosal surfaces
- Intractable or refractory epistaxis: recurrent or persistent despite appropriate packing or multiple episodes during a short period, each requiring medical attention
- Synonym(s): nosebleed

EPIDEMIOLOGY
Incidence
- Very common in the United States
- Estimated lifetime prevalence: ~60%
- Bimodal, with peaks in children up to 15 years and in adults >50 years, particularly ages 70 to 79 years
- Most common in males <49 years
- Rare in children age <2 years
- ~6% of patients require medical or surgical intervention; accounts for ~1 in 200 ER visits

ETIOLOGY AND PATHOPHYSIOLOGY
- Local versus systemic disease. Most nosebleeds are due to local causes.
- Anterior: 90–95% of all cases (Kiesselbach plexus)
- Posterior: 5–10% of cases (Woodruff plexus); usually branches of sphenopalatine arteries: may be asymptomatic or may present with other symptoms (hematemesis, hemoptysis)
- Idiopathic
- Local inflammation, irritation, and insult
  - Infection (viral URI, sinusitis, TB, syphilis)
  - Irritant inhalation (smoking, rhinitis, current or past cocaine use)
  - Topical steroid or antihistamine use
  - Chronic and excessive use of nasal vasoconstrictors
  - Septal deviation (disproportionate, unilateral air movement)
  - Low humidity, nasal oxygen use, CPAP
  - Tumors: benign, malignant
  - Vascular malformations, especially in context of prior trauma (e.g., carotid artery aneurysm)
- Trauma
  - Epistaxis digitorum (nose picking)
  - Foreign bodies
  - Septal perforation
  - Nasal fracture
  - Nasal surgery
  - Barotrauma
- Systemic
  - Thrombocytopenia
  - Congenital or acquired coagulopathies
  - Liver or renal disease
  - Chronic alcohol abuse
  - Leukemia
  - Anticoagulant drug use
  - CHF
  - Hereditary hemorrhagic telangiectasia (HHT)
  - Collagen abnormalities
  - Mitral valve stenosis
  - Multiple myeloma
  - Polycythemia vera
  - HIV

RISK FACTORS
- Local irritation from multiple causes
- Medications/supplements including aspirin, clopidogrel, ginseng, garlic, ginkgo biloba, sildenafil, warfarin, and other anticoagulants
- Prior septoplasty/turbinate procedures, anemia, and thrombocytopenia are risk factors for recurrent epistaxis.

GENERAL PREVENTION
- Humidification at night
- Cut fingernails and minimize picking.
- For topical-nasal medication users, direct spray laterally away from septum. Use opposite hand to spray (i.e., right hand to spray in left nostril).
- Petroleum jelly to prevent anterior mucosal drying
- Control hypertension (HTN) (controversial association with increased risk for recurrent epistaxis).

COMMONLY ASSOCIATED CONDITIONS
- Vascular malformation/telangiectasia (hereditary hemorrhagic telangiectasia-HHT)
- Neoplasm (rare; consider if persistent and unilateral)
- Systemic
  - Coagulopathy: primary or iatrogenic
  - Thrombocytopenia
  - Cirrhosis
  - Renal failure
  - Alcoholism
- No proven association with HTN but may make control of bleeding more difficult

DIAGNOSIS

HISTORY
- Assess for symptoms of anemia and cardiovascular compromise.
- Determine the side on which bleeding began as well as its severity and duration.
- Define trauma (including nose picking) and other possible precipitants (e.g., cocaine use).
- Ask about previous episodes of epistaxis and their frequency (if applicable).
- Identify comorbid conditions (e.g., cardiovascular compromise symptoms, cirrhosis, primary coagulopathies).
- Review current medications, including nasal sprays, anticoagulants, antiplatelets, and attempted treatments.
- Assess for nausea, hematemesis, and hemoptysis, which may indicate a posterior and more severe bleed.

PHYSICAL EXAM
- Assess for airway patency and cardiovascular stability.
- Focus on localizing site of bleeding to anterior versus posterior nasal cavity. Most cases are due to anterior nasal septal bleeding.
- When formally examining the nasal cavity, have patient seated in an upright or semiupright position.
- Utilize a nasal speculum, if available, with a reliable light source to increase visualization of the nasal cavities.
- Between exams, have the patient lean forward and pinch their nose (or use nasal clips) to avoid blood from draining into the posterior pharynx.

DIFFERENTIAL DIAGNOSIS
- Diagnosis usually apparent; the differential for the etiology is key.
- Posterior bleeding must be included in the differential for any chronic blood loss.

DIAGNOSTIC TESTS & INTERPRETATION
Lab testing is not indicated in most uncomplicated cases in which bleeding is easily controlled.

Initial Tests (lab, imaging)
- Mild cases, responsive to pressure: no labs
- For recurrent or intractable cases
  - CBC, PT/PTT, BMP
  - PT/PTT if on warfarin or other medications affecting coagulation
  - Cross-match when appropriate.
- Toxicology screen when nasal use of illicit drugs is suspected
- For most cases, imaging is not indicated.

Follow-Up Tests & Special Considerations
Consider neoplasm if recurrent unilateral epistaxis, especially if not responding to treatment.

Diagnostic Procedures/Other
Nasal endoscopy

Pediatric Considerations
More likely anterior, idiopathic, and recurrent

Geriatric Considerations
More likely to be posterior bleed

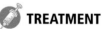

TREATMENT
- Most cases are managed as outpatient (1)[B].
- Home use—Nosebleed QR: a nonprescription powder of hydrophilic polymer with potassium salt; induces scab formation
- Patient applies direct pressure by pinching the lower part of the nose (nasal ala) for 5 to 20 minutes without a break. This stops bleeding in most patients.
- Cleanse nasal cavity of blood clots by blowing nose.
- An ice pack placed over the dorsum of the nose may help with hemostasis.
- Inspect the nasal septum for the bleeding site.

GENERAL MEASURES

Resuscitation, as indicated. Use universal "airway/breathing/circulation (ABC)" approach.

MEDICATION

First Line

If general measures fail, affected naris may be sprayed with topical vasoconstrictor, such as:

- Oxymetazoline: 0.05%
- Epinephrine: 1:1,000
- Phenylephrine: 0.5–1%
- Cocaine: 4%

Second Line

- Chemical (silver nitrate) or electrical cautery
- Nasal packing: ribbon gauze, nasal tampons, nasal balloon catheter
- For intractable/refractory: Consider surgical ligation, endoscopic ligation/cautery, endovascular embolization.

ISSUES FOR REFERRAL

- Posterior bleeding frequently requires an otolaryngology consultation.
- Anterior bleeding that fails conservative measures, packing, and cauterization
- Recurrent episodes
- HHT patients should establish care with ENT.
- Concurrent anticoagulation
  - If bleeding stops with packing, may continue same dose of warfarin if INR therapeutic; decrease dose if supratherapeutic INR.
  - If bleeding persists despite packing, stop anticoagulation and administer vitamin K 10 mg IV × 1, recheck INR in 30 minutes, if still >1.5, give PCC.
  - Novel anticoagulation may be associated with lower rates of epistaxis than warfarin. When epistaxis occurs, it may be harder to control.

ADDITIONAL THERAPIES

- Nasal packing: either with ribbon gauze or preformed nasal tampons. Systemic prophylactic antibiotics are unnecessary in the majority of patients with nasal packs; topical antibiotics may be as effective and cheaper (2)[B].
- FloSeal: A biodegradable hemostatic sealant (a thrombin-type gel) in one study is more effective and better tolerated than packing (3)[B].
- Local application of tranexamic acid may reduce bleeding time as compared to anterior packing (4).
- If an actively bleeding anterior septal site is visualized, this may be treated with gentle silver nitrate cautery for ~10 seconds for definitive treatment. 75% silver nitrate is preferred. Apply in a spiral fashion, starting around the bleeding vessel, moving inward.
- Limit cautery (silver nitrate) to one side of septum, or wait 4 to 6 weeks in between treatments to reduce risk of perforation.
- Posterior: Posterior packing or tamponade with balloon devices (Foley catheters have been used). Inpatient monitoring is generally required in these cases.

- Recurrent epistaxis: Cochrane review in children shows no difference in effectiveness between antiseptic nasal cream, petroleum jelly, silver nitrate cautery, or no treatment.
  - Silver nitrate cautery followed by 4 weeks of antiseptic cream may be better than antiseptic cream alone (5).

SURGERY/OTHER PROCEDURES

- Packing
  - Layering of Vaseline ribbon gauze (1/2 inch)
    ○ For gauze packing, be certain that both ends of the ribbon gauze protrude from the nostril.
    ○ Packing is layered from the floor upward.
    ○ Secure packing with gauze across the outside of the nostril.
  - Nasal tampon may be used after lubricating the tip with KY Jelly or antibiotic cream or ointment.
  - Additional saline may be needed to expand the tampon if the bleeding has slowed.
  - Merocel and Rapid Rhino packs are easier to use than gauze packing and are usually well tolerated.
- Posterior bleed
  - In the emergent setting, this may be attempted utilizing a Foley catheter or a specific posterior packing balloon.
  - With both methods, the tubing is introduced through the nose similar to the passage of a nasogastric tube. Once it reaches the posterior oral pharynx, the balloon is inflated and the tubing is pulled back outward to tamponade the posterior bleeding source.
    ○ If using a Foley catheter (10 to 14F catheter), the balloon can be inflated with 10 mL of saline.
    ○ Traction is maintained with an umbilical cord clamp with adequate padding between the clip and the nose to avoid injury.

ADMISSION, INPATIENT, AND NURSING CONSIDERATIONS

- Consider hospitalization for elderly or for patients with posterior bleeding or coagulopathy; may also consider if significant comorbidities
- Admission criteria/initial stabilization
  - Posterior bleed
  - Hemodynamic changes
  - Clotting dysfunction
  - Universal ABC approach. Stop blood loss.

 ONGOING CARE

FOLLOW-UP RECOMMENDATIONS

Patient Monitoring

- Hemodynamic monitoring if severe blood loss
- 24-hour minimum for leaving packing in place; some recommend 3 to 5 days. Rebleed usually occurs between 24 and 48 hours. Longer durations of packing have increased risk of mucosal injury and toxic shock syndrome.

PATIENT EDUCATION

- Demonstrate proper pinching pressure techniques.
- Avoidance of trauma or irritants is key.
- Management of systemic illness and proper use of medication

PROGNOSIS

- Most are self-limited.
- Good results with proper treatment

COMPLICATIONS

- Septal perforation
- Pressure-induced tissue necrosis of the nasal mucosa
- Toxic shock syndrome with packing
- Arrhythmias triggered by packing (particularly posterior)

REFERENCES

1. Tunkel DE, Anne S, Payne SC, et al. Clinical practice guideline: nosebleed (epistaxis) executive summary. *Otolaryngol Head Neck Surg.* 2020;162(1):8–25.
2. Biggs TC, Nightingale K, Patel NN, et al. Should prophylactic antibiotics be used routinely in epistaxis patients with nasal packs? *Ann R Coll Surg Engl.* 2013;95(1):40–42.
3. Escabasse V, Bequignon E, Vérillaud B, et al. Guidelines of the French Society of Otorhinolaryngology (SFORL). Managing epistaxis under coagulation disorder due to antithrombotic therapy. *Eur Ann Otorhinolaryngol Head Neck Dis.* 2017;134(3):195–199.
4. Clinkard D, Barbic D. Tranexamic acid for epistaxis—a promising treatment that deserves further study. *CJEM.* 2016;18(1):72–73.
5. Calder N, Kang S, Fraser L, et al. A double-blind randomized controlled trial of management of recurrent nosebleeds in children. *Otolaryngol Head Neck Surg.* 2009;140(5):670–674.

CODES

ICD10

R04.0 Epistaxis

CLINICAL PEARLS

- Most epistaxis is anterior and responds well to timed pressure over the anterior nares for 5 to 20 minutes.
- Most nosebleeds are idiopathic or as a result of digital trauma (nose picking).
- Posterior nosebleeds can be asymptomatic or present with nausea, hematemesis, or heme-positive stool.
- Consider evaluation for neoplasm in cases of recurrent unilateral epistaxis.

ERECTILE DYSFUNCTION

Katherine L. Rotker, MD • Christine M. Van Horn, MD, MS

 BASICS

DESCRIPTION
- Erectile dysfunction (ED): the consistent or recurrent inability to acquire or sustain an erection of sufficient rigidity and duration for sexual intercourse
- In the past, ED was assumed to be a symptom of the aging process in men, but it is more often the result of concurrent medical conditions of the patient or from medications that patients may be taking to treat those conditions.
- Sexual problems are frequent among older men and have a detrimental effect on their quality of life but are infrequently discussed with their physicians.
- Synonym(s): impotence

EPIDEMIOLOGY
Incidence
It is estimated that >600,000 new cases of ED will be diagnosed annually in the United States, although this may be an underestimation of the true incidence, as ED is vastly underreported.

Prevalence
Overall prevalence for some degree of ED:
- 52% in men age 40 to 70 years
- Age-related increase ranging from 12.4% in men age 40 to 49 years up to 46.6% in men age 50 to 69 years

ETIOLOGY AND PATHOPHYSIOLOGY
- Erections are neurovascular events.
  - With stimulation, there is release of nitrous oxide, which increases production of cyclic guanosine 3′,5′-monophosphate (cGMP).
  - This leads to relaxation of cavernous smooth muscle, leading to increased blood flow to penis.
  - As cavernosal sinusoids distend with blood, there is passive compression of subtunical veins, which decreases venous outflow, and this leads to an erection.
- Alterations in any of these events lead to ED.
- ED may result from problems with systems required for normal penile erection.
  - Vascular: diseases that compromise blood flow
    - Peripheral vascular disease, diabetes, arteriosclerosis, essential hypertension, and some medications that treat hypertension
  - Neurologic: diseases that impair nerve conduction to brain or penile vasculature
    - Spinal cord injury, stroke, diabetes
  - Endocrine: diseases associated with changes in testosterone, luteinizing hormone, prolactin levels
  - Structural: phimosis, lichen sclerosis, congenital curvature
  - Psychological: patients suffering from malaise, depression, performance anxiety
- Social habits such as smoking or excessive alcohol intake
- Medications may cause ED (see "Risk Factors").
- Prostate cancer treatment
- Structural injury or trauma (bicycling accident)

Genetics
Rarely related to chromosomal disorders

RISK FACTORS
- Advancing age
- Cardiovascular disease
- Diabetes mellitus
- Metabolic syndrome
- Sedentary lifestyle

- Cigarette smoking
- Pelvic surgery, radiation, trauma/injury to pelvic area or spinal cord
- Medications that induce ED
  - SSRIs, β-blockers, clonidine, digoxin, spironolactone, antiandrogens, corticosteroids, H₂ blockers, anticonvulsants
- Central neurologic and endocrinologic conditions
- Substance abuse (alcohol, cocaine, opioids, marijuana)
- Psychological conditions: stress, anxiety, or depression, sexual abuse, relationship problems

GENERAL PREVENTION
The two best ways to prevent ED are by the following:
- Making healthy lifestyle choices by exercising regularly, eating well-balanced meals, limiting alcohol, and avoiding smoking
- Treating existing health problems and working with your patients to manage diabetes, heart disease, and other chronic problems

ALERT
Aging alone is not a cause.

COMMONLY ASSOCIATED CONDITIONS
- Cardiovascular disease:
  - Men with ED have a greater likelihood of having angina, myocardial infarction, stroke, transient ischemic attack, congestive heart failure, or cardiac arrhythmia compared to men without ED (1).
- Diabetes
- Neurologic conditions
- Metabolic syndrome
- Psychiatric disorders

 DIAGNOSIS

Inability to achieve or maintain erection satisfactory for intercourse

HISTORY
- Identify concurrent medical illnesses or surgical procedures, history of trauma, and a list of current medications (e.g., antihypertensive meds).
- Psychosocial history: smoking, ethanol intake, recreational drug use, anxiety and depression, satisfaction with current relationship
- Presence or absence of morning erections
- Speed of onset and duration of symptoms
- Relationship of symptoms to libido
- Detailed sexual history important to rule out premature ejaculation, as this is frequently confused with ED
- International Index of Erectile Function (IIEF) patient questionnaire is a useful tool in the clinical assessment and measurement of effectiveness of ED treatments (1).

PHYSICAL EXAM
- Signs and symptoms of hypogonadism: gynecomastia, small testicles, decreased body hair
- Penile plaques (Peyronie disease)
- Detailed examination of the cardiovascular, neurologic, and genitourinary systems
  - Blood pressure, waist circumference, BMI
  - Check femoral and lower extremity pulses to assess vascular supply to genitals.
  - Check anal sphincter tone and genital reflexes, including cremasterics and bulbocavernosus.

DIFFERENTIAL DIAGNOSIS
- Premature ejaculation
- Decreased libido
- Anorgasmia
- Sudden versus chronic ED

DIAGNOSTIC TESTS & INTERPRETATION
Vascular and/or neurologic assessment and monitoring of nocturnal erections may be indicated in selected patients but not for routine workup (2)[C].

Initial Tests (lab, imaging)
- HbA1c, lipid panel, CBC, BMP, TSH, morning total and free testosterone level (1)[C]
- Doppler, angiogram, and cavernosogram are available radiologic modalities but not recommended in routine practice for the diagnosis of ED (2)[C].

Follow-Up Tests & Special Considerations
Other hormonal tests, such as prolactin, should only be ordered when there is suspicion for a specific endocrinopathy.

Diagnostic Procedures/Other
Questionnaires can be offered to assess the severity of ED, including the IIEF and its validated and more easily administered abridged version, the Sexual Health Inventory for Men (SHIM) (2)[C].

 TREATMENT

- Lifestyle modifications and managing medications contributing to ED is first-line therapy for ED (3)[C]. Use least invasive therapy first; reserve more invasive therapies for nonresponders.
- Cardiovascular risk stratification and risk-factor management is recommended in all men with vasculogenic ED (4).
- Current smoking is significantly associated with ED, and smoking cessation has a beneficial effect on the restoration of erectile function (1)[A].
- Phosphodiesterase type 5 (PDE-5) inhibitors are the first-line treatment for ED (1)[A].

GENERAL MEASURES
- Psychosexual therapy alone or in combination with psychoactive drugs may be helpful in men whose ED is related to depression or anxiety (5).
- Weight loss and increased physical activity for obese men with ED. Men with metabolic syndrome should be counseled to make lifestyle modifications to reduce the risk of cardiovascular events and ED (1)[B].

MEDICATION
First Line
PDE-5 inhibitors are effective in the treatment of ED in many men, including those with diabetes mellitus and spinal cord injury and sexual dysfunction associated with antidepressants (6). Choice should be based on patient's preference (cost, ease of use, and adverse effects). There is insufficient evidence to support the superiority of one agent over the others (3)[A]:
- Sildenafil (Viagra): usual daily on-demand dose: 50 to 100 mg at least 1 hour and up to 4 hours prior to sexual intercourse
- Vardenafil (Levitra): usual daily on-demand dose: 5 to 20 mg within at least 1 hour and up to 5 hours prior to sexual intercourse
- Vardenafil (Staxyn): (oral-dissolving tablet) usual daily on-demand dose: 10 mg within at least 1 hour and up to 5 hours prior to sexual intercourse

- Tadalafil (Cialis): usual daily dose 2.5 to 5.0 mg daily regardless of activity or on-demand dosing 5 to 20 mg at least 30 minutes and up to 36 hours prior to sexual intercourse
- Avanafil (Stendra): usual daily on-demand dose: 50 to 200 mg at least 15 to 30 minutes and up to 4 hours prior to sexual intercourse
  - Adverse effects of PDE-5 inhibitors: headache, facial flushing, dyspepsia, nasal congestion, dizziness, hypotension, increased sensitivity to light (sildenafil and vardenafil), vision changes, lower back pain (tadalafil), and priapism (with excessive doses)
  - Sildenafil and vardenafil should be taken on an empty stomach for maximum effectiveness.

Geriatric Considerations
Use doses at the lower end of the dosing range for elderly patients and evaluate exercise tolerance before prescribing.
- Sildenafil 25 mg daily
- Vardenafil 5 mg daily

Second Line
Intraurethral and intracavernosal injectables are second-line therapies shown to be effective and should be administered based on patient preference (1)[B]. Intraurethral suppositories are a less invasive treatment option than intracavernosal injections; however, they are not as effective (3)[C]. Alprostadil, also known as prostaglandin E1, causes smooth muscle relaxation of the arterial blood vessels and sinusoidal tissues in the corpora:
- Intraurethral alprostadil (Muse):
  - Intraurethral suppository: 125-, 250-, 500-, and 1,000-μg pellets. Administer 5 to 50 minutes before intercourse. No >2 doses in 24 hours are recommended.
- Intracavernosal alprostadil (available in 2 formulations):
  - Alprostadil (Caverject): usual dose: 10 to 20 μg, with max dose of 60 μg. Injection should be made at right angles into one of the lateral surfaces of the proximal 3rd of the penis using a 0.5-inch, 27- or 30-gauge needle. Do not use >3 times a week or more than once in 24 hours.
  - Alprostadil may also be combined with papaverine (Bimix) plus phentolamine (Trimix), plus atropine (QuadMix).
- Vacuum erection device (VED): noninvasive option, available over the counter
- Penile prosthesis (7)

ALERT
- Initial trial dose of second-line agents should be administered under supervision of a specialist or primary care physician with expertise in these therapies.
- Patient should notify physician if erection lasts >4 hours for immediate attention.
- Do not use vacuum devices in men with sickle cell anemia or blood dyscrasias.
- Testosterone supplementation in men with hypogonadism improves ED and libido (6)[B]. Available formulations include injectable depots, transdermal patches and gels, SC pellets, and oral therapy.
- Best practices in urology recommendation: Do not prescribe testosterone to men with ED who have normal testosterone levels (1).
- Contraindications:
  - Nitroglycerin (or other nitrates) and phosphodiesterase inhibitors: potential for severe, fatal hypotension

- Precautions/side effects:
  - Testosterone: precautions: Exogenous testosterone reduces sperm count and thus do not use in patients wishing to keep fertility; side effects: acne, sodium retention
  - Intraurethral suppository: local penile pain, urethral bleeding, dizziness, and dysuria
  - Intracavernosal injection: penile pain, edema and hematoma, palpable nodules or plaques, and priapism
  - Sildenafil: hypotension (caution for patients on nitrates)
  - PDE-5 inhibitors: Use caution with congenital prolonged QT syndrome, class Ia or II antiarrhythmics, nitroglycerin, α-blockers (e.g., terazosin, tamsulosin), retinal disease, unstable cardiac disease, liver and renal failure.
  - Significant possible interactions
  - PDE-5 inhibitor concentration is affected by CYP3A4 inhibitors (e.g., erythromycin, indinavir, ketoconazole, ritonavir, amiodarone, cimetidine, clarithromycin, delavirdine, diltiazem, fluoxetine, fluvoxamine, grapefruit juice, itraconazole, nefazodone, nevirapine, saquinavir, and verapamil). Serum concentrations and/or toxicity may be increased. Lower starting doses should be used in these patients.
  - PDE-5 inhibitor concentration may be reduced by rifampin and phenytoin.

ADDITIONAL THERAPIES
Men with relationship difficulties who received therapy plus sildenafil had more successful intercourse than those who received only sildenafil (8)[A].

SURGERY/OTHER PROCEDURES
Penile prosthesis should be reserved for patients who have failed or are ineligible for first- or second-line therapies.

COMPLEMENTARY & ALTERNATIVE MEDICINE
Trazodone, yohimbine, and herbal therapies are not recommended for the treatment of ED, as they have not proven to be efficacious. Low–intensity shock wave treatment is not FDA approved, but some studies have shown improvement particularly in younger, nondiabetic patients with milder cases of ED. Further research is needed (9).

ONGOING CARE

FOLLOW-UP RECOMMENDATIONS
Patient Monitoring
Treatment should be assessed at baseline and after the patient has completed at least 1 to 3 weeks of a specific treatment: Monitor the quality and quantity of penile erections and monitor the level of satisfaction patient achieves.

DIET
Diet and exercise recommended to achieve a normal body mass index; limit alcohol.

PROGNOSIS
- All commercially available PDE-5 inhibitors are equally effective. In the presence of sexual stimulation, they are 55–80% effective.
  - Lower success rates with diabetes mellitus and radical prostatectomy patients who suffer from ED
- Overall effectiveness is 70–90% for intracavernosal alprostadil and 43–60% for intraurethral alprostadil (2)[B].
- Penile prostheses are associated with an 85–90% patient satisfaction rate (2)[C].

REFERENCES
1. Rew KT, Heidelbaugh JJ. Erectile dysfunction. *Am Fam Physician*. 2016;94(10):820–827.
2. McVary KT. Clinical practice. Erectile dysfunction. *N Engl J Med*. 2007;357(24):2472–2481.
3. American Urological Association. Guideline on the management of erectile dysfunction: diagnosis and treatment recommendations. https://www.auanet.org/guidelines/guidelines/erectile-dysfunction-(ed)-guideline. Accessed January 13, 2017.
4. Miner M, Nehra A, Jackson G, et al. All men with vasculogenic erectile dysfunction require a cardiovascular workup. *Am J Med*. 2014;127(3):174–182.
5. Wiggins A, Tsambarlis PN, Abdelsayed G, et al. A treatment algorithm for healthy young men with erectile dysfunction. *BJU Int*. 2019;123(1):173–179.
6. Heidelbaugh JJ. Management of erectile dysfunction. *Am Fam Physician*. 2010;81(3):305–312.
7. Le TV, Tsambarlis P, Hellstrom WJG. Pharmacodynamics of the agents used for the treatment of erectile dysfunction. *Expert Opin Drug Metab Toxicol*. 2019;15(2):121–131.
8. Melnik T, Soares BG, Nasselo AG. Psychosocial interventions for erectile dysfunction. *Cochrane Database Syst Rev*. 2007;(3):CD004825.
9. Kitrey ND, Vardi Y, Appel B, et al. Low intensity shock wave treatment for erectile dysfunction—how long does the effect last? *J Urol*. 2018;200(1):167–170.

 CODES

ICD10
- N52.03 Combined arterial insufficiency and corporovenous occlusive erectile dysfunction
- N52.2 Drug-induced erectile dysfunction
- F52.21 Male erectile disorder

CLINICAL PEARLS
- Nitrates should be withheld for 24 hours after sildenafil or vardenafil administration and for 48 hours after use of tadalafil. PDE-5 inhibitors are contraindicated in patients taking concurrent nitrates of any form (regular or intermittent nitrate therapy), as it can lead to severe hypotension and syncope.
- Reserve surgical treatment for patients who do not respond to drug treatment.
- The use of PDE-5 inhibitors with α-adrenergic antagonists may increase the risk of hypotension. Tamsulosin is the least likely to cause orthostatic hypotension.
- Avanafil should not be used with strong CYP3A4 inhibitors and max dose should be 50 mg with moderate CYP3A4 inhibitors.
- ED may be a marker for subclinical cardiovascular disease. Thoroughly assess patients with nonpsychogenic ED for cardiovascular risks.

ERYSIPELAS
Barbara M. Kiersz Muller, DO

BASICS

DESCRIPTION
- Distinct form of cellulitis: an acute, well-demarcated, superficial bacterial skin infection (most commonly on face or leg) with lymphatic involvement almost always caused by *Streptococcus pyogenes*
- Usually acute, but a chronic recurrent form can also exist
- Nonpurulent
- System(s) affected: skin, exocrine

EPIDEMIOLOGY
- Predominant age: infants, children, and adults >45 years
- Greatest in elderly (>75 years)
- No gender/racial predilection

Incidence
- Erysipelas occurs in ~1/1,000 persons/year.
- Incidence on the rise since the 1980s (1)

Prevalence
Unknown

ETIOLOGY AND PATHOPHYSIOLOGY
- Group A streptococci induce inflammation and activation of the contact system, a proinflammatory pathway with antithrombotic activity, releasing proteinases and proinflammatory cytokines.
- The generation of antibacterial peptides and the release of bradykinin, a proinflammatory peptide, increase vascular permeability and induce fever and pain.
- The M proteins from the group A streptococcal cell wall interact with neutrophils, leading to the secretion of heparin-binding protein, an inflammatory mediator that also induces vascular leakage.
- This cascade of reactions leads to the symptoms seen in erysipelas: fever, pain, erythema, and edema.
- Group A β-hemolytic streptococci primarily; commonly *S. pyogenes*, occasionally, other *Streptococcus* groups C/G
- Rarely, group B streptococci/*Staphylococcus aureus* may be involved.

RISK FACTORS
- Disruption in the skin barrier (surgical incisions, insect bites, eczematous lesions, local trauma, abrasions, dermatophytic infections, intravenous drug user [IVDU])
- Chronic diseases (diabetes, malnutrition, nephrotic syndrome, heart failure)
- Immunocompromised (HIV)/debilitated
- Fissured skin (especially at the nose and ears)
- Toe-web intertrigo and lymphedema
- Leg ulcers/stasis dermatitis
- Venous/lymphatic insufficiency (saphenectomy, varicose veins of leg, phlebitis, radiotherapy, mastectomy, lymphadenectomy)
- Alcohol abuse
- Morbid obesity
- Recent streptococcal pharyngitis
- Varicella

GENERAL PREVENTION
- Good skin hygiene
- It is recommended that predisposing medical conditions, such as tinea pedis and stasis dermatitis, be appropriately managed first.
- Men who shave within 5 days of facial erysipelas are more likely to have a recurrence.
- With recurrences, search for other possible sources of streptococcal infection (e.g., tonsils, sinuses).
- Compression stockings should be encouraged for patients with lower extremity edema.
- Consider suppressive prophylactic antibiotic therapy, such as penicillin, in patients with >2 episodes in a 12-month period.

Pediatric Considerations
Group B *Streptococcus* may be a cause of erysipelas in neonates/infants.

DIAGNOSIS

Prodromal symptoms before the skin eruption of erysipelas may include:
- Moderate- to high-grade fever
- Chills
- Headache
- Malaise
- Anorexia, usually in the first 48 hours
- Vomiting
- Arthralgias

ALERT
It is important to differentiate erysipelas from a methicillin-resistant *S. aureus* (MRSA) infection, which usually presents with an indurated center, significant pain, and later evidence of abscess formation.

PHYSICAL EXAM
- Vital signs: moderate- to high-grade fever with resultant tachycardia. Hypotension may occur.
- The presence of a fever in erysipelas can be considered a differentiating factor from other skin infections.
- Headache and vomiting may be prominent.
- Acute onset of intense erythema; well-demarcated painful plaque (2)
- Peau d'orange appearance
- Milian ear sign (Erythema involves skin of ear as well as face implies erysipelas.)
- Vesicles and bullae may form but are not uniformly present.
- Desquamation may occur later.
- Lymphangitis
- Location (most commonly unilateral; bilateral presentation should prompt consideration of alternative diagnosis)
  - Lower extremity 70–80% of cases
  - Face involvement is less common (5–20%), especially nose and ears.
  - Chronic form usually recurs at site of the previous infection and may recur years after initial episode.

- Patients on systemic steroids may be more difficult to diagnose because signs and symptoms of the infection may be masked by anti-inflammatory action of the steroids.
- Systemic toxicity resolves rapidly with treatment; skin lesions desquamate on days 5 to 10 but usually heal without scarring.
- In geriatric patients, facial involvement presents in a butterfly pattern. Pustules characteristically absent and regional lymphadenopathy with lymphangitic streaking is seen.

Pediatric Considerations
- Abdominal involvement is more common in infants, especially around umbilical stump.
- Face, scalp, and leg involvement are common in older children due to the excoriations when scratching in atopic dermatitis, allowing an easy port of entry.

Geriatric Considerations
- Fever may not be as prominent.
- 80% of cases affect the lower extremities. The rest are usually on the face.
- High-output cardiac failure may occur in debilitated patients with underlying cardiac disease.
- More susceptible to complications

DIFFERENTIAL DIAGNOSIS
- Cellulitis (Margins are less clear and do not involve ear.)
- Necrotizing fasciitis (systemic illness and more pain)
- Skin abscess (feel for area of fluctuance)
- DVT (needs to rule out if clinically suspected)
- Acute gout (Check patient history.)
- Insect bite (Check patient history.)
- Dermatophytes
- Impetigo (blistered/crusted appearance; superficial)
- Ecthyma (ulcerative impetigo)
- Herpes zoster (dermatomal distribution)
- Erythema annulare centrifugum (raised pink-red ring/bull's-eye marks)
- Contact dermatitis (no fever, pruritic, not painful)
- Giant cell urticaria (transient, wheal appearance, severe itching)
- Angioneurotic edema (no fever)
- Scarlet fever (widespread rash with indistinct borders and without edema; rash is most common early in skin folds; develops generalized "sandpaper" feeling as it progresses)
- Toxic shock syndrome (diffuse erythema with evidence of multiorgan involvement)
- Lupus (of the face; less fever, positive antinuclear antibodies)
- Polychondritis (Common site is the ear.)
- Other bacterial infections to consider:
  - Meat, shellfish, fish, and poultry workers: *Erysipelothrix rhusiopathiae* (known as erysipeloid)
  - Human bite: *Eikenella corrodens*
  - Cat/dog bite: *Pasteurella multocida*/*Capnocytophaga canimorsus*
  - Salt water exposure: *Vibrio vulnificus*
  - Fresh/brackish water exposure: *Aeromonas hydrophila*

DIAGNOSTIC TESTS & INTERPRETATION

Reserve diagnostic tests for severely ill, toxic patients, patients who failed initial antibiotic therapy, or those who are immunosuppressed.

Initial Tests (lab, imaging)
- Leukocytosis
- Blood culture (<5% positive)
- Elevated erythrocyte sedimentation rate (ESR) and C-reactive protein (CRP)
- Streptococci may be cultured from exudate/noninvolved sites.

Test Interpretation
Biopsy is not needed; however, skin findings would show
- Dermal and epidermal edema, extending into the SC tissues
- Peau d'orange appearance caused by edema in the superficial tissue surrounding the hair follicles
- Vasodilation and enlarged lymphatics
- Mixed interstitial infiltrate mainly consisting of neutrophils and mononuclear cells
- Endothelial cell swelling
- Gram-positive cocci in lymphatics and tissue with rare invasion of local blood vessels
- Fibrotic thickening of lymphatic vessel walls with possible luminal occlusion may be seen in recurrent erysipelas.

 ## TREATMENT

GENERAL MEASURES
- Symptomatic treatment of myalgias and fever
- Adequate fluid intake
- Local treatment with cold compresses
- Elevation of affected extremity
- Appropriate therapy for any underlying predisposing condition

MEDICATION
- Antibiotics cure 50–100% of infections, but which regimen is most successful is unclear.
- Antibiotics may be as effective when given orally versus intravenously unless systemic symptoms are present (fever, chills).
- A 5-day course of antibiotics may be as effective as a 10-day course at curing.

First Line
- Adults
  - Extremities, nondiabetic
    ○ Primary
      ▪ Penicillin G: 1 to 2 million U IV q6h or cefazolin 1 g IV q8h
    ○ Alternative (if penicillin allergic)
      ▪ Vancomycin 15 mg/kg IV q12h
      ▪ When afebrile, change to oral regimen of TMP-SMX or clindamycin
  - Total 10 days, diabetics
    ○ Early mild:
      ▪ Trimethoprim-sulfamethoxazole (TMP-SMX)-DS: 1 to 2 tabs PO BID and penicillin VK 500 mg PO QID or cephalexin 500 mg PO QID
  - Severe disease
    ○ MP or MER or ERTA IV and linezolid 600 mg IV/PO BID or vancomycin IV or daptomycin 4 mg/kg IV q24h

  - Facial
    ○ Primary
      ▪ Vancomycin: 15 mg/kg (actual weight) IV q8–12h with target trough 15 to 20
    ○ Alternative
      ▪ Daptomycin 4 mg/kg IV q24h or linezolid 600 mg IV q12h
- Children
  - Penicillin G
    ○ 0 to 7 days, <2,000 g = 50,000 U/kg q12h
    ○ 8 to 28 days, <2,000 g = 75,000 U/kg q8h
    ○ 0 to 7 days, >2,000 g = 50,000 U/kg q8h
    ○ 8 to 28 days, >2,000 g = 50,000 U/kg q6h
    ○ >28 days = 50,000 U/kg/day
  - Cefazolin
    ○ 0 to 7 days, <2,000 g = 25 mg/kg q12h
    ○ 8 to 28 days, <2,000 g = 25 mg/kg q12h
    ○ 0 to 7 days, >2,000 g = 25 mg/kg q12h
    ○ 8 to 28 days, >2,000 g = 25 mg/kg q8h
    ○ >28 days = 25 mg/kg q8h
- No reported group A streptococci resistance to β-lactam antibiotics
- In chronic recurrent infections, prophylactic treatment after the acute infection resolves:
  - Penicillin G benzathine: 1.2 million U IM q4wk or penicillin VK 500 mg PO BID or azithromycin 250 mg PO QD
- If staphylococcal infection is suspected or if patient is acutely ill, consider a β–lactamase-stable antibiotic.
- Consider community-acquired MRSA, and depending on regional sensitivity, may treat MRSA with TMP-SMX DS 1 tablet PO BID or vancomycin 1 g IV q12h or doxycycline 100 mg PO BID.

ISSUES FOR REFERRAL
Recurrent infection, treatment failure

ADDITIONAL THERAPIES
Some patients may notice a deepening of erythema after initiating antimicrobial therapy. This may be due to the destruction of pathogens that release enzymes, increasing local inflammation. In this case, treatment with corticosteroids, in addition to antimicrobials, can mildly reduce healing time and antibiotic duration in patients with erysipelas. Consider prednisolone 30 mg/day with taper over 8 days.

ADMISSION, INPATIENT, AND NURSING CONSIDERATIONS
- Admission criteria/initial stabilization
  - Patient with systemic toxicity
  - Patient with high-risk factors (e.g., elderly, lymphedema, postsplenectomy, diabetes)
  - Failed outpatient care
- IV therapy if systemic toxicity/unable to tolerate PO
- Discharge criteria: no evidence of systemic toxicity with resolution of erythema and swelling

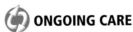 ## ONGOING CARE

FOLLOW-UP RECOMMENDATIONS
Bed rest with elevation of extremity during acute infection and then activity as tolerated

Patient Monitoring
Patients should be treated until all symptoms and skin manifestations have resolved.

PATIENT EDUCATION
Stress importance of completing prescribed medication regimen.

PROGNOSIS
- Patients should recover fully if adequately treated.
- May experience deepening of erythema after initiation of antibiotics
- Most respond to therapy after 24 to 48 hours.
- Mortality is <1% in patients receiving appropriate treatment.
- Bullae formation suggests longer disease course and often indicates a concomitant S. aureus infection that may require antibiotic coverage for MRSA.
- Chronic edema/scarring may result from chronic recurrent cases.
- Rarely, obstructive lymphadenitis may result from chronic recurrent cases.

COMPLICATIONS
- Recurrent infection
- Abscess (suggests staphylococcal infection)
- Necrotizing fasciitis
- Lymphedema (most prominent risk factor for recurrence) (3)
- Bacteremia, which may lead to sepsis
- Pneumonia (due to sepsis/toxin-producing organism)
- Meningitis (due to sepsis/toxin-producing organism)
- Embolism
- Gangrene
- Bursitis, septic arthritis, tendinitis, or osteitis

REFERENCES
1. Celestin R, Brown J, Kihiczak G, et al. Erysipelas: a common potentially dangerous infection. *Acta Dermatovenerol Alp Pannonica Adriat.* 2007;16(3):123–127.
2. Breen JO. Skin and soft tissue infections in immunocompetent patients. *Am Fam Physician.* 2010;81(7):893–899.
3. Inghammar M, Rasmussen M, Linder A. Recurrent erysipelas—risk factors and clinical presentation. *BMC Infect Dis.* 2014;14:270.

ADDITIONAL READING
Gilbert D, Chambers HF, Eliopoulos GM, et al, eds. *The Sanford Guide to Antimicrobial Therapy.* 44th ed. Sperryville, VA: Antimicrobial Therapy; 2014.

 ## CODES

ICD10
A46 Erysipelas

CLINICAL PEARLS
- Athlete's foot is the most common portal of entry.
- Erysipelas is distinguished from cellulitis by its sharp, shiny, fiery-red, raised border.
- In recurrent cases, search for other possible source of streptococcal infection (e.g., tonsils, sinuses, intertrigo).
- Most erysipelas infections now occur on the legs, rather than the face.

E

ERYTHEMA MULTIFORME

Niti N. Khambhati, MD • Rajasree Nair, MD

BASICS

- Erythema multiforme (EM) is an uncommon, self-limiting, immune-mediated, mucocutaneous disease.
  - Approximately 90% of cases are triggered by infectious agents (herpes simplex virus [HSV]-1 or -2 up to 50%), or less commonly, by drugs and vaccinations (1),(2).
  - Characteristic skin lesions are acrally distributed, distinct, targetoid papules with concentric color variation (three zones), occasionally accompanied by oral, genital, or ocular mucosal involvement (1),(3),(4).
  - EM needs to be differentiated from Steven-Johnson syndrome (SJS) and toxic epidermal necrolysis (TEN), which are characterized by truncal, flat lesions with or without blisters which can result in significant mortality (2),(3).
- There are no universal diagnostic criteria, but clinical history, clinical examination, skin biopsy, laboratory studies, and special consideration of persistent EM are all helpful in making a diagnosis (1).
- Treatment focuses on supportive care in addition to treating the underlying etiology and discontinuing causative agents (2).

DESCRIPTION

- There are two subtypes of EM: erythema multiforme minor (EMm), which involves ≤1 mucosal site, and erythema multiforme major (EMM), which involves ≥2 mucosal sites (4).
- EMM is now separate from SJS and TEN. Skin lesions that are predominantly truncal, flat (macular, nonpalpable), and atypical (less sharply demarcated with only two concentric zones) with or without blisters are more suggestive of SJS or TEN (2),(3).
- Recurrent EM is defined as ≥3 episodes but has a mean number of 6 episodes per year and a mean duration of 6 to 10 years.

EPIDEMIOLOGY

Incidence
Annual U.S. incidence is estimated at <1% (2).

Prevalence
- Predominant in young adults from age 20 to 40; rare <3 years and >50 years of age (2).
- Slight male predominance is observed (2).
- There is no apparent race predilection (2).

ETIOLOGY AND PATHOPHYSIOLOGY

- Etiology (1),(2),(4)
  - Viral infections: HSV-1 and -2 (most common etiology), Epstein-Barr, hepatitis C, coxsackievirus, echovirus, varicella, mumps, poliovirus, cytomegalovirus, HIV, molluscum contagiosum
  - Bacterial infections: *Mycoplasma pneumoniae* (2nd most common etiology), *Treponema pallidum*, *Mycobacterium tuberculosis*, and *Gardnerella vaginalis*
  - Drugs: NSAIDs, anti-epileptics, antibiotics (penicillin, sulfonamides, erythromycin, nitrofurantoin, tetracyclines), statin, TNF-α inhibitors, and barbiturates
  - Vaccines: stronger association with HPV, MMR, and small pox vaccines, but also associated with hepatitis B, meningococcal, pneumococcal, varicella, influenza, diphtheria-pertussis-tetanus, and *Haemophilus influenzae*
  - Occupational exposures: herbicides (alachlor and butachlor), iodoacetonitrile, heavy metals
  - Radiation therapy
  - Premenstrual hormone changes
  - Malignancy (e.g., lymphoma)
  - Inflammatory bowel disease
- Pathogenesis of EM (1)
  - In HSV-associated EM, peripheral mononuclear cells that phagocytose the virus transport fragmented HSV DNA to keratinocytes. Within the keratinocytes, the HSV DNA polymerase gene *(pol)* leads to a TH-1 mediated immune response. Activation of the HSV-specific CD4+ TH-1 cells then produces cytokines such as interferon (IFN)-γ and triggers an inflammatory cascade, which leads to the mucocutaneous findings.
  - Development of EM from other inciting factors such as drugs and vaccinations is not completely understood, but it appears that the pathway involves tumor necrosis factor (TNF)-α, perforin, and granzyme B rather than IFN-γ.

Genetics
- Genetic susceptibility may play a role in some patients with EM.
- Strong association with the HLA-DQB1*0301 allele is found among patients with herpes-associated EM (1).
- In recurrent EM, there is an association with HLA-B35, -B62, and -DR53 alleles (1).

RISK FACTORS
- Previous history of EM
- Age 20 to 40
- Male
- Use of causative agents or infection with causative pathogens

GENERAL PREVENTION
- Known etiologic agents or those with potential for cross-reactivity should be avoided.
- Oral acyclovir or valacyclovir may help prevent herpes-related recurrent EM (4),(5).

COMMONLY ASSOCIATED CONDITIONS
See "Etiology and Pathophysiology" earlier.

DIAGNOSIS

- Diagnosis is based on history and clinical findings, and most cases do not require further work-up.
- In unclear cases, histopathologic analysis including immunofluorescence microscopy and other laboratory studies can help in making a diagnosis (2).

HISTORY
- Acute, self-limiting episodic course
- Cutaneous rash with possible mucosal involvement, most commonly in mouth
- Prodromal symptoms are usually absent, but common in cases with mucosal involvement
- Signs and symptoms of infections associated with EM such as a HSV eruption (10 to 15 days prior to onset of EM lesions) or respiratory symptoms suggestive of *M. pneumoniae*
- History of new medication use or vaccination
- Exposure to other causative agents like radiation, herbicides, heavy metals, etc.

PHYSICAL EXAM
- Thorough skin exam should be completed, including of mucous membranes.
  - Typical cutaneous lesions with erythematous, papular, and targetoid appearance that has three concentric zones of varied color
  - Acral lesions with symmetric distribution and predilection for extensor surfaces
  - Mucosal involvement
- Mucosal involvement (1)
  - Oral involvement manifests as erythema, erosions, bullae, and ulcerations on both nonkeratinized and keratinized mucosal surfaces and on the vermilion of the lips
  - Minimal involvement in EMm, but if present, most commonly involves the mouth
  - At least two mucosal sites involved in EMM, including eyes (conjunctivitis, keratitis); mouth (stomatitis, cheilitis, characteristic blood-stained crusted erosions on lips); and probable trachea, bronchi, GI tract, or genital tract (balanitis and vulvitis)

DIFFERENTIAL DIAGNOSIS
- SJS (1),(3)
  - Medications are the most frequent cause.
  - Generalized distribution of lesions; concentrated on the trunk
  - Targetoid lesions are less sharply demarcated and atypical.
    - Atypical signifies macular (flat and nonpalpable) with only two concentric zones
  - Blisters and skin detachment <10% of the total body surface area
  - Nikolsky sign may be positive—applying gentle pressure to what appears to be intact skin will extend sloughing of epidermis.
  - 90% of patients have mucosal involvement, commonly at ≥2 sites.
  - Presence of constitutional symptoms with presence of high fever (>38.5°C)
  - Can be associated with anemia, lymphadenopathy, high C-reactive protein levels (>10 mg/dL), and hepatic dysfunction (1)
  - ~10% mortality
- TEN (3)
  - Similar to SJS but has full-thickness skin necrosis and skin detachment >30% of the total body surface area
  - Up to 50% mortality rate
- Urticaria (1)
  - Pruritic wheal-and-flare skin lesion
  - Each lesion is transient, lasting <24 hours, unlike in EM
- Fixed drug eruption
- Bullous pemphigoid, paraneoplastic pemphigoid
- Sweet syndrome, Rowell syndrome
- Polymorphous light eruption
- Cutaneous small-vessel vasculitis
- Mucocutaneous lymph
- Erythema annulare centrifugum
- Acute hemorrhagic edema of infancy
- Subacute cutaneous lupus erythematosus
- Contact dermatitis
- Pityriasis rosea, tinea corporis
- Secondary syphilis
- Dermatitis herpetiformis
- Herpes gestationis
- Septicemia
- Serum sickness, Rocky Mountain spotted fever
- Viral exanthem
- Meningococcemia
- Lichen planus
- Behçet syndrome, recurrent aphthous ulcers
- Herpetic gingivostomatitis

DIAGNOSTIC TESTS & INTERPRETATION
Laboratory studies and skin biopsies are not required for diagnosis. However, they can be useful in determining inciting factors, ruling out other conditions, and confirming a diagnosis of EM (1),(2).

Initial Tests (lab, imaging)
- Because HSV is the most common cause of EM, every patient should be evaluated for an underlying infection (1).
  - Evaluation can include serologic tests or checking skin biopsy samples for HSV infection by direct immunofluorescence (DIF), direct fluorescent antibody (DFA), polymerase chain reaction (PCR), viral culture, or Tzanck smear (1),(2).
- No imaging studies are indicated unless there is suspicion for *M. pneumoniae* in which case work-up should include CXR, PCR testing of throat swab, and serologic tests (1).

Follow-Up Tests & Special Considerations
- Antinuclear antibodies, rheumatoid factor, and anti-Ro and anti-La antibodies can be ordered if suspicious for Rowell syndrome (1).
- Presence of IgM antibodies or greater than 2-fold increase in IgG antibodies can confirm the diagnosis (1).
- Antibody staining to IFN-γ and TNF-α to differentiate HSV from drug-associated EM (1)
- Serum complement levels should be checked in cases of persistent EM as they are likely to be low (1).
- Erythrocyte sedimentation rate, white blood cell count, and liver function enzymes should be checked in severe cases with mucosal involvement as they are likely to be elevated.

Diagnostic Procedures/Other
- Skin biopsy: Histopathologic analysis of lesional and perilesional tissue can help with diagnosis in equivocal conditions.
- DIF and indirect immunofluorescence (IIF) can be used to differentiate EM from other vesiculobullous diseases. DIF is performed on a biopsy of perilesional tissue, and IIF is performed on a blood sample.

Test Interpretation
- Histopathology of EM lesions may demonstrate the following (3),(4):
  - Spongiosis (intercellular edema)
  - Necrotic keratinocytes resulting in dermal interface bullae formation
  - Inflammatory infiltrate including lymphocytes in the dermal-epidermal junction with perivascular accentuation
- DIF and IIF findings are usually either negative or nonspecific in EM. It may show lichenoid inflammatory infiltrate and epidermal necrosis including circulating immune complexes, deposition of C3, IgM, and fibrin around the dermal blood vessels (1).

TREATMENT

GENERAL MEASURES
- Treatment will depend on disease severity, underlying cause, and course of the disease.
- Determine the level of care: outpatient versus inpatient.
- Determine the cause of EM.
  - Drug-induced EM: Discontinue the inciting factor and avoid reexposure to the same drug or exposure to other drugs with potential for cross-reactivity (4).
  - Infectious: Treat the underlying condition as indicated.
- Some cases may require close follow-up.

MEDICATION
- Acute EM
  - Discontinue inciting factors and treat the underlying disease (1)[B].
    - *M. pneumoniae*–associated EM: may require antibiotics
    - HSV-induced EM: Most recent sources report no proven effect on the course of EM using antivirals with acute mild EM (1)[B].

- Mild cutaneous involvement
  - Medium potency topical steroids for lesions on trunk and extremities (2)[C]
  - Low potency topical steroids for lesions on the face and intertriginous skin (2)[C]
  - Oral antihistamines for pruritic lesions (2)[C]
- Mucous membrane EM
  - Ocular involvement
    - Urgent ophthalmology consultation (2)[C]
    - Ophthalmic preparations such as nonpreserved dexamethasone 0.1% and lubricants such as nonpreserved hyaluronate should be used under the guidance of ophthalmologists.
  - Oral involvement
    - Nondisabling
      - High-potency topical corticosteroid gel (e.g., fluocinonide 0.05% gel applied 2 to 3 times per day) (2)[C]
      - Mouthwashes that contain a combination of lidocaine 2%, antacids, and diphenhydramine 12.5 mg/5 mL (e.g., Maalox, swish and spit as needed up to 4 times per day) (2)[C]
    - Disabling
      - Hospitalization may be required for pain control and to ensure adequate hydration and nutrition if insufficient oral intake.
      - Systemic corticosteroids may be used for severe symptoms, but controlled studies have not been performed to validate efficacy of this approach (e.g., prednisone 40 to 60 mg per day, tapered over 2 to 4 weeks) (1)[C].
- Recurrent EM
  - First-line treatment with HSV-associated and idiopathic recurrent EM is antiviral prophylaxis for at least 6 months (1)[B]. Options include:
    - Acyclovir 400 mg BID
    - Valacyclovir 500 mg BID
    - Famciclovir 250 mg BID
    - If the patient is unresponsive to one antiviral, can double the dose or switch to a different antiviral regimen
  - Second-line therapy includes
    - Dapsone (100 to 150 mg/day)
    - Azathioprine (100 to 150 mg/day)
    - Mycophenolate mofetil (1,000 to 1,500 mg BID)
    - Thalidomide (100 to 200 mg/day)
    - Tacrolimus (0.1% ointment daily)
    - Hydroxychloroquine (400 mg/day)
    - Levamisole (75 to 200 mg/week)

> **ALERT**
> Levamisole can cause agranulocytosis, although the incidence is low (1–2%). The agranulocytosis is dose-dependent, hence, initiation of treatment with a lower dose and regular monitoring during treatment is recommended.

  - Once in remission, therapy should be continued for 6 to 12 months followed by a taper over 2 to 4 months to the lowest effective dose or cessation.

ISSUES FOR REFERRAL
Consider appropriate referrals when concerned about etiologies such as autoimmune disorders, recurrent HSV infections, or possible malignancy.

ADMISSION, INPATIENT, AND NURSING CONSIDERATIONS
Determining the level of care:
- Most cases can be managed outpatient.
- However, if lesions involve the oral mucosa thereby preventing sufficient oral intake, patients need to be hospitalized for IV hydration, electrolyte repletion, nutrition, and pain control.
- Wound care may also be indicated for cases with epidermal detachment.

 ONGOING CARE

FOLLOW-UP RECOMMENDATIONS
Patient Monitoring
- The disease is self-limiting.
- Complications are rare, with no mortality.

PATIENT EDUCATION
Avoid any identified etiologic agents.

PROGNOSIS
- Rash evolves over 1 to 2 weeks and subsequently resolves within 2 to 6 weeks, generally without scarring or sequelae.
- Following resolution, there may be some post-inflammatory hyper- or hypopigmentation.

COMPLICATIONS
Secondary infection, scarring, eye damage

REFERENCES
1. Sokumbi O, Wetter DA. Clinical features, diagnosis, and treatment of erythema multiforme: a review for the practicing dermatologist. *Int J Dermatol.* 2012;51(8):889–902.
2. Trayes KP, Love G, Studdiford JS. Erythema multiforme: recognition and management. *Am Fam Physician.* 2019;100(2):82–88.
3. Grünwald P, Mockenhaupt M, Panzer R, et al. Erythema multiforme, Stevens Johnson syndrome/toxic epidermal necrolysis—diagnosis and treatment. *J Dtsch Dermatol Ges.* 2020;18(6):547–553.
4. Lerch M, Mainetti C, Terziroli Beretta-Piccoli B, et al. Current perspectives on erythema multiforme. *Clin Rev Allergy Immunol.* 2018;54(1):177–184.
5. de Risi-Pugliese T, Sbidian E, Ingen-Housz-Oro S, et al. Interventions for erythema multiforme: a systematic review. *J Eur Acad Dermatol Venereol.* 2019;33(5):842–849.

 SEE ALSO

Cutaneous Drug Reactions; Dermatitis Herpetiformis; Pemphigoid Gestationis; Stevens-Johnson Syndrome; Toxic Epidermal Necrolysis; Urticaria

 CODES

ICD10
- L51.0 Nonbullous erythema multiforme
- L51.1 Stevens-Johnson syndrome
- L51.3 Stevens-Johnson syndrome-toxic epidermal necrolysis overlap syndrome

CLINICAL PEARLS
- EM is diagnosed clinically. No lab tests are required for the diagnosis.
- Typical lesions are targetoid or "iris." Lesions are symmetrically distributed on palms, soles, dorsum of the hands, and extensor surfaces of extremities and face. The oral mucosa is the most affected mucosal region in EM.
- Management of EM involves determining the etiology when possible.
- Recurrence risk may be as high as 30%.
- Recurrent cases are often secondary to HSV infection. Antiviral therapy may be beneficial in these patients.

ERYTHEMA NODOSUM

Lolwa Al-Obaid, MD • Faruq Pradhan, MD • Fredric D. Gordon, MD, FAASLD, AGAF

 BASICS

DESCRIPTION
- A delayed-type hypersensitivity reaction to various antigens, or an autoimmune reaction presenting as a panniculitis (1) that affects subcutaneous fat
- Clinical pattern of multiple, bilateral, erythematous, tender nodules in a typically pretibial distribution that undergo a characteristic pattern of color changes, similar to that seen in bruises. Unlike erythema induratum, the lesions of erythema nodosum (EN) do not typically ulcerate.
- Occurs most commonly on the shins; less commonly on the thighs, forearms, trunk, head, or neck
- Often associated with nonspecific prodrome including fever, weight loss, and arthralgia
- Often idiopathic but may be associated with a number of clinical entities
- Usually remits spontaneously in weeks to months without scarring, atrophy, or ulceration
- Uncommon to have recurrences after initial presentation

Pregnancy Considerations
May have repeat outbreaks during pregnancy

Pediatric Considerations
Rare pediatric variant has lesions only on palms or soles, often unilateral; typically has a shorter duration in children than adults

EPIDEMIOLOGY
Incidence
- 1 to 5/100,000/year
- Predominant age: 20 to 30 years
- Predominant sex: female > male (6:1) in adults

Prevalence
- Varies geographically depending on the prevalence of disorders associated with EN
- Reported 1 to 5/100,000

ETIOLOGY AND PATHOPHYSIOLOGY
- Idiopathic: up to 55%
- Infectious: 44%. Streptococcal pharyngitis (most common), mycobacteria, mycoplasma, chlamydia, mycoplasma, coccidioidomycosis, rarely can be caused by *Campylobacter* spp., rickettsiae, *Salmonella* spp., psittacosis, syphilis

- Sarcoidosis: 11–25%
- Drugs: 3–10%; sulfonamides amoxicillin, oral contraceptives, bromides, azathioprine, vemurafenib
- Pregnancy: 2–5%
- Enteropathies: 1–4%; ulcerative colitis, Crohn disease, Behçet disease, celiac disease, diverticulitis
- Rare causes: <1% (2)
  - Fungal: dermatophytes, coccidioidomycosis, histoplasmosis, blastomycosis
  - Viral/chlamydial: infectious mononucleosis, lymphogranuloma venereum, paravaccinia, HIV, hepatitis B, C
  - Malignancies: lymphoma/leukemia, sarcoma, myelodysplastic syndrome
  - Sweet syndrome

RISK FACTORS
See "Etiology and Pathophysiology."

COMMONLY ASSOCIATED CONDITIONS
See "Etiology and Pathophysiology."

 DIAGNOSIS

HISTORY
- Often a prodrome 1 to 3 weeks prior to onset of lesions; can consist of malaise, fever, weight loss, cough, and arthralgia
- Increasingly tender nodules on the legs, usually over the shins
- Fever, malaise, chills, fatigue
- Headache
- Can precede systemic process by weeks

PHYSICAL EXAM
- Lesions initially present as warm, tender, erythematous firm nodules and become fluctuant, gradually fading to resemble a bruise over 1 to 2 months (erythema contusiformis).
- Typically pretibial, although can extend proximally to involve thighs or trunk (atypically can involve extensor surface of forearms)
- Diameter varies from 1 to 10 cm with poor demarcation.

DIFFERENTIAL DIAGNOSIS
- Nodular vasculitis or erythema induratum (warm ulcerating calf nodules)
- Superficial thrombophlebitis
- Cellulitis
- Weber-Christian disease (violaceous, scarring nodules)
- Lupus panniculitis
- Cutaneous polyarteritis nodosa
- Sarcoidal granulomas
- Cutaneous T-cell lymphoma
- EN leprosum (clinically similar to EN but shows vasculitis on histopathology)
- Subcutaneous infection (including *Staphylococcus*, *Sporothrix schenckii*, *Nocardia brasiliensis*, *Mycobacterium marinum*, *Leishmania braziliensis*)

DIAGNOSTIC TESTS & INTERPRETATION
Diagnosis is made clinically, with support of testing.
- ESR or C-reactive protein (CRP): often elevated, but can be normal in up to 40% (3)[C]
- CBC: mild leukocytosis (3)
- Urine pregnancy test (3)
- Throat culture, antistreptolysin O titer (3)
- Blood and/or stool culture, stool ova and parasites (O&P)
- Tuberculin skin testing (3)
- Seronegative rheumatoid factor

Initial Tests (lab, imaging)
CXR for hilar adenopathy or infiltrates related to sarcoidosis or tuberculosis (3)[C]

Diagnostic Procedures/Other
Deep-incisional or excisional skin biopsy including subcutaneous tissue; rarely necessary except in atypical cases with ulceration, duration >12 weeks, or absence of nodules overlying lower limbs (4)[C]

Test Interpretation
- Septal panniculitis without vasculitis
- Neutrophilic infiltrate in septa of fat tissue early in course
- Actinic radial (Miescher) granulomas, consisting of collections of histiocytes around a central stellate cleft, may be seen.
- Fibrosis, paraseptal granulation tissue, lymphocytes, and multinucleated giant cells predominate late in course (5).

TREATMENT

- Condition usually self-limited within 1 to 2 months
- All medications listed as treatment for EN are off-label uses of the medications. There are no specific FDA-approved medications.

GENERAL MEASURES
- Mild compression bandages and leg elevation may reduce pain (wet dressings, hot soaks, and topical medications are not useful).
- Discontinue potentially causative drugs.
- If specific cause is identified, treatment of the condition typically leads to resolution of EN.
- Indication for treatment is poorly defined in literature; hence, therapy specifically for EN is directed toward symptom management.

MEDICATION
First Line
- NSAIDs:
  - Ibuprofen 400 mg PO q4–6h (not to exceed 3,200 mg/day)
  - Indomethacin 25 to 50 mg PO TID
  - Naproxen 250 to 500 mg PO BID
- Precautions
  - GI upset/bleeding (avoid in Crohn or ulcerative colitis)
  - Fluid retention
  - Renal insufficiency
  - Dose reduction in elderly, especially those with renal disease, diabetes, or heart failure
  - May mask fever
  - NSAIDs can increase cardiovascular (CV) risk.
- Significant possible interactions
  - May blunt antihypertensive effects of diuretics and β-blockers
  - NSAIDs can elevate plasma lithium levels.
  - NSAIDs can cause significant elevation and prolongation of methotrexate levels.

Second Line
- Potassium iodide 400 to 900 mg/day divided BID or TID for 3 to 4 weeks (for persistent lesions); need to monitor for hyperthyroidism with prolonged use; pregnancy class D (6)[B]
- Corticosteroids for severe, refractory, or recurrent cases in which an infectious workup is negative. Prednisone 1 mg/kg/day for 1 to 2 weeks is the recommended dose/duration. Potential side effects include hyperglycemia, hypertension, weight gain, worsening gastroesophageal reflux disease, mood changes, bone loss, osteonecrosis, and proximal myopathy (2).

- For EN related to Behçet disease, one can also consider colchicine 0.6 to 1.2 mg BID. Potential side effects include GI upset and diarrhea (7)[B].

ADMISSION, INPATIENT, AND NURSING CONSIDERATIONS
Occasionally, admission may be needed for the antecedent illness (e.g., tuberculosis).

 ONGOING CARE

FOLLOW-UP RECOMMENDATIONS
- Keep legs elevated.
- Elastic wraps or support stockings may be helpful when patients are ambulating.

Patient Monitoring
Monthly follow-up or as dictated by underlying disorder

DIET
No restrictions

PATIENT EDUCATION
- Lesions will resolve over a few weeks to months.
- Scarring is unlikely.
- Joint aches and pains may persist.
- <20% recur.

PROGNOSIS
- Individual lesions resolve generally within 2 weeks.
- Total time course of 6 to 12 weeks but may vary with underlying disease
- Joint aches and pains may persist for years.
- Lesions do not scar.
- Recurrences: occurs over variable periods, averaging several years; seen most often in sarcoid, streptococcal infection, pregnancy, and oral contraceptive use. If medication induced, avoid recurrent exposure.

COMPLICATIONS
- Vary according to underlying disease
- None expected from lesions of EN

REFERENCES
1. Chowaniec M, Starba A, Wiland P. Erythema nodosum—review of the literature. *Reumatologia*. 2016;54(2):79–82.
2. Schwartz RA, Nervi SJ. Erythema nodosum: a sign of systemic disease. *Am Fam Physician*. 2007;75(5):695–700.
3. Cribier B, Caille A, Heid E, et al. Erythema nodosum and associated diseases. A study of 129 cases. *Int J Dermatol*. 1998;37(9):667–672.
4. Requena L, Yus ES. Erythema nodosum. *Dermatol Clin*. 2008;26(4):425–438.
5. Sánchez Yus E, Sanz Vico MD, de Diego V. Miescher's radial granuloma. A characteristic marker of erythema nodosum. *Am J Dermatopathol*. 1989;11(5):434–442.
6. Horio T, Imamura S, Danno K, et al. Potassium iodide in the treatment of erythema nodosum and nodular vasculitis. *Arch Dermatol*. 1981;117(1):29–31.
7. Yurdakul S, Mat C, Tüzün Y, et al. A double-blind trial of colchicine in Behçet's syndrome. *Arthritis Rheum*. 2001;44(11):2686–2692.

ADDITIONAL READING
- Bartyik K, Várkonyi A, Kirschner A, et al. Erythema nodosum in association with celiac disease. *Pediatr Dermatol*. 2004;21(3):227–230.
- Chong TA, Hansra NK, Ruben BS, et al. Diverticulitis: an inciting factor in erythema nodosum. *J Am Acad Dermatol*. 2012;67(1):e60–e62.
- Harris T, Henderson MC. Concurrent Sweet's syndrome and erythema nodosum. *J Gen Intern Med*. 2011;26(2):214–215.
- Jeon HC, Choi M, Paik SH, et al. A case of assisted reproductive therapy-induced erythema nodosum. *Ann Dermatol*. 2011;23(3):362–364.
- Then C, Langer A, Adam C, et al. Erythema nodosum associated with myelodysplastic syndrome: a case report. *Onkologie*. 2011;34(3):126–128.

CODES

ICD10
- L52 Erythema nodosum
- A18.4 Tuberculosis of skin and subcutaneous tissue

CLINICAL PEARLS
- Lesions of EN appear to be erythematous patches, but when palpated, their underlying nodularity is appreciated.
- Evaluation for a concerning underlying etiology is necessary in EN, but most cases are idiopathic.
- EN in the setting of hilar adenopathy may be seen with multiple etiologies and does not exclusively indicate sarcoidosis.
- In patients with a history of Hodgkin lymphoma, EN may be an early sign of recurrence.

E

ESOPHAGEAL VARICES

Maximos Attia, MD, FAAFP • Marcelle Meseeha, MD

BASICS

DESCRIPTION
- Dilated submucosal esophageal veins connecting the portal and systemic circulations
- Most commonly results from portal hypertension (typically a result of cirrhosis)
- Variceal rupture: most common fatal complication of cirrhosis; severity of liver disease correlates with presence of varices and risk of bleeding.

EPIDEMIOLOGY
Incidence
- 30% of cirrhotic patients have varices at the time of diagnosis; 90% at 10 years
- 1-year rate of first variceal bleeding is 5% for small varices, 15% for large varices.

Prevalence
- 50% of patients with esophageal varices experience bleeding at some point.
- Variceal bleeding: 10–20% mortality in the 6 weeks following the episode
- Gender: male > female

ETIOLOGY AND PATHOPHYSIOLOGY
- Portal hypertension causes the formation of portacaval anastomoses to decompress the portal circulation. This leads to a congested submucosal venous plexus with tortuous dilated veins, particularly in the distal esophagus. Variceal rupture results in hemorrhage.
- Pathophysiology of portal hypertension:
  - Increased resistance to portal flow at the level of hepatic sinusoids caused by
    o Intrahepatic vasoconstriction due to decreased nitric oxide production and increased release of endothelin-1 (ET-1), angiotensinogen, and eicosanoids
    o Sinusoidal remodeling causes disruption of blood flow.
  - Increased portal flow caused by hyperdynamic circulation due to splanchnic arterial vasodilation through mediators such as nitric oxide, prostacyclin, and TNF
- Causes of portal hypertension:
  - Prehepatic:
    o Extrahepatic portal vein obstruction (EHPVO)
    o Massive splenomegaly with increased splenic vein blood flow
  - Posthepatic:
    o Severe right-sided heart failure, constrictive pericarditis, and hepatic vein obstruction (Budd-Chiari syndrome)
  - Intrahepatic:
    o Cirrhosis (accounts for most cases of portal hypertension)
  - Less frequent causes are schistosomiasis, massive fatty change, diseases affecting portal microcirculation as nodular regenerative hyperplasia, and diffuse fibrosing granulomatous disease as sarcoidosis.

Genetics
Cirrhosis is rarely hereditary.

RISK FACTORS
- Cirrhosis
- In cirrhotic patients, thrombocytopenia and splenomegaly are independent predictors of esophageal varices.

- Noncirrhotic portal hypertension
- Increased bleeding risk for known varices is associated with varix size, endoscopic signs (red wale marks, cherry-red spots), vessel wall thickness, and abrupt increase in variceal pressure (i.e., Valsalva maneuver).
- MELD/Child-Pugh score; presence of portal vein thrombosis; high hepatic venous pressure gradient (HVPG)

GENERAL PREVENTION
Prevent underlying causes: Prevent alcohol abuse, administer hepatitis B vaccine, needle hygiene, intravenous (IV) drug use (needle exchange programs reduce risk of hepatitis); specific screening and therapy for hepatitis B and C, hemochromatosis

COMMONLY ASSOCIATED CONDITIONS
- Portal hypertensive gastropathy; varices in stomach, duodenum, colon, rectum (causes massive bleeding, unlike hemorrhoids); rarely at umbilicus (caput medusae) or ostomy sites
- Isolated gastric varices can occur due to splenic vein thrombosis/stenosis from hypercoagulability/contiguous inflammation (most commonly, chronic pancreatitis).
- Other complications of cirrhosis: hepatic encephalopathy, ascites, hepatorenal syndrome, spontaneous bacterial peritonitis, hepatocellular carcinoma

DIAGNOSIS
- First indication of varices is often GI bleeding: hematemesis, hematochezia, and/or melena.
- Occult bleeding (anemia): uncommon

HISTORY
- Underlying history of cirrhosis/liver disease. Variceal bleed can be initial presentation of previously undiagnosed cirrhosis.
- Alcohol abuse, exposure to blood-borne viruses through IV drug use or sexual practices
- Hematemesis, melena, or hematochezia
- Rapid upper GI bleed can present as rectal bleeding.

PHYSICAL EXAM
- Assess hemodynamic stability: hypotension, tachycardia (active bleeding).
- Abdominal exam—liver palpation/percussion (often small and firm with cirrhosis)
- Splenomegaly, ascites (shifting dullness; fluid shift; puddle splash—physical maneuvers have limited sensitivity)
- Visible abdominal periumbilical collateral circulation (caput medusae)
- Peripheral stigmata of alcohol abuse: spider angiomata on chest/back, palmar erythema, testicular atrophy, gynecomastia
- Rectal varices
- Hepatic encephalopathy; asterixis
- Blood on rectal exam

DIFFERENTIAL DIAGNOSIS
- Upper GI bleeding: 10–30% are due to varices.
  - In patients with known varices, as many as 50% bleed from nonvariceal sources.
  - Peptic ulcer; gastritis
  - Gastric/esophageal malignancy
  - Congestive gastropathy of portal hypertension

  - Arteriovenous malformation
  - Mallory-Weiss tears
  - Aortoenteric fistula
  - Hemoptysis; nosebleed
- Lower GI bleeding
  - Rectal varices; hemorrhoids
  - Colonic neoplasia
  - Diverticulosis/arteriovenous malformation
  - Rapidly bleeding upper GI site
- Continued/recurrent bleeding risk: actively bleeding/large varix, high Child-Pugh severity score, infection, renal failure

DIAGNOSTIC TESTS & INTERPRETATION
Initial Tests (lab, imaging)
- Anemia: Hemoglobin may be normal in active bleeding; may require 6 to 24 hours to equilibrate; other causes of anemia are common in patients with cirrhosis.
- Thrombocytopenia: most sensitive and specific parameter, correlates with portal hypertension, large esophageal varices
- Abnormal aspartate aminotransferase (AST), alanine aminotransferase (ALT), alkaline phosphatase, bilirubin; prolonged PT; low albumin suggests cirrhosis.
- BUN, creatinine (BUN often elevated in GI bleed)
- Sodium level; may drop in patients treated with terlipressin (1)[A]
- Noninvasive tests are preferred to rule out high-risk varices (HRVs) in patients with compensated cirrhosis (2)[B].
- Esophagogastroduodenoscopy (1)[A]
  - Can identify actively bleeding varices as well as large varices and stigmata of recent bleeding
  - Can be used to treat bleeding with esophageal band ligation (preferred to sclerotherapy); prevent rebleeding; detect gastric varices, portal hypertensive gastropathy; diagnose alternative bleeding sites
  - Can identify and treat nonbleeding varices (protruding submucosal veins in the distal third of the esophagus)

Diagnostic Procedures/Other
- Transient elastography (TE) for identifying CLD patients at risk for developing clinically significant portal hypertension (CSPH) (1)[A]
- HVPG >10 mm Hg: gold standard to diagnose CSPH (normal: 1 to 5 mm Hg) (1)[A]
- HVPG response of ≥10% or to ≤12 mm Hg to IV propranolol identifies responders to nonselective β-blocker (NSBB) and is linked to a decreased risk of variceal bleeding (1),(3)[A].
- Video capsule endoscopy screening as an alternative to traditional endoscopy
- Doppler sonography (second line): demonstrates patency, diameter, and flow in portal and splenic veins, and collaterals; sensitive for gastric varices; documents patency after ligation or transjugular intrahepatic portosystemic shunt (TIPS)
- CT- or MRI-angiography (second line, not routine): demonstrates large vascular channels in abdomen, mediastinum; demonstrates patency of intrahepatic portal and splenic vein
  - Venous-phase celiac arteriography: demonstrates portal vein and collaterals; hepatic vein occlusion
  - Portal pressure measurement using retrograde catheter in hepatic vein

E

TREATMENT

GENERAL MEASURES
- Treat underlying cirrhotic comorbidities.
- Variceal bleeding is often complicated by hepatic encephalopathy and infection.
- Active bleeding (2)
  - IV access, hemodynamic resuscitation
  - Type and crossmatch packed RBCs. Overtransfusion increases portal pressure and increases rebleeding risk.
  - Treat coagulopathy as necessary. Fresh frozen plasma may increase blood volume and increase rebleeding risk.
  - Avoid sedation, monitor mental status, and avoid nephrotoxic drugs and β-blockers acutely.
  - IV octreotide to lower portal venous pressure as adjuvant to endoscopic management; IV bolus of 50 μg followed by drip of 50 μg/hr
  - Terlipressin (alternative): 2 mg q4h IV for 24 to 48 hours and then 1 mg q4h
  - Erythromycin 250 mg IV 30 to 120 minutes before endoscopy (1)[A]
  - Urgent upper GI endoscopy for diagnosis and treatment
    - Variceal band ligation preferred to sclerotherapy for bleeding varices; also for nonbleeding medium-to-large varices to decrease bleeding risk
    - Ligation: lower rates of rebleeding, fewer complications, more rapid cessation of bleeding, higher rate of variceal eradication
- Repeat ligation/sclerosant for rebleeding.
- If endoscopic treatment fails, consider self-expanding esophageal metal stents or per oral placement of Sengstaken-Blakemore–type tube up to 24 hours to stabilize patient for TIPS (1)[C].
- As many as 2/3 of patients with variceal bleeding develop an infection, most commonly spontaneous bacterial peritonitis, UTI, or pneumonia; antibiotic prophylaxis with oral norfloxacin 400 mg or IV ceftriaxone 1 g q24h for up to a week
- In active bleeding, avoid β-blockers, which decrease BP and blunt the physiologic increase in heart rate during acute hemorrhage.
- Prevent recurrence of acute bleeding.
  - Vasoconstrictors: terlipressin, octreotide (reduce portal pressure)
  - Endoscopic band ligation (EBL): if bleeding recurs/portal pressure measurement shows portal pressure remains >12 mm Hg
  - TIPS: second-line therapy if above methods fail; TIPS decreases portal pressure by creating communication between hepatic vein and an intrahepatic portal vein branch.

MEDICATION
Primary prevention of variceal bleeding (4)[A]

- Endoscopy: assesses variceal size, presence of red wale sign (longitudinal variceal reddish streak that suggests either a recent bleed or a pending bleed) to determine risk stratification. F1 varices are small and straight; F2 varices are enlarged and tortuous-occupying <1/3 of the esophageal lumen; F3 varices are enlarged, coiled in appearance and occupy over a third of the esophageal lumen. F2 and F3 varices are managed similarly.
  - Primary prophylaxis: (i) NSBB; (ii) endoscopic variceal ligation (EVL)

- Endoscopy every 2 to 3 years if cirrhosis but no varices; every 1 to 2 years if small varices and not receiving β-blockers (3)[A]

First Line
- Not actively bleeding. NSBB reduce portal pressure and decrease risk of first bleed from 25% to 15% when used as primary prophylaxis; beneficial in cirrhosis with small varices and increased hemorrhage risk as well as cirrhosis with medium-to-large varices (3),(4)[A]
- Carvedilol: 6.25 mg daily (3)[A] is more effective than NSBB in dropping HVPG (1)[A].
  - Propranolol: 20 mg BID increase until heart rate decreased by 25% from baseline
  - Nadolol 80 mg daily; increase as above
  - Contraindications: severe asthma
- Chronic prevention of rebleeding (secondary prevention): NSBBs and EBL reduce rate of rebleeding to a similar extent, but β-blockers reduce mortality, whereas ligation does not (5)[A].

Second Line
Obliterate varices with esophageal ligation if not tolerant of medication prophylaxis.

- During ligation: proton pump inhibitors, such as lansoprazole 30 mg/day, until varices obliterated
- Management of Budd-Chiari syndrome: anticoagulation, angioplasty/thrombolysis, TIPS, and orthotopic liver transplantation (1)[C]
- Management of EHPVO: anticoagulation (1)[B]; mesenteric-left portal vein bypass (meso-Rex procedure) (1)[C]

ISSUES FOR REFERRAL
Refer for endoscopy, liver transplant, and interventional radiology for TIPS.

ADDITIONAL THERAPIES
Pneumococcal and hepatitis A/B vaccine (HAV/HBV)

SURGERY/OTHER PROCEDURES
- Esophageal transection: in rare cases of uncontrollable, exsanguinating bleeding
- Liver transplantation

ONGOING CARE

FOLLOW-UP RECOMMENDATIONS
Patient Monitoring
- Endoscopic variceal ligation, every 1 to 4 weeks, until varices eradicated
- If TIPS, repeat endoscopy to assess rebleeding.
- Endoscopic screening in patients with known cirrhosis every 2 to 3 years; yearly in patients with decompensated cirrhosis (1)[C]
- Patients with a liver stiffness <20 kPa and with platelets >150,000 can avoid endoscopic screening (1)[A] and may follow up by annual TE and platelet count (1)[C].

PATIENT EDUCATION
National Digestive Diseases Information Clearinghouse (http://www.niddk.nih.gov/health -information/health-topics/digestive-diseases/Pages /default.aspx) or American Liver Foundation (http://www.liverfoundation.org/)

PROGNOSIS
- In cirrhosis, 1-year survival is 50% for those who survive at least 2 weeks following a variceal bleed.
- In-hospital mortality remains high and is related to severity of underlying cirrhosis, ranging from 0% in Child-Pugh class A disease to 32% in Child-Pugh class C disease.
- Prognosis in noncirrhotic portal fibrosis is better than for cirrhotic portal fibrosis.

COMPLICATIONS
- Formation of gastric varices after eradication of esophageal varices
- Esophageal varices can recur.
- Hepatic encephalopathy, renal dysfunction, hepatorenal syndrome
- Infections after banding/ligation of varices

REFERENCES
1. de Franchis R; and Baveno VI Faculty. Expanding consensus in portal hypertension: report of the Baveno VI Consensus Workshop: stratifying risk and individualizing care for portal hypertension. *J Hepatol*. 2015;63(3):743–752.
2. Jakab SS, Garcia-Tsao G. Evaluation and management of esophageal and gastric varices in patients with cirrhosis. *Clin Liver Dis*. 2020;24(3):335–350.
3. Simonetto DA, Liu M, Kamath PS. Portal hypertension and related complications: diagnosis and management. *Mayo Clin Proc*. 2019;94(4):714–726.
4. Simonetto DA, Shah VH, Kamath PS. Primary prophylaxis of variceal bleeding. *Clin Liver Dis*. 2014;18(2):335–345.
5. Albillos A, Tejedor M. Secondary prophylaxis for esophageal variceal bleeding. *Clin Liver Dis*. 2014;18(2):359–370.

CODES

ICD10
- I85.0 Esophageal varices
- I85 Esophageal varices
- I85.1 Secondary esophageal varices

CLINICAL PEARLS

- Thrombocytopenia is the most sensitive marker of increased portal pressure and large esophageal varices.
- Roughly half of all patients with cirrhosis will have esophageal varices. One in three of those patients with varices will experience a variceal bleed.
- The risk of bleeding relates directly to the size and appearance of the esophageal varices.
- β-Blockers (nadolol; propranolol; carvedilol) act to reduce pressure in the portal circulation and are the preferred pharmacologic choice for primary prevention of variceal bleeding.
- In acute bleeding, avoid β-blockers.
- In acute bleeding, overtransfusion can elevate portal pressure and increase bleeding risk.

ESSENTIAL TREMOR SYNDROME

Jennifer E. Svarverud, DO

BASICS

DESCRIPTION
- A postural (occurring with voluntary maintenance of a position against gravity) or kinetic (occurring during voluntary movement) flexion–extension tremor that is slow and rhythmic and primarily affects the hands, forearms, head, or voice with a frequency of 4 to 12 Hz
- Older patients tend to have lower frequency tremors, whereas younger patients exhibit frequencies in the higher range.
- May be familial, sporadic, or associated with other movement disorders
- Incidence and prevalence increase with age, but symptom onset can occur at any age.
- The tremor can be intermittent and exacerbated by emotional or physical stressors, fatigue, and caffeine.
- System(s) affected include neurologic, musculoskeletal, ear/nose/throat (ENT) (voice).

EPIDEMIOLOGY
Essential tremor is the most common pathologic tremor in humans.

Incidence
- Can occur at any age but bimodal peaks exist in the 2nd and 6th decades
- Incidence rises significantly after age 49 years.

Prevalence
The overall prevalence for essential tremor has been estimated between 0.4% and 0.9% but is increased in older patients with an estimated prevalence of 4.6% at age 65 years and up to 22% at age 95 years.

ETIOLOGY AND PATHOPHYSIOLOGY
- Suspected to originate from an abnormal oscillation within thalamocortical and cerebello-olivary loops, as lesions in these areas tend to reduce essential tremor
- Essential tremor is not a homogenous disorder; many patients have other motor manifestations and nonmotor features, including cognitive and psychiatric symptoms.

Genetics
- Positive family history in 50–70% of patients; autosomal dominant inheritance is demonstrated in many families with poor penetrance. Twin studies suggest that environmental factors are also involved.
- A link to genetic loci exists on chromosomes 2p22–2p25, 3q13, and 6p23. In addition, a Ser9Gly variant in the dopamine D_3 receptor gene on 3q13 has been suggested as a risk factor.

COMMONLY ASSOCIATED CONDITIONS
- Can be present in 10% of patients with Parkinson disease (PD); characteristics of PD that distinguish it from essential tremor include 3- to 5-Hz resting tremor; accompanying rigidity, bradykinesia, or postural instability; and no change with alcohol consumption

- Patients with essential tremor have a 4% risk of developing PD.
- Resting tremor, typically of the arm, may be seen in up to 20–30% of patients with essential tremor. Although action tremor is the hallmark feature of essential tremor, it is commonly found in patients with PD as well.

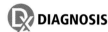

DIAGNOSIS

HISTORY
- Core criteria for diagnosis
  - Bilateral action (postural or kinetic) tremor of the hands and forearms that is most commonly asymmetric
  - Absence of other neurologic signs, with the exception of cogwheel phenomenon
  - May have tremor in other locations to include head, voice or lower limbs
  - Symptoms present for at least 3 years' duration
- Secondary criteria include positive family history and beneficial response to alcohol.

PHYSICAL EXAM
- Tremor can affect upper limbs (~95% of patients).
- Less commonly, the tremor affects head (~34%), lower limbs (~30%), voice (~12%), tongue (~7%), face (~5%), and trunk (~5%).

DIFFERENTIAL DIAGNOSIS
- PD
- Enhanced physiologic tremor
- Wilson disease
- Hyperthyroidism
- Multiple sclerosis
- Dystonic tremor
- Cerebellar tremor
- Asterixis
- Psychogenic tremor
- Orthostatic tremor
- Drug-induced or enhanced physiologic tremor (amiodarone, cimetidine, lamotrigine, itraconazole, valproic acid, SSRIs, steroids, lithium, cyclosporine, β-adrenergic agonists, ephedrine, theophylline, tricyclic antidepressants [TCAs], antipsychotics)

DIAGNOSTIC TESTS & INTERPRETATION
Initial Tests (lab, imaging)
- No specific biologic marker or diagnostic test is available.
- Ceruloplasmin and serum copper to rule out Wilson disease
- Thyroid-stimulating hormone to rule out thyroid dysfunction
- Serum electrolytes, blood urea nitrogen (BUN), creatinine
- Brain MRI usually is not necessary or indicated unless Wilson disease is found or exam findings imply central lesion.

Diagnostic Procedures/Other
- Accelerometry evaluates tremor frequency and amplitude; >95% of PD cases exhibit frequencies in the 4- to 6-Hz range, and 95% of essential tremor cases exhibit frequencies in the 5- to 8-Hz range.
- Surface electromyography is less helpful in distinguishing essential tremor from PD.

Test Interpretation
Posture-related tremor seen on exam

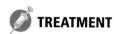

TREATMENT

MEDICATION
Pharmacologic treatment should be considered when tremor interferes with activities of daily living (ADLs) or causes psychological distress.

First Line
- Propranolol 60 to 320 mg/day in divided doses or in long-acting formulation reduces limb tremor magnitude by ~50%, and almost 70% of patients experience improvement in clinical rating scales. There is insufficient evidence to recommend propranolol for vocal tremor. Single doses of propranolol, taken before social situations that are likely to exacerbate tremor, are useful for some patients.
- Primidone 25 mg at bedtime, gradually titrated to 150 to 300 mg at bedtime, improves tremor amplitude by 40–50%. Maximum dose is 750 mg/day, with doses >250 mg/day typically divided to BID or TID. Low-dose therapy (<250 mg/day) is just as effective as high-dose (750 mg/day) therapy.
- Propranolol and primidone have similar efficacy when used as initial therapy for limb tremor; both carry a level A recommendation (1)[A].
- 30–50% of patients will not respond to either propranolol or primidone.

Second Line
- Topiramate at a mean dose of 292 mg/day demonstrated significantly greater reduction in Tremor Rating Scale (TRS) compared with placebo (7.70 vs. 0.08; $p < .005$; baseline TRS = 37.0) in a small study combining results of three double-blind, randomized, controlled trials following a common protocol. Use is limited by dropout rates as high as 40% due to appetite suppression, weight loss, paresthesias, and concentration difficulties (2)[B].
- Gabapentin up to 400 mg TID (3)[B]
- Sotalol, nadolol, and atenolol are alternative β-blockers; each has less evidence than propranolol to support use.
- Clonazepam and alprazolam should be used with caution because of potential abuse.
- Clozapine has shown efficacy at doses of 6 to 75 mg/day but is recommended only for refractory cases of limb tremor because of a 1% risk of agranulocytosis. The American Academy of Neurology (AAN) indicates that insufficient evidence exists to support or refute the efficacy of clozapine for chronic use (1)[A].

- Memantine, in a pilot study using doses up to 40 mg/day, showed significant benefit in a small subset of the study group. Adverse events at this dose included dizziness, somnolence, and poor energy (4)[B].
- Pramipexole, at a dose of 2.1 mg/day, demonstrated moderate efficacy in reducing severity of tremor in a pilot study of 29 patients. Immediate- and extended-release formulations were equally effective (5)[B].
- Levetiracetam and 3,4-diaminopyridine are probably ineffective at reducing limb tremor and should not be considered according to the AAN (1)[A].
- Other medications that have been evaluated for treatment of essential tremor, with limited data to support their use, include acetazolamide, clonidine, flunarizine, methazolamide, nimodipine, olanzapine, phenobarbital, pregabalin, quetiapine, sodium oxybate, and zonisamide (1)[A].
- Alcohol may provide transient improvement in symptoms, but its brief duration of action, subsequent rebound, and associated risk of developing alcohol addiction make it a less attractive option for longer term treatment. Alcohol may be an appropriate option for short-term, situation-specific improvement in symptoms.
- Botulinum toxin A injections should be offered as a treatment option for cervical dystonia (level A recommendation from AAN) and may be offered for blepharospasm, focal upper extremity dystonia, adductor laryngeal dystonia, and upper extremity essential tremor. Limited data support its use for head and vocal tremor (6)[B].

ISSUES FOR REFERRAL
Referral to a neurologist can help to differentiate those with dystonia, neuropathic tremor, PD, or drug-induced tremor.

SURGERY/OTHER PROCEDURES
- Deep brain stimulation provides a magnitude of benefit that is superior to all available medications and may be used to treat medically refractory limb tremor; it has fewer adverse effects than thalamotomy.
- Bilateral thalamic ventral intermediate nucleus stimulation is effective in reducing tremor and functional disability; however, paresthesias and dysarthria are possible complications.
- Unilateral thalamotomy may be used to treat limb tremor that is refractory to medical management.
- Bilateral thalamotomy is not recommended because of adverse side effects.
- There is growing interest in development of external neuromodulator devices for the treatment of essential tremor to include exoskeletons, orthosis and biomechanical loading. Currently evidence for these devices is limited, of low quality, and further research is needed.

COMPLEMENTARY & ALTERNATIVE MEDICINE
Physical therapy may be considered for strengthening and training in use of weighted utensils to help offset tremor. Although strength training has not been shown to have improvement in functional ability, no negative effects have been reported.

 ## ONGOING CARE

DIET
Avoid caffeine.

PATIENT EDUCATION
Although essential tremor can cause significant impairment in daily functioning, it does not decrease life expectancy.

PROGNOSIS
Tremor tends to worsen with age, increasing in amplitude.

REFERENCES

1. Zesiewicz TA, Elble RJ, Louis ED, et al. Evidence-based guideline update: treatment of essential tremor: report of the Quality Standards Subcommittee of the American Academy of Neurology. *Neurology*. 2011;77(19):1752–1755.
2. Connor GS, Edwards K, Tarsy D. Topiramate in essential tremor: findings from double-blind, placebo-controlled, crossover trials. *Clin Neuropharmacol*. 2008;31(2):97–103.
3. Gironell A, Kulisevsky J, Barbanoj M, et al. A randomized placebo-controlled comparative trial of gabapentin and propranolol in essential tremor. *Arch Neurol*. 1999;56(4):475–480.
4. Handforth A, Bordelon Y, Frucht SJ, et al. A pilot efficacy and tolerability trial of memantine for essential tremor. *Clin Neuropharmacol*. 2010;33(5):223–226.
5. Herceg M, Nagy F, Pál E, et al. Pramipexole may be an effective treatment option in essential tremor. *Clin Neuropharmacol*. 2012;35(2):73–76.
6. Simpson DM, Blitzer A, Brashear A, et al; for Therapeutics and Technology Assessment Subcommittee of the American Academy of Neurology. Assessment: botulinum neurotoxin for the treatment of movement disorders (an evidence-based review): report of the Therapeutics and Technology Assessment Subcommittee of the American Academy of Neurology. *Neurology*. 2008;70(19):1699–1706.

ADDITIONAL READING

- Bain P, Brin M, Deuschl G, et al. Criteria for the diagnosis of essential tremor. *Neurology*. 2000;54(11 Suppl 4):S7.
- Bhatia KP, Bain P, Bajaj N, et al. Consensus statement on the classification of tremors from the task force on tremor of the International Parkinson and Movement Disorder Society. *Mov Disord*. 2018;33(1):75–87.

- Buijink AW, Contarino MF, Koelman JH, et al. How to tackle tremor—systematic review of the literature and diagnostic work-up. *Front Neurol*. 2012;3:146.
- Castrillo-Fraile V, Peña EC, Gabriel Y Galán JMT, et al. Tremor control devices for essential tremor: a systematic literature review. *Tremor Other Hyperkinet Mov (NY)*. 2019;9:10.
- Deuschl G, Raethjen J, Hellriegel H, et al. Treatment of patients with essential tremor. *Lancet Neurol*. 2011;10(2):148–161.
- Elias WJ, Shah BB. Tremor. *JAMA*. 2014;311(9):948–954.
- Flora ED, Perera CL, Cameron AL, et al. Deep brain stimulation for essential tremor: a systematic review. *Mov Disord*. 2010;25(11):1550–1559.
- O'Connor RJ, Kini MU. Non-pharmacological and non-surgical interventions for tremor: a systematic review. *Parkinsonism Relat Disord*. 2011;17(7):509–515.
- Schuurman PR, Bosch DA, Bossuyt PM, et al. A comparison of continuous thalamic stimulation and thalamotomy for suppression of severe tremor. *N Engl J Med*. 2000;342(7):461–468.
- Sullivan KL, Hauser RA, Zesiewicz TA. Essential tremor Epidemiology, diagnosis, and treatment. *Neurologist*. 2004;10(5):250–258.
- Thenganatt MA, Louis ED. Distinguishing essential tremor from Parkinson's disease: bedside tests and laboratory evaluations. *Expert Rev Neurother*. 2012;12(6):687–696.
- Zeuner KE, Deuschl G. An update on tremors. *Curr Opin Neurol*. 2012;25(4):475–482.

 ## CODES

ICD10
G25.0 Essential tremor

CLINICAL PEARLS

- Core criteria for diagnosis of essential tremor include bilateral action or postural tremor of the hands, forearm, and/or head without a resting component present for at least 3 years.
- Beneficial response to alcohol and positive family history help to differentiate essential tremor from PD (PD is characterized by tremor at rest, bradykinesia, and rigidity, and it does not improve with alcohol use).
- 10% of patients with PD will have both resting tremors of PD and essential tremor.
- Wilson disease, thyroid disease, and medication effect should be ruled out.
- Brain MRI is usually not necessary or indicated.
- First-line treatments include propranolol and primidone. 30–50% of patients will not benefit from these first-line treatments.

EUSTACHIAN TUBE DYSFUNCTION

Roland W. Newman II, DO

BASICS

The eustachian tube (ET), also known as the auditory or pharyngotympanic tube, connects the posterior nasopharynx to the middle ear. The proximal two-thirds of the ET is composed of cartilage, whereas the distal third closest to the middle ear is made of bone. Its primary function is to equilibrate pressure within the middle ear to atmospheric pressure. It also ventilates and drains the middle ear space which prevents and clears infection and debris. When the ET malfunctions by either becoming too dilated (patulous dysfunction) or occluded (obstructive dysfunction), it results in ET dysfunction (ETD).

DESCRIPTION
- A spectrum of disorders involving impairment of the functional valve of the ET
- ETD can be classified as *patulous dysfunction*, in which the ET is excessively open, or *dilatory dysfunction*, in which there is failure of the tubes to dilate (i.e., open) appropriately.
- Pathophysiology related to pressure dysregulation, impaired protection secondary to reflux of irritating material into the middle ear, or impaired clearance by the mucociliary system
- May occur in the setting of pressure changes (e.g., scuba diving or air travel) or acute upper airway inflammation (e.g., allergic or infectious rhinosinusitis, acute otitis media [OM])
- Chronic ETD may lead to a retracted tympanic membrane, recurrent serous effusion, recurrent OM, adhesive OM, chronic mastoiditis, or cholesteatoma.
- Synonym(s): auditory tube dysfunction; ET disorder; blocked ET; patulous ET

ALERT
Sudden sensorineural hearing loss (SSNHL) can be misdiagnosed as ETD.

- A simple 512-Hz tuning fork test lateralizes to the opposite ear in SSNHL and to the affected ear in ETD with conductive hearing loss.
- Any SSNHL is a medical emergency and should be referred to an otolaryngologist immediately.

EPIDEMIOLOGY
Adults: >2 million health care visits annually
- Median age: 48
- Females > males
- Most common comorbidity is acute rhinitis.

ETIOLOGY AND PATHOPHYSIOLOGY
- Under normal circumstances, the ET is closed, opening to release a small amount of air to equilibrate middle ear pressure with surrounding atmospheric pressure.
- ETD is failure of the ET, palate, nasal cavities, and nasopharynx to regulate middle ear and mastoid pressure.
- ET functions:
  - Ventilation/regulation of middle ear pressure
  - Protection from nasopharyngeal secretions
  - Drainage of middle ear fluid
  - ET is closed at rest and opens with yawning, swallowing, and chewing.

- Cycle of dysfunction: structural or functional obstruction of the ET:
  - Negative pressure develops in middle ear.
  - Serous exudate is drawn to the middle ear by negative pressure or refluxed into the middle ear if the ET opens momentarily.
  - Infection of static fluid causes edema and release of inflammatory mediators, exacerbating the cycle of inflammation and obstruction.
- In children, a horizontal and shorter ET predisposes to difficulties with ventilation and drainage.
- Adenoid hypertrophy can block the torus tubarius (proximal opening of the ET).
- In adults, paradoxical closing of the ET with swallowing occurs in a majority of affected patients.
- Tumors that impair/occlude the ET or that invade the tensor veli palatini to impair normal swallow regulation can also lead to dysfunction.

Genetics
Twin studies show a genetic component. Specific genetic cause is undefined.

RISK FACTORS
Adult and pediatric:
- Allergic rhinitis, tobacco exposure, GERD, chronic sinusitis, adenoid hypertrophy or nasopharyngeal mass, neuromuscular disease, altered immunity
- Prematurity and low birth weight, young age, daycare, crowded living conditions, low socioeconomic status, prone sleeping position, prolonged bottle use, craniofacial abnormalities (e.g., cleft palate, Down syndrome)

Pregnancy Considerations
ETD may be exacerbated by rhinitis of pregnancy; symptoms resolve postpartum.

GENERAL PREVENTION
- Control of upper airway inflammation: allergies, infectious rhinosinusitis, GERD
- Autoinsufflation of middle ear (i.e., blow gently against pinched nostril and closed mouth)
- Avoid atmospheric pressure changes (e.g., plane flight, scuba diving) in the setting of acute allergy exacerbation or URI.
- Avoid exposure to environmental irritants: tobacco smoke and pollutants.

COMMONLY ASSOCIATED CONDITIONS
- Hearing loss
- OM: acute, chronic, and serous
- Chronic mastoiditis
- Cholesteatoma
- Allergic rhinitis
- Chronic sinusitis/URI
- Adenoid hypertrophy
- GERD
- Cleft palate
- Down syndrome
- Obesity
- Nasopharyngeal carcinoma or other tumor

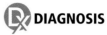

DIAGNOSIS

HISTORY
- Symptoms of ear pain, fullness, "plugging," hearing loss, tinnitus, popping or snapping noises, and vertigo
  - Unilateral or bilateral. Evaluate adults with persistent unilateral symptoms for nasopharyngeal tumor.
  - History of previous ear infections, surgeries, head trauma, recent flying or diving
  - Voice change (hypo- or hypernasal voice, consider NP mass or palatal dysfunction)
  - Differentiate patulous dysfunction, in which patient's own voice and breath sounds are amplified (autophony), from dilatory dysfunction, in which patient complains more of ear pain, "plugged" ear, hearing loss, and tinnitus.
- ETDQ-7 is a questionnaire that attempts to quantify ETD in adult patients. Based on presence and intensity of symptoms in past 1 month, severity is rated on 1 to 7 scale. A total score >14.5 categorizes patient as having ETD (1)[B],(2)[B].
  - Pressure in ears in past 1 month?
  - Pain in ears in past 1 month?
  - A feeling that ears are clogged or "under water"?
  - Ear symptoms when you have cold or sinusitis?
  - Crackling or popping sounds in the ears?
  - Ringing in ears?
  - A feeling that your hearing is muffled?

PHYSICAL EXAM
- Pneumatic otoscopy: retracted tympanic membrane, effusion, decreased drum movement
- Toynbee maneuver: View changes of the drum while patient autoinsufflates against closed lips and pinched nostrils; may show various degrees of retraction
  - Entire drum may be retracted and "lateralize" with insufflation.
  - Posterosuperior quadrant (pars flaccida) may form a retraction pocket.
- Tuning fork tests: 512-Hz fork placed on the forehead lateralizes to affected ear (Weber test); the fork will be louder behind the ear on the mastoid than in front of the ear (bone conduction > air conduction, Rinne test) in conductive hearing loss.
- Nasopharyngoscopy: adenoid hypertrophy or nasopharyngeal mass
- Anterior rhinoscopy: deviated nasal septum, polyps, mucosal hypertrophy, turbinate hypertrophy

DIFFERENTIAL DIAGNOSIS
- SSNHL (a medical emergency)
- Tympanic membrane perforation
- Barotrauma
- Temporomandibular joint disorder
- Ménière disease
- Superior semicircular canal dehiscence

DIAGNOSTIC TESTS & INTERPRETATION

Initial Tests (lab, imaging)

- No routine radiologic studies needed if clinical signs/symptoms suggest ETD
- CT scan (not necessary) may show changes related to OM or middle ear/mastoid opacification.
- Functional MRI might determine cause of ETD (in recalcitrant cases), as the ET opening can be visualized during Valsalva.

Diagnostic Procedures/Other

- Audiogram may show conductive hearing loss.
- Tympanometry: Type B or C tympanograms indicate fluid or retraction, respectively; negative middle ear peak pressures seen even with normal (type A) tympanograms

TREATMENT

- Due to limited high-quality evidence, it is difficult to recommend any one treatment option/intervention as superior (3).
- Use of a "nasal balloon" shown effective for clearing OM with effusion; unclear of benefit for ETD
- General principle is to remove or fix the underlying cause (e.g., infection, tumor, perforation of TM, restore tensor palatini muscle) and reduce or eliminate the cycle of infection/inflammation.
- Although no evidence exists, some consider antibiotics for acute OM; decongestants, nasal steroids, antihistamines (if allergic rhinitis is present), and surgery/procedures for recalcitrant cases
- Tympanostomy tubes ± adenoidectomy when indicated for recurrent ear infections or severe progressive retractions

MEDICATION

- Antibiotics only if infection is suspected as cause of ETD (4)[A]
- Few data support pharmacologic treatments such as decongestants, nasal steroids, or antihistamines for ETD.
- Medications treat comorbid conditions.
- Decongestants, topical, oral
  - Avoid prolonged use (>3 days); can cause rhinitis medicamentosa
  - Decongestants are most useful for acute ETD related to a resolving URI.
  - Decongestants are not typically used for relief of chronic ETD in children.
    - Phenylephrine
    - Pseudoephedrine
    - Oxymetazoline
- Nasal steroids (may be beneficial for those with allergic rhinitis) (5)[A]
  - Beclomethasone (Beconase, Vancenase)
  - Budesonide (Rhinocort)
  - Fluticasone propionate (Flonase)
  - Mometasone (Nasonex)
  - Triamcinolone (Nasacort)

- 2nd-generation H1 antihistamines (may be beneficial for those with ETD and chronic rhinitis)
  - Cetirizine (Zyrtec) (tablets, chewable tablets, liquid)
  - Desloratadine (Clarinex) (tablets, RediTabs, liquid)
  - Fexofenadine (Allegra) (tablets, RediTabs, liquid)
  - Levocetirizine (Xyzal) (tablets, liquid)
- Antihistamine nasal sprays (may be beneficial for those with ETD and chronic rhinitis)
  - Azelastine (Astepro or Astelin)
  - Olopatadine (Patanase)

ADDITIONAL THERAPIES

- Any activity that promotes swallowing, such as chewing gum, eating or drinking, can open the ET and promote relief of symptoms.
- Patients with ETD should refrain from flying during times of nasal congestion or ear infection. If the patient must fly, advise them to take oral and intranasal decongestants an hour prior to take off.
- Patients should refrain from scuba diving.

SURGERY/OTHER PROCEDURES

- Myringotomy and pressure equalization tube placement to ventilate middle ear, relieve pressure, and prevent sequelae of chronically retracted drum
- Patients with ETD during pressure changes may benefit from minimally invasive laser eustachian tuboplasty.
- Balloon tuboplasty (limited data in terms of efficacy, safety, and long-term outcomes) (6)[B]
- Adenoidectomy, if hypertrophied tissue is present
  - In children, first set of tubes are typically placed alone. Adenoidectomy is performed with second set of tubes if problems recur.
  - Some advocate adenoidectomy even in absence of excess tissue; reduces frequency and number of subsequent tubes

COMPLEMENTARY & ALTERNATIVE MEDICINE

Osteopathic manipulative treatment (OMT) can be utilized in the treatment of ETD.

- Galbreath technique
- Modified Muncie technique (7)

ONGOING CARE

FOLLOW-UP RECOMMENDATIONS

- Monitor pressure equalization tubes every 6 to 8 months in children and every 6 to 12 months in adults.
- Monitor tympanic membrane retraction pocket for progression every 6 to 12 months to allow for early intervention for progression in hearing loss, obvious ossicular erosion, or cholesteatoma.

DIET

Breastfeeding is associated with lower incidence of ETD and OM.

PROGNOSIS

If symptoms of ETD persist beyond age 7 years, patient is more likely to have long-term problems and requires regular monitoring.

COMPLICATIONS

Morbidity related to hearing compromise or associated sequela of chronic ear infections

REFERENCES

1. McCoul ED, Anand VK, Christos PJ. Validating the clinical assessment of eustachian tube dysfunction: the Eustachian Tube Dysfunction Questionnaire (ETDQ-7). Laryngoscope. 2012;122(5):1137–1141.
2. Van Roeyen S, Van de Heyning P, Van Rompaey V. Value and discriminative power of the seven-item Eustachian Tube Dysfunction Questionnaire. Laryngoscope. 2015;125(11):2553–2556.
3. Norman G, Llewellyn A, Harden M, et al. Systematic review of the limited evidence base for treatments of eustachian tube dysfunction: a health technology assessment. Clin Otolaryngol. 2014;39(1):6–21.
4. van Zon A, van der Heijden GJ, van Dongen TM, et al. Antibiotics for otitis media with effusion in children. Cochrane Database Syst Rev. 2012;(9):CD009163.
5. Simpson SA, Lewis R, van der Voort J, et al. Oral or topical nasal steroids for hearing loss associated with otitis media with effusion in children. Cochrane Database Syst Rev. 2011;(5):CD001935.
6. Gürtler N, Husner A, Flurin H. Balloon dilation of the eustachian tube: early outcome analysis. Otol Neurotol. 2015;36(3):437–443.
7. Channell MK. Modified Muncie technique: osteopathic manipulation for eustachian tube dysfunction and illustrative report of case. J Am Osteopath Assoc. 2008;108(5):260–263.

 SEE ALSO

Algorithm: Ear Pain/Otalgia

CODES

ICD10

- H69.90 Unspecified Eustachian tube disorder, unspecified ear
- H69.00 Patulous Eustachian tube, unspecified ear
- H68.109 Unspecified obstruction of Eustachian tube, unspecified ear

CLINICAL PEARLS

- ETD can be acute or chronic. Treatment is based on the underlying etiology.
- Rule out SSNHL (medical emergency), which can be misdiagnosed as ETD, especially in patients with unilateral symptoms.

FACTOR V LEIDEN

Elyas Parsa, DO • Viktor Limanskiy, MD

BASICS

DESCRIPTION
- Factor V Leiden is a genetic point mutation in the F5 gene at the activated protein C (APC) cleavage site on the factor V and Va molecule leading to increase in thrombin and as a result leads to clot formation. This is the most common form of inherited thrombophilia.
- System(s) affected: cardiovascular, gastrointestinal, hemo/lymphatic/immunologic, nervous, pulmonary, reproductive
- Synonym(s): factor V Leiden thrombophilia; factor V Leiden mutation, hereditary APC resistance

Pediatric Considerations
- The incidence of venous thrombosis in healthy children is extremely low (0.07/100,000 per year).
- Potential for increased thrombosis risk in patients with factor V Leiden and concomitant risks
- There is a weak, however significant, association between procoagulant states (including factor V Leiden) and coronary events in younger patients.

Pregnancy Considerations
- Recurrent pregnancy loss is a possible complication.
- Increased thrombotic risk in pregnancy and postpartum (additive) especially in homozygous state
- Possible increased risk of IUGR, preeclampsia, placental abruption: evidence mixed
- Women with a history of adverse pregnancy outcomes should be tested for thrombophilia if they are planning a future pregnancy (1).

EPIDEMIOLOGY
Prevalence
- Studies estimate ~5–8% occurrence of heterozygosity in Caucasians, Hispanic Americans ~2%, African American ~1%, and Asian Americans ~0.45% of those heterozygous for factor V Leiden small percentage of individuals develop venous thromboembolism (VTE), estimated 5–10%
- General population 4–5% without history of VTE. Higher prevalence 12–14% reported in parts of Greece, Sweden, and Lebanon. No reports seen in Chinese or Japanese.

ETIOLOGY AND PATHOPHYSIOLOGY
- Factor V is a protein that is part of the clotting cascade that circulates in the plasma. When exposed to tissue factor, factor V amplifies the production of thrombin, which further promotes clotting by activating factor V into procoagulant factor Va.
- For balance, thrombin also promotes APC production, which will cleave and inactivate factor V, Va, and VIII, thereby keeping the clotting cascade in check (negative feedback loop).
- In factor V Leiden, a point mutation at the binding site of APC (Arg506Glu) renders it less able to cleave factor V or Va. This, in turn, reduces the anticoagulant role of factor V as a cofactor to APC and increases the *procoagulant* role of activated factor V because there is now 20-fold slower degradation of factor Va.

RISK FACTORS
- Risk for VTE is ~7-fold in heterozygous and ~80-fold in homozygous factor V Leiden individuals, compared with individuals without the mutation. This risk is compounded/increased by the presence of the following:
  - Having non-O blood type (A, B, or AB): 2- to 4-fold
  - Oral contraceptives: homozygotes up to 100-fold; heterozygotes, 35-fold. The increased risk is halved when the patient uses desogestrel-containing oral contraceptives.

- Hormone replacement therapy (HRT) and selective estrogen receptor modulators (SERMs) both increase the risk of thrombosis; in patients with factor V Leiden, that risk is compounded.
  - In men with an underlying thrombophilia, testosterone therapy can promote VTE.
  - Pregnancy and *homozygous* factor V Leiden increase the risk of thrombosis 7- to 16-fold during pregnancy and the puerperium.
  - Those with combined thrombophilias and end-stage renal disease are at risk for developing calciphylaxis.
  - 30% of patients with VTE thrombosis is attributed to factor V Leiden and prothrombin G2021A mutation; however, the risk is weaker compared to antithrombin III, protein C, and protein S deficiency, which is around 1% in the general population.
- Data are conflicting with regard to risk for recurrent VTE for patients with factor V Leiden but trend toward an increased risk.
- It's been shown, factor V Leiden versus general population, a modest increase in the recurrence risk of VTE is seen.

GENERAL PREVENTION

ALERT
Patients with factor V Leiden without thrombosis do not require prophylactic anticoagulation.

COMMONLY ASSOCIATED CONDITIONS
Venous thrombosis

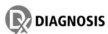

DIAGNOSIS

HISTORY
- It is critical to differentiate between provoked and unprovoked VTE and determine family history, risk factors, detailed symptoms.
- In up to 70% of patients suffering from VTE, a provoking factor is present.
- Isolated PE without evidence of DVT, however, is less common than general population; this phenomenon is known as "factor V Leiden paradox."
- There is no clinical feature specific for factor V Leiden. Most patient are asymptomatic until they develop thrombosis.
- Recurrent pregnancy loss
- Family history of thrombosis
- Family history of factor V Leiden mutation

PHYSICAL EXAM
- No physical exam finding specific to factor V Leiden
- Findings suggestive of VTE in any form (DVT, PE, cerebral thrombosis): 10–26% of patients with VTE are carriers of the factor V Leiden mutation.
- Thrombosis in unusual locations, such as the sagittal sinus or mesentery and portal systems, although these are less common in patients with factor V Leiden than in patients with deficiency of protein C or S

DIFFERENTIAL DIAGNOSIS
- Protein C deficiency
- Protein S deficiency
- Antithrombin deficiency
- Other causes of APC resistance (e.g., antiphospholipid antibodies)
- Dysfibrinogenemia

- Dysplasminogenemia
- Homocystinemia
- Prothrombin 20210 mutation
- Elevated factor VIII levels

DIAGNOSTIC TESTS & INTERPRETATION
Initial Tests (lab, imaging)
- For VTE diagnosis, tests and imaging refer to DVT/PE chapters.
- NICE guidelines specifies that the only clear indication for thrombophilia testing including factor V Leiden is when the consideration is being given to discontinuing anticoagulation therapy after an unprovoked VTE event.
- Factor V Leiden thrombophilia should be suspected in individuals with the following:
  - A history of first and recurrent VTE manifest as deep vein thrombosis (DVT) or pulmonary embolism (PE), especially in women with a history of VTE during pregnancy or in association with use of estrogen-containing contraceptives more particular 3rd generation
  - A family history of recurrent thrombosis
- Factor V Leiden molecular genetic test: DNA-based for factor V mutation, will be unaffected by anticoagulation and other drugs; recommended in individuals on direct thrombin inhibitors or direct factor Xa inhibitors, those with strong lupus inhibitors and significantly prolonged baseline aPTT.
- Functional assay for aPC resistance: plasma-based coagulation assay using factor V–deficient plasma to which patient plasma is added along with purified APC. The relative prolongation of the aPTT is used to assay for the defect. Heparin, direct thrombin inhibitors, and factor Xa inhibitor may cause false-negative results. In the absence of exposure to anticoagulants, functional testing is preferred to genetic testing due to cost and time to diagnosis.

Follow-Up Tests & Special Considerations
- Test individuals who develop VTE in unusual location, e.g., portal vein, cerebral vein, or recurrent VTE—especially <50 years old.
- For individuals with family history of factor V Leiden, genetic testing is preferred, especially if they have concomitant antiphospholipid syndrome or who are receiving anticoagulant—this will elucidate potential source of test interference for direct thrombin inhibitor or direct factor Xa inhibitor.
- Inherited genetic factors such as factor V Leiden, 20210A prothrombin mutation, antithrombin, protein C or protein S deficiencies, non-O blood group, as well as CYP2C9*2 and the rs4379368 mutations, have been shown to be genetic predictive risk factors for VTE in women. Therefore, consider testing for mutations prior implementing combined oral contraception and monitor for potential thrombogenicity induced by COC therapy.

Diagnostic Procedures/Other
- Suggest to perform thrombophilia testing in the pediatric group of patients, specifically those with recurrent central venous catheter (CVC) related VTE.
- If thrombophilia is suspected in children with VTE, include testing: factor V Leiden mutation, prothrombin 20210 mutation, antithrombin deficiency, protein C deficiency, protein S deficiency, and antiphospholipid.
- The thrombophilia screen consists of antithrombin III, protein c and s deficiency, PCR for factor V Leiden mutation and prothrombin G2021A mutation, testing for antiphospholipid antibodies and homocysteine level.

TREATMENT

Only indicated if with thrombotic event. For asymptomatic patients (no thrombotic event), prophylaxis is not recommended.

GENERAL MEASURES
- Initiation of anticoagulation therapy for acute venous thrombosis should be the same in patients with and without factor V Leiden or other inherited thrombophilia.
- The treatment for first VTE in patients with factor V Leiden or any other thrombophilias does not differ from those without it (2).
- VTE treatment should be a minimum of 3 months for the first episode.
- For those patients with recurrence, the risks and benefits of indefinite anticoagulation need to be assessed and considered.

MEDICATION
First Line
- See specific chapters for PE and DVT.
- First-line treatment for first VTE is the same for a patient with and a patient without factor V Leiden.
- In patients with proximal DVT or PE, anticoagulation therapy is recommended over no therapy (grade 1B).
- In patients with DVT or PE and no cancer, anticoagulation suggested are dabigatran, rivaroxaban, apixaban, or edoxaban over vitamin K antagonist (all Grade 2B).
- In patients with cancer-associated thrombosis, low-molecular-weight heparin (LMWH) is recommended.
- LMWH:
  - Enoxaparin (Lovenox): SC: 1 mg/kg every 12 hours (preferred) or 1.5 mg/kg once every 24 hours. Note: In select low-risk patients, may consider outpatient treatment using 1 mg/kg every 12 hours for the remainder of the course after first dose administered in hospital or urgent care center
  - Fondaparinux (Arixtra): 5 mg (body weight <50 kg), 7.5 mg (body weight 50 to 100 kg), or 10 mg (body weight >100 kg) SC daily
  - Tinzaparin (Innohep): 175 anti-Xa IU/kg SC daily for minimum of 5 days, and patient is adequately anticoagulated with warfarin (INR of at least 2 for 2 consecutive days)
  - Dalteparin (Fragmin): 200 IU/kg SC daily
- Oral anticoagulant
  - Apixaban (Eliquis): treatment dose: 10 mg BID × 7 days and then 5 mg BID × 3 to 6 months
  - Rivaroxaban (Xarelto): treatment dose: 15 mg BID × 7 days and then 20 mg daily × 3 to 6 months
  - Dabigatran (Pradaxa): After at least 5 days of initial therapy with a parenteral anticoagulant, transition to dabigatran in hemodynamically stable patients: 150 mg BID.
- Contraindications
  - Active bleeding precludes anticoagulation.
  - Risk of bleeding is a relative contraindication to long-term anticoagulation.
- Precautions
  - Observe patient for signs of embolization, further thrombosis, or bleeding.
  - Avoid IM injections. Periodically check stool and urine for occult blood; monitor CBCs, including platelets.
  - LMWH: Adjust dosage in renal insufficiency; may also need dose adjustment in pregnancy

- Significant possible interactions
  - Agents that intensify the response to oral anticoagulants: alcohol, allopurinol, amiodarone, anabolic steroids, androgens, many antimicrobials, cimetidine, chloral hydrate, disulfiram, all NSAIDs, sulfinpyrazone, tamoxifen, thyroid hormone, vitamin E, ranitidine, salicylates, acetaminophen
  - Agents that diminish the response to anticoagulants: aminoglutethimide, antacids, barbiturates, carbamazepine, cholestyramine, diuretics, griseofulvin, rifampin, oral contraceptives

Second Line
- Heparin 80 mg/kg IV bolus followed by 18 g/kg/hr continuous infusion
- Oral anticoagulant
  - Warfarin (Coumadin) PO with dose adjusted to an INR of 2 to 3
  - Contraindications
    ○ Active bleeding precludes anticoagulation.
    ○ Risk of bleeding is a relative contraindication to long-term anticoagulation.
    ○ Warfarin is contraindicated in patients with history of warfarin skin necrosis.
    ○ Warfarin is contraindicated in pregnancy.
  - Precautions
    ○ Heparin: thrombocytopenia and/or paradoxical thrombosis with thrombocytopenia
    ○ Warfarin: necrotic skin lesions (typically breasts, thighs, or buttocks

ISSUES FOR REFERRAL
- Recurrent thrombosis on anticoagulation
- Difficulty anticoagulating
- Genetic counseling
- Homozygous state in pregnancy

SURGERY/OTHER PROCEDURES
For most patients with DVT, recommendations are against routine use of inferior vena cava filter in addition to anticoagulation, except when there is contraindication for anticoagulation.

ADMISSION, INPATIENT, AND NURSING CONSIDERATIONS
- Admission criteria/initial stabilization: complicated thrombosis, such as PE
- Nursing
  - Teach LMWH and warfarin use.
- Discharge criteria: stable on anticoagulation

 ONGOING CARE

FOLLOW-UP RECOMMENDATIONS
Patient Monitoring
Warfarin use requires periodic (~monthly after initial stabilization) INR measurements, with a goal of 2 to 3.

DIET
Large amounts of foods rich in vitamin K may interfere with anticoagulation with warfarin.

PATIENT EDUCATION
- Patients should be educated about the following:
  - Use of oral anticoagulant therapy
  - Avoidance of NSAIDs while on anticoagulation
- The role of family screening is unclear because most patients with this mutation do not have thrombosis. In a patient with a family history of factor V Leiden, consider screening during pregnancy or if considering oral contraceptive use.

PROGNOSIS
- Most patients heterozygous for factor V Leiden do not have thrombosis.
- Homozygotes have about a 50% lifetime incidence of thrombosis.
- Recurrence rates after a first thrombosis are not clear; some estimate as high as 5%.
- Factor V Leiden does not increase overall mortality.

COMPLICATIONS
- Recurrent thrombosis
- Bleeding on anticoagulation

REFERENCES
1. Dłuski D, Mierzyński R, Poniedziałek-Czajkowska E, et al. Adverse pregnancy outcomes and inherited thrombophilia. *J Perinat Med*. 2018;46(4):411–417.
2. Guyatt GH, Akl EA, Crowther M, et al; for American College of Chest Physicians Antithrombotic Therapy and Prevention of Thrombosis Panel. Executive summary: Antithrombotic Therapy and Prevention of Thrombosis, 9th ed: American College of Chest Physicians Evidence-Based Clinical Practice Guidelines. *Chest*. 2012;141(2 Suppl):7S–47S.

 SEE ALSO

Deep Vein Thrombophlebitis

CODES

ICD10
D68.51 Activated protein C resistance

CLINICAL PEARLS
- Extremely rare in Asian and African populations
- Asymptomatic patients with factor V Leiden do not need anticoagulation.
- For pregnant women homozygous for factor V Leiden but no prior history of VTE, postpartum prophylaxis with prophylactic or intermediate-dose LMWH or vitamin K antagonists with target INR 2 to 3 for 6 weeks is recommended. Antepartum prophylaxis is added if there is positive family history of VTE.

F

FAILURE TO THRIVE

Durr-e-Shahwaar Sayed, DO

 BASICS

DESCRIPTION

- Failure to thrive (FTT) is not a diagnosis but a sign of inadequate nutrition in young children manifested by a failure of physical growth, usually affecting weight. In severe cases, decreased length and/or head circumference may develop.
- Various parameters are used to define FTT, but in clinical practice, it is commonly defined as either weight or BMI for age that falls below the 5th percentile on more than one occasion or weight that drops two or more major percentile lines on standard growth charts OR weight-for-length that falls below the 5th percentile.
- A combination of anthropometric criteria rather than one criterion should be used to identify children at risk of FTT.

Pediatric Considerations

- Children with genetic syndromes, intrauterine growth restriction (IUGR), or prematurity follow different growth curves.
- 25% of children will decrease their weight or height crossing ≥2 major percentile lines in the first 2 years of life. These children are failing to reach their genetic potential or demonstrating constitutional growth delay (slow growth with a bone age < chronologic age). After shifting down, these infants grow at a normal rate along their new percentile and do not have FTT.

EPIDEMIOLOGY

Incidence

- Predominant age: 6 to 12 months; 80% <18 months
- Predominant sex: male = female

Prevalence

- As many as 10% of children seen in primary care have signs of growth failure.
- 1–5% of pediatric inpatient admissions are for FTT.
- Occurs more frequently in children living in poverty

ETIOLOGY AND PATHOPHYSIOLOGY

- Mismatch between caloric intake and caloric expenditure
- Often grouped into four major categories:
  - Inadequate caloric intake (most frequent)
  - Inadequate caloric absorption
  - Excessive caloric expenditure
  - Defective utilization
- Traditionally, FTT was classified as organic or nonorganic, but most cases are multifactorial.
- FTT often begins with a specific event and may lead to persistent difficulties.
- Causes of FTT can be grouped by pathophysiology (including examples):
  - Inadequate intake: breastfeeding difficulty, incorrect formula preparation, poor transition to food (6 to 12 months), poor feeding habits (e.g., excessive juice, restrictive diets), mechanical problems (e.g., oromotor dysfunction, congenital anomalies, GERD, CNS, or PNS anomalies), oral aversion, poverty, neglect/abuse, poor parent–child interaction, caregiver feeding style
  - Inadequate absorption: necrotizing enterocolitis, short gut syndrome, biliary atresia, liver disease, cystic fibrosis, celiac disease, milk protein allergy, vitamin/mineral deficiency, environmental enteric dysfunction

- Increased expenditure: hyperthyroidism, congenital/chronic cardiopulmonary disease, HIV, immunodeficiencies, malignancy, renal disease, obstructive sleep apnea
- Defective utilization: metabolic disorders, congenital infections (TORCH: toxoplasmosis, other agents, rubella, cytomegalovirus, herpes simplex)

RISK FACTORS

- Psychosocial risks (1)
  - Poverty, parent(s) with mental health disorder or cognitive impairment, ineffective parenting skills or hypervigilant parents, families with unique health/nutritional beliefs, physical or emotional abuse, substance abuse, and social isolation
- Medical risks (1)
  - Intrauterine exposures, history of IUGR (symmetric or asymmetric), congenital abnormalities, oromotor dysfunction, premature or sick newborn, infant with physical deformity, acute or chronic medical conditions, developmental delay, lead poisoning, anemia

Pregnancy Considerations

FTT is linked to intrauterine exposures, IUGR, and prematurity.

GENERAL PREVENTION

- Educate parents on normal feeding and parenting skills.
- Access to supplemental feeding programs (Women, Infants, and Children [WIC])
- Consider more frequent visits for children at higher risk for FTT.

 DIAGNOSIS

HISTORY

- Successful treatment of FTT is almost always accomplished by a careful and detailed history because most cases are due to underfeeding or inappropriate feeding.
- Prenatal and developmental history/prenatal exposures
- Past medical history: acute/chronic disease affecting caloric intake, digestion, absorption, or causing increased energy need or defective utilization
- Medication history, including complementary and alternative medications
- Family history: stature of parents and growth trajectories of siblings, chronic diseases, genetic disorders, developmental delay, consanguinity
- Diet history from birth: breastfeeding or formula feeding; timing and introduction of solids; who feeds the child, when, and how often; placement of child during feeds; amounts consumed/caloric intake; beverages consumed; snacking; vomiting or stooling associated with feeds; oral aversions or unusual behaviors during feeding
- Social history: family composition, socioeconomic status, hygiene practices, child-rearing beliefs, stressors, parental depression, parental substance abuse, caretaker personal history of abuse/neglect
- Review of systems: anorexia, activity level, mental status, fevers, dysphagia, vomiting, gastroesophageal reflux, stooling pattern/consistency, dysuria, urinary frequency

PHYSICAL EXAM

- A combination of anthropometric criteria, rather than one criterion, should be used, and measurements over time are required for diagnosis.
- Accurate measurement of height, weight, and head circumference from the National Center for Health Statistics (NCHS) (https://www.cdc.gov/growthcharts/)
- The World Health Organization (WHO) growth charts may be more appropriate for breastfed infants (http://www.who.int/childgrowth/standards/en/).
- Exam should assess for the following:
  - Signs of dehydration or severe malnutrition
    - Severity of malnutrition estimated via Gomez classification: Compare current weight for age with expected weight for age (50th percentile): severe, <60% of expected; moderate, 61–75%; mild, 76–90%.
  - Dysmorphic features
  - Mental status (alert, responsive to stimuli)
  - Any signs of physical abuse and/or neglect
- Observe interaction with caregivers and feeding techniques, specifically bonding and social/psychological cues.

DIFFERENTIAL DIAGNOSIS

Differentiate based on growth patterns.

- FTT classically presents as low weight for age, with normal linear growth and head circumference OR low weight for age, followed by decreased linear growth OR low weight for age, leading to decreased linear growth and decreased head circumference (without neurologic signs).
- If low linear growth with normal weight for length or low linear growth and proportionately low weight and decreased head circumference:
  - Consider genetic potential (constitutional short stature or growth delay), genetic syndromes, teratogens, and endocrine disorders.
- If microcephaly with prominent neurologic signs, with poor growth secondary to presumed neurologic disorder:
  - Consider TORCH infections, genetic syndromes, teratogens, and brain injury (i.e., hypoxic/ischemic).

DIAGNOSTIC TESTS & INTERPRETATION

- Labs useful only in ~1% of cases and are generally not recommended
- A period of addressing nutritional causes is preferable prior to extensive labs and other workup.

Initial Tests (lab, imaging)

Labs should be ordered based on history and physical exam findings and the age of the patient.

- Tests often considered in initial evaluation:
  - CBC with differential, ESR, lead level
  - Electrolytes, BUN/creatinine, liver function tests, TSH, free T_4
  - Urinalysis and urine culture
- Other tests as dictated by the history and exam:
  - Amylase/lipase, serum zinc level, iron studies, IGF-1, karyotype, genetic testing, sweat chloride test, stool for ova and parasite or fat/reducing substances, guaiac, α_1-antitrypsin and elastase, radioallergosorbent test for IgE food allergies, tissue transglutaminase and total IgA (celiac sprue), p-ANCA and fecal calprotectin (for inflammatory bowel disease [IBD]), TB test, HIV, hepatitis A and B, other infections
  - X-ray of hand/wrist to assess bone age and for skeletal dysplasia

Follow-Up Tests & Special Considerations
- Prospective 3-day food diary for accurate record of caloric intake should be obtained.
- Home visit by a clinician to observe infant feeding, interaction of caretakers, and home environment
- Observe breastfeeding and/or formula preparation to ensure adequacy and offer instruction.
- Additional indicated evaluations may be performed by dietitians; occupational, physical, and speech therapists; social workers; developmental specialists; psychiatrists; psychologists; visiting nurses; lactation consultants; and/or child protective services.

Diagnostic Procedures/Other
Can consider
- Skeletal survey if suspicion of physical abuse
- Bone age if possible endocrine disorder
- Swallowing studies, small bowel follow-through if possible oromotor dysfunction, GERD, structural abnormalities
- Brain imaging if microcephalic and/or neurologic findings on examination
- Echocardiogram if murmur auscultated
- Consider referral to specialist based on results of initial evaluation (e.g., endocrinology, gastroenterology).

 TREATMENT

GENERAL MEASURES
- Treat underlying conditions.
- Caregiver and infant interaction should be evaluated in infants and children with FTT.
- Age-appropriate nutritional counseling should be provided.
  - The goal is to improve nutrition to allow catch-up growth (weight gain 2 to 3 times > average for age).
- Calculate energy needs based on recommended energy intake for age and then increase by 50%.
- Alternatively, may calculate caloric requirements for infants to achieve catch-up growth
  - kcal/kg/day required = RDA for age (kcal/kg) × ideal weight for height/actual weight, where ideal weight for height is the median weight for the patient's height
- Try various strategies to increase caloric intake, such as the following:
  - Optimize breastfeeding support; consider supplementation.
  - Higher calorie formulas
  - Addition of rice cereal or fats to current foods
  - Limit intake of milk to 24 to 32 oz/day.
  - Avoid juice and soda.
  - Vitamin and/or nutritional supplements
  - Assist with social and family problems (WIC, food stamps, and other transitional assistance).
- Rapid high-calorie intake can cause diarrhea, malabsorption, hypokalemia, and hypophosphatemia. Therefore, increasing formulas >24 kcal/oz is not recommended.
- The target energy intake should be slowly increased to goal over 5 to 7 days.
- Catch-up growth should be seen in 2 to 7 days.

- Accelerated growth should be continued for 4 to 9 months to restore weight and height.
- Consider Visiting Nurse Referral & Social Services evaluation to determine services family may qualify for.

ISSUES FOR REFERRAL
Multidisciplinary care is beneficial. Specialized multidisciplinary clinics may be of benefit for children with complicated situations, failure to respond to initial treatment, or when the PCP does not have access to specialized services such as nutrition, psychology, PT/OT, and speech therapy.

SURGERY/OTHER PROCEDURES
In severe cases nasogastric tube feedings or gastrostomy may be considered.

ADMISSION, INPATIENT, AND NURSING CONSIDERATIONS
- Most cases of FTT can be managed as outpatients.
- Hospitalization should be considered if:
  - Outpatient management fails
  - There is evidence of severe dehydration or malnutrition.
  - There are signs of abuse or neglect.
  - There are concerns that the psychosocial situation presents harm to child.
  - During catch-up growth, some children will develop nutritional recovery syndrome:
    - Symptoms include sweating, increased body temperature, hepatomegaly (increased glycogen deposits), widening of cranial sutures (brain growth > bone growth), increased periods of sleep, fidgetiness, and mild hyperactivity.
  - There may also be an initial period of malabsorption with resultant diarrhea.
- Catch-up growth should be seen in 2 to 7 days. If this is not seen, reevaluation of causes is needed.

 ONGOING CARE

FOLLOW-UP RECOMMENDATIONS
- Close (every 2 to 4 weeks at first and then 1 to 2 months if good progress), long-term follow-up with frequent visits
- Children with history of FTT are at increased risk of recurrent FTT.
- If the family fails to comply, child protection authorities must be notified.

DIET
Nutritional requirements for a "normal" child:
- Infant
  - 120 kcal/kg/day, decreased to 95 kcal/kg/day at 6 months; if breastfed, ensure appropriate frequency and duration of feeding.
  - Between 6 and 12 months, continue breast milk and/or formula, but pureed foods should be consumed several times a day during this period.
- Toddler
  - Three meals plus two nutritional snacks, 16 to 32 oz of milk per day; avoid juice and soda and feed in a social environment.

- Rate of weight gain expected for age:
  - 0 to 3 months: 26 to 31 g/day
  - 3 to 6 months: 17 to 18 g/day
  - 6 to 9 months: 12 to 13 g/day
  - 9 to 12 months: 9 g/day
  - 1 to 3 years: 7 to 9 g/day

PATIENT EDUCATION
- Counsel parents regarding the need to avoid "food battles," which can worsen the problem.
- Educate parents regarding infant social and physiologic cues, formula/food preparation, proper feeding techniques, and importance of relaxed and social mealtimes.
- "Failure to thrive: What this means for your child" available from AAFP at: https://www.aafp.org/afp/2011/0401/p837.html
- WIC provides grants to states for supplemental foods, health care referrals, and nutrition education for low-income pregnant, breastfeeding, and nonbreastfeeding postpartum women and to infants and children up to age 5 years at nutritional risk: https://www.fns.usda.gov/wic/women-infants-and-children-wic.

PROGNOSIS
- Many children with FTT show adequate improvement in dietary intake with intervention (1)[B].
- Children with FTT are at increased risk for future undernutrition, overnutrition, and eating disorders.

REFERENCE
1. Black MM, Tilton N, Bento S, et al. Recovery in young children with weight faltering: child and household risk factors. *J Pediatr*. 2016;170:301–306.

ADDITIONAL READING
Homan GJ. Failure to thrive: a practical guide. *Am Fam Physician*. 2016;94(4):295–299.

CODES

ICD10
- R62.7 Adult failure to thrive
- R62.51 Failure to thrive (child)
- P92.6 Failure to thrive in newborn

CLINICAL PEARLS
- FTT is a sign of inadequate nutrition. It is rarely due to a medical condition.
- Underlying medical and/or social issues are generally suggested by history and physical exam, and extensive laboratory or imaging tests are rarely needed.
- A multidisciplinary team approach to diagnosis and treatment is critical to help children with FTT and their families.

FEMALE ATHLETE TRIAD

Rahul Kapur, MD • Torb Morkeberg, DO

 BASICS

Syndrome of three interrelated clinical entities: low energy availability (with or without disordered eating, menstrual dysfunction, and low bone mineral density (LBMD) (1)

DESCRIPTION

- Female athlete triad first described in 1992 to include disordered eating, amenorrhea, osteoporosis
- In 2007, American College of Sports Medicine (ACSM) updated definition to the following: components including low energy availability (with or without disordered eating), menstrual dysfunction, LBMD with each component representing an inter-related spectrum ranging from health to dysfunction
- Low energy availability is fundamental to the triad and full recovery not possible without correction of it (1).
- 2014 Female Athlete Triad Coalition (TC) consensus statement largely agreed with ACSM update and included many recommendations (as later briefly outlined in this review) (1).
- 2014 International Olympic Committee's position statement from 2014 deviated to consider "Relative Energy Deficiency in Sport" (RED-S) (2).
  - Focus on energy deficiency and its broader physiologic effects beyond bone and menstrual health, ranging from growth to cardiovascular
  - Emphasized similar syndrome in males
- Since then, debate has ensued between the classic TC model and RED-S. TC authors assert that RED-S movement is simply "rebranding" 30+ years worth of triad research.
- TC authors have since released papers introducing the concept of the male athlete triad.
- Concept of energy deficiency in men that seem to be related to reproductive and bone abnormalities
  - Men seem to have a higher threshold to meet low energy availability.
  - Male triad needs to be further evaluated.

EPIDEMIOLOGY

Prevalence

- Overall prevalence: 3/3 criteria (EA, menstrual dysfunction, LBMD): 0–16%. 2/3 criteria: 3–27%. 1/3 criteria: 16–60%.
- Disordered eating higher than general population
- Menstrual dysfunction: Prevalence of secondary amenorrhea is as high as 60% in female athletes compared to 2–5% in the general population.
- LBMD: Using the WHO criteria for LBMD, prevalence of osteopenia (T-score between −1 and −2) ranges from 0% to 40% in female athletes, as compared to ~12% in the general population.
- Full triad more prevalent in lean sports (1.5–6.7%), including swimming and cross country, versus non-lean sports (0–2%), including volleyball and softball.

ETIOLOGY AND PATHOPHYSIOLOGY

- Energy availability is defined by energy intake minus exercise energy expenditure.
  - Low energy availability can occur either intentionally or inadvertently. Examples include increasing training or disordered eating (2).
- When there is low energy availability, energy is shunted from reproduction to more critical functions, such as thermoregulation cellular maintenance.
- Specifically, low energy availability leads to suppression of luteinizing hormone (LH) pulse frequency and thus menstrual dysfunction.
  - This process suppresses ovulation and estrogen concentrations, which can lead to decreased

bone formation and increased bone resorption, ultimately leading to LBMD.
- Triad elements exist along a bidirectional continuum of severity, ranging from "healthy" to "unhealthy." Importantly, elements exist as a triad, although, there is unidirectionally implied from one to another.
  - Low energy availability (with or without an eating disorder) can lead to both menstrual dysfunction and LBMD.
- Menstrual dysfunction (via hypoestrogenemia) can lead to LBMD.
- Other effects of low energy availability seem to include endothelial dysfunction and altered lipid profiles.
- RED-S considers low energy availability to lead to broader physiologic effects including metabolic rate, growth and development, immunity, protein synthesis, hematologic, gastrointestinal, cardiovascular, psychological (3).
- TC authors hold that there may be a basis for RED-S but it is insufficiently supported by evidence at the present time.

RISK FACTOR

- History of menstrual irregularities and amenorrhea; history of stress fractures and recurrent or nonhealing injuries; history of critical comments about eating or weight from parent or coach; history of depression; history of dieting; personality factors including perfectionism and/or obsessiveness, overtraining, and inappropriate coaching behaviors (1).
- Lean physique sports with an aesthetic component (ballet, figure skating, gymnastics, distance running, diving, and swimming) or sports with weight classifications (martial arts and wrestling). Frequent weigh-ins, consequences for weight gain, and win-at-all-cost attitude all increase risk.
- A lack of family or social support; intense training hours; social isolation or entering a new environment (boarding school or college); an athlete with comorbid psychological conditions (anxiety, depression, and/or obsessive-compulsive disorder)
- Age: Japanese study found stress fracture in teenagers with the Triad but no stress fractures in athletes in their 20s.

GENERAL PREVENTION

- Education of athletes (middle school through college), coaches, trainers, parents, and physicians. Young athletes are extremely impressionable and may turn negative comments and unhealthy advice into maladaptive eating and exercising habits.
- General screening during preparticipation exam (PPE) and annual physicals are endorsed by AAP, AAFP, ACSM, AOSSM, and AMSSM.
- Female Athlete Triad Coalition has 11-question screening to use during PPE (1).
- Screen athletes presenting with "red flag" conditions such as fractures, weight changes, fatigue, amenorrhea, bradycardia, orthostatic hypotension, syncope, arrhythmias, electrolyte abnormalities, or depression.
- Screen for other conditions that may accelerate bone loss, including steroid use, tobacco use, alcohol use, and hyperthyroidism.

COMMONLY ASSOCIATED CONDITIONS

- Anorexia nervosa, bulimia nervosa, avoidant or restrictive food intake disorder, and other psychological disorders, including low self-esteem, depression, and anxiety (3)
- LBMD predisposes athletes to stress fractures and may not be fully reversible. This may lead to a higher rate of fractures after menopause.

 DIAGNOSIS

The female athlete triad is a clinical diagnosis based primarily on patient history; screening for the female athlete triad at annual sports physicals or during routine exams and acute visits if there are concerns (1),(4)[A]

HISTORY

Assess menstrual history (including hormonal contraceptive use), fracture history, and symptoms of depression. Assess dietary practices, eating behaviors, and history of weight changes. Dietary intake logs and a nutritional assessment by a sports dietitian can help. Assess body image, fear of weight gain, fluctuations in weight, history of disordered eating, and use of laxatives, diet pills, or enemas.

PHYSICAL EXAM

- Height, weight, body mass index (BMI) <17.5% kg/m^2, <85% of expected body weight in adolescents, or ≥10% weight loss in 1 month (1)
- Common findings include bradycardia, orthostatic hypotension, hypothermia, cold or cyanotic extremities, lanugo, parotid gland enlargement or tenderness, epigastric tenderness, eroded tooth enamel, and knuckle or hand calluses (Russell sign).
- Patients with amenorrhea should undergo a pelvic exam to verify the presence of a uterus and evaluate for outflow tract abnormalities. Vaginal atrophy may be present if the patient is in a low estrogen state.

DIFFERENTIAL DIAGNOSIS

Screen for anorexia nervosa, bulimia nervosa, avoidant/restrictive food intake disorder, and rumination disorder using the *DSM-5* criteria. Rule out the following in amenorrheic patients:

- Pregnancy
- Endocrine abnormalities: thyroid dysfunction, Cushing syndrome
- Hypothalamic dysfunction: psychological stress-induced amenorrhea, medication-induced amenorrhea, Kallmann syndrome
- Pituitary dysfunction: prolactinoma, Sheehan syndrome, sarcoidosis, empty sella syndrome
- Ovarian dysfunction: polycystic ovarian syndrome, premature ovarian failure, menopause, gonadal dysgenesis, Turner syndrome, ovarian neoplasm, autoimmune disease
- Uterine dysfunction: Asherman syndrome, absence of uterus

DIAGNOSTIC TESTS & INTERPRETATION

Initial Tests (lab, imaging)

- Basic metabolic panel, magnesium, phosphorus, albumin, CBC with differential, ESR, thyroid-stimulating hormone (TSH), calcium, 25-OH vitamin D, and urinalysis (1),(4)
- Evaluation for secondary amenorrhea includes urine hCG and serum FSH, LH, prolactin, and TSH.
- Consider adding an alkaline phosphatase in patients with multiple metatarsal fractures to evaluate for possible underlying hypophosphatasia.
- Pelvic ultrasound in patients with hyperandrogenism to exclude polycystic ovaries or virilizing ovarian tumors
- ECG to rule out prolonged QT interval

Follow-Up Tests & Special Considerations

- BMD testing by DEXA is based on a risk stratification model (1). Risk factors include disordered eating, eating disorders >6 months, hypoestrogenism, amenorrhea, oligomenorrhea, and/or in patients with a history of stress fractures or fractures from minimal impact.

- If components of the triad persist, ISCD 2013 guidelines suggest reevaluation by the same DEXA machine every 1 to 2 years.

TREATMENT

- A multidisciplinary team including a physician, registered dietitian, and behavioral health provider. Build open lines of communication with coaches, trainers, and family.
- Cognitive-behavioral therapy (CBT) may have a role in treating low energy availability itself (1).
- Physically active females should strive for an EA of >45 kcal/kg of fat-free muscle mass per day (1)[A].
- Nonpharmacologic measures should be taken first and followed for at least 1 year (5)[B].
- First step is optimizing nutritional status to increase energy intake, which often encourages weight gain and increased BMI (1).
- Goal is body weight associated with normal menses (proving return of acceptable estrogen levels). This often correlates with BMI >18.5 or >90% predicted weight (1)[A].
- Encourage real food with proper balance of macro/micronutrients over supplements if possible (1).
- Calcium intake with goal of 1,000 to 1,300 mg/day. Encourage calcium-rich foods; supplementation to reach goal if dietary intake is insufficient (5)
- A minimum of 600 IU of vitamin D should be consumed/supplemented; may require 1,500 to 2,000 IU to keep serum levels between 32 and 50 ng/mL (5)
- There may be a role for iron, at least in athletes with iron-deficiency anemia if not others (5).
- Treat maladaptive behavioral disorders (1).

MEDICATION

First Line
First-line medication for failed nutrition intervention and/or worsening symptoms (particularly fractures): nonoral estrogen, specifically transdermal estrogen with oral cyclic progestin (5)[B]

Second Line
- Other postmenopausal medications, including bisphosphonates and denosumab, should not be recommended in reproductive-aged women, due to potential teratogenic effect (5).
- Experimental medications: recombinant insulin-like growth factor (rhIGF-1) and metreleptin (synthetic leptin analogue) (5).

ADMISSION, INPATIENT, AND NURSING CONSIDERATIONS
Evaluate patients with eating disorders for potentially life-threatening conditions requiring hospital admission, including bradycardia, severe orthostatic hypotension, significant electrolyte imbalances, hypothermia, arrhythmias, or prolonged QT interval.

ONGOING CARE

- Patients should have regular follow-up with a multidisciplinary treatment team (1)[A].
- Periodized (2 weeks on, 2 weeks off) training may be a safe, enjoyable way to build strength without exacerbating features of the Triad (6)[B].
- The Female Athlete TC consensus statement provided the first evidence-based clearance and return to play guidance, which considers the following factors: low energy availability (with emphasis on disordered eating), BMI, delayed menarche, oligo/amenorrhea, LBMD, stress fracture (1).

- RED-S released a clinical assessment tool (CAT) in 2014 (updated in 2015), which considers similar criteria as compared to the TC clearance guide, although classifies them into "green, yellow, red" categories.
- Both groups continue to debate the validity of the other group's CATs.

PATIENT EDUCATION
All young female patients should be counseled on the importance of proper nutrition, calcium and vitamin D intake, and the benefits of regular weight-bearing exercise. Patients presenting with ≥1 components of the triad should be educated about the short- and long-term effects of LBMD (1)[A].

PROGNOSIS
- The short- and long-term prognosis for patients with female athlete triad depends on time to diagnosis and response to treatment.
- It is estimated that amenorrheic women will lose 2–3% of bone mass per year without intervention.
- With early diagnosis and treatment using a multidisciplinary team, the prognosis for patients with the female athlete triad is good. Patients regain normal menstrual cycling and increase BMD.
- Because the triad often occurs within the age window of optimal bone strengthening, patients with a prolonged disease course may suffer from complications of decreased BMD throughout their adolescent and adult life.
- Patients with disordered eating behaviors often require long-term therapy to manage their disease.

REFERENCES

1. De Souza MJ, Nattiv A, Joy E, et al. 2014 Female Athlete Triad Coalition consensus statement on treatment and return to play of the female athlete triad: 1st International Conference held in San Francisco, CA, May 2012, and 2nd International Conference held in Indianapolis, IN, May 2013. *Clin J Sport Med*. 2014;24(2):96–119.
2. Mountjoy M, Sundgot-Borgen J, Burke L, et al. The IOC consensus statement: beyond the female athlete triad—relative energy deficiency in sport (RED-S). *Br J Sports Med*. 2014;48(7):491–497.
3. Mountjoy M, Sundgot-Borgen J, Burke L, et al. Internal Olympic Committee (IOC) consensus statement on relative energy deficiency in sport (RED-S): 2018 update. *Int J Sport Nutr Exerc Metab*. 2018;28(4):316–331. doi:10.1123/ijsnem.2018-0136.
4. Temme KE, Hoch AZ. Recognition and rehabilitation of the female athlete triad/tetrad: a multidisciplinary approach. *Curr Sports Med Rep*. 2013;12(3):190–199.
5. Southmayd EA, Hellmers AC, De Souza MJ. Food versus pharmacy: assessment of nutritional and pharmacological strategies to improve bone health in energy-deficient exercising women. *Curr Osteoporos Rep*. 2017;15:459–472. doi:10.1007/s11914-017-0393-9.
6. Wikström-Frisén L, Boraxbekk CJ, Henriksson-Larsén K. Increasing training load without risking the female athlete triad: menstrual cycle based periodized training may be an answer? *J Sports Med Phys Fitness*. 2017;57(11):1519–1525. doi:10.23736/S0022-4707.16.06444-6.

ADDITIONAL READING

- De Souza MJ, Koltun KJ, Williams NI. The role of energy availability in reproductive function in the female athlete triad and extension of its effects to men: an initial working model of a similar syndrome in male athletes. *Sports Medicine*. 2019;49:S125–S137.

- De Souza MJ, Williams NI, Nattiv A. Misunderstanding the female athlete triad: refuting the IOC consensus statement on relative energy deficiency in sport (RED-S). *Br J Sports Med*. 2014;48:1461–1465.
- Fink DA, Pasculli RM, Wright A, et al. Unexpected hurdle in the race: hypophosphatasia unmasked by the female athlete triad. *Curr Sports Med Rep*. 2019;18(12):434–436. doi:10.1249/JSR.0000000000000664.
- Joy EA, Nattiv A. Clearance and return to play for the female athlete triad: clinical guidelines, clinical judgment, and evolving evidence. *Curr Sports Med Rep*. 2017;16(6):382–385. doi:10.1249/JSR.0000000000000423.
- Nose-Ogura S, Yoshino O, Dohi M, et al. Risk factors of stress fractures due to the female athlete triad: differences in teens and twenties. *Scand J Med Sci Sports*. 2019;29(10):1501–1510. doi:10.1111/sms.13464.
- Petkus DL, Murray-Kolb LE, De Souza MJ. The unexplored crossroads of the female athlete triad and iron deficiency: a narrative review. *Sports Med*. 2017;47:1721–1737. doi:10.1007/s40279-017-0706-2.
- Raj MA, Creech JA, Rogol AD. Female athlete triad. National Center for Biotechnology Information Web site. https://www.ncbi.nlm.nih.gov/books/NBK430787/.
- The IOC relative energy deficiency in sport clinical assessment tool: doi:10.1136/bjsports-2015-094873.
- VanBaak K, Olson D. FACSM the female athlete triad. *Curr Sports Med Rep*. 2016;15(1):7–8. doi:10.1249/JSR.0000000000000222.
- Williams NI, Koltun KJ, Strock NCA, et al. Female athlete triad and relative energy deficiency in sport: a focus on scientific rigor. *Exerc Sport Sci Rev*. 2019;47(4):197–205.

SEE ALSO

Algorithms: Amenorrhea, Primary (Absence of Menarche by Age 16 Years); Amenorrhea, Secondary; Weight Loss, Unintentional

CODES

ICD10
- F50.9 Eating disorder, unspecified
- N91.2 Amenorrhea, unspecified
- R53.83 Other fatigue

CLINICAL PEARLS

- The female athlete triad consists of low EA (with or without disordered eating), menstrual dysfunction, and LBMD. Athletes may exhibit varying degrees of dysfunction in any of these three areas. There is emerging research regarding an expanded syndrome called RED-S.
- Screen at-risk women to allow for early diagnosis and intervention.
- Early intervention by a multidisciplinary team, including physicians, registered dietitians, mental health professionals, coaches, trainers, and parents, is the most successful strategy to minimize further bone loss, recover BMD, and regain normal menstrual function.
- Nonpharmacologic treatment with dietary recommendations for 1 year are first line.
- There are currently two main return to play tools that are continually being evaluated and improved.

FEVER OF UNKNOWN ORIGIN (FUO)

Daniel R. Matta, MD • Fabiola Puga Dueñas, MD

 BASICS

DESCRIPTION

- Classic definition
  - Repeated fever >38.3°C
  - Fever duration at least 3 weeks
  - Diagnosis remains uncertain (1) after 1 week of study in the hospital.
- In over 50% of cases, no etiology is determined. The three most common underlying mechanisms for fever of unknown origin (FUO) are infection, malignancy, and systemic rheumatic or connective tissue diseases (2).

EPIDEMIOLOGY

Incidence
The exact incidence is not known.

Prevalence
The definition of fever with unresolved cause (true FUO) is difficult, as it is a moving target, given the constant advancement of imaging and biomarker analysis. Therefore, the prevalence of fever of unknown origin is unknown.

ETIOLOGY AND PATHOPHYSIOLOGY

- True FUO are uncommon; most frequently, FUO is an atypical presentation of a common condition.
- Spectrum of causes varies widely.
  - Noninfectious inflammatory diseases are the most frequent causes in high-income countries. Common causes include temporal arteritis, poly-myalgia rheumatica, or rheumatoid arthritis.
- Infection
  - Abdominal or pelvic abscesses
  - Amebic hepatitis
  - Catheter infections
  - Cytomegalovirus
  - Dental abscesses
  - Endocarditis/pericarditis
  - HIV (advanced stage)
  - Mycobacterial infection (often with advanced HIV)
  - Osteomyelitis
  - Pyelonephritis or renal abscess
  - Sinusitis
  - Wound infections
  - Other miscellaneous infections
- Neoplasms
  - Atrial myxoma
  - Colorectal cancer and other GI malignancies
  - Hepatoma
  - Lymphoma
  - Leukemia
  - Solid tumors (renal cell carcinoma)
- Noninfectious inflammatory disease
  - Connective tissue diseases
    ○ Adult Still disease
    ○ Rheumatoid arthritis
    ○ Systemic lupus erythematosus
  - Granulomatous disease
    ○ Crohn disease
    ○ Sarcoidosis
  - Vasculitis syndromes
    ○ Giant cell arteritis
    ○ Polymyalgia rheumatica
- Other causes
  - Alcoholic hepatitis
  - Cerebrovascular accident
  - Cirrhosis
  - Medications
    ○ Allopurinol, captopril, carbamazepine, cepha-losporins, cimetidine, clofibrate, erythromycin, heparin, hydralazine, hydrochlorothiazide, isoniazid, meperidine, methyldopa, nifedipine, nitrofurantoin, penicillin, phenytoin, procain-amide, quinidine, sulfonamides
  - Endocrine disease
  - Factitious/fraudulent fever
  - Occupational causes
  - Periodic fever
  - Pulmonary emboli/deep vein thrombosis
  - Thermoregulatory disorders
- In up to 20–30% of cases, the cause of the fever is never identified despite a thorough workup.

RISK FACTORS

- Recent travel (malaria, enteric fevers)
- Exposure to biologic or chemical agents
- HIV infection (particularly in acute infection and advanced stages)
- Elderly
- Drug abuse
- Immigrants
- Young (typically) female health care workers (factitious fever)

Geriatric Considerations
Common infectious causes of FUO in geriatric populations include systemic rheumatic diseases (polymyalgia rheumatica, giant cell arteritis), sarcoidosis, intra-abdominal abscess, urinary tract infection, tuberculosis (TB), and endocarditis. Other common causes of FUO in patients >65 years include malignancies (particularly hematologic cancers) and drug-induced fever.

Pediatric Considerations
- One-third are self-limited undefined viral syndromes. ~50% of FUO in pediatric cases are infectious. Collagen vascular disease and malignancy are the next most common.
- Inflammatory bowel disease is a common cause of FUO in older children and adolescents.

℞ DIAGNOSIS

The initial approach should include a comprehensive history and physical examination as well as laboratory testing. The decision of what further testing should be gathered should be guided by the resulting information.

HISTORY

- Onset and pattern of fever
- Constitutional symptoms:
  - Chills, night sweats, myalgias, weight loss with an intact appetite (infectious etiology)
  - Arthralgias, myalgias, fatigue (inflammatory etiology)
  - Fatigue, night sweats, weight loss with loss of appetite (neoplastic etiology)
- Past medical history: chronic infections, abdominal diseases, transfusion history, malignancy, psychiatric illness, and recent hospitalization
- Past surgical history: type of surgery performed, postoperative complications, and any indwelling foreign material
- Comprehensive medication history, including over-the-counter and herbal products
- Family history, such as hereditary causes, periodic fever syndromes, and recent febrile illnesses in close contacts
- Social history: travel, animal exposure (e.g., pets, occupational, farms), living environment, sexual activity, recreational drug use

ALERT
Obtain a thorough travel, psychosocial, occupational, sexual, medication, and recreational drug use history.

PHYSICAL EXAM
Physical findings with high diagnostic yield generally involve skin, eyes, lymph nodes, liver, and spleen. Helpful clues can be found with:

- Funduscopic exam for choroid tubercles or Roth spots
- Temporal artery tenderness
- Oral-mucosal lesions
- Cardiac auscultation for bruits and murmurs
- Pulmonary exam: consolidation or effusion
- Abdominal palpation for masses or organomegaly and tenderness or peritoneal signs
- Rectal examination for blood, fluctuance, and/or tenderness
- Testicular examination
- Lymph node examination
- Skin and nail bed exam for clubbing, nodules, lesions, and erosions
- Focal neurologic signs
- Musculoskeletal exam for tenderness or effusion
- Serial exams help identify evolving physical signs (e.g., findings associated with endocarditis).

DIAGNOSTIC TESTS & INTERPRETATION

Initial Tests (lab, imaging)

- CBC, C-reactive protein, ESR, ANA
- Peripheral blood smear
- Electrolytes, BUN, and creatinine; LFT; calcium; lactate dehydrogenase
- Heterophile antibody testing
- HIV testing
- Three blood cultures drawn from different sites, within hours, without administering antibiotics
- Creatine phosphokinase
- Urinalysis and urine culture
- Chest x-ray
- CT or MRI of abdomen and pelvis (with directed biopsy, if indicated) (3)[C]

Follow-Up Tests & Special Considerations

- Rheumatoid factor and antinuclear antibody test
- Serologies: Epstein-Barr, hepatitis, syphilis, Lyme disease, Q fever, cytomegalovirus, brucellosis, amebiasis, coccidioidomycosis, histoplasmosis
- Serum ferritin; serum protein electrophoresis
- AFB smear; sputum and urine cultures for TB
- TB testing
  - Tuberculin skin test
    ○ May not be helpful if anergic or acute infection
    ○ If test negative, repeat in 2 weeks.
  - Interferon-γ release assay (IGRA)
    ○ Preferred in those likely to be infected with TB and/or who are BCG-vaccinated
- Thyroid function tests

- Technetium-based scan (infection tumor) (3)[B]
- FDG-PET/CT scan if infectious process, inflammatory process, or tumor suspected; PET scans have a high negative predictive value and good sensitivity (but may have false positives) (4)[A].
- Ultrasound of abdomen and pelvis (with directed biopsy, if indicated) if renal obstruction or biliary pathology suspected
- Echocardiogram if endocarditis, atrial myxomas, or pericardial effusion is suspected
- Lower extremity Doppler if deep vein thrombosis/pulmonary embolism suspected
- CT scan of chest if pulmonary embolism suspected
- Indium-labeled leukocyte scanning if inflammatory process or occult abscess suspected
- Bone scan if osteomyelitis or metastatic disease suspected

Diagnostic Procedures/Other
- Liver biopsy if granulomatous disease suspected (3)[C]
- Temporal artery biopsy, particularly in the elderly
- Lymph node, muscle, or skin biopsy, if clinically indicated
- Bone marrow aspiration biopsy with smear, culture, histologic examination, and flow cytometry
- Lumbar puncture, if clinically indicated
- Endoscopy procedures can be helpful for IBD or sarcoidosis.

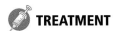 TREATMENT

GENERAL MEASURES
- Treatment depends on the specific etiology.
- Empiric therapy is not recommended in patients with prolonged fever because it may camouflage and therefore delay diagnosis and subsequently also hamper correct treatment decisions.
- Therapeutic trials are a last resort and should be as specific as possible based on available clinical evidence. Avoid "shotgun" approaches because they obscure the clinical picture, have untoward effects, and do not provide a diagnostic solution (3)[C].
- Empiric therapy is prudent in a few difficult-to-diagnose life-threatening cases, for example, CNS or miliary tuberculosis, or giant cell arteritis/temporal arteritis.

MEDICATION
First Line
- Antipyretic therapy as a symptomatic approach is a special form of empiric therapy, as it does not necessarily require understanding the cause of fever.
- First-line drugs depend on the diagnosis.
- Evidence does not support isolated treatment of fever (5)[C].

Second Line
Consider a therapeutic trial only if the patient has localizing symptoms associated with the fever or continues to decline. Consultation with appropriate specialists (infectious disease, rheumatology) is recommended in this case.
- Antibiotic trial based on patient's history and suspected culture negative endocarditis
- Antituberculous therapy if there is a high risk for TB pending definitive culture results

- Corticosteroid trial based on patient's history (once occult malignancy is ruled out) if temporal arteritis is suspected

ALERT
If a steroid trial is initiated, patient may have a relapse after treatment or if certain conditions (e.g., TB) have been undiagnosed.

ADDITIONAL THERAPIES
Febrile patients have increased caloric and fluid demands.

SURGERY/OTHER PROCEDURES
The need for exploratory laparotomy has been largely eliminated with the advent of more sophisticated tests and imaging modalities.

ADMISSION, INPATIENT, AND NURSING CONSIDERATIONS
- Reserved for the ill and debilitated
- Consider if factitious fever has been ruled out or an invasive procedure is indicated.

 ONGOING CARE

FOLLOW-UP RECOMMENDATIONS
Patient Monitoring
If the etiology of the fever remains unknown, repeat the history, physical exam, and screening lab studies.

DIET
No specific dietary recommendations have been shown to ameliorate undiagnosed fever.

PATIENT EDUCATION
Maintain an open line of communication between physician and patient/family as the workup progresses:
- The extended time required in establishing a diagnosis can be frustrating.

PROGNOSIS
- Depends on etiology and age
  – Patients with HIV have the highest mortality.
- Prognosis worse if delay in diagnosis
- Spontaneous remission is not uncommon in patients with unknown cause of FUO after a through workup including a negative FDG-PET/CT scan
- 1-year survival rates (reflecting deaths due to all causes)

Age	Survival
<35 y	91%
35–64 y	82%
>64 y	67%

COMPLICATIONS
Depends on etiology

Pregnancy Considerations
Fever increases the risk of neural tube defects in pregnancy and can also trigger preterm labor.

REFERENCES
1. Hayakawa K, Ramasamy B, Chandrasekar PH. Fever of unknown origin: an evidence-based review. *Am J Med Sci*. 2012;344(4):307–316.
2. Mulders-Manders C, Simon A, Bleeker-Rovers C. Fever of unknown origin. *Clin Med (Lond)*. 2015;15(3):280–284.
3. Kaya A, Ergul N, Kaya SY, et al. The management and the diagnosis of fever of unknown origin. *Expert Rev Anti Infect Ther*. 2013;11(8):805–815.
4. Takeuchi M, Dahabreh IJ, Nihashi T, et al. Nuclear imaging for classic fever of unknown origin: meta-analysis. *J Nucl Med*. 2016;57(12):1913–1919.
5. Hersch EC, Oh RC. Prolonged febrile illness and fever of unknown origin in adults. *Am Fam Physician*. 2014;90(2):91–96.

ADDITIONAL READING
- Cunha BA, Lortholary O, Cunha CB. Fever of unknown origin: a clinical approach. *Am J Med*. 2015;128(10):1138.e1–1138.e15.
- Santana LFE, Rodrigues MS, Silva MPA, et al. Fever of unknown origin—a literature review. *Rev Assoc Med Bras*. 2019;65(8):1109–1115.

 SEE ALSO

- Arteritis, Temporal; Arthritis, Juvenile Idiopathic; Colon Cancer; Cytomegalovirus (CMV) Inclusion Disease; Endocarditis, Infective; Hepatoma (Hepatocellular Carcinoma); HIV/AIDS; Lupus Erythematosus, Discoid; Osteomyelitis; Polyarteritis Nodosa; Polymyalgia Rheumatica; Pulmonary Embolism; Rectal Cancer; Rheumatic Fever; Sinusitis; Stroke, Acute (Cerebrovascular Accident [CVA])
- Algorithms: Fever in the First 3 Months of Life; Fever of Unknown Origin (FUO)

CODES

ICD10
R50.9 Fever, unspecified

CLINICAL PEARLS
- A sequential approach to FUO based on a careful history, physical examination, with targeted testing and imaging typically yields an appropriate diagnosis and avoids excessive nontargeted testing.
- Empiric therapy is indicated only for carefully defined circumstances.
- FUO cases that defy precise diagnosis after intensive investigation and prolonged observation generally have a favorable prognosis.
- FUO in older persons often presents as an atypical presentation of a common disease.
- The most common causes of FUO in high-income countries are noninfectious inflammatory diseases and idiopathic causes.

F

FIBROCYSTIC CHANGES OF THE BREAST
Sharon L. Koehler, DO, FACS

BASICS

DESCRIPTION
- Benign epithelial lesions are common findings in women and can be divided into nonproliferative and proliferative and with and without atypia.
- Fibrocystic changes (FCC) are not a disease but refers to a constellation of benign, nonproliferative histologic findings. It is the most frequent female benign epithelial lesion.
- FCC are seen clinically in up to 50% and histologically in up to 90% of women (1).
- FCC may also be described as aberrations of normal development and evolution.
- The most common symptoms are cyclic pain, tenderness, swelling, and fullness.
- The breast tissue may feel dense with areas of thicker tissue having an irregular, nodular, or ridge-like surface.
- Women may experience sensitivity to touch with a burning sensation. For some, the pain is so severe that it limits exercise or the ability to lie prone. Usually affects both breasts, most often in the upper outer quadrant where most of the milk-producing glands are located
- Histologically, in addition to macrocysts and microcysts, FCC may contain solid elements including adenosis, sclerosis, apocrine metaplasia, stromal fibrosis, and epithelial metaplasia and hyperplasia.
  - Depending on the presence of epithelial hyperplasia, FCC is classified as nonproliferative, proliferative without atypia, or proliferative with atypia (2).
  - Nonproliferative lesions are generally not associated with an increased risk of breast cancer.
- System(s) affected: endocrine/metabolic, reproductive
- Synonym(s): diffuse cystic mastopathy; fibrocystic disease; chronic cystic mastitis; or mammary dysplasia

EPIDEMIOLOGY
FCC occurs with great frequency in the general population. It affects women between the ages of 25 and 50 years, and it is rare below the age of 20 years.

Incidence
Unknown but very frequent

Prevalence
Up to 1/3 of women aged 30 to 50 years have cysts in their breasts (2). It most commonly presents in the 3rd decade, peaks in the 4th decade when hormonal function is at its peak, and sharply diminishes after menopause.
- With hormone replacement therapy, FCC may extend into menopause.

ETIOLOGY AND PATHOPHYSIOLOGY
- FCC originates from an exaggerated response of breast stroma and epithelium to a variety of circulating and locally produced hormones (mainly estrogen and progesterone) and growth factors.
- Cysts may form due to dilatation of the lobular acini possibly due to imbalance of fluid secretion and resorption or due to obstruction of the duct leading to the lobule.

RISK FACTORS
- In many women, methylxanthine-containing substances (e.g., coffee, tea, cola, and chocolate) can potentiate symptoms of FCC, although a direct causality has not been established.
- Diet high in saturated fats may increase risk of FCC.

COMMONLY ASSOCIATED CONDITIONS
FCC categorized as proliferative with atypia confers a higher risk of breast cancer.

DIAGNOSIS

HISTORY
- Obtain personal history of breast biopsy and family history of breast disease (benign or malignant). It is important to ascertain if the patient has a known family history of *breast, ovarian, and other cancers*.
- *Determine whether the patient has relatives any of the following deleterious mutations: BRCA1, BRCA2, PALB2, CHEK2, CDH1, PTEN, STK11, PT53,ATM, BARD1, BRIP1, CASP8, CTLA4, CYP19A1, FGFR2, H19, LSP1, MAP3K1, MRE11A, NBN, RAD51 and TERT.*
- Inquire regarding pertinent signs/symptoms, such as breast pain, swelling, nipple discharge, palpable lumps, retractions, skin changes, and tenderness.
  - Symptomatically, the condition is manifested as premenstrual cyclic mastalgia, with pain and tenderness to touch.

PHYSICAL EXAM
- The patient should be examined in the following positions while disrobed down to the waist:
  - With the patient standing with arms at sides, observe for elevation of the level of a nipple, dimpling, bulging, and peau d'orange.
  - With the patient's arms raised above her head, observe for dimpling and elevation/retraction of the nipple (may accentuate a mass fixed to the pectoral fascia). If so, have the patient push her hands down against her hips to flex and tense the pectoralis major muscles; move the mass to determine fixation to the underlying fascia.
  - If the patient has large and pendulous breasts, ask her to lean forward, so that her breasts hang free from the chest wall (retraction and masses may become more evident).
  - Axillary lymph nodes are evaluated with the patient sitting up, the arm supported by the examiner's arm while finger pads gently palpate the axilla from the posterior axillary line to the pectoralis.
  - With the patient lying supine, palpate with the pads of the three middle fingers (with varying pressures from light, to medium, to deep), rotating the fingers in small circular motions and moving in vertical overlapping passes from rostral to caudal and then back caudal to rostral in the next pass. The lateral half of the breast is best palpated with the patient rolled onto the contralateral hip and the medial half with the patient supine, both with the ipsilateral hand behind the head. The entire breast from the 2nd to 6th rib and from the left sternal border to the midaxillary line must be palpated against the chest wall.
- Be certain to examine the creases under and between the breasts. If the patient has noted a lump, ask her to point it out; always palpate the opposite breast first.
- Patients with FCC have clinical breast findings that range from mild alterations in texture to dense, firm breast tissue with palpable masses.

DIFFERENTIAL DIAGNOSIS
- Pain
  - Mastitis
  - Costochondritis
  - Pectoralis muscle strain
  - Neuralgia
  - Breast cancer
  - Angina pectoris
  - Gastroesophageal reflux (GERD)
  - Superficial phlebitis of the thoracoepigastric vein (Mondor disease)
- Masses
  - Breast cancer
  - Sebaceous cyst
  - Fibroadenoma
  - Lipoma
  - Fat necrosis
  - Phyllodes tumor
  - Granuloma
- Skin changes
  - Breast cancer (peau d'orange: thickened skin similar to peel of an orange)
  - Eczema
  - Infection
  - Fungus
  - Paget disease

DIAGNOSTIC TESTS & INTERPRETATION
- Evaluation should focus on excluding breast cancer.
- Testing may be conducted based on a level of clinical suspicion.
- FCC can be evaluated with mammogram, although dense breast tissue may appear normal in women <35 years of age.
- Ultrasound (US) is the most useful method for assessing a cyst.

Initial Tests (lab, imaging)
- On mammogram, FCC appears as nodular densities of breast tissue; solitary cysts can appear as round or ovoid or well-circumscribed masses, usually with low to intermediate density. FCC may also contain calcifications.
- On US, if a simple cyst is demonstrated as an anechoic structure with imperceptible wall and posterior acoustic enhancement, benign diagnosis is confirmed and no further imaging or intervention is indicated. However, if the cyst appears to be thick-walled and/or contains internal echoes, differential diagnosis should include a complicated cyst, an abscess, a galactocele, or a focal duct ectasia in the appropriate clinical contexts.
- MRI is indicated in patients with *BRCA1, BRCA2,* or other related deleterious mutation, or in any woman with ≥25% lifetime risk for breast cancer. Additionally, MRI may be indicated for extremely dense breasts as well as inconclusive findings on other breast imaging.
- On MRI, cystic changes are well-circumscribed lesions of high-signal intensity on T2-weighted sequences and of low-signal intensity on T1-weighted images (2).

Diagnostic Procedures/Other

- Fine-needle aspiration (FNA) biopsy:
  - Allows differentiation of cystic and solid lesions
  - Aspirate may be straw-colored, dark brown, or green.
  - Cells sent for cytology can reveal cancer with high accuracy.
  - Low morbidity
- If mass disappears, no further evaluation is necessary (including cytologic evaluation of aspirated fluid).
- On the basis of the presence and degree of epithelial hyperplasia, FCC is comprised of nonproliferative (approximately 65% of the total), proliferative without atypia (approximately 30% of the total), and proliferative with atypia (approximately 5–8% of the total) (3).

Test Interpretation

Certain histologic changes in the setting of FCC confer an increased risk for breast cancer:

- Nonproliferative changes: relative risk of 1.2 to 1.4
- Proliferative disease (PD) without atypia: relative risk of 1.7 to 2.1
- PD with atypia: relative risk ≥4 (4)[B]

TREATMENT

- After ruling out malignancy by means of examination and/or imaging and diagnostic procedures, FCC may not require treatment and often resolves with time.
- Cool compresses, avoiding trauma, and around-the-clock wearing of a well-fitting, supportive brassiere may be useful for symptom relief.
- Reduction in caffeine, additional supplementation with vitamin E, and/or evening primrose oil have been advocated. Trials have not proven benefit (2).

MEDICATION

First Line

Analgesics and anti-inflammatory drugs are used to reduce cyclic breast pain and swelling. This includes oral and topical NSAIDs or acetaminophen.

- Acetaminophen: 1,000 mg every 6 to 8 hours; maximum daily dose of 3,000 mg unless directed by health care provider
- Ibuprofen: 400 mg every 4 to 6 hours as needed
- Naproxen: 500 mg every 12 hours as needed

Second Line

- Oral contraceptives (OCPs) may be useful in modulating symptoms or in preventing the development of new changes in females with cyclic symptoms.
- For severe pain, consider the following (5)[B],(6)[B]:
  - Danazol is effective for reducing breast pain and tenderness but has androgenic effects and is associated with hepatotoxicity and teratogenicity, which limits its use. This drug is administered orally at a dosage of 100 to 400 mg/day in 2 divided doses.
  - Tamoxifen 10 mg/day for 3 to 6 months. Along with teratogenicity, this selective estrogen receptor modulator (SERM) can increase the risk of thromboembolism and endometrial carcinoma in treated females.
  - Several other medications, such as bromocriptine and GnRH agonists, have been studied but are associated with toxicities.

ISSUES FOR REFERRAL

- If discrete palpable lesion in a woman <30 years: US, then refer to a surgeon
- If discrete palpable lesion in a woman >30 years: diagnostic mammography ± US, then refer to surgeon

SURGERY/OTHER PROCEDURES

- Breast cyst aspiration can be both diagnostic and therapeutic.
- Core-needle biopsies performed under stereotactic guidance with vacuum assistance has similar accuracy in distinguishing between malignant and benign lesions compared to open surgical biopsy (7)[A].
- Biopsy results must be assessed for concordance.

COMPLEMENTARY & ALTERNATIVE MEDICINE

- The use of vitamin E has shown effectiveness in treating breast pain due to FCC (4)[B].
- Anecdotal evidence supports the use of evening primrose oil for FCC.

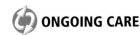

ONGOING CARE

FOLLOW-UP RECOMMENDATIONS

Condition is benign, chronic, and recurrent.

Patient Monitoring

- Follow-up times are variable, depending on the clinical situation and pertinent family history.
- US is useful to differentiate cysts from solid lesions and in evaluating women <35 years of age for FCC but is not useful for screening.
- Screening mammograms: Refer to the USPSTF, ACOG, or ACS recommendations for screening schedules.

DIET

The role of caffeine consumption in the development and treatment of FCC has never been proven; however, some patients report relief of symptoms after abstinence from coffee, tea, and chocolate.

PATIENT EDUCATION

- Patient information on fibrocystic breasts from the Mayo Foundation for Medical Education and Research: http://www.mayoclinic.com/health/fibrocystic-breasts/DS01070
- Information on breast cancer prevention from the National Cancer Institute: http://www.cancer.gov
- Information on fibrocystic breasts from the American Cancer Society: http://www.cancer.org/Healthy/FindCancerEarly/WomensHealth/Non-CancerousBreastConditions/non-cancerous-breast-conditions-fibrocystic-changes

REFERENCES

1. Guray M, Sahin AA. Benign breast diseases: classification, diagnosis & management. *Oncologist*. 2006;11(5):435–449.
2. Pearlman M, Griffin J, Swain M, et al; for American College of Obstetricians and Gynecologists' Committee on Practice Bulletins—Gynecology. Practice Bulletin No. 164: diagnosis and management of benign breast disorders. *Obstet Gynecol*. 2016;127(6):e141–e156.
3. Hartmann LC, Sellers TA, Frost MH, et al. Benign breast disease and the risk of breast cancer. *N Engl J Med*. 2005;353(3):229–237.
4. Horner NK, Lampe JW. Potential mechanisms of diet therapy for fibrocystic breast conditions show inadequate evidence of effectiveness. *J Am Diet Assoc*. 2000;100(11):1368–1380.
5. Srivastava A, Mansel RE, Arvind N, et al. Evidence-based management of mastalgia: a meta-analysis of randomised trials. *Breast*. 2007;16(5):503–512.
6. Mousavi SR, Mousavi SM, Samsami M, et al. Comparison of tamoxifen with danazol in the management of fibrocystic disease. *Int J Med Sci*. 2011;2:329–331.
7. Bruening W, Fontanarosa J, Tipton K, et al. Systematic review: comparative effectiveness of core-needle and open surgical biopsy to diagnose breast lesions. *Ann Intern Med*. 2010;152(4):238–246.

ADDITIONAL READING

- Amin AL, Purdy AC, Mattingly JD, et al. Benign breast disease. *Surg Clin North Am*. 2013;93(2):299–308.
- Hafiz SP, Barnes NLP, Kirwan CC. Clinical management of idiopathic mastalgia: a systematic review. *J Prim Health Care*. 2018;10(4):312–323.
- Salzman B, Collins E, Hersh L. Common breast problems. *Am Fam Physician*. 2019;99(8):505–514.
- Santen RJ, Mansel R. Benign breast disorders. *N Engl J Med*. 2005;353(3):275–285.

 CODES

ICD10

- N60.19 Diffuse cystic mastopathy of unspecified breast
- N60.09 Solitary cyst of unspecified breast
- N60.29 Fibroadenosis of unspecified breast

CLINICAL PEARLS

- FCC of the breast comprise a spectrum of histopathologic changes are a common finding in reproductive-aged women. The former term of fibrocystic disease is a misnomer.
- Atypia, as demonstrated histopathologically, confers an increased cancer risk.
- NSAIDs are the first-line treatment.
- OCPs, danazol, and tamoxifen are second-line treatments, with considerable adverse effects.
- Consultation with a breast specialist is recommended for symptomatic disease refractory to simple measures or for diagnostic issues.

F

FIBROMYALGIA

F. Stuart Leeds, MD, MS

BASICS

DESCRIPTION
- Chronic, widespread noninflammatory musculoskeletal pain syndrome with multisystem manifestations. Although the specific pathophysiology has not been fully elucidated, it is generally thought to be a disorder of altered central pain regulation.
- Synonym(s): FMS; fibrositis, fibromyositis (misnomers)

EPIDEMIOLOGY
Incidence
- Predominant sex: female (70–90%) > male
- Predominant age range: 20 to 65 years

Prevalence
2–5% of adult U.S. population (1); 8% of primary care patients

ETIOLOGY AND PATHOPHYSIOLOGY
- Idiopathic; appears to be a primary disorder of central pain processing (central sensitization) with afferent augmentation of peripheral nociceptive stimuli
- Alterations in neuroendocrine, neuromodulation, neurotransmitter, neurotransporter, biochemical, and neuroreceptor function/physiology
- Sleep abnormalities—α-wave intrusion
- Systemic inflammation is not a feature of fibromyalgia, although localized immunologic processes in the CNS may play a role.

Genetics
- Genetics
  - High familial aggregation
  - Inheritance is unknown but likely polygenic.
  - Odds ratio may be as high as 8.5 for a first-degree relative of a familial proband.
- Environmental—several triggers have been described:
  - Physical trauma or severe illness
  - Stressors (e.g., work, family, life events, and physical or sexual abuse)
  - Viral and bacterial infections

RISK FACTORS
- Female gender
- Poor functional status
- Negative/stressful life events
- Low socioeconomic status

GENERAL PREVENTION
No known strategies for prevention

COMMONLY ASSOCIATED CONDITIONS
- Often a comorbid condition with other rheumatologic or neurologic disorders
- Obesity is common and associated with increased severity of symptoms.

DIAGNOSIS

- Original 1990 ACR criteria, still widely used: (i) pain in all four quadrants > 3 months, (ii) axial (neck/spine) involvement, (iii) tender points ≥11 (1)
- 2010/2011 ACR criteria, revised in 2016 (1)
  - Based on Widespread Pain Index (WPI) and Symptom Score (SS)
    ○ Generalized pain present in 4/5 body regions
    ○ Must have WPI ≥7 + SS ≥5, or WPI 4–6 and SS ≥9
    ○ Symptoms for >3 months
    ○ Fibromyalgia may be diagnosed irrespective of other active disease entities (i.e., it need not be the only explanation for the patient's symptoms).
- WPI/SS patient scoring and diagnosis tool: https://www.prohealth.com/wp-content/uploads/2016/12/NewFibroCriteriaSurvey.pdf
- The Visual Analogue Scale Fibromyalgia Impact Questionnaire (VASFIQ) is recommended for initial and serial assessment of patient's functional status (2).

HISTORY
- Invariant symptoms include
  - Chronic widespread pain ≥3 months: bilateral limbs and in the axial skeleton
  - Fatigue and sleep disturbances
- Often present:
  - Mood disorders, including depression, anxiety, and panic symptoms
  - Cognitive impairment: qualitatively different from that seen in isolated mood disorders ("fibro fog")
  - Headaches: typically tension and migraine types
  - Other regional pain syndromes, such as irritable bowel syndrome, chronic pelvic pain, vulvodynia, and interstitial cystitis
  - Small-fiber neuropathies and "nonanatomic" paresthesias
  - Exercise intolerance, dyspnea, and palpitations
  - Sexual dysfunction
  - Ocular dryness
  - "Multiple chemical sensitivity" and an increased tendency to report drug reactions
  - Impaired social/occupational functioning
  - Symptoms can wax and wane on a day-to-day basis, varying in quality, intensity, and location.

PHYSICAL EXAM
- Classic fibromyalgia tender points (TPs): 9 symmetric pairs (5 anterior, 4 posterior).
- The presence of ≥11 TPs carries a sensitivity of 88% and specificity 81% for the disease (1)
- TPs in fibromyalgia are distinct from the "trigger points" found in myofascial pain syndromes and are not sites for therapeutic injection.
- Examine joints for swelling, tenderness, erythema, decreased range of motion, crepitus, and cystic or mass lesions. These are typically absent in fibromyalgia.

- Document absence of inflammatory features (e.g., no synovitis, enthesopathy, dermatologic, or ocular findings).
- Neurologic exam: may demonstrate generalized or "nonanatomic" dysesthesia, hyper- or hypesthesia

DIFFERENTIAL DIAGNOSIS
- RA, SLE, sarcoidosis, and other inflammatory connective tissue disorders
- Diffuse/advanced OA
- Seronegative spondyloarthropathies (AS, psoriatic arthritis, etc.)
- Polymyalgia rheumatica
- Inherited myopathies
- Drug-induced and endocrine myopathies
- Viral/postviral polyarthralgia
- Anemia and iron deficiency
- Sickle-cell anemia
- Electrolyte disturbances: Mg, Na, K, Ca
- Obstructive sleep apnea
- Restless leg syndrome
- Osteomalacia/vitamin D deficiency
- Joint hypermobility syndromes (Ehlers-Danlos et al)
- Complex regional pain syndromes (CRPS)
- Opioid-induced hyperalgesia
- Hypothyroidism
- Hyperparathyroidism
- Multiple sclerosis
- Lyme disease
- Hepatitis B and C (chronic)
- Inclusion-body myositis
- Generalized muscular deconditioning
- Peripheral vascular disease
- Central poststroke pain syndromes
- Spinal cord injury syndromes
- Inflammatory polyneuropathies
- Malignancies: metastatic and paraneoplastic syndromes
- Somatic symptom disorder and other psychiatric conditions with associated somatization symptoms
- Overlap syndromes
  - Chronic fatigue syndrome/chronic fatigue immune dysfunction syndrome (CFIDS)
  - Myofascial pain syndrome (more anatomically localized than fibromyalgia, but they may co-occur)

DIAGNOSTIC TESTS & INTERPRETATION
Initial Tests (lab, imaging)
- CBC with differential, ESR or CRP, CPK, TSH, comprehensive metabolic profile; consider 25-OH vitamin D, Mg, vitamin B_{12}, folate, and urine drug screen.
- ANA, RF, and other rheumatologic labs generally unnecessary, unless there is evidence of an inflammatory connective tissue disorder
- Imaging is not indicated, except to exclude other specific diagnoses.

Diagnostic Procedures/Other
- Sleep studies may be indicated to rule out obstructive sleep apnea or narcolepsy.
- Consider psychiatric or neuropsychiatric evaluation for mood disorders and cognitive disturbances.

TREATMENT

Evidence-based interventions:
- Includes both medication and nonpharmacologic interventions. In general, a partial or complete remission can only be achieved with committed changes in lifestyle, including regular exercise, proper sleep hygiene, and smoking cessation.
- Nonpharmacologic
  - Educate about diagnosis, signs, symptoms, and treatment options: Online resources include:
    - https://www.fmaware.net
    - https://www.fibromyalgiaforums.org/
    - https://fibroandpain.org/
  - VASFIQ for initial assessment and interval evaluation during treatment
  - Cognitive-behavioral therapy (CBT) improves mood, energy, pain, and functional status.
  - Acceptance and commitment therapy (ACT)
  - Aerobic exercise: moderately intense, with gradual titration to minimize symptom exacerbation ("start low and slow")
  - Strength/resistance training—mild to moderate
  - Tai chi—equal or superior to aerobic exercise (3)[A]
  - Aquatic exercise training
  - Mixed exercise training (combined aerobic, resistance, flexibility)
  - Weight loss may augment the benefits of exercise.
  - Sleep hygiene
  - Mitigate/eliminate tobacco, alcohol, and substance use.
- Pharmacologic
  - Three FDA-approved drugs: duloxetine, milnacipran, and pregabalin; others are off-label. Recent studies suggest that these agents, when used as monotherapy, only benefit a minority of responders.
  - **Caution**: Fibromyalgia patients are frequently treated with multidrug regimens; monitor closely for drug interactions, sedative, serotonergic, and anticholinergic effects.

MEDICATION
First Line
- Amitriptyline 10 to 50 mg PO at bedtime to treat pain, fatigue, and sleep disturbances (4)[A]. Other TCAs (imipramine, desipramine, nortriptyline) may be similarly effective.
- Duloxetine initially 30 mg/day for 1 week and then increase to 60 mg/day as tolerated. Taper if discontinued (4)[A].
- Milnacipran day 1: 12.5 mg/day; days 2 to 3, begin dividing doses: 12.5 mg BID; days 4 to 7: 25 mg BID; after day 7: 50 mg BID; max dose 100 to 200 mg BID. Taper if discontinued (4)[A].
- Pregabalin: Start with 75 mg BID, titrate over 1 week to 150 mg BID; max dose 450 mg/day (some authorities recommend up to 600 mg daily) divided BID–TID (4)[A].
- Cyclobenzaprine 5 mg qHS; titrate to 10 mg BID–TID as tolerated.

Second Line
- Gabapentin: Start at 300 mg HS, titrate to 1,200 to 2,400 mg/day divided BID–TID; max dose 3,600 mg daily
- Venlafaxine XR 37.5 to 225 mg; likely to be as effective as other SNRIs (duloxetine, milnacipran)

- Tramadol 50 to 100 mg q6h; likely more effective in combination with acetaminophen
- Quetiapine 25 to 100 mg qHS (5)[B]
- Several agents have shown some promise of benefit, albeit with limited evidence, including pramipexole, memantine, low-dose naltrexone, medical cannabis, and hyperbaric O_2 therapy.
- Cholecalciferol may be beneficial in patients with low 25-OH vitamin D levels.

ISSUES FOR REFERRAL
In cases of unclear diagnosis or poor response to therapy, refer to rheumatology, neurology, and/or pain management.

ADDITIONAL THERAPIES
- Trigger point (not tender point) injections for regional myofascial dysfunction may provide relief.
- Multidisciplinary rehab (specialized clinic with physical medicine and therapy, occupational therapy, and integrated pain management)
- Ineffective or dangerous treatment modalities
  - NSAIDs, full-agonist opioids (except in refractory cases), benzodiazepines, SSRIs (although may have efficacy in combination therapy with TCAs or pregabalin), magnesium, guaifenesin, thyroxine, corticosteroids, DHEA, valacyclovir, interferon, calcitonin, nabilone, and antiepileptic agents (other than those listed above) (5)[A]
  - *Fibromyalgia often presents concurrently with other pain syndromes that may respond to NSAIDs, corticosteroids, opioids, and other agents.*

COMPLEMENTARY & ALTERNATIVE MEDICINE
- Acupuncture and electroacupuncture, biofeedback, hypnotherapy
- Balneotherapy (mineral-rich baths)
- Yoga, tai chi, and qi gong
- Mindfulness-based meditation
- Low-level laser therapy
- Myofascial massage—short- to medium-term benefit
- Limited double-blind trials have shown effectiveness of supplementation with S-adenosyl-l-methionine and acetyl-L-carnitine.
- Weak evidence for transcranial direct current and other forms of cranial electrical stimulation
- Likely to be ineffective: chiropractic treatment, multivitamin therapy, homeopathy

ONGOING CARE

FOLLOW-UP RECOMMENDATIONS
Patient Monitoring
- For efficacy of initial therapy: at 2- to 4-week intervals, then every 1 to 6 months, tailored to patient's needs
- Advance exercise gradually to maintain tolerability.

DIET
Patient should make healthy choices and address negative dietary habits. Caloric or carbohydrate restriction may be helpful in obese patients. Reduction in pain has been reported in patients following hypocaloric and vegan diets, as well as a diets low in fermentable saccharides and polyols (FODMAP).

PROGNOSIS
- 50% with partial remission after 2 to 3 years of therapy; complete remission possible but rare
- Typically has fluctuating, chronic course
- Poorer outcomes tied to greater duration and severity of symptoms, depression, obesity, insufficient engagement and "ownership" of the treatment plan, advanced age, and lack of social support

REFERENCES
1. Wolfe F, Clauw DJ, Fitzcharles MA, et al. 2016 Revisions to the 2010/2011 fibromyalgia diagnostic criteria. *Semin Arthritis Rheum*. 2016;46(3):319–329.
2. Boomershine CS, Emir B, Wang Y, et al. Simplifying fibromyalgia assessment: the VASFIQ Brief Symptom Scale. *Ther Adv Musculoskelet Dis*. 2011;3(5):215–226.
3. Cheng C-A, Chiu Y-W, Wu D, et al. Effectiveness of tai chi on fibromyalgia patients: a meta-analysis of randomized controlled trials. *Complement Ther Med*. 2019;46:1–8.
4. Welsch P, Üçeyler N, Klose P, et al. Serotonin and noradrenaline reuptake inhibitors (SNRIs) for fibromyalgia. *Cochrane Database Syst Rev*. 2018;(2):CD010292.
5. Bair MJ, Krebs EE. Fibromyalgia. *Ann Intern Med*. 2020;172(5):ITC33–ITC48.

ADDITIONAL READING
- Bazzichi L, Giacomelli C, Consensi A, et al. One year in review 2020: fibromyalgia. *Clin Exp Rheumatol*. 2020;38(1 Suppl 123):3–8.
- Lowry E, Marley J, McVeigh JG, et al. Dietary interventions in the management of fibromyalgia: a systematic review and best-evidence synthesis. *Nutrients*. 2020;12(9):E2664.
- Sagy I, Bar-Lev Schleider L, Abu-Shakra M, et al. Safety and efficacy of medical cannabis in fibromyalgia. *J Clin Med*. 2019;8(6):807.
- Theadom A, Cropley M, Smith HE, et al. Mind and body therapy for fibromyalgia. *Cochrane Database Syst Rev*. 2015;(4):CD001980.

SEE ALSO

Algorithm: Fatigue

CODES
ICD10
M79.7 Fibromyalgia

CLINICAL PEARLS
- Fibromyalgia is a disease of central sensitization; it is not a somatoform disorder and is not merely a manifestation of depression or anxiety. As with all chronic pain syndromes, however, fibromyalgia is frequently associated with comorbid mood and anxiety disorders.
- Use ACR criteria to make the formal diagnosis of fibromyalgia.
- The best clinical outcomes occur in patients who understand their illness and actively engage in a multimodal treatment plan that includes exercise, sleep hygiene, and other lifestyle modifications, along with appropriate pharmacotherapy and CBT.

FOLLICULITIS
David C. Cadena Jr., MD

BASICS

DESCRIPTION
- Inflammation of a hair follicle (1). Subtypes include perifolliculitis and pseudofolliculitis, which occur around the follicle.
- Can occur anywhere on the body where hair is found
- Most frequent symptom is pruritus.
- Painless or tender pustules, vesicles, or pink/red papulopustules up to 5 mm in size
- Most commonly infectious in etiology:
  - *Staphylococcus aureus* bacteria
  - *Pseudomonas aeruginosa* infects areas of the body exposed to poorly sanitized hot tubs, pools, or contaminated water.
  - *Aeromonas hydrophila* with recreational water exposure
  - Fungal (dermatophytic, *Pityrosporum, Candida*)
  - Viral (VZV, herpes simplex virus [HSV])
  - Parasitic (*Demodex* spp. mites, schistosomes)
- Noninfectious types
  - Acneiform folliculitis
  - Actinic superficial folliculitis
  - Acne vulgaris
  - Keloidal folliculitis
  - Folliculitis decalvans
  - Perioral dermatitis
  - Fox-Fordyce disease
  - Pruritus folliculitis of pregnancy
  - Eosinophilic pustular folliculitis (three variants: Ofuji disease in patients of Asian descent, HIV positive/immunocompromised, infantile)
  - Toxic erythema of the newborn
  - Eosinophilic folliculitis (seen in HIV positive/ immunocompromised)
  - Follicular mucinosis
- Skin disorders that may produce a follicular eruption:
  - Pseudofolliculitis barbae: similar in appearance; occurs after shaving; commonly known as razor bumps, occurs more frequently in black men
  - Atopic dermatitis
  - Follicular psoriasis
  - Rosacea

EPIDEMIOLOGY
Affects persons of all ages, gender, and race; African ethnicities more predisposed to certain types of folliculitis

ETIOLOGY AND PATHOPHYSIOLOGY
Predisposing factors to folliculitis
- Chronic staphylococcal carrier
- Diabetes mellitus
- Malnutrition
- Pruritic skin disease (e.g., scabies, eczema)
- Exposure to poorly chlorinated swimming pools/ hot tubs or water contaminated with *P. aeruginosa, A. hydrophila*, or schistosomes
- Occlusive corticosteroid use (for multiple hours)
- Bacteria
  - Most frequently due to *S. aureus* (increasing number of methicillin-resistant *S. aureus* [MRSA] cases)
  - Also due to *Streptococcus* species, *Pseudomonas* (following exposure to water contaminated with the species), or *Proteus*
  - May progress to furunculosis (painful pustular nodule with central necrosis that leaves a permanent scar after healing)

- Fungal
  - Dermatophytic (tinea capitis, tinea corporis, tinea pedis)
  - *Pityrosporum* (Pityrosporum orbiculare) commonly affecting teenagers and men, predominantly on upper chest and back
  - *Candida albicans*, although rare, has been reported with broad-spectrum antibiotic use, glucocorticoid use, immunosuppression, and in those who abuse heroin, resulting in candidemia that leads to pustules and nodules in hair-bearing areas.
- Viral
  - HSV
  - Molluscum contagiosum
- Parasitic
  - *Demodex* mites (most commonly *Demodex folliculorum*), common around nasolabial area
  - Schistosomes (swimmer's itch)
- Acneiform type commonly drug induced (systemic and topical corticosteroids, lithium, isoniazid, rifampin), EGFR inhibitors
- Severe vitamin C deficiency, scurvy
- Actinic superficial type occurs within 24 to 48 hours of exposure to the sun, resulting in multiple follicular pustules on the shoulders, trunk, and arms.
- Acne vulgaris
- Keloidal folliculitis is a chronic condition affecting mostly black patients; involves the neck and occipital scalp, resulting in hypertrophic scars and hair loss; usually consequence of uncontrolled folliculitis barbae
- Folliculitis decalvans is a chronic folliculitis that leads to progressive scarring and alopecia of the scalp.
- Rosacea consists of papules, pustules, and/or telangiectasias of the face; individuals are genetically predisposed; *can be confused with folliculitis*
- Fox-Fordyce disease affects the skin containing apocrine sweat glands (i.e., axillae), resulting in chronic pruritic, annular, follicular papules.
- Eosinophilic pustular folliculitis has three variants: classic (Ofuji disease), associated with HIV infection, and infantile.
- Toxic erythema of the newborn is a self-limiting pustular eruption usually appearing during the first 3 to 4 days of life and subsequently fading in the following 2 weeks.
- *Malassezia* infections in adult males with lesions on trunk (2)

RISK FACTORS
- Hair removal (shaving, plucking, waxing, epilating agents)
- Other pruritic skin conditions: eczema, scabies
- Occlusive dressing or clothing
- Sweating
- Personal carrier or contact with MRSA-infected persons
- Diabetes mellitus
- Immunosuppression (medications, chemotherapy, HIV)
- Use of hot tubs or saunas
- Use of EGFR inhibitors
- Chronic antibiotic use (gram-negative folliculitis)
- Tattoo recipient

GENERAL PREVENTION
- Good hygiene practices
  - Wash hands frequently with antimicrobial soap.
  - Wash towels, clothes, and linens frequently with hot water to avoid reinfection.

- Good hair removal practices
  - Exfoliate beforehand.
  - Use witch hazel, alcohol, or Tend Skin afterward.
  - Shave in direction of hair growth; use shaving gel and moisturizer.
  - Decrease frequency of shaving.
  - Use clippers primarily or single-blade razors if straight shaving is desired.

COMMONLY ASSOCIATED CONDITIONS
- Impetigo
- Scabies
- Acne
- Follicular psoriasis
- Eczema
- Xerosis
- *Staphylococcus*/MRSA colonization

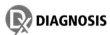
DIAGNOSIS

HISTORY
- Recent use of hot tubs, swimming pools, topical corticosteroids, certain hair styling and shaving practices, antibiotics or systemic steroids
- HIV status
- History of STDs (specifically syphilis)
- MRSA exposures/carrier status
- Home and work environment (risk/exposure potential)
- Pityrosporum folliculitis occurs more often in warm, moist climates.
- Inquire about the timeline in which the lesions have occurred, including previous similar episodes.

PHYSICAL EXAM
- Characteristic lesions are 1- to 5-mm–wide vesicles, pustules, or inflamed papules with surrounding erythema.
- Rash occurs on hair-bearing skin, especially the face (beard), proximal limbs, scalp, and pubis.
- Pseudomonal folliculitis appears as a widespread rash, mainly on the trunk and limbs.
- In pseudofolliculitis barbae, the growing hair curls around and penetrates the skin at shaved areas.

DIFFERENTIAL DIAGNOSIS
- Acne vulgaris/acneiform eruptions
- Arthropod bite
- Contact dermatitis
- Perioral dermatitis
- Cutaneous candidiasis
- Milia
- Atopic dermatitis
- Follicular psoriasis
- Hidradenitis suppurativa

DIAGNOSTIC TESTS & INTERPRETATION
Initial Tests (lab, imaging)
- Diagnosis can be made clinically, taking risk factors, history, and locations of lesions into account.
- Culture and Gram stain may be done for larger lesions lancing or unroofing the pustule.
- KOH preparation as well as Wood lamp fluorescence to identify *Candida* or yeast
- Tzanck smear where suspicion of herpetic simplex viral folliculitis is high
- Ultrasound can be performed for questionably deeper seeding infections.

Follow-Up Tests & Special Considerations
- If risk factors or clinical suspicion exist, consider serologies for HIV or syphilis.
- If recurrent, consider HIV testing and A1C/fasting blood sugar testing to evaluate for diabetes.
- Consider punch biopsy with uncertain diagnosis.
- Treat positive bacterial culture according to sensitivities.
- Positive HIV serology: Follow up with CD4 count and punch biopsy to rule out eosinophilic folliculitis.

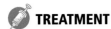 **TREATMENT**

GENERAL MEASURES
- Lesions usually resolve spontaneously.
- Avoid shaving and waxing affected areas (3)[C].
- Warm compresses may be applied TID.
- Systemic antibiotics are typically unnecessary.
- Topical mupirocin may be used in presumed *S. aureus* infection (4)[B].
- Topical antifungals for fungal folliculitis (2)[B]
- Preventive measures:
  - Antibacterial soaps (Dial soap, chlorhexidine, or benzoyl peroxide wash when showering/bathing)
  - Bleach baths (1/2 cup of 6% bleach per standard bathtub and soak for 5 to 15 minutes followed by water, rinse 1 to 2 times a week)
  - Keep skin intact; daily skin care with noncomedogenic moisturizers; avoid scratching.
  - Avoid trauma to skin: Use an electric razor as able.
  - Clean shaving instruments daily or use disposable razor, disposing after one use (5)[B].
  - Change washcloths, towels, and sheets daily.

MEDICATION
Antiseptic and supportive care is usually enough. Systemic antibiotics may be used but have questionable efficacy.

First Line
- Staphylococcal folliculitis
  - Mupirocin ointment applied TID for 10 days
  - Cephalosporin (cephalexin): 250 to 500 mg PO QID for 7 to 10 days
  - Dicloxacillin: 250 to 500 mg PO QID for 7 to 10 days
- For MRSA
  - Bactrim DS: 1 to 2 tablets (160 mg/800 mg) BID PO for 5 to 10 days
  - Clindamycin: 300 mg PO TID for 10 to 14 days
  - Minocycline: 200 mg PO initially and then 100 mg BID for 5 to 10 days
  - Doxycycline: 50 to 100 mg PO BID for 5 to 10 days
- *Pseudomonas* folliculitis
  - Topical dilute acetic acid baths
  - Ciprofloxacin: 500 to 750 mg PO BID for 7 to 14 days only if patient is immunocompromised or lesions are persistent
- Eosinophilic folliculitis/eosinophilic pustular folliculitis
  - HAART treatment for HIV-positive–related causes. Consider referral to appropriate treatment center.
  - High-potency topical corticosteroids for inflammation
  - Antihistamines (hydroxyzine, cetirizine) to control itching
  - Can consider: tacrolimus topically BID *or*
  - Isotretinoin 0.5 mg/kg/day PO with caution
  - Itraconazole or metronidazole

- Fungal folliculitis
  - Topical antifungals: ketoconazole 2% cream or shampoo or selenium sulfide shampoo daily *or*
  - Econazole cream applied to affected area BID for 2 to 3 weeks
    - Systemic antifungals for relapses fluconazole (100 to 200 mg/day for 3 weeks) *or* itraconazole (200 mg/day for 1 week) *or* griseofulvin (500 mg/day for 2 to 4 weeks)
    - Do not use oral ketoconazole due to risk of liver failure.
- Parasitic folliculitis
  - 5% permethrin: Apply to affected area, leave on for 8 hours, and wash off.
  - Ivermectin: 200 μg/kg PO and repeat in 1 to 2 weeks if topical application unsuccessful
- Herpetic folliculitis
  - Valacyclovir: 500 mg PO TID for 5 to 10 days *or*
  - Famciclovir: 500 mg PO TID for 5 to 10 days *or*
  - Acyclovir: 200 mg PO 5 times daily for 5 to 10 days

ISSUES FOR REFERRAL
Unusual or persistent cases should be biopsied and then referred to dermatology.

ADDITIONAL THERAPIES
- Stay informed: Testing strips can be used to test hot tubs and pools. This will help determine proper chlorine levels.
- Both hot tubs and pools should have a pH level of 7.2 to 7.8.

SURGERY/OTHER PROCEDURES
Incision and drainage is unlikely to be necessary and typically not preferred due to potential for scar formation.

 ONGOING CARE

FOLLOW-UP RECOMMENDATIONS
Patient Monitoring
- Resistant cases should be followed every 2 weeks until cleared.
- Consider prompt system therapy for worsening cases.

DIET
Caloric monitoring for obese patients; weight reduction will decrease risk of skin trauma and distension.

PATIENT EDUCATION
- Avoid shaving in involved areas.
- Monitor hot tub and pools.

PROGNOSIS
- Usually resolves with treatment; however, *S. aureus* carriers may experience recurrences.
- Mupirocin nasal treatment for carrier status and for family/household members might be helpful.
- Resistant or severe cases may warrant testing for diabetes mellitus or immunodeficiency (HIV).

COMPLICATIONS
- Primary complication is recurrent folliculitis.
- Extensive scarring with hyperpigmentation
- Progression to furunculosis or abscesses

REFERENCES
1. Laureano A, Schwartz RA, Cohen P. Facial bacterial infections: folliculitis. *Clin Dermatol.* 2014;32(6):711–714.
2. Song HS, Kim SK, Kim YC. Comparison between *Malassezia* folliculitis and non-*Malassezia* folliculitis. *Ann Dermatol.* 2014;26(5):598–602.
3. Khanna N, Chandramohan K, Khaitan BK, et al. Post waxing folliculitis: a clinicopathological evaluation. *Int J Dermatol.* 2014;53(7):849–854.
4. Lopez FA, Lartchenko S. Skin and soft tissue infections. *Infect Dis Clin North Am.* 2006;20(4):759–772.
5. Stevens DL, Bisno AL, Chambers HF, et al. Practice guidelines for the diagnosis and management of skin and soft tissue infections: 2014 update by the Infectious Diseases Society of America. *Clin Infect Dis.* 2014;59(2):147–159.

ADDITIONAL READING
- Böer A, Herder N, Winter K, et al. Herpes folliculitis: clinical, histopathological, and molecular pathologic observations. *Br J Dermatol.* 2006;154(4):743–746.
- Brooke RC, Griffiths CE. Folliculitis decalvans. *Clin Exp Dermatol.* 2001;26(1):120–122.
- Centers for Disease Control and Prevention. Rashes. https://www.cdc.gov/healthywater/swimming/swimmers/rwi/rashes.html. Accessed October 31, 2018.
- Ellis E, Scheinfeld N. Eosinophilic pustular folliculitis: a comprehensive review of treatment options. *Am J Clin Dermatol.* 2004;5(3):189–197.
- Fiorillo L, Zucker M, Sawyer D, et al. The *Pseudomonas* hot-foot syndrome. *N Engl J Med.* 2001;345(5):335–338.
- Fridkin SK, Hageman JC, Morrison M, et al; for Active Bacterial Core Surveillance Program of the Emerging Infections Program Network. Methicillin-resistant *Staphylococcus aureus* disease in three communities. *N Engl J Med.* 2005;352(14):1436–1444.
- Luelmo-Aguilar J, Santandreu MS. Folliculitis: recognition and management. *Am J Clin Dermatol.* 2004;5(5):301–310.
- Nervi SJ, Schwartz RA, Dmochowski M. Eosinophilic pustular folliculitis: a 40 year retrospect. *J Am Acad Dermatol.* 2006;55(2):285–289.
- Parsad D, Saini R, Negi KS. Short-term treatment of pityrosporum folliculitis: a double blind placebo-controlled study. *J Eur Acad Dermatol Venereol.* 1998;11(2):188–190.

 SEE ALSO

Algorithm: Rash

 CODES

ICD10
- L73.9 Follicular disorder, unspecified
- L66.2 Folliculitis decalvans
- L73.8 Other specified follicular disorders

CLINICAL PEARLS
- Folliculitis lesions are typically 1- to 5-mm clusters of pruritic erythematous papules and pustule surrounding hair follicles.
- Most commonly due to *S. aureus*. If community has increased incidence of MRSA, consider anti-MRSA treatment.
  - It is extremely important to educate patients on proper hygiene and skin care techniques to prevent chronic or recurrent cases.

FOOD ALLERGY

Stanley Fineman, MD • Brian P. Vickery, MD

 BASICS

Food allergy is defined as an adverse health effect arising from a specific immune response that occurs reproducibly on exposure to a given food.

DESCRIPTION
- Hypersensitivity reaction related to certain food exposures; can involve IgE-mediated and non–IgE-mediated mechanisms
- System(s) affected: gastrointestinal (GI), heme/lymphatic/immunologic, pulmonary, skin/exocrine
- Synonym(s): allergic bowel disease; dietary protein sensitivity syndrome

EPIDEMIOLOGY
- Predominant age: all ages but more common in infants and children
- Predominant sex: male > female (2:1)
- Disproportionate impact on underserved and minority patients

Incidence
~2.5% of infants experience hypersensitivity reactions to cow's milk in their 1st year of life (1)[B].

Prevalence
- The prevalence of IgE-mediated food allergy assessed by food challenge is 3% (1)[B].
- The self-reported prevalence of food allergy is 12% in children and 13% in adults (1)[B].
- In young children, the most common food allergies are cow's milk (2.5%), egg (1.3%), peanut (0.8%), and wheat (0.4%) (2)[B].
- Adults more commonly have allergies to shellfish (2%), peanuts (0.6%), tree nuts (0.5%), and fish (0.4%).
- Food allergy is frequently a transient phenomenon; only 3–4% of children >4 years of age have persisting food allergy (2)[B].
- 20% of children with peanut protein allergy may outgrow their sensitivity by school age.

ETIOLOGY AND PATHOPHYSIOLOGY
Allergic response triggered by immunologic mechanisms (e.g., IgE-mediated or non–IgE-mediated allergic responses) or non–immunologic-mediated mechanisms
- Any ingested substance can cause allergic reactions:
  – Most commonly implicated foods include cow's milk, egg whites, wheat, soy, peanuts, fish, tree nuts (e.g., walnut, cashew, and pecan), and shellfish.
- Several food dyes and additives may elicit non–IgE-mediated allergic-like reactions.

Genetics
- Although there is likely a heritable component to allergic diseases, the genetics are complex and not monogenic.
- Human leukocyte antigen (HLA) studies in peanut allergy have consistently failed to find associations.
- In families with a history of food hypersensitivity, the probability of food allergy in subsequent siblings may be as high as 50%.

RISK FACTORS
- Patients with allergic or atopic predisposition have increased risk of hypersensitivity reaction to food.
- Family history of food hypersensitivity

GENERAL PREVENTION
- High-risk infants fed peanut protein (6 g/week) have an 80% risk reduction in developing peanut allergy by age 5 years, and global infant feeding guidelines now recommend introducing peanut and other complementary foods starting at 5 months of age.
- In patients at risk for anaphylaxis, epinephrine autoinjectors should be readily available.

COMMONLY ASSOCIATED CONDITIONS
- Atopic dermatitis
- Eosinophilic esophagitis

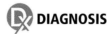 **DIAGNOSIS**

HISTORY
- Symptoms after food ingestion/exposure—usually within 30 minutes of ingestion but could be delayed 4 to 8 hours
- Document a temporal relationship between symptoms and suspected food. Include manner in which food was prepared and quantity of food ingested.
- Differentiate true food allergy/hypersensitivity from food intolerance which may present with similar symptoms.
- GI
  – More common: nausea, vomiting, diarrhea, abdominal pain, occult bleeding, flatulence, and bloating
  – Less common: malabsorption, protein-losing enteropathy, eosinophilic enteritis, colitis
- Skin
  – More common: urticaria/angioedema, atopic dermatitis, pallor, or flushing
  – Less common: contact rashes
- Respiratory
  – More common: allergic rhinitis, asthma and bronchospasm, stridor, cough, serous otitis media
  – Less common: pulmonary infiltrates (Heiner syndrome), pulmonary hemosiderosis
- Neurologic
  – Less common: migraine headaches
- Other
  – Systemic anaphylaxis, vasculitis, ocular injection, conjunctival edema, periorbital swelling
  – Associated factors—exercise; NSAID use; alcohol consumption

PHYSICAL EXAM
- Vital signs; growth parameters
- Signs of allergic disease—pulmonary, skin exam in particular
- Other exam findings based on clinical presentation

DIFFERENTIAL DIAGNOSIS
- Nonimmune food intolerance such as enzyme deficiencies (e.g., lactose intolerance)
- Toxic food exposures (e.g., scombroid fish, bacterial food poisoning)
- GI (irritable bowel syndrome, celiac sprue, dumping syndrome, inflammatory bowel diseases, etc.), dermatologic, respiratory, neurologic, psychiatric (generalized anxiety disorder, personality disorders, etc.)

- Oral allergy syndrome
  – The oral allergy syndrome is the result of cross-reacting proteins in pollens (e.g., patients sensitive to birch tree pollen frequently have cross-reactivity to fresh apples and pears).
- Galactose-α-1,3-galactose (α-gal)
  – Following a lone star tick bite, susceptible patients may develop an IgE sensitivity to α-gal which manifests as delayed anaphylaxis presenting 3 to 6 hours after ingestion of mammalian meat. Diagnosis is by history and confirmed by specific IgE to α-gal (3).

DIAGNOSTIC TESTS & INTERPRETATION
Initial Tests (lab, imaging)
- CBC with differential: Eosinophilia suggests atopy.
- Epicutaneous (prick or puncture) allergy skin tests document IgE-mediated immunologic hypersensitivity using commercially available extracts (variable sensitivities) or fresh food skin testing.
- Skin testing using the suspect food is helpful. If negative on skin test, an oral challenge may aid in diagnosis. The overall correlation between commercially available allergy skin testing and oral food challenge is 60%, increasing to 90% when fresh food skin testing is done (i.e., the positive skin test correlates with a positive challenge).
  – Skin testing has a high sensitivity (low false-negative rate) *but* a low specificity (high false-positive rate), so *only* skin test against antigens found on history (4)[C].
- Food-specific IgE assays (radioallergosorbent test [RAST] and fluorescent enzyme immunoassay [FEI]) detect specific IgE antibodies to offending foods and are less sensitive to skin testing.
  – Using a serum assay alone to diagnose food allergy can result in misdiagnosis of true food allergic sensitivity, particularly in children with atopic dermatitis. Do not use a panel. Test for specific IgE to foods based on patient history.
- Periodic monitoring of peanut-specific IgE levels every 2 years may be helpful. If the level of peanut-specific IgE falls to <0.5 kU/L, a supervised oral challenge can be helpful. Consider a fresh food skin test with peanut protein prior to the oral challenge (4)[B].
- Component-resolved diagnosis (CRD) is a new diagnostic tool that measures specific allergenic proteins in various foods to identify specific IgE to allergenic proteins rather than whole allergen; particularly helpful for certain nuts (e.g., peanuts) (5)[B].
- Patch testing for patients with eosinophilic esophagitis and atopic dermatitis to determine delayed-sensitivity immunologic reactions is of marginal benefit (1)[B].
- Widespread allergy skin testing or serum IgE tests are *not* recommended because of their poor predictive value without a clinical correlating history (2)[B].
- Leukocyte histamine release assays for circulating immune complexes are of limited clinical use (2)[B].
- Provocative injection and sublingual tests are of little benefit for diagnosis of food allergy.
- The leukocytotoxic assay is unproven (1)[B].
- Other unproven diagnostic procedures that are not recommended include provocative neutralization, lymphocyte stimulation, hair analysis, and applied kinesiology (2)[B].

Diagnostic Procedures/Other
Elimination and challenge testing is best for confirming food allergy:

- Eliminate the suspected food from the diet for 1 to 2 weeks.
- Monitor the patient's symptoms. If they disappear or substantially improve, perform an oral challenge with the suspected food under medical supervision.
- Optimally, this challenge should be performed in a double-blind, placebo-controlled manner, although open oral food challenges are most commonly utilized in routine practice.
- Patients with history of anaphylaxis should not have an oral challenge until a substantial period of time has elapsed since the reaction causing anaphylaxis and IgE sensitivity has declined or disappeared.
- Most allergic reactions occur within 30 minutes to 2 hours after challenge. Late reactions have been described up to 12 to 24 hours.
- Consider referral to gastroenterology for endoscopy and continue monitoring carefully if history and testing are inconclusive.

Test Interpretation
Pathologic findings on tissue biopsy are uncommon in food allergies; inflammatory changes can sometimes be seen in the GI tract. The diagnosis of eosinophilic esophagitis is defined by >15 to 20 eosinophils per high-power field on esophageal biopsy (2)[C].

 ## TREATMENT

GENERAL MEASURES
- Offending food avoidance is the most effective treatment.
- Patients with severe food allergy should be meticulous about food avoidance. They should carry epinephrine for self-administration in the event that the offending food is ingested unknowingly and an immediate reaction develops.
- Immunotherapy may be effective for certain food allergies. Peanut (*Arachis hypogaea*) allergen powder has recently been approved for oral immunotherapy (OIT) by the FDA for children with peanut allergy ages 4 to 17 years old. OIT to other foods, sublingual immunotherapy (SLIT), and epicutaneous immunotherapy (EPIT) are still considered experimental and are not recommended for patients who are not participating in appropriately controlled and monitored clinical trials.
- Subcutaneous immunotherapy or hyposensitization (e.g., "allergy shots") with food extracts are not recommended. Research studies are in progress, but any type of immunotherapy besides OIT is considered experimental at this time.

MEDICATION
- Patients with significant type 1, IgE-mediated hypersensitivity should have epinephrine available for autoinjection in case of an anaphylactic reaction.
- After receiving epinephrine for a systemic anaphylactic reaction to a food, patients should be monitored in a medical facility (15–25% of patients may require >1 dose of epinephrine).
- Symptomatic treatment for milder reactions with antihistamines is generally adequate.

- For patients aged 4 to 17 years with allergic sensitivity to peanut protein, consider using FDA-approved peanut allergy powder (Palforzia) to reduce the risk for anaphylaxis after accidental peanut protein exposure (6).
- Cromolyn is not recommended for use in most patients with food allergy.

COMPLEMENTARY & ALTERNATIVE MEDICINE
Benefits of herbal medicines in food allergy are inconclusive.

 ## ONGOING CARE

FOLLOW-UP RECOMMENDATIONS
Patient Monitoring
- As needed
- Many patients are routinely seen at least annually, with follow-up skin tests and/or serum IgE studies as clinically indicated in order to determine the likelihood of spontaneous resolution.

DIET
- As determined by tests and clinical evaluation
- Strict avoidance of offending food

PATIENT EDUCATION
- Dietary counseling is advised to maintain a nutritionally sound diet avoiding foods to which the patient is sensitive.
- Food Allergy Research & Education, Inc.: 7901 Jones Branch Drive, Suite 240, McLean, VA 22102 Toll-Free: 800-929-4040; website: https://www.foodallergy.org
- http://www.allergyasthmanetwork.org, https://college.acaai.org, and https://www.aaaai.org

PROGNOSIS
- Most infants outgrow food hypersensitivity by 2 to 4 years:
  - It may be possible to reintroduce the offending food cautiously into the diet (especially if a particular food is difficult to avoid). Check food-specific IgE by serum or food allergy skin test prior to oral challenge. Significant reductions in skin test wheal diameter or serum-specific IgE can indicate the development of tolerance.
  - 20% of peanut allergies resolve by age 5 years.
  - 42% of children with egg allergy and 48% of children with milk allergy develop clinical tolerance and lose their sensitivity over time (1)[C].
- Adults with food hypersensitivity (particularly to milk, fish, shellfish, or nuts) tend to maintain their allergy for many years (2)[B].

COMPLICATIONS
- Anaphylaxis
- Angioedema
- Bronchial asthma
- Enterocolitis
- Eosinophilic esophagitis
- Eczematoid lesions

REFERENCES
1. Sicherer SH, Sampson HA. Food allergy: epidemiology, pathogenesis, diagnosis, and treatment. *J Allergy Clin Immunol*. 2014;133(2):291–308.
2. Bird JA. Food allergy. *Immunol Allergy Clin North Am*. 2018;38(1):xv–xvi.
3. Steinke JW, Platts-Mills TAE, Commins SP. The alpha-gal story: lessons learned from connecting the dots. *J Allergy Clin Immunol*. 2015;135(3):589–597.
4. Sicherer SH, Sampson HA. Food allergy: a review and update on epidemiology, pathogenesis, diagnosis, prevention, and management. *J Allergy Clin Immunol*. 2018;141(1):41–58.
5. Iweala OI, Choudhary SK, Commins SP. Food allergy. *Curr Gastroenterol Rep*. 2018;20(5):17.
6. Vickery BP, Vereda A, Casale TB, et al; for PALISADE Group of Clinical Investigators. AR101 oral immunotherapy for peanut allergy. *N Engl J Med*. 2018;379(21):1991–2001.

ADDITIONAL READING
- Du Toit G, Roberts G, Sayre PH, et al; for LEAP Study Team. Randomized trial of peanut consumption in infants at risk for peanut allergy. *N Engl J Med*. 2015;372(9):803–813.
- Gernez Y, Nowak-Węgrzyn A. Immunotherapy for food allergy: are we there yet? *J Allergy Clin Immunol Pract*. 2017;5(2):250–272.
- Sampson HA, Aceves S, Bock SA, et al; for Joint Task Force on Practice Parameters. Food allergy: a practice parameter update—2014. *J Allergy Clin Immunol*. 2014;134(5):1016.e43–1025.e43.
- Scurlock AM, Jones SM. Advances in the approach to the patient with food allergy. *J Allergy Clin Immunol*. 2018;141(6):2002–2014.

 ### SEE ALSO

Anaphylaxis; Celiac Disease; Irritable Bowel Syndrome

 ## CODES

ICD10
- T78.1XXA Oth adverse food reactions, not elsewhere classified, init
- T78.00XA Anaphylactic reaction due to unspecified food, init encntr
- L27.2 Dermatitis due to ingested food

CLINICAL PEARLS
- Up to 20% of children with peanut allergy may outgrow their sensitivity. Most other common childhood food allergies are outgrown by adulthood.
- Oral itching following ingestion of fresh fruit may be a warning for anaphylaxis.
- Maternal dietary restrictions during pregnancy and lactation do not appear to prevent atopic disease in infants.
- Breastfeeding is recommended for the first 6 months of life, particularly when there is a family history of atopy and food allergy.
- Delaying the introduction of solid foods beyond 6 months does not appear to have a significant protective effect on the development of allergies.
- Children 4 to 11 months of age with eczema or other food allergy may benefit from early introduction of peanut protein. Consider allergy skin testing prior to introducing peanut protein.

F

FOOD POISONING, BACTERIAL

Irfan H. Siddiqui, MD • Rosario Bartolomeo, DO • Samantha Storti, MD

BASICS

DESCRIPTION

- Food poisoning or foodborne illness is caused by the consumption of food or water that is contaminated with bacterial, parasitic, or viral pathogens. Other causes can result from ingestion of molds, toxin, contaminants and/or allergens.
- Symptoms are most commonly gastrointestinal in nature.
- Foodborne illness is typically self-limited and resolves with supportive care, but in some cases can lead to severe dehydration and critical illness.

EPIDEMIOLOGY

- The cause is unclear in up to 80% of cases.
- Most foodborne illnesses are secondary to viral causes, with *Norovirus* being the most common (1). Other viral causes include hepatitis A, rotavirus, and adenovirus.
- Since 2013, *Campylobacter* and nontyphoidal *Salmonella* were the most common causes of bacterial foodborne illness in the United States.
- Other less common pathogens including Shiga toxin-producing *Escherichia coli* (STEC), *Shigella*, *Cyclospora*, *Yersinia*, *Listeria*, and *Vibrio*
- *Salmonella* (nontyphoidal) infections are the leading cause of foodborne illness associated with hospitalizations and deaths (2).

Incidence

- Roughly 1 in 6 Americans (48 million) and 1 in 10 across the world become ill from foodborne illness each year (3).
- In the United States, ~128,000 cases of foodborne illness require hospitalization and 3,000 result in death (3).

ETIOLOGY AND PATHOPHYSIOLOGY

- Short incubation period (1 to 6 hours)
  - *Bacillus cereus* toxin
    - Toxin can tolerate high temperatures.
    - Food sources: improperly cooked rice/fried rice and red meats
    - Symptoms: sudden onset of severe nausea; vomiting and diarrhea
  - *Staphylococcus aureus* (4)
    - Toxin mediated; toxin is heat stable.
    - Food sources: nonrefrigerated or improperly refrigerated meats and potato, mayonnaise and egg salads
    - Symptoms: sudden onset of severe nausea and vomiting; abdominal cramps and fever
- Medium incubation period (8 to 16 hours)
  - *B. cereus* (4)
    - Food sources: meat, stews, gravy, vanilla sauce
    - Symptoms: watery diarrhea, cramps, nausea
  - *Clostridium perfringens* (4)
    - Food sources: dry/precooked or undercooked meats, home-canned goods
    - Symptoms: watery diarrhea, nausea, cramps
- Long incubation period (>16 hours)
  - Toxin-producing organisms:
    - *Clostridium botulinum* (4)
      - Food source: commercially canned or improperly home-canned foods
      - Symptoms: vomiting, diarrhea, slurred speech, diplopia, dysphagia, and descending muscle weakness/flaccid paralysis
    - Enterohemorrhagic *E. coli* (e.g., 0157:H7) (4)
      - Food sources: undercooked ground beef, juice, unpasteurized milk; raw produce; and contaminated water (3)

- Risk factors: daycare centers, nursing homes, extremes of age
- Symptoms: severe diarrhea that often becomes bloody, abdominal pain, vomiting
  - Enterotoxigenic *E. coli* ("traveler's diarrhea") (5)
    - Food sources: food or water contaminated by human feces
    - Symptoms: watery diarrhea, abdominal cramps, tenesmus, fecal urgency, and vomiting
  - *Vibrio cholerae*
    - Food sources: contaminated water, fish, and shellfish, especially food sold by street vendors
    - Symptoms: profuse watery "rice water" diarrhea and vomiting, which can lead to severe dehydration and rapid death
- Invasive organisms
  - *Salmonella*, nontyphoidal (1),(4)
    - Food sources: contaminated eggs, poultry; unpasteurized milk or juice, cheese; contaminated raw fruit and vegetables; and contaminated peanut butter
    - Risk factors: contact with animals
    - Symptoms: small volume, mucopurulent/bloody diarrhea; fever; cramps; vomiting
  - *Campylobacter jejuni* (4)
    - Food sources: raw and undercooked poultry, unpasteurized milk, and contaminated meats
    - Symptoms: diarrhea (bloody), cramps, vomiting, fever
  - *Shigella* (4)
    - Food sources: contaminated water, raw produce, uncooked foods, foods handled by infected food workers
    - Risk factors: men who have sex with men
    - Symptoms: abdominal cramps, fever, mucopurulent and bloody diarrhea
  - *Vibrio parahaemolyticus* (4)
    - Food source: undercooked or raw seafood, especially shellfish
    - Risk factors: cirrhosis
    - Symptoms: nausea, vomiting, diarrhea, abdominal pain
  - *Vibrio vulnificus* (4)
    - Food source: undercooked or raw seafood, particularly oysters
    - Symptoms: vomiting, diarrhea, abdominal pain, bacteremia, wound infections; can be fatal in patients with liver disease or those who are immunocompromised
  - *Yersinia enterocolitica*
    - Food sources: undercooked beef and pork, unpasteurized milk, tofu, contaminated water
    - Risk factors: cirrhosis, hemochromatosis, blood transfusion
    - Symptoms: abdominal pain, fever, diarrhea (possibly bloody), vomiting
  - *Listeria monocytogenes* (4)
    - Food sources: unpasteurized/contaminated milk, soft cheese, and processed deli meats
    - Risk factors: pregnancy
    - Symptoms: nausea, vomiting, fever, watery diarrhea; pregnant women may have a flu-like illness leading to premature delivery or stillbirth; immunocompromised patients may develop meningitis and bacteremia

RISK FACTORS

- Recent travel to developing countries (1)
- Food handlers, daycare attendees, nursing home residents, recently hospitalized patients, or patients recently exposed to antibiotics

- Altered immunity due to underlying disease or use of certain medications, including antacids, H_2 blockers, and proton pump inhibitors (1)
- Cross-contamination and subsequent ingestion of improperly prepared and stored foods
- Pregnancy
- Children >5 years and adults age >65 years
- Immunocompromised patients

GENERAL PREVENTION

- When preparing food:
  - Wash hands, cutting boards, and preparation surfaces
  - Wash fresh produce thoroughly before consuming
  - Keep raw meat, poultry, fish, and their juices away from other food (e.g., salad). Wear gloves when handling raw meat (6).
  - Thoroughly cook the meat
  - Refrigerate leftovers within 2 to 3 hours in clean, shallow, covered containers. If the temperature is >90°F, refrigerate within 1 hour.
- When traveling to underdeveloped countries:
  - Eat only freshly prepared food.
  - Avoid beverages and foods prepared with nonpotable water.
  - Bottled, carbonated, and boiled beverages are safe to drink.
- Chemoprophylaxis for traveler's diarrhea is recommended for high-risk travelers (e.g., immunocompromised) (5).

COMMONLY ASSOCIATED CONDITIONS

- Botulism—potentially lethal neuroparalytic condition characterized by symmetric neurologic deficits and changes in mental status because of ingestion of toxin types A, B, and E produced by *C. botulinum*. Outbreaks typically involve home-canned foods such as fruits, vegetables, and meats.
- Neonatal meningitis—immunocompromised hosts, particularly neonates (<29 days old) can contract meningitis from systemic *L. monocytogenes* infection.
- Hemolytic uremic syndrome (HUS)—hematologic condition characterized by microangiopathic hemolytic anemia, renal impairment, and thrombocytopenia caused by both *Shigella* and STEC; can be precipitated in patients harboring enterohemorrhagic *E. coli* who are treated with antibiotics (1)
- Guillain-Barré syndrome—ascending paralysis strongly associated with *C. jejuni* infection
- Reactive arthritis—can occur after severe infections with *Salmonella*, *Shigella*, *Yersinia*, or *Campylobacter* species

DIAGNOSIS

HISTORY

- Onset, duration, frequency, severity, and character (i.e., watery, bloody, mucus-filled, etc.) of diarrhea
- The definition of diarrhea is >3 or more unformed stools daily or the passage of >250 g of unformed stool per day (1).
- Suspect bacterial food poisoning when multiple persons have rapid onset of symptoms after eating the same meal; high fever, blood, or mucus in stool; severe abdominal pain; signs of dehydration; or recent travel to a foreign country (1).
- Further evaluation and treatment with high fever (≥101.3°F), ≥6 stools per day, blood in the stools, elevated white blood cell count, signs of dehydration, or diarrheal illness that lasts >2 to 3 days (1)

PHYSICAL EXAM

- Key signs of dehydration: delayed capillary refill, decreased skin turgor, dry mucous membranes, and orthostatic hypotension (2)
- Fever may suggest invasive or toxin-producing bacteria.
- Abdominal exam: Assess for pain, peritoneal signs, and bowel activity to differentiate from other acute abdominal processes.
- Rectal exam for blood, rectal pain, stool consistency

DIFFERENTIAL DIAGNOSIS

Other infectious gastrointestinal illnesses (i.e., viral or parasitic), *Clostridium Difficile* colitis, inflammatory bowel disease, appendicitis, acute cholecystitis, acute choledocholithiasis, acute diverticulitis, acute hepatitis, malabsorption disorders (i.e., celiac disease, *Helicobacter pylori* infection, short bowel syndrome)

DIAGNOSTIC TESTS & INTERPRETATION
Initial Tests (lab, imaging)

- For mild, self-limiting illness, a stool culture is not typically necessary and is unlikely to change management unless there are signs of fever, blood, or severe diarrhea (4)[C].
- Testing for fecal leukocytes and fecal occult blood is not necessary unless patients have fever or bloody diarrhea (6) and consider ova and parasites if dehydration, history of foreign travel, or symptoms lasting >2 weeks (1).
- CBC, basic metabolic profile for severe cases with dehydration, inpatient, and nursing home exposure (1)
- Consider endoscopic evaluation for severe cases (1),(6),(7). Have a low threshold for endoscopy among patients with AIDS and persistent diarrhea (6).
- Abdominal CT may be helpful when intra-abdominal pathology is in the differential and clinical presentation is unclear (1),(6).

Follow-Up Tests & Special Considerations

Epidemiologic investigation may be warranted. Reporting requirements vary by state and organism (4).

 ## TREATMENT

Most cases of food poisoning are self-limited.

MEDICATION
First Line

- Oral rehydration is the first-line therapy for acute diarrheal illness (6).
- A balanced oral rehydration solution (ORS) is particularly recommended for elderly or pediatric patients with severe diarrhea, or for travelers with severe, cholera-like watery diarrhea (7)[B].
- Most patients with mild illness do not need formal ORS and can rehydrate with fluids and salt-rich foods (7).
- Empiric antibiotic therapy is not recommended for most cases of acute diarrhea (unless traveler's diarrhea is suspected) (7)[A].

Second Line

Consider antibiotics only for patients with severe illness requiring hospitalization and those with fever and hematochezia or when diagnostic testing confirms a bacterial source (4). Pathogen-specific therapy:

- *B. cereus*: supportive care only
- *C. jejuni* (1): mild: supportive care only—antibiotics may induce resistance. Severe: azithromycin 500 mg/day for 3 to 5 days. Fluoroquinolones are no longer recommended (4).

- *C. botulinum*: supportive care only. Antitoxin can be helpful early during illness.
- *C. perfringens*: supportive care only
- Enterohemorrhagic *E. coli* (e.g., 0157:H7) (1): supportive care only. Closely monitor renal function, hemoglobin, and platelets. Infection associated with HUS. Avoid antibiotics because this may increase risk of HUS.
- Enterotoxigenic *E. coli* (common cause of traveler's diarrhea) (1),(5): generally self-limited. Antibiotics shorten course of illness. Ciprofloxacin 500 mg BID or 750 mg daily for 1 to 3 days; azithromycin 1 g × single dose or daily for 3 days; or rifaximin 200 mg TID for 3 days
- *Salmonella* (nontyphoidal) (1),(5),(7): no therapy for mild disease (antibiotics may lengthen shedding). Moderate: ciprofloxacin 500 mg BID for 5 to 7 days, levofloxacin 500 mg daily for 7 to 10 days, or TMP/SMX DS 160/800 mg BID for 5 to 7 days. Severe diarrhea, immunocompromised, systemic signs, positive blood cultures: IV ceftriaxone 1 to 2 g daily for 7 to 10 days
- *Shigella* (1),(7): ciprofloxacin 500 mg BID or 750 mg daily for 3 days, or 2 g single dose; alternative options: azithromycin (drug of choice secondary to quinolone resistance) 500 mg BID for 3 days, TMP/SMX DS 160/800 mg BID for 5 days, or ceftriaxone 2 to 4 g single dose
- *S. aureus* (1): supportive care only
- Noncholeraic *Vibrio* (1): ciprofloxacin 750 mg daily for 3 days or azithromycin 500 mg daily for 3 days
- *V. cholerae* (1): doxycycline 300 mg 1-time dose in most cases, or tetracycline 500 mg QID for 3 days, or erythromycin 250 mg TID for 3 days, or azithromycin 1,000 mg as single dose or 500 mg/day for 3 days
- *Yersinia*: usually, supportive care only. Severe: doxycycline combine with aminoglycoside; TMP/SMX DS 160/800 mg BID for 5 days; or ciprofloxacin 500 mg BID for 7 to 10 days

ADDITIONAL THERAPIES

- For severe nausea and vomiting, promethazine is effective for adults. Ondansetron is effective in children (5).
- Loperamide 4 mg initially and then 2 mg after each loose stool to a maximum of 8 mg in a 24-hour period may be used *unless* high fever, bloody diarrhea, and/or severe abdominal pain present (signs of enteroinvasion) (5).
- Bismuth subsalicylate 525 mg QID is moderately effective in traveler's diarrhea (5),(7).
- Evidence for the effectiveness of probiotics and prebiotics is limited and inconsistent. Use is not currently recommended outside of postantibiotic-related infectious diarrhea (6),(7).
- Diligent hand washing throughout the course of illness decreases spread.

 ## ONGOING CARE

DIET

- Modify food intake when nausea is present or vomiting prevents intake. Drink plenty of fluids in frequent sips.
- As nausea subsides, drink adequate fluids; add in bland, low-fat meals; and rest. Avoid alcohol, coffee, nicotine, and spicy foods.
- Breastfeed nursing infants on demand. Infants and older children should be offered the usual food.
- For diarrhea, consider a bland diet.
- Limiting dairy to 24 hours after last diarrhea episode may assist in symptom reduction.

PROGNOSIS

Most infections are self-limited and resolve over several days. Antibiotics for moderate to severe traveler's diarrhea shorten duration by several days (5).

REFERENCES

1. DuPont HL. Acute infectious diarrhea in immunocompetent adults. *N Engl J Med*. 2014;370(16):1532–1540.
2. Sell J, Dolan B. Common gastrointestinal infections. *Prim Care*. 2018;45(3):519–532.
3. U.S. Department of Health & Human Services. Food poisoning. https://www.foodsafety.gov/food-poisoning. Published 2021. Accessed October 29, 2021.
4. Switaj TL, Winter KJ, Christensen SR. Diagnosis and management of foodborne illness. *Am Fam Physician*. 2015;92(5):358–365.
5. Steffen R, Hill DR, DuPont HL. Traveler's diarrhea: a clinical review. *JAMA*. 2015;313(1):71–80.
6. Shane AL, Mody RK, Crump JA, et al. 2017 Infectious Diseases Society of America clinical practice guidelines for the diagnosis and management of infectious diarrhea. *Clin Infect Dis*. 2017;65(12):1963–1973.
7. Riddle MS, DuPont HL, Connor BA. ACG clinical guideline: diagnosis, treatment, and prevention of acute diarrheal infections in adults. *Am J Gastroenterol*. 2016;111(5):602–622.

 ## SEE ALSO

Appendicitis, Acute; Botulism; Brucellosis; Dehydration; Diarrhea, Acute; Guillain-Barré Syndrome; Hypokalemia; Intestinal Parasites; *Salmonella* Infection; Typhoid Fever

 ## CODES

ICD10

- A05.9 Bacterial foodborne intoxication, unspecified
- A02.0 Salmonella enteritis
- A04.5 Campylobacter enteritis

CLINICAL PEARLS

- Consider bacterial food poisoning when multiple patients present with fever and blood/mucus in stool after ingesting the same food or having recently returned from a developing nation.
- Consider culture and antibiotics if there is persistent fever with blood/mucus in stool, concern for sepsis, and/or for symptoms lasting >7 days.
- Withhold antispasmodics and antidiarrheal agents if there is concern for enteroinvasion (high prolonged fever, bloody diarrhea, severe pain, septicemia).
- Consider empiric antibiotic therapy for traveler's diarrhea in cases of moderate to severe disease.

F

FROSTBITE
Sangili Chandran, MD • Aliyah Ahmed, DO

BASICS

DESCRIPTION
- A severe localized injury due to cold exposure, causing tissue to freeze, resulting in direct cellular injury and progressive dermal ischemia (most commonly of exposed hands, feet, face, and ears)
- Systems affected: integumentary, vascular, muscular, skeletal, nervous
- Synonym: dermatitis congelationis

EPIDEMIOLOGY
- Predominantly adults but can affect all ages
- Predominant sex: male ≤ female, potentially more common in females due to increased surface area in conjunction with less body mass though exposure rates in males may be higher (1)

ETIOLOGY AND PATHOPHYSIOLOGY
- Prolonged exposure to cold
- Refreezing thawed extremities
- Ice crystals form intracellularly and extracel-lularly. Vasoconstriction reduces blood flow and microvascular endothelial injury leads to ischemia. Cellular dehydration leads to abnormal electrolyte concentrations and cell death.
- In severe cases, tissue injury extends to muscle and bone leading to necrosis and mummification. Rewarming injured endothelium results in edema and bullae as the ice crystals melt. Inflammatory mediators such as prostaglandins and thromboxane A2 induce vasoconstriction and platelet aggrega-tion, worsening ischemia.
- In severe frostbite, the chronic inflammation can result in an imbalance of proinflammatory and antiinflammatory macrophages, which can lead to delayed healing (2).
- If refreezing occurs after thawing, cascade of events are more extreme (1).

RISK FACTORS
- Prolonged exposure to below freezing temperatures, especially combined with wind and/or water exposure
- High-altitude activities, such as mountaineering
- Military operations in cold environments
- Constricting or wet clothing with inadequate insulation
- Altered mental status due to alcohol, drugs, or psychiatric illness
- Homelessness
- Previous cold-related injury
- Dehydration and/or malnutrition
- Conditions that interfere with total heat production and/or thermoregulation (i.e., endocrine abnormalities) (1)
- Conditions that promote loss of body heat including chronic skin conditions, hyperhidrosis, burns (including sunburns) (1)
- Hypothermia
- Any condition that results in decreased vasoconstriction and/or vascular pathology as in (1):
  - Smoking, Raynaud phenomenon, peripheral vascular disease, diabetes

GENERAL PREVENTION
- Dress in layers with appropriate cold weather gear and avoid clothing that is too constricting.
- Cover exposed areas and extremities appropriately.
- Stay dry; avoid alcohol and minimize wind exposure.
- Ensure adequate hydration and caloric intake.

- Use supplemental oxygen at very high altitudes (>7,500 meters).
- Exercise can protect against frostbite by increasing core and peripheral temperatures. Note: Caution should be made that the exercise will not lead to exhaustion and inability to seek for shelter/warmth.
- Appropriate use of chemical or electric hand and foot warmers can help maintain peripheral warmth.
- Recognize expected temperatures and take into consideration wind chills prior to exposure and if possible avoid exposure.
- Avoid emollients on the skin as they can lead to a false sense of protection (1).
- Avoid alcohol, caffeine, and other medications that can cause vasoconstriction (1).

COMMONLY ASSOCIATED CONDITIONS
- Hypothermia
- Alcohol or drug abuse

DIAGNOSIS

HISTORY
- Significant cold exposure—determine length and severity.
- Throbbing pain
- Paresthesias
- Numbness
- Loss of coordination and dexterity

PHYSICAL EXAM
- Hands, feet, face, and ears are most commonly affected.
- Before rewarming, skin may be insensate, white or grayish-yellow in color, cyanotic, or hard and waxy to touch.
- After rewarming, immediate physical exam findings can be categorized as:
  - Grade 1: no cyanosis on the extremity
  - Grade 2: cyanosis isolated to the distal phalanx
  - Grade 3: intermediate and proximal phalangeal cyanosis
  - Grade 4: cyanosis over the carpal or tarsal bones (3)[C]
- Frostbite can alternatively be categorized into four degrees (similar to burn injuries):
  - 1st degree: numbness and erythema. A white or yellow, firm, slightly raised plaque develops. No gross tissue infarction occurs; there may be slight epidermal sloughing. Mild edema is common.
  - 2nd degree: superficial skin vesiculation; a clear or milky blisters, surrounded by erythema and edema
  - 3rd degree: deeper hemorrhagic blisters
  - 4th degree: extends through the dermis to involve subcutaneous tissues, with necrosis extending into muscle and bone
  - 1st- and 2nd-degree injuries are superficial.
  - 3rd- and 4th-degree injuries are deep (4)[C].

DIFFERENTIAL DIAGNOSIS
- Frostnip: a superficial cold injury that resolves spontaneously without tissue loss
- Chilblains (pernio): a localized inflammatory reaction to cold and wet exposure without tissue freezing; typically presents as edematous, erythematous to violaceous skin lesions
- Immersion foot (trench foot): inflammatory reaction of the feet to prolonged exposure to cold and moisture
- COVID toes, a SARS-CoV2 phenomenon related to pernio/chilblains (5)

DIAGNOSTIC TESTS & INTERPRETATION
Initial Tests (lab, imaging)
- Baseline labs: complete blood count, comprehensive metabolic panel, UA for myoglobinuria, culture wound if suspected infection
- Radiography can be an initial imaging to identify extent of soft tissue involvement versus bone involvement (2).
- Technetium (Tc)-99m scintigraphy can identify tissue viability at early stage and identify candidates for thrombolytic therapy.
- MRI/MRA, duplex ultrasonography, and standard or digital subtraction angiography are occasionally used.
- Consider serial photographs at time of injury, at 24 hours, and every several days until hospital discharge.
- For severe frostbite especially, angiography and bone scans, as well as MRI/MRA, US, and infrared thermal imaging, are useful to determine need for thrombolysis versus amputation (2).
- Angiography and bone scans can be used to deter-mine effectiveness of thrombolysis if done before and after treatment (2).
- There is some evidence that angiography has been shown to accurately determine the need for amputation, whereas bone scans cannot reveal this information (caution with angiography with renal insufficiency).
- SPECT/CT should be used to reveal clini-cal prognosis (2).

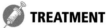

TREATMENT

GENERAL MEASURES
- Correct hypothermia.
- Assess for additional injuries.
- Remove jewelry from affected extremities.
- Initiate rewarming of affected body part only if there is no risk of refreezing. Warm affected parts of body in 37–39°C water for approximately 30 minutes until the involved part takes on a red or purple appearance and becomes pliable to touch. A whirlpool bath can help with rewarming and antiseptic. Avoid using other heat sources, such as a fire or space heater, to rewarm affected parts avoided.
- Apply topical aloe vera gel before dressing.
- Selectively drain clear or cloudy blisters; leave hemorrhagic blisters intact.
- Splint and elevate affected extremity.
- Tetanus prophylaxis
- Oral hydration if patient is alert and has no GI symptoms, otherwise IV hydration with warm normal saline in small boluses
- Daily bathing in warm water with active and passive mobilization
- Dry, loose bulky dressings, including in between fingers/toes (4)[C]
- Pain control (1)
- Antibiotics only if infectious complications become apparent (1)

ALERT
- Avoid rubbing the affected area as this can lead to further tissue damage.
- Patients should avoid weight bearing on frostbitten limbs prior to definitive care.

MEDICATION

First Line
- tPA for deep injury (grades 3 and 4) (6), administered (either IV or intra-arterially) within 24 hours of injury may prevent damage from microvascular thrombosis and reduce amputation rates (7)[B],(8)[B],(9)[B]; if administered, should be done so immediately after rewarming (6)
- **Precaution:** tPA should not be used with history of recent bleeding, stroke, peptic ulcer, or recent surgery.
- Heparin is recommended as adjunctive therapy in tPA protocols. Heparin is not recommended as monotherapy (9)[C].
- Consider low-molecular-weight dextran in patients not given other systemic treatments (e.g., tPA) (4)[C].
- Iloprost plus rTPA has little supporting evidence. Buflomedil has been withdrawn from use (6).
- Update tetanus toxoid (4)[C].
- Ibuprofen 400 mg q12h (inhibit prostaglandins) (4)[C]
- NSAIDs for mild to moderate pain; narcotic analgesia for moderate to severe pain
- Use systemic antibiotics for proven infection. Prophylactic antibiotics are not recommended (4)[C].

Second Line
Pentoxifylline 400 mg q8 hours (10)[C]

ADDITIONAL THERAPIES
- Heated oxygen
- Warm IV fluids
- Botulinum toxin injections to improve sequelae including chronic pain (11)

SURGERY/OTHER PROCEDURES
- Urgent surgery is rarely needed.
- Fasciotomy is indicated if the patient develops elevated compartment pressures (4)[C].
- Surgical débridement, as needed, to remove necrotic tissue
- Amputation only if tissues are necrotic: may take 4 to 12 weeks for the demarcation of tissue necrosis to become definitive
- Consider imaging with 99 mTc bone scan and/or MRA in severe cases to determine extent of injury; assess viability of surrounding tissue and determine need for surgery.

ADMISSION, INPATIENT, AND NURSING CONSIDERATIONS
- Hospitalization is generally recommended unless no blisters are present after rewarming (e.g., grade 1/1st-degree frostbite) (3)[C],(4)[C].
- Patients are typically best cared for in a hospital with experience treating frostbite injuries (trauma center or burn unit).
- Administer tPA in intensive care setting.
- Ensure proper hydration and nutrition.
- Treat pain (often requires narcotic analgesia).
- Wound care—clean dressings and twice daily whirlpool baths
- Apply aloe vera gel every 6 to 8 hours through resolution of blisters.
- Elevate injured extremities above heart level to minimize edema.
- Physical therapy and early mobilization
- If patient cannot tolerate oral fluids or has altered mental status, give warmed normal saline in small boluses (4)[C].

 ## ONGOING CARE

FOLLOW-UP RECOMMENDATIONS
- Protect injured body parts.
- Continue physical therapy.
- Avoid smoking and alcohol.
- Avoid recurrent cold exposure.
- Ensure properly fitting clothing and footwear.

Patient Monitoring
- Follow up for physical therapy progress, infection, and other complications listed below.
- Monitor growth of affected extremity in pediatric patients.

DIET
- As tolerated
- Warm oral fluids

PATIENT EDUCATION
Provide education on:
- Protection from cold injuries
- Risk factors for frostbite
- Early signs and symptoms of frostbite
- Field treatment of cold injuries
- Wound care grade 1: no amputation and no sequelae

PROGNOSIS
- Grade 2: potential soft tissue amputation and nail sequelae
- Grade 3: potential bone amputation of the digit and functional sequelae
- Grade 4: potential bone amputation of the limb with functional sequelae (3)[C]
- Other factors that attribute to poor prognosis include the following:
  – Severity of injury as seen above
  – Longer duration of exposure
  – Concomitant substance abuse (12)

COMPLICATIONS
- Tissue loss: distal parts of an extremity may undergo spontaneous amputation; tissue necrosis requiring amputation
- Gangrene
- Hyperhidrosis due to nerve injury
- Decreased hair and nail growth
- Raynaud phenomenon
- Changes in skin color
- Frostbite arthropathy and osteoarthritis (13)
- Chronic regional pain; neuropathy
- Localized osteoporosis
- Premature closure of epiphyses in pediatric patients

REFERENCES

1. Fudge J. Preventing and managing hypothermia and frostbite injury. *Sports Health.* 2016;8(2):133–139.
2. Gao Y, Wang F, Zhou W, et al. Research progress in the pathogenic mechanisms and imaging of severe frostbite. *Eur J Radiol.* 2021;137:109605.
3. Cauchy E, Chetaille E, Marchand V, et al. Retrospective study of 70 cases of severe frostbite lesions: a proposed new classification scheme. *Wilderness Environ Med.* 2001;12(4):248–255.
4. McIntosh SE, Hamonko M, Freer L, et al. Wilderness Medical Society practice guidelines for the prevention and treatment of frostbite. *Wilderness Environ Med.* 2011;22(2):156–166.
5. Volansky R. Diagnosing 'COVID toes' and other challenges in the derm-rheum overlap. https://www.healio.com/news/rheumatology/20210818/diagnosing-covid-toes-and-other-challenges-in-the-dermrheum-overlap. Accessed December 17, 2021.
6. Hickey S, Whitson A, Jones L, et al. Guidelines for thrombolytic therapy for frostbite. *J Burn Care Res.* 2020;41(1):176–183.
7. Cauchy E, Cheguillaume B, Chetaille E. A controlled trial of a prostacyclin and rt-PA in the treatment of severe frostbite. *N Engl J Med.* 2011;364(2):189–190.
8. Bruen KJ, Ballard JR, Morris SE, et al. Reduction of the incidence of amputation in frostbite injury with thrombolytic therapy. *Arch Surg.* 2007;142(6):546–553.
9. Twomey JA, Peltier GL, Zera RT. An open-label study to evaluate the safety and efficacy of tissue plasminogen activator in treatment of severe frostbite. *J Trauma.* 2005;59(6):1350–1355.
10. Hayes D Jr, Mandracchia V, Considine C, et al. Pentoxifylline. Adjunctive therapy in the treatment of pedal frostbite. *Clin Podiatr Med Surg.* 2000;17(4):715–722.
11. Norheim AJ, Mercer J, Musial F, et al. A new treatment for frostbite sequelae; Botulinum toxin. *Int J Circumpolar Health.* 2017;76(1):1273677.
12. Ghumman A, St Denis-Katz H, Ashton R, et al. Treatment of frostbite with hyperbaric oxygen therapy: a single center's experience of 22 cases. *Wounds.* 2019;31(12):322–325.
13. Irsay L, Ungur RA, Borda IM, et al. Frostbite arthropathy—a rare case of osteoarthritis, review of the literature and case presentation. *Rom J Morphol Embryol.* 2019;60(4):1337–1341.

 ## SEE ALSO

- Hypothermia
- Algorithm: Hypothermia

 ## CODES

ICD10
- T33.90XA Superficial frostbite of unspecified sites, init encntr
- T34.90XA Frostbite with tissue necrosis of unsp sites, init encntr
- T33.829A Superficial frostbite of unspecified foot, initial encounter

CLINICAL PEARLS

- Frostbite is a tetanus-prone injury. Provide appropriate tetanus prophylaxis.
- Avoid rewarming en route to the hospital if there is a chance of refreezing; rewarm only with water.
- Assess for additional injuries to areas which may be insensate.
- tPA can reduce amputation rates. Use within 24 hours of injury in appropriate clinical settings.
- Early assessment of the degree of tissue involvement is difficult. Delay surgery until a definite tissue demarcation of necrosis occurs (may take 4 to 12 weeks).

F

FURUNCULOSIS

Zoltan Trizna, MD, PhD

BASICS

DESCRIPTION
- Acute bacterial abscess of a hair follicle (often *Staphylococcus aureus*)
- System(s) affected: skin/exocrine
- Synonym(s): boils

EPIDEMIOLOGY

Incidence
- Predominant age
  - Adolescents and young adults
  - Clusters have been reported in teenagers living in crowded quarters, within families, or in high school athletes.
- Predominant sex: male = female

Prevalence
Exact data are not available.

ETIOLOGY AND PATHOPHYSIOLOGY
- Infection spreads away from hair follicle into surrounding dermis.
- Pathogenic strain of *S. aureus* (usually); most cases in United States are now due to community-acquired methicillin-resistant *S. aureus* (CA-MRSA), whereas methicillin-sensitive *S. aureus* (MSSA) is most common elsewhere (1)[A].

Genetics
Unknown

RISK FACTORS
- Carriage of pathogenic strain of *Staphylococcus* sp. in nares, skin, axilla, and perineum
- Rarely, polymorphonuclear leukocyte defect or hyperimmunoglobulin E–*Staphylococcus* sp. abscess syndrome
- Diabetes mellitus, malnutrition, alcoholism, obesity, atopic dermatitis
- Primary immunodeficiency disease and AIDS (common variable immunodeficiency, chronic granulomatous disease, Chédiak–Higashi syndrome, C3 deficiency, C3 hypercatabolism, transient hypogammaglobulinemia of infancy, immunodeficiency with thymoma, Wiskott-Aldrich syndrome)

- Secondary immunodeficiency (e.g., leukemia, leukopenia, neutropenia, therapeutic immunosuppression)
- Medication impairing neutrophil function (e.g., omeprazole)
- The most important independent predictor of recurrence is a positive family history.

GENERAL PREVENTION
Patient education regarding self-care (see "General Measures"); treatment and prevention are interrelated.

COMMONLY ASSOCIATED CONDITIONS
- Usually normal immune system
- Diabetes mellitus
- Polymorphonuclear leukocyte defect (rare)
- Hyperimmunoglobulin E–*Staphylococcus* sp. abscess syndrome (rare)
- See "Risk Factors."

DIAGNOSIS

HISTORY
- Located on hair-bearing sites, especially areas prone to friction or repeated minor traumas (e.g., underneath belt, anterior aspects of thighs, nape, buttocks)
- No initial fever or systemic symptoms
- The folliculocentric nodule may enlarge, become painful, and develop into an abscess (frequently with spontaneous drainage).

PHYSICAL EXAM
- Painful erythematous papules/nodules (1 to 5 cm) with central pustules
- Tender, red, perifollicular swelling, terminating in discharge of pus and necrotic plug
- Lesions may be solitary or clustered.

DIFFERENTIAL DIAGNOSIS
- Folliculitis
- Pseudofolliculitis
- Carbuncles
- Ruptured epidermal cyst
- Myiasis (larva of botfly/tumbu fly)
- Hidradenitis suppurativa
- Atypical bacterial or fungal infections

DIAGNOSTIC TESTS & INTERPRETATION

Initial Tests (lab, imaging)
Obtain culture if with multiple abscesses marked by surrounding inflammation, cellulitis, systemic symptoms such as fever, or if immunocompromised.

Follow-Up Tests & Special Considerations
- Immunoglobulin levels in rare (e.g., recurrent or otherwise inexplicable) cases
- If culture grows gram-negative bacteria or fungus, consider polymorphonuclear neutrophil leukocyte functional defect.

Test Interpretation
Histopathology (although a biopsy is rarely needed)
- Perifollicular necrosis containing fibrinoid material and neutrophils
- At deep end of necrotic plug, in SC tissue, is a large abscess with a Gram stain positive for small collections of *S. aureus*.

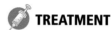

TREATMENT

GENERAL MEASURES
- Moist, warm compresses (provide comfort, encourage localization/pointing/drainage) 30 minutes QID
- If pointing or large, incise and drain: Consider packing if large or incompletely drained.
- Routine culture is not necessary for localized abscess in nondiabetic patients with normal immune system.
- Sanitary practices: Change towels, washcloths, and sheets daily; clean shaving instruments; avoid nose picking; change wound dressings frequently; do not share items of personal hygiene (2)[B].

MEDICATION

First Line
- Systemic antibiotics usually *unnecessary*, unless extensive surrounding cellulitis or fever. Other indications include a single abscess >2 cm, immunocompromise.
- If suspecting MRSA, see "Second Line."

- If multiple abscesses, lesions with marked surrounding inflammation, cellulitis, systemic symptoms such as fever, or if immunocompromised: Place on antibiotics therapy directed at *S. aureus* for 10 to 14 days.
  - Dicloxacillin (Dynapen, Pathocil) 500 mg PO QID *or* cephalexin 500 mg PO QID *or* clindamycin 300 mg TID, if penicillin-allergic

Second Line
- Resistant strains of *S. aureus* (MRSA): clindamycin 300 mg q6h or doxycycline 100 mg q12h or trimethoprim-sulfamethoxazole (TMP-SMX DS) 1 tab q8–12h or minocycline 100 mg q12h
- If known or suspected impaired neutrophil function (e.g., impaired chemotaxis, phagocytosis, superoxide generation), add vitamin C 1,000 mg/day for 4 to 6 weeks (prevents oxidation of neutrophils).
- If antibiotic regimens fail:
  - May try PO pentoxifylline 400 mg TID for 2 to 6 months
  - Contraindications: recent cerebral and/or retinal hemorrhage; intolerance to methylxanthines (e.g., caffeine, theophylline); allergy to the particular drug selected
  - Precautions: prolonged prothrombin time (PT) and/or bleeding; if on warfarin, frequent monitoring of PT

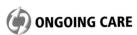

ONGOING CARE

FOLLOW-UP RECOMMENDATIONS
Patient Monitoring
Instruct patient to see physician if compresses are unsuccessful.

DIET
Unrestricted

PROGNOSIS
- Self-limited: usually drains pus spontaneously and will heal with or without scarring within several days
- Recurrent/chronic: may last for months or years

- If recurrent, usually related to chronic skin carriage of staphylococci (nares or on skin). Treatment goals are to decrease or eliminate pathogenic strain *or* suppress pathogenic strain.
  - Culture nares, skin, axilla, and perineum (culture nares of family members).
  - Mupirocin 2%: Apply to both nares BID for 5 days each month.
  - Culture anterior nares every 3 months; if failure, retreat with mupirocin or consider clindamycin 150 mg/day for 3 months.
  - Long-term efficacy of strategies to eliminate carrier state (decolonization) remains unclear.
- Especially in recurrent cases, wash entire body and fingernails (with nailbrush) daily for 1 to 3 weeks with povidone-iodine (Betadine), chlorhexidine (Hibiclens), or hexachlorophene (pHisoHex soap), although all can cause dry skin.

COMPLICATIONS
- Scarring
- Bacteremia
- Seeding (e.g., septal/valve defect, arthritic joint)

REFERENCES
1. Lin HS, Lin PT, Tsai YS, et al. Interventions for bacterial folliculitis and boils (furuncles and carbuncles). *Cochrane Database Syst Rev.* 2021;(2):CD013099.
2. Fritz SA, Camins BC, Eisenstein KA, et al. Effectiveness of measures to eradicate *Staphylococcus aureus* carriage in patients with community-associated skin and soft-tissue infections: a randomized trial. *Infect Control Hosp Epidemiol.* 2011;32(9):872–880.

ADDITIONAL READING
- Ibler KS, Kromann CB. Recurrent furunculosis—challenges and management: a review. *Clin Cosmet Investig Dermatol.* 2014;7:59–64.
- Nowicka D, Grywalska E. *Staphylococcus aureus* and host immunity in recurrent furunculosis. *Dermatology.* 2019;235(4):295–305.

SEE ALSO

Folliculitis; Hidradenitis Suppurativa

CODES

ICD10
- L02.92 Furuncle, unspecified
- L02.12 Furuncle of neck
- L02.429 Furuncle of limb, unspecified

CLINICAL PEARLS
- Pathogens may be different in different localities. Keep up-to-date with the locality-specific epidemiology.
- If few, furuncles/furunculosis do not need antibiotic treatment. If systemic symptoms (e.g., fever), cellulitis, or multiple lesions occur, oral antibiotic therapy is used.
- Other treatments for MRSA include linezolid PO or IV and IV vancomycin.
- Folliculitis, furunculosis, and carbuncles are parts of a spectrum of pyodermas.
- Other causative organisms include aerobic (e.g., *Escherichia coli, Pseudomonas aeruginosa,* and *Streptococcus faecalis*), anaerobic (e.g., *Bacteroides, Lactobacillus, Peptobacillius,* and *Peptostreptococcus*), and *Mycobacteria.*
- Decolonization (treatment of the nares with topical antibiotic) is only recommended if the colonization was confirmed by cultures because resistance is common and treatment is of uncertain efficacy.

F

GALACTORRHEA

Kelley V. Lawrence, MD, IBCLC • Morgan J. Parker, DO • Angela Baker, DO

 BASICS

DESCRIPTION
- Milky nipple discharge not associated with gestation or present >1 year after weaning. Galactorrhea does not include serous, purulent, or bloody nipple discharge.
- System(s) affected: endocrine/metabolic, nervous, reproductive

Pediatric Considerations
Can occur in infants secondary to maternal estrogen exposure

Pregnancy Considerations
- Pregnancy stimulates lactotroph cells, so pituitary prolactin-secreting macroadenomas may increase by 21% (1)[A].
- Milk production often begins during the 2nd trimester; milk leakage that occurs during pregnancy is not pathophysiologic galactorrhea.

EPIDEMIOLOGY
Predominant age: 15 to 50 years (reproductive age), most commonly ages 20 to 35

Incidence
Prolactinomas, as a cause of galactorrhea, have a 44.4 persons per 100,000 incidence in adults (2).

Prevalence
Third most common breast complaint in women. 20–25% of women experience galactorrhea in their lifetime (3)[C].

ETIOLOGY AND PATHOPHYSIOLOGY
- Oxytocin stimulates prolactin secretion, which induces lactation. Prolactin is secreted by the anterior pituitary and inhibited by dopamine produced in the hypothalamus.
- Galactorrhea results either from prolactin overproduction or from loss of inhibitory regulation by dopamine.
  - Physiologic galactorrhea is due to pregnancy or from nipple stimulation, piercing
  - Pathophysiologic galactorrhea
    ○ Hyperprolactinemia (craniopharyngiomas, other tumors; irradiation; traumatic brain injury; pituitary stalk compression; postbreast augmentation surgery [1%]; prolactinoma [sellar tumor, somatotroph adenoma, pituitary macroadenoma]; vascular malformations [aneurysms])
    ○ Hyperprolactinemia in systemic diseases (adrenal insufficiency, chronic kidney disease, cirrhosis, thyroid disease, lung cancer, renal cell cancer, sarcoidosis/histocytosis)
    ○ Nonhyperprolactinemia
      ■ Chest wall trauma; spinal cord injury
      ■ Chiari-Frommel, del Castillo, and Forbes-Albright syndromes
      ■ Herpes zoster

- Medications/substances:
  - Cardiovascular (α-methyldopa, reserpine, verapamil, spironolactone)
  - GI (domperidone, H_2 blockers, metoclopramide, proton pump inhibitors) (4)[C]
  - Herbal (anise [liquorice], barley, blessed thistle, fenugreek seed, fennel, goat's rue)
  - Illicit (cocaine, marijuana) (3)[C]
  - Anti-infectives (isoniazid, protease inhibitors)
  - Opioids
  - Psych/neuro (neuroleptics, antipsychotics, stimulants, SSRIs, SNRIs [prolactin not always elevated], tricyclic antidepressants)
  - Reproductive (estrogens, copper IUD)
- Normal prolactin levels (if patient has galactorrhea plus amenorrhea, likely can have microprolactinoma)

GENERAL PREVENTION
- Avoid frequent nipple stimulation.
- Avoid medications that can suppress dopamine.

COMMONLY ASSOCIATED CONDITIONS
See "Etiology and Pathophysiology."

 DIAGNOSIS

PHYSICAL EXAM
- Breast examination should be performed with attention to the presence of spontaneous or induced (with gentle hand expression) nipple discharge.
- Should observe bilateral, milky white, or brown nipple discharge
- Perform formal visual field testing if pituitary adenoma suspected.
- Look for physical signs of associated conditions:
  - Acromegaly
  - Adrenal insufficiency
  - Chest wall conditions
  - Hypogonadism
  - Hypothyroidism
  - Polycystic ovarian syndrome
  - Pituitary macroadenoma

DIFFERENTIAL DIAGNOSIS
- Pregnancy-induced lactation or recent weaning (Average duration of lactation after weaning is 40 days but can be longer in cases of prolonged duration of breastfeeding.)
- Nonmilky (straw colored, gray, yellow, green, brown) nipple discharge: intraductal papilloma; fibrocystic disease
- Purulent breast discharge: typically due to infection; may see breast redness, pain, warmth, and edema: mastitis; breast abscess; impetigo; eczema
- Bloody breast discharge: If palpable mass, edema, or axillary lymphadenopathy, consider malignancy (Paget disease, breast cancer).

DIAGNOSTIC TESTS & INTERPRETATION
Initial Tests (lab, imaging)
Prolactin level, thyroid-stimulating hormone, pregnancy test, liver and renal functions
- Lab evaluation of prolactin may be falsely elevated by a recent breast examination, vigorous exercise, sexual activity, or high-carbohydrate diet.
- Repeat prolactin if borderline elevation (30 to 40).
- Prolactin levels fluctuate (highest in early morning). Elevated levels should be confirmed with repeat level drawn in a fasting, nonexercised state, with no breast stimulation (5)[C].
- If a breast mass is palpated in the setting of nipple discharge, evaluate with mammogram and/or ultrasound (mammogram preferred if patient is >30).
- Pituitary MRI with gadolinium if the serum prolactin level is significantly elevated (>200 ng/mL) or if a tumor is otherwise suspected
- For pediatric patients, culture the breast fluid to better treat and evaluate and to rule out infectious cause.

Follow-Up Tests & Special Considerations
- Consider evaluation of follicle-stimulating hormone and luteinizing hormone if amenorrheic.
- Consider evaluation of growth hormone levels if acromegaly suspected (1)[A].
- Measure adrenal steroids if signs of Cushing disease present.

Diagnostic Procedures/Other
If diagnosis is in question, confirm by microscopic evaluation that nipple secretions are lipoid, with a stained smear.

TREATMENT
- Identify and treat the underlying cause.
- Avoid excess nipple stimulation.
- Discontinue causative medications, if possible.
- If SSRI/SNRI is implicated, trial of mirtazapine instead.
- Medication to lower prolactin levels is preferred.
- Consider surgery or radiotherapy for patients not responding to medication.
- For tumors >10 mm (even if asymptomatic), surgery should be performed to reduce pituitary tumor size or prevent progression to avoid neurologic sequelae.
- If microadenoma, watchful waiting can be appropriate because 95% do not enlarge.
- Idiopathic galactorrhea (normal prolactin levels) does not require treatment.

MEDICATION

- Dopamine agonists work to reduce prolactin levels and shrink tumor size. Therapy is not curative (5)[C].
- Treatment is discontinued when tumor size has reduced or regressed completely or after pregnancy has been achieved.
- Dopamine agonists are class B in pregnancy and may be resumed if a macroadenoma grows significantly (1)[A].
- Cabergoline (Dostinex)
  - Start at 0.25 mg PO twice weekly and increase by 0.25 mg monthly until prolactin levels normalize. Usual dose ranges from 0.25 to 1.00 mg PO once or twice weekly.
  - Equally efficacious and better tolerated than bromocriptine (6)[A]
  - Check ESR, creatinine, and ECG at baseline and every 6 to 12 months.
  - DC after prolactin level normal for 6 months
- Bromocriptine
  - Start at 1.25 mg QHS PO with food and increase every 3 to 7 days by 2.5 mg/day until therapeutic response achieved (usually 2.5 to 15.0 mg/day).
  - Long-term treatment can cause woody fibrosis of the pituitary gland.
  - Check creatinine, CBC, LFTs, cardiovascular evaluation; pregnancy test every 4 weeks during amenorrhea and after menses restored if period is >3 days late
- Contraindications are similar for all and include the following:
  - Uncontrolled hypertension
  - Sensitivity to ergot alkaloids
- Precautions
  - Dopamine antagonists may cause nausea, vomiting, psychosis, or dyskinesia.
- Significant possible interactions
  - H_2 blockers, CYP3A4; weak serotonin effect; hypotensive effect
  - For women with microadenomas who do not wish to become pregnant, oral contraceptives may be a treatment option.

First Line
Cabergoline (see above)

Second Line
Bromocriptine (see above)

ISSUES FOR REFERRAL
Neurology, endocrinology, and breast surgeon as indicated; dermatology if refractory skin changes

SURGERY/OTHER PROCEDURES
- Surgery
  - Macroadenomas need surgery if (i) medical management does not halt growth, (ii) neurologic symptoms persist, (iii) size >10 mm, or (iv) patient cannot tolerate medications; also considered in young patients with microadenomas to avoid long-term medical therapy
  - Transsphenoidal pituitary resection
  - 50% recurrence after surgery

- Radiotherapy is an alternative for macroprolactinoma not responsive to other modes:
  - Risk of optic nerve damage, hypopituitarism, neurologic dysfunction, and increased risk for stroke and secondary brain tumors
  - 50% risk of panhypopituitarism after radiation
  - 20–30% success rate

COMPLEMENTARY & ALTERNATIVE MEDICINE
Alternative modalities used to cease milk production include ingestion of peppermint, parsley, and/or sage on a regular basis and topical application of cabbage leaves over all breast tissue. These treat symptoms, not underlying causes.

ADMISSION, INPATIENT, AND NURSING CONSIDERATIONS
Severe mastitis/abscess

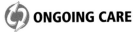 ONGOING CARE

FOLLOW-UP RECOMMENDATIONS
- Bromocriptine patients require adequate hydration.
- Discontinue dopamine agonist in pregnancy.

Patient Monitoring
- Check prolactin levels every 6 weeks until normalized and then every 6 to 12 months.
- Monitor visual fields and/or MRI at least yearly until stable for prolactinoma.

DIET
No restrictions; may include peppermint, parsley, and sage in diet for symptom management

PATIENT EDUCATION
- Warn about symptoms of mass enlargement in pituitary (vision changes, headaches).
- Inform patient that offending medications should be discontinued long term.
- Make new moms aware that this condition can be normal in baby boys and girls.

PROGNOSIS
- Symptoms can recur after discontinuation of a dopamine agonist.
- Surgery can have 50% recurrence.
- Prolactinomas <10 mm can resolve spontaneously.
- Postsurgical hyperprolactinemia is associated with better outcomes in node-negative breast cancer.

COMPLICATIONS
- If enlarging pituitary adenoma, risk of permanent visual field loss.
- Panhypopituitarism can complicate radiation or surgical therapy.
- Osteoporosis if amenorrhea persists without estrogen replacement.
- Hyperprolactinemia does not increase breast cancer risk.

REFERENCES

1. Molitch ME. Diagnosis and treatment of pituitary adenomas: a review. *JAMA.* 2017;317(5):516–524.
2. Frohlich DM, Caldwell KJ, Rohrs H, et al. A 17-year old female with secondary amenorrhea, galactorrhea, and headaches. *J Pediatr Health Care.* 2015;29(2):205–211.
3. Dawson RS. Sudden-onset galactorrhea in a teen-aged girl. *Contemporary OB/Gyn.* 2015;60(8):16–41.
4. Pipaliya N, Solanke D, Rathi C, et al. Esomeprazole induced galactorrhea: a novel side effect. *Clin J Gastroenterol.* 2016;9(1):13–16.
5. Huang W, Molitch ME. Evaluation and management of galactorrhea. *Am Fam Physician.* 2012;85(11):1073–1080.
6. Fachi MM, de Deus Bueno L, de Oliveira DC, et al. Efficacy and safety in the treatment of hyperprolactinemia: a systematic review and network meta-analysis [published online ahead of print June 16, 2021]. *J Clin Pharm Ther.* 2021;46(6):1549–1556. doi:10.1111/jcpt.13460.

ADDITIONAL READING
DiVasta AD, Weldon CB, Labow BI. The breast: examination and lesions. In: Emans SJ, Laufer MR, DiVasta AD, eds. *Emans, Laufer, Goldstein's Pediatric & Adolescent Gynecology.* 7th ed. Philadelphia, PA: Wolters Kluwer; 2020:781.

SEE ALSO

Hyperprolactinemia

CODES

ICD10
- N64.3 Galactorrhea not associated with childbirth
- N64.52 Nipple discharge

CLINICAL PEARLS

- Galactorrhea is a common disorder, affecting up to 50% of reproductive-age women.
- Galactorrhea is defined as bilateral milk production, usually milky, but can be varied.
- Common causes include idiopathic, nipple stimulation, dopamine-suppressing medications, systemic disease, or pituitary prolactinoma.
- In women >30 years old, consider imaging with mammography to rule out associated malignancy.
- Evaluate prolactin >200 ng/mL (or signs of suspicion for a pituitary macroadenoma) with a gadolinium-enhanced MRI.
- First-line medication treatment is cabergoline; second-line is bromocriptine.

G

GAMING DISORDER, INTERNET
Madhavi Singh, MD • Lawrence Go, MD

BASICS

DESCRIPTION

- Internet gaming disorder (IGD) is where the "gamers" play compulsively, to the exclusion of other interests resulting in clinically significant impairment or distress.
- For gaming disorder to be diagnosed, the behavior pattern must be of sufficient severity and would be evident for at least 12 months.
- IGD is identified in section III of *DSM-5* as a condition warranting more clinical research and experience before it might be considered for inclusion in the main book as a formal disorder.
- On June 18, 2018, WHO recognized gaming disorder as a mental health condition.
- Gaming disorder (digital or video) is included in ICD-11.

EPIDEMIOLOGY

Incidence
- Predominant age—adolescence
- Predominant sex—male

Prevalence
- Median prevalence of 2.0%
- Prevalence rates are highest in Eastern Asian countries and male adolescents aged 12 to 20 years (1).

ETIOLOGY AND PATHOPHYSIOLOGY

- On the molecular level, Internet addiction is characterized by an overall reward deficiency that entails decreased dopaminergic activity (2).
- On the level of neural circuitry, Internet and gaming addiction lead to neuroadaptation and structural changes that occur as a consequence of prolonged increased activity in brain areas associated with addiction (2).
- On a behavioral level, Internet and gaming addicts appear to be constricted with regards to their cognitive functioning in various domains (2).
- IGD shares multiple features with drug addictions, including elevated impulsivity, cognitive inflexibility, and attentional biases.

RISK FACTORS

The following risk factors were found to be significantly associated with IGD (3):

- Functional and dysfunctional impulsivity
- Belief self-control
- Anxiety
- Pursuit of desired appetitive goals
- Money spent on gaming
- Weekday game time
- Offline community meeting attendance
- Game community membership
- Gaming motives play a role as well.
- Gamers with psychiatric distress use it a coping strategy to improve their mood and/or attain emotional stability.
- Achievement-related motives may be related to the lack of real-life achievements that are compensated by virtual victories and successes.

COMMONLY ASSOCIATED CONDITIONS

- Anxiety disorder
- Mood disorder
- Autism spectrum disorder
- Attention deficit hyperactivity disorder
- Personality disorder
- Behavioral disorder

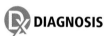

DIAGNOSIS

HISTORY

- Thorough history
- *DSM-5* section III proposed symptoms of IGD include:
  - Preoccupation with gaming
  - Withdrawal symptoms when gaming is taken away or not possible (sadness, anxiety, irritability)
  - Tolerance, the need to spend more time gaming to satisfy the urge
  - Inability to reduce playing, unsuccessful attempts to quit gaming
  - Giving up other activities, loss of interest in previously enjoyed activities due to gaming
  - Continuing to game despite problems
  - Deceiving family members or others about the amount of time spent on gaming
  - The use of gaming to relieve negative moods, such as guilt or hopelessness
  - Risk, having jeopardized or lost a job or relationship due to gaming
  - Under the proposed criteria, a diagnosis of IGD would require experiencing five or more of these symptoms within a year.
  - The condition can include gaming on the Internet or on any electronic device.
  - Most people who develop clinically significant gaming problems play primarily on the Internet.
  - 7-item Game Addiction Scale—GAS items such as relapse, conflict, withdrawal, and problems (loss of interests) were endorsed more frequently in more severe IGD stages, whereas items related to tolerance, salience (preoccupation), and mood modification (escape) were endorsed more widely among participants (including in less severe IGD stages) (4).

PHYSICAL EXAM

- Evaluate for signs related to excessive use of gaming devices:
  - Wrist, neck, and elbow pain, tenosynovitis ("nintendinitis")
  - Obesity
  - Skin blisters, calluses, sore tendons
- Mental status exam

DIFFERENTIAL DIAGNOSIS

- High-engagement Internet gaming, which is normal
- Social anxiety

DIAGNOSTIC TESTS & INTERPRETATION

- Internet Gaming Disorder test—20
- Gaming Disorder Test—brief four-item measure

TREATMENT

GENERAL MEASURES

- Cognitive-behavioral therapy (CBT) is considered efficacious (5)[A].
- Suggested psychotherapies (6)[C]:
  - CBT is suggested to improve inhibitory control ability, recognize maladaptive cognition, and employ adaptive decision making.
  - Cognitive enhancement therapy to help improve elevated impulsivity, impaired cognitive control, and cognitive inflexibility
  - Cognitive bias modification to target attention biases
  - Mindfulness-based stress reduction to address stress-induced association of IGD

MEDICATION

Methylphenidate, bupropion, and escitalopram have been studied but showed no added benefit.

ISSUES FOR REFERRAL

Therapist skilled in CBT

 ONGOING CARE

PATIENT EDUCATION

- American Academy of Pediatrics recommends no screen time for toddlers <18 months of age except video chatting.
- For children 2 to 5 years, limit are for 1 hr/day for high-quality content and parents should co-view.
- For children 6 years and older, should have consistent limits on screen time with designated media-free times
- For all ages, media should not be located in bedroom and video game play should not begin within half an hour before sleep.

PROGNOSIS

Fair

COMPLICATIONS

- Higher risk of mood disturbance, suicide ideation, and suicide planning in heavy gamers involved with screen times of >5 hours a day (1)
- Reduced sleep duration and disrupted sleep patterns
- Auditory hallucinations
- Enuresis
- Encopresis
- Wrist, neck, and elbow pain, tenosynovitis ("nintendinitis")
- Obesity
- Skin blisters, calluses, sore tendons
- Hand–arm vibration syndrome and peripheral neuropathy

REFERENCES

1. Paulus FW, Ohmann S, von Gontard A, et al. Internet gaming disorder in children and adolescents: a systematic review. *Dev Med Child Neurol.* 2018;60(7):645–659.
2. Griffiths MD, King DL, Demetrovics Z. *DSM-5* Internet gaming disorder needs a unified approach to assessment. *Neuropsychiatry.* 2014;4(1):1–4.
3. Rho MJ, Lee H, Lee TH, et al. Risk factors for Internet gaming disorder: psychological factors and Internet gaming characteristics. *Int J Environ Res Public Health.* 2017;15(1):40.
4. Khazaal Y, Breivik K, Billieux J, et al. Game addiction scale assessment through a nationally representative sample of young adult men: item response theory graded-response modeling. *J Med Internet Res.* 2018;20(8):e10058.
5. Torres-Rodríguez A, Griffiths MD, Carbonell X. The treatment of Internet gaming disorder: a brief overview of the PIPATIC program. *Int J Ment Health Addict.* 2018;16(4):1000–1015.
6. Dong G, Potenza MN. A cognitive-behavioral model of Internet gaming disorder: theoretical underpinnings and clinical implications. *J Psychiatr Res.* 2014;58:7–11.

ADDITIONAL READING

- Gentile D. Pathological video-game use among youth ages 8 to 18: a national study. *Psychol Sci.* 2009;20(5):594–602.
- Gentile DA, Bailey K, Bavelier D, et al. Internet gaming disorder in children and adolescents. *Pediatrics.* 2017;140(Suppl 2):S81–S85.
- Higuchi S, Nakayama H, Mihara S, et al. Inclusion of gaming disorder criteria in ICD-11: a clinical perspective in favor. *J Behav Addict.* 2017;6(3):293–295.
- Király O, Griffiths MD, Demetrovics Z. Internet gaming disorder and the *DSM-5*: conceptualization, debates, and controversies. *Curr Addict Rep.* 2015;2(3):254–262.

CLINICAL PEARLS

- IGD is considered a mental health disorder where the "gamers" play compulsively, to the exclusion of other interests resulting in clinically significant impairment or distress with symptoms presence of 12 months.
- Should be differentiated from high-engagement Internet gaming, which is normal
- Most prevalent in Southeast Asian countries in young adolescent males
- Gaming disorder (digital or video) is included in ICD-11.
- CBT is considered efficacious treatment.

G

GASTRITIS

Marie L. Borum, MD, EdD, MPH • Valeria A. Martinez-Lebron, MD

 BASICS

DESCRIPTION
- Inflammation of the gastric mucosa
- Can be classified by time course
  - Acute: neutrophilic infiltration on histology
  - Chronic: mixture of mononuclear cells, lymphocytes, macrophages on histology
- Subtypes of gastritis include:
  - Erosive gastritis
    ○ Mucosal injury by a noxious agent (especially nonsteroidal anti-inflammatory drugs [NSAIDs] or alcohol)
    ○ Vascular congestion due to portal hypertension (HTN) or gastric antral vascular ectasia (GAVE)
  - Reflux gastritis
    ○ A reaction to protracted reflux exposure to biliary and pancreatic fluid
  - Hemorrhagic gastritis (stress ulceration)
    ○ A reaction to hemodynamic disorder (e.g., hypovolemia or hypoxia [shock]). Common in intensive care unit (ICU) patients, particularly after severe burns and trauma
  - Infectious gastritis
    ○ Acute and/or chronic: *Helicobacter pylori* infection (most common cause of gastritis)
    ○ Viral infection (reaction to systemic infection) caused by cytomegalovirus or Epstein-Barr virus
    ○ Phlegmonous gastritis: a rapidly progressive and frequently fatal bacterial infection of the gastric wall
  - Atrophic gastritis
    ○ Metaplastic atrophic gastritis: autoimmune primary (pernicious) anemia
    ○ Frequent in elderly
    ○ Primarily from long-standing *H. pylori* infections
    ○ Prolonged proton pump inhibitor (PPI) use
    ○ Major risk factor for gastric cancer
  - Others
    ○ Granulomatous disease: sarcoidosis or Crohn disease

Geriatric Considerations
Persons age >60 years often harbor *H. pylori* infection.

Pediatric Considerations
Gastritis rarely occurs in infants or children; increases in prevalence with age. Most common etiology for pediatric gastritis is *H. pylori* infection.

EPIDEMIOLOGY
- Predominant age: all adult ages (more common in elderly)
- Predominant sex: male = female, although autoimmune gastritis is female > male

Incidence
1.8 to 2.1 million annual visits in the United States

Prevalence
- Gastritis is more prevalent in those born before 1950.
  - Roughly 50% of people >60 years are infected with *H. pylori* vs. 20% of people <40 years.
- In 2018, ~27% of U.S. adults were found to be infected with *H. pylori*.
  - Rates of infection are higher in minority groups and immigrants.
  - Prevalence higher in lower socioeconomic status

ETIOLOGY AND PATHOPHYSIOLOGY
- Noxious agents cause a breakdown in the gastric mucosal barrier, exposing underlying epithelial tissue to injury.
- Infection: *H. pylori* (most common cause), *Staphylococcus aureus* exotoxins, and viral infections (Epstein-Barr virus, human cytomegalovirus)
- Alcohol via cell DNA damage and subsequent pyroptosis
- Aspirin and other NSAIDs through inhibition of protective prostaglandin synthesis
- Bile reflux, pancreatic enzyme reflux
- Portal hypertensive gastropathy, causing erosion
- Emotional stress due to cortisol production
- Crohn-related gastritis, causing focally enhanced gastritis with histiocytes, lymphocytes, and granulomatous inflammation
- Hemodynamic instability (hypoxemia)

Genetics
There is difference in opinion regarding genome studies between the association of toll-like receptor 1 (TLR1) causing inflammation in *H. pylori*–infected gastric mucosa. Further research is warranted.

RISK FACTORS
- Age >60 years
- Exposure to potentially noxious drugs or chemicals (e.g., alcohol or NSAIDs)
- Hypovolemia, hypoxia (shock), burns, head injury, complicated postoperative course
- Autoimmune diseases (thyroiditis and type 1 diabetes mellitus, Addison disease, vitiligo, erosive oral lichen planus)
- Family history of *H. pylori* and/or gastric cancer
- Tobacco use
- Radiation, chemotherapy, ischemia, pernicious anemia, gastric mucosal atrophy

GENERAL PREVENTION
- Avoid injurious drugs or chemical agents, alcohol, and tobacco.
- Patients with hypovolemia or hypoxia (especially ICU patients) should receive prophylaxis with H_2 receptor antagonists, PPIs, prostaglandins, or sucralfate.
- Consider testing for *H. pylori* (and eradicating if present) in patients on long-term NSAID therapy, diagnosed with idiopathic thrombocytopenic purpura (ITP), or from endemic regions.

COMMONLY ASSOCIATED CONDITIONS
- Gastric or duodenal peptic ulcer
- Primary (pernicious) anemia—atrophic gastritis
- Portal HTN, hepatic failure
- Mucosa-associated lymphoid tissue (MALT) lymphoma

DIAGNOSIS

HISTORY
- Epigastric discomfort, often aggravated by eating
- Burning epigastric pain, anorexia
- Nausea, with or without vomiting
- Significant bleeding is unusual except in hemorrhagic gastritis.
- Rectal bleeding/melena
- Hiccups, belching
- Bloating or abdominal fullness, unintentional weight loss
- Generalized fatigue due to iron-deficiency anemia

- Neurologic symptoms related to vitamin B_{12} deficiency if atrophic gastritis
- History of smoking, consumption of alcohol, NSAID use, radiotherapy, gallbladder disorders, autoimmune disorders, IBD, vasculitis, or eosinophilic gastrointestinal (GI) disorders
- Can be asymptomatic

PHYSICAL EXAM
- Vital signs to assess hemodynamic stability
- Abdominal exam often normal
- Mild epigastric tenderness
- May have heme-positive stool
- Examine for stigmata of chronic alcohol abuse.
- May have pallor, slowing of capillary refill if patient is anemic

DIFFERENTIAL DIAGNOSIS
- Functional abdominal pain (dyspepsia)
- Peptic ulcer disease, viral gastroenteritis
- Gastric cancer (elderly), cholecystitis
- Pancreatic disease (inflammation vs. tumor)

DIAGNOSTIC TESTS & INTERPRETATION
Initial Tests (lab, imaging)
Usually normal
- Evaluate for iron deficiency anemia.
- Stool analysis for fecal *H. pylori* antigen
  - 95% specificity and sensitivity
  - Can be used for diagnosis and eradication
- ^{13}C-urea breath test for *H. pylori*
  - 95% specificity and sensitivity
- *H. pylori*, serology serum IgG
  - Inexpensive; 85% sensitivity, 79% specificity
  - Positive in history of colonization or prior infections; *cannot be used to assess eradication*
- Gastric acid analysis may be abnormal but is not a reliable indicator of gastritis.
- Patients with autoimmune chronic gastritis may have antibodies to intrinsic factor or parietal cells (the latter being the most sensitive biomarker), elevated serum fasting gastrin level, elevated serum pepsinogen I (PGI) level, and elevated PGI to PGII ratio.
- Patients with pernicious anemia may have macrocytic anemia with low serum vitamin B_{12} levels and intrinsic factor autoantibodies.
- Drugs that may alter lab results: Antibiotics, PPIs, and bismuth containing compounds may affect urea breath test for *H. pylori*.
  - Hold PPIs for 2 weeks, H_2 receptor antagonists for 24 hours, and antibiotics for 4 weeks prior to stool or breath tests (1)[B].

Follow-Up Tests & Special Considerations
Endoscopy for *H. pylori*
- Obtain biopsy for culture; polymerase chain reaction (PCR); histology with H&E plus second staining; rapid urease testing

Diagnostic Procedures/Other
- Gastroscopy with biopsy is first line in:
  - Age >50 years with new-onset symptoms
  - Weight loss, persistent vomiting, or GI bleed
- Consider for patients <50 years who are *H. pylori*–negative.
- Gastric biopsies (multiple) in both body and antrum recommended if there is a poor response to initial treatment. *Patients must discontinue PPIs for 2 weeks prior to endoscopy to improve diagnostic accuracy.*

Test Interpretation

- Acute or chronic inflammatory infiltrate in gastric mucosa, often with distortion or erosion of adjacent epithelium; presence of *H. pylori* often confirmed. Ulcers or bleeding may be present.
- Biopsies from antrum and body of the stomach

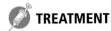 TREATMENT

GENERAL MEASURES

- *H. pylori* treatment is required to relieve symptoms.
- Parenteral fluid and electrolyte supplements if unable to tolerate oral intake
- Discontinue NSAID use.
- Abstinence from alcohol; smoking cessation
- Endoscopy in patients not responsive to treatment

MEDICATION

First Line

- Antacids: liquid form, 30 mL 1 hour after meals and at bedtime
- H_2 receptor antagonists oral cimetidine (Tagamet) 300 mg q6h or famotidine (Pepcid) 20 mg BID or nizatidine (Axid); 150 mg BID not shown to be clearly superior to antacids
- Sucralfate (Carafate): 1 g q4–6h on an empty stomach; rationale uncertain but empirically helpful
- Prostaglandins (misoprostol [Cytotec]): can help allay gastric mucosal injury; dosage 100 to 200 μg QID
- PPIs if no response to antacids or H_2 receptor blockers (e.g., omeprazole 20 mg daily or BID or esomeprazole 20 mg daily or BID)
- Treatment will depend on penicillin allergy and previous macrolide exposure or clarithromycin resistance of >15%.
  - Clarithromycin triple therapy (CTT)
    o Short course (14 days) of amoxicillin 1 g BID, standard-dose PPI BID (omeprazole 20 mg BID, etc.), and clarithromycin 500 mg BID
    o If PCN allergic: Substitute amoxicillin with metronidazole 500 mg TID.
    o 75–80% eradication per recent meta-analyses
    o Alternative: Prevpac combination pill (lansoprazole, amoxicillin, and clarithromycin)
  - Bismuth quadruple therapy (BQT)
    o PPI (omeprazole 20 mg) BID plus bismuth salicylate (Pepto-Bismol) 30 mL liquid or 2 tablets QID plus metronidazole 250 mg QID plus tetracycline 500 mg QID for 10 to 14 days (2)[A]
    o 75–90% eradication
    o Use as initial therapy in areas of high clarithromycin resistance (>15%).
    o Consider in penicillin-allergic patients.
    o Alternative: Pylera combination pill (bismuth subcitrate, metronidazole, and tetracycline)
- *H. pylori* treatment failure: Use a different regimen; avoid clarithromycin (unless resistance testing confirms susceptibility):
  - BQT for 7 to 14 days (3)[A]
  - Consider levofloxacin 250 mg BID, amoxicillin 1 g BID, and standard-dose PPI BID for 14 days in those who fail twice (2)[A].
  - In those allergic to penicillin, consider levofloxacin quadruple therapy with levofloxacin 500 mg QD, omeprazole QD 40 mg, nitazoxanide 500 mg BID, and doxycycline 100 mg QD for 7 to 10 days (3)[A].

- Consider probiotics in known symptomatic *H. pylori*; may decrease severity of gastritis, peptic ulcers; and possibly slow progression toward atrophic gastritis and gastric adenocarcinoma (4)[A]
  - Probiotics alone likely do not eradicate *H. pylori*.
  - Possible regimens as used in trials: *Bifidobacterium* spp BID × 14 days
- Contraindications: hypersensitivity
- Precautions:
  - Bismuth may turn stool black.

Pregnancy Considerations

- Avoid sodium carbonate and magnesium trisilicate–containing antacids.
- Women with hyperemesis gravidarum (HG) have a higher prevalence of *H. pylori* infection. Treatment can be deferred until after delivery. Routine testing for *H. pylori* is not recommended in those with HG (5).

SURGERY/OTHER PROCEDURES

Surgical intervention is not necessary, except in the case of phlegmonous gastritis or gastritis with high-grade dysplasia.

COMPLEMENTARY & ALTERNATIVE MEDICINE

Some studies suggest cranberry, garlic, curcumin, ginger, and Pistacia gum may prevent and/or reduce *H. pylori* infection due to their potent anti-inflammatory properties.

ADMISSION, INPATIENT, AND NURSING CONSIDERATIONS

- Prophylaxis in ICU patients
- Hemorrhagic gastritis

 ONGOING CARE

FOLLOW-UP RECOMMENDATIONS

- Usually no restrictions
- Confirm *H. pylori* eradication 4+ weeks after treatment.

Patient Monitoring

- Consider repeat endoscopy after 6 weeks if gastritis was severe or if poor treatment response.
- Surveillance endoscopy in patients with mild to moderate atrophic gastritis not currently recommended. Patients with advanced atrophic gastritis should receive endoscopy with biopsy sampling every 3 years.
- 25% of patients with high-grade dysplasia may progress to adenocarcinoma within a year, although this number is strongly influenced by geography, ethnicity, race, and family history.
- It is recommended patients with confirmed high-grade dysplasia undergo surgical or endoscopic resection.
- Surveillance may be suspended when two or more endoscopies are negative for dysplasia.

DIET

Diet restrictions (e.g., bland, light, soft foods) depend on symptom severity. In general, avoid caffeine, spicy foods, alcohol, peppermint, carbonated beverages, and high-fat content food.

PATIENT EDUCATION

- Smoking cessation; limit alcohol, dietary changes
- Relaxation therapy; avoid NSAIDs.

PROGNOSIS

- Phlegmonous gastritis has a 40–50% mortality even with treatment.
- Recurrence of *H. pylori* infection requires a repeated course of treatment.

COMPLICATIONS

- Bleeding from extensive mucosal erosion or ulceration
- Gastric outlet obstruction due to edema limiting adequate transfer of food from stomach to small intestine
- Gastric intestinal metaplasia, which puts patient at a 10-fold increase of developing gastric cancer.
- Clearing *H. pylori* before the development of chronic gastritis may prevent development of gastric cancer.
- Chronic autoimmune gastritis has increased risk for development of gastric neuroendocrine tumors and adenocarcinoma due to dysplasia.

REFERENCES

1. Shirin D, Matalon S, Avidan B, et al. Real-world *Helicobacter pylori* diagnosis in patients referred for esophagoduodenoscopy: the gap between guidelines and clinical practice. *United European Gastroenterol J*. 2016;4(6):762–769.
2. Malfertheiner P, Megraud F, O'Morain CA, et al; for European Helicobacter and Microbiota Study Group and Consensus panel. Management of *Helicobacter pylori* infection—the Maastricht V/Florence Consensus Report. *Gut*. 2017;66(1):6–30.
3. Chey WD, Leontiadis GI, Howden CW, et al. ACG clinical guideline: treatment of *Helicobacter pylori* infection [published correction appears in *Am J Gastroenterol*. 2018;113(7):1102]. *Am J Gastroenterol*. 2017;112(2):212–239.
4. Lü M, Yu S, Deng J, et al. Efficacy of probiotic supplementation therapy for *Helicobacter pylori* eradication: a meta-analysis of randomized controlled trials. *PLoS One*. 2016;11(10):e0163743.
5. Li L, Zhou X, Xiao S, et al. *Helicobacter pylori* infection is associated with an increased risk of hyperemesis gravidarum: a meta-analysis. *Gastroenterol Res Pract*. 2015;2015:278905.

 CODES

ICD10

- K29.5 Unspecified chronic gastritis
- K29.40 Chronic atrophic gastritis without bleeding
- K29.50 Unspecified chronic gastritis without bleeding

CLINICAL PEARLS

- *H. pylori* is the most common cause of gastritis; >50% of adult patients are colonized with *H. pylori* by age 60 years.
- *H. pylori* antibodies decline in the year after treatment and should not be used to determine eradication.
- *H. pylori* stool antigen tests can be used before and after therapy to assess for eradication and reinfection.
- Several courses of therapy may be necessary to eradicate *H. pylori*.
- In cases of suspected gastritis, discontinue PPI 2 weeks prior to endoscopy to improve diagnostic accuracy.

G

GASTROESOPHAGEAL REFLUX DISEASE

Sarah Burroughs, DO

 BASICS

DESCRIPTION
- Changes of the esophageal mucosa resulting from reflux of gastric contents into the esophagus
- Often described as "heartburn," "acid indigestion," and "acid reflux"

EPIDEMIOLOGY
Incidence
Incidence: 5/1,000 person-years
Prevalence
- 10–20% in the United States
- Chronic GERD is a risk factor for Barrett esophagus.
- Risk of adenocarcinoma without Barrett esophagus and no dysplasia: 0.1–0.5% per patient-year
- Risk of adenocarcinoma with Barrett esophagus and high-grade dysplasia: 6–19% per patient-year
- Pediatric population: Regurgitation occurs at least once a day in 2/3 of 4-month-old infants, decreasing to 21% at age 6 to 7 months, and 5% at 10 to 12 months.

ETIOLOGY AND PATHOPHYSIOLOGY
- The pattern and mechanism of reflux varies depending on the severity of disease.
- GERD begins when acidic stomach contents contact the squamous mucosal lining of the esophagus, at the esophagogastric junction (EGJ).
- Inappropriate transient lower esophageal sphincter (LES) relaxation. Foods that are spicy; acidic; and high in fat, caffeine, alcohol, tobacco, anticholinergic medications, nitrates, smooth muscle relaxants affect LES relaxation.
- Patients with severe GERD often have evidence of a hiatal hernia, which can:
  – Trap acid in the hernia sac
  – Impair acid emptying
  – Increase retrograde acid flow rate
  – Reduce the EGJ sphincter pressure
  – Increase frequency of transient LES relaxations

Genetics
Genetic heterogeneity has been associated with GERD.

RISK FACTORS
- Obesity
- Hiatal hernia
- Scleroderma
- Alcohol use
- Tobacco use
- Pregnancy

GENERAL PREVENTION
- Decrease consumption of food and beverage triggers such as spicy, fatty foods, alcohol, and caffeine.
- Weight loss
- Avoid lying down after meals.
- Eliminate tobacco and alcohol cessation.
- Elevate head of bed at night.
- Avoid meals close to bedtime.
- Infants: Use car seat for 2 to 3 hours after meals; thickened feedings

COMMONLY ASSOCIATED CONDITIONS
- Nonerosive esophagitis
- Erosive esophagitis
- Irritable bowel syndrome
- Peptic ulcer disease
- Extraesophageal reflux: aspiration, chronic cough, laryngitis, vocal cord granuloma, sinusitis, otitis media
- Halitosis
- Hiatal hernia: acid pocket (zone of high acidity in the proximal stomach above the diaphragm) (1)[B]
- Peptic stricture: 10% of patients with GERD
- Barrett esophagus
- Esophageal adenocarcinoma

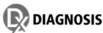 **DIAGNOSIS**

HISTORY
- Typical symptoms: acid regurgitation, heartburn, dysphagia (mostly postprandial)
- Atypical symptoms: epigastric fullness/pressure/pain, dyspepsia, nausea, bloating, belching, chest pain, lump in throat
- Extraesophageal signs and symptoms: chronic cough, bronchospasm, wheezing, hoarseness, sore throat
- Heartburn: retrosternal burning sensation
- Regurgitation; sour or acid taste in mouth ("water brash")
- Symptoms worse with bending or lying down
- Diet, alcohol and tobacco use

PHYSICAL EXAM
Often benign but look for potential:
- Epigastric tenderness or palpable epigastric mass
- Dental erosions

DIFFERENTIAL DIAGNOSIS
- Infectious esophagitis (*Candida*, herpes, HIV, cytomegalovirus)
- Chemical esophagitis; pill-induced esophagitis
- Eosinophilic esophagitis
- Nonulcer dyspepsia
- Biliary tract disease
- Radiation injury
- Crohn disease
- Angina/coronary artery disease
- Esophageal stricture or anatomic defect (ring, sling)
- Esophageal adenocarcinoma
- Achalasia; scleroderma
- Peptic ulcer disease

DIAGNOSTIC TESTS & INTERPRETATION
Diagnosis typically is based on history and clinical symptoms.

Initial Tests (lab, imaging)
- Indication for laboratory workup depends on clinical presentation. Check for anemia (history of bleeding; or possible poor vitamin B_{12} absorption due to chronic proton pump inhibitor [PPI] use).
- Appropriately evaluate patients who present with symptoms suspicious for cardiac disease.

Diagnostic Procedures/Other
- Upper endoscopy
  – First-line diagnostic test for those with alarm signs and uncontrolled symptoms (1)[B]
  – Indications for endoscopy:
    ○ Alarm symptoms such as dysphagia, bleeding, anemia, weight loss, recurrent vomiting
    ○ Persistent typical GERD symptoms despite treatment with twice-daily PPI for 4 to 8 weeks
    ○ New-onset dyspepsia in patients ≥60 years
    ○ Men >50 years with chronic GERD (>5 years) and other risk factors: hiatal hernia, high BMI, tobacco use, high abdominal fat distribution
    ○ History of severe erosive esophagitis (Assess healing and check for UGI pathology including Barrett esophagus.)
    ○ Surveillance (history of Barrett esophagus)
  – ~50–70% of patients with heartburn have negative endoscopic findings.
- High-resolution manometry (HRM), particularly in refractory cases
  – Used to evaluate peristaltic function and to record LES pressure (2)
  – Not recommended for primary GERD diagnosis; a second option for those with GERD and normal endoscopy (1)[B]
  – Diagnose motility disorders: functional heartburn, achalasia, and distal esophageal spasm.
- Ambulatory reflux (pH) monitoring
  – Evaluate excessive acid exposure in those with GERD symptoms, normal endoscopy, and no response to PPI (1)[B].
  – Used to document frequency of reflux
  – Discontinue PPI for 7 days prior to procedure.
- Barium swallow: not used for GERD diagnosis; used to evaluate complaints of dysphagia or to outline anatomic abnormalities (hiatal hernia)

 TREATMENT

GENERAL MEASURES
Lifestyle changes are first-line intervention:
- Elevate head of bed (1)[B].
- Avoid meals 2 to 3 hours before bedtime (1)[B].
- Avoid stooping, bending, and tight-fitting garments.
- Avoid medications that relax LES (anticholinergic drugs; calcium channel blockers).
- Promote weight loss (1)[B].
- Tobacco cessation and alcohol avoidance
- Limit consumption of patient-specific food triggers (global elimination of all reflux-causing foods is not necessary, practical, or beneficial).
- Stepwise approach to therapy
  – Phase I: lifestyle and diet modifications, antacids plus H_2 blockers or PPIs
  – Phase II: If symptoms persist, consider endoscopy.
  – Phase III: If symptoms still persist, consider surgery.

MEDICATION

First Line

- H_2 blockers in equipotent oral doses (e.g., ranitidine 150 mg BID, famotidine 20 mg BID
  - Renally dosed: Decrease dose to 50 mg and for creatinine clearance <50 mL/min.
  - Although less effective than PPIs, H_2 blockers given in divided doses provide symptomatic relief in patients with less severe symptoms (3)[A].
- PPIs: irreversibly bind proton pump (H^+/K^+ ATPase), effective onset within 4 days; omeprazole 20 to 40 mg/day, pantoprazole 40 mg/day, esomeprazole 40 mg/day, lansoprazole 15 to 30 mg/day, dexlansoprazole 30 mg/day, rabeprazole 20 mg/day
  - No major differences in efficacy among PPIs
  - Dose 30 to 60 minutes before meals with the exception of dexlansoprazole (1)[A].
  - PPIs may increase risk of hypomagnesemia, hip fracture, *Clostridium difficile* infection, vitamin B_{12} deficiency, and community-acquired pneumonia.
- PPI more effective than H_2 blocker and prokinetics for healing erosive and nonerosive esophagitis (4)[A].
- Erosive esophagitis: 8 weeks of PPI effective in 90%
- Reevaluate symptoms after 4 to 8 weeks of treatment.

Pediatric Considerations

Antacids or liquid H_2 blockers and PPIs are available. Prokinetics have a minimal role due to safety concerns and limited efficacy.

Second Line

- Antacids or barrier agents (sucralfate 1 g PO QID 1 hour before meals and at bedtime for 4 to 8 weeks) may relieve breakthrough symptoms.
- Prokinetics: metoclopramide 5 to 10 mg before meals
- Precautions
  - Blood dyscrasias and anemia with PPIs and H_2 blockers
  - Metoclopramide is a dopamine blocker; risk of dystonia and tardive dyskinesia
  - Tachyphylaxis may occur with H_2 blockers.
- Significant possible interactions
  - PPIs and H_2 blockers: multiple cytochrome P450 drug interactions; warfarin, phenytoin, antifungals, digoxin

ISSUES FOR REFERRAL

Persistent or severe disease

SURGERY/OTHER PROCEDURES

- Laparoscopic fundoplication (wrapping gastric fundus around distal esophagus) increases pressure gradient between stomach and esophagus.
- Bariatric surgery
  - Surgery indicated if patient desires to discontinue medical therapy, has side effects with medical therapy, has a large hiatal hernia, has esophagitis refractory to medical therapy, or has refractory symptoms. Gastric bypass is preferred (4)[A].
  - Manometry to rule out esophageal dysmotility, achalasia, or scleroderma prior to surgery (4)[A]

Pediatric Considerations

Surgery for severe symptoms (apnea, choking, persistent vomiting)

 ONGOING CARE

FOLLOW-UP RECOMMENDATIONS

Patient Monitoring

- Monitor symptoms over time. Consider additional workup and/or treatment if symptoms fail to improve after 8 weeks of PPI treatment.
- Repeat endoscopy in 4 to 8 weeks if there is a poor symptomatic response to medical therapy, especially in older patients.
- In patients with Barrett esophagus who would opt for treatment if cancer is detected, perform endoscopic surveillance every 2 to 3 years.

PATIENT EDUCATION

Lifestyle and dietary modifications: Eat small meals; avoid lying down after meals; elevate head of bed; weight loss; smoking cessation; avoid alcohol and caffeine.

PROGNOSIS

- Symptoms and esophageal inflammation often return promptly when treatment is withdrawn. To prevent relapse of symptoms, continue antisecretory therapy (in addition to lifestyle and dietary modifications).
  - PPI maintenance therapy likely improves quality of life more than H_2 blockers.
  - Full-dose PPIs are more effective than half-dose for maintenance (4)[A].
  - In erosive esophagitis, daily maintenance therapy with PPI prevents relapse; intermittent PPI therapy not as effective
- Medical and surgical therapy are equally effective for symptom reduction (4)[A].
- Antireflux surgery
  - 90–94% symptom response. Patients with persistent symptoms should have repeat anatomic evaluation (endoscopy or esophagram).
  - Some surgically treated patients eventually require medical therapy due to recurrence of symptoms.
- Regression of Barrett epithelium does not routinely occur despite aggressive medical or surgical therapy.

COMPLICATIONS

- Peptic stricture: 10–15%
- Barrett esophagus: 10%
  - Adenocarcinoma cancer develops at an annual rate of 0.5%.
  - Primary treatment for Barrett esophagus with high-grade dysplasia is endoscopic radiofrequency ablation.
- Extraesophageal symptoms: hoarseness, aspiration, (including pneumonia)
- Bleeding due to mucosal injury
- Noncardiac chest pain

Geriatric Considerations

Complications more likely (e.g., aspiration pneumonia)

REFERENCES

1. Patti MG. An evidence-based approach to the treatment of gastroesophageal reflux disease. *JAMA Surg.* 2016;151(1):73–78.
2. Patel A, Yadlapati R. Diagnosis and management of refractory gastroesophageal reflux disease. *Gastroenterol Hepatol (N Y).* 2021;17(7):305–315.
3. Kröner PT, Cortés P, Lukens FJ. The medical management of gastroesophageal reflux disease: a narrative review [published online ahead of print September 28, 2021]. *J Prim Care Community Health.* 2021 doi:10.1177/21501327211046736.
4. Katz PO, Gerson LB, Vela MF. Guidelines for the diagnosis and management of gastroesophageal reflux disease. *Am J Gastroenterol.* 2013;108(3):308–328.

ADDITIONAL READING

- Alimi Y, Azagury DE. Gastroesophageal reflux disease and the patient with obesity. *Gastroenterol Clin North Am.* 2021;50(4):859–870.
- Kellerman R, Kintanar T. Gastroesophageal reflux disease. *Prim Care.* 2017;44(4):561–573.
- Newberry C, Lynch K. Using diet to treat diseases of esophagus: back to the basics. *Gastroenterol Clin North Am.* 2021;50(4):959–972.

 SEE ALSO

Algorithms: Abdominal Pain, Upper; Dyspepsia

 CODES

ICD10

- K21.9 Gastro-esophageal reflux disease without esophagitis
- K21.0 Gastro-esophageal reflux disease with esophagitis

CLINICAL PEARLS

- GERD is diagnosed primarily by an accurate medical history.
- Consider GERD in nonsmokers with a chronic cough (>3 weeks).
- PPIs provide the most rapid symptomatic relief and healing of esophagitis.
- Consider additional workup and/or treatment if symptoms fail to improve after 8 weeks of PPI treatment.
- Endoscopy is recommended for patients with alarm symptoms, onset age >60 years, or prolonged severe symptoms.

G

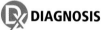
BASICS

- Men who have sex with men (MSM) are estimated to comprise 4% of the U.S. population, but this number is likely higher because many men don't disclose male-male sexual activity.
- MSM are less likely to have access to health care and are disproportionately impacted by mental health issues, smoking and substances abuse, and sexually transmitted infections (STIs).
- Health disparities exist between LGBT patients and heterosexuals. Sexual minority groups tend to fare worse across all realms.

DESCRIPTION

- Structural barriers of an unwelcoming healthcare system and minority stress (fear, stigma, internalized homophobia) experienced by LGBT people likely contribute to the development of health disparities. These disparities do not arise from innate characteristics of LGBT people.
- LGBT individuals may hide their orientation out of fear of stigma and discrimination, so it is important to ask all patients about sexual identity and behavior in a nonjudgmental environment.
- This chapter focuses on the diverse group of gay, bisexual, and other MSM. Men who have sex with transgender women may need many of the same screenings and prevention strategies as MSM.
- Although this chapter reviews the important topics that disproportionally effect this population, primary care of MSM is foremost about delivering the same care delivered to all patients.

GENERAL PREVENTION

- Centers for Disease Control and Prevention (CDC) recommends at least annual screening for HIV, syphilis, gonorrhea, and chlamydia as detailed below.
- CDC recommends testing for hepatitis B (1)[A].
- Annual screening for hepatitis C is only recommended in MSM with HIV (1)[A]. Screening for hepatitis A is not recommended.

DIAGNOSIS

- STIs
  - STIs among MSM are increasing. In 2018, MSM accounted for approximately 64% of reported primary and secondary syphilis cases. Behaviors that increase risk of non-HIV STIs also increase risk of HIV acquisition.
  - Physicians should screen for these high-risk behaviors such as:
    - Anonymous sexual encounters
    - Multiple active sex partners
    - Inconsistent barrier protection (condom) use
    - Substance use around and during sex
    - Receptive > insertive anal intercourse
  - Among adolescents, those who are unsure about their sexual identity report the highest rates of sexual risk-taking behavior.

- Annual screening of all asymptomatic sexually active MSM should include:
  - Syphilis serology using both nontreponemal and treponemal testing
  - Urine testing with nucleic acid amplification test (NAAT) for *Neisseria gonorrhoeae* and *Chlamydia trachomatis* if having insertive intercourse within the last year
  - Rectal swab NAAT for *N. gonorrhoeae* and *C. trachomatis* if having anal receptive intercourse within the last year
  - Pharyngeal swab NAAT for *N. gonorrhoeae* if having oral receptive intercourse within the last year. Pharyngeal swab for *C. trachomatis* is not recommended (1)[A].
  - Sexually active MSM should be screened at least annually for HIV.
- Screening should be increased to every 3 or 6 months in MSM at higher risk (see above) (1)[A].
- MSM are at risk for sexual transmission of enteric pathogens such as *Shigella*, hepatitis C, and others through oral-anal contact or through contact with fecally contaminated fingers or objects.
- HIV
  - 69% of new cases of HIV diagnosed in 2018 were among MSM. These disproportionately affected African American and Hispanic/Latino MSM, young MSM, and transgender women.
  - Up to 44% of MSM may not know their HIV status. This is more likely in men who are not open about their sexual identity and behavior (1).
  - Indications for PrEP
    - HIV negative (confirm with RNA viral load if exposure within last 4 weeks)
    - Sexually active but not in a monogamous relationship with an HIV-negative partner
    - *And* at least one of the following:
      - Anal sex without condoms in past 6 months (receptive or insertive)
      - Any STI diagnosed in past 6 months
      - In a sexual relationship with HIV-positive partner
  - There are two FDA-approved regimens for PrEP. Both are daily oral single-pill combinations and have similar efficacy:
    - Tenofovir disoproxil fumarate (TDF) 300 mg and emtricitabine (FTC) 200 mg; should not be used if CrCl <60 mL/min (2)[A]
    - Tenofovir alafenamide (TAF) 300 mg and emtricitabine (FTC) 200 mg. TAF is a version of tenofovir with less impact on bone and renal integrity; should not be used if CrCl <30 mL/min (2)[A].
    - Alternative dosing:
      - On-demand dosing (2-1-1 PrEP)—Take 2 doses of TDF/FTC within 2 to 24 hours before sex and 1 dose daily for 2 days afterward. Highly effective among MSM but not currently approved by the FDA or recommended by the CDC. On demand use of TAF/FTC has not been studied (2)[A].
      - Monitor HIV status and screen for STIs every 3 months. Monitor renal function at least every 6 months (2)[A].

  - Indications for PEP
    - ≤72 hours after exposure to known HIV-positive partner
  - PEP generally involves 28-day course of highly active antiretroviral therapy (HAART) in a three-drug combination:
    - Two nucleoside reverse transcriptase inhibitors (NRTIs) and an integrase inhibitor
    - Selection of medications is based on side effect profiles, patient compliance, and patient convenience.
    - "Preferred" regimens include the following:
      - Tenofovir 300 mg AND FTC 200 mg PLUS raltegravir 400 mg OR dolutegravir 50 mg in patients with CrCl >60 mL/min (3)[A]
      - Zidovudine AND lamivudine at renal doses PLUS raltegravir 400 mg OR dolutegravir 50 mg for patients with CrCl <60 mL/min (3)[A]
    - Counsel on safer sex and risk reduction for repeated exposures, including immediate transition to PrEP after completing PEP.
- Hepatitis C
  - HIV-negative MSM have a slightly higher prevalence of hepatitis C infection than the general population. However, HIV-positive MSM are at much higher risk for hepatitis C infection compared to both HIV negative MSM and the general population.
  - Annual screening for hepatitis C is recommended in MSM with HIV (1)[A].
- Cancer
  - Annual incidence of anal cancer is 5 times higher in HIV-negative MSM than the general population; increases to between 78 and 168 times higher in HIV-positive MSM
  - Anal carcinoma has been linked to certain high-risk subtypes of HPV, specifically types 16 and 18.
  - Screening for anal dysplasia with anal cytology may be considered for at-risk populations, especially HIV-infected MSM, but further research is needed for appropriate screening intervals (4)[A].
  - HPV vaccine is recommended for all boys age 11 to 12 years and young MSM through age 26 years to reduce the risk of anal cancer.
- Substance and tobacco abuse
  - Men who identify as gay and bisexual have significantly higher rates of use of nearly all substances as well as higher rates of substance use disorders than men who identify as heterosexual.
  - Many gay and bisexual men may find difficulty seeking aid in faith-based groups such as Alcoholics Anonymous due to the long history of religious discrimination of LGBT people.
  - "Chemsex" refers to use of drugs in conjunction with sexual intercourse by MSM. Inhaled nitrites ("poppers"), stimulants (methamphetamine and cocaine), GHB, ketamine, and alcohol are often used during or around sexual encounters to increase pleasure and performance (5).
    - The use of these substances may be associated with unprotected intercourse and other high-risk sexual behaviors which may increase risk of HIV and STI transmission.

○ Substance abuse treatment programs implementing cognitive behavioral intervention from a harm reduction perspective is beneficial in reducing stimulant use and sexual risk-taking behavior.

- Diabetes
  - Lifetime diabetes diagnoses are higher among MSM than among cisgender heterosexual men despite similar BMIs.
  - Higher rates of cigarette smoking and alcohol use may contribute to higher diabetes rates.
  - People living with HIV are more likely to have type 2 diabetes. This may be, in part, due to some HIV medications increasing insulin resistance.
- Mental health
  - Rates of mental illness or serious mental illness among MSM are 2–3× as high as rates among other men.
  - Risk of deliberate self-harm is also increased especially among youth due to stressors such as having an identity different than family and peers, isolation, bullying, family rejection, and self-nonacceptance.
- Social determinants of death
  - LGBT people are disproportionately affected by homelessness and unemployment.
  - Many patients report delaying necessary medical care in order to avoid experiencing stigma and bias from health care providers.
  - Sexual minority stress is thought to contribute to mental health problems and risky sexual behaviors.

Pediatric Considerations

- Normalizing nonheterosexual identities and behaviors during regular screening of sexual development during well adolescent visits could reduce stigma and decrease risk for negative mental health outcomes.
  - Rates of body image and eating disorders are increased in adolescent and young adult gay men.
  - Depression has been linked to increased sexual risk-taking behavior.
  - In addition to depression screenings recommended for all patients, regular assessments of mental health and suicide risk should include questions about family and peer support, experiences of stigma, connection to an LGBT community, and self-acceptance.
- Same-sex parenting
  - There is no causal relationship between parents' sexual orientation and children's emotional, psychosocial, and behavioral development.
  - The 2010 census reported that approximately 19% of same-sex couples are currently raising children and a 2013 national survey reported that 51% of LGBT adults have children or would like to have children in the future.
  - With changes in same-sex marriage laws, same-sex couples may feel more encouraged to start families.
  - Pathways to parenting for same-sex couples include adoption, IVF, and surrogacy.

- Intimate partner violence (IPV) (domestic violence)
  - Recent study reported ~21% of sexual minority men with a history of physical abuse and ~50% with psychological abuse; highest rates reported among bisexual men
  - Despite rates of IPV among male same-sex couples being equal to heterosexual couples, there is a lack of attention to IPV among LGBT people.
  - Same-sex IPV can be complex, involving worsening of the emotional and psychological minority stress of the victim, threats to "out" partner, abuse regarding HIV status.
  - Gay and bisexual victims are less likely to have support from family or the community.
  - Providers can stigmatize male same-sex IPV as not being as serious.
  - Screen for IPV with patients alone.
  - Be prepared to respond with compassion and connection to local LGBT-welcoming resources.

 ## ONGOING CARE

Obtaining a history
- Establish with patients that information related to sexual orientation is confidentially asked of all patients to assist in providing them the best care.
- Individualize regular discussions about substance and tobacco abuse, HIV/STIs, mental health, and IPV.
- Take an inclusive and complete sexual history.
- Creating a welcoming environment
  - Intake forms and waiting room and marketing materials inclusive of same-sex couples and identities
  - Displaying LGBT-friendly symbols and materials
    ○ Rainbow flags and pink triangles
    ○ Posters with same-sex couples
    ○ Brochures with LGBT health concerns such as safe sex, STIs, HIV/AIDS, mental health, and substance abuse
  - Language
    ○ Avoid labeling patients as gay, lesbian, bisexual, or transgender unless prompted by the patients. Many MSM identify as heterosexual rather than homosexual or bisexual. Some may not choose to label at all.
    ○ Understand significance of terms used in LGBT communities such as "bottom" partner (receptive sex) and "top" partner (insertive sex).

PATIENT EDUCATION
- Educate patients on risk-reduction strategies for safer sex such as avoiding or limiting substance use around sex, condoms, PrEP, and PEP.
- Educate patients on LGBT-specific or welcoming resources in your community for substance and tobacco abuse, IPV, mental health, and suicide prevention.

REFERENCES

1. Workowski KA, Bolan GA; for Centers for Disease Control and Prevention. Sexually transmitted diseases treatment guidelines, 2015. *MMWR Recomm Rep.* 2015;64(RR-03):1–137.
2. National LGBTQIA+ Health Education Center. PrEP action kit (updated 2020). https://www.lgbthealth education.org/publication/prep-action-kit/. Published June 3, 2020. Accessed November 15, 2021.
3. Dominguez KL, Smith DK, Vasavi T, et al. *Updated Guidelines for Antiretroviral Postexposure Prophylaxis after Sexual, Injection Drug Use, or Other Nonoccupational Exposure to HIV—United States, 2016.* Atlanta, GA: Centers for Disease Control and Prevention; 2016.
4. Clarke MA, Wentzensen N. Strategies for screening and early detection of anal cancers: a narrative and systematic review and meta-analysis of cytology, HPV testing, and other biomarkers. *Cancer Cytopathol.* 2018;126(7):447–460. doi:10.1002/cncy.22018.
5. Compton WM, Jones CM. Substance use among men who have sex with men. *N Engl J Med.* 2021;385(4):352–356.

ADDITIONAL READING

- Chou R, Evans C, Hoverman A, et al. *Pre-Exposure Prophylaxis for the Prevention of HIV Infection: A Systematic Review for the U.S. Preventive Services Task Force.* Philadelphia, PA: Agency for Healthcare Research and Quality; 2019.
- Gay & Lesbian Medical Association. *Guidelines for Care of Lesbian, Gay, Bisexual, and Transgender Patients.* San Francisco, CA: Gay & Lesbian Medical Association; 2006. http://www.glma.org/_data /n_0001/resources/live/GLMA%20guidelines%20 2006%20FINAL.pdf. Accessed November 15, 2021.

 ## CODES

ICD10
- Z11.59 Encounter for screening for other viral diseases
- Z11.4 Encounter for screening for human immunodeficiency virus
- Z72.52 High risk homosexual behavior

CLINICAL PEARLS

- Provide gay, bisexual, and MSM with the same comprehensive primary care delivered to all patients.
- All sexually active MSM should be offered annual screening for HIV, syphilis, rectal and urethral gonorrhea and chlamydia, and pharyngeal gonorrhea.
- Screen for HCV annually in HIV-positive MSM.
- Counsel patients on risk-reduction strategies for safer sex such as avoiding or limiting substance use around sex, condoms, PrEP, and PEP.

G

GENITO-PELVIC PAIN/PENETRATION DISORDER (VAGINISMUS)

Jeffrey D. Quinlan, MD, FAAFP

BASICS

Genito-pelvic pain/penetration disorder is the name of the conditions formally known as vaginismus and dyspareunia. Vaginismus results from involuntary contraction of the vaginal musculature. Primary vaginismus occurs in women who have never been able to have penetrative intercourse. Women with secondary vaginismus were previously able to have penetrative intercourse but are no longer able to do so.

DESCRIPTION
- Persistent or recurrent difficulties for 6 months or more with at least one of the following:
  - Inability to have vaginal intercourse/penetration on at least 50% of attempts
  - Marked genito-pelvic pain during at least 50% of vaginal intercourse/penetration attempts
  - Marked fear of vaginal intercourse/penetration or of genito-pelvic pain during intercourse/penetration on at least 50% of vaginal intercourse/penetration attempts
  - Marked tensing or tightening of the pelvic floor muscles during attempted vaginal intercourse/penetration on at least 50% of occasions
- The disturbance causes marked distress or interpersonal difficulty.
- Dysfunction is not as a result of:
  - Nonsexual mental disorder
  - Severe relationship stress
  - Other significant stress
  - Substance or medication effect
- Specify if with a general medical condition (e.g., lichen sclerosus, endometriosis)

Pregnancy Considerations
May first present during evaluation for infertility
- Pregnancy can occur in patients with genito-pelvic pain/penetration disorder when ejaculation occurs on the perineum.
- Vaginismus may be an independent risk factor for cesarean delivery.

EPIDEMIOLOGY

Incidence
The incidence of vaginismus is thought to be about 1–17% per year worldwide. In North America, 12–21% of women have genito-pelvic pain of varying etiologies (1).

Prevalence
- True prevalence is unknown due to limited data/reporting.
- Population-based studies report prevalence rates of 0.5–30%.
- Affects women in all age groups
- Approximately 15% of women in North America report recurrent pain during intercourse.

ETIOLOGY AND PATHOPHYSIOLOGY
Most often multifactorial in both primary and secondary vaginismus
- Primary
  - Psychological and psychosocial issues
    - Negative messages about sex and sexual relations in upbringing may cause phobic reaction.
    - Poor body image and limited understanding of genital area
    - History of sexual trauma
  - Abnormalities of the hymen
  - History of difficult gynecologic examination
- Secondary
  - Often situational
  - Often associated with dyspareunia secondary to:
    - Vaginal infection
    - Inflammatory dermatitis
    - Surgical or postdelivery scarring
    - Endometriosis
    - Inadequate vaginal lubrication
    - Pelvic radiation
    - Estrogen deficiency
  - Conditioned response to pain from physical issues previously listed

RISK FACTORS
- Most often idiopathic
- Although the exact role in the condition is unclear, many women report a history of abuse or sexual trauma.
- Often associated with other sexual dysfunctions

COMMONLY ASSOCIATED CONDITIONS
- Marital stress, family dysfunction
- Anxiety
- Vulvodynia/vestibulodynia

DIAGNOSIS

DSM-5 has combined vaginismus and dyspareunia in a condition called genito-pelvic pain/penetration disorder.

HISTORY
- Complete medical history
- Full psychosocial and sexual history, including the following:
  - Onset of symptoms (primary or secondary)
  - If secondary, precipitating events, if any
  - Relationship difficulty/partner violence
  - Inability to allow vaginal entry for different purposes
    - Sexual (penis, digit, object)
    - Hygiene (tampon use)
    - Health care (pelvic examination)
  - Infertility
  - Traumatic experiences (exam, sexual, etc.)
  - Religious beliefs
  - Views on sexuality

PHYSICAL EXAM
- Pelvic examination is necessary to exclude structural abnormalities or organic pathology.
- Educating the patient about the examination and giving her control over the progression of the examination is essential because genital/pelvic examination may induce varying degrees of anxiety in patients.
- Referral to a gynecologist, family physician, or other provider specializing in the treatment of sexual disorders may be appropriate.
- Contraction of pelvic floor musculature in anticipation of examination may be seen.
- Lamont classification system aids in the assessment of severity:
  - First degree: perineal and levator spasm relieved with reassurance
  - Second degree: perineal spasm maintained throughout the pelvic exam
  - Third degree: levator spasm and elevation of buttocks
  - Fourth degree: levator and perineal spasm and elevation with adduction and retreat

DIFFERENTIAL DIAGNOSIS
- Vaginal infection
- Vulvodynia/vestibulodynia
- Vulvovaginal atrophy
- Urogenital structural abnormalities
- Interstitial cystitis
- Endometriosis

DIAGNOSTIC TESTS & INTERPRETATION
No laboratory tests indicated unless signs of vaginal infection are noted on examination. When diagnosing of this disorder has been conducted, five factors should be considered.
- Partner factors
- Relationship factors
- Individual vulnerability factors
- Cultural/religious factors
- Medical factors

Test Interpretation
Not available; may be needed to check for secondary causes

TREATMENT
- Genito-pelvic pain/penetration disorder may be successfully treated (1)[B].
- Meta-analysis of RCTs documented a trend toward higher efficacy of active treatment versus controls, whereas the meta-analysis of observational studies indicated that women with vaginismus benefit from a range of treatments in almost 80% of cases (2)[A].

- Another meta-analysis of level 1 evidence found that 2/3 of the treatment effect for female sexual dysfunction is accounted for by placebo (3)[A]. These findings suggest that the current treatments for female sexual dysfunction are, overall, minimally superior to placebo, which emphasizes the ongoing need for more efficacious treatment for female sexual dysfunction.
- Outpatient care is appropriate.
- Treatment of physical conditions, if present, is first line (see "Secondary" under "Etiology and Pathophysiology").
- Most begin with pelvic floor physical therapy and myofascial release
- Some evidence suggests that cognitive-behavioral therapy may be effective, including desensitization techniques, such as gradual exposure, aimed at decreasing avoidance behavior and fear of vaginal penetration (4)[A].
- Based on a Cochrane review, a clinically relevant effect of systematic desensitization cannot be ruled out (5)[A].
- Evidence suggests that sex therapy may be effective (5)[B].
  - Involves Kegel exercises to increase control over perineal muscles
  - Stepwise vaginal desensitization exercises
    - With vaginal dilators that the patient inserts and controls
    - With woman's own finger(s) to promote sexual self-awareness
    - Advancement to partner's fingers with patient's control
    - Coitus after achieving largest vaginal dilator or three fingers; important to begin with sensate-focused exercises/sensual caressing without necessarily a demand for coitus
    - Female superior at first; passive (nonthrusting); female-directed
    - Later, thrusting may be allowed.
- Topical anesthetic or anxiolytic with desensitization exercises may be considered.
- Patient education is an essential component of treatment (see "Patient Education" section).

MEDICATION

- Antidepressants and anticonvulsants have been used with limited success. Low-dose tricyclic antidepressant (amitriptyline 10 mg) may be initiated and titrated as tolerated (4)[B].
- Topical anesthetics or anxiolytics may be used in combination with either cognitive-behavioral therapy or desensitization exercises as noted above (5)[B].
- Botulinum neurotoxin type A injections may improve vaginismus in patients who do not respond to standard cognitive behavioral and medical treatment for vaginismus (6)[B].
  - Dosage: 20, 50, and 100 to 400 U of botulinum toxin type A injected in the levator ani muscle have been shown to improve vaginismus (5)[B].
- Intravaginal botulinum neurotoxin type A injection (100 to 150 U) followed by bupivacaine 0.25% with epinephrine 1:400,000 intravaginal injection (20 to 30 mL) while the patient is anesthetized may facilitate progressive placement of dilators and ultimately resolution of symptoms (6)[B].

ISSUES FOR REFERRAL
For diagnosis and treatment recommendations, the following resources may be consulted:
- Obstetrics/gynecology
- Pelvic floor physical therapy
- Psychiatry
- Sex therapy
- Hypnotherapy

SURGERY/OTHER PROCEDURES
Contraindicated

COMPLEMENTARY & ALTERNATIVE MEDICINE
- Biofeedback
- Functional electrical stimulation

 ONGOING CARE

FOLLOW-UP RECOMMENDATIONS
Desensitization techniques of gentle, progressive, patient-controlled vaginal dilation

Patient Monitoring
General preventive health care

DIET
No special diet

PATIENT EDUCATION
- Education about pelvic anatomy, nature of vaginal spasms, normal adult sexual function
- Handheld mirror can help the woman to learn visually to tighten and loosen perineal muscles.
- Important to teach the partner that spasms are not under conscious control and are not a reflection on the relationship or a woman's feelings about her partner
- Instruction in techniques for vaginal dilation
- Resources
  - American College of Obstetricians and Gynecologists (ACOG), 409 12th St., SW, Washington, DC 20024-2188; 800-762-ACOG. http://www.acog.org/
  - Valins L. *When a Woman's Body Says No to Sex: Understanding and Overcoming Vaginismus.* New York, NY: Penguin; 1992.

PROGNOSIS
Favorable, with early recognition of the condition and initiation of treatment

REFERENCES

1. Landry T, Bergeron S. How young does vulvovaginal pain begin? Prevalence and characteristics of dyspareunia in adolescents. *J Sex Med*. 2009;6(4):927–935.
2. Maseroli E, Scavello I, Rastrelli G, et al. Outcome of medical and psychosexual interventions for vaginismus: a systematic review and meta-analysis. *J Sex Med*. 2018;15(12):1752–1764.
3. Weinberger JM, Houman J, Caron AT, et al. Female sexual dysfunction and the placebo effect: a meta-analysis. *Obstet Gynecol*. 2018;132(2):453–458.
4. Crowley T, Goldmeier D, Hiller J. Diagnosing and managing vaginismus. *BMJ*. 2009;338:b2284.
5. Melnik T, Hawton K, McGuire H. Interventions for vaginismus. *Cochrane Database Syst Rev*. 2012;(12):CD001760.
6. Pacik PT. Vaginismus: review of current concepts and treatment using Botox injections, bupivacaine injections, and progressive dilation with the patient under anesthesia. *Aesthetic Plast Surg*. 2011;35(6):1160–1164.

ADDITIONAL READING

- Basson R, Wierman ME, van Lankveld J, et al. Summary of the recommendations on sexual dysfunctions in women. *J Sex Med*. 2010;7(1, Pt 2):314–326.
- Pacik PT. Understanding and treating vaginismus: a multimodal approach. *Int Urogynecol J*. 2014;25(12):1613–1620.
- Simons JS, Carey MP. Prevalence of sexual dysfunctions: results from a decade of research. *Arch Sex Behav*. 2001;30(2):177–219.
- ter Kuile MM, van Lankveld JJ, de Groot E, et al. Cognitive-behavioral therapy for women with lifelong vaginismus: process and prognostic factors. *Behav Res Ther*. 2007;45(2):359–373.

 SEE ALSO

Dyspareunia; Sexual Dysfunction in Women

 CODES

ICD10
- N94.2 Vaginismus
- N94.1 Dyspareunia

CLINICAL PEARLS

- In a patient with suspected genito-pelvic pain/penetration disorder, a complete medical history, including a comprehensive psychosocial and sexual history and a patient-centric, patient-controlled educational pelvic exam should be conducted.
- This condition can be treated effectively. Further research into the most effective methods is needed.
- Cognitive-behavioral therapy may be effective for the treatment of this condition.
- Botox injection therapy is in the experimental stages but looks promising for the treatment of vaginismus. Bupivacaine and dilation under general anesthesia has also been tried as a treatment for vaginismus.

G

GERIATRIC CARE: GENERAL PRINCIPLES

Jeremy Golding, MD, FAAFP • Zahra Sardar Sheikh, MD, MPH, CMD

 BASICS

DESCRIPTION

The optimal approach to caring for our elderly patient population requires an understanding of the physiology of normal aging as well as unique geriatric considerations for access to care, diagnosis, treatment, and ongoing care. "First do no harm"; many well-intended diagnostic and therapeutic interventions (with efficacy established in younger patients) may not benefit the elder. Geriatric care, more than many other medical specialties, focuses on preserving and improving function and comfort, rather than on life extension.

EPIDEMIOLOGY

The percentage of the U.S. population anticipated to be >65 years by the year 2050 exceeds 20%, and the percentage of those who are >85 years may reach 24%.

ETIOLOGY AND PATHOPHYSIOLOGY

Physiology of aging

- Although patients age ≥65 years are typically considered elderly, there is variability in the rate of decline in organ function associated with aging dependent on genetic, environmental, socioeconomic factors as well as disease burden.
- The aging process is not pathologic but part of the developmental continuum. However, physiologic changes associated with aging tend to diminish the body's compensatory reserve and increase susceptibility to disease.
  - Aging increases body fat and decreases total body water and lean body mass. This results in hydrophilic drugs having a smaller apparent volume of distribution. Lipophilic drugs will have an increased volume of distribution and longer half-life.
  - Aging decreases renal elimination of drugs.
  - Declines in lung capacity, oxygen uptake, cardiac output, muscle mass, glomerular filtration rate as well as blood flow to the brain, liver, and kidneys are associated with aging and must be considered in the diagnosis and treatment of elderly patients.

RISK FACTORS

Access to care

- Despite Medicare, persistent barriers to care include:
  - A lack of provider responsiveness to patient concerns
  - Mounting medical bills
  - Transportation challenges
- Barriers tend to be more prevalent in the female population and with increasing age.
- Alternatives to the traditional face-to-face visit should be considered to enhance access to care:
  - Encrypted email or home telehealth for those who are technologically equipped
  - Phone visits for those with adequate hearing
  - Nurse visits at home to evaluate and plan care by reporting to provider

GENERAL PREVENTION

- Vaccination schedule for seniors: https://www.vaccines.gov/who_and_when/seniors/index.html
- Function is the heart of geriatric care. Assess and promote function at each encounter as changes in functional independence are common. Assess: activities of daily living (ADLs), instrumental ADLs (IADLs) (ability to use equipment such as a phone)
- Hearing assessment via hearing
  - Handicapped inventory
- Depression via:
  - Geriatric Depression Scale: https://consultgeri.org/try-this/general-assessment/issue-4.pdf

- Cognition via Mini Cognitive Assessment Instrument https://www.alz.org/media/Documents/mini-cog.pdf and Montreal Cognitive Assessment https://www.mocatest.org/
- Falls: Those with two or more falls in the past year, fall with injury requiring medical treatment, or fear of falling due to difficulty with gait or balance require a full fall risk assessment: https://www.cdc.gov/steadi/pdf/STEADI-Algorithm-508.pdf and https://www.cdc.gov/steadi/materials.html
- Urinary incontinence: Inquire if patient has lost urine >5 times in past year.
- Polypharmacy
  - Use pill bottles, pharmacy records, patient and caregiver input to reconcile medication lists.
  - Ask about use of over-the-counter and alternative medications.
  - Reconcile medications at each visit
  - Make an attempt to simplify medications at each encounter.
  - Engage patients and their caregivers in discussions regarding prescribing cascade and polypharmacy disadvantages
- Substance use: CAGE criteria: https://www.mdcalc.com/cage-questions-alcohol-use
- Advanced care planning

ALERT

Completion of an advanced directive among most important interventions

- Definition: Advanced directives are documents a person completes while still in possession of decisional capacity to ensure their values are reflected when considering how treatment decisions should be made on her or his behalf in the event she or he loses the capacity to make such decisions.
- Instruments:
  - Durable power of attorney: Patient (called the principal) appoints an agent to handle specific health, legal, and financial responsibilities.
  - Health care proxy: a durable power of attorney specifically for health care decisions; their role is to express the patient's wishes and make health care decisions if the patient cannot speak for themselves.
  - Living will: a legal document that allows patients to express their wishes for end-of-life medical care, in case they become unable to communicate their decisions
  - Discussions and completion of orders pertaining to end-of-life care, referred to as POLST (physician order for life-sustaining treatment) in most states and MOLST (medical orders for life sustaining treatment) in some northeastern states

℞ DIAGNOSIS

HISTORY

Optimizing communication

- Speak directly to your patient unless directed toward their surrogate.
- Assess and manage emotionally charged interactions. Refrain from taking negative energy personally.
- Assess patient and caregiver health literacy and adjust explanations accordingly.
- Gauge the degree of social and financial support.
- Establish patient's values, preferences, and goals of care.

PHYSICAL EXAM

Geriatric-specific considerations:

- Orthostatic hypotension: contributes to poor energy, diminished functional status, increased risk of falls, and decline in renal function due to ineffective organ perfusion
- Hypothermia/hyperthermia: increased susceptibility in the elderly; less likely to mount a fever in the setting of infection; consider thyroid derangement.
- Weight loss: Assess access to food; may be presenting feature in mood disorder, thyroid derangement, dementia, malignancy
- Hearing: Check for cerumen impaction; perform Whisper Test: https://www.youtube.com/watch?v=PzRzpW6JKzQ.
- Gait, balance, and proximal muscle strength: assessed via Timed Get up and Go Test (https://www.cdc.gov/steadi/materials.html), functional reach test and Tinetti balance assessment tool

DIFFERENTIAL DIAGNOSIS

Geriatric-specific presentations:

- Coronary artery disease: Elderly patients with coronary heart disease often present with atypical symptoms, including exertional dyspnea. Silent myocardial ischemia is also common.
- Constipation: In older adults, constipation due to slow transit is very common and may be associated with fecal impaction and overflow fecal incontinence.
- Delirium: Nearly 30% of older patients experience delirium at some time during hospitalization.
- Urinary tract infection (UTI): UTI is the most common infectious illness in adults age ≥65 years, but diagnosis of UTI is fraught with difficulty because of the high prevalence of asymptomatic bacteriuria and pyuria, neither of which should be treated unless symptomatic. Asymptomatic bacteriuria is a marker for debility, but treatment does not improve outcomes and may cause harm.
- Depression: It is more common in elderly females. If left untreated, is often the precursor of overt dementia.
- Insomnia: Late-life insomnia is often persistent and may prompt self-medication with over-the-counter sleep aids or alcohol.
- Hearing difficulties: Some studies showed increased incidence of dementia in patient with hearing difficulties.
- Visual impairment: Macular degeneration, glaucoma and cataracts are the most commonly encountered causes and a yearly eye exam is important.

DIAGNOSTIC TESTS & INTERPRETATION

Informed decision-making

- Decision-making capacity: Evaluate in four areas: ability to understand information about treatment, ability to appreciate how that information applies to their situation, ability to reason with that information, and ability to make a choice and express it: http://www.aafp.org/afp/2001/0715/p299.html.
- Surrogate decision maker
  - Patient-identified agent (durable power of attorney for health care, medical power of attorney, health care agent)
  - Court-appointed surrogate (legal guardian or conservator)

Diagnostic Procedures/Other

- Avoid unnecessary patient/caregiver burden if results will not significantly enhance the plan of

care. Consider risks/harms, cost, time, travel, pain/discomfort, anxiety, and recovery time for all testing under consideration.
- Take into consideration renal function for imaging studies involving contrast.
- Many lab results require comparison with age-specific reference values (e.g., thyroid-stimulating hormone, A1c, prostate-specific antigen, D-dimer).

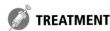 TREATMENT

GENERAL MEASURES
- Optimize nonpharmacologic options first.
- Align with patients' goals of care.
- Feasibility for patient and caregivers: Assess cost, availability, travel burden, and adherence.
- Compliance
- Nonpharmacologic (1)
  - Measures (1):
    ○ Occupational therapy (OT)/physical therapy (PT), speech therapy, hearing aids
    ○ Walking assist devices
    ○ Nonpharmacologic treatment of depression and insomnia
- Pharmacologic
  - Start low and go slow.
  - Adjust dose for renal and hepatic function, volume of distribution, decreased protein binding (more free/active drug available)
  - Be cognizant of pill burden, drug–drug interactions, and risks of polypharmacy. Anticoagulants and hypoglycemic medication (particularly insulin and sulfonylureas) are high-risk drugs in the elderly.
  - Beers criteria: assists in selecting medications with best geriatric benefit to risk ratio; https://geriatricscareonline.org/ProductAbstract/american-geriatrics-society-updated-beers-criteria-for-potentially-inappropriate-medication-use-in-older-adults/CL001#
- Deprescribing: AGA and Choosing Wisely suggest:
  - Don't recommend percutaneous feeding tubes in patients with advanced dementia; instead, offer oral-assisted feeding. Feeding tubes do not prolong life and may worsen suffering and thirst in this population.
  - Avoid antipsychotics as the first choice to treat behavioral and psychological symptoms of dementia.
  - Nonpharmacologic interventions are more efficacious than pharmacologic interventions for reducing aggression and agitation in adults with dementia (2)[A]. Antipsychotic medications increase risk of death. They may have a role in a carefully considered overall palliative plan that focuses on nonpharmacologic means of soothing agitation. And in individuals who are being cared for at home and lack of antipsychotics may add caregiver burden and hence hasten placement.
  - In diabetes care, meticulously avoid hypoglycemia, which is of far greater potential harm to the patient than is hyperglycemia. Metformin is generally safe. The major goal, especially in care of the older or more debilitated population is maintenance of glucose levels below those that cause symptomatic polyuria and polydipsia. This is not a specific A1c target.
  - Don't use benzodiazepines or other sedative hypnotics in older adults as first choice for insomnia, agitation, or delirium.
  - Don't use antimicrobials to treat bacteriuria in older adults unless specific urinary tract symptoms are present. Delirium in patients seen in the ED

and hospital is not likely caused by bacteriuria or lower UTI but usually by other causes.
  - Don't prescribe cholinesterase inhibitors for dementia without periodic assessment for perceived cognitive benefits and adverse gastrointestinal (GI) effects.
  - Don't recommend screening for breast, colorectal, prostate, or lung cancer without considering life expectancy and the risks of testing, overdiagnosis, and overtreatment.
  - Avoid using prescription appetite stimulants or high-calorie supplements for treatment of anorexia or cachexia in older adults; instead, optimize social supports, discontinue medications that may interfere with eating, provide appealing food and feeding assistance, and clarify patient goals and expectations.
  - Don't prescribe any medication without conducting a drug regimen review. Consider deprescribing as possible.
  - Don't use physical restraints to manage behavioral symptoms of hospitalized older adults with delirium.
- Geriatric pain management:
  - Treatment goal is to improve function.
  - Stepwise care, beginning with nonpharmacologic interventions such as PT, massage, environmental changes (e.g., music and aromatherapy), followed by cautious use of medication as necessary. Nonsteroidal anti-inflammatory medications (NSAIDs) involve significant risks in the elderly (renal, GI, cardiovascular). Use low doses of naproxen or ibuprofen preferentially, with GI-protective medication (e.g., omeprazole) if chronic therapy is needed. Low-dose opioid may be appropriate in some patients. A bowel regimen to prevent obstipation is needed for those using opioids.
  - Pharmacologic: Consider Beers criteria. Many commonly used adjunctive pain medications (e.g., gabapentin) offer little benefit and significant potential for harm in the elderly.
- Assess the home environment: Consider social work consultation, PT/OT evaluations as indicated, and diagnose and address social isolation (3). Home visitation, social activity, and group support may be of particular value. Consider adult day program enrollment.

MEDICATION
Nonpharmacologic pain management with modalities like weight reduction, PT, acupuncture, and massage therapy should be tried before medications. Biofeedback and CBT may be beneficial.

First Line
Acetaminophen <3 g dose over 24 hours.

Second Line
Use caution with pain treatment: Tramadol, narcotics, and NSAIDs need to have risk/benefit considerations before implementation. CBD is gaining popularity in the geriatric population but has limited efficacy.

ADDITIONAL THERAPIES
Acupuncture

SURGERY/OTHER PROCEDURES
- Does surgery align with goals of care?
- Explore alternatives thoroughly.
- Preop discharge planning with caregiver input

COMPLEMENTARY & ALTERNATIVE MEDICINE
Discuss potential risks and limitations.

ADMISSION, INPATIENT, AND NURSING CONSIDERATIONS
Inpatient prevention measures:
- Falls
- Acute delirium
- Skin breakdown, pain management, infections

 ONGOING CARE

Home nursing services and care at home with additional resources.

FOLLOW-UP RECOMMENDATIONS
- Realistic expectations
- Carefully review medications, eliminate hospital-prescribed unnecessary medications.

DIET
A well-balanced diet should be encouraged and caloric intake should be optimal.

PATIENT EDUCATION
- Caregiver support: screening for frustration, depression, social supports, financial burden, coping mechanisms, and need for help
  - Resources for caregivers:
    ○ Local agency on aging (Councils on Aging)
    ○ Respite care
    ○ Alzheimer's Association 800-272-3900
- Elder mistreatment, be aware of warning signs such as bruises and lacerations, fractures, malnutrition, and dehydration. Can also screen using:
  - Brief Abuse Screen for the Elderly (BASE)
  - Elder Assessment Instrument (EAI)
  - Interventions:
    ○ Prevention by supporting caregivers
    ○ Documentation
    ○ Reporting to adult protective or other agency
- Consider referral for palliative care evaluation.
- Consider referral for hospice.

REFERENCES
1. Abraha I, Cruz-Jentoft A, Soiza RL, et al. Evidence of and recommendations for non-pharmacological interventions for common geriatric conditions: the SENATOR-ONTOP systematic review protocol. *BMJ Open*. 2015;5(1):e007488.
2. Watt JA, Goodarzi Z, Veroniki AA, et al. Comparative efficacy of interventions for aggressive and agitated behaviors in dementia: a systematic review and network meta-analysis. *Ann Intern Med*. 2019;171(9):633–642.
3. Dickens AP, Richards SH, Greaves CJ, et al. Interventions targeting social isolation in older people: a systematic review. *BMC Public Health*. 2011;11:647.

 CODES

ICD10
Z71.89 Other specified counseling

CLINICAL PEARLS
- Establish patient goals of care and align all clinical decisions within the context of these goals.
- Use an interdisciplinary team approach to optimize holistic care for elders and their caregivers.

G

GIARDIASIS

Marie L. Borum, MD, EdD, MPH • Adam Jacobs, MD

BASICS

DESCRIPTION
- *Giardia lamblia* (also known as *Giardia duodenalis* or *Giardia intestinalis*) is a protozoan pathogen that leads to intestinal infection and is one of the most common causes of diarrhea worldwide.
- Life cycle consists of cysts and trophozoite stages. Transmission occurs via ingestion of infective cysts, followed by excystation in the duodenum with release of trophozoites, leading to symptoms.
  - Trophozoites pass to the large intestine, where they revert to the infectious cyst form, which are excreted in the stool back into the environment.
- Most infections result from ingestion of unfiltered surface water (e.g., contaminated swimming areas) or fecal-oral transmission; less commonly acquired through contaminated food

EPIDEMIOLOGY
- Age
  - Most commonly children <5 years old and adults aged 25–44 (1)
- Gender
  - More common in males
- Minimal seasonal variability: slight increase in cases reported in summer and early fall
- Highest risk areas include South and South East Asia, North Africa, the Caribbean, and South America (1).

Pediatric Considerations
- Most common in early childhood
- Chronic infection in children can lead to intestinal malabsorption (may also be associated with growth restriction/failure to thrive).

Incidence
- Estimated to cause 280 million diarrheal infections annually (2)
- In 2018, over 15,000 cases were reported in the United States, (~6 cases per 100,000) (3).
- In the United States, Giardiasis affects 1.2 million individuals annually, resulting in 3,584 hospitalizations per year (4).
- Actual rate of Giardiasis infection is likely much higher due to underreporting.

Prevalence
Occurs in about 2% of adults and 6–8% of children in developed countries, while 33% of people in developing countries have had Giardiasis (5).

ETIOLOGY AND PATHOPHYSIOLOGY
Giardia trophozoites colonize the surface of the proximal small intestine.
- Cellular attachment to host enterocytes via the ventral suction disc and the excretion of parasite products results in structural damage compromising intestinal epithelial cells and inhibiting the function of brush border enzymes. This causes electrolyte imbalances and increased intestinal permeability, leading to the production of diarrhea (2).

Genetics
G. lamblia has 8 defined genotypes (referred to as assemblages A–H), but only A and B are known to infect humans (2).

RISK FACTORS
- Daycare centers
- Anal intercourse
- Wilderness camping
- Travel to developing countries
- Children adopted from developing countries
- Drinking untreated water from lakes, streams, or wells
- Swimming in contaminated recreational water (pools, lakes, streams, rivers)
- Pets with *Giardia* infection/diarrhea
- Eating raw produce

GENERAL PREVENTION
- Hand hygiene
- Water purification when camping and when traveling to developing countries. Boiling is most effective.
- Properly cook all foods.
- Protect public water supply from fecal contamination.
- Sanitary disposal of feces
- Barrier protection during anal intercourse

COMMONLY ASSOCIATED CONDITIONS
Hypogammaglobulinemia, common variable immunodeficiency, IgA deficiency, and immunosuppression are associated with prolonged course of the disease and treatment failures.

DIAGNOSIS

HISTORY
- Acute giardiasis
  - 50–75% of infected people are asymptomatic (4).
  - Symptomatic infections occur more frequently in children than adults (4).
  - Symptoms usually appear 1 to 2 weeks after exposure and may last 2 to 4 weeks.
  - Diarrhea (90%)
  - Malaise (86%)
  - Foul-smelling and fatty stools (75%)
  - Flatulence (75%)
  - Abdominal cramps and bloating (71%)
  - Nausea (69%)
  - Weight loss (66%)
  - Vomiting (23%)
  - Fever (15%)
  - Constipation (13%)
  - Urticaria (10%)
- Chronic giardiasis
  - Loose stools
  - Steatorrhea
  - Profound weight loss
  - Malabsorption
  - Stunted growth
  - Malaise
  - Fatigue
  - Depression
  - Abdominal cramping
  - Borborygmi
  - Flatulence
  - Burping

PHYSICAL EXAM
- Vital signs are typically normal.
- Nonspecific; abdominal exam; may have bloating, tenderness, or increased bowel sounds
- Assess for weight loss, signs of dehydration, malabsorption or failure to thrive in children.

DIFFERENTIAL DIAGNOSIS
- Cryptosporidiosis, microsporidiosis, strongyloidiasis, cyclosporiasis, amebiasis, *Dientamoeba fragilis* infection
- Viral gastroenteritis or traveler's diarrhea caused by a range of pathogens, including *Escherichia coli* and *Campylobacter* spp.
- Other causes of malabsorption include lactose intolerance, celiac sprue, tropical sprue, bacterial overgrowth syndromes, and Crohn disease.
- Irritable bowel syndrome (diarrhea without weight loss)

DIAGNOSTIC TESTS & INTERPRETATION
Initial Tests (lab, imaging)
- Light microscopy of stool for ova and parasites:
  - Three serial stool specimens collected every 2 to 3 days; single stool specimen examination has 50–70% sensitivity, while three serial specimens increases sensitivity to >90% (4).
  - Cysts in fixed or fresh stools, and occasionally trophozoites are found in fresh diarrhea stools.
  - Test limitations: labor intensive; experienced operator for interpretation; intermittent shedding means that ova may not be present in stool sample.
- When available, gold standard test for diagnosis are direct fluorescent antibody (DFA) tests, which detect intact organisms with 92–100% sensitivity and 100% specificity. ELISA, which detect soluble antigens in the stools with sensitivity 85–100% and specificity ≥95% (1). These two methods have increased turn-around time compared to stool microscopy (4).
- PCR assays have replaced routine microscopy in some developed countries, showing sensitivity of 98% and specificity of 100% (4).
- Serologic tests for circulating IgG and IgM antibodies to *Giardia* are not appropriate for clinical diagnosis (1).

Follow-Up Tests & Special Considerations
String test (entero-test):
- A gelatin capsule on a string is swallowed and left in the duodenum for several hours or overnight. The string is removed and evaluated for presence of trophozoites by microscopy.

Diagnostic Procedures/Other
Esophagogastroduodenoscopy (EGD) with biopsy and sample of small intestinal fluid

Test Interpretation
Intestinal biopsy shows flattened, mild lymphocytic infiltration and trophozoites on the surface.

TREATMENT

Outpatient for mild cases; inpatient if symptoms are severe enough to cause dehydration warranting parenteral fluid replacement

GENERAL MEASURES
- No treatment required in asymptomatic patients
- Prophylactic therapy indicated for asymptomatic patients in close contact with pregnant or immunocompromised individuals
- Fluid replacement is first line for dehydration.

MEDICATION
First Line
Drugs of choice
- Tinidazole: 2 g PO single dose
- Nitazoxanide: 500 mg PO BID for 3 days

Second Line
Alternative agents
- Metronidazole: 250 mg PO TID for 5 to 7 days
- Albendazole: 400 mg PO daily for 5 days
- Mebendazole 200 mg PO TID for 5 days
- Paromomycin: 10 mg/kg PO TID for 5 to 10 days
- Furazolidone: 100 mg PO QID for 7 to 10 days
- Quinacrine: 100 mg PO TID for 5 days

Precautions
- Consumption of alcohol while on treatment with tinidazole or metronidazole has been associated with a disulfiram-like effect (4).
- Patient with refractory giardiasis who fail monotherapy may warrant combination therapy, high-dose therapy, and/or longer courses of therapy (4).
  - Confirmation of treatment failure is best provided by PCR (1).
  - Treatment failure might be due to host factors or to true drug resistance, which is increasingly common, particularly in travelers returning from South and South East Asia (1).

Pregnancy Considerations
- For patients with mild giardiasis, delay of treatment until second trimester may be reasonable to avoid adverse drug effects to the fetus.
- Medications to treat giardiasis are relatively contraindicated during pregnancy.
- Paromomycin is a nonaminoglycoside recommended in pregnancy due to lower risk of teratogenicity because systemic absorption is low; cure rate, however, is about 60%, which is lower than most other agents (4).

Pediatric Considerations
- For children <12 months of age, metronidazole is the drug of choice.
- For children 12 to 36 months of age, nitazoxanide is preferred.
- For children ≥36 months of age, tinidazole is preferred.

ISSUES FOR REFERRAL
Patients with treatment failure should be discussed with or referred to a specialist, who should exclude underlying problems such as celiac disease, inherited disaccharidase deficiency, and immunodeficiency disorders, particularly of total and IgA antibody production (1).

ADDITIONAL THERAPIES
Fluids to prevent dehydration

COMPLEMENTARY & ALTERNATIVE MEDICINE
Zinc and vitamin A have been associated with protective effect against giardiasis among children (6).

 ## ONGOING CARE

FOLLOW-UP RECOMMENDATIONS
Patient Monitoring
Monitor symptoms, weight, and stool exams, particularly if patients fail to improve.

DIET
Low lactose/lactose free for at least 1 month; low-fat diet generally helpful

PATIENT EDUCATION
- Hand washing is more important than water purification to prevent transmission in outdoor enthusiasts.
- Lactose intolerance may follow Giardia infection and cause persistent diarrhea posttreatment. Recommend patients adhere to a low-lactose/lactose-free diet to mitigate symptoms.
- CDC facts about Giardia and swimming pools: http://www.cdc.gov/healthywater/pdf/swimming /resources/giardia-factsheet.pdf
  - Don't swim if you have diarrhea.
  - Wash hands with soap after changing diapers before returning to the pool.
  - Do not ingest pool, lake, or river water.
  - Use chlorine to kill Giardia in water used for recreational activities.

PROGNOSIS
- Generally, prognosis is excellent; most patients are asymptomatic.
- Majority of infections resolve within a few weeks; occasionally may last for months and persist as chronic infections; patients with underlying immunodeficiency may experience more severe and prolonged illness.
- Mortality is rare, except in those cases of extreme dehydration that are untreated or inadequately treated, which occurs mainly in infants or malnourished children (4).

COMPLICATIONS
Malabsorption, impaired growth development, hypersensitivity reactions, weight loss, postinfectious IBS, and lactose intolerance. More rarely cholecystitis, cholangitis, granulomatous hepatitis, impaired exocrine pancreatic function

ALERT
Reportable disease to the CDC

REFERENCES

1. Minetti C, Chalmers RM, Beeching NJ, et al. Giardiasis. *BMJ*. 2016;355:i5369.
2. Einarsson E, Ma'ayeh S, Svärd SG. An up-date on *Giardia* and giardiasis. *Curr Opin Microbiol*. 2016;34:47–52.
3. Centers for Disease Control and Prevention. *Giardiasis Summary Report—National Notifiable Disease Surveillance System, United States, 2018*. Atlanta, GA: Centers for Disease Control and Prevention; 2019.
4. Leung AKC, Leung AAM, Wong AHC, et al. Giardiasis: an overview. *Recent Pat Inflamm Allergy Drug Discov*. 2019;13(2):134–143.
5. Kappus KD, Lundgren RG Jr, Juranek DD, et al. Intestinal parasitism in the United States: update on a continuing problem. *Am J Trop Med Hyg*. 1994;50(6):705–713.
6. Rogawski ET, Bartelt LA, Platts-Mills JA, et al. Determinants and impact of *Giardia* infection in the first 2 years of life in the MAL-ED birth cohort. *J Pediatric Infect Dis Soc*. 2017;6(2):153–160.

ADDITIONAL READING
- Fink MY, Singer SM. The intersection of immune responses, microbiota, and pathogenesis in Giardiasis. *Trends Parasitol*. 2017;33(11):901–913.
- Heymann D. *Control of Communicable Diseases Manual, 20th ed*. Washington, DC: American Public Health Association; 2015.
- Leung AKC, Leung AAM, Wong AHC, et al. Giardiasis: an overview. *Recent Pat Inflamm Allergy Drug Discov*. 2019;13(2):134–143.

 ## SEE ALSO

Algorithm: Diarrhea, Chronic

 ## CODES

ICD10
A07.1 Giardiasis [lambliasis]

CLINICAL PEARLS
- Daycare facilities and public swimming pools are common sources of *Giardia* transmission (a history of camping or recent travel is not required for the diagnosis).
- Abdominal bloating and loose, foul-smelling stool are common presenting symptoms.
- First-line treatment is tinidazole and nitazoxanide. Metronidazole is also highly effective (but is often poorly tolerated).
- Most treatment failures may warrant combination therapy, high-dose therapy, and/or longer courses of therapy (with same or other medication).
- Direct fluorescent antibody testing is the gold standard for diagnosis, while ELISA and PCR are also commonly used, replacing stool microscopy testing.

G

GILBERT SYNDROME
Alethea Y. Turner, DO, FAAFP

 BASICS

DESCRIPTION
A benign, inherited syndrome in which mild, intermittent unconjugated hyperbilirubinemia occurs in the absence of hemolysis or liver dysfunction

Pediatric Considerations
Rare for the disorder to be diagnosed before puberty

Pregnancy Considerations
The relative fasting that may occur with morning sickness can elevate bilirubin level.

EPIDEMIOLOGY
- Predominant age: present from birth but most often presents in the 2nd or 3rd decade of life
- Predominant sex: male > female (2 to 7:1)

Prevalence
Prevalence in the United States: ~8% of the population; ~1 in 3 of those affected are not aware that they have the disorder.

ETIOLOGY AND PATHOPHYSIOLOGY
Indirect hyperbilirubinemia in Gilbert syndrome (GS) results from impaired hepatic bilirubin clearance (~30% of normal) due to decreased levels of the enzyme uridine diphosphoglucuronate-glucuronosyltransferase (UDPGT). Hepatic bilirubin conjugation (glucuronidation) is thus reduced, although this may not be the only defect.

Genetics
- Inherited defects within the promoter region of the gene that encodes the enzyme UDPGT yields reduced conjugation of bilirubin with glucuronic acid.
- Once considered as an autosomal dominant condition, GS is now thought to be inherited in an autosomal recessive manner.

RISK FACTORS
- Male gender
- Family history; particularly first-degree relatives

COMMONLY ASSOCIATED CONDITIONS
GS is part of a spectrum of hereditary disorders that includes types I and II Crigler-Najjar syndrome (1). However, bilirubin levels in these cases will be >6 mg/dL.

 DIAGNOSIS

HISTORY
- In patients with GS, a nonpruritic jaundice can occur in the setting of stressors like fasting, dehydration, infection, lack of sleep, physical exertion, or surgery. Other symptoms that may present during an episode of jaundice, including fatigue, are caused by the triggering factor and are not directly a result of GS.
- Some medications may also trigger episodes of jaundice in patients with GS due to abnormal metabolism. These include drugs that inhibit glucuronyl transferase (i.e., gemfibrozil) as well as selective protease inhibitors (i.e., atazanavir and indinavir) (2). There is some evidence that tocilizumab (3), a monoclonal antibody used to treat rheumatoid arthritis, and ribavirin, an antiviral for hepatitis C treatment, may also induce jaundice (4). Note, the aforementioned drugs have not been associated with causing liver toxicity in patients with GS.

PHYSICAL EXAM
Occasional mild jaundice precipitated by the aforementioned triggers (fasting, dehydration, infection, lack of sleep, physical exertion, surgery, and some medications). Exam should be devoid of the stigmata of chronic liver disease.

DIFFERENTIAL DIAGNOSIS
- Hemolysis
- Ineffective erythropoiesis (megaloblastic anemias, certain porphyrias, thalassemia major, sideroblastic anemia, severe lead poisoning, congenital dyserythropoietic anemias)
- Cirrhosis
- Chronic persistent hepatitis
- Pancreatitis
- Biliary tract disease

DIAGNOSTIC TESTS & INTERPRETATION
Initial Tests (lab, imaging)
- Bilirubin: elevated but <6 mg/dL (103 μmol/L) and usually <3 mg/dL (51 μmol/L) (1)[C], virtually all unconjugated (indirect), with conjugated bilirubin within the normal range and/or <20% of the total bilirubin (2)

- CBC with peripheral smear is normal.
- Reticulocyte count, haptoglobin, and lactate dehydrogenase levels are normal.
- Liver function tests (LFTs) (aspartate aminotransferase [AST], alanine transaminase [ALT], alkaline phosphatase, and γ-glutamyl transpeptidase [GGT]) are normal.
- Direct Coombs test is normal.
- Up to 60% of patients with GS have a clinically insignificant mild hemolysis that frequently can only be detected with sophisticated red cell survival studies (1).
- Drugs that may alter lab results: Bilirubin level may be raised by nicotinic acid and some other medications and lowered by phenobarbital (1).
- Disorders that may alter lab results: Bilirubin levels increase during fasting and may increase during a febrile illness.

Follow-Up Tests & Special Considerations
GS should be suspected if unconjugated hyperbilirubinemia persists in the absence of hemolysis or other liver dysfunction. A definitive diagnosis may be reported after 3 to 12 months of follow-up if the exam and diagnostic workup is otherwise normal.

Diagnostic Procedures/Other
Confirmatory testing is often unnecessary.
- A 48-hour fast is impractical and nonspecific for GS (2).
- Provocation testing with rifampin (5)[C] could be employed if there is significant diagnostic doubt:
  - After 12 hours of fasting, an increase of total bilirubin to >1.9 mg/dL 2 hours after an oral dose of rifampin 900 mg distinguishes patients with GS with a sensitivity of 100% and a specificity of 100% (5).
- Genetic testing is available in the form of polymerase chain reaction (PCR) or DNA-fragment sequencing for DNA mutations in the *UGT1A1* gene.

ALERT
A liver biopsy is not usually needed to exclude other diagnoses, unless concomitant liver disease is present.

TREATMENT

- Outpatient
- Avoid unnecessary testing and procedures.
- Specific treatment is not necessary (1)[C].

 ONGOING CARE

FOLLOW-UP RECOMMENDATIONS
Patient Monitoring
Once GS has been confidently diagnosed, no further monitoring is required.

PATIENT EDUCATION
- Reassure patients that GS is benign.
- Educate patients on common triggers for jaundice.
- Recommend patients to inform medical providers of their diagnosis.
- Instruct patients to seek medical help if severe or prolonged jaundice occurs because these may be signs of a separate disease process.

PROGNOSIS
- GS is benign with an excellent prognosis.
- Patients with GS are able to serve as donors for right lobe of liver for transplantation (6)[B].
- Preliminary evidence suggests that patients with GS may have protective properties against cardiovascular disease, type 2 diabetes mellitus, some cancers such as Hodgkin lymphoma, and all-cause mortality (7).

COMPLICATIONS
There are no known complications from GS.

ALERT
- Caution before using irinotecan in patients with GS. Once metabolized, this colorectal cancer treatment affects the enzyme responsible for GS, significantly increasing risk of toxicity (7).
- The impact of UGT1A1 mutations on the metabolism of chemotherapy agents should be taken into consideration in patients with known or suspected GS; however, there are no current recommendations on specific dose adjustments to minimize risk of toxicity.

REFERENCES
1. Watson KJ, Gollan JL. Gilbert's syndrome. *Baillieres Clin Gastroenterol*. 1989;3(2):337–355.
2. Claridge LC, Armstrong MJ, Booth C, et al. Gilbert's syndrome. *BMJ*. 2011;342:d2293.
3. Lee JS, Wang J, Martin M, et al. Genetic variation in UGT1A1 typical of Gilbert syndrome is associated with unconjugated hyperbilirubinemia in patients receiving tocilizumab. *Pharmacogenet Genomics*. 2011;21(7):365–374.
4. Deterding K, Grüngreiff K, Lankisch TO, et al. Gilbert's syndrome and antiviral therapy of hepatitis C. *Ann Hepatol*. 2009;8(3):246–250.
5. Murthy GD, Byron D, Shoemaker D, et al. The utility of rifampin in diagnosing Gilbert's syndrome. *Am J Gastroenterol*. 2001;96(4):1150–1154.
6. Demirbas T, Piskin T, Dayangac M, et al. Right-lobe liver transplant from donors with Gilbert syndrome. *Exp Clin Transplant*. 2012;10(1):39–42.
7. Ha VH, Jupp J, Tsang RY. Oncology drug dosing in Gilbert syndrome associated with UGT1A1: a summary of the literature. *Pharmacotherapy*. 2017;37(8):956–972.

CODES

ICD10
- E80.4 Gilbert syndrome
- E80.6 Other disorders of bilirubin metabolism

CLINICAL PEARLS

- GS is a benign, inherited syndrome, in which mild, intermittent unconjugated hyperbilirubinemia causing jaundice occurs with otherwise normal liver function.
- Reduced hepatic bilirubin conjugation (glucuronidation) occurs due to altered *UDPGT1A1* gene promotion.
- GS is diagnosed when a mild, persistent or recurrent elevation in unconjugated hyperbilirubinemia persists in the absence of hemolysis or other liver dysfunction.
- Confirmatory tests are not frequently needed, and a liver biopsy is not recommended, unless there is serious concern for concomitant liver disease.
- Patient education and reassurance is essential, and unnecessary testing and procedures should be avoided.

G

GINGIVITIS

Karlynn Sievers, MD • Sheila O. Stille, DMD, MAGD

 BASICS

DESCRIPTION
Gingivitis is a reversible form of inflammation of the gingiva. It is a mild form of periodontal disease. Classification includes the following:
- Plaque induced
- Not plaque induced (bacterial, viral, or fungal; e.g., necrotizing ulcerative gingivitis, Vincent disease ["trench mouth"], denture related)
- Modified by systemic factors (e.g., pregnancy, puberty, HIV, diabetes, smoking, leukemia)
- Modified by medications (calcium channel blockers, antipsychotics, antiepileptics, antirejection medications, hormones)
- Modified by malnutrition (vitamin deficiencies)
- Acute or chronic
- System(s) affected: gastrointestinal; ears, nose, throat; dental
- Synonym(s): mild periodontal disease; gum disease

Geriatric Considerations
More frequent in this age group

Pediatric Considerations
Cases of plaque-induced gingivitis are common in children (most common form of pediatric periodontal disease) and usually require no specific interventions other than improved oral hygiene.

Pregnancy Considerations
- Very common in pregnant women; hormonal effect
- Self-limited

EPIDEMIOLOGY
- Predominant age: children, teenagers, and young adults
- 42% of adults in United States have periodontal diseases (1).

ETIOLOGY AND PATHOPHYSIOLOGY
Inflammation of the marginal gingiva. This can progress to deeper, destructive inflammation; if involving supporting bone, classified as periodontitis, not gingivitis (2)
- Inadequate plaque removal
- Medication induced (e.g., oral contraceptives, antiepileptics)
- Nutritional deficiencies
- Vasoconstriction (nicotine, methamphetamine)
- Endocrine/hormonal variations
  - Pregnancy, menses, menarche
- Chronic debilitating disease
- Vincent disease, necrotizing ulcerative gingivitis
  - Synergistic infection with fusiform bacillus (*Fusobacterium* spp.) and spirochete (*Borrelia vincentii*)
- Pathology
  - Acute or chronic inflammation
  - Hyperemic capillaries

- Polymorphonuclear infiltration
- Papillary projections in subepithelial tissue
- Fibroblasts

Genetics
Possible genetic link (up to 30% of population); rare condition called hereditary gingival fibromatosis, where severe gingival hyperplasia covers teeth, associated with hirsutism

RISK FACTORS
- Poor dental hygiene/plaque formation
- Pregnancy
- Uncontrolled diabetes mellitus
- Malocclusion, dental crowding, faulty dental restorations
- Smoking
- Mouth breathing
- Xerostomia
- HIV positive; AIDS
- Vitamin C deficiency; coenzyme Q10 deficiency
- Dental appliances (dentures, braces)
- Necrotizing ulcerative gingivitis
  - Stress
  - Lack of sleep
  - Malnutrition
  - Viral illness
  - Typically teens and young adults
- Bronchial asthma and other respiratory diseases
- Rheumatoid arthritis
- Epilepsy

GENERAL PREVENTION
- Good oral hygiene
  - Adults
    - Regular twice-daily brushing with fluoride toothpaste
    - Powered toothbrushes, especially the oscillating-rotating type, improve gingivitis (2),(3).
    - Daily "high-quality" flossing (studies show that flossing only helps when it is done correctly), water jets, and interdental brushes (2),(3)
    - Chlorhexidine with oral hygiene better than other oral rinse agents (2)
      - Use in acute phase (2).
  - Pediatrics
    - Regular twice-daily brushing with fluoride toothpaste under parental supervision until full manual dexterity (~8 years of age)
    - Regular flossing if no spaces between teeth
- Cleaning by a dentist or hygienist every 6 months or more frequently, as indicated (2)
- Mouth rinse with essential oils (menthol, thymol, eucalyptol; e.g., Listerine) combined with brushing (2),(3)

COMMONLY ASSOCIATED CONDITIONS
- Periodontitis
- Glossitis
- Pedunculated growths (pyogenic granulomata)

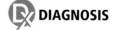 **DIAGNOSIS**

HISTORY
- Gingival erythema, edema, and bleeding
- Gingiva is tender to touch but otherwise painless.
- Bleeding of gingiva when brushing, flossing, or eating
- Inquire about HIV risk, pregnancy, nutritional deficiencies, diabetes, and other risk factors as indicated (see "Risk Factors").
- Smoking history
- Poor oral hygiene, infrequent dental visit history

PHYSICAL EXAM
- Normal gums should appear pink, firm, stippled, and scalloped.
- Gingivitis—marginal gingiva edematous with blunted papilla (usually painless, except to touch)
- Gingiva erythema: bright red or red-purple appearance
- Bleeding with manipulation of gingiva
- Biofilm of plaque (soft) and calculus (calcified, not easily removed)
- Edema of interdental papillae
- HIV gingivitis
  - Also called linear gingival erythema
  - Narrow band of bright red inflamed gum surrounding neck of tooth
  - Painful
  - Bleeds easily
  - Rapid destruction of gingival tissue and can progress to periodontitis with destruction of underlying support tissues (periodontal ligament, supporting alveolar bone)
- Vincent disease/necrotizing ulcerative gingivitis
  - Ulcers
  - Fever
  - Malaise
  - Regional lymphadenopathy
  - Pain
  - Mouth odor

DIFFERENTIAL DIAGNOSIS
- Periodontitis (deeper inflammation, causing destruction to connective tissue, ligaments, and alveolar bone)
- Glossitis
- Desquamative gingivitis (painful, persistent, usually middle-aged women)
- Pericoronitis (gum flap traps food and plaque over partially erupted 3rd molar), common in adolescence
- Gingival ulcers (aphthous, herpetic, malignancy, TB, syphilis)
- Specific forms of gingivitis: See "Description," including acute necrotizing ulcerative gingivitis (Vincent disease) and HIV gingivitis (linear gingival erythema), adrenal crisis, leukemia.

DIAGNOSTIC TESTS & INTERPRETATION
Initial Tests (lab, imaging)
- No tests usually needed
- Possible smear or culture to identify causative agent (HIV gingivitis includes gram-negative anaerobes, enteric strains, and yeast—*Candida*.)
- Labs for contributing conditions (HIV, pregnancy, diabetes, nutritional deficiencies)
- Increase in C-reactive protein

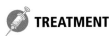 TREATMENT

GENERAL MEASURES
- Stop any contributing medications.
- Remove irritating factors (plaque, calculus, faulty dental restorations, or partial dentures).
- Good oral hygiene (see "General Prevention")
- Regular dental checkups (for scaling and polishing if plaque and/or tartar are present)
- Smoking cessation
- Special needs patients: use of tray-applied 10% carbamide peroxide gels

MEDICATION
First Line
- Chlorhexidine rinses or varnishes may be used. (Note: Prolonged use of chlorhexidine can lead to blackening of the tongue and taste alterations/metallic (4),(5)[B].)
- Essential oil mouthwash (EOMW) may be equally effective to chlorhexidine for reduction of gingival inflammation (2)[A],(3),(4).
- Antibiotics indicated *only* for acute necrotizing ulcerative gingivitis (Vincent disease):
  - Penicillin V: pediatric dose, 25 to 50 mg/kg/day divided q6h; adult dose, 250 to 500 mg q6h, *OR*
  - Metronidazole: pediatric dose, 30 mg/kg/day PO/IV divided q6h; maximum 4 g/day; adult dose, 500 mg BID or TID for 10 days *OR*
  - Amoxicillin/clavulanic acid: pediatric dose, 30 mg/kg/day PO divided q12h; information: use 125 mg/31.25 mg/5 mL suspension; adult dose, 875 mg/125 mg PO BID for 10 days
  - Erythromycin: pediatric dose, 30 to 40 mg/kg/day divided q6h; adult dose, 250 mg q6h
  - Clindamycin: penicillin allergy; pediatric dose, 8 to 20 mg/kg/day in 3 to 4 divided doses as hydrochloride; adults, 300 mg q6h (maximum 1.8 g/day)
  - Doxycycline: adult dose, 100 mg BID 1st day and then QD for 10 days
- Topical corticosteroids
  - Triamcinolone 0.1% in Orabase (spray or ointment), applied locally TID, QID
- Precautions
  - Erythromycin frequently causes GI issues.

Second Line
- Acetaminophen or ibuprofen for pain
- Other antibiotics or antifungal rinses or systemic according to culture or smear
- Decapinol oral rinse (surfactant that acts as a physical barrier, making it harder for bacteria to stick to the polysaccharide pellicle on tooth and mucosal surfaces) to reduce bacteria (not recommended for pregnant women or children <12 years); should be used in conjunction with traditional oral hygiene practices when those practices alone are not enough

ISSUES FOR REFERRAL
- Dental referral for acute gingivitis and routine cleanings and further treatment, as needed
- If gingivitis becomes periodontitis, deep root scaling, root planing, and antibiotics may be indicated.

SURGERY/OTHER PROCEDURES
- Débridement for acute necrotizing gingivitis
- Minor surgery may be necessary to correct tissue overgrowth for gingivitis caused by medicines/hereditary gingival fibromatosis.

COMPLEMENTARY & ALTERNATIVE MEDICINE
- Bilberry: potentially helpful in reducing inflammation and stabilizing collagen tissue
- Coenzyme Q10: topically, to restore coenzyme Q10 deficiency
- Replace any nutritional deficiencies (e.g., vitamins A, B_{12}, C).

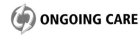 ONGOING CARE

FOLLOW-UP RECOMMENDATIONS
Patient Monitoring
Until clear; dental follow-up for continued cleanings and secondary prevention

DIET
- Well-balanced diet that includes fruits, vegetables, vitamin C
- Avoid sugary snacks and drinks, which contribute to plaque formation.
- Soft foods during flare, if significant inflammation/bleeding

PATIENT EDUCATION
- Good oral hygiene, including twice-daily brushing with circular oscillating electric brush, fluoridated toothpaste, and daily flossing; regular dental visits
- Printable and viewable patient information available from the American Dental Association at http://www.mouthhealthy.org/en.org/en/; American Academy of Periodontology under "Patient Resources" at http://www.perio.org/; and NIDCR at http://www.nidcr.nih.gov/oralhealth/Topics/GumDiseases/PeriodontalGumDisease.htm

PROGNOSIS
- Usual course: acute, relapsing, intermittent; chronic
- Prognosis: generally favorable, responds well to appropriate treatment
- Left untreated, may progress to periodontitis (controversial), which is a major cause of tooth loss

COMPLICATIONS
Severe periodontal disease (which is associated with supporting bone loss, tooth loss, heart disease, diabetes, dementia, and preterm birth)

REFERENCES
1. Eke PI, Thornton-Evans GO, Wei L, et al. Periodontitis in US adults: National Health and Nutrition Examination Survey 2009–2014. *J Am Dent Assoc*. 2018;149(7):576–588.e6.
2. Chapple IL, Van der Weijden F, Doerfer C, et al. Primary prevention of periodontitis: managing gingivitis. *J Clin Periodontol*. 2015;42(Suppl 16):S71–S76.
3. Kumar S. Evidence-based update on diagnosis and management of gingivitis and periodontitis. *Dent Clin N Am*. 2019;63(1):69–81.
4. Figuero E, Roldán S, Serrano J, et al. Efficacy of adjunctive therapies in patients with gingival inflammation: a systematic review and meta-analysis. *J Clin Periodontol*. 2020;47(Suppl 22):125–143.
5. James P, Worthington HV, Parnell C, et al. Chlorhexidine mouthrinse as an adjunctive treatment for gingival health. *Cochrane Database Syst Rev*. 2017;(3):CD008676.
6. Aarabi G, Heydecke G, Seedorf U. Roles of oral infections in the pathomechanism of atherosclerosis. *Int J Mol Sci*. 2018;19(7):1978.

 SEE ALSO

- Dental Infection; Glossitis
- Algorithm: Bleeding Gums

 CODES

ICD10
- K05.10 Chronic gingivitis, plaque induced
- K05.11 Chronic gingivitis, non-plaque induced
- K05.00 Acute gingivitis, plaque induced

CLINICAL PEARLS
- Gingivitis may be prevented and treated with regular dental cleanings, good oral hygiene, and use of certain mouth rinses including chlorhexidine.
- Untreated, gingivitis may progress to periodontitis, a possible contributor to systemic inflammation and its consequences (e.g., coronary artery disease and uncontrolled diabetes) (6).
- New-onset or difficult-to-treat gingivitis, consider differential of etiology: pregnancy, HIV, diabetes, medications, and vitamin deficiencies.

G

GLAUCOMA, PRIMARY CLOSED-ANGLE
Richard W. Allinson, MD • Alyce D. Alven, OD, MS

BASICS

DESCRIPTION

- Glaucoma is a progressive decline in vision from damage to the optic nerve and is usually associated with elevated intraocular pressure (IOP) in the eye. Angle-closure is a mechanical blockage of the trabecular meshwork (TM) by the peripheral iris.
- In primary angle-closure (PAC), there is an anatomic predisposition with no identifiable secondary pathologic condition.
- In secondary angle-closure, there is an identifiable pathologic cause, such as iris neovascularization or an enlarged cataractous lens.
- Angle-closure can be classified as the following:
  - Primary angle-closure suspect (PACS) is >180 degrees of iridotrabecular contact (ITC) but no evidence of TM or optic nerve damage.
  - PAC is >180 degrees of ITC with peripheral anterior synechiae (PAS) or elevated IOP but with no optic neuropathy.
  - Primary angle-closure glaucoma (PACG) is PAC with glaucomatous optic neuropathy.
  - Acute primary angle-closure (APAC) or acute angle-closure crisis (AACC) is when the angle is occluded with symptomatic high IOP. It is a medical emergency requiring prompt treatment.
  - Chronic angle-closure (CAC) may develop after APAC in which synechial closure persists. It can also develop when the angle gradually closes and the angle function becomes progressively compromised leading to a slow rise in IOP. Vision loss may be the presenting complaint because of the asymptomatic nature of the condition.

Geriatric Considerations
Increased risk with age and cataracts

Pregnancy Considerations
Medications used may cross the placenta and be excreted into breast milk. Majority of IOP-lowering medications are within class C, and the risk of adverse effects to the fetus must be balanced with risk of vision loss in the mother.

EPIDEMIOLOGY
- Older age
- Female sex. PAC is 2 to 4 times more common in women than in men. Women tend to have smaller anterior segments and shorter axial lengths.
- More likely in those of Inuit and East or South Asian descent

Prevalence
The prevalence of PACG in patients >40 years varies depending on race and ethnicity. The prevalence is 0.1%–0.2% in blacks, 0.1%–0.6% in whites, 0.3% in the Japanese, 0.4%–1.4% in other East Asians, 2.1%–5.0% in the Inuit. The burden of PACG is greater in Asian countries.

ETIOLOGY AND PATHOPHYSIOLOGY
- PAC happens when iris touches the TM in the anterior chamber angle. ITC causes obstruction of aqueous humor outflow through the TM, which causes elevation in IOP. Prolonged ITC can cause scarring, with formation of PAS.

- Most common underlying mechanism of angle-closure is pupillary blockage of the aqueous flow from posterior to anterior chamber. This causes increase in pressure in the posterior chamber as compared to the anterior chamber. The buildup of pressure in the posterior chamber leads to anterior bowing of the iris and closing of the angle.
  - One of the most important factors in closing the angle in an anatomically predisposed eye is dilation of the pupil. Dilation leading to closure of the angle may occur as a result of a variety of causes including darkness, emotion, and medications that can cause the pupil to dilate. Pupillary block is maximal when the pupil is in the mid-dilated position.
- Plateau iris syndrome is an atypical configuration of the anterior chamber angle that can result in acute or chronic PAC. Angle-closure in plateau iris is most often caused by anteriorly positioned ciliary processes that narrow the anterior chamber recess by pushing the peripheral iris forward. A component of pupillary block is often present.

Genetics
First-degree relatives have a 1–12% increased risk in whites; 6 times greater risk in Chinese patients with positive family history

RISK FACTORS
- Age >50 years
- Female gender
- Asian or Inuit descent
- Family history of angle-closure
- Shallow anterior chamber
- Hyperopia
- Short axial length
- Thick crystalline lens
- Anterior positioned lens
- Plateau iris
- Drugs that can induce angle-closure by dilating the pupil include:
  - Adrenergic agonists (albuterol, phenylephrine), anticholinergics (oxybutynin, atropine), antihistamines, antidepressants including selective serotonin reuptake inhibitors (SSRIs) and tricyclic antidepressants (TCAs), and cocaine
- Drugs that can induce angle-closure by causing a uveal effusion include:
  - Topiramate and other sulfonamides

GENERAL PREVENTION
- Routine eye exam with gonioscopy for high-risk populations
- Prophylactic laser peripheral iridotomy (LPI) may be considered in PACS patients for preventing PACG.
- Argon laser peripheral iridoplasty for plateau iris syndrome

COMMONLY ASSOCIATED CONDITIONS
- Cataract
- Hyperopia

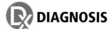

DIAGNOSIS

HISTORY
- Patient may be asymptomatic as in PACS or may have acute symptoms as in APAC.
- Acute symptoms commonly include unilateral:
  - Severe eye pain
  - Blurred vision
  - Eye redness
  - Halos around lights/objects
  - Headache
  - Nausea and vomiting
- Patients with PACG can be asymptomatic, have subacute symptoms (intermittent subacute attacks), or compromised peripheral vision.
- Family history of acute angle-closure glaucoma
- Obtain history of prescription, over-the-counter, and herbal medications.

PHYSICAL EXAM
Includes, but is not limited to, the following in the undilated eye:
- Visual acuity with refractive error (hyperopic eyes especially in older phakic patients)
- Visual field testing
- Pupil size and reactivity (mid-dilated, asymmetric or oval, minimally reactive, and may have relative afferent pupillary defect)
- Slit-lamp examination demonstrates conjunctival hyperemia (in acute cases), central and peripheral anterior chamber shallowing, corneal edema, iris abnormalities (diffuse and focal iris atrophy, posterior synechiae), lens changes (cataract and glaukomflecken-patchy localized anterior subcapsular lens opacities).
- IOP elevation. During an acute attack, the IOP may be high enough to cause glaucomatous optic nerve damage, ischemic nerve damage, and/or retinal vascular occlusion.
- The Van Herick assessment (VHA) is a noncontact estimate of the angle configuration based on comparison of peripheral anterior chamber depth to peripheral corneal thickness using a thin slit lamp beam of light. Even when performed by experienced ophthalmologists, VHA misses a substantial proportion of angle-closure.
- Gonioscopy allows visualization of anatomy of the angle of both eyes. Look for ITC and PAS.
- Anterior segment imaging with ultrasound (US) biomicroscopy and anterior segment optical coherence tomography (AS-OCT) to understand the angle anatomy

DIFFERENTIAL DIAGNOSIS
- Secondary angle closure due to iris membranes:
  - Neovascularization of the iris
  - Iridocorneal endothelial (ICE) syndrome
- Secondary pupillary block due to the following:
  - Uveitis with secondary posterior synechiae leading to iris bombe
  - Lens-related disorders, such as ectopia lentis or malpositioned intraocular lenses
- Retinal conditions leading to the forward shift of the lens-iris diaphragm (uveal effusion, hemorrhagic choroidal detachment, intraocular tumors)

- Topiramate is an oral medication prescribed for the treatment of epilepsy, depression, and headaches. In some patients, this medication may cause a syndrome characterized by acute myopic shift and acute bilateral angle closure. Treatment involves immediate discontinuation of the medication and initiation of medical therapy to lower the IOP. Cycloplegia may deepen the anterior chamber and relieve the attack. Because pupillary block is not an underlying mechanism of this syndrome, an LPI is not indicated.
- Malignant glaucoma (also called aqueous misdirection) is a rare form of glaucoma that usually presents following ocular surgery. Miotics can make malignant glaucoma worse and should not be used; instead, use cycloplegics.

DIAGNOSTIC TESTS & INTERPRETATION
Initial Tests (lab, imaging)
- Gonioscopy
- US biomicroscopy
- AS-OCT

Test Interpretation
Narrow or closed anterior chamber angle

 ## TREATMENT

ALERT
For patients with acute symptoms (severe eye pain, blurred vision, eye redness, halos around lights/objects, headache, nausea and vomiting) and asymmetric pupillary response, obtain immediate consultation with ophthalmology.

GENERAL MEASURES
Goals of treatment are to reverse or prevent angle-closure process, control IOP, and prevent damage to the optic nerve.

MEDICATION
- During acute attack, medical therapy lowers IOP to relieve symptoms and clear corneal edema so that LPI can be performed as soon as possible.
- Medical therapy aims at:
  - Reduction of aqueous production:
    - Carbonic anhydrase inhibitors (CAIs): acetazolamide 250 to 500 mg IV or 250 mg tab × 2 PO at once. Topical CAI such as dorzolamide 2%. CAIs are contraindicated in sulfa allergy and hepatic insufficiency.
    - Topical β-blockers such as timolol 0.5%. Use with caution in patients with lung disease.
    - Topical α_2-agonists such as brimonidine 0.2%
  - Prostaglandin analogues such as latanoprost 0.005% enhance uveoscleral outflow and increase aqueous outflow.
  - Pupillary constriction to open the chamber angle: topical pilocarpine 1% or 2% q15min × 3. Miotic therapy may be ineffective when IOP is markedly elevated due to iris sphincter ischemia.
  - Topical steroid such as prednisolone acetate 1% q15–30min × 4 and then hourly to treat the inflammation
  - Hyperosmotic agents which reduce the vitreous volume, which in turn reduces IOP:
    - Glycerin 50% solution administered orally, dosage is 1.0 to 1.5 g/kg. Use with caution if patient has nausea or emesis. To improve the taste, the solution may be mixed with a small amount of orange juice and poured over crushed ice.

- Mannitol 20% solution, administered IV at 1.5 to 2.0 g/kg of body weight over 30 minutes to 60 minutes
  - Hyperosmotic agent should be used with caution in patients with heart and kidney disease. Glycerin can increase blood sugar level and should not be given to diabetic patients.
- During acute attack, acetazolamide 500 mg IV is given followed by 500 mg PO BID. Topical therapy is initiated with 0.5% timolol maleate and 0.2% brimonidine drops 1 minute apart. Reduction of inflammation is accomplished with frequent topical steroids. In addition, systemic therapy with mannitol 20% 1.5 to 2.0 g/kg infused over 30 to 60 minutes or oral glycerol (Osmoglyn) (50%) 6 oz PO may be needed. Treat pain and nausea with analgesic and antiemetics. Initiate treatment with 3 doses of 1% or 2% pilocarpine drops administered 15 minutes apart to cause miosis in an attempt to open the angle.

SURGERY/OTHER PROCEDURES
- Definitive therapy for PAC, PACG, and AACC is Nd:YAG or argon LPI. LPI can be performed temporally or superiorly. Location of the LPI, does not seem to influence the occurrence of new postoperative dysphotopsias.
- Surgical iridectomy may be performed if cornea is cloudy and laser iridotomy cannot be performed.
- Plateau iris syndrome may be initially treated by either LPI or lensectomy if a cataract is present. Eyes with plateau iris syndrome remain predisposed to angle closure despite a patent iridotomy or lensectomy.
  - Argon laser peripheral iridoplasty may be needed to flatten and thin the peripheral iris.
- Growing evidence shows cataract extraction alone can lower IOP and reduce the risk of lens-induced angle closure. This can be considered as a treatment option in appropriate cases. Other procedures to reduce IOP include argon laser peripheral iridoplasty (especially for plateau iris syndrome), anterior chamber paracentesis, goniosynechialysis, and trabeculectomy.
  - APAC patients who underwent phacoemulsification with an intraocular lens (IOL) had better IOP control, deeper anterior chambers and required less glaucoma medications than those who underwent LPI alone. Performing phacoemulsification weeks to months after the initial LPI did not appear to adversely affect outcomes compared to early phacoemulsification (1)[B].
  - Clear lens extraction (CLE) can be considered for first-line treatment of eyes with more advanced angle-closure disease, such as APAC eyes with an IOP >30 mmHg (2)[C].

 ## ONGOING CARE

FOLLOW-UP RECOMMENDATIONS
Patient Monitoring
Half of the other eye of patients with APAC will develop APAC within 5 years. Hence, prophylactic LPI should be performed in the other eye as soon as possible.

PATIENT EDUCATION
- Advise patient to seek emergency attention if experiencing a change in visual acuity, blurred vision, eye pain, or headache.
- PACS patients and no LPI; avoid use of decongestants, motion sickness medications, adrenergic agents, antipsychotics, antidepressants, and anticholinergic agents.

PROGNOSIS
- Prognosis depends on ethnicity, underlying eye disease, and time to treatment.
- After LPI, most PACS subjects can be expected to have no further treatment.
- Many PAC and APAC eyes and most PACG eyes are given additional treatment to control IOP after LPI.

COMPLICATIONS
- Chronic angle closure
- Iris atrophy; cataract; optic atrophy
- Malignant glaucoma
- Central retinal artery/vein occlusion
- Permanent decrease in visual acuity; blindness
- Fellow (contralateral) eye attack

REFERENCES
1. Lin Y-H, Wu C-H, Huang S-M, et al. Early versus delayed phacoemulsification and intraocular lens implantation for acute primary angle-closure. J Ophthalmol. 2020;2020:8319570.
2. Tanner L, Gazzard G, Nolan WP, et al. Has the EAGLE landed for the use of clear lens extraction in angle-closure glaucoma? And how should primary angle-closure suspects be treated? Eye (Lond). 2020;34(1):40–50.

ADDITIONAL READING
Radhakrishnan S, Chen PP, Junk Ak, et al. Laser peripheral iridotomy in primary angle closure: a report by the American Academy of Ophthalmology. Ophthalmology. 2018;125(7):1110–1120.

CODES

ICD10
- H40.20X0 Unsp primary angle-closure glaucoma, stage unspecified
- H40.219 Acute angle-closure glaucoma, unspecified eye
- H40.2290 Chronic angle-closure glaucoma, unsp eye, stage unspecified

CLINICAL PEARLS
For patients with acute symptoms (severe eye pain, blurred vision, eye redness, halos around lights/objects, headache, nausea and vomiting) and asymmetric pupillary response, obtain immediate consultation with ophthalmology.

GLAUCOMA, PRIMARY OPEN-ANGLE

Richard W. Allinson, MD • Alyce D. Alven, OD, MS

BASICS

DESCRIPTION
Primary open-angle glaucoma (POAG) is a chronic, progressive optic neuropathy which causes loss of the optic nerve rim and retinal nerve fiber layer (RNFL) with associated visual field defects. POAG is associated with increased intraocular pressure (IOP). Normal IOP is 10 to 21 mm Hg.

Pregnancy Considerations
Prostaglandins should be avoided during pregnancy in the treatment of POAG.

EPIDEMIOLOGY
Incidence
Predominant age: usually >40 years

Prevalence
Prevalence in persons >40 years of age is ~1.8%.

ETIOLOGY AND PATHOPHYSIOLOGY
- Aqueous is produced by the ciliary epithelium of the ciliary body and is secreted into the posterior chamber of the eye. Aqueous then flows through the pupil and enters the anterior chamber to be drained by the trabecular meshwork (TM) in the iridocorneal angle of the eye. It then drains into the Schlemm canal and passes into the episcleral venous system. 5–10% of the total aqueous outflow leaves via the uveoscleral pathway.
- Impaired aqueous outflow through the TM leads to greater resistance in the aqueous drainage system and causes an increase in IOP.

Genetics
- A family history of glaucoma increases the risk for developing glaucoma.
- TMCO1 genotype has been found to increase the risk of developing glaucoma among non-Hispanic whites.
- The myocilin (MYOC) gene was the first gene associated with POAG.

RISK FACTORS
- Increased IOP
- Myopia
- Diabetes mellitus (DM)
- Elderly
- Hypothyroidism
- Positive family history
- Prolonged use of topical, periocular, inhaled, or systemic corticosteroids
- Systemic calcium-channel blockers
- Prior history pars plana vitrectomy
- Obstructive sleep apnea
- Hypertension
- Corneal hysteresis (CH): a measure of the viscoelastic damping of the cornea; lower CH associated with faster rates of visual field loss

GENERAL PREVENTION
Higher dietary nitrate and green leafy vegetable intake has been associated with a lower POAG risk. Evidence suggests that nitrate, a precursor of nitric oxide, is beneficial for blood circulation.
- The vascular endothelium regulates the microcirculation via vasoactive factors with nitric oxide being one of them. Nitric oxide reduces IOP by causing relaxation of the TM and the Schlemm canal, resulting in increased aqueous outflow.

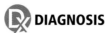

DIAGNOSIS

HISTORY
Painless, slowly progressive visual loss; patients are generally unaware of the visual loss until late in the disease. Central visual acuity remains unaffected until late in the disease.

PHYSICAL EXAM
- Visual acuity and visual field assessment
- Ophthalmoscopy to assess optic nerve for glaucomatous damage
- Tonometry to measure IOP. The IOP may be elevated or within the normal range.
- CDR >0.5: Normal eyes show a characteristic configuration for disc rim thickness of inferior ≥ superior ≥ nasal ≥ temporal (ISNT rule).
- Earliest visual field defects are paracentral scotomas and peripheral nasal steps.

DIFFERENTIAL DIAGNOSIS
- Normal-tension glaucoma
- Optic nerve pits
- Anterior ischemic optic neuropathy
- Compressive lesions of the optic nerve or chiasm
- Posthemorrhagic (shock optic neuropathy)

DIAGNOSTIC TESTS & INTERPRETATION
Initial Tests (lab, imaging)
Optical coherence tomography (OCT) can be useful in the detection of glaucoma.
- The RNFL is primarily composed of the axons of the retinal ganglion cells (RGCs).
- Glaucoma involves not only the RGC axons but also the bodies and dendrites.
- RGC axonal thickness is greatest at the peripapillary retina; therefore, OCT measures the peripapillary RNFL.
- RGCs are concentrated in the macula; therefore, OCT measurements of the macular ganglion cell–inner plexiform layer (mGCIPL) can determine glaucoma progression by the thinning of the mGCIPL.
- RNFL is thinner in patients with glaucoma.
- RNFL tends to be thinner with older age, in Caucasians, greater axial length, and smaller optic disc area.
- Significant RGC loss may occur at a specific location before corresponding visual field loss is detected.
- OCT angiography (OCTA) demonstrates a decrease in macular vessel density in eyes with POAG (1)[B].
- OCTA shows parapapillary choroidal microvasculature dropout (mvD) is associated with progressive RNFL thinning in POAG.

Diagnostic Procedures/Other
- Visual field testing: perimetry
- Tonometry to measure IOP: Thicker corneas resist the deformation inherent in most methods of tonometry, which may result in an overestimation of the IOP. Thinner corneas may give an artificially low reading.
  - IOP measured after photorefractive keratectomy (PRK) and laser in situ keratomileusis (LASIK) may be artificially low because of the thinning of the cornea induced by these refractive procedures.

Test Interpretation
- Atrophy and cupping of optic nerve
- Loss of RGCs and their axons produces defects and thinning in the RNFL. Assessment of RNFL thickness with OCT can detect glaucomatous damage before the appearance of visual field defects on standard automated perimetry.
- RNFL OCT utility declines in advanced glaucoma, whereas the mGCIPL OCT remains a sensitive progression detector from early to advanced glaucoma.
- mGCIPL OCT thickness is effective for predicting glaucoma progression regardless of the presence of high myopia (2)[B]. The peripapillary RNFL of highly myopic eyes tends to be thinner than that of normal eyes.

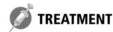

TREATMENT

GENERAL MEASURES
- Early Manifest Glaucoma Trial compared observation to treatment with betaxolol combined with argon laser trabeculoplasty (ALT) and found that early treatment delays progression, with the magnitude of initial IOP reduction influenced disease progression.
- Ocular Hypertension Treatment Study of patients with increased IOP of 24 to 32 mm Hg were treated with topical ocular hypotensive medication with a ~20% reduction in IOP. At 5 years, treatment reduced the incidence of POAG by >50%: 9.5% in the observation group versus 4.4% in the medication-treated group.
- Advanced Glaucoma Intervention Study randomized patients to laser trabeculoplasty or filtering surgery when medical therapy failed. In follow-up, if IOP was always <18 mm Hg, visual fields tended to stabilize. When IOP was >17 mm Hg, more than half the time, patients tended to have worsening of visual fields.
- Collaborative Initial Glaucoma Treatment Study demonstrated that both initial medical and surgical (trabeculectomy) treatment achieved significant IOP reduction, and both had little visual field loss over time.

MEDICATION
More than one medication, with different mechanisms of action, may be needed. Ocular hypotensive agent categories include the following:
- Prostaglandin analogues: generally used as first-line treatment. Enhance uveoscleral outflow and increase aqueous outflow through the TM: latanoprost 0.005% one drop at bedtime; travoprost 0.004% one drop at bedtime; bimatoprost 0.01% one drop at bedtime.
  - Latanoprostene bunod, 0.024% solution. This is a combination drug with one of the actions being the release of nitric oxide. Instill one drop at bedtime.
  - Contraindications/precautions
    ○ Prostaglandin analogues may cause increased pigmentation of the iris and periorbital tissue.
    ○ Increased pigmentation and growth of eyelashes
    ○ Should be used with caution in active intraocular inflammation (iritis/uveitis)

○ Caution is also advised in eyes with risk factors for herpes simplex, iritis, and cystoid macular edema.
○ Macular edema may be a complication associated with treatment.
○ Avoid during pregnancy.

- β-Adrenergic antagonists (nonselective and selective): decrease aqueous formation; best when used as an add-on therapy: timolol 0.25% (initial) to 0.5% one drop in affected eye q12h; gel-forming solution (0.25% or 0.5%) one drop in affected eye once daily (nonselective); betaxolol 0.5% one drop affected eye BID (selective)
  - Nonselective β-adrenergic antagonists: Avoid in asthma, chronic obstructive pulmonary disease (COPD), 2nd- and 3rd-degree atrioventricular (AV) block, and decompensated heart failure. Betaxolol is a selective β-adrenergic antagonist and is safer in patients with pulmonary disease.
  - β-Adrenergic antagonists: caution in patients taking calcium antagonists because of possible AV conduction disturbances, left ventricular failure, or hypotension
- Adrenergic agonists (selective α₂-adrenergic agonists)
  - Brimonidine tartrate 0.2%: One drop TID (α₂-adrenergic agonist) decreases aqueous formation and increases uveoscleral outflow.
    ○ Brimonidine should not be used in infants and young children because of the risk of CNS depression, apnea, bradycardia, and hypotension.
    ○ Monoamine oxidase inhibitors and tricyclic antidepressants may interfere with the metabolism of brimonidine and result in toxicity.
- Carbonic anhydrase inhibitors (oral, topical): Decrease aqueous formation.
  - Acetazolamide: 250 mg PO 1 to 4 times per day
  - Dorzolamide 2%: one drop TID
  - Brinzolamide 1%: one drop TID
  - Carbonic anhydrase inhibitors
    ○ Do not use with sulfa drug allergies.
    ○ Do not use if patient has cirrhosis because of the risk of hepatic encephalopathy.
- Rho kinase (Rock) inhibitors increase aqueous outflow through the trabecular outflow pathway by decreasing actomyosin-driven cellular contraction and reducing production of fibrotic extracellular matrix proteins.
  - Netarsudil 0.02%: one drop once daily in the evening
  - Corneal verticillata, or whorl keratopathy can occur with its usage.
- Parasympathomimetics (miotics), including direct-acting cholinergic agonists increase aqueous outflow
  - Pilocarpine 1–4%: one drop in affected eye BID–QID (direct-acting cholinergic agonist)
  - Parasympathomimetics (miotics): Cause pupillary constriction and may cause decreased vision in patients with a cataract; may cause eye pain or myopia due to increased accommodation. All miotics break down the blood–aqueous barrier and may induce chronic iridocyclitis.

- Hyperosmotic agents: Increase blood osmolality, drawing water from the vitreous cavity
  - Mannitol 20% solution is administered IV at 0.5 to 2 g/kg of body weight over a period of 45 minutes.
  - Glycerin 50% solution is administered orally; dosage is 1 to 1.5 g/kg, this is usually 4 to 7 oz. To improve the taste the solution may be mixed with a small amount of orange juice and poured over crushed ice.
  - Hyperosmotic agents: caution in diabetics; dehydrated patients; and those with cardiac, renal, and hepatic disease.
- Contact lenses wearers: Many glaucoma drops contain benzalkonium chloride; remove contact lenses prior to administration and wait 15 minutes before reinsertion.

SURGERY/OTHER PROCEDURES
- ALT
  - Improves aqueous outflow
  - The Glaucoma Laser Trial Research Group showed in newly diagnosed, previously untreated patients with POAG that ALT was as effective as topical glaucoma medication within the first 2 years of follow-up.
- Selective laser trabeculoplasty (SLT)
  - 532-nm Nd:YAG laser
  - Appears to be as effective as ALT in lowering IOP
  - May be repeated if necessary
- Trabeculectomy (glaucoma filtering surgery)
  - Usually reserved for patients needing better IOP control after maximal medical therapy and who may have previously undergone an ALT/SLT
- Shunt (tube) surgery
  - For example, Molteno and Ahmed devices
  - Generally reserved for difficult glaucoma cases in which conventional filtering surgery has failed or is likely to fail
  - Tube Versus Trabeculectomy (TVT) study showed after 5 years of follow-up, both procedures were associated with similar IOP reduction and the number of glaucoma medications needed.
- Ciliary body ablation: indicated to lower IOP in patients with poor visual potential or those who are poor candidates for filtering or shunt procedures
- Minimally invasive glaucoma surgery (MIGS) is frequently combined with cataract surgery; currently targeted at patients with mild to moderate glaucoma
  - Schlemm canal, suprachoroidal or subconjunctival stents
  - The Kahook Dual Blade performs an excisional goniotomy by removing a strip of TM.
  - Cataract extraction can decrease IOP in patients with ocular hypertension.

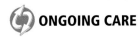

ONGOING CARE

FOLLOW-UP RECOMMENDATIONS
Patient Monitoring
- Monitor vision and IOP every 3 to 6 months.
- Visual field testing every 6 to 18 months

- Optic nerve evaluation every 3 to 18 months, depending on POAG control
- A worsening of the mean deviation by 2 dB on the Humphrey field analyzer and confirmed by a single test after 6 months had a 72% probability of progression.

PATIENT EDUCATION
POAG is a silent robber of vision, and patients may not appreciate the significance of their disease until much of their visual field is lost.

PROGNOSIS
- With standard glaucoma therapy, the rate of visual field loss in POAG is slow.
- Patients still may lose vision and develop blindness, even when treated appropriately.
- The structure of the mGCIPL was better preserved in surgically treated eyes than in medically treated eyes, even when the IOPs were similar during follow-up in cases of advanced glaucoma (3)[B].

COMPLICATIONS
Blindness

REFERENCES

1. Hou H, Moghimi S, Proudfoot J, et al. Ganglion cell complex thickness and macular vessel density loss in primary open-angle glaucoma. *Ophthalmology.* 2020;127(8):1043–1052.
2. Shin JW, Song MK, Sung KR. Longitudinal macular ganglion cell-inner plexiform layer measurements to detect glaucoma progression in high myopia. *Am J Ophthalmol.* 2021;223:9–20.
3. Inuzuka H, Sawada A, Yamamoto T. Comparison of changes in macular ganglion cell-inner plexiform layer thickness between medically and surgically treated eyes with advanced glaucoma. *Am J Ophthalmol.* 2018;187:43–50.

ADDITIONAL READING
Zhang X, Dastiridou A, Francis B, et al. Comparison of glaucoma progression detection by optical coherence tomography and visual field. *Am J Ophthalmol.* 2017;184:63–74.

 CODES

ICD10
H40.1190 Primary open-angle glaucoma, unspecified eye, stage unspecified

CLINICAL PEARLS
- Painless, slowly progressive visual loss; patients generally are unaware of the visual loss until late in the disease. Central visual acuity remains unaffected until late in the disease.
- Patients still may lose vision and develop blindness, even when treated appropriately.
- Topical or system steroids can cause the IOP to increase.

G

GLOMERULONEPHRITIS, ACUTE

Michael D. Kolman, DO • Daniel Kniaz, MD

BASICS

DESCRIPTION

- Acute glomerulonephritis (GN) is an inflammatory process involving the glomerulus of the kidney, resulting in a clinical syndrome consisting of sudden-onset of hematuria, proteinuria, and renal insufficiency, often in association with hypertension and edema.
- Acute GN may be caused by primary glomerular disease or secondary to systemic disease.
- Clinical severity ranges from self-limited asymptomatic microscopic or gross hematuria to a rapidly progressive loss of kidney function over days to weeks, termed rapidly progressive GN (RPGN).

ALERT
Urgent investigation and treatment are required to avoid irreversible loss of kidney function.

EPIDEMIOLOGY

- Infection-related GN
  - Postinfectious GN most commonly manifests after resolution of group A β-hemolytic *Streptococcus* infection.
  - Can also occur as a result of other bacterial infections, such as infective endocarditis, VP shunt nephritis, or less commonly with viral, helminthic, or parasitic infections
- IgA nephropathy
  - Most common primary GN in the world
  - Most common in the 2nd and 3rd decades
  - Incidence differs geographically: Asia > United States
  - HSP, the form with extrarenal manifestations, typically occurs in children <10 years old.
- Anti-GBM disease
  - Goodpasture syndrome: a notable cause of pulmonary–renal syndrome
  - Peak distribution in 3rd and 6th decades
- ANCA-associated GN
  - Often has a relapsing and remitting course
  - Four disease presentations:
    - Granulomatosis with polyangiitis (GPA), formerly Wegener granulomatosis
    - Microscopic polyangiitis (MPA)
    - Isolated pauci-immune GN—when isolated to kidneys
    - Eosinophilic GPA, formerly Churg-Strauss disease—GN relatively common but renal involvement rarely severe
- MPGN
  - May be primary or secondary to systemic diseases
  - Epidemiology varies depending on the mechanism of injury and is more often a subacute or chronic presentation
- Lupus nephritis
  - About 60% of systemic lupus patients will have renal involvement.
  - Incidence of lupus nephritis is higher among black and Hispanic populations in comparison to white populations.

- 6 classes
  - Minimal mesangial disease
  - Mesangial proliferation
  - Focal proliferative (active) and/or sclerosing (chronic) disease
  - Diffuse segmental or global proliferative (active) and/or sclerosing (chronic) disease
  - Membranous lupus nephritis
  - Advanced sclerosis lupus nephritis
- Cryoglobulin-associated vasculitis
  - 80% of cases with hepatitis C virus (HCV) infection
  - May also be associated with autoimmune disease or dysproteinemia

Prevalence

- In patients >65 years of age, with an average age of 75 years, about 1.2% of people are affected by either primary or secondary GN.
- In patients between the ages of 37 and 65 years of age, GN was much less commonly seen, with only about 0.12% of people affected by either primary or secondary GN (1).
- The incidence and prevalence of GN in children is unknown. Acute postinfectious GN is the most common type but has diminished over the years.

ETIOLOGY AND PATHOPHYSIOLOGY

- Systemic and/or local immune activation causes glomerular injury.
- Immune-complex mediated: antigen–antibody formation and deposition in the kidneys. Immune complexes are seen on immunofluorescence.
  - Postinfectious GN
  - IgA nephropathy
  - MPGN
    - Cryoglobulin-associated GN
  - Lupus nephritis
- Direct antibody-mediated injury, linear staining on immunofluorescence
  - Anti-GBM disease
- Pauci-immune GN, not seen on immunofluorescence staining
  - ANCA-associated GN
- Alternative complement pathway dysregulation
  - C3 glomerulopathy

RISK FACTORS

- Epidemics of nephritogenic strains of streptococci are triggers for postinfectious GN.
- Anti-GBM disease has been associated with prior pulmonary injury and inhalation exposures, such as hydrocarbon solvents.
- ANCA-associated GN may be drug induced (e.g., hydralazine, levamisole-contaminated cocaine) and is also associated with environmental exposures such as silica.
- Hepatitis B is associated with MPGN. Hepatitis C is associated with both MPGN and cryoglobulinemic GN.

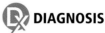

DIAGNOSIS

HISTORY

- Symptoms: cola- or tea-colored urine, decreased urine volume, blurry vision, dizziness, light-headedness, headache, altered mentation, edema, dyspnea, generalized malaise
- Timing
  - Poststreptococcal GN typically occurs 1 to 3 weeks after pharyngitis or 2 to 6 weeks after skin infection.
  - IgA nephropathy may present within several days after an acute infection.
- Patients may also present with complaints more specific to the associated disease:
  - Lupus nephritis: joint pain or rash
  - Pulmonary–renal syndromes: hemoptysis (see "Physical Exam")
  - ANCA-associated GN: sinusitis, pulmonary infiltrates, arthralgias
  - IgA–HSP: abdominal or joint pain and purpura
  - Cryoglobulinemia-associated GN: purpura and skin vasculitis

PHYSICAL EXAM

- Majority of patients will have normal exam but can often present with hypertension and signs of fluid overload.
- Sinus disease: ANCA-associated GN/GPA
- Pharyngitis or impetigo: postinfectious GN or IgA nephropathy
- Pulmonary hemorrhage (pulmonary–renal syndrome): anti-GBM disease/Goodpasture, ANCA-associated GN, or lupus nephritis
- Hepatomegaly or liver tenderness: cryoglobulinemia-associated GN or IgA nephropathy
- Purpura: ANCA-associated GN or HSP/IgA nephropathy

DIFFERENTIAL DIAGNOSIS
Nonglomerular hematuria: trauma, prostate diseases, urologic cancer, cystitis, nephrolithiasis, renal cysts, thrombotic microangiopathy

DIAGNOSTIC TESTS & INTERPRETATION

Initial Tests (lab, imaging)

- Urinalysis
  - Dysmorphic red blood cells (RBCs) or RBC casts on urine microscopy indicate glomerular hematuria and strongly suggest the diagnosis of an acute GN.
  - Pyuria and white blood cell casts may also be present.
- Proteinuria: 24-hour collection or random urine protein/creatinine ratio
- Electrolytes, blood urea nitrogen, creatinine, complete blood count
- Serologies may help clarify etiology:
  - Antistreptolysin O titer, streptozyme
  - Complement levels (C3, C4)
  - Antinuclear antibody (ANA) to rule out lupus nephritis

- ANCA screen: myeloperoxidase and anti-proteinase 3 antibodies
- Anti-GBM antibody
- Hepatitis B surface antigen and antibody
- Hepatitis C antibody
- Cryoglobulins
- Rheumatoid factor
- HIV testing
- Serum free light chain to assess for monoclonal gammopathies
- Renal ultrasound to rule out structural causes of glomerular disease
- Chest x-ray in the setting of hemoptysis or a suspected infiltrate

Diagnostic Procedures/Other
Definitive diagnosis is made via renal biopsy.

Test Interpretation
Renal biopsy

- Light microscopy
  - Diffuse hypercellularity suggests a proliferative disease such as IgA nephropathy, lupus nephritis, or postinfectious GN.
  - Presence of glomerular crescents correlates with RPGN and disease severity.
  - Significant overlap between endothelial, mesangial, and epithelial cell proliferation
- Immunofluorescence
  - Pattern of IgG, IgA, IgM, C3, and C4 staining may aid in characterizing the GN.
  - Lupus nephritis typically positive for all immuno-globulins and complements
  - Isolated mesangial IgA staining is pathognomonic for IgA nephropathy.
  - Crescentic GN in absence of immune complex staining suggests ANCA-associated GN.
  - Crescentic GN with linear staining of IgG is characteristic of anti-GB
- Electron microscopy: The location of immunoglobulin deposits is useful in pointing to a particular diagnosis.

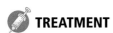

TREATMENT

GENERAL MEASURES
Treat the underlying condition if able.

MEDICATION
First Line
- Diuretics
- Calcium channel blockers
- Avoid ACE inhibitors or ARBs if acute renal dysfunction is present.

Second Line
- Supportive care is typically adequate in postinfectious GN.
- Crescents on renal biopsy may be an indication for steroids in postinfectious GN and, in other cases, are often an indication for additional potent immuno-suppressive medications (2)[C].
- Treatment with antiviral therapy for nephritic syndromes that have been shown to be secondary to underlying viral infections such as HCV and hepatitis B virus (HBV).

- Commonly used immunosuppressive medications include:
  - Corticosteroids—may consider initiation in high doses even prior to kidney biopsy (2)[C]
  - Cyclophosphamide
  - Mycophenolate mofetil (MMF)
  - Calcineurin inhibitors (cyclosporine, tacrolimus)
  - Rituximab
- Choice of immunosuppressive agent depends on patient characteristics and the disease process.
- Plasmapheresis may also be considered in some cases for RPGN or ANCA-associated renal disease with diffuse pulmonary hemorrhage (2)[C],(3),(4)[A].
- Dialysis may be needed for uremia, hyperkalemia refractory to medical management, intractable acidosis, and diuretic-resistant pulmonary edema.

ISSUES FOR REFERRAL
- Consultation with a nephrologist is usually required to assist with renal biopsy to confirm diagnosis and assist with management.
- Consultation with a rheumatologist may also be helpful in cases with systemic manifestations.

ADMISSION, INPATIENT, AND NURSING CONSIDERATIONS
- Consider admission for patients with no urine output, rapidly deteriorating renal function, significant hypertension, and suspicion of pulmonary hemorrhage or fluid overload that is compromising heart or respiratory function.
- Hemodynamically stable patients without complications may be managed as outpatients.

 ONGOING CARE

FOLLOW-UP RECOMMENDATIONS
Patient Monitoring
- Regular blood pressure checks and urinalysis to detect recurrence, assessment of renal function to detect acute or follow chronic renal disease as a result of the primary event, and regular clinical assessment to detect suspicious symptoms that may herald a recurrence (i.e., rash, joint complaint, hemoptysis)
- Periodic reassessment of serology tests to follow asymptomatic individuals

DIET
- Salt-restricted diet (<2 g/day) and fluid restriction until edema and hypertension clear
- Avoid foods that are high in potassium and phosphorus if significant renal dysfunction is present.

PATIENT EDUCATION
National Kidney Foundation:
https://www.kidney.org/atoz/content/glomerul

PROGNOSIS
- The GN may be self-limited or part of a chronic disease that makes the possibility of recurrence of acute disease likely, with the potential for progressive loss of renal function over time.
- Some forms of acute GN (including ANCA-associated and severe lupus) require long-term immunosuppression to prevent recurrence.

COMPLICATIONS
- Hypertensive retinopathy and encephalopathy
- Microscopic hematuria may persist for years.
- Chronic kidney disease
- Nephrotic syndrome (~10%)

REFERENCES

1. Wetmore JB, Guo H, Liu J, et al. The incidence, prevalence, and outcomes of glomerulonephritis derived from a large retrospective analysis. Kidney Int. 2016;90(4):853–860.
2. Beck L, Bomback AS, Choi MJ, et al. KDOQI US commentary on the 2012 KDIGO clinical practice guideline for glomerulonephritis. Am J Kidney Dis. 2013;62(3):403–441.
3. Walters G, Willis NS, Craig JC. Interventions for renal vasculitis in adults. Cochrane Database Syst Rev. 2008;(3):CD003232.
4. Jayne DR, Gaskin G, Rasmussen N, et al; for European Vasculitis Study Group. Randomized trial of plasma exchange or high-dosage methylprednisolone as adjunctive therapy for severe renal vasculitis. J Am Soc Nephrol. 2007;18(7):2180–2188.

 SEE ALSO

- Glomerulonephritis, Postinfectious; Henoch-Schönlein Purpura; Hyperkalemia; Hypertensive Emergencies; IgA Nephropathy; Lupus Nephritis; Nephrotic Syndrome; Vasculitis
- Algorithms: Acute Kidney Injury (Acute Renal Failure); Hematuria

 CODES

ICD10
- N00.9 Acute nephritic syndrome with unsp morphologic changes
- N00.2 Acute nephritic syndrome w diffuse membranous glomrlneph
- N00.8 Acute nephritic syndrome with other morphologic changes

CLINICAL PEARLS

- Dysmorphic RBCs and RBC casts are a key component of the urinalysis in GN.
- Postinfectious GN in children is typically a self-limited disease.
- Searching for other organ involvement is useful in establishing a definitive diagnosis.
- With the discovery of a GN, monitor the initial renal function labs frequently to identify an RPGN.
- Clinical course and treatment strategies depend on the underlying disease process.

G

GLOMERULONEPHRITIS, POSTINFECTIOUS

Theodore B. Flaum, DO • Ian Paul Persits, DO, MS

 BASICS

DESCRIPTION

Postinfectious glomerulonephritis (PIGN) is an immune complex disease associated with nonrenal infection by certain strains of bacteria, most commonly *Streptococcus* and *Staphylococcus*. The most common form of PIGN, poststreptococcal glomerulonephritis (PSGN), is preceded by infection with *Streptococcus* spp. and predominantly affects children. The clinical presentation can be asymptomatic or with an acute nephritic syndrome, characterized by gross hematuria, proteinuria, edema, hypertension (HTN), and acute kidney injury.

EPIDEMIOLOGY

PIGN is declining globally, especially in developed countries, in large part due to better hygiene and a decreased incidence of streptococcal skin infections. There are an estimated 470,000 new cases per annum of PSGN worldwide, and it remains the most common cause of acute nephritis in children globally, with 97% of cases occur in developing countries. PSGN is primarily a pediatric disease, but a recent increase in cases has been seen in nonstreptococcal GN in adults.

Incidence
- New cases of PSGN in developing countries ranges from 9.5 to 28.5 per 100,000 persons per year.
- Pediatrics: 24.3 cases/100,000 persons per year in developing countries; 6 cases/100,000 persons per year in developed countries
- Adults: 2 cases/100,000 persons per year in developing countries; 0.3 cases/100,000 persons per year in developed countries
- Worldwide: 34% of cases are now seen in adults with a global burden of 68,000 cases per year.
- Estimated incidence of 470,000 and 5,000 deaths per year globally
- Male > female (2:1)

ETIOLOGY AND PATHOPHYSIOLOGY
- Glomerular immune complex disease induced by specific nephritogenic strains of bacteria:
  - >95% of cases are caused by group A β-hemolytic *Streptococcus* (GAS) (1)
  - *Staphylococcus* (predominantly *Staphylococcus aureus*; more commonly methicillin-resistant *S. aureus* [MRSA], occasionally coagulase-negative *Staphylococcus*)
  - Gram-negative bacteria including *Escherichia coli*, *Yersinia*, *Pseudomonas*, and *Haemophilus* (2)
  - Occasionally viral, fungal, helminthic or protozoal causes
- Proposed mechanisms for the glomerular injury (3):
  - Deposition of circulating immune complexes with streptococcal or staphylococcal antigens—while these complexes can be detected in patients with streptococcal- or staphylococcal-related GN, they do not correlate to disease activity.
    - ○ Note: IgG is the most frequent immunoglobulin in PSGN (2).
  - In situ immune complex formation from deposition of antigens within the glomerular basement membrane (GBM) and subsequent antibody binding

- In situ glomerular immune complex formation promoted by antibodies to streptococcal or staphylococcal antigens
- Alteration of normal renal antigen leading to molecular mimicry that elicits an autoimmune response
- Glomerular immune complex causing complement activation and inflammation:
  - Nephritis-associated plasmin receptor (NAPlr): activates plasmin, contributes to activation of the alternative complement pathway
  - Streptococcal pyrogenic exotoxin B (SPE B): binds plasmin and acts as a protease; promotes the release of inflammatory mediators
- Activation of the alternative complement pathway causes initial glomerular injury as evidenced by C3 deposition and decreased levels of serum C3. The lectin pathway of complement activation has also been recently implicated in glomerular injury (1),(4).

RISK FACTORS
- Children 5 to 12 years of age
- Older patients (>65 years of age):
  - Patients with immunocompromising comorbid conditions
  - Diabetes
  - Alcohol abuse

GENERAL PREVENTION
- Early antibiotic treatment for streptococcal and staphylococcal infections, although efficacy in preventing GN is uncertain
- Improved hand hygiene and respiratory etiquette
- Prophylactic penicillin treatment to be used in closed communities and household contacts of index cases in areas where PIGN is prevalent

COMMONLY ASSOCIATED CONDITIONS
Streptococcal or staphylococcal infection

Ⓡ DIAGNOSIS

HISTORY
- Usually history of antecedent GAS skin/throat infection
- Patients present with acute nephritic syndrome, characterized by sudden onset of hematuria associated with edema and HTN for 1 to 2 weeks after an infection.
- A triad of edema (usually generalized), gross hematuria, and HTN is classic but not always seen.
- Urine described as "tea-colored" or "cola-colored"
- The latent period between GAS infection and PIGN depends on the site of infection: 1 to 3 weeks following GAS pharyngitis and 3 to 6 weeks following GAS skin infection.
- Adult PIGN most commonly follows staphylococcal infections (3 times more common than streptococcal infections) of the upper respiratory tract, skin, heart, lung, bone, or urinary tract. Studies show 7–16% of cases of adult PIGN have no preceding evidence of infection, and in 24–59%, the offending microorganism cannot be identified (5)[A].

PHYSICAL EXAM
- Constitutional:
  - Fever: 40–50% of patients
- Cardiovascular:
  - Edema: present in ~2 of 3 adult patients due to sodium and water retention; less common in pediatric patients
  - HTN: present in 80–90% of patients and varies from mild to severe; secondary to fluid retention. Hypertensive encephalopathy is an uncommon but serious complication.
- Pulmonary:
  - Respiratory distress: due to pulmonary edema (rare)
- Genitourinary:
  - Gross hematuria: present in 25–60% of patients
  - Microscopic hematuria: subclinical cases of PIGN
  - Oliguria: present in 18–51% of patients
  - Azotemia/impaired renal function: 44–70% of patients
  - Proteinuria: ~90% of patients
- Neuro:
  - Encephalopathy and seizures are rare

DIFFERENTIAL DIAGNOSIS

The diagnosis of PIGN is generally accomplished by history once the diagnosis of acute nephritis is made, with documentation of a recent infection and nephritis beginning to resolve 1 to 2 weeks after presentation. However, with progressive disease (>2 weeks, persistent hematuria/HTN >4 to 6 weeks, or no adequate documentation of a GAS or other infection) the differential diagnosis of GN needs to be considered and renal biopsy performed:

- Membranoproliferative glomerulonephritis (MPGN): Patients with MPGN have persistent nephritis and hypocomplementemia beyond 4 to 6 weeks. Patients with PIGN tend to have resolution of their disease and a return to normal C3 and CH50 levels within 2 to 4 weeks.
- Secondary causes of GN: Lupus nephritis and Henoch-Schönlein purpura nephritis have similar features to PIGN. Hypocomplementemia is not characteristic of Henoch-Schönlein purpura, and the hypocomplementemia that occurs in lupus nephritis usually results in reductions in both C3 and C4, whereas C4 levels are normal in PIGN.
- IgA nephropathy often presents after an upper respiratory infection. It can be distinguished from PIGN based on a shorter time frame between the upper respiratory illness and onset of hematuria, as well as history of gross hematuria, as PIGN recurrence is rare. IgA nephropathy is a chronic illness and will recur. Patients with IgA nephropathy have normal C3/C4 levels.
- IgA-dominant acute PIGN: a recently recognized form of PIGN occurring in poststaphylococcal GN. This differs from primary IgA nephropathy in that these patients do not have a history of renal disease (2)[A].
- Pauci-immune crescentic GN: In elderly with severe renal failure and active urine sediment, this is much more common, so antineutrophil cytoplasmic antibody (ANCA) testing should be done (2)[A].

DIAGNOSTIC TESTS & INTERPRETATION
Initial Tests (lab, imaging)
- Urinalysis
  - Hematuria with possible dysmorphic red cells
  - With/without RBC casts and pyuria
  - Proteinuria (nephrotic range proteinuria is uncommon in children)
- Renal function
  - Decreased glomerular filtration rate (GFR) with elevated creatinine to the point of renal insufficiency in 25–83% of cases, more commonly in adults (83%)

Follow-Up Tests & Special Considerations
- Culture: PSGN usually presents weeks after a GAS infection; only ~25% of patients will have either a positive throat or skin culture.
- Complement: 90% of pediatric patients (slightly fewer adult patients) will have depressed C3 and CH50 levels in the first 2 weeks of the disease, whereas C2 and C4 levels remain normal. C3 and CH50 levels return to normal within 4 to 8 weeks after presentation.
- Serology: Elevated titers of antibodies support evidence of a recent GAS infection. Streptozyme test measuring antistreptolysin O (ASO), antihyaluronidase (AHase), antistreptokinase (ASKase), anti–nicotinamide-adenine dinucleotidase (anti-NAD), and anti-DNAse B antibodies: positive in >95% of patients with PSGN due to pharyngitis and 80% with skin infections. In pharyngeal infection, ASO, anti-DNAse B, anti-NAD, and AHase titers are elevated. In skin infections, only the anti-DNAse and AHase titers are typically elevated.

Diagnostic Procedures/Other
Renal biopsy is rarely done in children; recommended in most adults to confirm the diagnosis and rule out other glomerulopathies with similar clinical presentations

Test Interpretation
- Light microscopy: diffuse proliferative glomerulonephritis with prominent endocapillary proliferation and numerous neutrophils within the capillary lumen. Deposits may also be found in the mesangium ("starry sky"). Severity of involvement varies and correlates with clinical findings. Crescent formation is uncommon and is associated with a poor prognosis.
- Immunofluorescence microscopy: deposits of C3 and IgG distributed in a diffuse granular pattern
- Electron microscopy: dome-shaped subepithelial electron-dense deposits that are referred to as "humps." These deposits are immune complexes, and they correspond to the deposits of IgG and C3 found on immunofluorescence. Rate of clearance of these deposits affects recovery time.

 TREATMENT

MEDICATION
- No specific therapy exists for PIGN, and no randomized controlled trials indicate that aggressive immunosuppressive therapy has a beneficial effect in patients with rapidly progressive crescentic disease. Despite this, patients with >30% crescents on renal biopsy are often treated with steroids (4)[A].
- Older patients often require hospitalization to treat complications of heart failure (HF) from volume overload (2).
- Management is mainly supportive, with focus on treating the clinical manifestations of PIGN (HTN; pulmonary edema):
  - Salt and water restriction and loop diuretics
  - Calcium channel blockers/angiotensin-converting enzyme (ACE) inhibitors may be used in cases of severe HTN (4)[A].
- Patients with evidence of persistent bacterial infection should be given a course of antibiotic therapy.

SURGERY/OTHER PROCEDURES
Acute dialysis is required in approximately 50% of elderly patients (1),(2).

ADMISSION, INPATIENT, AND NURSING CONSIDERATIONS
Admission may be necessary, specifically for elderly patients who are at greater risk for complications such as new onset or exacerbation of preexisting congestive HF (2).

 ONGOING CARE

FOLLOW-UP RECOMMENDATIONS
Patient Monitoring
- Repeat urinalysis to check for clearance of hematuria and/or proteinuria.
- Consider other diagnosis if no improvement within 2 weeks.

DIET
Renal diet if requiring instances of dialysis

PROGNOSIS
- Most children with PIGN have an excellent outcome, with >90% of cases achieving full recovery of renal function.
- Elderly patients, especially adults, develop HTN, recurrent proteinuria, and renal insufficiency long after the initial illness. Adults with multiple comorbid factors have the worst prognosis and highest incidence of chronic renal injury following PIGN (2).

- Complete remission in adult PIGN is only 26–56%. This has declined since the 1990s, suggesting prognosis is worsening (5).
- The presence of diabetes, higher creatinine levels, and more severe glomerular disease (e.g., crescents) on biopsy are all risk factors for developing end-stage renal disease (2).

REFERENCES
1. Hunt EAK, Somers MJG. Infection-related glomerulonephritis. *Pediatr Clin North Am*. 2019;66(1):59–72.
2. Nasr SH, Radhakrishnan J, D'Agati VD. Bacterial infection-related glomerulonephritis in adults. *Kidney Int*. 2013;83(5):792–803.
3. Nadasdy T, Hebert LA. Infection-related glomerulonephritis: understanding mechanisms. *Semin Nephrol*. 2011;31(4):369–375.
4. Ramdani B, Zamd M, Hachim K, et al. Acute postinfectious glomerulonephritis [in French]. *Nephrol Ther*. 2012;8(4):247–258.
5. Wen Y-K. Clinicopathological study of infection-associated glomerulonephritis in adults. *Int Urol Nephrol*. 2010;42(2):477–485.

ADDITIONAL READING
Balasubramanian R, Marks SD. Post-infectious glomerulonephritis. *Paediatr Int Child Health*. 2017;37(4):240–247.

 CODES

ICD10
- N05.9 Unsp nephritic syndrome with unspecified morphologic changes
- N00.9 Acute nephritic syndrome with unsp morphologic changes

CLINICAL PEARLS
- PIGN is an immune complex disease occurring after infection with certain strains of bacteria, most commonly group A *Streptococcus pyogenes*.
- The clinical presentation can be asymptomatic or with an acute nephritic syndrome, characterized by gross hematuria, proteinuria, edema, HTN, and acute kidney injury.
- Treatment is primarily supportive and includes treating HTN and edema, along with antibiotics for any ongoing bacterial infection.
- Persistent nephritis and low C3 levels for >2 weeks should prompt evaluation for other causes of GN, such as MPGN or systemic lupus erythematosus nephritis.

G

GLUCOSE INTOLERANCE

Mariya Milko, DO, MS

BASICS

DESCRIPTION
- Glucose intolerance is an intermediate stage between a normal glucose metabolism and diabetes. It occurs due to a gradual decline in β-cell function.
- Individuals with impaired fasting glucose (IFG) and/or impaired glucose intolerance (IGT) have been referred to as having prediabetes:
  - IFG: 100 to 125 mg/dL
  - IGT: 140 to 199 mg/dL 2 hours after ingestion of 75 g oral glucose load
  - Hemoglobin A1c (HbA1c) 5.7–6.4% (1)

EPIDEMIOLOGY
- As of 2010, it is estimated that one of every three U.S. adults $\geq$20 years of age have prediabetes (2).
- In the United States, an estimated 88 million people 18 years or older are living with prediabetes as of 2020, based on the National Diabetes Statistics Report.
- Only 11% of people with prediabetes are aware of their condition (3).
- Prediabetes has a 34.5% prevalence among adults >18 years old and 51% of adults $\geq$65 years in the United States (4).

Incidence
- Systematic review indicates a 5-year cumulative incidence of developing diabetes of 9–25% for people with an HbA1c of 5.5–6.0% and 25–50% with an HbA1c of 6.0–6.5% (1).
- Highest incidence in American Indians/Alaska Natives, non-Hispanic blacks, and Hispanics (2)

Prevalence
As of 2020, prevalence of prediabetes in the United States was 34.5% in adults >20 years old and 51% in adults >65 years old. According to ADA, in 2015, 84.1 million Americans >18 years old had prediabetes. As of 2010, worldwide prevalence was 8%.

ETIOLOGY AND PATHOPHYSIOLOGY
Progressive loss of insulin secretion on the background of insulin resistance (1)

Genetics
- Genetic heterogeneity is established by family, twin, immunologic, and HLA disease association studies.
- Variants in 11 genes have been shown to be significantly associated with future development of type 2 diabetes and IFG. Variants in 8 of these genes have been associated with impaired β-cell function.

RISK FACTORS
- Body mass index (BMI) $\geq$25: overweight
- History of gestational diabetes mellitus (GDM)
- Sedentary lifestyle
- Medications

GENERAL PREVENTION
- Lifestyle modification with weight reduction and increased physical activity
- A decrease in excess body fat provides the greatest risk reduction.

Pregnancy Considerations
- Screening for diabetes in pregnancy is based on risk factor analysis:
  - High risk: first prenatal visit
  - Average risk: 24 to 28 weeks' gestation
- Women with GDM should be screened for diabetes 6 to 12 weeks' postpartum with 75-g OGTT and then every 1 to 3 years via any method (5).

COMMONLY ASSOCIATED CONDITIONS
- Obesity (abdominal and visceral obesity)
- Dyslipidemia with high triglycerides (TG)
- PCOS
- GDM
- Congenital diseases (Down, Turner, Klinefelter, and Wolfram syndromes)

DIAGNOSIS

Who to screen
- BMI $\geq$25 or $\geq$23 for Asian Americans (1)[B]
- Age $\geq$45 years (1)[B]
- First-degree relative with diabetes
- High TG >250 mg/dL
- Low HDL <35 mg/dL
- HTN: BP >140/90 mm Hg or on treatment
- History of GDM
- History of cardiovascular disease
- Ethnic group at increased risk (non-Hispanic black, Native American, Hispanics, Asian American, Pacific Islander)
- PCOS
- Conditions associated with insulin resistance such as severe obesity or acanthosis nigricans

HISTORY
- No clear symptoms
- Polyuria
- Polydipsia
- Weight loss
- Blurred vision
- Polyphagia

PHYSICAL EXAM
- General physical exam
- BMI assessment

DIFFERENTIAL DIAGNOSIS
- Type A insulin resistance
- Leprechaunism
- Rabson-Mendenhall syndrome
- Lipoatrophic diabetes
- Pancreatitis
- Cushing syndrome
- Glucagonoma
- Pheochromocytoma
- Hyperthyroidism
- Somatostatinoma
- Aldosteronoma
- Drug-induced hyperglycemia
  - Thiazide diuretics (high doses)
  - β-Blockers
  - Corticosteroids (including inhaled corticosteroids)
  - Thyroid hormone
  - α-Interferon
  - Pentamidine
  - Protease inhibitors
  - Atypical antipsychotics
  - Selective serotonin reuptake inhibitors

DIAGNOSTIC TESTS & INTERPRETATION
Initial Tests (lab, imaging)
- Fasting glucose, 2-hour OGTT, or HbA1c is equally appropriate (1)[B].
- Repeat screen at 3-year intervals with normal results, sooner depending on risk status (1)[C].

Follow-Up Tests & Special Considerations
- Fasting lipid profile
- Creatinine and GFR
- Urinalysis
- Microalbumin-to-creatinine ratio
- Thyroid-stimulating hormone with free T_4
- Periodic measurement of vitamin B_{12} levels for patients on long-term metformin therapy especially those with anemia or peripheral neuropathy

TREATMENT

- Therapeutic lifestyle modification to include physical activity focused on weight loss and medical nutrition therapy (preferably via a registered dietitian)
- Mediterranean diet and diets high in fiber-rich foods such as vegetables, fruits, whole grains, seeds, and nuts plus white meat sources are protective against type 2 diabetes (6)[B].
- Consider referring patients with prediabetes to an intensive diet and physical activity behavioral counseling program adhering to the tenets of the Diabetes Prevention Program targeting a loss of 7% of body weight and should increase their moderate-intensity physical activity (such as brisk walking to at least 150 min/week) (6)[A].

- Resistance training and endurance exercise both reduce diabetes risk.
- Interrupt prolonged sitting every 30 minutes with short bouts of physical activity (6)[B].
- Diabetes prevention programs are cost-effective and often covered by third-party payers (6)[B].
- Screen and treat modifiable risk factors for cardiovascular disease (6)[B].
- Diabetes self-management education and support systems are appropriate venues for people with prediabetes to receive education and support to develop and maintain behaviors that can prevent or delay the onset of diabetes (6)[B].
- Technology-assisted tools including internet-based social networks, distance learning, DVD-based content, and mobile applications can be useful elements of effective lifestyle modification to prevent diabetes (6)[B].

MEDICATION

Consider metformin therapy for prevention of type 2 diabetes, especially in those with BMI >35, those aged <60 years, and women with prior GDM and/or rising HbA1c despite lifestyle intervention (6)[C].

First Line

Metformin (drug of choice): started at 500 mg BID or 500 mg XR. Observational data suggest it can be used safely down to GFR of 30 to 45 but may require dose adjustments.

Second Line

- Acarbose: started at 50 mg PO once daily and titrated to 100 mg PO TID; GI upset is common.
- GLP-1 agonists: Recent clinical trials in primarily obese patients, GLP-1 agonists have shown various benefits including weight loss, improvement in B-cell function, and a return to a normal glycemic state. Overall prediabetes incidence decreased by 84–96%. However, no GLP-1 inhibitors are FDA approved for prediabetes as of 2020 (7)[A].

ISSUES FOR REFERRAL

- Diabetes educator/registered dietitian upon diagnosis
- Exercise physiologist
- Lifestyle coaching
- Obesity specialist

ADDITIONAL THERAPIES

Alternative/botanical therapy:
- Although studies lack large sample size and ideal design, there is some evidence that fenugreek, bitter melon, and cinnamon can reduce hyperglycemia and improve insulin sensitivity (7).

 ONGOING CARE

FOLLOW-UP RECOMMENDATIONS

Patient Monitoring

- At least annual monitoring for development of diabetes with HbA1c, 2-hour OGTT, or fasting glucose
- BP should be routinely measured.
- Annual testing for lipid abnormalities and microalbuminuria (for detection and therapy modification of incipient diabetic nephropathy)
- Monitoring of BMI

DIET

- Mediterranean diet has been shown to be beneficial. One small cohort study showed that the addition of about 10 g of extra virgin olive oil to meals improved postprandial glucose by reducing DPP4 activity and increasing insulin and GLP-1. It also showed a significant decrease in TG and apolipoprotein B-48.
- Limit high glycemic carbohydrates and sucrose-containing foods.
- Diets high in fiber, vegetables, nuts, seeds, and whole grains
- Intermittent fasting has shown benefit in improving fasting glucose as well as postprandial hyperglycemia (8)[C].

PROGNOSIS

- Individuals with IFG and/or IGT have high risk for the future development of diabetes.
- Prediabetes increases the risk of developing type 2 diabetes, heart disease, and stroke.
- 20–70% of individuals with prediabetes who do not lose weight, change their dietary habits, and/or engage in moderate physical activity will progress to type 2 diabetes within 3 to 6 years.
- Lifestyle intervention reduced 3-year diabetes incidence by 58% compared to 31% with metformin.

COMPLICATIONS

- Cardiovascular and peripheral artery disease
- Stroke: 2 to 4 times higher risk
- Ketoacidosis
- Sexual dysfunction
- Gastroparesis
- Nephropathy and potential for renal failure
- Retinopathy and potential for loss of vision
- Peripheral and autonomic neuropathy

REFERENCES

1. American Diabetes Association. 2. Classification and diagnosis of diabetes. *Diabetes Care.* 2017;40(Suppl 1):S11–S24.
2. Centers for Disease Control and Prevention. *National Diabetes Statistics Report, 2014: Estimates of Diabetes and Its Burden in the United States.* Atlanta, GA: U.S. Department of Health and Human Services; 2014.
3. Centers for Disease Control and Prevention. Awareness of prediabetes—United States, 2005–2010. *MMWR Morb Mortal Wkly Rep.* 2013;62(11):209–212.
4. Centers for Disease Control and Prevention. Prediabetes. http://www.cdc.gov/diabetes/basics/prediabetes.html. Accessed January 18, 2017.
5. American Diabetes Association. 13. Management of diabetes in pregnancy. *Diabetes Care.* 2017;40(Suppl 1):S114–S119.
6. American Diabetes Association. 5. Prevention or delay of type 2 diabetes. *Diabetes Care.* 2017;40(Suppl 1):S44–S47.
7. Deng R. A review of the hypoglycemic effects of five commonly used herbal food supplements. *Recent Pat Food Nutr Agric.* 2012;4(1):50–60.
8. Arnason TG, Bowen MW, Mansell KD. Effects of intermittent fasting on health markers in those with type 2 diabetes: a pilot study. *World J Diabetes.* 2017;8(4):154–164.

ADDITIONAL READING

Papaetis GS. Incretin-based therapies in prediabetes: current evidence and future perspectives. *World J Diabetes.* 2014;5(6):817–834.

 CODES

ICD10

- E74.39 Other disorders of intestinal carbohydrate absorption
- R73.09 Other abnormal glucose
- R73.01 Impaired fasting glucose

CLINICAL PEARLS

- Patient education and lifestyle reinforcement should be emphasized in all clinical encounters as lifestyle optimization is essential for all patients with prediabetes.
- Research shows that you can lower your risk for type 2 diabetes by 58% by losing 7% of your body weight (or 15 lb if you weigh 200 lb).
- Recommend exercising moderately (such as brisk walking) 30 min/day, 5 days a week.
- Consider concurrent cardiovascular risks and further workup as indicated clinically.

G

GONOCOCCAL INFECTIONS

Melissa Jefferis, MD, FAAFP

BASICS

DESCRIPTION
A sexually or vertically transmitted bacterial infection caused by *Neisseria gonorrhoeae*:

- *N. gonorrhoeae* is a fastidious gram-negative intracellular diplococcus (1)[A].
- Presents as conjunctival, pharyngeal, urogenital, or anorectal infection. Urogenital infections are the most common (1)[A].
- Hematogenous dissemination leads to fever, cutaneous lesions, arthralgias, purulent or sterile arthritis, tenosynovitis, endocarditis, or (rarely) meningitis (1)[A].
- Asymptomatic carrier states occur in men and women.
- In newborns of infected mothers, gonococcal ophthalmia neonatorum, a purulent conjunctivitis, may occur after vaginal delivery; can lead to potential blindness if not treated promptly (1),(2)[A]
- System(s) affected: cardiovascular, musculoskeletal, nervous, reproductive, skin/exocrine
- Synonym(s): gonococcal infection; clap

EPIDEMIOLOGY
- Predominant age: 15 to 44 year olds account for 92% of cases; highest rate among those ages 20 to 24 years
- Predominant sex: men 213/100,000; women 146/100,000

Incidence
Centers for Disease Control and Prevention (CDC) 2018: 583,405 reported cases

Prevalence
Incidence and prevalence are roughly equal. The true prevalence is higher due to asymptomatic cases (2)[A]:
- Rates peaked in mid-1970s and fell 74% over the next 20 years with national control program. Rates have been slowly increasing since 2012 (2)[A].
- Rates in men now higher than women (2)[A]

ETIOLOGY AND PATHOPHYSIOLOGY
Infection requires four steps: (i) mucosal attachment—bacterial proteins bind to receptors on host cells, (ii) local penetration/invasion, (iii) local proliferation, (iv) inflammatory response or dissemination. *N. gonorrhoeae* spreads most commonly through sexual contact.

Genetics
Deficiency of late components of complement cascade (C7–C9) predisposes to disseminated disease.

RISK FACTORS
- History of previous gonorrhea infection or other STIs
- Sexual exposure to an infected individual without appropriate use of barrier protection (condom)
- New/multiple sexual partners
- Inconsistent condom use
- Commercial sex work or drug use
- Infants: infected mother
- Children: sexual abuse by infected individual
- Autoinoculation (finger to eye)

GENERAL PREVENTION
- Condoms offer partial protection and must be used appropriately during oral, anal, and vaginal sex.
- Treat sexual contacts; consider expedited partner therapy (EPT) (2)[A].

COMMONLY ASSOCIATED CONDITIONS
Other STIs: *Chlamydia*, syphilis, HIV, hepatitis B, herpes (2),(3)[A]

DIAGNOSIS

HISTORY
- Sexual history
  - Number of partners; age of onset of sexual activity; STI history
  - New/recent change in sexual partners
  - Contact with commercial sex workers
  - Condom use
  - Menses and possibility of pregnancy
- 10% of men and 20–40% of women are asymptomatic (2)[A].
- If symptomatic, explore onset, context, duration, timing, severity, and associated symptoms:
  - Symptoms (when present) typically appear within 1 to 14 days after exposure (1)[A].
- Ocular symptoms: discharge, itch, redness (1)[A]
- Pharyngeal symptoms: asymptomatic infection (98%), sore throat (1)[A]
- GI symptoms: acute diarrhea (1)[A]
- Urinary symptoms: frequency, urgency, dysuria (1)[A]
- Urethral symptoms: discharge (1),(2)[A]
  - Males: scant to copious purulent urethral discharge (82%), dysuria (53%), asymptomatic (10%), testicular pain (1%), proctitis
  - Females: endocervical discharge (96%), asymptomatic cervical infection (20%), vaginal discharge, Bartholin gland swelling, dysmenorrhea, menometrorrhagia, abdominal pain/tenderness, dyspareunia, cervical motion tenderness, rebound, infertility, chronic pelvic pain
- Either sex, with receptive anal intercourse: rectal discharge, tenesmus, rectal burning; can also be asymptomatic
- Disseminated syndromes (1),(2)[A]
  - Fever, chills, malaise, skin rash, arthralgia/arthritis
  - Endocarditis: high fevers
  - Meningitis: meningeal signs, headache, skin lesions, fever, altered mental status

PHYSICAL EXAM
- General: fever, chills (1)[A]
- Ocular: purulent discharge, conjunctivitis, chemosis, eyelid edema, corneal ulceration (1)[A]
- Pharynx: exudative pharyngitis (<1%) (1)[A]
- GI: acute diarrhea, hyperactive bowel sounds (1)[A]
- Genitourinary (GU) (1)[A]
  - Males: urethral discharge, testicular tenderness
  - Females: endocervical discharge, Bartholin gland abscess, abdominal pain/tenderness, cervical motion tenderness, rebound tenderness
- Either sex, for receptive anal intercourse: rectal discharge; rectal exam may be normal (1)[A].

- Disseminated syndromes (1)[A]:
  - Fever, chills, malaise, tenosynovitis, maculopapular–pustular rash, polyarthralgia—typically large joints (knee, wrist, ankle), purulent arthritis
  - Endocarditis: rapid cardiac valve destruction, heart murmurs, high fevers
  - Meningitis: meningeal signs, headache, skin lesions, fever, altered mental status

DIFFERENTIAL DIAGNOSIS
Chlamydia trachomatis, UTIs, other vaginitis, or urethritis (bacterial, viral, or parasitic)

DIAGNOSTIC TESTS & INTERPRETATION
Initial Tests (lab, imaging)
- The nucleic acid amplification test (NAAT) is the most sensitive and specific test for *N. gonorrhoeae* (2)[A].
- Other options:
  - Genital culture
  - Add pharyngeal culture in adolescents.
  - Gram stain (recommended for urethritis)
  - Urethral smear, sensitivity in symptomatic male: ≥95%; sensitivity of endocervical smear in infected woman: 40–60%; specificity: 100%
- DNA probes and polymerase chain reaction (PCR) sensitivity: 92–99% dependent on population; specificity: >97%; can replace culture
- Blood culture is 50% sensitive in disseminated disease. Joint fluid culture is 50% sensitive in septic arthritis. Screen for additional STIs, especially chlamydia, syphilis, and HIV.
- Imaging is not generally recommended.

Follow-Up Tests & Special Considerations
- Test of cure unnecessary for persons with uncomplicated urogenital or rectal gonorrhea who are treated with any of the recommended or alternative regimens (4)[A]:
  - Individuals treated for pharyngeal gonorrhea should have test of cure 7 to 14 days after treatment with NAAT or culture (4)[A].
- Reinfection within 12 months occurs in 7–12% of persons treated for gonorrhea. Patients should be retested 3 months after treatment regardless of whether they believe their sex partners were treated. If retesting at 3 months is not possible, clinicians should retest within 12 months after initial treatment (4)[A].

Diagnostic Procedures/Other
Culdocentesis may demonstrate free purulent exudate and provide material for Gram staining and culture. Gram staining material from unroofed skin lesions may show typical organisms. Pelvic ultrasound or CT scan may demonstrate thick, dilated fallopian tubes or abscess formation.

Test Interpretation
- Gram-negative intracellular diplococci
- Nonpathologic gram-negative diplococci may be found in extragenital locations. For this reason, Gram stain of pharyngeal or rectal swabs is not recommended.

TREATMENT

GENERAL MEASURES
- STI counseling and condom use
- In children and adolescents, suspect sexual abuse.

MEDICATION
- Dual therapy no longer recommended (4)[A]
- Quinolones are not recommended (2),(5)[A].
- *If treatment fails, check culture and sensitivities and report to CDC through local health authorities (2),(3)[A].*
- Treat with regimen that is also effective against uncomplicated genital chlamydial infection if chlamydial infection has not been ruled out (4)[A].

First Line
- Uncomplicated urogenital, anorectal, and pharyngeal gonorrheal infection (4)[A]
  - Ceftriaxone 500 mg IM in a single dose. For persons weighing ≥150 kg (300 lb), use 1 g IM in a single dose.
    - If IM ceftriaxone is not available, cefixime 800 mg PO once is an alternative. Cefixime has limited treatment efficacy for pharyngeal gonorrhea.
  - If chlamydial infection has not been excluded, also give doxycycline 100 mg orally BID for 7 days.
  - Alternative: gentamicin 240 mg IM once PLUS azithromycin 2 g PO once
- Conjunctivitis: ceftriaxone, 1 g IM single dose PLUS azithromycin 1 g PO once (1),(2)[A]
- Arthritis and arthritis–dermatitis syndrome (1),(2)[A]
  - Ceftriaxone 1 g IM or IV q24h until 24 to 48 hours after improvement begins and then switch to PO agent. Complete at least 1 week of antibiotic treatment, PLUS azithromycin 1 g PO once.
  - Alternative regimens:
    - Cefotaxime 1 g IV every 8 hours until 24 to 48 hours after improvement begins and then switch to PO agent. Complete at least 1 week of antibiotic treatment, PLUS azithromycin 1 g PO once.
    - Ceftizoxime 1 g IV every 8 hours until 24 to 48 hours after improvement begins and then switch to PO agent. Complete at least 1 week of antibiotic treatment, PLUS azithromycin 1 g PO once.
- Meningitis and endocarditis (1),(2)[A]
  - Ceftriaxone 1 to 2 g IV q12h 10 to 14 days for meningitis; 4 weeks for endocarditis PLUS azithromycin 1 g PO once
- Contraindications: Doxycycline is contraindicated in pregnancy and young children.

Pediatric Considerations
- Children >45 kg: same dosing as adults (1),(2)[A]
  - Bacteremia or arthritis: ceftriaxone 1 g IM or IV in single daily dose every 24 hours for 7 days
- Children <45 kg: uncomplicated urethral, cervical, rectal, or pharyngeal gonococcal infections (1),(2)[A]
  - Ceftriaxone 25 to 50 mg/kg IV or IM in a single dose, not to exceed 125 mg IM
  - Disseminated infections: ceftriaxone 50 mg/kg IV or IM daily (max dose 1 g) in single dose; bacteremia or arthritis: 7 days; meningitis: 10 to 14 days; endocarditis: 4 weeks
- Ophthalmic neonatorum prophylaxis: single application of erythromycin 0.5% ophthalmic ointment to each eye immediately after delivery (1),(2)[A]

- Neonatal conjunctivitis: ceftriaxone 25 to 50 mg/kg IV or IM in a single dose (not to exceed 125 mg) (1),(2)[A]
- *Conjunctival exudates should be cultured for definitive diagnosis (1),(2)[A].*
- Scalp abscesses (from scalp electrodes) (1),(2)[A]
  - Ceftriaxone 25 to 50 mg/kg/day IV or IM in a single daily dose for 7 days. Treat for a duration of 10 to 14 days if meningitis is documented.
  - Alternative: cefotaxime 25 mg/kg IV or IM every 12 hours for 7 days. Treat for a duration of 10 to 14 days if meningitis is documented.
- Asymptomatic infants born to mothers with untreated gonorrhea (1),(2)[A]
  - Ceftriaxone 25 to 50 mg/kg IV or IM, not to exceed 125 mg in a single dose

Pregnancy Considerations
- Pregnant women should be treated with the same treatments as listed above (2)[A].
- An alternative is treatment with spectinomycin. If spectinomycin or other regimens are not possible, consultation with an infectious disease specialist is recommended (2)[A].

Second Line
- A single 2-g oral dose of azithromycin has been used in the past, although should be avoided due to the potential to develop macrolide resistance (2)[A].
- For additional treatment options, see CDC STD treatment guidelines: http://www.cdc.gov/std/tg2015/.

ADMISSION, INPATIENT, AND NURSING CONSIDERATIONS
- Hematogenously disseminated infection
- Pneumonia or eye infection in infants

 ONGOING CARE

FOLLOW-UP RECOMMENDATIONS
Patient Monitoring
- U.S. Preventive Services Task Force (USPSTF) (6)[A]
  - Screen all sexually active women 24 years of age and younger and in older women at increased risk for infection for chlamydia and gonorrhea: grade B recommendation.
  - Insufficient evidence to recommend for or against screening for chlamydia and gonorrhea in men: grade I recommendation
  - Report cases of gonorrhea to public health (3),(6)[A].
- CDC
  - Screen annually for sexually active men who have sex with men (MSM) at sites of contact (urethra, rectum, pharynx), regardless of condom use. Increase screening to every 3 to 6 months if at increased risk.

PATIENT EDUCATION
- Counseling concerning risk reduction, condom use, future fertility, and full STI testing
- Encourage patient to notify partners (from past 60 days); consider EPT.

PROGNOSIS
Complete cure with return to normal function with adequate and timely treatment

---

COMPLICATIONS
- Infertility
- Ectopic pregnancy
- Urethral stricture
- Corneal scarring
- Destruction of joint articular surfaces
- Cardiac valvular damage

Pediatric Considerations
Vertical transmission is a significant risk among patients with gonococcal infection at the time of delivery (1),(2)[A].

REFERENCES
1. Mayor MT, Roett MA, Uduhiri KA. Diagnosis and management of gonococcal infections. *Am Fam Physician*. 2012;86(10):931–938.
2. Centers for Disease Control and Prevention. 2015 sexually transmitted diseases treatment guidelines: gonococcal infections. https://www.cdc.gov/std/tg2015/gonorrhea.htm. Accessed January 15, 2021.
3. Centers for Disease Control and Prevention. Update to CDC's sexually transmitted diseases treatment guidelines, 2010: oral cephalosporins no longer a recommended treatment for gonococcal infections. *MMWR Morb Mortal Wkly Rep*. 2012;61(31):590–594.
4. Centers for Disease Control and Prevention. Update to CDC's treatment guidelines for gonococcal infection, 2020. *MMWR Morb Mortal Wkly Rep*. 2020;69(50):1911–1916.
5. Committee on Gynecologic Practice. ACOG Committee Opinion No. 645: dual therapy for gonococcal infections. *Obstet Gynecol*. 2015;126(5):e95–e99.
6. U.S. Preventive Services Task Force. Final recommendation statement: chlamydia and gonorrhea: screening. http://www.uspreventiveservicestaskforce.org/Page/Document/UpdateSummaryFinal/chlamydia-and-gonorrhea-screening. Accessed December 8, 2019.

 SEE ALSO

Chlamydia Infection (Sexually Transmitted); HIV/AIDS; Pelvic Inflammatory Disease; Syphilis

 CODES

ICD10
- A54.9 Gonococcal infection, unspecified
- A54.03 Gonococcal cervicitis, unspecified
- A54.31 Gonococcal conjunctivitis

CLINICAL PEARLS
- Antibiotic resistance is a significant problem.
- Treatment for uncomplicated gonorrhea should include two drugs, one of which is effective against chlamydia.
- Screen patients with gonorrhea for chlamydia, syphilis, HIV, and hepatitis.

GOUT

Sangili Chandran, MD • Ahja D. Steele, MD

 BASICS

DESCRIPTION

- An inflammatory arthritis leading to an acutely red, hot, swollen joint, which can progress to a chronic tophaceous joint that is associated with pain, nodule formation, and cutaneous compromise
- Also characterized by deposition of monosodium urate (MSU) crystals that accumulate in joints and soft tissues, resulting in acute and chronic arthritis, soft-tissue masses called tophi, urate nephropathy, and uric acid nephrolithiasis
- The long limb, foot, ankle, and knee is preferentially involved.
- The involvement of the 1st metatarsophalangeal joint (podagra) is characteristic.
- Gout flares can occur in the elbows, wrists and hand joints, but the upper limb involvement is usually only in patients with long-standing, poorly controlled disease. Axial skeleton involvement occurs occasionally.
- Flares are usually monoarticular. Polyarticular flares can be associated with pronounced systemic symptoms, including fever, chills, and delirium.
- Gout is related to a hyperuricemia (serum uric acid level >6.8 mg/dL).

EPIDEMIOLOGY

Incidence
- Incidence ranges between 0.6 and 2.9 per 1,000 person-years.
- Gout has a higher incidence in males than females.

Prevalence
Prevalence ranges between 0.68% and 3.9% in adults.

ETIOLOGY AND PATHOPHYSIOLOGY
Four pathophysiologic stages:
- Development of hyperuricemia (from uric acid overproduction and/or renal underexcretion)
- Deposition of MSU crystals (Changes in uric acid solubility caused by local temperature decrease, trauma, or acidosis may precipitate out of solution and accumulate as crystals in joints and soft tissues.)
- Clinical presentation of gout flares due to an acute inflammatory response to deposited crystals
- Clinical presentation of advanced disease characterized by tophi and joint damage

Genetics
- Consider HLA-B*5801 mutation genotyping for people in Asian origin.
- Phosphoribosyl pyrophosphate (PRPP) deficiency and hypoxanthine guanine phosphoribosyltransferase (HGPRT) deficiency (Lesch-Nyhan syndrome) are inherited enzyme defects associated with overproduction of uric acid.
- Polymorphisms in the URAT1 and SLC2A9 (GLUT9) renal transporters are hereditary enzyme defects resulting in primary underexcretion of uric acid.

RISK FACTORS
- Age >40 years
- Male gender
- Excessive purine consumption from diet (alcohol [especially beer], red meat, seafood, sugar-sweetened beverages)

- Metabolic syndrome/obesity (BMI >30)
- Congestive heart failure
- Chronic kidney disease (CKD)
- Dyslipidemia, hypertension
- Smoking
- Dehydration (similar to diuretic effects)
- Diabetes mellitus
- Urate-elevating medications: thiazide diuretics, loop diuretics (less of a risk vs. thiazides), niacin, aspirin
- Transplant associated gout can happen in immunosuppressed solid organ transplant recipients on low dose prednisolone and calcineurin inhibitors (cyclosporine and tacrolimus) as these medications increase uric acid (1).
- Hyperuricemia from rapid cell turnover/tumor lysis syndrome (e.g., hemolysis, chemotherapy)

GENERAL PREVENTION
- Diet modification: Avoid purine rich foods like red meat and shellfish. Reduce alcohol consumption (beer and liquor).
- Maintain fluid intake and avoid dehydration.

COMMONLY ASSOCIATED CONDITIONS
- Nontraumatic joint disorders
- Metabolic syndrome, obesity (BMI >30)
- Renal disease

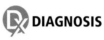 **DIAGNOSIS**

HISTORY
- Typical first presentation of gout (2):
  - Intensely painful acute inflammatory arthritis, usually a gout flare, affecting a lower limb joint, which can be self-limited over a period of 7 to 14 days if goes untreated
  - Lower limb and mono-articular arthritis are common early in course of disease—gout flares can occur in the joints or periarticular tissues (e.g., bursae, tendons, and entheses) while upper extremity and polyarticular presentations are usually seen in chronic cases.
  - Joint may be swollen, warm, erythematous and exquisitely tender to touch. The pain can be described as stabbing, gnawing, burning, or throbbing.
  - There is substantial limitation in using the affected areas, difficulty walking, and fear of even minimal physical contact.
  - Often awakes patients from sleep due to an intolerance to contact with clothing or bed sheets
  - There is a rapid onset of intense pain, often progressing rapidly over 12 to 24 hours.
  - Acute attacks are usually precipitated by infection, injury, dehydration, or excess alcohol or purine intake.
  - Fever can be present.
  - Subcutaneous or intraosseous nodules, referred to as tophi, can be seen after many recurrent attacks.
  - Rarely, pain with urination secondary to uric acid renal stones can be seen in chronic cases.
- Chronic manifestations of gout:
  - Subcutaneous tophi located in joints, ears, olecranon bursae, finger pads, tendon
  - Tophi are firm and hard, vary in size, can become acutely inflamed, but usually not tender.
  - Can ulcerate with thick/white discharge and superimposed infections

PHYSICAL EXAM
- Examine suspected joint(s) for tenderness, swelling, and range of motion (ROM).
- Tophi can be found in the affected joints, the helix of the ear, over the olecranon process, or on the Achilles tendon.

DIFFERENTIAL DIAGNOSIS
Septic arthritis, calcium pyrophosphate deposition disease (formerly "pseudogout"), cellulitis, osteoarthritis, rheumatoid arthritis and bursitis, traumatic arthritis, hemarthrosis

DIAGNOSTIC TESTS & INTERPRETATION
- Diagnostic compound score for patients presenting with monarthritis in primary care settings (3):
  - Male sex
  - Previous patient-reported arthritis attack
  - Onset within 1 day
  - Joint redness
  - First metatarsophalangeal joint involvement
  - Hypertension or cardiovascular disease
  - High concentration of serum urate
- Score <4 ruled out gout in 97%; score >8 ruled in 80% with gout.
- Initial acute gout episode
  - Uric acid (may be normal or low), CBC (WBC maybe elevated), ESR/CRP
- Synovial fluid analysis: urate crystals (negatively birefringent under polarizing microscopy), cell count (WBC usually 2,000 to 5,000 cells/mm³); gram stain and culture to rule out infection
- 24-hour urine to screen for uric acid overproduction (>800 mg/24 hr) in those with onset before the age of 25 years or with a history of urolithiasis
- Radiographs/plain x-rays are normal early in disease but can reveal periarticular erosions with periosteum overgrowth in chronic gout.
- Ultrasonography can show a double contour sign (reflecting MSU crystal deposition on the surface of hyaline articular cartilage), intra-articular or intra-bursal tophi, and a snowstorm appearance.
- Dual-energy CT (DECT) imaging can show urate deposition at articular or periarticular sites.

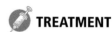 **TREATMENT**

GENERAL MEASURES
Supportive care including ice packs, rest, mobility assistance, and adequate nutrition and hydration

MEDICATION
- Acute treatment
  - Pharmacologic treatment should be initiated within 12 to 24 hours of acute gout attack and continued for 1 to 2 days after acute attack has subsided (1).
  - Urate-lowering therapy should not be interrupted during an acute gout attack.
  - Mild/moderate gout severity (≤6 of 10 on visual analog pain scale, particularly for an attack involving only one or a few small joints or one to two large joints)

- NSAIDs
  - Naproxen: 500 mg BID
  - Meloxicam: 7.5 to 15 mg/day
  - Indomethacin: 50 to 150 mg/day (generally less well tolerated than others)
  - Diclofenac: 75 mg twice daily
  - Ibuprofen: 800 mg every 8 hours
- Oral/intra-articular/intramuscular/intravenous corticosteroids
  - Consider intra-articular corticosteroids.
  - Corticosteroids are useful in patients with acute gout flare who cannot tolerate NSAIDs or have contraindications to NSAIDs and colchicine such as CKD.
  - When monotherapy is insufficient for acute flares, a combination of NSAIDs with either intra-articular corticosteroid, oral steroid, or colchicine may be used.
    - Oral corticosteroids:
      □ Medium dose (15 to 20 mg/day) to high dose (30 to 35 mg/day) for 5 days
    - Intra-articular/intramuscular/intravenous preparation (unable to take oral medications):
      □ Triamcinolone acetonide, dexamethasone, and methylprednisolone
- Colchicine
  - Used for gout attacks where the onset was <36 hours prior to treatment initiation
  - Begin a loading dose of 1.0 to 1.2 mg followed by 0.5 to 0.6 mg 1 hour later, after 12 hours, resume 0.5 to 0.6 mg every 8 hours with no more than 6 mg per course and at least 3 days between courses
- Interleukin 1 (IL-1) inhibitors
  - Reserved for patients who have intolerable side-effects or have contraindications to first-line anti-inflammatory therapy
    - Canakinumab 150 mg SQ X1 (Monitor for adverse events, including serious infections.)
    - Anakinra 100 mg SQ daily for 5 days
- Severe gout (≥7 of 10 pain scale, involving ≥4 joints with arthritis involving >1 region, or involving 3 separate large joints)
  - Initial combination therapy is an option and includes the use of full doses of the following:
    - Colchicine and NSAIDs
    - PO corticosteroids and colchicine
    - Intra-articular steroids
- For patients not responding to initial pharmacologic monotherapy, add a second agent.
- Chronic treatment
- Urate-lowering therapy for:
  - Tophus formation
  - Radiographic damage from gout or ≥1 attacks per year
  - CKD stage 2 or worse or urolithiasis
- Treat to the serum uric acid <6 mg/dL (may need <5 mg/dL to improve symptoms).
- Urate-lowering agents can be prescribed during an acute attack provided that effective anti-inflammatory prophylaxis has been initiated first such as:
  - Low-dose NSAIDs: naproxen 250 mg PO BID
  - Low-dose colchicine: 0.5 to 0.6 mg once or twice daily

- If colchicine and NSAIDs, contraindicated, or ineffective:
  - Low-dose prednisone at ≤10 mg/day
- Treatment duration of at least 6 months or 3 months after achieving serum urate target
- Urate-lowering agents
  - Allopurinol: xanthine oxidase inhibitor—does not reduce number of acute attacks.
    - Start no higher than 100 mg/day (50 mg/day in stage 4 or 5 CKD).
    - Titrate dose upward q2–5wk to maximum dose.
    - Monitor serum uric acid level and renal function 3 months in the first year and annually thereafter.
    - Monitor for allopurinol hypersensitivity syndrome (AHS), pruritus, rash, elevated hepatic transaminases, and eosinophilia. HLA-B*5801 allele for AHS should be performed in those of Korean, Chinese, or Thai.
  - Febuxostat: selective xanthine oxidase inhibitor
    - Start 40 mg/day; titrate to 80 mg/day.
  - Probenecid: uricosuric agent
    - Alternative if xanthine oxidase inhibitor is contraindicated.
    - May be used in addition to allopurinol or febuxostat if serum urate target not achieved
    - Increased risk of urolithiasis with this agent
    - Not recommended if CrCl <50 or if history of urolithiasis
    - Start 250 mg BID; titrate to 2,000 mg/day.

ADDITIONAL THERAPIES
Other treatment (4)

- Losartan possesses uricosuric properties; consider for hypertensive patients.
- Fenofibrate also possesses uricosuric properties and may be useful with lipid disorders.

SURGERY/OTHER PROCEDURES
Large tophi that are infected or interfering with joint motion may need to be surgically removed.

COMPLEMENTARY & ALTERNATIVE MEDICINE
Vitamin C (>500 mg every day) has been shown to reduce serum uric acid levels (1)[C].

 ONGOING CARE

FOLLOW-UP RECOMMENDATIONS
Patient Monitoring
- Serum uric acid measurements q2–5wk while titrating urate-lowering treatment to goal
- Regularly monitor CBC, renal function, liver function test, and urinalysis.

DIET
- Avoid:
  - Organ meats high in purine content (sweetbreads, liver, kidney)
  - High-fructose corn syrup–sweetened sodas, other beverages, or foods (reducing fructose to <1 g/kg/day)
  - Alcohol overuse (>2 servings per day for men and >1 serving per day for women)
- Limit:
  - Beef, lamb, pork, and seafood with high purine content such as sardines and shellfish
  - Servings of naturally sweetened fruit juices

- Sugar, sweetened beverages, and desserts
- Table salt, including in sauces and gravies
- Alcohol (particularly beer) in all patients (<1 to 2 units per day)
- Encourage:
  - Coffee intake of >4 cups per day reduced risk of gout by 57%.
  - Foods rich in dietary fiber, folate, vitamin C, dairy products decreased the incidence of gout
  - Cherry consumption may be of benefit in gout prophylaxis (5)[C].

PATIENT EDUCATION
- Dietary and lifestyle modifications
- Discussion on causes of gout and that effective urate-lowering therapy is often essential for treatment.

PROGNOSIS
Gout can usually be successfully managed with proper treatment and lifestyle modifications.

COMPLICATIONS
- Inflammatory arthritis and joint destruction
- Uric acid nephropathy and renal stones

REFERENCES
1. Abhishek A, Roddy E, Doherty M. Gout—a guide for the general and acute physicians. *Clin Med (Lond)*. 2017;17(1):54–59.
2. Rogenmoser S, Arnold MH. Chronic gout: barriers to effective management. *Aust J Gen Pract*. 2018;47(6):351–356.
3. Neogi T, Jansen T, Dalbeth N, et al. 2015 Gout classification criteria: an American College of Rheumatology/European League Against Rheumatism collaborative initiative. *Arthritis Rheumatol*. 2015;67(10):2557–2568.
4. Mirkov S. Reducing clinical risks associated with the pharmacological treatment of acute gout attacks. *Drugs Ther Perspect*. 2018;34:377–385.
5. Lamb KL, Lynn A, Russell J, et al. Effect of tart cherry juice on risk of gout attacks: protocol for a randomised controlled trial. *BMJ Open*. 2020;10(3):e035108.

CODES
ICD10
- M10.269 Drug-induced gout, unspecified knee
- M10.161 Lead-induced gout, right knee
- M10.221 Drug-induced gout, right elbow

CLINICAL PEARLS
- Acute gouty arthritis can affect ≥1 joint; the 1st metatarsophalangeal joint is most commonly involved at presentation (podagra).
- MSU crystals found in synovial fluid aspirate are pathognomonic for gout.
- Pharmacologic treatment should begin within 24 hours of acute gout flare. NSAIDs and/or corticosteroids are effective for mild/moderate attacks.
- Asymptomatic hyperuricemia does not require treatment.

G

GRANULOMA ANNULARE

Stephen C. Sears, DO • Adam K. Saperstein, MD

 BASICS

DESCRIPTION

Granuloma annulare (GA) is a benign skin condition characterized by groups of skin-colored to erythematous papules that are usually in an annular (ringlike) pattern and typically located on the dorsal aspects of the hands and feet. There are five types of GA: localized, generalized, subcutaneous, patch, and perforating.

EPIDEMIOLOGY

Incidence

- GA is a relatively common, noninfectious granulomatous disease. Population-based studies to determine the incidence and/or prevalence of GA are lacking. A single study in 1980 demonstrated that 0.1–0.4% of new patients presenting to dermatologists have GA but did not report similar descriptive statistics in the primary care arena (1).
- Although most lesions resolve spontaneously within 2 years, some persist for 10 years or more.
- Predominant sex: female > male (1 to 2.5:1)
- Onset of symptoms occurs at <30 years old in 2/3 of all patients. Typical ages for onset of each subtype are:
  – Localized: <30 years old
  – Generalized: bimodal: <10 years old, 30 to 60 years old
  – Subcutaneous: 2 to 14 years old
  – Patch: >30 years old
  – Perforating: children and young adults
- Distribution of subtypes:
  – Localized: 75%
  – Generalized: 10–15%
  – Subcutaneous: <5%
  – Patch type: <5%
  – Perforating: <5%

ETIOLOGY AND PATHOPHYSIOLOGY

The etiology of GA remains unknown. It is hypothesized to be a dermatologic manifestation of a delayed-type hypersensitivity reaction to an unknown antigen in the derm is mediated by tumor necrosis factor alpha (TNF-α) and interleukin factors 1 and 2 (IL-1 and IL-2) (2). Characteristic histopathologic features include lymphohistiocytic infiltrates, degeneration of collagen, palisading or interstitial granulomatous inflammation, and mucin deposition.

Genetics

There is some evidence for a genetic predisposition. Two studies reported an increased frequency of HLA-Bw35 in patients with generalized GA. Of note, HLA-Bw35 has also been associated with thyroid disease (1).

RISK FACTORS

No definite risk factors have been identified. There are reported associations between GA and diabetes mellitus (DM), autoimmune thyroid disease, dyslipidemia, HIV, Epstein-Barr virus, herpes simplex virus, systemic lupus erythematosus, tuberculosis, and hepatitis B and C, among others. There have also been associations with interferon-α therapy, trauma, sun exposure, insect bites, borreliosis, and malignancies (most commonly lymphoma) (2),(3).

GENERAL PREVENTION

There are no known preventive measures for GA.

COMMONLY ASSOCIATED CONDITIONS

- DM: The association between GA and DM is controversial. Early studies from the 1980s showed a possible link, but recent case-controlled studies have shown no statistically significant association between GA and DM (3).
- Autoimmune thyroid disease: Multiple case reports have linked thyroid disease with both generalized and localized GA. In one case-control study, 24 women with localized GA were compared to 100 age-matched women with non-GA dermatologic disease. A statistically significant increase in the incidence of autoimmune thyroid disease among those with localized GA as compared with those with other non-GA cutaneous disease was identified (12% vs. 1%, $p = .022$) (2),(3).
- Malignancy: There is no definitive relationship between GA and malignancy. A review of the literature found 14 case reports and two correlation studies in which patients who had one or more malignancies also had GA. In a majority of these cases, the malignancies were hematologic, primarily lymphoma (2),(3).
- Dyslipidemia: Dyslipidemia may be associated with GA. A single case-control study ($n = 140$) demonstrated a statistically significant increase in hyperlipidemia among patients with GA compared to controls (79.3% vs. 51.9%, $p < .001$).
- HIV: Among patients with GA, those who also have HIV appear more likely to have the generalized subtype. In one study of 34 patients with GA and HIV, 20 (59%) had generalized GA (2).
- Note: Conclusions regarding associations between GA and various diseases, including those listed above, are limited by both design and power. Consequently, in the absence of new research, definitive associations between GA and other diseases cannot be made.

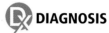 **DIAGNOSIS**

HISTORY

Cutaneous lesions of GA are generally asymptomatic. Lesions often persist for months or years, especially in patients who have generalized GA. In most cases, regardless of subtype, GA resolves spontaneously but may thereafter recur without obvious trigger.

PHYSICAL EXAM

- Localized: asymptomatic, flesh-colored or erythematous annular, or arciform plaque with a moderately firm, rope-like border and central clearing, ranging from 5 mm to 5 cm in diameter. Small 1- to 2-mm papules may be noted peripheral to the primary lesion. The most common locations are the dorsal aspects of the distal upper and lower extremities; involvement of palms is rare. It is common to have multiple lesions at the time of presentation.
- Generalized: Lesions have the same morphology as localized GA lesions, but tend to be larger, greater in number (usually >10), persist for a longer period of time, and are more widespread.
- Subcutaneous: firm, nontender nodules that tend to grow rapidly; usually solitary but may occur in groups; most common location is scalp and/or anterior aspect of the lower extremities, followed by upper extremities and buttocks.
- Patch: erythematous macules and patches distributed symmetrically on the extremities and trunk. The typical annular configuration may or may not be present; often involves proximal extremities
- Perforating: Damaged collagen from dermis is extruded onto skin surface. Papules may be up to 4 mm in diameter and display yellowish umbilication, crusting, or scale. Lesions are often widely distributed on the body and cause scaring.

DIFFERENTIAL DIAGNOSIS

- Localized: tinea corporis, annular lichen planus, necrobiosis lipoidica, pityriasis rosea, erythema migrans, leprosy
- Generalized: sarcoidosis, lichen planus, cutaneous metastases, mycosis fungoides (cutaneous T-cell lymphoma)
- Patch type: erythema migrans
- Subcutaneous: rheumatoid nodules
- Perforating: molluscum contagiosum, sarcoidosis, insect bites

DIAGNOSTIC TESTS & INTERPRETATION

Initial Tests (lab, imaging)

- Diagnosis is typically established by history and physical examination; laboratory investigations are rarely needed. Microscopic evaluation of skin cells using potassium hydroxide (KOH) preparation may be useful to exclude a fungal process.
- Consider laboratory testing to evaluate comorbid dyslipidemia, DM, thyroid disease, HIV, hepatitis B/C, and malignancy as clinically indicated.

Diagnostic Procedures/Other

Punch biopsy and histologic evaluation may aid in confirming the diagnosis and identifying the subtype. Immunohistochemical streptavidin-biotin–horseradish peroxidase (HRP) analysis for CD68/KP-1 (a marker for histiocytic differentiation) may also aid in the diagnosis.

Test Interpretation

Dermal infiltrate demonstrating foci of degenerative collagen associated with palisading granulomas around an anuclear dermis with mucin deposition. Histologic variants include interstitial (histiocytic infiltrate between collagen fibers), classic (palisading dermal granulomas), and epithelioid (tuberculoid and sarcoidal granulomas).

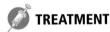 **TREATMENT**

GENERAL MEASURES

GA is a self-limited condition that is likely to regress spontaneously. The clinician's primary role after making the diagnosis is to educate the patient about the natural history of GA and to consider screening for conditions that may be associated with this disease. No specific treatment has been satisfactorily studied in reliable randomized controlled trials with most recommendations based on case reports, case series, and retrospective reviews (4).

MEDICATION

- The trauma induced by biopsy alone can cause involution of lesions through an unknown mechanism.
- Given the self-limited nature of the disease, it is incumbent on providers to assess the risk/benefit ratio of treatment. Reassurance is often all that is required for localized, asymptomatic disease.
- The following therapies have been tried with variable success (2),(3),(5),(6). Duration of therapy is often undefined and is based on clinical response.

First Line

Corticosteroids

- High-potency topical (class I or II), with or without occlusion (3)[C],(5)[C]
- Intralesional triamcinolone: concentration of 2.5 to 5.0 mg/mL (3)[C],(5)[C]. Technique: Insert the needle into the dermis at the elevated border and slowly inject while withdrawing the needle, with enough volume to cause the lesion to begin to blanch. Take care to avoid allowing the tip of the needle to push through to inserting the needle through the lesion.

Second Line

- Pimecrolimus cream: 1% BID (3)[C]
- Tacrolimus ointment: 0.1% BID (3)[C]
- Chloroquine: 250 mg/day (3)[C]
- Hydroxychloroquine: 9 mg/kg/day for 2 months, 6 mg/kg/day for month 3, 2 mg/kg/day for month 4 (3)[C]

- Doxycycline: 100 mg/day for 10 weeks (3)[C]
- Isotretinoin: 0.50 to 0.75 mg/kg/day (3)[C]
- Rifampin 600 mg, ofloxacin 400 mg, with minocycline 100 mg once daily (3)[C]
- Dapsone: 100 mg/day (3)[C]
- Cyclosporine: 3 to 4 mg/kg/day (3)[C]
- Methotrexate: 15 mg IM weekly (3)[C]
- Niacinamide: 500 mg TID (3)[C]
- Fumaric acid esters: variable dosing schemes (3)[C]
- Interferon gamma 1b: intralesional injection, 2.5 × 10^5 IU/lesion for 7 consecutive days followed by 3 times per week for 2 weeks (3)[C]
- TNF-α inhibitors, such as infliximab 5 mg/kg IV weeks 0, 2, and 6, then variable or adalimumab 80 mg SC at week 0, and then 40 SC at week 1 and every other week, or etanercept 50 mg twice weekly (3)[C]

ADDITIONAL THERAPIES

- Cryotherapy (one 10- to 60-second freeze thaw cycle) (3)[C]
- Fractional thermolysis (e.g., YAG fractionated laser) (3)[C]
- 585- to 595-nm pulsed dye laser (3)[C]
- Narrowband ultraviolet B (NBUVB) (6)[C]
- Psoralen ultraviolet A (PUVA) (6)[C]
- Surgical excision (for subcutaneous GA) (2)[C]

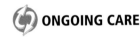 **ONGOING CARE**

FOLLOW-UP RECOMMENDATIONS

Routine follow-up is not required unless treatment is initiated. In such situations, follow-up is recommended to monitor for possible adverse effects of treatment. Referral to a dermatologist is prudent for patients who have generalized GA, cosmetic concerns, and for patients whose lesions persist despite conservative therapy.

PATIENT EDUCATION

Patients should be educated that GA is a benign, self-limited condition that may persist for months to years, spontaneously resolve, and spontaneously recur. Additionally, patients may benefit from knowing that GA is not thought to be of an infectious etiology and is not transmissible to others.

PROGNOSIS

>50% of cases resolve spontaneously within 2 months to 2 years after onset, although recurrence, typically at the original site, is common (>40%). Patients <39 years tend to have a shorter duration of illness.

COMPLICATIONS

Complications of treatment are much more likely than complications from GA.

REFERENCES

1. Piette EW, Rosenbach M. Granuloma annulare: clinical and histologic variants, epidemiology, and genetics. *J Am Acad Dermatol.* 2016;75(3): 457–465.
2. Piette EW, Rosenbach M. Granuloma annulare: pathogenesis, disease associations and triggers, and therapeutic options. *J Am Acad Dermatol.* 2016;75(3):467–479.
3. Keimig EL. Granuloma annulare. *Dermatol Clin.* 2015;33(3):315–329.
4. Wang J, Khachemoune A. Granuloma annulare: a focused review of therapeutic options. *Am J Clin Dermatol.* 2018;19(3):333–344.
5. Cyr PR. Diagnosis and management of granuloma annulare. *Am Fam Physician.* 2006;74(10): 1729–1734.
6. Cunningham L, Kirby B, Lally A, et al. The efficacy of PUVA and narrowband UVB phototherapy in the management of generalised granuloma annulare. *J Dermatolog Treat.* 2016;27(2):136–139.

ADDITIONAL READING

- De Paola MD, Batsikosta A, Feci L, et al. Granuloma annulare, autoimmune thyroiditis, and lichen sclerosus in a woman: randomness or significant association? *Case Rep Dermatol Med.* 2013;2013:289084.
- Duarte AF, Mota A, Pereira MA, et al. Generalized granuloma annulare—response to doxycycline. *J Eur Acad Dermatol Venereol.* 2009;23(1):84–85.
- Plotner AN, Mutasim DF. Successful treatment of disseminated granuloma annulare with methotrexate. *Br J Dermatol.* 2010;163(5):1123–1124.

 CODES

ICD10
L92.0 Granuloma annulare

CLINICAL PEARLS

- GA is benign, self-limited condition. Consider risk-to-benefit ratio when partnering with patients to determine treatment.
- When initiating therapy for localized GA, start with high-dose topical corticosteroids or intralesional corticosteroids followed by cryotherapy or other listed topical therapies. For widespread disease, consider initiating treatment with antimalarials or phototherapy.
- Consider GA in the differential diagnosis of lesions that appear to be tinea, especially when these lesions lack scale and are KOH negative.
- Consider fasting lipid panel, fasting blood glucose or HbA1C, TSH, free T_4, thyroid antibodies, hepatitis B and C panel, HIV screening test, and age-appropriate cancer screening, especially in those with generalized or atypical presentations of GA.

G

GRANULOMA, PYOGENIC

Cameron S. Gilbert, MD, USAF, CSARME

BASICS

DESCRIPTION
- Pyogenic granulomas (PG), also called lobular capillary hemangiomas, are benign vascular proliferations that can appear on the skin and mucus membranes. Most common sites are head and neck, the lips and oral cavity, the trunk, and the extremities (1),(2).
- They are friable and tend to bleed profusely due to the vascular nature of the lesion.
- Smooth, red to purple, sessile or pedunculated, grow rapidly over several weeks
- Rarely regress completely without intervention (2)

EPIDEMIOLOGY
- The peak incidence of PG occurs in children and young adults (2).
- Commonly seen in early pregnancy

ETIOLOGY AND PATHOPHYSIOLOGY
- Definitive cause unknown
- Thought to be associated with capillary proliferation resulting from aberrant healing response to minor trauma
- Associated with peripheral nerve injury, inflammatory systemic diseases, and drugs (retinoids, systemic steroids, protease inhibitors, epidermal growth factor receptor inhibitors)
- May be related to hormonal changes in pregnancy
- Not considered a hemangioma or neoplasm; no true granulomatous histology present

RISK FACTORS
- Pregnancy
- Trauma
- Intraoral trauma or surgery
- Inflammatory systemic diseases

GENERAL PREVENTION
Good oral hygiene may be helpful.

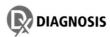**DIAGNOSIS**

HISTORY
- Solitary lesion that develops rapidly from days to weeks after minor trauma
- Tends to bleed easily
- Grows early in pregnancy and partially regresses postpartum

PHYSICAL EXAM
- Most commonly located at the head, neck, and upper extremities, especially in children
- Among oral lesions, gingiva is the most common location.
- Usually a bright red, friable papule; can also be purple, yellow, or brown
- Moist and sometimes scaly-appearing surface
- Usually <1 cm but ranges from a few millimeters to 2 to 3 cm in diameter
- Giant lesions may occur on areas such as the foot (rare).
- Soft; pedunculated or sessile
- Solitary red papule, grows rapidly, forming a stalk, may bleed, and ulcerate

- On diascopy, red structureless areas surrounded by a white collarette intersected by white lines
- Erythematous, soft compressible papule with serosanguineous crusting and sharp demarcation

DIFFERENTIAL DIAGNOSIS
- Benign lesions
  - Cherry/infantile hemangioma (3)
  - Fibrous papule (1),(3)
  - Bacillary angiomatosis, from by *Bartonella* (1)
- Malignant lesions
  - Basal cell carcinoma (1)
  - Squamous cell carcinoma (1)
  - Amelanotic melanoma (1)
  - Kaposi sarcoma (1)
  - Cutaneous metastases (1)

DIAGNOSTIC TESTS & INTERPRETATION
Initial Tests (lab, imaging)
No labs are necessary for the diagnosis.

Diagnostic Procedures/Other
- Excisional/shave biopsy
- Send for pathology.

Test Interpretation
Microscopic examination reveals
- Small, endothelial-lined vascular spaces
- Loose/dense connective tissue stroma
- Acute and chronic inflammatory cells
- No true granuloma formation
- Abundant mitotic activity
- Resembles granulation tissue in an edematous matrix, showing immature capillaries with interspersed tissue

TREATMENT

- Full thickness surgical excision is best to yield material for histopathologic analysis and avoid recurrence (4)[A]. Excision must be adequate to avoid recurrence. Even a small fragment of tissue left behind may lead to recurrence.
- CO_2 laser ablation results in less pain and allows for superficial dermal ablation (4)[A].
- Shave biopsy can be used for pedunculated lesions; can combine with cautery (5)[B]
- Punch biopsy acceptable for small lesions
- Electrosurgery: electrodesiccation and curettage (5)[B]

SURGERY/OTHER PROCEDURES
- Cryotherapy with liquid nitrogen (recur 2%) (5)[B]
- Pulsed dye laser or CO_2 laser (5)[B]
- Topical imiquimod (5)[B]
- Silver nitrate (5)[A]
- Topical 1.5% phenol solution may be used for periungual lesion (5)[B].
- Recurrence rate of up to 15% depending on treatment modality used

 ONGOING CARE

PATIENT EDUCATION
Patient should avoid trauma to area following excision.

PROGNOSIS
- Some lesions spontaneously resolve on their own (usually within 6 months).
- With treatment, recurrence rates are between 4% and 5% (2).

COMPLICATIONS
Recurrence: After removal or destruction of solitary lesion, multiple satellite lesions can form around original treatment site.

REFERENCES

1. Lin RL, Janniger CK. Pyogenic granuloma. *Cutis.* 2004;74(4):229–233.
2. Borden A, Harrington JW. Pyogenic granuloma: an overview of pathogenesis, diagnosis, and management. *Consultant.* 2018;58(6):e181.
3. Pagliai KA, Cohen BA. Pyogenic granuloma in children. *Pediatr Dermatol.* 2004;21(1):10–13.
4. Plachouri KM, Georgiou S. Therapeutic approaches to pyogenic granuloma: an updated review [published online ahead of print October 21, 2018]. *Int J Dermatol.* doi:10.1111/ijd.14268.
5. Lee J, Sinno H, Tahiri Y, et al. Treatment options for cutaneous pyogenic granulomas: a review. *J Plast Reconstr Aesthet Surg.* 2011;64(9):1216–1220.

ADDITIONAL READING

- Gilmore A, Kelsberg G, Safranek S. Clinical inquiries. What's the best treatment for pyogenic granuloma? *J Fam Pract.* 2010;59(1):40–42.
- Greene AK. Management of hemangiomas and other vascular tumors. *Clin Plast Surg.* 2011;38(1):45–63.
- Kroumpouzos G, Cohen LM. Dermatoses of pregnancy. *J Am Acad Dermatol.* 2001;45(1):1–19.

- Losa Iglesias ME, Becerro de Bengoa Vallejo R. Topical phenol as a conservative treatment for periungual pyogenic granuloma. *Dermatol Surg.* 2010;36(5):675–678.
- Piraccini BM, Bellavista S, Misciali C, et al. Periungual and subungual pyogenic granuloma. *Br J Dermatol.* 2010;163(5):941–953.
- Zalaudek I, Kreusch J, Giacomel J, et al. How to diagnose nonpigmented skin tumors: a review of vascular structures seen with dermoscopy: part II. Nonmelanocytic skin tumors. *J Am Acad Dermatol.* 2010;63(3):377–386.

 CODES

ICD10
- L98.0 Pyogenic granuloma
- K06.8 Oth disrd of gingiva and edentulous alveolar ridge
- K13.4 Granuloma and granuloma-like lesions of oral mucosa

CLINICAL PEARLS

- Benign, vascular tumor, usually rapidly growing, that involves exposed areas, such as distal extremities and face, as well as in the oral cavity
- Excision must be adequate to avoid recurrence.
- Excisional biopsy recommended to ensure proper diagnosis and rule out malignancy
- Excision with primary closure is superior to shave excision with cautery in terms of recurrence risk, but both are effective.

G

GRAVES DISEASE

Angela Pauline Patawaran Calimag, MD, BSN, RN, MAN • Ruchita Patel, DO

 BASICS

DESCRIPTION

Autoimmune disease in which thyroid-stimulating hormone receptor (TSHR) activation by thyrotropin receptor antibodies (TRAb) cause increased thyroid hormone secretion. Most common cause of hyperthyroidism. Classic findings are thyrotoxicosis, diffuse goiter, ophthalmopathy (orbitopathy), and occasionally localized dermopathy (pretibial myxedema).

EPIDEMIOLOGY

Incidence
- Annual incidence of 20 to 50 cases per 100,000 persons (1)
- Peaks between 30 and 50 years of age, but people can be affected at any age
- Occurs in 0.2% of pregnancies, of which 95% is due to Graves disease

Prevalence
- Overall prevalence of hyperthyroidism in United States: ~2% for women and 0.2% for men
- Graves disease accounts for 60–80% of all cases of hyperthyroidism
- Synonym(s): von Basedow disease

ETIOLOGY AND PATHOPHYSIOLOGY
- Excessive production of thyroid-stimulating hormone (TSH) receptor antibodies from B cells primarily within the thyroid, likely due to genetic clonal lack of suppressor T cells
- Binding of these antibodies to TSH receptors in the thyroid activates the receptor, stimulating thyroid hormone synthesis and secretion as well as thyroid growth (leading to goiter).
- Binding to similar antigen in retro-orbital connective tissue causes ocular symptoms.

Genetics
- Higher risk with personal or family history of any autoimmune disease, especially Hashimoto thyroiditis
- Twin studies show concordance rate as high as 20%.

RISK FACTORS
- Female gender (5 to 10 times more than men)
- Postpartum period
- Family history (15% of patients with Graves disease have an affected relative)
- Medications: iodine, amiodarone, lithium, highly active antiretroviral (HAART); rarely, immune-modulating medications (e.g., interferon therapy)
- Smoking (higher risk of developing ophthalmopathy)

GENERAL PREVENTION
Screening TSH in asymptomatic patients is not recommended.

COMMONLY ASSOCIATED CONDITIONS
- Mitral valve prolapse
- Type 1 diabetes mellitus
- Addison disease, hypokalemic periodic paralysis
- Vitiligo, alopecia areata
- Other autoimmune disorders

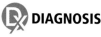 **DIAGNOSIS**

HISTORY
- Tachycardia, palpitations
- Tremor, restlessness

- Hyperactivity, anxiety, emotional lability, insomnia
- Sweating, heat intolerance
- Pruritus, skin changes
- Weight loss with increased appetite
- Fatigue, dyspnea (due to muscle weakness)
- Oligo-/amenorrhea (women), loss of libido, erectile dysfunction (men), gynecomastia
- Loose, frequent stools
- Blurred vision or diplopia, lacrimation, photophobia, gritty sensation in eyes (ocular dryness), retro-orbital discomfort, painful eye movement, loss of color vision or visual acuity
- Worsening of chronic medical conditions (anxiety, bipolar disorder, glucose intolerance, heart failure, or angina)

Geriatric Considerations
Elderly patients may not display classic symptoms; may present with atrial fibrillation, weight loss, or shortness of breath

PHYSICAL EXAM
- Ophthalmologic (present in 50% of cases): Grittiness/discomfort in the eyes, retrobulbar pressure/pain, lid lag/retraction, proptosis, ophthalmoplegia, papilledema, and loss of color vision may signify optic neuropathy.
- Thyroid: enlarged (goiter), nontender, and without nodules; possible bruit (increased blood flow)
- Integumentary: fine hair, warm skin, onycholysis, palmar erythema, brittle nails, clubbing of fingers, possible pretibial myxedema (orange peel appearance), possible hyperpigmented plaques (dermopathy)
- Cardiac: resting tachycardia, hyperdynamic circulation, possible atrial fibrillation
- Extremities: fine tremor, hyperreflexia, proximal myopathy; rarely, soft tissue edema of extremities and clubbing of digits (acropachy)

DIFFERENTIAL DIAGNOSIS
- Toxic multinodular goiter or toxic adenoma
- Thyroiditis (hormone leakage)
  - Subacute destructive thyroiditis, usually postviral (Thyroid will be tender.)
  - Lymphocytic, including postpartum
  - Hashimoto thyroiditis (Antithyroperoxidase [TPO] antibodies may stimulate TSH receptors.)
- Iatrogenic (treatment induced)
  - Iodine induced (dietary, radiographic contrast, or medications)
  - Amiodarone induced
  - Thyroid hormone overreplacement (accidental or intentional)
- Tumor
  - Pituitary adenoma–producing TSH
  - Human chorionic gonadotropin (hCG)-producing tumors (stimulate TSH receptors)
  - Extraglandular thyroid hormone production (e.g., struma ovarii or metastatic thyroid cancer)

DIAGNOSTIC TESTS & INTERPRETATION

Initial Tests (lab, imaging)
- TSH is initial test: suppressed (low or undetectable)
- TSH <0.1 mU/L has >98% sensitivity and >92% specificity in confirming suspected thyroid disease. Elevated free T_4 with low TSH confirms hyperthyroidism.
- T_3 maybe elevated as well in conjunction with free T_4 or isolated elevation, known as T_3 toxicosis.

Follow-Up Tests & Special Considerations
Thyroid peroxidase antibodies (present in 70–80% of patients with Graves disease) and TSH receptor antibodies (thyroid binding inhibitory immunoglobulin) may be useful in differentiating between Graves disease and toxic multinodular goiter.

Pregnancy Considerations
- Increase in serum T_4-binding globulin concentration and initial stimulation of TSH by hCG results in a total T_4 and T_3 rise during first half of pregnancy. The TSH level is decreased throughout pregnancy and should be compared to the trimester-specific ranges for pregnancy. Measurement of thyrotropin receptor autoantibody (TRAb) is positive in 95% of patients with Graves and should be used if diagnosis is unclear in pregnancy (2)[A].
- Ultrasonography is the primary modality of imaging during pregnancy.

Diagnostic Procedures/Other
- After confirming suppressed TSH and high T_4, perform radioactive iodine uptake (RAIU) and scan. Patients with Graves disease will have diffuse, elevated RAIU (vs. localized/nodular elevated uptake in adenoma and multinodular goiter and decreased uptake in thyroiditis or exogenous thyroid hormone).
- Thyroid ultrasound may be used to distinguish nodular forms of Graves disease from nodular nonautoimmune causes of hyperthyroidism.

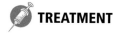 **TREATMENT**

GENERAL MEASURES
Choice of treatment modality is based on shared decision making between the medical provider and patient. The goal is to correct the hypermetabolic state with the fewest side effects and lowest incidence of posttreatment hypothyroidism.

MEDICATION

First Line
- Antithyroid drugs: methimazole (MMI) and propylthiouracil (PTU)
  - Compete with the thyroid for iodine, thereby decreasing the synthesis of thyroid hormone; propylthiouracil blocks peripheral conversion of T_4 to T_3.
  - Treatment of choice for children and for adults who refuse RAI
  - May use as pretreatment for older or cardiac patients before RAI or surgery
  - Methimazole is now almost exclusively used except during the 1st trimester of pregnancy. It has longer duration of action, allowing for once-daily dosing, more rapid efficacy, and lower incidence of side effects (3)[A].
  - Lowest effective dose of methimazole should be used (2)[B].
  - Minor side effects (<5% incidence): controlled by switching from one agent to another: skin rash (3–5%), fever, arthralgias, GI side effects
  - Major side effects necessitating change in treatment: polyarthritis (1–2%), idiopathic granulocytopenia (0.5%), and cholestasis/jaundice (rare)

- Optimal duration of antithyroid drugs is 12 to 18 months; no increased benefit to treatment beyond 18 months (4)[A].
- Relapse rates up to 50% in patients who respond initially; higher rates if smoker, large goiter, or positive thyroid-stimulating antibodies at end of treatment
- Radioactive Iodine (RAI)
  - Concentrates in the thyroid gland and destroys thyroid tissue
  - Radioiodine plus prednisone therapy might have the least probability of leading to an exacerbation or new appearance of ophthalmopathy, and radioiodine therapy might have the least probability of causing a recurrence (4)[A].
  - Treatment of choice for definitive therapy of hyperthyroidism, in the absence of moderate or severe orbitopathy (2)[A]
  - Risks: side effects (neck soreness, flushing, decreased taste); worsening ophthalmopathy (15% incidence, higher in smokers); posttreatment hypothyroidism (80% incidence, not dosage dependent); radiation thyroiditis (1% incidence); need to adhere to safety precautions until radiation is eliminated from the body
  - Pretreatment with antithyroid medication should be considered in patients with severe disease and the elderly, to reduce risk of posttreatment transient hyperthyroidism and posttreatment radiation thyroiditis.
  - May be repeated in as soon as 3 months if minimal response or after 6 months if not euthyroid (3)[A]

ISSUES FOR REFERRAL

- Endocrinologist for RAI therapy; if patient is pregnant or breastfeeding
- Ophthalmologist for Graves ophthalmopathy
- Surgeon if failed drug therapy or refusing RAI; obstruction or cosmesis

ADDITIONAL THERAPIES

- Graves hyperthyroidism
  - β-Blockers provide prompt control of adrenergic symptoms; start while workup is in progress (3)[A]. Long-acting propranolol is used most commonly and titrated to symptom control (40 to 160 mg/day).
  - Symptom control may be achieved with iodides, which block the conversion of T_4 to T_3 and inhibit TSH release. Use for pregnant patients who do not tolerate antithyroid medication or in conjunction with antithyroid medications; should not be used long term (may cause a paradoxical increase in TSH release) or in combination with RAI
  - IV corticosteroids are utilized when rapid control of thyrotoxicosis is needed, they inhibit deiodinase type 2 thereby inhibiting conversion of T_4 to T_3 (5).
  - Bile acid sequestrants are used as adjuncts with antithyroid drugs; its mechanism is binding of thyroid hormones in the enterohepatic circulation (5).
- Graves ophthalmopathy
  - For corneal protection: tinted glasses when outdoors, artificial tears, patching/taping the lids at night
  - For orbitopathy: Mild cases can be treated with lubricants, nocturnal ointments, botulinum toxin injection for upper lid retraction, and smoking cessation. Moderate to severe cases should be treated with pulse-dose IV glucocorticoid if no contraindications. Alternative is PO steroid (prednisone 60 to 80 mg/day for 2 to 4 weeks and then taper off).

- Newly approved by the FDA is the use of teprotumumab, which is a fully humanized monoclonal antibody inhibitor of insulin-like growth factor 1 receptor in patients with moderate to severe ophthalmopathy (5),(6),(7).
- Compressive optic neuropathy is a medical emergency managed with a combination of IV glucocorticoid, orbital irradiation, and surgical decompression (5),(6),(7).
- Graves dermopathy
  - For dermopathy, use medium- to high-potency topical corticosteroids with occlusive dressing.

SURGERY/OTHER PROCEDURES

- Indications for thyroidectomy include persistent or recurrent thyrotoxicosis, diffusely enlarged thyroid with compressive symptoms, concurrent hyperparathyroidism or thyroid cancer, nodular thyroid, active Graves ophthalmopathy, and 2nd-trimester pregnancy (5),(6),(7).
- Postoperative risks include ophthalmopathy progression, bleeding, permanent hypoparathyroidism, recurrent laryngeal nerve palsy—total thyroidectomy (TT) is consistent with subtotal thyroidectomy (ST) in patients with Graves disease. However, TT is associated with a reduced incidence of recurrent hyperthyroidism and results in an increase in temporary hypoparathyroidism (8)[A].

ADMISSION, INPATIENT, AND NURSING CONSIDERATIONS

ICU management for severe thyrotoxicosis with hemodynamic compromise (thyroid storm)

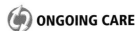 ONGOING CARE

FOLLOW-UP RECOMMENDATIONS

Patient Monitoring

Check TSH and T_4 levels every 1 to 2 months for the first 6 months after treatment, then every 3 months for a year, and then every 6 to 12 months thereafter. For patients on treatment with propylthiouracil and methimazole, check CBC yearly. Also, check anti-TSH receptor antibodies at 12 months of treatment to determine possibility of discontinuing medication.

Pregnancy Considerations

- RAI is contraindicated in pregnancy and during breastfeeding.
- Propylthiouracil is preferred in 1st trimester of pregnancy due to teratogenic effects of methimazole. Switch to methimazole in 2nd and 3rd trimesters due to risk of PTU-induced hepatotoxicity (9)[A].
- Postpartum exacerbation of hyperthyroidism is common for women not currently under treatment, so TSH and symptoms should be monitored.

PATIENT EDUCATION

Adherence to both follow-up surveillance and medication regimens

PROGNOSIS

- Generally good with treatment, although may have irreversible ocular, cardiac, and psychiatric consequences
- Increased morbidity and mortality due to osteoporosis, atherosclerotic disease, insulin resistance and obesity, and endothelial cell dysfunction (thromboembolic risk)

COMPLICATIONS

The percentage of patients with Graves disease who become hypothyroid within the 1st year after treatment varies with treatment modality.

REFERENCES

1. Smith T, Hegedus L. Graves' disease. *N Engl J Med*. 2016;375(16):1552–1565.
2. Ren Z, Qin L, Wang JQ, et al. Comparative efficacy of four treatments in patients with Graves' disease: a network meta-analysis. *Exp Clin Endocrinol Diabetes*. 2015;123(5):317–322.
3. Bahn Chair RS, Burch HB, Cooper DS, et al; for American Thyroid Association and American Association of Clinical Endocrinologists. Hyperthyroidism and other causes of thyrotoxicosis: management guidelines of the American Thyroid Association and American Association of Clinical Endocrinologists. *Thyroid*. 2011;21(6):593–646.
4. Abraham P, Avenell A, McGeoch SC, et al. Antithyroid drug regimen for treating Graves' hyperthyroidism. *Cochrane Database Syst Rev*. 2010;(1):CD003420.
5. Kotwal A, Stan M. Current and future treatments for Graves' disease and Graves' ophthalmopathy. *Horm Metab Res*. 2018;50(12):871–886.
6. Kahaly GJ. Management of Graves thyroidal and extrathyroidal disease: an update. *J Clin Endocrinol Metab*. 2020;105(12):3704–3720.
7. Dosiou C, Kossler AL. Thyroid eye disease: navigating the new treatment landscape. *J Endocr Soc*. 2021;5(5):bvab034.
8. Guo Z, Yu P, Liu Z, et al. Total thyroidectomy vs bilateral subtotal thyroidectomy in patients with Graves' diseases: a meta-analysis of randomized clinical trials. *Clin Endocrinol (Oxf)*. 2013;79(5):739–746.
9. Stagnaro-Green A, Abalovich M, Alexander E, et al; for American Thyroid Association Taskforce on Thyroid Disease During Pregnancy and Postpartum. Guidelines of the American Thyroid Association for the diagnosis and management of thyroid disease during pregnancy and postpartum. *Thyroid*. 2011;21(10):1081–1125.

 SEE ALSO

Algorithms: Anxiety; Cardiac Arrhythmias; Weight Loss, Unintentional

 CODES

ICD10

- E05.00 Thyrotoxicosis w diffuse goiter w/o thyrotoxic crisis
- E05.01 Thyrotoxicosis w diffuse goiter w thyrotoxic crisis or storm
- E05.20 Thyrotoxicosis w toxic multinod goiter w/o thyrotoxic crisis

CLINICAL PEARLS

- Graves disease accounts for 60–80% of all cases of hyperthyroidism.
- Potential morbidities of hyperthyroidism include ophthalmopathy, atrial fibrillation, congestive heart failure (CHF), stroke, seizure, and osteopenia/osteoporosis.

G

GUILLAIN-BARRÉ SYNDROME
Grant M. Reed, DO • John J. Whitney, BS

BASICS

DESCRIPTION
- A group of acquired autoimmune disorders causing acute peripheral neuropathy and ascending paralysis that progressively worsens for up to 4 weeks followed by a slow spontaneous recovery of function
- Subtypes classified by pattern of neural injury:
  - *Acute inflammatory demyelinating polyradiculoneuropathy (AIDP)*: progressive limb weakness with areflexia (~95% of GBS cases in Europe and North America)
  - Axonal subtypes:
    - *Acute motor axonal neuropathy (AMAN)*: pure motor neuropathy strongly associated with *Campylobacter jejuni* and a higher rate of respiratory failure (~5% of cases in Europe and North America but 30–47% of cases in China, Japan, and Central and South America)
    - *Acute motor-sensory axonal neuropathy (AMSAN)*: combined motor-sensory neuropathy; poor prognosis with prolonged course
  - Regional subtypes:
    - *Miller Fisher syndrome (MFS)*: triad with ophthalmoplegia, ataxia, and areflexia; antibodies to GQ1b present in 90% of patients with MFS
    - *Bickerstaff encephalitis*: possible variant of MFS with encephalopathy, ophthalmoplegia, ataxia, and hyperreflexia
    - *Pharyngeal-cervical-brachial GBS*: Parasympathetic and cholinergic dysfunction leads to neck, arm, and oropharyngeal weakness along with upper extremity areflexia.
  - Sensory subtypes:
    - *Acute pandysautonomia*: orthostatic hypotension, gastroparesis, ileus, constipation/diarrhea, sudomotor/pupillary abnormalities, and neuropathic pain
    - *Acute sensory ataxic neuropathy (ASAN)*: controversial variant with sensory loss and ataxia
- *Polyneuritis cranialis*: bilateral cranial nerve involvement and severe peripheral sensory loss associated with cytomegalovirus (CMV) infections
- Synonym(s): GBS, AIDP; Landry-Guillain-Barré-Strohl syndrome, acute inflammatory idiopathic polyneuritis; acute autoimmune neuropathy; Landry ascending paralysis

ALERT
Rapidly progressing paralysis and respiratory failure occur in 20–30% of patients. Some require mechanical ventilation within 48 hours.

ALERT
Areflexia is a red flag for GBS in patients with rapidly progressive limb weakness.

ALERT
A history of weakness preceded by respiratory or GI infection suggests GBS.

EPIDEMIOLOGY
Incidence
- Most common acute paralytic disease in Western countries
- 0.6 to 2.0/100,000 worldwide
- U.S. incidence: 0.9 to 1.8/100,000
- Increases with age: 0.8/100,000 in children <18 years of age; 3/100,000 in adults >60 years
- 1.5 times higher incidence in males

ETIOLOGY AND PATHOPHYSIOLOGY
- Postinfectious autoimmune process targets Schwann cell surface membrane, myelin, and/or gangliosides causing peripheral nerve destruction and demyelination.
- Pathogenesis thought to involve molecular mimicry (i.e., an immune response to antigenic targets that are coincidentally shared by infectious organisms and host peripheral nerve tissue). Antibodies cross-react with GM1 myelin ganglioside with resultant damage to peripheral nervous system.

Genetics
Host factors appear to play a role in GBS, but no clear genetic risk has been identified.

RISK FACTORS
- COVID-19 vaccinations
  - A systematic review study showed a GBS rate of 1.8 to 53 cases per 1 million doses with the Pfizer, Johnson & Johnson, and Sinovac coronavirus vaccines.
- Influenza vaccinations
  - Inactivated seasonal flu vaccines associated with an increase in GBS risk equivalent to one case/million vaccines above background incidence (far less than the 17 cases of GBS per million people *infected* with influenza virus).
  - Incidence of GBS associated with flu vaccine decreasing over time with no increase detected in 2017 to 2018 season
  - *Of historical note*: Increased incidence during 1976 National H1N1 Immunization Program had vaccine-attributable risk of 8.8 per million recipients compared to 1.6 per million recipients in the 2009 H1N1 vaccination campaign.

COMMONLY ASSOCIATED CONDITIONS
Infection of the respiratory (22–53%) or gastrointestinal (GI) tract (6–26%) in preceding 6 weeks
- *Campylobacter jejuni*: most common precipitant of GBS, (21–40% of cases):
  - Associated with axonal degeneration, slower recovery, more severe residual disability
- CMV: Primary CMV infection precedes 10–22% of cases.
- Rarely associated with *Mycoplasma pneumoniae*, influenza infection, Epstein-Barr virus, varicella-zoster virus, HIV infection, zika virus, and some arboviral infections

DIAGNOSIS

HISTORY
- AIDP presents with onset of progressive limb weakness that reaches its worst within 4 weeks (73% reach a functional nadir in 1 week; 98% by 1 month).
- Preceding respiratory or GI infection
- Earliest symptoms include pain, numbness, paresthesias, or proximal muscle weakness that can spread to involve cranial nerves and muscles of respiration.
- Cranial nerve symptoms: facial nerve palsy; diplopia; dysarthria; dysphagia; ophthalmoplegia
- Neuropathic pain, sometimes severe, occurs in 30–50%, most commonly in the back and lower extremities.
- Purely sensory symptoms exclude GBS.

PHYSICAL EXAM
Diagnostic criteria for typical GBS:
- Required for diagnosis:
  - Progressive weakness reaching nadir between 12 hours and 28 days
  - Affects >1 limb
  - Areflexia/hyporeflexia
- Strongly supportive:
  - Paresthesias with only mild changes in objective sensory function (e.g., pinprick, light touch)
  - Relative symmetry
  - Cranial nerve involvement, especially bilateral/symmetric weakness of facial muscles
  - Recovery beginning within 4 weeks after progression ceases
  - Autonomic dysfunction (tachycardia, bradycardia, facial flushing, hypertension, hypotension, anhidrosis, diaphoresis); urinary retention; diarrhea; constipation
  - Absence of fever at onset

DIFFERENTIAL DIAGNOSIS
Differential diagnosis of acute flaccid paralysis:
- Brain: basilar artery stroke, brainstem encephalitis
- Spinal cord: transverse myelitis, spinal cord compression
- Motor neuron: poliomyelitis, acute flaccid myelitis
- Peripheral neuropathy other than GBS: vasculitis, critical illness polyneuropathy, infectious disease (e.g., diphtheria, Lyme disease; HIV), chronic inflammatory demyelinating polyradiculoneuropathy (CIDP), acute intermittent porphyria
- Neuromuscular junction: myasthenia gravis, Eaton-Lambert syndrome, botulism, toxins (e.g., heavy metals, inhalant abuse, organophosphates)
- Muscle: electrolyte disturbance (hypokalemia, hypophosphatemia), inflammatory myopathy, critical illness myopathy, acute rhabdomyolysis, trichinosis, periodic paralysis
- Psychological causes of weakness

DIAGNOSTIC TESTS & INTERPRETATION
Initial Tests (lab, imaging)
- Studies to establish the diagnosis:
  - Lumbar puncture (LP): Increased CSF protein (most patients with GBS will have CSF protein >400 mg/L) without pleocytosis is present in ~80% of cases (Note: CSF protein is often normal within the first 48 hours of symptom onset).
  - Nerve conduction study (NCS): *Most useful confirmatory test*; conduction velocities abnormal in 85% of patients with demyelination, even early in the disease. If nondiagnostic, repeat after 1 to 2 weeks.
- Imaging generally not required. MRI demonstrates spinal nerve root and/or cauda equina enhancement.
- Studies to find underlying cause:
  - Stool culture and serology for *C. jejuni*
  - Acute and convalescent serology for CMV, EBV, HIV, and *M. pneumoniae*
  - Anti-GQ1b antibodies in MFS variant and anti-GM1 antibodies in AMAN
  - Peripheral neuropathy: TFT; rheumatoid factor, B12/folate; hemoglobin A1C; ESR; RPR; heavy metal assay

Follow-Up Tests & Special Considerations
- Analyze CSF prior to treatment with intravenous immunoglobulin (IVIG), which can cause aseptic meningitis.
- A repeat NCS 3 to 8 weeks after onset can classify the subtype of GBS.

Diagnostic Procedures/Other

Sural nerve biopsy not indicated except to rule out vasculitis or amyloidosis

 TREATMENT

GENERAL MEASURES
- Consider admission to ensure that disease does not progress (respiratory function; autonomic stability; paralysis).
- Supportive care is essential, paying close attention to complications of immobility, neurogenic bladder/ bowel, and pain management.
- Pain treatment: NSAIDs helpful but often insufficient. Gabapentin and carbamazepine decrease opioid requirements in patients with GBS. One is not superior to others (1)[A].
- DVT prophylaxis recommended in nonambulatory patients (2)[C]
- Neostigmine or erythromycin may be effective for ileus, if present (2)[C].

MEDICATION
First Line
- IVIG 0.4 g/kg/day for 5 days or (less commonly) 1 g/kg/day for 2 days
  - In severe disease, IVIG started within 2 weeks of onset hastens recovery as much as plasma exchange (PE) (3)[A].
  - In children, IVIG hastens recovery compared with supportive care alone (3)[A].
  - Combined treatment with IVIG and PE confers no clinically significant benefit (3)[A].
- PE:
  - Compared with supportive treatment alone, those treated with PE are quicker to recover walking (NNT 7), have less requirement and shorter duration for mechanical ventilation (NNT 8), recover full muscle strength more quickly (NNT 8), and have fewer severe sequelae at 1 year (NNT 17) (4)[A].
  - Higher risks of relapse found with PE versus supportive care with no difference in severe infection or mortality (4)[A]
  - In mild GBS, two sessions of PE are superior to none. In moderate GBS, four sessions are superior to two. In severe GBS, six sessions are not significantly better than four (4)[A].
  - PE is most beneficial if started within 7 days of disease onset. PE still helpful up to 30 days (4)[A].
  - Value of PE in children <12 is unknown.

Second Line
- Corticosteroids: not beneficial as monotherapy or as combined treatment. Low-quality evidence suggests steroids delay recovery (5)[A].
- CSF filtration is no different than PE (6)[B].
- Interferon-β and brain-derived neurotrophic factor no different than placebo (6)[B]

ADDITIONAL THERAPIES
- Physical and occupational therapy improves fatigue and functional abilities (2)[C].
- Speech and language therapy improves swallowing function, if affected (2)[C].

COMPLEMENTARY & ALTERNATIVE MEDICINE
Tripterygium polyglycoside hastened recovery significantly more than corticosteroids (NNT 4), in one small trial (6)[A].

ADMISSION, INPATIENT, AND NURSING CONSIDERATIONS
- Admit patients with suspected GBS.
- Closely monitor respiratory status with serial measurement of vital capacity (VC) and static inspiratory and expiratory pressures (PI_{max} and PE_{max}).
- Predictors of respiratory failure:
  - Rapid progression: ≥3 days between onset of weakness and hospital admission
  - Facial and/or bulbar weakness
  - VC decrease >30%
  - Medical Research Council (MRC) sum score indicating muscle weakness: 0 to 5/5 muscle strength grading for bilateral upper arm abductors, elbow flexors, wrist extensors, hip flexors, knee extensors, and foot dorsal flexors totaling 60 points
- Indications for intubation:
  - VC <20 mL/kg
  - PI_{max} <30 cm H_2O
  - PE_{max} <40 cm H_2O
- Prevent complications of immobilization with DVT prophylaxis and frequent turning.
- Respiratory care, aspiration precautions, pulmonary toilet
- Monitor bowel and bladder function for ileus and urinary retention.
- Begin immediate physical therapy to preserve passive range of motion.
- Mildly affected patients who can walk unaided and are stable for >2 weeks are unlikely to experience disease progression and may be managed as outpatients. Monitor bowel and bladder function for ileus and urinary retention.

 ONGOING CARE

FOLLOW-UP RECOMMENDATIONS
Patient Monitoring
- Patients require close monitoring of respiratory, cardiac, and hemodynamic function, typically in the ICU setting.
- Pulmonary function testing (VC, respiratory frequency) q2–6h in the progressive phase and q6–12h in the plateau phase
- Monitor bulbar weakness and ability to handle airway secretions.
- Telemetry in patients with severe disease

PATIENT EDUCATION
Emphasize expectation for significant recovery and explain phases of illness.

PROGNOSIS
- If untreated, three phases of illness:
  - Initial progressive phase up to 4 weeks with highest risk of death and complication
  - Variable plateau phase
  - Recovery phase (weeks to months): return of proximal then distal strength
- Most recovery occurs within the first year.
- 80% recover within 6 to 12 months with maximum 18 months past onset.
- 20–39% with residual disability after 1 year:
  - Bilateral footdrop, intrinsic hand muscle wasting, sensory ataxia, dysesthesia, fatigue, musculoskeletal pain
  - Half of these with severe disability

- Factors associated with poor functional outcome:
  - Age >60 years, rapid progression, severe disease, severe disability on either admission or discharge, preceding diarrhea, male sex, positive *C. jejuni* or CMV serology, axonal degeneration, need for mechanical ventilation

COMPLICATIONS
- 3–7% mortality in Europe and North America. Older patients, those with severe disease have highest risk.
- 20–30% require mechanical ventilation.
- 70% develop autonomic dysfunction with hemodynamic instability, urinary retention, ileus, and anhidrosis.
- 10% have relapse.
- ~2% develop relapsing CIDP.

REFERENCES
1. Liu J, Wang LN, McNicol ED. Pharmacological treatment for pain in Guillain-Barré syndrome. *Cochrane Database Syst Rev*. 2015;(4):CD009950.
2. Hughes RA, Wijdicks EF, Benson E, et al; for Multidisciplinary Consensus Group. Supportive care for patients with Guillain-Barré syndrome. *Arch Neurol*. 2005;62(8):1194–1198.
3. Hughes RA, Swan AV, van Doorn PA. Intravenous immunoglobulin for Guillain-Barré syndrome. *Cochrane Database Syst Rev*. 2014;(9):CD002063.
4. Chevret S, Hughes RA, Annane D, et al. Plasma exchange for Guillain-Barré syndrome. *Cochrane Database Syst Rev*. 2017;2(2):CD001798.
5. Hughes RA, Brassington R, Gunn AA, et al. Corticosteroids for Guillain-Barré syndrome. *Cochrane Database Syst Rev*. 2016;10(10):CD001446.
6. Pritchard J, Hughes RA, Hadden RD, et al. Pharmacological treatment other than corticosteroids, intravenous immunoglobulin and plasma exchange for Guillain-Barré syndrome. *Cochrane Database Syst Rev*. 2016;11(11):CD008630.

ADDITIONAL READING
- Shao S, Wang C, Chang KC, et al. Guillain-Barré syndrome associated with COVID-19 vaccination [published online ahead of print October 14, 2021]. *Emerg Infect Dis*. 2021;27(12):3175–3178. doi:10.3201/eid2712.211634
- Vellozzi C, Iqbal S, Broder K. Guillain-Barre syndrome, influenza, and influenza vaccination: the epidemiologic evidence. *Clin Infect Dis*. 2014;58(8):1149–1155.
- Willison HJ, Jacobs BC, van Doorn PA. Guillain-Barre syndrome. *Lancet*. 2016;388(10045):717–727.

CODES

ICD10
G61.0 Guillain-Barré syndrome

CLINICAL PEARLS
- Suspect GBS in cases of ascending flaccid paralysis with areflexia and an antecedent history of viral respiratory illness or gastroenteritis.
- When GBS is suspected, evaluate VC and inspiratory force for signs of respiratory compromise.
- Uncomplicated GBS has a slow spontaneous recovery. Treatment with IVIG or PE speeds rate of recovery and reduces disability.
- The most useful diagnostic tests for GBS are nerve conduction studies and lumbar puncture.
- GBS risk following native influenza virus infection is 40 to 70 times greater than after seasonal influenza vaccination.

G

GYNECOMASTIA

Franklyn C. Babb, MD, FAAFP

BASICS

DESCRIPTION
- Benign glandular proliferation of male breast tissue
- Increase in estrogen activity relative to androgen leads to the development of gynecomastia.
- Gynecomastia can be transient and may represent the normal physiologic changes that occur in utero or in adolescence. However, gynecomastia presenting or persisting in adulthood is typically pathologic in nature.
- Pseudogynecomastia which is lipomastia (subareolar fat)

EPIDEMIOLOGY
- 60–90% of infants and 50–60% of pubertal males have transient gynecomastia.
- Up to 70% of men between 50 and 69 years of age report gynecomastia.

Incidence
A study out of Bulgaria in 2007 put the incidence of pubertal gynecomastia at 3.9% in Caucasian boys ages 10 to 19 years.

Prevalence
Prevalence in adolescents varies from 22% to 69% and in adult males ranges from 36% to 57% (1).

ETIOLOGY AND PATHOPHYSIOLOGY
Multiple factors can alter the estrogen to androgen ratio and precipitate gynecomastia:
- Decrease in androgen production
- Increase in estrogen production
- Increase in peripheral conversion to estrogen
- Inhibition of the androgen receptor
- Increase in the level of sex hormone–binding globulin (SHBG) or the affinity of androgens to SHBG (decreases free or bioavailable testosterone)
- Displacement of estrogen relative to testosterone from SHBG due to medications

RISK FACTORS
Gynecomastia can be physiologic or pathologic in nature.
- Physiologic gynecomastia presents in infants and adolescent boys and resolves spontaneously.
  - Neonatal gynecomastia: The placenta converts dehydroepiandrosterone (DHEA) and dehydro-epiandrosterone sulfate (DHEA-S) to estrone and estradiol resulting in transient gynecomastia.
  - Adolescent gynecomastia: Transient increases in estradiol levels at the onset of puberty lead to gynecomastia.
- Pathologic gynecomastia: persistent or adult-onset gynecomastia. 25% of cases are idiopathic, most secondary to age-associated decline in free testosterone and adipose tissue–mediated aromatase activity.

ALERT
- Illicit drugs: marijuana, heroin, methadone, alcohol, amphetamines, and over-the-counter bodybuilding supplements
- Hormones: androgens, anabolic steroids, estrogens, estrogen agonist, and human chorionic gonadotropin (hCG)
- Antiandrogens or inhibitors of androgen synthesis: bicalutamide, flutamide, nilutamide, cyproterone, and GnRH agonists (leuprolide and goserelin)
- Anti-infectives: metronidazole, ketoconazole, minocycline, isoniazid
- Antiulcer medications: cimetidine, ranitidine, metoclopramide, and proton pump inhibitors
- Cytotoxic agents: methotrexate, alkylating agents, and vinca alkaloids
- Cardiovascular drugs: Digoxin, spironolactone, calcium channel blockers, ACE inhibitors, amiodarone, methyldopa, reserpine, minoxidil, and recently statins can be added to this list.
- Psychoactive drugs: antidepressants, benzodiazepines, phenothiazines, antipsychotics (typical and atypical) (i.e., haloperidol and risperidone)
- Medications: HIV medications like efavirenz, phenytoin, penicillamine, sulindac, or theophylline
- Causes to rule out:
  - Primary hypogonadism: androgen insensitivity syndromes (defect in the androgen receptor), Klinefelter syndrome
  - Testicular tumor: germ cell (secretes hCG), Leydig cell (secretes estrogen), Sertoli cell (excessive aromatization to estrogens)
  - Adrenal tumors (secrete DHEA-S and estrogens)
  - Ectopic hCG tumors (hepatoblastoma, gastric tumors, renal cell carcinomas)
  - Cirrhosis
  - Secondary hypogonadism: Kallmann syndrome or prolactinemia, which can also stimulate milk production in breast tissue
  - Hyperthyroidism
  - Renal disease or dialysis
  - Malnutrition/starvation
  - Rare (true hermaphroditism [both testicular and ovarian tissue present])

Pediatric Considerations
Transient gynecomastia is seen in neonates or pubertal boys; typically resolves within 6 to 24 months

Geriatric Considerations
Medications and age-associated decline in testosterone production and increase in SHBG production leads to low free testosterone levels. The increased ratio of fat mass to lean mass leads to adipose tissue–mediated peripheral conversion of androgens to estrogen.

COMMONLY ASSOCIATED CONDITIONS
- Prostate carcinoma—treatment estrogen and antiandrogen leads to gynecomastia in 50–75% of patients.
- Cirrhosis
- Primary hypogonadism; especially Klinefelter syndrome—primary hypogonadism; at risk for breast cancer
- Testicular tumors; Leydig or Sertoli cell tumors especially when associated with Peutz-Jeghers syndrome or Carney complex

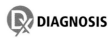 DIAGNOSIS

HISTORY
- If suspicious of hypogonadism, ask about erectile dysfunction, muscle mass, and decreased shaving frequency and libido.
- Obtain a family history including Carney complex and Peutz-Jeghers syndrome.
- Review medication list extensively and inquire about the use of illicit substances.
- Herbal supplements, marijuana use, and over-the-counter cimetidine or other H_2 antagonist use

PHYSICAL EXAM
- Careful breast exam to evaluate characteristics:
  - Firm, concentric glandular tissue beneath the nipple and areola palpable by pinching the thumb and forefinger together from either side of the breast toward the nipple. Diameter of this tissue for diagnostic purposes ranges from >0.5 to >2.0 cm, but the most recent large study recommended 1.0 cm as the diagnostic criteria.
  - May involve one or both breasts
  - Usually asymptomatic but may be painful or tender if it is of recent onset
  - Off center, hard, fixed mass is concerning for malignancy, although palpation of subareolar fat is more consistent with pseudogynecomastia.
  - Breast discharge should raise concern for malignancy or prolactinemia. In the latter, the discharge is typically clear or milky.
- Thyroid exam
- Abdominal exam (Evaluate for masses and liver size.)
- Genitourinary exam (Evaluate for testicular size, hair pattern, and presence of ovary or uterus.)
- Visual field exam (Evaluate for peripheral field defect.)

DIFFERENTIAL DIAGNOSIS
- Pseudogynecomastia—fat deposition without glandular proliferation often seen in obesity
- Breast cancer—typically unilateral; firm; eccentric to the nipple; skin dimpling, nipple retraction/discharge, and lymphadenopathy
- Lipomas, sebaceous cyst, dermoid cyst, mastitis, hematoma, hamartoma

DIAGNOSTIC TESTS & INTERPRETATION
Laboratory and radiologic investigations should be tailored to fit history and physical exam findings.

Initial Tests (lab, imaging)
- Luteinizing hormone (LH)—elevated in primary hypogonadism and decreased in secondary hypogonadism
- Morning total and free testosterone—decreased testosterone level in hypogonadism
- hCG—elevated in germ cell tumors and ectopic hCG tumors
- Estradiol —elevated in Leydig cell tumors, Sertoli cell tumors, adrenal tumors, and with increased aromatase activity
- DHEA-S levels, which can be increased in adrenal tumors
- Urine for drugs of abuse (UDA)
- Other tests to consider include creatinine, liver function test, thyroid function tests, and prolactin.

Diagnostic Procedures/Other
Consider biopsy to rule out malignancy (i.e., off center, hard, fixed, discharge).

Test Interpretation
- Elevated hCG: Check testicular ultrasound. If positive for a mass, likely a testicular germ cell tumor. If the ultrasound is negative, consider extragonadal germ cell tumor or hCG-secreting neoplasm and order a CXR and CT abdomen.
- Elevated LH: if in relation to low testosterone, likely primary hypogonadism. If elevated in relation to high testosterone, check thyroid-stimulating hormone (TSH) and free thyroxine (FT$_4$). If FT$_4$ is elevated and TSH is suppressed, likely hyperthyroidism; if TSH and FT$_4$ are normal, likely androgen resistance
- Normal or decreased LH in relation to low testosterone: Check prolactin level. If prolactin is elevated, likely due to a prolactin-secreting pituitary tumor (need MRI); if normal, likely due to secondary hypogonadism
- Normal or decreased LH in relation to increased estradiol: Check testicular ultrasound. If positive for a mass, likely Leydig or Sertoli cell tumor. If negative for mass, check CT abdomen to evaluate the adrenals. If mass is present, possible adrenal neoplasm versus adenoma; if no mass is detected, then likely due to increased aromatase activity in extraglandular tissue

 TREATMENT

GENERAL MEASURES
- Gynecomastia usually regresses spontaneously within 6 months of onset. Monitor for the first 6 months.
- Neonatal and pubertal gynecomastia spontaneously resolves within 6 to 24 months. Persistent pubertal gynecomastia (>24 months) occurs in 8% of pubertal boys. In adult males, 75% of gynecomastia is secondary to persistent pubertal gynecomastia, medications, and idiopathic conditions. Only 25% is related to an underlying medical condition.
- All illicit drug use and offending medications should be stopped if appropriate.
- Treat underlying medical conditions (i.e., testosterone replacement for hypogonadal men, dopamine agonist for prolactinoma, appropriate treatment for thyrotoxicosis, and tumor resection).

MEDICATION
There are no U.S. Food and Drug Administration–approved medications for the treatment of gynecomastia.
- SERMs: Clinical trials of both tamoxifen (10 to 20 mg/day) and raloxifene (60 mg/day) showed partial reduction in pubertal gynecomastia and successful resolution of idiopathic gynecomastia in 90% of study participants after 3 to 9 months.
- Aromatase inhibitors block peripheral conversion of androgens to estrogens. In prostate cancer patients, anastrozole prevented the development of gynecomastia in patients undergoing androgen deprivation therapy.

ADDITIONAL THERAPIES
In clinical trials, prophylactic radiotherapy prevented the development of gynecomastia in prostate cancer patients on androgen deprivation therapy.

SURGERY/OTHER PROCEDURES
Surgery can be recommended if gynecomastia does not regress within 12 months either spontaneously or after medical therapy, significant discomfort (i.e., pain, tenderness), it causes embarrassment or anxiety, and if biopsy is suspicious for malignancy.

 ONGOING CARE

FOLLOW-UP RECOMMENDATIONS
Patient Monitoring
Every 3 to 6 months for 24 months; consider medical therapy (i.e., tamoxifen) if severe, painful symptoms persist after 6 to 12 months and surgery after 12 to 24 months. In individuals with asymptomatic or mild disease, routine yearly breast and physical exam is recommended.

PATIENT EDUCATION
Patients should be reassured of the benign nature of gynecomastia in almost all cases.

PROGNOSIS
- Good in physiologic cases because they often regress spontaneously within 3 to 6 months
- Majority of patients experience regression once underlying disorder is treated or offending agents are eliminated.
- The majority of patients, who undergo surgery, are satisfied with the postoperative cosmetic appearance.

REFERENCE
1. Kanakis GA, Nordkap L, Bang AK, et al. EAA clinical practice guidelines-gynecomastia evaluation and management. *Andrology.* 2019;7(6):778–793.

 SEE ALSO

Algorithm: Gynecomastia

 CODES

ICD10
N62 Hypertrophy of breast

CLINICAL PEARLS
- Gynecomastia can be transient and may represent normal physiologic changes in neonates or adolescents. Gynecomastia presenting or persisting in adulthood is pathologic.
- Lab and radiologic studies associated with gynecomastia including thyrotoxicosis, prolactinemia, hypogonadism, testicular tumors, adrenal tumors, and ectopic hCG tumors.
- ~25% of gynecomastia is idiopathic in nature, and treatment should focus on symptom control.
- Clinical trials of SERMs, aromatase inhibitors, and radiation therapy seem promising. Surgery is the treatment of choice for refractory gynecomastia.

G

HAMMER TOES
Neil Feldman, DPM

BASICS

Contraction deformities of the toes

DESCRIPTION
- Hammer toes include three distinct types of deformity.
  - Hammer toe (as defined) involves a plantar flexion deformity of the proximal interphalangeal (PIP) joint with varying degrees of hyperextension of the metatarsophalangeal (MTP) and distal interphalangeal (DIP) joint, primarily in sagittal plane (1).
  - Claw toe involves a plantar flexion deformity of the PIP and DIP joint with varying degrees of hyperextension of the MTP.
  - Mallet toe involves a plantar flexion deformity of the DIP joint only.
- Each can be flexible, semirigid, or fixed.
  - Flexible: passively correctable to neutral position
  - Semirigid: partially correctable to neutral position
  - Fixed: not correctable to neutral position without intervention

EPIDEMIOLOGY
Most common deformity of lesser digits, typically affecting only one or two toes:
- 2nd toe is the most commonly involved.
- Hallux malleus is term used when the great toe (hallux) is involved.

Incidence
- Undefined
- Increases with age, duration of deformity (from flexible to rigid)

Prevalence
- Predominant sex: female > male (2)
  - Female predominance from 2.5:1 to 9:1, depending on age group
- Can range from 1% to 20% of population studied
- Blacks are more often affected than whites (2).

ETIOLOGY AND PATHOPHYSIOLOGY
- Can be congenital or acquired
- Three categories of acquired hammer toes:
  - Flexor stabilization (most common cause and occurs in pronated foot/foot with pes planus). The flexor digitorum longus (FDL) muscle remains overactive, overutilizing the toes to assist in relative foot instability.
  - Extensor substitution (most common with pes cavus). Occurs during the swing phase of gait. The extensor digitorum longus (EDL) muscle remains overactive, substituting for dysfunctional hip and ankle extensors.
  - Flexor substitution. Least common cause and seen commonly with pes cavus. The FDL muscle remains overactive with relative weakness/dysfunction to the Achilles and flexor hallucis longus (FHL), which are the main foot flexors.
- Biomechanical dysfunction results in muscle/tendon imbalance between the EDL tendon at the PIP joint and the FDL tendon at the MTP joint; the imbalance at the MTP joint level leads to the altering of the stabilizing force of the intrinsic muscles inserting into the extensor sling and wing apparatus of the MTP joint. In the case of classic hammer toes, the toe(s) sublux dorsally as the MTP hyperextends. This results in plantar flexion of the PIP joint and hyperextension of the MTP joint (2).

- Specific pathomechanics vary by etiology:
  - Toe length discrepancy or narrow footwear toe box induces PIP joint flexion by forcing digit to accommodate shoe.
    - May also lead to MTP joint synovitis secondary to overuse, with elongation of plantar plate and MTP joint hyperextension
    - 4th and 5th toes commonly assume an adducto-varus attitude, which can make the toes appear to sit on their side.
  - Rheumatoid arthritis (RA) causes MTP joint destruction and resultant subluxation.
  - Any condition that compromises intra-articular and periarticular tissues, such as second ray longer than first, inflammatory joint disease, neuromuscular conditions, improper-fitting shoes, and trauma (3)
  - Damage to joint capsule, collateral ligaments, or synovia leads to unstable PIP joint or MTP joint.

Genetics
- Significant heritability rates of 49–90% (4)
- Specific genetic markers are not identified.

RISK FACTORS
- Pes cavus, pes planus
- Hallux valgus
- Metatarsus adductus
- Ankle equinus
- Neuromuscular disease (rare)
- Trauma; improperly fitted shoes (narrow toe box) and/or tight hosiery
- Abnormal metatarsal and/or digit length
- Inflammatory joint disease (e.g., RA)
- Connective tissue disease
- Diabetes mellitus

GENERAL PREVENTION
- Proper fitting of shoes. Use of pressure-dispersive footwear helps reduce pain.
- Foot orthoses modulate biomechanical dysfunction and muscular imbalance, preventing progression (2).
- Limiting use of shoes in the growing foot. Use of zero drop shoes when necessary. Traditional shoes have an elevated heel relative to the ball of the foot (MTP joints). Therefore, at rest, the toes are positioned in dorsal subluxation at the MTP joints and forced to be contracted (termed toe spring).
- Perform toe strengthening exercises, which will help with prevention of imbalance between the extrinsic muscles of the calf and the intrinsic muscles of the foot.
- Control of predisposing factors (e.g., inflammatory joint disease) may also slow progression.

COMMONLY ASSOCIATED CONDITIONS
- Hallux valgus
- Cavus foot (pes cavus)
- Flat foot (pes planus)
- Metatarsus adductus
- Dorsal callus

DIAGNOSIS

History and physical exam are typically sufficient for diagnosis of hammer toes. Additional tests are available to exclude other conditions.

HISTORY
- Location, duration, severity, and rate of progression of foot deformity
- Type, location, duration of pain
  - Patients often relate sensation of lump on plantar aspect of MTP joint.
- Degree of functional impairment
- Improving/exacerbating factors
- Type of footwear and hosiery worn
- Peripheral neurologic symptoms
- Any prior treatment rendered

PHYSICAL EXAM
- Note MTP joint hyperextension, PIP joint flexion, and DIP joint extension or flexion.
- Observe any adjacent toe deformities (e.g., hallux valgus, flexion contractures).
- Assess degree of flexibility and reducibility of deformity in both weight-bearing and non–weight-bearing positions (2).
- Note any hyperkeratosis over the joint, ulcers, clavi (dorsal PIP joint, metatarsal head), adventitious bursa, erythema, or skin breakdown or ulceration (2).
- Palpate for pain over dorsal aspect of PIP joint or MTP joint.
- Drawer test of MTP joint
- Palpate web spaces to exclude interdigital neuroma.
- Neurovascular evaluation (e.g., pulses, sensation, muscle bulk)

DIFFERENTIAL DIAGNOSIS
- Hammer toe: hyperextension of the MTP and DIP joints and plantar flexion of the PIP joint
- Claw toe: dorsiflexion of MTP joint and plantar flexion of the DIP joint
- Mallet toe: fixed or flexible deformity of the DIP joint of the toe
- Overlapping 5th toe
- Interdigital neuroma
- Plantar plate rupture
- Nonspecific synovitis of MTP joint
- Fracture; exostosis
- Arthritis (e.g., rheumatoid, psoriatic)

DIAGNOSTIC TESTS & INTERPRETATION
Initial Tests (lab, imaging)
- Not required unless clinically indicated to rule out suspected metabolic or inflammatory arthropathies (2)[C]: rheumatoid factor, antinuclear antibodies (ANA), HLA-B27 serologies for inflammatory disease
- Weight-bearing x-rays of affected foot in anteroposterior (AP), lateral, and oblique views (2)[C]:
  - AP view superior for assessing transverse plane MTP subluxation or dislocation
  - Lateral view is best for the evaluation of hammer toe.

Follow-Up Tests & Special Considerations
MRI or bone scan if osteomyelitis is suspected

Diagnostic Procedures/Other
- Nerve conduction studies or EMG if neurologic disorder is suspected
- Doppler or plethysmography if impaired circulation and surgery is considered
- Computerized weight-bearing pressure testing is indicated only in setting of neuromuscular deficiencies.

Test Interpretation
Histologic evaluation is not necessary before treatment.

TREATMENT

- Goal of treatment is to relieve symptoms and help patients return to their normal activity level.
- Surgical and nonsurgical interventions are available.
- Mild and asymptomatic cases may not require treatment.

GENERAL MEASURES
Nonsurgical (conservative) treatments include
- Shoe modifications (wider and/or deeper toe box) to accommodate the deformity and decrease the pressure over osseous prominences. Avoid high-heeled shoes (2)[C].
- Toe sleeve or orthodigital padding of the hammer toe prominence (5)[C]
- Metatarsal pads in reducible deformities and crest pads in nonreducible deformities
- Dynamic toe splints for MTP joint subluxations or dislocations with (semi)reducible deformity
- Hammer toe–straightening orthotics or taping to reduce flexible deformities
- Débridement of hyperkeratotic lesions can reduce symptoms. Topical keratolytics may be helpful (2)[C].
- Shoe orthotics mitigates abnormal biomechanics.
- Physical therapy for stretching and strengthening of the toes helps preserve flexibility, which include intrinsic muscle strengthening (short foot exercises).

MEDICATION
For pain relief
First Line
NSAIDs may be helpful in managing symptoms of pain as well as soft tissue and joint inflammation.

ISSUES FOR REFERRAL
If nonsurgical (conservative) treatment is unsuccessful and/or impractical or patient has combined deformity of MTP joint, PIP joint, and/or DIP joint, then patient may be referred to a podiatric physician/surgeon or orthopedic surgeon.

SURGERY/OTHER PROCEDURES
- Surgical procedures for the correction of hammer toes depend on the degree and flexibility of the contracture(s) and related abnormalities.
- Surgical interventions for *flexible* hammer toes include (1),(3),(5),(6),(7)[C]
  - PIP joint arthroplasty or arthrodesis (most common)
  - Flexor tenotomy for reducible or mallet toe deformities with distal ulceration
  - Extensor tendon lengthening/tenotomy/MTP joint capsulotomy
  - Flexor tendon transfer with digital arthrodesis
  - Exostosectomy
  - Implant arthroplasty
- Surgical interventions for semirigid/rigid hammer toes include (1),(3),(5),(7)[C]
  - PIP joint resection arthroplasty or arthrodesis
  - Girdlestone-Taylor flexor-to-extensor transfer
  - Metatarsal shortening (Weil osteotomy)
  - Exostosectomy
  - Middle phalangectomy (more common in 5th toe)
  - Soft tissue releases/lengthening
  - Diaphysectomy of the proximal phalanx (less common)
  - Phalangeal base resection as part of Hoffman-Clayton procedure for RA mutilans
- Procedures may be performed as isolated operations or in conjunction with other procedures.
- Contraindications for surgery: active infection, inadequate vascular supply, and desire for cosmesis alone

COMPLEMENTARY & ALTERNATIVE MEDICINE
CBD oil and creams may also be helpful in managing symptoms of pain and inflammation.

 ## ONGOING CARE

FOLLOW-UP RECOMMENDATIONS
- Obtain radiographs immediately following surgery or at the first postoperative visit; subsequent x-rays as needed
- Full weight-bearing in a postoperative (surgical) shoe or other device based on the procedure(s) performed and the individual patient
- Pinning often used across the MTP joint, which requires limited to non–weight-bearing to the forefoot for 3 to 5 weeks
- Elevate the foot to minimize swelling.
- Return to regular shoe wear after pain is controlled, swelling has subsided, and wounds have healed.
- Role and efficacy of postoperative physical therapy unclear

Patient Monitoring
In the absence of complications, the patient should be seen initially within the 1st week following the procedure(s). Frequency of subsequent visits is determined based on the procedure(s) performed and the postoperative course.

PATIENT EDUCATION
- Patients should be aware of mild to moderate swelling and plantar foot discomfort that may persist for many (1 to 6) months after surgery and may limit footwear options until resolved.
- MTP joint and PIP joint may remain stiff for extended periods of time.
- "Molding" of the operative toe (assuming the contours of adjacent toes) is common.
- Encourage patients to wear shoes of adequate size with "roomy" (rounded or squared) toe box.

PROGNOSIS
- Nonoperative (conservative) treatment in mild deformities usually alleviates pain; however, the deformity may progress.
- Surgical treatment of flexible hammer toe deformity reliably corrects the deformity and alleviates pain. Recurrence and progression are common, especially if the patient continues to wear ill-fitting shoes.
- Surgical treatment of fixed hammer toe deformity provides reliable deformity correction and pain relief. Recurrence is uncommon.

COMPLICATIONS
- Common complications specific to digital surgery include but are not limited to
  - Persistent edema
  - Recurrence of deformity
  - Residual pain
  - Excessive stiffness
  - Metatarsalgia
- Less common complications include
  - Numbness (e.g., digital nerve palsy)
  - Flail toe
  - Symptomatic osseous regrowth
  - Malposition of toe
  - Malunion/nonunion
  - Infection
  - Sausage toe
  - Vascular impairment (e.g., toe ischemia, gangrene)

REFERENCES
1. Shirzad K, Kiesau CD, DeOrio JK, et al. Lesser toe deformities. *J Am Acad Orthop Surg.* 2011;19(8):505–514.
2. Thomas JL, Blitch EL IV, Chaney DM, et al; and Clinical Practice Guideline Forefoot Disorders Panel. Diagnosis and treatment of forefoot disorders. Section 1: digital deformities. *J Foot Ankle Surg.* 2009;48(3):418.e1–418.e9.
3. Zelen CM, Young NJ. Digital arthrodesis. *Clin Podiatr Med Surg.* 2013;30(3):271–282.
4. Hannan MT, Menz HB, Jordan JM, et al. High heritability of hallux valgus and lesser toe deformities in adult men and women. *Arthritis Care Res (Hoboken).* 2013;65(9):1515–1521.
5. Smith BW, Coughlin MJ. Disorders of the lesser toes. *Sports Med Arthrosc Rev.* 2009;17(3):167–174.
6. Kwon JY, De Asla RJ. The use of flexor to extensor transfers for the correction of the flexible hammer toe deformity. *Foot Ankle Clin.* 2011;16(4):573–582.
7. Sung W, Weil L Jr, Weil LS Sr. Retrospective comparative study of operative repair of hammertoe deformity. *Foot Ankle Spec.* 2014;7(3):185–192.

ADDITIONAL READING
- Marx RC, Mizel MS. What's new in foot and ankle surgery. *J Bone Joint Surg Am.* 2013;95(10):951–957.
- Miller JM, Blacklidge DK, Ferdowsian V, et al. Chevron arthrodesis of the interphalangeal joint for hammertoe correction. *J Foot Ankle Surg.* 2010;49(2):194–196.
- Schuberth JM. Hammer toe syndrome. American College of Foot and Ankle Surgeons. *J Foot Ankle Surg.* 1999;38(2):166–178.

 ## SEE ALSO

Algorithm: Foot Pain

CODES
ICD10
- M20.40 Other hammer toe(s) (acquired), unspecified foot
- M20.41 Other hammer toe(s) (acquired), right foot
- M20.42 Other hammer toe(s) (acquired), left foot

CLINICAL PEARLS
- Hammer toe is a plantar flexion deformity of the PIP joint. Claw toe and mallet toe are additional types of hammer toes.
- Initial management of hammer toe deformity is conservative. Consider surgery if pain persists or the deformity worsens.
- Properly fitting footwear helps minimize recurrence. Patients should be aware of mild to moderate swelling and plantar foot discomfort that may persist for months after surgery and may limit footwear options until resolved.

HAND-FOOT-AND-MOUTH DISEASE

Tyler S. Rogers, MD • Shelby L. Sheider, DO

 BASICS

DESCRIPTION
- Common clinical syndrome caused by enterovirus serotypes
- Classic appearance of oral enanthem along with exanthem of hands and feet (classically) and potentially located elsewhere
- Exanthem (rash) may be macular, maculopapular, and/or vesicular.
- Synonym(s): herpangina (when affecting oral mucosa and posterior pharynx)

EPIDEMIOLOGY
- Self-limiting illness resolves in 7 to 10 days
- Moderately contagious
- Infection is spread by direct contact with nasal secretions, saliva, blister fluid, or stool.
- Infected individuals are most contagious during the 1st week of the illness but may continue to spread illness for days to weeks after. Some exposed individuals (especially adults) may be asymptomatic but still contagious.
- The viruses that cause hand-foot-and-mouth disease (HFMD) can persist for weeks after symptoms have resolved, most commonly in stool, allowing transmission following resolution of symptoms.
- The incubation period is 3 to 7 days (1).

Incidence
- Children <5 years of age are most commonly affected, especially in daycare facilities (1),(2).
- Can occur as isolated cases, outbreaks, or epidemics
- Occurs worldwide
- Vertical transmission is possible.
- Most large outbreaks occur in Southeast Asia.

ETIOLOGY AND PATHOPHYSIOLOGY
- HFMD is not the same as foot (hoof) and mouth disease found in cattle, and there is no cross species infectious concern (3).
- Transmission by the fecal–oral route or contact with skin lesions or oral secretions; caused by viruses that belong to the *Enterovirus* genus and replicated in the GI tract, most commonly coxsackievirus A16 and enterovirus 71.
- Also coxsackie viruses A5, A7, A9, A10, B2, B5
- More severe cases are associated with enterovirus 71 (4).

GENERAL PREVENTION
- Hand washing, especially around food handling or diaper changes
- Exclusion of children from group settings during the first few days of the illness in the presence of open lesions in the mouth or on the skin may reduce the spread of infection.
- Hand hygiene measures are effective in reducing transmission.
- Pregnant woman should avoid contact with infected individuals.
- New vaccine showing promise in clinical trials to decrease the incidence and prevalence (5)

 DIAGNOSIS

HISTORY
- 1- to 2-day prodrome of fever, anorexia, malaise, abdominal pain, upper respiratory symptoms
- Fever may last 3 to 4 days.
- Maculopapular rash on hands, feet, and mouth. Oral lesions may precede skin.
- Sore throat (follows fever)
- Often history of sick contacts

PHYSICAL EXAM
- Oral enanthem along with tender vesicles becoming ulcers on buccal mucosa, sides of tongue, and palate
- May persist for up to 1 week
- Cutaneous vesicles 3 to 5 mm in diameter start as painful maculopapular eruptions, occur typically on dorsal aspect of fingers and toes.
- May also occur on the palms, soles, buttocks, and groin
- Adults are less likely to have cutaneous findings.
- Nail dystrophies are not uncommon and may persist for weeks following the acute infection.
- Be mindful of central nervous system (CNS) symptoms. Although rare, CNS involvement is possible.

DIFFERENTIAL DIAGNOSIS
- Herpetic gingivostomatitis
- Aphthous stomatitis
- Scabies
- Chickenpox
- Measles
- Rubella
- Scarlet fever
- Roseola infantum
- Fifth disease
- Other enteroviral infections
- Kawasaki disease
- Viral pharyngitis
- Varicella
- Rickettsial infection (RFSF)
- Behçet syndrome
- Pemphigus vulgaris
- Stevens-Johnson syndrome

DIAGNOSTIC TESTS & INTERPRETATION
Clinical diagnosis is typically adequate.

Initial Tests (lab, imaging)
Culture for responsible virus (virus isolation) can be obtained from oral lesions, cutaneous vesicles, nasopharyngeal swabs, stool, and CSF, although not typically performed. Polymerase chain reaction (PCR) of throat swabs and vesicle fluid is the most efficient test if enterovirus 71 is suspected (3).

TREATMENT
- Symptomatic
- Avoid spicy or acidic foods to limit oral pain.
- IV fluids may be required in more severe cases of dehydration.

MEDICATION
- Symptomatic care using ibuprofen or acetaminophen for pain from oral ulcers or fever
- Soothing mouthwashes ("magic mouthwash") containing lidocaine are not recommended as they do not appear to be superior to placebo and have risk of side effects when absorbed systemically (6)[B].
- Antiviral treatments are not available.

Pediatric Considerations
Avoid aspirin use in treating febrile illness in children due to concern of Reye syndrome—an encephalopathy associated with aspirin use in viral illness in children.

ADMISSION, INPATIENT, AND NURSING CONSIDERATIONS
- Patients with CNS manifestations or autonomic dysregulation should require hospitalization.
- Admit those with dehydration unable to maintain adequate oral hydration.
- Intravenous immunoglobulin is not recommended.

ONGOING CARE

DIET
- Encourage cold liquids (e.g., ice cream, popsicles) to prevent dehydration.
- Avoid acidic, salty, and spicy foods, as they will increase pain.

COMPLICATIONS
- Dehydration most common due to painful oral ulcerations
- CNS involvement (i.e., aseptic meningitis) is a rare complication, although it is on the rise globally.
- Fever >3 days and lethargy are associated with CSF pleocytosis.
- Enterovirus 71 has caused outbreaks and has been implicated in more severe disease associated with CNS infection.
- Cardiopulmonary complications include myocarditis, pneumonitis, and pulmonary edema.
- Nail dystrophies and desquamation (loss of nails, Beau lines) are common.

REFERENCES
1. Centers for Disease Control and Prevention. Hand, foot, and mouth disease (HFMD). http://www.cdc.gov/hand-foot-mouth/. Accessed October 19, 2021.
2. Centers for Disease Control and Prevention. Notes from the field: severe hand, foot, and mouth disease associated with coxsackievirus A6—Alabama, Connecticut, California, and Nevada, November 2011-February 2012. MMWR Morb Mortal Wkly Rep. 2012;61(12):213–214.
3. World Health Organization Western Pacific Region. A guide to clinical management and public health response for hand, foot and mouth disease (HFMD). https://iris.wpro.who.int/bitstream/handle/10665.1/5521/9789290615255_eng.pdf. Accessed October 19, 2021.
4. Saguil A, Kane SF, Lauters R, et al. Hand-Foot-and-Mouth Disease: Rapid Evidence Review. Am Fam Physician. 2019;100(7):408–414.
5. Han Y, Chen Z, Zheng K, et al. Epidemiology of hand, foot, and mouth disease before and after the introduction of enterovirus 71 vaccines in Chengdu, China, 2009-2018. Pediatr Infect Dis J. 2020;39(10):969–978.
6. Hopper SM, McCarthy M, Tancharoen C, et al. Topical lidocaine to improve oral intake in children with painful infectious mouth ulcers: a blinded, randomized, placebo-controlled trial. Ann Emerg Med. 2014;63(3):292–299.

ADDITIONAL READING
Jones E, Pillay TD, Liu F, et al. Outcomes following severe hand foot and mouth disease: a systematic review and meta-analysis. Eur J Paediatr Neurol. 2018;22(5):763–773.

 CODES

ICD10
- B08.4 Enteroviral vesicular stomatitis with exanthem
- B34.1 Enterovirus infection, unspecified
- B08.5 Enteroviral vesicular pharyngitis

CLINICAL PEARLS
- Most common: May to October
- Children <5 years of age tend to have worse symptoms than older children.
- HFMD is the most common cause of mouth sores in pediatric patients.
- Dehydration is a common problem secondary to swallowing aversions.
- Usually self-limiting, resolving in 7 to 10 days
- Careful hand washing to limit dissemination
- Counsel parents that nail desquamation may occur in the weeks following the infection.

H

HEADACHE, CLUSTER
Samuel C. Wang, MD • Sarah Ali, MD

 BASICS

DESCRIPTION
- A primary headache disorder characterized by multiple attacks of severe, unilateral sharp, searing, or piercing pain typically localized to the periorbital and/or temporal areas
- Accompanied by signs of ipsilateral parasympathetic autonomic activation as well as restlessness or agitation
- Autonomic symptoms: signs of parasympathetic hyperactivity (ipsilateral lacrimation, eye redness, nasal congestion) and sympathetic hypoactivity (ipsilateral ptosis and miosis)
- Patients often pace the floor during an acute attack because lying down seems to exacerbate the pain.
- Individual attacks occur from once every other day up to 8 times per day and can last 15 to 180 minutes per day if untreated.
- Attacks usually occur in series (cluster periods) that are often seasonal, lasting for weeks or months, and are separated by remission periods usually lasting months to years.
- About 10–15% of patients have chronic symptoms without remissions (i.e., chronic cluster headache [cCH]).

EPIDEMIOLOGY
Incidence
Incidence: 2 to 10/100,000
Prevalence
Prevalence: 53/100,000
- Gender: male > female; 4.3:1 overall
- Women often develop CH earlier in life (20s).
- Mean age of onset: 30 years
- Episodic/chronic ratio: 6:1

ETIOLOGY AND PATHOPHYSIOLOGY
- Complex and incompletely understood
- Possible mechanisms include the following:
  - Activation of the trigeminovascular system, which leads to the release of vasodilatory peptides including substance P, neurokinin, and calcitonin gene-related peptide (CGRP)
  - Posterior hypothalamus activation may trigger an attack by activating trigeminal nociceptive pathways through increased parasympathetic outflow.
  - Alterations in the descending pain modulation network and disordered pain modulation during cluster periods

Genetics
- Usually sporadic: autosomal dominant in 5% of cases; otherwise, autosomal recessive or multifactorial
- Evidence varies: First-degree relatives are 18 times more likely, and second-degree relatives are 1 to 3 times more likely to be affected by cluster headaches.
- >50% with migraine and 18% with CH in family history

RISK FACTORS
- Male gender
- Age: 70% onset before age 30 years
- Cigarette smoking or childhood exposure to cigarette smoke
- Family history of CH
- Personal history of head trauma

COMMONLY ASSOCIATED CONDITIONS
- Depression (24%)
- Increased risk of suicide secondary to the extreme nature of the pain
- Medication-overuse headache
- Asthma (9%)
- History of migraine, frequently in female patients
- Sleep apnea (30–80%)

 DIAGNOSIS

- Diagnosis is clinical.
- *International Classification of Headache Disorders* (3rd ed, 2018) criteria
- At least five attacks of severe or very severe unilateral orbital, supraorbital, and/or temporal pain lasting 15 to 180 minutes if untreated
- Either one or both of the following:
  - At least one of the following symptoms ipsilateral to the headache:
    - Conjunctival injection and/or lacrimation
    - Nasal congestion and/or rhinorrhea
    - Eyelid edema
    - Forehead and facial sweating/flushing
    - Miosis and/or ptosis
  - Restlessness or agitation during acute attack
- Attack frequency: one every other day to eight per day for more than half of the time during cluster periods
- Episodic CH (eCH): At least two cluster periods lasting 7 days to 1 year, separated by a pain-free interval of ≥3 months (80–90% of cases)
- Chronic CH (cCH): occurring for ≥1 year without remission period, or remission period lasting <3 months, for at least 1 year

HISTORY
- Episodic periods of headache described as excruciating, unilateral, sharp, searing, or piercing pain typically localized to the periorbital and/or temporal area.
- Conjunctival injection, tearing, nasal congestion, rhinorrhea, sweating
- Timing of headaches is often circadian in nature, occurring at the same time each day (usually at night).
- Presence of triggers such as vasodilators (e.g., alcohol, nitroglycerin, sildenafil), histamine, or strong odors
- Seasonal pattern of cluster periods, often recurring around the same time of the year

PHYSICAL EXAM
- Patients are usually seen between attacks, so physical exam is often unremarkable.
- Distress, crying spells, restlessness, and/or agitation during acute attack
- Ipsilateral lacrimation, conjunctival injection, ptosis, and miosis during an acute attack
- Edematous nasal mucosa or rhinorrhea during acute attack

DIFFERENTIAL DIAGNOSIS
- Other trigeminal autonomic cephalgias (e.g., paroxysmal hemicrania, short-lasting unilateral neuralgiform headache attacks with conjunctival injection and tearing [SUNCT], hemicrania continua), hypnic headaches, trigeminal and other facial neuralgias, migraine, temporal arteritis, herpes zoster, acute angle closure glaucoma

- Secondary CH:
  - Vertebral or carotid artery dissection, brain arteriovenous malformations, intracranial artery aneurysms
  - Pituitary tumors/meningiomas/carcinomas
  - Cavernous hemangioma or inflammation of the cavernous sinus (i.e., Tolosa-Hunt syndrome)

DIAGNOSTIC TESTS & INTERPRETATION
- Diagnosis is primarily clinical.
- Diagnosis is often delayed (>40% report 5-year delay in diagnosis).

Initial Tests (lab, imaging)
Neuroimaging (MRI/CT head with detailed study of pituitary and cavernous sinus) recommended for all trigeminal autonomic cephalgias in order to exclude other intracranial conditions that may mimic TACs

TREATMENT

Many of the medications discussed in the following section are used off-label in the treatment of CH.

GENERAL MEASURES
- Avoid major changes in sleep habits.
- Stop smoking.
- Avoid use of alcohol during cluster period.
- Avoid extreme changes in altitude which can cause changes in oxygen levels.
- Avoid exposure to chemical agents/solvents or other known triggers.

MEDICATION
- Avoid pain medications, especially narcotic analgesics, for acute attacks.
- Goal is abortion of acute attack and transitional prophylaxis for expected duration of the cluster period.
- Long-term prophylaxis used for cCH
- Assess cardiovascular risk before instituting vasoactive drugs, such as triptans or ergot derivatives.

First Line
- For acute attacks:
  - Oxygen: 100% at 12 to 15 L/min via nonrebreather mask or demand valve oxygen mask while sitting or standing provides relief within 15 minutes. High flow used if resistant to lower-flow oxygen; excellent side effect profile (1)[A]

ALERT
Avoid high-flow oxygen in patients with severe COPD.

- Sumatriptan
  - SubQ: 6 mg, up to 12 mg/24 h with at least 1 hour between injections is most effective medication for acute attacks; NNT = 2.4 and 3.3 for headache relief and pain free in 15 minutes, respectively
  - Intranasal: 20 mg once in single nostril contralateral to the side of the headache; may repeat in 2 hours, max dose 40 mg/24 hr; NNT = 3.2 for headache relief at 30 minutes (1),(2)[A]
- Zolmitriptan
  - Intranasal: 5- and 10-mg dosage both effective; may repeat in 2 hours, max 2 times per day; NNT = 12 and 4.9 for headache relief in 15 minutes for 5 and 10 mg, respectively
  - PO: 5- and 10-mg dosage both effective; may repeat in 2 hours, max dose 10 mg/24 hr; NNT = 6.7 and 4.5 for headache relief in 30 minutes for 5 and 10 mg, respectively (1),(2)[B]

ALERT

Adverse effects: paresthesias, flushing, tingling, chest pain, neck tightness ("Triptan sensations"). Triptans are contraindicated in ischemic cardiac disease, stroke, uncontrolled hypertension, Prinzmetal angina, basilar migraine, hemiplegic migraine, ischemic bowel disease, and peripheral vascular disease

- For prophylaxis:
  – Use as soon as possible at the start of cluster period to prevent and shorten further attacks.
  – Galcanezumab: 300 mg SC every month until cluster period ends. Only FDA-approved medication for eCH prophylaxis. Most common side effects are nasopharyngitis, hepatic enzyme elevation, and local injection site reaction and pain; NNT = 5.2 (3)[B]
  – Verapamil: Start at 80 mg TID and increase by 80 mg/week to 480 mg and then 80 mg every 2 weeks if needed. Short- or long-acting equivalent. Most patients respond to daily dose of 200 to 480 mg but up to 960 mg/day may be needed; NNT = 1.2 (1)[A]

ALERT

Baseline ECG and repeat monitoring with dosage increases is required for verapamil because of risk of bradycardia, prolonged PR interval, RBBB, or complete heart block. Avoid grapefruit juice due to CYP3A4 inhibition.

Second Line

- For acute attacks:
  – Noninvasive vagus nerve stimulation (nVNS): modest efficacy in short-term pain reduction for eCH was demonstrated in two double-blind, sham controlled trials (ACT-1, ACT-2). FDA-cleared for treatment of eCH. Contraindicated in those with implantable devices, carotid atherosclerosis, cervical vagotomy, and clinically significant hypertension or arrhythmias.
  – Lidocaine/cocaine: 10 mg (1 mL) of lidocaine or 40 to 50 mg of 10% cocaine intranasal. No well-controlled randomized controlled trials (RCTs) done. Most common side effects are nasal congestion and unpleasant taste.
  – Octreotide: S 100 μg. Can be considered in patients when triptans are contraindicated. Main side effect is GI upset.
- For prophylaxis:
  – Melatonin: 10-mg regular-release tablet in late evening has shown reduction in headache frequency versus placebo in small RCT. No side effects were reported.
  – Lithium: Start 300 mg BID; titrate to therapeutic range of 600–1500 mg/day. In a head-to-head trial with verapamil, lithium was shown to be comparable (4). Must monitor drug levels, liver, renal, and thyroid function. Caution with nephrotoxic drugs, diuretics. Monitor for CNS side effects.
  – Capsaicin: 0.025% ipsilateral nostril for 7 days showed benefit in one small RCT.
  – Topiramate: 100–200 mg/day showed efficacy in several small, open-label trials.

ISSUES FOR REFERRAL

Consider a neurology or headache center referral for refractory or complicated patients.

ADDITIONAL THERAPIES

Transitional prophylaxis:

- Used to rapidly reduce attack frequency until the effectiveness of longer term preventive treatment is reached. Longer term maintenance agents are started concurrently.

- Steroids: prednisolone 1 mg/kg/day (max 60 mg) with a taper no longer than 18 days to avoid side effects. Several open studies suggested benefit but no rigorous trials to prove efficacy. Adverse effects for short-term use: insomnia, psychosis, hyponatremia, edema, hyperglycemia, peptic ulcer.
- Suboccipital nerve or greater occipital nerve steroid injections: 3.75 mg of cortivazol injected into the suboccipital area on the ipsilateral side of the headache; single injection or series of three injections, given 48 to 72 hours apart, reduces attack frequency during cluster period when used as add-on therapy to verapamil; NNT = 2.5 (5)[B]

Pregnancy Considerations

- Collaboration between headache specialist, obstetrician, pediatrician, and lactation specialist is recommended.
- Patient should be informed of limited data on treatment efficacy versus safety.
- For acute treatment, oxygen is most appropriate first-line therapy. Intranasal triptans (pregnancy Category C), intranasal lidocaine (pregnancy Category B), and/or subcutaneous sumatriptan (pregnancy Category C) can be used as second-line therapy (6).
- For transitional prophylaxis, oral steroids (pregnancy Category C/D) or greater occipital nerve blockade can be used but should be used at the lowest dose and duration possible.
- For preventive therapy, verapamil (pregnancy Category C) remains the preferred option. If possible, avoid in third trimester. Avoid lithium (pregnancy Category D) and ergotamines (pregnancy Category X).

SURGERY/OTHER PROCEDURES

- No evidence for Botox or hyperbaric oxygen treatment
- Surgery may be considered for patients who are refractory to, or have contraindications to, medical therapy.
- Neurostimulation
  – Multicenter RCT showed efficacy of sphenopalatine ganglion stimulation (SPG) compared to sham treatment; CINTHA trial ongoing
  – Bilateral occipital nerve stimulation (ONS) has been shown to reduce severity and attack frequency in cCH patients.
  – Deep brain stimulation (DBS) of the hypothalamus has shown a positive response rate but carries risks of stroke, hemorrhage, and death.

ADMISSION, INPATIENT, AND NURSING CONSIDERATIONS

- Intractable, severe pain
- Suicidal ideation

ONGOING CARE

FOLLOW-UP RECOMMENDATIONS

Patient Monitoring

- Anticipate cluster bouts and initiate prophylaxis early.
- Monitor for depression and suicidal ideation, especially in those with cCH.
- Watch for adverse medication responses and side effects, such as unmasking of underlying cardiovascular disorder, when using medications to treat CH.

PROGNOSIS

- Unpredictable but often chronic course
- Attack frequency often decreases with increasing age.
- Possibility of transformation of eCH to cCH

COMPLICATIONS

- Depression and suicide
- Side effects of medication, including unmasking of coronary artery disease

REFERENCES

1. Robbins M, Starling A, Pringsheim T, et al. Treatment of cluster headache: the American Headache Society evidence-based guidelines. *Headache*. 2016;56(7):1093–1106.
2. Law S, Derry S, Moore RA. Triptans for acute cluster headache. *Cochrane Database Syst Rev*. 2013;(7):CD008042.
3. Yuan H, Spare N, Silberstein S. Targeting CGRP for the prevention of migraine and cluster headache: a narrative review. *Headache*. 2019;59:20–32.
4. Suri H, Ailani J. Cluster headache: a review and update in treatment. *Curr Neurol Neurosci Rep*. 2021;21(7):31.
5. Leroux E, Valade D, Taifas I, et al. Suboccipital steroid injections for transitional treatment of patients with more than two cluster headache attacks per day: a randomised, double-blind, placebo-controlled trial. *Lancet Neurol*. 2011;10(10):891–897.
6. Bjørk MH, Kristoffersen ES, Tronvik E, et al. Management of cluster headache and other trigeminal autonomic cephalalgias in pregnancy and breastfeeding. *Eur J Neurol*. 2021;28(7):2443–2455.

ADDITIONAL READING

- Ljubisavljevic S, Zidverc Trajkovic J. Cluster headache: pathophysiology, diagnosis and treatment. *J Neurol*. 2019;266(5):1059–1066.
- Magis D. Emerging treatments for cluster headache: hopes and disappointments. *Curr Opin Neurol*. 2019;32(3):432–437.

CODES

ICD10

- G44.009 Cluster headache syndrome, unspecified, not intractable
- G44.019 Episodic cluster headache, not intractable
- G44.029 Chronic cluster headache, not intractable

CLINICAL PEARLS

- CHs are present as severe, unilateral sharp, searing, or piercing pain typically localized to the periorbital and/or temporal areas, accompanied by autonomic symptoms such as ipsilateral lacrimation, miosis, ptosis, eye redness, and nasal congestion.
- Patients are often agitated and restless during acute attacks.
- High-flow oxygen and triptans, not narcotics, are first-line therapy for acute attacks.
- Among triptans, injected forms are more effective than nasal sprays, which are more effective than oral tablets.
- Abortive, transitional, and prophylactic treatment must all be considered.

H

HEADACHE, MIGRAINE

Karly Pippitt, MD • Seniha Ozudogru, MD

BASICS

DESCRIPTION

Recurrent headache disorder manifesting in attacks lasting 4 to 72 hours. Typically: unilateral location, pulsating quality, moderate to severe intensity, and associated nausea and/or photophobia and phonophobia (1)

- Most frequent subtypes of migraine (1):
  - Without aura: defines >80% of migraines, vomiting, photophobia, and/or phonophobia
  - With aura: visual or other (motor, sensory or brainstem symptoms, including previously known as basilar or hemiplegic migraine); fully reversible neurologic phenomenon, develop gradually over 5 minutes and last up to 60 minutes
  - Chronic migraine: >15 migraine days/month, >4 hours/attack, for ≥3 months
  - Menstrual migraine: migraine attacks in a menstruating person, onset 1 to 2 days prior to menses or up to day 3 of menstruation, occurring in 2 of 3 menstrual cycles and at no other time during cycle
  - Menstrually related migraine: menstrual migraine plus migraine attacks at other times during cycle
- Rare but important subtypes (1):
  - Status migrainosus: debilitating migraine lasting >72 hours
  - Prolonged aura: aura symptoms >60 minutes (can last up to 7 days), should prompt consideration of secondary causes
  - Ocular: repeated attacks of monocular visual disturbance, including scintillations, scotomata, or blindness, with migraine
  - Vertiginous: migraine with vertigo or dizziness
  - Acephalgic migraine (migraine aura without headache): typical aura symptoms not followed by a migraine headache

EPIDEMIOLOGY

- Female > male (3:1)
- Affects >28 million Americans

ETIOLOGY AND PATHOPHYSIOLOGY

- Trigeminovascular hypothesis: hyperexcitable trigeminal sensory neurons in brainstem are stimulated and release neuropeptides, such as substance P and calcitonin gene-related peptide (CGRP), leading to vasodilation and neurogenic inflammation
- Cortical spreading depression: mainly accepted hypotheses for migraine with aura; change in electrical activity with reduction of blood flow, leading to aura

Genetics

>80% of patients have a family history

RISK FACTORS

- Female sex (menstrual cycle)
- Sleep pattern disruption
- Diet: skipped meals (48%), alcohol (32%), chocolate (20%), cheese (13%), caffeine overuse (14%), monosodium glutamate (MSG) (12%), and artificial sweeteners
- Medications: estrogens, vasodilators

GENERAL PREVENTION

- Lifestyle modifications are the cornerstone: sleep hygiene, stress management, healthy diet, adequate hydration, and regular exercise.
- Prophylactic medication for frequent attacks

COMMONLY ASSOCIATED CONDITIONS

- Depression, anxiety, PTSD
- Sleep disturbance (e.g., sleep apnea)
- Cerebral vascular disease
- Seizure disorders
- Irritable bowel syndrome
- Medication overuse headache (MOH)

DIAGNOSIS

Clinical diagnosis; recommend thorough history and neurologic examination

HISTORY

- Validated migraine screening tool: ID migraine (2)
- In the last 3 months did you have the following symptoms with your headaches: Nauseated or sick to your stomach? Light bothered you (more than when you didn't have a headache)? Headaches limited your ability to work, study, or do what you needed for a day?
  - Yes to 2 questions: 81% migraine probability; yes to 3 questions increases probability of migraine to 93% (2).
- Headache usually begins with mild pain escalating into unilateral (30–40% bilateral) throbbing (40% nonthrobbing) pain lasting 4 to 72 hours. If side locked headache, never shifts sides, or there are potential secondary causes (e.g., tumor, systemic illnesses), this should prompt evaluation for alternative diagnosis.
- Intensified by movement and associated with: nausea, vomiting, diarrhea, photophobia, phonophobia, muscle tenderness, light-headedness, and vertigo
- May be preceded by aura
  - Visual disruptions most common: scotoma, hemianopsia, fortification spectra, geometric visual patterns, and occasionally hallucinations
  - Somatosensory disruption in face or arms
  - Speech difficulties
- Headache diary: episodes per month, HA days per month, frequency, and amount and effect of medications used
- Identify possible triggers (e.g., stress, sleep disturbance, food, caffeine, alcohol)
- Migraine disability assessment (MiDAS) is a useful tool to assess level of disability and correlates well with headache diaries.

PHYSICAL EXAM

Neurologic exam, including funduscopy, to rule out other causes:

- Gait abnormalities, other cerebellar findings
- Loss of gross and/or fine motor function
- Altered mental status
- Short-term memory loss
- Papilledema

DIFFERENTIAL DIAGNOSIS

- Other primary headache syndromes (e.g., idiopathic intracranial hypertension [IIH], trigeminal autonomic cephalgia [TAC])
- Secondary headaches: MOH, tumor, infection, inflammation, vascular pathology, drug use

DIAGNOSTIC TESTS & INTERPRETATION

Neuroimaging is appropriate with suspicious symptomatology and/or an abnormality on exam (3). Other red flags include the following:

- New onset in patient >50 years of age
- Change in established headache pattern
- Atypical pattern or unremitting/progressive neurologic symptoms
- Prolonged or different/change in typical aura
- CT head for concern of brain bleed; brain MRI more common imaging study
- EEG NOT indicated unless evaluating LOC, AMS
- Consider systemic disease (i.e., hypothyroidism, SLE, and vitamin deficiencies) in appropriate clinical scenario and evaluate accordingly.

Pediatric Considerations

- NSAIDs and triptans are effective for acute treatment; NSAIDs first line
- Rizatriptan is FDA-approved for children >6 years; sumatriptan succinate, almoptriptan, and zolmitriptan nasal spray FDA-approved for >12 years (4)[A]

Pregnancy Considerations

- Frequency may decrease in 2nd, 3rd trimesters.
- For new-onset headaches in pregnancy, consider preeclampsia and venous sinus thrombosis.
- No migraine drug has FDA approval in pregnancy and breastfeeding.
  - Acetaminophen, antiemetics, and short-acting opioids can be considered for acute headaches.
  - Data does not find increased teratogenicity with triptans (most data for sumatriptan). When triptans compellingly needed, they are acceptable.
  - Ergotamines are contraindicated.
  - Avoid herbal remedies.
  - β-Blockers and calcium channel blockers are effective prophylaxis.
  - Occipital nerve blocks and trigger point injections (lidocaine and bupivacaine) are safe.

TREATMENT

GENERAL MEASURES

- Consistent sleep hours and eating habits
- Cold compresses to area of pain

MEDICATION

- First-line abortive treatments
  - Mild to moderate attacks:
    - Acetaminophen is effective; when combined with metoclopramide has relief rates similar to triptans (5)[A]
    - NSAIDs are effective in up to 60% of cases (5)[B].
    - Aspirin-acetaminophen-caffeine (Excedrin Migraine) (5)[B]

- Moderate to severe attacks:
  - ○ Triptans when OTC agents fail for mild to moderate attacks OR first line for moderate to severe attacks (5)[C]
    - ▪ Sumatriptan 100 mg PO. Can repeat after 2 hours; max 200 mg/24 hr; sumatriptan 3 or 4 or 6 mg SC. Can repeat after 1 hour; max 12 mg/24 hr; rapid onset, should consider for wake up headache and migraine with severe GI upset; Sumatriptan intranasal 20 mg. Can repeat after 2 hours; max 40 mg/24 hr
    - ▪ Rizatriptan 10 mg PO (dose is 5 mg if using propranolol for prophylaxis). Can repeat after 2 hours; max 30 mg/24 hr
    - ▪ Naratriptan 2.5 mg PO. Can repeat after 4 hours; max 5 mg/24 hr
    - ▪ Zolmitriptan 2.5 mg PO; 5 mg intranasal. Can repeat after 2 hours; max 5 mg for oral, 10 mg for nasal spray/24 hr
    - ▪ Frovatriptan 2.5 mg PO. Can repeat after 4 hours; max 5 mg/24 hr
    - ▪ Eletriptan 40 mg PO. Can repeat after 2 hours; max 80 mg/24 hr
      - □ Frovatriptan and naratriptan have slow onset but long half-lives—best for long migraine duration and menstrual migraine.
  - ○ Antiemetics: dopamine antagonists add-ons (5)[B]
  - – Contraindications: Avoid triptans and ergots in coronary artery or uncontrolled hypertension.
  - – Precautions
    - ○ Frequent use of acute-treatment drugs can result in MOH (especially Excedrin, triptans, butalbital).
    - ○ Triptan common adverse reactions: chest pain, flushing, weakness, dizziness, and paresthesias. Recommend trying more than one triptan before considered a class failure.
- Second-line abortive treatment
  - – Dihydroergotamine: drug of choice in status migrainosus and triptan resistance or failure. Ergotamine oral tablets and dihydroergotamine nasal sprays are more convenient and safer than intramuscular injections.
  - – Lasmitidan 50 and 100 mg: 5-HT1F receptor agonist. Schedule V controlled substance. Patient should not drive following 8 hours; safe with CV risk factors
  - – Ubrogepant 50 and 100 mg: can repeat after 2 hours; max 200 mg/24 hr
  - – Rimegepant 75 mg ODT: 1 daily PRN dose; max 75 mg/24 hr
- First-line preventive treatment (6)[A]: lifestyle modifications, trigger reduction, CBT
  - – Consider prophylactic treatment if:
    - ○ Quality of life is severely impaired
    - ○ ≥6 headache days per month, ≥4 headache days per month of moderate severity, or ≥2 headache days per month of severe impairment
    - ○ Migraines not responding to abortives
    - ○ Frequent, long, or uncomfortable auras
- Preventive treatment of *migraine*: divalproex, topiramate, metoprolol, and propranolol to reduce frequency. Amitriptyline, venlafaxine, lisinopril, and candesartan are other options (6)[A].
  - – NSAIDs can be effective prevention if predictable triggers (menses, etc.).

- CGRP monoclonal antibodies:
  - ○ Erenumab 70 and 140 mg, complete CGRP receptor antagonist; 1 SC/month
  - ○ Fremanezumab-vfrm partial CGRP receptor antagonist; 225 mg monthly SC injections or 675 mg quarterly SC injections
  - ○ Galcanezumab-gnlm partial CGRP receptor antagonist. 240 mg loading dose, then 120 mg monthly SC injections
  - ○ Eptinizumab-jjmr 100 mg/mL: Dilute with 0.9% NaCl; infuse over 30 minutes.
- CGRP small molecule antagonists:
  - ○ Rimegepant 75 mg ODT: 1 tablet every other day
  - ○ Atogepant 10, 30, and 60 mg: 1 tablet daily
- For *chronic migraine*, onobotulinum toxin A (Botox) (6)[A]

ISSUES FOR REFERRAL
Obscure diagnosis, unresponsive to usual treatment, significant comorbid medical diagnoses

COMPLEMENTARY & ALTERNATIVE MEDICINE
- Riboflavin (vitamin B_2): 400 mg/day (6)[B]
- Magnesium: 400 mg/day (6)[B]
- MIG-99 (Feverfew): 6.25 mg TID (6)[B]
- Acupuncture is as effective as prophylactic drug treatment with fewer adverse effects.

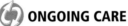 ONGOING CARE

FOLLOW-UP RECOMMENDATIONS
Patient Monitoring
- Quarterly or more frequent appointments when headaches not well controlled
- Monitor frequency of attacks and medication usage via headache diary.
- Migraine (especially with aura) is a risk factor for stroke; consider lipid assessment and other risk reduction such as tobacco cessation. Women with migraine with aura should avoid estrogens due to increased risk of stroke (2)[A].

PATIENT EDUCATION
- Trigger identification and modification can significantly improve headache frequency.
- Setting expectations critical, especially with prophylactic medications where success is 50% reduction in severity of headaches or decrease in disability from headaches
- Benefits may be seen from prophylactic medications after many weeks of treatment.

PROGNOSIS
- With increasing age (including menopause), there is a reduction in severity, frequency, and disability.
- Most attacks subside within 72 hours.

COMPLICATIONS
- Status migrainosus (>72 hours)
- MOH: headache 10 or more days per month for >3 months due to regular overuse of a rescue headache medication; likelihood with butalbital > opiates > triptans > NSAIDs
- Cerebral ischemic events (rare)

REFERENCES
1. Headache Classification Committee of the International Headache Society. The International Classification of Headache Disorders, 3rd edition. *Cephalalgia*. 2018;38(1):1–211.
2. Sacco S, Merki-Feld GS, Ægidius KL, et al. Hormonal contraceptives and risk of ischemic stroke in women with migraine: a consensus statement from the European Headache Federation (EHF) and the European Society of Contraception and Reproductive Health (ESC). *J Headache Pain*. 2017;18(1):108.
3. Loder E, Weizenbaum E, Frishberg B, et al; for American Headache Society Choosing Wisely Task Force. Choosing wisely in headache medicine: the American Headache Society's list of five things physicians and patients should question. *Headache*. 2013;53(10):1651–1659.
4. Patterson-Gentile C, Szperka CL. The changing landscape of pediatric migraine therapy: a review. *JAMA Neurol*. 2018;75(7):881–887.
5. Becker WJ. Acute migraine treatment in adults. *Headache*. 2015;55(6):778–793.
6. Loder E, Burch R, Rizzoli P. The 2012 AHS/AAN guidelines for prevention of episodic migraine: a summary and comparison with other recent clinical practice guidelines. *Headache*. 2012;52(6):930–945.

 SEE ALSO

Algorithm: Headache, Chronic

 CODES

ICD10
- G43.909 Migraine, unsp, not intractable, without status migrainosus
- G43.109 Migraine with aura, not intractable, w/o status migrainosus
- G43.409 Hemiplegic migraine, not intractable, w/o status migrainosus

CLINICAL PEARLS
- Migraine is a chronic headache disorder of unclear etiology often characterized by unilateral, throbbing pain that may be associated with additional neurologic symptoms.
- Consider OTC analgesics for mild attacks; migraine-specific treatments for more severe attacks or those not responding to OTC medications
- Avoid opiates and barbiturates or frequent (>8 per month) triptan or NSAID use to avoid MOH.
- Counsel on lifestyle modifications and trigger identification.
- Consider prophylactic treatment if frequent or debilitating migraines.

H

HEADACHE, TENSION

Afreen N. Papa, MD • Joseph Francis Urbanik, DO

 BASICS

DESCRIPTION
- A bilateral mild to moderate, nonthrobbing head pain or pressure, without other associated symptoms. Three types of tension-type headache (TTH):
  - Infrequent episodic TTH: <1 day per month
  - Frequent episodic TTH: ≥1 but <15 days per month
  - Chronic TTH: ≥15 days per month for >3 months
- TTHs replaced older terms: muscle contraction headache, stress or tension headache, and psychogenic headache.

EPIDEMIOLOGY
The most common type of primary headache, and the second-most prevalent disorder in the world

Prevalence
- Peak age of prevalence in the United States: the 4th decade
- Lifetime prevalence: men (69%); women (88%)
- Prevalence of episodic TTH decreases with age, whereas the prevalence of chronic TTH increases with age.

ETIOLOGY AND PATHOPHYSIOLOGY
- Multifactorial: peripheral and/or central mechanisms
- Activation of peripheral nociceptors leads to myofascial pain in episodic TTH.
- Prolonged stimulation of nociceptors sensitizes the central pain pathways leading to chronic TTH.
- Nitric oxide may play an important role in TTH.

RISK FACTORS
Associated with triggers/precipitating factors:
- Stress (mental or physical): the most common
- Change in sleep regimen
- Skipping meals
- Certain foods (caffeine, alcohol, chocolate)
- Dehydration
- Physical exertion
- Environmental factors (sun glare, odors, smoke, noise, lighting)
- Poor or sustained posture
- Female hormonal changes
- Medications (e.g., nitrates, SSRIs, antihypertensives)
- Overuse of abortive headache medication

GENERAL PREVENTION
- Identify and avoid triggers/precipitating factors.
- Minimize physical and emotional stress.
- Relaxation techniques: biofeedback, relaxation therapy, and physical therapy

COMMONLY ASSOCIATED CONDITIONS
- 83% of patients with migraine headaches also suffer from TTHs.
- Debatable: increased prevalence of comorbid anxiety and depression

 DIAGNOSIS

HISTORY
Obtain a thorough pain history to rule out other headache disorders, including onset, location, radiation, quality of pain, severity, associated symptoms; concurrent medical conditions and medications; and recent trauma or other procedures.
- Diagnosis is based on clinical assessment.
- Pain may be described in many ways, such as "dull," "band-like," pressure.
- Diagnostic criteria by the International Headache Society (ICHD-3) (1):
  - Episodic TTH: ≥10 headache episodes that meet all of the following criteria:
    - Headache lasting 30 minutes to 7 days
    - At least two of the following:
      - Bilateral location
      - Pressing/tightening (nonpulsating) quality
      - Mild or moderate intensity
      - Not aggravated by routine physical activity
    - Not associated with:
      - Nausea or vomiting
      - No more than one of photophobia or phonophobia
    - Headache not due to another ICHD-3 diagnosis
  - Chronic TTH: ≥15 days per month (on average) for >3 months that meet all of the following criteria:
    - Headache lasting hours to days, or unremitting
    - At least two of the following:
      - Bilateral location
      - Pressing/tightening (nonpulsating) quality
      - Mild or moderate intensity
      - Not aggravated by routine physical activity
    - Both of the following:
      - No more than one of photophobia, phonophobia, or mild nausea
      - Neither moderate or severe nausea nor vomiting

PHYSICAL EXAM
- Usually unremarkable
- Head and neck: palpation of myofascial tissues for pericranial muscle tenderness
- Neurologic exam: mental status, pupillary responses, motor-strength testing, deep tendon reflexes, sensation, cerebellar function, gait testing, signs of meningeal irritation

DIFFERENTIAL DIAGNOSIS
- Migraine headache
- Cluster headache
- Head trauma
- Subarachnoid hemorrhage (SAH), subdural hematoma, unruptured vascular malformation
- Ischemic cerebrovascular disease, cerebral venous thrombosis
- Temporal arteritis
- Arterial hypertension (HTN), benign intracranial HTN
- Intracranial neoplasm, infection, or meningitis
- Low cerebrospinal fluid pressure
- Medication (nonprescription analgesic dependency, nitrates)
- Caffeine dependency

- Metabolic disorders (hypoxia, hypercapnia, hypoglycemia)
- Temporomandibular joint syndrome
- Eyes: glaucoma, refractive errors
- Sinusitis or middle ear infection
- Cervical spondylosis
- Severe anemia or polycythemia
- Paget disease of bone

DIAGNOSTIC TESTS & INTERPRETATION
- Most primary headaches with typical features do not require lab testing or diagnostic imaging.
- Labs and neuroimaging (CT or MRI) should be considered when a secondary cause is suspected:
  - Atypical pattern of headache (does not fit specific category such as migraine, cluster, or tension)
  - Rapid increase in frequency
  - Unexplained focal neurologic findings
  - New onset after age 35 years
  - Sudden onset or worsening with exertion
- MRI with and without contrast is the test of choice. However, head CT is preferred in emergency settings.
- If acute SAH is suspected, head CT should be performed before lumbar puncture (1)[B].

TREATMENT

- Nonsteroidal anti-inflammatory drugs (NSAIDs), aspirin, or acetaminophen is effective for short-term relief of episodic TTH (2),(3)[B].
- Amitriptyline should be considered first line for prophylaxis of chronic TTH (2),(3)[B].

GENERAL MEASURES
Relief measures: relaxation routines; rest in quiet, dark room; hot bath or shower; massage of back of neck and temples

MEDICATION
Choice of simple analgesic is based on patient-specific parameters:
- NSAIDs may be more effective than acetaminophen for episodic TTH (2)[C]: Ibuprofen and naproxen may be preferred due to better gastrointestinal (GI) tolerability.
- Acetaminophen should be considered for patients unable to tolerate NSAIDs or allergic to aspirin or NSAIDs.

First Line
- For acute treatment in episodic TTH:
  - NSAIDs:
    - Ibuprofen (Motrin, Advil): 200 to 400 mg; may repeat q8h PRN (max 3.2 g/day)
    - Naproxen sodium (Naprosyn): 220 to 550 mg BID PRN (max 1,250 mg base per day)
    - Contraindications: aspirin or NSAID allergy or bronchospasm, renal disease, bleeding disorders, increased risk of cardiovascular events (myocardial infarction [MI], stroke, new onset or worsening of HTN)
    - Drug interactions: antihypertensives, anticoagulants, antiplatelet drugs, aspirin, lithium, methotrexate
    - Adverse effects: epigastric distress, peptic ulcer

– Aspirin: 650 to 1,000 mg; may repeat q6h PRN (max 4 g/day):
  ○ Contraindication: aspirin or NSAID allergy or bronchospasm, bleeding disorders, peptic ulcer
  ○ Drug interactions: anticoagulants, antiplatelet drugs, angiotensin-converting enzyme inhibitors, β-blockers, corticosteroids, NSAIDs, sulfonylureas
  ○ Adverse effects: GI irritation/bleeding, thrombocytopenia
– Acetaminophen (Tylenol): 1,000 mg; may repeat q6h PRN (max 3 to 4 g/day):
  ○ Adverse effects (rare): rash, pancytopenia, liver damage
  ○ Precaution: hepatic impairment, consumption of ≥3 per day alcoholic beverages
• For prophylaxis in frequent episodic and chronic TTH:
– Tricyclic antidepressants (TCAs): Amitriptyline [Elavil]: Start at 10 mg, may slowly up-titrate to 100 mg QHS.
  ○ Not U.S. Food and Drug Administration (FDA)-approved for chronic TTH
  ○ Consider if patient has depression, anxiety, or insomnia.
  ○ Contraindications: acute recovery phase (within 30 days) of MI, use of monoamine oxidase inhibitors (MAOIs) within 14 days
  ○ Drug interactions: clonidine, MAOIs, quinolone antibiotics, SSRIs, sympathomimetics, azole antifungals, valproic acid
  ○ Adverse effects: weight gain, drowsiness, dry mouth, tachycardia, heart block, blurred vision, urinary retention, seizure

Second Line
• For acute treatment in episodic TTH:
– Caffeine combinations: 130-mg caffeine with 500-mg acetaminophen and/or 500-mg aspirin q6h PRN (2)[C]
– Ketorolac: 60 mg IM once, for severe episodes
– Opioids (e.g., codeine), butalbital, or their combination: not recommended. Consider secondary causes of headache or secondary gain such as drug-seeking behavior for personal use or diversion/sale.
• For prophylaxis in frequent episodic and chronic TTH:
– Mirtazapine: 15 to 30 mg/day (not FDA-approved for chronic TTH) (2),(3)[B].

ALERT
Use of abortive agents >2 days/week may lead to *medication-overuse headaches*; must withdraw acute treatment to diagnose

ADDITIONAL THERAPIES
• The combination of stress management therapy and a TCA (amitriptyline) may be most effective for chronic TTH.
• Topiramate: 100 mg/day (limited clinical evidence for prevention of chronic TTH; not FDA-approved for chronic TTH)
• Alternative TCAs: limited evidence of benefit (4)[B].
– Nortriptyline (Pamelor): 25 to 50 mg/day (mild-moderately sedating, causes weight gain)
– Protriptyline (Vivactil): 25 mg/day (nonsedating, causes weight loss)
• Tizanidine: conflicting clinical evidence for use in chronic TTH, thus should not be considered

SURGERY/OTHER PROCEDURES
• Trigger point lidocaine injections: may reduce headache frequency in frequent episodic or chronic TTH (5)[B]
• Botulinum toxin injection: conflicting clinical evidence for use in chronic TTH.

COMPLEMENTARY & ALTERNATIVE MEDICINE
• Tiger Balm or peppermint oil (not FDA-approved for TTH) applied topically to the forehead may be effective for episodic TTH (6)[B].
• Cognitive-behavioral therapy may be helpful (2),(6)[C].
• Electromyography (EMG) biofeedback may be effective and is enhanced when combined with relaxation therapy (2),(5)[C].
• Physical therapy, including positioning, ergonomic instruction, massage, transcutaneous electrical nerve simulation, and application of heat/cold, may help.
• Chiropractic spinal manipulation has equivocal evidence in the management of episodic and chronic TTH (6)[B].
• Acupuncture may decrease symptoms frequency; NNT = 3 to have at least 50% reduction in headache frequency, compared to routine care (7)[B].

ADMISSION, INPATIENT, AND NURSING CONSIDERATIONS
Typical symptoms usually managed in the outpatient setting. However, red flag symptoms may prompt emergent evaluation (thunderclap onset, fever and meningismus, papilledema with focal signs); or urgent management (temporal arteritis, relevant systemic illness, papilledema without focal signs, elderly patient with new headache and cognitive changes).

 ONGOING CARE

FOLLOW-UP RECOMMENDATIONS
• Keep headache diary to identify triggers, monitor progress, and prevent medication-overuse headache.
• Regular exercise and sleep schedule

DIET
• Identify and avoid dietary triggers.
• Regulate meal schedule.

PATIENT EDUCATION
• National Headache Foundation: http://www.headaches.org/resources
• Family Doctor by American Academy of Family Physicians: https://familydoctor.org/condition/headaches

PROGNOSIS
• Usually follows a chronic course when life stressors are not changed
• Most cases are intermittent and decrease with age.

COMPLICATIONS
• Lost days of work and productivity (more with Chronic TTH)
• Medication-overuse headache
• Dependence/addiction to narcotic analgesics
• GI bleeding from NSAID use

REFERENCES

1. Headache Classification Committee of the International Headache Society (IHS) The International Classification of Headache Disorders, 3rd edition. *Cephalalgia*. 2018;38(1):1–211.
2. Bendtsen L, Jensen R. Treating tension-type headache—an expert opinion. *Expert Opin Pharmacother*. 2011;12(7):1099–1109.
3. Becker WJ, Findlay T, Moga C, et al. Guideline for primary care management of headache in adults. *Can Fam Physician*. 2015;61(8):670–679.
4. Verhagen AP, Damen L, Berger MY, et al. Lack of benefit for prophylactic drugs of tension-type headache in adults: a systematic review. *Fam Pract*. 2010;27(2):151–165.
5. Karadaş Ö, Gül HL, Inan LE. Lidocaine injection of pericranial myofascial trigger points in the treatment of frequent episodic tension-type headache. *J Headache Pain*. 2013;14(1):44.
6. Sun-Edelstein C, Mauskop A. Complementary and alternative approaches to the treatment of tension-type headache. *Curr Pain Headache Rep*. 2012;16(6):539–544.
7. Linde K, Allais G, Brinkhaus B, et al. Acupuncture for the prevention of tension-type headache. *Cochrane Database Syst Rev*. 2016;(4):CD007587.

 SEE ALSO

Algorithm: Headache, Chronic

CODES

ICD10
• G44.209 Tension-type headache, unspecified, not intractable
• G44.219 Episodic tension-type headache, not intractable
• G44.229 Chronic tension-type headache, not intractable

CLINICAL PEARLS
• Typically characteristics include bilateral mild to moderate, nonthrobbing head pain or pressure, without other associated symptoms.
• Consider secondary causes and obtain further testing, such as neuroimaging, if there are unexplained focal signs, atypical presentation, late onset (>50 years of age), or when usual treatment fails.
• Medication-overuse headaches can be minimized by limiting use of abortive agents to no more than 2 days/week.
• Chronic TTH is difficult to treat, and these patients are more likely to develop medication-overuse headache.
• Avoid the use of opioids or butalbital-containing medications as first-line treatment for recurrent headaches.

H

HEARING LOSS
Daniel Jason Frasca, DO

BASICS

DESCRIPTION
- Decrease in the ability to perceive and comprehend sound. It can be partial, complete, unilateral, and/or bilateral.
  - Typically defined as a deficit of >25 dB
- Types of hearing loss include conductive hearing loss (CHL or air–bone gap), sensorineural hearing loss (SNHL), or mixed hearing loss.
- System(s) affected: auditory; outer and middle ear (CHL) or inner ear, auditory nerve, and/or brainstem (SNHL).
- Sudden hearing loss is defined as rapid-onset, subjective sensation of hearing impairment in one or both ears (1).

EPIDEMIOLOGY
- All ages affected; common in children (CHL) and elderly (SNHL)
- Usually more severe at an earlier age in men

Incidence
- Increases with age
- Sudden sensorineural hearing loss (SSHL) occurs in 5 to 27 per 100,000 persons per year.

Prevalence
Geriatric Considerations
- 24.7% of 60 to 69 year olds in United States have bilateral speech-frequency hearing loss.
- ~80% of people aged >85 years have hearing loss.
- Loss of communication is a source of emotional stress and a physical risk for the elderly.
- Consider auditory rehabilitation (facing people when talking, improving lighting, minimizing background noise).

Pediatric Considerations
- Early diagnosis and treatment improve outcome.
- 60% of childhood hearing loss is secondary to preventable causes.
- Mandatory screening in >97% of newborns with otoacoustic emission (OAE) and auditory brainstem response (ABR) testing

ETIOLOGY AND PATHOPHYSIOLOGY
- CHL: Hearing loss can result from middle ear effusion, obstruction of canal (cerumen/foreign body, osteomas/exostoses, cholesteatoma, tumor), loss of continuity (ossicular discontinuity), stiffening of the components (myringosclerosis, tympanosclerosis, and otosclerosis), and loss of the pressure differential across the tympanic membrane (TM) (perforation).

- SNHL: damage along the pathway from oval window, cochlea, auditory nerve, and brainstem. Examples include vascular/metabolic insult, mass effect, infection and inflammation, and acoustic trauma.
  - Noise-induced hearing loss is caused by acoustic insult that affects outer hair cells in the organ of Corti, causing them to be less stiff. Over time, severe damage occurs with fusion and loss of stereocilia. Eventually this may progress to inner hair cells and auditory nerve as well.
- Large vestibular aqueduct or superior canal dehiscence: Third mobile window shunts acoustic energy away from cochlea.

Genetics
- Connexin 26 (13q11–13q12): most common cause of nonsyndromic genetic hearing loss
- Otosclerosis: familial
- There are several congenital syndromes (e.g., Alport syndrome, Stickler syndrome).

RISK FACTORS
- Loud noise/acoustic trauma
- Medications (aminoglycosides, loop diuretics, aspirin, nonsteroidal anti-inflammatory drugs [NSAIDs], quinine, chemotherapeutic agents, especially cisplatin, vancomycin)
- Tobacco, alcohol use
- Vestibular schwannoma/skull base neoplasm
- Previous ear surgery
- Sensorineural, pediatric specific
  - Perinatal asphyxia
  - Mechanical ventilation lasting ≥5 days
  - Congenital infections (toxoplasmosis, other agents, rubella, cytomegalovirus, herpes simplex [TORCH] syndrome)
  - Toxemia of pregnancy
  - Maternal diabetes
  - Rh incompatibility
  - Prematurity or birth weight <1,500 g
  - Severe hyperbilirubinemia; exchange transfusions
  - Anomalous temporal bone (Mondini or large vestibular aqueduct)
  - Infectious diseases (chickenpox, measles, encephalitis, influenza, mumps, bacterial meningitis)
  - Vasculitis (Kawasaki disease)

GENERAL PREVENTION
- Limit noise exposure; use hearing protection.
- Avoid ear canal instrumentation (e.g., cotton swabs).
- Avoid or limit ototoxic medications.

COMMONLY ASSOCIATED CONDITIONS
Tinnitus: common for patients to experience both tinnitus and hearing loss

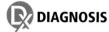

DIAGNOSIS

HISTORY
- Social problems and comments from friends and family are often the first presentation of presbycusis (age-related hearing loss); patients are often not aware of the degree of hearing loss they experience and how it affects their life; insidious onset and progression
- Difficulty hearing
  - Rapid versus gradual decline: Rapid loss (<3 days) is a medical emergency. Urgent ear/nose/throat referral and steroid therapy are recommended.
  - Difficulty with discrimination of sounds, hearing in crowds, or turning up the volume of television sets
  - Frequently having to ask speakers to repeat
  - Friends/family complain of hearing loss
- Tinnitus, bilateral or unilateral
- Otalgia
- Otorrhea, clear or purulent
- Dizziness or vertigo
- Aural fullness
- Autophony (hearing own voice louder or echoing)
- History of ear infections or ear surgeries
- History of trauma or noise exposure
- Family history of hearing loss
- History of recent viral infection

PHYSICAL EXAM
- Whispered voice test: A whisper heard from ~2 feet away is a good screen for intact hearing. Patients with SNHL have difficulty with this because their hearing loss is usually in the high frequency range.
- A simple 512-Hz tuning fork test lateralizes to unaffected ear in sudden SNHL (emergency) and lateralizes to the affected ear in CHL (not an emergency).
- 512-Hz tuning fork tests:
  - Sensorineural loss
    - Placed on the forehead: lateralizes to unaffected ear (Weber test)
    - Base of tuning fork placed on the mastoid and then fork end placed next to ear; heard louder next to ear—air > bone (+ Rinne test)
  - Conductive loss
    - Placed on the forehead or teeth lateralizes to affected or symptomatic ear
    - Placed on the mastoid and then next to ear; heard louder behind the ear on the side of conductive deficit bone > air (− Rinne test)
- Otoscopy: Assess for deformity, canal patency, and otorrhea; TM integrity/retraction/mobility with insufflation, canal, or middle ear mass, cerumen impaction.
- Facial symmetry

- Cranial nerve exam
- Nasopharyngoscopy: adenoid hypertrophy or nasopharyngeal mass (mandatory in adult patient with new unilateral serous effusion)

DIFFERENTIAL DIAGNOSIS
- Conductive loss secondary to mechanical issues (e.g., cerumen impaction/foreign body, perforation of TM, acoustic neuroma)
- Sensorineural loss:
  - Presbycusis (age-related hearing loss)
  - Noise induced (recreational, occupational)
  - Ménière disease
  - Ototoxicity (aspirin, NSAIDs, aminoglycosides)
  - Viral labyrinthitis
  - Cerebellopontine angle (CPA) tumor
  - Temporal bone fracture
  - Metabolic (hyper-/hypothyroidism)
  - Paget disease
  - Perilymphatic (inner ear) fistula
  - Vasculitis (including giant cell arteritis, Takayasu arteritis, polyarteritis nodosa, granulomatous with polyangiitis, microscopic polyangiitis, eosinophilic granulomatosis with polyangiitis, systemic lupus erythematosus, immune-complex associated vasculitis, and others) (2)

DIAGNOSTIC TESTS & INTERPRETATION
Consider as clinically indicated:
- MRI of the brain and brainstem with gadolinium to evaluate SNHL in congenital, early-onset, and asymmetric hearing loss
- Fine-cut CT temporal bones without contrast may help in the evaluation of CHL.
- Newborn screening with OAE and/or ABR
- Consider genetic testing for connexin 26, mitochondrial studies for children with SNHL.
- TORCH screening (congenital infection)
- Rapid plasma reagin (RPR) or venereal disease research laboratory (VDRL) confirmed by fluorescent treponemal antibody absorption (FTA-ABS)
- Lyme titer in endemic areas
- Antinuclear antibodies and sedimentation rate as a screen for autoimmune disease
- Pendred syndrome (goiter, mental retardation + SNHL): perchlorate test, thyroid function tests
- Alport syndrome (nephritis + SNHL): urinalysis, renal function tests
- Jervell and Lange-Nielsen syndrome (syncope, family history of sudden death + profound SNHL): ECG

Diagnostic Procedures/Other
- Audiometry: pure tone (air and bone), speech testing, and impedance (middle ear pressure) testing
- Tympanometry: Type B or C tympanograms indicate fluid or retraction, respectively. Negative middle ear peak pressures were seen even with normal (type A) tympanograms.
- Other tests: ABR, OAEs: "echo" of the cochlea, behavioral audiometry for children 6 months to 5 years old
- Myringotomy and tubes can be considered for persistent fluid with hearing loss.

 TREATMENT

MEDICATION
- Clinical practical guidelines for sudden hearing loss include the following:
  - Distinguishing SNHL from CHL; testing for bilateral sudden hearing loss in patients with unilateral sudden hearing loss; obtaining an MRI, ABR, or audiometric follow-up to evaluate for retrocochlear pathology; offer intratympanic steroid perfusion for refractory cases after initial management fails to treat idiopathic sudden SNHL (ISSNHL).
  - May offer corticosteroids as initial therapy to patients with ISSNHL and hyperbaric oxygen therapy (HBOT) within 2 weeks of onset; may consider HBOT within 1 month of onset as salvage therapy
  - Recommend against prescribing antivirals, thrombolytics, vasodilators, vasoactive substances, or antioxidants to patients with ISSNHL.
  - Recommend against routine laboratory tests in patients with ISSNHL.
- Treatment should begin ASAP, within 1 to 2 weeks of onset with high-dose oral steroids: 1 mg/kg or 60 to 100 mg/day prednisone or 12 to 16 mg/day dexamethasone for 7 to 14 days, followed by a taper.
- Intratympanic steroids show similar efficacy to oral steroids and reduce systemic side effects.
- Some studies suggest benefit of combined oral and intratympanic steroids for first-line treatment of sudden SNHL.

ISSUES FOR REFERRAL
- Failure of newborn screen
- Audiology for suspected hearing loss for formal evaluation
- Speech therapist: if speech delay or speech impediment is present
- Neurology and neurosurgery: CPA lesion, intracranial complication of middle ear disease

ADDITIONAL THERAPIES
Aural rehabilitation: interdisciplinary approach involving audiologists, speech language pathologists, otologist, family physician, and other members of health care team as needed

SURGERY/OTHER PROCEDURES
- Surgical options for CHL:
  - Tympanostomy and tube placement, tympanoplasty, mastoidectomy
  - Ossicular chain reconstruction, stapedectomy/ stapedotomy, canaloplasty
- Surgical options for SNHL
  - Cochlear implantation (in those with profound, bilateral hearing loss)

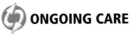 **ONGOING CARE**

FOLLOW-UP RECOMMENDATIONS
Patient Monitoring
Audiogram and clinical exam are the primary means of monitoring patient.

DIET
- Salt restriction to 2 g/day is helpful for patients with Ménière disease.
- Reduce alcohol consumption.

PATIENT EDUCATION
- To prevent damage that leads to noise-induced hearing loss:
  - Avoid excessive and prolonged noise exposure.
  - Use protective devices.
- National Institute on Deafness and Other Communication Disorders (NIDCD): http://www.nidcd.nih.gov/health/hearing/Pages/Default.aspx

PROGNOSIS
- SNHL is usually permanent and may be progressive.
- ISSNHL may recover spontaneously in 32–70% of cases, but urgent referral and treatment is recommended to maximize recovery.

COMPLICATIONS
Acute middle ear problems may become chronic (perforations, cholesteatoma).

REFERENCES
1. Michels TC, Duffy MT, Rogers DJ. Hearing loss in adults: differential diagnosis and treatment. *Am Fam Physician*. 2019;100(2):98–108.
2. Rahne T, Plontke S, Keyßer G. Vasculitis and the ear: a literature review. *Curr Opin Rheumatol*. 2020;32(1):47–52.

ADDITIONAL READING
Michaudet C, Malaty J. Cerumen impaction: diagnosis and management. *Am Fam Physician*. 2018;98(8):525–529.

 CODES

ICD10
- H91.11 Presbycusis, right ear
- H91 Other and unspecified hearing loss
- H91.09 Ototoxic hearing loss, unspecified ear

CLINICAL PEARLS
- In sudden hearing loss, if a 512-Hz tuning fork test (Weber test) lateralizes to the *unaffected ear*, suspect sensorineural causes (emergent evaluation needed), but if it lateralizes to the *affected ear*, the diagnosis is CHL (not an emergency).
- ~80% of people aged >85 years have hearing loss; encourage screening and treatment, especially in patients with early dementia.
- Best way to prevent noise-induced hearing loss is to protect against noise exposure.
- Consider auditory rehabilitation in all patients.

H

HEART FAILURE, ACUTELY DECOMPENSATED

Muhammad I. Durrani, DO, MS • Akash Ray, DO • Kayla Hempel, MD

BASICS

DESCRIPTION
Acute decompensated heart failure (ADHF) is a heterogenous group of related syndromes with new-onset or recurrence of cardiac pump function impairment. ADHF may be due to complications arising from the pericardium, myocardium, endocardium, or the heart valves. This leads to a wide variety of symptoms that are secondary to pulmonary congestion with elevated left atrial pressure, excessive fluid accumulation and reduction in cardiac output. ADHF can be a new diagnosis or represent worsening of preexisting chronic heart failure (HF). A number of terms have been used to describe this pathology including acute HF, acute HF syndrome, as well as acute decompensation of chronic HF.

EPIDEMIOLOGY
Incidence
- Incidence, prevalence, and costs of HF are discussed in the chapter "Heart Failure: Chronic."
- Medicare spends more to diagnose and treat HF than any other medical condition. HF is the most common cause of admission and readmission in the United States in those >65 years of age, responsible for >1 million annual hospitalizations.
- About half of people who have HF die within 5 years of diagnosis. 90% of patients who have HF die within 10 years. Newer studies have cited a 37% mortality rate within 1 year in the elderly population.

ETIOLOGY AND PATHOPHYSIOLOGY
- Two potential pathophysiologic conditions lead to the clinical findings of HF, namely systolic and/or diastolic heart dysfunction. See "Heart Failure: Chronic." Systolic dysfunction: an *inotropic* abnormality, and diastolic dysfunction: a *compliance* abnormality
  - The terms HF with reduced, midrange, preserved, or improved LVEF (HFrEF, HFmrEF, HFpEF, and HFimpEF respectively) have been adopted recently.
  - Recent American HF guidelines have also described three clinical profiles of patients with ADHF that take into account the patient's clinical manifestations, hemodynamics, and systemic perfusion:
    - Patients with volume overload: evidenced by pulmonary and/or systemic congestion and often triggered by an acute hypertensive crisis
    - Patients with depression of cardiac output: evidenced by hypotension, renal hypoperfusion, and/or shock
    - Patients with signs and symptoms of both volume overload and shock
- ADHF can result from the following conditions:
  - Myocardial disease: exacerbation of preexisting chronic HF heralded by noncompliance or infection or some other acute trigger, such as coronary artery disease (CAD), MI, toxic damage, immune-mediated and inflammatory damage, infiltrative diseases, metabolic derangements, and genetic abnormalities
  - Abnormal loading conditions: HTN, valvular and myocardial structural defects, pericardial and endomyocardial pathologies, high-output states, volume overload
  - Arrhythmias: atrial fibrillation, tachyarrhythmias, high-grade heart block, bradyarrhythmias

Genetics
See "Heart Failure: Chronic."

RISK FACTORS
See "Heart Failure: Chronic."

GENERAL PREVENTION
See "Heart Failure: Chronic."

COMMONLY ASSOCIATED CONDITIONS
Dysrhythmia followed by pump failure is the leading cause of death in ADHF. Most patients have >5 comorbidities (especially CAD, chronic kidney disease, and diabetes) and take >5 medications.

DIAGNOSIS
Requires a multifaceted clinical approach with no gold standard diagnostic test: No single historical, physical exam (PE), ECG, or radiographic finding can rule out HF. See "Heart Failure: Chronic."

HISTORY
- Patients typically have a history of HF, MI, uncontrolled HTN, and other risk factors mentioned above.
- Dyspnea on exertion and orthopnea are the only symptoms with high sensitivity but suffer from low specificity.
- Other symptoms: See "Heart Failure: Chronic."

PHYSICAL EXAM
- S_3 has the highest likelihood ratio (LR) in respect to PE with positive LR ranging from 1.6 to 13.0. No PE finding has sensitivity >70%.
- Lung exam: rales (crackles) and sometimes wheezing, Cheyne-Stokes respirations

DIFFERENTIAL DIAGNOSIS
Rule out life-threatening diagnoses first: pulmonary embolism, MI, tamponade, pneumothorax, acute respiratory distress syndrome, sepsis, chronic obstructive pulmonary disease (COPD), pneumonia, constrictive pericarditis, high-output states (anemia, hyperthyroidism).

DIAGNOSTIC TESTS & INTERPRETATION
Laboratory data are adjunctive and help with prognostication and clinical course.

Initial Tests (lab, imaging)
- See also "Heart Failure: Chronic." First, assess blood pressure (BP) and other vital signs and rule out hemodynamic instability and signs of cardiogenic shock.
- ECG and cardiac troponins to evaluate for ACS. Note that elevated troponins are detected in the majority of HF patients, often without obvious myocardial ischemia.
- BUN, creatinine, electrolytes, liver function tests, TSH (new onset), glucose, and CBC
- Transthoracic echocardiogram: recommended immediately in hemodynamically unstable ADHF patients and within 48 hours when cardiac structure and function are either not known or may have changed since previous studies

- BNP and/or N-terminal fragment pro-BNP (NT-proBNP): Measurement of BNP or NT-proBNP is recommended in all patients with acute dyspnea and suspected ADHF when the cause of dyspnea is unclear and may be related to ADHF.
  - BNP <100 essentially will rule out HF with negative LR of 0.2 and sensitivity of 93.5%. BNP >500 have a specificity of 89.8%. BNP 100 to 400 may indicate HF or may be related to other cardiac conditions, noncardiac (e.g., pulmonary) conditions, or multiple conditions.
- NT-proBNP values >450 pg/mL for people age <50 years, >900 pg/mL ages 50 to 75 years, and >1,800 pg/mL ages >75 years are highly suggestive of HF (sensitivity 90%, specificity of 84%) in the correct clinical setting.
- Chest x-ray: to assess for pulmonary congestion and to detect other cardiac or noncardiac diseases that may cause or contribute to the patient's symptoms
- Lung ultrasound (LUS): emerging as a diagnostic tool for ADHF with a positive LUS defined by the presence of >3 B lines in two bilateral lung zones yielding a specificity of 92.7% and LR of 7.4

Follow-Up Tests & Special Considerations
Please see "Heart Failure, Chronic."

Diagnostic Procedures/Other
Cardiac catheterization may be considered when CAD is suspected. Pulmonary artery catheterization may be performed to guide therapy in severe cases with cardiogenic shock.

Test Interpretation
Cardiac pathology depends on the etiology of HF. Please refer to "Heart Failure, Chronic."

TREATMENT
The goal of treatment is to improve hemodynamics and organ perfusion, alleviate symptoms, limit cardiac and renal damage, restore oxygenation, and minimize hospital length of stay as well as identify the etiology or precipitating factors. See "Heart Failure: Chronic." Below recommendations are all derived from the 2017 ACC guideline for the management of heart failure (1).

MEDICATION

ALERT
- Many therapies do not favorably impact morbidity or mortality. Diuretics are used initially in fluid overload ADHF, with nitrates added as needed during initial stabilization.
- Precipitating factors should be recognized and chronic oral therapy should be optimized during the patient's hospitalization after they are stabilized. Patients who could potentially benefit from revascularization should also be identified. Lastly, education must be provided concerning dietary sodium restriction, self-assessment of volume status, and medications.

- Once ADHF is stabilized, the guideline suggests an ACE inhibitor, ARB, or ARNI and β-blocker be started in patients with reduced systolic function. Use of a new agent ivabradine has also been touted in select patients but has not been shown to reduce cardiovascular mortality. Avoid NSAIDs and COX-2 inhibitors. There are no class IA drug recommendations for ADHF.

First Line

- Vasodilators: Consider in ADHF with systolic blood pressure (SBP) >90 mm Hg. Patients with hypertensive ADHF should get IV vasodilators as initial therapy to reduce congestion if no contraindications exist. Use in chronic HF is not effective. Vasodilators lower ventricular filling pressure and systemic vascular resistance to indirectly improve cardiac function.
  - IV nitroglycerin may be of short-term benefit by decreasing preload and afterload by dilating peripheral capacitance and resistance vessels on vascular smooth musculature (IV 10 to 20 μg/min, increase up to 200 μg/min).
  - IV nitroprusside: Administer with caution, start with 0.3 μg/kg/min, and increase up to 5.0 μg/kg/min.
  - IV ACE inhibitors evidence unclear and recommendations vary. They are thought to work by reducing both preload and afterload.
- IV loop diuretics recommended for all patients with ADHF and symptoms of fluid overload in hemodynamically stable patients (contraindicated if SBP <90 mm Hg, severe hyponatremia, acidosis); be cautious of electrolyte abnormalities if kidney disease is present. Diuresis should be instituted early in ADHF, continuous infusion is no better than bolus, and high dose is not significantly better than low dose.
  - Furosemide (Lasix): New-onset ADHF patients should get boluses of 20 to 40 mg IV.
  - If on furosemide (Lasix) chronically, initial IV dose should be equal or exceed chronic oral daily dose (1.0 to 2.5 times home dose). Monitor for appropriate urine output.
  - Bumetanide and torsemide are alternative loop diuretics.
  - When congestion fails to improve with initial diuretic therapy, consideration should be given to addition of second type of diuretic orally (metolazone or spironolactone) or intravenously (chlorothiazide).
- Thiazides in combination with loop diuretics may be useful if ineffective diuresis. Hydrochlorothiazide [HCTZ] 25 mg PO) and spironolactone or eplerenone (25 to 50 mg PO) may be used in combination with loop diuretics if excessive volume overload.
- Metolazone (Zaroxolyn): 2.5 to 20.0 mg/day PO, can be added as the second, synergistic diuretic to a loop diuretic in cases of ineffective diuresis and may be more effective than other thiazides in patients with renal insufficiency
- Bilevel positive airway pressure (BIPAP)/NPPV: NPPV decreases symptom severity, rate of intubation, and early mortality in ADHF. With clinical evidence of pulmonary edema, this is a level A recommendation. See "Additional Therapies" section.

Second Line

- Tolvaptan for severe hypervolemic hyponatremia refractory to water restriction and medical therapy is being studied.
- Inotropes: reserved for patients with severe systolic dysfunction occurring most often in hypotensive ADHF.
  - Phosphodiesterase inhibitors (milrinone, enoximone) decrease pulmonary resistance; may be used for patients on β-blockers but may increase medium-term mortality in CAD patients. Milrinone specifically produces ionotropic and vasodilatory effects without β-adrenergic stimulation of the heart.
  - Dobutamine infusion 2 to 20 μg/kg/min requires close BP monitoring; avoid in cardiogenic shock or with tachyarrhythmias. Low-dose dopamine infusion may be considered (3 to 5 μg/kg/min).
  - Levosimendan (calcium sensitizer) improves hemodynamic parameters but not survival compared to placebo.
- Vasopressors: Consider in patients with cardiogenic shock despite treatment with another inotrope.
- Nesiritide, a BNP analog, is not recommended secondary to higher rates of hypotension, no benefit on death, or rehospitalization rates.
- Ultrafiltration renal replacement therapy: Routine use of ultrafiltration is not recommended.
- Extracorporeal membrane oxygenation (ECMO): venoarterial ECMO for the sickest cohort of ADHF patients. ECMO has been used as a bridge to transplant or to long-term mechanical support.

ADDITIONAL THERAPIES

- Oxygen: Begin treatment early; ideally titrate to an arterial oxygen saturation >92% (90% if COPD). Treat anemia with transfusion: conservative trigger Hgb <8; target Hgb 10.
- Cochrane review shows that one death can be avoided for every 14 ADHF patients treated with NPPV and one death for every 9 ADHF patients treated with CPAP. Avoid mechanical ventilation for patients with right HF if possible.
- See "Heart Failure: Chronic" for maintenance treatments.

SURGERY/OTHER PROCEDURES

Heart valve surgery if valvular disease is responsible, PCI/CABG for patients with CAD/MI if applicable

ADMISSION, INPATIENT, AND NURSING CONSIDERATIONS

- Admission criteria considerations:
  - Evidence of severely decompensated HF: hypotension, worsening renal function, altered mental status, dyspnea at rest, concomitant arrhythmia, acute coronary syndrome
  - Consider observation unit stay for stable patients with preexisting HF and the following: no acute interventions needed for comorbid condition, SBP >120 mm Hg, RR <32 breaths/min, BUN <40 mg/dL, creatinine <3.0 mg/dL, no evidence of ischemia or elevated troponins, and BNP <1,000, N-type pro-BNP <5,000, and the clinical impression that the patient could be discharged in the next 24 hours.

- 1.5 to 2.0 L/day fluid restriction may be useful to reduce congestive symptoms.
- Discharge criteria: improved symptoms, SBP normalized at 100 to 120 mm Hg, good urine output, serum sodium >135 mEq/L, HF outpatient education

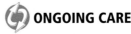

ONGOING CARE

FOLLOW-UP RECOMMENDATIONS

Patient Monitoring
Early follow-up and multidisciplinary care to reduce hospitalization and mortality.

DIET
See "Heart Failure: Chronic" (1).

PATIENT EDUCATION
Monitoring and self-care; teach: medication, activity, daily weight (and how to adjust diuretic). See "Heart Failure: Chronic."

PROGNOSIS
See "Heart Failure: Chronic."

COMPLICATIONS
Arrhythmia, pulmonary edema, hyponatremia, death

REFERENCE

1. Yancy CW, Jessup M, Bozkurt B, et al. 2017 ACC/AHA/HFSA Focused Update of the 2013 ACCF/AHA guideline for the management of heart failure: a report of the American College of Cardiology/American Heart Association Task Force on Clinical Practice Guidelines and the Heart Failure Society of America. *Circulation*. 2017;136(6):e137–e161.

CODES

ICD10
- I50.9 Heart failure, unspecified
- I50.21 Acute systolic (congestive) heart failure
- I50.31 Acute diastolic (congestive) heart failure

CLINICAL PEARLS

- BNP in ADHF is helpful in situations in which the diagnosis of ADHF is unclear.
- Look for an underlying cause of each episode of ADHF.

H

HEART FAILURE, CHRONIC

Afsha Rais Kaisani, MD • Mohamad Elzaim, MD • Niyomi De Silva, MD

 BASICS

DESCRIPTION

- Heart failure (HF) results from inability of the heart to fill and/or pump blood sufficiently to meet tissue metabolic needs. HF may occur when adequate cardiac output can be achieved only at the expense of elevated filling pressures. It is the principal complication of heart disease. For acute HF, see "Heart Failure, Acutely Decompensated."
- HF is the preferred term over congestive HF as patients are not always congested (fluid overloaded). HF may involve the left heart, the right heart, or be biventricular. It is progressive—manifested by the remodeling (altered heart geometry) process.
- The New York Heart Association (NYHA) classification is a subjective grading scale used for classifying a patient's functional status: NYHA class I: asymptomatic; NYHA class II: symptomatic with moderate exertion; NYHA class III: symptomatic with mild exertion and may limit activities of daily living; NYHA class IV: symptomatic at rest.
- The American Heart Association (AHA)/American College of Cardiology (ACC) stages are a system to delineate the progression of HF: stage A: at risk for HF, no structural disease; stage B: structural disease, no HF symptoms; stage C: structural disease, HF symptoms; stage D: end-stage disease.

EPIDEMIOLOGY

HF accounts for close to 1 million hospitalizations a year with 25% readmitted within 30 days. The annual direct and indirect cost of HF in the United States is ~$34.4 billion.

Incidence

In the United States, 550,000 new cases are diagnosed annually with >250,000 deaths/year.

Prevalence

- An estimated 23 million individuals have HF worldwide. ~6.5 million people in the United States have HF; <1% in those age <50 years, increasing to 10% of those age >80 years
- Primarily a disease of the elderly; 75% of hospital admissions for HF are for persons >65 years of age.

ETIOLOGY AND PATHOPHYSIOLOGY

- Two physiologic components explain most of the clinical findings of HF and result in classifications in four general categories:
  - HF with reduced ejection fraction (HFrEF) or systolic HF: an *inotropic* abnormality, often from myocardial infarction (MI) or dilated cardiomyopathy (CM), resulting in diminished systolic emptying (ejection fraction [EF] ≤40%)
  - HF with preserved EF (HFpEF) or diastolic HF: a *compliance* abnormality, often due to hypertensive CM, in which the ventricular relaxation is impaired (EF ≥50%)
  - Borderline HFpEF (EF 41–49%): mild systolic dysfunction, clinically behaves like HFpEF
  - Improved HFpEF (EF >40%): previously HFrEF, with improvement in systolic function

- Most common etiologies: coronary artery disease (CAD)/MI and hypertension (HTN). Others:
  - Myocarditis and CM: alcoholic, viral, drugs, muscular dystrophy, infiltrative (e.g., amyloidosis, sarcoidosis), postpartum, infectious (e.g., Chagas disease, HIV), hypertrophic CM (HCM), inherited familial dilated CM
  - Valvular and vascular abnormalities: valvular stenosis or regurgitation, rheumatic heart; renal artery stenosis, usually bilateral, may cause recurrent "flash" pulmonary edema.
  - Chronic lung disease and pulmonary HTN
  - Arrhythmias (atrial fibrillation [AF] and other tachyarrhythmias, high-grade heart block, frequent PVCs)
  - Other: high-output states: hyperthyroidism, anemia; cardiac depressants (β-blocker overdose), stress induced; iatrogenic volume overload (extreme overload in patients with normal hearts and kidneys); idiopathic: 20–50% of idiopathic dilated CM are familial.

Genetics

Multiple genetic abnormalities responsible for a variety of phenotypes have been identified. Consider genetic screening for first-degree relatives of HCM and arrhythmogenic RV dysplasia.

RISK FACTORS

CAD/MI, HTN, valvular heart disease, diabetes, cardiotoxic medications, obesity, older age

GENERAL PREVENTION

Control HTN and other risk factors.

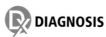 DIAGNOSIS

HISTORY

- Dyspnea on exertion: *cardinal sign of left-sided HF.* Deteriorating exercise capacity: easy fatigued, general weakness
- Nocturnal nonproductive cough, orthopnea, and paroxysmal nocturnal dyspnea; sometimes frothy or pink sputum. Wheezing, especially nocturnal, in absence of history of asthma or infection (cardiac asthma); Cheyne-Stokes respirations
- Anorexia and/or fullness or dull pain in right upper quadrant (hepatic congestion). Nausea and poor appetite may indicate advanced HF.

PHYSICAL EXAM

- Increased filling pressures: rales and sometimes wheezing, peripheral edema, S_3 gallop, hepatomegaly, jugular venous distention, hepatojugular reflux, ascites
- Remodeling: enlarged or displaced point of maximal impulse
- Poor cardiac output: hypotension, pulsus alternans, tachycardia, narrow pulse pressure, cool extremities, cyanosis

DIFFERENTIAL DIAGNOSIS

Simple dependent edema, pulmonary embolism, exertional asthma, cardiac ischemia, asthma/chronic obstructive pulmonary disorder, constrictive pericarditis, nephrotic syndrome, cirrhosis, venous occlusive disease

DIAGNOSTIC TESTS & INTERPRETATION

Diagnosis should be primarily clinical, with laboratory data as adjunctive and indicative of complications.

Initial Tests (lab, imaging)

- β-Type natriuretic peptide (BNP) and N-terminal pro-BNP (NT-proBNP): helpful in acute setting to differentiate the cause of dyspnea (<100 essentially rules out HF). A BNP level in those with risk factors for developing HF or with structural heart disease but no symptoms of HF can help predict the development of symptomatic HF (1)[A]. Pulmonary embolism, renal failure, and acute coronary syndromes may elevate BNP. Sacubitril/valsartan can raise BNP levels but has less impact on NT-proBNP levels. Obesity may lower BNP levels. The use of BNP-guided therapy in chronic HF and acutely decompensated HF is not well established, although a predischarge BNP can predict risk of readmission and survival (1)[A].
- Lab findings: respiratory alkalosis, azotemia, decreased erythrocyte sedimentation rate, proteinuria, elevated creatinine (cardiorenal syndrome), dilutional hyponatremia (poor prognosis), hyperbilirubinemia
- Chest x-ray (changes lag clinical symptoms): increased heart size, vascular redistribution (cephalization) with "butterfly" pattern of pulmonary edema, interstitial and alveolar edema, Kerley B lines, and pleural effusions. Findings of pulmonary edema may be absent in long-standing HF.

Diagnostic Procedures/Other

- Echocardiogram: most useful test to determine LVEF, which is critical for proper diagnosis and management of HF, as well as RV function, diastolic dysfunction, ventricular size, wall thickness, and valvular abnormalities; repeated if change suspected in underlying cardiac status
- Other tests: nuclear imaging to estimate ventricular size, assess for ischemia or infarction, amyloidosis, and systolic function. Cardiac MRI in select circumstances: suspicion of cardiac sarcoidosis, arrhythmogenic RV CM, acute myocarditis, amyloidosis, and hemochromatosis. Cardiac catheterization is important for excluding CAD as an etiology in the setting of risk factors; endomyocardial biopsy only in special circumstances (e.g., suspected giant cell myocarditis)

 TREATMENT

GENERAL MEASURES

Treatment is focused on improving hemodynamics, relieving symptoms, and blocking the neurohormonal response to improve survival.

MEDICATION

Diuretics and nitrates are used in acute HF management. ACE-I and aldosterone antagonists (especially for HFrEF) can be added at any time. β-Blocker should be started once acute HF resolved. Avoid nonsteroidal anti-inflammatory drugs (NSAIDs), which worsen HF. Avoid the use of diltiazem and verapamil with systolic dysfunction due to increase mortality and negative inotropic effects.

First Line

- ACE-I: used to decrease afterload, increase survival, improve symptoms, and exercise capacity in all NYHA classifications; benefit greatest for patients with systolic dysfunction and post-MI. Number needed to treat (NNT) ~25 per year for mortality. All ACE-Is are considered equally effective. Initiate at low doses and titrate as tolerated to target doses.
  - Starting dose: captopril: 6.25 mg PO TID; enalapril: 2.5 mg PO BID; lisinopril: 2.5 to 5.0 mg daily; ramipril: 1.25 mg daily
- Angiotensin receptor blockers (ARBs): indicated if intolerant to ACE-Is. Avoid combination of ACE-I and ARB.
  - Starting dose: candesartan: 4 to 8 mg PO daily; losartan: 25 to 50 mg PO daily; valsartan: 40 mg PO BID
- β-Blockers: used in systolic or diastolic HF. Initiate in hemodynamically stable/compensated patients at low dose and titrate upward slowly. NNT = 25/year for mortality. Mortality decreased in systolic HF; evidence for titration to heart rate (HR) rather than specific dose
  - Starting dose: carvedilol: 3.125 mg PO BID; metoprolol succinate ER: 12.5 mg/day PO; bisoprolol: 1.25 to 10.00 mg once daily
- Sacubitril/valsartan (Entresto): an angiotensin receptor and neprilysin inhibitor (ARNI), shown to reduce the risk of CV death and HF hospitalizations in patients with HFrEF. Recommended dose: 24/26 mg or 49/51 mg PO BID to a target of 97/103 mg PO BID. Patients with HFrEF and NYHA class II and III who tolerate an ACE-I or ARB with CrCl >30, replacement by an ARNI is recommended to reduce morbidity and mortality (NNT to prevent one CV death over 3.5 years: 31). ACE-Is should be discontinued at least 36 hours prior to starting ARNIs. Most common adverse effects: hypotension, angioedema, renal insufficiency
- Serum glucose cotransporter-2 (SGLT-2) inhibitors, dapagliflozin and empagliflozin, medications used for type 2 diabetes mellitus, showed improvement in worsening HF or CV death in patients with EF ≤40% and NYHA class II/IV, irrespective of diabetes, and may decrease overall death (NNT 50 to 60/year) based on randomized clinical trials, DAPA-HF and EMPEROR-Reduced. Recommended dose for both is 10 mg PO daily. Based on evidence, FDA approved the use of SGLT-2 inhibitors for the treatment of HFrEF. Adverse effects: urogenital infections, ketoacidosis, reduced blood pressure, enhanced diuresis (2)[A]
- Vericiguat, a guanylate cyclase simulator, shown to reduce the risk of death from CV causes or hospitalization for HF with a hazard ration of 0.9 (95% CI 0.82–0.98); FDA approved in patients with an EF ≤45%, recent HF hospitalization, or need for IV diuretics based on the VICTORIA trial (1)[B]
- Diuretics are helpful to manage volume overload/reduce preload.
  - Furosemide (Lasix): 40 to 120 mg/day PO divided dose; bumetanide (Bumex): 0.5 to 10.0 mg/day IV/PO divided dose; torsemide (Demadex): 10 to 200 mg/day PO divided dose
  - Metolazone (Zaroxolyn): 2.5 to 20.0 mg/day PO divided dose; hydrochlorothiazide: 12.5 to 100.0 mg/day PO divided dose; chlorothiazide (Diuril): 250 to 2,000 mg/day IV/PO divided dose
  - Spironolactone, eplerenone (improve mortality when added to standard therapy in NYHA class II to IV + EF <35%): spironolactone 12.5 to 25.0 mg/day PO; maximum 50 mg/day PO; eplerenone 25 to 50 mg/day; caution regarding hyperkalemia and chronic kidney disease (CKD)

- Digoxin: reduces symptoms, without positive effect on mortality. In patients with preserved renal function (CrCl >50 mL/min), the recommended dose is 0.125 mg/day.
- Combination of isosorbide dinitrate and hydralazine (20 mg/37.5 mg PO TID) is effective for improving survival and reducing hospitalizations in African Americans and can be used if the patient is unable to take an ACE-I/ARB.
- Ivabradine (Corlanor) can be considered in NYHA class II and III HF, EF ≤35%, on maximally tolerated β-blockers with HR >70 to reduce hospitalization (1)[B]. Contraindication: ADHF, hypotension (<90/50 mm Hg), severe hepatic impairment, pacemaker dependence, bradyarrhythmias, or strong CYP3A4 inhibitors. Do not administer to patients currently in AF and discontinued if AF develops.
- In HFpEF, no therapy has improved survival. ARBs and spironolactone can be used to potentially reduce hospitalizations (1)[A].

ADDITIONAL THERAPIES

Device therapy including implantable cardioverter-defibrillators (ICDs) and cardiac resynchronization therapy (CRT) are shown to improve outcomes.

- CRT recommendation: sinus rhythm with a QRS width ≥150 ms due to left bundle branch block (LBBB), LVEF ≤35%, persistent mild to moderate HF despite goal directed medical therapy (GDMT), reduced LVEF and chronic RV pacing or with bradyarrhythmias, and an anticipated need for a pacemaker
- CRT consideration: LVEF ≤35%, sinus rhythm, QRS width >150 ms, non-LBBB pattern, and NYHA class II or ambulatory NYHA class IV symptoms. If QRS width >150 ms due to LBBB pattern, consider CRT in ambulatory NYHA class IV patients. If QRS width is between 120 and 150 ms with LBBB pattern, consider CRT in NYHA class II to IV, despite GDMT.
- ICDs recommendation: primary prevention in patients with *nonischemic* and *ischemic* CM, at least 40 days post-MI; LVEF ≤35%, NYHA class II or III HF, or LVEF ≤30%, NYHA class I HF; and on optimal medical therapy and >1 year estimated survival; generally not indicated in end-stage HF

SURGERY/OTHER PROCEDURES

- Heart valve surgery for defective heart valve; mitral valve repair if mitral regurgitation (MR) is the primary issue and not functional
- Advanced therapies such as cardiac transplantation and LV assist device (LVAD) implantation can be considered in patients with HF refractory. Cardiac transplantation: considered for patients ≤70 years old with a predicted 1-year survival worse than that afforded by transplantation. LVAD implantation indications are similar but evolving.

ADMISSION, INPATIENT, AND NURSING CONSIDERATIONS

- Admission: hemodynamic/respiratory compromise, mental status change, acute renal injury, significant volume overload, electrolyte abnormalities (e.g., hyponatremia)
- Discharge: subjective improvement, euvolemia on assessment, improved vitals, outpatient education performed

 ONGOING CARE

FOLLOW-UP RECOMMENDATIONS
Close outpatient follow-up after hospitalization to decrease frequency of readmission

DIET
Reduce sodium load; optimal level unknown

PATIENT EDUCATION
AHA: https://www.heart.org/

PROGNOSIS
After diagnosis: 1-year survival ~75%, 5-year survival <50%, and 10-year survival <25%

COMPLICATIONS
Sudden death, progressive pump failure

REFERENCES

1. Yancy CW, Jessup M, Bozkurt B, et al. 2017 ACC/AHA/HFSA focused update of the 2013 ACCF/AHA guideline for the management of heart failure: a report of the American College of Cardiology/American Heart Association Task Force on Clinical Practice Guidelines and the Heart Failure Society of America. *Circulation*. 2017;136(6):e137–e161.
2. Cardoso R, Graffunder FP, Ternes CMP, et al. SGLT2 inhibitors decrease cardiovascular death and heart failure hospitalizations in patients with heart failure: a systematic review and meta-analysis. *EClinicalMedicine*. 2021;36:100933.

ADDITIONAL READING

Maddox TM, Januzzi JL Jr, Allen LA, et al. 2021 Update to the 2017 ACC Expert Consensus Decision Pathway for optimization of heart failure treatment: answers to 10 pivotal issues about heart failure with reduced ejection fraction: a report of the American College of Cardiology Solution Set Oversight Committee. *J Am Coll Cardiol*. 2021;77(6):772–810.

 SEE ALSO

Algorithm: Congestive Heart Failure: Differential Diagnosis

 CODES

ICD10
- I50.9 Heart failure, unspecified
- I50.1 Left ventricular failure
- I50.22 Chronic systolic (congestive) heart failure

CLINICAL PEARLS

- Have patients weigh themselves and report weight gains of >2 lb in a day or 5 lb above dry weight.
- β-Blockers, ACE-I, and aldosterone antagonists are the core medications for management.

H

HEAT ILLNESS: HEAT EXHAUSTION AND HEAT STROKE

Sean C. Robinson, MD, CAQSM

 BASICS

DESCRIPTION
- A continuum of increasingly severe illness caused by dehydration, electrolyte losses, and failure of thermoregulatory mechanisms when exposed to elevated environmental temperatures
  - Heat exhaustion is a mild to moderate form of heat illness displaying dehydration type symptoms with a normal to elevated temperature (1).
  - Heat stroke is characterized by an elevated core temperature >104°F with central nervous system (CNS) abnormalities and is a true medical emergency (1),(2).
- Can be exertional (related to activity) or nonexertional
- System(s) affected: endocrine/metabolic, nervous, hepatic, hematologic
- Synonym(s): heat illness; heat injury; hyperthermia; heat collapse; heat prostration

Geriatric Considerations
Elderly persons are more susceptible.

Pediatric Considerations
Children are more susceptible.

Pregnancy Considerations
Pregnant women may be more susceptible to volume depletion with heat stress.

EPIDEMIOLOGY
- Predominant age: more likely in children or elderly
- Predominant sex: male = female

Incidence
- Depends on intensity of heat; estimate of 20/100,000 persons per season
- Concern for increasing incidence because ambient environmental temperatures continue to rise

Prevalence
- Depends on predisposing conditions in combination with environmental factors
- Roughly 600 deaths per year in the United States

ETIOLOGY AND PATHOPHYSIOLOGY
- Excess heat has direct cellular toxicity. Excess heat also leads to an imbalance between inflammatory and anti-inflammatory cytokines, vascular endothelial damage, and end-organ dysfunction.
- Interplay between failure of heat-dissipating mechanisms, an overwhelming heat stress, and an exaggerated acute-phase inflammatory response

RISK FACTORS
- Poor acclimatization to heat
- Poor physical conditioning
- Salt or water depletion
- Obesity

- Acute febrile or GI illnesses
- Chronic illnesses: uncontrolled diabetes mellitus, hypertension, cardiac disease
- Alcohol and other substance abuse
- High heat and humidity, poor environmental air circulation
- Heavy, restrictive clothing
- Nutritional supplements (e.g., ephedra) (2)
- Medications (α-adrenergics, anticholinergics, antihistamines, antipsychotics, benzodiazepines, β-blockers, calcium channel blockers, clopidogrel, diuretics, laxatives, neuroleptics, phenothiazines, thyroid agonists, tricyclic antidepressants) (1)

GENERAL PREVENTION
- The most important factor in preventing heat illness is prevention. Activity modification and adequate fluid replacement are key preventive measures.
- Allow acclimatization through proper conditioning and activity modification.
- Dress appropriately with loose-fitting, open-weaved, light-colored clothing.
- Consume a proper volume of fluids, particularly during physical activity in hot environments.
- Never leave children (or pets) unattended in cars during hot weather.
- Try to gain access to air-conditioned environments during hot weather.

 DIAGNOSIS

- Heat exhaustion: Symptoms are milder than in heat stroke, and there are no CNS derangements:
  - Fatigue, lethargy, weakness, dizziness, nausea, vomiting, myalgias, headache, profuse sweating, tachycardia, hypotension, thirst, hyperventilation
  - Core temperature usually elevated but can be normal; if elevated, <104°F (40°C)
- Heat stroke: marked by mental status changes and elevated core temperature
  - *Classic (nonexertional)*: caused by environmental exposure, primarily in elderly or chronically ill patients, and may develop gradually over days
    - Delirium
    - Confusion
    - Coma
    - Core temperature >104°F (>40°C)
    - Hot, flushed, dry skin
  - *Exertional*: typically younger, active patients; rapid onset
    - Exhaustion
    - Confusion, disorientation
    - Delirium
    - Coma
    - Hot, flushed skin, typically with sweating
    - Core temperature >104°F (>40°C) (1),(2)

HISTORY
- Heat cramps: sweating; muscle cramps/spasms
- Heat exhaustion: sweating; fatigue, light-headedness/dizziness; cramping; nausea, vomiting; headache
- Heat stroke: altered mental status

PHYSICAL EXAM
- Rectal temperature (*Don't rely on oral temperature.*)
- Heat exhaustion: tachycardia; cool/clammy skin;
- Heat stroke: rectal (core temperature) elevated (>103); hot/dry skin (compensatory sweating impaired)

DIFFERENTIAL DIAGNOSIS
- Febrile illnesses, sepsis
- Drug-induced fluid loss
- Cardiac arrhythmia or infarction
- Acute cocaine intoxication
- Neuroleptic malignant syndrome
- Malignant hyperthermia (an autosomally inherited disorder of skeletal and cardiac muscle in which patients have abnormal muscle metabolism on exposure to halothane or skeletal muscle reactants)

DIAGNOSTIC TESTS & INTERPRETATION
Detect end-organ damage

Initial Tests (lab, imaging)
- Creatinine, BUN, electrolytes (sodium in particular)
- Liver enzymes, muscle enzymes (creatine phosphokinase)
- CBC—hemoconcentration
- Urinalysis: increased urine specific gravity
- Drugs that may alter lab results: diuretics

 TREATMENT

GENERAL MEASURES
- For heat stroke: immediate body immersion in ice water to cool core temperature. Monitor hemodynamics and airway status (1)[C].
- Careful fluid and electrolyte replacement with normal saline; avoid hypotonic fluids. Follow serum sodium (1),(2)[C].
- Consider CVP monitoring.
- For heat exhaustion, consider:
  - Evaporative cooling: spraying water over the patient and using fans to facilitate evaporative and convective heat loss (1)[C]
  - Immerse hands and forearms in cold water.
  - Ice or cold packs on the neck, groin, and axillae (1),(2)[C]
- No clear superiority of any one method for heat exhaustion (1)

MEDICATION

First Line
- No medications are required in the initial management. Use isotonic saline solution to rehydrate (1)[C].
- Do not use antipyretics to lower core temperature in heat illness.

Second Line
- For severely ill, consider immunomodulators such as corticosteroids (patients in ICU setting).
- Iced gastric, bladder, or peritoneal lavage
- If disseminated intravascular coagulation (DIC), consider appropriate replacement therapy.

ADMISSION, INPATIENT, AND NURSING CONSIDERATIONS
- *Cool patient immediately* (prior to transport even) if heat stroke is suspected or once diagnosed.
- Rapid cooling: Remove clothing, wet patient down, and apply ice packs.
- Emergency treatment; best in a hospital setting

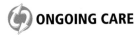 ONGOING CARE

FOLLOW-UP RECOMMENDATIONS
Rest with legs elevated.

Patient Monitoring
- Rectal temperature monitoring: Cooling may be discontinued when the core temperature drops to 102°F (38.9°C) and stabilizes.
- Heat stroke patients may require airway management, hemodynamic monitoring, and careful fluid and electrolyte administration and monitoring.
- Consider CVP monitoring.

DIET
- Cool or cold clear liquids only (noncarbonated)
- Avoid caffeine.
- Unrestricted sodium

PATIENT EDUCATION
- Proper hydration is the key to prevention.
- Proper conditioning and acclimatization
- Recognize signs and symptoms of heat stress—fatigue and headache.
- Skin exposure facilitates heat loss in hot, humid conditions (use proper sun protection).

PROGNOSIS
- If mental function is not altered and serum chemistries are normal, the prognosis is good and recovery within 24 to 48 hours is typical.
- The mortality rate for heat stroke (10–80%) is directly related to the duration and intensity of hyperthermia as well as to the speed and effectiveness of diagnosis and treatment.
- The priority in heat-related illness is early recognition and intervention. The faster the patient is cooled to below 40°C, the lower the patient mortality (3).

COMPLICATIONS
- May involve failure of any major organ system
- Cardiac arrhythmias or infarction
- Pulmonary edema, acute respiratory distress syndrome
- Coma, seizures
- Acute renal failure
- Rhabdomyolysis
- DIC
- Hepatocellular necrosis

REFERENCES

1. Lipman GS, Eifling KP, Ellis MA, et al. Wilderness Medical Society practice guidelines for the prevention and treatment of heat-related illness: 2014 update. *Wilderness Environ Med*. 2014;25(Suppl 4): S55–S65.
2. Gauer R, Meyers BK. Heat-related illnesses. *Am Fam Physician*. 2019;99(8):482–489.
3. Nye EA, Edler JR, Eberman LE, et al. Optimizing cold-water immersion for exercise-induced hyperthermia: an evidence-based paper. *J Athl Train*. 2016;51(6):500–501.

ADDITIONAL READING

- Armstrong LE, Casa DJ, Millard-Stafford M, et al. American College of Sports Medicine position stand. Exertional heat illness during training and competition. *Med Sci Sports Exerc*. 2007;39(3):556–572.
- Atha WF. Heat-related illness. *Emerg Med Clin North Am*. 2013;31(4):1097–1108.
- O'Connor FG. Sports medicine: exertional heat illness. *FP Essent*. 2019;482:15–19.

 CODES

ICD10
- T67.5XXA Heat exhaustion, unspecified, initial encounter
- T67.0XXA Heatstroke and sunstroke, initial encounter
- T67.3XXA Heat exhaustion, anhydrotic, initial encounter

CLINICAL PEARLS
- Exertional heat stroke is a life-threatening medical emergency that requires immediate whole-body cooling (cold/ice water immersion preferred).
- The diagnosis of heat stroke includes an elevated core temperature and signs of CNS dysfunction (e.g., mental status changes, irritability, ataxia, confusion, seizures, or coma).
- Start the cooling process immediately when heat exhaustion is recognized, beginning with wetting the skin with a cool mist and giving oral rehydration solutions if the patient is alert and oriented.
- If in the field (e.g., sporting events, wilderness), cooling should begin immediately (prior to transport if possible).
- Do not rely on oral temperature—a rectal temperature is always preferred.

H

HEMATURIA
Jyothi R. Patri, MD, MHA, FAAFP, HMDC • Vinay Krishna Pulusu, MD, MHA

BASICS

DESCRIPTION
Gross (visible) or microscopic (nonvisible) blood in the urine, either symptomatic or asymptomatic

EPIDEMIOLOGY
Prevalence
Children: gross: 0.13%; asymptomatic microscopic hematuria (AMH): 0.4–4.1%. Adults: AMH: 0.9–17%

ETIOLOGY AND PATHOPHYSIOLOGY
- Trauma
  - Exercise-induced (resolves within 24 hours of ceasing activity)
  - Abdominal trauma or pelvic fracture with renal, bladder, or ureteral injury
  - Iatrogenic from abdominal or pelvic surgery, indwelling catheters, or foreign body
  - Physical/sexual abuse
- Neoplasms
  - Urologic malignancies or benign tumors
  - Endometriosis of the urinary tract (suspect in females with cyclic hematuria)
- Inflammatory/infectious causes
  - UTI: most common cause of hematuria in adults
  - Renal diseases: radiation nephritis and cystitis, acute/chronic tubulointerstitial nephritis (due to drugs, infections, systemic disease)
  - Glomerular disease
    - Goodpasture syndrome (antiglomerular basement membrane disease; autoimmune; associated pulmonary hemorrhage)
    - IgA nephropathy
    - Lupus nephritis
    - Henoch-Schönlein purpura
    - Membranoproliferative, poststreptococcal, or rapidly progressive glomerulonephritis (GN)
    - Wegener granulomatosis
  - Endocarditis/visceral abscesses
  - Other infections: schistosomiasis, tuberculosis (TB), syphilis
- Metabolic causes
  - Stones (85% have hematuria)
    - Hypercalciuria: a common cause of both gross and microscopic hematuria in children
    - Hyperuricosuria
    - Drugs that cause calculi such as acyclovir
- Congenital/familial causes
  - Cystic disease: polycystic kidney disease, solitary renal cyst
  - Benign familial hematuria or thin basement membrane nephropathy (autosomal dominant)
  - Alport syndrome (X-linked in 80%; hematuria, proteinuria, hearing loss, corneal abnormalities)
  - Fabry disease (X-linked recessive inborn error of metabolism; vascular kidney disease)
  - Nail–patella syndrome (autosomal dominant; nail and patella hypoplasia; hematuria in 33%)
  - Renal tubular acidosis type 1 (autosomal dominant or autoimmune)
- Hematologic causes
  - Bleeding dyscrasias (e.g., hemophilia)
  - Sickle cell anemia/trait (renal papillary necrosis)

- Vascular causes
  - Hemangioma
  - Arteriovenous malformations (rare)
  - Nutcracker syndrome: compression of left renal vein with renal parenchymal congestion
  - Renal artery/vein thrombosis
  - Arterial emboli to kidney
- Chemical causes
  - Aminoglycosides, cyclosporine, analgesics, oral contraceptives, Chinese herbs, cyclophosphamide, anticoagulants (Coumadin, Eliquis, Xarelto), sulfa drugs, penicillins
- Obstruction
  - Strictures or posterior urethral valves
  - Hydronephrosis from any cause
  - Benign prostatic hyperplasia: Rule out other causes of hematuria.
- Other causes: loin pain hematuria (most often in young women on oral contraceptives)

RISK FACTORS
- Smoking
- Occupational exposures (dyes, rubber, or tire manufacturing, petrochemicals)
- Medications (e.g., cyclophosphamide, pioglitazone therapy >1 year)
- Pelvic radiation
- Chronic infection, especially with calculi
- Recent upper respiratory tract infection
- Positive family history of stones, GN, or cancer
- Chronic indwelling foreign body

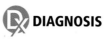

DIAGNOSIS

HISTORY
Considerations
- Burning, urgency, frequency: UTI
- Dark cola-colored urine: glomerular origin
- Clots: extraglomerular bleeding
- Arthritis/arthralgias/rash: lupus, vasculitis, Henoch-Schönlein purpura
- Flank pain: stones, infarction, pyelonephritis
- Recent upper respiratory infection (URI): poststreptococcal GN, membranoproliferative GN
- Concurrent URI: IgA nephropathy
- Excessive vitamin use: stones
- Marathon runner: traumatic, rhabdomyolysis
- Travel: schistosomiasis, TB
- Painless hematuria and/or weight loss: malignancy
- Family history: Alport disease (hereditary nephritis), sickle cell, polycystic, IgA nephropathy, thin basement membrane disease, von Willebrand
- Any episode of visible hematuria (VH) in the urine, even if transient, is associated with an OR of 7.2 for urologic cancers.

PHYSICAL EXAM
Considerations
- Elevated BP, edema, and weight gain: glomerular disease
- Fever: infection
- Palpable kidney: neoplasm, polycystic
- Genitalia: Look for meatal erosion, lesions.

DIFFERENTIAL DIAGNOSIS
Menstrual/vaginal bleeding, rectal bleeding, drugs such as rifampin and phenazopyridine can turn urine orange/red mistaking for hematuria.

DIAGNOSTIC TESTS & INTERPRETATION
A hematuria risk index may assist in stratifying patients at risk for urothelial malignancies who require more intensive testing. High-risk indicators are VH, age >50 years, male gender, family history of urological malignancies, and smoking.

Initial Tests (lab, imaging)
- If acute cystitis/UTI is ruled out, guidelines recommend evaluating AMH with upper urinary tract imaging and cystoscopy; none recommend cytology or urine markers for initial AMH evaluation (1)[C].
- Urine dipstick (sensitivity 91–100%; specificity 65–99%)
  - False negatives are rare but can be caused by high-dose vitamin C.
  - False positives: oxidizers used to cleanse the perineum, alkaline urine (>9), semen; free hemoglobin (hemolysis) and myoglobin (rhabdomyolysis)
  - Heme-negative red urine: Food dyes, beets, blackberries, rhubarb, porphyria, rifampin, phenytoin, phenazopyridine may discolor the dipstick, making interpretation difficult.
  - Any proteinuria >2+ raises concern for glomerular disease.
- Microscopic urinalysis should always be done to confirm dipstick findings and quantify RBCs (1)[C].
  - American Urological Association (AUA) defines clinically significant microscopic hematuria as ≥3 RBCs/HPF on a properly collected urinary specimen when there is not an obvious benign cause (1).
  - Positive dipstick, but a negative microscopic exam should be followed by three repeat tests. If anyone is positive, proceed with a workup (1).
  - Exclude factitious or nonurinary causes, such as menstruation, mild trauma, exercise, poor collection technique, or chemical/drug causes, through cessation of activity/cause and a repeat urinalysis (1)[C].
  - RBC casts are pathognomonic for glomerular origin; dysmorphic cells are also suggestive.
- Renal function tests (eGFR, BUN, creatinine), albumin, and electrolytes to differentiate intrinsic renal disease and to evaluate for risks for imaging with contrast (1)[C]
  - Indicators of renal disease are significant (>500 mg/day) proteinuria, red cell casts, dysmorphic RBCs, increased creatinine, and albumin:creatinine ratio ≥30 mg/mmol (1).
- Urine culture if suspected infection/pyuria
- Multidetector CT urography (MDCTU); sensitivity 95%, specificity 92%
  - The initial imaging of choice in nonpregnant adults without contraindications to contrast or radiation with unexplained hematuria per the AUA and the American College of Radiology (ACR) (1)
  - Normal does not obviate the need for cystoscopy, particularly in high-risk patients.
  - Presence of calculi on noncontrast does not exclude another diagnosis or need for contrast phase.

- CT
  - Noncontrast CT is preferred first line in adult patients with acute flank pain suspicious of stones.
  - Perform unenhanced helical CT for suspected stone disease in children if US is negative.
  - Perform CT abdomen and pelvis with contrast in children with traumatic hematuria.
- Renal and bladder US (RBUS)
  - Best for differentiating cystic from solid masses
  - Sensitive for hydronephrosis; point of care US may help avoid CT with suspected stones.
  - No radiation or iodinated contrast exposure and cost-efficient
  - US can be used first line in patients with contraindications to CTU or at low risk of malignancy.
  - Sensitivity and NPV: for renal cancer = 85.7% and 99.9% and for upper tract urothelial cancer = 14.3% and 99.7%
  - Poor sensitivity for renal masses <3 cm
  - Main disadvantage is inability to fully evaluate the urothelium for transitional cell cancer.
- Magnetic resonance urography (MRU)
  - High sensitivity/specificity for renal parenchyma; less useful for collecting system or stones
  - Can be used in patients with contraindications to MDCTU
- MRI
  - Similar to CT in sensitivity for renal masses
  - No radiation exposure but least cost-efficient
  - Limited ability to reliably detect urinary tract calcifications
  - Can be combined with retrograde pyelogram (RPG) for patients who cannot tolerate MDCTU or MRU

Follow-Up Tests & Special Considerations
- Other tests depend on suspected etiology: STD testing, antineutrophil cytoplasmic antibody (ANCA), C3, C4, antistreptolysin O (ASO) titer, hemoglobin electrophoresis, prothrombin time (PT)/international normalized ratio (INR) for patients on warfarin.
- Consider genetic testing in patients suspected of having familial hematuria.
- Voided urine cytology (sensitivity 43.5%; specificity 95.7%; positive predictive value 47.6%; negative predictive value 94.9%)
  - Not recommended for routine evaluation of AMH; may be considered in those with significant risk factors for urinary malignancy (1)
- Insufficient evidence to recommend routine use of urinary tumor markers
- Malignancies are more likely in patients with VH than in patients with nonvisible hematuria (13.8% vs. 3.1%).
- Summary positive predictive value of VH for bladder/renal cancer in age >15 years is 5.1%; risk increases with age and male gender.
- VCUG in children with frequent UTIs requiring workup

Diagnostic Procedures/Other
- Flexible cystoscopy (sensitivity 62%; specificity 43–98%)
  - Best for evaluation of bladder, especially small urothelial lesions; NPV for bladder tumors is 99%.
  - AUA recommends all patients with hematuria who are ≥35 years of age, and all patients with risk factors for bladder cancer regardless of age to receive cystoscopy in addition to imaging (1).

- Renal biopsy
  - Not routine but may be necessary to diagnose GN or in the face of increasing renal insufficiency
- RPG
  - Reserved when MDCTU equivocal or in addition to US or noncontrast studies in patients who are contraindicated for contrast or MRI
  - Sensitive for small lesions of supravesicular collecting system
  - Requires cystoscopy
- Ureteroscopy/pyeloscopy
  - For visualization of suspected supravesical collecting system lesions
  - Biopsy, excision, fulguration, or extraction of lesions/stones possible
  - Requires anesthesia and cystoscopy
  - Risk of injury to collecting system

Pregnancy Considerations
US is initial imaging choice for pregnant patients. MRU or RPG combined with either MRI or US are alternatives.

Pediatric Considerations
- Consider UTI, GN, Wilms tumor, child abuse, hyperuricemia, hypercalciuria, and familial causes.
- The AAP recommends workup for hematuria should not be initiated for hematuria in a pediatric patient before repeating a dipstick urinalysis. In patients with persistent ASM, most common diagnoses on renal biopsy are hypercalciuria (30–35%), hyperuricemia (5–20%), and glomerulonephritides, such as IgAN and thin basement membrane disease.
- Gross or symptomatic hematuria needs a full workup.
  - If eumorphic RBCs, consider UTI, hypercalciuria, familial causes, or masses, stones, or cysts. Obtain a family history, urine culture, US and urinary Ca:Cr ratio. Urine Ca:Cr ratio >0.2 (mg/mg) is suggestive of hypercalciuria in children >6 years of age.
  - If dysmorphic RBCs, consider renal consult, especially if associated proteinuria, elevated blood pressure, edema, or a positive family history.
- Renal US identifies most congenital and malignant conditions; CT is reserved for cases of suspected trauma (with contrast) or stones (without contrast).

 TREATMENT

MEDICATION
First Line
Treatment of the underlying cause of hematuria is the first line. Discontinue drugs that cause hematuria.

ISSUES FOR REFERRAL
- Nephrology referral for proteinuria, red cell casts, elevated serum creatinine, and albumin:creatinine ratio ≥30 mg/mmol
- Urology referral for stones, vascular/anatomic anomalies, or nutcracker syndrome

ADDITIONAL THERAPIES
Surgery for removal of endometriosis if causing hematuria with symptoms

 ONGOING CARE

Close follow-up by specialists indicated based on the underlying cause. Primary care physicians play a critical role in identifying secondary causes of hematuria and ensuring multidisciplinary care when indicated.

FOLLOW-UP RECOMMENDATIONS
Patient Monitoring
Some experts still recommend periodic urinalysis; recent literature suggests that, after thorough initial negative investigations (imaging, cystoscopy), no follow-up is indicated for the patient with AMH unless symptoms or frank hematuria develop. AUA recommends annual urinalyses in these patients, until two consecutive are negative and the consideration for a repeat workup at 3 to 5 years if hematuria is persistent (1).

DIET
Increased fluids for stones or clots

PROGNOSIS
- Generally excellent for common causes of hematuria
- Poorer for malignant tumors and certain types of nephritis
- Persistent AMH is associated with an increased risk of end-stage renal disease in patients aged 16 to 25 years.

REFERENCE
1. Linder BJ, Bass EJ, Mostafid H, et al. Guideline of guidelines: asymptomatic microscopic haematuria. *BJU Int.* 2018;121(2):176–183.

 SEE ALSO

Algorithm: Hematuria

CODES

ICD10
- R31.9 Hematuria, unspecified
- R31.1 Benign essential microscopic hematuria
- R31.0 Gross hematuria

CLINICAL PEARLS
- Screening asymptomatic patients for microscopic hematuria is an "I" recommendation from the USPSTF.
- AMH and hematuria persisting after treatment of UTIs must be evaluated.
- Patients with bladder cancer can have intermittent microscopic hematuria; a thorough evaluation in high-risk patients is needed after just one episode.
- In patients with AMH, a history of anticoagulant use does not preclude the need for an evaluation and any new hematuria in patients on anticoagulants requires full evaluation including imaging and cystoscopy (1)[C].
- Signs of underlying renal disease indicate the need for a nephrologic workup, but a urologic evaluation is still needed in the presence of persistent hematuria.

H

HEMOCHROMATOSIS

Alethea Y. Turner, DO, FAAFP • Nikita Mathew, DO

 BASICS

DESCRIPTION

Hereditary hemochromatosis (HH) is a common genetic disease with autosomal recessive inheritance that results in iron overload and subsequent deposition into various tissues.

- HH includes at least four types of iron overload conditions, which involve gene mutations that alter iron metabolism.
- There is no mechanism to excrete excess iron, so the surplus is stored in tissue, including the liver, pancreas, and heart, eventually resulting in severe damage to the affected organ(s).
- Patients are often asymptomatic, but early clinical features can include fatigue, malaise, arthralgia, and decreased libido.
- Late effects may include diabetes, liver cirrhosis, hypermelanotic pigmentation of the skin, porphyria cutanea tarda, cardiomyopathy, and cardiac arrhythmias.
- Cirrhosis may ultimately result in hepatocellular carcinoma.
- Synonym(s): bronze diabetes; Troisier-Hanot-Chauffard syndrome

EPIDEMIOLOGY

Incidence

- Predominant age: Metabolic abnormality is congenital, but symptoms typically present between the 3rd and 5th decades for HH types 1, 3, and 4; type 2 juvenile hemochromatosis typically presents between the 1st and 3rd decades of life, and neonatal presentation is exceedingly rare.
- Predominant sex: Gene frequency is equal between male and female, although clinical signs are more frequent in men.

Prevalence

- Prevalence in the United States for carrying an *HFE* gene mutation (type 1 HH) is 5.4% for the *C282Y* gene and 13.5% for the *H63D* gene; prevalence for homozygosity is 0.3% for *C282Y* and 1.9% for *H63D* (1).
- Type 1 accounts for >90% of HH cases in the United States and primarily occurs in people of northern European descent; ~1 in 200 white adults in the United States are *C282Y* homozygous (1).

Pediatric Considerations

Juvenile (type 2) HHC is rare but can present in young patients (between 1st and 3rd decades of life) with hypogonadism and cardiomyopathy.

ETIOLOGY AND PATHOPHYSIOLOGY

- HH type 1 is caused by mutations in the *HFE* gene (most frequently *C282Y* and/or *H63D*), and it is the most common form of HH overall. Other variations include type 2 which is caused by mutations in either the *HJV* or *HAMP* gene, type 3 by mutations in the *TFR2* gene, and type 4 by mutations in the *SLC11A3* gene.
- Types 1 to 3 involve a deficiency in an iron-regulating hormone named hepcidin, which causes increased intestinal absorption of iron through excessive expression of ferroportin (a transmembrane protein that transports iron out of the cell and into the bloodstream).
- Type 4 is caused by an insensitivity of ferroportin to hepcidin (4a) or an inactivity of ferroportin itself (4b); the latter leads to iron accumulation within mesenchymal tissue.

- Other rare types of HH exist as a result of different gene mutations.
- Increased plasma iron and transferrin saturation (TS) leads to elevated levels of unbound iron, which are then absorbed into various tissue, eventually causing organ dysfunction.

Genetics

- Genetically heterogeneous disorder of iron overload; types 1, 2, and 3 are autosomal recessive; type 4 is autosomal dominant.
- Biochemical penetrance is incomplete and expressivity is variable; in type 1 HH, the penetrance for developing clinically significant iron overload is rare, but approximately 75% of men with type 1 HH and 50% of women will have an increase in TS (with or without elevated serum ferritin [SF]).
- Factors contributing to variable expressivity include different mutations in the same gene, mitigating or exacerbating genes, and environmental factors.

RISK FACTORS

- Family history
- White men between the ages of 30 and 50 years (particularly for HFE-related HH)
- Loss of blood, such as that which occurs during menstruation and pregnancy, delays the onset of symptoms in women
- Alcohol consumption because it increases the absorption of iron and synergistically damages the liver along with the oxidative effects of iron

GENERAL PREVENTION

- First-degree relatives of those with HH should be screened; typically, with fasting TS and ferritin levels.
- Children of a diagnosed parent, HFE testing of the other parent is recommended with no further testing required if the results are normal.

> **ALERT**
> Screening of the general population is *not* recommended because only a small subset of patients with HH will develop symptoms or advanced disease.

COMMONLY ASSOCIATED CONDITIONS
See "Complications."

DIAGNOSIS

HISTORY

- Fatigue
- Weakness
- Arthralgias
- Abdominal pain
- Loss of libido or impotency
- Symptoms of diabetes
- Skin pigmentation or blistering
- Dyspnea on exertion

PHYSICAL EXAM

- Hepatomegaly and/or splenomegaly
- Increased skin pigmentation
- Hepatic tenderness
- Peripheral edema
- Jaundice
- Gynecomastia
- Ascites
- Testicular atrophy
- Hepatic tenderness

DIFFERENTIAL DIAGNOSIS

- Inflammatory syndromes
- Various causes of hepatitis
- Biliary or alcoholic cirrhosis
- Repeated transfusions
- Sideroblastic anemia
- β-Thalassemia major

DIAGNOSTIC TESTS & INTERPRETATION

Initial Tests (lab, imaging)

There is currently no evidence to support a concrete relationship between symptoms and the degree of iron overload (1).

- SF: $\geq$300 μg/L for men and postmenopausal women and 200 μg/L for premenopausal women; may be elevated for a number of other reasons including but not limited to inflammation (consider checking inflammatory markers); if elevated with suspicion of hemochromatosis, obtain fasting TS.
- Fasting TS (serum iron concentration ÷ total iron-binding capacity × 100) is the earliest biochemical marker to be increased in HH: $\geq$45% is suspicious for HH but warrants further evaluation because it can be elevated in other disease processes including chronic anemias.
- Confirmatory testing should be done through HFE gene mutation analysis.

Follow-Up Tests & Special Considerations

- After the diagnosis is established, check the following to determine need for phlebotomy:
  - ALT and AST
  - Hematocrit and hemoglobin
- Assess for complications of HH and order testing as deemed appropriate; for instance:
  - HbA1c to rule out diabetes
  - ECG to evaluate an arrhythmia
  - Echocardiogram if concerned for cardiomyopathy
  - Total testosterone if symptoms of hypogonadism are present
- Consider screening for osteoporosis in patients >50 years with additional risk factors (i.e., alcohol or tobacco use).
- Test for viral hepatitis if transaminitis exists to rule out concomitant disease.
- Monitor for liver lesions with an abdominal ultrasound every 6 months if severe liver fibrosis or cirrhosis is present.

Diagnostic Procedures/Other

- Hepatic MRI or liver biopsy should be done to measure liver iron content if hepatomegaly is present, SF is >1,000 μg/L, and/or ALT/AST are elevated.
- Consider liver biopsy only if there is a need to determine the degree of liver fibrosis for staging or to confirm the etiology of liver damage.

Test Interpretation

- Hepatic MRI without contrast (T2-weighted imaging) can effectively rule out iron overload within the liver (negative predictive value 0.88) and diagnose it as well, but with slightly less accuracy (positive predictive value 0.74).
- Liver biopsy will reveal increased hepatic parenchymal iron stores and evidence of any fibrosis or cirrhosis.

TREATMENT

GENERAL MEASURES

Due to a lack of evidence-based data, there is debate regarding when treatment should be initiated (particularly in asymptomatic patients) as well as what the target serum indices and frequency of phlebotomy should be. American and European liver associations recommend initiating treatment when SF is above the normal limit (see "Initial Tests [lab, imaging]"). The American College of Gastroenterology further outlines their recommendations regarding initiation of treatment based on whether the patient is C282Y homozygote or C282Y/H63D heterozygote. If HH diagnosis is confirmed, there is no liver involvement, SF remains normal, and the patient is asymptomatic, it is reasonable to monitor SF at least annually.

- Phlebotomy (~500 mL per session) is the mainstay of therapy and is performed once or twice weekly in the initial treatment phase and may take up to 2 to 3 years to deplete iron stores (1).
- When the patient finally becomes iron deficient, a lifelong maintenance program of ~2 to 6 phlebotomies a year is required to keep iron storage normal or below normal.
- Erythrocytapheresis (~600 mL per session) is an alternative to phlebotomy and only removes red cells from the blood; it is expensive and not widely available. However, there is limited evidence that erythrocytapheresis in the maintenance phase of treatment can reduce the frequency of treatments (1.9 vs. 3.3 treatments annually when compared to phlebotomy).
- Adverse effects of phlebotomy and erythrocytapheresis are mild and are typically secondary to hypovolemia, so pre-hydration is recommended.

MEDICATION

- If phlebotomy is not feasible or if it is contraindicated (severe anemia or heart failure), a second tier option is chelation therapy with parenteral deferoxamine (monitor patients for auditory or visual changes), oral deferasirox (contraindicated in renal or hepatic failure, and can increase risk of gastrointestinal hemorrhage in some patients) or oral deferiprone (can cause agranulocytosis and neutropenia); of these options, deferoxamine is preferred in most patients.
- Proton pump inhibitor (PPI) use for a minimum of 1 year may reduce the absorption of iron in patients with HH and decrease the overall number of phlebotomies needed. Consider adding a PPI as adjunct therapy to phlebotomy.
- Testosterone replacement in men with HH may improve symptoms of erectile dysfunction, but risks of hepatotoxicity
- Hepatitis A and hepatitis B immunizations should be provided if no evidence of previous exposure.
- Pneumococcal vaccination (PPSV23) should be given if cirrhosis is present.

ALERT

Caution is advised for prescribing androgens in the setting of hypogonadism secondary to risk of hepatotoxicity.

First Line

Phlebotomy, as outlined above

Second Line

Chelation therapy, as outlined above

ISSUES FOR REFERRAL

- Refer to a gastroenterologist if liver biopsy is indicated and for the management of concomitant liver disease.
- Refer to a cardiologist if cardiac involvement is suspected.
- Refer to endocrinology if male infertility is present.

ADDITIONAL THERAPIES

Experimental treatments with hepcidin mimetics to decrease intestinal iron absorption and to reduce levels of iron from the reticuloendothelial system are being researched.

SURGERY/OTHER PROCEDURES

Liver transplant is indicated in end-stage liver disease.

ADMISSION, INPATIENT, AND NURSING CONSIDERATIONS

Need for hospitalization is typically rare and necessary only for the management of severe complications including need for organ transplant.

ONGOING CARE

FOLLOW-UP RECOMMENDATIONS

Patient Monitoring

- Measure hemoglobin and hematocrit before each phlebotomy; skip phlebotomy if hemoglobin is <11 g/dL.
- During the initiation phase of treatment, check SF every 1 to 3 months.
- Once iron stores are depleted, the maintenance phase of treatment should include phlebotomy every 1 to 6 months (adjusted based on patient's need) to maintain SF levels near 50 μg/L.
- During maintenance therapy, measure TS and SF yearly.

DIET

- Avoid consumption of iron-fortified foods, oysters, uncooked shellfish, vitamin C supplements, and iron-containing supplements.
  - Natural sources of vitamin C and iron are considered safe.
- Black tea chelates iron and may be consumed with meals.
- Minimize alcohol use; consumption of >60 g/day increases the risk of developing cirrhosis by 9-fold.

PATIENT EDUCATION

- Adequate hydration prior to phlebotomy
- Blood phlebotomy may be donated.
- http://www.hemochromatosis.org/

PROGNOSIS

- The presence or absence of cirrhosis is a critical factor for prognosis.
- Type 2 HH is associated with earlier onset and increased disease severity that type 1 HH.
- SF <1,000 μg/L, normal AST, and the absence of hepatomegaly have a negative predictive value of 95% for severe fibrosis or cirrhosis.
- Patients diagnosed and treated before the development of cirrhosis or diabetes have a normal life expectancy.
- Life expectancy is reduced in patients with cirrhosis and/or diabetes.

- Cirrhosis is associated with an increased risk of hepatocellular carcinoma (annual incidence of 3–4%) and mortality.
- Cirrhosis is irreversible; diabetes, arthralgias, and symptoms of hypogonadism may not improve with phlebotomies, but other complications and symptoms may be averted with successful management.

COMPLICATIONS

Complications develop as a result of untreated HH.

- Arthritis, chondrocalcinosis
- Diabetes mellitus
- Hypogonadism
- Arrhythmia
- Congestive heart failure
- Cirrhosis (prevalence of 20–45% in C282Y homozygotes with SF >1,000 μg/L)
- Hepatocellular carcinoma (One study suggests carcinoma risk is higher in men with p.C282y homozygosity.)
- Osteoporosis
- Infection from Listeria monocytogenes, Escherichia coli, Yersinia enterocolitica, or Vibrio vulnificus is rare, but those with iron overload are at increased risk.

REFERENCE

1. Buzzetti E, Kalafateli M, Thorburn D, et al. Interventions for hereditary haemochromatosis: an attempted network meta-analysis. Cochrane Database Syst Rev. 2017;3(3):CD011647.

ADDITIONAL READING

U.S. Preventive Services Task Force. Screening for hemochromatosis: recommendation statement. Ann Intern Med. 2006;145(3):204–208.

CODES

ICD10

- E83.110 Hereditary hemochromatosis
- E83.118 Other hemochromatosis
- E83.111 Hemochromatosis due to repeated red blood cell transfusions

CLINICAL PEARLS

- Types 1 to 3 involve a deficiency in an iron-regulating hormone (hepcidin), which causes increased intestinal absorption of iron.
- Type 4 is caused by an insensitivity of ferroportin to hepcidin (4a) or an inactivity of ferroportin itself (4b); the latter leads to iron accumulation within mesenchymal tissue.
- Screening of the general population for hemochromatosis is not recommended, but testing is recommended if there is clinical suspicion or family history.
- Although fatigue and arthralgias are the most common symptoms in early disease, some patients with iron overload may remain asymptomatic.
- Genetic testing is recommended to confirm type 1 HH, which is the most common type.
- Initiate once or twice weekly phlebotomy when SF levels are elevated, especially when symptoms or clinical findings are present.
- Goal is to achieve and then maintain SF levels near 50 μg/L.
- Monitor hemoglobin and ensure it does not fall below 11 g/dL.
- PPI as adjuvant therapy for at least 1 year.

H

HEMOPHILIA

Toussaint L. Mears-Clarke, MD

BASICS

DESCRIPTION

- Deficiency of factor VIII (hemophilia A) or factor IX (hemophilia B) coagulation proteins leading to bleeding tendencies in affected individuals. The majority of cases are due to inherited genetic mutations in factor VIII or factor IX coagulation proteins. However, an estimated 30% of all hemophilia cases result from spontaneous mutations.
- Hemophilia A and B are clinically indistinguishable but can be differentiated by assays that detect levels of factors VIII and IX, respectively.
- Disease severity correlates with the relative levels of coagulation factors present in serum analysis:
  - Severe: frequent spontaneous bleeding (factor activity <1%)
  - Moderate: occasional spontaneous bleeding; prolonged bleeding with minor trauma or surgery (factor activity 1–5%)
  - Mild: rare spontaneous bleeding, severe bleeding with major trauma, or surgery (factor activity 5–40%)
- Bleeding frequency is similar in hemophilia A and B with similar levels of factor deficiency (1)[A].

EPIDEMIOLOGY

- Worldwide, an estimated 1,125,000 people are affected with hemophilia (1)[A].
- Hemophilia A represents 80–85% of the total hemophilia population; hemophilia B comprises the remaining 15–20%.

Prevalence

- Estimated prevalence of hemophilia A at birth is 24.6 per 100,000 males (9.5 cases for severe hemophilia A).
- Estimated prevalence of hemophilia B at birth is 5 cases per 100,000 males (1.5 cases for severe hemophilia B) (1)[A].

ETIOLOGY AND PATHOPHYSIOLOGY

- Damage to vascular endothelium leads to exposure of subendothelial tissue factors, which interact with platelets, plasma proteins, and coagulation factors to produce a localized platelet plug contributing to hemostasis. Complexes involving factors VIII and IX participate in the intrinsic coagulation pathway to activate factor X, FXa. Downstream interactions involving FXa culminate in the conversion of prothrombin to thrombin, mediating platelet activation and fibrin deposition necessary for stabilization of the platelet plug.
- Deficiencies of factor VIII or factor IX result in decreased production of FXa, leading to an unstable platelet plug and impaired hemostasis.

Genetics

- Exhibits an X-chromosome linked inheritance pattern. Males are almost exclusively affected; females are usually asymptomatic carriers. Females with hemophilia have both X chromosomes affected, or one X chromosome is affected and the other is inactivated.
- Carriers may have symptomatically low clotting factor levels:
  - May bleed at the time of surgery
- Males within the same family share similar deficiencies and level of severity owing to the same genetic defect.

GENERAL PREVENTION

- Patients should carry medical ID tags listing their factor deficiency, inhibitor status, type of treatment products used, and initial treatment doses for mild, moderate, or severe bleeding.
- Immediate family members of affected patients should have factor VIII and IX levels checked prior to invasive procedures, childbirth, and if bleeding tendencies occur.
- Genetic testing should be offered to at-risk female family members to facilitate genetic counseling.
- Regular dental care and good oral hygiene are recommended to prevent gum bleeding.

DIAGNOSIS

- History and initial presentation
  - 2/3 of presenting hemophilic patients have a positive family history. All male infants born to known carriers should have factor level testing.
  - Prolonged bleeding with circumcision, dental work, surgery, or injury
  - Excessive or easy bruising in early childhood
  - Spontaneous bleeding, especially in joints, muscle, or soft tissue
  - Typical age of presentation: mild (36 months), moderate (8 months), severe (1 month)
  - *Pregnancy considerations*: Genetic counseling should be provided to asymptomatic carriers either prior to or during pregnancy. Treat all males born to a carrier as if they have hemophilia; recommend planned cesarean delivery if male infant is potentially affected. Avoid fetal scalp electrode placement, vacuum/forceps deliveries (1)[A].
  - Test infant clotting factor levels at birth and again at 6 months of age if mild hemophilia A/B is suspected (in cases of mild hemophilia, factor levels may be normal at birth). Cord blood can be used for testing.
- Life-threatening bleeds
  - Intracranial hemorrhage: generally resulting from trauma
  - Hematomas of bowel wall can cause obstruction or intussusception and pain mimicking appendicitis.
  - Neck or throat bleeds: can lead to airway obstruction
- Serious bleeds
  - Hemarthrosis, most commonly of ankles, elbows, and knees
    - Infants may present with irritability or decreased use of limb.
    - Adults may have prodromal stiffness, acute pain, and swelling of joint.
    - Arthropathy results from repeated bleeding into joints, damaging cartilage, and subchondral bone:
      - Can result in fixed joints, muscle wasting, and significantly impaired mobility
  - Muscular hematomas most commonly occur in quadriceps, iliopsoas, and forearm:
    - May result in compartment syndrome and ischemic nerve damage, such as femoral nerve neuropathy due to undetected retroperitoneal hemorrhage
  - Mucous membrane bleeding, such as in the genitourinary tract, leading to hematuria
  - Pseudotumor syndrome: untreated hemorrhage causing a hematoma, which calcifies (named because it can be mistaken for cancer)

DIFFERENTIAL DIAGNOSIS

- von Willebrand disease
- Vitamin K deficiency, anticoagulant (i.e., warfarin, rivaroxaban, heparin) therapy (Factor IX is vitamin K dependent.)
- Other factor deficiencies (i.e., hemophilia C, acquired hemophilia A), afibrinogenemia, dysfibrinogenemia, fibrinolytic defects, platelet disorders
- Child abuse

DIAGNOSTIC TESTS & INTERPRETATION

Initial Tests (lab, imaging)

- Screening tests: CBC with platelet count, PT, aPTT, platelet function (preferred), or bleed time
  - aPTT usually prolonged. aPTT may be normal in patients with mild hemophilia.
  - PT, platelet count, and function are normal.
- Follow-up tests: mixing study, vWF, factor activity levels (factor VIII:C and factor IX)
  - Mixing study: Patient's plasma is mixed with pooled normal plasma. Prolonged aPTT corrects in absence of inhibitors, that is, lupus anticoagulant and acquired factor inhibitors.
  - vWF is normal.
- Diagnosis based on factor VIII:C or IX activity
  - Normal factor levels: 50 to 150 IU/dL
  - Mild: 5 to 40 IU/dL
  - Moderate: 1 to 5 IU/dL
  - Severe: <1 IU/dL

Follow-Up Tests & Special Considerations

- Genetic counseling, and participation in genotyping to identify specific underlying variant for affected individuals and family, is recommended; the information may help predict inhibitor risk/bleeding severity, and individualize treatment.
- Inhibitors to factor VIII and IX (see "Complications"):
  - Should be periodically measured using the Nijmegen or Bethesda assay, which quantifies the alloantibody titer
  - Screen before invasive procedures and at regular intervals.

Diagnostic Procedures/Other

Prenatal diagnosis should be offered to pregnant female carriers via genetic testing of a sample of chorionic villus or fluid obtained via amniocentesis (1)[A].

Test Interpretation

Pathology of affected joints: synovial hemosiderosis, articular cartilage degeneration, thickening of periarticular tissues, bony hypertrophy

TREATMENT

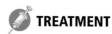

GENERAL MEASURES

- Optimal care is provided via an integrated, multidisciplinary, comprehensive care model, including hematologist, physical therapist, nurse, and social worker (1)[A].
- Treat early; acute bleeds should be treated as quickly as possible.
- For surgical prophylaxis
  - If major surgery is undertaken, factor levels should be maintained at >30–50% for approximately 2 weeks after the procedure:
    - Fibrin glue products may be beneficial for oozing.
  - Dental extractions: Antifibrinolytics (aminocaproic acid, tranexamic acid) may be used.
  - Minor procedures: may use desmopressin (DDAVP) in hemophilia A
- Patients and caregivers should be taught how to manage their care at home including bleed recognition, self-infusion skills, self-care, and pain management.
- Pain management associated with chronic hemophilic arthropathy may include acetaminophen, selective COX-2 inhibitors (other NSAIDs should be avoided), and opioids.
- Hepatitis A and B vaccinations are recommended.
- Encourage physical activity: Patients should avoid high-impact contact sports. Organized sports should be encouraged (1)[A].

MEDICATION

First Line

- Principles of therapy
  - Prophylaxis: administration of specific factor replacement therapy in the absence of bleeding to maintain adequate baseline plasma levels sufficient for hemostasis in all categories of severity or administration of nonfactor hemostatic agents (1)[A]
    - Lower frequency of acute bleeds and episodes of life-threatening hemorrhage compared to on-demand therapy
    - Standard of care for children with severe hemophilia A or B to prevent joint bleeds and joint degeneration
    - Emicizumab, a nonfactor hemostatic agent, is a bispecific monoclonal antibody for FIXa and FX used for prophylaxis for hemophilia A with/without inhibitors.
    - Dosing, frequency, duration of therapeutic regimens tailored to individual patient needs in clinical practice
    - Gene therapy, extended half-life recombinant factor VIIa, and other nonfactor agents such as fitusiran (RNAi therapy), and antitissue factor pathway inhibitor agents are currently under development to reduce the risk of bleeding (1)[A].
  - On-demand therapy: treatment administered in response to occurrence of bleeding
    - Amount and duration of factor replacement depends on location and severity of bleeding:
      - Mild bleeds correct to a factor level of approximately 30–50%. Major hemorrhages and large muscle bleeds require correction to levels between 50% and 100%.
      - Life-threatening bleeds require levels between 50% and 100%, sustained with bolus dosing or continuous infusion (1)[A].
- Specific agents:
  - Hemophilia A: Replacement with factor VIII concentrates is the treatment of choice: two sources for the factor available (1)[A]:
    - Recombinant factor VIII
      - Dosing: 1 IU of factor VIII (the amount in 1 mL of plasma)/kg body weight administered will raise the plasma level of the recipient by 2%.
    - Purified plasma-derived factor VIII: Donor pool is screened, and the plasma-derived factor is treated to inactivate viruses (HIV, hepatitis B, and hepatitis C); theoretical risks still exist.
  - Hemophilia B: Replacement with factor IX concentrates is the treatment of choice:
    - Plasma-derived factor IX and recombinant factor IX (preferred) are commercially available.
      - Dosing: 1 IU/kg body weight administered will raise plasma factor IX levels by 1%.
- Hemophilia patients with inhibitors (neutralizing alloantibodies to factors VIII or IX) (1)[A]
  - Inhibitor formation should be suspected when replacement with the deficient factor fails to correct coagulopathy.
  - Low-titer patients: Replace with high doses of the deficient factor to overcome the circulating inhibitor concentration.
  - High-titer patients: Treat using products that *bypass* the factor neutralized by the alloantibody or emergently with high doses of the specific deficient factor:
    - Two bypassing agents are available:
      - Activated prothrombin complex concentrate (known to have increased thromboembolic risks when administered in patients receiving emicizumab for prophylaxis)
      - Recombinant activated factor VII (preferred agent in patients with hemophilia B and allergy/anaphylaxis to factor IX therapy)

- Immune tolerance induction (ITI): protocols to eradicate inhibitors, and promote immune tolerance through repeated exposure to high-dose factor VIII therapy over 12 to 18 months, with or without immunosuppressive therapy (mycophenolate mofetil, rituximab). Success rates are 70–80% in patients with severe hemophilia A. Inhibitor prevalence is low in hemophilia B, thus limited evidence is available on the use of ITI in hemophilia B patients.
  - Home therapy allows immediate access to clotting factor, resulting in improved quality of life, decreased pain, dysfunction, and long-term disability (1)[A].

Second Line

- Cryoprecipitate and fresh frozen plasma (FFP) can be used in instances where the specific factor concentrate is unavailable for *emergent hemostasis*.
  - FFP: contains all coagulation factors but generally difficult to attain high levels of factors VIII or IX.
    - Starting dose: 15 to 20 mL/kg
  - Cryoprecipitate: derived from precipitates of cooled FFP; contains significant levels of factor VIII (up to 100 IU/bag) but *not* factor IX:
    - Dosing: 1 mL cryoprecipitate has ~3 to 5 IU factor VIII
- DDAVP: synthetic vasopressin; stimulates endogenous release of factor VIII (and vWF) from endothelial stores; used in mild hemophilia A
  - IV or SC: 0.3 μg/kg infused 30 minutes prior to procedure; may repeat if needed
  - Intranasal (150 μg/spray): adult dose, 1 spray to each nostril (300 μg total). Alternate dose if <50 kg: 150 μg once
  - DDAVP use is limited to 3 consecutive days due to tachyphylaxis and the association with adverse side effects with prolonged use.
  - Adverse effect: hyponatremic seizures, especially in children; restrict fluids and watch sodium levels and urine output.
  - DDAVP therapeutic use is recommended only in patients with a clinically significant rise in factor VIII levels observed in prior testing.
- Antifibrinolytic agents: inhibit plasminogen activation, thereby stabilizing the clot
  - Effective in controlling mucosal bleeding, such as bleeding in oral cavity, epistaxis, and menorrhagia; can also be used prophylactically (e.g., prior to tooth extractions) or in combination with first-line agents of treatment.
    - Tranexamic acid (25 mg/kg PO q6–8h or 10 mg/kg IV q8–12h)
    - Amicar is less frequently used

ISSUES FOR REFERRAL

Patients with disabling pain from chronic hemophilic arthropathy should be referred to a physical therapist, and an orthopedic surgeon for consideration of surgery (1)[A].

COMPLEMENTARY & ALTERNATIVE MEDICINE

Pain management associated with chronic hemophilic arthropathy may benefit from the use of complementary pain management techniques such as mindfulness, meditation, or music therapy (1)[A].

ONGOING CARE

FOLLOW-UP RECOMMENDATIONS

Patient Monitoring

Regular evaluations every 6 to 12 months, including a musculoskeletal evaluation, an inhibitor screen, liver tests, and tests for antibodies to hepatitis viruses and HIV

PATIENT EDUCATION

- National Hemophilia Foundation: http://www.hemophilia.org/
- World Federation of Hemophilia: http://www.wfh.org/
- Centers for Disease Control and Prevention: https://www.cdc.gov/ncbddd/hemophilia/index.html

PROGNOSIS

- Prognosis is excellent for those with mild disease and access to medical care; mortality is increased in those with moderate to severe disease.
- Liver failure is a leading cause of death in hemophilia.
- Hemophilic arthropathy is the main cause of morbidity in patients with severe hemophilia.

COMPLICATIONS

- Hemophilic arthropathy: Symptoms include pain, limitation of motion, and contractures.
- Theoretical transmission of blood-borne infections, such as hepatitis A, B, C, and D and HIV; this risk has been greatly reduced with current testing of blood products.
- Development of inhibitor autoantibodies
  - More common in hemophilia A (20–30% of patients with severe hemophilia compared to 5% in hemophilia B) and in patients with severe disease requiring multiple transfusions
  - Risk of inhibitor development in hemophilia B associated with family history and/or specific genetic defects
  - Severe allergic reactions, including anaphylaxis, is associated with factor IX administration in hemophilia B patients with inhibitors.
  - No increased risk of bleeding, but when bleeding occurs, it is more difficult to achieve hemostasis due to decreased response to factor replacement.

REFERENCE

1. Srivastava A, Santagostino E, Dougall A, et al; for WFH Guidelines for the Management of Hemophilia panelists and co-authors. WFH guidelines for the management of hemophilia, 3rd edition. *Haemophilia*. 2020;26 Suppl 6:1–158.

ADDITIONAL READING

Hartmann J, Croteau S. 2017 Clinical trials update: innovations in hemophilia therapy. *Am J Hematol*. 2016;91(12):1252–1260.

CODES

ICD10

- D66 Hereditary factor VIII deficiency
- D68.1 Hereditary factor XI deficiency
- D67 Hereditary factor IX deficiency

CLINICAL PEARLS

- Deficiency of factor VIII (hemophilia A) or factor IX (hemophilia B) coagulation proteins leading to bleeding tendencies in affected individuals
- The majority of hemophilia cases are due to inherited genetic mutations in factor VIII or factor IX.
- An estimated 30% of all hemophilia cases result from spontaneous mutations.
- Exhibits an X-chromosome linked inheritance pattern. Males are almost exclusively affected.
- Diagnosis based on decreased factor VIII:C or IX activity
- Initial site of bleeding and bleeding severity dependent on coagulation factor levels
- Prognosis is excellent for those with mild disease and access to medical care; mortality is increased in those with moderate to severe disease.

HEMORRHOIDS

Donna I. Meltzer, MD

BASICS

DESCRIPTION
- Varicosities of the hemorrhoidal venous plexus
- External hemorrhoids
  - Located below (distal to) the dentate line; somatic innervation (painful)
  - Covered by squamous epithelium
- Internal hemorrhoids
  - Located above (proximal to) the dentate line; visceral innervation (painless)
  - Covered by columnar epithelium
  - Classification of internal hemorrhoids (1):
    - Grade I: Hemorrhoid vessel bulges without prolapse.
    - Grade II: Hemorrhoid prolapses with straining but reduces spontaneously.
    - Grade III: Hemorrhoid prolapses with straining and requires manual reduction.
    - Grade IV: chronically prolapsed—cannot be reduced
- Internal and external hemorrhoids often coexist.
- Although often asymptomatic, hemorrhoids can present with itching, bleeding, soilage, prolapse, or pain.
- Pain and thrombosis more common with external than internal hemorrhoids

Geriatric Considerations
Hemorrhoids and rectal prolapse are more common in elderly.

Pediatric Considerations
- Uncommon in infants and children; most common cause is chronic liver failure; other findings (rectal polyps, skin tags, condyloma) often misdiagnosed as hemorrhoids.
- In adolescents, chronic constipation and prolonged toilet time can result in hemorrhoids.

Pregnancy Considerations
- Common in pregnancy
- Usually resolves after delivery
- No treatment required, unless extremely painful

EPIDEMIOLOGY
- Predominant age: adults; peak from 45 to 65 years (2)
- Predominant sex: male = female

Incidence
Common; over 3.5 million office visits in United States per year are related to hemorrhoidal disease (1).

Prevalence
- ~4–5% in general population in the United States
- 39% prevalence on routine screening colonoscopy (2)

ETIOLOGY AND PATHOPHYSIOLOGY
- Exact pathophysiology is unknown.
- There are three primary hemorrhoidal cushions—typically located in left lateral, right anterior, and right posterior positions. Hemorrhoidal cushions augment anal closing pressure and protect the anal sphincter during stool passage. During Valsalva, increased intra-abdominal pressure raises pressure within the hemorrhoidal cushions. Mechanisms implicated in symptomatic hemorrhoidal disease include the following:
  - Dilated veins of hemorrhoidal plexus
  - Tight internal anal sphincter
  - Abnormal distention of the arteriovenous anastomosis
  - Prolapse of the cushions and the surrounding connective tissues

Genetics
No known genetic pattern

RISK FACTORS
- Pregnancy
- Pelvic space-occupying lesions
- Liver disease; portal HTN
- Constipation (prolonged straining)
- Occupations that require prolonged sitting
- Loss of perianal muscle tone due to old age, rectal surgery, birth trauma/episiotomy, anal intercourse
- Obesity
- Chronic diarrhea

GENERAL PREVENTION
- Avoid constipation by consuming high-fiber diet (>30 g/day) and ensuring proper hydration.
- Avoid prolonged sitting or straining on the toilet.

COMMONLY ASSOCIATED CONDITIONS
- Liver disease; cirrhosis, ascites
- Pregnancy
- Constipation

DIAGNOSIS

Diagnosis is typically straightforward through history and inspection of the perineum, rectal exam, and anoscopy.

HISTORY
- Symptoms
  - Bleeding (~60%)
  - Classically, bright red blood per rectum, may range from scant blood on toilet paper to copious blood in the toilet bowl
  - Pruritus (~55%)
  - Perianal discomfort (~20%)
  - Soiling (~10%)
  - Constipation or diarrhea
  - Straining with defecation
- More extensive internal hemorrhoids
  - Feeling of incomplete evacuation
- External hemorrhoids
  - Episodic bleeding on stool or toilet paper, pruritus, and irritation from compromised hygiene and pain
- Thrombosed hemorrhoids present as acute painful mass.
- Ask about diet (fiber, fluid intake), bowel patterns (frequency, consistency, incontinence), bowel habits (prolonged sitting), change in stools, systemic symptoms (weight loss, pain, fever).
- Ask about past medical history and family history (gastrointestinal disease, colorectal cancer).

PHYSICAL EXAM
- Visual anorectal inspection at rest and with Valsalva maneuver
- Digital exam with anoscopy
  - Internal hemorrhoid appears as purple mass on lumen wall.
  - Examine for additional anorectal pathology (skin tags, mass, abscess, fissure, fistula).
- Attempt to reduce prolapsed hemorrhoids.
- Abdominal exam to exclude mass
- Peripheral stigmata of cirrhosis and portal HTN (caput, telangiectasias, palmar erythema)

DIFFERENTIAL DIAGNOSIS
- Rectal or anal neoplasia
- Condyloma
- Skin tag
- Inflammatory bowel disease
- Anal fistula, fissure, or abscess
- Rectal polyp
- Rectal prolapse

DIAGNOSTIC TESTS & INTERPRETATION
Initial Tests (lab, imaging)
Not indicated unless anemia is suspected

Diagnostic Procedures/Other
Sigmoidoscopy or colonoscopy depending on risk factors for malignancy in patients with rectal bleeding

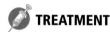**TREATMENT**

Prevention
- Fiber supplements and adequate fluid intake
- Stool softeners
- Anal hygiene

GENERAL MEASURES
- Hemorrhoids are a recurrent disease, even after surgical excision. Preventive measures should be continued indefinitely.
- For mild symptoms or prevention
  - Avoid prolonged sitting during bowel movements; effect of squatting is unknown.
  - Avoid straining.
  - Avoid constipation by eating a high-fiber diet or by taking fiber supplements; if necessary, take regular stool softeners.
  - Regular exercise, weight loss if indicated
- Pruritus or mild discomfort after stooling might respond to topical corticosteroid ointment, anesthetic ointments or sprays, and warm sitz baths.
- Constipation relief, anal hygiene, local ointments, and sitz baths are effective through the stage of easy reduction (grade II). More severe stages often require ligation or surgery.

MEDICATION
First Line
- Dietary modification with adequate fluid (generally ≥2 L water per day) and high fiber (25 to 35 g/day) is first-line, nonoperative therapy for symptomatic hemorrhoids (2); fiber supplementation (psyllium husk) to complement diet
- Fiber supplementation helps relieve overall symptoms and bleeding (3)[A],(4)[A].
- Stool softener or bulk-forming laxative to soften stool
- Sitz bath with warm water for pain relief
- Topic anesthetics (benzocaine, lidocaine, pramoxine), steroids, emollients to alleviate symptoms; these over-the-counter (OTC) products have been traditionally used but lack strong evidence for long-term use.
  - Local anesthetics for relief of pain and itch; applied to perianal area (not inserted into rectum)
  - Dibucaine 1% ointment (Nupercainal), lidocaine 5% (Preparation H, Tucks), pramoxine 1% foam, ointment, wipe (Proctofoam); benzocaine 20% spray, ointment. Use sprays with caution as alcohol in product may cause burning sensation.

- Anti-inflammatory agents (corticosteroids) to decrease swelling and for discomfort and itch
  – Hydrocortisone ointment, cream (0.25–2.5%) (Anusol HC, Cortifoam). Rectal suppositories are for short-term use only.
- Astringents to help dry skin
  – Witch hazel solution, wipes, pads (Preparation H, Tucks) after stooling
- Vasoconstrictors to shrink hemorrhoids and ameliorate bleeding, pain, itch
  – 0.25% phenylephrine ointment, suppository, gel (Preparation H, Rectacaine)

Second Line
Treatment for special cases
- Thrombosed external hemorrhoids: if present within 72 hours after pain onset, recommend incision and clot evacuation or excision of hemorrhoid complex. Early surgical excision may resolve symptoms faster and lower incidence of recurrence (3)[C].
- Strangulated hemorrhoid: untreated irreducible hemorrhoid can progress to thrombosis and necrosis. Treatment requires urgent or emergent hemorrhoidectomy.
- Acute hemorrhoidal bleeding associated with portal HTN: treatment depends on degree of hemorrhoids and amount of bleeding. Differentiate from more serious anorectal varices which require medical management (correct coagulopathy) and surgical interventions (suture ligation and shunts if necessary).

SURGERY/OTHER PROCEDURES
- Indications: failure of medical and nonoperative therapy, symptomatic grade III or IV hemorrhoids in presence of a concomitant anorectal condition requiring surgery, or patient preference
- Office-based procedures for patients with grade I or II (or III) internal hemorrhoids who have failed conservative management
  – Rubber band ligation (RBL) most common and most effective office-based procedure for symptomatic internal hemorrhoids. Avoid if on anticoagulants (3)[A],(4),(5).
  – Infrared photocoagulation: Infrared light waves cause necrosis within hemorrhoid; similar or slightly higher recurrence rates compared to RBL; less postoperative pain and fewer complications (1),(2)[A],(3)[B].
  – Sclerotherapy: submucosal injections causing local thrombosis; might be best for patients at increased bleeding risk (anticoagulated, advanced liver disease); care must be taken to inject proper site; not for advanced disease or if evidence of infection, inflammation, and ulceration is present
  – Cryotherapy is no longer recommended due to high rate of complications.
- Surgery for patients with symptomatic grade III or IV disease who have failed nonoperative treatments (3)[A]
  – Conventional hemorrhoidectomy
  – Closed hemorrhoidectomy—closure of mucosal defect
  – Open hemorrhoidectomy—tissue removed and mucosal defect left open
  – Different technologies are now used to excise hemorrhoidal tissue: diathermy, lasers, ultrasonic dissectors; associated with less pain

- Newer techniques reduce surgical time, early postoperative pain, urinary retention, and time to return to normal activity.
  – Doppler guided/assisted hemorrhoidal artery ligation (HAL): Anoscope or proctoscope with Doppler probe identifies hemorrhoidal artery which is then ligated; faster return to work than open hemorrhoidectomy (6)[A]
  – Stapled hemorrhoidopexy—for advanced internal hemorrhoidal disease. Excises submucosa; shorter recovery but more recurrent disease than conventional hemorrhoidectomy (2),(5)[A],(6)[A]
  – LigaSure hemorrhoidectomy: reduces operating time, is superior in terms of patient tolerance, and is equal to conventional hemorrhoidectomy in long-term symptom control (2)[A],(5)[A]
  – Laser treatment for grade 2 and 3 hemorrhoids has acceptable outcomes with less postoperative pain and bleeding compared to open hemorrhoidectomy (7)[A]
- No gold standard surgical treatment; need to individualize based on symptoms and risks/benefits of each procedure

COMPLEMENTARY & ALTERNATIVE MEDICINE
- Oral bioflavonoids have shown beneficial effect on bleeding, pruritus, and recurrence (3)[A].
- Topical nifedipine (compounded by pharmacist) can relieve pain of thrombosed hemorrhoids.
- Topical nitroglycerin (0.4%) has been used to decrease anal sphincter spasm in thrombosed hemorrhoids; headache is primary side effect.
- Botulinum toxin injection into anal sphincter to relieve spasm and pain of thrombosed hemorrhoid
- Aloe vera cream on the surgical site after hemorrhoidectomy reduces postoperative pain and decreases healing time and analgesic requirements.

 ## ONGOING CARE

FOLLOW-UP RECOMMENDATIONS
- Encourage physical fitness, weight management, and dietary compliance.
- Avoid prolonged sitting and straining on the toilet.

Patient Monitoring
As needed, depending on treatment

DIET
High fiber with a target of 30 g of insoluble fiber per day through sources such as wheat bran cereals, oatmeal, peanuts, artichokes, beans, corn, peas, spinach, potatoes, apples, apricots, blackberries, raspberries, prunes, pears, bananas; adequate fluids (6 to 8 glasses of water per day); avoid excessive caffeine.

PATIENT EDUCATION
Increasing dietary fiber: https://familydoctor.org/fiber-how-to-increase-the-amount-in-your-diet/

PROGNOSIS
- Spontaneous resolution
- Recurrence

COMPLICATIONS
- Thrombosis
- Ulceration
- Anemia (rare)
- Incontinence
- Pelvic sepsis following hemorrhoidectomy

REFERENCES

1. Cengiz TB, Gorgun E. Hemorrhoids: A range of treatments. *Cleve Clin J Med*. 2019;86(9):612–620.
2. Mott T, Latimer K, Edwards C. Hemorrhoids: diagnosis and treatment options. *Am Fam Physician*. 2018;97(3):172–179.
3. Davis BR, Lee-Kong SA, Migaly J, et al. The American Society of Colon and Rectal Surgeons clinical practice guidelines for the management of hemorrhoids. *Dis Colon Rectum*. 2018;61(3):284–292.
4. Gardner IH, Siddharthan RV, Tsikitis VL. Benign anorectal disease: hemorrhoids, fissures and fistulas. *Ann Gastroenterol*. 2020;33(1):9–18.
5. Lohsiriwat V. Treatment of hemorrhoids: a coloproctologist's view. *World J Gastroenterol*. 2015;21(31):9245–9252.
6. Aibuedefe B, Kling SM, Philp MM, et al. An update on surgical treatment of hemorrhoidal disease: a systematic review and meta-analysis. *Int J Colorectal Dis*. 2021;36(9):2041–2049.
7. Lakmal K, Basnayake O, Jayarajah U, et al. Clinical Outcomes and Effectiveness of Laser Treatment for Hemorrhoids: A Systematic Review. *World J Surg*. 2021;45(4):1222–1236.

ADDITIONAL READING
- Guttenplan M. The evaluation and office management of hemorrhoids for the gastroenterologist. *Curr Gastroenterol Rep*. 2017;19(7):30.
- Jacobs DO. Hemorrhoids: what are the options in 2018? *Curr Opin Gastroenterol*. 2018;34(1):46–49.
- Sandler RS, Peery AF. Rethinking what we know about hemorrhoids. *Clin Gastroenterol Hepatol*. 2019;17(1):8–15.
- Wald A, Bharucha AE, Cosman BC, et al. ACG clinical guideline: management of benign anorectal disorders. *Am J Gastroenterol*. 2014;109(8):1141–1157.
- Yeo D, Tan K-Y. Hemorrhoidectomy—making sense of the surgical options. *World J Gastroenterol*. 2014;20(45):16976–16983.

 ## SEE ALSO

Colon Cancer; Portal Hypertension; Rectal Cancer

CODES

ICD10
- K64.9 Unspecified hemorrhoids
- K64.4 Residual hemorrhoidal skin tags
- K64.1 Second degree hemorrhoids

CLINICAL PEARLS
- Hemorrhoids are common. Internal hemorrhoids are typically painless. External hemorrhoids are typically painful.
- Many cases can be managed conservatively.
- All patients should be encouraged to consume 25 to 35 g of fiber per day.
- More advanced hemorrhoidal disease requires intervention with ligation or surgery.

H

HENOCH-SCHÖNLEIN PURPURA

Jonathan A. Phillips, DO • Laura B. Bishop, MD

 BASICS

Increasingly referred to as immunoglobulin A vasculitis (IgAV)

DESCRIPTION
- Henoch-Schönlein purpura (HSP) is a nonthrombocytopenic, predominantly IgA-mediated, small vessel vasculitis that affects multiple organ systems and occurs in both children and adults.
- HSP is often self-limited, with the greatest morbidity and mortality attributable to long-term renal damage.
- Characterized by a tetrad of purpuric skin lesions, arthralgia, abdominal pain, and nephropathies

EPIDEMIOLOGY
Incidence
- Annual incidence: ranges from 3 to 27/100,000 children and 0.8 to 1.8/100,000 adults
- Mean age: 6 years; 90% of patients with HSP are <10 years of age; however, has been reported in patients age 6 months to 75 years old
- Gender: Male-to-female ratio is between 1.2:1 and 1.8:1.
- Race/ethnicity: most common in Caucasians and Asians, less common among African Americans

Prevalence
- Annual prevalence: 10 to 22/100,000 persons
- Year-round occurrence; more common in fall

ETIOLOGY AND PATHOPHYSIOLOGY
- Autoimmune disorder in which IgA production is increased in response to trigger(s), IgA1 immune complexes then activate the complement pathway, leading to production of inflammatory cytokines and chemokines.
- IgA-containing immune complex deposition results in small vessel inflammation which leads to fibrosis and necrosis within skin, intestinal mucosa, joints, and kidneys.
- No single etiologic agent has been identified; however, there are some associations (listed below) and a popular theory is one of a multihit model leading to HSP-associated glomerulonephropathy.
  - Infections are suggested by prevalence in the fall and a common upper respiratory infection (URI) prodrome. Associated pathogens include (but are not limited to) group A *Streptococcus* (may be present in up to 30% of HSP-associated nephritis), parvovirus B19, *Bartonella henselae*, *Helicobacter pylori*, *Haemophilus parainfluenzae*, coxsackievirus, adenovirus, hepatitis A and B viruses, *Mycoplasma*, Epstein-Barr virus, herpes simplex, varicella, *Campylobacter*, methicillin-resistant *Staphylococcus aureus*.
  - Drugs are most often associated with adults with HSP: acetaminophen, angiotensin-converting enzyme inhibitors (ACEI), angiotensin II receptor antagonists (ARB), some antibiotics including clarithromycin quinolones, etanercept, codeine, nonsteroidal anti-inflammatory drugs.
  - Vaccinations are rarely reported in association with HSP; however, there are some reports surrounding administration of MMR (measles, mumps, rubella), pneumococcal, meningococcal, influenza and hepatitis B immunizations.

Genetics
Associated with α_1-antitrypsin deficiency, familial Mediterranean fever, HLA-A2, HLA-A11, HLA-B35, HLA-DRB1, renin-angiotensin and nitric oxide synthase polymorphisms

COMMONLY ASSOCIATED CONDITIONS
- Malignancy: this is rare and the greatest association is with solid tumors, including lymphoma, prostate cancer, and non–small cell lung cancer, but also multiple myeloma.
- Studies suggest a possible relationship with *H. pylori* infection (1) and immune-related disorders (food allergy, drug allergy, inflammatory bowel disease).

DIAGNOSIS

Palpable purpura/petechiae without thrombocytopenia and *at least one* of the following:
- Diffuse abdominal pain
- Biopsy with predominant IgA deposition
- Arthralgia or arthritis
- Renal involvement (hematuria or proteinuria)
- Direct immunofluorescence showing IgA deposition (2)[A]

HISTORY
- Exposure to possible trigger, including recent infection (particularly URI) or offending drug
- Rash (most common presenting symptom): purpuric, palpable; predominant distribution often symmetric on dependent areas (lower extremities and buttocks); may spread elsewhere, typical duration 3 to 10 days with no definitive temporal association with other symptoms
- Gastrointestinal (GI) (about 50–75% of cases)
  - Nausea/vomiting
  - Abdominal pain (diffuse, colicky, may be transient or constant)
  - Hematochezia/melena
- Polyarthritis (about 75% of cases)
  - Often symmetric involvement of knees and ankles
- Renal (about 20–55% of cases)
  - Gross hematuria (higher in adults than children)
  - Oliguria or anuria
- Fatigue
- Low-grade fever
- Rare symptoms: periorbital or scrotal swelling, headache, seizures, neuropathy, behavioral changes, hemoptysis

PHYSICAL EXAM
- Rash (96% of cases, 74% primary presenting symptom):
  - May start as urticaria, develops into nonblanching, palpable purpura, with or without petechiae, ecchymoses and bullae
  - Distribution usually symmetric, most commonly involving the lower extremities but may involve the face and trunk
- Abdominal tenderness (66% of cases, 12% primary presenting symptom):
  - Evidence of GI hemorrhage (28% of cases), recommend rectal examination to assess for hematochezia
- Joint tenderness (64% of cases, 15% primary presenting symptom):
  - Mainly affects knees or ankles; may have associated warmth and limited range of motion, less commonly effusion; erythema is absent.
  - Mostly nonmigratory, transient, and nondeforming
- Orchitis (5%):
  - Presents as scrotal swelling and tenderness, may have associated torsion
- Renal disease (<1% primary presenting symptom):
  - Hypertension may be present.

- Rarely, patients present with central nervous system (CNS) or pulmonary involvement, which may manifest as signs of cerebral hemorrhage or diffuse interstitial pneumonia, respectively.
- Lower extremity edema is more common in adults than children.

DIFFERENTIAL DIAGNOSIS
- Infection:
  - Meningococcemia
  - Rocky Mountain spotted fever
  - Bacterial endocarditis
  - Rheumatic fever
  - Epstein-Barr virus
  - Sepsis
- Vasculitides:
  - Polyarteritis nodosa
  - Granulomatosis with polyangiitis
  - Microscopic polyangiitis
  - Systemic lupus erythematosus
  - Kawasaki disease
  - Urticarial vasculitis
  - Cryoglobulinemia-associated vasculitis
- Other:
  - Acute poststreptococcal glomerulonephritis
  - Inflammatory bowel disease
  - Idiopathic thrombocytopenic purpura/thrombotic thrombocytopenic purpura
  - Juvenile idiopathic arthritis/mixed connective tissue disease/juvenile dermatomyositis
  - Leukemia/lymphoma
  - Hereditary hemorrhagic telangiectasia
  - Acute surgical abdomen
  - Child abuse

DIAGNOSTIC TESTS & INTERPRETATION
- No single lab test confirms the diagnosis of HSP.
- Labs directed toward excluding other illnesses and assessing degree of renal involvement

Initial Tests (lab, imaging)
The following are generally accepted as initial labs for HSP:
- Complete blood count:
  - Leukocytosis and thrombocytosis may occur. Eosinophilia is common. Thrombocytopenia indicates an alternative cause of purpura.
  - Hemoglobin is variable, depending on whether GI hemorrhage occurs.
- Basic serum chemistry panel:
  - Electrolyte imbalances or elevated creatinine indicate renal dysfunction.
- Urinalysis:
  - Gross or microscopic hematuria, proteinuria, and red cell casts indicate renal dysfunction.
- Prothrombin time/international normalized ratio and partial thromboplastin time:
  - Normal in HSP. Abnormal coagulation studies may indicate an alternative cause of purpura.
- Imaging is not part of the routine workup for HSP but may be performed to rule out alternative etiologies or for evaluation of suspected complications, particularly in cases of GI and renal involvement. Initial imaging modalities to consider include the following:
  - Abdominal radiographs, with or without barium enema: to evaluate for free abdominal air suggestive of bowel perforation
  - Abdominal ultrasound: sensitive for the detection of intramural bleeding in HSP and may also show thickened bowel wall, reduced peristalsis, intussusception
- Renal ultrasound: evaluates for hydronephrosis in cases of renal failure

Follow-Up Tests & Special Considerations

The following labs are also useful in diagnosing HSP:

- Blood culture:
  - To rule out sepsis/bacteremia when diagnosis is unclear
- Acute phase reactants (erythrocyte sedimentation rate (ESR)/C-reactive protein):
  - Expect mild elevation
- IgA level:
  - Often elevated, although nonspecific and nonsensitive
- Complement levels:
  - Normal; sometimes decreased
- Antinuclear antibody/antineutrophil cytoplasmic antibody:
  - Negative but helps with narrowing ddx
- Antistreptolysin-O titer:
  - Evaluates for preceding streptococcal infection
- Stool guaiac if suspected GI hemorrhage
- CT arteriography may be necessary to identify the location of bleeding in patients with GI hemorrhage.

Diagnostic Procedures/Other

- Renal biopsy: Obtain if diagnosis is uncertain or if urinalysis shows nephrotic range proteinuria. Biopsy may show mesangial IgA deposition, mesangial proliferation, or, in severe cases, crescentic glomeru- lonephritis (3)[A].
- Skin biopsy of purpura: IgA deposition in the dermis on immunofluorescence
- Endoscopy may be considered in cases of GI hemorrhage given symptomatic overlap of HSP with inflammatory bowel disease.
- Barium enema may be therapeutic in some instances of intussusception, although surgical correction is commonly needed.

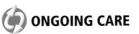 **TREATMENT**

GENERAL MEASURES

Rest and elevation of affected areas may limit purpura. Hydration and nutrition play a supportive role in treatment.

MEDICATION

- In the absence of renal dysfunction or complication, HSP is usually self-limited and best managed with supportive care as it resolves in 94% of children and 89% of adults.
- NSAIDs effective for symptomatic joint pain. Caution is advised in cases of renal involvement and con- sider acetaminophen as an alternative.
- Steroids useful early in disease for patients with severe joint and abdominal pain and in those with glomerulonephritis with severe renal involvement. Oral prednisone (1 to 2 mg/kg) may decrease both duration of abdominal pain and severity of joint pain. This may have benefit in preventing GI bleed- ing and causes of surgical abdomen, including intussusception (3)[B].
  - Steroids have benefit in treatment of severe and/ or bullous purpura.
  - Steroids given early in disease are effective for the acute treatment of crescentic nephritis and may prevent chronic renal disease in such patients.
  - Early steroids have no effect on prevention or development of renal involvement after 1 year.
- Immunosuppressive (cyclosporine [Sandimmune] and mycophenolate [Cellcept]) therapy may be ben- eficial for patients with evidence of severe renal in- volvement and those with steroid-resistant disease.

There have been many small case studies and case reports showing benefit in these patients. High-dose IV pulse steroids, cyclophosphamide, rituximab, mycophenolate, and plasmapheresis, have all been described in small studies. Consensus for when to definitively use these agents is still controversial and the subject of further research (4)[B].

- ACEI or ARB may be helpful in patients with HSP and persistent proteinuria.

ISSUES FOR REFERRAL

- Consider nephrology referral for possible renal biopsy if nephrotic range proteinuria at any time or proteinuria >100 mg/mmol for 3 months after diagnosis.
- Could consider dermatology referral for skin biopsy if diagnosis is unclear

ADMISSION, INPATIENT, AND NURSING CONSIDERATIONS

- Admission criteria/initial stabilization
  - Insufficient oral intake
  - Renal insufficiency
  - Severe abdominal pain
  - Severe GI bleeding
  - Altered mental status
  - Mobility restriction due to arthritis
  - HTN
  - Nephrotic syndrome
- IV fluids: Hydration should be maintained.

 ONGOING CARE

FOLLOW-UP RECOMMENDATIONS

Patient Monitoring

- Patients should be seen weekly during the acute illness. Visits should include history, physical exam (include BP measurement), and urinalysis.
- Because ~100% of patients who develop renal involvement will do so within 6 months of HSP diagnosis, all patients should be followed at least monthly with BP and urinalysis for a duration of at least 6 months.
- Women with a history of HSP should be monitored for proteinuria and HTN during pregnancy.
- Consider workup for occult malignancy in patients with adult-onset HSP.

PATIENT EDUCATION

National Kidney and Urologic Diseases Information Clearinghouse (NKUDIC): condition/HSP

PROGNOSIS

- Long-term prognosis heavily dependent on presence and severity of nephritis
- HSP is self-limited in 94% of children and 89% of adults.
- Most cases of HSP resolve within 4 weeks of diag- nosis. Recurrence rate within 6 months of diagnosis is 33%.
- Factors associated with poorer prognosis include age >8 years, fever at presentation, purpura above the waist, elevated ESR or IgA concentration, and increasing severity of renal histology grade.
- Chronic renal disease occurs in up to 20% of children with nephritic and nephrotic syndrome compared with 50% of adults who had any renal involvement. Risk of long-term renal failure is ≤5%.
- Risk factors that may result in renal failure include old age, HTN, elevated serum creatinine, and nephrotic and mixed nephritic/nephrotic syndrome at the onset of disease.

COMPLICATIONS

- Nephrotic/nephritic syndrome and renal failure
- HTN
- Hemorrhagic cystitis
- Ureteral obstruction
- Intestinal infarction, perforation, obstruction, stricture
- GI hemorrhage
- Intussusception
- Alveolar hemorrhage
- CNS complications, including cerebral hemorrhage and seizure
- Anterior uveitis
- Myocarditis
- Orchitis
- Testicular torsion

REFERENCES

1. Kutlubay Z, Zara T, Engin B, et al. Helicobacter pylori infection and skin disorders. *Hong Kong Med J*. 2014;20(4):317–324.
2. Ozen S, Pistorio A, Iusan SM, et al; for Paediatric Rheumatology International Trials Organisation (PRINTO). EULAR/PRINTO/PRES criteria for Henoch–Schönlein purpura, childhood polyarteritis nodosa, childhood Wegener granulomatosis and childhood Takayasu arteritis: Ankara 2008. Part II: final classification criteria. *Ann Rheum Dis*. 2010;69(5):798–806.
3. Trnka P. Henoch–Schönlein purpura in children. *J Paediatr Child Health*. 2013;49(12):995–1003.
4. Pohl M. Henoch-Schönlein purpura nephritis. *Pediatr Nephrol*. 2015;30(2):245–252.

ADDITIONAL READING

- Batu ED, Ozen S. Pediatric vasculitis. *Curr Rheumatol Rep*. 2012;14(2):121–129.
- Boulis E, Majithia V, McMurray R. Adult-onset Henoch-Schonlein purpura with positive c-ANCA (anti-proteinase 3): case report and review of litera- ture. *Rheumatol Int*. 2013;33(2):493–496.
- Heineke MH, Ballering AV, Jamin A, et al. New insights in the pathogenesis of immunoglobulin A vasculitis (Henoch-Schönlein purpura). *Autoimmun Rev*. 2017;16(12):1246–1253.
- Jithpratuck W, Elshenawy Y, Saleh H, et al. The clini- cal implications of adult-onset Henoch-Schonelin purpura. *Clin Mol Allergy*. 2011;9(1):9.
- Kawasaki Y. The pathogenesis and treatment of pediatric Henoch-Schönlein purpura nephritis. *Clin Exp Nephrol*. 2011;15(5):648–657.

CODES

ICD10

D69.0 Allergic purpura

CLINICAL PEARLS

- HSP is a systemic small vessel vasculitis character- ized by clinical tetrad of palpable purpura, abdomi- nal pain, arthralgia, and renal dysfunction.
- The main form of treatment is supportive care, but oral corticosteroids may be beneficial if there ap- pears to be severe renal involvement.
- In all patients with HSP, regardless of renal involve- ment at presentation, it is reasonable to check BP and urinalysis at weekly to monthly intervals for at least 6 months after diagnosis to monitor for developing renal dysfunction.

HEPARIN-INDUCED THROMBOCYTOPENIA

Dureshahwar Ali, DO

 BASICS

DESCRIPTION

- A potentially life-threatening complication of heparin use
  - Platelet count falls 50% or more from baseline.
  - 5–10% daily risk for thromboembolism, amputation, and death
- Antibody-mediated prothrombotic disorder initiated by heparin administration
- Unlike other thrombocytopenias, heparin-induced thrombocytopenia (HIT) is an idiosyncratic reaction that results in thrombosis rather than bleeding.
- Two types: nonimmune heparin-associated thrombocytopenia (previously called HIT type I) and heparin-induced thrombocytopenia/thrombosis (HITT) (immune induced; previously called HIT type II)
  - Nonimmune heparin-associated thrombocytopenia (HIT): more common, onset 1 to 4 days after starting heparin, mild thrombocytopenia ($>100,000/mm^3$), few complications, platelet count may normalize spontaneously
  - Immune HITT: less common, onset 5 to 14 days after primary exposure to heparin, thrombocytopenia often $<100,000/mm^3$, but usually $>20,000/mm^3$; high risk of thrombosis and mortality.
- HIT has three different patterns of onset: rapid, typical, and delayed. HIT has three different patterns of onset: rapid, typical, and delayed.
  - Typical pattern is exhibited in 60% of the cases, resulting in fall in platelet decline 5 to 10 days after exposure.
  - Rapid pattern is seen in 30% of the cases with decline in platelet count immediately after exposure to any heparin product
  - Delayed-onset pattern occurs at an average of 9.2 days from initiation of heparin products. It can develop even after cessation of heparin.

EPIDEMIOLOGY

Incidence

- 0.1–5% of heparin-treated patients will experience thrombocytopenia, regardless of dose, schedule, or route of administration.
- 25–50% of these patients will develop HITT (1)[B].

ETIOLOGY AND PATHOPHYSIOLOGY

- Nonimmune heparin-associated thrombocytopenia: potentially a result of direct platelet membrane binding with heparin
- HITT: Heparin can cause an increase in the blood concentration of platelet factor 4 (PF4), a chemokine. PF4 will form a complex with heparin, which acts as a substrate for immunoglobulin (IgG) antibodies. IgG antibodies recognize neoepitopes on PF4 and the resulting complex activates monocytes and platelets, resulting in increased production of thrombin and platelet-fibrin thrombi.
- Heparin/PF4 complex can, in turn, stimulate the production of specific antiheparin/PF4 complex antibodies. These antibodies cause platelet activation and a prothrombotic state. Ultimately, this hypercoagulable state leads to thromboembolic complications in many patients.

- Sources of heparin
  - Heparin flushes (e.g., for arterial lines or heparin locks)
  - Heparin-bonded catheters
  - Unfractionated heparin (UFH)
  - Low-molecular-weight heparin (LMWH) (enoxaparin, dalteparin)

RISK FACTORS

- Postsurgical > medical > obstetric
  - Postcardiopulmonary bypass (CPB) is the most significant risk factor.
  - Surgical or trauma patients have a greater risk than medical or intensive care unit patients.
- Bovine UFH > porcine UFH > LMWH; UFH carries a risk 10 times greater than LMWH.
- Female > male
- Heparin duration >5 days
- Therapeutic anticoagulation doses result in a greater reduction in platelet count compared to prophylactic dose.
- Rare in pregnant females

GENERAL PREVENTION

- Inquire about recent heparin exposure and any history of HIT.
- Use of LMWH (vs. unfractionated), for a shorter duration, can reduce the risk of developing HIT.
- Properly document past HIT reactions in patient's medical record. Develop a HIT recognition and treatment protocol.
- No form of heparin should be administered once the diagnosis of HIT is confirmed.

COMMONLY ASSOCIATED CONDITIONS

- Venous thrombosis: deep venous thrombosis (DVT), pulmonary embolism (PE), adrenal vein thrombosis with hemorrhagic infarction; seen more frequently among medical and postoperative orthopedic surgery patients
- Arterial thrombosis: myocardial infarction, stroke, mesenteric infarction, limb ischemia; seen more frequently among vascular and cardiac surgery patients
- Skin lesions (skin necrosis at site of injection)
- Acute systemic reactions

DIAGNOSIS

- Nonimmune heparin-associated thrombocytopenia (HIT): asymptomatic drop in platelet count
- HITT: thrombocytopenia or thrombosis with the presence of heparin-dependent antibodies
  - The foundation for diagnosis is based on both clinical and serologic findings.

HISTORY

- Duration of current heparin therapy
- Previous exposure to heparin, including heparin flushes and heparin-coated catheters
- In patients being treated with heparin for thrombosis, in which thrombosis recurs during therapy, consider HITT as a potential cause.

- Clinical scoring systems:
  - The commonly used "4 Ts" methodology, a risk stratification:
    - Thrombocytopenia of new onset
    - Timing of thrombocytopenia (5 to 10 days after exposure)
    - Thrombosis of new onset
    - Thrombocytopenia by other causes is ruled out.
    - Low 4Ts score is associated with a high negative predictive value for HIT.
    - Intermediate (4–5) and high (>6) have predictive positive values for HIT
  - The HIT Expert Probability score is an effective pretest probability tool.
  - The post-CPB scoring system

PHYSICAL EXAM

- Signs of venous or arterial thrombosis
- Skin necrosis (begins with erythema, progresses to ecchymosis and necrosis)
- Ischemic changes (signs of limb, renal, splenic, mesenteric ischemia)
- Bleeding (less common)
- Acute systemic reactions after IV bolus of heparin (e.g., signs of anaphylaxis)

DIFFERENTIAL DIAGNOSIS

Other potential causes of thrombocytopenia include (list is not all inclusive)

- Sepsis and other infections
- Drug reactions
- Autoimmune
- Transfusion reactions
- Physical destruction (e.g., during CPB)

DIAGNOSTIC TESTS & INTERPRETATION

- Serial platelet counts in patients receiving heparin who have a possible risk of HITT >1%: Check platelets at baseline and then every 2 to 3 days from days 4 to 14 of heparin therapy:
  - Withhold platelet monitoring for patients receiving heparin with risk of HITT <1%.
- Confirmatory lab tests needed for a clinical diagnosis can be divided into two major categories:
  - Antigen assay to detect presence of anti-PF4 antibodies:
    - ELISA: up to 99% sensitive, poor specificity; has a high negative predictive value for HIT
  - Functional assay to detect evidence of platelet activation in the presence of heparin:
    - Serotonin release assay (SRA), gold standard for diagnosis: high specificity and high sensitivity
    - Heparin-induced platelet activation (HIPA): high specificity and low sensitivity
- Antigenic assay should be the initial test.
  - Either a functional assay or an antigenic assay alone may not be adequate for clinical diagnosis; their use in combination is usually recommended.
- The diagnostic interpretation of these laboratory tests must be made in the context of the clinical estimation of the pretest probability because HIT is a clinicopathologic syndrome. Patients may form heparin-dependent antibodies and still not develop HIT.

TREATMENT

Treatment is by prompt discontinuation of heparin and replacement with a suitable alternative anticoagulant. LMWH is NOT indicated in the treatment of HIT.

GENERAL MEASURES

- Discontinue all heparin products, including flushes and heparin-coated catheters.
- All patients with a diagnosis of HIT should receive alternative anticoagulation because they are of high thrombotic risk.
- Nonimmune heparin-associated thrombocytopenia generally resolves when heparin is stopped.

ALERT

- Platelet transfusions can increase thrombosis. Give platelet transfusions only if bleeding or during an invasive procedure with a high risk of bleeding.
- Warfarin should not be administered until platelet recovery. If warfarin has been administered, vitamin K should be given due to depletion of proteins S and C and increased risk for venous limb gangrene.
- Adverse reaction to heparin should be clearly documented in the patient's medical record with instruction to avoid all heparin products.
- For patients with a documented history of HIT, under special circumstances only (such as the need for CPB), the use of heparin for a short duration may be acceptable if the absence of heparin /PF4 complex antibodies can be documented. Patients who develop antibodies to the heparin/PF4 complex have a significantly higher rate of postoperative thrombotic events than patients who lack these antibodies (1)[B].

MEDICATION

- Most patients require anticoagulation because of
  - Preexisting thrombosis or
  - Risk of thrombosis during 30 days after HIT diagnosis (Consider anticoagulation for 30 days.)
- Dosing of anticoagulant depends on indication (prophylaxis vs. treatment):
  - In cases with a clinically low suspicion/pretest probability of HIT and laboratory confirmation is pending, it may be appropriate to continue antithrombotic prophylaxis using nonheparin anticoagulants.
  - In cases with high suspicion/pretest probability of HITT and laboratory confirmation is pending, it is appropriate to begin anticoagulation treatment with a nonheparin product (1)[B],(2)[A].
- Direct thrombin inhibitors (DTIs) (argatroban and bivalirudin)
  - Reduce relative risk of thrombosis by 30% and are associated with a 5–10% risk of bleeding.
  - Can produce misleading elevation in international normalized ratio (INR) (most likely an in vitro reaction)
    - Argatroban > bivalirudin
  - Argatroban
    - Currently approved for treatment of HITT or in patients undergoing percutaneous coronary intervention when heparin is contraindicated
    - Initial dose, 2 μg/kg/min by continuous IV infusion; decrease dose (0.5 to 1.2 μg/kg/min) for patients with reduced hepatic function or with critical illness.
    - Relatively short half life
    - Dose adjustments based to achieve activated partial thromboplastin time (aPTT) 1.5 to 3 times the baseline. The activated partial-thromboplastin time may be falsely high when argatroban is given to patients who have additional coagulopathies.
    - Dose adjustment required for patients with hepatic dysfunction. Dose adjustment not required for renal function
  - Bivalirudin
    - Off-label use for HIT, complicated by thrombosis
    - Reduced risk of bleeding in patients undergoing percutaneous artery interventions (PCIs) and other cardiac procedures
    - Initial dose of 0.15 to 0.20 mg/kg/hr; adjust aPTT 1.5 to 2.5 times the baseline.
    - Drug elimination is relative to GFR. The half life is 25 to 30 minutes in a patient with normal renal function and 3.5 hour in a patient with end-stage renal disease.
- Factor Xa inhibitors (2)[A]
  - Reports of factor Xa treatment are theorized to be useful; however, minimal data support its efficacy for HIT, and an ideal dose has yet to be determined.
  - Rivaroxaban has been frequently studied and provides evidence for HIT management
  - Fondaparinux has not been recommended due to lack of evidence.
- Warfarin transition
  - Must anticoagulate with an immediate-acting agent before starting warfarin
  - Begin warfarin after platelet count is >150,000/mm³.
  - Discontinue other anticoagulant and continue only warfarin after INR is therapeutic (2 to 3) for at least 5 days. This management differs from the normal heparin-to-warfarin transition in other conditions requiring anticoagulation (1)[A].
- LMWH
  - Although LMWH has a lower risk of initiating a HIT reaction, it should not be used when antibodies are already present, which cross-react with LMWH and induce thrombosis and thrombocytopenia.

ADMISSION, INPATIENT, AND NURSING CONSIDERATIONS

- Avoid heparin flushes.
- Avoid platelet transfusion.
- HIT in pregnancy is rare. Safety of therapeutic agents has not been established but may be effective in the prevention of thrombotic complications.

ONGOING CARE

FOLLOW-UP RECOMMENDATIONS

- The transition period of anticoagulation with a DTI and warfarin in patients with HIT can be problematic.
- The INR while administering both a DTI and warfarin should be therapeutic (2 to 3) for at least 5 days before discontinuing the DTI.

- Warfarin therapy should not be commenced until the platelet count has stabilized within a normal range. Therapy should continue for a minimum of 3 months.
- DTIs can prolong INR; therefore, if INR is <4 while on both warfarin and a DTI, temporarily hold the DTI for 4 to 6 hours and recheck INR; this second INR will represent only the anticoagulant effect of warfarin.

Patient Monitoring

- Serial platelet counts
- Monitor PTT or INR as determined by the anticoagulation agent.

PATIENT EDUCATION

Patient should inform all health care providers of any previous adverse reaction to heparin.

PROGNOSIS

- Thrombosis in HIT has 20–30% mortality, with additional morbidity from stroke and limb ischemia.
- Platelet counts normalize within weeks after stopping heparin.

REFERENCES

1. Salter BS, Weiner MM, Trinh MA, et al. Heparin-induced thrombocytopenia: a comprehensive clinical review. *J Am Coll Cardiol.* 2016;67(21):2519–2522.
2. Cuker A, Arepally GM, Chong B, et al. American Society of Hematology 2018 guidelines for management of venous thromboembolism: heparin-induced thrombocytopenia. *Blood Adv.* 2018;2(22):3360–3392.

 CODES

ICD10
D75.82 Heparin induced thrombocytopenia (HIT)

CLINICAL PEARLS

- Heparin exposure through any preparation (including LMWH), any dose, or any route can cause HITT, a life-threatening condition which is associated with arterial or venous thromboembolic complications such as stroke, pulmonary embolism, mesenteric ischemia, or myocardial infarction.
- LMWH, warfarin, and prophylactic platelet transfusion are contraindicated in HIT, although LMWH is less likely to cause HIT. Once HIT is present, the antibodies will cross-react and continue to cause a HIT reaction.
- If a patient is suspected of HIT (with or without confirmatory testing), immediately discontinue all forms of heparin.
- Patients will require anticoagulation either because of preexisting thrombosis or the risk of thrombosis in first 30 days after HIT. Prophylactic dose of anticoagulation is not sufficient due to large amount of thrombin production, even in the absence of apparent thrombosis.
- A DTI should be used until a patient's INR is therapeutic (2 to 3) on warfarin for at least 5 days.

HEPATIC ENCEPHALOPATHY

Walter M. Kim, MD, PhD • Kevin Hoang, MD

BASICS

DESCRIPTION
- Reversible altered mental and neuromotor functioning in association with acute or chronic liver disease and/or portosystemic shunting
- Wide spectrum of neurologic/psychiatric abnormalities ranging from subclinical alterations to coma: prominent features are confusion, impaired arousability, and a "flapping tremor" (asterixis)
- System(s) affected: gastrointestinal (GI); hepatic; nervous
- Synonym(s): portosystemic encephalopathy (PSE); hepatic coma; liver coma

EPIDEMIOLOGY
Male = female (reflects prevalence of underlying liver disease)

Incidence
- Risk of first episode of overt hepatic encephalopathy (HE) is 5–25% within 5 years of cirrhosis diagnosis.
- Posttransjugular intrahepatic portosystemic shunt (TIPS), median cumulative 1-year incidence of overt HE is 10–50%.

Prevalence
- May occur at any age
- Parallels the age predominance of fulminant liver disease: peaks in the 40s (Cirrhosis peaks in the late 50s.)
- Occurs in all cases of fulminant hepatic failure or acute liver failure (ALF)
- Overt HE occurs in 30–40% of cirrhotic patients.
- Present in ~50% of patients requiring liver transplantation

ETIOLOGY AND PATHOPHYSIOLOGY
- There is no defined pathophysiology for the development of HE. Classifications based on 4 factors have been proposed (1):
  – According to the underlying disease:
    ○ Type A: resulting from acute liver failure (ALF)
    ○ Type B: resulting from portosystemic bypass or shunting
    ○ Type C: resulting from cirrhosis
  – According to severity of manifestation:
    ○ West Haven classification:
      ▪ Minimal: psychometric or neuropsychological alterations without mental status changes
      ▪ Grade I: lack of awareness, anxiety, shortened attention span, impaired arithmetic, altered sleep rhythm
      ▪ Grade II (overt): asterixis, lethargy, disorientation to time, personality change, inappropriate behavior
      ▪ Grade III: somnolence to stupor, confusion, gross disorientation, bizarre behavior
      ▪ Grade IV: coma
  – According to time course:
    ○ Episodic HE
    ○ Recurrent HE = bouts occurring within 6 months
    ○ Persistent HE = persistent behavioral alterations interspersed with relapses of overt HE
  – According to precipitating factors:
    ○ Nonprecipitated
    ○ Precipitated
- Several metabolic factors implicated in HE based on the failure of the liver to detoxify noxious CNS agents (e.g., ammonia, mercaptan, octopamine, tyramine, fatty acids, lactate, manganese)
- Increased aromatic and reduced branched chain amino acids in blood may act as false neurotransmitters, possibly interacting with the γ-aminobutyric acid (GABA) receptor to cause clinical symptoms.

- HE presents most commonly in patients with long-standing cirrhosis and spontaneous shunting of intestinal blood through collateral vessels or surgical portacaval shunts.
- Asterixis is the inability to maintain a particular posture due to metabolic encephalopathy. Abnormal diencephalic function leads to the characteristic liver flap noted when the arms and wrists are held in extension. Asterixis is also present in patients with uremia, barbiturate toxicity, and some cases of pulmonary disease. As such, asterixis is not pathognomonic for HE.

Genetics
- Unknown
- Conditions that predispose an individual to developing chronic liver disease such as cystic fibrosis, α_1-antitrypsin deficiency, hemochromatosis, and Wilson disease can contribute to the development of HE.

RISK FACTORS
In patients with underlying liver disease, precipitating factors include:
- Infection (overt or occult, including spontaneous bacterial peritonitis [SBP])
- GI hemorrhage
- Use of sedative (e.g., benzodiazepines) or opiate drugs
- Electrolyte disturbance (Na$^+$, K$^+$, Mg^{2+} most common)
- Fluid abnormalities including from diuretic overdose
- Transjugular intrahepatic portosystemic shunt (TIPS—a radiologically inserted shunt to lower portal pressure): Elderly patients and those with worse liver function are at increased risk for developing HE following TIPS.

GENERAL PREVENTION
- Recognize early signs and seek prompt treatment.
- Avoid nonessential medications, particularly opiates, benzodiazepines, and sedatives.
- Consider lactulose therapy as secondary prophylaxis for recurrence of HE (2)[B].
- For patients who have already experienced bouts of overt HE while on lactulose, lactulose + rifaximin is the best-documented agent to maintain remission (1).

COMMONLY ASSOCIATED CONDITIONS
- Cirrhosis
- Portal hypertension
- May occur as a complication of acute fatty liver of pregnancy
- Occurs rarely in patients with a portacaval shunt accompanied by normal liver function

DIAGNOSIS

HISTORY
- Preexisting liver disease
- Confusion; altered mental status
- Impaired arousability
- Constipation

PHYSICAL EXAM
- Age 10 to 60 years
  – Five grades of confusion and degree of obtundation (West Haven classification) (1):
    ○ Minimal: psychometric or neuropsychological alterations without mental status changes
    ○ Grade I: lack of awareness, anxiety, shortened attention span, impaired arithmetic, altered sleep rhythm
    ○ Grade II: asterixis, lethargy, disorientation to time, personality change, inappropriate behavior

    ○ Grade III: somnolence to stupor, confusion, gross disorientation, bizarre behavior
    ○ Grade IV: coma
  – Prominent signs of underlying liver disease (50%); jaundice is most common, ascites is second most common.
  – GI bleeding with hematemesis or melena (20%)
  – Systemic infection, urinary tract infection, or pulmonary infection (20%)
- Age >60 years
  – Signs of underlying liver disease diminish (25%).
  – Confusion more prominent
  – Precipitating GI hemorrhage or infection is less often identified.
  – Progression is slower.
- Age <10 years
  – Signs of underlying liver disease are prominent; fulminant hepatic failure or advanced cirrhosis
  – Progression is very rapid, often over hours.
  – Wilson disease can imitate HE.
- Vital signs:
  – Bradycardia
  – Increased blood pressure suggestive of increased intracranial pressure
- Jaundice, ascites, other correlates of liver disease (e.g., spider telangiectasias, muscle wasting)
- CNS exam: Assess short-term memory and presence of asterixis ("liver flap"—a flapping of the wrist when arms and wrists are extended).
- Pupillary reaction regresses from normal to sluggish and then absent with worsening HE.

DIFFERENTIAL DIAGNOSIS
- Metabolic encephalopathy related to anoxia, hypoglycemia, hypokalemia, hypo- or hypercalcemia, or uremia
- Head trauma, concussion, subdural hematoma; transient ischemic attack (TIA), ischemic stroke
- Increased intracranial pressure (ICP), intracranial hemorrhage (ICH)
- Alcohol intoxication; alcohol withdrawal syndrome
- Confusion due to medications or illicit drugs
- Meningitis, encephalitis
- Wilson disease without cirrhosis; Reye syndrome; Wernicke-Korsakoff syndrome

DIAGNOSTIC TESTS & INTERPRETATION
- Clinical findings diagnostic in 80% of cases
- Response to treatment often confirms the diagnosis
- EEG (limited utility): symmetric slowing of basic (α) rhythm (also common with other metabolic encephalopathies)
- Visual evoked potential: specific in grades II to IV
- Number connection test (NCT), line drawing test, critical flicker frequency (CFF) test, digit symbol test (DST), continuous reaction time (CRT) test, inhibitory control test (ICT), repeatable battery for the assessment of neuropsychological status (RBANS), and other psychometric tests may be used to assess minimal HE.

Initial Tests (lab, imaging)
- Serum ammonia level is elevated in 90% of patients with HE however is not diagnostic nor correlative with disease severity; levels are affected by infusion of amino acid solutions, opiate administration (constipation), uremia, tissue breakdown, burns, trauma, or infection.
- A normal ammonia value calls for diagnostic reevaluation
- Liver function tests, including aspartate aminotransferase (AST), alanine aminotransferase (ALT), and serum albumin
- Prothrombin time (PT) and international normalized ratio (INR) often elevated

- CBC: anemia and leukocytosis
- Complete metabolic profile to identify hypokalemia, hyperbilirubinemia, altered calcium concentration, hypomagnesemia, and hypoglycemia. BUN: creatinine >20 suggests dehydration or GI bleeding.
- Diagnostic paracentesis to rule out SBP
- Blood, urine, sputum, and ascitic fluid cultures to identify infection, as clinically indicated
- Consider arterial blood gas measurement.
- Toxicology screen
- Head CT to identify frontal cortical atrophy and/or edema; MRI may demonstrate increased T1 signal within the globus pallidus.

Follow-Up Tests & Special Considerations
Clinicians should not rely on serial monitoring of serum ammonia levels when evaluating severity of HE.

Test Interpretation
- Brain edema is seen in 100% of fatal cases.
- Glial hypertrophy in chronic encephalopathy

 # TREATMENT

GENERAL MEASURES
- Identify and treat precipitating causes: electrolyte imbalance, GI bleeding, infection
- Avoid sedatives, benzodiazepines, opiates, diphenoxylate, and atropine.
- Grade I or higher: Ensure adequate fluid and caloric ≥1,000 kcal (4.19 MJ) intake; avoid hypoglycemia.
- Consider lactulose enema for patients without diarrhea.
- If clumsiness and poor judgment are prominent, institute fall precautions.

MEDICATION
First Line
- Lactulose syrup (nonabsorbable disaccharide with laxative action that decreases colonic transit time and bacterial digestion that acidifies the colon to promote conversion of ammonia [NH_3] to ammonium [NH_4^+] which decreases ammonia absorption and reduces plasma ammonia levels): 30 to 45 mL PO up to every hour for goal of 3 to 6 bowel movements per day. Decrease to 15 to 30 mL BID when ≥3 bowel movements per day (3)[A].
- Lactulose enema (for patients who cannot tolerate oral lactulose or have suspected ileus): 300 mL lactulose plus 700 mL tap water, retained for 1 hour
- If worsening occurs acutely or there is no improvement in 2 days, add antibiotics:
  – Rifaximin: 400 mg PO TID or 550 mg PO BID (nonabsorbable antibiotic); highly effective in reversing minimal HE (4)[B]
- Contraindications:
  – Total ileus; hypersensitivity reaction
- Precautions:
  – Hypokalemia; other electrolyte imbalance; dehydration and renal failure

Second Line
- Neomycin: 1 to 2 g/day PO divided q6–8h, if renal function is within normal limits.
- Polyethylene glycol may be effective as an alternative to lactulose in management of acute HE (5)[B].
- Metronidazole and vancomycin are alternative antibiotics, though use limited by adverse side effect profile and risk of antimicrobial resistance.
- Flumazenil may be of benefit in select patients.
- Oral L-ornithine-L-aspartate (LOLA), a drug composed of two amino acids substrates, is not available in the United States but used commonly in Europe to promote urea cycle and subsequent loss of ammonia (6).

ISSUES FOR REFERRAL
Refer early to experienced transplant center, especially if refractory to drug therapies.

SURGERY/OTHER PROCEDURES
- Artificial liver perfusion devices are useful in fulminant hepatic failure as a bridge to transplantation.
- Liver failure with recurrent, intractable overt HE is indication for liver transplant.
- Consider liver transplant in grade II to IV HE.

COMPLEMENTARY & ALTERNATIVE MEDICINE
Probiotics and prebiotics have been associated with improvement of HE through modulation of gut flora (1)[C].

ADMISSION, INPATIENT, AND NURSING CONSIDERATIONS
- Monitor clinical status closely in grades I and II when diagnosis is clear and watch for progression.
- Evaluate patients with grades II to IV HE in fulminant hepatic failure for liver transplantation.

 # ONGOING CARE

FOLLOW-UP RECOMMENDATIONS
Activity as tolerated once resolved

Patient Monitoring
- Asterixis and using the trail-making test (ask patient to connect-the-dots according to numbers) helps monitor HE patients. Periodic evaluation helps determine maintenance treatment and diet. Test daily at first and then at each visit when changes in drugs and diet are made.
- See patients biweekly if there are changes on the trail-making test. Stable patients should be seen monthly.
- NCT or line drawing test at each office visit can also help with patient monitoring.
- In cirrhosis, evaluate for transplantation and periodically monitor Model for End-Stage Liver Disease (MELD) score.
- Uncontrolled diabetes and malnutrition are associated with precipitation of overt HE in cirrhotic patients.

DIET
- Weight loss with sarcopenia may worsen HE.
- Regular protein diet (1.2 to 1.5 g/kg/day); protein-limited diets are avoided as patients are typically malnourished. Vegetable protein diets are better tolerated than animal protein diets in patients with advanced cirrhosis; special IV/enteral formulations with increased branched chain amino acids are available.
- Grades III to IV patients need parenteral nutrition or jejunal feeds.

PATIENT EDUCATION
American Association for the Study of Liver Diseases, 1729 King St., Suite 200, Alexandria, VA 22314; 703-299-9766; www.aasld.org

PROGNOSIS
- With appropriate treatment, acute HE often resolves.
- Chronic liver disease
  – HE recurs
  – With each recurrence, HE is more difficult to treat—the degree of improvement with treatment is reduced and the mortality rate approaches 80%.

COMPLICATIONS
- Recurrence
- With many recurrences, permanent basal ganglion injury (non-Wilsonian hepatolenticular degeneration)
- Hepatorenal syndrome

REFERENCES
1. Vilstrup H, Amodio P, Bajaj J, et al. Hepatic encephalopathy in chronic liver disease: 2014 practice guideline by the American Association for the Study of Liver Diseases and the European Association for the Study of the Liver. *Hepatology.* 2014;60(2):715–735.
2. Agrawal A, Sharma BC, Sharma P, et al. Secondary prophylaxis of hepatic encephalopathy in cirrhosis: an open-label, randomized controlled trial of lactulose, probiotics, and no therapy. *Am J Gastroenterol.* 2012;107(7):1043–1050.
3. Gluud LL, Vilstrup H, Morgan MY. Non-absorbable disaccharides versus placebo/no intervention and lactulose versus lactitol for the prevention and treatment of hepatic encephalopathy in people with cirrhosis. *Cochrane Database Syst Rev.* 2016;(5):CD003044.
4. Kandia PA, Kumar G. Hepatic encephalopathy—the old and the new. *Crit Care Clin.* 2016;32(3):311–329.
5. Rahimi RS, Singal AG, Cuthbert JA, et al. Lactulose vs polyethylene glycol 3350—electrolyte solution for treatment of overt hepatic encephalopathy: the HELP randomized clinical trial. *JAMA Intern Med.* 2014;174(11):1727–1733.
6. Butterworth RF, Kircheis G, Hilger N, et al. Efficacy of L-ornithine L-aspartate for the treatment of hepatic encephalopathy and hyperammonemia in cirrhosis: systematic review and meta-analysis of randomized controlled trials. *J Clin Exp Hepatol.* 2018;8(3):301–313.

ADDITIONAL READING
- Acharya C, Bajaj JS. Current management of hepatic encephalopathy. *Am J Gastroenterol.* 2018;113(11):1600–1612.
- Konerup LS, Gluud LL, Vilstrup H, et al. Update on the therapeutic management of hepatic encephalopathy. *Curr Gastroenterol Rep.* 2018;20(5):21.
- Wijdicks EFM. Hepatic encephalopathy. *N Engl J Med.* 2016;375(17):1660–1670.

 ## SEE ALSO

Algorithm: Delirium

 ## CODES

ICD10
- K72.91 Hepatic failure, unspecified with coma
- K72.11 Chronic hepatic failure with coma
- K70.40 Alcoholic hepatic failure without coma

CLINICAL PEARLS
- HE includes a spectrum of neuropsychiatric findings that occur in patients with significant alterations in hepatic function.
- Lactulose helps reduce serum ammonia levels and is a cornerstone of therapy for HE.
- Asterixis ("liver flap") is the classic physical finding associated with HE.
- Serum ammonia level is not diagnostic nor correlative with the severity of HE.

HEPATITIS A
Marie L. Borum, MD, EdD, MPH • Justin Paul Canakis, DO

BASICS

DESCRIPTION
Hepatitis A infections are caused by the hepatitis A virus (HAV), a member of the *Hepatovirus* genus. This virus is one of the world's most common infections and primarily involves the liver. HAV is one of several types of hepatitis viruses that can lead to liver injury. However, compared to the other hepatitis viruses, HAV has distinct features that set it apart.

EPIDEMIOLOGY
Incidence
- 1.4 million cases globally each year
- Since the release of the HAV vaccine in 1995, the incidence of HAV in the United States decreased by 95% from 1996 to 2011.
- Regional outbreaks have contributed to the increasing number of reported cases in the United States (1).
- 12,474 cases were documented in 2018 in the United States (2).
- Incidence was approximately 4.0/100,000 in 2018 in the United States (2).
- No difference in infection rates based on sex
- As many as 1/2 of current HAV infections in the United States are acquired during travel to endemic countries.
- Incubation period of 28 days (range 15 to 50 days)

Prevalence
Serologic evidence of prior HAV infection is present in approximately 1/3 of the U.S. population. Anti-HAV prevalence relates to age, ranging from 9% in children ages 6 to 11 years to 75% of those >70 years.

Pediatric Considerations
- Often, milder or asymptomatic in children; severity increases with age.
- Infections asymptomatic in 70% of children <6 years
- >75% of 13- to 17-year-olds in the United States are vaccinated.

Pregnancy Considerations
- Increased risk of complications including preterm labor, premature rupture of membranes, antepartum hemorrhage, and placental abruption
- Vertical transmission has been reported; fecal–oral transmission during birth is possible.
- Breastfeeding is not contraindicated.

ETIOLOGY AND PATHOPHYSIOLOGY
- HAV is a single-stranded linear RNA enterovirus of the Picornaviridae family. Infection is limited to hepatocytes and macrophages.
- HAV is excreted into the bile and then stool, providing major route of spread. Primary transmission is fecal–oral. Can also transmit through sexual intercourse (particularly anal-oral contact) and intravenous drug use. Humans are the only natural host.
- Incubation is 2 to 6 weeks (mean 4 weeks). Greatest infectivity is the 2 weeks before and 1 week after onset of clinical illness.
- Infection occurs primarily after consuming food or water contaminated with HAV or via direct contact.
- Virus is stable in water and on surfaces but is easily killed with high heat or cleaning agents.
- Shellfish (clams and oysters) may be contaminated if harvested from waters contaminated with HAV.
- Blood-borne transmission is rare.
- HAV is not a chronic disease.

Genetics
Autoimmune hepatitis is rarely associated with HLA class II DR3 and DR4 after infection with HAV.

RISK FACTORS
- Person-to-person contact:
  - Intimate exposure, particularly among men who have sex with men
  - Residential institutional transmission
  - Employment in health care
  - Household exposure
  - Child care centers, schools
- Contaminated food or water contact:
  - Travel to developing countries accounts for >50% of cases in North America and Europe.
  - Consumption of raw/undercooked shellfish, vegetables, or other foods
  - Consumption of improperly handled food
- Other modes of transmission:
  - Injection of illicit drugs
  - Clotting factor disorders, such as hemophilia
  - Blood exposure or transfusion (rare)
  - No identifiable risk factor in 50%

GENERAL PREVENTION
- Proper sanitation and personal hygiene (hand washing), especially for food handlers, health care, and daycare workers
- Active immunization through HAV vaccines:
  - Havrix and Vaqta—inactivated vaccine
  - Twinrix—combination HAV and HBV
- Vaccine provides protection for 20+ years (2).
- Vaccine is recommended for (3)[A]:
  - All children aged 12 to 23 months, with catch-up administration until 18 years old
  - All travelers to countries with high endemic rate of hepatitis A (parts of Africa, Central and South America, and South and Southeast Asia)
  - Men who have sex with men
  - Individuals using injection and noninjection drugs
  - Individuals with occupational risks
  - Pregnant women, if risk of infection or severe outcomes is present
  - All individuals ≥1 year of age with HIV
  - Chronic liver disease (including pre– and post–liver transplant patients)
  - Household members and close contacts of children adopted from countries with a high HAV prevalence (prior to arrival)
  - Individuals experiencing homelessness or unstable housing
  - Unvaccinated individuals exposed during an outbreak
- Routine vaccination is no longer routinely recommended for individuals who receive blood products for treatment clotting disorders (3)[A].
- Do not delay vaccination in individuals with HIV until CD4 count surpasses a certain threshold (3)[A].
  - Vaccination response may be reduced in individuals with HIV. Postvaccination serologic testing should be conducted ≥1 month after HAV series.
  - Individuals with HIV who do not respond should consider revaccination and Ig prophylaxis.
- HAV is *not* killed by freezing; HAV is killed by:
  - Heating to >185°F for 60 seconds
  - Chlorine, iodine

COMMONLY ASSOCIATED CONDITIONS
HAV can sometimes be associated with more rare extrahepatic manifestations such as (4):
- Glomerulonephritis, cryoglobulinemia, optic neuritis
- Myocarditis, pericardial effusion, Guillain-Barré syndrome, pancreatitis
- Pneumonitis, pleural effusion
- Thrombocytopenia, aplastic anemia, or red cell aplasia, leukocytoclastic vasculitis

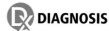

DIAGNOSIS

HISTORY
- Onset is often abrupt. Common initial symptoms include nausea, emesis and diarrhea, and headache.
- Symptom severity increases with age.
- Pediatric cases (<6 years) frequently asymptomatic
- Other presenting historical findings:
  - Fever, malaise, fatigue, myalgias, anorexia, joint pain
  - Dark urine (bilirubinuria)
  - Right upper abdominal pain
  - Pruritus (can suggest cholestasis)

PHYSICAL EXAM
- Fever (variable)
- Jaundice and icterus present in >70% of adults and older children.
- Hepatomegaly is common; splenomegaly is less common.
- Right upper quadrant abdominal tenderness
- Rare: lymphadenopathy (cervical), arthritis, or rash
- Asterixis suggests acute hepatic failure.

DIFFERENTIAL DIAGNOSIS
- Hepatitis B, C, D, E. Not clinically distinguishable from other forms of viral hepatitis; diagnosis may be suspected with typical symptoms during an outbreak.
- HIV infection
- Drug-induced hepatitis; toxin-induced hepatitis, alcoholic hepatitis; autoimmune hepatitis
- Hemochromatosis (adults) or Wilson disease
- Malarial infection; adenovirus infection; Epstein-Barr virus (EBV), cytomegalovirus (CMV), herpes simplex virus, yellow fever
- Primary or secondary hepatic malignancy
- Ischemic hepatitis or Budd-Chiari syndrome
- Nonhepatobiliary disease (elevated AST/ALT): celiac disease, congestive heart failure, thyroid disease
- Bacterial infections (Q fever, leptospirosis, syphilis, Rocky Mountain spotted fever)
- Parasites (liver flukes or toxocariasis)

DIAGNOSTIC TESTS & INTERPRETATION
Initial Tests (lab, imaging)
- Anti-HAV IgM: positive at time of onset of symptoms sensitivity and specificity >95%; primary test used to diagnose acute infection
- Anti-HAV IgG: appears soon after IgM and generally persists from years to lifetime
- AST/ALT elevated ~500 to 5,000: ALT usually > AST
- Alkaline phosphatase: mildly elevated
- Bilirubin: conjugated and unconjugated fractions usually increased. Bilirubin rises typically following rise in ALT/AST, consistent with hepatocellular injury pattern.
- Prothrombin time and partial thromboplastin time usually remain normal or near normal.
  - Significant rises should raise concern for acute hepatic failure or coexisting chronic liver disease.
- CBC: mild leukocytosis; aplasia and pancytopenia
  - Thrombocytopenia may predict illness severity.
  - Autoimmune hemolytic anemia (rare)
- Albumin, electrolytes, and glucose to evaluate for hepatic and renal function (rare renal failure)
- Urinalysis (not clinically necessary): bilirubinuria
- Consider ultrasound (US) to rule out biliary obstruction only if lab pattern is cholestatic.

Follow-Up Tests & Special Considerations
- Illness usually resolves within 4 weeks of onset.
- Repeat labs are not indicated unless symptoms persist or new symptoms develop.

Diagnostic Procedures/Other
- Liver biopsy is usually not necessary.
- US can evaluate other causes (e.g., thrombosis or concurrent cirrhosis).

Test Interpretation
- Positive serum markers in hepatitis A
  - Acute disease: anti-HAV IgM only
  - Recent disease (last 6 months): anti-HAV IgM and IgG positive
  - Previous disease or prior vaccination: anti-HAV IgM negative and IgG positive
- If liver biopsy obtained, shows portal inflammation; immunofluorescent stains for HAV antigen positive

 TREATMENT

GENERAL MEASURES
- Maintain appropriate nutrition/hydration.
- Avoid alcohol.
- Universal precautions to prevent spread
- Monitor coagulation defects, fluid, electrolytes, acid–base imbalance, hypoglycemia, and renal function.
- Report cases to local public health department.
- Laboratory evaluation including coagulation factors to rule out hepatic failure
- Referral to liver transplant center for fulminant failure (rare)

MEDICATION
- Preexposure vaccination per recommended guidelines. Both hepatitis A vaccines in the United States (Havrix, Vaqta) require 2 doses at least 6 months apart (5)[C].
- The ACIP recommends administering the first dose as soon as possible in travelers to endemic areas (3)[A].
  - For healthy individuals aged 12 months to 40 years, administer a single dose as soon as possible and complete the series within the recommended time frame.
  - In addition to a single dose of vaccine, consider administration of Ig to those >40 years, with chronic liver disease, or with immunosuppression if <2 weeks from planned departure. Vaccination series should also be completed within recommended time frame.
  - Infants <6 months should receive IG, with dose determined by length of travel.
  - Infants between 6 and 11 months should receive 1 dose of the vaccine, although this dose does not provide long-term protection; infant will require vaccine series at 12 months.
- Give postexposure prophylaxis to persons who have not previously received HAV vaccine within 2 weeks of exposure to HAV (3)[A].
  - Administer hepatitis A vaccine series as soon as possible to healthy persons between the ages of 1 and 40 years. Consider IG for individuals >40 years of age. A second dose of vaccine is not needed if patient has previously received at least 1 dose of vaccine.
  - Administer IG (0.1 mL/kg) to persons <1 year of age.
  - Vaccine and immunoglobulin should be administered to individuals with significant comorbidities (immunosuppression, liver disease) who have not previously completed the vaccination series. A second dose of vaccine is not needed if the patient has previously received at least 1 dose of vaccine.
- Use Ig for passive preexposure prophylaxis if not eligible for the vaccine (3)[A].
  - 0.1 and 0.2 mL/kg provide 1 and 2 months of coverage, respectively.
  - Long-term (≥2 months) prophylaxis should be with 0.2 mL/kg every 2 months for sustained risk (e.g., travelers).
  - Infants age <6 months, those with immunocompromise or chronic liver disease, or those in whom vaccination is contraindicated should receive 1 dose of 0.1 to 0.2 mL/kg.
  - Use Ig alone in children <1 year.
  - Do not give Ig within 6 months of administration of the MMR or varicella vaccines.

First Line
- No antiviral medications indicated; spontaneous resolution occurs in nearly 99% of patients.
- Caution with acetaminophen; if used, limit to 2 g/day or less.
- Avoid hepatotoxic agents.

Second Line
- Antiemetics (e.g., ondansetron)
- IV fluids
- Pruritus: diphenhydramine 50 mg PO IM q6h; consider cholestyramine 4 g BID if cholestasis.

ISSUES FOR REFERRAL
- Dictated by severity of illness
- Hepatic failure, refer to a high-volume liver transplant program.

SURGERY/OTHER PROCEDURES
Liver transplant in fulminant hepatic failure—only rare indications

COMPLEMENTARY & ALTERNATIVE MEDICINE
Avoid potentially hepatotoxic botanicals including barberry, comfrey, golden ragwort, groundsel, huang qin, kava kava, pennyroyal, sassafras, senna, valerian, wall germander, and wood sage.

ADMISSION, INPATIENT, AND NURSING CONSIDERATIONS
- Treatment is usually outpatient unless signs of liver failure; dictated by severity of illness.
- Treat dehydration and electrolyte imbalances.
- Enteric isolation. Private rooms, gowns, and masks are not necessary.
- Frequent hand washing. Use gloves when handling potentially contaminated material.
- 1:100 bleach dilution can be used to clean surfaces.

 ONGOING CARE

FOLLOW-UP RECOMMENDATIONS
Return to work/school 10 to 14 days after onset of symptoms with diligence to hygiene (patients remain infectious for up to 4 weeks from symptom onset).

Patient Monitoring
Monitor:
- Coagulation defects, fluid and electrolytes, acid–base imbalance, hypoglycemia, renal function

DIET
Adequate balanced nutrition; avoid alcohol.

PATIENT EDUCATION
- Segregate food handlers with HAV.
- HAV immunity persists after infection.
- CDC hepatitis A FAQs link: http://www.cdc.gov/hepatitis/hav/afaq.htm

PROGNOSIS
- Excellent; case-fatality ratio ranges from 0.1% to 5.4% depending on age and study (4)
- Risk increased with underlying chronic liver disease and in the elderly (1.8% mortality age >50 years)

COMPLICATIONS
- Coagulopathy, encephalopathy, and renal failure
- Relapsing HAV: usually milder than the initial case
- Positive anti-HAV IgM; total duration typically <9 months
- Prolonged cholestasis: characterized by protracted periods of jaundice and pruritus (>3 months); resolves with supportive care only
- Autoimmune hepatitis: can be seen after HAV infection; however, responds well to steroids
- Hepatic failure is rare (1–2%).
- Postviral encephalitis, Guillain-Barré syndrome, pancreatitis, aplastic or hemolytic anemia, agranulocytosis, thrombocytopenic purpura, pancytopenia, arthritis, vasculitis, and cryoglobulinemia (all rare)

REFERENCES
1. Abutaleb A, Kottilil S. Hepatitis A: epidemiology, natural history, unusual clinical manifestations, and prevention. *Gastroenterol Clin North Am.* 2020;49(2):191–199.
2. Centers for Disease Control and Prevention. Hepatitis A questions and answers for health professionals. https://www.cdc.gov/hepatitis/hav/havfaq.htm. Accessed January 27, 2021.
3. Nelson NP, Weng MK, Hofmeister MG, et al. Prevention of hepatitis A virus infection in the United States: recommendations of the Advisory Committee on Immunization Practices, 2020. *MMWR Recomm Rep.* 2020;69(No. RR-5):1–38.
4. Lemon SM, Ott JJ, Van Damme P, et al. Type A viral hepatitis: a summary and update on the molecular virology, epidemiology, pathogenesis and prevention. *J Hepatol.* 2018;68(1):167–184.
5. Desai AN, Kim AY. Management of hepatitis A in 2020–2021. *JAMA.* 2020;324(4):383–384.

ADDITIONAL READING
- Langan RC, Goodbred AJ. Hepatitis A. *Am Fam Physician.* 2021;104(4):368–374.
- Seto MT, Cheung KW, Hung IFN. Management of viral hepatitis A, C, D and E in pregnancy. *Best Pract Res Clin Obstet Gynaecol.* 2020;68:44–53.

 SEE ALSO

- Hepatitis B; Hepatitis C
- Algorithms: Cirrhosis; Hyperbilirubinemia and Jaundice

CODES

ICD10
B15.9 Hepatitis A without hepatic coma

CLINICAL PEARLS
- HAV vaccine is indicated for all children, travelers (particularly to endemic areas), those at elevated risk of disease, and patients with liver impairment.
- Check HAV IgG in all HIV-positive patients; provide HAV vaccine if results are negative.
- HAV disease severity directly correlates with age; children are often asymptomatic.
- Treatment of acute HAV is supportive.
- Eligible patients should receive postexposure prophylaxis within 14 days of exposure.

H

HEPATITIS B

Niyomi De Silva, MD • Heran Abiye, MD, BS • Afsha Rais Kaisani, MD

BASICS

DESCRIPTION
Infections caused by the hepatitis B virus (HBV), a DNA virus that is in the Hepadnaviridae family. HBV can lead to a spectrum of liver disease ranging from acute hepatitis to chronic conditions such as cirrhosis or hepatocellular carcinoma (HCC).

EPIDEMIOLOGY
Incidence
- Can infect patients of all ages, 80% of cases are in persons aged 30 to 59 (1)
- Predominant sex: fulminant HBV: male > female (2:1)
- In the US, ~3,200 cases of acute HBV in 2019 (2)
- White, non-Hispanic people have the highest rate of acute HBV infection in the United States (2).
- Overall rate of new infections is down over 80% since 1991 (due to national immunization strategy). There has been a slight increase in new infections since 2014 (associated with increased IV drug use).
- Vaccine coverage for the birth dose ~72% in US

Prevalence
- In the United States, 1.59 million persons (range 1.25 to 2.49 million) with chronic HBV (3)
- Asia, the Pacific Islands, and people born in Africa have the largest populations at risk for HBV (4).
- Chronic HBV worldwide: 350 to 400 million persons
  - 1 million deaths annually
    - Second most important carcinogen (behind tobacco)
    - Of chronic carriers with active disease, 25% die due to complications of cirrhosis or HCC.
    - Of chronic carriers, 75% are Asian.

ETIOLOGY AND PATHOPHYSIOLOGY
HBV is a DNA virus of the Hepadnaviridae family; highly infectious via blood and secretions

Genetics
Family history of HBV and/or HCC

RISK FACTORS
- Screen the following high-risk groups for HBV with HBsAg/sAb. Vaccinate if seronegative:
  - Persons born in endemic areas (45% of world)
  - End-stage renal disease (dialysis)
  - IV drug users (IVDUs), past or present
  - Men who have sex with men (MSM)
  - HIV- and HCV-positive patients
  - Individuals with chronic liver disease
  - Household members of HBsAg carriers
  - Sexual contacts of HBsAg carriers
  - Inmates of correctional facilities
  - Patients with chronically elevated AST/ALT levels
- Additional risk factors:
  - Needle stick/occupational exposure
  - Recipients of blood/products; organ transplants
  - Intranasal drug use; body piercing/tattoos
  - Survivors of sexual assault

Pediatric Considerations
- Shorter acute course; fewer complications
- 90% of vertical/perinatal infections become chronic.

Pregnancy Considerations
- Screen all prenatal patients for HBsAg.
- If HBsAG (+), obtain HBV DNA.
- Consider treating patients with high viral load at 28 weeks or history of previous HBV (+) infant with oral nucleos(t)ide medication beginning at 32 weeks to reduce perinatal transmission.

- Infants born to HBV-infected mothers require hepatitis B immune globulin (HBIg) (0.5 mL) and HBV vaccine within 12 hours of birth.
- Breastfeeding is safe if HBIg and HBV vaccines are administered and the areolar complex is without fissures or open sores. Oral nucleos(t)ide medications are not recommended during lactation.
- HIV increases risk of vertical transmission.
- Continue medications if pregnancy occurs while on an oral antiviral therapy to prevent acute flare.

GENERAL PREVENTION
- Vaccination
  - Three IM injections at 0, 1, and 6 months in infants or healthy adults
  - All infants at birth and during well-child care visits (age 1 and 6 months)
  - All at-risk patients (see "Risk Factors")
  - Health care and public safety workers
  - Sexual contacts of HBsAg carriers
  - Household contacts of HBsAg carriers
- Proper hygiene/sanitation by health care workers, IVDUs, and tattoo/piercing artists
  - Barrier precautions, needle disposal, sterilize equipment, cover open cuts
- Do not share personal items exposed to blood (e.g., nail clipper, razor, toothbrush).
- Safe sexual practices (condoms)
- HBsAg carriers cannot donate blood or tissue.
- Postexposure (e.g., needle stick):
  - HBIg 0.06 mL/kg in <24 hours in addition to vaccination (no more than 7 days after exposure)
  - Second dose of HBIg should be administered 30 days after exposure.

COMMONLY ASSOCIATED CONDITIONS
- HIV, hepatitis C coinfection
- Extrahepatic manifestations include:
  - Serum sickness-like syndrome (fever, erythematous skin rash, myalgias, arthralgias, fatigue)
  - Glomerulonephritis (membranous or membranoproliferative glomerulonephritis, IgA-mediated nephropathy)
  - Polyarteritis nodosa (primary systemic necrotizing vasculitis, high fever, weakness, malaise, loss of weight and appetite)
  - Dermatologic conditions (bullous pemphigoid, lichen planus, Gianotti-Crosti syndrome)
  - Cryoglobulinemia (Raynaud phenomenon, arthritis, sicca syndrome)
  - Neurologic/psychological condition (Guillain-Barré syndrome, altered mental status, depression/psychosis)

DIAGNOSIS

HISTORY
- Exposure: detailed family history, such as HBV infection and liver disease, and social history including alcohol use, drug use, and sexual history
- Acute HBV
  - Fever, malaise, fatigue, arthralgias, myalgias
  - Anorexia, nausea, vomiting
  - Jaundice, scleral icterus; dark urine, pale stools
  - Right upper quadrant (RUQ) abdominal pain
- Chronic HBV: typically asymptomatic

PHYSICAL EXAM
Acute disease: anorexia, jaundice/scleral icterus, RUQ tenderness, hepatomegaly

DIFFERENTIAL DIAGNOSIS
- Epstein-Barr virus (EBV); cytomegalovirus (CMV); hepatitis A, C, or E
- Drug-induced, alcoholic, or autoimmune hepatitis
- Wilson disease; hemochromatosis

DIAGNOSTIC TESTS & INTERPRETATION
Initial Tests (lab, imaging)
- AST/ALT:
  - Markedly elevated in acute HBV, ALT typically higher than AST
  - Transaminases may be normal or mildly elevated in chronic HBV:
    - Transaminases elevate before bilirubin.
- Bilirubin (conjugated/unconjugated): normal to markedly elevated in acute HBV
  - Last test to normalize as acute infection resolves
- Alkaline phosphatase: mild elevation
- HBcAb IgM may be the only early finding ("window period," before HBsAg turns positive).
- For acute hepatitis:
  - PT/INR, albumin, electrolytes, glucose, and CBC
  - If severe acute HBV, check for superinfection with hepatitis D (HDV Ag and HDV Ab).
  - Hepatitis B serologic markers
- Hepatitis B e-antigen (HBeAg+) indicates high replication/infectivity; confirmed with high HBV DNA ($\geq 10^5$ copies/mL); benefit from medical therapy
- Screen for HDV, HIV, HCV, and immunity to hepatitis A virus (HAV Ab total/IgG).
  - Acute HBV and HDV coinfection tends to be more severe than acute HBV infection alone.
- Ultrasound to document ascites, organomegaly, signs of portal hypertension, hepatic or portal obstruction, and to screen for HCC

Follow-Up Tests & Special Considerations
- HBsAg+ persistence >6 months defines chronic HBV:
  - Measure HBV DNA level and ALT q3–6mo.
  - If age >40 years and ALT borderline or mildly elevated, consider liver biopsy.
  - Measure baseline AFP.
  - Follow HBeAg for elimination q6–12mo.
  - Lifetime monitoring for progression
- Screening for HCC (5):
  - HCC surveillance recommended for all patients with viral load >100,000 copies/mL
  - Abdominal ultrasound alone can be used every 6 months as screening for HCC; addition of AFP increases sensitivity for early detection.

Diagnostic Procedures/Other
- Liver biopsy
- Noninvasive tests (Hepascore, FibroTest) or elastography (FibroScan) to assess fibrosis

Test Interpretation
Liver biopsy in chronic HBV may show interface hepatitis and inflammation, necrosis, cholestasis, fibrosis, cirrhosis, or chronic active hepatitis.

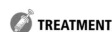

TREATMENT

GENERAL MEASURES
- Vaccinate for HAV if seronegative.
- Monitor CBC, coagulation, electrolytes, glucose, renal function, and phosphate.
- Monitor ALT and HBV DNA; increased ALT and reduced DNA imply response to therapy.
- Screen for HCC if HBsAg+.

Marker	Acute Infection	Chronic Infection	Inactive Carrier	Resolved Infection	Susceptible to Infection	Vaccinated
HBsAg	+	+	+	−	−	−
HBsAb	−	−	−	+	−	+
HBcAb	+IgM	−IgM; +total/IgG	+	+	−	−
HBeAg	+	±	−	−	−	−
HBeAb	−	±	+	±	−	−
HBV DNA	Present	Present	Low negative	−	−	−
ALT	Marked elevation	Normal to mildly elevated	Normal	Normal	Normal	Normal

MEDICATION

First Line

- Acute HBV
  - Supportive care; spontaneously resolves in 95% of immunocompetent adults
  - Antiviral therapy not indicated except for fulminant liver failure or immunosuppressed
  - Treat patients with severe or protracted course and those with acute liver failure.
    - Treatment options include monotherapy with tenofovir or entecavir.
- Chronic HBV: Treatment is based on HBeAg status:
  - FDA-approved drugs: lamivudine 100 mg, adefovir 10 mg, entecavir 0.5 to 1.0 mg, telbivudine 600 mg, or tenofovir alafenamide 25 mg, all given PO every day (dose based on renal function); pegylated interferon (peg-IFN) α2a, α2b SC weekly
- Extended oral regimens are indicated:
  - If HBeAg+, treat 6 to 12 months post disappearance of HBeAg and gain of HBeAb.
  - If HBeAg−, treat indefinitely or until HBsAg clearance and HBsAb development.
- Change/add drug based on resistance:
  - Confirm medication adherence prior to assuming drug resistance.
- Adjust dosing for renal function.
- Peg-IFN preferred to standard interferon:
  - Weekly peg-IFN (Pegasys) injections for 48 weeks
- Goals of therapy: undetectable HBV DNA, normal ALT, loss of HBeAg, gain of HBeAb; loss of HBsAg and gain of HBsAb
- Precautions:
  - Oral drugs: renal insufficiency
  - Peg-IFN: coagulopathy, myelosuppression, depression/suicidal ideation

Second Line

In persons with confirmed or suspected antiviral resistance, meaning a history of prior exposure or primary nonresponse to lamivudine, entecavir, adefovir, or telbivudine, a switch to tenofovir is recommended (6).

ISSUES FOR REFERRAL

- Refer all persistent HBsAg+ patients.
- Immediate referral for liver transplant if fulminant acute hepatitis, end-stage liver disease or HCC

SURGERY/OTHER PROCEDURES

Liver transplantation, operative resection, radiofrequency ablation for HCC

ADMISSION, INPATIENT, AND NURSING CONSIDERATIONS

- Worsening course (marked increase in bilirubin, transaminases, or symptoms)
- Hepatic failure (high PT, encephalopathy)

 ## ONGOING CARE

FOLLOW-UP RECOMMENDATIONS

Patient Monitoring

- Serial ALT and HBV DNA:
  - High ALT + low HBV DNA associated with favorable response to therapy
- CBC for WBC and platelets if on interferon therapy
- Monitor HBV DNA q3–6mo during therapy:
  - Undetectable DNA at week 24 of oral drug therapy associated with low resistance at year 2
- Monitor for complications (ascites, encephalopathy, variceal bleed) in cirrhosis.
- Vaccinate household contacts and sexual partners.
- Ultrasound q6–12mo to screen for HCC starting at age 40 years in men and 50 in women (5)

DIET

Alcohol increases risk of cirrhosis or HCC.

PATIENT EDUCATION

- Acute HBV: Review transmission precautions.
- Chronic HBV, alcohol and tobacco use accelerate progression.
  - Emphasize medication compliance to prevent flare.
- Counsel chronic HBV carriers regarding risk of transmission to others.
- Immunizations, especially against hepatitis A
- http://www.cdc.gov/hepatitis/Resources/PatientEdMaterials.htm

PROGNOSIS

Chronic hepatitis B:

- Once HBV diagnosed, the 5-year cumulative incidence of developing cirrhosis is ~8–20% in those with untreated chronic HBV.

- Of the patients with chronic HBV, 2–5% will progress to HCC with or without presence of cirrhosis.

COMPLICATIONS

- Hepatic necrosis; cirrhosis; hepatic failure
- HCC (all chronic HBV patients are at risk)
- Severe flare of chronic HBV with corticosteroids and other immunosuppressants
- Reactivation of infection if immunosuppressed. Premedicate prophylactically if HBsAg+ or if HBcAb+ and receiving systemic chemotherapy.

REFERENCES

1. Schillie S, Vellozzi C, Reingold A, et al. Prevention of hepatitis B virus infection in the United States: recommendations of the Advisory Committee on Immunization Practices. *MMWR Recomm Rep.* 2018;67(1):1–31.
2. Centers for Disease Control and Prevention. 2019 Viral hepatitis surveillance report. https://www.cdc.gov/hepatitis/statistics/2019surveillance/index.htm. Published July 2021. Accessed November 4, 2021.
3. Lim JK, Nguyen MH, Kim WR, et al. Prevalence of chronic hepatitis B virus infection in the United States. *Am J Gastroenterol.* 2020;115(9):1429–1438.
4. Centers for Disease Control and Prevention. People born outside of the United States and viral hepatitis. https://www.cdc.gov/hepatitis/populations/Born-Outside-United-States.htm. Updated September 24, 2020. Accessed October 31, 2021.
5. Tzartzeva K, Obi J, Rich NE, et al. Surveillance imaging and alpha fetoprotein for early detection of hepatocellular carcinoma in patients with cirrhosis: a meta-analysis. *Gastroenterology.* 2018;154(6):1706–1718.e1.
6. World Health Organization. Policy brief: Guidelines for the prevention, care and treatment of persons with chronic hepatitis B infection. March 2015. https://apps.who.int/iris/rest/bitstreams/690439/retrieve. Accessed November 28, 2021.

 SEE ALSO

Cirrhosis of the Liver; Hepatitis A; Hepatitis C

 CODES

ICD10

- B19.10 Unspecified viral hepatitis B without hepatic coma
- B16.9 Acute hepatitis B w/o delta-agent and without hepatic coma
- B18.1 Chronic viral hepatitis B without delta-agent

CLINICAL PEARLS

- Screen all patients born in countries with endemic disease for HBV infection using HBsAg.
- Chronic HBV is present if HBsAg persists for >6 months. Patients with chronic HBV need lifetime monitoring for disease progression and HCC.
- Acute HBV is diagnosed with HBsAg and IgM anti-HBc. Treatment is mainly supportive.
- Antiviral therapy is based on the presence or absence of cirrhosis, the ALT level, and HBV DNA levels. HBeAg indicates the immunologic response to infection. Goals of antiviral therapy are loss of HBsAg, suppression of HBV DNA, and loss of HBeAg (if positive).
- HBV is the second most common worldwide carcinogen (behind tobacco).

H

Chronic Hepatitis B Therapy

HBeAg	HBV DNA Viral Load	ALT*	Recommend
+	≥20,000 IU/mL	Elevated	Treat with antiviral or interferon.
−	≥2,000 IU/mL	Elevated	Consider biopsy or serum fibrosis marker and treatment.
+	≤20,000 IU/mL	Any	Monitor q6–12mo.
−	≥2,000 IU/mL	Normal	Biopsy; treat if disease.
+	≥20,000 IU/mL	Normal	Observe, consider treatment if ALT elevated. Biopsy if age >40 y or ALT is high normal to mild elevation.
−	≤2,000 IU/mL	Any	Monitor q6–12mo.
Cirrhosis	Any	Any	Treat with mono or combination treatment.
Liver failure	Any	Any	Treat and refer for transplant.

*ALT elevated if >2 × ULN; ULN for male = 30 IU/mL and for female = 19 IU/mL

HEPATITIS C

Anqi Li, DO • Alhang Konyak, MD, FAAFP

BASICS

DESCRIPTION
Systemic viral infection involving the liver

EPIDEMIOLOGY
Geriatric Considerations
Patients >60 years are less responsive to therapy (1),(2).

Pregnancy Considerations
- Routine prenatal HCV testing
- Vertical transmission rate is ~6/100 births; risk doubles with HIV coinfection.
- Breastfeeding is safe if there are no cracks or fissures (3).

Pediatric Considerations
- Prevalence: 0.3%
- Test children born to HCV-positive mothers.
- 20% of infants clear HCV; 30% have chronic active HCV.
- HCV-positive children have no restrictions for participation in regular childhood activities.
- Treatment starts ≥3 years of age (2),(3).

Incidence
- Highest incidence is between 20 and 39 years of age.
- Most common in males and non-Hispanic whites
- IV drug use accounts for ~60–70% of new cases.

Prevalence
- HCV is the most common cause of chronic liver disease and transplantation in the United States.
- HCV-related deaths are more common than HIV-related deaths.
- Eight known genotypes (GT) with 86 subtypes. GT 1 is the predominant form, 75% in United States, ~46% worldwide. GT predicts response to treatment (1),(2),(4),(5).

ETIOLOGY AND PATHOPHYSIOLOGY
Single-stranded RNA virus of Flaviviridae family (4)

Genetics
- No known predisposing genetic factors
- Transmission occurs primarily via parenteral exposure to infected blood.

RISK FACTORS
- Exposure risks
  - Chronic hemodialysis
  - Blood/blood product transfusion or organ transplantation before July 1992
  - Household or health care–related exposure
  - Children born to HCV-positive mothers
- Other risks:
  - Prior/current history of injection drug use
  - High-risk sexual behaviors, intra-nasal illicit drug use
  - HIV and hepatitis B infection, history of incarceration
  - Tattooing in unregulated settings
  - Sharing personal hygiene products—razor, toothbrush, nail clippers
  - Needle stick injury in health care setting (3)

GENERAL PREVENTION
- Primary prevention
  - Do not share hygiene products.
  - Use clean needles and dispose of needles properly.
  - Do not share needles; cover cuts and sores.
  - Practice safe sex (condoms).
- Secondary prevention
  - No vaccine or postexposure prophylaxis available
  - Substance abuse treatment
  - Barrier contraception
  - Assess for degree of liver fibrosis/cirrhosis (3).

COMMONLY ASSOCIATED CONDITIONS
Extrahepatic manifestations/associated diseases (3)

- Hepatitis B coinfection, HIV coinfection
- Mixed cryoglobulinemia
- HCV-related renal disease—most commonly membranoproliferative glomerulonephritis
- Diabetes mellitus/insulin resistance
- Dermatologic manifestations: necrotizing vasculitis, mixed cryoglobulinemia, porphyria cutanea tarda, lichen planus, erythema multiforme, erythema nodosum
- Autoimmune conditions
- Lymphoma—most commonly non-Hodgkin
- Depression, substance abuse/recovery

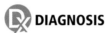

DIAGNOSIS

HISTORY
- Determine exposure risk: detailed social history, including alcohol and IV drug use, psychiatric and medical comorbidities, and coinfections.
- Chronic HCV: Most cases are mildly symptomatic (nonspecific fatigue, depression) or asymptomatic (isolated elevation in ALT, AST).
- Acute HCV: if symptoms develop (rare)
  - Onset typically 2 to 12 weeks postexposure
  - Fatigue, jaundice, dark urine, steatorrhea, nausea, abdominal pain, low-grade fevers, myalgias, arthralgias (2),(3),(6)

PHYSICAL EXAM
- May have RUQ tenderness/hepatomegaly and/or jaundice
- Signs of advanced fibrosis/cirrhosis: spider angioma, caput medusa, palmar erythema, jaundice, gynecomastia, Terry nails
- HCV-associated conditions with pertinent physical exam findings: arthralgias/myalgias, neuropathy (decreased sensation), sun-exposed skin blisters (PCT), livedo reticularis, lichen planus (palpable purpura), acanthosis nigricans, enlarged lymph node

DIFFERENTIAL DIAGNOSIS
Hepatitis A or B; EBV, CMV; alcoholic hepatitis; non-alcoholic steatohepatitis (NASH); hemochromatosis; Wilson disease, α_1-antitrypsin deficiency; ischemic, drug-induced, or autoimmune hepatitis

DIAGNOSTIC TESTS & INTERPRETATION
Initial Tests (lab, imaging)
Screening
- One-time, routine HCV antibody (Ab) screening for all adults aged 18 to 79 years of age
- Routine prenatal HCV testing
- Screen patients <18 years of age or >79 years of age if high risk:
  - Current or former IV drug users, HIV+ individuals
  - High-risk sexual behaviors; patients with persistently elevated ALT
  - Chronic hemodialysis
  - Blood transfusion or organ transplant before July 1992
  - Needle sticks or mucosal exposure to HCV+ blood
  - Children born to HCV-positive mother

Follow-Up Tests & Special Considerations
- Anti-HCV Ab
  - If nonreactive, no further action unless exposure within the last 6 months (Test with HCV RNA.)
  - If reactive, test for HCV RNA. If not detected, no current HCV infection and no further action required.
- Anti-HCV Ab detected 4 to 10 weeks after infection
  - ~97% of patients with HCV will develop Abs by 6 months after exposure.
- HCV RNA detected as early as 1 to 2 weeks after infection

Diagnostic Procedures/Other
Evaluate for hepatic fibrosis:
- Models to assess for the presence of fibrosis include AST to Platelet Ratio Index (APRI), Fibrosis-4 (FIB-4) score, FibroIndex, Forns index, HepaScore, and FibroSURE. Most guidelines recommend calculating FIB-4 score prior to initiation of treatment.
- Liver imaging: ultrasound (US), CT scan, MRI, transient US elastography, MR elastography
- Liver biopsy (gold standard)

Test Interpretation
- FIB-4 scoring: https://www.hepatitisc.uw.edu/page/clinical-calculators/fib-4
  - Score >3.25 indicates advanced fibrosis.
- Patient is presumed to have cirrhosis if they have: FIB-4 score >3.25.
- Child-Pugh scoring: https://www.mdcalc.com/child-pugh-score-cirrhosis-mortality
- Sustained virologic response (SVR): undetectable HCV RNA after 12 weeks; considered a virologic cure of HCV infection

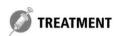

TREATMENT

GENERAL MEASURES
- Goal is to achieve SVR, reduce adverse events and all-cause mortality.
- Report acute HCV to state health department.
- Treat all patients with virologic evidence of HCV.
- Exceptions: children <3 years of age, pregnancy

MEDICATION
First Line
- Chronic HCV treatment with traditional agents, pegylated interferon (PEG-IFN) and ribavirin, is often poorly tolerated, which limits consideration as first-line treatment.
- Patients are first divided into those without cirrhosis and those with compensated cirrhosis, these groups are then divided into simplified and nonsimplified treatment plans.

ISSUES FOR REFERRAL
- If a patient fails to achieve SVR with initial first-line treatment
- Refer to liver transplant program if fulminant acute hepatitis, complication of end-stage disease, or HCC.

COMPLEMENTARY & ALTERNATIVE MEDICINE
No strong evidence or guidelines to support effective complementary/alternative therapy in HCV/cirrhosis/HCC

ADMISSION, INPATIENT, AND NURSING CONSIDERATIONS
Standard precautions

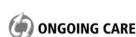

ONGOING CARE

FOLLOW-UP RECOMMENDATIONS
- Monitor serial viral load only if on antiviral therapy.
- AASLD and IDSA now recommend an abdominal US every 6 months, with or without serum α-fetoprotein (AFP) to monitor for HCC.

Medications*	Standard Dose	Common Side Effects; Contraindications
A: Elbasvir-grazoprevir (Zepatier)	50 mg/100 mg daily	Fatigue, headaches, nausea; avoid with OATPIB1/3 inhibitors or CYP3A inducers.
B: Glecaprevir-pibrentasvir (Mavyret)	300 mg/120 mg daily	Fatigue, headaches, nausea, diarrhea; avoid with atazanavir or rifampin; must take with food.
C: Ledipasvir-sofosbuvir (Harvoni)	90 mg/400 mg daily	Fatigue, headaches, weakness, irritability, insomnia, dizziness, depression, nausea, diarrhea, myalgia, cough, dyspnea
D: Sofosbuvir-velpatasvir (Epclusa)	400 mg/100 mg daily	Fatigue, headaches, irritability, insomnia, depression, rash, nausea, weakness

Simplified regimen for noncirrhotic patients: B for 8 weeks OR D for 12 weeks

Simplified regimen for compensated cirrhotic patients:

- **For GT 1 to 6: regimen B for 8 weeks**

OR

- **For GT 1, 2, 4, 5, 6: regimen D for 12 weeks**
- **For GT 3—NS5A RAS testing results dictate treatment regimen:**
  - **If NO Y93H: can be treated with regimen D for 12 weeks**

Genotype-Directed, Nonsimplified Treatment Regimens for Treatment-Naive Patients: Genotype, Regimen, Duration, Evidence

1A—without cirrhosis: A for 12 weeks [A], B for 8 weeks [A], C for 12 weeks [A], C for 8 weeks[‡] [B], D for 12 weeks [A]
1A—with compensated cirrhosis: A for 12 weeks [A], B for 8 weeks [B], C for 12 weeks [A], D for 12 weeks [A]
1B—without cirrhosis: A for 12 weeks [A], B for 8 weeks [A], C for 12 weeks [A], C for 8 weeks[‡] [B], D for 12 weeks [A]
1B—with compensated cirrhosis: A for 12 weeks [A], B for 8 weeks** [B], C for 12 weeks [A], D for 12 weeks [A]
2—without cirrhosis: B for 8 weeks [A], D for 12 weeks [A]
2—with compensated cirrhosis: B for 12 weeks** [B], D for 12 weeks [A]
3—with compensated cirrhosis: B for 8 weeks** [A], D for 12 weeks*** [A]
4—without cirrhosis: B for 8 weeks [A], D for 12 weeks [A], A for 12 weeks [B], C for 12 weeks [B]
4—with compensated cirrhosis: A for 12 weeks [B], B for 8 weeks** [A], C for 12 weeks [B], D for 12 weeks [A]
5 or 6—without cirrhosis: B for 8 weeks [A], C for 12 weeks [B], D for 12 weeks [B]
5 or 6—with compensated cirrhosis: B for 8 weeks [B], C for 12 weeks [B], D for 12 weeks [B]

*Other medications still in use, although recommended for specific circumstances include ombitasvir, paritaprevir, ritonavir, and dasabuvir, ribavirin, simeprevir, daclatasvir, and voxilaprevir.
**If HIV/HCV-coinfected, duration recommendation is 12 weeks.
***Only without baseline NS5A RAS Y93H.
[‡]If HIV noninfected and HCV RNA <6 m IU/mL.

- If cirrhosis is present, patients need endoscopic screening for varices.
  - Compensated cirrhosis without known varices: endoscopic evaluation every 2 to 3 years
  - Cirrhosis with known varices: endoscopic surveillance every 1 to 2 years (3)

Patient Monitoring
- Serial ALT/AST, renal function, and CBCs
- 12-week course of therapy
  - Follow up 4 weeks after starting therapy, and follow up 12 weeks after completing therapy.
  - 4-week HCV RNA: If detectable, recheck at week 6. If RNA has increased >10 times, stop therapy.
  - SVR12: Undetectable HCV RNA 12 weeks after completing therapy generally translates to long-term cure (goal of therapy).
  - If no evidence of cirrhosis once SVR is achieved, there is no recommendation for continued surveillance. The AASLD and IDSA guidelines currently recommend treating the patient as if they have never had HCV.
- SVR decreases risk of portal hypertension, hepatic decompensation, and HCC. Monitor for decompensation (low albumin, ascites, encephalopathy, GI bleed, etc.).
- Monitor for HBV reactivation.

DIET
- Low-fat, high-fiber diet and exercise to treat obesity/fatty liver
- Extra protein and fluids while on IFN therapy
- Avoid alcohol.

PATIENT EDUCATION
- Avoid alcohol, tobacco, and illicit drugs (including marijuana); refer to rehabilitation/12-step program and monitor for relapse as appropriate.
- Education on risk of transmission to sexual partners and with sharing personal hygiene items
- Caution with nutritional supplements and herbal medications (may contain hepatotoxins)
- Online educational resources for patients:
  - http://www.cdc.gov/knowmorehepatitis/
  - https://www.niddk.nih.gov/health-information/liver-disease/viral-hepatitis/hepatitis-c
  - https://familydoctor.org/condition/hepatitis-c/

PROGNOSIS
- Only 50% of patients with chronic HCV are diagnosed. 43% are linked to medical care. 16% are prescribed treatment, and 9% achieve SVR (4).
- Modern treatment regimens have SVR of >95% in most circumstances.
- 3–6% annual risk of hepatic decompensation
- Patients with HCV have a 1–4% annual risk of HCC.
- Cirrhosis increases risk of HCC with 2–8% annual incidence.
- There is an approximate 70% reduction in risk of HCC following successful HCV SVR (2),(3),(7).

COMPLICATIONS
- Fibrosis and cirrhosis typically develop within the first 5 to 10 years of infection if untreated.

- Risk factors for cirrhosis: age, white race, hypertension, alcohol use, anemia; risk for decompensation: diabetes, hypertension, anemia

REFERENCES
1. Hofmeister MG, Rosenthal EM, Barker LK, et al. Estimating prevalence of hepatitis C virus infection in the United States, 2013–2016. *Hepatology.* 2019;69(3):1020–1031.
2. Schillie S, Wester C, Osborne M, et al. CDC recommendations for hepatitis C screening among adults—United States, 2020. *MMWR Recomm Rep.* 2020;69(2):1–17.
3. Ghany MG, Morgan TR. Hepatitis C guidance 2019 update: American Association for the Study of Liver Diseases–Infectious Diseases Society of America recommendations for testing, managing, and treating hepatitis C virus infection. *Hepatology.* 2020;71(2):686–721.
4. Hedskog C, Parhy B, Chang S, et al. Identification of 19 novel hepatitis C virus subtypes–further expanding HCV classification. *Open Forum Infect Dis.* 2019;6(3):ofz076.
5. Centers for Disease Control and Prevention. Viral hepatitis surveillance report 2018—hepatitis C. https://www.cdc.gov/hepatitis/statistics/2018surveillance/HepC.htm. Accessed January 28, 2021.
6. Owens DK, Davidson KW, Krist AH, et al. Screening for hepatitis C virus infection in adolescents and adults: US Preventive Services Task Force recommendation statement. *JAMA.* 2020;323(10):970–975.
7. Marrero JA, Kulik LM, Sirlin CB, et al. Diagnosis, staging, and management of hepatocellular carcinoma: 2018 practice guidance by the American Association for the Study of Liver Diseases. *Clin Liver Dis (Hoboken).* 2019;13(1):1.

 SEE ALSO

- Cirrhosis of the Liver; Hepatitis A; Hepatitis B; HIV/AIDS
- Algorithm: Hyperbilirubinemia and Jaundice
- http://www.hepatitisc.uw.edu/
- Scoring calculators: http://www.mdcalc.com/

 CODES

ICD10
- B19.20 Unspecified viral hepatitis C without hepatic coma
- B17.10 Acute hepatitis C without hepatic coma
- B18.2 Chronic viral hepatitis C

CLINICAL PEARLS
- HCV is the most common cause of HCC in the western world.
- GT 1 is the most common GT of HCV in the United States
- 1 of 10 patients with HCV has no identifiable risk factors; 15–25% of HCV-infected persons clear the infection without specific treatment.
- ~50% of patients infected with HCV are unaware; ~60% of patients with anti-HCV Abs are positive for HCV RNA.
- Coinfections with HBV/HIV and comorbid substance abuse in patients with HCV are common.
- One-time routine HCV screening in all adults age 18 to 79 and HCV testing as part of routine prenatal care are recommended.
- Half of all patients with acute HCV develop chronic HCV, 25% of those develop cirrhosis within 20 years (7).

H

HERNIA
Yuhamy Curbelo-Peña, MD • Yulibeth Curbelo Peña, MD • Nolberto Adrián Medina-Gallardo, MD, PhD

 ## BASICS

DESCRIPTION
Areas of weakness or disruption of the abdominal wall through which structures can pass
- Types
  - Inguinal
    - Direct: acquired; herniation through defect in transversalis fascia of abdominal wall medial to inferior epigastric vessels; increased frequency with age as fascia weakens
    - Indirect: congenital; herniation lateral to the inferior epigastric vessels through internal inguinal ring into inguinal canal. A "complete hernia" descends into the scrotum, an "incomplete hernia" remains in the inguinal canal.
  - Pantaloon: combination of direct and indirect inguinal hernia with protrusion of abdominal wall on both sides of the epigastric vessels
  - Femoral: herniation descending through the femoral canal deep to the inguinal ligament; has a narrow neck and is especially prone to incarceration and strangulation
  - Incisional or ventral: herniation through a defect in the anterior abdominal wall at the site of a prior surgical incision
  - Congenital: herniation through defect in abdominal wall fascia due to collagen deficiency disease
  - Umbilical: defect at umbilical ring
  - Epigastric: protrusion through the middle line above the level of the umbilicus
  - Spigelian hernia: herniation through Spigelian line (lateral border of the rectus abdominis) for a lateral ventral hernia result
  - Sports hernia (not a true hernia): strain or tear of soft tissue of groin or lower abdomen
  - Others: obturator, sciatic, perineal
- Definitions
  - Reducible: Extruded sac and its contents can be returned to intra-abdominal position spontaneously or with gentle manipulation.
  - Irreducible/incarcerated: Extruded sac and its contents cannot be returned to original intra-abdominal position.
  - Strangulated: Blood supply to hernia sac contents is compromised.
  - Richter: Partial circumference of the bowel is incarcerated or strangulated. Partial wall damage may occur, increasing potential for bowel rupture and peritonitis.
  - Sliding: Wall of a viscus forms part of the wall of the inguinal hernia sac (i.e., right side–cecum, left side–sigmoid colon).

Geriatric Considerations
Abdominal wall hernias increase with advancing age, with significant increase in risk during surgical repair.

Pregnancy Considerations
- Increased intra-abdominal pressure and hormone imbalances with pregnancy may contribute to increased risk of abdominal wall hernias.
- Umbilical hernias are associated with multiple, prolonged deliveries.

EPIDEMIOLOGY
Incidence
- 75–80% groin hernias: inguinal and femoral
- 2–20% incisional/ventral, depends if prior surgery was associated with infection or contamination
- 3–10% umbilical, considered congenital
- Groin
  - 6–27% lifetime risk in adult men
  - Two peaks: most inguinal hernias present before 1 year of age or after 55 years of age
  - ~50% of children <2 years of age have a patent processus vaginalis, decreasing to 40% after age 2 years. Only between 25% and 50% are clinically significant.
  - Inguinal hernia in <5% of newborns male-to-female ratio 10:1
  - Increased incidence in premature infants
  - Increased incidence in patients with abdominal aortic aneurysms
  - Femoral <10% of all groin hernias, 40% present as a surgical emergency
- Incisional/ventral: ~10–23% of abdominal surgeries complicated by an incisional hernia, most common in upper midline incisions
- Incidence ratio: male = female
- Umbilical: 10–20% of newborns; most close by age 5 years

Prevalence
- Groin and inguinal hernias are more prevalent in men; femoral and umbilical more prevalent in women
- Most inguinal hernias are indirect in men and women.
- Incisional/ventral hernias (IVH) are more prevalent in smokers and obese individuals.

ETIOLOGY AND PATHOPHYSIOLOGY
Loss of tissue strength and elasticity (especially with aging or congenital defect in abdominal fascia) results in a fascial defect of the abdominal wall. Most pediatric hernias are congenital (e.g., patent processus vaginalis). Most adult hernias are a result of acquired weakness in the tissues of the anterior abdominal wall.

Genetics
No known genetic pattern

RISK FACTORS
- Increased abdominal pressure, coughing, heavy lifting, constipation, pregnancy, ascites, prostatism, obesity, advancing age (loss of tissue turgor), smoking, steroid use, low birth weight, prematurity
- Age: Femoral and scrotal hernias, along with recurrent groin hernias, are associated with increased risk for acute hernia surgery.

COMMONLY ASSOCIATED CONDITIONS
Obesity, chronic obstructive pulmonary disease, multiple abdominal surgeries, pregnancy, advanced age, Ehlers-Danlos syndrome, Marfan syndrome, polycystic kidney disease (PKD), osteogenesis imperfecta, Down syndrome, abdominal aortic aneurysm

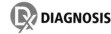 ## DIAGNOSIS

HISTORY
- May observe protrusion through abdominal wall during increased intra-abdominal pressure (Valsalva maneuver or cough)
- Pain, nausea, vomiting, bloating; relieved with reclining; may signal complication (e.g., strangulation)

PHYSICAL EXAM
- Examine initially with patient standing. During palpation, the patient should cough, strain, or perform Valsalva maneuver to determine the extent of intracavitary content movement. Repeat exam with patient in supine position.
- Inguinal (superior to inguinal ligament)
  - Direct inguinal hernia: Finger in inguinal canal finds defect of the transversalis fascia as a deep (posterior to anterior) bulge palpated with increased intra-abdominal pressure.
  - Indirect inguinal hernia: Finger in inguinal canal finds a persistent process vaginalis as a bulge (lateral to medial) that may extend into scrotum.
- Femoral (inferior to inguinal ligament): bulge in upper middle thigh; neck of the sac protrudes lateral to and below a finger placed on the pubic tubercle.
- Umbilical: palpable protrusion at umbilicus
- Incisional/ventral: palpable protrusion at site of prior abdominal incision or midline superior to the umbilicus
- Epigastric: palpable protrusion off midline above umbilicus

DIFFERENTIAL DIAGNOSIS
Lymphadenopathy, hydrocele, lipoma, varices, cryptorchidism, abscess, tumor, sports hernia (athletic pubalgia), pelvic fractures, adductor tears, omphalomesenteric duct, urachal cyst

DIAGNOSTIC TESTS & INTERPRETATION
Imaging rarely required; reserve for suspected abdominal hernia or unclear diagnosis; plain radiographs to rule out obstruction
- Ultrasound (US) can assess inguinal hernias.
- CT or tangential radiography for incisional and abdominal wall hernias and postsurgical patients with complaints of abdominal pain
- Herniography is no longer recommended.

Follow-Up Tests & Special Considerations
Diagnostic laparoscopy may be beneficial for occult hernias poorly appreciated on exam or with imaging.

 ## TREATMENT

- Elective
  - Elective surgical repair is associated with significantly lower morbidity and mortality.
- Acute setting
  - Pain management for symptomatic hernias
  - Strangulated hernias should be surgically repaired early to prevent complications such as necrosis and viscus perforation.

– Manual reduction of incarcerated hernias improves outcomes by allowing for elective repair after swelling and inflammation subside.

– Complication rate is greater with emergent pediatric inguinal hernia repairs compared to elective procedures.

– Acute hernia repair carries a higher morbidity and lower survival rate.

– Laparoscopic repair of IVH is safe, has fewer complications, shorter hospital stays, and possibly a shorter surgical time. Postoperative pain and recurrence rates are similar to open repair.

– For patients undergoing repair, operative times are shorter for extraperitoneal laparoscopic repair compared to open mesh repair with no difference in complication rates (1)[B].

– Mesh is generally preferred for hernia repairs; there have been numerous FDA product recalls in the past—primarily related to complications of bowel perforation and obstruction (https://www.fda.gov/medicaldevices/productsandmedical procedures/implant).

MEDICATION

- Antibiotics: Prophylaxis does not reduce wound infections after groin hernia repairs.
- Pain: Local anesthetic during surgical repair results in significant reduction of postoperative pain. Tension-free procedures (e.g., Lichtenstein) may be performed under local anesthesia.

ISSUES FOR REFERRAL

Warn patients of symptoms or signs of incarceration or strangulation (acute abdominal pain, fever, bloody bowel movements), which mandate immediate evaluation.

ADDITIONAL THERAPIES

Geriatric Considerations
Use of a truss (external supportive device) for direct inguinal hernias is common; no data regarding efficacy

SURGERY/OTHER PROCEDURES

All inguinal hernias should be surgically repaired. Watchful waiting in asymptomatic patients is safe if the patient has significant comorbidities that may compromise urgent repair.

- Incarceration and strangulation are absolute indications for hernia repair.
- Contraindications: patients who are not surgical candidates based on risk factors
  – Avoid elective repair in pregnant patients or patients with active infections.
- Special considerations
  – Umbilical hernias <0.5 cm can usually be followed clinically.
  – Umbilical hernias in children age 2 to 4 years typically close spontaneously.
  – Operative times and complication rates are similar when comparing single-incision laparoscopic inguinal hernia repair versus traditional multiport laparoscopic repair (2)[B].
  – "Watchful waiting" is recommended in pregnancy. Elective postpartum repair has similar outcomes and no increased risk of incarceration or strangulation before or during delivery.

– Women have lower recurrence rates using laparoscopic compared with open method.

– Ascites is not a strict contraindication for repair.

- Gold standard
  – Inguinal hernia
    ○ Open: Lichtenstein with mesh (37%): decreased recurrence rates
    ○ Laparoscopic (14%) with mesh: decreased hospital stay and postoperative pain
      ▪ Requires general anesthesia
      ▪ Transabdominal preperitoneal (TAPP) versus total extraperitoneal (TEP)
    ○ Pediatric: Laparoscopic percutaneous repair is an efficient, safe, and effective alternative to open repair. It is associated with reduced operative times and no increase in complication or recurrence rates. Avoid mesh in pediatric patients (3)[B].
  – Incisional/ventral
    ○ Laparoscopic repair is effective for most patients with primary or recurrent ventral hernias; there is <10% recurrence rate.
  – Umbilical
    ○ Pediatric: open excision with suture closure
    ○ Adult: Open repair with mesh may reduce hernia recurrence.
- Complications
  – Recurrence
  – Seromas
  – Postoperative pain, temporary or chronic: less with laparoscopic versus open technique
  – Wound infection
  – Injury to cord structures in inguinal herniorrhaphy; with nerve injury, most symptoms will resolve.

ONGOING CARE

PATIENT EDUCATION

Cleveland clinic: http://my.clevelandclinic.org/disorders/hernia/hic_hernia.aspx

PROGNOSIS

- Groin (pediatric): low recurrence rates (<3%) with surgery; may spontaneously resolve in infants
- Groin (adult): ≥1% per year risk of bowel strangulation without surgical treatment; 0–10% postoperative recurrence rates, depending on surgeon experience and procedure type
- Incisional/ventral: 3–5% postoperative occurrence: 2–17% postrepair recurrence, increased to 20–46% in larger hernias
- Umbilical (pediatric)
  – High rate of spontaneous resolution
  – Hernia less likely to close further in older children and in children with larger defects
- Umbilical (adult): up to 11% postoperative recurrence
- Epigastric: most ultimately become incarcerated and/or strangulated without surgical treatment. Recurrence is high due to frequency of missed defects during repair.

REFERENCES

1. Lockhart K, Dunn D, Teo S, et al. Mesh versus non-mesh for inguinal and femoral hernia repair. *Cochrane Database Syst Rev.* 2018;(9):CD011517.
2. Buckley FP III, Vassaur H, Monsivais S, et al. Comparison of outcomes for single-incision laparoscopic inguinal herniorrhaphy and traditional three-port laparoscopic herniorrhaphy at a single institution. *Surg Endosc.* 2014;28(1):30–35.
3. Timberlake MD, Sukhu TA, Herbst KW, et al. Laparoscopic percutaneous inguinal hernia repair in children: review of technique and comparison with open surgery. *J Pediatr Urol.* 2015;11(5):262.e1–262.e6.

ADDITIONAL READING

- Pereira JA, López-Cano M, Hernández-Granados P, et al. Initial results of the National Registry of Incisional Hernia. *Cir Esp.* 2016;94(10):595–602.
- Schmidt L, Öberg S, Andresen K, et al. Recurrence rates after repair of inguinal hernia in women: a systematic review [published online ahead of print October 31, 2018]. *JAMA Surg.* doi:10.1001/jamasurg.2018.3102.

SEE ALSO

Algorithms: Abdominal Pain, Lower; Intestinal Obstruction; Pelvic Pain

CODES

ICD10
- K46.9 Unspecified abdominal hernia without obstruction or gangrene
- K40.90 Unil inguinal hernia, w/o obst or gangr, not spcf as recur
- K41.90 Unil femoral hernia, w/o obst or gangrene, not spcf as recur

CLINICAL PEARLS

- Inguinal hernias are either direct or indirect:
  – Direct: acquired herniation through defect in transversalis fascia of abdominal wall medial to inferior epigastric vessels
  – Indirect: congenital herniation lateral to the inferior epigastric vessels; a "complete hernia" descends into the scrotum; an "incomplete hernia" remains within the inguinal canal.
- Pantaloon: combined direct and indirect inguinal hernia
- Femoral: descends through the femoral canal deep to the inguinal ligament
- Incisional or ventral: iatrogenic, herniation through a defect at site of a prior surgical incision
- Umbilical: Defect occurs at umbilical ring tissue. Most pediatric umbilical hernias close spontaneously within the first few years of life.
- Incarceration and strangulation are the primary complications associated with hernias.

HERPES EYE INFECTIONS
Stephanie L. Conway-Allen, PharmD, RPh • Kathleen A. Barry, MD

 BASICS

DESCRIPTION
- Eye infection (blepharitis, conjunctivitis, keratitis, stromal keratitis, uveitis, retinitis, glaucoma, or optic neuritis) caused by herpes simplex virus (HSV) types 1 or 2 or varicella-zoster virus (VZV, also known as human herpes virus type 3 [HHV3]).
  - HSV: most often affects the cornea (herpes keratoconjunctivitis); HSV1 > HSV2; can be further divided into primary and recurrent
  - VZV: When VZV is reactivated and affects the ophthalmic division of the 5th cranial nerve, this is known as herpes zoster ophthalmicus (HZO), a type of shingles
- System(s) affected: eye, skin, central nervous system (CNS) (neonatal)

EPIDEMIOLOGY
Predominant age: HSV—mean age of onset 37.4 years but can occur at any age, including primary infection in newborns; VZV usually advancing age (>50 years)

Incidence
- HSV keratitis: In the United States, approximated at 18.2 per 100,000 person-years. Incidence is 1.5 million per year worldwide (1).
- VZV: 1 million new cases of shingles per year in the US; 25–40% develop ophthalmic complications. Temporary keratitis is most common.

Prevalence
- Ocular HSV prevalence estimated at 500,000 in the United States (1)
- VZV: Prevalence of herpes zoster infection is 20–30%. Ocular involvement in 50% if not treated with antivirals (2); overall lifetime prevalence of HZO: 1%

ETIOLOGY AND PATHOPHYSIOLOGY
- HSV and VZV are Herpesviridae dsDNA viruses.
- HSV: primary infection from direct contact with infected person via saliva, genital contact, or birth canal exposure (neonates)
  - Primary infection may lead to severe disease in neonates, including eye, skin, CNS, and disseminated disease.
  - Recurrent infection is more common overall cause of herpetic eye infections.
- VZV: Primary infection from direct contact with infected person may cause varicella ("chickenpox") and/or lead to a latent state within trigeminal ganglia.
  - Reactivation of the virus may affect any dermatome (resulting in herpes zoster or "shingles"), including the ophthalmic branch (HZO).

RISK FACTORS
- HSV: personal history of HSV or close contact with HSV-infected person
  - General risk factors for reactivation: stress, trauma, fever, UV light exposure, other viral infections
  - Risk factors for HSV keratitis: UV laser eye treatment, some topical ocular medications such as prostaglandin analogues and primary/secondary immunosuppression

- HZO
  - History of varicella infection, advancing age (>50 years), sex (female > male), acute/painful prodrome, trauma, stress, immunosuppression (1),(3)

ALERT
Consider primary/secondary immunodeficiency disorders in all zoster patients <40 years of age (e.g., AIDS, malignancy).

GENERAL PREVENTION
- Contact precautions with active lesions (HSV and VZV)
- VZV can be spread to those who have not had chickenpox, are not immunized, or are not immune.
- Varicella recombinant zoster vaccine (Shingrix) (VZV only): 2 doses 2 to 6 months apart recommended by the CDC for all persons age 50 years and older; preferred over older vaccine (Zostavax), which can still be used for persons age >60 years unable to take Shingrix, although no longer available in the United States (4)
  - Do not give varicella vaccine during an acute infection.
- Acyclovir can be used prophylactically to prevent recurrence of ocular HSV.
- HSV immunization currently being researched (1)

ALERT
Zoster vaccination with live vaccine (Zostavax) is contraindicated if HIV positive or other immunocompromised state, pregnancy, or in active untreated tuberculosis (TB).

Pregnancy Considerations
- Pregnant women without history of chickenpox should avoid contact with persons with active zoster.
- Pregnancy increases risk of recurrence of HSV/VZV.
- Shingrix and Zostavax vaccinations are both contraindicated during pregnancy.

COMMONLY ASSOCIATED CONDITIONS
Primary and secondary immunocompromised states

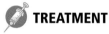 **DIAGNOSIS**

HISTORY
- Varies according to the virus and the ocular structures involved
- History of varicella or herpes simplex infection
- Acute onset, eye pain, headache, photophobia, tearing, ocular redness, decreased or blurry vision (3)
- May present with a prodromal period of fever, malaise, headache, and eye pain before skin eruptions and eye lesions (HZO) (3)

PHYSICAL EXAM
- Varies according to the virus and ocular structures involved
  - HSV most commonly affects the corneal epithelium (1).
  - VZV most commonly affects corneal stroma and uvea (3).
- Typically unilateral in presentation
  - HZO presents as early as 1 to 2 days after unilateral vesicular eruption in a dermatomal pattern (3).

- Decreased visual acuity
- Conjunctival injection near the limbus
- Decreased corneal sensation
- Dendritic pattern seen with conjunctival florescence staining

ALERT
Unilateral dermatomal vesicular rash most commonly in ophthalmic branch (V$_1$) of trigeminal nerve (VZV):

- Hutchinson sign: Vesicular lesion on nose from VZV indicates an increased risk of HZO due to involvement of nasociliary branch of trigeminal nerve, which also innervates the eye (3)[A].

DIFFERENTIAL DIAGNOSIS
- Any other cause of red, painful eye
  - Bacterial, fungal, allergic, or other viral conjunctivitis
  - Acute angle-closure glaucoma
- Corneal abrasion, recurrent corneal erosion, toxic conjunctivitis
- Temporal arteritis; trigeminal neuralgia

DIAGNOSTIC TESTS & INTERPRETATION
Initial Tests (lab, imaging)
Typically none needed, as diagnosis is based on history and physical exam (3)[C]
- Corneal swab for HSV DNA by polymerase chain reaction (PCR) (PPV = 96%)
- If vesicle present, can perform a Tzanck smear for VZV or HSV (multinucleated giant cells)
- Antibody titers to assess exposure only; direct fluorescent antibody (DFA); tissue culture

ALERT
Urgent ophthalmology referral necessary for slit-lamp exam, dilated fundus exam, and intraocular pressure measurement

TREATMENT

GENERAL MEASURES
- Avoid contact with nonimmune people.
- No contact lenses should be worn during treatment period.
- Cool compresses; artificial tears; oral pain medications

MEDICATION
First Line
- HSV corneal epithelial disease
  - Trifluridine 1%: Apply 1 drop q2h while awake to a max of 9 drops daily until reepithelialization occurs and then 1 drop q4h for an additional 7 days.
  - Acyclovir: 400 mg PO 5 times per day for 10 days
  - Ganciclovir: 0.15% gel: Apply 1 drop in eye q3h while awake, ~5× daily, until reepithelialization occurs, and then 1 drop q8h for 7 days.
  - Trifluridine and acyclovir cure about 90% of treated eyes within 2 weeks with no significant differences in effectiveness (5)[A].
  - Evidence conflicting as to whether ganciclovir is as good as or better than acyclovir (5)[A].

- Epithelial débridement by an ophthalmologist: may accelerate healing in combination with treatment as above (5)[A]
- Avoid topical steroids.
- Utility of PO antivirals unclear HSV stromal keratitis or uveitis (without epithelial disease): combination of antiviral and steroid treatment; requires ophthalmology evaluation
  - Prednisolone acetate: 1% drops QID with slow taper (6)[A]
  - Consider systemic steroids in severe uveitis (6)[A].
  - Trifluorothymidine: 1% drops QID for prophylaxis while on topical steroids
- HZO
  - Valacyclovir (Valtrex) 1 g PO TID for 7 to 10 days or famciclovir (Famvir) 500 mg PO TID for 7 to 10 days or acyclovir 800 mg PO 5 times a day for 7 to 10 days
  - Valacyclovir and famciclovir result in significant reduction in PHN compared to acyclovir (number needed to treat [NNT] = 3) with equivalent efficacy (7)[A].
  - Topical antibiotic ophthalmic ointment to protect ocular surfaces (e.g., bacitracin, polymyxin B): 0.5-inch ribbon BID to TID for 7 to 10 days (8)[C]
  - If immunocompromised: acyclovir 10 to 15 mg/kg IV q8h for 10 days
  - Prednisolone acetate: 1% drops QID with slow taper with an ophthalmologist (8)[C]
- Cycloplegic agent if anterior uveitis present; intraocular pressure-lowering agent if necessary

Second Line
- HSV: acyclovir 2 g/day PO in divided doses over 10 days in patients intolerant of topical antivirals
- Topical idoxuridine, acyclovir, brivudine, although approved internationally, are not approved for use in the United States.
- Concomitant treatment with interferon may also improve outcomes but is not currently available.

ALERT
HZO: Antiviral therapy is most effective within the first 72 hours of rash onset but should still be initiated >72 hours after onset because of the possible complications of HZO (2)[C].

- Topical antiviral agents
  - Toxic to corneal epithelium, especially after 10 to 14 days of continuous use
- Acyclovir: Reduce dosage in renal insufficiency.
- Topical steroids
  - Prescribe only in consultation with an ophthalmologist
  - Contraindicated with active corneal epithelial disease, which is best monitored with a slit lamp
  - Can increase intraocular pressure; cause corneal thinning; and, with long-term use, cause cataracts
- Prednisone: caution in immunocompromised patients

ISSUES FOR REFERRAL
Emergent or urgent ophthalmology referral, depending on severity of disease

ADDITIONAL THERAPIES
- Recurrent HSV requires suppressive therapy.
- HZO leading to PHN is common and can be treated with gabapentin or pregabalin, TCAs, opioids, and/or lidocaine gel.

SURGERY/OTHER PROCEDURES
Corneal transplantation for severe scarring or perforation

ADMISSION, INPATIENT, AND NURSING CONSIDERATIONS
- Severe systemic VZV disease
- Systemic HSV in neonates—see "Herpes Simplex Virus, Pediatric."

 ONGOING CARE

FOLLOW-UP RECOMMENDATIONS
Patient Monitoring
- Monitor with slit-lamp exam q1–2d until improvement and then q3–4d until epithelial defect resolves.
- Weekly after epithelial disease resolves until off topical antivirals

PATIENT EDUCATION
Educate about the importance of early recognition of recurrent symptoms and need for prompt evaluation and treatment.

PROGNOSIS
- Many cases are self-limited but, depending on the ocular structure involved, can lead to permanent blindness, especially in the setting of recurrent disease.
- Ocular HSV is the number one cause of infectious blindness worldwide (1).
- Recurrent ocular HSV
  - HSV epithelial disease without treatment
  - Without sequelae, 40% resolve.
  - With treatment, 90–95% resolve without complication.

Pediatric Considerations
- Neonatal primary HSV often disseminated, with high mortality rate; 37% develop vision worse than 20/200.
- Pediatric cases more likely to be bilateral (26%), recurrent (48% in 15 months), and may cause amblyopia.

COMPLICATIONS
- Recurrence
- Corneal neovascularization and scarring resulting in poor vision
- Neurotrophic ulcer with perforation
- Secondary bacterial or fungal infection
- Secondary glaucoma in 10%
- PHN in 20–40% with VZV, typically longer lasting in older patients
- Vision loss from optic neuritis or chorioretinitis

REFERENCES
1. Farooq AV, Shukla D. Herpes simplex epithelial and stromal keratitis: an epidemiologic update. *Surv Opththalmol*. 2012;57(5):448–462.
2. Carter WP III, Germann CA, Baumann MR. Ophthalmic diagnoses in the ED: herpes zoster ophthalmicus. *Am J Emerg Med*. 2008;26(5):612–617.
3. Liesegang TJ. Herpes zoster ophthalmicus natural history, risk factors, clinical presentation, and morbidity. *Ophthalmology*. 2008;115(Suppl 2):S3–S12.
4. Dooling KL, Guo A, Patel M, et al. Recommendations of the Advisory Committee on Immunization Practices for use of herpes zoster vaccines. *MMWR Morb Mortal Wkly Rep*. 2018;67(3):103–108. doi:10.15585/mmwr.mm6703a5.
5. Wilhelmus KR. Antiviral treatment and other therapeutic interventions for herpes simplex virus epithelial keratitis. *Cochrane Database Syst Rev*. 2015;(1):CD002898.
6. Knickelbein JE, Hendricks RL, Charukamnoetkanok P. Management of herpes simplex virus stromal keratitis: an evidence-based review. *Surv Ophthalmol*. 2009;54(2):226–234.
7. McDonald EM, de Kock J, Ram FS. Antivirals for management of herpes zoster including ophthalmicus: a systematic review of high-quality randomized controlled trials. *Antivir Ther*. 2012;17(2):255–264.
8. Dworkin RH, Johnson RW, Breuer J, et al. Recommendations for the management of herpes zoster. *Clin Infect Dis*. 2007;44(Suppl 1):S1–S26.

 SEE ALSO
- Herpes Simplex; Herpes Simplex Virus, Pediatric; Herpes Zoster (Shingles)
- Algorithm: Eye Pain

 CODES

ICD10
- B00.50 Herpesviral ocular disease, unspecified
- B02.30 Zoster ocular disease, unspecified
- B00.52 Herpesviral keratitis

CLINICAL PEARLS
- HSV and VZV can lead to a wide array of ocular manifestations, ranging from self-limited disease to potentially vision-threatening disease and complications.
- An exam with fluorescein stain should be performed on all patients with possible HSV keratitis or HZO.
- Topical antiviral treatment is appropriate for HSV, but systemic PO antiviral treatment is necessary for HZO.
- An ophthalmologist should be consulted before prescribing topical steroids. All HZO patients should be referred to an ophthalmologist.
- Hutchinson sign (vesicular lesion on nose from VZV) is a strong indicator of HZO.
- Shingrix is effective at preventing zoster and HZO as well as decreasing the duration of PHN.

HERPES SIMPLEX
Simone Prioli, PA-C • Ekaterina Brodski-Quigley, MD, EdM

BASICS

DESCRIPTION
- Characteristic vesicular rash primarily located in oral and genital regions caused by infection with:
  - HSV-1: blisters mostly on lips, in mouth, face, eyes
  - HSV-2: blisters primarily on the genitals
- Historically, HSV-1 and HSV-2 caused infection in different areas. More recently, the incidence of primary genital infection with HSV-1 is as common as with HSV 2 (HSV-1 can cause genital sores through oral–genital contact).
- Associated with a wide range of sequelae, depending on the age and immune status of host, whether the infection is primary or recurrent, and the degree of dissemination
- Viral shedding is typically greatest in the first (primary) infection and lessens with recurrences.
- Meningitis, encephalitis, and pneumonia are serious systemic manifestations associated with HSV infection.

EPIDEMIOLOGY
- Affects all ages; most HSV-1 is acquired in childhood, and most HSV-2 is acquired in young–middle adulthood.
- Predominant sex: male = female

Incidence
- >1 million new cases of HSV per year
- HSV can reactivate, causing recurrent disease.

Prevalence
- Widespread; 1–25% of adults may shed HSV-1 or HSV-2 at any given time. Many are unaware of their infection status.
- Prevalence of antibodies to HSV-1 is 90% by adulthood in the general population; 33% of the population infected by age 5 years
- 30% of adults have antibodies to HSV-2.
- According to the World Health Organization, about 417 million people in the world age ranging from 15 to 49 years are affected by HSV-1.
- 400 million people have genital herpes caused by HSV-2.
- 1 in 5 pregnant women are seropositive for HSV-2.

ETIOLOGY AND PATHOPHYSIOLOGY
HSV-1 and HSV-2 are double-stranded DNA viruses from the family *Herpesviridae*. HSV-1 and HSV-2 are transmitted by contact with infected skin during periods of viral shedding. Transmission can occur vertically during childbirth.

RISK FACTORS
- Immunocompromised state: advanced age, chemotherapy, malignancy, or chronic diseases such as diabetes or AIDS
- Atopic eczema, especially in children
- Prior HSV infection
- Sexual intercourse with infected person (Condoms help minimize HSV transmission, but lesions outside condom-protected areas can spread virus.)
- Occupational exposure: dental professionals at higher risk for HSV-1 and resulting herpetic whitlow
- Neonatal herpes simplex: usually acquired by vaginal birth to an infected mother; risk is greatest in mothers with primary genital herpes infection; incubation is usually from 5 to 7 days (rarely 4 weeks); cutaneous, mucous membrane, or ocular signs seen in only 70%
- Herpes gladiatorum: contact with abrasion sites, often acquired through sports with high levels of physical contact (such as rugby and wrestling)

- People with HSV-2 have a higher risk of developing HIV infection due to open ulcers or lymphocytes at lesions, facilitating HIV invasion during sexual contact.

GENERAL PREVENTION
- If active lesions are present, avoid direct contact with immunocompromised people, elderly, and newborns.
- Hand hygiene
- Avoid kissing, sharing beverages, sharing utensils, and sharing toothbrushes.
- Genital herpes: Avoid sexual contact if active lesions are present (although transmission can occur when disease appears inactive); discuss condom benefits and limits, and encourage safe sex; and consider antiviral therapy to reduce viral shedding.

COMMONLY ASSOCIATED CONDITIONS
- Erythema multiforme: 50% of cases associated with HSV-1 or HSV-2
- Herpetic whitlow, Bell palsy
- Screen all severe, treatment-resistant, or unusual HSV for concurrent HIV infection.

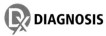

DIAGNOSIS

HISTORY
- Many patients are unaware of a known exposure.
- Prodrome of fatigue, low-grade fever, itching, tingling, or hot skin for several days prior to primary outbreak of characteristic vesicular rash
- Prodrome of pain, burning, tingling, and itching commonly occurs 6 to 48 hours before vesicles appear in subsequent outbreaks.
- Outbreak precipitated by sunlight, fever, trauma, menses, and stress

PHYSICAL EXAM
- Vesicles are often clustered and become painful ulcerated lesions with erythematous base.
- For more information on genital herpes: See "Herpes, Genital."
- Primary herpetic gingivostomatitis and pharyngitis: usually in early childhood; incubation from 2 to 12 days, followed by fever, sore throat, pharyngeal edema, and erythema
  - Small vesicles develop on pharyngeal and oral mucosa, rapidly ulcerate, and increase in number to involve soft palate, buccal mucosa, tongue, floor of mouth, lips, and cheeks; tender, bleeding gums; cervical adenopathy; fever, poor oral intake, and excess salivation contribute to dehydration; autoinoculation of other sites may occur; resolves in 10 to 14 days
  - Children usually present with blisters and fever, whereas adults present with sore throat and cervical lymphadenopathy during the primary outbreak.
- Primary herpes keratoconjunctivitis: unilateral conjunctivitis with regional adenopathy, blepharitis with vesicles on lid marginal keratitis with dendritic lesions or with punctate opacities; lasts 2 to 3 weeks; systemic involvement prolongs process.
- Eczema herpeticum: painful diffuse pox-like eruption complicating atopic dermatitis; sudden appearance of lesions in typical atopic areas (upper trunk, neck, head); high fever, localized edema, adenopathy
- Herpetic whitlow: localized infection of a finger with intense itching and pain, followed by vesicles that may coalesce with swelling and erythema. Mimics pyogenic paronychia; neuralgia and axillary adenopathy are possible; heals in 2 to 3 weeks

- Congenital infection through transplacental transfer may present with jaundice, hepatosplenomegaly, disseminated intravascular coagulation (DIC), encephalitis, seizures, temperature instability, chorioretinitis, and conjunctivitis with/without vesicles.
- Recurrent diseases from endogenous reactivation
  - Herpes labialis: recurrent lesions with HSV-1; usually <1 recurrence per 6 months, but 5–25% may have >1 attack per month; vesicles often at vermilion border, ulcerate and crust within 48 hours; heal within 8 to 10 days; may have local adenopathy
  - Ocular herpes: may recur as keratitis, blepharitis, or keratoconjunctivitis; dendritic ulcers, decreased corneal sensation, decreased visual acuity; uveitis may cause permanent visual loss.

DIFFERENTIAL DIAGNOSIS
- Impetigo: honey-crusted vesicles
- Aphthous stomatitis: grayish, shallow erosions with ring of hyperemia of anterior in mouth and lips
- Herpes zoster: unilateral dermatome distribution
- Syphilitic chancre: painless genital ulcer
- Folliculitis: "shave bumps" in genital area
- Herpangina: Vesicles predominate on anterior tonsillar pillars, soft palate, uvula, and oropharynx but not more anteriorly on lips/gums (usually caused by group A coxsackievirus).
- Stevens-Johnson syndrome
- Fungal infection
- Secondary bacterial infection
- Lymphogranuloma venereum

DIAGNOSTIC TESTS & INTERPRETATION
- Screen for other sexually transmitted infections (STIs) in patients with primary genital herpes.
- Viral: HIV, hepatitis B and C, and human papillomavirus (HPV) have crossover.
- Bacterial: Screen for concurrent gonorrhea, chlamydia in new primary genital outbreaks.

Initial Tests (lab, imaging)
- Usually a clinical diagnosis. Testing should be reserved for atypical presentation and immunocompromised patients.
- Tzanck smear shows multinucleated giant cells often with eosinophilic intranuclear inclusions (scrape material from lesion to slide, fix with ethanol/methanol, stain with Giemsa or Wright stain); varicella (herpes zoster) has identical findings.
- HSV culture: gold standard of diagnosis. Unroof vesicle, soak swab with fluid, and use swab to scrape the base of the vesicle. Must have correct viral swab and media. Highest yield if swab collected within 48 hours of outbreak. Sample may need to be refrigerated and can take up to 6 days to be positive; highly specific (reliable if positive) but has 20% false-negative rate
- HSV type–specific antibody tests distinguish between HSV-1 and HSV-2.
  - Polymerase chain reaction (PCR), direct fluorescent antibody (DFA), ELISA, and Western blot
  - 3 weeks after infection, 50% of those infected test positive; 70%, 6 weeks after infection; by 16 weeks, nearly all infected test positive
- HSV IgM testing is not clinically useful; can be positive during initial or recurrent infection

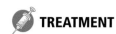

TREATMENT

GENERAL MEASURES
- Symptom management while lesions heal
- Cool dressings moistened with aluminum acetate solution

- For genital lesions: Pour a cup of warm water over genitals while urinating or by sit in a warm bath while urinating (sitz baths) if lesions are causing urinary difficulty.
- Children with gingivostomatitis who resist oral intake due to pain or extensive skin disease (eczema herpeticum) may require IV hydration.

MEDICATION

First Line
- Begin promptly, preferably in prodromal phase.
- Treat outbreak as close to the onset of symptoms as possible.
- For episodic treatment of recurrent HSV infection, start treatment within 1 day of symptom onset.
- Offer suppressive therapy to individuals who have severe psychological distress from outbreaks, severe physical pain from outbreaks, or pregnant women after 36 weeks of gestation.
- Topical therapy:
  – Penciclovir (Denavir): 1% cream. Apply to oral lesions q2h during waking hours for 4 days.
- Acyclovir (generic)
  – Mucocutaneous (or genital) HSV
    ○ Primary/first infection: 400 mg 5 times per day for 5 days
    ○ If severe, start with IV q8h dosing for the first few days, then complete 10-day course PO route.
    ○ Recurrence: days
      ▪ 200 mg orally 5 times daily for 5 days
      ▪ 400 mg orally 3 times daily for 5 days
      ▪ 800 mg orally twice daily for 5 days
      ▪ 800 mg orally 3 times daily for 2 days
    ○ Suppression: 400 mg BID daily (1)[B]
    ○ Keratitis HSV: 400 mg PO 5 times per day; topical treatment is preferred as first line.
  – Pediatric dosing: neonatal herpes simplex or encephalitis: 60 mg/kg/day IV divided q8h for 14 to 21 days (2)[B]
    ○ Older (>3 months of age) immunocompetent is weight-based dosing (40 to 80 mg/kg/day [max 1,000 mg/day] divided q8h for 5 to 7 days).
  – Safe in pregnancy and lactation—Category B (3),(4)[B]
- Valacyclovir (Valtrex)
  – Herpes labialis: 2,000 mg PO q12h for 1 day
  – Primary genital herpes: 1 g PO BID for 10 days, started within 48 hours of symptoms
  – Recurrent genital herpes: 500 mg PO BID for 3 days, started within 24 hours of symptoms; 500 to 1,000 mg PO daily (depending on frequency of outbreaks
  – Suppression: 500 to 1,000 mg daily dose
- Famciclovir (Famvir)
  – Primary genital herpes: 250 mg PO TID for 7 to 10 days
  – Recurrence: 125 mg PO BID for 5 days or 1,000 mg PO BID for 1 day
  – Suppression: 250 mg PO BID
- Precautions
  – Renal dosing for all oral antivirals
  – Significant possible interactions: Probenecid with IV acyclovir and possibly probenecid with valacyclovir may reduce renal clearance and elevate antiviral drug levels.

Second Line
- Foscarnet
  – Drug of choice for acyclovir resistance in immunocompromised persons with systemic HSV
  – 40 mg/kg IV q8h (Assume valacyclovir and famciclovir resistance also if acyclovir resistance occurs.)

- Other topicals
  – Ophthalmic preparations for herpes keratoconjunctivitis; acyclovir, vidarabine (Vira-A), ganciclovir, trifluridine
  – Topical acyclovir and penciclovir improve recurrent herpes labialis healing times by ~10% (3)[B].
  – Topical analgesics: Lidocaine 2% or 5% helps reduce pain associated with vulvar and penile outbreaks.
- Over-the-counter topical antivirals: docosanol

ISSUES FOR REFERRAL
Refer recurrent cases of herpes keratoconjunctivitis to an ophthalmologist.

ADMISSION, INPATIENT, AND NURSING CONSIDERATIONS

Pregnancy Considerations
- Cesarean section and/or acyclovir are indicated if any active genital lesions (or prodrome) present at time of delivery; consider cesarean delivery if primary genital herpes is suspected within previous 4 weeks (5),(6)[B].
- Daily oral antivirals after 36 weeks of pregnancy in women with history of genital herpes help to prevent outbreak around the time of delivery.
- Avoid fetal scalp electrodes, forceps, vacuum extractor, and artificial rupture of membranes if mother has history of genital HSV.
- Risk of viral shedding at delivery from asymptomatic recurrent genital HSV is low (~1.6%).
- Primary maternal HSV-1 or HSV-2 infection carries a 60% risk of neonatal infection at time of delivery.

Pediatric Considerations
Neonates with likely exposure (high index of suspicion) at birth or those who exhibit signs of HSV infection should have body fluids cultured and immediately start treatment (IV acyclovir).

 ### ONGOING CARE

FOLLOW-UP RECOMMENDATIONS
- For most routine cases, follow-up is not necessary. Lesions and symptoms resolve rapidly within 10 days. Extensive cases should be rechecked in 1 week; monitor for secondary bacterial infections.
- Consider long-term suppression.

DIET
If oral lesions are present, avoid salty, acidic, or sharp foods (e.g., snack chips, orange juice).

PATIENT EDUCATION
- Counsel patients on the natural course of the virus, that timing of exposure is difficult to determine, and that the virus will remain in the body indefinitely. Acknowledging and discussing psychological impact of the diagnosis helps to reduce stigmatization.
- Emphasize personal hygiene to avoid self-spreading to other body areas or exposing others. Frequent hand washing; avoid scratching; cover active, moist lesions.
- Reinforce safe sexual practices.
- Inform sex partners of infection before starting sexual relationship.

PROGNOSIS
- Usual duration of primary disease is 5 days to 2 weeks.
- Antiviral treatment shortens duration, reduces complications, and mitigates recurrences (if used for suppression).
- Viral shedding during recurrence is briefer than with primary disease; frequency of recurrence is variable and depends on individual host factors.

- Newborns/immunocompromised individuals are at highest risk for major morbidity/mortality.
- HSV is never eliminated from the body but stays dormant in dorsal root ganglia and can reactivate, causing recurrent symptoms and lesions.

COMPLICATIONS
- Herpes encephalitis: Brain biopsy may be needed for diagnosis.
- Herpes pneumonia, pneumonitis
- New research suggested that recurrent reactivation of latent HSV-1 infection may lead to neurodegeneration and Alzheimer disease.
- Pelvic inflammatory disease
- Hepatitis
- Disseminated herpes
- Acute urinary retention
- Neonatal infection

REFERENCES

1. Sauerbrei A. Optimal management of genital herpes: current perspectives. *Infect Drug Resist.* 2016;9:129–141.
2. Pinninti SG, Kimberlin DW. Neonatal herpes simplex virus infections. *Pediatr Clin North Am.* 2013;60(2):351–365.
3. Rahimi H, Mara T, Costella J, et al. Effectiveness of antiviral agents for the prevention of recurrent herpes labialis: a systematic review and meta-analysis. *Oral Surg Oral Med Oral Pathol Oral Radiol.* 2012;113(5):618–627.
4. Sawleshwarkar S, Dwyer DE. Antivirals for herpes simplex viruses. *BMJ.* 2015;351:h3350.
5. Lee R, Nair M. Diagnosis and treatment of herpes simplex 1 virus infection in pregnancy. *Obstet Med.* 2017;10(2):58–60.
6. Obiero J, Mwethera PG, Wiysonge CS. Topical microbicides for prevention of sexually transmitted infections. *Cochrane Database Syst Rev.* 2012;(6):CD007961.

ADDITIONAL READING
Groves MJ. Genital herpes: a review. *Am Family Physician.* 2016;93(11):928–934.

 ### SEE ALSO

- Herpes, Genital
- Algorithm: Genital Ulcers

 ### CODES

ICD10
- B00 Herpesviral [herpes simplex] infections
- B00.0 Eczema herpeticum
- B00.1 Herpesviral vesicular dermatitis

CLINICAL PEARLS
- Up to 25–30% of the U.S. population has serologic evidence of genital herpes (HSV-2), and >80% is seropositive for HSV-1.
- Most individuals are unaware they are infected, allowing for asymptomatic viral transmission.
- Viral suppression for patients with frequent recurrences reduces transmission and decreases outbreak frequency.

HERPES ZOSTER (SHINGLES)

Shane L. Larson, MD • Eva Fremaint, MPAS, DMSc

BASICS

DESCRIPTION
- Results from reactivation of latent varicella-zoster virus (VZV) (human herpesvirus type 3) infection
- Postherpetic neuralgia (PHN) is defined as pain persisting at least 1 month after rash has healed. The term *zoster-associated pain* is more clinically useful.
- Usually presents as a painful unilateral vesicular eruption with a dermatomal distribution
- System(s) affected: nervous; integumentary; exocrine
- Synonym(s): shingles

EPIDEMIOLOGY
Incidence
- Incidence increases with age—2/3 of cases occur in adults age ≥50 years. Incidence is increasing overall as the U.S. population ages.
- Herpes zoster: 4/1,000 person-years
- PHN: 18% in adult patients with herpes zoster; 33% in patients ≥79 years of age
- Individual lifetime risk of 30% in the United States

Prevalence
~1 million new cases of herpes zoster annually in the United States

Pregnancy Considerations
May occur during pregnancy

Geriatric Considerations
- Increased incidence of zoster outbreaks
- Increased incidence of PHN

Pediatric Considerations
- Occurs less frequently in children
- Has been reported in newborns infected in utero

ETIOLOGY AND PATHOPHYSIOLOGY
Reactivation of VZV from dorsal root/cranial nerve ganglia. Upon reactivation, the virus replicates within neuronal cell bodies, and virions are carried along axons to dermatomal skin zones, causing local inflammation and vesicle formation.

RISK FACTORS
- Increasing age
- Immunosuppression (malignancy or chemotherapy)
- Physical trauma
- Female
- HIV infection
- Spinal surgery

GENERAL PREVENTION
- Recombinant herpes zoster vaccination (Shingrix) is approved and recommended by the CDC for adults 50 years and older (1).
- Shingrix is recommended for adults who previously received Zostavax (live attenuated) and is the preferred vaccine.

- Live VZV vaccine (Zostavax) is contraindicated in immunosuppressed persons, patients with HIV and CD4 counts <200, patients undergoing cancer treatment, and patients with hematologic or lymphatic cancer (1),(2).
- Patients with active zoster may transmit disease-causing varicella virus—typically through direct contact.

COMMONLY ASSOCIATED CONDITIONS
Immunocompromised states, HIV infection, posttransplantation, immunosuppressive drugs, and malignancy

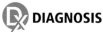

DIAGNOSIS

HISTORY
- Prodromal phase (sensory changes over involved dermatome prior to rash)
  - Tingling, paresthesias
  - Itching
  - Boring "knife-like" pain
  - Allodynia and hyperalgesia
- Acute phase
  - Constitutional symptoms (e.g., fatigue, malaise, headache, low-grade fever) are variable.
  - Dermatomal rash

PHYSICAL EXAM
- Acute phase
  - Rash: initially erythematous and maculopapular; evolves to characteristic grouped vesicles usually in one dermatome but may affect two to three adjacent dermatomes
  - Thoracic and lumbar dermatomes are most commonly involved sites (2).
  - Vesicles become pustular and/or hemorrhagic in 3 to 4 days.
  - Weakness in distribution of rash (1%)
  - Rash crusts and resolves by 14 to 21 days.
- Possible sine herpete (zoster without rash) and other chronic disorders associated with VZV without the typical rash
  - Herpes zoster ophthalmicus (HZO). Vesicles on tip of the nose (Hutchinson sign) indicate involvement of the external branch of cranial nerve V and are associated with increased incidence of HZO.
- Chronic phase
  - PHN is the most common complication (15% overall; increases with age).
  - 1–5% of cases may affect the motor nerves, causing weakness (*zoster motorius*), facial nerve involvement (Ramsay Hunt syndrome), spinal motor radiculopathies
  - Lesions usually heal 2 to 4 weeks after onset, but scarring and pigmentation changes are common (2).

DIFFERENTIAL DIAGNOSIS
Rash
- Herpes simplex virus
- Coxsackievirus
- Contact dermatitis
- Superficial pyoderma

DIAGNOSTIC TESTS & INTERPRETATION
Initial Tests (lab, imaging)
Rarely necessary. Clinical appearance is distinct.

Follow-Up Tests & Special Considerations
- Viral culture
- Tzanck smear (does not distinguish from herpes simplex, and false-negative results occur)
- Polymerase chain reaction
- Immunofluorescent antigen staining
- Varicella-zoster–specific IgM

Test Interpretation
- Multinucleated giant cells with intralesional inclusion
- Lymphatic infiltration of sensory ganglia with focal hemorrhage and nerve cell destruction

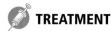

TREATMENT

GENERAL MEASURES
- Treat to control symptoms and prevent complications.
- Antiviral therapy decreases viral replication, lessens inflammation and nerve damage, and reduces the severity and duration of long-term pain.
- Prompt analgesia may shorten the duration of zoster-associated pain.
- Calamine and colloidal oatmeal may help reduce itching and burning.

MEDICATION
First Line
- Acute treatment
  - Antiviral agents initiated within 72 hours of skin lesions help relieve symptoms, speed resolution, and prevent or mitigate PHN (3)[A].
  - Antivirals do not significantly reduce the incidence of PHN (4)[A].
  - Valacyclovir: 1,000 mg PO TID for 7 days
  - Famciclovir: 500 mg PO TID for 7 days
  - Acyclovir: 800 mg q4h (5 doses daily) for 7 days
  - In children, oral acyclovir is the drug of choice.
- Analgesics (acetaminophen, NSAIDs)

- Corticosteroids do not prevent PHN but may accelerate resolution of acute neuritis.
  - Tricyclic antidepressants (TCAs); amitriptyline 10 to 25 mg at bedtime and other low-dose TCAs relieve pain acutely and may reduce pain duration; dose may be titrated up to 75 to 150 mg/day as tolerated.
  - Lidocaine patch 5% (Lidoderm) applied over painful areas (limit three patches simultaneously or trim a single patch) for up to 12 hours may be effective.
  - Gabapentin: 300 to 600 mg TID for pain; limited by adverse effects
  - Capsaicin cream and other analgesics may be useful adjuncts. Use opioids sparingly.
  - Capsaicin 8% patch or plaster provides pain relief for patients with PHN (5)[C]; better tolerated when initially applied with topical anesthetic
  - Pregabalin: 150 to 300 mg/day divided BID or TID reduces pain; use is limited by side effects.
- Prevention of PHN and zoster-associated pain: There are no treatments to prevent PHN. Treatment may, however, shorten duration and/or reduce severity of symptoms.
  - Antiviral therapy with valacyclovir, famciclovir, or acyclovir given during acute skin eruption may decrease the duration of pain.
  - Low-dose amitriptyline (25 mg at bedtime) started within 72 hours of rash onset and continued for 90 days may reduce PHN incidence/duration.
  - Paravertebral blockade: Nerve blocks during the acute phase shorten the duration of pain; somatic blocks, paravertebral blocks, and repeated/continuous epidural blocks can be used to prevent PHN (6)[A].
  - Insufficient evidence to suggest that corticosteroids reduce incidence, severity, or duration of PHN
- Precautions
  - Assess renal function prior to using valacyclovir, famciclovir, acyclovir, gabapentin, and pregabalin.
  - Valacyclovir, famciclovir, and acyclovir are pregnancy Category B.

Second Line
Numerous therapies have been advocated, but supporting evidence to routinely recommend is lacking.

COMPLEMENTARY & ALTERNATIVE MEDICINE
Cupping therapy (traditional Chinese medicine) shows potential benefit, but evidence is conflicting.

ADMISSION, INPATIENT, AND NURSING CONSIDERATIONS
- Outpatient treatment, unless disseminated or occurring as complication of serious underlying disease requiring hospitalization
- Consultation with ophthalmology for ophthalmic involvement (VZO)

 ## ONGOING CARE

FOLLOW-UP RECOMMENDATIONS
Refer to ophthalmology if concern that ophthalmic branch of the trigeminal nerve is involved.

Patient Monitoring
Follow duration of symptoms—particularly PHN. Consider hospitalization if symptoms are severe; patients are immunocompromised; >2 dermatomes are involved; serious bacterial superinfection, disseminated zoster, ophthalmic involvement, or meningoencephalitis develops.

DIET
No special diet

PATIENT EDUCATION
- The rash typically lasts 2 to 3 weeks.
- Encourage good hygiene and proper skin care.
- Warn of potential for dissemination (dissemination must be suspected with constitutional illness signs and/or spreading rash).
- Warn of potential PHN.
- Warn of potential risk of transmitting illness (chickenpox) to susceptible persons.
- Seek medical attention if any eye involvement.

PROGNOSIS
- Immunocompetent individuals should experience spontaneous and complete recovery within a few weeks.
- Acute rash typically resolves within 14 to 21 days.
- PHN may occur in patients despite antiviral treatment.

COMPLICATIONS
- PHN
- HZO: 10–20%
- Superinfection of skin lesions
- Meningoencephalitis
- Disseminated zoster
- Hepatitis; pneumonitis; myelitis
- Cranial and peripheral nerve palsies
- Acute retinal necrosis

REFERENCES
1. Centers for Disease Control and Prevention. Shingles (herpes zoster). https://www.cdc.gov/shingles/vaccination.html. Accessed October 2, 2021.
2. Saguil A, Kane S, Mercado M, et al. Herpes zoster and postherpetic neuralgia: prevention and management. *Am Fam Physician*. 2017;96(10):656–663.
3. McDonald EM, de Kock J, Ram FS. Antivirals for management of herpes zoster including ophthalmicus: a systematic review of high-quality randomized controlled trials. *Antivir Ther*. 2012;17(2):255–264.
4. Harbecke R, Cohen JI, Oxman MN. Herpes zoster vaccines. *J Infect Dis*. 2021;224(Supp 4): S429–S442.
5. Massengill JS, Kittredge JL. Practical considerations in the pharmacological treatment of postherpetic neuralgia for the primary care provider. *J Pain Res*. 2014;7:125–132.
6. Kim HJ, Ahn HS, Lee JY, et al. Effects of applying nerve blocks to prevent postherpetic neuralgia in patients with acute herpes zoster: a systematic review and meta-analysis. *Korean J Pain*. 2017;30(1):3–17.

ADDITIONAL READING
- Forbes HJ, Bhaskaran K, Grint D, et al. Incidence of acute complications of herpes zoster among immunocompetent adults in England: a matched cohort study using routine health data. *Br J Dermatol*. 2021;184(6):1077–1084.
- Tartari F, Spadotto A, Zengarini C, et al. Herpes zoster in COVID-19-positive patients. *Int J Dermatol*. 2020;59(80):1028–1029.
- Tseng HF, Bruxvoort K, Ackerson B, et al. The epidemiology of herpes zoster in immunocompetent, unvaccinated adults 50 years old: incidence, complications, hospitalization, mortality, and recurrence. *J Infect Dis*. 2020;222(5):798–806.

 ## SEE ALSO

- Bell Palsy; Chickenpox (Varicella Zoster); Herpes Eye Infections; Herpes Simplex
- Algorithm: Genital Ulcers

 ## CODES

ICD10
- B02.9 Zoster without complications
- B02.29 Other postherpetic nervous system involvement

CLINICAL PEARLS
- Initiate antiviral therapy within 72 hours of the onset of rash for maximal effect.
- Patients with active herpes zoster can transmit clinically active disease (chickenpox) to susceptible individuals.
- Shingrix (recombinant) is the recommended vaccine for healthy adults 50 years and older, including those who previously received Zostavax (live attenuated), to prevent shingles and related complications.

H

HERPES, GENITAL

Cecilia M. Kipnis, MD, FAAFP

BASICS

DESCRIPTION
- Chronic, recurrent herpes simplex virus (HSV) type 1 or 2 infection of any area innervated by the sacral ganglia
- HSV-1 causes anogenital and orolabial lesions.
- HSV-2 causes anogenital lesions.
- Primary episode: occurs in the absence of preexisting antibodies to HSV-1 or HSV-2 (may be asymptomatic)
- First episode, nonprimary: initial genital eruption; preexisting antibodies are present.
- Reactivation: recurrent episodes
- Synonym(s): herpes genitalis

EPIDEMIOLOGY
- Most commonly infected from age 15 to 30 years; prevalence increases with age due to cumulative likelihood of exposure.
- Predominant sex: female > male
- Predominant race: non-Hispanic blacks

Incidence
True incidence is unknown because genital herpes is not a reportable disease. Studies have estimated the incidence in the United States to be 572,000 to 1.6 million new cases per year and highest in 18- to 24-year-olds.

Prevalence
- Overall prevalence of HSV-2 is 10–40% in the general population and up to 60–95% in the HIV-positive population (1).
- Between the ages of 14 and 49 years, the prevalence of HSV-1 in the United States is ~48% and the prevalence of HSV-2 is ~12%. The prevalence of HSV-1 was highest (72%) in Mexican Americans and HSV-2 was highest (35%) in non-Hispanic blacks.
- Up to 90% of those who are seropositive lack formal diagnosis.
- Globally, it is estimated that 3.7 billion people are infected with HSV-1 and 140 million with HSV-2.

ETIOLOGY AND PATHOPHYSIOLOGY
- HSV is a double-stranded DNA virus of the *Herpetoviridae* family (1).
- Spread via genital-to-genital contact, oral-to-genital contact, and via maternal–fetal transmission (2)
- Incubation is 4 to 7 days after exposure.
- Risk of transmission highest when lesions are present
- Viral shedding is possible in the absence of lesions, increasing the risk of transmission (precautions— abstinence, condom use—may not be followed). Viral shedding occurs intermittently, unpredictably, and more commonly with HSV-2.
- HSV infection increases the risk for HIV.

RISK FACTORS
- Risk increases with age, number of lifetime partners, history of sexually transmitted infections (STIs), history of HIV, sexual encounters before the age of 17 years, and partner with HSV-1 or HSV-2.
- Infection with HSV-1 confers 3-fold risk of infection with HSV-2.
- Immunosuppression, fever, stress, and trauma increase risk of reactivation.

GENERAL PREVENTION
- Use barrier contraception and avoid sexual contact when symptoms/lesions are present.
- Abstinence is the only means of complete protection.

COMMONLY ASSOCIATED CONDITIONS
Syphilis, HIV, chlamydia, gonorrhea, and other STIs

DIAGNOSIS

HISTORY
- Many patients are asymptomatic (74% of HSV-1 and 63% of HSV-2) or do not recognize clinical manifestations of disease (2).
- If symptoms are present during primary episode, they are often more severe, longer in duration, and associated with constitutional symptoms.
- Common presenting symptoms (primary episode): multiple genital ulcers, dysuria, pruritus, fever, tender inguinal lymphadenopathy, headache, malaise, myalgias, cervicitis/dyspareunia, urethritis (watery discharge)
- First episode, nonprimary: In general, symptoms are less severe than primary episode.
- Common presenting symptoms for recurrent episodes: prodrome of tingling, burning, or shooting pain (2 to 24 hours before lesion appears); single ulcer; lesion can be atypical in appearance; dysuria; pruritus (lasting 4 to 6 days on average)
- Recurrent episodes are more frequent with HSV-2 than with HSV-1, especially the 1st year after infection. Recurrences are less frequent over time.
- Less common presentations: constipation (from anal involvement causing tenesmus), proctitis, stomatitis, pharyngitis, sacral paresthesias

PHYSICAL EXAM
- Lesions around groin/perineum and within anus, vagina, and on cervix
- Lesion may appear as papular, vesicular, pustular, ulcerated, or crusted; can be in various stages
- Inguinal lymphadenopathy
- Extragenital manifestations include meningitis, recurrent meningitis (Mollaret syndrome), sacral radiculitis/paresthesias, encephalitis, transverse myelitis, and hepatitis.

Pediatric Considerations
- Neonatal infection occurs in 20 to 50/100,000 live births; 80% of infections result from asymptomatic maternal viral shedding during an undiagnosed primary infection in the 3rd trimester.
- Transmission ranges from 30% to 50% if the primary episode is near time of delivery. This risk is higher with HSV-1 than with HSV-2. Neonatal disease is associated with high morbidity and mortality.
- Suspect sexual abuse with genital lesions in children.

DIFFERENTIAL DIAGNOSIS
- HIV; syphilis; chancroid
- Herpes zoster
- Ulcerative balanitis
- Granuloma inguinale; lymphogranuloma venereum
- Cytomegalovirus; Epstein-Barr virus
- Drug eruption; trauma
- Behçet syndrome
- Neoplasia

DIAGNOSTIC TESTS & INTERPRETATION
Initial Tests (lab, imaging)
- Confirm clinical diagnosis with laboratory testing.
- Viral isolation (swab or scraping) for culture or PCR
  - Use Dacron or polyester-tipped swabs with plastic shafts (cotton tips/wood shafts inhibit viral growth and/or replication) (1).
  - Culture by unroofing vesicle to obtain fluid sample. Specificity >99%; sensitivity depends on sample: 52–93% for vesicle, 41–72% for ulcer, 19–30% for crusted lesion (1),(3).
  - Culture requires timely transport of live virus to the laboratory in appropriate medium at 4°C.
  - PCR has the greatest sensitivity (98%) and specificity (>99%) but is also expensive and not readily available. It can increase detection rates by up to 70% (4); used primarily for CSF (1)
- Type-specific serologic assays
  - Seroconversion occurs 10 days to 4 months after infection (3). *Antibody testing is not necessary if a positive culture or PCR has been obtained.*
  - *IgM antibody testing is not useful because HSV IgM is often present with recurrent disease and does not distinguish new from old infection.*
  - Western blot (gold standard) and type-specific IgG antibody (glycoprotein G) enzyme-linked immunosorbent assay (ELISA) are used to discriminate between HSV-1 and HSV-2 (3)[B].
  - Western blot is >97–99% sensitive and specific but labor intensive and not readily available (1),(3).
  - ELISA 81–100% sensitive; 93–100% specific (1) for HSV-2 but lower for HSV-1 detection. False positives are possible.
  - Screening with type-specific antibody is not generally recommended for (3):
    - Asymptomatic patients with HIV infection
    - Discordant couples (one partner with known HSV, the other without)
    - Recurrent symptoms but no active lesions

TREATMENT

GENERAL MEASURES
- Ice packs to perineum, sitz baths, topical anesthetics
- Analgesics, NSAIDs

MEDICATION
Start antiviral medications within 72 hours of onset of symptoms (including prodrome). After 3 days, antivirals may help if new lesions form or for significant pain. Persons with HIV will require higher doses for longer duration.

First Line
- Acyclovir (4)[A]: the most studied antiviral in genital herpes; decreases pain, duration of viral shedding, and time to full resolution
  - Primary episode
    - 400 mg PO TID for 7 to 10 days
    - Longer if needed for incomplete healing

– Episodic therapy
  ○ 800 mg BID for 5 days
  ○ 800 mg TID for 2 days
  ○ For persons with HIV, 400 mg TID for 5 to 10 days
– Daily suppression
  ○ 400 mg BID
  ○ For persons with HIV, 400 to 800 mg 2 to 3 times per day
– Severe, complicated infections (IV therapy)
  ○ 5 to 10 mg/kg/dose q8h until clinical improvement; switch to PO therapy to complete a 10-day course (14 days for CNS involvement).
– HIV infection: 400 mg PO 3 to 5 times per day until clinical resolution is attained
– Precautions
  ○ Modify dose in renal insufficiency.
• Valacyclovir (Valtrex) (4)[A]: prodrug of acyclovir, improved bioavailability, less frequent dosing
  – Primary episode
    ○ 1 g PO BID for 7 to 10 days
  – Episodic therapy
    ○ 500 mg PO BID for 3 days
    ○ 1 g PO daily for 5 days
    ○ For persons with HIV, 1 g PO daily for 5 to 10 days
  – Daily suppression
    ○ 500 mg PO daily
    ○ 1 g PO daily
    ○ For persons with HIV, 500 mg PO BID
• Famciclovir (Famvir) (4)[A]
  – Primary episode
    ○ 250 mg PO TID for 7 to 10 days
  – Episodic therapy
    ○ 125 mg PO BID for 5 days
    ○ 1 g PO BID for 1 day
    ○ 500 mg PO once, followed by 250 mg PO BID for 2 days
    ○ For persons with HIV, 500 mg PO BID for 5 to 10 days
  – Daily suppression 250 mg PO BID
    ○ 250 mg PO BID
    ○ For persons with HIV, 500 mg PO BID

ISSUES FOR REFERRAL
For acyclovir-resistant HSV, in consultation with infectious disease specialist (4)[A]:

• Foscarnet: 40 to 80 mg/kg/dose IV q8h until clinical resolution
  – First-line treatment
  – Associated with significant nephrotoxicity
• Cidofovir: 5 mg/kg IV once weekly

Pregnancy Considerations
ACOG clinical management guidelines (4)[A]:

• Screening: Pregnant women negative for HSV-1 and HSV-2 antibodies should avoid sexual contact in the 3rd trimester if their partner is antibody positive.
• Suppressive therapy: Pregnant women with a history of genital herpes should be offered suppression treatment starting at 36 gestational weeks until delivery to decrease reactivation rate and reduce the risk of neonatal infection:
  – Acyclovir 400 mg PO TID
  – Valacyclovir 500 mg PO BID
• Monitor for outbreaks during pregnancy and examine for any lesions at the onset of labor. C-section is recommended if prodromal symptoms or lesions are present at onset of labor.

Pediatric Considerations
• High-risk infants include those with active symptoms or lesions, those delivered vaginally with maternal lesions present, and those born during a primary maternal episode. Monitor closely; obtain diagnostic laboratory specimens (HSV PCR and ocular, nasal, anal, and oral cultures). If symptomatic, require prolonged treatment:
  – Acyclovir 20 mg/kg IV q8h for 14 days if skin or mucosal lesions, 21 days if disseminated or CNS disease (4)[A]
• Low-risk infants who are asymptomatic can be observed while obtaining serum HSV PCR and ocular, nasal, anal, and oral cultures.
• Infants with possible HSV infection should be isolated from other neonates; maternal separation is not necessary, and breastfeeding is not contraindicated.

 ## ONGOING CARE

FOLLOW-UP RECOMMENDATIONS
Patient Monitoring
Test for HIV and other STIs.

PATIENT EDUCATION
• Patient education helps in treatment of subsequent outbreaks and to reduce risk of transmission:
  – Options include daily suppressive therapy and episodic therapy.
  – Alert partners of history prior to sexual activity.
  – Avoid sexual contact when symptoms or lesions are present.
  – Viral shedding and transmission can occur when symptoms/lesions are NOT present.
    ○ Shedding increased with HSV-2 and HIV
  – 100% condom use reduces HSV-2 transmission risk by 30%.
  – Sexual activity between concordant couples (i.e., both partners with the same type of herpes [HSV-1 or HSV-2]) does not increase risk of outbreaks.
  – Ensure maternity care team knows HSV status.
• Herpes Resource Center: http://www.ashasexualhealth.org/stdsstis/herpes/
• Centers for Disease Control and Prevention: http://www.cdc.gov/

PROGNOSIS
• Resolution of signs/symptoms: 3 to 21 days
• Average recurrence rate is 1 to 4 episodes per year (2).
• Antivirals do not eliminate virus from body but can reduce transmission, shedding, and outbreaks.

Pediatric Considerations
Neonatal infection survival rates: localized >95%, CNS 85%, systemic 30%

COMPLICATIONS
• Behavioral issues include lowered self-esteem, guilt, anger, depression, fear of rejection, and fear of transmission to partner.
• The risk of being infected with HIV is 2- to 3-fold with HSV-2.
• Hepatitis with disseminated HSV, especially in pregnancy

REFERENCES

1. Nath P, Kabir MA, Doust SK, et al. Diagnosis of herpes simplex virus: laboratory and point-of-care techniques. *Infect Dis Rep.* 2021;13(2):518–539.
2. Hofstetter AM, Rosenthal SL, Stanberry LR. Current thinking on genital herpes. *Curr Opin Infect Dis.* 2014;27(1):75–83.
3. Groves MJ. Genital herpes: a review. *Am Fam Physician.* 2016;93(11):928–934.
4. Workowski KA, Bachmann LH, Chan PA, et al. Sexually transmitted infections treatment guidelines, 2021. *MMWR Recomm Rep.* 2021;70(RR-4):1–187.

ADDITIONAL READING

• Dhankani V, Kutz JN, Schiffer JT. Herpes simplex virus-2 genital tract shedding is not predictable over months or years in infected persons. *PLoS Comput Biol.* 2014;10(11):e1003922.
• Gnann JW Jr, Whitley RJ. Clinical practice. Genital herpes. *N Engl J Med.* 2016;375(7):666–674.
• Management of genital herpes in pregnancy: ACOG Practice Bulletin, Number 220. *Obstet Gynecol.* 2020;135(5):e193–e202.
• McQuillan G, Kruszon-Moran D, Flagg EW, et al. Prevalence of herpes simplex virus type 1 and type 2 in persons aged 14–49: United States, 2015–2016. *NCHS Data Brief.* 2018;(304):1–8.
• Spicknall IH, Flagg EW, Torrone EA. Estimates of the prevalence and incidence of genital herpes, United States, 2018. *Sex Transm Dis.* 2021;48(4):260–265.
• Whitley R, Baines J. Clinical management of herpes simplex virus infections: past, present, and future. *F1000Res.* 2018;7:F1000.

 ## SEE ALSO

Algorithm: Genital Ulcers

CODES

ICD10
• A60 Anogenital herpesviral [herpes simplex] infections
• A60.02 Herpesviral infection of other male genital organs
• A60.0 Herpesviral infection of genitalia and urogenital tract

CLINICAL PEARLS

• Genital herpes is caused by HSV-1 and/or HSV-2.
• Many seropositive individuals are unaware that they are infected.
• Most primary episodes are asymptomatic.
• Viral shedding occurs in the absence of lesions.
• Meticulous (100%) condom use decreases transmission of HSV.

H

HICCUPS

Ravishankar E. Rao, MD • Stephanie M. Bouwer, DO

BASICS

DESCRIPTION
- Hiccups are caused by a repetitive sudden involuntary contraction of the inspiratory muscles (predominantly the diaphragm) and terminated by the abrupt closure of the glottis, which stops the inflow of air and produces a characteristic sound.
- Hiccups are classified based on their duration: Hiccup bouts last up to 48 hours; persistent hiccups last >48 hours but <1 month; intractable hiccups last for >1 month.
- System(s) affected: nervous, pulmonary
- Synonym(s): hiccoughs; singultus

Geriatric Considerations
Can be a serious problem, particularly among the elderly

Pregnancy Considerations
- Fetal hiccups are rhythmic fetal movements (confirmed sonographically) that can be confused with contractions.
- Fetal hiccups are a sign of normal neurologic development (1).

EPIDEMIOLOGY
- Predominant age: all ages (including fetus)
- Predominant sex: male > female (4:1)

Prevalence
Self-limited hiccups are extremely common, as are intraoperative and postoperative hiccups.

ETIOLOGY AND PATHOPHYSIOLOGY
- Results from stimulation of ≥1 limbs of the hiccup reflex arc (vagus and phrenic nerves) with a "hiccup center" located in the upper spinal cord and brain (2)
- In men, >90% have an organic basis; in women, psychogenic causes are more common.
- Specific underlying causes include the following:
  - CNS disorders: vascular lesions (AV malformation), infectious causes (meningitis, encephalitis), structural lesions (intracranial/brainstem mass lesions, multiple sclerosis, hydrocephalus, syringomyelia), posterior inferior cerebellar artery (PICA) aneurysm; seizure disorder
  - Diaphragmatic irritation (tumors, pericarditis, eventration, splenomegaly, hepatomegaly, peritonitis)
  - Irritation of the tympanic membrane
  - Nerve irritation: pharyngitis, laryngitis, neck tumors
  - Mediastinal and other thoracic lesions (pneumonia, aortic aneurysm, tuberculosis [TB], myocardial infarction [MI], lung cancer, rib exostoses)
  - Esophageal lesions (reflux esophagitis, achalasia, Candida esophagitis, carcinoma, obstruction)
  - Gastrointestinal disorders (gastritis, GERD, PUD, distention, cancer)

- Hiccups have been reported as an initial presentation of COVID-19
- Cardiovascular disorders (MI, pericarditis) (3)
- Hepatic lesions (hepatitis, hepatoma); pancreatic lesions (pancreatitis, pseudocysts, cancer)
- Inflammatory bowel disease; cholelithiasis, cholecystitis
- Prostatic disorders
- Appendicitis; postoperative, particularly with abdominal procedures
- Metabolic causes (uremia, hyponatremia, gout, diabetes)
- Drug-induced (dexamethasone, methylprednisolone, anabolic steroids, benzodiazepines, α-methyldopa, propofol, levofolinate, oxaliplatin, fluorouracil, carboplatin, cisplatin, tramadol) (4)
- Toxic (alcohol-induced)
- Psychogenic causes (anorexia, conversion, grief, malingering, schizophrenia, stress)
- Idiopathic

RISK FACTORS
- Overeating
- Consuming carbonated beverages
- Excessive alcohol consumption
- Excitement or emotional stress
- Changes in ambient or gastrointestinal temperature

GENERAL PREVENTION
- Identify and correct relevant underlying cause(s).
- Avoid gastric distention.
- Acupuncture shows promise compared to chronic drug therapy for controlling hiccups (5).

DIAGNOSIS

- Hiccup attacks usually occur at brief intervals and last seconds or minutes. Persistent bouts lasting >48 hours often imply an underlying physical or metabolic disorder.
- Intractable hiccups may occur continuously for months or years (6).
- Hiccups usually have a frequency of 4 to 60 per minute (6).
- Persistent and intractable hiccups warrant further evaluation.

HISTORY
- Severity and duration of hiccup bouts
- Associated medical conditions that could be causative—gastrointestinal, cardiac, neurologic, or pulmonary disorders
- Recent surgery (especially genitourinary)
- Behavioral health history
- Review of medications
- Alcohol and illicit drug use

PHYSICAL EXAM
- Correlate exam with potential etiologies (e.g., rales with pneumonia; organomegaly with splenic or hepatic disease).
- Examine the ear canal for foreign bodies.
- Head and neck masses and lymphadenopathy
- Complete neurologic exam

DIFFERENTIAL DIAGNOSIS
Hiccups are rarely confused with burping (eructation).

DIAGNOSTIC TESTS & INTERPRETATION
- When an underlying etiology is suspected, consider condition-specific testing (e.g., CBC, electrolytes, BUN, creatinine, LFTs, amylase/lipase, metabolic panel, chest x-ray) for hiccups lasting longer than 48 hours.
- Fluoroscopy can evaluate hemidiaphragm movement.

Diagnostic Procedures/Other
- Upper endoscopy; CT scan (or other imaging) of brain, thorax, abdomen, and pelvis to look for underlying causes
- Head MRI with contrast, lumbar puncture
- The extent of the workup is often in proportion to the duration and severity of the hiccups (2).

TREATMENT

- Outpatient (usually)
- Inpatient (if elderly, debilitated, or intractable hiccups)
- Many hiccup treatments are purely anecdotal.

GENERAL MEASURES
- Evaluate frequent bouts or persistent hiccups.
- Treat underlying cause when identified (2)[C],(6)[C],(7).
  - Dilate esophageal stricture or obstruction.
  - Treat ulcers or reflux disease.
  - Remove hair or foreign body from ear canal.
  - Angostura bitters for alcohol-induced hiccups
  - Catheter stimulation of pharynx for operative and postoperative hiccups
  - Antifungal treatment for Candida esophagitis
  - Correct electrolyte imbalance.
- Medical measures
  - Relieve gastric distention (gastric lavage, nasogastric aspiration, induced vomiting).
  - Cautious counterirritation of the vagus nerve (supraorbital pressure, carotid sinus massage, digital rectal massage)
  - Respiratory center stimulants (breathing 5% CO_2)
  - Behavioral health modification (hypnosis, meditation, paced respirations)
  - Phrenic nerve block or electrical stimulation (or pacing) of the dominant hemidiaphragm
  - Acupuncture
  - Miscellaneous (cardioversion)

MEDICATION

First Line
- Physical maneuvers: breath holding, Valsalva maneuver, breathing into a bag, fright, ice water gargles
- Others: swallowing granulated sugar, hard bread, or peanut butter; biting on a lemon, pulling knees to chest, or leaning forward to compress chest
- Drug therapy if physical maneuvers have failed or treatment is directed toward a specific cause of hiccups
- Pharmacologic therapy
  - Chlorpromazine (FDA-approved for hiccups): 25 to 50 mg PO/IV TID
  - Metoclopramide: 5 to 10 mg PO QID
  - Baclofen: 5 to 10 mg PO TID (2)[B],(6)[B],(8)[B]
  - Haloperidol: 2 to 5 mg PO/IM followed by 1 to 2 mg PO TID
  - Phenytoin: 200 to 300 mg PO HS
  - Nifedipine: 10 to 20 mg PO daily to TID
  - Amitriptyline: 10 mg PO TID
  - Viscous lidocaine 2%: 5 mL PO daily to TID
  - Gabapentin (Neurontin): 300 mg PO HS; may increase up to 1,800 mg/day PO in divided doses (6)[B]; 1,200 mg/day PO for 3 days and then 400 mg/day PO for 3 days in patients undergoing stroke rehabilitation or in the palliative care setting where chlorpromazine adverse effects are undesirable (6)[B]
  - Combination of lansoprazole 15 mg PO daily, clonazepam 0.5 mg PO BID, and dimenhydrinate 25 mg PO BID
  - Contraindications: Refer to manufacturer's literature.
    - Chlorpromazine is not recommended in elderly patient with dementia.
  - Baclofen is not recommended in patients with stroke or other cerebral lesions or in severe renal impairment. Avoid abrupt withdrawal of baclofen.
- Other possible drug therapies (2)[C],(8)[C]
  - Amantadine, carbidopa and levodopa in Parkinson disease
  - Steroid replacement in Addison disease
  - Antifungal agent in *Candida* esophagitis
  - Ondansetron in carcinomatosis with vomiting
  - Nefopam (a nonopioid analgesic with antishivering properties related to antihistamines and antiparkinsonian drugs) is available outside the United States in both IV and oral formulations.
  - Olanzapine 10 mg QHS
  - Pregabalin 375 mg/day

ISSUES FOR REFERRAL
For acupuncture or phrenic nerve crush, block, or electrostimulation; continuous cervical epidural block; cardioversion

SURGERY/OTHER PROCEDURES
- Phrenic nerve crush or transaction or electrostimulation of the dominant diaphragmatic leaflet
- Resection of rib exostoses

COMPLEMENTARY & ALTERNATIVE MEDICINE
- Acupuncture is increasingly used to manage persistent or intractable hiccups, especially in cancer patients (5)[A],(6)[A].
- Home remedies (2)[C]
  - Swallowing a spoonful of sugar
  - Sucking on hard candy or swallowing peanut butter
  - Holding breath and increasing pressure on diaphragm (Valsalva maneuver)
  - Tongue traction
  - Lifting the uvula with a cold spoon
  - Inducing fright
  - Smelling salts
  - Rebreathing into a paper (not plastic) bag
  - Sipping ice water
  - Rubbing a wet cotton-tipped applicator between hard and soft palate for 1 minute

ADMISSION, INPATIENT, AND NURSING CONSIDERATIONS
Most patients can be managed as outpatients; those with severe intractable hiccups may require rehydration, pain control, IV medications, or surgery.

 ONGOING CARE

FOLLOW-UP RECOMMENDATIONS
Patient Monitoring
Until hiccups cease

DIET
Avoid gastric distension from overeating, carbonated beverages, and aerophagia.

PATIENT EDUCATION
See "General Measures."

PROGNOSIS
- Hiccups often cease during sleep.
- Most acute benign hiccup bouts resolve spontaneously or with home remedies.
- Intractable hiccups may last for years or decades.
- Hiccups have persisted despite bilateral phrenic nerve transection.

COMPLICATIONS
- Inability to eat
- Weight loss
- Exhaustion, debility
- Insomnia
- Cardiac arrhythmias
- Wound dehiscence
- Death (rare)

REFERENCES

1. Witter F, Dipietro J, Costigan K, et al. The relationship between hiccups and heart rate in the fetus. *J Matern Fetal Neonatal Med*. 2007;20(4):289–292.
2. Calsina-Berna A, García-Gómez G, González-Barboteo J, et al. Treatment of chronic hiccups in cancer patients: a systematic review. *J Palliat Med*. 2012;15(10):1142–1150.
3. Brañuelas Quiroga J, Urbano García J, Bolaños Guedes J. Hiccups: a common problem with some unusual causes and cures [published correction appears in *Br J Gen Pract*. 2017;67(654):13]. *Br J Gen Pract*. 2016;66(652):584–586.
4. Hosoya R, Uesawa Y, Ishii-Nozawa R, et al. Analysis of factors associated with hiccups based on the Japanese Adverse Drug Event Report database. *PLoS One*. 2017;12(2):e0172057.
5. Ge AX, Ryan ME, Giaccone G, et al. Acupuncture treatment for persistent hiccups in patients with cancer. *J Altern Complement Med*. 2010;16(7):811–816.
6. Thompson DF, Brooks KG. Gabapentin therapy of hiccups. *Ann Pharmacother*. 2013;47(6):897–903.
7. Steger M, Schneemann M, Fox M. Systemic review: the pathogenesis and pharmacological treatment of hiccups. *Aliment Pharmacol Ther*. 2015;42(9):1037–1050.
8. Moretto EN, Wee B, Wiffen PJ, et al. Interventions for treating persistent and intractable hiccups in adults. *Cochrane Database Syst Rev*. 2013;(1):CD008768.

ADDITIONAL READING

- Chang F-Y, Lu CL. Hiccup: mystery, nature and treatment. *J Neurogastroenterol Motil*. 2012;18(2):123–130.
- Choi T-Y, Lee MS, Ernst E. Acupuncture for cancer patients suffering from hiccups: a systematic review and meta-analysis. *Complement Ther Med*. 2012;20(6):447–455.
- Rizzo C, Vitale C, Montagnini M. Management of intractable hiccups: an illustrative case and review. *Am J Hosp Palliat Care*. 2014;31(2):220–224.

CODES

ICD10
- R06.6 Hiccough
- F45.8 Other somatoform disorders

CLINICAL PEARLS
- Most hiccups resolve spontaneously.
- An organic cause is more likely in men and individuals with intractable hiccups.
- Rule out foreign body in the ear canal as a trigger.
- Baclofen and gabapentin are the only pharmacologic agents proven to be clinically effective.
- Acupuncture may be effective for persistent hiccups.

HIDRADENITIS SUPPURATIVA

Christopher A. Zagar, MD, FAAFP • James T. Chapman, DO

 BASICS

DESCRIPTION
- Chronic inflammatory skin disease manifested as recurrent inflammatory nodules, abscesses, sinus tracts, and complex scar formation
- Areas affected are tender, malodorous, often with exudative drainage.
- Common in intertriginous skin regions: axillae, groin, perianal, perineal, inframammary skin
- System affected: skin, psychosocial
- Synonym(s): acne inversa; Verneuil disease; apocrinitis; hidradenitis axillaris

Geriatric Considerations
Rare after menopause

Pediatric Considerations
Rarely occurs before puberty; occurrence in children is associated with premature adrenarche.

Pregnancy Considerations
No Accutane (isotretinoin) or tetracycline treatment during pregnancy. Disease may ease during pregnancy and rebound after parturition.

EPIDEMIOLOGY
- Predominant sex: female > male (3:1)
  - Adolescents: female > male (3.8:1) (1)
- African Americans

Incidence
Peak onset during 2nd and 3rd decades of life

Prevalence
0.05–4.10% (2)

ETIOLOGY AND PATHOPHYSIOLOGY
- Not fully understood; previously considered a disorder of apocrine glands but more recently thought to be due to a follicular epithelium defect. Deregulation of the local immune system may also play a role.
- Inflammatory disorder of the hair follicle triggered by follicular plugging within apocrine gland–bearing skin
- Hormonally induced ductal keratinocyte proliferation leads to a failure of follicular epithelial shedding, causing follicular occlusion.
- Mechanical stress on skin (intertriginous regions) precipitates follicular rupture and immune response.
- Bacterial involvement is a secondary event.
- Rupture and reepithelialization cause sinus tracts to form.

Genetics
- Familial occurrences suggest single gene transmission (autosomal dominant), but the condition may also be polygenic.
- Estimated 40% of patients have an affected family member.

RISK FACTORS
- Obesity
- Smoking
- Hyperandrogenism
- Lithium may trigger onset of or exacerbate this condition.

GENERAL PREVENTION
- Lose weight if overweight or obese.
- Smoking cessation
- Avoid constrictive clothing/synthetic fabrics, frictional trauma, heat exposure, excessive sweating, shaving, depilation, and deodorants.
- Use of antiseptic soaps

COMMONLY ASSOCIATED CONDITIONS
- Acne vulgaris, acne conglobate
- Perifolliculitis capitis abscedens et suffodiens (dissecting cellulitis of scalp)
- Pilonidal disease
- Metabolic syndrome/obesity
- Polycystic ovary syndrome (PCOS) and androgen dysfunction
- Thyroid disease
- Arthritis and spondyloarthritis (seronegative)
- Inflammatory bowel disease (Crohn disease and ulcerative colitis) (3)
- Squamous cell carcinoma
- PAPASH syndrome (pyogenic arthritis, pyoderma gangrenosum, acne, and suppurative hidradenitis)
- Type 2 diabetes mellitus (4)

 DIAGNOSIS

HISTORY
- Diagnostic criteria adopted by the 2nd International Conference on Hidradenitis Suppurativa, 2009 (5)
- All three criteria (morphology, location, progression) must be present for diagnosis:
  - Typical lesions: painful nodules, abscesses, draining sinus, bridged scars, and "tombstone" double-ended pseudocomedones in secondary lesions
  - Typical topography: axillae, groins, perineal and perianal region, buttocks, infra- and intermammary folds
  - Chronicity and recurrences, commonly refractory to initial treatments

PHYSICAL EXAM
- Tender dome-shaped nodules 0.5 to 3.0 cm in size are present.
  - Location corresponds with the distribution of apocrine-related mammary tissue and terminal hair follicles dependent on low androgen concentrations.
  - Sites ordered by frequency of occurrence: axillary, inguinal, perianal and perineal, mammary and inframammary, buttock, pubic region, chest, scalp, retroauricular, eyelid
  - Large lesions are often fluctuant; comedones may be present.
- Possible malodorous discharge
- Hurley clinical staging system
  - **Stage I**: nodule/abscess formation without sinus tracts or scarring
  - **Stage II**: more than one lesion widely spaced with tract and scar formation
  - **Stage III**: diffuse, multiple interconnected tracts and abscesses with scarring
- Sartorius clinical staging system (points attributed)
  - Anatomic region involved
  - Quantity and quality of lesions
  - Distance between lesions
  - Presence or absence of normal skin between lesions

DIFFERENTIAL DIAGNOSIS
- Acne vulgaris, conglobate
- Furunculosis/carbuncles
- Infected Bartholin or sebaceous cysts
- Lymphadenopathy/lymphadenitis
- Cutaneous Langerhans cell histiocytosis
- Actinomycosis
- Granuloma inguinale
- Lymphogranuloma venereum

- Apocrine nevus
- Crohn disease with anogenital fistula(s) (may coexist with hidradenitis suppurativa)
- Fox-Fordyce disease

DIAGNOSTIC TESTS & INTERPRETATION
Initial Tests (lab, imaging)
- Cultures of skin or aspirates of boils are most commonly negative. When positive, cultures are often polymicrobial and commonly grow *Staphylococcus aureus* and *Staphylococcus epidermidis*.
- Lesion biopsy usually unnecessary; useful to rule out other disorders such as squamous cell carcinoma
- May note increased erythrocyte sedimentation rate (ESR), leukocytosis, decreased serum iron, normocytic anemia, or changes in serum electrophoresis pattern

Follow-Up Tests & Special Considerations
- Consider biopsy of concerning lesions due to increased risk of squamous cell carcinoma.
- If the patient is female, overweight, and/or hirsute, consider evaluating the following:
  - Dehydroepiandrosterone sulfate
  - Testosterone: total and free
  - Sex hormone–binding globulin
  - Progesterone

Diagnostic Procedures/Other
- Incision and drainage, culture and biopsy
- Ultrasound may be useful in planning an excision to identify the full extent of sinus tracts.

Test Interpretation
- Dermis shows granulomatous inflammation and inflammatory cells, giant cells, sinus tracts, subcutaneous abscesses, and extensive fibrosis.
- Hair follicular dilatation and occlusion by keratinized stratified squamous epithelium

 TREATMENT

Despite the prevalence of this condition, most trials have been small and underpowered. Evidence is therefore generally of poor quality (6)[A]. Treatment goals: Reduce extent of disease, prevent new lesions, remove chronic disease, and limit scar formation.

- Conservative treatment includes all items under "General Prevention," plus use of warm compresses, sitz baths, topical antiseptics for inflamed lesions, and nonopioid analgesics.
- Weight loss and smoking cessation result in marked improvement (2).
- Corticosteroids, isotretinoin, and zinc gluconate
- For stages I and II, attempt medical treatment.
- Short medical trial may be appropriate in stage III prior to moving on to surgical therapies.
- Only FDA-approved medication for this condition is adalimumab. Other biologics may be effective. No medications are curative; relapse is almost inevitable, but the disease may be controlled. Usually must fail other treatments before starting biologics. They can be a costly option.

GENERAL MEASURES
- Education and psychosocial support
- Appropriate hygiene including avoidance of shearing stress to skin (light clothing), daily cleansing with antibacterial soap
- Diet: Avoid dairy, high glycemic loads.

- Symptomatic treatment for acute lesions
- Improve environmental factors that cause follicular blockage (see "General Prevention").
- Smoking cessation and weight loss

MEDICATION

First Line

- Stage I disease: Consider either systemic or topical antibiotics.
  - Topical antibiotics (clindamycin was studied in clinical trials) (2)[B]
    - Clindamycin 0.1% solution BID for 12 weeks with or without benzoyl peroxide 5–10% solution
    - Chlorhexidine 4% solution
  - Systemic antibiotics (initial 7- to 10-day course)
    - Tetracycline 500 mg BID
    - Doxycycline 100 mg q12h
    - Augmentin 875 mg q8–12h
    - Clindamycin 300 mg BID (7)[B]
  - Intralesion corticosteroids: limited evidence; possible reduction in pain, erythema, edema, and lesion size (2) (triamcinolone acetonide 10 mg/mL usually 0.2 to 2.0 mL injection)
- Stages II and III disease
  - Address overlying bacterial infection with broad-spectrum coverage. Base antibiotic selection on disease location and characteristics; best evidence for antibiotic treatment with combinations of clindamycin and rifampicin, or ertapenem followed by combination rifampin, moxifloxacin, and metronidazole for 6 months (2)[A]
  - Minor surgical procedures (punch débridement, local unroofing) to treat individual lesions or sinus tracts
- Other modalities (rarely used)
  - Hormonal therapy: antiandrogenic therapy such as cyproterone acetate (may not be available in the United States), estrogen/norgestrel oral contraceptive, finasteride (5 mg daily)

Second Line

- Dapsone 50 to 150 mg daily
- Metformin: significant reduction in Sartorius score
- Spironolactone: significant reduction in amount of lesions and pain (8)
- Oral retinoids (isotretinoin): poor efficacy, limited therapeutic effect
- TNF-α inhibitors:
  - Adalimumab 40 mg weekly (a high dose) produces statistically significant differences versus placebo in treated patients, but clinical effect size is small (Cochrane) (2)[A], and long-term safety is unknown (9)[A].
  - Infliximab: A majority of patients in the treatment group had a 50% or greater decrease in disease, improving quality of life (9)[A].
  - Etanercept: no difference versus placebo

ISSUES FOR REFERRAL

- Lack of response to treatment, stages II and III disease, or concern for malignancy (squamous cell carcinoma) is a reason to refer for surgical excision or radiation/laser treatment (stage II).
- If significant psychosocial stress exists secondary to disease, refer for stress management or psychiatric evaluation.
- Suspicion of hyperandrogenic states (e.g., PCOS) should prompt investigation or referral.
- Severe perianal/perivulvar disease or otherwise very extensive disease may prompt referral to plastic surgeon or reconstructive urologist.

SURGERY/OTHER PROCEDURES

- Important mode of treatment; necessary if wanting to permanently remove tunnels and scarring
- Could be used in conjunction with antibiotics or if first-line therapy fails
- Various surgical approaches have been used for stages II and III disease.
  - Incision and drainage: necessary to treat acute flare-ups when abscess is present
  - Deroofing of sinus tracts and skin tissue–sparing excision with electrosurgical peeling (STEEP) allow for healing by secondary intention. Recurrences remain common but usually are smaller than original lesions.
  - Wide full-thickness excision with healing by granulation or flap placement is the most definitive treatment and rarely has local recurrence if all sinus tracts are excised with a clear 1- to 2-cm margin. Rates of local recurrence (within 3 to 72 months): axillary (3%), perianal (0%), inguino-perineal (37%), submammary (50%)
- Laser therapy for Hurley stages I and II disease (rarely used); no consensus on the benefit
  - Monthly treatments with neodymium-doped yttrium aluminum garnet (Nd:YAG) laser for 3 to 4 months
  - CO_2 laser ablation with healing by secondary intention
- Cryotherapy and photodynamic therapy have shown variable results; they are not routinely recommended.
- Potential role for combined therapy consisting of radical resection plus biologic in advanced cases

 ONGOING CARE

FOLLOW-UP RECOMMENDATIONS

Follow up monthly or sooner to evaluate progress and to assist with symptom management.

DIET

- Avoid dairy and high glycemic loads.
- Healthy diet that promotes weight loss
- May benefit from zinc supplementation

PATIENT EDUCATION

- Severity can range from only two to three papules per year to extensive draining sinus tracts.
- Medications are temporizing measures, rarely curative. Attempts at local surgical "cures" do not affect recurrence at other sites.
- Smoking cessation and weight loss can improve symptoms significantly.
- Hidradenitis Suppurativa Foundation: www.hs-foundation.org

PROGNOSIS

- Individual lesions heal slowly in 10 to 30 days.
- Recurrences may last for several years.
- Relentlessly progressive scarring and sinus tracts are likely with severe disease.
- Radical wide-area excision, with removal of all hair-bearing skin in the affected area, shows the greatest chance for cure.
- Increased all-cause mortality

COMPLICATIONS

- Contracture and stricturing of the skin after extensive abscess rupture, scarring, and healing; or at sites of surgical excisions
- Lymphatic obstruction, lymphedema
- Psychosocial: anxiety, malaise, depression, self-injury

- Anemia, amyloidosis, and hypoproteinemia (due to chronic suppuration)
- Lumbosacral epidural abscess, sacral bacterial osteomyelitis
- Squamous cell carcinoma may develop in indolent sinus tracts.
- Disseminated infection or septicemia (rare)
- Urethral, rectal, or bladder fistula (rare)

REFERENCES

1. Garg A, Wertenteil S, Baltz R, et al. Prevalence estimates for hidradenitis suppurativa among children and adolescents in the United States: a gender- and age-adjusted population analysis. J Invest Dermatol. 2018;138:2152.
2. Saunte D, Jemec G. Hidradenitis suppurativa: advances in diagnosis and treatment. JAMA. 2017;318(20):2019–2032.
3. Chen WT, Chi CC. Association of hidradenitis suppurativa with inflammatory bowel disease: a systematic review and meta-analysis. JAMA Dermatol. 2019;155(9):1022–1027.
4. Garg A, Birabaharan M, Strunk A. Prevalence of type 2 diabetes mellitus among patients with hidradenitis suppurativa in the United States. J Am Acad Dermatol. 2018;79:71.
5. Rambhatla PV, Lim HW, Hamzavi I. A systematic review of treatments for hidradenitis suppurativa. Arch Dermatol. 2012;148(4):439–446.
6. van der Zee HH, Boer J, Prens EP, et al. The effect of combined treatment with oral clindamycin and oral rifampicin in patients with hidradenitis suppurativa. Dermatology. 2009;219(2):143–147.
7. Wang S, Wang S, Sibbald R. Hidradenitis suppurativa: a frequently missed diagnosis, part 1: a review of pathogenesis, associations, and clinical features. Adv Skin Wound Care. 2015;28(7):325–332.
8. Golbari NM, Porter ML, Kimball AB. Antiandrogen therapy with spironolactone for the treatment of hidradenitis suppurativa. J Am Acad Dermatol. 2019;80:114.
9. Falola R, DeFazio M, Anghel E, et al. What heals hidradenitis suppurativa: surgery, immunosuppression, or both? Plast Reconstr Surg. 2016;138(Suppl 3):219S–229S.

CODES

ICD10

L73.2 Hidradenitis suppurativa

CLINICAL PEARLS

- Chronic inflammatory disease of the skin, often difficult to control with behavior changes and medication alone
- First-line treatment for mild disease is topical and/or systemic antibiotics.
- For patients with refractory or severe disease, wide local excision provides the only chance at a cure. Success rates depend on the location and extent of excision.
- This is a difficult to treat disease that can greatly affect the patient's quality of life.

H

HIRSUTISM

Ruchita Patel, DO • Natasha S. Kadakia, DO

BASICS

DESCRIPTION
- Presence of excessive terminal (coarse, pigmented) hair of body and face, in a male pattern
- May be present in normal adults as an ethnic characteristic or may develop as a result of androgen excess
- Often seen in polycystic ovary syndrome (PCOS), which is characterized by hirsutism, acne, menstrual irregularities, and obesity
- System(s) affected: dermatologic, endocrine, metabolic, reproductive

EPIDEMIOLOGY
Prevalence
5–10% of reproductive age women

ETIOLOGY AND PATHOPHYSIOLOGY
- Due to increased androgenic (male) hormones, either from increased peripheral binding (idiopathic) or increased production from the ovaries, adrenals, or body fat
- Exogenous medications
- Can be a symptom of multiple etiologies such as clinical evidence of PCOS, androgen-secreting tumors, virilizing disorders, or androgenic medication use

Genetics
Multifactorial

RISK FACTORS
- Family history/ethnicity (e.g., Ashkenazi Jews and Mediterranean backgrounds)
- Obesity

GENERAL PREVENTION
Women with late-onset congenital adrenal hyperplasia (CAH) should be counseled that they may be carriers for the severe early-onset childhood disease.

COMMONLY ASSOCIATED CONDITIONS
- PCOS: the most common cause of premenopausal hirsutism (1)
- Insulin resistance, common
- Prolonged amenorrhea and anovulation, common
- Emotional distress and depression, common
- Acne, common
- Central obesity
- Hypothyroidism/hyperthyroidism, rare
- Hyperprolactinemia, rare
- Risk for endometrial hyperplasia or carcinoma, rare
- Virilization (rapid onset, clitoromegaly, balding, deepening voice) (2)
- Cushing syndrome: characterized by moon facies, striae, hypertension, rare
- Acromegaly, rare
- Vitamin D deficiency

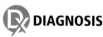

DIAGNOSIS

HISTORY
- Severity, time course, and age of onset of hirsutism
- Weight
- Psychosocial impact on patient

- Menstrual and fertility history, anovulation (defined as ovulatory cycle >35 days)
- Severe acne, especially if treatment resistant
- Presence of virilization
- Medication history: Look for use of valproic acid, testosterone, danazol, glucocorticoids, topical androgen use by partner, and athletic performance drugs.
- The presence of galactorrhea

PHYSICAL EXAM
- Increased hair growth in premenopausal women, particularly over the chin, neck, sideburns, lower back, sternum, abdomen, shoulders, buttocks, perineal area, and inner thighs
- Check skin for acne, striae, acanthosis nigricans (velvety black skin in the axillae or neck).
- Virilization: deep voice, male pattern balding, increased muscle mass, and clitoromegaly indicate risk of tumor
- The Ferriman-Gallwey scale (an instrument that rates hair growth in nine areas on a scale of 0 to 4, with >8 being positive) may be used for diagnosis but underrates patient's perception of hirsutism and altered by previous cosmetic treatment. Scores between 8 and 15 are considered to be mild hirsutism, 16 to 25 moderate, and >25 severe (1),(2).

DIFFERENTIAL DIAGNOSIS
- PCOS (72–82%)—irregular menses, elevated androgens, polycystic ovaries on US, infertility, insulin resistance
- Idiopathic hyperandrogenemia (6–15%)—hirsutism with normal ovaries on US, elevated androgen levels, no other explainable cause
- Idiopathic hirsutism (4–7%)—hirsutism with normal menses, androgen levels, and ovaries on ultrasonography, no other explainable cause
- Late-onset CAH (2–4%), a genetic enzyme deficiency associated with more severe and earlier-onset hirsutism in amenorrheic patients, presents in adolescence with severe hirsutism and irregular menses.
- Androgen-secreting tumor (0.2%)—ovaries (benign or malignant) or adrenals (commonly malignant); have rapid onset, virilization, resistance to treatment
- Ovarian hyperthecosis—increase in testosterone by theca cells. Gradual onset of hirsutism, frank virilization; mostly affects postmenopausal women
- Thyroid dysfunction
- Hyperprolactinemia if accompanied by galactorrhea or amenorrhea
- Rare endocrine disorders—Cushing, acromegaly

DIAGNOSTIC TESTS & INTERPRETATION
- Assess androgen levels in all women with an abnormal hirsutism score. Guidelines recommend screening hyperandrogenemic women for NCCAH due to 21-hydroxylase deficiency by measuring early morning 17-hydroxyprogesterone levels (2).
- PCOS diagnosed with two out of three signs: menstrual dysfunction, clinical or biochemical hyperandrogenemia, polycystic ovaries on US (2)[C]
- Lab testing is to rule out underlying tumor and pituitary diseases (rare).

Initial Tests (lab, imaging)
- Basic workup of moderate hirsutism is a total testosterone level +/− thyroid screen (TSH) (1)[C].
- Testosterone: Random total testosterone level is usually sufficient.

- Normal upper limit for serum total testosterone in adult women is approximately 40 to 60 ng/dL (1.4 to 2.1 nmol/L). Patients who have clinical features consistent with PCOS but have normal total testosterone should have repeat testing, preferably an early morning serum free testosterone level calculated from sex hormone—binding globulin (SHBG). A morning free testosterone is 50% more sensitive (1),(3).
- If testosterone is >150 (some use 200) ng/dL, consider ovarian or adrenal tumor (2),(4). Testosterone is made by both the ovaries and adrenals, so both areas should be imaged. US is best for the ovaries, and CT is best for the adrenals.
- The workup for PCOS recommended by the American College of Obstetricians and Gynecologists (ACOG) includes the above plus:
  - Screening for metabolic syndrome with a fasting and 2-hour glucose after 75-g glucose load, lipid panel, waist circumference, and blood pressure (4)[C]
- Ovarian US to look for polycystic ovaries
- If the patient is amenorrheic, check prolactin, FSH, LH, TSH, and a pregnancy test (5)[C]. An LH/FSH ratio >2 indicates PCOS.

Follow-Up Tests & Special Considerations
- 17α-Hydroxyprogesterone (17α-OHP)
  - Elevations of 17α-OHP (>300) can indicate late-onset CAH.
  - Consider in patients with onset in early adolescence or high-risk group (Ashkenazi Jews) (2)[C].
  - If elevated, order corticotropin stimulation test.
- If prolactin level is high, MRI the pituitary
- If PCOS is diagnosed, ACOG recommends screening for dyslipidemia and DM type 2 (4)[C].
- New studies show an inverse correlation between vitamin D levels and insulin resistance in women with PCOS. Screening women who are at risk for vitamin D deficiency and supplementation with vitamin D could be considered (6)[B].
- Suggests against testing for elevated androgen levels in eumenorrheic women with unwanted local hair growth
- Dehydroepiandrosterone sulfate (DHEA-S) should be checked in virilization (5)[C].
  - Levels >700 may indicate adrenal tumor.

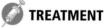

TREATMENT

GENERAL MEASURES
- Treatment depends on patient preference and psychosocial effect.
- Treatment goal is to decrease new hair growth and improve metabolic disorders.
- If patient desires pregnancy, induction of ovulation may be necessary.
- Provide contraception, as needed.
- A calorie-restricted diet is recommended in all overweight patients with PCOS. Weight loss has positive effects on fertility, metabolic profile, and may improve hirsutism (5).
- Treat accompanying acne.

MEDICATION

First Line

- Direct hair removal or pharmacologic therapy recommended for mild hirsutism (2)[B]
- Oral contraceptives are first line to manage menstrual abnormalities and hirsutism/acne (3)[A]; they will suppress ovarian androgen production and increase SHBG, improve metabolic syndrome, and slow but not reverse hair growth.
  - Doses of 20 to 35 μg ethinyl estradiol effectively decrease ovarian androgen production. Those containing the progestins, norgestimate, desogestrel, or drospirenone have more androgen-blocking effects, but desogestrel and drospirenone are associated with more DVTs especially in severely obese patients (3),(4)[C].
  - They take 6 months to show effect and are continued for years.
  - Oral preparations, compared to vaginal or transdermal, are better at controlling hirsutism and acne; by passing through the liver, they induce SHBG production (1).
  - For patients with high risk for VTE, it is recommended to use the lowest dose of an ethinyl estradiol–based oral contraceptive and a low-risk, progesterone-based oral contraceptive (2).
- Progesterone (depot or intermittent oral) can be used if estrogens are contraindicated (4).
- Eflornithine (Vaniqa) HCl cream: Apply BID at least 8 hours apart; reduces facial hair in 40% of women (must be used indefinitely to prevent regrowth); only FDA-approved hirsutism treatment
- Laser therapy with eflornithine cream shown to have a more rapid response.
- Combination oral contraceptives and antiandrogen is contraindicated first line unless those with severe hirsutism and significant emotional distress or no success with oral contraceptives alone (failure of therapy after 6 months) (2)[B].

Second Line

- Antiandrogenic drugs will further reduce hirsutism to 15–25%. Usually begun 6 months after first-line therapy if results are suboptimal. Must be used in combination with oral contraceptives to prevent menorrhagia and potential fetal toxicity. All should be avoided in pregnancy (2),(5)[C].
  - Spironolactone, 50 to 200 mg/day: Onset of action is slow; use with oral contraceptives to prevent menorrhagia. Watch for hyperkalemia, especially with drospirenone-containing OCP (Yasmin); avoid use in pregnancy (7)[B].
  - Finasteride: 5 mg/day decreases androgen binding; not approved by FDA. Use with contraception (pregnancy Category X).
  - Cyproterone, not available in the United States: 12.5 to 100.0 mg/day for days 5 to 15 of cycle combined with ethinyl estradiol 20 to 50 μg for days 5 to 25 of cycle
  - Flutamide is not recommended due to potential hepatotoxicity (2)[C].
  - Topical antiandrogen therapy is not recommended.

- It is suggested against using insulin-lowering drugs as the sole indication of treating hirsutism (2).
- Steroids: used in late-onset CAH
  - Dexamethasone: 2 mg/day
- Cosmetic treatment: includes many methods of hair removal
  - Temporary: shaving, chemical depilation, plucking, waxing
  - Permanent: Laser epilation and photoepilation are preferred to electrolysis (4)[C].
  - For direct hair removal, electrolysis rather than photoepilation is recommended in women with blonde or white hair (6).
  - Pharmacologic therapy is suggested to minimize regrowth.

Pregnancy Considerations

- May have related infertility
- As hormone balance improves, fertility may increase; provide contraception, as needed.
- Several medications used for treatment are contraindicated in pregnancy.

COMPLEMENTARY & ALTERNATIVE MEDICINE

Several herbals including spearmint tea, saw palmetto, licorice, fennel, and soy have been shown in small (<50 people) and short (<12 weeks) studies to decrease hair size or lower androgen levels (5)[C].

 ONGOING CARE

FOLLOW-UP RECOMMENDATIONS

Patient Monitoring

Monitor for known side effects of medications.

DIET

Diet consisting of low-calorie, low-glycemic index foods improve fertility in obese PCOS patients with anovulatory infertility.

PATIENT EDUCATION

- Hormonal treatment stops further hair growth and will improve but not reverse present hair.
  - Treatment takes 6 months to take effect and may need to be lifelong.
- Cosmetic measures may be needed for the already present hair.

PROGNOSIS

- Good (with long-term therapy) for halting further hair growth
- Moderate to poor for reversing current hair growth

COMPLICATIONS

- If PCOS is present, dysfunctional uterine bleeding may lead to anemia.
- If PCOS is present, anovulation may increase endometrial hyperplasia and uterine cancer risk.
- Androgenic excess may adversely affect lipid status, cardiac risk, and bone density.

REFERENCES

1. Azziz R, Carmina E, Dewailly D, et al; for Task Force on the Phenotype of the Polycystic Ovary Syndrome of the Androgen Excess and PCOS Society. The Androgen Excess and PCOS Society criteria for the polycystic ovary syndrome: the complete task force report. *Fertil Steril*. 2009;91(2):456–488.
2. Martin KA, Anderson RR, Chang RJ, et al. Evaluation and treatment of hirsutism in premenopausal women: an Endocrine Society clinical practice guideline. *J Clin Endocrinol Metab*. 2018;103(4):1233–1257.
3. Goodman NF, Cobin RH, Futterweit W, et al; for American Association of Clinical Endocrinologists, American College of Endocrinology, Androgen Excess and PCOS Society. American Association of Clinical Endocrinologists, American College of Endocrinology, and Androgen Excess and PCOS Society disease state clinical review: guide to the best practices in the evaluation and treatment of polycystic ovary syndrome—part 1. *Endocr Pract*. 2015;21(11):1291–1300.
4. Rosenfield RL. Clinical practice. Hirsutism. *N Engl J Med*. 2005;353(24):2578–2588.
5. Williams T, Mortada R, Porter S. Diagnosis and treatment of polycystic ovary syndrome. *Am Fam Physician*. 2016;94(2):106–113.
6. Krul-Poel YHM, Snackey C, Louwers Y, et al. The role of vitamin D in metabolic disturbances in polycystic ovary syndrome: a systematic review. *Eur J Endocrinol*. 2013;169(6):853–865.
7. Brown J, Farquhar C, Lee O, et al. Spironolactone versus placebo or in combination with steroids for hirsutism and/or acne. *Cochrane Database Syst Rev*. 2009;(2):CD000194.

 SEE ALSO

Acne Vulgaris; Infertility; Polycystic Ovarian Syndrome (PCOS)

CODES

ICD10

- L68.0 Hirsutism
- E28.2 Polycystic ovarian syndrome

CLINICAL PEARLS

- PCOS is the most common cause of hirsutism (diagnosed with two out of three: menstrual dysfunction, clinical or biochemical hyperandrogenemia, polycystic ovaries on US).
- Diagnosis is based on androgen level in all women with abnormal hirsutism score; total testosterone and TSH for initial testing
- Virilization (clitoromegaly, balding, deepening voice): Suspect if testosterone >150 ng/dL; look for adrenal and ovarian tumor.
- Lifestyle modification and OCPs are first-line therapy for hirsutism, menstrual irregularities, and acne.

H

HIV/AIDS

Pamela R. Hughes, MD • Kyler M. Douglas, DO

 BASICS

DESCRIPTION
- HIV is a retrovirus (subgroup lentivirus) that integrates into CD4 T lymphocytes, altering cell-mediated immunity and causing cell death, severe immunodeficiency, opportunistic infections, and malignancies if not treated.
- The natural history of untreated HIV infection includes viral transmission, acute retroviral syndrome, recovery and seroconversion, asymptomatic chronic HIV infection, and symptomatic HIV infection or AIDS.
- Without treatment, the average patient progresses to AIDS ~10 years after acquiring HIV.
- HIV-infected persons with CD4 <200 cells/mm^3 or with AIDS-defining illnesses are categorized as persons living with AIDS.

EPIDEMIOLOGY
Incidence
United States ~37,000 new cases in 2019, a decrease in incidence of 9% between 2015 and 2019. There were approximately 1.7 million new cases of HIV worldwide in 2018 (1).

Prevalence
- ~1.2 million persons in the United States have HIV, ~13% are not aware they are infected (1).
- ~38 million people are living with HIV worldwide. ~43% of new diagnoses are in sub-Saharan Africa (1).
- In 2019, 690,000 people died from AIDS-related illnesses (1).

ETIOLOGY AND PATHOPHYSIOLOGY
- HIV primarily infects CD4+ cells. HIV is a single-stranded, positive-sense, enveloped RNA virus. After entering target cells, viral RNA is transcribed to DNA (through reverse transcription), imported to the host cell nucleus and incorporated into host DNA. The virus can become latent or produce new viral RNA with proteins that are released to infect other CD4+ cells. Host CD8+ cells are activated as part of the seroconversion response.
- There are two types of HIV. HIV-1 causes the majority of HIV infections. HIV-2 is less infectious and seen primarily in West Africa.

RISK FACTORS
- Sexual activity (>90% of transmission): Receptive anal sex is highest risk. Ulcerative urogenital lesions promote transmission (1).
- Injection drug use
- Children of HIV-infected women: Maternal HIV-1 RNA level predicts transmission.
  - HIV can also be transmitted in breast milk. HIV+ women should not breastfeed unless there is no alternative. In this case, consider antiretroviral therapy (ART) (2).
- Recipients of blood products prior to 1985
- Occupational exposure (health care workers)

GENERAL PREVENTION
- Avoid unprotected, high-risk sex, and injection drug use, especially shared needles.
- Preexposure prophylaxis (PrEP) is recommended by WHO and USPSTF for persons at high risk of acquiring HIV.
  - General guidelines for PrEP: (i) exclude acute or chronic HIV infection before initiating therapy, (ii) repeat HIV testing every 3 months during therapy, (iii) renal and liver function testing at baseline, 2 to 8 weeks after initiating PrEP, and every 6 months.
- Postexposure prophylaxis (PEP) should be started within 72 hours of exposure and continued for 28 days with a three-drug regimen (3)[A].
- For HIV+ patients using ART, maintaining HIV RNA levels <200 copies/mL prevents risk of transmission to sexual partners (treatment as prevention) (4)[A].
- CDC and USPSTF recommend screening for HIV at least once in patients ages 15 to 65.
- At least annual screening is recommended for patients at higher risk (4).

COMMONLY ASSOCIATED CONDITIONS
- Syphilis is more aggressive in HIV-infected persons.
- Tuberculosis (TB) is coepidemic with HIV; test all patients for TB. Dually infected patients (TB and HIV) have 100 times greater risk of developing active TB.
- Patients coinfected with hepatitis B or C have a more rapid progression to cirrhosis.
- Increased risk for cervical cancer, lymphoma, and skin malignancies

DIAGNOSIS

- Acute retroviral syndrome: CD4 lymphocyte count declines with increase in viral load 1 to 4 weeks after transmission; confirmed by high-HIV RNA in the absence of HIV antibody
- Acute retroviral syndrome presents as a mononucleosis-like syndrome: fever, adenopathy, pharyngitis, rash, myalgias/arthralgias.
- Clinical latency (asymptomatic): variable duration (average is 8 to 10 years) accompanied by a gradual decline in CD4 cell counts and relatively stable HIV RNA levels (the viral "set point"). Patients often develop persistent generalized lymphadenopathy and may develop fever, weight loss, myalgias, and gastrointestinal problems if unrecognized.
- AIDS: defined by a CD4 cell count <200, a CD4 cell percentage of total lymphocytes <14%, or an AIDS-related opportunistic infection: *Pneumocystis jiroveci* (*carinii*) pneumonia, cryptococcal meningitis, recurrent bacterial pneumonia, Candida esophagitis, CNS toxoplasmosis, TB, non-Hodgkin lymphoma (NHL), progressive multifocal encephalopathy, HIV nephropathy, Kaposi sarcoma, Hodgkin lymphoma, and invasive cervical cancer
- Advanced HIV disease: CD4 cell count <50. Most AIDS-related deaths occur at this time.

HISTORY
- Complete medical history, including risk exposures, sexual, social and occupational histories, injection drug use, receipt of blood products (prior to 1985), prior use of PrEP or PEP, and medications
- Comprehensive review of systems
- Review immunizations record.

PHYSICAL EXAM
- No physical examination findings are specific to HIV.
- Focus on weight (weight loss is common), skin, retinal exam, oropharynx, lymph nodes (generalized lymphadenopathy is common), lung, liver, spleen, mental status, neurologic, genital, and rectal examinations.

DIFFERENTIAL DIAGNOSIS
Burkitt lymphoma, candidiasis, CMV, coccidioidomycosis, Cryptococcus, EBV, herpes simplex, influenza, lymphoma, mononucleosis, TB, toxoplasmosis

DIAGNOSTIC TESTS & INTERPRETATION
Initial Tests (lab, imaging)
- 4th-generation HIV testing combines antibody/antigen immunoassay for HIV-1/HIV-2 (4)[A].
  - Can be positive within 2 to 3 weeks of exposure
  - Considered a confirmatory test, Western blot confirmation no longer recommended
- Obtain HIV RNA if acute HIV infection is suspected using quantitative PCR; detects infection within 12 days of exposure
- CD4 cell count and percentage (4)[A]
- Plasma HIV RNA viral load (4)[A]
- CBC with differential, lipid levels, fasting blood glucose, creatinine (Cr), blood urea nitrogen (BUN), chemistry, transaminase levels, total bilirubin
- Screen for hepatitis A/B/C and STIs (chlamydia, gonorrhea, syphilis).
- Cervical cytology
- PPD or interferon-γ release assay (IGRA) to screen for latent TB infection; chest x-ray (CXR) if pulmonary symptoms or positive PPD
- HLAB*5701 testing if abacavir planned for treatment (4)[A]
- Genotypic tests for resistance to antiretrovirals for patients with pretreatment HIV RNA level <1,000 copies/mL; transmitted resistance to at least one drug seen in 6–16% of patients (4)[A]

Follow-Up Tests & Special Considerations
PEP
- Nonoccupational PEP (nPEP) is recommended if care sought within 72 hours of possible exposure and substantial risk of exposure (3)[A]:
  - Source known to be HIV+, exposure to blood, semen, vaginal or rectal secretions, breast milk
- 28 days of a three-drug regimen should be started if nPEP indicated (3)[A].
  - Tenofovir disoproxil fumarate 300 mg + emtricitabine 200 mg daily plus:
    - Raltegravir 400 mg BID OR dolutegravir 50 mg daily
- Counsel patients with more than one course of nPEP on prevention and consider PrEP (3)[A].
- For nPEP: complete HIV, hepatitis B, and hepatitis C testing at baseline, 4 to 6 weeks, 3 months, and 6 months after exposure (3)[A].
- For persons exposed via sexual contact: Obtain syphilis serology, gonorrhea, chlamydia, and pregnancy tests at time of presentation and 4 to 6 weeks after exposure; syphilis serology 6 months postexposure (3)[A]

TREATMENT

- Initiate ART in eligible patients. Select/change regimens based on resistance testing.
- Consider dosing frequency, pill burden, adverse toxic effect profiles, comorbidities, and drug interactions.
- Pregnancy, AIDS-defining conditions, acute opportunistic infections, CD4 count <200, HIV-associated nephropathy, acute/early infection, hepatitis B or C coinfection, rapidly declining CD4 counts (>100 cells/mm³ per year), and high viral loads (>100,000 copies/mL) increase urgency for immediate therapy (4)[A].

GENERAL MEASURES
- The goal of ART is to reduce viral load (below limits of detection; HIV RNA <200) and delay immune suppression. Viral load is the most important indicator of response to ART.
- Genotypic testing is recommended to guide therapy in patients who are naive to ART.
- Assess drug resistance before starting ART (4).
- Assess substance abuse, economic factors (unstable housing, food insecurity), social support, mental illness, comorbidities, and high-risk behaviors.
- In women of childbearing age, use ART regimen that decreases viral load with minimal teratogenicity (2)[A].
- Prophylactic antimicrobials and vaccines:
  - *P. jiroveci* prophylaxis: trimethoprim/sulfamethoxazole (TMP-SMX) if CD4 <200 cells/mm³, prior *P. jiroveci*, thrush, or unexplained fever for >2 weeks
  - *Mycobacterium tuberculosis*: Treat for latent TB if positive PPD or positive IGRA if no prior prophylaxis or treatment, negative CXR, no recent TB contact, and no history of inadequately treated TB.
  - *Toxoplasma gondii* prophylaxis: 33% per year risk of infection in untreated patients with CD4 <100 cells/mm³; prophylaxis: TMP-SMX 1 DS tab daily
  - *Mycobacterium avium* complex prophylaxis: 20–40% risk with CD4 <50 and no ART. Azithromycin 1,200 mg PO weekly is preferred.
  - *Streptococcus pneumoniae*: 50 to 100 times increased risk of invasive infection compared with general population; pneumococcal conjugate vaccine (Prevnar) and pneumococcal vaccine polyvalent (Pneumovax 23) at least 8 weeks apart, repeat every 5 years.
  - Influenza vaccine annually (no live vaccine), hepatitis A and B vaccines, human papilloma virus vaccine, at least three Tdap vaccines in lifetime and Td vaccination every 10 years

MEDICATION
First Line
- Recommended regimens for most people with HIV (4)[A]
  - Integrase strand transfer inhibitor plus two nucleoside reverse transcriptase inhibitors:
    - Bictegravir/tenofovir alafenamide/emtricitabine (50 mg/25 mg/200 mg PO daily)
    - Dolutegravir/abacavir/lamivudine (50 mg/600 mg/300 mg PO daily)—only for patients who are HLA-B*5701 negative
    - Dolutegravir (50 mg PO daily) plus, tenofovir disoproxil fumarate (300 mg PO daily) or tenofovir alafenamide (25 mg PO daily), plus emtricitabine (200 mg PO daily) or lamivudine (300 mg PO daily) (right parenthesis)

- Integrase strand transfer inhibitor plus one nucleoside reverse transcriptase inhibitors
  - Dolutegravir/lamivudine (50 mg/300 mg PO daily) except if HIV RNA >500,000, hepatitis B coinfection or genotypic resistance testing results not available
  - Dolutegravir is the preferred treatment for women who are pregnant or trying to conceive (4)[A].
- Tenofovir/emtricitabine (Truvada) 300 mg/200 mg PO daily is FDA approved for PrEP in adults at high risk (3)[A].

 ONGOING CARE

FOLLOW-UP RECOMMENDATIONS
Patient Monitoring
- Monitor HIV RNA viral load 2 to 8 weeks after starting therapy; if detectable, repeat testing every 4 to 8 weeks until viral load is suppressed to <200 copies/mL. Then, repeat testing every 3 to 6 months (4).
  - A 3-fold decrease in HIV RNA viral load is considered a significant response.
- Monitor HIV RNA viral load, CD4, and CBC every 3 to 4 months for first 2 years of ART or if the CD4 count is <300 cells/mm³ (4).
- Confirm CD4 count level has increased 50 to 150 cells/mm³ within the 1st year of ART.
- HIV RNA monitoring can be spaced to every 6 months in patients adherent to ART with consistently suppressed viral load and immunologically stable for >2 years (4).
- Monitor CBC with every CD4 count (4).
- Space CD4 monitoring to 12 months if suppressed viral load and CD4 >300 cells/mm³ (4).
- Once viral load has been suppressed consistently for >2 years and CD4 cell counts are consistently >500/μL, monitoring CD4 cell counts is optional unless virologic failure occurs (or there are intercurrent immunosuppressive treatments or conditions).
- Annual fasting lipids and fasting glucose if normal at baseline (4)
- Basic metabolic panel, AST/ALT, total/direct bilirubin every 6 months (4)
- Annual cervical cytology (regardless of age) until three negative screens and then every 3 years (4)
- Urinalysis every 6 to 12 months or as indicated (4)
- β-hCG in women of childbearing age (4)

DIET
- Encourage good nutrition; avoid raw eggs and unpasteurized dairy products.
- Discuss unknown and potentially harmful effects of supplement use including drug–drug interactions.

PATIENT EDUCATION
Provide nonjudgmental, sex-positive prevention counseling, reviewing high-risk behaviors and viral transmission.

PROGNOSIS
- Untreated HIV infection leading to the diagnosis of AIDS has an associated life expectancy of about 3 years. If the patient has an opportunistic infection, the life expectancy is about 1 year.
- AIDS-defining opportunistic infections usually do not develop until CD4 <200.
- Adherence failure—not drug resistance—is the most common cause of treatment failure.

COMPLICATIONS
- Immunodeficiency and opportunistic infections
- Lymphoma, cervical, or anal cancer

REFERENCES

1. Centers for Disease Control and Prevention. Statistics overview. https://www.cdc.gov/hiv/statistics/overview/index.html. Accessed December 7, 2021.
2. Panel on Treatment of Pregnant Women with HIV Infection and Prevention of Perinatal Transmission. Recommendations for the use of antiretroviral drugs in pregnant women with HIV infection and interventions to reduce perinatal HIV transmission in the United States. https://clinicalinfo.hiv.gov/en/guidelines/perinatal/whats-new-guidelines. Updated February 10, 2021. Accessed October 16, 2021.
3. Centers for Disease Control and Prevention. Updated guidelines for antiretroviral postexposure prophylaxis after sexual, injection drug use, or other nonoccupational exposure to HIV—United States, 2016. https://stacks.cdc.gov/view/cdc/38856. Updated May 23, 2018. Accessed October 16, 2021.
4. Panel on Antiretroviral Guidelines for Adults and Adolescents. Guidelines for the use of antiretroviral agents in adults and adolescents living with HIV. https://clinicalinfo.hiv.gov/sites/default/files/guidelines/documents/AdultandAdolescentGL.pdf. Updated August 16, 2021. Accessed October 16, 2021.

ADDITIONAL READING
Kim J, Vasan S, Kim JH, et al. Current approaches to HIV vaccine development: a narrative review. *J Int AIDS Soc.* 2021;24(Suppl 7):e25793.

H

CODES

ICD10
- Z21 Asymptomatic human immunodeficiency virus infection status
- B20 Human immunodeficiency virus [HIV] disease
- R75 Inconclusive laboratory evidence of human immunodef virus

CLINICAL PEARLS
- Acute HIV seroconversion illness mimics mononucleosis and is characterized by fever, sore throat, adenopathy, myalgias, and rash.
- Transmitted drug resistance is increasing. Evaluate for resistance prior to initiating ART.
- Provide necessary vaccinations and prophylactic antibiotics to HIV+ patients based on clinical history and CD4 count.
- Discuss prevention strategies, including PrEP, with individuals who are at high risk of HIV infection.
- Routine screening for HIV should be completed in adults and adolescents.
- Consider HIV testing in at-risk patients reporting unintended weight loss, fatigue, night sweats, or rash.

HODGKIN LYMPHOMA

Prarthna V. Bhardwaj, MBBS

BASICS

Hodgkin lymphoma (HL) is a neoplasm of the lymphatic system representing one of the common cancers in young adults; characterized by a low number of malignant cells deriving from B lymphocytes and an extensive inflammatory microenvironment

DESCRIPTION
- Historical background:
  - Described first in 1832 by Thomas Hodgkin about a series of six patients with clinical findings different from those with tuberculosis, syphilis, and inflammation
  - German pathologist Carl Sternberg (1898) and American pathologist Dorothy Reed (1902) independently provided accounts of the giant "Reed-Sternberg" (RS) cells—the microscopic hallmarks of Hodgkin lymphoma.
  - Initially treated with herbs, surgery, and arsenic in the 19th century; noted to shrink upon exposure to x-rays in the beginning of the 20th century
  - Chemotherapy instituted as first-line treatment in the early 1970s with the introduction of two different regimen—MOPP (mechlorethamine, vincristine [Oncovin], procarbazine, prednisone) and ABVD (doxorubicin [Adriamycin], bleomycin, vinblastine, and dacarbazine); noted to have 80–90% remission rates
- Subtypes:
  - Two subtypes:
    - Classical Hodgkin lymphoma (cHL)—95% of cases; includes nodular sclerosing, mixed cellularity, lymphocyte rich, and lymphocyte depleted
    - Nodular lymphocyte predominant Hodgkin lymphoma (NLPHL)—5% of cases

EPIDEMIOLOGY
- Incidence: 2 to 3 per 100,000 per year
- Predominance: 11% of all lymphoid malignancies
- Has a bimodal age distribution—between 20 and 40 years and a second peak at around 55 years; typically diagnosed at age 20 to 34 years with median age 39 years at diagnosis given decreasing bimodal age distribution
- 1.3:1 male-to-female ratio

ETIOLOGY AND PATHOPHYSIOLOGY
- cHL is a B-cell lymphoma of germinal center origin that has lost its B-cell phenotype.
- RS cells harbor clonal rearrangements of hypermutated, class-switched immunoglobulin genes resulting in nonfunctional immunoglobulin genes lacking the expression of the cell surface B-cell receptor. In a healthy B cell, this should lead to apoptosis; however, in HL, these cells appear to be "rescued" from apoptosis by additional oncogenic events.
- NLPHL lacks typical RS cells but has lymphocytic and histiocytic cells, characterized by larger cells with folded multilobulated nuclei ("popcorn cells" or LP cells)—show a nucleus with multiple nucleoli that are basophilic and smaller than RS cells.
- Genome-wide association studies identified 19p13.3 at intron 2 of *TCF3*.

Genetics
- First-degree relative: 3 to 9 times risk
- Siblings of younger patients: 7 times risk
- Weak correlation between familial HL and HLA class I regions containing HLA-A1, HLA-B5, HLA-B8, HLA-B18 alleles

RISK FACTORS
- HIV: increased risk of HL in patients who are HIV positive
- Epstein-Barr virus (EBV): detected in nearly 45% patients with HL
- Genetic predisposition: significantly increased risk in identical twins indicating role of genetics in HL

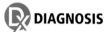

DIAGNOSIS

HISTORY
- Painless lymphadenopathy (cervical/supraclavicular)
- Pel-Ebstein (cyclic) fever—high-grade fever every 7 to 10 days
- Constitutional symptoms or "B symptoms": drenching night sweats, profound weight loss, fatigue, anorexia
- Chronic pruritus may be encountered.
- If mediastinal lymphadenopathy large, can cause chest pain and shortness of breath
- Can present with a mass on chest radiograph

PHYSICAL EXAM
- Lymphadenopathy 70% (cervical > supraclavicular > axillary)—firm, rubbery consistency
- Splenomegaly may be present.
- Hepatomegaly may be present.
- Tonsillar enlargement may be present.

DIFFERENTIAL DIAGNOSIS
Non-HL, infections like HIV, syphilis, tuberculosis, solid tumor metastases, sarcoidosis, autoimmune disease, drug reaction

DIAGNOSTIC TESTS & INTERPRETATION
Initial Tests (lab, imaging)
- CBC with differential—may be associated with eosinophilia
- Comprehensive metabolic panel
- LFT, LDH
- ESR
- HIV, EBV, HCV
- Pregnancy test for women of childbearing age
- Echocardiogram—in anticipation of treatment with anthracycline
- Pulmonary function tests (PFTs)—DLCO measurement in anticipation of treatment with bleomycin
- Chest x-ray
- Computed tomography (CT) with contrast of chest, abdomen, and pelvis
- Positron emission tomography (PET): for initial staging, midtreatment decision-making, and end-of-treatment evaluation

Follow-Up Tests & Special Considerations
- Fertility considerations:
  - Semen cryopreservation if chemotherapy or pelvic radiation therapy (RT)
  - In vitro fertilization or ovarian tissue/oocyte cryopreservation
- RT considerations:
  - Splenic RT: pneumococcal, *Haemophilus influenzae*, meningococcal vaccine

Geriatric Considerations
Advise careful selection of treatment as poorer prognosis if present at ≥60 years:
- Less likely to tolerate intensive chemotherapy
- Less likely to be included in clinical trial

Pediatric Considerations
Young females (<30 years of age) treated with thoracic radiation are at high risk for breast cancer, and early breast cancer screening is recommended.

Pregnancy Considerations
Abdominal ultrasonography to detect subdiaphragmatic disease
- Treatment:
  - Delay until after delivery if asymptomatic and early stage.
  - ABVD more likely to cause fetal malformations in first trimester; malformation risk is lower when used in 2nd and 3rd trimesters.
  - Vinblastine monotherapy to control symptoms

Diagnostic Procedures/Other
- Excisional/incisional lymph node biopsy
- Immunohistochemistry
- Bone marrow biopsy if cytopenia with negative PET
- Lumbar puncture and MRI of the brain if neurologic symptoms

Test Interpretation
- Morphology: RS cells in cHL described as "owl eye" appearance—two nucleoli in two separate nuclear lobes, abundant slightly basophilic cytoplasm; popcorn cells noted in NLPHL
- Immunophenotype: CD15+, CD30+, CD45−, CD3− (T-cell marker), and typically CD20−
- Cytogenetics: no consistent or specific karyotypic findings

TREATMENT
- Ann Arbor staging with Cotswold modification
  - Stage I: single lymph node or of a single extralymphatic organ or site
  - Stage II: ≥2 lymph node regions on the same side of diaphragm alone or with involvement of extralymphatic organ or tissue
  - Stage III: node groups on both sides of the diaphragm

– Stage IV: dissemination involving extranodal organs (except the spleen, which is considered lymphoid tissue)

– Subclasses: A = no systemic symptoms; B = systemic symptoms (fever, night sweats, weight loss >10% body weight); X = bulky disease (>1/3 intrathoracic, diameter, or >10-cm nodal mass)

- Intent of treatment: curative
- All subsequent treatment and follow-up care recommendations based on National Comprehensive Cancer Network (NCCN) consensus. Please refer to NCCN Practice Guidelines in Oncology for Hodgkin lymphoma.

MEDICATION

First Line

- Early stage disease: combined modality treatment with chemotherapy/radiotherapy or chemotherapy
- Advanced stage disease: chemotherapy
- PET/CT used after cycle 2 (PET-2) to guide either escalation or de-escalation of therapy (1)
- Chemotherapy:
  – ABVD:
    ○ Severe phlebitis—need for central line to administer treatment
    ○ Highly emetogenic
    ○ Vinblastine: risk of neuropathy
    ○ Bleomycin: risk of pulmonary toxicity, death; test dose may be administered prior to first cycle.
    ○ Doxorubicin: risk of cardiotoxicity; monitor LVEF.
  – AAVD (doxorubicin, brentuximab vedotin [anti-CD30 chimeric antibody conjugated to synthetic antimicrotubule agent monomethyl auristatin E], vinblastine, dacarbazine):
    ○ Superior to ABVD per ECHELON-1 trial (2)
    ○ Preferred especially if abnormal PFTs
    ○ Brentuximab vedotin: peripheral neuropathy, nausea, fatigue, neutropenia, diarrhea

Second Line

- Reserved for patients with relapsed/refractory (R/R) disease
- Therapeutic strategy and sequencing of treatment influenced by: eligibility for autologous stem cell transplant (ASCT), functional response to salvage chemotherapy, duration of remission, prior therapy, and comorbidities
- Standard: chemotherapy agents not used for initial treatment followed by high-dose therapy (HDT) with ASCT +/− ISRT.
- Pembrolizumab (anti-PD1) FDA approved for patients with R/R cHL who have failed two or more lines of therapy
- Nivolumab (anti-PD1) in a phase 2 study of R/R cHL showed ORR 69% with durable response and favorable safety profile (3).
- Third-line novel agents undergoing studies: proteosome inhibitors (bortezomib), mammalian target of rapamycin (mTOR) inhibitors (everolimus), immunomodulators (lenalidomide). CAR T-cell therapy directed to CD30 noted high rates of durable response in heavily pretreated patients.
- Median survival <3 years if fail second-line therapy, including HDT/ASCT
- NLPHL
  – Treated with rituximab + CHOP (CD20 positive)

SURGERY/OTHER PROCEDURES

An excisional lymph node biopsy is recommended for initial diagnosis.

ADMISSION, INPATIENT, AND NURSING CONSIDERATIONS

Placement of a central venous catheter for chemotherapy administration

 ## ONGOING CARE

Patients treated with ABVD become neutropenic. Treatment is continued despite neutropenia with no clear increased risk of infection with or without growth factors.

FOLLOW-UP RECOMMENDATIONS

Patient Monitoring

- During therapy: CBC, nutrition, and hydration
- Restage with PET after 2 cycles of chemotherapy: sensitive prognostic indicator
- Posttreatment surveillance:
  – History and physical: q3–6mo for first 2 years, then q6–12mo for next 1 year, and then annually
  – Laboratory studies
    ○ CBC, platelets, BMP, ESR (if elevated at time of diagnosis), as indicated clinically
    ○ Thyroid-stimulating hormone (TSH) annually if radiation to neck
  – Imaging:
    ○ PET-CT to demonstrate negativity within 3 months following completion of treatment to document "Complete Response"; no role for annual surveillance PET
    ○ CT scan no often than every 6 months for the first 2 years or as clinically indicated
    ○ Annual breast mammogram beginning 8 to 10 years after therapy or at age 40 years (whichever first) if chest or axillary irradiation (annual breast MRI as well if initially radiated between ages 10 and 30 years) according to the American Cancer Society
  – Annual influenza vaccine
  – Referral for cancer survivorship with psychosocial support
  – Smoking cessation: Combination of smoking and chest irradiation dramatically increases risk of lung cancer.

PATIENT EDUCATION

- Reproductive impact
- Risks of secondary malignancy

PROGNOSIS

- Cure rate for cHL: 85%
- Relapse or progression of disease rate: 5–20%
- Overall survival rates:
  – 1-year survival: 92%
  – 5-year survival: 87% (93% if localized)
  – 10-year survival: 80%
- International prognostic score for advanced disease:
  – Age >45 years
  – Male gender
  – Albumin <4 g/dL
  – Hemoglobin <10.5 g/dL
  – Lymphocytopenia: <600 lymphocyte cells/dL or lymphocytes <8% of WBC
  – WBC ≥15,000 cells/dL
  – Stage IV disease

COMPLICATIONS

Late complications:

- Patients can develop peripheral neuropathy after treatment.
- Anthracycline use and radiation exposure increase the risk of cardiovascular and valvular disease.
- Irreversible pulmonary toxicity secondary to bleomycin use
- Risk of secondary malignancies like myeloid neoplasms (due to alkylating agents) and breast cancer (radiation exposure)

REFERENCES

1. Barrington SF, Kirkwood AA, Franceschetto A, et al. PET-CT for staging and early response: results from the Response-Adapted Therapy in Advanced Hodgkin Lymphoma study. *Blood.* 2016;127(12):1531–1538.
2. Connors JM, Jurczak W, Straus DJ, et al. Brentuximab vedotin with chemotherapy for stage III or IV Hodgkin's lymphoma. *N Engl J Med.* 2018;378(4):331–344.
3. Armand P, Engert A, Younes A, et al. Nivolumab for relapsed/refractory classic Hodgkin lymphoma after failure of autologous hematopoietic cell transplantation: extended follow-up of the multicohort single-arm phase II CheckMate 205 trial. *J Clin Oncol.* 2018;36(14):1428–1439.

ADDITIONAL READING

- National Cancer Institute. Cancer stat facts: Hodgkin lymphoma. http://seer.cancer.gov/statfacts/html/hodg.html. Accessed July 7, 2017.
- National Comprehensive Cancer Network. NCCN clinical practice guidelines in oncology. Hodgkin lymphoma. http://www.nccn.org/. Accessed July 8, 2017.

 ## CODES

ICD10

- C81.96 Hodgkin lymphoma, unspecified, intrapelvic lymph nodes
- C81.44 Lymphocyte-rich Hodgkin lymphoma, lymph nodes of axilla and upper limb
- C81.75 Other Hodgkin lymphoma, lymph nodes of inguinal region and lower limb

CLINICAL PEARLS

- HL mainly affects young people.
- It is a potentially curable lymphoma. Treatment includes chemotherapy +/− RT.
- If patient develops neutropenia during treatment of HL with ABVD regimen, chemotherapy should be continued provided there is no concern for an infection without delays.
- Long-term effects of chemotherapy should be discussed with patients.
- Close collaboration between oncologist and PCP required for future monitoring

H

HOMELESSNESS

Dana Sprute, MD, MPH, FAAFP • Jocelyn Worley, DO

BASICS

DESCRIPTION
- Homelessness is defined as the condition in which (i) an individual or family lacks a fixed, regular, and adequate nighttime residence; or (ii) an individual or family who has a primary nighttime residence that is (a) a public or private place not meant for human habitation, (b) living in a publicly or privately operated shelter designated to provide temporary living arrangements, or (c) exiting an institution where they have resided for 90 days or less and who resided in an emergency shelter or place not meant for human habitation immediately before entering that institution (1).
- Chronic homelessness is defined as an individual who has experienced homelessness for at least 1 year, or experienced homelessness at least 4 times in the past 3 years. These people typically have complex and chronic medical illnesses such as mental illness, substance use disorders, physical disabilities, and other medical conditions that further hinder their ability to obtain or maintain housing (1).

EPIDEMIOLOGY
Incidence
In 2020, homelessness increased by 2%, marking the 4th year in a row of nation-level increases. However, when compared with 2007, homelessness is down by 12% (1).

Prevalence
As of January 2019, 0.17% of the total United States population, or approximately 580,466 individuals, experienced homelessness on any given night: 63% in sheltered locations such as emergency shelters or transitional housing and 37% in unsheltered locations such as on the street, in abandoned buildings, or any place unfit for human habitation. The 2020 Annual Homeless Assessment Report examines trends within subpopulations of the homeless.

- Around 40,000 (7%) of homeless individuals are veterans. This group has experienced the greatest decrease in homelessness over the last decade as a result of prioritized policy making.
- 96,000 (17%) are chronically homeless.
- 34,000 (6%) are unaccompanied youth.
- 226,000 (40%) are African Americans, a group disproportionately affected because they make up 13% of the U.S. population.
- The COVID-19 crisis is expected to exacerbate homelessness across the board; however, data is not available at time of update. For 2021, COVID-19–related health concerns disrupted counts of unsheltered people.

RISK FACTORS
- Economic factors
  - Poverty
    - 2021 Federal poverty definition: $26,500 annual income for four-person household in the lower 48 states and District of Columbia, slightly higher in Alaska and Hawaii
    - In 2020, 11.4% of the U.S. population fell below federal poverty definition (U.S. Census Bureau); this represents a 1% increase from 2019.
  - Unemployment: U.S. rate 4.8% in September 2021 (U.S. Bureau of Labor Statistics)

- Lack of affordable health care: In 2020, 9.7% of people in the United States (31.6 million) were uninsured for the entire calendar year.
  - Working age adults (ages 19 to 64 years) had a lower rate of health insurance when compared to children and older adults. Those aged 26 to 34 years were least likely to be insured. The uninsured rate for ages 19 to 25 years decreased by 12% between 2009 and 2016, following The Affordable Care Act provision allowing individuals in this age group to stay on parental insurance plans.
- Lack of affordable housing. Affordable housing is defined as housing in which the occupant(s) is paying no more than 30% of gross income for housing costs, including utilities. An estimated 37.8 million U.S. households face cost burdens in housing (>30% of income is spent on housing) and 18.2 million households are "severely housing cost burdened" (≥50% of income is spent on housing).
- Additional at-risk populations: intimate partner violence (IPV), victims of violence; youth (particularly those aging out of foster care); veterans; rural; addiction; psychiatric illness; disabled due to chronic medical disease, psychiatric illness, or substance use disorder; reentry after incarceration/prison
  - IPV: 12% of overall persons experiencing homelessness, and as many as 1 in 5 families experiencing homelessness will have reported experiencing IPV; IPV leads directly to homelessness in many cases (1).
  - Youth: On a single night in 2019, approximately 35,000 unaccompanied youth <25 years of age experienced homelessness. This is a 4% decrease since the 2018 data collection. 89% were ages 18 to 24 years. 51% of homeless unaccompanied youth were unsheltered.
  - Veterans: The number of homeless veterans decreased by 2% from 2018 to 2019 and by 50% since 2009.
  - Transgender individuals: In 2019, 0.6% of all persons experiencing homelessness identified as transgender and 0.2% identified as gender nonconforming.
  - Addiction disorders: 46% of homeless individuals report alcohol and/or drug use as a major factor contributing to homelessness (1).
  - Psychiatric illness: 25% of adults experiencing homelessness suffer from chronic mental illness (1).
  - Reentry after incarceration: Up to 50,000 people each year enter homeless shelters from jails or prisons (1).
- Fundamental issues in homelessness and health care that require ongoing consideration:
  - Unstable housing, limited access to nutritious food and water, lack of transportation
  - Higher risk for abuse and violence
  - Physical/cognitive impairments, behavioral health problems
  - Developmental discrepancies for children: speech delay, chronic ear infection, insufficient opportunity to practice gross and fine motor skills
  - Higher risk for communicable disease
  - Lack of health insurance/resources, discontinuous/inaccessible health care, lack of a medical home, barriers to disability assistance
  - Cultural/linguistic barriers: racial and ethnic groups overrepresented in homeless population
  - Limited education/literacy
  - Lack of social supports: Alienation from family and friends precipitates homelessness.
  - Criminalization of homelessness: frequent arrests for loitering, sleeping in public places

GENERAL PREVENTION
- Policy and funding for community programs to provide emergency/rapid housing, housing stabilization, and case management services. The CARES ACT of 2020 and the American Rescue Plan Act of 2021 provide funding for permanent housing. Over the past 5 years, the fastest growing forms of assistance include rapid rehousing and "other permanent housing."
- Increased Medicaid eligibility, expanded home and community-based services and case management for people experiencing homelessness
- HUD: increasing permanent supportive housing units, increasing services for veterans, families with children and those with disabilities
- Social justice policy recommendations: permanent affordable housing, foreclosure and homelessness prevention, increased funds for HUD McKinney-Vento programs (emergency, transitional, and permanent housing) and National Housing Trust Fund, rural homeless assistance, universal health care, universal livable income, employment/workforce services, prevention of hate crimes against the homeless, decriminalization of homelessness

COMMONLY ASSOCIATED CONDITIONS
- Hunger and malnutrition
- Exposure-related conditions (frostbite, heatstroke)
- Substance use disorders and their associated conditions
  - Liver disease (alcohol, hepatitis B and C)
  - Abscesses (intravenous drug use)
  - Overdose
- Dental problems
- Psychiatric illness
- Trauma (increased risk of assault, victims of hate crime)
- Infectious diseases
  - Skin/nail infection and infestation (lice, bedbugs, and scabies)
  - Tuberculosis (TB), HIV/AIDS, STI
- Worsening of chronic medical conditions: lack of healthy food, places to store medications, or medical equipment; lack of restful sleep; decreased health literacy; limited transportation to appointments

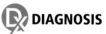

DIAGNOSIS

HISTORY
- Living conditions: location, access to food, restrooms, place to store medicines, safety
- Prior homelessness: causes and circumstances
- Individual/family history of reactive airway disease (RAD), chronic otitis media, anemia, diabetes, cardiovascular disease (CVD), TB, HIV/STIs, hospitalizations
- Family members, especially dependent children
- Medications: include OTC medication, dietary supplements, medication "borrowed" from others
- Prior providers: oral health, primary and specialty care, current medical home
- Mental health: stress, anxiety, appetite, sleep, concentration, mood, speech, memory, thought process and content, auditory/visual hallucinations, suicidal/homicidal ideation, insight, judgment, impulse control, social interactions; symptoms of brain injury (headaches, seizures, memory loss, irritability, dizziness, insomnia, poor organizational/decision-making skills), trauma history
- Alcohol/nicotine/drug use: amount, frequency, duration
- Gender identity/orientation, behaviors, rape, pregnancies, hepatitis, HIV, other STIs

- History of or current abuse: emotional, physical, sexual; patient safety
- Legal problems/violence: history of incarceration
- Activities: routines (treatment feasibility); level of strenuous activity
- Work: previous types of jobs, length held, veteran status, occupational injuries/toxic exposures; vocational skills, interest
- Education: highest level; in special education; assess ability to read/language skills/English fluency.
- Nutrition/hydration: diet, food resources, preparation skills, liquid intake
- Cultural heritage/affiliations: family, friends, faith community, other sources of support
- Strengths: coping skills, job skills, resourcefulness, abilities, interests

PHYSICAL EXAM
- Comprehensive exam: height; weight; BMI; especially abdominal, cardiopulmonary, dermatologic, oral, feet, neurologic, mental status
- Focused exams: for patients uncomfortable with full-body, unclothed exam at first visit
- Dental assessment: age-appropriate teeth, obvious caries, dental/referred pain, diabetes, CVD

DIAGNOSTIC TESTS & INTERPRETATION
Initial Tests (lab, imaging)
- Mental health: Patient Health Questionnaire (PHQ-9, PHQ-2), MHS-III, MDQ, GAD-7
- Cognitive assessment: Mini-Mental State Examination (MMSE), Traumatic Brain Injury Questionnaire (TBIQ), Repeatable Battery for the Assessment of Neuropsychological Status (RBANS)
- Developmental assessment: Ages & Stages Questionnaires, Parents' Evaluation of Developmental Status (PEDS), Denver II, or other screening tool
- Interpersonal violence: IPV, sexual assault, TBI
- Forensic evaluation: if indicated by history
- Baseline labs: as needed to address suspected medical concerns
- TB screening: PPD or T-SPOT/QuantiFERON-TB Gold if available
- STI screening: HIV, chlamydia, gonorrhea, syphilis, hepatitis B, hepatitis C, trichomonas
- Substance abuse: Simple Screening Instrument for Alcohol and Other Drugs (SSI-AOD), urine drug screen

Follow-Up Tests & Special Considerations
- Reproductive health care and STIs: Obtain detailed sexual history (sexual identity, orientation, behaviors/sexual practices, number of partners). Consider patient exploitation, especially if mental illness/developmental disability suspected. Communicate willingness to initiate contraception first visit without exam. Genital exam recommended, but be sensitive to patient, especially if possible sexual abuse history. If pelvic exam is refused, consider self-collected testing and/or empiric treatment for STI (and possibility of multiple orifice infection). Dispense medications on site; facilitate partner treatment.
- Access to facilities is highly variable, even if residing at a shelter. For example, patient may not have access to restroom for colonoscopy bowel prep.
- Pediatric care: complete exam every visit; use each visit to identify/address problems and provide vaccinations because homeless families may not see a medical provider unless child is sick. Vision and hearing screening at every visit. Facilitate referrals as able.

 TREATMENT
- Establish rapport: Many patients will have had negative health care experiences.
- Enlist community resources: mental health and substance abuse programs, free clinics, case management.
- Health care maintenance: vaccinations (hepatitis A and B, Pneumovax, Tdap, influenza), cancer and chronic disease screening for adults; Early and Periodic Screening, Diagnosis, and Treatment (EPSDT) program screening and vaccinations for children
- Care plan
  - Basic needs: Food, clothing, and housing may be higher priorities than health care.
  - Patient goals and priorities: immediate/long-term health needs. Address patient concerns first.
  - Action plan: simple language, pocket card
  - After hours: extended clinic hours and access
  - Safety plan: violence and abuse; mandatory reporting requirements
  - Emergency plan: location of nearest emergency department (ED), preparation for evacuation
  - Adherence plan: use of interpreter; identification of potential barriers

MEDICATION
- Simple regimen: low pill count, once-daily dosing
- Dispensing: small amounts on site to promote follow-up, decrease loss/theft/misuse. Determine resources for written prescriptions.
- Storage of medications: If no access, avoid medications requiring refrigeration.
- Patient assistance: free/low-cost drugs depending on available local options
- Aids to adherence: harm reduction, outreach/case management, directly observed therapy
- Side effects: Primary reason for medication nonadherence are drugs causing diarrhea, polyuria, nausea, and/or disorientation.
- Analgesia/symptomatic treatment: Consider pain contract, single provider for pain medication refills.
- Dietary supplements: multivitamins with minerals, nutritional supplements
- Managed care: generics, if possible; assistance getting prescription filled
- Lab monitoring: Monitor patients on antipsychotic medications for metabolic disorders using available laboratory resources.

ADDITIONAL THERAPIES
- Associated problems/complications
  - Fragmented care: multiple providers. Use electronic medical record (EMR) as possible; list prescribed medication on wallet-sized card.
  - Masked symptoms/misdiagnosis: for example, weight loss, dementia, edema, lactic acidosis
  - Focus on immediate concerns, not possible future consequences.
  - Integrated treatment for concurrent mental illness/substance use disorders
  - Support for parent of child abused by others and for abused parent
  - Large appointment burdens: For those individuals who suffer from multiple chronic illnesses, specialty care may be difficult to obtain due to the many barriers to care listed above.
- Follow-up
  - Reliable phone/e-mail contact for patient/friend/family/case manager
  - Frequent follow-up, incentives, nonjudgmental care regardless of adherence
  - Anticipate/accommodate unscheduled clinic visits.

- Provide car fare, tokens, and help with transportation services.
- Monitor school attendance and address health/developmental problems with family/school.

ADMISSION, INPATIENT, AND NURSING CONSIDERATIONS
- Persons experiencing homelessness are likely to benefit from admission if living conditions are suboptimal to treat medical, psychiatric, and substance use disorders.
- Discharge considerations:
  - Acute or chronic wound care: Bed rest, extended periods of elevation, rest, or icing are not feasible in most instances.
  - Need for durable medical equipment (DME): Portable oxygen tanks and nebulizers may not be covered by the hospital and may be cumbersome to use in absence of stable housing.
  - Medications: It is preferable to fill prescriptions at hospital outpatient pharmacy.
  - Outpatient follow-up: Transportation to appointments should be arranged if possible.

 ONGOING CARE

FOLLOW-UP RECOMMENDATIONS
- Patients with a history of nonadherence need additional support (e.g., case manager, outreach) to succeed in ongoing care after hospital discharge.
- Limited telephone access to schedule appointments; may be unable to receive telephone messages with test results or rescheduled appointment times. Some social service agencies will provide phone, mail, e-mail, Internet, and laundry services.
- Arrange appointments prior to discharge.
- Document the best way to contact the individual.
- Work with experienced health care agency designed to address physical/mental health services and substance use treatment.

PATIENT EDUCATION
- https://www.nhchc.org/
- http://www.endhomelessness.org/

PROGNOSIS
Mortality rates for homeless adults are 3 to 4 times higher compared with general U.S. population.

REFERENCES
1. National Alliance to End Homelessness. State of homelessness: 2021 edition. https://www.endhomelessness.org./homelessness-in-america/homelessness-statistics/state-of-homelessness-2021/. Accessed October 22, 2021.

 CODES

ICD10
- Z59.0 Homelessness
- Z59.1 Inadequate housing
- Z59.8 Other problems related to housing and economic circumstances

CLINICAL PEARLS
- Permanent supportive housing is an important step toward ending homelessness, in accordance with a Housing First approach.
- Assistance in gaining access to benefits or providing help to support basic needs decreases stress, improves therapeutic relationship, and allows individuals to focus on physical and mental health.

HORDEOLUM (STYE)

Konstantinos E. Deligiannidis, MD, MPH, FAAFP

BASICS

DESCRIPTION
- An acute inflammation or infection of the eyelid margin involving the sebaceous gland of an eyelash (external hordeolum) or a meibomian gland (internal hordeolum)
- System(s) affected: skin/exocrine
- Synonym(s): internal hordeolum; external hordeolum; zeisian stye; meibomian stye; stye

EPIDEMIOLOGY
- Predominant age: none
- Predominant sex: male = female

Incidence
Unknown: Although external hordeolum is common, internal hordeolum is rare.

ETIOLOGY AND PATHOPHYSIOLOGY
- Bacterial infection of sweat or sebaceous glands, causing an acute inflammatory reaction
- In an internal hordeolum, the meibomian gland may become obstructed, leading to a pustule on the conjunctival surface as opposed to the margin of the eyelid.
- Most commonly caused by *Staphylococcus aureus* (~90–95% of all cases) or by *Staphylococcus epidermidis*
- Seborrhea can predispose to infections of the eyelid.

Genetics
No known genetic pattern

RISK FACTORS
- Poor eyelid hygiene
- Previous hordeolum
- Contact lens wearers
- Application of makeup
- Seborrheic dermatitis
- Predisposing blepharitis (low-grade infections of the eyelid margin)
- Ocular rosacea

GENERAL PREVENTION
Eyelid hygiene

COMMONLY ASSOCIATED CONDITIONS
- Acne
- Seborrhea
- An association may exist between hordeolum during childhood and developing rosacea in adulthood.

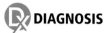

DIAGNOSIS

HISTORY
- Localized inflammation (vs. involvement of the entire eyelid or surrounding skin)
- Foreign body sensation in the eye
- Symptoms may start as vague eyelid pain and inflammation and then localize 1 to 2 days later.
- Prior episodes are common.

PHYSICAL EXAM
- Localized inflammation of the eyelashes or a small pustule at the margin of the eyelid
- Localized swelling and tenderness on the internal or external aspect of the eyelid with an opening to either side
- To determine if an internal hordeolum is obstructed, the eyelid should be gently everted to examine for a pustule on the tarsal conjunctiva.
- Itching or scaling of the eyelids; collection of discharge, redness, and irritation leading to localized tenderness and pain
- The size of the swelling usually correlates to the severity of the hordeolum.

DIFFERENTIAL DIAGNOSIS
- Chalazion
- Blepharitis
- Eyelid neoplasms
- Periorbital cellulitis
- Dacryocystitis
- Squamous cell carcinoma

DIAGNOSTIC TESTS & INTERPRETATION
Culture of the eyelid margins usually is not necessary.

Diagnostic Procedures/Other
History and eye exam

Test Interpretation
Bacterial contamination and white cells in eyelid discharge

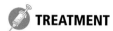

TREATMENT

GENERAL MEASURES
- The hordeolum should not be expressed.
- Warm compresses to the area of inflammation can help increase blood supply and encourage spontaneous drainage.
- Good personal hygiene with attention to cleansing the eyelids on a daily basis helps to prevent recurrent infections.

MEDICATION
First Line
- A Cochrane review found no evidence for or against nonsurgical treatment of internal hordeolum. External hordeola were not considered (1)[A].
- Usually, a hordeolum spontaneously drains, aided by warm compresses to the area.
- Also, lid scrubs, digital massage, and alternative medicine have been used to reduce healing time and to relieve symptoms.
- Application of an antibiotic ointment (e.g., erythromycin) to the margin of the eyelid after proper cleansing (except in children age <12 years, in whom there is a risk of blurred vision and amblyopia) helps reduce bacterial proliferation. There is little evidence that any topical therapy is effective. Erythromycin ophthalmic ointment may be applied up to 6 times per day for 7 to 10 days or an antibiotic ointment containing bacitracin (2),(3)[C].
- Treat underlying dry eye with artificial tears.

Second Line

- Occasionally, the use of an aminoglycoside ophthalmic ointment, such as gentamicin or tobramycin, may be necessary if condition is refractory to simpler treatment (case reports).
- Oral dicloxacillin or cephalexin for 2 weeks if refractory to topical antibiotics

ISSUES FOR REFERRAL

Consider referral if unresponsive to oral antibiotics.

SURGERY/OTHER PROCEDURES

- If the infection becomes localized to a single gland, incision, drainage, or curettage sometimes is necessary. This is an in-office procedure with a local anesthetic: Exercise caution because ocular perforation has been reported with the injection of an anesthetic to an infected lid.
- Use of combined antibiotic ointment (neomycin sulfate, polymyxin B sulfate, and gramicidin) after surgery was not shown to have any statistically significant benefit compared with artificial tears.

COMPLEMENTARY & ALTERNATIVE MEDICINE

- Broncasma berna is a polyvalent antigen vaccine that may be useful in the treatment of recurrent hordeolum.
- A Cochrane review found low-quality evidence that acupuncture (with or without antibiotics and/or warm compresses) may increase the chance of improvement of hordeolum compared to antibiotics and/or warm compresses (4)[A].

ADMISSION, INPATIENT, AND NURSING CONSIDERATIONS

Outpatient

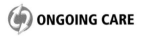 ONGOING CARE

FOLLOW-UP RECOMMENDATIONS

No restrictions

Patient Monitoring

The patient should be seen within several weeks to assess the effectiveness of therapy or should at least call the physician's office with a progress report.

DIET

No special diet

PATIENT EDUCATION

- The patient should be instructed in proper cleansing of the eyelids using a solution of tap water and baby shampoo or a commercially prepared hypoallergenic cleanser.
- The stye should not be squeezed or incised.

PROGNOSIS

- Usually responds well to good hygiene and warm compresses
- Inflammation usually improves within a week.
- Hordeolum tends to recur in some patients, usually due to incomplete elimination of bacteria.

COMPLICATIONS

An internal hordeolum, if untreated, may lead to chalazion, infections of adjacent glands, or generalized cellulitis of the lid.

REFERENCES

1. Lindsley K, Nichols JJ, Dickersin K. Non-surgical interventions for acute internal hordeolum. *Cochrane Database Syst Rev*. 2017;(1):CD007742.
2. Wald ER. Periorbital and orbital infections. *Pediatr Rev*. 2004;25(9):312–320.
3. Mueller JB, McStay CM. Ocular infection and inflammation. *Emerg Med Clin North Am*. 2008;26(1):57–72.
4. Cheng K, Law A, Guo M, et al. Acupuncture for acute hordeolum. *Cochrane Database Syst Rev*. 2017;(2):CD011075.

ADDITIONAL READING

- Bamford JT, Gessert CE, Renier CM, et al. Childhood stye and adult rosacea. *J Am Acad Dermatol*. 2006;55(6):951–955.
- Hirunwiwatkul P, Wachirasereechai K. Effectiveness of combined antibiotic ophthalmic solution in the treatment of hordeolum after incision and curettage: a randomized, placebo-controlled trial: a pilot study. *J Med Assoc Thai*. 2005;88(5):647–650.
- Kim JH, Yang SM, Kim HM, et al. Inadvertent ocular perforation during lid anesthesia for hordeolum removal. *Korean J Ophthalmol*. 2006;20(3):199–200.
- Nakatani M. Treatment of recurrent hordeolum with broncasma berna. *Eye (Lond)*. 1999;13(Pt 5):692.
- Wald ER. Periorbital and orbital infections. *Infect Dis Clin North Am*. 2007;21(2):393–408, vi.

 CODES

ICD10

- H00.019 Hordeolum externum unspecified eye, unspecified eyelid
- H00.029 Hordeolum internum unspecified eye, unspecified eyelid
- H00.039 Abscess of eyelid unspecified eye, unspecified eyelid

CLINICAL PEARLS

- A hordeolum should not be expressed.
- Warm compresses to the area of inflammation can encourage spontaneous drainage.
- Application of an antibiotic ointment (e.g., erythromycin) to the margin of the eyelid after proper cleansing helps reduce bacterial proliferation but may have no effect on the healing of the stye.
- Good personal hygiene with attention to cleansing the eyelids on a daily basis can prevent recurrent infections.

H

HORNER SYNDROME

Iain W. Decker, DO • Zaiba Malik, MD

 BASICS

DESCRIPTION
- Horner syndrome is a constellation of neurological signs and symptoms manifested as a classic triad of ipsilateral miosis, eyelid ptosis, and anhidrosis of the ipsilateral face and/or neck (with iris heterochromia in children).
- It is caused by the interruption of sympathetic nervous system innervation to the head, neck, and eye.
- System(s) affected: nervous, skin/exocrine
- Synonym(s): Bernard-Horner syndrome; Bernard syndrome; Horner syndrome; cervical sympathetic syndrome; oculosympathetic syndrome; oculosympathetic paralysis; oculosympathetic deficiency; oculosympathetic paresis

EPIDEMIOLOGY
- Predominant age: none
- Predominant sex: male = female

Incidence
- Estimated incidence of pediatric Horner syndrome is 1.42 per 100,000 in patients younger than 19 years of age, with a birth prevalence of 1 in 6,250 for those with congenital onset of Horner syndrome.
- Incidence in adults is not known.

Prevalence
Unknown

ETIOLOGY AND PATHOPHYSIOLOGY
- Oculosympathetic pathway anatomy:
  - First-order neuron: Sympathetic nerve fibers originate in the hypothalamus, descend through the brainstem, and synapse at the ciliospinal center (of Budge-Waller) located at approximately the C8–T2 levels of the spinal cord.
  - Second-order neuron: exits the spinal column, arches over the apex of the lung and under the subclavian artery, ascending to the superior cervical ganglion at the level of the carotid bifurcation and angle of the jaw (C2)
  - Third-order neuron: ascends along the adventitia of the internal carotid artery, through the cavernous sinus in proximity to cranial nerve (CN) VI and the trigeminal ganglion, and joins the nasociliary branch of CN V1 to enter the orbit—innervating the iris dilator muscle, Müller muscle in the upper eyelid, and inferior retractors in the lower eyelid.
- A lesion affecting the neurons in the sympathetic chain (first, second, or third order) may produce signs and symptoms of Horner syndrome as a result of a lack of sympathetic input to the orbit.
  - Ptosis: Sympathetic innervation to the Müller muscle in the upper eyelid and the lower eyelid retractors helps to maintain normal eyelid position. When sympathetic innervation to these structures is interrupted, a subtle ptosis of both the upper lid (ptosis) and lower lid (reverse ptosis) may result. This ptosis may be subtle, often 2 mm or less.
  - Meiosis: The radially oriented pupillary dilator muscle produces pupillary dilation in response to stimulation by the sympathetic nervous system. Aniscoria will be more pronounced in dim lighting, reflecting impairment of dilation in the affected eye. The affected eye will constrict normally in response to light but will be slower to dilate than the unaffected pupil.
  - Anhidrosis: When present, anhidrosis may assist in localizing a lesion. Sympathetic fibers innervating sweat glands of the lower face and vasodilatory muscles branch off before the superior cervical sympathetic ganglion and travel along the external carotid artery. Lesions affecting primary and secondary neurons are more likely to produce anhidrosis of both the upper and lower face.
- Etiologies of Horner syndrome are best classified by which neuron in the sympathetic chain is affected (first/second/third order) and by age (pediatric vs. adult).
- Etiologies in adults:
  - First-order neuron lesions located in hypothalamus/brainstem (lateral medulla)/spinal cord (cervico-thoracic) include:
    ◦ Arnold-Chiari malformation, basal meningitis (e.g., syphilis), cerebral vascular accident: lateral medullary (Wallenberg) syndrome, cervical cord trauma, cervical spondylosis, demyelinating disease (multiple sclerosis), Intrapontine hemorrhage, neck trauma, syringomyelia/syringobulbia, tumor (basal skull, pituitary), unintended subdural placement of lumbar epidural catheter
  - Second-order neuron pulmonary or cervico-thoracic lesions include:
    ◦ Aneurysm/dissection of aorta, central venous catheterization, chest tubes, 1st rib fracture, lymphadenopathy (Hodgkin, leukemia, tuberculosis, sarcoid), mandibular tooth abscess, neuroblastoma, Pancoast tumor or infection of lung apex, proximal common carotid artery dissection, thoracic outlet obstruction (cervical rib, subclavian artery aneurysm), trauma/surgical injury, tumor (thyroid, mediastinum)
  - Third-order neuron lesions located in superior cervical ganglion, internal carotid artery, skull base, cavernous sinus, or orbit include:
    ◦ Carotid cavernous fistula or other pathology, carotid endarterectomy or carotid artery stenting, cluster headaches/paroxysmal hemicrania, internal carotid artery dissection, herpes zoster, lesions of the middle ear (acute otitis media), Lyme disease, tumor (nasopharyngeal, pituitary, paratrigeminal, metastasis, skull base), tonsillectomy, trauma/surgical injury, raeder paratrigeminal syndrome
- Etiologies in children:
  - Birth trauma/neck trauma (injury to the brachial plexus)—most common. Brainstem glioma, neuroblastoma, vascular anomalies, surgical interventions in the neck/chest, Idiopathic

Genetics
Rare autosomal dominant inheritance

RISK FACTORS
- Recent trauma to the head/neck/thorax (e.g., motor vehicle accidents)
- Smoking (Pancoast tumor)
- Known aneurysm of the carotid or subclavian arteries
- Known malignancy/tumor/mass
- Previous surgery (Neck/thoracic)
- Previous instrument of the head/neck/thoracic regions (chest tube, central venous catheterization)
- Cluster headache

 DIAGNOSIS

HISTORY
- When did symptoms begin? (acute vs. chronic)
- Any visual symptoms? (blurred vision, field loss, transient visual loss, diplopia)
- Previous ophthalmic history? (eye trauma, surgery)
- Are symptoms associated with pain? (ipsilateral head/neck/face)
- Recent head/neck trauma?
- Recent surgical procedures?
- Any associated headaches?
- Any other neurologic signs?
- Does the degree of ptosis vary over the course of the day or with fatigue?
- Any sweating abnormalities or flushing on one side of the face?

Pediatric Considerations
In infants and children, loss of facial flushing is appreciated more than anhidrosis (harlequin sign—affected side will appear pale secondary to denervation supersentivity to circulating adrenaline). New onset, non-traumatic Horner syndrome in a child necessitates workup for neuroblastoma.

> **ALERT**
> Horner syndrome in the presence of pain merits urgent evaluation and referral to the emergency room.

- Acute-onset, ipsilateral facial or neck pain: Consider carotid artery dissection until proven otherwise, even in the absence of obvious head/neck trauma.
  - Pain from dissection is usually located around the temple and orbit. Patients may also experience amaurosis fugax and dysgeusia. If missed, stroke is a potential complication.
- Axial, shoulder, scapula, arm, or hand pain may be related to Pancoast tumor or cervical cord lesion.
- Paratrigeminal syndromes:
  - Raeder paratrigeminal syndrome type I: orbital pain, miosis, ptosis, with associated ipsilateral lesions of CN III to VI; suspect middle cranial fossa mass or cavernous sinus lesion.
  - Raeder paratrigeminal syndrome type II: episodic retrobulbar or orbital pain, miosis, ptosis with no CN lesions; suspect migraine variant.

PHYSICAL EXAM
- Evaluate pupillary function:
  - Measure pupillary diameter under both dim and bright lighting to determine presence of anisocoria. In Horner syndrome, anisocoria will be greater in dim/dark lighting conditions.
  - Evaluate pupil reactivity to light and accommodative response.
  - A pupillary dilation lag may be present, and the affected pupil may gradually dilate 5–15 seconds after exposure to light.
- Evaluate for lid ptosis:
  - Examine the upper lids for ptosis (often <2 mm).
  - A "reverse ptosis" of the lower lid may also be visible in the form of a slight elevation of the lower lid relative to the unaffected eye.
- Evaluate for anhidrosis:
  - This may be difficult. Subtle signs of anhidrosis include flushing of the skin on the involved side.
- Additional acute features of sympathetic disruption may include ipsilateral conjunctival injection and nasal congestion.
- Biomicroscopic/slit lamp exam of the eye, including iris structure and color (if available)
  - In congenital Horner syndrome, the affected iris shows reduced pigmentation, blue-gray, and mottling of the affected eye (heterochromia iridis) because formation of iris pigment early in life is under sympathetic control.
- Observe for the presence of nystagmus, facial swelling, lymphadenopathy, or vesicular eruptions.
- A full cranial nerve exam with special attention to extraocular movements
- Palpation and inspection of the neck for any masses or evidence of trauma
- Neurologic and chest exams for associated physical findings

DIFFERENTIAL DIAGNOSIS

- Physiologic anisocoria (~20% population)
  - Physiologic variation often varies by less than 1mm and may fluctuate throughout the day.
- Neurologic diseases versus neuromuscular junctional disease (myasthenia gravis, botulinum toxin)
- 3rd nerve palsy
- Aponeurotic ptosis
- Congenital ptosis
- Adie tonic pupil
- Intermittent unilateral pupillary mydriasis (sympathetic vs. parasympathetic form)
- Damage to the iris sphincter muscle
- Pharmacologic causes including unilateral use of miotics or mydriatics, acetophenazine, alseroxylon, bupivacaine, butaperazine, carphenazine, chloroprocaine, deserpidine, diacetylmorphine, diethazine, ethopropazine, etidocaine, guanethidine, influenza virus vaccine, levodopa, lidocaine, mepivacaine, mesoridazine, methdilazine, methotrimeprazine, oral contraceptives, perazine, prilocaine, procaine, prochlorperazine, promazine, propoxycaine, reserpine, thioproperazine, thioridazine, trifluoperazine

DIAGNOSTIC TESTS & INTERPRETATION

Initial Tests (lab, imaging)

- Lab: CBC, FTA-ABS, VDRL, purified protein derivative; vanillylmandelic acid (VMA), homovanillic acid I (HVA) to rule out neuroblastoma in pediatric patients
- Imaging considerations are unique because of the long pathway traveled by the sympathetic nervous system. A lesion at any point along this pathway, extending from the hypothalamus down to T2, may contribute to the onset of Horner syndrome.
- Clinicians should attempt to follow 3 steps in the evaluation of a patient with Horner syndrome:
  - Clinical diagnosis of Horner Syndrome
  - Pharmacologic confirmation of Horner Syndrome
  - In the chronic setting, a single neuroimaging study of the oculosympathetic pathway extending from the hypothalamus down to T2 with a contrast-enhanced MRI, with or without MRA of the head and neck
  - In the acute setting (or for patients unable to tolerate MRI), an initial CT scan of the head/neck and computed tomography angiography (CTA) of the neck followed by HS MRI if initial CT/CTA are negative. Life-threatening causes of Horner syndrome including carotid artery dissection may be ruled out with this initial CT/CTA to avoid delay in treatment (1)[B].

Pediatric Considerations

In a child of any age without contributory history, MRI brain, neck, and chest as outlined above is appropriate. Clinicians may consider MRI abdomen as well if clinical suspicion of neuroblastoma is high.

Pregnancy Considerations

In the pregnant population, the safety of MRI for the fetus has not yet been established. Most authors believe that pregnant patients may undergo MRI safely, but it should be noted that contrast material (e.g., gadolinium) is FDA category C (1)[B].

Diagnostic Procedures/Other

- To diagnose Horner syndrome, a confirmation test is required. The first two of these tests (apraclonidine and cocaine) help to confirm the presence of Horner syndrome, whereas the third (hydroxyamphetamine) attempts to localize the lesion. It is usually not necessary to test with both apraclonidine and cocaine,

and most choose apraclonidine due to the challenge associated with obtaining cocaine drops.
  - Topical 0.5% apraclonidine drops: (2)[A],(3),(4)[B]
    - Apraclonidine is a strong alpha-2 agonist and weak alpha-1 agonist with little to no effect on the normal pupil. Instillation tests for denervation supersensitivity of the dilator muscle of the pupil. This develops after an interruption in sympathetic input. This weak alpha-1 agonist activity is enough to dilate the supersensitive Horner pupil. To test for Horner syndrome, 1 drop of apraclonidine is placed in each eye, and the patient is re-assessed after 60 minutes.
    - A positive test result occurs when both pupils become equally sized, or if the affected pupil becomes the larger one. Note: The apraclonidine test may be negative in cases of acute trauma, as there has not been enough time for denervation hypersensitivity to develop (2–5 days).
    - Caution: Do not use in infants <6 months, as alpha-2 activity can cause respiratory depression. May consider cocaine testing in this age group
  - 4–10% topical cocaine drops:
    - Cocaine blocks reuptake of norepinephrine from the synaptic cleft. To test for Horner syndrome, two drops of 4% or 10% cocaine are instilled in both eyes 5 minutes apart and after 40–60 minutes the pupils are re-evaluated.
    - Cocaine drops will dilate the normal pupil. The miotic pupil in Horner syndrome (regardless of location of lesion) will not dilate or will dilate poorly after 45 minutes because of the absence of norepinephrine at the nerve endings of the third-order neuron (2)[A]. Positive test is anisocoria of ≥1 mm.
  - Topical 1% hydroxyamphetamine drops (2)[A]
    - Used to differentiate between preganglionic (first and second order neurons) and postganglionic (third order neuron) Horner syndrome. Hydroxyamphetamine causes release of endogenous norepinephrine stored in the postganglionic neuron, causing pupillary dilation.
    - One hour after instillation of 1% hydroxyamphetamine drops, the pupils should be evaluated. Dilation of both pupils indicates a lesion of the first or second order neurons. Failure of the pupil to dilate, or poor dilation, indicates a third-order neuron lesion (test considered positive when anisocoria increases by ≥1 mm).
    - No pharmacologic test exists to differentiate between a first- and second-order neuron lesion.
- Must wait 24 to 72 hours between the cocaine and hydroxyamphetamine tests as cocaine may inhibit uptake of hydroxyamphetamine and alter the accuracy of the test.

Pediatric Considerations

Due to transsynaptic degeneration in children, the hydroxyamphetamine test is not reliable.

 TREATMENT

GENERAL MEASURES

- Treatment generally revolves around addressing any underlying etiologies.
- Once life-threatening etiologies have been excluded, cosmesis or functional vision impairment due to ptosis may be addressed if symptoms have persisted for 12 months.

MEDICATION

Carotid artery dissection: Pharmacologic treatment options include thrombolysis, antithrombotic therapy with anticoagulation, or antiplatelet therapy. No randomized control trials have compared these treatment options (5)[C].

ISSUES FOR REFERRAL

Depending on etiology of Horner syndrome, referrals may include neurosurgery, oncology, interventional radiology, pulmonology, neurology/neuro-ophthalmology, and oculoplastic surgery.

SURGERY/OTHER PROCEDURES

- Surgical intervention depending on etiology
- Consider ptosis repair for cosmesis or functional vision impairment secondary to ptosis if symptoms have persisted for 12 months (oculoplastics).

 ONGOING CARE

PROGNOSIS

- Postganglionic: usually benign
- Central and preganglionic: poorer prognosis

COMPLICATIONS

- Chronic pupillary constriction
- Cosmesis

REFERENCES

1. Chen Y, Morgan ML, Barros Palau AE, et al. Evaluation and neuroimaging of the Horner syndrome. Can J Ophthalmol. 2015;50(2):107–111.
2. Antonio-Santos AA, Santo RN, Eggenberger ER. Pharmacological testing of anisocoria. Expert Opin Pharmacother. 2005;6(12):2007–2013.
3. Koc F, Kavuncu S, Kansu T, et al. The sensitivity and specificity of 0.5% apraclonidine in the diagnosis of oculosympathetic paresis. Br J Ophthalmol. 2005;89(11):1442–1444.
4. Chen PL, Chen JT, Lu DW, et al. Comparing efficacies of 0.5% apraclonidine with 4% cocaine in the diagnosis of Horner syndrome in pediatric patients. J Ocul Pharmacol Ther. 2006;22(3):182–187.
5. Sadaka A, Schockman SL, Golnik KC. Evaluation of Horner syndrome in the MRI era. J Neuroophthalmol. 2017;37(3):268–272.

ADDITIONAL READING

- Lyrer PA, Brandt T, Metso TM, et al. Clinical import of Horner syndrome in internal carotid and vertebral artery dissection. Neurology. 2014;82(18):1653–1659.
- Mahoney NR, Liu GT, Menacker SJ, et al. Pediatric Horner syndrome: etiologies and roles of imaging and urine studies to detect neuroblastoma and other responsible mass lesions. Am J Ophthalmol. 2006;142(4):651–659.
- Reede DL, Garcon E, Smoker WR, et al. Horner's syndrome: clinical and radiographic evaluation. Neuroimaging Clin N Am. 2008;18(2):369–385.

 CODES

ICD10

- G90.2 Horner's syndrome
- S14.5XXA Injury of cervical sympathetic nerves, initial encounter

CLINICAL PEARLS

- Horner syndrome triad: ipsilateral miosis, eyelid ptosis, and anhidrosis caused by a lesion of the oculosympathetic pathway
- Red flag: Horner syndrome in the presence of acute-onset, ipsilateral facial or neck pain: Consider carotid artery dissection until proven otherwise.
- Ptosis is mild, usually <2 mm.

H

HYDROCELE

Jared M. Patton, MD, MS

BASICS

DESCRIPTION
A collection of fluid between the parietal and visceral layers of the tunica vaginalis within the scrotum
- Communicating hydrocele (patent processus vaginalis)
  - Direct communication with the peritoneal cavity
  - Contains peritoneal fluid
  - Almost always with associated indirect inguinal hernia
  - Decreases in size with recumbent position
- Noncommunicating hydrocele (The processus vaginalis is not patent.)
  - No direct connection to the peritoneal cavity
  - Fluid contained is from the mesothelial lining.
  - Can be isolated to the cord with the distal and proximal portions of the processus vaginalis closed
- Acute hydrocele: fluid collection resulting from an acute process within the tunica vaginalis, typically involving only the scrotum
- Although this disorder is found nearly exclusively in male patients, there is a rare hydrocele into the canal of Nuck in females which results from a fluid collection in an abnormal open pouch of peritoneum extending into the labia majora.
- System(s) affected: urogenital

Pediatric Considerations
Most congenital communicating hydroceles resolve spontaneously by 2 years of age.

EPIDEMIOLOGY
Predominant age: childhood

Incidence
Estimated at 0.7–4.7% of male infants

Prevalence
- 1,000/100,000
- Estimated at 1% of adult men

ETIOLOGY AND PATHOPHYSIOLOGY
- Incomplete closure of the processus vaginalis trapping peritoneal fluid anywhere along the length of the tunica vaginalis
- Failure of closure of the processus vaginalis maintaining a communication to the peritoneal cavity

- Imbalance of the secretion and reabsorption of fluid from the lining of the tunica vaginalis
- Infection
- Tumors
- Trauma
- Ipsilateral renal transplantation (due to disruption of the spermatic cord during the procedure)

RISK FACTORS
- For adult-acquired hydroceles:
  - Ventriculoperitoneal shunt
  - Ehlers-Danlos syndrome
  - Peritoneal dialysis
  - History of scrotal surgery to include varicocelectomy
- For congenital hydroceles:
  - Exstrophy of the bladder
  - Cloacal exstrophy

COMMONLY ASSOCIATED CONDITIONS
- For adult-acquired hydroceles:
  - Testicular tumors
  - Scrotal trauma
  - Ventriculoperitoneal shunt
  - Nephrotic syndrome
  - Renal failure with peritoneal dialysis

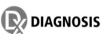**DIAGNOSIS**

HISTORY
- Acute, subacute, or chronic swelling of the scrotum or inguinal canal
- Frequent changes in size of the hydrocele with position change or activity (indicative of communicating)
- Usually painless unless acute onset
- Sensation of heaviness or pressure in the scrotum
- Pain radiating to the flank/back

PHYSICAL EXAM
- Swelling in the scrotum or inguinal canal
- Scrotal mass, usually fluctuant
- Fluctuation in size with change of position (communicating hydrocele)
- Scrotal mass that transilluminates

- A fluctuant mass that is reducible with gentle pressure can identify a communicating hydrocele versus noncommunicating.

DIFFERENTIAL DIAGNOSIS
- Indirect inguinal hernia
- Orchitis
- Epididymitis
- Varicocele
- Traumatic testicular injury
- Testicular torsion or torsion of appendix testes
- Testicular neoplasm

DIAGNOSTIC TESTS & INTERPRETATION
Initial Tests (lab, imaging)
- Inguinoscrotal ultrasound (US): can demonstrate the presence of bowel (e.g., distinguish incarcerated hernia from a hydrocele of the cord) as well as the presence of testicular torsion
- Testicular MRI when US is unable to distinguish etiology
- Doppler US or testicular nuclear scan can distinguish testicular torsion.

> **ALERT**
> Aspiration of a hydrocele for diagnosis is not indicated and may lead to severe complications if herniated bowel is present.

Diagnostic Procedures/Other
Trans-illumination of the hemiscrotum along with history and exam are usually sufficient in making the diagnosis, but a formal US may be needed to confirm.

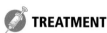**TREATMENT**

ISSUES FOR REFERRAL
- Urology referral for symptomatic adults or if underlying diagnosis is unclear
- Pediatric urology/surgery referral for children with symptomatic noncommunicating hydrocele
- Pediatric urology/surgery referral if not resolved by 2 years of age

SURGERY/OTHER PROCEDURES

- Children: For congenital hydrocele, surgical treatment is generally deferred until 2 years of age because many hydroceles will spontaneously resolve. Some evidence shows that delaying longer than 2 years may be appropriate and decreases unnecessary surgery (1)[C]. When surgery is indicated, children with communicating hydroceles may undergo either open or laparoscopic approach.
  - Laparoscopic repair offers the benefit of contralateral exploration.
  - Open scrotal approach involves ligation and removal of the processus vaginalis. The benefit of this approach is improved cosmesis and decreased operative time (2)[B].
  - Open inguinal approach involves ligation of the processus vaginalis and excision, distal splitting, or drainage of hydrocele sac (in a hydrocele of cord, the sac can be completely removed).
- Adults: No therapy is needed unless the hydrocele causes discomfort or unless there is a significant underlying cause such as a tumor.
  - Aspiration of the hydrocele with instillation of a sclerosing agent has been successfully used in adults (3)[A].
  - If resection is indicated, all of the open surgical techniques have the same 6% rate of recurrence; however, the overall rate of complications and the rate of postoperative hematoma were lowest with the "Lord's" repair (4)[B].
  - Postoperative complications as well as cost and time to work resumption were less in treatment by aspiration and sclerotherapy versus resection, but the recurrence rate was higher (RR 9.43) (5)[A].

ADMISSION, INPATIENT, AND NURSING CONSIDERATIONS

- Open inguinal or scrotal approach is typically performed as an outpatient.
- Laparoscopic approach in pediatric patients may require 24-hour admission for postoperative monitoring.
- Sclerotherapy is a same-day office procedure.

 ONGOING CARE

FOLLOW-UP RECOMMENDATIONS
Patient Monitoring
- Depending on method of treatment, initial follow-up is generally in the first 4 to 6 weeks.
- With sclerotherapy, follow-up is for confirmation of resolution or to proceed with retreatment.
- Postoperative follow-up at 2 to 4 weeks and subsequent 2- to 3-month intervals until resolution of any postoperative complications

PROGNOSIS
- Children/infants: As stated above, most congenital hydroceles resolve spontaneously with no intervention by age 2. For those that do need treatment, nearly all patients have resolution of symptoms after surgical intervention with very low long-term morbidity.
- Adults: low risk of long-term morbidity with either treatment method with eventual resolution of symptoms in nearly all cases depending on the underlying etiology (e.g., peritoneal dialysis)

COMPLICATIONS
- Complication rate for a scrotal approach may reach 30%.
- Postoperative traumatic hydrocele is common and usually resolves spontaneously.
- Injury to vas deferens or spermatic vessels
- Suture granuloma
- Hematoma
- Wound infection
- Recurrence

REFERENCES

1. Hall NJ, Ron O, Eaton S, et al. Surgery for hydrocele in children—an avoidable excess? *J Pediatr Surg*. 2011;46(12):2401–2405.
2. Alp BF, Irkilata HC, Kibar Y, et al. Comparison of the inguinal and scrotal approaches for the treatment of communicating hydrocele in children. *Kaohsiung J Med Sci*. 2014;30(4):200–205.
3. Lund L, Kloster A, Cao T. The long-term efficacy of hydrocele treatment with aspiration and sclerotherapy with polidocanol compared to placebo: a prospective, double-blind, randomized study. *J Urol*. 2014;191(5):1347–1350.
4. Tsai L, Milburn PA, Cecil CL, et al. Comparison of recurrence and postoperative complications between 3 different techniques for surgical repair of idiopathic hydrocele. *Urology*. 2019;125:239–242.
5. Shakiba B, Heidari K, Jamali A, et al. Aspiration and sclerotherapy versus hydrocelectomy for treating hydroceles. *Cochrane Database Syst Rev*. 2014;(11):CD009735. doi:10.1002/14651858.CD009735.pub2.

CODES

ICD10
- N43.0 Encysted hydrocele
- N43.3 Hydrocele, unspecified
- N43.2 Other hydrocele

CLINICAL PEARLS

- A hydrocele can usually be diagnosed by physical exam and transillumination. If there is any concern for other underlying process, a formal US is recommended.
- Aspiration alone is not indicated as the primary treatment of a hydrocele due to high recurrence rate.
- Attempted aspiration of an unconfirmed hydrocele could lead to bowel injury in an undiagnosed inguinal hernia and should not be attempted.
- Expectant management of children with hydrocele until >2 years of age is acceptable to allow sufficient time for spontaneous resolution, decreasing the likelihood of an unnecessary procedure.
- In adults, surgical resection costs more and has more complications but has a much lower recurrence rate and a much higher patient satisfaction rate.

H

HYDROCEPHALUS, NORMAL PRESSURE

Dennis E. Hughes, DO, FACEP

BASICS

DESCRIPTION

- Normal pressure hydrocephalus (NPH) is a clinical triad of gait instability, incontinence, and dementia (mnemonic: *wet, wobbly, wacky*); originally described by Hakim in 1957
- Two forms of the disorder: idiopathic and obstructive (the latter usually due to physical insult—posttrauma, meningitis, or subarachnoid hemorrhage)
- There is an absence of papilledema on clinical exam and normal cerebrospinal fluid (CSF) pressures at lumbar puncture

ALERT

- Idiopathic NPH (iNPH) primarily affects persons >60 years; extremely rare before 40 years
- Consider NPH in ground level falls of patients >60 years. In one study, over 10% had findings of NPH (1).

EPIDEMIOLOGY

- iNPH form primarily affects elderly, at least >40 years of age.
- Secondary form can occur at any age.
- Estimated to be a contributing factor in 6% of all cases of dementia

Incidence

Varies from 1.1% to 2.2%. Arriving at accurate data is hampered by uncertain diagnosis (2).

Prevalence

Ranges from 1.3% in the >65 years age group and increases to 5.9% in those 80 years and older. It is estimated that approximately 700,000 are affected in the United States (compared with 400,000 with multiple sclerosis) and 2,000,000 in Europe (2).

ETIOLOGY AND PATHOPHYSIOLOGY

- Idiopathic form is a communicating hydrocephalus, a disorder of decreased CSF absorption (not overproduction). In iNPH, the leading theory suggests that poor venous compliance impairs the subarachnoid granulations' ability to maintain baseline removal of CSF. In secondary NPH, scarring is likely.
- The result is a pressure gradient between the subarachnoid space and ventricular system.
- CSF production decreases in the face of an increased pressure set point (but still in excess of the amount of CSF absorbed).
- Elevated pressure distends ventricles and compresses the brain parenchyma, disrupting the normal cerebral blood flow with resulting ischemic changes leading to subsequent tissue damage and loss.

- Some believe that the idiopathic form is a result of persistently insufficient removal of CSF by immature subarachnoid granulations from childhood.
- Secondary NPH may result from the following:
  – Head trauma (most common)
  – Subarachnoid hemorrhage
  – Resolved acute meningitis
  – Chronic meningitis (tuberculosis, syphilis)
  – Paget disease of the skull

RISK FACTORS

Secondary form is due to head trauma, subarachnoid hemorrhage, meningitis, or encephalitis.

DIAGNOSIS

Detailed history and careful examination is the key to early diagnosis.

HISTORY

- Insidious and usually progressive; gait instability usually manifests initially, followed by changes in mentation, and, eventually, urinary incontinence.
- Behavioral changes noted in many cases: Depression, mania, and psychotic features in many cases precede the physical findings and respond poorly to usual treatment.
- Difficulty with initiation of movement: Feet appear "glued to the floor." Gait is wide based and shuffling, and turning appears "en bloc."
- Inattention, forgetfulness, and lack of spontaneity often are seen with the subcortical dementia of NPH.
- Urinary urgency initially, followed by lack of inhibition and then frank incontinence
- A minimum duration of at least 3 to 6 months of symptoms and progression over time
- A remote trauma or infection suggests secondary versus the idiopathic form.
- A lack of psychiatric, neurologic, or other medical conditions to explain the symptoms (including structural reasons for CSF flow restriction)
- Because memory impairment may be present, it is important to include a knowledgeable informant who is familiar with the patient's premorbid state.
- Frontal lobe function is affected disproportionately to the memory impairment (objective testing may lead to an early diagnosis).
- Many exhibit symptoms of Parkinsonism such as bradykinesia and rigidity.

PHYSICAL EXAM

- Decreased step height and length
- Reduced speed of walking (cadence)
- Widened standing base
- Swaying of trunk during walking
- Decreased fine motor speed and accuracy
- Recall impaired for recent events
- Impaired ability to do multistep tasks or interpret abstractions
- "Get up and go" testing (rise from chair, walk 10 steps, turn and return to start) useful

DIFFERENTIAL DIAGNOSIS

- Alzheimer disease (may be a comorbid condition in as many as 75%)
- Parkinson disease
- Chronic alcoholism
- Intracranial infection
- Multi-infarct dementia
- Subdural hematoma
- Carcinomatous meningitis
- Collagen vascular disorders
- Depression
- Syphilis
- Vitamin B_{12} deficiency
- Urologic disorders
- Case report suggesting Lyme disease may cause similar imaging and clinical characteristics (reversible with antibiotic treatment) (3)

DIAGNOSTIC TESTS & INTERPRETATION

Initial Tests (lab, imaging)

- Thyroid-stimulating hormone (TSH), syphilis serology, complete blood count, vitamin B_{12}, folate, metabolic profile
- Blood alcohol, analysis for drugs of abuse
- Urinalysis
- CSF analysis, including an opening pressure <245 mm H_2O (a value greater than this rules out iNPH by definition)
- Imaging is essential.
  – Either computed tomography (CT) or magnetic resonance imaging (MRI) (preferred imaging study) shows the ventriculomegaly (particularly lateral and 3rd ventricles) with preservation of the cerebral parenchyma (as opposed to ventricular enlargement seen in other forms of dementia where brain atrophy is present). A narrow subarachnoid space ("tight convexity") was recently shown to correlate to probable or definite iNPH.
  – Use of T1-weighted MRI images and combining Evans index (ratio of width of lateral ventricles/maximum internal diameter of skull) and the callosal angle gives good accuracy in differentiating NPH from other conditions (AUC = 0.96). Evans index of >0.3 suggestive of NPH (1).

Diagnostic Procedures/Other

CSF removal aids in the definitive diagnosis as well as predicting response to surgical treatment.

- High-volume (30 to 70 mL) CSF removal via spinal tap ("tap test") (4)
- Comparison of gait analysis before and after CSF removal should be performed within 24 hours (a ≥20% improvement indicates a positive test) especially when combined with coexisting executive function improvement. Testing should be done with a quantifiable gait scale (Berg Balance Scale, Timed Get Up and Go Test, etc.) (5).

 TREATMENT

MEDICATION

- No medication is significantly helpful.
- Use of carbonic anhydrase inhibitors (acetazolamide) with repeat lumbar punctures has provided mild and transient relief but is only supported by anecdotal evidence.
- Use of levodopa to rule out Parkinson disease may be helpful (NPH will display little, if any, significant improvement to dopamine agonist).

ISSUES FOR REFERRAL

- Neurology or neurosurgical consultation is helpful in suspected cases when other reversible medical conditions are ruled out.
- Recent cohort studies have demonstrated clinical improvement after surgical shunts. Perimeters of urinary continence, gait stability, and cognitive scores all improved at 1 year postshunt.

ADDITIONAL THERAPIES

Gait training and use of ambulation assist devices, as indicated, but limited efficacy

SURGERY/OTHER PROCEDURES

- Current therapy is limited to placement of ventricle-peritoneal or ventricle-atrial shunt from a lateral ventricle tunneled subcutaneous and drained into the peritoneal cavity (or right atrium). Recent work demonstrated that use of a lumbar-peritoneal shunt to be noninferior is technically easier and associated with less complications.

- Patients whose symptoms have been present for a shorter period (<2 years) have a greater chance of improvement with shunting. Age has not been shown to negatively affect response to shunting. Improvement has been seen in patients with symptoms present for many years and previously undiagnosed.
- Endoscopic 3rd ventriculostomy gaining attention as it obviates the shunt-related postoperative issues (late shunt infection, blocking, etc.) (2)

ADMISSION, INPATIENT, AND NURSING CONSIDERATIONS

For planned surgical treatment

 ONGOING CARE

FOLLOW-UP RECOMMENDATIONS

- Assessment and modification of environment for fall risks
- Evaluation for ability to operate a motor vehicle safely (if driving)

Patient Monitoring

- Repeat neuropsychological testing to evaluate the status of the dementia after treatment.
- Improvement in the incontinence and walking speed can also be objectively measured.

PATIENT EDUCATION

Information at https://www.ninds.nih.gov/Disorders/All-Disorders/Normal-Pressure-Hydrocephalus-Information-Page

PROGNOSIS

Natural history is progressive deterioration. Patient's axial skeletal stability worsens with inability to walk, stand, sit, or turn over in bed.

COMPLICATIONS

- In patients treated surgically, cerebral infarcts, hemorrhage, infection, and seizures (in addition to the usual surgical risks): all usual age-related illnesses (as NPH is a condition affecting those age >65 years)
- Shunt malfunction (especially when symptoms recur after successful shunt placement)

- Falls due to gait instability
- Urinary tract infections
- Skin breakdown, pressure ulcers, infections as movement dysfunction progresses

REFERENCES

1. Oike R, Inoue Y, Matsuzawa K, et al. Screening for idiopathic normal pressure hydrocephalus in the elderly after falls. *Clin Neurol Neurosurg*. 2021;205:106635.
2. Wang Z, Zhang Y, Hu F, et al. Pathogenesis and pathophysiology of idiopathic normal pressure hydrocephalus. *CNS Neurosci Ther*. 2020;26(12):1230–1240.
3. Gimsing LN, Hejl AM. Normal pressure hydrocephalus secondary to Lyme disease, a case report and review of seven reported cases. *BMC Neurol*. 2020;20(1):347.
4. Lee S-M, Kwon K-Y. Clinical tips in diagnosing idiopathic normal pressure hydrocephalus: a new concept beyond the cerebrospinal fluid tap test. *J Integr Neurosci*. 2021;20(2):471–475.
5. Allali G, Laidet M, Armand S, et al. Brain comorbidities in normal pressure hydrocephalus. *Eur J Neurol*. 2018;25(3):542–548.

 SEE ALSO

Algorithm: Ataxia

 CODES

ICD10

- G91.2 (Idiopathic) normal pressure hydrocephalus
- G91.0 Communicating hydrocephalus
- G91.3 Post-traumatic hydrocephalus, unspecified

CLINICAL PEARLS

- Consider in unexplained dementia or behavioral change.
- Insidious and usually progressive; gait instability usually manifests initially, followed by changes in mentation, and eventually, urinary incontinence.

H

HYDRONEPHROSIS
Pang-Yen Fan, MD • Mwangi Kamau, MD

 BASICS

DESCRIPTION
- Hydronephrosis refers to a structural finding: dilatation of the renal calyces and pelvis.
- Can be accompanied with hydroureter (dilatation of the ureter)
- Hydronephrosis should not be used interchangeably with obstructive uropathy, which refers to the damage to renal parenchyma resulting from urinary tract obstruction (UTO).

EPIDEMIOLOGY
- More common in children than adults due to congenital anomalies.
- Hydronephrosis is more common in women for adults <60 years old and in men for adults >60 years old.

ETIOLOGY AND PATHOPHYSIOLOGY
- Hydronephrosis develops with increased pressure in the urinary collecting system, most commonly from some form of obstruction.
- Nonobstructive hydronephrosis can occur in the setting of very high urinary output such as with diabetes insipidus or as a physiologic change in pregnancy.
- Hydronephrosis may be acute/chronic, partial/complete, and uni-/bilateral.
- Obstruction may occur at an level of the GU system:
  - Kidney: nephrolithiasis, transitional cell carcinoma, sloughed renal papillae, congenital ureteropelvic junction (UPJ) obstruction, blood clot, fungal ball
  - Ureter: nephrolithiasis, transitional cell carcinomas, strictures, sloughed renal papillae, retroperitoneal fibrosis, extrinsic compression
  - Bladder: neurogenic bladder, extrinsic compression, posterior urethral valves
  - Urethra: prostatic hypertrophy or cancer, strictures
- Hydronephrosis in a transplanted kidney is more common than in native kidneys, due to ureteral reflux, strictures, ureteral compression (from peritransplant lymphoceles, hematomas) and bladder dysfunction.

Pediatric Considerations
- Antenatal hydronephrosis is diagnosed in 1–5% of pregnancies, usually by US, as early as the 12th to 14th week of gestation.
- Children with antenatal hydronephrosis are at greater risk of postnatal pathology.
- Postnatal evaluation begins with US exam; further studies, such as voiding cystourethrogram (VCUG), based on the severity of postnatal hydronephrosis
- In neonates, it is the most common cause of abdominal mass.
- Common etiologies in children are VUR, congenital UPJ obstruction, neurogenic bladder, and posterior urethral valves.
- Pediatric diagnostic algorithm differs from adult due to different differential diagnosis necessitating age-appropriate testing.

Pregnancy Considerations
- Physiologic hydronephrosis in pregnancy is more prominent on the right than left and can be seen in up to 80% of pregnant women.
- Dilatation is caused by hormonal effects, external compression from expanding uterus, and intrinsic changes in the ureteral wall.
- Despite high incidence, most cases are asymptomatic.
- If symptomatic and refractory to medical management, ureteric calculus should be considered and urinary infection must be excluded.

 DIAGNOSIS

HISTORY
- Symptoms vary according to cause, chronicity, location, and degree of obstruction.
- Although often asymptomatic, hydronephrosis can be associated with pain ranging from vague, intermittent discomfort to severe renal colic.
- Can be associated with hematuria
- Nausea and vomiting may be associated with pain or infection.
- Fever and chills suggest coexisting urinary infection.
- Anuria suggests complete obstruction bilaterally or unilateral obstruction of a solitary kidney.
- Polyuria may occur due to impaired urinary concentration in partial obstruction.
- Symptoms of chronic kidney disease (CKD): anorexia, malaise, weight gain, edema, shortness of breath, mental state changes, tremors from long-standing obstruction
- Symptoms of bladder outlet obstruction: weak urine stream, nocturia, straining to void, overflow incontinence, urgency, and frequency
- General medical and surgical history: malignancy (extrinsic compression), radiotherapy (ureteric stricture/fibrosis), surgery (iatrogenic obstruction), trauma hematoma or fibrosis), gynecologic disease (extrinsic compression from endometriosis, ovarian masses, uterine prolapse), smoking (urothelial cancer), drugs (methysergide-induced retroperitoneal fibrosis)

PHYSICAL EXAM
- General signs
  - Volume overload (edema, rales, hypertension [HTN]) from renal failure
  - Diaphoresis, tachycardia, tachypnea with pain
  - High-grade fever, if infection
- Abdominal exam: CVA tenderness, palpable bladder, rarely palpable abdominal mass (may be visible, particularly in thin children)
- Pelvic exam: pelvic mass, uterine prolapse, palpable enlarged prostate (cancer or benign), urethral meatal stenosis, phimosis

DIAGNOSTIC TESTS & INTERPRETATION
- Urinalysis with microscopy: hematuria, proteinuria, crystalluria, pyuria
- Midstream urine culture and sensitivity: Exclude UTI.
- Basic metabolic panel: Elevated urea and creatinine may indicate obstructive uropathy. Hyperkalemic nonanion gap metabolic acidosis may indicate type 4 distal RTA due to obstruction.
- CBC: anemia of CKD, leukocytosis; if infection, check platelet count prior to considering ureteral instrumentation.
- Prostate-specific antigen (PSA): adult males age >50 years or with abnormal digital rectal exam or bladder outlet obstruction signs or symptoms
- Urine cytology: for malignant cells in urothelial malignancies
- US and noncontrast CT scanning are effective in diagnosing presence and cause of obstruction in most cases.
- US: screening test of choice for hydronephrosis
  - Sensitivity 90%, specificity 84.5%. Does not assess function and rarely detects cause and level of obstruction. Degree of hydronephrosis does not correlate with duration or severity of the obstruction.
  - Advantages: detects renal parenchymal disease (decreased renal size, increased cortical echogenicity, cortical thinning, cysts); no exposure to radiation or contrast; safe in pregnancy, contrast allergy, and renal dysfunction
  - False-positive findings 15.5%: normal extrarenal pelvis, parapelvic cysts, VUR, excessive diuresis
  - False-negative findings 10%: dehydration, acute obstruction, calyceal dilatation misinterpreted as renal cortical cysts, and retroperitoneal fibrosis
- Noncontrast helical CT (NHCT): test of choice for suspected nephrolithiasis
  - Reported sensitivity 94–96%, specificity 94–100%. Stone is most commonly found at levels of ureteric luminal narrowing: UPJ, pelvic brim, and the vesicoureteric junction.
  - Typical findings in acute obstruction are hydronephrosis with hydroureter proximal to the level of obstruction, perinephric stranding, and renal swelling. If chronic, renal atrophy may be noted.
  - Advantages: no contrast exposure, time-saving, cost-effective, identifies extraurinary pathology (1)
  - Disadvantages: does not assess function or degree of obstruction; higher radiation exposure, although low radiation dose protocols have shown comparable accuracy
- DTPA or MAG-3 radionuclide renal scan (diuretic renal scintigraphy)
  - Indicated only for evaluation of hydronephrosis without apparent obstruction
  - Determines presence of true obstruction as well as total and split (right vs. left) renal function
  - Furosemide is given 20 minutes after the tracer and the T1/2 for the tracer's washout is measured. T1/2; <10 minutes is unobstructed, >20 minutes

is obstructed, and 10 to 20 minutes is equivocal; some experts consider <15 minutes normal.
- Advantages: no contrast exposure, safe in contrast allergy and renal dysfunction
- False-positive findings: delayed excretion due to renal failure, massive dilatation causing a water-reservoir effect of delayed excretion without obstruction
- False-negative findings: dehydration or inadequate diuretic challenge
- Multiphase contrast-enhanced CT
  - Nonenhanced phase detects stones and swelling.
  - Parenchymal phase demonstrates decreased enhancement of renal parenchyma with acute obstruction; can identify extraurinary causes of obstruction and determine the relative glomerular filtration rate (GFR) of each kidney with accuracy equal to radionuclide renal scan
  - Delayed phase allows visualization of the collecting system and soft tissue filling defects (e.g., urothelial cancer).
- Magnetic resonance urography (MRU): indicated when US and NHCT are nondiagnostic
  - Provides anatomic, functional, and prognostic information; sensitivity not superior to US or NHCT for nephrolithiasis (70%) but superior for soft tissue causes including strictures
  - Advantages: no radiation exposure, safe in pregnancy
  - Disadvantages: more expensive and time-consuming (35 minutes vs. 5 minutes) and less available compared with CT. Gadolinium is contraindicated in renal failure especially when GFR is <30 mL/min due to risk of nephrogenic systemic fibrosis.

Follow-Up Tests & Special Considerations
The presence of fever in the setting of hydronephrosis should be considered a medical emergency due to the risk of bacteremia from urinary infection in an obstructed urinary system.

Diagnostic Procedures/Other
Cystoscopy, retrograde pyelogram ± ureteroscopy, and biopsy are occasionally used to determine the cause of obstruction (e.g., small urothelial cancer missed on imaging) or to confirm a normal distal ureter prior to pyeloplasty. In addition, such procedures are often needed to establish a definitive pathologic diagnosis for mass lesions.

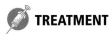 **TREATMENT**

GENERAL MEASURES
- Medical treatment: correction of fluid and electrolyte abnormalities, pain control, antibiotics as an adjunct to drainage if infection present
- Relief of obstruction: prompt drainage indicated in the presence of UTI, compromised renal function, or uncontrollable/persistent pain
  - Bladder outlet obstruction: urethral or suprapubic catheter
  - Ureteric obstruction: retrograde (cystoscopic) or antegrade (percutaneous) stenting (2)

- VUR is often managed conservatively with antibiotics; surgical management may be required in severe cases in children or women of childbearing age.
- Medical expulsive therapy (MET) with α-blockers or calcium channel blockers indicated for urethral stones <10 mm in patients with controlled pain, no signs of sepsis, with good renal function (3)[C]

SURGERY/OTHER PROCEDURES
- Hydronephrosis due to obstruction
  - Congenital UPJ obstruction: Pyeloplasty (open or laparoscopic) and minimally invasive stricture incision (endopyelotomy) are used with comparable results.
  - Nephrolithiasis: Extracorporeal shock wave lithotripsy (ESWL) is the initial treatment of choice for management of impacted upper urethral stones ≤2 cm. Ureteroscopy with or without intracorporeal lithotripsy has lower retreatment but higher complication rates and longer hospital stay; ureteral stenting pre-ESWL or postureteroscopy associated with no additional benefit and more discomfort and morbidity (4)[A],(5)
  - Transitional cell cancer: nephroureterectomy
  - Idiopathic retroperitoneal fibrosis: ureterolysis (frees ureters from inflammatory mass)
  - Prostate disorders: various treatment modalities, including transurethral resection of the prostate (TURP) and radical prostatectomy
- Nonobstructed hydronephrosis
  - VUR: ureteric reimplantation, endoscopic suburethral injection

ADMISSION, INPATIENT, AND NURSING CONSIDERATIONS
Obstruction coexisting with infection (pyonephrosis) is a true urologic emergency requiring urgent drainage. Typically, this requires placement of percutaneous nephrostomy tube(s) because retrograde (cystoscopic) stenting is often difficult, but both are equally effective.

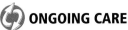 **ONGOING CARE**

FOLLOW-UP RECOMMENDATIONS
- Serial monitoring of kidney function (electrolytes, BUN, and creatinine) and BP until renal function stabilizes. Frequency of monitoring depends on severity of renal dysfunction.
- Follow-up US after stabilization of renal function to assess for resolution of hydronephrosis. If hydronephrosis persists, consider diuretic radionuclide study to rule out persistent obstruction.

PROGNOSIS
- Recovery of renal function depends on etiology, presence or absence of UTI, and degree and duration of obstruction.
- Significant recovery can occur despite days of complete obstruction, although some irreversible injury may develop within 24 hours. Delays in therapy can lead to irreversible renal damage (6).
- Diagnostic testing is of poor predictive value. Course of incomplete obstruction is highly unpredictable.

COMPLICATIONS
- Urine stasis: increased risk of infection and stones formation
- Obstruction causes progressive atrophy of kidney with irreversible loss of function.
- Spontaneous rupture of a calyx may occur with urine extravasation in the perinephric space.
- Postobstructive diuresis: marked polyuria after relief of obstruction:
  - Caused mostly by fluid and solute overload but may be exacerbated by impaired renal tubular concentrating ability. Urine output may be >500 mL/hr.
  - Replace urine losses with hypotonic fluid (usually with 0.45% NaCl) and only enough to avoid volume depletion. Replacement of urine output with equal amounts of saline will perpetuate the diuresis.

REFERENCES
1. Worster A, Preyra I, Weaver B, et al. The accuracy of noncontrast helical computed tomography versus intravenous pyelography in the diagnosis of suspected acute urolithiasis: a meta-analysis. *Ann Emerg Med.* 2002;40(3):280–286.
2. Ramsey S, Robertson A, Ablett MJ, et al. Evidence-based drainage of infected hydronephrosis secondary to ureteric calculi. *J Endourol.* 2010;24(2):185–189.
3. Seitz C, Liatsikos E, Porpiglia F, et al. Medical therapy to facilitate the passage of stones: what is the evidence? *Eur Urol.* 2009;56(3):455–471.
4. Aboumarzouk OM, Kata SG, Keeley FX, et al. Extracorporeal shock wave lithotripsy (ESWL) versus ureteroscopic management for ureteric calculi. *Cochrane Database Syst Rev.* 2011;(12):CD006029.
5. Shen P, Jiang M, Yang J, et al. Use of ureteral stent in extracorporeal shock wave lithotripsy for upper urinary calculi: a systematic review and meta-analysis. *J Urol.* 2011;186(4):1328–1335.
6. Cohen EP, Sobrero M, Roxe DM, et al. Reversibility of long-standing urinary tract obstruction requiring long-term dialysis. *Arch Intern Med.* 1992;152(1):177–179.

 CODES

ICD10
- N13.2 Hydronephrosis with renal and ureteral calculous obstruction
- N13.30 Unspecified hydronephrosis
- Q62.0 Congenital hydronephrosis

CLINICAL PEARLS
- US and noncontrast CT identify most causes of hydronephrosis.
- Relief of obstruction, when present, is the primary treatment.

H

HYPERCHOLESTEROLEMIA
Michelle Nelson, MD • Egle Klugiene, MD

BASICS

DESCRIPTION
- Elevated cholesterol is a significant risk factor for atherosclerotic cardiovascular disease (ASCVD).
- Lipoprotein subtypes:
  - Low-density lipoproteins (LDL): atherogenic; primary target of therapy
  - High-density lipoproteins (HDL): atheroprotective
  - Triglycerides (TG)
- System(s) affected: cardiovascular (CV)

EPIDEMIOLOGY
- 28% of U.S. adults >20 years old have hypercholesterolemia.
- 7% of U.S. children and adolescents between the ages of 6 and 19 years have hypercholesterolemia.

Prevalence
Disease incidence and prevalence increases with age.

ETIOLOGY AND PATHOPHYSIOLOGY
- Pathophysiology
  - Deposition of cholesterol in vascular walls creates fatty streaks that become fibrous plaques.
  - Inflammation causes plaque instability, leading to plaque rupture.
  - Atherosclerosis, inflammation, and vascular reactivity have a multifactorial etiology.
- Etiology of hypercholesterolemia
  - Primary: genetic causes (familial dyslipidemia)
  - Secondary: obesity, diet, excessive alcohol intake, hypothyroidism, diabetes, inflammatory disease, liver disease, nephrotic syndrome, chronic renal failure, medications (thiazide diuretics, carbamazepine, cyclosporine, progestins, anabolic steroids, corticosteroids, protease inhibitors, antipsychotics, isotretinoin)

Genetics
- Familial hypercholesterolemia (FH)
  - Elevated LDL levels from birth
  - Prevalence is 1:300 worldwide for heterozygous FH.
  - Predisposition to atherosclerotic disease in early adulthood and high coronary heart disease risk at younger ages. Individuals with homozygous FH typically die before 20 years old.
  - Early lipid-lowering drug therapy has been shown to reduce ASCVD risk.
- Early lipid screening of first-degree relatives is recommended.

RISK FACTORS
Obesity, physical inactivity, family history, cigarette smoking, excessive alcohol use. The relationship between dietary saturated fat and hypercholesterolemia and coronary artery disease is complex.

GENERAL PREVENTION
- Regular physical activity
- Weight control (see "Ongoing Care")
- Diet lower in saturated fats (grade 1B)

COMMONLY ASSOCIATED CONDITIONS
Hypertension, diabetes mellitus (DM), obesity

DIAGNOSIS

Screening recommendations:
- U.S. Preventive Services Task Force (USPSTF) (1)[A]: total cholesterol and HDL cholesterol (HDL-C) every 5 years
  - Men and women ≥40 years
  - No recommendation for or against screening in adults aged 21 to 39 years
  - No recommendation for or against screening in children and adolescents
- American Diabetes Association: yearly dyslipidemia screening for patients with diabetes

Pediatric Considerations
- National Heart, Lung, and Blood Institute: Recommend universal lipid screening on all children between 9 and 11 years and between 17 and 21 years old. This was endorsed by the American Academy of Pediatrics.
- Screening recommended for children with a family history of premature coronary artery disease or familial hypercholesterolemia.

HISTORY
- Review possible secondary etiologies (see "Etiology and Pathophysiology").
- Assess other ASCVD risk factors.

PHYSICAL EXAM
Nonspecific findings; may calculate BMI and examine for xanthomas

DIAGNOSTIC TESTS & INTERPRETATION
Initial Tests (lab, imaging)
- Lipid panel (nonfasting preferred). LDL is usually a calculated value and is accurate if TG <350 mg/dL. Perform fasting labs in hypertriglyceridemia (TG >440 mg/dL) or conditions that can elevated TG such as pancreatitis.
- Consider genetic etiology in very high LDL (>190 mg/dL) or TG (>500 mg/dL).

TREATMENT

ALERT
Multiple guidelines exist. The 2018 American College of Cardiology/American Heart Association (ACC/AHA) cholesterol guidelines return to targeting LDL goals. Risk stratifying patients should be reserved for primary prevention as patients with established CV disease should be considered high risk (secondary prevention).

- United States: ACC/AHA cholesterol guidelines (2)
  - According to the ACC/AHA, four groups benefit from statin therapy:
    ○ Primary elevation of LDL-C >190 mg/dL: high-intensity statin
    ○ Patients with diabetes ages 40 to 75 years with LDL-C >70 mg/dL: moderate-intensity statin
    ○ ASCVD risk based on Pooled Cohort Equations: http://tools.acc.org/ASCVD-Risk-Estimator (see below comment on calculator)
      ■ 10-year ASCVD risk <5%: lifestyle modifications with Mediterranean diet and exercise

- 10-year ASCVD risk 5–7.5%: moderate-intensity statin, discuss with patient
- 10-year ASCVD risk 7.5–20%: moderate-intensity statin with goal to reduce LDL-C by 30–49%
- 10-year ASCVD risk >20%: high-intensity statin with goal to reduce LDL-C >50%
  ○ Secondary ASCVD prevention
    ■ Age <75 years: high-intensity statin with goal to reduce LDL-C >50%. Add ezetimibe if LDL is >70 mg/dL after maximal statin therapy in very high-risk ASCVD patients.*
    ■ Age >75 years: moderate- or high-intensity statin as tolerated
  - *Definition of very high-risk ASCVD is at least one major ASCVD event and multiple high-risk conditions:
    ○ Major ASCVD events
      ■ Acute coronary syndrome or history of myocardial infarction, history of ischemic stroke, symptomatic peripheral arterial disease
    ○ High-risk conditions: age >65 years, heterozygous FH, history of CABG or PCI, diabetes mellitus, HTN, chronic kidney disease, current smoker, history of congestive heart failure, LDL-C >100 mg/dL despite maximum medical therapy
    ○ Controversy exists regarding the threshold calculated risk with which to treat patients: The Pooled Cohort Equations significantly *overestimates* 10-year ASCVD risk (50% or more). Therefore, discuss with patients the benefits and harms of statin therapy. Factor in patient longevity.
- United States: USPSTF statin recommendations (1)[A]
  - Adults aged 40 to 75 years with no history of CVD, one or more CVD risk factors (dyslipidemia, hypertension, diabetes, or smoking), and a calculated 10-year CVD event risk of 10% or greater: low- to moderate-intensity statin (grade B recommendation)
  - Adults aged 40 to 75 years with no history of CVD, one or more CVD risk factors, and a calculated 10-year CVD event risk of 7.5–10%: low- to moderate-dose statin (grade C recommendation)
  - Adults ≥76 years with no history of CVD: insufficient evidence to make recommendation
- United Kingdom: National Institute for Health and Care Excellence (NICE) cholesterol guidelines (3)
  - 10-year risk to be calculated using QRISK2: https://qrisk.org/three/
  - NICE recommends lifestyle modifications prior to starting any statin therapy in candidates under primary prevention consideration.
  - If 10-year risk of CVD >10% and no history of CVD, start atorvastatin 20 mg.
  - If 10-year risk of CVD >10% in presence of known CVD, start atorvastatin 80 mg.
  - Consider atorvastatin 20 mg if age ≥85 years to reduce the risk of nonfatal myocardial infarctions, though this is controversial due to uncertain benefit.
  - If estimated glomerular rate <60 or type I diabetes, start atorvastatin 20 mg.

MEDICATION

- Therapeutic lifestyle changes are cornerstone therapies to be attempted before drug therapy.
- Available data do not support initiation of statin therapy for primary prevention in most adults age >75 years (ALLHAT-LLT).
- Check lipid panel 4 to 12 weeks after starting medication to evaluate response and/or adherence.
  - Subsequent monitoring not generally indicated unless there is a question of patient adherence

First Line
HMG-CoA reductase inhibitors (statins)

- Categorized based on intensity
  - High intensity (reduces LDL-C by >50%): atorvastatin 40 to 80 mg/day, rosuvastatin 20 to 40 mg/day
  - Moderate intensity (reduces LDL-C by 30–49%): atorvastatin 10 to 20 mg/day, rosuvastatin 5 to 10 mg/day, simvastatin 20 to 40 mg/day, pravastatin 40 to 80 mg/day, lovastatin 40 mg/day, fluvastatin XL 80 mg/day, fluvastatin 40 mg BID, pitavastatin 2 to 4 mg/day
  - Low intensity (reduces LDL-C by <30%): simvastatin 10 mg/day, pravastatin 10 to 20 mg/day, lovastatin 20 mg/day, fluvastatin 20 to 40 mg/day, pitavastatin 1 mg/day
- Effect is greatest in lowering LDL-C; shown to decrease coronary heart disease incidence and all-cause mortality (1).
- Contraindications: pregnancy, lactation, or active liver disease
- Adverse reactions:
  - Mild myalgia is common.
  - Liver transaminase elevations: alanine aminotransferase (ALT) before therapy to establish baseline; if ALT >3 times upper limit of normal, do not start statin; routine monitoring is not recommended.
  - Association with increased cases of diabetes: 0.1 excess cases of diabetes per 100 persons on moderate-intensity statin and 0.3 excess cases per 100 persons on high-intensity statin
  - Myopathies (considered rare but not well studied)
  - Statin intolerance
    - Consider using a different statin.
    - Dose reduction
    - Alternate day therapy
    - A majority of patients who had previously discontinued statins due to side effects are able to restart the same or another statin and tolerate them.

- Do not exceed simvastatin 10 mg/day with amiodarone, verapamil, and diltiazem.
- Do not exceed simvastatin 20 mg/day with amlodipine and ranolazine.
- Drug interactions: Some HMG-CoA reductase inhibitors can interact with hepatitis C antiviral medications. Interactions can be checked at https://www.hep-druginteractions.org/checker.
- Avoid grapefruit juice with statins as it can increase the risk of statin myopathy.

Pregnancy Considerations
- Statins contraindicated during pregnancy.
- Lactation: possibly unsafe

Second Line
- Second-line drugs are now recommended in primary prevention if LDL-C is >70 mg/dL on maximal statin therapy.
- Ezetimibe
  - Can be taken by itself or in combination with a statin: monotherapy (10 mg/day) or ezetimibe/simvastatin
  - Effect: lowers LDL-C; one randomized controlled trial shows combination therapy with statin has small benefit in reducing CV events and CV-related mortality after acute coronary syndromes.
- Fibrates
  - Types: gemfibrozil, fenofibrate
  - Effect: most effective in lowering TG with moderate effect in lowering LDL and raising HDL. More recent studies fail to show mortality benefit in most patients.
- Niacin raises HDL but no evidence for improved outcomes; should not be used routinely.
- PCSK9 inhibitors (e.g., alirocumab, evolocumab)
  - Monoclonal antibody. Current evidence shows decreased incidence of CVD in secondary prevention without affecting incidence of all-cause mortality; VERY expensive

COMPLEMENTARY & ALTERNATIVE MEDICINE
Omega-3 fatty acids and fish oil intake:

- Sources—fatty fish, plants (flaxseed, canola oil, soybean oil, nuts)
- Effect—decreases TG and LDL level and increases HDL. Overall CV benefit and mortality reduction is uncertain.

ADMISSION, INPATIENT, AND NURSING CONSIDERATIONS
If lipid panel was checked while inpatient due to myocardial infarction, recommend rechecking a fasting lipid panel in 4 to 12 weeks after discharge as the first lab may not be as accurate.

 ## ONGOING CARE

FOLLOW-UP RECOMMENDATIONS
Moderate intensity exercise for 150 minutes per week: increases HDL, lowers TC, and helps control weight

Patient Monitoring
Routine monitoring of liver function tests is no longer recommended if initial ALT is within normal range.

DIET
Plant-based diets and the Mediterranean diet, which are high in legumes, fruits, vegetables, nuts, fish, and olive oil reduce the risk of CV disease.

PATIENT EDUCATION
From the American Heart Association on the Mediterranean diet: https://www.heart.org/en/healthy-living/healthy-eating/eat-smart/nutrition-basics/mediterranean-diet

COMPLICATIONS
Myocardial infarction, peripheral artery disease, cerebrovascular accident

REFERENCES
1. U.S. Preventive Services Task Force. Final recommendation statement: statin use for the primary prevention of cardiovascular disease in adults: preventive medication. https://uspreventiveservicestaskforce.org/uspstf/recommendation/statin-use-in-adults-preventive-medication. Accessed September 28, 2021.
2. Grundy SM, Stone NJ, Bailey AL, et al. 2018 AHA/ACC/AACVPR/AAPA/ABC/ACPM/ADA/AGS/APhA/ASPC/NLA/PCNA guideline on the management of blood cholesterol: executive summary: a report of the American College of Cardiology/American Heart Association Task Force on Clinical Practice Guidelines. *J Am Coll Cardiol*. 2019;73(24):3168–3209.
3. National Institute for Health and Care Excellence. Cardiovascular disease: risk assessment and reduction, including lipid modification. https://www.nice.org.uk/guidance/cg181/chapter/1-recommendations. Accessed September 28, 2021.

 SEE ALSO

Diabetes Mellitus, Type 2; Hypertension, Essential; Obesity

CODES

ICD10
E78.0 Pure hypercholesterolemia

CLINICAL PEARLS

- A plant-based diet, or the Mediterranean diet, and exercise should be tried before pharmaceutical interventions.
- Decision to initiate statins in primary prevention should be based on risk and patient preferences.

H

HYPEREMESIS GRAVIDARUM

Lorena Likaj, MD, MPH • Robert A. Monteleone, MD

 BASICS

- Nausea and vomiting in pregnancy is a common condition that affects approximately 70–80% of pregnancies.
- A more severe form of nausea and vomiting, hyperemesis gravidarum, affects 0.5–2% of pregnancies, and can have significant adverse physical and psychological sequela.
- Hyperemesis gravidarum remains a diagnosis of clinical judgement and is one of the most common indications for hospitalization during pregnancy.
- Hyperemesis gravidarum is associated with several adverse fetal outcomes including preterm delivery, low birth weight, small for gestation age, low 5-minute Apgar scores, and neurodevelopmental delay.

DESCRIPTION

- Although morning sickness is common during pregnancy, hyperemesis gravidarum is a rare condition.
- Hyperemesis gravidarum is intractable vomiting in a pregnant woman that interferes with fluid and electrolyte balance as well as nutrition:
  – Usually associated with the first 8 to 20 weeks of pregnancy
  – Believed to have biomedical and behavioral aspects
  – Associated with high estrogen and human chorionic gonadotropin (hCG) levels
  – Symptoms usually begin ~2 weeks after first missed period, peak around the 12th week, and resolve by the 20th week
- System(s) affected: endocrine/metabolic, gastrointestinal (GI), reproductive

EPIDEMIOLOGY

- Generally affects young women, primiparous, non-smokers, and non-Caucasians
- Other risk factors include prior history of hyperemesis, preexisting diabetes, hyperthyroid disorder, psychiatric illness, asthma, and GI disorders.

Incidence

Hyperemesis gravidarum occurs in 0.5–2% of pregnancies.

Prevalence

Hyperemesis gravidarum is the most common cause of hospitalization in the first half of pregnancy and the second most common cause of hospitalization of all pregnant women.

ETIOLOGY AND PATHOPHYSIOLOGY

Etiology unknown. Proposed influences include:
- Hyperthyroidism
- Hyperparathyroidism
- Pregnancy hormones
- Liver dysfunction
- Autonomic nervous system dysfunction
- CNS neoplasm
- Addison disease
- Possible psychological factors

Genetics

Increased risk if maternal family history of hyperemesis gravidarum

RISK FACTORS

- Nulliparity
- Multiple gestations
- History of migraines
- History of motion sickness
- Black or Asian women
- Gestational trophoblastic disease
- Fetus with trisomy 21
- Female fetus
- Possible association with *Helicobacter pylori* infection

GENERAL PREVENTION

Anticipatory guidance regarding dietary habits to avoid dehydration and nutritional depletion
- Small, frequent meals
- Avoiding an overly empty or full stomach

 DIAGNOSIS

The definition of hyperemesis gravidarum varies but often includes intractable nausea and vomiting in pregnancy, signs of dehydration, electrolyte imbalances after the exclusion of other causes of severe nausea and vomiting.

HISTORY

- Nausea
- Vomiting with retching >3 times per day
- Decreased urine output
- Fatigue
- Dizziness with standing
- Poor appetite

PHYSICAL EXAM

- >5% weight loss from prepregnancy weight
- Thyroid evaluation
- Signs of dehydration, such as orthostatic hypotension, large ketonuria, high urine specific gravity

DIFFERENTIAL DIAGNOSIS

Other common causes of vomiting must be considered:
- Gastroenteritis
- Gastritis
- Reflux esophagitis
- Peptic ulcer disease
- Cholelithiasis
- Cholecystitis
- Pyelonephritis
- Appendicitis
- Pancreatitis
- Anxiety
- Hyperparathyroidism
- Hypercalcemia
- Thyrotoxicosis
- *H. pylori* infection

DIAGNOSTIC TESTS & INTERPRETATION

Initial laboratory studies for hyperemesis gravidarum are used to evaluate maternal clinical status and rule out other possible causes of nausea and vomiting.

Initial Tests (lab, imaging)

- Urinalysis: may see glucosuria, albuminuria, granular casts, and hematuria (rare); ketosis more common
- Thyroid-stimulating hormone (TSH), free T_4
- Electrolytes, BUN, creatinine:
  – Electrolyte abnormalities due to nausea and vomiting and subsequent dehydration
  – Acidosis
- Liver enzymes and bilirubin levels
- Hematocrit
- Hepatitis panel
- Calcium
- Albumin

Follow-Up Tests & Special Considerations

No imaging is indicated unless there is a concern for hydatidiform mole or multiple gestation, in which case ultrasound may be obtained.

Diagnostic Procedures/Other

Indicated only if it is necessary to rule out other diagnoses, as listed in the following section:
- Upper abdominal ultrasound if pancreatitis or cholecystitis is suspected to be the cause of nausea and vomiting.
- Abdominal MRI of appendicitis is the suspected cause of nausea and vomiting.

Test Interpretation

- Urinalysis: When positive for ketones and high specific gravity, indicate starvation ketosis and volume depletion.
- TSH, free T_4: A transient hyperthyroidism (suppressed TSH with normal free T_4) may be present in approximately 50% of hyperemesis gravidarum; if TSH is suppressed with elevated free T_4, further investigation needed for overt hyperthyroidism
- Electrolytes, BUN, creatinine: Dehydration can cause low potassium, low sodium, and elevated BUN and creatinine.
- Liver enzymes and bilirubin levels: Mild elevation of AST and ALT occurs in approx 50% of cases and self-resolves. Other etiologies of must be considered with significantly elevated liver enzymes.
- Hematocrit: Dehydration causes increase (volume contraction).
- Hepatitis panel: Hepatitis A, B, and C may present similarly to hyperemesis; consider and rule out.
- Calcium: Hypercalcemia resulting from hyperparathyroidism occurs rarely.
- Albumin: Decreased albumin may indicate malnutrition secondary to nausea and vomiting.

 TREATMENT

Pyridoxine and doxylamine (pregnancy Category A) are first-line treatments for hyperemesis gravidarum (1)[C]. This is followed by metoclopramide or ondansetron (pregnancy Category B) and then prochlorperazine (pregnancy Category C), methylprednisolone (pregnancy Category C), or promethazine (pregnancy Category C).

GENERAL MEASURES

- First, treat dehydration and electrolyte imbalances and then treat nausea.
- IV fluids, either normal saline or 5% dextrose normal saline (with consideration for potential thiamine deficiency)
- For severe cases, consider PO thiamine 25 to 50 mg TID or IV 100 mg in 100 mL of normal saline over 30 minutes once weekly and potential parental nutrition if needed.
- Ondansetron carries an FDA warning for concerns of QT prolongation. It has unclear risk in the setting of pregnancy. The majority of the current studies appear to show no increased risk of fetal malformation, but this is still an area of controversy.

MEDICATION

- Pyridoxine (vitamin B_6) 25 mg PO or IV every 8 hours, max dose of 200 mg/day
- Antihistamines (e.g., diphenhydramine [25 to 50 mg q4–6h], doxylamine [12.5 mg PO BID], meclizine [25 mg PO q4–6h], and dimenhydrinate [25 to 50 mg PO q4–6h]) (2)[C]
- Combination product Diclegis (sustained-release pyridoxine 10 mg and doxylamine 10 mg) dosed (start 2 tabs PO QHS; if symptoms persist, increase to 1 tab in AM and 2 QHS; if symptoms still persist, take 1 tab every AM, 1 midday, and 2 QHS; max 4 tablets/day) or doxylamine 12.5 mg and pyridoxine 25 mg
- Phenothiazines (e.g., promethazine or prochlorperazine):
  – Precautions: Phenothiazines are associated with prolonged jaundice, extrapyramidal effects, and hyper- or hyporeflexia in newborns.
- Metoclopramide 10 mg PO q6–8h
- Methylprednisolone 16 mg PO/IV q8h for 2 to 3 days and then taper over 2 weeks if initial 3-day treatment is effective; reserved for severe cases with unclear benefit
- Ondansetron 4 to 8 mg PO q8h

Pregnancy Considerations
All medications taken during pregnancy should balance the risks and benefits both to the mother and the fetus.

First Line
- For women with mild to moderate nausea, pyridoxine (vitamin B_6) 10 to 25 mg PO or IV q8h can improve symptoms and has a good safety profile. Maximum dose is 200 mg/day.
- If nausea and vomiting continue, combination doxylamine succinate 12.5 mg and pyridoxine 25 mg PO q8h. This combination is more effective than either drug alone.
- Ginger capsules 350 mg PO TID can be added with refractory vomiting.

Second Line
- Antihistamines such as diphenhydramine, meclizine, and dimenhydrinate. Doxylamine-pyridoxine should be discontinued before starting a different antihistamine.
- Metoclopramide 10 mg PO q8h
- Promethazine 12.5 mg PO or rectally q8h
- Ondansetron 4 to 8 mg PO or IV q8h

ISSUES FOR REFERRAL
- Inpatient management required for IV antiemetics and fluids for symptoms refractory to outpatient management
- Referral to gastroenterology or surgery if the etiology of nausea and vomiting is more consistent with alternate diagnosis.
- May also consider psychiatry or psychology referral if psychological assessment is warranted

ADDITIONAL THERAPIES
- Glucocorticoids (methylprednisolone 16 mg IV q8h for 48 to 72 hours) of uncertain benefit but may be considered for severe and refractory cases
- H_2 receptor antagonists (cimetidine and ranitidine) as adjunctive therapy to reduce heartburn/acid reflux

SURGERY/OTHER PROCEDURES
Rarely, if all pharmacologic and nonpharmacologic interventions fail and weight loss continues, tube feeding or parenteral nutrition is initiated. Enteral nutrition, either through a gastric or duodenal route, is preferred to the parenteral route, as it may relieve nausea and vomiting.

COMPLEMENTARY & ALTERNATIVE MEDICINE
- Ginger 350 mg PO q6h may help (3)[A].
- Mixed evidence for acupressure and acupuncture. Acupressure bands at the Neiguan point are effective adjuvant treatment in severe hyperemesis (4)[A].
- Medical hypnosis may be a helpful adjunct to the typical medical treatment regimen, but further study is needed.

ADMISSION, INPATIENT, AND NURSING CONSIDERATIONS
- Typically outpatient therapy
- In some severe cases, parenteral therapy in the hospital or at home may be required.
- Enteral volume and nutrition repletion may be indicated, but early enteral tube feeding does not improve maternal or perinatal outcomes (5)[A].

 ONGOING CARE

Approximately 10% of patients with hyperemesis gravidarum will be affected throughout the pregnancy.

FOLLOW-UP RECOMMENDATIONS
Overall quality of life and future fertility plans can be impacted by severity of nausea and vomiting (6)[B].

Patient Monitoring
- In severe cases, follow-up on a daily basis for weight monitoring
- Special attention should be given to monitor for ketosis, hypokalemia, or acid–base disturbances due to hyperemesis.

DIET
- Bland or liquid diet as tolerated
- For outpatient: a diet rich in carbohydrates and protein, such as fruit, cheese, cottage cheese, eggs, beef, poultry, vegetables, toast, crackers, rice. Patients should avoid spicy meals and high-fat foods. Encourage small amounts at a time every 1 to 2 hours.

PATIENT EDUCATION
- Attention should be given to psychosocial issues, such as possible ambivalence about the pregnancy.
- Patients should be instructed to take small amounts of fluid frequently to avoid volume depletion.
- Avoid individual foods known to be irritating to the patient.
- Wet-to-dry nutrients (sherbet, broth, gelatin to dry crackers, toast)

PROGNOSIS
- Self-limited illness with good prognosis if patient's weight is maintained at >95% of prepregnancy weight.
- With complication of hemorrhagic retinitis, mortality rate of pregnant patient is 50%.

COMPLICATIONS
- Maternal complications:
  – Vitamin deficiency, dehydration, and malnutrition
  – In severe cases, Wernicke encephalopathy secondary to thiamine deficiency, coma, and even death
- Fetal complications:
  – Patients with >5% weight loss are associated with intrauterine growth retardation and fetal anomalies.
  – Poor weight gain is associated with slightly increased risk for small for gestational age infant <2,500 g and premature birth <37 weeks (7)[A].
  – Hemorrhagic retinitis
  – Liver damage

REFERENCES

1. Maltepe C, Koren G. The management of nausea and vomiting of pregnancy and hyperemesis gravidarum—a 2013 update. *J Popul Ther Clin Pharmacol.* 2013;20(2):e184–e192.
2. Boelig RC, Barton SJ, Saccone G, et al. Interventions for treating hyperemesis gravidarum. *Cochrane Database Syst Rev.* 2016;(5):CD010607.
3. Viljoen E, Visser J, Koen N, et al. A systematic review and meta-analysis of the effect and safety of ginger in the treatment of pregnancy-associated nausea and vomiting. *Nutr J.* 2014;13:20.
4. Adlan AS, Chooi KY, Mat Adenan NA. Acupressure as adjuvant treatment for the inpatient management of nausea and vomiting in early pregnancy: a double-blind randomized controlled trial. *J Obstet Gynaecol Res.* 2017;43(4):662–668.
5. Grooten IJ, Koot MH, van der Post JA, et al. Early enteral tube feeding in optimizing treatment of hyperemesis gravidarum: the Maternal and Offspring outcomes after Treatment of HyperEmesis by Refeeding (MOTHER) randomized controlled trial. *Am J Clin Nutr.* 2017;106(3):812–820.
6. Heitmann K, Nordeng H, Havnen GC, et al. The burden of nausea and vomiting during pregnancy: severe impacts on quality of life, daily life functioning and willingness to become pregnant again—results from a cross-sectional study. *BMC Pregnancy Childbirth.* 2017;17(1):75.
7. Veenendaal MVE, van Abeelen AFM, Painter RC, et al. Consequences of hyperemesis gravidarum for offspring: a systematic review and meta-analysis. *BJOG.* 2011;118(11):1302–1313.

ADDITIONAL READING

- Boelig RC, Barton SJ, Saccone G, et al. Interventions for treating hyperemesis gravidarum: a Cochrane systematic review and meta-analysis. *J Matern Fetal Neonatal Med.* 2018;31(18):2492–2505.
- Jarvis S, Nelson-Piercy C. Management of nausea and vomiting in pregnancy. *BMJ.* 2011;342:d3606.
- Matthews A, Haas DM, O'Mathúna DP, et al. Interventions for nausea and vomiting in early pregnancy. *Cochrane Database Syst Rev.* 2015;2015(9):CD007575.

CODES

ICD10
- O21.9 Vomiting of pregnancy, unspecified
- O21.0 Mild hyperemesis gravidarum
- O21.1 Hyperemesis gravidarum with metabolic disturbance

CLINICAL PEARLS

- Do not allow patients to become volume depleted. Once this occurs, it is more difficult to interrupt the process.
- Do not be hesitant to use medications to assist the patient, as this may help avoid volume depletion.
- Consider secondary causes of hyperemesis if it develops after 12 weeks of gestation.

HYPERKALEMIA

Waiz Wasey, MD • Sarah Hutchings, MD • Rebecca Dix, MD

 BASICS

DESCRIPTION
- Hyperkalemia is a common electrolyte disorder defined as a plasma potassium (K) concentration >5.5 mEq/L (>5 mmol/L).
- Hyperkalemia depresses cardiac conduction and can lead to fatal arrhythmias.
- Normal K regulation
  - Ingested K enters portal circulation; pancreas releases insulin in response. Insulin facilitates K entry into cells.
  - K in renal circulation causes renin release from juxtaglomerular cells, leading to activation of angiotensin I, which is converted to angiotensin II in lungs. Angiotensin II acts in adrenal zona glomerulosa to stimulate aldosterone secretion. Aldosterone, at the renal collecting ducts, causes K to be excreted and sodium to be retained.
- Four major causes
  - Increased load: either endogenous from tissue release or exogenous from a high intake, usually in association with decreased excretion
  - Decreased excretion: due to decreased glomerular filtration rate or impaired aldosterone secretion
  - Cellular redistribution: shifts from intracellular space (majority of K is intracellular) to extracellular space
  - Pseudohyperkalemia: related to red cell lysis during collection or transport of blood sample, thrombocytosis, or leukocytosis

Geriatric Considerations
Increased risk for hyperkalemia because of decreases in renin and aldosterone as well as comorbid conditions

EPIDEMIOLOGY
Incidence
Incidence is higher in patients of older age, male sex, worse kidney function, comorbidities, and use of renin angiotensin-aldosterone system inhibitors (1).

Prevalence
- 1–10% of hospitalized patients
- 2–3% in general population but as high as 50% in patients with chronic kidney disease (2)

ETIOLOGY AND PATHOPHYSIOLOGY
- Pseudohyperkalemia
  - Hemolysis of red cells in phlebotomy tube (spurious result is most common)
  - Thrombolysis
  - Leukocytosis (reverse pseudohyperkalemia)
  - Thrombocytosis
  - Hereditary spherocytosis
  - Infectious mononucleosis
  - Traumatic venipuncture or fist clenching during phlebotomy (spurious result)
  - Familial pseudohyperkalemia
- Increased K intake (3)
  - Banana, potatoes, melons, citrus juice, and avocados
  - Salt substitutes given to chronic kidney patients
  - Clay ingestion
  - Consuming burn match heads

- Transcellular shift (redistribution)
  - Metabolic acidosis
  - Insulin deficiency
  - Hyperglycemia (diabetic ketoacidosis or hyperosmolar hyperglycemic state)
  - Tissue damage (rhabdomyolysis, burns, trauma)
  - Cocaine abuse
  - Exercise with heavy sweating
- Impaired K excretion
  - Renal insufficiency/failure
  - Addison disease
  - Mineralocorticoid deficiency
  - Primary hyporeninemia, primary hypoaldosteronism
  - Type IV renal tubular acidosis (hyporeninemic hypoaldosteronism)
  - Obstructive uropathy
  - Cirrhosis
  - Congestive heart failure
  - Sickle cell disease
  - Amyloidosis
  - Gordon syndrome
  - Systemic lupus erythematosus
- Medication-induced (numerous)

Genetics
Associated with some inherited diseases and conditions
- Familial hyperkalemic periodic paralysis
- Congenital adrenal hyperplasia

RISK FACTORS
- Impaired renal excretion of K
- Acidemia
- Massive cell breakdown (rhabdomyolysis, burns, trauma)
- Use of K-sparing diuretics
- Excess K supplementation
- Comorbid conditions: chronic kidney disease, diabetes, heart failure, liver disease

GENERAL PREVENTION
Low K diet and oral supplement compliance in those at risk

COMMONLY ASSOCIATED CONDITIONS
- Chronic kidney disease
- End-stage renal disease
- Congestive heart failure
- Myocardial infarction
- Rhabdomyolysis
- Liver disease
- Use of medications such as ACE inhibitors or angiotensin II receptor blockers

 DIAGNOSIS

Serum K level greater than the normal range (3.5 to 5.0 mEq/L)

HISTORY
- Neuromuscular cramps, myalgias, muscle weakness or paralysis
- Abdominal pain
- Palpitations
- Numbness

PHYSICAL EXAM
- Decreased deep tendon reflexes
- Muscle weakness or flaccid paralysis of extremities

DIAGNOSTIC TESTS & INTERPRETATION
- Serum electrolytes
- Renal function: BUN, creatinine
- Urinalysis: K, creatinine, osmoles (to calculate fractional excretion of K and transtubular K gradient; both assess renal handling of K)
- Disorders that may alter lab results
  - Acidemia: K shifts from the intracellular to extracellular space.
  - Insulin deficiency
  - Hemolysis of sample
- Cortisol, aldosterone, and renin levels to check for mineralocorticoid deficiency when other causes are ruled out

Diagnostic Procedures/Other
ECG abnormalities usually occur when K ≥7 mEq/L.
- Peaked T wave with shortened QT interval in precordial leads (most common, usually earliest ECG change; however, neither sensitive nor specific) (4)[C]
- Lengthening of PR interval, loss of P wave, widened QRS
- Sine wave at very high K
- Can eventually lead to arrhythmias including bradycardia, ventricular fibrillation, and asystole

 TREATMENT

MEDICATION
- Stabilize myocardial membranes; initial treatment with calcium gluconate IV 1,000 mg (10 mL of 10% solution) over 2 to 3 minutes (5)[A]
  - With constant cardiac monitoring
  - Can repeat after 5 minutes if needed
  - Effect begins within minutes, but only lasts 30 to 60 minutes and should be used in conjunction with definitive therapies
  - Can also use calcium chloride (3 times as concentrated; however, central or deep vein administration is necessary to avoid tissue necrosis).
- Drive extracellular K into cells.
  - Nebulized albuterol (at 10 to 20 mg/4 mL saline >10 minutes—4 to 8 times bronchodilation dose) and other β-agonists have an additive effect with insulin and glucose (5)[B].
  - Dextrose 50% 1 amp (if plasma glucose <250 mg/dL) and insulin 10 U IV may drive K intracellularly but does not decrease total body K and may result in hypoglycemia (close monitoring advised, especially 1 to 2 hours postinjection) (5)[B].
  - Sodium bicarbonate not routinely recommended but some possible benefits in severe metabolic acidosis (6)[C]

- Remove excess K from body.
  - Cation exchange resins definitive treatment but require several doses and best used with rapidly acting transient therapies above and when dialysis not readily available (7)[A]
  - Gastrointestinal cation exchangers, patiromer calcium (Veltassa), sodium polystyrene sulfonate (Kayexalate), and zirconium cyclosilicate bind K in the intestinal tract. Patiromer in particular is favored for improved tolerance and decreased side effects in both acute and chronic settings (8)[C].
  - Patiromer calcium (Veltassa): 8.4 g PO daily (dose may vary 4.2 to 16.8 g BID in studies)
    - This requires ~7 to 24 hours to lower K. This may be repeated q12h, if necessary (9)[C].
  - Sodium polystyrene sulfonate (Kayexalate): 15 g PO or 30 g rectally
    - This requires 1 to 4 hours to lower K. This may be repeated q6h, if necessary.
    - Enema has faster effect than PO (5)[C].
  - Loop diuretics (furosemide): 40 mg IV q12h or continuous infusion
  - Hemodialysis is the definitive therapy when other measures are not effective. This may be required particularly when conditions, such as digitalis toxicity, rhabdomyolysis, end-stage renal disease, severe chronic kidney disease, or acute kidney injury, are present; should watch for postdialysis rebound (5)[A]
  - Little clinical evidence for the use of diuretics (loop and thiazides), however, can consider for control of chronic hyperkalemia (5)[B]
- Chronic hyperkalemia treatment
  - Review medication and discontinue those that can be contributing to hyperkalemia.
  - Dietary counseling of K-rich food
  - Diuretic therapy using thiazide and loop diuretics

ALERT
- Sodium polystyrene sulfonate (Kayexalate) provides a sodium load that may exacerbate fluid overload in patients with cardiac or renal failure.
- Avoid sodium polystyrene sulfonate use in patients who are postoperative or with a bowel obstruction or ileus due to high risk of intestinal necrosis.
- Rapid administration of calcium in patients with suspected digitalis toxicity may result in a fatal dysrhythmia. Calcium should be administered slowly over 20 to 30 minutes in 5% dextrose with extreme caution. Preferred therapy is digoxin-specific antibody fragments.

ADDITIONAL THERAPIES
Mineralocorticoid replacement (10)
- If the patient does not have a contraindication (greater than stage 1 HTN, volume overload, history of heart failure) to mineralocorticoid administration then
  - Consider a trial of fludrocortisone 0.1 mg daily × 3 to 5 days (10) (in patients with moderately advanced chronic kidney disease, consider maintaining or increasing diuretics in tandem with the assistance of nephrology consulting service).

ADMISSION, INPATIENT, AND NURSING CONSIDERATIONS
- If hyperkalemia is severe, treat first, and then do diagnostic investigations.
- IV calcium to stabilize myocardium (caution in setting of digoxin toxicity/digoxin-induced hyperkalemia, as this treatment can induce heart block)
- Insulin (usually 10 U IV, given with 50 mL of 50% glucose [if serum glucose <250 mg/dL] to avoid hypoglycemia); consider repeating if elevation persists.
- Inhaled β_2-agonist (nebulized albuterol)
- Discontinue any medications that may increase K (e.g., K-sparing diuretics, exogenous K).
- Admit for cardiac monitoring if ECG changes are present or if K is >6 mEq/L (6 mmol/L).

 ONGOING CARE

FOLLOW-UP RECOMMENDATIONS
Patient Monitoring
Serum K levels should be rechecked every 2 to 4 hours until the patient has stabilized, and recurrent hyperkalemia is no longer a threat.

DIET
Recommend ≤80 mEq (≤80 mmol) of K per 24 hours. Many foods contain K. Those that are particularly high in K (>6.4 mEq/serving) include bananas, orange juice, other citrus fruits and their juices, figs, molasses, seaweed, dried fruits, nuts, avocados, lima beans, bran, tomatoes, tomato juice, cantaloupe, honeydew melon, peaches, potatoes, and salt substitutes. Multiple herbal medications can also increase K levels, including alfalfa, dandelion, horsetail nettle, milkweed, hawthorn berries, toad skin, oleander, foxglove, and ginseng.

PATIENT EDUCATION
Consult with a dietitian about a low-K diet.

PROGNOSIS
- Associated with poor prognosis in patients with heart failure and chronic kidney disease
- Associated with poor prognosis in disaster medicine, with trauma, tissue necrosis, K^+ supplementation, metabolic acidosis, if calcium gluconate administered for treatment of hyperkalemia, if AKI, or if prolonged duration of hyperkalemia (6)

COMPLICATIONS
- Life-threatening cardiac arrhythmias
- Potential complications of the use of ion-exchange resins for the treatment of hyperkalemia include volume overload and intestinal necrosis (8)[C].

REFERENCES
1. Nilsson E, Gasparini A, Ärnlöv J, et al. Incidence and determinants of hyperkalemia and hypokalemia in a large healthcare system. *Int J Cardiol*. 2017;245:277–284.
2. Palmer BF, Clegg DJ. Hyperkalemia. *JAMA*. 2015;314(22):2405–2406.
3. Palmer BF, Clegg DJ. Diagnosis and treatment of hyperkalemia. *Cleve Clin J Med*. 2017;84(12):934–942.
4. Wong R, Banker R, Aronowitz P. Electrocardiographic changes of severe hyperkalemia. *J Hosp Med*. 2011;6(4):240.
5. Viera AJ, Wouk N. Potassium disorders: hypokalemia and hyperkalemia. *Am Fam Physician*. 2015;92(6):487–495.
6. Khanagavi J, Gupta T, Aronow WS, et al. Hyperkalemia among hospitalized patients and association between duration of hyperkalemia and outcomes. *Arch Med Sci*. 2014;10(2):251–257.
7. Sterns RH, Rojas M, Bernstein P, et al. Ion-exchange resins for the treatment of hyperkalemia: are they safe and effective? *J Am Soc Nephrol*. 2010;21(5):733–735.
8. Ingelfinger JR. A new era for the treatment of hyperkalemia? *N Engl J Med*. 2015;372(3):275–277.
9. Bushinsky DA, Williams GH, Pitt B, et al. Patiromer induces rapid and sustained potassium lowering in patients with chronic kidney disease and hyperkalemia. *Kidney Int*. 2015;88(6):1427–1433.
10. Montford JR, Linas S. How dangerous is hyperkalemia? *J Am Soc Nephrol*. 2017;28(11):3155–3165.

 SEE ALSO

- Addison Disease; Hypokalemia
- Algorithm: Hyperkalemia

 CODES

ICD10
E87.5 Hyperkalemia

CLINICAL PEARLS
- Emergency and urgent management of hyperkalemia takes precedent to a thorough diagnostic workup. Urgent treatment includes stabilization of the myocardium with calcium gluconate to protect against arrhythmias and pharmacologic strategies to move K from the extracellular (vascular) space into cells.
- Calcium and dextrose/insulin are only temporizing measures and do not actually lower total body K levels. Definitive treatment with either dialysis or cation exchange resin (sodium polystyrene sulfonate) is necessary.
- To lower a patient's risk of developing hyperkalemia, have the patient follow a low-K diet, use selective β_1-blockers, such as metoprolol or atenolol, instead of nonselective β-blockers such as carvedilol. Avoid NSAIDs. Concomitant use of kaliuretic loop diuretics may be useful.

H

HYPERNATREMIA
Pang-Yen Fan, MD • Rajarshi Bhadra, MD

 BASICS

DESCRIPTION
- Defined as serum sodium (Na) concentration >145 mEq/L, which usually represents a state of hypertonicity (1),(2)
- Na concentration reflects balance between total body water (TBW) and total body Na. Hypernatremia occurs from deficit of water relative to Na.
- Dehydration refers to hypernatremia from water loss.
- Hypovolemia refers to concomitant water and salt loss.
- Hypernatremia commonly results from net water loss or, more rarely, from primary Na gain (1).
- Hypernatremia will not develop in patients with intact thirst mechanisms who are able to access water.

EPIDEMIOLOGY
Incidence
- More common in elderly and very young
- Occurs in 1% of hospitalized elderly patients (3)
- Seen in about 9% of ICU patients (3)

ETIOLOGY AND PATHOPHYSIOLOGY
- Due to the powerful effect of the thirst mechanism, hypernatremia typically occurs only in patients who cannot readily access water such as infants, intubated patients, and those with altered mental status or patients with hypodipsia (4).
- Water loss out of proportion to salt loss is the most common cause of hypernatremia. The following conditions lead to excessive water loss:
  - Transdermal loss such as burns or excessive sweating (e.g., fever, infants under radiant heaters, heat exposure, extreme exercise)
  - Urinary loss
    ○ Nephrogenic diabetes insipidus (DI) (congenital or due to renal dysfunction, hypercalcemia, hypokalemia, medication-related, e.g., lithium)
    ○ Central DI (due to head trauma, stroke, meningitis) (3)
    ○ Osmotic diuresis: glucose, urea, and mannitol
    ○ Post-ATN diuresis
  - Gastrointestinal loss
    ○ Osmotic diarrhea: lactulose, malabsorption, and some types of infectious diarrhea
    ○ Enterocutaneous fistula
    ○ Vomiting, NG suction
- Disorders of the thirst mechanism can result in hypernatremia due to reduced water intake (e.g., intracranial lesions, primary hypodipsia, chronic volume expansion in mineralocorticoid excess).

- Excess Na (increase in total body Na) less commonly leads to hypernatremia. The following condition may result in excessive total body Na:
  - IV infusion of hypertonic NaCl or $NaHCO_3$ during treatment of brain injury, metabolic acidosis, or hyperkalemia (3)
  - Sea water ingestion
  - Excessive use of $NaHCO_3$ antacid
  - Incorrect infant formula preparation, tube feeding
  - Excessive Na in dialysate solutions
- With acute hypernatremia, the rapid decrease in brain volume can cause rupture of the cerebral veins, leading to focal intracerebral and sub-arachnoid hemorrhages and possibly irreversible neurologic damage (2).

Genetics
Some forms of DI may be hereditary.

RISK FACTORS
- Infants/children
- Elderly patients (may also have a diminished thirst response to osmotic stimulation via an unknown mechanism)
- Patients who are intubated/have altered mental status
- Acute gastrointestinal illness
- Poorly controlled diabetes mellitus
- Prior brain injury
- Surgery
- Diuretic therapy, especially loop diuretics
- Lithium treatment

GENERAL PREVENTION
- Treatment/prevention of underlying cause
- Properly prepare infant formula and never add salt to any commercial infant formula.
- Keep patients well hydrated.

COMMONLY ASSOCIATED CONDITIONS
- Gastroenteritis
- Altered mental status
- Burns
- Head injury

DIAGNOSIS

HISTORY
- History of conditions leading to water loss or impaired thirst: nausea, vomiting, diarrhea, polyuria, fever, heat exposure, extreme exercise, brain injury
- Neurologic symptoms are common:
  - Mild: thirst, anorexia
  - Moderate: altered mental status, myalgia, muscle weakness, twitching, lethargy, irritability
  - Severe: seizure (especially if rapid development of hypernatremia), coma

- Severity of symptoms correlate with rapidity of the increase in Na as well as the degree of hypernatremia.
- Severe symptoms are likely to occur with sudden increases in plasma Na levels or at concentrations >160 mEq/L.

PHYSICAL EXAM
- Signs of water or volume loss: tachycardia, hypotension, orthostatic hypotension, dry mucous membranes, poor skin turgor
- Neurologic abnormalities: lethargy, weakness, tremor, focal deficits (in cases of intracerebral bleeding/lesion), confusion, coma, seizures

DIFFERENTIAL DIAGNOSIS
- DI
- Hyperosmotic coma
- Salt ingestion
- Hypertonic dehydration
- Hypothyroidism
- Cushing syndrome

DIAGNOSTIC TESTS & INTERPRETATION
Initial Tests (lab, imaging)
- Serum Na, potassium, BUN, creatinine, glucose, calcium, and osmolality (serum lithium if appropriate)
- Hemoglobin/hematocrit (may be elevated above baseline due to hemoconcentration)
- Urine Na and osmolality
  - Low urine osmolality: urine osmolality (usually <300 mOsm/kg) < serum osmolality suggests DI.
  - Intermediate urine osmolality (300 to 800 mOsm/kg) may be from hypovolemia, osmotic diuresis, partial DI.
  - High urine osmolality (>800 mOsm/kg) suggests extrarenal water loss or, rarely, salt ingestion.
- Urine Na
  - Low urine Na (<10): usually suggests volume depletion, although may also be from dilution in the setting of high urine output with DI
  - Intermediate urine Na may be from osmotic diuresis.
  - High urine Na suggests salt ingestion.

Follow-Up Tests & Special Considerations
- Special tests for DI
  - Antidiuretic hormone (ADH) stimulation: distinguishes central versus nephrogenic DI
    ○ Urine osmolality does not increase after ADH or desmopressin in nephrogenic DI.
- Head CT/MRI in patients with central DI or hypodipsia to rule out intracranial lesions

TREATMENT

GENERAL MEASURES
- The treatment of hypernatremia involves treating the underlying cause and correcting the water deficit.
- Determine the duration of hypernatremia because speed of correction depends on symptom severity and rate of development of hypernatremia.
- Acute hyponatremia: relatively uncommon, may occur in acute DI, severe hyperglycemia, or salt ingestion
  - D5W infusion at 3 to 6 mL/kg/hr to lower the serum Na by 1 to 2 mEq/L/hr
  - Check serum Na every 1 to 2 hours to confirm correction at desired rate.
  - When serum Na decreases to 145 mEq/L, reduce D5W infusion to 1 mL/kg/hr until serum Na normalizes.
  - Aim to correct hypernatremia in 24 to 48 hours.
- Chronic hypernatremia (>48 hours): Avoid rapid correction to prevent development of cerebral edema.
- D5W infusion at 1.35 mL/kg/hr
- Check serum Na every 4 to 6 hours to determine correction at desired rate.
- Correct at maximum of 0.5 mEq/L/hr or 10 to 12 mEq/L/day.
- Often need to adjust infusion rate to account for ongoing water losses
- Hypernatremia with hyponatremia: Correct severe volume depletion with isotonic IV fluids first and then address hypernatremia:
  - Once hemodynamically stable, can correct hypovolemia and hypernatremia simultaneously with 0.45% saline as every 2 mL of this solution will provide 1 mL of saline and 1 mL of water
- Hypernatremia with hypervolemia: can treat hypervolemia with diuretics while simultaneously correcting hypernatremia
  - Concomitant diuretic treatment will increase urinary water losses and may necessitate increased water repletion.
- Consider oral water repletion for mild hypernatremia.
- High infusion rates of D5W may cause hyperglycemia.
- Hyperglycemia-induced osmotic diuresis will increase urinary water losses and necessitate increased water repletion.
- Dialysis can be considered if acute kidney injury and conventional treatment has failed (5)[B].

MEDICATION
First Line
- See "General Measures" for overall approach because treatment is generally done with water or hypotonic IV fluids rather than medication.
- May use medication in treatment of DI

- Central DI
  - Desmopressin acetate (DDAVP): Use parenteral form for acute symptomatic patients, and use intranasal or oral form for chronic therapy (4).
  - Free water replacement: may use 2.5% dextrose in water if giving large volumes of water in DI to avoid glycosuria
  - May consider sulfonylureas/thiazide diuretics for chronic but not acute treatment
- Nephrogenic DI
  - Treat with diuretics and NSAIDs.
  - Lithium-induced nephrogenic DI: hydrochlorothiazide 25 mg PO BID or indomethacin 50 mg PO TID, or amiloride hydrochloride 5 to 10 mg PO BID

Second Line
- Consider NSAIDs in nephrogenic DI.
- Continuous renal replacement therapy (CRRT): Multiple case reports and case series have shown success and safety in using CRRT to treat hypernatremia in critically ill patients with CHF and severe burns (5).

ISSUES FOR REFERRAL
Underlying renal involvement associated with hypernatremia would benefit from a nephrology referral.

ADMISSION, INPATIENT, AND NURSING CONSIDERATIONS
- Symptomatic patient with serum Na >155 mEq/L requires IV fluid therapy.
- Discharge criteria: stabilization of serum Na level and resolution of symptoms

ONGOING CARE

FOLLOW-UP RECOMMENDATIONS
Patient Monitoring
- Frequent neurologic checks during acute correction
- Daily weight, electrolytes, and blood glucose for a period immediately after correction
- Periodic monitoring of urine osmolality and urine output in DI

DIET
- Ensure proper nutrition during acute phase.
- After resolution of acute phase, may consider Na-restricted diet for patient
- Low-salt, low-protein diet in nephrogenic DI

PATIENT EDUCATION
Patients with nephrogenic DI must avoid salt and drink large amounts of water.

PROGNOSIS
Most recover but neurologic impairment can occur.

COMPLICATIONS
- More common if rapid development of hypernatremia
- CNS thrombosis/hemorrhage
- Seizures
- Chronic hypernatremia: >2 days duration has higher mortality.
- Serum Na >180 mEq/L (>180 mmol/L): often results in residual CNS damage

REFERENCES
1. Adrogué HJ, Madias NE. Hypernatremia. *N Engl J Med*. 2000;342(20):1493–1499.
2. Sterns RH. Disorders of plasma sodium—causes, consequences, and correction. *N Engl J Med*. 2015;372(1):55–65.
3. Bagshaw SM, Townsend DR, McDermid RC. Disorders of sodium and water balance in hospitalized patients. *Can J Anaesth*. 2009;56(2):151–167.
4. Hannon MJ, Finucane FM, Sherlock M, et al. Clinical review: disorders of water homeostasis in neurosurgical patients. *J Clin Endocrinol Metab*. 2012;97(5):1423–1433.
5. Huang C, Zhang P, Du R, et al. Treatment of acute hypernatremia in severely burned patients using continuous veno-venous hemofiltration with gradient sodium replacement fluid: a report of nine cases. *Intensive Care Med*. 2013;39(8):1495–1496.

SEE ALSO
- Diabetes Insipidus
- Algorithm: Hypernatremia

CODES

ICD10
- P74.21 Hypernatremia of newborn
- E87.0 Hyperosmolality and hypernatremia

CLINICAL PEARLS
- Occurs from water deficit in comparison to total body Na stores
- Common causes include dehydration, DI, impaired access to fluids.
- Avoid rapid correction of chronic hypernatremia to prevent development of cerebral edema (goal rate is 10 mEq/L in 24 hours).
- Monitor serum Na and adjust water repletion to achieve desired rate of correction as available formulas for calculating water deficit and estimating ongoing water losses have limited accuracy.

H

HYPERPARATHYROIDISM

Jonathan A. Phillips, DO • Bradly J. Thrasher, DO

BASICS

DESCRIPTION
A dysfunction of the body's normal regulatory feedback mechanisms resulting in excess production of parathyroid hormone (PTH)

- Primary hyperparathyroidism (HPT): intrinsic parathyroid gland dysfunction resulting in excessive secretion of PTH with a lack of response to feedback inhibition by elevated calcium
- Secondary HPT: appropriate increased secretion of PTH in response to potential hypocalcemia and/or hyperphosphatemia. This is can be caused by vitamin D deficiency, kidney dysfunction, decreased calcium intake, decreased calcium absorption, and/or phosphate loading.
- Tertiary HPT: autonomous hyperfunction of the parathyroid gland in the setting of long-standing secondary HPT

EPIDEMIOLOGY
Incidence
- Predominantly postmenopausal females
- Female > male (3:1)

Prevalence
Primary HPT is 1 in 500 to 1 in 1,000 in the United States.

ETIOLOGY AND PATHOPHYSIOLOGY
- PTH is mostly regulated by calcium levels.
- PTH is synthesized by the four parathyroid glands, which are located behind the four poles of the thyroid gland (locations can vary).
- Ectopic (abnormal locations and most common is the thymus) or supernumerary glands (more than four glands)
- PTH releases calcium from bone by osteoclastic stimulation (increasing bone resorption).
- PTH increases reabsorption of calcium in the distal tubules of the kidneys.
- PTH increases phosphorus excretion by decreasing reabsorption.
- PTH stimulates conversion of 25-hydroxycholecalciferol (25[OH]D) to 1,25-dihydroxycholecalciferol (1,25[OH]$_2$D or active vitamin D) in the kidneys. 1,25(OH)$_2$D increases calcium and phosphate absorption from the GI tract and kidneys, and stimulates osteoclastic activity and bone resorption.
- Primary HPT: unregulated PTH production and release due to the loss of normal feedback control by extracellular calcium, causing increase in serum calcium
  - Solitary adenoma (80–85%)
  - Diffuse hyperplasia (10–15%) of the four parathyroid glands, either sporadically or in association with multiple endocrine neoplasia (MEN) type I or MEN type IIA
  - Parathyroid carcinoma (<1%), a very rare and severe form
- Secondary HPT: adaptive parathyroid gland hyperplasia and hyperfunction from decreased calcium
  - Dietary
    - Vitamin D deficiency causes decreased calcium absorption.
    - Calcium deficiency
  - Chronic renal disease resulting in the following:
    - Renal parenchymal loss causing hyperphosphatemia
    - Impaired calcitriol production causing hypocalcemia
    - General skeletal and renal resistance to PTH

- Tertiary HPT: autonomous oversecretion of PTH following prolonged parathyroid stimulation

Genetics
- MEN type I and MEN type IIA: Patients with multiple gland hyperplasia in the absence of renal disease should be screened for MEN-I gene mutation.
- Neonatal severe primary HPT: infants born without both calcium-sensing receptor (CaSR) gene alleles
- HPT—jaw tumor syndrome
- Familial hypocalciuric hypercalcemia (FHH): loss of one CaSR gene alleles
- Familial isolated HPT

RISK FACTORS
Chronic kidney disease, increasing age, poor nutrition, radiation, and/or family history

GENERAL PREVENTION
Adequate intake of calcium and vitamin D may help prevent secondary HPT.

COMMONLY ASSOCIATED CONDITIONS
- Vitamin D deficiency
- Chronic renal failure
- MEN syndromes: MEN I and MEN IIA

DIAGNOSIS

HISTORY
- History of present illness
  - Almost 80% of patients are asymptomatic.
  - Kidney stones (15–20%)
  - Osteitis fibrosa cystica (<5%) characterized by subperiosteal resorption of phalanges, tapering of distal clavicles, bone cysts, brown tumors of long bones, and "salt and pepper" appearance of the skull
  - Symptoms due to hypercalcemia like mental fogginess, memory impairment, polyuria, polydipsia, constipation, bone pain, decreased concentration, altered mental status, fatigue, and muscle weakness
- Past medical history
  - The following conditions may be associated with HPT:
    - MEN syndrome (MEN I associated with pituitary adenomas, pancreatic cancers and parathyroid hyperplasia; MEN IIA associated with medullary thyroid cancer, pheochromocytoma, and parathyroid hyperplasia), nephrolithiasis (in 20–30%), nephrocalcinosis, pancreatitis, gastroduodenal ulcer, hypertension, short QT interval, left ventricular hypertrophy, osteitis fibrosa cystica, cystic bone lesions, spontaneous fracture, vertebral collapse, osteoporosis, gout, pseudogout, anxiety, depression, psychosis, coma, conjunctivitis, band keratopathy, conjunctival calcium deposits, radiation to the neck
- Medications: hydrochlorothiazide or lithium (decreases parathyroid sensitivity to calcium in small subset of patients)

PHYSICAL EXAM
- Limited usefulness; 70–80% of patients have no obvious symptoms or signs of disease.
- Physical findings related to the underlying cause of HPT may be found.

DIFFERENTIAL DIAGNOSIS
- Increased PTH: Ectopic PTH production is rare. In most of the cases, it establishes the diagnosis of primary HPT, but first rule out:
  - FHH: Rule out FHH with a 24-hour urine calcium:creatinine ratio.
  - Thiazide diuretics and lithium
- Nonparathyroid causes
  - Malignancy: lung (squamous cell) carcinoma, breast carcinoma, multiple myeloma, lymphoma, leukemia, prostate cancer, Paget disease
  - Granulomatous diseases: sarcoidosis, tuberculosis, berylliosis, histoplasmosis, coccidioidomycosis
  - Drugs: vitamin D intoxication, milk-alkali syndrome
  - Endocrine: hyperthyroidism, acute adrenal insufficiency

DIAGNOSTIC TESTS & INTERPRETATION
Initial Tests (lab, imaging)
- Often detected by incidental hypercalcemia on routine labs. The best modality is to check ionized calcium.
- Calculate corrected calcium: [serum calcium in mg/dL + 0.8 × (4 − patient's albumin in g/dL)]. Some patients will have mild hypercalcemia for years, and it won't be detected because the uncorrected calcium is normal.
- If hypercalcemia is confirmed, follow with intact PTH level (1)[B].
  - PTH-dependent: High or (abnormally) normal PTH suggests primary HPT.
  - PTH-independent: Undetectable or low PTH suggests PTH-independent hypercalcemia.
- Other findings may include low serum phosphate and high 24-hour urine calcium excretion.
- In secondary HPT, an elevated phosphorus suggests chronic renal failure; a low phosphorus suggests another cause, commonly 25(OH)D deficiency. Both are common causes of elevated PTH levels while having normal corrected calcium levels.

Follow-Up Tests & Special Considerations
- A 24-hour urine calcium concentration to creatinine clearance ratio >0.02 suggests primary HPT; a ratio <0.01 may be normal or indicate FHH; an important finding because FHH does not require surgery (1)[C].
- Routine measurement of 25(OH)D levels is recommended in all patients with primary HPT. In case of vitamin D deficiency (<20 ng/mL or <50 nmol/L), defer management decisions until levels are maintained >20 ng/mL (50 nmol/L) (1)[C].

Diagnostic Procedures/Other
- Imaging is not required for diagnosis. It is required for surgical planning, especially for minimally invasive parathyroidectomy (MIP) (2)[C].
  - Imaging is also indicated to localize hyperplasia or an ectopic parathyroid gland in repeat surgery.
- Imaging options for presurgical localization
  - Technetium-99m sestamibi with or without single-photon emission computed tomography (SPECT): It has the greatest reported success in localizing single parathyroid adenomas but often inaccurate in multigland disease (3)[B].
  - Neck ultrasound (US): painless, noninvasive, and does not expose the patient to radiation; however, its accuracy is operator-dependent (4)[C].

- Four-dimensional CT (4D-CT) may be more effective for primary localization than both US and sestamibi-SPECT (4)[B].
- Positron emission tomography (PET) using C-methionine (MET-PET) is comparable to US and technetium-99m sestamibi with SPECT in terms of diagnostic use (2)[B].
- CT and MRI are mostly used to localize ectopic mediastinal glands.

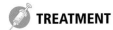 **TREATMENT**

MEDICATION
- Primary HPT: Operative management is curative; indications for surgical intervention are mentioned below. For those awaiting or unable to have surgery:
  - Bisphosphonates (alendronate): Reduce bone turnover and help to maintain bone density; avoid in kidney disease (GFR ≤35).
  - Calcimimetics (cinacalcet) (1)[B]: activates CaSR in parathyroid gland thereby inhibiting PTH secretion. FDA-approved for symptomatic patients who are unfit for surgery; no long-term data on its effect on constitutional, neuropsychological symptoms or fractures
  - Selective estrogen receptor modulator therapy (raloxifene): antagonizes PTH-mediated bone resorption
  - Hormone replacement therapy with estrogens is not recommended as first-line treatment; must weigh benefit with risks of known systemic effects
    ○ Can be used in postmenopausal women who do not undergo or refuse surgery
- Secondary HPT: Treatment is often aimed at underlying etiology.
  - Calcium replacement
  - Vitamin D analogues (paricalcitol and calcitriol)
  - Phosphorus-binding agents (sevelamer)
  - Calcimimetic (cinacalcet)
- Tertiary HPT
  - Medical treatment is not curative and generally not indicated.

SURGERY/OTHER PROCEDURES
- Operative management is curative for patients with primary HPT in 95–98% of patients. It is the first-line treatment for pediatrics. It is also usually the first-line treatment for young adults up to 50 years of age (5)[C].
- Indications for parathyroidectomy
  - Symptomatic primary HPT
    ○ Nephrolithiasis
    ○ Fragility fractures
    ○ Osteitis fibrosa cystica
  - Asymptomatic primary HPT (1)[C]
    ○ Serum Ca$^+$ level >1 mg/dL above normal
    ○ Age <50 years
    ○ Creatinine clearance <60 mL/min
    ○ 24-hour urine for calcium >400 mg/day (>10 mmol/day) and increased stone risk by biochemical stone risk analysis
    ○ Presence of nephrolithiasis or nephrocalcinosis by x-ray, US, or CT
    ○ Bone density loss with a T-score <−2.5 at the lumbar spine, femoral neck, total hip, or distal 1/3 radius

- Surgical removal of diseased gland or tissue is only proven curative therapy for HPT.
- Surgical options include the following:
  - Bilateral open neck exploratory surgery
  - MIP using preoperative sestamibi scan with SPECT/US/4D-CT and intraoperative PTH levels (high sensitivity 79–95% to predict location of single parathyroid adenoma) (6), which result in decreased pain, smaller incisions, improved cosmetic results, lower morbidity, and decreased length of hospital stay when compared with open neck exploratory surgery
- Follow postoperative serum calcium, magnesium, and phosphorus levels; monitor closely for hypocalcemia "hungry bone" syndrome.
- Patients may need IV calcium infusion postoperatively with oral calcitriol and calcium supplementation initially. Hungry pain syndrome can be severe, although less common now.
- Patients also at risk for bleeding and airway compromise
- Monitor renal function closely.

ADMISSION, INPATIENT, AND NURSING CONSIDERATIONS
Critical hypercalcemia requires IV fluid rehydration, IV bisphosphonate therapy, and SC calcitonin (4 U/kg q12h) for severe symptoms.

 ONGOING CARE

FOLLOW-UP RECOMMENDATIONS
Asymptomatic patients with primary HPT require serial monitoring of calcium and PTH.

Patient Monitoring
In patients with primary HPT who are asymptomatic, measurement of serum calcium and creatinine annually and bone density scan every 1 to 2 years is sufficient (1)[C].

DIET
- In the presence of hypercalciuria or elevated 1,25(OH)$_2$D levels, dietary calcium restriction is recommended. Otherwise, daily calcium intake should be maintained at up to 1,000 mg.
- Restrict dietary phosphate in secondary HPT.

PATIENT EDUCATION
- Importance of periodic lab testing
- Signs of severe hypercalcemia

PROGNOSIS
Prognosis after surgery is excellent in primary HPT, with resolution of many of the preoperative symptoms.

COMPLICATIONS
Related to high levels of PTH and/or elevated calcium

REFERENCES
1. Bilezikian JP, Brandi ML, Eastell R, et al. Guidelines for the management of asymptomatic primary hyperparathyroidism: summary statement from the Fourth International Workshop. *J Clin Endocrinol Metab*. 2014;99(10):3561–3569.
2. Caldarella C, Treglia G, Isgrò MA, et al. Diagnostic performance of positron emission tomography using ^{11}C-methionine in patients with suspected parathyroid adenoma: a meta-analysis. *Endocrine*. 2013;43(1):78–83.
3. Caldarella C, Treglia G, Pontecorvi A, et al. Diagnostic performance of planar scintigraphy using ^{99}mTc-MIBI in patients with secondary hyperparathyroidism: a meta-analysis. *Ann Nucl Med*. 2012;26(10):794–803.
4. Cheung K, Wang TS, Farrokhyar F, et al. A meta-analysis of preoperative localization techniques for patients with primary hyperparathyroidism. *Ann Surg Oncol*. 2012;19(2):577–583.
5. Markowitz ME, Underland L, Gensure R. Parathyroid disorders. *Pediatr Rev*. 2016;37(12):524–535.
6. Kunstman JW, Kirsch JD, Mahajan A, et al. Clinical review: parathyroid localization and implications for clinical management. *J Clin Endocrinol Metab*. 2013;98(3):902–912.

ADDITIONAL READING
Bilezikian JP. Primary hyperparathyroidism. *J Clin Endocrinol Metab*. 2018;103(11):3993–4004. doi:10.1210/jc.2018-01225.

 CODES

ICD10
- E21.3 Hyperparathyroidism, unspecified
- N25.81 Secondary hyperparathyroidism of renal origin
- E21.1 Secondary hyperparathyroidism, not elsewhere classified

CLINICAL PEARLS
- 80% of patients with primary HPT are asymptomatic.
- HPT is often detected by an incidental finding of hypercalcemia on a routine serum chemistry analysis.
- Classic symptoms of HPT include painful bones, renal stones, abdominal pain, and behavioral changes (stones, bones, moans, and groans).
- Repeat calcium (elevated), correct for serum albumin, and obtain intact PTH levels to make an initial diagnosis.
- Secondary HPT is due to excessive secretion of PTH in response to hypocalcemia, which can be caused by vitamin D deficiency or renal failure.
- In patients with primary HPT who are asymptomatic, measurement of serum calcium and creatinine annually and bone density scan every 1 to 2 years is sufficient.

H

HYPERPROLACTINEMIA
William E. Somerall Jr., MD, MAEd • D'Ann Wilson Somerall, FAANP, FNP-BC, DNP, CRNP, MAEd

 BASICS

DESCRIPTION
Hyperprolactinemia is an abnormal elevation in the serum prolactin level, from either physiologic or pathologic influences of the lactotroph cells of the pituitary gland.

EPIDEMIOLOGY
Prevalence
- Predominant age: reproductive age
- Predominant sex: female (70%) > male (30%)
- More readily detected in females because a slight elevation in prolactin causes changes in menstruation and galactorrhea; men present with headache, visual disturbances, and erectile dysfunction (1)
- Adenomas in men are typically larger because of delayed onset of symptoms (1).

ETIOLOGY AND PATHOPHYSIOLOGY
- Prolactin, which is produced by lactotrophs in the anterior pituitary, is regulated by:
  - Inhibitory factors, primarily dopamine, are produced in the hypothalamus and delivered via the hypothalamic-pituitary vessels in the pituitary stalk.
  - Stimulatory factors, primarily thyrotropin-releasing hormone (TRH)
- Causes of hyperprolactinemia include the following:
  - Physiologic
  - Pregnancy due to increased estrogen
  - Breastfeeding or nipple stimulation
  - Stress, including postoperative state
  - Medications: Concentrations are typically in the 20 to 100 ng/mL range (2)[A].
    - Dopamine (D_2) blockers: prochlorperazine, metoclopramide
    - Dopamine depleters: α-methyldopa, reserpine
    - Antidepressants: tricyclic antidepressants (TCAs); paroxetine (an SSRI) causes transient hyperprolactinemia—usually resolves in 7 to 10 days
    - Verapamil (but no other calcium channel blockers; thought to decrease the hypothalamic synthesis of dopamine)
    - Older antipsychotics (category is the most common cause of medication induced): haloperidol, fluphenazine, risperidone (level of elevation with risperidone greater than with other antipsychotics)
    - Newer antipsychotics (asenapine, iloperidone, lurasidone) may cause elevation but less than the older antipsychotics (1).
  - Hypothyroidism (due to elevated TRH)
  - Chest wall conditions such as herpes zoster, trauma, or post-thoracotomy
  - Prolactin-secreting adenoma in the anterior pituitary (microadenoma: <1 cm; macroadenoma: >1 cm)

- Pituitary stalk compression/disruption:
  - Craniopharyngioma, Rathke cleft cyst
  - Meningioma, astrocytoma
  - Metastases
  - Head trauma
  - Infiltrative/inflammatory disorders
- Diminished prolactin clearance (chronic renal failure, cirrhosis, cocaine)
- Idiopathic hyperprolactinemia—a substantial number of cases where the serum levels are between 20 and 100 ng/mL and the cause cannot be found (3)[A]

 DIAGNOSIS

Based on clinical history, physical exam, and laboratory findings

HISTORY
- Galactorrhea
- Amenorrhea or oligomenorrhea
- Infertility
- Osteoporosis/osteopenia
- Decreased libido, impotence
- Weight gain
- Also may have signs and symptoms of pituitary enlargement:
  - Headache
  - Visual field impairment (bitemporal hemianopia)
  - Hypopituitarism (secondary to tumor pressure on surrounding structures)
- Also may have signs and symptoms of associated conditions:
  - Hypothyroidism
  - Cushing disease
  - Acromegaly
  - Multiple endocrine neoplasia (MEN)-1 syndrome

PHYSICAL EXAM
- Visual field testing
- Cranial nerve exam
- Examination of chest wall for lesions

DIFFERENTIAL DIAGNOSIS
Macroprolactinemia: Macroprolactin, a polymer of several units of prolactin, is detected by immunologically based lab tests but is not biologically active. If the patient is asymptomatic but found to have elevated prolactin (PRL), consider this diagnosis and notify the lab. No treatment is required.

DIAGNOSTIC TESTS & INTERPRETATION
- Serum prolactin (most accurate results if checked fasting, in morning; food only has a small effect on concentrations, thus fasting is not required, but if elevated levels repeat on a fasting specimen) <25 μg/L normal; >25 μg/L abnormal; >30 in postmenopausal women; >250 μg/L often indicates a prolactinoma (4)[A].
- Pregnancy test

- Thyroid-stimulating hormone (TSH)
- Luteinizing hormone (LH)/follicle-stimulating hormone (FSH) if amenorrheic
- Chem panel

Initial Tests (lab, imaging)
A single measurement of serum prolactin; a level above the upper limit of normal confirms the diagnosis.
- Pituitary MRI: single best imaging
- CT scan if MRI is contraindicated
- Levels should be drawn prior to a breast exam.

Follow-Up Tests & Special Considerations
Formal visual field testing if pituitary adenoma is suspected

 TREATMENT

GENERAL MEASURES
- Discontinue offending medications, if any (4)[A].
- Treat underlying causes (4)[A].
- For asymptomatic patients with mild prolactin elevations, observation alone may be considered (4)[A],(5)[A].
- Medications indicated for (4)[A]:
  - Symptoms of hypogonadism, such as decreased libido
  - Galactorrhea (if bothersome to patient)
  - Restoration of fertility
  - Pituitary adenoma
  - Prevention of osteoporosis

MEDICATION
Dopamine agonists: Decrease serum prolactin concentrations and decrease the size of most lactotroph adenomas.

- Cabergoline (Dostinex): This is now the first-line choice due to efficacy and favorable side effect profile (4)[A],(6)[A]: dosed 0.25 mg twice weekly or 0.50 once a week. While more expensive, cabergoline was more effective than bromocriptine in reducing persistent hyperprolactinemia, galactorrhea, and amenorrhea/oligomenorrhea (5)[A]. Has recently been reported to be associated with significant improvements in the body mass index, total HDL and LDL cholesterol levels, and insulin sensitivity (7); decrease in proinflammatory markers; and carotid intima-media thickness, indicated with bromocriptine failure or resistance; has been shown to reduce erectile dysfunction in hyperprolactinemic men (4)[A]
  - Adverse effects (better tolerated if start with low dose, slow titration, given at night with food):
    - Nausea/vomiting
    - Headache, dizziness, fatigue
    - Postural hypotension (5)[A]

– Contraindications
  ○ Uncontrolled hypertension
  ○ Cardiac valvular disorders
  ○ Pulmonary, pericardial, or retroperitoneal fibrotic disorders
- Bromocriptine (Parlodel): This has the longest clinical history: dosed BID; begin at 1.25 mg once at bedtime or after dinner for 1 week then increase to BID; preferred by some clinicians when infertility is an indication for treatment (2)[A],(5)[A]
- Both are effective for reducing tumor size and improving symptoms (5)[A].
- SE less with cabergoline than bromocriptine (5)[A]. Pergolide (Permax) is no longer used in the United States. If patient is still on med, do not withdraw abruptly.

ADDITIONAL THERAPIES
Patients with medically and surgically refractory prolactinomas; radiotherapy produced a reduction in prolactin levels in nearly all patients and normalization in over a quarter of patients with low complication rates (5)[A].

SURGERY/OTHER PROCEDURES
- For adenomas, medical treatment will be successful in 80–90% of patients. In some cases, surgery is indicated (4):
  – Intolerance or resistance to medical treatment
  – Headache
  – Visual field loss
  – CSF leak due to tumor apoplexy or shrinkage
  – Cranial nerve deficit
- Risks include a high recurrence rate (up to 40%), CSF leakage, meningitis, pituitary insufficiency, and transient diabetes insipidus (8).

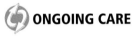 ONGOING CARE

FOLLOW-UP RECOMMENDATIONS
Reevaluate lab levels after 1 month; if normal, continue the initial dose. If lab levels do not decrease, but patient experiences no side effects increase cabergoline to 1.25 mg 2 to 3 times/week or bromocriptine to 5 mg twice a day.

Patient Monitoring
- After at least 2 years of treatment, no tumor, and prolactin levels normal may consider decreasing and stopping medication; must be followed closely, as the tumor may grow back (4)
- Consider:
  – Formal visual field testing yearly (2)[A]
  – Serial MRIs if clinically indicated (2)[A]

Pregnancy Considerations
- If pregnancy is desired in a woman with hyperprolactinemia, dopamine agonists are not approved during pregnancy and should be discontinued once pregnancy is confirmed, but their use is recommended if neurologic findings are present (4)[A].
- With microprolactinoma: Treat with bromocriptine if symptomatic; monthly pregnancy tests; discontinue bromocriptine when pregnancy is confirmed.
- With macroprolactinomas: a definitive, individualized plan is made. Options include discontinuation of bromocriptine at conception and careful monitoring of prolactin levels and VS, with or without MRI scan evidence of tumor enlargement; prepregnancy transsphenoidal surgery with debulking of tumor; continuation of bromocriptine throughout gestation, with a risk to the fetus.
- Careful monitoring of visual fields in each trimester; no need to monitor prolactin levels, as they are normally high due to pregnancy (4)[A]

PATIENT EDUCATION
Discuss risks of untreated hyperprolactinemia:
- Headache
- Visual field loss
- Decreased bone density
- Infertility

PROGNOSIS
- Following treatment for 1 to 2 years, if PRL levels have remained normal, consider stopping meds.
- 5–10% of macroadenomas may progress to macroadenomas.
- Follow-up imaging not needed unless signs or symptoms of enlarging tumor
- >10 years, 7% chance of progression of prolactin-secreting microadenoma (2)

COMPLICATIONS
- If pituitary adenoma, risk of permanent visual field loss
- For patients with high doses of cabergoline, suggest cardiac US every 2 years.

REFERENCES
1. Somerall WE Jr, Somerall DW. Hyperprolactinemia: the ABCs of diagnosis and management. *Women Healthc*. 2020;8(6):6–12.
2. Casanueva FF, Molitch ME, Schlechte JA, et al. Guidelines of the Pituitary Society for the diagnosis and management of prolactinomas. *Clin Endocrinol (Oxf)*. 2006;65(2):265–273.
3. Inder WJ, Castle D. Antipsychotic-induced hyperprolactinaemia. *Aust N Z J Psychiatry*. 2011;45(10):830–837.
4. Hoffman AR, Melmed S, Schlechte J. Patient guide to hyperprolactinemia diagnosis and treatment. *J Clin Endocrinol Metab*. 2011;96(2):35A–36A.
5. Wang AT, Mullan RJ, Lane MA, et al. Treatment of hyperprolactinemia: a systematic review and meta-analysis. *Syst Rev*. 2012;1:33.
6. Wong A, Eloy JA, Couldwell WT, et al. Update on prolactinomas. Part 2: treatment and management strategies. *J Clin Neurosci*. 2015;22(10):1568–1574.
7. Inancli SS, Usluogullari A, Ustu Y, et al. Effect of cabergoline on insulin sensitivity, inflammation, and carotid intima media thickness in patients with prolactinoma. *Endocrine*. 2013;44(1):193–199.
8. Bloomgarden E, Molitch ME. Surgical treatment of prolactinomas: cons. *Endocrine*. 2014;47(3):730–733.

ADDITIONAL READING
Klibanski A. Clinical practice. Prolactinomas. *N Engl J Med*. 2010;362(13):1219–1226.

 CODES

ICD10
E22.1 Hyperprolactinemia

CLINICAL PEARLS
- If a cause for hyperprolactinemia cannot be found by history, examination, and routine laboratory testing, an intracranial lesion might be the cause, and brain MRI with specific pituitary cuts and intravenous contrast media should be performed.
- Treatment of hyperprolactinemia should be targeted at correcting the cause (hypothyroidism, discontinuation of offending medications, etc.).
- There is a difference among antipsychotics in influencing prolactin levels. In general, those with the highest potency D_2 antagonism are most likely to elevate prolactin levels. Among the newer atypical antipsychotics, risperidone has been identified as more likely to elevate prolactin.
- High prolactin levels decrease testosterone by inhibiting gonadotropin-releasing hormone (GnRH), LH, and FSH secretion and by decreasing central dopamine activity, both of which are important in mediating sexual arousal.

H

HYPERSENSITIVITY PNEUMONITIS

Han Q. Bui, MD, MPH

 BASICS

DESCRIPTION
- Hypersensitivity pneumonitis (HP) is also called extrinsic allergic alveolitis (EAA).
- HP is a diffuse inflammatory disease of the lung parenchyma caused by an immunologic reaction to aerosolized antigenic particles found in a variety of environments. Classification depends on time frame involved:
  - Acute: fever, chills, diaphoresis, myalgias, nausea; cough and dyspnea common but not necessarily present. Occurs 4 to 12 hours after heavy exposure to an inciting agent. Symptoms subside within 12 hours to several days after removal from exposure. Complete resolution occurs within weeks.
  - Subacute: mainly caused by continual low-level antigen exposure, could have a low-grade fever in 1st week; cough, dyspnea, fatigue, anorexia, weight loss—develops over days to weeks
  - Chronic: from recurrent exposure either acute or subacute cases; prolonged and progressive cough, dyspnea, fatigue, weight loss; could lead to fibrosis and respiratory failure
- Farmer's lung is an old term of this disease, a type of HP, particular to the farmer population; causative agent is a bacterium found in moldy hay or straw. Farmer's lung now has new and different etiologies due to modernization of farming practices (1),(2).

EPIDEMIOLOGY
- Not well defined; tends to occur in adults as a result of occupation-related exposure, but some home environmental exposures are also seen
- HP is increasingly recognized as an important cause of fibrotic interstitial lung disease (3).

Incidence
0.9/100,000

Prevalence
- Farmers: 1–19% exposed farmers
- Bird fanciers: 6–20% exposed individuals
- Others: 1–8% exposed

ETIOLOGY AND PATHOPHYSIOLOGY
- Hypersensitivity reaction involving immune complexes: Inhaled antigens bind to IgG, triggering complement cascade (types III and IV immunologic reactions) (3).
- Cellular-mediated reaction: T cell–mediated immune inflammatory response
- Farming, vegetable, or dairy cattle workers (1),(2)
  - Moldy hay, grain, silage: thermophilic actinomycetes, such as *Faenia rectivirgula*
  - Mold on pressed sugar cane: *Thermoactinomyces sacchari, Thymus vulgaris*
  - Tobacco plants: *Aspergillus* sp., *Scopulariopsis brevicaulis*
  - Mushroom worker's lung: *Saccharopolyspora rectivirgula, T. vulgaris, Aspergillus* spp.
  - Potato riddler's lung: thermophilic actinomycetes, *T. vulgaris, F. rectivirgula, Aspergillus* sp.

- Wine maker's lung: *Mucor stolonifer*
- Cheese washer's lung: *Penicillium caseifulvum, Aspergillus clavatus*
- Coffee worker's lung: coffee bean dust
- Tea grower's lung: tea plants
- Ventilation and water-related contamination (1),(2)
  - Contaminated humidifiers and air conditioners: amoebae, nematodes, yeasts, bacteria
  - Unventilated shower: *Epicoccum nigrum*
  - Hot-tub lung: *Cladosporium* sp., *Mycobacterium avium complex*
  - Sauna taker's lung: *Aureobasidium* sp.
  - Summer-type pneumonitis: *Trichosporon cutaneum*
  - Swimming pool lifeguard's lung: aerosolized endotoxin and *M. avium complex*
  - Contaminated basement pneumonitis: *Cephalosporium* and *Penicillium* spp.
- Bird and poultry handling (1)
  - Bird fancier's lung: droppings, feathers, serum proteins
  - Poultry worker's lung: serum proteins
  - Turkey-handling disease: serum proteins
  - Canary fancier's lung: serum proteins
  - Duck fever: feathers, serum proteins
- Veterinary work and animal handling (1),(2)
  - Laboratory worker's lung: urine, serum, pelts, proteins
  - Pituitary snuff taker's disease: dried, powdered neurohypophysis
  - Furrier's lung: animal pelts
  - Bat lung: bat serum protein
  - Fish meal worker's lung: fish meal
  - Coptic lung: cloth wrapping of mummies
  - Mollusc shell HP: sea-snail shell
  - Pearl oyster shell pneumonitis: oyster shells
- Grain and flour (1),(2)
  - Grain measurer's lung: cereal grain, grain dust
  - Miller's lung: *Sitophilus granarius*
  - Malt worker's disease: *Aspergillus fumigatus, A. clavatus*
- Lumber milling, construction, wood stripping, paper, wallboard manufacture (1),(2)
  - Wood dust pneumonitis: *Alternaria* sp., *Bacillus subtilis*
  - Sequoiosis: *Graphium, Pullularia, Trichoderma* sp., *Aureobasidium pullulans*
  - Maple bark disease: *Cryptostroma corticale*
  - Wood trimmer's disease: *Rhizopus* sp., *Mucor* sp.
  - Wood pulp worker's disease: *Penicillium* sp.
  - Suberosis: *Trogon viridis, Penicillium glabrum*
- Plastic manufacturing, painting, electronics, chemicals (1)
  - Chemical HP: diphenyl diisocyanate, toluene diisocyanate
  - Detergent worker's lung: *B. subtilis* enzymes
  - Pauli reagent alveolitis: sodium diazobenzene sulfate
  - Vineyard sprayer's lung: copper sulfate
  - Pyrethrum: *Pyrethrum*
  - Epoxy resin lung: phthalic anhydride
  - Bible printer's lung: moldy typesetting water
  - Machine operator's lung: *Pseudomonas fluorescens*, aerosolized metal working fluid

- Textile workers
  - Byssinosis: cotton mill dust
  - Velvet worker's lung: nylon, tannic acid, potato starch
  - Upholstery fabric: aflatoxin-producing fungus, *Fusarium* sp.
  - Lycoperdonosis: puffball spores

Genetics
No evidence of clear genetic susceptibility; possible genetic predisposition involving tumor necrosis factor alpha (TNF-α) and major histocompatibility complex (MHC) class II genes (1),(3)[B]

RISK FACTORS
- Contact with organic antigens increases risk of developing HP. Viral infection at time of exposure may increase risk.
- Nonsmokers have an increased incidence of HP compared with smokers. The mechanisms that account for the "protective" effect of smoking are poorly understood, but nicotine is thought to inhibit macrophage activation and lymphocyte proliferation and function (3).
  - Smokers have a diminished antibody response to inhaled antigens.
  - However, smokers who develop disease tend to have the chronic form, and mortality is higher.

GENERAL PREVENTION
Avoidance of offending antigen and/or use of protective equipment

COMMONLY ASSOCIATED CONDITIONS
Constrictive bronchiolitis

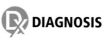 **DIAGNOSIS**

- Diagnosis criteria most widely used but not validated: (i) history and physical and pulmonary function tests (PFTs) indicating restriction or diffusion disease. DL_{co} is the most frequently affected lung parameter but may be normal in up to 22% of patients, (ii) radiologic imaging consent with interstitial lung disease, (iii) exposure to a recognized cause, (iv) proof of sensitization in bronchoalveolar lavage (BAL) fluids (serum precipitins and/or lymphocytosis) (2)
- Six significant predictors: exposure to a known antigen, positive antibodies precipitating (if identified), recurrent episodes of symptoms, inspiratory crackles, symptoms 4 to 8 hours after exposure, weight loss (3)
- Acute form: develops 4 to 12 hours following exposure. Cough, dyspnea without wheezing, fever, chills, diaphoresis, headache, nausea, malaise, chest tightness. Symptoms last hours to days.
- Sequela (prior subacute, chronic): gradual or progressive productive cough, dyspnea, fatigue, anorexia, weight loss can lead to respiratory failure; develops over days, weeks to months
- Symptomatic improvement when away from work or home

PHYSICAL EXAM
- Acute: fever, tachypnea, diffuse fine rales
- Sequela or chronic: inspiratory crackles, progressive hypoxia, weight loss, diffuse rales, clubbing, rarely wheezing

DIFFERENTIAL DIAGNOSIS

- Acute: acute infectious pneumonia: influenza (or other viral pneumonia), mycoplasma, *Pneumocystis jiroveci* pneumonia, asthma, aspiration
- Chronic: sarcoidosis, chronic bronchitis, chronic obstructive pulmonary disease, tuberculosis, collagen vascular disease, idiopathic pulmonary fibrosis, lymphoma, fungal infections, *P. jiroveci* pneumonia

DIAGNOSTIC TESTS & INTERPRETATION

- Testing for positive precipitating antibodies is NOT diagnostic because up to 40% may have positive antibody without disease; antigens that cover most cases: pigeon and parakeet sera, dove feather, *Aspergillus* sp., *Penicillium*, *S. rectivirgula*, and *Thalassomonas viridans*
- PFTs: Typical profile is a restrictive pattern with low diffusing capacity; could also have an obstructive pattern (4)
- BAL with serum precipitins and lymphocytosis (greater than 50%) and a relative predominance of CD8—low CD4-to-CD8 ratio; findings not unique to HP (1),(4)
- Positive antigen–specific inhalation challenge testing: reexposure to the environment, inhalation challenge to the suspected antigen in a hospital setting, but it lacks standardization (3)
- Chest x-ray (CXR): used to rule out other diseases
  – Acute: ground-glass infiltrates, nodular or striated patchy opacities, interstitial pattern in a variety of distributions in lung field. Up to 20% could be normal.
  – Sequela/chronic: upper lobe fibrosis, nodular or ground-glass opacities, volume loss, emphysematous changes
- CT scan of chest; patterns not specific to HP:
  – Acute: ground-glass opacities, poorly defined centrilobular nodules, and ground-glass opacities and air trapping on expiratory images (3),(5)
  – Chronic: fibrosis, ground-glass attenuation, irregular opacities, bronchiectasis, loss of lung volume, honeycombing, emphysematous changes (3),(5)
- High-resolution CT (HRCT) mid-to-upper zone predominance of centrilobular ground glass or nodular opacities with signs of air trapping (3)
- Usually start with CXR; may progress to HRCT based on findings (3)

Diagnostic Procedures/Other

Lung biopsy:
- Transbronchial: reveals small, poorly formed noncaseating granulomas near respiratory or terminal bronchioles, large foam cells, peribronchial fibrosis
- Open lung biopsy: highest yield in advanced disease; reveals varying patterns of organizing pneumonia, centrilobular and perilobular fibrosis, multinucleated giant cells with clefts

ALERT

HP in farmers must be distinguished from febrile, toxic reactions to inhaled dusts (organic dust toxic syndrome [ODTS]). Nonimmunologic reactions occur 30–50% more commonly than HP in farmers. ODTS is associated with intense exposure occurring on a single day.

TREATMENT

GENERAL MEASURES

- Outpatient, except for acute pneumonitis cases and admission for workup (BAL, lung biopsy)
- Every effort should be made to remove the patient completely from repeated exposure to the causative antigen. This action offers the best outcome of disease.

MEDICATION

First Line

- Avoidance of offending antigen is primary therapy and results in disease regression (3).
- Corticosteroids: help control the symptoms of exacerbations but do not improve long-term outcomes
  – Prednisone: 20 to 50 mg daily (3),(4)
  – For severe symptomatic patients, initial course of 1 to 2 weeks with taper (3),(4)[C]

Second Line

- Bronchodilators and inhaled corticosteroids may symptomatically improve patients with wheeze and chest tightness (4)[C].
- Oxygen may be needed in advanced cases.
- Lung transplantation may be the last resort in severe cases unresponsive to therapy.

ISSUES FOR REFERRAL

Referral to pulmonologist/immunologist

ADMISSION, INPATIENT, AND NURSING CONSIDERATIONS

Supportive management, as needed, to maintain oxygenation and ventilation:
- Unstable ventilation, oxygen requirement, mental status changes
- Need for invasive evaluation (lung biopsy)

ONGOING CARE

FOLLOW-UP RECOMMENDATIONS

Patient Monitoring

- Initial follow-up should be weekly to monthly, depending on severity and course.
- Follow treatments with serial CXR, PFTs, and circulating antibody levels.

DIET

No dietary restrictions

PATIENT EDUCATION

Note that chronic exposure may lead to a loss of acute symptoms with exposure (i.e., the patient may lose awareness of exposure–symptom relationship).

PROGNOSIS

- Presence of fibrosis is a poor prognosis factor (3).
- Acute: good prognosis with reversal of pathologic findings if elimination of offending antigen early in disease (2)
- Sequela/chronic: Corticosteroids have been found to improve lung function acutely but offer no significant difference in long-term outcome (3)[C].

COMPLICATIONS

- Progressive interstitial fibrosis with eventual respiratory failure
- Cor pulmonale and right-sided heart failure

REFERENCES

1. Girard M, Cormier Y. Hypersensitivity pneumonitis. *Curr Opin Allergy Clin Immunol*. 2010;10(2):99–103.
2. Costabel U, Bonella F, Guzman J. Chronic hypersensitivity pneumonitis. *Clin Chest Med*. 2012;33(1):151–163.
3. Spagnolo P, Rossi G, Cavazza A, et al. Hypersensitivity pneumonitis: a comprehensive review. *J Investig Allergol Clin Immunol*. 2015;25(4):237–250.
4. Lacasse Y, Girard M, Cormier Y. Recent advances in hypersensitivity pneumonitis. *Chest*. 2012;142(1):208–217.
5. D'souza RS, Donato A. Hypersensitivity pneumonitis: an overlooked cause of cough and dyspnea. *J Community Hosp Intern Med Perspect*. 2017;7(2):95–99.

CODES

ICD10

- J67.9 Hypersensitivity pneumonitis due to unspecified organic dust
- J67.0 Farmer's lung
- J67.2 Bird fancier's lung

CLINICAL PEARLS

- Skin testing is not useful for the diagnosis of HP.
- Diagnosis should be suspected in every patient with unexplained cough and dyspnea on exertion, functional impairment (restriction or diffusion defect), and unclear fever, especially if exposure to potential antigens is known (workplace, domestic bird keeping, moldy walls in the home) (2).
- HP may mimic viral upper respiratory illness or asthma exacerbation. Misdiagnosis has critical therapeutic and prognostic implications because it may delay proper treatment, result in significant morbidity, unnecessary hospitalizations, and irreversible fibrosis to the lungs (3).
- Once the disease is established, smoking does not appear to attenuate its severity, and it may predispose to more chronic and severe course.
- Use of protective gear on individual with high-risk exposure occupations can prevent HP.
- Chronic HP is increasingly recognized as an important mimic of other fibrotic lung diseases (3).

H

HYPERSPLENISM

Shadi Hamdeh, MD • Adil Abdalla, MD

 BASICS

DESCRIPTION
- Hypersplenism is defined as overactivity of the spleen and presents as the following:
  - Splenomegaly (commonly but not always)
  - Cytopenias with respective bone marrow hyperplasia of precursors
  - Resolution of cytopenias with splenectomy
- Splenomegaly is not synonymous with hypersplenism. Overactivity of the spleen can occur without enlargement, as is seen in immune thrombocytopenic purpura (ITP) and autoimmune hemolytic anemia. Similarly, splenomegaly is not always associated with hypersplenism.

EPIDEMIOLOGY
May be as common as 30–70% in patients with cirrhosis and portal hypertension (HTN)

ETIOLOGY AND PATHOPHYSIOLOGY
- Enlargement of the spleen results in sequestration of formed blood elements, leading to peripheral cytopenias and concomitant bone marrow precursor hyperplasia.
- Many of the common etiologies are listed below. Almost any process involving the spleen or the hematologic system can result in hypersplenism:
  - Infectious
    - Tuberculosis
    - Brucellosis
    - Malaria
    - Leishmaniasis
    - Ehrlichiosis
    - Schistosomiasis
    - Histoplasmosis
    - Candidiasis
    - Viral
    - Syphilis
    - Infective endocarditis
  - Hematologic
    - Myeloproliferative disorders
    - Polycythemia vera
    - Primary hypersplenism
    - ITP
    - Hemolytic anemias
  - Neoplastic
    - Hematologic malignancies
    - Melanoma
    - Various carcinomas
    - Metastatic cancers
  - Storage diseases
    - Gaucher disease
    - Niemann-Pick disease
    - Amyloidosis
    - Glycogen storage disease
  - Inflammatory
    - Sarcoidosis
    - Systemic lupus erythematosus
    - Felty syndrome
  - Congestive
    - Cirrhosis
    - Heart failure
    - Portal or splenic vein thrombosis
    - Congenital malformations of the portal vein

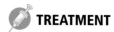 **DIAGNOSIS**

HISTORY
- Patients may complain of abdominal fullness or protrusion of the spleen through the abdominal wall; may complain of early satiety if the spleen is compressing stomach
- Patients may complain of tenderness in the left upper quadrant, especially with viral infections. In lymphoproliferative disorders, spleen may be enlarged but asymptomatic unless there is splenic infarction. Given location of the spleen next to the diaphragm, a sense of fullness may be referred through the phrenic nerve to the C3–C5 dermatomes in the left shoulder.
- Symptoms related to the underlying cause of hypersplenism may be present.

PHYSICAL EXAM
Splenomegaly

- The normal spleen is not palpable. A palpable spleen always indicates underlying abnormality such as splenomegaly and, in turn, hypersplenism in the appropriate clinical context or may indicate a wandering spleen. Also, spleen can be palpated in chronic obstructive pulmonary disease and acute asthma exacerbation, without coexisting splenomegaly.
- Begin by percussing Traube semilunar space, demarcated laterally by left anterior axillary line, inferiorly by the left costal margin, and superiorly by the left 6th rib. This space is usually hollow. Splenic enlargement may cause dullness to percussion in this area. Other processes that may cause dullness include pleural or pericardial effusions. Additionally, if the patient recently ate a large meal, this area may be dull to percussion.
- With patient supine, rest hand gently on the abdomen to prevent sudden tensing of the abdominal musculature, which may obscure palpation. Better abdominal relaxation can be obtained by flexing the knees toward the abdomen. As the spleen enlarges, it moves caudally and medially. Start by palpating in the right lower quadrant and moving toward the umbilicus, toward the left upper quadrant. If there is doubt about whether the spleen has moved beyond the costal margin, ask patient to take a large breath, which will push the diaphragm, and, in turn, the spleen toward the examiner's hands.
- Jaundice: if hemolytic anemia is present or in advanced cirrhosis
- Petechiae, purpura, or ecchymosis: if thrombocytopenia is present
- Lymphadenopathy: in hematologic or solid organ malignancies. It also can be seen in infectious etiologies.

DIAGNOSTIC TESTS & INTERPRETATION
On CBC, any and all cell lines may be decreased, resulting in the following:
- Anemia
- Leukopenia
- Thrombocytopenia

Initial Tests (lab, imaging)
- CBC
- If anemia, reticulocyte count, haptoglobin

- If there is hemolysis, there should be an elevated reticulocyte count, elevated LDH, decreased haptoglobin, along with evidence of hyperbilirubinemia (unconjugated).
- US
- CT
- Tc-99m sulfur colloid scintigraphy
- PET
- MRI

Follow-Up Tests & Special Considerations
Based on other historical and exam findings, testing for specific infectious etiologies may be warranted:
- Blood parasite smear for malaria and other parasitic infections
- EBV serologies
- HIV ELISA with Western blot
- JAK2 mutation in polycythemia vera
- PPD for tuberculosis
- Hgb electrophoresis in hereditary hemoglobinopathies

Diagnostic Procedures/Other
- Bone marrow biopsy
- Liver biopsy for cirrhosis and storage diseases

Test Interpretation
Hyperplasia of bone marrow precursors, especially those correlating with the patient's individual cytopenias

TREATMENT

MEDICATION
- No specific medication can be recommended for patients with hypersplenism. The most important intervention is to treat the underlying disorder.
- If ITP is the cause, the patient may benefit from the following:
  - Prednisone or methylprednisolone
  - IVIG
  - Rituximab
- If an infectious cause is discovered, treatment with appropriate antibiotic therapy may help to improve the cytopenias.

SURGERY/OTHER PROCEDURES
- Many patients with severe uncontrolled cytopenias undergo splenectomy.
- Laparoscopic splenectomy is preferred over open splenectomy (1)[A].

ALERT
Splenectomized patients should receive immunization to pneumococcus, meningococcus, *Haemophilus influenzae*, and influenza at least 14 days prior to splenectomy (2)[A].

- If this cannot be done (i.e., in cases of emergent splenectomy), wait at least 14 days postsplenectomy to immunize.
  - Pneumococcal vaccine
    - Pneumococcal polyvalent-23 vaccine (PPSV23) for use in adults and fully immunized children ≥2 years of age

- Pneumococcal polyvalent-13 vaccine (PCV13) for infants and young children ≥2 months of age as part of routine immunization schedule (3)[A]
- PCV13 for children >2 years of age, adolescents and adults in addition to PPSV23; refer to CDC for timing of administration.
- Current guidelines recommend single revaccination of PPSV23 5 years after the initial dose and again at age of ≥65 years, at least 5 years after the previous dose.

– *H. influenzae* vaccine
  - All unvaccinated individuals ≥5 years of age should be given 1 dose of *H. influenzae* type B (Hib) conjugate vaccine.
  - Children <5 years old should also be vaccinated. Refer to CDC for timing.
  - Vaccinated individuals can also be given additional dose of vaccine (4)[A].
– Meningococcal vaccine (5)[A]
  - Meningococcal conjugate vaccine (MCV4) for use in patients between 2 and 55 years
  - Meningococcal polysaccharide vaccine (MPSV4) for use in patients >55 years of age
  - Revaccination is recommended every 5 years.
– Influenza vaccine should be administered yearly based on prevalent circulating strains. Although patients are not at higher risk from influenza itself, infection with influenza may place patients at higher risk for secondary bacterial infections.
- Radiofrequency ablation (RFA) is becoming more available and can be successful at preventing recurrence of hypersplenism. It is not currently known whether there are differences between RFA and splenectomy in terms of postprocedure infectious risks. Other alternatives to splenectomy include total and partial splenic embolization and shunting, although these techniques are evolving and additional studies are needed to evaluate efficacy and morbidity as compared to splenectomy.

ADMISSION, INPATIENT, AND NURSING CONSIDERATIONS
- Hypersplenism alone generally does not warrant admission. However, all patients should be monitored closely for complications of the resulting cytopenias, including bleeding and infection, as well as complications of splenomegaly, including increased risk of splenic rupture. In some patients, the large spleen compresses the stomach and prevents adequate oral intake.
- Splenectomized patients are at increased risk of infection and postsplenectomy sepsis, especially with *Streptococcus pneumoniae*. Fevers, chills, or pain concerning for underlying infection warrant immediate attention because clinical decompensation can occur within hours. Empiric broad-spectrum antibiotics should not be delayed while evaluation is ongoing. Common empiric regimens include the following:
– Ceftriaxone: 2 g IV q24h and vancomycin 1 g IV q12h
– Levofloxacin: 750 mg IV q24h and vancomycin 1 g IV q12h in β-lactam–allergic patients

 ## ONGOING CARE

- Adult patients who are splenectomized should be advised to monitor closely for fever or rigors at home, which may be an early sign of bacteremia. They should be instructed to begin antibiotics immediately prior to proceeding to a medical facility for evaluation. Early antibiotics have been shown to reduce the mortality from overwhelming postsplenectomy sepsis.
- Controlled trials have not been performed, but some regimens include the following:
– Amoxicillin-clavulanate: 875 mg PO BID
– Cefuroxime axetil: 500 mg PO BID
- Patients allergic to β-lactam antibiotics can be given an extended-spectrum fluoroquinolone such as levofloxacin 750 mg PO *or* moxifloxacin 400 mg PO daily.
- In children with splenectomy, daily antibiotic prophylaxis for overwhelming postsplenectomy sepsis with penicillin VK or amoxicillin is recommended until age 5 years or at least 3 years after splenectomy:
– Age 2 months to 5 years: 125 mg PO BID
– >5 years old: 250 mg PO BID

PATIENT EDUCATION
Patients who are splenectomized should be counseled extensively about the risk of overwhelming postsplenectomy sepsis and the need to obtain prompt medical evaluation in the event of fevers, chills, or any other concerning symptoms.

REFERENCES

1. Bai YN, Jiang H, Prasoon P. A meta-analysis of perioperative outcomes of laparoscopic splenectomy for hematological disorders. *World J Surg*. 2012;36(10):2349–2358.
2. Advisory Committee on Immunization Practices. Recommended adult immunization schedule: United States, 2012. *Ann Intern Med*. 2012;156(3):211–217.
3. American Academy of Pediatrics. Children with asplenia or functional asplenia. In: Pickering LK, Baker CJ, Kimberlin DW, et al, eds. *Red Book: 2009 Report of the Committee on Infectious Diseases*. 28th ed. Elk Grove Village, IL: American Academy of Pediatrics; 2009:72.
4. American Academy of Pediatrics Committee on Infectious Diseases: *Haemophilus influenzae* type b conjugate vaccines: recommendations for immunization with recently and previously licensed vaccines. *Pediatrics*. 1993;92(3):480–488.
5. Centers for Disease Control and Prevention. Updated recommendations for use of meningococcal conjugate vaccines—Advisory Committee on Immunization Practices (ACIP), 2010. *MMWR Morb Mortal Wkly Rep*. 2011;60(3):72–76.

ADDITIONAL READING

- Abdella HM, Abd-El-Moez AT, Abu El-Maaty ME, et al. Role of partial splenic arterial embolization for hypersplenism in patients with liver cirrhosis and thrombocytopenia. *Indian J Gastroenterol*. 2010;29(2):59–61.
- Di Sabatino A, Carsetti R, Corazza GR. Postsplenectomy and hyposplenic states. *Lancet*. 2011;378(9785):86–97.
- Feng K, Ma K, Liu Q, et al. Randomized clinical trial of splenic radiofrequency ablation versus splenectomy for severe hypersplenism. *Br J Surg*. 2011;98(3):354–361.
- Iriyama N, Horikoshi A, Hatta Y, et al. Localized, splenic, diffuse large B-cell lymphoma presenting with hypersplenism: risk and benefit of splenectomy. *Intern Med*. 2010;49(11):1027–1030.
- Jandl JH, Aster RH, Forkner CE, et al. Splenic pooling and the pathophysiology of hypersplenism. *Trans Am Clin Climatol Assoc*. 1967;78:9–27.
- Kapoor P, Singh E, Radhakrishnan P, et al. Splenectomy in plasma cell dyscrasias: a review of the clinical practice. *Am J Hematol*. 2006;81(12):946–954.
- Mourtzoukou EG, Pappas G, Peppas G, et al. Vaccination of asplenic or hyposplenic adults. *Br J Surg*. 2008;95(3):273–280.
- Shatz DV, Schinsky MF, Pais LB, et al. Immune responses of splenectomized trauma patients to the 23-valent pneumococcal polysaccharide vaccine at 1 versus 7 versus 14 days after splenectomy. *J Trauma*. 1998;44(5):760–766.

 ## SEE ALSO

Anemia, Autoimmune Hemolytic; Malaria; Polycythemia Vera; Tuberculosis

 ## CODES

ICD10
D73.1 Hypersplenism

CLINICAL PEARLS

- Splenectomy is not necessary to make the diagnosis.
- Avoid splenectomy in patients unless absolutely necessary. Splenectomized patients are at lifelong risk for overwhelming postsplenectomy infection and sepsis.
- If splenectomy is to be performed, give immunization for pneumococcus, meningococcus, *H. influenzae*, and influenza at least 14 days prior to surgery. Otherwise, wait until the 14th postoperative day to immunize.

H

HYPERTENSION, ESSENTIAL

Ronald N. Adler, MD, FAAFP • Jeremy Golding, MD, FAAFP

 BASICS

DESCRIPTION

- Essential hypertension (HTN) is HTN without an identifiable cause; also known as primary HTN and (inappropriately) as benign HTN. Although its importance as a risk factor for cardiovascular and other morbidity and mortality is well established, there is persistent controversy regarding recommended thresholds for diagnosis and treatment.
- HTN is defined (Joint National Committee [JNC] 8) (1) and the International Society of Hypertension) as (all pressures in mm Hg):
  – Age <60 years: systolic BP (SBP) ≥140 and/or diastolic BP (DBP) ≥90 at ≥2 visits
  – Age ≥60 years: SBP ≥150 and/or DBP ≥90 at ≥2 visits
  – With diabetes or chronic kidney disease (CKD): SBP ≥140 and/or DBP ≥90
  – The American College of Cardiology (ACC)/American Heart Association (AHA) uses SBP ≥130 and/or DBP ≥80 as "stage 1 hypertension" which should be treated with exercise and lifestyle modification and reserve medication for when the patient is at "higher risk" which is defined as age ≥65 years, CKD, diabetes, or known cardiovascular disease (CVD).

Geriatric Considerations
Isolated systolic HTN is common. Therapy has been shown to be effective and beneficial at preventing stroke and cardiovascular morbidity and all-cause mortality (2)[A], although target SBP for seniors is higher than in younger patients (~150 mm Hg systolic), and adverse reactions to medications are more frequent. The benefit of therapy has been conclusively demonstrated in older patients for SBP ≥160. Very elderly patients may be at particularly high risk of adverse events associated with pharmaceutical treatment of HTN. Strongest evidence of benefit has been shown with use of thiazide diuretics.

Pediatric Considerations
Defined as SBP or DBP ≥95th percentile on repeated measurements. Measure BP during routine exams beginning at age 3 years. Pre-HTN: SBP or DBP between 90th and 95th percentile

Pregnancy Considerations
- Elevated BP during pregnancy may represent chronic HTN, pregnancy-induced HTN, or preeclampsia. Angiotensin-converting enzyme (ACE) inhibitors and angiotensin II receptor blockers (ARBs) are contraindicated.
- Maternal and fetal mortality are reduced with treatment of severe HTN (see topic "Preeclampsia and Eclampsia (Toxemia of Pregnancy)"); preferred agents: labetalol, nifedipine, methyldopa, or hydralazine

EPIDEMIOLOGY

Prevalence
Depending on the definition used, 32–46% of adults in the United States have HTN; incidence and prevalence higher in men

ETIOLOGY AND PATHOPHYSIOLOGY
>90% of cases of HTN have no identified cause. For differential diagnosis and causes of secondary HTN, see "Hypertension, Secondary and Resistant."

Genetics
BP levels are strongly familial. Familial risk for CVD should be considered.

RISK FACTORS
Family history, obesity, alcohol use, excess dietary sodium, stress, physical inactivity, tobacco use, insulin resistance, obstructive sleep apnea (OSA)

 DIAGNOSIS

- Despite more aggressive guidelines issued by the ACC/AHA in 2017, many experts consider recommendations from JNC 8 (1) to retain primacy.
- Critics of the ACC/AHA guidelines note multiple methodologic concerns. Thresholds of <130/80 (as endorsed by ACC/AHA) compared to JNC 8 would result in the diagnosis of and treatment for HTN of millions more people, with unclear benefits and some inevitable harms.
- This chapter uses JNC 8 as its basis but recommendations are relevant regardless of the specific guideline being applied. We recommend assessment of overall CV risk and joint decision-making.

HISTORY
HTN is asymptomatic except in extreme cases or after related cardiovascular complications develop. Headache can be seen with higher BP, often present on awakening and occipital in location.

PHYSICAL EXAM
- Body mass index (BMI), waist circumference. Measure BP in both arms (see below for correct technique—essential to accurate diagnosis and treatment). Incorrect BP determination is a common cause of overdiagnosis.
- Complete cardiac and peripheral pulse exam: Compare radial and femoral pulse for differences in volume and timing (evaluation for aortic coarctation [especially in young persons], subclavian stenosis). Funduscopic exam for arteriolar narrowing, AV compression, hemorrhages, exudates, and papilledema

DIFFERENTIAL DIAGNOSIS
- Secondary HTN: Consider workup only if the history, physical exam, or basic laboratory evaluation suggests a higher likelihood. Also consider for patients who prove nonresponsive to treatment (see "Hypertension, Secondary and Resistant").
- White coat HTN: elevation of BP in office setting and normal BP outside office

DIAGNOSTIC TESTS & INTERPRETATION

ALERT
- Measuring BP: caffeine, exercise, and smoking avoided >30 minutes before measurement. Patient should be seated with back supported quietly for at least 5 minutes with feet on floor and patient's arm supported at heart level. Use correct cuff size. Deflate cuff slowly or use an automated device. Average two or more measurements, avoid "rounding" results. May leave patient alone to obtain in-office readings using an automated or patient-activated cuff.

- 2021 United States Preventive Services Taskforce (USPSTF) statement (Grade A): A diagnosis of HTN should be confirmed with BP measurements outside the clinical setting. Home BP measurements (HBPM) correlate better with CV outcomes than office values and also help to mitigate the errors of clinic measurement (3)[A]. Home BP measurement for diagnosis and for monitoring should be encouraged. For HBPM results, ≥135/85 should be used as a diagnostic threshold, and <135/85 should be the treatment target.
- Ambulatory BP monitoring (ABPM) is the ideal method, but this is not widely available in the United States.

Initial Tests (lab, imaging)
- Hemoglobin or hematocrit or complete blood count; potassium, calcium, creatinine, and uric acid; complete urinalysis (proteinuria, hematuria)
- Lipid panel. Fasting blood glucose or hemoglobin A1c. Consider possibility of sleep apnea with high BMI (2).
- ECG to evaluate possible presence of left ventricular hypertrophy (LVH) or rhythm abnormalities

Follow-Up Tests & Special Considerations
- ABPM or HBPM if "white coat" HTN is suspected, episodic HTN, or autonomic dysfunction. Ambulatory measurement may be especially helpful if there is suspected autonomic dysfunction.
- Perform CV risk assessment. The ACC/AHA risk tool overestimates risk (by 50% or more, especially in older patients). A definition of "low risk" excludes patients with a history of CVD, diabetes mellitus, CKD, and familial hypercholesterolemia or familial premature coronary artery disease.

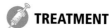 TREATMENT

GENERAL MEASURES
- The treatment discussed follows JNC 8 guidelines. Recent systematic reviews and meta-analyses of randomized trials do not support recommendations for lower-than-standard targets for the average-risk population. Potential harms of therapy must be weighed against the potential benefits.
- Treatment goals:
  – Age <60 years: SBP <140 and DBP <90 (for HBPM <135/85)
  – Age ≥60 years: SBP <150 and DBP <90 (for HBPM <140/90)
  – Age ≥60 years with CKD or diabetes: SBP <140 and DBP <90 (for HBPM <135/85)
- More aggressive treatment may be considered in high-risk patients meeting enrollment criteria for SPRINT because aggressive treatment shows improvement in outcomes, but 61 nondiabetic patients would need to be treated (NNT) for 3 years to a goal SBP of <120 mm Hg to prevent one major cardiovascular outcome and 90 such patients treated over 3 years to prevent one death (NNT 90).
- Even in secondary prevention, no firm conclusions can yet be drawn regarding the comparative effectiveness of intensive versus standard therapy.
- Individual treatment goals should be jointly established with patients after discussion of the anticipated potential benefits and harms (shared decision making) (2).

- Recommend lifestyle improvements, including diet, exercise, and reducing or eliminating tobacco/alcohol.
- Benefit of pharmacologic treatment of low-risk patients with class I HTN (140 to 150/90 to 99) remains uncertain, with harms including syncope, kidney injury, and electrolyte abnormalities. Individualize decisions.
- Treating patients with CKD or diabetes to lower-than-standard BP targets, <140/90, does not appear to further reduce mortality or morbidity. Individualize goal BP based on risk factors and patient preferences.
- The majority of treatment benefit is attained by lowering very high SBP (e.g., from 190 to 150, as compared with the benefit of lowering from 150 to 136). Striving for small additional drops in BP by adding fourth or fifth medications to achieve a "target" is less clinically beneficial and more likely to cause adverse effects. Lower-than-standard JNC-8 DBP targets are not associated with decreased morbidity/mortality.

MEDICATION
- Multiple drugs at submaximal dose may achieve target BP with fewer side effects. However, these benefits must be balanced against adherence challenges associated with increased pill burden and more complicated dosing regimens.
- In patients on >1 medication, give nondiuretic medications at bedtime for better 24-hour antihypertensive effect.
- Sequential monotherapy attempts should be tried with different classes because individual responses vary.
- Many patients will require multiple medications.
- For initial monotherapy, choose from 1 of 4 classes of medications: ACE inhibitors, ARBs, calcium channel blockers (CCBs), or diuretics; thiazide diuretics or CCB preferred as first line in the general black population
- β-Blockers such as atenolol had been strongly recommended until recent meta-analyses. However, β-blockers may benefit patients with ischemic heart disease, atrial fibrillation, CHF, migraine, and patients with history of ST-segment elevation myocardial infarction (STEMI).
- ACE inhibitors should be used in patients with diabetes, proteinuria, atrial fibrillation, or heart failure with reduced ejection fraction (HFrEF) but *not in pregnancy*.
- α-Adrenergic blockers are not a first choice for monotherapy but remain as second line after combination therapy of first-line agents; might benefit males with benign prostatic hypertrophy (BPH)
- CCB could be considered in patients with isolated systolic HTN, atherosclerosis, angina, migraine, or asthma; well-documented to reduce risk of stroke

First Line
- Thiazide diuretics may not be effective with creatinine clearance <30.
  - Chlorthalidone: 12.5 to 25.0 mg/day (longer half-life and more potent than hydrochlorothiazide but causes more hyponatremia and hypokalemia); strongest evidence base for this medication
  - Hydrochlorothiazide: 12.5 to 50.0 mg/day; indapamide: 1.25 to 2.50 mg/day; metolazone: 2.5 to 5.0 mg daily is more effective in patients with impaired renal function than other thiazides, but outcomes studies lacking.

- ACE inhibitors: lisinopril: 5 to 40 mg/day; enalapril: 5 to 40 mg/day; ramipril: 2.5 to 20.0 mg/day; benazepril: 10 to 40 mg/day
- CCB: amlodipine: 2.5 to 10 mg/day; nifedipine (sustained release): 30 to 90 mg/day; diltiazem CD: 180 to 360 mg/day; verapamil (sustained release): 120 to 480 mg/day
- ARBs: losartan: 25 to 100 mg in 1 or 2 doses, has unique but modest uricosuric effect; valsartan: 80 to 320 mg/day; irbesartan: 75 to 300 mg/day; candesartan: 4 to 32 mg/day; telmisartan: 20 to 80 mg/day; renin inhibitor: aliskiren 150 to 300 mg daily
- Contraindications: Thiazide diuretics may worsen gout. β-Blockers (relative) in asthma, heart block, diabetes, and peripheral vascular disease; probably should be avoided in patients with metabolic syndrome or insulin-requiring diabetes. Diltiazem or verapamil: Do not use with systolic dysfunction or heart block. Amlodipine causes peripheral edema.

Second Line
- Before escalating therapy, ensure that patient is adherent to prescribed regimen. Most classes may be combined. Choose additional medications with complementary effects (i.e., ACE inhibitors/ARBs with diuretic or a vasodilator with a diuretic or β-blocker). Don't combine ACE inhibitor and ARB.
- Medication-refractory HTN (see "Hypertension, Secondary and Resistant" topic): spironolactone 25 to 100 mg/day or eplerenone 50 mg once to twice daily are especially effective.
- β-Blockers may be effective in patients with resting tachycardia. Metoprolol succinate allows for once-daily dosing over a wide dosage range (25 to 400 mg daily). Carvedilol and labetalol combine α- and β- blockade.
- Centrally acting α₂-agonists: clonidine 0.1 to 1.2 mg BID or weekly patch 0.1 to 0.3 mg/day, guanfacine 1 to 3 mg daily, or methyldopa 250 to 2,000 mg BID
- α-Adrenergic antagonists: prazosin 1 to 10 mg BID, terazosin 1 to 20 mg/day, or doxazosin 1 to 16 mg/day
- Vasodilators: hydralazine: 10 to 25 mg QID; risk of tachycardia, so generally combined with β-blocker; also drug-induced systemic lupus erythematosus (SLE). Minoxidil: rarely used due to adverse effects; may be more effective than other medications in renal failure and refractory HTN
- Metolazone and loop diuretics may be used with more severe renal impairment, but outcomes data are absent; loop diuretics (for volume overload): furosemide 20 to 320 mg/day or bumetanide 0.5 to 2.0 mg/day
- K₊-sparing diuretics in patients with hypokalemia while taking thiazides: amiloride 5 to 10 mg/day or triamterene 50 to 150 mg/day

COMPLEMENTARY & ALTERNATIVE MEDICINE
Biofeedback and relaxation exercise

 ## ONGOING CARE

FOLLOW-UP RECOMMENDATIONS
Patient Monitoring

ALERT
Repeat electrolytes, BUN/creatinine about 3 to 6 weeks after initiating thiazide diuretics, ARB, or ACE inhibitor, to evaluate for drug-induced complications. Reevaluate patients q3–6mo until stable and then q6–12mo. Consider BP self-monitoring; monitor quality-of-life issues including sexual function.

- Poor medication adherence is a leading cause of apparent medication failure.
- At least annual creatinine and potassium for patients on diuretics, ACE inhibitors, and ARBs

DIET
- ~20% of patients will respond to reduced-salt diet (<6 g NaCl or <2.4 g Na per days). Limit alcohol consumption to <1 oz/day.
- Consider Dietary Approaches to Stop Hypertension (DASH) diet: http://www.nhlbi.nih.gov/files/docs/public/heart/hbp_low.pdf.

COMPLICATION
Heart and renal failure, LVH, myocardial infarction, retinal hemorrhage, stroke, hypertensive heart disease, drug side effects, erectile dysfunction

REFERENCES
1. James PA, Oparil S, Carter BL, et al. 2014 Evidence-based guideline for the management of high blood pressure in adults: report from the panel members appointed to the Eighth Joint National Committee (JNC 8). *JAMA*. 2014;311(5):507–520.
2. Qaseem A, Wilt TJ, Rich R, et al. Pharmacologic treatment of hypertension in adults aged 60 years or older to higher versus lower blood pressure targets: a clinical practice guideline from the American College of Physicians and the American Academy of Family Physicians. *Ann Intern Med*. 2017;166(6):430–437.
3. U.S. Prevention Services Task Force. Hypertension in adults: screening. https://www.uspreventiveservicestaskforce.org/uspstf/recommendation/hypertension-in-adults-screening. Published April 27, 2021. Accessed November 16, 2021.

 ## SEE ALSO

Hypertension, Secondary and Resistant; Hypertensive Emergencies; Polycystic Kidney Disease

 ## CODES

ICD10
I10 Essential (primary) hypertension

CLINICAL PEARLS
- Treatment of HTN reduces risk of major adverse CV events (MACE). The NNT to prevent a MACE from 10 to 50 per year in patients with severe HTN, but hundreds or thousands per year for patients with mild HTN.
- Measure BP outside the office.
- Overly aggressive treatment may cause significant harms, especially in the elderly.

H

HYPERTENSION, SECONDARY AND RESISTANT

George Maxted, MD

BASICS

DESCRIPTION

Uncontrolled hypertension (HTN) comprises the following entities (see "Alert" below):

- Resistant HTN: defined as blood pressure (BP) that remains above goal in spite of the concurrent use of three antihypertensive agents of different classes. Ideally, one of the three agents should be a diuretic, and all agents should be prescribed at optimal dose amounts. The diagnosis should not include "white-coat effect" or medication nonadherence, although these are common mimics.
- Secondary HTN: elevated BP that results from an identifiable underlying mechanism
- The 2017 revised ACC/AHA guideline recommends a change in the classification of HTN. For the purposes of this chapter, we are considering stage 2 HTN: systolic blood pressure (SBP) ≥140 mm Hg or diastolic blood pressure (DBP) ≥90 mm Hg. The guideline is quite controversial (1). See "Hypertension, Essential" topic. Many experts still adhere to the JNC 8 guideline, which allows for a goal of <150/90 mm Hg for patients age >60 years, and do not agree with a diagnosis or class of HTN for pressures below 140/90 (2)[C].

Geriatric Considerations
- Onset of HTN in adults >60 years of age is a strong indicator of secondary HTN.
- In patients >80 years of age, consider a higher target SBP of ≥150 mm Hg. Be cautious to avoid excessive diastolic lowering.
- Elderly may be particularly responsive to diuretics and dihydropyridine calcium channel blockers.
- Systolic HTN is particularly problematic in the elderly.
- Secondary causes more common in the elderly include sleep apnea, renal disease, atherosclerotic renal artery stenosis, and primary aldosteronism (PA).
- Noncompressible arteries (Osler phenomenon)—mostly in elderly with arteriosclerosis: Brachial and radial artery pulsations are present at high cuff pressures.

ALERT
Pseudoresistance:

- Inaccurate measurement of BP
  - Cuff too small
  - Patient not at rest; sitting quietly for 5 minutes
- Poor adherence: In primary care settings, this has been estimated to occur in 40–60% of patients with HTN.
- White coat effect: prevalence 20–40%. Do not make clinical decisions about HTN based solely on measurement in the clinic setting. Home BP monitoring and/or ABPM is more reliable. See USPSTF and AHA recommendations (3).
  - Automated office blood pressure (AOBP) is the preferred method of measurement. If AOBP is not possible, home blood pressure measurement (HBPM) is preferred when making decisions about treatment.
- Inadequate treatment

EPIDEMIOLOGY
- Predominant age: In general, HTN has its onset between ages 30 and 50 years. Patients with resistant HTN are more likely to experience the combined outcomes of death, myocardial infarction, congestive heart failure (CHF), stroke, or chronic kidney disease.
- Depending on etiology, age of onset can vary. Age of onset <20 or >50 years increases likelihood of a secondary cause for HTN.

- The strongest predictors for resistant HTN are age (>75 years), presence of left ventricular hypertrophy (LVH), obesity (body mass index [BMI] >30), and high baseline SBP. Other predictors include chronic kidney disease, diabetes, living in the Southeastern United States, African American race (especially women), and excessive salt intake.

Incidence
The age-standardized incidence in the United Kingdom is 0.4 cases per 100 person-years in 2015. Information in the United States is less clear (4).

Prevalence
- Prevalence of resistant HTN is estimated to be 10–15% in clinic-based reports (5). NHANES analysis indicates only 53% of adults are controlled to a BP of <140/90 mm Hg. The most common cause of apparently resistant hypertension is likely medication nonadherence.
- Secondary HTN occurs in about 5–10% of adults with chronic HTN.

ETIOLOGY AND PATHOPHYSIOLOGY
- Obstructive sleep apnea (25–50%): Results of interventions have been mixed.
- Primary hyperaldosteronism (8–20% of resistant HTN cases)
- Chronic renal disease (1–2% of hypertensives)
- Renovascular disease (0.2–0.7%, up to 35% of elderly, 20% of patients undergoing cardiac catheterization)
- Cushing syndrome (<0.1%)
- Pheochromocytoma (0.04–0.1% of hypertensives)
- Other rare causes: hyperthyroidism, hyperparathyroidism, aortic coarctation, intracranial tumor
- Drug-related causes
  - Medications, especially NSAIDs (may also blunt effectiveness of ACE inhibitors), decongestants, stimulants (e.g., amphetamines, attention deficient hyperactivity disorder [ADHD] medications), anorectic agents (e.g., modafinil, ephedra, guarana, ma huang, bitter orange), erythropoietin, natural licorice (in some chewing tobacco), yohimbine, glucocorticoids
  - Oral contraceptives (OCP): Women taking oral contraceptives may have more severe HTN and poorer BP control, primarily correlated with the estrogen content. Cessation of OCP may result in normalization of the BP. Postmenopausal estrogen does not appear to correlate as strongly (5).
  - Cocaine, amphetamines, other illicit drugs; drug and alcohol withdrawal syndromes
- Lifestyle factors: Obesity and dietary salt may negate the beneficial effect of diuretics. Excessive alcohol may cause or exacerbate HTN. Physical inactivity also contributes.

Genetics
BP has a genetic basis: It is heritable and more prevalent in certain families. Genetic variants have been detected in patients with resistant HTN but are estimated to account for <3% of BP variance (5).

RISK FACTORS
A large cohort study revealed that those with resistant HTN (16.2%) were more likely to be male, Caucasian, older, and diabetic. They were also more likely to be taking β-blockers, calcium channel blockers, and α-adrenergic blockers compared with other drug classes. Factors predictive of resistant or secondary HTN: obesity, diabetes, worsening of control in previously stable hypertensive patient, onset in patients age <20 years or >50 years, lack of family history of HTN, significant target end-organ damage,

stage 2 HTN (SBP >160 mm Hg or DBP >100 mm Hg), renal disease, and alcohol or drug use

GENERAL PREVENTION
The prevention of resistant and secondary HTN is thought to be the same as for primary or essential HTN: Adopting a Dietary Approaches to Stop Hypertension (DASH) diet, a low-sodium diet, weight loss in obese patients, exercise, limitation of alcohol intake, and smoking cessation may all be of benefit. Relaxation techniques may be of help, but data are limited.

COMMONLY ASSOCIATED CONDITIONS
Sleep disorders; obesity

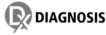

DIAGNOSIS

HISTORY
- Ask or review at every visit: SANS mnemonic: (i) Salt intake, (ii) Alcohol intake, (iii) NSAID use, (iv) Sleep (author's suggestion, based on reference listed) (1)
- Ask about medication adherence. Estimates are that during the 1st year of treatment for HTN, 20% of patients have sufficiently high adherence to achieve clinical benefit (5).
- Review home BP readings; consider ambulatory BP ABMP.
- History will vary with etiology of secondary HTN.
  - OSA: loud snoring while asleep, daytime somnolence
  - Pheochromocytoma: episodes of headache, palpitations, sweating
  - Cushing syndrome: weight gain, fatigue, weakness, easy bruising, amenorrhea
  - Increased intravascular volume: swelling

PHYSICAL EXAM
- Ensure that the BP is measured correctly. The patient should be sitting quietly with back supported for at least 5 minutes before measurement. Proper cuff size: bladder encircling at least 80% of the arm. Support arm at heart level. Minimum of two readings at least 1 minute apart. Check BP in both arms. Also check standing BP for orthostasis.
- The USPSTF recommends "obtaining measurements outside of the clinical setting for diagnostic confirmation." Attention to findings related to possible etiologies: renovascular HTN: systolic/diastolic abdominal bruit; pheochromocytoma: diaphoresis, tachycardia; Cushing syndrome: hirsutism, moon facies, dorsal hump, purple striae, truncal obesity; thyroid disease: enlarged thyroid, tremor, exophthalmos, tachycardia; coarctation of the aorta: upper limb HTN with decreased or delayed femoral pulses
- Check pulses, heart auscultation, legs for edema, funduscopic exam

DIFFERENTIAL DIAGNOSIS
Pseudoresistance

DIAGNOSTIC TESTS & INTERPRETATION
- ECG performed as part of the initial workup; LVH is an important marker of resistant HTN.
- Sleep study if history and physical indicate. The Epworth Sleepiness Scale is recommended.
- Home-based polysomnography has been shown to be accurate in screening for OSA. Overnight oximetry is not helpful.

Initial Tests (lab, imaging)
Initial limited diagnostic testing should include urinalysis, CBC, potassium, sodium, glucose, creatinine, lipids, thyroid-stimulating hormone (TSH), and calcium. 50%

of patients with hyperaldosteronism may have normal potassium levels.

- Imaging tests listed are necessary only if history, physical, or lab data indicate.
- Abdominal US: if renal disease is suspected
- Duplex ultrasonography may be the preferred test for renovascular disease. MR angiography (MRA) of renal vasculature is sensitive but has low specificity and potentially more harmful. Conventional catheter angiography or CT angiography may be required to confirm the diagnosis.
- Adrenal "incidentaloma" frequently arises in this era of multiple CT studies. If present in the setting of resistant HTN, consider hyperaldosteronism or hyperadrenal corticoid states.

Follow-Up Tests & Special Considerations

Further testing for PA may be considered.

- Empiric treatment with an aldosterone antagonist may be preferable and more clinically relevant: spironolactone or eplerenone (less estrogenic than spironolactone). Amiloride may be an option for potassium sparing but has not been shown to affect the aldosterone level.
- Plasma aldosterone-to-renin ratio (ARR) is the preferred lab test, but the test is difficult to perform and interpret properly. Consult your reference lab and interpret results with caution.
  – Further testing (screening) for pheochromocytoma: plasma metanephrines
  – Other tests to consider for resistant or secondary HTN: 24-hour urine for free cortisol, calcium, parathyroid hormone (PTH), overnight 1-mg dexamethasone suppression test, urine toxicology screen

Diagnostic Procedures/Other

Consider 24-hour ambulatory BP monitoring (ABPM), especially if white coat effect is suspected. Home BP monitor results predict mortality, stroke, and other target organ damage better than office BP. Optimal protocol involves two paired measurements: morning and evening (four measurements) over 4 to 7 days.

- Oscillometric, electronic, upper arm, fully automatic device with memory: average multiple readings over several days
- See http://www.dableducational.org/ for validated monitors.

 TREATMENT

- Treatment modality depends on etiology of HTN. Please see each etiology listed for information on proper treatment.
- The National Institute for Health Care and Excellence (5) offers a useful management algorithm emphasizing lifestyle modification: diet, less sodium, exercise, alcohol in moderation.
- Emphasize adherence to JNC 8 and/or AHA/ACC guidelines, with emphasis on lifestyle modification (1),(2)[C].
  – Obese patients and elderly may be particularly responsive to diuretics.
  – Tolerance to diuretics may occur: long-term adaptation to thiazides or the "braking effect." Consider increasing the dose of thiazide or adding an aldosterone inhibitor.
- Treatment specific to certain secondary etiologies
  – PA: aldosterone receptor antagonist: spironolactone or eplerenone (latter has less estrogenic effect)
  – Cushing syndrome: aldosterone receptor antagonist
  – OSA: continuous positive airway pressure (CPAP) ± oxygen, surgery, weight loss
    ○ Mandibular advancement devices may be equally effective in some patients.
  – Nocturnal hypoxia: oxygen supplementation

– Renal sympathetic denervation is controversial as current approaches have largely failed to demonstrate clinical benefit. A recent study on catheter-based renal denervation showed a modest decrease in SBP, but larger studies are needed to determine overall benefit (6).

- The treatment of atherosclerotic renal artery stenosis (ARAS) is controversial. A recent meta-analysis again questions the value of percutaneous stenting. ACEi and ARB medications may confer long-term mortality benefit (5)[C].

MEDICATION

- Follow treatment guidelines and algorithms by JNC 8 and AHA/ACC/CDC, understanding the differences between them (1)[C],(2)[C].
- Adding a medication to the regimen may have greater efficacy than increasing the dose of medications (see JNC 8 management algorithm option B) (2).
- Nighttime dosing of nondiuretic medications may increase efficacy and reduce adverse HTN outcomes (7)[A].
- Empiric use of aldosterone antagonists is often effective.
- Central-acting agents (e.g., clonidine) are effective at reducing BP, but outcome data are lacking.

ALERT

- Agents specific for treatment of HTN emergencies should be initiated in those situations, in which immediate BP reduction will prevent or limit endorgan damage (see "Hypertensive Emergencies").
- Renovascular HTN: Angioplasty is the treatment of choice for fibromuscular dysplasia of a renal artery.
- The CORAL study concluded that in patients with atherosclerotic renovascular disease and HTN, renal artery stenting did not improve outcomes over medical therapy alone.
- Referral to an HTN specialist or clinic: Retrospective studies indicate improved control rates for patients with resistant HTN referred to special HTN clinics.

First Line

- For non-black patients: thiazide diuretics, ACEi or ARB (not both), CCB
- For black patients: thiazide diuretics, CCBs. Hydralazine and isosorbide mononitrate or dinitrate are options. Note: Race-based prescribing has lately been called into question. People of African descent may, however, not respond to ACEi or ARB medications.

Second Line

Combine thiazide diuretic with ACEi, ARB, or CCB or add a K$^+$-sparing diuretic. β-Blockers—especially if compelling indication such as ischemic heart disease or CHF—migraine and tachyarrhythmias may also be indications.

Third Line

Add agent not used in second line; if this does not adequately lower BP, initiate workup for secondary causes (chronic NSAID use, alcohol abuse, RAS, etc.).

ISSUES FOR REFERRAL

If control is not successful, consider referral to a hypertension center or nephrology. If a secondary cause is identified, refer to the appropriate specialty.

ADDITIONAL THERAPIES

Nondrug interventions, other than standard lifestyle modifications, may be helpful.

COMPLEMENTARY & ALTERNATIVE MEDICINE

The University of Wisconsin Integrative Medicine program has an excellent handout and patient information.

ADMISSION, INPATIENT, AND NURSING CONSIDERATIONS

Hypertensive urgency or emergency general measures

 ONGOING CARE

FOLLOW-UP RECOMMENDATIONS

Encourage aerobic activity of 30 min/day, depending on patient's condition.

DIET

- Reduced salt may lower BP in some patients.
- Recommend the Mediterranean diet or DASH.

PATIENT EDUCATION

Home BP monitoring is recommended.

REFERENCES

1. Whelton PK, Carey RM, Aronow WS, et al. 2017 ACC/AHA/AAPA/ABC/ACPM/AGS/APhA/ASH/ASPC/NMA/PCNA guideline for the prevention, detection, evaluation, and management of high blood pressure in adults: executive summary: a report of the American College of Cardiology/American Heart Association Task Force on Clinical Practice Guidelines. *Hypertension*. 2018;71(6):1269–1324.
2. James PA, Oparil S, Carter BL, et al. 2014 Evidence-based guideline for the management of high blood pressure in adults: report from the panel members appointed to the Eighth Joint National Committee (JNC 8). *JAMA*. 2014;311(5):507–520.
3. Muntner P, Shimbo D, Carey RM, et al. Measurement of blood pressure in humans: a scientific statement from the American Heart Association. *Hypertension*. 2019;73(5):e35–e66.
4. Sinnott SJ, Smeeth L, Williamson E, et al. Trends for prevalence and incidence of resistant hypertension: population based cohort study in the UK 1995-2015. *BMJ*. 2017;358:j3984.
5. Carey RM, Calhoun DA, Bakris GL, et al. Resistant hypertension: detection, evaluation, and management: a scientific statement from the American Heart Association. *Hypertension*. 2018;72(5):e53–e90.
6. Böhm M, Kario K, Kandzari DE, et al. Efficacy of catheter-based renal denervation in the absence of antihypertensive medications (SPYRAL HTN-OFF MED Pivotal): a multicentre, randomised, sham-controlled trial. *Lancet*. 2020;395(10234):1444–1451.
7. National Institute for Health and Care Excellence. Hypertension in adults: diagnosis and management. https://www.nice.org.uk/guidance/ng136/chapter/recommendations. Published August 28 2019. Accessed January 27, 2021.

 SEE ALSO

Aldosteronism, Primary; Coarctation of the Aorta; Cushing Disease and Cushing Syndrome; Hyperparathyroidism; Hypertension, Essential; Hyperthyroidism; Pheochromocytoma

 CODES

ICD10

- I15.9 Secondary hypertension, unspecified
- I15.8 Other secondary hypertension
- I15.0 Renovascular hypertension

CLINICAL PEARLS

- Onset of HTN in adults >60 years of age is a strong indicator of secondary HTN.
- Aldosterone inhibitors should be considered in all cases of resistant HTN.
- Home BP monitoring predicts outcomes better than office monitoring of BP.

H

HYPERTHYROIDISM

Anup Sabharwal, MD, MBA, FACE, FASPC, FNLA

BASICS

- Hyperthyroidism or thyrotoxicosis is a spectrum of clinical findings consistent with thyroid hormone excess. The former describes excess from the thyroid gland, whereas the latter can also be produced from another source.
- In general, patients with thyrotoxicosis have hyperthyroidism. However, this is not always the case. Patients could suffer from thyrotoxicosis subacute thyroiditis, exogenous thyrotoxicosis, and radiation-induced thyroiditis.

DESCRIPTION

- Graves disease (GD): the most common form; diffuse goiter and thyrotoxicosis are common characteristics. Infiltrative orbitopathy is seen in up to 50% of patients. Infiltrative dermopathy is rare (1). Autoantibodies are directed at the thyroid-stimulating hormone (TSH) receptors.
- Toxic multinodular goiter (TMNG): second most common; most common cause of hyperthyroidism in patients age >65 years; patients >40 years, insidious onset, frequent in iodine-deficient areas
- Toxic adenoma (Plummer disease): younger patients, autonomously functioning nodules
- Iodine-induced hyperthyroidism
- Thyroiditis: transient autoimmune process:
  - Subacute thyroiditis/de Quervain: granulomatous giant cell thyroiditis, benign course; viral infections have been involved.
  - Postpartum thyroiditis
  - Drug-induced thyroiditis: amiodarone, interferon-α, interleukin-2, lithium
  - Miscellaneous: thyrotoxicosis factitia, TSH-secreting pituitary tumors, and functioning trophoblastic tumors (2)[B]
- Subclinical hyperthyroidism: suppressed TSH with normal thyroxine (T_4). There are two grades based on level of TSH. Grade 1 reflects a mild suppression of TSH in the range of (0.1–0.39 mU/L), and grade 2 reflecting a greater suppression with TSH <0.1 mU/L.
- Thyroid storm: rare hyperthyroidism; fever, tachycardia, gastrointestinal (GI) symptoms, CNS dysfunction (e.g., coma); up to 50% mortality

Geriatric Considerations

- Characteristic symptoms and signs may be absent.
- Atrial fibrillation is common when TSH <0.1 mIU/L (3)[A].

Pediatric Considerations

- Neonates and children are treated with antithyroid medications for 12 to 24 months.
- Radioactive iodine treatment is controversial in patients <15 to 18 years.

Pregnancy Considerations

Propylthiouracil is currently the drug of choice during 1st trimester of pregnancy, and methimazole is preferred in the 2nd and 3rd trimester (4)[A]. Treat with lowest effective dose. Avoid treatment-induced hypothyroidism. Radioiodine therapy is contraindicated.

EPIDEMIOLOGY

- 1.3% of population
- Predominant sex: female > male (7 to 10:1)
- Predominant age: autoimmune thyroid disease (GD) in 2nd and 3rd decades; TMNG more common in patients >40 years

Prevalence

The prevalence of hyperthyroidism is 1.3% and can increase in older women to 4–5%.

ETIOLOGY AND PATHOPHYSIOLOGY

- GD: autoimmune disease
- TMNG: 60% TSH receptor gene abnormality; 40% unknown
- Toxic adenoma: point mutation in TSH receptor gene with increased hormone production
- Thyroiditis:
  - Hashitoxicosis: autoimmune destruction of the thyroid; antimicrosomal antibodies present
  - Subacute/de Quervain thyroiditis: granulomatous reaction; genetic predisposition in specific human leukocyte antigens; viruses, such as coxsackievirus, adenovirus, echovirus, and influenza virus, have been implicated; self-limited course, 6 to 12 months
  - Suppurative: infectious
  - Drug-induced thyroiditis: Amiodarone produces an autoimmune reaction and a destructive process. Lithium, interferon-α, and interleukin-2 cause an autoimmune thyroiditis.
  - Postpartum thyroiditis: autoimmune thyroiditis that lasts up to 8 weeks, and in 60% of patients, hypothyroidism manifests in the future

Genetics

Concordance rate for GD among monozygotic twins is 35%.

RISK FACTORS

- Positive family history, especially in maternal relatives
- Other autoimmune disorders
- Iodide repletion after iodide deprivation, especially in TMNG

COMMONLY ASSOCIATED CONDITIONS

- Autoimmune diseases
- Down syndrome
- Iodine deficiency

℞ DIAGNOSIS

HISTORY

- Thyrotoxicosis is a hypermetabolic state in which energy production exceeds needs, causing increased heat production, diaphoresis, and even fever.
- Thyrotoxicosis affects several different systems:
  - Constitutional: fatigue, weakness, increased appetite, weight loss
  - Neuropsychiatric: agitation, anxiety, emotional lability, psychosis, coma, and poor concentration and memory
  - GI: increased appetite, hyperdefecation
  - Gynecologic: oligomenorrhea, amenorrhea
  - Cardiovascular: tachycardia (most common) and chest discomfort that mimics angina

Geriatric Considerations

Apathetic hyperthyroidism in the elderly

PHYSICAL EXAM

- Adults:
  - Skin: warm, moist, pretibial myxedema (GD only)
  - Head, eye, ear, nose, throat (HEENT): exophthalmos, lid lag
  - Endocrine: hyperhidrosis, heat intolerance, goiter, gynecomastia, and spider angiomata (males)
  - Cardiovascular: tachycardia, atrial fibrillation, cardiomegaly
  - Musculoskeletal: fractures
  - Neurologic: tremor, proximal muscle weakness, anxiety and lability, brisk deep tendon reflexes
  - Rarely: thyroid acropathy (clubbing), localized dermopathy
- Children:
  - Linear growth acceleration
  - Ophthalmic abnormalities more common

DIFFERENTIAL DIAGNOSIS

- Anxiety; depression
- Malignancy
- Diabetes mellitus
- Pregnancy
- Menopause
- Pheochromocytoma; carcinoid syndrome

DIAGNOSTIC TESTS & INTERPRETATION

- 95% have suppressed TSH and elevated free T_4. Total T_4 and triiodothyronine (T_3) represent the bound hormone and can be affected by pregnancy and hepatitis (2)[A].
- T_3: elevated, especially in T_3 toxicosis or amiodarone-induced thyrotoxicosis (AIT): Presence of TSH receptor antibody or thyroid-stimulating immunoglobulin is diagnostic of GD.
- Free thyroxine index (FTI): calculated from T_4 and thyroid hormone–binding ratio; corrects for misleading results caused by pregnancy and estrogens
- Inappropriately normal or elevated TSH with high T_4 suspicious for pituitary tumor or thyroid hormone resistance
- Drugs may alter lab results: estrogens, heparin, iodine-containing compounds (including amiodarone and contrast agents), phenytoin, salicylates, and steroids (e.g., androgens, corticosteroids).
- Exogenous biotin supplements can interfere with immunoassays for thyroid hormones, TSH, thyroglobulin, and TSH receptor binding inhibiting antibody (5)[B].
- Drug precautions: Amiodarone and lithium may induce hyperthyroidism; methimazole may cause warfarin resistance.
- Other findings that can occur: anemia, granulocytosis, lymphocytosis, hypercalcemia, transaminase, and alkaline phosphate elevations

Initial Tests (lab, imaging)

- TSH, free T_4, total T_4, and T_3 will establish the hyperthyroid diagnosis (6)[A].
- Thyrotropin receptor antibody (TRAb) (7)[A]
- TSH receptor antibodies (TSH-R Abs): The routine assay is the TSH-binding inhibitor immunoglobulin assay (TBII). TSH-R Abs are useful in the prediction of postpartum Graves thyrotoxicosis and neonatal thyrotoxicosis (6)[A].
- T_4/T_3 ratio: The T_4-to-T_3 ratio may be a useful tool when the iodine uptake testing is not available/contraindicated. ~2% of thyrotoxic patients have "T_3 toxicosis."

- Nuclear medicine uptake and scanning (^{123}I or ^{131}I): The reference-range value for 24-hour radioiodine uptake is between 5% and 25%.
- Increased thyroid iodine uptake is seen with TMNG, toxic solitary nodule, and GD.
- GD shows a diffuse uptake and can have a paradoxical finding of high uptake at 4 to 6 hours but normal uptake at 24 hours because of the rapid clearance.
- TMNG will show a heterogeneous uptake, whereas solitary toxic nodule will show a warm or "hot" nodule.
- In iodine-deficient areas, an increased uptake is associated with low urine iodine levels.
- Causes of thyrotoxicosis with low iodine uptake:
  – Acute thyroiditis, thyrotoxicosis factitia, and iodine intoxication with amiodarone or contrast material can cause low-uptake transient thyrotoxicosis. After thyroiditis resolves, the patient can become euthyroid or hypothyroid.
  – Iodine loading can cause iodine trapping and decreased iodine uptake (Wolff-Chaikoff effect).
  – Thyrotoxicosis factitia: Thyroglobulin levels are low in exogenous intake and high in endogenous production.
  – Other extrathyroidal causes include ovarian and metastatic thyroid carcinoma.
  – Technetium-99m scintigraphy: controversial because it has a 33% discordance rate with radioactive iodine scanning

Follow-Up Tests & Special Considerations
In severe cases, such as thyroid storm, hospitalize until stable, especially if >60 years of age, because of the risk of atrial fibrillation.

Diagnostic Procedures/Other
Neck ultrasound will show increased diffuse vascularity in GD.

Test Interpretation
- GD: hyperplasia
- Toxic nodule: nodule formation

 TREATMENT

- Observation may be appropriate for patients with mild hyperthyroidism (TSH >0.1 or no symptoms) especially those who are young and with low risk of complications (atrial fibrillation, osteoporosis).
- Antithyroid medication is contraindicated in patients with thyroiditis. Treatment for subacute thyroiditis is supportive with NSAIDs and β-blockers. Steroids can be used for 2 to 3 weeks (4). GD or TMNG can be managed by either antithyroid medication, radioactive iodine therapy (RAIT), or thyroidectomy.
- RAIT: most common definitive treatment used in United States for GD and TMNG
- Pretreatment with antithyroid drugs is preferred to avoid worsening thyrotoxicosis after RAIT. Methimazole is preferred over propylthiouracil as pretreatment because of decreased relapse, but it is held 3 to 5 days before therapy (4)[A].
- Usually, patients become hypothyroid 2 to 3 months after RAIT; therefore, antithyroid medications are continued after ablation.
- Glucocorticoids: reduce the conversion of active T_4 to the more active T_3. In Graves ophthalmopathy, the use of prednisone before and after RAIT prevents worsening ophthalmopathy (4)[B].
- For GD, due to the chance of remission, 12- to 18-month trial of antithyroid medications may be considered prior to offering RAIT.

- For TMNG, the treatment of choice is RAIT. Medical therapy with antithyroid medications has shown a high recurrence rate. Surgery is considered only in special cases (4)[B].
- For AIT type I, the treatment is antithyroid drugs and β-blockers. Thyroidectomy is the last option. AIT type II is self-limited but may use glucocorticoids.
- β-Blockers can aid in mitigating palpitations and reducing heart rate in those with accelerated sinus rhythm.

MEDICATION
First Line
- Antithyroid drugs: Methimazole and propylthiouracil are thioamides that inhibit iodine oxidation, organification, and iodotyrosine coupling. Propylthiouracil can block peripheral conversion of T_4 to active T_3. Both can be used as primary treatment for GD and prior to RAIT or surgery (2)[A].
- Duration of treatment: 12 to 18 months; 50–60% relapse after stopping; treatment beyond 18 months did not show any further benefit on remission rate. The most serious side effects are hepatitis (0.1–0.2%), vasculitis, and agranulocytosis; baseline CBC recommended:
  – Methimazole (preferred): adults: 10 to 15 mg q12–24h; children aged 6 to 10 years: 0.4 mg/kg/day PO once daily
  – Propylthiouracil: adults (preferred in thyroid storm and 1st trimester of pregnancy): 100 to 150 mg PO q8h, not to exceed 200 mg/day during pregnancy
- β-Adrenergic blocker: Propranolol in high doses (>160 mg/day) inhibits T_3 activation by up to 30%. Atenolol, metoprolol, and nadolol can be used and are also useful in relieving palpitations and in slowing the heart rate in patients with sinus tachycardia (1)[A].
- Glucocorticoids: reduce the conversion of active T_4 to the more active T_3
- Cholestyramine: anion exchange resin that decreases thyroid hormone reabsorption in the enterohepatic circulation; dose: 4 g QID (2)[B]
- Other agents:
  – Lithium: inhibits thyroid hormone secretion and iodotyrosine coupling; use is limited by toxicity.
  – Lugol solution or saturated solution of potassium iodide (SSKI); blocks release of hormone from the gland but should be administered at least 1 hour after thioamide was given; otherwise, acts as a substrate for hormone production (Jod-Basedow effect)
  – RAIT: See "Treatment" section.

ISSUES FOR REFERRAL
Refer patients with Graves ophthalmopathy to an experienced ophthalmologist.

SURGERY/OTHER PROCEDURES
Thyroidectomy for compressive symptoms, masses, and thyroid malignancy may be performed in the 2nd trimester of pregnancy only.

 ONGOING CARE

FOLLOW-UP RECOMMENDATIONS
Smoking cessation in GD patients as this is a risk factor for ophthalmopathy, especially after RAIT

Patient Monitoring
- Repeat thyroid tests q3mo, CBC, and liver function tests (LFTs) on thioamide therapy; continue therapy with thioamides for 12 to 18 months.
- After RAIT, thyroid function tests at 6 weeks, 12 weeks, 6 months, and annually thereafter if euthyroid; TSH may remain undetectable for months even after patient is euthyroid; follow T_3 and T_4.

DIET
Sufficient calories to prevent weight loss

PROGNOSIS
Good (with early diagnosis and treatment)

COMPLICATIONS
- Surgery: hypoparathyroidism, recurrent laryngeal nerve damage, and hypothyroidism
- RAIT: postablation hypothyroidism
- GD: high relapse rate with antithyroid drug as primary therapy
- Graves ophthalmopathy, worsening heart failure if cardiac condition, atrial fibrillation, muscle wasting, proximal muscle weakness, increased risk of cerebrovascular accident (CVA), and cardiovascular mortality

REFERENCES
1. Ross DS, Burch HB, Cooper DS, et al. 2016 American Thyroid Association guidelines for diagnosis and management of hyperthyroidism and other causes of thyrotoxicosis. *Thyroid*. 2016;26(10):1343–1421.
2. Bahn Chair RS, Burch HB, Cooper DS, et al. Hyperthyroidism and other causes of thyrotoxicosis: management guidelines of the American Thyroid Association and American Association of Clinical Endocrinologists. *Thyroid*. 2011;21(6):593–646.
3. Cappola AR, Fried LP, Arnold AM, et al. Thyroid status, cardiovascular risk, and mortality in older adults. *JAMA*. 2006;295(9):1033–1041.
4. Bahn RS, Burch HB, Cooper DS, et al. Hyperthyroidism and other causes of thyrotoxicosis: management guidelines of the American Thyroid Association and American Association of Clinical Endocrinologists. *Endocr Pract*. 2011;17(3):456–520.
5. Barbesino G. Misdiagnosis of Graves' disease with apparent severe hyperthyroidism in a patient taking biotin megadoses. *Thyroid*. 2016;26(6):860–863.
6. Abraham P, Avenell A, Park CM, et al. A systematic review of drug therapy for Graves' hyperthyroidism. *Eur J Endocrinol*. 2005;153(4):489–498.
7. Abraham-Nordling M, Törring O, Hamberger B, et al. Graves' disease: a long-term quality-of-life follow up of patients randomized to treatment with antithyroid drugs, radioiodine, or surgery. *Thyroid*. 2005;15(11):1279–1286.

 CODES

ICD10
- E05.81 Other thyrotoxicosis with thyrotoxic crisis or storm
- E05.80 Other thyrotoxicosis without thyrotoxic crisis or storm
- E05.1 Thyrotoxicosis with toxic single thyroid nodule

CLINICAL PEARLS
- Not all thyrotoxicoses are secondary to hyperthyroidism.
- GD presents with hyperthyroidism, ophthalmopathy, and goiter.
- Medical treatment for GD has a high relapse rate after stopping medications.
- Thyroid storm is a medical emergency that needs hospitalization and aggressive treatment.
- Serum TSH level may be misleading and remain low in the early period after initiating treatment, even when T_4 and T_3 levels have decreased.

H

HYPERTRIGLYCERIDEMIA
S. Lindsey Clarke, MD, FAAFP

BASICS

DESCRIPTION
- Hypertriglyceridemia (HTG) is a common form of dyslipidemia characterized by an excess fasting plasma concentration of triglycerides (TGs).
  - TGs are fatty molecules that occur naturally in vegetable oils and animal fats and are major sources of dietary energy.
  - Absorbed TGs are packaged into very low-density lipoproteins (VLDL) and chylomicrons.
- HTG is a risk factor for acute pancreatitis at levels ≥500 mg/dL and especially ≥1,000 mg/dL.
  - Risk is 10–20% at these TG levels.
  - Third leading cause of acute pancreatitis
- HTG also is independently associated with cardio-vascular disease (atherosclerotic cardiovascular disease [ASCVD]) at levels ≥175 mg/dL.
  - The American Heart Association (AHA) and the American College of Cardiology (ACC) consider persistent HTG a risk-enhancing factor.
  - A large Danish population study in 2018 showed that TG ≥264 mg/dL conferred a 10-year risk of major adverse cardiovascular events comparable to that of statin eligible individuals.
  - However, a causal relationship between HTG and ASCVD has not been firmly established.
  - Moreover, lowering TG has not been proven to reduce cardiovascular risk.
- AHA and ACC classify HTG into two categories:
  - Moderate: 175 to 499 mg/dL (2.0 to 5.6 mmol/L), characterized mainly by excess VLDL
  - Severe: ≥500 mg/dL (≥5.6 mmol/L), characterized by excess VLDL and chylomicrons

EPIDEMIOLOGY
- Predominant gender: male > female
- Predominant race: Hispanic, white > black

Prevalence
- 25–33% of U.S. population has TG levels ≥150 mg/dL.
- 1.7% has TG levels ≥500 mg/dL.
- Highest prevalence at age 50 to 70 years
- The most common genetic syndromes with HTG, familial combined hyperlipidemia and familial HTG, each affect ≤1% of general population.

ETIOLOGY AND PATHOPHYSIOLOGY
- Primary
  - Familial
  - Acquired (sporadic)
- Secondary
  - Lifestyle factors
    - Obesity and overweight
    - Physical inactivity
    - Cigarette smoking
    - Excess alcohol intake
    - Very high carbohydrate diets (>60% of total caloric intake)
  - Medical conditions
    - Type 2 diabetes mellitus
    - Metabolic syndrome/insulin resistance
    - Hypothyroidism
    - Chronic liver disease
    - Chronic kidney disease, nephrotic syndrome
    - Autoimmune disorders (e.g., systemic lupus erythematosus)
    - Paraproteinemias (e.g., macroglobulinemia, myeloma, lymphoma, lymphocytic leukemia)
    - Pregnancy (usually physiologic and transient)
  - Certain medications
    - Atypical antipsychotics (e.g., quetiapine)
    - Nonselective β-blockers
    - Bile acid sequestrants
    - Cyclophosphamide
    - Cyclosporine
    - Glucocorticoids
    - Interferon
    - Oral estrogens
    - Protease inhibitors (e.g., ritonavir, darunavir)
    - Retinoids
    - Rosiglitazone
    - Tamoxifen and raloxifene
    - Thiazides

Genetics
- Familial chylomicronemia (type 1 dyslipidemia): autosomal recessive inheritance of lipoprotein lipase deficiency; 0.0001% population prevalence
- Familial combined hyperlipidemia (type IIb): usually autosomal dominant, caused by overproduction of apolipoprotein (APO) B-100; approximately 1% prevalence
- Familial dysbetalipoproteinemia (type III): usually autosomal recessive, caused by lipoprotein overproduction due to inheritance of two APOE2 variants; 0.01% prevalence
- Familial HTG (type IV): autosomal dominant, caused by an inactivating mutation of the lipoprotein lipase gene; 1% prevalence
- Primary mixed HTG (type V)

RISK FACTORS
- Genetic susceptibility
- Obesity, overweight
- Lack of exercise
- Type 2 diabetes mellitus
- Alcoholism
- Certain medical conditions and drugs (see "Etiology and Pathophysiology")

GENERAL PREVENTION
- Maintain healthy body weight.
- Moderation of dietary fat and refined carbohydrates
- Regular aerobic exercise
- Avoid excess alcohol.

COMMONLY ASSOCIATED CONDITIONS
- Pancreatitis
- Coronary artery disease
- Type 2 diabetes mellitus and insulin resistance
- Dyslipidemias
  - Decreased high-density lipoprotein (HDL) cholesterol
  - Increased LDL, non-HDL, and total cholesterol
  - Small, dense LDL particles
- Metabolic syndrome (three of the following):
  - Abdominal obesity (waist circumference >40 inches in men, >35 inches in women)
  - TG ≥150 mg/dL
  - Low levels of HDL cholesterol (<40 mg/dL in men, <50 mg/dL in women)
  - BP ≥130/85 mm Hg
  - Fasting glucose ≥100 mg/dL
- Nonalcoholic steatohepatitis (NASH)
- Polycystic ovarian syndrome

DIAGNOSIS

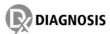

HISTORY
- Usually asymptomatic
- Patients with chylomicronemia syndrome can have memory loss, headache, vertigo, dyspnea, and paresthesias.
- Pancreatitis: epigastric pain, nausea, and vomiting
- Assess for other cardiac risk factors.
- Family history of coronary artery disease

PHYSICAL EXAM
- Obesity, overweight (body mass index ≥25 kg/m²)
- Eruptive cutaneous, tuberous, and striate palmar xanthomas
- Lipemia retinalis
- Epigastric tenderness in pancreatitis
- Hepatomegaly in NASH and chylomicronemia

DIFFERENTIAL DIAGNOSIS
Primary and secondary HTG

DIAGNOSTIC TESTS & INTERPRETATION

Initial Tests (lab, imaging)
- Serum: turbid with milky supernatant
- Fasting (12 hours) or nonfasting lipid profile
  - USPSTF recommends screening adults aged 40 to 75 years to identify dyslipidemia and to calculate 10-year ASCVD risk; repeat every 5 years.
  - American Academy of Pediatrics recommends screening all children for dyslipidemia at 9 to 11 years and 17 to 21 years of age, but USPSTF found insufficient evidence for screening in children and adolescents.
  - Statin therapy may be indicated for LDL and ASCVD risk reduction in some adults (e.g., clinical ASCVD, diabetes) regardless of lipid levels.
  - Confirm severe HTG with fasting measurement.
  - For interpretation, see "Description."
- Evaluation for secondary causes
  - Glycosylated hemoglobin, fasting or postprandial glucose for type 2 diabetes mellitus
  - Creatinine, urinary protein measurement for nephrotic syndrome, renal failure
  - Thyroid-stimulating hormone for hypothyroidism
  - Human chorionic gonadotropin for pregnancy
- Pancreatitis: serum lipase; US and/or CT of pancreas
- Atherosclerosis: cardiac stress testing, coronary CT angiography, cardiac catheterization, and coronary angiography

Follow-Up Tests & Special Considerations
- Repeat lipid panel after 2 months of therapy.
- High levels of apoB (>130 mg/dL) are a strong predictor of coronary death in patients whose LDL cannot be calculated because of very high TGs. But evidence for routine clinical measurement of apoB is lacking.

 TREATMENT

GENERAL MEASURES
- Cardiovascular risk reduction through LDL lowering should be prioritized over TG lowering unless patient is at risk for pancreatitis due to severe HTG (TG ≥500 mg/dL) (1)[C].
- Therapeutic lifestyle changes are first-line interventions for all patients and can reduce TG by as much as 50%:
  – Dietary modification (by decreasing carbohydrate intake to <50% of calories and limiting alcohol intake)
  – Moderate-intensity physical activity can reduce TG by 20–30%.
  – Weight loss of 5–10% can reduce TG by as much as 20%.
  – Persons with very high TG should abstain from alcohol.
- Search for correctable secondary causes, treat underlying illness, or remove offending drug.
- Improve glycemic control if diabetic.
- Control other cardiac risk factors, such as hypertension, diabetes mellitus, and smoking.
- Primary HTG: Screen other family members.

MEDICATION
First Line
- Statins: the most effective agents for reducing cardiovascular risk; primarily affect LDL but also may lower TG 15–30% (2)[A]. 2018 ACC/AHA guidelines recommend initiating therapy for 10-year ASCVD risk ≥7.5% and other clinical factors (1)[C], but AHA/ACC calculator overestimates risk significantly. Dosing depends on intensity of statin desired based on ASCVD risk. See "Coronary Artery Disease and Stable Angina" and "Hypercholesterolemia."
  – Rosuvastatin: 5 to 40 mg/day
  – Atorvastatin: 10 to 80 mg/day
  – Adverse reactions: myalgias, myopathy, rhabdomyolysis (especially if combined with fibrates); contraindicated in pregnancy and lactation
- Fibrates: the most effective agents for reducing TG up to 50%; used primarily to reduce risk of pancreatitis in severe HTG; have been shown to decrease nonfatal myocardial infarction but not all-cause mortality (3)[A]:
  – Fenofibrate: 30 to 200 mg daily (preferred)
  – Gemfibrozil: 600 mg BID; avoid in combination with statins due to high risk of muscle injury
  – Adverse reactions: GI upset, hepatotoxicity, cholelithiasis, myalgias, rhabdomyolysis (when combined with a statin), gemfibrozil-warfarin interaction (enhanced anticoagulation)

Second Line
Marine omega-3 fatty acids
- Icosapent ethyl (Vascepa) 2 g BID; preferred add-on therapy for HTG in patients with high ASCVD risk (4)[A]
- Omega-3-acid ethyl esters (Lovaza, other fish oils): 4 g daily or 2 g BID
- May lower TG 30–50%
- Limited tolerability due to adverse GI effects (diarrhea in up to 15%; also nausea, abdominal pain, dysgeusia, eructation, dyspepsia)
- Conflicting outcomes data (5)[A]

ISSUES FOR REFERRAL
- HTG refractory to treatment
- Familial HTG syndromes

ADMISSION, INPATIENT, AND NURSING CONSIDERATIONS
- Acute pancreatitis
- Acute coronary syndrome
- In acute hypertriglyceridemic pancreatitis with TG >1,000 mg/dL, the following interventions can be used to lower TG rapidly and safely to <500 mg/dL:
  – Apheresis (therapeutic plasma exchange) for 1 to 3 days
  – Insulin infusion
    ○ Regular insulin 0.1 to 0.3 U/kg/hr IV for 2 to 4 days
    ○ Administer separate infusion of dextrose 5% if blood glucose <200 mg/dL.
- Discharge criteria: stabilization of acute complicating illness

 ONGOING CARE

FOLLOW-UP RECOMMENDATIONS
2 months after initiation or modification of therapy (repeat fasting lipid profile)

Patient Monitoring
- Fasting lipid profile every 6 to 12 months
- Maintain TG <500 to 1,000 mg/dL to reduce risk of acute pancreatitis.
- Hepatic transaminases
- Creatine phosphokinase if patient has myalgias

DIET
- Restrict dietary fat to 30% of total caloric intake; restrict further to 15% of caloric intake if TG ≥1,000 mg/dL.
- Limit carbohydrates (especially simple carbohydrates and sugars) to 60% of total caloric intake.
- Mediterranean-style diet reduces TG 10–15% more than a low-fat diet.
- Increase marine-derived omega-3 polyunsaturated fatty acids. Eat fatty fish such as salmon, mackerel, sardines, and trout.
- Eliminate trans fatty acids.
- Increase dietary fiber.
- Avoid refined carbohydrates.
- Moderate alcohol intake (<1 oz/day) or complete abstinence if TGs are very high.

PATIENT EDUCATION
Smoking cessation for cardiovascular risk reduction

PROGNOSIS
- Good with correction of TG levels
- Patients with primary HTG usually require lifelong treatment.

COMPLICATIONS
- Atherosclerosis
- Chylomicronemia syndrome
- Pancreatitis

REFERENCES
1. Grundy SM, Stone NJ, Bailey AL, et al. 2018 AHA/ACC/AACVPR/AAPA/ABC/ACPM/ADA/AGS/APhA/ASPC/NLA/PCNA guideline on the management of blood cholesterol: a report of the American College of Cardiology/American Heart Association Task Force on Clinical Practice Guidelines. *J Am Coll Cardiol*. 2019;73(24):e285–e350.
2. Karlson BW, Palmer MK, Nicholls SJ, et al. A VOYAGER meta-analysis of the impact of statin therapy on low-density lipoprotein cholesterol and triglyceride levels in patients with hypertriglyceridemia. *Am J Cardiol*. 2016;117(9):1444–1448.
3. Wang D, Liu B, Tao W, et al. Fibrates for secondary prevention of cardiovascular disease and stroke. *Cochrane Database Syst Rev*. 2015;2015(10):CD009580.
4. Bhatt DL, Steg PG, Miller M, et al. Cardiovascular risk reduction with icosapent ethyl for hypertriglyceridemia. *N Engl J Med*. 2019;380(1):11–22.
5. Aung T, Halsey J, Kromhout D, et al. Associations of omega-3 fatty acid supplement use with cardiovascular disease risks: meta-analysis of 10 trials involving 77917 individuals. *JAMA Cardiol*. 2018;3(3):225–234.

ADDITIONAL READING
- Oh RC, Trivette ET, Westerfield KL. Management of hypertriglyceridemia: common questions and answers. *Am Fam Physician*. 2020;102(6):347–354.
- Simha V. Management of hypertriglyceridemia. *BMJ*. 2020;371:m3109.

 SEE ALSO

- Hypercholesterolemia; Pancreatitis, Acute
- Algorithm: Hypertriglyceridemia

 CODES

ICD10
E78.1 Pure hyperglyceridemia

CLINICAL PEARLS
- HTG is likely a risk factor for atherosclerosis at levels ≥175 mg/dL and for acute pancreatitis at levels ≥500 to 1,000 mg/dL.
- Therapeutic lifestyle interventions (diet and exercise) are recommended for all patients who have HTG and for all patients at risk for ASCVD.
- Address reversible secondary causes of HTG.
- In patients with TG levels <500 mg/dL, the primary pharmacologic strategy for cardiovascular risk management is statins.
- For patients with TG levels ≥500 mg/dL, the greatest amount of TG lowering is achieved with fibrates; however, the magnitude of clinical benefit is uncertain, so statin use is generally recommended first for cardiovascular risk reduction, with additional use of marine omega-3 fatty acids and/or cautious use of fibrates, if needed.

H

HYPOGLYCEMIA, DIABETIC

Niyomi De Silva, MD • Afsha Rais Kaisani, MD

BASICS

DESCRIPTION
- Abnormally low concentration of glucose in circulating blood of a patient with diabetes mellitus (DM); often referred to as an *insulin reaction*
- Classification of hypoglycemia (1):
  – Level 1: hypoglycemia alert value; <70 mg/dL (3.9 mmol/L): may or may not be accompanied by symptoms; asymptomatic hypoglycemia if symptoms not present
  – Level 2: clinically significant hypoglycemia; <54 mg/dL (3.0 mmol/L)
  – Level 3: severe hypoglycemia. No specific glucose threshold: hypoglycemia associated with severe cognitive impairment requiring external assistance for recovery
- Pseudohypoglycemia: typical symptoms but glucose ≥70 mg/dL (3.9 mmol/L)
- Hypoglycemia is the leading limiting factor in the glycemic management of type 1 DM (T1DM) and type 2 DM (T2DM). Severe or frequent hypoglycemia requires modification of treatment regimens, including higher treatment goals.

EPIDEMIOLOGY
Incidence
- Most commonly found in patients with long-standing T1DM and children age <7 years
- From the ACCORD study, the annual incidence of hypoglycemia was the following:
  – 3.14% in the intensive treatment group
  – 1.03% in the standard group
  – Increased risk among women, African Americans, those with less than high school education, aged participants, and those who used insulin at trial entry
- From the RECAP-DM study: Hypoglycemia was reported in 35.8% of patients with T2DM who added a sulfonylurea or thiazolidinedione to metformin therapy during the past year.

ETIOLOGY AND PATHOPHYSIOLOGY
Loss of hormonal counterregulatory mechanism in glucose metabolism
- Impaired insulin, glucagon, and epinephrine secretion

RISK FACTORS
- Nearly 3/4 of severe hypoglycemic episodes occur during sleep.
- Severe hypoglycemia is associated with comorbid conditions in patients aged ≥65 years.
- Intensive insulin therapy (further lowering HbA1c from 7% to 6%) is associated with higher rate of hypoglycemia.
- Comorbidities: renal/liver disease, congestive heart failure (CHF), hypothyroidism, hypoadrenalism, gastroenteritis, gastroparesis (unpredictable CHO delivery), autonomic neuropathy, pregnancy, anxiety, depression, disordered eating behavior, illness/stress, and unplanned life events
- Duration of DM >5 years
- Young children with type 1 diabetes
- Advanced age
- Reduced cognitive function, dementia

- Starvation, prolonged fasting, weight loss, or food insecurity
- Current smokers with T1DM
- Alcoholism: Alcohol consumption may increase risk of delayed hypoglycemia, especially if on insulin or insulin secretagogues. Evening consumption of alcohol is associated with an increased risk of nocturnal and fasting hypoglycemia, especially in patients with T1DM.
- Insulin secretagogues: Sulfonylureas (glyburide, glimepiride, glipizide, etc.) and glinide derivatives (repaglinide, nateglinide) stimulate insulin secretion.
- Hypoglycemia is rare in diabetics not treated with insulin or insulin secretagogues.
- Other antidiabetes medications such as dipeptidyl peptidase 4 (DPP-4) inhibitors, glucagon-like peptide-1 (GLP-1) agonists, and sodium-glucose cotransporter-2 (SGLT-2) agents carry a lower but present risk of hypoglycemia, which may increase when combining agents from different categories.

Geriatric Considerations
- American Geriatric Society Beers Criteria recommend avoiding glyburide and chlorpropamide due to their prolonged half-life in older adults and risk for prolonged hypoglycemic episodes. Medications should be dosed for age and renal function.
- Individualize pharmacologic therapy in older adults to reduce the risk of hypoglycemia, avoid overtreatment, and simplify complex regimens if possible while maintaining the HbA1c target (1)[A].

Pediatric Considerations
Children may not realize when they have hypoglycemia, needing increased supervision during times of higher activity. Children may have higher glycemic goals for this reason. Caregivers should be instructed in use of glucagon (2)[A].

Pregnancy Considerations
Hypoglycemia management and avoidance education should be reemphasized and blood glucose monitoring increased due to more stringent glycemic goals and increased risk in early pregnancy (1)[A].

GENERAL PREVENTION
- Maintain routine schedule of diet (consistent CHO intake), medication, and exercise (1)[A].
- Regular self-monitoring of blood glucose (SMBG) or continuous glucose monitoring (CGM)
  – Particularly helpful for asymptomatic hypoglycemia
  – Use if taking insulin or secretagogue.
  – Utilize ≥3 times daily testing if multiple injections of insulin, insulin pump therapy, or pregnant diabetic; frequency and timing dictated by needs and treatment goals
- Diabetes treatment and teaching programs (DTTPs) especially for high-risk type 1 patients, which teach flexible insulin therapy to enable dietary freedom
- Hypoglycemia may be decreased with use of insulin analogs, continuous SC insulin infusion (CSII) pumps, and CGM systems (1)[A].

COMMONLY ASSOCIATED CONDITIONS
- Neuropathies
- Cardiomyopathies

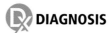

DIAGNOSIS

HISTORY
- Discuss timing of episodes, awareness, frequency, and causes (1).
- Symptoms vary considerably between individuals.
- Adrenergic symptoms
  – Hunger, trembling, pallor, sweating, shaking, pounding heart, anxiety, urinary incontinence
- Neurologic symptoms
  – Dizziness, poor concentration, drowsiness, weakness, confusion, light-headedness, slurred speech, blurred vision, double vision, unsteadiness, poor coordination
  – Hypoglycemia causes a significant deterioration in reading span and subject-verb agreement, demonstrating that language processing is impaired during moderate hypoglycemia (3).
- Behavioral symptoms: tearfulness, confusion, fatigue, irritability, aggressiveness
- If altered cognition, consider hypoglycemia.

PHYSICAL EXAM
- General: confusion, lethargy
- HEENT: diplopia
- Coronary: tachycardia
- Neurologic: tremulousness, weakness, paresthesia, stupor, seizure, or coma
- Mental status: irritability, anxiety, inability to concentrate, or short-term memory loss
- Skin: pale, diaphoresis
- End-organ damage: microvascular, macrovascular, ophthalmologic, neurologic, renal

DIFFERENTIAL DIAGNOSIS
Hypoglycemia not associated with DM may be seen in:
- Chronic alcoholics and binge drinkers
- GI dysfunction causing postprandial hypoglycemia or alimentary reactive hypoglycemia
- Hormonal deficiency states (hormonal reactive hypoglycemia)
- Hypoglycemia of sepsis
- Islet cell tumors
- Factitious hypoglycemia from surreptitious injection of insulin

DIAGNOSTIC TESTS & INTERPRETATION
- Plasma, serum, or whole-blood glucose
- SMBG and CGM are especially useful for asymptomatic hypoglycemia (2)[A].
- A hypoglycemic reading from a CGM sensor should be verified by SMBG fingerstick glucose testing prior to treatment, unless specific device is approved otherwise (1)[A].
- Low HbA1c level may be due to chronic hypoglycemia.
- Disorders that may alter lab results
  – Conditions that affect erythrocyte turnover, such as hemolysis or blood loss, and hemoglobin variants may alter HbA1c (1)[A].

TREATMENT

GENERAL MEASURES

- Glucose: pure glucose preferred; any form of CHO that contains glucose should be effective (see "Medication" section below) (1)[A].
- Glucagon should be prescribed proactively to patients at risk for clinically significant hypoglycemia. People in close contact with these individuals should be instructed on how to use an emergency glucagon kit (1)[A].
- Insulin-treated patients with hypoglycemia unawareness or an episode of clinically significant hypoglycemia should have glycemic targets raised to strictly avoid hypoglycemia (1)[A].
- α-Glucosidase inhibitors (acarbose) prevent digestion of complex CHOs; therefore, hypoglycemia must be treated with monosaccharides, such as glucose tablets.
- Patients with T1DM should use insulin analogs to reduce hypoglycemia risk (1)[A].
- Address medications (i.e., insulin, sulfonylureas, GLP-1 agonists, thiazolidinediones) that may induce hypoglycemia.
- CGM-augmented CSII with automated insulin suspension when blood glucose falls below a threshold value reduces the combined rate of severe and moderate hypoglycemia in T1DM and reduces nocturnal hypoglycemia without increasing HbA1c levels in patients >16 years old (4)[A].

MEDICATION

- Conscious patients (1)[A]:
  – Glucose (15 to 20 g) is preferred, although any form of CHO may be used.
    ○ Any sugar-containing food or beverage that can be rapidly absorbed: juice or nondiet soda (4 to 5 oz), candy (5 to 6 pieces of hard candy), or OTC glucose tablets (4 tablets = 16 g CHO)
    ○ Takes ~15 minutes for CHOs to be digested and enter bloodstream as glucose
    ○ "Rule of 15": 15 to 20 g CHO (~60 to 80 calories simple CHO) repeated q15min until blood sugar is ≥70 mg/dL
- Loss of consciousness at home (4)[A]:
  – Administer glucagon.
  – IM or SC in the deltoid or anterior thigh
    ○ Age <6 years and/or weight <20 to 25 kg: 0.50 mg
    ○ Age ≥6 years and/or weight >20 to 25 kg: 1 mg
    ○ May repeat dose in 15 minutes if needed
- In unconscious, with emergency medical personnel present or patient hospitalized (4)[A]:
  – Give 25 g IV 50% dextrose every 5 to 10 minutes until patient awakens.
  – Then, feed orally and/or administer 5% dextrose IV at level that will maintain blood glucose >100 mg/dL.
  – Patients with hypoglycemia secondary to oral hypoglycemics should be monitored for 24 to 48 hours because hypoglycemia may recur after apparent clinical recovery.
- Nasal glucagon—currently in developmental stage—comes in a ready-to-use device (5).

ADMISSION, INPATIENT, AND NURSING CONSIDERATIONS

- A hypoglycemia prevention and management protocol should be adopted and implemented by each hospital or hospital system (1)[A].
- Admission criteria/initial stabilization
  – Any doubt of cause
  – Expectation of prolonged hypoglycemia (e.g., caused by sulfonylurea drug)
  – Inability to drink
  – Treatment has not resulted in prompt sensory recovery.
  – Seizures, coma, or altered behavior (e.g., ataxia, disorientation, unstable motor coordination, dysphasia) secondary to documented or suspected hypoglycemia
- Discharge criteria: Normoglycemia and risk of severe hypoglycemia are negligible (1).

 ONGOING CARE

DIET

- Alcohol consumption may place patients with diabetes at increased risk for delayed hypoglycemia (1)[A].
- CHO sources high in protein should not be used to treat or prevent hypoglycemia (1)[A].
- Fats may slow absorption of CHOs and may prolong the acute glycemic response (1)[A].
- Food insecurity increases risk of hypoglycemia due to inadequate or erratic carbohydrate consumptions following administration of sulfonylureas or insulin (1)[A].

PATIENT EDUCATION

- Always have access to quick-acting CHO.
- For exercise, consider ingestion of added CHO if preexercise blood sugar <100 mg/dL or a reduced insulin dose.
- Educate patients and their relatives, close friends, teachers, and supervisors to be aware of DM diagnosis and signs/symptoms of hypoglycemia and treatment.
- Teach SMBG and self-adjustment for insulin therapy, diet control, and exercise regimen.
- Wear medical alert identification bracelet or necklace.

COMPLICATIONS

- Coma, seizure, myocardial infarction, stroke (especially in elderly)
- Prolonged or severe hypoglycemia may cause permanent neurologic damage and/or cognitive impairment.
- Children with T1DM have a greater vulnerability to neurologic manifestations of hypoglycemia.

ALERT
The ACCORD trial (adults with T2DM) demonstrated that intensively lowering blood glucose below current recommendations increased the risk of death versus standard treatment strategy.

REFERENCES

1. American Diabetes Association. 6. Glycemic targets: standards of medical care in diabetes—2021. *Diabetes Care*. 2021;44(Suppl 1):S73–S84.
2. Seaquist ER, Anderson J, Childs B, et al; for American Diabetes Association, Endocrine Society. Hypoglycemia and diabetes: a report of a workgroup of the American Diabetes Association and the Endocrine Society. *J Clin Endocrinol Metab*. 2013;98(5):1845–1859.
3. Allen KV, Pickering MJ, Zammitt NN, et al. Effects of acute hypoglycemia on working memory and language processing in adults with and without type 1 diabetes. *Diabetes Care*. 2015;38(6):1108–1115.
4. Cryer PE, Axelrod L, Grossman AB, et al; for Endocrine Society. Evaluation and management of adult hypoglycemic disorders: an Endocrine Society clinical practice guideline. *J Clin Endocrinol Metab*. 2009;94(3):709–728.
5. Beato-Víbora PI, Arroyo-Díez FJ. New uses and formulations of glucagon for hypoglycaemia. *Drugs Context*. 2019;8:212599.

ADDITIONAL READING

Thompson AE. JAMA patient page. Hypoglycemia. *JAMA*. 2015;313(12):1284.

 SEE ALSO

- Diabetes Mellitus, Type 1
- Algorithm: Hypoglycemia

 CODES

ICD10
- E11.649 Type 2 diabetes mellitus with hypoglycemia without coma
- E10.649 Type 1 diabetes mellitus with hypoglycemia without coma
- E13.649 Oth diabetes mellitus with hypoglycemia without coma

CLINICAL PEARLS

- Abnormally low concentration of glucose in patients with DM; often referred to as an *insulin reaction*
- Best treatment includes:
  – Immediate administration of glucose—in form of CHO (oral) IM or IV glucagon
  – Patient education and empowerment—address hypoglycemia in every visit with patients at risk
  – Frequent SMBG or CGM with flexible insulin (or other drug) regimens
  – Individualized glycemic goals based in part on the risk of hypoglycemia
- Using the "rule of 15" is an easy way to teach patients to manage hypoglycemia at home. "Rule of 15": 15 to 20 g CHO (~60 to 80 calories simple CHO) SMBG and repeated q15min until blood sugar is ≥70 mg/dL

H

HYPOGLYCEMIA, NONDIABETIC

Matthew A. Silva, PharmD, RPh, BCPS • Pablo I. Hernandez Itriago, MD, MHCM, FAAFP

BASICS

DESCRIPTION
- Hypoglycemia is defined by the Whipple triad:
  - Low plasma glucose level (≤60 mg/dL) with hypoglycemic symptoms that are relieved when glucose is corrected
  - Occurs commonly in patients with diabetes receiving insulin secretagogues (sulfonylureas, meglitinides) or insulins; is less common in patients without diabetes
- Postprandial or reactive hypoglycemia occurs in response to a meal, drugs, herbal substances, or nutrients and may occur 2 to 3 hours postprandially or later. This is noncongenital, beta-islet dysregulation with or without hyperplasia and insulin secretion.
  - Autonomic symptoms are generally observed with a serum glucose ≤60 mg/dL, and neuroglycopenic symptoms at a serum glucose of ≤50 mg/dL, or lower in patients with hypoglycemic unawareness.
  - Hypoglycemia is also seen after GI or bariatric surgery (in association with dumping syndrome in some).
- Spontaneous (fasting) hypoglycemia may be associated with primary conditions including hypopituitarism, Addison disease, myxedema, or disorders related to critical illness, heart failure, hepatic or renal failure.
  - If hypoglycemia presents as a primary disorder, consider hyperinsulinism and extrapancreatic tumors.

EPIDEMIOLOGY
Incidence
- 0.5–8.6% of hospitalized patients ≥65 years without diabetes (1),(2)
- Asymptomatic in 25% of cases

Prevalence
True prevalence is unknown:
- Predominant age: older adult
- Predominant sex: female > male

ETIOLOGY AND PATHOPHYSIOLOGY
- Reactive, postprandial
  - Alimentary hyperinsulinism
  - Meals including refined or processed carbohydrates, liquid forms of fructose, sucrose, or glucose
  - Certain nutrients, including galactose, leucine
  - Glucose intolerance (prediabetes)
  - GI surgery, especially bariatric surgery (i.e., Roux-en-Y gastric bypass)
  - Idiopathic (unknown causes)
- Spontaneous
  - Fasting
  - Situations or housing with restricted food access (i.e., unhoused persons, those in hospitals, prisons)
  - Alcohol or prescription medication–associated (insulin, sulfonylureas, meglitinides, thiazolidinediones, incretin mimetics, sodium-glucose cotransporter-2 (SGLT-2) inhibitors, DPP-IV inhibitors, angiotensin-converting enzyme inhibitors, β-blockers, salicylates, quinine, hydroxychloroquine, fluoroquinolones, doxycycline and tetracycline derivatives, linezolid, sertraline, disopyramide, pentamidine, gabapentin, tramadol) (3)

- Nonprescription over-the-counter (OTC) agents, including performance-enhancing agents. Adulterated versions of phosphodiesterase inhibitors and performance-enhancing agents are routinely imported and may contain sulfonylureas and other hypoglycemic agents.
- Consider medication administration errors as a source of unexplained hypoglycemia in persons without diabetes, especially those with polypharmacy (6 or more medications).
  - This includes accidental, surreptitious, or malicious use of insulin or oral hypoglycemics.
- Natural medicines or herbs (bitter melon, caffeine, cassia cinnamon, chromium, fenugreek, ginseng, guarana, mate, stevia, vanadium)
- Postsurgical (e.g., Roux-en-Y bariatric surgery, gastrectomy) hypoglycemia/dumping syndrome
- Islet cell hyperplasia or tumor (insulinomas)
- Extrapancreatic insulin-secreting tumors and other large tumors secreting insulin-like growth factor 2 (IGF-2)
- Autoimmune hypoglycemia (Hirata disease) and insulin receptor mutations
- Heart failure with or without SGLT-2 inhibitors (empagliflozin, dapagliflozin, canagliflozin)
- Hepatic disease or failure; renal disease or failure
- Renal glycosuria
- Glucagon deficiency
- Adrenal insufficiency
- Catecholamine deficiency
- Hypopituitarism
- Hypothyroidism
- Eating disorders
- Exercise or physical activity (i.e., manual labor)
- Fever
- Pregnancy
- Ketotic hypoglycemia of childhood
- Severe nutrient deficiencies (i.e., selenium)
- Congenital disorders
- Sepsis, cachexia, anorexia

Genetics
- Monogenic and congenital hyperinsulinism (i.e., channelopathies, enzyme and transport anomalies, transcription factor or enzyme abnormalities) (4),(5)
- Inborn errors of metabolism including the glycogenoses, fructose intolerance, neoglucogenesis, and fatty acid or beta-oxidation disorders (5)

RISK FACTORS
Refer to "Etiology and Pathophysiology."

GENERAL PREVENTION
- Follow dietary and exercise guidelines.
- Patient recognition of early symptoms and knowledge of corrective action

Pediatric Considerations
- Usually divided into two syndromes:
  - Transient neonatal hypoglycemia
  - Hypoglycemia of infancy and childhood
- Screening infants for hypoglycemia is appropriate when pregnancy was complicated by maternal diabetes.
- Cases of hypoglycemia observed in children taking propranolol for infantile hemangioma
- Associated with indomethacin when treating patent ductus arteriosus

Geriatric Considerations
- More likely to have underlying disorders or be caused by medications
- Iatrogenic hypoglycemia is common in the hospitalized elderly with renal insufficiency.

COMMONLY ASSOCIATED CONDITIONS
- Heart failure; severe, chronic hepatic and renal disease; alcoholism
- Addison disease; adrenocortical insufficiency
- Myxedema
- Malnutrition (patients with renal failure)
- GI and bariatric surgery
- Panhypopituitarism
- Insulinoma

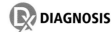

DIAGNOSIS

HISTORY
- Adrenergic symptoms are prominent with acute drop in glucose ≤60 mg/dL.
  - Anxiety
  - Tremulousness
  - Dizziness
  - Diaphoresis
  - Warmth/flushing
  - Heart palpitations
- CNS (neuroglycopenic) symptoms appear at a serum glucose ≤50 mg/dL.
  - Headache
  - Confusion
  - Light-headedness
  - Fatigue and weakness
  - Visual disturbances
  - Changes in personality
- GI symptoms
  - Hunger
  - Nausea
  - Belching

PHYSICAL EXAM
- CNS (neuroglycopenic) symptoms predominate with gradual glucose reduction:
  - Convulsions
  - Coma
  - Hypotension
- Adrenergic symptoms: more prominent in acute drop in glucose
  - Tremulousness
  - Diaphoresis
  - Warmth/flushing
  - Heart palpitations

DIFFERENTIAL DIAGNOSIS
CNS disorders
- Psychogenic
- Pseudohypoglycemia: Symptoms of hypoglycemia or self-diagnosis in patients in whom low blood glucose may not be detectable and may be impossible to convince that they do not suffer from hypoglycemia after all tests are found to be normal.

DIAGNOSTIC TESTS & INTERPRETATION

Initial Tests (lab, imaging)

- Blood glucose ≤45 mg/dL (≤2.5 mmol/L) when symptomatic followed by symptom resolution with feeding (6)[C]
- Plasma glucose overnight fasting: ≤60 mg/dL (≤3.33 mmol/L); confirm on ≥2 occasions (6)[C].
- Plasma glucose 72-hour fasting: ≤45 mg/dL (≤2.5 mmol/L) for females; ≤55 mg/dL (≤3.05 mmol/L) for males; fasting may be ended when Whipple triad is achieved or hypoglycemia is demonstrated (6)[C].
- Imaging (abdominal) using transabdominal ultrasound, CT, MRI, or PET (4)[C]

Follow-Up Tests & Special Considerations

- Misinterpretation of glucose tolerance tests may lead to misdiagnosis of hypoglycemia; ≥1/3 of normal patients have hypoglycemia, with or without symptoms, during the 4-hour glucose tolerance test. These patients may be at future risk for type 2 diabetes.
- C-peptide measurement (6)[C]
- Check liver studies, serum insulin, adrenocorticotropic hormone (ACTH), and cortisol. Serum insulin should be suppressed when glucose is <60 mg/dL (4)[C].
- Serum β-hydroxybutyrate <2.7 mg/dL in the presence of high-serum insulin, C-peptide, and low serum glucose suggests excessive insulin production (6)[C]
- Insulin radioimmunoassay: Elevated insulin levels suggest islet cell hyperplasia or tumor.
- Drugs that may alter lab results: Many drugs can affect glucose levels; review drugs individually and refer to drug or laboratory reference.

Diagnostic Procedures/Other

For definitive diagnosis, patient should have (4),(6)[C]

- Documented low glucose levels
- Symptoms when glucose levels are low
- Evidence that symptoms are relieved specifically by ingestion of glucose or food
- Identification of the specific type of hypoglycemia (4),(5),(6)[C]

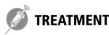

TREATMENT

GENERAL MEASURES

- Oral carbohydrate for alert patient without drug overdose (2 to 3 tbsp of sugar in glass of water or fruit juice, 1 to 2 cups of milk, piece of fruit, or several soda crackers)
- If unable to swallow: Use glucagon IM or SC.
- If caused by medication or nutrients: Avoid or control causative agents.
- If triggered by meals: Try high-protein diet with carbohydrate restriction.

- Nonhypoglycemic hypoglycemia or pseudohypoglycemia
  - Many patients (often women aged 20 to 45 years) present with diagnosis of reactive or post-prandial hypoglycemia (self-diagnosed or misinterpretation of tests).
  - Symptoms may pertain to chronic fatigue and somatic complaints (stress often plays a role in these symptoms).
  - Management difficult; listening is important. Try 120 g carbohydrate diet.
  - Counseling may be useful for stress and other problems.

MEDICATION

- Once diagnosis is established, begin therapy appropriate for underlying disorder (6)[C].
- If unable to swallow: glucagon 1 mg (1 unit) IV, IM, or SC. If no response, give IV bolus of 25 to 50 g of 50% glucose solution followed by continuous infusion until patient able to take by mouth. Intranasal glucagon is 3 mg (one actuation per device) into a single nostril; may repeat one time after 15 minutes if there is no response using a second intranasal device (4)[C].
- Postsurgical gastrectomy patients unresponsive to dietary changes may benefit from propantheline, psyllium, fiber, or oat bran to delay gastric emptying.

SURGERY/OTHER PROCEDURES

If islet cell tumor (insulinoma) or other insulin-secreting tumor, surgery is treatment of choice; if inoperable, diazoxide may relieve symptoms (4),(5)[C].

ADMISSION, INPATIENT, AND NURSING CONSIDERATIONS

Hypoglycemia unresponsive to oral intake

 ONGOING CARE

FOLLOW-UP RECOMMENDATIONS

- Exercise routine or daily activity may need to be reevaluated and readjusted.
- Patients with recurrent hypoglycemia should have glucose source at hand for immediate ingestion during symptoms.

Patient Monitoring

- Depends on type and severity of symptoms and treatment of underlying cause
- Hypoglycemia from sulfonylureas can last for hours to days depending on half-life and renal function.

DIET

- High protein, high fiber, complex carbohydrates from plant and multigrain sources with some fat by using whole foods in moderation
- Frequent small feedings (six daily); avoid liquid calories (4)[C].
- Avoid fasting.

PATIENT EDUCATION

- Dietary instruction
- Counseling for stress, if appropriate
- Recognition of early symptoms of hypoglycemia and how to take corrective action

PROGNOSIS

Favorable, with appropriate treatment

COMPLICATIONS

- Insulinoma: If tumor identified and removed, some surgical risk is involved.
- Organic brain syndrome: may occur with extensive, prolonged hypoglycemia

REFERENCES

1. Mannucci E, Monami M, Mannucci M, et al. Incidence and prognostic significance of hypoglycemia in hospitalized non-diabetic elderly patients. *Aging Clin Exp Res*. 2006;18(5):446–451.
2. Leibovitz E, Khanimov I, Wainstein J, et al. Documented hypoglycemia is associated with poor short and long term prognosis among patients admitted to general internal medicine departments. *Diabetes Metab Syndr*. 2019;13(1):222–226.
3. Ben Salem C, Fathallah N, Hmouda H, et al. Drug-induced hypoglycaemia: an update. *Drug Saf*. 2011;34(1):21–45.
4. Kittah NE, Vella A. MANAGEMENT OF ENDOCRINE DISEASE: Pathogenesis and management of hypoglycemia. *Eur J Endocrinol*. 2017;177(1):R37–R47.
5. Douillard C, Jannin A, Vantyghem MC. Rare causes of hypoglycemia in adults. *Ann Endocrinol (Paris)*. 2020;81(2–3):110–117.
6. Cryer PE, Axelrod L, Grossman AB, et al. Evaluation and management of adult hypoglycemic disorders: an Endocrine Society clinical practice guideline. *J Clin Endocrinol Metab*. 2009;94(3):709–728.

 SEE ALSO

- Hypoglycemia, Diabetic; Insulinoma
- Algorithm: Hypoglycemia

 CODES

ICD10

- E16.2 Hypoglycemia, unspecified
- E16.1 Other hypoglycemia
- P70.4 Other neonatal hypoglycemia

CLINICAL PEARLS

- Symptoms coincide with low blood glucose levels and resolve with PO/IV glucose or glucagon.
- Avoid known agents/nutrients that trigger hypoglycemia.
- Treat underlying cause.

H

HYPOKALEMIA
Jason Chao, MD, MS • Sibley Strader, MD

 BASICS

DESCRIPTION
Hypokalemia is defined as a serum potassium concentration <3.5 mEq/L (normal range, 3.5 to 5.0 mEq/L).
- Mild hypokalemia (serum potassium 3.0 to 3.5 mEq/L)
- Moderate hypokalemia (serum potassium 2.5 to 3.0 mEq/L)
- Severe hypokalemia (serum potassium <2.5 mEq/L)

EPIDEMIOLOGY
Predominant sex: male = female

Prevalence
- Commonly encountered in clinical practice
- >20% of hospitalized patients (when defined as potassium <3.6 mEq/L)
- >10% of inpatients with alcoholism
- 80% of patients receiving diuretics
- 12–18% of patients with chronic kidney disease
- Higher (5–20%) in individuals with eating disorders
- Higher in patients with AIDS
- Associated risk after bariatric surgery

ETIOLOGY AND PATHOPHYSIOLOGY
Most common causes:
- Decreased intake: deficient diet in alcoholics and elderly; anorexia nervosa
- GI loss: vomiting, diarrhea, nasogastric tubes, laxative abuse, fistulas, colorectal tumor, bowel diversion, ureterosigmoidostomy, malabsorption, chemotherapy, radiation enteropathy, bulimia
- Intracellular shift of potassium: metabolic alkalosis, insulin excess, β-adrenergic catecholamine excess (acute stress, β_2-agonists), hypokalemic periodic paralysis, intoxications (theophylline, caffeine, barium, toluene), refeeding syndrome (1), intensive exercise
- Renal potassium loss
  - Drugs: diuretics especially loop and thiazides, amphotericin B, aminoglycosides, antipseudomonal penicillins (carbenicillin), high-dose penicillin, clay (bentonite)
  - Mineralocorticoid excess: primary hyperaldosteronism (Conn syndrome); secondary hyperaldosteronism (congestive heart failure, cirrhosis, nephrotic syndrome, malignant hypertension, renin-producing tumors); renovascular hypertension
  - Exogenous mineralocorticoids (glycyrrhizic acid in licorice, carbenoxolone, nasal steroids)
  - Osmotic diuresis (e.g., poorly controlled diabetes)
  - Types I and II renal tubular acidosis
- Magnesium depletion
- Glucocorticoid excess: Cushing syndrome, exogenous steroids, ectopic adrenocorticotrophic hormone production, refeeding syndrome
- Diabetic ketoacidosis (DKA) treatment with delayed/inadequate potassium replenishment

Genetics
Some rare, familial disorders that can cause hypokalemia
- 11-β-Hydroxysteroid dehydrogenase deficiency
- Apparent mineralocorticoid excess
- Congenital adrenogenital syndromes
- Familial glucocorticoid resistance
- Familial hypokalemic periodic paralysis
- Familial interstitial nephritis
- Fanconi syndrome
- Geller syndrome
- Sodium channel mutations: Bartter, Gitelman, Liddle syndrome

RISK FACTORS
- Higher systolic BP
- Thiazide/loop diuretic use; ACE
- Low serum cholesterol/low BMI
- Higher albumin-to-creatinine ratio

GENERAL PREVENTION
When initiating a diuretic, monitor potassium level

COMMONLY ASSOCIATED CONDITIONS
- Acute GI illnesses with severe vomiting or diarrhea
- Increased risk of cardiac arrhythmias
- Predictor of development of severe alcohol withdrawal syndrome

 DIAGNOSIS

- Usually asymptomatic until serum potassium is below 3.0 mEq/L, unless it falls rapidly or patient has potentiating factor, for example, disposition to arrhythmia
- Signs and symptoms mainly involve neuromuscular, cardiovascular, renal, and endocrine system.

HISTORY
- Diuretic use, malnutrition, vomiting, diarrhea
- Easy fatigability, leg cramps, muscle weakness
- Polyuria, polydipsia, nocturia; hyperglycemia, alkalosis/acidosis
- Heart failure, shortness of breath

PHYSICAL EXAM
- Neuromuscular—skeletal muscle weakness (proximal > distal), ascending paralysis
  - Smooth muscle—GI hypomobility
  - Respiratory muscle—respiratory acidosis, respiratory arrest
- Cardiovascular—hypotension, orthostasis, peripheral edema; auscultate for arrhythmias and rales.
- Renal—metabolic acidosis, rhabdomyolysis, myoglobinuria; chronic kidney disease (tubular interstitial nephritis, nephrogenic diabetes insipidus, renal cyst)

DIFFERENTIAL DIAGNOSIS
Hypokalemia is a laboratory diagnosis that does not require distinction from other entities once laboratory error has been excluded.

DIAGNOSTIC TESTS & INTERPRETATION
- Serum potassium <3.5 mEq/L (<3.5 mmol/L)
- Disorders that may alter lab results: leukemia and leukocytosis

Initial Tests (lab, imaging)
- ECG
- Start workup if history rules out GI or iatrogenic causes (2).
  - Serum and urinary potassium level to evaluate the severity of hypokalemia
  - Basic metabolic panel (serum sodium, potassium, glucose, chloride, bicarbonate, BUN, creatinine);

serum magnesium, calcium, and/or phosphorus to exclude associated electrolyte abnormality especially if alcoholism is suspected
  - Spot urine electrolytes (potassium and chloride) to differentiate renal versus nonrenal cause
  - Arterial blood gas to detect metabolic acidosis or alkalosis
  - Urinalysis and urine pH for renal tubular acidosis
  - Serum digoxin level for patient on digitalis
  - Creatinine kinase for rhabdomyolysis in severe hypokalemia
  - Clinical suspicion is high: urine/serum drug screen for amphetamines and other sympathomimetic stimulants; TSH in case of tachycardia or suspicion of hypokalemic periodic paralysis

Follow-Up Tests & Special Considerations
- Two major components (2)
  - Urine potassium excretion to distinguish renal loss versus other causes
  - Acid–base status
- 24-hour urinary potassium excretion (best method): >15 mEq/day = inappropriate renal loss; if unavailable:
  - Spot urine potassium-to-creatinine ratio >13 mEq/g (1.5 mEq/mmol) can indicate inappropriate renal loss; or
  - Transtubular potassium gradient (TTKG) >4 can also suggests renal loss.
    - TTKG = (urine K^+/plasma K^+) / (urine Osm/plasma Osm)
- Metabolic acidosis + low urinary excretion → GI loss
- Metabolic acidosis + urinary potassium wasting → DKA, renal tubular acidosis type 1 or 2
- Metabolic alkalosis + low urinary excretion → vomiting or diuretic use
- Metabolic alkalosis + urine potassium wasting →
  - Normotensive: vomiting (low urine chloride); Gitelman/Bartter syndrome (normal urine chloride), diuretics (Urine chloride varies with types.)
  - Hypertensive: primary aldosteronism, Liddle syndrome, Geller syndrome, glucocorticoid resistance
- If excessive renal potassium loss (>20 mEq/day) and hypertension, obtain plasma renin and aldosterone levels to differentiate adrenal from nonadrenal causes of hyperaldosteronism.

Diagnostic Procedures/Other
- Consider imaging in cases with high clinical index of suspicion (2).
  - MRI/CT of adrenal gland with suspicion of mineralocorticoid, glucocorticoid, or catecholamine excess
  - MRI of pituitary gland to exclude Cushing syndrome
  - Abdominal CT for VIPoma

Test Interpretation
- ECG
  - T-wave flattening, ST-segment changes
  - U waves (small, positive deflection after T wave, best seen in V_2 and V_3)
  - Arrhythmias include sinus bradycardia, PAC/PVC, paroxysmal atrial or junctional tachycardia, atrioventricular block, ventricular tachycardia or fibrillation.

TREATMENT

- Reduce potassium loss.
- Replenish stored potassium.
- Evaluate potential toxicities.
- Determine cause.

GENERAL MEASURES
- Manage underlying disease or eliminate causative factor.
  - Discontinue laxative, use potassium-neutral or potassium-sparing diuretics.
  - Treat diarrhea and vomiting.
  - Use H_2 blockers in patient with nasogastric suction.
  - Control hyperglycemia if glucosuria is present.

MEDICATION
- Nonemergent conditions (serum potassium >2.5 mEq/L [>2.5 mmol/L], no cardiac manifestations)
  - Oral therapy preferred: 40 to 120 mEq/day (40 to 120 mmol/day) in divided doses
  - Ensure adequate hydration (100 to 250 mL of water), better if given with or after meal.
  - IV potassium only when oral administration is not feasible (e.g., vomiting, postoperative state)
    - Rate should not exceed 10 mEq/hr, and concentration should not exceed 40 mEq/L to lessen burning and discomfort at IV site and to avoid phlebitis.
    - A central line is recommended for rate over 10 mEq/hr; up to 40 mEq in 100 mL can be safely given via central access.
    - Potassium chloride (KCl) is suitable for all forms of hypokalemia.
    - Potassium bicarbonate or precursor (gluconate, acetate, or citrate) in metabolic acidosis
    - Potassium phosphate in phosphate deficiency as in DKA (3)[C]
- Emergent situations (serum potassium <2.5 mEq/L [<2.5 mmol/L], arrhythmias) (2)[A]
  - IV replacement—standard infusion rate: 10 mmol/hr; maximum infusion rate: 20 mmol/hr
  - Central line preferred
- If patient is hypomagnesemic (2)[A]
  - First, give 4 mL MgSO4 50% (8 mmol) in 10 mL of NaCl 0.9% over 20 minutes and then start first 40 mmol KCl infusion followed by magnesium replacement.
- Precautions
  - Any form of potassium replacement carries the risk of hyperkalemia.
  - Serum potassium should be checked more frequently in groups at higher risk: the elderly, diabetic patients, and patients with renal insufficiency.
  - Patients receiving insulin for DKA require more timely and aggressive potassium replacement in order to account for the intracellular shift (4)[A].
  - Dietary potassium is almost entire coupled to phosphate, rather than chloride, and does not correct potassium loss from chloride depletion (e.g., diuretics or vomiting).
- Significant possible interactions: Concomitant administration of potassium-sparing diuretics (spironolactone, triamterene, amiloride, ACE inhibitors) magnifies risk of hyperkalemia.

Geriatric Considerations
- Younger patient has a higher prevalence for hypokalemia, but elderly develop hypokalemia more rapidly.
- Low serum potassium can induce limb paralysis, myonecrosis, and increase fall risk.

ISSUES FOR REFERRAL
Patient with unexplained hypokalemia, refractory hyperkalemia, or features suggesting alternative diagnosis (e.g., aldosteronism or hypokalemic periodic paralysis) should be referred to endocrinology or nephrology.

ADMISSION, INPATIENT, AND NURSING CONSIDERATIONS
- Outpatient follow-up is sufficient for asymptomatic patients treated with oral replacement.
- Patients with cardiac manifestations require IV replacement with continuous cardiac monitoring in an inpatient setting.
- Patient with life-threatening complications such as arrhythmias or respiratory failure requires ICU admission.

 ONGOING CARE

FOLLOW-UP RECOMMENDATIONS
Patient Monitoring
- Patients receiving IV therapy should have continuous cardiac monitoring and serum potassium level monitored q4–6h.
- Patients requiring potassium supplements should have serum potassium and magnesium levels repeated at intervals dictated by clinical judgment and patient compliance (5)[C].

DIET
- Ensure adequate intake: potassium-rich food including oranges, bananas, cantaloupes, prunes, raisins, dried beans, dried apricots, and squash.
- Reduce sodium intake: High-sodium diet can cause urinary potassium loss.

PATIENT EDUCATION
- Instructions for appropriate diet
- Emphasis the risk of nonadherence to potassium supplement.
- Potassium Fact Sheet for Consumers. NIH Office of Dietary Supplements: https://ods.od.nih.gov/pdf /factsheets/Potassium-Consumer.pdf

PROGNOSIS
- Most hypokalemia will correct with replacement after 24 to 72 hours.
- If primary cause is eliminated, hypokalemia will likely resolved with no further treatment needed.
- Associated with higher morbidity and mortality because of cardiac arrhythmias

COMPLICATIONS
- Hyperkalemia during the course of treatment
- Increased risk of digoxin toxicity
- Increased risk of arrhythmias by increasing myocyte's resting potential and in turn its refractory period

REFERENCES
1. Palmer BF. A physiologic-based approach to the evaluation of a patient with hypokalemia. *Am J Kidney Dis*. 2010;56(6):1184–1190.
2. Kardalas E, Paschou SA, Anagnostis P, et al. Hypokalemia: a clinical update. *Endocr Connect*. 2018;7(4):R135–R146.
3. Asmar A, Mohandas R, Wingo CS. A physiologic-based approach to the treatment of a patient with hypokalemia. *Am J Kidney Dis*. 2012;60(3): 492–497.
4. Kovesdy CP, Matsushita K, Sang Y, et al. Serum potassium and adverse outcomes across the range of kidney function: a CKD Prognosis Consortium meta-analysis. *Eur Heart J*. 2018; 39(17):1535–1542.
5. Unwin RJ, Luft FC, Shirley DG. Pathophysiology and management of hypokalemia: a clinical perspective. *Nat Rev Nephrol*. 2011;7(2):75–84.

ADDITIONAL READING
- Osadchii OE. Mechanisms of hypokalemia-induced ventricular arrhythmogenicity. *Fundam Clin Pharmacol*. 2010;24(5):547–559.
- Skogestad J, Aronsen JM. Hypokalemia-induced arrhythmias and heart failure: new insights and implications for therapy. *Front Physiol*. 2018;9:1500.
- Viera A, Wouk N. Potassium disorders: hypokalemia and hyperkalemia. *Am Fam Physician*. 2015;92(6):487–495.

 SEE ALSO

- Hyperkalemia
- Algorithm: Hypokalemia

CODES

ICD10
E87.6 Hypokalemia

CLINICAL PEARLS
- In patients with cardiac ischemia, heart failure, or left ventricular hypertrophy, even mild to moderate hypokalemia can cause arrhythmias. These patients should receive potassium repletion as well as cardiac monitoring.
- Uncorrected hypomagnesemia can hinder the correction of hypokalemia.
- Hypokalemia in an otherwise healthy young woman should prompt evaluation for bulimia nervosa.
- Supplement potassium when prescribing drugs that cause hypokalemia; minimize dosage of non–potassium-sparing diuretics.

H

HYPONATREMIA
Cassandra Q. White, MD, FACS • Caitlin E. Jones, MD • Patricia Martinez Quinones, MD, PhD

BASICS

DESCRIPTION
- Hyponatremia is a plasma sodium (Na^+) concentration of ≤ 135 mEq/L.
- Hyponatremia itself does not provide information about the total body water (TBW) state of the patient. Patients with hyponatremia may be hypervolemic, hypovolemic, or euvolemic.
- System(s) affected: endocrine/metabolic, renal, cardiovascular, central nervous system (CNS)

EPIDEMIOLOGY
Incidence
- Most common electrolyte disorder seen in the general hospital population
- Predominant age: all ages
- Predominant sex: male = female
Prevalence
- 2.5% of hospitalized patients
- 20–30% in hospitalized patients (1)
- 7.7% outpatients (1)

Geriatric Considerations
Elderly patients have a decreased renal mass placing them at risk decreased urinary concentration and decreased response to antidiuretic hormone. Additionally, they have a lower TBW state, a decreased thirst mechanism, and decreased renal blood flow, which will also affect the glomerular filtration rate. Presenting symptoms may be frequent falls and gait disturbances.

Pediatric Considerations
Children <16 years of age have less intracranial space and are at increased risk of brain herniation from cerebral edema.

ETIOLOGY AND PATHOPHYSIOLOGY
- Volume status and serum osmolality must be ascertained to determine etiology in order to direct management.
- Hypertonic hyponatremia: serum osmolarity (Osm) > 295 mOsmol/kg
  - Water shifts from intracellular fluid (ICF) to extracellular fluid (ECF), resulting in dilution.
    - Unchanged TBW and Na^+
    - Causes: hyperglycemia, mannitol, sorbitol, radiologic contrast
- Isotonic hyponatremia ("pseudohyponatremia"): serum Osm 275 to 295 mOsmol/kg
  - Excessive osmoles leading to dilution
  - Unchanged TBW and Na^+
  - Causes: hyperlipidemia, hyperproteinemia (e.g., multiple myeloma), laboratory artifact, irrigant solutions
- Hypotonic hyponatremia: serum Osm <275 mOsmol/kg
  - Subdivided by volume status into hypovolemic, euvolemic, or hypervolemic
  - Hypovolemic hyponatremia: low TBW and low Na^+
- Signs include orthostatic hypotension, decreased skin turgor, dry mucous membranes.
- If urine Na^+ <30 mmol/L, it indicates extrarenal loss such as GI loss (vomiting, diarrhea), third-spacing (pancreatitis, burns), skin loss (burns, cystic fibrosis, sweating), and heat-related illnesses.
- If urine Na^+ >30 mmol/L, it indicates renal loss such as cerebral salt wasting, adrenal insufficiency, diuretics, and osmotic diuresis.

- Euvolemic hyponatremia: mild to moderate increase in TBW, normal Na^+ (most common subtype)
- Signs include a nonedematous state.
- If urine Osm >100 mOsm/kg, causes include syndrome of inappropriate antidiuretic hormone (SIADH), hypothyroidism, adrenal insufficiency, medications (e.g., thiazide diuretics, loop diuretics, carbamazepine, clofibrate, cyclosporine, levetiracetam, oxcarbazepine, SSRIs, TCAs, vincristine).
- If urine Osm <100 mOsm/kg, causes include primary polydipsia, beer potomania, and exercise induced hyponatremia.
- Hypervolemic hyponatremia: increased TBW and Na^+
- Signs include edematous state.
- Urine Na^+ <30 mmol/L
- Causes include congestive heart failure (CHF), cirrhosis, nephrotic syndrome, hypoalbuminemia, and psychogenic polydipsia.

Genetics
- Polymorphisms have been demonstrated.
- Mutations have been associated with nephrogenic syndrome of inappropriate antidiuresis (NSIAD; SIADH).

GENERAL PREVENTION
Depends on underlying etiology

COMMONLY ASSOCIATED CONDITIONS
- Hypothyroidism
- Hypopituitarism
- Cirrhosis
- CHF
- Nephrotic syndrome
- Adrenocortical hormone deficiency
- HIV patients
- SIADH is associated with cancers, pneumonia, tuberculosis, encephalitis, meningitis, head trauma, cerebrovascular accident, and HIV infection.
- Traumatic brain injury
- Marathon runners in hot environments
- Beer potomania
- Tea-and-toast diet
- Ecstasy use

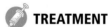
DIAGNOSIS

- Symptoms are related to the rate of fall in serum Na^+, onset, and degree of hyponatremia (1),(2)[C].
- Acute (≤ 48 hours): no time for full adaptation, more likely to present with moderate or severe symptoms
- Chronic (>48 hours): develops gradually, organ systems adapt to Na^+ concentration, associated with minimal symptoms
- Mild (serum Na^+ 130 to 135 mEq/L): usually asymptomatic, fatigue, loss of appetite
- Moderate (serum Na^+ 120 to 130 mEq/L): nausea, vomiting, lethargy
- Severe (serum Na^+ 115 to 120 mEq/L): headache, lethargy, restlessness, disorientation
- Severe/rapid decrease in serum Na^+ can cause seizures, coma, brain herniation, respiratory arrest, and may be fatal.
- Other signs and symptoms: weakness, muscle cramps, anorexia, hiccups, depressed deep tendon reflexes, hypothermia, positive Babinski responses, cranial nerve palsies, orthostatic hypotension

ALERT
Low Na^+ creates an osmotic gradient between plasma and cells, resulting in fluid shift into cells. This causes cerebral edema and increased intracranial pressure; eventually, this can lead to hyponatremic encephalopathy and brain herniation.

HISTORY
- Symptoms include headache, nausea, vomiting, muscle cramps.
- Can progress to lethargy or restlessness and disorientation

PHYSICAL EXAM
- Volume status: skin turgor, jugular venous pressure, heart rate, orthostatic blood pressure measurement
- Evaluate for underlying illness: signs of CHF, cirrhosis, hypothyroidism.
- Decreased reflexes may be seen.

DIFFERENTIAL DIAGNOSIS
See "Etiology and Pathophysiology."

DIAGNOSTIC TESTS & INTERPRETATION
Initial Tests (lab, imaging)
- Comprehensive metabolic profile (BUN, creatinine, glucose, electrolytes, liver function studies, etc.)
- Thyroid-stimulating hormone (TSH)
- Lipid panel
- Serum osmolality
- Urine Na^+ and osmolality
- Chest x-ray to rule out pulmonary pathology if SIADH is diagnosed

Follow-Up Tests & Special Considerations
CT scan of head if pituitary problem is suspected or if SIADH from CNS problem is suspected.

TREATMENT

GENERAL MEASURES
- Assess all medications patient is taking.
- Institute seizure precautions.
- Institute fluid restriction for hypervolemic patients.
- Fluid resuscitation in hypovolemic patients. Indications for 3% hypertonic saline versus normal saline solution include acute hyponatremia, symptomatic hyponatremia, association with intracranial pathology already at risk for cerebral edema (1),(2)[C].

MEDICATION
ALERT
Rapid correction of severe symptomatic hyponatremia has been associated with central pontine myelinolysis, a neurologic disorder of loss of myelin and supportive structures in pons and occasionally in other areas of the brain (3)[A]. This results in irreversible injury. Symptoms are apparent 2 to 6 days after injury and include seizure, coma, spastic paraparesis, dysarthria, and dysphagia. Patients at increased risk are those with Na^+ <105 mEq/L, alcoholism, hypokalemia, malnutrition, and advanced liver disease liver transplant recipients. MRI is not required for diagnosis because it may not be positive until 4 weeks after symptom onset.

- Treatment is tailored to etiology, degree of hyponatremia, onset, and symptomatology.

- Some general principles apply:
  - Expected change in serum Na^+ with selected infusate: $\Delta Na = [(\text{infusate } Na^+ + \text{infusate } K^+ - \text{serum } Na^+) / (TBW + 1)]$
  - TBW = a coefficient $\times$ weight (kg) as in the following table:

Total Body Water	
Children	$0.6 \times$ weight
Women	$0.5 \times$ weight
Men	$0.6 \times$ weight
Elderly women	$0.45 \times$ weight
Elderly men	$0.5 \times$ weight

  - Formula to determine correction available at http://www.medcalc.com/sodium.html
- Asymptomatic, euvolemic patients can be treated with fluid restriction; etiology must be addressed.
- For severely hyponatremic/symptomatic patients, administer 3% hypertonic saline, 2 mL/kg up to 100 mL, over a 20-minute period. Check serum Na^+ levels after infusion. Repeat as necessary until a 5 mmol/L increase in serum Na^+ is seen. Admit to ICU and check Na^+ every 2 hours.
  - If symptoms improve after a 5 mmol/L increase, discontinue the hypertonic saline and switch to 0.9% isotonic saline solution. Increase serum Na^+ with a limit of 10 mmol/L during the first 24 hours and then 8 mmol/L every day afterward until serum Na^+ is 130 mmol/L.
  - If symptoms do not improve after a 5 mmol/L increase, continue the hypertonic saline infusion until 1 mmol/L/hr increase in serum Na^+ is achieved. Discontinue infusion if symptoms improve, serum Na^+ increases by 10 mmol/L, or serum Na^+ is 130 mmol/L.
- For mild to moderate hyponatremia, use isotonic saline solution (0.9%). For moderate to severe hyponatremia, consider specialist consultation for use of hypertonic saline (3%) via central venous access at a rate of 1 to 2 mL/kg/hr; increasing serum Na^+ levels by 0.5 mmol/L/hr and monitoring frequently the plasma Na^+ level (approximately every 2 hours)
- In patients with severe hyponatremia (euvolemic and hypervolemic state) who do not respond to the aforementioned approach, consider the use of vasopressin V2-receptor antagonists, such as tolvaptan or conivaptan (4)[A].
- Treat underlying etiology.
- Chronic hyponatremia resulting from SIADH (5)[A]: demeclocycline (inhibits ADH action at the collecting duct) if fluid restriction alone is not effective.
  - Contraindications: drug allergy, pregnancy, children <8 years old; caution in renal and hepatic disease
  - In doses of 600 to 1,200 mg/day, the drug produces nephrogenic diabetes insipidus.
  - Significant possible interactions: oral anticoagulants, oral contraceptives, penicillin
  - In case of overcorrection, re-lower Na^+ concentration. Begin with infusion of 3 mL/kg of 5% dextrose in water over 1 hour. Repeat Na^+ measurement. Be cautious, dextrose infusion rates >250 to 300 mL/hr can cause significant hyperglycemia in both diabetic and nondiabetic patients and may lead to osmotic diuresis and subsequent free water loss with increased serum Na^+ concentration. Consider 2 to 4 μg IV desmopressin every 8 hours to prevent overcorrection.

ALERT
Caution: If severe, consider hypertonic saline (3% Na^+ chloride) with central line access, exercise extreme caution, and monitor serum Na^+ as frequently as every 1 to 2 hours.

First Line
- Fluid resuscitation (hypovolemia)
- Fluid restriction (euvolemia/hypervolemia)

Second Line
Vasopressin V2-receptor antagonists

ADMISSION, INPATIENT, AND NURSING CONSIDERATIONS
- Admission is mandatory if the patient is symptomatic or has acute hyponatremia (developing over <48 hours), which increases the risk of cerebral edema.
- Admission is advised if patient is asymptomatic and has a serum Na^+ <125 mEq/dL.

 ## ONGOING CARE

DIET
- Euvolemic hyponatremia: Restrict water to 1 to 1.5 L/day.
- Hypervolemic hyponatremia: water and Na^+ restriction

PROGNOSIS
- In hospitalized patients, hyponatremia is associated with an elevated risk of adverse clinical outcomes and higher mortality (1).
- Recently, in community-dwelling, middle-aged, and elderly adults, mild hyponatremia has been shown to be an independent predictor of death.
- Associated with poor prognosis in patients with acute pulmonary embolism
- Associated with poor prognosis in patients with liver cirrhosis and those waiting for liver transplant. It is associated with significant postoperative risk and short-term graft loss.

COMPLICATIONS
- Occult tumor may be present if SIADH is identified.
- Hypervolemia if isotonic saline solution is used.
- Osmotic demyelination (central pontine and extrapontine irreversible myelinolysis) if the Na^+ is corrected too quickly (1)
- Hyponatremia is the cause of 30% new-onset seizures in intensive care settings.
- Can cause hyponatremic encephalopathy and brain herniation if severe and untreated, especially in young women and children (2)
- Chronic hyponatremia is associated with increased risk of osteoporosis, attention deficit, gait disturbances, falls, and fractures.

REFERENCES

1. Rondon-Berrios H, Agaba EI, Tzamaloukas AH. Hyponatremia: pathophysiology, classification, manifestations and management. *Int Urol Nephrol*. 2014;46(11):2153–2165.
2. Williams DM, Gallagher M, Handley J, et al. The clinical management of hyponatraemia. *Postgrad Med J*. 2016;92(1089):407–411.
3. Singh TD, Fugate JE, Rabinstein AA. Central pontine and extrapontine myelinolysis: a systematic review. *Eur J Neurol*. 2014;21(12):1443–1450.
4. Rozen-Zvi B, Yahav D, Gheorghiade M, et al. Vasopressin receptor antagonists for the treatment of hyponatremia: systematic review and meta-analysis. *Am J Kidney Dis*. 2010;56(2):325–337.
5. Basu A, Ryder RE. The syndrome of inappropriate antidiuresis is associated with excess long-term mortality: a retrospective cohort analyses. *J Clin Pathol*. 2014;67(9):802–806.

ADDITIONAL READING

- Abraham WT, Hensen J, Gross PA, et al; for LIBRA Study Group. Lixivaptan safely and effectively corrects serum sodium concentrations in hospitalized patients with euvolemic hyponatremia. *Kidney Int*. 2012;82(11):1223–1230.
- De Picker L, Van Den Eede F, Dumont G, et al. Antidepressants and the risk of hyponatremia: a class-by-class review of literature. *Psychosomatics*. 2014;55(6):536–547.
- Friedman B, Cirulli J. Hyponatremia in critical care patients: frequency, outcome, characteristics, and treatment with the vasopressin V2-receptor antagonist tolvaptan. *J Crit Care*. 2013;28(2):219.e1–219.e12.
- Krisanapan P, Vongsanim S, Pin-on P, et al. Efficacy of furosemide, oral sodium chloride, and fluid resuscitation for treatment of syndrome of inappropriate antidiuresis (SIAD): an open-label randomized controlled study (The EFFUSE-FLUID Trial). *Am J Kidney Dis*. 2020;76(2):203–212.
- Sood L, Sterns RH, Hix JK, et al. Hypertonic saline and desmopressin: a simple strategy for safe correction of severe hyponatremia. *Am J Kidney Dis*. 2013;61(4):571–578.
- Zieg J. Pathophysiology of hyponatremia in children. *Front Pediatr*. 2017;5:213.

 ### SEE ALSO

Algorithm: Hyponatremia

 ### CODES

ICD10
E87.1 Hypo-osmolality and hyponatremia

CLINICAL PEARLS
- Assess all medications patient is taking because many are associated with hyponatremia.
- Alcohol-dependent individuals with vitamin deficiencies, elderly women taking thiazide diuretics, and people with hypokalemia or burns are at increased risk of central pontine myelinolysis from too rapid correction of hyponatremia. Chronic hyponatremia is also a risk factor.
- Bronchogenic carcinoma and pancreatic, duodenal, and prostate cancer, as well as thymoma, lymphoma, and mesothelioma, are neoplastic diseases associated with SIADH.
- Formulas have been developed (Adrogue and Madias) for safe correction of hyponatremia and are available online (see http://www.medcalc.com/sodium.html).

H

HYPOPARATHYROIDISM

Luay Sarsam, MD • Carrie Valenta, MD, FACP, FHM

BASICS

DESCRIPTION

- Deficient or absent secretion of parathyroid hormone (PTH), a major hormone regulator of serum calcium and phosphorus levels in the body (1)
- Acute hypoparathyroidism: tetany that is mild (muscle cramps, perioral numbness, paresthesias of hands and feet) or severe (carpopedal spasm, laryngospasm, heart failure, seizures, stridor)
- Chronic: often asymptomatic; lethargy, anxiety/depression, urolithiasis and renal impairment, dementia, blurry vision from cataracts or kerato-conjunctivitis, parkinsonism or other movement disorders, mental retardation, dental abnormalities, and dry, puffy, coarse skin
- System(s) affected: endocrine/metabolic, musculoskeletal, nervous, ophthalmologic, renal

Pediatric Considerations
- May occur in premature infants
- Neonates born to hypercalcemic mothers may experience suppression of developing parathyroid glands.
- Congenital absence of parathyroids
- May appear later in childhood as autoimmune

Geriatric Considerations
Hypocalcemia is fairly common in elderly, however, rarely secondary to hypoparathyroidism.

Pregnancy Considerations
- Use of magnesium as a tocolytic may induce functional hypoparathyroidism.
- For women with hypoparathyroidism, calcitriol requirements decrease during lactation.

EPIDEMIOLOGY
More common in women; affects all ages

Incidence
- Most common after surgical procedure of the anterior neck, particularly when the surgeon performs few anterior neck dissections (<50–100 thyroidectomies/parathyroidectomies per year).
- Transient hyperparathyroidism is common (6.9–46% of thyroidectomies), whereas permanent hypoparathyroidism differs depending on surgeon and facility expertise.

Prevalence
- Affects 24 to 37/100,000 persons per year in the United States (1)
- Genetic disorders account for <10% of all hypoparathyroidism, but represent a large proportion of cases in children.

ETIOLOGY AND PATHOPHYSIOLOGY
- PTH aids in regulating calcium homeostasis:
  - Mobilizes calcium and phosphorus from bone stores
  - Increases calcium absorption from the intestine by stimulating formation of 1,25-dihydroxy vitamin D
  - Stimulates reabsorption of calcium in the distal convoluted tubule and phosphate excretion in proximal tubule
- Reduced or absent PTH action results in hypocalcemia, hyperphosphatemia, and hypercalciuria.

- Acquired hypoparathyroidism
  - Surgical: removal or damage to parathyroid glands or their blood supply/enervation during neck surgery for thyroidectomy/parathyroidectomy, or neck surgery for head and neck cancers (2)
  - Autoimmune: isolated or combined with other endocrine deficiencies in polyglandular autoimmune (PGA) syndrome
  - Deposition of heavy metals in gland: copper (Wilson disease) or iron (hemochromatosis, thalassemias), radiation-induced destruction, and metastatic infiltration
  - Functional hypoparathyroidism: may result from hypomagnesemia or hypermagnesemia because magnesium is crucial for PTH secretion and activation of the PTH receptor
  - Congenital
    ○ Calcium-sensing receptor (CaSR) abnormalities: hypocalcemia with hypercalciuria
    ○ HDR or Barakat syndrome: deafness, renal dysplasia
    ○ Familial: mutations of the *TBCE* gene; abnormal PTH secretions
    ○ 22q11.2 deletion syndrome
- Autoimmune: genetic gain-of-function mutation in CaSR
- Infiltrative: metastatic carcinoma, hemochromatosis, Wilson disease, granulomas

Genetics
- X-linked or in autosomal recessive mutations in the transcription factor glial cell missing B (GCMB)
- Mutations in transcription factors or regulators of parathyroid gland development
  - Component of a larger genetic syndrome (APS-1 or DiGeorge syndrome) or in isolation (X-linked hypoparathyroidism) (3)
  - May be autosomal dominant (DiGeorge), autosomal recessive (APS-1), or X-linked recessive (X-linked hypoparathyroidism) (3)
  - Congenital syndromes
    ○ 22q11.2 deletion syndrome, familial hypomagnesemia, hypoparathyroidism with lymphedema (3)
    ○ Hypoparathyroidism with sensorineural deafness
    ○ ADHH: mutations gain-of-function of the CaSR gene suppressing the parathyroid gland, without elevation of PTH
  - PGA syndrome type I: mucocutaneous candidiasis, hypoparathyroidism, and Addison disease

RISK FACTORS
Neck surgery and neck trauma, neck malignancies, family history of hypocalcemia, PGA syndrome

GENERAL PREVENTION
Intraoperative identification and preservation of parathyroid tissue

COMMONLY ASSOCIATED CONDITIONS
- DiGeorge syndrome
- Bartter syndrome
- PGA syndrome type I
- Multiple endocrine deficiency autoimmune candidiasis (MEDAC) syndrome
- Juvenile familial endocrinopathy
- Addison disease
- Moniliasis (HAM) syndrome: a polyglandular deficiency syndrome, possibly genetic, characterized by hypoparathyroidism

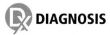

DIAGNOSIS

HISTORY
Often asymptomatic; ask about previous neck trauma or surgery, head or neck irradiation, family history of hypocalcemia, or presence of other autoimmune endocrinopathies.

- Cardinal clinical feature: neuromuscular hyperexcitability
- Also includes: fatigue, circumoral or distal extremity paresthesias, muscle spasm, seizures, neuropsychiatric symptoms

PHYSICAL EXAM
- Surgical scar on neck
- Chvostek sign: ipsilateral twitching of the upper lip on tapping the facial nerve on the cheek. 15% of normocalcemic people have positive sign (1).
- Trousseau sign: painful carpal spasm after 3-minute occlusion of brachial artery with BP cuff. BP cuff inflation to above systolic BP for 3 minutes leads to carpal spasm (flexion of metacarpophalangeal [MCP] joints, extension of interphalangeal [IP] joints, adduction of fingers and thumb).
- Tetany, laryngo- or bronchospasm, cardiac arrhythmias, refractory heart failure, dyspnea, edema
- Dry, coarse, puffy hair; brittle nails
- Loss of deep tendon reflexes
- Dysrhythmias (secondary hypocalcemia)
- Cataracts or ectopic calcifications
- Tooth enamel defects
- Vitiligo

DIFFERENTIAL DIAGNOSIS
- Vitamin D deficiency/resistance
- Pseudohypoparathyroidism, which presents in childhood; kidney and bone unresponsiveness to PTH; characterized by hypocalcemia, hyperphosphatemia, and, in contrast to hypoparathyroidism, elevated rather than reduced PTH concentrations
- Hypoalbuminemia, renal failure, malabsorption, familial hypocalcemia, hypomagnesemia

DIAGNOSTIC TESTS & INTERPRETATION

Initial Tests (lab, imaging)
- Calcium: low ionized and total (Correct serum calcium level for albumin.)
  - Corrected serum calcium = total serum calcium + 0.8 (4 − serum albumin)
- Phosphorus: high
- Intact or "whole" PTH: low; distinguish from pseudohypoparathyroidism or secondary causes
- Magnesium: low or normal
- BUN, creatinine: Monitor renal function, especially in the elderly.
- 25-OH vitamin D level: Vitamin D deficiency can worsen hypoparathyroidism.
- Urinary calcium: normal or high
- Calcium should be monitored after thyroid or parathyroid surgery, including intraoperatively
- Radiographs may show absent tooth roots, calcification of cerebellum, choroid plexus, or cerebral basal ganglia.

Follow-Up Tests & Special Considerations

- ECG: prolongation of ST and QTc intervals, nonspecific repolarization changes, dysrhythmias
- Urine calcium: Creatinine ratio (normal 0.1 to 0.2) may be low before treatment but should be monitored to prevent stones due to hypercalciuria.
- Gene sequencing: Evaluation of other hormone levels may be required to diagnose APS-1.
- Hungry bone syndrome (transient hypoparathyroidism after parathyroid surgery)
  - Hypocalcemia due to hungry bone syndrome may persist despite recovery of PTH secretion from the remaining normal glands. Thus, serum PTH concentrations may be low, normal, or even elevated.
- Osteoblastic metastasis of prostate, breast, or lung cancer; consider appropriate imaging.
- Autoantibodies against NACHT leucine-rich-repeat protein 5 (NALPS) found in 49% of 73 patients with APS-1 and hypoparathyroidisms

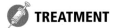 TREATMENT

GENERAL MEASURES

- Monitor ECG during calcium repletion.
- Maintenance therapy: may require lifelong treatment with calcium and calcitriol
  - Maintain serum calcium in low normal range: 8 to 8.5 mg/dL (2.00 to 2.12 mmol/L).
- If hypercalcemia occurs, hold therapy until calcium returns to normal. Treat magnesium deficiency if present.
- Phosphate binders are required if high calcium-phosphate product.
- Thiazide diuretics combined with a low-salt diet may be used to prevent hypercalciuria, nephrocalcinosis, and nephrolithiasis.
- Oral calcium administration and vitamin D supplementation after thyroidectomy may reduce the risk for symptomatic hypocalcemia after surgery.

MEDICATION

- Acute hypoparathyroidism
  - Hypoparathyroid with severe symptoms (tetany, seizures, cardiac failure, laryngospasm, bronchospasm)
    - IV calcium gluconate: 1 or 2 g, each infused over a period of 10 minutes. Central venous catheter is preferred because calcium-containing solutions can irritate surrounding tissues. Follow with infusion of 10 g calcium gluconate in 1 L 5% dextrose water at a rate of 1 to 3 mg calcium gluconate per kg body weight per hour (2)[B].
  - Hypomagnesemia: acutely: 1 to 2 g IV q6h; long-term magnesium oxide tablets (600 mg) once or twice per day
  - Maintenance: See "First Line" treatment for chronic hypoparathyroidism.
- Chronic hypoparathyroidism

First Line

- Adults
  - Oral calcium carbonate: preferred due to high elemental calcium concentration; take with meals and stop PPI for better absorption.
- Oral calcium citrate: preferred for patients on PPI therapy and those with constipation on calcium carbonate
- Starting dose: 1 to 3 g/day of elemental calcium, although doses vary widely; divided doses preferred

- Calcitriol (vitamin D 1, 25-dihydroxycholecalciferol): preferred form of vitamin D replacement; start at 0.25 μg/day; doses 0.5 to 2.0 μg/day are usually required (3)[A].
- For hypercalciuria, consider a thiazide diuretic.
- For phosphate level well above normal (>6.5 mg/dL), use low phosphate diet or phospate binder.
- Children
  - Oral elemental calcium: 25 to 50 mg/kg daily
  - Calcitriol: 0.25 μg daily for age >1 year

ISSUES FOR REFERRAL

- Endocrinologist.
- Refer to nephrologist for renal impairment or recurrent stones; ophthalmologist for eye involvement; geneticist for inherited concerns

ADDITIONAL THERAPIES
PTH peptides 1–34 and 1–84 SC

- rhPTH 1-84—FDA-approved, 50 μg SC daily
- For patients with frequent episodes of hyper- and hypocalcemia, nephrolithiasis, nephrocalcinosis, GFR <60 mL/min, persistently high phosphate (4)[B]
- Treatment goal: Eliminate use of active vitamin D₃, reduce supplemental calcium to 500 mg daily; maintain consistent calcium level in low normal range.
- Improved well-being and increased bone mineral density have been shown for these patients.

SURGERY/OTHER PROCEDURES
Autotransplantation of cryopreserved parathyroid tissue: restores normocalcemia in 23% of cases

ADMISSION, INPATIENT, AND NURSING CONSIDERATIONS

- Admission criteria/initial stabilization: laryngospasm, seizures, tetany, QT prolongation
- Discharge criteria: resolution of hypocalcemic symptoms, patient educated on hypoparathyroidism and treatment

 ONGOING CARE

FOLLOW-UP RECOMMENDATIONS
Patient Monitoring

- Goal is a total corrected serum calcium level in low normal range (8.0 to 8.5 mg/dL or 2.00 to 2.12 mmol/L), 24-hour urine calcium <300 mg, and calcium-phosphate product <55. If calcium <2.0 mmol/L or <8.0 mg/dL, then treat even if asymptomatic (4)[B].
- Outpatient measurement of serum calcium, phosphate, magnesium, and creatinine weekly to monthly during initial management; for changes in medication, check weekly or every other week; when stable, measure every 6 months (4)[B].
- 24-hour urine for calcium and Cr secretion yearly
- If symptoms of renal stone disease or increasing Cr, get renal imaging every 5 years (4)[B].
- Annual slit-lamp and ophthalmologic evaluations are recommended.
- DEXA scan: standard monitoring recommended (4)[B]

DIET
Low-phosphate diet in patients with hyperphosphatemia

PATIENT EDUCATION
https://www.hypopara.org/

PROGNOSIS
Hypoparathyroidism following neck surgery is often transient. Length of required treatment may vary depending on origin.

COMPLICATIONS
- Reversible: due to low calcium levels, most likely to improve with adequate treatment
  - Neuromuscular symptoms: paresthesias (circumoral, fingers, toes), tetany, seizures, parkinsonian symptoms; pseudotumor cerebri has been described.
  - Renal: hypercalciuria, nephrocalcinosis, nephrolithiasis
  - Cardiovascular: heart failure, arrhythmias
- Irreversible: when condition starts early in childhood and will not improve with calcium and vitamin D treatment
  - Stunting of growth
  - Enamel defects and hypoplasia of teeth
  - Atrophy, brittleness, and ridging of nails
  - Cataracts and basal ganglia calcifications

REFERENCES
1. Abate E, Clarke B. Review of hypoparathyroidism. *Front Endocrinol (Lausanne).* 2017;7:172.
2. Al-Azem H, Khan A. Hypoparathyroidism. *Best Pract Res Clin Endocrinol Metab.* 2012;26(4):517–522.
3. Bilezikian JP, Khan A, Potts JT Jr, et al. Hypoparathyroidism in the adult: epidemiology, diagnosis, pathophysiology, target-organ involvement, treatment, and challenges for future research. *J Bone Miner Res.* 2011;26(10):2317–2337.
4. Brandi M, Bilezikian D, Shoback D, et al. Management of hypoparathyroidism: summary statement and guidelines. *J Clin Endocrinol Metab.* 2016;101(6):2273–2283.

ADDITIONAL READING
- Bollerslev J, Rejnmark L, Marcocci C, et al. European Society of Endocrinology clinical guideline: treatment of chronic hypoparathyroidism in adults. *Eur J Endocrinol.* 2015;173(2):G1–G20.
- Michels TC, Kelly KM. Parathyroid disorders. *Am Fam Physician.* 2013;88(4):249–257.
- Stack BC Jr, Bimston DN, Bodenner DL, et al. American Association of Clinical Endocrinologists and American College of Endocrinology disease state clinical review: postoperative hypoparathyroidism—definitions and management. *Endocr Pract.* 2015;21(6):674–685.

 CODES

ICD10
- E20 Hypoparathyroidism
- E20.8 Other hypoparathyroidism
- E20.0 Idiopathic hypoparathyroidism

CLINICAL PEARLS
Often asymptomatic; consider if hypocalcemic with fatigue and circumoral or distal extremity paresthesias.
- Correct the serum calcium level for albumin level.
- Monitor calcium after thyroid or parathyroid surgery.
- Distinguish hypoparathyroidism from pseudohypoparathyroidism and secondary causes by PTH level.
- Not much clinical difference between 2nd- and 3rd-generation PTH assays
- Serum levels of magnesium and 25-OH should be measured to rule out deficiency that could contribute to reduced serum calcium levels.

HYPOTHERMIA
Scott T. Henderson, MD

 BASICS

DESCRIPTION
- Accidental hypothermia is the result of an unanticipated environmental exposure to cold temperatures. It is manifested as a core temperature of <35°C (95°F).
- May take several hours to days to develop
- While patients with cold-water immersion may appear dead, they can sometimes still be resuscitated.
- System(s) affected: all body systems
- Synonym(s): accidental hypothermia

EPIDEMIOLOGY
- Predominant age: very young and the elderly
- Predominant sex: male > female

Geriatric Considerations
More common in elderly due to lower metabolic rate, impaired ability to maintain normal body temperature, and impaired ability to detect temperature changes

Incidence
From 1999 to 2011, the CDC reported 16,911 deaths due to hypothermia.

Prevalence
Estimates vary widely; typically a secondary issue

ETIOLOGY AND PATHOPHYSIOLOGY
Core temperature is typically tightly maintained between 36.5°C and 37.5°C. Accidental hypothermia is most often the result of overwhelming environmental cold stress. Other contributing factors include:
- Decreased heat production (e.g., hypopituitarism; hypothyroidism; adrenal insufficiency)
- Increased heat loss (e.g., immersion—this is the most commonly encountered form of hypothermia in emergency situations—or burns)
- Alcohol consumption (found to contribute in up to 68% of cases)
- Impaired thermoregulation (e.g., stroke, CNS tumors)

Pediatric Considerations
- Children, especially young children and infants, are at greater risk for hypothermia than adults because younger children have a larger ratio of surface area to body mass.
- Young infants cannot increase heat production through shivering. Children and infants have limited glycogen stores to maintain heat production.
- Children and infants have a decreased ability to recognize, avoid, or escape hypothermic exposure. Also, the history may not suggest hypothermia. Hypothermia does not require extreme exposure in children. Nonaccidental trauma may be also be contributory.

RISK FACTORS
- Alcohol consumption; drug intoxication
- Bronchopneumonia
- Cardiovascular disease; cardiac arrest
- Cold-water immersion; prolonged environmental exposure
- Dermal dysfunction (burns, erythrodermas)
- Endocrinopathies (myxedema, severe hypoglycemia)
- Excessive fluid loss
- Hepatic failure; renal failure/uremia; sepsis
- Hypothalamic and central nervous system (CNS) dysfunction
- Malnutrition
- Mental illness; Alzheimer disease
- Trauma (especially head)

GENERAL PREVENTION
- Appropriate clothing, with particular attention to head, feet, and hands
- For outdoor activities, carry survival bags with rescue foil blanket for use if stranded or injured.
- Avoid alcohol.
- Remain alert to early symptoms and initiate preventive steps (e.g., drinking warm fluids; getting out of the cold).
- Identify medications that may predispose to hypothermia (e.g., neuroleptics, sedatives, hypnotics, tranquilizers).

COMMONLY ASSOCIATED CONDITIONS
- Addison disease; hypothyroidism; hypopituitarism; diabetes; ketoacidosis
- CNS dysfunction
- Congestive heart failure
- Pulmonary infection; sepsis
- Uremia

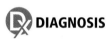 **DIAGNOSIS**

HISTORY
- Presentation varies with the temperature of the patient at the time of presentation.
- The history is often apparent in the setting of outdoor environmental exposures. It may be less clear with cold indoor environments. Patients can present with confusion, dizziness, dyspnea, alterations in judgement. Taking a careful history is particularly important in cases of "indoor hypothermia."

ALERT
History of prolonged exposure to cold may make the diagnosis obvious, but hypothermia may be overlooked in other situations, especially in comatose patients. Always obtain a core temperature if hypothermia is suspected.

PHYSICAL EXAM
- Esophageal temperature is most accurate, minimally invasive method of assessing core temperature.
  - Must have secure airway
  - Probe inserted into lower 3rd of esophagus
  - Peripheral thermometers (tympanic membrane, temporal artery, axillary, or oral) associated with reduced accuracy
- Exam findings vary with the temperature of the patient at the time of presentation.
  - Mild (32–35°C)
    - Lethargy and mild confusion
    - Shivering
    - Tachypnea; tachycardia; elevated BP
    - Hyperventilation
    - Loss of fine motor coordination
    - Peripheral vasoconstriction
    - Hyperactive reflexes
  - Moderate (28–32°C)
    - Delirium
    - Bradycardia; hypotension; hypoventilation
    - Cyanosis
    - Arrhythmias (prolonged PR interval, AV junctional rhythm, accelerated idioventricular rhythm, prolonged QT interval, altered T waves)
    - CNS depression
    - Muscular rigidity
    - Generalized edema
    - Slowed reflexes
  - Severe (<28°C)
    - Very cold skin
    - Rigidity
    - Apnea

- Bradycardia; hypotension
- No pulse: ventricular fibrillation or asystole
- Areflexia
- Unresponsive
- Pupils (dilated <27°C; fixed and dilated <27°C)

ALERT
Use specially designed thermometers that can record low temperatures and measure core temperatures.

Pediatric Considerations
- Infants may present with bright red, cold skin, and very low energy.
- A child's body temperature drops faster than an adult does when immersed in cold water.
- Altered mental status is the most important clue to significant hypothermia in children.

DIFFERENTIAL DIAGNOSIS
- Cerebrovascular accidents
- Intoxication
- Drug overdose
- Complications of diabetes, hypothyroidism, hypopituitarism

DIAGNOSTIC TESTS & INTERPRETATION
Initial Tests (lab, imaging)
- Arterial blood gases (corrected for temperature)
- CBC and platelet counts
- Serum electrolytes; BUN/creatinine; glucose; calcium; magnesium
- Urinalysis
- Coagulation studies; fibrinogen level
- Blood culture
- Liver function studies; amylase
- Cardiac enzymes
- Alcohol level and toxicology screen
- Cervical spine, chest, and abdomen x-rays, if appropriate
- Bedside ultrasound to assess hemodynamics
- CT of the head for any concern regarding mental status

Follow-Up Tests & Special Considerations
Serum cortisol and TSH if underlying endocrine dysfunction (Hypothalamus stimulates release of hormones in response to hypothermia.)

Diagnostic Procedures/Other
ECG

Test Interpretation
Serum potassium >12 mmol/L in adults is associated with nonsurvival.

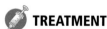 **TREATMENT**

GENERAL MEASURES
- Prehospital (1)[C]
  - Factors to guide treatment (While helpful, core temperature should not be the sole basis to guide treatment.)
    - Level of consciousness
    - Shivering intensity
    - Cardiovascular stability based on blood pressure and cardiac rhythm
  - Treatment
    - Basic life support
    - Remove wet garments and dry the patient.
    - Protect against heat loss and wind chill.
    - If mildly hypothermic, with significant endogenous heat production from shivering, will likely be able to rewarm themselves with insulation

and a vapor barrier; active rewarming will provide comfort and save energy (2)[A].
- For colder, nonshivering patients, add active warming—a nonshivering patient will not rewarm spontaneously (2)[A].
  - Warm intravenous fluids before infusion.
  - Give warm, humidified oxygen if available.
  - If far from definitive care, begin active rewarming but do not delay transport.
- See "Admission, Inpatient, and Nursing Considerations."

MEDICATION

- For sepsis or bacterial infections, begin antibiotics based on site and etiology of underlying infection.
- For hypoglycemia: D50W at a dose of 1 mg/kg
- Thiamine: 100 mg, if alcoholic or cachectic
- Naloxone: 2 mg if opioid use suspected
- Levothyroxine: 150 to 500 μg for myxedema
- For severe acidosis: Consider sodium bicarbonate.
- Precautions
  - Medications including epinephrine, lidocaine, and procainamide can accumulate to toxic levels if used repeatedly; avoid until core temperature is >30°C:
    - When temperature reaches >30°C, IV medications are indicated. Administer slowly.
  - Consider vasopressors according to standard ACLS algorithm with concurrent rewarming in setting of cardiac arrest.
- Significant possible interactions:
  - Use all drugs cautiously due to impaired metabolism and renal elimination.
- Once rewarming has occurred, there is mobilization of depot stores.
- Routine use of steroids or antibiotics does not increase survival or decrease postresuscitative damage.

ADMISSION, INPATIENT, AND NURSING CONSIDERATIONS

- Rewarming depends on severity of hypothermia and presence of cardiac arrest.
  - If no cardiac arrest, consider active external rewarming.
  - If cardiac arrest is present, consider active internal rewarming (3)[B].
- Warm core first (4)[C].
  - Don't rewarm frostbitten extremities until core temperature is >34°C.
- The rate of rewarming is determined by whether perfusing cardiac output is present.
  - If a perfusing cardiac output is present, 1–2°C/hr is appropriate.
  - If not, use a faster rate of >2°C/hr.
- Monitor core temperature, BP, cardiac rhythm.
- Correct metabolic acidosis.
- Evaluate for frostbite and other trauma.
- Mild hypothermia
  - Passive rewarming
  - Administration of heated IV solutions
  - Provide warm fluids by mouth if fully alert.
- Moderate hypothermia
  - Active external rewarming
  - Administration of heated IV solutions
- Severe hypothermia (active internal [core] rewarming)
  - Heated IV fluids
  - Heated humidified oxygen
  - Extracorporeal life support (preferred method in cardiac arrest (5)[C])
    - Cardiopulmonary bypass
    - Extracorporeal membrane oxygenation
  - Body cavity lavage (second options)
    - Thoracic cavity lavage (40–45°C)
    - Peritoneal lavage (40–45°C)
    - Continuous arteriovenous rewarming
    - Hemodialysis and hemofiltration

- Cardiac arrhythmias
  - Atrial fibrillation and sinus bradycardia are common—patients usually convert to normal sinus rhythm with rewarming.
  - If ventricular fibrillation is present, treat with one shock. If patient does not respond, consider deferring further attempts until rewarm has occurred.
  - Do not treat transient ventricular arrhythmias.
  - If cardiac pacing required, preferable to use external noninvasive pacemaker.
- Admit patients, preferably to the ICU, with underlying disease, physiologic abnormalities, or core temperature <32°C.
- Normal saline is preferred as fluid of choice (1)[C].
- IV bolus preferred over continuous infusion, when practical (1)[C].
- Heat IVs from 40°C to 42°C if possible—should at least be no colder than patient core temperature.

ALERT
- Avoid fluid overload.
- Avoid overheating dextrose solutions; dextrose caramelizes at 60°C.
- Avoid lactated Ringer solution because of decreased lactate metabolism.
- Heart is irritable and susceptible to arrhythmias; take care transporting.
- Electrolytes may fluctuate with rewarming, check electrolytes (particularly potassium) frequently.
- Discharge from emergency department once normothermic, if mild hypothermia and no predisposing conditions or complications and has suitable place to go. All others require admission.

 ## ONGOING CARE

FOLLOW-UP RECOMMENDATIONS
Patient Monitoring
- During acute episode
  - Monitor cardiac rhythm.
  - Monitor electrolytes and glucose frequently.
  - Monitor urinary output.
  - Follow blood gases.
- Following acute episode
  - Continued therapy for any underlying disorder

DIET
Warm fluids only if alert and able to swallow
- Alcohol intake increases risk of becoming hypothermic in cold conditions.
- Encourage persons with cardiovascular disease to avoid outdoor exercise in cold weather.
- Refer to social service agency for help with adequate housing, heat, and/or clothing, if appropriate.

PROGNOSIS
- Mortality rates are decreasing due to increased recognition and advanced therapy.
- Mortality usually depends on age and the severity of underlying cause and comorbidities.
  - Mortality rate in healthy patients is <5%.
  - Mortality rate with coexisting illness is >50%.
  - Alcohol or drug poisoning seen in 10% of deaths

Geriatric Considerations
Mortality rates increase with increasing age. Over half of deaths are seen in patients >65 years.

COMPLICATIONS
- Core temperature after drop
- Cardiac arrhythmias
- Hypotension
- Hyperkalemia, hypoglycemia
- Rhabdomyolysis

- Sepsis
- Pneumonia (aspiration and bronchopneumonia), pulmonary edema
- Acute respiratory distress syndrome
- Pancreatitis, peritonitis, GI bleeding, ileus
- Acute tubular necrosis, bladder atony
- Intravascular thromboses/disseminated intravascular coagulation
- Metabolic acidosis
- Gangrene of extremities
- Compartment syndromes
- Seizures, cerebral ischemia, delirium

REFERENCES

1. Dow J, Giesbrecht GG, Danzl DF, et al. Wilderness Medical Society clinical practice guidelines for the out-of-hospital evaluation and treatment of accidental hypothermia: 2019 update. *Wilderness Environ Med*. 2019;30(4S):S47–S69.
2. Haverkamp FJ, Giesbrecht GG, Tan ECTH. The prehospital management of hypothermia—an up-to-date overview. *Injury*. 2018;49(2):149–164.
3. Kempainen RR, Brunette DD. The evaluation and management of accidental hypothermia. *Respir Care*. 2004;49(2):192–205.
4. van der Ploeg G-J, Goslings JC, Walpoth BH, et al. Accidental hypothermia: rewarming treatments, complications and outcomes from one university medical centre. *Resuscitation*. 2010;81(11):1550–1555.
5. Paal P, Gordon L, Strapazzon G, et al. Accidental hypothermia—an update: the content of this review is endorsed by the International Commission for Mountain Emergency Medicine (ICAR MEDCOM). *Scand J Trauma Resusc Emerg Med*. 2016;24(1):111.

ADDITIONAL READING

- Rathjen NA, Shahbodaghi SD, Brown JA. Hypothermia and cold weather injuries. *Am Fam Physician*. 2019;100(11):680–686.
- Rischall ML, Rowland-Fisher A. Evidence-based management of accidental hypothermia in the emergency department. *Emerg Med Pract*. 2016;18(1):1–19.

 ## SEE ALSO

- Frostbite; Nonfatal Drowning
- Algorithm: Hypothermia

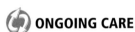 ## CODES

ICD10
- T68.XXXA Hypothermia, initial encounter
- T68.XXXD Hypothermia, subsequent encounter
- T68.XXXS Hypothermia, sequela

CLINICAL PEARLS

- The most common cause of hypothermia in the United States is cold exposure associated with alcohol intoxication.
- With a severely decreased core temperature, begin resuscitation (if possible) unless there are obvious lethal injuries. Continue resuscitation and rewarm to 33–35°C ("not dead until warm and dead").
- ECG changes associated with hypothermia: slowing of sinus rate with T-wave inversion; QT, QRS, and PR interval prolongation; atrial and ventricular arrhythmias; J waves (Osborn waves)
- Hypothermia, coagulopathy, and acidosis are the trauma triad associated with higher rates of death.

H

HYPOTHYROIDISM, ADULT

Faraz Ahmad, MD, MPH • Hiba Ahmad, PharmD, BCOP • Kathryn E. Anderson, DO

BASICS

DESCRIPTION

- Clinical and metabolic state resulting from decreased levels of free thyroid hormone or from resistance to hormone action
- Primary (intrinsic thyroid disease) or central (secondary or tertiary resulting from hypothalamic-pituitary disease)
- Subclinical: serum TSH above the upper reference limit with a normal free thyroxine (T_4) and normal hypothalamic-pituitary-thyroid axis (1)
- Overt: elevated TSH, typically 4 to 5 mIU/L with a subnormal free T_4

EPIDEMIOLOGY

Incidence
- Women: 3.5/1,000 persons per year
- Men: 0.6/1,000 persons per year

Prevalence
- The National Health and Nutrition Examination Survey III (NHANES III), subclinical hypothyroidism 4.3%, overt 0.3% in an unselected U.S. population age >12 years, with upper limit TSH 4.5
- In Framingham Study, 5.9% of women and 2.3% of men age >60 years had a serum TSH >10 mIU/L.

ETIOLOGY AND PATHOPHYSIOLOGY

- Primary: abnormality at the thyroid gland (>95% of cases)
- Most common cause worldwide: environmental iodine deficiency (1)[A]
- Most common cause in the United States: Hashimoto thyroiditis (chronic autoimmune thyroiditis)
  - Hashimoto is characterized by loss of thyroid function secondary to autoimmune-mediated destruction from thyroid antibodies.
  - The typical course of the disease is gradual loss of thyroid function.
- Postablative/posttherapeutic: follows radioactive iodine therapy or total subtotal thyroidectomy for hyperthyroidism; radiotherapy or surgery for thyroid cancer, benign nodular thyroid disease, or neck malignancies
- Transient hypothyroidism: de Quervain syndrome (viral), postpartum, silent thyroiditis (2)
- Drug use: propylthiouracil, methimazole, lithium, amiodarone, antiepileptic drugs, and newer chemo-therapeutic agents such as tyrosine kinase inhibitors (sunitinib), interleukin-2, or interferon-α
- Central: hypothyroidism due to insufficient stimulation by TSH of an otherwise normal thyroid gland; can be secondary (level of the pituitary) or tertiary (level of the hypothalamus)
- Consumptive: triiodothyronine (T_3) and T_4 excessively degraded by ectopically produced type 3 iodothyronine deiodinase (rare)
- Other etiologies include involves genetic defects, tumors, vascular, empty sella syndrome, inflammatory, infiltrative, iatrogenic, posttrauma, or drug related.

RISK FACTORS

- Personal or family history of autoimmune diseases
- Pregnant women or those with previous postpartum thyroiditis
- External head or neck irradiation

- Past history of thyroid dysfunction, radioiodine therapy or thyroid surgery
- Abnormal thyroid examination, presence of goiter and/or TPOAb positivity
- Treatment with amiodarone, lithium, interferon-α, sunitinib, or sorafenib
- Down syndrome or Turner syndromes

COMMONLY ASSOCIATED CONDITIONS

- Diabetes mellitus type 1 and 2
- Pernicious anemia
- Celiac disease
- Primary adrenal failure (Addison disease)
- Myasthenia gravis
- Rheumatoid arthritis
- Systemic lupus erythematosus
- Depression
- Genetic syndromes that have multiple autoimmune endocrinopathies

DIAGNOSIS

HISTORY

Symptoms can vary and can be nonspecific.
- Lethargy, fatigue
- Cold intolerance
- Hearing impairment
- Constipation
- Dry skin
- Muscle cramps, arthralgias, paresthesias
- Modest weight gain (4 to 11 lb [2.0 to 4.5 kg])
- Menstrual disturbances, infertility, subfertility
- Depression
- Change in voice (hoarseness)
- Sleep apnea
- Carpal tunnel syndrome

PHYSICAL EXAM

- Dry, thickened skin
- Hair loss/brittle hair
- Periorbital edema
- Nonpitting swelling of hands and feet (myxedema)
- Bradycardia
- Reduced systolic BP; increased diastolic BP
- Delayed relaxation of deep tendon reflexes
- Macroglossia
- Goiter (particularly in patients with Hashimoto thyroiditis)

Geriatric Considerations
- Frequently nonspecific signs and symptoms
- Normal serum thyrotropin ranges increase with age.

DIFFERENTIAL DIAGNOSIS

- Chronic fatigue syndrome
- Depression
- Anemia
- Congestive heart failure
- Obstructive sleep apnea
- Dementia
- Primary adrenal insufficiency

DIAGNOSTIC TESTS & INTERPRETATION

Initial Tests (lab, imaging)
- Primary hypothyroidism
  - Elevated TSH (>4.5 mIU/L)
  - Decreased serum free T_4 (2)[A]
- Central (secondary or tertiary) hypothyroidism (decreased TSH)
  - Assess free T_4 or free T_4 index (1)[A].
  - Decreased serum free T_4
  - Antithyroid antibodies absent
  - TRH stimulation test, especially if free T_4 and/or TSH is low-normal and patient has hypothalamo-pituitary pathology
  - Imaging of the hypothalamus and pituitary gland
- Subclinical hypothyroidism
  - Elevated serum TSH (>4.5 mIU/L)
  - Normal serum free T_4 (3)[A]
  - Note: Serum free T_3 or total T_3 should not be done to diagnose hypothyroidism (1)[A].

Follow-Up Tests & Special Considerations
- Antithyroid antibodies (primarily thyroid peroxidase antibodies and antithyroglobulin antibodies) may define the cause of primary hypothyroidism but are not necessary in all settings.
- Drugs that may alter lab results:
  - Drugs that decrease TSH:
    ○ Thyroid supplement, glucocorticoids, dopamine agonists, octreotide
  - Drugs that increase TSH:
    ○ Phenytoin, amiodarone, dopamine antagonist (metoclopramide/domperidone), oral cholecys-tographic dyes (sodium ipodate), or estrogen or androgen in excess
  - Drugs that increase free T_4:
    ○ Heparin, high intake of biotin
- Disorders that may alter lab results
  - Any severe illness, pregnancy, chronic protein mal-nutrition, hepatic failure, or nephrotic syndrome

Test Interpretation
Screening
- Patient with risk factors as described above (1)[A]
- Patient with imaging abnormalities of thyroid or laboratory abnormalities including
  - Substantial hyperlipidemia or change in lipid pattern
  - Hyponatremia, often resulting from inappropriate production of antidiuretic hormone
  - High serum muscle enzyme concentrations
  - Macrocytic anemia
  - Pericardial or pleural effusion
  - Pituitary or hypothalamic disorder
- Pregnant women
  - Personal or family history of thyroid disease
  - Diabetes mellitus type 1
  - H/o recurrent miscarriage, morbid obesity, or infertility; TPOAb should be considered (1)[A].
  - Universal screening not recommended for patients pregnant or planning pregnancy
- U.S. Preventive Services Task Force found insufficient evidence for or against screening nonpregnant, asymptomatic children or adults (2)[A].
  - ACOG recommends women with h/o autoimmune disease or strong family h/o thyroid disease should be screened at age 19 years.

TREATMENT

MEDICATION

First Line

- Levothyroxine (Synthroid, Levothroid)
  - 1.5 to 1.8 μg/kg/day (use ideal body weight) (2)[A]; titrate by 12.5 to 25.0 μg/day every 4 to 8 weeks until TSH in normal range.
  - Dosage requirements may vary with age, gender, residual secretory capacity of thyroid gland, other drugs being taken by patient, and intestinal function (1)[A].
  - Use caution when changing between capsule, tablet, and liquid because formulations may be absorbed differently.
  - Elderly patients may require 2/3 of dose used in young adults because clearance is decreased.
  - Levothyroxine should be taken on an empty stomach, ideally an hour before breakfast. Administering at bedtime may result in higher levels of T4 than administering in the morning if taken at least 2 hours after last meal (4)[A].
  - Medications that interfere with its absorption should be taken 4 hours after the T_4 dose; these include ferrous sulfate, proton pump inhibitors, calcium carbonate, bile acid resins.
- Contraindications
  - Overt thyrotoxicosis
  - Uncorrected adrenocorticoid insufficiency
  - MI, acute
  - TSH suppression, preexisting
- Precautions
  - If elderly or known coronary artery disease, start with lower doses, such as 12.5 to 25.0 μg.
  - Diabetic patients may need readjustment of hypoglycemic agents with institution of T_4.
  - Dosage of vitamin K antagonists may need adjustment; monitor prothrombin time while initiating treatment.
  - Patients on digoxin may need close monitoring.
  - Elderly patients more susceptible to AFib and osteoporotic fracture with thyroid hormone excess
  - Patients requiring doses that are higher than expected should be evaluated for GI disorders that may lead to decreased thyroid hormone absorption (Helicobacter pylori, celiac disease).
- Possible interactions with the following medications:
  - Vitamin K antagonists, insulin, oral hypoglycemic agents, estrogen
  - Ferrous sulfate, calcium carbonate, antacids, colestipol, sucralfate, PPI, OCPs, ciprofloxacin, and cholestyramine may decrease absorption.
- Controversy exists whether subclinical hypothyroidism should be treated. Cochrane Review found no improvement in survival, cardiovascular morbidity, or health-related quality of life. Subclinical hypothyroidism should be treated in patients with iron deficiency anemia and in patients with TSH >10 (3),(5)[B],(6).
- If elective surgery: Achieve euthyroid state prior to procedure.
- If urgent surgery: Proceed with individualized replacement therapy preoperatively and postoperatively.
- Brand and generic T_4 formulations available. Likely equivalent efficacy of preparation when switching between manufactures; can measure serum TSH 6 weeks after changing manufactures if concerns

Pregnancy Considerations

- Replacement therapy may need adjustment; average dose increases from 25% to 50% (6)[A].
- TSH levels should be monitored monthly during first half of pregnancy and at least once in second half; goal TSH of 2.0 to 2.5 mIU/L for 1st trimester and <3.0 mIU/L for 2nd and 3rd trimester (6)[A].
- Postpartum: Check TSH levels at 6 weeks (6)[A].
- Painless subacute thyroiditis may occur in postpartum period, leading to transient hypothyroidism lasting 2 weeks to 6 months. Treatment with replacement therapy may be warranted. Up to 30% of these individuals develop permanent hypothyroidism.

Second Line

- No benefit to adding T_3 to T_4 (6)[A]
- Desiccated thyroid hormone is not recommended for the treatment of hypothyroidism (1).
- Liothyronine (T_3) or desiccated thyroid hormone (T_3 and T_4) may be an alternative for patients who do not tolerate T_4 alone.

ISSUES FOR REFERRAL

- Children and infants
- Pregnancy or women planning conception
- Presence of goiter, nodule, or other structural changes in the thyroid gland
- Presence of adrenal or pituitary disorders (1)[C]

ADMISSION, INPATIENT, AND NURSING CONSIDERATIONS

- Myxedema coma (decompensated severe untreated hypothyroidism)
- Hypotension or potentially fatal arrhythmias
- Pericardial or pleural effusion

ONGOING CARE

FOLLOW-UP RECOMMENDATIONS

Patient Monitoring

- Monitor TSH and free T_4 every 4 to 8 weeks after initiating treatment or after change in dose. Once stabilized, periodic TSH level should be done after 6 months and then at 12-month intervals or more frequently if clinically indicated (1)[B].
- Monitor cardiac function in older patients.
- Check TSH more frequently during pregnancy, initiation of estrogen supplementation, or after large changes in body weight.
- In central hypothyroidism, TSH is unreliable; must monitor free T_4
- Thyroid hormones should not be used to treat obesity in euthyroid patients (1)[A].

PATIENT EDUCATION

- Explain need for lifelong treatment with thyroid replacement therapy.
- Further education required for patients taking multiple medications that may interact
- Instruct to report to physician any signs of infection or heart associated symptoms.
- Describe signs of thyrotoxicity.

PROGNOSIS

- Return to normal state is the rule.
- Relapses will occur if treatment is interrupted.
- If untreated, severe cases may progress to myxedema coma.

COMPLICATIONS

- Mortality and complication rates from surgery are similar between euthyroid patients and patients with mild to moderate hypothyroidism.
- Myxedema coma: mortality 30–60%
- Increased susceptibility to infection
- Megacolon
- Sexual dysfunction, infertility
- Organic psychosis, depressed mood, apathy
- Hypersensitivity to opiates
- Treatment over long periods can lead to decreased bone mineral density.
- Iatrogenic thyrotoxicosis can lead to AFib and osteoporosis.
- Can precipitate adrenal crisis if levothyroxine initiated prior to steroids in patients with untreated adrenal insufficiency
- Treatment-induced congestive heart failure in people with coronary artery disease (small risk)

REFERENCES

1. Garber JR, Cobin RH, Gharib H, et al. Clinical practice guidelines for hypothyroidism in adults: cosponsored by the American Association of Clinical Endocrinologists and the American Thyroid Association. Endocr Pract. 2012;18(6):988–1028.
2. Chaker L, Bianco AC, Jonklaas J, et al. Hypothyroidism. Lancet. 2017;390(10101):1550–1562.
3. Cooper DS, Biondi B. Subclinical thyroid disease. Lancet. 2012;379(9821):1142–1154.
4. Khandelwal D, Tandon N. Overt and subclinical hypothyroidism: who to treat and how. Drugs. 2012;72(1):17–33.
5. Jonklaas J, Bianco AC, Bauer AJ, et al. Guidelines for the treatment of hypothyroidism: prepared by the American Thyroid Association Task Force on Thyroid Hormone Replacement. Thyroid. 2014;24(12):1670–1751.
6. Alexander EK, Marqusee E, Lawrence J, et al. Timing and magnitude of increases in levothyroxine requirements during pregnancy in women with hypothyroidism. N Engl J Med. 2004;351(3):241–249.

CODES

ICD10

- E03.9 Hypothyroidism, unspecified
- E06.3 Autoimmune thyroiditis
- E89.0 Postprocedural hypothyroidism

CLINICAL PEARLS

- Screening test: Order TSH levels; serum free T_4 should be obtained only if TSH is abnormal and not as part of initial screening test (1)[A].
- Monitor TSH and free T_4 every 4 to 8 weeks after initiating treatment or after change in dose. Once stabilized, periodic TSH level should be done after 6 months and then at 12-month intervals or more frequently if clinically indicated.

H

ID REACTION

Sahil Mullick, MD • Diana V. Steau, MD

 BASICS

DESCRIPTION

A generalized skin reaction associated with various infectious (fungal, bacterial, viral, or parasitic) or inflammatory cutaneous conditions distant from the primary disease site (1)

- "Id" is often combined with a root to reflect the causative factor (i.e., bacterid, syphilid, and tuberculid). Dermatophytid is the most frequently referenced id reaction. A dermatophytid is an autosensitization reaction in which a secondary cutaneous reaction occurs at a site distant to a primary fungal infection. The eruption typically begins within 1 to 2 weeks of the onset of the main lesion or following exacerbation of the main lesion.
- Most commonly localized vesicular lesions, erythema nodosum, and erythema multiforme. More uncommonly, can cause presence of vesicles and pustules.
- System(s) affected: skin/exocrine
- Synonym(s): dermatophytid, trichophytid, autoeczematization

EPIDEMIOLOGY

- Predominant age: all ages
- Predominant sex: male = female
- Predominant race: all races

Incidence
Unknown

Prevalence
Common

ETIOLOGY AND PATHOPHYSIOLOGY

Precise pathophysiology is uncertain. Circulating antigens may react with antibodies at sensitized areas of the skin. An abnormal immune recognition of autologous skin antigens may also occur. Inflammation may lower the irritation threshold of the skin, and hematogenous spread of cytokines from the primary site of inflammation may also play a role (1).

- Etiology
  - Infectious
    - Fungal infections: *Trichophyton mentagrophytes*, *Trichophyton rubrum*, *Epidermophyton floccosum*, and *Candida* spp.
    - Bacterial infections: *Streptococcus pyogenes*, *Staphylococcus aureus*, and *Mycobacterium tuberculosis*

- Viral infections: HSV, *Molluscum contagiosum*, orf, and milker's nodules
- Parasitic infections: *Sarcoptes scabiei* and *Leishmania* spp.
  - Allergic
    - Id reactions occur in patients with nickel and aluminum allergy.
  - Miscellaneous
    - Id reaction rarely develops due to retained postoperative sutures, cyanoacrylate application, ionizing radiation, blunt trauma, and red tattoo ink.
    - Rarely, id reaction has been documented in patients receiving intravesical BCG live therapy for transitional cell carcinoma.

RISK FACTORS
- Fungal infection of the skin, especially tinea pedis
- Stasis dermatitis

GENERAL PREVENTION
- Good skin hygiene (particularly in intertriginous areas) to minimize risk of developing fungal infections
- Promptly treat any developing fungal infection.

COMMONLY ASSOCIATED CONDITIONS
- Primary fungal infection
- Stasis dermatitis

 DIAGNOSIS

HISTORY

Itchy rash: Inquire about presence of lesions (typically fungal or bacterial) that could have incited the id reaction in the preceding days to weeks.

PHYSICAL EXAM
- Common
  - Symmetric, pruritic vesicles on the palms and, most commonly, on lateral aspects of fingers
  - Tinea infection on the feet; contact or other eczematous dermatitis; bacterial, fungal, or viral infection of the skin
- Less common
  - Papules
  - Lichenoid eruption
- Eczematoid eruption

DIFFERENTIAL DIAGNOSIS
- Pompholyx (dyshidrotic eczema)
- Contact dermatitis
- Drug eruptions
- Pustular psoriasis
- Folliculitis
- Scabies

DIAGNOSTIC TESTS & INTERPRETATION
- Potassium hydroxide (KOH) or fungal culture of primary lesion
- No fungal elements are present at the site of the id reaction.
- Special tests: Skin shows a positive trichophyton reaction. A wheal >10 mm at 20 minutes and induration >5 mm at 72 hours is a positive response.

Follow-Up Tests & Special Considerations
- The id reaction resolves with successful eradication of the primary skin condition.
- It is important to distinguish dermatophytids from drug-induced allergic reactions because continued treatment is essential to clear the underlying infection.

Test Interpretation
Histology
- Vesicles in the upper dermis
- Superficial perivascular lymphohistiocytic infiltrate with small numbers of eosinophils and increased granular cell layer
- No infectious agents present in biopsy specimen.

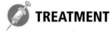 **TREATMENT**

GENERAL MEASURES
- Outpatient treatment of the underlying infection or eczematous dermatitis
- Symptomatic treatment of pruritus with antihistamines and/or topical steroids if needed (may require class 1 or 2 steroid)
- Treatment for secondary bacterial infection

MEDICATION

First Line

- PO antihistamines for pruritus (2)
  - Chlorpheniramine: 4 mg PO q4–6h PRN; max 24 mg/24 hr (pediatric: 6 to 11 years 2 mg PO q4–6h PRN; max 12 mg/24 hr; ≥12 years, refer to adult dosing)
  - Diphenhydramine: 25 to 50 mg PO q4–6h PRN; max 400 mg/24 hr (pediatric: 5 mg/kg/24 hr divided q6h PRN; 2 to 5 years max 37.5 mg/24 hr; 6 to 11 years max 150 mg/24 hr; ≥12 years, refer to adult dosing)
  - Hydroxyzine: 25 to 100 mg PO q6–8h PRN; max 600 mg/24 hr (pediatric: 2 mg/kg/24 hr divided q6h PRN)
- Topical treatments for pruritus
  - Triamcinolone 0.1% ointment TID
  - Hydrocortisone 0.5%, 1%, 2.5%: up to QID
  - Capsaicin 0.025%, 0.075% cream: Apply TID–QID; EMLA (2.5% lidocaine + 2.5% prilocaine) applied 30 to 60 minutes prior to capsaicin may minimize burning.
  - Doxepin 5% cream: Apply QID for up to 8 days (to max of 10% of the body).
  - Permethrin 5% cream (for scabies)
    - Apply from neck down after bath.
    - Wash off thoroughly with water in 8 to 12 hours.
    - May repeat in 7 days
  - Permethrin 1% cream rinse (for lice)
    - Shampoo, rinse, towel dry, saturate hair and scalp (or other affected area), leave on 10 minutes and then rinse.
    - May repeat in 7 days
  - White petroleum emollients: Apply after short bath/shower in warm (not hot) water.
- Systemic steroids only if reaction is severe or generalized (e.g., prednisone 20 mg)

Second Line

- Topical and/or systemic antifungals for identified associated fungal infection (common)
  - Tinea cruris/corporis
    - Topical azole antifungal compounds econazole (Spectazole) and ketoconazole (Nizoral): usually applied BID for 2 to 4 weeks

- Terbinafine (Lamisil): over-the-counter (OTC) compound; can be applied daily or BID for 1 to 2 weeks
- Butenafine (Mentax): applied once daily for 2 weeks; also very effective
  - Tinea capitis
    - PO griseofulvin for *Trichophyton* and *Microsporum* spp.; microsized preparation available; dosage 20 to 25 mg/kg/day divided BID or as a single dose daily for 6 to 12 weeks
    - PO terbinafine can be used for *Trichophyton* spp. at 62.5 mg/day in patients weighing 10 to 20 kg, 125 mg/day if weight 20 to 40 kg, 250 mg/day if weight >40 kg, and use for 4 to 6 weeks.
- Topical or systemic antibiotics for any secondary bacterial infection
- Treatment with antiviral agents for erythema multiforme associated with HSV is required.

 ONGOING CARE

PATIENT EDUCATION

Avoid hot, humid conditions that promote fungal growth. Aerate susceptible body areas (e.g., wear sandals or open footwear). If possible, wear loose-fitting clothing and undergarments, dry wet skin after bathing, and use powders and antiperspirants to discourage fungal growth. Treat primary dermatitis promptly.

PROGNOSIS

After appropriate treatment, complete resolution in days to weeks

COMPLICATIONS

- Secondary bacterial infection (cellulitis)
- After resolution of dermatophytid, postinflammatory hyperpigmentation is common and disappears without treatment in 1 month.

REFERENCES

1. Ilkit M, Durdu M, Karakaş M. Cutaneous id reactions: a comprehensive review of clinical manifestations, epidemiology, etiology, and management. *Crit Rev Microbiol*. 2012;38(3):191–202.

2. Cotes ME, Swerlick RA. Practical guidelines for the use of steroid-sparing agents in the treatment of chronic pruritus. *Dermatol Ther*. 2013;26(2):120–134.

ADDITIONAL READING

- Elmariah SB, Lerner EA. Topical therapies for pruritus. *Semin Cutan Med Surg*. 2011;30(2):118–126.
- Huerth KA, Glick PL, Glick ZR. Cutaneous id reaction after using cyanoacrylate for wound closure. *Cutis*. 2020;105(03):E11–E13.
- Jordan L, Jackson NAM, Carter-Snell B, et al. Pustular tinea id reaction. *Cutis*. 2019;103(06): E3–E4.
- Paulsen LL, Geller DD, Guggenbiller M. Symmetrical vesicular eruption on the palms. *Am Fam Physician*. 2012;85(8):811–812.
- Prince A, Tavazole M, Meehan SA, et al. Id reaction associated with red tattoo ink. *Cutis*. 2018;102(5):E32–E34.
- Stachler RJ, Al-khudari S. Differential diagnosis in allergy. *Otolaryngol Clin North Am*. 2011;44(3): 561–590, vii–viii.
- Veien NK. Acute and recurrent vesicular hand dermatitis. *Dermatol Clin*. 2009;27(3):337–353, vii.
- Yosipovitch G, Bernhard JD. Clinical practice. Chronic pruritus. *N Engl J Med*. 2013;368(17):1625–1634.

CODES

ICD10

- L30.2 Cutaneous autosensitization
- B35.9 Dermatophytosis, unspecified

CLINICAL PEARLS

- When one skin eruption follows another closely in time, consider an id reaction.
- When assessing an itchy rash, inquire about potential fungal or bacterial lesions in the preceding days to weeks as a potential prelude to the id reaction.

I

IMMUNE THROMBOCYTOPENIA (ITP)

Cristhiam Rojas-Hernandez, MD • Nathaniel R. Wilson, MD

 BASICS

DESCRIPTION

- Immune thrombocytopenia (ITP) is a condition characterized by the immunologic destruction of normal platelets and/or impaired thrombopoiesis in response to an unknown stimulus.
- It is defined as a platelet count <100 × 10^9/L, once other causes of thrombocytopenia have been ruled out (1).
- ITP nomenclature:
  - Newly diagnosed (<3 months), persistent (3 to 12 months), and chronic (>12 months)
  - Primary when it presents in isolation; secondary when associated with other disorders
- ITP is a relatively common disease of childhood that typically follows a viral infection. Onset is within 1 week, and spontaneous resolution occurs within 2 months in >80% of patients.
- In adults, ITP is usually a chronic disease and spontaneous remission is rare.
- Synonym(s): idiopathic thrombocytopenic purpura; immune thrombocytopenic purpura; and Werlhof disease

EPIDEMIOLOGY

- Peak age
  - Pediatric ITP: 2 to 4 years
  - Chronic ITP: >50 years with incidence 2 times higher in persons 60 years than those <60 years of age
- Predominant gender
  - Pediatric ITP: male = female
  - Chronic ITP: female > male (1.2 to 1.7:1)

Incidence

- Pediatric acute ITP: 1.9 to 6.4/100,000 children per year
- Adult ITP: 1.6/100,000 per year (1)

Prevalence

Limited data; in one population (in Oklahoma):
- Overall prevalence of 11.2/100,000 persons
- In children (<16 years): 8.1/100,000 with average age of 6 years
- In adults (>16 years): 12.1/100,000 persons with average age of 55 years

ETIOLOGY AND PATHOPHYSIOLOGY

- Accelerated platelet uptake and destruction by reticuloendothelial phagocytes results from action of IgG autoantibodies against platelet membrane glycoproteins IIb/IIIa. There is also cell-mediated platelet destruction by CD8$^+$ T cells.
- Autoantibodies interfere with megakaryocyte maturation, resulting in decreased production.
- Fc-independent desialylated platelet clearance has been proposed as the mechanism of refractoriness to therapies that target the classic FC-dependent pathway.
- Association in patients receiving immune checkpoint inhibitor therapy (2)

RISK FACTORS

- Autoimmune thrombocytopenia (e.g., Evans syndrome)
- Common variable immunodeficiency (CVID)
- Drug side effect (e.g., quinidine, vancomycin, penicillin, sulfonamides)
- Infections: *Helicobacter pylori*, hepatitis C, HIV, CMV, varicella zoster, measles, rubella, influenza, EBV, Whipple disease

- Vaccination side effect. Live virus vaccinations carry a lower risk than natural viral infection: 2.6/100,000 cases MMR vaccine doses versus 6 to 1,200/100,000 cases of natural rubella or measles infections.
- Bone marrow transplantation side effect
- Connective tissue disease, such as systemic lupus erythematosus, antiphospholipid antibody syndrome
- Lymphoproliferative disorders

 DIAGNOSIS

A careful history, physical exam, and review of CBC and peripheral blood smear remain the key components of the diagnosis of ITP.

HISTORY

- Often asymptomatic; found incidentally on routine CBC
- Posttraumatic bleeding occurs at counts of 40 to 60 × 10^9/L. With counts <30 × 10^9/L, bruising tendency, epistaxis, menorrhagia, and gingival bleeding are common. Spontaneous bleeding may occur with platelet count <20 × 10^9/L. Intracerebral bleeding is rare and may occur with counts <20 × 10^9/L and associated trauma or vascular lesions, resulting in neurologic symptoms.
- Female sex and exposure to NSAIDs have been associated with bleeding.

PHYSICAL EXAM

- Ecchymoses, petechiae, epistaxis, and gingivorrhagia are common.
- Abnormal uterine bleeding may be present.
- Hemorrhagic bullae on buccal mucosa reflect acute, severe thrombocytopenia.
- Absence of splenomegaly, hepatomegaly, lymphadenopathy, stigmata of congenital disease

DIFFERENTIAL DIAGNOSIS

- Acute leukemia
- Thrombotic thrombocytopenic purpura
- Hemolytic uremic syndrome
- Factitious: platelet clumping on peripheral smear
- Thrombocytopenia secondary to sepsis
- Myelodysplastic syndrome, particularly in older patients
- Decreased marrow production: malignancy, drugs, viruses, megaloblastic anemia
- Posttransfusion
- Gestational thrombocytopenia
- Isoimmune neonatal purpura
- Congenital thrombocytopenias
- Disseminated intravascular coagulation
- Alcohol-induced thrombocytopenic purpura

DIAGNOSTIC TESTS & INTERPRETATION

Initial Tests (lab, imaging)

- CBC with differential and peripheral smear:
  - Isolated decreased platelet count <100 × 10^9/L
  - Giant platelets are usually present.
  - Normal red and white blood cell morphology
- For patients with history, exam, CBC, and peripheral smear typical of ITP, consider the following:
  - PT/PTT is normal.
  - In adults, serologies for hepatitis B, hepatitis C, and HIV infections are recommended (1)[B].
  - In pediatric ITP, immunoglobulin levels to exclude CVID are commonly obtained (1)[B].
  - Other tests are not necessary for patients with typical ITP presentation: antiplatelet, antinuclear, antiphospholipid antibodies; *H. pylori* testing;

thrombopoietin; platelet parameters; direct antiglobulin test; reticulocyte count; urinalysis; and thyroid function tests (1)[C].
- Further studies should be considered if the patient with thrombocytopenia also presents with:
  - Fever, arthralgia, lymphadenopathy, family history of bleeding disorder, risk factors for HIV, or abnormalities in other cell lines
- Other tests not currently recommended in the guidelines:
  - Analyzing reticulated platelets or immature platelet function (RP/IPF) to make a differential diagnosis in cases of ITP yields a sensitivity and specificity of 83% and 75%, respectively (3).
  - In equivocal cases, testing for platelet antibodies such as GPIIb/IIIa and GPIb/IX yield sensitivity and specificity of 90% and 78%, respectively (4).

Diagnostic Procedures/Other

- Imaging is not necessary.
- Bone marrow aspiration/biopsy
  - Not necessary for diagnosis in children (1)[B] and adults (1)
  - Can be considered for a patient with atypical symptoms, such as fever and weight loss and multiple abnormalities in blood count

Test Interpretation

- Peripheral smear: normal red and white cells with large or giant platelets but diminished in number
- Marrow reveals normal to abundant megakaryocytes with normal erythroid and myeloid precursors.

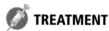 **TREATMENT**

GENERAL MEASURES

- Management is based on both platelet count and hemorrhagic manifestations.
- Current evidence-based guidelines recommend treatment should be administered for newly diagnosed patients with a platelet count <30 × 10^9/L (1).
- The main goal is to achieve a platelet count associated with adequate hemostasis, rather than a normal count (1).
- Outpatient management unless patient has platelet count <20 × 10^9/L and is at risk for bleeding
- Admit patients with active bleeding.

MEDICATION

First Line

- Pediatric
  - First-line treatment:
    - For children with no or mild bleeding (bruising and petechiae only with no mucosal bleeding), observation alone regardless of platelet count (1)[B]
    - For children with significant bleeding
      - Single-dose intravenous immunoglobulin (IVIG) 0.8 to 1.0 g/kg, especially when a more rapid increase in platelet count is desired (1)[B]. Do not administer in patients with IgA deficiencies because of anaphylaxis risk.
      - A short course of corticosteroids (e.g., PO prednisone 2 mg/kg/day for 2 weeks with 3 weeks taper) (1)[B]
      - Single dose of anti-Rho(D) immunoglobulin (anti-D), 50 to 75 g/kg for nonsplenectomized children who are Rh-positive, with negative direct antiglobulin test (1). Do not use in children with low hemoglobin or evidence of hemolysis (1)[C].

- Second and other treatments for pediatric and adolescent with ITP
  - Splenectomy for chronic or persistent ITP (1)[B]
  - Rituximab (Rituxan) 375 mg/m² weekly for 4 weeks (1)
  - High-dose dexamethasone 0.6 mg/kg/day for 4 days every 4 weeks (1)
  - Others without adequate data: azathioprine, cyclosporin A, danazol, mycophenolate mofetil, anti-CD52 monoclonal antibody, and interferon
  - Phase 3 clinical trials have shown that thrombopoietin receptor agonists induce good response in children with chronic ITP.
- Adult
  - First line, adult ITP
    - Treatment is recommended for newly diagnosed patients with platelet count $<30 \times 10^9$/L (1).
    - 4 days of dexamethasone 40 mg/day for 4 consecutive days is preferred over longer courses of steroids or IVIG, as shorter course of corticosteroids has equivalent efficacy without as many adverse effects (5).
    - If corticosteroids are contraindicated:
      - IVIG: 1 to 2 g/kg once, repeating as necessary (1) OR
      - Anti-D: 50 to 75 μg/kg once, repeating as necessary for Rh⁺, nonsplenectomized patients. Do not use anti-D in patients with low hemoglobin or evidence of hemolysis (1).
  - Second line, adult ITP
    - Splenectomy for patients who failed corticosteroid therapy (1)[B]
    - For patients for whom splenectomy is contraindicated and have risk of bleeding, thrombopoietin receptor agonists: eltrombopag (Promacta), 50 mg/day PO OR romiplostim (Nplate), 1 μg/kg SC weekly
    - Rituximab, 375 mg/m² IV weekly for 4 weeks, for patients at high risk of bleeding who have failed one line of therapy or postsplenectomy (1)
    - Others to consider: azathioprine, cyclosporine A, cyclophosphamide, danazol, dapsone, mycophenolate mofetil, and vincristine
    - Asymptomatic patients after splenectomy, with platelet counts $>30 \times 10^9$/L, do not require treatment (1)[C].
    - FDA has recently approved:
    - Avatrombopag (Doptelet), 5 daily doses (60 mg if baseline platelet count below 40×10^9/L or 40 mg if 40 to below 50×10^9/L) and
    - Fostamatinib (Tavalisse), 100 mg twice daily
- ITP in pregnancy
  - Preeclampsia or gestational thrombocytopenia may cause thrombocytopenia unrelated to ITP.
  - Corticosteroids or IVIG are considered safe and are considered first line (1)[C].
  - Do not use danazol or cyclophosphamide.
  - ITP management at time of delivery is based on maternal bleeding risks, and mode of delivery should be based on obstetric indications. Platelet autoantibodies can cross the placenta and cause neonatal thrombocytopenia.
  - Cesarean section can be considered if platelet count $>50 \times 10^9$/L.
  - Prednisone and/or IVIG may be considered 2 to 3 weeks prior to delivery.
- ITP secondary to HIV
  - Antivirals should be considered before other treatment (1)[A].
  - If treatment is required, corticosteroids, IVIG, or anti-D are first-line options, and splenectomy is a second-line option (1).
- ITP secondary to HCV
  - Antivirals should be considered before other treatment (1).

- If treatment required, IVIG is initial treatment (1).
- Based on recent studies, TPO mimetics are approved for HCV-related ITP because they increase platelets to a level required to initiate antiviral therapy.
- ITP and *H. pylori*
  - Screen for *H. pylori* in patients in whom eradication therapy would be considered if result is positive (1).
- ITP secondary to immune checkpoint inhibitor therapy
  - When suspected, first, stop the offending agent and treat with first-line therapy for ITP in adults as outlined above (2).
- Emergency treatment
  - Patients with intracranial or GI bleeding, massive hematuria, internal hematoma, or who need emergent surgery
  - IV corticosteroids (e.g., IV methylprednisolone, 1 g/day for 3 doses) with caution in patients with GI bleeding and/or IVIG 1 g/kg; repeat following day for count $<50 \times 10^9$/L (1)[B].
  - Platelet transfusions with IVIG may also be considered for significant bleeding (1)[C].
  - Other agents that may be considered: Recombinant factor VIIa not only promotes hemostasis but also increases risk of thrombosis. Efficacy of antifibrinolytic agents, aminocaproic acid and tranexamic acid, is unproved in randomized trials; they may be used as adjunctive treatments only. Emergent splenectomy has been reported.

ISSUES FOR REFERRAL
Hematology consultation is recommended for acute bleeding or for those who fail to respond to first-line therapies.

SURGERY/OTHER PROCEDURES
Splenectomy

- Mortality rate is very low (<1%) even in patients with severe thrombocytopenia.
- Necessary vaccinations prior to splenectomy: polyvalent pneumococcal vaccine and quadrivalent meningococcal vaccine every 3 to 5 years and one-time *Haemophilus influenzae* type b (Hib)
- Consider lifelong prophylactic antibiotics with penicillin or erythromycin.
- Should raise the platelet count to at least 20×10^9/L prior to surgery
- Reported 5- to 10-year efficacy is ~65% for all patients.
- Laparoscopic splenectomy has similar long-term outcomes compared to open splenectomy and has better short-term outcomes in medically suitable patients (1)[C].

 ONGOING CARE

FOLLOW-UP RECOMMENDATIONS
Patient Monitoring
Platelet counts weekly for patients on steroids and monthly for stable patients are reasonable. If short-course of dexamethasone is selected, platelet counts are recommended after 10 days of initiation of therapy. A second course of short course is recommended if platelet count increment is below target goal (5).

DIET
- Evidence demonstrating benefit of an anti-inflammatory diet in ITP is lacking.
- The following foods and supplements can cause significant bleeding: garlic, ginger, *Ginkgo biloba*, and saw palmetto.
- Some foods and supplements that may inhibit platelets: evening primrose oil, fish oil, feverfew, ginseng, licorice, soy, vitamin C, vitamin E, and wintergreen

- Partial list of foods and supplements with coumarin or salicylate components: alfalfa, angelica, anise, asafetida, aspen bark, birch, black cohosh, celery, chamomile, cinnamon, dandelion, fenugreek, heartsease, horse chestnut, meadowsweet, poplar, prickly ash, *Quassia*, sarsaparilla, sweet birch, sweet clover, and willow bark

PATIENT EDUCATION
- Modified activity to prevent injury or bruising; avoid contact sports.
- Avoid anticoagulants, aspirin and other platelet-inhibiting drugs, and NSAIDs.

PROGNOSIS
- Acute ITP
  - ~80–85% of patients completely recover within 2 months.
  - 15% proceed to chronic ITP.
- Chronic ITP
  - ~10–20% of the patients recover spontaneously.
  - Remainder with diminished platelets for months to years
  - May see spontaneous remissions (5%) and relapses
- ~10% are refractory (fail medical therapy and splenectomy).

COMPLICATIONS
- Related to thrombocytopenia: 1% mortality due to intracranial hemorrhage and severe blood loss
- Related to treatment: for example, corticosteroid adverse effects, anaphylaxis and renal failure with IVIG, hepatotoxicity with eltrombopag, reports of progressive multifocal leukoencephalopathy with rituximab, hemolysis with anti-D, and septicemia for splenectomized patients

REFERENCES

1. Neunert C, Terrell DR, Arnold DM, et al; American Society of Hematology 2019 guidelines for immune thrombocytopenia. *Blood Adv.* 2019;3(23):3829–3866.
2. Brahmer JR, Lacchetti C, Schneider BJ, et al; for National Comprehensive Cancer Network. Management of immune-related adverse events in patients treated with immune checkpoint inhibitor therapy: American Society of Clinical Oncology clinical practice guideline. *J Clin Oncol.* 2018;36(17):1714–1768. doi:10.1200/JCO.2017.77.6385.
3. Buttarello M, Mezzapelle G, Freguglia F, et al. Reticulated platelets and immature platelet fraction: clinical applications and method limitations. *Int J Lab Hematol.* 2020;42(4):363–370. doi:10.1111/ijlh.13177.
4. Al-Samkari H, Rosovsky RP, Karp Leaf RS, et al. A modern reassessment of glycoprotein-specific direct platelet autoantibody testing in immune thrombocytopenia. *Blood Adv.* 2020;4(1):9–18. doi:10.1182/bloodadvances.2019000868.
5. Wei Y, Ji XB, Wang YW, et al. High-dose dexamethasone vs prednisone for treatment of adult immune thrombocytopenia: a prospective multicenter randomized trial. *Blood.* 2016;127(3):296–370.

CODES

ICD10
D69.3 Immune thrombocytopenic purpura

CLINICAL PEARLS
- Pediatric ITP: relatively common, with spontaneous remission in 2 months
- Adult ITP: usually persistent; requires treatment, with rare spontaneous remission
- Goal of treatment is to achieve adequate hemostasis.

IMPETIGO

Elisabeth L. Backer, MD

BASICS

DESCRIPTION
- A contagious, superficial, intraepidermal infection occurring prominently on exposed areas of the face and extremities, most often seen in children
- Primary impetigo (pyoderma): invasion of previously normal skin
- Secondary impetigo (impetiginization): invasion at sites of minor trauma (abrasions, insect bites, underlying eczema)
- Infected patients usually have multiple lesions.
- Cultures are positive in >80% cases for *Staphylococcus aureus* either alone or combined with group A β-hemolytic streptococci; *S. aureus* is the more common pathogen since the 1990s.
- Nonbullous impetigo: most common form of impetigo. Formation of vesiculopustules that rupture, leading to crusting with a characteristic golden appearance; local lymphadenopathy may occur.
- Bullous impetigo: staphylococcal impetigo that progresses from small to large flaccid bullae (newborns/young children) caused by epidermolytic toxin release; ruptured bullae leaving brown crust; less lymphadenopathy; trunk more often affected; <30% of patients
- Folliculitis: considered by some to be *S. aureus* impetigo of hair follicles
- Ecthyma: a deeper, ulcerated impetigo infection often with lymphadenitis
- System(s) affected: skin/exocrine
- Synonym(s): pyoderma; impetigo contagiosa; impetigo vulgaris

EPIDEMIOLOGY
Incidence
- Predominant sex: male = female
- Predominant age: children ages 2 to 5 years

Prevalence
In the United States: not reported but common

Pediatric Considerations
- Poststreptococcal glomerulonephritis may follow impetigo (in young children).
- Impetigo neonatorum may occur due to nursery contamination.

ETIOLOGY AND PATHOPHYSIOLOGY
- Coagulase-positive staphylococci: pure culture ~50–90%; more contagious via contact
- β-Hemolytic streptococci: pure culture only ~10% of the time (primarily group A)

- Mixed infections of streptococci and staphylococci are common; data suggest increasing importance of staphylococci over the past decades.
- Methicillin-resistant *S. aureus* (MRSA) detected in some cases
- Direct contact or insect vector
- Can result from contamination at trauma site
- Regional lymphadenopathy

RISK FACTORS
- Warm, humid environment
- Tropical or subtropical climate
- Summer or fall season
- Minor trauma, insect bites, breaches in skin
- Poor hygiene, poverty, crowding, epidemics, wartime
- Familial spread
- Poor health with anemia and malnutrition
- Complication of pediculosis, scabies, chickenpox, eczema/atopic dermatitis
- Contact dermatitis (*Rhus* spp.)
- Burns
- Contact sports
- Children in daycare
- Carriage of group A *Streptococcus* and *Staphylococcus aureus*

GENERAL PREVENTION
- Close attention to family hygiene, particularly hand washing among children
- Covering of wounds
- Avoidance of crowding and sharing of personal items
- Treatment of atopic dermatitis

COMMONLY ASSOCIATED CONDITIONS
- Malnutrition and anemia
- Crowded living conditions
- Poor hygiene
- Neglected minor trauma
- Any chronic/underlying dermatitis
- Can occur as coinfection with scabies

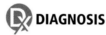

DIAGNOSIS

HISTORY
- Lesions are often described as painful.
- May be slow and indolent or rapidly spreading
- Most frequent on face around mouth and nose or at site of trauma

PHYSICAL EXAM
- Tender red macules or papules as early lesions (contact dermatitis presents with pruritic lesions)
- Thin-roofed vesicles to bullae: usually nontender
- Pustules
- Weeping, shallow, red ulcers
- Honey-colored crusts
- Satellite lesions
- Often multiple sites
- Bullae on buttocks, trunk, face

DIFFERENTIAL DIAGNOSIS
- Nonbullous
  - Contact dermatitis
  - Chickenpox
  - Herpes
  - Folliculitis
  - Erysipelas
  - Insect bites
  - Severe eczematous dermatitis
  - Scabies
  - Tinea corporis
- Bullous
  - Burns
  - Pemphigus vulgaris
  - Bullous pemphigoid
- Stevens-Johnson syndrome

DIAGNOSTIC TESTS & INTERPRETATION
Initial Tests (lab, imaging)
- None usually necessary in typical presentations; cultures of pus/bullae fluid may be helpful if no response to empiric therapy.
  - Culture: taken from the base of lesion after removal of crust; will grow both staphylococci and group A streptococci
  - Antistreptolysin-O (ASO) titer: can be weak positive for streptococci but overall not useful
  - Antideoxyribonuclease B (anti-DNase B) and antihyaluronidase (AHT) response more reliable than ASO response
  - Streptozyme: positive for streptococci
- Disorders that may alter lab results: Streptococcal pharyngitis will alter streptococcal enzyme tests.

Follow-Up Tests & Special Considerations
- Monitor for spread of disease and systemic manifestations.
- Serologic testing is helpful in context of impetigo with subsequent poststreptococcal glomerulonephritis.

TREATMENT

GENERAL MEASURES
- Treatment speeds healing, improves cosmetic appearance, and avoids spread of disease.
- Prevent with mupirocin ointment TID to sites of minor skin trauma.
- Remove crusts; clean with gentle washing 2 to 3 times daily; and clean with antibacterial soap, chlorhexidine, or Betadine.
- Washing of entire body may prevent recurrence at distant sites.

MEDICATION
- In 2014, the Infectious Diseases Society of America (IDSA) recommended topical treatment for limited lesions and oral medication when the disease is more severe/extensive (1)[A]. A 2017 Canadian systematic review found that topical mupirocin is equally, or more effective than oral treatments for nonextensive impetigo (2)[A]. Penicillin and macrolide therapy is no longer recommended. Fluoroquinolones are not indicated due to resistance patterns.
- Consult the local hospital or health department for microbial resistance information.
- Nonbullous (minor spread, treat 7 days; widespread, treat 10 days); bullous (treat 10 days)
  – Mupirocin (Bactroban) 2% topical ointment applied TID for 5 to 7 days (nonbullous only); not as effective on scalp as around mouth
  – Retapamulin 1% ointment to be applied BID for 5 days (very expensive)
  – Dicloxacillin: adult 250 mg PO QID; pediatric <40 kg: 12 to 25 mg/kg/day divided q6h; >40 kg: 125 to 250 q6h
- Dicloxacillin, cephalexin, topical mupirocin, and fusidic acid are effective, unless local staphylococcal strains are resistant. For MRSA infections, treatment options include clindamycin, tetracyclines, or trimethoprim-sulfamethoxazole. Oral doses given for 7 days are usually sufficient (3)[C].
- 1st-generation cephalosporins
  – Children
    ○ Cephalexin 25 to 50 mg/kg/day divided, q6–12h
    ○ Cefaclor 20 to 40 mg/kg/day divided q8h
    ○ Cephradine 25 to 50 mg/kg/day divided q6–12h
    ○ Cefadroxil 30 mg/kg/day divided BID
  – Adults
    ○ Cephalexin 250 mg up to QID
    ○ Cefaclor 250 mg TID
    ○ Cephradine 500 mg BID
    ○ Cefadroxil 1 g/day in divided doses

- Clindamycin 300 mg q6–8h
- Severe bullous disease may require IV therapy such as nafcillin or cefazolin.

ISSUES FOR REFERRAL
If resistant or extensive infections occur, especially in immunocompromised patients

ADDITIONAL THERAPIES
Monitor for microbial resistance patterns.

 ONGOING CARE

FOLLOW-UP RECOMMENDATIONS
- Athletes are restricted from contact sports.
- School and daycare contagious restrictions
- Children can return to school 24 hours after initiation of antimicrobial treatment.

Patient Monitoring
If not clear within 7 to 10 days, culture the lesions.

PATIENT EDUCATION
Avoidance of infection spread is the key; hand washing is vital, especially for reducing spread in children.

PROGNOSIS
- Complete resolution in 7 to 10 days with treatment
- Antibiotic treatment will not prevent or halt glomerulonephritis, as it will in rheumatic fever.
- If not clear within 7 to 10 days, culture is necessary to find resistant organism.
- Recurrent impetigo: Evaluate for carriage of *S. aureus* in nares (also perineum, axillae, toe web). Apply mupirocin ointment to nares BID for 5 days for decolonization.

COMPLICATIONS
- Ecthyma
- Erysipelas
- Poststreptococcal acute glomerulonephritis
- Cellulitis
- Bacteremia
- Osteomyelitis
- Septic arthritis
- Pneumonia
- Lymphadenitis

REFERENCES

1. Stevens DL, Bisno AL, Chambers HF, et al. Practice guidelines for the diagnosis and management of skin and soft tissue infections: 2014 update by the Infectious Diseases Society of America. *Clin Infect Dis*. 2014;59(2):147–159.

2. Edge R, Argáez C. *Topical Antibiotics for Impetigo: A Review of the Clinical Effectiveness and Guidelines*. Ottawa, Ontario, Canada: Canadian Agency for Drugs and Technologies in Health; 2017.
3. Del Giudice P, Hubiche P. Community-associated methicillin-resistant *Staphylococcus aureus* and impetigo. *Br J Dermatol*. 2010;162(4): 905–906.

ADDITIONAL READING

- Bowen AC, Mahé A, Hay RJ, et al. The global epidemiology of impetigo: a systematic review of the population prevalence of impetigo and pyoderma. *PLoS One*. 2015;10(8):e0136789.
- George A, Rubin G. A systematic review and meta-analysis of treatments for impetigo. *Br J Gen Pract*. 2003;53(491):480–487.
- Koning S, van der Sande R, Verhagen AP, et al. Interventions for impetigo. *Cochrane Database Syst Rev*. 2012;(1):CD003261.
- Parish LC, Jorizzo JL, Breton JJ, et al; for SB275833/032 Study Team. Topical retapamulin ointment (1%, wt/wt) twice daily for 5 days versus oral cephalexin twice daily for 10 days in the treatment of secondarily infected dermatitis: results of a randomized controlled trial. *J Am Acad Dermatol*. 2006;55(6):1003–1013.
- Stanley JR, Amagai M. Pemphigus, bullous impetigo, and the staphylococcal scalded-skin syndrome. *N Engl J Med*. 2006;355(17):1800–1810.

 SEE ALSO

Algorithm: Rash

 CODES

ICD10
- L01.00 Impetigo, unspecified
- L01.01 Non-bullous impetigo
- L01.03 Bullous impetigo

CLINICAL PEARLS
- Superficial, intraepidermal infection
- Predominantly staphylococcal in origin
- Microbial resistance patterns need to be monitored.
- Topical treatment is recommended for limited lesions and oral medication only when the disease is more severe/extensive.

I

INCONTINENCE, FECAL

Kalyanakrishnan Ramakrishnan, MD

 BASICS

Continuous or recurrent involuntary passage of fecal material through the anal canal for >1 month in an individual at least 4 years of age
- Involves recurrent, involuntary loss of stool
- Requires careful rectal exam to assess rectal tone, voluntary squeeze, and rule out overflow incontinence from fecal impaction
- Endorectal ultrasound (EUS) is the simplest, most reliable, and least invasive method to detect anatomic anal sphincter defects.
- The goal of treatment is to restore continence and/or improve quality of life.

DESCRIPTION
Major incontinence is the involuntary evacuation of feces. Minor incontinence (fecal soilage) includes incontinence due to flatus and/or occasional seepage of liquid stool.

Geriatric Considerations
- The prevalence of fecal incontinence increases with age. It is an important cause for nursing home placement among the elderly.
- Idiopathic fecal incontinence is more common in older women.

EPIDEMIOLOGY
Incidence
Patients often do not report fecal incontinence unless specifically queried ("silent affliction"). The number of affected patients is likely significantly underestimated.

Prevalence
- Women > men
- 7% of adults; 15% of adults age >90 years
- 56–66% of hospitalized older patients and >50% of nursing home residents
- 50–70% of patients who have urinary incontinence also suffer from fecal incontinence.

Pregnancy Considerations
Obstetric injury to the pelvic floor may result in either temporary or persistent incontinence.

Geriatric Considerations
- Fecal impaction and overflow diarrhea leading to fecal incontinence is common in older patients.
- Surgical history—particularly anal surgery, including hemorrhoidectomy, anal fissure repair (sphincterotomy), anal dilatation, or prior pelvic floor surgeries

ETIOLOGY AND PATHOPHYSIOLOGY
- Continence requires the complex orchestration of pelvic musculature, nerves, and reflex arcs.
- Stool volume and consistency, colonic transit time, anorectal sensation, rectal compliance, anorectal reflexes, external and internal sphincter muscle tone, puborectalis muscle function, and mental capacity each play a role in maintaining fecal continence.
- Disease processes or structural defects impacting any of these factors may contribute to incontinence.
- Diabetes is the most common metabolic disorder leading to fecal incontinence through pudendal nerve neuropathy.
- Congenital: spina bifida and myelomeningocele with spinal cord damage
- Trauma: anal sphincter damage from vaginal delivery or surgical procedures
- Medical: diabetes mellitus, stroke, spinal cord trauma, degenerative disorders of the nervous system, inflammatory bowel disorders, rectal neoplasia

RISK FACTORS
- Poor functional status—older age, female sex, obesity, limited physical activity
- Neuropsychiatric conditions (dementia, depression)
- Multiple sclerosis, spinal cord injury, stroke, diabetic neuropathy
- Prostatectomy, radiation
- Trauma: Risk factors for perineal trauma at the time of vaginal delivery include occipitoposterior presentation, prolonged second stage of labor, assisted vaginal delivery (forceps or vacuum-assist), and episiotomy.
- Diarrhea, inflammatory bowel disease (IBD), irritable bowel syndrome (IBS), menopause, smoking, constipation
- Potential association with child abuse and sexual abuse
- Congenital abnormalities, such as imperforate anus/rectal prolapse
- Fecal impaction

GENERAL PREVENTION
- Behavioral and lifestyle changes: Obesity, limited physical activity/exercise, poor diet, and smoking are modifiable risk factors.
- Postmeal bowel regimen—defecate regularly after meals to leverage maximal impact of gastrocolic reflex.
- Pelvic floor muscle training during and after pregnancy and pelvic surgery
- Increase fiber intake (>30 g/day).

COMMONLY ASSOCIATED CONDITIONS
- Increasing age (>65 years)
- Urinary incontinence/pelvic organ prolapse
- Chronic medical conditions—diabetes mellitus, dementia, stroke, spinal cord compression, depression, immobility, chronic obstructive pulmonary disease, IBS, and IBD
- Perineal trauma (obstetric); anorectal surgery; history of pelvic/rectal irradiation

 DIAGNOSIS

Diagnosis is based on history and physical findings.

HISTORY
- Patients seldom volunteer information about fecal incontinence. Direct questioning is important.
- Problem-specific history includes (1)[C]:
  - Severity of soiling by liquid stool or gross incontinence of solid stool
  - Onset and duration (recent onset vs. chronic)
  - Frequency, presence of constipation/diarrhea
- Thorough medication review
- Review diet, medical and obstetric history, lifestyle, and mobility.
- Evaluate for social withdrawal and depression.

PHYSICAL EXAM
- Inspect the perineum for chemical dermatitis, hemorrhoids, fistula, surgical scars, skin tags, rectal prolapse, soiling, and ballooning of the perineum (sarcopenia of pelvic musculature).
- A patulous anal orifice may indicate myopathy or a neurologic disorder.
- Evaluate the external sphincter response to perineal skin stimulation (anal wink). Absence suggests neuropathy.

- Ask the patient to bear down, preferably in standing position, to assess for rectal prolapse.
- Digital rectal exam to assess anal canal pressure sphincter tone, rectal bleeding, hemorrhoids, neoplasm, fecal consistency, and diarrhea/distal fecal impaction
- General neurologic examination, including perianal sensation (1)[C]
- Evaluate mental status.

DIFFERENTIAL DIAGNOSIS
- Anorectal disorders
  - Inflammatory/infectious gastrointestinal disorders
  - Bowel neoplasms, radiation proctitis, ischemic colitis, fistulas
  - Prolapsed internal hemorrhoids; rectal prolapse
  - Trauma: obstetric, surgical, radiation, accidental, sexual
- Neurologic disorders
  - Stroke, dementia, neoplasms, spinal cord injury, and/or diseases causing altered level of consciousness
  - Pudendal neuropathy, neurosyphilis, multiple sclerosis, diabetes mellitus
- Miscellaneous causes
  - Infectious diarrhea, fecal impaction and overflow, IBS, laxative abuse, IBD, short bowel syndrome, myopathies, senescence and frailty, collagen vascular disease, psychological and behavioral problems

DIAGNOSTIC TESTS & INTERPRETATION
The approach to fecal incontinence in older patients should be individualized, minimally invasive, and practically feasible. History and physical examination are generally sufficient for diagnosis. If uncertainty remains, consider the following:
- EUS is the most reliable and least invasive test for defining anatomic defects in the external and internal anal sphincters, rectal wall, and the puborectalis muscle (1)[B]. EUS can reliably predict therapeutic response to sphincteroplasty.
- Plain abdominal x-ray (fecal impaction, constipation)
- Sigmoidoscopy/anoscopy/colonoscopy (hemorrhoids, colitis, neoplasm)

Initial Tests (lab, imaging)
- If history of travel, antibiotics, tube feedings, or signs and symptoms of sepsis, consider stool studies:
  - Culture
  - Ova and parasites
  - *Clostridium difficile* toxin assay
- Thyroid-stimulating hormone (TSH), electrolytes, and BUN in elderly patients
- EUS may demonstrate structural abnormalities of the anal sphincters, rectal wall, or puborectalis muscle.
- EUS may detect a sphincter injury in over 1/3 of primiparous vaginal deliveries and nearly half of multiparous vaginal deliveries.

Follow-Up Tests & Special Considerations
- Defecography can measure the anorectal angle, evaluate pelvic descent, and detect occult/overt rectal prolapse.
- MRI defecography (dynamic MRI) can further define pelvic floor anatomy.

- Anorectal manometry measures parameters such as maximal resting anal pressure, amplitude and duration of squeeze pressure, the rectoanal inhibitory reflex, threshold of conscious rectal sensation, rectal compliance, and anorectal pressures during straining.
- Pudendal nerve terminal motor latency (PNTML) measures neuromuscular integrity between the pudendal nerve and the anal sphincter; is operator-dependent and has poor correlation with clinical and histologic findings
- Electromyography can assess neurogenic/myopathic damage.

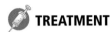 **TREATMENT**

GENERAL MEASURES

- In ambulatory patients, scheduled (or prompted) defecation is effective, particularly in those with overflow incontinence.
- Kegel exercises to strengthen pelvic floor
- If bed-bound, scheduled osmotic or stimulant laxatives for constipation
- Enemas, laxatives, and suppositories may help promote more complete bowel emptying in impacted patients and minimize postdefecation leakage.
- Use of stool deodorants (Peri-Wash, Derifil, Devrom)

MEDICATION

There is limited evidence that antidiarrheals (loperamide, codeine) and drugs enhancing sphincter tone (phenylephrine gel, sodium valproate) are of benefit (2)[B]. Cholestyramine, colestipol are useful in diarrhea following malabsorption or cholecystectomy; alosetron can be used in diarrhea associated with IBS; amitriptyline is sometimes useful in idiopathic fecal incontinence.

First Line

Specific treatment of underlying disorder (e.g., infectious diarrhea/IBD) may improve fecal continence.

Second Line

- Increasing dietary fiber in milder forms of fecal incontinence reduces symptoms (1)[B]. Stool-bulking agents include high-fiber diet, psyllium products, or methylcellulose.
- Antidiarrheal agents, such as adsorbents or opium derivatives, may reduce diarrhea-associated incontinence (1)[C].
- Disimpacting patients with fecal impaction and overflow incontinence and treating with a bowel regimen to prevent recurrence

ADDITIONAL THERAPIES

- Biofeedback: initial treatment modality in motivated patients with some voluntary sphincter control (1)[C]; teaches patients to recognize rectal distension and contract the external anal sphincter while keeping intra-abdominal pressure low
- Biofeedback plus electrical stimulation of the anal sphincters is more effective than either alone.
- Patients with systemic neurologic disorders, anal deformities, or frequent episodes of incontinence respond poorly.

SURGERY/OTHER PROCEDURES

- Surgery should be considered only when nonsurgical approaches have failed.
- Sphincter repair should be offered for highly symptomatic patients with well-defined defect of external anal sphincter (1)[A].

- Injectable therapy (tissue-bulking agent injected into the anorectal submucosa or the intersphincteric space) appears safe and effective (40% efficacy) for patients with internal anal sphincter dysfunction (3)[A].
- Artificial anal sphincter implantation/dynamic graciloplasty (where gracilis muscle transposed into anus as modified sphincter) considered in patients with severe fecal incontinence and irreparable sphincter damage (4)[B]
- Stoma (colostomy/ileostomy) creation may be appropriate in patients with disabling fecal incontinence when other available therapeutic options have failed or if preferred by patient (1)[B]. A continent stoma created using the appendix or the cecum as the point of entry is a less radical option and enables using antegrade continence enema to flush the colon in these patients.
- Anal plugs minimize fecal leakage in patients who do not benefit from other treatment modalities, especially immobilized, institutionalized, or neurologically disabled patients; plugs often poorly tolerated (1)[C]
- Sacral nerve stimulation (neuromodulation) via implantation of SC electrodes delivering low-amplitude electrical stimulation to sphincter muscles improves overall rectal tone, especially in patients with a coexistent sphincter defect (5)[B].
- SECCA procedure (radiofrequency anal sphincter remodeling)—temperature-controlled radiofrequency energy delivered to the anorectal junction distal to the dentate line causing tissue damage, scarring, and anal canal narrowing. Minimally invasive, ambulatory procedure useful in mild-to-moderate fecal incontinence (1)[C].
- Magnetic anal sphincter (MAS) devices—series of interlinked titanium beads (14 to 20) with internal magnetic cores placed to form a flexible ring that encircles the external anal sphincter 3 to 5 cm from the anal verge. During expulsion of feces, the beads separate allowing evacuation. After evacuation, the beads approximate closing the canal (5)[C]; useful in moderate and severe incontinence
- A vaginally placed bowel control device that the patient inflates to control leakage and deflates to defecate is well tolerated and effective in 86% (5)[B].
- Percutaneous posterior tibial nerve stimulation at the ankle for 30 minutes weekly for 12 weeks (50% efficacy) and the TOPAS pelvic floor repair system (self-fixating polypropylene mesh placed behind the anorectum to support the puborectalis) (55% efficacy) are other recent advances in controlling fecal incontinence (5)[B].

ADMISSION, INPATIENT, AND NURSING CONSIDERATIONS

- If secondary to fecal impaction, manual evacuation of fecal mass (after lubrication with lidocaine jelly)
- Avoid catharsis.
- No hot water, soap, or hydrogen peroxide enemas
- Outpatient care

 ONGOING CARE

FOLLOW-UP RECOMMENDATIONS

Periodic rectal exam

Patient Monitoring

Consider impaction if there is <1 bowel movement every other day in patients with fecal incontinence.

DIET

- High fiber (20 to 30 g/day) and at least 1.5 L fluid daily
- Avoid precipitants (caffeine).

PATIENT EDUCATION

Kegel/sphincter training exercises are helpful but not sufficient for treating fecal incontinence.

PROGNOSIS

- Reimpaction likely if bowel regimen discontinued
- 50% failure rate over 5 years following overlapping sphincteroplasty

COMPLICATIONS

- Depression and social isolation
- Skin ulcerations
- Artificial bowel sphincter: infection, erosion, mechanical failure

REFERENCES

1. Tjandra JJ, Dykes SL, Kumar RR, et al. Practice parameters for the treatment of fecal incontinence. *Dis Colon Rectum*. 2007;50(10):1497–1507.
2. Omar MI, Alexander CE. Drug treatment for faecal incontinence in adults. *Cochrane Database Syst Rev*. 2013;(6):CD002116.
3. Hong KD, Kim JS, Ji WB, et al. Midterm outcomes of injectable bulking agents for fecal incontinence: a systematic review and meta-analysis. *Tech Coloproctol*. 2017;21(3):203–210.
4. Rao SSC. Current and emerging treatment options for fecal incontinence. *J Clin Gastroenterol*. 2014;48(9):752–764.
5. Rosenblatt P. New developments in therapies for fecal incontinence. *Curr Opin Obstet Gynecol*. 2015;27(5):353–358.

ADDITIONAL READING

- Menees SB. My approach to fecal incontinence: it's all about consistency (stool, that is). *Am J Gastroenterol*. 2017;112(7):977–980.
- Wellmark. Fecal continence management. https://www.wellmark.com/Provider/MedpoliciesAndAuthorizations/MedicalPolicies/policies/Fecal_Incontinence_Management.aspx. Published May 2021. Accessed June 30, 2021.

CODES

ICD10

- R15.9 Full incontinence of feces
- R15.2 Fecal urgency
- R15.0 Incomplete defecation

CLINICAL PEARLS

- Scheduled defecation after meals, bulking agents, and scheduled enemas minimize impaction and are helpful in managing mild/moderate fecal incontinence.
- Differentiate true incontinence from pseudoincontinence (overflow or functional incontinence).
- New-onset fecal incontinence may indicate spinal cord compression if accompanied by other neurologic signs or symptoms.

INCONTINENCE, URINARY ADULT FEMALE

Alyssa Anderson, MD • Jennifer Grana, DO

BASICS

DESCRIPTION

- Stress incontinence: associated with increased intra-abdominal pressure, such as coughing, laughing, sneezing, or exertion
- Urge incontinence: sudden uncontrollable loss of urine, preceded or accompanied by urgency, or a sudden compelling desire to urinate that is difficult to delay. Urge incontinence may be associated with overactive bladder or detrusor overactivity.
- Mixed incontinence: loss of urine from a combination of stress and urge incontinence
- Overflow incontinence: high residual or chronic urinary retention leading to urinary spillage from an overdistended bladder
- Functional incontinence: loss of urine due to deficits of cognition and/or mobility
- Continuous incontinence: continuous leakage of urine; leakage without awareness.

EPIDEMIOLOGY

- Overall prevalence: Studies have shown prevalence rates as high as 44–57% in middle-aged and postmenopausal women (1). Of these, one-third of the cases were classified by women as moderate to severe and one-quarter of these women feel the symptoms affect their daily lives.
- Underreporting by women is likely. A survey of U.S. women found only approximately 45% of women experiencing these symptoms brought them up to their healthcare provider, underscoring the importance of screening for these conditions (1).

ETIOLOGY AND PATHOPHYSIOLOGY

- Stress incontinence: occurs with increased intra-abdominal pressure. There are two types of stress incontinence: anatomic, which is due to urethral hypermobility from lack of pelvic support, and intrinsic sphincter deficiency (ISD), which is impaired closure of urethra secondary to surgical scarring, radiation, or hormonal and age-related changes.
- Urge incontinence: may be due to detrusor overactivity, neurologic causes (such as spinal cord injury), or idiopathic
- Overflow incontinence: detrusor underactivity ("neurogenic bladder") or bladder outlet obstruction. Bladder outlet obstruction could be caused by fibroids, pelvic organ prolapse, and less commonly masses/tumors.
- Mixed incontinence: combination of urgency and stress incontinence features.
- Continuous incontinence: constant involuntary loss of urine. Ectopic ureters in females usually open in the urethra distal to the sphincter or in the vagina, causing continuous leakage; may also occur with fistulous connections between bladder, ureters, or urethra and vagina or uterus.

RISK FACTORS

Advanced age, menopause/vaginal atrophy, impaired functional status, obesity (BMI >30), diabetes mellitus, parity, vaginal childbirth, pelvic surgery or radiation, urethral diverticula, pelvic organ prolapse, neurologic disease such as stroke, smoking, chronic obstructive pulmonary disease (COPD), cognitive impairment, constipation, caffeine, high impact exercises, and pelvic floor dysfunction

GENERAL PREVENTION

Obesity and caffeine avoidance, smoking cessation, high-fiber diet to reduce constipation

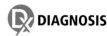

DIAGNOSIS

HISTORY

- Age: Stress incontinence is more common in women aged 19 to 64 years, whereas mixed incontinence is more common in women >65 years. Onset from childhood indicates congenital causes (e.g., ectopic ureter). Amount and frequency of leakage; pad usage. Pain: Suprapubic pain with dysuria implies urinary infection or interstitial cystitis.
- Stress incontinence: occurs in small spurts; patients typically remain dry at night in bed. Concomitant pelvic floor symptoms such as bulging, dyspareunia, or pressure. Urge incontinence: sudden urge followed by leakage of large amounts, usually associated with frequency and nocturia. Sensory stimuli may trigger (e.g., cold). Continuous slow leakage in between regular voiding indicates ectopic ureter or urinary fistula.
- Surgical history: Pelvic surgery, including gynecologic and bowel surgery, can injure the pelvic floor musculature and affect neurologic function.
- Medications: Sympatholytic α-blockers (terazosin, prazosin, doxazosin, tamsulosin, alfuzosin, silodosin) can cause or worsen incontinence. Sympathomimetic agents, tricyclic antidepressants, anticholinergics, and opioids can cause retention with overflow incontinence.
- International Consultation on Incontinence Questionnaire (ICIQ) is highly recommended for assessment of patient's perspective of symptoms of incontinence and his or her impact on quality of life. Consider a 3-day voiding diary to evaluate fluid intake, caffeine intake, timing of leakage, and patient habits.

PHYSICAL EXAM

- General status including BMI and general neurologic examination including sensory status looking for impairment of perineal–sacral area sensation
- Urologic examination with attention to: Abdomen: masses, incisional scars of previous surgeries; Suprapubic tenderness: may indicate cystitis; and palpable, distended bladder: chronic urinary retention
- Pelvic examination including examination of the perineum and external genitalia, including tissue quality and sensation. Do a vaginal (half-speculum) examination for prolapse. Bimanual pelvic and anorectal examination for pelvic masses, fecal impaction, pelvic floor function. Assessment of pelvic floor resting tone and function (ability to isolate and contract pelvic floor musculature); can use Oxford scale to grade strength. Cystocele: if evident, should stage (grade 0 to 4). Rectocele: if evident, should stage (stage 0 to 4).
- Urethral mobility (cotton swab test): little utility in diagnosis when added to urodynamics but may help in predicting response to midurethral sling surgery (1)
- Stress test: positive with involuntary loss of urine from urethral meatus with cough or Valsalva maneuver. Ensure that patient has a comfortably full bladder. Positive predictive value for this test ranges from 78% to 97%.

DIFFERENTIAL DIAGNOSIS

- Nocturnal enuresis: idiopathic, detrusor overactivity, neurogenic, cardiogenic, or sleep apnea
- Continuous leakage: ectopic ureter, urinary fistulas
- Postvoid dribbling: urethral diverticulum, idiopathic, iatrogenic, surgical
- Pelvic pain/dyspareunia: interstitial cystitis, STI
- Pelvic organ prolapse
- Hematuria/recurrent UTI/pelvic mass: malignancy
- Functional: neurologic, cognitive, psychological, physical impairment (1)

DIAGNOSTIC TESTS & INTERPRETATION

Initial Tests (lab, imaging)

- Urinalysis and urine culture
- Renal function assessment: recommended if renal impairment is suspected. TSH if constipation is present
- Imaging is unnecessary in uncomplicated patients.
- Bladder scan to evaluate postvoid residual (PVR) if overflow suspected (>150 mL)
- Upper tract imaging if upper tract involvement is suspected, such as presence of microscopic hematuria: renal ultrasound or CT urogram

Follow-Up Tests & Special Considerations

With a positive urine culture, initial treatment is reasonable. However, treatment of asymptomatic bacteriuria will not improve UI in the elderly.

Diagnostic Procedures/Other

Urodynamic studies and cystoscopy are not indicated in initial workup and should only be performed after failing conservative treatment; this includes cystometric study of detrusor function and pressure flow studies looking at bladder emptying (2)[B]. Cystoscopy should be performed in women with microscopic hematuria and may be helpful in evaluating recurrent UTIs. Results of urodynamic testing are not predictive of treatment success (1)[A] and are not necessary prior to surgery for uncomplicated patients with known SUI (1)[C].

TREATMENT

GENERAL MEASURES

- Treat correctable causes such as infection and/or constipation.
- Begin with conservative options as first line.
- Surgical options may be offered sooner for women with moderate to severe stress stress incontinence.
- Pharmacologic treatments should be reserved for urge or mixed urinary incontinence and can include anticholinergics, β-agonists, topical estrogens, and onabotulinumtoxinA.

MEDICATION

First Line

- Lifestyle changes: Moderate weight loss can improve urinary incontinence symptoms in overweight or obese females (1)[B]. Decrease fluid intake before bedtime, <2 L of fluid per day. Reduce caffeine to <1 cup coffee per day. Aggressive treatment of constipation. Smoking cessation is strongly recommended.

- Pelvic floor muscle training with Kegel exercises may be used alone or in combination with bladder training, biofeedback, or electrical stimulation (1)[A].
- Incontinence pessaries or vaginal inserts for stress and mixed urinary incontinence are options for women wishing to pursue nonsurgical options but evidence regarding their effectiveness is limited (1).
- Bladder training: scheduled voiding, urge suppression between voids. Increased benefit is seen when training is supervised by a healthcare provider.

Second Line
- Medication treatment for stress incontinence is not effective and not recommended; there are no FDA-approved medications for stress incontinence.
- Anticholinergics are effective treatment options for urge urinary incontinence and overactive bladder resulting in statistically significant improvement in symptoms and is associated with a modest increase in quality of life. Studies demonstrating similar efficacy of tolterodine and oxybutynin with respect to efficacy and tolerability.
  - Contraindications to anticholinergic medications include narrow angle glaucoma, prolonged QT intervals. Recent literature raises the question of dementia risk associated with long-term exposure (1)[B].
- There is weak evidence to support α-adrenergic agents for stress incontinence. Contraindications in patients with uncontrolled high blood pressure or end-stage renal or liver disease
- You can consider dual therapy with mirabegron and low-dose anticholinergics in combination.
- Duloxetine (Cymbalta) 40 mg is effective for stress and mixed urinary incontinence.
- Estrogen may be beneficial in topical form for symptoms of urgency and frequency in postmenopausal women with vaginal atrophy, but transdermal or PO estrogen may worsen symptoms (1)[B].
- OnabotulinumtoxinA for urge incontinence results in similar reduction in incontinence episodes as antimuscarinic (anticholinergic) options with more patients reporting complete resolution of symptoms. Risks include urinary retention, incomplete bladder emptying, and urinary tract infections.
- Urge incontinence:
  - Anticholinergic agents (inhibit involuntary detrusor contractions). No single agent has been shown to be overall superior. Extended-release and transdermal medications cause fewer side effects. Dry mouth, dry eyes, constipation, impaired cognitive function, and other anticholinergic side effects can limit use. Avoid with narrow-angle glaucoma, urinary retention (PVR >250 mL), impaired gastric emptying, frail elders; may worsen existing cardiac arrhythmias
- Higher doses are more effective but have higher risk of side effects.
- β_3-Agonist (mirabegron [Myrbetriq ER] 25–50 mg/day). Avoid in patients with end-stage renal or liver disease. Avoid in patients with uncontrolled hypertenion; consider rechecking blood pressures a few weeks after initiation. Not associated with increased risk of cognitive decline.

Third Line
Surgical options (may be offered as first or second line for moderate to severe stress incontinence as below)
- Stress incontinence
  - Mesh midurethral sling (most common, most studied surgical intervention), autologous fascia PVS, Burch colposuspension and bulking agents; decision should be individualized based on patient symptoms, goals, and expectations.
  - Women with moderate to severe stress incontinence have better outcomes at 1 year with midurethral slings than pelvic floor muscle training.
  - Pelvic organ prolapse may unmask incontinence in up to 40% of women; consider repair of both during same surgery.
  - Periurethral bulking agents (silicone polymers, collagen) can increase periurethral resistance in women who have recurrent symptoms after surgery or who cannot tolerate surgery but often require further injections.
- Urge incontinence
  - Sacral nerve stimulation: invasive with frequent complications but is not more effective than onabotulinumtoxinA, posterior tibial nerve stimulation. Bladder augmentation: should be offered when patients have failed all other treatment options

Geriatric Considerations
- Anticholinergics should be used in caution in the geriatric population. Anticholinergics (oxybutynin, in particular) can worsen cognition and delirium; the effects are cumulative and increase with length of exposure. Evidence is being reviewed as to long-term dementia risks.
- Physicians may offer synthetic MUS, in addition to other slings, to the geriatric populations after appropriate evaluation and shared decision making.
- Incontinence surgery has similar outcomes in older patients >65.
- Consider polypharmacy or patient's current medications as a contributing factor to LUTS or urinary incontinence.
- β_3-Agonist: mirabegron (Myrbetriq ER) 25–50 mg/day can increase blood pressure and should not be used in patients with liver or end-stage renal disease; however, studies do not indicate a concern in the geriatric population regarding cognition and dementia.

 ONGOING CARE

FOLLOW-UP RECOMMENDATIONS
Patient Monitoring
Periodic long-term follow-up with outcome-based questionnaire surveys

PATIENT EDUCATION
Instructions on self-care and warning signs are available at PubMed Health: Urinary incontinence: https://medlineplus.gov/urinaryincontinence.html.

PROGNOSIS
Significant improvements are usually obtained with most patients.

COMPLICATIONS
- Prolonged exposure to urine causes skin breakdown and dermatitis, which may lead to ulceration and secondary infection.
- Inability to self-care (including toileting) is the precipitating factor for many nursing home admissions.
- Social isolation/depression
- Weight gain (due to self-limiting exercise from fear of leakage)
- Impaired sexual function
- Impaired quality of life

REFERENCES
1. Committee on Practice Bulletins—Gynecology and the American Urogynecologic Society. ACOG Practice Bulletin No. 155: urinary incontinence in women. *Obstet Gynecol*. 2015;126(5):e66–e81.
2. Lightner DJ, Gomelsky A, Souter L, et al. Diagnosis and treatment of overactive bladder (non-neurogenic) in adults: AUA/SUFU guideline amendment 2019. *J Urol*. 2019;202(3):558–563.

ADDITIONAL READING
Riemsma R, Hagen S, Kirschner-Hermanns R, et al. Can incontinence be cured? A systematic review of cure rates. *BMC Med*. 2017;15(1):63.

CODES

ICD10
- R32 Unspecified urinary incontinence
- N39.3 Stress incontinence (female) (male)
- N39.41 Urge incontinence

CLINICAL PEARLS
- Most urinary incontinence diagnoses can be made via history and exam in conjunction with urinary stress tests, PVR, and urinalysis. Urodynamics do not add value beyond this in uncomplicated patients.
- Rule out infection (UTI or STI) and hematuria.
- Try lifestyle changes first for all types of urinary incontinence.
- Pelvic floor muscle training is a safe an effective first-line treatment for stress and urge urinary incontinence, which can also improve quality of life.
- If lifestyle changes do not work for stress incontinence, mesh midurethral sling surgery has high success rates.
- If lifestyles changes do not work for urge incontinence, anticholinergic medications and/or mirabegron could be trialed.

INCONTINENCE, URINARY ADULT MALE

Jason R. Ramos, MD, FAAFP

 BASICS

DESCRIPTION

- Urinary incontinence (UI) is a pathologic condition of an acute or chronic nature that refers to the involuntary loss of urine leading to medical, financial, social, or hygienic problems. Five main types of UI have been described: stress, urge, mixed, overflow (urinary retention), and functional UI (1).
- Stress incontinence: involuntary urine leaks secondary to increased intra-abdominal pressure being greater than the sphincter can control; may be precipitated by sneezing, laughing, coughing, exertion
- Urge incontinence: Involuntary leakage of urine associated with urgency is believed to be secondary to uncontrolled contraction of the urinary bladder. It is also called detrusor overactivity.
- Mixed incontinence: involuntary leakage of urine with urgency and with stress, such as sneezing, laughing, coughing, exertion
- Overflow incontinence: also known as urinary retention; this occurs with bladder overdistention due to impaired detrusor contraction or bladder outlet obstruction (due to benign prostatic hyperplasia [BPH], bladder stones, bladder tumors, pelvic tumors, urethral strictures, or spasms).
- Functional UI: urine leakage variable, often due to environmental or physical barriers to toileting (i.e., reduced mobility)
- Polyuria is defined by excessive amounts of urine (≥2.5 to 3.0 L) >24 hours.
- Nocturnal polyuria is where >33% of total daily urine output occurs during sleeping hours.

EPIDEMIOLOGY

- Stress incontinence in men is rare and is often attributable to prostate surgery, neurologic disease, or trauma.
- Reported rates of incontinence range from 1% after transurethral resection to 2–66% after radical prostatectomy and 1–15% following transvesical prostatectomy, although rates decline with time (1).

Prevalence

- 12.4% prevalence of UI in community-dwelling adult men in the United States
- 4.5% reported moderate to severe UI, of which 48.6% experienced urge, 23.5% experienced other UI, 15.4% experienced mixed, and 12.5% experienced stress incontinence as per the National Health and Nutrition Examination Survey (NHANES) report in 2010 (1).

ETIOLOGY AND PATHOPHYSIOLOGY

- Incontinence secondary to bladder abnormalities
  - Detrusor overactivity results in urge incontinence.
  - Detrusor overactivity commonly is associated with bladder outlet obstruction from BPH.
  - Medications that increase bladder contractility or exacerbate obstructive effects
- Incontinence secondary to outlet abnormalities
  - Sphincteric damage secondary to pelvic surgery or radiation
  - Sphincteric dysfunction secondary to neurologic disease
  - Commonly associated with BPH due to compression of the urethra, affecting urinary flow

- Mixed incontinence is caused by abnormalities of both the bladder and the outlet overflow or by enlarged prostate/bladder neck contracture from prostate surgery.
- Stress incontinence is caused by weakened urethral sphincter and/or pelvic floor weakness.

RISK FACTORS

- Age
- Diseases: diabetes, BPH, hypertension (HTN), major depression, neurologic disease
- History of urinary tract infections (UTIs)
- Pelvic trauma, including prostate surgery
- Polypharmacy

GENERAL PREVENTION

Proper management of conditions, such as symptomatic bladder outlet obstruction caused by BPH early in the course, may prevent continence problems later in life (2).

DIAGNOSIS

HISTORY

- 3 Incontinence Questions tool questionnaire:
  - During the last 3 months, have you leaked urine (even a small amount)? If no, end quiz.
  - During the last 3 months, did you leak urine (check all that apply):
    - When you were performing some physical activity, such as coughing, sneezing, lifting, or exercise?
    - When you had the urge or the feeling that you needed to empty your bladder, but you could not get to the toilet fast enough?
    - Without physical activity and without a sense of urgency?
  - During the last 3 months, did you leak urine most often (check only one):
    - When you were performing some physical activity, such as coughing sneezing, lifting, or exercise?
    - When you had the urge or the feeling that you needed to empty your bladder, but you could not get to the toilet fast enough?
    - Without physical activity and without a sense of urgency?
    - About equally as often with physical activity as with a sense of urgency?
- Voiding symptoms
  - Duration and characteristics of incontinence
  - Precipitants, severity, timing, and associated symptoms (BPH, fluid intake, etc.)
  - Use of pads, briefs, diapers
  - Alteration in bowel habits
  - Previous treatments and effect on incontinence
- Transient causes: UTI, delirium, medications, constipation, immobility
- Geriatric patients: Assess cognitive levels (dementia/delirium), psychological disorders, mobility problems.
- Medication use: diuretics, drugs for BPH, opioids, muscle relaxants, anticholinergics, antidepressants
- Alcohol and drug use, including caffeine

- Surgery: pelvic surgery or radiation, bowel, back, genitourinary procedures, abdominoperineal resection, prostatectomy: radical for cancer, open/transurethral for benign disease
- Red flag symptoms requiring rapid referral to specialist management
  - Pain, hematuria, recurrent UTI, history of prostate irradiation, history of radical pelvic surgery (i.e., prostate surgery), constant leakage suggesting fistula, voiding difficulty, suspected neurologic disease

PHYSICAL EXAM

- Abdominal examination
  - Suprapubic tenderness suggests UTI.
  - Surgical scars suggesting prior pelvic surgery
  - Suprapubic mass may be a palpable bladder and suggest retention.
  - Suprapubic mass may also be an abdominal mass applying pressure on a normal bladder.
  - Increased abdominal girth
- Genitourinary examination: external genitalia, DRE (prostate)
- Musculoskeletal (Look for neurogenic or functional causes.)
  - Extremities, spine, skeletal deformities, scars from previous spinal surgery
  - Sacral abnormalities may be associated with neurogenic bladder dysfunction.
- Neurologic
  - Motor, sensory, reflexes

DIFFERENTIAL DIAGNOSIS

- Transient (infections, meds, constipation, etc.)
- Chronic
  - Urge incontinence
  - Stress incontinence
  - Mixed incontinence
  - Overflow incontinence
  - Functional UI

DIAGNOSTIC TESTS & INTERPRETATION

Initial Tests (lab, imaging)

- Urinalysis and urine culture to check for glucosuria, pyuria, proteinuria, and/or blood
  - If UTI is present, treat and then reassess need for further workup because this frequently causes UI.
- Voiding diary, the 3 Incontinence Questions (1)[C]
- Pad test if quantity of leakage or objective outcome measure is desired (low sensitivity)
- Postvoid residual (PVR) volume if difficulty voiding or other lower urinary tract symptoms using ultrasound (US) to measure PVR: PVR persistently ≥100 mL indicates voiding dysfunction (1)[C].
- PVR >200 mL suggests overflow incontinence. A patient whose PVR is <200 mL does not have overflow incontinence.
- Uroflowmetry
- PSA only if diagnosis of prostate cancer will influence treatment or if levels can help decision making for patients at risk for BPH
- Renal function
- Voiding cystogram in select cases

Diagnostic Procedures/Other

- Prostate US and biopsy if indicated by physical exam or PSA level
- Urethrocystoscopy to exclude suspected bladder or urethral pathology or before invasive therapies
- Imaging of upper and lower urinary tract is not routinely indicated as part of UI assessment.

TREATMENT

Conservative, nonmedication interventions, such as behavioral modification, timed voiding, bladder training, and pelvic floor muscle training, should be considered *first-line therapies*, prior to initiating any pharmacologic therapy.

GENERAL MEASURES

- Bladder diaries (2)[A]
- Bladder training and timed voiding are effective.
- Pelvic floor muscle training speeds recovery of continence following radical prostatectomy
- Weight loss may improve UI symptoms.
- Constipation is associated with UI, but treatment may not improve UI.
- Reduction in caffeine intake does not improve UI but may improve urgency and frequency (2)[B].
- Pads may be used for urine containment in UI as well as external sheaths (1)[B]—external sheaths may have similar rates of UTIs with indwelling catheters but result in better QoL (1)[B].
  - Men with UI should be counseled that leakage is not a normal part of aging and that goals of treatment include elimination of the need for these.

MEDICATION

First Line

- Urge incontinence: There is no consistent evidence that drug therapy is better than behavioral therapy in UUI (1)[B], and behavioral therapy results in higher patient satisfaction (1)[B].
- Antimuscarinic agents are first-line drug therapy in UUI (1)[B], and there is no evidence that any one agent is superior for UUI (1)[A].
- Oxybutynin (Ditropan XL) 5 to 15 mg PO every day
- Tolterodine (Detrol LA) 2 to 4 mg PO every day
- Darifenacin (Enablex) 7.5 to 15.0 mg PO every day
- Solifenacin (VESIcare) 5 to 10 mg PO every day
- Trospium chloride (Sanctura XR) 60 mg PO every day
- Transdermal oxybutynin (Gelnique) 10% apply daily (EAU Grade B)—no dry mouth
- Fesoterodine (Toviaz) 4 to 8 mg PO every day
- Mirabegron, a β_3-agonist, has been shown in some trials and systematic reviews to be as efficacious as antimuscarinics.
- Mirabegron (Myrbetriq): 25 to 50 mg PO daily. *caution*: HTN
- Review efficacy and side effects 4 to 6 weeks after treatment initiation.

- Most patients will stop antimuscarinic therapy within 3 months due to adverse effects, nonefficacy, or cost (2).
- Caution in those with bladder outlet obstruction and PVR >250 to 300 mL: In men with urgency associated with BPH, consider α-blockers (i.e., tamsulosin, alfuzosin, silodosin) as monotherapy or in combination with antimuscarinic for residual overactive bladder.
- Stress incontinence
  - No generally accepted drug therapy
  - Mixed stress and urge incontinence; ER formulations are preferred due to reduced side effects.

Second Line

- Urge incontinence
- Tricyclic antidepressants
  - Imipramine 10 to 25 mg PO BID/TID
- Desmopressin (DDAVP) for occasional short-term relief of UI
  - 25 to 50 μg PO or intranasal at bedtime
- Intradetrusor botulinum toxin injections 100 U intravesical injections (not FDA-approved)
- Duloxetine for temporary improvements of incontinence with dose titration (mixed stress/urge)

Geriatric Considerations

Anticholinergics and tricyclics may result in significant cognitive impairment in elderly patients.

ISSUES FOR REFERRAL

- Prior pelvic surgery/invasive procedure or radiation of the prostate or urethra
- PVR >300 mL
- Neurologic disease
- Recurrent bladder or prostate infections
- Pelvic pain
- Severe incontinence requiring multiple heavy pads or diapers each day

ADDITIONAL THERAPIES

- Pelvic floor rehabilitation (Kegel exercises) may significantly reduce both stress and urge incontinence in male patients and should be considered a part of initial management for stress UI.
- Overflow incontinence is usually caused by poor bladder contractility with urinary retention.
  - Indwelling or intermittent catheterization, evaluate for outlet obstruction.

SURGERY/OTHER PROCEDURES

- Urge incontinence
  - Sacral nerve stimulation with behavioral therapy
  - Augmentation cystoplasty and urinary diversion
  - Botulinum toxin injection via cystoscopy
- Stress incontinence
  - Urethral bulking agents: modest success rates with low cure rates
  - Male sling procedures: promising short-term and intermediate results but no long-term studies

- Artificial urinary sphincter implant has excellent long-term continence rates and is considered gold standard.
  - Success rates have been defined as use of <1 pad a day and have ranged from 59% to 90% at follow-up intervals from 1 to 8 years. Surgical intervention has very high patient satisfaction rate, but revision is often required due to urethral erosion, infection, or atrophy. Foley catheter trauma is a common cause of late urethral erosion.

ONGOING CARE

FOLLOW-UP RECOMMENDATIONS

- To assess associated symptoms, severity, and hassles of incontinence, there are:
  - Michigan Incontinence Symptom Index (M-ISI) (3).
- International Consultation on Incontinence Questionnaire Short Form
- To assess severity of UI, there are:
  - Sandvik questionnaire—used to assess frequency and amount of leakage
  - 24-hour pad weight
  - Bladder diary

COMPLICATIONS

- Dermatitis, candidiasis, skin breakdown
- Social isolation
- Avoidance of sex
- Weight gain

REFERENCES

1. Khandelwal C, Kistler C. Diagnosis of urinary incontinence. *Am Fam Physician*. 2013;87(8):543–550.
2. Gravas A, Bachmann A, Descazeaud A, et al. *EAU Guidelines on Management of Non-Neurogenic Male Lower Urinary Tract Symptoms (LUTS), Including Benign Prostatic Obstruction (BPO)*. Arnhem, The Netherlands: European Association of Urology; 2014.
3. Suskind AM, Dunn RL, Morgan DM, et al. The Michigan Incontinence Symptom Index (M-ISI): a clinical measure for type, severity, and bother related to urinary incontinence. *Neurourol Urodyn*. 2014;33(7):1128–1134.

CODES

ICD10

- R32 Unspecified urinary incontinence
- N39.3 Stress incontinence (female) (male)
- N39.41 Urge incontinence

CLINICAL PEARLS

- Think "outside" the lower urinary tract: Comorbid medical illness and impairments are independently associated with UI; treat contributing comorbidities and rule out secondary causes.
- Always check PVR to rule out overflow incontinence.

INFECTIOUS MONONUCLEOSIS, EPSTEIN-BARR VIRUS INFECTIONS

Dennis E. Hughes, DO, FACEP

 BASICS

DESCRIPTION

- Epstein-Barr virus (EBV) is a member of the herpes-virus family; human herpesvirus type 4.
  - Two subtypes: ST1 predominates in Western Hemisphere, Southeast Asia; ST1 and ST2 equally prevalent in Africa
- Primary infection typically occurs in childhood. The majority of individuals seroconvert by 2 years of age with little clinical manifestation of illness. A second peak occurs in adolescence and young adulthood (1).
- WHO classified EBV as "tumor virus" (group I carcinogen) due to cancer association.

EPIDEMIOLOGY

Incidence

- Military recruits, college students, and others living in cloistered and crowded populations have highest symptomatic infection rate. Overall rate in United States is 500/100,000.
- Predominant age of symptomatic primary infection is 15 to 24 years; 200 to 800/100,000 affected
- Incidence increases during the summer months.

Prevalence

- Worldwide 95% of population has been infected by adulthood. By age 5, 50% of children have been infected, the vast majority of those without manifesting symptoms (2).
- Seroconversion occurs later in childhood in developed countries; there is suggestion of race/ethnicity disparity in the United States with higher seroprevalence in non-Hispanic black, Asian, and Hispanic populations. Also higher prevalence in larger households and lower levels of parental education (3)

ETIOLOGY AND PATHOPHYSIOLOGY

- After inoculation, the virus replicates in the naso-pharyngeal epithelium with resulting cell lysis, virion spread, and viremia. EBV exhibits dual tropism for B-cells and epithelial cells. The reticuloendothelial system is affected, resulting in a host response and the appearance of atypical lymphocytes in the peripheral blood. Viral genome can be detected in the oral cavity 1 week prior to symptoms.
- A polyclonal B-cell proliferative response follows. Relatively few (<0.1%) of the circulating lympho-cytes are infected by EBV in the acute illness.
- A persistent (asymptomatic) state ensues with the EBV genome invisible to the immune system. The maintenance of the invisible state (to host immunity) is thought to be due to EBV particles wrapping themselves in host cell-derived membranes.
- Either through B-cell stimulation or diminished EBV-specific immune modulation, the previously latent EBV-infected B cells replicate and enter a "lytic" phase, allowing clinical expression of the EBV genome. Risk of this occurring may be linked to host genetic factors, smoking, increased BMI, and low vitamin D/sunlight exposure. The proteins produced may either modify host response to or contribute directly to malignancy (1),(3).
- Immunosuppression (organ transplant/acquired immune deficiency) can result in transformation and lymphoproliferative disorders.

RISK FACTORS

- Age (highest incidence of symptomatic infection in adolescent, young adults)
- Sociohygienic level ("crowded conditions")
- Geographic location
- Close, intimate contact; especially "deep kissing" in adolescents and young adults
- Immunosuppression
- Possibly some risk of transmission by fomites (e.g., shared toys) (4)

GENERAL PREVENTION

- Avoid close physical contact with symptomatic EBV/IM patients.
- Meticulous hand washing and hygiene
- General precautions with potential blood exposure (EBV can be transmitted via blood contamina-tion as well as hematopoietic cell and solid organ transplant)
- EBV vaccines under investigation (lack of intimate knowledge of mechanism of immune response has impaired ability to develop an effective vaccine) (4)

COMMONLY ASSOCIATED CONDITIONS

- Infectious mononucleosis (IM): Symptomatic primary EBV infection is common in otherwise healthy adolescents and young adults.
  - Clinical features vary in severity and duration: In children age <10 years, generally mild; in adolescents and adults, symptoms can be more severe and protracted (are dependent on intensity of T-cell response) (2).
  - Incubation period is 30 to 50 days (extremely long for a viral infection).
- X-linked lymphoproliferative syndrome (XLP—rare, inherited extreme vulnerability to EBV infection)
- Lymphoproliferative syndromes due to EBV infections in transplant recipients
- Lymphomas (B-cell lymphoblastic, T cell)
- Lymphocytic interstitial pneumonitis
- Hairy leukoplakia of the tongue, leiomyosarcoma, and CNS lymphomas in patients with AIDS
- Burkitt lymphoma (most common childhood tumor in Africa and Papua New Guinea where malaria is also endemic and may be a cofactor); much higher prevalence than other areas of the world
- Nasopharyngeal carcinoma (seen worldwide but highest prevalence in Africa and Asia)
- Parotid carcinoma
- Hodgkin lymphoma (most common EBV-associated malignancy in United States, European Union)
- Postulated to be associated with multiple sclerosis (2 to 3 times incidence in EBV-positive individuals)
- Chronic active Epstein-Barr virus (CAEBV) due to loss of host control of viral replication

DIAGNOSIS

HISTORY

- May be either abrupt or insidious in onset
- Syndrome of fatigue, malaise, and sore throat
- In adults, temperature may rise to 103°F (39.4°C) and gradually fall over a variable period of 7 to 10 days; in severe cases, temperature elevations of 104 to 105°F (40.0 to 40.6°C) may persist for 2 weeks.
- Children typically have low-grade fever or are afebrile.

- Rash, red eye
- Chest pain (myocarditis and pericarditis)

PHYSICAL EXAM

- Fever, lymphadenopathy, pharyngitis in >50%, with palatal petechiae and hepatosplenomegaly in ~10%
- Diffuse hyperemia and hyperplasia of oropharyngeal lymphoid tissue
- Gelatinous, grayish-white exudative tonsillitis persists for 7 to 10 days in 50%.
- Petechiae at border of hard and soft palates in 60%
- Bilateral upper eyelid edema (Hoagland sign)
- Axillary, epitrochlear, popliteal, inguinal, mediastinal, and mesenteric lymphadenopathy (95% of patients)
- Lymph node enlargement subsides over days/weeks.
- Tender lymphadenopathy (Cervical nodes are most commonly enlarged.)
- Splenomegaly in 50%
- Skin manifestations in 3–16%
  - Erythematous macular/maculopapular rash
  - Petechial and purpuric exanthems reported
  - Rash typically on trunk and upper arms; occasion-ally, the face and forearms are involved.

DIFFERENTIAL DIAGNOSIS

- Streptococcal pharyngitis and tonsillitis
- Diphtheria
- Blood dyscrasias
- Rubella
- Measles
- Viral hepatitis
- Cytomegalovirus
- Toxoplasmosis
- Acute HIV infection

DIAGNOSTIC TESTS & INTERPRETATION

Initial Tests (lab, imaging)

- CBC with differential
- Lymphocytes and atypical lymphocytes
  - Increased numbers of lymphocytes (especially atypical lymphocytes; may be up to 70% of leuko-cytes) in peripheral blood
  - In 1st week after onset, WBC count is normal/moderately decreased. Due to EBV-related neutro-phil fragility, automated processing can result in pseudoneutropenia.
    - By week 2, atypical lymphocytosis develops.
  - During early illness, atypical lymphocytes are B cells transformed by the EBV; later, atypical cells are activated CD8 T lymphocytes.
- Antibodies
  - Heterophile antibodies in 80–90% of adults. Monospot (latex agglutination) test highly specific, but sensitivity varies from 70% to 90%.
  - Heterophile antibody is an IgM response, which appears during the first 2 weeks of illness; disap-pears in 4 to 6 weeks (higher false-negative rate in children <4 years of age).
  - In general, agglutinin titer is higher in IM than other disorders; an unabsorbed heterophile titer >1:128 and ≥1:40 is significant.
- Specific antibodies to EBV-associated antigens
  - Develop regularly in IM
  - Viral capsid-specific IgM and IgG are present early in illness.
  - Viral capsid-IgM disappears after several weeks; viral capsid-IgG persists for life.

- Liver tests: Transaminitis, hyperbilirubinemia are common; jaundice is rare.
- Atypical lymphocytes are not specific for EBV infections and may be present in other clinical conditions, including rubella, infectious hepatitis, allergic rhinitis, asthma, and atypical pneumonia.
- Routine abdominal ultrasound to monitor for splenic enlargement is not necessary.
- Consider ultrasound for those wishing to return to strenuous activity/contact sports at day 21 of illness to exclude splenomegaly.

Follow-Up Tests & Special Considerations
- Abnormal hepatic enzymes persist in 80% of patients for several weeks; hepatomegaly in 15–20%
- In transplant recipients, quantitative polymerase chain reaction (PCR) used to monitor EBV loads

Diagnostic Procedures/Other
Chest x-ray
- Hilar adenopathy may be observed in IM with extensive lymphoid hyperplasia.

Test Interpretation
- Mononuclear infiltrations of lymph nodes, tonsils, spleen, lungs, liver, heart, kidneys, adrenal glands, skin, and CNS
- Bone marrow hyperplasia with small granulomas formation may be present; these findings are non-specific and have no prognostic significance.

TREATMENT
- Treatment is primarily supportive.
- NSAIDs or acetaminophen
- During acute stage, limit activity for 4 weeks to reduce potential complications (e.g., splenic rupture).
- Transplant recipients who develop EBV infection may require alteration of immunosuppressive therapy and administration of monoclonal anti-CD20 (rituximab).

MEDICATION
- In primary infections:
  - Antimicrobial agents (usually penicillin) only if throat culture is positive for group A β-hemolytic streptococci. Incidence of rash following beta-lactam antibiotic therapy (previously is much lower than historically thought.
  - Warm saline gargles for oropharyngeal pain
  - Corticosteroids
    ○ May provide some symptomatic relief but no improvement in resolution of illness
    ○ Consider in severe pharyngotonsillitis with oropharyngeal edema and airway encroachment. Dexamethasone 0.3 mg/kg/day may be used for 1 to 3 days.
    ○ Also for patients with marked toxicity/major complications (e.g., hemolytic anemia, thrombocytopenic purpura, neurologic sequelae, myocarditis, pericarditis) (5)[B]
- Antiviral medications (acyclovir) have been found to shorten recovery time and improve subjective symptoms in acute EBV infection in small studies.

ISSUES FOR REFERRAL
Most cases can be managed as an outpatient without the need for specialty referral. Consider referral for complications such as oropharyngeal edema with airway compromise.

SURGERY/OTHER PROCEDURES
- Splenectomy may be necessary with profound thrombocytopenia that is refractory to corticosteroids.
- Only current effective treatment for XLP is hematopoietic stem cell transplantation. There is some use of mono-clonal antibody to delay progression pre-HST or treat relapse post transplant.
- Splenic rupture

ONGOING CARE

FOLLOW-UP RECOMMENDATIONS

ALERT
Rupture of the spleen may be fatal if not recognized; it requires blood transfusions, treatment for shock, and splenectomy. Occurrence is estimated at 0.1%.

Patient Monitoring
- Avoid contact sports, heavy lifting, and excess exertion until spleen and liver have returned to normal size (ultrasound can verify). Current consensus is that if after 3 weeks and normal exam, no fever, and no constitutional symptoms, patients may return to contact sport activities.
- Eliminate alcohol/exposure to other hepatotoxic drugs until LFTs return to normal.
- Rates of complications are highest during the first 3 weeks of illness.
- Symptoms (malaise, fatigue, intermittent sore throat, lymphadenopathy) may persist for months.

DIET
No restrictions. Hydration is important.

PROGNOSIS
- Most recover in ~4 weeks.
- Fatigue may persist for months.

COMPLICATIONS
- Neurologic (rare)
  - Aseptic meningitis, meningoencephalitis
  - Bell palsy, Guillain-Barré syndrome
  - Transverse myelitis
  - Cerebellar ataxia
  - Acute psychosis
- Hematologic (rare)
  - Thrombocytopenia, early in illness
  - Hemolytic anemia with neutropenia (early)
  - Hemophagocytic syndrome (splenomegaly, fever, cytopenia)
  - Agammaglobulinemia
- Pneumonitis
- Airway obstruction
- Splenic rupture
  - Rare but most often occurs in first 21 days of illness

REFERENCES

1. Frappier L. Epstein-Barr virus: current questions and challenges. *Tumour Virus Res*. 2021;12:200218.
2. Guidry JT, Birdwell CE, Scott RS. Epstein-Barr virus in the pathogenesis of oral cancers. *Oral Dis*. 2018;24(4):497–508.
3. Houen G, Trier NH. Epstein-Barr virus and systemic autoimmune diseases. *Front Immunol*. 2021;11:587380.
4. Dunmire SK, Verghese PS, Balfour HH Jr. Primary Epstein-Barr virus infection. *J Clin Virol*. 2018;102:84–92.
5. Odumade O, Hogquist K, Balfour HH Jr. Progress and problems in understanding and managing primary Epstein-Barr virus infections. *Clin Microbiol Rev*. 2011;24(1):193–209.

ADDITIONAL READING
- Arai A. Chronic active Epstein–Barr virus infection: the elucidation of the pathophysiology and the development of therapeutic methods. *Microorganisms*. 2021;9(1):180.
- Hoover K, Higginbotham K. *Epstein Barr Virus (EBV)*. In: StatPearls [Internet]. Treasure Island, FL: StatPearls Publishing; 2020. https://www.ncbi.nlm.nih.gov/books/NBK559285/.
- Kanda T, Yajima M, Ikuta K. Epstein-Barr virus strain variation and cancer. *Cancer Sci*. 2019;110(4):1132–1139.

CODES

ICD10
- B27.00 Gammaherpesviral mononucleosis without complication
- B27.09 Gammaherpesviral mononucleosis with other complications
- B27.01 Gammaherpesviral mononucleosis with polyneuropathy

CLINICAL PEARLS
- 98% of patients with acute IM present with some combination of fever, sore throat, cervical node enlargement, and tonsillar hypertrophy.
- False-negative monospot (heterophile antibody) is common in the first 10 to 14 days of illness. 90% will have heterophile antibodies by week 3 of illness.
- Lymphocytosis (not monocytosis) is common in IM.
- Treatment of IM is primarily supportive.

INFERTILITY
Sahil Mullick, MD • Ravneet Kaur, MD

BASICS

DESCRIPTION
Definition: failure to conceive after 1 year of regular sexual intercourse without the use of contraception in women <35 years of age or failure to conceive after 6 months of regular intercourse without contraception in women >35 years of age. Primary infertility: Couple has never been pregnant. Secondary infertility: Couple has been pregnant.

EPIDEMIOLOGY
Incidence
Incidence is the probability of achieving a pregnancy within 1 year. The incidence of infertility increases with age, with a decline in fertility in the early 30s, accelerating in the late 30s. ~85% of couples will conceive within 12 months of unprotected intercourse. ~95% of couples will conceive within 24 months of unprotected intercourse.

Prevalence
- About 25% of couples experience infertility at some point in their reproductive lives.
- ~9% of couples between ages 15 and 34 years, 25% between ages 35 and 39 years, ~30% couples between the ages of 40 and 44 years meet the criteria for being infertile, according to the National Survey of Family Growth.
- May increase as more women delay childbearing.

ETIOLOGY AND PATHOPHYSIOLOGY
- Most cases multifactorial: approximately 35% of cases due to female factors (of which 21% are due to ovulatory dysfunction and 14% due to tubal damage); ~26% due to male factors; 28% unknown etiology
- Acquired: Most common cause of infertility in the United States is pelvic inflammatory disease (PID) secondary to sexually transmitted infections (STIs), endometriosis, polycystic ovary syndrome (PCOS), premature ovarian failure, and increased maternal age.
- Diminished ovarian reserve (DOR): low fertility due to low quantity or functional quality of oocytes
- Congenital: anatomic and genetic abnormalities

Genetics
- Higher incidence of genetic abnormalities among infertile population, including Klinefelter syndrome (47,XXY), Turner syndrome (45X or mosaic), and fragile X syndrome
- Y chromosomal microdeletions are associated with isolated defects of spermatogenesis → found in 16% of men with azoospermia/severe oligozoospermia.
- Cystic fibrosis transmembrane conductance regulator (CFTR) gene mutation causing congenital bilateral absence of vas deferens (CBAVD)

RISK FACTORS
- Female
  - Gynecologic history: irregular/abnormal menses, STIs, dysmenorrhea, fibroids, prior pregnancy
  - Medical history: advanced age, endocrinopathy, autoimmune disease, undiagnosed celiac disease, collagen vascular diseases, thrombophilia, obesity, and cancer

- Surgical history: appendicitis, pelvic surgery, intrauterine surgery, tubal ligation
- Social history: smoking, alcohol/substance abuse, eating disorders, exercise, advanced maternal age
- Male
  - Medical history: STI, prostatitis, medication use (i.e., β-blockers, calcium channel blocker, antiulcer medication), endocrinopathy, cancer
  - Surgical history: orchiopexy, hernia repair, vasectomy with/without reversal
  - Social: smoking, alcohol/substance abuse, anabolic steroids, environmental exposures, occupations leading to increased scrotal temperature (frequent use of saunas, hot tubs, or tight underwear), prescription drugs that impair male potency

GENERAL PREVENTION
Normal diet and exercise, avoid smoking and other substance abuse, prevention of STIs

COMMONLY ASSOCIATED CONDITIONS
Pelvic pathology, endocrine dysfunction, and anovulation (hyperandrogenism, PCOS)

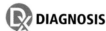

DIAGNOSIS

HISTORY
- Complete reproductive history:
  - Age of female
  - Complete female reproductive history
    - Age at menarche, regularity of menstrual cycle, physical development (Tanner stages), previous methods of contraception, history of abnormal Pap smears and treatment
    - History of abortion, dilation and curettages, bilateral tubal ligation, vasectomy, or other pelvic/abdominal surgery
- Coital frequency and timing
- History of sexual dysfunction
- History of STI, endocrine abnormalities, malignancy or chronic illness
- Family history of reproductive issues
- Medications: drug abuse, allergies, and exposure to environmental hazards

PHYSICAL EXAM
- Body mass index (BMI), distribution of body fat, and waist circumference
- Female
  - Pubertal development with Tanner staging
  - Signs of PCOS: androgen excess, obesity, signs of insulin resistance
  - Vaginal exam: Describe rugation, discharge, anatomic variation.
  - Uterine size/shape, mobility, tenderness
- Male
  - Abnormalities of the penis or urethral meatus
  - Testes: volume, symmetry, masses (varicocele, hydrocele), presence/absence of vas deferens

DIAGNOSTIC TESTS & INTERPRETATION
Initial Tests (lab, imaging)
Evaluation is directed by history:
- Assessment of ovulation
  - Irregular or infrequent menses
  - Elevated follicle-stimulating hormone (FSH) and luteinizing hormone (LH) but low estradiol indicate ovarian insufficiency. High LH alone suggests PCOS.
    - Use of basal body temperature (BBT) charts to confirm ovulation is not a reliable method for ovulation prediction but is low-cost and may be useful for some couples to guide the timing of intercourse.
- Assessment of ovarian reserve
  - Women >35 years old need to have ovarian reserve assessed. On day 3 of menses, an FSH >15 to 20 IU/L is suggestive of impaired reserve.
  - Anti-müllerian hormone (AMH) and antral follicle counts (AFCs): The number of antral follicles measured by transvaginal ultrasound (US) is termed the "antral follicle count." AMH decreases as a woman approaches menopause. AMH can be measured any time during the cycle and is not affected by hormones.
  - Clomiphene challenge test: After administration of clomiphene from day 5 to 9, measure FSH of ≥10 mIU/mL on day 10 to help confirm the diagnosis of DOR.
- Semen analysis
  - Warranted in all infertile couples. Semen analysis alone is not used to predict male fertility potential.
  - Semen collection: collected after 2 to 5 days of abstinence. Repeat test 2 to 3 times due to inherent variability within the same individual.
  - Parameters for normal male values: semen volume 1.5 mL or more, pH 7.2 or more, sperm concentration 15 million spermatozoa per mL or more, total sperm number 39 million spermatozoa per ejaculate or more, total motility: 40% or more motile or 32% or more with progressive motility, vitality 58% or more live spermatozoa, sperm morphology (percentage of normal forms) 4% or more
- Additional labs
  - Prolactin, thyroid-stimulating hormone, 17-hydroxyprogesterone, androgen levels
  - HIV, herpes simplex virus 1 and 2, chlamydia, gonorrhea, rapid plasma reagin, hepatitis B, and CMV
  - Genetic testing based on family history
- Transvaginal US for anatomic abnormality
- Hysterosalpingogram (HSG) to evaluate patency of tubes and contour of the cavity; may be both diagnostic and therapeutic

Follow-Up Tests & Special Considerations
Abnormal imaging may require surgical evaluation.

Diagnostic Procedures/Other
- Hysteroscopy: gold standard, used to directly visualize the endometrial cavity; may be indicated to evaluate filling defects on HSG or SHG
- Laparoscopy: used to directly visualize the peritoneal cavity and may be indicated to evaluate abnormal findings on HSG. Laparoscopy is the only way to definitively diagnose endometriosis.

Test Interpretation
Refer to section "Initial Tests (lab, imaging)."

TREATMENT

GENERAL MEASURES
- Lifestyle changes that may improve fertility:
  - Achieving an ideal BMI, cessation of smoking, limiting exposure to caffeine and alcohol, wait for at least 12 months before initiating the infertility evaluation.
- Couples may wish to begin with simpler methods for determining ovulation. BBT tracking and/or detection of LH surge may be helpful for some. BBT is not as reliable as other methods for ovulation prediction.
- Be aware of insurance coverage for each patient. Be mindful of the couple's emotional state: Depression, anger, anxiety, and marital discord are common. Many patients benefit from counseling and support measures.
- All female fertility patients should be given folate supplementation 1 mg/day by mouth. Dietary carotenoids in males may improve sperm quality.
- In vitro fertilization (IVF) is the most effective infertility treatment available for women with unexplained infertility who have not conceived after 2 years of regular unprotected sexual intercourse:
  - Eggs are removed from the female and fertilized outside the body. The embryo is monitored for 3 to 5 days and then implanted into the uterus on day 3 or day 5.
  - Anatomic causes should be referred immediately for IVF, although surgical consult may be required.
  - Fewer complications have been reported for individuals undergoing IVF for anatomic causes rather than ovulatory dysfunction (low APGAR scores, diabetes mellitus).
  - As compared to the general population, an increased risk of preterm birth and low birth weight has also been seen among subfertile women who conceived naturally without IVF.
  - Donor eggs may be obtained.
  - Women <40 years of age or those who have not conceived after 2 years of unprotected intercourse or 12 cycles of artificial insemination should be offered 3 full cycles of IVF.
  - Women ages 40 to 42 years with no evidence of previous IVF or low ovarian reserve should be offered 1 full cycle of IVF.
- Intrauterine insemination (IUI) without ovarian stimulation can be considered in special circumstances: physical disabilities limiting vaginal intercourse or psychosexual issues, people in same-sex relationships, etc. (please refer to "Male factors").
- Male factors
  - Consider lifestyle changes.
  - IUI: Sperm is placed via a catheter directly in the uterus. IUI effectively increases the sperm count.
  - Intracytoplasmic sperm injection (ICSI) is performed in conjunction with IVF for males with severe abnormalities (i.e., <5 million sperm) or those who have failed to conceive with IUI. A single sperm is injected directly into the cytoplasm of the egg. Fertilization occurs ~70% of the time.
  - Donor sperm may be obtained.

MEDICATION
First Line
- Treatment of infertility depends on the etiology.
- Achieving optimal BMI >17 kg/m² and <29 kg/m²

- Women:
  - Anovulation: must determine if HYPOgonadotropic or NORMOgonadotropic
    - Hypogonadotropic patients: Standard treatment to induce ovulation consists of daily injections of both FSH and LH, which need to be carefully monitored to avoid overstimulation, resulting in ovarian hyperstimulation syndrome (OHSS).
    - Normogonadotropic patients: most commonly due to PCOS. Ovulation induction with letrozole (aromatase inhibitor) is possibly superior to clomiphene for patients with PCOS; clomiphene citrate (Clomid)
    - Unexplained infertility: The first-line therapy might be controlled ovarian hyperstimulation, as with clomiphene citrate and IUI. IVF may be recommended as second line.
  - Coital or cervical problems: IUI
  - Endometriosis: either IVF or surgery; medical therapy does not increase pregnancy rates.
  - Lifestyle changes: increasing frequency and timing of intercourse
- Male:
  - Lifestyle changes: increasing frequency and timing of intercourse
  - Medications changes to improve sperm count, testicular function, sperm production and quality by discontinuing or changing certain selective serotonin reuptake inhibitor, calcium channel blocker, and highly active antiretroviral therapy medications
  - Surgery: reversal of sperm blockage (e.g., vasectomy, varicocele)
  - Sperm retrieval when ejaculation is problematic.

Second Line
If clomiphene and letrozole fail to induce ovulation:
- Metformin beneficial in anovulatory women with PCOS, especially those with glucose intolerance; initiate with 500 mg daily and increase to ~1,500 mg/day; monitor renal function; might take up to 3 months to be effective
- Consider also oral contraceptive pills (OCPs) for ≥2 cycles and then retry the clomiphene immediately after stopping the OCPs.
- Cabergoline or bromocriptine used if prolactin is elevated or if no withdrawal bleed after progesterone administration. Once pregnancy has occurred, the medication can be stopped.
- Human menopausal gonadotropins (hMGs) or recombinant FSH is indicated if there is resistance to clomiphene or if there is hypogonadotropism.

ISSUES FOR REFERRAL
Reproductive endocrinology and/or urology

ADDITIONAL THERAPIES
Consider using surrogate pregnancy if female cannot conceive.

SURGERY/OTHER PROCEDURES
Reproductive surgery may be necessary in those with anatomic causes of infertility. Polypectomy, myomectomy, and salpingectomy for hydrosalpinx. Consider treatment of varicocele and aspiration of sperm using.

COMPLEMENTARY & ALTERNATIVE MEDICINE
Acupuncture may increase live birth rates with IVF.

ONGOING CARE

FOLLOW-UP RECOMMENDATIONS
Specialist if not successful after 3 to 6 cycles of oral ovulation induction

Patient Monitoring
Cycle monitoring may decrease risks. US can show the number of developing follicles per cycle.

DIET
Low-caffeine diet, limit alcohol intake

PATIENT EDUCATION
- American Society for Reproductive Medicine (http://www.asrm.org)
- Resolve: patient advocacy group (http://www.resolve.org)

PROGNOSIS
Most couples (80–90%) will achieve a pregnancy within 12 months of attempting pregnancy with regular unprotected sexual intercourse. Fecundability progressively decreases over time (1).

COMPLICATIONS
Anxiety, multiple pregnancy, OHSS, a slight increased risk of congenital abnormalities; women diagnosed with infertility and women receiving fertility treatment are at a higher risk of maternal morbidity than are fertile women (2).

REFERENCES

1. American College of Obstetricians and Gynecologists Committee on Gynecologic Practice and Practice Committee. Female age-related fertility decline. Committee Opinion No. 589. *Fertil Steril.* 2014;101(3):633–634.
2. Murugappan G, Li S, Lathi RB, et al. Increased risk of severe maternal morbidity among infertile women: analysis of US claims data. *Am J Obstet Gynecol.* 2020;223(3):404.e1–404.e20.

SEE ALSO

- Amenorrhea; Endometriosis; Metabolic Syndrome; Polycystic Ovarian Syndrome (PCOS); Pelvic Inflammatory Disease
- Algorithm: Infertility

CODES

ICD10
- N97.9 Female infertility, unspecified
- N46.9 Male infertility, unspecified
- N97.1 Female infertility of tubal origin

CLINICAL PEARLS
- Women <35 years of age should be evaluated for infertility after failing to conceive after 1 year of unprotected intercourse, those ≥35 years should receive evaluation after 6 months, and those ≥40 years should receive assistance immediately.
- Infertility is often multifactorial.

INFLUENZA

Alice Yang, MD

BASICS

DESCRIPTION
Acute, typically self-limited, febrile infection caused by orthomyxovirus influenza types A and B marked by inflammation of nasal mucosa, pharynx, conjunctiva, and respiratory tract

EPIDEMIOLOGY
- Outbreaks of influenza occur annually during the fall-winter months in the Northern and Southern Hemispheres.
- Influenza virus can undergo antigenic shift (abrupt change) leading to viral strains with little immunologic resistance in a population, resulting in pandemic outbreaks. Minor seasonal variations are called *antigenic drift*.
- Persons of all ages are susceptible to infection. Notable demographics at risk for complications and hospitalization include:
  - Those between <2 and >65 years
  - Immunocompromised states, including pregnancy up to 2 weeks postpartum
  - Individuals with cardiovascular or pulmonary disease, Addison disease, or diabetes
  - Residents of nursing homes or other long-term care facilities
  - Individuals who identify as American Indian or Alaska Native

Incidence
Incidence is difficult to ascertain as most individuals do not seek medical care and are therefore not diagnosed.

Prevalence
- In the United States, the Centers for Disease Control and Prevention (CDC) provides yearly surveillance data. During the 2019 to 2020 season, prevalence was estimated to be at 38,000,000 positive tests with 18,000,000 related medical visits, 400,000 hospitalizations, and 22,000 deaths, 199 of these in the pediatric population. The proportion of positive tests ranged from 26% to 30%.
- The 2020 to 2021 season was historic due to its setting during the COVID-19 pandemic. The CDC reported a positive test rate of just 0.2%. A single influenza-related pediatric death was reported. A record number of vaccinations were given, at least 25 million more doses than previous seasons. Concurrent COVID-19 precautionary measures such as social distancing, face masking, and school closures likely contributed to the mitigation of influenza spread.

ETIOLOGY AND PATHOPHYSIOLOGY
Orthomyxovirus (influenza types A [majority] and B); influenza A virus subtypes HxNx based on hemagglutinin and neuraminidase
- Incubation is 1 to 4 days; infected persons are most contagious during peak symptoms.
- Spread by aerosolized droplets or contact with respiratory secretions
- Hemagglutinin binds to columnar respiratory epithelium where replication occurs, and neuraminidase protein facilitates spread along respiratory epithelium (1).

RISK FACTORS
- For contracting disease:
  - Crowded environments such as nursing homes, barracks, schools, and correctional facilities

- For complications:
  - Neonates, infants, elderly
  - Pregnancy, especially in 3rd trimester
  - Chronic pulmonary diseases
  - Cardiovascular diseases, including valvular pathology and congestive heart failure (CHF)
  - Metabolic disease, morbid obesity
  - Hemoglobinopathies
  - Malignancy; immunosuppression
  - Neuromuscular diseases that limit respiratory function and ability to handle secretions

GENERAL PREVENTION
- Vaccination: all persons ≥6 months should be vaccinated annually unless contraindication present. The CDC does not express preference for any type of vaccine over another.
- Live attenuated influenza vaccine (LAIV) is a quadrivalent intranasal vaccine approved for healthy, nonpregnant individuals between 2 and 49 years of age.
- Inactivated influenza vaccine (IIV) is available either as trivalent (IIV3) or quadrivalent (IIV4) with either three or four strains of influenza. IIV also is available as high-dose, intradermal, cell culture–based (ccIIV3), MF59-adjuvanted (aIIV3), and recombinant hemagglutinin vaccine (RIV3).
  - LAIV is an intranasal quadrivalent vaccine.
- IIV recommended annually for the following:
  - All persons aged ≥6 months
  - Vaccine should be administered annually as soon as the vaccine is available.
  - Protection occurs 1 to 2 weeks after immunization.
  - Typically, mild side effects include low-grade fever and local reaction at vaccination site.
  - Inactivated IM dose: ≥3 years of age: 0.5 mL; children 6 to 35 months of age: 0.25 mL
  - Intradermal formulation for 18- to 64-year-olds uses a short 30-gauge needle in a single-use prefilled syringe with 0.1 mL vaccine; somewhat higher local reactions when given intradermal
  - Single annual dose except for children <9 years of age, who should receive 2 doses (4 weeks apart) the 1st year they receive influenza vaccine
  - Vaccine contraindication: Severe allergy such as anaphylaxis to IIV components, allergies from eggs are not considered a contraindication; observe all patients for 15 minutes after vaccination; no skin testing with influenza vaccine is needed in egg-allergic patients. RIV is safe in patients with an egg allergy.
- IIV-HD: high-dose quadrivalent IIV
  - Contains 4 times the antigen concentration of IIV
  - Licensed for persons ≥65 years of age
  - Results in higher antibody levels but somewhat higher rates of local reactions
  - Advisory Committee on Immunization Practices does not express a preference for/against IIV-HD.
- Antiviral prophylaxis depends on current resistance patterns each year; see https://www.cdc.gov/flu/ for patterns or check with local health department.
  - In high-risk groups that have not been vaccinated or need additional control measures during epidemics; *not* a substitute for vaccination unless vaccine is contraindicated
  - During influenza season, for those with contraindications to vaccine who have been exposed to the virus
  - For staff and residents in nursing home outbreaks
  - For immune-deficient persons who are expected not to respond to vaccination after viral exposure

Pediatric Considerations
- Vaccinate children >6 months annually.
- Recommend all household members with children <6 months be vaccinated.
- For children who need 2 doses, administer first dose as soon as available for second dose to be given before the end of October.
- For prophylaxis, oseltamivir dosage varies by weight and is recommended by the CDC for prophylaxis for children ≥3 months; zanamivir is approved for prophylaxis for children ≥5 years of age at a dosage of 2 inhalations per day. Prophylaxis treatment duration is 7 days. For prophylaxis, the dosage of amantadine and of rimantadine is 5 mg/kg/day up to 150 mg in 2 divided doses. Currently, amantadine and rimantadine are not recommended due to resistance.

Pregnancy Considerations
- The CDC recommends vaccinating all women who will be pregnant during influenza season.
- If unvaccinated at the time of flu season, pregnant women should receive IIV or RIV.
- Oseltamivir, zanamivir, peramivir, rimantadine, and amantadine are pregnancy Category C.

COMMONLY ASSOCIATED CONDITIONS
Bacterial pneumonia

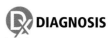 DIAGNOSIS

Look for:
- Systemic symptoms
- Cough
- Not being able to cope with daily activities
- Being confined to bed

HISTORY
Sudden onset of:
- Fever (37.7–40.0°C), especially within 3 days of illness onset
- Anorexia
- Chills, sweats, malaise, myalgia, arthralgia
- Headache
- Sore throat/pharyngitis
- Nonproductive cough
- Rhinorrhea, nasal congestion

PHYSICAL EXAM
- Physical exam is not specific for influenza.
- Physical examination should exclude complications such as otitis media, pneumonia, sinusitis, and tracheobronchitis.

DIFFERENTIAL DIAGNOSIS
- Respiratory viral infections including, SARS-CoV-2, respiratory syncytial virus, parainfluenza, adenovirus, enterovirus ("influenza-like illness")
- Infectious mononucleosis
- Coxsackievirus infections
- Viral or streptococcal tonsillitis
- Atypical mycoplasmal pneumonia
- *Chlamydia pneumoniae*
- Q fever
- Less likely possibilities include severe acute respiratory syndrome, primary HIV infection, acute myeloid leukemia, tuberculosis, anthrax, and malaria (2).

DIAGNOSTIC TESTS & INTERPRETATION

Initial Tests (lab, imaging)

During influenza season, decision to pursue diagnostic testing is based on clinical findings. Various testing modalities are discussed below:

- Antigen detection
  - Known as rapid influenza diagnostic tests (RIDTs)
  - Modality of all outpatient office-based testing by recommendation of the Infectious Disease Society of America
  - Detects viral antigens within 10 to 15 minutes
  - Moderate sensitivity (80%), high specificity
- Molecular assay
  - Reverse transcription polymerase chain reaction (RT-PCR)
  - High sensitivity (90–95%) and specificity
- Immunofluorescence
  - Commercial rapid enzyme-linked immunosorbent assay antigen tests are available. Some rapid tests diagnose influenza A, others diagnose A and B. Sensitivity and specificity vary by manufacturer, strain of influenza, and age of patient. False-negative results are common, particularly during peak influenza activity.
  - Viral culture is reserved for surveillance of antigenic and genetic characteristics of circulating influenza viruses for vaccine planning and does not play a role in clinical management.

Follow-Up Tests & Special Considerations

- In patient with severe symptoms at presentation, consider the additional tests:
  - Complete blood count: typically shows normal WBC count or mild leukopenia. Leukocytosis may indicate bacterial complication.
  - Comprehensive metabolic panel: elevations of liver enzymes or creatinine may indicate severe disease.
  - Chest x-ray if pneumonia is suspected
- The concurrent SARS-CoV-2 pandemic poses a diagnostic challenge during the 2020 to 2021 influenza season given the wide overlap of symptoms. It is not yet known how common coinfection is. The FDA has granted Emergency Use Authorization for developing commercially available combination tests for both SARS-CoV-2 and influenza A and B.

Test Interpretation

Positive and negative predictive values of the above-mentioned tests are dependent on local community prevalence. As prevalence increases (as influenza peaks), a positive test is more likely to reflect true infection, whereas a negative test is more likely to be false.

TREATMENT

- Symptomatic treatment (saline nasal spray, analgesic gargle, antipyretics, analgesics)
- Cool-mist or ultrasonic humidifier to increase moisture of inspired air
- Counsel on droplet precautions: wearing a disposable surgical mask around others.
- 5 days is the average period of viral shedding in immunocompetent hosts.
- Hospitalized patients may require oxygen or ventilatory support.
- Tobacco cessation

MEDICATION

- Antiviral treatment depends on yearly resistance patterns; check https://www.cdc.gov/flu/ or with local health department. Antivirals are most effective if administered within first 48 hours in laboratory-confirmed (or highly suspected based on clinical findings) influenza cases.

- Antivirals within 48 hours of symptom onset are recommended for patients at risk for complications (i.e., diabetes, CHD, COPD, asthma, etc.).
- Antivirals are recommended if hospitalized.
- Antivirals include baloxavir, oseltamivir, zanamivir, and peramivir. Amantadine *and* rimantadine *currently are not recommended due to resistance*.
- Consider antivirals for patients whose onset of symptoms is within the past 48 hours and who wish to shorten the duration of illness and further reduce their relatively low risk of complications.
- Symptomatic treatment is preferred for those patients *without risk factors* and *without* signs of lower respiratory tract infection.
- Effect is 24-hour reduction of symptoms and a reduction in complication rates.
  - Baloxavir dose: oral, 1-time dose
    - 40 to <80 kg, 40 mg
    - >80 kg, 80 mg
    - For children >12 years, use adult dosing.
  - Zanamivir dose: 2 inhalations BID for 5 days (age ≥7 years)
  - Oseltamivir dose: 75 mg PO BID for 5 days (age ≥13 years)
  - If severe renal impairment, 75 mg/day PO
  - Oseltamivir for children ≥1 year of age
    - <15 kg, 30 mg BID
    - >15 to 23 kg, 45 mg BID
    - >23 to 40 kg, 60 mg BID
    - >40 kg, 75 mg BID
  - Oseltamivir for children <1 year of age: 3 mg/kg/dose BID
  - Peramivir dose: 600 mg IV infusion over 15 to 30 minutes for adults ≥18 years of age
- Antipyretics
  - Acetaminophen: in children
- Precautions
  - Zanamivir may cause bronchospasm if the patient has COPD or asthma; the patient should have a bronchodilator available.
  - Amantadine has anticholinergic properties and should be used with caution in those with psychiatric, addiction, or neurologic disorders because it may increase risk for suicide attempts or increase neurologic symptoms.
  - Rimantadine may increase the risk of seizures in those with an underlying seizure disorder.
  - Oseltamivir may cause nausea and vomiting; may be less severe if taken with food
  - Peramivir may cause serious skin reactions.
- Decrease dose of certain antivirals if creatinine clearance <60 mL/min.
- Ibuprofen or other NSAIDs for symptomatic relief
- Aspirin: should not be used in children <16 years due to risk of Reye syndrome
- Outpatient treatment is sufficient except for cases with severe complications or in high-risk groups (3).

ADMISSION, INPATIENT, AND NURSING CONSIDERATIONS

- Initiate droplet precautions for both confirmed or suspected influenza.
- Initiate prompt antiviral therapy for patients hospitalized with influenza-related illness, regardless of prior duration of symptoms.

ONGOING CARE

FOLLOW-UP RECOMMENDATIONS

- Mild cases: follow-up typically not required
- Moderate or severe cases: Follow up until symptoms and any secondary sequelae resolve.

PROGNOSIS

Good

COMPLICATIONS

- Sepsis
- Pneumonia (primary viral or secondary bacterial)
- Myocarditis
- Encephalitis
- Myositis, rhabdomyolysis
- Otitis media; acute sinusitis
- Croup; bronchitis
- Apnea in neonates
- Reye syndrome
- Postinfluenza asthenia
- COPD or CHF exacerbation
- Encephalopathy, death

Geriatric Considerations

Complications requiring hospitalization are more likely in elderly patients.

REFERENCES

1. Centers for Disease Control and Prevention. Background and epidemiology. https://www.cdc.gov/flu/professionals/acip/background-epidemiology.htm. Published September 10, 2019. Accessed January 28, 2021.
2. Erlikh IV, Abraham S, Kondamudi VK. Management of influenza. *Am Fam Physician*. 2010;82(9):1087–1095.
3. Gaitonde DY, Moore FC, Morgan MK. Influenza: diagnosis and treatment. *Am Fam Physician*. 2019;100(12):751–758.

ADDITIONAL READING

- Centers for Disease Control and Prevention. 2020-2021 Flu season summary. https://www.cdc.gov/flu/season/faq-flu-season-2020-2021.htm. Published July 22, 2021. Accessed November 17, 2021.
- Centers for Disease Control and Prevention. Influenza antiviral medications: summary for clinicians. https://www.cdc.gov/flu/professionals/antivirals/summary-clinicians.htm. Published January 25, 2021. Accessed November 17, 2021.

 CODES

ICD10

- J10.08 Influenza due to other identified influenza virus with other specified pneumonia
- J11.89 Influenza due to unidentified influenza virus with other manifestations
- J10.81 Influenza due to other identified influenza virus with encephalopathy

CLINICAL PEARLS

- Influenza is an acute, (typically) self-limited, febrile infection caused by influenza virus types A and B.
- All persons >6 months should be vaccinated against influenza on an annual basis (there are rare exceptions).
- Recommend concurrent administration of pneumonia vaccine if indicated per CDC guidelines.
- Complications from influenza are most common in the very young, very old, and individuals with comorbid disease.
- Hand hygiene either with soap and water (slightly superior) or with alcohol-based hand rubs and covering coughs are simple ways to reduce the spread of influenza.

INGROWN TOENAIL

Sally-Ann L. Pantin, MD, FAAFP • Thomas A. Waller, MD

BASICS

DESCRIPTION
- In an ingrown toenail, the distal margin of the nail plate grows into the lateral nail fold, causing irritation, inflammation, and sometimes bacterial or fungal infection:
  - Stage 1 (inflammation): erythema, edema, tenderness to palpation of lateral nail fold
  - Stage 2 (abscess): increased pain, erythema, and edema as well as drainage (purulent or serous)
  - Stage 3 (granulation): Chronic inflammation leads to further erythema, edema, and pain, often with granulation tissue growing over the nail plate and significant nail fold hypertrophy.
- Can reoccur
- Synonym(s): onychocryptosis, unguis incarnatus

EPIDEMIOLOGY
- Great toenail is most often affected.
- Lateral edge of nail is more commonly affected than the medial edge.
- Most common in males aged 14 to 25 years
- Infrequent, but more often in elderly females than in elderly males
- More common in those with lower incomes

Prevalence
- 24.5/1,000 overall
- 50/1,000 ≥65 years

ETIOLOGY AND PATHOPHYSIOLOGY
- Nail plate penetrates the nail fold, causing a foreign body reaction (inflammation).
- Bacteria or fungi may enter through the opening in the nail fold, causing infection and abscess formation.
- The inflamed and infected area leads to granulation tissue and hypertrophy of the nail fold.

RISK FACTORS
- Genetic factors
  - Increased nail fold width
  - Decreased nail thickness
  - Medial rotation of the toe
- Many others proposed; none proven, including the following:
  - Distorted, thickened nail (onychogryphosis)
  - Fungal infection (onychomycosis)
  - Hyperhidrosis
  - Improper trimming of the lateral nail plate
  - Poorly fitting shoes
  - Trauma to nail or nail fold
  - Conditions that predispose to pedal edema (i.e., thyroid dysfunction, diabetes, obesity, heart failure, renal disease)

GENERAL PREVENTION
- Properly fitting shoes
- Proper nail trimming (see "Patient Education")

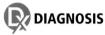

DIAGNOSIS

HISTORY
- Patients most often present with pain, redness, and swelling in the toe along one or both sides of the nail.
- Drainage can occur as inflammation and/or infection develop.

PHYSICAL EXAM
- Nail fold tenderness
- Erythema and edema
- Drainage (serous or purulent)
- Granulation tissue
- Lateral nail fold hypertrophy

DIFFERENTIAL DIAGNOSIS
- Cellulitis
- Felon (pulp abscess on plantar aspect of toe)
- Onychogryphosis (gross thickening and hardening of the nail)
- Onycholysis (separation of nail from nail bed)
- Onychomycosis (fungal infection of the nail)
- Osteomyelitis
- Paronychia (infection or inflammation around the nail fold)
- Subungual exostosis (bony projection from distal phalanx)
- Subungual osteochondroma (benign bone tumor)

DIAGNOSTIC TESTS & INTERPRETATION
Initial Tests (lab, imaging)
None usually needed
- Consider MRI, x-ray, or bone scan if osteomyelitis is suspected.
- Consider x-ray if subungual exostosis or osteochondroma is suspected.

TREATMENT

GENERAL MEASURES
- Majority of cases respond to conservative therapy.
- Warm, soapy water or Epsom salt soaks for 10 to 20 minutes 3 times per day until symptoms resolve (1)
- Bluntly insert a cotton wisp or dental floss underneath the ingrown portion of the nail. The patient can continue to replace the insert until the nail grows beyond the fold.

- Use tape to pull the lateral nail fold away from the nail plate until the nail grows beyond the fold.
- Stage 2 ingrown nails often respond to conservative treatment, as above, especially cotton wool, or a trial of cryotherapy.

MEDICATION
- NSAIDs are usually adequate for analgesia.
- Topical antibiotic can be applied after soaking (1).
- Neither oral nor topical antibiotics are useful as an adjunct to surgical treatment.

SURGERY/OTHER PROCEDURES
- Surgical interventions are more effective than nonsurgical interventions in preventing recurrence (2),(3)[A].
- Nail avulsion techniques are more effective than nail fold debulking techniques (not described in this topic) (3)[A].
  - Partial avulsion of the nail with phenol nail matrix ablation
    - Obtain surgical consent after explaining the risks, benefits, and alternatives.
    - Achieve local anesthesia with a digital wing or ring block.
    - May consider placing a tourniquet around the base of the toe to assist with hemostasis (caution in patients with diabetes or peripheral vascular disease)
    - Elevate the ingrown part of the nail from the nail bed with a periosteal (Freer) elevator or hemostat.
    - Incise the nail longitudinally with scissors or a nail splitter a few millimeters from the ingrown border, starting at the distal edge and proceeding to the matrix.
    - Grasp, down to the cuticle, the avulsed fragment with a hemostat and pull this portion gently out with a hemostat, utilizing longitudinal traction, as well as rotation to the lateral nail fold if needed.
    - Remove the tourniquet once hemostasis is attained.
    - Dip a urethral swab in 80–88% phenol solution (phenol use is contraindicated in pregnancy).
    - Apply the phenol 3 times for 30 seconds to the nail matrix under the proximal nail fold. Wash the area with 70% isopropyl (rubbing) alcohol to neutralize phenol.
- Nonsurgical interventions, such as a flexible gutter splint, are another option for treatment of stage 2 or 3 ingrown nails (4),(5)[B].
  - J Flexible gutter splint
    - Cut a 1- to 2-cm long piece of sterilized plastic tube, such as IV tubing, 2 to 3 mm in diameter (alternatively, you may use a cap from a 29-gauge needle).

○ Make a slit in the tubing lengthwise and cut the end off at an angle.
○ Apply local anesthesia with a digital wing or ring block.
○ Release the ingrown edge of the nail from the nail fold with a hemostat.
○ Slide the tube, angled end first, along the ingrown edge of the nail.
○ Consider fixing the tube in place with self-curing formable acrylic resin (used for dentures and sculptured nails), tape, or a single suture through the nail plate.
○ Leave the tube in place until nail has grown beyond the nail fold.
- Bilateral partial matricectomy should be considered in patients with severe ingrown toenail or recurrence.
- Permanent destruction of the germinal matrix can be used to prevent recurrence. The use of phenol for nail bed ablation is probably more effective than nail avulsion alone in preventing recurrence (2),(3)[A].
  - Other options for nail bed ablation:
    ○ Sodium hydroxide (NaOH)
    ○ Cryotherapy
    ○ Electrocautery with a special flattened tip coated with Teflon on one side to protect the proximal nail fold
    ○ Carbon dioxide laser
    ○ Surgical excision of the nail matrix

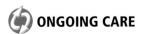 **ONGOING CARE**

FOLLOW-UP RECOMMENDATIONS
- Dress with antibiotic ointment or sterile petroleum jelly; cover with sterile gauze and tube gauze.
- Postop instructions should include the following:
  - Rest and elevate the foot for 12 to 24 hours.
  - Take NSAIDs for discomfort.
  - Change dressing and wash with soap and water at least daily for 1 to 2 weeks following procedure.
  - Expect a sterile exudate for 2 to 6 weeks.
  - Avulsed nails may take 6 to 12 months to grow completely out (if no matrix ablation).
  - Call for increasing pain, redness, or swelling.
  - Average time to return to normal activities is 2 weeks.
- Patients treated conservatively should be followed up in the office every 7 to 10 days until marked improvement is noted.

PATIENT EDUCATION
- Trim nails straight across perpendicular to long axis of the nail (do not round corners) and not too short.
- Wear properly fitting, comfortable shoes.

COMPLICATIONS
- Cellulitis after surgical procedure (uncommon)
- Damage to fascia or periosteum from overly aggressive matrix ablation
- Damage to nail bed
- Distal toe ischemia due to prolonged use of a tourniquet during surgery (rare)
- Nail plate deformity (due to nail matrix damage)
- Osteomyelitis (rare)
- Permanent narrowing of nail (if partial matrix ablation is performed)
- Persistent postoperative wound drainage particularly with excessive phenolization of adjacent tissues
- Recurrence (40–80% with avulsion alone, 0.6–14% with matrix ablation, 6–13% with gutter splint)

REFERENCES
1. Heidelbaugh J, Lee H. Management of the ingrown toenail. *Am Fam Physician*. 2009;79(4):303–308.
2. Eekhof JA, Van Wijk B, Knuistingh Neven A, et al. Interventions for ingrowing toenails. *Cochrane Database Syst Rev*. 2012;(4):CD001541.
3. Park DH, Singh D. The management of ingrowing toenails. *BMJ*. 2012;344:e2089.
4. Arai H, Arai T, Nakajima H, et al. Formable acrylic treatment for ingrowing nail with gutter splint and sculptured nail. *Int J Dermatol*. 2004;43(10):759–765.
5. Nazari S. A simple and practical method in treatment of ingrown nails: splinting by flexible tube. *J Eur Acad Dermatol Venereol*. 2006;20(10):1302–1306.

ADDITIONAL READING
- Bos AM, van Tilburg MW, van Sorge AA, et al. Randomized clinical trial of surgical technique and local antibiotics for ingrowing toenail. *Br J Surg*. 2007;94(3):292–296.
- Bryant A, Knox A. Ingrown toenails: the role of the GP. *Aust Fam Physician*. 2015;44(3).102–105.

- Chapeskie H. Ingrown toenail or overgrown toe skin? Alternative treatment for onychocryptosis. *Can Fam Physician*. 2008;54(11):1561–1562.
- Reyzelman AM, Trombello KA, Vayser DJ, et al. Are antibiotics necessary in the treatment of locally infected ingrown toenails? *Arch Fam Med*. 2000;9(9):930–932.
- Richert B. Basic nail surgery. *Dermatol Clin*. 2006;24(3):313–322.
- Woo SH, Kim IH. Surgical pearl: nail edge separation with dental floss for ingrown toenails. *J Am Acad Dermatol*. 2004;50(6):939–940.

 SEE ALSO

For a video of this Nail Avulsion and Matrixectomy procedure, go to http://5minuteconsult.com/procedure/1508006.

 CODES

ICD10
L60.0 Ingrowing nail

CLINICAL PEARLS
- The best treatment for a stage 1 ingrown toenail is to insert a wisp of cotton or dental floss between the nail plate and lateral nail fold.
- The best treatment for a stage 3 ingrown toenail is partial nail avulsion with phenol matrix ablation.
- Patients can prevent ingrown toenails by trimming nails properly and wearing properly fitting shoes.
- Oral and topical antibiotics are not useful in the treatment of ingrown nails in conjunction with surgical treatment.

INJURY AND VIOLENCE

Tisha K. Johnson, MD, MPH • Jonathan R. Ballard, MD, MPH, MPhil, FACPM

BASICS

DESCRIPTION
- Injury, intentional or not, is often predictable and preventable.
- Unintentional injuries are no longer considered "accidents" given that most injuries are preventable.
- As of 2017, unintentional injury is the 3rd leading cause of death, and suicide is the 10th leading cause of death in the United States.
- Injury is the leading cause of death for people aged 1 to 44 years and a leading cause of disability for people of all ages, regardless of sex, race/ethnicity, or socioeconomic status.
- Violence-related deaths accounted for over 66,500 deaths in the United States in 2017 (over 47,000 suicides and over 19,500 homicides).

EPIDEMIOLOGY
Incidence

Leading Cause of Death by Age Group, United States, 2017

Age	Most Common	Number of Deaths
<1 y	Congenital anomalies	4,580
1–44 y	Unintentional injury	64,783
45–64 y	Malignant neoplasm	154,076
≥65 y	Heart disease	519,052

Source: Centers for Disease Control and Prevention (CDC) Web-based Injury Statistics Query and Reporting System (WISQARS)

- Children mostly die of unintentional injuries: motor vehicle traffic (MVT), drowning, poisoning, and suffocation.
- MVT is the most common type of unintentional injury deaths in adolescents.

ALERT
Poisoning, which includes drug overdose, has been the leading cause of injury deaths in the United States overall since 2011 and is particularly deadly for persons ages 15 to 64 years, as the leading cause of injury deaths among 25 to 64 years and the second leading cause of unintentional injury deaths for 15 to 24 years.

- Approximately 5.8 million people worldwide die yearly from injuries, of which all forms of violence combine to cause nearly 1/3 of these deaths (World Health Organization [WHO]).
- Unintentional MVT deaths rank second in the United States for overall injury deaths, first in those aged 5 to 24 years and second in those aged 1 to 4 years and 25 to >65 years.
- Among leading causes of injury deaths in the United States, unintentional falls rank third overall. Firearms are related to the fourth and fifth leading causes of injury deaths in the United States, suicide and homicide, respectively.
- Homicide is the third leading cause of death in 2016 for persons 15 to 34 years in the United States.

ALERT
Consider homicide as cause of unexplained death in young children.

ETIOLOGY AND PATHOPHYSIOLOGY
Multifactorial

RISK FACTORS
- Motor vehicle accident (MVA):
  - MVT deaths accounted for 40,231 deaths in 2017 with an age-adjusted rate of 12.4 deaths per 100,000 persons (CDC).
  - Each year, approximately 3 million people are nonfatally injured in the United States from motor vehicle crashes (CDC).
  - The leading cause of death for U.S. teens is MVAs (CDC).
  - In the United States, 1 in 3 deaths involved drunk driving and almost 1 in 3 deaths implicated speeding (CDC).
  - Motorcyclists are more likely to die in a motor vehicle crash than car occupants. The risk of death is reduced by 37% with helmets (CDC).
  - Risk factors for involvement in an MVA include high speed, teenage drivers, consumption of alcohol or drugs affecting the central nervous system, fatigue, and distracted driving (handheld mobile phones and inadequate visibility).
  - Increased risk of death by MVA in the United States: not using seat belts, car seats, and booster seats; drunk driving; speeding (CDC)
- Pedestrians:
  - 5,977 pedestrians were killed by motor vehicles and an estimated 137,000 were treated in EDs for nonfatal injuries in the United States (2017; CDC, National Center for Injury Prevention and Control [NCIPC]).
- Bicycles:
  - In the United States, >1,000 bicyclists died and nearly 467,000 bicycle-related injuries occurred in 2015 (CDC, NCIPC).
  - Risk factors for cyclist injury include age (5 to 19 years for nonfatal injury, 50 to 59 years highest bicycle death rates), male sex, urban area at nonintersection location, and alcohol involvement.
- Sports- and recreation-related injury (CDC):
  - >2.6 million children (0 to 19 years) treated in EDs each year
  - Prevention tips include the following: Use protective gear that is in good condition, fits properly, and worn correctly; sports program and/or school has instituted action plan to teach athletes ways to lower risk of getting a concussion and other injuries; monitor temperature to prevent heat-related injuries; and serve as a role model of safe behavior.
- Drowning: a leading cause of unintentional injury death among all children, particularly those 1 to 4 years of age
  - Children at increased risk include African Americans and those unattended in bathtubs, swimming pools, and recreational water activities (CDC, NCIPC).
- Suffocation: increased risk for children <1 year, unsafe sleeping environments (CDC)
- Falls (CDC, NCIPC):
  - The leading cause of nonfatal injuries accounting for over 8 million nonfatal injuries in the United States in 2017
  - Most common cause of traumatic brain injuries (TBIs)
  - Risk factors for falls include lower body weakness, vitamin D deficiency, difficulties with walking and balance, use of medications (tranquilizers, sedatives, antidepressants, some over-the-counter medicines), vision problems, foot pain or poor footwear, home hazards (broken/uneven steps, throw rugs, clutter).

- **Violence**: Risk factors include the following: adverse childhood exposures (ACEs); lack of access to social capital, community organization, and economic resources; familial instability; community and family violence; access to firearms; mental health; personal or household member alcohol and drug use; exposure to suicidal behavior; history of aggressive behavior; cognitive deficits; poor supervision; poor peer-to-peer interaction; academic failure; poverty; lower socioeconomic class (CDC).
- Homicide and gun violence: Homicide is the third leading cause of death for persons aged 15 to 34 years in the United States (CDC). Most common victims are young males. Firearms are used in more than half of U.S. homicides.
- Suicide: Females are more likely to have suicidal thoughts, but males are 4 times more likely to complete suicide. Most common methods are firearms for males and poisoning for females (CDC, NCIPC).
- Adolescent violence (CDC):
  - In 2015, nearly 8% of students participated in a physical fight at school in the last year.
  - >5% of high schoolers reported not going to school on ≥1 day(s) in the last 30 days because they felt unsafe at school or on their way to or from school.
  - 4% of students have carried a weapon to school; 6% of students have been threatened or injured by a weapon at school.
- Bullying (CDC):
  - In 2015, 20% of 9th- to 12th-grade students bullied on school property in the last year.
  - 15% of students report cyberbullying.
  - Bullying is associated with social, emotional, and academic difficulties.
- Interpersonal and intimate partner violence (IPV):
  - WHO reports about 38% of female homicides globally were killed by male partners, similar to CDC reports of nearly half of female homicide victims in the United States are killed by a current or former male intimate partner.
  - Approximately 1 in 4 women and almost 1 in 10 men have experienced sexual violence, physical violence, and/or stalking in their lifetime from an intimate partner (CDC).
  - Dating violence among teens:
    ○ Almost 1 in 11 female and approximately 1 in 15 male high school students report physical dating violence in the last year (CDC).
    ○ Approximately 1 in 9 female and 1 in 36 male high school students report sexual dating violence in the last year (CDC).
  - Risk factors include individual risk factors (such as low income, young age, heavy alcohol and drug use, depression and suicide attempts, unemployment, being a victim of physical or psychological abuse, witnessing IPV between parents as child, unplanned pregnancy), relationship factors (such as marital conflict, economic stress, association with antisocial and aggressive peers), community factors (such as poverty, low social capital), and societal factors (such as traditional gender norms or gender inequality, societal income inequality).
  - Protective factors include high friendship quality, social support, neighborhood collective efficacy (community cohesiveness, mutual trust, willingness to intervene for the common good), coordination of resources and services among community agencies.

Poisonings (CDC):

- The U.S. epidemic of drug overdoses (poisonings) includes nearly 450,000 deaths from 1999 to 2018 from an overdose involving any opioid (prescription and illicit).
- In 2018, >67,000 drug overdose deaths occurred in the United States.
- Opioids, primarily synthetic fentanyl and fentanyl derivatives, are the main cause of drug overdose deaths.
  – In 2018, opioids were involved in almost 70% of all drug overdose deaths; two out of three opioid-involved overdose deaths involved synthetic opioids.
- Preventive measures of opioid deaths include the following: Improve opioid prescribing, reduce exposure to opioids, prevent misuse, and access to naloxone and treat opioid use disorder.
- Consider opioid-induced poisonings in unexplained altered mental status.

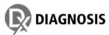 **DIAGNOSIS**

HISTORY

- Mechanism, timing, and location of injury:
  – Blunt versus penetrating; intentional versus unintentional; others injured versus isolated injury; circumstances (weather, substance use, restrained vs. unrestrained)
  – Does history correlates with level of injury (i.e., level of suspicion for abuse [elderly, child, or partner])?
  – Is further evaluation required (blood and/or urine testing, response to opioid receptor antagonists, imaging)?
- IPV: neurologic deficits, seizures, chronic pain, GI, STI, pregnancy, psychiatric presentations
  – Screen women of childbearing age for IPV and intervene if screening results are positive.

 TREATMENT

- Prevention: The primary focus for reducing injury and violence is individually tailored prevention based on risk factors combined with population-level prevention (1). The "three Es": education, engineering strategies, and enforcement of laws (1). The "Haddon Matrix" describes injury events in terms of three influencing factors (host, agent/vector, environment) and three phases (preevent, event, postevent) (1).
- Primary (i.e., prevent crash), secondary (i.e., prevent injury from crash), and tertiary (i.e., prevent poor outcomes from injury) prevention (1)[C]
- Acute setting: Follow basic life support (BLS), advanced trauma life support (ATLS), advanced cardiovascular life support (ACLS), and pediatric advanced life support (PALS) guidelines (1)[C]
- Motor vehicle injuries (CDC):
  – Infants, toddlers, and children: age-appropriate child safety seats and passenger restraints with distribution programs, education programs for parents and caregivers, safety seat checkpoints, penalties for drivers transporting children under the influence of drugs and/or alcohol, legislation regarding restraint of motor vehicle occupants
  – Adolescents and adults: seat belts, air bags, graduated driver licensing programs, blood alcohol concentration laws, minimum drinking age laws, sobriety checkpoints, ignition interlocks, programs for alcohol servers, zero-alcohol tolerance laws for young drivers, school-based education programs on drinking and driving. Emergency medical

services (EMS) response times, engineering cars for rapid extraction, organized trauma systems; collapsible automobile steering columns have been shown to decrease injury mortality and morbidity; texting and driving penalties
  – Older adults: alternative transportation programs, screening for high-risk drivers, gradual curtailment of driving privileges, more frequent license renewal process
  – Bicycle helmets can reduce risk of head injury by 63–88%. Canadian helmet legislation decreased mortality by 52%.
  – Pedestrian injury: pedestrian safety education, reflective clothing, use of crosswalks, limit mobile phone use while crossing roads, street lighting for pedestrians, fluorescent clothing for pedestrians and cyclists
  – Cyclists injury: flashing lights and reflectors at night (1)[B], helmet use and laws, cyclists separation for motor vehicles
- Sports-related injuries:
  – Proper equipment: Helmets can prevent bicyclist head injuries and mortality.
  – Plan of action for dealing with concussion and head injury in young athletes, with guidelines regarding if or when it is safe to return to play (CDC)
- Drowning:
  – Improved supervision of young children, especially for those with epilepsy; swimming lessons; trained lifeguard supervision; fencing; locked gates and pool alarms; no use of alcohol in recreation aquatic activities; personal flotation devices and boating safety awareness; parental and caregiver certification in CPR
- Falls:
  – Home safety assessments, installation of handrails and grab bars, removal of tripping hazards, nonslip mats, exercise programs such as tai chi to improve strength and balance, night lights, cataract surgery, gradual withdrawal of psychotropic medication
  – In April 2018, USPSTF recommends exercise interventions to prevent falls in community-dwelling adults aged 65 years or older who are at increased risk for falls.
- Violence (homicide, suicide, assaults) (CDC):
  – Primary prevention: Most effective strategies focus on younger age groups to change individual attitudes and behaviors.
  – Secondary prevention: Detect and identify violence in early stages. The USPSTF recommends that clinicians screen women of childbearing age for IPV, such as domestic violence, and provide or refer women who screen positive to intervention services.
  – Gun and school violence prevention among youth: social and emotional learning via CDC Whole School, Whole Community, Whole Child model (CDC)
  – Tertiary prevention: IPV reduced by alcoholism treatment for partner; intense advocacy interventions of >12 hours
  – Suicide: access to mental health services, improved family and community support, development of healthy coping and problem-solving skills, reduced access to lethal means (CDC)
  – USPSTF recommends screening adults for depression when depression care supports are in place to assure accurate diagnosis, effective treatment, and follow-up.
  – Dating violence: self-reported dating violence reduced by school- and community-based programs for prevention of dating violence

Poisonings (CDC): In response to the opioid epidemic, the *CDC Guideline for Prescribing Opioids for Chronic Pain—United States, March 2016* was released to **improve prescribing practices**, to aid in early identification of those at high risk for addiction, and to prevent opiate and heroin addiction and deaths.

- Prevent and treat opioid abuse: prescribing practice quality improvement programs; substance abuse counseling and medication for the treatment of opioid use disorders (MOUD) such as buprenorphine and methadone.
- In April 2018, the U.S. Surgeon General issued an advisory emphasizing the importance of the overdose-reversing drug naloxone.
- *Consider use of naloxone to counter the effects of opioid overdose.*
- *Multiple doses of naloxone may be required because the duration of many opioids is greater than that of naloxone.*
- Follow acute care guidelines and call 911; may contact Poison Control Center hotline after discovered ingestion of toxin for recommendations (2)

 ONGOING CARE

COMPLICATIONS
Social burden of injury: loss of productivity, emotional loss, nonmedical expenditures, reduced quality of life, litigation, rehabilitation, mental health costs, altered family and peer relationships, chronic pain, substance use and abuse, changes in lifestyle (CDC)

REFERENCES

1. Sleet DA, Dahlberg LL, Basavaraju SV, et al; for Centers for Disease Control and Prevention. Injury prevention, violence prevention, and trauma care: building the scientific base. *MMWR Suppl*. 2011;60(4):78–85.
2. Mowry JB, Spyker DA, Brooks DE, et al. 2015 Annual report of the American Association of Poison Control Centers' National Poison Data System (NPDS): 33rd annual report. *Clin Toxicol (Phila)*. 2016;54(10):924–1109.

ADDITIONAL READING

- National Center for Injury Prevention and Control: https://www.cdc.gov/injury
- WHO Violence and Injury Prevention: http://www.who.int/violence_injury_prevention/en

 CODES

ICD10
- T14.90 Injury, unspecified
- T14.8 Other injury of unspecified body region
- R29.6 Repeated falls

CLINICAL PEARLS

- Injury and violence are predictable and preventable.
- MVT cause most deaths in children and adolescents.
- Gun violence and school violence have evidenced-based prevention strategies.
- Opioid overdose is a serious cause of unintentional injury and death.

I

INSOMNIA

Susanne Wild, MD

 BASICS

DESCRIPTION
- Difficulty initiating or maintaining sleep or non-restorative sleep despite adequate opportunity and circumstances for sleep
- Causes at least one of the following forms of day-time impairment related to nighttime sleep difficulty:
  - Fatigue or malaise
  - Attention, concentration, or memory impairment
  - Social or vocational dysfunction or poor school performance
  - Mood disturbance or irritability
  - Daytime sleepiness
  - Motivation, energy, or initiative reduction
  - Proneness for errors or accidents at work or while driving
  - Tension, headaches, or GI symptoms in response to sleep loss
  - Concerns or worries about sleep

EPIDEMIOLOGY
- Predominant age: increases with age
- Predominant sex: female > male (5:1)

Prevalence
- Most common sleep disorder
- Insomnia (transient and chronic): 5–35% of the population; 10–15% associated with daytime impairment
- Chronic insomnia: 10% middle-aged adults; 1/3 of people >65 years

ETIOLOGY AND PATHOPHYSIOLOGY
- Transient/intermittent (<30 days) and short-term (<3 months)
  - Usually caused by an identifiable stressor
    - Stress/excitement/bereavement
    - Shift work
    - Medical illness
    - High altitude
  - Can lead to chronic insomnia
- Chronic (>3 months)
  - Usually not due to one single cause
  - Medical: gastroesophageal reflux disease, sleep apnea, chronic pain, congestive heart failure, Alzheimer disease, Parkinson disease, chronic fatigue syndrome, irritable bowel syndrome
  - Psychiatric: mood, anxiety, psychotic disorders
  - Primary sleep disorder: idiopathic, psychophysiologic (heightened arousal and learned sleep-preventing associations), paradoxical (sleep state misperception)
  - Circadian rhythm disorder: irregular pattern, jet lag, delayed/advanced sleep phase, shift work
  - Environmental: light (liquid crystal display [LCD] clocks), noise (snoring, household, traffic), movements (partner/young children/pets)
  - Behavioral: poor sleep hygiene, adjustment sleep disorder
  - Substance induced
  - Medications: antihypertensives, antidepressants, corticosteroids, levodopa-carbidopa, phenytoin, quinidine, theophylline, thyroid hormones

RISK FACTORS
- Age
- Female gender
- Medical comorbidities
- Unemployment
- Psychiatric illness
- Impaired social relationships
- Lower socioeconomic status
- Shift work
- Separation from spouse or partner
- Drug and substance abuse
- Family or personal history of insomnia

GENERAL PREVENTION
- Practice consistent sleep hygiene:
  - Fixed wake-up times and bedtimes regardless of amount of sleep obtained (weekdays and weekends)
  - Go to bed only when sleepy.
  - Avoid naps.
  - Sleep in a cool, dark, quiet environment.
  - No activities or stimuli in bedroom associated with anything but sleep or sex
  - 30-minute wind-down time before sleep
  - If unable to sleep within 20 minutes, move to another environment and engage in quiet activity until sleepy.
- Limit caffeine intake to mornings.
- No alcohol after 4 PM
- Fixed eating times
- Avoid medications that interfere with sleep.
- Regular moderate exercise (>4 hours prior to bedtime)

COMMONLY ASSOCIATED CONDITIONS
- Psychiatric disorders
- Painful musculoskeletal conditions
- Obstructive sleep apnea
- Restless leg syndrome
- Drug or alcohol addiction/dependence

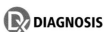 **DIAGNOSIS**

HISTORY
- Daytime sleepiness and napping
- Unintended sleep episodes (e.g., dozing at a stop-light while driving, working)
- Insomnia history
  - Duration, time of problem
  - Sleep latency, difficulty in maintaining sleep (repeated awakening), early morning awakening, nonrestorative sleep, or patterns (weekday vs. weekend, with or without bed partner, home vs. away)
- Sleep hygiene
  - Bedtime/wakening time
  - Physical environment of sleep area: LED clocks, TV, room lighting, ambient noise
  - Activity: nighttime eating, exercise, sexual activity
  - Intake: caffeine, alcohol, herbal supplements, diet pills, illicit drugs, prescriptions, over-the-counter (OTC) sleep aids
- Symptoms or history of depression, anxiety, obsessive-compulsive disorder, or other major psychological symptomatology
- Symptoms of restless leg syndrome and periodic limb movement disorder
- Symptoms of heightened arousal
- Snoring and other symptoms of sleep apnea
- Symptoms or history of drug or alcohol abuse
- Current medication use
- Chronic medical conditions
- Acute change or stressors such as travel or shift work
- Sleep diary: sleep log for 7 consecutive days

PHYSICAL EXAM
No association with specific findings on physical examination

DIFFERENTIAL DIAGNOSIS
- Sleep-disordered breathing such as obstructive sleep apnea
- CNS hypersomnias (e.g., narcolepsy)
- Circadian rhythm sleep disturbances
- Sleep-related movement disorders (e.g., restless leg syndrome)
- Substance abuse
- Insomnia due to medical or neurologic disorder
- Mood and anxiety disorders such as depression or anxiety

DIAGNOSTIC TESTS & INTERPRETATION
Diagnostic testing usually not required; consider polysomnography if sleep apnea or periodic limb movement disorder is suspected (1)[C].

Initial Tests (lab, imaging)
Routine laboratory testing not recommended; testing to consider based on history and physical exam to evaluate for comorbid conditions

Diagnostic Procedures/Other
Polysomnography or multiple sleep latency test not routinely indicated but may be considered if
- Initial diagnosis is uncertain
- Treatment interventions have proven unsuccessful

 TREATMENT

- Transient and short-term insomnia
  - May use medications for short-term use only; hypnotic sedatives favored
  - Self-medicating with alcohol can increase awakenings and sleep-stage changes.
- Chronic insomnia
  - Treatment of underlying condition (major depressive disorder, generalized anxiety disorder, medications, pain, substance abuse)
  - Advise good sleep hygiene.
  - Cognitive-behavioral therapy is first-line treatment for chronic insomnia (2).
  - Behavioral therapy is an effective treatment for insomnia and a potentially more effective long-term treatment than pharmacotherapy (3)[B].
  - Ramelteon is the only agent without known abuse potential (4)[B].

MEDICATION
- Reserved for transient and short-term insomnia such as with jet lag, stress reactions, transient medical condition
- Nonbenzodiazepine hypnotics
  - Act on benzodiazepine receptor, so have abuse potential
    - Zaleplon (Sonata) 5 to 20 mg; half-life 1 hour
    - Zolpidem (Ambien) 5 to 10 mg (males); 5 mg (females); half-life 2.5 to 3.0 hours

○ Zolpidem (Ambien CR) 6.25 to 12.50 mg (males); 6.25 mg (females); half-life 2.5 to 3.0 hours
○ Eszopiclone (Lunesta) 1 to 3 mg; half-life 6 hours
• Benzodiazepine hypnotics
  – Short acting
    ○ Triazolam (Halcion) 0.25 mg; half-life 1.5 to 5.5 hours
  – Intermediate acting
    ○ Temazepam (Restoril) 7.5 to 30.0 mg; half-life 8.8 hours
    ○ Estazolam (Prosom) 1 to 2 mg; half-life 10 to 24 hours
  – Long acting
    ○ Flurazepam (Dalmane) 15 to 30 mg; half-life 40 to 100 hours
    ○ Quazepam (Doral) 7.5 to 15.0 mg; half-life 39 hours (parent drug), 73 hours (active metabolite)
• Contraindications/precautions are as follows:
  – Not indicated for long-term treatment due to risks of tolerance, dependency, daytime attention and concentration compromise, incoordination, rebound insomnia
  – Long-acting benzodiazepines associated with higher incidence of daytime sedation and motor impairment
  – Avoid in elderly, pregnant, breastfeeding, substance abusers, and patients with suicidal or parasuicidal behaviors.
  – Avoid in patients with untreated obstructive apnea and chronic pulmonary disease.
  – No good evidence for benzodiazepines for patients undergoing palliative care (4)[A]
  – Nonbenzodiazepine receptor agonists may occasionally induce parasomnias (sleepwalking, sleep eating, sleep driving).
• Melatonin receptor agonist
  – Ramelteon (Rozerem) 8 mg; half-life 1.0 to 2.6 hours
    ○ Effective to reduce sleep time onset for short- and long-term use in adults, without abuse potential; no comparative studies with older agents have been completed. Onset of effect may take up to 3 weeks.
• Sedating antidepressants
  – Doxepin (Silenor) 3 to 6 mg; half-life 15 hours (the only antidepressant with FDA approval for insomnia)
  – Trazodone (Oleptro) 25 to 200 mg; half-life 3 to 9 hours
  – Mirtazapine (Remeron) 7.5 to 15.0 mg; half-life 20 to 40 hours
  – Amitriptyline (Elavil) 25 to 100 mg; half-life 10 to 26 hours
• Orexin receptor agonists
  – Suvorexant (Belsomra) 10 to 20 mg; half-life 12 hours
• Sedating antihistamines are not recommended and should be used conservatively for insomnia due to insufficient evidence of efficacy and significant concerns about risks of these medications.
• Evidence for use of antipsychotics is weak. They should only be prescribed if the patient has a concurrent psychiatric diagnosis warranting their use.

Geriatric Considerations
Caution (risk of falls and confusion) when prescribing benzodiazepines or other sedative hypnotics; if absolutely necessary, use short-acting nonbenzodiazepine agonists at half the dosage or melatonin agonists for short-term treatment.

COMPLEMENTARY & ALTERNATIVE MEDICINE
• Melatonin: decreases sleep latency when taken 30 to 120 minutes prior to bedtime, but there is no good evidence for efficacy in insomnia, and long-term effects are unknown (5)[B]
• Valerian: Inconsistent evidence supporting efficacy and its slow onset of action (2 to 3 weeks) makes it unsuitable for the acute treatment of insomnia.
• Acupuncture: may improve sleep quality
• Antihistamines: insufficient evidence; should not be recommended for use
• Cognitive-behavioral therapy (including relaxation therapy): effective and considered more useful than medications; recommended initial treatment for patients with chronic insomnia; no improvement of efficacy when combined with medication
• Mindfulness awareness practices: improved sleep quality and sleep-related daytime impairment for older adults per small randomized trial
• Behavioral interventions such as stimulus control therapy, sleep restriction, relaxation training may all be effective.

 ## ONGOING CARE

FOLLOW-UP RECOMMENDATIONS
• Daily exercise improves quality of sleep and may be more effective than medication.
• Avoid exercise within 4 hours of bedtime.

Patient Monitoring
• Reassess need for medications periodically; avoid standing prescriptions. Treatment response should be measured by using patient self-report (e.g., sleep diary); wearable sleep monitors are often inaccurate.
• Caution patients that nonbenzodiazepine agonists (zolpidem, zaleplon, eszopiclone), as well as benzodiazepines, can be habit forming.
• Studies suggest an association between receiving a hypnotic prescription and a >3-fold increase in hazards of death, even when prescribed <18 pills per year (6)[B].

DIET
• Avoid caffeine or reserve for morning only.
• Avoid heavy late-night snacks (light snack at bedtime may help).
• Avoid alcohol within 6 hours of bedtime.

PROGNOSIS
• Situational insomnia should resolve with time.
• Treatment of underlying etiology and consistent sleep hygiene are the mainstays of treatment.

COMPLICATIONS
• Transient insomnia can become chronic.
• Daytime sleepiness, cognitive dysfunction

• Pulmonary hypertension if chronic sleep apnea left untreated
• Sleep apnea may lead to hypertension, stroke, or cardiac ischemia.

REFERENCES
1. Kushida CA, Littner MR, Morgenthaler T, et al. Practice parameters for the indications for polysomnography and related procedures: an update for 2005. *Sleep.* 2005;28(4):499–521.
2. Quaseem A, Kansagara D, Forciea MA, et al; for Clinical Guidelines Committee of the American College of Physicians. Management of chronic insomnia disorder in adults: a clinical practice guideline from the American College of Physicians. *Ann Intern Med.* 2016;165(2):125–133.
3. Ebben MR, Spielman AJ. Non-pharmacological treatments for insomnia. *J Behav Med.* 2009;32(3):244–254.
4. Hirst A, Sloan R. Benzodiazepines and related drugs for insomnia in palliative care. *Cochrane Database Syst Rev.* 2002;(4):CD003346.
5. Verster GC. Melatonin and its agonists, circadian rhythms and psychiatry. *Afr J Psychiatry (Johannesbg).* 2009;12(1):42–46.
6. Kripke DF, Langer RD, Kline LE. Hypnotics' association with mortality or cancer: a matched cohort study. *BMJ Open.* 2012;2(1):e000850.

ADDITIONAL READING
Glass J, Lanctôt KL, Herrmann N, et al. Sedative hypnotics in older people with insomnia: meta-analysis of risks and benefits. *BMJ.* 2005;331(7526):1169.

 ## SEE ALSO

• Anxiety (Generalized Anxiety Disorder); Depression; Fibromyalgia; Sleep Apnea, Obstructive
• Algorithms: Anxiety; Insomnia, Chronic; Restless Legs Syndrome

 ## CODES

ICD10
• G47.00 Insomnia, unspecified
• F51.02 Adjustment insomnia
• F51.01 Primary insomnia

CLINICAL PEARLS
• Treatment of underlying etiology of the insomnia and consistent sleep hygiene are key.
• Most medications are indicated for short-term use only.
• Sedative hypnotics are not recommended in the elderly because risks may outweigh benefits.
• Patients with chronic insomnia benefit from sleep hygiene education and cognitive-behavioral therapy.

INTELLECTUAL DISABILITY (INTELLECTUAL DEVELOPMENTAL DISORDER)
Jennifer L. Ayres, PhD

BASICS

- A global deficit in cognitive functioning evidenced by a significant difference in mental and chronologic ages (IQ) and significantly impaired adaptive functioning (1)
- The term "*mental retardation*" was deleted from the *DSM-5* and replaced with "intellectual disability" (ID) or "intellectual developmental disorder." The term "mental retardation" is pejorative and insensitive and should be avoided.
- Although cognitive issues typically have a pervasive impact, patients with ID display highly variable levels of functioning and subsequent service needs.
- Tailor evaluation and treatment to individual needs.

DESCRIPTION

- ID is defined as an IQ ≤70 + 5 and a significant impairment in intellectual functioning. This includes verbal and nonverbal reasoning, planning, academic learning, problem solving, and experiential learning. Intellectual function is confirmed by IQ testing and clinical assessment (1).
- A diagnosis of ID also requires deficits in adaptive functioning, such as communication, socialization, and independent living (1).
- By definition, ID is a neurodevelopmental disorder that is typically present from birth or recognized during early childhood because developmental milestones are delayed (1).
- ID is currently subgrouped according to adaptive function and level of needed support: *mild* (typical development in some domains, mild impairment in others), *moderate* (skills are markedly behind typically developing, same-age peers), *severe* (skills quite limited compared to peers), *profound* (limited awareness of concepts, language; dependent on others for adaptive functioning) (1).
- The three most common causes of ID are Down syndrome, fragile X syndrome, and fetal alcohol syndrome (FAS).
- If ID reflects a loss of previously acquired intellectual skills, consider a comorbid neurocognitive disorder.
- Stereotypes of people with ID (e.g., always happy, poor prognosis, unable to function independently) have been categorically refuted. People with ID show levels of functional variability that parallels the non-ID population.
- Under the Individuals with Disabilities Education Act (IDEA), caregivers should familiarize themselves with their child's legal rights to facilitate coordination of services with the school district.
- Under the Americans with Disabilities Act (1990), people with ID cannot be discriminated against based on their disability, and employers are legally required to ensure that appropriate accommodations are in place.

ALERT
For some causes of ID, prenatal testing is available.

EPIDEMIOLOGY

Incidence
- 1 of 6 children (2)
- Predominant sex: male > female: 1.6:1 for mild ID, 1.2:1 for severe ID (1)

Prevalence
In the United States, 1% of the general population. The prevalence of severe ID is 6/1,000 (1).

ETIOLOGY AND PATHOPHYSIOLOGY
- Causes:
  - Maternal substance abuse (e.g., alcohol); FAS is a leading environmental cause of ID.
  - Maternal infections: TORCH viruses (toxoplasma, other infections, rubella, cytomegalovirus, and herpes simplex virus)
  - Down syndrome
  - Sex chromosome abnormalities: fragile X, Turner syndrome, Klinefelter syndrome
  - Autosomal dominant conditions: neurocutaneous syndromes (e.g., neurofibromatosis, tuberous sclerosis)
  - Autosomal recessive conditions:
    ○ Amino acid metabolism (e.g., phenylketonuria, maple syrup urine disease)
    ○ Carbohydrate metabolism (e.g., galactosemia, fructosuria)
    ○ Lipid metabolism
    ○ Tay-Sachs disease
    ○ Gaucher disease
    ○ Niemann-Pick disease; mucopolysaccharidosis
    ○ Purine metabolism (e.g., Lesch-Nyhan disease)
    ○ Other (e.g., Wilson disease)
- Maternal medications (e.g., isotretinoin, phenytoin [Dilantin])
- Perinatal factors:
  - Prematurity
  - Birth injuries
  - Perinatal anoxia
- Postnatal factors:
  - Childhood diseases (e.g., meningitis, encephalitis, hypothyroidism, seizure disorders)
  - Trauma (e.g., accidents, physical abuse, hypoxia)
  - Severe deprivation
  - Poisoning (e.g., lead, carbon monoxide, household products)

Genetics
A number of genetic and epigenetic causes are known, and more are under investigation.

RISK FACTORS
- Maternal substance abuse during pregnancy
- Maternal infection during pregnancy
- For some causes, family history

GENERAL PREVENTION
- Reduce alcohol and drug use by pregnant women.
- Prenatal folic acid supplementation

COMMONLY ASSOCIATED CONDITIONS
- Seizures
- Mood disorders
- Behavioral disorders
- Constipation

DIAGNOSIS

The diagnosis of ID requires a thorough assessment conducted by an appropriately credentialed mental health professional who is formally trained and licensed to conduct appropriate psychodiagnostic testing.

HISTORY
- Children with profound/severe ID are typically diagnosed at birth or during the newborn period. They may have pathognomonic dysmorphic features.
- Children with ID are often identified because they fail to meet motor/language milestones.

PHYSICAL EXAM
Certain morphologic features suggest a specific etiology for ID (e.g., microcephaly).

DIFFERENTIAL DIAGNOSIS
- Auditory, visual, and/or speech/language impairment
- Autism spectrum disorder (language and social skills are more affected than other cognitive abilities); however, 75% of individuals with an autistic disorder may meet criteria for a comorbid diagnosis of ID.
- Expressive/receptive language disorders
- Cerebral palsy
- Brain tumors
- Emotional/behavioral disturbance
- Learning disorders (reading, math, written expression)
- Auditory/sensory processing difficulties
- Lack of environmental opportunities for appropriate development

DIAGNOSTIC TESTS & INTERPRETATION
- Visual and hearing tests to rule these out as the cause of impairment and to provide an assessment of visual and auditory functioning (often impaired in children and adults with ID)
- Formal testing of intellectual and adaptive functioning:
  - A child's communication skills must be considered in test selection. For example, a patient with auditory processing issues/limited expressive/receptive language skills may need to be assessed using a nonverbal IQ test, such as the Leiter-R, *Test of Nonverbal Intelligence*, or other nonverbal measures.
  - Commonly used intelligence tests (e.g., Bayley Scales of Infant Development, Stanford-Binet Intelligence Scale, Wechsler Intelligence Scales) are determined by age/developmental level.
  - Common tests of adaptive functioning include the *Vineland Adaptive Behavior Scales, 2nd ed.* and *Adaptive Behavior Assessment System, 2nd ed.* These tests assess areas of functioning such as age-appropriate communication, social skills, activities of daily living, and motor skills.
- Metabolic screening as indicated by history and physical exam or if no newborn screening was previously performed (3).

Initial Tests (lab, imaging)
- Lead levels (3)[B]
- Thyroid-stimulating hormone if systemic features are present or no newborn screening was done (3)[B]
- Routine cytogenetic testing (karyotype) (3)[B]:
  - Fragile X screening (*FMR1* gene), particularly with a family history of ID
  - Rett syndrome (*MECP2* gene) in women with unexplained moderate to severe ID (3)
- Molecular screening (e.g., array comparative genomic hybridization) is increasing in use.
- Neuroimaging (MRI more sensitive than CT) is routinely recommended. The presence of physical findings (microcephaly, focal motor deficit) increase yield (3)[B].
- MRI may show mild cerebral abnormalities but is unlikely to establish etiology of ID.

Follow-Up Tests & Special Considerations
Electroencephalography is not routinely used, unless a specific epileptiform diagnosis is present (3)[C].

 ## TREATMENT
- Tailor early intervention services to individual needs.
- Caregiver support, including:
  - Train caregiver(s) to address behavioral issues, discipline, and social development.
  - Encourage caregivers to create a structured home environment based on the child's developmental level and specific needs rather than routine age-appropriate expectations.
  - Offer caregiver(s) an opportunity to address their reactions to the diagnosis and their child's special needs.
  - Inform caregivers about advocacy groups and available resources (4).
  - Encourage caregiver(s) to seek social support to increase their own overall sense of well-being.
  - Encourage caregivers to intermittently seek respite care to promote self-care.
- Individualized education plans, social skills, and behavioral plans/training
- Refer to job training programs and independent living opportunities, if appropriate.
- Note changes in behavior, which may be indicative of pain/illness, particularly in individuals with limited communication skills.
- Assess for abuse and neglect.

MEDICATION
Medication may be appropriate for comorbid conditions (e.g., anxiety, ADHD, depression).

 ## ONGOING CARE
Match provider communication of procedures, results, and treatment recommendations to patient level of cognitive functioning and receptive language skills.
- Most patients with mild ID are fully capable of understanding information when provided at the appropriate level.
- Provide oral and written explanations directly to the patient instead of solely to caregivers. Respect patient dignity at all times. Provide honest information, respond to patient's questions with respect, and do not infantilize the patient due to the ID.

FOLLOW-UP RECOMMENDATIONS
Link to community-based resources for job training, independent living, caregiver support, school-based services

Patient Monitoring
- A quality of life assessment provides information about a patient's general sense of well-being and life satisfaction. Quality of life may be difficult to assess when significant behavioral issues confound an individual's self-report and socialization.
- Vision testing at least once before age 40 years (age 30 years in Down syndrome) and every 2 years thereafter
- Hearing evaluations every 5 years after age 45 years (every 3 years throughout life in Down syndrome)
- Screen for sexual activity and offer contraception and testing for STIs as appropriate.
- Screen annually for abuse and neglect, more frequently if behavior change is noted. Report abuse/neglect to appropriate protective agencies.
- Dysphagia and aspiration are common; consider speech pathology evaluation and swallowing study.

DIET
No restrictions, except in cases of metabolic and storage disorders (e.g., phenylketonuria)

PATIENT EDUCATION
- The Arc: www.thearc.org
- American Association on Intellectual and Developmental Disabilities: www.aaidd.org
- Family support groups (Parent to Parent, Local Down Syndrome, or Autism Association)
- Special Olympics: www.specialolympics.org

PROGNOSIS
- Although ID is a lifelong diagnosis, most individuals with ID are capable of fulfilling, purposeful lives that include career, independent living, participating in a committed relationship, and becoming a parent.
- The level of severity and support needed may vary over the course of the individual's life.

COMPLICATIONS
- Constipation is a commonly overlooked problem and can lead to significant morbidity.
- Polypharmacy, often associated with psychotropic medication use to control behaviors, should be addressed to minimize adverse side effects.

REFERENCES
1. American Psychiatric Association. *Diagnostic and Statistical Manual of Mental Disorders*. 5th ed. Arlington, VA: American Psychiatric Association; 2013.
2. Centers for Disease Control and Prevention. Developmental disabilities. http://www.cdc.gov/ncbddd/developmentaldisabilities/index.html. Accessed December 27, 2020.
3. Shevell M, Ashwal S, Donley D, et al. Practice parameter: evaluation of the child with global developmental delay: report of the Quality Standards Subcommittee of the American Academy of Neurology and the Practice Committee of the Child Neurology Society. *Neurology*. 2003;60(3):367–380.
4. Shogren KA, Bradley VJ, Gomez SC, et al. Public policy and the enhancement of desired outcomes for persons with intellectual disability. *Intellect Dev Disabil*. 2009;47(4):307–319.

ADDITIONAL READING
- Kripke C. Adults with developmental disabilities: a comprehensive approach to medical care. *Am Fam Physician*. 2018;97(10):649–656.
- Verdugo MA, Aguayo V, Arias VB, et al. A systematic review of the assessment of support needs in people with intellectual and developmental disabilities. *Int J Environ Res Public Health*. 2020;17(24):9494.

 ## CODES

ICD10
- F79 Unspecified intellectual disabilities
- F70 Mild intellectual disabilities
- F71 Moderate intellectual disabilities

CLINICAL PEARLS
- "Mental retardation" is an insensitive and disrespectful term that should not be used. ID or intellectual developmental disorder is preferred.
- Multiple factors (including appropriateness of school placement/special education services, exposure to early intervention, behavioral therapy, parent training, self-esteem, and social skills) influence overall functional ability for individuals with ID.
- Children with developmental disabilities are at higher risk of abuse.
- The diagnosis of ID should be confirmed through psychodiagnostic testing by an appropriately licensed professional.

I

INTERSTITIAL CYSTITIS

Dmitry Bisk, MD • Daniel S. Smoots, MD

 BASICS

DESCRIPTION

- A condition characterized by pain, pressure, or discomfort of the bladder or pelvic region associated with one or more of the following urinary symptoms: increased frequency, urgency, or nocturia
- A chronic inflammatory disease of unknown etiology, with associated urinary symptoms for >6 weeks without other identifiable causes such as infection or other pathology
- The symptoms in many patients are insidious, and the disease progresses for years with relapsing and remitting symptoms often before diagnosis is established.
- Types include ulcerative (classic) and nonulcerative
- System(s) affected: renal/urologic
- Synonym(s): urgency frequency syndrome; IC/bladder pain syndrome; chronic cystitis; Hunner ulcer

Pregnancy Considerations
Unpredictable symptom improvement or exacerbation during pregnancy; may be associated with increased risk of preeclampsia and preterm birth but further prospective studies are needed; usual problems of unknown effect on fetus with medications taken during pregnancy

EPIDEMIOLOGY

- Occurs predominantly among white patients
- Predominant sex: female > male (5:1) in patients 25 to 80 years of age
- Most common in adults >30 years of age and diagnosis increases with age

Incidence
Difficult to estimate due to different diagnostic criteria and regional differences but 1-year incidence has been reported as:
- 21 per 100,000 female patients
- 4 per 100,000 male patients

Prevalence
In the United States:
- Prevalence is variable.
- Up to 1.2 million female and 82,000 male patients affected, but many cases likely are undiagnosed.
- 0.052% but may be higher up to 10%

ETIOLOGY AND PATHOPHYSIOLOGY

- Etiology is unclear; pathophysiology likely multifactorial
- Potential causes include:
  – Disruption of urothelium, production of antiproliferative factor, and diminished glycosaminoglycan layer
  – Afferent nerve plasticity
  – Pelvic floor dysfunction
  – Mast cell infiltration, bladder nitric oxide
  – Reduced vascularization
  – Neurogenic inflammation
  – Autoimmune

RISK FACTORS
Unclear but some reported risks include:
- Female
- Recent UTI
- IBS
- Allergies
- History of sexual abuse

COMMONLY ASSOCIATED CONDITIONS
- Fibromyalgia
- Allergies
- Chronic fatigue syndrome
- Depression and panic disorder
- Vulvodynia
- Sexual dysfunction
- Sleep disturbance
- Migraines
- Syncope
- Dyspepsia
- Chronic prostatitis
- Chronic pelvic pain and pelvic floor dysfunction
- IBS
- Anal/rectal disease
- Chronic scrotal pain
- Trauma
- Autoimmune conditions such as SLE and Sjögren syndrome

 DIAGNOSIS

- Many diagnostic criteria exist that are dependent on patient symptoms and the exclusion of other overlapping pathology.
- A clinical diagnosis in uncomplicated cases can be characterized by symptoms that have been present for >6 weeks without other causes such as infection or other disorders.
  – Pain, pressure, or discomfort of the bladder or pelvic area and at least one of the following urinary symptoms:
    ○ Increased daytime frequency, urgency, or nocturia
- Cystoscopy with hydrodistension or urodynamic studies should not be used to establish a diagnosis but can be considered if diagnosis is unclear or the presentation is complex (1).

HISTORY
- Thorough history detailing bladder/pelvic pain and urinary symptoms (with voiding patterns)
- Variable symptoms that may be progressive over time
- Common urinary symptoms at presentation are urgency and frequency.
- Symptoms occur in flares with remission.
- Episodes may be related to menses, stress, sexual activity, IBS, endometriosis, vulvodynia, fibromyalgia, chronic fatigue syndrome, autoimmune conditions.
- Common food triggers: caffeine, sodas and other carbonated drinks, alcohol, and acidic foods (citrus, tomatoes)
- Use of validated questionnaires:
  – O'Leary/Sant Voiding and Pain Indices (http://www.ichelp.org/wp-content/uploads/2015/06/OLeary_Sant.pdf)

PHYSICAL EXAM
- Exams can be nonspecific but most common findings include dysphoric mood, bladder neck tenderness, suprapubic tenderness, and levator ani tenderness.
- Abdominal exam
  – Rule out masses or hernias.
  – Findings of interstitial cystitis can include suprapubic tenderness and costovertebral tenderness.
- Female pelvic exam
  – Findings suggesting interstitial cystitis can include pelvic floor spasms, suprapubic tenderness, rectal spasms, urethral tenderness, and bladder base tenderness when examining the anterior vaginal wall.
- Male digital rectal exam
  – Tenderness of the prostate can occur but may lead to a false diagnosis of chronic prostatitis.
  – Findings suggesting interstitial cystitis can include spasms of the sphincter.

DIFFERENTIAL DIAGNOSIS
- UTI
- Acute and chronic prostatitis
- Overactive bladder
- Urge incontinence
- Bladder neoplasm
- Bladder or ureteral stone
- Chronic pelvic pain
- Urogenital prolapse
- Urethral diverticulum
- Neurologic bladder disease
- Nonurinary pelvic disease (STIs, endometriosis, pelvic relaxation, pudendal neuralgia)

DIAGNOSTIC TESTS & INTERPRETATION

Initial Tests (lab, imaging)
- Voiding diary to record symptoms and to establish baseline symptoms when evaluating treatment
- Urinalysis and urine culture to rule out infection
- Gonorrhea and chlamydia testing in patients with pyuria or at high risk for STI
- Urine biomarkers are not recommended.
- Urine cytology
  – Not recommended for routine evaluation. Testing can be considered in patients at high risk for urologic malignancy in addition to the recommended work-up for malignancy.

Diagnostic Procedures/Other
- Cystoscopy with hydrodistension can be used to help differentiate other pathology but should not be used to establish the diagnosis of interstitial cystitis (1).
- Urodynamic studies are not recommended for routine evaluation but can be used to differentiate other coexisting disorders that will affect management such as overactive bladder, stress urinary incontinence, or voiding dysfunction (1).
- Intravesical lidocaine (anesthetic bladder challenge) can help to pinpoint the bladder as the source of pain in patients with pelvic pain.
- Potassium sensitivity test is not recommended for clinical use as it is nonspecific, painful, and does not change the treatment approach.
- Bladder biopsy is not recommended for the diagnosis but is performed if there is a suspicion for malignancy.

Test Interpretation
- When bladder biopsies are performed, findings include nonspecific chronic inflammation and/or high levels of mast cells.
- Urine cytology negative for dysplasia and neoplasia

TREATMENT

GENERAL MEASURES
- The goal of treatment should be symptom control and to increase patient's quality of life.
- There is no universally effective treatment plan. There is also no strong evidence that any treatment method is effective and more large trials are needed. However, conservative general measures can be considered for all patients which can include (1)[C]:
  – Patient education on normal bladder function, disease course, lack of cure, expectant management, and treatment strategies
  – Diet changes
    ○ Food and fluid elimination diets with specific focus on common triggers such as caffeine, alcohol, sodas (and other carbonated beverages), foods high in citrus, tomatoes, and bananas
  – Meditation, counseling, and stress management
  – Regular exercise
  – Pelvic floor relaxation
  – Avoidance of activity that exacerbates the pain

MEDICATION
- Randomized controlled trials of most medications for interstitial cystitis demonstrate limited benefit over placebo; there are no clear predictors of what will benefit an individual. Prepare the patient that treatment may involve trial and error.
- A systemic review of treatment options including antidepressants, pentosan polysulfate sodium, and neuromuscular blockade did not demonstrate conclusive evidence that they are effective for the treatment of symptoms (2)[A].
- Conservative therapies should be trialed first and more aggressive therapies can be started based on patient's symptoms and quality of life (1)[C].
- Treatments should be based on symptoms, symptom severity, and patient preferences (1)[C].
- Multiple simultaneous treatments may be considered if it is in the patient's best interest and patient's symptoms are followed and assessed carefully (1)[C].

First Line
Note: AUA consensus states patient education, pain management, general relaxation, stress reduction, behavior modification, and self-care are first line (1)[C].

Second Line
There is no consensus on which medications should be started first. Choices should be based off patient's symptoms and preferences. The following treatment methods are considered second line by the AUA (1)[C]:
- Amitriptyline: 25 to 100 mg daily, most effective at higher doses (≥50 mg/day); however, initiate with lower doses to minimize side effects (1)[C].
- Cimetidine 400 mg BID. Side effects are rare (1)[C].
- Hydroxyzine 25 to 75 mg HS. Common side effects include drowsiness and xerostomia (1)[C].
- Pentosan polysulfate 100 mg TID on empty stomach; may take several months (3 to 6) to become effective (only FDA-approved treatment for interstitial cystitis). Side effects can include headache, nausea, diarrhea, dizziness, rash, edema, and hair loss. Routine eye exams recommended for patients who use chronically due to increased rare atypical maculopathy risk (1)[C].
- Intravesical treatment (1)[C]
  – Dimethyl sulfoxide (DMSO) every 1 to 2 weeks for 3 to 6 weeks and then PRN (only FDA-approved intravesical treatment). Side effects include pain with instillation, unpleasant odor, and exacerbation of long-term pain.

– Heparin 10 to 20,000 units in 2 to 5 mL of solution, 3 times a week
– Lidocaine 1% 20 to 30 mL considered a short-term treatment option

Third Line
- Cystoscopy under anesthesia with low-pressure hydrodistention (1)[C]
- Treatment of Hunner lesions if found with laser, electrocautery, and/or injection of triamcinolone (1)[C]

Fourth Line
Neurostimulation: A permanent neurostimulation device can be placed if other treatments have not been effective in providing the patient with improvement of symptoms or quality of life (1)[C].

ISSUES FOR REFERRAL
- Need for clarity with respect to diagnosis
- Surgical intervention

ADDITIONAL THERAPIES
- Manual physical therapy (targeted pelvic, hip girdle, abdominal trigger point massage) is considered a second-line therapy by the AUA (1)[C],(3)[B].
- Oral cyclosporine A (considered as fifth line by the AUA), intravesical hyaluronic acid, and/or intravesical chondroitin sulfate may be offered as a treatment option if other therapies outline above have not been effective in improving symptoms and quality of life (1)[C].
- Sildenafil 25 mg: small, randomized trial demonstrated urinary symptom improvement at 3 and 6 months

SURGERY/OTHER PROCEDURES
- Hydraulic distention of bladder under anesthesia: symptomatic but transient relief
- Sacral neuromodulation
- Transurethral electro- or laser fulguration (effective for Hunner lesions). Pain relief may persist from several months to years.
- Augmentation cystoplasty to increase bladder capacity and decrease pressure with or without partial cystectomy. Expected results in severe cases: much improved, 75%; with residual discomfort, 20%; unchanged, 5%
- Urinary diversion with total cystectomy only if disease is completely refractory to medical therapy

COMPLEMENTARY & ALTERNATIVE MEDICINE
- There has been suggested therapy of glycerophosphate and acupuncture, but no clinical trials completed to demonstrate efficacy.
- One small trial of 21 patients undergoing hyperbaric oxygen therapy showed a 28% decrease in pain at 3 months.

ONGOING CARE

FOLLOW-UP RECOMMENDATIONS
Patient Monitoring
Tailored to severity, duration, and response to intervention

DIET
- Dietary modification, elimination diet
- Common irritants include caffeine, chocolate, citrus, tomatoes, carbonated beverages, potassium-rich foods, soybean, spicy foods, acidic foods, and alcohol.

PATIENT EDUCATION
- Interstitial Cystitis Association, 110 Washington St. Suite 340, Rockville, MD 20850; 1-800-HELPICA: http://www.ichelp.org/
- Given overlap with chronic pelvic pain syndrome, patients may benefit from home exercises—examples: https://youtu.be/NnqAkM9r2a8 or https://youtu.be/R3Rydb1nZU4

PROGNOSIS
- Patients often report decreased quality of life.
- Potential symptom plateau after approximately 5 years of symptoms.
- Mild: exacerbations and remissions of symptoms; may not be progressive; does not predispose to other diseases
- Severe: progressive problems, often require surgery to control symptoms

REFERENCES
1. Hanno PM, Erickson D, Moldwin R, et al; for American Urological Association. Diagnosis and treatment of interstitial cystitis/bladder pain syndrome: AUA guideline amendment. *J Urol.* 2015;193(5):1545–1553.
2. Imamura M, Scott NW, Wallace SA, et al. Interventions for treating people with symptoms of bladder pain syndrome: a network meta-analysis. *Cochrane Database Syst Rev.* 2020;7(7):CD013325.
3. FitzGerald MP, Payne CK, Lukacz ES, et al; for Interstitial Cystitis Collaborative Research Network. Randomized multicenter clinical trial of myofascial physical therapy in women with interstitial cystitis/painful bladder syndrome and pelvic floor tenderness. *J Urol.* 2012;187(6):2113–2118.

SEE ALSO

- Urinary Tract Infection (UTI) in Females
- Algorithm: Pelvic Girdle Pain (Pregnancy or Postpartum Pelvic Pain)

CODES

ICD10
- N30.10 Interstitial cystitis (chronic) without hematuria
- N30.11 Interstitial cystitis (chronic) with hematuria

CLINICAL PEARLS
- In most cases, this is a clinical diagnosis that is characterized by symptoms that have been present for >6 weeks without other underlying causes. Symptoms include pain, pressure, or discomfort of the bladder or pelvic area and at least one of the following urinary symptoms: increased daytime frequency, urgency, or nocturia.
- At present, there is no definitive treatment for interstitial cystitis.
- Most patients with severe disease receive multiple treatment approaches. Regular multidisciplinary follow-up, pharmacologic therapy, avoidance of symptom triggers, and psychological and supportive therapy are all important because this disease tends to wax and wane. Monitor patients for comorbid depression.
- Empower patients to manage their symptoms, communicate regularly with their physicians, and learn as much as they can about this disease, which may help them to optimize their outcome.

INTERSTITIAL NEPHRITIS

Gemma Kim, MD • Yea Ping Lin, MD, PhD, MPH, MS, BS

BASICS

DESCRIPTION

- Acute and chronic tubulointerstitial diseases result from the interplay of renal cells and inflammatory cells. Injury to renal cells leads to new local antigen expression, inflammatory cell infiltration, and proinflammatory activation and cytokines. The outcome is acute interstitial nephritis (AIN) or chronic interstitial nephritis (CIN).
- Central component in AIN is altered tubular function, which precedes decrements in filtration rate.
- AIN presents as acute kidney injury (AKI) after the use of offending drugs or agents (OFA) and associated with findings of proteinuria, hematuria, and white cell casts.

EPIDEMIOLOGY

- Observed in approximately 20% of patients with AKI or CKD who undergo biopsy
- AIN is the primary cause of 3–4% of patients with ESRD.

Incidence

- Accounts for 15–20% of AKI
- Peak incidence in women 60 to 70 years of age

Pediatric Considerations

- Children with history of lead poisoning are more likely to develop CIN as young adults.
- Tubulointerstitial nephritis with uveitis (TINU) presents in adolescent females with mean age of 15 years.

Geriatric Considerations

Elderly (≥65 years) have severe disease and increased risk of permanent damage given polypharmacy, specifically drug-induced AIN (87% vs. 64%), proton pump inhibitor–induced AIN (18% vs. 6%), but less AIN from autoimmune or systemic causes (7% vs. 27%) than younger adults (1)[B].

ETIOLOGY AND PATHOPHYSIOLOGY

- AIN
  - T-cell activation by an antigen leads to delayed drug hypersensitivity reactions, which leads to interstitial inflammatory infiltrates that damage tubules.
  - Renal dysfunction generally is partially or completely reversible.
  - Hypersensitivity to drugs (75%): not dose dependent. The top three were omeprazole (12%), amoxicillin (8%), and ciprofloxacin (8%) (2)[C].
    ○ NSAIDs
    ○ Antibiotics
    ○ Proton pump inhibitors
    ○ Diuretics
    ○ AEDs
    ○ Antivirals
    ○ Anticancer drugs
    ○ Miscellaneous (allopurinol, H_2 blockers, diphenylhydantoin, sulfasalazine, and mesalamine)
  - Infections (10–15%): streptococci, *Legionella*, *Leptospira*, *Leishmania*, *Escherichia coli*, *Campylobacter*, *Salmonella*, *Treponema pallidum*, *Mycobacterium tuberculosis*, *Histoplasma*, *Coccidioides*, *Toxoplasma*, CMV, EBV, and HSV, HIV, and SARS-CoV-2 (COVID-19) virus (3)

- Autoimmune (10–15%): sarcoidosis, SLE, Sjögren syndrome, granulomatosis with polyangiitis, cryoglobulinemia
- Toxins (e.g., snake bite venom)
- Idiopathic (5–10%): TINU syndrome and anti–tubular basement membrane (anti-TBM) disease
- CIN
  - Follows long-term exposure to OFA (e.g., heavy metals, especially lead)
  - Often found on routine labs
  - Characterized by interstitial scarring, fibrosis, and tubular atrophy, resulting in progressive CKD

GENERAL PREVENTION

- Early recognition and prompt discontinuation of OFA
- Avoid nephrotoxic substances.

COMMONLY ASSOCIATED CONDITIONS

- Chronic pyelonephritis
- Abuse of analgesics
- Lithium use
- Gout and gout therapy
- Immune disorders
- Malignancy (lymphoma, multiple myeloma)
- Amyloidosis
- Exposure to heavy metals (e.g., lead, cadmium)
- Renal papillary necrosis
- Uveitis

DIAGNOSIS

- Renal biopsy is the gold standard diagnostic method.
- AIN: suspected in a patient with nonspecific signs and vague symptoms of AKI (e.g., malaise, fever, nausea, vomiting) with an elevated serum creatinine and an abnormal UA
  - AKI
    ○ Elevated creatinine, BUN, and electrolyte abnormalities
    ○ Decreased urine output (oliguria in 51%)
    ○ Signs of fluid overload or depletion
  - Signs of systemic allergy (e.g., fever [27%], maculopapular rash [15%], peripheral eosinophilia [23%], arthralgias [45%] but less commonly found when NSAIDs are the OFA)
  - Urine—WBC, RBC, and white cell casts (sterile pyuria, <1 g proteinuria per day except if caused by NSAIDs)
- CIN
  - HTN
  - Decreased urine output or polyuria
  - Inability to concentrate urine
  - Polydipsia
  - Metabolic acidosis
  - Anemia
  - Fanconi syndrome

HISTORY

- Medications: Onset of AIN following drug exposure ranges from 3 to 5 days to as long as several weeks to many months or years (the latter more with NSAIDs) (2).
- Infection
- TINU patients present with interstitial nephritis and uveitis.
- Exposure to heavy metals
- Postorgan transplant

PHYSICAL EXAM

- Increased BP
- Fluid retention/extremity swelling/weight gain
- Rash accompanying renal findings in acute AIN
- Lung crackles/rales
- Pericardial rub in uremic pericarditis

DIFFERENTIAL DIAGNOSIS

- AKI secondary to other causes:
  - Prerenal
  - Intrarenal
  - Postrenal
  - Aminoglycosides can cause acute tubular necrosis.
  - NSAIDs can exacerbate prerenal disease.
- CKD secondary to long-standing HTN, diabetes, and chronic pyelonephritis

DIAGNOSTIC TESTS & INTERPRETATION

Initial Tests (lab, imaging)

- Chemistry
  - Elevated creatinine, with 40% requiring dialysis
  - Hyperkalemia and acidosis
- CBC
  - Eosinophilia (80%) but NSAID-induced AIN is associated with eosinophilia in ~15%.
  - Anemia
- Urinalysis with urine electrolytes
  - Hematuria (95%)
  - Mild and variable proteinuria: usually <1 g/24 hr, except in AIN associated with NSAIDs where it is higher
  - Urine sediment: WBC, RBC, white cell casts
  - Eosinophiluria but has no clinical utility specific for AIN (4)[C]
  - Urinary α_1- and β_2-microglobulin, TNF-α, and IL-9 may help in the diagnosis and monitoring of tubulointerstitial nephritis.
  - Normal urinalysis does not rule out AIN.
- CXR to evaluate for pulmonary tuberculosis, sarcoidosis, and infections
- Serologies for immunologic disease (e.g., sarcoidosis, Sjögren syndrome, granulomatosis with polyangiitis, Behçet syndrome) or infectious causes
  - Serum levels of ACE and Ca^+ for sarcoidosis
  - ANA and dsDNA to exclude SLE
  - ANCA
  - Urinary *Legionella* antigen
  - C3 and C4 to evaluate for SLE and IgG4-related disease
  - Serum protein electrophoresis
  - Anti-Ro/SSA, anti-La/SSB antibodies, CRP, and RF to exclude Sjögren syndrome

- Liver function tests elevated in patients with associated drug-induced liver injury
- Renal US may demonstrate kidneys that are normal to enlarged in size but no reliable confirmatory US findings for AIN.
- IV pyelography and CT scans with contrast are relatively contraindicated given nephrotoxicity and limited diagnostic yield. Gallium-67 imaging has limited sensitivity and specificity for AIN.

Diagnostic Procedures/Other
- Renal biopsy is the definitive method of establishing the diagnosis of AIN.
  - Patients on an OFA known to cause AIN but have normal UA
  - Patients considered for steroid therapy
  - Patients not on glucocorticoid therapy and no recovery following cessation of the OFA
  - Patients with advanced renal failure with onset <3 months
  - Patients with any features (e.g., high-grade proteinuria) that makes AIN diagnosis uncertain
- Biopsy is contraindicated in bleeding diathesis, solitary kidney, ESRD, uncontrolled HTN, sepsis, or renal parenchymal infection.

Test Interpretation
- AIN
  - Biopsy shows marked interstitial infiltrate consisting of T lymphocytes and monocytes, eosinophils, plasma cells, and neutrophils may be found.
- CIN is characterized by tubular atrophy, fibrosis, and cellular infiltration with mononuclear cells.

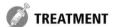 **TREATMENT**

GENERAL MEASURES
- Discontinue offending agent, including topical NSAIDs.
- Reduce exposure to nephrotoxic agents.
- Supportive measures:
  - Maintain adequate hydration.
  - Symptomatic relief for fever and rash
  - Control of BP and anemia
  - Correct acidosis and electrolyte imbalances.
  - Short-term dialysis until renal recovery
  - Renally dose meds
- Renal biopsy at 4 to 7 days
- Consider steroid if no improvement within 7 days of removing OFA. For AIN, data on corticosteroids' efficacy have been limited (5)[C], but steroids are commonly used.

MEDICATION
- Mainstay is supportive therapy.
- If AKI persists after removing OFA, attempt medication therapy.

First Line
- There are no evidence-based guidelines about management of patients with AIN.
- Withdrawal of OFA is the best first step.
- Immunosuppression if no improvement within 3 to 7 days after OFA discontinuation

- Need renal biopsy to confirm AIN and to exclude others or CIN before starting immunosuppressive therapy or when diagnosis is not clear
- Prednisone 1 mg/kg/day PO or equivalent IV (max of 40 to 60 mg/day) for 1 to 2 weeks, beginning a gradual taper after serum creatinine has returned to near baseline for 2 to 3 months, followed by a gradual taper over 4 to 8 weeks (5)[C]. Complete recovery is noted in 49% and partial in 39% (1)[C].
  - Steroids started within 7 days of withdrawal of OFA more likely to recover than those who started later.
  - NSAID-induced AIN does not generally respond to steroid therapy.

Second Line
- Limited evidence with treating AIN in patients who are steroid dependent
- Mycophenolate mofetil may be considered in biopsy-proven AIN patients. Prescription may need to be continued for 1 to 3 years (6)[C].
- Lead toxicity: Chelation may improve function.
  - Succimer 10 mg/kg (max 500 mg) PO q8h for 5 days, then q12h for 14 days, or
  - EDTA 2 g IV/IM; if IM, use with 2% lidocaine.
- SLE nephritis: steroids + cyclophosphamide or azathioprine
- Urate nephropathy: urate-lowering agents
  - Allopurinol starting at 100 mg/day, increasing to 300 mg/day to achieve serum urate level <6 mg/dL
  - Dose need to be adjusted depending on level of renal impairment.
  - Allopurinol itself can be a cause of AIN.
  - Discontinue thiazide.
- Lithium-induced nephritis: Use amiloride as adjunct.
- Indinavir-induced nephritis: Use probenecid as adjunct.

ISSUES FOR REFERRAL
Patients presenting with AKI, proteinuria, and acid–base and/or electrolyte disorders require consultation with a nephrologist.

ADMISSION, INPATIENT, AND NURSING CONSIDERATIONS
Patients with AKI and/or with serious electrolyte or acid–base disorders require hospitalization.

 ONGOING CARE

FOLLOW-UP RECOMMENDATIONS
Patient Monitoring
If patients must remain on nephrotoxic agents, measure renal function, electrolytes, and phosphorus frequently.

DIET
Low potassium (<2 g/day), sodium, and protein

PATIENT EDUCATION
National Kidney Disease Education Program, (866) 4-KIDNEY, http://www.niddk.nih.gov/health-information/health-communication-programs/nkdep/Pages/default.aspx

PROGNOSIS
- If AIN is detected early (within 1 week of the rise in serum creatinine) and the OFA is discontinued promptly, the long-term outcome is favorable; however, it is often incomplete with persistent serum creatinine noted in up to 40% of patients, especially in NSAID-induced AIN.
- Renal biopsy reveals extent of damage.
- For AIN, recovery within weeks to months; 65% recover, whereas 23% remain with long-term impairments.
- Acute dialysis is needed for 1/3 of patients before resolution.
- Progresses to ESRD in 12% patients
- CIN: can progress to ESRD
- Untreated severe AKI has 45–70% mortality.

COMPLICATIONS
- Chronic tubulointerstitial disease may progress to ESRD, requiring dialysis or transplantation.
- Analgesics increase the risk of transitional cell cancers of the uroepithelium.

REFERENCES
1. Muriithi AK, Leung N, Valeri AM, et al. Clinical characteristics, causes and outcomes of acute interstitial nephritis in the elderly. *Kidney Int.* 2015;87(2):458–464.
2. Muriithi AK, Leung N, Valeri AM, et al. Biopsy-proven acute interstitial nephritis, 1993–2011: a case series. *Am J Kidney Dis.* 2014;64(4):558–566.
3. Ng JH, Zaidan M, Jhaveri KD, et al. Acute tubulointerstitial nephritis and COVID-19. *Clin Kidney J.* 2021;14(10):2151–2157.
4. Muriithi AK, Nasr SH, Leung N. Utility of urine eosinophils in the diagnosis of acute interstitial nephritis. *Clin J Am Soc Nephrol.* 2013;8(11):1857–1862.
5. Clarkson MR, Giblin L, O'Connell FP, et al. Acute interstitial nephritis: clinical features and response to corticosteroid therapy. *Nephrol Dial Transplant.* 2004;19(11):2778–2783.
6. Preddie DC, Markowitz GS, Radhakrishnan J, et al. Mycophenolate mofetil for the treatment of interstitial nephritis. *Clin J Am Soc Nephrol.* 2006;1(4):718–722.

CODES

ICD10
- N12 Tubulo-interstitial nephritis, not spcf as acute or chronic
- N10 Acute tubulo-interstitial nephritis
- N11.9 Chronic tubulo-interstitial nephritis, unspecified

CLINICAL PEARLS
- First step in treatment is to remove offending agents. Most common in elderly are proton pump inhibitors and antibiotics.
- A renal biopsy is preferred to confirm AIN.
- Immunosuppressive therapy is employed if no subsequent improvement within 3 to 7 days after discontinuation of OFA.

IRRITABLE BOWEL SYNDROME

Marie L. Borum, MD, EdD, MPH • Andrew F. Boylan, MD

BASICS

DESCRIPTION
- A gastrointestinal (GI) disorder characterized by chronic and recurrent abdominal pain, discomfort, bloating, distension, and alteration in bowel habits in the absence of an organic cause
- May be characterized as diarrhea-predominant (IBS-D),constipation-predominant (IBS-C), mixed (IBS-M), or unknown (IBS-U); may alternate between symptoms
- Synonym(s): spastic colon; irritable colon

EPIDEMIOLOGY
Irritable bowel syndrome (IBS) accounts for 30–50% of visits to gastroenterologists and ~2 million primary care visits annually in United States with estimated cost of $1.5 to $10 billion dollars a year.

Incidence
2 per 1,000 person years

Prevalence
Pooled estimate of ~4% globally using Rome IV criteria or 9% globally using Rome III criteria
- Predominant age: 20 to 39 years
- If age >50 years, consider other diagnoses.
- In the United States, female > male (3:1)
- More common in low socioeconomic communities

ETIOLOGY AND PATHOPHYSIOLOGY
- The etiology is unknown; associated with abnormalities of intestinal motility and enhanced sensitivity to visceral stimuli. The trigger may be luminal or environmental.
- PI-IBS (post-infectious) develops in roughly 10% with infectious enteritis.
- The role of food sensitivity, microbiome dysbiosis, genetic, and psychosocial causes including early childhood stress are under investigation.
- Increase in mast cell density and activity has been demonstrated on biopsy from terminal ileum, jejunum, and colon in patients with IBS and may correlate with visceral hypersensitivity (1).
- Current investigation is ongoing regarding low-grade mucosal and neuroinflammation, and the contribution of this inflammation in the dysregulation of the "brain-gut" axis (1).

Genetics
Unknown. IBS tracks in some families, relatives of someone with IBS are 2 to 3 times more likely to have IBS.

RISK FACTORS
- Female sex, odds ratio 1.67
- Other family members with similar GI disorder
- Psychological factors: stress, abuse history, anxiety, depression or somatization
- Somatic factors: GI infection, pain syndromes, obesity, antibiotic use, and abdominal surgery
- Social factors: socioeconomic status in childhood, family history

Pediatric Considerations
No risk to mother or fetus

GENERAL PREVENTION
See "Diet."

COMMONLY ASSOCIATED CONDITIONS
- Other functional GI disorders (heartburn, dyspepsia, gastroesophageal reflux disease, nausea, diarrhea, incontinence, pelvic floor dyssynergia, and constipation)
- Chronic conditions including migraines, fibromyalgia, chronic pelvic pain, temporomandibular joint dysfunction, chronic fatigue syndrome, sleep disorders, and overactive bladder
- Psychiatric disorders: major depression, anxiety, somatoform disorders, and posttraumatic stress

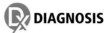

DIAGNOSIS

HISTORY
- Rome IV criteria: abdominal pain >1 day/week, on average, in the previous 3 months with an onset >6 months before diagnosis
- Abdominal pain and at least two of the following:
  – Improvement or worsening of pain with defecation
  – Change in frequency of stools
  – Change in form (appearance) of stools
- Four bowel patterns in the Rome IV classification:
  – IBS-D: diarrhea predominant: >25% diarrhea with Bristol stool types 6 or 7 and <25% constipation
  – IBS-C: constipation predominant: >25% constipation with Bristol stool types 1 or 2 and <25% diarrhea
  – IBS-M: mixed bowel habits: >25% constipation and >25% diarrhea
  – IBS-U: unclassified-symptoms: meets Rome IV criteria but not subtypes
- Patient has no warning signs (red flags):
  – Age >50 years, no previous colon cancer screening and presence of symptoms
  – Recent change in bowel habit
  – Evidence of overt GI bleeding (melena or hematochezia)
  – Nocturnal pain or passage of stools
  – Unintentional weight loss (>10% in 3 months)
  – Family history of colorectal cancer, inflammatory bowel disease or celiac disease
  – Palpable abdominal mass or lymphadenopathy
  – Evidence of iron deficiency anemia on blood testing
  – Positive fecal occult blood
  – Fever in association with the bowel symptoms

PHYSICAL EXAM
- Complete exam to exclude other causes including digital rectal exam; vital signs and exam typically unremarkable
- There is an absence of peritoneal signs, ascites, lymph node enlargement, jaundice, and organomegaly.

DIFFERENTIAL DIAGNOSIS
- Inflammatory bowel disease (Crohn and ulcerative colitis)
- Endocrine disorders (hyper/hypothyroidism, Addison disease, diabetes mellitus)
- Lactose intolerance; fructose malabsorption
- Infections (*Giardia lamblia, Entamoeba histolytica, Salmonella, Campylobacter, Yersinia, Clostridium difficile*)
- Celiac sprue; microscopic colitis
- Medication induced: opioid constipation, laxative abuse; magnesium antacids
- Pancreatic insufficiency
- Small bowel bacterial overgrowth
- Somatization; depression
- Villous adenoma, endocrine tumors (gastrinoma or carcinoid)
- Radiation damage to colon or small bowel

DIAGNOSTIC TESTS & INTERPRETATION
- Use a positive diagnostic strategy rather than making a diagnosis of exclusion.
- With a typical history and no warning signs (anemia or weight loss), only obtain baseline labs (CBC; basic metabolic profile; stool O&P; fecal leukocytes; Giardia antigen; *Clostridium difficile* toxin) and begin treatment.
- Plasma anti-cytolethal distending toxin B (anti-CdtB) and anti-vinculin antibodies are elevated in IBS-D and IBS-M but not IBS-C (2).

Initial Tests (lab, imaging)
Rule out pathology specific to the patient's symptoms:
- Diarrhea-predominant: CRP, CBC, IgA tissue transglutaminase (rule out celiac disease) with IgA level, fecal calprotectin or fecal lactoferrin, thyroid-stimulating hormone (TSH), and stool for ova and parasites
- Constipation-predominant: TSH, electrolytes, calcium (hyperparathyroidism)
- Abdominal pain: LFTs, lipase or amylase
- In the absence of alarm symptoms, labs such a fecal calprotectin (<40 μg/g) are considered sufficient to effectively rule out IBD. CRP (<0.5 mg/dL) and fecal lactoferrin (<7 μg/g) can be used as an alternative (3).
- Consider hydrogen breath testing to exclude bacterial overgrowth.
- In patients who do not respond to treatment, consider further evaluation with imaging (ultrasound or CT), endoscopy, video capsule endoscopy, or sitz marker study. These will generally be unremarkable in IBS.

Follow-Up Tests & Special Considerations
- Consider lactulose breath test to assess for small intestinal bacterial overgrowth associated with IBS.
- Consider colonoscopy in patients at high risk for microscopic colitis (female gender, >60 years old, and more intense diarrhea).

Diagnostic Procedures/Other
- Sigmoidoscopy/colonoscopy may be used to rule out inflammatory bowel disease or microscopic colitis.
- Abdominal radiograph can be considered to assess for severity of stool burden in IBS-C.
- Physiologic testing (anorectal manometry and balloon expulsion) can be done to rule out dyssynergic defecation in patients with severe constipation refractory to dietary change and osmotic laxative therapy.

Test Interpretation
None

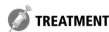

TREATMENT

- Goals: Relieve symptoms, improve quality of life (4). Therapy should be aimed at specific subtype of IBS.
- Lifestyle modification
  - Exercise 3 to 5 times per week decreases severity (4).
  - Food diary to determine triggers (4)

MEDICATION

- Soluble fiber supplementation (psyllium) increases stool bulk; does not typically relieve abdominal pain; may be used for all types (3)[B]
- For all types of IBS:
  - Antispasmodics such as hyoscyamine 0.125 to 0.250 mg PO/SL q4h PRN and dicyclomine 20 to 40 mg PO BID. Adverse effects include dry mouth, dizziness, and blurred vision (4)[C].
  - TCAs starting at the lowest dose. Multimodal mechanism of action in IBS. Common adverse effects include dry mouth, insomnia, flushing, and palpitations. Numbers needed to treat (NNT) is 4.5. Numbers need to harm (NNH) ranges 9 to 18 (5)[A].
  - Probiotics such as *Lactobacillus*, *Bifidobacterium*, and *Streptococcus* (6)[C]
- Diarrhea-predominant (IBS-D)
  - Loperamide 4 to 8 mg/day divided 1 to 3 times per day as needed to decrease stool frequency and increase stool consistency may also use diphenoxylate and atropine (4)[B]
  - Bile acid sequestrants in patients with suspicion of bile acid malabsorption; these include cholestyramine, colestipol, and colesevelam.
  - Rifaximin (2-week course) has been shown to improve bloating, pain, and stool consistency. Favorable safety profile with an NNH of 8,971 (5)[A].
  - Alosetron (Lotronex; 0.5 to 1.0 mg PO BID) is a 5-HT$_3$ antagonist, slows intestinal transit indicated for women with severe symptoms; associated with ischemic colitis, constipation, and death in a small number of patients (5)[C]
  - Ondansetron was found to reduce symptoms severity other than pain (5)[C].
  - Eluxadoline (75 to 100 mg BID) is a mixed opioid receptor agonist and antagonist. Adverse effects include nausea, constipation, abdominal pain, sphincter of Oddi spasm, and pancreatitis. Contraindicated in patients with history of alcoholism, pancreatitis, cholecystectomy, and alcohol use (5)[A].
- Constipation-predominant (IBS-C)
  - Laxatives such as polyethylene glycol may improve stool frequency but not pain.
  - Antibiotics such as neomycin
  - Lubiprostone (8 μg BID with meals) prostaglandin E1 analogs with high affinity for type 2 chloride channels, which increases intestinal secretion and peristalsis. NNT of 12.5, adverse effects include nausea and diarrhea (5)[A].
  - Linaclotide (290 μg qd) is a guanylate cyclase 2C agonist that has been shown to improve bowel function and reduces abdominal pain and overall severity in adults only; NNT of 6 (5)[A]
  - Plecanatide (3 mg qd) is approved for patients with constipation-predominant IBS; acts by increasing intestinal transit and fluid content and is comparable to linaclotide; NNT of 9 (5)[A]
  - Tenapanor (50 mg BID) is a NHE3 inhibitor that reduces absorption of sodium and phosphate and increases intestinal fluid volume and transit.
  - Tegaserod FDA-approved Serotonin 5-HT$_4$ receptor agonist increases colonic motility. Also reduces abdominal pain. Only approved for women <65. Contraindicated in patients with >1 CV risk factors, history of bowel obstruction, gallbladder disease, sphincter of Oddi dysfunction, abdominal adhesions or history of ischemic colitis
- Mixed
  - Use medications to match symptoms (4)[B].

ISSUES FOR REFERRAL

- Behavioral health referral may help with management of affective or personality disorders.
- Gastroenterology referral for difficult to control cases

ADDITIONAL THERAPIES

- Probiotics use may result in reducing IBS symptoms and decreasing pain and flatulence. Multistrain probiotics tend to be more effective in symptom improvement than monostrain (6).
- Peppermint oil is used as a first-line therapy for IBS-D in Europe, as it has antispasmodic, anti-inflammatory, and serotonin 5-HT3 receptor antagonism that can help slow motility and may decrease visceral hypersensitivity while having minimal adverse effects.

ONGOING CARE

FOLLOW-UP RECOMMENDATIONS
Patient Monitoring
The IBS Severity Scoring System is a validated measure to assess the severity of IBS symptoms and can help monitor response to treatment. This includes severity of pain and distension, frequency of bowel movements, satisfaction with bowel habits, and level of impact IBS is having on quality of life.

DIET

- A low FODMAP diet
- Increase fiber slowly to avoid excess intestinal gas production.
- Initially, consider 2 weeks of lactose-free diet to rule out lactose intolerance.
- Avoid large meals, fatty foods, and caffeine, which can exacerbate symptoms.
- A gluten-free diet can resolve symptoms for some patients despite negative testing for celiac disease.

PATIENT EDUCATION
IBS is not a psychiatric illness but is a chronic condition with no increased risk of malignancy.

PROGNOSIS

- IBS is a disorder that reduces quality of life but does not increase mortality.
- Recurrences common
- Evidence suggests that "symptom shifting" occurs in some patients, whereby resolution of functional bowel symptoms is followed by the development of functional symptoms in another system.

REFERENCES

1. Ng QX, Soh AYS, Loke W, et al. The role of inflammation in irritable bowel syndrome (IBS). *J Inflamm Res*. 2018;11:345–349.
2. Rezaie A, Park SC, Morales W, et al. Assessment of anti-vinculin and anti-cytolethal distending toxin B antibodies in subtypes of irritable bowel syndrome. *Dig Dis Sci*. 2017;62(6):1480–1485.
3. Kurin M, Cooper G. Irritable bowel syndrome with diarrhea: treatment is a work in progress. *Cleve Clin J Med*. 2020;87(8):501–511.
4. Chey WD, Kurlander J, Eswaran S. Irritable bowel syndrome: a clinical review. *JAMA*. 2015;313(9):949–958.
5. Lacy BE, Pimentel M, Brenner DM, et al. ACG Clinical Guideline: management of irritable bowel syndrome. *Am J Gastroenterol*. 2021;116(1):17–44.
6. Dale HF, Rasmussen SH, Asiller ÖÖ, et al. Probiotics in irritable bowel syndrome: an up-to-date systematic review. *Nutrients*. 2019;11(9):2048.

ADDITIONAL READING

Gastroenterologic Society of Australia. Low FODMAP diet. https://cart.gesa.org.au/membes/files/Consumer%20Information/Low%20FODMAP%20Diet.pdf.

SEE ALSO

Algorithm: Diarrhea, Chronic

CODES

ICD10

- K58.9 Irritable bowel syndrome without diarrhea
- K58.0 Irritable bowel syndrome with diarrhea
- K58 Irritable bowel syndrome

CLINICAL PEARLS

- Use Rome IV criteria to establish the diagnosis of IBS.
- Goals of treatment are to relieve symptoms and improve quality of life.
- If patients do not respond to initial treatment, consider further evaluation (including imaging and/or referral for endoscopy) to exclude organic pathology.

KAWASAKI SYNDROME

Khadija Kabani, DO, FAAFP • Katherine E. Bouchard, DO

 BASICS

DESCRIPTION

- Kawasaki syndrome (KS) is a self-limited acute, febrile, systemic vasculitis of small- and medium-sized arteries that predominantly affects patients age 6 months to 5 years.
- The most prominent cause of acquired coronary artery disease in children in developed countries (1).
  - Vasculitis of coronary arteries results in aneurysms/ectasia, leading to myocardial infarction (MI)/ischemia or sudden death
- System(s) affected: cardiovascular, gastrointestinal, hematologic/lymphatic/immunologic, musculoskeletal, nervous, pulmonary, renal/urologic, skin/exocrine
- Synonym(s): mucocutaneous lymph node syndrome (MCLS), infantile polyarteritis, Kawasaki disease

ALERT
KS should be considered in any child with extended high fever unresponsive to antibiotics or antipyretics, rash, and nonexudative conjunctivitis.

EPIDEMIOLOGY

Incidence
- Worldwide: affects all races but most prevalent in Asia; Japan annual incidence rate 265/100,000 in children <5 years old
- In the United States, the annual incidence in children <5 years is 19/100,000. In comparison to Caucasians, African Americans have a 1.5 times risk, and Asian Americans have a 2.5 times increased risk. Highest state incidence is in Hawaii.
- Leading cause of acquired heart disease in children in developed countries
  - Predominant age: 1 to 5 years, median age of diagnosis is 1.5 years of age.
  - 85% of cases are children <5 years of age and 50% <2 years of age.
  - Male-to-female ratio = 1.5:1

Prevalence
- Highest to lowest prevalence: Asians > Black Americans > Hispanics > Caucasians
- Seasonal variation: peaks in winter and early spring (January to March) in temperate places; peaks in summer in Asia
- Outbreaks at 2- to 3-year intervals

ETIOLOGY AND PATHOPHYSIOLOGY
- Infectious agent triggers abnormal inflammatory reaction in children with genetic predisposition.
- Acute KS causes a necrotizing arteritis in the smooth muscle layer of medium extraparenchymal arteries, destroying arterial walls into the adventitia, especially in coronary arteries.
- Inflammatory cells secrete cytokines (TNF-α), interleukins 1 and 6, and matrix metalloproteases that cause fragmentation of the internal elastic lamina.
- As the acute process resolves, active neutrophilic inflammatory cells are succeeded by a subacute/chronic, lymphocytic vasculitis; fibroblasts and monocytes cause tissue repair/remodeling that may cause vascular fibrosis and stenosis.

Genetics
- Populations at higher risk and family link suggest a genetic predisposition.
- Siblings of patients in Japan have a 10- to 30-fold increased risk, and >50% develop KS within 10 days of first case; increased occurrence of KS in children whose parents also had illness in childhood

- Single-nucleotide polymorphisms in six different genes have been implicated in KS (Fcγ receptor 2A, CASP3, HLA class II, B-cell lymphoid kinase, IPTKC, CD40).
- Coronary aneurysms are associated with variants in TGF-β signaling pathways.

RISK FACTORS
- Male to female prevalence 1.5:1 in United States
- Black Americans at 1.5 times risk; Asian Americans at 2.5 times risk
- Sibling with Kawasaki

GENERAL PREVENTION
No preventive measures available

 DIAGNOSIS

- ≥5 days of fever ≥4 of the following five principal clinical features (1); OR <4 features and presence of coronary artery disease on 2D echocardiography:
  - Bilateral, nonpurulent conjunctival injection with limbic sparing
  - Erythematous changes to mouth, pharynx, tongue, and lips
  - A polymorphous, generalized, erythematous rash
  - Changes in the skin of the peripheral extremities (edema of hands/feet; erythema of palms/soles; desquamation of fingers/toes)
  - Cervical lymphadenopathy (>1 node >1.5 cm in diameter)
- Note: Diagnosis can be made at day 4 of fever in a patient with >4 principal clinical features, especially if redness/swelling of hands/feet is present.

Pediatric Considerations
- Prolonged fever without rash that is treated with antibiotics may cause clinicians to believe that a subsequent rash is due to a drug reaction.
- Incomplete KS (atypical KS)
  - ≥5 days of fever, 2 to 3 principal clinical features, labs indicating systemic inflammation, and exclusion of other diseases
  - Incomplete cases that exhibit <4 clinical criteria often occur in infants ≤6 months of age or older children/adolescents. The frequency of coronary artery aneurysms (CAAs) is often higher in patients with missed diagnosis/delayed treatment. Therefore, in infants with prolonged fever and few or no clinical features, consider echocardiography and inflammatory labs.

HISTORY
- Fever is the first sign during the acute phase.
- Symptoms may not occur all at once but usually occur in close proximity.

PHYSICAL EXAM
- High-spiking and remittent fever for ≥5 days
  - Fever is high (102–105°F [39.4–40.5°C]) and unresponsive to antibiotics/antipyretics.
  - May be prolonged up to 10 to 12 days with more rare cases lasting 3 to 4 weeks (1)
  - Extreme irritability is a common feature.
- Bilateral, painless, nonpurulent, conjunctival injection without corneal ulceration or edema. Limbic sparing is usually seen.
- Changes in lips and oral cavity
  - Redness and swelling of lips in the acute stage; cracking, fissuring, bleeding in subacute phase
  - Strawberry/erythematous tongue

- Extensive erythematous polymorphous rash: within 5 days of fever
  - Morbilliform is most common. May be maculo-papular, scarlatiniform; can resemble erythema multiforme, erythroderma, urticarial exanthem; rarely micropustular
  - Perineal desquamation, especially in skin folds
- Extremity changes
  - Reddened palms and soles on days 3 to 5
  - Edema of hands and feet on days 4 to 7; painful induration
  - Desquamation of fingers and toes that begins in periungual area at 2 to 3 weeks
- Acute, unilateral cervical lymphadenopathy (least common symptom)
  - ≥1 lymph nodes >1.5 cm, firm, nonfluctuant, and usually with no to slight tenderness
- Cardiac exam: tachycardia, gallop rhythms, hyperdynamic precordium, innocent flow murmurs, depressed contractility
- Other organ system involvement
  - Cardiovascular: myocarditis; pericarditis (often subclinical), CAAs, and other medium-sized arterial aneurysms
  - Gastrointestinal: anorexia, abdominal pain, vomiting/diarrhea, acute gallbladder hydrops, hepatic enlargement, jaundice
  - Renal: proteinuria, sterile pyuria
  - Joints: polyarthritis of small joints in acute phase; weight-bearing joints affected after 10th day from onset of fever
  - Neurologic: irritability, aseptic meningitis, peripheral neuropathy (unilateral facial palsy), transient high-frequency hearing loss

DIFFERENTIAL DIAGNOSIS
- Bacterial: scarlet fever, bacterial cervical lymphadenitis, *Mycoplasma* infection, leptospirosis, Lyme disease, Rocky Mountain spotted fever
- Toxin mediated: staphylococcal scalded-skin syndrome, streptococcal scarlet fever, toxic shock syndrome (1)
- Viral: measles, adenovirus, Epstein-Barr virus, SARS-CoV-2
  - Multisystem inflammatory syndrome in children (MIS-C): important consideration given similar presentation; linked with SARS-CoV-2
- Toxoplasmosis
- Reiter syndrome
- Hypersensitivity drug reactions (erythema multiforme minor, Stevens-Johnson syndrome)
- Juvenile rheumatoid arthritis
- Acrodynia (mercury poisoning)

DIAGNOSTIC TESTS & INTERPRETATION
- Initial workup: CBC with differential, urinalysis (UA)/culture, blood culture; lumbar puncture if signs of meningitis or if <90 days old
  - Leukocytosis (12,000 to 40,000 cells/mm³) with immature and mature granulocytes
  - Anemia: normochromic, normocytic
  - Thrombocytosis (500,000 to >1,000,000/mm³) in 2nd and 3rd week. Thrombocytopenia during acute phase is associated with CAA and MI.
- Elevated C-reactive protein (CRP) (>35 mg/L in 80% cases), erythrocyte sedimentation rate (ESR) (>60 mm/hr in 60% cases), and α_1-antitrypsin
- Normal ESR, CRP, and PLTs after day 7 suggest diagnosis other than KS.

ALERT
ESR can be artificially high after intravenous immunoglobulin (IVIG) therapy.

- Hyponatremia
- Moderately elevated AST, ALT, GGT, and bilirubin
- Decreased albumin and protein
- CSF pleocytosis may be seen (lymphocytic with normal protein and glucose).
- *N*-terminal brain natriuretic peptide might be elevated in acute phase, but definitive cut-off values have not been established.
- Sterile pyuria but not seen in suprapubic collection
- Nasal swab to rule out adenovirus, coronavirus (SARS-CoV-2)

Initial Tests (lab, imaging)
- If KS is suspected, obtain ECG and echocardiogram.
  - ECG may show arrhythmias, prolonged PR interval, and ST/T wave changes.
  - Echocardiography has a high sensitivity and specificity for detection of abnormalities of proximal left main coronary artery, and right coronary artery may show perivascular brightening, ectasia, decreased left ventricular contractility, pericardial effusion, or aneurysms.
  - Repeat echocardiography frequency determined by degree of abnormal more significant findings should be followed twice weekly until aneurysmal progression halts.
  - Cardiac stress test if CAA seen on echocardiogram
- Baseline chest x-ray may show pleural effusion, atelectasis, and congestive heart failure (CHF).
- Hydrops of the gallbladder may be associated with abdominal pain or may be asymptomatic.

Diagnostic Procedures/Other
- No laboratory study is diagnostic; diagnosis rests on constellation of clinical features and exclusion of other illnesses.
- Magnetic resonance coronary angiography is noninvasive modality to visualize coronary arteries for stenosis, thrombi, and intimal thickening.
- Patients with complex coronary artery lesions (CALs) may benefit from coronary angiography after the acute inflammatory process has resolved; generally recommended in 6 to 12 months

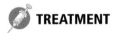 **TREATMENT**

GENERAL MEASURES
Use antibiotics until bacterial etiologies are excluded (e.g., sepsis or meningitis).

MEDICATION
- Optimal therapy is IVIG 2 g/kg IV over 10 to 12 hours with high-dose aspirin preferably within 7 to 10 days of fever, followed by low-dose aspirin until follow-up echocardiograms indicate a lack of coronary abnormalities.
  - IVIG lowers the risk of CAA and may shorten fever duration.
  - The extreme irritability often resolves very quickly after IVIG is given.
  - CALs develop in 3–5% of children treated with IVIG. CALs develop in up to 25% of untreated children (1).
- Retreatment with IVIG if clinical response is incomplete or fever persists/returns >36 hours after start of IVIG treatment
  - ≥10% of patients do not respond to initial IVIG treatment. 2/3 of nonresponders respond to the second dose of IVIG.
  - Nonresponders tend to have ↑ bands, ↓ albumin, and an abnormal echocardiogram.

- Aspirin 80 to 100 mg/kg/day in 4 doses beginning with IVIG administration. Switch to low-dose aspirin (3 to 5 mg/kg/day) when afebrile for 48 to 72 hours, or continue until day 14 of illness. Maintain low dose for 6 to 8 weeks until follow-up echocardiogram is normal and CRP and/or ESR are normal. Continue salicylate regimen in children with coronary abnormalities, long term or until documented regression of aneurysm.
- Aspirin does not appear to reduce CAA.
- Corticosteroids have conflicting evidence for use and:
  - Should not be used as first-line agent in all KS patients; reserve for IVIG resistant cases.
  - Should be used in conjunction with IVIG and aspirin as initial treatment to decrease risk of CAAs in those at highest risk of IVIG failure
- Contraindications
  - IVIG: documented hypersensitivity, IgA deficiency, anti-IgE/IgG antibodies, severe thrombocytopenia, coagulation disorders
  - Aspirin: vitamin K deficiency, bleeding disorders, liver damage, documented hypersensitivity, hypoprothrombinemia
- Precautions
  - No statistically significant difference is noted between different preparations of IVIG.
  - High-dose aspirin therapy can result in tinnitus, decreased of renal function, and increased transaminases.
  - Do not use ibuprofen in children with CAAs who are taking aspirin for antiplatelet effects.
  - Significant possible interactions: Aspirin therapy has been associated with Reye syndrome in children who develop viral infections, especially influenza B and varicella. Yearly influenza vaccination thus is recommended for children requiring long-term treatment with aspirin. Delay any live vaccines for 11 months after IVIG treatment.

First Line
High-dose IVIG and aspirin should be instituted promptly upon confirmed diagnosis (1).

Second Line
- In patients refractory to IVIG and steroids, consider infliximab or cyclosporine.
- Plasma exchange may decrease likelihood of CAA in IVIG nonresponders.

ISSUES FOR REFERRAL
Pediatric cardiologist if abnormalities on echocardiogram or if extensive stenosis

ADDITIONAL THERAPIES
- Treatment and prevention of thrombosis are crucial.
- Antiplatelet agents (clopidogrel, dipyridamole), heparin, low-molecular-weight heparin, or warfarin are sometimes added to the low-dose aspirin regimen, depending on severity of CAAs.
- Clarithromycin given with IVIG may reduce relapse rates and length of hospital stay; does not reduce duration of fever or improve cardiac outcomes

SURGERY/OTHER PROCEDURES
- Rarely needed; coronary artery bypass grafting for severe obstruction/recurrent MI. Younger patients have a higher mortality rate.
- Coronary revascularization via percutaneous coronary intervention for patients with evidence of ischemia on stress testing

ADMISSION, INPATIENT, AND NURSING CONSIDERATIONS
- Normal saline (NS) for rehydration and 1/2 NS for maintenance
- Discharge if afebrile after IVIG treatment for 24 hours.

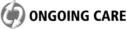 **ONGOING CARE**

FOLLOW-UP RECOMMENDATIONS
With aneurysms, contact and high-risk sports should be avoided.

Patient Monitoring
- Repeat ECG and echocardiogram at 6 to 8 weeks. If abnormal, repeat at 6 to 12 months.
- Patients with complex CALs may require a combination of β-blockers to decrease oxidative stress and antithrombotic therapy (1). These patients may benefit from coronary angiography at 6 to 12 months and will require close follow-up.
- Patients receiving long-term ASA who are not fully vaccinated should receive immunizations. Measles and varicella-containing immunizations are contraindicated for 11 months after administration of IVIG for Kawasaki disease (1).

PROGNOSIS
- Usually self-limited
- Relates entirely to the extent and severity of cardiac disease (1)
- Moderate-sized aneurysms usually regress in 1 to 2 years, resolving in 50–66% of cases.
- Recurrence (3% in Japan, <1% in the United States)
- Sudden death in early adulthood (rare)

COMPLICATIONS
- 15–25% of untreated patients develop CAAs in convalescent phase.
- 2–7% of treated patients develop aneurysms. 1% develop giant aneurysms.
- Risk factors for aneurysm
  - Male, <1 year of age, ↑ ESR >4 weeks, fever >2 weeks, fever >48 hours after IVIG treatment
- Mortality of 0.08–0.17% is due to cardiac disease.

REFERENCE
1. Son MBF, Newburger JW. Kawasaki disease. *Pediatr Rev.* 2018;39(2):78–90.

ADDITIONAL READING
- Most ZM, Hendren N, Drazner MH, et al. Striking similarities of multisystem inflammatory syndrome in children and a myocarditis-like syndrome in adults: overlapping manifestations of COVID-19. *Circulation.* 2021;143(1):4–6.
- Oates-Whitehead RM, Baumer JH, Haines L, et al. Intravenous immunoglobulin for the treatment of Kawasaki disease in children. *Cochrane Database Syst Rev.* 2003;2003(4):CD004000.
- Saguil A, Fargo M, Grogan S. Diagnosis and management of Kawasaki disease. *Am Fam Physician.* 2015;91(6):365–371.

 CODES

ICD10
M30.3 Mucocutaneous lymph node syndrome [Kawasaki]

CLINICAL PEARLS
- The diagnosis of KS rests on a constellation of clinical features.
- Once KS is suspected, all patients need an inpatient cardiac evaluation, including ECG and echocardiogram.
- Expert recommendation for optimal therapy is IVIG 2 g/kg IV over 10 hours, with high-dose aspirin 80 to 100 mg/kg/day in 4 doses.

K

KERATOACANTHOMA

Patrick M. Zito, DO, PharmD • Daniel Rivlin, MD • Richard Scharf, DO

BASICS

DESCRIPTION
- Most common is a solitary, rapidly proliferating, dome-shaped, erythematous or flesh-colored papule or nodule with a central keratinous plug, typically reaching 1 to 2 cm in diameter.
- Clinically and microscopically resemble squamous cell carcinoma (SCC)
- Other presentations include grouped, multiple, keratoacanthoma (KA) centrifugum marginatum, intraoral, subungual, regressing, nonregressing, generally eruptive (1).
- Majority are benign and resolve spontaneously, but lesions do have the potential for invasion and metastasis, therefore require treatment.
- Three clinical stages of KAs (1):
  - Proliferative: rapid growth of the lesion over weeks to several months
  - Maturation/stabilization: Lesion stabilizes and growth subsides.
  - Involution: spontaneous resolution of the lesion, leaving a hypopigmented, depressed scar; most but not all lesions will enter this stage.
- System(s) affected: integumentary

EPIDEMIOLOGY
- Greatest incidence age >50 years but may occur at any age
- Presentation increased during summer and early fall seasons
- Most frequently on sun-exposed, hair-bearing skin but may occur anywhere
- Predominant sex: male > female (2:1)
- Most commonly in fair-skinned individuals; highest rates in Fitzpatrick I to III
- 104 cases per 100,000 individuals

ETIOLOGY AND PATHOPHYSIOLOGY
- Derived from an abnormality causing hyperkeratosis within the follicular infundibulum
- Squamous epithelial cells proliferate to extend upward around the keratin plug and proceed downward into the dermis; followed by invasion of elastic and collagen fibers
- Cellular mechanism responsible for the hyperkeratosis is currently unknown; role of human papillomavirus (HPV) has been discussed but has no established causality (2).
- Regression may be due to immune cytotoxicity or terminal differentiation of keratinocytes.
- Multiple etiologies have been suggested:
  - UV radiation
  - May be provoked by surgery, cryotherapy, chemical peels, or laser therapy
  - Viral infections: HPV or Merkel cell polyomavirus
  - Genetic predisposition: Muir-Torre syndrome, xeroderma pigmentosum, Ferguson-Smith syndrome
  - Immunosuppression
  - BRAF inhibitors (1)
  - Chemical carcinogen exposure

Genetics
- Mutation of *p53* or H-*ras*
- Ferguson-Smith (AD)
- Witten-Zak (AD)
- Muir-Torre (AD)
- Xeroderma pigmentosum (AR)
- Grzybowski (sporadic)
- Incontinentia pigmenti (XLD)

RISK FACTORS
- UV exposure/damage: outdoor and/or indoor tanning
- Fitzpatrick skin type I to III
- Trauma (typically appears within 1 month of injury): laser resurfacing, surgery, cryotherapy, tattoos
- Chemical carcinogens: tar, pitch, and smoking
- Immunocompromised state
- Discoid lupus erythematosus
- HPV infection

GENERAL PREVENTION
Sun protection

COMMONLY ASSOCIATED CONDITIONS
- Frequently, the patient has concurrent sun-damaged skin: solar elastosis, solar lentigines, actinic keratosis, nonmelanoma skin cancers (basal cell carcinoma, SCC).
- In Muir-Torre syndrome, KAs are found with coexisting sebaceous neoplasms and malignancy of the GI and GU tracts; may have sebaceous differentiation known as a seboacanthoma

DIAGNOSIS

HISTORY
- Lesion begins as a small, solitary, pink macule that undergoes a rapid growth phase; classically reaching a diameter of 1 to 2 cm; size may vary.
- Once the proliferative stage has subsided, lesion size remains stable.
- May decrease in size, indicating regression
- Asymptomatic, occasionally tender
- If multiple lesions present, important to elicit a family history and recent therapies or treatments
- If sebaceous neoplasms present, must review history for signs/symptoms of GI or GU malignancies

PHYSICAL EXAM
- Firm, solitary, erythematous or flesh-colored, dome-shaped papule or nodule with a central keratin plug, giving a crateriform appearance
- Surrounding skin and borders of lesion may show telangiectasia, atrophy, or dyspigmentation.
- Usually solitary; multiple lesions can occur.
- Most commonly seen on sun-exposed areas: face, neck, scalp, dorsum of upper extremities, and posterior legs
- May also be seen on areas without sun exposure: buttocks, anus, subungual, mucosal surfaces
- Subungual KAs are very painful and seen on the first 3 digits of the hands.
- Examine for regional lymphadenopathy due to chance of lesion invasion and metastasis.
- Dermoscopy (3)
  - Central keratin highest sensitivity to distinguish from SCC (4)
  - White circles, blood spots; white circles highest specificity (4)
  - Cannot reliably distinguish between KA and SCC

DIFFERENTIAL DIAGNOSIS
- SCC
- Nodular or ulcerative basal cell carcinoma
- Cutaneous horn
- Hypertrophic actinic keratosis
- Amelanotic melanoma
- Merkel cell carcinoma
- Metastasis to the skin
- Molluscum contagiosum
- Prurigo nodularis
- Verruca vulgaris
- Verrucous carcinoma
- Sebaceous adenoma
- Hypertrophic lichen planus
- Hypertrophic lupus erythematosus
- Deep fungal infection
- Atypical mycobacterial infection
- Nodular Kaposi sarcoma

DIAGNOSTIC TESTS & INTERPRETATION
- Excisional biopsy, including the center of the lesion as well as the margin, is the best diagnostic test (2)[C].
- A shave biopsy may be insufficiently deep to distinguish KA from an SCC.
- If unable to perform an excisional biopsy, a deep shave (saucerization) of the entire lesion, extending into the subcutaneous fat, can be done.
- Punch biopsies should be avoided because they give an insufficient amount of tissue to represent the entire lesion.

Initial Tests (lab, imaging)

- Subungual KA: radiograph of the digit to monitor for osteolysis (cup-shaped radiolucent defect)
- Aggressive tumors may need CT with contrast for evaluation of lymph nodes and MRI if there is concern of perineural invasion.
- Most lesions do not need any form of imaging.

Test Interpretation

- Pathology of biopsy: a well-demarcated central core of keratin surrounded by well-differentiated, mildly pleomorphic, atypical squamous epithelial cells with a characteristic glassy eosinophilic cytoplasm
- Histopathology: keratin-filled crater encompassed with epithelial lips
- May see elastic and collagen fibers invading into the squamous epithelium
- Histologic differentiation of a KA from an SCC may be difficult and unreliable, although immunochemical staining for cellular protein Ki-67 may help do this (4).
- KAs have a greater tendency than SCC to display fibrosis and intraepidermal abscesses of neutrophils and eosinophils.
- Regressing KA shows flattening and fibrosis at base of lesion.

 TREATMENT

- Treatment of choice is an excisional procedure plus electrodesiccation and curettage (ED&C); however, there are many treatment options available (2)[C].
- Aggressive tumors (>2 cm) or lesions in cosmetically sensitive areas (face, digits, genitalia) that require tissue sparing; consider Mohs micrographic surgery.
  - Mohs micrographic surgery is the treatment of choice in cases with perineural or perivascular invasion.
- Small lesions (<2 cm) of the extremities may undergo ED&C.
- Immunocompromised patients should receive immediate surgical treatment.

MEDICATION

- Nonsurgical management is a viable and relatively cost-effective option in these select cases not amenable to surgery due to lesion number, size, or location; also for patients with multiple comorbidities who are unwilling or unable to withstand surgery
- Evidence for the following treatments based on case reports and retrospective reviews:
  - Intralesional methotrexate 12.5 to 25.0 mg in 0.5 mL normal saline every 2 to 3 weeks for 1 to 4 treatment sessions (5)[B]
    - Monitor for pancytopenia with complete blood count (5)[C].
  - 5% imiquimod cream 3 times per week for 11 to 13 weeks (5)[B]
  - Topical 5% 5-fluorouracil cream daily, 61–92% cure rate (5)[B]
  - Intralesional 5-fluorouracil of 50 mg/mL on a weekly basis for 3 to 8 treatment sessions—98% cure rate (5)[B]
  - Intralesional IFN α-2a or α-2b (83%, 100% cure rate, respectively) (5)[B]
  - Intralesional bleomycin—100% cure rate (5)[B]
  - Isotretinoin oral 0.5 to 1.0 mg/kg/day

ISSUES FOR REFERRAL

Dermatology referral if lesions are >2 cm, numerous, mucosal, or subungual

ADDITIONAL THERAPIES

- Photodynamic therapy with methyl aminolevulinic acid and red light, successful case reports (1)[B] but also reported aggravation following treatment
- Cryotherapy (1)
- Argon or YAG lasers
- Radiotherapy, primary or adjuvant: KAs may regress with low doses of radiation but may require doses up to 25 to 50 Gy in low-dose (5 to 10 Gy) fractions for possible SCC (1)[B].
- Erlotinib (EGFR inhibitor) 150 mg daily for 21 days, single case report (1)[B]

SURGERY/OTHER PROCEDURES

Excisional and office-based procedures as discussed above

 ONGOING CARE

FOLLOW-UP RECOMMENDATIONS

After the surgical site has healed or lesion has resolved, patient should be seen every 6 months due to increased risk of developing new lesions or skin cancers, annually at minimum (3)[C].

Patient Monitoring

- Skin self-exams should be routinely performed with detailed instructions (see "Additional Reading").
- If multiple KAs are present in patient or family members, evaluate for Muir-Torre syndrome and obtain a colonoscopy beginning at age 25 years, as well as testing for genitourinary cancer (3)[C].

PATIENT EDUCATION

- Sun protection measures: sun block with SPF >30, wide-brimmed hats, long sleeves, dark clothing, avoiding indoor tanning
- Arc welding may produce harmful UV radiation and skin should not be exposed.
- Tar, pitch, and smoking should be avoided.

PROGNOSIS

- Atrophic scarring and hypopigmentation can occur with self-resolution but may be significantly reduced by intervention.
- 52 of 445 cases (12%) spontaneously regressed without treatment and none of these recurred (2).
- 393 (88%) regressed following medical or excisional treatment (2).
- 445 cases reported with no metastases or deaths attributable to the KA (2)

- 4–8% recurrence
- Mucosal and subungual lesions do not regress; must undergo treatment

REFERENCES

1. Kwiek B, Schwartz RA. Keratoacanthoma (KA): an update and review. *J Am Acad Dermatol.* 2016;74(6):1220–1233.
2. Savage JA, Maize JC Sr. Keratoacanthoma clinical behavior: a systematic review. *Am J Dermatopathol.* 2014;36(5):422–429.
3. Cavicchini S, Tourlaki A, Lunardon L, et al. Amelanotic melanoma mimicking keratoacanthoma: the diagnostic role of dermoscopy. *Int J Dermatol.* 2013;52(8):1023–1024.
4. Scola N, Segert HM, Stücker M, et al. Ki-67 may be useful in differentiating between keratoacanthoma and cutaneous squamous cell carcinoma. *Clin Exp Dermatol.* 2014;39(2):216–218.
5. Chitwood KL, Etzkorn J, Cohen G. Topical and intralesional treatment of nonmelanoma skin cancer: efficacy and cost comparisons. *Dermatol Surg.* 2013;39(9):1306–1316.

ADDITIONAL READING

The Skin Cancer Foundation: http://www.skincancer.org/

 SEE ALSO

Squamous Cell Carcinoma, Cutaneous

 CODES

ICD10

- D23.9 Other benign neoplasm of skin, unspecified
- D48.5 Neoplasm of uncertain behavior of skin
- L85.8 Other specified epidermal thickening

CLINICAL PEARLS

- Suspect KA with a solitary, dome-shaped, erythematous or flesh-colored papule or nodule with a central keratinous plug.
- If KA is in the differential diagnosis, elicit time frame of onset during patient encounter; rapid onset supports diagnosis.
- Due to the broad differential diagnosis of a suspected KA and unreliable clinical differentiation between these, strongly consider surgical excision as first-line diagnostic test and therapy.
- Medical and radiation therapies are reasonable and effective options available for patients who are not surgical candidates or for lesions that are not amenable for surgery.

K

KERATOSIS, ACTINIC

Zoltan Trizna, MD, PhD

 BASICS

DESCRIPTION

- Common, usually multiple, premalignant lesions of sun-exposed areas of the skin. Many resolve spontaneously, and a small proportion progresses to squamous cell carcinoma (SCC).
- Common consequence of excessive cumulative ultraviolet (UV) light exposure
- Synonym(s): solar keratosis

Geriatric Considerations
Frequent problem

Pediatric Considerations
Rare (if child, look for freckling and other stigmata of xeroderma pigmentosum)

EPIDEMIOLOGY

Incidence
- Rates vary with age group and exposure to sun.
- Predominant age: ≥40 years; progressively increases with age
- Predominant sex: male > female
- Common in those with blonde and red hair; rare in darker skin types

Prevalence
- Age-adjusted prevalence rate for actinic keratoses (AKs) in U.S. Caucasians is 6.5%.
- For 65- to 74-year-old males with high sun exposure: ~55%; low sun exposure: ~18%

ETIOLOGY AND PATHOPHYSIOLOGY

- The epidermal lesions are characterized by atypical keratinocytes at the basal layer with occasional extension upward. Mitoses are present. The histopathologic features resemble those of SCC in situ or SCC, and the distinction depends on the extent of epidermal involvement.
- Cumulative UV exposure

Genetics
The p53 chromosomal mutation has been shown consistently in both AKs and SCCs. Many new genes have been shown recently to have similar expression profiles in AKs and SCCs.

RISK FACTORS

- Exposure to UV light (especially long-term and/or repeated exposure due to outdoor occupation or recreational activities, indoor or outdoor tanning)
- Skin type: burns easily, does not tan
- Immunosuppression, especially organ transplantation

GENERAL PREVENTION
Sun avoidance and protective techniques are helpful.

COMMONLY ASSOCIATED CONDITIONS

- SCC
- Other features of chronic solar damage: lentigines, elastosis, and telangiectasias

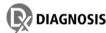 **DIAGNOSIS**

HISTORY

- The lesions are frequently asymptomatic; symptoms may include pruritus, burning, and mild hyperesthesia.
- Lesions may enlarge, thicken, or become more scaly. They also may regress or remain unchanged.
- Most lesions occur on the sun-exposed areas (head and neck, hands, forearms).

PHYSICAL EXAM

- Usually small (<1 cm), often multiple red, pink, or brown macules, papules, or plaques that are rough to palpation
- Yellow or brown adherent scale is often present on top of the lesion.
- Several clinical variants exist.
  - Atrophic: dry, scaly macules with indistinct borders and an erythematous base
  - Hypertrophic: Overlying hyperkeratosis (in an extreme form, cutaneous horn) may be impossible to differentiate from SCC clinically.
  - Pigmented: smooth tan/brown plaque, spreading centrifugally
  - Bowenoid: red scaly plaques with distinct borders
  - Actinic cheilitis: inflammatory lesion involving usually the lower lip

DIFFERENTIAL DIAGNOSIS

- SCC (hypertrophic type)
- Keratoacanthoma
- Bowen disease
- Basal cell carcinoma
- Verruca vulgaris
- Less likely: verrucous nevi, warty dyskeratoma, lichenoid keratoses, seborrheic keratoses, porokeratoses, seborrheic dermatitis or psoriasis (near hairline), lentigo maligna, solar lentigo, discoid lupus erythematosus

DIAGNOSTIC TESTS & INTERPRETATION

Diagnostic Procedures/Other
- The diagnosis is usually made clinically, except where there is a suspicion of carcinoma.
- Skin biopsy is especially recommended if large, ulcerated, indurated, or bleeding, or if the lesions are nonresponsive to treatment.

Test Interpretation
- Dysplastic keratinocytes in lower levels of epidermis with a dermal lymphocytic infiltrate
- Neoplastic cells, mostly found in the lower epidermal layers, are cytologically identical to those of SCCs.
- If neoplastic cells extend throughout entire epidermis or into the dermis, the lesions will qualify as an SCC in situ or invasive SCC, respectively.
- Malignant cells are sparse except of the bowenoid variety.
- Hypertrophic, atrophic, bowenoid, acantholytic, and pigmented varieties show the corresponding epidermal findings.

 TREATMENT

- First-line treatment is cryotherapy (technically, this is considered surgery, especially by insurance companies) (1),(2)[A]. Medical therapy is usually reserved for multiple or extensive AKs ("field therapy").
- Cryotherapy combined with a topical approach resulted in significantly higher complete clearance rates than monotherapy (3)[A].

GENERAL MEASURES
- Sun-protective techniques
- Sunscreens and physical sun protection recommended

MEDICATION

First Line
- Topical treatments target both visible and subclinical lesions.
- With the exception of generic 5-fluorouracil, medication cost is high ($600 to $1,200 per course).
- Topical fluorouracil (Efudex, Carac, Fluoroplex cream, Fluoroplex solution)
  - Every day—BID for 3 to 6 weeks, depending on the brand, concentration, and formulation
  - Can be very irritating
  - Likely the most effective of the topical treatments listed in this section (3)[A],(4)[A]
- Topical imiquimod (Aldara) 5% cream
  - Apply 2 days per week at HS for up to 16 weeks to an area not larger than the forehead or one cheek.
  - Can be irritating
- Topical imiquimod (Zyclara) 3.75% cream
  - Apply once a day for 2 weeks, followed by no treatment for the next 2 weeks, and then apply once a day for another 2 weeks.
  - Can be irritating
- Topical ingenol mebutate (Picato) 0.015% and 0.05% gel
  - Apply to the face and scalp once a day for 3 consecutive days.
  - Apply to the trunk and extremities once a day for 2 consecutive days.
    - It should only be used on one contiguous skin area of not >25 cm^2.
    - Cases of severe allergic reactions (including anaphylaxis) and herpes zoster reactivation unrelated to application errors have been reported.
  - Picato is no longer authorized in the EU because the marketing authorization was withdrawn on February 11, 2020 at the request of LEO Laboratories Ltd.
- Diclofenac (Solaraze) 3% gel
  - Apply BID for 60 to 90 days.

Second Line
- Topical tretinoin (Retin-A) or tazarotene (Tazorac): may be used to enhance the efficacy of topical fluorouracil
- Systemic retinoids: used infrequently

ADDITIONAL THERAPIES
Close monitoring with no treatment is an appropriate option for mild lesions.

SURGERY/OTHER PROCEDURES
- Cryosurgery ("freezing," liquid nitrogen)
  - Most common method for treating AK
  - Cure rate: 75–98.8%
  - May cause atrophy and hypopigmentation
  - May be superior to photodynamic therapy for thicker lesions
- Photodynamic therapy with a photosensitizer (e.g., aminolevulinic acid) and "blue light"
  - May clear >90% of AKs
  - Less scarring than cryotherapy
  - May be superior to cryotherapy, especially in the case of more extensive skin involvement
- Curettage and electrocautery (electrodesiccation and curettage [ED&C]; "scraping and burning")
- Medium-depth peels, especially for the treatment of extensive areas
- CO_2 laser therapy
- Dermabrasion
- Surgical excision (excisional biopsy)

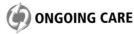 ONGOING CARE

FOLLOW-UP RECOMMENDATIONS

Patient Monitoring
Depends on associated malignancy and frequency with which new AKs appear

PATIENT EDUCATION
- Teach sun-protective techniques.
  - Limit outdoor activities between 10 AM and 4 PM.
  - Wear protective clothing and wide-brimmed hat.
  - Proper use (including reapplication) of sunscreens with SPF >30, preferably a preparation with broad-spectrum (UV-A and UV-B) protection
- Teach self-examination of skin (melanoma, squamous cell, basal cell).
- Patient education materials
  - http://dermnetnz.org/lesions/solar-keratoses.html

PROGNOSIS
Very good. A significant proportion of the lesions may resolve spontaneously (5), with regression rates of 20–30% per lesion per year.

COMPLICATIONS
- AKs are premalignant lesions that may progress to SCCs. The rate of malignant transformation is unclear; the reported percentages vary but range from 0.1% to a few percent per year per lesion.
- Patients with AKs are at increased risk for other cutaneous malignancies.
- Approximately 60% of SCCs arise from an AK precursor.

REFERENCES
1. Helfand M, Gorman AK, Mahon S, et al. *Actinic Keratoses: Final Report*. Rockville, MD: Agency for Healthcare Research and Quality; 2001.
2. de Berker D, McGregor JM, Hughes BR; for British Association of Dermatologists Therapy Guidelines and Audit Subcommittee. Guidelines for the management of actinic keratoses. *Br J Dermatol*. 2007;156(2):222–230.
3. Heppt MV, Steeb T, Ruzicka T, et al. Cryosurgery combined with topical interventions for actinic keratosis: a systematic review and meta-analysis. *Br J Dermatol*. 2019;180(4):740–748.
4. Jansen MHE, Kessels JPHM, Nelemans PJ, et al. Randomized trial of four treatment approaches for actinic keratosis. *N Engl J Med*. 2019;380(10): 935–946.
5. Criscione VD, Weinstock MA, Naylor MF, et al; for Department of Veterans Affairs Topical Tretinoin Chemoprevention Trial Group. Actinic keratoses: natural history and risk of malignant transformation in the Veterans Affairs Topical Tretinoin Chemoprevention Trial. *Cancer*. 2009;115(11):2523–2530.

ADDITIONAL READING
Feldman SR, Fleischer AB Jr. Progression of actinic keratosis to squamous cell carcinoma revisited: clinical and treatment implications. *Cutis*. 2011;87(4): 201–207.

CODES

ICD10
L57.0 Actinic keratosis

CLINICAL PEARLS
- AKs are premalignant lesions, although most will not progress to SCC and many will regress with time.
- Often more easily felt than seen
- Therapy-resistant lesions should be biopsied, especially on the face.

K

KERATOSIS, SEBORRHEIC

Michael T. Partin, MD • Karl T. Clebak, MD, MHA, FAAFP • Christopher Davis, MD, MPH

 BASICS

DESCRIPTION
- Common benign tumor of the epidermis formed from proliferation of keratinocytes
- Frequently appears in multiples on the head, neck, and trunk (sparing the palms and soles) of older individuals but may occur on any hair-bearing area of the body
- Typically presents as multiple, well-circumscribed, yellow to brown raised lesions that feel greasy, velvety, or warty; usually described as having a "stuck-on" appearance
- Clinical variants include the following:
  - Common seborrheic keratosis
  - Dermatosis papulosa nigra
  - Stucco keratosis
  - Flat seborrheic keratosis
  - Pedunculated seborrheic keratosis
- System(s) affected: integumentary
- Synonym(s): SK, verruca seborrhoica; seborrheic wart; senile wart; basal cell papilloma; verruca seni-lis; basal cell acanthoma; benign acanthokeratoma; barnacles of aging

EPIDEMIOLOGY
Incidence
- Predominant age: appear most commonly in those aged 31 to 50, and incidence increases with age, peaking at age 60 (1)
- Predominant sex: slightly more common and more extensive involvement in males
- Most common among Caucasians, except for the dermatosis papulosa nigra variant, which usually presents in darker skinned individuals

Prevalence
- 69–100% in patients >50 years of age
- The prevalence rate increases with advancing age.

ETIOLOGY AND PATHOPHYSIOLOGY
- Etiology remains largely unclear with ultraviolet (UV) light and genetics thought to be involved.
- The role of human papillomavirus is uncertain.

Genetics
An autosomal dominant inheritance pattern is suggested.

RISK FACTORS
- Advanced age
- Exposure to UV light and genetic predisposition are possible factors.

GENERAL PREVENTION
Sun protection methods may help prevent seborrheic keratoses from developing.

COMMONLY ASSOCIATED CONDITIONS
- Sign of Leser-Trélat: a paraneoplastic syndrome characterized by a rapid outbreak of multiple seborrheic keratoses often associated with an internal malignancy, most commonly adenocarcinoma (2). Seborrheic keratosis may resolve with treatment of the malignancy and reappear with neoplasm recurrence.
- Documentation of other cutaneous lesions, such as basal cell carcinoma, malignant melanoma, or squamous cell carcinoma, growing adjacent to or within a seborrheic keratosis, has been reported. The exact relationship between lesions is unclear.

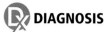 DIAGNOSIS

HISTORY
Generally asymptomatic, but trauma or irritation of the lesion may result in pruritus, erythema, bleeding, pain, and/or crusting.

PHYSICAL EXAM
- Typically begin as oval- or round-shaped, flat, dull, sharply demarcated patches
- As they mature, may develop into thicker, elevated, uneven, verrucous-like papules, plaques, or peduncles with a waxy or velvety surface and appear "stuck on" to the skin
- Commonly appear on sun-exposed areas of the body, predominately the head, neck, or trunk but may appear on any hair-bearing skin
- Surface tends to crumble when scratched.
- Vary in color (black, brown, tan, gray to white, or skin-colored) as well as size, ranging from several millimeters to several centimeters, but the average diameter is 0.5 to 1.0 cm
- Usually occur as multiples; patients having >100 is not uncommon.
- If irritated, may be bleeding, inflamed, painful, pruritic, or crusted
- Common clinical variants include:
  - Common seborrheic keratoses: on hair-bearing skin, usually on the face, neck, and trunk; verrucous-like, waxy, or velvety lesions that appear "stuck on" to the skin
  - Dermatosis papulosa nigra: small black papules that usually appear on the face, neck, chest, and upper back; symmetric distribution most common in darker skinned individuals, more common in females; most have a positive family history
  - Stucco keratoses: small gray-white, rough, verrucous papules; usually occur in large numbers on the lower extremities or forearms; more common in men
  - Flat seborrheic keratoses: oval-shaped, tan to brown patches or macules on face, chest, and upper extremities; increases with age
  - Pedunculated seborrheic keratoses: Hyperpigmented peduncles appear on areas of friction (neck, axilla).

DIFFERENTIAL DIAGNOSIS
Consider the following diagnoses if the seborrheic keratosis is:
- Pigmented
  - Malignant melanoma
  - Melanocytic nevus
  - Angiokeratoma
  - Pigmented basal cell carcinoma
- Lightly pigmented
  - Basal cell carcinoma
  - Bowen disease
  - Condyloma acuminatum
  - Fibroma
  - Verruca vulgaris
  - Eccrine poroma
  - Invasive squamous cell carcinoma
  - Acrochordon
  - Acrokeratosis verruciformis of Hopf
  - Follicular infundibulum tumor
- Flat
  - Solar lentigo
  - Verrucae planae juveniles
- Hyperkeratotic
  - Actinic keratosis

DIAGNOSTIC TESTS & INTERPRETATION
Initial Tests (lab, imaging)
Testing is generally not indicated unless diagnosis is unclear or malignancy is suspected.

Diagnostic Procedures/Other
- Diagnosis is generally made clinically.
- Biopsy and histologic exam should be performed if the seborrheic keratosis is atypical or has recently been inflamed or changed in appearance.
- Dermoscopy
  - Can assist in confirmation if diagnosis is uncertain
    - Common findings are pigment networks, pigmented globules, streaks, homogenous blue patterns, milia-like cysts, blotches, blue-whitish veils, hairpin vessels (3),(4).

Test Interpretation
Several histologic variants exist and can include the following:
- Acanthosis and papillomatosis due to basaloid cell proliferation
- "Squamous eddies" or squamous epithelial cell clusters
- Hyperpigmentation
- Hyperkeratosis
- Horn cysts
- Pseudocysts

 TREATMENT

- Treatment is typically performed for cosmetic concerns but is usually not required.
- Removal of seborrheic keratoses may be indicated if:
  - They are aesthetically displeasing or undesirable (common patient concern, although removal for this reason not always covered by insurance).
  - They are symptomatic (e.g., easily irritated, gets caught on clothing or jewelry).
  - There is a concern for their association with malignancy.

MEDICATION
- Generally, medical therapies are not considered first line, with surgical approaches being favored.
- The FDA recently approved HP40 (Eskata) as the first topical treatment for raised seborrheic keratosis, consisting of a 40% hydrogen peroxide solution. The treatment may require two office visits for application and has not shown better cosmetic results than other treatments (5)[C].
- Some reports exist regarding successful treatment of seborrheic keratoses using tazarotene, diclofenac gel, imiquimod, calcitriol, and dobesilate (1).
- Topical vitamin D analogs do not seem to be effective (1).

ISSUES FOR REFERRAL

- New seborrheic keratoses that appear abruptly, particularly if many occur within a short time frame concerning for Leser-Trélat sign
- A seborrheic keratosis becomes inflamed or changes in appearance.

SURGERY/OTHER PROCEDURES

- A surgical approach to treatment is generally preferred with the selected therapy depending on physician preference and availability of the treatment.
- The following procedures can be utilized in practice:
  - Cryotherapy (liquid nitrogen)
    - Spray flat lesions for 5 to 10 seconds; may require more time or additional treatments if the seborrheic keratosis is thicker
    - Possible complications include scarring, hypopigmentation, recurrence.
  - Curettage
    - Curette (metal hand tool with small scoop at the tip) is used to scrape off the lesion.
    - Requires local anesthesia
  - Electrodessication
    - Tool with needle-like metal tip that uses electric current to destroy affected tissue
    - Requires local anesthesia
  - Shave excision
    - Scalpel or flexible razor blade is used to remove lesion.
    - Requires local anesthesia
  - Laser
    - Intense beams of light are used to burn and vaporize the lesion.
    - Requires local anesthesia
  - Chemical peel
    - An application of chemical solution (e.g., Trichloroacetic acid) is used to remove the top layer of skin.
- In a small study of 25 patients, there were no statistically significant differences in patient's ratings of cosmetic appearance between cryotherapy and curettage, although a majority of patients preferred cryotherapy over curettage due to decreased wound care after the procedure (6)[B].

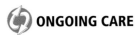 ONGOING CARE

FOLLOW-UP RECOMMENDATIONS

Patient Monitoring

After initial diagnosis, follow-up is not usually required unless

- Inflammation or irritation develops.
- There is a change in appearance.
- New seborrheic keratoses suddenly appear.

PATIENT EDUCATION

- Sun-protective methods may help reduce seborrheic keratosis development.
- Patient education materials
  - http://www.aad.org/public/diseases/bumps-and-growths/seborrheic-keratoses
  - http://www.cdc.gov/cancer/skin/basic_info/prevention.htm

PROGNOSIS

- Seborrheic keratoses generally do not become malignant.
- Sign of Leser-Trélat usually represents a poor prognosis.

COMPLICATIONS

- Irritation and inflammation due to mechanical irritation (e.g., from clothing, jewelry)
- Possible complications of surgical treatment include hypopigmentation, hyperpigmentation, scarring, incomplete removal, and recurrence.
- Misdiagnosis (rare)

REFERENCES

1. Wollina U. Recent advances in managing and understanding seborrheic keratosis. *F1000Res.* 2019;8:F1000 Faculty Rev-1520.
2. Husain Z, Ho JK, Hantash BM. Sign and pseudo-sign of Leser-Trélat: case reports and a review of the literature. *J Drugs Dermatol.* 2013;12(5):e79–e87.
3. Marghoob AA, Usatine RP, Jaimes N. Dermoscopy for the family physician. *Am Fam Physician.* 2013;88(7):441–450.
4. Yélamos O, Braun RP, Liopyris K, et al. Dermoscopy and dermatopathology correlates of cutaneous neoplasms. *J Am Acad Dermatol.* 2019;80(2):341–363. doi:10.1016/j.jaad.2018.07.073.
5. Hydrogen peroxide 40% (Eskata) for seborrheic keratoses. *Med Lett Drugs Ther.* 2018;60(1556):157–158.
6. Wood LD, Stucki JK, Hollenbeak CS, et al. Effectiveness of cryosurgery vs curettage in the treatment of seborrheic keratoses. *JAMA Dermatol.* 2013;149(1):108–109.

ADDITIONAL READING

- Culbertson GR. 532-nm diode laser treatment of seborrheic keratoses with color enhancement. *Dermatol Surg.* 2008;34(4):525–528.
- Draelos ZD, Rizer RL, Trookman NS. A comparison of postprocedural wound care treatments: do antibiotic-based ointments improve outcomes? *J Am Acad Dermatol.* 2011;64(Suppl 3):S23–S29.
- Garcia MS, Azari R, Eisen DB. Treatment of dermatosis papulosa nigra in 10 patients: a comparison trial of electrodesiccation, pulsed dye laser, and curettage. *Dermatol Surg.* 2010;36(12):1968–1972.
- Georgieva IA, Mauerer A, Groesser L, et al. Low incidence of oncogenic EGFR, HRAS, and KRAS mutations in seborrheic keratosis. *Am J Dermatopathol.* 2014;36(8):635–642.

- Herron MD, Bowen AR, Krueger GG. Seborrheic keratoses: a study comparing the standard cryosurgery with topical calcipotriene, topical tazarotene, and topical imiquimod. *Int J Dermatol.* 2004;43(4):300–302.
- Higgins JC, Maher MH, Douglas MS. Diagnosing common benign skin tumors. *Am Fam Physician.* 2015;92(7):601–607.
- Husain Z, Ho JK, Hantash BM. Sign and pseudo-sign of Leser-Trélat: case reports and a review of the literature. *J Drugs Dermatol.* 2013;12(5):e79–e87.
- Krupashankar DS; and IADVL Dermatosurgery Task Force. Standard guidelines of care: CO_2 laser for removal of benign skin lesions and resurfacing. *Indian J Dermatol Venereol Leprol.* 2008;74(Suppl 7):S61–S67.
- Luba MC, Bangs SA, Mohler AM, et al. Common benign skin tumors. *Am Fam Physician.* 2003;67(4):729–738.
- Rajesh G, Thappa DM, Jaisankar TJ, et al. Spectrum of seborrheic keratoses in South Indians: a clinical and dermoscopic study. *Indian J Dermatol Venereol Leprol.* 2011;77(4):483–488.
- Saeed AK, Salmo N. Epidermal growth factor receptor expression in mice skin upon ultraviolet B exposure—seborrheic keratosis as a coincidental and unique finding. *Adv Biomed Res.* 2012;1:59.
- Taylor SC, Averyhart AN, Heath CR. Postprocedural wound-healing efficacy following removal of dermatosis papulosa nigra lesions in an African American population: a comparison of a skin protectant ointment and a topical antibiotic. *J Am Acad Dermatol.* 2011;64(Suppl 3):S30–S35.

 CODES

ICD10

- L82.1 Other seborrheic keratosis
- L82.0 Inflamed seborrheic keratosis

CLINICAL PEARLS

- Seborrheic keratoses are one of the most common benign tumors of the epidermis, and frequency increases with age.
- While seborrheic keratoses do not need to be removed, there are many options for doing so if patients request this (with surgical methods generally being preferred).
- Underlying internal malignancy should be considered if large numbers of seborrheic keratoses appear suddenly.

K

KNEE PAIN

Lee A. Mancini, MD, CSCS*D, CSN • Emily J. Eshleman, DO, MS • Michael J. Maddaleni, MD

 BASICS

DESCRIPTION

A common outpatient complaint with a broad differential

- Knee pain may be acute, chronic, or an acute exacerbation of a chronic condition.
- Trauma, overuse, and degenerative change are frequent causes.
- A detailed history, including patient's age, pain onset and location, mechanism of injury, and associated symptoms can help narrow the differential diagnosis.
- A thorough and focused examination of the knee (as well as the back, hips, and ankles) helps to establish the correct diagnosis and appropriate treatment.

EPIDEMIOLOGY

Incidence
- Knee complaints account for 12.5 million primary care visits annually.
- The incidence of knee osteoarthritis (OA) is 240 cases per 100,000 person-years.

Prevalence
- The knee is a common site of lower extremity injury.
  - Patellar tendinopathy and patellofemoral syndrome are the most common causes of knee pain in runners.
- OA of the hip/knee is 11th cause of global disability and 38th most common cause of disability-adjusted life years (DALYs).

ETIOLOGY AND PATHOPHYSIOLOGY
- Trauma (ligament or meniscal injury, fracture, dislocation)
- Overuse (tendinopathy, patellofemoral syndrome, bursitis, apophysitis)
- Age (arthritis, degenerative conditions in older patients; apophysitis in younger patients)
- Rheumatologic (rheumatoid arthritis [RA], systemic lupus erythematosus [SLE])
- Crystal arthropathies (gout, pseudogout)
- Infectious (bacterial, postviral, Lyme disease)
- Referred pain (hip, back)
- Vascular (popliteal artery aneurysm, deep vein thrombosis)
- Others (tumor, cyst, plica)

RISK FACTORS
- Obesity
- Malalignment
- Poor flexibility, muscle imbalance, or weakness
- Rapid increases in training frequency and intensity
- Improper footwear, training surfaces, technique
- Activities that involve cutting, jumping, pivoting, deceleration, kneeling
- Previous injuries

GENERAL PREVENTION
- Maintain normal body mass index.
- Proper exercise technique, volume, and equipment; avoid overtraining.
- Correct postural strength and flexibility imbalances.

COMMONLY ASSOCIATED CONDITIONS
- Fracture, contusion
- Effusion, hemarthrosis
- Patellar dislocation/subluxation
- Meniscal or ligamentous injury
- Tendinopathy, bursitis
- Osteochondral injury
- OA, septic arthritis
- Muscle strain

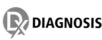 **DIAGNOSIS**

HISTORY
- Pain location, quality, and mechanism of injury guide diagnostic reasoning (also see "Differential Diagnosis"):
  - Diffuse pain: OA, patellofemoral pain syndrome, chondromalacia
  - Pain ascending/descending stairs: meniscal injury, patellofemoral pain syndrome
  - Pain with prolonged sitting, standing from sitting: patellofemoral pain syndrome
  - Mechanical symptoms (locking): meniscal injury
- Mechanism of injury:
  - Hyperextension, deceleration, cutting: anterior cruciate ligament (ACL) injury
  - Hyperflexion, fall on flexed knee, "dashboard injury": posterior cruciate ligament (PCL) injury
  - Lateral force (valgus load): medial collateral injury
  - Twisting on planted foot: meniscal injury
- Effusion:
  - Rapid onset (2 hours): ACL tear, patellar subluxation/dislocation, large meniscal tear, tibial plateau fracture. Hemarthrosis is common.
  - Slower onset (24 to 36 hours), smaller: meniscal injury, ligament sprain, arthritis
  - Swelling behind the knee: popliteal (Baker) cyst

PHYSICAL EXAM
- Observe gait (antalgia); patellar tracking
- Inspect for malalignment, atrophy, swelling, ecchymosis, or erythema.
- Palpate for effusion, warmth, and tenderness.
- Evaluate active and passive range of motion (ROM) and flexibility of quadriceps and hamstrings.
- Evaluate strength and muscle tone.
- Note joint instability, locking, and catching.
- Evaluate hip ROM, strength, and stability.
- Special tests:
  - Patellar apprehension test: patellar instability; patellar grind test: patellofemoral pain or OA (1)
  - Lachman test (more sensitive and specific), pivot shift, anterior drawer, lever sign: ACL integrity
  - Posterior drawer, posterior sag sign: PCL integrity

- Valgus/varus stress test: medial/lateral collateral ligament (MCL/LCL) integrity
- McMurray test, Apley grind test, Thessaly test: meniscal injury
- Ober test: iliotibial band (ITB) tightness
- Dial test: positive with posterolateral corner laxity
- Patellar tilt test and squatting may help suggest patellofemoral pain syndrome.
- Patella facet tenderness suggests OA or patellofemoral pain syndrome (1).

DIFFERENTIAL DIAGNOSIS
- Acute onset: fracture, contusion, cruciate or collateral ligament tear, meniscal tear, patellar dislocation/subluxation; if systemic symptoms: septic arthritis, gout, pseudogout, Lyme disease, osteomyelitis
- Insidious onset: patellofemoral pain syndrome/chondromalacia, ITB syndrome, OA, RA, bursitis, tumor, tendinopathy, loose body, bipartite patella, degenerative meniscal tear
- Anterior pain: patellofemoral pain syndrome, patellar injury, patellar tendinopathy, pre- or suprapatellar bursitis, tibial apophysitis, fat pad impingement, quadriceps tendinopathy, OA (1)
- Posterior pain: PCL injury, posterior horn meniscal injury, popliteal cyst or aneurysm, hamstring or gastrocnemius injury, deep venous thrombosis (DVT)
- Medial pain: MCL injury, medial meniscal injury, pes anserine bursitis, medial plica syndrome, OA
- Lateral pain: LCL injury, lateral meniscal injury, ITB syndrome, OA

DIAGNOSTIC TESTS & INTERPRETATION

Initial Tests (lab, imaging)
- Suspected septic joint, gout, pseudogout:
  - Arthrocentesis with cell count, Gram stain, culture, protein/glucose, synovial fluid analysis
- Suspected RA:
  - CBC, erythrocyte sedimentation rate (ESR), rheumatoid factor
- Consider Lyme titer.
- Radiographs to rule out fracture in patients with acute knee trauma (Ottawa Rules):
  - Age >55 years or
  - Tenderness at the patella or fibular head or
  - Inability to bear weight four steps or
  - Inability to flex knee to 90 degrees
- Radiographs help diagnose OA, osteochondral lesions, patellofemoral pain syndrome:
  - Weight-bearing, upright anteroposterior, lateral, merchant/sunrise, notch/tunnel views

Follow-Up Tests & Special Considerations
- MRI is "gold standard" for soft tissue imaging.
- Ultrasound may help diagnose tendinopathy.
- CT can further elucidate fracture.

Diagnostic Procedures/Other
Arthroscopy may be beneficial in the diagnosis of certain conditions, including meniscus and ligament injuries.

Geriatric Considerations

OA, degenerative meniscal tears, and gout are more common in middle-aged and elderly populations.

Pediatric Considerations

- 3 million pediatric sports injuries occur annually.
- Look for physeal/apophyseal and joint surface injuries in skeletally immature:
  - Acute: patellar subluxation, avulsion fractures, ACL tear
  - Overuse: patellofemoral pain syndrome, apophysitis, osteochondritis dissecans, patellar tendonitis, stress fracture
  - Others: neoplasm, juvenile RA, infection, referred pain from slipped capital femoral epiphysis

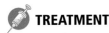 TREATMENT

GENERAL MEASURES

Acute injury: PRICEMM therapy (**p**rotection, **r**elative rest, **i**ce, **c**ompression, **e**levation, **m**edications, **m**odalities)

MEDICATION

First Line

- Oral medications:
  - Acetaminophen: up to 3 g/day; safe and effective in OA
  - Nonsteroidal anti-inflammatory drugs (NSAIDs):
    - Ibuprofen: 200 to 800 mg TID
    - Naproxen: 250 to 500 mg BID:
      - Useful for acute sprains, strains
      - Useful for short-term pain reduction in OA. Long-term use is not recommended due to side effects.
      - Not recommended for fracture, stress fracture, chronic muscle injury; may be associated with delayed healing; low dose and brief course only if necessary
  - Tramadol/opioids: not recommended as first-line treatment; can be used with acute injuries for severe pain
  - Celecoxib: 200 mg QD may be effective in OA with less GI side effects than NSAIDs (2)[A].
- Topical medications:
  - Topical NSAIDs provide pain relief in OA and may be more tolerable than oral medications (3)[A].
  - Topical capsaicin may be an adjuvant for pain management in OA.
- Injections:
  - Intra-articular corticosteroid injection may provide short-term benefit in knee OA stage 2 or 3.
  - Viscosupplementation may reduce pain and improve function in patients with OA. Peak effectiveness is 5 to 13 weeks.
  - Equivocal evidence for platelet-rich plasma (PRP) compared to viscosupplementation
  - Prolotherapy injections can provide some long-term relief.
  - Stem cell therapy with insufficient data

ISSUES FOR REFERRAL

- Acute trauma, young athletic patient
- Joint instability
- Lack of improvement with conservative measures
- Salter-Harris physeal fractures (pediatrics)

ADDITIONAL THERAPIES

- Physical therapy is recommended as initial treatment for patellofemoral pain and tendinopathies.
- Muscle strengthening improves outcome in OA.
- Foot orthoses, taping, acupuncture
- May need bracing for stability

SURGERY/OTHER PROCEDURES

- Surgery may be indicated for certain injuries (e.g., ACL tear in competitive athletes or grade IV OA).
- Chronic conditions refractory to conservative therapy may require surgical intervention.

COMPLEMENTARY & ALTERNATIVE MEDICINE

May reduce pain and improve function in early OA:

- Glucosamine sulfate (500 mg TID)
- Chondroitin (400 mg TID)
- Turmeric or curcumin 1,000 mg/day
- Collagen hydrolysates 10 g daily
- S-adenosyl-l-methionine (SAMe), ginger extract, methylsulfonylmethane: less reliable improvement with inconsistent supporting evidence
- Acupuncture: need to do 4 weeks or 10 sessions

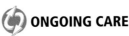 ONGOING CARE

FOLLOW-UP RECOMMENDATIONS

- Activity modification in overuse conditions
- Rehabilitative exercise in OA:
  - Low-impact exercise: walking, swimming, cycling
  - Strength, ROM, and proprioception training

Patient Monitoring

- Rehabilitation after initial treatment of acute injury
- In chronic and overuse conditions, assess functional status, rehabilitation adherence, and pain control at follow-up visit.

DIET

Weight reduction by 10% improved function by 28%.

PATIENT EDUCATION

- Review activity modifications.
- Encourage active role in the rehabilitation process.
- Review medication risks and benefits.

PROGNOSIS

Varies with diagnosis, injury severity, chronicity of condition, patient motivation to participate in rehabilitation, and whether surgery is required

COMPLICATIONS

- Disability
- Arthritis
- Chronic joint instability
- Deconditioning

REFERENCES

1. Hong E, Kraft MC. Evaluating anterior knee pain. *Med Clin North Am*. 2014;98(4):697–717.
2. Bijlsma JW, Berenbaum F, Lafeber FP. Osteoarthritis: an update with relevance for clinical practice. *Lancet*. 2011;377(9783):2115–2126.
3. Zeng C, Wei J, Persson MSM, et al. Relative efficacy and safety of topical non-steroidal anti-inflammatory drugs for osteoarthritis: a systematic review and network meta-analysis of randomised controlled trials and observational studies. *Br J Sports Med*. 2018;52(10):642–650.

ADDITIONAL READING

Collins NJ, Bisset LM, Crossley KM, et al. Efficacy of nonsurgical interventions for anterior knee pain: systematic review and meta-analysis of randomized trials. *Sports Med*. 2012;42(1):31–49.

 SEE ALSO

Algorithms: Knee Pain; Popliteal Mass

 CODES

ICD10

- M25.569 Pain in unspecified knee
- M17.9 Osteoarthritis of knee, unspecified
- M76.50 Patellar tendinitis, unspecified knee

CLINICAL PEARLS

- A careful history (location/quality of pain and mechanism of injury) targets diagnosis for most causes of knee pain.
- Consider ligamentous injury, meniscal tear, and fracture for patients presenting with acute knee pain.
- Consider OA, patellofemoral pain syndrome, tendinopathy, bursitis, and stress fracture in patients presenting with more chronic symptoms.
- Consider physeal, apophyseal, or articular cartilage injury in young patients presenting with knee pain.
- The presence of an effusion in a patient <30 years of age indicates a significant injury.
- Referred pain from the hip (slipped capital femoral epiphysis, Legg-Calvé-Perthes disease) can present as knee pain.

K

LABYRINTHITIS

Joseph D. Hogue, MD, MBA • Esha Rajiv Sharma, MD, MPH

 BASICS

DESCRIPTION

- The sudden onset of vertigo, accompanied by sensorineural hearing loss and tinnitus, lasting hours to days, and caused by acute inflammation or infection of the labyrinth
- Can be categorized as suppurative or serous/toxic labyrinthitis (1)
- Labyrinthitis is a clinical diagnosis in absence of neurologic deficits.
- Typically presents with a subjective sense of motion or room-spinning vertigo lasting for hours or days and often sudden unilateral sensorineural hearing loss
- Often associated with vestibular hypofunction of the involved ear. Peripheral vertigo improves over time with central compensation. Hearing loss generally improves in the case of serous labyrinthitis but is permanent in the case of suppurative labyrinthitis.
- System(s) affected: nervous, special sensory (auditory and vestibular)

ALERT

- "Vertigo" and "dizziness" are commonly used terms. Clarify symptoms by giving options of alternative descriptions such as light-headedness, disequilibrium, room-spinning vertigo, or imbalance.
- Hearing loss and duration of symptoms can help narrow the differential diagnosis in patients with vertigo.
- Vestibular neuritis/neuronitis occurs due to inflammation of the vestibular nerve causing vertigo lasting hours to days without the auditory symptoms of labyrinthitis (2).
- Benign paroxysmal positional vertigo (BPPV) is the most common cause of vertigo. Unlike labyrinthitis, BPPV is episodic, with severe symptoms lasting <1 minute. BPPV is diagnosed using the Dix-Hallpike maneuver. Unlike labyrinthitis, it is not associated with hearing loss.
- Ménière disease is more episodic than labyrinthitis; it comes and goes, rather than remaining continuous, and is associated with the triad of episodic vertigo, tinnitus, and hearing loss.
- Vestibular migraine is the second most common cause of recurrent vertigo, lasting hours and usually with a history of migraine. Up to 10% of cases can occur without headaches (2).

EPIDEMIOLOGY

- Data is lacking for labyrinthitis alone.
- Most common in 30 to 50 years of age (3)
- 10% of all patients seen for dizziness, if vestibular neuritis is included (4)
- Predominant sex: female = male

Incidence

- Estimated incidence of 3.5 per 100,000 if including vestibular neuritis (3)
- Viral labyrinthitis is the most common etiology.
- Suppurative labyrinthitis secondary to otitis media or meningitis is increasingly rare.

Prevalence

20–30% of adults see a health care provider for vertigo in their lifetimes (3). True labyrinthitis is rare.

ETIOLOGY AND PATHOPHYSIOLOGY

- Acute inflammation and damage to the labyrinth, involving both the vestibular apparatus and cochlea
- Viral or bacterial toxins may pass into the labyrinth directly from the middle ear to labyrinth via the round or oval window, in the case of serous labyrinthitis.
- Bacterial invasion of the inner ear, either from a middle ear infection or meningitis, occurs in suppurative labyrinthitis (1).
- Infections
  - Common viral: *cytomegalovirus*, mumps, varicella zoster, rubeola, influenza, parainfluenza, herpes simplex, adenovirus, *coxsackievirus*, respiratory syncytial virus, HIV
  - Common bacterial: *Streptococcus pneumoniae*, *Haemophilus influenzae*, *Moraxella catarrhalis*, *Neisseria meningitidis*, *Streptococcus* spp., *Staphylococcus* spp., *Borrelia burgdorferi*
  - Treponemal: *Treponema pallidum*

Genetics

No known genetic link

RISK FACTORS

- Viral upper respiratory infection
- Otitis media
- Cholesteatoma
- Head trauma
- Meningitis

GENERAL PREVENTION

- Early treatment of acute otitis media to prevent complications
- Scheduled immunizations (to prevent common viral pathogens)
- Prevent maternal transmission of pathogens, including syphilis and HIV.

COMMONLY ASSOCIATED CONDITIONS

- Viral upper respiratory infection
- Otitis media
- Cholesteatoma
- Head injury

Rx **DIAGNOSIS**

HISTORY

- Vertigo *AND* sensorineural hearing loss in one ear
- Vertigo is acute in onset and lasts hours to days.
- Nausea and vomiting are common.
- Fullness of affected ear
- Tinnitus of affected ear (roaring, ringing)
- Upper respiratory tract infection symptoms
- Otorrhea or otalgia (not common with viral causes)
- Severe headache, fever, and nuchal rigidity in the setting of meningitis
- Recurrent symptoms should raise suspicion for autoimmune causes.
- Profound imbalance or associated focal neurologic signs are not typical and should prompt imaging.

PHYSICAL EXAM

- Nystagmus
  - Fast-beating nystagmus toward affected ear during the acute phase
  - Fast-beating nystagmus away from affected ear during the convalescent phase, 48 to 72 hours later
- Symptoms abate with eyes open and visual fixation.
- Otologic exam may be unremarkable in the setting of viral labyrinthitis.
- Serous/purulent effusion may be present in the middle ear.
- Retraction of the tympanic membrane and keratinaceous debris may be present with cholesteatoma.

DIFFERENTIAL DIAGNOSIS

- Vestibular neuritis/neuronitis (vertigo without hearing loss)
- BPPV: episodic, vertigo lasting seconds/minutes, worse when lying down or looking up
- Ménière disease associated with the triad of episodic vertigo, tinnitus, and hearing loss
- Vestibular migraine
- Autoimmune inner ear disease
- Postconcussive syndrome
- Acute otitis media
- Ototoxicity
- Cardiovascular accident (CVA)/brainstem infarct
- Cerebellopontine-angle tumors (e.g., vestibular schwannoma)
- Less common etiologies: parainfectious encephalomyelitis or cranial polyneuritis, Ramsay Hunt syndrome, HIV infection, syphilis, temporal lobe epilepsy, perilymphatic fistula, superior canal dehiscence, idiopathic sudden single-sided deafness, multiple sclerosis, vasculitis (cerebral or systemic)

DIAGNOSTIC TESTS & INTERPRETATION

- Routine lab studies are not helpful unless an autoimmune cause is suspected.
- Consider culture of otorrhea or middle ear fluid to direct antibiotic choice.
- CT of the temporal bone may be indicated in the setting of complicated otitis media or cholesteatoma.
- Consider lumbar puncture only if meningitis is suspected.
- Consider screening for syphilis or HIV when clinically indicated by risk factors or clinical history.
- Imaging is not required for the diagnosis of acute labyrinthitis.
- With acute sensorineural hearing loss or other associated neurologic symptoms, an MRI of the internal auditory canals and/or MRA of the brain and brainstem are recommended.

Follow-Up Tests & Special Considerations

Labyrinthitis ossificans is fibrosis of the internal auditory canal following bacterial meningitis and is thought to occur due to a suppurative labyrinthitis. This can occur rapidly, especially after *S. pneumoniae* meningitis.

Diagnostic Procedures/Other
- Audiogram should be obtained.
- Vestibular tests are not typically indicated in the acute setting. If vertigo and dizziness persist after expected resolution of symptoms, videonystagmography should be used.

Test Interpretation
- Audiogram may show varying degrees of both sensorineural hearing loss and discrimination loss.
- Caloric testing may show relative weakness of the horizontal semicircular canal of the affected side. Sensitivity and specificity of this test are variable within literature.

 TREATMENT

- Symptom management and reassurance in the acute phase
- Vestibular suppressants as needed (see "Medication") for severe acute attacks of vertigo only. Patients should be advised *NOT* to use these medications as scheduled medications or for prophylaxis without symptoms because this can delay central compensation (2)[B].
- Sudden single-sided sensorineural hearing loss should be managed with high-dose steroids (oral and/or intratympanic) as soon as possible, ideally within 2 weeks. Steroids have not been found to definitively improve vestibular symptoms (5)[B].
- Vestibular rehabilitation is the mainstay of treatment for persistent vertigo and dizziness and has been shown to be safe and effective management for unilateral peripheral vestibular dysfunction (6)[A].
- Patients should begin exercises as soon as the acute phase resolves and movement is tolerable, generally within 2 to 3 days of onset (4).
- For suppurative labyrinthitis, appropriate antibiotics to eradicate infection. Surgical intervention may also be required with tympanostomy tubes or mastoidectomy, depending on the extent of middle ear involvement.

GENERAL MEASURES
Vestibular exercises for prolonged symptoms and unilateral vestibular loss have been shown to alleviate postural control.

MEDICATION
Use of the following drugs should be on a PRN basis. Benzodiazepines can also assist with the anxiety associated with vertigo. No patient should take vestibular suppressants as a chronic medication because they can block central compensation.
- Vestibular suppressants
  - Lorazepam (Ativan) 0.5 to 2.0 mg SL/PO BID PRN or diazepam (Valium) 2 to 5 mg QID PO PRN
  - Meclizine (Antivert, Bonine, Zentrip [dissolvable]) 12.5 to 25.0 mg PO BID–TID PRN
  - Dimenhydrinate (Dramamine) 25 to 50 mg PO q4–6h PRN
- Antiemetics
  - Ondansetron (Zofran) 4 to 8 mg PO TID PRN or granisetron (Kytril) 1 mg PO TID PRN
  - Meclizine (Antivert, Bonine) 12.5 to 25.0 mg PO q4h PRN

- Promethazine (Phenergan) 12.5 to 25.0 mg PO/PR QID PRN or prochlorperazine (Compazine) 25 mg PR BID PRN
- Metoclopramide (Reglan) 10 mg PO TID PRN
- Antivirals
  - Acyclovir 800 mg PO 5 times per day for 7 days can be used in cases associated with herpes.
- Steroids
  - Prednisone 1 mg/kg/day up to maximum 60 mg daily for 1 week, followed by 1 week taper
  - Methylprednisolone initially 100 mg PO daily and then tapered to 10 mg PO daily over 3 weeks
  - Dexamethasone 0.4 to 0.8 mL of 24 mg/mL strength given via transtympanic injection for three to four sessions; can be used for salvage therapy
  - Given early in the setting of bacterial meningitis, may decrease the otologic sequelae, specifically labyrinthitis ossificans
  - Used in treatment of labyrinthitis for associated sudden sensorineural hearing loss, ideally within the first 2 weeks

Geriatric Considerations
- Avoid excessive use of scopolamine, meclizine, and other vestibular suppressants following the initial event because this will delay central compensation.
- Benzodiazepines are the preferred vestibular suppressant treatment but do increase the risk of falls in older persons.

Pregnancy Considerations
Dimenhydrinate, diphenhydramine, ondansetron, granisetron, and metoclopramide are pregnancy Category B.

First Line
- Benzodiazepines, which are better vestibular suppressants, are preferred over antihistamine/anticholinergics such as meclizine. Sublingual benzodiazepines are very effective for vertigo and should be considered first-line therapy.
- Urgent steroid treatment in acute setting

ISSUES FOR REFERRAL
- Consider neurology referral for suspected central causes of vertigo or dizziness.
- Consider otolaryngology/neurotology referral for progressive hearing loss and vertigo, or in cases of suppurative labyrinthitis requiring surgical intervention.

ADMISSION, INPATIENT, AND NURSING CONSIDERATIONS
Patients with systemic infection or intractable nausea and vomiting may need to be hospitalized for intravenous fluids and medications.

 ONGOING CARE

FOLLOW-UP RECOMMENDATIONS
Patient Monitoring
Follow hearing loss weekly with audiograms until hearing stabilizes. Acute vertiginous symptoms may last up to 6 weeks. Residual symptoms have been documented to last years.

DIET
Avoid alcohol because this may exacerbate symptoms.

PATIENT EDUCATION
Opening eyes with visual fixation should improve symptoms, whereas closing eyes may make symptoms worse. Minimize rapid head movement until symptoms resolve. Avoid vestibular suppressants long term because this can inhibit central compensation.

COMPLICATIONS
Permanent hearing loss, more common with bacterial causes, and chronic impairment of balance

REFERENCES
1. Kaya S, Schachern PA, Tsuprun V, et al. Deterioration of vestibular cells in labyrinthitis. *Ann Otol Rhinol Laryngol*. 2017;126(2):89–95.
2. Sandhu JS, Rea PA. Clinical examination and management of the dizzy patient. *Br J Hosp Med (Lond)*. 2016;77(12):692–698.
3. Neuhauser HK, Lempert T. Vertigo: epidemiologic aspects. *Semin Neurol*. 2009;29(5):473–481.
4. Wipperman J. Dizziness and vertigo. *Prim Care*. 2014;41(1):115–131.
5. Yoo MH, Yang CJ, Kim SA, et al. Efficacy of steroid therapy based on symptomatic and functional improvement in patients with vestibular neuritis: a prospective randomized controlled trial. *Eur Arch Otorhinolaryngol*. 2017;274(6):2443–2451.
6. McDonnell M, Hillier SL. Vestibular rehabilitation for unilateral peripheral vestibular dysfunction. *Cochrane Database Syst Rev*. 2015;(1):CD005397.

 SEE ALSO

Ménière Disease; Postconcussion Syndrome (Mild Traumatic Brain Injury); Tinnitus

CODES
ICD10
- H83.02 Labyrinthitis, left ear
- H83.01 Labyrinthitis, right ear
- H83.09 Labyrinthitis, unspecified ear

CLINICAL PEARLS
- Ask patients to describe symptoms in their own words; alternative symptoms include light-headedness, vertigo, disequilibrium, or imbalance.
- Benzodiazepines are better vestibular suppressants and are preferred over antihistamine/anticholinergics such as meclizine. Vestibular suppressants should be used for short duration only because these will delay central compensation.
- Episodic vertigo tends to be caused by BPPV or Ménière disease, whereas persistent vertigo with sensorineural hearing loss and tinnitus is more consistent with labyrinthitis.
- Vestibular neuritis would be considered if there was no hearing involvement.

L

LACTOSE INTOLERANCE

Nihal K. Patel, MD

BASICS

DESCRIPTION

- Lactose intolerance is a syndrome of abdominal pain, bloating, and flatulence after the ingestion of lactose.
- Lactose malabsorption results from a reduction in lactase activity in the brush border of the small intestinal mucosa.
- Lactase activity peaks at birth then decreases after the first few months of life, declining continuously throughout life. 75% of adults worldwide exhibit a decline in lactase activity after birth. *Only 50% of lactase activity is needed to digest lactose without causing symptoms of lactose intolerance.*
  - Congenital lactose intolerance: very rare
  - Primary lactose intolerance: common in adults who develop low lactase levels after childhood
  - Secondary lactose intolerance: inability to digest lactose caused by any condition injuring the intestinal mucosa (e.g., infectious enteritis, celiac disease, eosinophilic gastroenteritis, or inflammatory bowel disease) or a reduction of available mucosal surface (e.g., resection).
- Lactose malabsorption may be asymptomatic and is equally common in healthy patients and in those with functional bowel disorders.
- System(s) affected: endocrine/metabolic, gastrointestinal

Pediatric Considerations

- Primary lactose intolerance begins in late childhood.
- No consensus on whether young children (<5 years of age) should avoid lactose following diarrheal illness
- Lactose-free formulas are available.
- Exclude milk protein allergy.

EPIDEMIOLOGY

Incidence

- ≥50% of infants with acute or chronic diarrheal disease have lactose intolerance; particularly common with rotavirus infection
- Lactose intolerance is common with giardiasis, ascariasis, irritable bowel syndrome (IBS), tropical and nontropical sprue, and AIDS malabsorptive syndrome.

Prevalence

- In South America, Africa, and Asia, rates of lactose intolerance are >50%.
- In the United States, the prevalence is 15% among whites, 53% among Hispanics, and 80% among African Americans.
- In Europe, lactose intolerance varies from 15% in Scandinavian countries to 70% in Italy.
- Predominant age:
  - Primary: teenage and adult
  - Secondary: depends on underlying condition
- Predominant sex: male = female

ETIOLOGY AND PATHOPHYSIOLOGY

- Primary lactose intolerance: The normal decline in lactase activity in the intestinal mucosa is genetically determined and permanent after weaning from breast milk.
- Secondary lactose intolerance: associated with gastroenteritis in children; also associated with any gastrointestinal infection or inflammation of the small intestine with resultant lactose malabsorption in both adults and children

Genetics

- In whites, lactase deficiency is associated with a single nucleotide polymorphism (SNP) consisting of a nucleotide switch of T for C 13910 bp on chromosome 2. This results in variants of CC-13910 (lactase nonpersistence) OR CT-13910/TT-13910 (lactase persistence) (1).
- SNP (C/T-13910) is associated with lactase persistence in northern Europeans.
- Other SNPs (G/C-14010, T/G-13915, and C/G-13907) have been linked to lactase persistence in some patients of African descent.

RISK FACTORS

- Adult-onset lactase deficiency has wide geographic variation.
- Age:
  - Signs and symptoms usually do not become apparent until after age 6 to 7 years.
  - Symptoms may not be apparent until adulthood, depending on dietary lactose intake and rate of decline of intestinal lactase activity.
  - Lactase activity correlates with age, regardless of symptoms.

GENERAL PREVENTION

Lactose avoidance relieves symptoms. Patients can learn what level of lactose is tolerable in their diet.

COMMONLY ASSOCIATED CONDITIONS

- Tropical or nontropical sprue
- Giardiasis
- IBS or other functional bowel disorders
- Small intestinal bacterial overgrowth (SIBO)
- Celiac disease

Ⓡ DIAGNOSIS

- Lactose intolerance can be presumed in patients manifesting mild symptoms after ingestion of significant amounts of lactose (such as >2 servings of dairy per day), with resolution of symptoms after avoidance of lactose-containing foods for 1 week.
- A positive lactose hydrogen breath test is confirmatory.
- Lactose intolerance can mimic symptoms of functional gastrointestinal disorders. Lactose intolerance can also be a coexisting condition.

HISTORY

- Assess daily lactose consumption.
- A single dose of lactose (12 g, equivalent to 1 cup of milk) consumed alone produces no or minor symptoms in persons with lactose intolerance.
- Lactose doses of 15 to 18 g are well tolerated with other nutrients. Doses >18 g cause progressively more symptoms, and quantities >50 g elicit symptoms in most individuals.
- Symptoms arise 30 minutes to 2 hours after consumption of lactose-containing products.
- Symptoms include bloating, flatulence, cramping abdominal discomfort, and diarrhea or loose stools. Vomiting may be noted in adolescents.
- Abdominal pain may be crampy in nature and often is localized to the periumbilical area or lower quadrant.
- Stools usually are bulky, frothy, and watery, although diarrhea may be rare in adults.
- Only 20–30% of individuals with lactose malabsorption develop symptoms.

PHYSICAL EXAM

- Vital signs and general appearance are typically normal.
- Audible bowel sounds (borborygmi) on physical examination (may be particularly bothersome to the patient). The exam is otherwise typically normal or nonspecific.

DIFFERENTIAL DIAGNOSIS

- Functional GI disorder (e.g., IBS)
- SIBO
- Celiac disease
- Inflammatory bowel disease
- Infectious enteritis such as giardiasis
- Drug or radiation induced enteritis
- Sucrase deficiency
- Cow's milk protein allergy

DIAGNOSTIC TESTS & INTERPRETATION

Initial Tests (lab, imaging)

- The lactose breath test (LBT) is a confirmatory for lactose intolerance. It is noninvasive, easy to perform (sensitivity 78%; specificity 98%) (2).
- Intestinal bacteria digest carbohydrates and produce measurable hydrogen and methane in expired breath:
  - Administer lactose when fasting (2 g/kg; max dose 25 g in children; 50 g in adults). Note any symptoms; sample breath hydrogen at baseline and at 30-minute intervals for 3 hours. Compare postlactose and baseline values. A rise in hydrogen concentration value of 20 ppm over baseline is diagnostic for lactose malabsorption. An early peak (15 to 30 minutes) suggests SIBO.
- Small bowel biopsy for histology and direct measurement of lactase activity (rarely needed)
- A positive LBT confirms lactose malabsorption but does not determine etiology.

Diagnostic Procedures/Other

- Lactose tolerance test is an alternative to LBT in adults and measures lactose absorption through serum glucose measurements. Following oral administration of a 50-g test dose in adults (2 g/kg in children), blood glucose levels are monitored at 0, 60, and 120 minutes. An increase in blood glucose of <20 mg/dL (1.1 mmol/L) with the concurrent development of symptoms is diagnostic. False-negative results may occur in patients with diabetes or bacterial overgrowth.
- Stool electrolyte testing, if done, may indicate a stool osmotic gap >125 mOsm/kg, although this is not specific to lactose intolerance.

Test Interpretation

Low lactase enzyme activity in intestinal mucosa, tested by small bowel biopsy, may be patchy or focal.

 TREATMENT

There is insufficient evidence to recommend any particular treatment (including probiotics, colonic adaptation, and other supplements) as definitive first line.

- In the absence of a correctable underlying disease, treatment includes four general principles (3)[B].
  - Avoid milk/dairy products to improve symptoms.
  - Up to 12 to 15 g of lactose can be tolerated in without significant symptoms (1 cup of milk).
  - Gradually reintroduce lactose as symptoms allow. Spreading lactose servings throughout the day improves tolerance.
  - If symptoms persist, substitute fermented and matured milk products for lactose.
- Certain strains, concentrations, and preparations of probiotics may alleviate symptoms.
- Incrementally increasing doses of lactose to induce adaptation have limited success.
- Insufficient evidence to routinely recommend lactose-reduced or hydrolyzed milk, lactase supplements taken with milk or probiotics
- Maintain calcium and vitamin D intake.

MEDICATION

First Line

Lactase (Lactaid, Lactrase):

- Commercially available "lactase" preparations are bacterial or yeast β-galactosidases.
- Take 1 to 2 capsules or tablets prior to ingesting dairy products.
- Effectiveness at preventing symptoms varies.
- Can add tablets or contents of capsules to milk (1 to 2 caps/tabs per quart of milk) before drinking; also commercially available in milk in some areas
- Not effective for all people with lactose intolerance

COMPLEMENTARY & ALTERNATIVE MEDICINE

Certain probiotic formulations taken with meals may alleviate some symptoms of lactose intolerance (4)[B].

 ONGOING CARE

DIET

- Reduce or restrict dietary lactose to control symptoms—patient-specific "trial and error."
- Yogurt and fermented products such as hard cheese are often better tolerated than milk.
- Supplement calcium (e.g., calcium carbonate).
- Prehydrolyzed milk (Lactaid) is available.

PATIENT EDUCATION

- Read labels on commercial products—milk sugar is used in many products and may cause symptoms.
- Patients may tolerate whole milk or chocolate milk better than skim milk (slower rate of gastric emptying)
- Lactose consumed with other food products is better tolerated than when consumed with milk alone.
- Primary lactase deficiency is permanent; secondary lactose intolerance usually is temporary, although it may persist for months after the inciting event.
- 20% of prescription drugs and 6% of over-the-counter (OTC) medicines may contain lactose as a base.
- Most patients with lactose intolerance or malabsorption can tolerate 12 to 15 g of lactose per day.

PROGNOSIS

- Normal life expectancy
- Symptoms can be controlled through diet alone if lactase tablets are ineffective.

COMPLICATIONS

Calcium deficiency: Avoidance of milk and other dairy products can lead to reduced calcium intake, which may increase the risk for osteoporosis and fracture.

REFERENCES

1. Jansson-Knodell CL, Krajicek EJ, Savaiano DA, et al. Lactose intolerance: a concise review to skim the surface. *Mayo Clin Proc.* 2020;95(7):1499–1505. doi:10.1016/j.mayocp.2020.04.036.
2. Gasbarrini A, Corazza GR, Gasbarrini G, et al; and 1st Rome H2-Breath Testing Consensus Conference Working Group. Methodology and indications of H2-breath testing in gastrointestinal diseases: the Rome Consensus Conference. *Aliment Pharmacol Ther.* 2009;29(Suppl 1):1–49.
3. Shaukat A, Levitt MD, Taylor BC, et al. Systematic review: effective management strategies for lactose intolerance. *Ann Intern Med.* 2010;152(12):797–803.
4. Deng Y, Misselwitz B, Dai N, et al. Lactose intolerance in adults: biological mechanism and dietary management. *Nutrients.* 2015;7(9):8020–8035.

ADDITIONAL READING

- Almeida CC, Lorena SL, Pavan CR, et al. Beneficial effects of long-term consumption of a probiotic combination of *Lactobacillus casei* Shirota and *Bifidobacterium breve* Yakult may persist after suspension of therapy in lactose-intolerant patients. *Nutr Clin Pract.* 2012;27(2):247–251.
- Facioni MS, Raspini B, Pivari F, et al. Nutritional management of lactose intolerance: the importance of diet and food labeling. *J Transl Med.* 2020;18(1):260. doi:10.1186/s12967-020-02429-2.
- Tan-Dy CR, Ohlsson A. Lactase treated feeds to promote growth and feeding tolerance in preterm infants. *Cochrane Database Syst Rev.* 2013;(3):CD004591.

 CODES

ICD10

- E73.9 Lactose intolerance, unspecified
- E73.1 Secondary lactase deficiency
- E73.8 Other lactose intolerance

CLINICAL PEARLS

- The diagnosis of lactose intolerance is based on clinical history and confirmed by hydrogen breath testing.
- Most lactose-intolerant patients can tolerate up to 12 to 15 g of lactose per day (equivalent to 1 cup of milk).
- Lactose-intolerant patients may tolerate yogurt and fermented products better than milk and cheese.
- A diary helps identify problematic foods.
- Patients should read ingredient labels to look for milk, lactose, whey, and curd.
- Lactose-intolerant patients may tolerate whole milk or chocolate milk better than skim milk due to a slower rate of gastric emptying.
- Many patients with lactose intolerance unnecessarily avoid all dairy products, potentially causing an inadequate intake of calcium and vitamin D.

L

LARYNGITIS

Karlynn Sievers, MD • Bethany Price, DO

 BASICS

DESCRIPTION

- Laryngitis is inflammation, erythema, and edema of the mucosa of the larynx and/or vocal cords characterized by hoarseness, loss of voice, throat pain, coughing, and often a negative impact on a person's quality of life and daily activities.
- There is a range of severity, but most cases are acute and are associated with viral upper respiratory infection, irritation, or acute vocal strain.
- System(s) affected: pulmonary; ears, nose, throat
- Synonym(s): acute laryngitis; chronic laryngitis; croup or laryngotracheitis (in children)

EPIDEMIOLOGY

Children more susceptible than adults due to increased risk of symptomatic inflammation from smaller airways

Incidence
Common

Prevalence
Common; approximately 1.7% of population have dysphonia with 50% of this being caused by acute laryngitis. Prevalence rates are increasing but difficult to calculate because many patients do not seek medical attention.

ETIOLOGY AND PATHOPHYSIOLOGY

- Misuse or abuse of voice
- Infectious
  - Viral: influenza A, B; parainfluenza; adenovirus; coronavirus; rhinovirus; human papillomavirus; cytomegalovirus; varicella-zoster virus; herpes simplex virus; respiratory syncytial virus; coxsackievirus
  - Fungal: uncommon but thought to be underdiagnosed, potentially accounting for up to 10% of presentations in both immunocompromised and immunocompetent patients; risk factors include recent antibiotic or inhaled corticosteroid use (1): histoplasmosis, blastomycosis, *Coccidioides*, *Cryptococcus*, and *Candida*.
  - Bacterial (uncommon): β-hemolytic streptococcus, *Streptococcus pneumoniae*, *Haemophilus influenzae*, tuberculosis (TB), leprosy, *Moraxella catarrhalis*, *Mycoplasma pneumoniae*, *Chlamydophila pneumoniae*. In patients with chronic laryngitis, methicillin-resistant *Staphylococcus aureus* (MRSA) should be considered as a potential cause (2).
  - Secondary syphilis if left untreated
  - Leprosy (in 30–55% of those with leprosy, larynx is affected; in tropical and warm countries)
- Irritants
  - Inhalation of irritating substances (e.g., air pollution, cigarette smoke)
  - Aspiration of caustic chemicals
  - Gastroesophageal reflux disease (GERD)/laryngopharyngeal reflux disease (LPRD)
  - Excessively dry environment
  - Allergy exposures (including pollens)

- Anatomic
  - Aging changes: muscle atrophy, loss of moisture in larynx, and bowing of vocal cords
  - Vocal cord nodules/polyps ("singer's nodes")
  - Local cancer
- Iatrogenic: inhaled steroids such as those used to treat asthma, surgical injury, endotracheal intubation injury
- Idiopathic
- Neuromuscular disorder (e.g., myasthenia gravis); stroke
- Rheumatoid arthritis
- Trauma (e.g., blunt or penetrating trauma to neck)

RISK FACTORS

- Acute:
  - Infection or trauma
  - Upper respiratory tract viral infection (e.g., influenza, rhinovirus, adenovirus, parainfluenza)
  - Voice overuse—excess talking, singing, or shouting
  - Pneumonia—viral or bacterial
  - Coughing
  - Lack of immunization against pertussis or diphtheria
  - Immunocompromised
  - Recent endotracheal intubation or local surgery
- Chronic (persists beyond 3 weeks):
  - Allergic laryngitis (3)
  - Chronic rhinitis/sinusitis with postnasal drip (PND)
  - Voice abuse
  - GERD/LPRD (1)
  - Smoking: primary or secondhand
  - Excessive alcohol use
  - Autoimmune disorders (e.g., rheumatoid arthritis) (1)
  - Granulomatous diseases (e.g., sarcoidosis) (1)
  - Stroke
  - Environmental pollution; constant exposure to dust or other irritants such as chemicals at workplace
  - Medications: inhaled steroids, anticholinergics, antihistamines, anabolic steroids

Geriatric Considerations
May be more ill, slower to heal; need to consider neoplasm

Pediatric Considerations
- Common
- Consider congenital/anatomic causes.

GENERAL PREVENTION

- Avoid overuse of voice (speech therapy/voice training is helpful for vocal musicians/public speakers).
- Influenza virus vaccine is recommended as well as other routine vaccines.
- Quit smoking and avoid secondhand smoke.
- Limit or avoid alcohol/caffeine/acidic foods.
- Control GERD/LPRD.
- Maintain proper hydration status.
- Avoid allergens.
- Wear mask around chemical/environmental irritants.
- Good hand washing (infection prevention)

COMMONLY ASSOCIATED CONDITIONS

- Viral pharyngitis
- Diphtheria (rare): Membrane can descend into the larynx.
- Pertussis: larynx involved as part of the respiratory system
- Bronchitis
- Pneumonitis
- Croup, epiglottitis, in children

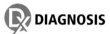 **DIAGNOSIS**

HISTORY

- Hoarseness, throat "tickle," dry cough, and rawness (4)
- Dysphonia (abnormal-sounding voice)
- Constant urge to clear the throat
- Possible fever
- Malaise
- Dysphagia/odynophagia
- Regional cervical lymphadenopathy
- Stridor or possible airway obstruction in children (1)
- Cough may be worse at night in children.
- Hemoptysis
- Laryngospasm or sense of choking
- Allergic rhinitis/rhinorrhea/PND (4)
- Occupation or other reasons for voice overuse
- Smoking history
- Blunt or penetrating trauma to neck
- GERD/LPRD

PHYSICAL EXAM

- Head and neck exam, including airway patency, cervical nodes; cranial nerve exam
- Visualization of the larynx: preferably with a flexible or rigid endoscope or with an indirect mirror examination as a screening technique to dictate further appropriate testing (4)
- Note quality of voice (i.e., hoarse, breathy, wet, "hot potato like," asthenic [weak], strained) (3).

DIFFERENTIAL DIAGNOSIS

- Diphtheria
- Vocal nodules or polyps
- Laryngeal malignancy
- Thyroid malignancy
- Upper airway malignancy (3),(4)[A]
- Epiglottitis
- Pertussis
- Laryngeal nerve trauma/injury
- Foreign body (in children)
- Autoimmune (rheumatoid arthritis)

DIAGNOSTIC TESTS & INTERPRETATION

- Rarely needed
- WBCs elevated in bacterial laryngitis
- Viral culture (seldom necessary)

Follow-Up Tests & Special Considerations
- Barium swallow, only if needed for differential diagnosis
- CT scan if foreign body suspected
- Do not offer CT imaging before visualization of the larynx with laryngoscopy (5)

Diagnostic Procedures/Other
- Fiber-optic or indirect laryngoscopy: looking for red, inflamed, and occasionally hemorrhagic vocal cords; rounded edges and exudate (Reinke edema)
- Consider otolaryngologic evaluation and biopsy: laryngitis lasting >2 weeks in adults with history of smoking or alcohol abuse, to rule out malignancy.
- pH probe (24-hour): no difference in incidence of pharyngeal reflux as measured by pH probe between patients with chronic reflux laryngitis and healthy adults (3)[A]
- Strobo video laryngoscopy for diagnosis of subtle lesions (e.g., vocal cord nodules or polyps) (4)[A]

 TREATMENT

- Limited but good evidence that treatment beyond supportive care is ineffective (4)[A]
- Supportive care consists of hydration, voice rest, humidification, and limitation of caffeine (1)[A].
- Antibiotics appear to have no benefit in acute laryngitis because etiologies are predominantly viral (1),(6)[A]. In chronic laryngitis, consider bacterial sources such as MRSA (2),(5).
- Corticosteroids in severe cases of laryngitis to reduce inflammation such as croup
- May need voice training, if voice overuse (5)
- Nebulized epinephrine reduces croup symptoms 30 minutes posttreatment; evidence does not favor racemic epinephrine or L-epinephrine or IPPB over simple nebulization. Racemic epinephrine reduces croup symptoms at 30 minutes, but effect lasts only 2 hours (6)[A].
- Botulinum toxin injections for spasmodic dysphonia (5)

GENERAL MEASURES
- Acute:
  - Usually a self-limited illness lasting <3 weeks and not severe
  - Antibiotics of no value (6)[A]
  - Avoid excessive voice use, including whispering.
  - Steam inhalations or cool-mist humidifier
  - Increase fluid intake, especially in cases associated with excessive dryness.
  - Avoid smoking (or secondhand exposure).
  - Warm saltwater gargles
- Chronic:
  - Symptomatic treatment as above
  - Voice therapy (for patients with intermittent dysphagia and vocal abuse)
  - Smoking cessation
  - Reduction or cessation of alcohol intake
  - Occupational change or modification, if exposure driven

- Allergen avoidance
- Consider discontinuing offending medication (e.g., inhaled steroids) (6)[A].
- Reflux laryngitis:
  - Elevate head of bed.
  - Diet changes
  - Other antireflux lifestyle change management
  - Proton pump inhibitors (1)[A]

MEDICATION
Usually none

First Line
- Analgesics
- Antipyretics (rare)
- Cough suppressants
- Throat lozenges
- Plenty of fluids

Second Line
- Inhaled corticosteroids (consider only if allergy induced) (3)
- Oral corticosteroids: only if urgent need in adults (presenter, singer, actor)
- Oral corticosteroids: Evidence of benefit has been studied with single-dose dexamethasone in children ages 6 months to 5 years for moderate-severity croup; reduces symptoms within 6 hours; reduces hospitalizations, hospital length of stay, and revisits to office (6)[A]
- Standard of care is to prescribe proton pump inhibitors for chronic laryngitis if GERD or LPRD is suspected; however, evidence suggests only a modest benefit, if any (1)[A].
- Treat nonviral infectious underlying causes.
- Candidal laryngitis:
  - Mild cases: oral antifungal (fluconazole)
  - Amphotericin B or echinocandin can be given in life-threatening cases (1)[A].

ISSUES FOR REFERRAL
- Immediate emergency ENT referral for patients with stridor or respiratory distress (1)[A]
- ENT referral for persistent symptoms (>2 to 3 weeks) or concern for foreign body
- Consider otolaryngologic evaluation and biopsy for laryngitis lasting >3 weeks in adults, especially in those with history of smoking or alcohol abuse to rule out malignancy.
- Consider GI consult to rule out GERD/LPRD.

SURGERY/OTHER PROCEDURES
- Vocal cord biopsy of hyperplastic mucosa and areas of leukoplakia if cancer or TB is suspected
- Removal of nodules or polyps if voice therapy fails

COMPLEMENTARY & ALTERNATIVE MEDICINE
Some experts, although not well studied, have recommended the following:
- Barberry, black currant, *Echinacea*, *Eucalyptus*, German chamomile, goldenrod, goldenseal, warmed lemon and honey, licorice, marshmallow, peppermint, saw palmetto, slippery elm, vitamin C, zinc

 ONGOING CARE

PATIENT EDUCATION
- Educate on the importance of voice rest, including whispering.
- Provide assistance with smoking cessation.
- Help the patient with modification of other predisposing habits or occupational hazards.

PROGNOSIS
Complete clearing of the inflammation without sequelae

COMPLICATIONS
Chronic hoarseness

REFERENCES
1. Wood JM, Athanasiadis T, Allen J. Laryngitis. *BMJ.* 2014;349:g5827.
2. Carpenter P, Kendall K. MRSA chronic bacterial laryngitis: a growing problem. *Laryngoscope.* 2018;128(4):921–925.
3. Platt MP, Brook CD, Kuperstock J, et al. What role does allergy play in chronic ear disease and laryngitis? *Curr Allergy Asthma Rep.* 2016;16(10):76.
4. Reiter R, Hoffmann TK, Pickhard A, et al. Hoarseness—causes and treatments. *Dtsch Arztebl Int.* 2015;112(19):329–337.
5. Francis D, Smith L. Hoarseness guidelines redux: toward improved treatment of patients with dysphonia. *Otolaryngol Clin North Am.* 2019;52(4): 597–605.
6. Reveiz L, Cardona AF. Antibiotics for acute laryngitis in adults. *Cochrane Database Syst Rev.* 2015;(5):CD004783.

ADDITIONAL READING
Benninger MS, Holy CE, Bryson PC, et al. Prevalence and occupation of patients presenting with dysphonia in the United States. *J Voice.* 2017;31(5):594–600.

 CODES

ICD10
- J37.0 Chronic laryngitis
- J04.0 Acute laryngitis
- J05.0 Acute obstructive laryngitis [croup]

CLINICAL PEARLS
- Laryngitis is usually self-limited and needs only comfort care. Standard treatment is voice rest, hydration, humidification, and limit caffeine intake.
- Refer to ENT for direct visualization of vocal cords for prolonged laryngitis.
- Corticosteroids have some benefits for children with moderately severe croup.
- Voice training useful for chronic laryngitis

L

LEAD POISONING

Jason Chao, MD, MS

BASICS

DESCRIPTION
- Disease resulting from a high body burden of lead (Pb)—an element with no known physiologic purpose
- Synonym(s): lead poisoning, inorganic

EPIDEMIOLOGY
- Predominant age: 1 to 5 years, adult workers
- Predominant sex: male > female (1:1 in childhood)

Prevalence
- Centers for Disease Control and Prevention (CDC) estimates half a million U.S. children aged 1 to 5 years have blood Pb levels >5 μg/dL. Levels vary among communities and populations.
- In 2017, 11,097 children in the United States were noted with a blood Pb level ≥10 μg/dL, down from 17,246 in 2012.
- CDC estimates suggest that Pb poisoning prevention has significantly reduced the number of children with blood Pb levels over 1 μg/dL.

ETIOLOGY AND PATHOPHYSIOLOGY
- Inhalation of Pb dust or fumes, or ingestion of Pb
- Pb replaces calcium in bones. Pb interferes with heme synthesis, causes interstitial nephritis, and interferes with neurotransmitters, especially glutamine. High Pb levels can lead to encephalopathy, seizures, and coma.
- Pb crosses blood–brain barrier by displacing calcium ions—the developing nervous system is particularly vulnerable to the toxic effects of Pb.
- Pb exposure early in life causes methylation changes leading to epigenetic alterations that may predispose to brain dysfunction.

RISK FACTORS
- Children with pica or with iron deficiency anemia
- Residence in or frequent visitation to deteriorating pre-1978 housing with Pb-painted surfaces or recent renovation
- Soil/dust exposure near older homes, Pb industries, or urban roads
- Sibling or playmate with current or past Pb poisoning
- Dust from clothing of Pb worker or hobbyist
- Pb dissolved in water from Pb or Pb-soldered plumbing (e.g., Flint, Michigan 2014 to 2015)
- Pb-glazed ceramics leachate (especially with acidic food or drink)
- Folk remedies, spices, and cosmetics
  - Mexico: Azarcon, Greta
  - Dominican Republic: litargirio, a topical agent
  - Asia and Middle East: chuifong tokuwan, pay-loo-ah, ghasard, bali goli, kandu, ayurvedic herbal medicine from South Asia, kohl (alkohl, ceruse), surma, saoott, cebagin
- Hobbies: target shooting, glazed pottery making, Pb soldering, preparing Pb shot or fishing sinkers, stained-glass making, car/boat repair, home remodeling
- Occupational exposure: plumbers, pipe fitters, Pb miners, auto repairers, glass manufacturers, ship builders, printer operators, plastic manufacturers, Pb smelters and refiners, steel welders or cutters, construction workers, rubber product manufacturers, battery manufacturers, bridge reconstruction workers, firing range workers, military and law enforcement

- Dietary: zinc or calcium deficiency
- Imported toys or jewelry with Pb
- Retained bullet fragments, especially if multiple fragments, associated with fracture, or in joints

Pediatric Considerations
- Children are at increased risk because of incomplete development of the blood–brain barrier prior to 3 years of age (allowing more Pb into the CNS).
- Ingested Pb 40% bioavailable in children (10% in adults)
- Common childhood behaviors such as frequent hand-to-mouth activity and pica (repeated ingestion of nonfood products) increase the risk of Pb ingestion.

Pregnancy Considerations
Cross-sectional studies suggest an association between elevated blood Pb and preeclampsia.

GENERAL PREVENTION
- Counsel families on sources of Pb and how to decrease exposure. Screen high-risk children (1)[C].
- Warn parents about unsafe home renovations.
- Wet mopping and dusting with a high-phosphate solution (e.g., powdered automatic dishwasher detergent with 1/4 cup per gallon of water) helps control Pb-bearing dust. High-phosphate detergent is no longer available in some states.
- If tap water is potentially Pb contaminated, use cold water instead of hot water and run for 30 to 60 seconds to flush pipes. Use Pb-free water source if possible (bottled or distilled water).
- Consider screening at-risk pregnant women (2)[C].

COMMONLY ASSOCIATED CONDITIONS
Iron-deficiency anemia

DIAGNOSIS

HISTORY
- Often asymptomatic
- Mild-to-moderate toxicity
  - Myalgias, paresthesias, fatigue, irritability, lethargy
  - Abdominal discomfort, arthralgia, difficulty concentrating, headache, tremor, vomiting, weight loss, muscular exhaustibility
- Severe toxicity: three major clinical syndromes:
  - Alimentary type: anorexia, metallic taste, constipation, severe abdominal cramps due to intestinal spasm and sometimes associated with abdominal wall rigidity
  - Neuromuscular type (characteristic of adult plumbism): peripheral neuritis, usually painless and limited to extensor muscles
  - Cerebral type or Pb encephalopathy (more common in children): seizure, coma, and long-term sequelae, including neurologic defects, delayed mental development, and chronic hyperactivity (or other behavioral changes)
- Chronic exposure may cause renal failure.

PHYSICAL EXAM
Often normal, but abdominal tenderness may be severe. Neurologic exam may reveal neuropathy or encephalopathy.

DIFFERENTIAL DIAGNOSIS
- Alimentary type may present as acute abdomen.
- Neuromuscular type presents similar to other polyneuropathies.
- May be confused with ADD, intellectual disability, autism, dementia, and other causes of seizures
- Elevated erythrocyte protoporphyrin may be caused by iron-deficiency anemia or (less commonly) hemolytic anemia.
- Erythropoietic protoporphyria produces a very high erythrocyte protoporphyrin level.

DIAGNOSTIC TESTS & INTERPRETATION
- Venous blood reference value Pb >5 μg/dL (0.24 μmol/L). CDC is considering lowering the reference value to >3.5 μg/dL (0.17 μmol/L). Confirm screening capillary Pb levels >5 μg/dL (0.24 μmol/L) with a venous sample.
- Hemoglobin and hematocrit slightly low; eosinophilia; basophilic stippling on peripheral smear (not diagnostic)
- Renal function is decreased in late stages.
- Abdominal radiograph for Pb particles in gut if recent ingestion is suspected
- Radiograph of long bones may show metaphyseal changes (resulting from growth arrest). Films are not routinely recommended.

Initial Tests (lab, imaging)
Screening questionnaires are only 60% sensitive to identify children with elevated blood levels.

TREATMENT

Blood Level (μg/dL)	Time to Confirmation Testing
≥ref value–9	1–3 mo
10–44	1 wk–1 mo
45–59	48 hr
60–69	24 hr
≥70	Urgently as emergency test

ALERT
- For Pb levels above 5 μg/dL, confirm with repeat testing according to the table.
- For blood Pb levels persistently >15 μg/dL, contact local public health department for home inspection.
- For any elevated level, educate on sources of Pb exposure.
- Pb level 5 to 45: complete history and physical exam, follow-up Pb monitoring; complete inspection of home or workplace to determine source of Pb and Pb-hazard reduction; neurodevelopmental monitoring: iron status, hemoglobin, or hematocrit (3)[C]
- Pb level 45 to 69 μg/dL: treatment to lower level plus free erythrocyte protoporphyrin, oral chelation therapy, or hospitalization if Pb-safe environment cannot be ensured (3)[C]
- Pb >70 μg/dL: Hospitalize for chelation therapy (4)[C]

GENERAL MEASURES

Remove child from source of exposure.

MEDICATION

- Consider oral chelation for asymptomatic and Pb >45 and <70; chelation (preferably parenteral) for Pb >70 or symptomatic Pb <70 (4)[C].
- If evidence of Pb in GI tract, withhold chelation until bowel is decontaminated, because all chelating agents increase absorption of lead by the gut (3)[C].

First Line

- Oral chelation: succimer (Chemet), dimercaptosuccinic acid (DMSA) 350 mg/m^2 or 10 mg/kg q8h for 5 days and then q12h for 2 weeks. This may be repeated after 2 weeks off if Pb levels are not stabilized at <15 μg/dL (<0.72 μmol/L) (4)[C].
- Parenteral chelation (begin after establishment of adequate urine output):
  - Dimercaprol (British anti-Lewisite [BAL]) 75 mg/m^2 given deep IM, then BAL 450 mg/m^2/day divided q4h for 5 days plus Ca edetate calcium disodium (EDTA) 1,500 mg/m^2/day continuous IV infusion for 5 days. If rebound Pb level ≥45 μg/dL (≥2.17 μmol/L), chelation may be repeated after 2-day interval if symptomatic or after 5-day interval if asymptomatic.
  - Ca EDTA 1,000 mg/m^2/day for 5 days; may be repeated after 5 to 7 days
  - In adults, dimercaprol had greater impact on reducing Pb levels than CaEDTA
  - Contraindications: Do not give BAL to patients with a peanut allergy (the drug solution contains peanut oil).
- Diazepam for initial control of seizures; further control maintained with paraldehyde
- Precautions
  - Succimer: GI upset, rash, nasal congestion, muscle pains, elevated liver function tests
  - BAL: nausea, vomiting, fever, headache, transient hypertension, hepatocellular damage
  - Ca EDTA: renal failure; increased excretion of zinc, copper, and iron
- Significant possible interactions
  - Do not give vitamins with minerals while giving chelation.
  - BAL may precipitate hemolytic crisis in a patient with glucose-6-phosphate dehydrogenase deficiency.

Second Line

Oral chelation with penicillamine (D-penicillamine, Depen, Cuprimine) (4)[C]

- Penicillin-allergic patient should not receive penicillamine (cross-sensitivity is common).
- 10 to 15 mg/kg/day given BID mixed in apple juice/sauce on empty stomach (*not* FDA-approved)
- Penicillamine may cause GI upset, renal failure, granulocytopenia, liver dysfunction, iron deficiency, and drug-induced lupus-like syndrome.

ISSUES FOR REFERRAL

Consider consultation if parenteral chelation is required.

ADDITIONAL THERAPIES

Remove patient from potential source of Pb if Pb level >45 until complete home inspection is performed.

COMPLEMENTARY & ALTERNATIVE MEDICINE

Garlic has been used to treat mild to moderate Pb poisoning in adults.

ADMISSION, INPATIENT, AND NURSING CONSIDERATIONS

- Blood Pb level >70 μg/dL
- If symptomatic, blood Pb level >35 μg/dL
- Outpatient care unless parenteral chelation or immediate removal from contaminated environment is required.
- If Pb source is in the home, the patient must reside elsewhere until the abatement process is completed.
- Avoid visit to any site of potential contamination.

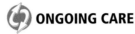 ONGOING CARE

FOLLOW-UP RECOMMENDATIONS

Patient Monitoring

- Expect rebound after chelation, due to release of Pb from bone stores.
- Check for rebound Pb level 7 to 10 days after chelation therapy. Monitor biweekly or monthly thereafter.
- Correct iron or other detected nutritional deficiencies.
- Once Pb <35 μg/dL, repeat testing every 1 to 3 months until level <25 μg/dL is achieved. Then, monitor every 3 to 6 months until level <10 μg/dL. Once <9 μg/dL, test every 6 to 9 months (3)[C].

DIET

- If symptomatic, avoid excessive fluids.
- Avoid pica.
- Adequate calcium, iron, zinc, magnesium, and vitamins C and D to reduce absorption of Pb (5)[B]

PATIENT EDUCATION

- National Lead Information Center, 422 South Clinton Avenue, Rochester, NY 14620; 800-424-5323; https://www.epa.gov/lead
- National Safety Council, 1121 Spring Lake Drive, Itasca, IL 60143-3201; 800-621-7615; https://www.nsc.org/home-safety/safety-topics /other-poisons/lead
- Centers for Disease Control and Prevention. Lead Poisoning Prevention Program. https://www.cdc.gov /nceh/lead/default.htm

PROGNOSIS

- Symptomatic Pb poisoning without encephalopathy generally improves with chelation, but subtle CNS toxicity may be long-lasting or permanent.
- Preschool children with higher Pb levels have lower reading and math scores in elementary school.
- Children with high Pb levels at age 11 years have lower IQ score and socioeconomic status in adulthood.
- With Pb encephalopathy, permanent sequelae (e.g., mental retardation, seizure disorder, blindness, and hemiparesis) occurs in 25–50%.

COMPLICATIONS

- CNS toxicity may be long-lasting or permanent.
- Long-term Pb exposure may cause chronic renal failure (Fanconi-like syndrome), gout, or Pb line (blue–black) on gingival tissue.
- Pb exposure in pregnancy is associated with reduced birth weight and premature birth.

REFERENCES

1. Council on Environmental Health. Prevention of childhood lead toxicity. *Pediatrics*. 2016;138(1):e20161493.
2. United States Preventive Services Task Force. Screening for elevated blood lead levels in children and pregnant women, US Preventive Services Task Force recommendation statement. *JAMA*. 2019;321:1502–1509.
3. Centers for Disease Control and Prevention. *Recommended Actions Based on Blood Lead Level*. Atlanta, GA: Centers for Disease Control and Prevention; 2018. https://www.cdc.gov/nceh/lead /advisory/acclpp/actions-blls.htm
4. American Academy of Pediatrics Committee on Environmental Health. Lead exposure in children: prevention, detection, and management. *Pediatrics*. 2005;116(4):1036–1046.
5. Hauptman M, Bruccoleri R, Woolf AD. An update on childhood lead poisoning. *Clin Pediatr Emerg Med*. 2017;18(3):181–192.

ADDITIONAL READING

- Alzer A, Currie J, Simon P, et al. Do low levels of blood lead reduce children's future test scores? *Am Econ J Appl Econ*. 2018;10(1):307–341.
- Reuben A, Caspi A, Belsky DW, et al. Association of childhood blood lead levels with cognitive function and socioeconomic status at age 38 years and with IQ change and socioeconomic mobility between childhood and adulthood. *JAMA*. 2017;317(12):1244–1251.

 SEE ALSO

Anemia, Iron Deficiency

 CODES

ICD10

- T56.0X4A Toxic effect of lead and its compounds, undetermined, init
- T56.0X1A Toxic effect of lead and its compounds, accidental, init

CLINICAL PEARLS

- Screen children 6 to 11 months of age with ≥1 risk factors: living near industry likely to release Pb; living with adult with job or hobby involving Pb; sibling/playmate with elevated Pb; living in or frequently visits a building built before 1978 with peeling paint or recent renovation; children living in high-risk communities (>12% elevated Pb) should be tested annually from 1 to 5 years of age; newly arrived refugees.
- There is no clear safe Pb level. Many experts consider levels >3.5 μg/dL to be elevated.
- There are no studies that show benefit of chelation for asymptomatic children with Pb <45. Environmental removal of Pb sources is critical.

LEGIONNAIRES' DISEASE

Kenneth A. Ballou, MD

BASICS

DESCRIPTION
- *Legionnaires' disease* was named for an epidemic of lower respiratory tract disease at the 1976 American Legion convention in Philadelphia. The previously unrecognized causative bacterium was isolated, identified, and named *Legionella pneumophila*. The organism primarily causes pneumonia and flulike illness. *Legionella* preferentially colonizes commercial water systems (e.g., hotels, hospitals, apartment buildings, air conditioning cooling towers).
  - It is one of the three most common causes of pneumonias and the most common atypical pneumonia.
- System(s) affected: pulmonary, gastrointestinal (GI)
- Synonym(s): *Legionella* pneumonia; legionellosis; Pontiac fever (self-limited flulike illness without pneumonia caused by *Legionella* species)

EPIDEMIOLOGY
- Predominant age: 15 months to 84 years; 74–91% of patients are >50 years old.
- Predominant gender: male > female

Incidence
- Cases of Legionnaires' disease have increased 4-fold in the United States since 2000; almost 10,000 cases reported in 2018 (1)[C]
- Outbreaks most common in late summer/early fall
- ~2–9% of all cases of pneumonia in the United States. Legionnaires' disease is fatal in 1 of every 10 cases.

ETIOLOGY AND PATHOPHYSIOLOGY
- *L. pneumophila* is a weak gram-negative aerobic saprophytic freshwater bacterium. It is widely distributed in soil and water. Bipolar flagella provide motility; grow optimally at 40–45°C
- Exists in nature as a protozoan parasite, often within fresh water biofilms
- Serogroups 1 to 6 account for clinical disease.
- Serogroup 1 represents 70–92% of all clinical cases of *Legionella* in the United States.
- In the lung, *Legionella* infects alveolar macrophages.
- The organism is transmitted by breathing in contaminated water droplets or by aspiration of contaminated water (e.g., contaminated shower water was responsible for the inaugural Philadelphia outbreak).
- Community outbreaks have been associated with whirlpools, spas, fountains, and aboard cruise ships.

RISK FACTORS
- Impaired cellular immunity (*Legionella* are intracellular pathogens.)
- Male gender
- Smoking; alcohol abuse
- Immunosuppression; HIV; diabetes; organ transplant recipients; chronic or high-dose corticosteroid use
- Chronic cardiopulmonary disease
- Advanced age
- Use of antimicrobials within the past 3 months

GENERAL PREVENTION
- *Not transmitted person to person* (Respiratory isolation is unnecessary.)
- Superheat and flush water systems: Heat water to at least 70°C and flush for 30 minutes (2)[C].
- Ultraviolet light and copper–silver ionization are bactericidal.
- Monochloramine disinfection of municipal water supplies decreases risk for *Legionella* infection.
- 0.2 micron water filters—must change regularly
- Keep water heaters >60°C, cold water <20°C.

DIAGNOSIS
- Illness ranges from asymptomatic seroconversion and mild febrile illness to severe pneumonia.
- Wound infections with *Legionella* also reported
- Incubation period is 2 to 14 days.

HISTORY
- Signs and symptoms (with associated percentage):
  - Cough: 92% (typically dry; rarely productive)
  - Fever/chills: 90%
  - Dyspnea: 62%
  - Pleuritic chest pain: 35%
  - Headache: 48%
  - Myalgia/arthralgia: 40%
  - Watery diarrhea: 50%
  - Nausea and vomiting: 49%
  - Neuropsychiatric symptoms include encephalopathy, confusion, disorientation, obtundation, depression, hallucinations, insomnia, and seizure: 53%.
- History of immunosuppression increases risk.

PHYSICAL EXAM
- Fever
- Relative bradycardia (key sign)
  - Temperature ≥102°F with an inappropriately low pulse pressure <100 beats/min (Normal compensatory reaction to fever is >110 beats/min.)
- Rales and signs of consolidation (i.e., pectoriloquy, egophony, or tactile fremitus)

DIFFERENTIAL DIAGNOSIS
- Other bacterial pneumonias, especially atypical pneumonias: *Mycoplasma pneumoniae*, Q fever (*Coxiella burnetii*), *Chlamydophila pneumoniae*, *Chlamydophila psittaci*, *Francisella tularensis*
- Viral pneumonias, such as adenovirus, influenza (human, avian, swine), cytomegalovirus (CMV)
- Must be differentiated from COVID-19 pulmonary disease; COVID-19 testing recommended

DIAGNOSTIC TESTS & INTERPRETATION
Indications for *Legionella* testing:
- Failed outpatient antibiotic treatment for community-acquired pneumonia (CAP)
- Severe pneumonia, particularly those requiring intensive care
- Immunocompromised patients with pneumonia
- Patients with a history of traveling away from their home within 10 days of illness onset, especially with a history of commercial lodging such as hotel or cruise ship stay within the last 2 weeks

- Pneumonia in the setting of a known Legionnaires' disease outbreak
- Pneumonia beginning ≥48 hours after hospital admission

Initial Tests (lab, imaging)
Diagnosis:
- *Legionella* PCR detects ~100% of all *Legionella* species from lower respiratory secretions (3)[C].
- Urinary antigen test (UAT) detects serogroup 1 (which causes 80% of disease). UATs are highly specific (95–100%) but of variable sensitivity.
- *Legionella* culture (gold standard) requires an adequate sputum sample and special media (buffered charcoal yeast extract [BCYE] agar). Culture has variable sensitivity (10–80%) and time delays of up to 7 days for results (4)[C].
- Other lab abnormalities:
  - Hyponatremia
  - Hypophosphatemia (transient)
  - Lymphopenia
  - Mildly elevated serum transaminases; elevated LDH; elevated creatine kinase
  - Microscopic hematuria
  - Highly elevated C-reactive protein (CRP) (>30)
  - Highly elevated ferritin (≥2 times normal)
- Chest radiograph
  - Not specific for *Legionella*
  - Commonly shows unilateral lower lobe patchy alveolar infiltrate with consolidation
  - Cavitation and abscess formation are more common in immunocompromised patients.
  - Pleural effusion occurs in up to 50%.
  - May take 1 to 4 months for radiographic findings to resolve. Progression of infiltrate on x-ray can be seen despite antibiotic therapy.

Diagnostic Procedures/Other
Transtracheal aspiration/bronchoscopy occasionally necessary to obtain sputum/lung samples

Test Interpretation
- Multifocal pneumonia with alveolitis and bronchiolitis and fibrinous pleuritis; may have serous or serosanguineous pleural effusion
- Abscess formation occurs in up to 20% of patients.
- Progression of infiltrates on x-ray (despite appropriate therapy) suggests Legionnaires' disease. Radiographic improvement may not correlate with clinical findings (longer lag times).
- Use of procalcitonin levels of limited value as it is not as sensitive in atypical pathogens such as Legionalla

TREATMENT
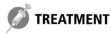

GENERAL MEASURES
- Supportive care:
  - Oxygenation, hydration, and electrolyte balance with antibiotic therapy
- Extrapulmonary complications and higher mortality may be seen in patients with AIDS.
- In severe pneumonia, obtain UAT and start empiric antibiotics to include coverage for *Legionella* (5)[C].

MEDICATION

First Line

- Antibiotics that achieve high intracellular concentrations (e.g., macrolides, tetracyclines, fluoroquinolones) are most effective; first-line treatment is levofloxacin; no prospective randomized controlled trials have compared fluoroquinolones to macrolides for the treatment of *Legionella*; levofloxacin associated with more rapid defervescence, fewer complications, decreased hospital stay by 3 days, and decreased mortality (4% vs. 10.9%) compared with macrolide antibiotics (5)[A]
- Start antibiotics parenterally if sufficiently ill due to the GI symptoms associated with *Legionella*:
  - Levofloxacin is the preferred agent:
    ○ Levofloxacin 750 mg/day IV (switch to PO when patient is afebrile/tolerating PO) for 5 days or 750 mg/day for 7 to 10 days
  - Azithromycin may also be used first line. It requires a shorter duration of treatment than levofloxacin due to a longer half-life:
    ○ Azithromycin 500 mg/day IV (switch to PO when afebrile/tolerating PO) for 7 to 10 days
- Contraindications: hypersensitivity reactions
- Precautions: liver disease
- Significant drug interactions:
  - Can increase theophylline, carbamazepine, and digoxin levels; can increase activity of oral anticoagulants
  - May decrease the effectiveness of digoxin, quinidine, oral contraceptives, and hypoglycemic agents
- Longer courses of treatment (up to 21 days) may be needed in immunocompromised patients or valvular heart disease.

Second Line

- Doxycycline 100 mg IV/PO q12h for 14 days; for severe infections, initial dose is 200 mg IV/PO q12h.
- Doxycycline should not be used in pregnant patients and is not approved for children <8 years.

ADMISSION, INPATIENT, AND NURSING CONSIDERATIONS

- Inability to tolerate oral antibiotics
- Hypoxemia
- Criteria for direct admission to the ICU:
  - Any major criteria for severe CAP:
    ○ Septic shock requiring vasopressor support
    ○ Acute respiratory failure requiring intubation and/or mechanical ventilation
  - Three or more minor criteria for severe CAP:
    ○ RR ≥30 breaths/min, PaO$_2$:FiO$_2$ ratio ≤250, multilobular infiltrates, confusion/disorientation, uremia (BUN ≥20 mg/dL), leukopenia (WBC <4,000 cells/mm^3), thrombocytopenia (PLT <100,000 cells/mm^3), hypothermia (temperature <36°C), hypotension requiring aggressive fluid resuscitation
- Discharge criteria
  - Afebrile
  - Able to tolerate oral antibiotics
  - Return to normal/baseline room-air oxygen saturation

ONGOING CARE

FOLLOW-UP RECOMMENDATIONS

Patient Monitoring

- Monitor respiratory status, hydration, and electrolyte status closely.
- Chest radiography lags behind the clinical status and may not help with monitoring clinical response.

PATIENT EDUCATION

- Disease prevention: Eliminate pathogens from water supplies, low-emission cleaning of cooling towers with control measurements of water and air samples.
- *Legionella* is not spread person to person.

PROGNOSIS

- Improved prognosis when appropriate antibiotics are started early in the disease course
- Recovery is variable:
  - Patients may clinically worsen despite appropriate initial treatment (first 1 to 2 days of therapy).
  - Improvement with defervescence in 3 to 5 days and complete recovery in 6 to 10 days is typical. Some have a more protracted course.
- Mortality in nosocomial infections as high as 15–34%

COMPLICATIONS

- Dehydration
- Hyponatremia
- Respiratory insufficiency requiring ventilator support
- Bacteremia/lung abscess formation in up to 20%
- Extrapulmonary diseases:
  - Endocarditis (most common extrapulmonary site); cellulitis; sinusitis; pancreatitis; pyelonephritis; encephalitis; pericarditis; perirectal abscess
- Renal failure
- Disseminated intravascular coagulation
- Multiple organ dysfunction syndrome (MODS)
- Coma
- Death occurs in 8–12% of treated immunocompetent patients and in up to 80% of untreated immunocompromised patients.

REFERENCES

1. Adams DA, Thomas KR, Jajosky RA, et al; for Nationally Notifiable Infectious Conditions Group. Summary of notifiable infectious diseases and conditions—United States, 2015. *MMWR Morb Mortal Wkly Rep*. 2017;64(53):1–143.
2. Walser SM, Gerstner DG, Brenner B, et al. Assessing the environmental health relevance of cooling towers—a systematic review of legionellosis outbreaks. *Int J Hyg Environ Health*. 2014;217(2–3):145–154.
3. Botelho-Nevers E, Grattard F, Viallon A, et al. Prospective evaluation of RT-PCR on sputum versus culture, urinary antigens and serology for Legionnaire's disease diagnosis. *J Infect*. 2016;73(2):123–128.
4. Cristovam E, Almeida D, Caldeira D, et al. Accuracy of diagnostic tests for Legionnaires' disease: a systematic review. *J Med Microbiol*. 2017;66(4):485–489.
5. Burdet C, Lepeule R, Duval X, et al. Quinolones versus macrolides in the treatment of legionellosis: a systematic review and meta-analysis. *J Antimicrob Chemother*. 2014;69(9):2354–2360.

ADDITIONAL READING

- Bellew S, Grijalva C, Williams D, et al. Pneumococcal and *Legionella* urinary antigen tests in community-acquired pneumonia: prospective evaluation of indications for testing. *Clin Infect Dis*. 2019;68(12):2026–2033.
- Jomehzadeh N, Moosavian M, Saki M, et al. *Legionella* and legionnaires' disease: an overview. *J Acute Disease*. 2019;8(6):221–232.
- Mercante JW, Winchell JM. Current and emerging *Legionella* diagnostics for laboratory and outbreak investigations. *Clin Microbiol Rev*. 2015;28(1):95–133.
- Metlay JP, Waterer GW, Long AC, et al. Diagnosis and treatment of adults with community-acquired pneumonia. An official clinical practice guideline of the American Thoracic Society and Infectious Diseases Society of America. *Am J Respir Crit Care Med*. 2019;200(7):e45–e67.
- Palazzolo C, Malffongelli G, D'Abramo A, et al. *Legionella* pneumonia: increase risk after COVID-19 lockdown? Italy, May to June 2020. *Eurosurveillance*. 2020;25(30):2001372.
- Phin N, Parry-Ford F, Harrison T, et al. Epidemiology and clinical management of Legionnaires' disease. *Lancet Infect Dis*. 2014;14(10):1011–1021.

SEE ALSO

Pneumonia, Bacterial

CODES

ICD10

- A48.2 Nonpneumonic Legionnaires' disease [Pontiac fever]
- A48.1 Legionnaires' disease

CLINICAL PEARLS

- *Legionella* is an intracellular organism that can only be grown on BCYE agar.
- Consider Legionnaires' disease in patients with pneumonia who have GI and other extrapulmonary findings (atypical CAP) and a relative bradycardia. Relative lymphopenia, mildly elevated serum transaminases (aspartate aminotransferase/alanine aminotransferase), highly increased ferritin levels, or hypophosphatemia are other laboratory clues to *Legionella* infection.
- Serology is not useful in early stages of the disease (an increase in *Legionella* antibody titers cannot be detected until 3 to 4 weeks after symptom onset).
- UAT and *Legionella* sputum PCR are the most sensitive and practical initial tests. Sputum culture is definitive but can take up to 7 days.
- Consider Legionnaires' disease in cases of nosocomial pneumonia.
- Levofloxacin and azithromycin are first-line agents.

L

LESBIAN HEALTH

Tina D'Amato, DO

BASICS

DESCRIPTION
- A lesbian is a woman who has her primary emotional and sexual relationships with women.
- Sexual behaviors
  - May be celibate, sexually active only with women or with men, women and/or nonbinary partners
  - ~75% of self-reported lesbians have reported prior or ongoing sexual contact with men.
- Sexual orientation and gender are complex concepts and defining them can be challenging.

EPIDEMIOLOGY
Prevalence
- Estimated to be between 1% and 5%
- Approximately 1.4 million women living in the United States identify as lesbians. Another 2.6 million women identify as bisexual. 2020 Gallup Poll results had 1.3% of women identifying as lesbian, 4.3% as bisexual, and 1.3% as something else.
- 2016 American Community Survey from United States Census Bureau estimates 451,594 households are headed by female same-sex couples.

RISK FACTORS
Higher incidence for the following risk factors compared to heterosexual women:
- Elevated BMI
  - Lesbian women have a higher prevalence of overweight/obesity than all other female sexual orientation groups.
  - Higher prevalence rates of obesity have been found among lesbians who are:
    - African American
    - Live in urban or rural areas
    - Have lower levels of education
    - Lower socioeconomic status
- Alcohol use
  - More common use than reported in heterosexual women
  - Age 20 to 34 years is at highest risk for daily use and heavy use of alcohol. Those numbers decline in older age groups, but even 1 drink per day can increase risks for cancer, hepatic, and heart disease.
- Tobacco use
  - 1.5 to 2 times more likely to smoke than heterosexual women
  - Aggressive marketing by tobacco industry to LGBT individuals
- Sexual minority stress (1)
  - Increased risk for health issues secondary to greater exposure to social stresses related to prejudice and stigma
  - Many of the increased health risks in lesbians can be attributed to behaviors that are the result of dealing with the stress and stigma of homophobia and discrimination.
- The above factors can increase risks for cardiovascular disease (CVD), type 2 diabetes, hepatic disease, cancers.

COMMONLY ASSOCIATED CONDITIONS
- Cervical cancer
  - Lesbians are equally at risk for developing cervical cancer compared to heterosexual women.
  - HPV can be transmitted genitally skin to skin, oral to genitals, and digital to genitals.
  - Risk of cervical cancer is highest in lesbians:
    - With prior HPV infection/abnormal Pap smear
    - Who have had a history of heterosexual intercourse
  - Lesbian and bisexual women are 10 times less likely to have adequate cervical cancer screening compared to heterosexual women.
  - Tobacco use influences cervical cell atypia.
- Breast cancer
  - Risk factors same as heterosexual women
    - Moderate or heavy alcohol consumption
    - Obesity
    - Nulliparity or first child born after age 30 years
  - Mammogram screening rates lower among lesbians
  - Data suggest lesbians have increased mortality rate compared to heterosexual women.
- Ovarian cancer
  - Elevated BMI and tobacco use increases risks.
  - Lesbians less likely to have been on hormonal contraception for 5 years or longer
  - Lesbians less likely to have been pregnant or breastfed an infant before age 30 years
  - Lesbians at increased risk for ovarian cancer may want to explore potential benefits of long-term progestin-containing contraception to reduce risk.
- Endometrial cancer
  - Elevated BMI and tobacco use increases risks.
  - Lesbians less likely to have been pregnant
  - Lesbians with polycystic ovarian syndrome should be asked about sustained amenorrhea and consider use of progestin-containing contraception or regular schedule of induced "withdrawal bleeds" to reduce risks.
- CVD—lesbians have higher rates of obesity, alcohol use, smoking, and stress, which increase risks for CVD
- Mental health diagnoses
  - 2 times more likely to see general physician for mental/emotional complaint compared to heterosexual women
  - More likely to seek care if physician is aware of their sexual orientation
    - Depression
      - Discrimination stress proposed factor
      - Double the rate compared to heterosexual women
    - Suicide
      - "Out" lesbian women 2 to 2.5 times more likely to have had suicidal ideation in last 12 months compared to heterosexual women
      - Lesbian women who were not "out" were more likely to have attempted suicide compared to heterosexual women.

- Anxiety disorders
  - 3 times risk, multiple diagnoses
  - Higher rates of PTSD, panic, phobia, and 2- to 4-fold higher rate of generalized anxiety disorder
  - Alcohol abuse
    - Greatest in lesbians ages 20 to 34 years
    - Bar culture
    - May not feel comfortable in traditional Alcoholics Anonymous environment
    - Sexual minority females more likely than heterosexual counterparts to be current alcohol users, binge drinkers, and heavy drinkers (2)
  - Substance abuse
    - Sexual minority women at higher rates of all substance abuse compared to heterosexual counterparts (3)
      - Bisexual women have highest rates of substance abuse compared to lesbian and heterosexual women.
    - Higher levels of socioeconomic instability were associated with increased odds for substance abuse.
      - Household Pulse Survey from United States Census Bureau showed COVID-19 pandemic impacted LGBTQ population significantly greater than heterosexual counterparts.
- Sexually transmitted infections (STI)
  - Many lesbians underestimate their STI risks.
  - Difficult to ascertain accurate statistics because of lack of research and the confounding factors of relying on identifiers of sexual orientation versus sexual behaviors
  - Increased risk during menstruation and activities causing friction
  - Lesbian sexual practices include the following:
    - High risk: oral–vaginal contact, genital–genital contact, oral–anal contact, digital stimulation/penetration, and sharing of sex toys
    - Lower risk: kissing, rubbing genitals against partner's body/clothing
- Bacterial vaginosis
  - Higher rate than heterosexual women; estimated 25–52% prevalence
  - Increased incidence with smoking, receptive oral sex, symptomatic partner, and new partner
  - Often found in monogamous lesbian couples suggesting it can be sexually transmitted. Consider treating asymptomatic partner especially in recurrent cases.
- Chlamydia, gonorrhea, hepatitis B, syphilis, trichomonas, and herpes—can all be transmitted woman to woman (WTW)
- HPV
  - Can be transmitted WTW
  - Up to 30% of women who have sex with women (WSW) have genital HPV.
  - 12% of WSW report genital warts.
  - 25% of WSW report cervical abnormalities.
  - WSW may not get HPV vaccine due to perceived decreased risk.

- HIV—transmission between women rare but possible; WSW more likely to have sexual contact with men having sex with men (MSM) than heterosexual women
- STI screening and prevention
  - Screen based on woman's history.
  - Encourage safer sex practices:
    - Avoid menstrual blood/open sores.
    - Dental dams for oral sex, condoms on sex toys, and cleaning immediately after use
    - Vinyl/latex gloves for manual sex, limit friction with lubricants
- Psychosocial considerations
  - Sexual abuse
    - 3 times more likely than heterosexual women to report having been sexually assaulted
    - 43% of lesbians reported at least one sexual assault in their lifetime.
    - History of childhood sexual abuse can be associated with more complicated and difficult "coming out."
  - Intimate partner violence: 17–45% of lesbians report at least one act of physical violence at the hands of a lesbian partner.
  - Parenthood: A reported 41% of lesbians desire to have a child. Perinatal depression is common and may be more common than in heterosexual women.
    - >30% have biologic children.
      - Often from previous heterosexual relationship
      - Adoption
      - Assisted reproductive technology/donor insemination
      - Some will engage in high-risk sexual behaviors (MSM, "one-night stand") in an attempt to get pregnant.
      - Providers should discuss parenting with their lesbian patients.
      - Encourage both partners or nonbiologic parent to adopt child to ensure permanent legal relationship to child.
      - Discuss durable power of attorney for health care and finances in the event of death or separation.
      - Adolescents who have been reared in lesbian mother families since birth demonstrate healthy psychological adjustment.
  - Adolescent lesbians
    - Increased risk for eating disorders
    - Higher rates of substance use particularly polysubstance abuse
    - If also having sexual contact with males, higher rates of pregnancy compared to heterosexual counterparts due to (4)
      - High rates of early sexual initiation
      - Greater number of partners
      - Less contraceptive use
    - Higher rates of physical and/or sexual abuse—childhood sexual abuse does not cause children to become LGBTQ

- Aging lesbians
  - Elders aging "back into the closet"
    - Discrimination by religious and other groups that own nursing homes
    - Fear of discrimination by caregivers/health care workers
    - Few elder care programs specifically directed at LGBT persons

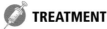 **TREATMENT**

GENERAL MEASURES
- Create a safe practice environment for lesbian patients.
  - Have nondiscrimination policy posted where it is visible to patients.
  - Educate staff to be comfortable dealing with the needs of lesbian patients and their families.
  - Brochures/photos should feature both same-sex and heterosexual couples.
  - Intake forms should include options for patient to indicate sexual preference and include options for partnered status.
  - Use "gender-neutral" language. For example, "Do you have a significant other?"
  - Avoid heterosexist assumptions ("What do you use for birth control?" asking instead "Do you plan to become pregnant or have a child? Do you need birth control?").
- Ask about sexual orientation.
  - Many physicians do not ask.
  - Intake/annual physical forms should include questions about orientation/activity.
  - Twice as likely to identify as a sexual minority if questions asked in an indirect way
- Take a detailed sexual history.
  - Sexual identity and sexual behaviors not always strongly correlated
  - Ask about behaviors ("Do you have sex with women, men, or both?"); do not just assume current/past sexual activity with women.
  - STI screening based on reported history/activity
  - Address contraception when appropriate.
  - Some physicians may create barriers by believing a patient's sexual self-identity and behaviors are not pertinent to competent care (5).
- Respect the partners.
  - Treat them as you would any other spouse/partner.
  - Assure access if partner hospitalized.
  - Recommend durable power of attorney if couple is not legally married.
- Follow same preventive screening guidelines and lifestyle recommendations as for heterosexual women (Pap smear, mammography, colonoscopy screening, safer sex, exercise, diet, alcohol moderation, and tobacco avoidance).
- Legal/U.S. government
  - Healthy People 2010 identified lesbian/gay Americans as 1 of 6 population groups affected by health care disparities.

- Healthy People 2020 goals to increase routine data collection efforts on LGBT populations via health care surveys
  - Questions about sexual orientation and gender identity added to many population surveys
- Healthy People 2030 focus is on collecting data on specific health needs of LGBT population and improving health in LGBT adolescents.
  - Goal to add questions about gender and sexual identity on more state and national surveys
- Access to health insurance was increased with supreme court decisions on *United States v. Windsor* in 2013 and *Obergefell v. Hodges* in 2015. Some states still recognize same-sex civil union, but access to health insurance varies by state.
- Affordable Care Act (ACA): prohibits discrimination based on sexual orientation in any program receiving federal funds (Medicare/Medicaid). Increased emphasis on research and data collections in LGBT population. National Health Interview Survey (NHIS): In 2013, survey added a question about sexual orientation.

REFERENCES
1. Frost DM, Lehavot K, Meyer IH. Minority stress and physical health among sexual minority individuals. *J Behav Med.* 2015;38(1):1–8.
2. Medley G, Lipari RBN, Bose J, et al. Sexual orientation and estimates of adult substance use and mental health: results from the 2015 National Survey on Drug Use and Health. https://www.samhsa.gov/data/sites/default/files/NSDUH-SexualOrientation-2015/NSDUH-SexualOrientation-2015/NSDUH-SexualOrientation-2015.htm. Accessed November 29, 2021.
3. Rosner B, Neicun J, Yang JC, et al. Substance use among sexual minorities in the US—linked to inequalities and unmet need for mental health treatment? Results from the National Survey on Drug Use and Health (NSDUH). *J Psychiatr Res.* 2021;135:107–118.
4. Committee on Adolescence. Office-based care for lesbian, gay, bisexual, transgender, and questioning youth. *Pediatrics.* 2013;132(1):198–203.
5. Knight DA, Jarrett D. Preventive health care for women who have sex with women. *Am Fam Physician.* 2017;95(5):314–321.

 CODES

ICD10
- E66.3 Overweight
- Z72.0 Tobacco use
- F10.10 Alcohol abuse, uncomplicated

CLINICAL PEARLS
- Create a safe health care environment for all patients. Use gender-neutral language. Do not assume heterosexuality or sexual practices.
- Discuss durable power of attorney for health care needs to ensure partner's involvement in care.

L

LEUKEMIA, ACUTE LYMPHOBLASTIC (ALL) IN ADULTS
Afsha Rais Kaisani, MD • Nivas Govindarajan, MD, BS • Niyomi De Silva, MD

 BASICS

DESCRIPTION
- ALL in adults is the result of a clonal proliferation, survival, and impaired differentiation of immature lymphocytes. The World Health Organization (WHO) defines ALL as the presence of ≥25% lymphoblasts in the bone marrow, and the National Comprehensive Cancer Network (NCCN) uses a ≥20% as cutoff.
- ALL and lymphoblastic lymphoma (LBL) can arise from same precursor cell line and be considered diseases along the same spectrum:
  – LBL presents as a mass, possibly, but not limited to, the mediastinum, with <25% blasts in the bone marrow.
  – ALL may present with a mass lesion but contains ≥25% bone marrow involvement.
- Any organ can be affected.

Pregnancy Considerations
Many chemotherapy (CTX) drugs are teratogenic.

Pediatric Considerations
ALL is the most common malignancy in children—it accounts for 30% of all pediatric malignancies and 80% of pediatric leukemias (see "Acute Lymphoblastic Leukemia, Pediatric").

Geriatric Considerations
Patients >60 years with ALL have a 42% mortality during induction CTX. The cause of death is usually CTX-related complications or relapse. Survival is often reduced due to poor tolerance of CTX, thus leading to dose reductions and ineffective medication delivery.

EPIDEMIOLOGY
Incidence
- Incidence of ALL is 1.8/100,000 per year.
- Higher incidence in older age, males, whites, those with history of radiation, CTX, or certain genetic disorders

Prevalence
- Prevalence of ALL can range from 15% to 50% and increases with age.
- Bimodal distribution: early peak in childhood, second peak at around age 50
- 75–80% of cases occur in children, approximately 20% in adults.

ETIOLOGY AND PATHOPHYSIOLOGY
The pathophysiology of ALL involves the abnormal proliferation and differentiation of clonal lymphoid cells.

Genetics
- Higher rates in monozygotic and dizygotic twins
- Increased risk of ALL with diseases related to chromosomal instability and inherited chromosomal abnormalities

RISK FACTORS
- Age >70 years, radiation and CTX exposure, and infection with HIV are risk factors for developing ALL.
- Human T-cell lymphotropic virus type 1 is associated with adult T-cell ALL.
- Epstein-Barr virus is associated with mature B-cell ALL.

DIAGNOSIS

HISTORY
- Symptoms arise from sequelae of bone marrow suppression and/or from leukemic cell organ infiltration.
- B symptoms: fever, weight loss, night sweats
- Anemia: fatigue, shortness of breath, light-headedness, angina, headache
- Thrombocytopenia: easy bruising or bleeding
- Neutropenia: fever, infection
- Lymphocytosis: bone pain
- CNS: confusion

PHYSICAL EXAM
- Thrombocytopenia: petechiae, ecchymoses, epistaxis, retinal hemorrhages
- Anemia: pallor
- Neutropenia: fever, infections
- Lymphocytosis: lymphadenopathy; splenomegaly; less often, hepatomegaly
- CNS: cranial nerve palsies, meningeal signs
- Testicular invasion: abnormal testicular exam

DIFFERENTIAL DIAGNOSIS
- Malignant disorders: other leukemias, AML, chronic myeloid leukemia in lymphoid blast phase, prolymphocytic leukemia, malignant lymphomas; multiple myeloma, bone marrow metastases from solid tumors (breast, prostate, lung, renal), and myelodysplastic syndromes
- Nonmalignant disorders: aplastic anemia, myelofibrosis, autoimmune diseases (Felty syndrome, lupus), infectious mononucleosis, pertussis, autoimmune thrombocytopenic purpura, leukemoid reaction to infection

DIAGNOSTIC TESTS & INTERPRETATION
Initial Tests (lab, imaging)
- CBC with platelets and differential: evidence of leukocytosis, may also present with anemia and thrombocytopenia
- Peripheral blood smear: lymphoblasts (B cell or T cell)
- Hepatitis B/C, HIV, CMV, HSV testing
- Pregnancy test in female patients; testicular examination and scrotal US if indicated in male patients
- Human leukocyte antigen (HLA) typing if posttreatment hematopoietic stem cell transplant might be indicated
- CT of the neck, chest, abdomen, and pelvis with IV contrast and PET/CT if suspicion of lymphomatous involvement

- CT/MRI of head with contrast if neurologic symptoms are present
- Evaluate patients for opportunistic infections.

Follow-Up Tests & Special Considerations
- Immunophenotyping of marrow/blood lymphoblasts: B lineage (CD19, CD20, CD22, CD24), T lineage (CD2, CD3, CD5, CD7), common ALL antigen (CD10); HLA-DR, terminal deoxynucleotidyl transferase (TdT), aberrant myeloid antigens (CD13, CD33), and stem cell antigen (CD34)
- Cytochemical stains: myeloperoxidase negative; Sudan black B usually negative; TdT positive; periodic acid–Schiff ± is variable, depending on subtype.
- Cytogenetics: Specific chromosomal abnormalities have independent diagnostic and prognostic significance.
- Reverse transcriptase–polymerase chain reaction for rapid diagnosis of BCR/ABL1+ ALL
- Genomic analysis by next-generation sequencing: detection of mutations associated with Ph-like ALL
- HLA typing of patient and siblings for hematopoietic stem cell transplantation

Diagnostic Procedures/Other
- Bone marrow aspiration/biopsy with immunohistochemistry, immunophenotyping, cytogenetics, and molecular diagnostics
- Lymph node biopsy if available
- Lumbar puncture (LP) for CNS involvement and for intrathecal (IT) CTX. First LP should be performed at time of IT CTX unless symptomatic earlier. Repeat LP after bone marrow remission is achieved to evaluate occult CNS involvement.

Test Interpretation
Diagnosis is based on the presence of lymphoblasts in the bone marrow. In some cases, the diagnosis can be made based on the presence of certain mutations, even if the percentage of blasts is lower. Bone marrow biopsy typically shows diffuse replacement of marrow and lymph node architecture by sheets of malignant lymphoblasts, T-cell or B-cell lineage determined by CD expression.

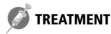 TREATMENT

GENERAL MEASURES
Three phases to CTX, given with CNS prophylaxis at intervals throughout therapy:
- Induction, consolidation, prolonged maintenance

MEDICATION
- Induction: Goal is to achieve complete remission and restore normal hematopoiesis.
  – Mainstay of treatment is a regimen called hyper-CVAD (1)[A]: hyperfractionated cyclophosphamide, vincristine, anthracycline, and dexamethasone, and is the most widely used regimen.
  – Hyper-CVAD consists of eight alternating treatment cycles of parts A and B:
    ○ Part A: hyper-CVAD
    ○ Part B: high-dose methotrexate and cytarabine

○ Granulocyte colony-stimulating factors given after each cycle to prevent delay in treatment and hasten bone marrow recovery (1)[A]

○ CNS prophylaxis: IT CTX consistent—methotrexate or cytarabine or 6-mercaptopurine (6-MP) (1)[A]

○ CNS leukemia at diagnosis needs twice a week IT therapy until CSF is cleared on three subsequent LP (1)[A].

– <40 years of age with complete remission after the first induction; the next step is either consolidation CTX or allogeneic stem cell transplant based on risk donor availability.

– Minimal residual disease (MRD), measured by flow cytometry in the US, signifies CTX refractory disease, usually in 8 months from start of treatment with continued CTX. These patients should be evaluated for an allogeneic bone marrow transplant (1)[A].

- Consolidation: Goal is to eliminate residual leukemic cells after induction therapy.
  – Induction phase drugs are used.
  – Peg-asparaginase is used in children but has poor outcomes and toxicities in adults.
- Prolonged maintenance: Goal is to prevent relapse and prolong remission.
  – Consist of POMP: daily 6-MP, weekly methotrexate, monthly vincristine, with pulses of prednisone for 2 to 3 years. Little benefit has been shown for >3 years of prolonged maintenance (1),(2)[A].
  – Dexamethasone can be substituted for prednisone, a.k.a DOMP.
- Special considerations
  – Besides hyper-CVAD, some pediatric ALL regimens have shown superior remission outcomes for adults from 15 to 39 years. These usually contain vincristine and peg-asparaginase, nonmyelosuppressive agents.
  – Allogeneic stem cell transplantation is recommended with relapsed ALL during the first remission or for high-risk genetic features.
  – Burkitt leukemia requires 18 weeks of treatment, has better outcomes with methotrexate and alkylating agents in the initial therapy.
  – Rituximab improves outcomes if CD20 expression is >20% of blast cells in ALL.
  – Immunotherapy: Bispecific anti-CD19/anti-CD3 antibody blinatumomab is approved for relapse/refractory ALL.
  – Ofatumumab, a 2nd-generation anti-CD20 monoclonal antibody, is an alternative frontline therapy for CD20+ pre-B-ALL and option for patients who failed a rituximab-based regimen.
  – Ph-positive ALL have improved prognosis with tyrosine kinase inhibitors (TKIs) targeting BCR-ABL1 translocation. Consolidation/maintenance with a TKI may be used instead of allogeneic stem cell transplant in these patients.
  – Adult T-cell ALL is much less common than B-cell ALL and has a relapse rate up to 50% with traditional hyper-CVAD therapy. Nelarabine, a T cell–specific purine nucleoside, is approved for relapsed T-cell ALL, with additional clinical trials studying a combination of hyper-CVAD and nelarabine as part of induction therapy.

– Patients with unfavorable cytogenetic subtypes should undergo allogeneic stem cell transplantation on first remission if an HLA-identical donor is available.

– Inotuzumab-ozogamicin (InO) combination has shown higher rates of complete remission and longer progression free and overall survival in patients with relapsed or refractory ALL when compared to standard therapy (1).

ISSUES FOR REFERRAL
Patients should be referred to and treated by an oncologist, preferably at a comprehensive cancer center where medication regimen can be tailored as appropriate with a combination of multiple modalities.

SURGERY/OTHER PROCEDURES
In some centers, patients may undergo surgical placement of a port for CTX. Nevertheless, PICC lines are preferred as they can be easily removed after treatment to decrease the risk of infections, which is important as these patients can get neutropenic.

COMPLEMENTARY & ALTERNATIVE MEDICINE
Unproven

 ## ONGOING CARE

FOLLOW-UP RECOMMENDATIONS
Patient Monitoring
- Inpatient admission during induction CTX for continuous infusion and monitoring of complications
- Weekly clinic visits with remission consolidation CTX
- Monthly clinic visits during maintenance therapy
- Outpatient follow-up every 3 months thereafter

DIET
- Nutritional support; avoid alcohol.
- Calcium/vitamin D for steroid-induced osteoporosis

PATIENT EDUCATION
- Neutropenic precautions
- Physical rehabilitation for deconditioning
- Emphasize smoking cessation.

PROGNOSIS
About 80–90% of adults <60 years will achieve a complete remission; however, only 40–50% will remain cured due to relapses. Only 30–40% of adults have a 5-year overall survival as opposed to in children.

COMPLICATIONS
- Hyperleukocytosis: WBC >50,000 to 100,000 can lead to leukostasis, a medical emergency with microvascular white cell plugs; presents with neurologic deficits or respiratory distress, treated with fluids, and cytoreductive therapy
- Tumor lysis syndrome (high uric acid, potassium, phosphate, decreased calcium, leading to renal failure and cardiac arrhythmias) may be prevented by administering allopurinol prior to CTX. Doses should be reduced if used with 6-MP or azathioprine. Increase fluids; IV urate oxidase (rasburicase) can be used to treat hyperuricemia rapidly (if not G6PD deficient).

- Neutropenia from myelosuppression
- High-dose cyclophosphamide causes severe nausea and vomiting. Use appropriate antiemetic regimen.
- Vincristine can cause neurotoxicity and ileus.
- Alkylating agents and corticosteroids can cause AVN or osteonecrosis.
- Steroid-induced hyperglycemia
- Anthracyclines causes cardiotoxicity; obtain transthoracic echocardiography before hyper-CVAD initiation with monitoring during treatment to assessment left ventricular ejection fraction.
- Asparaginase therapy increases risks for deep vein thromboses and veno-occlusive disease.
- Infections (*Pneumocystis carinii* pneumonia, bacterial and fungal pneumonia or sepsis)
- CTX can cause sterility, pancreatitis and liver dysfunction, arachnoiditis, and CNS effects.
- Relapse of ALL in marrow or extramedullary sites (CNS, testis)

REFERENCES
1. Kantarjian HM, O'Brien S, Smith TL, et al. Results of treatment with hyper-CVAD, a dose-intensive regimen, in adult acute lymphocytic leukemia. *J Clin Oncol*. 2000;18(3):547–561.
2. Jabbour E, O'Brien S, Konopleva M, et al. New insights into the pathophysiology and therapy of adult acute lymphoblastic leukemia. *Cancer*. 2015;121(15):2517–2528.

ADDITIONAL READING
Davis AS, Viera AJ, Mead MD. Leukemia: an overview for primary care. *Am Fam Physician*. 2014;89(9):731–738.

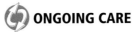 ## CODES

ICD10
- C91.00 Acute lymphoblastic leukemia not having achieved remission
- C91.01 Acute lymphoblastic leukemia, in remission
- C91.02 Acute lymphoblastic leukemia, in relapse

CLINICAL PEARLS
- ALL diagnosis is based on the presence of lymphoblasts or characteristic mutations in the bone marrow.
- Hyper-CVAD is the main therapy.
- Treatment at an appropriate cancer center for tailored therapy based on mutations in ALL cells
- Patients need to be monitored closely for CTX toxicities and progression of disease.

L

LEUKEMIA, ACUTE MYELOID

Jan Cerny, MD, PhD

BASICS

DESCRIPTION
- Acute myeloid leukemia (AML) is characterized by proliferation of abnormal immature myeloid progenitors (blasts) with reduced capacity to differentiate leading to bone marrow failure and a variety of systemic symptoms.
- Historically, the French–American–British (FAB) classification system divided AML based on the cell morphology with the addition of cytogenetics (subtypes M0 to M7).
- The World Health Organization (WHO) classification attempts to provide more meaningful prognostic information.
  - AML with characteristic genetic abnormalities: translocation t(8;21), t(15;17), and inversion in chromosome 16 inv(16)
  - AML with multilineage dysplasia: presence of a prior myelodysplastic syndrome (MDS) or myeloproliferative neoplasm (MPN) that transformed into AML
  - AML and MDS, therapy related
  - AML not otherwise categorized
  - Acute leukemias of ambiguous lineage (*biphenotypic acute leukemia*)

EPIDEMIOLOGY
- ~19,940 cases estimated in 2020, making it the most common type of leukemia in adults
- Predominant sex: male ≥ female

Incidence
The incidence of AML increases with age, and median age is 67 years.

ETIOLOGY AND PATHOPHYSIOLOGY
Precise causes unknown, but some risk factors have been identified (see "Risk Factors").

Genetics
- Three risk groups
  - Good risk: inv(16), t(8;21), t(15;17)
  - Standard risk: normal karyotype
  - Poor risk: monosomy 5 and 7 (typically secondary AML), deletion 5q, abnormalities of 11q23, or complex karyotype
- *FLT3* gene mutations, especially internal tandem duplications (FLT3-ITD), have been associated with poor survival in AML. These and growing list of (onco)gene (e.g., *NPM1*, *IDH1/2*, *DNMT3A*, and *P53*) mutations have been studied to further risk-stratify patients (1).

RISK FACTORS
- Genetic predisposition (e.g., Down syndrome); Bloom syndrome (~25% develop AML), Fanconi anemia (52%), neurofibromatosis, Li-Fraumeni syndrome, Wiskott-Aldrich syndrome, Kostmann syndrome, and Diamond-Blackfan anemia
- Radiation exposure
- Immunodeficiency states
- Chemical and drug exposure (nitrogen mustard and alkylating agents; benzene)
- MDS
- Cigarette smoking

GENERAL PREVENTION
None currently identified, but treatment of high-risk MDS with hypomethylating agents (5-azacitidine [Vidaza]) has been shown to prolong time to transformation from MDS into AML

COMMONLY ASSOCIATED CONDITIONS
- Disseminated intravascular coagulopathy (DIC) especially in acute promyelocytic leukemia (APL) but may be seen in any AML
- Leukostasis (high blast number and increased adhesive ability of blasts)
- Tumor lysis syndrome (TLS): spontaneous or in response to chemotherapy

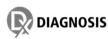

DIAGNOSIS

HISTORY
Fatigue (anemia or tumor burden); bleeding (low platelets or DIC); difficulty clearing infections (neutropenia or immune dysregulation)

PHYSICAL EXAM
- Mostly nonspecific and related to marrow or tissue infiltration
  - Fever, bleeding, pallor, splenomegaly, hepatosplenomegaly
  - Lymphadenopathy (usually reactive)
- If CNS is involved, symptoms of increased intracranial pressure can be present.
- Occasionally, patients will present with prominent extramedullary sites of leukemia (e.g., skin infiltration or ultimately as a myeloid sarcoma).

DIFFERENTIAL DIAGNOSIS
- Virus-induced cytopenia, lymphadenopathy, and organomegaly
- Immune cytopenias (including systemic lupus erythematosus [SLE])
- Drug-induced cytopenias
- Other marrow failure and infiltrative diseases (e.g., aplastic anemia, paroxysmal nocturnal hemoglobinuria, MDS, Gaucher disease)

DIAGNOSTIC TESTS & INTERPRETATION
- CBC shows subnormal RBCs, neutrophils, and platelets.
- Bone marrow for histology, flow cytometry, and cytogenetics to establish diagnosis and prognosis
- ESR
- Lactate dehydrogenase (LDH) and uric acid can be elevated (e.g., TLS).
- Coagulation profile can be normal or prolonged (e.g., DIC).
- Drugs that may alter lab results: chemotherapy agents, corticosteroids
- Other special tests: Spinal tap may reveal fluid with leukemic cells.
- Ultrasonography or CT scan of the abdomen may discover organomegaly.

Diagnostic Procedures/Other
Bone marrow studies are usually necessary to make the diagnosis.
- Aspirates: for cell morphology, cytochemistries, immunophenotyping (can confirm differentiation stage of AML); cytogenetics: chromosomal aberration (prognostic value; see "Genetics")

- Biopsies provide valuable information for cellularity, architecture, and so forth.

Test Interpretation
- Marrow is usually hypercellular and the normal architecture effaced; leukemic blast count is 20% or more.
- Liver and spleen may be infiltrated with leukemic cells.

TREATMENT
- Classical (cytotoxic) chemotherapy has been the backbone of AML therapy; it consists of induction and consolidation phase ± maintenance (APL), but more recently, other transplant-ineligible AML patients can be treated with hypomethylating agent (oral) azacitidine.
- Bone marrow transplantation (BMT) for high-risk AML
- Relatively modest improvements have been made in AML induction chemotherapy. Supportive care had improved significantly.

GENERAL MEASURES
- Close monitoring of bone marrow, liver, heart, renal function, and coagulation parameters (risk for DIC)
- Supportive therapy with
  - Good hydration
  - Transfusions of packed RBCs and platelets based on patient's needs (threshold as for platelets as low as 5,000); use leukoreduced, irradiated blood products because all patients can be considered for BMT.
  - Avoid antiplatelet agents (e.g., aspirin products).
  - Follow febrile neutropenic guidelines in neutropenic patient who becomes febrile (even low-grade fever).

Geriatric Considerations
- Older patients (>60 to 65 years of age) remain a therapeutic challenge. These patients are offered so-called reduced-intensity or nonmyeloablative BMT.
- Adding growth factors (granulocyte colony-stimulating factor [G-CSF]) may reduce toxicity in older patients (but is not broadly accepted).
- Hypomethylating agent, such as 5-azacitidine or decitabine, with or without Venetoclax have been broadly adopted and prolong survival in older adults ineligible for classical chemotherapy.

Pregnancy Considerations
Chemotherapy is a viable option in the 2nd and 3rd trimesters.

MEDICATION
First Line
- APL (APL, AML with t[15;17])
  - All-trans retinoic acid (ATRA) and arsenic trioxide both promote maturation to granulocytes. Their combination can be used in low- and intermediate-risk APL for (chemotherapy) free treatment.
  - Idarubicin is often added to induction therapy, in high-risk group.
  - Monoclonal anti-CD33 (Myelotarg) is being added as well in order to minimize chemotherapy use in this curable leukemia.

- Treatment of AML in younger adults: AML (other than APL)
  - Induction (daunorubicin or idarubicin [anthracycline and cytarabine]): The generally accepted combination is 3 + 7 (anthracycline is given for 3 days and cytarabine for 7 days) or more intensive regimens with high-dose cytarabine (HiDAC) or high dose of anthracycline.
  - Liposomal preparation of daunorubicin and cytarabine (Vyxeos) is now available for AML with MDS changes or therapy-related AML.
- Remission is typically consolidated in younger patients by the following:
  - In good-risk AML, 3 to 4 cycles of HiDAC and BMT is reserved for time of recurrence.
  - In poor-risk patients, 1 to 2 cycles of HiDAC (until donor is identified) are followed by allogeneic BMT.
  - Intermediate-risk AML should be treated based on individual patient's features, donor availability, and access to clinical trials. A meta-analysis showed that even intermediate-risk patients benefit from allogeneic BMT.
- Treatment of AML in older adults (>65 years of age) remains a challenge. These patients have poor performance status, more likely secondary AML, higher incidence of unfavorable cytogenetics, comorbidities, shorter remissions, and shorter overall survival. Liposomal daunorubicin and cytarabine is an agent approved for secondary and therapy related AML.
  - Intensive chemotherapy may be feasible for patients with good performance status; alternative regimens with mitoxantrone, fludarabine, and clofarabine
  - Newly diagnosed patients who are 75 years or older or who have conditions that preclude them from receiving intense induction therapy have following options of novel (targeted) agents.
    - Low-dose cytarabine with glasdegib (DAURISMO, Pfizer Labs)
    - Hypomethylating agents (azacitidine [Vidaza], decitabine [Dacogen]) with ivosidenib (Tibsovo; IDH1 inhibitor)
    - Hypomethylating agents (azacitidine [Vidaza], decitabine [Dacogen]) with venetoclax (Venclexta; BCL-2 inhibitor)
- FLT-3 inhibitors such as midostaurin (Rydapt) are approved as addition to induction and consolidation chemotherapy, and gilteritinib (Xospata) is approved for relapsed/refractory AML.
- Ivosidenib (Tibsovo; IDH1 inhibitor) and enasidenib (Idhifa; IDH2 inhibitor) are approved for relapsed/refractory AML. Both of these agents can cause differentiation syndrome similar to the one seen in ATRA or arsenic treated APL patients.
- Contraindications: comorbidities; therapy has to be individualized.
- Precautions
  - If organ failure, some drugs may be avoided or dose reduced (e.g., no anthracyclines in patients with preexisting cardiac problems).
  - Patients will be immunosuppressed during treatment. Avoid live vaccines. Administer varicella-zoster or measles immunoglobulin as soon as exposure of patient occurs.
- Significant possible interactions: Allopurinol accentuates the toxicity of 6-mercaptopurine.

- Targeted therapies: midostaurin for AML with FLT3 mutations (both ITD and TKD). Ivosidenib (IDH1 inhibitor) and enasidenib (IDH2 inhibitor) for relapsed/refractory AML with respective IDH mutations; gemtuzumab ozogamicin (anti-CD33 monoclonal antibody) for relapsed/refractory AML with CD33 expression

Second Line
- Healthy, younger patients usually are offered reinduction chemotherapy and allogeneic BMT.
- Older patients would receive hypomethylating agent with or without venetoclax or targeted agent (FLT3 or IDH 1/2 inhibitor).

ISSUES FOR REFERRAL
Refer patient to a transplant center early because a search for a donor may be necessary.

SURGERY/OTHER PROCEDURES
- BMT: Decision between myeloablative and nonmyeloablative approach should be based on patient's performance status, comorbidities, and AML risk factors.
  - Allogeneic BMT is usually indicated in first remission in intermediate- or high-risk AML or in second remission in all other AML patients. Matched related donor used to be preferred over matched unrelated donor (lower risk of graft versus host disease); recent data suggest equal outcomes because allogeneic transplant regimens and post-transplant care have improved significantly.
- Haploidentical transplants and cord blood have emerged as alternative sources of hematopoietic stem cells for adults that show comparable outcomes as well.
- Autologous BMT may be acceptable in specific situations (e.g., no donor is available).

ADMISSION, INPATIENT, AND NURSING CONSIDERATIONS
- Induction treatment for AML requires inpatient care, usually on a specialized ward. Episodes of febrile neutropenia typically require admission and IV antibiotics.
- Appropriate hydration to prevent TLS
- IV may lead to chemical burns in the event of extravasation.

 ONGOING CARE

FOLLOW-UP RECOMMENDATIONS
Patient Monitoring
- Repeat bone marrow studies to document remission and also if a relapse is suspected.
- Follow CBC with differential, coagulation studies, uric acid level, and other chemistries related to TLS (creatinine, potassium, phosphate, calcium); monitor urinary function at least daily during induction phase and less frequently later.
- Physical evaluation, including weight and BP, should be done frequently during treatment.

DIET
Total parenteral nutrition (TPN) in case of severe mucositis

PATIENT EDUCATION
Leukemia Society of America, 600 Third Avenue, New York, NY 10016, 212-573-8484

PROGNOSIS
AML remission rate is 60–80%, with only 20–40% long-term survival. The wide variable prognosis is due to prognostic group (age, cytogenetics, and genetics).

COMPLICATIONS
- Acute side effects of chemotherapy, including febrile neutropenia
- TLS
- DIC
- Late-onset cardiomyopathy in patients treated with anthracyclines
- Chronic side effects of chemotherapy (secondary malignancies)
- Graft versus host disease in patients who have received allogeneic BMT

REFERENCE
1. Döhner H, Estey EH, Amadori S, et al; for European LeukemiaNet. Diagnosis and management of acute myeloid leukemia in adults: recommendations from an international expert panel, on behalf of the European LeukemiaNet. *Blood.* 2010;115(3): 453–474.

ADDITIONAL READING
O'Donnell MR, Appelbaum FR, Coutre SE, et al. Acute myeloid leukemia. *J Natl Compr Canc Netw.* 2008;6(10):962–993.

 SEE ALSO

Disseminated Intravascular Coagulation; Leukemia, Acute Lymphoblastic (ALL) in Adults; Leukemia, Chronic Myelogenous; Myelodysplastic Syndromes (MDS); Myeloproliferative Neoplasms

CODES

ICD10
- C92.00 Acute myeloblastic leukemia, not having achieved remission
- C92.01 Acute myeloblastic leukemia, in remission
- C92.02 Acute myeloblastic leukemia, in relapse

CLINICAL PEARLS
- Acute myeloid leukemia (AML) is a proliferation and accumulation of abnormal immature myeloid progenitors (blasts) with reduced capacity to differentiate into more mature cellular elements. This leads to bone marrow failure and results in a variety of systemic symptoms.
- AML is most common leukemia in adults
- Prognosis of leukemia depends on the cytogenetic and molecular profile of the disease.
- Allogeneic transplant remains the only therapy with curative potential for patients with intermediate- and high-risk AML.

L

LEUKEMIA, CHRONIC LYMPHOCYTIC

Jan Cerny, MD, PhD

BASICS

DESCRIPTION
- Chronic lymphocytic leukemia (CLL) is a monoclonal disorder characterized by a progressive accumulation of mature but functionally incompetent lymphocytes.
- Based on percentage of prolymphocytes, the disease may be regarded as CLL (<10% prolymphocytes), prolymphocytic leukemia (PLL; >55%), or CLL/PLL (>10% and <55%).
- Small lymphocytic lymphoma is a lymphoma variant of CLL.
- System(s) affected: hematologic, lymphatic, immunologic

EPIDEMIOLOGY
Incidence
- CLL represents the most common form of leukemia in adults in the United States with an estimated 21,050 new cases diagnosed in 2021.
- In 2021, an estimated 4,320 adults in the United States died from CLL, which makes it the second leading cause of death among adults with leukemia in the United States after acute myeloid leukemia.
- CLL primarily affects elderly individuals, median age of diagnosis being 70 years. Incidence continues to rise in those age >55 years.
- Predominant sex: male > female (1.6:1)
- The incidence is higher among Caucasians than among African Americans.

ETIOLOGY AND PATHOPHYSIOLOGY
- The cell of origin in CLL is a clonal B cell arrested in the B-cell differentiation pathway, intermediate between pre–B cells and mature B cells. In the peripheral blood, these cells resemble mature lymphocytes.
- Genetic mutations leading to disrupted function and prolonged survival of affected lymphocytes are suspected but not well known. The BCL2 proto-oncogene (suppressor of apoptosis or programmed cell death) is overexpressed in CLL.

Genetics
Truly familial cases are exceedingly rare. CLL has been shown, however, to occur at higher frequency among first-degree relatives of patients with the disease, and several somatic gene mutations have been identified at significantly higher rates among CLL patients (1).

RISK FACTORS
The exact cause of CLL is uncertain. Possible chronic immune stimulation is suspected but is still being evaluated. Monoclonal B-cell lymphocytosis: 1% risk progression to CLL

GENERAL PREVENTION
Unknown

COMMONLY ASSOCIATED CONDITIONS
- Immune system dysregulation is common.
- Autoimmune hemolytic anemia (AIHA)
- Immune thrombocytopenia purpura (ITP)
- Pure red cell aplasia (PRCA)

DIAGNOSIS

HISTORY
- Insidious onset. CLL is often discovered incidentally (up to 40% of patients are asymptomatic at the time of diagnosis).
- Others may have the following symptoms:
  - B symptoms: fevers, night sweats, >10% weight loss
  - Fatigue and/or other symptoms of anemia
  - Enlarged lymph nodes (lymphadenopathy = LAD)
  - Mucocutaneous bleeding and/or petechiae
  - Early satiety and/or abdominal discomfort related to an enlarged spleen
  - Recurrent infection(s)

PHYSICAL EXAM
- Lymphadenopathy (localized or generalized)
- Organomegaly (splenomegaly, hepatomegaly)
- Mucocutaneous bleeding (thrombocytopenia)
- Skin: petechiae (thrombocytopenia), pallor (anemia), rash (leukemia cutis)

DIFFERENTIAL DIAGNOSIS
- Infectious:
  - Bacterial (tuberculosis, pertussis)
  - Viral (mononucleosis)
- Neoplastic:
  - Leukemic phase of non-Hodgkin lymphomas
  - Hairy cell leukemia
  - PLL
  - Large granular lymphocytic leukemia
  - Waldenström macroglobulinemia

DIAGNOSTIC TESTS & INTERPRETATION
Initial Tests (lab, imaging)
- CBC with differential: B cell absolute lymphocytosis with >5,000 B lymphocytes/μL; often also shows anemia and/or thrombocytopenia in advanced stage
- Blood smear: ruptured lymphocytes ("smudge" cells) and morphologically small mature-appearing lymphocytes
- Confirm diagnosis with immunophenotyping on peripheral blood via flow cytometry or lymph node biopsy: CLL cells are positive for CD19, CD20 (dim), CD23, and CD5; low levels of surface membrane immunoglobulin (Ig)—either IgM or IgM and IgD; only a single Ig light chain is expressed (κ or λ) confirming monoclonality.
- Additional labs:
  - Hemolysis labs (in cases associated with high disease activity or AIHA): high LDH and indirect bilirubin, low haptoglobin, +/– elevated reticulocyte count (bone marrow infiltration)
  - High plasma β_2-microglobulin (poor prognosis)
  - Hypogammaglobulinemia
- Liver/spleen ultrasound: may demonstrate organomegaly and enlarged abdominal lymph nodes (not required for initial workup)
- CT scan of chest/abdomen/pelvis: not necessary for staging but may identify compression of organs or internal structures from enlarged lymph nodes
- Positron emission tomography (PET) scan: not recommended unless Richter transformation (RT) is suspected

Follow-Up Tests & Special Considerations
Frequency and type of follow-up depend on severity of symptoms as well as risk factors (see "Prognosis").

Diagnostic Procedures/Other
- Bone marrow biopsy: not performed routinely but may be helpful to assess etiology of cytopenia found in conjunction with CLL diagnosis
- Lymph node biopsy: Consider if lymph node(s) begins to rapidly enlarge in a patient with known CLL to assess the possibility of transformation to a high-grade lymphoma (RT), especially when accompanied by fever, weight loss, and painful lymphadenopathy.

Test Interpretation
- Bone marrow biopsy aspirate usually shows >30% lymphocytes.
- Cytogenetics (fluorescence in situ hybridization) may show chromosomal changes, which are prognostic:
  - Unfavorable: del(17p) or TP53 mutation, del(11q), unmutated immunoglobulin heavy-chain variable (IGHV)
  - Neutral: normal, trisomy 12
  - Favorable: del(13q), mutated IGHV

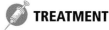

TREATMENT

GENERAL MEASURES
- Patients with frequent infections due to hypogammaglobulinemia are likely to benefit from infusions of intravenous immunoglobulin (IVIG).
- Genetic risk stratification in therapy selection for advanced or symptomatic CLL
  - Very high-risk disease: del (17p) and/or TP53 mutations
  - High-risk disease: IGHV unmutated (without 17p del or TP53 mutation)
  - Standard risk disease: IGHV mutated (without 17p del or TP53 mutation)

MEDICATION
First Line
- Standard of care for new diagnosis with no symptoms or early stage disease: observation
- Standard of care for new diagnosis with symptoms (B symptoms, symptomatic anemia and/or thrombocytopenia as a result of progressive marrow failure, AIHA and/or thrombocytopenia poorly responsive to corticosteroids, progressive organomegaly), steroid-refractory autoimmune cytopenias, or progressive lymphocytosis (increase >50% in 2 months or a doubling time of <6 months): Initiate treatment.
- Low-risk disease, Rai stage 0: observation with periodic follow-up
- Intermediate-risk group, Rai stages I and II: Observe until evidence of disease progression or development of symptoms.
- High-risk patients, Rai stage III and IV: Initiate treatment. Selection of first-line therapy depends on patient functional status (age, performance status, and medical comorbidities), as well as genetic risk stratification their CLL (above).

- Main groups of therapeutic agents:
  - Targeted therapies: preferred especially for very high and high-risk patients
    - Bruton tyrosine kinase (BTK) inhibitor: ibrutinib, acalabrutinib, and zanubrutinib
    - BCL2 inhibitor: venetoclax
  - Immunotherapy:
    - Monoclonal anti-CD20 antibodies (immunotherapy): rituximab (R), obinutuzumab, ofatumumab
  - Chemotherapy:
    - Alkylators: cyclophosphamide (C), chlorambucil, and bendamustine (B)
    - Purine analogs: fludarabine (F), cladribine, and pentostatin (P)
- Ibrutinib or acalabrutinib (newer agents have fewer side effects) can be used with rituximab or obinutuzumab (2).
- Venetoclax in combination with obinituzumab and BTK inhibitor offer very effective regimens fixed duration.
- Combinations with venetoclax are being evaluated for the possibility of time-limited treatment for CLL patients that achieved complete response at the molecular level.
- Combination regimens: FC, FR (lower toxicity), BR, PCR, and FCR are used less often, but FCR with BTK inhibitor can offer time-limited and highly effective therapy in IGHV-mutated CLL).
- Steroids, high dose: useful in autoimmune manifestations of CLL (AIHA, ITP)

Second Line
- Second-line therapy depends on time to progression and previous therapy.
- Early relapse (within 1 year after chemoimmunotherapy, 2 to 3 years after FCR), treatment with targeted therapy is favored.
  - Alternative BTK inhibitor
  - Venetoclax: as monotherapy and with rituximab in relapsed/refractory CLL and in patients with 17p deletion (2)
  - PI3K kinase inhibitors: idelalisib (PI3Kδ) with rituximab in patients with comorbidities. Duvelisib (PI3Kδ and PI3Kγ): approved as single agent for patients (PJP prophylaxis is recommended.) (2)
  - Obinutuzumab alone or with chlorambucil in patients with comorbidities and previously untreated CLL, ofatumumab
- Other options:
  - Lenalidomide, a thalidomide derivative, can be useful in some situations.
- Allogenic (nonmyeloablative conditioning) hematopoietic stem cell transplant (hSCT) may be considered in high-risk and younger patients, particularly those with refractory or RT.

ISSUES FOR REFERRAL
- Surgical consultation for splenectomy in patients with progressive splenomegaly +/− refractory cytopenias
- Radiation oncology consultation for large or bulky lymphadenopathy, particularly those causing compressive symptoms

ADDITIONAL THERAPIES
- Patients requiring therapy who are high risk for tumor lysis syndrome should be given allopurinol to prevent uric acid nephropathy.

- Vaccinations (avoid live vaccines):
  - Annual influenza vaccine
  - Pneumococcal vaccine every 5 years
  - Zoster vaccine recombinant, adjuvanted for treatment-naïve patients, or those treated with BTK inhibitor
  - COVID-19 vaccination

SURGERY/OTHER PROCEDURES
See "Issues for Referral" above.

ADMISSION, INPATIENT, AND NURSING CONSIDERATIONS
Complications of disease (AIHA) or of therapy (febrile neutropenia, tumor lysis syndrome). Venetoclax can be associated with tumor lysis syndrome and monitoring inpatient may be needed.

ONGOING CARE

FOLLOW-UP RECOMMENDATIONS
Patient Monitoring
Patients with low-risk CLL and/or patients in remission:
- CBC with differential (lymphocytosis), LDH, and β_2-microglobulin every 3 to 6 months
- Physical exam (lymphadenopathy, organomegaly)

DIET
- Ensure adequately balanced calorie/vitamin intake.
- Follow weights.

PATIENT EDUCATION
Leukemia and Lymphoma Society has educational pamphlets: https://www.lls.org/resource-center/download-or-order-free-publications?language=English&category=Leukemia&sortby=alpha

PROGNOSIS
- Rai system used in the United States and Binet system in Europe. There is also an International Prognostic Score for Early-Stage CLL (IPS-E) for predicting time to first treatment.
- Rai staging system:
  - Stage 0: lymphocytosis only; low-risk status
  - Stage I: lymphocytosis and adenopathy; intermediate-risk status
  - Stage II: lymphocytosis +/− adenopathy and splenomegaly and/or hepatomegaly; intermediate-risk status
  - Stage III: lymphocytosis and anemia (hemoglobin <11 g/dL); high-risk status
  - Stage IV: lymphocytosis and thrombocytopenia (platelets $<100 \times 10^9$/L); high-risk status
- IPS-E is helpful to identify patients who are at risk of needed therapy sooner.
  - The IPS-E is calculated by giving 1 point for each of the following
    - Unmutated IGHV
    - Lymphocytes $>15 \times 10^9$/L
    - Palpable lymph nodes
    - A score of 0 indicated low risk, 1 intermediate risk, and 2 to 3 high risk of progressing to symptomatic disease requiring treatment.

- Adverse risk factors:
  - Advanced stage, peripheral lymphocyte doubling time <12 months, diffuse marrow infiltration, increased number of prolymphocytes or cleaved cells, poor response to chemotherapy, high β_2-microglobulin and thymidine kinase levels and low micro-RNAs (miRNAs), abnormal karyotyping: del(17p) and del(11q), IGHV genes (expression of ZAP-70 >20% or CD38 >30% evaluated by immunophenotyping are surrogate markers.), NOTCH1 mutation (associated with unmutated IgVH), increased CIRS (Cumulative Illness Rating Scale)

COMPLICATIONS
Acute or long-term effects of chemotherapy and targeted therapy, RT, AIHA (some cases may be related to the use of fludarabine), slightly increased risk of solid tumors (especially Kaposi sarcoma, malignant melanoma, laryngeal, lung and colon cancer), infection, membranoproliferative glomerulonephritis (MPGN)

REFERENCES
1. Yan H, Tian S, Kleinstern G, et al. Chronic lymphocytic leukemia (CLL) risk is mediated by multiple enhancer variants within CLL risk loci. *Hum Mol Genet*. 2020;29(16):2761–2774.
2. Burger J. Treatment of chronic lymphocytic leukemia. *N Engl J Med*. 2020;383(5):460–473.

ADDITIONAL READING
National Comprehensive Cancer Network. National Comprehensive Cancer Network guidelines. https://www.nccn.org/guidelines/nccn-guidelines.

CODES

ICD10
- C91.12 Chronic lymphocytic leukemia of B-cell type in relapse
- C91.11 Chronic lymphocytic leukemia of B-cell type in remission
- C91.10 Chronic lymphocytic leukemia of B-cell type not having achieved remission

CLINICAL PEARLS
- CLL is the most common form of leukemia in adults in the United States.
- CLL primarily affects elderly individuals, median age of diagnosis being 70 years. Incidence continues to rise in those age >55 years.
- Clinical monitoring of asymptomatic and low-risk patients is a reasonable approach ("watch and wait").
- High-risk patients, patients with bulky disease, and patients who fail fludarabine- and rituximab-based therapies typically have poor prognoses and may require intensive therapies, including allogeneic hSCT.
- Several novel agents are being developed to improve therapeutic approaches to CLL.

L

LEUKEMIA, CHRONIC MYELOGENOUS

Jan Cerny, MD, PhD • Erin Thomas, MD, BS

BASICS

DESCRIPTION
- Chronic myelogenous leukemia (CML) is a myeloproliferative neoplasm characterized by clonal proliferation of myeloid precursors in the bone marrow with continuing differentiation into mature granulocytes.
- Hallmark of CML is Philadelphia chromosome (translocation t[9;22]).
- Natural history of the disease evolves in three clinical phases: a chronic phase, an accelerated phase, and a blast phase or crisis (can transform to acute myeloid leukemia [80%] or acute lymphoblastic leukemia [20%]).

EPIDEMIOLOGY
Incidence
- Per year, 1.9 cases/100,000 persons
- Median age at diagnosis: 65
- Predominant sex: male > female (1.7:1)

Prevalence
Accounts for 15–20% of adult leukemias

ETIOLOGY AND PATHOPHYSIOLOGY
Philadelphia chromosome is a balanced translocation between *BCR* (on chromosome 22) and *ABL* (on chromosome 9) genes t(9;22)(q34;q11). This fusion gene, *BCR-ABL*, codes for an abnormal, constitutively active tyrosine kinase that affects numerous signal transduction pathways, resulting in uncontrolled cell proliferation and reduced apoptosis.

Genetics
Acquired genomic changes

RISK FACTORS
Ionizing radiation exposure (uncommon)

GENERAL PREVENTION
None currently identified

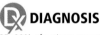

DIAGNOSIS

85–90% of patients present in the chronic phase, and the disease can be found incidentally during routine screening (up to 50%).

HISTORY
- Chronic phase: fatigue, weight loss, night sweats, abdominal fullness owing to enlarged spleen, early satiety, dyspnea, and bleeding. Rare: bruising, left upper quadrant abdominal pain, sternal pain (owing to expanding bone marrow), and gouty arthritis; up to 30% of patients are asymptomatic.
- Accelerated phase: progressive splenomegaly and left upper quadrant abdominal pain occasionally referred to the left shoulder (owing to splenic infarction or rupture), progressive weight loss and sweats, unexplained fever or bone pain, chloromas (extramedullary tumors)
- Blast phase: bleeding, bruising, infections, prominent constitutional symptoms

PHYSICAL EXAM
- Splenomegaly (50–90%), hepatomegaly (<10%)
- Less common: splenic friction rub, lymphadenopathy, lower sternal tenderness

DIFFERENTIAL DIAGNOSIS
- Chronic myelomonocytic leukemia, chronic neutrophilic leukemia, chronic eosinophilic leukemia, juvenile myelomonocytic leukemia, infectious mononucleosis, leukemoid reaction, polycythemia vera, and treatment with granulocyte-stimulating factors
- Acute myelogenous leukemia resembles blast crisis with myeloid blasts, and acute lymphoblastic leukemia resembles blast crisis with lymphoid blasts.
- Atypical CML is a chronic myeloproliferative disorder with a clinical hematologic picture similar to CML, but it lacks the Philadelphia chromosome and *BCR-ABL* rearrangement. A hallmark feature is dysplastic granulopoiesis.

DIAGNOSTIC TESTS & INTERPRETATION
- CBC
  - WBC count: markedly increased (50,000 to 100,000/μL), with granulocytes in all stages of maturation, including occasional (<10%) blasts in chronic phase, basophilia, eosinophilia
  - Hematocrit: may be normal, slightly increased, or decreased
  - Platelets: may be normal, elevated, or occasionally low
  - In accelerated phase: anemia, >20% basophils, thrombocytopenia
- Bone marrow biopsy: hypercellular marrow, myeloid hyperplasia. In accelerated phase: 10–19% blasts, > or = 20% blasts in blood or marrow indicates blast phase
- Genetics
  - Demonstration of the Philadelphia chromosome, t(9;22), by cytogenetic techniques, fluorescence in situ hybridization (FISH), or reverse transcription-polymerase chain reaction (RT-PCR)
  - Additional cytogenetic abnormalities occur in the accelerated and blast phases (monosomy 7; t[3,21]; trisomies 8 and 19; Philadelphia chromosome duplication; abnormalities of chromosome 17 such as monosomy, trisomy, and isochromosome mutations). These may contribute to resistance to tyrosine kinase inhibitors (TKIs; e.g., imatinib). Further molecular testing (mutations within *BCR-ABL*) is suggested in case of loss of response to therapy.
- Others:
  - Low or absent leukocyte alkaline phosphatase in neutrophils
  - High lactate dehydrogenase (LDH)
  - Elevated uric acid

Initial Tests (lab, imaging)
- CBC, LDH, uric acid, LFTs, bone marrow biopsy and aspiration, cytogenetics on bone marrow, FISH for *BCR-ABL*, and baseline RT-PCR (quantitative as well as qualitative analysis to identify BCR-ABL transcript type)
- Abdominal ultrasound or CT scan shows splenomegaly; not mandatory

Follow-Up Tests & Special Considerations
- Serial monitoring of BCR-ABL by RT-PCR is used to evaluate response to treatment.
- Mutation analysis of tyrosine kinase domain of *ABL* kinase can predict resistance to therapy with TKIs.
- HLA-A*02 positive is associated with CML, and a protective effect is seen with the HLA-B*35 allele (pooled odds ratio 0.64, 95% CI 0.48–0.86).

Diagnostic Procedures/Other
Bone marrow aspiration and biopsy

Test Interpretation
Myeloid hyperplasia with elevated myeloid: erythroid ratio, normal maturation, marrow basophilia, and increased reticulin fibrosis

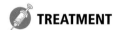

TREATMENT

MEDICATION
- TKIs (e.g., imatinib) provide durable, long-term control of disease.
- The response to TKIs is assessed at specific time points from the beginning of treatment and is categorized as follows:
  - Complete hematologic response (CHR): normalization of peripheral counts, no disease symptoms, no immature cells
  - Complete cytogenetic response (CCR): no Philadelphia-positive metaphases on chromosome analysis
  - Major molecular response (MMR): decreased level of *BCR-ABL* transcript by PCR 3-log
  - Complete molecular response (CMR): *BCR-ABL* transcript is undetectable by PCR.
  - Failure to achieve CHR in 3 months is an indication to change therapy.
  - Hematologic, cytogenetic, and molecular response to TKIs are most important prognostic indicators or predictors of outcome.

First Line
- Imatinib mesylate (Gleevec), an oral TKI, 400 mg/day
- Side effects: thrombocytopenia, anemia, elevated liver enzymes, edema, GI disturbances, rash
- International Randomized Study of Interferon versus STI571 (IRIS) established imatinib as first-line therapy (1)[A], and it has shown long-term efficacy after 10-year follow-up (2)[A].
- Imatinib dose can be increased to 600 and 800 mg/day if only suboptimal response is achieved with standard dose.
- 2nd-generation TKIs have shown higher efficacy and fewer side effects and are approved for first-line therapy of chronic phase CML: nilotinib (Tasigna), dasatinib (Sprycel), and bosutinib (Bosulif) (3),(4),(5)[A].

Second Line
- 2nd-generation TKIs; active against most of *BCR-ABL* mutants; not active in *T315I* mutation
  - Dasatinib
    - 100 mg/day in patients resistant or intolerant to imatinib and 70 mg BID or 140 mg/day for patients in accelerated or blastic phase
    - Side effects: pleural effusions, cytopenias, pulmonary arterial hypertension

- Nilotinib
  - 400 mg PO BID in patients resistant or intolerant to imatinib in chronic or accelerated phase
  - Side effects: cytopenias, QTc prolongation, pancreatitis, hyperglycemia, risk of thrombotic events
- Bosutinib
  - 400 mg PO daily, 500 mg in patients resistant or intolerant to prior therapy in chronic or accelerated phase
  - Side effects: GI toxicity, myelosuppression, hepatotoxicity, fluid retention
- 3rd-generation TKI
  - Ponatinib has restricted approval due to the risk of thrombotic events, but in addition to omacetaxine (below), they are the only effective agents in patients with *T315I* mutation approved by the FDA.
- Other approved agents or in development:
  - Omacetaxine is approved for patient with resistance or intolerance to two TKIs.
  - Asciminib (a STAMP inhibitor, Specifically Targeting the ABL Myristoyl Pocket) is showing promise patients with chronic phase CML who have been treated previously with 2 or more TKIs, or who have the *T315I* mutation.

ISSUES FOR REFERRAL
All patients with CML should be referred to a hematologist. Patients with inadequate response to TKIs or with *T315I* mutation should consult with a bone marrow transplant (BMT) physician.

ADDITIONAL THERAPIES
Agents targeting leukemic stem cells are being developed for clinical use. Emerging agents being studied: PF-114 (4th-generation oral TKI), HQP1351 (3rd-generation oral TKI)

SURGERY/OTHER PROCEDURES
Allogeneic BMT

- It is the only known cure; however, 71% of patients who achieve CCR with imatinib maintain that response beyond 7 years, and no patient progressed on the trial between years 5 and 6 of treatment.
- Most effective in patients <50 years of age who are in the chronic phase
- Initial mortality is higher (related to the use of myeloablative regimens) than medical management but provided higher rates of survival in pre-TKI era.
- Significant improvement in transplant techniques leading to better outcomes, such as alternative sources of stem cells; nonmyeloablative regimens have shown improvements in transplant-related mortality.
- Transplant option should be thoroughly discussed with young patients in chronic phase and considered an alternative to TKIs, especially if the patient does not tolerate TKIs or disease is not responding.
- Can be considered in blast phase CML patients in remission, accelerated phase CML with suboptimal or resistant response to TKIs, and chronic phase patients who fail to achieve CHR by 3 months, have no cytogenetic response or cytogenetic relapse, have *T315I* mutation, or have extramedullary disease with chronic phase CML cells.

ADMISSION, INPATIENT, AND NURSING CONSIDERATIONS
- Acute abdominal symptoms (infarcted or ruptured spleen); tumor lysis syndrome owing to initial therapy; complications of BMT
  - Hydroxyurea might be given, with the goal of reduction of the WBC count, but it has minimal impact on patient response to TKIs.
  - Induction chemotherapy (for acute leukemia) in setting of blastic phase
  - Allopurinol to prevent tumor lysis syndrome in patients with very high counts; however, probably not necessary when TKIs are used
- Discharge criteria: abatement of acute symptoms

 ONGOING CARE

FOLLOW-UP RECOMMENDATIONS
- Frequency depends on stage at presentation and response to first-line therapy.
- Although splenomegaly persists, avoid contact sports or trauma to abdomen.

Patient Monitoring
- CBC with differential: weekly until blood counts stable and then every 2 to 4 weeks during CHR; once in CCR and stable, patient can be followed less frequently (3-month intervals).
- Bone marrow cytogenetics (evaluation for clonal evolution) every 6 months while in CHR, every 12 to 18 months while in CCR, MMR, CMR
- Quantitative RT-PCR every 3 months (peripheral blood)
- ECGs (concern for QT prolongation), LFTs while on TKIs. Nilotinib, bosutinib, and ponatinib can cause pancreatitis.
- Blood pressure monitoring because several TKIs have been associated with elevated blood pressure and related cardiovascular complications

PROGNOSIS
- With treatment and good response, the survival is similar to the normal population.
- Without treatment: CML invariably will progress to accelerated phase within 2 to 5 years and blast phase within several months of the accelerated phase.
- Poor prognosis: patients presenting in accelerated or blastic phase or presenting with very large spleen size, platelets >700,000/μL, and patients resistant to TKIs (*T315I* mutation)

COMPLICATIONS
- Splenic infarct or rupture
- Progression to accelerated or blastic phase
- Thrombotic events owing to elevated platelets
- Bleeding owing to low or dysfunctional platelets
- Sequelae of anemia

REFERENCES
1. O'Brien SG, Guilhot F, Goldman JM, et al. International Randomized Study of Interferon versus STI571 (IRIS) 7-year follow-up: sustained survival, low rate of transformation and increased rate of major molecular response (MMR) in patients (pts) with newly diagnosed chronic myeloid leukemia in chronic phase (CMLCP) treated with imatinib (IM). *Blood*. 2008;112(11):186.
2. Hochhaus A, Larson RA, Guilhot F, et al. Long-term outcomes of imatinib treatment for chronic myeloid leukemia. *N Engl J Med*. 2017;376(10):917–927.
3. Saglio G, Kim DW, Issaragrisil S, et al; for ENESTnd Investigators. Nilotinib versus imatinib for newly diagnosed chronic myeloid leukemia. *N Engl J Med*. 2010;362(24):2251–2259.
4. Kantarjian H, Shah NP, Hochhaus A, et al. Dasatinib versus imatinib in newly diagnosed chronic-phase chronic myeloid leukemia. *N Engl J Med*. 2010;362(24):2260–2270.
5. Corte JE, Gambacorti-Passerini C, Deininger MW, et al. Bosutinib versus imatinib for newly diagnosed chronic myeloid leukemia: results from the randomized BFORE trial. *J Clin Oncol*. 2018;36(3):231–237.

ADDITIONAL READING
- Jabbour E, Kantarjian HM. Chronic myeloid leukemia: 2020 update on diagnosis, therapy and monitoring. *Am J Hematol*. 2020;95(6):691–709.
- Kantarjian HM, Baccarani M, Jabbour E, et al. Second-generation tyrosine kinase inhibitors: the future of frontline CML therapy. *Clin Cancer Res*. 2011;17(7):1674–1683.
- Kantarjian HM, Pasquini R, Hamerschlak N, et al. Dasatinib or high-dose imatinib for chronic-phase chronic myeloid leukemia after failure of first-line imatinib: a randomized phase 2 trial. *Blood*. 2007;109(12):5143–5150.
- Naugler C, Liwski R. Human leukocyte antigen class I alleles and the risk of chronic myelogenous leukemia: a meta-analysis. *Leuk Lymphoma*. 2010;51(7):1288–1292.

CODES

ICD10
- C92.2 Atypical chronic myeloid leukemia, BCR/ABL-negative
- C92.12 Chronic myeloid leukemia, BCR/ABL-positive, in relapse
- C92.22 Atypical chronic myeloid leukemia, BCR/ABL-negative, in relapse

CLINICAL PEARLS
- CML belongs to the myeloproliferative disorders group.
- The gold standard for diagnosis of CML is detection of the Philadelphia chromosome or its products, *BCR-ABL* mRNA, and fusion protein.
- TKIs provide durable, long-term control of the disease and have dramatically altered treatment.
- Atypical CML is a form of clinically typical CML but without the presence of the typical *BCR-ABL* translocation.
- Blast crisis is a form of acute leukemia that is a possible complication of CML.

L

LEUKOPLAKIA, ORAL

Kathya M. Chartre, MD • Kelsey Gallagher, DO • Samuel Michael Leschisin, MD

BASICS

DESCRIPTION
- Leukoplakia is defined by the World Health Organization (WHO) as "a white plaque of questionable risk having excluded (other) known diseases or disorders that carry no increased risk for cancer."
- System(s) affected: gastrointestinal
- Hyperplasia of squamous epithelium

EPIDEMIOLOGY
Most common where more people smoke and chew tobacco and areca nuts (Asian populations)

Incidence
250,000 annual cases worldwide

Prevalence
- Age of onset is >40 years old with peak in the 60s (1).
- Males 3 times more likely to be affected as females (1)
- Smokers 6 times more likely to be affected than nonsmokers (1)

Geriatric Considerations
Malignant transformation to carcinoma is more common in older patients.

ETIOLOGY AND PATHOPHYSIOLOGY
Hyperkeratosis or dyskeratosis of the oral squamous epithelium. Tissue cell exposure to carcinogens spurs adaptive changes including hyperplasia. Continued irritant exposure can lead to cellular degeneration of the epithelium and eventually apoptosis or malignant transformation.
- Tobacco use in any form
- Alcohol consumption/alcoholism
- Periodontitis
- *Candida albicans* infection may induce dysplasia and increase malignant transformation.
- Human papillomavirus types 16 and 18
- Sunlight
- Vitamin deficiency
- Syphilis
- Dental restorations/prosthetic appliances
- Estrogen therapy
- Chronic trauma or irritation
- Epstein-Barr virus (oral hairy leukoplakia)
- Areca nut/betel (Asian populations)
- Mouthwash preparations and toothpaste containing the herbal root extract sanguinaria

Genetics
- Dyskeratosis congenital and epidermolysis bullosa increase the likelihood of oral malignancy.
- P53 overexpression, PTEN allelic loss correlates with leukoplakia and particularly squamous cell carcinoma.
- Changes in expression of p53, p16INK4a and 3p, 9p, and 17 (especially TP53) gene mutations can have greater cancer risk (2).
- Biomarkers: IL-6, IL-8, and TNF-α have been detected in leukoplakia, and there is new research showing possible use of Hsp27 and PTHRP/PTHLH as biomarkers (2).

RISK FACTORS
- 70–90% of oral leukoplakia is related to tobacco, particularly smokeless tobacco or areca/betel nut use.
- Similar to risk factors for squamous cell carcinoma
- Alcohol increases risk 1.5-fold.
- Repeated or chronic mechanical trauma from dental appliances or cheek biting
- Chemical irritation to oral regions
- Diabetes
- Age
- Socioeconomic status
- Risk factors for malignant transformation of leukoplakia
  - Female
  - Long duration of leukoplakia
  - Nonsmoker (idiopathic leukoplakia)
  - Located on tongue or floor of mouth
  - Size >200 mm^2
  - Nonhomogenous type
  - Presence of epithelial dysplasia
  - New research shows possible shift of oral microbiome in those with malignant transformation (3).

GENERAL PREVENTION
- Avoid tobacco of any kind, alcohol, habitual cheek biting, tongue chewing, betel nut ingestion.
- Use well-fitting dental equipment.
- Regular dental check-ups to avoid bad restorations
- Diet rich in fresh fruits and vegetables may help to prevent cancer.
- HPV vaccination may be preventive.

COMMONLY ASSOCIATED CONDITIONS
- HIV infection is closely associated with hairy leukoplakia.
- Erythroplakia in association with leukoplakia, "speckled leukoplakia," or erythroleukoplakia is a marker for underlying dysplasia.

DIAGNOSIS

Leukoplakia is an asymptomatic white patch on the oral mucosa.

HISTORY
- Usually asymptomatic
- History of tobacco or alcohol use or oral exposure to irritants
- Elicit timing of onset, progression, and presence of pain or sensitivity.
- Identify sources of friction or chronic irritation.

PHYSICAL EXAM
- Location
  - Can develop on any oral mucosal surface
  - Floor of mouth, ventrolateral tongue, and soft palate complex are more likely to have dysplastic lesions.
- Appearance
  - Varies from homogeneous, nonpalpable, faintly translucent white areas to thick, fissured, papillomatous, indurated plaques
  - May feel rough or leathery
  - Lesions can become exophytic or verruciform.
  - Color may be white, gray, yellowish white, or brownish gray.
  - Cannot be wiped or scraped off
- WHO classification
  - Homogeneous refers to color.
    - Flat, corrugated, wrinkled, or pumice
  - Nonhomogeneous refers to color and texture (more likely to be dysplastic or malignant).
    - Erythroleukoplakia (mixture of red and white)
    - Proliferative verrucous leukoplakia (PVL) (multifocal, mostly women)

DIFFERENTIAL DIAGNOSIS
- White oral lesions that can be rubbed off: acute pseudomembranous candidiasis
- White oral lesions that cannot be rubbed off (2):
  - Developmental/genetic (rare):
    - Cannon white sponge nevus (diffuse bilateral white plaques of buccal mucosa, tongue)
    - Hereditary benign intraepithelial dyskeratosis
    - Pachyonychia congenita
    - Genodermatoses
    - Darier-White disease
    - Geographic tongue
  - Reactive/frictional:
    - Leukoedema (delicate gray-white lines, disappear with stretching)
    - Contact desquamation
    - Morsicatio mucosae oris (cheek/gum biting)
    - Benign alveolar ridge keratosis (ill-fitting dentures)
    - Hairy tongue (elongated filiform papillae, may become pigmented from food/bacteria)
    - Nicotinic stomatitis and smokeless tobacco keratosis (South Asian "paan" or "gutka"; American/Swedish snuff; Ethiopian "toombak")
    - Glassblower's white patch
    - Actinic cheilitis
    - Aspirin burn
    - Cinnamon-induced contact stomatitis
    - Epithelial peeling
    - Keratotic lesions
    - Linea alba
  - Infectious:
    - Candidiasis
    - Hairy leukoplakia (associated with EBV and HIV-infected individuals)
    - Syphilis
  - Immune-mediated:
    - Lichen planus (typically symmetric, bilateral, reticular white lesions)
    - Lichenoid lesions
    - Benign migratory glossitis
  - Autoimmune:
    - SLE
    - Chronic graft versus host disease

DIAGNOSTIC TESTS & INTERPRETATION
Biopsy with histopathologic examination is the gold standard.

Initial Tests (lab, imaging)
- Laboratory tests generally are not indicated.
  - Consider saliva culture if *C. albicans* infection is suspected.
- No imaging is indicated.

Follow-Up Tests & Special Considerations

- Biopsy is necessary to rule out carcinoma if lesion is persistent, changing, or unexplained.
- Consider CBC, rapid plasma reagin (RPR).

Diagnostic Procedures/Other

- Oral cytology is superior to conventional oral examination (4)[A].
- Computer-assisted cytology or liquid-based cytology is not superior to oral cytology (4)[A].
- Noninvasive brush biopsy and analysis of cells with DNA–image cytometry constitute a sensitive and specific screening method.
- Patients with dysplastic or malignant cells on brush biopsy should undergo more formal excisional biopsy.
- Excisional biopsy is definitive procedure.

Test Interpretation

- Biopsy specimens range from hyperkeratosis to keratosis of unknown significance (KUS) to dysplasia to invasive carcinoma.
- At initial biopsy, 6% are invasive carcinoma.
- 0.13–6% subsequently undergo malignant transformation.
- Location is important: 60% on floor of mouth or lateral border of tongue are cancerous; buccal mucosal lesions are generally not malignant but require biopsy if not resolving.

TREATMENT

- All oral leukoplakias should be treated because they are potentially malignant.
- Treatment may include the following:
  - For 2 to 3 circumscribed lesions, surgical excision is treatment of choice (5)[C].
  - For multiple or large lesions where surgery would cause unacceptable deformity, consider cryosurgery or laser surgery (5)[C].
  - Abstinence from predisposing habits (alcohol and tobacco)
- Complete excision is standard treatment for dysplasia or malignancy.
- After treatment, up to 30% of leukoplakia recurs, and some leukoplakia still transforms to squamous cell carcinoma (5)[B].
- Oral hairy leukoplakia may be treated with podophyllin with acyclovir cream.

GENERAL MEASURES

- Eliminate habitual lip biting.
- Correct ill-fitting dental appliances, bad restorations, or sharp teeth.
- Stop smoking and using alcohol.
- Some small lesions may respond to cryosurgery.
- β-Carotene, lycopene, retinoids, and cyclooxygenase 2 (COX-2) inhibitors may cause partial regression.
- For hairy tongue: tongue brushing

MEDICATION

Carotenoids; vitamins A, C, and K; bleomycin; and photodynamic therapy ineffective to prevent malignant transformation and recurrence. No generally approved standard systemic pharmacotherapy regimen at this time, but there is new research being done on chemoprevention (3).

ISSUES FOR REFERRAL

Consider otolaryngologist or oral surgery referral for extensive disease.

ADDITIONAL THERAPIES

Systemic therapies that may reduce progression include retinoids, cyclooxygenase-2 inhibitors, epidermal growth factor inhibitors, and peroxisome proliferator–activated receptor-γ agonists.

SURGERY/OTHER PROCEDURES

- Scalpel excision, laser ablation, electrocautery, or cryoablation
- Cryotherapy slightly less effective than photodynamic therapy response (73% vs. 90%) and recurrence (27% vs. 24%) (6)[A]
- Biopsy/excision algorithm (2)[C]:
  - KUS that is poorly demarcated and likely frictional: Rebiopsy and follow up.
  - KUS that is well demarcated and >3 cm: Follow up every 3 months; rebiopsy every 12 months.
  - KUS that is <3 cm: Excise/ablate with narrow margins; follow up every 3 months; if recurs, excise with wider margins.
  - PVL: Follow up every 3 months; excise verrucous or nodular areas.
  - Dysplastic/SCC: Excise.

COMPLEMENTARY & ALTERNATIVE MEDICINE

Low or very low evidence for systemic β-carotene, herbal extracts, freeze-dried black raspberry gel, and Bowman-Birk inhibitor

ADMISSION, INPATIENT, AND NURSING CONSIDERATIONS

- Eliminate etiologic factors.
- Reevaluate in 7 to 14 days.
- Biopsy if lesion is persistent

ONGOING CARE

FOLLOW-UP RECOMMENDATIONS

Patient Monitoring

- 3–6 monthly follow-up appointments are the norm based on anticipated risk and patient preference.
- Biopsy as needed

DIET

Regular

PATIENT EDUCATION

- If biopsy is negative, stress importance of periodic and careful follow-up.
- Initiate a dental referral to eliminate dental factors.
- Stress importance of stopping tobacco and alcohol use.
- Encourage participation in smoking cessation program.

PROGNOSIS

- Most leukoplakia is benign.
- Leukoplakia may regress, remain stable, or progress.
- 0.13–6% of initially benign lesions subsequently develop into cancer.
- Lack of treatment generally results in malignant development at an annual rate of 2–3%.
- Size >200 mm^2 increases risk of malignant transformation (7).
- 5-year survival rate of oral cancer is 50%.

COMPLICATIONS

- New lesions may develop after treatment.
- Larger lesions and nonhomogeneous leukoplakia are associated with higher rates of malignant transformation.

REFERENCES

1. Nadeau C, Kerr A. Evaluation and management of oral potentially malignant disorders. *Dent Clin North Am*. 2018;62(1):1–27.
2. Villa A, Woo S. Leukoplakia—a diagnostic and management algorithm. *J Oral Maxillofac Surg*. 2017;75(4):723–734.
3. Gopinath D, Kunnath Menon R, Chun Wie C, et al. Salivary bacterial shifts in oral leukoplakia resemble the dysbiotic oral cancer bacteriome. *J Oral Microbiol*. 2020;13(1):1857998.
4. Fuller C, Camilon R, Nguyen S, et al. Adjunctive diagnostic techniques for oral lesions of unknown malignant potential: systematic review with meta-analysis. *Head Neck*. 2015;37(5):755–762.
5. Feller L, Lemmer J. Oral leukoplakia as it relates to HPV infection: a review. *Int J Dent*. 2012;2012:540561.
6. Kawczyk-Krupka A, Waśkowska J, Raczkowska-Siostrzonek A, et al. Comparison of cryotherapy and photodynamic therapy in treatment of oral leukoplakia. *Photodiagnosis Photodyn Ther*. 2012;9(2):148–155.
7. Chaturvedi AK, Udaltsova N, Engels EA, et al. Oral leukoplakia and risk of progression to oral cancer: a population-based cohort study. *J Natl Cancer Inst*. 2020;112(10):1047–1054.

ADDITIONAL READING

Reamy BV, Derby R, Bunt CW. Common tongue conditions in primary care. *Am Fam Physician*. 2010;81(5):627–634.

SEE ALSO

HIV/AIDS; Infectious Mononucleosis, Epstein-Barr Virus Infections

CODES

ICD10

- K13.21 Leukoplakia of oral mucosa, including tongue
- K13.3 Hairy leukoplakia

CLINICAL PEARLS

- White plaque or patches on the oral mucosa that cannot be rubbed or easily scrapped off
- Excisional biopsy is indicated for any undiagnosed leukoplakia.
- After treatment, up to 30% of leukoplakia recurs, and some leukoplakia still transforms to squamous cell carcinoma; thus, long-term surveillance is essential.
- To lessen risk of malignant transformation, encourage tobacco and alcohol cessation, HPV vaccination, and consider *C. albicans* eradication.

L

LICHEN PLANUS

Dongsheng Jiang, MD, MSc • Joanna Jiang, MD

BASICS

Lichen planus (LP) is an idiopathic eruption with characteristic shiny, flat-topped (Latin: *planus*, "flat"), purple (violaceous) papules and plaques on the skin, often accompanied by characteristic mucous membrane lesions. Itching may be severe.

DESCRIPTION

- Classic (typical) LP is a relatively uncommon inflammatory disorder of the skin and mucous membranes; hair and nails may also be affected.
  - Skin lesions are small, flat, angular, red-to-violaceous, shiny, pruritic papules and/or plaques with overlying fine, white lines (called Wickham striae), or gray-white puncta; most commonly seen on the flexor surfaces of the upper extremities, extensor surfaces of the lower extremities, the genitalia, and the mucous membranes
  - On the oral mucosa, lesions typically appear as raised white lines in a lacelike pattern seen most often on the buccal mucosa.
  - Onset is abrupt or gradual. Course is unpredictable; may resolve spontaneously, recur intermittently, or persist for many years
- Drug-induced LP
  - Clinical and histopathologic findings may mimic those of classic LP. Lesions usually lack Wickham striae (see in the following text) and oral involvement is rare.
  - There is generally a latent period of months from drug introduction until lesions appear.
  - Lesions resolve when the inciting agent is discontinued, often after a prolonged period.
- LP variants
  - Follicular: also called lichen planopilaris; typically seen on the scalp, can lead to scarring alopecia
  - Annular: papules spread centrifugally as central area resolves; occur on glans penis, axillae, and oral mucosa
  - Linear: may be an isolated finding
  - Hypertrophic: itchy, hyperkeratotic, thick plaques on dorsal legs and feet
  - Atrophic: rare, most often the result of resolved lesions
  - Bullous LP: Intense inflammation in the dermis leads to blistering of epidermis.
  - LP pemphigoides: a combination of LP and bullous pemphigoid (IgG autoantibodies to collagen 17)
  - Nail LP: affects the nail matrix, lateral thinning, longitudinal ridging, and fissuring
- System(s) affected: skin/exocrine
- Synonym(s): lichenoid eruptions

EPIDEMIOLOGY

- Predominant age: 30 to 60 years old; rare in children and the geriatric population
- Predominant sex: female > male

Prevalence

In the United States, 450/100,000

ETIOLOGY AND PATHOPHYSIOLOGY

LP is considered to be a T cell–mediated autoimmune response to self-antigens on damaged keratinocytes.

RISK FACTORS

Exposure to certain drugs or chemicals

- Thiazides, furosemide, β-blockers, sulfonylureas, antimalarials, penicillamine, gold salts, and angiotensin-converting enzyme inhibitors
- Rarely: photo-developing chemicals, dental materials, tattoo pigments

COMMONLY ASSOCIATED CONDITIONS

- An association has been noted between LP and hepatitis C virus infection, particularly in certain geographic regions (Asia, South America, the Middle East, Europe). Hepatitis should be considered in patients with widespread presentations of LP and those with primarily oral disease.
- In addition, chronic active hepatitis, lichen nitidus, and primary biliary cirrhosis have been noted to coexist with LP.
- Association with dyslipidemia has been reported.
- LP has also been reported in association with other diseases of altered immunity, more often than would be expected by chance.
  - Bullous pemphigoid
  - Alopecia areata
  - Myasthenia gravis
  - Vitiligo
  - Ulcerative colitis
  - Graft-versus-host reaction
  - Lupus erythematosus (lupus erythematosus–LP overlap syndrome)
  - Morphea and lichen sclerosus et atrophicus

DIAGNOSIS

- LP is most commonly diagnosed by its appearance despite its range of clinical presentations.
- Dermoscopy: Most common findings are polymorphic pearly white structures, radial capillaries, and blue-gray granules (1).
- A skin biopsy should be performed if the diagnosis is in doubt.

HISTORY

A minority of patients have a family history of LP. Affected families have an increased frequency of human leukocyte antigen B7 (HLA-B7). A thorough drug history should be performed.

PHYSICAL EXAM

- Skin (often severe pruritus)
  - Papules: 1 to 10 mm, shiny, flat-topped (planar) lesions that occur in crops; lesions may have a fine scale.
  - Evidence of scratching (i.e., crusts and excoriations) is usually absent.
  - Color: violaceous, with white lacelike pattern (Wickham striae) on surface of papules. Wickham striae are best seen after topical application of mineral oil and, if present, are virtually pathognomonic for LP.
  - Shape: polygonal or oval. Annular lesions may appear on trunk and mucous membranes. Various shapes and sizes may be noted (polymorphic).
  - Arrangement: may be grouped, linear, or scattered individual lesions
  - Koebner phenomenon (isomorphic response): New lesions may be noted at sites of minor injuries, such as scratches or burns.

- Distribution: ventral surface of wrists and forearms, dorsa hands, glans penis, dorsa feet, groin, sacrum, shins, and scalp. Hypertrophic (verrucous) lesions may occur on lower legs and may be generalized.
  - Postinflammatory hyperpigmentation: Lesions typically heal, leaving darkly pigmented macules in their wake.
- Mucous membranes (40–60% of patients with skin lesions; 20% have mucous membrane lesions without skin involvement)
  - Most commonly asymptomatic, nonerosive, milky-white lines with an elegant, lacy, netlike streaked pattern
  - Usually seen on buccal mucosa but may appear on tongue, gingiva, palate, or lips
  - Less commonly, LP may be erosive; rarely bullous
  - Painful, especially if ulcers present
  - Lesions may develop into squamous cell carcinoma (1–3%).
  - Glans penis, labia minora, vaginal vault, and perianal areas may be involved.
- Hair/scalp
  - LP of the hair follicle (lichen planopilaris) presents with keratotic plugs at the follicle orifice with a violaceous rim; may result in atrophy and permanent destruction of hair follicles (scarring alopecia)
- Nails (10%)
  - Involvement of nail matrix may cause proximal-to-distal linear grooves and partial or complete destruction of nail bed with pterygium formation.

DIFFERENTIAL DIAGNOSIS

- Skin
  - Lichen simplex chronicus
  - Eczematous dermatitis
  - Psoriasis
  - Discoid lupus erythematosus
  - Other lichenoid eruptions (those that resemble LP)
  - Pityriasis rosea
  - Lichen nitidus
  - Self-induced dermatoses
- Oral mucous membranes
  - Leukoplakia
  - Oral hairy leukoplakia
  - Candidiasis
  - Squamous cell carcinoma (particularly in ulcerative lesions)
  - Aphthous ulcers
  - Herpetic stomatitis
  - Secondary syphilis
- Genital mucous membranes
  - Psoriasis (penis and labia)
  - Nonspecific balanitis, Zoon balanitis
  - Fixed drug eruption (penis)
  - Candidiasis (penis and labia)
  - Pemphigus vulgaris, bullous pemphigoid, and Behçet disease (all rare)
- Hair and scalp
  - Scarring alopecia (central centrifugal cicatricial alopecia)

DIAGNOSTIC TESTS & INTERPRETATION

If suggested by history

- Serology for hepatitis
- Liver function tests

Diagnostic Procedures/Other
- Skin biopsy
- Direct immunofluorescence helps to distinguish LP from discoid lupus erythematosus.

Test Interpretation
- Dense, bandlike (lichenoid) lymphocytic infiltrate of the upper dermis
- Vacuolar degeneration of the basal layer
- Hyperkeratosis and irregular acanthosis, increased granular layer
- Basement membrane thinning with "saw-toothing"
- Degenerative keratinocytes, known as colloid or Civatte bodies, are found in the lower epidermis.
- Melanin pigment in macrophages

TREATMENT

Although LP can resolve spontaneously, treatment is usually requested by patients who may be severely symptomatic or troubled by its cosmetic appearance.

GENERAL MEASURES
- Goal is to relieve itching and resolve lesions.
- Asymptomatic oral lesions require no treatment.
- For oral LP (2):
  - No treatment is curative.
  - Goal of treatment is to resolve pain, heal ulcerative lesions, decrease the risk for oral cancer.

MEDICATION
First Line
- Skin (3),(4)
  - Ultrahigh-potency and high-potency topical steroids: 0.05% clobetasol propionate or 0.1% betamethasone valerate, twice daily, for 2 to 4 weeks
  - Triamcinolone acetonide 0.1% or fluocinonide 0.05% under occlusion
  - Intralesional corticosteroids (e.g., triamcinolone [Kenalog] 5 to 10 mg/mL) for recalcitrant and hypertrophic lesions
  - "Soak and smear" technique: can lead to a rapid improvement of symptoms in even 1 to 2 days and may obviate the need for systemic steroids. Soaking allows water to hydrate the stratum corneum and allows the anti-inflammatory steroid in the ointment to penetrate more deeply into the skin. Smearing of the ointment traps the water in the skin because water cannot move out through greasy materials.
    - Soaking is done in a bathtub using lukewarm plain water for 20 minutes and then, without drying the skin, the affected area is immediately smeared with a thin film of the steroid ointment containing clobetasol or another superpotent topical steroid.
    - Soak and smear may be done for 4 to 5 days or longer, if necessary. The treatments are best done at night because the greasy ointment applied to the skin gets on pajamas (instead of on daytime clothes) and the ointment is on the skin during sleep. A topical steroid cream is applied thereafter during the daytime hours, if necessary.
- Mucous membranes
  - For oral, erosive, painful LP
    - Topical corticosteroids (0.1% triamcinolone [Kenalog] in Orabase) or 0.05% clobetasol propionate ointment BID
    - Intralesional corticosteroids BID

Pediatric Considerations
Children may absorb a proportionally larger amount of topical steroid because of larger skin surface-to-weight ratio.

Second Line
Skin and mucous membranes
- Oral steroids: Reserved for acute exacerbation, severe or widespread, or unresponsive to topical steroids. Prednisone at 0.5 to 1 mg/kg body weight per day (30 to 60 mg/day) for 3 to 6 weeks, taper over 4 to 6 weeks
- Isotretinoin 10 mg, or acitretin 30 mg, or alitretinoin 30 mg PO daily in some refractory cases. Observe carefully for resultant dyslipidemia.
- Topical calcineurin inhibitors: 0.1% tacrolimus (Protopic ointment) BID or 1% pimecrolimus (Elidel) cream BID
- Topical retinoids: tretinoin 0.05% twice a day; isotretinoin 0.1% twice a day
- Topical calcipotriol
- Metronidazole
- Sulfasalazine
- Methotrexate
- Cyclosporine
- Hydroxychloroquine
- Dapsone
- Thalidomide
- Narrow-band UVB (NBUVB) and broad-band UVB (BBUVB): especially when systemic steroids and immunnosuppresive drugs are contraindicated
- Psoralen plus ultraviolet A (PUVA) therapy
- Low-level laser therapy and photodynamic therapy
- Griseofulvin
- Azathioprine
- Mycophenolate mofetil

ALERT
Avoid oral and topical retinoids during pregnancy.

ADDITIONAL THERAPIES
Antihistamines (e.g., hydroxyzine 25 mg PO q6h) have limited benefit for itching but may be helpful for sedation at bedtime.

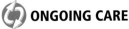

ONGOING CARE

FOLLOW-UP RECOMMENDATIONS
Patient Monitoring
Serial oral examinations for erosive/ulcerative lesions

PATIENT EDUCATION
- Oral, erosive, or ulcerative LP: annual follow-up to screen for malignancy
- Maintain good oral hygiene and dental status.
- Avoid hot, salty, acidic or spicy foods, alcohol, smoking and use of tobacco products especially in patients with atrophic and erosive lesions.
- Avoid mucosal trauma: Avoid dry, crispy foods such as corn chips, pretzels, and toast.

PROGNOSIS
- Spontaneous resolution in weeks is possible, but disease may persist for years, especially oral lesions and hypertrophic lesions on the shins.
- There is a tendency toward relapse.
- Recurrence in 12–20%, especially in those with generalized involvement

COMPLICATIONS
- Alopecia
- Nail destruction
- Squamous cell carcinoma of the mouth or genitals

REFERENCES
1. Cook LC, Hanna C, Foulke GT, et al. Dermoscopy in the diagnosis of inflammatory dermatoses: systematic review findings reported for psoriasis, lupus, and lichen planus. *J Clin Aesthet Dermatol*. 2018;11(4):41–42.
2. Rotaru D, Chisnoiu R, Picos AM, et al. Treatment trends in oral lichen planus and oral lichenoid lesions (Review). *Exp Ther Med*. 2020;20(6):198.
3. Thandar Y, Maharajh R, Haffejee F, et al. Treatment of cutaneous lichen planus (part 1): a review of topical therapies and phototherapy. *Cogent Med*. 2019;6(1):1582467.
4. Thandar Y, Maharajh R, Haffejee F, et al. Treatment of cutaneous lichen planus (part 2): a review of systemic therapies. *J Dermatolog Treat*. 2019;30(7):633–647. doi:10.1080/09546634.2018.1544411.

ADDITIONAL READING
Arnold DL, Krishnamurthy K. *Lichen Planus*. In: StatPearls [Internet]. Treasure Island, FL: StatPearls Publishing; 2021. https://www.ncbi.nlm.nih.gov/books/NBK526126/.

 CODES

ICD10
- L43.9 Lichen planus, unspecified
- L43.0 Hypertrophic lichen planus
- L43.1 Bullous lichen planus

CLINICAL PEARLS
- 7 P's of LP: **p**urple, **p**lanar, **p**olygonal, **p**olymorphic, **p**ruritic (not always), **p**apules that heal with **p**ostinflammatory hyperpigmentation.
- Serial oral or genital exams are indicated for erosive/ulcerative LP lesions to monitor for the development of squamous cell carcinoma.
- An association has been noted between LP and hepatitis C virus infection, chronic active hepatitis, and primary biliary cirrhosis.
- The "soak and smear" technique can lead to a rapid improvement of symptoms in 1 to 2 days and may obviate the need for systemic steroids.

L

LICHEN SIMPLEX CHRONICUS

Dongsheng Jiang, MD, MSc • Joanna Jiang, MD

BASICS

DESCRIPTION
- Lichen simplex chronicus (LSC) is a chronic dermatitis resulting from chronic, repeated rubbing or scratching of the skin. Skin becomes thickened with accentuated lines ("lichenification").
- System(s) affected: skin
- Synonym(s): LSC; lichen simplex; localized neurodermatitis; neurodermatitis circumscripta

EPIDEMIOLOGY
Geriatric Considerations
Most common in middle aged and elderly

Pediatric Considerations
Rare in preadolescents

Incidence
- Common
- Peak incidence 35 to 50 years
- Predominant sex: females > males (2:1)

Prevalence
Common

ETIOLOGY AND PATHOPHYSIOLOGY
- Itch–scratch cycle leads to a chronic dermatosis. Repeated scratching or rubbing causes inflammation and pruritus, which leads to continued scratching.
- Primary LSC: scratching secondary to nonorganic pruritus, habit, or a conditioned response to stress/anxiety
- Common triggers are excess dryness of skin, heat, sweat, and psychological stress.
- Secondary LSC: begins as a pruritic skin disease that evolves into neurodermatitis, which persists after resolution of the primary condition. Precursor dermatoses include atopic dermatitis, contact dermatitis, lichen planus, stasis dermatitis, psoriasis, tinea, and insect bites.
- There is a possible relation between disease development and underlying neuropathy, particularly radiculopathy or nerve root compression.
- Pruritus-specific C neurons are temperature sensitive, which may explain itching that occurs in warm environments.

RISK FACTORS
- Anxiety disorders
- Dry skin
- Insect bites
- Pruritic dermatosis

GENERAL PREVENTION
Avoid common triggers such as psychological distress, environmental factors such as heat and excessive dryness, skin irritation, and the development of pruritic dermatoses.

COMMONLY ASSOCIATED CONDITIONS
- Prurigo nodularis is a nodular variety of the same disease process.
- Atopic dermatitis
- Anxiety, depression, and obsessive-compulsive disorders

DIAGNOSIS

HISTORY
- Gradual onset
- Begins as a localized area of pruritus
- Most patients acknowledge that they respond with vigorous rubbing, itching, or scratching, which brings temporary satisfaction.
- Pruritus is typically paroxysmal, worse at night, and may lead to scratching during sleep.
- Can be asymptomatic with patient scratching at night while asleep

PHYSICAL EXAM
- Well-circumscribed lichenified plaques with varying amounts of overlying excoriation or scaling
- Lichenification: accentuation of normal skin lines
- Hyperpigmentation or hypopigmentation can be seen.
- Scarring is uncommon with typical LSC; can be seen following ulcer formation or secondary infection
- Most commonly involves easily accessible areas
  - Lateral portions of lower legs/ankles
  - Nape of neck (lichen simplex nuchae)
  - Vulva/scrotum/anus
  - Extensor surfaces of forearms
  - Palmar wrist
  - Scalp
- Dermoscopic criteria (in genital disease) (1)
  - Rich vascularization, linear, serpentine, and dotted in shape
  - Diffuse arrangement
  - White-grayish background

DIFFERENTIAL DIAGNOSIS
- Lichen sclerosis
- Psoriasis
- Atopic dermatitis
- Contact, irritant, or stasis dermatitis
- Extramammary Paget disease
- Lichen planus
- Lichen amyloidosis
- Tinea
- Nummular eczema
- Other systemic disease:
  - T-cell lymphoma
  - Lymphoma
  - Multiple myeloma
  - Lung cancer
  - Leukemia
  - GI tract cancer

DIAGNOSTIC TESTS & INTERPRETATION
Initial Tests (lab, imaging)
- No specific diagnostic test
- Microscopy (i.e., KOH prep) and culture preparation may be helpful in identifying possible bacterial or fungal infection.

Diagnostic Procedures/Other
- Skin biopsy if diagnosis is in question
- Patch testing may be used to rule out a contact dermatitis.

Test Interpretation
- Hyperkeratosis
- Acanthosis
- Lengthening of rete ridges
- Hyperplasia of all components of epidermis
- Mild to moderate lymphohistiocytic inflammatory infiltrate with prominent lichenification

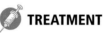

TREATMENT

GENERAL MEASURES
- Patient education is critical.
- Low likelihood of resolution if patient unable to avoid scratching
- Treatment aimed at reducing inflammation and pruritus.

MEDICATION
First Line
- Reducing inflammation
  - Topical steroids are first-line agents (2)[C].
  - High-potency steroids alone, such as 0.05% betamethasone dipropionate cream or 0.05% clobetasol propionate cream, can be used initially but should be avoided on the face, anogenital region, or intertriginous areas. They should be used on small areas only, for no longer than 2 weeks except under the close supervision of a physician.
  - Switch to intermediate- or low-potency steroids as response allows.
  - An intermediate-potency steroid, such as 0.1% triamcinolone cream, may be used for initial, brief treatment of the face and intertriginous areas, and for maintenance treatment of other areas.
  - A low-potency steroid, such as 1% hydrocortisone cream, should be used for maintenance treatment of the face and intertriginous areas.
  - Steroid tape, flurandrenolide, has optimized penetration and provides a barrier to continued scratching. Change tape once daily.
  - Intralesional steroids, such as triamcinolone acetate, are also safe and effective for severe cases.

- Preventing scratching
  - Topical antipruritic agents
  - 1st-generation oral antihistamines such as diphenhydramine and hydroxyzine for antipruritic and sedative effects
  - Sedating tricyclics, such as doxepin and amitriptyline, for nighttime itching
  - Itching may occur at night while the patient is asleep; occlusive dressings may be helpful in these cases.

ALERT
High-dose and prolonged treatment with topical steroids can cause dermal/epidermal atrophy as well as pigmentary changes and should not be used on the face, intertriginous areas, or anogenital region. Duration of treatment on other parts of the body should not exceed 3 weeks without close physician supervision.

Second Line
All recommendations

- Topical aspirin has been shown to be helpful in treating neurodermatitis (3)[C].
- Topical 5% doxepin cream has significant antipruritic activity (3)[C].
- Topical capsaicin cream can be helpful for treatment of early disease manifestations (3)[C].
- 0.1% tacrolimus applied twice daily over 6 weeks as an effective alternative treatment (4)[C]
- Gabapentin was found to decrease symptoms in patients who are nonresponsive to steroids.
- Topical lidocaine can be effective in decreasing neuropathic pruritus (3)[C].
- Intradermal botulinum toxin injections have been reported to improve symptoms in patients with recalcitrant pruritus.
- Transcutaneous electrical nerve stimulation may relieve pruritus in patients for whom topical steroids were not effective (5)[C].
- A case report showed NB-UVB as a possible off-label treatment of refractory LSC (6)[C].
- SSRIs may be effective in controlling compulsive scratching secondary to psychiatric diagnosis.

ISSUES FOR REFERRAL
- No response to treatment
- Presence of signs and symptoms suggestive of a systemic cause of pruritus
- Consultation with a psychiatrist for patients with severe stress, anxiety, or compulsive scratching
- Consultation with an allergist for patients with multisystem atopic symptoms

ADDITIONAL THERAPIES
- Psychotherapy
- Cooling of the skin with ice or cold compresses
- Soaks and lubricants to improve barrier layer function
- Occlusion of lesion with bandages or Unna boots
- Nail trimming
- Silk underwear to decrease friction in genital LSC

COMPLEMENTARY & ALTERNATIVE MEDICINE
- Acupuncture has been shown as an effective treatment for pruritus (7)[C].
- Cognitive-behavioral therapy may improve awareness and help to identify coping strategies.
- Hypnosis may be beneficial in decreasing pruritus and preventing scratching.
- Homeopathic remedies (i.e., thuja and graphite) have been used.

 ONGOING CARE

FOLLOW-UP RECOMMENDATIONS
Patient Monitoring
Patients should be followed for response to therapy, complications from therapy (especially topical steroids), and secondary infections.

DIET
Regular balanced diet

PATIENT EDUCATION
- Patients should understand the cause of this disease and the critical role they play in its resolution:
  - Emphasize that scratching and rubbing must stop for lesions to heal; medications ineffective if scratching continues
- Stress reduction techniques can be useful for patients for whom stress plays a role.
- Avoid exposure to known triggers.

PROGNOSIS
- Often chronic and recurrent; can be persistent on genitals
- Good prognosis if the itch–scratch cycle can be broken
- After healing, the skin should return to normal appearance but may also retain accentuated skin markings or postinflammatory pigmentary changes that may be slow to resolve.

COMPLICATIONS
- Secondary infection
- Scarring is rare without ulceration or secondary infection.

- Complications related to therapy, as mentioned in medication precautions
- Squamous cell carcinoma within affected regions is rare.

REFERENCES
1. Borghi A, Virgili A, Corazza M. Dermoscopy of inflammatory genital diseases: practical insights. *Dermatol Clin.* 2018;36(4):451–461.
2. Lynch PJ. Lichen simplex chronicus (atopic/neurodermatitis) of the anogenital region. *Dermatol Ther.* 2004;17(1):8–19.
3. Patel T, Yosipovitch G. Therapy of pruritus. *Expert Opin Pharmacother.* 2010;11(10):1673–1682.
4. Tan ES, Tan AS, Tey HL. Effective treatment of scrotal lichen simplex chronicus with 0.1% tacrolimus ointment: an observational study. *J Eur Acad Dermatol Venereol.* 2015;29(7):1448–1449.
5. Mohammad Ali BM, Hegab DS, El Saadany HM. Use of transcutaneous electrical nerve stimulation for chronic pruritus. *Dermatol Ther.* 2015;28(4):210–215.
6. Virgili A, Minghetti S, Borghi A, et al. Phototherapy for vulvar lichen simplex chronicus: an "off-label use" of a comb light device. *Photodermatol Photoimmunol Photomed.* 2014;30(6):332–334.
7. Ma C, Sivamani RK. Acupuncture as a treatment modality in dermatology: a systematic review. *J Altern Complement Med.* 2015;21(9):520–529.

CODES

ICD10
L28.0 Lichen simplex chronicus

CLINICAL PEARLS
- LSC is a chronic inflammatory condition that results from repeated scratching and rubbing.
- Primary LSC originates de novo, whereas secondary LSC occurs in the setting of a preexisting pruritic dermatologic condition.
- LSC is a clinical diagnosis based on history and skin examination with biopsy only indicated in difficult or unclear cases.
- Stopping the itch–scratch cycle through patient education, skin lubrication, and topical medications is key.
- Treatment aimed at decreasing both inflammation and pruritus utilizing topical steroids and antipruritics

L

LONG QT INTERVAL

Alec M. Wilhelmi, MD • Leigh A. Romero, MD, CAQSM

BASICS

DESCRIPTION
- QT interval: the interval from the beginning of the QRS complex to the end of the T wave on the surface electrocardiogram (ECG). This represents the period from the onset of ventricular depolarization to completion of repolarization of the ventricular myocardium, or ventricular systole. The QT interval is normal if it is <50% of the RR interval.
- Corrected QT interval (QTc): The QT interval has an inverse relationship with heart rate. The QTc is the QT interval corrected for heart rate, and it estimates the QT interval at a heart rate of 60 beats/min. See formulas.
- Prolonged QTc is generally defined as >450 ms for adult males and >470 ms for adult females (1):
  - 430 to 450 ms considered borderline in men
  - 450 to 470 ms considered borderline in women (1),(2),(3)
  - 440 to 460 ms considered borderline in children aged 1 to 15 years old
- Most cases of prolonged QT are acquired, but several genetic mutations cause inherited long QT syndrome (LQTS) (3).
- Prolonged QTc from any cause can precipitate polymorphic ventricular tachycardia (VT) called torsade de pointes (TdP), leading to dizziness, syncope, and sudden cardiac death from ventricular fibrillation (VF).

EPIDEMIOLOGY
Incidence
Incidence of medication-induced QTc prolongation and TdP varies with medication and a host of other factors. Exact incidences are difficult to estimate but may be 1/2,000 to 1/2,500 (2).

Prevalence
- Hereditary LQTS is estimated to occur in 1/2,500 to 1/7,000 births.
- Five thousand people across the United States may die yearly due to LQTS-related cardiac arrhythmia.

ETIOLOGY AND PATHOPHYSIOLOGY
- Acquired
  - Demographics: increasing age, female sex
  - Electrolyte abnormalities: hypokalemia, hypocalcemia, and hypomagnesemia
  - Noncardiac disease: hypothyroidism, renal impairment, and hepatic impairment
  - Cardiac disease: heart failure, LVH, and myocardial ischemia (2)
  - Scenarios: rapid increase in the QT interval >60 ms, conversion from atrial fibrillation/bradycardia (4)
  - Medications (*denote "high-risk" medication for TdP 25) (2),(3),(4)
    - Antiarrhythmic medications (quinidine, procainamide, dronedarone, dofetilide, sotalol, disopyramide, and amiodarone)
    - Antipsychotic medications: especially if given IV (haloperidol*, chlorpromazine*, thioridazine*, pimozide*)
    - Antidepressants: most commonly used drugs responsible (SSRIs, SNRIs, trazodone, TCAs)
    - Antibiotics/antivirals/antifungals/antiprotozoals/antimalarials: macrolides (clarithromycin*, erythromycin* also CYP3A4 inhibitors), fluoroquinolones, quinine, and chloroquine
    - Antiemetics: metoclopramide, ondansetron, promethazine
    - Opioids: methadone*, buprenorphine
    - Antihistamines: cetirizine, hydroxyzine, diphenhydramine
    - Decongestants: pseudoephedrine, phenylephrine
    - Stimulants: albuterol, phentermine
    - Misc: chloroquine*, pentamidine*, various antimuscarinics, and anticonvulsants
- Congenital
  - Loss of function mutations in several potassium ion membrane channels or gain of function mutations in the sodium or calcium ion membrane channels in cardiac myocytes
- Pathophysiology
  - Depolarization (phase 0) of the myocardium results from the rapid influx of sodium through sodium channels (I_{Na}) causing myocyte contraction during systole; seen on ECG as the QRS complex
  - Repolarization occurs through the efflux of potassium from the cell (phases 2 and 3) by rapid (I_{Kr}) and slow (I_{Ks}) components of the delayed rectifier; represented by the T wave on an ECG
  - Drug-induced QT prolongation most often due to blockade of the I_{Kr} channel leading to delay in phase 3 rapid repolarization (2).
  - In both cases, deviation from normal ion channel function leads to transmural dispersion of repolarization currents across the myocardium, triggering early after depolarizations which may devolve into TdP (3).
  - Prolonged QT interval alone does not denote imminent risk for TdP; TdP is often self-limited, but TdP can cause syncope or degrade to VF (2).

Genetics
- 13+ distinct genotypes are linked to LQTS (1).
- Penetrance is highly variable making both diagnosis and management challenging (3).
- LQT1 (40–55%) is the most common cause of LQTS. Loss of function in the KCNQ1 gene coding for the I_{Ks} transport protein; arrhythmias triggered by sympathetic activation (stress/exercise—especially swimming), leading to shorter ventricular repolarization
- LQT2 (30–45%) results from a mutation in the KCNH2 gene causing a defect in the I_{Kr} transport protein; at risk for cardiac events due to abrupt catecholamine surges like auditory stimuli/emotional arousal (postpartum)
- LQT3 (5–10%) is caused by a mutation in the SCN5A gene leading to a gain of function in the alpha subunit of the I_{Na} transport protein. Excessive sodium accumulates in the cell, increasing repolarization time; prominent during sleep due to amplified inward flow of sodium at low heart rates (1),(3).
- LQT4 to LQT13—<1% of the total frequency
- Jervell and Lange-Nielsen syndrome (JLNS): autosomal recessive inheritance through homozygous or compound heterozygous mutations of the KCNQ1 or KCNE1 genes. Reduced function in the I_{Ks} transport protein; associated with sensorineural hearing loss
- Romano-Ward syndrome (RWS): most common. Results from any of the 13 identified gene mutations; autosomal dominant with variable penetrance and normal hearing
- Others: Andersen-Tawil syndrome (LQT7), Timothy syndrome (LQT8). Both are very rare (3).

RISK FACTORS
For the feared complication, TdP, risk factors include the following (2),(4):
- Female (~2 times increased risk)
- QTc >500 ms (2 to 3 times increased risk)
- QTc >60 ms over previous baseline
- For every 10 ms increase in the QTc, there is a 5–7% increased risk for developing TdP.
- History of syncope or presyncope
- History of TdP

- Bradycardia
- Liver or kidney disease (by increasing blood levels of QT-prolonging medications)
- Medications that cause QTc prolongation
  - High doses
  - Fast infusions
  - Combination of medications
- Medications that inhibit CYP3A4
- Electrolyte abnormalities
  - Hypokalemia
  - Hypomagnesemia
  - Hypocalcemia
- For hereditary LQTS
  - Catecholamine surges from exercise, emotional stress, loud noises, postpartum

GENERAL PREVENTION
- Avoid (or use with caution) causative medications, including combinations with potentially additive effects (1)[C],(2)[C],(4)[C].
- Replete electrolytes (goal Mg >2, K 4.5 to 5.0) (2)[C].
- Treat underlying diseases.
- Avoid strenuous sports and other stimulating activities, like amusement park rides or jumping into cold water, in LQTS.
- Avoid sudden loud noises in LQTS (alarm clocks, doorbells, telephones).
- The 36th Bethesda Conference recommends restriction of athletes with LQTS from participation to class 1A activities (e.g., bowling, golf, riflery), although evidence of safe participation is emerging (3)[C].

COMMONLY ASSOCIATED CONDITIONS
- Illnesses with associated severe vomiting and/or diarrhea leading to electrolyte disturbances
- Eating disorders—anorexia nervosa, bulimia
- RWS
- Andersen-Tawil syndrome (LTQS type 7)—prolonged QT interval, muscle weakness, facial dysmorphism
- Timothy syndrome (LQTS type 8)—prolonged QT interval, hand/foot, facial, and neurodevelopment
- JLNS—associated with profound sensorineural hearing loss

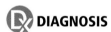

DIAGNOSIS

HISTORY
- Incidental finding on ECG in asymptomatic patients
- Evaluate for syncope, presyncopal episodes, palpitations, and associated precipitating events (emotional triggers, swimming, diving).
- Family history of syncope or sudden cardiac death
- History of seizures in patient or family members (tonic–clonic movement may be due to cerebral hypoperfusion during episodes of ventricular arrhythmia or syncope)
- Detailed medication history
- Congenital deafness

PHYSICAL EXAM
- The physical exam is typically unremarkable.
- Signs of underlying cardiac disease
- Signs of hypothyroidism, liver, or renal impairment
- Congenital deafness present in many forms of LQTS

DIFFERENTIAL DIAGNOSIS
- When evaluating Long QT interval, differential should also include: QT-prolonging drugs, hypokalemia, hypomagnesemia, hHypocalcemia, neurologic conditions leading to subarachnoid bleed, structural heart disease

- When evaluating other causes of syncope or sudden death, differential should also include:
  - Sudden infant death syndrome (SIDS), vasovagal (neurally mediated) syncope, orthostatic hypotension, seizures, familial VF, cardiomyopathies (HCM, DCM, ARVC), Brugada syndrome, anomalous coronary artery, catecholaminergic polymorphic VT

DIAGNOSTIC TESTS & INTERPRETATION
Initial Tests (lab, imaging)
- ECG
- Metabolic panel: especially calcium, magnesium, and potassium. TSH

Follow-Up Tests & Special Considerations
- Echocardiogram to evaluate for cardiomyopathy
- Outpatient cardiac rhythm monitoring (Holter, Event, or Implantable monitoring)
- Consider provocative testing (epinephrine infusion, exercise stress testing) to evaluate for QTc interval changes and/or for coronary artery disease (2)[C].
- Genetic testing for LQTS mutations

Test Interpretation
- The QT interval is best measured from the onset of the QRS to the completion of the T wave; most commonly measured in lead II or V_2
- QTc calculation can be performed in several ways using RR interval immediately preceding the QT interval for calculation. The Bazett formula is most commonly used method (1),(2).
  - Framingham formula: QT + 0.154 (1 − RR)
  - Bazett formula: QTc = QT / √(RR) (all measurements in seconds, and RR obtained by direct measurement or 60/heart rate)
  - Fridericia formula is similar to Bazett but uses the cube root RR interval: QTc = QT / (RR)$^{1/3}$.

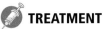 TREATMENT

GENERAL MEASURES
- Treat VT, TdP, and VF emergently per ACLS guidelines.
- Withdraw offending agents and correct electrolytes (2)[C].
- Treat underlying disorder in the setting of gastrointestinal illness, eating disorder, or neurologic conditions involving subarachnoid bleed.
- Avoid triggers, if known.
- Transvenous cardiac pacing or isoproterenol may be used for drug-induced TdP to prevent bradycardia. Maintain heart rate 90 to 110 beats/min.

MEDICATION
First Line
- For TdP: magnesium sulfate 2 g infused over 2 to 5 minutes, followed by continuous infusion of 2 to 4 mg/min if needed. Flushing is a normal side effect of bolus injections. Monitor for magnesium toxicity in those with renal insufficiency (1)[C],(2)[C].
- For hereditary LQTS, to prevent life-threatening arrhythmias: propranolol or nadolol generally regarded as the best β-blockers for management of LQTS, although rigorous studies are lacking
- β-Blockers are effective in decreasing but not eliminating the risk of fatal arrhythmias.
- For high-risk patients who remain symptomatic on a β-blocker, implantable cardiac defibrillators (ICDs) with or without pacemaker may be indicated (2)[B].

Second Line
Atenolol or metoprolol may be used, although switching β-blockers may precipitate lethal or near-lethal events.

ISSUES FOR REFERRAL
- Refer to cardiologist to establish diagnosis, especially for congenital or hereditary LQTS.
- Referral should also be made in patients with symptomatic prolonged QT.
- If patient has history of sudden cardiac death in family, congenital LQTS should be on the differential and, if suspected, patient should be referred to cardiology for further workup and diagnosis.

ADDITIONAL THERAPIES
Trials are currently being conducted on medicines that block cardiac sodium channels for LQTS type 3.

SURGERY/OTHER PROCEDURES
- ICD for those with a history of major cardiac events (whether treated with appropriate medical therapy or not)
  - ICDs do not prevent TdP, so patients should continue optimal medical therapy in conjunction to ICD.
- Left cervical–thoracic sympathetic denervation was used for symptomatic LQTS prior to the advent of β-blockers. It is still an option for those patients with LQTS who are refractory to β-blocker therapy (3)[B].

COMPLEMENTARY & ALTERNATIVE MEDICINE
- Not much research has been done on this modality of treatment in those with LQTS
- In general, many dietary supplements and herbal remedies can be harmful to patients with LQTS.
- Many such over-the-counter treatments have been linked to cardiac arrhythmias and should be avoided in this population.

ADMISSION, INPATIENT, AND NURSING CONSIDERATIONS
- Treat TdP, VT, and VF promptly as per ACLS guidelines. Correct electrolytes on an emergent basis. Evaluate for acquired QT prolongation. If no cause is found, consider hereditary LQTS.
- Patients with prolonged QTc and syncope/near syncope should be monitored on telemetry.
- Obtain a baseline ECG if initiating or combining medications with QT-prolonging medications, then when the drug reaches steady state, at 30 days, and annually thereafter.
- Avoid QT-prolonging medications in patients with congenital LQTS.
- Patients at risk for LQTS should be educated on symptoms of arrhythmia.
- Monitor electrolytes, urgently treat hypomagnesemia and hypokalemia, and discontinue/change offending medications (1)[C],(2)[C].
- Avoid sudden loud noises or emotional stress for those who have LQTS.
- Review adherence to β-blocker therapy.
- Clinical decision support systems may be useful to assess the risk of drug-induced risk of QT prolongation while considering clinical scenario (4).

 ONGOING CARE

FOLLOW-UP RECOMMENDATIONS
Patient Monitoring
- On routine visits, ask about syncope, presyncope, and palpitations in those who have QTc prolongation.
- Consider ECG and/or outpatient cardiac rhythm monitoring with medication additions or dosage changes.
- Prompt evaluation is warranted for symptomatic QTc prolongation of any cause. This may include ECG and/or outpatient cardiac rhythm monitoring.
- Check and correct for electrolyte imbalances.

DIET
- Those with known LQTS often benefit from additional potassium in their diet, whether through diet or supplementation.
- Avoiding caffeinated products, supplements with stimulant properties (such as ginseng), alcohol, and illicit/recreational drugs is also recommended as these can all increase the risk of life-threatening arrhythmias.
- QT prolongation has been noted in the setting of ketogenic diet and diabetic ketoacidosis irrespective of electrolyte disturbances.

PATIENT EDUCATION
- Educate patients with QTc prolongation about medications side effects and medication interactions.
- Patients with congenital forms of LQTS should be aware of and avoid triggers (depending on their specific gene mutation).
- Consider the emotional and psychological impacts. Additional reading by Fortescue shares the personal impact of LQTS.

PROGNOSIS
Acquired LQTS will resolve after withdrawal of offending agents and normalization of metabolic abnormalities. Patients with underlying cardiovascular disease may be at increased risk of mortality and require further intervention. Prognosis for congenital LQTS if untreated is quite poor. Perhaps 20% of untreated patients presenting with syncope die within 1 year, 50% within 10 years.

COMPLICATIONS
TdP resulting in ventricular fibrillation, sudden cardiac death, seizures, loss of consciousness, drowning and other accidents

REFERENCES
1. Kramer DB, Zimetbaum PJ. Long-QT syndrome. *Cardiol Rev.* 2011;19(5):217–225.
2. Kallergis EM, Goudis CA, Simantirakis EN, et al. Mechanisms, risk factors, and management of acquired long QT syndrome: a comprehensive review. *ScientificWorldJournal.* 2012;2012:212178.
3. Abrams DJ, Macrae CA. Long QT syndrome. *Circulation.* 2014;129(14):1524–1529.
4. Schwartz PJ, Woosley RL. Predicting the unpredictable: drug-induced QT prolongation and torsades de pointes. *J Am Coll Cardiol.* 2016;67(13):1639–1650.

 SEE ALSO

Algorithms: Cardiac Arrhythmias; Torsade de Pointes (TdP): Variant Form of Polymorphic Ventricular Tachycardia (VT)

CODES
ICD10
I45.81 Long QT syndrome

CLINICAL PEARLS
- Evaluate for acquired causes before making a diagnosis of hereditary LQTS.
- For accurate diagnosis, calculate QTc manually.
- Magnesium sulfate is the treatment of choice during ACLS for TdP.

L

LUNG, PRIMARY MALIGNANCIES

Abdel-Rahman Zakieh, MD, BS • Arvey Stone, MD • Phillip Knouse, MD

BASICS

DESCRIPTION

- Primary lung cancers are the leading cause of cancer-related deaths in the United States (estimated 154,050 deaths in 2018, 25.3% of all cancer-related deaths).
- Divided into two broad categories
  - Non–small cell lung cancer (NSCLC) (>85% of all lung cancers); normally originate in periphery
    - Adenocarcinoma (~40% of NSCLC): most common type in the United States and occurs in both smokers and nonsmokers; metastasizes earlier than squamous cell; lepidic growth, a subtype of adenocarcinoma has better prognosis.
    - Squamous cell carcinoma (SCC) (also known as epidermoid carcinoma) (~25% of NSCLC): dose-related effect with smoking; slower growing than adenocarcinoma
    - Large cell (~10% of NSCLC): prognosis similar to adenocarcinoma
  - Small cell lung cancer (SCLC) (16% of all lung cancers): centrally located, early metastases, aggressive
- Others: mesothelioma and carcinoid tumor
- Staging
  - Both NSCLC and SCLC: staged from I to IV based on: primary tumor (T), lymph node status (N), and presence of metastasis (M)
  - SCLC further staged by:
    - Limited disease: confined to ipsilateral hemithorax
    - Extensive disease: beyond ipsilateral hemithorax (stages IIIB and IV), which may include malignant pleural or pericardial effusion or hematogenous metastases (stage IV)
    - Tumor locations: upper: 60%; lower: 30%; middle: 5%; overlapping and main stem: 5%
    - May spread by local extension to chest wall, diaphragm, pulmonary vessels, vena cava, phrenic nerve, esophagus, or pericardium
    - Most commonly metastasize to lymph nodes (pulmonary, mediastinal), then liver, adrenal glands, bones, brain

EPIDEMIOLOGY

Incidence

- There are >230,000 new cases of lung cancer and 130,000 deaths annually in the United States in 2021.
- Overall, lung cancer causes more deaths than breast, prostate, colorectal, and brain cancers combined.
- Usual age of diagnosis: between 65 and 74 years; peak at 70 years
- Due to decreases in smoking, lung cancer deaths are declining in both men and women.
- Nearly one-half of all lung cancer deaths occur in women.

Prevalence

- Mortality from SCLC declined almost entirely as a result of declining incidence, with no improvement in survival
- Population-level mortality from NSCLC in the United States fell sharply from 2013 to 2016, and survival after diagnosis improved substantially.

ETIOLOGY AND PATHOPHYSIOLOGY

Multifactorial; see "Risk Factors."

Genetics

NSCLC

- Oncogenes: Ras family (H-ras, K-ras, N-ras), EGFR, NTRK, ALK, etc.
- Tumor suppressor genes: retinoblastoma, *p53*

RISK FACTORS

- Smoking
- Secondhand smoke exposure
- Radon
- Environmental and occupational exposures
  - Air pollution
  - Asbestos exposure (synergistic increase in risk for smokers)
  - Ionizing radiation
  - Mutagenic gases (halogen ethers, mustard gas, aromatic hydrocarbons)
  - Metals (inorganic arsenic, chromium, nickel)
- Lung scarring from tuberculosis
- Radiation therapy to the breast or chest

GENERAL PREVENTION

- Smoking cessation and prevention programs
- Screening recommended by National Comprehensive Cancer Network (NCCN) and shown to reduce mortality in National Lung Screening Trial (NLST) (1)[A].
- As of March 9, 2021, the USPSTF recommends annual screening for lung cancer with low-dose computed tomography (LDCT) in adults aged 50 to 80 years who have a 20 pack-year smoking history and currently smoke or have quit within the past 15 years (2).
- Screening should be discontinued once a person has not smoked for 15 years or develops a health problem that substantially limits life expectancy or the ability or willingness to have curative lung surgery.
- Prevention via aggressive smoking cessation counseling and therapy; a 20–30% risk reduction occurs within 5 years of cessation.

COMMONLY ASSOCIATED CONDITIONS

- Paraneoplastic syndromes: hypertrophic pulmonary osteoarthropathy, Lambert-Eaton syndrome (LES), Cushing syndrome, hypercalcemia from ectopic parathyroid-releasing hormone (PTHrP), syndrome of inappropriate antidiuretic hormone (SIADH)
- Hypercoagulable state
- Pancoast syndrome
- Superior vena cava (SVC) syndrome
- Pleural effusion
- Chronic obstructive pulmonary disease (COPD), other sequelae of cigarette smoking

DIAGNOSIS

HISTORY

- May be asymptomatic for most of course
- Respiratory
  - Cough (new or change in chronic cough)
  - Wheezing and stridor
  - Dyspnea
  - Hemoptysis
  - Pneumonitis (fever and productive cough)
- Constitutional
  - Malaise
  - Bone pain (metastatic disease)
  - Fatigue
  - Weight loss, anorexia
  - Fever
  - Anemia
- Other presentations
  - Chest pain (dull, pleuritic)
  - Shoulder/arm pain (Pancoast tumors)
  - Dysphagia
  - Plethora (redness of face or neck)
  - Hoarseness (involvement of recurrent laryngeal nerve)
  - Horner syndrome

- Neurologic abnormalities (e.g., headaches, syncope, weakness, cognitive impairment)
- Pericardial tamponade (pericardial invasion)

PHYSICAL EXAM

- General: fever, chills, night sweats, weight loss
- Head, eye, ear, nose, throat (HEENT): Horner syndrome, dysphonia, stridor, scleral icterus, dysphagia
- Neck: supraclavicular/cervical lymph nodes, mass
- Lungs: effusion, wheezing, airway obstruction, dyspnea
- Abdomen/groin: hepatomegaly or lymphadenopathy
- Extremities: signs of hypertrophic pulmonary osteoarthropathy, deep venous thrombosis (DVT), fingernail clubbing
- Neurologic: headache, syncope, weakness, cognitive impairment

DIFFERENTIAL DIAGNOSIS

- COPD (may coexist)
- Granulomatous (tuberculosis, sarcoidosis)
- Cardiomyopathy
- Congestive heart failure (CHF)

DIAGNOSTIC TESTS & INTERPRETATION

Initial Tests (lab, imaging)

- Serum
  - Complete blood count (CBC)
  - Comprehensive metabolic panel (CMP): Check for hyponatremia (SIADH).
  - Serum calcium: Check for hypercalcemia (paraneoplastic syndrome).
  - Lactate dehydrogenase (LDH)
- Sputum cytology
- Chest x-ray (CXR) (Compare with prior XRs.)
  - Nodule or mass, especially if calcified
  - Persistent infiltrate
  - Atelectasis
  - Mediastinal widening
  - Hilar enlargement
  - Pleural effusion
- CT scan of chest (with IV contrast)
  - Nodule or mass (central or peripheral)
  - Lymphadenopathy
- Evaluation for metastatic disease
  - Positron emission tomography (PET) scan to evaluate metastasis mediastinal lymphadenopathy (replacing CT abdomen/pelvis and bone scan)
  - Brain MRI: Lesions may be necrotic, bleeding.

Follow-Up Tests & Special Considerations

CBC, BUN, serum creatinine, LFTs prior to each cycle of chemotherapy

Diagnostic Procedures/Other

- Biopsy with pathology review using
  - Bronchoscopy with transbronchial biopsy (WANG needle); usually for centrally located tumors
  - CT-guided biopsy of lung mass or metastatic site; usually for peripherally located tumors
  - Endobronchial ultrasound (EBUS)-guided fine-needle aspiration
  - Enlarged mediastinal lymph nodes necessitate staging by mediastinoscopy, video-assisted thoracoscopy, EBUS-guided fine-needle aspiration.
- Video-assisted thoracoscopy (associated pleural disease and suspected mediastinal nodal spread)
- Pulmonary function tests (PFTs)
- In patients with advanced NSCLC, screening for mutations in EGFR, BRAF, *KRAS G12C*, NTRK, *ALK, ROS1, MET exon 14, and RET* non-SCC (NSCC) or mixed squamous histology
- PD-L1 testing
- Bone marrow aspirate (small cell)

Test Interpretation

Pathologic changes from smoking are progressive: basal cell proliferation, development of atypical nuclei, stratification, metaplasia of squamous cells, carcinoma in situ, and then invasive disease.

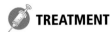 TREATMENT

GENERAL MEASURES

- NSCLC
  - Stage I, stage II, and selected stage III tumors are surgically resectable. Neoadjuvant or adjuvant therapy is recommended for select patients with high-risk IB, II, and IIIA NSCLC. Patients with resectable disease but who are not surgical candidates may receive radiation therapy.
  - Patients with unresectable or N2, N3 disease are treated with concurrent chemoradiation followed by maintenence immunotherapy. Select patients with T3 or N2 disease can be treated effectively with surgical resection and either pre- or postoperative chemotherapy or chemoradiation therapy.
  - Patients with distant metastases (M1B) can be treated with chemotherapy, targeted therapy, immunotherapy, or radiation therapy for palliation or best supportive care alone.
- SCLC
  - Limited stage: concurrent chemoradiation
  - Extensive stage: combination chemotherapy and immunotherapy
  - Consider prophylactic cranial irradiation (PCI) in patients achieving a complete or partial response (3)[A].
- Quality-of-life assessments: Karnofsky Performance Status (KPS) scale (4); Eastern Cooperative Oncology Group (ECOG)
- Discussions with patient and family about end-of-life care

MEDICATION

- Chemotherapies, targeted therapies, and immunotherapies are the mainstay of treatment.
- Adjuvant chemotherapy following surgery improves survival in patients with fully resected stages II and III NSCLC.
- Palliative measures: analgesics
- Dyspnea: oxygen, morphine

First Line

- NSCLC
  - Stages II and III: neoadjuvant or adjuvant chemotherapy
    - Cisplatin-based doublets (combination with paclitaxel, etoposide, vinorelbine, docetaxel, gemcitabine)
    - Carboplatin alternative for patients unlikely to tolerate cisplatin
    - Cisplatin plus pemetrexed (NSCC)
  - Unresectable stages IIA, IIIB
    - Concurrent chemoradiation
      - Cisplatin plus etoposide, vinblastine, or pemetrexed (NSCC) plus concurrent radiation
      - Carboplatin plus paclitaxel plus concurrent radiation
      - Carboplatin plus pemetrexed (NSCC) plus concurrent radiation
    - Durvalumab consolidation post chemoradiation for stage III
  - Stage IV
    - No chemotherapy regimen can be recommended for routine use.
    - Cisplatin- or carboplatin-based doublets are standard of care in the absence of targetable mutations.
    - Pembrolizumab with pemetrexed and carboplatin for adenocarcinoma without EGFR, ROS, or ALK mutations regardless of PD-L1 expression

- Pembrolizumab, atezolizumab, or cemiplimab monotherapy for NSCLC with PD-L1 expression ≥50% of tumor cells
- Osimertinib first line for most patients with EGFR mutations
- Dabrafenib with trametinib for untreated patients with BRAF V600E mutations
- Alectinib, lorlatinib, crizotinib, brigatinib, ceritinib, or crizotinib for untreated ALK-positive NSCLC
- Crizotinib, ceritinib, or entrectinib for patients with ROS1-positive NSCLC
- Sotorasib for KRAS G12C mutated tumors
- Larotrectinib or entrectinib for NTRK fusion positive tumors
- Capmatinib, crizotinib, or tepotinib for tumors with MET exon 14 skipping mutations
- Selpercatinib, pralsetinib, cabozantinib, or vandetanib for tumors with RET rearrangements
- SCLC
  - Cisplatin or carboplatin plus etoposide with addition of atezolizumab in extensive stage disease

Second Line

- NSCLC
  - Cisplatin-based doublets +/− bevacizumab (NSCC) if not previously used
  - Docetaxel +/− ramucirumab, pemetrexed if not previously used (NSCC), gemcitabine, or nivolumab (squamous cell)
  - Immunotherapy may be considered if progressed during or after first-line platinum-based drug.
- SCLC
  - Lurbinectedin, topotecan, or clinical trial. Alternatives include CAV (cyclophosphamide, doxorubicin, vincristine), gemcitabine, docetaxel, paclitaxel, nivolumab, and temozolomide

ADDITIONAL THERAPIES

- Smoking cessation counseling
- Consider IV bisphosphonates or denosumab in patients with bone metastases to reduce skeletal-related events.

SURGERY/OTHER PROCEDURES

- Resection for NSCLC, for stages I, II, and IIIA, if medically fit to undergo surgery
- Resection of isolated, distant metastases has been achieved and may improve survival.
- Resection involves lobectomy in 71%, wedge in 16%, and complete pneumonectomy in 18%.
- Resection should be accompanied by lymph node dissection for pathologic staging.

 ONGOING CARE

FOLLOW-UP RECOMMENDATIONS

Patient Monitoring

- Depends on clinical history; in general, postoperative visits every 3 to 6 months in the first 2 years after surgery with physical exam and CT scan
- Follow-up usually lifelong with CT scans, following NCCN criteria

PATIENT EDUCATION

- National Cancer Institute: https://www.cancer.gov/
- Smokefree.gov: https://smokefree.gov/

PROGNOSIS

- For combined, all types and stages, 5-year survival rate is 18.6%.
- NSCLC 5-year survival
  - Localized disease: for stages IA1, IA2, and IA3 is 92%, 83%, and 77%, respectively; stages IB and IIA is 68% and 60%, respectively

- Regional disease: for stages IIIA, IIIB, and IIIC is 36%, 26%, and 13%, respectively
- Distant metastatic disease: for stages IVA and IVB is 10% and <1%, respectively
- SCLC
  - Without treatment: median survival from diagnosis of only 2 to 4 months
  - 5-year survival rate: ranges from 2% (stage IV) to 31% (stage I)
  - Extensive-stage disease: median survival of 6 to 12 months; long-term disease-free survival is rare.

COMPLICATIONS

- Development of metastatic disease
- Local recurrence of disease
- Postoperative complications
- Side effects of chemotherapy or radiation

REFERENCES

1. Aberle DR, Adams AM, Berg CD, et al; for National Lung Screening Trial Research Team. Reduced lung-cancer mortality with low-dose computed tomographic screening. N Engl J Med. 2011;365(5):395–409.
2. Krist AH, Davidson KW, Mangione CM, et al; for U.S. Preventive Services Task Force. Screening for lung cancer: US Preventive Services Task Force recommendation statement. JAMA. 2021;325(10):962–970.
3. Slotman B, Faivre-Finn C, Kramer G, et al; for EORTC Radiation Oncology Group and Lung Cancer Group. Prophylactic cranial irradiation in extensive small-cell lung cancer. N Engl J Med. 2007;357(7):664–672.
4. Conill C, Verger E, Salamero M. Performance status assessment in cancer patients. Cancer. 1990;65(8):1864–1866.

ADDITIONAL READING

- National Cancer Institute. Lung cancer—health profession version. https://www.cancer.gov/types/lung/hp. Accessed October 29, 2021.
- Wender R, Fontham ET, Barrera E Jr, et al. American Cancer Society lung cancer screening guidelines. CA Cancer J Clin. 2013;63(2):107–117.

CODES

ICD10

- C34.90 Malignant neoplasm of unsp part of unsp bronchus or lung
- C34.10 Malignant neoplasm of upper lobe, unsp bronchus or lung
- C34.30 Malignant neoplasm of lower lobe, unsp bronchus or lung

CLINICAL PEARLS

- Two types: NSCLC and SCLC
  - NSCLC (>85% of all lung cancers); normally originate in periphery
    - Adenocarcinoma (~40% of NSCLC)
    - SCC (~25% of NSCLC)
    - Large cell (~10% of NSCLC)
  - SCLC centrally located, early metastases, aggressive
- Prognosis and treatment of lung cancer differ greatly between non–small cell and small cell histologies.
- Adjuvant cisplatin-based chemotherapy improves survival in patients with completely resected stages II and III NSCLC.
- Chemotherapy, with or without radiation, can be offered to patients with advanced NSCLC or SCLC.
- There is little role for surgery in the treatment of SCLC.

L

LUPUS ERYTHEMATOSUS, SYSTEMIC (SLE)
Jonathan Triantafyllou, MD • Erin Cathcart, MD, MPH

BASICS

DESCRIPTION
- Multisystem autoimmune inflammatory disorder with variable presentation, disease course, and prognosis
- May manifest in any organ system, especially dermatologic, renal, hematologic, musculoskeletal, cardiovascular, pulmonary, immunologic, and reproductive
- Synonyms: systemic lupus erythematosus (SLE), lupus

EPIDEMIOLOGY
Incidence
- Overall incidence in United States is 5 to 7 per 100,000 person-years.
- Significant variation based on ethnicity: black 16.0, American Indian/Alaska Native 7.4, Hispanic 5.6, Asian/Pacific Islander 4.6, white 3.3 per 100,000 person-years
- Strong female predominance compared to male: 9.8 versus 0.8 per 100,000 person-years (about 12-fold higher)
- Peak incidence in females ranges from 3rd to 7th decades of life.
- Peak incidence in males later, from 5th to 7th decades of life

Prevalence
- Overall prevalence in United States ranges from 70 to 100 cases per 100,000.
- Increasing due to better recognition and increased survival
- Highest prevalence in black women: 498 per 100,000
- Strong female predominance compared to male: 179 versus 21 cases per 100,000 (about 9-fold higher)

ETIOLOGY AND PATHOPHYSIOLOGY
Complex and multifactorial: Genetic, environmental, immunoregulatory, hormonal, and epigenetic factors all play a role in pathogenesis.

Genetics
- More than 30 susceptibility loci for SLE in genome-wide association studies
- Heritability, the proportion of phenotypic variance explained by genetics, between 40% and 70%
- Previous criteria from American College of Rheumatology (ACR) and Systemic Lupus International Collaborating Clinics (SLICC) still used widely in clinical practice

RISK FACTORS
- Ethnicity: highest risk in black populations; intermediate risk in Asian, Hispanic, and American Indian/Alaska Native populations
- Hormonal: female sex, early menarche, endometriosis, surgical menopause, earlier age at menopause
- Family history of SLE or other autoimmune disease
- Environmental: cigarette smoking, crystalline silica exposure, exogenous female hormones, certain medications (drug-induced lupus)

COMMONLY ASSOCIATED CONDITIONS
- Antiphospholipid syndrome
- Depression
- Fibromyalgia
- Thyroid disease
- Overlap connective tissue disease syndromes: rheumatoid arthritis (RA), Sjögren syndrome, systemic sclerosis, polymyositis, dermatomyositis

DIAGNOSIS

- Suspect in multisystem disease including fever, fatigue, and signs of inflammation
- New classification criteria from European League Against Rheumatism (EULAR) and ACR in 2019: sensitivity 96%, specificity 93% (1)[C]
- Note: Do not exclude clinically-appropriate patients from treatment solely based on classification criteria (1)[C].

HISTORY
- Symptoms frequently nonspecific, may involve any organ system, and need not present simultaneously
- Common presenting symptoms: fatigue, joint pains, fever, oral ulcers, hair loss, rash, photosensitivity
- Examples of other presentations that may raise suspicion: unprovoked venous thromboembolism, cerebrovascular accident at young age, acute pericarditis, recurrent pregnancy loss, new-onset seizure or psychosis, unexplained cytopenias or renal failure

PHYSICAL EXAM
- Constitutional (common): weight loss, fever, lymphadenopathy
- Skin (common)
  - Nonspecific: nonscarring alopecia, painless oral or nasal ulcers, photosensitivity, vasculitis, Raynaud phenomenon
  - Lupus-specific
    ○ Acute cutaneous lupus erythematosus (ACLE)
      ■ Includes classic malar or "butterfly" rash that spares nasolabial folds
      ■ Also generalized maculopapular form that is photodistributed
    ○ Subacute cutaneous lupus erythematosus (SCLE)
      ■ Annular or papulosquamous eruptions, photodistributed, frequently found on shoulders, neck, forearms, torso
    ○ Chronic cutaneous lupus erythematosus (CCLE)
      ■ Includes discoid lupus
      ■ Erythematous-violaceous lesions with secondary changes of atrophic scarring and dyspigmentation
      ■ When found on scalp, causes follicular hyperkeratosis and plugging, scarring alopecia
    ○ All have characteristic changes on skin biopsy (see "Test Interpretation").
- Musculoskeletal (common)
  - Synovitis, especially symmetric polyarthritis
  - Periarticular involvement (tendons, joint capsule), leading to nonerosive joint deformities (Jaccoud arthropathy)
- Other
  - Nonspecific findings possible in any organ system
  - Cardiopulmonary findings in pericarditis, pleural effusion, pneumonitis, venous thromboembolism
  - Edema or anasarca in advanced renal disease
  - Pallor, jaundice, splenomegaly in hematologic disease
  - Seizures, psychosis, delirium, mononeuritis multiplex, peripheral or cranial neuropathies, and cognitive impairment in central nervous system disease

DIFFERENTIAL DIAGNOSIS
- Extremely broad due to variable presentation and widespread disease manifestations
- Consider other rheumatologic conditions, thyroid disease, fibromyalgia, or organ-specific diagnoses based on presenting symptoms.
- Consider drug-induced lupus with commonly implicated drugs (hydralazine, procainamide, isoniazid, methyldopa, quinidine, chlorpromazine).

DIAGNOSTIC TESTS & INTERPRETATION
Initial Tests (lab, imaging)
- Initial testing based on presentation and level of suspicion
- Low suspicion: Limited initial laboratory evaluation may include complete blood count (CBC), complete metabolic panel (CMP), thyroid-stimulating hormone (TSH), and urinalysis.
- Higher suspicion: include immunologic testing
  - Lupus-specific:
    ○ ANA (titer 1:80 by indirect immunofluorescence): sensitivity 97.8%, specificity 74.7%
    ○ Anti-dsDNA: sensitivity 70%, specificity 95%
    ○ Anti-Smith: sensitivity 39.7%, specificity 98.6%
  - Supporting:
    ○ Complement levels (low C3 and/or C4)
    ○ Antiphospholipid antibodies (anti-cardiolipin, anti-β2GP1, lupus anticoagulant)
- Imaging studies based on specific signs/symptoms

Follow-Up Tests & Special Considerations
- 24-hour urine collection or spot protein/creatinine ratio to quantify proteinuria (1)[C]
- Anemia: reticulocyte count, indirect bilirubin, haptoglobin, direct Coombs to evaluate for hemolysis (1)[C]
- Screen for antiphospholipid syndrome at diagnosis if not already done (2)[C].
- Baseline metabolic labs: lipid panel, fasting glucose or hemoglobin A1c, vitamin D level, TSH

Diagnostic Procedures/Other
- Renal biopsy for urine protein >500 mg/24 hr (1)[C]
- Skin biopsy if necessary to confirm clinical findings of cutaneous lupus (1)[C]
- Other diagnostic modalities as needed based on specific manifestations

Test Interpretation
- Skin biopsy: Typical findings include interface vacuolar dermatitis consisting of perivascular lymphohistiocytic infiltrate, often with dermal mucin; may have immune-complex deposition at dermoepidermal junction
- Renal biopsy: per International Society of Nephrology/Renal Pathology Society classification

TREATMENT

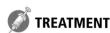

GENERAL MEASURES
- Requires a multidisciplinary, individualized approach to treatment
- General treatment goals: achieving remission or low disease activity, preventing flares and end-organ damage, increasing survival, improving quality of life (2)[C]
- Supportive measures (2)[C]
  - Sun protection
  - Smoking cessation
  - Adequate exercise
  - Managing cardiovascular risk factors (lipids, glucose, blood pressure, weight)
  - Preconception counseling and family planning
  - Immunizations: 2019 EULAR guidelines for vaccination in autoimmune inflammatory rheumatic disease (see "Additional Reading")

MEDICATION
First Line
- Hydroxychloroquine
  - Recommended for all patients with SLE unless contraindicated (3)[A]
  - Reduces flares, improves skin and musculoskeletal manifestations, reduces thrombosis and bone

mass loss, prevents organ damage, increases survival (3)[A]
- Safe to continue through pregnancy (3)[A]
- Dosing:
  - 200 to 400 mg/day as single daily dose or 2 divided doses
  - Limit to 5 mg/kg/day (actual body weight) (2)[C].
- Contraindications: known hypersensitivity to hydroxychloroquine
- Most common adverse reactions are gastrointestinal (nausea, vomiting, diarrhea, abdominal pain) and cutaneous (rash), and usually mild (3)[A].
- Precautions
  - Retinal damage
    - Less common at doses <5 mg/kg/day
    - Risk factors: higher doses, renal insufficiency, concurrent macular disease, concurrent tamoxifen use
    - Ophthalmologic screening at baseline (2)[C]
    - Yearly screening may start after 5 years in the absence of other risk factors (2)[C].
  - Cardiomyopathy: conduction abnormalities including prolonged QT interval
  - Proximal myopathy and neuropathy
  - Neuropsychiatric changes
  - Hypoglycemia
  - Caution in hepatic and/or renal disease (no specific dose reductions given)
- Interactions
  - Caution with insulin and other antidiabetic medications
  - Caution with medications that affect cardiac conduction, especially QT prolonging agents
- Glucocorticoids
  - Dose and route of administration depend on organ involvement and severity.
    - Topical steroids have a role in cutaneous disease.
    - Oral steroids frequently required for initial management, flares, and/or maintenance therapy
    - Life-/organ-threatening flares frequently require pulsed intravenous (IV) methylprednisolone (250 to 1,000 mg/day for 1 to 3 days) (2)[C]
  - Dose of chronic maintenance therapy should be minimized to <7.5 mg/day (prednisone equivalent) and discontinued if possible (2)[C].
  - Early initiation of immunomodulatory therapy may help minimize glucocorticoid needs (2)[C].

Second Line
- Choice of agent depends on disease manifestations, patient characteristics (such as age and childbearing potential), safety, and cost.
- Consider methotrexate, azathioprine, or mycophenolate for patients not controlled on hydroxychloroquine, unable to adequately taper glucocorticoids, or for initial treatment in more severe disease (2)[C].
- Consider belimumab as add-on for high residual disease activity or frequent flares despite standard treatments (2)[C].
- Consider cyclophosphamide or rituximab for severe life-/organ-threatening or refractory disease (2)[C].

ISSUES FOR REFERRAL
- Mild disease without significant end-organ involvement may be appropriate for treatment in primary care.
- Generally requires a multidisciplinary team in coordination with rheumatology
- Severe disease best managed in dedicated lupus center

SURGERY/OTHER PROCEDURES
Renal transplant for end-stage renal disease

COMPLEMENTARY & ALTERNATIVE MEDICINE
Supplements with some evidence of benefit: vitamin D, omega-3 fatty acids, *N*-acetylcysteine, and turmeric (4)[C]

ADMISSION, INPATIENT, AND NURSING CONSIDERATIONS
- Difficult to differentiate SLE flare from infection; may need to treat both pending full evaluation
- IV pulse methylprednisolone (250 to 1,000 mg/day for 1 to 3 days) for life-/organ-threatening flares

 ONGOING CARE

FOLLOW-UP RECOMMENDATIONS
Patient Monitoring
- Intensity of monitoring depends on specific manifestations, disease severity, medication regimen, and comorbidities.
- Stable, inactive disease without significant organ involvement or comorbidities may be followed every 6 to 12 months (5)[C].
- Evaluation should include at least one validated measure of disease activity (i.e., Systemic Lupus Erythematosus Disease Activity Index) (5)[C].
- Vigilant monitoring for development of kidney disease (i.e., every 3 months) in high-risk ethnicity, male sex, juvenile-onset, high serologic activity, positive anti-C1q antibodies (2)[C]
- Atherosclerotic cardiovascular disease (ASCVD)
  - Monitor and treat traditional risk factors per established guidelines.
  - Standard ASCVD risk calculators may underestimate risk in SLE—take into account SLE-specific factors (i.e., high disease activity, high doses of glucocorticoids, lupus nephritis, antiphospholipid antibodies) (5)[C].
- Osteoporosis
  - All patients: adequate calcium/vitamin D intake, smoking cessation, weight-bearing exercise, limited alcohol intake (5)[C]
  - Long-term treatment with glucocorticoids: clinical fracture risk assessment +/− bone mineral density measurement (5)[C]
  - 2017 ACR guideline for prevention and treatment of glucocorticoid-induced osteoporosis (see "Additional Reading")
- Ophthalmologic evaluation with hydroxychloroquine (retinal damage) and/or glucocorticoids (cataracts, glaucoma)
- Malignancy: Follow routine cancer-screening guidelines for general population (5)[C].
- Neuropsychiatric: Consider screening for mood disorders and cognitive impairment (5)[C].

DIET
- Although dietary factors likely affect immune system function, evidence insufficient to recommend specific dietary pattern for patients with SLE
- Complications/comorbidities may require dietary modification (renal failure, diabetes, cardiovascular disease, osteoporosis, or high-dose glucocorticoids).

PATIENT EDUCATION
- Centers for Disease Control and Prevention (https://www.cdc.gov/lupus/index.htm)
- Lupus Foundation of America (https://www.lupus.org/)

PROGNOSIS
- Permanent, treatment-free remission is rare.
- Increased all-cause mortality in SLE compared to the general population, with standardized mortality ratio (SMR) of 2.6
- 10-year survival about 90%

COMPLICATIONS
- Medication toxicity, including osteoporosis and osteonecrosis
- Obstetric complications
- Malignancy (especially hematologic, cervical, breast, lung)
- Renal failure, cardiovascular and thromboembolic events, infections, and death

REFERENCES
1. Aringer M, Costenbader K, Daikh D, et al. 2019 European League Against Rheumatism/American College of Rheumatology classification criteria for systemic lupus erythematosus. *Arthritis Rheumatol*. 2019;71(9):1400–1412. doi:10.1002/art.40930.
2. Fanouriakis A, Kostopoulou M, Alunno A, et al. 2019 Update of the EULAR recommendations for the management of systemic lupus erythematosus. *Ann Rheum Dis*. 2019;78(6):736–745. doi:10.1136/annrheumdis-2019-215089.
3. Ruiz-Irastorza G, Ramos-Casals M, Brito-Zeron P, et al. Clinical efficacy and side effects of antimalarials in systemic lupus erythematosus: a systematic review. *Ann Rheum Dis*. 2010;69(1):20–28.
4. Furer V, Rondaan C, Heijstek MW, et al. 2019 Update of EULAR recommendations for vaccination in adult patients with autoimmune inflammatory rheumatic diseases. *Ann Rheum Dis*. 2020;79(1):39–52. doi:10.1136/annrheumdis-2019-215882.
5. Greco CM, Nakajima C, Manzi S. Updated review of complementary and alternative medicine treatments for systemic lupus erythematosus. *Curr Rheumatol Rep*. 2013;15(11):378. doi:10.1007/s11926-013-0378-3.

ADDITIONAL READING
- Buckley L, Guyatt G, Fink HA, et al. 2017 American College of Rheumatology guideline for the prevention and treatment of glucocorticoid-induced osteoporosis. *Arthritis Rheumatol*. 2017;69(8):1521–1537. doi:10.1002/art.40137.
- Mosca M, Tani C, Aringer M, et al. European League Against Rheumatism recommendations for monitoring patients with systemic lupus erythematosus in clinical practice and in observational studies. *Ann Rheum Dis*. 2010;69(7):1269–1274. doi:10.1136/ard.2009.117200.

 SEE ALSO

Antiphospholipid Antibody Syndrome

 CODES

ICD10
- M32.0 Drug-induced systemic lupus erythematosus
- M32.14 Glomerular disease in systemic lupus erythematosus
- M32.19 Other organ or system involvement in systemic lupus erythematosus

CLINICAL PEARLS
- Multisystem disease with variable presentation—must maintain high index of suspicion for diagnosis
- Increased all-cause mortality, particularly related to renal disease, infections, and cardiovascular disease
- Low threshold for renal biopsy— lupus nephritis is a major risk factor for poor outcomes
- Aggressiveness of therapy should reflect intensity of disease.

L

LUPUS NEPHRITIS
Neena R. Gupta, MD

 BASICS

DESCRIPTION
- Renal disease associated with systemic lupus erythematosus (SLE)
- American College of Rheumatology (ACR) criteria: persistent proteinuria >500 mg/day or ≥3 on dipstick and/or presence of cellular casts; alternatively, spot urine protein-to-creatinine ratio (UPCR) >0.5 and "active urinary sediment" (>5 RBC/HPF, >5 WBC/HPF in absence of infection, or cellular casts—RBC or WBC casts) (1)
- Clinical manifestations primarily due to immune complex–mediated glomerular disease. Tubulointerstitial and vascular involvement often coexist. Diagnosis is based on clinical findings, urine abnormalities, autoantibodies, and renal biopsy.
- Treatment and prognosis depend on International Society of Nephrology/Renal Pathology Society (ISN/RPS) histologic class.
- Early diagnosis improves renal outcomes.

EPIDEMIOLOGY
- Peak incidence of SLE is 15 to 45 years of age. Mean age of diagnosis is between 25 and 30 years of age.
- Predominant sex: female > male (10:1)
- Once SLE develops, lupus nephritis (LN) affects both genders equally; it is more severe in children and men and less severe in older adults.
- More common in African American and Asian populations.

Incidence
- SLE: 1 to 22/100,000
- Up to 60% of SLE patients develop LN over time; 25–50% of SLE patients have nephritis as the initial presentation.

Pediatric Considerations
LN is more common and more severe in children: 60–80% of children have LN at or soon after SLE onset.

Prevalence
SLE: 7 to 159/100,000

ETIOLOGY AND PATHOPHYSIOLOGY
- Immune complex–mediated inflammation injures glomeruli, tubules, interstitium, and vasculature.
- Glomeruli: Varying degrees of mesangial proliferation, crescent formation, and fibrinoid necrosis cause reduced glomerular filtration rate (GFR).
- Persistent inflammation (chronicity) leads to sclerosis and glomerular loss.
- Tubulointerstitial injury (edema, inflammatory cell infiltrate acutely; tubular atrophy in chronic phase) with or without tubular basement membrane immune complex deposition leads to reduced renal function.
- Vascular lesions: immune complex deposition and noninflammatory necrosis in arterioles
- SLE is a multifactorial disease, with multigenic inheritance; exact etiology remains unclear.
- Defective T-cell autoregulation and polyclonal B-cell hyperactivity contribute to dysregulated apoptosis. Impaired clearance of apoptotic cells inhibits self-tolerance to nuclear antigen.

- Anti-DNA, anti-C1q, anti–α-actin, and other nuclear component autoantibodies develop.
- Deposition of circulating immune complexes or autoantibodies attaching to local nuclear antigens leads to complement activation, inflammation, and tissue injury.
- Interaction of genetic, hormonal, and environmental factors leads to great variability in LN severity.

Genetics
- Polygenic inheritance; clustering in families, ~25% concordance in identical twins
- Interaction of general SLE susceptibility genes with more renal-specific genes and epigenetic changes

RISK FACTORS
Younger age, African American or Hispanic race, more ACR criteria for SLE, longer disease duration, hypertension, lower socioeconomic status, family history of SLE, anti-dsDNA antibodies, low albumin to globulin ratio

COMMONLY ASSOCIATED CONDITIONS
Other organ systems often involved in SLE.

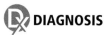 **DIAGNOSIS**

HISTORY
- Assess for signs/symptoms of SLE.
- Active nephritis is often accompanied by fever, peripheral edema, nausea, vomiting, headache and dizziness.

PHYSICAL EXAM
- Hypertension, fever
- Pleural/pericardial rub (serositis)
- Skin rash
- Edema
- Arthritis
- Alopecia
- Oral ulcers
- Signs of synovitis

DIFFERENTIAL DIAGNOSIS
- Primary glomerular disease
- Secondary renal involvement in other systemic disorders such as antineutrophil cytoplasmic antibody (ANCA)-associated vasculitis, Henoch-Schönlein purpura (HSP), antiglomerular basement membrane disease, polyarteritis nodosa, and viral infections

DIAGNOSTIC TESTS & INTERPRETATION
- Renal biopsy is the gold standard for diagnosing and classifying LN.
- Active urine sediment suggests nephritis.
- Autoantibodies, low C3, C4, and CH50 complement levels support LN.

Initial Tests (lab, imaging)
- Urinalysis, serum electrolytes, BUN, creatinine, albumin, routine serologic markers of SLE such as antinuclear antibody (ANA), anti-dsDNA, anti-Ro, anti-La, anti-RNP, anti-Sm, antiphospholipid (aPL) antibody, C3, C4, CH50, CBC with differential, and C-reactive protein (CRP) (2)[C]
- Renal ultrasound

Follow-Up Tests & Special Considerations
- Monitor disease activity q3mo (2)[C]: urinalysis for hematuria and proteinuria; blood for C3, C4, anti-dsDNA, serum albumin, and creatinine.
- Manage patients with estimated glomerular filtration rate (eGFR) of <60 mL as per National Kidney Foundation guidelines for chronic kidney disease (CKD): https://kdigo.org/guidelines/ckd-evaluation-and-management/.
- Biomarker panel: α_1-acid glycoprotein (AGP); ceruloplasmin; lipocalin-like prostaglandin synthase (LPGDS); transferring correlates with disease activity in children.

Pregnancy Considerations
- Pregnancy leads to worsening of renal function. Risk factors include renal impairment at baseline, active disease, hypertension, and proteinuria.
- Risk factors for fetal loss include elevated serum creatinine, heavy proteinuria, hypertension, and anticardiolipin antibodies.
- Renin-angiotensin system blockade and mycophenolate mofetil (MMF) are contraindicated in pregnancy; azathioprine can be used, FDA pregnancy category D.

Test Interpretation
- On renal biopsy immunofluorescence microscopy: Immune complex deposits consisting of IgG, IgA, IgM, C1q, and C3 ("full house") are highly suggestive of LN.
- Revised ISN/RPS 2003 histologic classification guides therapeutic decisions: https://jasn.asnjournals.org/content/jnephrol/15/2/241.full.pdf?with-ds=yes. Revised 2008 classification awaits endorsement.
- LN is classified as purely mesangial (class I-minimal mesangial LN and II-mesangial proliferative LN), focal proliferative LN: <50% glomeruli (class III), diffuse proliferative LN: ≥50% (class IV), membranous LN (class V), and advanced sclerosis LN (class VI); subdivisions for activity (A) and chronicity (C) in class III/IV and for segmental (S) or global (G) glomerular involvement in class IV (class III A, C, A/C and class IV S[A], G[A], S[A/C], S[C], G[C]); LN class may change with or without therapy.
- Focal and diffuse proliferative LN (classes III and IV) are common and most likely to progress to ESRD.

 TREATMENT

GENERAL MEASURES
- Monitor bone density; optimize vitamin D and calcium intake, BMI, and regular exercise.
- Low-salt diet
- Avoid sun or ultraviolet light exposure.

MEDICATION
Note: Other than methylprednisolone, prednisone, and belimumab, no other medications listed below are FDA approved for LN.

First Line
- Class I + II LN: no specific therapy. Monitor UPCR; renin-angiotensin system blockade (ACEI or ARB) to manage BP and proteinuria (e.g., lisinopril 5 to 40 mg/day PO, losartan 25 to 100 mg/day PO)

- Proliferative LN (class III or IV [±V]) (2),(3)
- Principles of treatment:
  - Avoid delay; proteinuria reduction of at least 25% by 3 months, 50% by 6 months, and UPCR target <0.5 to 0.7 by 12 months (3)
  - Patients with baseline nephrotic range proteinuria may need an additional 6 to 12 months.
- INDUCTION: steroids + immunosuppressive agent (for mild class III, high-dose steroids may be sufficient):
  - Glucocorticoids: methylprednisolone pulses, (total dose 500 to 2,500 mg) followed by oral prednisone (0.3 to 0.5 mg/kg/day) for up to 4 weeks, tapered to ≤7.5 mg/day by 3 to 6 months (3)[A] AND
  - Cyclophosphamide: IV cyclophosphamide (low dose = 0.5 g every 2 weeks for total 6 doses) OR
  - MMF: Target dose 2 to 3 g/day for 6 months. MMF is as effective as cyclophosphamide in achieving remission with fewer side effects (3)[A].
  - MMF (target dose 1 to 2 g/day) with calcineurin inhibitor (CNI) is an alternative to patients with nephrotic range proteinuria.
  - High-dose IV cyclophosphamide (0.50 to 0.75 g/m^2) monthly for 6 doses is an option for patients at high risk for kidney failure.
  - In Asian population, combination of tacrolimus, MMF, and glucocorticoids found to be superior to cyclophosphamide and glucocorticoids (4).
- MAINTENANCE:
  - Glucocorticoids: low-dose oral prednisone (2.5 to 5.0 mg/day) AND
  - MMF 1 to 2 g/day especially if used as initial agent OR azathioprine: 2 mg/kg/day PO (3)[A]
  - Optimum duration is unclear but gradual withdrawal (glucocorticoids first) after at least 3 to 5 years therapy in complete clinical response
- Pure class V LN: good prognosis, no standardized treatment
  - MMF (2 to 3 g/day) with IV methylprednisolone pulse (500 to 2,500 mg) followed by oral prednisone (20 mg/day tapered to ≤5 mg/day by 3 months) (3)
  - Options for nephrotic range proteinuria patients include CNI (especially tacrolimus) or IV cyclophosphamide, either as monotherapy or in combination with MMF (3).
- Belimumab in combination with standard initial and subsequent therapy as 10 mg/kg IV every 2 weeks for 3 doses followed by maintenance dosing every 4 weeks for total 100 weeks has been shown to improve outcome (5).
- Hydroxychloroquine: All LN of any class unless contraindicated; maximum daily dose not to exceed 5 mg/kg/day and adjust for GFR with regular ophthalmologic follow-up

Second Line
Refractory LN: No response to initial treatment within 3 to 4 months. Multitarget therapy recommended. Change either cyclophosphamide to MMF or vice versa, rituximab, CNI, belimumab, stem cell transplantation, IVIG, plasma exchange (6)[C].

ISSUES FOR REFERRAL
Nephrology consults for initial management and relapses

ADDITIONAL THERAPIES
- RAS blockade beneficial because of antiproteinuric and antihypertensive effects
- Vaccination review
- Treat hypertension and other modifiable cardiovascular risk factors.
- Low-dose aspirin for high-risk aPL profile

SURGERY/OTHER PROCEDURES
- Renal transplant for ESRD when indicated
- Patient and graft survival rates similar to non-SLE patients
- Recurrent LN ranges between 0% and 30%; graft loss due to recurrence is rare.

ADMISSION, INPATIENT, AND NURSING CONSIDERATIONS
Admission criteria/initial stabilization
- Uncontrolled hypertension, acute kidney injury
- Severe extrarenal manifestation
- Nephrology input for management and renal biopsy

 ## ONGOING CARE

FOLLOW-UP RECOMMENDATIONS
Patient Monitoring
- UPCR, urine microscopy, serum albumin, creatinine, antibody titers (especially anti-dsDNA), C3, C4, BP at least every 3 months for first 2 to 3 years followed by 6 to 12 months if no active disease (2)[C]
- CBC, LFT, and hydration per immunosuppressive regimen

DIET
Low-salt diet. For eGFR <60 mL: Follow National Kidney Foundation guidelines for CKD.

PATIENT EDUCATION
- Medication adherence and self-monitoring for relapse
- Preconception counseling

PROGNOSIS
- 10-year survival of 88% and 94% in SLE patients with and without renal involvement
- Relapse rate is ~35%. 10–20% of patients progress to ESRD within 10 years.
- 5-year renal survival of class IV LN <30% before 1970 has improved to >80% in last 2 decades.
- Remission of proteinuria is the best prognostic factor. Others include low baseline proteinuria, normal creatinine, Caucasian race, and treatment initiated within 3 months of diagnosis.
- Poor prognosis: crescentic diffuse proliferative LN, higher activity/chronicity index, APOL 1 risk alleles, African American race, lower socioeconomic status, poor response to treatment, high creatinine at baseline, uncontrolled hypertension, and relapse

COMPLICATIONS
- Risks of immunosuppressive therapy: infections, malignancy, GI upset, primary amenorrhea with cyclophosphamide, teratogenic effect of MMF
- Vascular thromboses with aPL antibodies
- About 10–20% of patients develop ESRD requiring dialysis/kidney transplantation.

REFERENCES
1. Hahn BH, McMahon MA, Wilkinson A, et al. American College of Rheumatology guidelines for screening, treatment, and management of lupus nephritis. *Arthritis Care Res (Hoboken)*. 2012;64(6):797–808.
2. Tunnicliffe DJ, Singh-Grewal D, Kim S, et al. Diagnosis, monitoring, and treatment of systemic lupus erythematosus: a systematic review of clinical practice guidelines. *Arthritis Care Res*. 2015;67(10):1440–1452.
3. Fanouriakis A, Kostopoulou M, Cheema K, et al. 2019 Update of the Joint European League Against Rheumatism and European Renal Association-European Dialysis and Transplant Association (EULAR/ERA-EDTA) recommendations for the management of lupus nephritis. *Ann Rheum Dis*. 2020;79(6):713–723.
4. Zhou T, Lin S, Yang S, et al. Efficacy and safety of tacrolimus in induction therapy of patients with lupus nephritis. *Drug Des Devel Ther*. 2019;13:857–869.
5. Furie R, Rovin BH, Houssiau F, et al. Two-year, randomized, controlled trial of belimumab in lupus nephritis. *N Engl J Med*. 2020;383(12):1117–1128.
6. Kronbichler A, Brezina B, Gauckler P, et al. Refractory lupus nephritis: when, why and how to treat. *Autoimmun Rev*. 2019;18(5):510–518.

ADDITIONAL READING
- Gasparotto M, Gatto M, Binda V, et al. Lupus nephritis: clinical presentations and outcomes in the 21st century. *Rheumatology (Oxford)*. 2020;59(Suppl 5):v39–v51.
- Kidney Disease: Improving Global Outcomes Glomerulonephritis Work Group. KDIGO clinical practice guideline for glomerulonephritis. *Kidney Int Suppl*. 2012;2(2):139–274.

CODES

ICD10
M32.14 Glomerular disease in systemic lupus erythematosus

CLINICAL PEARLS
- Early diagnosis, correct classification (based on renal biopsy), and rapid treatment improve renal survival.
- Treat proliferative/progressive LN with a short induction course followed by maintenance therapy using glucocorticoids and immunosuppressants.
- Due to advances in diagnosis and treatment, survival rates for patients have improved dramatically over the past several decades.

L

LYME DISEASE

Felix B. Chang, MD, DABMA, ABIHM, ABIM

 BASICS

Lyme disease is caused by the bacterium *Borrelia burgdorferi*.

DESCRIPTION
- An infection caused by *Borrelia* spirochetes, transmitted primarily by ixodid ticks
- *Ixodes scapularis* (deer ticks) in the Northeast and Great Lakes areas
- *Ixodes pacificus* in the West (black-legged ticks and Western black-legged ticks)

EPIDEMIOLOGY
In 2019, a total of 34,945 confirmed and probable cases of Lyme disease where reported to CDC. Approximately 300,000 people may get Lyme disease each year in the United States.

Incidence
High incidence U.S. states: Wisconsin, West Virginia, Virginia, Vermont, Rhode Island, Pennsylvania, New York, New Jersey, New Hampshire, Minnesota, Massachusetts, Maryland, Maine, District of Columbia, Delaware, Connecticut

Prevalence
Predominant age: most common in children ages 5 to 14 years and in adults aged 55 to 70 years of age

ETIOLOGY AND PATHOPHYSIOLOGY
- Average incubation period 7 to 10 days after tick bite
- Most transmissions occur in May to September when nymphal tick activity is highest.
- If a tick is infected, the chance of transmission increases with time attached: 12% at 48 hours, 79% at 72 hours, and 94% at 96 hours of attachment.
- Primary animal reservoir is the white-footed mouse.
- Spirochetes multiply and spread within dermis, resulting in characteristic (erythema multiforme [EM]) rash. Hematogenous dissemination results in involvement of central nervous system (CNS), cardiovascular, or other organ stems.

Genetics
Human leukocyte antigen haplotype DR4 or DR2 increases susceptibility to prolonged arthritis.

RISK FACTORS
Lyme endemic area. Ixodid ticks are common on deer; hunters at increased risk

GENERAL PREVENTION
- Wear appropriate clothing when outdoors in endemic areas during times of high tick activity. Clothing should cover the ankles and pretreat clothes, shoes, and tents with 0.5% permethrin.
- "Tick checks": Examine skin after outdoor activities.
- Remove ticks as soon as possible to limit transmission.
- To prevent of tick bites: N,N-diethyl-meta-toluamide (DEET), picaridin ethyl-3-(N-n-butyl-N-acetyl) aminopropionate (IR3535), oil of eucalyptus (OLE), p-menthane-3,8-diol (PMD), 2-undecanone
- Prophylactic treatment with 1 dose of 200 mg of doxycycline within 72 hours of a tick that has been attached for at least 36 hours is indicated in endemic areas. Number needed to treat = 50 to 53

COMMONLY ASSOCIATED CONDITIONS
- Coinfection with other tick borne illness (e.g., babesiosis, ehrlichiosis, anaplasmosis)
- Comorbid human granulocytic anaplasmosis and/or babesiosis in patients living in endemic regions

DIAGNOSIS
Test with a sensitive enzyme immunoassay (EIA) or immunofluorescence assay, followed by Western immunoblot assay for specimens yielding positive or equivocal results.

HISTORY
- History of a tick bite followed by EM and/or illness (fever, fatigue, headache, myalgias)
- EM = round, flat or raised, erythematous bull's-eye lesion that expands in diameter over days to weeks that has an area of central clearing
  - Common sites: axilla, back, abdomen, groin, or popliteal fossa
  - 75–80% presenting with EM having a single lesion
- Early Lyme disease: incubation period 3 to 30 days; patients may be asymptomatic. Fever; headache; myalgias; arthralgias, regional lymphadenopathy
- Early disseminated Lyme disease:
  - Carditis: pleuritic chest pain, palpitations, light headaches, fainting, shortness of breath
  - Facial palsies or other cranial neuropathies
  - Joint pain (polyarthritis/polyarthralgia
  - Late disease: monoarthritis, iritis, conjunctivitis, migratory musculoskeletal pain
- Late Lyme disease arises months after exposure.
  - Recurrent synovitis; recurrent tendonitis and bursitis
  - Encephalopathic symptoms: severe headaches and neck stiffness; confusion; facial palsy on one or both sides of the face
  - Peripheral nerve involvement: radiculoneuropathy, numbness, tingling, shooting pain, or weakness in the arms or legs
  - Symptoms mimicking other CNS diseases: multiple sclerosis–like symptoms; stroke-like symptoms; transverse myelitis

PHYSICAL EXAM
- Early Lyme disease:
  - EM in 70–80% of patients. Expanding erythema arising 7 to 14 days after tick detaches. Lesions are often >5 cm, flat or raised, may be homogeneous or have an area of central clearing (classic target session).
- Disseminated Lyme disease:
  - Skin: multiple EM lesions
  - Neurology: facial palsies (uni- or bilateral) or other cranial neuropathies
  - Cardiovascular: irregular pulse, bradycardia (heart block); friction rub (pericarditis)

DIFFERENTIAL DIAGNOSIS
- Other tick-borne illnesses: Rocky Mountain spotted fever (RMSF), ehrlichiosis, babesiosis
- Autoimmune process: juvenile rheumatoid arthritis (RA); systemic lupus erythematosus (SLE); RA
- Viral syndromes
- Contact dermatitis, cellulitis
- Granuloma annulare (mimic EM)
- Syphilis

DIAGNOSTIC TESTS & INTERPRETATION
- A tick bite is considered to be high risk only if the tick bite was from an identified *Ixodes* spp. vector species, it occurs in a highly endemic area, the tick was attached for ≥36 hours (1)[A],(2)[A],(3)[A].
- Patients who have a typical EM lesion and who live in or have traveled to a Lyme-endemic area can be diagnosed with acute Lyme disease without laboratory testing.
- Serologic testing of patients presenting with EM lesions is not recommended due to insensitivity of serologic assays during the acute stage of infection.
- Health care providers should order Lyme testing only when there is existing clinical and epidemiologic support for diagnosis.

Initial Tests (lab, imaging)
- Potential tick exposure in a Lyme disease endemic area who have one or more skin lesions compatible with EM, recommended clinical diagnosis rather than laboratory testing
- Testing for IgM or IgG-class antibodies to *B. burgdorferi* solely by immunoblot, without a prior positive or equivocal first-tier immunoassay, is strongly discouraged due to an increase frequency of false-positive result.
- CDC recommends two-tier testing
  - Tier 1 is an antibody screening assay.
  - Tier 2 is an immunoblot.
    ○ If the immunoassay(s) are negative, no further test is necessary.
    ○ If the immunoassays are positive or equivocal, reflex testing by immunoblot is required.
    ○ For patients with symptoms lasting ≤30 days, both IgM and IgG specific anti-*B. burgdorferi* immunoblots should be performed.
    ○ For patients with symptoms >30 days, only anti-*B. burgdorferi* Ig immunoblot should be performed.
- Modified two-tiered Lyme disease serologic testing
  - Both tiers are immunoassays, done concurrently or sequentially.
  - Results are faster and simpler to interpret.

Follow-Up Tests & Special Considerations
- Arthritis: serology + PCR of synovial fluid is both sensitive and specific.
- Neuroborreliosis: serology + CSF pleocytosis (PCR of CSF has a very low sensitivity.)

Diagnostic Procedures/Other
Lumbar puncture when neurologic findings are present.

TREATMENT

Prophylactic antibiotic therapy should be given only to adults and children within 72 hours of removal of an identified high-risk tick bite—not for bites that are equivocal risk or low risk (1)[A],(2)[A],(3)[A]; doxycycline 200 mg PO for adults and 4.4 mg/kg up to 200 mg for children (1)[A],(2)[A],(3)[A]

MEDICATION

For people intolerant of amoxicillin, doxycycline, and cefuroxime, macrolides (azithromycin, clarithromycin, or erythromycin) may be used. Macrolides have lower efficacy, so patients treated with them should be monitored to ensure that symptoms resolve.

First Line

- Early Lyme disease (1)[A],(2)[A],(3)[A]: doxycycline 100 mg PO BID for 10 to 14 days (do not use in children <8 years old or in pregnant women); *or* amoxicillin 500 mg PO TID for 14 days (pediatric dose 50 mg/kg/day); *or* cefuroxime axetil 500 mg PO BID for 14 days. Alternative: azithromycin 500 mg QD for 7 to 10 days or clarithromycin 500 mg BID for 14 to 21 days
- Early disseminated Lyme
  - Neurologic disease:
    ○ In patients age ≥16 years with acute facial nerve palsy but without other evidence of Lyme disease, corticosteroid treatment should be administered within 72 hours. Treat with appropriate Lyme therapy.
    ○ Adults: doxycycline 100 mg PO for 14 to 21 days
    ○ Children: doxycycline 4.4 mg/kg/day divided into 2 doses; 14 to 21 days
    ○ Lyme meningitis or radiculoneuritis: adults doxycycline 200 mg PO divided into 1 or 2 doses for 14 to 21 days or ceftriaxone 2 g IV once a day 14 to 21 days
  - Cardiac disease:
    ○ Mild (1st-degree AV block, PR <300 ms): adults doxycycline 100 mg PO BID or amoxicillin 500 mg PO TID for 14 to 21 days; children: doxycycline 4.4 mg/kg/day PO, divided BID for 14 to 21 days or amoxicillin 50 mg/kg/day PO, divided TID for 14 to 21 days or cefuroxime 30 mg/kg/day PO, divided BID for 14 to 21 days
    ○ Severe (symptomatic, 1st-degree AV block with PR interval ≥ 300 ms, 2nd- or 3rd-degree AV block): adults: ceftriaxone 2 g IV QD for 14 to 21 days; children: ceftriaxone 50 to 75 mg/kg IV QD for 14 to 21 days
  - Arthritis:
    ○ Adults: doxycycline 100 mg BID PO for 28 days or amoxicillin 500 mg TID PO for 28 days or cefuroxime 500 mg BID PO for 28 days
    ○ Children ≥ 8 years old: doxycycline 4.4 mg/kg/day PO, divided BID for 28 days, or amoxicillin 50 mg/kg PO daily divided TID for 28 days or cefuroxime 30 mg/kg/day PO, divided BID for 28 days
    ○ Children <8 years old: amoxicillin 50 mg/kg/day PO for 28 days or cefuroxime 30 mg/kg/day PO, divided into 2 doses for 28 days
    ○ Parenteral treatment: adults: ceftriaxone 2 g IV QD for 14 to 28 days; children: ceftriaxone 50 to 75 mg/kg IV QD for 14 to 28 days
- Contraindications:
  - Allergies to specific medications
  - Doxycycline is contraindicated in children and in women who are pregnant or breastfeeding.
- Precautions:
  - ~15% of patients treated with IV therapy, a Jarisch-Herxheimer–type reaction develops within 24 hours.
  - Significant interactions: oral anticoagulants and oral contraceptives

Pregnancy Considerations

Because *B. burgdorferi* can cross the placenta, pregnant patients with active disease should be treated with parenteral antibiotics.

SURGERY/OTHER PROCEDURES

Temporary pacemaker with carditis and high-grade heart block

ADMISSION, INPATIENT, AND NURSING CONSIDERATIONS

Admit patients with Lyme carditis and symptoms of chest pain, syncope, or dyspnea and those with 2nd- or 3rd-degree heart block or 1st-degree heart block of ≥300 ms or symptoms of meningitis.

 ONGOING CARE

FOLLOW-UP RECOMMENDATIONS

Do not retest patient to determine whether antibody titers have declined after treatment because seroreactivity often persists for months after treatment of early infection and years after treatment of late infection.

PATIENT EDUCATION

- In endemic areas, protect against tick exposure. Avoid "painting" the tick with nail polish or petroleum jelly, or using heat, detach ticks from skin.
- Prevention: Use repellents that contain 20–30% DEET. Bathe as soon as possible after coming indoors (within 2 hours) and perform regular tick checks.

PROGNOSIS

Early treatment with antibiotics can shorten the duration of symptoms and prevent later disease. Late-stage disease to treatment is variable. Symptoms may take weeks to resolve. Untreated rash usually resolves in 3 to 4 weeks. Excellent long-term prognosis with early antibiotics. Neurologic symptoms arise in about 15% of untreated Lyme disease patients.

COMPLICATIONS

- Posttreatment Lyme disease syndrome (PTLDS): pain, fatigue, or difficulty thinking that last for >6 months after they finish treatment; no proven treatment for PTLDS
- PTLDS: 10–20% lingering symptoms of fatigue, pain, or joint and muscle aches; can last for 6 months
- Lyme carditis >40% syncopal presentation

REFERENCES

1. Lantos PM, Rumbaugh J, Bockenstedt LK, et al. Clinical practice guidelines by the Infectious Diseases Society of America (IDSA), American Academy of Neurology (AAN), and American College of Rheumatology (ACR): 2020 guidelines for the prevention, diagnosis and treatment of Lyme disease. *Clin Infect Dis*. 2021;72(1):1–8.
2. Association of Public Health Laboratories. Suggested reporting language, interpretation and guidance regarding Lyme disease serologic test results. https://www.aphl.org/aboutAPHL/publications/Documents/ID-2021-Lyme-Disease-Serologic-Testing-Reporting.pdf. Accessed January 6, 2022.
3. Branda JA, Steere AC. Laboratory diagnosis of Lyme borreliosis. *Clin Microbiol Rev*. 2021;34(2):e00018–19.

 SEE ALSO

https://www.cdc.gov/lyme/index.html

 CODES

ICD10

- A69.20 Lyme disease, unspecified
- A69.2 Lyme disease

CLINICAL PEARLS

Steps to prevent Lyme disease include using insect repellent, removing ticks promptly, applying pesticides, and reducing tick habitat. There is no test that can "prove cure." Antibodies can persist long after the infection is gone.

L

LYMPHANGITIS

Lindsay N. Moy, MD • Thomas Holmes, MD

BASICS

DESCRIPTION
Acute or chronic inflammation of lymphatic channels that typically presents as red, tender streaks extending (often quickly) to regional lymph nodes
- May be infectious or noninfectious
- Commonly occurs on an extremity secondary to a skin infection that extends into the lymphatic vessels
- May result from compromised lymphatic drainage following surgical procedures, trauma, or malignancy

ETIOLOGY AND PATHOPHYSIOLOGY
- Acute infection
  - Usually caused by group A β-hemolytic *Streptococcus*
  - Immunocompromised patients often infected with gram-negative bacteria or fungi; usually secondary to lower extremity cellulitis
  - Less commonly caused by:
    - *Staphylococcus aureus*
    - *Pasteurella multocida*
    - *Erysipelothrix* (fish exposure)
    - *Spirillum minus* (rat bite disease)
    - *Pseudomonas*
    - Other *Streptococcus* sp.
    - In fresh water exposures, *Aeromonas hydrophila*
    - Bacillus anthracis
    - Parapoxvirus (occupational milker's nodule)
    - Herpes simplex virus (lymphogranuloma venereum)
- Nodular lymphangitis
  - Also known as sporotrichoid lymphangitis
  - Painful or painless nodular subcutaneous swellings along lymphatic vessels
  - Lesions may ulcerate with accompanying regional lymphadenopathy.
  - Usually does not develop as rapidly as acute lymphangitis and may not present with systemic symptoms
  - Typical of infections from *Sporothrix schenckii*, *Nocardia brasiliensis*, *Mycobacterium marinum*, *Leishmania* sp., *Francisella tularensis*, and systemic mycoses
  - Pathology may show granulomas.
- Noninfectious granulomatous lymphangitis
  - Rare, acquired lymphedema of the genitalia in children
  - May be due to atypical Crohn disease or sarcoidosis (1)[C]
- Filarial lymphangitis
  - Mosquito bites transmit parasites causing lymphatic inflammation and dilatation; can predispose to secondary bacterial infection
  - Usually caused by nematodes *Wuchereria bancrofti*; less commonly, *Brugia malayi* and *Brugia timori*
- Lymphangitis can occur after surgical procedures and lymph node dissection.

- Cutaneous lymphangitis carcinomatosa is rare. Represents ~5% of all skin metastases; caused by neoplastic occlusion of dermal lymphatic vessels (2)
  - Associated cancers include breast, lung, stomach, pancreas, and rectal.
- Sclerosing lymphangitis of the penis
  - Swelling around coronal sulcus of penis as a result of vigorous sexual activity or masturbation

RISK FACTORS
- Impaired lymphatic drainage due to surgery, nodal dissection, or irradiation
- Diabetes mellitus
- Chronic steroid use
- Peripheral venous catheter
- Varicella infection
- Immunocompromising condition
- Human, animal, or insect bites; skin trauma
- Fungal, bacterial, or mycobacterial skin infections
- IV drug abuse
- Residence in endemic areas of filariasis

GENERAL PREVENTION
- Reduce chronic lymphedema with compression devices or by treating underlying processes.
- Insect repellant; arthropod bite precautions
- Proper wound and skin care

COMMONLY ASSOCIATED CONDITIONS
- Lymphedema
- Prior lymph node dissection
- Tinea pedis (athlete's foot)
- Sporotrichosis
- Cellulitis, erysipelas
- Filarial infection (*W. bancrofti*)

DIAGNOSIS

HISTORY
- Trauma to skin, cut, abrasion, or fungal infection
- Erythematous streaks that can spread within a few hours (3)
- Systemic symptoms:
  - Malaise
  - Fever and chills
  - Loss of appetite
  - Headache
  - Muscle aches
- Travel to a tropical zone or region with filariasis

PHYSICAL EXAM
Local signs:
- Erythematous, macular linear streaks from site of infection toward regional lymph nodes
- Tenderness and warmth over affected skin or lymph nodes
- Blistering of affected skin
- Fluctuance, swelling, or purulent drainage
- Nodular lymphangitis can present with subcutaneous swellings along the lymphatic channels.
- Sporotrichosis may present with papulonodular lesions that may ulcerate.
- Sites may be painless.

DIFFERENTIAL DIAGNOSIS
- Superficial thrombophlebitis
  - Thrombus or infection within the thrombosis (septic thrombophlebitis)
- Contact dermatitis
- Cellulitis
- Erysipelas
- Allergic reaction: less likely to be allergic if >24 hours after exposure (e.g., insect bite)
- Lymphangitis carcinomatosa
- Malignancy-related inflammation

DIAGNOSTIC TESTS & INTERPRETATION
- CBC may show leukocytosis; blood smear may show filarial infection.
- Blood or wound cultures
- Biopsy or aspiration cultures for nodular lymphangitis
- FNAC for filariasis of testiculoscrotal swelling but not for other superficial locations (4)

Initial Tests (lab, imaging)
Plain films are unnecessary; consider lymphangiography and lymphoscintigraphy for lymphedema (5)[C].

Diagnostic Procedures/Other
- Swab, aspirate, and/or biopsy primary site; purulent discharge; nodule or distal ulcer for culture; acid fast staining; histology; and microscopy
- Blood cultures if systemically ill
- Serology (e.g., *F. tularensis*, histoplasma)
- Blood film/smear (e.g., filaria)
- Lymphangiography or lymphoscintigraphy to determine lymphedema or lymphatic obstruction

TREATMENT

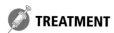

GENERAL MEASURES
- Hot, moist compresses to affected area
- Compression garments and weight loss may help lymphedema.
- Abstinence from sexual activity for sclerosing lymphangitis

MEDICATION
- Treat common organisms empirically. Use culture and susceptibility to guide antibiotic treatment.
- If mild disease, outpatient oral antibiotics
- If no improvement after 48 hours of oral antibiotics, reassess and consider IV antibiotics and/or hospitalization.
- IV antibiotics if systemically ill
- If necrotizing fasciitis is suspected, treat aggressively with antibiotics and surgical intervention.

First Line
Antibiotics for group A streptococcal infection
- Amoxicillin (if known group A *Streptococcus*)
  - Dosing
    - Adults
      - Mild to moderate: 500 mg PO q12h
      - Severe: 875 mg PO q12h or 500 mg PO q8h
    - Children <3 months: 30 mg/kg/day PO divided q12h

○ Children ≥3 months, ≤40 kg
- Mild to moderate: 25 mg/kg/day PO divided q12h or 20 mg/kg/day divided q8h
- Severe: 45 mg/kg/day PO divided q12h or 40 mg/kg/day divided q8h
○ Children ≥40 kg same as adult dosing
– Common adverse effects
○ Diarrhea
– Serious adverse effects
○ Anaphylaxis, Stevens-Johnson syndrome (SJS), toxic epidermal necrolysis (TEN)
– Drug interactions
○ Methotrexate, venlafaxine, warfarin, hormonal contraceptives
– Contraindications
○ Hypersensitivity to penicillin
• Ampicillin/sulbactam
– Dosing
○ Adults and children ≥40 kg: 1.5 to 3.0 g IV/IM q6h
○ Children <40 kg: 200 mg/kg/day IV infusion, in divided doses q6h; maximum 8 g ampicillin per day
– Common adverse effects
○ Diarrhea, injection site reactions
– Serious adverse effects
○ *Clostridium difficile* diarrhea, pseudomembranous enterocolitis
– Drug interactions
○ Hormonal contraceptives
– Contraindications
○ Hypersensitivity reactions
• Ceftriaxone
– Dosing
○ Adults: 1 to 2 g IV/IM q24h
○ Children: 50 to 75 mg/kg/day IV/IM once daily or in divided doses q12h; maximum 2 g/day
– Common adverse effects
○ Injection site reactions, diarrhea
– Serious adverse effects
○ Same as amoxicillin or ampicillin
– Drug interactions
○ Do not administer calcium-containing solutions in the same IV line.
– Contraindications
○ Hypersensitivity to cephalosporins
○ Concurrent calcium-containing IV fluids
○ Increased risk of kernicterus, salt precipitation in lungs and kidneys in neonates <28 days (use cefotaxime instead)
• Cephalexin
– Dosing
○ Adults: 500 mg PO q12h or up to q6h for severe infection or wider involvement
○ Children: 25 to 50 mg/kg/day divided q12h
– Common adverse effects
○ Diarrhea
– Serious adverse effects
○ SJS, TEN, interstitial nephritis, renal failure, pseudomembranous enterocolitis, anaphylaxis
– Contraindications
○ Hypersensitivity to cephalosporins

• Azithromycin (if penicillin or cephalosporin allergy)
– Dosing
○ Adults: 500 mg PO on day 1 followed by 250 mg/day PO on days 2 to 5
○ Children ≥2 years: 12 mg/kg/day PO (maximum dose: 500 mg/day) once daily for 5 days (FDA off-label use for skin infections in children)
– Common adverse effects
○ Abdominal pain, nausea, vomiting, diarrhea, headache
– Serious adverse effects
○ Prolonged QT interval, torsade de pointes, liver failure, Lambert-Eaton syndrome, myasthenia gravis, corneal erosion, anaphylaxis
– Drug interactions
○ Nelfinavir, warfarin, other medications with potential to prolong QT interval
– Contraindications
○ Hepatic dysfunction or cholestatic jaundice with prior treatment
○ Hypersensitivity to macrolide (azithromycin, erythromycin, clarithromycin)
• Diethylcarbamazine, ivermectin, albendazole, and doxycycline are used to treat filarial infection.
• Acetaminophen or ibuprofen (NSAIDs) for pain and fever

SURGERY/OTHER PROCEDURES
• Incision and drainage of abscess if present
• Necrotizing fasciitis requires surgical evaluation and likely débridement.
• Nodular lymphangitis may benefit from I&D.

ADMISSION, INPATIENT, AND NURSING CONSIDERATIONS
• Admit for signs of serious illness: fluids if in hypotensive shock.
• Fever, chills, systemic toxicity
• IV antibiotics, ICU, or surgery as indicated
• Discharge on oral antibiotics after systemic symptoms resolve. Home IV antibiotics are an option depending on clinical setting.

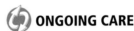 **ONGOING CARE**

FOLLOW-UP RECOMMENDATIONS
• Elevate affected area.
• 48-hour follow-up to ensure improvement
• Work up recurrent lymphangitis to ascertain underlying cause (other infectious organism, anatomic abnormality, etc.).

Patient Monitoring
Close follow-up to ensure decreasing inflammation

PATIENT EDUCATION
Instruct patients on proper wound and skin care.

PROGNOSIS
• Good prognosis for uncomplicated cases
• Antimicrobial therapy is effective in 90% of patients.
• Untreated, can spread rapidly, especially group A *Streptococcus*

COMPLICATIONS
Sepsis, cellulitis, necrotizing fasciitis, myositis

REFERENCES
1. Taylor MJ, Hoerauf A, Bockarie M. Lymphatic filariasis and onchocerciasis. *Lancet.* 2010;376(9747):1175–1185.
2. Prat L, Chouaid C, Kettaneh A, et al. Cutaneous lymphangitis carcinomatosa in a patient with lung adenocarcinoma: case report and literature review. *Lung Cancer.* 2013;79(1):91–93.
3. Kano Y, Momose T. Acute lymphangitis. *Cleve Clin J Med.* 2020;87(3):129–130.
4. Khare P, Kala P, Jha A, et al. Incidental diagnosis of filariasis in superficial location by FNAC: a retrospective study of 10 years. *J Clin Diagn Res.* 2014;8(12):FC05–FC08.
5. Falagas ME, Bliziotis IA, Kapaskelis AM. Red streaks on the leg. Lymphangitis. *Am Fam Physician.* 2006;73(6):1061–1062.

ADDITIONAL READING
• Babu AK, Krishnan P, Andezuth DD. Sclerosing lymphangitis of penis—literature review and report of 2 cases. *Dermatol Online J.* 2014;20(7): 13030/qt7gq9h1v9.
• Cohen BE, Nagler AR, Pomeranz MK. Nonbacterial causes of lymphangitis with streaking. *J Am Board Fam Med.* 2016;29(6):808–812.
• Raja A, Seshadri RA, Sundersingh S. Lymphangitis carcinomatosa: report of a case and review of literature. *Indian J Surg Oncol.* 2010;1(3):274–276.
• Tirado-Sánchez A, Bonifaz A. Nodular lymphangitis (sporotrichoid lymphocutaneous infections). Clues to differential diagnosis. *J Fungi (Basel).* 2018;4(2):56.

 CODES

ICD10
• I89.1 Lymphangitis
• L03.91 Acute lymphangitis, unspecified
• N48.29 Other inflammatory disorders of penis

CLINICAL PEARLS
• Lymphangitis classically presents with erythematous linear streaks of the skin from site of entry (e.g., bite, cut, abrasion) to regional lymph nodes.
• Patients with prior surgical lymph node dissection are predisposed to lymphangitis.
• Patients with severe systemic symptoms should be admitted for treatment with IV antibiotics.
• Parasitic or fungal infections can cause acute or chronic lymphangitis.
• Treatment of underlying skin infection (such as tinea pedis) may prevent recurrence.

L

LYMPHEDEMA
Khalid Bashir, MD

BASICS

DESCRIPTION
- Accumulation of lymphatic fluid in the interstitial tissue causing swelling
- Lymphedema can develop when lymphatic vessels are missing or impaired (primary) or when lymph vessels are damaged or lymph nodes are removed (secondary).
- Most common in the lower limb(s) (80%) but also can occur in the arm(s), face, trunk, and external genitalia

EPIDEMIOLOGY
Incidence
- Predominant sex: female > male
- 13% of patients with breast cancer treated with surgery; 42% of those treated with surgery and radiation therapy; 25% after GYN cancer surgery
- Milroy disease presents at birth; estimated to be between 1/6,000 and 1/300 live births
- Meige disease develops during puberty.

Prevalence
- 120 million people worldwide are affected with primary lymphatic filariasis.
- 10 million people are affected by nonfilarial secondary lymphedema in the United States.

ETIOLOGY AND PATHOPHYSIOLOGY
Secondary lymphedema:
- Postoperative: gradual failure of distal lymphatics, which have to "pump" lymph at a greater pressure through damaged proximal ducts
- Risk is higher with postoperative radiation because radiation reduces regrowth of ducts due to fibrous scarring.
- Trauma; recurrent infection; malignancy, including metastatic disease, and marked obesity
- Lymphangiogenesis inhibition and tissue fibrosis promotion by T cells appear to promote lymphedema.
- Developing countries: Most common cause is filariasis (*Wuchereria bancrofti*).

Genetics
- Milroy disease: autosomal dominant; diagnosed either at birth or the 1st year of life
- Lymphedema praecox has onset between the ages of 1 and 35 years.
- Lymphedema tarda occurs in those >35 years of age.
- Genetics referral: primary and lymphedema tarda

RISK FACTORS
- Filariasis: most common cause worldwide
- Lymphadenectomy or radiation therapy for malignancy (mastectomy, melanoma)
- Prior trauma, serious burns, infection of affected limb
- Obesity (>50 body mass index)
- Inflammatory disorders: arthritis, sarcoidosis, dermatitis

GENERAL PREVENTION
Healthy body weight; treatment of congestive heart failure, early recognition of infection and cancer, and venous insufficiency

COMMONLY ASSOCIATED CONDITIONS
Venous disease, morbid obesity, regional cancer, filarial disease (Africa and Asia)

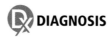

DIAGNOSIS

HISTORY
Recent surgery: Vein stripping can significantly exacerbate mild lymphedema.
- First symptom: painless swelling
- Feeling of heaviness in the limb, especially at the end of the day and in hot weather

PHYSICAL EXAM
- Initial: pitting edema; can spread proximally or distally
- Later: nonpitting; after 1st year, does not spread proximally/distally but spreads radially
- Hyperkeratosis (thicker skin)
- Papillomatosis (rough skin)
- Increase in skin turgor
- Positive Stemmer sign (inability to pinch the skin of the dorsum of the 2nd toe between the thumb and forefinger); false positives are rare.

DIFFERENTIAL DIAGNOSIS
- CHF, renal failure, lipedema
- Hypoalbuminemia, protein-losing nephropathy
- DVT, chronic venous disease
- Postoperative complications following ipsilateral surgery
- Cellulitis, Baker cyst, idiopathic edema

DIAGNOSTIC TESTS & INTERPRETATION
- Lack of response to elevation or diuretic therapy may indicate a lymphatic insufficiency.
- Diuretics increase excretion of salt and water, thereby decreasing plasma volume, venous capillary pressure, and filtration. Diuretics improve filtration edema but do not improve lymph drainage over the long term.
- Some relevant protein biomarkers for lymphedema have been identified and show promise for early- and latent-stage diagnosis.

Initial Tests (lab, imaging)
- Comprehensive chemistry panel: hepatic or renal impairment
- TSH: hypothyroidism
- Urinalysis: protein-losing nephropathy
- Ultrasound: evaluates for acute/chronic DVT; gives information about soft tissue changes but does not inform about truncal anatomy of the lymphatics
- Duplex ultrasound: Lymphedema causes gradual impedance of venous return that aggravates the edema; 82% of patients with unexplained limb edema were diagnosed using a combination of duplex ultrasound and lymphoscintigram.

Follow-Up Tests & Special Considerations
- Lymphangiogram: direct cannulation of lymphatics through the skin; risk for infection, local inflammation; rarely used now
- Fluorescence microlymphography may be highly sensitive (91.4%) and specific (85.7%), atraumatic, and is without radiation in diagnosis of leg lymphedema.
- Lymphoscintigram: radiolabeled protein technetium-99m–labeled colloid
  - Measures lymphatic function, lymph movement, lymph drainage, and response to treatment
  - Sensitivity, 73–97%; specificity, 100%
  - Best to use 1 hour and delayed images together
- Indocyanine green lymphography: reported
  - Superior to lymphoscintigraphy in early diagnosis of arm
  - Accurately screens postsurgically for subclinical lymphedema (1)[B]
- CT scan: calf skin thickening, thickening of the SC compartment, increased fat density, thickened perimuscular aponeurosis; typical honeycomb appearance
- MRI: circumferential edema, increased volume of SC tissue, honeycomb pattern above the fascia between the muscle and subcutis; cannot differentiate primary from secondary lymphedema

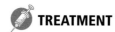

TREATMENT

GENERAL MEASURES
- Seek optimal weight; early treatment of cellulitis; avoid trauma to affected area (direct injury, venipunctures, inept nail care, extreme heat/cold).
- Achieve mechanical reduction and maintenance of limb size: compression garments via professionals.
- Elevate affected limb/area, but avoid stasis.
- Avoid BP cuffs and other focal constriction in affected limbs.
- Prevent skin infection with daily cleansing, inspection, and skin care (with emollients).
- Nonsurgical treatment of varicose veins in some
- Doubtful that air travel is associated with increased limb volumes

MEDICATION

> **ALERT**
> No medications, including diuretics, have been shown to be effective to treat lymphedema.

ISSUES FOR REFERRAL
- Refer to physical therapist with lymphedema training for manual decongestive therapy.
  - In patients with recurrent or metastatic disease, discuss with oncologist prior to initiation of complete decongestive therapy in order not to promote the spread of cancer.
- Provide education for patient/family for self-administration of therapy in future.
- Education for family about bandaging
- Fitting for compression garments (2)[A]

ADDITIONAL THERAPIES

- Exercise: Lymph flow occurs as a result of inspiratory reduction in the intrathoracic pressure associated with inspiration. Best results are achieved with combination of flexibility, strength, and aerobic training.
- Compression with custom-made elastic stocking (minimum pressure is 40 mm Hg)
  - Protection against external incidental trauma
  - Decreases the intrinsic trauma on the skin due to chronically increased interstitial pressures, which cause stretch of the skin and SC tissues
  - No data on preference of custom made versus prefabricated
  - Replace every 3 to 6 months or when starting to lose elasticity.
- Multilayer bandaging: inner layer of tubular stockinette followed by foam and padding to protect the joint flexures and to even out the contours of the limb so that pressure is distributed evenly; outer layer of at least two short-stretch extensible bandages; more effective than hosiery alone
- Pneumatic pumps develop high pressures like systolic BP and can reduce limb girth significantly; wear a compression sock afterward (2)[A].
- Advanced pneumatic compression devices (APCDs) are programmable, offer a more individualized fit, reduce rates of cellulitis by at least 75%, and reduce early treatment costs by 37–54% depending on health care setting (3)[B].

SURGERY/OTHER PROCEDURES

- Bypass procedures: Creation of lymphatic–venous anastomosis or lymph node transplantation (most effective) via microsurgery showed a reduction in use of conservative compression therapy (4)[C]; reserved for refractory cases only
- Low-level laser therapy in smaller studies was shown to be noninferior to manual lymphatic drainage or in combination in arm volume reduction among breast cancer patients in half the treatment time (4)[C].
- Axillary reverse mapping during axillary node dissection in selected preclinical breast cancer can significantly reduce lymphedema incidence (5)[A].
- Thoracic sympathetic ganglion block for breast cancer–related lymphedema, a new treatment showed better life quality and arm size reduction >50%, especially in patients with high-grade lymphedema.
- Debulking procedures (Charles procedure): radical excision of SC tissue with primary or staged skin grafting
  - Men had less improvement than women.
  - Main risk is infection and necrosis of the skin graft.
  - Liposuction is cosmetically preferred to debulking (4)[C].

ADMISSION, INPATIENT, AND NURSING CONSIDERATIONS

- Systemic signs of infection
  - May admit to specialized rehabilitation unit for combination treatment in patients with heart failure or severe pulmonary disease
  - IV antibiotics for infection; cellulitis is most common.
- Affected extremity positioning with some distal elevation
- Encourage patient mobilization/exercise.
- Patient education for bandaging/wound care
- Discharge criteria
  - Improved signs/symptoms of infection (e.g., elevated WBC count, fever, abnormal vital signs)
  - Clinical improvement in wound appearance

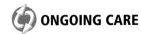 ONGOING CARE

FOLLOW-UP RECOMMENDATIONS

Lymphedema will return in several days if patient stops wearing compression garments during the day and bandaging at night.

Patient Monitoring

- Daily visit to therapist for acute treatment
- Monthly visits for maintenance care

DIET

Lower sodium, healthy protein, and weight loss-oriented (if needed)

PATIENT EDUCATION

- Use compression garments, especially when exercising.
- Avoid affected limb(s) being dependent for long periods of time: Patient should perform daily skin examination.
- http://www.nlm.nih.gov/medlineplus/lymphedema.html

PROGNOSIS

No cure, but treatment can produce good results with daily care.

COMPLICATIONS

- Infection (local vs. systemic): common
- Risk of wound formation (punctures/abrasions) that are difficult to heal: common
- Lymphangiosarcoma: found in lymphedematous arms of patients following radical mastectomy, also in patients with Milroy disease. Treatment is radiotherapy with surgery; reserved for patients with discrete nonmetastatic disease

REFERENCES

1. Keo HH, Husmann M, Groechenig E, et al. Diagnostic accuracy of fluorescence microlymphography for detecting limb lymphedema. *Eur J Vasc Endovasc Surg.* 2015;49(4):474–479.
2. Rogan S, Taeymans J, Luginbuehl H, et al. Therapy modalities to reduce lymphoedema in female breast cancer patients: a systematic review and meta-analysis. *Breast Cancer Res Treat.* 2016;159(1):1–14.
3. Karaca-Mandic P, Hirsch AT, Rockson SG, et al. The cutaneous, net clinical, and health economic benefits of advanced pneumatic compression devices in patients with lymphedema. *JAMA Dermatol.* 2015;151(11):1187–1193.
4. Merchant SJ, Chen SL. Prevention and management of lymphedema after breast cancer treatment. *Breast J.* 2015;21(3):276–284.
5. Han C, Yang B, Zuo W-S, et al. The feasibility and oncological safety of axillary reverse mapping in patients with breast cancer: a systematic review and meta-analysis of prospective studies. *PLoS One.* 2016;11(2):e0150285.

ADDITIONAL READING

Choi E, Nahm FS, Lee PB. Sympathetic block as a new treatment for lymphedema. *Pain Physician.* 2015;18(4):365–372.

 CODES

ICD10

- I89.0 Lymphedema, not elsewhere classified
- I97.2 Postmastectomy lymphedema syndrome
- Q82.0 Hereditary lymphedema

CLINICAL PEARLS

- Affected skin has a heavy feeling, with painless swelling initially, later nonpitting swelling.
- No medications, including diuretics, are useful.
- Rule out DVT if unilateral limb or CHF if bilateral.
- Early referral to lymphedema therapist for manual therapy, compression devices/wrappings
- Aggressive weight loss and health promotion as needed
- High risk for cutaneous-sourced infections, so promote therapeutic skin care.
- Lymphoscintigram is standard diagnostic if clinically diagnosis is uncertain and refer primary lymphedema and lymphedema tarda to genetics.

L

MACULAR DEGENERATION, AGE-RELATED

Richard W. Allinson, MD • Alyce D. Alven, OD, MS

BASICS

DESCRIPTION
- Age-related macular degeneration (AMD) is the leading cause of irreversible, severe visual loss in persons age >65 years.
- AMD can be classified as:
  - Atrophic/nonexudative, such as drusen or macular pigmentary changes
  - Neovascular/exudative or neovascular age-related macular degeneration (nAMD)

EPIDEMIOLOGY
- nAMD form is rare in blacks and more common in whites.
- Predominant sex: female

Incidence
- In the Framingham Eye Study (FES), drusen were noted in 25% of all participants who were ≥52 years of age. AMD-associated visual loss was noted in 5.7%.
- Atrophic/nonexudative stage accounts for 20% of cases of severe visual loss.
- nAMD stage accounts for 80% of cases of severe visual loss.

Prevalence
Per FES study:
- People 65 to 74 years old: 11%
- People ≥75 years old: 27.9%

ETIOLOGY AND PATHOPHYSIOLOGY
- Atrophic/nonexudative
  - Drusen and/or pigmentary changes in the macula. Drusen are deposits of hyaline material between the RPE and Bruch's membrane (the limiting membrane between the RPE and the choroid).
  - Visible light can result in the formation and accumulation of metabolic by-products in the retinal pigment epithelium (RPE), a pigment layer underneath the retina that normally helps remove metabolic by-products from the retina. Excess accumulation of these metabolic by-products interferes with the normal metabolic activity of the RPE and can lead to the formation of drusen.
  - Most do not progress beyond the atrophic/nonexudative stage; however, those who do are at a greater risk for severe visual loss.
- nAMD
  - nAMD stage generally arises from the atrophic stage.
    - In type 1 neovascularization, breaks in Bruch's membrane allow choroidal neovascular membranes (CNVMs) to grow into the sub-RPE space. This corresponds to occult CNVMs. Fluid leakage and bleeding can produce a vascularized serous or fibrovascular RPE detachment.
    - In type 2 neovascularization, the CNVM passes through the RPE and is located in the subretinal space. Typically appears as a lacy or gray-green lesion. This corresponds to classic CNVM.
    - Type 3 neovascularization, also known as retinal angiomatous proliferations (RAPS), the neovascularization develops from the deep capillary plexus of the retina and grows downward toward the RPE.

- Polypoidal choroidal vasculopathy (PCV) is a subtype of nAMD and often presents with multiple, recurrent serosanguineous RPE detachments. An RPE detachment is also known as a pigment epithelial detachment (PED). Optical coherence tomography (OCT) features of PCV include multiple PEDs, sharply peaked PED, notched or multilobulated PED, and a hyperreflective ring surrounding an internal hyporeflective lumen beneath a PED.

Genetics
- Genetic susceptibility may be a factor in AMD: ~25% genetically determined.
- Complement factor H Y402H genotype is an important susceptibility gene for AMD.
- Although the development of AMD may be predicted by specific alleles, the clinical response to anti–vascular endothelial growth factor (anti-VEGF) is not.

RISK FACTORS
- Obesity
- Cigarette smoking
- *Chlamydia pneumoniae* infection
- Family history
- Excess sunlight exposure
- Blue or light iris color
- Hyperopia
- Short stature
- High plasma high-density lipoprotein cholesterol levels are associated with an increased risk for AMD.
- Physical activity is associated with lower risk of early and late AMD in white populations.

GENERAL PREVENTION
- Ultraviolet (UV) protection for eyes
- Routine ophthalmologic visits
  - Every 2 to 4 years for patients age 40 to 64 years
  - Every 1 to 2 years after age 65 years

DIAGNOSIS

HISTORY
Patients frequently notice distortion of central vision. On Amsler grid testing, the horizontal or vertical lines may become broken, distorted, or missing.

PHYSICAL EXAM
- Atrophic/nonexudative stage
  - Drusen (small yellowish white lesions)
    - Subtypes: hard drusen and soft drusen
  - Atrophy of the RPE
    - When the area of absent or attenuated RPE is contiguous, the condition is termed geographic atrophy (GA) of the RPE.
- nAMD
  - Blood vessels growing underneath the retina from the choroid are called CNVMs or subretinal neovascularization (SRN). The choroid is the vascular layer underneath the RPE.
  - Subretinal fluid or hemorrhage
  - Exudates
- Disciform scar: an advanced stage resulting in a fibrovascular scar

DIFFERENTIAL DIAGNOSIS
- Idiopathic SRN
- Presumed ocular histoplasmosis syndrome
- Diabetic or hypertensive retinopathy
- Central serous chorioretinopathy
- Topiramate can cause a macular neurosensory retinal detachment.

DIAGNOSTIC TESTS & INTERPRETATION
Diagnostic Procedures/Other
- Fluorescein angiography (FA): differentiates between atrophic and nAMD
- Indocyanine green video angiography: may identify occult or hidden CNVMs
- OCT: useful in determining the presence of subretinal fluid, the degree of retinal thickening, and the presence of a PED. Newer generation OCT modalities, including spectral-domain OCT (SD-OCT), swept-source OCT (SS-OCT), and OCT angiography (OCTA), are preferred for evaluating AMD.
  - OCTA-visualized anatomic subtypes of neovascularization include type 1 (sub-RPE), type 2 (subretinal), and type 3 (intraretinal vascular proliferation).

TREATMENT

GENERAL MEASURES
Low-vision aids may be helpful.

MEDICATION
First Line
- Ranibizumab (Lucentis)
  - Antibody fragment that inhibits all active forms of VEGF
  - Injected intravitreally, at a dose of 0.5 mg, every 4 weeks
  - 1 year after treatment, up to 40% of patients treated with ranibizumab gained at least three lines of vision, and ~95% maintained vision.
  - The PrONTO study demonstrated OCT-guided, variable-dosing regimen with ranibizumab resulted in similar results to the MARINA (minimally classic/occult CNVM trial) and ANCHOR (predominantly classic CNVM trial) studies with monthly injections of ranibizumab.
  - When comparing ranibizumab and bevacizumab in a multicenter study, both treatments were effective in stabilizing visual loss, and no difference was found in the visual outcome between the two treatment groups.
    - In this study, treatment as needed resulted in less gain in visual acuity, whether instituted at enrollment or after 1 year of monthly treatment.
    - Visual gains during the first 2 years were not maintained at 5 years. At the 5-year visit, 50% of eyes had vision of 20/40 or better and 20% had vision of 20/200 or worse.
  - Eyes with ≥50% of the lesion composed of blood had a similar visual prognosis compared to other treated eyes in the Comparison of Age-related Macular Degeneration Treatments Trials (CATT). nAMD lesions composed of >50% blood can be managed similarly to those with less or no blood.
  - The treat and extend regimen (TER) is commonly used to decrease the treatment burden. Once no signs of CNVM activity are detected, patient follow-ups and treatments are then extended by intervals of 2 weeks as long as no signs of CNVM activity are present, up to a maximum interval of 12 weeks. If examination shows any sign of recurrence, the interval is shortened by 2 weeks at a time, until the disease is considered to be inactive. Interval extension is then restarted, with the maximum final interval being 2 weeks less than the period when the previous recurrence was observed.

- Aflibercept (Eylea)
  - A VEGF receptor decoy that binds both VEGF and placental-like growth factor
  - Injected intravitreally, at a dose of 2 mg, every 4 weeks for 12 weeks and then every 8 weeks
  - Dosed as needed after the 12-week fixed dosing schedule resulted in a 5.3-letter gain in best corrected visual acuity at 52 weeks.
  - Routine use of prophylactic antibiotics after intravitreal injections (IVIs) may be unnecessary.
  - May be beneficial in patients who are not responding to ranibizumab or bevacizumab.
  - Anti-VEGF treatment with either ranibizumab or aflibercept has limited efficacy for the complete resolution of PEDs.
    - Patients with a PED tend to have worse outcomes when switched from a fixed regimen to a PRN strategy.
  - Brolucizumab (Beovu)
    - It is a humanized single-chain antibody fragment that inhibits all isoforms of VEGF-A. It is the smallest of the anti-VEGF antibodies.
    - Injected intravitreally, at a dose of 6 mg monthly for the first 3 doses, followed by one dose every 8 to 12 weeks.
    - A 12-week treatment cycle may be a viable option, which would help reduce the frequency of IVIs. Greater than 50% of brolucizumab-treated eyes were maintained on q12wk dosing.
    - There have been some reports of retinal vasculitis and/or retinal vascular occlusion after Beovu was approved by the FDA. There have been cases reported with severe visual loss with brolucizumab treatment.

Second Line
- Bevacizumab (Avastin) is a full-length antibody to VEGF, administered intravitreally at a dose of 1.25 mg; widely used off-label because of its lower cost
- Faricimab neutralizes angiopoietin-2 and vascular endothelial growth factor A. It has the potential advantage of being administered every 16 weeks. It is being investigated for the treatment of nAMD.
- Avacincaptad pegol is an inhibitor of complement C5. Complement is believed to play an important role in retinal degeneration secondary to AMD. Avacincaptad pegol is being investigated for the treatment of GA.
- No FDA-approved stem cell therapies for AMD exist.

SURGERY/OTHER PROCEDURES
- Laser treatment for CNVMs located ≥200 microns from the center of the macula have been evaluated in the Macular Photocoagulation Study (MPS).
  - Anti-VEGF treatment is first-line therapy for subfoveal CNVMs.
- Vitrectomy has been used to remove CNVMs, but this is generally not recommended.
- CNVMs can bleed spontaneously, leaving blood underneath the retina. Vitrectomy to remove subretinal blood may be of benefit and should be performed within 7 days of the bleed. Tissue plasminogen activator (tPA) instilled into the eye may help remove a subretinal hemorrhage. In some cases, intravitreal gas with or without tPA may displace submacular blood.
  - Intravitreal anti-VEGF monotherapy may be helpful in the treatment of nAMD associated with a submacular hemorrhage.

- Photodynamic therapy (PDT) with verteporfin is not frequently used anymore.
  - Patients should be informed of a <4% risk of acute, severe vision loss after PDT.
  - Ranibizumab has greater clinical efficacy than PDT.
  - Combination treatment with intravitreal ranibizumab and PDT appears to offer similar gain in visual acuity when compared with ranibizumab monotherapy.

COMPLEMENTARY & ALTERNATIVE MEDICINE
Free radical formation in the retina, induced by visible light, may play a role in cellular damage that results in atrophic/nonexudative macular degeneration. The Age-Related Eye Disease Study (AREDS) found that a high-dose regimen of antioxidant vitamins and mineral supplements reduced progression of AMD in some cases.
- Recommended daily doses: vitamin C 500 mg, vitamin E 400 IU, β-carotene 15 mg, zinc oxide 80 mg, and cupric oxide 2 mg
  - Exercise caution with β-carotene use in smokers due to potential link to lung cancer.
- The AREDS2 found the addition of lutein with zeaxanthin alone or in combination with omega-3 fatty acids had no overall effect in further reducing the risk of progression to advanced AMD. The recommended daily doses: vitamin C 500 mg, vitamin E 400 IU, lutein 10 mg, zeaxanthin 2 mg, zinc 80 mg

 ONGOING CARE

FOLLOW-UP RECOMMENDATIONS
Patient Monitoring
- Amsler grid can aid in discovering visual disturbances.
- Patients with soft drusen or pigmentary changes in the macula are at an increased risk of visual loss. They should monitor their vision, by doing daily Amsler grid testing, and by following subjective measures of visual acuity, such as reading ability; if no new symptoms, follow-up examination in 6 to 12 months

DIET
- Eating dark green, leafy vegetables (spinach/collard greens), which are rich in carotenoids, may decrease the risk of developing the nAMD.
- Fish consumption with omega-3 fatty acid intake may reduce the risk of AMD.
- A Western-type diet characterized by higher intake of red meat, processed meat, high-fat dairy products, fried foods, refined grains, and eggs increases the risk of AMD as compared to an Oriental-type diet characterized by higher intake of vegetables, legumes, fruit, whole grains, tomatoes, and seafood which decreases the risk of AMD.
  - A Mediterranean-type diet may reduce the risk of developing AMD. A Mediterranean-type diet was associated with lower risk of progression to late AMD, particularly GA, and to large drusen (1)[A].

PROGNOSIS
- Patients with bilateral soft drusen and pigmentary changes in the macula, but no evidence of exudation, have an increased likelihood of developing nAMD and subsequent visual loss.
- Patients with bilateral drusen carry a cumulative risk of 14.7% over 5 years of suffering significant visual loss in one eye from nAMD.
- Patients with nAMD in one eye and drusen in the opposite eye are at an annual risk of 5–14% of developing nAMD in the opposite eye with drusen.

- Macular atrophy progression and severity were the primary anatomic determinants of visual outcomes 7 years after treatment with ranibizumab. Macular atrophy can occur in eyes treated with anti-VEGF therapy.
- Attainment of good vision by the fourth injection of a VEGF inhibitor was strongly associated with 3-year visual outcomes (2)[B].
- Patients with nAMD with stable preoperative fluid on OCT generally do not have worsening of their nAMD after cataract surgery.
- Aspirin use is not significantly associated with progression to late AMD. When aspirin is medically indicated, patients with AMD do not need to avoid taking it (3)[A].
- Anti-VEGF treatment for nAMD was associated with preserved useful vision in almost 20% of patients over their average remaining lifetime (4)[B].

COMPLICATIONS
- Blindness
- The intraocular pressure should be monitored in eyes receiving intravitreal anti-VEGF injections.
  - Seven or more IVIs annually is associated with a higher risk of glaucoma surgery compared to less frequent administration.

REFERENCES
1. Keenan TD, Argon E, Mares J, et al. Adherence to the Mediterranean diet and progression to late age-related macular degeneration in the Age-Related Eye Disease Studies 1 and 2. *Ophthalmology*. 2020;127(11):1515–1528.
2. Nguyen V, Daien V, Guymer R, et al. Projection of long-term visual acuity outcomes based on initial treatment response in neovascular age-related macular degeneration. *Ophthalmology*. 2019;126(1):64–74.
3. Keenan TD, Wiley HE, Argrón E, et al. The association of aspirin use with age-related macular degeneration progression in the Age-Related Eye Disease Studies: Age-Related Eye Disease Study 2 Report No. 20. *Ophthalmology*. 2019;126(12):1647–1656.
4. Finger RP, Puth M-T, Schmid M, et al. Lifetime outcomes of anti-vascular endothelial growth factor treatment for neovascular age-related macular degeneration. *JAMA Ophthalmol*. 2020;138(12):1234–1240.

ADDITIONAL READING
Starr MR, Mahr MA, Barkmeier AJ, et al. Outcomes of cataract surgery in patients with exudative age-related macular degeneration and macular fluid. *Am J Ophthalmol*. 2018;192:91–97.

CODES

ICD10
- H35.32 Exudative age-related macular degeneration
- H35.31 Nonexudative age-related macular degeneration
- H35.3290 Exudative age-related macular degeneration, unspecified eye, stage unspecified

CLINICAL PEARLS
- Patients may notice straight lines appear crooked (e.g., telephone poles).
- The ARED Study found that a high-dose regimen of antioxidant vitamins and mineral supplements reduces progression of AMD in some cases.

M

MALARIA
Kathrine R. Tan, MD, MPH • Francisca Abanyie-Bimbo, MD, MPH

 BASICS

DESCRIPTION
- Potentially deadly infection with *Plasmodium* species protozoa, transmitted to humans by *Anopheles* mosquitoes
- System(s) affected: cardiovascular, hematologic, renal, respiratory, cerebral, lymphatic, immunologic, hepatic

EPIDEMIOLOGY
- Cases imported to the United States: 79% *Plasmodium falciparum*; 11% *Plasmodium vivax*; 6% *Plasmodium ovale*; 3% *Plasmodium malariae*
- About 229 million cases annually worldwide; with ~400,000 deaths/year (primarily children in sub-Saharan Africa)
- Most prevalent in rural tropics

Incidence
~2,000 cases (>99% are imported) and 7 deaths per year in the United States

Prevalence
- Predominant age: all ages
- Predominant sex: male = female

ETIOLOGY AND PATHOPHYSIOLOGY
- Plasmodia are transmitted via saliva from an infected Anopheles mosquito to the human during a blood meal. Circulating plasmodia enter red blood cells (RBC), digest RBC proteins and alter the RBC membrane, causing hemolysis, increased splenic clearance, and anemia.
- RBC lysis stimulates release of cytokines and TNF-α causing fever and systemic symptoms.
- *P. falciparum* alters RBC viscosity, causing obstruction and end-organ ischemia.

Genetics
Inherited conditions may affect disease severity and susceptibility (e.g., sickle cell disease or trait)

RISK FACTORS
- Travel to or migration from endemic areas
- In nonendemic areas, rarely: blood transfusion, congenital transmission, and autochthonous transmission

GENERAL PREVENTION
- Mosquito avoidance: Use insect repellent, wear clothing to cover exposed skin, use mosquito nets treated with insecticides such as permethrin, and avoid outdoor activity from dusk to dawn, when feeding activity of Anopheles mosquito is the greatest.
- *Malarial chemoprophylaxis in endemic areas*
  - Atovaquone/proguanil: Begin 1 to 2 days before arrival, take daily until 1 week after leaving area. Adults, 1 adult tablet QD; children 5 to 8 kg, 1/2 pediatric tablet QD; children 9 to 10 kg, 3/4 pediatric tablet QD; children >10 to 20 kg, 1 pediatric tablet QD; children >20 to 30 kg, 2 pediatric tablets QD; children >30 to 40 kg, 3 pediatric tablets QD; children >40 kg, 1 adult tablet QD
    ○ Contraindicated in pregnant women and infants <5 kg
  - Chloroquine: Begin 1 to 2 weeks before arrival, take weekly until 4 weeks after leaving area. Adults, 500-mg salt (300-mg base) weekly; children, 8.3 mg/kg salt (5 mg/kg base) weekly up to 500-mg salt
    ○ Caution: can make psoriasis worse

- Doxycycline: Begin 1 to 2 d before arrival, take daily until 4 weeks after leaving area. Adults, 100 mg QD; children >8 years old, 2 mg/kg up to 100 mg QD
  ○ Caution: Don't use in pregnant women and children ≤8 years old.
- Hydroxychloroquine: Begin 1 to 2 weeks before arrival, take weekly until 4 weeks after leaving area. Adults, 400-mg salt (310-mg base)/week; children, 6.5 mg/kg salt (5-mg base/kg)/week up to 400-mg salt
- Mefloquine: Begin at least 2 weeks before arrival, take weekly until 4 weeks after leaving area. Adults, 250 mg (1 tablet) weekly; children ≤9 kg, 5 mg/kg weekly; children >9 to 19 kg, 1/4 tablet weekly; children >19 to 30 kg, 1/2 tablet weekly; children >30 to 45 kg, 3/4 tablet weekly; children >45 kg, 1 tablet weekly
  ○ Caution: mefloquine-resistant areas; don't use if history of psychiatric disorders.
- Primaquine: Begin 1 to 2 d before arrival, take daily until 1 week after leaving area; adults, 30 mg QD; children, 0.5 mg/kg/day up to adult dose
  ○ Use only in areas endemic for *P. vivax*
  ○ Caution: Exclude G6PD deficiency prior to first use; don't use in pregnant women or breast-feeding women if infant hasn't been tested for G6PD deficiency.
- Tafenoquine: Begin 3 days before arrival, take daily until 1 week after leaving area; adults 200 mg QD
  ○ Caution: Exclude G6PD deficiency prior to first use; don't use if history of psychiatric disorders; don't use in children or in pregnant or breast-feeding women.

COMMONLY ASSOCIATED CONDITIONS
- Bacterial coinfections sometimes occur.
- Sickle cell trait confers an element of protection.

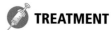 **DIAGNOSIS**

HISTORY
- Initial symptoms are nonspecific. Suspect malaria in ill patients returning from endemic area with:
  - Fever, malaise, myalgias, chills, headache, nausea, splenomegaly (chronic infection), hypotension, anemia, thrombocytopenia, jaundice, vomiting, and/or diarrhea
- *P. falciparum*
  - Incubation period 7 to 14 days, symptoms usually within 1 month of infection (Partially immune individuals may become ill up to 1 year after last exposure.)
  - Severe disease and complications: vascular collapse, central nervous system impairment, renal failure, and acute respiratory distress syndrome
- *P. vivax* and *P. ovale*
  - Incubation period 9 to 18 d for primary infection; up to 12 months or longer for relapses
- *P. malariae*
  - Incubation period 18 to 40 days
  - Case reports of asymptomatic persistence in untreated individuals
- *P. knowlesi*
  - Incubation period 9 to 12 days

PHYSICAL EXAM
- Often not specific
- General: elevated temperature, fatigue, tachycardia, tachypnea, jaundice

- Neurologic: change in mental status and motor-sensory findings (cerebral malaria)
- Cardiopulmonary exam: hemodynamic instability and signs of vascular leak (effusion; pulmonary edema)
- Skin exam: pallor, rash
- Abdominal exam: organomegaly

DIFFERENTIAL DIAGNOSIS
- Infections (disseminated or localized): abscess, viral, gastroenteritis, typhoid/paratyphoid, other bacteremias, rickettsial disease, mycobacteria
- Collagen vascular disease
- Neoplasms (lymphoma, leukemia, other blood dyscrasias, other tropical causes of splenomegaly)
- Severe malaria infection may mimic hepatitis, pneumonia, meningitis, stroke, or sepsis

DIAGNOSTIC TESTS & INTERPRETATION
- Malaria microscopy, thick and thin blood smears (1)[A]
  - Thick smear used to determine presence of parasite (rings, trophozoites, schizonts)
  - Thin smear used to determine species and quantify the percentage of infected RBCs
- Rapid antigen testing: can detect the presence of malaria parasites within minutes
- Other tests: PCR for species confirmation
- General laboratory findings (nonspecific)
  - Thrombocytopenia, anemia, and leukopenia
  - Elevated liver function tests and LDH
- Note: Low to low-normal platelet count or slightly high bilirubin after travel to endemic area should increase suspicion for malaria.

Initial Tests (lab, imaging)
- Complete blood count with differential
- Basic chemistry panel, including bilirubin
- Malaria thick and thin blood films (If negative, repeat q12–24h for at least three sets.)
- Imaging necessary only for respiratory disease (chest x-ray) or cerebral malaria (CT scan prior to lumbar puncture)

Follow-Up Tests & Special Considerations
Request diagnostic confirmation, speciation, and drug resistance testing from CDC.

Test Interpretation
- Microscopy: confirms diagnosis including species of plasmodium and quantifies percentage of red cells infected
- Rapid diagnostic test: preliminary determination. Perform smears to confirm results, determine species, and quantify percentage of red cells infected.

 TREATMENT

MEDICATION
First Line
- Oral therapy for uncomplicated chloroquine-resistant *P. falciparum* (most *P. falciparum*), chloroquine-resistant *P. vivax*, or unknown species:
  - Artemether-lumefantrine (Coartem): Tablet (tab) contains 20-mg artemether and 120-mg lumefantrine. 6 doses over 3 days. On day 1, the initial dose and then second dose 8 hours later. On days 2 and 3, BID. Persons 5 to <15 kg: 1 tablet per dose; persons 15 to <25 kg: 2 tablets per dose;

persons 25 to <35 kg: 3 tablets per dose; persons ≥35 kg: 4 tablets per dose (Call 1-855-COARTEM to locate pharmacy with stock.)
- Caution: not recommended in infants <5 kg or in pregnant women in 1st trimester
– Atovaquone-proguanil (Malarone): adult tablet: 250-mg atovaquone and 100-mg proguanil. Pediatric tablet: 62.5-mg atovaquone and 25-mg proguanil. Adults: 4 adult tablets QD for 3 days. Children 5 to 8 kg: 2 pediatric tablets QD for 3 days; children >8 to 10 kg: 3 pediatric tablets QD for 3 days; children >10 to 20 kg: 1 adult tablet QD for 3 days; children >20 to 30 kg: 2 adult tablets QD for 3 days; children >30 to 40 kg: 3 adult tablets QD for 3 days; children >40 kg: 4 adult tablets QD for 3 days
  - Caution: not recommended in pregnant women and infants <5 kg
– Quinine sulfate plus doxycycline or for those unable to take doxycycline, clindamycin: adults: quinine sulfate 650 mg (salt) TID for 3 days (extend to 7 days for infections from Southeast Asia). Doxycycline 100 mg BID for 7 days. Clindamycin 20 mg (base)/kg/day divided TID for 7 days; children: quinine sulfate 10 mg (salt)/kg TID for 3 days (extend to 7 days for infections from Southeast Asia) plus doxycycline 2.2 mg/kg BID for 7 days if ≥8 years old, or clindamycin dosed as above if <8 years old
  - Caution: doxycycline not recommended in pregnant women and children ≤8 years old
– Mefloquine: adults: 750 mg, then 500 mg 8 hours later; children: 15 mg/kg, then 10 mg/kg 8 hours later (max total dose: 1,250 mg)
  - Caution: not recommended in infections from SE Asia due to drug resistance or in patients with neuropsychiatric history
- Oral therapy for uncomplicated chloroquine-sensitive *P. vivax*, *P. ovale*, *P. malariae*, and chloroquine-sensitive *P. falciparum* (rare); in addition to the treatment regimens listed above, other options include:
– Chloroquine: adults: 1 g (600-mg base), then 500 mg (300-mg base) at 6, 24, and 48 hours after first dose; children: 16.7 mg/kg (10-mg base/kg) on day 1 (max 1,000 mg [600-mg base]) and then 8.3 mg/kg (5 mg/kg base) at 6, 24, and 48 hours after first dose
  - Caution: can make psoriasis worse
– Hydroxychloroquine sulfate: adult: 800-mg salt (620-mg base), then 400-mg salt (310-mg base) at 6, 24, and 48 hours after first dose; children: 13 mg/kg salt (10 mg base/kg), then 6.5 mg/kg salt (5 mg base/kg) at 6, 24, and 48 hours after first dose
  - Caution: can make psoriasis worse
– For *P. vivax* or *P. ovale*, add primaquine or tafenoquine to treat dormant parasites. Tafenoquine must be coadministered with chloroquine or hydroxychloroquine:
  - Primaquine: adults: 30-mg base (52.6-mg salt) QD for 2 weeks; children: 0.6 mg base/kg/day for 2 weeks
    - Caution: Exclude G6PD prior to first use; do not use in pregnant women.

- Tafenoquine: patients age ≥16; 300 mg single dose
  - Caution: Exclude G6PD deficiency prior to first use; do not use in pregnant or breast-feeding women.
- Parenteral therapy required for severe malaria
– Criteria for severe malaria (at least one):
  - Parasitemia ≥5%, impaired level of consciousness (LOC), repeated convulsions, respiratory distress, shock, renal failure, severe anemia (Hb <7), acidosis, disseminated intravascular coagulation, jaundice
– Intravenous artesunate (IVAS): 2.4 mg/kg per dose. Dose at 0, 12, and 24 hours. Reassess parasite density, and continue once daily dose until parasite density is ≤1%, then give a full oral regimen as described above for uncomplicated chloroquine-resistant *P. falciparum*.
– IVAS is commercially available. If not locally available within 24 hours, contact CDC to request artesunate: 770-488-7100; http://www.cdc.gov/Malaria/.

ISSUES FOR REFERRAL
Infectious disease or tropical medicine consultation. Report https://www.cdc.gov/malaria/report.html.

ADDITIONAL THERAPIES
None

Pediatric Considerations
- Children are susceptible to severe disease and are prone to hypoglycemia. Use IV fluids with glucose for maintenance.
- All children and infants should receive chemoprophylaxis if traveling to endemic area.
- Can resemble acute gastroenteritis.

Pregnancy Considerations
- Artesunate, chloroquine, mefloquine, quinine, and clindamycin: safe at recommended doses
- Coartem: safe in 2nd and 3rd trimesters at recommended doses; some evidence of safety in 1st trimester
- Malarone: limited evidence of safety
- Do not use primaquine, tafenoquine, or tetracyclines in pregnant or lactating women.

SURGERY/OTHER PROCEDURES
Rarely, splenectomy with splenic rupture

ADMISSION, INPATIENT, AND NURSING CONSIDERATIONS
- Inpatient care for all cases of *P. falciparum* malaria or signs of severe illness, regardless of species; outpatient care for others
- Follow up all treated as outpatient within 24 hours.
- Observe for fluid excess, renal insufficiency, and hypoglycemia.
- Add glucose to maintenance IV fluids.
- Discharge criteria: clinical improvement with documented decreasing parasite levels

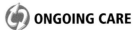 **ONGOING CARE**

PATIENT EDUCATION
- Malaria chemoprophylaxis prior to travel
- Travel information: http://www.cdc.gov/travel

PROGNOSIS
Malaria infection (particularly *P. falciparum*) can be deadly. If diagnosed early and treated appropriately, the prognosis is excellent.

COMPLICATIONS
- If not treated early: cerebral malaria, acute renal failure, respiratory distress syndrome, disseminated intravascular coagulation, and hemolysis and anemia
- Other complications: seizures, anuria, delirium, coma, dysentery, hyperpyrexia
- *P. malariae*: Nephrotic syndrome may develop in patients with chronic infection

REFERENCE
1. Centers for Disease Control and Prevention. Malaria diagnosis & treatment in the United States. https://www.cdc.gov/malaria/diagnosis_treatment/index.html. Accessed October 5, 2021.

ADDITIONAL READING
- Bonam SR, Rénia L, Tadepalli G, et al. *Plasmodium falciparum* malaria vaccines and vaccine adjuvants. *Vaccines (Basel)*. 2021;9(10):1072.
- Forgie EME, Brooks HM, Barton M, et al. Pediatric malaria: global and north american perspectives. *Pediatr Clin North Am*. 2022;69(1):47–64.
- Mace KE, Lucchi NW, Tan KR. Malaria surveillance—United States, 2017. *MMWR Surveill Summ*. 2020;70(SS-2):1–35.
- Milner DA Jr. Malaria pathogenesis. *Cold Spring Harb Perspect Med*. 2018;8(1):a025569.

 CODES

ICD10
- B51.9 Plasmodium vivax malaria without complication
- B50.9 Plasmodium falciparum malaria, unspecified
- B52 Plasmodium malariae malaria

CLINICAL PEARLS
- Consult CDC guidance for appropriate chemoprophylactic agent when traveling to endemic areas.
- Test for malaria in travelers returning from endemic areas who present with fever or flulike illness.
- Timely diagnosis and treatment of persons with malaria is key to good outcomes.
- Treat malaria patients with a different medication than what was used for chemoprophylaxis.
- *P. falciparum* malaria can be rapidly fatal; inpatient treatment is recommended.

M

MARIJUANA (CANNABIS) USE DISORDER

Jason Edward Lambrecht, MD, FHM, FACP, PharmD • Paul G. Millner, MD

 BASICS

DESCRIPTION
- Marijuana use leading to clinically significant impairment or distress, manifested by two or more of the following symptoms within a 12-month period:
  - Consumption of larger amounts over a longer period of time than intended
  - Persistent desire or inability to cut down or control amount used
  - Inordinate amount of time spent in activities is necessary to obtain, use, or recover from use
  - Presence of craving for cannabis
  - Recurrent use resulting in failure to fulfill major role obligations at work, school, or home
  - Continued use despite having persistent or recurrent social or interpersonal problems due to cannabis use
  - Important social, occupational, or recreational activities are given up or reduced
  - Recurrent use in physically hazardous situations
  - Continued use despite knowledge of a persistent physical or psychological problem caused or exacerbated by cannabis
  - Tolerance defined by using increased amounts of cannabis to achieve the desired effect or intoxication or diminished effect with continued use of the same amount
  - Withdrawal occurs following cessation of prolonged use and has at least three behavioral symptoms such as anxiety, restlessness, depression, irritability, insomnia, odd dreams or physical symptoms such as tremors and/or decreased appetite.
- According to *DSM-5*, marijuana or cannabis use disorder is defined as being mild, moderate, or severe depending on how many symptoms are present. Mild: 2 to 3; moderate: 4 to 5; severe: 6+ (1)

EPIDEMIOLOGY
- The WHO ranks the United States first among 17 European and North American countries for the prevalence of marijuana use.
- It is estimated that 4.5 to 7 million persons in the United States meet criteria for cannabis use disorder (CUD) annually (2).
- The prevalence of daily cannabis use in the United States has doubled in the past 2 decades.
- Cannabis use disorder applies to a subset of marijuana users; ~20% of lifetime marijuana users meet criteria for cannabis use disorder; 23% of these individuals meet criteria for severe use.
- Risk of CUD is estimated to be 1 in 11 (9%) in adults and 1 in 6 (17%) in adolescents (2).
- Cannabis is the most widely used illicit psychoactive substance in the United States (22.2 million monthly users) (3).
- Approximately 30% of students have used marijuana by the time of college entry.
- In the United States, 10% of marijuana users become daily users, 20–30% become weekly users.
- In the general population of young people, individuals who use high-potency cannabis are more likely to use cannabis regularly, have cannabis-related problems, use other illicit drugs, and have general anxiety disorder.

- The landscape is changing rapidly. Many states have legalized marijuana in some form. In 1969, only 12% of people approved of legalizing marijuana; by 2019, 67% approved of legalization.

ETIOLOGY AND PATHOPHYSIOLOGY
- The two most known therapeutically active cannabinoids in marijuana are δ9-tetrahydrocannabinol (THC) and cannabidiol (CBD). While CBD has become much more widely available, it remains prohibited by the FDA.
- THC is the psychoactive component responsible for marijuana's analgesic, antiemetic, and intoxicating properties.
- Cannabidiol is the nonpsychoactive component responsible for marijuana's antianxiety, antidepressant, antipsychotic, antispastic, anticonvulsant, and antineoplastic properties.
- THC concentrations in marijuana have risen over the past 20 years from 4% to 12–20% (2).
- Smoking marijuana results in 25–50% absorption of THC, which rapidly passes into the circulation. The oral bioavailability of THC is much less (3–10%).
- Effects of smoked marijuana occur within minutes and last several hours; effects from marijuana consumed in foods or beverages appear after 30 minutes to 1 hour and can last up to 4 hours.
- Frequent users are likely to experience withdrawal.
- Use in men is reported at 3.5% and women 1.7%; females have a faster transition from recreational use to cannabis use disorder (4).
- An emerging area of study involved cannabis-related drug interactions and adverse events, which have been noted to be increasing in frequency.
- Evidence for the use of cannabis to treat pain remains mixed.

RISK FACTORS
- Young individuals, especially 18- to 29-year-olds, are at more risk for severe cannabis use disorder (4).
- Cigarette smokers are at higher risk for cannabis use disorder compared to nonsmokers.
- Higher potency marijuana increases risk of cannabis use disorder and increases severity of symptoms (5).
- Family history of chemical dependence
- Comorbid psychiatric disorders (i.e., antisocial personality disorder)
- Other substance use (i.e., alcohol, tobacco)
- Lower educational achievement (rates of dependence are lowest among college graduates)
- Low socioeconomic status
- Ease of acquisition of marijuana
- Among youths with mood disorders, CUD is a risk marker for self-harm, all-cause mortality, and death by unintentional overdose and homicide.

 DIAGNOSIS

- In 2020, the USPSTF encouraged all primary care physicians to screen adults for drug use (2).
- Screen for marijuana (similar to tobacco and alcohol).
- Ask for frequency and amount used (e.g., "How often do you use marijuana? Daily? Weekly?"; "How long does a typical 'eighth' [1/8 oz] last?").

- Usage is defined by occasional = 1/8 oz/week, moderate = 1/4 oz/week, heavy = 1/2 oz/week (1 oz = 28.5 g which is equivalent to about 50 to 60 cigarettes).
- Unexplained deterioration in school or work performance is a red flag for abuse.
- Problems with, or changes in, social relationships (e.g., spending more time alone or with persons suspected of using drugs) and recreational activities (e.g., giving up activities that were once pleasurable) may also indicate abuse.
- If possible, obtain information from concerned parents or significant others.

HISTORY
- Clinical presentation of acute intoxication:
  - Euphoria, elation, laughter, heightened sensory perception, altered perception of time, increased appetite
  - Poor short-term memory, concentration
  - Fatigue, depression
  - Occasionally, distrust, fear, anxiety, panic
  - With large doses, acute psychosis: delusions, hallucinations, loss of sense of identity (6)
- Withdrawal symptoms include:
  - Irritability; anxiety
  - Restlessness
  - Nausea; weight loss; decreased appetite
  - Insomnia; depressed mood
  - Tremors

PHYSICAL EXAM
- Evaluate for:
  - Conjunctival injection
  - Xerostomia
  - Nystagmus
  - Increased heart rate
  - Decreased coordination
  - Altered mental status
- Withdrawal findings (nonspecific-similar to other drugs of abuse) include:
  - Restlessness/agitation
  - Irritability
  - Tremor
  - Diaphoresis
  - Increased body temperature

DIAGNOSTIC TESTS & INTERPRETATION
- Urine drug screen.
- Cannabinoids can be detected in urine weeks to months after marijuana use. Blood testing is preferred for interpreting acute effects and levels. In the United States, there is no consensus for acceptable legal limits for marijuana levels while driving. Hair testing can be unreliable and may reflect second-hand exposure. In general, testing identifies cannabis use (not necessarily cannabis use disorder).

🩹 **TREATMENT**

- Currently, there are no FDA-approved medications for the treatment of CUD (2).
- No specific treatment guidelines for cannabis use disorder are currently available. No intervention has proved consistently effective for marijuana abuse. Users often have a hard time quitting (1)[A].

- A Cochrane review showed that CBT and MET in combination had the most consistent evidence for decreasing cannabis use and dependence.
- Only 5% of those with cannabis use disorder seek treatment from a health care provider.
- Behavioral interventions include:
  - Cognitive-behavioral therapy; motivational interviewing; contingency management
  - Social network behavior therapy; 12-step approach; family-oriented therapy
  - Brief intervention; relapse prevention; community reinforcement approach
- The addition of a comprehensive parenting training curriculum does not enhance efficacy.
- Treating comorbid behavioral health disorders may help reduce use, particularly among heavy users.
- To help manage withdrawal:
  - Reduce amount used before quitting entirely.
  - Delay first use of marijuana until later in the day.
  - Consider nicotine replacement therapy if concomitant tobacco use is present.
  - Avoid cues and triggers associated with use.
- Prescribe short-term analgesia and sedation for withdrawal symptoms, if required; keep in mind potential for abuse with these agents as well.
- With marked irritability and restlessness, consider very low-dose diazepam for 3 to 4 days.
- Provide user and family members with information regarding abuse and withdrawal to increase understanding of abuse and reduce likelihood of relapse.
- Withdrawal symptoms peak on day 2 or 3; generally subside by day 7. Vivid dreams can continue for 2 to 3 weeks.

MEDICATION
- No effective medication currently exists to treat marijuana abuse.
- A recent review of medication options for treatment of CUD include:
  - SSRI (low strength evidence—did not reduce cannabis use or assist with cravings)
  - Antipsychotics (insufficient evidence for benefit)
  - Anxiolytics (low strength evidence that buspirone has no benefit over placebo)
  - Mood stabilizers (insufficient evidence for any benefit)
  - Cannabinoids (no benefit for achieving abstinence)
  - Gabapentin (insufficient evidence)
- Oral FDA-approved cannabinoids such as dronabinol or nabiximol may help abate marijuana withdrawal symptoms in individuals who are trying to quit.
- Options to assist with cravings include naltrexone 50 mg PO daily or N-acetylcysteine 1200 mg PO TID (2).
- Treatment of withdrawal is targeted toward symptom management such as anxiety, insomnia, and nausea.

ONGOING CARE

FOLLOW-UP RECOMMENDATIONS
- Monitor cessation by testing urine over several weeks for the inactive cannabis metabolites (carboxy-THC).
- Drug screening of heavy smokers may remain positive for marijuana up to 6 weeks after last use.

PATIENT EDUCATION
National Institute on Drug Abuse (NIDA):
- http://www.drugabuse.gov
- https://drugpubs.drugabuse.gov/promotions/back-to-school
- http://www.drugabuse.gov/drugs-abuse/marijuana
- https://teens.drugabuse.gov/

COMPLICATIONS
- Acute adverse effects:
  - Acute panic or paranoid reactions can occur, especially in drug-naive individuals or those with a history of psychosis or other behavioral health conditions.
  - Marijuana use is an independent risk factor for heart failure (6).
  - The American Heart Association (AHA) recently released a statement outlining the cardiovascular effects of cannabis use, noting that in states where cannabis has been legalized, there has been an increase in ED visits for acute myocardial infarction.
  - Psychotic symptoms with high doses
  - Driving under the influence of marijuana increases the risk for motor vehicle accidents.
- Chronic adverse effects:
  - Abnormal brain development; diminished lifetime achievement
  - Chronic bronchitis and impaired respiratory function in regular smokers
  - Smoking marijuana is harmful in transplant patients and other immunosuppressed individuals (increased risk of inhaled aspergillosis and other infections).
  - Marijuana use is associated with an increased risk of fibrosis in hepatitis C patients.
  - Marijuana may contribute to or result in pancreatitis.
  - Psychotic symptoms in heavy users, especially those with a personal or family history of schizophrenia
  - Marijuana use increases the risk for addiction to other substances.
  - An increased risk of heart failure, hypertension, ischemic stroke, and overall mortality in heavy cannabis users
  - Cannabinoid hyperemesis syndrome is characterized by episodes of cyclic nausea and vomiting in association with chronic cannabis use.

REFERENCES

1. American Psychiatric Association. Substance-related and addictive disorders. In: *Diagnostic and Statistical Manual of Mental Disorders*. 5th ed. Arlington, VA: American Psychiatric Association; 2013.
2. Williams AR, Hill KP. Care of the patient using cannabis. *Ann Intern Med*. 2020;173(9):ITC65–ITC80.
3. Substance Abuse and Mental Health Services Administration. Results from the 2015 National Survey on Drug Use and Health: detailed tables, SAMHSA, CBHSQ. http://www.samhsa.gov/data/sites/default/files/NSDUH-DetTabs-2015/NSDUH-DetTabs-2015/NSDUH-DetTabs-2015.pdf. Accessed November 5, 2020.
4. Kerridge BT, Pickering R, Chou P, et al. DSM-5 cannabis use disorder in the National Epidemiologic Survey on Alcohol and Related Conditions-III: gender-specific profiles. *Addict Behav*. 2018;76:52–60.
5. Arterberry BJ, Treloar Padovano H, Foster KT, et al. Higher average potency across the United States is associated with progression to first cannabis use disorder symptom. *Drug Alcohol Depend*. 2019;195:186–192.
6. Abayomi O, Adelufosi AO. Psychosocial interventions for cannabis abuse and/or dependence among persons with co-occurring cannabis use and psychotic disorders. *Cochrane Database Syst Rev*. 2015;(1):CD011488.

ADDITIONAL READING

- Hasin DS, Sarvet AL, Cerda M, et al. US adult illicit cannabis use, cannabis use disorder, and medical marijuana laws 1991–1992 to 2012–2013. *JAMA Psychiatry*. 2017;74(6):579–588.
- National Institute on Drug Abuse. What is the scope of marijuana use in the United States? https://www.drugabuse.gov/publications/research-reports/marijuana/what-scope-marijuana-use-in-united-states. Accessed November 5, 2020.

CODES

ICD10
- F12.10 Cannabis abuse, uncomplicated
- F12.20 Cannabis dependence, uncomplicated
- F12.288 Cannabis dependence with other cannabis-induced disorder

CLINICAL PEARLS
- It is estimated that 4.5 to 7 million persons in the United States meet criteria for CUD (2).
- Acute marijuana intoxication is manifested by conjunctival injection, increased heart rate, euphoria, heightened sensory perception, altered perception of time, increased appetite, poor short-term memory and concentration, and fatigue. Large doses may result in acute psychosis, panic or paranoid reactions, delusions, or hallucinations.
- Withdrawal symptoms include weight loss, decreased appetite, insomnia, and depressed mood. These symptoms peak on day 2 or 3 and resolve by day 7.
- Treatment of withdrawal is targeted toward symptom management such as anxiety, insomnia, and nausea.
- Cognitive-behavioral therapy, motivational interviewing, motivational enhancement therapy, and contingency management are four methods of behavioral-based interventions used to treat marijuana use disorder.

MASTITIS

Preeya Patel, DO • Kelley V. Lawrence, MD, IBCLC • Adeem Tahira, DO

 BASICS

DESCRIPTION
- Mastitis is an inflammation of the breast parenchyma and possibly associated tissues (areola, nipple, subcutaneous [SC] fat).
- Usually associated with bacterial infection (and milk stasis in the postpartum mother)
- Can be lactational or nonlactational
- Usually an acute condition but can become chronic cystic mastitis

EPIDEMIOLOGY
- Predominantly affects females
- Mostly in the puerperium; epidemic form rare in the age of reduced hospital stays for mothers and newborns
- Neonatal form
- Posttraumatic: ornamental nipple piercing increases risk of transmission of bacteria to deeper breast structures; *Staphylococcus aureus* is the predominant organism.

Incidence
- 3–20% of breastfeeding mothers develop nonepidemic mastitis, with greatest incidence among breastfeeding mothers 2 to 6 weeks postpartum.
- Neonatal form occurs at 1 to 5 weeks of age, with equal gender risk and unilateral presentation.
- Pediatric form occurs at or around or after puberty, with 82% of cases in girls.

ETIOLOGY AND PATHOPHYSIOLOGY
- Microabscesses along milk ducts and surrounding tissues
- Inflammatory cell infiltration of breast parenchyma and surrounding tissues
- Nonpuerperal (infectious) *S. aureus* (*including methicillin-resistant* S. aureus [MRSA]), *Bacteroides* spp., *Peptostreptococcus*, *Staphylococcus* (coagulase negative), *Enterococcus faecalis*, *Histoplasma capsulatum*, *Salmonella enterica*, rare case of *Actinomyces europaeus*
- Puerperal (infectious) *S. aureus* (*including MRSA*), *Streptococcus pyogenes* (group A or B), Enterobacteriaceae, *Corynebacterium* spp., *Bacteroides* spp., *Staphylococcus* (coagulase negative), *Escherichia coli*, *Salmonella* spp. (1)
- Rare secondary site for tuberculosis in endemic areas (1% of mastitis cases in these areas): single breast nodule with mastalgia
- Tuberculosis mastitis in nonendemic areas has also been reported in patients with exposure to TNF-α inhibitors and other immunomodulating compounds (2)[C].
- *Corynebacterium* spp. associated with greater risk for development of chronic cystic mastitis
- Granulomatous mastitis
  - Idiopathic
    - Predilection for Asian and Hispanic women
    - Association with α_1-antitrypsin deficiency, hyperprolactinemia with galactorrhea, oral contraceptive use, *Corynebacterium* spp. infection, and breast trauma
    - Most women have a history of lactation in previous 5 years.
    - New cases have been reported in male-to-female transgender patients in setting of exogenous progesterone and estrogen treatment (3)[B].
  - Lupus; autoimmune

- Puerperal
  - Retrograde migration of surface bacteria up milk ducts
  - Bacterial trapping behind plugged milk in the ductal outflow tracts
  - Bacterial migration from nipple fissures to breast lymphatics
  - Secondary monilial infection in the face of recurrent mastitis or diabetes
  - Seeding from mother to neonate in cyclical fashion
- Nonpuerperal—a variety of causes including: ductal ectasia, breast carcinoma, inflammatory cysts, chronic recurring SC or subareolar infections, parasitic infections (*Echinococcus*, filariasis, guinea worm in endemic areas), herpes simplex, cat-scratch disease, and, in older patients, smoking. Lupus is a rare cause.

RISK FACTORS
- Breastfeeding
- Milk stasis: inadequate emptying of breast (scarring due to previous breast surgery [breast reduction, biopsy, or partial mastectomy], scarring of breast due to prior mastitis), breast engorgement: interruption of breastfeeding, milk oversupply, plugged ducts
- Nipple trauma increases risk of transmission of bacteria to deeper breast structures: *S. aureus* predominant organism.
- Neonatal colonization with epidemic *Staphylococcus*
- Neonatal—occurs more commonly in bottle-fed babies; may be related to manual expression of "witch's milk" and can lead to lethal necrotizing fasciitis
- Maternal diabetes
- Maternal HIV
- Smoking

GENERAL PREVENTION
Regular emptying of both breasts and nipple care to prevent fissures when breastfeeding; also good hygiene including hand washing and washing breast pumps after each use

COMMONLY ASSOCIATED CONDITIONS
Breast abscess

 DIAGNOSIS

- Fever >38.5°C, malaise, and myalgia
- Nausea ± vomiting
- Localized breast tenderness, firmness, heat, swelling, and redness
- Possible breast mass

HISTORY
Breast pain, "hot cords burning in chest wall"

PHYSICAL EXAM
- Breast tenderness
- Localized breast induration, redness, and warmth
- Peau d'orange appearance to overlying skin

DIFFERENTIAL DIAGNOSIS
- Abscess (bacterial, idiopathic granulomatous mastitis, fungal, tuberculosis)
- Tumor, including inflammatory breast cancer
- Idiopathic granulomatous mastitis
- Wegener granulomatosis
- Sarcoidosis
- Foreign-body granuloma

- Vasospasm (may be presentation for Raynaud): Consider yeast infection if nipple pain and burning and/or infant with thrush.
- Ductal cyst (ductal ectasia)
- Consider monilial infection in lactating mother, especially if mastitis is recurrent.
- Mondor disease—thrombophlebitis of the superficial veins of the breast and anterior chest wall.

DIAGNOSTIC TESTS & INTERPRETATION
Initial Tests (lab, imaging)
Mastitis is typically a clinical diagnosis. Labs rarely needed. In those ill enough to need hospitalization, consider the following:
- CBC, blood culture
- In epidemic puerperal mastitis: milk leukocyte count, milk culture (or if recurrent outpatient mastitis), neonatal nasal culture
- No imaging required for postpartum mastitis in a breastfeeding mother that responds to antibiotic therapy
- Mammography for women with nonpuerperal mastitis
- Breast ultrasound to rule out abscess formation in women with a mass or fluctuance on palpation; special consideration for this in women with breast implants who have mastitis

Follow-Up Tests & Special Considerations
Lactating mothers produce salty milk from affected side (higher Na and Cl concentrations) as compared with unaffected side. Consider breast milk culture if suspect MRSA. Also consider testing for tuberculosis as may be initial presentation.

Diagnostic Procedures/Other
Options if further progression to abscess formation: needle aspiration, incision and drainage, excisional biopsy, ultrasound (US)-guided core needle biopsy is diagnostic method of choice for idiopathic granulomatous mastitis

 TREATMENT

- A Cochrane review found that insufficient evidence exists to confirm or refute the effectiveness of antibiotic therapy for the treatment of lactational mastitis (4)[A]. If present <24 hours and symptoms are mild, conservative management with milk removal and supportive measures is recommended.
- For patients with early idiopathic granulomatous mastitis and mild symptoms or those concerned for surgical scarring, close surveillance or observation alone is acceptable nonsurgical management.

GENERAL MEASURES
- Supportive care including analgesia, warm compress, and effective, frequent milk removal from the affected breast via breastfeeding, pumping, or hand expression
- Smoking cessation for patients with periductal mastitis

MEDICATION
- Prioritized on the basis of likelihood of MRSA as etiologic factor and clinical severity of condition. Treat for 10 to 14 days.
- For idiopathic granulomatous mastitis and localized infection, usually resolves with antibiotics and drainage

First Line

- Outpatient
  - Effective milk removal is most important management step.
  - Dicloxacillin 500 mg QID *or* cephalexin 500 mg QID
  - Trimethoprim/sulfamethoxazole (TMP/SMX); DS BID (If mastitis not improving within 48 hours after starting first-line treatment, consider MRSA.)
  - Doxycycline 100 mg BID; consider MRSA (if clinical course <3weeks).
  - *Lactobacillus fermentum* or *Lactobacillus salivarius* 9 log 10 CFU/day
- Inpatient
  - Nafcillin 2 g q4h *or* oxacillin 2 g q4h *or* vancomycin 1 g q12h (MRSA possible)
  - Daptomycin 1 g q24h
- If idiopathic granulomatous mastitis, consider corticosteroids ± methotrexate (5)[A]. May consider mycophenolate mofetil in patient refractory to treatment with antibiotics, steroids, and methotrexate (6)[C].
- To prevent recurring plugs and mastitis, can use sunflower lecithin 1,200 mg three to four times per day.

Pediatric Considerations

- TMP/SMX given to breastfeeding mothers with mastitis can potentiate jaundice for neonates.
- Treatment with doxycycline is limited to <3 weeks; long-term therapy (over 3 to 4 weeks) is not recommended because it may cause damage of infant's growth cartilage, teeth discoloration, and imbalance of intestinal flora.

Second Line

- If mastitis is odoriferous and localized under areola, add metronidazole 500 mg TID IV or PO.
- If yeast is suspected in recurrent mastitis, add topical and oral nystatin. Consider testing nipple tissue and milk for presence of yeast. Oral treatment can be considered for mother as well.

ISSUES FOR REFERRAL

- Abscess formation
- Need for breast biopsy (suspected abscess or IGM)

ADDITIONAL THERAPIES

- Warm packs to improve blood flow and milk letdown and/or ice packs to reduce inflammation to affected breast for comfort
- The use of a breast pump may aid in breast emptying, especially if the infant is unable to assist in doing this.
- Wear supporting bra that is not too tight.

SURGERY/OTHER PROCEDURES

In cases of biopsy-proven idiopathic granulomatous mastitis, the most effective and fastest way for complete eradication is surgical removal. The addition of steroids increases the rate of complete remission and decreases remission rate compared to surgery alone; NNT 3.84.

COMPLEMENTARY & ALTERNATIVE MEDICINE

- Breast lift technique for lymphatic breast drainage (can reduce engorgement and relieve plugging)
- Cold cabbage leaf compress to be applied up to 15 minutes twice per day. (Avoid long or frequent application of cabbage leaves as milk production can be diminished with this.)
- To prevent recurring plugs and mastitis, can use sunflower lecithin 1,200 mg three to four times per day.

ADMISSION, INPATIENT, AND NURSING CONSIDERATIONS

- If a new mother is admitted to the hospital for treatment of her mastitis, rooming-in of the infant with the mother is highly recommended so that breastfeeding can continue. In some hospitals, rooming-in may require hospital admission of the infant.
- Admission criteria/initial stabilization: Failure or outpatient/oral therapy (patient unable to tolerate oral therapy, nonadherent to oral therapy, or severe illness without adequate supportive care at home). Neonatal mastitis also requires admission.
  - Administer antibiotics.
  - Empty breasts frequently, if breastfeeding.
  - Give analgesics for pain: ibuprofen or acetaminophen.
  - Breastfeeding/pumping of breasts encouraged; baby and/or breast pump to bedside
- Start infant with feedings on affected side.
- Abscess drainage is not a contraindication for breastfeeding.
- Massage in direction from blocked area toward nipple.
- Positioning infant at breast with chin or nose pointing to blockage might help drain affected area.
- Discharge criteria: Patients should be afebrile and tolerating oral antibiotics well.

 ## ONGOING CARE

FOLLOW-UP RECOMMENDATIONS

Patient Monitoring

- Rest for lactating mothers, up to bathroom. Admit to medical floor. If concern for sepsis or hemodynamic instability, admit to intermediate level of care or intensive care unit.
- Follow up with breast imaging such as mammography or ultrasound in women >40 years of age after resolution of acute pathology to exclude underlying breast cancer.

DIET

- Encourage oral fluids.
- Multivitamin, including vitamin A

PATIENT EDUCATION

- Encourage oral fluids. Rest is essential.
- Regular emptying/draining of both breasts with breastfeeding
- Nipple care (simply with breastmilk or with hypoallergenic nipple balm) to prevent fissures
- Best nipple/areola health comes with optimized latch—seek help with latch if needed from a lactation professional.

PROGNOSIS

- Puerperal
  - Good with prompt (within 24 hours of symptom onset) antibiotic treatment and breast emptying; 96% success rate
  - 11% risk of abscess if left untreated with antibiotics
  - Antibodies develop in breast glands within first few days of infection, which may provide protection against infection or reinfection.
- Rare risk of abscess formation beyond 6 weeks postpartum if no recurrent mastitis
- Idiopathic granulomatous mastitis recurrence rates high, encourage close follow-up

COMPLICATIONS

Breast abscess 3% of women with puerperal mastitis, recurrent mastitis with resumption of breastfeeding or with breastfeeding after next pregnancy, cessation of breastfeeding, bacteremia, sepsis

REFERENCES

1. Wilson E, Woodd S, Benova L. Incidence of and risk factors for lactational mastitis: a systematic review. *J Hum Lact*. 2020;36(4):673–686.
2. Qiao Y, Hayward JH, Balassanian R, et al. Tuberculosis mastitis presenting as bilateral breast masses. *Clin Imaging*. 2018;52:28–31.
3. Sam KQ, Severs FJ, Ebuoma LO, et al. Granulomatous mastitis in a transgender patient. *J Radiol Case Rep*. 2017;11(2):16–22.
4. Jahanfar S, Ng CJ, Teng CL. Antibiotics for mastitis in breastfeeding women. *Sao Paulo Med J*. 2016;134(3):273.
5. Ma X, Min X, Yao C. Different treatments for granulomatous lobular mastitis: a systematic review and meta-analysis. *Breast Care (Basel)*. 2020;15(1):60–66.
6. Di Xia F, Ly A, Smith GP. Mycophenolate mofetil as a successful therapy for idiopathic granulomatous mastitis. *Dermatol Online J*. 2017;23(7): 13030/qt51g1k0zm.

 ## SEE ALSO

Algorithms: Breast Discharge; Breast Pain

CODES

ICD10

- O91.11 Abscess of breast associated with pregnancy
- O91.211 Nonpurulent mastitis associated with pregnancy, first trimester
- O91.113 Abscess of breast associated with pregnancy, third trimester

CLINICAL PEARLS

- Emptying/draining of the breasts on a regular schedule (recommend following baby's cues, but going no more than 3 to 4 hours between feeds), avoiding constrictive clothing or bras that might obstruct breast ducts, attention to good latch technique for mom and baby, "adequate rest," and a liberal intake of oral fluids for the mother can all reduce the risk of a breastfeeding mother's developing mastitis.
- Reassure mothers that it is safe (and imperative for healing) to feed baby and/or pump the affected breast.
- Among breastfeeding mothers, if the symptoms of mastitis fail to resolve within several days of appropriate management, including antibiotics, nonsteroidal anti-inflammatory drug, and breast emptying, further investigations may be required to confirm resistant bacteria, abscess formation, an underlying mass, or inflammatory or ductal carcinoma.
- More than two recurrences of mastitis in the same location or with associated axillary lymphadenopathy warrant evaluation with US and/or mammography to rule out an underlying mass.

M

MASTOIDITIS
Megan Finneran, DO, MS • Emilio Nardone, MD

BASICS

Mastoiditis is an inflammatory process of the mastoid bone. It is most commonly seen as a complication of acute otitis media (AOM).

DESCRIPTION
- Clinical manifestations of mastoiditis typically appear days to weeks after the first middle ear symptoms.
- Subdivided according to pathologic stage:
  - Acute mastoiditis with periostitis (incipient mastoiditis): purulent material in the mastoid cavities. Symptom duration typically 1 month or less
  - Coalescent mastoiditis (acute mastoid osteitis): destruction of the thin bony septae between air cells; followed by the formation of abscess cavities with pus dissecting into adjacent areas
- Masked mastoiditis (subacute mastoiditis): low-grade, persistent infection with destruction of the bony septae between air cells; occurs in patients with persistent middle ear effusion or recurrent episodes of inadequately treated AOM
- Chronic mastoiditis: associated with failed treatment of chronic otitis media. Often associated with cholesteatoma; symptoms last months to years.

EPIDEMIOLOGY
Highest incidence in children <2 years
- Similar to population susceptible to AOM (male, daycare attendance)
- Less common if immunizations up-to-date and antibiotics used to treat suppurative AOM

Incidence
1 to 2 cases per 100,000 children per year in United States (1)

ETIOLOGY AND PATHOPHYSIOLOGY
- Subclinical stage begins with AOM and inflammation of mastoid air cells.
- Mastoid is part of petrous temporal bone composed of air-filled cells.
- Mastoid aditus and antrum form a narrow connection between middle ear and mastoid air cells.
  - Fluid in the middle ear can cause obstruction at aditus or antrum, blocking outflow tract of mastoid air cells.
  - Edema and accumulation of purulent material most commonly spreads from mastoid air cells to periosteum via mastoid emissary veins with penetration of periosteum (acute mastoiditis with periosteitis) (1).
- Increased pressure from fluid within the air cells leads to destruction of bony septae (acute mastoid osteitis/acute coalescent mastoiditis).
- Acute mastoid osteitis can spread to adjacent areas in head and neck with abscess formation:
  - Subperiosteal abscess (most common complication), Bezold abscess, suppurative labyrinthitis, suppurative CNS complications
- AOM: *Streptococcus pneumoniae*, nontypeable *Haemophilus influenzae*
- Acute mastoiditis: *Streptococcus pneumoniae* (most common), group A streptococci—*Streptococcus pyogenes*, *Staphylococcus aureus* (including methicillin-resistant *S. aureus* [MRSA]), *H. influenzae*, *Fusobacterium necrophorum*
- Chronic mastoiditis: *Pseudomonas aeruginosa*, *S. aureus*, anaerobic bacteria, polymicrobials (organisms present in external ear canal), rarely *Mycobacterium tuberculosis*

- Abscess: *S. aureus*, mycobacteria, *Aspergillus*
- Increased incidence of penicillin-resistant *S. pneumoniae* infections has gradually lead to higher incidence of mastoiditis as complication of AOM (2).

Genetics
No known genetic pattern

RISK FACTORS
- Cholesteatoma appears as squamous pearl in anterosuperior area of middle ear near tympanic membrane.
- Recurrent AOM or chronic suppurative otitis media
- Immunocompromised state

GENERAL PREVENTION
- Ensure immunizations (particularly pneumococcal vaccine) are up-to-date.
- Referral to ENT for chronic otitis media
- Appropriate diagnosis and treatment of AOM; prevent recurrent AOM.
  - Chemoprophylaxis for AOM is controversial. Historically, consider in children with two episodes of AOM in first 6 months of life or in older children, three episodes in 6 months, or four episodes in 1 year. Chemoprophylaxis not currently recommended by American Academy of Pediatrics due to concern for multidrug resistance
- Wear ear plugs when swimming or showering to keep water out of the ears with AOM.
- Treat chronic eustachian tube dysfunction (pressure equalization tubes).
- Early diagnosis of cholesteatoma

COMMONLY ASSOCIATED CONDITIONS
Acute otitis media

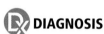

DIAGNOSIS

HISTORY
- Most common symptoms in infancy
  - Lethargy/malaise/irritability
  - Fever
  - Poor feeding/decreased appetite
- Recent ear infection
- Otorrhea (drainage from an ear infection)
- Otalgia and/or pain on mastoid bone behind the ear
- Swelling or redness over mastoid
- Swelling of the ear lobe
- Headache
- Hearing loss
- Chronic: persistent ear drainage, persistent ear pain
- Chronic: AOM nonresponsive to antibiotic
- Suspicion for mastoiditis increases when symptoms of AOM persist >2 weeks.

PHYSICAL EXAM
- Acute:
  - Fever
  - Erythema, tenderness, and/or edema overlying mastoid (postauricular)
  - Palpable postauricular fluctuance (later finding): most commonly postauricular in children >1 year and above ear in children < 1 year
  - Displaced pinna up and outward in children >1 year or down and outward in children <1 year (2)
  - Otoscopic exam: AOM present, may have perforation of TM with or without purulent discharge

- Chronic mastoiditis:
  - Persistent or intermittent mucopurulent drainage
  - Decreased hearing
  - May be painless from chronic process
  - Otoscopic exam: may have mucopurulent discharge, perforation of TM

DIFFERENTIAL DIAGNOSIS
- Scalp infection
- Mumps, parotitis
- Severe otitis externa
- Periauricular cellulitis
- Benign neoplasm: aneurysmal bone cyst, fibrous dysplasia
- Malignant neoplasm: acute lymphocytic leukemia, acute myelogenous leukemia, Burkitt lymphoma, non-Hodgkin lymphoma, rhabdomyosarcoma, neuroblastoma
- Deep neck space infections (2)

DIAGNOSTIC TESTS & INTERPRETATION
Initial Tests (lab, imaging)
- CBC with differential: elevated WBC count
- Elevated erythrocyte sedimentation rate (ESR) and C-reactive protein (CRP) in acute but may be normal in chronic
- Blood cultures
- Myringotomy/tympanocentesis: send for cultures, Gram stain, acid-fast stain.
- Aspiration if postauricular fluctuance is present: send for cultures.
- Plain films of mastoid has low diagnostic yield but may show loss of sharpness of mastoid outline, clouding of mastoid air cells, or demineralization of bony septa (3). These changes are not diagnostic and can also be seen in AOM.
- Preferred: CT of the temporal bone (97% sensitivity; 94% positive predictive value for identifying intracranial complications) (4)
  - Clouding/opacification of air cells (also in AOM)
  - Mastoid air cell coalescence
  - Cortical bone erosion
  - Rim-enhancing fluid collections
  - Absence of mastoid opacification excludes the diagnosis
- Use CT with contrast if complications are suspected (suppurative extension).
- Due to radiation, CT in children should be performed when clinically appropriate. Indications include:
  - Neurologic signs
  - Vomiting/lethargy
  - Suspected cholesteatoma
  - Fever after 48 to 72 hours of therapy
- Technetium-99m bone scan is more sensitive to osteolytic changes than CT.
- MRI: partial-to-complete opacification of the mastoid air cells ± middle ear cleft
  - Needed to evaluate for intracranial complications if clinical or radiographic suspicion
- Consider MRA if venous sinus thrombosis suspected.

Follow-Up Tests & Special Considerations
- Send all cultures for aerobic and anaerobic growth.
- Interpret normal WBC with caution in symptomatic, immunocompromised patients.
- Lumbar puncture if meningitis suspected
- Consider immunologic evaluations in children with recurrent episodes of OM leading to mastoiditis.

Diagnostic Procedures/Other

- Tympanocentesis to obtain middle ear fluid for culture and sensitivity
- Myringotomy with culture (also therapeutic)
- Audiography if hearing loss suspected
- Obtain CSF if intracranial extension suspected.
- Biopsy tissue protruding through TM or tympanostomy tube

 ## TREATMENT

- IV antibiotics and myringotomy (± tympanostomy tubes) is the preferred treatment for uncomplicated acute mastoiditis (reflecting a shift away from more invasive surgical treatment).
- To avoid intracranial complications, simple mastoidectomy is recommended if patients do not respond to treatment after 3 to 5 days.
- Myringotomy or incision and drainage may be necessary if an abscess is present in mastoid air cells.

GENERAL MEASURES
Inpatient care during acute phase for IV antibiotics

MEDICATION

First Line

- Empiric antibiotics against most common organisms: *S. pneumoniae* (including multiple resistant strains), *S. pyogenes*, *S. aureus* (including MRSA), *P. aeruginosa*
- Use combination therapy with 3rd-generation cephalosporin (ceftriaxone or cefotaxime) plus clindamycin with coverage for resistant strains.
- Ceftriaxone 2 g IV q24h
  - Pediatric dosing: 50 to 75 mg/kg/day IV divided q12–24h
  - Precaution: Adjust dose with renal impairment.
  - Consider levofloxacin 750 mg IV q24h if severe β-lactam allergy.
- Clindamycin for coverage of ceftriaxone-resistant *S. pneumoniae* in pediatric patients:
  - Clindamycin pediatric dosing: 20 to 40 mg/kg/day IV divided q6–8h
- Cefotaxime 1 to 2 g IV q4–8h, depending on severity
  - Pediatric dosing: 100 to 200 mg/kg/day q6–8h
- Add vancomycin 30 to 60 mg/kg/day divided q8–12h if concerned for MRSA or acute on chronic exacerbation:
  - Pediatric dosing: 15 mg/kg/dose q6–8h
  - Precaution: Adjust dose with renal impairment.
- For patients with a history of recurrent AOM or recent antibiotic administration, treat with piperacillin and tazobactam 3.375 g IV q6h:
  - Pediatric dosing: 300 mg/kg/day based on piperacillin component divided q6–8h
- Once culture results are available, target treatment based on antibiotic sensitivities.

Second Line

- Oral antibiotics after 7 to 10 days of IV antibiotics and once myringotomy/blood cultures identify pathogen and sensitivities. Common oral antibiotics:
  - Amoxicillin-clavulanate (Augmentin) or clindamycin + 3rd-generation cephalosporin for 3 weeks or total treatment duration of 4 weeks or longer for intracranial complications (5)
- For chronic mastoiditis: Use topical drops, ofloxacin otic solution (0.3%) or neomycin, polymyxin B, hydrocortisone 3 drops, 3 to 4 times per day.

ISSUES FOR REFERRAL

- Consult ENT for mastoiditis in adults and children.
- Consult neurosurgery for intracranial complications.
- Consider infectious disease consult for assistance with antibiotic management.

SURGERY/OTHER PROCEDURES

- Perform tympanocentesis to obtain cultures and guide antibiotic choice.
- Myringotomy and tympanostomy tubes allow for middle ear drainage.
- Clean ear canal under microscopic guidance to ensure pressure-equalization tube patency and adequate drainage of middle ear.
- Simple mastoidectomy is most effective for management of subperiosteal abscesses if trial of conservative therapy (drainage, myringotomy, and IV antibiotics) fails.

COMPLEMENTARY & ALTERNATIVE MEDICINE
No known home remedies

ADMISSION, INPATIENT, AND NURSING CONSIDERATIONS

- Admission criteria/initial stabilization
  - Clinical or imaging evidence of acute mastoiditis
  - Hospitalize patients with acute mastoiditis and start IV antibiotics immediately.
- Avoid getting affected ear wet.
- Discharge criteria
  - Afebrile for 48 hours before IV antibiotics are discontinued
  - Clinical improvement
  - Able to tolerate oral antibiotics

 ## ONGOING CARE

FOLLOW-UP RECOMMENDATIONS

- Oral antibiotics for 3 weeks following course of IV antibiotics (Total duration of antibiotics is 4 weeks or longer for intracranial complications.)
- For chronic mastoiditis, consider several months of antimicrobial prophylaxis with amoxicillin.

Patient Monitoring

- Assess for hearing loss postoperatively (audiogram) after acute condition has subsided.
- Follow-up with ENT and/or neurosurgery, particularly patients with hearing loss and/or intracranial complications

PATIENT EDUCATION

- Avoid getting the affected ear wet.
- Complete full course of antibiotics.

PROGNOSIS

- Depends on severity and stage of disease
- Most cases of mastoiditis recover fully if diagnosis is made early and treated appropriately.
- Conductive hearing loss may require reconstructive surgery; hearing loss may be permanent.

COMPLICATIONS
Complication rate 5–29% (5)

- Extracranial
  - Subperiosteal abscess (most common); Bezold abscess (abscess of sternocleidomastoid muscle, insidious, risk of mediastinitis); Citelli abscess (osteomyelitis of the calvaria)
  - Osteomyelitis of the temporal bone; suppurative labyrinthitis
  - Permanent hearing loss
  - Facial nerve paralysis (2)
- Intracranial
  - Intracranial abscess: epidural/subdural/cerebral
  - Meningitis/cerebritis/periostitis
  - Hearing loss

  - Otitis hydrocephalus: decreased venous drainage causes benign intracranial hypertension, manifesting as increased intracranial pressure, headache, papilledema, and sixth nerve palsy
  - Encephalitis; brain abscess
  - Gradenigo syndrome (sixth nerve palsy, severe pain in distribution of fifth nerve, and suppurative OM) (2)
  - Sigmoid sinus thrombophlebitis or thrombosis
  - Lateral sinus thrombosis; central venous sinus thrombosis (3)

REFERENCES

1. Psarommatis IM, Voudouris C, Douros K, et al. Algorithmic management of pediatric acute mastoiditis. *Int J Pediatr Otorhinolaryngol*. 2012;76(6):791–796.
2. Alkhateeb A, Morin F, Aziz H, et al. Outpatient management of pediatric acute mastoiditis. *Int J Pediatr Otorhinolaryngol*. 2017;102:98–102.
3. Loh R, Phua M, Shaw CL. Management of paediatric acute mastoiditis: systematic review. *J Laryngol Otol*. 2018;132(2):96–104.
4. Bakhos D, Trijolet JP, Morinière S, et al. Conservative management of acute mastoiditis in children. *Arch Otolaryngol Head Neck Surg*. 2011;137(4):346–350.
5. Mansour T, Yehudai N, Tobia A, et al. Acute mastoiditis: 20 years of experience with a uniform management protocol. *Int J Pediatr Otorhinolaryngol*. 2019;125:187–191.

ADDITIONAL READING

- Cherry JD, Vahabzadeh-Hagh AM, Shapiro NL. Mastoiditis. In Cherry J, Demmler-Harrison GJ, Kaplan SL, et al, eds. *Feigin and Cherry's Textbook of Pediatric Infectious Diseases*. 8th ed. Philadelphia, PA: Elsevier; 2019:169–175.
- Pelton SI. Otitis externa, otitis media, and mastoiditis. In Bennett JE, Dolin R, Blaser MJ, eds. *Mandell, Douglas, and Bennett's Principles and Practice of Infectious Diseases*. 9th ed. Philadelphia, PA: Elsevier; 2020:835–843.

 ## CODES

ICD10

- H70.90 Unspecified mastoiditis, unspecified ear
- H70.009 Acute mastoiditis without complications, unspecified ear
- H70.099 Acute mastoiditis with other complications, unspecified ear

CLINICAL PEARLS

- Suspect mastoiditis if symptoms of AOM persist >2 weeks despite a normal-appearing TM.
- Temporal bone CT is best diagnostic tool; use only when mastoiditis is suspected to limit radiation exposure in children.
- Hospitalize patients with acute mastoiditis for IV antibiotics. Consult ENT for drainage procedure.
- Treat with broad-spectrum IV antibiotics; collect middle ear fluid cultures to guide specific therapy. Total duration of antibiotics is 4 weeks or longer for intracranial complications.
- If conservative treatment fails after 3 to 5 days, perform mastoidectomy to avoid intracranial complications.

M

MEASLES (RUBEOLA)

Jason Chao, MD, MS • Wail Yar, MD, MPH

 BASICS

DESCRIPTION

- A highly communicable, acute viral illness characterized by an exanthematous maculopapular rash that begins at the head and spreads inferiorly to the trunk and extremities
- Rash is preceded by fever and the classic triad of cough, coryza, and conjunctivitis (3 Cs). Koplik spots are pathognomonic lesions of the oral mucosa early in the course of the infection.
- Public health problem in the developing world, with significant morbidity and mortality; rising incidence in developed nations with declining vaccination rates
- One dose of MMR vaccine is 93% effective, and 2 doses are 97% effective against measles.
- System(s) affected: hematologic; lymphatic; immunologic; pulmonary; skin
- Synonym(s): rubeola

EPIDEMIOLOGY

- Transmission: direct contact with infectious droplets; highly contagious; 90% of nonimmune close contacts likely to become infected on exposure
  - Droplets can remain airborne for hours.
- Infectivity is greatest during the prodromal phase.
  - Patients are considered contagious from 4 days before symptoms until 4 days after rash appears.
  - Immunocompromised patients are considered contagious for the entire duration of disease.
- Incubation period: averages 12.5 days from exposure to onset of prodromal symptoms
- Predominant age: varies based on local vaccine practices and disease incidence. In developing countries, most cases occur in children <2 years.

Incidence

- No longer considered an endemic disease in the United States; isolated outbreaks still occur.
- In 2019, measles cases surged worldwide to the highest number of cases in 23 years with over 850,000 cases globally, and global deaths climbed 50% since 2016.
- Although the number of measles cases was going down in 2020 due to COVID-19 control measures, measles campaigns in 26 countries were suspended due to the COVID-19 pandemic with 94 million children missing scheduled measles vaccine doses in 2020.
- The WHO and UNICEF are expecting more child deaths from measles than COVID-19 in Africa due to the measles campaigns disruption.
- Unvaccinated subpopulations and vaccine hesitancy have contributed to persistence of measles in the United States (1).

ETIOLOGY AND PATHOPHYSIOLOGY

The measles virus enters through the respiratory mucosa and replicates locally. It spreads to regional lymphatic tissues and other reticuloendothelial sites via the bloodstream.

- Measles virus is a spherical, enveloped, nonsegmented, single-stranded, negative-sense RNA virus of genus *Morbillivirus*, family *Paramyxoviridae*.
- Humans are the only natural host.

RISK FACTORS

- For developing measles:
  - Lack of adequate vaccination (2 doses)
  - Travel to countries where measles is endemic
  - Contact with exposed individuals

- For severe measles or measles complications:
  - Immunodeficiency
  - Malnutrition
  - Pregnancy
  - Vitamin A deficiency
  - Age <5 years or >20 years

GENERAL PREVENTION

- 100% preventable with proper vaccination
- Measles vaccine (active immunization)
  - Vaccine is usually given in combination with MMR or with added varicella (MMRV; ProQuad).
  - Primary vaccination requires 2 doses.
    - First dose at 12 to 15 months of age; 95% develop immunity.
    - Second dose at the time of school entry (4 to 6 years of age) or any time >4 weeks after first measles vaccine; the 5% of initial nonresponders almost always develop immunity after the second dose.
    - Health care workers should have immunity verified and, if not immune, should receive the vaccine if not contraindicated.
  - Common adverse reactions to the vaccine
    - Fever
    - Febrile seizures are rare (<5%) and occur 6 to 12 days after vaccination. Risk of febrile seizures increases if initial immunization is delayed past age 15 months (2).
    - Transient, mild, measles-like rash 7 to 10 days after vaccination (2%, with decreasing incidence during second vaccination)
    - If hypersensitivity reaction occurs, test for immunity; if immune, second dose not needed
    - *There is no substantiated link between MMR vaccine and autism.*
  - Contraindications
    - Live viral vaccines are contraindicated in immunosuppressed patients. For MMR, vaccinate asymptomatic HIV-infected children with adequate CD4 count.
    - Live vaccine is contraindicated in pregnancy (risk of fetal infection).
    - Anaphylactic reaction to gelatin or neomycin; consult an allergist before vaccination.
    - Egg anaphylaxis is not a contraindication.

COMMONLY ASSOCIATED CONDITIONS

- Immunosuppression
- Malnutrition

 DIAGNOSIS

HISTORY

- Prodromal period: usually 2 to 3 days before rash (may be up to 8 days)
  - Fever
    - May begin 8 to 12 days after exposure; can persist until 2 to 3 days after rash onset
    - Temperature often >102°F (39–40.5°C); can precipitate febrile seizures
    - Fever onset >3 days after rash suggests a complicated course.
  - "3 Cs": cough, coryza, and conjunctivitis
  - Cough may persist for 2 weeks.
  - Prodromal symptoms typically intensify over 2 to 4 days, peaking on 1st day of rash before subsiding.
- Other symptoms: loose stools, malaise, irritability, photophobia (from iridocyclitis), sore throat, headache, and abdominal pain

PHYSICAL EXAM

- Koplik spots
  - Pathognomonic of prodromal measles
  - 2- to 3-mm, gray-white, raised lesions on an erythematous base on buccal mucosa
  - Occur ~48 hours before measles exanthem
- Exanthematous rash (characteristic but not pathognomonic)
  - Maculopapular blanching rash
  - Begins at ears and hairline and spreads head to toe, reaching hips by day 2
  - Discrete erythematous patches become confluent over time, particularly on the upper body
  - Clinical improvement usually occurs within 48 hours after rash appears.
  - Rash fades in 3 to 4 days changing to a brownish color, followed by fine desquamation.
- Lymphadenopathy and pharyngitis may be seen during exanthematous period.

DIFFERENTIAL DIAGNOSIS

- Drug eruptions
- Rubella
- *Mycoplasma pneumoniae* infection
- Infectious mononucleosis
- Parvovirus B19 infection, roseola
- Enteroviruses
- Rocky Mountain spotted fever, dengue
- Toxic shock syndrome
- Meningococcemia
- Kawasaki disease

DIAGNOSTIC TESTS & INTERPRETATION

Initial Tests (lab, imaging)

- Obtain serum sample and throat (or nasopharyngeal) swab. Molecular testing of serum and respiratory specimens is the most accurate method to confirm measles infection by real-time polymerase chain reaction (RT-PCR) detection of RNA.
- Measles virus–specific IgM assay from serum and saliva. Antibodies may be undetectable on 1st day of exanthem but are usually detectable by day 3.
  - Sensitivity: 77% within 72 hours of rash onset; 100% within 4 to 11 days after rash onset. If negative but rash lasts >72 hours, repeat.
  - IgM falls to undetectable levels 4 to 8 weeks after rash onset.
- Measles virus–specific IgG may be undetectable up to 7 days after exanthem; levels peak 14 days after exanthem.
  - A 4-fold increase in IgG titers 14 days after an initial titer that was measured at least 7 days after rash onset is confirmatory.
- Viral cultures for measles are not usually performed.
- Mild neutropenia is common.
- Liver transaminases and pancreatic amylase may be elevated, particularly in adults.
- Chest x-ray if concern for secondary pneumonia

ALERT

Report suspected measles cases to public health authorities.

TREATMENT

GENERAL MEASURES

- Place all patients with measles in respiratory isolation until 4 days after onset of rash; immunocompromised patients should be isolated for duration of illness.
- Supportive therapy (i.e., antipyretics, antitussives, humidification, increased oral fluid consumption)
- Outbreak control
  - A single case of measles constitutes an outbreak. Report all suspected (and/or confirmed) cases to public health authorities.
  - Measles may remain active for several hours in the air. Airborne spread precautions (masking, physical distancing).
  - Immunize contacts (individuals exposed or at risk of having been exposed) within 72 hours.
    - Monovalent vaccine may be given to infants 6 months to 1 year of age, but 2 further doses of vaccine after 12 months must be given for adequate immunization.
    - Monovalent or combination vaccine may be given to all measles-exposed susceptible individuals age >1 year if not contraindicated.
    - Individuals not immunized within 72 hours of exposure should be excluded from school, child care, and health care settings (social quarantine) for at least until 2 weeks after onset of rash in last case of measles.

MEDICATION

- Vitamin A: WHO recommends daily dosages for 2 consecutive days (3)[B]:
  - Children <6 months of age 50,000 IU
  - Children 6 to 12 months of age 100,000 IU
  - Children >12 months of age 200,000 IU
- No approved antiviral therapy is available.
  - Measles virus is susceptible to ribavirin in vitro.
  - In one randomized trial including 100 children with measles treated with ribavirin or supportive care, ribavirin group had a shorter duration of fever, constitutional symptoms, and length of hospitalization.
  - Immunosuppressed children with severe measles have been treated with IV or aerosolized ribavirin. Use is not FDA-approved.
- Antibiotics
  - Reserve for patients with clinical signs of bacterial superinfection (pneumonia, purulent otitis, pharyngitis/tonsillitis) (3)[A].
  - A small trial resulted in an 80% (number needed to treat [NNT] = 7) decrease in measles-associated pneumonia with prophylactic antibiotics; consider in patients with a high risk of complications.
- Immunoglobulin therapy (passive immunity) for high-risk individuals exposed to measles for whom vaccine is inappropriate:
  - Children age <1 year (infants 6 to 12 months of age may receive MMR vaccine in place of immunoglobulin if given within 72 hours of exposure)
  - Pregnant women
  - Severe immunosuppression
  - Give IM immunoglobulin within 6 days of measles exposure; CDC recommends 0.25 mL/kg to maximum of 15 mL for infants and pregnant women; dose for immunocompromised is 0.5 mL/kg to a maximum of 15 mL.

ADMISSION, INPATIENT, AND NURSING CONSIDERATIONS

- Inpatient setting: airborne transmission precautions for 4 days after the onset of rash in otherwise healthy patients and for the duration of illness in immunocompromised patients
- Outpatient care is appropriate, except where complications develop (e.g., encephalitis, pneumonia).

ONGOING CARE

FOLLOW-UP RECOMMENDATIONS

Signs of complications needing close follow-up:
- Difficulty breathing or noisy breathing
- Changes in vision
- Changes in behavior, confusion
- Chest or abdominal pain

PATIENT EDUCATION

- Adhere to recommended immunization schedules.
- Avoid exposure, particularly to unimmunized children and adults, pregnant women, and immunocompromised persons, until 4 days after rash onset.
- Avoid contact with potential pathogens until respiratory symptoms resolve.
- Centers for Disease Control and Prevention: Measles: http://www.cdc.gov/measles/about/index.html

PROGNOSIS

- Typically self-limited; prognosis good
- About 3% of adults will develop pneumonia that will require hospitalization.
- High fatality rates may be seen among malnourished or immunocompromised children, particularly in developing countries.
- Pregnant women, immunocompromised patients, children age <5, and adults >20 are at the greatest risk of developing measles complications.

COMPLICATIONS

- GI complications: Diarrhea (may lead to dehydration) is the most common complication.
- Otitis media (5–15%), which may lead to hearing loss
- Respiratory complications:
  - Bronchopneumonia (5–10%)
    - Accounts for most measles-related deaths
    - May be viral or bacterial
  - Interstitial pneumonitis (immunocompromised patients)
  - Laryngotracheobronchitis ("measles croup"): occurs in younger age group (<2 years)
- Neurologic complications
  - Acute disseminated encephalomyelitis with seizures and neurologic abnormalities (occurs in 1/1,000 cases): presents within 2 weeks of rash, probably an autoimmune response
  - Inclusion body encephalitis is rare but fatal in those with defective cellular immunity.
  - Subacute sclerosing panencephalitis
    - Rare degenerative CNS disease resulting from persistent measles infection following natural disease; usually fatal
    - Presents 5 to 15 years after infection
    - Most often in persons infected before age 2 years
- The immune response to measles infection paradoxically depresses response to non–measles-virus antigens for years, rendering individuals more susceptible to pneumonia and diarrhea.
- There is a decrease in humoral immunity memory cells after native measles infection. This has not been observed in vaccinated individuals.
- Ocular complications
  - Keratitis
    - Can lead to permanent scarring, blindness
    - Vitamin A deficiency predisposes to more severe keratitis and its complications.
- Cardiac complications include myocarditis and pericarditis.
- Secondary bacterial infections: Measles can cause systemic secondary infection especially in developing countries.
- Death: results from complications, mainly pneumonia, rather than the virus itself. CDC statistics show that for every 1,000 children who get measles, 1 or 2 will die.
- Febrile seizures within 7–10 days of immunization; risk might increase if given as a combination with the varicella vaccine.

REFERENCES

1. Dimala CA, Kadia BM, Nji MAM, et al. Factors associated with measles resurgence in the United States in the post-elimination era. *Sci Rep.* 2021;11(1):51.
2. Rowhani-Rahbar A, Fireman B, Lewis E, et al. Effect of age on the risk of fever and seizures following immunization with measles-containing vaccines in children. *JAMA Pediatr.* 2013;167(12):1111–1117.
3. Kabra SK, Lodha R. Antibiotics for preventing complications in children with measles. *Cochrane Database Syst Rev.* 2013;(8):CD001477.

ADDITIONAL READING

- Dimala CA, Kadia BM, Nji MAM, et al. Factors associated with measles resurgence in the United States in the post-elimination era. *Sci Rep.* 2021;11(1):51.
- Moss WJ. Measles. *Lancet.* 2017;390(10111): 2490–2502.
- Mulholland K, Kretsinger K, Wondwossen L, et al. Action needed now to prevent further increases in measles and measles deaths in the coming years. *Lancet.* 2020;396(10265):1782–1784.
- Papania MJ, Wallace GS, Rota PA, et al. Elimination of endemic measles, rubella, and congenital rubella syndrome from the Western hemisphere: the US experience. *JAMA Pediatr.* 2014;168(2):148–155.

CODES

ICD10

- B05.9 Measles without complication
- B05.2 Measles complicated by pneumonia
- B05.89 Other measles complications

CLINICAL PEARLS

- There is no substantiated link between MMR vaccine and autism.
- A single case of measles constitutes an outbreak; report suspected measles cases to state or local health departments immediately.
- Immunization requires 2 doses: one at 12 to 15 months of age and one at school age (4 to 6 years of age).
- The clinical presentation of measles includes a prodrome of fever, cough, coryza, and conjunctivitis, followed by a descending maculopapular rash beginning on the face and progressing to the chest and lower body (centrifugal)
- Consider measles in the differential diagnosis of a febrile rash illness (especially in unvaccinated individuals with recent international travel).
- Measles-associated pneumonia is the most common cause of mortality.
- Measles cases and deaths are expected to rise after 2021 due to the COVID-19 pandemic disruption of measles vaccine campaigns globally.

M

MEASLES, GERMAN (RUBELLA)

Brittany L. Wiles, MD • Nathaniel John Irvine, MD

BASICS

DESCRIPTION

- A generally self-limited viral infection of children and adults, characterized by a mild, maculopapular rash, lymphadenopathy, and slight fever. Complications in normal, immunocompetent populations are rare. Nonimmune women infected with rubella while pregnant may have devastating fetal effects.
- As many as 50% of all rubella infections are asymptomatic (1),(2).
- System(s) affected: hematologic; nervous; pulmonary; exocrine; ophthalmologic; skeletal
- Synonym(s): German measles; 3-day measles

Pregnancy Considerations

- Pregnancy-associated rubella infection may lead to congenital rubella syndrome (CRS) with potentially devastating fetal outcomes. CRS most commonly manifests as sensorineural deafness, eye abnormalities, and/or congenital heart disease.
- Exposure during the 1st trimester presents highest risk for development of CRS (2).
- Screening pregnant women for rubella immunity and vaccinating nonimmune women is the most effective strategy to prevent CRS (1),(2),(3).
- Although no case of vaccine-associated CRS has been reported, women should not become pregnant for at least 28 days after vaccination because vaccine-type virus can cross the placenta (4).
- Polymerase chain reaction (PCR) can be used for rapid fetal diagnosis by detection of viral RNA from multiple samples such as amniotic fluid or fetal blood (5).

EPIDEMIOLOGY

- RNA togavirus of genus *Rubivirus* (1)
- Multiple genotypes have been identified without significant antigenic differences (2),(3).
- A live attenuated vaccine has been available in the United States since 1969. Primary use is to prevent CRS.
- Since 2004, all U.S. cases of rubella have been imported; most cases are inadequately immune travelers.
- Average incubation: 17 days; ranges 12 to 23 days (1).
- Infectious period between 7 days before and 7 days after rash appears
- Transmitted primarily via respiratory droplets
- Most common in late winter and early spring (2)
- Humans are only natural hosts (5).

Incidence

- U.S. incidence: <1/10,000,000 since 2001
- Declared eliminated (no endemic transmission for 12+ months) from the United States in 2004. However, primarily due to disease in international travelers, vaccine avoidance, and lack of routine pediatric care in migrant populations, cases are still reported annually.
- From 2005 to 2015, only 94 cases of rubella and 8 cases of CRS were reported in the United States.
- Still occurs in developing countries with 100,000 cases of CRS reported annually worldwide (1)

ETIOLOGY AND PATHOPHYSIOLOGY

- Virus invades the respiratory epithelium, replicates in nasopharynx and regional lymph nodes, and spreads hematogenously. Infected patients start shedding virus from the nasopharynx 7 days before the rash appears. Shedding lasts 7 or more days after onset of the rash (2).
- Disease typically progresses from a prodromal stage (1 to 5 days) to lymphadenopathy (5 to 10 days) to an exanthematous, maculopapular rash. Petechiae on the soft palate (Forchheimer spots) may precede or accompany the rash. Rash starts on the face and spreads outward to the trunk and extremities, sparing the palms and soles (14 to 17 days after onset of prodromal symptoms). The rash typically lasts an average of 3 days (1),(2).
- Rubella first described by German scientists in the early 1800s as a variant of measles or scarlet fever (2).
- 1964 to 1965: epidemic resulting in an estimated 12.5 million cases in the United States, with 2,000 cases of encephalitis; 11,250 cases of therapeutic or spontaneous abortions; 2,100 neonatal deaths; and 20,000 infants born with CRS (1)

Genetics

- Polymorphisms in HLA genes are associated with different rubella antibody levels and with vaccine side effects.
- HLA-DPB1 homozygosity has been associated with higher levels of rubella antibody.
- Arthritis-like joint vaccination side effect has been weakly connected with HLA-DR (3).

RISK FACTORS

Inadequate immunization, inadequate immunity after prior vaccination, immunodeficiency states, immunosuppressive therapy, crowded living/working conditions, international travel (1),(2)

GENERAL PREVENTION

- Vaccination is the most effective preventive strategy.
- Available combined with mumps, measles, rubella (MMR) or with varicella (MMR-V). Isolated rubella vaccine is not available in the United States.
  - Adults: 1- or 2-dose MMR vaccine schedule is recommended for those born after 1957. When 2 doses are used, each must be ≥28 days apart.
  - Pediatric: A 2-dose MMR vaccine schedule is recommended with the first dose given at ages 12 to 15 months; second dose recommended at 4 to 6 years of age.
  - MMR-V is approved for use in children aged 12 months to 12 years and is the vaccine of choice for the second dose and the first dose at ≥48 months old.
  - Special pediatric cases: In special circumstances (e.g., upcoming international travel), the second dose may be given prior to 4 years of age but no sooner than 28 days since the initial dose.
  - Children 6 to 11 months of age may also receive a single dose prior to international travel but should be revaccinated with a full 2-dose schedule starting at 12 months of age.
  - Children with HIV should receive MMR vaccine at 12 months of age if no contraindications exist.
  - In the event of an outbreak, immediate vaccination of infants 6 to 11 months old is recommended.
  - Vaccination is recommended for nonimmune people in the following groups: prepubertal boys and girls, all women of reproductive age, college students, daycare personnel, health care workers, and military personnel.

- Contraindications to vaccine: pregnancy, immunodeficiency (except HIV infection without significant immunosuppression), first-degree relative with congenital or genetic immunodeficiency, recent IVIG or blood administration (wait 3 to 11 months to vaccinate; based on product received), severe febrile illness, or hypersensitivity to vaccine components. Patients who receive rubella vaccine do not transmit rubella to others, although the virus can be isolated from the pharynx. Breastfeeding is not a contraindication to vaccination (2),(4).
- During outbreaks, serologic screening before vaccination is *not* recommended because rapid mass vaccination is needed to stop disease spread.
- MMR vaccine *is not associated with autism*.
- Children who receive the MMR-V vaccine have a 2-fold increase in risk of febrile seizures compared with those who receive MMR and varicella vaccines separately.
- Routine rubella antibody (IgG) screening is recommended during pregnancy (4).

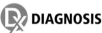
DIAGNOSIS

Council of State and Territorial Epidemiologists (CSTE) case definition of rubella (1)[A],(2)[A]:

- Clinical case definition
  - Acute maculopapular rash that is generalized
  - Temperature >99°F (37.2°C; if measured)
  - Arthralgia or arthritis, lymphadenopathy, or conjunctivitis
- Laboratory criteria for diagnosis
  - Isolation of virus from throat or nasopharynx, serum, CSF, or urine
  - Notable rise in acute- and convalescent-phase titers of serum IgG Ab
  - Positive serologic test for IgM Ab
  - PCR positive for virus

HISTORY

- Most cases of postnatal rubella in the United States are inadequately immunized travelers returning from endemic areas.
- Rubella spreads quickly when individuals are in close proximity.
- Postnatal rubella: low-grade fever, lymphadenopathy (postcervical, occipital, and postauricular), maculopapular rash, conjunctivitis, sore throat, arthritis, arthralgia, malaise. Thrombocytopenic purpura and encephalitis are rare. Up to 50% are asymptomatic.
- CRS: Defects can occur in all organs to include hearing or vision impairment, developmental delay, cardiac defects.
- Deafness, the most common manifestation of CRS, may not be noticed for several years (4)[A],(2)[A],(5)[B].

PHYSICAL EXAM

- Postnatal rubella: low-grade fever, lymphadenopathy (posterior auricular, occipital, posterior cervical), exanthem (mild, pink, noncoalescent maculopapular rash), soft palate petechiae (Forchheimer sign), conjunctivitis (2)[A]
- CRS: microcephaly, hearing loss, cataracts, glaucoma, microphthalmia, pigmentary retinopathy, purpura, murmur consistent with patent ductus arteriosus (PDA), hepatosplenomegaly, bone disease (2)[A],(5)[B]

DIFFERENTIAL DIAGNOSIS

- Postnatal rubella (1)[A],(2)[A],(6)[B]:
  - Measles virus (rubeola)
  - Scarlet fever (strep A)
  - Erythema infectiosum (parvovirus B19)
  - Roseola infantum (i.e., exanthem subitum)
  - Epstein-Barr virus
  - Cytomegalovirus
  - Drug eruptions
  - Other exanthematous enteroviral or adenoviral infections
- Congenital rubella (1)[A],(2)[A],(6)[B]:
  - Measles
  - Parvovirus B19
  - Human herpesvirus 6
  - Other exanthematous entero- or arboviruses

DIAGNOSTIC TESTS & INTERPRETATION

Initial Tests (lab, imaging)

- Because 50% of cases are subclinical, laboratory testing to confirm the diagnosis is preferred (1)[A],(2)[A],(6)[B].
- Detection of wild-type virus and of rubella specific antibodies in the serum is the standard for diagnosis (1)[A],(6)[B].
- Enzyme-linked immunosorbent assay (ELISA): sensitive and available. Most testing performed uses a form of ELISA. Will give positive result for 10 IU/mL (1)[A],(3)[B].
- Hemagglutination inhibition (HAI) test: once the most commonly used test and was used in development of many different tests that are used today (3)[B]
- Immunofluorescence, RT-PCR, and immunocolorimetric assays can be used by detection of viral RNA or proteins for affirmation that the virus has been isolated (3)[B],(6)[B].
- Avidity test: not routinely used; distinguishes recent versus past infections
- Samples from oral secretions and serum are usually used to detect rubella antibodies, and samples from the throat and oral secretions are often utilized to identify viral RNA (3)[B].
- Ideal window for testing: Most rubella cases are virus positive on the day of the rash onset and remain positive for the next 7 to 10 days. Perform serum collection during this period. IgM antibodies may not be identified in the serum until 5 days after rash onset. Repeat testing for confirmation 7 to 21 days after initial testing. When testing for seroconversion, collect a second IgG sample 2 to 3 weeks after the first (acute to convalescent phase) (1)[A],(2)[A],(3)[B],(6)[B].
- Detection of the virus in patients with CRS is often from urine. Will be able to detect the virus for months in CRS patients (3)[B]
- Epidemiologically, viral genotyping is important to fully understand the virus and to identify elimination. CDC should be notified as it is a reportable disease in the United States (1)[A],(6)[B].
- If a pregnant female tests positive, a sample can be taken from amniotic fluid, placenta, or blood from the umbilical cord via amniocentesis, chorionic villu sampling, or cordocentesis. The fetus should be monitored closely by an obstetric provider for any defects reflective of CRS (5)[B].
- As the incidence of rubella decreases, the positive predictive value (PPV) of IgM results decreases. False-positive findings occur in patients with other infections such as parvovirus, enterovirus, or adenovirus, and positive rheumatoid factor (2)[A],(6)[B].

- Important to differentiate between primary infection, rare reinfection, and persistent antibodies from prior infection as IgM antibodies may be present from 8 weeks to >6 months. CRS has not been reported when reinfection occurred >12 weeks' gestation (4)[A],(6)[B].

Follow-Up Tests & Special Considerations

- Rubella and CRS are notifiable diseases in the United States. The jurisdiction or state health department should report a rubella case quickly to the CDC (preferred within 24 hours) (1)[A],(2)[A].
- Infants with CRS may shed virus up to 1 year (2)[A].

 ## TREATMENT

- Treatment is based on symptoms (5)[B].
- Patients with postnatal rubella and CRS complications such as encephalitis and thrombocytopenic purpura may need hospitalization (2)[A].
- Isolate patients for 7 days after rash onset (1)[A].
- CRS-related long-term complications may require multidisciplinary management (2)[A],(5)[B].

MEDICATION

No pharmacologic therapy that is specific to rubella exists (5)[B].

First Line

- Any medication used is to treat symptoms such as NSAIDs can be used for pain and fever.
- Immune globulin may be administered 72 hours after exposure to pregnant patients to limit symptoms; it does not prevent CRS (5)[B].

 ## ONGOING CARE

FOLLOW-UP RECOMMENDATIONS

Patient Monitoring

- Individuals immune to rubella through natural infection or vaccine may be reinfected when reexposed. Reinfection could occur in previously vaccinated patients with low antibody levels (2)[A],(4)[A].
- Close monitoring for symptoms of mild CRS in exposed infants is important as they may not be present for years (4)[A].

PATIENT EDUCATION

http://www.cdc.gov/rubella/

PROGNOSIS

- Postnatal rubella: Complete recovery is typical.
- CRS
  - Varied and unpredictable spectrum, ranging from stillbirth/fetal death to normal infancy/childhood (1)[A],(2)[A]
  - If an infant with CRS survives past the neonatal period, may have significant disabilities such as deafness and developmental issues such as autism (3)[B]
  - Prognosis is excellent if only minor congenital defects are present (2)[A],(5)[B].

COMPLICATIONS

- Arthralgia/arthritis in up to 70% of women (1)[A]
- Encephalitis (1/6,000 cases)
- Hemorrhagic diseases such as thrombocytopenic purpura (1/3,000 cases)
- Less common: neuritis, progressive panencephalitis, orchitis
- CRS: incidence dependent on trimester exposed (2)[A]
- MMR vaccine may rarely cause encephalitis, anaphylaxis, or ITP (self-limited) (4)[A].

REFERENCES

1. Lanzieri T, Redd S, Abernathy E, et al. Chapter 14: rubella. In: Roush SW, Baldy LM, Hall MAK, eds. *Manual for the Surveillance of Vaccine-Preventable Diseases*. Atlanta, GA: Centers for Disease Control and Prevention; 2020. http://www.cdc.gov/vaccines/pubs/surv-manual/chpt14-rubella.html. Accessed July 29, 2021.
2. Lanzieri T, Haber P, Icenogle JP, et al. Rubella. In: Hamborsky J, Kroger A, Wolfe C, eds. *Epidemiology and Prevention of Vaccine-Preventable Diseases*. 13th ed. Atlanta, GA: Centers for Disease Control and Prevention; 2015:325–338. https://www.cdc.gov/vaccines/pubs/pinkbook/rubella.html. Accessed July 29, 2021.
3. Lambert N, Strebel P, Orenstein W, et al. Rubella. *Lancet*. 2015;385(9984):2297–2307.
4. McLean HQ, Fiebelkorn AP, Temte JL, et al; and Centers for Disease Control and Prevention. Prevention of measles, rubella, congenital rubella syndrome, and mumps, 2013: summary recommendations of the Advisory Committee on Immunization Practices (ACIP). *MMWR Recomm Rep*. 2013;62(RR-04):1–34.
5. White SJ, Boldt KL, Holditch SJ, et al. Measles, mumps, and rubella. *Clin Obstet Gynecol*. 2012;55(2):550–559.
6. Hübschen JM, Bork SM, Brown KE, et al. Challenges of measles and rubella laboratory diagnostic in the era of elimination. *Clin Microbiol Infect*. 2017;23(8):511–515.

ADDITIONAL READING

- Essential Programme on Immunization, Immunization, Vaccines and Biologicals. *Global Strategy for Comprehensive Vaccine-Preventable Disease Surveillance*. Geneva, Switzerland: World Health Organization; 2020. https://www.who.int/publications/m/item/global-strategy-for-comprehensive-vaccine-preventable-disease-(vpd)-surveillance. Accessed July 29, 2021.
- Lanzieri T, Redd S, Abernathy E, et al. Chapter 15: congenital rubella syndrome. In: Roush SW, Baldy LM, Hall MAK, eds. *Manual for the Surveillance of Vaccine-Preventable Diseases*. Atlanta, GA: Centers for Disease Control and Prevention; 2020. https://www.cdc.gov/vaccines/pubs/surv-manual/chpt15-crs.html. Accessed October 29, 2021.
- Papania MJ, Wallace GS, Rota PA, et al. Elimination of endemic measles, rubella, and congenital rubella syndrome from the Western hemisphere: the US experience. *JAMA Pediatr*. 2014;168(2):148–155.

CODES

ICD10

- B06.9 Rubella without complication
- B06.00 Rubella with neurological complication, unspecified
- P35.0 Congenital rubella syndrome

CLINICAL PEARLS

- Rubella is typically a self-limited viral exanthem in children and adults.
- Congenital rubella syndrome (CRS) in nonimmune women may have devastating fetal effects.
- Immunization is the key prevention strategy.

M

MEDIAL TIBIAL STRESS SYNDROME (MTSS)/SHIN SPLINTS

Vasilios Chrisostomidis, DO

 BASICS

DESCRIPTION

- The term medial tibial stress syndrome (MTSS) is currently preferred to "shin splints." MTSS is aching pain along the inner edge of the tibial shaft that develops when the musculature and/or periosteum in the (lower) leg become irritated by repetitive activity. The condition is part of a continuum of stress-related injuries to the lower leg. MTSS does not encompass pain from ischemia (compartment syndrome) or stress fractures.
- Tendonitis/periostitis of the medial soleus muscles, anterior tibialis, and posterior tibialis muscles
- Synonyms: tibial stress reaction, anterior muscle syndrome, tibial periostitis, perimyositis, soleus syndrome, shin splints

EPIDEMIOLOGY

Incidence
Common, can account for between 5% and 35% of novice-running injuries; frequently occurs bilaterally (1)

Pediatric Considerations
MTSS may account for up to 31% of all overuse injuries in high school athletes.

ETIOLOGY AND PATHOPHYSIOLOGY

- Multifactorial anatomic and biomechanical factors
  - Overuse injuries causing or limited by
    - Microtrauma from repetitive motion leading to periosteal inflammation
    - Overpronation of the subtalar joint and tight gastrocnemius/soleus complex with increased eccentric loading of musculature inserting along the medial shin
    - Interosseous membrane pain
    - Periostitis
    - Tears of collagen fibers
    - Enthesopathy
  - Anatomic structures affected include
    - Flexor hallucis longus
    - Tibialis anterior
    - Tibialis posterior
    - Soleus
    - Crural fascia
- Pathogenesis: theorized to be due to (i) calf muscle traction on periosteum and (ii) persistent repetitive loading on tibia, which leads to inadequate bone remodeling with subsequent tibial cortex changes and possible microfissures causing pain without evidence of fracture or ischemia

RISK FACTORS

- Intrinsic (personal) risk factors
  - Greater ranges of internal and external (>65 degrees) hip rotation
  - Significant overpronation at the ankle
  - Imbalance of musculature of the ankle and foot (inversion/eversion misbalance)
  - Female gender
  - Lean calf girth
  - Femoral neck anteversion
  - Navicular drop
  - Genu varum
  - History of previous MTSS
- External (environmental) risk factors
  - Lack of physical fitness
  - Inexperienced runners—particularly those with rapid increases in mileage and inadequate prior conditioning
  - Excessive overuse or distance running, particularly on hard or inclined (crowned) surfaces
  - Prior injury
  - Equipment (shoe) failure
- Other risk factors
  - Elevated BMI
  - Lower bone mineral density
  - Tobacco use
- Those typically affected by MTSS include
  - Runners
  - Military personnel—common in recruit/boot camp
  - Gymnasts, soccer, and basketball players
  - Ballet dancers

GENERAL PREVENTION

- Proper technique for guided calf stretching and lower extremity strength training, although supplementary gastrocnemius and soleus stretching has no statistical significance in reducing risk of shin splints
- Rehabilitate prior injuries adequately.
- Other recommendations
  - Gait analysis and retraining, particularly for overpronation
  - Orthotic footwear inserts were found to be preventative in naval recruits.

COMMONLY ASSOCIATED CONDITIONS

- Rule out stress fracture and compartment syndrome: Pain often persists at rest.
- Pes planus (flat feet)

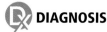 DIAGNOSIS

HISTORY

- Patients typically describe dull, sharp, or deep pain along the lower leg that is resolved with rest.
- Patients are often able to run through the pain in early stages.
- Pain is commonly associated with exercise (also true with compartment syndrome), but in severe cases, pain may persist with rest.

PHYSICAL EXAM

- Tenderness to palpation is typically elicited along the posteromedial border of the middle to distal 3rd of the tibia.
- Pain with plantar flexion
- Preservation of neurovascular integrity via palpable distal pulses, intact sensation, reflexes, and muscular strength

DIFFERENTIAL DIAGNOSIS

- Bone
  - Tibial stress fractures
    - Typically, pain persists at rest or with weight-bearing activities.
    - Focal tenderness over the anterior tibia
    - Hopping on involved leg will reproduce pain (less likely with MTSS).
- Muscle/soft tissue injury
  - Strain, tear, tendinopathy
  - Muscle hernia
- Fascial
  - Chronic exertional compartment syndrome (2)[C]
    - Pain without direct tenderness on exam
    - Pain increases with exertion and resolves at rest.
    - Pain is described as cramping or squeezing.
    - Pain with possible weakness or paresthesias on exam
  - Interosseous membrane tear
- Nerve
  - Spinal stenosis
  - Lumbar radiculopathy
  - Common peroneal nerve entrapment
- Vascular
  - DVT
  - Popliteal arterial entrapment
    - Rare but limb-threatening disease
    - History of intermittent unilateral claudication
    - MRI reveals compression of the artery by the medial head of the gastrocnemius muscle.
- Infection
  - Osteomyelitis
- Malignancy
  - Bone tumors

DIAGNOSTIC TESTS & INTERPRETATION

- Plain radiographs help rule out stress fractures if >2 weeks of symptoms (3).
- Bone scintigraphy
  - Diffuse linear vertical uptake in the posterior tibial cortex on the lateral view
  - Stress fractures demonstrate a focal ovoid uptake.
- High-resolution MRI reveals abnormal periosteal and bone marrow signals, which are useful for early discrimination of tibial stress fractures.
- Increased pain and localized tenderness warrant further imaging with MRI due to concern for tibial stress fracture.
- Exclude compartment syndrome using intracompartmental pressure testing.

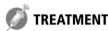

TREATMENT

GENERAL MEASURES

- Activity modification with a gradual return to training based on improvement of symptoms
- Running on flat and firm surfaces can help minimize pain.
- Patients should maintain fitness with low-impact activities such as swimming and cycling.
- Continue activity modification until pain free on ambulation.

MEDICATION

- Analgesia with acetaminophen or other oral nonsteroidal anti-inflammatory agent
- Cryotherapy (ice massage) is also advised to relieve acute-phase symptoms (4)[C].

ADDITIONAL THERAPIES

- Orthotics may be beneficial.
- Calf stretch, peroneal stretch, TheraBand exercises, and eccentric calf raises may improve endurance and strength (5)[A].
- Compression stockings have been used to treat MTSS with mixed results.
- Structured running programs with warm-up exercises have not been demonstrated to reduce pain in young athletes (6)[B].
- CAM boot for people with significant pain with weight-bearing

SURGERY/OTHER PROCEDURES

- Surgical intervention includes a posterior medial fascial release in individuals with both
  - Severe limitation of physical activity and
  - Failure of 6 months of conservative treatment
    - Counsel patients that complete return of activity to sport may not be always achieved postoperatively. Surgical risks include infection and hematoma formation.
- Extracorporeal shock wave therapy (ESWT) may decrease recovery time when added to a running program (5)[A].

COMPLEMENTARY & ALTERNATIVE MEDICINE

- Individualized polyurethane orthoses may help chronic running injuries.
- Special insoles, low-energy laser treatment, pulsed electromagnetic field, and knee braces have not been shown to improve outcomes (5)[A].
- Ultrasound, acupuncture, aquatic therapy, electrical stimulation, whirlpool baths, cast immobilization, taping, and steroid injection may help improve pain.
- Physical therapy approaches including Kinesio tape and fascial distortion massage may yield quicker return to activity.
- Osteopathic manipulative treatment may yield quicker return to athletic/activity as well.

ONGOING CARE

FOLLOW-UP RECOMMENDATIONS
Patient Monitoring

- Once well, recommend gradual return to preinjury running pace.
- Maintain stretching and strengthening exercises.
- Identify and correct preinjury training errors.
- Good supportive footwear is recommended as is replacing running shoes every 350 to 450 miles.
- Allow a gradual return to activity dictated by symptoms (pain).

PROGNOSIS

The condition is usually self-limiting, and most patients respond well with rest and nonsurgical intervention.

COMPLICATIONS

- Stress fractures and compartment syndrome
- Undiagnosed MTSS or chronic exertional compartment syndrome can lead to a complete fracture or tissue necrosis, respectively.

REFERENCES

1. Fullem BW. Overuse lower extremity injuries in sports. *Clin Podiatr Med Surg.* 2015;32(2):239–251.
2. Hutchinson M. Chronic exertional compartment syndrome. *Br J Sports Med.* 2011;45(12):952–953.
3. Chang GH, Paz DA, Dwek JR, et al. Lower extremity overuse injuries in pediatric athletes: clinical presentation, imaging findings, and treatment. *Clin Imaging.* 2013;37(5):836–846.
4. Fields KB, Sykes JC, Walker KM, et al. Prevention of running injuries. *Curr Sports Med Rep.* 2010;9(3):176–182.
5. Winters M, Eskes M, Weir A, et al. Treatment of medial tibial stress syndrome: a systematic review. *Sports Med.* 2013;43(12):1315–1333.
6. Moen MH, Holtslag L, Bakker E, et al. The treatment of medial tibial stress syndrome in athletes; a randomized clinical trial. *Sports Med Arthrosc Rehabil Ther Technol.* 2012;4:12.

ADDITIONAL READING

- Abelson B. The tibialis anterior stretch–kinetic health. https://www.youtube.com/watch?v=iaA5PT85azU. Accessed June 19, 2014.
- Hamstra-Wright KL, Bliven KCH, Bay C. Risk factors for medial tibial stress syndrome in physically active individuals such as runners and military personnel: a systematic review and meta-analysis. *Br J Sports Med.* 2015;49(6):362–369.
- Reshef N, Guelich DR. Medial tibial stress syndrome. *Clin Sports Med.* 2012;31(2):273–290.
- Yeung SS, Yeung EW, Gillespie LD. Interventions for preventing lower limb soft-tissue running injuries. *Cochrane Database Syst Rev.* 2011;(7):CD001256.

CODES

ICD10

- S86.899A Other injury of other muscle(s) and tendon(s) at lower leg level, unspecified leg, initial encounter
- S86.891A Other injury of other muscle(s) and tendon(s) at lower leg level, right leg, initial encounter
- S86.892A Other injury of other muscle(s) and tendon(s) at lower leg level, left leg, initial encounter

CLINICAL PEARLS

- MTSS is the preferred term for "shin splints."
- Diagnosis is based on a reliable history of repetitive overuse accompanied by characteristic shin pain; imaging only if strong suspicion for stress fracture
- MTSS pain is typically along the middle and distal 3rd of the posteromedial tibial surface, worsened with activity and relieved with rest.
- Treatment includes ice, activity modification, analgesics, eccentric stretching, gait retraining, and a gradual return to activity.
- Symptoms recur if return to activity is "too much too fast."

M

MEDICAL MARIJUANA

Teresa Bormann, MD

 BASICS

Medical marijuana or medical cannabis refers to the use of pharmacologic agents derived from the flowering plant genus Cannabis to treat disease or alleviate symptoms.

DESCRIPTION

- Marijuana plants contain >100 phytocannabinoids.
- Phytocannabinoids are naturally occurring molecules with an affinity for the mammalian cannabinoid receptors.
- The main cannabinoids are Δ-9-tetrahydrocannabinol (THC) and cannabidiol (CBD). Most of the psychoactive properties come from THC.
- Cannabis interacts with the endocannabinoid system (ECS) in our bodies. The ECS plays critical roles in body homeostasis.
- The ECS has two main receptors:
  - CB1—highly expressed in the central nervous system
  - CB2—expressed in the periphery including the immune system
  - Our body synthesizes two endogenous cannabinoids: N-arachidonoylethanolamine (anandamide) and 2-arachidonoylglycerol. Both are agonists at the cannabinoid receptors.
- Routes of external cannabinoid administration include inhalation (smoking and vaporized), oral ingestion of edible products, and topical (oral mucosa or skin).

EPIDEMIOLOGY

- 36 states and 4 territories allow for the medical use of cannabis products, although it remains illegal under federal law.
- 49 countries worldwide have legalized the medical use of cannabis.

Prevalence

Prevalence of medical cannabis in U.S. primary care population is 1–2%.

 TREATMENT

- Conditions that are qualified for medical cannabis varies by state, but most common conditions approved by states include chronic pain, cancer-related weight loss, cancer-related nausea and vomiting, and epilepsy.
- Recent reviews of the literature reveal conclusive or substantial evidence that cannabis or cannabinoids are effective for symptom control in (1)[A]:
  - Chronic pain in adults
  - As antiemetics in chemotherapy-induced nausea and vomiting
  - Improving muscle spasticity syndromes in multiple sclerosis (MS)

- Chronic pain (1)[A]
  - Most common condition cited by patients for medical use of cannabis
  - May benefit in refractory pain, neuropathic pain, and pain associated with cancer. In a recent meta-analysis of 27 randomized trials, there is low-strength evidence that cannabis alleviates neuropathic pain but insufficient evidence in treating other types of pain.
  - Meta-analysis suggests 40% greater improvement in pain with plant-derived cannabinoids compared to placebo.
- Chemotherapy-induced nausea and vomiting
  - Conclusive evidence suggests that oral THC preparations are associated with improvements in nausea and vomiting due to chemotherapy (dronabinol and nabiximols) (2)[A].
  - Despite abundant anecdotal evidence of the benefits of plant based and inhaled preparations for nausea and vomiting, there are no good randomized trials examining this option.
- MS muscle spasticity
  - Substantial evidence that oral cannabinoids are an effective treatment of patient-reported spasticity symptoms but not clinician-measured spasticity (1)[A]
- Anorexia or cachexia due to HIV/AIDS or cancer
  - Low-quality evidence showed some weight gain on dronabinol, although the effect was similar to megestrol (2)[A].
  - Studies done in the 1980s that showed that inhaled cannabis increased caloric intake by 40% have not been replicated due to the difficulties in investigating the cannabis plant (3)[A].
- Posttraumatic stress disorder (PTSD)
  - Single small crossover trial suggests potential benefit from oral cannabinoid, Nabilone. This contrasts with nonrandomized trials that showed worsened symptoms of PTSD on plant-based medical cannabis (3)[A].
- Seizures (3)[B]
  - Insufficient evidence to support or refute cannabis as an effective treatment of epilepsy
  - In 2018, FDA approved cannabinoid oral solution (Epidiolex) for treatment of seizures related to two rare conditions: Lennox-Gastaut syndrome and Dravet syndrome.
- Others
  - Limited evidence for cannabis use in acute pain, glaucoma, other neurologic conditions: tremor, Tourette syndrome, Huntington disease, and inflammation

GENERAL MEASURES

- States with medical cannabis laws:
  - May require a registry of patients
  - May require patients to carry an ID card
  - May require provider education on the risks and benefits of medical cannabis
- For non–FDA-approved medical cannabis: Certifying providers do not prescribe medical cannabis but only certify the qualifying condition according to state laws.

MEDICATION

FDA-approved medical cannabis products:

- Dronabinol (Marinol [capsule] and Syndros [oral solution]). Synthetic THC. Indications include the following:
  - Refractory chemotherapy-induced nausea and vomiting
  - Anorexia resulting in weight loss in patients with AIDS
- Nabilone (Cesamet): a capsule; synthetic cannabinoid
  - Indications above as dronabinol
- Cannabidiol (Epidiolex): oral solution
  - Lennox-Gastaut syndrome and Dravet syndrome
- Nabiximols (Sativex): an oromucosal spray containing THC and CBD in 1:1 ratio; investigational in the United States
  - Used for treating spasticity in MS, cancer-related pain, and neuropathic pain

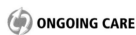 **ONGOING CARE**

Pediatric Considerations

- Between 2000 and 2013, annual rate of poison center calls related to cannabis exposures among children younger than 6 years was 2.82 times higher in states that had legalized medical cannabis compared to those that had not legalized medical cannabis.
- Pediatric cannabis exposure is associated with potentially serious symptoms:
  - Respiratory depression or failure
  - Tachycardia
  - Temporary coma
- Adolescents have increased vulnerability to adverse long-term outcomes (4)[C].
- Brain ECS actively develops during adolescence.
- Initial use during adolescence is associated with long-term brain changes:
  - Increased school dropout
  - Lower IQ
  - Diminished life satisfaction

Pregnancy and Lactation Considerations

- The data on marijuana use during pregnancy is heavily confounded by tobacco use and socioeconomic factors, but concern for impaired fetal neurodevelopment should be as high as for tobacco use or alcohol use during pregnancy.
- There are no pregnancy indications for medical cannabis.
- Pregnancy women should be discouraged from using medical cannabis in any form, around conception, during pregnancy, and throughout breastfeeding.
- There are insufficient data to evaluate the effects of marijuana use (nonmedical or medical) on infants during lactation and breastfeeding. American College of Obstetricians and Gynecologists (ACOG) has recommended that marijuana use be discouraged for breastfeeding mothers.

COMPLICATIONS

- Any data on complications of marijuana use is in reference to nonmedical use. There is no data on complications of medical cannabis use. If the route of medical cannabis dosing is inhalation, some inferences could be made because most studies are done in populations of nonmedical cannabis smokers.
- Short-term complications
  - Intoxication and withdrawal
    - Intoxication may cause:
      - Acute physiologic effects including conjunctival injection, orthostatic hypotension, tachycardia, dry mouth, and poor motor coordination
      - Acute psychologic effects relaxation, euphoria, altered sensory perception
    - Withdrawal may cause (mainly psychological symptoms), irritability, depression, restlessness, insomnia, and less likely physiologic symptoms of GI distress, hypertension, chills, diaphoresis.
  - Increased motor vehicle accidents, relative risk (RR) = 2, compared to RR = 5 for blood alcohol level >.08
  - Driving under the influence of cannabis as confirmed by presence of THC metabolite, was associated with a 20–30% higher odds of having a motor vehicle accident.
- Long-term complications
  - Respiratory (4)[C]
    - Substantial evidence of worsened respiratory symptoms and more frequent bronchitis in regular cannabis smokers
    - Overall acute cannabis smoking is associated with bronchodilation, but any benefit is offset by chronic use.

- Several studies noted increased FVC in regular cannabis smokers, which is of unclear significance.
- With limited data, it is unclear if there is an association between regular cannabis use and increased risk of developing COPD. Certainly regular cannabis smoking is less significant than regular tobacco smoking in development of COPD.
- Cardiovascular risk
  - Limited data to support increased risk of cannabis triggering an acute MI with case study of 9 patients with RR of 3.2
  - A retrospective cohort study showed an RR of acute MI in current users of marijuana as 1.1.
  - Limited quality data that shows small insignificant increase risk of stroke with current use of cannabis
- Cancer risk
  - Limited quality evidence that shows no statistical evidence of association between cannabis smoking and incidence of lung cancer
  - Recent cohort studies did not find any association between cannabis use and head and neck cancers.
  - Limited quality evidence that shows possible association between chronic cannabis smoking and nonseminoma-type testicular germ cell tumors
  - Insufficient evidence to support or refute an association between cannabis smoking and esophageal cancer
  - Insufficient evidence to support or refute association between cannabis smoking and prostate cancer, cervical cancer, malignant gliomas, non-Hodgkin lymphoma, penile cancer, anal cancer, Kaposi sarcoma, or bladder cancer
- Psychological (4)[C]
  - Increased anxiety, psychosis, and depression (noncausal association)
  - Increased risk of schizophrenia in early chronic users
  - Based on data for nonmedical users of cannabis, addiction occurs in 9% of all users, with higher rates among adolescents (17%) and daily users (20–25%). There are no studies that examine the risk of addiction with medical cannabis.
  - Interference with cognitive function and short-term memory results in difficulty learning
  - "Gateway drug" phenomenon persists even in states where marijuana use is legal.
    - Concurrent use primes brain for enhanced response to other drug
  - Marijuana reduces dopamine activity in reward centers, increasing susceptibility to drug abuse.
- Gastrointestinal
  - Cannabis-induced hyperemesis syndrome
  - Cannabis use has been associated with hepatotoxicity.

REFERENCES

1. Ebbert JO, Scharf EL, Hurt RT. Medical cannabis. *Mayo Clin Proc*. 2018;93(12):1842–1847.
2. Whiting PF, Wolff RF, Deshpande S, et al. Cannabinoids for medical use: a systematic review and meta-analysis. *JAMA*. 2015;313(24):2456–2473.
3. National Academies of Sciences, Engineering, and Medicine. *The Health Effects of Cannabis and Cannabinoids: The Current State of Evidence and Recommendations for Research*. Washington, DC: National Academies Press; 2017.
4. Gloss D, Vickrey B. Cannabinoids for epilepsy. *Cochrane Database Syst Rev*. 2014;2014(3):CD009270.

ADDITIONAL READING

- American College of Obstetricians and Gynecologists Committee on Obstetric Practice. Committee Opinion No. 637: marijuana use during pregnancy and lactation. *Obstet Gynecol*. 2015;126(1):234–238.
- Khalsa JH, Bunt GC, Galanter M, et al. Medicinal uses of cannabis and cannabinoids. In: Miller SC, Fiellin DA, Rosenthal RN, et al, eds. *The ASAM Principles of Addiction Medicine*. 6th ed. Philadelphia, PA: Wolters Kluwer; 2019:1742–1750.
- Matson TE, Carrell DS, Bobb JF, et al. Prevalence of medical cannabis use and associated health conditions documented in electronic health records among primary care patients in Washington State. *JAMA Netw Open*. 2021;4(5):e219375.
- National Conference of State Legislatures. State medical marijuana laws. https://ncsl.org/research/health/state-medical-marijuana-laws.aspx.
- Noel W, Wang J. *Is Cannabis a Gateway Drug? Key Findings and Literature Review*. Washington, DC: U.S. National Institute of Justice; 2018.

 ## CODES

ICD10

F12.90 Cannabis use, unspecified, uncomplicated

CLINICAL PEARLS

- The clinical evidence supporting benefits of medical cannabis are lacking. Current evidence shows modest benefit in a limited number of conditions.
- In adults with chemotherapy-induced nausea and vomiting, oral cannabinoids are effective antiemetics.
- Medical cannabis may be a useful adjunctive chronic pain medication in selected patients.

M

MELANOMA
Lloyd A. Runser, MD, MPH, FAAFP • Mary E. Cox, DO

BASICS

DESCRIPTION
- Melanoma is a tumor arising from malignant transformation of pigment-containing cells called melanocytes, which are found in the stratum basale of the epidermis.
  - Most arise in the skin but may also present as a primary lesion in any tissue: ocular (uvea), GI, GU, lymph node, paranasal sinuses, nasal cavity, anorectal mucosa, and leptomeninges.
  - Extracutaneous sites have an adverse prognosis.
  - Metastatic spread to any site in the body
- Types of invasive cutaneous melanomas include the following:
  - Superficial-spreading melanoma: approximately 70% of cases; occurs in sun-exposed areas (trunk, back, and extremities); most <1 mm thick at diagnosis; when seen in younger patients, presents as a flat, slow growing, irregularly bordered lesion
  - Nodular: 15–30% of cases; present in older patients; tendency to ulcerate and hemorrhage; most commonly thick and pigmented; most common melanoma >2 mm
  - Lentigo maligna (subtype of melanoma in situ): slowest growing; older population; occurs in sun-exposed areas (head, neck, forearms). Lentigo maligna melanoma (LMM) is its invasive counterpart seen in 10–15% of cases; it is most commonly seen in elderly patients most often in the head and neck regions.
  - Acral lentiginous: <5% of all melanomas; however, most common melanoma in black or Asian patients; found in palmar, plantar, and subungual areas; can mimic other skin abnormalities, including warts, calluses, tinea pedis, or ingrown toenails
    - An important subtype of acral lentiginous melanoma is subungual melanoma. From the nail matrix, presents as dark stripe under the nail plate; Hutchinson nail sign when brown or black pigment extends from the nail to the cuticle and proximal or lateral nail folds
  - Amelanotic melanoma: <5% of cases; can be missed and diagnosed at a later stage because it can mimic benign skin conditions, and thus is referred to as a "great pretender"
  - Desmoplastic melanoma: ~1% of cases; "neurotropic melanoma" or "spindled melanoma" with an abundance of fibrous tissue; demonstrates sarcoma-like tendencies with increased hematogenous spread; presents as a slow-growing lesion that is scar-like (no history of injury at the site is noted); often seen in the head and neck
- System(s) affected: skin/exocrine

Geriatric Considerations
Lentigo maligna is most common in elderly patients. This type is usually found on the face, beginning as a circumscribed macular patch of mottled pigmentation showing shades of dark brown, tan, or black.

Pediatric Considerations
Large congenital nevi (>5 cm) are risk factors and have a >2% lifetime risk of malignant conversion. Blistering sunburns in childhood significantly increase risk.

Pregnancy Considerations
No increased risk of melanoma in pregnancy. In the case of recent melanoma treatment, it is recommended to wait 1 to 2 years prior to becoming pregnant because melanoma can spread to the placenta.

EPIDEMIOLOGY

Incidence
- In 2020, 100,350 Americans are estimated to be newly diagnosed with melanoma, with approximately 6,850 expected deaths (1).
- Predominant age: median age at diagnosis 65 years (https://www.cancer.gov/)
- Predominant sex: male > female (1.5 times)
- Melanoma is >20 times more common in whites than in African Americans (1).
- Minority groups demonstrate increased rates of metastasis, advanced stages at diagnosis, thicker initial lesions, earlier age at diagnosis, and overall poorer outcomes.
- Low socioeconomic status associated with higher incidence of melanoma

Prevalence
- Melanoma is the fifth most common type of cancer in the United States
- Lifetime risk: men: 1/28; female: 1/4 1 (1)
- 1.2% of all cancer deaths (1)

ETIOLOGY AND PATHOPHYSIOLOGY
- DNA damage by UVA/UVB exposure
- Tumor progression: initially may be confined to epidermis with lateral growth, may then grow into dermis with vertical growth

Genetics
- Dysplastic nevus syndrome is a risk factor for development of melanoma. Close surveillance is warranted.
- 8–12% of patients with melanoma have a family history of disease.
- Mutations in *BRAF (V600E)* implicated in 50–60% of cutaneous melanomas
- Familial atypical mole malignant melanoma (FAMMM) syndrome characterized by >50 atypical moles, +FH of melanoma, clinical diagnosis (2)

RISK FACTORS
- Genetic predisposition, personal/family history of melanoma
- UVA and UVB exposure
- History of >5 sunburns during lifetime, blistering sunburns in childhood
- Previous pigmented lesions (especially dysplastic melanocytic nevi)
- Fair complexion, freckling, blue eyes, blond/red hair
- Highest predictor of risk is increased number of nevi (>50).
- 70% of melanomas are de novo, not existing from previous nevi (2)
- Tanning bed use: 75% increased risk if first exposure before age 35 years
- Changing nevus (see "ABCDE" criteria)
- Large (>5 cm) congenital nevi
- Chronic immunosuppression (chronic lymphocytic leukemia, non-Hodgkin lymphoma, AIDS, or posttransplant)
- Living at high altitude (>700 meters or 2,300 feet above sea level)
- Occupational exposure to ionizing radiation

GENERAL PREVENTION
- Avoidance of sunburns, especially in childhood. Seek shade and avoid midday sun.
- Use of broad-spectrum sunscreen with at least SPF 30 to all skin exposed to sunlight reapplying regularly and after toweling or swimming
- Avoid tanning beds; class 1 carcinogen by World Health Organization (WHO)

- Screening of high-risk individuals, especially males >50 years
- Education for proper diagnosis plays a large factor in prevention.
- Any suspicious lesions should be biopsied with a narrow excision with 1- to 3-mm margins that encompass the entire breadth plus sufficient depth of the lesion. Options include elliptical excisions, punch, or deep shave biopsies.

COMMONLY ASSOCIATED CONDITIONS
- Dysplastic nevus syndrome
- >50 nevi. These individuals have higher lifetime risk of melanoma than the general population because 30% of all melanoma arise in preexisting nevi.
- Giant congenital nevus: 6% lifetime incidence of melanoma
- Xeroderma pigmentosum is a rare condition associated with an extremely high risk of skin cancers, including melanoma.
- Psoriasis after psoralen-UV-A (PUVA) therapy

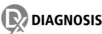

DIAGNOSIS

HISTORY
- Change in a pigmented lesion: either hypo- or hyperpigmentation, bleeding, scaling, ulceration, or changes in size or texture
- Obtain family and personal history of melanoma or nonmelanoma skin cancer.
- Obtain social history including occupation, sunbathing, tanning, and other sun exposure.

PHYSICAL EXAM
- ABCDE: Asymmetry, Border irregularity, Color variegation (especially red, white, black, blue), Diameter >6 mm, Evolution over time
- Any new and/or changing nevus, bleeding/ulcerated
- Location on Caucasians is primarily back and lower leg; on African Americans, it is the hands, feet, and nails.
- May include mucosal surfaces (nasopharynx, conjunctiva)
- Individuals at high risk for melanoma should have careful ocular exam to assess for presence of melanoma in the iris and retina.

DIFFERENTIAL DIAGNOSIS
- Dysplastic and blue nevi
- Vascular skin tumor
- Pigmented actinic keratosis
- Traumatic hematoma
- Pigmented basal cell carcinomas, seborrheic keratoses, other changing nevi
- Common or atypical melanocytic nevi
- Lentigo
- Pyogenic granuloma

DIAGNOSTIC TESTS & INTERPRETATION
- Lactate dehydrogenase (LDH), chest/abdomen/pelvic CT with or without PET/CT at baseline and in monitoring progression in metastatic disease (stage IV); brain MRI if any CNS symptoms or physical findings
- Imaging studies only helpful in detecting and evaluating for progression of metastatic disease

Diagnostic Procedures/Other
- Dermoscopy allows for magnification of lesions; evidence limited on utility (2)[C]
- Full-thickness excisional biopsy remains the gold standard for diagnosis. Any suspicious nevus should be excised, either by elliptical excision, punch biopsy,

or a scoop shave (saucerization) biopsy . Avoid superficial shave of suspicious lesion. Goal for full-thickness excision with 1- to 3-mm margins. Orient excisional biopsy to optimize future treatment.
- Sentinel lymph node biopsy, a staging procedure, remains an important factor for prognosis.

Test Interpretation
- Nodular melanoma is primarily vertical growth, whereas the other three types are horizontal.
- Estimated that 1/10,000 dysplastic nevi become melanoma annually.
- Immunohistochemical testing increases sensitivity of lymph node biopsies.
- Staging is based on the tumor-node-metastasis (TNM) criteria by current American Joint Committee on Cancer (AJCC) criteria, including:
  – (T) thickness (mm) and ulceration
  – (N) number of regional lymph nodes involved
  – (M) distant metastases and serum LDH
  – See https://www.cancer.org/cancer/melanoma-skin-cancer/detection-diagnosis-staging/melanoma-skin-cancer-stages.html for more information.

 ## TREATMENT

GENERAL MEASURES
Full surgical excision of melanoma is the standard of care and primary treatment recommended for resectable/nonmetastatic melanomas. See below for recommended surgical margins.
- For stages I and II, surgical excision is curative in most cases

MEDICATION
- Treatment within the context of a clinical trial always recommended
- FDA-approved medication for unresectable or metastatic melanoma include the following:
  – Anti PD-1 monotherapy
    ○ Pembrolizumab (Keytruda)
    ○ Nivolumab (Opdivo)
    ○ Nivolumab with ipilimumab
      ■ Combo therapy demonstrated 61% response versus ipilimumab alone.
  – If BRAF V600 activating mutation is present, can opt for target therapy with combinations of:
    ○ Dabrafenib/trametinib
    ○ Vemurafenib/cobimetinib + atezolizumab (new FDA approval)
    ○ Encorafenib/binimetinib
- Adjuvant medical therapy for certain high-risk patients after undergoing complete surgical excision with lymph node involvement or metastasis
  – Stage IIIA with sentinel lymph node metastases
    ○ Pembrolizumab (Keytruda)
    ○ Dabrafenib/trametinib for BRAF V600-activating mutation
  – Stage IIB/C and IV with nodal recurrence
    ○ Pembrolizumab (Keytruda)
    ○ Nivolumab (Opdivo)
    ○ Dabrafenib/trametinib for BRAF V600-activating mutation
  – Stage IV complete resected
    ○ Nivolumab (Opdivo)
  – Stage IV with nodal recurrence
    ○ Iplimumab recommended only if prior exposure to anti PD-1 therapy
- Additional active regimens (e.g., dacarbazine [DTIC], temozolomide, paclitaxel, carmustine [BCNU], cisplatin, carboplatin, vinblastine) often limited to those who are not candidates to preferred regimens
- Imatinib (Gleevec) in tumors with c-KIT mutation

- Interferon-α as adjuvant therapy received FDA approval in 1995 (high dose) and 2011 (pegylated) to treat stage IIB to III melanoma; shown to improve 4-year relapse rate but no overall effect on survival; 1/3 of patients will discontinue due to toxicity (granulocytopenia, hepatotoxicity).

ISSUES FOR REFERRAL
- Consultation with oncologist for consideration of chemotherapeutic options
- Surgical specialties may be required based on the extent of nodal and/or metastatic disease, if present.

ADDITIONAL THERAPIES
Local therapy for stage III in-transit disease for the patient's when resection not possible, prior resection unsuccessful, or refuse surgery and seek conservative management include intralesional injections, topical imiquimod, laser ablation, and radiation therapy.
- Talimogene laherparepvec (T-VEC) intralesional injection is the recommended option for intralesional injection.
- Other injections include IL-2, BCG, or IFN.

SURGERY/OTHER PROCEDURES
- Standard of care for melanoma includes early surgical excision with the following recommended margins:
  – In situ tumors: 0.5- to 1.0-cm margin
  – Thickness of ≤1 mm (T1): 1-cm margin
  – Thickness of 1.01 to 2.00 mm (T2): 1- to 2-cm margins
  – Thickness of 2 to 4 mm (T3): 2-cm margins
  – Thickness of >4 mm (T4): 2-cm margins
- Sentinel lymph node biopsy is indicated in patients with T1b, T2-, T3-, and T4-staged melanomas.
  – Not recommended in melanoma in situ or T1a
- Mohs micrographic surgery is being increasingly used for melanoma in situ, but in general, it is not considered a treatment modality for melanoma because it relies on frozen section technique.
- Radiotherapy can be used to treat lentigo maligna in addition to certain head and neck lesions.
- Palliative radiation therapy can be used with metastatic melanoma.
- Stage IIIB/C—intralesional injections in certain cases if limited number of in-transit metastasis or not amenable to complete surgical excision

ADMISSION, INPATIENT, AND NURSING CONSIDERATIONS
Most monitoring and treatment completed in the outpatient setting

 ## ONGOING CARE

FOLLOW-UP RECOMMENDATIONS
After diagnosis and treatment, close follow-up and skin protection (i.e., sunblock, UV protective clothing) are highly advised.

Patient Monitoring
- Routine screening clinical skin examination annually for all persons >40 years is controversial and without proven benefit.
- Total body photography and dermoscopy should be used for surveillance of skin lesions, most commonly used for patients with >5 atypical nevi.
- For patients with a history of cutaneous melanoma, NCCN guidelines recommend screening every 3 to 12 months depending on recurrence risk, with annual examinations if there is no disease progression for 5 years.
- Surveillance chest x-ray, CT, brain MRI, and/or PET/CT scan every 3 to 12 months for 3 to 5 years

at discretion of physician with more frequent brain MRI recommended for patients with history of brain metastasis
- Lab and imaging tests after diagnosis and treatment of stage I to II melanoma are low yield, have high false-positive rates, and are not recommended.

PATIENT EDUCATION
- Teach all patients to perform regular full-body skin examinations looking for ABCDEs, especially those at high risk, or who have had melanoma.
- High-risk patients should perform monthly skin self-examinations and be taught to examine inaccessible areas.
- Patients with a history of melanoma or dysplastic nevus syndrome should have regular total body examinations by a dermatologist.

PROGNOSIS
- Breslow depth (thickness) in millimeters remains among strongest predictors of prognosis.
- Median age at death is 70 years.
- Highest survival seen in women <45 years of age at diagnosis
- Metastatic melanoma has an average survival of 6 to 9 months; 15–20% 5-year survival with current treatment
- Stages I and II, appropriately treated, have 20-year survival rates of 90% and 80%, respectively.

COMPLICATIONS
- Metastatic spread and subsequent death
- Often referred to as the "great imitator," given that metastatic disease may present in a variety of ways
- Unsatisfactory cosmetic results

REFERENCES
1. Siegel RL, Miller KD, Jemal A. Cancer statistics, 2020. *CA Cancer J Clin*. 2020;70(1):7–30. doi:10.3322/caac.21590.
2. Swetter SM, Tsao H, Bichakjian CK, et al. Guidelines of care for the management of primary cutaneous melanoma. *J Am Acad Dermatol*. 2019;80(1):208–250.

ADDITIONAL READING
Melanoma Prediction Tools:
http://www.melanomaprognosis.net/

 ## SEE ALSO

Atypical Mole (Dysplastic Nevus) Syndrome

CODES

ICD10
- C43.9 Malignant melanoma of skin, unspecified
- C43.30 Malignant melanoma of unspecified part of face
- C43.4 Malignant melanoma of scalp and neck

CLINICAL PEARLS
- Remember that amelanotic melanomas exist; pigmentation is not required.
- 70% of melanomas are de novo, not from preexisting nevi. Still, any changing nevi should be biopsied, preferably utilizing an excisional method to ensure that complete margins are taken (2).
- The prognosis is excellent with early detection and treatment.

M

MÉNIÈRE DISEASE

Sangili Chandran, MD • Jay B. Shah, DO

 BASICS

- An inner ear (labyrinthine) disorder characterized by recurrent attacks of hearing loss, tinnitus, vertigo, and sensations of aural fullness
- The international diagnostic criteria define Ménière Disease as a condition with at least two spontaneous episodes of vertigo lasting longer than 20 minutes but less than 12 hours, an audiogram showing evidence of low- to medium-frequency sensorineural hearing loss in one ear at any point in time, and fluctuating aural symptoms such as hearing loss, tinnitus, or aural fullness (1).
- Clinically, it involves the triad of:
  - Vertigo lasting 20 minutes to 12 hours
  - Audiometrically documented sensorineural hearing loss (predominantly low frequency)
  - Fluctuating aural symptoms (tinnitus or aural fullness)

DESCRIPTION
- Often unilateral initially; nearly half become bilateral over time.
- Severity and frequency of vertigo may diminish with time, but hearing loss is often progressive and/or fluctuating.
- Usually idiopathic (Ménière disease) but may be secondary to another condition causing endolymphatic hydrops (Ménière syndrome)
- There are 5 clinical subtypes of both unilateral and bilateral disease (1).
  - Type 1: refers to classic unilateral MD and metachronic bilateral MD (symptom onset in one ear followed by the other)
  - Type 2: refers to delayed unilateral MD (hearing loss onset preceding vertigo onset by months or years) or synchronic bilateral MD (simultaneous symptom onset in both ears)
  - Type 3: familial MD (Most families have bilateral hearing loss, but unilateral patient may coexist in the same family.)
  - Type 4: sporadic MD with migraine
  - Type 5: sporadic MD with an autoimmune disease
- System(s) affected: nervous
- Synonym(s): Ménière syndrome; endolymphatic hydrops

EPIDEMIOLOGY
- Predominant age of onset: 40 to 60 years
- Predominant gender: female > male (2:1)
- Race/ethnicity: white, Northern European > blacks

Incidence
Estimates 1 to 150/100,000 per year

Prevalence
Varies from 7.5 to >200/100,000

ETIOLOGY AND PATHOPHYSIOLOGY
- Not fully understood; theories include increased pressure of the endolymph fluid due to increased fluid production or decreased resorption. This may be caused by endolymphatic sac pathology, abnormal development of the vestibular aqueduct, or inflammation caused by circulating immune complexes. Increased endolymph pressure may cause rupture of membranes and changes in endolymphatic ionic gradient.
- Other major theories include vascular compromise, cochlear trauma, and viral infection or reactivation.

- Ménière syndrome may be secondary to injury or other disorders (e.g., reduced middle ear pressure, allergy, endocrine disease, lipid disorders, vascular, viral, syphilis, autoimmune). Any disorder that could cause endolymphatic hydrops could be implicated in Ménière syndrome.

Genetics
Some families show increased incidence, but genetic and environmental influences are incompletely understood.

RISK FACTORS
May include
- Stress
- Allergy
- Increased salt intake
- Caffeine, alcohol, or nicotine
- Chronic exposure to loud noise
- Family history and genetic predisposition is found in 10% of cases with an autosomal dominant inheritance pattern (2).
- Certain vascular abnormalities (including migraines)
- Certain viral exposures (especially herpes simplex virus [HSV])

GENERAL PREVENTION
Reduce known risk factors: stress; salt, alcohol, and caffeine intake; smoking; noise exposure; ototoxic drugs (e.g., aspirin, quinine, aminoglycosides).

COMMONLY ASSOCIATED CONDITIONS
- Anxiety (secondary to the disabling symptoms)
- Migraines
- Hyperprolactinemia
- Hypothyroidism

 DIAGNOSIS

Diagnosis is clinical.

HISTORY
- Symptomatic episodes are typically spontaneous but may be preceded by an aura of increasing fullness in the ear and tinnitus. These may occur in clusters, with long periods of symptom-free remissions.
- Formal criteria for diagnosis from American Academy of Otolaryngology–Head and Neck Surgery:
  - At least two episodes of vertigo >20 minutes in duration (usually described as rotatory spinning or rocking sensations)
  - Tinnitus or aural fullness
  - Hearing loss: Low frequency (sensorineural) is confirmed by audiometric testing.
  - Other causes (e.g., acoustic neuroma) excluded
  - During severe attacks: Pallor, sweating, nausea, vomiting, falling, prostration may occur.

PHYSICAL EXAM
- Physical exam rules out other conditions; no finding is unique to Ménière disease.
- Horizontal nystagmus may be seen during attacks.
- Otoscopy is typically normal.
- Triggering of attacks in the office with Dix-Hallpike maneuver suggests diagnosis of benign paroxysmal positional vertigo (BPPV), not Ménière disease as vertigo is typically of shorter duration and triggered by head movements in BPPV.

DIFFERENTIAL DIAGNOSIS
- Acoustic neuroma or other CNS tumor
- Syphilis
- Endolymphatic sac tumor
- Viral labyrinthitis
- Transient ischemic attack (TIA), migraine
- Vertebrobasilar disease
- Other labyrinthine disorders (e.g., Cogan syndrome, benign positional vertigo, temporal bone trauma)
- Diabetes or thyroid dysfunction
- Vestibular neuronitis
- Medication side effects
- Otitis media

DIAGNOSTIC TESTS & INTERPRETATION
Testing is done to rule out other conditions but does not necessarily confirm or exclude Ménière disease.

Initial Tests (lab, imaging)
- Consider serologic tests specific for *Treponema pallidum* in at-risk populations.
- Thyroid, fasting blood sugar, and lipid studies
- Consider MRI to rule out acoustic neuroma or other CNS pathology, including tumor, aneurysm, and multiple sclerosis (MS).

Diagnostic Procedures/Other
- Auditory
  - Audiometry using pure tone and speech to show low-frequency sensorineural (nerve) loss and impaired speech discrimination; usually shows low-frequency sensorineural hearing loss
  - Tuning fork tests (i.e., Weber and Rinne), ABR, or MRI to rule out acoustic neuroma
  - Electrocochleography may be useful to confirm etiology.
- Vestibular
  - Caloric testing: Reduced activity on either side is consistent with Ménière diagnosis but is not itself diagnostic.
  - Head-impulse testing (3)[C]

Test Interpretation
- Histologic temporal bone analysis (at autopsy); dilation of inner ear fluid system, neuroepithelial damage with hair cell loss, basement membrane thickening, and perivascular microvascular damage
- Cytochemical analysis can reveal altered AQP4 and AQP6 expression in the supporting cell, altered cochlin, and mitochondrial protein expression (4)[B].
- Familial Ménière disease has been associated with DTNA and FAM136A genes (5)[B].

 TREATMENT

- A paucity of evidence-based guidelines exists.
- Medications are primarily for symptomatic relief of vertigo and nausea.
- During attacks, bed rest with eyes closed prevents falls. Attacks rarely last >4 hours.

GENERAL MEASURES
Since Dederding's and Mygind's publications in 1929 and Furstenberg's trial in 1934, the salt restriction diet has remained the primary first-line treatment for MD. Since the 1950s, various publications have both supported and argued this treatment, and the evidence of its validity remains inconclusive (6).

MEDICATION

First Line

- Acute attack: Initial goal is stabilization and symptom relief; for severe episodes
  - Benzodiazepines (such as diazepam): decrease vertigo and anxiety
  - Antihistamines (meclizine/dimenhydrinate): decrease vertigo and nausea
  - Anticholinergics (transdermal scopolamine): reduce nausea and emesis associated with motion sickness
  - Antidopaminergic agents (metoclopramide, promethazine): decrease nausea, anxiety
  - Rehydration therapy and electrolyte replacement
  - Steroid taper for acute hearing loss
- Maintenance (goal is to prevent/reduce attacks)
  - Lifestyle changes (e.g., low-salt diet) are needed.
  - Diuretics may help reduce attacks by decreasing endolymphatic pressure and volume; there is insufficient evidence to recommend routine use:
    ○ Hydrochlorothiazide; hydrochlorothiazide/triamterene (Dyazide, Maxzide)
    ○ Acetazolamide (Diamox)
  - In Europe, betahistine, a weak histamine H1 agonist and a stronger H3 antagonist, is routinely used (unavailable in the United States) (7). Other vasodilators, such as isosorbide dinitrate, niacin, and histamine, have also been used; evidence of their effectiveness is incomplete.
- Contraindications/warnings:
  - Atropine: cardiac disease, especially supraventricular tachycardia and other arrhythmias, prostatic enlargement
  - Scopolamine: children and elderly, prostatic enlargement
  - Diuretics: electrolyte abnormalities, renal disease
- Precautions:
  - Sedating drugs should be used with caution, particularly in the elderly. Patients are cautioned not to operate motor vehicles or machinery. Atropine and scopolamine should be used with particular caution.
  - Diuretics: Monitor electrolytes.
- Significant possible interactions: transdermal scopolamine: anticholinergics, antihistamines, tricyclic antidepressants, other

Second Line

- Steroids, both intratympanic and systemic (PO or IV), have been used for longer treatment of hearing loss:
  - Addition of prednisone 30 mg/day to diuretic treatment reduced severity and frequency of tinnitus and vertigo in one pilot study.
  - Dexamethasone is practical to use due to better tolerance by patients, as methylprednisone creates burning sensation in the middle ear mucosa.
- Evidence is lacking for routine use of Famvir; may improve hearing more than balance

ISSUES FOR REFERRAL

- Consider ear, nose, throat/neurology referral.
- Patients should have formal audiometry to confirm hearing loss.

ADDITIONAL THERAPIES

- Application of intermittent pressures via a myringotomy using a Meniett device has been shown to relieve vertigo (8)[B]:
  - Safe; requires a long-term tympanostomy tube

- Vestibular rehabilitation may be beneficial for patients with persistent vestibular symptoms
  - Safe and effective for unilateral vestibular dysfunction
  - International consensus on treatment of MD suggests that vestibular rehabilitation should be offered as treatment option for patients between vertigo crises (9).

SURGERY/OTHER PROCEDURES

- Interventions that preserve hearing:
  - Endolymphatic sac surgery shown to be effective in controlling vertigo in 75% of patients with Ménière disease who failed medical therapy
  - Vestibular nerve section (intracranial procedure)
    ○ More invasive
    ○ Decreases vertigo and preserves hearing
    ○ Tympanostomy tube: may decrease symptoms by decreasing the middle ear pressure
- Interventions for patients with no serviceable hearing:
  - Labyrinthectomy: very effective at controlling vertigo but causes deafness
  - Vestibular neurectomy
  - Endoscopic vestibular nerve section
  - Cochlear implantation

COMPLEMENTARY & ALTERNATIVE MEDICINE

Insufficient evidence to support effectiveness, but many integrative techniques have been tried, including:

- Acupuncture, acupressure, tai chi
- Niacin, bioflavonoids, Lipo-flavonoid, ginger, *Ginkgo biloba*, and other herbal supplements

 ONGOING CARE

FOLLOW-UP RECOMMENDATIONS

Patient Monitoring

Due to the possibility of progressive hearing loss despite decrease in vertiginous attacks, it is important to monitor changes in hearing and to monitor for more serious underlying causes (e.g., acoustic neuroma).

DIET

Diet is usually not a factor, unless attacks are brought on by certain foods.

PROGNOSIS

- Alert patients about the nature of alternating attacks and remission.
- Between attacks, patient may be fully active but is often limited due to fear or lingering symptoms. This can be severely disabling.
- 50% resolve spontaneously within 2 to 3 years.
- Some cases last >20 years.
- Severity and frequency of attacks diminish, but hearing loss is often progressive.
- 90% can be treated successfully with medication; 5–10% of patients require surgery for incapacitating vertigo.

COMPLICATIONS

Loss of hearing; injury during attack; inability to work

REFERENCES

1. Borowiec E, Crossley J, Hoa M. Understanding fluctuating hearing loss. *Hear J.* 2020;73(6):12–13.
2. Perez-Carpena P, Lopez-Escamez JA. Current understanding and clinical management of Ménière's disease: a systematic review. *Semin Neurol.* 2020;40(1):138–150.
3. Lee SU, Kim HJ, Koo JW, et al. Comparison of caloric and head-impulse tests during the attacks of Meniere's disease. *Laryngoscope.* 2017;127(3):702–708.
4. Ishiyama G, Lopez IA, Sepahdari AR, et al. Meniere's disease: histopathology, cytochemistry, and imaging. *Ann N Y Acad Sci.* 2015;1343:49–57.
5. Frejo L, Giegling I, Teggi R, et al. Genetics of vestibular disorders: pathophysiological insights. *J Neurol.* 2016;263(Suppl 1):S45–S53.
6. Shim T, Strum DP, Mudry A, et al. Hold the salt: history of salt restriction as a first-line therapy for Meniere's disease. *Otol Neurotol.* 2020;41(6):855–859.
7. Casani AP, Guidetti G, Schoenhuber R; for Consensus Conference Group. Report from a Consensus Conference on the treatment of Ménière's disease with betahistine: rationale, methodology and results. *Acta Otorhinolaryngol Ital.* 2018;38(5):460–467.
8. Ahsan SF, Standring R, Wang Y. Systematic review and meta-analysis of Meniett therapy for Meniere's disease. *Laryngoscope.* 2015;125(1):203–208.
9. Dunlap PM, Holmberg JM, Whitney SL. Vestibular rehabilitation: advances in peripheral and central vestibular disorders. *Curr Opin Neurol.* 2019;32(1):137–144.

 SEE ALSO

- Hearing Loss; Labyrinthitis; Tinnitus
- Algorithm: Dizziness

 CODES

ICD10

- H81.03 Ménière's disease, bilateral
- H81.09 Ménière's disease, unspecified ear
- H81.0 Ménière's disease

CLINICAL PEARLS

- Ménière disease is characterized by vertigo (lasting 20 minutes to 12 hours), with associated hearing loss, tinnitus +/− aural fullness.
- There is a wide differential diagnosis for Ménière disease; therefore, one must fully investigate symptoms.
- Multiple medical, surgical, and rehabilitative treatments are available to decrease the severity and frequency of attacks.

M

MENINGITIS, BACTERIAL

Felix B. Chang, MD, DABMA, ABIHM, ABIM

BASICS

DESCRIPTION
Bacterial infection of the meninges resulting in inflammation, pain, and systemic illness

EPIDEMIOLOGY
Predominant age: neonates, infants, and elderly; predominant sex: male = female

Incidence
Varies by age and pathogen
- 18 to 34 years: 0.66/100,000. 35 to 49 years: 0.95/100,000. 50 to 64 years: 1.73/100,000. ≥65 years: 1.92/100,000
- Group B *Streptococcus*: 0.25/100,000. *Neisseria meningitidis*: 0.19/100,00
- *Haemophilus influenzae type B*: 0.08/100,000. *Listeria monocytogenes*: 0.05/100,000

Prevalence
15,000 to 25,000 cases occur annually in United States.

ETIOLOGY AND PATHOPHYSIOLOGY
Community-acquired bacterial meningitis is most commonly due to *Streptococcus pneumoniae* (50%) and *N. meningitidis* (30%). Nosocomial or postsurgical meningitis occurs after manipulation of the central nervous system (CNS) space allowing for entry of pathogens. Newborns (<2 months): Group B *Streptococcus, Escherichia coli, L. monocytogenes.* Infants and children: *S. pneumoniae, N. meningitidis, H. influenzae.* Adolescents and young adults: *N. meningitidis, S. pneumoniae.* Immunocompromised adults: *S. pneumoniae, L. monocytogenes,* gram-negative bacilli such as *Pseudomonas aeruginosa.* Mixed bacterial infection in <1% of cases. Older adults: *S. pneumoniae* 50%, *N. meningitidis* 30%, *L. monocytogenes* 5%. 10% gram-negatives bacilli: *E. coli, Klebsiella, Enterobacter, P. aeruginosa*

Genetics
Some Native American populations appear to have genetic or acquired susceptibility to invasive disease.

RISK FACTORS
- Household or close contacts of case patients. Immunocompromised, alcoholism, diabetes, chronic disease. Neurosurgical procedure/head injury, close living quarters. Neonates: prematurity, low birth weight, premature rupture of membranes, maternal peripartum infection, and urinary tract abnormalities. Abnormal communication between nasopharynx and subarachnoid space (congenital, trauma), dural fistula. Parameningeal source: otitis, sinusitis, mastoiditis; trauma: skull fracture. Adults age >65 years, immunocompromised patients, and pregnant women are at risk for listeriosis; complement component deficiencies C3, C5 to C9, properdin, factor H, and factor D
- HIV infection. Functional or anatomic asplenia. Patients taking eculizumab and ravulizumab are at increased risk for meningococcal disease; microbiologists who are routinely exposed to isolates of *N. meningitidis*
- Military recruits, young college students living in crowded residence halls

GENERAL PREVENTION
- Consider CSF fistula in cases of recurrent meningitis; aseptic techniques for head wounds or skull fractures

- Meningitis caused by *H. influenzae* type B has decreased 55% with routine vaccination. Conjugate vaccines against *S. pneumoniae* may reduce the burden of disease in childhood; chemoprophylaxis for close contacts of meningococcal meningitis patients

COMMONLY ASSOCIATED CONDITIONS
Factors associated with a worse prognosis: alcoholism, old age, infancy, diabetes mellitus, multiple myeloma, head trauma, seizures, immunocompromised, coma, sepsis, sinusitis

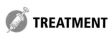

DIAGNOSIS

HISTORY
- Antecedent upper respiratory infection; fever, headache, vomiting, photophobia; seizures, confusion
- Nausea, rigors, sweats, weakness. Elderly: subtle findings including confusion
- Infants: irritability, lethargy, poor feeding. Altered mental status; food exposures (e.g., *L. monocytogenes*)

PHYSICAL EXAM
- The triad of fever, neck stiffness, and altered mental status has low sensitivity (44%).
- 95% of patients present with at least two of the following: headache, fever, neck stiffness, and altered mental status.
  - Meningismus; focal neurologic deficits. Meningococcal rash: macular and erythematous at first, then petechial or purpuric. Purpura fulminans (suspect meningococcus). Papilledema. Brudzinski sign: Passive flexion of neck elicits involuntary flexing of knees in supine position. Kernig sign: resistance or pain with passive knee extension following 90-degree hip flexion in supine position. Late signs and symptoms: hemiparesis, stroke, cognitive impairment, coma, epilepsy, hearing loss, permanent visual impairment

DIFFERENTIAL DIAGNOSIS
- Bacteremia, sepsis, brain abscess. Seizures, other nonbacterial meningitides; aseptic meningitis
- Inflammatory noninfectious: Behçet disease, systemic lupus erythematosus (SLE), sarcoidosis, migraine
- Stroke. Viral meningitis, Lyme disease, leptospirosis. Subarachnoid hemorrhage; central nervous vasculitides

DIAGNOSTIC TESTS & INTERPRETATION
Initial Tests (lab, imaging)
- Prompt lumbar puncture (1)[A]
  - Head CT first if focal neurologic findings, papilledema, or altered mentation. CSF appearance: turbid; CSF Gram stain and cultures
  - Adults: >500 cells/mL WBCs, glucose <40 mg/dL, <2/3 blood-to-glucose ratio, CSF protein >200 mg/dL
    - CSF opening pressure >30 cm. Suspect ruptured brain abscess when WBC count is unusually high (>100,000); polymerase chain reaction (PCR) of CSF (particularly in suspected viral meningitis)
- Reserve bacterial antigen tests for cases where initial CSF Gram stain is negative and CSF culture is negative at 48 hours.
- Serum blood cultures, serum electrolytes. Evaluate clotting function if petechiae or purpura is present. Chest radiograph may reveal pneumonitis or abscess. C-reactive protein (CRP): Normal CRP has high negative predictive value.

- Later in course, head CT if hydrocephalus, brain abscess, subdural effusions, and subdural empyema are suspected or if no clinical response after 48 hours of appropriate antibiotics. Lactate concentration not recommended for suspected community-acquired bacterial meningitis. Elevated CSF protein concentration plus hypoglycorrhachia suggest ventriculitis or meningitis.

Follow-Up Tests & Special Considerations
Consider initiation of empiric antibiotics once the blood cultures are drawn if lumbar puncture is delayed.

Diagnostic Procedures/Other
Lumbar puncture
- Noncontrast head CT is recommended prior to lumbar puncture to assess the risk of herniation if the patient is immunocompromised, has papilledema, a history of CNS disease, focal neurologic deficit on exam, visual field cut, new-onset seizure 1 week or less prior to presentation, or an abnormal level of consciousness.
- Lumbar puncture contraindications: signs of increased intracranial pressure (decerebrate posturing, papilledema), skin infection at site of lumbar puncture, CT or MRI evidence of obstructive hydrocephalus, cerebral edema, herniation
- Symptoms of infection plus positive CSF culture and CSF pleocytosis indicate ventriculitis or meningitis.

Test Interpretation
Bacterial meningitis: opening pressure >180 mm $H_2$0; CSF protein, usually high; CSF glucose, usually low; cell counts >1×10^9/L.

TREATMENT

GENERAL MEASURES
Initiate empiric antibiotic therapy immediately after lumbar puncture (lumbar puncture > Abx). If head CT scan is needed, initiate antibiotic therapy immediately after blood cultures (Abx > CT > lumbar puncture) (1)[A]. Watch for seizures and aspiration precautions.

MEDICATION
Empiric antibiotic IV therapy with dexamethasone for known or suspected *S. pneumoniae* meningitis) until culture results are available (1)[A].

First Line
- Neonates: ampicillin: 150 mg/kg/day divided q8h and cefotaxime: 150 mg/kg/day divided q8h
- Infants >4 weeks of age: ceftriaxone: 100 mg/kg/day divided q12–24h or cefotaxime 225 to 300 mg/kg/day divided q6–8h and vancomycin: 60 mg/kg/day divided q6h
- Adults (1)[A]
  - Immunocompetent: cefotaxime: 2 g IV q4–6h or ceftriaxone: 2 g IV q12h.
    - In countries with ceftriaxone resistance rates >1%, vancomycin 15 to 20 mg/kg IV q8–12h (target level 15 to 20 μg/mL), plus in adults >50 years of age, ampicillin 2 g IV q4h
  - Immunocompromised: vancomycin 15 to 20 mg/kg IV q8–12h, plus ampicillin 2 g IV q4h, plus either cefepime 2 g IV q8h or meropenem 2 g IV q8h (If meropenem is used, ampicillin is not required.)

– >50 years, add ampicillin: 2 g IV q4h for *Listeria* plus either cefotaxime: 2 g IV q4–6h or ceftriaxone: 2 g IV q12h or meropenem 2 g IV q8h (ampicillin not needed). If *Listeria* is identified as the causative agent, the regimen should be modified to include ampicillin or penicillin in combination with gentamicin.

– Penicillin-allergic patients:
  ○ Without severe *β*-lactam allergy: Meropenem should be use instead of ceftriaxone in patients with mild hives to a cephalosporin without other signs of anaphylaxis.
  ○ Severe allergy: vancomycin: loading dose 25 to 30 mg/kg IV and then 15 to 20 mg/kg q8–12h (goal trough of 15 to 20) plus moxifloxacin 400 mg IV once daily

- Treatment duration: *S. pneumoniae*: 10 to 14 days (2)[A]
  – *N. meningitidis*, *H. influenzae*: 7 to 10 days. Group B *Streptococcus* organisms, *E. coli*, *L. monocytogenes*: 14 to 21 days. Neonates: 12 to 21 days or at least 14 days after a repeated culture is sterile
  – No reliable evidence to support the use preadmission antibiotics for suspected cases of nonsevere meningococcal disease

- Corticosteroids pediatrics: Corticosteroids are associated with lower rates of hearing loss and neurologic sequelae.
  – Early treatment with dexamethasone (0.15 mg/kg IV q6h for 2 to 4 days) decreases mortality and morbidity for patients >1 month of age with acute bacterial meningitis with no increased risk of GI bleeding.
  – Adults: Initiate in adults and continue only if CSF Gram stain shows gram-positive diplococcus or if blood or CSF positive for *S. pneumoniae*.
    ○ Associated with increased recurrence of fever (RR 1.27, 95% CI 1.09–1.47); decreased mortality in *S. pneumoniae* (RR 0.8, 95% CI 0.20–0.59) but not in *H. influenzae* or *N. meningitidis* (2)[A]
    ○ Lower rates of severe hearing loss (RR 0.67, 95% CI 0.51–0.88), any hearing loss (RR 0.74, 95% CI 0.63–0.87), and neurologic sequelae (RR 0.83, 95% CI 0.69–1.00). Nonsignificant reduction in mortality (RR 0.90, 95% CI 0.53–1.05); *p* value = .009
  – Dexamethasone: 0.15 mg/kg IV q6h (start 15 to 20 minutes before or with antibiotic) for 2 to 4 days. Dexamethasone should only be continued if the CSF Gram stain and/or CSF or blood culture reveal *S. pneumoniae*.

Second Line
Antipseudomonal penicillins should be given in combination with other appropriate agents.

- Aztreonam 2 g IV q6–8h. Fluoroquinolones (e.g., ciprofloxacin) IV 400 mg q8–12h; meropenem IV 2 g q8h

ISSUES FOR REFERRAL
Consultation from infectious disease and/or critical care specialist

ADDITIONAL THERAPIES
Chemoprophylaxis in close contacts include household members, roommates, intimate contacts, contacts at a childcare center, young adults exposed in dormitories, military recruits exposed in training centers. Travelers who had direct contact with respiratory secretions from an index patient or who were seated directly next to an index patient on a prolonged flight (≥8 hours); individuals exposed to oral secretions from an index patient

SURGERY/OTHER PROCEDURES
Postsurgical bacterial meningitis or associated with head trauma or shunt: empiric cover for MRSA and aerobic gram-negative organisms, such as *Pseudomonas* spp., and Enterobacteriaceae (3)[A]

ADMISSION, INPATIENT, AND NURSING CONSIDERATIONS
- Bacterial meningitis requires hospitalization. ICU monitoring may be needed. Patients with suspected meningococcal infection require respiratory isolation for 24 hours.
- Droplet precautions of hospitalized patients as soon as diagnosis is suspected through the first 24 hours of antimicrobial therapy.

 ONGOING CARE

FOLLOW-UP RECOMMENDATIONS
Patient Monitoring
- Brainstem auditory—evoked response hearing test for infants before hospital discharge
- Vaccinations
  – **Meningococcal vaccination:**
    ○ All 11 to 12 years old should get a MenACWY vaccine, with a booster dose at 16 years old. Teens and young adult (16 through 23 years old) also may get a MenB vaccine. CDC also recommends meningococcal vaccination for other children and adults who are at increased risk for meningococcal disease.
    ○ CDC recommends routine MenACWY vaccination for: all preteens and teens at 11 to 12 years old with a booster dose at 16 years old, children and adults at increase risk for meningococcal disease
    ○ Routine MenB vaccination for: people 10 years or older at increased risk for meningococcal disease
  – Pneumococcal vaccination:
    ○ PCV13: Infants and young children usually need 4 doses of pneumococcal conjugate vaccine, at 2, 4, 6, and 12 to 15 months of age. In some cases, a child might need fewer than 4 doses to complete PCV13 vaccination. A dose of PCV13 is also recommended for anyone ≥2 years with certain medical conditions if they did not already receive PCV13. This vaccine may be given to adults ≥65 years based on discussions between the patient and health care provider.
    ○ Per CDC, PPSV23 for all adults ≥65 years. People 2 through 64 years old with certain medical conditions; adults 19 to 64 years old who smoke cigarettes
- Prophylaxis: During 2019 to 2020, 11 meningococcal isolates from U.S. patients had mutations conferring penicillin resistance and also ciprofloxacin resistance.
  – Most isolates in the United States are susceptible to recommended antibiotics.
  – Rifampin: 600 mg PO BID for 2 days; ciprofloxacin: 500 mg PO for 1 dose; ceftriaxone: 250 mg IM for 1 dose; azithromycin 500 mg PO single dose for ciprofloxacin-resistance *N. meningitidis* exposure (not first agent); chemoprophylaxis for close contacts of patients with confirmed meningococcal meningitis

DIET
Regular, as tolerated, except with syndrome of inappropriate secretion of antidiuretic hormone

PROGNOSIS
- Mortality: *S. pneumoniae* meningitis 19–37%; meningococcal meningitis: 5%
- Deaths associated with *N. meningitidis* usually occur within 12 to 24 hours of the first symptoms. Mortality rate of untreated disease approaches 100%.

COMPLICATIONS
- Up to 50% develop long-term neurologic complications (cognitive impairment) after pneumococcal meningitis
- Seizures: 20–30% focal neurologic deficit. 15–20% cerebrovascular complications: subdural effusion or empyema, septic sinus thrombosis, intracraneal hypertension, cerebral edema, temporal lobe or cerebellar herniation, hydrocephalus
- Cranial nerve palsies (III, VI, VII, VIII) in 10–20% of cases; usually transient. Sensorineural hearing loss: 10% in children. Permanent visual impairment. Neurodevelopmental sequelae: 30% with subtle learning deficits
- Obstructive hydrocephalus, subdural effusion; syndrome of inappropriate secretion of antidiuretic hormone (SIADH)
- Elevated intracranial pressure: herniation, brain swelling; purpura fulminans, septic shock
- Meningococcal-induced microvascular thrombosis and DIC; depression, subarachnoid bleed, stroke

REFERENCES
1. Mount HR, Boyle SD. Aseptic and bacterial meningitis: evaluation, treatment, and prevention. *Am Fam Physician*. 2017;96(5):314–322.
2. Tunkel AR, Hartman BJ, Kaplan SL, et al. Practice guidelines for the management of bacterial meningitis. *Clin Infect Dis*. 2004;39(9):1267–1284.
3. Tunkel AR, Hasbun R, Bhimraj A, et al. 2017 Infectious Diseases Society of America's clinical practice guidelines for healthcare-associated ventriculitis and meningitis. *Clin Infect Dis*. 2017;64(6):e34–e65.

ADDITIONAL READING
- Mbaeyi SA, Bozio CH, Duffy J, et al. Meningococcal vaccination: recommendations of the Advisory Committee on Immunization Practices, United States, 2020. *MMWR Recomm Rep*. 2020;69(9):1–41.
- Roberts L. Plan aims to slash toll from bacterial meningitis. *Science*. 2021;374(6564):140–141.
- van de Beek D, Cabellos C, Dzupova O, et al. ESCMID guideline: diagnosis and treatment of acute bacterial meningitis. *Clin Microbiol Infect*. 2016;22 Suppl 3:S37–S62.

CODES

ICD10
- G00.9 Bacterial meningitis, unspecified
- G00.2 Streptococcal meningitis
- G00.8 Other bacterial meningitis

CLINICAL PEARLS
- Monitor prophylaxis failures and antimicrobial resistance among meningococcal isolates to inform prophylaxis recommendations.
- Empirical therapy for suspected meningococcal disease should include an extended-spectrum cephalosporin, such as cefotaxime or ceftriaxone. Once microbiologic diagnosis is established, definitive treatment with penicillin G, ampicillin, or an extended-spectrum cephalosporin (cefotaxime or ceftriaxone) is recommended.

M

MENINGITIS, VIRAL

Zoe Foster, MD, FAAFP • Jesse Miller, MD

BASICS

DESCRIPTION
- A clinical syndrome characterized by fever with signs/symptoms of acute meningeal inflammation (including but not limited to headache, photophobia, neck stiffness, and/or nausea/vomiting)
- Viral meningitis (VM) is the most common cause of aseptic (nonbacterial) meningitis.
- System(s) affected: nervous

EPIDEMIOLOGY
Incidence
- Estimated 75,000 VM cases caused by enterovirus annually in the United States
- Most common form of meningitis
- Peaks summer to fall in temperate climates (but is year round in subtropical or tropical climates)
  - Nonpolio enteroviruses are the most common cause of viral meningitis.

ETIOLOGY AND PATHOPHYSIOLOGY
- In immunocompetent hosts, VM is a rare complication of an acute viral infection like gastroenteritis, mumps, HSV, VZV, and arthropod-borne viruses.
  - Case reports in the literature indicate that SARS-CoV-2 can also cause VM as a rare complication.
  - In immunocompromised hosts, viral pathogens may also include CMV and EBV.
- 23–61% of VM cases are caused by nonpolio human enteroviruses. These viruses are typically transmitted via the fecal-oral route.
- Mosquito-borne viruses include West Nile, Zika, chikungunya, dengue, St. Louis encephalitis virus, and Eastern equine encephalitis virus. Tick-borne viruses include Powassan virus, Colorado tick fever virus, tick-borne encephalitis virus.
- Recurrent benign lymphocytic (Mollaret) meningitis is generally associated with HSV-2 (80% of cases).

Genetics
None identified

RISK FACTORS
- Close contacts of people with VM are unlikely to get VM but may get the primary viral syndrome.
- Age (most common in children <5 years)
  - Babies <1 month of age are more likely to have severe disease.
- Immunocompromised host (patients more susceptible to CMV, HSV, and EBV)

Geriatric Considerations
Cases of VM in the elderly are rare (most common cause is VZV, HSV); consider alternative diagnoses (e.g., cancer, medication-induced aseptic meningitis).

GENERAL PREVENTION
- Practice hand washing and general hygiene procedures.
- Avoid sharing drinks/cups and silverware with others, especially those who are ill.
- Avoid exposure to mosquitos and ticks; if outdoors, recommend use of appropriate clothing, DEET, and mosquito nets.

COMMONLY ASSOCIATED CONDITIONS
Encephalitis; myopericarditis; neonatal enteroviral sepsis; meningoencephalitis; flaccid paralysis

DIAGNOSIS

HISTORY
- Predominant adult symptoms include acute onset (hours to days) of:
  - Fever (incidence varies by virus; 65–83% in enterovirus, 54–98% in mumps, 6–52% in HSV) (1)[C]
  - Headache (prominent early symptom)
  - Photophobia (mainly with enterovirus, 79–85% of cases; 33–64% in HSV; 7% in mumps) (1)[C]
  - Myalgias/arthralgias (88% in enterovirus; 50% in HSV; 14–21% in mumps) (1)[C]
  - Nausea/vomiting, malaise
  - Nuchal rigidity (55–69% in enterovirus; 22–71% in HSV; 8–85% in mumps) (1)
    - Altered mental status, seizure, or focal neurologic deficits should prompt consideration of alternative diagnoses.
- In infants, nonspecific symptoms are more common, including poor feeding, vomiting, lethargy, fever (most common), and irritability (most common) (2)[B].
- Additional historical elements:
  - Travel history and outdoor activities
  - Sexual history (e.g., HSV, HIV)
  - Immunocompromised host, including solid-organ transplant and HIV (CMV, HSV, adenovirus)
  - History of VZV infection
  - Immunization status (mumps, influenza, VZV)

PHYSICAL EXAM
- Vital signs: fever, tachycardia, tachypnea, hypotension
- Neurologic:
  - Lack of mental status changes (if present, consider alternative diagnoses)
  - Photophobia
  - Meningeal signs
    - Nuchal rigidity
    - Brudzinski sign (neck flexion elicits involuntary hip and knee flexion in supine patient) and Kernig sign (resistance to knee extension following flexion of hips to 90 degrees) are poorly sensitive (~5%) in patients with meningitis (1)[C]
    - Jolt accentuation test: rapid horizontal rotation of the head accentuates headache (of questionable utility in diagnosis of meningitis given low sensitivity and specificity) (1)[C],(3)[C]
  - Asymmetric flaccid paralysis is seen in West Nile virus infection (1)[C].
- HEENT:
  - Parotitis (in mumps infection)
  - Herpangina (coxsackievirus A)
  - Bulging fontanelle (in infants)
  - Generalized lymphadenopathy (EBV, HIV)
- Dermatology:
  - Vesicular rash of hand, foot, and mouth disease (coxsackievirus)
  - Generalized maculopapular rash
    - Presence of a palpable petechial/purpuric rash should prompt consideration of bacterial meningitis
- Abdomen:
  - Splenomegaly (in EBV)
  - Abdominal pain

DIFFERENTIAL DIAGNOSIS
- Bacterial meningitis (BM)
- Fungal meningitis (consider if immunocompromised; agents include *Coccidioides* and *Cryptococcus neoformans*) (4)[C]
- Other infectious agents include tuberculosis, syphilis, leptospirosis, Lyme disease, ehrlichiosis, amebiasis (4)[C].
- Parameningeal infections (e.g., subdural empyema)
- Encephalitis
- Postinfectious encephalomyelitis
- Viral syndrome (e.g., influenza)
- Leukemia, lymphoma, or other neoplastic disease (including metastasis) (5)[C]
- Migraine/tension headache
- Acute metabolic encephalopathy
- Postoperative aseptic meningitis
- Drug-induced (chemical) meningitis (NSAIDs, TMP/SMX, amoxicillin, TNF-α inhibitors, lamotrigine, IVIG, and monoclonal antibodies) (1)[C]
- Brain/epidural abscess
- Inflammatory disorders (e.g., Behçet, sarcoidosis, SLE) (1)[C]

DIAGNOSTIC TESTS & INTERPRETATION
Initial Tests (lab, imaging)
- Serum labs: CBC, BMP, procalcitonin/C-reactive protein, blood cultures (4)[C]
  - CBC: normal or mildly elevated WBC
  - BMP: CSF glucose levels should be compared to plasma levels.
  - Procalcitonin/C-reactive protein: should be normal in VM (consider bacterial meningitis in adults when serum PCT is elevated)
  - Blood cultures: should be negative in VM
- Lumbar puncture (5)[C]:
  - LP is the essential diagnostic tool in the differentiation between VM and BM
    - Do not delay empiric antibiotics if there is concern for bacterial meningitis
    - Consider use of a validated clinical decision-making tool, like the Bacterial Meningitis Score (BMS) in children to calculate risk of bacterial meningitis.
  - Contraindications/risks:
    - Signs/symptoms of increased intracranial pressure (focal neurologic findings, papilledema, altered mental status, new-onset seizure), impaired cellular immunity, local infection over potential LP site, suspected epidural abscess, use of anticoagulation or potential coagulopathy, and possibility of cardiorespiratory compromise due to patient positioning during procedure
      - Consider CT if clinical concern for increased intracranial pressure.
    - Procedural risks include cerebral herniation, post-LP headache, bleeding, infection, and pain.

– CSF analysis:
  ○ Opening pressure: should be normal
  ○ Cell count/differential:
    ▪ 100–1,000 WBC/μL (can be higher in entero-viral meningitis)
    ▪ Lymphocyte predominance (in early infection, may be PMN predominance)
    ▪ RBCs suggest traumatic tap but may be seen in HSV meningitis/encephalitis
  ○ CSF glucose: usually normal (may have mild decrease in mumps or HIV)
  ○ CSF protein: normal to mildly elevated
  ○ CSF lactate: normal (if elevated >4.2 mmol/L, highly suggestive of bacterial meningitis; differential diagnosis also includes TB, seizures, hemorrhage, and ischemia if elevated; lactate levels less reliable if antibiotics have been started prior to LP)
- Gram stain: should be negative for bacteria
- CSF culture:
  – Gold standard for diagnosis of bacterial meningitis
  – Should be negative for bacterial pathogens in VM
- PCR/NAAT (4)[C]:
  – Becoming more commonplace with improving sensitivities/specificities
  – Subject to institutional availability
  – Useful for rapid identification of multiple possible pathogens (bacteria, viruses, fungi)—sensitivity for pathogens varies by test
  – May allow early discontinuation of empiric therapies
- CSF IgM antibodies for arboviruses (1)[C]

Follow-Up Tests & Special Considerations
Disorders that may alter lab results:
- Diabetes: Consider current blood sugar level to correlate with CSF glucose level (5)[C].
- Neurologic diseases (e.g., history of stroke or transient ischemic attack, intracranial neoplasm, demyelinating disease) (5)[C]

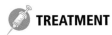

TREATMENT

GENERAL MEASURES
Management includes supportive care (e.g., pain control, IV fluids) and low threshold for empiric antibiotics for BM pending laboratory results (1),(3)[C].

MEDICATION
First Line
- Antipyretics/analgesics (Adult doses are presented; titrate doses to pain relief.)
  – Acetaminophen (Tylenol) 500 to 1,000 mg PO q8h; 325 to 650 mg PR q4–6h (limit 3 g/24 hr)
  – Ibuprofen 400 to 800 mg PO q8h
  – Naproxen 550 mg PO BID
  – Consider short-term opioids if pain uncontrolled.
- Antiemetics
  – Ondansetron (Zofran) 4 to 8 mg IV q8h
  – Promethazine (Phenergan) 12.5 to 25 mg PO/PR/IM/IV q4–6h (Consider maximum dose of 50 mg/24 hr to limit side effects.)

- Antiviral agents (1),(3)[C]
  – Empiric acyclovir at 10 mg/kg IV q8h (adult dose) for patients with CSF pleocytosis, negative Gram stain, and suspicion for HSV while awaiting results of definitive (e.g., HSV or VZV PCR) testing
    ○ Immunocompetent patients with HSV meningitis improve with or without antiviral therapy and can be treated with supportive care alone.
- Antibiotics (targeted to most likely pathogen)
  – Not indicated for treatment of VM
  – Empiric treatment reasonable while ruling out BM. Initiate following blood cultures and LP if possible. Consider especially in elderly, those pretreated with antibiotics, ill-appearing, and immunocompromised patients (1),(3)[C].
    ○ If very low risk for BM, treat symptomatically and observe in the inpatient setting pending laboratory results.
- Corticosteroids (1),(3)[C]
  – Not recommended in VM (recommended as adjunctive treatment in BM)

ISSUES FOR REFERRAL
For patients with known CSF shunts/drains, recent neurosurgery/trauma, or intrathecal pumps in the setting of possible VM or BM, an emergent neurosurgical referral is warranted (4)[C].

ADMISSION, INPATIENT, AND NURSING CONSIDERATIONS
- Initial inpatient management includes:
  – Pain management and empiric therapies (pending lab results)
  – IV fluids (based on hydration status and clinical presentation)
  – Neurologic monitoring for changes in mental status, fever, neck stiffness, headache
  – Contact precautions and private room until BM ruled out
- Discharge depends on clinical parameters (dehydration, emesis, pain control, functional level, social circumstances, and ability to follow up). VM in stable patients can be managed in the outpatient setting (3)[C].

ONGOING CARE

FOLLOW-UP RECOMMENDATIONS
- Close follow-up to ensure resolution of all symptoms.
  – A small portion of adult patients suffer from ongoing neuropsychological morbidities following VM, with the degree of disability dependent on the causative virus.
- Developmental surveillance after VM in children as children are more likely to have severe complications of disease.

Patient Monitoring
- Monitor for relapse or exacerbation of symptoms.
- Monitor for neurologic complications:
  – Seizures, altered mental status, new onset weakness
  – Assess ability to have companion monitor change in mental/neurologic status if patient discharged.

DIET
Push fluids. Diet as tolerated

PATIENT EDUCATION
- Discuss very low probability of transmission to close contacts. Encourage hand washing.
- Recurrence of headache, myalgia, and weakness is possible over 2 to 3 weeks.

PROGNOSIS
- Recovery generally within 7 to 10 days
  – In some patients, return to work may be delayed and quality of life may take months to return to baseline, as headaches and other neurologic symptoms may intermittently persist for weeks to months.
- There is a low mortality rate from VM.
- Very young children and some adults suffer from prolonged neuropsychological disabilities as a result of VM.

COMPLICATIONS
- Common: fatigue, irritability, muscle weakness
- Rare: neuropsychological problems and developmental delay

REFERENCES
1. Wright WF, Pinto CN, Palisoc K, et al. Viral (aseptic) meningitis: a review. J Neurol Sci. 2019;398:176–183.
2. Hudson JA, Broad J, Martin NG, et al. Outcomes beyond hospital discharge in infants and children with viral meningitis: a systematic review. Rev Med Virol. 2020;30(2):e2083.
3. Kohil A, Jemmieh S, Smatti MK, et al. Viral meningitis: an overview. Arch Virol. 2021;166(2):335–345.
4. Poplin V, Boulware DR, Bahr NC. Methods for rapid diagnosis of meningitis etiology in adults. Biomark Med. 2020;14(6):459–479.
5. Shahan B, Choi EY, Nieves G. Cerebrospinal fluid analysis. Am Fam Physician. 2021;103(7):422–428.

 SEE ALSO

Meningitis, Bacterial

CODES

ICD10
- A87.9 Viral meningitis, unspecified
- A87.1 Adenoviral meningitis
- A87.0 Enteroviral meningitis

CLINICAL PEARLS
- VM often cannot be reliably distinguished from BM based on clinical findings alone.
- Hospitalize potential cases of BM for evaluation and treatment with broad-spectrum antibiotics until BM has been ruled out.
- VM is more common than BM, especially when vaccination rates are high.
- Morbidity and mortality with VM is low

M

MENINGOCOCCAL DISEASE

Han Q. Bui, MD, MPH

BASICS

DESCRIPTION
- Meningococcemia is a blood-borne infection caused by *Neisseria meningitidis*.
- Bacteremia without meningitis: Patient is acutely ill and may have skin manifestations (rashes, petechiae, and ecchymosis) and hypotension.
- Bacteremia with meningitis: sudden onset of fever, nausea, vomiting, headache, decreased ability to concentrate, and myalgias
- Disease progresses rapidly (within hours).
- Skin findings and hypotension may be present.
  - A petechial rash appears as discrete lesions 1 to 2 mm in diameter; most frequently on the trunk and lower portions of the body; seen in >50% of patients on presentation
  - Purpura fulminans is a severe complication of meningococcal disease and occurs in up to 25% of cases. It is characterized by acute onset of cutaneous hemorrhage and necrosis due to vascular thrombosis and disseminated intravascular coagulopathy.

EPIDEMIOLOGY
Incidence
- The mortality rate is ~13%.
  - 11–19% of survivors suffer serious sequelae, including deafness, neurologic deficits, or limb loss due to peripheral ischemia.
- Disease is seasonal, peaks in December/January.
- Atypical clinical presentations include abdominal symptoms, septic arthritis, and bacteremic pneumonia.
- Peak incidence occurs in the first year of life; 35–40% of cases occur in children <5. A second peak occurs in adolescence.
- In 2017 (most recent CDC data), there were <350 cases of reported meningococcal disease (incidence rate of 0.18 cases per 100,000 persons) (1).
  - Most common in adolescents and young adults, followed by infants <1 year

ETIOLOGY AND PATHOPHYSIOLOGY
- *N. meningitidis* is a fastidious, aerobic, gram-negative diplococcus with at least 13 serotypes.
- *N. meningitidis* has an outer coat that produces disease-causing endotoxin. Bacterial virulence factors promote invasive disease.
- Humans are the only known reservoir for *N. meningitidis*.
- Major serogroups in the United States are B, C, Y, and W-135.
  - Serogroup B is the predominant cause of meningococcemia in children <1 year.
  - Serogroup C is the most common cause of meningococcal disease in the United States.
  - Serogroup Y is the predominant cause of meningococcemia in the elderly (2).
- Major serogroups worldwide are A, B, C, Y, and W-135.
  - W-135 is the major cause of disease in the "meningitis belt" of sub-Saharan Africa.

Genetics
Late complement component deficiency has an autosomal recessive inheritance.

RISK FACTORS
- Age: 3 months to 1 year
- Late complement component deficiency (C5, C6, C7, C8, or C9)
- Asplenia (1)

- Living in close quarters (e.g., household contacts, nursery/daycare, dormitories, military barracks)
- Exposure to active (and/or) passive tobacco smoke (1)

GENERAL PREVENTION
- Two vaccines are currently licensed for use in the United States. Each contains antigens to serogroups A, C, Y, and W-135. Neither provides immunity against serotype B, which is responsible for 1/3 of U.S. cases (3).
  - Meningococcal polysaccharide vaccine (MPSV-4): recommended for patients ≥55 years at elevated risk (1)
    - Short duration of protection: 1 to 3 years for patients age <5 years; 3 to 5 years for adolescents and adults (3)
    - Often used for patients requiring short duration of protection—traveling to endemic areas, college freshmen, community outbreaks (3)
  - Meningococcal conjugate vaccine (MCV-4; MenACWY) (1):
    - Routine immunization recommended for all children 11 to 18 years
    - Immunization recommended for those 2 to 55 years with increased risk for meningococcal disease
    - Guillain-Barré syndrome has been associated with the MCV-4 vaccine; therefore, a personal history of Guillain-Barré is a relative contraindication for this vaccine.
- The FDA has licensed two serogroup B meningococcal (MenB) vaccines. The first (MenB-FHbp) is a 3-dose series. The second (MenB-4C) is a 2-dose series. Both vaccines were approved for use in persons aged 10 to 25 years. Individuals aged ≥10 years who are at increased risk for meningococcal disease due to persistent complement component deficiencies, anatomic or functional asplenia, should receive MenB vaccine (3).
- Protective levels of antibody are achieved ~7 to 10 days after primary immunization (2).
- CDC international travel advisory
  - Vaccine is required by the government of Saudi Arabia for Hajj pilgrims >2 years of age.
  - The vaccine should be given to travelers to sub-Saharan Africa ("meningitis belt").

DIAGNOSIS

HISTORY
Symptoms
- Sudden onset of fever, nausea, vomiting, headache, myalgias, chills, rigor, and/or sore throat (nonsuppurative)
  - Pharyngitis may be mistaken for streptococcal disease (strep throat).
  - Myalgia may be mistaken for severe "flu," which also has a peak incidence in winter.
- Changes in mental status, decreased ability to concentrate, stiff neck, convulsions
- Assess possible exposures.
- Other

PHYSICAL EXAM
- Fever, hypotension, tachycardia
- Neurologic: nuchal rigidity, focal neurologic findings, coma, seizure
  - Focal neurologic findings and seizures are more commonly seen with *Haemophilus influenzae* or *Streptococcus pneumoniae*.
- Cardiopulmonary: signs of heart failure with pulmonary edema—gallop, rales

- Dermatologic: maculopapular rash, petechiae, ecchymosis, purpura
- Onset of specific meningitis symptoms (e.g., neck stiffness, photophobia, bulging fontanelle) can occur within 12 to 15 hours (4).
- Late signs of meningitis (e.g., unconsciousness, delirium, or seizures) occur after ~15 hours in infants <1 year and after ~24 hours in older children.

DIFFERENTIAL DIAGNOSIS
- Sepsis; bacterial meningitis (other organisms)
- Gonococcemia
- Acute bacterial endocarditis
- Rocky Mountain spotted fever
- Hemolytic uremic syndrome
- Gonococcal arthritis dermatitis syndrome
- Influenza

DIAGNOSTIC TESTS & INTERPRETATION

> **ALERT**
> - Isolation of *N. meningitidis* from a sterile site (blood or CSF) is the gold standard for diagnosing systemic meningococcal infection.
> - Antibiotic administration may render blood and/or CSF culture negative within 2 hours.

Initial Tests (lab, imaging)
- Definitive diagnosis is through culture (blood, CSF, or other sterile site).
- CBC with differential
  - Leukocytosis (left shift; toxic granulation) or leukopenia, thrombocytopenia
- Lactic acidosis
- Procalcitonin; often elevated in bacterial meningitis (5)
- Coagulation studies
  - Prolonged prothrombin time/partial thromboplastin time
  - Low fibrinogen
  - Elevated fibrin degradation products
- Blood culture
  - Blood culture positive for *N. meningitidis*
  - Cultures positive in 50–60% of cases
- CSF
  - Grossly cloudy
  - Increased WBCs with polymorphonuclear predominance
  - Gram stain showing gram-negative diplococci
  - Glucose-to-blood glucose ratio <0.4
  - Protein >45 mg/dL
  - Positive for *N. meningitidis* antigen (MAT or PCR)
  - CSF culture positive in 80–90% of cases
- Head CT prior to lumbar puncture (LP) if concern for space-occupying lesions or if focal findings on neurologic examination

Test Interpretation
- Disseminated intravascular coagulation (DIC)
- Meningeal exudates
- Polymorphonuclear infiltration of meninges
- Hemorrhage of adrenal glands

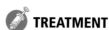

TREATMENT

MEDICATION
First Line
- Antibiotics (5)[A]
  - Begin treatment as soon as meningococcal meningitis is suspected.

– Age guides empiric treatment.
  ○ Preterm to <1 month: ampicillin plus cefotaxime or ampicillin plus gentamicin
    ▪ Cefotaxime
      □ 0 to 7 days: 50 mg/kg q12h
      □ 8 to 28 days: 50 mg/kg q8h
    ▪ Ampicillin
      □ >2,000 g
        ● 0 to 7 days: 50 mg/kg q8h
        ● 8 to 28 days: 50 mg/kg q6h
      □ <2,000 g
        ● 0 to 7 days: 50 mg/kg q12h
        ● 8 to 28 days: 50 mg/kg q8h
  ○ 1 month to 50 years: cefotaxime or ceftriaxone plus vancomycin
    ▪ If severe penicillin allergy: chloramphenicol plus trimethoprim-sulfamethoxazole (TMP-SMX) plus vancomycin
  ○ >50 years of age or patients with significant comorbidity, alcohol abuse, or impaired immunity: ampicillin plus ceftriaxone plus vancomycin
    ▪ Ampicillin: 2 g IV q4h
    ▪ Ceftriaxone: 2 g IV q12h
    ▪ Vancomycin: 30 to 45 mg/kg/day IV divided q6h
    ▪ If severe penicillin allergy: TMP-SMX plus vancomycin
– Penicillin G
  ○ Effective if the isolate is penicillin-sensitive (minimum inhibitory concentration [MIC] <0.1 μg/mL)
  ○ Penicillin can be used if the isolate has a penicillin MIC of <0.1 μg/mL.
  ○ For isolates with a penicillin MIC of 0.1 to 1.0 μg/mL, a 3rd-generation cephalosporin is preferred.
  ○ Penicillin G: 4 million units IV q4h (pediatric dose: 0.25 mU/kg/day IV divided q4–6h) *OR* ampicillin: 2 g IV q4h (pediatric dose: 200 to 300 mg/kg/day IV divided q6h)
  ○ Duration of treatment: 7 days (4)
• Dexamethasone
  – Indications
    ○ Known or suspected pneumococcal meningitis in selected adults
    ○ Children with *H. influenzae* type B meningitis
  – Dexamethasone is often given initially in adults and children with suspected bacterial meningitis while awaiting microbiologic study results.
  – Dexamethasone has not been shown to be of benefit in meningococcal meningitis and should be discontinued once the diagnosis is established.
  – Dosage
    ○ Infants and children >6 weeks: IV 0.15 mg/kg/dose q6h for the first 2 to 4 days of antibiotic treatment
    ○ Start 10 to 20 minutes before or with the first dose of antibiotic.
• Chemoprophylaxis
  – Indications
    ○ Close contacts: those with prolonged (>8 hours) close contact (<3 feet) to the patient or those directly exposed to the patient's oral secretions between 1 week before the onset of the patient's symptoms and until 24 hours after initiation of appropriate antibiotic therapy (2)
      ▪ Examples: household members; close contacts in nursery, daycare centers, nursing homes, dormitories, military barracks, correctional facilities, and other closed institutional settings
    ○ No chemoprophylaxis is indicated for casual contacts, including most health care workers, unless exposed to respiratory secretions.

– Timing
  ○ Ideally <24 hours after case identification
  ○ Chemoprophylaxis should not be administered if >14 days since exposure.
– Prophylactic regimens. Ciprofloxacin-resistant, β-lactamase-producing *N. meningitidis* serogroup Y cases are on the rise in the United States (1), the CDC recommends considering antimicrobial susceptibility testing on meningococcal isolates to inform prophylaxis decisions if there has been a case of meningococcal disease caused by ciprofloxacin-resistant strains in that state within the past 2 years.
  ○ Rifampin, ciprofloxacin, and ceftriaxone
    ▪ Ceftriaxone
      □ Recommended for pregnant women
      □ Adults: 250 mg IM as a single dose; <15 years of age: 125 mg IM as a single dose
    ▪ Rifampin (meningococcal prophylaxis)
      □ Adult: 600 mg IV or PO q12h for 2 days
      □ Pediatric
        ● <1 month: 10 mg/kg/day in divided doses q12h for 2 days
        ● Infants and children: 20 mg/kg/day in divided doses q12h for 2 days (max 600 mg/dose)
    ▪ Ciprofloxacin
      □ Adults: 500 mg PO as a single dose
• Vaccination
  – For household contacts (if the case is from a vaccine-preventable serogroup)
• Precautions
  – Adjust the dosage of medications in patients with severe renal dysfunction.

Second Line
• For meningitis
  – Chloramphenicol: 1 g IV q6h (pediatric dose: 75 to 100 mg/kg/day divided q6h) or ceftriaxone 2 g IV q12h (pediatric dose: 80 to 100 mg/kg/day divided q12–24h)
  – In large outbreaks, a single dose of long-acting chloramphenicol has been used. Single-dose ceftriaxone shows equal efficacy in one randomized controlled trial.
• Precautions
  – Ceftriaxone should not be used in patients with a history of anaphylactic reactions to penicillin (e.g., hypotension, laryngeal edema, wheezing, hives).
  – Chloramphenicol may cause aplastic anemia.

ISSUES FOR REFERRAL
Potential complications
• Seizure activity
• DIC
• Acute respiratory distress syndrome
• Renal failure
• Adrenal failure
• Multisystem organ failure

ADMISSION, INPATIENT, AND NURSING CONSIDERATIONS
• Begin antibiotics (± corticosteroids) and obtain LP immediately if meningitis is suspected.
• Droplet isolation for 24 hours after starting antibiotics
• IV fluids: Replace volume as needed; with septic shock, large volumes of crystalloid may be required.

ONGOING CARE

PATIENT EDUCATION
Educate family and close contacts regarding the risk of contracting meningococcal infection.

PROGNOSIS
Overall mortality is 13%. Factors associated with poor prognosis include young age, hypotension, thrombocytopenia, altered mental status, and leukopenia.

COMPLICATIONS
• DIC
• Acute tubular necrosis
• Neurologic: sensorineural hearing loss, cranial nerve palsy, seizures
• Obstructive hydrocephalus
• Subdural effusions
• Acute adrenal hemorrhage
• Waterhouse-Friderichsen syndrome

REFERENCES
1. Centers for Disease Control and Prevention. Meningococcal disease: technical and clinical information. https://www.cdc.gov/meningococcal/clinical-info.html. Accessed November 25, 2020.
2. Deghmane A-E, Taha S, Taha M-K. Global epidemiology and changing clinical presentations of invasive meningococcal disease: a narrative review [published online ahead of print August 28, 2021]. *Infect Dis (Lond)*. doi:1080/23744235.2021.1971289.
3. Folaranmi T, Rubin L, Martin SW, et al. Use of serogroup B meningococcal vaccines in persons aged ≥10 years at increased risk for serogroup B meningococcal disease: recommendations of the Advisory Committee on Immunization Practices, 2015. *MMWR Morb Mortal Wkly Rep*. 2015;64(22):608–612.
4. Wei T-T, Hu Z-D, Qin B-D, et al. Diagnostic accuracy of procalcitonin in bacterial meningitis versus nonbacterial meningitis: a systematic review and meta-analysis. *Medicine (Baltimore)*. 2016;95(11):e3079.
5. Fitzgerald D, Waterer GW. Invasive pneumococcal and meningococcal disease. *Infect Dis Clin North Am*. 2019;33(4):1125–1141.

ADDITIONAL READING
• Visintin C, Mugglestone MA, Fields EJ, et al; for Guideline Development Group, National Institute for Health and Clinical Excellence. Management of bacterial meningitis and meningococcal septicaemia in children and young people: summary of NICE guidance. *BMJ*. 2010;340:c3209.
• Wright C, Wordsworth R, Glennie L. Counting the cost of meningococcal disease: scenarios of severe meningitis and septicemia. *Paediatr Drugs*. 2013;15(1):49–58.

CODES

ICD10
• A39.4 Meningococcemia, unspecified
• A39.0 Meningococcal meningitis
• A39.2 Acute meningococcemia

CLINICAL PEARLS
• Invasive meningococcal disease can be rapidly fatal. Rapid identification and early treatment with antibiotics is essential to promote good clinical outcomes. Treat then test in suspected cases.
• Provide chemoprophylaxis to close contacts.
• All adolescents and children in high-risk groups should receive MenACWY vaccine. Meningitis B vaccines are recommended for high-risk children age >10 years.

M

MENISCAL INJURY

Jennifer Schwartz, MD

 BASICS

DESCRIPTION

- The menisci are fibrocartilaginous structures between the femoral condyles and tibial plateaus.
- The menisci help stabilize the knee and distribute forces across the joint.
- Meniscal tears can lead to knee pain and disability and, ultimately, are a risk factor for the development of knee osteoarthritis (OA).

Pediatric Considerations

- Meniscal injuries are rare in children <10. In this population, they are often due to a discoid meniscus and not trauma (1).
- MRI is still the study of choice but is less sensitive and specific for diagnosing meniscal tears in children <12.
- Meniscal repair is an effective treatment option with good clinical outcomes in the pediatric/adolescent population.

EPIDEMIOLOGY

Bimodal age distribution—young athletes (traumatic) and older patients (degenerative)

Incidence

Medial meniscus more commonly injured

Prevalence

One of the most common musculoskeletal injuries, affecting 0.6 to 8 per 1000 patients each year (2)

ETIOLOGY AND PATHOPHYSIOLOGY

- Traumatic tears are acute. They generally occur due to a twisting motion of the knee with foot planted.
- Degenerative tears are chronic. They generally occur with overuse and minimal trauma.

Genetics

No specific gene locus has been identified.

RISK FACTORS

- Traumatic tear:
  - High degree of physical activity (especially cutting sports)
  - Younger patients
  - Anterior cruciate ligament (ACL) insufficiency
  - Underlying meniscal degeneration—can still increase risk of meniscal tear even in traumatic event (2)
- Degenerative tear:
  - Increased age (>60 years)
  - Obesity
  - Work-related kneeling/squatting/climbing stairs

GENERAL PREVENTION

- Treatment and rehabilitation of previous knee injuries, particularly ACL injuries
- Strengthening and increased flexibility of quadriceps and hamstring muscles
- Weight management

COMMONLY ASSOCIATED CONDITIONS

- Traumatic tear:
  - ACL concomitantly torn in 1/3 of cases
- Degenerative tear:
  - Baker cyst—greater association with medial meniscal tears
  - Osteoarthritis (OA)

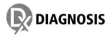 **DIAGNOSIS**

HISTORY

- Medial or lateral knee pain and swelling—increased with knee flexion, walking down stairs
- Noncontact twisting mechanism of injury (if trauma present)
- ± Locking, catching
  - Limited association between self-reported mechanical symptoms and presence of meniscal tear on arthroscopy

PHYSICAL EXAM

- Effusion—typically >24 hours postinjury
- Joint line tenderness (medial and/or lateral)
- Decreased range of motion of knee
  - Pain with full flexion (posterior horn tear) or extension (anterior horn tear)
- Accuracy of special tests (McMurray, Apley grind test) varies.

DIFFERENTIAL DIAGNOSIS

- ACL or collateral ligament tear
- Pathologic plica
- Osteochondritis dissecans
- Loose body or fracture
- OA
- Patellofemoral syndrome

DIAGNOSTIC TESTS & INTERPRETATION

- Plain radiographs can detect fractures, loose bodies, or arthritic changes.
- Ultrasound may help identify meniscal tears.
- MRI is the primary imaging study for detecting meniscal tears.

Follow-Up Tests & Special Considerations

Meniscal tears are often found incidentally on MRI and may not always be the cause of a patient's symptoms—important to correlate history, physical exam, and imaging findings.

- Incidental tears found on MRI in 60% asymptomatic patients (3)[C]
- Asymptomatic tears more common in older patients, those with OA

Diagnostic Procedures/Other

Arthroscopy may be needed if the MRI is indeterminate.

 TREATMENT

GENERAL MEASURES

- For traumatic tears (with locking sensation, implying bucket handle tear):
  - Consider surgery—these patients generally have greater improvement after surgery compared to patients with degenerative tears (4)[C].
- For degenerative tears:
  - Nonsurgical management is appropriate first-line treatment for symptomatic meniscal tears without mechanical symptoms (3)[C]. These include:
    - Rest, ice, activity modification
    - OTC medications
    - Physical therapy (PT)
    - Intra-articular corticosteroid injection
- Recommend supportive care first—there is no increased benefit from surgery versus PT in patients >40 years old with degenerative meniscal tears (5)[B],(6).
  - Clinically favorable outcomes are seen over a 5-year period for both conservative and surgical treatment options—decreased pain, improved quality of life, improved knee function (7)[C].
  - Arthroscopic partial meniscectomy can be a reasonable option in those who do not respond to initial PT.
  - There may a slightly higher rate of total knee replacement in those treated with surgery (7).
  - PT is more cost-effective than surgery and preferred from an economic standpoint (8).
  - In one study, 90% of patients with degenerative meniscal tears had symptom improvement over 2 years regardless of treatment choice. Predictors of poor improvement included elevated BMI, higher pain, decreased mental health, concurrent OA, decreased quadriceps/hamstring strength (9).

MEDICATION

First Line

- NSAIDs (i.e., ibuprofen 800 mg PO TID or naproxen [Naprosyn] 500 mg PO BID) or acetaminophen [Tylenol]
- Corticosteroid injection (5 mL lidocaine plus methylprednisolone acetate [Depo-Medrol] [80 mg/mL] or equivalent)

ISSUES FOR REFERRAL

Surgical consult for patients meeting operative criteria or wishing surgical repair

ADDITIONAL THERAPIES

- Rehabilitation is required for both surgical and nonsurgical patients.
- Weight control
- Platelet-rich plasma (PRP) injections may improve symptoms from degenerative meniscal tears.

SURGERY/OTHER PROCEDURES

- Consider surgical intervention if:
  - Young/active patient with traumatic tear and no underlying OA
  - Concurrent injuries (i.e., ACL tear)
  - Mechanical symptoms (knee "catching" or "locking")
  - No symptom improvement after 3 to 6 months of conservative treatment with degenerative tear
- Meniscal preservation surgery (i.e., meniscal repair or replacement) is preferred and may have better outcomes.
- Meniscectomy removes injured portion of meniscus. Both partial and total meniscectomy can lead to articular cartilage degeneration and OA.
  - Higher risk if age >40 years, high BMI, valgus malalignment

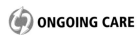 ONGOING CARE

FOLLOW-UP RECOMMENDATIONS

- Return to play requires the athlete be pain free, have full range of motion, and full strength.
- Following meniscal repair, patients can generally return to activities in 3 to 6 months.

PATIENT EDUCATION

Patients should be aware of the risks and benefits of surgery compared with conservative treatment.

PROGNOSIS

Prognosis better if surgery is done within 8 weeks (acute tear), patient is <30 years of age, or tear is peripheral/lateral and <2.5 cm

COMPLICATIONS

- Meniscectomies may eventually lead to OA.
- Risk of developing OA increases 6-fold 20 years after a meniscectomy.

REFERENCES

1. Geffroy L. Meniscal pathology in children and adolescents. *Orthop Traumatol Surg Res*. 2021; 107(1 Suppl):102775.
2. Wesdorp MA, Eijgenraam SM, Meuffels DE, et al. Traumatic meniscal tears are associated with meniscal degeneration. *Am J Sports Med*. 2020;48(10):2345–2352.
3. van de Graaf VA, Bloembergen CH, Willigenburg NW, et al. Can even experienced orthopaedic surgeons predict who will benefit from surgery when patients present with degenerative meniscal tears? A survey of 194 orthopaedic surgeons who made 3880 predictions. *Br J Sports Med*. 2020;54(6):354–359.
4. Thorlund JB, Rodriguez Palomino J, Juhl CB, et al. Infographic. Exercise therapy for meniscal tears: evidence and recommendations. *Br J Sports Med*. 2019;53(3):315–316.

5. Lizaur-Utrilla A, Miralles-Munoz FA, Gonzalez-Parreño S, et al. Outcomes and patient satisfaction with arthroscopic partial meniscectomy for degenerative and traumatic tears in middle-aged patients with no or mild osteoarthritis. *Am J Sports Med*. 2019;47(10):2412–2419.
6. Lubowitz JH, Brand JC, Rossi MJ. Nonoperative management of degenerative meniscus tears is worth a try. *Arthroscopy*. 2020;36(2):327–328.
7. Katz JN, Shrestha S, Losina E, et al. Five-year outcome of operative and nonoperative management of meniscal tear in persons older than forty-five years. *Arthritis Rheumatol*. 2020;72(2):273–281.
8. van de Graaf VA, van Dongen JM, Willigenburg NW, et al. How do the costs of physical therapy and arthroscopic partial meniscectomy compare? A trial-based economic evaluation of two treatments in patients with meniscal tears alongside the ESCAPE study. *Br J Sports Med*. 2020;54(9):538–546.
9. Berg B, Roos EM, Kise NJ, et al. On a trajectory for success—9 in every 10 people with a degenerative meniscus tear have improved knee function within 2 years after treatment: a secondary exploratory analysis of a randomized controlled trial. *J Orthop Sports Phys Ther*. 2021;51(6):289–297.

ADDITIONAL READING

- Abram SGF, Beard DJ, Price AJ; for BASK Meniscal Working Group. Arthroscopic meniscal surgery: a national society treatment guideline and consensus statement. *Bone Joint J*. 2019;101-B(6):652–659.
- Bernard CD, Kennedy NI, Tagliero AJ, et al. Medial meniscus posterior root tear treatment. A matched cohort comparison of nonoperative management, partial meniscectomy, and repair. *Am J Sports Med*. 2020;48(1):128–132.
- Bruno F, Goderecci R, Barile A, et al. Comparative evaluation of meniscal pathology: MRI vs arthroscopy. *J Biol Regul Homeost Agents*. 2019;33(2):9–14.
- DeFroda AF, Yang DS, Donnelly JC, et al. Trends in the surgical treatment of meniscal tears in patients with and without concurrent anterior cruciate ligament tears. *Phys Sportsmed*. 2020;48(2):229–235.
- Hagmeijer MH, Hevesi M, Desai VS, et al. Secondary meniscal tears in patients with anterior cruciate ligament injury: relationship among operative management, osteoarthritis, and arthroplasty at 18-year mean follow-up. *Am J Sports Med*. 2019;47(7):1583–1590.
- Jacquet C, Moutin C, Becker R, et al. Does practice of meniscus surgery change over time? A report of the 2021 'THE MENISCUS' Webinar. *J Esp Ortop*. 2021;8(1):46.
- Lee D-Y, Park Y-J, Kim H-J, et al. Arthroscopic meniscal surgery versus conservative management in patients aged 40 years and older: a meta-analysis. *Arch Orthop Trauma Surg*. 2018;138(12):1731–1739.

- Lee SH, Lee OS, Kim ST, et al. Revisiting arthroscopic partial meniscectomy for degenerative tears in knees with mild or no osteoarthritis: a systematic review and meta-analysis of randomized controlled trials. *Clin J Sports Med*. 2020;30(3):195–202.
- Pan H, Zhang P, Zhang Z, et al. Artrhoscopic partial meniscectomy combined with medical exercise therapy versus isolated medical exercise therapy for degenerative meniscal tear: a meta-analysis of randomized control trials. *Int J Surg*. 2020;79:222–232.
- Pihl K, Turkiewicz A, Englund M, et al. Association of specific meniscal pathologies and other structural pathologies with self-reported mechanical symptoms: a cross-sectional study of 566 patients undergoing meniscal surgery. *J Sci Med Sport*. 2019;22(2):151–157.
- Ronnblad E, Barenius B, Engstrom B, et al. Predictive factors for failure of meniscal repair: a retrospective dual-center analysis of 918 consecutive cases. *Orthop J Sports Med*. 2020;8(3):2325967120905529.
- Siemieniuk RAC, Harris IA, Agoritsas T, et al. Arthroscopic surgery for degenerative knee arthritis and meniscal tears: a clinical practice guideline. *Br J Sports Med*. 2018;52(5):313.
- Smith BE, Thacker D, Crewesmith A, et al. Special tests for assessing meniscal tears within the knee: a systematic review and meta-analysis. *Evid Based Med*. 2015;20(3):88–97.

 SEE ALSO

Algorithm: Knee Pain

 CODES

ICD10

- S83.209A Unsp tear of unsp meniscus, current injury, unsp knee, init
- S83.249A Oth tear of medial meniscus, current injury, unsp knee, init
- S83.289A Oth tear of lat mensc, current injury, unsp knee, init

CLINICAL PEARLS

- Chronic/degenerative meniscal tears are common in patients >40 years old and are generally managed conservatively.
- Acute/traumatic meniscal tears are more common in young athletes and may require surgery.
- MRI is imaging modality of choice to identify meniscal tears.
- In patients opting for surgery, meniscal repairs have a better functional outcome and decreased risk of OA compared with meniscectomy.

M

MENOPAUSE

Nicole Monk, DO • Lawrence M. Gibbs, MD, MSEd

 BASICS

DESCRIPTION
- Natural menopause: 12 consecutive months of amenorrhea in a nonpregnant woman ≥40 years of age; mean age of 51 years; resulting from loss of ovarian activity
- Perimenopause/menopausal transition (MT): the period from the onset of irregular menses to the final menstrual cycle. Begins on average 4 years before menopause; starts at mean age of 47 years
- Postmenopause: usually >1/3 of a woman's life
- Primary ovarian insufficiency: irregularity or cessation of ovulatory cycles before age 40 years
- Surgical menopause: removal of functioning ovaries leading to immediate menopause

EPIDEMIOLOGY
- The median age of menopause is 51 years.
- 5% of women undergo menopause after age 55 years; another 5% between ages 40 and 45 years
- Occurs earlier in Hispanic women and later in Japanese American women as compared with Caucasians

Incidence
In the United States, 1.3 million women reach menopause annually.

ETIOLOGY AND PATHOPHYSIOLOGY
- As women age, the number of ovarian follicles decreases: Ovarian production of estrogen varies and then decreases. Follicle-stimulating hormone (FSH) production varies and then increases.
- Insufficient estradiol production leads to the absence of the luteinizing hormone (LH) surge, resulting in anovulation. Anovulation causes lack of progesterone production.
- Failure to produce estradiol leads to thinning of endometrial lining and eventually menstruation ceases.
- Estrone (produced by adipose tissue) becomes the dominant form of estrogen during menopause.

RISK FACTORS
- Aging
- Oophorectomy/hysterectomy
- Sex chromosome abnormalities (e.g., Turner syndrome and fragile X syndrome)
- Family history of early menopause
- Smoking (earlier age of onset by 2 years)
- Chemotherapy and/or pelvic radiation
- Low body mass index

GENERAL PREVENTION
Menopause is a physiologic event and cannot be prevented. It is associated with increased risk of long-term medical issues, including cardiovascular disease (CVD) and osteoporotic fractures.
- Decrease risk of CVD by:
  - Increasing exercise
  - Maintaining healthy diet and a healthy weight
  - Avoiding tobacco use
  - Treating hypertension, hyperlipidemia, and diabetes mellitus
- Decrease risk of osteoporotic fractures with:
  - Weight-bearing exercise and fall prevention
  - Avoidance of smoking and excessive alcohol intake
  - Dietary calcium of 1,200 mg/day
  - Adequate vitamin D intake (800 to 1,200 IU daily)

DIAGNOSIS

Clinical diagnosis—12 consecutive months of amenorrhea in a nonpregnant woman ≥40 years of age

HISTORY
- Cessation of menses:
  - Generally preceded by a period of irregular cycles with heavy vaginal bleeding followed by diminished vaginal bleeding
- Vasomotor symptoms reported by 80%:
  - Sudden unpleasant feeling of heat and sweating, most commonly over face, neck, and chest, typically lasting 1 to 5 minutes; intervals unpredictable
  - Generally begin 2 years before the final menstrual period, peak during 1 year after the final menstrual period, and then diminish
  - Frequency and duration varies: 87% of women who report flushes experience them daily; ~33% have >10 per day. Mean duration of symptoms lasts 4 to 10.2 years and may begin during MT and extend well past menopause.
  - Varies with ethnicity: greatest in African and Hispanic women and least in Asian women
  - More common in obese women
- Genitourinary syndrome of menopause:
  - Vulvovaginal atrophy in 50%:
    - Vaginal/vulvar dryness, itching, dyspareunia, and possible sexual dysfunction
    - Alkaline vaginal pH and atrophy increases risk of vaginal infections and UTIs.
    - Persists or worsens with aging
  - Urologic symptoms (urgency, frequency, dysuria, incontinence) not clearly correlated with MT
- Anxiety/depression: Some studies show a new diagnosis of depression is 2.5 times more likely to occur during the MT as compared to premenopause.
- Sleep disturbance: arousal from sleep, chronic sleep disruption, and chronic insomnia linked with menopause
- Change in intensity and severity of migraines
- Skin thinning, mild hirsutism, brittle nails

Geriatric Considerations
Vaginal bleeding in postmenopausal women is abnormal; thus, endometrial cancer/endometrioid adenocarcinoma (EAC) must be ruled out.

PHYSICAL EXAM
- Decrease in breast size and change in breast texture
- Genitourinary exam:
  - Atrophic vulva and vaginal mucosa
  - Increased risk for uterine prolapse

DIFFERENTIAL DIAGNOSIS
Pregnancy, thyroid diseases, pituitary adenoma, Sheehan syndrome, hypothalamic dysfunction, anorexia nervosa, Asherman syndrome, and obstruction of uterine outflow tract

DIAGNOSTIC TESTS & INTERPRETATION
Initial Tests (lab, imaging)
- Lab testing for menopause is not required; the patient's age and symptoms establish the diagnosis.
- Lab tests appropriate in age <45 if premature/early menopause suspected or to rule out other causes of oligo-/amenorrhea:
  - Elevated serum FSH level >30 mIU/mL indicates ovarian failure.
  - Symptoms may precede lab changes.

- Infertility evaluation: may use elevated day 3 FSH, decreased anti-müllerian hormone levels, and decreased antral follicle count to predict decreased ovarian reserve
- Estrogens, androgens, and oral contraceptive pills (OCPs) may alter lab results.

Follow-Up Tests & Special Considerations
- Pregnancy test
- TSH and prolactin level if pituitary disease is suspected
- Abnormal uterine bleeding, including postmenopausal bleeding, should be evaluated by TVUS and/or EMB. If endometrial stripe is <5 mm on TVUS, EAC is unlikely.
- U.S. Preventive Services Task Force (USPSTF) recommends mammogram every 2 years from ages 50 to 74 years.
- USPSTF recommends bone mineral density (BMD) screening with dual energy x-ray absorptiometry (DEXA) scan in postmenopausal women >65 years or <65 years if the risk for fracture is equivalent to that of a 65-year-old woman (using the FRAX tool to assess, https://www.sheffield.ac.uk/FRAX/). Risk factors include a previous history of fractures, low body weight, cigarette smoking, and family history of osteoporotic fracture.

Test Interpretation
- Abnormal BMD and DEXA scan results:
  - T-score on DEXA of −1 to −2.5 = osteopenia
  - T-score <−2.5 = osteoporosis
  - Defer to femoral neck T-score over spine T-score.
- Z-score measures age-matched mean bone density (not clinically useful).

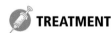 **TREATMENT**

MEDICATION
First Line
Hormone therapy (HT): HT is the most effective treatment for vasomotor symptoms and genitourinary symptoms of menopause and has been shown to prevent bone loss and fracture (1). Developing an individual risk-benefit profile is essential. Treatment goal is to minimize menopausal symptoms to improve quality of life (1).

- Long-term use of hormone replacement therapy (HRT) has more risks than benefits, including breast, ovarian, and endometrial cancer; venous thromboembolism; CVD; and gallbladder disease.
- If, after a discussion of risks and benefits, shared decision-making leads to initiation of HRT, benefits are more likely to outweigh risks in women <60 years or who are within 10 years of menopause onset (1).
- The primary indication for HT is the treatment of moderate to severe vasomotor symptoms.
  - Oral estrogen or estrogen-progestin mix can reduce weekly hot flush frequency ~75%.
- HT may help with disrupted sleep, urogenital atrophy, and lowers risk of osteoporotic fractures.
- In women with an intact uterus, give estrogen with progestin because unopposed estrogen carries an increased risk of EAC.

- Treatment regimens include but are not limited to:
  - Standard dose: conjugated equine estrogen (CEE) 0.625 mg/day OR micronized estradiol 17β 1.0 mg/day OR transdermal estradiol 17β 0.0375 to 0.050 mg/day
  - Low dose: CEE 0.30 to 0.45 mg/day OR micronized estradiol 17β 0.5 mg/day OR transdermal estradiol 17β 0.025 mg/day
  - Ultra-low dose: micronized estradiol 17β 0.025 mg/day OR transdermal estradiol 17β 0.014 mg/day
  - Micronized progesterone 100 mg/day can be used as progestin. Alternative: medroxyprogesterone acetate (MPA) 2.5 mg/day. Combination estradiol/progestin transdermal treatments have either levonorgestrel or norethindrone as progestin source. Although NOT approved for postmenopausal women, the levonorgestrel intrauterine system (IUS) has been used.
  - Tissue-selective estrogen complex: bazedoxifene (selective estrogen receptor modulator [SERM])+ conjugated estrogens; provides endometrial protection without need for progesterone for relief of vasomotor symptoms and bone loss prevention
- Less worrisome side effects include breast tenderness, vaginal bleeding, bloating, and headaches.
- MenoPro app is free for iPhones and iPad from The North American Menopause Society (NAMS). It has two modes: one for clinicians and one for patients to aid in shared decision-making. It allows users to progress through questions to evaluate cardiovascular and reproductive organ cancer risk.
- American College of Obstetricians and Gynecologists (ACOG) recommends HT should be individualized with lowest effect dose given for the shortest duration of time needed to relieve vasomotor symptoms. Lower doses have similar symptom reduction profiles for many patients. Results of ultra-low-dose regimens are mixed.
- Precautions:
  - Women's Health Initiative (WHI) study demonstrate women who take CEE with MPA versus placebo had increased CHD events, invasive breast cancer, stroke, pulmonary embolism, dementia, gallbladder disease, urinary incontinence; benefits included decreased hip fractures, diabetes, and vasomotor symptoms.
  - Breast cancer risk not seen until 5 years of use
  - Women on estrogen alone had no increased risk of invasive breast cancer but did increase abnormal mammograms requiring follow-up investigations.
  - HRT should NOT be used for cardioprotective benefit as risk outweighs benefit.
  - Higher doses of estrogen can cause hypercoagulability, breast tenderness, gallbladder disease, and hypertension.
  - Contraindications to HT:
    - Estrogen-dependent malignancies
    - Unexplained uterine bleeding or untreated endometrial hyperplasia
    - History of thromboembolism or stroke
    - CAD
    - Active liver disease
    - Untreated hypertension
    - Current or past breast cancer
- For osteoporosis: It is recommended to treat postmenopausal women at high risk for fractures, especially those who have experienced a recent fracture, with pharmacologic therapies, because the benefits outweigh the risks.

- Women with a history of hip or vertebral fracture or personal history of osteoporosis should be treated with one of the following:
  - Bisphosphonates to inhibit osteoclast action and resorption of bone:
    - Alendronate: 70 mg/week or 10 mg/day
    - Risedronate: 35 mg once a week or 5 mg/day
    - Zoledronic acid: 5 mg IV annually
    - Ibandronate: 150 mg/month PO or 3 mg IV q3mo
  - SERMs selectively inhibit or stimulate estrogen-like action with stimulation of osteoblasts:
    - Raloxifene: 60 mg/day
      - Decreases the risk of vertebral fracture
    - Bazedoxifene + conjugated estrogens (0.45 mg/20 mg)
      - FDA-approved for moderate to severe vasomotor symptoms and osteoporosis
  - Denosumab (60 mg SC every 6 months) is a monoclonal antibody that prevents receptor activator of nuclear factor–κB ligand (RANKL) from accelerating osteoclast generation; reduces incidence of vertebral and hip fractures in postmenopausal women
  - Parathyroid hormone—rarely used due to the adverse effect on bone but shown to reduce fracture risk in menopausal women with osteoporosis
- For vulvar/vaginal atrophy:
  - Topical estrogen therapy (ET) reverses vaginal atrophy, enhances blood flow, and reduces UTI. Continue for as long as distressing symptoms remain. Initiate treatment daily for 1 to 2 weeks and then decrease to 2 times weekly. Comes as estradiol cream, tablet, or ring. No evidence of difference in efficacy between various intravaginal estrogenic preparations. Apply vaginally:
    - Estradiol cream 0.01% (1 g), conjugated estrogen 0.625 mg/g (0.5 g), vaginal tablet (10 μg) used twice weekly, or vaginal ring (7.5 μg daily lasting for 3 months)
    - Ospemifene: 60 mg PO daily; SERM for moderate to severe dyspareunia associated with vaginal atrophy
  - Nonestrogen vaginal lubricant may be as effective as topical estrogen for some.

Second Line
Nonhormonal treatments may be helpful to treat vasomotor symptoms:
- Paroxetine (10 to 25 mg/day) is approved for treatment of vasomotor symptoms. This SSRI demonstrated modest decrease in hot flushes.
- Other SSRI/SRNIs: venlafaxine (37.5 to 100.0 mg/day) or fluoxetine (20 mg/day) and citalopram (20 mg/day) shown to reduce hot flushes as compared to placebo
- Gabapentin (300 to 900 mg/day) shown to have an effect on lowering hot flushes compared to placebo
- Clonidine (0.05 mg BID) may be used to treat mild hot flashes, less effective than SSRI/SRNIs.
- Note that most trials of second-line therapies have been brief (i.e., a few months).

COMPLEMENTARY & ALTERNATIVE MEDICINE
- Phytoestrogens, herbs, and other supplements do not have clear benefit in relieving menopause symptoms compared to placebo. Some may interact with anticoagulants, like warfarin, so should be used with caution.
- Hypnotherapy and mindfulness meditation may provide relief for some.
- Acupuncture has not been shown to be more effective than simulated acupuncture for relieving hot flashes.

- Yoga has not been shown to relieve hot flashes but may be helpful for some symptoms associated with menopause.
- Compounded bioidentical HT should be avoided, given concerns about safety, including possibility of overdosing or underdosing, lack of efficacy and safety studies, and lack of a label providing risks (1).
- Overall, most data involves short-term trials, so little is known about their long-term safety. But, mind-body practices such as acupuncture, hypnosis, meditation, and yoga generally have good safety records.

ONGOING CARE

FOLLOW-UP RECOMMENDATIONS
Patient Monitoring
- A DEXA scan in women at age ≤65 years with risk equivalent to age 65 years
- If HRT initiated, consider decrease or discontinuation after 3 to 5 years to minimize risks. ACOG recommends decision to stop/continue HT be individualized, based on patient's symptoms and medical history.

DIET
Calcium-rich diet and vitamin D supplementation (800 to 1,200 IU/day). Calcium supplements may increase risk of kidney stone and cardiac events.

PATIENT EDUCATION
- Smoking cessation, reducing alcohol intake
- Exercise >30 minutes, 3 times weekly
- Healthy diet to maintain appropriate weight
- Address cardiovascular risk factor modification.

PROGNOSIS
If untreated:
- Ultimate disappearance of vasomotor symptoms
- Worsening of vaginal/vulvar atrophy
- Osteoporosis

COMPLICATIONS
- Osteoporosis: Accelerated bone loss up to 3–5% per year for 5 to 7 years.
- Increased risk of CVD following menopause

REFERENCE
1. The NAMS 2017 Hormone Therapy Position Statement Advisory Panel. The 2017 hormone therapy position statement of the North American Menopause Society. *Menopause*. 2017;24(7):728–753.

CODES

ICD10
- E28.310 Symptomatic premature menopause
- N95.1 Menopausal and female climacteric states
- Z78.0 Asymptomatic menopausal state

CLINICAL PEARLS
- Menopause is usually diagnosed by history alone.
- HT can be used short term for relief of moderate to severe vasomotor symptoms but should not be used for long-term prevention of CVD.

M

MENORRHAGIA (HEAVY MENSTRUAL BLEEDING)

Daniel R. Matta, MD • Thandi Walters, MD

 BASICS

DESCRIPTION

- The term menorrhagia has fallen out of favor and the terminology "abnormal uterine bleeding" (AUB) is now preferred.
- AUB describes a range of symptoms, such as heavy menstrual bleeding (HMB), intermenstrual bleeding (IMB) and a combination of both heavy and prolonged menstrual bleeding (1).
- Due to inconsistent use of terminology and definitions to characterize AUB, the International Federation of Gynecology and Obstetrics (FIGO) has developed two systems to assist with the major challenge of determining the cause of AUB for clinicians. These include:
  - FIGO AUB system 1: standardized nomenclature and defined the parameters of normal and abnormal menstrual bleeding
  - FIGO AUB system 2: focused on classifications of AUB etiology into structural and nonstructural causes using the PALM-COEIN classification system (see below)

EPIDEMIOLOGY

- AUB is a common problem that leads to increased health care costs and decreased quality of life.
- It is one of the leading causes of outpatient gynecologic visits, with 20–30% of patients presenting with this complaint annually.

Prevalence

- AUB has a profound impact on women in their reproductive years and has a prevalence of 3–30%.
- The prevalence varies with age and is higher in adolescence and the fifth decade.

ETIOLOGY AND PATHOPHYSIOLOGY

- The pathophysiology of AUB is as diverse as the classification of the disease.
- Structural causes include (PALM acronym)
  - P—polyp (AUB-P)
  - A—adenomyosis (AUB-A)
  - L—leiomyoma (AUB-L)
    - Submucosal leiomyoma (AUB-LSM)
    - Other myoma (AUB-LO)
  - M—malignancy/hyperplasia (AUB-M)
- Nonstructural causes (COIEN acronym) include:
  - C—coagulopathy (AUB-C)
  - O—ovulatory (AUB-O)
  - E—endometrial (AUB-E)
  - I—iatrogenic (AUB-I)
  - N—not yet classified (AUB-N)

Pediatric Considerations

- Genital bleeding before puberty is, by definition, not menstrual bleeding and requires further evaluation.
- Due to immaturity of the hypothalamic-pituitary-ovarian axis, adolescents are at risk of irregular bleeding and HMB.
- Adolescents with HMB should be evaluated for possible bleeding disorders, especially von Willebrand disease and qualitative platelet dysfunction.

Pregnancy Considerations

Bleeding in pregnancy is, by definition, not menstrual bleeding and requires further evaluation. Pregnancy test should be obtained as part of the evaluation of AUB.

GENERAL PREVENTION

- Combined oral contraceptives may prevent HMB, particularly when progesterone is dominant. Lower estrogen doses result in less menstrual bleeding.
- Progesterone-only contraceptives may reduce overall blood loss but often result in irregular bleeding.

 DIAGNOSIS

HISTORY

- It is important to obtain a proper understanding of the patient's bleeding episode and to ask questions focused on PALM-COEIN etiologies to determine the patient's cause of abnormal bleeding.
- Menstrual history should include:
  - Menstrual cycle length, duration, variability, quantity of blood loss. To determine the quantity of blood loss, ask about how frequently pads are changed or if pads need to be changed overnight. Women who change pads every 2 to 3 hours would have lost at least 80 mL per cycle. One can also ask about the presence and size of clots or the sensation of "flooding."
- The clinician should obtain the patient's gynecologic, obstetric, sexual, medical, surgical, family, and medication history.
- To identify possible coagulopathy, the following screening tool for women with HMB can be used:
  - HMB since menarche
    - Plus one of the following conditions:
      - Postpartum hemorrhage
      - Surgery-related bleeding
      - Bleeding associated with dental work
    - Two or more of the following:
      - Bruising 2× per month
      - Epistaxis 1 to 2 times per month
      - Frequent gum bleeding
      - A family history of bleeding symptoms

- The screen is positive if the patient answered yes to any of the above categories and warrants further testing and hematology referral.
- Symptoms that suggest bleeding is ovulatory include regular menstrual interval, midcycle pain, and premenstrual symptoms.
  - Abdominal pain or cramps at other times of the cycle may be associated with structural causes.
  - Evaluate for symptoms of anemia and impact of bleeding on patient's well-being.

PHYSICAL EXAM

- If the patient has acute blood loss, the exam should begin by assessing for life-threatening signs of hemodynamic instability. Orthostatic vitals should be obtained which can indicate hypovolemia.
- One can look for other possible causes of AUB by observing obesity; assessing the thyroid gland; and examining the skin for signs of bleeding disorders such as petechiae and ecchymoses, signs of hyperandrogenism such as hirsutism and acne.
- Perform a speculum examination looking for other sites of bleeding by thoroughly inspecting the vulva, urethra, vagina, anus, and perineum. Note signs of trauma like lacerations. It is also prudent to note any hemorrhoids as a possible source of bleeding.
- Bimanual exam is done to feel for uterine or cervical abnormalities or enlargement. Pelvic and adnexal masses would also be palpated during this exam.

DIFFERENTIAL DIAGNOSIS

- Normal menses
- Complications of pregnancy
- Other sources of bleeding (e.g., cervical, vaginal, gastrointestinal)

DIAGNOSTIC TESTS & INTERPRETATION

Initial Tests (lab, imaging)

- Initial testing on all patients should include pregnancy test and CBC.
- If the patient is acutely bleeding, type and cross-match is necessary.
- Other tests may include:
  - PT/INR, PTT
  - TSH with reflex T_4
  - CMP
  - Iron studies
  - STI panel

- Labs to consider in select cases:
  - Suspected coagulopathy: plasma vWF antigen, plasma vWF activity (ristocetin cofactor activity, vWF:RCo activity and vWF collagen binding), factor VIII, and other factor testing (2)
  - Ovulatory dysfunction: thyroid function testing, human chorionic gonadotropin, prolactin, and follicle-stimulating hormone
  - Endocervical cultures to rule out infections
  - Pap smear
- Imaging should be obtained based on clinician judgment and should begin with transvaginal ultrasound.

Follow-Up Tests & Special Considerations
- Saline infusion sonohysterography, diagnostic hysterography, hysterosalpingography can be performed to diagnose endometrial polyps and submucosal leiomyoma (2).
  - Polyp removal and endometrial sampling can be done at the time of hysteroscopy.
- MRI can be performed to better visualize the changes of adenomyosis and determine if uterine-sparing treatment is an option in patients with leiomyoma (2). MRI can also detect leiomyosarcoma.

Diagnostic Procedures/Other
If a patient is >40 years or <40 years with high-risk factors endometrial biopsy with or without hysteroscopy is performed for possible endometrial hyperplasia or carcinoma (1).

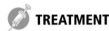

TREATMENT

MEDICATION

First Line
- Hormonal
  - OCP normally used to regulate and decrease bleeding.
  - Progesterone and estrogen
- Nonhormonal. These are normally chosen by women who wish to conceive and decrease hormonal side effects.
  - NSAIDS
  - Antifibrinolytics
- Acute heavy bleeding
  - Conjugated equine estrogen 25 mg IV every 4 to 6 hours for 24 hours with IV antiemetic agents
  - Monophasic 35-mg estrogen-containing OCP 3 times daily for 7 days and then 1 daily
  - Medroxyprogesterone 20 mg or norethindrone 20 mg 3 times daily for 7 days
  - Tranexamic acid 10 mg/kg IV (maximum, 600 mg/dose) or 1.5 g orally every 8 hours for 5 days

- Chronic bleeding
  - Ibuprofen 600 mg every 6 hours or 800 mg every 8 hours; naproxen 500 mg initially and repeat 3 to 5 hours later and then 250 to 500 mg twice daily; mefenamic acid 500 mg 3 times daily (with food)
  - Monophasic 30- to 35-mg estrogen-containing OCP daily with or without inert pills
  - Medroxyprogesterone 5 to 10 mg or norethindrone 5 to 10 mg daily
  - Depot medroxyprogesterone 150 mg subcutaneously every 3 months. Levonorgestrel 19.5- to 52-mg intrauterine devices for 5 years (19.5-mg LNG-IUS is a slightly smaller device); etonogestrel subdermal implant for 3 years

Second Line
Danazol, GnRH agonists, aromatase inhibitors, selective estrogen receptor modulators (SERMs), and selective progesterone receptor modulators (SPRMs) are used as second-line agents in management of HMB caused by leiomyoma and adenomyosis. Of note, SPRMs are not currently available in the United States.

ISSUES FOR REFERRAL
- Patients in whom a coagulopathy is suspected or diagnosed should be referred to hematology.
- Refer to gynecology if a primary care physician is uncomfortable placing an intrauterine device, performing endometrial sampling, there is persistent bleeding despite treatment or malignancy is suspected.

ADDITIONAL THERAPIES
- Iron replacement therapy oral and intravenous for anemia
- MRI-guided focused ultrasound (MgFUS) had been approved by the FDA for the treatment of uterine fibroids and has been used with success in decreasing bleeding in patients with adenomyosis (3).

SURGERY/OTHER PROCEDURES
- Dilation and curettage can be considered in the setting of acute severe bleeding.
- Surgical procedures are directed to the specific identified pathology.
  - Polypectomy for endometrial and cervical polyps
  - Adenomyosis—hysterectomy
  - Leiomyoma—for women who do not desire fertility laparoscopic radiofrequency ablation, uterine artery embolization or hysterectomy can be performed. For women who desire fertility, myomectomy is preferred.
  - Malignancy—hysterectomy with or without adjuvant therapy and radiotherapy

- Conservative surgery (i.e., myomectomy, endometrial ablation, or uterine artery embolization) is more effective for controlling bleeding symptoms at 1 and 2 years than oral medications or the levonorgestrel-releasing IUD, but by 5 years, there is no difference in long-term results or patient satisfaction.
- Hysterectomy is curative but with more severe adverse effects and is typically reserved for failure of medical management or presence of another indication such as malignancy.

ONGOING CARE

COMPLICATIONS
- Iron deficiency anemia
- Acute severe blood loss
- Impaired quality of life

REFERENCES
1. Cheong Y, Cameron IT, Critchley HO. Abnormal uterine bleeding. *Br Med Bull.* 2019;131(1):119.
2. Marnach ML, Laughlin-Tommaso SK. Evaluation and management of abnormal uterine bleeding. *Mayo Clin Proc.* 2019;94(2):326–335.
3. Munro MG, Critchley HOD, Fraser IS; for FIGO Menstrual Disorders Committee. The two FIGO systems for normal and abnormal uterine bleeding symptoms and classification of causes of abnormal uterine bleeding in the reproductive years: 2018 revisions. *Int J Gynaecol Obstet.* 2018;143(3):393–408.

CODES

ICD10
- N92.0 Excessive and frequent menstruation with regular cycle
- N92.3 Ovulation bleeding
- N92.2 Excessive menstruation at puberty

CLINICAL PEARLS

- HMB is often associated with a structural uterine disorder.
- A thorough history and physical examination is a key part of determining the cause of AUB.
- The treatment of AUB should take the cause of the bleeding into consideration as well as the severity of symptoms and the patient's desire for fertility.
- The goal of initial therapy is to stop bleeding, treat anemia, and restore quality of life.

MESOTHELIOMA

Khalid Bashir, MD

BASICS

DESCRIPTION
- Mesothelioma is a rare, aggressive malignancy of the mesothelial or serous tissues primarily found in the pleura (65–70%), peritoneum (20–33%), tunica vaginalis (1–2%), or pericardium (1–2%) (1).
- Inhalation of asbestos is the predominant cause of mesothelioma, most often from occupational exposure.

EPIDEMIOLOGY
Incidence
- The incidence in the United States is decreasing, but it is increasing in other countries, particularly Great Britain and Australia.
- It is expected that rates of mesothelioma will start to drop after 2025, related to reduced exposure and better understanding of the process of development of mesothelioma after exposure to asbestos (2).
- The incidence increases with age, peaking in the 6th decade, with 70% of pleural disease occurring in males. Peritoneal involvement is slightly higher in women.
- Main risk factor is asbestos exposure, but tumors have arisen after prior radiation or exposure to talc, erionite, or mica or in patients with familial Mediterranean fever and diffuse lymphocytic leukemia.

Prevalence
There are 3,300 cases of mesothelioma diagnosed in the United States annually (3).

ETIOLOGY AND PATHOPHYSIOLOGY
- The predominant cause of mesothelioma is exposure to asbestos (hydrated magnesium silicate fibrous minerals).
- There is a long latent period of up to 44 years between exposure and development of mesothelioma (2).
- Inhaled or ingested asbestos fibers become trapped in pleural or peritoneal membranes, causing changes of irritation and inflammation.

Genetics
Loss of nuclear deubiquitinase BAP1 is associated with incidence of mesothelioma in some families as well as with other cancers such as melanoma.

RISK FACTORS
- The predominant risk factor is exposure to asbestos.
- Occupational exposures involve mining or milling of fibers, work with textiles, cement, friction materials, insulation, or shipbuilding.
- Nonoccupational exposures include renovation or destruction of asbestos-containing buildings, exposure to industrial sources in the community or natural geologic sources, or exposure to soiled clothing of asbestos workers (1),(3),(4).
- Radiation exposure, smoking, proximity to naturally occurring asbestos deposits, or inhalation of other fibrous silicates can contribute to malignant mesothelioma.

GENERAL PREVENTION
- Avoidance of asbestos exposure
- Strict adherence to protective protocols for workers in buildings where asbestos is found
- Continued aggressive remediation of asbestos-affected buildings and homes

DIAGNOSIS

HISTORY
- Symptoms are usually nonspecific and occur when disease is advanced. General fatigue, night sweats, and weight loss may be present.
- Pleural mesothelioma presents with gradual onset of pulmonary symptoms, chest pain, dyspnea, and cough.
- Peritoneal disease presents with vague abdominal pain, increased abdominal girth, nausea, anorexia, and weight loss.

PHYSICAL EXAM
- Pulmonary findings consistent with pleural effusion, including decreased breath sounds, dullness to percussion, and asymmetric chest wall expansion, are found.
- Abdominal findings consistent with ascites, including abdominal distension, fluid wave, and tenderness, are found.

DIFFERENTIAL DIAGNOSIS
- Pleural mesothelioma's differential diagnosis includes inflammatory reactions (empyema, pleural effusion), metastatic tumor from other sites, fibrosarcoma, malignant fibrous histiocytoma, sarcomatoid carcinoma, and synovial sarcoma.
- Peritoneal mesothelioma's differential diagnosis includes peritoneal carcinomatosis, serous peritoneal carcinoma, ovarian carcinoma in women, lymphomatosis, and tuberculous peritonitis.

DIAGNOSTIC TESTS & INTERPRETATION
Initial Tests (lab, imaging)
- At present, there is no tumor marker or serum chemistry that is of value in establishing the diagnosis of mesothelioma.
- Biomarkers that may be elevated in mesothelioma include fibulin-3, mesothelin, and osteopontin. However, they do not have an established role in diagnosis or monitoring response to therapy (2)[A].
- Pleural mesothelioma diagnosis requires tissue. Thoracentesis for cytology and closed pleural biopsy may be adequate, but often, more invasive procedures such as video-assisted thoracoscopic surgery (VATS) is needed to obtain an adequate specimen (1),(2)[A].

Follow-Up Tests & Special Considerations
Seeding of biopsy sites and tracks may occur in mesothelioma, which can be prevented with prophylactic radiation therapy to the scar or biopsy site (5)[A].

Diagnostic Procedures/Other
- CT, MRI, PET, or integrated PET-CT helps with clinical staging in pleural and peritoneal disease (1),(2),(3),(4),(5)[A].
- Mediastinoscopy, bronchoscopy, and laparoscopy can assist in full surgical staging of pleural disease (2)[A].
- Endobronchial ultrasound for staging is under investigation for pleural disease.

Test Interpretation
- The tumor, node, metastasis (TNM) staging system is most commonly used, although some centers use other staging systems.
- Butchart staging system is the oldest and still used in some parts of the world.
- Brigham staging system attempts to define resectability and lymph node involvement.

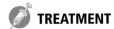

TREATMENT

GENERAL MEASURES
- A multidisciplinary team is important in management and should include thoracic surgery, oncology, pathology, pulmonary, and radiology for patient-specific planning of management.
- Pain assessment and control should follow principles of cancer pain management (5).

MEDICATION

First Line
- In pleural disease, combined therapy with cisplatin + gemcitabine or cisplatin + pemetrexed are associated with longer median survival than cisplatin alone (2),(4)[A].
- Addition of bevacizumab to cisplatin and pemetrexed in pleural disease has also been looked at as an alternative strategy in select populations.
- Vinflunine is showing some potential for first-line treatment in pleural disease (2)[A].
- Hyperthermic intraoperative or early postoperative intraperitoneal chemotherapy can increase drug concentration in the peritoneum and decrease systemic side effects. Use cisplatin, mitomycin C, fluorouracil, doxorubicin, and/or paclitaxel (1),(2),(3)[A].

Second Line
- Palliative benefit in pleural disease with mitomycin C, vinblastine, cisplatin, and pemetrexed alone or in combination with carboplatin (2),(3),(4)[A]
- Systemic therapy for peritoneal disease may include pemetrexed + cisplatin; vinorelbine or gemcitabine alone or in combination (1),(5)[A].

ISSUES FOR REFERRAL
- Pulmonary, oncology, and surgical follow-up after discharge as indicated
- Anger and depression may require psychological or psychiatric services (5).

ADDITIONAL THERAPIES
Immunotherapy in pleural disease uses humanized anti-CB3 AB (OKT3), cytotoxic T lymph (CTL), interferon α-2a, and autovaccine in advanced disease (1),(2),(3),(4),(5).
- Gene therapy
- Photodynamic therapy
- Radiotherapy in some cases of pleural disease
- Vascular endothelial growth factor (anti-VEGF-2) in combination with chemotherapy (2)
  – Vaccines are under study (5).

SURGERY/OTHER PROCEDURES
- For pleural mesothelioma, the role of surgery is not as clear cut. Pleurectomy with tumor decortication and extrapleural pneumonectomy reduces the tumor load, but there remains no clear effect on mortality (2),(4),(5).
- Radical resection of the peritoneum and cytoreductive surgery is associated with a better prognosis (1).

ADMISSION, INPATIENT, AND NURSING CONSIDERATIONS
- Based on overall clinical condition
- IV fluids as indicated by level of hydration
- Nursing as indicated by medical needs and clinical status
- Discharge criteria as indicated by general condition

 ONGOING CARE

FOLLOW-UP RECOMMENDATIONS
- Smoking cessation
- Immunization for pneumococcal pneumonia and influenza

Patient Monitoring
Monitor for paraneoplastic phenomenon, including fever, thrombocytosis, malignancy-related thrombosis, hypoglycemia, and rare Coombs-positive hemolytic anemia.

DIET
No specific restrictions

PROGNOSIS
- Prognosis is based on gender, stage, and level of completeness of cytoreduction.
- Poorly differentiated tumor grade, failure to undertake surgical resection, advanced age, and male gender are all independent predictors of poorer prognosis (2),(3).
- Average survival is 17 to 92 months, with 5-year survival rate at 63%.

COMPLICATIONS
Relapses and progression, infection and dysphagia

Geriatric Considerations
Age >65 years is associated with significantly increased morbidity and mortality.

Pediatric Considerations
Rarely a pediatric issue because most disease occurs after the 5th decade of life

Pregnancy Considerations
Rarely an issue with pregnancy because most disease occurs after the 5th decade of life

REFERENCES

1. Bridda A, Padoan I, Mencarelli R, et al. Peritoneal mesothelioma: a review. *MedGenMed*. 2007;9(2):32.
2. Weder W. Mesothelioma. *Ann Oncol*. 2010;21(Suppl 7):vii326–vii333.
3. Mott FE. Mesothelioma: a review. *Ochsner J*. 2012;12(1):70–79.
4. Fuhrer G, Lazarus AA. Mesothelioma. *Dis Mon*. 2011;57(1):40–54.
5. van Meerbeeck JP, Scherpereel A, Surmont VF, et al. Malignant pleural mesothelioma: the standard of care and challenges for future management. *Crit Rev Oncol Hematol*. 2011;78(2):92–111.

CODES

ICD10
- C45.1 Mesothelioma of peritoneum
- C45.2 Mesothelioma of pericardium
- C45.0 Mesothelioma of pleura

CLINICAL PEARLS
- Mesothelioma remains a rare but universally fatal disease in part due to long latency.
- Multimodal treatment has decreased recurrence rates and has extended survival time.
- Main risk factor is asbestos exposure, but tumors have arisen after prior radiation or exposure to talc, erionite, or mica or in patients with familial Mediterranean fever and diffuse lymphocytic leukemia.

M

METABOLIC SYNDROME
Naomi Parrella, MD, FAAFP, Dipl. ABOM

BASICS

DESCRIPTION

- Rather than a distinct disease, metabolic syndrome (MetS) represents a cluster of risk factors that together, correlate with an increased risk of premature morbidity including complications associated with COVID-19, type 2 diabetes mellitus (T2DM), cardiovascular disease, stroke, nonalcoholic fatty liver disease (NAFLD), certain cancers, and all-cause mortality.
- Multiple definitions for MetS; the most commonly accepted from WHO 1999, National Cholesterol Education Program (NCEP) ATP3 2005, and International Diabetes Federation (IDF) 2006 (1)
- A cluster of progressive metabolic abnormalities demonstrating insulin resistance, a proinflammatory and prothrombotic state that manifest with at least three of:
  - Increased waist circumference (WC) (required criteria, IDF; optional NCEP; waist:hip ratio >0.9 men, > 0.85 women or BMI >30 kg/m² WHO)
  - Elevated blood pressure (BP) (>130/85, NCEP and IDF; >140/90, WHO)
  - Elevated triglycerides (TG) ≥150 mg/dL or treatment (consistent WHO, NCEP, IDF)
  - Decreased high-density lipoprotein (HDL-C) (men <35 mg/dL, women 30 mg/dL, WHO; men <40 mg/dL, women <50 mg/dL, NCEP, IDF)
  - Elevated fasting glucose ≥100 mg/dL

EPIDEMIOLOGY

Incidence
Parallels the incidence of obesity and T2DM.

Prevalence
Global prevalence is estimated at approximately one-quarter of the world population as of 2015 (1) and over one-third of the U.S. adult population as of 2016 (2).

ETIOLOGY AND PATHOPHYSIOLOGY

- Increase in intra-abdominal and visceral adipose tissue
- Adipose tissue dysfunction, hormone dysregulation, insulin resistance, and leptin resistance
- Decreased levels of adiponectin, an adipocytokine, known to protect against T2DM, HTN, atherosclerosis, and inflammation; decreased levels of ghrelin, that is associated with T2DM, insulin resistance and obesity
- Abnormal fatty acid metabolism, vascular endothelial dysfunction, systemic inflammation (increased IL-6, tumor necrosis factor-α [TNF-α], resistin, CRP), oxidative stress, elevated renin-angiotensin system activation, and a prothrombotic state (increased tissue plasminogen activator inhibitor-1) are also associated.
- The main etiologic factors are the following:
  - Central obesity (particularly abdominal)/excess visceral adipose tissue
  - Endocrine imbalances, insulin resistance, leptin resistance
  - Other contributing factors:
    - Advancing age and associated hormonal changes
    - Proinflammatory state
    - Genetics, epigenetics, parental obesity
    - Sedentary lifestyle
    - Disordered sleep
    - Dietary patterns with high levels of ultraprocessed foods and sugar sweetened beverages (SSB)
    - Prescription medications (e.g., corticosteroids, antipsychotics, β-blockers)

Genetics
Genetic factors appear to contribute to predisposition promoting obesity and MetS. Most identified genes are transcription factors or regulators of transcription and translation with evidence of complex interactions between genetics and environment. Parental obesity at the time of conception and epigenetic changes may play a significant role in promoting MetS in offspring.

RISK FACTORS

- Childhood obesity; intra-abdominal obesity, insulin resistance, gestational diabetes mellitus
- Older age, postmenopausal status
- Family history; ethnicity
- Physical inactivity
- Diet high in processed or excessive carbohydrates
- High consumption of sugar, fructose, and SSB
- Smoking
- Low socioeconomic status
- High level of chronic stress
- Alteration of gut microbiome
- Poor sleep, disrupted circadian rhythm, obstructive sleep apnea

GENERAL PREVENTION

- Maintenance of healthy weight
- Built environment to promote healthy lifestyle choices and reduce sedentary time
- Regular and sustained physical activity (3)[A]
- Limiting processed carbohydrates and sugars (4)[A]; avoidance of SSB; limiting alcohol consumption

COMMONLY ASSOCIATED CONDITIONS

- PCOS
- Acanthosis nigricans
- Nonalcoholic fatty liver disease (NAFLD), nonalcoholic steatohepatitis
- Obstructive sleep apnea (OSA)
- Asthma
- Osteoarthritis
- Depression and anxiety
- Cognitive impairment, Alzheimer dementia
- Heartburn and gastroesophageal reflux disease
- Gallstones
- Chronic renal disease
- Erectile dysfunction
- Hyperuricemia and gout
- Vitamin D deficiency
- Subclinical hypothyroidism

DIAGNOSIS

HISTORY
Identifying risk factors

- Family history of MetS, T2DM, stroke, and cardiovascular disease
- Symptoms indicating cardiovascular disease or diabetes or PCOS or sleep apnea
- Comprehensive lifestyle history:
  - Diet, including timing (night eating), frequency (snacking/grazing), and intake of proteins, fats, carbohydrates, especially processed foods, added sugars, and caloric beverages
  - Weight history, including onset of obesity and previous weight loss attempts
  - Comprehensive medication history
  - Exercise regimen, daily activity level
  - Alcohol intake, tobacco, cannabis, and illicit substance use history
  - Sleep patterns, duration, and quality
  - Perceived stressors and social support
- Cardiovascular risk assessment tool

PHYSICAL EXAM

- Waist circumference with abdominal obesity: men ≥102 cm, women ≥88 cm in white, African, Hispanic, and Native American populations and ≥90 cm and ≥80 cm, respectively, in East Asian and South Asian populations
- BP ≥130/85 mm Hg or treatment
- Additional exam findings suggestive of insulin resistance such as acanthosis nigricans, hirsutism, acrochordons

DIFFERENTIAL DIAGNOSIS

- Prediabetes, T2DM are associated with MetS
- OSA, PCOS, thyroid abnormalities, Cushing syndrome, medication effect (especially psychotropic, some anticonvulsants, chronic steroids, β-blockers, and thiazide diuretic medications) should be considered in the differential.

DIAGNOSTIC TESTS & INTERPRETATION

Initial Tests (lab, imaging)

- Fasting TGs ≥150 mg/dL or treatment
- HDL: men <40 mg/dL, women <50 mg/dL or treatment
- Fasting glucose ≥100 mg/dL or treatment or hemoglobin A1C >5.7%

Follow-Up Tests & Special Considerations

- Body composition measurements to assess lean tissue and fat mass. Athletes and bodybuilders may demonstrate elevated BMI despite low body fat. Older and more frail individuals with sarcopenic obesity may demonstrate normal BMI.
- Formal 75-mg oral glucose tolerance test or hemoglobin A1C for diagnosis of impaired glucose tolerance (IGT) or prediabetes
- Consider measurement of fasting insulin levels and/or calculation of TGA:HDL ratio (elevated in insulin resistance) or HOMA-IR.
- Liver function tests to assess for NAFLD
- Consider evaluation for OSA.
- Consider evaluation for hyperuricemia, hs-CRP, and microalbuminuria.
- Consider detailed lipid analysis and APOE-4 genotype testing.

Diagnostic Procedures/Other

- Home BP monitoring or 24-hour BP monitoring may be used to rule out white coat HTN.
- ECG, stress test, coronary calcium score
- Ultrasound of liver to evaluate for fatty liver

Test Interpretation

Evaluations are for further cardiometabolic risk factor assessment and management.

 TREATMENT

Primary therapeutic goal is to prevent or reduce obesity and risk factors. Aggressive lifestyle modification (diet and exercise and sleep) is considered first-line therapy and most clinically effective >7% weight loss and/or significant dietary carbohydrate restriction can improve/reverse risk factors associated with MetS (4)[A],(5). There is evidence that time-restricted feeding may also help the individual components of MetS (6),(7)[A].

GENERAL MEASURES

- Increase daily physical activity (3)[A].
- Stop smoking.
- Avoid excess alcohol intake.
- Promote a Mediterranean and/or a low-carbohydrate diet, low glycemic load diet, avoiding sugars and starchy carbohydrates.
- Avoid sugar-sweetened beverages. Note that some nonnutritive sweeteners may also alter sweet-taste receptors, gut hormone secretion, and promote gut microbiome imbalance and insulin resistance (8)[C].
- Consider use of time-restricted feeding (6)[A],(7). (Avoid in individuals with history of eating disorders.)
- Maintain healthy sleep patterns and regular stress management.

MEDICATION

Optional: Metformin (Glucophage) to prevent T2DM and GLP1 receptor agonists (GLP1RA) may also be effective in treating insulin resistance. If CAD or T2DM is already evident, treat as per guidelines. With metformin (Glucophage), consider vitamin B_{12} supplementation as needed.

First Line

Lifestyle modification alone can be an initial strategy in individuals with low 10-year risk for coronary artery disease (CAD). In individuals with higher 10-year risk, more aggressive risk factor–based approach is recommended in addition to lifestyle modifications:

- Obesity: Aim for a ≥5–10% weight reduction, which is associated with significant benefits.
- Physical activity: 30 to 60 minutes of moderate-intensity aerobic activities such as brisk walking 5 to 7 days/week; increase in daily lifestyle activities and resistance training 1 to 2 days/week. In patients with established CAD, assess detailed history of physical activity and exercise tolerance to guide activity prescription. Advise medically supervised programs for high-risk population. Shorter bursts of exercise several times a day also contributes to health benefit.
- Smoking cessation
- Evaluate suspected obstructive sleep apnea.
- Treat cardiac risk factors associated with MetS including elevated triglycerides and low HDL.
- Aim for similar BP targets to patients with diabetes if hypertension.
- For IGT and/or prediabetes, intensive lifestyle interventions including low-carbohydrate diets (5)+/− metformin +/− GLP1RA to decrease the risk of progression to T2DM.

ISSUES FOR REFERRAL

- Obesity management, nutrition therapy
- Decreasing mobility, impaired mobility
- Liver function tests suggesting liver disease
- Suspected OSA

SURGERY/OTHER PROCEDURES

Bariatric surgery can treat MetS in severely obese patients who have failed trials of lifestyle modification and pharmacotherapy if body mass index (BMI) >40 or BMI >35 with obesity-related comorbidities.

COMPLEMENTARY & ALTERNATIVE MEDICINE

Insufficient or no evidence on the use of garlic, cinnamon, green tea, L-carnitine, plant sterols, or zinc supplementation for improved insulin sensitivity

 ONGOING CARE

FOLLOW-UP RECOMMENDATIONS

- Regular exercise will improve all components of MetS. Cumulative small periods of exercise over the day provide significant health benefits. Encourage small increases in physical activity over time (3)[A].
- Encourage replacing sedentary activity choices (e.g., sitting at desk, driving car, taking elevator, and the like) to more active ones (e.g., standing desk, walking, cycling, stationary walking during commercials). Interrupt sedentary times with physical activity like getting up from a chair or walking or stretching.
- Regular monitoring of weight, WC, and BP. Fasting TG, HDL, and sugar levels may be routinely monitored to assess progress and to focus treatment efforts.
- Long-term regular follow-up and monitoring may result in increased adherence to healthy behavior changes.

Patient Monitoring

Especially with significant weight loss, intermittent fasting (6)[A], or low-carbohydrate diet (4)[A],(5), monitor for low blood sugars, and blood pressure, and deescalate medications, as necessary.

DIET

- Dietary recommendations may include limiting sugars and simple carbohydrates in diet; intermittent fasting or time-restricted feeding (6)[A]; eating a low-carbohydrate (4)[A],(5), Mediterranean, or DASH (Dietary Approaches to Stop Hypertension) diet.
- To reduce risk of developing T2DM, encourage increasing intake of vegetables and fiber, limit fruit, and keep alcohol in moderation.
- Avoid processed grains, fruit juice, and sugar-sweetened beverages (5).

PATIENT EDUCATION

Diet and exercise are crucial. This is a reversible condition.

COMPLICATIONS

Progression of CVD and T2DM, an increased risk of NAFLD, stroke, chronic kidney disease, cognitive decline, and an increased risk of developing certain cancers, including breast cancer in women, pancreatic cancer, colon cancer, among others

REFERENCES

1. Saklayen MG. The global epidemic of the metabolic syndrome. *Curr Hypertens Rep.* 2018;20(2):12.
2. Hirode G, Wong RJ. Trends in the prevalence of metabolic syndrome in the United States, 2011–2016. *JAMA.* 2020;323(24):2526–2528.
3. Myers J, Kokkinos P, Nyelin E. Physical activity, cardiorespiratory fitness, and the metabolic syndrome. *Nutrients.* 2019;11(7):1652.
4. Fechner E, Smeets ETHC, Schrauwen P, et al. The effects of different degrees of carbohydrate restriction and carbohydrate replacement on cardiometabolic risk markers in humans—a systematic review and meta-analysis. *Nutrients.* 2020;12(4):991.
5. Hyde PN, Sapper TN, Crabtree CD, et al. Dietary carbohydrate restriction improves metabolic syndrome independent of weight loss. *JCI Insight.* 2019;4(12):e128308.
6. Harris L, Hamilton S, Azevedo LB, et al. Intermittent fasting interventions for treatment of overweight and obesity in adults: a systematic review and meta-analysis. *JBI Database System Rev Implement Rep.* 2018;16(2):507–547.
7. Świątkiewicz I, Woźniak A, Taub PR. Time-restricted eating and metabolic syndrome: current status and future perspectives. *Nutrients.* 2021;13(1):221.
8. Schiano C, Grimaldi V, Scognamiglio M, et al. Soft drinks and sweeteners intake: possible contribution to the development of metabolic syndrome and cardiovascular diseases. Beneficial or detrimental action of alternative sweeteners? *Food Res Int.* 2021;142:110220.

 SEE ALSO

Diabetes; Hypertension; Obesity; Obstructive Sleep Apnea; Polycystic Ovarian Syndrome (PCOS); Prediabetes

 CODES

ICD10

E88.81 Metabolic syndrome

CLINICAL PEARLS

- Consider further evaluation for MetS when history and/or physical exam demonstrates findings consistent with sedentary lifestyle, sleep apnea, increasing WC, elevation of BP, increased TG:HDL ratio, evidence of insulin resistance, or abnormal screening labs or treatment for lipids or blood glucose.
- Reduction of obesity and cardiovascular risk factors is the cornerstone of management of MetS.
- Consider alternatives for medications known to increase risk of weight gain and/or MetS such as atypical antipsychotic medications and chronic steroids.
- Aggressive lifelong lifestyle modification is the first-line and most potent treatment for all patients (limiting daily sugars and carbohydrates, regular 30- to 60-minute exercise regiments). Advance interventions early to prevent progression and further complications. Add medications and/or refer to obesity medicine specialists or endocrinologists early if no improvement despite initial efforts.

M

METATARSALGIA

Ammar Shahid, MD • Marc McKenna, MD, CAQSM

BASICS

DESCRIPTION
- Metatarsalgia is defined as pain in the forefoot under one or more metatarsal heads.
- There are three groups:
  - Primary: due to anatomical issues between the MT and other parts of the foot
  - Secondary: due to conditions that increase metatarsal loading via indirect mechanisms, such as chronic synovitis or fracture or injury to the MTP joint
  - Iatrogenic usually after a prior forefoot surgery

EPIDEMIOLOGY
Incidence
The overall incidence is in the general population is 5–36%; especially common in athletes engaging in high-impact sports (running, jumping, dancing), in rock climbers (12.5%), and in older active adults

Prevalence
Common

ETIOLOGY AND PATHOPHYSIOLOGY
- The 1st metatarsal head bears significant weight when walking or running. A normal metatarsal arch ensures this balance. The 1st metatarsal head normally has adequate padding to accommodate increased forces.
- Reactive tissue can build a callus around the metatarsal head, compounding the pain.
  - Excessive or repetitive stress. Forces are transmitted to the forefoot during several stages (midstance and push off) of walking and running. These forces are translated across the metatarsal heads at nearly 3 times the body weight.
  - A pronated splayfoot disturbs this balance, causing equal weight-bearing on all metatarsal heads.
  - Any foot deformity changes distribution of weight, impacting areas of the foot that do not have sufficient padding.
  - Soft tissue dysfunction: intrinsic muscle weakness, laxity in the Lisfranc ligament
  - Abnormal foot posture: forefoot varus or valgus, cavus or equinus deformities, loss of the metatarsal arch, splayfoot, pronated foot, inappropriate footwear
  - Dermatologic: warts, calluses (1)[C]
- Great toe
  - Hallux valgus (bunion), either varus or rigidus
- Lesser metatarsals
  - Freiberg infraction (i.e., aseptic necrosis of the metatarsal head usually due to trauma in adolescents who jump or sprint)
  - Hammer toe or claw toe
  - Morton syndrome (i.e., long 2nd metatarsal)

RISK FACTORS
- Obesity
- Forefoot surgery or trauma

- High heels, narrow shoes, or overly tight-fitting shoes (rock climbers typically wear small shoes)
- Competitive athletes in weight-bearing sports (e.g., ballet, basketball, running, soccer, baseball, football)
- Foot deformities or changes in range of motion (e.g., pes planus, pes cavus, tight Achilles tendon, tarsal tunnel syndrome, hallux valgus, prominent metatarsal heads, excessive pronation, hammer toe deformity, tight toe extensors) (1)[C]

Geriatric Considerations
- Concomitant arthritis
- Metatarsalgia is common in older athletes.
- Age-related atrophy of the metatarsal fat pad may increase the risk for metatarsalgia.

Pediatric Considerations
- Muscle imbalance disorders (e.g., Duchenne muscular dystrophy) causing foot deformities in children.
- In adolescent girls, consider Freiberg infraction.
- Salter I injuries may affect subsequent growth and healing of the epiphysis.

Pregnancy Considerations
- Forefoot pain during pregnancy usually results from change in gait, center of mass, and joint laxity.
- Wear properly fitted low-heeled shoes.

GENERAL PREVENTION
- Wear properly fitted shoes with good padding.
- Start weight-bearing exercise programs gradually.
- Adequate stretching, particularly of the calf muscles
- Weight loss if overweight

COMMONLY ASSOCIATED CONDITIONS
- Arthritis
- Morton neuroma
- Sesamoiditis
- Plantar keratosis—callous formation

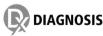

DIAGNOSIS

HISTORY
- Pain gradually develops and persists over the heads of one or more metatarsals. Pain is usually on the plantar surface and worse during midstance gait phase.
- Pain is often chronic.
- Predisposition with pes cavus and hyperpronation
- Pain often described as walking with a pebble in the shoe; aggravated during midstance or propulsion phases of walking or running

PHYSICAL EXAM
- Point tenderness over plantar metatarsal heads
- Pain in the interdigital space or a positive metatarsal squeeze test suggests Morton neuroma.
- Plantar keratosis
- Tenderness of the metatarsal head(s) with pressure applied by the examiner's finger and thumb
- Erythema and swelling (occasionally)

DIFFERENTIAL DIAGNOSIS
- Stress fracture (most commonly 2nd metatarsal)
- Morton neuroma (i.e., interdigital neuroma)
- Tarsal tunnel syndrome
- Sesamoiditis or sesamoid fracture
- Salter I fracture in children
- Arthritis (e.g., gouty, rheumatoid, inflammatory, osteoarthritis, septic, calcium pyrophosphate dihydrate [CPPD] crystal deposition disease)
- Lisfranc injury
- Avascular necrosis of the metatarsal head
- Ganglion cyst
- Foreign body
- Vasculitis (diabetes)
- Bony tumors

DIAGNOSTIC TESTS & INTERPRETATION
Initial Tests (lab, imaging)
- Weight-bearing radiographs: anteroposterior, lateral, and oblique views:
  - Occasionally, metatarsal or sesamoid axial films (to rule out sesamoid fracture) or skyline view of the metatarsal heads to assess the plantar declination of the metatarsal heads: obtained with the metatarsophalangeal (MTP) joints in dorsiflexion (to evaluate alignment)
- Ultrasound and MRI in recalcitrant cases especially if concern for stress fracture (2)[C]
- MR arthrography of the MTP joint can delineate capsular tears, typically of the distal lateral border of the plantar plate (an often underrecognized cause of metatarsalgia).
- Only if diagnosis is in question
  - Erythrocyte sedimentation rate or C-reactive protein
  - Rheumatoid factor
  - Uric acid
  - Glucose
  - CBC with differential

Diagnostic Procedures/Other
Plantar pressure distribution analysis may help distinguish pressure distribution patterns due to malalignment.

TREATMENT

Treatment for metatarsalgia is typically conservative.
- Relieve pain.
- Ice initially
- Rest: temporary alteration of weight-bearing activity; use of cane or crutch. For more physically active patients, suggest an alternative exercise or cross-training:
  - Moist heat later
  - Taping or gel cast
  - Stiff-soled shoes will act as a splint.
  - Gastrocnemius stretching exercises

- Relieve the pressure beneath the area of maximal pain by redistributing the pressure load of the foot, which can be achieve through orthotics.
- Weight loss, if overweight

MEDICATION
Nonsteroidal anti-inflammatory medications for 7 to 14 days if no contraindications toward use

ISSUES FOR REFERRAL
High-level athletes may benefit from early podiatric or orthopedic evaluation.

ADDITIONAL THERAPIES
- Physical therapy to restore normal foot biomechanics
- Low-heeled (<2 cm height) wide-toe-box shoes
- Metatarsal bars, pads, and arch supports. Metatarsal bars are often more effective than pads; if hallux valgus present, may try a valgus splint
- Orthotics/rocker bar (Prescriptive orthotics have been shown to be effective treatment.)
- Thick-soled shoes
- Shaving the callus may provide temporary relief. Callus excision is not recommended.
- Corticosteroid injection may benefit interdigital neuritis but should be used with caution because it may cause MTP instability and fat pad atrophy.
- Improve flexibility and strength of the intrinsic muscles of the foot with:
  – Exercises (e.g., towel grasps, pencil curls)
  – Physical therapy to maintain range of motion and restore normal biomechanics

SURGERY/OTHER PROCEDURES
- If no improvement with conservative therapy for 3 months, refer to foot/ankle orthopedic surgeon or podiatrist.
- Surgery may help correct anatomic abnormality: bunionectomy, partial osteotomy, or surgical fusion. Success rates vary depending on procedure.
- Direct plantar plate repair (grade II tear) combined with Weil osteotomy can restore normal alignment of the MTP joint, leading to diminished pain with improved functional scores.
- Callus removal is generally not recommended.
- Morton neurectomy and ultrasound-guided alcohol ablation of Morton neuroma are options (3)[C].
- Surgery only as a last resort if no anatomic abnormality is present.

COMPLEMENTARY & ALTERNATIVE MEDICINE
Magnetic insoles are not effective for chronic nonspecific foot pain.

ADMISSION, INPATIENT, AND NURSING CONSIDERATIONS
Patients generally admitted only for surgery

ONGOING CARE

FOLLOW-UP RECOMMENDATIONS
Patient Monitoring
If stress fracture has been ruled out and patient's condition has not improved >3 months of conservative treatment, consider surgical evaluation or corticosteroid injection (depending on the condition).

PATIENT EDUCATION
- Instruct about wearing proper shoes and gradual return to activity.
- Cross-training until symptoms subside. Goal is to restore normal foot biomechanics, relieve abnormal pressure on the plantar metatarsal heads, and relieve pain (4)[C].

PROGNOSIS
Outcome depends on the severity of the problem and whether surgery is required to correct it.

COMPLICATIONS
- Back, knee, and hip pain due to change in gait
- Transfer metatarsalgia following surgical intervention, which subsequently transfers stress to other areas.

REFERENCES

1. DiPreta JA. Metatarsalgia, lesser toe deformities, and associated disorders of the forefoot. *Med Clin North Am.* 2014;98(2):233–251.
2. Besse JL. Metatarsalgia. *Orthop Traumatol Surg Res.* 2017;103(Suppl 1):S29–S39.
3. Musson RE, Sawhney JS, Lamb L, et al. Ultrasound guided alcohol ablation of Morton's neuroma. *Foot Ankle Int.* 2012;33(3):196–201.
4. Espinosa N, Brodsky JW, Maceira E. Metatarsalgia. *J Am Acad Orthop Surg.* 2010;18(8):474–485.

ADDITIONAL READING

- Birbilis T, Theodoropoulou E, Koulalis D. Forefoot complaints—the Morton's metatarsalgia. The role of MR imaging. *Acta Medica (Hradec Kralove).* 2007;50(3):221–222.
- Burns J, Landorf KB, Ryan MM, et al. Interventions for the prevention and treatment of pes cavus. *Cochrane Database Syst Rev.* 2007;(4):CD006154.

- Deshaies A, Roy P, Symeonidis PD, et al. Metatarsal bars more effective than metatarsal pads in reducing impulse on the second metatarsal head. *Foot (Edinb).* 2011;21(4):172–175.
- Pace A, Scammell B, Dhar S. The outcome of Morton's neurectomy in the treatment of metatarsalgia. *Int Orthop.* 2010;34(4):511–515.
- Park CH, Chang MC. Forefoot disorders and conservative treatment. *Yeungnam Univ J Med.* 2019;36(2):92–98.
- Thomas JL, Blitch EL IV, Chaney DM, et al; and Clinical Practice Guideline Forefoot Disorders Panel. Diagnosis and treatment of forefoot disorders. Section 2. Central metatarsalgia. *J Foot Ankle Surg.* 2009;48(2):239–250.

SEE ALSO

Morton Neuroma (Interdigital Neuroma)

CODES

ICD10
- M77.40 Metatarsalgia, unspecified foot
- G57.60 Lesion of plantar nerve, unspecified lower limb
- M77.42 Metatarsalgia, left foot

CLINICAL PEARLS
- Metatarsalgia refers to pain of the plantar surface of the forefoot in the region of the metatarsal heads.
- Metatarsalgia is common in athletes who participate in high-impact sports involving the lower extremities.
- Patients describe as "walking with a pebble in the shoe." Pain is worse during midstance or propulsion phases of walking or running. The most common physical finding is point tenderness over the plantar metatarsal heads.
- Typical treatment is conservative, including rest and ice, activity modification, and ensuring proper padding under the foot.
- Pregnant patients should wear properly fitted, low-heeled shoes to reduce incidence of metatarsalgia.

M

MILD COGNITIVE IMPAIRMENT

Birju B. Patel, MD, FACP • N. Wilson Holland, MD, FACP

BASICS

DESCRIPTION
- Mild cognitive impairment (MCI) is defined as significant cognitive impairment in the absence of dementia, as measured by standard memory tests:
  - Concern regarding change in cognition
  - Preservation of independence in functional activities (ADLs)
  - Impairment in ≥1 cognitive domains (attention, executive dysfunction, memory, visuospatial, language)
  - Other terms used in the literature relating to MCI: Cognitive impairment not dementia (CIND); mild cognitive disorder. Some of these conditions do not progress to dementia. *DSM-5* mentions "mild neurocognitive disorder" (mNCD), which may be a precursor to Alzheimer disease and has many of the same features as MCI.
- Older adults with MCI are 3 times more likely to progress to dementia in 2 to 5 years than age-matched cohorts (1)[A].

EPIDEMIOLOGY

Incidence
- Predominant sex: male > female
- Predominant age:
  - Higher in older persons and in those with less education
  - 12 to 15/1,000 person-years in those age ≥65 years
  - 50 to 75/1,000 person-years in those age ≥75 years

Prevalence
- MCI is more prevalent than dementia in the United States.
- 12–18% for those age ≥60 years. ~25% for age 80–84 years. Prevalence increases with age and for those with lower educational level (2).

ETIOLOGY AND PATHOPHYSIOLOGY
- Subtypes of MCI:
  - Single-domain amnestic
  - Multiple-domain amnestic
  - Nonamnestic single-domain
  - Nonamnestic multiple-domain
- The amnestic subtype is higher risk for progression to Alzheimer disease.
- Vascular, neurodegenerative, traumatic, metabolic, psychiatric, or a combination

Genetics
In certain subsets of MCI where the disease will progress to Alzheimer dementia one must consider apolipoprotein (APO) E4 genotype: Various pathways exist leading to amyloid accumulation and deposition thought to be associated with dementia.

RISK FACTORS
- Diabetes; hypertension; hyperlipidemia; cerebrovascular disease
- Smoking
- Sleep apnea
- APO E4 genotype

- Low educational levels
- Depression
- Sedentary lifestyle

GENERAL PREVENTION
Optimize vascular risk factors and focus on a healthy, active lifestyle.

COMMONLY ASSOCIATED CONDITIONS
See "Risk Factors."

DIAGNOSIS

HISTORY
- Focus on cognitive deficits and impairment. MCI is meant to reflect a change in cognition and not lifelong impaired cognition.
- Review all medications that may affect cognition with emphasis given to anticholinergic medications (patients on these may mistakenly be classified as having MCI).
- Rule out depression. The prevalence of depression in patients with MCI is higher than age-matched cohorts.
- Assess function (ADLs, instrumental ADLs) and subtle changes in daily function (e.g., in the workplace).
- Impact on interpersonal relationships and caregiver stress
- Assess vascular risk factors (hypertension, diabetes, hyperlipidemia, and cerebrovascular disease).
- Assess behavioral changes.
- Olfactory dysfunction may be associated with amnestic MCI and progression to Alzheimer dementia. This can be easily evaluated in patients with memory impairment (3)

PHYSICAL EXAM
- A general exam focusing on clinical clues to identifying vascular disease (e.g., bruits, abnormal BP)
- Neurologic exam to rule out reversible CNS causes cognitive impairment or other causes of cognitive impairment
- Office measures of cognitive function, depression, and functional status

DIFFERENTIAL DIAGNOSIS
- Normal aging (age related cognitive impairment, age associated memory impairment)
- Delirium; dementia; depression
- "Reversible" cognitive impairment
  - Medications (anticholinergics and medications with anticholinergic properties)
  - Hypothyroidism
  - Vitamin B$_{12}$ deficiency
- Give consideration to sleep conditions, especially sleep apnea, that can contribute to cognitive deficits.

DIAGNOSTIC TESTS & INTERPRETATION
- Formal screening with standardized cognitive tests is important (e.g., Montreal Cognitive Assessment [MoCA] and Saint Louis University Mental Status [SLUMS]); MoCA may be more sensitive for detecting and following MCI.
- Neuropsychological testing is recommended for all patients with confirmed MCI.

Initial Tests (lab, imaging)
- Complete blood count
- Comprehensive metabolic profile
- Thyroid-stimulating hormone
- Vitamin B$_{12}$
- Imaging tests are helpful when there are focal neurologic deficits or rapid or atypical presentations:
  - CT scan can detect structural CNS conditions leading to cognitive impairment:
    - Subdural hematoma; normal pressure hydrocephalus; metastatic disease; cerebrovascular accident
  - MRI further evaluates vascular, infectious, neoplastic, and inflammatory conditions.

Follow-Up Tests & Special Considerations
- Document progression of functional impairment, cognitive decline, concurrent depression, and comorbid conditions.
- Advanced care planning while patient is competent
- Early education of caregivers on safety, maintaining structure, managing stress, and future planning
- Focus on driving ability and safety.
- Work-related issues should be explored and optimized as best possible.
- Neuropsychological testing should be done at 1- to 2-year intervals depending on subjective concerns and ongoing diagnosis of MCI.

Test Interpretation
- Little is known about MCI pathology due to a lack of longitudinal studies and heterogeneity of population studied.
- Alzheimer dementia pathophysiology:
  - Neurofibrillary tangles in hippocampus
  - Senile plaques (amyloid deposition)
  - Neuronal degeneration
- Those with MCI have intermediate amounts of pathologic findings of Alzheimer disease with amyloid deposition and neurofibrillary tangles in the mesial temporal lobes compared with those with dementia.
- Amnestic MCI is associated with white matter hyperintensity volume on MRI, whereas nonamnestic MCI is associated with infarcts.

TREATMENT

GENERAL MEASURES
Atherosclerotic risk factors should be treated aggressively.

MEDICATION
The use of cholinesterase inhibitors (ChEIs) in MCI is not associated with any delay in the onset of Alzheimer disease or dementia. Moreover, the safety profile showed that the risks associated with ChEIs are significant. Therefore, ChEIs are not routinely recommended (1)[B].

ISSUES FOR REFERRAL

Consider referral to a memory specialist (i.e., geriatrician, neurologist, geropsychiatric, neuropsychologist) to evaluate and differentiate subtypes of MCI and specific cognitive deficits.

ADDITIONAL THERAPIES

There may be benefit in terms of improvement in performance on tests for global cognitive functioning with cognitive training and physical exercise. Exercise training for 6 months is likely to improve cognitive measures.

COMPLEMENTARY & ALTERNATIVE MEDICINE

- No evidence suggests the efficacy of vitamin E in the prevention or treatment of people with MCI.
- Long-term use of *Ginkgo biloba* extract has shown to have no benefit in the treatment of MCI and in terms of progression to dementia. In addition, *Ginkgo biloba* can be associated with increase in bleeding risk including CNS bleeds (4)[B].

ADMISSION, INPATIENT, AND NURSING CONSIDERATIONS

Delirium is more common in patients hospitalized with all forms of cognitive impairment.

- Avoid medications that may worsen or precipitate cognitive decline (e.g., anticholinergics, antihistamines, and sedatives).
- Patients may be extremely sensitive to the hospital environment:
  - Moderate level of stimulation is best.
  - Avoid sensory deprivation. Make sure that patients have access to hearing aids and eyeglasses.
  - Use frequent cueing and have caregivers or family in the room whenever possible with patient.
  - Frequently orient patients to date and time.

ONGOING CARE

FOLLOW-UP RECOMMENDATIONS

Reevaluate every 6 to 12 months to determine if symptoms are progressing.

Patient Monitoring

Appropriate cognitive and functional testing should be used to evaluate progression, along with clinical history and exam. If a medication is started, patients need to be followed more frequently to evaluate for efficacy, side effects, dose titration, and so forth. Declining executive function may be an early marker to progression of MCI to dementia, and clinicians should monitor and advise patients and families proactively to look for this. Impairments in ADL function is a good clue to progression to dementia from MCI. Attempts should be made to wean medications that can impact cognition.

DIET

Diet to minimize atherosclerotic risk factors should be emphasized.

PATIENT EDUCATION

- Long-term planning topics should be discussed including advanced directives, firearm safety, driving safety, finances, and estate planning.
- Encourage lifestyle changes:
  - Physical activity, such as walking 30 minutes daily on most days of the week, as exercise modestly improved some measures of cognition in some studies
  - Mental activity that stimulates language skills and psychomotor coordination should be encouraged. Computer activities, reading books, crafts, crossword puzzles, and games may be linked to decreased risk of development of MCI (5)[C].
- Cognitive rehabilitation strategies may be beneficial in helping with daily activities relating to memory tasks in MCI.
- Treatment of vascular risk factors (hypertension, diabetes, cerebrovascular disease, and hyperlipidemia) is important in lowering risk of progression to dementia (e.g., intensive blood pressure lowering in the Sprint Mind Study reduced incidence of MCI with target SBP of 120 mm Hg).
- There are no FDA-approved medications or dietary agents currently for MCI shown to have benefit.
- In those with sleep apnea, compliance with CPAP improves cognition.
- Good dental hygiene and regular dental evaluation must be maintained. Significant periodontal disease is associated with MCI.
- Excessive alcohol consumption, above recommended limits, worsens cognition.

PROGNOSIS

- Older adults with MCI have 3 times higher risks of progression to dementia in 2 to 5 years.
- Amnestic subtypes of MCI are most likely to progress to dementia.
- Neuropsychological testing measures, cerebrospinal fluid (CSF) biomarkers, and neuroimaging studies are being used in specialty settings to predict conversion to dementia. These are not widely available or cost-effective and are not used in general use.
- Women are more likely to progress to dementia.
- Olfactory dysfunction can be higher risk for progression to dementia.
- Patients with neuropsychiatric symptoms, such as anxiety or depression, are higher risk for progression to Alzheimer disease. This may be helpful in identifying higher risk MCI patients (6)[C].

REFERENCES

1. Petersen RC, Lopez O, Armstrong MJ, et al. Practice guideline update summary: mild cognitive impairment: report of the Guideline Development, Dissemination, and Implementation Subcommittee of the American Academy of Neurology. *Neurology*. 2018;90(3):126–135.
2. Petersen RC. Mild cognitive impairment. *Continuum (Minneap Minn)*. 2016;22(2 Dementia):404–418.
3. Roberts RO, Christianson TJ, Kremers WK, et al. Association between olfactory dysfunction and amnestic mild cognitive impairment and Alzheimer disease dementia. *JAMA Neurol*. 2016;73(1): 93–101.
4. Vellas B, Coley N, Ousset PJ, et al; for GuidAge Study Group. Long-term use of standardised *Ginkgo biloba* extract for the prevention of Alzheimer's disease (GuidAge): a randomised placebo-controlled trial. *Lancet Neurol*. 2012;11(10):851–859.
5. Marshall GA, Rentz DM, Frey MT, et al. Executive function and instrumental activities of daily living in mild cognitive impairment and Alzheimer's disease. *Alzheimers Dement*. 2011;7(3):300–308.
6. Roberto N, Portella MJ, Marquié M, et al. Neuropsychiatric profiles and conversion to dementia in mild cognitive impairment, a latent class analysis. *Sci Rep*. 2021;11(1):6448.

 CODES

ICD10

G31.84 Mild cognitive impairment, so stated

CLINICAL PEARLS

- Amnestic MCI affects primarily memory and is more likely to progress to Alzheimer dementia.
- Screen for reversible factors, particularly anticholinergic medications, depression, and sleep disorders.
- Look closely at vascular risk factors and modify them as best as possible.
- ChEIs should not be used routinely unless memory complaints are affecting quality of life in patients. Potential side effects of these medications should be thoroughly discussed with patients and their families. A baseline ECG should be done prior to initiation of ChEIs due to risk of bradycardia and syncope.
- Neuropsychological testing is recommended in individuals suspected of having MCI. Patients with MCI and with prominent subjective complaints should have follow-up testing to evaluate for progression between 1 and 2 years after the initial assessment.

M

MISCARRIAGE (EARLY PREGNANCY LOSS)

Clara M. Keegan, MD

BASICS

DESCRIPTION
- Miscarriage, also known as early pregnancy loss (EPL) or spontaneous abortion (SAb), is the failure or loss of a pregnancy before 13 weeks' gestational age (WGA).
- Related terms
  - Anembryonic gestation: gestational sac on ultrasound (US) without visible embryo after 6 WGA
  - Complete abortion: entire contents of uterus expelled
  - Ectopic pregnancy: pregnancy outside the uterus
  - Embryonic or fetal demise: cervix closed; embryo or fetus present in the uterus without cardiac activity
  - Incomplete abortion: abortion with retained products of conception, generally placental tissue
  - Induced or therapeutic abortion: evacuation of uterine contents or products of conception medically or surgically
  - Inevitable abortion: cervical dilatation or rupture of membranes in the presence of vaginal bleeding
  - Recurrent abortion: ≥3 consecutive pregnancy losses at <15 WGA
  - Threatened abortion: vaginal bleeding in the 1st trimester of pregnancy
  - Septic abortion: a spontaneous or therapeutic abortion complicated by pelvic infection; common complication of illegally performed induced abortions
- Synonym(s): spontaneous abortion
  - Missed abortion and blighted ovum are used less frequently in favor of terms representing the sonographic diagnosis.

EPIDEMIOLOGY
Predominant age: increases with advancing age, especially >35 years; at age 40 years, the loss rate is twice that of age 20 years.

Incidence
- Threatened abortion (1st-trimester bleeding) occurs in 20–25% of clinical pregnancies.
- Between 10% and 15% of all clinically recognized pregnancies end in EPL, with 80% of these occurring within 12 weeks after last menstrual period (LMP) (1).
- When both clinical and biochemical (β-hCG detected) pregnancies are considered, about 30% of pregnancies end in EPL.
- One in four women will have an EPL during her lifetime (1).

ETIOLOGY AND PATHOPHYSIOLOGY
- Chromosomal anomalies (50% of cases)
- Congenital anomalies
- Trauma
- Maternal factors: uterine abnormalities, infection (toxoplasma, other viruses, rubella, cytomegalovirus, herpesvirus), maternal endocrine disorders, hypercoagulable state

Genetics
Approximately 50% of 1st-trimester EPLs have significant chromosomal anomalies, with 50% of these being autosomal trisomies and the remainder being triploidy, tetraploidy, or 45X monosomies.

RISK FACTORS
Most cases of EPL occur in patients without identifiable risk factors; however, risk factors include the following:
- Chromosomal abnormalities
- Advancing maternal age

- Uterine abnormalities
- Maternal chronic disease (antiphospholipid antibodies, uncontrolled diabetes mellitus, polycystic ovarian syndrome, obesity, hypertension, thyroid disease, renal disease)
- Other possible contributing factors include smoking, alcohol, cocaine use, infection, and luteal phase defect.

GENERAL PREVENTION
- Insufficient evidence supports the use of aspirin and/or other anticoagulants, bed rest, hCG, immunotherapy, uterine muscle relaxants, or vitamins for general prevention of EPL, before or after threatened abortion is diagnosed.
- By the time hemorrhage begins, half of pregnancies complicated by threatened abortion already have no fetal cardiac activity.
- In threatened abortion, oral progestogens may reduce the risk of EPL (RR 0.73, 95% CI 0.59–0.92) and increase the rate of live birth (RR 1.07, 95% CI 1.00–1.15) (2)[B].
- Antiphospholipid syndrome: The combination of unfractionated heparin and aspirin reduces risk of EPL in women with antiphospholipid antibodies and a history of recurrent abortion (3)[C].

DIAGNOSIS

HISTORY
- The possibility of pregnancy should be considered in a reproductive-age woman who presents with nonmenstrual vaginal bleeding.
- Vaginal bleeding
  - Characteristics (amount, color, consistency, associated symptoms), onset (abrupt or gradual), duration, intensity/quantity, and exacerbating/precipitating factors
  - Document LMP if known: allows calculation of estimated gestational age
- Abdominal pain/uterine cramping as well as associated nausea/vomiting/syncope
- Rupture of membranes
- Passage of products of conception
- Prenatal course: toxic or infectious exposures, family or personal history of genetic abnormalities, past history of ectopic pregnancy or EPL, endocrine disease, autoimmune disorder, bleeding/clotting disorder

PHYSICAL EXAM
- Orthostatic vital signs to estimate hemodynamic stability
- Abdominal exam for tenderness, guarding, rebound, bowel sounds (peritoneal signs more likely with ectopic pregnancy)
- Speculum exam for visual assessment of cervical dilation, blood, and products of conception (confirms diagnosis of EPL)
- Bimanual exam to assess for uterine size–dates discrepancy and adnexal tenderness or mass

DIFFERENTIAL DIAGNOSIS
- Ectopic pregnancy: potentially life-threatening; must be considered in any woman of childbearing age with abdominal pain and vaginal bleeding
- Physiologic bleeding in normal pregnancy (implantation bleeding)
- Subchorionic bleeding
- Cervical polyps, neoplasia, and/or inflammatory conditions

- Hydatidiform mole pregnancy
- hCG-secreting ovarian tumor

DIAGNOSTIC TESTS & INTERPRETATION
Initial Tests (lab, imaging)
- Quantitative hCG
  - Particularly useful if intrauterine pregnancy (IUP) has not been documented by US
  - Serial quantitative serum hCG measurements can assess viability of the pregnancy. Serum hCG should rise at least 53% every 48 hours through 7 weeks after LMP. An inappropriate rise, plateau, or decrease of hCG suggests abnormal IUP or possible ectopic pregnancy.
- Complete blood count (CBC) with differential
- Rh type
- Cultures: gonorrhea/chlamydia
- US exam to evaluate fetal viability and to rule out ectopic pregnancy (4)[A]
  - hCG >2,000 mIU/mL necessary to detect IUP via transvaginal US (TVUS), >5,500 mIU/mL for abdominal US
  - TVUS criteria for nonviable intrauterine gestation: 7-mm fetal pole without cardiac activity or 25-mm gestational sac without a fetal pole, IUP with no growth over 1 week, or previously seen IUP no longer visible
  - Structures and timing: with TVUS, gestational sac of 2 to 3 mm generally seen around 5 WGA; yolk sac by 5.5 WGA; fetal pole with cardiac activity by 6 WGA

Follow-Up Tests & Special Considerations
- In the case of vaginal bleeding with no documented IUP and hCG <2,000 mIU/mL, follow serum hCG levels weekly to zero.
- If levels plateau, consider ectopic pregnancy or retained products of conception. If levels are very high, consider gestational trophoblastic disease.
- If initial hCG level does not permit documentation of IUP by TVUS, follow serum hCG in 48 hours to document appropriate rise.
- Repeat US once hCG is at a level commensurate with visualization on US (see above).
- Provide patient with ectopic precautions in interim: worsening abdominal pain, dizziness/syncope, nausea/vomiting.
- In a pregnancy of unknown location with hCG rise <53% in 48 hours, offer methotrexate for treatment of presumed ectopic pregnancy.

Diagnostic Procedures/Other
- Fetal heart tones can be auscultated with Doppler starting between 10 and 12 WGA in a viable pregnancy.
- In threatened abortion, fetal cardiac activity at 7 to 11 WGA is 90–96% predictive of continued pregnancy (1).

TREATMENT

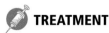

GENERAL MEASURES
- Discuss contraception plan at the time of diagnosis of EPL, as ovulation can occur prior to resumption of normal menses.
- Expectant management ("watchful waiting") is 90% effective for incomplete abortion, although it may take several weeks for the process to be complete (1). This approach is only recommended in the 1st trimester and is more effective in women with symptoms of impending pregnancy loss (3)[C].

MEDICATION

- Rates of complete miscarriage and of need for surgical evacuation are equivalent with expectant management and medication (5)[A].
- Long-term conception rate and pregnancy outcomes are similar for women who undergo expectant management, medical treatment, or surgical evacuation.
- Infection rates are lower with medical versus surgical management.

First Line

- Misoprostol: most common agent for inducing passage of tissue in incomplete abortion or embryonic demise
  - Off-label use; has not been submitted to the FDA for consideration for use in treatment of early pregnancy failure; recognized by the World Health Organization (WHO) as a life-saving medication for this indication
  - Efficacy: complete expulsion of products of conception in 71% by day 3, 84% by day 8
  - Efficacy depends on route of administration, gestational age of pregnancy, and dose.
  - Recommended dose is 800 μg vaginally; alternate regimens include the WHO regimen of 600 μg sublingually q3h for up to 3 doses; multidose regimens and oral dosing (including buccal and sublingual) may result in increased side effects.
  - The addition of mifepristone 200 mg, if available, given 24 hours before misoprostol increases the efficacy to 83.8% (ARR 16.7%, 95% CI 7.1–26.3%) (6)[A].
- Common adverse effects include abdominal pain/cramping, nausea, and diarrhea. Pain increases at higher doses but is manageable with oral analgesia.
- Recommended for stable patients who decline surgery but do not want to wait for spontaneous passage of products of conception.

Second Line

- Rh-negative patients should be given Rh immunoglobulin (RhoGAM) 50 μg IM following an EPL.
- Women with evidence of anemia should receive iron supplementation.

ISSUES FOR REFERRAL

Patients should be monitored for up to 1 year for the development of pathologic grief. There is insufficient evidence to support counseling to prevent development of anxiety or depression related to grief following EPL.

SURGERY/OTHER PROCEDURES

- Uterine aspiration (suction dilation and curettage [D&C] or manual uterine aspiration [MUA]), also known as manual vacuum aspiration (MVA), is the conventional treatment.
- Indications: septic abortion, heavy bleeding, hypotension, persistent IUP after medical or expectant management, patient choice
- Risks (all rare): anesthesia (usually local), uterine perforation, intrauterine adhesions, cervical trauma, infection that may lead to infertility or increased risk of ectopic pregnancy
- When compared with expectant management, surgical intervention leads to fewer days of vaginal bleeding, with a lower risk of incomplete abortion and heavy bleeding and a similar risk of infection, but a higher cost (7)[A]. It is appropriate to prioritize the patient's preference in determining management.

- Vacuum aspiration (manual or electric) is considered preferable to sharp curettage, as aspiration is less painful, takes less time, involves less blood loss, and does not require general anesthesia. The WHO supports use of suction curettage over rigid metal curettage.
- Although data from induced abortions suggest that antibiotic prophylaxis with doxycycline 200 mg in a single dose reduces the already rare risk of postprocedure infection, data are insufficient to support use of antibiotics before aspiration for EPL.

COMPLEMENTARY & ALTERNATIVE MEDICINE

A systematic review of Chinese herbal medicine alone and in conjunction with Western medicine showed benefit over Western medicine alone in achieving continued viability at 28 weeks (number needed to treat [NNT] = 4.8 pregnancies with combined therapy). However, the available studies did not meet international standards for reporting quality.

ADMISSION, INPATIENT, AND NURSING CONSIDERATIONS

- If the patient has orthostatic vital signs, initiate resuscitation with IV fluids and/or blood products, if needed.
- Hemodynamically unstable patients may require IV fluids and/or blood products to maintain BP.

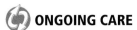 ONGOING CARE

FOLLOW-UP RECOMMENDATIONS

All patients should be offered follow-up in 2 to 6 weeks to monitor for resolution of bleeding, return of menses, and symptoms related to grief, as well as to review the contraception plan.

Patient Monitoring

- If EPL occurs in setting of previously documented IUP and abortion is completed with resumption of normal menses, it is not necessary to check or follow serum hCG to 0.
- After medical management, confirm complete expulsion with US or serial serum β-hCG.
- If pregnancy is not immediately desired, offer effective contraception. Immediate insertion of an intrauterine device is both acceptable and safe.
- If pregnancy is desired, provide preconception counseling. There is no evidence that it is necessary to wait a certain number of cycles before attempting conception again.

DIET

NPO if patient is to undergo D&C under general anesthesia

PATIENT EDUCATION

- Pelvic rest for 1 week after D&C or MUA
- Advise patients to call with excessive bleeding (soaking two pads per hour for 2 hours), fever, pelvic pain, or malaise, which could indicate retained products of conception or endometritis.
- A patient fact sheet on miscarriage is available through the American Academy of Family Physicians at http://www.aafp.org/afp/2011/0701/p85.html.

PROGNOSIS

- Prognosis is excellent once bleeding is controlled.
- Recurrent miscarriage: Prognosis depends on etiology; up to 70% rate of success with subsequent pregnancy

COMPLICATIONS

- D&C or MUA: uterine perforation, bleeding, adhesions, cervical trauma, and infection that may lead to infertility or increased risk of ectopic pregnancy. Bleeding and adhesions more common with D&C than with MUA; all complications rare
- Retained products of conception

REFERENCES

1. Prine LW, MacNaughton H. Office management of early pregnancy loss. *Am Fam Physician*. 2011;84(1):75–82.
2. Li L, Zhang Y, Tan H, et al. Effect of progestogen for women with threatened miscarriage: a systematic review and meta-analysis. *BJOG*. 2020;127(9):1055–1063.
3. Committee on Practice Bulletins-Gynecology. The American College of Obstetricians and Gynecologists Practice Bulletin No. 200. Early pregnancy loss. *Obstet Gynecol*. 2018;132(5):1311–1313.
4. Doubilet PM, Benson CB, Bourne T, et al; for Society of Radiologists in Ultrasound Multispecialty Panel on Early First Trimester Diagnosis of Miscarriage and Exclusion of a Viable Intrauterine Pregnancy. Diagnostic criteria for nonviable pregnancy early in the first trimester. *N Engl J Med*. 2013;369(15):1443–1451.
5. Kim C, Barnard S, Neilson JP, et al. Medical treatments for incomplete miscarriage. *Cochrane Database Syst Rev*. 2017;(1):CD007223.
6. Schreiber CA, Creinin MD, Atrio J, et al. Mifepristone pretreatment for the medical management of early pregnancy loss. *N Engl J Med*. 2018;378(23):2161–2170.
7. Nanda K, Lopez LM, Grimes DA, et al. Expectant care versus surgical treatment for miscarriage. *Cochrane Database Syst Rev*. 2012;(3):CD003518.

ADDITIONAL READING

MacNaughton H, Nothnagle M, Early J. Mifepristone and misoprostol for early pregnancy loss and medication abortion. *Am Fam Physician*. 2021;103(8):473–480.

 SEE ALSO

- Ectopic Pregnancy
- Algorithm: Recurrent Pregnancy Loss

 CODES

ICD10

- O03.9 Complete or unspecified spontaneous abortion without complication
- O03.4 Incomplete spontaneous abortion without complication
- O02.1 Missed abortion

CLINICAL PEARLS

- Any pregnant woman with abdominal pain and/or vaginal bleeding must be evaluated to rule out ectopic pregnancy, which is potentially life threatening.
- As all options have similar long-term outcomes, patient preference should determine whether management is expectant, medical, or surgical.

M

MITRAL REGURGITATION

Yongkasem Vorasettakarnkij, MD, MSc

BASICS

DESCRIPTION

- Disorder of mitral valve (MV) closure, either primary, secondary (functional), or mixed, resulting in a backflow of the left ventricular (LV) stroke volume into the left atrium (LA); uncompensated, this leads to LV and LA enlargement, elevated pulmonary pressures, atrial fibrillation (AF), heart failure (HF), and sudden cardiac death.
- Types of mitral regurgitation (MR):
  – Acute versus chronic
  – Primary versus secondary (functional) and mixed
    ○ Primary: abnormalities at any level of the MV structures (annulus, leaflets, chordae tendineae, and papillary muscles)
    ○ Secondary: no valvular abnormalities are found. The abnormal and dilated LV causes papillary muscle displacement, resulting in leaflet tethering with annular dilatation that prevents coaptation.
    ○ Mixed: mixed abnormalities of both primary and secondary types
- System(s) affected: cardiac; pulmonary

EPIDEMIOLOGY

Moderate to severe MR affects 2.5 million people in the United States (2000 data). It is the most common valvular disease and is expected to double by 2030 (1).

Prevalence

- By severity on echocardiography:
  – Mild MR: 19% (up to 40% if trivial jets included)
  – Moderate MR: 1.9%
  – Severe MR: 0.2%
- By category (1)
  – Degenerative (myxomatous disease, annular calcification): 60–70%
  – Ischemic: 20%
  – Endocarditis: 2–5%
  – Rheumatic: 2–5%

ETIOLOGY AND PATHOPHYSIOLOGY

- Acute MR
  – Leaflet perforation: infective endocarditis, trauma
  – Chordae tendineae rupture: trauma, spontaneous rupture, infective endocarditis, or rheumatic fever
  – Papillary muscle rupture or dysfunction: acute myocardial infarction (MI), severe myocardial ischemia, or trauma
- Chronic MR
  – Primary
    ○ Degenerative: mitral annular calcification, MV prolapse (MVP)
    ○ Infective endocarditis
    ○ Rheumatic heart disease (RHD)
    ○ Inflammatory diseases: lupus, eosinophilic endocardial disease
    ○ Toxin-induced valvulopathy: anorectic drugs
    ○ Congenital (cleft leaflet)
  – Secondary (functional)
    ○ Ischemic: coronary artery disease (CAD)/MI
    ○ Nonischemic: cardiomyopathy from any cause, annular dilatation from chronic AF, dyssynchrony from right ventricular pacing
- Acute MR: Acute MV damage leads to sudden LA and LV volume overload. Sudden rise in LV volume load without LV remodeling results in impaired forward cardiac output and possible cardiogenic shock.
- Chronic MR: LV eccentric hypertrophy compensates for increased regurgitant volume to maintain forward cardiac output and alleviate pulmonary congestion. However, LV remodeling can result in LV dysfunction. LA compensatory dilatation for the larger regurgitant volume predisposes patients to develop AF.

- Ischemic MR: papillary muscle rupture, ischemia during acute MI, and incomplete coaptation of leaflets or restricted valve movement from chronic ischemia

RISK FACTORS

Age, hypertension, RHD, endocarditis, anorectic drugs

GENERAL PREVENTION

- Risk factor modification for CAD
- Antibiotic prophylaxis for poststreptococcal RHD
- Endocarditis prophylaxis is no longer recommended.

COMMONLY ASSOCIATED CONDITIONS

MVP with MR common in Marfan syndrome

DIAGNOSIS

HISTORY

- Associated conditions: RHD, prior MI, connective tissue disorder
- Acute MR
  – Sudden onset of dyspnea
  – Orthopnea, paroxysmal nocturnal dyspnea
- Chronic MR
  – Exertional dyspnea, fatigue
  – Palpitation: paroxysmal/persistent AF

PHYSICAL EXAM

- Acute MR
  – Rapid and thready pulses
  – Signs of poor tissue perfusion with peripheral vasoconstriction
  – Hyperdynamic precordium without apical shift
  – S_3 and S_4 (if in sinus rhythm)
  – Systolic murmur at left sternal border and base
    ○ Early, middle, or holosystolic murmur
    ○ Often soft, low-pitched decrescendo murmur
  – Rales
- Chronic MR
  – Brisk upstroke of arterial pulse
  – Leftward displaced LV apical impulse
  – Systolic thrill at the apex (suggests severe MR)
  – Soft S_1 and widely split S_2, S_3 gallop
  – Loud P_2 (if pulmonary hypertension)
  – Holosystolic murmur at apex that radiates to axilla or to left parasternal border
  – Ankle edema, jugular venous distension, and ascites, if development of right-sided HF

DIFFERENTIAL DIAGNOSIS

- Aortic stenosis (AS): usually midsystolic but can be long; difficult to distinguish from holosystolic, at apical area, and radiating to the carotid arteries (unlike MR)
- Tricuspid regurgitation: holosystolic but at left lower sternal border, does not radiate to axilla, and may increase in intensity with inspiration (unlike MR)
- Ventricular septal defect (VSD): harsh holosystolic murmur at lower left sternal border but radiates to right sternal border (not axilla)

DIAGNOSTIC TESTS & INTERPRETATION

Initial Tests (lab, imaging)

- Chest x-ray (CXR)
  – Acute MR: pulmonary edema, normal heart size
  – Chronic MR: LA and LV enlargement
- ECG
  – Acute MR: varies depending on etiologies (e.g., AMI)
  – Chronic MR
    ○ P mitrale from LA enlargement, AF
    ○ LV hypertrophy
    ○ Q waves from prior MI

- Cardiac enzymes brain natriuretic peptide, if appropriate
- Transthoracic echocardiogram (TTE)
  – Indications for TTE (2)
    ○ Baseline evaluation of LV size and function, right ventricular function and LA size, pulmonary artery pressure, and severity of MR
    ○ Delineation of the mechanism of MR
    ○ Surveillance of asymptomatic moderate to severe LV dysfunction (ejection fraction [EF] and end-systolic dimension [ESD])
    ○ Evaluate MV apparatus and LV size and function after a change in sign/symptom in MR patient.
    ○ Evaluate after MV repair or replacement.
  – Findings in acute MR
    ○ Evidence of etiology: flail leaflet or vegetations
    ○ Normal LA and LV size
  – Findings in chronic MR
    ○ Evidence of degenerative, rheumatic, ischemic, congenital, and other causes
    ○ Enlarged LA and LV

Follow-Up Tests & Special Considerations

- Intervals for follow-up TTE: See "Follow-Up Recommendations."
- Cardiovascular magnetic resonance (CMR):
  – TTE results are not satisfactory to assess LV and RV volumes, function, or MR severity (2)[B].
- Transesophageal echocardiogram (TEE)
  – Intraoperatively to define the anatomic basis of MR and to guide repair (2)[B]
  – Nondiagnostic information about severity, mechanism of MR, and/or status of LV function from noninvasive imaging (2)[C]
- Exercise hemodynamics with either Doppler echocardiography or cardiac catheterization (2)[B].
  – Discrepancy between symptoms and the severity of MR from resting TTE in symptomatic patients with chronic primary MR
- Exercise treadmill testing (2)[C]
  – To establish symptom status and exercise tolerance in asymptomatic patients with chronic primary MR
- Noninvasive imaging (stress nuclear/positron emission tomography, CMR, stress echocardiography, cardiac CT angiography)
  – To establish etiology of chronic secondary MR and/or to assess myocardial viability (2)[C]

Diagnostic Procedures/Other

Cardiac catheterization (2)[C]

- Left ventriculography and hemodynamic measurement
  – Noninvasive tests are inconclusive regarding the severity of MR, LV function, and the need for surgery.
- Coronary angiography: prior to MV surgery in patients at risk for CAD

Test Interpretation

Quantification of severe MR requires an integration of the following structural parameters:

- LA size: dilated, unless acute
- LV size: dilated, unless acute
- MV morphology: flail leaflet, ruptured papillary muscle
- Doppler parameters: large central jet (>50% of LA), pulmonary vein systolic flow reversal
- Quantitative parameter: effective regurgitant orifice area ≥ 0.40 cm^2, regurgitation volume ≥ 60 mL, regurgitation fraction $\geq 50\%$

TREATMENT

MEDICATION

- Acute, severe MR
  - Medical therapy has a limited role and is aimed to stabilize hemodynamics preoperatively.
  - Vasodilators (nitroprusside, nicardipine): to improve hemodynamic compensation but is often limited by systemic hypotension (2),(3)[C]
- Chronic MR
  - Primary
    - Asymptomatic: no proven long-term medical therapy
    - Symptomatic: diuretics, β-blockers, angiotensin-converting enzyme inhibitors (ACE-I) or angiotensin receptor blockers (ARBs), and possibly aldosterone antagonists as indicated in standard therapy for HF (2)[B],(3)[C]
  - Secondary: LV dysfunction or symptomatic (stages B to D)
    - ACE-I or ARBs, β-blockers, and/or aldosterone antagonists as indicated in standard therapy for HF (2)[B],(3)[C]

SURGERY/OTHER PROCEDURES

- Isolated MV surgery is not indicated for patients with mild to moderate MR.
- Acute, severe MR secondary to acute MI
  - Acute rupture of papillary muscle: emergency MV repair/replacement
  - Papillary muscle displacement
    - Aggressive medical stabilization and intra-aortic balloon pump
    - Valve surgery usually required in addition to revascularization
- Chronic severe MR
  - Severe primary MR (2),(3),(4)
    - MV surgery
      - Symptomatic patients (stage D)
        - Absence of severe LV dysfunction (EF >30%) (2),(3)[B]
        - May be considered if presence of severe LV dysfunction (EF ≤30%) (2),(3)[C]
      - Asymptomatic patients
        - Mild/moderate LV dysfunction (EF 30–60% and/or ESD ≥40 mm, stage C2) (2)[B]
        - MV repair is reasonable for asymptomatic patients (stage C1) with preserved LV function (EF >60% and ESD <40 mm):
          - The likelihood of a successful and durable repair without residual MR is >95% and expected mortality <1% when performed at a heart valve center of excellence (2)[B].
      - Progressive increase in LV size or decrease in EF on serial imaging studies (4)[B]
      - Nonrheumatic MR with new onset of AF or resting pulmonary hypertension (pulmonary artery systolic pressure >50 mm Hg) and the likelihood of a successful and durable repair is high (2),(3)[B].
    - MV repair is recommended over MV replacement in patients with
      - MR limited to the posterior leaflet (2)[B]
      - MR involving the anterior leaflet or both leaflets when a successful and durable repair can be accomplished (2)[B]
    - Transcatheter MV repair:
      - May be considered for severely symptomatic patients (NYHA class III/IV) despite optimal GDMT for HF, who have favorable anatomy for the repair, and a reasonable life expectancy but a prohibitive surgical risk from severe comorbidities (2)[B]

  - Severe secondary MR (2),(3),(4)
    - MV surgery
      - Undergoing coronary artery bypass graft (CABG) (2),(3)[C]
      - Undergoing aortic valve replacement (2)[C]
      - May be considered for severely symptomatic patients (NYHA classes III and IV) despite optimal GDMT for HF (2)[B],(3)[C]
      - Chordal-sparing MVR is preferred over downsized annuloplasty repair in ischemic MR patients (4)[B].
    - Cardiac resynchronization therapy is recommended for symptomatic patients (stages B to D) who meet the indications for device therapy (2)[C].
    - Transcatheter MV repair:
      - May be considered for persistent symptoms despite maximally tolerated GDMT as assessed by a multidisciplinary experienced team in the evaluation and treatment of HF and MV disease, who have moderately severe or severe secondary MR, LVEF 20–50%, and LV end-systolic diameter <7.0 cm (5)[C]

Geriatric Considerations
- Medical therapy alone for patients >75 years of age with MR is preferred, owing to increased operative mortality and decreased survival (compared with those with AS), especially with preexisting CAD or need for MV replacement.
- MV repair is preferable than MV replacement.

ADMISSION, INPATIENT, AND NURSING CONSIDERATIONS

Acute MR: Stabilize airway, breathing, circulation (ABCs). Initiate IV, O₂, and monitoring. Nitroprusside (plus dobutamine and/or aortic balloon counterpulsation if hypotensive). Treat underlying causes (e.g., MI). Treat acute pulmonary edema with furosemide and morphine. Obtain urgent surgical consultation.

 ONGOING CARE

FOLLOW-UP RECOMMENDATIONS
Chronic MR: asymptomatic

- Mild MR with normal LV size and function and no pulmonary hypertension: annual clinical evaluation and TTE every 3 to 5 years or more frequently depending on course
- Moderate MR: annual clinical evaluation and TTE every 1 to 2 years
- Severe MR: clinical evaluation and TTE every 6 to 12 months
- Consider serial CXRs and ECGs and consider stress test if exercise capacity is doubtful.

PATIENT EDUCATION
- Exercise after MV repair: Avoid sports with risk for bodily contact or trauma. Low-intensity competitive sports are allowed.
- Competitive athletes with MR
  - Asymptomatic with normal LV size and function, normal pulmonary artery pressures, and sinus rhythm: no restrictions
  - Mildly symptomatic and those with LV dilatation: activities with low to moderate dynamic and static cardiac demand allowed
- AF and anticoagulation: no contact sports

PROGNOSIS
- Acute, severe MR: Mortality risk with surgery is 50%; mortality risk with medical therapy alone is 75% in the first 24 hours and 95% at 2 weeks.

- Chronic MR: asymptomatic severe MR with normal LVEF: 10% yearly rate of progression to symptoms and subnormal resting LVEF. Symptomatic severe MR: 8-year survival rate, 33% without surgery; mortality rate, 5% yearly

Pregnancy Considerations
MR with NYHA functional classes III and IV at high risk for maternal and/or fetal risk

COMPLICATIONS
Acute pulmonary edema, CHF, AF, bleeding risk with anticoagulation, endocarditis, sudden cardiac death

REFERENCES
1. Enriquez-Sarano M, Akins CW, Vahanian A. Mitral regurgitation. *Lancet*. 2009;373(9672): 1382–1394.
2. Nishimura RA, Otto CM, Bonow RO, et al. 2014 AHA/ACC guideline for the management of patients with valvular heart disease: a report of the American College of Cardiology/American Heart Association Task Force on Practice Guidelines. *Circulation*. 2014;129(23):e521–e643.
3. Baumgartner H, Falk V, Bax JJ, et al; for European Society of Cardiology Scientific Document Group. 2017 ESC/EACTS guidelines for the management of valvular heart disease. *Eur Heart J*. 2017;38(36): 2739–2791.
4. Nishimura RA, Otto CM, Bonow RO, et al. 2017 AHA/ACC focused update of the 2014 AHA/ACC guideline for the management of patients with valvular heart disease: a report of the AHA/ACC Task Force on Clinical Practice Guidelines. *Circulation*. 2017;135(25):e1159–e1195.
5. Bonow RO, O'Gara PT, Adams DH, et al. 2020 Focused update of the 2017 ACC expert consensus decision pathway on the management of mitral regurgitation: a report of the American College of Cardiology Solution Set Oversight Committee. *J Am Coll Cardiol*. 2020;75(17):2236–2270.

ADDITIONAL READING
- El Sabbagh A, Reddy YNV, Nishimura RA. Mitral valve regurgitation in the contemporary era: insights into diagnosis, management, and future directions. *JACC Cardiovasc Imaging*. 2018;11(4):628–643.
- Obadia JF, Messika-Zeitoun D, Leurent G, et al. Percutaneous repair or medical treatment for secondary mitral regurgitation. *N Engl J Med*. 2018;379(24):2297–2306.
- Stone GW, Lindenfeld J, Abraham WT, et al. Transcatheter mitral-valve repair in patients with heart failure. *N Engl J Med*. 2018;379(24):2307–2318.

 CODES

ICD10
- I34.0 Nonrheumatic mitral (valve) insufficiency
- I05.1 Rheumatic mitral insufficiency
- Q23.3 Congenital mitral insufficiency

CLINICAL PEARLS
- Follow-up for mild to moderate MR: serial exam and/or echo (mild, every 3 to 5 years, moderate 1 to 2 years) unless LV structural changes
- Severe MR is usually managed with MV repair.
- Endocarditis prophylaxis is not recommended.

M

MITRAL STENOSIS

Matthew A. Tunzi, DO • Laith Rommel Dinkha, DO

 BASICS

DESCRIPTION

- Mitral stenosis (MS) is the narrowing of the valve area causing obstruction of the left ventricular (LV) inflow, resulting in increased left atrial (LA) pressures and consequent elevation of pulmonary venous pressure.
- Normal valve orifice is 4 to 5 cm^2; symptoms typically seen when orifice is <2.5 cm^2 (1).
- Staging of the disease is used to guide appropriate treatment regimen (1).
  - Stage A: "at risk of MS"—mild valve doming with normal flow velocity and NO hemodynamic obstruction or symptoms
  - Stage B: "progressive MS"—increased diastolic doming, increased flow velocity, but MVA >1.5 cm^2, diastolic pressure 1/2 time <150 ms
  - Stage C: "asymptomatic severe MS"—diastolic doming, MVA <1.5 cm^2, diastolic pressure half time >150 ms, severe LA enlargement, PASP >30 mm Hg, but NO symptoms
  - Stage D: "symptomatic severe MS"—stage C with dyspnea on exertion and decreased exercise tolerance
- The most common etiology for MS is rheumatic heart disease (RHD), and MS is the most common valvular disease secondary to RHD.
- Other etiologies are discussed below.

EPIDEMIOLOGY

- Global incidence of RHD remains significant with 282,000 new cases of RHD annually and 305,000 deaths attributed to RHD annually.
- Incidence of rheumatic disease in the continental United States remains low. Annual incidence of acute rheumatic fever (ARF) in the continental United States is unknown because it is no longer nationally reportable but is higher in Hawaii and American Samoa.
- Predominant age: Symptoms primarily occur in 3rd to 4th decades.
  - In North America and Europe, prevalence is 1 case per 100,000 population, and patients present with severe valve obstruction in 6th decade of life. In Africa, disease prevalence is 35 per 100,000, and severe disease can often present in teens.
- Predominant sex: female > male (3:1)

ETIOLOGY AND PATHOPHYSIOLOGY

- Narrowing of the mitral valve (MV) orifice leads to obstruction of blood flow between LA and LV. This impairs LV filling during diastole and causes increased LA pressure.
- Increased LA pressure is transmitted passively ("back pressure") to the pulmonary circulation causing pulmonary hypertension (HTN) and pulmonary congestion over time.
- Chronic LA pressure overload results in atrial dilation and fibrosis, resulting in atrial fibrillation.
- Rheumatic fever: most common cause (see "Risk Factors")
  - Pathognomonic commissural fusion, leaflet thickening, and "fish mouth appearance" seen with RHD
  - The anatomic changes of severe MS is thought to be secondary to recurrent episodes of ARF as well as a chronic autoimmune process caused by cross-reactivity between a streptococcal protein and valve tissue.
- Aging (extension of mitral annular calcification)

- Rare causes: congenital (associated with mucopolysaccharidoses); autoimmune: systemic lupus erythematosus (SLE), rheumatoid arthritis, malignant carcinoid, Whipple disease, methysergide therapy; and other acquired: LA myxoma, LA thrombus, endomyocardial fibrosis

RISK FACTORS

- ARF and RHD are the greatest risk factors.
  - ARF occurs 2 to 3 weeks after an episode of untreated pharyngitis caused by rheumatogenic group A streptococci (GAS) organism in a genetically susceptible host.
  - RHD refers to the chronic valvular damage caused by a single severe episode of ARF, multiple recurrent episodes of ARF, and/or the chronic autoimmune process from cross-reactivity between streptococcal protein and valve tissue.
  - 30–40% of rheumatic fever patients eventually develop MS, presenting 20 years after diagnosis of ARF.
  - Recurrent infections can accelerate the progression of the disease.
  - Low socioeconomic status (i.e., crowded conditions) favors the spread of streptococcal infection.
- Aging (increasing valvular calcification)
- Chest irradiation (increasing tissue fibrosis)

GENERAL PREVENTION

- Prompt recognition and treatment of GAS infection in at-risk populations; recognition of cardinal signs and symptoms of ARF via Jones criteria
- Echocardiographic screening has been shown to increase diagnosis of RHD in asymptomatic patients residing in areas of high prevalence.

COMMONLY ASSOCIATED CONDITIONS

- Atrial fibrillation (30–40% of symptomatic patients)
- Associated valve lesions due to chronic inflammation (aortic stenosis, aortic insufficiency)
- Pulmonary HTN and right heart failure
- Systemic embolism, stroke, pulmonary embolism (10%)
- Infection, including infective endocarditis (1–5%)

DIAGNOSIS

HISTORY

- History of ARF or RHD
- Severity depends on valve area; most early cases will be asymptomatic.
- Mean age of symptom onset in rheumatic valvular disease is in the late 30s to 40s. Latent period 20 to 40 years after infection. Rapid progression can be seen in some high prevalence areas.
- Presenting features usually include dyspnea on exertion, decrease exercise tolerance, chest pain, palpitations, hoarseness, hemoptysis, fatigue, paroxysmal nocturnal dyspnea, atrial fibrillation, and embolic events.
- In advanced disease, symptoms of pulmonary HTN and right heart failure predominate: jugular venous distention, hepatomegaly, ascites, and peripheral edema.
- Other presentations: hemoptysis (due to pulmonary vein rupture and bronchial circulation causing intra-parenchymal hemorrhage), hoarseness (compression of recurrent laryngeal nerve by enlarged pulmonary artery or LA, Ortner syndrome), dysphagia (compression of esophagus), chronic cough (due to LA compressing the bronchi), and infective endocarditis
- Not infrequently, symptoms are first noted in pregnancy: mitral facies, plethoric cheeks, and bluish patches.

PHYSICAL EXAM

- Elevated jugular venous pressure, diastolic thrill in the left lateral decubitus position. A right ventricle (RV) lift may be felt in the left parasternal area in patients with pulmonary HTN.
- Auscultation
  - Classic murmur: accentuated S_1, opening snap, apical early decrescendo diastolic rumble with presystolic accentuation (presystolic accentuation of murmur is lost with atrial fibrillation). Murmur is low pitch and best heard at the apex in the left lateral decubitus position.
  - Murmur is accentuated with exercise and decreased with rest and Valsalva.
    - With mobile, noncalcified valve, murmur persists throughout diastole and S_1, and the opening snap remains loud.
    - With increasing severity of MS, murmur often is difficult to hear. Duration of murmur reflective of severity. S_1 and the opening snap may be soft to absent.
    - A shorter S_2 to O_2 interval indicates more severe MS.
    - Further evaluation is required while looking for concomitant murmurs.
- If pulmonary HTN is present: Increased P_2, high-pitched decrescendo diastolic murmur of pulmonic insufficiency is heard (Graham Steell murmur); may have signs of right heart failure. RV lift can also be seen.
- May also find associated aortic or tricuspid murmurs due to involvement from RHD

DIAGNOSTIC TESTS & INTERPRETATION

Initial Tests (lab, imaging)

- ECG
  - LA enlargement, atrial fibrillation, and right ventricular hypertrophy (RVH) may be seen
- Chest radiograph
  - LA enlargement, straightening of the left heart border, a "double density," in the cardiac silhouette, and elevation of the left main stem bronchus
  - Prominent pulmonary arteries at the hilum with rapid tapering, RVH, and edema pattern with Kerley A and B lines (late presentation)
- Transthoracic echo (TTE) recommended in all patients with signs or symptoms of MS (1)[C]
  - Used for diagnosis of MS
  - Assess for concomitant valvulopathies.
- TEE should be performed if TTE images are nondiagnostic or if being considered for a PMBC to exclude thrombus in LA and evaluate severity of MR (1)[C].
- Exercise stress testing with Doppler echocardiography can also be considered in patients with MS who have a discrepancy in their symptoms and signs and resting echo findings (1)[C].
- Cardiac catheterization indications and use of Gorlin formula to assess LA and LV pressures (1):
  - Routine diagnostic cardiac cath is not recommended for evaluation of MS.
- Class I recommendations
  - When echo is inconclusive
  - Discrepancy between echo, symptoms, and severity
- Class II recommendations
  - Assess cause of severe pulmonary HTN that out of proportion to echo results.
- Class III recommendations: satisfactory result of echo
- CT imaging: may provide MVA estimates, LA cavity size; useful prior to surgery, particularly to evaluate for concomitant coronary artery disease (CAD)

Follow-Up Tests & Special Considerations

- If valve area >1.5 cm^2 and mean pressure gradient <5 mm Hg, clinical follow-up in 3 to 5 years is recommended.

- Otherwise, follow-up is usually symptom based. Symptomatic patients with severe MS need further evaluation for interventional/surgical treatment.
- Holter monitor placement in order to rule out paroxysmal atrial fibrillation

Diagnostic Procedures/Other
- Exercise testing is recommended for those with clinical discrepancy.
- Wilkins score evaluates valvular anatomy from a TTE in order to see if patient is a candidate for surgery.

Test Interpretation
- Rheumatic fever–induced pathologic changes: leaflet thickening, leaflet calcification, commissural fusion, chordal shortening
- MVA defined (1)
  – Normal: 4 to 6 cm^2, progressive MS: >1.5 cm^2, asymptomatic severe MS: <1.5 cm^2, severe MS: <1.5 cm^2, very severe MS: <1.0 cm^2

 TREATMENT

GENERAL MEASURES
- Treatment is dependent on severity of stenosis and symptoms.
- Patients who have a valvular area >1.5 cm^2 and no symptoms can be managed medically.
- MS is generally progressive, and medical therapy only delays the need for definitive therapy. It entails:
  – Treatment to prevent recurrence of rheumatic fever
  – Treatments aimed at improving dyspnea and exercise tolerance
  – Controlling the ventricular rate whether in sinus rhythm or atrial fibrillation
  – Anticoagulation for prevention of thromboembolic events

MEDICATION
First Line
- Use of anticoagulation for prevention of thromboembolism (1)[C]
  – Class I recommendations
    ○ MS and atrial fibrillation or history of atrial fibrillation, MS and prior embolic event, or MS and LA thrombus
  – Class IIB recommendations
    ○ Patients with enlarged LA and spontaneous contrast on echo
- Warfarin is the accepted modality for anticoagulation in patients with rheumatic MV disease (international normalized ratio range 2 to 3). The new oral anticoagulants (factor Xa inhibitor and direct thrombin inhibitor) are not approved for use in atrial fibrillation with patients that have moderate-to-severe MS (2),(3).
- Heparin is used for anticoagulation with atrial fibrillation.
- Antibiotic prophylaxis against rheumatic fever and/or carditis is recommended for patients with history of rheumatic fever (1)[C]. Secondary prophylaxis is dependent on many factors: number of previous attacks, time since previous infection, risk for getting GAS, age of patient, and absence or presence of cardiac involvement.
- Antibiotic prophylaxis against infective endocarditis is not routinely recommended, unless there are other indications (1)[C].
- Diuretics for congestive symptoms and symptomatic heart failure (1)[A]
- β-Blockers or nondihydropyridine calcium channel blockers used for controlling heart rate both in sinus rhythm and atrial fibrillation to allow adequate diastolic filling and decrease LA diastolic pressure tachycardia or exertional symptoms (class IIa) (1)
- Ivabradine *helpful because it doesn't affect myocardial contraction*

- Consider cardioversion, especially in patients with mild MS and recent diagnosis of atrial fibrillation (<6 months).

Second Line
One can also consider amiodarone or digitalis if β-blockers and calcium channel blockers are not beneficial in controlling rapid ventricular rate . Consider digitalis in patients with symptomatic systolic dysfunction.

SURGERY/OTHER PROCEDURES
- Surgical techniques include balloon valvotomy, open mitral commissurotomy, or closed mitral commissurotomy and MV replacement.
- Patients with severe MS and symptoms consistent with NYHA classes III and IV are candidates for surgery.
- Any patient with a valve area >1.5 cm^2, LA thrombus, moderate or severe MR, severe or bicommissural calcifications, severe aortic valve disease, moderate TR or TS, and concomitant CAD requiring bypass surgery are NOT candidates for PMBC.
- Per the 2014 AHA/ACC valvular heart disease guidelines (1) (which is similar to the 2017 European Society of Cardiology guidelines [4]), PMBC is recommended for patients with the following:
  – Symptomatic severe MS (MVA <1.5 cm^2) and favorable valve morphology (1)[C]
  – Symptomatic severe MS with severe (NYHA III/IV) symptoms who have suboptimal valve anatomy and are not candidates or are high risk for surgery (1)[C]
  – Asymptomatic very severe MS (MVA <1.0 cm^2) and favorable valve anatomy in the absence of contraindications (1)[C]
  – Asymptomatic severe MS and favorable valve morphology with new-onset atrial fibrillation in absence of contraindications (1)[C]
  – Symptomatic patients with MVA >1.5 cm^2 if there is evidence of hemodynamically significant MS during exercise (1)[C]
- MV surgery is recommended for patients with the following:
  – Severe MS with severe symptoms (NYHA classes III and IV), who are not high-risk surgical candidates, and balloon valvotomy is contraindicated or failed PMBC (1)[C]
  – Severe MS and recurrent embolic events while receiving adequate anticoagulation that requires LA appendage excision (1)[C]
  – Severe MS in patients undergoing other cardiac surgery or possibly in patients with moderate MS undergoing other cardiac surgery (1)[C]
- Patient's age, bleeding risk, and other comorbidities prior to deciding if patient should have a prosthetic versus mechanical valve

Pregnancy Considerations
- Volume expansion during pregnancy can exacerbate heart failure symptoms. Patients with known severe MS, prepregnancy discussions should be pursued with a cardiologist.
- Warfarin (Coumadin) is considered relatively safe in the 2nd and 3rd trimesters if anticoagulation is required. However, unfractionated heparin is preferred prior to labor and delivery.

 ONGOING CARE

FOLLOW-UP RECOMMENDATIONS
- Counsel patients that MS usually is slowly progressive but can have sudden onset of atrial fibrillation, which could become rapidly fatal. Call 911 for marked worsening of symptoms.
- Echocardiographic surveillance in asymptomatic patients in any degree of MS: very severe (MVA <1.0 cm^2) MS: yearly, severe (MVA ≤1.5 cm^2)

MS: every 1 to 2 years, mild or moderate MS (MVA >1.5 cm^2): every 3 to 5 years
- Follow-up will depend on the severity of the MS and the patient's symptoms.
  – Asymptomatic patients: annual history and examination
  – Symptomatic patients are followed closely based on clinical response to adjust therapy and plan definitive treatment (1)[C].

DIET
Salt restriction for pulmonary congestion

PROGNOSIS
Natural history
- Asymptomatic latent period after rheumatic fever for 10 to 30 years. 10-year survival for asymptomatic or minimally symptomatic patients is 80%. 10-year survival after onset of debilitating symptoms is only 0–15%. Mean survival with significant pulmonary HTN is <3 years.
- Commissurotomy is an effective means of reducing stenosis but is not curative. Restenosis sometimes occurs and can be early (<5 years) or late (>20 years).

COMPLICATIONS
Left and right heart failure, atrial fibrillation and systemic embolization, pulmonary HTN, pulmonary vasoconstriction hepatic congestion, and bacterial endocarditis

REFERENCES
1. Nishimura RA, Otto CM, Bonow RO, et al. 2014 AHA/ACC guideline for the management of patients with valvular heart disease: a report of the American College of Cardiology/American Heart Association Task Force on Practice Guidelines. *J Thorac Cardiovasc Surg.* 2014;148(1):e1–e132.
2. January CT, Wann LS, Calkins H, et al. 2019 AHA/ACC/HRS focused update of the 2014 AHA/ACC/HRS guideline for the management of patients with atrial fibrillation: a report of the American College of Cardiology/American Heart Association Task Force on Clinical Practice Guidelines and the Heart Rhythm Society. *J Am Coll Cardiol.* 2019;74(1):104–132.
3. Nishimura RA, Otto CM, Bonow RO, et al. 2017 AHA/ACC focused update of the 2014 AHA/ACC guideline for the management of patients with valvular heart disease: a report of the American College of Cardiology/American Heart Association Task Force on Clinical Practice Guidelines. *J Am Coll Cardiol.* 2017;70(2):252–289.
4. Baumgartner H, Falk V, Bax JJ, et al. 2017 ESC/EACTS guidelines for the management of valvular heart disease. *Eur Heart J.* 2017;38(36):2739–2791.

CODES

ICD10
- I01.1 Acute rheumatic endocarditis
- Q23.2 Congenital mitral stenosis
- I34.2 Nonrheumatic mitral (valve) stenosis

CLINICAL PEARLS
- Asymptomatic patients may be followed clinically with yearly exams for development of symptoms with periodic echo to evaluate valve area.
- Once symptoms of MS develop, initiate appropriate medical therapy, but advise patient that, for most, surgical therapy will be needed to prolong survival. Almost all cases of MV stenosis progress in severity over time.

M

MITRAL VALVE PROLAPSE

Justin T. Ertle, MD • Timothy A. Scully, DO

BASICS

DESCRIPTION
- Mitral valve prolapse (MVP) is the billowing of one or both mitral valve leaflets into the left atrium (LA) during ventricular systole.
- MVP can be classified in different ways, including by etiology (primary or secondary; see "Etiology and Pathophysiology") or by morphology (classic MVP and nonclassic MVP; see "Test Interpretation").
- MVP is often asymptomatic and often has a benign clinical course; however, it may occasionally be associated with symptoms, such as palpitations, or complications, such as mitral regurgitation (MR) (see "Complications").
- Synonyms include systolic click-murmur syndrome, billowing mitral cusp syndrome, myxomatous mitral valve, floppy valve syndrome, redundant cusp syndrome, Barlow syndrome.

EPIDEMIOLOGY
Prevalence
- The prevalence of MVP is estimated at 2–3% of the general population and is equally distributed by gender and across the age spectrum (1).
- Prior to current echocardiographic criteria, earlier studies estimated the prevalence at 5–15% and indicated a higher prevalence among women and with increased age.

ETIOLOGY AND PATHOPHYSIOLOGY
- The pathophysiology of MVP typically involves myxomatous degeneration of the mitral valve leaflets. Myxomatous degeneration is characterized by expansion of the valve spongiosa layer, structural alterations in collagen, and structurally abnormal chordae (1).
- Papillary muscle or chordae disruption, dysfunction, or rupture may also cause MVP; this can occur without a process causing myxomatous degeneration, or as part of the natural history of a process causing myxomatous degeneration.
- The etiology of MVP is multifactorial and includes the following (1),(2):
  - Primary MVP: sporadic, familial
  - Secondary MVP
    - "Syndromic" MVP: myxomatous degeneration associated with connective tissue disorders: Marfan syndrome, Ehlers-Danlos syndrome, osteogenesis imperfecta, pseudoxanthoma elasticum, Loeys-Dietz syndrome
    - Associated with congenital heart disease: atrial septal defect, Ebstein anomaly
- Papillary/chordae disruption, dysfunction or rupture (infarction, endocarditis, rheumatic fever, trauma, hypertrophic cardiomyopathy)

Genetics
- The genetics of MVP is an active area of research (1),(2).
- In primary MVP, both autosomal dominant and X-linked familial MVP have been identified.
- Autosomal dominant: variable penetrance. Multiple genetic loci have been identified (1).
  - *MMVP1* on chromosome 16 p11.2–p12.1
  - *MMVP2* on chromosome 11 p15.4
  - *MMVP3* on chromosome 13 q31.3–q32.1

- X-linked: One gene has been identified (1): filamin A gene, Xq28.
- Connective tissue disorders, which often have a genetic basis, are associated with secondary MVP (see "Etiology and Pathophysiology" above).

RISK FACTORS
- Medical conditions implicated in the development of MVP include both heritable and sporadic congenital abnormalities as well as other disease processes (see "Etiology and Pathophysiology" above).
- MVP appears to be more common with a leaner body mass (1).

COMMONLY ASSOCIATED CONDITIONS
- Conditions implicated in the development of MVP include both heritable and sporadic congenital abnormalities as well as other disease processes (see "Etiology and Pathophysiology" above).
- MVP is implicated in the development of other medical conditions/complications, such as MR and stroke (see "Complications" below).
- Some associated conditions that are less clearly either (i) a cause of MVP or (ii) caused by MVP include (3) von Willebrand disease; primary hypomastia; thoracic skeletal abnormalities; prolapse of the tricuspid, pulmonic, or aortic valves.

DIAGNOSIS

HISTORY
- Most patients with MVP are asymptomatic.
- If patients are symptomatic, the most commonly associated symptom is palpitations.
- Symptoms may be related to MVP itself, to MR as a result of MVP, or to other complications of MVP such as stroke, arrhythmia, etc.
  - Symptoms related to MVP include palpitations, atypical chest pain, fatigue, exercise intolerance, orthostasis/syncope/presyncope, and neuropsychiatric symptoms such as panic attacks.
  - Symptoms related to progression of MR: fatigue, dyspnea, exercise intolerance, orthopnea, paroxysmal nocturnal dyspnea

PHYSICAL EXAM
- The principal auscultatory finding is a midsystolic click, although this is not heard in all cases.
- This may also be followed by mid- to late-systolic murmur, loudest at the apex.
- Dynamic auscultation may help differentiate between similar systolic sounds (3).
- Maneuvers that decrease end-diastolic volume move the click and murmur toward S1: standing up, Valsalva.
- Maneuvers that increase end-diastolic volume move the click and murmur toward S2: squatting, leg raise.
- Note: Valsalva maneuver may help differentiate hypertrophic obstructive cardiomyopathy (HOCM) from MVP as it increases the intensity of the murmur in HOCM, whereas it increases the duration of the murmur in MVP.
- Exam findings may also reflect the presence of MR as a result of MVP.
  - MR holosystolic murmur best heard at the apex, with radiation to the left axilla
  - The duration of the murmur corresponds with the severity of MR. Presence of an S3 may indicate severe regurgitation.

DIFFERENTIAL DIAGNOSIS
- Ejection clicks (do not change timing with systole)
- Papillary muscle dysfunction
- MR
- Tricuspid regurgitation
- Hypertrophic cardiomyopathy

DIAGNOSTIC TESTS & INTERPRETATION
Initial Tests (lab, imaging)
- Transthoracic echocardiogram (TTE) is the diagnostic modality of choice after an appropriate physical exam; echocardiogram is required for definitive diagnosis (3)[C].
  - In asymptomatic patients with physical signs of MVP, echocardiography is indicated for the diagnosis of MVP and assessment of MR, leaflet morphology, and ventricular compensation (3)[C].
  - Echocardiography is not indicated to exclude MVP in asymptomatic patients with ill-defined symptoms in the absence of a constellation of clinical symptoms or physical findings suggestive of MVP, or a positive family history (3)[C].
- Electrocardiogram (ECG) is not required in the workup of MVP, without other indication.
  - Palpitations are a common symptom prompting ECG.
  - ECG in MVP is typically normal; however, ECG findings in MVP can include nonspecific ST- to T-wave changes; T-wave inversions, prominent Q waves, and even prolonged QT in some cases (3).

Follow-Up Tests & Special Considerations
- Transesophageal echocardiography (TEE), particularly with 3D imaging, may be considered to further visualize anatomy if intervention is planned or there is limited visibility of the mitral valve on TTE (2).
- Angiography is rarely used for diagnostic purposes but may be recommended for hemodynamic assessment when noninvasive options are inconclusive.
- Patients with MVP and severe MR may require coronary angiography and TEE if cardiac surgical referral is planned (3)[C] (see "Issues for Referral").
- Ambulatory ECG monitoring/event monitor may be considered if patient has palpitations but is not indicated for MVP alone (3)[C].

Test Interpretation
- MVP is defined as anterior, posterior, or bileaflet prolapse of at least 2-mm superior displacement into the LA during systole on the parasternal long-axis annular plane of the valve on echocardiogram, with or without associated leaflet thickening (1).
  - Morphologic classification (1):
    - Classic MVP (a.k.a. Barlow syndrome): prolapse with >5 mm of leaflet thickening
    - Nonclassic MVP (fibroelastic deficiency): prolapse with <5 mm of leaflet thickening
- "Flail" mitral prolapse is the term for a severe form in which a segment or segments of a leaflet protrude into the LA during systole; typically this is associated with torn chordae or ruptured papillary muscle (2).

TREATMENT

GENERAL MEASURES
- Reassurance is appropriate for patients with milder forms of prolapse and low symptom burden; normal lifestyle and regular exercise is encouraged (3)[C].
- If MVP is associated with palpitations, fatigue, or anxiety, patients may be encouraged to discontinue alcohol, cigarettes, and caffeine (3)[C].
- MVP with orthostatic symptoms may be managed by liberalizing fluid and salt intake. Support stockings may also be beneficial (3)[C].

MEDICATION
- Aspirin (75 to 325 mg daily) may be considered for MVP with "high-risk" echocardiographic features (thickening >5 mm or valve redundancy) (3)[C].
- Aspirin (75 to 325 mg daily) is recommended for patients with MVP and transient ischemic attacks (TIAs) (3)[C].
- Warfarin may be considered for patients with MVP and transient ischemic attacks who continue to experience TIAs despite aspirin (3)[C].
- Aspirin (75 to 325 mg daily) is considered for patients with MVP and history of stroke, without high-risk echocardiographic features (thickening >5 mm or valve redundancy), MR, atrial fibrillation, or left atrial thrombus (3)[C].
- Warfarin is considered for patients with MVP and history of stroke, who do have either high-risk echocardiographic features (thickening >5 mm or valve redundancy), MR, atrial fibrillation, or left atrial thrombus (3)[C].
- Patients with MVP and palpitations may be treated with β-blockers (3)[C].
- Note: MVP alone is no longer considered an indication for infectious endocarditis (IE) antibiotic prophylaxis (2)[C].

ISSUES FOR REFERRAL
- Cardiology referral is indicated in MVP with significant symptoms, high-risk features, or concomitant cardiac diagnoses.
- Cardiothoracic surgery referral is indicated in patients with indication for surgical repair.
- Genetic counselling may be considered for patients where a heritable condition is suspected.

SURGERY/OTHER PROCEDURES
- MVP and myxomatous valve degeneration is the most common cause of chronic primary MR requiring surgery in high-income countries (2).
- Referral for mitral valve repair is indicated for the following (3)[C]:
  – In symptomatic patients with severe primary MR
  – In asymptomatic MR patients with left ventricular (LV) systolic dysfunction (left ventricular ejection fraction [LVEF] ≤60%, left ventricular end-systolic diameter [LVESD] ≥40 mm)
  – Asymptomatic patients with atrial fibrillation or pulmonary hypertension may be considered for surgical intervention as well (3)[C].
- In general, if surgery is indicated for MR, mitral valve repair is preferred over replacement when possible due to lower rates of operative mortality and long-term complications (4)[C],(5).
- Minimally invasive surgery and surgery for asymptomatic patients without LV systolic dysfunction is an area of ongoing research (5).

 ONGOING CARE

FOLLOW-UP RECOMMENDATIONS
- Asymptomatic MVP patients with no significant MR can be followed clinically every 3 to 5 years (3)[C].
- Periodic monitoring with TTE is recommended in asymptomatic patients with known valvular heart disease, at intervals depending on valve lesion, severity, ventricular size, and ventricular function (4)[C].
- Patients who are symptomatic or have high-risk features on initial echocardiogram, including moderate to severe MR, may need serial echocardiograms and should be followed clinically at least once per year (3)[C].

DIET
Patients with MVP and symptoms of palpitations should be cautioned to limit caffeine, alcohol, and smoking (3)[C].

PATIENT EDUCATION
- Patients can be counselled that MVP is often a benign condition.
- Patients should be counselled that there is no contraindication to pregnancy based on the diagnosis of MVP alone (3)[C].
- Patients should be counselled to promptly report any change in symptom status, which may require repeat echocardiography (3)[C].
- Educate patients on occasional familial MVP occurrence.
- Restriction from high-intensity competitive sports is recommended if a patient has MVP with any one of the following features (3)[C]:
  – Moderate LV enlargement or LV dysfunction
  – Uncontrolled tachyarrhythmias
  – Prolonged QT interval
  – Unexplained syncope
  – Prior resuscitation from cardiac arrest
  – Aortic root enlargement

PROGNOSIS
- Prognosis is excellent for asymptomatic patients without complications; MVP is often benign with a normal life expectancy.
- Overall, the prognosis of MVP is closely tied to whether MR develops and how it progresses as well as occurrence of other serious complications (1),(3).

COMPLICATIONS
- MR—MVP and myxomatous valve degeneration is the most common cause of chronic primary MR in high-income countries (2).
- Many additional complications may arise as a consequence of severe MR:
  – Heart failure secondary to progressive or acute MR
  – Pulmonary hypertension with associated RV dysfunction
  – Left atrial dilatation with associated paroxysmal supraventricular tachycardias (including atrial fibrillation)
- Arrhythmias, including premature atrial complexes, supraventricular tachycardias, ventricular premature beats (3)

- Sudden cardiac death (SCD) occurs more often with MVP than in the general population but is still rare, with an incidence of 0.14 SCD events per 100 patient-years in patients with MVP.
- Risk factors for SCD in MVP may include bileaflet prolapse, ventricular fibrosis, complex ventricular ectopy, and ST-T wave abnormalities.
- Cerebrovascular ischemic events (stroke and TIAs)
- Infective endocarditis (3)

REFERENCES
1. Delling FN, Vasan RS. Epidemiology and pathophysiology of mitral valve prolapse: new insights into disease progression, genetics, and molecular basis. *Circulation*. 2014;129(21):2158–2170.
2. Guy TS, Hill A. Mitral valve prolapse. *Annu Rev Med*. 2012;63:277–292.
3. Bonow RO, Carabello BA, Chatterjee K, et al. 2008 Focused update incorporated into the ACC/AHA 2006 Practice Guideline Guidelines for the Management of Patients with Valvular Heart Disease. *Circulation*. 2008;118(15):e523–e661.
4. Otto CM, Nishimura RA, Bonow RO, et al. 2020 ACC/AHA Guideline for the Management of Patients with Valvular Heart Disease: a report of the American College of Cardiology/American Heart Association Joint Committee on Clinical Practice Guidelines. *Circulation*. 2021;143(5):e35–e71.
5. Nishimura RA, Vahanian A, Eleid MF, et al. Mitral valve disease—current management and future challenges. *Lancet*. 2016;387(10025):1324–1334.

 CODES

ICD10
- I34.1 Nonrheumatic mitral (valve) prolapse
- I05.8 Other rheumatic mitral valve diseases

CLINICAL PEARLS
- MVP is the billowing of one or both mitral valve leaflets into the LA during ventricular systole.
- The principal auscultatory finding is a midsystolic click, although this is not heard in all cases; the click may also be followed by mid- to late-systolic murmur, loudest at the apex.
- Echocardiogram is required for definitive diagnosis.
- The etiology of MVP is multifactorial and can be secondary to a diverse range of other conditions such as connective tissue disorders, congenital heart disease, infarction, endocarditis, rheumatic fever, and trauma.
- MVP often has a benign clinical course; it is associated with MR, and confers a higher risk of arrhythmias, strokes and TIAs, endocarditis, and even SCD (although this is still exceedingly rare).

M

MOLLUSCUM CONTAGIOSUM

Dongsheng Jiang, MD, MSc • Joanna Jiang, MD

BASICS

DESCRIPTION

Molluscum contagiosum is a common, benign, viral (poxvirus) skin infection, characterized by small (2 to 5 mm), waxy white or flesh-colored, dome-shaped papules often with central umbilication. Lesions contain a cheesy grayish white material. Molluscum contagiosum is highly contagious and spreads by autoinoculation, skin-to-skin contact, sexual contact, and shared clothing/towels. Molluscum contagiosum is a self-limited infection in immunocompetent patients but can be difficult to treat and disfiguring in immunocompromised patients.

EPIDEMIOLOGY

Prevalence

- 1% in the United States, occurring mainly in children 2 to 15 years and sexually active young adults
- 5–18% HIV population

ETIOLOGY AND PATHOPHYSIOLOGY

- DNA virus; *Poxviridae* family
- Four genetic virus types, clinically indistinguishable
- Virions invade and replicate in cytoplasm of epithelial cells causing abnormal cell proliferation.
- Genome encodes proteins to evade host immune system.
- Incubation period: 2 to 6 weeks
- Time to resolution: 6 to 24 months
- Not associated with malignancy
- No cross-hybridization or reactivation by other poxviruses

RISK FACTORS

- Skin-to-skin contact with infected person
- Contact sports
- Swimming
- Atopic dermatitis
- Sexual activity with infected partner
- Immunocompromised: HIV, chemotherapy, corticosteroid therapy, transplant patients, patients on biologics

GENERAL PREVENTION

- Avoid skin-to-skin contact with host (e.g., contact sports, sexual activity).
- Avoid sharing clothing and towels.

COMMONLY ASSOCIATED CONDITIONS

- Atopic dermatitis
- Immunosuppression medications: corticosteroids, biologics, chemotherapy, etc.
- HIV/AIDS

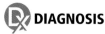

DIAGNOSIS

HISTORY

- Contact with known infected person
- Participation in contact sports
- Sexual activity

PHYSICAL EXAM

- Perform thorough skin exam including conjunctiva and anogenital area.
- Discrete, firm papules with a central umbilication
- White curd-like core under umbilicated center
- Lesions are flesh, pearl, or red in color and frequently located in intertriginous areas.
- May have surrounding erythema or dermatitis
- Immunocompetent hosts: average of 11 to 20 lesions, 2 to 5 mm diameter (range: 1 to 10 mm)
- Immunocompromised hosts may have hundreds of widespread lesions or "giant" molluscum (lesions >1 cm)
- Sexually active: inner thighs, anogenital area

Pediatric Considerations

- Infants <3 months: Consider vertical transmission. If vertical transmission, lesions often located on scalp
- Children: fever, >50 lesions, limited response to therapy; consider immunodeficiency.
- Children: anogenital lesions; most likely autoinoculation if lesions present elsewhere on body. However, provider should consider possible sexual abuse.

DIFFERENTIAL DIAGNOSIS

- Verruca vulgaris
- Chickenpox
- Milia
- AIDS patients: *Cryptococcus neoformans*, penicilliosis, histoplasmosis, coccidioidomycosis
- Basal cell carcinoma
- Benign appendageal tumors: syringomas, hidrocystomas, ectopic sebaceous glands
- Condyloma acuminatum
- Dermatofibroma
- Eyelid: abscess, chalazion, foreign-body granuloma
- Folliculitis/furunculosis
- Keratoacanthoma
- Oral squamous cell carcinoma
- Trichoepithelioma
- Warty dyskeratoma
- Amelanotic melanoma
- Papular urticaria

DIAGNOSTIC TESTS & INTERPRETATION

Initial Tests (lab, imaging)

- Virus cannot be cultured.
- Culture lesion if concern is secondary infection.
- Sexual transmission: Test for other sexually transmitted infections, including HIV.
- Microscopy: scrape lesion
  - Core material has characteristic Henderson-Paterson intracytoplasmic viral inclusion bodies.
  - Crush prep with 10% potassium hydroxide will show characteristic inclusion bodies as well.
  - Alternatively, hematoxylin-eosin-stained formalin-fixed tissue shows same confirmatory features.

Diagnostic Procedures/Other

Clinical exam generally diagnostic, but dermatoscopy can be helpful.

Test Interpretation

Characteristic dermoscopic findings (1):

- Central pore or umbilication, white-to-yellow polylobular structure, and crown vessels

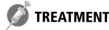

TREATMENT

GENERAL MEASURES

- In healthy patients, molluscum contagiosum is generally self-limited and resolves spontaneously; therefore, treatment is optional (2)[A].
- No single intervention is shown to be convincingly more effective than any other in treating molluscum contagiosum (2)[A].
- There are no FDA-approved treatments for molluscum contagiosum.

- Treatment decision is typically based on patient's age, location, number of lesions, comorbidities, availability, and cost.
- Three categories of treatment: destructive, immune-enhancing, and antiviral

MEDICATION

First Line
Cantharidin 0.7–0.9% solution: In office application to lesions, cover with dressing; wash off in 2 to 6 hours or sooner if blistering. Repeat treatment every 2 to 4 weeks until lesions resolve (2)[B].

- Not commercially available in the United States but may be prepared in United States by compounding pharmacy from powder; might be available as solution from Canada
- Adverse effects: blistering, erythema, pain, pruritus
- Precautions: Do not use on face or on genital mucosa.

Second Line
- Benzoyl peroxide 10% cream: Apply to each lesion twice daily for 4 weeks (2)[B].
  - Inexpensive, available over the counter
  - Adverse effects: mild dermatitis
- Imiquimod 5% cream: 3 to 5 times per week for 12 weeks
  - Adverse effects: mucositis, leukopenia, vitiligo (3)
- Other topicals reported: podophyllotoxin, trichloroacetic acid, salicylic acid, lactic acid, glycolic acid, and tretinoin (1)
- Cimetidine: oral. 25 to 40 mg/kg/day (1)
- For immunocompromised patients (including HIV) with refractory lesions, consider
  - Cidofovir: topical cream or IV

ISSUES FOR REFERRAL
Immunocompromised patients not responding to first- or second-line treatment

SURGERY/OTHER PROCEDURES
- Cryotherapy: 1 or 2 cycles of 10 to 20 seconds (1); repeat every 3 to 4 weeks as needed until lesions disappear.
  - Adverse effects: erythema, edema, pain, blistering
  - Contraindications: cryoglobulinemia, Raynaud disease
- Curettage under local or topical anesthesia (2)[A]
  - Adverse effects: pain, scarring
- Intralesional immunotherapy (4)[C]:
  - Candida antigen, PPD, vitamin D, MMR
  - Benefits: low to no recurrence
  - Adverse effects: erythema, edema, allergic reaction, anaphylaxis

COMPLEMENTARY & ALTERNATIVE MEDICINE
- Australian lemon myrtle oil: Apply 10% solution once daily for 21 days (2)[B].
- Potassium hydroxide 5–10% solution: Apply 1 to 2 times a day until the lesions disappeared completely (2)[B].

Pediatric Considerations
- Treatment is optional for immunocompetent children.
- Surgical interventions: second line in small children due to associated pain
- Pain control: Pretreat with topical lidocaine or EMLA before surgical treatment.
- Note: adverse effect:
  - Lidocaine or EMLA over large body surface area: methemoglobinemia and CNS toxicity. Refer to manufacturer's recommendations on dosing and use in children.

Pregnancy Considerations
Treatments safe in pregnancy: curettage, cryotherapy, incision, and expression

ONGOING CARE

FOLLOW-UP RECOMMENDATIONS

Patient Monitoring
Depends on type of treatment

PATIENT EDUCATION
- Cover lesions to prevent spread.
- Avoid scratching to prevent autoinoculation.
- Avoid sharing towels and clothing.
- Practice safe sex or avoid sexual activity when lesions present.

PROGNOSIS
- Immunocompetent: self-limited, resolves in 3 to 12 months (range: 2 months to 4 years)
- Immunocompromised: lesions difficult to treat; may persist for years

COMPLICATIONS
- Secondary infection
- Scarring, hyper-/hypopigmentation (generally only occurs as a result of treatment, not when lesions resolve spontaneously)

REFERENCES

1. Meza-Romero R, Navarrete-Dechent C, Downey C. Molluscum contagiosum: an update and review of new perspectives in etiology, diagnosis, and treatment. *Clin Cosmet Investig Dermatol*. 2019;12:373–381.
2. van der Wouden JC, van der Sande R, Kruithof EJ, et al. Interventions for cutaneous molluscum contagiosum. *Cochrane Database Syst Rev*. 2017;(5):CD004767.
3. DiBiagio JR, Pyle T, Green JJ. Reviewing the use of imiquimod for molluscum contagiosum. *Dermatol Online J*. 2018;24(6):13030/qt3b4606qt.
4. Wells A, Saikaly SK, Schoch JJ. Intralesional immunotherapy for molluscum contagiosum: a review. *Dermatol Ther*. 2020;33(6):e14386.

ADDITIONAL READING

- Clebak KT, Malone MA. Skin infections. *Prim Care*. 2018;45(3):433–454.
- Nowicka D, Bagłaj-Oleszczuk M, Maj J. Infectious diseases of the skin in contact sports. *Adv Clin Exp Med*. 2020;29(12):1491–1495.

CODES

ICD10
B08.1 Molluscum contagiosum

CLINICAL PEARLS

- Observation is preferred treatment in healthy patients as lesions will spontaneously resolve.
- Reassure parents that a child's lesions will heal naturally and generally resolve without scarring.
- No specific treatment has been identified as superior to any other, and no treatment is FDA approved.
- Consider topical corticosteroids for pruritus or associated dermatitis.

M

MORTON NEUROMA (INTERDIGITAL NEUROMA)

J. Herbert Stevenson, MD • James McKee, DO, MS

BASICS

DESCRIPTION
- Painful condition of the webbed spaces of the toes
- Features perineural fibrosis of the common digital nerve as it passes between metatarsals
  - The interspace between the 3rd and 4th metatarsals is most commonly affected.
  - The interspace between the 2nd and 3rd metatarsals is the next most common site.
- Systems affected: musculoskeletal, nervous
- Synonyms: plantar digital neuritis; Morton metatarsalgia; intermetatarsal neuroma

EPIDEMIOLOGY
Prevalence
- Unknown
- Mean age: 45 to 50 years
- Predominant sex: female > male (8:1)

ETIOLOGY AND PATHOPHYSIOLOGY
- Lateral plantar nerve joins a portion of medial plantar nerve, creating a nerve with a larger diameter than those going to other digits.
- Etiology not fully understood. Four main theories:
  - Chronic traction damage
  - Inflammatory environment due to intermetatarsal bursitis
  - Compression by the deep transverse intermetatarsal ligament
  - Ischemia of vasa nervorum
- Nerve lies in SC tissue, deep to the fat pad of foot, just superficial to the digital artery and vein.
- Superficial to the nerve is the strong, deep transverse metatarsal ligament that holds the metatarsal bones together.
- With each step the patient takes, the inflamed nerve becomes compressed between the ground and the deep transverse metatarsal ligament. This can generate perineural fibrotic reaction with subsequent neuroma formation.

RISK FACTORS
- High-heel shoes
  - Transfer more weight to the forefoot.
- Shoes with tight toe boxes
  - Cause lateral compression
- Pes planus (flat feet)
  - Pulls nerve medially, increasing irritation
- Obesity
- Female gender
- Ballet dancing, particularly associated with the demi-pointe position

- Basketball, aerobics, tennis, running, and similar activities
- Hyperpronation

GENERAL PREVENTION
- Wear properly fitting shoes.
- Avoid high heels and shoes with narrow toe boxes.

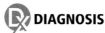

DIAGNOSIS

HISTORY
- Most common complaint is pain localized to interspace between 3rd and 4th toes.
- Pain is less severe when not bearing weight.
- Pain, cramping, or numbness of the forefoot during weight bearing or immediately after strenuous foot exertion
- Radiation of pain to the toes
- Pain is relieved by removing shoes and massaging the foot.
- Patients often complain of "walking on a marble."
- Burning pain in the ball of the foot radiating to the toes
- Tingling or numbness in the toes
- Aggravated by wearing tight or narrow shoes

PHYSICAL EXAM
- Intense pain when pressure applied between metatarsal heads, sometimes with a palpable nodule
- Assess midfoot motion and digital motion to determine if arthritis or synovitis.
- Palpate along metatarsal shafts to assess for metatarsalgia or stress fractures.
- Special testing (see "Diagnostic Procedures/Other")

DIFFERENTIAL DIAGNOSIS
- Stress fracture
- Hammer toe
- Metatarsophalangeal synovitis
- Metatarsalgia
- Arthritis
- Traumatic neuroma
- Osteomyelitis
- Bursitis
- Foreign body
- Freiberg infraction (avascular necrosis of the metatarsal head, most commonly in adolescent females at the 2nd metatarsal)
- Neoplasm (malignancy, osteochondroma, neurofibroma)
- Gout

DIAGNOSTIC TESTS & INTERPRETATION
Initial Tests (lab, imaging)
- Predominantly a clinical diagnosis; imaging should be reserved for when the diagnosis is unclear (1)[A].
- Imaging may be helpful if more than one web space is involved.
- Radiographs may help to rule out osseous pathology if diagnosis is in question, but plain films usually are normal in patients with a Morton neuroma (1)[A].
- Ultrasound (US) has 79% specificity and 99% sensitivity for Morton neuromas but is poor at assessing the size of the lesion. Specificity declines to 50% for lesions <6 mm (1)[A].
- MRI can rule out an osseous tumor and help with surgical planning; MRI has a sensitivity of 83% and a specificity of 99% for diagnosis of Morton neuroma (1)[A].

Diagnostic Procedures/Other
- Five special tests have been described: thumb index finger squeeze test, Mulder sign, foot squeeze test, plantar percussion test, and toe tip sensation deficit.
  - Thumb index finger squeeze test is the most sensitive and specific (96% and 96%, respectively). Positive when pain elicited by squeezing the symptomatic intermetatarsal space between the index finger and thumb (2)[B].
  - Mulder sign is a painful "click" produced by squeezing the metatarsal heads together while compressing the neuroma between the thumb and index finger of the other hand; sensitivity 40–84% (1)[A]
  - Foot squeeze test is positive when pain is induced in the symptomatic web space when the metatarsal heads are compressed by grasping the foot; sensitivity 40% (2)[B]
  - Plantar and dorsal percussion tests are positive when percussion of the affected webspace elicits pain.
  - Toe tip sensation deficit exists when the sensation of the toe distal to the affected web space is decreased relative to the other toes.
- More than one of the above tests being positive increases the diagnostic accuracy (3)[B].

Test Interpretation
Pathologic examination shows chronic fibrosis and thickening within and around the digital nerve. Arterial thickening and thrombosis of the common digital artery is sometimes present.

TREATMENT

GENERAL MEASURES

- Stepwise treatment, with typical progression from conservative measures followed by infiltrative treatment and ultimately surgical treatment
- Surgical treatments are the most successful (89%) followed by infiltrative (84%), then conservative (48%), as assessed by patient satisfaction with pain reduction at 6 months or greater (4)[A].
- Conservative treatments include
  - Flat shoes with a roomy toe box
  - Plantar pads or metatarsal bar may help with alignment of metatarsal heads to provide relief.
  - There is no role for varus or valgus footwear padding (5).
  - There is no role for Extracorporeal Shock Wave Therapy (ESWT) (5).
- NSAIDs for temporary symptom relief (6)[A]

MEDICATION

First Line

- Injectable steroids (e.g., betamethasone phosphate/acetate or methylprednisolone): number needed to treat (NNT) for significant benefit over conservative measures at 6 months = 2.3 (4)[A],(7)[A]
- One study demonstrated clinically significant improvement in use of US guidance versus palpation for corticosteroid injection (8).

Second Line

US-guided alcohol ablation therapy to sclerose the nerve is effective and has a lower complication rate than surgery (4)[A].

ISSUES FOR REFERRAL

- Continued pain despite conservative treatments and injections
- Large interdigital neuromas (>5 mm diameter) or young patients who may benefit from earlier operative intervention
- One study demonstrated that a cut-off value of 6.3 mm or larger Morton neuroma was associated with failure of corticosteroid injection (9)[B].

SURGERY/OTHER PROCEDURES

- Surgical removal of the neuroma or shortening of the metatarsals, with or without release of the transverse metatarsal ligament, has an 89% success rate at 6 months defined by satisfaction scores (4)[A].
- Small trials have been conducted using other invasive, nonsurgical techniques including injection with botulinum toxin, cryoablation, radiofrequency ablation, and platelet-rich plasma, but evidence is limited at this time.

ONGOING CARE

FOLLOW-UP RECOMMENDATIONS

At diagnosis, or if no improvement after 3 months of conservative treatment, consider corticosteroid injection.

- May repeat injection if no improvement after 2 to 4 weeks, or consider referring for surgical management.
- 21–51% of patients receiving a single corticosteroid injection require surgical intervention within 2 to 4 years (10)[B].
- Size >5 mm and younger patients are more likely to undergo invasive treatment (10)[B].

PATIENT EDUCATION

Wear properly fitting comfortable shoes.

PROGNOSIS

- 48% satisfaction rate with conservative treatment
- 85% satisfaction rate with infiltrative treatment
- 89% satisfaction rate with operative treatment (4)[A]

COMPLICATIONS

- Hip and knee pain can develop secondary to gait changes.
- Complications vary by treatment type.
- Failure rate is 47% with conservative treatment; 9–23% with invasive, nonsurgical treatment; 4% with surgical treatment (4)[A].
- Surgical complications vary by specific procedure and include keloid, CRPS, and stiffness. There was a global complication rate of 21% with operative treatment (4)[A].

REFERENCES

1. Sharp RJ, Wade CM, Hennessy MS, et al. The role of MRI and ultrasound imaging in Morton's neuroma and the effect of size of lesion on symptoms. *J Bone Joint Surg Br*. 2003;85(7):999–1005.
2. Mahadevan D, Venkatesan M, Bhatt R, et al. Diagnostic accuracy of clinical tests for Morton's neuroma compared with ultrasonography. *J Foot Ankle Surg*. 2015;54(4):549–553.
3. Owens R, Gougoulias N, Guthrie H, et al. Morton's neuroma: clinical testing and imaging in 76 feet, compared to a control group. *Foot Ankle Surg*. 2011;17(3):197–200.
4. Valisena S, Petri GJ, Ferrero A. Treatment of Morton's neuroma: a systematic review. *Foot Ankle Surg*. 2018;24(4):271–281.
5. Matthews BG, Hurn SE, Harding MP, et al. The effectiveness of non-surgical interventions for common plantar digital compressive neuropathy (Morton's neuroma): a systematic review and meta-analysis. *J Foot Ankle Res*. 2019;12:12.
6. Thomson CE, Gibson JN, Martin D. Interventions for the treatment of Morton's neuroma. *Cochrane Database Syst Rev*. 2004;(3):CD003118.
7. Saygi B, Yildirim Y, Saygi EK, et al. Morton neuroma: comparative results of two conservative methods. *Foot Ankle Int*. 2005;26(7):556–559.
8. Ruiz Santiago F, Prados Olleta N, Tomás Muñoz P, et al. Short term comparison between blind and ultrasound guided injection in Morton neuroma. *Eur Radiol*. 2019;29(2):620–627.
9. Park YH, Lee JW, Choi GW, et al. Risk factors and the associated cutoff values for failure of corticosteroid injection in treatment of Morton's neuroma. *Int Orthop*. 2018;42(2):323–329.
10. Mahadevan D, Salmasi M, Whybra N, et al. What factors predict the need for further intervention following corticosteroid injection of Morton's neuroma? *Foot Ankle Surg*. 2016;22(1):9–11.

ADDITIONAL READING

- Jain S, Mannan K. The diagnosis and management of Morton's neuroma: a literature review. *Foot Ankle Spec*. 2013;6(4):307–317.
- Schreiber K, Khodaee M, Poddar S, et al. Clinical inquiry. What is the best way to treat Morton's neuroma? *J Fam Pract*. 2011;60(3):157–158, 168.

CODES

ICD10

- G57.60 Lesion of plantar nerve, unspecified lower limb
- G57.61 Lesion of plantar nerve, right lower limb
- G57.62 Lesion of plantar nerve, left lower limb

CLINICAL PEARLS

- Morton neuroma is usually a clinical diagnosis but can be further evaluated with US or MRI.
- Typical treatment is stepwise with conservative, then infiltrative, and then operative treatment.
- Morton neuromas with >5 mm diameter are more likely to require operative treatment.
- Younger patients are more likely to require operative treatment.
- Neurectomy is the definitive treatment. Patients should be aware of surgical complications.

M

MOTION SICKNESS

Andrew J. Richardson, MD

 BASICS

DESCRIPTION

- Motion sickness is a physiologic response in affected individuals to a situation in which sensory conflict about body motion exists among visual receptors, vestibular receptors, and body proprioceptors.
- Often induced when patterns of motion differ from those previously experienced or expected
- Differs from "cybersickness" or "virtual reality sickness" (symptoms, including dizziness, that result from exposure to computer based stimuli) in the fact that some form of actual movement is generally required to diagnose motion sickness
- Systems affected: nervous, gastrointestinal
- Synonym(s): car sickness; sea sickness; air sickness; space sickness; physiologic vertigo; kinetosis

EPIDEMIOLOGY

Incidence
Predominant sex: female > male

Prevalence
Estimation is complex; syndrome occurs in ~25% due to travel by air, ~29% by sea, and ~41% by road. Estimates for vomiting are 0.5% by air, 7% by sea, and 2% by road.

ETIOLOGY AND PATHOPHYSIOLOGY
- Precise etiology unknown; thought to be due to a mismatch of vestibular and visual sensations
- Rotary, vertical, and low-frequency motions produce more symptoms than linear, horizontal, and high-frequency motions.
- Nausea and vomiting occur as a result of increased levels of dopamine and acetylcholine, which stimulate chemoreceptor trigger zone and vomiting center in CNS. Other signals which can be involved in this process include histamine, norepinephrine, and γ-aminobutyric acid (1).

Genetics
Heritability estimates range from 55% to 75%.

RISK FACTORS
- Motion (auto, plane, boat, amusement rides)
- Visual stimuli (e.g., moving horizon)
- Poor ventilation (fumes, smoke, carbon monoxide)
- Emotions (fear, anxiety)
- Zero gravity
- Pregnancy, menstruation, oral contraceptive use
- History of migraine headaches, especially vestibular migraine

GENERAL PREVENTION
See "General Measures."

Pediatric Considerations
- Rare in children <2 years of age
- Incidence peaks between 6 and 12 years of age.
- Antihistamines may cause excitation in children.

Geriatric Considerations
- Age confers some resistance to motion sickness.
- Elderly are at increased risk for anticholinergic side effects from treatment.

Pregnancy Considerations
- Pregnant patients are more likely to experience motion sickness.
- Treatment with medications is thought to be safe during morning sickness (e.g., meclizine, dimenhydrinate).
- Scopolamine, meclizine, diphenhydramine, and promethazine generally considered safe during breastfeeding

COMMONLY ASSOCIATED CONDITIONS
- Migraine headache
- Vestibular syndromes

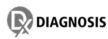 **DIAGNOSIS**

HISTORY
Presence of the following signs and symptoms in the context of a typical stimulus (2):
- Nausea
- Vomiting
- Stomach awareness (feeling of fullness in epigastrium)
- Diaphoresis
- Facial and perioral pallor
- Hypersalivation
- Yawning, hyperventilation
- Anxiety, panic
- Malaise/fatigue/lethargy
- Weakness
- Confusion
- Dizziness

PHYSICAL EXAM
No specific findings

DIFFERENTIAL DIAGNOSIS
- Mountain sickness
- Vestibular disease, central and peripheral
- Gastroenteritis
- Metabolic disorders
- Toxin exposure
- Concussion
- Hypoglycemia

DIAGNOSTIC TESTS & INTERPRETATION
None usually indicated; can consider pregnancy test or fingerstick glucose to rule out hypoglycemia

Follow-Up Tests & Special Considerations
Multiple online questionnaires (such as the Motion Sickness Susceptibility Questionnaire) are available to help patients recognize their susceptibility to motion sickness and what situations are most likely to cause symptom development.

 TREATMENT

- Follow guidelines under "General Measures" section to prevent motion sickness (2)[C].
- Premedicate before travel with antidopaminergic, anticholinergic, or antihistamine agents (2)[A]:
  - For extended travel, consider treatment with scopolamine transdermal patch (3)[A].
- Benzodiazepines suppress vestibular nuclei but would not be considered first line due to sedation and addiction potential (4)[C].
- Serotonin receptor agonist (rizatriptan) may be effective for migraineurs with motion sickness (5)[C].

GENERAL MEASURES
- Avoid noxious types of motions; travelling in inclement weather may exacerbate symptoms.
- Improve ventilation; avoid noxious stimuli.
- Eat before travel (light, soft, bland, low-fat, and low-acid foods); avoid alcohol; avoid empty stomach.
- Increase airflow around face.
- Use semirecumbent seating or lay supine.
- Fix vision on horizon; avoid fixation on moving objects; keep eyes fixed on still, distant objects.
- Avoid reading while actively traveling.
- Frequent and graded exposure to stimulus that triggers nausea (habituation)
- Counsel patient on minimizing motion (airplanes: sit over the wing; automobiles: driver or sit in front passenger seat, facing forward; boat: sit facing toward the waves, away from rocking bow, near surface of the water; buses: sit near the front, at lowest level, facing forward; trains: sit at the lowest level, facing forward).

MEDICATION

First Line

- Scopolamine transdermal patch (Transderm Scop): Apply 2.5-cm^2 (4 mg) patch behind ear over the mastoid at least 4 hours (preferably 6 to 12 hours) before travel and replace every 3 days (3)[A].
- Promethazine (Phenergan): Take 30 to 60 minutes before travel.
  – Adults: 25 mg q12h; 25 to 50 mg IM if already developed severe motion sickness
  – Children and adolescents: 0.5 mg/kg q12h, maximum 25 mg BID; *caution*: increased risk of dystonic reaction in this age group
- Dimenhydrinate (Dramamine): Take 30 to 60 minutes before travel.
  – Adults and adolescents: 50 to 100 mg q4–6h, maximum 400 mg/day
  – Children 6 to 12 years of age: 25 to 50 mg q6–8h, maximum 150 mg/day
  – Children 2 to 5 years of age: 12.5 to 25.0 mg q6–8h, maximum 75 mg/day
- Meclizine (Travel Ease): Take 60 minutes before travel.
  – Adults and adolescents >12 years of age: 25 to 50 mg q24h
  – Children <12 years of age: not recommended
- Diphenhydramine (Benadryl): Take 30 minutes before travel.
  – Adults and adolescents: 25 to 50 mg q6–8h, maximum 300 mg/day
  – Children 6 to 12 years of age: 5 mg/kg or 12.5 to 25.0 mg q4–6h, maximum 150 mg/day
- Contraindications: patients at risk for acute angle-closure glaucoma
- Precautions:
  – Young children
  – Elderly
  – Pregnancy
  – Urinary obstruction
  – Pyloric duodenal obstruction
- Adverse reactions:
  – Drowsiness
  – Dry mouth
  – Blurred vision
  – Confusion/delirium
  – Headache
  – Urinary retention
  – Constipation

- Significant possible interactions:
  – Sedatives (antihistamines, alcohol, antidepressants)
  – Anticholinergics (belladonna alkaloids)

Second Line

- Benzodiazepines: Take 1 to 2 hours before travel.
  – Diazepam 2 to 10 mg PO q6–12h
  – Lorazepam 1 to 2 mg PO q8h
- Contraindications:
  – Severe respiratory or liver dysfunction
- Precautions:
  – Alcohol/drug abuse
  – Elderly
  – Sedation
  – Addiction is possible.

COMPLEMENTARY & ALTERNATIVE MEDICINE

- Acupressure on point PC6 (*Neiguan* on pericardium meridian) has been shown to reduce feelings of nausea and vomiting during pregnancy, after surgery, and in cancer chemotherapy. However, limited evidence of efficacy has been found for motion sickness; point PC6: 2 cm proximal of transverse crease of palmar side of wrist between tendons of the palmaris longus and the flexor carpi radialis (6)[B].
- Ginger: 1.0 to 1.5 g per 24 hours (250 mg 4 times a day); take 4 hours before travel; studies have shown ginger to be an effective treatment for nausea and vomiting (7)[B].

 ONGOING CARE

DIET

- Eat before travel, avoid empty stomach; eat light, soft, bland, low-fat, and low-acid foods.
- Avoid alcohol.

PROGNOSIS

- Symptoms should resolve when motion exposure ends.
- Resistance to motion sickness seems to increase with age.

COMPLICATIONS

- Hypotension
- Dehydration
- Depression
- Panic
- Syncope

REFERENCES

1. Leung AK, Hon KL. Motion sickness: an overview. *Drugs Context*. 2019;8:2019-9-4.
2. Brainard A, Gresham C. Prevention and treatment of motion sickness. *Am Fam Physician*. 2014;90(1):41–46.
3. Spinks AB, Wasiak J. Scopolamine (hyoscine) for preventing and treating motion sickness. *Cochrane Database Syst Rev*. 2011;(6):CD002851.
4. Soto E, Vega R. Neuropharmacology of vestibular system disorders. *Curr Neuropharmacol*. 2010;8(1):26–40.
5. Furman JM, Marcus DA, Balaban CD. Rizatriptan reduces vestibular-induced motion sickness in migraineurs. *J Headache Pain*. 2011;12(1):81–88.
6. Lee EJ, Frazier SK. The efficacy of acupressure for symptom management: a systematic review. *J Pain Symptom Manage*. 2011;42(4):589–603.
7. Marx W, Kiss N, Isenring L. Is ginger beneficial for nausea and vomiting? An update of the literature. *Curr Opin Support Palliat Care*. 2015;9(2):189–195.

 SEE ALSO

Algorithm: Dizziness

 CODES

ICD10
T75.3XXA Motion sickness, initial encounter

CLINICAL PEARLS

- The scopolamine transdermal patch is first line for prevention of motion sickness. It should be applied at least 4 hours before travel, although it is most effective if placed 12 hours before departure.
- First-generation antihistamines are also effective, although sedating. They should be administered 30 to 60 minutes before departure.
- Nonsedating antihistamines, ondansetron, and ginger root are not effective in the prevention or treatment of motion sickness.
- Although acupressure wristbands have been found to be effective by systematic reviews in postoperative and chemotherapy-induced nausea and vomiting, as well as hyperemesis gravidarum, conflicting data exist for use with motion sickness.

M

MULTIPLE MYELOMA

Michael Haddadin, MD • Jan Cerny, MD, PhD

BASICS

DESCRIPTION
- Multiple myeloma (MM) involves a malignant proliferation of a single clone of plasma cells.
- The malignant plasma cells produce monoclonal protein (immunoglobulin [Ig]) in the blood and urine as it is filtered in the kidneys.
- MM is characterized by bony lytic lesions, hypercalcemia, increased susceptibility to infections, and renal impairment.
- Monoclonal gammopathy of undetermined significance (MGUS) is a common disorder with limited monoclonal plasma cell proliferation that can progress to smoldering MM (SMM) or symptomatic MM at rate of ~1% per year.

EPIDEMIOLOGY
- MM affect the older adults with a median age of 65 to 74 years.
- Accounts for nearly 2% of all cancers and 17% of hematologic malignancies in the United States.
- African Americans about 2 to 3 times more commonly affected than Caucasians; less common in Asians

Incidence
7 cases per 100,000 in the United States annually

Prevalence
In 2018, there were nearly ~160,000 recognized cases worldwide (1)[A].

ETIOLOGY AND PATHOPHYSIOLOGY
- It is most likely related to genetic alteration involving chromosomal abnormalities and sporadic mutations.
- Genetic damage in developing B lymphocytes occur at time of isotype switching.
- Chromosomal abnormalities involve Ig heavy chain translocations, with cyclin D1 t(11;14) the most common and deletion of 17p13 (p53 locus) (2)[C].

Genetics
It occurs rarely in familial clusters. A rare form of paratarg-7 protein might have pathogenic role.

RISK FACTORS
- Most cases have no known risks associated.
- Old age; immunosuppression; and exposure to chemicals, heavy metals, and ionizing radiation increase the risk of MM.

COMMONLY ASSOCIATED CONDITIONS
Secondary amyloidosis commonly due to MM and polyneuropathy, organomegaly, endocrinopathy, M protein, skin changes (POEMS)

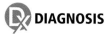

DIAGNOSIS

HISTORY
- 34% of patients are asymptomatic at the time of presentation.
- Anemia (73%) is the most common presentation of MM.
- Hypercalcemia (28%): anorexia, abdominal pain, somnolence, polydipsia, polyuria, dehydration
- Elevated creatinine (48%), acute kidney injury in MM can occur due to multiple different mechanisms.

- Bony lesions (80%): lytic lesions causing bone pain (58%) (3)[C], osteoporosis, or pathologic fracture (26–34%)
- Other symptoms: fatigue (32%), peripheral neuropathy (PN), weight loss (24%), recurrent infections, hyperviscosity syndrome, and cord compression

PHYSICAL EXAM
- Dehydration, pallor, and bone tenderness
- Hyperviscosity syndrome in 7%: retinal hemorrhages, prolonged bleeding, neurologic changes
- Extramedullary plasmacytomas can present as large, purplish, subcutaneous masses.
- Skin findings of amyloidosis: waxy papules, or plaques that may be evident in the eyelids, retro-auricular region, neck, or inguinal and anogenital regions

DIFFERENTIAL DIAGNOSIS
- MGUS
- SMM: no end-organ damage (CRAB: hypercalcemia, renal insufficiency, anemia, bone lesions) features
- Metastatic carcinoma (kidney, breast, non–small cell lung cancer)
- Waldenström macroglobulinemia
- Reactive plasmacytosis
- AL amyloidosis
- Solitary plasmacytoma
- POEMS syndrome

DIAGNOSTIC TESTS & INTERPRETATION
Criteria for diagnosis: The diagnosis of MM requires the following (4)[C]:
- BM involvement with ≥10% of plasma cells or the presence of a plasmacytoma and any one or more of the following myeloma-defining events:
  - Evidence of end-organ damage that can be attributed to the underlying plasma cell proliferative disorder, specifically:
    - Hypercalcemia: serum calcium >0.25 mmol/L (>1 mg/dL) higher than the upper limit of normal or >2.75 mmol/L (>11 mg/dL)
    - Renal insufficiency: creatinine clearance <40 mL/min or serum creatinine >177 μmol/L (>2 mg/dL)
    - Anemia: hemoglobin value of >2 g/dL below the lower limit of normal or a hemoglobin value <10 g/dL
    - Bone lesions: one or more osteolytic lesions on skeletal radiography, CT, or PET-CT
  - Any one or more of the following findings is considered a MM-defining event:
    - Clonal BM plasma cell percentage ≥60%
    - Involved: uninvolved serum free light chain (FLC) ratio ≥100
    - >1 focal lesion on MRI studies or PET-CT

Initial Tests (lab, imaging)
- CBC with differential to evaluate anemia and other cytopenias
- BUN, creatinine, serum electrolytes, albumin, and calcium
- Serum lactate dehydrogenase (LDH), β_2-microglobulin
- Serum protein electrophoresis (SPEP), serum immunofixation electrophoresis (SIFE): M protein level elevated
- Quantitative serum Ig levels: IgG, IgA, and IgM

- Quantitative serum FLC levels: κ and λ chains
- ESR, C-reactive protein: elevated
- Urine analysis: 24-hour urine for protein, urine protein electrophoresis (UPEP), urine immunofixation electrophoresis (UIFE); 20% positive urine protein (3)[C]:
  - Urinalysis dip is often negative for protein because this test identifies albumin, and the protein in MM is Bence Jones (BJ) monoclonal protein.
- Cross-sectional imaging (whole body low-dose CT) is preferred over plain radiographs for the detection of bone involvement (4)[C].
- Skeletal surveys are reserved for patients who are unable to undergo low-dose whole body CT, MRI, and PET.
- Bone marrow (BM) biopsy: plasma cell percentage, histology, immunohistochemistry, flow cytometry, cytogenetics, and fluorescence in situ hybridization (FISH)

Follow-Up Tests & Special Considerations
- For patients with suspected SMM, a whole body MRI or MRI of the spine and pelvis is recommended to evaluate for cord compression.
- For patients with suspected extramedullary disease outside of the spine, a whole body PET/CT is recommended.
- Baseline bone densitometry may be indicated (5)[A].
- BM aspiration and biopsy to monitor response to treatment
- SPEP with SIFE: M protein helps to track progression of myeloma and response to treatment.
- Serum Igs and FLCs can be used to monitor response or relapse.

Diagnostic Procedures/Other
Staging to determine disease burden (2)[C]; multiple staging systems are used. The most common one is the Revised International Staging System (R-ISS). Durie-Salmon staging system is rarely used nowadays.
- International Staging System (ISS)
  - Stage I: albumin ≥3.5 g/dL and β_2-microglobulin <3.5 μg/mL
  - Stage II: neither stage I nor stage III
  - Stage III: β_2-microglobulin ≥5.5 μg/mL
- Mayo Stratification of Myeloma and Risk-Adapted Therapy (mSMART)
  - Standard risk: >t(11;14), t(6;14), and hyperdiploidy
  - Intermediate risk: t(4;14), del(13q) by cytogenetics, hypodiploidy
  - High risk: t(14;16), t(14;20), del(17 p)
- R-ISS combines ISS information with chromosomal abnormalities and LDH to provide better prognostic information for MM.

TREATMENT

- Treatment varies by risk, stage of MM, patient characteristics.
- Key determinant factor in choosing chemotherapy regimen is to establish transplant candidacy; if the patient is an autologous stem cell transplant (ASCT) candidate or not
- ASCT following induction chemotherapy is standard of care for eligible patients.

GENERAL MEASURES

Maintain adequate hydration to prevent renal insufficiency (5)[A]. Most patients will require some form of antimicrobial prophylaxis during treatment.

MEDICATION

- Treatment for MM consists of three different phases: induction phase, consolidation (often ASCT) eligible patients (6)[C], and maintenance.
- Agents include chemotherapy, proteasome inhibitors, immunomodulatory agents, steroids, and monoclonal antibodies.
- Induction phase for ASCT eligible patient can be composed of a 3- or 4-drug combination, such as bortezomib/lenalidomide/dexamethasone, bortezomib/cyclophosphamide/dexamethasone, or carfilzomib/lenalidomide/dexamethasone.
- Induction chemotherapy for ASCT-ineligible patients is similar either with doublet or triplet (e.g., lenalidomide/low-dose dexamethasone or daratumumab/lenalidomide/dexamethasone).
- Maintenance treatment: Lenalidomide is approved for maintenance therapy after induction or transplant. Additional agents are being investigated.

First Line

- Proteasome inhibitors (6)
  - Blocks ubiquitin-proteasome catalytic pathway in cells by binding to the 20S proteasome complex
  - Consider herpes simplex virus (HSV) prophylaxis with acyclovir.
  - Bortezomib: IV or SC; SC has lower risk of PN. Toxicity: PN, cytopenia, nausea, anorexia, leukopenia, thrombocytopenia, rash
  - Carfilzomib: IV, 2nd-generation proteasome inhibitor. Toxicity: cardiomyopathy and other cardiac adverse events, fever, diarrhea, thrombotic microangiopathy, fatigue; can have hypersensitivity reaction after infusion
  - Ixazomib—oral proteasome inhibitor. Toxicity: PN, diarrhea, thrombocytopenia, neutropenia, back pain, edema
- Cyclophosphamide
  - Nitrogen mustard–derivative alkylating agent
  - Toxicity: cytopenia, anaphylaxis, interstitial pulmonary fibrosis, hemorrhagic cystitis, impaired fertility
- Immunomodulators: thalidomide, lenalidomide, and pomalidomide
  - Works by antiangiogenesis inhibition, immunomodulation, and inhibition of tumor necrosis factor
  - Toxicity: birth defects (thalidomide), deep vein thrombosis (DVT), neuropathy, rash, nausea, bradycardia
- Dexamethasone: dose (40 mg/week)
- Daratumumab: IgGκ1 monoclonal Ab against CD38. Toxicity: fatigue, back pain, lymphocytopenia, neutropenia, anemia including Coombs positive hemolytic anemia, thrombocytopenia, cough, flu-like symptoms, and infusion-related reaction
- Bisphosphonates (5)[A]
  - No effect on mortality but decrease pain, pathologic vertebral fractures, and fractures of other bones
  - Dose-adjust/monitor renal function.
  - Monitor for osteonecrosis of jaw.

Second Line

- Progression of MM is usually identified by a rise in monoclonal M protein in the serum or the urine or in the serum FLC ratio with new or worsening end-organ damage.
- Multiple regimens can be used as salvage therapy to treat relapsed or refractory myeloma (6).
- Most patients with relapsed or refractory MM should undergo transplant if not attempted previously.
- Regimen of choice depends on the previously failed lines; if relapse occurs >6 months after completing initial primary treatment, can use same regimen for retreatment
- Regimens can include, but not limited to daratumumab if not previously used, pomalidomide (immunomodulator) or elotuzumab.
- Several others have been developed recently that can be used for second and subsequent relapses. Options include: selinexor, melphalan flufenamide, isatuximab, and the recently approved chimeric antigen receptor T-cell (CAR-T) therapy agent idecabtagene vicleucel.

ISSUES FOR REFERRAL

For spinal or other bone pathology, refer to orthopedics for support.

ADDITIONAL THERAPIES

- Local radiation therapy for uncontrolled bone pain or plasmacytoma
- Effective pain management; avoid NSAIDs due to nephrotoxicity.
- Aspirin 81 to 325 mg is recommended for patients treated with immunomodulators for DVT prophylaxis.
- Erythropoietin for selected patients with anemia
- IVIG infusion for patients with recurrent life-threatening infections
- Patients should receive vaccines for pneumococcus, influenza, and SARS-CoV-2.
- Do not administer live-virus vaccines (3).

SURGERY/OTHER PROCEDURES

Kyphoplasty/vertebroplasty: Consider for symptomatic vertebral compressions.

ADMISSION, INPATIENT, AND NURSING CONSIDERATIONS

Indications: pain, infections, cytopenia, renal failure, bone complications, spinal cord compression

- Adequate hydration and practice caution for contrast-induced nephropathy
- Manage hypercalcemia.

 ONGOING CARE

PATIENT EDUCATION

- http://myeloma.org/Main.action
- https://www.nccn.org/patients/guidelines/content/PDF/myeloma-patient.pdf

PROGNOSIS

- The 5-year survival rate is around 50%.
- Median survival by R-ISS stage:
  - Stage I: has not been reached
  - Stage II: 83 months
  - Stage III: 43 months

COMPLICATIONS

Patients with MM are prone to many complications related to the disease itself and the treatment options. Complications include infections, pain, fractures, hypercalcemia, hyperuricemia, spinal cord compression, hyperviscosity syndrome, amyloidosis, and dialysis.

REFERENCES

1. Siegel RL, Miller KD, Jemal A. Cancer statistics, 2019. *CA Cancer J Clin*. 2019;69(1):7–34.
2. Palumbo A, Avet-Loiseau H, Oliva S, et al. Revised international staging system for multiple myeloma: a report from International Myeloma Working Group. *J Clin Oncol*. 2015;33(26):2863–2869.
3. Palumbo A, Anderson K. Multiple myeloma. *N Engl J Med*. 2011;364(11):1046–1060.
4. Rajkumar SV, Dimopoulos MA, Palumbo A, et al. International Myeloma Working Group updated criteria for the diagnosis of multiple myeloma. *Lancet Oncol*. 2014;15(12):e538–e548.
5. Mhaskar R, Kumar A, Miladinovic B, et al. Bisphosphonates in multiple myeloma: an updated network meta-analysis. *Cochrane Database Syst Rev*. 2017;12(12):CD003188.
6. National Comprehensive Cancer Network. NCCN guidelines insights: multiple myeloma, version 1.2020. https://jnccn.org/view/journals/jnccn/17/10/article-p1154.xml. Accessed December 1, 2019.

CODES

ICD10

- C90.0 Multiple myeloma
- C90.00 Multiple myeloma not having achieved remission
- C90.01 Multiple myeloma in remission

CLINICAL PEARLS

- MM is a plasma cell malignancy that causes end-organ damage.
- Look for presence of "CRAB."
- Suspect MM if high total protein-to-albumin ratio is present.
- Avoid nephrotoxins (radiographic contrast material, NSAIDs, dehydration).
- Patients with MM are immunocompromised.

M

MULTIPLE SCLEROSIS

Niyomi De Silva, MD • Peter Kim, MD • Afsha Rais Kaisani, MD

BASICS

DESCRIPTION

- An autoimmune disease directed against components of the neural myelin sheath causing demyelination often leading to progressive axonal loss and eventual CNS atrophy affecting primarily white matter but may also damage grey matter and overlying meninges
- Four clinical subtypes of multiple sclerosis (MS):
  - Clinically isolated syndrome (CIS): a patient's initial symptom characteristic of CNS demyelination that may be due to MS but does not fulfill the criteria of dissemination in time. Approximately 60% of individuals diagnosed with CIS will later relapse and be diagnosed with MS.
  - Relapsing-remitting MS (RRMS): episodic flare-ups occurring over days to weeks between periods of neurologic stability. During attacks, new symptoms may present, whereas previous symptoms may worsen. Complete recovery of residual deficits may ensue following each bout (~90% of patients).
  - Secondary progressive MS (SPMS): a gradual decline in disease status after an initial relapsing-remitting disease course. Progressive phase may be associated with acute exacerbations. SPMS is often diagnosed retrospectively.
  - Primary progressive MS (PPMS): a progressive decline in disease status and accumulation of disability from onset of disease without an initial relapsing-remitting disease course (~10% of patients) (1)

Pregnancy Considerations

- In most cases, MS treatment should be discontinued during pregnancy. If treatment is clinically necessary during pregnancy, preferred treatments include interferon-β and glatiramer acetate (2).
- For patients where there is a high risk of relapse of symptoms, natalizumab may be continued until 34 weeks (2).
- A majority of patients experience reduced disease exacerbations during pregnancy, but frequency of relapse typically increases in the postpartum period.
- MS therapy should be promptly resumed after delivery, particularly for individuals with very active disease prior to conception.
- All drugs licensed for MS treatment are contraindicated during breastfeeding. Patients desiring to breastfeed should carefully consider risk of delaying MS treatment (3).

EPIDEMIOLOGY

MS is a complex condition that is multifactorial, and although advances in genomics and immunology have increased our understanding of the disease process, much is yet to be discovered. It most often affects Caucasian women in their 2nd and 3rd generations of life and is more common in those with first-degree relatives with the disease.

Incidence

- Women (worldwide): 3.6 cases per 100,000 person-years
- Men (worldwide): 2.0 cases per 100,000 person-years

Prevalence

- Americas: 117.49 per 100,000 people
- Worldwide: 35.9 per 100,000 people (4)

ETIOLOGY AND PATHOPHYSIOLOGY

- Predominately an autoimmune process driven by T cells and B cells against the myelin sheath. Dysregulation and mistaken antigen identity lead CD4 T cells to cross the blood–brain barrier and recognize proteins on the surface of the myelin sheath. Cytokines, interferon-γ, and tumor necrosis factor-α are subsequently released, and activation of macrophages and B cells leads to oligodendrocyte and myelin destruction.
- Following demyelination, faster salutatory nerve conduction velocities (impulses jumping between nodes of Ranvier) are replaced with considerably slower continuous nerve velocities. These changes in the acute setting lead to the focal neurologic deficits associated with MS.
- Oligodendrocytes, which have survived, or ones formed from precursor cells, are able to partially remyelinate stripped axons, producing scars which overtime can lead to irreversible axonal loss and brain atrophy.
- The majority of axons are typically lost from the lateral corticospinal (motor) tracts of the spinal cord. MS was once thought to be a disease of strictly affecting white matter tracts; however, there is increasing evidence of inflammatory damage within the cortical grey matter and overlying meninges (1).

Genetics

- MS is polygenic and does not follow a mendelian inheritance pattern. Those with affected first-degree relatives are 5 to 7 times more likely to be diagnosed.
- Over 100 genetic loci have been associated with MS suggesting that it is ultimately an antigen-specific autoimmune process. Most commonly, these are mapped to the class II region of the HLA gene cluster. The most common being the HLA-DRB1 locus on chromosome 6. These produce major histocompatibility complexes with high-binding affinity for myelin basic proteins.
- Although not fully understood, variations of natural killer cells and their polymorphic killer-immunoglobulin-like receptors are thought to play a major role in the MS disease process (1).

RISK FACTORS

- Age: peak incidence ages 15 to 45 years, mean age 28 to 31 years (slightly earlier in women than men)
- Race: Caucasian > Afro-Caribbean > East Asian
- Gender: 2 to 3 times more common in women
- Infectious: prior infections with Epstein-Barr virus and history of infectious mononucleosis
- Substance: tobacco smoking
- Geographic: Historically, proximity to the equator and its correlation with increased vitamin D exposure were inversely proportional to MS incidence. However, recently this association has been less obvious and may be due to lifestyle changes that have led to decreased sun exposure in these locations (1).

COMMONLY ASSOCIATED CONDITIONS

- Internuclear ophthalmoplegia: Injury to the medial longitudinal fasciculus causes impaired adduction of the affected eye.
- Optic neuritis: inflammation of optic nerve resulting in loss of vision
- Associated with numerous other autoimmune processes

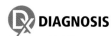

DIAGNOSIS

A person with MS can present with a number of neurologic signs and symptoms depending on the locations of the lesion. The essential means of diagnoses is to demonstrate evidence of CNS lesions that are separated by both time and space that are not more likely due to a separate disease process.

HISTORY

Symptoms can vary widely but may include fatigue, epilepsy, dizziness, visual disturbances, facial palsy, dysphagia, muscle weakness or spasms, hyperesthesia or paresthesia, pain, bowel or bladder incontinence, urinary frequency or retention, or impotence (1).

PHYSICAL EXAM

- Weakness, internuclear ophthalmoplegia, gait disturbance, foot drop
- Hyperesthesia or paresthesia, cerebellar dysarthria (scanning speech), spasticity (especially in lower extremities)
- Uhthoff phenomenon: Symptoms worsen with exposure to higher than usual temperature.
- Lhermitte sign: electric-like shocks extending down the spine caused by neck movement, especially flexion

DIFFERENTIAL DIAGNOSIS

- Infectious: Lyme disease, neurosyphilis, acute disseminated encephalomyelitis, progressive multifocal, Guillain-Barré syndrome, leukoencephalopathy, primary cerebral angiitis
- Autoimmune: systemic lupus erythematosus, antiphospholipid antibody syndrome, neurosarcoidosis, Behçet disease
- CNS: neuromyelitis optica, epilepsy, CNS neoplasms, stroke, normal pressure hydrocephalus
- Genetic: metachromatic leukodystrophy
- Other: cobalamin (vitamin B$_{12}$) deficiency

DIAGNOSTIC TESTS & INTERPRETATION

- MRI of head/spine: Periventricular and callosal lesions are relatively specific for MS. The additions of gadolinium can help identify active lesions.
- Lumbar puncture: Cerebrospinal fluid can reveal elevated or normal total protein levels. Oligoclonal immunoglobulin G bands are seen in approximately 90% of MS but may be absent early in the disease process. Positive findings are not diagnostic for MS but may be beneficial if other diagnostic criteria are equivocal.
- Blood tests: Antinuclear antibody, antineutrophil cytoplasmic antibody, anti–double-stranded DNA antibody, extractable nuclear antigen, antiphospholipid antibody, compliment, erythrocyte sedimentation rate, immunoglobulin G, immunoglobulin M, rheumatoid factor, and Lyme disease antibody can be used to rule out alternative diagnosis (1)[B],(5).

- McDonald criteria for diagnosing MS: must demonstrate dissemination in space and time of CNS lesions
  - Dissemination in space: ≥1 T_2 lesion on MRI in at least 2 of 4 CNS regions typically affected by MS: periventricular, juxtacortical, infratentorial, or spinal cord or by waiting for another clinical event implying a different CNS location
  - Dissemination in time: simultaneous presentation of asymptomatic gadolinium-enhanced and nonenhancing lesions at any moment or a new T_2 and/or gadolinium-enhanced lesion on an MRI when compared baseline scans

Diagnostic Procedures/Other
Evoked potentials: Assess function of visual, auditory, and somatosensory motor CNS pathways by measuring CNS electric potentials evoked by neural stimulation. A marked delay, without a clinical manifestation, is suggestive of a demyelinating disorder. Visual evoked potentials are delayed in 80–90% of individuals with MS (1).

TREATMENT

GENERAL MEASURES
- Holistic multidisciplinary team approach is paramount.
- Three main categories currently exist for MS treatment: treatment for acute relapses, reducing MS-related activity using disease-modifying agents, and symptomatic therapy
- The use of disease-modifying treatments early in the disease process is likely to slow overall disease progression and should be managed by an MS specialist (1)[C].

MEDICATION
- Acute relapse treatment (1)[A]
  - Methylprednisolone 0.5 g PO daily for 5 days or 1 g IV daily for 3 to 5 days; without subsequent oral tapering; a second course may be given.
    - Side effects: increased infection risk, adrenal insufficiency, Cushing syndrome, fluid retention, hypokalemia, GI disturbances, headache, emotional lability
  - ACTH gel 80 U IM or SC daily for 5 to 15 days
    - Side effects: similar to methylprednisolone
  - Plasmapheresis
- Disease-modifying treatment (1)[B]
  - IFN-β_{1a} (Avonex) 30 μg IM weekly or IFN-β_{1a} (Rebif) 22 or 44 μg SC 3 times per week or IFN-β_{1b} (Betaseron/Betaferon/Extavia) 250 μg SC every other day
    - Monitoring: CBC, LFTs, TSH
    - Side effects: flu-like symptoms, depression, skin site reactions, thyroid dysfunction, liver enzyme abnormalities
  - Glatiramer acetate (Copaxone) 20 mg SC daily
    - Monitoring: none
    - Side effects: skin site reactions, immediate postinjection reaction, lipoatrophy
  - Dimethyl fumarate (Tecfidera) 120 to 240 mg PO twice daily
    - Monitoring: CBC, LFTs
    - Side effects: diarrhea, cramps, LFT elevation, nausea, flushing

- Teriflunomide (Aubagio) 7 to 14 mg PO daily
  - Monitoring: CBC, LFTs, UA
  - Side effects: nasopharyngitis, headache, diarrhea, fatigue, back pain, influenza, hair thinning, LFT elevation, nausea, UTI
- Natalizumab (Tysabri) 300 mg IV every 28 days
  - Monitoring: CBC, LFTs
  - Side effects: headache, fatigue, UTI, hypersensitivity reaction
- Alemtuzumab (Lemtrada) 12 to 24 mg IV for 5 days then 3 days 12 months after initial treatment
  - Monitoring: CBC, LFTs, TSH
  - Side effects: immune thrombocytopenic purpura, autoimmune thyroid-related problems, headaches, flushing
- Fingolimod (Gilenya) 0.5 mg PO daily
  - Monitoring: ECG, CBC, LFTs, eye exam
  - Side effects: 1st-degree AV block, bradycardia, macular edema, shingles, worsening pulmonary function, skin cancer, back pain
- Symptomatic therapies (1)[B]
  - Spasticity: baclofen, dantrolene, diazepam, tizanidine, cannabis extract (nabiximols), botulinum toxin, physiotherapy
  - Pain: amitriptyline, pregabalin, gabapentin, cannabis extract (nabiximols)
  - Bladder dysfunction: oxybutynin, tolterodine, cannabis extract (nabiximols), catheterization, intravesical botulinum toxin
  - Fatigue: amantadine, modafinil
  - Tremors: clonazepam, primidone, β-blockers
  - Depression: SSRI (citalopram), SNRI (venlafaxine), TCA (amitriptyline)
  - Walking: fampridine

ONGOING CARE

FOLLOW-UP RECOMMENDATIONS
Patient Monitoring
Assessing the severity of neurologic impairment from MS can be done using the Kurtzke Expanded Disability Status Scale (EDSS): The EDSS quantifies severity of disability using eight functional systems (FS): pyramidal, cerebellar, brainstem, sensory, bowel and bladder, visual, and cerebral. EDSS scoring system:

- 1.0—no disability, minimal signs in 1 FS
- 2.0—minimal disability in 1 FS
- 3.0—moderate disability in 1 FS or mild disability in 3 to 4 FS but fully ambulatory
- 4.0—ambulatory without aid or rest for ~500 m
- 5.0—ambulatory without aid or rest for ~200 m
- 6.0—intermittent/constant unilateral assistance (cane, crutch, or brace); must be able to walk 100 m
- 7.0—unable to walk beyond 5 m even with aid; essentially restricted to wheelchair, wheels self and transfers alone; active in wheelchair for ~12 hr/day
- 8.0—essentially restricted to bed, chair, or wheelchair; may be out of bed most of the day; retains self-care functions, generally effective use of arms
- 9.0—helpless, bedbound; but patient can communicate, eat
- 10.0—death due to MS

PROGNOSIS
- Average life expectancy is 5 to 10 years less than the unaffected population (1).
- Using optical coherence tomography (OCT) to measure thinning of peripapillary retinal nerve fiber layer or the ganglion cell layer plus inner plexiform layer in patients without prior optic neuritis has shown an association with increased disability progression in patients with MS; however, at this time, unsure of clinical significance (6)

COMPLICATIONS
Mortality secondary to MS relapse is unusual; death more commonly associated with a complication of MS such as infection in a person with more disability

REFERENCES
1. Raffel J, Wakerley B, Nicholas R. Multiple sclerosis. *Medicine*. 2016;44(9):537–541.
2. Varytė G, Arlauskienė A, Ramašauskaitė D. Pregnancy and multiple sclerosis: an update. *Curr Opin Obstet Gynecol*. 2021;33(5):378–383.
3. Amato MP, Bertolotto A, Brunelli R, et al. Management of pregnancy-related issues in multiple sclerosis patients: the need for an interdisciplinary approach. *Neurol Sci*. 2017;38(10):1849–1858.
4. Walton C, King R, Rechtman L, et al. Rising prevalence of multiple sclerosis worldwide: insights from the Atlas of MS, third edition. *Mult Scler*. 2020;26(14):1816–1821.
5. Dendrou CA, Fugger L, Friese MA. Immunopathology of multiple sclerosis. *Nat Rev Immunol*. 2015;15(9):545–558.
6. Britze J, Frederiksen JL. Optical coherence tomography in multiple sclerosis. *Eye (Lond)*. 2018;32(5):884–888.

 CODES

ICD10
G35 Multiple sclerosis

CLINICAL PEARLS
- MS is an immune-mediated inflammatory disease causing demyelination, neuronal loss, and scarring within the CNS.
- Diagnosis is made with the McDonald criteria and must demonstrate damage to the CNS disseminated in space and time.
- Disease treatments consist of acute relapse, disease-modifying agents, and symptomatic therapies.
- MS treatment modalities are complex and rapidly changing. A patient's treatment should be guided by an MS specialist, but multiprofessional therapy is necessary.
- New approaches to manipulate inflammation, neurodegeneration, and remyelination such as hematopoietic stem cell transplants are being testing in clinical trials and may dramatically alter treatment and prevention of MS in the future (1).

M

MUMPS

Frances Yung-tao Wu, MD

BASICS

An acute, self-limited, generalized paramyxovirus infection typically presenting with unilateral or bilateral parotitis

DESCRIPTION

- Can be asymptomatic in 30% of nonimmune individuals and 60% of previously vaccinated cases
- Painful parotitis in 95% of symptomatic mumps cases
- Epidemics in late winter and spring; transmission by respiratory droplets or contact with saliva
- Incubation period is 12 to 25 days.
- System(s) affected: hematologic/lymphatic/immunologic, reproductive, skin, exocrine
- Synonym(s): epidemic parotitis; infectious parotitis

EPIDEMIOLOGY

- 85% of mumps cases occur prior to 15 years of age.
- Adult cases are typically more severe.
- Predominant sex: male = female
- Geriatric population: Most U.S. adults are immune.
- Acute epidemic mumps: highly contagious in susceptible populations, R0 =10
  - Most cases occur in unvaccinated children 5 to 15 years of age.
  - Multiple recent outbreaks in U.S. college students
- Mumps is unusual in children <2 years of age.
- Period of maximal communicability is 24 hours before to 72 hours after onset of parotitis.

Incidence

- Worldwide, 169,799 cases of mumps were reported in 2019. In the United States, 2019, 3474 cases of mumps were reported. In 2020, the COVID-19 pandemic year, only 616 cases were reported in the United States.
- Since 1967 (start of U.S. national vaccination program), case rate has dropped from 100/100,000 to 1.1/100,000.
- Occasional regional epidemic outbreaks

Prevalence

- 0.0064/100,000 persons in United States
- 90% of adults in the United States are seropositive.

ETIOLOGY AND PATHOPHYSIOLOGY

Mumps is an RNA virus (*Rubulavirus*) of the paramyxovirus genus. Mumps virus replicates in glandular epithelium of parotid gland, pancreas, and testes, leading to interstitial edema and inflammation.

- Interstitial glandular hemorrhage may occur.
- Pressure caused by testicular edema against the tunica albuginea can lead to necrosis and loss of function.

RISK FACTORS

- Global travel: One-third of countries in regions including Africa, South Asia, Southeast Asia, and Japan do *not* mandate mumps vaccination and continue to have pediatric epidemics every 4 years. Many areas of South and Central America do not have high mumps vaccine coverage. Travel from an area of recent epidemic should be noted.
- Crowded environments such as dormitories, barracks, or detention facilities increase risk of transmission. It is considered a human-only virus, but infectious viral particles have been found in bats.
- Immunity wanes rapidly after single-dose vaccination. With a 2-dose schedule, immunity drops slowly from 95% to 86% after 9 years.

GENERAL PREVENTION

- Vaccination
  - 2 doses of live mumps vaccine or mumps, measles, rubella (MMR, or with varicella MMR-V) vaccine recommended, first at 12 to 15 months and second at 4 to 6 years. May start early at 6 months of age if travel is planned.
  - 95% effective in clinical studies; field trials show 68–95% efficacy, which may be insufficient for herd immunity to prevent spread due to high contagiousness of mumps.
  - Prevention may require 95% first dose and >80% second-dose adherence. Vaccine failure may increase 10–27% each year after vaccination.
  - Adverse effects of vaccine: fever 8/100,000; seizure 25/100,000; thrombocytopenic purpura 3/100,000
  - *No relationship between MMR vaccine and autism celiac disease or multiple sclerosis. Recent data show a reduced autism risk in girls after MMR vaccination (aHR 0.79, overall for both genders aHR 0.93)* (1).
- Immunoglobulin (Ig) post exposure does not prevent mumps.
- Postexposure vaccination does not protect from recent exposure (2)[B].
- Institute respiratory droplet isolation for hospitalized patients for 5 days after onset of parotitis.
- Isolate nonimmune individuals for 26 days after last case onset (social quarantine) due to incubation period as long as 25 days.
- In an epidemic situation, a third dose of MMR is indicated to decrease the attack rate (3)[A]. The boosted immunity from a third dose only seems to last about 1 year.
- Vaccine neutralizing antibodies are still effective against variant strains of mumps virus.
- Although there are no reports of disseminated mumps from MMR vaccine in HIV patients, live vaccines (MMR) are contraindicated in immunocompromised patients (e.g., HIV with CD4 <200).

Pregnancy Considerations

- Live viral vaccines are typically contraindicated in pregnancy; however, vaccination of children should not be delayed if a family member is pregnant. MMR given to breastfeeding mothers has not shown adverse effects in their infants.
- Immunization of contacts protects against future (but not current) exposures.

DIAGNOSIS

HISTORY

- Parotid swelling peaks in 1 to 3 days; lasts 3 to 7 days
- Clinical diagnosis: swelling of one or both parotid glands possibly 12–25 days after exposure. Ask about travel or crowded environments.
  - Parotid pain lasting ≥2 days
  - Meningitis without parotitis (rare; 1–10%)
- 30% of individuals with mumps may be asymptomatic.
- Rare prodrome of fever, neck ache, and malaise
- Sour foods cause pain in parotid gland region.
- Moderate fever, usually not >104°F (40°C):
  - High fever frequently is associated with complications.

PHYSICAL EXAM

- Painful parotid swelling (95% bilateral) obscures angle of mandible and elevates earlobe.
- Meningeal signs (15%); encephalitis (<1%), rare bilateral optic neuritis
- 20–30% orchitis, polyarthritis, thyroiditis, mastitis, 4% pancreatitis, oophoritis, myocarditis, profound hearing loss. Complications may occur after days to weeks.
- Rare maculopapular, erythematous rash
- Up to 50% of cases are mild.
- Redness at opening of Stensen duct without pus
- Sternal swelling (rare and pathognomonic for mumps)

DIFFERENTIAL DIAGNOSIS

- If not epidemic, consider other viruses to test for in addition to mumps such as influenza, parainfluenza parotitis, Epstein-Barr virus, coxsackievirus, adenovirus, parvovirus B19, influenza parotitis—several hundred reported in 2016.
- Suppurative parotitis: often associated with *Staphylococcus aureus* (Presence of pus within Wharton duct with parotid massage essentially excludes diagnosis of mumps.)
- Recurrent allergic parotitis
- Salivary calculus with intermittent swelling (usually unilateral)
- Lymphadenitis from any cause, including HIV infection
- Cytomegalovirus parotitis (immunocompromised)
- Mikulicz syndrome: chronic, painless parotid and lacrimal gland swelling of unknown cause that occurs in tuberculosis, sarcoidosis, lupus, leukemia, lymphosarcoma, and salivary gland tumors
- Sjögren syndrome, diabetes mellitus, uremia, malnutrition
- Drug-related parotid enlargement (iodides, guanethidine, phenothiazine)
- Mumps orchitis must be differentiated from testicular torsion and from chlamydial or bacterial orchitis.

DIAGNOSTIC TESTS & INTERPRETATION

Buccal swab and serum tests recommended: https://www.cdc.gov/mumps/lab/specimen-collect.html

- Swab of fluid from parotid duct or other affected salivary ducts after gland massage for rRT-PCR plus viral culture—send to state lab or CDC; most sensitive day 1 to day 3 of parotitis, especially important for vaccinated persons
- IgM titer (positive by day 5 in 100% of nonimmunized patients), rapid EIA for IgM, low sensitivity in previously immunized persons
- Rise in IgG titer samples; if not previously immunized: first, sample within 5 days of onset and second, 2 weeks later. Previously vaccinated persons may not mount a 4-fold IgG increase, nor a significant IgM.
- Urine for PCR (not as sensitive as oral specimens). May not be positive until 4 days or more after symptom onset. 50 mL in sterile container. Send to state lab (or recognized public health lab).
- Other potential findings: elevated serum amylase; CSF leukocytosis, or leukopenia
- Testicular ultrasound may help differentiate mumps orchitis from testicular torsion.

Initial Tests (lab, imaging)

Buccal swab for mumps is recommended, especially in an epidemic setting. If not epidemic, consider testing for influenza in addition to mumps virus.

Follow-Up Tests & Special Considerations

Mumps is a reportable disease to your local health department.

Diagnostic Procedures/Other

If meningitis symptoms present, lumbar puncture to exclude bacterial process; CSF pleocytosis, usually lymphocytic, in 65% of patients with parotitis

Test Interpretation

Periductal edema and lymphocytic infiltration of affected glands would be expected for mumps on biopsy.

 TREATMENT

- No specific antiviral therapy; supportive care (3)[A]
- Immediately place mask on patients with any suspected mumps exposures who present for evaluation to decrease transmission.
- Analgesics to relieve pain
- Avoid corticosteroids for mumps orchitis because they can reduce testosterone and increase testicular atrophy.
- IVIG can reduce certain autoimmune-based sequelae:
  – Postinfectious encephalitis; Guillain-Barré syndrome; ITP
- Interferon-α2b improves bilateral orchitis but not testicular atrophy (4)[B].

GENERAL MEASURES

- Hospitalize patients with high fever, pancreatitis, or CNS symptoms for supportive care, steroids, or interferon. Mask the patient and use respiratory droplet isolation precautions.
- Orchitis
  – Ice packs to scrotum can help to relieve pain.
  – Scrotal support with adhesive bridge while recumbent and/or athletic supporter while ambulatory

MEDICATION

First Line

- Analgesics and anti-inflammatory medications (acetaminophen, nonsteroidal anti-inflammatory drugs [NSAIDs]) may diminish pain and swelling in acute orchitis and arthritis of mumps.
- May use acetaminophen for fever and/or pain
- Precautions: Avoid aspirin for pain in children as previously associated with Reye syndrome.

Second Line

Interferon-α2b (4)[B]

COMPLEMENTARY & ALTERNATIVE MEDICINE

Medicinal herbs or acupuncture have not shown benefit in randomized controlled trials.

ADMISSION, INPATIENT, AND NURSING CONSIDERATIONS

- Hospitalize only if CNS symptoms or severe complications occur. Use respiratory droplet precautions.
- Outpatient supportive care if no complications
- IV fluids if severe nausea or vomiting accompanies pancreatitis

 ONGOING CARE

FOLLOW-UP RECOMMENDATIONS

Mumps orchitis:

- Bed rest and local supportive clothing (e.g., two pairs of briefs) or adhesive-tape bridge
- Withhold from school until no longer contagious (5 days after onset of pain).
- Any unvaccinated school contacts should be excluded for 26 days.

Patient Monitoring

Most cases will be mild. Monitor hydration status.

DIET

Liquid diet if unable to chew

PATIENT EDUCATION

Orchitis is common in older children but rarely results in sterility, even if bilateral.

PROGNOSIS

- Complete recovery is typical; immunity is lifelong.
- Transient sensorineural hearing loss in 4% of adults. Some degree of permanent unilateral hearing loss 1/1000 children. Mumps is the most common cause of pediatric hearing loss in some countries.
- Recurrence after 2 weeks may be nonepidemic nonmumps viral parotitis, but mumps RNA has been found in some recurrent parotitis swabs.

COMPLICATIONS

- May precede, accompany, or follow salivary gland involvement and may occur (rarely) without primary involvement of the parotid gland
- Orchitis more common (20–30%) in postpubertal boys:
  – Starts within 8 days of onset of parotitis
  – Impaired fertility in 13%; absolute sterility is rare.
- Meningitis may present 5 to 10 days after first symptoms. Aseptic meningitis is typically mild, but meningoencephalitis may lead to seizures, paralysis, hydrocephalus, or death (in 2% of encephalitis cases).
- Acute cerebellar ataxia has been reported after mumps infections; self-resolving in 2 to 3 weeks
- Oophoritis in 7% of postpubertal females; no decreased fertility. Mastitis has been reported in females.
- Pancreatitis, usually mild
- Nephritis, thyroiditis, and arthralgias are rare.
- Myocarditis: usually mild but may depress ST segment; may be linked to endocardial fibroelastosis
- Deafness: 1/15,000 unilateral nerve deafness unrelated to encephalitis; may be permanent
- Inflammation about the eye (keratouveitis), and dacryoadenitis is rare. Transient bilateral blindness due to optic neuritis has been reported.

Pediatric Considerations

- Orchitis is more common in adolescents.
- Young children are less likely to develop complications.
- Most complications occur in postpubertal group.
- Avoid aspirin use in children with viral symptoms.

Pregnancy Considerations

May increase risk of spontaneous pregnancy loss in first trimester. Perinatal mumps often has a benign course.

REFERENCES

1. Hvild A, Hansen JV, Frisch M, et al. Measles, mumps, rubella vaccination and autism, a nationwide cohort study. *Ann Int Med*. 2019;170(8):513–520.
2. Fiebelkorn AP, Lawler J, Curns AT, et al. Mumps postexposure prophylaxis with a third dose of measles-mumps-rubella vaccine, Orange County, New York, USA. *Emerg Infect Dis*. 2013;19(9):1411–1417.
3. Lam E, Rosen JB, Zucker JR. Mumps: an update on outbreaks, vaccine efficacy, and genomic diversity. *Clin Microbiol Rev*. 2020;33(2):e00151-19.
4. Rubin S, Eckhaus M, Rennick LJ, et al. Molecular biology, pathogenesis and pathology of mumps virus. *J Pathol*. 2015;235(2):242–252.

ADDITIONAL READING

- Khan B, Nasir S, Hanif S. Bilateral optic neuritis: a rare complication of mumps. *Cureus*. 2020;12(4):e7768.
- Kitano T. Close the gap for routine mumps vaccination in Japan. *Hum Vaccin Immunother*. 2021;17(1):205–210.
- Morita S, Fujiwara K, Fukuda A, et al. The clinical features and prognosis of mumps-associated hearing loss: a retrospective, multi-institutional investigation in Japan. *Acta Otolaryngol*. 2017;137(Suppl 565):S44–S47.
- Tiffany A, Shannon D, Mamtcheung W, et al. Notes from the field: mumps outbreak—Alaska, May 2017–July 2018. *MMWR Morb Mortal Wkly Rep*. 2018;67(33):940–941.

 SEE ALSO

CDC Surveillance Manual

 CODES

ICD10

- B26.3 Mumps pancreatitis
- B26.2 Mumps encephalitis
- B26.81 Mumps hepatitis

CLINICAL PEARLS

- Mumps is a clinical diagnosis based on swelling of ≥1 parotid glands for ≥2 days without other obvious cause. Confirm with buccal swab PCR, viral culture, and IgM and IgG serology to identify early in epidemic setting. Work with local health authorities to ensure appropriate specimen collection and report positive results to public health authorities.
- Ultrasound helps distinguish testicular torsion from testicular pain related to mumps orchitis.
- A history of vaccination with MMR does not exclude mumps.
- The MMR vaccine is 68–95% effective after two immunizations. Immunity wanes over time.

M

MUSCULAR DYSTROPHY

George G.A. Pujalte, MD, FACSM, FAMSSM, FAAFP • Mantavya Punj, MD

 BASICS

- Primary inherited myopathies caused by dysfunctional proteins of muscle fibers and extracellular matrix
- Distribution of weakness, other associated symptoms, and disease prognosis depend on specific gene affected and severity of the mutation.

DESCRIPTION

- Duchenne muscular dystrophy (DMD)
  - Highest incidence muscular dystrophy, X-linked inheritance, early onset, progressive
  - Patients are wheelchair-dependent by age 13 years.
- Becker muscular dystrophy (BMD)
  - Less severe phenotype compared to DMD; also caused by mutation in *DMD* gene; later onset and milder clinical course
  - Distinction from DMD is clinical: Patients are usually wheelchair-dependent at age 16 years.
- Myotonic muscular dystrophy (MMD)
  - Myotonia (slow relaxation after muscle contraction), distal and facial weakness
  - Second most common inherited muscle disease
- Facioscapulohumeral muscular dystrophy (FSHMD)
  - Facial and shoulder muscles most affected
  - Third most common inherited muscle disease
- Limb-girdle muscular dystrophy (LGMD)
  - Proximal weakness and atrophy, variable prognosis with many different identified mutations
- Oculopharyngeal muscular dystrophy (OPMD)
  - Usually adult-onset, affects extraocular and pharyngeal muscles; presents with ptosis and dysphagia
- Emery-Dreifuss muscular dystrophy (EDMD)
  - Triad of early development of joint contractures, slowly progressive muscle wasting, and cardiomyopathy; can present as sudden death in apparently healthy, young adults
- Congenital muscular dystrophies (CMD)
  - Heterogeneous group of autosomal recessive myopathic diseases presenting in infancy, with generally poor prognosis

EPIDEMIOLOGY

Incidence

- Duchenne: 1/3,600 male births (1)
- Myotonic dystrophy: 1/10,000 births
- CMD: 0.99 per 100,000
- Other muscular dystrophies vary widely by population but are generally rare.

ETIOLOGY AND PATHOPHYSIOLOGY

Mutations affect proteins connecting cytoskeleton to cell membrane and extracellular matrix, causing muscle fibers to become fragile and easily damaged; muscle weakness and atrophy result.

- DMD/BMD
  - Defective protein is dystrophin, product of the largest human gene, *DMD*; Duchenne phenotype results from mutations that cause profound loss of dystrophin, the protein involved in calcium transport in muscle cells and stabilizing fibers during contraction.

- Becker phenotype results from less severe mutations in *DMD* gene; patients have low but detectable levels of functional dystrophin.
- MMD: trinucleotide repeat expansion in the untranslated region of the gene *DMPK* on chromosome 19; encodes myotonin–protein kinase
- LGMD: mutations in genes encoding proteins associated with dystrophin: calpain-, dysferlin-, and fukutin-related proteins are affected most commonly.
- EDMD: dysfunctional proteins are associated with the nuclear membrane in muscle fibers; emerin in X-linked form, lamin A/C in autosomal forms
- OPMD: Trinucleotide repeat expansion in *PABPN1* results in nuclear inclusions in muscle cells by hampering normal transport of mRNA from the nucleus.
- FSHMD: deletion in untranslated region of chromosome 4; function of deleted genes is unclear, although the most accepted concept is that they likely affect the expression of multiple genes by epigenetic effects.

Genetics

- X-linked
  - Duchenne and Becker muscular dystrophies
  - Gene located at Xp21
    - 30% of affected males have a de novo mutation (mother is not a carrier).
    - 20% of female carriers have some manifestation of the mutation (usually mild muscle weakness or cardiomyopathy).
- Autosomal dominant
  - Generally later onset and less severe than diseases with recessive or X-linked inheritance
  - FSHMD, OPMD, some forms of LGMD and EDMD
  - Myotonic dystrophy
    - Trinucleotide repeat expansion with more severe phenotype in subsequent generations due to accumulation of repeats
- Autosomal recessive
  - Most types of CMD

GENERAL PREVENTION

Genetic counseling for carriers and prenatal diagnosis

COMMONLY ASSOCIATED CONDITIONS

- Decreased IQ: on average, 1 *SD* below the mean in DMD; speech and language delay
- Dilated cardiomyopathy and conduction abnormalities
  - Can be severe in EDMD
  - Can affect otherwise asymptomatic female carriers of DMD
  - Progressive scoliosis

DIAGNOSIS

HISTORY

- DMD: normal attainment of early motor milestones with subsequent abnormal gait and slowing gross motor development: clumsiness, waddling gait, frequent falls, difficulty running, or climbing stairs
- BMD: progressive difficulty with ambulation and frequent falls in later childhood
- MMD: slurred speech, muscle wasting, difficulty with ambulation; often with family history

- LGMD: back pain, lordosis/inability to rise from a chair, climb stairs, and use arms overhead
- FSHMD: facial weakness, inability to close eyes completely
- EDMD: contractures of elbows and ankles, difficulty with ambulation in teenage years
- OPMD: ptosis and dysphagia; often with family history

PHYSICAL EXAM

- DMD/BMD
  - Proximal muscle weakness; Gower sign: use of arms to push upper body into standing posture from lying prone
  - Trendelenburg gait (asymmetric hip waddling)
  - Hyporeflexia/areflexia
  - Winged scapulae and lordosis
  - Pseudohypertrophy of the calf (caused by replacement of muscle with fibroadipose tissue)
  - Contractures of lower extremity joints and elbows
- MMD
  - Characteristic facial appearance: narrow face, open triangular mouth, high-arched palate, concave temples, drooping eyelids, frontal balding in males
  - Myotonia: inability to relax muscles after contraction
  - Distal muscle weakness and wasting
- CMD
  - Arthrogryposis (multiple joint contractures); diffuse hypotonia and muscle wasting in an infant

DIFFERENTIAL DIAGNOSIS

- Glycogen storage diseases and other metabolic myopathies
- Mitochondrial myopathies: MELAS (**M**itochondrial **E**ncephalopathy, **L**actic **A**cidosis, and **S**troke-like episodes), MERRF (**M**yoclonus with **E**pilepsy and **R**agged-**R**ed **F**ibers)
- Inflammatory myopathies: polymyositis, dermatomyositis, inclusion-body myositis
- Neuromuscular junction diseases: myasthenia gravis, Lambert-Eaton syndrome
- Motor neuron diseases: amyotrophic lateral sclerosis, spinal muscular atrophy
- Charcot-Marie-Tooth disease
- Friedreich ataxia

DIAGNOSTIC TESTS & INTERPRETATION

Initial Tests (lab, imaging)

- Creatine kinase (CK): initial screening test if MD is suspected
- Elevated in DMD (10 to 100 times); elevated at birth, peaks at time of presentation, and falls during illness
- Elevated aspartate transaminase/alanine transaminase (AST/ALT) from muscle
- Genetic testing/molecular diagnosis
  - For definitive diagnosis in patient with characteristic presentation and elevated CK
  - Deletion and duplication analysis (MLPA or CGH) will identify most patients (70–80%); followed by genomic sequencing of *DMD* gene for point mutations (20–30% of patients) (2)[A]
  - Genetic testing is available clinically for most other muscular dystrophies.

Diagnostic Procedures/Other
- Muscle biopsy: rarely performed in DMD (dystrophin protein absent); can be used for dystrophin analysis if genetic testing fails to find a mutation
- Electromyography and nerve conduction studies are not necessary unless considering alternative diagnoses.
- ECG: abnormalities found in >90% of males and up to 10% of female carriers of DMD

Test Interpretation
- Heterogenic muscle fibers: atrophy and hypertrophy of fibers with proliferation of connective tissue in muscle
- Immunohistochemical staining for dystrophin protein
  - DMD: no detectable dystrophin in most fibers; occasional revertant fibers with normal dystrophin
  - BMD: highly variable staining for dystrophin throughout muscle

TREATMENT

Glucocorticoid treatment is the only available therapy that affects disease progression. Novel drugs that affect gene expression are now available but clinical benefit unclear.

GENERAL MEASURES
- Ambulation prolonged by knee-ankle-foot orthoses
- Serial casting to treat contractures
- Diagnose sleep apnea with polysomnography; treat with noninvasive ventilation.
- Adaptive devices to improve function
- Avoid overexertion and strenuous exercise.

MEDICATION
Glucocorticoids:

- Prednisone (0.75 mg/kg/day) or deflazacort (0.9 mg/kg/day) a synthetic oral corticosteroid, which has been found to cause less weight gain than prednisone
- Slows the decline in muscle function, progression to scoliosis and degradation of pulmonary function; prolongs functional ambulation; prolongs lifespan; improves cardiac outcomes
- Therapy should be initiated when there is no longer progress in motor skills but prior to decline.
- Monitor adverse effects.
  - Add dietary calcium and vitamin D supplementation. Yearly DEXA scanning and bisphosphonates should be considered; annual exam for cataracts; hypertension should be monitored; no NSAIDs due to risk of peptic ulcer disease (PUD); stress-dose steroids during surgeries and illnesses
  - Patients should be aware of immune suppression and notify emergency providers.

- ACE inhibitors
  - Treatment of cardiomyopathy; may be used in conjunction with β-blockers

ISSUES FOR REFERRAL
- Refer to neuromuscular diseases center for definitive diagnosis and coordinated multidisciplinary care.
- Cardiology for management of cardiomyopathy
- Pulmonology for monitoring of pulmonary function and clearance regimen
- Physical medicine and rehabilitation for management of adaptive devices
- Nutrition/swallowing: for normal weight gain, attention to dysphagia
- Psychosocial: learning/behavior and coping assessment, social development
- Orthopedics: for surgical correction of scoliosis

ADDITIONAL THERAPIES
Dissociative steroids like vamorlone possible benefit. Golodirsen received FDA approval in 2019 for increasing dystrophin production.

SURGERY/OTHER PROCEDURES
- Spinal surgery for scoliosis diminishes rate of deformity progression.
- Scapular fixation for scapular winging may be beneficial; however, also lacking clinical trials
- Consider surgical treatment of ankle/knee contractures.

COMPLEMENTARY & ALTERNATIVE MEDICINE
Whole body vibration exercises

ONGOING CARE

FOLLOW-UP RECOMMENDATIONS
Patient Monitoring
- Electrocardiogram (ECG), echocardiogram, and consultation with a cardiologist at diagnosis and annually after age 10 years
  - Female carriers of DMD mutation should be monitored every 5 years.
- Annual spinal radiography for scoliosis
- Dual-energy x-ray absorptiometry (DEXA) scanning and serum marker testing for osteoporosis
- Pulmonary function testing twice yearly if no longer ambulatory
- Psychosocial: coping, emotional adjustment, depression

DIET
Diet may be limited by dysphagia; swallow evaluation can determine appropriate foods; may require gastrostomy

PATIENT EDUCATION
- Muscular Dystrophy Association: http://www.mda.org
- Parent Project Muscular Dystrophy: http://www.parentprojectmd.org
- Cure Duchenne: https://www.cureduchenne.org/

PROGNOSIS
DMD/BMD
- Progressive weakness, contractures, inability to walk
- Kyphoscoliosis and progressive decline in respiratory vital capacity with recurrent pulmonary infections
- Significantly shortened lifespan (DMD: 16 ± 4 years; BMD: 42 ± 16 years). Respiratory failure cause of death in 90%; remaining due to myocardial disease (heart failure and dysrhythmia)

COMPLICATIONS
- Cardiac arrhythmia, cardiomyopathy
- Dysphagia, gastroesophageal reflux disease (GERD), constipation
- Scoliosis, joint contractures
- Obstructive sleep apnea
- Malignant hyperthermia–like reaction to anesthesia
- Respiratory failure and early death

REFERENCES
1. Chung J, Smith AL, Hughes SC, et al. Twenty-year follow-up of newborn screening for patients with muscular dystrophy. *Muscle Nerve*. 2016;53(4):570–578.
2. Falzarano MS, Scotton C, Passarelli C, et al. Duchenne muscular dystrophy: from diagnosis to therapy. *Molecules*. 2015;20(10):18168–18184.

CODES

ICD10
- G71.0 Muscular dystrophy
- G71.11 Myotonic muscular dystrophy
- G71.2 Congenital myopathies

CLINICAL PEARLS
- Primary care providers should have a low threshold to obtain serum CK as a screening test in the face of gross motor delay/muscular weakness, especially in boys.
- Steroids should be initiated in patients with DMD when gross motor function ceases to progress.
- High-quality care of patients requires a medical home; a multidisciplinary team of physicians, therapists, and other providers; and extensive patient and family support.

M

MYALGIC ENCEPHALOMYELITIS/CHRONIC FATIGUE SYNDROME (CFS)

Grant M. Reed, DO • Siddharth Jain, BA

 BASICS

DESCRIPTION

- A chronic and complex physical illness characterized by a new or definitive onset of debilitating fatigue that persists for >6 months with moderate to severe intensity at least half of the time, which significantly reduces a person's ability to perform preillness activities
- Key features include (1):
  - Impaired memory or concentration
  - Joint and muscle pain, unrefreshing sleep
  - Postexertional malaise (PEM), orthostatic intolerance
- Synonyms: myalgic encephalomyelitis (ME)/chronic fatigue syndrome (CFS), chronic Epstein-Barr virus syndrome, postviral fatigue syndrome, chronic fatigue immune dysfunction, and systemic exertion intolerance disease
- Fatigue is not relieved by rest and results in >50% reduction in preillness activities (occupational, educational, social, and personal).
- Other commonly associated symptoms include heart rate variability; excessive sweating; muscle and joint pain; and light, sound, and chemical sensitivity (2).
- Other causes such as schizophrenia, manic-depressive illness, substance abuse, eating disorder, or proven organic brain disease must be ruled out (3).

EPIDEMIOLOGY

- Can affect all ages; incidence peaks at 10 to 19 years and 30 to 39 years (1).
- Females are twice as likely to be affected (3).
- Up to 70% of patients are unable to return to work, and one quarter remain bedridden or housebound (2).

Prevalence

- Affects all racial and ethnic groups; more prevalent in minority and low socioeconomic groups
- Estimated at 519 to 1,038 diagnosed per 100,000; 1.7 to 3.4 million patients may suffer from ME or CFS.
- Up to 90% of cases may remain undiagnosed (2).

ETIOLOGY AND PATHOPHYSIOLOGY

Cause is unknown and likely multifactorial

- Suspected initiating stressors:
  - Viral, bacterial, or parasitic infection: Epstein-Barr virus (EBV), retroviruses, Lyme disease, Q fever, human herpesvirus type 6, enteroviruses, Ross river virus, Borna disease virus
  - Significant physical or emotional trauma
  - Recent vaccination
  - Overexertion, chronic sleep deprivation
  - Toxin exposure (e.g., organophosphate pesticides) or an atypical adverse reaction to a medication
- Suspected perpetuating factors:
  - Delay in diagnosis
  - Overexertion
  - Stress, inadequate sleep
- Hypothesized contributing systems and factors (4):
  - Cellular metabolism (e.g., reduced oxidative phosphorylation and mitochondrial function)
  - Neuroendocrine system (e.g., diminished cortisol response to increased corticotropin)
  - Immune system (e.g., increased proinflammatory cytokines, C-reactive protein, and β_2-microglobulin)
  - Muscular system (e.g., reduced oxygen uptake)
  - Autonomic system (e.g., orthostatic hypotension)
  - Serotonergic system (e.g., upregulation of serotonin receptors)
  - Gastrointestinal system (e.g., increased wall permeability, altered gut microbiota, irritable bowel syndrome [IBS] comorbidity)

Genetics

- Higher concordance in monozygotic twins
- Genetic polymorphisms in several neuroimmunoendocrine-related genes may contribute to developing disease (4).

RISK FACTORS

- Family history of ME or CFS
- Personality characteristics (neuroticism and introversion)
- Comorbid depression or anxiety
- Long-standing medical and/or mental health conditions in childhood
  - Childhood inactivity or overactivity
  - Childhood trauma (emotional, physical, or sexual abuse)
- Prolonged idiopathic chronic fatigue

COMMONLY ASSOCIATED CONDITIONS

- Fibromyalgia (more common in women)
- IBS
- Gynecologic conditions (pelvic pain, endometriosis) and surgeries (hysterectomy, oophorectomy)
- Anxiety disorders and/or major depressive disorders
- Posttraumatic stress disorder (PTSD), including physical and/or past sexual abuse; domestic violence
- Attention deficit hyperactivity disorder (ADHD)
- Postural orthostatic tachycardia syndrome (POTS)
- Sleep disorders, including obstructive sleep apnea (OSA)
- Reduced left ventricular size and mass; prolapsed mitral valve
- Temporomandibular joint syndrome
- Multiple chemical sensitivities
- Migraines, myofascial pain syndrome
- Hashimoto thyroiditis, Raynaud phenomenon
- Interstitial cystitis, sicca syndrome, allergies

 DIAGNOSIS

HISTORY

A thorough medical history and psychosocial history is required for an accurate diagnosis. The 2015 diagnostic criteria proposed by the Institute of Medicine (IOM) (1) require three symptoms and at least one of two additional manifestations:

- A substantial reduction or impairment in the ability to engage in preillness levels of activity (occupational, educational, social, or personal life) that:
  - Lasts for 6 months
  - Is accompanied by fatigue that is:
    ○ Often profound
    ○ Of new onset (not lifelong)
    ○ Not the result of ongoing or unusual excessive exertion
    ○ Not substantially alleviated by rest
- PEM*—worsening of symptoms after physical, mental, or emotional exertion that would not have caused a problem before the illness. PEM often puts the patient in relapse that may last days, weeks, or even longer. Obtaining patient's response to activities that they were able to previously tolerate can be helpful in determining PEM along with a 2-day cardiopulmonary test (2).
- Unrefreshing sleep*—Patients with ME/CFS may not feel better or less tired even after a full night of sleep despite the absence of specific objective sleep alterations. Sleep studies may help identify underlying sleep apnea if present (2).

- At least one of the following two additional manifestations must be present:
  - Cognitive impairment*—Patients have problems with thinking, memory, executive function, and information processing as well as attention deficit and impaired psychomotor functions. Each can be exacerbated by exertion, effort, prolonged upright posture, stress, or time pressure and may have serious consequences on a patient's ability to maintain a job or attend school full time.
  - Orthostatic intolerance—Patients develop a worsening of symptoms upon assuming and maintaining upright posture as measured by objective heart rate and blood pressure abnormalities during standing, bedside orthostatic vital signs, or head-up tilt testing. Orthostatic symptoms, including light-headedness, fainting, increased fatigue, cognitive worsening, headaches, or nausea, are worsened with quiet upright posture (either standing or sitting) during day-to-day life and are improved (although not necessarily fully resolved) with lying down.

*The frequency and severity of these symptoms need to be evaluated.

PHYSICAL EXAM

Complete physical exam to rule out other medical causes for symptoms. A complete mental status examination should be performed as well.

DIFFERENTIAL DIAGNOSIS

- Idiopathic chronic fatigue (i.e., fatigue of unknown cause for >6 months without meeting criteria for CFS)
- Psychiatric disorders: depression, anxiety, somatization disorder, substance abuse
- Physiologic fatigue: poor sleep hygiene, menopause, pregnancy until 3 months postpartum
- Sleep disorders (e.g., insomnia, sleep apnea, narcolepsy)
- Endocrine disorders (e.g., hypothyroidism, Addison disease, Cushing syndrome, diabetes mellitus)
- Chronic infections
  - Lyme disease, chronic hepatitis B/C
  - Fungal disease (e.g., histoplasmosis, coccidioidomycosis)
  - Parasitic disease (e.g., amebiasis, giardiasis, helminth infestation)
  - HIV or related diseases, tuberculosis
  - Chronic or subacute bacterial diseases (e.g., endocarditis, occult abscess)
- Iatrogenic (e.g., medication side effects)
- Toxic agent exposure
- Obesity
- Malignancy, autoimmune diseases
- Chronic inflammatory diseases (e.g., sarcoidosis, Wegener disease, celiac disease, inflammatory bowel disease)
- Neuromuscular diseases (e.g., multiple sclerosis, myasthenia gravis, Parkinson disease)
- Cardiovascular diseases (e.g., cardiomyopathy or other causes of heart failure)

DIAGNOSTIC TESTS & INTERPRETATION

No validated diagnostic test is available. Note that an abnormal result is not always the same as discovering the cause of fatigue. Renew the search if the suspected problem is treated and the patient remains fatigued.

Initial Tests (lab, imaging)

Standard laboratory tests are recommended to rule out other causes for symptoms:

- CBC; complete metabolic panel
- Urinalysis
- Thyroid-stimulating hormone (TSH) and free thyroxine (free T_4)
- ESR or C-reactive protein
- Magnesium and phosphorus level; Vitamin B_{12}; serum folate; creatine kinase (CK)
- 25-hydroxy-cholecalciferol (vitamin D); serum iron, iron-binding capacity, ferritin
- Screen for domestic violence:
  - "Have you been hit, kicked, punched, or otherwise, hurt by someone within the past year? If so, by whom?"
  - "Do you feel safe in your current relationship?"
  - "Is there a partner from a previous relationship who is making you feel unsafe now?"

Follow-Up Tests & Special Considerations

- Additional laboratory studies, based on clinical features:
  - Antinuclear antibodies and rheumatoid factor
  - Tuberculin skin test
  - Serum cortisol
  - HIV; RPR; VDRL; Lyme serology
  - IgA tissue transglutaminase
- Consider age/gender-appropriate cancer screening.
- Consider an electroencephalogram and/or magnetic resonance imaging if central nervous system symptoms.
- Consider polysomnography and/or multiple sleep latency test (MSLT) if features of a sleep disorder.
- Consider urine drug screening in those with concerning historical features.
- Assess for personality and psychosocial factors and maladaptive coping styles.

TREATMENT

- No treatment has been proven effective by large randomized trials; recommendations are based on expert opinion and standard symptom management (e.g., sleep disturbances, depression, and pain).
- Patients commonly use earplugs, earphones, sunglasses, and eye glasses to relieve sensitivity to light and sound (2).
- Focus on changes in lifestyle and insight with a goal to avoid complicating treatments (e.g., addictive medications, invasive testing) or interventions that support secondary gain.
- A multidisciplinary approach is recommended.
- Evidence suggests cognitive-behavioral therapy (CBT), and graded exercise therapy (GET) may be beneficial (3).

GENERAL MEASURES

Treatment involves symptom control and guided self-management. The aim is to reduce symptoms and improve quality of life. Identify the most troublesome symptoms (typically pain and insomnia) and address those first.

- Individual CBT: not curative; may improve coping strategies and/or assist in rehabilitation (e.g., social, occupational)
- GET: Track amount of exercise patient can do without exacerbating symptoms and gradually increase intensity and duration. Strike a balance between activity and rest. GET should only be performed in the presence of a trained professional to prevent illness exacerbation.

MEDICATION

- There are no established pharmacologic treatments. Medications used are primarily for specific symptoms.
- Use the lowest effective dose and increase cautiously.
  - Studies have been conducted with antivirals, antidepressants, immunoglobulins, hydrocortisone, modafinil, staphylococcus toxoid, methylphenidate, melatonin, and galantamine. None show clear benefit.
  - Agomelatine, an antidepressant with agonist activity at melatonin receptors, has been promising in early studies.
  - If insomnia is present, use of nonaddicting sleep aids (hydroxyzine, trazodone, doxepin, etc.) may improve outcomes.

ISSUES FOR REFERRAL

- Psychiatrist for comorbid behavioral disorders
- Rehabilitative medicine
- Sleep or pain management specialist

COMPLEMENTARY & ALTERNATIVE MEDICINE

- Acupuncture, massage, and chiropractic have been shown to be benefit pain for some patients.
- Other helpful nonpharmacologic interventions may include physical therapy, stretches, hydrotherapy, yoga, tai chi, and meditations. Hot or cold packs, warm baths, electrical massagers, transcutaneous electrical nerve stimulations may help.
- Equivocal evidence for homeopathy and biofeedback

ONGOING CARE

FOLLOW-UP RECOMMENDATIONS

Patient Monitoring

Although no consensus exists, periodic reevaluation is appropriate for support, relief of symptoms, and assessment for other possible causes of symptoms.

DIET

- Well-balanced diet, including recommended daily allowance of vitamins and minerals
- No particular diet program has been shown to be effective for treatment of CFS.
- Whether weight loss improves symptoms in obese CFS patients is unknown.

PATIENT EDUCATION

- Gradually increase exercise tolerance.
- Explain PEM and aerobic metabolism impairment for patients to not exceed their "energy envelope" (2).
- "Paced" activity management can help patients not exceed their energy limits (2).
- Avoid extended periods of rest, but ensure adequate rest between sessions.
- Relaxation techniques may also be helpful (3).
- Promote the benefits of cognitive therapies, lifestyle changes, and pharmacologic therapy.
- Educate patient's family on the condition and assist with applications for disability (2).
- Chronic Fatigue and Immune Dysfunction Syndrome Association of America: http://solvecfs.org/
- CDC, Chronic Fatigue Syndrome: http://www.cdc.gov/cfs/

PROGNOSIS

- A fluctuating course with relapse is common.
- Improvement is generally slow over months to years.
- An estimated 15% achieve full recovery.
- Patients with poor social adjustment, a strong belief in an organic etiology, financial secondary gain, or age >50 years are less likely to improve.

COMPLICATIONS

- CFS patients may reduce physical activity out of fear that it may worsen symptoms.
- Depression; polypharmacy
- Unemployment: Although studies document improvement with treatment, <1/3 of patients in trials return to work.
- The Social Security Administration considers CFS to be a disability.
- Receipt of third-party disability pay (secondary gain) has been associated with treatment nonresponse.
- Chronic immune activation or an associated infection may increase risk for non-Hodgkin lymphoma in elderly (>80 years) CFS patients.

REFERENCES

1. Committee on the Diagnostic Criteria for Myalgic Encephalomyelitis/Chronic Fatigue Syndrome, Board on the Health of Select Populations, Institute of Medicine. *Beyond Myalgic Encephalomyelitis/Chronic Fatigue Syndrome: Redefining an Illness.* Washington, DC: National Academies Press; 2015.
2. Kim DY, Lee JS, Son CG. Systematic review of primary outcome measurements for chronic fatigue syndrome/myalgic encephalomyelitis (CFS/ME) in randomized controlled trials. *J Clin Med.* 2020;9(11):3463.
3. Yancey JR, Thomas SM. Chronic fatigue syndrome: diagnosis and treatment. *Am Fam Physician.* 2012;86(8):741–746.
4. Cortes Rivera M, Mastronardi C, Silva-Aldana CT, et al. Myalgic encephalomyelitis/chronic fatigue syndrome: a comprehensive review. *Diagnostics (Basel).* 2019;9(3):E91.

 SEE ALSO

Algorithm: Fatigue

 CODES

ICD10

R53.82 Chronic fatigue, unspecified

CLINICAL PEARLS

- No pharmacologic agents (e.g., antidepressants, immune modulators) are consistently effective in treating CFS.
- There are many more patients with idiopathic chronic fatigue than true CFS.
- Use the IOM criteria to diagnose CFS.
- Standardized instruments (SF-36, symptom index, and Multidimensional Fatigue Inventory [MFI]) help to follow patient progress.

M

MYASTHENIA GRAVIS

Melody A. Jordahl-Iafrato, MD, FAAFP • Jennifer R. Collins, PharmD

BASICS

DESCRIPTION
Primary disorder of neuromuscular transmission characterized by fluctuating muscle weakness:
- Ocular myasthenia gravis (MG) (15%): weakness limited to eyelids and extraocular muscles
- Generalized MG (85%): commonly affects ocular as well as a variable combination of bulbar, proximal limb, and respiratory muscles
- 50% of patients who present with ocular symptoms develop generalized MG within 2 years.
- Onset may be sudden and severe, but it is typically mild and intermittent over many years, maximum severity reached within 3 years for 85%.
- System(s) affected: neurologic, hematologic, lymphatic, immunologic, musculoskeletal

EPIDEMIOLOGY
Occurs at any age but a bimodal distribution to the age of onset:
- Female predominance: 20 to 40 years
- Male predominance: 60 to 80 years

Incidence
Estimated annual incidence 7 to 23/1 million

Prevalence
In the United States, 70 to 320/1 million; increasing over the past 5 decades

Pediatric Considerations
A transient form of neonatal MG seen in 10–20% of infants born to mothers with MG. It occurs as a result of the transplacental passage of maternal antibodies that interfere with function of the neuromuscular junction; resolves in weeks to months. Autoimmune juvenile MG makes up 10–15% of cases of MG in North America.

ETIOLOGY AND PATHOPHYSIOLOGY
- Reduction in the function of acetylcholine receptors (AChRs) at muscle end plates, resulting in insufficient neuromuscular transmission
- Antibody-mediated autoimmune disorder
- Antibodies are present in most cases of MG.
  - Seropositive/antiacetylcholine receptor (anti-AChR): a humoral, antibody-mediated, T-cell–dependent attack of the AChRs or receptor-associated proteins at the postsynaptic membrane of the neuromuscular junction. Found in 85% of generalized MG and 50% of ocular MG; thymic abnormalities common (1)
  - Muscle-specific kinase (MuSKs): 5% of generalized MG patients. Typically females. Is a severe form, respiratory and bulbar muscles involved. Thymic abnormalities are rare (1).
  - In remainder of seronegative, 12–50% with anti-LRP4, a molecule that forms a complex with MuSK, mild generalized weakness most common (1)
  - Seronegative MG (SNMG): 5%; may have anti-AChR detectable by cell-based assay. Clinically similar to anti-AChR; thymic hyperplasia may be present (1).
- Also documented immediately after viral infections (measles, Epstein-Barr virus [EBV], HIV, and human T-lymphotropic virus [HTLV])

Genetics
- Congenital MG syndrome describes a collection of rare hereditary disorders. This condition is not immune-mediated but instead results from the mutation of a component of the neuromuscular junction (autosomal recessive).
- Familial predisposition is seen in 5% of cases.

RISK FACTORS
- Familial MG
- D-penicillamine (drug-induced MG)
- Other autoimmune diseases

COMMONLY ASSOCIATED CONDITIONS
- Thymic hyperplasia (60–70%)
- Thymoma (10–15%)
- Autoimmune thyroid disease (3–8%)

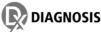

DIAGNOSIS

Myasthenia Gravis Foundation of America clinical classification (2)[C]:
- Class I: any eye muscle weakness, possible ptosis, no other evidence of muscle weakness elsewhere
- Class II: eye muscle weakness of any severity; mild weakness of other muscles:
  - Class IIa: predominantly limb or axial muscles
  - Class IIb: predominantly bulbar and/or respiratory muscles
- Class III: eye muscle weakness of any severity; moderate weakness of other muscles:
  - Class IIIa: predominantly limb or axial muscles
  - Class IIIb: predominantly bulbar and/or respiratory muscles
- Class IV: eye muscle weakness of any severity; severe weakness of other muscles:
  - Class IVa: predominantly limb or axial muscles
  - Class IVb: predominantly bulbar and/or respiratory muscles (can also include feeding tube without intubation)
- Class V: intubation needed to maintain airway

HISTORY
The hallmark of MG is fatigability.
- Fluctuating weakness, often subtle, that worsens during the day and after prolonged use of affected muscles; may improve with rest
- Early symptoms are transient with asymptomatic periods lasting days or weeks.
- With progression, asymptomatic periods shorten, and symptoms fluctuate from mild to severe.
- >50% of patients present with ocular symptoms (ptosis and/or diplopia). Eventually, 90% of patients with MG develop ocular symptoms.
- Ptosis might be unilateral, bilateral, or shifting from eye to eye.
- 15% present with bulbar symptoms.
- <5% present with proximal limb weakness alone.

ALERT
Myasthenic crisis: respiratory muscle weakness producing respiratory insufficiency and pending respiratory failure

PHYSICAL EXAM
- Ptosis may worsen with propping of opposite eyelid (curtain sign) or sustained upward gaze.
- "Myasthenic sneer," in which the midlip rises but corners of mouth do not move

- Muscle weakness is usually proximal and symmetric.
- Test for muscle fatigability by repetitive or prolonged use of individual muscles.
- Important to test and monitor respiratory function

DIFFERENTIAL DIAGNOSIS
- Thyroid ophthalmopathy
- Oculopharyngeal muscular dystrophy
- Myotonic dystrophy
- Kearns-Sayre syndrome
- Chronic progressive external ophthalmoplegia
- Brainstem and motor cranial nerve lesions
- Botulism
- Motor neuron disease (e.g., amyotrophic lateral sclerosis [ALS])
- Lambert-Eaton myasthenic syndrome
- Drug-induced myasthenia
- Congenital myasthenic syndrome
- Dermatomyositis/polymyositis
- Neurosarcoidosis
- Tolosa-Hunt syndrome

DIAGNOSTIC TESTS & INTERPRETATION
Initial Tests (lab, imaging)
- Anti-AChR antibody (74–85% are seropositive):
  - Generalized myasthenia: 75–85%
  - Ocular myasthenia: 50%
  - MG and thymoma: 98–100%
  - Poor correlation between antibody titer and disease severity (1)[C]
  - False-positive results in thymoma without MG, Lambert-Eaton myasthenic syndrome, small cell lung cancer, and rheumatoid arthritis treated with penicillamine
- Anti-MuSK antibody:
  - Used if MG is suspected and patient seronegative for AChR antibodies
  - Strong correlation between titer and disease severity (1)[C]
- LRP4 and clustered anti-AChR:
  - Used if MG suspected and patient seronegative for AChR antibodies
- Thyroid and other autoimmune testing anti-striated muscle (anti-SM) antibody:
  - Present in 84% of patients with thymoma who are <40 years of age
  - Can be present without thymoma in patients >40 years of age
- Chest radiographs or CT scans may identify a thymoma.
- MRI of brain and orbits to rule out other causes of cranial nerve deficit

Diagnostic Procedures/Other
- Tensilon (edrophonium) test:
  - Rarely done as edrophonium no longer available in United States and many other countries
  - A positive test shows improvement of strength within 30 seconds of administration.
  - Sensitivity 80–90% (3)[C]
  - Cardiac disease and bronchial asthma are relative contraindications, especially in elderly.
  - Atropine: 0.4 to 0.6 mg IV may rarely be required as antidote; must be available
- Ice pack test:
  - Ice pack applied to closed eyelid for 60 seconds, then removed; extent of ptosis immediately assessed
  - Ice will decrease the ptosis induced by MG.
  - Sensitivity 80% in patients with prominent ptosis

- Electrophysiology testing:
  - Repetitive nerve stimulation (RNS):
    - Widely available, most frequently used
    - Sensitivity generalized MG 76%; ocular MG 50% (3)[C]
  - Single-fiber electromyogram (SFEMG):
    - Assesses temporal variability between two muscle fibers within same motor unit (jitter)
    - Sensitivity 99%
    - Technically difficult to perform; limited availability, use if suspected and negative RNS (3)[C]

Test Interpretation
- Lymphofollicular hyperplasia of thymic medulla occurs in 65% of patients with MG, thymoma in 15%.
- Immunofluorescence: immunoglobulin (Ig) G antibodies and complement on receptor membranes in seropositive patients

TREATMENT

GENERAL MEASURES
- Treatment based on age, gender, and disease severity and progression
- Three basic approaches: symptomatic, immunosuppressive, and supportive. Few should receive a single therapeutic modality; most should receive symptomatic treatment along with immunosuppressive and/or supportive.

MEDICATION
First Line
Symptomatic treatments (anticholinesterase agents)
- Pyridostigmine bromide (Mestinon):
  - *Most commonly prescribed because available in oral tablet*
  - Starting dose of 60 mg PO TID with food
  - Maximum dose: 120 mg q3–4h
  - Long acting available but effect not consistent
  - Side effects common, which can result in dose reduction or slower titration of dose: gastrointestinal disturbances, hypotension, syncope, urinary frequency (4)
- Neostigmine methylsulfate (Prostigmin):
  - Starting dose of 0.5 mg SC or IM q3h
  - Titrate dosage to clinical need
  - Useful for patients who cannot absorb medications orally
  - May cause excessive salivary secretions, which may exacerbate swallowing difficulties (4)
- Patients with anti-MuSK may not respond well to these medications.

Second Line
- Immunosuppressants: Oral corticosteroids are the first choice of drugs when immunosuppression is necessary.
  - Prednisone:
    - May exacerbate symptoms short-term in up to 50% of patients
    - If inpatient and on other acute treatment, start with 60 mg/day PO
    - If outpatient, start at lower dose (10 to 20 mg/day PO)
    - Titrate dose by 5 mg every 3 to 7 days to attain lowest effective dose (5)[B].
    - Use caution regarding long-term side effects from corticosteroids, including but not limited to weight gain, fluid retention, gastritis, ulcer formation, hyperglycemia, risk of infection, and osteoporosis (4).

- Azathioprine: 100 to 200 mg/day PO (5)[B]
  - *Most frequently used for long-term immunomodulation*, similar efficacy to steroids and IVIG
  - Consider screening for thiopurine S-methyltransferase (TPMT) levels prior to initiation of azathioprine.
  - Benefit may not be apparent for up to 18 months after initiation of therapy.
  - Prednisolone + azathioprine may be effective when used as a corticosteroid-sparing agent.
- Mycophenolate: 1 g PO or IV BID
- Cyclosporine: dosing varies; may give IV or PO (use caution due to nephrotoxicity and drug interactions) [B]
- Acute immunomodulating treatments:
  - Plasmapheresis: bulk removal of 2 to 3 L of plasma 3 times per week, repeated until rate of improvement plateaus (6)[B]
    - Improves weakness in nearly all and can last up to 3 months
  - Ig: 2 g/kg IV over 2 to 5 days (5)[B]
  - *Plasmapheresis and Ig have comparable efficacy in treating moderate to severe MG* (6)[C].
  - Rapid onset of effect but short duration of action
  - Used for acute worsening of MG to improve strength prior to surgery, prevent acute exacerbations induced by corticosteroids, and as a chronic intermittent treatment to provide relief in refractory MG
- Other immunosuppressant therapies, typically used in refractory cases:
  - Eculizumab
  - Rituximab:
    - Seronegative MuSK-antibody positive MG patients may have better response to rituximab than conventional therapies.
  - Tacrolimus
  - Cyclophosphamide

ALERT
Use caution with drugs that can precipitate weakness: aminoglycosides, fluoroquinolones, β-blockers, calcium channel blockers, neuromuscular blockers, statins, diuretics, oral contraceptives, gabapentin, phenytoin, lithium, among others.

SURGERY/OTHER PROCEDURES
- Thymectomy recommended for patients with thymic abnormalities
- May be beneficial for patients without thymic abnormalities in those <60 years of age especially in patients with elevated anti-AChR

Pediatric Considerations
Infants with severe weakness from transient neonatal myasthenia may be treated with oral pyridostigmine; general support is necessary until the condition clears.
- Corticosteroids limited only to severe disease
- Side effects of many medications must be closely monitored in juvenile patients especially because some may affect long-term fertility or are consider carcinogenic.

ADMISSION, INPATIENT, AND NURSING CONSIDERATIONS
- Management of pulmonary infections
- Myasthenic/cholinergic crises
- Plasmapheresis
- IV γ-globulin

 ONGOING CARE

PATIENT EDUCATION
Myasthenia Gravis Foundation of America (MGFA): http://www.myasthenia.org/

PROGNOSIS
- Overall good but highly variable
- Myasthenic crisis associated with substantial morbidity and 4% mortality
- Seronegative patients are more likely to have purely ocular disease, and those with generalized SNMG have a better outcome after treatment.

COMPLICATIONS
Acute respiratory arrest; chronic respiratory insufficiency

REFERENCES
1. Berrih-Aknin S, Frenkian-Cuvelier M, Eymard B. Diagnostic and clinical classification of autoimmune myasthenia gravis. *J Autoimmun*. 2014; 48–49:143–148.
2. Jaretzki A III, Barohn RJ, Ernstoff RM, et al. Myasthenia gravis: recommendations for clinical research standards. Task Force of the Medical Scientific Advisory Board of the Myasthenia Gravis Foundation of America. *Neurology*. 2000;55(1): 16–23.
3. Pasnoor M, Dimachkie MM, Farmakidis C, et al. Diagnosis of myasthenia gravis. *Neurol Clin*. 2018;36(2):261–274.
4. Farrugia ME, Goodfellow JA. A practice approach to managing patients with myasthenia gravis—opinions and a review of the literature. *Front Neurol*. 2020;11(604):1–16.
5. Gotterer L, Li Y. Maintenance immunosuppression in myasthenia gravis. *J Neurol Sci*. 2016;369: 294–302.
6. Barth D, Nabavi Nouri M, Ng E, et al. Comparison of IVIg and PLEX in patients with myasthenia gravis. *Neurology*. 2011;76(23):2017–2023.

ADDITIONAL READING
- Angelini C. Diagnosis and management of autoimmune myasthenia gravis. *Clin Drug Investig*. 2011;31(1):1–14.
- Menon D, Barnett C, Bril V. Novel treatments in myasthenia gravis. *Front Neurol*. 2020;11(538):1–12.
- Meriggioli MN. Myasthenia gravis: immunopathogenesis, diagnosis, and management. *Continuum Lifelong Learn Neurol*. 2009;15(1):35–62.

 CODES

ICD10
- G70.01 Myasthenia gravis with (acute) exacerbation
- G70.00 Myasthenia gravis without (acute) exacerbation
- G70.0 Myasthenia gravis

CLINICAL PEARLS
- An autoimmune disease, marked by abnormal fatigability and weakness of selected muscles, which is relieved by rest
- >50% of patients present with ocular symptoms (ptosis and/or diplopia).
- Anticholinesterase medication and a thymectomy lessen symptom severity.
- Steroid therapy, plasma exchange, or Ig can be used in severely affected patients.

M

MYELODYSPLASTIC SYNDROMES (MDS)

Kartik Sidhar, MD • Michael Ibrahem, MD

 BASICS

DESCRIPTION
- Myelodysplastic syndromes (MDS) are a heterogeneous group of clonal stem cell disorders characterized by peripheral blood cytopenias: anemia, thrombocytopenia, and/or neutropenia.
- Dysplasia refers to an abnormality of development or differentiation in specific cell lines. In MDS, these changes take place in the bone marrow and confer a tendency for transformation to acute myelogenous leukemia (AML).

EPIDEMIOLOGY
Incidence
The incidence in the United States is approximately 3 to 4 cases per 100,000 population per year, expanding to 35 cases per 100,000 population per year, for patients age >60 years.

Prevalence
>60,000 people with MDS resided in the country, which continues to increase as population ages

ETIOLOGY AND PATHOPHYSIOLOGY
- MDS arises from mutations in hematopoietic blood cell lines.
- MDS is clinically characterized by peripheral cytopenias, consequence of ineffective marrow hematopoiesis (premature cell death).
- Nongenetic mechanisms encompass apoptosis, pyroptosis, deregulated immunity, and inflammatory cytokine amplification (see "Genetics" for genetic mechanisms) (1),(2).
- Low-risk MDS (LR-MDS) are characterized by deregulated immunity and apoptosis, whereas high-risk MDS (HR-MDS) are characterized by clonal expansion and transformation to AML.
- A changing interplay of proapoptotic versus antiapoptotic signals is central in the progression of the disease.
- In LR-MDS, stem cell programmed death occurs by different mechanisms: apoptosis, pyroptosis, and potentially autophagy.
  - *Apoptosis*: Tumor necrosis factor-α (TNF-α), TNF-related apoptosis-inducing ligand (TRAIL), Fas ligand, and proapoptotic cytokines (TNF-α and IL-6) play a major role in stem cell apoptosis in LR-MDS.
  - *Pyroptosis*: It is an inflammatory cell death different from apoptosis.
    - Activation of nod-like receptors leads to formation of the inflammasome complex and caspase 1 activation that leads to pore formation in the plasma membrane of the cells; creates ionic gradients, water influx, cell swelling, and cell death (3)
    - This potentially also explains the morphologic changes seen in MDS (macrocytosis, enlarged cells).

- Evolution to AML has been associated with upregulation of NFκB and enhanced activity of the Bcl2 and the inhibitors of apoptosis protein (IAP) families.
  - This is thought to be a mechanism of bypassing the apoptotic phenomenon in the bone marrow microenvironment.

Genetics
- Recurrent somatic mutations are observed in >90% of MDS patients.
- Mutated genes are involved in:
  - Epigenetic regulation: TET2, EZH2, IDH1, IDH2, DNMT3A, ASXL1
  - DNA repair: TP53
  - Transcriptional regulation: BCOR, ETV6, RUNX1
  - RNA splicing: U2AF35, ZRSR2, SF3B1, SRSF2
  - Cohesin complex: STAG2
  - Signal transduction: JAK2, CBL, NRAS
- Mutations in the epigenetic modifiers: The concept is that any gain of function mutations in the DNA methyltransferases (DNMT3A and DNMT3B) leads to hypermethylation (a gene silencing mechanism that contributes to clonal evolution).
- It is unclear how these different molecular and genetic mechanisms translate into the same phenotypic manifestation of myelodysplasia and cytopenias.

RISK FACTORS
- Age: increased risk in patients >60 years old
- Tobacco use
- Chronic exposure to chemicals: benzene, pesticides, insecticides, and petroleum
- Prior chemotherapy or radiation therapy
- Inherited disorders: Fanconi anemia, Shwachman-Diamond syndromes, severe congenital neutropenia, and familial platelet disorder
- An association has been noted in patients with end stage renal disease on dialysis (4).

GENERAL PREVENTION
Avoiding known cancer-causing industrial chemicals, such as benzene and also tobacco, might lower the risk of developing MDS.

COMMONLY ASSOCIATED CONDITIONS
Myeloproliferative disorders and hematologic conditions such as paroxysmal nocturnal hemoglobinuria

DIAGNOSIS

HISTORY
- The clinical course of MDS patients is driven by the type and degree of cytopenias.
- Recurrent infections, bleeding issues, fatigue, weight loss and exertional dyspnea, are common symptoms reported.
- Fatigue is the most common symptom and tends to be out of proportion to anemia.
- Fevers, night sweats, and weight loss are uncommon.
- Evaluate for toxin exposure, including alcohol or previous chemotherapy.

PHYSICAL EXAM
- Generalized pallor and ecchymosis as result of the anemia and thrombocytopenia, respectively
- Rarely hepatosplenomegaly as consequence of extramedullary hemopoiesis is present, especially in MDS/MPN overlapping syndromes
- Lymphadenopathies are uncommon.

DIFFERENTIAL DIAGNOSIS
- Acute leukemia: AML
- Vitamin B_{12} and folate deficiencies can manifest as a hypoproliferative anemia.
- HIV
- Chronic liver disease
- Excessive alcohol use
- Infections of the bone marrow: HIV, tuberculosis, atypical mycobacterium, and Epstein-Barr virus
- Indolent myeloid hematopoietic disorders that do not fulfill diagnostic criteria for MDS: idiopathic cytopenia of unknown significance, idiopathic dysplasia of unknown significance, clonal hematopoiesis of indeterminate potential (CHIP), and clonal cytopenia of unknown significance

DIAGNOSTIC TESTS & INTERPRETATION
Initial Tests (lab, imaging)
- A complete blood count with peripheral smear, chemistry, viral studies (HIV and hepatitis panel), and vitamin levels (B_{12} and folate) should be evaluated.
- The International Working Group (IWG) recommended minimal diagnostic prerequisites:
  - Stable cytopenia for ≥6 months or for 2 months with karyotype or bilineage dysplasia
  - Exclusion of other potential reasons for dysplasia/cytopenia
- Diagnosis of MDS includes:
  - Dysplasia (≥10% in ≥1 of the 3 major bone marrow lineages)
  - Blast cell count of 5–19%
  - Chromosomal abnormalities consistent with MDS

Diagnostic Procedures/Other
- *Histopathology*. A bone marrow evaluation is essential to distinguish MDS from AML and to perform karyotype studies, fluorescent in situ hybridization (FISH), and mutational studies.
  - Blast %: <20% is consistent with MDS; ≥20% is diagnostic of AML.
- *Cytogenetics*. Clonal chromosome abnormalities are observed in 30–80% of MDS patients. In the rest of the patients (20–70%), submicroscopic alterations (microdeletions, point mutations) provide diagnostic evidence.
- In cases of uncertainty, analysis of somatic mutations and flow cytometry of bone marrow can evidence clonal disease.

Test Interpretation

- Hematologic findings in the blood smear include macrocytic anemia with possible basophilic stippling, hyposegmented neutrophils (pseudo Pelger-Huet), and thrombocytopenia.
- A low reticulocyte index reflects the hypoproliferative nature of the disease.

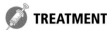 TREATMENT

GENERAL MEASURES

- LR-MDS: observation until patients develop symptoms from anemia, neutropenia, and/or thrombocytopenia given early treatment does not improves long-term survival
  - Initial treatment is tailored based on the specific cytopenia.
- In higher risk, the only curative therapy is allogeneic stem cell transplant (SCT).
- An accurate assessment of prognosis becomes critical for therapeutic decision making. For this aim, multiple scoring system have been developed:
  - The World Health Organization (WHO) guidelines identify six entities: MDS with single lineage dysplasia; MDS with ring sideroblasts; MDS with excess blasts; MDS with multilineage dysplasia; MDS with isolated del(5q); and MDS unclassifiable.
  - The International Prognostic Scoring System (IPSS) score assigns patients to four groups (low, intermediate 1, intermediate 2, high) on the basis of number of cytopenias, karyotype, and blast percentage in the bone marrow.
  - The MDAS (Global MD Anderson) score refines prognostic precision as complementary to the IPSS.

MEDICATION

First Line

- MDS-related anemia
  - Blood transfusions and erythropoiesis-stimulating agents (ESA)
    - ESA have a 30–60% response rate in LR-MDS; indications: hemoglobin <10 g/dL and erythropoietin level <500; uncommon complications: worsening hypertension and thromboembolism
  - Lenalidomide; used in anemia in MDS with isolated del(5q) (5); results in decreased need for transfusions and can lead to a median rise of hemoglobin by 5.4 g/dL
- MDS-related thrombocytopenia and neutropenia
  - In selected cases, thrombopoietin receptor agonists (romiplostim, eltrombopag) may be used for thrombocytopenia (with close monitoring owing its potential for leukemic transformation). Neutropenia may be managed with G-CSF and antibiotics, if clinically indicated.
- Low-intensity chemotherapy
  - In LR-MDS patients who lost response to the first line, the use of hypomethylating agents (HMA) is approved by the U.S. Food and Drug Administration.
    - HMA are disease-modifying agents. Examples are azacitidine and decitabine.
    - HMA cause DNA hypomethylation via DNMT1 sequestration.

- Immune therapy
  - Currently alemtuzumab is not recommended, additional clinical trials needed (5)
- High-intensity chemotherapy
  - Induction chemotherapy in combination with allogenic SCT can result in prolonged remission in 30–50% of patients (6).
- SCT
  - Allogenic SCT remains the only curative treatment option but is reserved for high-risk disease in patients who are stable enough to tolerate treatment due to its toxicity.
    - Patients <70 years of age with an available donor and reasonable comorbidity should be considered.
    - Mortality after the procedure is attributable to transplant-related complication or relapse.

Second Line

Clinical trials can be considered for patients depending on their severity (low vs. high risk), cytopenias, and potential for transplantation.

ISSUES FOR REFERRAL

- Patients with persistent cytopenias with unknown etiology should be evaluated by a hematologist–oncologist.
- Evaluation of bone marrow with a hematopathologist is recommended.
- Referral to a bone marrow transplant team for evaluation for SCT

ADDITIONAL THERAPIES

- *Management of iron overload.* Iron chelation is often considered in patient with transfusion dependency.
- *Promising agents.* Clinical trials for immune therapy including CD52 monoclonal antibody antagonist are ongoing.

SURGERY/OTHER PROCEDURES

Allogenic SCT, as discussed previously

ADMISSION, INPATIENT, AND NURSING CONSIDERATIONS

Complications, such as bleeding, neutropenic fever, and undergoing SCT, warrant a hospital admission.

 ONGOING CARE

FOLLOW-UP RECOMMENDATIONS

Patient Monitoring

- Follow-up of MDS is based on regular complete blood counts to detect the need for transfusions. Severe neutropenia may warrant antibiotic use if infection occurs.
- Bone marrow examination is generally triggered by worsening of cytopenias.

DIET

Alcohol consumption, meat, vegetable, and fruit intake do not appear to have significant influence in the risk of developing disease.

PATIENT EDUCATION

- Regular follow-up and compliance with medications; smoking cessation
- Instruct about symptoms that should prompt the patient to receive blood transfusion or commence antibiotics.

PROGNOSIS

Overall, the outcome of MDS patients is variable, with medial survival ranging from 6 months to >5 years depending on MDS classification.

COMPLICATIONS

- Infection and bleeding are the leading causes of death, rather than AML conversion.
- Increased risk of cardiovascular disease either secondary to iron overload or chronic anemia
- Possibility of hepatic dysfunction from iron overload

REFERENCES

1. Visconte V, Tiu RV, Rogers HJ. Pathogenesis of myelodysplastic syndromes: an overview of molecular and non-molecular aspects of the disease. *Blood Res.* 2014;49(4):216–227.
2. Kerbauy DB, Deeg HJ. Apoptosis and antiapoptotic mechanisms in the progression of myelodysplastic syndrome. *Exp Hematol.* 2007;35(11):1739–1746.
3. Walker AR. Dying a fiery death: pyroptosis in MDS. *Blood.* 2016;128(25):2875–2877.
4. Ayari H, Pasquier F, El Karoui K, et al. Myelodysplastic syndrome in hemodialysis patients. *Kidney Int Rep.* 2019;4(8):1175–1178.
5. Garcia-Manero G, Chien KS, Montalban-Bravo G. Myelodysplastic syndromes: 2021 update on diagnosis, risk stratification and management. *Am J Hematol.* 2020;95(11):1399–1420.
6. Greenberg PL, Stone RM, Al-Kali A, et al. Myelodysplastic syndromes, version 2.2017, NCCN Clinical Practice Guidelines in Oncology. *J Natl Compr Canc Netw.* 2017;15(1):60–87.

CODES

ICD10

- D46.9 Myelodysplastic syndrome, unspecified
- D46.4 Refractory anemia, unspecified
- D46.B Refract cytopenia w multilin dysplasia and ring sideroblasts

CLINICAL PEARLS

- MDS are a heterogeneous group of clonal stem cell disorders characterized by blood cytopenias and tendency for leukemic transformation.
- Different molecular and genetic mechanisms of pathogenesis translate into the same phenotypic manifestation of the disease.
- Infection and bleeding are the leading causes of death.
- Allogeneic SCT is ultimately the only curative treatment.

M

MYELOPROLIFERATIVE NEOPLASMS

Justin T. Ertle, MD • James Evan Davidson, MD

BASICS

DESCRIPTION
- Myeloproliferative neoplasms (MPNs) are a group of clonal disorders that share a common cell of origin in the pluripotent hematopoietic stem cell.
- This topic focuses on chronic myelogenous leukemia (CML), polycythemia vera (PV), essential thrombocythemia (ET), and primary myelofibrosis (PMF).
- The 2016 World Health Organization (WHO) MPN classification also includes chronic neutrophilic leukemia (CNL), chronic eosinophilic leukemia not otherwise specified (CEL-NOS), and MPN unclassifiable, all significantly more rare (1); mastocytosis reclassified out of MPN (1)
- CML is characterized by uninhibited proliferation of myeloid precursor cells.
- PV is characterized by erythrocytosis, ET is characterized by thrombocytosis, and PMF is characterized by bone marrow fibrosis and extramedullary hematopoiesis.
- The natural history can last decades, but each MPN carries the risk of complications, such as thrombotic events, as well as transformation into acute leukemia or bone marrow fibrosis.

EPIDEMIOLOGY
Increasing age. MPNs median age of diagnosis is >60 years.

Incidence
- CML: 1.6/100,000/year
- PV: 0.84/100,000/year
- ET: 1.03/100,000/year
- PMF: 0.47/100,000/year

ETIOLOGY AND PATHOPHYSIOLOGY
MPNs result from genetic mutations activating hematopoiesis, resulting in proliferation of cells of myeloid, erythroid, and/or megakaryocyte lineages.

Genetics
- CML is characterized by a 9:22 translocation (the Philadelphia chromosome) resulting in the oncogenic BCR-ABL1 fusion gene. The BCR-ABL1 fusion protein is a constitutively active tyrosine kinase leading to cell proliferation, particularly of granulocytes.
- PV, ET, and PMF share "driver" mutations, most often of JAK2, MPL, and CALR genes, that activate hematopoiesis. Mutation in one of these three genes is found in >90% of BCR-ABL negative MPNs.
- Janus kinase 2 (JAK2) mutations: JAK2 specifically regulates hematopoiesis via erythropoietin (EPO), GM-CSF, thrombopoietin, growth hormone, leptin, IL-3 and IL-5 signaling. JAK2 mutations constitutively activating the JAK2 protein lead to cell proliferation and prolonged survival.
  - JAK2 V617F mutations: 95% of PV, 55% of ET, and 65% of PMF cases
  - JAK2 exon 12 mutations: 4% of PV cases
- Myeloproliferative leukemia protein (MPL) gene mutations: The MPL gene encodes the thrombopoietin receptor, which regulates hematopoietic stem cells, especially megakaryocytes; thrombopoietin receptor mutations can cause cell overproduction.
  - MPL mutations: 3% of ET and 5% of PMF cases
- Calreticulin (CALR) gene mutations: specific frameshift mutations in the CALR gene, which encodes calreticulin protein, lead to activated hematopoiesis, particularly of the megakaryocyte lineage. The mechanism may be via constitutive activation of the

thrombopoietin receptor; this is an active area of research.
  - CALR mutations: 25% of ET and PMF cases
- As more driver mutations have been identified, they have been classified into mutations that appear "restricted," in that they only result in MPNs, and mutations that are "unrestricted," in that they can also be implicated in other myeloid neoplasms. JAK2, MPL, and CALR are considered "restricted" mutations.

RISK FACTORS
- Any factor that increases risk of somatic mutations, such as ionizing radiation
- The large majority of MPNs are due to somatic mutations, familial cases have been described.
- PV, ET, and PMF share mutations and can transform into one another.

COMMONLY ASSOCIATED CONDITIONS
- Thrombotic events (CVA, DVT, etc.)
- Major and minor hemorrhagic events (acquired von Willebrand disease)
- Anemia, bone marrow fibrosis, osteosclerosis
- Blast transformation into acute leukemia
- Extramedullary hematopoiesis

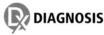

DIAGNOSIS

PHYSICAL EXAM
- Constitutional symptoms are common, although a minority are asymptomatic.
- All MPNs may share the following symptoms:
  - Constitutional: fatigue, weakness, night sweats, fevers, weight loss
  - Gastrointestinal: abdominal fullness, discomfort, or pain; early satiety
  - Musculoskeletal: bone pain
  - Neurologic: headaches, dizziness, trouble concentrating, transient visual disturbances
  - Psychiatric: depression, sexual dysfunction, insomnia
- More common with certain MPNs:
  - CML: excess sweating, gout
  - PV: aquagenic pruritus, erythromelalgia, facial plethora, gout, tinnitus
  - PMF: abdominal fullness or pain, early satiety, gastrointestinal bleeding, weight loss, arthralgias, bone pain
  - ET: light-headedness/syncope, transient visual disturbance, atypical chest pain, erythromelalgia, livedo reticularis, pregnancy loss
- All MPNs may have the following physical findings:
  - Pallor, splenomegaly, hepatomegaly
- More common with certain MPNs:
  - CML: gouty tophi
  - PMV: gouty tophi, increased blood pressure, conjunctival injection, facial plethora
  - ET: petechiae, livedo reticularis
  - PMF: petechiae, lymphadenopathy, marked splenomegaly (Splenomegaly tends to be especially prominent in PMF.)

DIAGNOSTIC TESTS & INTERPRETATION

Initial Tests (lab, imaging)
- Complete blood count (CBC) with differential
- Peripheral smear
- Metabolic panel (renal function, liver function, electrolytes)
- Lactate dehydrogenase (LDH)
- Uric acid

Follow-Up Tests & Special Considerations
- Testing for BCR-ABL (1)[A]
- Karyotype to detect the 9;22 translocation/ Philadelphia chromosome
- Detecting the BCR-ABL gene
  - Fluorescence in situ hybridization (FISH)
  - Reverse transcription polymerase chain reaction (RT-PCR)
- Testing for JAK2, MPL, CALR gene mutations (1)[A]
- Bone marrow biopsy (BMBx) and aspiration (1)
- Depending on the clinical scenario, consider:
  - EPO level, for detecting secondary causes of polycythemia
  - Iron studies (ferritin, transferrin, iron level)
  - von Willebrand factor, for detecting acquired von Willebrand disease, and assessing for increased bleeding risk

Diagnostic Procedures/Other
BMBx and aspiration is often used in establishing an MPN diagnosis.

Test Interpretation
- The WHO classification of myeloid neoplasms and acute leukemia, revised in 2016, establishing criteria for diagnosis of each MPN (1)
  - MPNs share many features, may present with multiple cell lineages increased, and can transform into one another, but treatment and prognosis for each varies significantly.
- CML
  - Leukocytosis, granulocytosis (neutrophil predominant), with mature and immature forms
    ○ Myelocytes > metamyelocytes is common finding.
  - The Philadelphia chromosome/BCR-ABL fusion gene establishes the diagnosis.
  - Chronic CML can progress to an accelerated phase or a blast crisis phase.
    ○ CML blast phase—WHO criteria (1)[A]
      ▪ 20% or more blasts in PB or BM, or
      ▪ Infiltrative proliferation of blasts at an extramedullary site
- PV—WHO criteria (1)[A]
  - Diagnosis requires either all three major criteria, or the first two major criteria and the minor criterion
  - Major criteria
    ○ Hemoglobin >16.5 g/dL in men / >16.0 g/dL in women OR
    ○ Hematocrit >49%/48% OR
    ○ Increased red cell mass (RCM)
    ○ BMBx showing hypercellularity for age with trilineage growth prominent erythroid, granulocytic, and megakaryocytic proliferation with pleomorphic, mature megakaryocytes
    ○ Presence of JAK2V617F or JAK2 SH2
  - Minor criterion:
    ○ Subnormal serum EPO level
- ET—WHO criteria (1)[A]
  - Diagnosis requires either all four major criteria or the first 3 major criteria and the minor criterion
  - Major criteria
    ○ Platelet count ≥450 × 10⁹/L
    ○ BMBx showing proliferation mainly of the megakaryocyte lineage with increased numbers of enlarged, mature megakaryocytes with hyperlobulated nuclei; no significant increase or left shift in neutrophil granulopoiesis or erythropoiesis and very rarely minor (grade 1) increase in reticulin fibers

○ Not meeting WHO criteria for BCR-ABL1+ CML, PV, PMF, myelodysplastic syndromes, or other myeloid neoplasms

○ Presence of JAK2, CALR, or MPL mutation

– Minor criterion:

○ Presence of a clonal marker or absence of evidence for reactive thrombocytosis

- PMF
  – PMF has been subdivided into prefibrotic/early stage and overt fibrotic stage. Criteria for overt fibrotic stage is presented here.
  – Overt PMF—WHO criteria (1)[A]
    ○ Diagnosis requires all three major criteria, and at least one minor criterion.
    ○ Major criteria
      ▪ Presence of megakaryocytic proliferation and atypia, accompanied by either reticulin and/or collagen fibrosis grades 2 and 3
      ▪ Not meeting WHO criteria for ET, PV, BCR-ABL1+ CML, MPNs, or other myeloid neoplasms
      ▪ Presence of JAK2, CALR, or MPL mutation or in the absence of these mutations, presence of another clonal marker, or absence of reactive myelofibrosis
    ○ Minor criteria
      ▪ Presence of at least one of the following, confirmed in two consecutive determinations:
        □ Anemia not attributed to a comorbid condition
        □ Leukocytosis ≥11 × 10⁹/L
        □ Palpable splenomegaly
        □ LDH above upper limit of normal
        □ Leukoerythroblastosis

TREATMENT

Management strategies include observation, phlebotomy/transfusion, medications, and stem cell transplantation.

GENERAL MEASURES

- PV:
  – Phlebotomy is first line for PV, with goal hematocrit <45% in men and <42% in women.
    ○ Achieving goal hematocrit decreases mortality from cardiovascular or thrombotic events 4-fold.
- PMF:
  – Transfusions for symptomatic anemia and thrombocytopenia
- As MPN confers increased risk of thromboembolic events, manage overall cardiovascular risk (address hypertension, hyperlipidemia, diabetes, smoking, etc.).

MEDICATION

- CML:
  – First-line medications:
    ○ Tyrosine kinase inhibitors (TKIs) are first line for chronic phase, accelerated phase, and in the blast phase while evaluating for stem cell transplant.
    ○ The first-generation TKI (1GTKI) is imatinib; second-generation TKIs (2GTKI) include nilotinib, dasatinib, bosutinib; third-generation TKI (3GTKI) is ponatinib.
    ○ In low-risk chronic phase, 1GTKI or 2GTKI is recommended.
    ○ In high-risk chronic phase, 2GTKI is preferred.
    ○ In accelerated phase, 2GTKI or 3GTKI is preferred while evaluating for stem cell transplant.
    ○ In blast phase, TKIs may be used while waiting for induction chemotherapy/stem cell transplant.
  – Second-line medications
    ○ Adding pegylated interferon-α to TKI therapy is an active area of research.

- PV:
  – First-line medications:
    ○ All patients: aspirin (81 to 100 mg); aids in prevention of thrombotic complications and treatment of microvascular episodes such as ocular migraine, transient ischemic attacks, and erythromelalgia
    ○ High-risk PV patients (older age or history of thrombosis): cytoreduction with hydroxyurea of pegylated interferon-α
  – Second-line medications:
    ○ For low-risk patients who do not tolerate phlebotomy for cytoreduction, consider hydroxyurea.
    ○ For high-risk patients with inadequate response to cytoreductive medication, consider JAK2 inhibitor ruxolitinib.

- ET:
  – First-line medications:
    ○ Aspirin (81 to 100 mg) is indicated in patients with prior history of thrombosis, JAK2 mutation, microvascular complications, or vasomotor symptoms.
    ○ Cytoreduction in hydroxyurea is indicated for high-risk ET patients (thrombosis, or age >60 years + JAK2 mutation), or patients with progressive thrombocytosis, acquired von Willebrand syndrome, significant bleeding, or splenomegaly
  – Second-line medications
    ○ When cytoreduction is indicated and an alternative to hydroxyurea is warranted, consider pegylated interferon-α or anagrelide.
    ○ For symptoms not controlled with aspirin alone, cytoreduction with hydroxyurea can be considered.

- PMF:
  – First-line medications:
    ○ If transplant is not planned, and platelets ≥50 × 10⁹/L, consider the JAK2 inhibitor ruxolitinib.
  – Second-line medication therapy:
    ○ Low-risk patients with bothersome symptoms may consider ruxolitinib, hydroxyurea, or pegylated interferon-α.
    ○ Patients with disease progression on ruxolitinib may be considered for a newer JAK2 inhibitor.
    ○ Patients with anemia who are not adequately responsive to nutrient repletion and/or transfusion
    ○ EPO <500 mUmL
    ○ Erythropoiesis-stimulating agents
    ○ EPO >500 mUmL
    ○ Consider danazol, prednisone, lenalidomide, thalidomide.

ISSUES FOR REFERRAL

Patients with MPNs, or suspected MPNs, are referred to hematology/oncology for expert consultation.

SURGERY/OTHER PROCEDURES

- Allogeneic stem cell transplant may be considered in CML accelerated phase and blast crisis, as well as in high-risk PMF.
- Splenectomy may be considered in severe cases, most often in PMF.

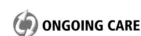

ONGOING CARE

PATIENT EDUCATION

- Avoid situations increasing their risk of thrombosis, such as prolonged immobility.
- With splenomegaly, patients may be advised to avoid high-contact sports and other activities increasing risk of rupture.

PROGNOSIS

- The natural history of MPNs can last decades.
- Prognosis of CML is strongly tied to phase of disease (chronic, accelerated, blast).
  – Patients in blast phase have a median overall survival of 1 year.
- CML prognosis is also closely correlated with response to TKI therapy.
  – After 3 months of therapy:
    ○ Patients with BCR-ABL suppressed to <10% had overall survival of 97%.
    ○ Patients with >10% BCR-ABL expression confers an overall survival of 87%.
- Although PV, ET, and PMF share driver mutations, prognosis among them varies considerably:
  – PV—median survival 14 years (24 years if age <60 years)
  – ET—median survival 20 years (33 years if age <60 years)
  – PMF—median survival 6 years (15 years if age <60 years)
    ○ Driver mutation affects prognosis as well; CALR generally confers a better prognosis, whereas JAK2 or "triple-negative" (no identified JAK2, MPL, or CALR mutation) status confers worse prognoses.
  – Transformation into acute leukemia confers a poor prognosis, which occurs most often in PMF and least often in ET.
  – Transformation into overt PMF with fibrotic marrow also confers a poor prognosis and may occur more often in PV than ET.

REFERENCE

1. Arber DA, Orazi A, Hasserjian R, et al. The 2016 revision to the World Health Organization classification of myeloid neoplasms and acute leukemia. *Blood.* 2016;127(20):2391–2405.

ADDITIONAL READING

Spivak JL. Myeloproliferative neoplasms. *N Engl J Med.* 2017;376(22):2168–2181.

 SEE ALSO

Leukemia, Chronic Myelogenous; Polycythemia Vera

 CODES

ICD10

- D47.1 Chronic myeloproliferative disease
- C92.10 Chronic myeloid leukemia, BCR/ABL-positive, not having achieved remission
- D45 Polycythemia vera

CLINICAL PEARLS

- MPNs result from mutations that activate hematopoiesis, resulting in proliferation of cells of myeloid, erythroid, and/or megakaryocyte lineages.
- CML is characterized by granulocytosis, PV is characterized by erythrocytosis, ET is characterized by thrombocytosis, and PMF is characterized by bone marrow fibrosis and extramedullary hematopoiesis, often also with thrombocytosis.
- As MPNs share common mutational origins, multiple cell lines may be increased, they often share common symptoms (such as constitutional symptoms) and clinical features, and they can transform into one another.

M

NARCOLEPSY

Waiz Wasey, MD • Maria Rossi, MD, MS • Naila Manahil, MD

 BASICS

DESCRIPTION
- Narcolepsy is a neurologic sleep disorder characterized by excessive daytime sleepiness (EDS) and may be associated with cataplexy (sudden loss of muscle control), hypnagogic hallucinations (vivid perceptual experiences while falling asleep), hypnopompic (vivid perceptual experiences while waking up from sleep), or sleep paralysis (temporary inability to move or speak that happens during transition from sleeping to awake state).
- Mainly two types identified by American Academy of Sleep Medicine:
  - Type 1 (60–70%) (formerly narcolepsy with cataplexy) and type 2 (formerly narcolepsy without cataplexy) (1)
- No cure, symptomatic management

EPIDEMIOLOGY
Incidence
- Affects 0.03 to 0.16% general population with incidence 1/2,000 worldwide (2)
- Bimodal distribution; age of onset peak at 15 years and again at 35 years of age.
- Predominant sex: male > female (1.6:1)
- 5% familial cases (1)
- African Americans are more likely to present without cataplexy and at a younger age.

Prevalence
- Narcolepsy type 1: 25 to 50/100,000 people
- Narcolepsy type 2: 20 to 34/100,000 people (1)

ETIOLOGY AND PATHOPHYSIOLOGY
- Primarily caused by degeneration of hypothalamic neurons that produce orexin (hypocretin). Postmortem studies show 85% loss of these neurons in type 1 and about 33% loss in type 2 (1).
- Orexin is crucial to promote wakefulness, it stimulates the RAS (reticular activating system) and inhibits rapid eye movement.
- Neurodegeneration may be caused by autoimmune process, probably stimulated by infections (such as influenza A or group A *Streptococcus*) or environmental factors (occurs commonly in late spring).
- Alterations in the L-PGDS (lipocalin-type prostaglandin D synthase) level also seem to be involved in causing EDS in narcolepsy (1).
- *International Classification of Sleep Disorders*, 3rd edition (ICSD-3) classification:
  - Narcolepsy
  - Narcolepsy type 1
  - Narcolepsy type 2
  - Narcolepsy due to medical conditions

Genetics
- Usually sporadic but increased incidence in families with positive history: 1–2% in first-degree relative of the index case (10 to 40 times the general population)
- 98% of patients with narcolepsy type 1 have human leukocyte antigen (HLA) DQB1*0602; 40–50% of patients with narcolepsy type 2 express this antigen. HLA DQB1*0602 is present in 12–30% of the general population.
- Autosomal recessive inheritance pattern
- Affects 12% of Asians and 25% of whites, and 38% of African Americans are gene carriers.

RISK FACTORS
- Age (peaks at 15 and 35 years), usually underdiagnosed before age of 18
- Obesity
- Head trauma
- Central nervous system infectious disease
- Anesthesia
- Psychological stress
- Positive family history
- Recent influenza A, streptococcal infection, or H1N1 vaccine (no evidence of COVID leading to narcolepsy yet) (3)

COMMONLY ASSOCIATED CONDITIONS
Obstructive sleep apnea (OSA) (up to 25%), obesity, anxiety

 DIAGNOSIS

HISTORY
- Classic pentad of EDS, cataplexy, sleep paralysis, and hypnagogic/hypnopompic hallucinations, and disrupted nocturnal sleep (five most common symptoms): Only 10–20% have all five.
- EDS and sleep attacks (cardinal symptom):
  - EDS is present in 100% of patients, usually the first initial symptom.
  - ICSD-3 classification for both type 1 and 2 requires EDS occurring almost daily for at least 3 months (1).
  - Patients may report refreshing daytime naps, with a possible return of EDS in 1 to 2 hours.
  - Sudden sleep attacks (seconds) during stimulating situations such as driving and walking
- Cataplexy (65–75% patients):
  - Mainly associated with type 1 narcolepsy (1)
  - Sudden transient (seconds to minutes) episodes of total or partial loss of motor tone (buckling of knees, head dropping, sagging of jaw or weakness in arms, slurred speech, facial droop or grimace, etc.), triggered by strong emotions (such as laughing, anger, or fright)
  - Consciousness and memory are not impaired.
- Sleep paralysis
  - Transient (several minutes) inability to move, speak, or open the eyes either while falling asleep or upon awakening
  - During the event, breathing may be difficult because intercostal muscles are paralyzed and chest feels heavier.
  - Patients are aware of their surroundings and are able to recall the event.
  - Seen in 67% of patients who have narcolepsy with cataplexy and 49% narcolepsy without cataplexy
- Hypnagogic or hypnopompic hallucinations:
  - Vivid dreamlike experience in 30–60% patients with type 1 narcolepsy occurs during awakening (hypnopompic hallucinations) or at sleep onset (hypnagogic). Hypnopompic hallucinations are more indicative of narcolepsy than hypnagogic.
  - Hallucination commonly visual, tactile, or auditory.
  - Characteristic hallucinations include being attacked by animals or feeling that someone else is in the room.
  - 15% of type 2 patients experience these as well.
- Other reported history
  - Nocturnal insomnia and sleep fragmentation (difficulty maintaining sleep rather than initiating sleep)
  - Retrograde amnesia
  - Increased periodic limb movements
  - Depression, anxiety, social phobia
  - Dream enactment behaviors
  - Weight gain seen with progression

PHYSICAL EXAM
- Unremarkable, but complete exam may help rule out other causes
- Deep tendon reflexes are either diminished or absent during an episode of cataplexy.

DIFFERENTIAL DIAGNOSIS
EDS is present in 4–28% of the general population, although most individuals are not narcoleptic:
- Sleep apnea syndromes
- Epileptic seizures and syncope
- Idiopathic hypersomnia (5–10% with EDS)
- Psychiatric (depression, bipolar 2 and substance abuse/withdrawal)
- Sleep-related movement disorders (restless leg syndrome, periodic limb movements of sleep)
- Iatrogenic/secondary to medication (benzodiazepines; barbiturates; opioids; antihistamines; β-blockers; and some antipsychotics, antidepressants, and anticonvulsants)
- Poor sleep hygiene and habits leading to sleep deficit and chronic sleep deprivation (1)
- Circadian rhythm disorders (jet lag, shift work, delayed or advanced sleep phase disorders)
- Cataplexy disorders (Niemann-Pick type C, Prader-Willi syndrome, Norrie disease) (1)
- Hypersomnia in Parkinson disease
- Menstrual-associated hypersomnia
- Stroke (slurred speech and facial sagging seen in partial cataplexy)

Pediatric Considerations
Narcolepsy is rare before the age of 5 years. EDS is more often attributable to OSA, poor sleep hygiene, and the increased sleep requirements early in life. The recommended amount of sleep decreases with age: newborns 16 to 18 hr/day; preschool-aged children 11 to 12 hr/day; school-aged children and teens 10 hr/day; adults 7 to 8 hr/day. Children can gain excessive weight, from 20 to 40 lb (2). Symptoms of EDS, sleep paralysis, and cataplexy might last longer than compared to adult population.

DIAGNOSTIC TESTS & INTERPRETATION
- Sleep log/actigraphy: First, ensure patient is getting 6 hours of sleep at night for at least 7 to 14 days.
- Prerequisites for valid multiple sleep latency test (MSLT) → normal polysomnography (PSG) with at least 360 minutes of sleep, free of drugs that may alter sleep for at least 2 weeks, standardized sleep schedule for 7 days
- Primary diagnostic tool
  - An overnight PSG to rule out other causes of EDS
  - MSLT: performed the day after PSG if at least 6 hours of sleep and no sleep disorder explained by PSG
    - Four to five 20-minute naps at 2-hour intervals
    - Positive if rapid onset of REM (<15 minutes) in at least 2 of 5 sleeps (including baseline PSG) and shortened mean sleep latency (<8 minutes)
    - If MSLT negative, but strong clinical suspicion, repeat the test.
    - Antidepressants and stimulants should be discontinued for at least 2 weeks prior.
- Scoring tools
  - Epworth Sleepiness Scale (ESS): scored 0 to 24: >10 is suggestive of a sleep disorder rather than generalized fatigue; helpful for detecting response to medications
  - Fatigue Severity Scale: 9-item scale, measuring the severity of fatigue (helps differentiate between fatigue and sleep disorder)

- Stanford Sleepiness Scale: Patients select 1 of 7 statements that best describe energy level, concentration, and sleepiness. Statements 4 to 7 may indicate excessive sleepiness.
- Narcolepsy Severity Scale: a 15-item scale to assess the frequency, severity, and consequences of symptoms of narcolepsy type 1
- Pediatric scoring tool: Epworth Sleepiness Scale for Children and Adolescents (a modified version of ESS) and Pediatric Daytime Sleepiness Scale

Follow-Up Tests & Special Considerations
- Lumbar puncture for orexin level; 110 pg/mL or less in the cerebrospinal fluid (CSF) is indicative of narcolepsy; rarely performed
- HLA typing: particularly in children. It is supportive of diagnosis, lacks specificity

Diagnostic Procedures/Other
- Narcolepsy type 1
  - EDS daily for ≥3 months
  - One of the following:
    ○ Cataplexy with positive MSLT
    ○ Low CSF orexin level <110 pg/mL or <1/3 of mean values in normal subjects
- Narcolepsy type 2
  - All of the above (with or without cataplexy) and normal CSF orexin level
- It is a diagnosis of exclusion.

 TREATMENT

GENERAL MEASURES
- Medications do not cure, but the goal is to minimize EDS and cataplectic episodes.
- Drug therapy, if used, should be supplemented by various behavioral strategies.
- Proper sleep hygiene and a regular sleep schedule.
- Well-timed 20-minute naps may be helpful.
- Avoid stimulants (alcohol, heavy meals, caffeine, nicotine).
- Maneuvers such as altering thoughts, placing tension on muscles, or pressing against a firm support might rapidly terminate cataplectic episodes.
- Maintaining warmer body temperature and consuming warm meals/drinks may improve wakefulness.
- Use safety precautions, particularly when driving. Untreated patients are at 10-fold at risk of accidents.

MEDICATION
First Line
- EDS
  - Modafinil (Provigil):
    ○ For mild to moderate EDS
    ○ Works on dopaminergic, adrenergic, and histaminergic receptors of hypothalamus
    ○ Dose: 200 mg/day. Start with 100 mg; max dose 400 mg/day
    ○ Half-life of 15 hours
    ○ Adverse effects: headache, GI upset, increased metabolism of oral contraceptives with less rebound hypersomnia and does not affect blood pressure (BP); tolerance limited
    ○ Caution with cardiac diseases, may cause tachycardia and with oral contraceptive use as it decreases the efficacy
    ○ Not FDA-approved for children
  - Armodafinil (Nuvigil):
    ○ Enantiomeric form of modafinil with the same half-life, but lower adverse effect profile
    ○ Dose: 150 to 250 mg every morning

- Less adverse effects in comparison to modafinil: headache, xerostomia, Stevens-Johnson syndrome, and toxic epidermal necrolysis
  ○ Not FDA-approved for children
- Pitolisant (Wakix): FDA-approved for narcolepsy and cataplexy approved. Doses up to 35.6 mg demonstrated effectiveness (4).
- Clarithromycin: acts on GABA-A receptor, can be used for hypersomnia if alternative primary medication fails. Dose 500 mg BID (start with a 2-week trial period). Adverse effect: GI distress
- Levothyroxine (25mcg/day): in euthyroid patients without cataplexy, improved EDS in 12 weeks
- Cataplexy:
  - Sodium oxybate (Xyrem):
    ○ Only medication FDA-approved for both EDS and cataplexy. Now approved for ages 7 years and up.
    ○ For moderate to severe cases
    ○ Best option for improving nighttime sleep
    ○ Dose: 6 to 9 g/day divided BID; start with 2.25 g and increase by 1.5 g/day qwk; max dose: 9 g/day
    ○ May take 8 to 12 weeks for a full response
    ○ Is a date rape drug; abuse potential
    ○ May worsen sleep-disordered breathing in patients with OSA
    ○ Overdose may lead to coma.
  - Solriamfetol (Sunosi):
    ○ Start with 75 mg qD, increased based on response every 3 days to the max dose of 150 mg/day
    ○ Contraindicated with concomitant or recent MAO-I use
    ○ Abuse potential: Use caution in patients with a history of drug use.
  - Tricyclic antidepressants
    ○ Protriptyline: dose: 5 to 60 mg/day. Taper dose.
    ○ Clomipramine: dose: 25 to 75 mg/day
    ○ Anticholinergic side effect profile: dry mouth, sedation, urinary retention, impotence
  - Serotonin-norepinephrine reuptake inhibitors
    ○ Venlafaxine: dose: 75 to 300 mg/day. Start at 37.5 mg, max dose 375 mg/day. Taper dose to discontinue.
    ○ Fluoxetine: dose: 20 to 80 mg/day
    ○ Work by suppressing REM sleep
    ○ Not FDA-approved
  - The patient may develop a tolerance to the anticataplectic drugs and can have rebound cataplexy when a drug is withdrawn. Taper to discontinue.
- Auxiliary symptoms (e.g., hypnagogic hallucination, sleep paralysis) require treatment less often than EDS and cataplexy, but anticataplectics are useful when symptoms are problematic.

Second Line
- EDS
  - Amphetamines: used if first line fail or patient unable to tolerate
    ○ Methylphenidate (Ritalin): dose: initial dose 5 to 10 mg/day divided BID or TID; max dose 60 mg/day, short acting, most potent amphetamine available; can be used in combination with modafinil and armodafinil
    ○ Dextroamphetamine: dose: initial dose 10 mg/day; can increase by 10 mg qwk to a max dose 60 mg/day divided BID or TID
    ○ Contraindicated in patients with hypertension (HTN)
    ○ Adverse reactions: headaches, irritability, HTN, psychosis, anorexia, habituation, rebound hypersomnia
    ○ If the patient develops a tolerance to stimulants, switch drug or drug holidays rather than increasing dose.
    ○ Addictive; high doses associated with frequent hospitalizations, arrhythmias, and psychiatric disturbances

- Cataplexy
  - Selegiline: selective MAO-B inhibitor
    ○ Anticataplectic effective for EDS; 20 to 40 mg/day divided morning and noon
    ○ Doses >20 mg require a low-tyramine diet because the drug begins to lose selectivity.
- Frequent nocturnal awakenings
  - Temazepam: benzodiazepam
    ○ Dose 15–30 mg at bedtime once helps with preventing frequent nocturnal awakenings and improving daytime sleepiness.

ISSUES FOR REFERRAL
Unresponsive to primary medication and severe cataplexy may benefit from neurology referral.

 ONGOING CARE

FOLLOW-UP RECOMMENDATIONS
Patient Monitoring
- Monitoring using scoring tools to gauge treatment effectiveness and symptom control
- Frequent BP checks and regular follow-ups recommended for those on medication.

DIET
Those taking high doses of Selegiline (>20 mg) require a low-tyramine diet.

PATIENT EDUCATION
- http://www.ninds.nih.gov/Disorders/Patient-Caregiver-Education/Fact-Sheets/Narcolepsy-Fact-Sheet
- http://narcolepsynetwork.org

PROGNOSIS
Narcolepsy is a lifelong disease. Improvements seen in 60–80% of patients. Symptoms can worsen with aging. In women, symptoms can improve after menopause.

COMPLICATIONS
Patients with cataplexy are more prone to binge eating.

REFERENCES
1. Zhang J, Han F. Sleepiness in narcolepsy. *Sleep Med Clin*. 2017;12(3):323–330.
2. Calik MW. Update on the treatment of narcolepsy: clinical efficacy of pitolisant. *Nat Sci Sleep*. 2017;9:127–133.
3. Mignot E, Black S. Narcolepsy risk and COVID-19. *J Clin Sleep Med*. 2020;16(10):1831–1833.
4. Meskill G, Davis C, Zarycranski D, et al. Assessment of the clinical benefits of pitolisant on excessive daytime sleepiness and cataplexy in adults with narcolepsy. *Sleep*. 2021;44(2):A189–A199.

 CODES

ICD10
- G47.429 Narcolepsy in conditions classified elsewhere w/o cataplexy
- G47.411 Narcolepsy with cataplexy
- G47.419 Narcolepsy without cataplexy

CLINICAL PEARLS
- Narcolepsy is an incurable, REM disorder.
- The classic tetrad includes EDS, cataplexy, sleep paralysis, and hypnagogic hallucinations; only cataplexy is pathognomonic for the disorder.

N

NASAL POLYPS
Tharani Ravi, MD • Carolina Sanchez, MD

 BASICS

- Chronic benign inflammatory lesion of nasal mucosa
- Arise from near the ethmoid sinus but can infrequently arise from maxillary sinus mucosa

DESCRIPTION
- Appearance of edematous pedunculated mass in the nasal cavity or within the paranasal sinus
- Often causes symptoms of blockage, discharge, or loss of smell
- Most commonly bilateral; if unilateral, malignancy should be on differential.

EPIDEMIOLOGY
Incidence
- Typical age at diagnosis ranges from 40 to 60 years.
- Increases with age to a peak in the sixth decade

Prevalence
- ~4% in general population
- Much rarer in children: ~0.1% and associated with cystic fibrosis
- Asthma is present in up to 65% of patients.

ETIOLOGY AND PATHOPHYSIOLOGY
- Separate T helper 1- and T helper 2-driven pathways
- White patients who have chronic rhinosinusitis with nasal polyps: Majority have type 2 pattern of inflammation.
  - Characterized by eosinophilia and elevated levels of interleukin-4, interleukin-5, and interleukin-13 cytokines

Genetics
Patients with nasal polyps are more likely than controls to report having a first-degree relative with nasal polyps (1)[B].

RISK FACTORS
An increased prevalence of nasal polyps has been described among textile workers who have been exposed to occupational dust, particularly among those with longer-duration exposure (1)[B].

GENERAL PREVENTION
Use of intranasal corticosteroids after polyp removal surgery has shown effectiveness against recurrence.

COMMONLY ASSOCIATED CONDITIONS
- Asthma
- Bronchiectasis
- Aspirin hypersensitivity
- Allergic rhinitis
- Chronic sinusitis
- Allergic fungal sinusitis
- Cystic fibrosis (pediatric patients)
- Primary ciliary dyskinesia (Kartagener syndrome)
- Laryngopharyngeal reflux
- Sleep apnea

 DIAGNOSIS

Made on the basis of the presence of sinonasal symptoms for more than 3 months and the visualization of polyps in the nasal cavity

HISTORY
Symptoms
- Rhinorrhea
- Nasal congestion
- Postnasal drainage
- Hyposmia/anosmia
- Inability to breathe through nose
- Dull headaches
- Facial pain/pressure over the middle third of the face
- Sleep disturbance
- In some cases, there may be no symptoms.

PHYSICAL EXAM
Besides rhinorrhea, sinus tenderness to palpation and/or visualization of polyp, there are no definitive physical exam findings.

DIFFERENTIAL DIAGNOSIS
- Chronic rhinosinusitis without nasal polyps, rhinitis, structural abnormalities of the nose, and neurologic causes of hyposmia
- Other benign or malignant tumors. e.g. fibroma, hemangioma, osteoma, chondroma, encephalocele
- Squamous cell carcinoma
- Malignant melanoma

DIAGNOSTIC TESTS & INTERPRETATION
Initial Tests (lab, imaging)
- Anterior rhinoscopy shows pale, translucent mass
  - Most commonly on lateral wall of middle meatus

Follow-Up Tests & Special Considerations
- If large posterior nasal polyps, examine tympanic membrane for Eustachian tube dysfunction.
- If unilateral polyp, consider histologic exam to exclude malignancy.
- Test for cystic fibrosis in children with polyps.
- Sinus CT scan (2)[C]:
  - May be helpful to corroborate history and endoscopic findings
  - Unable to differentiate polyp from other soft tissue masses
  - Reveals extent of disease and is necessary to formulate a plan for surgical intervention if indicated
- MRI (2)[C]:
  - May aid in diagnosis if concern for neoplasia, mycetoma, or encephalocele

Diagnostic Procedures/Other
Flexible/rigid endoscopy is required to assess the nasal cavity fully.
- Gold standard for diagnosis

 TREATMENT

GENERAL MEASURES
Goal is to reduce the size or eliminate nasal polyps because they can obstruct the nasal cavity and impair sense of smell, restrict breathing ability through nose, and obstruct drainage of sinuses.

MEDICATION
First Line
Daily intranasal corticosteroid use with saline irrigation is first-line therapy (3)[A].
- In patients who do not have significant nasal blockage by polyps, intranasal saline and intranasal glucocorticoids can be administered for 1 to 3 months.
- Intranasal corticosteroids shown to decrease nasal polyp size, lessen sinonasal symptoms, and improve quality of life
  - Budesonide 256 μg/day (one 64 μg spray in each nostril twice daily)
  - Beclomethasone dipropionate 168 to 320 μg/day (1 to 2 sprays per nostril twice daily)
  - Fluticasone propionate 400 to 744 μg/day (1 to 2 sprays per nostril twice daily)
  - Mometasone furoate 400 μg/day (2 sprays per nostril twice daily)
  - For children, mometasone furoate is preferred.

Second Line
In patients with severe symptoms or those who cannot tolerate intranasal steroids, consider short course of oral corticosteroids (14 to 21 days) and/or doxycycline (21 days).
- Prednisone 30 to 50 mg daily (taper when indicated)
- Prednisolone 20 to 60 mg daily (taper when indicated) (4)
- Doxycycline 200 mg once, followed by 100 mg daily

ISSUES FOR REFERRAL
- If unilateral polyp for biopsy evaluation
- Consider referral to otorhinolaryngologist for endoscopic sinus surgery if severe obstruction symptoms or conservative management ineffective.

ADDITIONAL THERAPIES
Patients with persistent symptoms and have concurrent allergic rhinitis, consider:
- Systemic antihistamine
- Leukotriene pathway antagonist
- Allergy immunotherapy
- Biologics:
  - Based on two multicentered randomized double-blinded studies, adding dupilumab to daily mometasone furoate nasal spray reduced polyp size, sinus opacification and symptom severity; it was well-tolerated and decreased systemic corticosteroid treatment and surgery (5).

- Dupilumab works by blocking interleukin-4 and interleukin-13.
- Dupilumab also improved lung function and symptoms in patients with comorbid asthma (5)[B].
- Other biologics that have efficacy and/or relief of symptoms: omalizumab, mepolizumab

SURGERY/OTHER PROCEDURES
- Most surgeries are approached endonasally.
  - The external (Caldwell-Luc) approach is used for more difficult cases but carries higher risk of complications.
- Functional endonasal sinus surgery has slightly lower revision rate than intranasal polypectomy. Both modalities provide effective symptom relief.
- Postoperative use of nasal corticosteroids delay the recurrence of nasal polyps and hence the timing of revision surgery.
- Postoperative use of steroid-releasing stents to prevent polyp recurrence by decreasing mucosal inflammation (6)

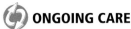 ONGOING CARE

- Recurrence up to ~40% (1)
- Use of intranasal corticosteroids after polyp removal surgery has shown effectiveness against recurrence.
- Recurrence twice as likely in those with asthma

PROGNOSIS
Persons who undergo surgery have great improvements in symptoms, but recurrence rate is high (7),(8)[B].

COMPLICATIONS
- Acute/chronic sinus infections
- Heterotrophic bone formation within the sinus cavity may occur.

REFERENCES
1. Hopkins C. Chronic rhinosinusitis with nasal polyps. *N Engl J Med*. 2019;381:55–63.
2. DeMarcantonio MA, Han JK. Nasal polyps: pathogenesis and treatment implications. *Otolaryngol Clin North Am*. 2011;44(3):685–695.
3. Rudmik L, Soler ZM. Medical therapies for adult chronic sinusitis: a systematic review. *JAMA*. 2015;314(9):926–939.
4. Rudmik L, Schlosser RJ, Smith TL, et al. Impact of topical nasal steroid therapy on symptoms of nasal polyposis: a meta-analysis. *Laryngoscope*. 2012;122:1431–1437.
5. Bachert C, Han JK, Desrosiers M, et al. Efficacy and safety of dupilumab in patients with severe chronic rhinosinusitis with nasal polyps (LIBERTY NP SINUS-24 and LIBERTY NP SINUS-52): results from two multicentre, randomised, double-blind, placebo-controlled, parallel-group phase 3 trials. *Lancet*. 2019;394(10209):1638–1650.
6. Forwith KD, Chandra RK, Yun PT, et al. ADVANCE: a multisite trial of bioabsorbable steroid-eluting sinus implants. *Laryngoscope*. 2011;121(11):2473–80.
7. Sharma R, Lakhani R, Rimmer J, et al. Surgical interventions for chronic rhinosinusitis with nasal polyps. *Cochrane Database Syst Rev*. 2014;(11):CD006990.
8. Rimmer J, Fokkens W, Chong LY, et al. Surgical versus medical interventions for chronic rhinosinusitis with nasal polyps. *Cochrane Database Syst Rev*. 2014;(12):CD006991.

 CODES

ICD10
- J33.9 Nasal polyp, unspecified
- J33.0 Polyp of nasal cavity
- J33.8 Other polyp of sinus

CLINICAL PEARLS
- Intranasal corticosteroid use has been demonstrated to reduce polyp size and recurrence as well as to improve nasal congestion.
- Short-course oral corticosteroids may be considered in those with persistent symptoms.
- Asthma is a common concomitant diagnosis and is often previously undiagnosed.
- Aggressive medical and surgical treatment improves asthma outcomes.
- Allergy testing can be helpful.
- If unilateral nasal polyp, refer for biopsy.

N

NEPHROTIC SYNDROME
Hanadi Abou Dargham, MD

BASICS

DESCRIPTION
- A constellation of clinical and laboratory features defined by the presence of heavy proteinuria (>3.5 g/1.73 m²/24 hr), hypoalbuminemia (<3 g/dL), severe hyperlipidemia (total cholesterol often >10 mmol/L) (380 mg/dL), and peripheral edema, with risk for thrombotic disease
- Includes both primary (idiopathic) and secondary forms
- Associated with many types of kidney disease

EPIDEMIOLOGY
Based on definitive diagnosis
- Diabetic nephropathy: most common cause of secondary nephrotic syndrome (1)
- Minimal change disease (MCD)
  - Most common cause of nephrotic syndrome in children <10 years (90%)
  - Peaks at 2 to 8 years of age
  - Idiopathic condition is adults associated with NSAID use or Hodgkin lymphoma.
- Amyloidosis: 4–17%% of idiopathic nephrotic syndrome—two renal types primary (AL) and secondary (AA)
- Lupus nephropathy (LN): Adult women are affected about 10 times more often than men.
- Focal segmental glomerulosclerosis (FSGS)
  - 35% of nephrotic syndrome in adults
  - Most common primary nephrotic syndrome in African Americans
  - Has both primary (idiopathic) and secondary forms (associated with HIV, morbid obesity, reflux nephropathy, previous glomerular injury)
- Membranous nephropathy
  - Most common cause of primary nephrotic syndrome in adults (40%)
  - Most often primary (idiopathic) but can be secondary associated with malignancy, hepatitis B, autoimmune diseases, thyroiditis, and certain drugs including NSAIDs, penicillamine, gold, and captopril
- Membranoproliferative glomerulonephritis (MGN)
  - May be primary or secondary
  - May present in the setting of a systemic viral or rheumatic illness

Incidence
Approximately 3 cases per 100,000 per year in adults and 2 to 7 per 100,000 in Caucasian children. There is higher incidence in children of South Asian descent.

Prevalence
- 16 in 100,000 children
- More common in women than in men with a ratio of 2:1 (2)

ETIOLOGY AND PATHOPHYSIOLOGY
- Increased glomerular permeability to protein macromolecules, especially albumin
- Podocytes injury is the most common finding in diseases that cause primary nephrotic syndrome.
- Edema results primarily from renal salt retention, with arterial underfilling from decreased plasma oncotic pressure playing an additional role.
- Hyperlipidemia is thought to be a consequence of increased hepatic synthesis resulting from low oncotic pressure and urinary loss of regulatory proteins.

- The hypercoagulable state that can occur in some nephrotic states is likely due to loss of antithrombin III in urine.
- Primary renal disease (e.g., MCD, FSGS, MGN, IgA nephropathy)
- Secondary renal disease (e.g., diabetic nephropathy, amyloidosis and paraproteinemias, infections, cancer, drugs)

Genetics
Mutations in number of genes regulating podocyte proteins were identified in families with inherited nephrotic syndrome.

RISK FACTORS
- Drug addiction (e.g., heroin [FSGS])
- Hepatitis B and C, HIV, other infections
- Immunosuppression
- Nephrotoxic drugs
- Vesicoureteral reflux (FSGS)
- Cancer (usually MGN, may be MCD)
- Chronic analgesic use/abuse (NSAIDs)
- Preeclampsia
- Diabetes mellitus

GENERAL PREVENTION
In general, there are few preventive measures, including avoidance of known causative medications including NSAIDs, gold, penicillamine, and captopril; avoidance of heroin abuse and tight glycemic control

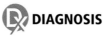
DIAGNOSIS

HISTORY
The history is key in looking for risk factors and the cause of nephrotic syndrome.
- Inquire about signs or symptoms of systemic disease: joint complaint, rash, edema, infectious complaint, fevers, anorexia, oliguria, foamy urine, acute flank pain, and hematuria.
- Obtain a recent drug history for medications that may be causative, especially NSAIDs.

PHYSICAL EXAM
A complete physical exam may discover clues to systemic disease as a potential cause and/or may suggest the severity of disease.
- Fluid retention: abdominal distention, abdominal fluid shift, extremity edema, puffy eyelids, scrotal swelling, weight gain, shortness of breath. Pericardial rub and decreased breath sounds with pleural effusions may develop.
- Arterial hypertension is found in 25% of the cases.
- Orthostatic hypotension
- Macroscopic hematuria is rare, but microscopic hematuria is present in 20% of the cases.

ALERT
The potential for thromboembolic disease leading to pulmonary embolism is one of the most life-threatening aspects of a patient who is actively nephrotic.

DIFFERENTIAL DIAGNOSIS
- Edema and proteinuria: see "Etiology and Pathophysiology."
- Edema alone: congestive heart failure, cirrhosis, hypothyroidism, nutritional hypoalbuminemia, protein-losing enteropathy

DIAGNOSTIC TESTS & INTERPRETATION
No guidelines are available for the investigation of nephrotic syndrome. Blood workup should be based on the clinical presentation.

Initial Tests (lab, imaging)
- Confirm proteinuria if present: by urine dipstick initially (3+ or 4+ readings) and then quantitate by 24-hour urine or spot urine protein-to-creatinine ratio.
- Rule out urine infection with urine culture.
- Full blood count and coagulation screen
- Renal function tests: BUN, creatinine with estimated glomerular filtration rate (GFR)
- Glucose to rule out overt diabetes
- Serum albumin that is often <2.5 g/dL in NS.
- Consider blood cultures to rule out a postinfectious process.
- Lipid panel
- Liver function tests to exclude liver disease or infection
- Look for autoimmune disease.
  - Antinuclear antibody and/or antidouble-stranded DNA positivity suggest lupus.
  - Complement levels (C3/C4 and total hemolytic complement): A low C3 may suggest a postinfectious or membranoproliferative process, whereas both low C3 and C4 point to lupus.
- Serum protein electrophoresis/urine immune electrophoresis to rule in a paraproteinemia
- Hepatitis B and C screen
- Measurement of cryoglobulins
- HIV and syphilis serology
- Urinalysis to evaluate for the presence of cellular casts
- Renal US to verify the presence of two kidneys of normal shape and size
- Chest x-ray to detect presence of pleural effusion or infection
- If thrombosis is suspected, obtain a Doppler US of the legs.

Follow-Up Tests & Special Considerations
Consider genetic testing for the NPHS1 and NPHS2 mutations for infants and testing for NPHS2 in children who are resistent to steroid therapy.

Diagnostic Procedures/Other
Renal biopsy is standard in determining the underlying cause of nephrotic syndrome.
- Rarely done in children with first episode of nephrotic syndrome because MCD is common and empiric steroid therapy is the standard of care
- Required to confirm the clinical diagnosis in adults and assist with making a treatment plan (1)[C]
- Contraindications to renal biopsy include small kidneys, renal tumor or bilateral renal cysts, active infection, severe malignant hypertension, hydronephrosis, bleeding diathesis, uncooperative patient.

Test Interpretation
- Light microscopy
  - May see nothing (e.g., MCD)
  - Sclerosis (e.g., FSGS or diabetic nodules in diabetes)
  - Diffuse hypercellularity suggests a proliferative disease such as IgA nephropathy, LN, or postinfectious GN.
- Immunofluorescence: Mesangial IgA suggests IgA nephropathy, Henoch-Schönlein purpura; other staining patterns are specific for other disease processes.

TREATMENT

The treatment for nephrotic syndrome depends on the type of renal pathology and varies between children and adults. KDIGO issued guidelines in 2012 on the treatment for nephrotic syndrome in adults and children (3).

MEDICATION

First Line

- Edema: salt restriction and salt-wasting diuretics (loop and thiazide diuretics) (4)[A]:
  - Salt restriction to <2 to 3 g sodium per day
  - Restrict fluid intake to <1.5 L/day if hyponatremic.
  - Target weight loss of 0.5 to 1.0 kg/day (1 to 2 lb/day)
- Edema should be corrected slowly to avoid acute hypovolemia, electrolyte disturbances, acute renal failure, and thromboembolism as a result of hemoconcentration.
- Hyperlipidemia is often reversed with resolution of the disease.
  - Statins have been shown to improve endothelial function (4)[A] and may decrease proteinuria (5)[A] with the exception of rosuvastatin that can worsen proteinuria, but effect on GFR and preservation of renal function is small. The major role for statin use is in cardiovascular risk reduction.
- Proteinuria:
  - ACE inhibitors or angiotensin II receptor blockers are thought to reduce proteinuria, hyperlipidemia, thrombotic tendencies, progression of renal failure, and to control hypertension, if present (6)[A].
  - Protein restriction can slow the progression of the disease but evidence is unclear.
- For steroid-responsive disease (MCD and FSGS), steroids dosed in consultation with nephrologist

Second Line

- Many of the nephrotic diseases will require escalation in therapy above steroids. These include rapidly relapsing forms as well as MGN, LN, and IgA nephropathy. Bolus steroids and other immunosuppressives are required in this circumstance (cyclophosphamide, mycophenolate mofetil, chlorambucil, cyclosporine) (7)[A].
- Rituximab, anti-CD20 and abatacept, anti–B7-1, combined with steroids or other immunosuppressive agents, has demonstrated early promise in the treatment of refractory nephrotic syndrome (8)[B].
- Randomized controlled data have been insufficient to determine which patients require prophylactic anticoagulation (9)[A] and for how long. Common practice is to anticoagulate with heparin and then warfarin in patients who have persistent nephrotic-range proteinuria. This decision is made based on the patient's history of edema, hypoalbuminemia, thromboembolism, or immobility.
- Corticotropin injection is a potential treatment for steroid-resistant nephrotic syndrome; however, data is only based on retrospective and observational studies.
- Hypocalcemia from vitamin D loss should be treated with oral vitamin D.

ISSUES FOR REFERRAL

Consultation with a nephrologist is often required to assist with renal biopsy to confirm diagnosis and to assist with management of edema. Cytotoxic medications may be called for, depending on the disease process, and this may best be handled by a nephrologist.

ADDITIONAL THERAPIES

Ambulation or range of motion exercises to lower risk of deep vein thrombosis (DVT)

ADMISSION, INPATIENT, AND NURSING CONSIDERATIONS

Admission criteria/initial stabilization: respiratory distress, sepsis/severe infection, thrombosis, renal failure, hypertensive urgency/emergency, or other complications

 ONGOING CARE

Adjustment in the doses of diuretics and angiotensin antagonists depends on the degree of edema and proteinuria.

FOLLOW-UP RECOMMENDATIONS

Patient Monitoring

- Frequent monitoring is required for relapse, disease progression, and for detecting signs of toxicity of medical management.
- Reevaluate for azotemia, urine protein, hypertension, edema, loss of renal function, cholesterol, and weight.

DIET

Muscle wasting and malnutrition are major problems in severe nephrotic syndrome. Optimal diet include the following:

- Normal protein (1 g/kg/day)
- Low fat (cholesterol)
- Reduced sodium (<2 g/day)
- Supplemental multivitamins and minerals, especially vitamin D and iron
- Fluid restriction if hyponatremic

PATIENT EDUCATION

- www.niddk.nih.gov/health-information/kidney-disease/children/childhood-nephrotic-syndrome
- Psychological counseling and peer support can be helpful.
- A diary that includes a plan for the management of relapses can be helpful.

PROGNOSIS

- Nephrotic syndrome in children (MCD) is typically self-limited and carries a good prognosis. In the adult, the prognosis is variable.
- Complete remission is expected if the basic disease is treatable (infection, malignancy, drug induced); otherwise, a relapsing and remitting course is possible, with progression to dialysis seen in more aggressive forms (diabetic glomerulosclerosis and FSGS).

COMPLICATIONS

- Deep vein, renal vein, or central venous thrombosis may occur.
- Pleural effusion
- Ascites
- Hyperlipidemia, cardiovascular disease
- Acute renal failure, progressive renal failure
- Protein malnutrition/muscle wasting
- Infection secondary to low serum IgG concentrations, reduced complement activity, and depressed T-cell function
- Proximal tubular dysfunction resulting in glucosuria, aminoaciduria, phosphaturia, bicarbonaturia, and vitamin D deficiency

REFERENCES

1. Kodner C. Diagnosis and management of nephrotic syndrome in adults. *Am Fam Physician*. 2016;93(6):479–485.
2. Varner J, Matory A, Gbadegesin R. Genetic basis of heath disparity in childhood nephrotic syndrome. *Am J Kidney Dis*. 2018;72(5 Suppl 1):S22–S25.
3. Kidney Disease Improving Global Outcomes. KDIGO clinical practice guideline for glumerulonephritis. *Kidney Inter Suppl*. 2012;2(2):1–143.
4. Crew RJ, Radhakrishnan J, Appel G. Complications of the nephrotic syndrome and their treatment. *Clin Nephrol*. 2004;62(4):245–259.
5. Fried LF, Orchard TJ, Kasiske BL. Effect of lipid reduction on the progression of renal disease: a meta-analysis. *Kidney Int*. 2001;59(1):260–269.
6. Kunz R, Friedrich C, Wolbers M, et al. Meta-analysis: effect of monotherapy and combination therapy with inhibitors of the renin angiotensin system on proteinuria in renal disease. *Ann Intern Med*. 2008;148(1):30–48.
7. Hodson EM, Willis NS, Craig JC. Interventions for idiopathic steroid-resistant nephrotic syndrome in children. *Cochrane Database Syst Rev*. 2010;(11):CD003594.
8. Kamei K, Okada M, Sato M, et al. Rituximab treatment combined with methylprednisolone pulse therapy and immunosuppressants for childhood steroid-resistant nephrotic syndrome. *Pediatr Nephrol*. 2014;29(7):1181–1187.
9. Kulshrestha S, Grieff M, Navaneethan SD. Interventions for preventing thrombosis in adults and children with nephrotic syndrome (protocol). *Cochrane Database Syst Rev*. 2006;(2):CD006024.

 SEE ALSO

Acute Kidney Injury; Amyloidosis; Diabetes Mellitus, Type 1; Diabetes Mellitus, Type 2; Glomerulonephritis, Acute; HIV/AIDS; Lupus Erythematosus, Discoid; Multiple Myeloma

 CODES

ICD10

- N04.0 Nephrotic syndrome with minor glomerular abnormality
- N04 Nephrotic syndrome
- N04.3 Nephrotic syndrome with diffuse mesangial proliferative glomerulonephritis

CLINICAL PEARLS

- Nephrotic syndrome is a clinical syndrome of >3.5 g/day proteinuria, hypoalbuminemia, hyperlipidemia, and edema often associated with diabetes and NSAIDs use.
- Pediatric nephrotic syndrome typically carries a good prognosis and is more easily treated with steroids, although recurrences are common.
- Nondiabetic adults with nephrotic syndrome will require a renal biopsy to determine cause.
- Have a high index of suspicion for symptoms that may represent an embolic event in patients with nephrotic syndrome.

N

NEUROFIBROMATOSIS TYPE 1

Marvin H. Sineath Jr., MD, FAAFP, CAQSM • Erik C. Shaw, DO, MBMS

BASICS

DESCRIPTION

- Neurofibromatosis types 1 (NF1) and 2 (NF2) are neurocutaneous syndromes (phakomatoses). Although they share a name, they are unrelated.
  - NF1, the most common of the phakomatoses, is a multisystem disorder that may affect any organ: the defining feature of NF1 is the neurofibroma, a nerve sheath tumor that forms in intimate association with spinal, peripheral or cranial nerves (1). It is also characterized by café au lait macules (CALM), axillary and inguinal freckling, Lisch nodules, choroidal freckling.
  - NF2 is a rare condition that causes bilateral vestibular schwannomas.
- System(s) affected: musculoskeletal; nervous; skin/exocrine; cardiovascular; neuro-ophthalmologic
- Synonym(s): von Recklinghausen disease, formerly peripheral NF

EPIDEMIOLOGY

Incidence
- Predominant sex for NF1: male = female
- Birth incidence NF1: 1:2,500 to 3,000

Prevalence
1:3,000 to 1:4,000

ETIOLOGY AND PATHOPHYSIOLOGY
- Neurofibromin is a GTPase–activating protein that acts as a tumor suppressor by down regulating p21-ras, a cellular proto-oncogene that enhances cell growth and proliferation.
- Some clinical manifestations of NF1, such as CALMs, require biallelic inactivation of NF1. Others, such as malignant peripheral nerve sheath tumors (MPNSTs), result from haploinsufficiency in combination with mutations in other genes, such as *TP53*.
- Neurofibromas are benign tumors composed of Schwann cells, fibroblasts, mast cells, and vascular components that develop along nerves.

Genetics
- Caused by a mutation in the *NF1* gene on chromosome 17q11.2; autosomal dominant inheritance; protein product is called *neurofibromin*.
- 50% of cases are due to de novo mutations, mostly paternal; likelihood increases with paternal age.
- Prenatal diagnosis is possible if mutation is known.
- Gene is large (~60 exons), with >3,000 different germline mutations causing NF1. Molecular technology can detect 95% of clinically important *NF1* mutations, but clinical diagnosis frequently can be made in childhood.
- Although expressivity is extremely variable, even within a family, the p.Arg1038Gly missense substitution correlates with a mild phenotype without neurofibromas or other complications.

RISK FACTORS
- Having an affected first-degree relative is a diagnostic criterion for NF1, although relatives may be unaware that they have NF1.
- Affected individuals with a positive family history (or a new mutation) have a 50% risk of transmitting NF1 to each offspring; 1 in 12 will be severely affected.

COMMONLY ASSOCIATED CONDITIONS
- Congenital heart disease, pulmonary stenosis, hypertension, renal artery stenosis
- Learning disabilities (50–75%)

DIAGNOSIS

- NF1 is diagnosed based on the presence of clinical features. A diagnosis can be made through routine exam usually by age 4 with special attention to skin stigmata. At least two of the following clinical features must be present to make a diagnosis of NF1:
  - ≥6 café au lait (light brown) macules (CALMs), ≥5 mm in prepubertal individuals or ≥15 mm in adults
  - ≥2 neurofibromas of any type or 1 plexiform (uncircumscribed) neurofibroma
  - Axillary or inguinal freckling
  - ≥2 Lisch nodules (benign iris hamartomas)
  - Optic glioma by MRI
  - Characteristic osseous lesions: sphenoid dysplasia, long-bone cortical thinning, ribbon ribs, angular scoliosis
  - First-degree relative with NF1 by above criteria
- Prenatal diagnosis is possible with known mutation or by linkage testing (with positive family history), although not predictive of clinical course.

HISTORY
- Family history of a first-degree relative with NF1
- Manifestations generally are not visible at birth, although plexiform neurofibromas are usually congenital, and tibial bowing is congenital.
- In addition to cutaneous lesions, NF1 may present with painful neurofibromas, pathologic fractures, or headaches secondary to hypertension caused by pheochromocytomas.
- Optic gliomas may present as involuntary eye movement, squinting, loss of vision, or as diencephalic syndrome.

PHYSICAL EXAM
- Skin
  - CALMs, usually the presenting feature of NF1, develop before age 3 years. Evenly pigmented, irregularly shaped (coast of California), light-brown macules seen in 97% of patients with NF1; many unaffected individuals have 1 to 3 such macules.
  - Neurofibromas: can be soft or firm, cutaneous, subcutaneous, or plexiform; buttonhole invagination is pathognomonic. Cutaneous neurofibromas usually appear during late childhood or adolescence.
  - Plexiform neurofibromas present in up to 50%.
    - Usually congenital; may be subtle in infancy
    - Freckling or hypertrichosis may be present over plexiform neurofibromas; may affect underlying structures or focal hyperplasia
    - Many are internal, not obvious on exam.
    - Most grow slowly but can have rapid growth, especially in early childhood.
  - Evaluate for new or progressive lesions. Rapidly growing cutaneous lesions should be evaluated.
  - Axillary freckling (Crowe sign) or inguinal freckling (91%)
- Ophthalmologic
  - Lisch nodules in 30%: well-defined, dome-shaped, gelatinous hamartomatous lesions projecting from the iris, varying from clear yellow to brown
  - Essentially unique to NF, Lisch nodules are asymptomatic; significant only for diagnosis
  - Pallor or atrophy of optic disc, bulging of orbit, loss of vision may be signs of optic glioma.
  - Choroidal freckling
- Skeletal
  - Scoliosis and vertebral angulation
  - Localized bone hypertrophy, especially of the face

- Limb abnormalities:
  - Pseudoarthrosis of the tibia
  - Tibial dysplasia (anterolateral bowing of the tibia)
  - Nonossifying fibromas of the long bones in adolescents and adults are uncommon but can increase risk of fracture.
- Pay particular attention to neurologic examination (asymmetry) or new focal pain.
- Measure BP yearly. Hypertension is more common in patients with NF1 and could be secondary to renal artery stenosis, aortic stenosis, pheochromocytoma.
- Evaluate neurodevelopmental progress in children. Learning disabilities occur in 50–75%.

DIFFERENTIAL DIAGNOSIS
Familial café au lait spots (autosomal dominant, no other NF1 features), Legius syndrome, constitutional mismatch repair deficiency syndrome (CMMRD), NF2, Watson syndrome, LEOPARD syndrome, McCune-Albright syndrome, neurocutaneous melanosis, proteus syndrome, lipomatosis, Jaffe–Campanacci syndrome

Geriatric Considerations
In NF1, cutaneous lesions and tumors increase in size and number with age.

Pediatric Considerations
- Children who have inherited the *NF1* gene of an affected parent usually are identified by age 1 year, but external stigmata may be subtle.
- If no stigmata noted by age 2 years, NF is unlikely, but the child should be reexamined. Diagnosis usually can be made by age 4 years using NIH criteria, although young children may have multiple CALMs but no other stigmata.
- Periodic ophthalmologic evaluations at increasing intervals after 10 years of age (1)[C].
- Molecular confirmation may be appropriate, especially with atypical presentation.
- There may be some association between NF1 and lower urinary tract dysfunction in pediatric populations. Therefor children exhibiting symptoms of lower urinary tract dysfunction (urgency, daytime frequency, nocturia, weak or slow stream, incomplete bladder emptying) should be considered for a thorough urologic evaluation.
- Cerebrovascular diseases (migraine, aneurysm, stroke, cognitive deficits) have been observed in children with NF1. There may be some prognostic value to screen for cerebrovascular abnormalities early in the diagnostic evaluation.

DIAGNOSTIC TESTS & INTERPRETATION
- Molecular genetic testing often not necessary for diagnosis
- Confirmatory genetic testing is appropriate in those suspected of having NF1 but do not fulfill diagnostic criteria or for prenatal diagnosis or preimplantation genetic diagnosis (PGD).
- Molecular genetic testing of the *NF1* gene can identify mutations in ~95% of those with a diagnosis.
- Multistep pathogenic variant detection with cDNA and gDNA sequence analysis recommended if molecular genetic testing is indicated. NF1 is caused by a wide variety of mutations in the NF1 gene.

Initial Tests (lab, imaging)
- Characteristic radiographic findings: sphenoid dysplasia, long bone cortical thinning, ribbon ribs, angular scoliosis. Screening radiographs of the knees in adolescents is controversial. CT can demonstrate bony changes.

- MRI findings of the orbits, brain, or spine (86%). Routine head MRI scanning in asymptomatic individuals is controversial. Optic gliomas (on MRI, 11–15%) may lead to blindness. Although areas of increased T_2 signal intensity (unidentified bright objects) are common on brain MRI, they are not diagnostic of NF1 and likely of no clinical significance.
- The NIH Consensus Development Conference does not recommend routine neuroimaging as a means of establishing a diagnosis, although modification of diagnostic criteria is discussed.

Diagnostic Procedures/Other

- Ophthalmologic evaluation, including slit-lamp exam of the irides; visual field testing to evaluate optic gliomas
- Neuropsychological testing: intelligence usually normal but may have significant deficits in language, visuospatial skills, and neuromotor skills
- Annual screening mammography and surveillance of breast lesions

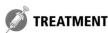 TREATMENT

MEDICATION

First Line

No specific therapeutic agents; symptoms are treated as they arise (e.g., anticonvulsants for seizures, medications for ADHD, management of blood pressure, vitamin D supplementation for osteopenia in those with low vitamin D levels).

Second Line

- Several biologically targeted therapies (e.g., mTOR inhibitors, imatinib, selective MEK inhibitors) that inhibit pathways responsible for tumor growth have been evaluated in clinical trials (1).
- Clinical trials with farnesyltransferase inhibitors, multikinase inhibitors, and antifibrotic agents have not been successful (1).
- A phase II trial of selumetinib is underway in adults and children with NF1 and symptomatic plexiform neurofibromas (1).
- Multiple clinical trials for NF1 are recruiting patients.

ISSUES FOR REFERRAL

- Patients with more than minimal manifestations of NF1: Refer to a multidisciplinary NF clinic.
- Referral for psychosocial issues
- Educational intervention for children with learning disabilities or ADHD (40%)
- Early referral to orthopedics for congenital tibial bowing

ADDITIONAL THERAPIES

- Occupational therapy for children with NF1 who present with fine motor difficulties
- Laser therapy not recommended for CALMs
- The Children's Tumor Foundation (CTF) has established the NF Clinical Trials Consortium and the CTF NF Clinic Network to facilitate clinical trials.

SURGERY/OTHER PROCEDURES

- Dermal neurofibromas can cause itching, stinging, pain, tenderness, bleeding, and cosmetic problems. Management may involve surgical removal, laser ablation of small lesions, electrodessication, emollients, camouflage make-up, psychological support (1).
- Plexiform neurofibromas, usually benign, can cause pain, disfigurement, neurologic deficit, difficulty swallowing and breathing, and severe hemorrhage, and are at risk for malignant transformation. Treatment is surgical (1)[C].
- Surgical treatment for dystrophic scoliosis (although nondystrophic scoliosis frequently can be managed conservatively, with bracing) or malignancy (especially MPNST).

ONGOING CARE

FOLLOW-UP RECOMMENDATIONS

NF1 health supervision 2008 guidelines:

- Infancy to 1 year
  - Growth and development: mild short stature, macrocephaly (increased brain volume); aqueductal stenosis/obstructive hydrocephalus
  - Check for focal neurologic signs or asymmetric neurologic exam.
  - Skeletal abnormalities, especially spine and legs
  - Neurodevelopmental progress
- 1 to 5 years
  - CALMs and axillary freckling have no clinical significance.
  - Annual ophthalmologic exam
  - Brain MRI for visual changes, persistent headaches, seizures, marked increase in head size, plexiform neurofibroma of the head
  - Assess speech and language: hypernasal speech due to velopharyngeal insufficiency and delayed expressive language development.
  - Developmental evaluation of learning and motor abilities; may benefit from speech/language and/or motor therapy, and special education
  - Monitor BP annually.
- 5 to 13 years
  - Evaluate for skin tumors causing disfigurement and obtain consultation if surgery is desired to improve appearance or function.
  - Evaluate for premature or delayed puberty. If sexual precocity is noted, evaluate for an optic glioma or hypothalamic lesion. Review the effects of puberty on NF.
  - Evaluate for learning disabilities and ADHD.
  - Evaluate social adjustment, development, and school placement.
  - Monitor ophthalmologic status yearly until age 8 years; complete eye exam every 2 years.
  - Monitor BP annually.
  - Refer patient to a clinical psychologist or child psychiatrist for problems with self-esteem.
  - Discuss growth of neurofibromas during adolescence and pregnancy.
  - Counsel parents about discussing diagnosis with child.
- 13 to 21 years
  - Examine the adolescent for abnormal pubertal development.
  - Skin examination for plexiform neurofibromas and neurologic exam for findings suggestive of deep plexiform neurofibromas; surgical consultation for signs of pressure on deep structures
  - Continue to monitor BP yearly.
  - Ophthalmologic exam every 2 years until age 18 years
  - Discuss genetics of NF1 or refer for genetic counseling.
  - Discuss sexuality, contraception, and reproductive options.
  - Discuss effects of pregnancy on NF1, if appropriate. Neurofibromas may enlarge, and new tumors may develop during pregnancy.
  - Review prenatal diagnosis or refer to a geneticist.

PATIENT EDUCATION

- Genetic counseling and patient education regarding future complications and family planning. Support groups are important.
- Children's Tumour Foundation, Washington University NF Center, Neuro Foundation

PROGNOSIS

Variable; most patients have a mild expression of NF1 and lead normal lives. Life expectancy may be reduced by ~8 to 21 years, with an excess of deaths in individuals <40 years of age (1).

COMPLICATIONS

- Disfigurement: Skin neurofibromas develop primarily on exposed areas. The number tends to increase with puberty or pregnancy.
- Scoliosis: 10–30% (most cases mild); bowing of long bones, 2%; osteopenia and osteoporosis
- A large head is common but rarely associated with hydrocephalus.
- Increased risk of malignancy: MPNST (5–10%) usually in adults, especially within the field of previous radiotherapy for plexiform neurofibroma
- CNS tumors (5–15%), optic pathway glioma most common, most often asymptomatic but usually presents before age 6 years if symptomatic; symptomatic lesions usually stable or slowly progressive
- High relative risk (RR) for uncommon malignancies
- Increased risk for pheochromocytoma, rhabdomyosarcoma, leukemia, Wilms tumor
- RR for cancer of the esophagus (3.3), stomach (2.8), colon (2.0), liver (3.8), lung (3.0), bone (19.6), thyroid (4.9), malignant melanoma (3.6), non-Hodgkin lymphoma (3.3), chronic myeloid leukemia (6.7), female breast (2.3), and ovary (3.7)
- Learning disability: ~50%; reduction in average IQ (~85) may be associated with ADHD; cognitive impairment in 4–8%.
- Neuropsychological phenotype: behavioral problems, executive dysfunction, reduced working memory; literacy, numeracy, and visual spatial difficulties
- GI neurofibromas may cause GI disturbances.
- Seizures: 6–7%. Focal, tonic-clonic are the most common type of seizure observed (60.9%).
- Hypertension frequent in adults, may occur in childhood
- Disorders of puberty

Pregnancy Considerations

Increased risk of perinatal complications, stillbirth, intrauterine growth constriction; risk of cord compression and outlet obstruction by pelvic neurofibromas

REFERENCE

1. Gutmann DH, Ferner RE, Listernick RH, et al. Neurofibromatosis type 1. *Nat Rev Dis Primers*. 2017;3:17004.

SEE ALSO

Tuberous Sclerosis Complex; Von Hippel-Lindau Syndrome

CODES

ICD10

Q85.01 Neurofibromatosis, type 1

CLINICAL PEARLS

- NF1 manifests marked clinical variability. External stigmata may be subtle or absent in young children. Minimally affected children may become severely affected adults.
- A single CALM is of no concern in a child, but having ≥6 is a diagnostic criterion for NF1.

N

NEUROPATHIC PAIN

Ying Tang, DO • Marilyn Hines, DO

BASICS

DESCRIPTION
- The term "neuropathic pain" represents a broad spectrum of pain syndromes and encompasses a wide variety of peripheral and central disorders.
- Defined as injury of the nociceptive pathway in the central or peripheral nervous system (CNS and PNS) that result in either impairment, absence, or paradoxically augmentation of pain sensation
- Symptoms are usually burning, tingling, sharp, stabbing, shooting, and electric shock-like quality.
- Often severe and resistant to standard treatments for pain.

EPIDEMIOLOGY
Incidence
There is insufficient evidence on the general incidence rate of neuropathic pain as most studies target a single type of neuropathic pain. In a Dutch study targeted between 1996 and 2003, 9,135 new cases of neuropathic pain out of 362,693 persons contributing to the study were identified, yielding 8.2 new cases per 1,000 person-years (PY). The study approximates an annual incidence of almost 1% of the general population, affecting more women and middle-aged population.

Prevalence
Includes chronic conditions that affect up to 10% of the population, accounting for 20–25% of individuals with chronic pain.
- Malignancy—up to 20% have neuropathic pain from either cancer or treatment
- Post-stroke patients—up to 8%
- Spinal cord injury—60–69%, a large majority of whom present with a syringomyelia
- Herpes zoster—lifetime incidence ~25%. Up to 10% develop chronic postherpetic neuralgia.
- HIV—up to 50% have neuropathic pain
- Diabetes—~50% will eventually develop neuropathy; 34% will develop neuropathic pain.

ETIOLOGY AND PATHOPHYSIOLOGY
- A variety of mechanisms contribute to neuropathic pain and many are still poorly understood.
- One proposed mechanism suggests that damaged primary afferents, including nociceptors, become highly sensitive to mechanical stimuli and may generate impulses in the absence of stimulation. This increase in sensitivity and spontaneous activation without apparent stimulation is thought to be caused by an increase in the density of sodium channels in the damaged nerve fibers, leading to increased excitability and signal transduction.

Genetics
There is growing evidence of genetic factors in neuropathic pain. Human genetics studies have demonstrated that $Na_v1.7$ and $Na_v1.8$, two types of voltage-gated sodium channels encoded by the *SCN9A* and *SCN10A* genes, respectively, are expressed at high levels on the peripheral nociceptive neurons in the dorsal root ganglion. Thus, therapeutics aimed at these channels with specific genetic mutations can play a role in patient care.

RISK FACTORS
- General risk factors include older age, female, physical inactivity, and manual occupation.
- Diabetes mellitus I and II, multiple sclerosis, Guillain-Barré syndrome, herpes zoster, trigeminal neuralgia, HIV, Lyme disease, malignancy/chemotherapy, nutrition (B_6 and B_{12} deficiencies), medications (isoniazid, ethambutol, chloroquine, paclitaxel, cisplatin, amiodarone, vincristine).

GENERAL PREVENTION
- Use of herpes zoster vaccines, which reduces both herpes zoster infections in patients >50 of age and postherpetic neuralgia
- Use of antiviral or analgesic treatment in patients with herpes zoster infection
- Perioperative treatment of surgical patients to prevent chronic postsurgical pain. Use of multimodal analgesia with gabapentin and local anesthetics to prevent acute and chronic pain after breast surgery for cancer
- Proper management of health conditions, such as DM

COMMONLY ASSOCIATED CONDITIONS
Depression and anxiety, sleep disturbances, substance abuse, impaired cognition, polypharmacy, and suicidal ideation

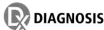

DIAGNOSIS

Diagnosis is based primarily on clinical history and the findings on physical examination.

HISTORY
- Onset and duration of symptoms, location, intensity (0–10), exacerbating factors
- Pain often described as burning, shooting, tingling, or electric shock-like
- Temporal profile: Symptoms become worse toward the end of the day.
- Sensory descriptors: numbness; weakness; reduced sensation to touch, pinprick, temperature, or vibration; decreased proprioception
- Effect on function: effect on sleep, ambulation, self-care, and sexual function
- Past medical, surgical, and psychosocial history, substance use (especially alcohol)
- Previous treatments: Neuropathic pain is generally resistant to acetaminophen or NSAIDs.
- Different screening tools in the form of questionnaires have emerged: Leeds Assessment of Neuropathic Symptoms and Signs, Douleur Neuropathique 4 questions, Neuropathic Pain Questionnaire, PainDETECT, Neuropathic Pain Symptom Inventory

PHYSICAL EXAM
- Positive symptoms
  - Hyperalgesia (abnormally increased pain response to stimulus) evoked by sharp or blunt pressure, heat or cold
  - Allodynia (pain from nonpainful stimulus) evoked by light touch, clothing, or bed sheets
- Negative symptoms
  - Hypoesthesia (abnormally reduced sensation of a tactile stimulus) to touch or temperature

- Gross motor examination
  - Weakness, fatigue, decreased range of motion, stiffness, and muscle spasm
  - Hypotonia, tremor, dystonia, ataxia, hypo-/hyperreflexia, motor neglect
- Sensory examination
  - Light touch, pinprick, vibration sense, and proprioception may be either diminished or amplified
  - Sensory disturbance may extend beyond a discrete nerve territory.
- Skin examination
  - Alterations in temperature, color, sweating, and hair growth suggestive of sympathetic nervous system involvement, such as in complex regional pain syndrome (CRPS)
  - Residual dermatomal scars can indicate previous herpes zoster infection.
  - Acanthosis nigricans can indicate diabetes.

DIFFERENTIAL DIAGNOSIS
- Nociceptive pain due to actual tissue damage
- Somatic symptom disorder
- Conversion disorder

DIAGNOSTIC TESTS & INTERPRETATION
Neurologic testing establishes distribution but does not yet provide benefit in determining treatment (1)[C].
- Confirmatory tests include the following (in order of increasing invasiveness):
  - Sensory assessment—touch, pinprick, pressure, cold, heat, vibration, temporal summation
  - Quantitative sensory testing—uses standardized mechanical and thermal stimuli to test the afferent nociceptive and nonnociceptive systems
  - Blink reflex testing—assesses trigeminal afferent system
  - Nerve conduction study/electromyography—assesses nonnociceptive large fiber function of the peripheral nerves.
  - Somatosensory-evoked potentials and laser-evoked potentials (LEP)—assess afferent fibre function
  - Skin biopsy—assesses quantification of the intraepidermal nerve fiber
  - Corneal confocal microscopy—assesses corneal innervation and small nerve fibres
- CT/MRI—facilitates specific diagnosis such as herniated disc, nerve compression by tumor

Initial Tests (lab, imaging)
None specifically for neuropathic pain but can rule in or out a possible cause: serum vitamin B_{12}, TSH, syphilis screening, fasting glucose/HbA1C, CBC, CMP, Lyme serology, HIV testing

TREATMENT

GENERAL MEASURES
- Due to multiple neuropathic pain pathways, all medications have limited efficacy and minority of patients have significant benefit at tolerable doses.
- Physical and occupational therapy can help with functional goals.

MEDICATION

- The efficacy of systemic drug treatments is generally not dependent on the etiology of the underlying disorder.
- Combined therapy likely more effective than increasing dose of single medicine
- Thought to be resistant to acetaminophen and NSAIDs but often used with some benefit in treatment of acute pain (2)[C]

First Line

- Calcium channel $\alpha 2\delta$ ligands
  - Gabapentin: number needed to treat (NNT) = 7 for significant pain improvement (3)[A]
    - Dosing: up to 3,600 mg in 3 divided doses
    - Precautions: requires renal dosing
    - Common side effects: sedation, dizziness, peripheral edema, weight gain
    - Also in the form of extended release or enacarbil
  - Pregabalin: NNT = 8 (3)[A]
    - Dosing: up to 600 mg in 2 doses
    - Precautions: requires renal dosing
    - Common side effects: sedation, dizziness, peripheral edema, weight gain
- Tricyclic antidepressants: NNT = 4 (3)[A]
  - Nortriptyline, desipramine, amitriptyline clomipramine, imipramine
    - Dosing: Start 10 to 25 mg at bedtime and then increase by 10 to 25 mg every 4 to 7 days up to 150 mg/day as tolerated.
    - Precautions: cardiac disease, glaucoma, prostatic adenoma, seizure, tramadol use
    - Geriatric: falls; limit dose to <75 mg.
    - Common side effects: somnolence, weight gain, anticholinergic effects, cardiac conduction block
    - Increased suicidality warning in children, adolescents, and young adults
- Serotonin norepinephrine reuptake inhibitors (SNRIs): NNT = 6 (3)[A]
  - Duloxetine
    - Dosing: 20 mg once daily to 60 mg twice daily; effective doses 60 to 120 mg daily
    - Precautions: hepatic disorder, tramadol use, hypertension
    - Common side effect: nausea, constipation; relatively the safest medication for neuropathic pain
  - Venlafaxine
    - Dosing: 37.5 to 225.0 mg daily
    - Effective doses: 150 to 225 mg daily
    - Precautions: cardiac disease, tramadol use, hypertension
    - Common side effects: nausea, hypertension at higher doses

Second Line

- Lidocaine, 5% patches (3)[B]
  - As effective as pregabalin for localized neuropathic pain from diabetes or herpes
  - Dosage: 1 to 3 patches for 12 hours daily to cover the painful area
  - Common side effects: local erythema, itch, rash

- Capsaicin high-concentration patches (8%): NNT = 11 (3)[A]
  - Dosing: 1 to 4 patches to cover the painful area; 30 minutes application to feet, 60 minutes application to remainder of body; avoid use on face; benefits for up to 3 months
  - Common side effects: pain (initial increase), erythema, itching, rare cases of hypertension, progressive neuropathy
  - No benefit from low-concentration capsaicin cream

Third Line

- Botulinum toxin type A (3)[B]
  - Limited evidence based on small studies, no quality of life improvement
    - Dosage: 50 to 200 units subcutaneously to the painful area; repeat every 3 months.
    - Common side effects: pain and infection at injection site, weakness
- Cannabinoids (dronabinol and nabilone): low-quality evidence (4)[B]
  - NNT = 20 for 50% improvement in pain
  - Number needed to harm (NNH) = 3 for adverse events
    - NNH = 25 for withdrawal due to adverse events
- Opioids (including tramadol): no proven long-term benefit; utility for neuropathic pain questioned (5)[A]
  - Chronic opioids decrease number and sensitivity of μ-opioid receptors, increasing hyperalgesia.

ISSUES FOR REFERRAL

Refer to pain clinic if refractory to initial treatment for trial of additional therapies.

ADDITIONAL THERAPIES

- Interventional pain management (epidural or peripheral nerve injections) will provide partial, lasting relief in 40–60% of patients (1)[B].
- Spinal cord stimulation (SCS): Pain that is continuous and unchanging responds best. Best evidence for failed back surgery syndrome with leg pain (1)[B].
- Intrathecal drug delivery: reserved for refractory pain; ziconotide has demonstrated efficacy (1)[B].
- Transcutaneous electrical nerve stimulation is widely used; evidence shows slight benefit (1)[B],(3)[B].
- Cognitive-behavioral and mindfulness therapies have some benefit as an adjunct to other therapies, especially in postherpetic neuropathy (1)[B],(3)[B].

SURGERY/OTHER PROCEDURES

Nerve destructive procedures haven't shown effectiveness and may cause additional insult/injury (an exception is treatment of terminal cancer) (1)[B].

- Sympathectomy dorsal root entry zone lesion (dorsal rhizotomy)
- Lateral cordotomy
- Trigeminal nerve ganglion ablation

COMPLEMENTARY & ALTERNATIVE MEDICINE

Acupuncture: limited evidence for improvement in pain

 ONGOING CARE

PROGNOSIS

Chronic course of pain symptoms often requires management with numerous medications and adjunctive therapies. Pain management requires ongoing evaluation, patient education, and reassurance. Complete pain relief is rare.

COMPLICATIONS

Long-term disability and drug addiction are possible.

REFERENCES

1. Jones RC III, Lawson E, Backonja M. Managing neuropathic pain. *Med Clin North Am.* 2016;100(1):151–167.
2. Gilron I, Baron R, Jensen T. Neuropathic pain: principles of diagnosis and treatment. *Mayo Clin Proc.* 2015;90(4):532–545.
3. Moisset X, Bouhassira D, Avez Couturier J, et al. Pharmacological and non-pharmacological treatments for neuropathic pain: systematic review and French recommendations. *Rev Neurol (Paris).* 2020;176(5):325–352.
4. Mücke M, Phillips T, Radbruch L, et al. Cannabis-based medicines for chronic neuropathic pain in adults. *Cochrane Database Syst Rev.* 2018;3(3):CD012182.
5. Zhang Y, Ahmed S, Vo T, et al. Increased pain sensitivity in chronic pain subjects on opioid therapy: a cross-sectional study using quantitative sensory testing. *Pain Med.* 2015;16(5):911–922.

ADDITIONAL READING

- Colloca L, Ludman T, Bouhassira D, et al. Neuropathic pain. *Nat Rev Dis Primers.* 2017;3:17002.
- Fornasari D. Pharmacotherapy for neuropathic pain: a review. *Pain Ther.* 2017;6(Suppl 1):25–33.

CODES

ICD10

- M79.2 Neuralgia and neuritis, unspecified
- E10.40 Type 1 diabetes mellitus with diabetic neuropathy, unsp
- E11.40 Type 2 diabetes mellitus with diabetic neuropathy, unsp

CLINICAL PEARLS

- Neuropathic pain is a common syndrome, affecting up to 10% of the population with major impacts on quality of life.
- Due to numerous mechanisms in neuropathy, potential benefit from any single treatment is limited.
- Narcotics likely have more harm than benefit; chronic use will likely increase pain.
- Functional goals and realistic pain targets are essential.

N

NEUROPATHY, PERIPHERAL

Christine S. Persaud, MD, MBA • Terry SeeToe, MD

BASICS

DESCRIPTION
- A functional or structural disorder of the peripheral nervous system (PNS), affecting any combination of motor, sensory, or autonomic nerves
- Peripheral motor involvement causes muscle atrophy, weakness, cramps, and fasciculations.
- Disorders of sensory nerves produce negative phenomena (loss of sensibility, lack of balance) or heightened phenomena (tingling or pain). Large sensory fiber dysfunction impairs touch and vibration sensation, whereas small fiber sensory neuropathy (SFSN) affects pin and thermal sensation and causes neuropathic pain.
- The autonomic nervous system (ANS) includes the sympathetic and parasympathetic systems. ANS dysfunction causes cardiovascular, gastrointestinal, and sudomotor symptoms.
- The PNS can be affected from the cell body (sensory ganglionopathy or motor neuronopathy), root (radiculopathy), or plexus (plexopathy) to the nerve (demyelinating or axonal neuropathy).
- Peripheral neuropathy (PN) can be subdivided as mononeuropathies, multifocal neuropathies, and polyneuropathies.

EPIDEMIOLOGY
Prevalence
- Prevalence of PN is estimated to be 1% and increases to 7% among people 65 years and older (1).
- Among adults with diabetes, the prevalence of peripheral neuropathy is estimated to be between 6% and 51%, depending on age, duration of diabetes, glucose control, and type 1 versus type 2 diabetes (2).

ETIOLOGY AND PATHOPHYSIOLOGY
PN occurs due to demyelination or axonal degeneration.
- 30% of PN cases are idiopathic.
- The most common cause of acquired PN is diabetes mellitus, which manifests most commonly at approximately 75% in the pattern of a distal sensory polyneuropathy (DSP).
- Other categories of acquired PN with examples are the following:
  - Vascular: ischemia, vasculitis
  - Infectious: HIV, hepatitis C, cryoglobulinemia, Lyme disease, varicella zoster
  - Traumatic: compression, crush, stretch, or transection (e.g., due to broken or dislocated bones, slipped disks between vertebrae, or arthritis)
  - Autoimmune: rheumatoid arthritis, Sjögren, lupus
  - Metabolic: renal failure, hypothyroidism, vitamin B_{12} deficiency, celiac disease, porphyria
  - Iatrogenic/toxic: chemotherapy, platinum, taxanes, metronidazole, colchicine, infliximab, lead, alcoholism
  - Neoplastic/paraneoplastic: paraproteinemia, Waldenström macroglobulinemia, multiple myeloma, amyloidosis, neurofibromatosis
- Acquired polyneuropathies typically present with distal onset of symptoms.

Genetics
Approximately 50% of undiagnosed PN is hereditary.

RISK FACTORS
Systemic disorders predispose to PN, such as diabetes and alcoholism.

COMMONLY ASSOCIATED CONDITIONS
Diabetes, alcoholism, and other conditions related to acquired forms of PN

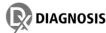
DIAGNOSIS

HISTORY
- A detailed inquiry for symptoms of sensory, motor, or autonomic dysfunction:
  - Numbness, tingling, prickling, burning pain, a "tightly wrapped" sensation, and an "unsteady gait"
  - Distal weakness manifests as foot drop (tripping, foot slapping) or difficulty with grip; proximal weakness (e.g., difficulty arising from a chair) is less common.
  - Orthostatic dizziness, abnormal sweating, constipation, erectile dysfunction, or voiding difficulties
- Symptom onset:
  - Acute: Consider infection (e.g., Lyme disease), postinfectious dysimmune process (e.g., GBS), ischemia (e.g., vasculitis), toxin, or trauma.
  - Subacute: Consider metabolic, neoplastic, paraneoplastic, or dysimmune processes.
  - Chronic: Consider dysimmune process (CIDP), idiopathic, or hereditary.
- Progression: stable or indolent; slowly or rapidly progressive; monophasic or relapsing or remitting
- Anatomic pattern: focal, multifocal, diffuse
- Inquire about family history and comorbidities to help determine if condition is inherited.

PHYSICAL EXAM
- Based on exam, a functional (*sensory*: small fiber vs. large fiber vs. mixed, *sensorimotor*, *motor*, *autonomic*) and anatomic pattern of PN (*distal symmetric*, *multifocal*, or *focal*) should be established.
- Cognition is preserved in isolated PN.
- Cranial nerves may be involved with focal or multifocal PN (e.g., bifacial weakness may occur with GBS, Lyme disease, sarcoidosis, among other causes).
- Stocking/glove sensory loss is typical of distal symmetric sensory PN (e.g., diabetes).
- Isolated reduced pin or thermal sensation or allodynia suggests a pure SFSN.
- Reduced vibration and proprioception suggest large-fiber sensory neuropathy; when severe, a Romberg sign is present, and gait is wide based or ataxic.
- Distal muscle atrophy and weaknesses of toe extension and finger abduction are often present with distal symmetric axonal PN.
- In acquired demyelinating PN (e.g., GBS or CIDP), weakness is commonly both proximally and distally.
- Deep tendon reflexes may be reduced or absent, distally at the ankles in large-fiber axonal PN, or diffusely in demyelinating PN.
- High arched or flat feet or hammer toes suggest hereditary PN.

DIFFERENTIAL DIAGNOSIS
- Pure sensory neuropathy (SFN, sensory ganglionopathy, polyradiculopathy)
- Distal symmetric sensorimotor axonal PN (distal acquired demyelinating symmetric [DADS] PN)
- Motor predominant PN (motor neuron disease, polyradiculopathy, immune-mediated multifocal motor neuropathy (MMN))
- Mononeuropathy most likely due to compression, entrapment, or trauma
- Mononeuropathy multiplex (plexopathy, polyradiculopathy)

DIAGNOSTIC TESTS & INTERPRETATION
Initial Tests (lab, imaging)
- CBC, Cr, HbA1C, vitamin B_{12} with methylmalonic acid, LFTs, serum protein immunofixation electrophoresis, TSH
- Nerve conduction studies (the gold standard for the diagnosis of diabetic painful neuropathy [DPN]) (3) and electromyography (NCS/EMG) delineate axonal versus demyelinating, anatomic pattern, chronicity, and severity of PN.
- Autonomic reflex screen, testing of sweat function, quantitative sensory testing, and epidermal skin biopsy to evaluate small nerve fiber function (4)
- Specialized epidermal skin biopsy if suspected SFN and NCS/EMG is normal
- Neuroimaging generally not indicated in evaluation of PN but useful in evaluation of brachial plexopathies, radiculopathies, or where findings are attributable to the CNS

Follow-Up Tests & Special Considerations
- Additional blood tests are done based on the medical history, the PN type, and NCS/EMG findings such as vitamins A, D, E; zinc; copper; ESR; CRP; ANA; Hep B/C; antitissue transglutaminase.
- Consider genetic testing for diagnosis of hereditary PN.
- Screen patients with distal symmetric PN for unhealthy alcohol use.

Diagnostic Procedures/Other
- Nerve biopsy (sural or superficial peroneal nerve): useful if vasculitis, amyloidosis, granulomatous disorders, or neoplastic infiltration is suspected; rarely helpful in late-onset chronic, slowly progressive distal symmetric PN
- Lumbar puncture

Test Interpretation

- Demyelinating PN: disproportionate slowing of conduction velocities, conduction block, increased temporal dispersion, or prolonged distal latencies on NCS. EMG findings include decreased recruitment and myokymia.
- Axonal PN: reduced amplitude in sensory or motor responses, with relatively preserved conduction velocities and distal latency on NCS. EMG findings include abnormal spontaneous activity, decreased recruitment, increased duration and amplitude, and polyphasicity.
- Reduced ENFD on distal leg skin biopsies is supportive of SFN.

 TREATMENT

GENERAL MEASURES

- Counsel on foot care and properly fitted footwear.
- Monitor feet for early signs of skin breakdown and injury.
- Targeted treatment for underlying systemic conditions

MEDICATION

First Line

Treatment of neuropathic pain: evidence of efficacy derived from clinical trials in DPN, postherpetic neuralgia (PHN), or trigeminal neuralgia:

- Anticonvulsants: gabapentin for PHN; pregabalin for DPN and PHN; gabapentin (off-label) for DPN; oxcarbazepine for DPN; carbamazepine for trigeminal neuralgia
- SNRI: duloxetine or venlafaxine for DPN
- Tricyclic antidepressants (TCA): amitriptyline or nortriptyline
- Patches: lidocaine 5%, capsaicin 8%
- Supplements: α-lipoic acid, acetyl-L-carnitine

Second Line

- Mexiletine
- Tramadol: off-label for DPN

Third Line

Tapentadol: for DPN

ISSUES FOR REFERRAL

- Neurology referral for rapidly progressive symptoms, suspected demyelinating PN, or hereditary PN
- Rheumatology referral for vasculitic PN
- Hematology referral and skeletal survey for patients with paraproteinemia
- Physical therapy for gait and balance training

ADDITIONAL THERAPIES

- Combination therapy (e.g., gabapentin with TCA or venlafaxine or tramadol) can be more effective than monotherapy for neuropathic pain.
- Botulinum toxin subcutaneous, intradermal, or direct nerve injections can be considered for trigeminal neuralgia, DPN, or complex regional pain syndrome (CRPS) (5)[A].
- Additional immunosuppressant agents (e.g., cyclophosphamide) may be used in refractory chronic dysimmune PN.

- Immunotherapy for dysimmune PN
  - Intravenous immunoglobulin (IVIG): within the first 2 weeks of GBS to hasten recovery (6)[A], as a first-line alternative to corticosteroids for treatment of CIDP (7)[A], and for prevention of secondary axonal loss in MMN (8)[A]
    - Loading dose 2 g/kg body weight divided into 2 to 5 days; maintenance regimen variable for CIDP and MMN
    - Adverse effects (AE): headache, fever, hypertension, and rarely pulmonary embolism
  - Plasma exchange: first agent shown to improve functional outcome for patients with GBS (9)[A]; short-term benefit in CIDP (9)[A]
    - AE: catheter complication, hypotension, and others
  - Corticosteroids: a first-line option in treatment of CIDP (9)[C]; oral or pulsed IV regimen can induce remission.
- Treatment of autonomic symptoms
  - Compression stockings, abdominal binder, hydration, midodrine, and fludrocortisone for orthostatic hypotension
  - Pyridostigmine for immune-mediated dysautonomia (off-label)

SURGERY/OTHER PROCEDURES

- Decompressive surgery for entrapment neuropathy (e.g., carpal tunnel syndrome)
- Foot and ankle surgery to improve symptoms or function in hereditary PN
- Radiation, surgery, or bone marrow transplantation for plasmacytoma or osteosclerotic myeloma or POEMS syndrome
- Liver transplantation for amyloidotic PN

COMPLEMENTARY & ALTERNATIVE MEDICINE

Low-intensity transcutaneous electrical nerve stimulation (TENS), acupuncture, meditation, supplements (G-agmatine, methylcobalamin, inositol) may be helpful.

ALERT

Vitamin B_6 supplementation may cause peripheral neurotoxicity and should be avoided except for a deficiency state.

ADMISSION, INPATIENT, AND NURSING CONSIDERATIONS

Patients with suspected GBS should be admitted for monitoring (30–60% may develop cardiovascular or respiratory failure) and treatment.

 ONGOING CARE

FOLLOW-UP RECOMMENDATIONS

- Strengthening exercises improved muscle strength, which may assist in function.
- Flu vaccination should be avoided in the 1st year following GBS.

DIET

Assess for B_{12} deficiency, ingestion of heavy metal toxins, thiamine deficiency in those with alcohol use disorder, and high carbohydrate intake for those with diabetes.

PROGNOSIS

- Late-onset idiopathic distal symmetric axonal PNs are indolent.
- 80% of GBS have a near complete or good recovery. 80% of CIDP have moderate or good response with treatment but can be relapsing.

COMPLICATIONS

PN is related to an increase in fall risk.

REFERENCES

1. Hanewinckel R, Ikram MA, Van Doorn PA. Peripheral neuropathies. *Handb Clin Neurol*. 2016;138:263–282.
2. Hicks CW, Selvin E. Epidemiology of peripheral neuropathy and lower extremity disease in diabetes. *Curr Diab Rep*. 2019;19(10):86.
3. Selvarajah D, Kar D, Khunti K, et al. Diabetic peripheral neuropathy: advances in diagnosis and strategies for screening and early intervention. *Lancet Diabetes Endocrinol*. 2019;7(12):938–948.
4. Barrell K, Smith AG. Peripheral neuropathy. *Med Clin North Am*. 2019;103(2):383–397.
5. Park J, Park HJ. Botulinum toxin for the treatment of neuropathic pain. *Toxins (Basel)*. 2017;9(9):260.
6. Hughes RAC, Swan AV, van Doorn PA. Intravenous immunoglobulin for Guillain-Barré syndrome. *Cochrane Database Syst Rev*. 2014;2014(9):CD002063.
7. Nobile-Orazio E, Cocito D, Jann S, et al; for IMC Trial Group. Intravenous immunoglobulin versus intravenous methylprednisolone for chronic inflammatory demyelinating polyradiculoneuropathy: a randomised controlled trial. *Lancet Neurol*. 2012;11(6):493–502.
8. Cats EA, van der Pol WL, Piepers S, et al. Correlates of outcome and response to IVIg in 88 patients with multifocal motor neuropathy. *Neurology*. 2010;75(9):818–825.
9. Nobile-Orazio E, Gallia F. Update on the treatment of chronic inflammatory demyelinating polyradiculoneuropathy. *Curr Opin Neurol*. 2015;28(5):480–485.

CODES

ICD10

- G62.9 Polyneuropathy, unspecified
- G60.9 Hereditary and idiopathic neuropathy, unspecified
- G60.8 Other hereditary and idiopathic neuropathies

CLINICAL PEARLS

- Diagnosis is made by history and physical exam, targeted laboratory testing, NCS/EMG, skin biopsy, or ANS testing.
- Consider hereditary neuropathy if patient has an early age of PN symptom onset, family history of PN, or foot deformity.
- GBS is monophasic and progresses for up to 4 weeks; CIDP progresses beyond 8 weeks, and if untreated, usually has a progressive course.

N

NICOTINE ADDICTION

Sarah E. Nickolich, MD • Meghan E. Reeves, MD

 BASICS

DESCRIPTION
Nicotine addiction is characterized by the compulsive use of nicotine products coupled with a lack of control over using, withdrawal symptoms, and/or continued use despite knowledge of or experiencing adverse consequences.

EPIDEMIOLOGY
Prevalence
- In 2018, there were an estimated 47.8 million U.S. adults who currently used any tobacco products, of which 41.1 million smoked combustible tobacco products and 9.0 million used two or more tobacco products. This included 34.3 million who smoked cigarettes, 9.3 million who smoked cigars, 6.9 million who used electronic cigarettes, 5.1 million who used smokeless tobacco, and 2.6 million who smoked pipes and hookahs.
- In 2020, an estimated 3.57 million middle and high school students currently used e-cigarettes. E-cigarette use among youth has increased 10-fold for high school and middle school students from 2011 to 2015 and has been associated with nicotine addiction in adulthood, and e-cigarettes have been the most commonly used tobacco product among youth since 2014. However, from 2019 to 2020, "current use" has declined among middle and high school students.

ETIOLOGY AND PATHOPHYSIOLOGY
- Similar to other addictive drugs, nicotine affects neural pathways that control reward and pleasure.
- Nicotine exerts its biologic effects through nicotinic acetylcholine receptors (nAChRs), which modulate neurotransmission with acetylcholine and other chemical messengers including glutamate, GABA, dopamine, serotonin, acetylcholine, and norepinephrine. In this way, it induces euphoria, assists in information processing, reduces anxiety, and mitigates fatigue.
- Upregulation of these receptors occurs over time, leading to tolerance and dependence.
- Polymorphisms in neuronal nAChR genes are associated with increased susceptibility to dependence.
- Nicotine is metabolized by cytochrome P450 2A6 (CYP2A6). Individuals who are fast metabolizers tend to smoke more cigarettes, are more likely to suffer intense withdrawal symptoms, and have a lower probability of quitting than slow metabolizers.
- Nicotine withdrawal involves the release of corticotropin-releasing factor in the amygdala, which induces the perception of anxiety and stress.

Pregnancy Considerations
- Smoking is a risk factor associated with placenta previa, abruptio placentae, decreased maternal thyroid function, preterm premature rupture of membranes, and ectopic pregnancy.
- Carbon monoxide and nicotine interfere with fetal oxygen supply, resulting in decreased birth weights and intrauterine growth restriction.
- Maternal smoking adversely affects fetal lung development, with lifelong decreases in pulmonary function and increased risk of asthma.
- Maternal smoking is associated with increased risk for sudden infant death syndrome, learning and behavioral problems, and obesity.

RISK FACTORS
- Mental illness (depression, posttraumatic stress disorder, bipolar disorder, and schizophrenia)
- Low socioeconomic status

- Low educational status
- Early firsthand nicotine experience
- Concurrent substance abuse
- Home and peer influence

GENERAL PREVENTION
- The U.S. Preventive Services Task Force (USPSTF) strongly recommends:
  - Screening all adults for tobacco use, providing cessation interventions for those who screen positive
  - Screening all pregnant women for tobacco use and providing pregnancy-tailored counseling to those who screen positive
- The USPSTF recommends that clinicians provide interventions, including education or brief counseling to prevent initiation of tobacco use among school-age children and adolescents.

 DIAGNOSIS

HISTORY
- Identify types, amount, and duration of nicotine products used.
- Review previous attempts to quit (methods used and duration of cessation).

PHYSICAL EXAM
- Pulmonary exam: wheezing, decreased breath sounds, prolonged expiration
- Cardiovascular exam: tachycardia, hypertension
- HEENT exam: epithelial dysplasia, squamous cell carcinoma, leukoplakia, stained teeth, hoarseness
- Skin exam: In combustible tobacco users, yellow-brown staining of the digits, "Harlequin nail" (bicolor nail seen after acute illness cause cessation of tobacco consumption, as unstained nail bed grows in), and clubbing may be seen.

DIAGNOSTIC TESTS & INTERPRETATION
- Lung cancer screening with low-dose CT is recommended annually by USPSTF for patients between 55 and 80 years old with a history of 30+ pack-years of tobacco use who are currently smoking or have quit within the past 15 years (except those with life-limiting comorbidities).
- Neither spirometry nor regular chest x-rays are recommended for routine screening.

 TREATMENT

Counseling (1)[A]
- Counseling interventions (individual, telephone, or group) improve quit rates compared to minimal support (relative risk [RR] of 1.76 [95% CI 1.58–1.96]).
- Combined behavioral and pharmaceutical interventions increased cessation (RR, 1.82 [95% CI 1.66–2.00]).
- More intensive interactions (i.e., motivational interviewing, close follow-up) may result in higher rates of quitting.
- Brief strategies to help the patient willing to quit tobacco use—the "5 As" (1)[A]
  - Ask patient if he or she uses nicotine.
  - Advise him or her to quit.
  - Assess willingness to make a quit attempt.
  - Assist those willing to make a quit attempt.
  - Arrange follow-up contact to prevent relapse.
- Enhancing motivation to quit: the "5 Rs" (1)[A]
  - Relevance: Encourage patient to indicate why quitting is personally relevant.

  - Risks: Ask patient to identify potential negative consequences of use.
  - Rewards: Ask patient to identify potential benefits of cessation.
  - Roadblocks: Ask patient to identify barriers to quitting and provide treatment (e.g., problem-solving counseling or medication) that could address barriers.
  - Repetition: Repeat motivational intervention each visit.
- Users should be given a choice of methods to quit.
- Quit rates appear to be higher with abrupt quitting rather than gradual reduction prior to the quit date (49% vs. 39% at 4 weeks and 22% vs. 15% at 6 months). Over 4 weeks, there was no significant difference between groups in withdrawal symptoms or urge intensity, both of which declined over time (2)[B].

MEDICATION
- There are currently seven FDA-approved medications: nicotine replacement therapy (NRT), both long-acting (i.e., patch) and short-acting (i.e., gum, inhaler, lozenge, nasal spray) types, and non-NRT meds, bupropion SR and varenicline.
- With few exceptions, the choice of a first-line medication depends on patient preference.
- Duration of nicotine addiction controller therapy is strongly recommended to be >12 weeks (3).
- Varenicline (RR, 2.27 [95% CI 2.02–2.55]) is a nicotinic acetylcholine partial agonist (pregnancy Category C). It is probably the single most effective pharmacologic intervention for smoking cessation. Contraindications: known history of skin reactions or hypersensitivity. Associated neuropsychiatric symptoms may include vivid dreams, sleepwalking, depression, suicidal ideation/attempts in patients with and without preexisting psychiatric conditions—close monitoring recommended.
  - Starter pack: 0.5 mg/day for 3 days, 0.5 mg BID for 4 days, 1 mg/day starting day 7
  - Maintenance pack of 1 mg BID for 12 weeks; if successful, may continue for another 12 weeks
  - Varenicline is strongly recommended over nicotine patch or bupropion monotherapy (3).
  - Varenicline + NRT is more effective at 6 months than varenicline alone (NNT 6) (3).
  - Clinicians should start varenicline in adults even if there are not yet ready to quit (3).
- Varenicline + bupropion is not more effective than either alone and confers increased side effects.
- Bupropion SR (RR, 1.62 [95% CI 1.49–1.76]) is an atypical antidepressant and norepinephrine-dopamine reuptake inhibitor (pregnancy Category C). Contraindications: history of seizure, stroke, brain injury, brain tumors, anorexia/bulimia, recent use of MAOI (within 14 days)
  - Start 1 week before target quit date due to time needed to reach steady state.
  - Use 150 mg/day for 3 days and then 150 mg BID for 7 to 12 weeks.
- Nortriptyline (off-label use) is a tricyclic antidepressant (pregnancy Category D). Contraindications: narrow-angle glaucoma, heart disease (CAD, heart block, long QT)
  - Start 25 mg/day, gradually increase to 75 to 100 mg/day and continue for 12 weeks.
  - Set quit date 2 to 4 weeks after initiation.
- NRT (RR, 1.60 [95% CI 1.53–1.68]) (Gum: pregnancy Category C. All other formulations are Category D.)
  - Patch: For <10 cigarettes per day or <2 cans per pouches of smokeless tobacco, start with 14 mg/day for 6 weeks and then 7 mg/day for 2 weeks;

for 10 to 29 cigarettes per day or 2 to 3 cans per pouches of tobacco, start 21 mg/day for 6 weeks, then 14 mg/day for 2 weeks, and then 7 mg/day for 2 weeks; for 30 to 39 cigarettes per day or 3+ pouches per cans of tobacco, start 35 mg (21 mg/day + 14 mg/day patch) for 4 weeks and then 21 mg/day for 2 weeks, 14 mg/day for 2 weeks, 7 mg/day for 2 weeks; for 40+ cigarettes per day, start 42 mg (21 mg/day patch for 2 weeks) for 4 weeks and then 21 mg/day for 2 weeks, 14 mg/day, 7 mg/day for 2 weeks. Extending use of the patch beyond 8 to 10 weeks may improve abstinence rates.
  – Gum: For >25 cigarettes per day, start 4 mg gum q1–2h for 6 weeks; for <25 cigarettes per day, start 2 mg gum q1–2h for 6 weeks; then double dosing interval every 3 weeks (i.e., q2–4h and then q4–8h). Chew then tuck between cheek and gingiva once nicotine flavor is released, repeat for up to 30 minutes and then discard. Avoid using with acidic foods (i.e., coffee, soda), which decrease nicotine absorption.
  – Lozenges: For patients who smoke their first cigarette within 30 minutes of waking, start 4 mg lozenge PO q1–2h for 6 weeks; if first cigarette >30 minutes after waking, start 2 mg lozenge PO q1–2h for 6 weeks; then double dosing interval every 3 weeks (i.e., q2–4h and then q4–8h).
  – Nasal spray: Start 1 to 2 sprays (0.5 mg per spray) each nostril q1h for 8 weeks and then taper; max 10 sprays per hour and 80 sprays per day
  – Inhaler: 6 to 16 cartridges inhaled (4 mg per cartridge) per day for 6 to 12 weeks and then taper; incorporates the behavioral and sensory aspects of smoking
- Combination NRT: All forms of NRT increase quit rate 50–70% (4)[A]. Combining long-acting maintenance with short-acting breakthrough NRTs is more effective than using any single method alone. If combining patch with lozenge or gum, limit to one to three 2 mg. Avoid combined NRT use for patients with serious arrhythmias, unstable angina, MI within the prior 2 weeks, or those age <18 years old.
- E-cigarette is an electronic device that delivers aerosolized liquid with or without nicotine and includes various flavorings and other chemicals. Insufficient evidence exists regarding this product's safety and efficacy. Low-quality evidence suggests that e-cigarettes can help patients cut down on the number of cigarettes smoked but not nicotine consumption. Other research demonstrates poor efficacy of abstinence with long-term follow-up. Long-term safety has not been established (5).

Pregnancy Considerations
- Tobacco cessation prior to 15 weeks' gestation provides the greatest benefit for both the woman and fetus, but quitting any time is beneficial.
- ACOG recommends that pregnant and breastfeeding women be offered behavioral therapy and education as first-line treatment. NRT and medications should be reserved for patients in need of additional assistance given limited safety data.
- NRT is metabolized faster in pregnant women, which may lead to higher dose requirements.
- Pregnant women may perceive e-cigarettes to be safer than conventional cigarettes; however, given limited evidence regarding this NRT and concerns regarding fetal nicotine exposure, e-cigarettes are not recommended in pregnancy.

Pediatric Considerations
- Behavioral therapy (including CBT) is recommended as first-line treatment. There is evidence that group counseling is superior to individual counseling and group messaging for tobacco cessation in youth (RR, 1.35 [95% CI 1.03–1.77]) (6)[A].

- There are currently no FDA-approved pharmacologic treatments for youth.
- AAP recommends using NRT only for youth with moderate to severe substance use disorder.
- Risk of long-term addiction is much higher when smoking is initiated in adolescence than later in life, likely reflecting changes induced by nicotine in the developing brain. The biology of addiction, including withdrawal, occurs with fewer daily cigarettes in teens than in adults. Explanation of these biologic factors may help adolescents to stop or defer smoking.
- E-cigarette use in adolescents is reliably associated with subsequent smoking. An intervention to reduce smoking initiation was found to reduce the likelihood of ever smoking, suggesting there is a role for interventions to reduce smoking initiation even in adolescents who use e-cigarettes.

COMPLEMENTARY & ALTERNATIVE MEDICINE
- Acupuncture: no consistent evidence of efficacy
- Hypnotherapy: no consistent evidence of efficacy

ADMISSION, INPATIENT, AND NURSING CONSIDERATIONS
- Consider NRT for inpatients who use nicotine to decrease withdrawal symptoms (use with caution in patients with unstable angina, serious arrhythmias, or MI within the previous 2 weeks).
- Bupropion may not adequately control acute withdrawal symptoms.

ONGOING CARE

FOLLOW-UP RECOMMENDATIONS
- Patients who have initiated therapy should follow up after 1 to 2 weeks to monitor response and side effects.
- Monitor for signs of nicotine withdrawal syndrome and start medication-assisted treatment or adjust dosage:
  – Increased appetite/weight gain (4 to 5 kg over 10 years)
  – Dysphoric, depressed mood, or anhedonia
  – Insomnia
  – Irritability, frustration, or anger
  – Anxiety
  – Difficulty concentrating
  – Restlessness
- Follow-up should continue periodically in person or via telephone, especially during the first 3 months.
- Pharmacotherapy is generally recommended for 2 to 3 months duration.

PATIENT EDUCATION
- http://smokefree.gov
- http://women.smokefree.gov/
- http://teen.smokefree.gov
- http://www.nicotine-anonymous.org
- 1-800-QUIT-NOW (1-800-784-8669)

PROGNOSIS
- Roughly 50% of all smokers will die from a tobacco-related illness.
- Former smokers have a 50% reduction in risk of CAD 1 year after quitting, a 50% reduction in head and neck cancers by 2 to 5 years, and a 50% reduction in lung cancer mortality by 10 years. The risk of stroke is reduced to that of nonsmokers 2 to 5 years after quitting.
- 22% of smokers relapse within 3 months of quitting. Multiple attempts are often required.
- Approximately 50% of women who quit smoking in pregnancy resume smoking by 6 months postpartum.
- Individuals receiving support from significant others are more likely to quit.

COMPLICATIONS
- Chronic obstructive pulmonary disease (COPD) (emphysema and chronic bronchitis)
- Cancers (i.e., lung, oral/pharyngeal, kidney, bladder, cervical, anal, squamous cell)
- Atherosclerotic disease
- Insulin resistance
- Periodontal disease
- Osteoporosis and hip fracture (in women)
- Peptic ulcer disease
- Delayed wound healing
- Pregnancy and neonatal complications (discussed elsewhere)

REFERENCES
1. Stead LF, Buitrago D, Preciado N, et al. Physician advice for smoking cessation. *Cochrane Database Syst Rev*. 2013;2013(5):CD000165.
2. Lindson-Hawley N, Banting M, West R, et al. Gradual versus abrupt smoking cessation: a randomized, controlled noninferiority trial. *Ann Intern Med*. 2016;164(9):585–592.
3. Leone FT, Zhang Y, Evers-Casey S, et al. Initiating pharmacologic treatment in tobacco-dependent adults. An official American Thoracic Society clinical practice guideline. *Am J Respir Crit Care Med*. 2020; 202(2):e5–e31. doi:10.1164/rccm.202005-1982ST.
4. Hartmann-Boyce J, Chepkin S, Ye W, et al. Nicotine replacement therapy versus control for smoking cessation. *Cochrane Database Syst Rev*. 2018;5(5):CD000146.
5. Malas M, van der Tempel J, Schwartz R, et al. Electronic cigarettes for smoking cessation: a systematic review. *Nicotine Tob Res*. 2016;18(10):1926–1936.
6. Fanshawe TR, Halliwell W, Lindson N, et al. Tobacco cessation interventions for young people. *Cochrane Database Syst Rev*. 2017;11(11):CD003289.

ADDITIONAL READING
- Centers for Disease Control and Prevention. Youth and tobacco use. https://www.cdc.gov/tobacco /data_statistics/fact_sheets/youth_data/tobacco _use/index.htm. Accessed September 25, 2020.
- Civiletto CW, Hutchison J. *Electronic Vaping Delivery of Cannabis and Nicotine*. In: StatPearls [Internet]. Treasure Island, FL: StatPearls Publishing; 2021. https://www.ncbi.nlm.nih.gov/books/NBK545160/.

CODES

ICD10
- F17.200 Nicotine dependence, unspecified, uncomplicated
- F17.201 Nicotine dependence, unspecified, in remission
- F17.203 Nicotine dependence unspecified, with withdrawal

CLINICAL PEARLS
- Nicotine dependence is a chronic disease and will often require repeated interventions and multiple cessation attempts.
- Follow-up is key to continuing engagement and providing additional support as needed.
- Treatments, including but not limited to medications, can significantly increase rates of long-term abstinence.
- No single type of medication is best; thus, the choice should be based on patient preference and risk factors for side effects.

NONALCOHOLIC FATTY LIVER DISEASE (NAFLD)

Jill T. Wei Doherty, MD • Anita Wong, MD • Daniel T. Lee, MD, MA

 BASICS

- A spectrum of fatty liver diseases ranging from nonalcoholic fatty liver (NAFL), to nonalcoholic steatohepatitis (NASH), to fibrosis and cirrhosis, not due to other cause of fatty infiltration of liver (such as alcohol use)
- Most common chronic liver disease in the United States and other industrialized nations; implicated in up to 90% of patients with asymptomatic, mild aminotransferase elevation not caused by alcohol, viral hepatitis, or medications

DESCRIPTION
- NAFL (1)
  - Reversible condition in which large vacuoles of triglyceride fat accumulate in hepatocytes
  - Liver biopsy: fatty deposits in cells without hepatocellular injury (no hepatocyte ballooning, no necrosis, no fibrosis)
  - ALT and AST normal or <3 to 4 times ULN
  - Minimal risk of progressing to cirrhosis or liver failure
  - Synonym: steatosis
- NASH: progressive form of NAFL (1)
  - Liver biopsy: fatty deposits in cells with hepatocellular injury (ballooning, acute/chronic inflammation, ± fibrosis); may be histologically indistinguishable from alcoholic steatohepatitis
  - ALT and AST elevated, generally <3 to 4 times ULN
  - 30% with NASH may progress to fibrosis over 5 years and may progress to cirrhosis, liver failure, and rarely hepatocellular cancer.
- NASH cirrhosis
  - Presence of cirrhosis with current or previous histologic evidence of steatosis or steatohepatitis

EPIDEMIOLOGY
- Most common chronic liver disease in industrialized Western countries
- Predicted to become the most frequent indication for liver transplantation by 2030 (2)
- Predominant age: 40s to 50s; can occur in children
- Predominant sex: male = female

Incidence
Estimates vary widely from 31 to 86 cases of NAFLD per 10,000 person-years to 29/100,000 person-years (1).

Prevalence
- United States estimate: 10–40%
- Present in 58–74% of obese persons (BMI ≥30); 90% of morbidly obese (BMI ≥40); 69–87% with type 2 diabetes mellitus; 50% with dyslipidemia (1)

ETIOLOGY AND PATHOPHYSIOLOGY
Primary mechanism is thought to be *insulin resistance*, leading to increased lipolysis, triglyceride synthesis, and increased hepatic uptake of fatty acids. Thus, there is an international momentum to rename this condition to metabolic-associated fatty liver disease (MAFLD).
- NAFL: excessive triglyceride accumulation in the liver and impaired ability to remove fatty acids
- NASH: multiple hit theory (insulin resistance, adipose tissue hormones, oxidative stress damage, genetic factors) that cause inflammation and act on liver parenchymal cells leading to steatohepatitis (3)

Genetics
- Largely unknown: some familial clustering and increased heritability
- NAFL: more first-degree relatives with cirrhosis than matched controls
- NASH: 18% with affected first-degree relative (1)

RISK FACTORS
- Obesity (BMI >30), visceral obesity (waist circumference >102 cm for men or >88 cm for women), hypertension, high triglycerides and low high-density lipoprotein (HDL) levels, metabolic syndrome
- Type 2 diabetes mellitus, cardiovascular disease, and chronic kidney disease
- Protein-calorie malnutrition; total parenteral nutrition (TPN) >6 weeks
- Severe weight loss (starvation, bariatric surgery)
- Organic solvent exposure (e.g., chlorinated hydrocarbons, toluene); vinyl chloride; hypoglycin A
- Gene for hemochromatosis/other conditions with increased iron stores
- Smoking
- Drugs: tetracycline, glucocorticoids, tamoxifen, methotrexate, amiodarone, antiretroviral agents for HIV, valproic acid, fialuridine, many chemotherapy regimens, nucleoside analogues
- History of cholecystectomy
- Increasing age associated with increased prevalence, severity, advanced fibrosis, and mortality

Pregnancy Considerations
Acute fatty liver of pregnancy: rare but serious complication in 3rd trimester
- 50% of cases are associated with preeclampsia.

Pediatric Considerations
- Pediatric NAFLD
  - Increasing prevalence of NAFLD among children parallels rise in pediatric obesity, with prevalence of 9.6% (1).
  - Vitamin E of possible benefit
- Reye syndrome: fatty liver syndrome with encephalopathy usually following viral illness

GENERAL PREVENTION
- Avoid excess alcohol: ≤2 units per day (men), ≤1 unit per day (women).
- Maintain appropriate BMI.
- Prevention and optimal management of diabetes
- Avoid hepatotoxic medications.
- HAV and HBV vaccination if not immune
- Pneumococcal and annual influenza vaccinations

COMMONLY ASSOCIATED CONDITIONS
Central obesity; hypertension; type 2 diabetes; insulin resistance; hyperlipidemia; preeclampsia in pregnancy; CVD and arrhythmias; hypothyroidism; hypogonadism; OSA (1)

DIAGNOSIS

- Routine screening not recommended because of lack of effective drug treatment and unclear long-term benefits of screening (2)
- Consider NAFLD in patients with asymptomatic aminotransferase elevations (1)[A].

- NAFLD has no distinguishing historical/lab features to distinguish from other chronic liver disorders.
- Index of suspicion is higher with risk factors, such as metabolic syndrome or obesity.
- May present as cryptogenic cirrhosis
- Noninvasive biomarkers of steatosis/fibrosis are not sufficiently reliable.
- Liver biopsy is the definitive diagnostic test but should only be considered if results will change management.

HISTORY
- Typically asymptomatic
- Possible fatigue and/or abdominal fullness
- Vague right upper quadrant pain
- History of medications, alcohol use, family history

PHYSICAL EXAM
Usually asymptomatic, but some signs may include:
- Liver tenderness
- Mild to marked hepatomegaly
- Splenomegaly
- In advanced cases: cutaneous stigmata of chronic liver disease or portal hypertension (e.g., palmar erythema, spider angiomata, ascites); jaundice

DIFFERENTIAL DIAGNOSIS
- Viral hepatitis
- Alcoholic liver disease
- Drug- or toxin-induced hepatitis
- Autoimmune hepatitis
- Celiac disease
- Muscle disease, if nonhepatic cause of elevated enzymes is possible
- Hemochromatosis
- Wilson disease
- Lipodystrophy

DIAGNOSTIC TESTS & INTERPRETATION
The diagnosis of NAFLD (2) requires:
- Evidence of hepatic steatosis by imaging or histology
- No history of significant alcohol consumption
- No competing causes to explain hepatosteatosis
- No coexisting causes to explain chronic liver disease

Initial Tests (lab, imaging)
- ALT and AST may be elevated.
  - Nonalcoholic, usually AST/ALT <1
  - If alcohol induced, usually AST/ALT ≥2
  - Nonspecific enzyme abnormalities may exist or may be normal with advanced cirrhosis (1),(3).
  - Level of enzyme elevation does NOT correlate with degree of fibrosis (1).
- Elevated ferritin (1.5 times normal)
- Elevated alkaline phosphatase, total/direct bilirubin
- Lipid abnormalities: elevated total cholesterol, elevated LDL, elevated triglycerides, decreased HDL
- If cirrhosis present: decreased serum albumin, elevated PT, thrombocytopenia
- Serum labs to exclude other causes of liver disease: celiac, α_1-antitrypsin, iron, copper, hepatitis serologies, anti-smooth muscle antibody, ANA, serum gammaglobulin (1)[B]
- Ultrasound (US) is first-line imaging: Fatty liver appears hyperechogenic (1)[B].

Follow-Up Tests & Special Considerations

Other modalities can help noninvasively quantify fibrosis by estimating liver stiffness, but no modality accurately distinguishes simple steatosis from steato-hepatitis (1).

- Clinical decision aids: NAFLD fibrosis score, FIB-4 index, APRI score (2)
- Serum biomarkers: enhanced liver fibrosis panel, FibroTest, HepaScore
- Imaging: vibration controlled transient elastography (VCTE) or FibroScan, acoustic radiation force impulse (ARFI), magnetic resonance elastography (MRE) (4)[B]

Diagnostic Procedures/Other

Liver biopsy: gold standard for diagnosis and prognosis—must have likelihood of changing management prior to biopsy (1)[B]

Test Interpretation

- The NAFLD activity score (NAS): used to grade diagnosis, based on three histologic features: steatosis (0 to 3), inflammation (0 to 3), and hepatocyte ballooning (0 to 2), for score between 0 and 8. NASH is very likely with scores ≥5 (3).
- Steatosis Activity Fibrosis: staging scale (0 to 4) based on degree of fibrosis (1),(3)

 TREATMENT

Emphasis on early management of metabolic risk factors, NAFLD associated with increased cardiovascular morbidity and mortality

GENERAL MEASURES

- Weight loss for those who are overweight or obese is the only therapy that has good evidence of benefits and safety. Aim for sustained weight loss (5–10% body weight) (1).
- Aerobic exercise 3 to 5 times per week for 20 to 45 minutes with reduced calorie intake/diet modifications (1)[B]
- Tight diabetes control (1)
- Treat metabolic syndrome—hypertension, dyslipidemia, and obesity (1).
- Avoid or limit alcohol consumption.
- Avoid hepatotoxic medications (1)[B].

MEDICATION

- Currently no definitively effective medication treatment to treat NAFL or NASH (1)
- Some promising agents include:
  - Thiazolidinediones (pioglitazone): improves liver histology, only use with biopsy-proven NASH (1)[B], can use in patients with and without type 2 diabetes mellitus
  - Vitamin E 400 to 800 IU daily: long-term safety concerns at high doses; only use with biopsy-proven NASH and those without diabetes (1)[C]
  - GLP-1 receptor agonists (exenatide and liraglutide). Early studies show benefit in patients with type 2 diabetes mellitus and NASH (2).
  - Pentoxifylline

- Agents that have shown +/− benefit:
  - Metformin
  - Ursodeoxycholic acid
  - Statins
  - Probiotics
  - Obeticholic acid (bile acid derivative)
  - Omega-3 fatty acids
  - Aspirin
  - Caffeine/coffee

ISSUES FOR REFERRAL

Refer to hepatology if persistent AST/ALT elevations, advanced fibrosis (stage F3 or greater) on liver scan, or fibrosis on liver biopsy (1)[A].

SURGERY/OTHER PROCEDURES

- Bariatric procedures: NAFLD is not a contraindication in eligible obese patients. There is a lack of data to definitively assess benefits and harms of surgery in treating patients with NASH (1)[B].
- Liver transplant: NAFLD is second most common cause for liver transplant; however, NAFLD will recur in the transplanted liver in 80–100% of patients.

 ONGOING CARE

FOLLOW-UP RECOMMENDATIONS

- Annual monitoring of LFTs (1)
- Surveillance with US or CT to evaluate for disease progression every 2 to 3 years or sooner if increasing metabolic risk factors
- Routine liver biopsy is not recommended but may be repeated 5 years after baseline biopsy if progression of fibrosis is suspected (1).
- Hepatic fibrosis staging is the strongest predictor for mortality in patients with histologically confirmed NAFLD (2).
- Screening for hepatocellular carcinoma in noncirrhotic NAFLD is yet to be determined (2).

DIET

Low in saturated and trans fat; low in simple carbohydrates; avoid excessive alcohol (protective or worsening effect of light/moderate consumption inconclusive).

PATIENT EDUCATION

Extensive counseling on sustained lifestyle changes in nutrition, exercise, and alcohol use.

PROGNOSIS

Within the spectrum of NAFLD, only NASH has been shown to be progressive, potentially leading to cirrhosis, hepatocellular carcinoma, cholangiocarcinoma, and/or liver failure.

- Cirrhosis develops in up to 20% of patients. Up to 42% of patients develop hepatocellular carcinoma without showing cirrhosis (3).
- Transplantation is effective, but NASH often recurs after transplantation due to ongoing risk factors.

COMPLICATIONS

Progressive disease may lead to decompensated cirrhosis and portal hypertension with complications such as ascites, encephalopathy, bleeding varices, and hepatorenal or hepatopulmonary syndromes.

REFERENCES

1. Chalasani N, Younossi Z, Lavine JE, et al. The diagnosis and management of nonalcoholic fatty liver disease: practice guidance from the American Association for the Study of Liver diseases. *Hepatology.* 2018;67(1):328–357.
2. Ando Y, Jou JH. Nonalcoholic fatty liver disease and recent guideline updates. *Clin Liver Dis (Hoboken).* 2021;17(1):23–38.
3. Borrelli A, Bonelli P, Tuccillo FM, et al. Role of gut microbiota and oxidative stress in the progression of non-alcoholic fatty liver disease to hepatocarcinoma: current and innovative therapeutic approaches. *Redox Biol.* 2018;15:467–479.
4. Miele L, Zocco MA, Pizzolante F, et al. Use of imaging techniques for non-invasive assessment in the diagnosis and staging of non-alcoholic fatty liver disease. *Metabolism.* 2020;112:154355.

ADDITIONAL READING

- Kumar R, Priyadarshi RN, Anand U. Non-alcoholic fatty liver disease: growing burden, adverse outcomes and associations. *J Clin Transl Hepatol.* 2020;8(1):76–86.
- Oseini AM, Sanyal AJ. Therapies in non-alcoholic steatohepatitis (NASH). *Liver Int.* 2017;37(Suppl 1):97–103.
- Spengler EK, Loomba R. Recommendations for diagnosis, referral for liver biopsy, and treatment of nonalcoholic fatty liver disease and nonalcoholic steatohepatitis. *Mayo Clin Proc.* 2015;90(9):1233–1246.

 SEE ALSO

Alcohol Use Disorder (AUD); Cirrhosis of the Liver; Diabetes Mellitus, Type 2; Metabolic Syndrome

 CODES

ICD10

K76.0 Fatty (change of) liver, not elsewhere classified

CLINICAL PEARLS

- NAFLD is a major cause of liver disease and is increasing every year with increasing rates of overweight and obesity.
- Spectrum ranges from NAFL to NASH, advanced fibrosis, and cirrhosis.
- NAFLD is the most common chronic liver disease in children; there has been a parallel rise in childhood obesity and NAFLD.
- Lifestyle changes with targeted weight loss are the cornerstones of therapy for NAFLD.

NONFATAL DROWNING

Tauhid Mahmud, MD, MPH • Amoreena Ranck Howell, MD, MSPH

BASICS

DESCRIPTION
- Respiratory impairment resulting from submersion in liquid (1)
- System(s) affected: cardiovascular, nervous, pulmonary, renal
- Synonym(s): submersion injury; terms such as "near drowning," "secondary drowning," and "wet drowning" should be avoided.

EPIDEMIOLOGY
Incidence
- From 2010 to 2019, an average of 3,957 fatal unintentional drownings in the United States (2)
- Three age-related peaks: toddlers and young children (1 to 5 years), adolescents and young adults (15 to 25 years), and the elderly (3)
- Nearly 80% of people who die from drowning are male (2).
- Black children ages 10 to 14 years drown at rates 7.6 times higher than white children (2).

Prevalence
- Most common injury-related cause of death for children 1 to 4 years in the United States (4)
- Second most common injury-related cause of death for children 1 to 14 years in the United States after motor vehicle crashes (2)
- For every child age <15 years who dies from drowning, 8 more children are seen in the emergency room for nonfatal submersion injuries (2).

ALERT
Proper water supervision and safety techniques are critical in avoiding morbidity and mortality from drowning.

ETIOLOGY AND PATHOPHYSIOLOGY
Hypoxemia via aspiration and/or reflex laryngospasm causing cerebral hypoxia and multisystem organ dysfunction
- 10–20% of victims drown without aspiration; likely due to prolonged laryngospasm
- Bathtub and bucket drowning in children <1 year
- Swimming pool drowning in children and young adults
- Motor vehicle accidents (vehicle submerged in water)
- Head trauma while swimming or diving
- Suicide
- Pulmonary: morbidity primarily caused by hypoxia. Aspiration causes dilution of surfactant with decreased gas transfer across alveoli, atelectasis, development of intrapulmonary right-to-left shunting; acute respiratory distress syndrome (ARDS); obstruction due to laryngospasm and bronchospasm
- Cardiac: hypoxic-ischemic injury and arrhythmia (primary or secondary)
- Renal: acute tubular necrosis from hypoxemia, shock, hemoglobinuria, myoglobinuria
- Neurologic: hypoxic-ischemic brain injury with damage especially to the hippocampus, insular cortex, and basal ganglia; cerebral edema
- Coagulation: hemolysis and coagulopathy

RISK FACTORS
- Inadequate physical barriers surrounding pools
- Alcohol ingestion; male sex
- Low socioeconomic status
- Use of illicit drugs
- Seizure disorder
- Inability to swim

- Hyperventilation prior to underwater swimming
- Boating mishaps and trauma during water sports, particularly when not wearing a life jacket
- Scuba diving
- Inadequate adult supervision of children; lack of appropriate instruction on how to swim
- Concomitant stroke or myocardial infarction (MI)
- Hypothermia
- Cardiac arrhythmias: familial long QT and polymorphic ventricular tachycardia (VT)

GENERAL PREVENTION
- Periodic education regarding proper supervision and drowning prevention for caretakers of young children
- Proper adult supervision of children, particularly around water
- Pool alarms, buddy system
- Knowledge of water safety guidelines
- Mandatory physical barriers surrounding pools; four-sided fencing, self-closing gate at least 48 inches above the ground (2)
- Avoid alcohol or recreational drugs around water.
- Swimming instruction at an early age
- Cardiopulmonary resuscitation (CPR) instruction for pool owners and parents
- Boating safety knowledge
- Personal flotation device and rescue equipment (e.g., preserver, if necessary)

Pediatric Considerations
Children should never be left alone near water. Young children can drown in very small amounts of water (bathtubs, buckets, and toilets).

COMMONLY ASSOCIATED CONDITIONS
- Trauma
- Seizure disorder
- Alcohol or illicit drug use
- Hypothermia
- Concomitant stroke or MI
- Cardiac arrhythmias: familial long QT and familial polymorphic VT
- Hyperventilation

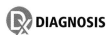

DIAGNOSIS

HISTORY
The revised Utstein-style approach provides a standardized template for evaluating drowning incidents and provides guidance for the history, physical exam, and appropriate management by categorizing information into core (considered important and feasible to be reported in most systems worldwide) and supplemental data (5):
- Victim information core data: (i) victim identifier—unique number or code; (ii) sex; (iii) age; (iv) incident date and time of day; (v) precipitating event; (vi) Was the face submerged at any time before or at the time of rescue? (vii) preexisting illness; supplemental: (viii) race/ethnicity
- Scene information core data: (i) water temperature, (ii) Who witnessed the drowning? (iii) Was bystander (non-EMS) CPR performed? (iv) Was bystander ventilation given? (v) Did a trained first responder perform CPR of ventilation only? (vi) Vital status at first trained responder assessment: Was the victim responsive? Breathing normally? Pulse palpable? (vii) Initial cardiac rhythm. Supplementary data: (viii) vital signs at first EMS assessment, (ix) pulmonary status at first EMS assessment, (x) type of water/liquid, (xi) body of water

- Time points and intervals from EMS Core data: (i) time face was first seen to be underwater, (ii) time victim was removed from water, (iii) duration underwater (submersion duration), (iv) time of first trained responder treatment, (v) time trained responder started CPR on scene, (vi) time return of spontaneous circulation achieved, (vii) time first conscious/awake, (viii) interval from face first submerged to first treatment/CPR

PHYSICAL EXAM
- Airway status and degree of respiratory distress
- Pulse: absent, weak, or normal
- Vital signs, including pulse oximetry
- Glasgow Coma Scale (GCS)
- Pulmonary: rales, wheezing
- Cardiac: rate, rhythm
- Neurologic examination

DIFFERENTIAL DIAGNOSIS
Syncopal event, head trauma, arrhythmia, seizure, MI, stroke, alcohol or other substance overdose, nonaccidental trauma

DIAGNOSTIC TESTS & INTERPRETATION
Initial Tests (lab, imaging)
Unnecessary if initial GCS and pulse oximetry are normal (and remain so for 6 to 8 hours). Otherwise consider:
- CBC with differential
- Arterial blood gas (ABG): hypoxia, hypercarbia, acidosis
- Electrolytes: hypokalemia, hyponatremia, hypernatremia
- Blood glucose: Increased levels may impair neurologic recovery after ischemic brain injury.
- BUN, creatinine: acute tubular necrosis
- ECG, cardiac monitoring, and serial troponin: MI
- Creatine kinase (CK) and urine myoglobin: rhabdomyolysis
- Coagulation studies: coagulopathy
- Toxicology screen
- Blood alcohol level
- Chest x-ray (CXR) unnecessary if all of the following:
  – Normal initial GCS and pulse oximetry
  – No evidence of respiratory distress
  – No change after 4 to 6 hours of observation
- CXR may show evidence of aspiration, atelectasis, pneumothorax, or ARDS in more severe cases.
- Head CT and/or C-spine imaging for trauma

Follow-Up Tests & Special Considerations
- Observe patients with an initial GCS of 15 and pulse oximetry >95% for 4 to 6 hours in the emergency department (ED) (6).
- CXR findings may be minimal or absent early on.

Diagnostic Procedures/Other
- Continuous cardiac monitoring and pulse oximetry
- Continuous core temperature monitoring if hypothermic
- 12-lead ECG
- Central venous pressure (CVP) monitoring for critically ill with hypotension refractory to IV fluids
- Electroencephalogram (EEG) if seizure suspected

TREATMENT

Early resuscitation and reversal of hypoxemia/acidosis are key.

GENERAL MEASURES

- Prehospital
  - Never approach a struggling victim alone.
  - Initiate basic life support (BLS) and advanced cardiovascular life support (ACLS) evaluation (7).
  - Rescue breathing may be helpful if the victim is in the water and cannot be removed; chest compressions not as effective while in the water and may harm the rescuer and the victim (7)[C]
  - Remove the victim from the water and begin effective resuscitation as quickly as possible (8).
  - Immediate CPR (airway, breathing, and circulation [ABC] sequence) (7)[A]
  - Start CPR if pulse is not definitely felt within 10 seconds, even in the hypothermic victim whose heart rate may be severely bradycardic (7)[C].
  - Routine cervical collar use and spinal precautions are not needed unless trauma is suspected (8)[C].
  - Supplemental oxygen and early intubation with mechanical ventilation, if needed (1)[A]
  - Rapid crystalloid infusion if there is hypotension that is not corrected by oxygenation (1)[A]
  - Ventricular fibrillation is rare in drowning, but if an AED is available, use during the initial resuscitation phase; AED use is not contraindicated in a wet environment (6).
  - If patient is breathing on his or her own and does not need spinal precautions, consider placing in the right lateral decubitus position to prevent aspiration of vomit or gastric contents (1).
  - Evacuate patients with abnormal lung sounds, severe cough, frothy sputum, foamy material in the airway, depressed mentation, or hypotension to advanced medical care (6).
  - An asymptomatic patient with normal lung exam can be considered for release from the scene if another person can be with them for the next 4 to 6 hours for symptom monitoring (6).
- ED
  - Oxygen, as needed, to maintain saturation between 92% and 96% (1)
  - Continuous positive airway pressure (CPAP), bilevel positive airway pressure (BiPAP), or intubation if supplemental oxygen alone is inadequate
  - If intubation is indicated, employ lung-protective ventilator settings (lower end-inspiratory airway pressures, lower tidal volumes of 6 mL/kg, higher positive end-expiratory pressures of 6 to 12 cm H_2O) to avoid barotrauma (7)[A].
  - Indications for intubation
    ○ Neurologic deterioration
    ○ Inability to protect the airway
    ○ Inability to maintain oxygen saturation >90% or PaO_2 >60 mm Hg on high-flow supplemental oxygen
    ○ $PaCO_2$ >50 mm Hg
  - Remove wet clothing and initiate rewarming.
  - Obtain core temperature to rule out hypothermia.
  - If hypothermic, rewarm with minimally invasive core techniques such as warm IV fluids, warm/ humidified oxygen, and external blanketing.
  - Active core rewarming only for refractory cases

MEDICATION

First Line

- High-flow oxygen, as needed (1)[A]
- For bronchospasm: aerosolized bronchodilator (4)[C]: albuterol (Proventil, Ventolin), 3 mL of 0.083% solution or 0.5 mL of 0.5% solution diluted in 3 mL of saline

- Vasopressors, as needed, for hypotension refractory to IV fluid resuscitation
- Prophylactic antibiotics are not recommended (1)[B].

Second Line

For pneumonia: antibiotics based on sputum or endotracheal lavage culture (1)[A]

ADMISSION, INPATIENT, AND NURSING CONSIDERATIONS

- Admit all symptomatic patients or patients with abnormal vital signs, mental status, oxygenation, CXR, or laboratory analysis.
- Monitor vital signs and reassess neurologic status, continuous cardiac, and pulse oximetry monitoring.
- After initial resuscitation, induce hypothermia with core temp maintained between 32°C and 34°C for 24 hours; may be neuroprotective for patients that remain comatose or have neurologic deterioration (1)
- Patients can be discharged from the ED after 4 to 6 hours if they have a normal mental status and respiratory function with no further deterioration (6).

ONGOING CARE

FOLLOW-UP RECOMMENDATIONS

Appropriate follow-up with primary care provider, orthopedic, neurologic, cardiac, pulmonary, and additional specialists as indicated

Patient Monitoring

- ABG monitoring, as indicated
- A pulmonary artery catheter may be needed for hemodynamic monitoring in unstable patients (4)[C].
- Intracranial pressure monitoring in selected patients (4)[C]
- Serum electrolyte determinations

DIET

NPO until mental status normalizes

PATIENT EDUCATION

Reemphasize preventive measures on discharge from hospital and educate parents regarding supervision and preventive practices.

PROGNOSIS

- 75% of drowning victims survive; 6% will have residual neurologic deficits (1).
- Patients with an initial GCS ≥13 and an oxygen saturation ≥95% have a low risk of complications and an excellent chance for a full recovery (1).
- Patients who are comatose or receiving CPR at the time of presentation and those who have dilated and fixed pupils and no spontaneous respiratory activity have a poor prognosis.
- Neurogenic pulmonary edema may occur within 48 hours of initial presentation.

COMPLICATIONS

- Early
  - Bronchospasm, vomiting, aspiration
  - Hypoglycemia, hypothermia, seizures
  - Hypovolemia, electrolyte abnormalities
  - Arrhythmia from hypoxia or hypothermia (rarely from electrolyte imbalance)
  - Hypotension
- Late
  - ARDS, pneumonia, lung abscess, empyema
  - Anoxic encephalopathy, barotrauma, seizure
  - Renal failure, coagulopathy, sepsis

REFERENCES

1. Szpilman D, Bierens JJLM, Handley AJ, et al. Drowning. *N Engl J Med*. 2012;366(22): 2102–2110.
2. Centers for Disease Control and Prevention. Drowning facts. http://www.cdc.gov/Homeand RecreationalSafety/Water-Safety/waterinjuries -factsheet.html/. Accessed January 12, 2021.
3. Peden AE, Mahony AJ, Barnsley PD, et al. Understanding the full burden of drowning: a retrospective, cross-sectional analysis of fatal and non-fatal drowning in Australia. *BMJ Open*. 2018;8(11):e024868.
4. Mott T, Latimer K. Prevention and treatment of drowning. *Am Fam Physician*. 2016;93(7):576–582.
5. Idris AH, Bierens JJLM, Perkins GD, et al. 2015 Revised Utstein-style recommended guidelines for uniform reporting of data from drowning-related resuscitation: an ILCOR advisory statement. *Resuscitation*. 2017;118:147–158.
6. Schmidt AC, Sempsrott JR, Hawkins SC, et al. Wilderness Medical Society Clinical Practice Guidelines for the Treatment and Prevention of Drowning: 2019 update. *Wilderness Environ Med*. 2019;30(4S):S70–S86.
7. Idris AH, Bierens JJLM, Perkins GD, et al. 2015 Revised Utstein-style recommended guidelines for uniform reporting of data from drowning-related resuscitation: an ILCOR advisory statement. *Circ Cardiovasc Qual Outcome*. 2017;10(7):e000024.
8. Sutherasan Y, Vargas M, Pelosi P. Protective mechanical ventilation in the non-injured lung: review and meta-analysis. *Crit Care*. 2014;18(2):211.

ADDITIONAL READING

Conover K, Romero S. Drowning prevention in pediatrics. *Pediatr Ann*. 2018;47(3):e112–e117.

CODES

ICD10

- T75.1XXA Unsp effects of drowning and nonfatal submersion, init
- T75.1XXD Unsp effects of drowning and nonfatal submersion, subs
- T75.1XXS Unsp effects of drowning and nonfatal submersion, sequel

CLINICAL PEARLS

- The most important treatment for near-drowning victims is prompt reversal of hypoxia.
- Water safety education (physical and behavioral modifications) helps prevent drowning.
- Encourage pool owners and parents with young children to become CPR certified.
- Patients remain at risk for ARDS for hours after submersion. All resuscitated patients require careful monitoring.
- Use lung-protective ventilator settings for intubated patients to prevent barotrauma.
- Patients with an initial GCS ≥13 and an oxygen saturation ≥95% have a low risk of complications and an excellent chance for a full recovery.

N

OBESITY

Justin Chu, DO • Jennifer Daily, MD

 BASICS

DESCRIPTION

- A serious, progressive, and chronic disease characterized by excess adipose tissue, typically quantified in adults by body mass index (BMI) (kg/m^2), $\geq$30 kg/m^2
- Overweight: BMI 25.0 to 29.9 kg/m^2
- Obesity is categorized into three classes:
  - Class 1 obesity is BMI 30.0 to 34.9 kg/m^2.
  - Class 2 obesity is BMI 35.0 to 39.9 kg/m^2.
  - Class 3 obesity (also called severe obesity) is BMI $\geq$40 kg/m^2.
- Obesity is associated with negative health outcomes. Abdominal obesity increases the risk of morbidity and mortality.

Geriatric Considerations
Aging is associated with changes in body composition including sarcopenia, decreased bone mineral density, and accumulation of visceral fat.

EPIDEMIOLOGY
Predominant age: Incidence rises in the early 20s and peaks at middle-aged adults 40 to 59 years old.

Prevalence
- 42% of U.S. adults classify as obese, and 68.5% classify as overweight or obese (1).
- 17% of children and adolescents (2 to 19 years old) in the United States are obese, and 32% classify as overweight or obese.

Pediatric Considerations
- The U.S. Preventive Services Task Force (USPSTF) recommends screening for obesity in children and adolescents $\geq$6 years old and refer them to comprehensive, intensive behavioral interventions (grade B recommendation).
- Pediatric classifications by age- and sex-specific WHO or CDC growth curves:
  - Overweight: BMI $\geq$85th to 94th percentile
  - Obesity (class I): BMI $\geq$95th percentile
  - Severe obesity:
    - Class II: BMI $\geq$120th percentile of the 95th percentile
    - Class III: BMI $\geq$140th percentile of the 95th percentile
- Obesity during adolescence is strongly associated with obesity in adulthood.
- Obesity in children is associated with mental health and psychological issues, low self-esteem, and impaired quality of life (2).

ETIOLOGY AND PATHOPHYSIOLOGY
- Multifactorial process where genetic, environmental, behavioral, and psychosocial issues lead to an imbalance between energy intake and expenditure
- After obesity has developed, an individual's neuronal signaling is altered to decrease satiety (3).
- Adipocytes (fat cells) produce peptides called adiponectin and leptin. Adiponectin improves insulin sensitivity and the absence of leptin has been associated with severe obesity.

Genetics
- Genetic syndromes such as Prader-Willi and Bardet-Biedl are found in a minority of people with obesity.
- Multiple genes are implicated in obesity and certain genotypes may account for differences in weight loss response following dietary changes (4).

RISK FACTORS
- Parental obesity
- Sedentary lifestyle and lack of regular physical activity
- Poor nutrition, especially consumption of calorie-dense food, and limited access to fresh produce/foods
- Stress and mental illness

GENERAL PREVENTION
- Encourage regular physical activity with a goal of at least 150 minutes of moderate activity per week (e.g., 30 minutes of exercise, 5 days per week), and a well-balanced diet with appropriate portion sizes.
- Avoid calorie-dense and nutrient-poor foods such as sugar-sweetened beverages and processed foods.
- Early preventive counseling, especially in children and young adults

COMMONLY ASSOCIATED CONDITIONS
- Type 2 diabetes, HTN, hyperlipidemia
- Coronary artery disease (CAD), congestive heart failure
- Obstructive sleep apnea
- Osteoarthritis
- Nonalcoholic fatty liver disease
- Mood disorders: anxiety, depression
- Polycystic ovarian syndrome

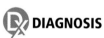 **DIAGNOSIS**

HISTORY
- Diet and exercise habits
- Reported readiness to change lifestyle and previous attempts at weight loss
- Life stressors, social support, and resources

PHYSICAL EXAM
- Physical activity vital sign
  - Assess if patient achieves minimum goal of 150 minutes of moderate physical activity per week.
- Waist circumference:
  - May be more important than BMI to assess obesity-associated health risks, especially in the elderly (sarcopenia)
  - Recommend measuring in patients with BMI 25 to 35 kg/m^2.
  - Measure at the level of the umbilicus. Elevated:
    - Male: >40 inches (102 cm)
    - Female: >35 inches (88 cm)
- Common abnormal findings: large neck habitus, acanthosis nigricans, striae

DIFFERENTIAL DIAGNOSIS
- Cushing syndrome
- Hypothyroidism
- Undiagnosed concomitant primary psychiatric disorder

DIAGNOSTIC TESTS & INTERPRETATION
- Screen for underlying physiologic causes as well as associated comorbid conditions.
- Fasting blood glucose, hemoglobin A1C, lipid panel
- Thyroid function tests
- LFTs (nonalcoholic fatty liver disease)

Follow-Up Tests & Special Considerations
Fatigue may be related to underlying obstructive sleep apnea and may warrant further investigation with sleep study.

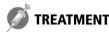 **TREATMENT**

GENERAL MEASURES
- Assess:
  - Motivation to lose weight and patient-specific goals of therapy
  - Nutritional intake and physical activity habits
- Goal is to achieve and sustain loss of at least $\geq$5% of body weight.
  - Weight loss is curvilinear with rapid weight loss at first and then slows until plateau.
- USPSTF recommendation: "Encourage clinicians to promote behavioral interventions as the primary focus of the effective interventions for weight loss in adults."
- Treat obesity-related comorbidities.

MEDICATION
- Guidelines suggest at least 3 to 6 months of non-pharmacologic treatment with comprehensive lifestyle intervention alone prior to starting medications.
- Consider pharmacotherapy in patients with a history of failure to achieve clinically meaningful weight loss ($\geq$5% total body weight) and to sustain lost weight in patients who meet the following criteria:
  - BMI $\geq$30
  - BMI $\geq$27 + comorbidities (e.g., CAD, diabetes, sleep apnea, HTN, hyperlipidemia)
- Meta-analyses of randomized trials comparing pharmacologic therapy with placebo demonstrated that all active drug interventions are effective at reducing weight compared with placebo (5).
- USPSTF found that pharmacotherapy combined with behavioral interventions was associated with greater weight loss and maintenance over 12 to 18 months than behavioral treatment alone (6)[A].

First Line
- There are 9 FDA-approved medications for weight loss (5 for long-term use and 4 for short-term use).
- The most common side effects are GI related (nausea, vomiting, diarrhea, abdominal pain), unless otherwise specified.
- Long-term treatment:
  - Liraglutide (Saxenda, Victoza):
    - GLP-1 agonist; preferred drug for patients with diabetes and cardiovascular disease; can be prescribed for adolescents $\geq$12 years old
    - Dose: 0.6 mg subcutaneously daily for 1 week and then increase at weekly intervals to target dose of 3 mg daily

- Semaglutide (Ozempic, Rybelsus, Wegovy):
  - GLP-1 agonist FDA approved for obesity in addition to diabetes
  - Dose: 0.25 mg subcutaneously once weekly ×4 weeks and then increase dose at 4 week intervals to a target dose of 2.4 mg once weekly
- Phentermine/topiramate (Qsymia) likely most effective medication available:
  - Phentermine reduces appetite through increasing norepinephrine in the hypothalamus, and topiramate reduces appetite through its effect on GABA receptors. Schedule IV medication.
  - Dose: phentermine 3.75 mg/topiramate 23 mg once daily for 14 days and then titrate up to 15 mg/92 mg once daily
  - Adverse effects: misuse potential, tachycardia, mood disorders, dry mouth; and topiramate is associated with fetal toxic effects (oral clefts).
- Orlistat (Xenical):
  - Inhibitor of pancreatic lipase that reduces intestinal absorption of fat and increases excretion; FDA approved for ≥12 years old
  - Dose: 120 mg 3 times daily with fat-containing meals
  - Adverse effects: GI (cramps, flatus, fecal incontinence, oily spotting); should be taken with vitamin supplements because of slight decrease in fat-soluble vitamins (A, D, E, and K)
- Naltrexone/bupropion (Contrave):
  - Naltrexone is an opioid antagonist that blocks effects of β-endorphins to reduce food intake. Bupropion reduces food intake by acting on adrenergic and dopaminergic receptors in the hypothalamus.
  - Dose: naltrexone 8 mg/bupropion 90 mg once daily for the first week and up titrate to a goal of 16 mg/180 mg twice daily by week 4
  - Adverse effects: increased blood pressure, dry mouth, headache, insomnia
- Plenity—oral hydrogel of cellulose and citric acid creates feeling of fullness. Taken twice daily, 30 minutes before lunch and dinner with at least 16 oz of water; relatively inexpensive

Second Line
- Short-term use medications (<12 weeks) are older, sympathomimetic drugs that reduce food intake by causing early satiety. Adverse effects include increase in heart rate, blood pressure, insomnia, and dry mouth.
  - Phentermine (schedule IV medication)
    - Dose: 15.0 to 37.5 mg daily or divided twice daily
  - Diethylpropion (schedule IV medication)
    - Dose: 25 mg 3 to 4 times daily before meals
  - Benzphetamine (schedule III medication)
    - Dose: Start at 25 mg once daily and may titrate up to max dose of 50 mg 3 times daily.
  - Phendimetrazine (schedule III medication)
    - Dose: 17.5 to 35.0 mg 2 or 3 times daily taken 1 hour before meals

ADDITIONAL THERAPIES
- Physical activity
  - Results in additional 1.0 to 1.5 kg weight loss over 1 year in addition to dietary intervention alone (7)
  - Aerobic versus resistance or high intensity versus low intensity does not seem to affect overall weight loss.

- Cognitive-behavioral therapy (CBT)
  - Components: (i) prescription of a moderately reduced calorie diet, (ii) program of increased physical activity, and (iii) behavioral strategies to facilitate adherence to diet and activity recommendations
  - Most effective in-person with high intensity (≥14 sessions in 6 months) by a trained interventionist

SURGERY/OTHER PROCEDURES
- A referral for bariatric surgery is considered when other treatments have failed, BMI ≥35 + comorbidities, or BMI ≥40.
- Associated with significant improvement in diabetes, sleep apnea, quality of life, depression, pain, and physical function (8)
- Requires complex presurgical evaluation and follow-up in a skilled treatment center
- Surgical procedures include biliopancreatic diversion, Roux-en-Y gastric bypass, sleeve gastrectomy, laparoscopic adjustable gastric banding, vagal blocking therapy, and gastric aspiration (AspireAssist).

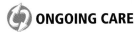 ONGOING CARE

FOLLOW-UP RECOMMENDATIONS
- Continue to discuss weight, lifestyle modifications, and address both current and new goals.
- A new treatment plan should be implemented if no clinical meaningful weight loss after 3 to 4 months.

DIET
- Long-term studies suggest net calorie reduction (~500 kcal/day) with a diet that a patient can adhere to is the best. Goal for women: 1,200 to 1,500 kcal/day, men: 1,500 to 1,800 kcal/day
  - A reduction of 500 kcal/day can result in ~1 lb (0.45 kg) weight loss per week.
- Very low calorie diet (200 to 800 kcal/day)
  - Produced significantly greater short-term weight loss but had similar long-term weight loss compared to low-calorie diets; requires medical supervision
- Mediterranean
  - Primarily plant-based foods, olive oil, nuts, legumes, whole grain, fruits, and vegetables; fish and poultry multiple times per week
  - Meta-analysis showed decrease in bodyweight, BMI, hemoglobin A1C, fasting glucose, and cardiovascular disease risk.
- Balanced-nutrient, moderate calorie
  - Usually 1,200 to 1,800 kcal/day; e.g., DASH diet
  - Based on MyPyramid food guide with emphasis on low saturated fat and ample fruits, vegetables, and fiber

PATIENT EDUCATION
Recommended website for FDA nutritional content in common foods: www.nal.usda.gov/fnic/foodcomp/search

PROGNOSIS
- Patients who are obese compared to those with a normal weight are at an increased risk for many serious health conditions.
- Patient motivation is associated with successful weight loss.

COMPLICATIONS
- Cardiovascular disease
- Osteoarthritis
- Hypoventilation syndrome
- Slipped capital femoral epiphysis (SCFE) in children
- Higher death rates from cancer: colon, breast, prostate, endometrial, gallbladder, liver, kidney

REFERENCES

1. Ogden CL, Carroll MD, Flegal KM. Prevalence of obesity in the United States. *JAMA*. 2014;312(2):189–190.
2. Grossman DC, Bibbins-Domingo K, Curry SJ, et al; for U.S. Preventive Services Task Force. Screening for obesity in children and adolescents: US Preventive Services Task Force recommendation statement. *JAMA*. 2017;317(23):2417–2426.
3. Curry SJ, Krist AH, Owens DK, et al; for U.S. Preventive Services Task Force. Behavioral weight loss interventions to prevent obesity-related morbidity and mortality in adults: US Preventive Services Task Force recommendation statement. *JAMA*. 2018;320(11):1163–1171.
4. Bray GA, Heisel WE, Afshin A, et al. The science of obesity management: an Endocrine Society scientific statement. *Endocr Rev*. 2018;39(2):79–132.
5. Khera R, Murad MH, Chandar AK, et al. Association of pharmacological treatments for obesity with weight loss and adverse events: a systematic review and meta-analysis. *JAMA*. 2016;315(22):2424–2434.
6. Yanovski SZ. Weight management in adults with obesity: what is a primary care clinician to do? *JAMA*. 2018;320(11):1111–1113.
7. Bray GA, Frühbeck G, Ryan DH, et al. Management of obesity. *Lancet*. 2016;387(10031):1947–1956.
8. LeBlanc EL, Patnode CD, Webber EM, et al. *Behavioral and Pharmacotherapy Weight Loss Interventions to Prevent Obesity-Related Morbidity and Mortality in Adults: An Updated Systematic Review for the U.S. Preventive Services Task Force* [Internet]. Rockville, MD: Agency for Healthcare Research and Quality; 2018. Report No.: 18-05239-EF-1.

 CODES

ICD10
- E66.9 Obesity, unspecified
- E66.3 Overweight
- R63.5 Abnormal weight gain

CLINICAL PEARLS
- A majority of American adults are overweight or obese.
- Modification in dietary and physical activity patterns remains the cornerstone of therapy. Consider bariatric surgery in patients with a BMI >40 who have failed more conservative treatment, particularly if there are associated risk factors.
- Medication may be indicated when nonpharmacologic treatment for 3 to 6 months has been ineffective and the patient has a BMI >30 or a BMI >27 with associated risk factors.

OBSESSIVE-COMPULSIVE DISORDER (OCD)

Saeed Ahmed, MD • Huma Baqir, MD

 BASICS

DESCRIPTION
- An anxiety disorder characterized by pathologic obsessions (recurrent intrusive thoughts, ideas, or images) and compulsions (repetitive, ritualistic behaviors or mental acts) causing significant distress
- Not to be confused with obsessive-compulsive personality disorder

EPIDEMIOLOGY
Incidence
- Predominant age: mean age of onset is 19.5 years (1).
  - Three subtypes: child/adolescent-onset (<18 years), adult-onset (18 to 39 years) and late-onset (≥40 years)
  - Child/adolescent-onset in 50% of cases (usually by age 18 years) (2)
  - Diagnosis rarely made at >50 years of age
- Predominant gender: females > males
  - Childhood-onset obsessive-compulsive disorder (OCD) (age <10 years) is more prevalent in males, more likely to be heritable and associated with co-morbid tic disorder.
  - Adolescent-onset OCD is more prevalent in females, although OCD can be precipitated in the peripartum or postpartum period as well.

Pediatric Considerations
Insidious onset; consider brain insult in acute presentation of childhood OCD.

Geriatric Considerations
Consider neurologic disorders in new-onset OCD.

Prevalence
- 2.3% lifetime in adults
- 1–2.3% prevalence in children/adolescents (3)

ETIOLOGY AND PATHOPHYSIOLOGY
Exact pathophysiology/etiology unknown. Potential role of:
- Cognitive-affective dysfunction
- Dysregulation of serotonergic, catecholaminergic, and glutamatergic pathways
- Dysfunction of cortico-striatal-thalamo-cortical (CSTC) circuit, involving the orbitofrontal cortex (OFC) and anterior cingulate cortex (ACC)
- Brain injury (physical trauma, stroke, etc.)
- Autoimmune insult to basal ganglia, as seen in Pediatric Autoimmune Neuropsychiatric Disorder Associated with Streptococcus (PANDAS); controversial

Genetics
- Polygenic disorder, with variants in serotonergic, catecholaminergic, and glutamatergic genes
- Positive family history: prevalence rates of 7–15% in first-degree relatives of children/adolescents with OCD
- Greater concordance in monozygotic twins

RISK FACTORS
Combination of biologic and environmental factors:
- Family history of OCD
- Advanced paternal and maternal age
- Coexisting psychiatric disorders, most commonly anxiety disorders and schizophrenia
- Low serotonin levels (Antipsychotics with greater anti-serotoninergic mechanism, such as clozapine and olanzapine, have been associated with onset of OCD.)
- Brain insult (i.e., encephalitis, pediatric streptococcal infection, or head injury)
- Perinatal insults (birth complications)
- History of childhood traumatic events, including social isolation and physical abuse

GENERAL PREVENTION
- Early diagnosis and treatment can decrease patient's distress and impairment.

COMMONLY ASSOCIATED CONDITIONS
- Major depressive disorder
- Panic disorder/phobia/social phobia
- Tourette syndrome/tic syndromes
- Substance abuse/eating disorder/body dysmorphic disorder

 DIAGNOSIS

HISTORY
- Patients present with obsessions, compulsions or both, which cause marked distress, are time-consuming (>1 hr/day), and cause significant occupational/social impairment.
- Two criteria support the diagnosis of obsessions:
  - Presence of recurrent, persistent, intrusive and inappropriate thoughts, causing significant anxiety and distress
  - The individual makes attempts to suppress or neutralize such thoughts with some other thought or activity (i.e., by performing a compulsion).
- Two criteria support the diagnosis of compulsions:
  - Repetitive, rigid behaviors (e.g., hand washing) or mental acts (e.g., counting silently), performed in response to an obsession
  - Although aimed at reducing stress, the response is either not realistically connected with the obsession or is excessive.
- In children, check for precedent streptococcal infection.

PHYSICAL EXAM
The following may be observed in affected individuals:
- Chapped hands caused by excessive hand washing
- Hair loss caused by compulsive pulling/twisting of hair
- Weight loss from food restriction due to contamination fears

DIFFERENTIAL DIAGNOSIS
- Obsessive-compulsive personality disorder (traits are pervasive, often ego-syntonic and include perfectionism and preoccupation with detail, trivia, or procedure and regulation. Patients tend to be rigid, moralistic and stingy.)
- Impulse-control disorders, involving compulsive gambling, sex, or substance use
- Major depressive disorder (depressive ruminations, with themes of self-criticism, guilt, failure, and regret; without compulsion)
- Eating disorder (limited to ritualized eating behavior)
- Tic disorder and stereotypic movement disorder (Tics are often preceded by premonitory sensations and not aimed at neutralizing the obsession.)
- Schizophrenia disorder
- Generalized anxiety disorder, phobic disorders, separation anxiety (excessive worry/anxious rumination, but without compulsion)
- Hoarding disorder (difficulty discarding or parting with the possession; not secondary to obsession)
- Body dysmorphic disorder (concerns limited to physical appearance)
- Trichotillomania (limited to hairpulling)
- Excoriation disorder (limited to excessive skin picking)
- Paraphilic disorder (limited to sexual urges or fantasies)

DIAGNOSTIC TESTS & INTERPRETATION
According to *DSM-5*, diagnostic criteria for OCD is as follows (4)[C]:
- Presence of obsessions, compulsions, or both
- Obsessions are defined by:
  - Recurrent or persistent thoughts, urges, or images that are experienced as intrusive and unwanted, and that cause marked anxiety or distress
  - The individual attempts to ignore or suppress such thoughts, urges, or images or to neutralize them with some other thought or actions (i.e., by performing compulsion).
- Compulsions are defined by the following:
  - Repetitive behavior (e.g., hand washing, ordering, checking) or mental acts (e.g., praying, counting, repeating words silently) that the individual feels driven to perform in response to an obsession or according to rules that must be applied rigidly
  - The behavior or mental acts are aimed at preventing or reducing anxiety or distress or preventing some dreaded event or situation. However, these behavior or mental acts are not connected in a realistic way with what they are designed to neutralize or prevent or are clearly excessive.
- The obsessions or compulsions are time-consuming (e.g., take >1 hr/day) or cause clinically significant distress or impairment in social, occupational, or other important areas of functioning.
- The OCD symptoms are not attributable to the physiologic effects of a substance (e.g., a drug of abuse, a medication, or other medical condition).
- The disturbance is not better explained by the symptoms of another mental disorder (e.g., excessive worries, as in generalized anxiety disorder, preoccupation with appearance, as in body dysmorphic disorder or skin picking).
- Specify if:
  - With good or fair insight: The individual recognizes the OCD beliefs are definitely or probably not true or that they may or may not be true.
  - With poor insight: The individual thinks that OCD beliefs are probably true.
  - With absent insight/delusional beliefs: The individual is completely convinced that OCD beliefs are true.
- Specify if:
  - Tic related: The individual has a current or past history of tic disorder.

Diagnostic Procedures/Other
- Free-form interviews are the most common method for determining an OCD diagnosis, standardized interviews are generally used to supplement assessment and management.
- Yale-Brown Obsessive-Compulsive Scale (Y-BOCS) to assess severity of OCD and monitor progress (5).

Test Interpretation
- Common obsessive themes
  - Harm (i.e., being responsible for an accident)
  - Doubt (i.e., whether doors/windows are locked or the iron is turned off)
  - Blasphemous thoughts (i.e., in a devoutly religious person)
  - Sexual obsessions (i.e. unwanted, forbidden sexual thoughts)
  - Contamination, dirt, or disease
  - Symmetry/orderliness
- Common rituals or compulsions
  - Hand washing, cleaning
  - Checking, counting, ordering, arranging
  - Hoarding
  - Repeating

- Neither obsessions nor compulsions are related to another mental disorder (i.e., thoughts of food and presence of eating disorder).
- 80–90% of patients with OCD have obsessions and compulsions.
- 10–19% of patients with OCD are pure obsessional.

 TREATMENT

GENERAL MEASURES
- Cognitive-behavioral therapy (CBT) composed of exposure with response prevention and cognitive therapy is recommended as first-line treatment (3)[A].
- Five phases of treatment for CBT:
  - Family and individual psychoeducation
  - Cognitive training
  - Mapping OCD
  - Graded exposure and response training
  - Relapse prevention and generalization training
- Combined use of medications and CBT is most effective (3),(4)[A].
- Brain modulation available for severe OCD includes electroconvulsive therapy and transcranial magnetic stimulation in small groups of patients.

MEDICATION
First Line
- Adequate trial of antidepressants for at least 10 to 12 weeks
- Doses may exceed typical doses for depression.
- Dosing: usually high FDA-indicated dose or even higher
- Optimal duration for pediatrics unknown but recommended minimum of maintenance treatment: 6 months
- Varying degrees of efficacy between agents (3); no one SSRI is superior to the other.
- SSRIs are recommended first-line agents (3),(6),(7)[A].
  - Fluoxetine (Prozac)
    - Adults: 20 mg/day; increase by 10 to 20 mg every 4 to 6 weeks until response (20 to 80 mg/day).
    - Children (7 to 17 years of age): 10 mg/day; increase gradually every 4 to 6 weeks until response (20 to 60 mg/day).
  - Sertraline (Zoloft)
    - Adults: 50 mg/day; increase by 50 mg every 4 to 7 days until response; range: 50 to 200 mg/day; may divide if >100 mg/day
    - Children (6 to 17 years of age): 25 mg/day; increase by 25 mg every 7 days until response (50 to 200 mg/day).
  - Paroxetine (Paxil)
    - Adults: 20 mg/day; increase by 10 mg every 4 to 7 days until response (40 to 60 mg/day).
    - Children: Safety and effectiveness in patients <18 years have not been established.
  - Citalopram (Celexa)
    - Not approved by the FDA for use in OCD but used due to good tolerability, black box warning—max 40 mg/day due to arrhythmia risk
- Absolute SSRI contraindications
  - Concomitant use within 14 days of monoamine oxidase inhibitor (MAOI)
- Relative SSRI contraindications
  - Severe liver impairment; seizure disorder
- Precautions
  - Watch for suicidal behavior/worsening depression during first few months of therapy/after dosage changes with antidepressants, particularly in children, adolescents, and young adults.
  - May cause drowsiness and dizziness when therapy is initiated.

Pregnancy Considerations
All SSRIs are pregnancy Category C, except paroxetine, which is Category D.

Second Line
- Try switching to another SSRI.
  - 40–70% of patients show an adequate response to a trial of SSRI, with a remission rate of 10–40%.
- If no response, switch to tricyclic acid (TCA), clomipramine (Anafranil) or SSRI plus clomipramine or IV medications: clomipramine or citalopram.
  - Adults: 25 mg/day; increase gradually over 2 weeks to 100 mg/day and then to 250 mg/day (max dose) over next several weeks, as tolerated.
  - Children (10 to 17 years of age): 25 mg/day; titrate as needed and tolerated up to 3 mg/kg/day or 200 mg/day (whichever is less).
  - Absolute clomipramine contraindications
    - Within 6 months of a myocardial infarction (MI)
    - Hypersensitivity to clomipramine or other TCA
    - Concomitant use within 14 days of a MAOI
    - 3rd-degree atrioventricular (AV) block
  - Relative clomipramine contraindications
    - Narrow-angle glaucoma
    - Prostatic hypertrophy
    - 1st- or 2nd-degree AV block, bundle branch block, and congestive heart failure
    - Pregnancy Category C
  - Precautions
    - Pretreatment ECG for patients >40 years of age; potential arrhythmia (6)
    - Watch for suicidal behavior/worsening depression during first few months of therapy or after dosage changes with antidepressants, particularly in children, adolescents, and young adults.
    - May cause drowsiness and dizziness when therapy is initiated (6).

ISSUES FOR REFERRAL
- Referral for CBT (in vivo exposure and prevention of compulsions)
- Psychiatric evaluation if obsessions and compulsions significantly interfere with patient's functioning

ADDITIONAL THERAPIES
- Antipsychotic agents alone are not effective in treatment of OCD. They can be used to augment SSRI therapy for treatment-resistant OCD; however, they also can worsen OCD symptoms (6)[C]. Some evidence show that addition of low-dose quetiapine or risperidone to antidepressants will increase efficacy (6)[A].
  - Risperidone (Risperdal): initial dose: 0.5 mg/day; target dose: 0.5 to 2.0 mg/day for at least 8 weeks
    - Aripiprazole (Abilify): initial dose: 5 mg/day; target dose: 10 mg/day for at least 8 weeks
  - If no response still, consider switching to serotonin-norepinephrine reuptake inhibitor (SNRI), venlafaxine.

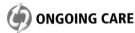 ONGOING CARE

FOLLOW-UP RECOMMENDATIONS
- Y-BCOS survey to track progress (5)
- Continue medication 1 to 2 years at full dose, the taper of 12–25% q1–2mo.

Patient Monitoring
Monitor for decrease in obsessions and time spent performing compulsions.

PATIENT EDUCATION
- International OCD Foundation: https://iocdf.org/
- Obsessive Compulsive Anonymous: http://obsessivecompulsiveanonymous.org

PROGNOSIS
- Chronic waxing and waning course in most patients:
  - 24–33% fluctuating course
  - 11–14% phasic periods of remission
  - 54–61% chronic progressive course
  - Suicide risk: elevated; 50% have suicidal thoughts.
- Early onset is a poor predictor.
- Few studies address how long to continue pharmacotherapy, although this is usually recommended for 1 to 2 years after remission is achieved.
- Discontinuation of medication is associated with high relapse rate (53% for those who switched to placebo compared to 23% on stable escitalopram) (6).

COMPLICATIONS
- Depression in 1/3 patients with OCD
- Avoidant behavior (Children may drop out of school; adults may become homebound.)
- Anxiety and panic-like episodes

REFERENCES
1. Fenske JN, Petersen K. Obsessive compulsive disorder: diagnosis and management. *Am Fam Physician*. 2015;92(10):896–903.
2. Goodman WK, Grice DE, Lapidus KA, et al. Obsessive-compulsive disorder. *Psychiatr Clin North Am*. 2014;37(3):257–267.
3. Skarphedinsson G, Weidle B, Thomsen PH, et al. Continued cognitive-behavior therapy versus sertraline for children and adolescents with obsessive-compulsive disorder that were non-responders to cognitive-behavior therapy: a randomized controlled trial. *Eur Child Adolesc Psychiatry*. 2015;24(5):591–602.
4. American Psychiatric Association. *Diagnostic and Statistical Manual of Mental Disorders*. 5th ed. Arlington, VA: American Psychiatric Association; 2013.
5. Goodman WK, Price LH, Rasmussen SA, et al. The Yale-Brown Obsessive Compulsive Scale. I. development, use, and reliability. *Arch Gen Psychiatry*. 1989;46(11):1006–1111.
6. Pittenger C, Bloch M. Pharmacological treatment of obsessive-compulsive disorder. *Psychiatr Clin North Am*. 2014;37(3):375–391.
7. Komossa K, Depping AM, Meyer M, et al. Second-generation antipsychotics for obsessive compulsive disorder. *Cochrane Database Sys Rev*. 2010;(12):CD008141.

 CODES

ICD10
- F42 Obsessive-compulsive disorder
- F42.2 Mixed obsessional thoughts and acts
- F42.3 Hoarding disorder

CLINICAL PEARLS
- CBT is the initial treatment of choice for mild OCD.
- CBT plus an SSRI or an SSRI alone is the treatment choice for more severe OCD.
- The majority of patients with OCD respond to first SSRI treatment.
- Improvement in symptoms, however, is often incomplete, ranging from 25% to 60%.

OCULAR CHEMICAL BURNS

Jonathan Tsui, MD

BASICS

DESCRIPTION
- Chemical exposure to the eye can result in rapid, devastating, and permanent damage and is one of the true emergencies in ophthalmology.
  - Alkali burns: more severe. Alkaline compounds are lipophilic, penetrating rapidly into eye tissue; saponification of cell membranes leads to necrosis and may produce injury to lids, conjunctiva, cornea, sclera, iris, and lens (cataracts).
  - Acid burns: Acid usually does not damage internal structures because its associated anion causes protein denaturation, creating a barrier to further acid penetration (hydrofluoric acid is an exception to this rule; see below). Injury is often limited to lids, conjunctiva, and cornea.
- System(s) affected: nervous, skin/exocrine
- Synonym(s): chemical ocular injuries

EPIDEMIOLOGY
- Predominant age: can occur at any age, peak from 20 to 40 years of age
- Predominant sex: male > female

Incidence
- Estimated 300/100,000 per year
- Chemical burns account for 11.5–22.1% of all ocular injuries.
- Alkali burns are twice as common as acid burns.

ETIOLOGY AND PATHOPHYSIOLOGY
- Alkaline compounds
  - Lipophilic compounds that penetrate into deep structures on disassociation into cations and hydroxide
  - Hydroxide causes saponification of fatty acids in cell membranes, leading to cell death.
  - Cation causes hydration of glycosaminoglycans, leading to corneal opacification and hydration of collagen, resulting in rapid shortening and thickening of collagen fibrils that leads to an acute elevation in intraocular pressure (IOP) secondary to shrinking and contraction of the cornea and sclera.
  - Long-term elevation in IOP may occur from accumulation of inflammatory debris within the trabecular meshwork.
  - Penetration into deep structures may also affect perfusing vessels, leading to ischemia of affected area.
- Acidic compounds
  - Anion leads to protein denaturing and protective barrier formation by coagulation necrosis forming an eschar. This more superficial mechanism of injury tends to have prominent scarring that may lead to vision loss:
    - Hydrofluoric acid is an exception. In its nonionized form, it behaves like an alkaline substance, capable of penetrating the corneal stroma and leading to extensive anterior segment lesions. When ionized, it may combine with intracellular calcium and magnesium to form insoluble complexes, leading to potassium ion movements and cell death. Once systemically absorbed, severe hypocalcemia can occur.

Sources of Alkaline and Acidic Compounds

Alkaline Compounds	Typical Sources
Calcium hydroxide (lime)	Cement, plaster, mortar, whitewash
Sodium/potassium hydroxide (lye)	Drain cleaner, airbags
Ammonia	Cleaning agents
Ammonium hydroxide	Fertilizers
Acidic Compounds	**Typical Sources**
Sulfuric acid	Car batteries
Sulfurous acid	Bleach, refrigerant
Hydrochloric acid	Chem labs, swimming pools
Acetic acid	Vinegar
Hydrofluoric acid	Glass polish

RISK FACTORS
- Construction work (plaster, cement, whitewash)
- Use of cleaning agents (drain cleaners, ammonia)
- Automobile battery explosions (sulfuric acid)
- Industrial work, including work in industrial chemical laboratories
- Alcoholism
- Any risk factor for assault (~10% of injuries due to deliberate assault)

GENERAL PREVENTION
- Safety glasses/goggles to safeguard eyes
- Safe handling training for occupational exposures

COMMONLY ASSOCIATED CONDITIONS
Facial (including eyelids) cutaneous chemical or thermal burns

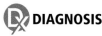

DIAGNOSIS

HISTORY
- Pain, photophobia, blurred vision, and foreign body sensation
- Chemical involved, duration of exposure, velocity of impact, and involved area
- In alkali burns, can have initial pain that later diminishes
- Mild burns: pain and blurred vision
- Moderate to severe burns: severe pain and markedly reduced vision

PHYSICAL EXAM
- Alkaline compounds may present with corneal opacification secondary to glycosaminoglycan hydration; however, severe acid burns may also present with this finding.
- Acidic compound may present with a ground-glass appearance secondary to superficial scar formation.
- Mild burns
  - Blurry vision
  - Eyelid skin erythema and edema
  - Corneal epithelial defects or superficial punctate keratitis
  - Conjunctival chemosis, hyperemia, and hemorrhages without perilimbal ischemia
  - Mild anterior chamber reaction
- Moderate to severe burns
  - Decreased visual acuity
  - 2nd- and 3rd-degree burns of eyelid skin
  - Corneal edema and opacification
  - Corneal epithelial defects
  - Marked conjunctival chemosis and perilimbal blanching
  - Moderate anterior chamber reaction
  - Increased IOP
  - Local necrotic retinopathy

DIFFERENTIAL DIAGNOSIS
- Thermal burns
- Ocular cicatricial pemphigoid
- Infectious keratitis
- Ultraviolet radiation keratitis
- Foreign body
- Acute angle glaucoma
- Conjunctivitis

DIAGNOSTIC TESTS & INTERPRETATION
Not necessary unless suspicion of intraocular or orbital foreign body is present. In this case, CT should be used—MRI is contraindicated.

Diagnostic Procedures/Other
- Measure pH of tear film with litmus paper or electronic probe:
  - Irrigating fluid with nonneutral pH (e.g., normal saline has pH of 4.5) may alter results.
- Careful slit-lamp exam, fundus ophthalmoscopy, tonometry, and measurement of visual acuity
- Full extent of damage from alkali burns may not be apparent until 48 to 72 hours after exposure.

Test Interpretation
- Corneal epithelial defects or superficial punctate keratitis, edema, opacification
- Corneal neurotrophic keratopathy
- Conjunctival chemosis, hyperemia, and hemorrhages
- Perilimbal ischemia
- Anterior chamber reaction
- Increased IOP

TREATMENT

Copious irrigation and removal of corneal or conjunctival foreign bodies are always the initial treatment and paramount to minimizing long-term sequelae (1),(2),(3),(4)[A]:
- Passively open patient's eyelid and have patient look in all directions while irrigating.
- Be sure to remove all reservoirs of chemical from the eyes via lid eversion.
- Continue irrigation until the tear film and superior/inferior cul-de-sac is of neutral pH (7.2 ± 0.1) and stable, testing every 30 minutes (1),(3)[A]:
  - Severe burns should be irrigated for at least 15 to 30 minutes to as much as 2 to 4 hours; this irrigation should not be interrupted during transportation to hospital (1),(3)[B].
  - Irrigation via Morgan lens (polymethylmethacrylate scleral lens) is a good way to achieve continuous irrigation over a prolonged period of time.

- Initial pH testing should be done on both eyes even if the patient claims to only have unilateral ocular pain/irritation so that a contralateral injury is not neglected.
- Use whatever nontoxic fluid is available for irrigation on scene. In hospital, sterile water, normal saline, normal saline with bicarbonate, balanced salt solution (BSS), lactated Ringer solution, Diphoterine or Cederroth eye wash may be used (5)[B].
  – Diphoterine or Cederroth eye wash has shown better patient comfort and healing but should not prevent prompt irritation if not readily available (2)[B].
- A topical anesthetic can be used to provide patient comfort (e.g., proparacaine, tetracaine).
- Sweep the conjunctival fornices every 12 to 24 hours to prevent symblepharon formation and adhesions (3)[C].

MEDICATION
First Line
- Further treatment aims to decrease inflammation and collagen degradation and aid in collagen synthesis and recovery of corneal epithelium. Selection depends on severity and associated conditions.
  – Topical prophylactic antibiotics: any broad-spectrum agent (e.g., bacitracin–polymyxin B ointment q2–4h, ciprofloxacin drops q2–4h)
    ○ Some experts suggest adding systemic tetracycline 250 mg PO q6h and especially derivatives such as doxycycline 100 mg PO BID may be beneficial to encourage healing and prevent corneal ulceration (1),(2)[C].
  – Tear substitutes: carboxymethylcellulose (Refresh Plus) drops q4h
    ○ Promotes reepithelialization, reduces recurrent erosion risk, and increases visual rehab (1),(2)[A]
  – Cycloplegics for photophobia and/or uveitis: cyclopentolate 1% TID or scopolamine 1/4% BID (3),(4)[C]
  – Topical corticosteroids for intraocular inflammation: prednisolone 1% or equivalent q1–2h for 7 to 10 days; if severe, prednisone 20 to 60 mg PO daily for 5 to 7 days. Taper rapidly if epithelium is intact, by day 10 to 14 (1),(3)[C]:
    ○ Using vitamin C in conjunction with steroids reduces incidence of corneal thinning, ulceration, and perforation (1),(2),(3)[A].
  – Vitamin C (ascorbic acid) 500 mg PO QID and topical 10% q2h ascorbate solution in artificial tears
  – Acetylcysteine (Mucomyst) 10–20% topically q4h may promote wound healing (1),(3)[B].
  – Ocular antihypertensives for IOP >30 to reduce risk of optic nerve damage: latanoprost 0.005% qhs, timolol 0.5% BID or levobunolol 0.5% BID, and/or acetazolamide 125 to 250 mg PO q6h or methazolamide 25 to 50 mg PO BID (2),(3)[B]
  – Bandage contact lens: Lenses with high oxygen permeability and hydrophilic properties aid in epithelial migration/adhesion and basement membrane regeneration (3),(4)[B].
- Precautions
  – Timolol and levobunolol: history of cardiac/pulmonary disease including bradycardia and asthma/COPD
  – Acetazolamide and methazolamide: history of nephrolithiasis or metabolic acidosis
  – Mannitol: history of HF, renal failure, or sickle cell
  – Scopolamine: history of urinary retention

  – Ascorbic acid: history of renal impairment
  – Tetracycline/doxycycline: Avoid systemic use in children <8 years old and pregnant patients.
  – Topical corticosteroids must be used with caution in the presence of damaged corneal epithelium because iatrogenic infection can occur. Use of corticosteroids >6 days may inhibit repair and cause corneoscleral melt (1)[B]. Daily follow-up or consultation with an ophthalmologist is recommended.
- Consider adjunctive treatments and corneal subspecialty referral in advanced cases.
  – Biologic fluids with consultation to ophthalmology: umbilical cord serum 20% q2–3h, autologous serum 20% q2–3h, platelet-rich plasma q2–3h, or amniotic membrane suspension 30–50% q1h. These consist of growth factors, vitamins, cytokines, and anti-inflammatory factors to improve dry eyes, reduce pain, persistent epithelial defects, recurrent erosion syndrome, and neurotrophic ulcers (1),(2)[B],(6).

SURGERY/OTHER PROCEDURES
- Goal of subacute treatment is restoration of the normal ocular surface anatomy, control of glaucoma, and restoration of corneal clarity.
- Surgical options include the following:
  – Debridement of necrotic tissue and inflammatory debris (1),(4)[A]
  – Conjunctival/tenon advancement (tenoplasty) to restore vascularity in severe burns
  – Tissue adhesive (e.g., cyanoacrylate) for impending or actual corneal perforation
    ○ Tectonic keratoplasty for acute perforation >1 mm
  – Limbal autograft transplantation for epithelial stem cell restoration
  – Amniotic membrane transplantation or umbilical cord serum drops to promote faster epithelial regeneration and improvement in visual acuity (1)[B]
  – Conjunctival or mucosal membrane transplant to restore ocular surface in severe injury
  – Corneal transplant (penetrating keratoplasty, anterior lamellar keratoplasty)
  – Enucleation for blind, painful eyes

ADMISSION, INPATIENT, AND NURSING CONSIDERATIONS
Based on ophthalmologic consultation, therapy compliance assessment, and concomitant burn injuries

 ONGOING CARE

FOLLOW-UP RECOMMENDATIONS
Patient Monitoring
- Depending on severity of ocular injury
  – From daily to weekly visits initially
- May be inpatient if concern for noncompliance or pediatric
- If on mannitol or prednisone, consider frequent serum electrolytes.

PATIENT EDUCATION
- Shield at all times during acute care
- Safety glasses
- Need for immediate ocular irrigation with water following ocular chemical exposure

PROGNOSIS
- Depends on severity of initial injury: increased limbal involvement in clock hours and greater percentage of conjunctival involvement correlate with poorer prognosis (Dua classification system)
- For mildly injured eyes, complete recovery is common.
- For severely injured eyes, permanent loss of vision is not uncommon.

COMPLICATIONS
- Orbital compartment syndrome
- Persistent epitheliopathy
- Keratoconjunctivitis sicca (dry eye)
- Corneal ulcer/perforation/scarring
- Progressive symblepharon
- Neurotrophic keratitis
- Cicatricial ectropion/entropion
- Glaucoma
- Cataract
- Phthisis bulbi
- Blindness

REFERENCES
1. Sharma N, Kaur M, Agarwal T, et al. Treatment of acute ocular chemical burns. *Surv Ophthalmol.* 2018;63(2):214–235.
2. Baradaran-Rafii A, Eslani M, Haq Z, et al. Current and upcoming therapies for ocular surface chemical injuries. *Ocul Surf.* 2017;15(1):48–64.
3. Singh P, Tyagi M, Kumar Y, et al. Ocular chemical injuries and their management. *Oman J Ophthalmol.* 2013;6(2):83–86.
4. Eslani M, Baradaran-Rafii A, Movahedan A, et al. The ocular surface chemical burns. *J Ophthalmol.* 2014;2014:196827.
5. Chau JP, Lee DT, Lo SH. A systematic review of methods of eye irrigation for adults and children with ocular chemical burns. *Worldviews Evid Based Nurs.* 2012;9(3):129–138.
6. Sharma N, Lathi SS, Sehra SV, et al. Comparison of umbilical cord serum and amniotic membrane transplantation in acute ocular chemical burns. *Br J Ophthalmol.* 2015;99(5):669–673.

 SEE ALSO

Burns

CODES

ICD10
- T26.50XA Corrosion of unsp eyelid and periocular area, init encntr
- T26.60XA Corrosion of cornea and conjunctival sac, unsp eye, init
- S05.00XA Inj conjunctiva and corneal abrasion w/o fb, unsp eye, init

CLINICAL PEARLS
- Prompt irrigation of all chemical burns, with any available nontoxic fluid on scene, even prior to arrival to the emergency department, is essential to ensure the best outcomes.
- All patients with ocular chemical injuries should have urgent ophthalmology evaluation.

ONYCHOMYCOSIS

Karl T. Clebak, MD, MHA, FAAFP • Matthew J. Kor, MD

BASICS

DESCRIPTION
- Fungal infection of fingernails/toenails
- Caused mostly by dermatophytes but also yeasts and nondermatophyte molds
- Toenails are more commonly affected than fingernails.
- Synonym: tinea unguium

EPIDEMIOLOGY

Prevalence
- Occurs in 2–10% of general population
- Predominant age: 20% in adults >60 years of age, 50% in adults >70 years of age (1)
- Rare before puberty
- Prevalence 15–40% in persons with human immunodeficiency infection
- Estimated 50% of all nail disorders in the outpatient setting (1)

ETIOLOGY AND PATHOPHYSIOLOGY
- Dermatophytes: *Trichophyton* (*Trichophyton rubrum* most common), *Epidermophyton*, *Microsporum*
- Yeasts: *Candida albicans* (most common), *Candida parapsilosis, Candida tropicalis, Candida krusei*
- Molds: *Scopulariopsis brevicaulis, Hendersonula toruloidea, Aspergillus* sp., *Alternaria tenuis, Cephalosporium, Scytalidium hyalinum*
- Dermatophytes cause 90% of toenail and most of fingernail onychomycoses.
- Yeasts, especially *Candida*, may involve fingernails (not uncommonly) or toenails.
- Dermatophytes can invade normal keratin, whereas nondermatophyte molds invade altered keratin (dystrophic/injured nails).

RISK FACTORS
- Older age
- Tinea pedis
- Occlusive footwear
- Cancer/diabetes/psoriasis
- Peripheral vascular disease
- Cohabitation with others with onychomycosis
- Immunodeficiency
- Communal swimming pools
- Smoking
- Peripheral vascular disease
- History of nail trauma
- Autosomal dominant genetic predisposition

GENERAL PREVENTION
- Keeping feet cool and dry
- Avoiding occlusive footwear
- Using sandals in public locker rooms and swimming pools
- Discarding or treating of infected footwear and socks (2)

COMMONLY ASSOCIATED CONDITIONS
- Immunodeficiency/chronic metabolic disease (e.g., diabetes)
- Tinea pedis/manuum

DIAGNOSIS

PHYSICAL EXAM
- Dermatophytes: commonly preceded by dermatophyte infection at another site; 80% involve toenails, especially hallux; simultaneous infection of fingernails and toenails is rare. Five clinical forms occur:
  – Distal/lateral subungual onychomycosis (most common): mainly due to *T. rubrum*. Spreads from distal/lateral margins to nail bed to nail plate; subungual hyperkeratosis; onycholysis; nail dystrophy; discoloration—yellow-white or brown-black, *bois vermoulu* ("worm-eaten wood"); onychomadesis
  – Proximal subungual onychomycosis (rare <1% of cases): hands/feet; leukonychia—begins at proximal part of nail plate, appearing to occur from the proximal underside of the nail (or direct invasion of the nail plate from above); spreads to nail plate and lunula; seen with immunosuppressive conditions
  – Superficial (formerly known as superficial white onychomycosis) about 10% of cases: infection of outer surface of nail plate, merging opaque white spots on nail plate eventually merge to involve entire surface of the nail, most commonly due to *Trichophyton mentagrophytes*
  – Endonyx onychomycosis involves interior of nail plate, sparing nail bed. Nail develops milky white appearance with indentations. Subungual hyperkeratosis is absent.
  – Totally dystrophic onychomycosis causes complete destruction of nail plate by fungus, resulting in thickened and ridged nail bed covered with keratotic debris.
- Candidal
  – Hands, 70% of all candida nail infections, especially for the dominant hand; middle finger is most common.
  – Pain is mild, unless secondarily infected. Increases on prolonged contact with water
  – Primarily affects tissue surrounding nail
  – Begins with cuticle detachment and produces white or white-yellow nail discoloration
  – Secondary ungual changes: convex, irregular, striated nail plate with dull, rough surface
  – Onycholysis, especially on hands. Distal subungual onychomycosis may occur.
  – Primary involvement of the nail plate is uncommon (thin, crumbly, opaque, brownish nail plate deformed by transverse grooves).
  – Periungual edema/erythema may occur (club-shaped, bulbous fingertips).
- Molds (nondermatophyte)
  – More common in those >60 years of age, more common in nails of hallux
  – Resembles distal and lateral onychomycosis

Pediatric Considerations
- Candidal infection presents more commonly as superficial onychomycosis.
- The U.S. Food and Drug Administration (FDA) has not approved any systemic antifungal agents for treatment of onychomycosis in children. Efficacy and safety profiles in children for some systemic antifungals are similar to those previously reported in adults (3).

DIFFERENTIAL DIAGNOSIS
- Psoriasis (most common alternate diagnosis)
- Traumatic dystrophy
- Lichen planus
- Onychogryphosis ("ram's horn nails")
- Eczematous conditions
- Hypothyroidism
- Drugs and chemicals
- Yellow nail syndrome
- Neoplasms (0.7–3.5%) of all melanoma cases are subungual. In a brownish yellow nail, if dark pigment extends into periungual skin fold, consider subungual melanoma.
- Alopecia areata
- Chronic paronychia
- Pemphigus vulgaris

DIAGNOSTIC TESTS & INTERPRETATION
- Accurate diagnosis requires both laboratory and clinical evidence. Diagnostic accuracy ranges from 66% to 75%.
- About 50% of nail dystrophy seen on visual inspection is not fungal in origin, so laboratory assessment improves diagnostic accuracy.
- A nail plate biopsy or partial/full removal of nail with culture is needed to diagnose proximal subungual onychomycosis.

Initial Tests (lab, imaging)
- Direct microscopy with potassium hydroxide (KOH) preparation from nail sample
- Cultures: False-negative finding in 30%; results may take 3 to 6 weeks.
- In-office dermatophyte test, medium culture indicates dermatophyte growth with yellow-to-red color change of the medium; results in 3 to 7 days; limited studies
- Histologic examination of nail clippings/nail plate punch biopsy: proximal lesions; stain both with periodic acid–Schiff (PAS) stain.
- Polymerase chain reaction (PCR) increases sensitivity of detection of dermatophytes in nail specimen; results available within 3 days can be used as complementary to direct microscope exam and fungal culture; not widely available
- Fluorescence microscopy can be used as a rapid screening tool for identification of fungi in nail specimens.
- Commercial laboratories may use KOH with calcofluor white stain to improve view of fungal elements in fluorescent microscopy.
- Discontinue all topical medication for at least 1 week before obtaining a sample.

Test Interpretation
Pathogens within the nail keratin

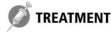

TREATMENT

GENERAL MEASURES
- Avoid factors that promote fungal growth (i.e., heat, moisture, occlusion, tight-fitting shoes).
- Treat underlying disease risk factors.
- Treat secondary infections.

MEDICATION

Pregnancy Considerations

Oral antifungals and ciclopirox are pregnancy Category B (terbinafine, ciclopirox) or C (itraconazole, fluconazole, and griseofulvin). Griseofulvin is not advised in pregnancy due to risks of teratogenicity and conjoined twins. Ideally postpone treatment of onychomycosis until after pregnancy.

First Line

- Oral antifungals are preferred due to higher rates of cure but have systemic adverse effects and many drug–drug interactions.
- Terbinafine: 250 mg/day PO for 6 weeks for fingernails and 12 weeks for toenails; most effective in cure and prevention of relapse compared with other antifungals and with itraconazole pulse in meta-analysis for toenail onychomycosis (4)[A]
- Alternative therapies for terbinafine resistant infections includes posaconazole, voriconazole, and itraconazole (5).
- Itraconazole pulse: 200 mg PO BID for 1 week and then 3 weeks off, repeat for two cycles for fingernails and three to four cycles for toenails; does not need to monitor liver function tests (LFTs) with pulse dosing
- Itraconazole continuous: 200 mg/day PO for 6 weeks for fingernails and 12 weeks for toenails (less effective than itraconazole pulse for dermatophytes, more effective than terbinafine for *Candida* and molds)

Second Line

- Fluconazole pulse: 150 to 300 mg PO weekly for 6 months; not FDA-approved for onychomycosis
- Griseofulvin: 500 to 1,000 mg/day PO for up to 18 months
- Posaconazole: 100, 200, or 400 mg once daily for 24 weeks; 400 mg once daily for 12 weeks; higher cost
- Topical agents: Use limited to disease not involving the lunula (proximal nail plate). Topical therapy does not cause systemic toxicity but is much less effective than oral therapy.
- Efinaconazole solution 10%, apply directly to affected nails once daily for 48 weeks; complete or almost-complete cure after 48 weeks in range of 15–18%
- Ciclopirox: 8% nail lacquer (available generically): Apply once daily to affected nails (if without lunula involvement) for up to 48 weeks; remove lacquer with alcohol every 7 days and then file away loose nail material and trim nails. Application after PO treatment may reduce recurrences; systematic review >60% failure rate after 48 weeks of use (6)[A]
- Tavaborole 5% solution, indicated for onychomycosis of the toenails due to *T. rubrum* or *T. mentagrophytes*; complete or almost-complete cure 15–18% after 48 weeks
- Contraindications for oral antifungals
  - Hepatic disease
  - Pregnancy
  - Current/history of congestive heart failure (CHF) (itraconazole)
  - Ventricular dysfunction (itraconazole)
  - Porphyria (griseofulvin)

- Precautions/adverse effects
  - Oral antifungals
    ○ Hepatotoxicity/neutropenia
    ○ Hypersensitivity
    ○ Photosensitivity, lupus-like symptoms, proteinuria (griseofulvin)
    ○ Chronic kidney disease (avoid terbinafine for patients with creatinine clearance [CrCl] <50 mL/min, decrease fluconazole dose)
    ○ CHF, peripheral edema, pulmonary edema (itraconazole)
    ○ Rhinitis (itraconazole)
- Ciclopirox topical: side effects: rash, nail disorders; avoid contact with skin except along nail edge; caution with broken skin or vascular compromise
- Oral agents: numerous significant drug–drug interactions; need to check each medication.

SURGERY/OTHER PROCEDURES

- Nail débridement to remove infected keratin. Use for few nails involved or if not, for candidate of systemic therapy.
  - Mechanical: File with abrasive stone or curette.
  - Chemical: Protect peripheral tissue with adhesive strips; apply ointment of 30% salicylic acid, 40% urea, or 50% potassium iodide under occlusive dressing.
  - Débridement may be combined with topical antifungal therapy.
  - Surgical avulsion if few nails are involved for pain control
- Laser treatment has shown some positive results but poor statistical power and limited efficacy or safety data (7)[A].
- Limited data with using photodynamic therapy using topical photosensitizing agents and irradiation
- Keratolytic agents including urea, salicylic acid, and papain applied to the nail prior to topical agents have been proposed as agents that enhance penetration.

COMPLEMENTARY & ALTERNATIVE MEDICINE

Melaleuca alternifolia (tea tree oil): Cochrane review found no evidence of benefit (6)[A]. Vicks VapoRub application to nails daily for 48 weeks has been found safe, but efficacy is uncertain.

 ## ONGOING CARE

FOLLOW-UP RECOMMENDATIONS

Formation of a new fingernail takes 4 to 6 months, and a new toenail takes 12 to 18 months.

Patient Monitoring

- Topical agents: Slow response is expected; visits every 6 to 12 weeks
- Terbinafine, griseofulvin: baseline, and as needed, LFTs and CBC
- Itraconazole continuous: baseline, and as needed, LFTs

PATIENT EDUCATION

Advise patient to: Keep affected area clean and dry, avoid occlusive footwear, wear absorbent socks, discard old sneakers, and avoid sharing nail implements and using on both infected and uninfected nails. Cure may not be attainable.

PROGNOSIS

- Complete clinical cure in 25–50% (higher mycologic cure rates) with oral therapy
- Recurrence is 10–50% (relapse/reinfection).
- Poor prognostic factors
  - Areas of nail involvement >50%
  - Significant proximal/lateral disease
  - Subungual hyperkeratosis >2 mm
  - White/yellow or orange/brown streaks in the nail (includes dermatophytoma)
  - Total dystrophic onychomycosis (with matrix involvement)
  - Nonresponsive organisms (e.g., *Scytalidium* mold)
  - Patients with immunosuppression
  - Diminished peripheral circulation

COMPLICATIONS

- Secondary infections with progression to soft tissue infection/osteomyelitis
- Toenail discomfort/pain that can limit physical mobility or activity
- Anxiety, negative self-image

REFERENCES

1. Stewart CR, Algu L, Kamran R, et al. Effect of onychomycosis and treatment on patient-reported quality-of-life outcomes: a systematic review. *J Am Acad Dermatol.* 2021;85(5):1227–1239.
2. Lipner SR, Scher RK. Onychomycosis: treatment and prevention of recurrence. *J Am Acad Dermatol.* 2019;80(4):853–867.
3. Gupta AK, Paquet M. Systemic antifungals to treat onychomycosis in children: a systematic review. *Pediatr Dermatol.* 2013;30(3):294–302.
4. Gupta AK, Ryder JE, Johnson AM. Cumulative meta-analysis of systemic antifungal agents for the treatment of onychomycosis. *Br J Dermatol.* 2004;150(3):537–544.
5. Gupta AK, Renaud HJ, Quinlan EM, et al. The growing problem of antifungal resistance in onychomycosis and other superficial mycoses. *Am J Clin Dermatol.* 2021;22(2):149–157.
6. Crawford F, Hollis S. Topical treatments for fungal infections of the skin and nails of the foot. *Cochrane Database Syst Rev.* 2007;(3):CD001434.
7. Ameen M, Lear JT, Madan V, et al. British Association of Dermatologists' guidelines for the management of onychomycosis 2014. *Br J Dermatol.* 2014;171(5):937–958.

CODES

ICD10

- B35.1 Tinea unguium
- B37.2 Candidiasis of skin and nail

CLINICAL PEARLS

- Psoriasis and chronic nail trauma are commonly mistaken for fungal infection.
- Diagnosis should be based on both clinical and mycologic laboratory evidence.

OPIOID USE DISORDER

Laurel Banach, MD • Pamela R. Tsinteris, MD, MPH

 BASICS

DESCRIPTION
Opioids are a class of medication that are commonly used for analgesia or pain relief with the concurrent potential for central nervous system (CNS) depression and/or feelings of euphoria. The diagnosis of opioid use disorder (OUD) refers to the misuse of prescription opioids or use of illicit opioids, such as heroin that may result in self-harm including death. OUD is considered a chronic illness.

EPIDEMIOLOGY
Prevalence
In 2018, an estimated 10,250,000 people reported opioid misuse (3.7% of population ≥12 years old)
- 2,028,000 of those reported a diagnosis of OUD (0.7% of population ≥12 years old) (1)

RISK FACTORS
- Prior history of substance use disorder
- More severe reported pain
- Co-occurring mental disorders (2)

GENERAL PREVENTION
- Opioid prescriptions have been reduced by 29% between 2006 and 2018, which reduces access to prescription opioids.
- Harm reduction practices can prevent complications from OUD such as clean needle exchanges and safe injection sites.
- Access to intranasal naloxone can prevent opioid-related deaths.

COMMONLY ASSOCIATED CONDITIONS
- Mood disorders
- Personality disorders
- Posttraumatic stress disorder (PTSD)
- Other substance use disorders
- Sexually transmitted infections
- Hepatitis A, B, C
- HIV

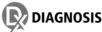 **DIAGNOSIS**

HISTORY
A majority of the diagnostic criteria can be obtained by history alone. Diagnosis of OUD is outlined in the *Diagnostic and Statistical Manual of Mental Disorders, 5th edition (DSM-5)* by exhibiting at least two of the following criteria in a 12-month period:
- Opioids are often taken in larger amounts or over a longer period than was intended.
- There is a persistent desire or unsuccessful efforts to cut down or control opioid use.
- A great deal of time is spent in activities necessary to obtain the opioid, use the opioid, or recover from its effects.
- Craving, or a strong desire or urge to use opioids
- Recurrent opioid use resulting in a failure to fulfill major role obligations at work, school, or home
- Continued opioid use despite having persistent or recurrent social or interpersonal problems caused or exacerbated by the effects of opioids
- Important social, occupational, or recreational activities are given up or reduced because of opioid use.
- Recurrent opioid use in situations in which it is physically hazardous
- Continued opioid use despite knowledge of having a persistent or recurrent physical or psychological problem that is likely to have been caused or exacerbated by the substance
- Exhibits tolerance
- Exhibits withdrawal

PHYSICAL EXAM
- Physical exam is of use for distinguishing between a substance use disorder and dependence. Numbers 10 and 11 from the diagnostic criteria, exhibiting tolerance and withdrawal, alone cannot be used for diagnosis of OUD because these represent signs of dependence. These signs may be exhibited on physical exam or found through history taking.
- Tolerance is either:
  – The need for increasing doses or frequency of opioid medication to achieve similar effect
  – Decreasing effectiveness with the same dose of prescription opioid
- Withdrawal is defined as the experience of pain or undesired symptoms with the absence of the opioid. Common undesired symptoms include sweating, restlessness, body aches, pupil dilation, tremor, anxiety, and diarrhea.

DIFFERENTIAL DIAGNOSIS
- Physical dependence on an opioid
- Disorders causing psychosis
- Mood disorders
- Effects of trauma including PTSD
- Another substance use disorder
- Polysubstance use disorder

DIAGNOSTIC TESTS & INTERPRETATION
One could make the diagnosis of OUD without additional testing; however, a medical professional may choose to obtain data from a prescription drug monitoring program or by urine or saliva drug testing.

GENERAL MEASURES
- Treatment mainstays include both medication-assisted treatment (MAT) and a variety of therapy interventions performed by trained professionals.
- Intranasal naloxone (Narcan) should be prescribed to all patients.
  - Family, friends, bystanders can administer in the setting of an overdose with a brief training.
  - Narcan reverses the effects of opioids causing respiratory and CNS depression almost immediately.
  - Narcan given to a person without experiencing an opioid overdose has minimal side effects.

MEDICATION
First Line
- Opioid agonists act by binding the opioid receptors stronger than prescription or illicit opioids. These medications include the following:
  - Methadone: a long-acting, full opioid agonist whose half-life allows for once daily dosing; available in an oral solution or tablet, methadone for maintenance MAT is only available at designated distribution sites but can also be used as a chronic pain agent.
  - Buprenorphine: available in transmucosal films or tablets as well as newer products including implants and injectable solutions; buprenorphine works as a partial mu-opioid agonist and is often paired with naloxone (Suboxone), to discourage abuse of buprenorphine
- Opioid antagonists are also a potential therapy and include naltrexone, which comes in both injectable and oral forms. As full antagonists, these medications have the potential to send patients into withdrawal if they have not been off of opioids for roughly 1 week.

ISSUES FOR REFERRAL
Pregnancy Considerations
- Will face challenges with pain management and potential for neonatal abstinence syndrome (NAS) in newborns
- The American College of Obstetricians and Gynecologists recognizes usual prenatal guidelines may need adjustment for women with co-occurring OUD and therefore may benefit from a provider with more experience caring for pregnant women with OUD.
- Newborns born to mothers with OUD even on MAT should be monitored by a provider trained in evaluating for NAS.

ADMISSION, INPATIENT, AND NURSING CONSIDERATIONS
Pain management is challenging with patients diagnosed with OUD or who have a history of opioid misuse and may require higher doses of opioid analgesia or alternative medications.

 ONGOING CARE

PATIENT EDUCATION
- All patients with OUD should discuss harm reduction practices to reduce chronic illnesses, including utilizing needle exchanges or pharmacies to obtain clean needles for injecting and intranasal or oral opioid use as opposed to IV administration.
- Intranasal naloxone (Narcan) prescriptions should be sent to all patients with OUD and close acquaintances.

PROGNOSIS
Mortality is high due to death by unintentional overdose and significant medical complications.

- In the United States in 2017, 47,600 died of an opioid-related overdose (age-adjusted rate being 14.9 per 100,000 people)
  - 43,036/47,600 were considered unintentional overdoses.

REFERENCES
1. Centers for Disease Control and Prevention. *Annual Surveillance Report of Drug-Related Risks and Outcomes—United States, 2019*. Atlanta, GA: Centers for Disease Control and Prevention, U.S. Department of Health and Human Services; 2019.
2. Kaye AD, Jones MR, Kaye AM, et al. Prescription opioid abuse in chronic pain: an updated review of opioid abuse predictors and strategies to curb opioid abuse: part 1. *Pain Physician*. 2017;20(Suppl 2):S93–S109.

ADDITIONAL READING
Kapman K, Jarvis M. American Society of Addiction Medicine (ASAM) national practice guideline for the use of medications in the treatment of addiction involving opioid use. *J Addict Med*. 2015;9(5):358–367.

 CODES

ICD10
- F11.10 Opioid abuse, uncomplicated
- F11.90 Opioid use, unspecified, uncomplicated
- F11.1 Opioid abuse

CLINICAL PEARLS
- Treatment includes both MAT and therapy interventions performed by trained professionals.
- Intranasal naloxone (Narcan) should be prescribed to all patients and close acquaintances.

OPTIC NEURITIS

Elyas Parsa, DO • Jose Alejandro Castellanos, MD

BASICS

DESCRIPTION

- Inflammation of the optic nerve (cranial nerve II)
- Most common form is acute demyelinating optic neuritis (ON), but other causes include infectious disease and systemic autoimmune disorders.
- Optic disc may be normal in appearance at onset (retrobulbar ON, 67%) or swollen (papillitis, 33%).
- Key features:
  – Abrupt visual loss (typically monocular)
  – Periorbital pain with eye movement (90%)
  – Pain in the distribution of the first division of the trigeminal nerve
  – Dyschromatopsia: color vision deficits
  – Relative afferent pupillary defect (RAPD)
- Usually unilateral in adults; bilateral disease more common in children
- Associated with multiple sclerosis (MS), presenting complaint (25% MS patients)
- In children, headaches are common.
- System(s) affected: nervous
- Synonym(s): papillitis, demyelinating optic neuropathy; retrobulbar ON

EPIDEMIOLOGY

Incidence

- 5/100,000 cases per year
- More common in whites than in other races
- Predominant age: 18 to 45 years; mean age 30 years
- Predominant sex: female > male (3:1)

ETIOLOGY AND PATHOPHYSIOLOGY

- In both MS-associated and isolated monosymptomatic ON, the cause is presumed to be a demyelinating autoimmune reaction.
- Neuromyelitis optica (NMO) IgG autoantibody, which targets the water channel aquaporin-4
- Viral infections: measles, mumps, varicella-zoster, coxsackievirus, adenovirus, hepatitis A and B, HIV, herpes simplex virus, cytomegalovirus, SARS-CoV-2 (myelin oligodendrocyte glycoprotein (MOG) antibody-associated ON and myelitis in COVID-19) (1)
- Nonviral infections: syphilis, tuberculosis, meningococcus, cryptococcosis, cysticercosis, bacterial sinusitis, *Streptococcus B*, *Bartonella*, typhoid fever, Lyme disease, fungus
- Systemic inflammatory disease: sarcoidosis, systemic lupus erythematosus, vasculitis
- Local inflammatory disease: intraocular or contiguous with the orbit, sinus, or meninges
- Toxic: lead, methanol, arsenic, radiation
- Medications: ethambutol, chloroquine, isoniazid, chronic high-dose chloramphenicol, tumor necrosis factor α-antagonist, infliximab (Remicade), adalimumab (Humira), etanercept (Enbrel)

Genetics

Genetics: Some people have genetic mutations that increase their chance of ON (i.e., MS) and several immune-mediated inflammatory diseases (IMIDs).

COMMONLY ASSOCIATED CONDITIONS

- MS (common): ON is associated with an increased risk of MS.
- Other demyelinating diseases: Guillain-Barré syndrome, Devic NMO, multifocal demyelinating neuropathy, acute disseminated encephalomyelitis

DIAGNOSIS

HISTORY

- *Decreased visual acuity*, deteriorating in hours to days, usually reaching lowest level after 1 week
- Usually unilateral but can also be bilateral
- Brow ache, globe tenderness, deep orbital *pain* exacerbated by *eye movement* (92%)
- Retro-orbital pain may precede visual loss.
- Desaturation of color vision (dull or faded colors), especially red tones
- Apparent dimness of light intensities
- Impairment of depth perception (80%); worse with moving objects (*Pulfrich phenomenon*)
- Transient increase in visual symptoms with increased body temperature and exercise (*Uhthoff phenomenon*)
- *Phosphenes*: fleeting colors and flashes of light (30%)
- May present with a recent flulike viral syndrome
- Detailed history and review of systems, looking for a history of demyelinating, infectious, or systemic inflammatory disease

PHYSICAL EXAM

Complete general exam, full neurologic exam, and ophthalmologic exam (with vision testing) looking for the following:

- Decreased visual acuity and color perception
- Central, cecocentral, arcuate, or altitudinal visual field deficits
- Papillitis: (1/3) swollen disc ± peripapillary flame-shape hemorrhage or often (2/3) normal disc exam
- Temporal disc pallor seen later *at 4 to 6 weeks* (2)[A]
- *RAPD*: The pupil of the affected eye dilates with a swinging light test unless disease is bilateral.

DIFFERENTIAL DIAGNOSIS

- Demyelinating disease, especially MS, the distribution and appearance of inflammatory lesions on orbital MRI have been reported to show significant differences between ON associated with AQP4-IgG-seropositive NMO spectrum disorders (NMOSD-ON), MOG-IgG encephalomyelitis (MOG-ON), and seronegative MS-ON (3).
- MOG-antibody disease (MOG-AD)
- Infectious/systemic inflammatory disease

- Acute papilledema (bilateral disc edema)
- Compression from a tumor/abscess compressing the optic nerve
- Temporal arteritis or other vasculitides
- Diabetic papillopathy

DIAGNOSTIC TESTS & INTERPRETATION

Initial Tests (lab, imaging)

- In typical presentations, erythrocyte sedimentation rate (ESR) is standard, but other labs are unnecessary. Antinuclear antibodies (ANAs), angiotensin-converting enzyme (ACE) level, fluorescent treponemal antibody absorption (FTA-ABS), and chest x-ray (CXR) have been shown to have no value in typical cases (2),(4)[A].
- In atypical presentations, including absence of pain, a very swollen optic nerve, >30 days without recovery, or retinal exudates, labs (CBC, ANA, rapid plasma reagin [RPR], SARS-CoV-2 PCR) may be indicated to rule out underlying disorders.
- MRI of brain and orbits to evaluate risk of etiology of ON from MS
- Lumbar puncture (LP): to evaluate cerebrospinal fluid (CSF) composition and oligoclonal bands (OCBs)
- CT scan of chest to rule out sarcoidosis if clinical suspicion is high

Follow-Up Tests & Special Considerations

- Optical coherence tomography (OCT) of the retinal nerve fiber layer (RNFL); a noninvasive imaging technique of the optic nerve; may serve as a diagnostic tool to quantify thickness of the nerve fiber layer objectively and thus, monitor structural change (axonal loss) of the optic nerve in the course of the disease
- Antibody testing: Serum NMO antibody testing is suggested for individuals with recurrent ON, particularly if the MRI brain is negative for any abnormal T2/FLAIR lesions outside of the affected optic nerve(s) (5).
- Visual field test (Humphrey 30–2) to evaluate for visual field loss: diffuse and central visual loss more predominant in the affected eye at baseline (2)[A]
- OCT of the optic nerve RNFL to detect and monitor axonal loss in the anterior visual pathways
- Low-contrast visual acuity (as a measure of disease progression)
- A blood test serum marker: *NMO-IgG* checks for antibodies for NMO

Diagnostic Procedures/Other

- In atypical cases, including bilateral deficits, young age, or suspicion of infectious etiology, LP with neurology consultation is indicated.
- LP for suspected MS is a physician-dependent decision. Some studies indicate that it may not add value to MRI for MS detection (2)[A], but no consensus on the subject exists.

TREATMENT

Most recover spontaneously.

MEDICATION

First Line

- IV methylprednisolone has been shown to speed up the rate of visual recovery but without significant long-term benefit; consider for patients who require fast recovery (i.e., monocular patients or those whose occupation requires high-level visual acuity). For significant vision loss, parenteral corticosteroids may be considered on an individualized basis: Optic Neuritis Treatment Trial (ONTT):
  - Observation and corticosteroid treatment are both acceptable courses of action.
  - High-dose IV methylprednisolone (250 mg q6h for 3 days) followed by oral corticosteroids (1 mg/kg/day PO for 11 days, taper over 1 to 2 weeks) (4),(6)[A]
- Others use IV Solu-Medrol infusion (1 g in 250 mL D_5 1/2 normal saline infused over 1 hour daily for 3 to 5 days):
  - No evidence of long-term benefit (6)[A]
  - May decrease recovery time (6)[A]
  - May decrease risk of MS at 2 years but not 5 years (6)[A]
- Discuss benefits and potential side effects of corticosteroids with patient (i.e., weight gain, osteoporosis, mood changes, gastrointestinal disturbances, hyperglycemia, insomnia).

ALERT

Avoid oral prednisone alone, as the primary treatment because this may increase the risk for recurrent ON.

Second Line

- Disease-modifying agents, such as interferon-β1a (IFN-β1a; Avonex, Rebif) and IFN-β1b (Betaseron), are used to prevent or delay the development of MS in people with ON who have ≥2 brain lesions evident on MRI (7)[B].
- *SOLIRIS® (Eculizumab)* is FDA approved for NMOSD in patients who are anti-aquaporin-4 (AQP4) antibody positive. The most common symptoms of NMOSD are ON and transverse myelitis.
- Vitamin D3 supplements for ON patients with low serum vitamin 25 (OH) D levels may delay the onset of a second clinical attack and the subsequent conversion to MS (8).

Pediatric Considerations

- Optic disc swelling and bilateral disease are more common in children as is severe loss of visual acuity (20/200 or worse).
- Obtain serologic marker for antibodies to MOG antibody (MOG-Ab) (9)
- No systematic study defining high-dose corticosteroids in children with pediatric ON (PON) has been conducted.
  - Consensus recommends: 3 to 5 days of IV methylprednisolone (4 to 30 mg/kg/day), followed by a 2- to 4-week taper of oral steroids
- Consider infectious and postinfectious causes of optic nerve impairment.

ISSUES FOR REFERRAL

Referral to a neurologist and/or ophthalmologist

ADMISSION, INPATIENT, AND NURSING CONSIDERATIONS

In acute visual loss, admit to expedite workup for initial diagnostic testing and referral to ophthalmology.

ONGOING CARE

FOLLOW-UP RECOMMENDATIONS

Patient Monitoring

Monthly follow-up to monitor visual changes and steroid side effects

PATIENT EDUCATION

North American Neuro-Ophthalmology Society (NANOS): http://www.nanosweb.org/files/Patient%20Brochures/English/OpticNeuritis_English.pdf (available in other languages)

PROGNOSIS

- Orbital pain usually resolves within 1 week.
- Improvement of visual acuity begins over 2 to 4 weeks and steadily continues over 6 to 12 weeks (10). Visual acuity often returns to normal or near-normal levels (20/40 or better) within 1 year (90–95%), even after near blindness.
- Other visual disturbances (e.g., contrast sensitivity, stereopsis) often persist after acuity returns to normal.
- Recurrence risk of 35% within 10 years: 14% affected eye, 12% contralateral, 9% bilateral; recurrence is higher in MS patients (48%).
- ON is associated with an increased risk of developing MS: 35% risk at 7 years, 58% at 15 years (11)[A].
- Poor prognostic factors:
  - Absence of pain
  - Low initial visual acuity
  - Involvement of intracanalicular optic nerve
- Children with bilateral visual loss have a better prognosis than adults.

COMPLICATIONS

Permanent loss of vision

REFERENCES

1. Benito-Pascual B, Gegúndez JA, Díaz-Valle D, et al. Panuveitis and optic neuritis as a possible initial presentation of the novel coronavirus disease 2019 (COVID-19). *Ocul Immunol Inflamm.* 2020;28(6):922–925.
2. Balcer LJ. Clinical practice. Optic neuritis. *N Engl J Med.* 2006;354(12):1273–1280.
3. Horton L, Bennett JL. Acute management of optic neuritis: an evolving paradigm. *J Neuroophthalmol.* 2018;38(3):358–367.
4. Vedula SS, Brodney-Folse S, Gal RL, et al. Corticosteroids for treating optic neuritis. *Cochrane Database Syst Rev.* 2007;(1):CD001430.
5. Petzold A, Pittock S, Lennon V, et al. Neuromyelitis optica-IgG (aquaporin-4) autoantibodies in immune mediated optic neuritis. *J Neurol Neurosurg Psychiatry.* 2010;81(1):109–111.
6. Keltner JL, Johnson CA, Cello KE, et al; for Optic Neuritis Study Group. Visual field profile of optic neuritis: a final follow-up report from the Optic Neuritis Treatment Trial from baseline through 15 years. *Arch Ophthalmol.* 2010;128(3):330–337.
7. Balk LJ, Cruz-Herranz A, Albrecht P, et al. Timing of retinal neuronal and axonal loss in MS: a longitudinal OCT study. *J Neurol.* 2016;263(7):1323–1331.
8. Derakhshandi H, Etemadifar M, Feizi A, et al. Preventive effect of vitamin D3 supplementation on conversion of optic neuritis to clinically definite multiple sclerosis: a double blind, randomized, placebo-controlled pilot clinical trial. *Acta Neurol Belg.* 2013;113(3):257–263.
9. Zhou S, Jones-Lopez EC, Soneji DJ, et al. Myelin oligodendrocyte glycoprotein antibody-associated optic neuritis and myelitis in COVID-19. *J Neuroophthalmol.* 2020;40(3):398–402.
10. Vaphiades MS, Kline LB. Optic neuritis. *Compr Ophthalmol Update.* 2007;8(2):67–75; discussion 77–78.
11. Optic Neuritis Study Group. Visual function 15 years after optic neuritis: a final follow-up report from the Optic Neuritis Treatment Trial. *Ophthalmology.* 2008;115(6):1079.e5–1082.e5.

SEE ALSO

Multiple Sclerosis

CODES

ICD10

- H46.9 Unspecified optic neuritis
- H46.00 Optic papillitis, unspecified eye
- H46.10 Retrobulbar neuritis, unspecified eye

CLINICAL PEARLS

- Key features include an abrupt visual loss (typically monocular), with periorbital pain with eye movement.
- MRI is the procedure of choice for determining relative risk and possible therapy for MS prevention.
- The ONTT showed that high-dose IV methylprednisolone followed by oral prednisone accelerated visual recovery but did not improve the 6-month or 1-year visual outcome, whereas treatment with oral prednisone alone did not improve the outcome and was associated with an increased rate of recurrence of ON.

OSGOOD-SCHLATTER DISEASE (TIBIAL APOPHYSITIS)

David P. Sealy, MD, CAQSM, FAAFP, FAMSSM • Robert J. Tiller, MD, FAAFP

 BASICS

DESCRIPTION
- Osgood-Schlatter disease (OSD) is a syndrome associated with traction apophysitis and patellar tendinosis that is most common in adolescent boys and girls.
  - Patients present with pain and swelling of the anterior tibial tubercle.
- System(s) affected: musculoskeletal
- Synonym: tibial tubercle apophysitis

EPIDEMIOLOGY
Incidence
Incidence in girls increasing with increased participation in organized youth sports; almost equal to boys in the United States

Prevalence
- A common apophysitis in childhood and adolescence affecting athletes more frequently than nonathletes (1)
- Up to 60% of patients will remain symptomatic into adulthood (2).
- 10% of all adolescent knee pain is due to OSD.

ETIOLOGY AND PATHOPHYSIOLOGY
Traction apophysitis of the tibial tubercle due to repetitive strain on the secondary ossification center of the tibial tuberosity, concurrent patellar tendinosis, and disruption of the proximal tibial apophysis leading to tendinosis and apophysitis. Some data suggest that avulsion microfractures occur at the tibial tuberosity.
- Basic etiology incompletely understood, multifactorial but likely secondary to repetitive microtrauma leading to tendinosis and multiple microfractures
  - Jumping and pivoting sports place highest strain on the tibial tubercle. Repetitive trauma is the most likely inciting factor.
- Possible association with tight hip flexors and tight quadriceps; increased quadriceps strength in adolescence relative to hamstring strength
- Early sports specialization increases the risk for OSD 4-fold (1)[B].

RISK FACTORS
- Affects children and adolescents most commonly from the ages of 8 to 18 years
  - Girls 8 to 13 years
  - Boys 10 to 15 years
- OSD is slightly more common in boys than girls but likely equally common with similar sports participation.
- Rapid skeletal growth
- Weak core stabilizers muscles
- Increased weight/BMI/height
- Patellofemoral malalignment
- Overload training volume
- Quadriceps tightness and/or shortening
- Participation in repetitive-jumping sports and sports with heavy quadriceps activity (football, volleyball, basketball, hockey, soccer, skating, gymnastics)
- Ballet (2-fold risk compared with nonathletes)

GENERAL PREVENTION
- Avoid sports with heavy quadriceps loading (especially deceleration activities—eccentric loading).
- Patients may compete if pain is minimal.
- Increase hamstring and quadriceps flexibility.
- Reduce sports specialization.
- Increase cross-training.

COMMONLY ASSOCIATED CONDITIONS
- Shortened (tight) rectus femoris found in 75% with OSD
- Hamstring tightness
- Possible association with ADD/ADHD; adolescents with ADD/ADHD are at risk for other musculoskeletal injuries.
- Sinding-Larsen-Johansson apophysitis

 DIAGNOSIS

HISTORY
- Unilateral or bilateral (30%) pain of the tibial tuberosity
- Pain exacerbated by exercise, especially jumping and landing after jumping
- Pain upon kneeling on the affected side(s)
- Antalgic or straight-legged gait
- Heavy or increasing intensity of jumping/cutting sports

PHYSICAL EXAM
- Knee pain with squatting or crouching
- Absence of effusion or condyle tenderness
- Tibial tuberosity swelling and tenderness
- Pain increased with resisted knee extension or kneeling
- Erythema over tibial tuberosity
- Hamstring/quadriceps tightness
- Core muscle weakness
- Functional testing: Single-leg squat (SLS) and standing broad jump reproduce pain.

DIFFERENTIAL DIAGNOSIS
- Stress fracture of the proximal tibia
- Pes anserinus bursitis
- Quadriceps tendon avulsion
- Patellofemoral stress syndrome
- Chondromalacia patellae (retropatellar pain)
- Proximal tibial neoplasm
- Osteomyelitis of the proximal tibia
- Tibial plateau fracture
- Sinding-Larsen-Johansson syndrome (patellar apophysitis)—pain over inferior patellar tendon
- Patellar fracture or stress fracture
- Infrapatellar bursitis
- Patellar tendinitis—pain over inferior patellar tendon and inferior pole of patella
- Osteochondroma of the tibial tubercle
- Tibial tuberosity fracture
- Patellar tendon lipoma
- Bacterial apophysitis
- Osteosynchondroses
- Osteochondritis dissecans
- Iliotibial band syndrome
- Hoffa disease (infrapatellar fat pad syndrome)
- Saphenous neuritis

DIAGNOSTIC TESTS & INTERPRETATION
Initial Tests (lab, imaging)
- Generally a clinical diagnosis. No tests are indicated unless other diagnoses are under consideration.
- Radiographic imaging of the proximal tibia and knee may show heterotopic calcification in the patellar tendon and primarily serves to rule out other pathology:
  - X-rays are rarely diagnostic, but appearance of a separate fragment at the tibial tuberosity identifies candidates for potential surgical intervention.
  - Calcified thickening of the tibial tuberosity with irregular ossification at tendon insertion on the tibial tubercle, fragmentation of the apophysis (1)[B]

Diagnostic Procedures/Other
- Bone scan may show increased uptake in the area of the tibial tuberosity:
  - Increased uptake in apophysitis is normal in children, but with OSD, there *may be more uptake on the affected side.*
- Ultrasound is an excellent alternative, showing thickening of the distal patellar tendon, occasional infrapatellar bursa effusion, and neovascularity of the patellar tendon insertion (1)[B].
- MRI shows fragmentation of the tibial tubercle and hyperintense T2 signal of the apophysis and patellar tendon insertion in more advanced cases.

Test Interpretation
Biopsy is not necessary but would show osteolysis and fragmentation of the tibial tubercle.

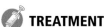 **TREATMENT**

GENERAL MEASURES
- Frequent ice applications 2 to 3 times per day for 15 to 20 minutes
- No randomized controlled studies have been published to demonstrate clear benefit of any treatment over another.
- Rest and activity modification: Avoid activities that increase pain and/or swelling.
- Physical therapy helps with hamstring and quadriceps strengthening and stretching.

- Open- and closed-chain eccentric quadriceps strengthening
- Avoid aggressive stretching if pain is significant to avoid risk of tibial tubercle avulsion.
- Consult orthopedic surgery for tibial tuberosity fracture or complete avulsion.
- Electrical stimulation and iontophoresis have been reported (1)[B].
- Patients with marked midfoot pronation may benefit from orthotics.
- Various bracing and straps have been used.
- With more severe disease, longer term removal from sports may be indicated.

MEDICATION

First Line

- Common OTC analgesics may be considered.
- NSAIDs may be beneficial for pain relief.
- Opioids are not recommended as first line.

Second Line

- More potent analgesics, such as opioids, may ONLY be considered for short-term use in extreme situations.
- Corticosteroid injections are not recommended.
- Hypertonic glucose and/or Xylocaine injections have shown recent benefit (3)[C].
- Autologous platelet injections (PRP) have shown benefit in one study (4)[C].
- Acupuncture

ISSUES FOR REFERRAL

When conservative therapy is unsuccessful and symptoms persist into adulthood, consider surgical referral.

SURGERY/OTHER PROCEDURES

- Débridement of a thickened, cosmetically unsatisfactory tibial tubercle (rare) or removal of mobile heterotopic bone
- Surgical excision of a painful tibial tubercle is rarely needed (<5%) and may be successfully done with bursoscopy instead of an open procedure (3)[C].
- Recent report of successful pain elimination in OSD with percutaneous screw fixation of the tibial tuberosity (1)[C]
- Reduction wedge osteotomy has been recently reported as 100% successful in a small case series (5)[C].

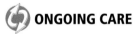 **ONGOING CARE**

FOLLOW-UP RECOMMENDATIONS

- Athletes may return to play if pain is controlled.
- Presence of pain does not preclude competition.

Patient Monitoring

With worsening of symptoms only

PATIENT EDUCATION

- Avoid jumping sports or reduce activities that increase pain and swelling.
- Assure patients and their family that symptoms and physical findings will diminish with time and rest.
- Patients can safely play sports with mild pain.
- Quadriceps stretching and strengthening are important.
- Surgical options are rarely needed, but good results can be expected.

PROGNOSIS

- Usually, this is a self-limiting illness that resolves within 2 years of full skeletal maturation. However, recent data suggest that many are affected into adulthood and must reduce sports and physical activity (2).
- Up to 60% of patients with OSD as adolescents may have symptoms in adulthood. Up to 60% of adults with prior OSD report occasional symptoms and pain with kneeling (2).
- Most patients with OSD will have residual "knots" on their tibial tubercles that never completely resolve.

COMPLICATIONS

- Rarely, a heavily fragmented and inflamed tibial ossicle will avulse and require surgery.
- Although 90% are reported to resolve, recent studies suggest that chronic pain and reduction of activity may continue into adulthood.
- Rare complications in adulthood include pseudarthrosis of the tibial tubercle, genu recurvatum, patella alta, and ossicle fragmentation possibly leading to osteoarthritis of the knee.

REFERENCES

1. Ladenhauf HN, Seitlinger G, Green DW. Osgood-Schlatter disease: a 2020 update of a common knee condition in children. *Curr Opin Pediatr.* 2020;32(1):107–112.
2. Guldhammer C, Rathleff MS, Jensen HP, et al. Long-term prognosis and impact of Osgood-Schlatter disease 4 years after diagnosis: a retrospective study. *Orthop J Sports Med.* 2019;7(10):2325967119878136.
3. Topol GA, Podesta LA, Reeves KD, et al. Hyperosmolar dextrose injection for recalcitrant Osgood-Schlatter disease. *Pediatrics.* 2011;128(5):e1121–e1128.
4. Danneberg D. Successful treatment of Osgood-Schlatter disease with autologous-conditioned plasma in two patients. *Joints.* 2017;5(3):191–194.
5. Pagenstert G, Wurm M, Gehmert S, et al. Reduction osteotomy of the prominent tibial tubercle after Osgood-Schlatter disease. *Arthroscopy.* 2017;33(8):1551–1557.

ADDITIONAL READING

- Kaya DO, Toprak U, Baltaci G, et al. Long-term functional and sonographic outcomes in Osgood-Schlatter disease. *Knee Surg Sports Traumatol Arthrosc.* 2013;21(5):1131–1139.
- Morris E. Acupuncture in Osgood-Schlatter disease. *BMJ Case Rep.* 2016;2016:bcr2015214129.
- Narayan N, Mitchell PD, Latimer MD. Complete resolution of the symptoms of refractory Osgood-Schlatter disease following percutaneous fixation of the tibial tuberosity. *BMJ Case Rep.* 2015;2015:bcr2014206734.
- Nierenberg G, Falah M, Keren Y, et al. Surgical treatment of residual Osgood-Schlatter disease in young adults: role of the mobile osseous fragment. *Orthopedics.* 2011;34(3):176.
- Sailly M, Whiteley R, Johnson A. Doppler ultrasound and tibial tuberosity maturation status predicts pain in adolescent male athletes with Osgood-Schlatter's disease: a case series with comparison group and clinical interpretation. *Br J Sports Med.* 2013;47(2):93–97.

 CODES

ICD10

- M92.50 Juvenile osteochondrosis of tibia and fibula, unsp leg
- M92.51 Juvenile osteochondrosis of tibia and fibula, right leg
- M92.52 Juvenile osteochondrosis of tibia and fibula, left leg

CLINICAL PEARLS

- Infrapatellar pain in an adolescent athlete undergoing a rapid growth spurt is OSD, patellar tendinosis, or Sinding-Larsen-Johansson syndrome.
- Always consider lumbar disc disease, osteogenic sarcoma, or hip pathology in the differential diagnosis of OSD.
- OSD is generally self-limited. Athletes should modify activity based on pain. Mild pain is not a contraindication to athletic participation.
- Treatment focuses on strengthening and stretching of the hamstrings and quadriceps.
- 10% or more of adolescents with OSD will be symptomatic as adults.
- Persistent employment hampering symptoms in adults often require surgery.

OSTEOARTHRITIS

Patrick Wakefield Joyner, MD, MS

BASICS

DESCRIPTION
- Progressive loss of articular cartilage with reactive changes at joint margins and in subchondral bone
- Primary osteoarthritis (OA)
  - Idiopathic: categorized by clinical features (localized, generalized, erosive)
- Secondary OA
  - Posttraumatic (e.g., ACL rupture, distal radius fracture, shoulder dislocation, etc.)
  - Childhood anatomic abnormalities (e.g., congenital hip dysplasia, slipped capital femoral epiphysis [SCFE])
  - Inheritable metabolic disorders (e.g., Wilson disease, alkaptonuria, hemochromatosis)
  - Neuropathic arthropathy (Charcot joints)
  - Endocrinopathies: acromegalic arthropathy, hyperparathyroidism, hypothyroidism
  - Paget disease
  - Noninfectious inflammatory arthritis (e.g., rheumatoid arthritis [RA], spondyloarthropathies)
  - Gout, calcium pyrophosphate deposition disease (pseudogout)
- Synonym(s): osteoarthrosis; degenerative joint disease (DJD)

EPIDEMIOLOGY
- Most common joint disease in United States
- Symptomatic OA most common in patients >40 years
- Leading cause of disability in patients >65 years
- Predominant sex: male = female
- Predominantly impacts weight-bearing joints

Incidence
- Hip (symptomatic)—88 per 100,000 per year
- Knee (symptomatic)—240 per 100,000 per year

Prevalence
- >30 million patients affected in United States
- Increases with age; radiographic evidence of OA is present in many patients >65 years old.
- Moderate to severe hip OA in 3–6% of whites; <1% in East Indians, blacks, Chinese, and Native Americans

ETIOLOGY AND PATHOPHYSIOLOGY
Failure of chondrocytes to maintain the balance between degradation and synthesis of extracellular collagen matrix. Collagen loss results in alteration of proteoglycan matrix and increased susceptibility to degenerative change.

Genetics
- Up to 65% of OA cases may have a genetic component.
- The heritability of end-stage hip OA is up to 27%.

RISK FACTORS
- Increasing age: >50 years
- Age as a risk factor is greatest for hip and knee OA.
- Obesity (weight-bearing joints); BMI >35
- Trauma, infection, or inflammatory arthritis
- Female gender (knee and hand)

GENERAL PREVENTION
Weight management; regular physical activity, perijoint muscle strengthening—"prehabbing"

COMMONLY ASSOCIATED CONDITIONS
- Obesity
- History of trauma
- Shoulder arthritis can be associated with a rotator cuff tear.

DIAGNOSIS

HISTORY
- Distinguish OA from other types of arthritis by:
  - Absence of systemic findings
  - Minimal articular inflammation
  - Distribution of involved joints (e.g., distal and proximal interphalangeal joints)
- OA characterized by slowly developing joint pain. Pain often described as aching or burning in nature. Anecdotally, many patients describe pain changes with alterations in weather conditions.
- Transient stiffness (especially after awakening in morning and after sitting) that tends to lessen 10 to 15 minutes after joint movement
- Most common joints in hand are as follows:
  - Distal interphalangeal > thumb carpometacarpal > proximal interphalangeal > MCP

PHYSICAL EXAM
- Joint bony enlargement
- Decreased range of motion of affected joints
- Mechanical symptoms (clicking, locking) may be present, especially in knees with degenerative meniscal injury.
- Meniscus tear in the setting of severe/end-stage knee OA is an OA problem, and should be treated as an OA ailment, in the absence of the mechanical symptoms.
- Local pain and stiffness with OA of spine; radicular pain (if compression of nerve roots)
- Changes in joint alignment (genu varum [bowlegs] and genu valgum [knock-knees])

DIFFERENTIAL DIAGNOSIS
- Crystalline arthropathies (gout; pseudogout): inflammatory arthritides (RA), spondyloarthropathies (reactive arthritis; psoriatic arthritis), septic arthritis
- Fibromyalgia; avascular necrosis; Lyme disease

DIAGNOSTIC TESTS & INTERPRETATION
Initial Tests (lab, imaging)
- Routine chemistries are not helpful in diagnosis.
- X-rays are usually normal early in disease process.
- As OA progresses, plain films show:
  - Narrowed, asymmetric joint space, osteophyte formation, subchondral bony sclerosis, subchondral cyst formation
- MRI may particularly demonstrate chondral degeneration and associated meniscal tears. 5–10% weight loss is associated with slowing of arthritic changes and decreased chondral loss on follow-up studies, subchondral bone edema (1).

Follow-Up Tests & Special Considerations
- Monitor treatment with NSAIDs (renal insufficiency and GI bleeding).
- In secondary OA, abnormal lab results associated with underlying disorder (e.g., hemochromatosis [abnormal iron studies])

Diagnostic Procedures/Other
Joint aspiration (not usually necessary for diagnosis)
- OA: cell count usually <500 cells/mm^3, predominantly mononuclear
- Inflammatory: cell count usually >2,000 cells/mm^3, predominantly neutrophils
- Birefringent crystals in gout (−) and pseudogout (+)

Test Interpretation
- Patchy cartilage damage and bony hypertrophy
- Histologic phases:
  - Extracellular matrix edema and cartilage microfissures, subchondral fissuring and pitting, erosion and formation of osteocartilaginous loose bodies
- Subchondral bone trabecular microfractures and sclerosis with osteophyte formation

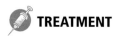

TREATMENT

GENERAL MEASURES
- Weight management combined with exercise/physical therapy to maintain or regain joint motion and muscle strength
  - Quadriceps strengthening for knee OA
  - Periscapular strengthening and range of motion for shoulder OA
  - Abductor and core strengthening as well as gait mechanics for hip OA
- Transition to non–weight-bearing exercises (i.e., elliptical, stationary bike, swimming)
- Exercise must be maintained; benefits are lost 6 months after exercise cessation.
- Protect joints from overuse; ambulatory aides are beneficial as is proper-fitting footwear.
- Bracing, joint supports, or insoles in patients with biomechanical instability:
  - Bracing is more beneficial in patients with unicompartmental disease of the knee.
- For knee OA in particular, several nonpharmacologic modalities are strongly recommended: aerobic, aquatic, and/or resistance exercise and weight loss.

MEDICATION
First Line
- Manage pain and inflammation:
  - Acetaminophen up to 1,000 mg TID: effective for pain relief in OA of knee and hip
  - Topical NSAID gels, creams have short-term (<4 weeks) benefits. Topical NSAIDs are a core treatment for hand and joints with minimal soft tissue—coverage (i.e., hand) OA.
  - If acetaminophen or topical NSAIDs are insufficient, consider an oral NSAID/COX-2 inhibitor. Use the lowest effective dose for the shortest time possible.
  - May use nonacetylated salicylates (e.g., salsalate, choline-magnesium salicylate) or low-dose ibuprofen ≤1,600 mg/day. Consider a once-daily NSAID, if necessary, to help maintain compliance.
  - Glucosamine sulfate and chondroitin sulfate are safe alternatives; however, their efficacy is still debatable (2).

- NSAID contraindications:
  - All PO NSAIDs/COX-2 inhibitors have analgesic effects of a similar magnitude but vary in their potential GI and cardiorenal toxicity.
  - Avoid NSAIDs in patients with renal disease, CHF, HTN, active peptic ulcer disease, and previous hypersensitivity to an NSAID or aspirin.
  - Combination of NSAIDs and full-strength aspirin (325 mg) is contraindicated.
  - In patients at high cardiovascular risk: Combination of a nonselective NSAID and low-dose aspirin (81 mg) is recommended.
  - Oral or parenteral corticosteroids are contraindicated.

ALERT

NSAIDS are associated with an increased risk of adverse cardiovascular events. The absolute risk is dependent on patient age, comorbidities, particular NSAID used, dose, and duration of use.

- Precautions:
  - If PO NSAID/COX-2 inhibitor use is necessary for a patient aged >65 years or a patient <65 years with increased GI-bleeding risk factors, proton pump inhibitors are recommended.
  - Significant possible interactions:
    ○ NSAIDs reduce effectiveness of ACE inhibitors and diuretics.
    ○ Aspirin and NSAIDs (except COX-2 inhibitors) may increase effects of anticoagulants.
    ○ Salicylates reduce effectiveness of spironolactone (Aldactone) and uricosurics.
    ○ Corticosteroids and some antacids increase salicylate excretion, whereas ascorbic acid and ammonium chloride reduce salicylate excretion and may cause toxicity.

Pregnancy Considerations

- ASA and NSAIDs have reported fetal risk during 1st and 3rd trimesters of pregnancy.
- Compatible with breastfeeding

Second Line

- Topical NSAIDs and capsaicin can lower gastric and renal risks associated with oral NSAIDs.
- Bracing; medial and lateral unloader braces are effective; long leg alignment x-rays can help determine the appropriate brace.
- TENS modalities for pain may be more beneficial than hyaluronic acid (HA) injection (3)[A].

Third Line

- Intra-auricular corticosteroid injections can be used for acute flares and for patients failing first- and second-line treatments. Minimize injections (≤3 per joint per year).
- Platelet-rich plasma (PRP) is a safe alternative for early knee OA but does not appear to offer any clinical advantage when compared to HA (4).
- When compared to HA or PRP alone, HA and PRP together provided long-term relief and better outcomes at 6 months in knee arthritis (5).
- Bone marrow aspirate concentrate (BMAC) injections demonstrate no difference in patient outcome in knee OA when compared to saline injections.
- Cryotherapy with physical therapy is better than physical therapy alone for knee arthritis (6).

ISSUES FOR REFERRAL

- Disease that fails conservative management
- Concern for a septic joint or gout
- Musculoskeletal injury as a result of OA

ADDITIONAL THERAPIES

Address psychosocial factors (i.e., self-efficacy, coping skills). Screen for and appropriately treat anxiety and depression. Improve social support.

SURGERY/OTHER PROCEDURES

- Total knee arthroplasty (TKA)
- Total hip arthroplasty (THA), total shoulder arthroplasty (TSA), reverse total shoulder arthroplasty (RTSA), and total ankle arthroplasty (TAA) all remain options for patients that fail conservative management for these respective joints.
- Ligament reconstruction and tendon interposition (LRTI) is an option for patients failing conservative treatment of the carpometacarpal joints.
- Knee arthroscopy is not routinely recommended for the treatment of OA in the absence of clear mechanical symptoms (i.e., locking, clicking, etc.).

COMPLEMENTARY & ALTERNATIVE MEDICINE

- Nutritional supplements (glucosamine and chondroitin sulfate) may benefit some patients and have low toxicity. There is lack of standardized outcome assessments. Trial results using glucosamine and chondroitin have been mixed. If no response is apparent within 6 months, discontinue use.
- TENS, yoga, and acupuncture have shown benefit.

 ## ONGOING CARE

FOLLOW-UP RECOMMENDATIONS

- Follow-up at 3-month intervals for assessment of conservative management treatment and future options
- Recommend plain films of effected joint annually.

Patient Monitoring

- Regularly assess range of motion and functional status.
- Monitor for GI blood loss and cardiac, renal, and mental status in older patients on NSAIDs or aspirin.
- Periodic CBC, renal function tests, stool for occult blood in patients on chronic NSAID therapy

DIET

Continue to ensure patients have adequate Vitamin D intake and levels to maximize bone health.

PATIENT EDUCATION

- American College of Rheumatology: http://www.rheumatology.org/public/factsheets/index.asp?aud=pat
- Arthritis Foundation: http://www.arthritis.org

PROGNOSIS

- Progressive and chronic disease: early in course, pain relieved by rest; later, pain may persist at rest and at night.
- Joint effusions and enlargement may occur (especially in knees) as disease progresses.
- Osteophyte (spur) formation, especially at joint margins

COMPLICATIONS

- Leading cause of musculoskeletal pain and disability
- Decompensated CHF, GI bleeding, decreased renal function on chronic NSAID or aspirin therapy

REFERENCES

1. Gersing AS, Schwaiger BJ, Nevitt MC, et al. Is weight loss associated with less progression of changes in knee articular cartilage among obese and overweight patients as assessed with MR imaging over 48 months? Data from the Osteoarthritis Initiative. *Radiology*. 2017;284(2):508–520.
2. Honvo G, Reginster J-Y, Rabenda V, et al. Safety of symptomatic slow-acting drugs for osteoarthritis: outcomes of a systematic review and meta-analysis. *Drugs Aging*. 2019;36(Suppl 1):65–99.
3. Chen WL, Hsu WC, Lin YJ, et al. Comparison of intra-articular hyaluronic acid injections with transcutaneous electric nerve stimulation for the management of knee osteoarthritis: a randomized controlled trial. *Arch Phys Med Rehabil*. 2013;94(8):1482–1489.
4. Lizis P, Manko G, Kobza W, et al. Manual therapy with cryotherapy versus kinesiotherapy with cryotherapy for knee osteoarthritis: a randomized control trial. *Altern Ther Health Med*. 2019;25(4):40–45.
5. Shapiro SA, Kazmerchak SE, Heckman MG, et al. A prospective, single-blind, placebo-controlled trial of bone marrow aspirate concentrate for knee osteoarthritis. *Am J Sports Med*. 2017;45(1):82–90.
6. Lizis P, Manko G, Kobza W, et al. Manual therapy with cryotherapy versus kinesiotherapy with cryotherapy for knee osteoarthritis: a randomized control trial. *Altern Ther Health Med*. 2019;25(4):40–45.

CODES

ICD10

- M19.239 Secondary osteoarthritis, unspecified wrist
- M19.9 Osteoarthritis, unspecified site
- M19.212 Secondary osteoarthritis, left shoulder

CLINICAL PEARLS

- Patients with OA typically have morning stiffness lasting for <15 minutes.
- OA most commonly affects the hips, knees, and hands (proximal interphalangeal and distal interphalangeal joints).
- NSAID use is associated with increase risk of cardiovascular events.
- If used, intra-articular steroid injections should be limited to no more than 2 per joint per year.
- Biologics are (higher cost) options for early-stage knee OA.
- PRP and PRP + HA appear to be more clinically effective than BMAC and other biologics for knee OA. PRP is currently the most cost-effective biologic option.
- Long-term OA therapy is individualized to patient pain management and activity goals.

OSTEOMYELITIS

Rebecca Wadlinger, DO, MS, ATC

 BASICS

DESCRIPTION

- An acute or chronic bone infection with associated inflammation; can occur as a result of hematogenous seeding, contiguous spread of infection, or direct inoculation into intact bone (trauma or surgery)
- Two major classification systems:
  - Lew and Waldvogel
    - Classified according to duration (acute or chronic) and source of infection (hematogenous or contiguous)
  - Cierny-Mader classification
    - Based on the portion of bone affected, physiologic status of the host, and risk factors
- Special situations
  - Vertebral osteomyelitis
    - Results from hematogenous seeding (most common), direct inoculation, or contiguous spread
    - Back pain is most common initial symptom.
    - Lumbar spine is most commonly involved, followed by thoracic spine.
    - Neurologic symptoms occur in 1/3 of patients (1)[C].
    - Surgery indicated with presence of neurologic symptoms or infection of spinal implant. Uncomplicated acute hematogenous vertebral osteomyelitis can be treated with 6 weeks of antibiotics (1)[C].
  - Prosthetic joint infections
    - X-ray and three-phase bone scan. MRI/CT is of limited use with prostheses.
    - Treat with pathogen-directed antibiotic therapy; may include rifampin (4 to 6 weeks) for higher success rate—penetrates biofilm
  - Posttraumatic infections
    - Risk factors include type and severity of fracture as well as contamination.
    - Tibia is the most common location.

EPIDEMIOLOGY

- Predominant age: more common in older adults
- Predominant sex: male > female
- Hematogenous osteomyelitis
  - Adults (most >50 years of age): vertebral
  - Children: long bones
- Contiguous osteomyelitis: related to diabetic foot infections (DFIs), decubitus ulcers, and infected total joint arthroplasties in older adults; trauma and surgery in younger adults
- *Mycobacterium tuberculosis* is the most common cause of vertebral osteomyelitis worldwide. It is more likely to involve multiple vertebral bodies—especially of the thoracic spine—and is associated with paraspinal abscess formation.

Incidence

Generally low; normal bone is resistant to infection.

Prevalence

Up to 66% of diabetics with foot ulcerations

ETIOLOGY AND PATHOPHYSIOLOGY

- Acute: suppurative infection of bone with edema and vascular compromise leading to sequestrum (segments of necrotic bone, may contain pus)
- Chronic: presence of necrotic bone or sequestrum or recurrence of previous infection
- Hematogenous osteomyelitis (typically monomicrobial)
  - *Staphylococcus aureus* (most common)
  - Coagulase-negative staphylococci and aerobic gram-negative bacteria

- *Pseudomonas aeruginosa* (intravenous [IV] drug user)
  - *Salmonella* sp. (sickle cell disease)
  - M. tuberculosis and fungal (rare; in endemic areas or in immunocompromised hosts)
- Contiguous focus osteomyelitis (polymicrobial)
  - Diabetes or vascular insufficiency
    - Coagulase-positive and coagulase-negative staphylococci
    - Streptococci, gram-negative bacilli, anaerobes (*Peptostreptococcus* sp.)
  - Sacral decubitus ulcer
    - Pressure-related skin ulceration and necrosis
    - May require débridement to healthy bone and/or soft tissue coverage/surgical flap procedure (2)[C]
  - Puncture wound through shoe
    - P. aeruginosa
- Prosthetic device
  - Coagulase-negative staphylococci and *S. aureus*

RISK FACTORS

- Diabetes mellitus (particularly, diabetic foot ulcer)
- Recent trauma/surgery
- Foreign body (e.g., prosthetic implant)
- Neuropathy and vascular insufficiency
- Immunosuppression (including dialysis)
- Sickle cell disease
- Injection drug use
- Previous osteomyelitis
- Bacteremia

GENERAL PREVENTION

- Comprehensive annual foot exam for diabetic patients
- Screen for peripheral artery disease.
- Optimize glycemic control in diabetes.
- Antibiotic prophylaxis for posttraumatic infection
  - Clean bone surgery
    - Administer IV antibiotics within an hour of skin incision, keep at therapeutic level throughout surgery, and continue ≤24 hours postprocedure.
  - Closed fractures
    - Cefazolin, cefuroxime, clindamycin (β-lactam allergy), or vancomycin (β-lactam allergy or MRSA infection)
  - Open fractures
    - In patients who can receive antibiotics within 3 hours of injury with prompt operative treatment, 1st-generation cephalosporins are preferred (clindamycin or vancomycin if allergic). Ceftriaxone for type III fractures. Add metronidazole if associated with soil or fecal matter contamination.

DIAGNOSIS

HISTORY

- Fever, chills, pain, swelling, and erythema, particularly in acute osteomyelitis. These features may be absent in chronic osteomyelitis.
- Hematogenous osteomyelitis
  - Elicit a history of conditions predisposing to bacteremia (diabetes, hemodialysis, invasive procedures, IV drug use, immunosuppression).
- Contiguous osteomyelitis and vascular insufficiency
  - Recent trauma/surgery within 1 to 2 months
  - Presence of prosthetic device
  - History of diabetes/DFI

- Chronic osteomyelitis
  - History of acute osteomyelitis
  - Draining sinus tract

PHYSICAL EXAM

- Fever, restricted range of motion, tenderness, signs of localized inflammation
- Motor and sensory deficits (vertebral infection)
- Probe to bone test in DFI has high pooled sensitivity and specificity for osteomyelitis of 0.87 (95% CI 0.75–0.93) and 0.83 (95% CI 0.65–0.93), respectively (3)[A].
- Exposed bone in the setting of DFI (4)[A]
- Ulcer >2-cm wide and >2-cm deep increases likelihood for osteomyelitis in DFI (4)[A].
- Positive probe to bone test and ulcer area >2 cm^2 are physical exam findings that best support osteomyelitis in the setting of DFI (4)[A].
- Classic signs and symptoms of infection may be masked in diabetics due to vascular disease and neuropathy.

DIFFERENTIAL DIAGNOSIS

- Systemic infection from other source
- Aseptic bone infarction
- Localized inflammation or infection of overlying skin and soft tissues (e.g., gout)
- Brodie abscess (subacute osteomyelitis)
- Neuropathic joint disease (Charcot foot)
- Fractures/trauma
- Tumor

DIAGNOSTIC TESTS & INTERPRETATION

Initial Tests (lab, imaging)

Labs

- WBC is not reliable (can be normal) (1)[A].
- CRP is usually elevated (nonspecific).
- ESR is high in most cases:
  - ESR >70 mm/hr increases likelihood >10-fold (4)[A].
- Procalcitonin may also be elevated.
- Antibiotics given prior to culture may alter results.
- Other disorders that may alter lab results: immunosuppression (including diabetes), chronic inflammatory disease, other sites of infection
- Routine radiography is first-line imaging: Classic triad for osteomyelitis is demineralization, periosteal reaction, and bone destruction.
  - Bone destruction is not apparent on plain films until after 10 to 21 days of infection.
  - Bone scan is first test after plain x-ray for evaluation of prosthesis-related infection.
- Radionuclide scanning (e.g., technetium, indium, or gallium) helps if diagnosis is ambiguous or unsure of extent of disease; limited by low sensitivity/specificity
- MRI
  - Best for visualization of septic arthritis, spinal infection, and DFI (1)[C],(4)[A]
  - T1-weighted image: low signal intensity
  - T2-weighted image: high signal intensity
  - MRI: sensitivity 90% and specificity 80% for osteomyelitis in diabetic foot ulcers (4)[A]
  - Not as accurate for diagnosis of osteomyelitis with presence of Charcot neuroarthropathy joint disease or after recent surgery (4)[A]
  - MRI does not help assess the response to therapy due to persistence of bony edema.
- CT
  - Better than standard radiography to evaluate bony fragments and sequestration; inferior to MRI for soft tissue and bone marrow assessment

Follow-Up Tests & Special Considerations

- A persistently elevated CRP (4 to 6 weeks) can be associated with osteomyelitis but is nonspecific. CRP decreases faster than ESR, but a decrease in ESR after treatment is a good prognostic sign.
- Monitor patients receiving prolonged antimicrobial therapy with weekly labs.

Diagnostic Procedures/Other

Blood cultures and bone biopsy

- For vertebral/hematogenous osteomyelitis, definitive diagnosis is made by vertebral disc aspiration or blood culture.
- Patients with positive blood cultures (with a pathogen likely to cause vertebral/hematogenous osteomyelitis) and with radiographic evidence of osteomyelitis do not need bone biopsy.
- For contiguous osteomyelitis, definitive diagnosis is made by bone biopsy for culture and histology.
- Avoid wound swabs or needle aspiration in DFI and decubitus ulcers because these do not correlate well with bone biopsy culture (2)[A],(4)[C].
- Can obtain bone biopsy at same time as surgical débridement

Test Interpretation

Pathology of bone revealing inflammatory process with pyogenic bacteria and necrosis is diagnostic.

 # TREATMENT

GENERAL MEASURES

Adequate nutrition, smoking cessation, glycemic control, foot care, IV drug use cessation

MEDICATION

- In clinically stable patients, delay initiation of empiric antibiotics until biopsy and/or blood cultures have been obtained.
- Direct empiric therapy toward probable organism and tailor according to culture results.
- Optimal antimicrobial concentration at infected site is essential (consider vascular perfusion).
- Adjust antibiotic dosing according to renal function.
- 4 to 6 weeks of therapy is appropriate for most cases of acute osteomyelitis. In the setting of amputation or complete removal of infected bone, a 2-week course of pathogen-directed antibiotics may be adequate (2)[C].
- If a prosthetic joint or other orthopedic hardware cannot be removed or completely débrided, a prolonged 6-week course of parenteral antibiotics is indicated. Some patients may subsequently require long-term oral antimicrobial suppression.
- Consider longer treatment courses for chronic osteomyelitis or MRSA infection (minimum 8 weeks).
- Empiric therapy:
  - For vertebral/hematogenous osteomyelitis, include coverage for MRSA and gram-negative organisms.
  - IV vancomycin plus 3rd- or 4th-generation IV cephalosporin +/− metronidazole for DFI/contiguous osteomyelitis

First Line

- *S. aureus* or coagulase-negative staphylococci
  - MSSA: β-lactam at high dose (nafcillin or oxacillin 2 g IV q4h) *or* cefazolin 1 to 2 g IV q8h (Use 2 g for patients >80 kg.)
  - MRSA: vancomycin 15 to 20 mg/kg IV q8–12h (use q8h interval if CrCl >70 mL/min) with target trough of 15 to 20 μg/mL, not to exceed 2 g/dose
- *Streptococcus* sp.
  - Ceftriaxone 2 g IV q24h or cefazolin 2 g IV q8h

- *Enterobacter* sp.
  - Ciprofloxacin 750 mg PO q12h (or 400 mg IV q12h) or cefepime 2 g IV q12h
- *P. aeruginosa*
  - Cefepime 2 g IV q8h or ciprofloxacin 750 mg PO q12h (or 400 mg IV q8h)

Second Line

- *S. aureus*
  - MSSA: ceftriaxone 2 g IV q24h
  - MRSA: linezolid 600 mg PO/IV q12h *or* daptomycin 6 mg/kg IV q24h
- *Streptococcus* sp.
  - Penicillin G 4 million U q4–6h
- *Enterobacter* sp. (quinolone-resistant, including extended-spectrum β-lactamase–producing *Escherichia coli*)
  - Carbapenem (imipenem/cilastatin) 500 mg IV q6h
- *P. aeruginosa*
  - Piperacillin-tazobactam 3.375 g IV q6h

ALERT
The combination of vancomycin plus piperacillin-tazobactam can increase risk of acute renal failure (number needed to harm 11) (5)[A].

ADDITIONAL THERAPIES

Evidence does not currently support the use of hyperbaric oxygen therapy, growth factors, maggots, or topical negative pressure for diabetic foot osteomyelitis.

SURGERY/OTHER PROCEDURES

- Surgical drainage, minimizing dead space, adequate soft tissue coverage, restoration of blood supply, and removal of necrotic tissues improve cure rates.
- Débridement of necrotic bone was once thought to be the cornerstone to management; however, recent evidence suggests antibiotics alone may be sufficient for DFI (4)[A]. There is still much research to be done on this topic.
- Use of antibiotic-loaded cement during surgery has been used for decades and shown success in patients with vascular insufficiency to manage dead space and help control the infection.

ADMISSION, INPATIENT, AND NURSING CONSIDERATIONS

- Off-load pressure
- Discharge criteria: clinical and laboratory evidence of resolving infection and appropriate outpatient therapy

 # ONGOING CARE

FOLLOW-UP RECOMMENDATIONS

Patient Monitoring
Blood levels of antimicrobial agents, ESR, CRP, and repeat plain radiography as clinical course dictates. CRP correlates more closely with clinical response to therapy than ESR.

DIET

- Glycemic control for diabetics
- Proper nutrition for malnourished patients

PATIENT EDUCATION

- Diabetic glycemic control and foot care
- IV drug use cessation

PROGNOSIS

- Superficial and medullary osteomyelitis treated with antimicrobial and surgical therapy have a response rate of 90–100%.
- Up to 36% recurrence rate in diabetics
- Increased mortality after amputation

COMPLICATIONS

- Abscess formation
- Bacteremia
- Fracture/nonunion
- Loosening of prosthetic implant
- Postoperative infection
- Sinus tract formation can be associated with neoplasms (e.g., Marjolin ulcer), especially in presence of long-standing infection.

REFERENCES

1. Zimmerli W. Clinical practice. Vertebral osteomyelitis. *N Engl J Med*. 2010;362(11):1022–1029.
2. Schmitt SK. Osteomyelitis. *Infect Dis Clin North Am*. 2017;31(2):325–338.
3. Lam K, van Asten SA, Nguyen T, et al. Diagnostic accuracy of probe to bone to detect osteomyelitis in the diabetic foot: a systematic review. *Clin Infect Dis*. 2016;63(7):944–948.
4. Malhotra R, Chan CS, Nather A. Osteomyelitis in the diabetic foot. *Diabet Foot Ankle*. 2014;5. doi:10.3402/dfa.v5.24445.
5. Luther MK, Timbrook TT, Caffrey AR, et al. Vancomycin plus piperacillin-tazobactam and acute kidney injury in adults: a systematic review and meta-analysis. *Crit Care Med*. 2018;46(1):12–20.

ADDITIONAL READING

- Nickerson EK, Sinha R. Vertebral osteomyelitis in adults: an update. *Br Med Bull*. 2016;117(1):121–138.
- Wong D, Holtom P, Spellberg B. Osteomyelitis complicating sacral pressure ulcers: whether or not to treat with antibiotic therapy. *Clin Infect Dis*. 2019;68(2):338–342.

CODES

ICD10
- M86.03 Acute hematogenous osteomyelitis, radius and ulna
- M86.032 Acute hematogenous osteomyelitis, left radius and ulna
- M86.01 Acute hematogenous osteomyelitis, shoulder

CLINICAL PEARLS

- Hematogenous osteomyelitis is usually monomicrobial. Osteomyelitis due to contiguous spread or direct inoculation is usually polymicrobial.
- Pain associated with acute osteomyelitis is typically gradual in onset.
- Treatment of chronic osteomyelitis often requires both surgical débridement and at least 6 weeks of antimicrobial therapy.
- Unlike diabetic foot ulcers, a positive probe-to-bone test (or frankly exposed bone) and abnormal MRI findings are not diagnostic of osteomyelitis in stage IV sacral pressure ulcers.
- Definitive treatment of osteomyelitis in stage IV sacral pressure ulcers often requires surgical débridement to healthy bone.
- Follow-up MRI is not needed for patients who are clinically improving with appropriate treatment.
- In diabetic foot wounds, if there are no signs or symptoms of soft tissue or bone infection, antibiotic therapy is unnecessary.

OSTEOPOROSIS AND OSTEOPENIA

Rahul Kapur, MD • Jennifer Oberstar, MD

BASICS

DESCRIPTION
A skeletal disease characterized by low bone mass, with disruption of bone architecture leading to compromised bone strength and risk of fracture

EPIDEMIOLOGY
- Predominant age: elderly >60 years of age
- Predominant sex: female > male (80%/20%)

Incidence
There are >2 million fractures annually attributed to osteoporosis in the United States.

Prevalence
- >9.9 million Americans have osteoporosis.
- >43.1 million Americans have osteopenia.
- Women >50 years of age: osteoporosis 15.4% and osteopenia 51.4%
- Men >50 years of age: osteoporosis 4.3% and osteopenia 35.2%

ETIOLOGY AND PATHOPHYSIOLOGY
- Imbalance between bone resorption/formation
- Hypoestrogenemia

Genetics
- Familial predisposition
- More common in Caucasians and Asians than in African Americans and Hispanics

RISK FACTORS
- Nonmodifiable:
  - Age >65 years
  - Female gender and menopause
  - Caucasian or Asian race
  - Family history of osteoporosis
  - History of fragility fracture
- Modifiable:
  - Low body weight (<58 kg or BMI <21)
  - Calcium/vitamin D deficiency
  - Inadequate physical activity
  - Cigarette smoking
  - Excessive alcohol intake (>3 drinks per day)
  - Various medications

GENERAL PREVENTION
- Regularly perform weight-bearing exercise.
- A diet with adequate calcium (1,000 mg/day for men aged 50 to 70 years and 1,200 mg/day for women aged 51+ years and men 70+ years) and vitamin D (800 to 1,000 IU/day)
- Avoid smoking.
- Limit alcohol consumption (<3 drinks per day).
- Fall prevention (home safety assessment, correction of visual impairment)
- Screen (USPSTF recommendations):
  - All women ≥65 years of age
  - Women >50 years of age with a 10-year risk of major osteoporotic fracture (using the World Health Organization's [WHO] Fracture Risk Assessment [FRAX] Tool) >8.4%
  - Evidence is insufficient to recommend screening men; however, the National Osteoporosis Foundation recommends screening men age >70 years, especially if at increased risk.
  - No clear benefit in predicting fractures from repeating bone mineral density (BMD) testing 4 to 8 years after initial screening.

COMMONLY ASSOCIATED CONDITIONS
- Malabsorption syndromes: gastrectomy, inflammatory bowel disease, celiac disease
- Hypoestrogenism: menopause, hypogonadism, eating disorders, etc.
- Endocrinopathies: hyperparathyroidism, hyperthyroidism, hypercortisolism, diabetes mellitus
- Hematologic disorders: sickle cell disease, multiple myeloma, thalassemia, hemochromatosis
- Other chronic diseases: multiple sclerosis, end-stage renal disease, rheumatoid arthritis, lupus, COPD, HIV/AIDS
- Medications: chemotherapy agents, antiepileptics, aromatase inhibitors (raloxifene), chronic corticosteroids (equivalent to at least 5 mg prednisone daily for at least 3 months), medroxyprogesterone acetate, heparin, SSRIs, thyroid hormone (in supraphysiologic doses), PPIs

DIAGNOSIS

HISTORY
- Review modifiable and nonmodifiable risk factors.
- Online risk factor assessment tool (FRAX): http://www.shef.ac.uk/FRAX/
- Assess for commonly associated conditions.

PHYSICAL EXAM
- Thoracic kyphosis, poor balance, deconditioning
- Historical height loss >4 cm (difference between current height and peak height at age 20 years)
- Prospective height loss >2 cm (difference between current height and previously documented height)

DIFFERENTIAL DIAGNOSIS
- Multiple myeloma/other neoplasms
- Osteomalacia; type I collagen mutations

DIAGNOSTIC TESTS & INTERPRETATION
Initial Tests (lab, imaging)
- Dual energy x-ray absorptiometry (DEXA) of the lumbar spine/hip is considered the gold standard for measuring BMD and for diagnosing osteoporosis
  - A BMD at the hip or lumbar spine that is >2.5 standard deviations below the mean BMD reference is diagnostic of osteoporosis.
  - A minimum of 2 years may be needed to reliably measure a change in BMD.
  - BMD is expressed in terms of T-scores and Z-scores:
    ○ T-score is the number of standard deviations a patient's BMD deviates from the mean.
    ○ The WHO defines normal BMD as a T-score ≥−1; osteopenia as a T-score between −1 and −2.5; osteoporosis as a T-score ≤−2.5; and established or severe osteoporosis as a T-score ≤−2.5 with an associated history of a fragility fracture.
    ○ WHO thresholds can be used for postmenopausal women and men >50 years of age. The Z-score is a comparison of the patient's BMD with an age-matched population.
    ○ A Z-score <−2 should prompt evaluation for causes of secondary osteoporosis.
- Consider screening for secondary osteoporosis causes:
  - Serum 25-hydroxyvitamin D and parathyroid hormone, with TSH
  - Complete blood count, calcium, phosphorus, magnesium, total protein, albumin, liver enzymes, creatinine, alkaline phosphatase
  - 24-hour urine calcium, sodium, and creatinine to identify hypercalciuria

- Plain radiographs lack sensitivity to diagnose osteoporosis, but an abnormality (e.g., widened intervertebral spaces, rib fractures, vertebral compression fractures) should prompt evaluation.

Follow-Up Tests & Special Considerations
Consider further lab work based on initial evaluation, Z-score −2.5 or lower, or young age:
- Iron and ferritin (hemochromatosis)
- Testosterone levels (hypogonadism in men)
- Serum protein electrophoresis and free κ and λ light chains (multiple myeloma)
- Urinary free cortisol (Cushing disease)
- Tissue transglutaminase antibodies (celiac disease)

Diagnostic Procedures/Other
Bone biopsy may be considered.

Test Interpretation
In osteoporosis, can see reduced skeletal mass; trabecular bone thinned or lost more than cortical bone

TREATMENT

- Criteria for patients who benefit from treatment for their osteoporosis includes the following:
  - Patients' T-score ≤−2.5 with no risk factors
  - All postmenopausal women and men >50 years old with an osteoporotic vertebral/hip fracture
  - All postmenopausal women who have BMD values consistent with osteoporosis (T-score ≤2.5) at the lumbar spine, femoral neck, or total hip region
  - Postmenopausal women and men >50 years with osteopenia (T-scores from −1.0 to −2.5) and a 10-year fracture risk of ≥20% or risk of hip fracture ≥3%, based on FRAX calculator or history of a fragility fracture
  - All men >50 years of age who present with a hip or vertebral fracture or a T-score ≤−2.5 after appropriate evaluation; however, evidence for the effectiveness of treatment in men is limited.
- Osteopenia, treatment focused on risk modification: weight-bearing exercise, vitamin D supplementation (2,000 to 4,000 IU/day), limiting alcohol, and smoking cessation

MEDICATION
Vitamin D 2,000 to 4,000 IU/day for all patients with osteoporosis

First Line
Bisphosphonates:
- Mechanism: inhibition of bone resorption by osteoclasts in skeletal tissue, reducing the incidence of vertebral and nonvertebral fractures
  - Alendronate 10 mg PO daily or 70 mg PO weekly
  - Risedronate 5 mg PO daily, 35 mg PO weekly, or 150 mg PO monthly
  - Zoledronic acid 5 mg IV yearly or 5 mg IV every 18 months
- For primary prevention, zoledronate (once every 18 month) reduced both vertebral (RR 0.46, 95% CI 0.28–0.74) and nonvertebral (HR 0.66, 95% CI 0.51–0.85) fractures (1)[A].
- For secondary prevention of mild/moderate osteoporosis, oral bisphosphonates preferred (1)[A]
- Side effects are similar for all bisphosphonates and include gastrointestinal problems: inflammation of the esophagus and stomach.

- Osteonecrosis of the jaw is a risk, particularly in patients with cancer who receive high doses and those who receive IV treatment (2)[C].
- There is a possible risk of atypical femur fractures in patients receiving bisphosphonates for >5 years (3)[A].
- Avoid oral bisphosphonates in patients with:
  – Delayed esophageal emptying
  – Inability to stand/sit upright for at least 30 to 60 minutes after taking the bisphosphonates
  – Hypocalcemia (Correct prior to initiating therapy.)
  – Severe renal impairment (creatinine clearance [CrCl] ≤30 for risedronate and ≤35 mL/min for alendronate and zoledronic acid)

Second Line

- Monoclonal antibody therapy:
  – Denosumab 60 mg SC every 6 months
    ○ Human monoclonal antibody receptor activator of nuclear factor κ-B ligand (RANKL) receptor, blocking, inhibiting osteoclast formation and decreasing bone resorption
    ○ Can be considered as an initial therapy option for postmenopausal women with higher fracture risk or who are not candidates for an oral bisphosphonate (4)[B]
    ○ Denosumab is the agent of choice in patients with renal insufficiency (4)[B].
    ○ Side effects can include dermatologic reactions (dermatitis, eczema, rashes), musculoskeletal pain, hypocalcemia and less commonly osteonecrosis of the jaw, atypical femur fracture, and serious infections (cellulitis and endocarditis).
    ○ Recommend reevaluation after 5 years of treatment, if low risk, therapy can be discontinued. If still high risk, then therapy can be continued for up to 10 years (4)[B].
    ○ Additionally, there is a potentially an increased risk for rebound bone turnover following discontinuation; therefore, consideration of subsequent bisphosphonate or alternative therapy is recommended.
  – Romosozumab 210 mg (split in two separate injections) once monthly
    ○ Monoclonal antibody that inhibits sclerostin, leading to increased bone formation
    ○ Romosozumab therapy (12 months) followed by alendronate for women with severe osteoporosis or at high risk for fractures (1)[B]
    ○ May increase risk of adverse cardiovascular events (although pairing with bisphosphonate therapy may reduce this risk)
- Recombinant formulations of PTH (anabolic agents that stimulate bone through osteoblastic activation):
  – Preferred in severe osteoporosis patients due to their capability of reducing fracture risk more quickly
    ○ Teriparatide 20 mg SC daily
      ■ Studies have shown a reduction in the incidence of vertebral fractures by 65% and nonvertebral fractures by 53%.
      ■ Although effective, use is limited to high risk for fractures (or previous therapy unsuccessful) as only approved for use up to 2 years in duration (4)[B].
      ■ Fractures and bone loss may rapidly occur after discontinuation; therefore, sequential therapy with antiresorptive agent (bisphosphonate) is recommended (1)[A].
    ○ Abaloparatide 80 μg SC daily
      ■ Similar safety profile to teriparatide

ISSUES FOR REFERRAL

- Endocrinology for recurrent bone loss/fracture or atypical cases of osteoporosis
- Dental professional for oral examinations

ADDITIONAL THERAPIES

- Weight-bearing exercise 30 minutes 3 times per week, physical therapy, and fall prevention strategies
- Smoking cessation

SURGERY/OTHER PROCEDURES

Options for patients compression fractures:

- Vertebroplasty: Orthopedic cement is injected into the compressed vertebral body.
- Kyphoplasty: A balloon is expanded within the compressed vertebral body; cement is injected.

ADMISSION, INPATIENT, AND NURSING CONSIDERATIONS

Inpatient care for pain control of acute fractures

ONGOING CARE

- Shared decision-making with the patient regarding treatment
- Drug holidays may be considered.

FOLLOW-UP RECOMMENDATIONS

- Lifestyle modifications
- Exercises including strength and balance
- Optimization of calcium and vitamin D
- Repeat analysis with DEXA.

Patient Monitoring

- Weight-bearing exercises such as walking, jogging, stair climbing, and tai chi have been shown to decrease falls and fracture risk.
- Yearly height measurement assists treatment efficacy. Patients who lose >2 cm in height should have repeat vertebral imaging (5)[C].
- Most recommendations suggest repeating a DEXA scan to assess BMD 2 years after starting bisphosphonate therapy.
- Perform a risk assessment after 3 to 5 years of treatment. If BMD T-score at the hip is ≥2.5 and there has not been a hip or vertebral fracture, consider stopping treatment. If BMD remains low or high risk for fractures, the patient may benefit by continuing treatment beyond 5 years (6)[B].
- Patients on bisphosphonates for 5 years (3 years of IV of zoledronic acid) and if a stable BMD, no prior fracture, and a low risk for fracture, can be considered for a drug holiday (4)[B]
- Patients on bisphosphonates for 5 years at high fracture risk (prior fragility fracture, older age, frailty, and high fall risk) should be continued on therapy and a drug holiday can be reconsidered after 6 to 10 years (4)[B].
- Physicians prescribing bisphosphonates should advise patients of the small risk of osteonecrosis of the jaw and encourage dental examinations (6)[C].

DIET

- Maintain normal body weight.
- Adequate calcium and vitamin D

PATIENT EDUCATION

- Bone Health and Osteoporosis Foundation (formerly the National Osteoprorosis Foundation): https://www.bonehealthandosteoporosis.org/
- International Osteoporosis Foundation: https://www.osteoporosis.foundation/educational-hub/topic/calcium-calculator

PROGNOSIS

- With treatment, 80% increase bone mass, mobility, and have reduced pain.
- 15% of vertebral and 20–40% of hip fractures may lead to chronic care and/or premature death.

COMPLICATIONS

Severe, disabling pain, and recurrent fractures

REFERENCES

1. Wen F, Du H, Ding L, et al. Clinical efficacy and safety of drug interventions for primary and secondary prevention of osteoporotic fractures in postmenopausal women: network meta-analysis followed by factor and cluster analysis. PLoS ONE. 2020;15(6):e0234123.
2. Cosman F, de Beur SJ, LeBoff MS, et al; for National Osteoporosis Foundation. Clinician's guide to prevention and treatment of osteoporosis. Osteoporos Int. 2014;25(10):2359–2381.
3. Zhou J, Ma X, Wang T, et al. Comparative efficacy of bisphosphonates in short-term fracture prevention for primary osteoporosis: a systematic review with network meta-analyses. Osteoporos Int. 2016;27(11):3289–3300.
4. Anthamatten A, Parish A. Clinical update on osteoporosis. J Midwifery Womens Health. 2019;64(3):265–275.
5. Qaseem A, Forciea MA, McLean RM, et al; for Clinical Guidelines Committee of the American College of Physicians. Treatment of low bone density or osteoporosis to prevent fractures in men and women: a clinical practice guideline update from the American College of Physicians. Ann Intern Med. 2017;166(11):818–839.
6. McClung M, Harris ST, Miller PD, et al. Bisphosphonate therapy for osteoporosis: benefits, risks, and drug holiday. Am J Med. 2013;126(1):13–20.

CODES

ICD10

- M85.80 Other specified disorders of bone density and structure, unspecified site
- M81.0 Age-related osteoporosis w/o current pathological fracture
- M80.00XA Age-rel osteopor w current path fracture, unsp site, init

CLINICAL PEARLS

- Screen all women ≥65 years of age with DEXA scans.
- Premenopausal women with osteoporosis and those not responding to treatment should be screened for secondary causes.
- Bisphosphonates are first line for treatment of osteoporosis.

OTITIS EXTERNA

Douglas S. Parks, MD

 BASICS

DESCRIPTION
Inflammation of the external auditory canal:

- Acute diffuse otitis externa: the most common form; an infectious process; usually bacterial; occasionally fungal (10%)
- Acute circumscribed otitis externa: synonymous with furuncle; associated with infection of the hair follicle, a superficial cellulitic form of otitis externa
- Chronic otitis externa: same as acute diffuse but of longer duration (>6 weeks)
- Eczematous otitis externa: may accompany typical atopic eczema or other primary skin conditions
- Necrotizing malignant otitis externa: an infection that extends into the deeper tissues adjacent to the canal; may include osteomyelitis and cellulitis; rare in children
- System(s) affected: skin/exocrine
- Synonym(s): swimmer's ear

EPIDEMIOLOGY

Incidence
- Unknown; higher in the summer months and in warm, wet climates
- Predominant age: all ages

Prevalence
- Acute, chronic, and eczematous: common
- Necrotizing: uncommon

ETIOLOGY AND PATHOPHYSIOLOGY
- Acute diffuse otitis externa
  - Traumatized external canal (e.g., from use of cotton swab)
  - Bacterial infection (90%): *Pseudomonas* (67%), *Staphylococcus*, *Streptococcus*, gram-negative rods
  - Fungal infection (10%): *Aspergillus* (90%), *Candida*, *Phycomycetes*, *Rhizopus*, *Actinomyces*, *Penicillium*
- Chronic otitis externa: bacterial infection: *Pseudomonas*
- Eczematous otitis externa (associated with primary skin disorder)
  - Eczema, seborrhea, psoriasis
  - Neurodermatitis
  - Contact dermatitis
  - Purulent otitis media
  - Sensitivity to topical medications
- Necrotizing otitis externa
  - Invasive bacterial infection: *Pseudomonas*, increasing incidence of methicillin-resistant *Staphylococcus aureus* (MRSA)
  - Associated with immunosuppression

RISK FACTORS
- Acute and chronic otitis externa
  - Traumatization of external canal
  - Swimming
  - Hot, humid weather
  - Hearing aid use
- Eczematous: primary skin disorder

- Necrotizing otitis externa in adults
  - Advanced age
  - Diabetes mellitus (DM)
  - Debilitating disease
  - AIDS, immunosuppression
- Necrotizing otitis externa in children (rare)
  - Leukopenia
  - Malnutrition
  - DM
  - Diabetes insipidus

GENERAL PREVENTION
- Avoid prolonged exposure to moisture.
- Use preventive antiseptics (acidifying solutions with 2% acetic acid [white vinegar] diluted 50/50 with water or isopropyl alcohol or 2% acetic acid with aluminum acetate [less irritating]) after swimming and bathing.
- Treat predisposing skin conditions.
- Eliminate self-inflicted trauma to canal with cotton swabs and other foreign objects.
- Treat underlying systemic conditions.
- Ear plugs when swimming

 DIAGNOSIS

HISTORY
Variable length history of itching, plugging of ear, ear pain, and discharge from ear

PHYSICAL EXAM
- Ear canal: red, containing purulent discharge and debris
- Pain on manipulation of the pinnae
- Possible periauricular adenitis
- Possible eczema of pinna
- Cranial nerve (VII, IX to XII) involvement (extremely rare)

DIFFERENTIAL DIAGNOSIS
- Otitis media with perforation
- Cranial nerve (VII, IX to XII) palsy with necrotizing otitis externa
- Wisdom tooth eruption
- Basal cell or squamous cell carcinoma

DIAGNOSTIC TESTS & INTERPRETATION
- Gram stain and culture of canal discharge (occasionally helpful)
  - Antibiotic pretreatment may affect results.
- Radiologic evaluation of deep tissues in necrotizing otitis externa with high-resolution CT scan, MRI, gallium scan, and bone scan

Test Interpretation
- Acute and chronic otitis externa: desquamation of superficial epithelium of external canal with infection
- Eczematous otitis externa: pathologic findings consistent with primary skin disorder; secondary infection on occasion
- Necrotizing otitis externa: vasculitis, thrombosis, and necrosis of involved tissues; osteomyelitis

 TREATMENT

GENERAL MEASURES
- Cleaning the external canal may facilitate recovery.
- Analgesics as appropriate for pain
- Antipruritic and antihistamines (eczematous form)
- Ear wick (Pope) for nearly occluded ear canal to assist with antibiotic droplet penetration

MEDICATION
- Trial data is of generally poor quality and may not be fully relevant to primary care settings (1)[A].
- *Pseudomonas* is the most common bacteria, and it is more susceptible to fluoroquinolones such as ciprofloxacin or ofloxacin, with increasing resistance to aminoglycocide. *Staphylococcus* is equally susceptible to both fluoroquinolones and polymyxin B combinations (2)[A]. If a patient has recurring episodes or is not improved in 2 weeks, change the class of antibacterial and consider cultures and sensitivities.
- There is evidence that using of a topical antibiotic with a corticosteroid shortens time to symptom resolution, although there is no evidence that it increases overall cure rate. There is not enough evidence to demonstrate that any antibiotic regimen is clearly superior to any other (3)[B].
- Oral antibiotics are indicated only if there is associated otitis media. Oral antibiotics alone are not effective and markedly increase the risk of progressing to chronic otitis externa.
- Analgesics as needed.
- Recurrent otitis externa may be prevented by applying equal parts white vinegar and isopropyl alcohol (over-the-counter [OTC] rubbing alcohol) to external auditory canals after bathing and swimming.
- Emerging evidence suggests that all topical quinolone antibiotics may have an increased risk of tympanic membrane perforation (4)[A].

First Line
- Acute bacterial and chronic otitis externa (a wick may be helpful in severe cases by keeping the canal open and keeping antibiotic solution in contact with infected skin).
  - Ciprofloxacin 0.3% and dexamethasone 0.1% suspension (expensive as brand): 4 drops BID for 7 days or ofloxacin 0.3% solution (inexpensive generic): 10 drops once a day for 7 days (1)[A]; less ototoxicity and reported antibiotic resistance (5)[A]
  - Neomycin/polymyxin B/hydrocortisone (Cortisporin, generics): 5 drops QID. If the tympanic membrane is ruptured, use the suspension; otherwise, the solution may be used; may be ototoxic and resistance-developing in *Staphylococcus* and *Streptococcus* sp.; not expensive
  - Acetic acid 2% with hydrocortisone 1%: 3 to 5 drops q4–6h for 7 days; may cause minor local stinging. An inexpensive generic. This is as effective as neomycin–polymyxin B. It may take up to 2 days longer to achieve resolution of symptoms (3)[A].

- Fungal otitis externa
  - Topical therapy, antiyeast for *Candida* or yeast: 2% acetic acid 3 to 4 drops QID; clotrimazole 1% solution; itraconazole oral
  - Parenteral antifungal therapy: amphotericin B
  - Patients with Ramsay Hunt syndrome: acyclovir IV
- Eczematous otitis externa: topical therapy
  - Acetic acid 2% in aluminum acetate
  - Aluminum acetate (5%; Burow solution)
  - Steroid cream, lotion, ointment (e.g., triamcinolone 0.1% solution)
  - Antibacterial, if superinfected
- Necrotizing otitis externa
  - Parenteral antibiotics: antistaphylococcal and antipseudomonal
  - 4 to 6 weeks of therapy
  - Fluoroquinolones PO for 2 to 4 weeks

Second Line
- Acute bacterial and chronic otitis externa
  - Betamethasone 0.05% solution may be as effective as a polymyxin B combination without the risk of ototoxicity or antibiotic resistance. However, the data are not very robust, and more study is needed (3)[A].
- Azole antifungals for fungal otitis externa

ISSUES FOR REFERRAL
Resistant cases or those requiring surgical intervention

SURGERY/OTHER PROCEDURES
For necrotizing otitis externa or furuncle

COMPLEMENTARY & ALTERNATIVE MEDICINE
- OTC white vinegar; 3 drops in affected ear for minor case
- Tea tree oil in various concentrations has been used as an antiseptic. Ototoxicity has been reported in animal studies at very high doses.
- Grapefruit seed extract in various concentrations has been described as useful in the lay literature.

ADMISSION, INPATIENT, AND NURSING CONSIDERATIONS
Necrotizing otitis media requiring parenteral antipseudomonal antibiotics

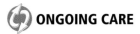 ONGOING CARE

FOLLOW-UP RECOMMENDATIONS
Patient Monitoring
- Chronic otitis externa
  - Every 2 to 3 weeks for repeated cleansing of canal
  - May require alterations in topical medication, including antibiotics and steroids

- Necrotizing otitis externa
  - Daily monitoring in hospital for extension of infection
  - Baseline auditory and vestibular testing at beginning and end of therapy

PROGNOSIS
- Acute otitis externa: rapid response to therapy with total resolution
- Chronic otitis externa: With repeated cleansing and antibiotic therapy, most cases will resolve. Occasionally, surgical intervention is required for resistant cases.
- Eczematous otitis externa: Resolution will occur with control of the primary skin condition.
- Necrotizing otitis externa: usually can be managed with débridement and antipseudomonal antibiotics; recurrence rate is 100% when treatment is inadequate. Surgical intervention may be necessary in resistant cases or if there is cranial nerve involvement. Mortality rate is significant, probably secondary to the underlying disease (6)[C].

COMPLICATIONS
- Necrotizing otitis externa may spread to infect contiguous bone and CNS structures.
- Acute otitis externa may spread to pinna, causing chondritis.

REFERENCES
1. Kaushik V, Malik T, Saeed SR. Interventions for acute otitis externa. *Cochrane Database Syst Rev.* 2010;(1):CD004740.
2. Heward E, Cullen M, Hobson J. Microbiology and antimicrobial susceptibility of otitis externa: a changing pattern of antimicrobial resistance. *J Laryngol Otol.* 2018;132(4):314–317.
3. Rosenfeld RM, Schwartz SR, Cannon CR, et al. Clinical practice guideline: acute otitis externa. *Otolaryngol Head Neck Surg.* 2014;150(Suppl 1):S1–S24.
4. Wang X, Winterstein AG, Alrwisan A, et al. Risk for tympanic membrane perforation after quinolone ear drops for acute otitis externa. *Clin Infec Dis.* 2020;70(6):1103–1109.
5. Mösges R, Nematian-Samani M, Hellmich M, et al. A meta-analysis of the efficacy of quinolone containing otics in comparison to antibiotic-steroid combination drugs in the local treatment of otitis externa. *Curr Med Res Opin.* 2011;27(10):2053–2060.
6. Sylvester MJ, Sanghvi S, Patel VM, et al. Malignant otitis externa hospitalizations: analysis of patient characteristics. *Laryngoscope.* 2017;127(10):2328–2336.

ADDITIONAL READING
Wipperman J. Otitis externa. *Prim Care.* 2014;41(1):1–9.

SEE ALSO
Algorithm: Ear Pain/Otalgia

CODES
ICD10
- H60.523 Acute chemical otitis externa, bilateral
- H60.593 Other noninfective acute otitis externa, bilateral
- B37.84 Candidal otitis externa

CLINICAL PEARLS
- Acute diffuse otitis externa is the most common form: bacterial (90%), occasionally fungal (10%).
- *Pseudomonas* is the most common bacteria, and it is more susceptible to fluoroquinolones such as ciprofloxacin or ofloxacin, with increasing resistance to aminoglycocide. *Staphylococcus* is equally susceptible to both fluoroquinolones and polymyxin B combinations.
- Ear wick (Pope) for nearly occluded ear canal to assist with antibiotic droplet penetration
- Oral antibiotics are indicated only if there is associated otitis media. Oral antibiotics alone are not effective and markedly increase the risk of progressing to chronic otitis externa.
- Eczematous otitis externa may accompany typical atopic eczema or other primary skin conditions.
- Necrotizing malignant otitis externa is an infection that extends into the deeper tissues adjacent to the canal. It may include osteomyelitis and cellulitis; it is rare in children.

OTITIS MEDIA

Sahil Mullick, MD • Paul J. Sliskovich, MD

BASICS

DESCRIPTION
- Inflammation of the middle ear; usually accompanied by fluid collection
- Acute otitis media (AOM): inflammation of the middle ear. Rapid onset; cause may be infectious, either viral (AOM-v) or bacterial (AOM-b), also known as suppurative otitis media, but there is also a sterile etiology (AOM-s)
- Recurrent AOM: ≥3 episodes in 6 months or ≥4 episodes in 1 year with ≥1 in the past 6 months
- Otitis media with effusion (OME): fluid in the middle ear without signs or symptoms of infection. This is also referred to as serous, secretory, or nonsuppurative otitis media.
- Chronic otitis media (COM): recurrent or chronic ear infections; with or without cholesteatoma
- System(s) affected: nervous

EPIDEMIOLOGY
Incidence
- AOM
  - Predominant age: 6 to 24 months; declines >7 years; rare in adults
  - Predominant gender: male > female
  - 50%–85% of children have had at least 1 episode of AOM by age 3; 24% have had 3 or more episodes.
  - Placement of tympanostomy tubes is second only to circumcision as the most frequent surgical procedure in infants.
  - Increased incidence in the fall and winter
- OME
  - 90% of children have had at least one episode by age 4.

Prevalence
- Most common infection for which antibacterial agents are prescribed in the United States
- >5 million cases diagnosed per year in the United States.

ETIOLOGY AND PATHOPHYSIOLOGY
- AOM-b (bacterial): Usually, a preceding viral upper respiratory infection (URI) can produce eustachian tube dysfunction, leading to reduced clearance.
  - *Streptococcus pneumoniae, Haemophilus influenzae, Moraxella catarrhalis* are most frequent pathogens. *Streptococcus pyogenes, Mycoplasma spp* are less frequent.
- AOM-v (viral): 15–44% of AOM infections are caused primarily by viruses (e.g., rhinovirus, respiratory syncytial virus, parainfluenza, influenza, enteroviruses, adenovirus, human metapneumovirus, and bocavirus).
- AOM-s (sterile/nonpathogens): 25–30%
- OME: middle ear inflammation and eustachian tube dysfunction; allergic causes are rarely substantiated.

Genetics
- Strong genetic component in twin studies for recurrent and prolonged AOM
- Immunologic defects and genetic disorders (e.g., Down syndrome) can predispose changes in physical anatomy (e.g., more horizontal and ear canals) that increase likelihood in developing otitis media.

RISK FACTORS
- Age—developing AOM prior to 1 year of age is a risk for recurrent AOM
- Male gender
- Race and ethnicity
- Bottlefeeding while supine; pacifier use
- Routine daycare attendance
- Family history of AOM
- Environmental smoke exposure
- Absence of breastfeeding during first 6 months of life
- Low socioeconomic status
- Atopy
- Underlying ENT disease (e.g., cleft palate, allergic rhinitis)

GENERAL PREVENTION
- PCV-7 and PCV-13 vaccines have lead to a decrease incidence of streptococcal pneumonia induced otitis media (1).
- Influenza vaccine (2)[B]
- Breastfeeding for ≥6 months is protective (2)[B].
- Avoiding supine bottlefeeding, passive smoke, and pacifiers >6 months may be helpful.
- Secondary prevention: Adenoidectomy and adenotonsillectomy for recurrent AOM have limited short-term efficacy and are associated with their own adverse risks. Xylitol is effective at preventing AOM but requires dosing 5 times daily making it impractical as a common preventative treatment.

COMMONLY ASSOCIATED CONDITIONS
URI

DIAGNOSIS

HISTORY
- AOM:
  - Otalgia
  - Preceding or accompanying URI symptoms
  - Decreased hearing
- AOM in adults can present with only otalgia without fever or unilateral hearing loss.

ALERT
- AOM in infants and toddlers may present with only irritability in early months of life.
- OME: usually asymptomatic and may only present with decreased hearing

PHYSICAL EXAM
- AOM:
  - Fever (not required for diagnosis)
  - Decreased eardrum mobility (with pneumatic otoscopy)
  - Moderate to severe bulging of tympanic membrane
  - Red, yellow, or cloudy tympanic membrane
  - Otorrhea
- OME:
  - Eardrum often dull but not bulging
  - Decreased eardrum mobility (pneumatic otoscopy)
  - Presence of air-fluid level
  - Weber test lateralizes to affected ear for an ear with effusion.
  - Tympanometry if pneumatic otoscopy has no findings

DIFFERENTIAL DIAGNOSIS
- Tympanosclerosis
- Trauma
- Referred pain from the jaw, teeth, or throat; TMJ in adults
- Otitis externa
- Otitis-conjunctivitis syndrome
- Temporal arteritis in adults

DIAGNOSTIC TESTS & INTERPRETATION
Initial Tests (lab, imaging)
AOM is largely a clinical diagnosis requiring middle ear effusion (MEE) and signs of middle ear inflammation on exam. Laboratory testing is generally not helpful. WBC count may be elevated in bacterial AOM compared with sterile AOM, but this is almost never useful.

Diagnostic Procedures/Other
- Otoscopy—to document the presence of middle ear fluid
- Pneumatic otoscopy—to detect middle ear fluid (can be supplemented with tympanometry and acoustic reflex measurement). Pneumatic otoscopy is contraindicated with known tympanic perforation.
- Hearing testing is recommended when hearing loss persists for ≥3 months or at any time suspecting language delay, significant hearing loss, or learning problems.
- Language testing should be performed for children with hearing loss.
- Tympanocentesis for microbiologic diagnosis warranted if the child appears toxic, is immunocompromised, or has failed previous courses of antibiotic therapy; may be followed by myringotomy

Test Interpretation
Pneumatic otoscopy—tympanic mobility will be impaired if middle ear fluid is present.

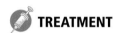

TREATMENT

GENERAL MEASURES
- Assess pain and, if present, recommend treatment to decrease otalgia.
- Minimize any risk factors.
- Two-thirds of children will recover without any antibiotic treatment.
- AOM: Observation with watchful waiting for those >6 months with mild acute otitis media. Prescribe antibiotics if no improvement or clinical worsening within 24–48 hours (3)[C].
- OME watchful waiting for 3 months and if no improvement, then refer to ENT for possible surgery. Antibiotics, decongestants, antihistamines, and steroids are not recommended.

MEDICATION
First Line
- Controversy exists about the usefulness of antibiotic treatment for this often self-resolving condition. Studies suggest number needed to treat for an additional beneficial outcome (NNTB) is 20 when looking at relief of pain at 2 to 3 days after start of antibiotics; the number needed to harm (primarily diarrhea and vomiting) is 9.
- AAP/AAFP recommends:
  - Treatment for <6 months of age: Treat with amoxicillin if >2 weeks old.
  - >6 months: Antibacterial therapy is recommended with severe otitis media (i.e., moderate to severe otalgia, otalgia >48 hours or fever ≥39°C) (4)[B] or otorrhea or bilateral otitis media between 6 months and 2 years of age.
- Observation is an option with nonsevere otitis media at >6 months to 2 years (otalgia <48 hours, temperature <39°C). However, there is a high risk of treatment failure, and antibiotics are recommended (5)[C].
- Immunocompetent children >2 can be observed. Parents/guardians must understand risks/benefits of observation.

- AOM: AAP/AAFP consensus guideline recommends treating with antibiotics if:
  - Between 2 weeks and 6 months OR
  - >6 months with severe otitis media (e.g., moderate to severe otalgia, otalgia > 48 hours, or fevers >39°C) OR
  - Otorrhea OR
  - Bilateral otitis media in infants between 6 and 23 months of age without severe signs/symptoms
- Treat with:
  - Amoxicillin, 90 mg/kg/day in 2 divided doses (maximum of 3 g/day) in those without risk of antibiotic resistance (4)[B]
- Treatment duration:
  - 10-day course for children <2 years
  - 5- to 7-day course for children ≥2 years (6)[C]
- If penicillin allergic:
  - Cefdinir, 14 mg/kg/day in 1 to 2 doses (maximum 600 mg/day) for 10 days OR
  - Cefpodoxime, 10 mg/kg/day in 2 divided doses (maximum 400 mg/day) for 10 days OR
  - Cefuroxime 30 mg/kg/day in 2 divided doses (maximum 1 g/day) for 10 days; OR
  - Ceftriaxone 50 mg/kg IM/IV per day for 1 to 3 days depending on symptomatic improvement (4)
  - Azithromycin 10 mg/kg on day 1 and 5 mg/kg days 2 to 5
- OME: No apparent benefit to medications which promote transitory resolution in 10–15%, but the effect is short-lived (7)[B].

Second Line
- Alternative antibiotics are indicated for the following AOM patients:
  - Persistent symptoms after 48 to 72 hours of amoxicillin
  - AOM within 1 month of amoxicillin therapy
  - Severe earache
  - Age <6 months with high fever
  - Immunocompromised
    - Amoxicillin-clavulanate; 90 mg/kg/day of amoxicillin, with 6.4 mg/kg/day of clavulanate in 2 divided doses; recommended in children who have taken amoxicillin in the previous 30 days and those with concurrent purulent conjunctivitis or history of AOM unresponsive to amoxicillin
    - Ceftriaxone, 50 mg/kg IM or IV q24h for 2 to 3 consecutive days can be reserved for those who are too sick to take oral medications or who unsuccessfully took amoxicillin-clavulanate.
- Neither erythromycin nor trimethoprim-sulfamethoxazole should be used as a second-line agent in treatment failures.
- Recurrent AOM: Antibiotic prophylaxis for recurrent AOM (>3 distinct, well-documented episodes in 6 months) is not recommended (2)[B].

ISSUES FOR REFERRAL
- If hearing loss occurs for >2 weeks after AOM resolution, follow up with audiogram.
- If >2 episodes in a 6-month period, consider ENT referral for fiberoptic nasopharyngoscopy to rule out malignancy.
- Refer to ENT for recurrent COM for consideration of tympanostomy tubes.

ADDITIONAL THERAPIES
Pain control: Acetaminophen, ibuprofen, topical procaine or lidocaine for children >2 years but should not be used in with tympanic perforation

SURGERY/OTHER PROCEDURES
- Recurrent AOM: No definitive guidelines agreed on as indications for surgery. Can consider referral for surgery if ≥3 episodes of well-documented AOM within 6 months, ≥4 episodes within 12 months with ≥1 episode in previous 6 months, or AOM episodes occur while on chemoprophylaxis
- Tympanostomy tubes may be effective in selective patients, particularly children age <2 years with recurrent AOM (8)[A].
- Adenotonsillectomy reduced the rate of AOM by 0.7 episode per child only in the 1st year after surgery and had a 15% complication rate.
- COM: Referral for surgery for tympanostomy should be individualized. It can be considered if >4 to 6 months of bilateral OME and/or >6 months of unilateral OME and/or hearing loss >25 dB or for high-risk individuals at any time.
- Tympanostomy tubes may reduce recurrence of AOM minimally, but it does not lower the risk of hearing loss (4)[B].

COMPLEMENTARY & ALTERNATIVE MEDICINE
Limited evidence for: acupuncture, herbal therapy, osteopathy, ear candling, and probiotics. Further studies required.

ADMISSION, INPATIENT, AND NURSING CONSIDERATIONS
Outpatient management is appropriate, except AOM in febrile infants age <2 months or children requiring ceftriaxone who also require monitoring for 24 hours.

ONGOING CARE

FOLLOW-UP RECOMMENDATIONS
Patients with otitis media who do not respond within 48 to 72 hours should be reevaluated:
- If therapy was initiated, consider changing the antibiotic; options are limited because macrolides have limited benefit against *H. influenzae* over amoxicillin, and most oral cephalosporins have no improved outcomes.

Patient Monitoring
- AOM: Up to 40% may have persistent middle ear effusion at 1 month, with 10–25% at 3 months.
- OME/COM: Repeat otoscopic or tympanometric exams at 3 months, as indicated, as long as OME persists or sooner if there are red flags (see earlier discussion).

PROGNOSIS
Most cases of uncomplicated, nonsevere AOM resolve without antibiotics.

COMPLICATIONS
- AOM: tympanic membrane perforation/otorrhea, acute mastoiditis, facial nerve paralysis, otitic hydrocephalus, meningitis, labyrinthitis and hearing impairment, myringosclerosis, petrositis, brain abscess, epidural or subdural abscess, lateral or cavernous sinus thrombosis, or cholesteatoma.
- COM: Speech and language disabilities may occur. Hearing loss is not caused by OME, but in children who are at risk for speech, language, or learning problems (e.g., autism spectrum, syndromes, craniofacial disorders, developmental delay, and children already with speech/language delay), it could lead to further problems because they are less tolerant of a hearing impairment.
- Recurrent AOM and COM: atrophy and scarring of eardrum, chronic perforation and otorrhea, cholesteatoma, permanent hearing loss, chronic mastoiditis, other intracranial suppurative complications

REFERENCES
1. Ben-Shimol S, Givon-Lavi N, Leibovitz E, et al. Impact of widespread introduction of pneumococcal conjugate vaccines on pneumococcal and nonpneumococcal otitis media. *Clin Infect Dis.* 2016;63(5):611–618.
2. Lieberthal A, Carroll A, Chonmaitree T, et al. The diagnosis and management of acute otitis media. *Pediatrics.* 2013;131(3):e964–e999.
3. Sakulchit T, Goldman RD. Antibiotic therapy for children with acute otitis media. *Can Fam Physician.* 2017;63(9):685–687.
4. Harmes K, Blackwood A, Burrows HL, et al. Otitis media: diagnosis and treatment. *Am Fam Physician.* 2013;88(7):435–440.
5. Hoberman A, Ruohola A, Shaikh N, et al. Acute otitis media in children younger than 2 years. *JAMA Pediatr.* 2013;167(12):1171–1172.
6. Hoberman A, Paradise J, Rockette H, et al. Shortened antimicrobial treatment for acute otitis media in young children. *N Engl J Med.* 2016;375(25):2446–2456.
7. Venekamp RP, Burton MJ, van Dongen TM, et al. Antibiotics for otitis media with effusion in children. *Cochrane Database Syst Rev.* 2016;(6):CD009163.
8. Kujala T, Alho O-P, Luotonen J, et al. Tympanostomy with and without adenoidectomy for the prevention of recurrences of acute otitis media: a randomized controlled trial. *Pediatr Infect Dis J.* 2012;31(6):565–569.

 SEE ALSO

Algorithm: Ear Pain/Otalgia

CODES

ICD10
- H65 Nonsuppurative otitis media
- H65.0 Acute serous otitis media
- H65.00 Acute serous otitis media, unspecified ear

CLINICAL PEARLS
- Pneumatic otoscopy is the single most specific and clinically useful test for diagnosis.
- Consider a delay of antibiotics for 24 to 48 hours in uncomplicated presentations (>6 months of age) who do not have severe illness or otorrhea.
- First-line treatment is amoxicillin, 80 to 90 mg/kg/day for 10 days for children age <2 years; consider a 5- to 7-day course in >2 years of age.
- Erythema and effusion can persist for weeks.
- Antibiotics, antihistamines, and steroids are not indicated for COM.
- OME rarely develops in adults. Persistent unilateral effusion should be investigated to rule out neoplasm, particularly if there is a cranial nerve palsy.

OTITIS MEDIA WITH EFFUSION
Hobart Lee, MD, FAAFP

 BASICS

DESCRIPTION
- Also called serous otitis media, secretory otitis media, nonsuppurative otitis media, "ear fluid," or "glue ear"
- Otitis media with effusion (OME) is defined as the presence of fluid in the middle ear in the absence of acute signs or symptoms of infection.
- More commonly, a pediatric disease
- May occur spontaneously from poor eustachian tube function or as an inflammatory response after acute otitis media (AOM)

EPIDEMIOLOGY
Approximately 90% of children have OME before school age, mostly between the ages of 6 months and 4 years.

Incidence
Approximately 2.2 million new cases annually in the United States

Prevalence
Less prevalent in adults and is usually associated with an underlying disorder

ETIOLOGY AND PATHOPHYSIOLOGY
- Chronic inflammatory condition where an underlying stimulus causes an inflammatory reaction with increased mucin production creating a functional blockage of the eustachian tube and thick accumulation of mucin-rich middle ear effusion
- Young children are more prone to OME due to shorter and more horizontal eustachian tubes, which become more vertical around 7 years of age.
- Biofilms, anatomic variations, and AOM caused by viruses or bacteria have been implicated as stimuli causing OME. The common pathogens causing AOM include nontypeable *Haemophilus influenzae*, *Streptococcus pneumoniae*, and *Moraxella catarrhalis*.
- In adults, OME is often associated with paranasal sinus disease (66%), smoking-induced nasopharyngeal lymphoid hyperplasia and adult-onset adenoidal hypertrophy (19%), or head and neck tumors (4.8%).

RISK FACTORS
- Risk factors include a family history of OME, early daycare, exposure to cigarette smoke, bottle-feeding, and low socioeconomic status (1).
- Eustachian tube dysfunction may be a predisposing factor, although the evidence is unclear (2).
- Gastroesophageal reflux is associated with OME (2).

GENERAL PREVENTION
OME is generally not preventable, although lowering smoke exposure, breastfeeding, and avoiding daycare centers at an early age may decrease the risk.

 DIAGNOSIS

HISTORY
- OME is transient and asymptomatic in many pediatric patients.
- Most common reported symptom is hearing loss (2). There may be mild discomfort present in the ear, fullness, or "popping."
- Infants may have ear rubbing, excessive irritability, sleep problems, or failure to respond appropriately to voices or sounds.
- Clinical features may include "a history of hearing difficulties, poor attention, behavioral problems, delayed speech and language development, clumsiness, and poor balance" (2).
- There may be a history of recent or recurrent episodes of AOM or a recent upper respiratory tract infection (2).

PHYSICAL EXAM
- Cloudy tympanic membrane (TM) with distinctly impaired mobility. Air-fluid level or bubble may be visible in the middle ear (1),(2).
- Color may be abnormal (yellow, amber, or blue), and the TM may be retracted or concave (2).
- Distinct redness of the TM may be present in approximately 5% of OME cases (1).
- Clinical signs and symptoms of acute illness should be absent in patients with OME (1).

DIFFERENTIAL DIAGNOSIS
- AOM
- Bullous myringitis
- Tympanosclerosis (may cause decreased/absent motion of the TM)
- Sensorineural hearing loss

DIAGNOSTIC TESTS & INTERPRETATION
Initial Tests (lab, imaging)
The primary standard to make the diagnosis is pneumatic otoscopy, which demonstrates reduced/absent mobility of the TM secondary to fluid in the middle ear. Pneumatic otoscopy has 94% sensitivity and 80% specificity for diagnosing OME. Accuracy of diagnosis with an experienced examiner is between 70% and 79% (1)[C].

Follow-Up Tests & Special Considerations
- Tympanometry may also be used to support or exclude the diagnosis in infants >4 months old, especially when the presence of middle ear effusion is difficult to determine (1)[C].
- Acoustic reflectometry (64% specificity and 80% sensitivity) may be considered instead of tympanometry (3)[B].
- Audiogram may show mild conductive hearing loss (2)[C].
- Hearing tests are recommended for OME lasting >3 months (1)[C].
- Language testing is recommended for children with abnormal hearing tests (1)[C].

Diagnostic Procedures/Other
Myringotomy is the gold standard but is not practical for clinical use (2)[C].

 TREATMENT

- OME improves or resolves without medical intervention in most patients within 3 months, especially if secondary to AOM (1)[C].
- Current guidelines support a 3-month period of observation with optional serial exams, tympanometry, and language assessment during that wait time (1),(2)[C].
- Adults found to have OME should be screened for an underlying disorder and treated accordingly (2)[C].

MEDICATION
- The 2016 AAOHNS guideline recommends against routine use of antibiotics in treatment of OME. A 2016 Cochrane review, however, found that children treated with oral antibiotics were more likely to have tympanogram confirmed OME resolution in 2 to 3 months (number needed to treat = 5). Adverse events included diarrhea, vomiting, skin rash, and allergic reactions (number needed to harm = 20). Importantly, there were no reported patient-oriented outcomes (e.g., cognitive development, language, quality of life, or speech). Outcomes regarding short-term hearing, reduction of AOM infections, or need for ventilation tubes are unknown (1)[C],(4)[A].
- The 2016 AAOHNS and a 2006 Cochrane review found that antihistamines and decongestants have no benefit over placebo in OME treatment with possible adverse side effects such as insomnia, hyperactivity, and drowsiness (5)[A].

- The 2016 AAOHNS guideline recommends against administering oral or intranasal corticosteroids. No long-term benefit was shown, and adverse side effects such as weight gain and behavioral changes are possible (1)[C].
- In adults, eustachian tube dysfunction secondary to allergic rhinitis or recent upper respiratory infection can be the cause of OME. It is unknown whether decongestants, antihistamines, or nasal steroids improve outcomes in adults.

ISSUES FOR REFERRAL
The following are indications for referral to a surgeon for evaluation of tympanostomy tube placement:
- Chronic bilateral OME (≥3 months) with hearing difficulty
- Chronic OME with symptoms (e.g., vestibular problems, poor school performance, behavioral issues, ear discomfort, or reduced quality of life)
- At-risk children (speech, language, or learning problems due to baseline sensory, physical, cognitive, or behavioral factors) with chronic OME or type B (flat) tympanogram

ADDITIONAL THERAPIES
Hearing aids may be an acceptable alternative to surgery (2)[C].

SURGERY/OTHER PROCEDURES
- Tympanostomy tubes are recommended as initial surgery. Risks include purulent otorrhea, myringosclerosis, retraction pockets, and persistent TM perforations (1)[C].
- Adenoidectomy with myringotomy has similar efficacy to tympanostomy tubes in children >4 years of age but with added surgical and anesthetic risks (1)[C],(6).
- Adenoidectomy should not be performed in children with persistent OME alone unless there is a distinct indication for the procedure for another problem (e.g., adenoiditis/chronic sinusitis/nasal obstruction) (1)[C].
- Adenoidectomy (and concurrent tube placement) may be considered when repeat surgery for OME is necessary (e.g., when effusion recurs after tubes have fallen out or are removed). In these cases, adenoidectomy has been shown to decrease the need for future procedures for OME (1),(2)[C].
- Tonsillectomy or myringotomy alone is not recommended for treatment (1)[C].

COMPLEMENTARY & ALTERNATIVE MEDICINE
Autoinflation, which refers to the process of opening the eustachian tube by raising intranasal pressure (e.g., by forced exhalation with closed mouth and nose), may be beneficial in improving patients' tympanogram or audiometry and quality of life scores.

 ONGOING CARE

FOLLOW-UP RECOMMENDATIONS
Patient Monitoring
- Children who are at risk for developmental difficulties should be evaluated for OME at the time of diagnosis and at 12 to 18 months (if initial diagnosis occurred <12 months). At-risk conditions include permanent hearing loss independent of OME, suspected or confirmed speech and language delay, autism spectrum disorder or other pervasive developmental disorder, Down syndrome or other craniofacial disorder, blindness or other uncorrectable visual impairment, cleft palate, and unspecified developmental delay (1)[C].
- For patients diagnosed with OME, reevaluation and repeat hearing tests should be performed every 3 to 6 months until the effusion has resolved or until the child develops an indication for surgical referral (1)[C].

PROGNOSIS
Approximately 50% of children >3 years of age have OME resolution within 3 months.

COMPLICATIONS
- The most significant complication of OME is permanent hearing loss, leading to possible language, speech, and developmental delays.
- Underventilation of the middle ear can cause a cholesteatoma (1)[C].

REFERENCES
1. Rosenfeld RM, Shin JJ, Schwartz SR, et al. Clinical practice guideline: otitis media with effusion executive summary (update). *Otolaryngol Head Neck Surg.* 2016;154(2):201–214.
2. Qureishi A, Lee Y, Belfield K, et al. Update on otitis media—prevention and treatment. *Infect Drug Resist.* 2014;7:15–24.
3. Shekelle P, Takata G, Chan LS, et al. Diagnosis, natural history, and late effects of otitis media with effusion. *Evid Rep Technol Assess (Summ).* 2002;(55):1–5.
4. Venekamp RP, Burton MJ, van Dongen TM, et al. Antibiotics for otitis media with effusion in children. *Cochrane Database Syst Rev.* 2016;(6):CD009163.
5. Griffin G, Flynn CA. Antihistamines and/or decongestants for otitis media with effusion (OME) in children. *Cochrane Database Syst Rev.* 2011;(9):CD003423.
6. Casselbrant ML, Mandel EM, Rockette HE, et al. Adenoidectomy for otitis media with effusion in 2–3-year-old children. *Int J Pediatr Otorhinolaryngol.* 2009;73(12):1718–1724.

ADDITIONAL READING
Cheng X, Sheng H, Ma R, et al. Allergic rhinitis and allergy are risk factors for otitis media with effusion: a meta-analysis. *Allergol Immunopathol (Madr).* 2017;45(1):25–32.

CODES

ICD10
- H65.90 Unspecified nonsuppurative otitis media, unspecified ear
- H65.00 Acute serous otitis media, unspecified ear
- H65.20 Chronic serous otitis media, unspecified ear

CLINICAL PEARLS
- OME is defined as the presence of a middle ear effusion in the absence of acute signs of infection.
- In children, OME most often arises following an AOM. In adults, it often occurs in association with eustachian tube dysfunction.
- The primary standard for diagnosis is pneumatic otoscopy.
- There is no benefit in antihistamines, decongestants, or corticosteroids for the treatment of OME in children.
- Management usually includes watchful waiting and surgery (when indicated); which strategy is chosen depends on many factors, including the risk/presence of any associated speech, language, or learning delays, and on the severity of any associated hearing loss.

OVARIAN CANCER

Susan Zweizig, MD • Aashna Saini, MD

 BASICS

Ovarian cancer accounts for 4% of cancers occurring in women. According to the CDC, there are >19,000 new cases of ovarian cancer annually in the United States, and approximately 14,000 deaths annually; thus, this the most lethal of gynecologic cancers, which accounts for 2.3% of all cancer deaths nationally.

DESCRIPTION
Malignancy that arises from the epithelium (90–95%), sex cord stromal (5–8%), or germ cells (5%) of the ovary as well as tumors metastatic to the ovary. Histologic types include the following:
- Epithelial: serous (most common, 70–80%), mucinous, endometrioid, clear cell
- Sex cord stromal: granulosa, Sertoli-Leydig
- Germ cell: dysgerminoma (most common), teratoma, yolk sac
- Metastatic from: GI (Krukenberg, colon), melanoma, lymphoma

EPIDEMIOLOGY
Incidence
- In 2018, there were 19,679 new cases per year in the United States; 13,748 deaths per year
- Represents 1.1% of all new cancer cases in the United States
- Leading cause of gynecologic cancer death in women, fourth most common cause of death overall cancer death in women
- Majority of ovarian cancer is diagnosed at an advanced stage.
- Average age of diagnosis
  - Epithelial: 63 years
  - Sex cord stromal: 50 years
  - Germ cell: 10 to 30 years

Prevalence
- In 2018, there were approximately 235,081 women living with ovarian cancer in the United States.
- Without a significant family history or known genetic mutation, women have a 1–2% lifetime risk of developing this disease. Although 5–10% of ovarian cancers may be attributed to hereditary syndromes, most ovarian cancers are sporadic in the general population.

ETIOLOGY AND PATHOPHYSIOLOGY
- Reproductive history and duration of reproductive career are the strongest predictors (low parity/infertility, early menarche, late menopause). Suppression of ovulation may prevent repetitive disruption of the epithelial lining and thereby preclude spontaneous mutations that unmask germline mutations.
- A higher percentage of ovarian cancers are now known to originate in the fallopian tube and other components of the secondary müllerian system, including primary peritoneal cancers.

Genetics
- Hereditary breast ovarian cancer syndrome: early-onset breast or ovarian cancer, autosomal dominant transmission with variable penetrance, usually associated with *BRCA-1* or *BRCA-2* mutation. 10–14% of patients with ovarian cancer have BRCA-1 or BRCA-2. Lifetime risk of ovarian cancer with BRCA-1: 39%, BRCA-2: 11%
- Lynch syndrome: autosomal dominant inheritance; increased risk for colorectal, endometrial, stomach, small bowel, breast, pancreas, and ovarian cancers; defect in DNA mismatch repair genes. Lifetime risk of ovarian cancer with Lynch syndrome: 6–12%

RISK FACTORS
- 90% is sporadic, but family history is the most significant risk factor. Multiple relatives with breast or ovarian cancer: Refer these patients for genetic counseling. Individuals with familial cancer syndromes have 20–60% risk of developing ovarian cancer.
- Risk factors: older age, white race, infertility, nulligravidity, early menarche or late menopause, endometriosis, postmenopausal estrogen replacement therapy, residence in an industrialized Western country
- Association between fertility medications and risk of ovarian cancer is controversial, but women with infertility who have a successful live birth do not have an increased risk of ovarian cancer.
- Obesity as a risk factor for ovarian cancer remains inconclusive; some studies do suggest an increased risk with BMI >30 and increased mortality related to BMI >35.

GENERAL PREVENTION
- Long-term use of oral contraceptives: 5 years of use decreases risk by 20%; 15 years of use decreases risk by 50%.
- Multiparity
- Breastfeeding
- Tubal ligation, salpingectomy, or hysterectomy
- Risk-reducing salpingo-oophorectomy (estimated to reduce the risk of BRCA-related gynecologic cancer by 96%)
- Protective effect of aspirin and NSAIDs in ovarian cancer is controversial.
- Recommendations for high-risk (family history of a hereditary ovarian cancer syndrome) population
  - Women should undergo pelvic examinations, CA-125 level measurement, and transvaginal US every 6 to 12 months beginning at age 30 or 10 years prior to the earliest age of diagnosis of ovarian cancer in the family—although efficacy of this approach has not been established.
  - Women with family histories of ovarian cancer or premenopausal breast cancer should be referred for genetic counseling.
  - Prophylactic oophorectomy is advised for mutation carriers after childbearing is completed or by age 35 years.
    - Risk of primary peritoneal carcinoma remains 1–2% after prophylactic oophorectomy.
- Screening: No effective screening exists for ovarian cancer in the general population.
  - Routine use of CA-125 and transvaginal US for screening in women of average risk is NOT recommended. Annual pelvic examinations may be performed, particularly in postmenopausal women. An adnexal mass in a premenarchal female or a palpable adnexa in a postmenopausal female warrants further evaluation.

COMMONLY ASSOCIATED CONDITIONS
- Pelvic pain, ascites, pleural effusion
- Carcinomatosis, bowel obstruction
- Breast cancer, endometrial cancer

DIAGNOSIS

HISTORY
- Vague, nonspecific abdominal symptoms
- Acute presentation:
  - Shortness of breath (pleural effusion)
  - Nausea, vomiting, decreased oral intake (bowel obstruction)
  - Calf pain, shortness of breath (venous thromboembolism)
  - Severe abdominal or pelvic pain (ovarian torsion or rupture)
- Subacute presentation:
  - Abdominal or pelvic pain/cramping
  - Bloating, sense of abdominal fullness, increased abdominal size (ascites)
  - Early satiety, anorexia, dyspepsia
  - Dyspareunia
  - Urinary frequency or urgency in absence of infection
  - Fatigue, weight loss
  - Precocious puberty (sex cord stromal or germ cell tumors)

PHYSICAL EXAM
- General appearance: cachexia, hirsutism (androgen-secreting tumors)
- Pelvic: pelvic mass: solid, irregular, fixed mass
- Rectovaginal: cul-de-sac nodularity
- Abdominal: fluid wave (ascites), mass, omental caking
- Pulmonary: decreased breath sounds (pleural effusion)
- Lymphatics: lymphadenopathy, firm immobile enlarged lymph nodes (supraclavicular, inguinal)

DIFFERENTIAL DIAGNOSIS
- Benign conditions of reproductive tract:
  - Uterine fibroids
  - Endometriomas
  - Physiologic cysts
  - Tubo-ovarian abscess or hydrosalpinx
  - Pelvic inflammatory disease (PID)
- GI or endometrial malignancies
- Benign or borderline neoplasms
- IBS, diverticulitis, colitis
- Hepatic failure with ascites
- Pelvic kidney

DIAGNOSTIC TESTS & INTERPRETATION
Diagnosis of ovarian cancer requires histologic examination of tissue pathology (often the resected ovary).

Initial Tests (lab, imaging)
- CBC
- Liver function tests (LFTs) to rule out hepatic disease
- Urinalysis
- Serum albumin
- Tumor markers:
  - Epithelial tumors: CA-125, CA 19-9, CEA
    - CA-125 (normal <35 unit/dL): elevated in 90% of women with malignant nonmucinous tumors. 50% of stage I ovarian cancers with falsely negative CA-125. Common benign gynecologic conditions (PID, endometriosis, fibroids, pregnancy, menstruation) can cause elevations. CA-125 levels can be elevated with non-gynecologic conditions, including ascites, pleural effusion, congestive heart failure, pancreatitis, systemic lupus erythematosus, and liver disease.
    - CA 19-9 and CEA: better indicators of disease in mucinous tumors, helpful if GI primary suspected
  - Nonepithelial tumors: inhibin A/B (granulosa cell tumor), HCG (dysgerminoma, choriocarcinoma, embryonal carcinoma), AFP (endodermal sinus tumor, embryonal carcinoma), LDH (dysgerminoma)
- Transvaginal US (better than transabdominal US or CT to evaluate pelvic masses): complex masses (irregular borders, echogenic, septae)

734

- CT abdomen and pelvis with contrast (Evaluate metastasis and preoperative planning.)
- CXR or CT chest (to evaluate for pleural effusions or lung nodules)

Follow-Up Tests & Special Considerations
- Patients with ovarian cancer should be up-to-date with screening: mammograms, Pap smear, colonoscopy.
- Colonoscopy (or other test to evaluate the colon) is needed if a colonic primary is suspected.

Diagnostic Procedures/Other
- Do not biopsy ovarian masses due to concern for tumor seeding.
- Consider paracentesis or thoracentesis (or IR biopsy of pelvic mass) if patient not an operative candidate.
  - IR biopsy: Epithelial ovarian cancer commonly involves the peritoneal surfaces of the abdomen and pelvis.

Test Interpretation
Pathologic diagnosis (with surgery, IR biopsy, or cytology) is necessary for definitive diagnosis.

 ## TREATMENT

Treatment determined by stage of disease

GENERAL MEASURES
- Surgical exploration with staging and debulking is critical. Optimal cytoreduction of tumor burden enhances effectiveness of adjuvant therapy and is associated with longer survival.
- In patients with bulky advanced disease in epithelial ovarian cancer where optimal cytoreduction with primary surgery is unlikely, it is reasonable to consider neoadjuvant chemotherapy (NACT), preoperative chemotherapy, after consultation with a gynecologic oncologist (1)[A].

MEDICATION
First Line
- After surgery, most patients will require chemotherapy or adjuvant therapy.
- Stage IA or IB and grade 1 or 2 who are optimally staged do not require adjuvant therapy (2)[A].
- Clear cell histology, grade 3 tumors, or stage IC or worse tumors require adjuvant therapy.
- Early stage epithelial ovarian cancer adjuvant chemotherapy regimen: carboplatin and paclitaxel (Taxol) for 6 cycles
- PARP inhibitors: target DNA repair pathway of tumor cells thereby targeting tumor cells while sparing normal cells. Particularly effective in BRCA-1 and BRCA-2 patients; often used as maintenance treatment for platinum sensitive or homologous recombination deficiency (HRD)-positive status
- Germ cell or sex cord–stromal cancers: bleomycin, etoposide, and cisplatin
- Contraindications to chemotherapy: poor functional status, excessive toxicity, hypersensitivity
- Adverse reactions: All regimens cause bone marrow suppression. Cisplatin is associated with ototoxicity, renal toxicity, and peripheral neuropathy. Paclitaxel (Taxol) can cause neuropathy and alopecia.
- Patients should be encouraged to participate in clinical trials whenever possible.
- Antiemetics: ondansetron (Zofran), aprepitant (Emend), metoclopramide (Reglan), prochlorperazine (Compazine), promethazine (Phenergan)

Second Line
Liposomal doxorubicin (Doxil), carboplatin/gemcitabine, topotecan, etoposide, bevacizumab, cyclophosphamide, tamoxifen

ADDITIONAL THERAPIES
- NACT followed by interval debulking surgery for disease if there is a good response to treatment followed by additional cycles of chemotherapy after surgery
- Given high risk of recurrence, patients with a known BRCA-1 or BRCA-2 mutation are placed on FDA-approved PARP inhibitor olaparib after completion of primary treatment for maintenance therapy.

SURGERY/OTHER PROCEDURES
- Goal of surgery is optimal cytoreduction (<1 cm of maximum tumor diameter remaining).
- Staging for epithelial cancer:
  - Cytologic evaluation of peritoneal fluid (free fluid or peritoneal washings)
  - Total hysterectomy, bilateral salpingo-oophorectomy with tumor reductive surgery
  - Omentectomy
  - Inspection, palpation, and biopsy of peritoneal surfaces
  - Biopsy of adhesions or any suspicious areas
  - Lymph nodes: bilateral pelvic and para-aortic lymph node biopsies
  - Appendectomy for mucinous tumors or if appendix appears abnormal
- Germ cell or sex cord–stromal cancers: salpingo-oophorectomy (unilateral if only one ovary involved) in young patient for fertility sparing management

COMPLEMENTARY & ALTERNATIVE MEDICINE
CAM (complementary and alternative medicine) treatments (cognitive distraction, exercise, hypnosis, and relaxation) may mitigate effects of chemotherapy such as nausea, diarrhea, fatigue, and hair loss. However, these lack quality evidence regarding their true effectiveness.

 ## ONGOING CARE

FOLLOW-UP RECOMMENDATIONS
- Surgical patients should follow-up within 4 weeks for postoperative assessment and for further treatment planning.
- Patient undergoing chemotherapy should have regular visits to assess toxicity and disease progression.

Patient Monitoring
- Physical exam every 2 to 4 months for the first 2 years, every 3 to 6 months for next 3 years and then annually
- If tumor markers elevated at diagnosis, follow levels after treatment to detect recurrence. CBC, BMP as indicated
- Germ cell/sex cord–stromal: physical exam and tumor markers every 3 months for the first 2 years and then annually
  - Tumor markers for sex cord–stromal cancers should be checked every 6 months for 10 years because recurrences can occur remote from initial diagnosis.
- CT scan of chest, abdomen, and pelvis and/or PET scan when clinically indicated (i.e., recurrence suspected)
  - Routine screening with imaging not recommended

PATIENT EDUCATION
Patients should be educated on signs/symptoms of recurrence, including pelvic or abdominal pain/discomfort, bloating, and early satiety.

PROGNOSIS
- Recurrence rates for epithelial cancer
  - Early-stage disease: 20%
  - Advanced disease: >80%
- 5-year survival rates for ovarian cancer (invasive epithelial) based on SEER data 2010 to 2016
  - Localized (confined to ovaries): 92.6%
  - Regional (spread to regional lymph nodes): 74.8%
  - Distant (metastasized to liver/lungs): 30.3%
- 5-year survival rates for ovarian cancer by stage based on International Federation of Gynecology and Obstetrics (FIGO)

Stage I	A 90%	B 86%	C 83%
Stage II	A 78%	B 73%	—
Stage III	A 47%	B 42%	C 33%
Stage IV	19%	—	—

COMPLICATIONS
- Bowel obstruction mechanical obstruction or carcinomatous ileus (often with recurrence)
- Malnutrition, electrolyte disturbances
- Fistula formation
- Pleural effusion, ascites
- Pseudomyxoma peritonei
- Toxicity of chemotherapy

REFERENCES
1. Morrison J, Haldar K, Kehoe S, et al. Chemotherapy versus surgery for initial treatment in advanced ovarian epithelial cancer. *Cochrane Database Syst Rev.* 2012;(8):CD005343.
2. Trimbos JB, Vergote I, Bolis G, et al. Impact of adjuvant chemotherapy and surgical staging in early-stage ovarian carcinoma: European Organisation for Research and Treatment of Cancer-Adjuvant ChemoTherapy in Ovarian Neoplasm trial. *J Natl Cancer Inst.* 2003;95(2):113–125.

ADDITIONAL READING
Olsen CM, Green AC, Whiteman DC, et al. Obesity and the risk of epithelial ovarian cancer: a systematic review and meta-analysis. *Eur J Cancer.* 2007;43(4):690–709.

CODES

ICD10
- C56.9 Malignant neoplasm of unspecified ovary
- C56.1 Malignant neoplasm of right ovary
- C56.2 Malignant neoplasm of left ovary

CLINICAL PEARLS
- Family history of ovarian cancer or early-onset breast cancer is the most significant risk factor for the development of ovarian cancer, yet the vast majority of cases remain sporadic.
- Ovarian cancer should be suspected in women with persistent bloating, upper abdominal discomfort, or GI symptoms of unknown etiology.
- Surgery is the mainstay of diagnosis and treatment for ovarian cancer. Many patients benefit from adjuvant chemotherapy.
- The prognosis of advanced ovarian cancer is poor and requires close follow-up by physical exam, tumor markers, and imaging when indicated.

OVARIAN CYST, RUPTURED

John Motley Alford, DO • Anna R. Peyton, DO

BASICS

- Ovarian cysts are frequent in reproductive-aged women.
- Most ovarian cysts are benign physiologic follicles created by the ovary at the time of ovulation.
- Ovarian cysts can cause symptoms when they become enlarged and exert a mass effect on surrounding structures, or when they rupture and the cyst contents irritate the peritoneum or nearby pelvic organs.
- Patients with a symptomatic ruptured cyst usually complain of acute onset unilateral lower abdominal pain.
- Rupture can be caused by sexual intercourse, luteal phase, exercise, trauma, pregnancy, or be idiopathic.
- Evaluation of the patient should include exclusion of other emergent causes: ectopic pregnancy, ovarian torsion, and nongynecologic sources of acute unilateral lower abdominal pain.
- Once the diagnosis of a ruptured cyst is confirmed, most patients can be managed conservatively as outpatients with adequate pain control. Surgical intervention is rarely indicated.

DESCRIPTION
A suspected ruptured ovarian cyst should be treated as an unknown adnexal mass (mass of the ovary, fallopian tube, and surrounding tissue) until proven otherwise.

EPIDEMIOLOGY
- The actual incidence of ovarian cysts is difficult to calculate as many ruptured cysts are asymptomatic or found incidentally.
- Ovarian cysts can be seen on transvaginal ultrasounds in nearly all premenopausal women and in up to 18% of postmenopausal women. The vast majority of these cysts are benign or functional.
- Most ruptured ovarian cysts are physiologic events and self-limited. Expectant management with pain control is usually sufficient.
- About 13% of ovarian masses in reproductive-aged women are malignant, as opposed to 45% in postmenopausal women. About 70% of ovarian malignancies are diagnosed at a late stage.
- Ruptured ovarian cysts most commonly affect the right ovary, 63%.

Incidence
About 7% of women worldwide experience a symptomatic cyst during their lifetime.

Prevalence
During pregnancy, prevalence varies from 1 to 5.3%; of those, just 0.63% are symptomatic and 1% malignant.

ETIOLOGY AND PATHOPHYSIOLOGY
Normal ovulation occurs when a follicle matures and ruptures, releasing an oocyte, leaving a corpus luteum, which subsequently involutes. If the follicle fails to rupture and continues growing, a follicular cyst is formed. If a corpus luteum fails to involute and continues growing, then a corpus luteum cyst occurs. These are the most common cysts. Both types are physiologic (termed "functional") without malignant potential. Other cyst types include endometriomas (filled with menstrual blood), dermoid cysts that contains mature tissue of ectodermal, mesodermal, and/or endodermal origin, and ovarian malignancy originating from any of the structures of the ovary.

RISK FACTORS
Medications or conditions associated with increased ovulation and/or increased risk of cyst rupture

- Ovulation induction agents (i.e., Clomid, aromatase inhibitors, GnRH agonists)
- Tamoxifen increases the risk of ovarian cysts in reproductive-aged women.
- Polycystic ovarian syndrome (common), fibrous dysplasia/McCune-Albright syndrome (rare)
- Ovarian endometriosis

GENERAL PREVENTION
Ovulation suppression with combined hormonal contraceptives is the mainstay therapy for prevention of recurrent ovarian cyst.

COMMONLY ASSOCIATED CONDITIONS
- Endometriomas located on or adjacent to the ovaries are found in 20–55% of women with endometriosis.
- PCOS

DIAGNOSIS

- The characteristic symptoms of ruptured cyst may resemble ectopic pregnancy. Ectopic pregnancy should be ruled out when a ruptured cyst is suspected (1)[C].
- Sonographic imaging along with computed tomography (CT) and magnetic resonance imaging (MRI) can aid in diagnosis of gynecologic emergencies (2)[C].
- CT is useful to confirm a hemoperitoneum, and MRI can assist when the diagnosis remains unclear after CT and ultrasound (2)[C].
- Ultrasound and CT imaging for diagnosis has decreased the need for diagnostic surgical intervention (3)[B].
- Additionally, ultrasound is useful in confirming normal Doppler flow to the affected ovary and adnexa (1)[C].

HISTORY
- Questions that should be addressed if a ruptured ovarian cyst is suspected include:
  - Onset and characteristics of pain
  - Pain associated with timing of sexual intercourse, strenuous activity, or trauma
  - Date of last menstrual period
  - Presence or absence of vaginal bleeding
  - Nausea or vomiting
  - Shoulder or upper abdominal pain due to subphrenic extravasation
- Symptoms of hypotension/hypovolemia, including palpitations, shortness of breath, sensation of being hot or clammy, dizziness
- Additional information that will guide diagnosis should include patient age, known or previous ovarian cysts, and reproductive history

ALERT
Patients with bleeding diathesis or undergoing anticoagulation therapy may experience significant bleeding from hemorrhagic cysts.

PHYSICAL EXAM
- Vital signs are usually normal unless significant blood loss has occurred.
- Rupture characterized by significant blood loss may be present in the form of pallor, pale mucosal membranes, and tachycardia.
- Patients will have significant tenderness to palpation or an acute abdomen if the peritoneum is irritated or inflamed.
- On some occasions, a palpable adnexal mass can be felt on bimanual exam. Care should be taken not to cause further injury with a forceful exam.

DIFFERENTIAL DIAGNOSIS
Includes all causes of acute abdominal pain, both gynecologic and nongynecologic

- Ectopic pregnancy should always be excluded with a negative pregnancy test (1)[C].
- Common gynecologic etiologies include:
  - Functional ovarian cysts
  - Ovarian torsion
  - Tubo-ovarian abscess
  - Teratomas
  - Degenerating fibroids
  - Endometrioma
  - Cystadenoma (mucinous or serous)
  - Hydrosalpinx
- Malignant gynecologic etiologies can usually be attributed to the various gynecologic cancers of the reproductive tract.
- Benign nongynecologic causes of acute lower abdominal pain include:
  - Appendicitis
  - Diverticulitis
  - Infections of the urinary tract
  - Renal colic
- Malignant nongynecologic causes of acute lower abdominal pain can be attributed to neoplastic processes of the lower GI tract.

DIAGNOSTIC TESTS & INTERPRETATION
- In all premenopausal women, pregnancy must be ruled out by a urine test. Serial quantitative β-hCG tests are helpful in evaluating an ectopic pregnancy (1)[C].
- Complete blood count (CBC) may reveal a significant drop in hematocrit if there is ongoing hemorrhage (3)[B]. Leukocytosis should raise the suspicion of an infectious process (1)[C].

- Urinalysis and STD testing should be obtained to evaluate for infectious causes, PID, or symptomatic renal stones (1)[C].
- A type and screen is indicated if surgical intervention is planned or blood products are being considered.
- Ultrasound is the first-line imaging modality (1)[C].
- CA-125 may assist in evaluation but can be elevated in a number of conditions (1)[C].

Initial Tests (lab, imaging)
- Ultrasound
- Serial quantitative β-hCG
- CBC
- Urinalysis and STD testing

Follow-Up Tests & Special Considerations
CT and MRI may narrow the differential diagnosis when ultrasound is indeterminate.

Diagnostic Procedures/Other
Laparoscopy may be diagnostic and therapeutic in emergent cases.

 ## TREATMENT

GENERAL MEASURES
- For many patients, pain associated with a ruptured cyst will be transient and self-limiting.
- Cyst rupture in a stable healthy patient can be managed conservatively in 80% of cases (3)[B].
- Patient with anticoagulation can also be managed conservatively with cyst rupture using a multidisciplinary team (4)[C].
- Scheduled NSAIDs or oral narcotics can be prescribed depending on pain severity.
- For patients with multiple episodes or a single severe occurrence, OCPs can be considered for ovulation suppression and prevention. They are not effective for treatment of ovarian cysts which are already present (5)[A].
- Unstable patients with hemodynamic compromise or patients with significant hemoperitoneum should be resuscitated, and laparoscopy or a laparotomy should be considered. Surgical exploration should also be considered if there is a concern for malignancy.

ISSUES FOR REFERRAL
- Obstetrician (OB)/GYN
  - Consider referral to an OB if an adnexal mass is diagnosed during pregnancy. Such masses have a low risk of malignancy or acute complication for the pregnancy.
  - Most cysts resolve without intervention within 2 to 3 weeks; those that do not resolve in 12 weeks require prompt referral for surgical assessment (5)[A].
- Gynecologic oncology
  - Referral to a gynecologic oncologist should be considered for complex adnexal masses with an elevated CA-125 and associated symptoms concerning for malignancy such as ascites, thick septation noted on ultrasound, early satiety, pleural effusion, enlarging abdominal mass, or bowel obstruction.

- General surgery
  - Acute lower abdominal pain that is nongynecologic and suspicious for bowel involvement should be referred to general surgery or a gastroenterologist.

ADDITIONAL THERAPIES
Guided cyst aspiration is not recommended for either diagnosis or treatment but could be considered in patients at high risk who are not good surgical candidates.

SURGERY/OTHER PROCEDURES
- Although the need for surgical intervention is rare, it is usually of an emergent nature.
- Patients with a low diastolic blood pressure and a large amount of hemoperitoneum often need surgery (3)[B].
- In most cases, laparoscopy is diagnostic and therapeutic. The decision to proceed with cystectomy or oophorectomy should be made intraoperatively after a thorough evaluation of the intra-abdominal environment has been completed.
- The advantages of a laparoscopic approach include a shorter length of stay, faster recovery, small scar, and few adhesions. Postoperative recovery time as well as patient satisfaction is significantly improved with a minimally invasive approach.
- Laparotomy should be performed in cases of critical hemodynamic instability or lack of laparoscopically trained surgeons. If there is concern for malignancy or metastases, laparotomy may be the preferred method of surgery.

ADMISSION, INPATIENT, AND NURSING CONSIDERATIONS
Patients who require inpatient management should be managed with serial abdominal exams, analgesia, and intravenous resuscitation as indicated by their initial presentation.

 ## ONGOING CARE

FOLLOW-UP RECOMMENDATIONS
- Follow-up for patients managed conservatively should be scheduled in 72 hours from the initial onset of symptoms. Patients should present sooner for new or worsening symptoms.
- Patients with complete resolution of symptoms within a few days can follow up as needed. However, these patients should be counseled on risk of reoccurrence and options for prevention.
- In patients who had surgery, postop follow-up should be scheduled 2 weeks from the date of surgery.
- Patients in whom an ovarian cyst was diagnosed incidentally should follow-up based on the size of their cyst.

Pregnancy Considerations
- The management of adnexal masses during pregnancy is controversial.
- Most adnexal masses in pregnancy can be managed expectantly because the risk of malignancy is low (1)[C]. If there is a risk for ruptured endometriotic cyst, early surgical intervention can reduce the risk of cyst fluid leakage, thus preventing adhesions and preserving fertility. MRI can help further characterize a mass safely in pregnancy (1)[C]. However, the possible risk of torsion or rupture should not be considered as an indication for surgery.

PATIENT EDUCATION
Reassurance of the benign nature of most ovarian cysts is an important cornerstone of patient education.

COMPLICATIONS
- Surgical procedure complications related to any laparoscopic surgery
- Ovarian reserve reduction may occur following any ovarian surgery. Desire for future fertility should be factored into surgical decisions. Cysts with a diameter of 5 cm or more can themselves cause compromise in ovarian reserve. It is unclear if the effect is temporary or permanent.

REFERENCES
1. Biggs WS, Marks ST. Diagnosis and management of adnexal masses. *Am Fam Physician*. 2016;93(8):676–681.
2. Iraha Y, Okada M, Iraha R, et al. CT and MR imaging of gynecologic emergencies. *Radiographics*. 2017;37(5):1569–1586.
3. Kim JH, Lee SM, Lee JH, et al. Successful conservative management of ruptured ovarian cysts with hemoperitoneum in healthy women. *PLoS One*. 2014;9(3):e91171.
4. Gupta A, Gupta S, Manaktala U, et al. Conservative management of corpus luteum haemorrhage in patients on anticoagulation: a report of three cases and review of literature. *Arch Gynecol Obstet*. 2015;291(2):427–431.
5. Seehusen DA, Earwood JS. Oral contraceptive are not an effective treatment for ovarian cyst. *Am Fam Physician*. 2014;90(9):623.

ADDITIONAL READING
American College of Obstetricians and Gynecologists Committee on Practice Bulletins—Gynecology. Practice Bulletin No. 174: evaluation and management of adnexal masses. *Obstet Gynecol*. 2016;128(5):e210–e226.

 ## CODES

ICD10
- N83.20 Unspecified ovarian cysts
- N83.0 Follicular cyst of ovary
- N83.1 Corpus luteum cyst

CLINICAL PEARLS
- Functional ovarian cysts are very common in reproductive-age women and are usually self-limiting.
- Always exclude ectopic pregnancy.
- Management of symptomatic ruptured cysts is usually accomplished with outpatient pain control and follow-up.
- Combined hormonal contraception is the mainstay of preventive treatment.

PALLIATIVE CARE

Erika Zimmons, DO, MS

BASICS

Palliative care focuses on preventing and alleviating the suffering of patients (and their families) living at any stage of a life-limiting illness.

DESCRIPTION

- The principal goal of palliative care is to prevent and alleviate suffering—whether physical (pain, breathlessness, nausea, etc.), emotional, social, or spiritual regardless of the underlying diagnosis.
- Palliative care is an interdisciplinary approach to caring for patients and families.
- Palliative care aims to improve or maintain quality of life for patients and families despite serious illness.
- The palliative care team often helps to identify the goals of care for the patient based on their preferences and values.
- Palliative care is available for patients with serious, life-limiting illness, at any stage of their disease, with or without concurrent curative care.
- Patients and their families may access palliative care services in the hospital, rehabilitation or skilled nursing facility, and ambulatory setting.
- Hospice: In the United Sates, hospice is available for patients whose average life expectancy is 6 months or less and whose principal goal is to stay at home (including long-term care or assisted living facility), avoid hospitalizations, and forego disease-directed care with a curative intent. Unlike regular home nursing services, hospice does not require a patient to be homebound. Hospice offers backup support for patients 24 hours a day and 7 days per week.

EPIDEMIOLOGY

- 67% of U.S. hospitals with >50 beds reported a palliative care program in data from 2012 to 2013 (1).
- It is estimated that between 69% and 82% of those who die in high-income countries need palliative care.

COMMONLY ASSOCIATED CONDITIONS

Common symptoms/syndromes encountered in palliative care:

- Pain
  - Chronic pain
  - Neuropathic pain
  - Pain from bone metastases

- GI symptoms (~60% incidence)
  - Ascites
  - Anorexia/cachexia
  - Bowel obstruction
  - Constipation and impaction of stool
  - Diarrhea
  - Dysphagia
  - Mucositis/stomatitis
  - Nausea (and vomiting)
    - Consider underlying etiology and treat accordingly.
      - GI causes: constipation, bowel (full or partial) obstruction, ileus, heart burn, reflux, inflammation
      - Intrathoracic causes: cardiac, effusions (cardiac, pulmonary), mediastinal causes, esophageal disease
      - Autonomic dysfunction
      - Centrally mediated: intracranial pressure change, inflammation, cerebellar, vestibular, medication or metabolic cause stimulating vomiting center, and/or chemoreceptor trigger zone
- Sialorrhea
- Xerostomia
- General medical
  - Delirium (40–85%)
- Pulmonary symptoms
  - Cough, chronic
  - Breathlessness or dyspnea (60%): which may be due to heart failure, COPD, lung cancer, etc.
- Psychological symptoms
  - Anxiety
  - Depression
  - Insomnia
- Skin
  - Decubitus ulcer
  - Pruritus
  - Complex wounds (fungating tumors, etc.)

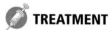**DIAGNOSIS**

A useful tool in palliative care is the PEACE tool. This tool evaluates (2):

- **P**hysical symptoms
- **E**motive and cognitive symptoms
- **A**utonomy and related issues
- **C**ommunication: contribution to others and closure of life affairs–related issues
- **E**conomic burden and other practical issues, including transcendent and existential concerns

HISTORY

A comprehensive palliative care assessment includes:

- Underlying medical conditions and associated physical symptoms
- Communication with empathic inquiry and open-ended questions
- Comprehensive pain assessment and review of systems (e.g., Edmonton Symptom Assessment Scale)
- Psychological symptom assessment
- Cultural, social, financial, and practical concerns
- Spiritual and existential issues
  - FICA assessment (**F**aith, **I**mportance and influence, **C**ommunity, **A**ddress—how does the patient wish these items to be addressed?) (3)
  - HOPE (sources of **H**ope/strength/comfort, **O**rganized religion's role, **P**ersonal spirituality and practices, **E**ffects on medical care and end-of-life care) (4)
- Presence and sources of suffering
- Goals of care: posthospital care, practical needs, hopes, and fears
- Prognosis: functional status and interest in knowing prognosis

PHYSICAL EXAM

The physical examination is directed by underlying diagnosis, symptoms, and functional decline in the context of meeting the goals of the patient and family to maximize function, comfort, and support.

DIAGNOSTIC TESTS & INTERPRETATION

Initial Tests (lab, imaging)

Laboratory and radiology testing depends on the underlying diagnosis and any associated symptoms. It is important to avoid unnecessary testing.

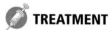**TREATMENT**

GENERAL MEASURES

- Targeted interventions to maximize quality of life and minimize symptom burden considering patient values, goals, fears, and social setting
- Treatment should involve an interdisciplinary team to address potential and realized suffering (physical, emotional, social, and/or spiritual).

MEDICATION

- Minimize polypharmacy; discontinue medications that offer little improvement in the quality of life.
- Focus the use of medications on symptom management.
- Continue use of disease-modifying medications especially if they lessen symptom burden and enhance immediate quality of life.
- Improve compliance by addressing
  - *Pain*
    - Use immediate-release opioids—titrate to adequate control.
    - Once pain is controlled, convert to long-acting opioids with short-acting agents made available because tolerance develops and/or patient develops breakthrough pain.
  - Bone pain: NSAIDs added to narcotics are more effective than narcotics alone.
  - Neuropathic pain: may use adjuvant treatment, such as gabapentin or other anticonvulsants.

ALERT

Avoid morphine in patients with renal failure; can induce delirium, hyperalgesia, agitation, and seizures

- *Vomiting* associated with a particular opioid may be relieved by substitution with an equianalgesic dose of another opioid or a sustained-release formulation (5).
  - Dopamine receptor antagonists (metoclopramide, prochlorperazine) may improve nausea symptoms.
  - Droperidol: insufficient evidence on the use for the management of nausea and vomiting
- *Constipation*: Consider prophylactic stimulants (bisacodyl or senna), or osmotic laxatives. Avoid nonessential medications that may cause constipation.

ALERT

Consider laxatives with opioid treatment to avoid constipation.

- Subcutaneous methylnaltrexone may be used for inducing bowel movements without inducing withdrawal in opioid-induced constipation.

- Dyspnea: Consider oxygen. Consider benzodiazepines if increased anxiety.
  - Treat the underlying cause of breathlessness. In addition, as the disease advances, low-dose opioids may be beneficial to patients (6)[C]. Immediate-release opioids PO/IV treat dyspnea effectively and typically at doses lower than necessary for the relief of moderate pain.
- *Delirium*: lowest doses necessary of benzodiazepines or antipsychotics (haloperidol or risperidone, etc.)
  - Monitor patient safety and use nonpharmacologic strategies to assist orientation (clocks, calendars, environment, and redirection). Consider review of medications or other causes that may be contributing to delirium.
- Pruritus: no optimal therapy. General measures include moisturizing skin and avoiding irritants.
- Anxiety: insufficient data for recommendations of specific medication
- Megestrol acetate improves appetite and slight weight gain in patients with anorexia-cachexia syndrome.

ISSUES FOR REFERRAL

- Referral to palliative care
  - Any patient with a serious, life-limiting illness who could use help with burdensome symptoms or suffering and/or complex goals of care discussion
  - Early referral to palliative care may improve quality of life and longevity for patients with advanced cancer.
- Referral to hospice care
  - Any patient with an average life expectancy of 6 months or less
  - Consider patients who have multiple hospitalizations and/or emergency department visits in the prior 6 months.
  - Refer to local hospice guidelines for additional disease-specific criteria.

REFERENCES

1. Dumanovsky T, Augustin R, Rogers M, et al. The growth or palliative care in U.S. hospitals: a status report. *J Palliat Med*. 2016;19(1):8–15.
2. Okon TR, Evans JM, Gomez CF, et al. Palliative educational outcome with implementation of PEACE tool integrated clinical pathway. *J Palliat Med*. 2004;7(2):279–295.
3. Borneman T, Ferrell B, Puchalski CM. Evaluation of the FICA Tool for Spiritual Assessment. *J Pain Symptom Manage*. 2010;40(2):163–173.
4. Anandarajah G, Hight E. Spirituality and medical practice: using the HOPE questions as a practical tool for spiritual assessment. *Am Fam Physician*. 2001;63(1):81–89.
5. Smith HS, Smith JM, Smith AR. An overview of nausea/vomiting in palliative medicine. *Ann Palliat Med*. 2012;1(2):103–114.
6. Ben-Aharon I, Gafter-Gvili A, Paul M, et al. Interventions for alleviating cancer-related dyspnea: a systematic review. *J Clin Oncol*. 2008;26(14):2396–2404.

ADDITIONAL READING

El Mokhallalati Y, Bradley SH, Chapman E, et al. Identification of patients with potential palliative care needs: a systematic review of screening tools in primary care. *Palliat Med*. 2020;34(8):989–1005.

 CODES

ICD10
Z51.5 Encounter for palliative care

CLINICAL PEARLS

- Palliative care is a holistic approach to providing comfort patients with life-limiting illness.
- Early referral to palliative care helps enhance the quality of life of patients living with serious illness.
- The addition of adjuvant treatments may be more effective than narcotics alone for managing pain.
- Use laxatives with opioid treatment to avoid constipation.

PANCREATIC CANCER

Marcelle Meseeha, MD • Maximos Attia, MD, FAAFP

BASICS

DESCRIPTION

- Adenocarcinoma of the exocrine pancreas (90% of pancreatic cancers) is the fourth most common cause of cancer death in the United States.
- Rarely curable: overall 5-year relative survival rate of 10.8%, the lowest of all cancers
- 60% occur in the head, 20% in the body and tail, and 20% diffusely involve the gland
- As few as 11% are localized at diagnosis. For localized, small cancers (<2 cm) with no lymph node metastases and no extension beyond the capsule, surgical resection has 5-year survival of about 41.6%.
- Majority of tumors have metastasized at diagnosis and are thus largely incurable and have a 5-year survival rate of 3%.
- Ampullary, duodenal, or distal bile duct tumors may mimic pancreatic carcinoma.

EPIDEMIOLOGY

During 2003 to 2007, median age at diagnosis was 70 years; rare <40 years; after 45 years of age, occurrence rises.

Incidence

- According to the American Cancer Society, an estimated 60,430 diagnoses and 48,220 deaths in the United States in 2021
- About 3.2% of all cancers and about 7% of cancer deaths; lifetime risk is about 1 in 64 (1.6%).
- More common in black and white races, 17 and 15.2 in 100,000 men and 14.3 and 11.7 in 100,000 women, respectively. Among Hispanic and Asian/Pacific Islanders, there is an incidence of 12.8 and 10.9 in 100,000 men and 11.1 and 9.3 in 100,000 women, respectively.

Prevalence

In the US, in 2018, ~83,777 people were living with pancreatic cancer.

RISK FACTORS

- Smoking: relative risk (RR) 2 to 3
- Diabetes: RR 2.1
- Prior partial gastrectomy or cholecystectomy: 2- to 5-fold increased risk 15 to 20 years after gastrectomy
- Familial aggregation/genetic factors: 5–10% of patients have a first-degree relative with the disease, which confers a 9-fold increase in risk versus the general population; subgroup may carry germline mutations of DNA repair genes (*BRCA2*).
- Hereditary chronic pancreatitis (autosomal dominant, highly penetrant): Cumulative risk by ages 50 and 75 years is 10% and 54%, respectively.
- Peutz-Jeghers syndrome: RR 30 to 40
- Familial atypical multiple mole and melanoma syndrome (p16): RR 10 to 20
- Hereditary nonpolyposis colon cancer (Lynch syndrome): RR 4
- Sporadic chronic pancreatitis
- Non–O blood type: RR 1 to 2

- High dietary fat, red meat, obesity, *Helicobacter pylori*
- Alcohol: in heavy consumers

GENERAL PREVENTION

- Clinicians should NOT screen average-risk individuals for pancreatic cancer.
- Screening should be considered in high-risk patients, including first-degree relatives of patients with pancreatic cancer with at least 2 affected genetically related relatives, in patients with genetic syndromes (Peutz-Jeghers syndrome, hereditary pancreatitis, patients with CDKN2A gene mutation, and patients with one or more first-degree relatives with pancreatic cancer with Lynch syndrome, and mutations in *BRCA1*, *BRCA2*, *PALB2*, and *ATM* genes).
- Screening in high-risk individuals should begin at age 50 years or <10 years the initial age of familial onset. Screening should be initiated at age 40 years in CKDN2A and PRSS1 mutation carriers with hereditary pancreatitis and at age 35 years in the setting of Peutz-Jeghers syndrome.

COMMONLY ASSOCIATED CONDITIONS

- Chronic pancreatitis, diabetes mellitus, cystic fibrosis
- KRAS mutations are present in >90% of pancreatic ductal adenocarcinomas.
- Mutation inactivation of tumor suppressors (SMAD4, p53, *CDKN2A*) allows for tumor progression.
- Subsets of familial pancreatic cancer involve germline cationic trypsinogen or *PRSS1* mutations (hereditary pancreatitis), *BRCA2* mutations (usually with hereditary breast-ovarian cancer syndrome), *CDKN2* mutations (familial atypical mole, multiple melanoma), or DNA repair gene mutations (e.g., *ATM* and *PALB2*, apart from *BRCA2*).
- Majority of familial pancreatic cancers have no genetic underpinnings.
- Precursor lesions are potentially curable—pancreatic intraepithelial neoplasia, intraductal papillary mucinous neoplasm, and mucinous cystic neoplasms.

DIAGNOSIS

HISTORY

- Depends on tumor location; majority become symptomatic late in disease. About 60–70% of pancreatic cancers develop in the pancreatic head and block the periampullary bile duct, causing obstructive jaundice.
- Weight loss 90%; pain 75% (progressive midepigastric dull ache that often radiates to the back); malnutrition 75%; jaundice 70%; anorexia 60%; pruritus 40%; diabetes mellitus 50%; weakness, fatigue, malaise 30–40%; back pain, alcoholic stools, dark urine, steatorrhea; depression is common.
- Pancreatic cancer is a consideration in acute pancreatitis in the elderly and with new-onset diabetes.
- Uncommon: unexplained thrombophlebitis; acute pancreatitis; duodenal obstruction or GI bleeding

PHYSICAL EXAM

- Muscle wasting and malnutrition
- Palpable abdominal mass or ascites in 20%
- Jaundice: 70% if tumor obstructs bile duct; 10% with body or tail carcinoma
- Courvoisier sign, hepatomegaly
- Virchow node (left supraclavicular) and Sister Mary Joseph node (umbilical) in metastatic disease; palpable rectal shelf
- Migratory thrombophlebitis (Trousseau sign)
- GI bleeding from tumor erosion; portal hypertension-related bleeding
- Pancreatic panniculitis: subcutaneous areas of nodular fat necrosis

DIFFERENTIAL DIAGNOSIS

- Chronic pancreatitis, duodenal cancer, cholangiocarcinoma, lymphoma, islet cell tumor, sarcoma, cystic neoplasms, tumor metastatic to pancreas (rare)
- Nonmalignant conditions: choledocholithiasis, acute or chronic pancreatitis, biliary tract stricture, adenoma; chronic mesenteric ischemia

DIAGNOSTIC TESTS & INTERPRETATION

- Cross-sectional imaging (usually CT scan as first-line choice) (1)[B]
- EUS-guided biopsy: best modality for tissue; sensitivity 75–90%; specificity ~100% for diagnosis of a mass (1)[A]
- Routine laboratory tests may reveal elevated serum bilirubin and alkaline phosphatase (cholestasis), anemia, or decreased serum albumin (malnutrition).

Initial Tests (lab, imaging)

- Most patients do not require measurement of serum tumor markers (CA19-9) for diagnosis or management. Some evidence suggests use in predicting outcome and response to adjuvant chemotherapy.
- CEA and CA19-9 are not recommended as screening tests.
- Elevated CA19-9 antigen: 80% sensitivity; 90% specificity; individuals with Lewis-negative blood group antigen phenotype (5–10%) are unable to synthesize CA19-9; elevations can occur in benign pancreatic or biliary diseases and in nonpancreatic malignancy.
- *MUC5AC* helps in differentiation.

Follow-Up Tests & Special Considerations

- CA19-9 may identify progressive tumor growth. Normal CA19-9 does not exclude recurrence.
- CT scan (pancreatic protocol) using thin section, multiphase multidetector helical CT with a pancreatic protocol is the choice for diagnosis and staging: 85–90% sensitivity; 90–95% specificity; for evaluation of distant metastasis and prediction of resectability
- Abdominal ultrasound (US): common initial test to assess jaundice and duct dilatation; less sensitive than CT for pancreatic masses
- EUS is accurate for tissue biopsy, local tumor and node staging, predicting vascular invasion (90%

specificity; 73% sensitivity), and when no mass is identified on CT.
- Endoscopic retrograde cholangiopancreatography (ERCP): 90% sensitivity; 95% specificity for ductal cancer; useful if endoscopic stent is indicated for biliary obstruction
- MRI: no advantage over contrast-enhanced CT
- MR cholangiopancreatography: 90% sensitivity; 95% specificity. Preferred in specific settings: gastric outlet or duodenal stenosis or after surgical rearrangement (Billroth II) or ductal disruption; to detect bile duct obstruction, after unsuccessful ERCP

Diagnostic Procedures/Other
- Percutaneous fine-needle biopsy with US or CT guidance: 80–90% sensitivity; 98–100% specificity
- EUS-guided biopsy: 85–90% sensitivity; virtually 100% specificity for pancreatic mass
- Staging laparoscopy and US: 92% sensitivity; 88% specificity; 89% accuracy
- Positive peritoneal cytology has a positive predictive value of 94%, specificity of 98%, and sensitivity of 25% for determining unresectability.
- PET scan: 90% sensitivity but 70% specificity; limited anatomic information
- Tumor staging
  - Stage Ia: T1 N0 M0 (tumor ≤2 cm)
  - Stage Ib: T2 N0 M0 (tumor >2 cm and ≤4 cm)
  - Stage IIa: T3 N0 M0 (tumor >4 cm)
  - Stage IIb: T1–T3 N1 M0 (N1 is metastasis in 1 to 3 regional lymph nodes.)
  - Stage III: T1–T3 N2 M0 (N2 is metastasis in ≥4 regional lymph nodes), T4 any N M0 (Tumor involves celiac axis, superior mesenteric artery, and/or common hepatic artery, regardless of size.)
  - Stage IV: any T any N M1 (distant metastases)

Test Interpretation

ALERT

Chronic pancreatitis can present with similar pain, weight loss, jaundice, and an inflammatory mass on imaging.

 ## TREATMENT
- Surgical resection: only chance of cure; no role for pancreatic resection in metastatic disease
- Nonmetastatic pancreatic cancer is classified as resectable, borderline resectable, or locally advanced (2).
- Criteria for unresectability: extrapancreatic spread, encasement or occlusion of major vessels, distant metastases
- Refer patients for clinical trials.

MEDICATION
- Stages I and II
  - Radical pancreatic resection plus chemotherapy
  - ESPAC-3 trial after resection: no significant difference between 5-fluorouracil (5-FU)/folinic acid and gemcitabine in overall survival
  - ESPAC-4: Gemcitabine combined with capecitabine is superior to gemcitabine alone.

- Currently, postoperative gemcitabine alone or in combination with 5-FU–based chemoradiation is the current standard of care; preoperative neoadjuvant treatment trials are in progress (1)[A].
  - Consider preoperative chemoradiotherapy in cases of borderline resectable pancreatic cancer.
- Stage III
  - Standard: 6 months of chemotherapy with gemcitabine-based regimens (1)[A]; added chemoradiation (capecitabine and radiotherapy) is controversial (1)[B].
  - FOLFIRINOX (leucovorin, fluorouracil, irinotecan, and oxaliplatin) and gemcitabine plus nab-paclitaxel. These regimens are used for patients with no or minimal performance restrictions (1).
  - Intraoperative radiation therapy and/or implantation of radioactive substances
- Stage IV
  - First-line treatment
    ○ FOLFIRINOX
    ○ Gemcitabine plus nab-paclitaxel/capecitabine/erlotinib
    ○ Gemcitabine alone is recommended for patients who have ECOG PS of 2 or a comorbidity that prevents aggressive approaches.
  - Second-line treatment
    ○ Pain-relieving procedures (celiac or intrapleural block); supportive care; palliative decompression
    ○ Duodenal obstruction: endoscopic expandable metal stent placement rather than surgery (1)[C]
    ○ Biliary obstruction: Endoscopic biliary stenting is safer than percutaneous insertion and is as successful as surgical hepaticojejunostomy (1)[A].
    ○ In tumors with NTRK fusions, treatment with larotrectinib or entrectinib is recommended.
    ○ Pembrolizumab is recommended for patients positive for mismatch repair deficiency or microsatellite instability high.
    ○ In patients with BRCA1 or BRCA2 mutation and who already had first-line platinum-based chemotherapy without disease progression for at least 16 weeks, options for continued treatment include chemotherapy or PARP inhibitor olaparib.
    ○ Gemcitabine plus nab-paclitaxel
    ○ Fluorouracil plus irinotecan
    ○ Fluorouracil plus oxaliplatin

SURGERY/OTHER PROCEDURES
- Standard treatment options
  - Pancreaticoduodenectomy, Whipple procedure, en bloc resection of the head of the pancreas, distal common bile duct, duodenum, jejunum, and gastric antrum
  - Total pancreatectomy
  - Distal pancreatectomy for body and tail tumors
- Nonstandard surgeries
  - Pylorus-preserving pancreaticoduodenectomy, regional pancreatectomy
  - Palliative bypass
    ○ Biliary decompression; gastrojejunostomy for gastric outlet obstruction; duodenal endoprosthesis for obstruction

 ## ONGOING CARE

FOLLOW-UP RECOMMENDATIONS
Assessment of treatment at 2 to 3 months from the initiation of therapy. CT with contrast is preferred. Routine PET scan is not recommended. CA19-9 is not substitute for imaging.

DIET
Fat-soluble vitamins and pancreatic enzymes may require replacement.

PROGNOSIS
- 90% diagnosed with pancreatic cancer die from the disease, predominantly from metastatic disease.
- 5-year survival: ~30% if node-negative; 10% if node-positive. Median survival: 10 to 20 months
- For localized disease and small cancers (<2 cm) with no lymph node involvement and no extension beyond the capsule, complete surgical resection can yield a 5-year survival of 18–24%.
- Cystadenocarcinomas have better prognoses than typical pancreatic cancers.

REFERENCES

1. Ducreux M, Cuhna AS, Caramella C, et al; for ESMO Guidelines Committee. Cancer of the pancreas: ESMO clinical practice guidelines for diagnosis, treatment and follow-up. *Ann Oncol*. 2015;26(Suppl 5):v56–v68.
2. National Comprehensive Cancer Network. NCCN clinical practice guidelines in oncology. https://www.nccn.org/professionals/physician_gls/pdf/pancreatic.pdf. Accessed November 23, 2021.

 ## CODES

ICD10
- C25.3 Malignant neoplasm of pancreatic duct
- C25.0 Malignant neoplasm of head of pancreas
- C25.2 Malignant neoplasm of tail of pancreas

CLINICAL PEARLS
- Sudden onset of diabetes mellitus in nonobese adults aged >40 years may warrant consideration of pancreatic cancer.
- Presence of occult peritoneal tumor cells denotes a worse survival in resectable pancreatic cancer patients.
- Diagnostic laparoscopy may decrease the rate of unnecessary laparotomy in pancreatic cancer found to be resectable on CT.

PANCREATITIS, ACUTE

Robert L. Frachtman, MD, FACG • Marni L. Martinez, APRN

 BASICS

DESCRIPTION

Acute inflammation of the pancreas with variable involvement of regional tissue or remote organ systems

- Symptoms relate to intrapancreatic activation of enzymes with pain, nausea and vomiting, and associated intestinal ileus
- Complete structural and functional recovery if there is no necrosis or pancreatic ductal disruption

EPIDEMIOLOGY

Incidence
1 to 5/10,000, with no predominant age or sex

Prevalence
- 19/10,000
- It is the most common gastrointestinal diagnosis for inpatient hospitalization.

ETIOLOGY AND PATHOPHYSIOLOGY

- Alcohol—most common in adults (ages 30 to 50)
- Gallstones (including microlithiasis)—most common in adults (median age of 69)
- Trauma/surgery—most common in adults (median age of 65)
- Acute discontinuation of medications for diabetes or hyperlipidemia
- Following endoscopic retrograde cholangiopancreatography (ERCP)
- Medications (most common, not an exhaustive list)
  - ACE inhibitors; angiotensin receptor blockers (ARBs); thiazide diuretics and furosemide
  - Antimetabolites (mercaptopurine and azathioprine)
  - Corticosteroids; glyburide; exenatide
  - Mesalamine; sulfamethoxazole/trimethoprim, pentamidine; valproic acid; statins
- Metabolic causes
  - Hypertriglyceridemia (classically >1,000 mg/dL); even nonfasting levels as low as ~≥177 mg/dL)
  - Hypercalcemia; acute renal failure
  - Diet with high glycemic load
  - Systemic lupus erythematosus/polyarteritis/other vascular disease
  - Autoimmune; type I with elevated IgG4 and type II with normal IgG4
  - Infections
    ○ Mumps, coxsackie, CMV, EBV, cryptosporidiosis, ascaris, clonorchis
- Penetrating peptic ulcer (rare)
- AIDS
- Cystic fibrosis, CFTR gene mutations, and other mutations
- Tumors (e.g., pancreatic, ampullary)
- Miscellaneous obstruction
  - Celiac disease; Crohn disease; pancreas divisum; sphincter of Oddi dysfunction; choledochocele
- Scorpion venom
- Acute fatty liver of pregnancy
- Idiopathic
- Associated coexisting risk factors
  - Obesity; type II diabetes; smoking
- Pathophysiology—enzymatic autodigestion of the pancreas with interstitial edema and third spacing of fluid. Possible sequelae include necrosis, pseudocyst formation, pancreatic ductal disruption, pancreatic ascites, multiorgan failure (early or late), walled off necrosis (late), and injury to surrounding vascular structures such as splenic vein thrombosis and splenic artery pseudoaneurysm.

- Cellular injury alters membrane trafficking, which alters lysosomal function leading to trypsin formation and zymogen activation. A robust inflammatory response ensues resulting in increased vascular permeability, hemorrhage, edema and necrosis.
- The severity of the first episode of acute pancreatitis, alcohol abuse, and smoking all increase the risk of acute recurrent pancreatitis, which, in turn, increases the risk of progression to chronic pancreatitis.
- Clinical features associated with an increasing severity of acute pancreatitis: age ≥60 years; obesity; long-term, heavy alcohol use

Genetics
- Hereditary pancreatitis is rare; autosomal dominant
- Polymorphisms and mutations in multiple genes

GENERAL PREVENTION
- Avoid excess alcohol consumption.
- Tobacco cessation
- Correct underlying metabolic processes (hypertriglyceridemia or hypercalcemia).
- Discontinue offending medications.
- Cholecystectomy (symptomatic cholelithiasis)
- Diet: There is an increased risk of gallstone pancreatitis with diets high in saturated fats, cholesterol, red meat, and eggs. Decreased risk of gallstone pancreatitis with diet high in fiber and vitamin D. There is a decreased risk of nongallstone pancreatitis with diets high in fiber, coffee, and caffeine.

COMMONLY ASSOCIATED CONDITIONS
- Alcohol withdrawal, alcoholic hepatitis, diabetic ketoacidosis, and ascending cholangitis
- Morbid obesity, a proinflammatory state, increases severity and adverse outcomes (organ failure, mortality).

 DIAGNOSIS

Symptoms don't always correlate with objective findings.

HISTORY
- Acute onset of "boring" epigastric pain, which may radiate posteriorly
- Nausea/vomiting
- Alcohol use
- Personal or family history of gallstones
- Medication use—look for inciting medications
- Abdominal trauma
- Recent significant rapid weight loss

PHYSICAL EXAM
- Vital signs—assess hemodynamic stability, fever, tachycardia, hypotension
- Abdominal findings: epigastric tenderness, loss of bowel sounds, peritoneal signs
- Other findings: jaundice, rales/percussive dullness
- Rare (with hemorrhagic pancreatitis)
  - Flank discoloration (Grey Turner sign) or umbilical discoloration (Cullen sign)

DIFFERENTIAL DIAGNOSIS
- Penetrating peptic ulcer
- Acute cholecystitis or cholangitis
- Macroamylasemia, macrolipasemia
- Mesenteric vascular occlusion and/or infarction
- Intestinal obstruction, perforated viscus
- Aortic aneurysm (dissecting or rupturing)
- Inferior wall myocardial infarction
- Lymphoma

DIAGNOSTIC TESTS & INTERPRETATION
- Interpret laboratory and radiographic findings in the context of the clinical history—false-positive and false-negative findings are common.
- Bedside Index for Severity in Acute Pancreatitis (BISAP) score
  - Patients receive 1 point for each element in the first 24 hours: BUN >25 mg/dL, impaired mental status, systemic inflammatory response syndrome (SIRS)—a score of 0 predicts mortality of <1%, and a score of 5 correlates with a mortality rate of 22%.
- Ranson criteria is an older model of predicting severity of pancreatitis. It includes 11 criteria, 5 of which are measured at admission, and 6 are measured in the following 48 hours. A score of 3 or less represents mild pancreatitis, and as the score increases, the mortality rises sharply.
- American College of Gastroenterology requires at least two of the three following elements to make a diagnosis of acute pancreatitis: characteristic abdominal pain, specific radiographic findings, and lipase level 3 times the upper limit of normal (ULN).
- Elevated serum amylase >3 times ULN (Severity is not related to degree of elevation. Amylase is not specific to pancreatitis.)
- Elevated serum lipase >3 times ULN (may stay elevated longer than amylase in mild cases. Lipase is more specific to the pancreas than amylase.)
- Elevated total bilirubin. If >3 mg/dL, consider common bile duct obstruction.
- A 3-fold elevation in the alanine aminotransferase (ALT) in the setting of acute pancreatitis has a 95% positive predictive value for gallstone pancreatitis. Triglyceride levels >1,000 mg/dL suggest hypertriglyceridemia as the cause.
- Glucose and calcium increased in severe disease.
- WBC elevation to 10,000 to 25,000/μL possible and not indicative of active infection
- Elevated baseline hematocrit >44 or rising hematocrit is poor prognostic sign (severe third spacing with associated hemoconcentration).
- Rising BUN and creatinine imply volume depletion or acute renal failure.
- Elevated D-dimer is predictive of organ failure.

Initial Tests (lab, imaging)
- Use follow-up labs to assess renal function, hydration, sepsis, biliary obstruction, and tissue oxygenation.
- Chest x-ray (CXR) to evaluate for early acute respiratory distress syndrome (ARDS) and pleural effusion; can also rule out subdiaphragmatic air (perforated viscus)
- Ultrasound to look for gallbladder/biliary stones
- CT scan
  - Confirms the diagnosis, assesses severity, establishes a baseline, provides prognostic information, and rules out most other pathologies (excluding noncalcified cholelithiasis)
  - IV contrast is not essential for the initial CT scan; avoid contrast in volume-depleted patients.
  - If not contraindicated, a CT scan with IV contrast on day 3 can assess the degree of necrosis if necrotizing pancreatitis is suspected.
  - The presence of gas in the peripancreatic collection is strong evidence for infection, but its absence does not rule it out.
- Magnetic resonance cholangiopancreatography (MRCP) helps assess choledocholithiasis, pancreas divisum, dilated pancreatic duct, and ductal changes.

- Esophagogastroduodenoscopy (EGD) may be necessary to rule out a penetrating duodenal ulcer or an obstructing ampullary neoplasm.
- ERCP may be necessary to decompress common bile duct due to an impacted stone.
- Endoscopic ultrasonography (EUS) is useful if patients present with "idiopathic pancreatitis."
- EUS-guided fine needle aspiration if autoimmune pancreatitis is suspected

Follow-Up Tests & Special Considerations
If renal function is stable, a contrast-enhanced CT scan at day 3 to assess for necrosis. CT guidance assists aspiration and drainage of abscess—mainly recommended if a fungal or drug-resistant infection is suspected.

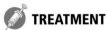 TREATMENT

GENERAL MEASURES
- The management of acute pancreatitis continues to evolve. Early feeding, careful use of antibiotics, and fewer interventions have changed the medical management of acute pancreatitis (1).
- Many cases of acute pancreatitis require hospitalization; ICU if multiorgan dysfunction or hypotension/respiratory failure; 15–20% of cases of acute pancreatitis progress from mild to severe (including persistent organ failure).
  - Fluid resuscitation
    - Significant volume deficit due to third spacing
    - Infuse bolus of 500 mL/hr × 4 hours (lactated Ringer may be better than normal saline, unless hypercalcemic), with follow-up rate adjusted on the basis of age, weight, hemodynamic response, and comorbid conditions (2)[A].
    - Target urine output should be 0.5 to 1.0 mL/kg/hr. Lower the infusion rate when this goal is achieved or once BUN decreases; 4 L should be the maximum total fluid on day 1.
    - Fluid resuscitation is of limited value after 24 hours, and fluid overload results in significant complications (3)[A].
  - Eliminate unnecessary medications, especially those implicated as causes of pancreatitis.
  - Nasogastric (NG) tube for intractable emesis
  - Follow renal function, volume status, calcium, and oxygenation. Organ failure is more important prognostic indicator than pancreatic necrosis.
  - DVT prophylaxis
  - Begin oral alimentation after pain, tenderness, and ileus have resolved; small amounts of high-carbohydrate, low-fat, and low-protein foods; advance as tolerated; NPO or NG tube if vomiting persists. In cases of mild pancreatitis, a soft low-fat diet may be started even before enzymes elevation and pain have completely resolved (3)[A].
  - Enteral nutrition at level of ligament of Treitz if oral feeding not possible within 5 to 7 days (preferable to total parenteral nutrition [TPN] due to decreased infection rate and decreased mortality). Discontinue with increases in pain, increases in amylase/lipase levels, or fluid retention.
  - TPN (without lipids if triglycerides are elevated) if oral or nasoenteric feedings are not tolerated (4)[A]

MEDICATION
First Line
- Analgesia: no consensus; guidelines vary: hydromorphone (Dilaudid) 0.5 to 1.0 mg IV q1–2h PRN
  - AVOID meperidine (Demerol) due to the potential of accumulation of a toxic metabolite.

- Antibiotics
  - In the clear absence of infection, the use of prophylactic antibiotics is no longer recommended (even with necrotizing pancreatitis).
  - In patients with ascending cholangitis or necrotizing pancreatitis, if there is a strong suspicion of active infection, consider empiric imipenem class or β-lactam/β-lactamase inhibitor (e.g., piperacillin/tazobactam 4.5 g IV q8h) for initial treatment before cultures (especially aspirates) return.
  - Levofloxacin 500 mg QD IV if cholangitis and there is an allergy to penicillin
  - Watch for fungal superinfections when giving prophylactic antibiotics.

ISSUES FOR REFERRAL
Refer to a tertiary center if pancreatitis is severe or actively evolving and when advanced imaging or endoscopic therapy is being considered.

SURGERY/OTHER PROCEDURES
- Consider cholecystectomy before discharge in patients with cholelithiasis and nonnecrotizing pancreatitis to reduce risk of recurrence.
- Necrosectomy should be performed nonsurgically for either infected or noninfected necrosis. Walled-off necrosis should be observed for 4 weeks (treated with antibiotics if infected), followed by percutaneous or dual-modality drainage if available. Drainage may not be required if there are no signs of infection. Aspiration and culture are not required if infection is suspected and if patient is responding to appropriate antibiotic therapy (3)[A].
- ERCP early if evidence of acute cholangitis or at 72 hours if evidence of ongoing biliary obstruction; ERCP with pancreatic ductal stent placement, if ductal disruption persists longer than 1 to 2 weeks
- Resection or embolization for bleeding pseudoaneurysms
- Plasma exchange with insulin within 24 hours of presentation if severe necrotizing pancreatitis secondary to hypertriglyceridemia (5)

ADMISSION, INPATIENT, AND NURSING CONSIDERATIONS
Discharge criteria
- Pain controlled
- Tolerating oral diet
- Alcohol rehabilitation and tobacco cessation
- Low-grade fever and mild leukocytosis do not necessarily indicate infection and may take weeks to resolve. Infections may occur even after 10 days (33% of patients with necrotizing pancreatitis) due to secondary infection of necrotic material, requiring surgical debridement.

 ONGOING CARE

FOLLOW-UP RECOMMENDATIONS
- Follow-up imaging in several weeks if the original CT scan showed a fluid collection or necrosis or if the amylase/lipase continues to be elevated. Follow-up findings may include:
  - Pseudocyst (occurs in 10%) or abscess (sudden onset of fever): Conservative management is an option for asymptomatic pseudocysts up to 6 cm in diameter.
  - Splenic vein thrombosis in 16–18% with necrotizing pancreatitis
  - Pseudoaneurysm (splenic, gastroduodenal, intrapancreatic) hemorrhage can be life-threatening.
- Mild exocrine and endocrine dysfunction is usually subclinical. Patients with necrotizing pancreatitis, steatorrhea, or ductal obstruction, however, should receive enzyme supplementation.

- After the first episode of acute pancreatitis, the risk of lifetime diabetes doubles.
- After the first episode of acute pancreatitis, the risk of developing acute recurrent pancreatitis is ~17%. The risk for developing chronic pancreatitis is ~8%.

DIET
Advance diet as tolerated; reduce fat, alcohol, and added sugars.

PROGNOSIS
85–90% of cases of acute pancreatitis resolve spontaneously; 3–5% mortality (17% in necrotizing pancreatitis)

REFERENCES
1. Vishnupriya K, Chanmugam A. Acute pancreatitis: the increasing role of medical management of a traditionally surgically managed disease [published online ahead of print September 21, 2021]. *Am J Med*. doi:10.1016/j.amjmed.2021.08.021.
2. Habtezion A, Gukovskaya AS, Pandol SJ. Acute pancreatitis: a multifaceted set of organelle and cellular interactions. *Gastroenterology*. 2019;156(7):1941–1950.
3. Forsmark CE, Vege SS, Wilcox CM. Acute pancreatitis. *N Engl J Med*. 2016;375(20):1972–1981.
4. Crockett SD, Wani S, Gardner TB, et al; for American Gastroenterological Association Institute Clinical Guidelines Committee. American Gastroenterological Association Institute guideline on initial management of acute pancreatitis. *Gastroenterology*. 2018;154(4):1096–1101.
5. Gulati A, Papachristou GI. Update on the management of acute pancreatitis and its complications. *New Gastroenterol*. 2017;2017:12–17.

ADDITIONAL READING
- Baron TH, DiMaio CJ, Wang AY, et al. American Gastroenterological Association clinical practice update: management of pancreatic necrosis. *Gastroenterology*. 2020;158(1):67–75.e1.
- Vivian E, Cler L, Conwell D, et al. Acute Pancreatitis Task Force on Quality: development of quality indicators for acute pancreatitis management. *Am J Gastroenterol*. 2019;114(8):1322–1342.

CODES

ICD10
- K85.9 Acute pancreatitis, unspecified
- K85.8 Other acute pancreatitis
- K85.2 Alcohol induced acute pancreatitis

CLINICAL PEARLS
- Pancreatitis is a common cause of hospitalization.
- Gallstones and alcohol misuse are the leading causes of pancreatitis.
- The BISAP score is easier to apply than Ranson criteria and just as accurate for predicting mortality in patients with acute pancreatitis.
- Review all medications and discontinue any that may cause (or contribute to) pancreatitis.
- Start oral feeding as soon as possible in the absence of severe pain, vomiting, or ileus.
- Patients with mild pancreatitis can progress to severe pancreatitis over the initial 48 hours, often due to inadequate fluid replacement.
- Refer to tertiary center if acute pancreatitis is severe or evolving/worsening.

PANIC DISORDER
Jay Winner, MD, FAAFP

 BASICS

DESCRIPTION
- A classic panic attack is characterized by rapid onset of a brief period of sympathetic nervous system hyperarousal accompanied by intense fear.
- In panic disorder, multiple panic attacks occur (including at least two without a recognizable trigger). Patients experience at least 1 month of worried anticipation of additional attacks and/or maladaptive (e.g., avoidance) behaviors.

EPIDEMIOLOGY
Incidence
- Median age of onset 24 years. Prevalence significantly decreases after 60 years.
- Predominant sex: female > male (2:1)

Prevalence
- Lifetime prevalence: 4.7%
- Of patients presenting with chest pain in the emergency room, 25% have panic disorder.
- Chest pain is more likely due to panic if atypical, younger age, female, and known problems with anxiety.

ETIOLOGY AND PATHOPHYSIOLOGY
Patients resist the initial surge of adrenaline which exacerbates the symptoms—in essence, they get anxious about being anxious.

Genetics
There is a higher incidence of panic disorder among family members, and there are a few genes associated with it; however, there is no specific known gene pattern that can fully explain the syndrome.

RISK FACTORS
- Life stressors of any kind can precipitate attacks.
- History of sexual or physical abuse
- Substance abuse, smoking, bipolar disorder, major depression, obsessive-compulsive disorder (OCD), and simple phobia

GENERAL PREVENTION
Healthy lifestyle, with stress reduction techniques and mindfulness are useful.

COMMONLY ASSOCIATED CONDITIONS
- Other psychiatric diagnoses: PTSD, social phobia, simple phobia, major depression, bipolar disorder, substance abuse, OCD, separation anxiety disorder
- More common in patients with asthma, migraine headaches, hypertension, mitral valve prolapse, reflux esophagitis, interstitial cystitis, irritable bowel syndrome, fibromyalgia, nicotine dependence
- Panic disorder increases the risk of suicide attempts and ideation.

DIAGNOSIS

- Panic attack: an abrupt surge of intense fear, reaching a peak within minutes in which ≥4 of the following symptoms develop abruptly: (i) palpitations, pounding heart, or accelerated heart rate; (ii) sweating; (iii) trembling or shaking; (iv) sensation of shortness of breath or smothering; (v) a choking sensation; (vi) chest pain or discomfort; (vii) nausea or abdominal distress; (viii) feeling dizzy, unsteady, light-headed, or faint; (ix) derealization (feelings of unreality) or depersonalization (feeling detached from oneself); (x) fear of losing control or going crazy; (xi) fear of dying; (xii) paresthesias; (xiii) chills or hot flashes (1)[C]
- Panic disorder: recurrent unexpected panic attacks not better accounted for by another psychiatric condition (e.g., PTSD, OCD, separation anxiety disorder, social anxiety disorder, or specific phobia) *and* not induced by drugs of abuse, medical conditions, or prescribed drugs *and* with >1 month of at least one of the following: (i) worry about additional attacks or worry about the implications of the attack (e.g., losing control, having a heart attack, "going crazy"), (ii) a significant maladaptive change in behavior related to the attacks (1)[C]

HISTORY
- Obtain a good history through tactful, nonjudgmental questioning. Information should be elicited about physical and emotional symptoms, current life stress, separations, recent deaths, patient's concerns and fears, interpersonal problems.
- A thorough medication and substance abuse history is important.
- Review *DSM-5* diagnostic criteria. Ask for avoidance patterns that have developed since the onset of panic attacks.

PHYSICAL EXAM
- During an attack, there can be tachycardia, hyperventilation, and diaphoresis.
- Thyroid exam for fullness or nodules. Look for exophthalmos or lid lag.
- Cardiac exam for murmur or arrhythmias
- Lung exam to rule out asthma (limited airflow, wheezing)

DIFFERENTIAL DIAGNOSIS
- Medication use may mimic panic disorder and create anxiety: Paradoxically, antidepressants used to treat panic may, initially, worsen panic; antidepressants in bipolar patients can cause anxiety/mania/panic; short-acting benzodiazepines (alprazolam), β-blockers (propranolol), and short-acting opioids can cause interdose rebound anxiety; benzodiazepine treatment causes panic when patients take too much and run out of these medicines early; bupropion, levodopa, amphetamines, steroids, albuterol, sympathomimetics, fluoroquinolones, and interferon can cause panic.
- Substance withdrawal or abuse: alcohol withdrawal, benzodiazepine withdrawal, opioid withdrawal, caffeine, marijuana (panic with paranoia), amphetamine abuse, MDMA, hallucinogens (PCP, LSD), dextromethorphan abuse, synthetic cathinones (bath salts) abuse

- Medical conditions: cardiovascular (tachyarrhythmias, myocardial infarction, mitral valve prolapse), pulmonary (asthma, COPD, hypoxia, pulmonary embolism), endocrine (hypo-/hyperthyroidism, premenstrual dysphoric disorder, menopause, pregnancy, hypoglycemia [in diabetes], carcinoid syndrome, pheochromocytoma, Cushing syndrome, hyperaldosteronism, hyperparathyroidism), neurologic (transient ischemic attacks [TIAs], pre- and postictal states, e.g., in TLE), miscellaneous (autoimmune disease, e.g., SLE; inner ear disturbances, e.g., labyrinthitis, anaphylaxis, heavy metal poisoning), sleep apnea (when nocturnal panic attacks). Note: It is unusual to have a first panic attack after the age for 40, making it more important to consider other medical conditions for those patients.
- Psychiatric conditions that have overlapping symptomatology include mood, anxiety, and personality disorders such as major depression, bipolar disorder, PTSD, borderline personality disorder, social phobia, OCD, and generalized anxiety disorder. In PTSD, there is always a recollection or visual image that precedes the panic attack. In social phobia, fear of scrutiny precedes the panic attack. In bipolar disorder, major depression, borderline personality disorder, and particularly substance abuse, the patient often complains first of panic symptoms and anxiety and minimizes other potentially relevant symptoms and behaviors.

DIAGNOSTIC TESTS & INTERPRETATION
No specific lab tests are indicated except to rule out conditions in the differential diagnosis.
- If chest discomfort, do appropriate workup. Electrocardiogram and pulse oximetry; consider Holter monitoring, stress testing, and/or chest CT in select patients.
- Fingerstick blood sugar in acute setting in a diabetic patient
- Thyroid-stimulating hormone (TSH), complete metabolic panel, CBC
- If nocturnal panic attacks, consider sleep study to evaluate for possible sleep apnea.

Diagnostic Procedures/Other
- If a medical cause of anxiety is strongly suspected, do the workup appropriate for that condition.
- Panic Disorder Severity Scale (PDSS) is a physician or self-administered instrument for monitoring changes in severity of symptoms and response to treatment (2).

 TREATMENT

Combined antidepressant therapy and psychotherapy is superior to either alone during initial treatment for panic disorder (3)[A]. Most effective therapy includes cognitive-behavioral therapy (CBT), mindfulness-based therapy, and exposure therapy. Psychotherapy provides long-lasting treatment, often without subsequent need for medications.

GENERAL MEASURES

Patient education is a vital part of treatment. A useful mnemonic is HR BET (think of Babe Ruth as the person you would have betted on to get a home run or your "HR BET").

- Harmless: Explain to patients why they are having their symptoms. For instance, hyperventilation may change the acid/base balance of the blood causing dizziness, extremity tingling, and odd out of body sensations.
- Resistance: Explain how resistance can prolong the panic and make it worse. People get anxious about being anxious.
- Breathing: Teach mindful diaphragmatic breathing.
- Energy: Discuss that adrenaline can be felt as anxiety or excitement. Instead of calling it a panic attack, reframe it as an energy burst and see if patients can feel the energy flowing through their veins.
- Thoughts: Develop the skill of noticing thoughts without believing them all. People can be taught to dispute irrational thoughts and beliefs (e.g., disputing "I'm dying now," with "I've had many of these attacks before; they have been thoroughly evaluated by my doctor and they are not harmful; if I don't resist them and just do my diaphragmatic breathing, they resolve more quickly").

MEDICATION

- Medication management is indicated if psychotherapy is not successful and may be combined with psychotherapy.
- Selective serotonin reuptake inhibitor (SSRI), serotonin-norepinephrine reuptake inhibitor (SNRI), tricyclic antidepressant (TCA), monoamine oxidase inhibitor (MAOI), and benzodiazepines have shown efficacy in treating panic disorder.
- It is recommended that medications be maintained for at least 1 year after symptom control to reduce risk of relapse.

First Line

- SSRIs and SNRIs are first line given efficacy, relatively benign side effect profile, and lack of abuse potential.
- Start a low-dose SSRI, for example, fluoxetine 5 mg, paroxetine 10 mg, sertraline 25 mg, citalopram 10 mg, and escitalopram 5 mg once daily in the morning. (If sedation occurs, this can be changed to night time dosing.) Titrate up slowly every 1 to 2 weeks to therapeutic doses over a period of 6 weeks. If indicated, further dose increases usually happen no more frequently than monthly. Side effects include irritability, diarrhea, and sexual dysfunction, with less frequent side effects such as hyponatremia, GI bleeding, manic episodes (if patient is bipolar), elevated LFTs, QT prolongation (more often with citalopram), and serotonin syndrome. Warn people starting escitalopram that nausea is very frequent but usually resolves after 1 week of treatment. Suicidality can be seen in young patients. When stopping SSRI, taper over few months because of risk of discontinuation syndrome. This is more important for medications with a shorter half-life like paroxetine compared with medications such as fluoxetine.

- Among SNRIs, venlafaxine extended release (ER) is effective. Start at 37.5 mg/day and titrate up to 75 mg/day after 7 days (maximum dose of 225 mg/day). Taper slowly over weeks to discontinue; risk of hypertension at higher doses. Other side effects are similar to SSRIs. SNRIs such as desvenlafaxine or duloxetine can also be tried.

Second Line

- Mirtazapine can be used started at 15 mg QHS and potentially increasing to 30 mg QHS. Side effects of sedation and weight gain may limit use, but for people suffering from weight loss and insomnia, this medication could be helpful.
- TCAs, particularly imipramine, may be an option, but are seldom used (because of difficulty in dosing, more side effects, and greater risk associated with overdose compared with SSRIs) (4)[A]. Screen for cardiac conduction system in patients >40 years of age with an ECG.
- MAOIs like phenelzine and tranylcypromine are also efficacious compared to placebo. Avoid with serotonergic agents given risk for serotonin syndrome. There are also dietary restrictions and multiple other drug interactions that limit use of these medications.
- Benzodiazepines should be used just for crisis and short-term relief of severe symptoms. Alprazolam (start 0.25 mg TID PRN) and clonazepam (start at 0.5 mg BID PRN) are FDA-approved for panic disorder. Clonazepam has a longer half-life, less interdose anxiety, and lower abuse potential than alprazolam. Benzodiazepines are associated with sedation, dependence, increased falls, increased car accidents, and increased mortality. Prescribing benzodiazepines to patients on opiates increases risk of overdose.

ISSUES FOR REFERRAL

- Refer for CBT, mindfulness-based therapy, and/or exposure therapy.
- Consider psychiatrist referral for comorbid bipolar disorder, borderline personality disorder, schizophrenia, suicidality, alcohol, substance abuse, or for patients unresponsive to initial treatment.

ADDITIONAL THERAPIES

- Aerobic exercise, yoga, or tai chi may reduce symptoms.
- Mindfulness meditation can be learned with stress reduction classes such as Mindfulness-Based Stress Reduction (MBSR), apps such as Ten Percent Happier, Headspace, and UCLA Mindful. Free meditations also at http://stressremedy.com/audio

COMPLEMENTARY & ALTERNATIVE MEDICINE

There is limited data supporting the use of supplements for the treatment of anxiety disorders. Kava kava should be avoided because of the risks of liver failure. A 2018 meta-analysis did show potential reduction in anxiety from omega-3 fatty acids 2 g daily with EPA <60% (would start at 1 g daily) (4)[C].

ADMISSION, INPATIENT, AND NURSING CONSIDERATIONS

- If certain life-threatening mimics of panic disorder have not been ruled out, such as an myocardial infarction or pulmonary embolus, hospitalize patient to complete the evaluation.
- If a panic disorder patient has concrete suicidal ideation, a psychiatric admission is indicated.

 ONGOING CARE

FOLLOW-UP RECOMMENDATIONS

Full therapeutic effect of antidepressants often does not occur until 4 to 6 weeks. Monitor (usually within 1 to 2 weeks) for suicidal ideation when starting antidepressants in patients aged 24 or younger.

DIET

A primarily whole food, plant-based diet and limiting caffeine may be helpful.

PATIENT EDUCATION

- Video on "Dealing with Panic and Anxiety" at http://stressremedy.com/videos
- http://www.nimh.nih.gov/health/publications/panic-disorder-when-fear-overwhelms/index.shtml

PROGNOSIS

Remission occurs in 64.5% of patients with a mean time to remission of about 5.7 months. Recurrence does occur in 21.4% in those who achieved remission. Predictors of remission are female gender, absence of ongoing stressors, and a low initial frequency of attacks.

COMPLICATIONS

- Iatrogenic benzodiazepine dependence
- Iatrogenic mania in bipolar patients treated for panic with unopposed antidepressants

REFERENCES

1. American Psychiatric Association. *Diagnostic and Statistical Manual of Mental Disorders*. 5th ed. Arlington, VA: American Psychiatric Association; 2013.
2. Shear MK, Brown TA, Barlow DH, et al. Multicenter collaborative panic disorder severity scale. *Am J Psychiatry*. 1997;154(11):1571–1575.
3. Furukawa TA, Watanabe N, Churchill R. Combined psychotherapy plus antidepressants for panic disorder with or without agoraphobia. *Cochrane Database Syst Rev*. 2007;2007(1):CD004364.
4. Su KP, Tseng PT, Lin PY, et al. Association of use of omega-3 polyunsaturated fatty acids with changes in severity anxiety symptoms: a systematic review and meta-analysis. *JAMA Netw Open*. 2018;1(5):e182327.

 SEE ALSO

Algorithm: Anxiety

 CODES

ICD10

F41.0 Panic disorder [episodic paroxysmal anxiety]

CLINICAL PEARLS

Evaluate a patient with panic for suicidality because patients with panic disorder are at increased risk for suicide, particularly if depressed.

PARKINSON DISEASE
Elyas Parsa, DO • Natasha S. Khokhar, DO, MPH

BASICS

DESCRIPTION
- A progressive neurodegenerative disorder caused by loss of dopaminergic neurons in the substantia nigra and other dopaminergic regions of the brain.
- Cardinal symptoms include resting tremor, rigidity, bradykinesia, and postural instability.

EPIDEMIOLOGY
Incidence
- 21 per 100,000 person-years
- Average age of onset: ~60 years
- Slightly more common in men than women

Prevalence
- Second most common neurodegenerative disease after Alzheimer disease
- 1 to 2/1,000 persons
- 0.3% of general population and 1–2% of those ≥60 years of age and up to 4% of those ≥80 years of age
- Affects 1 million people in the United States and 5 million worldwide

ETIOLOGY AND PATHOPHYSIOLOGY
Dopamine depletion in the substantia nigra and the nigrostriatal pathways results in the major motor complications of PD.
- Pathologic hallmark: selective loss of dopamine-containing neurons in the pars compacta of the substantia nigra
- Loss of neurons accompanied by presence of Lewy bodies (hyaline inclusion bodies) and Lewy neuritis

Genetics
Mutations in multiple autosomal dominant and autosomal recessive genes are linked to PD/parkinsonian syndrome particularly when the age at symptom onset is <50 years.

RISK FACTORS
- Age and family history of PD or tremor.
- Lifelong pesticide use by farmers, especially of rotenone and other carbamate, is associated with risk of developing PD.
- Repeated head trauma and living in rural areas, drinking well water, working in a wood pulp mill

GENERAL PREVENTION
Physical activity that has been linked to decreased risk of development of PD include weight training, running, dancing, yoga, and traditional Chinese martial arts (1).

COMMONLY ASSOCIATED CONDITIONS
Cognitive abnormalities, autonomic dysfunction (e.g., constipation, urinary urgency), sleep disturbances, mental status changes (depression, psychosis, hallucinations, dementia), orthostatic hypotension, and pain

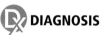

DIAGNOSIS

- Diagnosis is based on clinical features and response to dopaminergic therapy.
- Gold standard for diagnosis is neuropathologic exam.
- Generally, bradykinesia plus either tremor or rigidity must be present in order to make the diagnosis of idiopathic PD.

- African American patients with PD are less likely to receive standard of care compared to white counterparts (2).
- Idiopathic rapid eye movement sleep behavior disorder is considered a possible prodrome for PD (3).

HISTORY
Symptoms often subtle or attributed to aging
- Decreased emotion displayed in facial features
- General motor slowing and stiffness (One or both arms do not swing with walk.)
- Resting tremor (often initially one hand)
- Speech soft/mumbling
- Falls/difficulty with balance; seen with disease progression
- Psychiatric symptoms including depression, anxiety, hallucinations, and dementia
- Urinary symptoms including increased frequency and urgency

PHYSICAL EXAM
- Tremor
  - Resting tremor (4 to 6 Hz) that is often asymmetric
  - Disappears with voluntary movement
  - Frequently emerges in a hand while walking and may present as pill rolling
  - May also present in jaw, chin, lips, tongue
- Bradykinesia
- Rigidity: cogwheel (catching and releasing) or lead pipe (continuously rigid)
- Postural instability

DIFFERENTIAL DIAGNOSIS
- Essential tremor: Bradykinesia is not present; often symmetric and occurs mostly during action or when holding hands outstretched, nonresponsive to levodopa
- Depression can cause psychomotor slowing that may appear similar to bradykinesia in PD.
- Dementia with Lewy bodies: characterized clinically by visual hallucinations, fluctuating cognition, and parkinsonism; dementia occurs concomitantly with or before the development of parkinsonism.
- Multiple system atrophy: presets with parkinsonism and varying degrees of dysautonomia, cerebellar involvement, and pyramidal signs
- Progressive supranuclear palsy: impairment in vertical eye movements (particularly down gaze), hyperextension of neck, and early falling; pseudobulbar palsy
- Associated neurodegenerative disorders: late stages of Alzheimer disease, Huntington disease, frontotemporal dementia, spinocerebellar ataxias
- Secondary parkinsonism (drug induced: reversible; may take weeks/months after offending medication is stopped; often bilateral symptoms):
  - Neuroleptics (most common cause)
  - Antiemetics (e.g., prochlorperazine and promethazine), metoclopramide
  - SSRIs
  - Calcium channel blockers (e.g., flunarizine and cinnarizine)
  - Amiodarone
  - Lithium/valproic acid
  - Amphotericin B
  - Estrogens

DIAGNOSTIC TESTS & INTERPRETATION
Initial Tests (lab, imaging)
- Diagnosis is mainly clinical, and there are no confirmatory physiologic or blood tests.
- Reduction in α-synuclein and DJ-1 protein can act as a qualitative feature in PD diagnosis.
- MRI of brain is nondiagnostic but can be used to rule out structural abnormalities.

Follow-Up Tests & Special Considerations
Note that single-photon emission computerized tomography (SPECT) can be used to differentiate PD from parkinsonism (3).

Diagnostic Procedures/Other
PET and MR spectroscopy are not recommended (3).

Test Interpretation
Diagnosis is clinical and no tests are recommended to confirm diagnosis of PD.

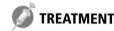

TREATMENT

GENERAL MEASURES
Multidisciplinary rehabilitation with standard physical and occupational therapy components to improve functional outcomes

MEDICATION
- PD goal: Improve motor and nonmotor deficits.
- Agents are chosen based on patient age and symptoms present.
- "Off" periods describe the development of symptoms (often dyskinesias) while patient is on PD medication. This especially occurs among elderly patients taking levodopa medications (3).

First Line
- First-line agents in early PD: levodopa, dopamine agonists, monoamine oxidase B (MAO-B) inhibitors (4)[A]
  - Levodopa combined with carbidopa is still the most effective treatment for symptoms of PD, particularly bradykinesia.
  - Levodopa versus dopamine agonist is controversial:
    - Most patients eventually will develop involuntary motor fluctuations or dyskinesias with levodopa.
    - Older patients often are less able to tolerate the adverse events of dopamine agonists.
    - All patients eventually will require levodopa.
  - For patients who experience dyskinesias while on levodopa, can consider MAO-B inhibitors (rasagiline) or catechol O-methyltransferase (COMT) inhibitors (entacapone) as adjuvants (3)
- Carbidopa + levodopa (Carbidopa inhibits peripheral conversion of levodopa.)
  - Immediate release (Sinemet)
  - Orally disintegrating (Parcopa)
- Carbidopa + levodopa + entacapone (Stalevo)
  - Addition of entacapone as a single agent should be initiated prior to use of this combination:
    - Once daily dose of carbidopa/levodopa has been identified, may convert to Stalevo
  - Side effects are the same, plus diarrhea and brownish orange urine.

- Dopamine-receptor agonists (nonergot): side effects: nausea, vomiting, hypotension, sedation, edema, vivid dreaming, compulsive behavior, confusion, light-headedness, and hallucinations:
  – Pramipexole (Mirapex)
  – Ropinirole (Requip)
- Selective MAO-B inhibitors: side effects: insomnia, jitteriness, hallucinations; mostly found with selegiline; rasagiline similar adverse events as placebo in clinical trials. Rasagiline is metabolized via *CYP1A2*; caution with other medications using this enzyme system (e.g., ciprofloxacin):
- Selegiline (Eldepryl)
- Rasagiline (Azilect)

Second Line
- Second-line agents in early PD: β-adrenergic antagonists (postural tremor), amantadine, anticholinergics (young patients with tremor); lack of good evidence for symptom control (4)[A]
- Dopamine agonists (ergot): Increased adverse event profile makes these agents nonpreferred to nonergot dopamine agonists; bromocriptine (Parlodel) (3)
- Treatment of levodopa-induced motor complications
  – End of dose wearing off (i.e., decreased responsiveness to PD medication resulting in return of PD symptoms)
  – Entacapone (with each levodopa dose) or rasagiline preferred
  – Dyskinesias: typically occur at peak dopamine level
  – Amantadine may be considered; however, efficacy is questionable (4)[B].
  – The FDA has approved istradefylline (Nourianz) as the first adenosine A2A receptor antagonist to be approved in the United States an oral agent for use as an adjunct to carbidopa/levodopa in adults with PD who experience "off" episodes.
- Anticholinergic agents: avoided due to lack of efficacy (only useful for tremor) and increased adverse event profile
  – Trihexyphenidyl
  – Benztropine (Cogentin)
- *N*-methyl-D-aspartic acid antagonist: exact mechanism unknown, efficacy is questionable; may be useful for dyskinesias. Side effects: confusion, dizziness, dry mouth, livedo reticularis, and hallucinations
  – Amantadine (Symmetrel)
- COMT inhibitors: entacapone preferred due to hepatotoxicity associated with tolcapone. Adverse events include nausea and orthostatic hypotension:
  – Entacapone (Comtan)
  – Tolcapone (Tasmar)
    ○ Requires LFT monitoring
- Apomorphine (Apokyn): nonergot-derived dopamine agonist given SC for off episodes in advanced disease; adverse events: nausea, vomiting, dizziness, hallucinations, orthostatic hypotension, somnolence
  – Only for "off" episodes with levodopa therapy

ISSUES FOR REFERRAL
Early specialty referral (neurology) for patients with suspected PD to receive a more thorough clinical assessment and for treatment recommendations

ADDITIONAL THERAPIES
- Emotional and psychological support of patient family
- Physical therapy and endurance exercise has been shown to improve balance, muscle strength, walking speed.
- Speech therapy: may be helpful in improving speech volume and maintaining voice quality
- Treatment of nonmotor symptoms
  – Psychosis
    ○ In 2016, the FDA approved pimavanserin (Nuplazid) as the first drug specifically designed to treat Parkinson disease psychosis.
    ○ Quetiapine (Seroquel) had been widely used for people with PDP before pimavanserin.
  ○ Insomnia
    ■ Rotigotine: FDA approved in transdermal form to treat insomnia in PD
  ○ Orthostatic hypotension: in addition to increasing salt and fluid intake, can also use FDA-approved droxidopa
    ■ Can also consider midodrine, fludrocortisone, use of compression stockings (3)
  ○ Dementia
    ■ Rivastigmine can be considered for cognitive impairment (i.e., mild to moderate dementia in PD)
  ○ Depression in PD
    ■ Can consider pramipexole, nortriptyline, desipramine, venlafaxine, and CBT (3)

SURGERY/OTHER PROCEDURES
Deep brain stimulation is an effective therapeutic option for patients with motor complications refractory to best medical treatment who are healthy, have no significant comorbidities, are responsive to levodopa, and do not have depression or dementia.

COMPLEMENTARY & ALTERNATIVE MEDICINE
Music therapy may help to improve quality of life and motor symptoms in PD patients (5).

ADMISSION, INPATIENT, AND NURSING CONSIDERATIONS
- Fall risk precaution when admitted
- Note that small variation in medication dosage can impact PD symptoms. Make sure patient has home PD medications.

 ONGOING CARE

FOLLOW-UP RECOMMENDATIONS
- Avoid drug holidays if patient is having "off" time on levodopa.
- Consider switching to dopamine agonist (nonergot preferred), MAO-B inhibitors, or COMT inhibitors if patient develops dyskinesias on levodopa/carbidopa therapy.
- Severe motor symptoms. At this point, patient should not be allowed to drive self. This should be noted and reported to licensing agency (3).

Patient Monitoring
If on dopamine agonists—monitor for development of impulse control behaviors (3).

DIET
- For dysphagia, consider soft food, swallowing evaluation, and increased time for meals.
- Avoid large, high-fat meals that slow digestion and interfere with medication absorption.

PATIENT EDUCATION
- www.parkinson.org
- For caregivers to patients with PD: https://www.caregiver.org/resource/parkinsons-disease-caregiving/

PROGNOSIS
- PD is a chronic progressive disease; prognosis varies based on patient-specific symptoms.
- Increased mortality in PD; on average, survival is reduced by 5% every year of follow-up.

REFERENCES
1. Fan B, Jabeen R, Bo B, et al. What and how can physical activity prevention function on Parkinson's disease? *Oxid Med Cell Longev.* 2020;2020:4293071.
2. Bailey M, Anderson S, Hall DA. Parkinson's disease in African Americans: a review of the current literature. *J Parkinsons Dis.* 2020;10(3):831–841.
3. DynaMed. Parkinson disease. EBSCO Information Services. https://www.dynamed.com/condition/parkinson-disease. Updated December 4, 2018. Accessed September 24, 2021.
4. Diaz NL, Waters CH. Current strategies in the treatment of Parkinson's disease and a personalized approach to management. *Expert Rev Neurother.* 2009;9(12):1781–1789.
5. García-Casares N, Martín-Colom JE, García-Arnés JA. Music therapy in Parkinson's disease. *J Am Med Dir Assoc.* 2018;19(12):1054–1062.

 SEE ALSO

American Academy of Neurology practice parameter on initiation of treatment of PD: https://n.neurology.org/content/58/1/11.long

CODES

ICD10
- G21.11 Neuroleptic induced parkinsonism
- G21.8 Other secondary parkinsonism
- G21.4 Vascular parkinsonism

CLINICAL PEARLS
- The classic description for PD is shaky (pill-rolling tremor at rest), stiff (cogwheel rigidity), slow (bradykinesia), and stumbling (shuffling gait).
- No cure—goals are to delay disease progression and relieve symptoms.
- Emphasize the importance of exercise and movement to help preserve function.
- Pharmacotherapeutic regimens need to be individualized based on age/specific symptoms.

PARONYCHIA

Nancy Nguyen, DO

 BASICS

DESCRIPTION

- Superficial inflammation of the lateral and posterior nail folds surrounding the fingernail or toenail; develops after breakdown of barrier between nail plate and the adjacent nail fold
- Acute: characterized by pain, erythema, and swelling (1) lasting <6 weeks; usually a bacterial infection appearing after nail biting, trauma, manicures, ingrown nails, and hangnail manipulation. It can progress to abscess formation.
- Chronic: characterized by swelling, tenderness, cuticle elevation, and nail dystrophy and separation lasting at least 6 weeks, or recurrent episodes of acute eponychial inflammation and drainage
- May be considered work-related among bartenders, restaurant servers, dishwashers, nurses, and others who often wash their hands
- Usually involves one finger but drug-induced paronychia may involve multiple fingers
- Relevant anatomy: nail bed, nail plate, and perionychium
- Synonym(s): eponychia, perionychia

Pediatric Considerations
Less common in pediatric age groups. Thumb/finger-sucking is a risk factor (anaerobes and *Escherichia coli* may be present).

EPIDEMIOLOGY

Incidence
- One of the most common hand infections in the United States
- Predominant age: all ages
- Predominant sex: female > male

ETIOLOGY AND PATHOPHYSIOLOGY

- Acute: mixed aerobic and anaerobic bacterial flora in 50% of cases. *Staphylococcus aureus* most common and *Streptococcus pyogenes*; less frequently, *Pseudomonas pyocyanea* and *Proteus vulgaris*
- Chronic: eczematous reaction with secondary *Candida albicans* (~95%)
- Pediatric age groups: mixed anaerobic (*Fusobacterium, Peptostreptococcus*) and aerobic infections (*Eikenella corrodens, S. aureus*, streptococci) from oral flora
- A paronychial infection commonly starts in the lateral nail fold.
- Acute paronychia of the fingers is often due to trauma; acute paronychia of the toes is often due to ingrown nails (2).
- Recurrent inflammation, persistent edema, and fibrosis of nail folds cause nail folds to round up and retract, exposing nail grooves to irritants, allergens, and pathogens.
- Inflammation compromises ability of proximal nail fold to regenerate cuticle leading to decreased vascular supply. This can cause decrease efficacy of topical medications.
- Early in the course, cellulitis alone may be present.
- An abscess can form if the infection does not resolve quickly.

RISK FACTORS

- Acute: direct or indirect trauma to cuticle or nail fold, manicured/sculptured nails, nail biting, thumb sucking, manipulating a hang nail
- Chronic: frequent immersion of hands in water with excoriation of the lateral nail fold (e.g., chefs, bartenders, housekeepers, swimmers, dishwashers, nurses)
- Predisposing conditions such as diabetes mellitus and immunosuppression
- Medications such as EGFR inhibitors, systemic retinoids, chemotherapy and antiretroviral agents

GENERAL PREVENTION

- Acute: Avoid trauma such as nail biting or manipulating a hangnail.
- Chronic: Avoid exposure to allergens and contact irritants; keep fingers/hands dry; wear rubber gloves with a cotton liner. Prevent excoriation of the skin.
- Keep nails short.
- Avoid manicures.
- Apply moisturizer after washing hands.
- Good glycemic control in diabetic patients

COMMONLY ASSOCIATED CONDITIONS

- Diabetes mellitus
- Eczema or atopic dermatitis
- Immunosuppression

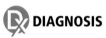 **DIAGNOSIS**

HISTORY

- Localized pain or tenderness, swelling, and erythema of posterior or lateral nail folds
  - Acute: fairly rapid onset (2 to 5 days after trauma)
  - Chronic: at least 6 weeks' duration
- Previous trauma (i.e., bitten nails, ingrown nails, manicured nails)
- Contact with herpes infections
- Contact with allergens or irritants (frequent water immersion, latex)
- Immunosuppressive therapy

PHYSICAL EXAM

- Acute: red, warm, tender, tense posterior or lateral nail fold ± abscess
- Chronic:
  - Initially appears as swollen, tender, boggy nail fold ± abscess
  - Later appears as retraction of nail fold and absence of adjacent healthy cuticle, thickening of nail plate with prominent transverse ridges known as Beau lines and discoloration; multiple digits typically involved
- Occasional elevation of nail bed or separation of nail fold from nail plate
- Fluctuance, purulence at the nail margin, or purulent drainage
- An untreated infection of the toe may lead to the formation of granulation tissue around the nail fold (2).
- Secondary changes of nail platelike discoloration
- Suspect *Pseudomonas* if with green changes in nail (chloronychia).

DIFFERENTIAL DIAGNOSIS

- Felon (abscess of fingertip pulp; urgent diagnosis required)
- Cellulitis
- Eczema
- Herpetic whitlow (similar in appearance, very painful, often associated with vesicles)
- Allergic contact dermatitis (latex, acrylic)
- Psoriasis (especially acute flare)
- Proximal/lateral onychomycosis (nail folds not predominantly involved)
- Retronychia
- Pemphigus vulgaris
- Acute osteomyelitis of the distal phalanx
- Reiter disease
- Pustular psoriasis
- Dermatomyositis
- Malignancy: squamous cell carcinoma of the nail, malignant melanoma, metastatic disease

DIAGNOSTIC TESTS & INTERPRETATION
None required unless condition is severe; resistant to treatment or if recurrence or methicillin-resistant *S. aureus* (MRSA) is suspected, then

- Gram stain
- Culture and sensitivity
- Potassium hydroxide wet mount plus fungal culture especially in chronic paronychia
- Drugs that may alter lab results: use of over-the-counter antimicrobials or antifungals

Initial Tests (lab, imaging)
Consider ultrasonography if uncertain about presence of an abscess.

Diagnostic Procedures/Other
- Incision and drainage recommended for suppurative cases or cases not responding to conservative management or empiric antibiotics
- Tzanck testing or viral culture in suspected viral cases
- Biopsy in cases not responding to conservative management or when malignancy suspected

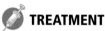 **TREATMENT**

GENERAL MEASURES

- Acute inflammation without abscess: warm water soaks or antiseptic soaks and topical antibiotics. Consider oral antibiotics for more severe cases that do not respond to topical treatment alone.
- Abscesses should be drained.
- Antibiotics may not be necessary for successful I&D of uncomplicated infections.
- Chronic: Keep fingers dry; apply moisturizing lotion after hand washing; avoid exposure to irritants; improved diabetic control

MEDICATION

First Line

- Acute paronychia (mild cases, no abscess formation):
  - Warm water soaks or antiseptic soaks (chlorhexidine, povidone-iodine) multiple times a day for 10 to 15 minutes each time, and topical antibiotics with *S. aureus* coverage (triple antibiotic ointment, mupirocin, bacitracin)
  - Antibiotic cream applied TID–QID after warm soak for 5 to 10 days
  - If eczematous: high-potency topical steroid applied BID (e.g., betamethasone 0.05% cream) for 7 to 14 days
- Acute paronychia (no abscess formation, not responding to topical treatment). Treat for 5 to 7 days.
  - Dicloxacillin 250 mg QID
  - Cephalexin 500 mg TID–QID
- Acute paronychia (exposure to oral flora, no abscess formation). Treat for 7 days. Cover for *Eikenella*.
  - Amoxicillin-clavulanate: 875 mg/125 mg BID; pediatric, 45 mg/kg q12h (for <40 kg) OR
  - One of the following for *Eikenella* coverage:
    ○ Doxycycline 100 mg BID
    ○ Trimethoprim/sulfamethoxazole BID
    ○ Ciprofloxacin 500 to 750 mg BID (Reserve fluoroquinolones for severe infection due to risks from this class of antibiotic.)
  - *PLUS* one of the following for anaerobic coverage:
    ○ Clindamycin 300 to 450 mg TID–QID (pediatric, 10 mg/kg q8h)
    ○ Metronidazole 500 mg TID
- Acute paronychia (with risk factors for MRSA including but not limited to: recent hospitalization, recent surgery, ESRD on hemodialysis, HIV/AIDS, IVDU, resident of long-term care facility). Treat for 7 days.
  - Trimethoprim/sulfamethoxazole 160 mg/800 mg BID
  - Doxycycline 100 mg BID
  - Clindamycin 300 to 450 mg TID–QID
- Acute paronychia with abscess formation:
  - Incision and drainage
    ○ Consider digital block anesthesia. Then, insert nail elevator, no. 11 scalpel blade, or hypodermic needle along nail plate at junction of the affected nail fold and nail to facilitate drainage. If no drainage occurs, use a needle or scalpel to open skin directly above abscess.
  - If ingrown nail involved or abscess extends to nail bed, consider partial nail removal.
  - Consider oral antibiotics for extension of cellulitis; otherwise, usually no antibiotics indicated after I&D
- Chronic paronychia: Stop source of irritation, control inflammation, and restore natural protective barrier.
  - Topical high-potency steroids: betamethasone 0.05%; applied BID for 7 to 14 days (3)[B]
  - Topical antifungal: clotrimazole or nystatin; applied topically TID for up to 30 days
  - Topical calcineurin inhibitor: Tacrolimus 0.1% ointment BID for up to 21 days has been shown to be more effective than betamethasone but is more expensive.
- For paronychia caused by antiepidermal growth factor receptor antibodies, use doxycycline 100 mg BID.
- For paronychia caused by oncology pharmacotherapy, treat with corticosteroid ointment and phenol chemical matricectomy. Prompt treatment enables patients to continue anticancer drug treatment without impairing their quality of life.

Second Line

- Systemic antifungals (rarely needed, use if topical fails)
  - Itraconazole 200 mg for 90 days (may have longer action because it is incorporated into nail plate); pulse therapy may be useful (i.e., 200 mg BID for 7 days, repeated monthly for 2 months).
  - Terbinafine 250 mg/day for 6 weeks (fingernails) or 12 weeks (toenails)
  - Fluconazole 100 mg daily for 7 to 14 days
  - Ciclopirox 0.77% topical suspension BID for 2 to 4 weeks along with strict irritant avoidance (4)[B]
- Antipseudomonal drugs (e.g., ceftazidime, aminoglycosides) when pseudomonas is suspected

ISSUES FOR REFERRAL

- Acute: Severe infection may spread to underlying tendons, requiring evaluation and treatment by a hand surgeon as it often involves débridement, washout, or amputation, based on the severity of the infection.
- Chronic: In treatment failure, consider biopsy and/or, in cases of chronic paronychia, referral for possible partial excision of the nail fold or eponychial marsupialization with or without complete nail removal or Swiss roll technique.
- Failure to respond to therapy or chronic redness, tenderness, and swelling of nail folds without abscess can be concerning for malignancy. Consider biopsy (2).

ADDITIONAL THERAPIES

Topical betaxolol 0.25% eye drops once daily on paronychia and pyogenic granuloma-like lesions covered with bandage

SURGERY/OTHER PROCEDURES

- Incision and drainage of abscess, if present
- A subungual abscess or ingrown nail requires partial or complete removal of nail with phenolization of germinal matrix.
- Swiss roll technique for chronic and severe acute paronychia with runaround abscess involving both nail folds (3)[B]
- May also use square flap technique or en bloc excision
- Recalcitrant cases may also need nail removal.

COMPLEMENTARY & ALTERNATIVE MEDICINE

Nail braces as a noninvasive alternative to nail extraction for patients with severe paronychia induced by EGFR inhibitors

 ## ONGOING CARE

FOLLOW-UP RECOMMENDATIONS

- Acute: Postdrainage care consists of warm soaks or antiseptic soaks. Follow up in 24 to 48 hours after I&D to monitor for worsening infection.
- Chronic: Avoid frequent immersion, triggers, allergens, nail biting, or finger sucking.

DIET

If patient is diabetic, consider appropriate dietary and medication changes for better control.

PATIENT EDUCATION

- Avoid trimming cuticles; avoid nail trauma; and stress importance of good diabetic control and diabetic education
- Avoid contact irritants; use rubber gloves with cotton liners to avoid exposure to excess moisture.
- Use moisturizing lotion after washing hands; do not bite nails/suck on fingers.

PROGNOSIS

- With adequate treatment and prevention, healing can be expected in 1 to 2 weeks.
- Chronic paronychia may respond slowly to treatment, taking weeks to months.
- If no response in chronic lesions, rarely benign or malignant neoplasm may be present and referral to dermatology should be considered.

COMPLICATIONS

- Acute: subungual abscess
- Chronic: nail thickening, discoloration of nail, and nail loss

REFERENCES

1. Leggit JC. Acute and chronic paronychia. *Am Fam Physician*. 2017;96(1):44–51.
2. Lomax A, Thornton J, Singh D. Toenail paronychia. *Foot Ankle Surg*. 2016;22(4):219–223.
3. Relhan V, Goel K, Bansal S, et al. Management of chronic paronychia. *Indian J Dermatol*. 2014;59(1):15–20.
4. Daniel CR III, Daniel MP, Daniel J, et al. Managing simple chronic paronychia and onycholysis with ciclopirox 0.77% and an irritant-avoidance regimen. *Cutis*. 2004;73(1):81–85.

ADDITIONAL READING

Iorizzo M. Tips to treat the 5 most common nail disorders: brittle nails, onycholysis, paronychia, psoriasis, onychomycosis. *Dermatol Clin*. 2015;33(2):175–183.

 ## SEE ALSO

Onychomycosis

CODES

ICD10

- L03.019 Cellulitis of unspecified finger
- L03.039 Cellulitis of unspecified toe
- L03.011 Cellulitis of right finger

CLINICAL PEARLS

- Consider incision and drainage when appropriate.
- For chronic paronychia, topical steroid is first-line treatment. Consider other differentials in nonresponders (e.g., rare causes: Raynaud, metastatic cancer, psoriasis, drug toxicity).
- Consider retronychia (nail embedded into proximal nail fold) for repeated episodes of proximal paronychia or treatment failure with antibiotics and antifungals. Treatment of choice is avulsion of the nail plate; often misdiagnosed as paronychia resulting in delay of treatment
- Consider presence of more than one nail disease at the same time (e.g., paronychia and onychomycosis).

PAROTITIS, ACUTE AND CHRONIC
Tamara L. Gayle, MD, MEd • Lemaat Michael, MD

BASICS

DESCRIPTION
- Parotitis is caused by inflammation of the parotid gland due to infection, systemic illnesses, mechanical obstruction, or medications.
- The parotid gland is the largest salivary gland, located lateral and anterior to the masseter muscle, and extends posteriorly over the sternocleidomastoid muscle behind the angle of the mandible. It produces serous secretions, which lack bacteriostatic properties, making it more susceptible to infection than other salivary glands.
- The parotid duct, also called the Stensen duct, pierces the buccinator muscle and enters the buccal mucosa opposite the second maxillary molar.
- The branches of the facial nerve bisect the gland into lobes.

EPIDEMIOLOGY
- Viral parotitis is the most common cause of parotitis in children; incidence has decreased since the advent of the mumps vaccine.
- Acute bacterial parotitis is less common, but occurs more frequently in elderly patients, neonates, and postoperative patients.
- Juvenile recurrent parotitis (JRP): second most common inflammatory cause of parotitis in children in the United States; first episode usually occurs between ages 3 and 6 years.
- Chronic parotitis primarily affects adults; typically presents between ages 40 and 60 years
- Chronic bilateral parotid enlargement is a common manifestation of HIV infection.

ETIOLOGY AND PATHOPHYSIOLOGY
- Acute viral parotitis begins as a systemic infection that localizes to the parotid gland, resulting in inflammation and swelling.
  - Mumps, or paramyxovirus, has a predilection for the parotid gland and classically has been linked to parotitis 16 to 18 days after infection. Mumps is a nationally reportable disease.
  - Other viral pathogens: parainfluenza, enterovirus, echovirus, influenza A, coxsackievirus, Epstein-Barr virus (EBV), human herpesvirus 6 (HHV-6)
  - Cytomegalovirus (CMV) and adenovirus have been seen in patients with HIV.
  - Case reports demonstrate that parotitis can be a manifestation of SARS-CoV-2 infection.
- Acute bacterial parotitis results from stasis of salivary flow that allows retrograde introduction of bacterial pathogens into the gland, resulting in localized infection.
  - *Staphylococcus aureus* is most common, followed by *Streptococcus pneumoniae* and anaerobes. Less common are *Streptococcus viridans*, *Escherichia coli*, and *Haemophilus influenzae*.
  - *Klebsiella*, *Enterobacter*, and *Pseudomonas* can be seen in chronically ill or hospitalized patients.
  - Consider *Bartonella henselae* with cat exposure.
  - May be a manifestation of late-onset group B *Streptococcus* (rare)
  - *Mycobacterium tuberculosis* has been seen in immunocompromised patients.

- Fungal
  - *Candida* has been isolated in chronically ill or hospitalized patients.
  - *Actinomyces* in patients with a history of trauma or dental caries
- Acute, recurrent parotitis
  - Mechanical: Repeated sialolith formation leads to ductal wall damage, fibrosis, and stricture formation.
  - Pneumoparotitis occurs when air is trapped in the parotid gland ducts; seen in wind instrument players, glass blowers, scuba divers, and rarely with dental cleaning
- "Anesthesia mumps": may be due to transient mechanical compression of the Stensen duct by airway devices, loss of muscle tone around the Stensen orifice after neuromuscular relaxants, increased salivary secretion, and increased flexion or rotation of the head during general anesthesia
- Chronic parotitis in patients with HIV can be due to presence of benign lymphoepithelial cysts, follicular hyperplasia of parotid lymph nodes, or diffuse infiltrative lymphocytosis syndrome, causing infiltration of the parotid gland by CD8 cells. Parotitis may be secondary to immune reconstitution after initiation of antiretroviral therapy.
- There are case reports of acute parotitis as a symptom of Kawasaki disease.

RISK FACTORS
- Immunosuppression, HIV, chemotherapy, radiation, malnutrition, alcoholism
- Acute viral parotitis: lack of mumps, measles, rubella (MMR) vaccination
- Acute bacterial parotitis: dehydration, debilitation, poor oral hygiene, Sjögren syndrome, cystic fibrosis, bulimia/anorexia, sialolithiasis (stones), ductal stenosis, trauma
- Neonatal parotitis: prematurity, dehydration, low birth weight, ductal obstruction, oral trauma, structural abnormalities
- JRP: dental malocclusion, congenital duct malformation, immunologic anomalies, disrupted enzyme activity
- Drug-induced parotitis: anticholinergics, ACE inhibitors (captopril), antihistamines, tricyclic antidepressants, antipsychotics (phenylbutazone, thioridazine, clozapine), iodine (contrast media), and L-asparaginase
- Chronic parotitis: ductal stenosis, HIV, tuberculosis, Sjögren syndrome, sarcoidosis, uremia, diabetes, gout, and atopy

GENERAL PREVENTION
- Completing MMR vaccine series; childhood vaccination does not guarantee prevention, possibly due to waning immunity with time.
  - Those without documented mumps immunity should receive 2 doses of the MMR vaccine, 28 days apart.
  - Pregnant women should not receive the mumps vaccine. Pregnancy should be avoided for 4 weeks after vaccination.
- Maintain adequate hydration, good dental hygiene, smoking cessation, abstinence from alcohol, and avoidance of chronic purging.

COMMONLY ASSOCIATED CONDITIONS
Mumps, HIV, Sjögren syndrome, sarcoidosis, sialolithiasis

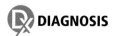

DIAGNOSIS

HISTORY
- Acute parotitis presents with sudden-onset pain and swelling of the cheek.
  - Viral parotitis is usually bilateral and accompanied by malaise, anorexia, headaches, myalgias, arthralgias, and fever.
  - Bacterial parotitis is associated with fever.
- JRP is usually unilateral, with pain and swelling resolving within 2 weeks.
- Other symptoms: trismus, pain exacerbated by chewing or worsened by foods that stimulate production of saliva, dry mouth with abnormal taste, difficulty with drinking/eating, anorexia, or dehydration
- Sialolithiasis is characterized by recurrent acute swelling and pain, exacerbated by eating. It may be associated with swelling around the Stensen duct.
- Chronic parotitis presents with recurrent or chronic nontender swelling of one or both parotid glands.

PHYSICAL EXAM
- Swelling or enlargement of the parotid gland(s); it may obscure the angle of the mandible or cause the ear to protrude upward and outward.
- Palpate with one hand starting at the attachment of the earlobe and proceed anteriorly and inferiorly along the mandibular ramus while the other hand simultaneously palpates the Stensen duct inside the oral cavity.
  - Bilateral tenderness suggests viral etiology, whereas unilateral tenderness, erythema, and warmth suggests a bacterial etiology.
  - Chronic parotitis is typically nontender.
- Trismus, halitosis, and dental decay may be noted.
- Drainage from the Stensen duct suggests bacterial parotitis or superinfection. The opening of the duct may appear edematous and erythematous in bacterial and viral cases.
- In JRP, the Stensen duct is often enlarged, dilated, erythematous, and swollen.
- Facial nerve palsy can be seen in severe cases.

DIFFERENTIAL DIAGNOSIS
Lymphoma, neoplasm, lymphangitis, cervical adenitis, otitis externa, odontogenic infections, Ludwig angina, and cellulitis

DIAGNOSTIC TESTS & INTERPRETATION
- History and exam are sufficient for diagnosis.
- Perform aerobic culture of purulent drainage from Stensen duct or aerobic and anaerobic culture from needle aspiration of gland or abscess.
  - Anaerobic culture from the Stensen duct will likely contain oropharyngeal contamination, thus perform anaerobic cultures only from needle aspirate fluid.

- Acute bacterial parotitis can be associated with leukocytosis and elevated amylase.
- For suspected mumps, the CDC recommends collecting a buccal swab for mumps RT-PCR if <3 days of symptom onset. If >3 days since onset of symptoms, obtain both buccal swab and a serum specimen for IgM.
  - Mumps RT-PCR is best obtained from a buccal swab performed after massaging the parotid gland for 30 seconds. In areas of high vaccination rates, IgM may be falsely negative necessitating correlation with clinical symptoms.
  - If initial IgM and RT-PCR obtained <3 days of symptom onset are negative, and there is strong clinical suspicion for mumps, consider repeating serum testing, as IgM response may not be detectable for 5 days after symptom onset.
- Send CMV titers in immunocompromised patients.
- For chronic, recurrent, or nontender parotitis, obtain HIV testing, PPD, SS-A/SS-B antibodies, rheumatoid factor, and antinuclear antibodies to evaluate for underlying etiology.

Initial Tests (lab, imaging)
- Imaging may be used to assess for abscess, masses, ductal stenosis, or sialolithiasis.
- Ultrasound is the first-line diagnostic modality for detecting sialadenitis and has high sensitivity for identifying abscess and ductal lithiasis (1)[B]. CT or MRI may also be used.

Follow-Up Tests & Special Considerations
Consider sialography in chronic parotitis to assess the anatomy and functional integrity of the gland (diagnostic and therapeutic) (1)[C].

Diagnostic Procedures/Other
- Consider biopsy or fine-needle aspiration if there is suspicion for tuberculosis, Sjögren syndrome, or sarcoidosis.
- Noncaseating granulomas may be seen in sarcoidosis. Caseating granulomas may be seen in tuberculosis and *B. henselae* infections.

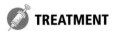 **TREATMENT**

GENERAL MEASURES
- Usually a self-limited course. Treat with supportive care: rest, hydration, analgesia, and antipyretics.
  - Stimulate saliva production by eating hard candies.
  - Local heat application and gentle massage.
  - Chronic parotitis: Encourage good dental hygiene and treat the underlying etiology.
- Patients with mumps should be isolated with standard and droplet precautions for 5 days after onset of parotid swelling.
- During a mumps outbreak, the CDC recommends administration of MMR vaccine even in fully vaccinated individuals, as a 3rd vaccine dose can decrease risk of mumps and improve outbreak control, especially in those whose second MMR was >13 years ago (2)[A].

MEDICATION
- Viral parotitis: no evidence for the use of immunoglobulin for postexposure prophylaxis or treatment; may initiate antibiotics if patient is toxic appearing
- Acute bacterial parotitis
  - Outpatient: amoxicillin/clavulanate or ciprofloxacin and clindamycin
  - Chronically ill or hospitalized: ampicillin/sulbactam or cefuroxime and metronidazole ; if MRSA is probable, consider vancomycin or linezolid.
- Sjögren syndrome recurrent parotitis: Pilocarpine and cevimeline can stimulate saliva production and inhibit ascending infection and provide symptomatic relief. Alternatively, botulism toxin injection may be a consideration in these patients because it limits production of saliva and sialectasis (3)[B].

ISSUES FOR REFERRAL
- For sialolithiasis, ductal stenosis, chronic obstruction due to Sjögren syndrome, or >1 recurrence per year, consult otolaryngologist for possible sialendoscopy, duct ligation, ductoplasty, or parotidectomy (4)[B].
- Refer to otolaryngology if parotid mass is seen, malignancy is suspected, or no improvement with antibiotics.

SURGERY/OTHER PROCEDURES
- Consider needle aspiration for bacterial parotitis with abscess, or clinical deterioration with increasing pain, erythema, and swelling not responding to medication.
- Consider superficial parotidectomy for severe recurrent parotitis in patients with underlying predisposing etiology.
- JRP: sialography; sialendoscopy with steroid irrigation is effective and safe for the treatment; performing US is recommended first to differentiate JRP from ductal stones (4)[A].
- Sclerotherapy with methyl violet or tetracycline is effective in the treatment of cysts in HIV parotitis and is also considered definitive treatment for chronic parotitis (5)[C].

ADMISSION, INPATIENT, AND NURSING CONSIDERATIONS
Admit those with comorbidities, systemic involvement, inability to tolerate PO, neonates, or those for whom close outpatient follow-up is not feasible.

 ONGOING CARE

FOLLOW-UP RECOMMENDATIONS
Antibiotic therapy for bacterial parotitis combined with adequate hydration should result in improvement within 48 hours; if not, patient should be reevaluated.

DIET
Ensure adequate fluid intake and promote salivary flow with hard or sour candy.

PROGNOSIS
- Viral infection in immunocompetent individuals often resolves with excellent prognosis.
- Parotid cysts in patients with HIV are usually benign lymphoepithelial lesions with infrequent malignant transformation.
- There is an increased incidence of malignant lymphoma or lymphoepithelial carcinoma in patients with Sjögren syndrome.

COMPLICATIONS
- Complications of mumps may include orchitis, oophoritis, mastitis, aseptic meningitis, encephalitis, pancreatitis, myocarditis, sensorineural hearing loss, and nephritis.
- Untreated bacterial parotitis can lead to abscess formation and facial paralysis.
- Neoplasm can result from chronic autoimmune parotitis.
- Facial nerve paralysis can result from chronic inflammatory parotitis.

REFERENCES
1. Nation J, Panuganti B, Manteghi A, et al. Pediatric sialendoscopy for recurrent salivary gland swelling: workup, findings, and outcomes. *Ann Otol Rhinol Laryngol.* 2019;128(4):338–344.
2. Cardemil CV, Dahl RM, James L, et al. Effectiveness of a third dose of MMR vaccine for mumps outbreak control. *N Engl J Med.* 2017;377(10):947–956.
3. O'Neil LM, Palme CE, Riffat F, et al. Botulinum toxin for the management of Sjögren syndrome-associated recurrent parotitis. *J Oral Maxillofac Surg.* 2016;74(12):2428–2430.
4. Wood J, Toll EC, Hall F, et al. Juvenile recurrent parotitis: review and proposed management algorithm. *Int J Pediatr Otorhinolaryngol.* 2021;142:110617.
5. Berg EE, Moore CE. Office-based sclerotherapy for benign parotid lymphoepithelial cysts in the HIV-positive patient. *Laryngoscope.* 2009;119(5):868–870.

ADDITIONAL READING
- Armstrong MA, Turturro MA. Salivary gland emergencies. *Emerg Med Clin North Am.* 2013;31(2):481–499.
- Brook I. The bacteriology of salivary gland infections. *Oral Maxillofac Surg Clin North Am.* 2009;21(3):269–274.
- Hamborsky J, Kroger A, Wolfe S. *Epidemiology and Prevention of Vaccine-Preventable Diseases.* 13th ed. Washington, DC: Public Health Foundation; 2015.
- Hernandez S, Busso C, Walvekar RR. Parotitis and sialendoscopy of the parotid gland. *Otolaryngol Clin North Am.* 2016;49(2):381–393.

CODES

ICD10
- K11.20 Sialoadenitis, unspecified
- K11.21 Acute sialoadenitis
- K11.23 Chronic sialoadenitis

CLINICAL PEARLS
- History and physical exam are sufficient for diagnosis (parotid swelling, tenderness, with or without purulent drainage from the Stensen duct).
- *S. aureus*, strep, and anaerobes are the most common organisms isolated in acute bacterial parotitis.
- In recurrent or chronic cases, consider other underlying etiologies, such as HIV.
- Usually self-limited with supportive care (local heat and gentle massage of gland, adequate hydration, analgesia, and antipyretics)
- Encouraging good oral hygiene and hydration in chronically ill, debilitated, and hospitalized patients can reduce risk of occurrence.

PARVOVIRUS B19 INFECTION

Christina Conrad, DO

 BASICS

DESCRIPTION

- Human parvovirus B19 is the cause of erythema infectiosum (fifth disease, morbus quintus).
- Individuals with increased RBC turnover (sickle-cell anemia, spherocytosis, thalassemia) are more susceptible to transient aplastic crisis (TAC). In immunocompromised individuals, pure red cell aplasia may lead to transfusion-dependent anemia. In immunocompetent individuals, arthritis and arthralgias are common complications of parvovirus B19 infection.
- Systems affected: hematologic/lymphatic/ immunologic, musculoskeletal, skin/exocrine, central nervous system, cardiac, renal, hepatobiliary

Pregnancy Considerations
Documented acute infection during pregnancy should prompt referral to maternal–fetal medicine specialist. There is 30% chance of fetal transmission with acute maternal infection- this may be higher during epidemic outbreaks. Fetal death is thought to occur in 5–10% of cases of fetal infection, with highest risk prior to 20 weeks of gestation (1).

EPIDEMIOLOGY

- Common in childhood; may be asymptomatic
- Erythema infectiosum has an extremely low mortality rate.
- Peak age for erythema infectiosum is 4 to 12 years.
- Males and females are equally affected.
- Women more likely to develop postinfectious arthritis
- No known racial predilection
- In temperate climates, infections often occur from late winter to early summer.
- Local outbreaks may occur every 2 to 5 years.
- Parvovirus B19 DNA has been isolated from human remains over 6900 years old
- The incidence of erythema infectiosum decreased with social isolation and physical distancing associated with the COVID pandemic (2).

Prevalence
Based on serologic studies, infection with parvovirus B19 is extremely common. By age 5, 2–15% of individuals in the United States and Western Europe are IgG positive. This steadily increases to 70–85% seropositivity by >40 years of age.

ETIOLOGY AND PATHOPHYSIOLOGY

- First described in 1974, parvovirus B19 is a small (20 to 25 nm) nonenveloped, single-stranded DNA virus in the *Erythrovirus* genus of the *Parvoviridae* family
  - Only known parvovirus to infect humans
- Natural host of B19 is human erythroid progenitor.
- Respiratory, transfusion-related, and vertical transmission are sources of human infection.
- Incubation period is usually 4 to 14 days but may rarely extend to 21 days.
- Prodromal symptoms include coryza, fever, headache, and nausea. However, infection may be asymptomatic.
- Rash and joint symptoms usually occur 2 to 3 weeks after initial infection. These are thought to be due to immune complex formation and are associated with viral clearance (and decreased risk of transmission).

- Patients infected with parvovirus B19 are most contagious 5 to 10 days after exposure, well before the rash typically manifests.
- Cytotoxic infection of erythroid progenitor cells decreases RBC production.

Genetics
Erythrocyte P antigen–negative individuals (approximately 1 in 200,000 people) are resistant to infection.

RISK FACTORS

- School-related epidemic and nonimmune household contacts have a secondary attack rate of 20–50%.
- Highest secondary attack rates are for daycare providers and school personnel in contact with affected children.
- Conditions with increased RBC turnover (spherocytosis, sickle-cell anemia, thalassemia) increase the risk of transient aplastic crisis.
- Immunodeficiency (congenital, due to HIV or malignancy) increases risk of pure red cell aplasia and chronic anemia.
- As many as 40% of pregnant women are not immune; 1.5% seroconversion rate per year

GENERAL PREVENTION

- Respiratory spread; hand washing, cough/sneeze hygiene, and barrier precautions
- Droplet precautions are recommended around patients with transient aplastic crisis and in immunocompromised patients.
- Difficult to eliminate exposure because the period of maximal contagion occurs prior to the onset of the typical rash
- No significant risk of infection based on occupational exposure if proper isolation precautions are followed. Exclusion from the workplace is neither necessary nor recommended.
- No preventive vaccine is currently available.

COMMONLY ASSOCIATED CONDITIONS

- Nondegenerative arthritis
  - In children, joint symptoms are uncommon, and typically involve the knees and ankles (may be symmetric or asymmetric joint involvement).
  - In adults, joint symptoms are much more common, usually symmetric, usually involve the hands, with less frequent involvement of larger joints. Women are affected with joint symptoms more often than men.
  - Joint symptoms generally resolve within 3 weeks but may persist for months or years. Longer duration symptoms are more common in women. Routine radiography is not necessary.
- Transient aplastic crisis
  - Involves patients with increased RBC turnover (sickle-cell disease, spherocytosis, thalassemia) or decreased RBC production (iron deficiency anemia)
  - Presents with fatigue, weakness, lethargy, and pallor (symptoms of anemia); may have dyspnea/ shortness of breath
  - Aplastic event may be life-threatening but is typically self-limited. Reticulocytes typically reappear in 7 to 10 days with full recovery in 2 to 3 weeks.
  - In children with sickle cell hemoglobinopathies and hereditary spherocytosis, fever is the most common symptom (73%); rash uncommon in these patients

- Chronic anemia
  - Seen in immunocompromised individuals (HIV, cancer, transplant) with poor antibody response
  - Usually no clinical manifestations (fever, rash, or joint symptoms)
  - Patients may be transfusion-dependent.
- Fetal/neonatal infection (1)
  - Risk of transplacental spread of virus is ~30% in infected mothers.
  - Up to 50% of infected pregnant women may be asymptomatic; vertical transmission can still occur.
  - Check IgM and IgG levels in pregnant women with symptoms consistent with parvovirus B19 infection.
  - Test pregnant women with known exposure to individuals with acute parvovirus B19.
    - If IgG positive and IgM negative, consider immune, and no further intervention is needed.
    - If IgM and IgG negative, repeat serologic testing in several weeks to look for seroconversion.
    - If IgM positive, test further to determine if acute infection is present (false-positive result).
  - Overall fetal death may occur in 5–10% of fetal infections, can occur with or without fetal hydrops.
  - Parvovirus B19 infection may account for 8–20% of cases of nonimmune fetal hydrops.
  - Fetal bone marrow is primarily impacted. RBC survival is shortened resulting in anemia and (potentially) high-output cardiac failure. Other complications can result from fetal hypoalbuminemia, myocarditis, hepatitis, and placentitis.
  - Risk of fetal loss is highest in 1st trimester (19%) and decreases as pregnancy progresses (15% at 13 to 20 weeks and 6% after 20 weeks).
  - Intrauterine fetal red blood cell transfusion can decrease fetal loss rate if fetal hydrops is present.
  - Infants who have undergone intrauterine transfusions are at risk for risk for delays in psychomotor development.
- Parvovirus has also been associated with a gloves and socks syndrome (3).
  - Typically in younger adults, there is symmetric painful erythema and edema of feet and hands.
  - Gradually progresses to petechiae/purpura/ vesicles/bullae and then skin sloughing
  - May have no other symptoms but can have fevers or arthralgias
  - Generally resolves in 1 to 3 weeks without scarring

 DIAGNOSIS

HISTORY

- May have a prodrome of fever, coryza, pharyngitis, headache, rhinorrhea, nausea
- Rash and arthralgias develop after these symptoms
- Arthralgias may last for weeks or longer.

PHYSICAL EXAM

- Typical "slapped cheek" appearance that spares the nasolabial folds
- A secondary lacy, reticular rash on the trunk, buttocks, and limbs often follows 1 to 4 days later, may last 1 to 6 weeks. This secondary rash may be pruritic and recurrent, exacerbated by bathing, exercise, sun exposure, heat, or emotional stress.
- B19 may manifest as painful pruritic papules and purpura on the hands and feet (glove and sock distribution).

DIFFERENTIAL DIAGNOSIS
- Rubella
- Measles
- Enteroviral disease
- Systemic lupus erythematosus
- Drug reaction
- Rheumatoid arthritis

DIAGNOSTIC TESTS & INTERPRETATION
Initial Tests (lab, imaging)
- No need for routine lab studies in typical cases. Diagnosis is clinical, and the illness is mild and self-limiting.
- IgG and IgM serology in immunocompetent patients
- B19-specific DNA polymerase chain reaction (PCR) testing for fetal infection (via cord blood or amniotic fluid) as well as for patients with chronic infection or those who are immunocompromised
- For patients with transient aplastic crisis, anemia and reticulocytopenia are present. IgM antibodies are noted by day 3, and IgG antibodies are detectable at time of clinical recovery. PCR shows high levels of viremia.
- Pregnant women exposed to B19 require serologic testing to assess fetal risk.

Follow-Up Tests & Special Considerations
Fetal/neonatal infection (4)[C]
- To exclude congenital B19 in infants with negative B19 IgM, follow IgG serology over the 1st year of life.
- Maternal serum α-fetoprotein may be increased with hydrops fetalis.
- Serial fetal ultrasound to assess for hydrops in cases of documented acute maternal infection in the 1st trimester, looking for ascites, pericardial effusion, oligohydramnios, cardiomegaly, and placental thickening.
- Weekly peak systolic velocity measurements of the middle cerebral artery by Doppler US is recommended to evaluate for heart failure, fetal anemia, and the potential need for intrauterine transfusion (>1.5 MoM).
- Cerebral MRI to assess for CNS damage in infected neonates with prolonged hydrops fetalis or hematocrit <15%.

TREATMENT

GENERAL MEASURES
- No therapy is usually needed (5)[C].
- Cessation of immunosuppressive therapy allows some patients to clear chronic infections.
- B19-associated anemia in HIV-positive patients may resolve with antiretroviral therapy and immune reconstitution.

MEDICATION
First Line
- Anti-inflammatory agents for arthritic symptoms
- Antipyretics for fever

Second Line
- May require RBC transfusions for transient aplastic crisis
- Intravenous immunoglobulin (IVIG) for B19-related refractory anemia or PRAC, especially in immunodeficient states (6)
- Intrauterine RBC transfusions reduce mortality in cases of fetal hydrops.

ISSUES FOR REFERRAL
- Acute infection during pregnancy should prompt referral to a maternal–fetal medicine specialist.
- Patients with chronic or abnormal B19 infections may benefit from consultation with immunology or infectious disease specialists.

ADMISSION, INPATIENT, AND NURSING CONSIDERATIONS
- Outpatient management is typical for erythema infectiosum.
- Inpatient management for aplastic crisis, which may require RBC transfusions
- In the inpatient setting, droplet isolation is appropriate for acute infections, transient aplastic crisis, and chronic infections in the immunocompromised.

 ONGOING CARE

FOLLOW-UP RECOMMENDATIONS
Patient Monitoring
Periodic blood counts for anemic patients until they have reticulocyte recovery

PATIENT EDUCATION
- Parvovirus B19 (fifth disease): http://www.cdc.gov/parvovirusB19/fifth-disease.html
- Parvovirus B19 and Fifth Disease: http://www.cdc.gov/parvovirusB19/pregnancy.html
- HealthyChildren.org: Parvovirus: https://www.healthychildren.org/English/health-issues/conditions/skin/Pages/fifth-disease-parvovirus-b19.aspx
- March of Dimes: Fifth Disease and Pregnancy: http://www.marchofdimes.org/complications/fifth-disease-and-pregnancy.aspx
- Children with typical rash are no longer infectious and may attend childcare or school.

PROGNOSIS
- Usually self-limited
- Joint symptoms usually subside within 3 weeks but may last months to years.
- ~20% of infections result in delayed virus elimination and viremia persisting for several months to years.
- Full recovery from aplastic crisis in 2 to 3 weeks

COMPLICATIONS
Conditions associated with B19 but where causality is unconfirmed
- Hepatitis—may predispose to acute fulminant hepatic failure
- Neurologic manifestations (meningoencephalitis, peripheral nervous system manifestations, myalgic encephalomyelitis/chronic fatigue syndrome)
- Myocarditis, pericarditis
- Membranoproliferative glomerulonephritis, focal segmental glomerulosclerosis, nephrotic syndrome
- Henoch-Schönlein purpura, idiopathic thrombocytopenic purpura, vasculitis, lymphocytic histiocytosis/hemophagocytic syndrome

REFERENCES
1. Ornoy A, Ergaz Z. Parvovirus B19 infection during pregnancy and risks to the fetus. *Birth Defects Res*. 2017;109(5):311–323.
2. Kataoka SY, Kataoka Y, Tochitani K, et al. Influence of anti-COVID-19 policies on 10 pediatric infectious diseases [published online ahead of print August 13, 2021]. *Pediatr Int*. doi:10.1111/ped.14958.
3. Servey J, Reamy B, Hodge J. Clinical presentations of parvovirus B19 infection. *Am Fam Physician*. 2007;75(3):373–376.
4. De Jong EP, Lindenburg IT, van Klink JM, et al. Intrauterine transfusion for parvovirus B19 infection: long-term neurodevelopmental outcome. *Am J Obstet Gynecol*. 2012;206(3):204.e1–204.e5.
5. Gallinella G. Parvovirus B19 achievements and challenges. *ISRN Virol*. 2013;2013:898730.
6. Landry ML. Parvovirus B19. *Microbiol Spectr*. 2016;4(3).

ADDITIONAL READING
- Barah F, Whiteside S, Batista S, et al. Neurologic aspects of human parvovirus B19 infection: a systematic review. *Rev Med Virol*. 2014;24(3):154–168.
- Dollat M, Chaigne B, Cormier G, et al. Extrahaematological manifestations related to human parvovirus B19 infection: retrospective study in 25 adults. *BMC Infect Dis*. 2018;18:302.

CODES

ICD10
- B34.3 Parvovirus infection, unspecified
- B08.3 Erythema infectiosum [fifth disease]

CLINICAL PEARLS
- Parvovirus B19 infection is usually a benign, self-limited illness with no long-term effects.
- Patients are no longer infectious by the time the rash of erythema infectiosum, a "slapped cheek" appears.
- Patients with increased RBC turnover (sickle cell disease, thalassemia, spherocytosis) are at risk for transient aplastic crisis.
- Immunocompromised patients are at risk for chronic anemia, which may be transfusion-dependent.
- Documentation of acute infection in pregnant women merits maternal–fetal consultation.

PATELLOFEMORAL PAIN SYNDROME (PFPS)

David L. Lee, MD • Rondy Michael Lazaro, MD

BASICS

DESCRIPTION
- Pain in or around the patella that is aggravated with increased patellar loading (e.g., prolonged sitting, squatting, kneeling, or ascending/descending stairs); not attributable to other causes
- Synonyms: anterior knee or retropatellar pain syndrome, chondromalacia patellae, runner's knee
- System(s) affected: musculoskeletal

EPIDEMIOLOGY
Prevalence
- Incidence between 2007 and 2011 in the United States was approximately 6%.
  - 55% of patients were female
  - More cases were identified in the Southern portion of the United States, compared to other regions of the country (1).
- In a military population, prevalence of 12% in males and 15% in females (2).

ETIOLOGY AND PATHOPHYSIOLOGY
Increased patellofemoral joint loading, which is often multifactorial (3):
- Patellar malalignment or maltracking (3)
- Abnormal anatomy (e.g., patella alta, trochlear dysplasia) (3)
- Quadriceps asymmetry, weakness and/or tightness (3)
- Hamstring tightness (3)
- Laxity of the patellofemoral joint or a tight lateral retinaculum (3)
- Increased hip joint internal rotation (3)
- Altered tibiofemoral joint mechanics (3)

RISK FACTORS
- Activities such as running, squatting, and climbing up and down stairs
- Sudden increase in activities
- Female gender
- Dynamic valgus
- Patellar instability
- Quadriceps weakness
- Foot abnormalities (e.g., pes pronatus, rearfoot eversion) (1)
- In adolescents: increased hip adduction strength, although this may represent increased activity level

- Previously considered risk factors, now of uncertain significance: age, height, weight, body mass index, body fat, Q angle, and hip weakness

GENERAL PREVENTION
Strengthening and stretching exercises, particularly hip abductors and terminal extension of the quadriceps

COMMONLY ASSOCIATED CONDITIONS
- Overuse
- Knee ligament injury/surgery
- Patellar tendinopathy
- Prolonged synovitis
- Iliotibial band friction syndrome

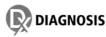

DIAGNOSIS

HISTORY
- An accurate history to differentiate between pain and instability (pain quality, location, swelling, giving way, locking, grinding, inciting events, overuse, changes in activity/training, and history of trauma)
- Most common symptom: diffuse anterior knee pain exacerbated during or after physical activity
- Pain with squatting, descending or ascending stairs, ambulating over uneven surfaces, or running (2)

PHYSICAL EXAM
- Evaluate knee range of motion (ROM) and for effusion.
- Palpation: pain on palpation of the patellar edges (medial or lateral)
- Compression/patellar grind test: With patient supine, place one hand superior to the patella and push the patella inferiorly. Ask the patient to contract the quadriceps; pain upon contraction is consistent with PFPS; grinding may indicate chondromalacia of the patellofemoral joint.
- Single-leg squat: 80% of patients with PFPS will demonstrate pain with this maneuver (2)[A]. Also helpful in assessing for dynamic valgus
- Patellar apprehension test: With the patient supine with the knee flexed to 30 degrees, medial pressure is applied to the patella (to displace it laterally); pain or apprehension with passive patellar displacement is a positive test. Not sensitive for PFPS (7–32%) but specific (86–92%)

- Passive patellar tilt test: With the patient supine with the knee extended, the patella is grasped, and the examiner lifts the lateral edge of the patella from the lateral femoral condyle, assessing for a tight lateral retinacular restraint. Not sensitive for PFPS (42%) but specific (92%)
- Gait and posture may indicate any imbalances (e.g., femoral internal rotation, hip height, scoliosis, quadriceps atrophy) that may contribute to PFPS.
- Footwear evaluation may detect pes pronatus or rearfoot eversion, which could contribute to PFPS (1).

DIFFERENTIAL DIAGNOSIS
- Prepatellar bursitis
- Patellar and quadriceps tendinopathy
- Chondromalacia patellae
- Patellofemoral arthrosis
- Patellar subluxation and dislocation
- Knee ligamentous and meniscal pathology
- Iliotibial band syndrome
- Plica syndrome
- Osteochondral defect
- Osteochondritis dissecans
- Sinding-Larsen-Johansson syndrome
- Osgood-Schlatter disease
- Knee infection
- Neuroma or nerve entrapment
- Benign or malignant tumors
- Referred pain from hip or spine

DIAGNOSTIC TESTS & INTERPRETATION
- None indicated. In general, imaging is not necessary for the diagnosis of PFPS. If imaging is indicated because of severity, atypical symptoms, or persistence of symptoms despite treatment, plain films with four views of the knee are recommended to view patellar tilt and to rule out other etiologies of anterior knee pain:
  - Lateral
  - Merchant or sunrise
  - Standing anteroposterior
  - Posteroanterior tunnel views
- CT can be used to grade patellar malalignment.
- Radiographic findings may not correlate with symptoms.

Follow-Up Tests & Special Considerations

Radiographic images may be normal until late stages, when the posterior patellar surface becomes irregular and cartilage erosion is radiographically detectable.

 ## TREATMENT

GENERAL MEASURES

- Conservative therapy of physical therapy, rehabilitation, and NSAIDs is the gold standard (4)[A].
- Initial goal of therapy is to increase strength, flexibility, and ROM to enable practice of correct motion.
- Supervised therapy should focus on hip abductors and external rotators, knee extensors, and core muscles (4)[A].
- Stretching of the muscles surrounding the hip and knee, particularly proprioceptive neuromuscular facilitation stretches (4)[A].

MEDICATION

- Acetaminophen or NSAIDs for pain management
- The evidence for oral glucosamine and chondroitin sulfate and hyaluronic acid injections is lacking and is not routinely recommended for treatment of patellofemoral pain.

ISSUES FOR REFERRAL

- Referral for surgery after all conservative measures fail. Surgery is rarely needed.
- Recalcitrant cases can be associated with psychosocial issues including depression and abuse. Referral to a mental health care professional may be necessary in these cases.

ADDITIONAL THERAPIES

- Combination therapy in addition to an exercise program with other modalities such as patellar taping or manual therapy may be beneficial (5)[A].
- Ankle and foot orthoses may offer some relief in the short term, but there is lack of strong evidence to support its use, particularly in the long term (4)[B],(5).

SURGERY/OTHER PROCEDURES

- Exercise therapy is first line.
- For patients with a tight lateral retinaculum and lateral patellar tilt: operative realignment of the patella
- For patients with a defect in the cartilage of the patellofemoral joint: cartilage resurfacing/restoration

 ## ONGOING CARE

PATIENT EDUCATION

- Educate patient on importance of participation and compliance in a specialized exercise program with a physical therapist.
- Provide a list of physical therapy locations for the patient.

PROGNOSIS

- PFPS may not be self-limiting and can become chronic (6).
- Patellofemoral pain for longer than 12 months duration is associated with long-term pain (6).
- Long-term PFPS is not associated with structural patellofemoral joint OA (6).

REFERENCES

1. Gaitonde D, Ericksen A, Robbins RC. Patellofemoral pain syndrome. *Am Fam Physician*. 2019;99(2): 88–94.
2. Crossley KM, Stefanik JJ, Selfe J, et al. 2016 Patellofemoral pain consensus statement from the 4th International Patellofemoral Pain Research Retreat, Manchester. Part 1: terminology, definitions, clinical examination, natural history, patellofemoral osteoarthritis and patient-reported outcome measures. *Br J Sports Med*. 2016;50(14):839–843.
3. Powers CM, Witvrouw E, Davis IS, et al. Evidence-based framework for a pathomechanical model of patellofemoral pain: 2017 patellofemoral pain consensus statement from the 4th International Patellofemoral Pain Research Retreat, Manchester, UK: part 3. *Br J Sports Med*. 2017;51(24): 1713–1723.
4. van der Heijden RA, Lankhorst NE, van Linschoten R, et al. Exercise for treating patellofemoral pain syndrome. *Cochrane Database Syst Rev*. 2015;(1):CD010387.
5. Collins NJ, Barton CJ, van Middelkoop M, et al. 2018 Consensus statement on exercise therapy and physical interventions (orthoses, taping and manual therapy) to treat patellofemoral pain: recommendations from the 5th International Patellofemoral Pain Research Retreat, Gold Coast, Australia, 2017. *Br J Sports Med*. 2018;52(18):1170–1178.
6. Lankhorst NE, van Middelkoop M, Crossley KM, et al. Factors that predict a poor outcome 5–8 years after the diagnosis of patellofemoral pain: a multicentre observational analysis. *Br J Sports Med*. 2016;50(14):881–886.

ADDITIONAL READING

- Bolgla LA, Boling MC, Mace KL, et al. National Athletic Trainers' Association position statement: management of individuals with patellofemoral pain. *J Athl Train*. 2018;53(9):820–836.
- Gulati A, McElrath C, Wadhwa V, et al. Current clinical, radiological and treatment perspectives of patellofemoral pain syndrome. *Br J Radiol*. 2018;91(1086):20170456.
- Saltychev M, Dutton RA, Laimi K, et al. Effectiveness of conservative treatment for patellofemoral pain syndrome: a systematic review and meta-analysis. *J Rehabil Med*. 2018;50(5):393–401.

 ## SEE ALSO

Algorithm: Knee Pain

CODES

ICD10

- M25.569 Pain in unspecified knee
- M25.561 Pain in right knee
- M25.562 Pain in left knee

CLINICAL PEARLS

- PFPS is the most common cause of anterior knee pain in active adults.
- The clinical diagnosis is made by an accurate history and physical exam.
- Well-designed exercises geared at core, hip, and lower extremity flexibility and strength are the most effective evidence-based treatments.

PEDICULOSIS (LICE)
Sangili Chandran, MD • Timothy D. Prajka, DO

BASICS

DESCRIPTION
- A contagious parasitic infection caused by ectoparasitic blood-feeding insects (lice)
- Two species of lice infest humans:
  - *Pediculus humanus* has two subspecies: the head louse (var. *capitis*) and the body louse (var. *corporis*). Both species are 1 to 3 mm long, flat, and wingless and have three pairs of legs that attach closely behind the head.
  - *Pthirus pubis* (pubic or crab louse): resembles a sea crab and has widespread claws on the 2nd and 3rd legs
- System(s) affected: skin/exocrine
- Synonym(s): lice; crabs

EPIDEMIOLOGY
Incidence
- In the United States: 6 to 12 million new cases per year
- Predominant age
  - Head lice: most common in children 3 to 12 years of age; more common in girls than boys
  - Pubic lice: most common in adults

Prevalence
Head lice: 1–3% in industrialized countries

ETIOLOGY AND PATHOPHYSIOLOGY
- Characteristics of lice:
  - Adult louse is dark grayish and moves quickly but does not jump or fly.
  - Eggs (nits) camouflage with the individuals' hair color and are cemented to the base of the hair shaft (within 4 mm of the scalp).
  - Nits (empty egg casings) appear white (opalescent) and remain cemented to the hair shaft.
  - Lice feed solely on human blood by piercing the skin, injecting saliva (anticoagulant properties to allow for blood meal), and then ingesting blood.
  - Itching is a delayed hypersensitivity reaction to the saliva of the feeding louse, which may take 4 to 6 weeks to develop after the first exposure. Subsequent exposures may take 1 to 2 days for symptoms to develop (1).
- Transmission: direct human-to-human contact
  - Head lice: direct head-to-head contact or contact with infested fomite (less likely)
  - Body lice: contact with contaminated clothing or bedding
  - Pubic lice: typically transmitted sexually (fomite transmission much less likely)

RISK FACTORS
- General: overcrowding and close personal contact
- Head lice
  - School-aged children, gender (girls; longer hair)
  - Sharing combs, hats (including helmets), clothing, and bed linens
  - African Americans rarely have head lice; theories include twisted hair shaft and increased use of pomades.
- Body lice: poor hygiene, homelessness
- Pubic lice: promiscuity (very high transmission rate)

GENERAL PREVENTION
- Environmental measures: Wash, dry-clean, or vacuum items that may have contacted infected individuals.
- Screen and treat affected household contacts.

- Head lice: Follow-up by school nurses may help to prevent recurrence and spread.
- Pubic lice: Limit the number of sexual partners (condoms do not prevent transmission nor does shaving pubic hair).
- Body lice: proper body hygiene

COMMONLY ASSOCIATED CONDITIONS
Up to 1/3 of patients with pubic lice have at least one concomitant STI.

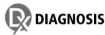

DIAGNOSIS

HISTORY
- Pruritus is common, often worse at night.
- Often associated with "outbreak" in school settings
- Investigate contacts of infected individuals.

PHYSICAL EXAM
- Diagnosis is confirmed by visualization of live lice.
- *P. capitis* (head lice)
  - Found most often on the back of the head and neck and behind the ears (warmer areas)
  - Eyelashes may be involved.
  - Eggs, found cemented on the base of a hair shaft, are difficult to remove.
  - Pruritus may be accompanied by local erythema and small papules.
  - May see excoriations around hairline
  - Scratching can cause inflammation and secondary bacterial infection.
  - Pyoderma and lymphadenopathy may occur in severe infestation.
- *P. humanus* (body lice)
  - Poor general hygiene
  - Adult lice and nits in the seams of clothing
  - Intense pruritus involving area covered by clothing (trunk, axillae, and groin)
  - Uninfected bites present as erythematous macules, papules, and wheals.
  - Pyoderma and excoriation may be seen.
  - Transmit *Bartonella quintana* (trench fever) and *Borrelia recurrentis* (louse-borne relapsing fever) and *Rickettsia prowazekii* (epidemic typhus).
- *P. pubis* (pubic lice)
  - Pubic hair is the most common site, but lice may spread to hair around anus, abdomen, axillae, chest, beard, eyebrows, and eyelashes.
  - Eggs are present at the base of hair shafts.
  - Anogenital pruritus
  - Blue macules may be seen in surrounding skin.
  - Delay in treatment may lead to development of groin infection and regional adenopathy.

DIFFERENTIAL DIAGNOSIS
- Scabies and other mite species that can cause cutaneous reactions in humans
- Dandruff and other hair debris sometimes look like head lice eggs and nits but are less adherent.

DIAGNOSTIC TESTS & INTERPRETATION
- Diagnosis is based on visualization of live louse.
- Head lice: Comb hair thoroughly with a fine-toothed louse comb (0.2 to 0.3 mm between teeth) to identify live lice (2)[C]. Wet the hair to limit static electricity, which repels lice. Simple visual inspection has same sensitivity as wet combing but is only ~25% as effective as dry combing with a metal comb (3).

- Body lice: Examine the seams of clothing to locate lice and eggs (4).
- Lice and eggs are more easily visualized with a microscope.
- In contrast to dandruff, eggs and nits cannot be removed easily from a hair shaft.

Follow-Up Tests & Special Considerations
- Empty nits remain on hair shafts for months after eradication of the live infestation. Wood lamp exam: Live nits fluoresce white and empty nits fluoresce gray.
- Pubic lice: Evaluate for concurrent STIs.

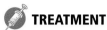

TREATMENT

GENERAL MEASURES
- Head lice: Clean items that have been in contact with the head of the infected individual within 48 hours.
- Wash all bedding, towels, clothes, headgear, combs, brushes, and hair accessories in hot water (>60°C).
- Vacuum furniture and carpets.
- Seal any personal articles that cannot be washed in hot water, dry-cleaned, or vacuumed in a plastic bag and store for at least 2 weeks.
- Examine and treat household members and close contacts concurrently.
- Insecticide sprays are not necessary.
- Pubic lice: Avoid sexual activity until all partners are successfully treated.
- Nit and egg removal
  - Remove eggs within 1 cm of the scalp to prevent reinfestation.
  - After treatment with shampoo or lotion, eggs and nits remain in the scalp or pubic hair until mechanically removed. Hair conditioner facilitates nit removal.
  - Eggs and nits best removed with a fine nit comb

MEDICATION
Permethrin (over the counter [OTC]), synergized pyrethrin (OTC), spinosad (Rx), benzyl alcohol (Rx), malathion (Rx), and topical ivermectin (Rx) are all effective for head lice (2)[A],(3)[C] Permethrin, synergized pyrethrin, and malathion are effective for pubic lice (3)[C]:
- Permethrin generally preferred because it may have residual activity for up to 3 weeks. However, use of newer shampoos and conditioners may reduce the residual effect (2)[C].
- Malathion and spinosad are considered second line for head lice but may not require a second application due to ovicidal activity (2)[B],(3)[C].
- Ivermectin 0.5% lotion and benzyl alcohol 5% lotion are also effective for head lice (2),(3)[C].

First Line
- Head and pubic lice:
  - Pyrethrum insecticides: Permethrin 1% cream rinse (Nix) or pyrethrins 0.33% with piperonyl butoxide 4% (synergized pyrethrin, Rid, Pronto) are first line unless there is proven resistance in the community.
    - Apply for 10 minutes and then wash.
    - Reapply synergized pyrethrin in 7 to 10 days (day 9 is optimal); also be necessary with permethrin, if live lice are observed
    - Side effects: application-site erythema, ocular erythema, and application-site irritation

- Body lice: best treated with synergized pyrethrin lotion applied once and left on for several hours
- Eyelash infestation: Apply petroleum jelly BID for 10 days.
- Precautions:
  – Pyrethrin: Avoid in patients with ragweed allergy (may cause respiratory symptoms).
  – Pediculicides should never be used to treat eyelash infections.

Second Line
- Head lice and pubic lice
  – Malathion 0.5% lotion (Ovide)
    ○ Apply for 8 to 12 hours and then wash off.
    ○ Excipients isopropyl alcohol (78%) and terpineol (12%) may contribute to its efficacy:
      ■ Flammable and has a bad odor
      ■ Despite ovicidal activity, a second application may be necessary after 7 to 10 days (day 9 is optimal) if live lice are observed.
  – Lindane 1% shampoo, no longer recommended
    ○ Apply for 4 minutes and then wash (do not repeat).
    ○ Side effects: neurotoxicity (seizures, muscle spasms), aplastic anemia
    ○ Contraindications: uncontrolled seizure disorder, premature infants
    ○ Precautions: Do not use on excoriated skin, in immunocompromised patients, conditions that increase seizure risk, or with medications that decrease seizure threshold.
    ○ Possible interactions: concomitant use with medications that lower the seizure threshold
- Head lice
  – Spinosad 0.9% lotion (Natroba)
    ○ Apply to dry hair and scalp for 10 minutes and then rinse with warm water. Repeat in 7 days if live lice are observed.
    ○ Side effects: application-site erythema, ocular erythema, and application-site irritation
  – Benzyl alcohol 5% lotion (Ulesfia)
    ○ Apply to dry hair using enough to saturate scalp and hair (amount depends on hair length), rinse after 10 minutes; repeat in 1 week.
    ○ Side effects: pruritus, erythema, pyoderma, ocular irritation, application-site irritation
  – Ivermectin 0.5% lotion (Sklice)
    ○ Apply to dry hair by using enough to saturate the scalp and hair (max 4 oz) and then rinse after 10 minutes.
    ○ Side effects: burning sensation at application site, dandruff, dry skin, eye irritation
- Mechanical removal of lice and nits by wetting hair and then systematically combing with a fine-toothed comb every 3 to 4 days for 2 weeks to remove all lice as they hatch

ALERT
Lindane: FDA black box warning of severe neurologic toxicity (use only when first-line agents have failed). The National Pediculosis Association strongly advises against using lindane at all.

Pediatric Considerations
- Avoid synergized pyrethrin and permethrin in infants <2 months of age. Avoid benzyl alcohol, topical ivermectin, and spinosad in children <6 months of age and avoid malathion in children <2 years of age.
- Lindane: not recommended

Pregnancy Considerations
Permethrin, synergized pyrethrin, malathion, spinosad, and benzyl alcohol are pregnancy Category B. Lindane and topical ivermectin are pregnancy Category C.

ADDITIONAL THERAPIES
- For "difficult to treat" cases of head lice, oral ivermectin 400 μg/kg (not approved by the FDA for lice), given twice at a 7-day interval, is superior to topical 0.5% malathion lotion (5),(6)[B].
- Ivermectin: 200 μg/kg PO repeated after 10 days or 300 μg/kg PO repeated after 7 days
  – Should not be used in children <15 kg; pregnancy Category C
  – Not approved by the FDA for lice
- Dual therapy with permethrin 1% and oral trimethoprim/sulfamethoxazole (TMP/SMX) only for cases of multiple treatment failures or suspected cases of lice-related resistance to therapy (TMP/SMX is not approved by the FDA for lice)
- Permethrin 5% cream (Rx) is not FDA-approved for lice and is unlikely to be effective for lice that are resistant to 1% cream rinse (2)[B].

COMPLEMENTARY & ALTERNATIVE MEDICINE
- Cetaphil lotion: dry-on, suffocation-based pediculicide (not approved by the FDA for lice)
  – Apply thoroughly to hair, comb, and then dry with hair dryer; shampoo after 8 hours.
  – Repeat once a week until cured, up to a maximum of three applications.
- Dimethicone 4% lotion: Apply to hair for 8 hours; repeat in 1 week (not approved by the FDA for lice).
- No home remedies (e.g., vinegar, isopropyl alcohol, olive oil, ylang ylang oil, mayonnaise, melted butter, and petroleum jelly) are proven as effective.
- Herbal shampoos and pomades have not been evaluated in clinical trials.
- Lavender oil and tea tree oil have been implicated in triggering prepubertal gynecomastia in boys and should not be used to treat lice.
- Electronic louse combs have not proven effective and are not approved by the FDA.

ONGOING CARE

FOLLOW-UP RECOMMENDATIONS
Children may return to school after completing topical treatment, even if nits remain in place. No-nit policies are unnecessary.

Patient Monitoring
Drug resistance should be suspected if no dead lice are observed 8 to 12 hours after treatment.

PATIENT EDUCATION
- National Pediculosis Association: http://www.headlice.org/
- CDC: https://www.cdc.gov/parasites/lice/
- http://www.guideline.gov/content.aspx?id=46429&search=lice

PROGNOSIS
- With appropriate treatment, >90% cure rate
- Recurrence is common, mainly from reinfection or treatment nonadherence. Resistance to synthetic pyrethroids is increasing.

COMPLICATIONS
- Poor sleep due to pruritus
- Persistent itching may be caused by too frequent use of the pediculicide.

- Missed school; social stigma
- Secondary bacterial infections
- Body lice can transmit typhus and trench fever.

REFERENCES
1. Gunning K, Pippitt K, Kiraly B, et al. Pediculosis and scabies: treatment update. Am Fam Physician. 2019;99(10):896–905.
2. Devore CD, Schutze GE; for Council on School Health and Committee on Infectious Diseases, American Academy of Pediatrics. Head lice. Pediatrics. 2015;135(5):e1355–e1365.
3. Coates SJ, Thomas C, Chosidow O, et al. Ectoparasites: pediculosis and tungiasis. J Am Acad Dermatol. 2020;82(3):551–569.
4. Gunning K, Pippitt K, Kiraly B, et al. Pediculosis and scabies: treatment update. Am Fam Physician. 2012;86(6):535–541.
5. Chosidow O, Giraudeau B, Cottrell J, et al. Oral ivermectin versus malathion lotion for difficult-to-treat head lice. N Engl J Med. 2010;362(10):896–905.
6. Feldmeier H. Treatment of pediculosis capitis: a critical appraisal of the current literature. Am J Clin Dermatol. 2014;15(5):401–412.

ADDITIONAL READING
- Cole SW, Lundquist LM. Spinosad for treatment of head lice infestation. Ann Pharmacother. 2011;45(7–8):954–959.
- Sanchezruiz WL, Nuzum DS, Kouzi SA. Oral ivermectin for the treatment of head lice infestation. Am J Health Syst Pharm. 2018;75(13):937–943.
- Webber E, McConnell S. Lice update: management and treatment in the home. Home Healthc Now. 2018;36(5):289–294.

SEE ALSO

Arthropod Bites and Stings; Scabies

CODES

ICD10
- B85.0 Pediculosis due to Pediculus humanus capitis
- B85.1 Pediculosis due to Pediculus humanus corporis
- B85.3 Phthiriasis

CLINICAL PEARLS
- School-based no-nit policies are not necessary because empty nits may remain on hair shafts for months after successful eradication.
- Improper product application is a common cause of treatment failure.
- Prevalence of resistant infestations is increasing; if no dead lice are observed 8 to 12 hours after treatment, suspect resistance and use an alternative agent.
- Routine retreatment on day 9 is recommended for nonovicidal products (permethrin and synergized pyrethrin).
- With all treatment options, reinspect hair after 7 to 9 days, and if live lice are detected, repeat treatment on day 9.

PELVIC INFLAMMATORY DISEASE

Erin Fredrickson, DO, MPH • Jeanne M. Cawse-Lucas, MD • Jenell Stewart, DO, MPH

 BASICS

DESCRIPTION

- Pelvic inflammatory disease (PID) is an infectious and inflammatory disorder of the upper female genital tract, including the uterus, fallopian tubes, ovaries, and adjacent pelvic structures. PID is most commonly an ascending polymicrobial infection acquired from sexually transmitted organisms (1).
- Salpingitis is the most clinically critical diagnostic component due to its consequences for future fertility.
- Mild to moderate PID is infection and inflammation in the absence of a tubo-ovarian abscess (TOA). Severe disease is defined as severe systemic symptoms OR the presence of a TOA (2).
- Diagnosis may be challenging due to nonstandardized definitions and guidelines, lack of a single definitive diagnostic test, and variation in signs and symptoms. Many patients with PID have subtle or nonspecific symptoms (3).

EPIDEMIOLOGY
Predominant age: 15 to 29 years

Incidence
PID is the most common gynecologic reason for admission in the United States accounting for 18 per 10,000 recorded hospital discharges (2).

Prevalence
The estimated prevalence of self-reported lifetime PID is 4.4% in sexually active cisgender women ages 18 to 44 years.

- Lifetime prevalence has decreased steadily since 1995 (4).
- Among those with no history of prior STI, lifetime prevalence higher in black versus white women (6% vs. 2.7%). Among patients with a prior STI, lifetime prevalence was similar across race (10% vs. 10.3%). This disparity suggests black patients might be more likely to have had an undiagnosed STI or not received care for a symptomatic infection, subsequently developing PID (4).

ETIOLOGY AND PATHOPHYSIOLOGY
Multiple organisms cause PID. Most cases begin with cervicitis and progress to polymicrobial infection. <50% of women with acute PID test positive test for a microbe.

- Mixed infections are common. *Chlamydia trachomatis, Neisseria gonorrhoeae*, genital tract mycoplasmas (particularly *Mycoplasma genitalium*), aerobic and anaerobic (*Bacteroides fragilis*), and vaginal microbes (e.g., *Prevotella*, peptostreptococci, *Gardnerella vaginalis, Escherichia coli, Haemophilus influenzae*) are common flora (1),(5),(6).
- Many nongonococcal, nonchlamydial microorganisms recovered from the upper genital tract in acute PID are associated with bacterial vaginosis.
- Possible mechanisms for ascent from the lower genital tract include (i) travel from cervix to endometrium to salpinx to peritoneal cavity; (ii) lymphatic spread via infection of the parametrium (from an IUD); and (iii) hematogenous route, although this is rare.
- Of cases, 75% occur within 7 days of menses, when cervical mucus favors ascent of organisms.

RISK FACTORS
- Sexually active and age <25 years
- First sexual activity at younger age (<15 years)
- New/multiple sexual partners

- Inconsistent condom use
- Gynecologic procedures that break the cervical barrier such as endometrial biopsy, curettage, hysterosalpingography, hysteroscopy, in vitro fertilization, and insertion of IUD in the last 6 weeks
- Other factors associated with PID:
  - Certain contraceptive methods, such as oral contraceptive pills and spermicidal creams, disrupt vaginal pH/microbiome and increase risk for STIs
  - Previous history of PID; 20–25% will have a recurrence.
  - Cervical ectopy
  - History of *C. trachomatis*; 10–40% will develop PID.
  - History of gonococcal cervicitis; 10–20% will develop PID.

GENERAL PREVENTION
- Educational programs about safe sex practices such as barrier contraceptives, especially condoms
- The U.S. Preventive Services Task Force recommends annual screening for chlamydia in all sexually active women <25 years and in those ≥25 years at increased risk (new sex partner/multiple sex partners). Moderate-quality evidence suggests that chlamydia screening reduces cases of PID (3)[A].
- Routine STI screening in pregnancy
- Early medical care with occurrence of genital lesions or abnormal discharge

COMMONLY ASSOCIATED CONDITIONS
- In a patient with an IUD and a pelvic abscess, suspect *Actinomyces* infection requiring penicillin treatment.
- Rupture of an adnexal abscess is rare but life-threatening. Early surgical exploration is mandatory (5).
- Chlamydial or gonococcal perihepatitis, called Fitz-Hugh-Curtis (FHC) syndrome, may occur with PID. FHC syndrome is characterized by severe pleuritic right upper quadrant pain and complicates 10% of PID cases.
- Plasma cell endometritis in women with PID: seen in majority of women with PID; density of plasma cell infiltration correlates to severity of symptoms (5).

℞ DIAGNOSIS

- The diagnosis of PID is primarily clinical.
- The positive predictive value of clinical diagnosis is 65–90% compared with laparoscopy (2).
- The CDC recommends empiric treatment for PID in females at risk with pelvic/lower abdominal pain of unknown etiology and one or more of the following:
  - Cervical motion tenderness
  - Uterine tenderness
  - Adnexal tenderness
- Additional criteria enhance specificity: fever >101°F, new/abnormal cervical mucopurulent discharge or cervical friability, presence of abundant WBCs on wet prep, elevated C-reactive protein (CRP), elevated ESR, and laboratory documentation of genitourinary infection with *N. gonorrhoeae* or *C. trachomatis* (1),(7)
- Most specific for diagnosing PID: Endometrial biopsy reveals endometritis, transvaginal ultrasound showing thickened, fluid-filled salpinges, or laparoscopic abnormalities consistent with PID (1),(3).

HISTORY
- Lower abdominal/pelvic pain: dull, aching or crampy, bilateral, constant; exacerbated by motion, exercise, or coitus
- New/abnormal vaginal discharge (~75% of cases)
- Fever, chills, cramping, dyspareunia
- Low back pain
- Urinary discomfort
- Unanticipated vaginal bleeding, often postcoital, is reported in about 40% of cases.
- Recent hysterosalpingogram (HSG) or other procedure breaking uterine barrier
- IUD insertion within the past 21 days (1)

PHYSICAL EXAM
- Fever
- Lower abdominal pain
- Cervical motion tenderness
- Evidence of cervicitis with/without vaginal discharge (1)

DIFFERENTIAL DIAGNOSIS
- Appendicitis
- Constipation
- Gastroenteritis
- Ectopic pregnancy
- Ovarian tumor/torsion
- Hemorrhagic/ruptured ovarian cyst
- Endometriosis/dysmenorrhea
- Functional pelvic pain
- Inflammatory bowel disease
- Diverticulitis
- UTI/pyelonephritis
- Nephrolithiasis (1)

DIAGNOSTIC TESTS & INTERPRETATION
Initial Tests (lab, imaging)
- Pregnancy test to rule out ectopic pregnancy and complications of an intrauterine pregnancy
- Chlamydia and gonorrhea testing (urine or cervical swab nucleic acid amplification test [NAAT] and/or ligase chain reaction); a negative result does not exclude PID.
- Urinalysis
- Saline microscopy of vaginal fluid (for WBC)
- HIV test and syphilis screening test
- Transvaginal ultrasound not necessary for diagnosis, but may show thickened, fluid-filled tubes (hydrosalpinges) ± free fluid, or TOA.

Pediatric Considerations
Consider sexual abuse in children presenting with symptoms of PID.

Follow-Up Tests & Special Considerations
Follow-up ultrasound as outpatient for resolution of adnexal abscess

Diagnostic Procedures/Other
- Laparoscopy only in the following situations:
  - Ill patient with competing diagnosis (e.g., appendicitis)
  - Ill patient who has failed outpatient treatment
  - Any patient not improving after 72 hours of inpatient treatment
- Endometrial biopsy (rarely indicated): reveals endometritis/plasma cells (5)

TREATMENT

- Patient education: Avoid intercourse until patient and partner(s) have been treated due to risk of reinfection. Counsel patients and partners on possible long-term implications.
- Outpatient treatment recommended, if clinically appropriate
- Criteria for hospitalization and parenteral treatment are described below.

GENERAL MEASURES
- IUD removal is NOT required for mild PID.
- Treatment should cover principal pathogens (CT, NG, and polymicrobial infections with anaerobic coverage), regardless of the test results.

MEDICATION
First Line
Outpatient treatment regimen: long-acting cephalosporin, macrolide or tetracycline, and metronidazole
- Ceftriaxone 500 mg IM single dose *plus* doxycycline 100 mg PO BID for 14 days ± metronidazole 500 mg twice daily for 14 days. Patients weighing >300 lb need 1 g ceftriaxone.
- Due to fluoroquinolone-resistant gonococci, CDC no longer recommends fluoroquinolones for the treatment of gonococcal infections including PID.

Second Line
- Because of emerging resistance in gonococci, collecting a culture swab for resistance testing and repeat CT/NG testing for confirmation of treatment success 2 weeks after completion of treatment is advisable (5).
- Outpatient treatment regimen
  - Cefoxitin 2 g IM single dose and probenecid 1 g PO, or cefotaxime (1 g IM) or ceftizoxime (1 g IM) administered concurrently in single dose *plus* doxycycline 100 mg PO BID for 14 days AND metronidazole 500 mg PO BID for 14 days
- In persons with documented severe allergic reactions to penicillin:
  - Skin testing is important to confirm or refute penicillin allergy.
  - Third-generation cephalosporins have low cross-reactivity with penicillin.
  - Clindamycin 900 mg IV q8h PLUS gentamicin loading dose IV or IM (2 mg/kg body weight), followed by a maintenance dose (1.5 mg/kg body weight) q8h; single daily dosing (3 to 5 mg/kg body weight) can be substituted.
- Special consideration
  - Refer sex partners for treatment if they had sexual contact with patient during preceding 60 days. Expedited partner therapy should be administered where available (5).
  - HIV-infected patients with acute PID should be treated similar to non–HIV-infected patients (6), although they are at higher risk for TOA.

SURGERY/OTHER PROCEDURES
Reserved for failures of medical treatment and for suspected ruptured adnexal abscess with resulting acute surgical abdomen

ADMISSION, INPATIENT, AND NURSING CONSIDERATIONS
- Criteria for hospitalization if any of following (5)[C]:
  - Surgical emergencies (e.g., appendicitis) cannot be excluded.
  - Pregnancy
  - Failure to respond clinically within 72 hours of oral antibiotics

- For inpatient treatment of PID, the CDC recommends following treatment regimens (7):
  - Parenteral regimen A
    - Cefotetan 2 g IV q12h or cefoxitin 2 g IV q6h + doxycycline 100 mg PO or IV q12h
    - Parenteral therapy for 24 hours after clinical improvement. Doxycycline should be preferred orally when possible as oral and IV provides similar bioavailability. Continue doxycycline for a total of 14 days (3).
  - Parenteral regimen B
    - Clindamycin 900 mg IV q8h plus gentamicin loading dose IV or IM (2 mg/kg of body weight) followed by a maintenance dose (1.5 mg/kg) q8h or single daily dosing at 3 to 5 mg/kg can be substituted (3).
    - Parenteral therapy may be discontinued 24 hours after clinical improvement, and oral therapy with doxycycline as aforementioned or clindamycin 450 mg PO QID for a total of 14 days should be continued.
  - Parenteral regimen C
    - Ampicillin/sulbactam 3 g IV q6h plus doxycycline 100 mg PO or IV q12h
- PID is rare in pregnant patients, but requires hospitalization. Change doxycycline to azithromycin + 2nd-generation cephalosporin (7).

ONGOING CARE

FOLLOW-UP RECOMMENDATIONS
Patient Monitoring
- Follow up 72 hours after initiation of treatment, particularly for patients with moderate or severe clinical presentation (3).
- Observe for worsening symptoms (fever, abdominal pain, and cervical motion tenderness).
- Retest for gonorrhea and chlamydia in 3 to 6 months.
- Follow adnexal abscess size and position with serial ultrasounds.

PATIENT EDUCATION
- Abstinence from any type of sexual contact until treatment of patient/partner is complete.
- Consistent and correct condom use should be encouraged.
- Hepatitis B and human papilloma virus (HPV) vaccines should be given to patients who meet criteria.
- Advise comprehensive STI screening (7).
- Offer HIV preexposure prophylaxis (PrEP) to patients presenting with new STI or PID.
- IUD insertion presents a low risk of PID in the setting of prior/current STI diagnosis.

PROGNOSIS
- PID has a high morbidity; about 20% of affected patients become infertile, 40% develop chronic pelvic pain, and 1% have an ectopic pregnancy (1).
- Good prognosis if early effective therapy and further infection is avoided.
- Poor prognosis with delayed treatment
- Nongonococcal, nonchlamydial PID is associated with severe PID and worse prognosis for future fertility.

COMPLICATIONS
- TOA in 7–16% of patients before presentation; 1/3 of patients hospitalized with PID
- Recurrent infection occurs in 20–25% of patients.
- Risk of ectopic pregnancy is increased 7- to 10-fold among patients with a history of PID.
- Tubal infertility in 8%, 19.5%, and 40% of patients after 1, 2, and 3 episodes of PID, respectively.
- Chronic pelvic pain in 20% of cases is related to adhesions, chronic salpingitis, or recurrent infection (1),(4).
- Hydrosalpinx: After PID resolves, fallopian tube fills with sterile fluid and becomes blocked; associated with pain and infertility

REFERENCES
1. Brunham RC, Gottlieb SL, Paavonen J. Pelvic inflammatory disease. *N Engl J Med*. 2015;372(21):2039–2048.
2. Ross J. Pelvic inflammatory disease. *Am Fam Physician*. 2014;90(10):725–726.
3. Low N, Redmond S, Uusküla A, et al. Screening for genital chlamydia infection. *Cochrane Database Syst Rev*. 2016;9(9):CD010866.
4. Kreisel K, Torrone E, Bernstein K, et al. Prevalence of pelvic inflammatory disease in sexually experienced women of reproductive age—United States, 2013–2014. *MMWR Morb Mortal Wkly Rep*. 2017;66(3):80–83.
5. Judlin P. Current concepts in managing pelvic inflammatory disease. *Curr Opin Infect Dis*. 2010;23(1):83–87.
6. Ross J, Guaschino S, Cusini M, et al. 2017 European guideline for the management of pelvic inflammatory disease. *Int J STD AIDS*. 2018;29(2):108–114.
7. Workowski KA, Bolan GA; for Centers for Disease Control and Prevention. Sexually transmitted diseases treatment guidelines, 2015. *MMWR Recomm Rep*. 2015;64(RR-03):1–137.

 CODES

ICD10
- N70.0 Acute salpingitis and oophoritis
- N70 Salpingitis and oophoritis
- N71.0 Acute inflammatory disease of uterus

CLINICAL PEARLS
- PID often starts with gonorrhea or chlamydia infection, but it is can be polymicrobial.
- Treat based on clinical suspicion (pelvic pain, cervical motion, or adnexal or uterine tenderness) without waiting for confirmatory testing.
- PID is a common cause of infertility.
- Complications include hydrosalpinx, adhesions, pelvic pain, and 10-fold increased risk of ectopic pregnancy.
- Three major predictors of preserved post-PID fertility: (i) short duration of symptoms (<72 hours) before treatment, (ii) first episode of PID, and (iii) nongonococcal PID

PEPTIC ULCER DISEASE

Apaar Dadlani, MBBS • Thomas L. Abell, MD

 BASICS

Peptic ulcer disease is characterized by defects in the stomach and/or duodenal mucosa, leading to inflammation of the underlying tissue by gastric acid and pepsin.

DESCRIPTION
- Duodenal ulcer
  - Most common form of peptic ulcer
  - Usually located in the proximal duodenum
  - Multiple ulcers or ulcers distal to the second portion of duodenum and/or jejunum raise possibility of gastrinoma (Zollinger-Ellison syndrome).
- Gastric ulcer: less common than duodenal ulcer in absence of NSAID use; often located along lesser curvature of the antrum
- Esophageal ulcers: located in the distal esophagus; usually secondary to gastroesophageal reflux disease (GERD); also seen with gastrinoma
- Ectopic gastric mucosal ulceration: may develop with Meckel diverticulum

EPIDEMIOLOGY
Incidence
- Predominant sex: male = female
- Predominant age
  - 70% of ulcers occur between ages 25 and 64 years.
  - Duodenal/gastric ulcer incidence increases with age.
- Peptic ulcer: 500,000 new cases per year
- Recurrence: 4 million per year
- Global incidence rate: 0.1–0.19%

Prevalence
- <10% in the general population
- The lifetime prevalence is higher (10–20%) in *Helicobacter pylori*–positive patients, compared to the general population (5–10%).
- The incidence and prevalence of peptic ulcer disease have decreased in high-income countries including the United States (1).

ETIOLOGY AND PATHOPHYSIOLOGY
Genetics
Increased incidence of PUD in families is likely due to familial clustering of *H. pylori* infection and inherited genetic factors reflecting response to the organism.

RISK FACTORS
- *H. pylori* infection (95% of duodenal and 70% of gastric ulcers)
- Chronic use of NSAIDs, including aspirin and COX-2 inhibitors. People who take NSAIDs regularly have been found to have concomitant *H. pylori* infection.
- Tobacco use
- Stress (such as acute illness, ventilator support, extensive burns, head injury)
- Hypersecretion syndromes: gastrinoma (Zollinger-Ellison), systemic mastocytosis, carcinoid syndrome; alcohol use
- Medications: corticosteroids (high-dose and/or prolonged therapy), bisphosphonates, potassium chloride, clopidogrel, sirolimus chemotherapeutic agents
- Radiation therapy

GENERAL PREVENTION
- NSAID ulcers: Discontinue NSAIDs and use acetaminophen instead when appropriate, or add a proton pump inhibitor [PPI]) in patients with previous NSAID-related ulcer.
  - If NSAIDs are absolutely necessary, use lowest possible dose and use in combination with a PPI or misoprostol.
  - To reduce ulcer risk, consider testing for and eradicating *H. pylori*.
- Maintenance therapy with PPIs or H_2 blockers is indicated for patients with a history of ulcer complications, recurrences, refractory ulcers, or persistent *H. pylori* infection.
- Consider maintenance PPI treatment in patients with *H. pylori*–negative, non–NSAID-induced ulcer.
  - *H. pylori* infection: present in 95% of duodenal and 70% of gastric ulcers; annual risk of duodenal ulcer in those with *H. pylori* infection: ≤1%

COMMONLY ASSOCIATED CONDITIONS
- Gastrinoma (Zollinger-Ellison syndrome)
- Multiple endocrine neoplasia type 1
- Carcinoid syndrome
- Chronic illness: Crohn disease, chronic obstructive pulmonary disease (COPD), chronic renal failure, hepatic cirrhosis, cystic fibrosis
- Hematopoietic disorders (rare): systemic mastocytosis, myeloproliferative disease, hyperparathyroidism, polycythemia rubra vera

 DIAGNOSIS

HISTORY
- Signs and symptoms:
  - Duodenal ulcer
    - Midepigastric pain
    - Gnawing or burning, nonradiating, recurring pain that is often is episodic
    - Relieved by food or antacids
  - Gastric ulcer
    - Midepigastric pain
    - Gnawing or burning, nonradiating, recurring pain that is often is episodic
    - Aggravated by food, relieved by antacids
- Nonspecific dyspeptic symptoms: indigestion, nausea, vomiting, loss of appetite, heartburn, and epigastric fullness
- Red flag or alarm symptoms
  - Onset of symptoms after age 55 years
  - Progressive dysphagia
  - Blood in stool, melena, hematemesis, anemia
  - Persistent or recurrent vomiting
  - Severe abdominal pain
  - Weight loss, anorexia, or family history of gastric malignancy
- NSAID-induced ulcers are often silent; perforation or bleeding may be the initial presentation.

PHYSICAL EXAM
May be nonspecific: Check vital signs for hemodynamic stability, conjunctival pallor (anemia); epigastric tenderness (absent in at least 30% of older patients); guaiac-positive stool from occult blood loss

DIFFERENTIAL DIAGNOSIS
Functional dyspepsia, gastritis, GERD, biliary colic, gastroenteritis, pancreatitis, cholecystitis, Crohn disease, intestinal ischemia, cardiac ischemia, GI malignancy

DIAGNOSTIC TESTS & INTERPRETATION
Initial Tests (lab, imaging)
- Lab tests to consider:
  - CBC: Rule out anemia.
  - Fecal occult blood test
  - Liver function tests
  - Lipase
  - *H. Pylori* testing
  - If multiple/refractory ulcers: Consider fasting serum gastrin to rule out gastrinoma.
- Indications for *H. pylori* testing: new-onset PUD, prior history of PUD, persistent symptoms after empiric antisecretory therapy, gastric mucosa–associated lymphoid tissue (MALT) lymphoma, noninvestigated dyspepsia in patients <50 years of age without alarm symptoms
- *H. pylori* diagnostic tests:
  - False-negative results may occur if patient was recently treated with antibiotics, bismuth, or PPIs, or in patients with active bleeding.
  - Noninvasive tests:
    ○ Stop antibiotics and bismuth for at least 4 weeks and PPIs for 1 week prior to testing.
    ○ Stool antigen: identifies active infection; can be used for screening and posttreatment testing; high positive and negative predictive value (sensitivity, 87%; specificity, 70%); patients might not want to collect stool
    ○ Urea breath test: identifies active infection; can be used for screening and posttreatment testing; high positive and negative predictive value (sensitivity, 93%; specificity, 92%); variable availability and reimbursement
    ○ Serology: inexpensive; can be used only in untreated patients and cannot be used to document successful eradication (sensitivity, 88%; specificity, 69%)
    ○ Invasive tests:
      ■ Upper endoscopy (sensitivity, >95%; specificity, >95%) is most accurate for diagnosing PUD and active *H. pylori* infection. Endoscopy is costly, invasive, and recommended only for patients with "red flag" symptoms (1)[B].
      ■ Rapid urease test: conducted on gastric biopsies (sensitivity, 93–97%; specificity, 95%)
- Barium or Gastrografin contrast radiography (double-contrast hypotonic duodenography): indicated when endoscopy is unsuitable or not feasible

Diagnostic Procedures/Other
- Upper endoscopy (sensitivity, >95%; specificity, >95%) is most accurate for diagnosing PUD and active *H. pylori* infection. Endoscopy is costly, invasive, and recommended only for patients with "red flag" symptoms (1)[B].
- Rapid urease test: conducted on gastric biopsies (sensitivity, 93–97%; specificity, 95%)

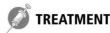 **TREATMENT**

MEDICATION
First Line
- Acid suppression
  - PPIs have higher efficacy than H_2 blockers. 95% of duodenal ulcers heal on PPI therapy within 4 weeks.
    ○ Omeprazole 20 mg/day PO; lansoprazole 30 mg/day PO; rabeprazole 20 mg/day PO; esomeprazole 40 mg/day PO; pantoprazole 40 mg/day PO; dexlansoprazole 30 mg/day PO
    ○ Length of treatment: 4 to 8 weeks

– H$_2$ blockers
  ○ Ranitidine or nizatidine 150 mg PO BID or 300 mg PO at bedtime; cimetidine 400 mg PO BID or 800 mg PO at bedtime; famotidine 20 mg PO BID or 40 mg PO at bedtime
  ○ Length of treatment: 4 to 8 weeks
- Precautions:
  – Decrease H$_2$ blocker dosage by 50% if CrCl <50 mL/min.
  – PPIs may decrease bone density. Obtain interval bone densitometry with long-term PPI use (2).
  – PPIs may cause hypomagnesemia.
  – PPIs may be associated with increased risk of *Clostridium difficile* infection (2).
  – Short-term PPI use associated with development of community-acquired pneumonia; long-term use does not appear to have an increased risk.
  – Despite earlier concerns, PPIs do not appear to decrease the efficacy of clopidogrel (2).
- NSAID-induced ulcers
  – Discontinue NSAID use.
  – Treat with PPIs for 4 to 8 weeks; may use as maintenance for patients with recurrent, complicated, or idiopathic ulcers; or in patients who require long-term aspirin or NSAID use.
- *H. pylori*–induced ulcers
  – *H. pylori* eradication regimens
    ○ Clarithromycin-based triple therapy for 14 days: standard dose PPI PO BID plus clarithromycin 500 mg PO BID plus amoxicillin 1 g PO BID
    ○ Bismuth-based quadruple therapy for 14 days: standard dose PPI PO BID plus clarithromycin 500 mg PO BID plus amoxicillin 1 g PO BID
    ○ Metronidazole-based therapy for patients with amoxicillin allergy: standard dose PPI PO BID plus metronidazole 500 mg PO BID plus clarithromycin 500 mg PO BID
    ○ Sequential therapy: standard dose PPI PO BID plus 1 g amoxicillin PO BID for 5 days followed by PPI PO BID plus clarithromycin 500 mg PO BID and tinidazole 500 mg PO BID for 5 days

Second Line

- For *H. pylori* eradication: Use second-line therapy if first-line fails:
  – Bismuth quadruple therapy for 14 days
    ○ Bismuth subsalicylate 525 mg PO QID plus
    ○ Metronidazole 250 mg PO QID plus
    ○ Tetracycline 500 mg PO QID plus
    ○ Standard dose PPI PO BID
  – Another alternative salvage therapy:
    ○ PPI orally BID
    ○ Amoxicillin 1,000 mg PO BID plus
    ○ Rifabutin 300 mg PO daily plus
- Alternative ulcer-healing drugs:
  – Sucralfate and antacids
- Significant possible interactions:
  – Cimetidine inhibits cytochrome P450 isozymes (avoid with theophylline, warfarin, phenytoin, and lidocaine).
  – Omeprazole may prolong elimination of diazepam, warfarin, and phenytoin.
  – Sucralfate reduces absorption of tetracycline, norfloxacin, ciprofloxacin, and theophylline; it leads to subtherapeutic levels.

Pregnancy Considerations

PPIs *not* associated with increased risk of major birth defects, spontaneous abortions, or preterm delivery

- Breastfeeding: Both ranitidine and esomeprazole are secreted in breast milk at considerably lower doses than used for treatment in infants with reflux disease. Use in breastfeeding women is generally safe.

ISSUES FOR REFERRAL

Refer for endoscopy if red flag signs are present:
- Onset of symptoms after age 55 years
- Progressive dysphagia
- Recurrent vomiting
- Heme positive stool, melena, hematemesis, anemia
- Progressive dysphagia or persistent/recurrent vomiting
- Severe abdominal pain
- Weight loss, anorexia, or family history of gastric malignancy

SURGERY/OTHER PROCEDURES

- Endoscopy is indicated for patients age >55 years with new onset of dyspeptic symptoms, those who do not respond to treatment, and patients of any age with alarm/red flag symptoms (3)[B].
- During endoscopy:
  – Biopsy stomach for *H. pylori* testing (CLO test)
  – Biopsy ulcer margin to exclude malignancy
  – Interventions to stop active bleeding or prevent rebleeding in those with certain stigmata include injection with epinephrine, heater probe treatment, or placement of endoscopic clips (2).
- Emergent surgery is the treatment for ulcer perforation.
- Surgery is rarely needed due to effective medical treatment of ulcers and *H. pylori* infection.
- Nonemergent indications for surgery: ulcers that are refractory to treatment; patients at high risk for complications (e.g., transplant recipients, patients dependent on steroids/NSAIDs); bleeding not responding to endoscopic therapy (4)
- Surgical options:
  – Duodenal ulcers: truncal vagotomy and drainage (pyloroplasty/gastrojejunostomy), selective vagotomy (preserving the hepatic and/or celiac branches of the vagus) and drainage, or highly selective vagotomy (1)
  – Gastric ulcers: partial gastrectomy, Billroth I or II
  – Perforated ulcers: laparoscopy/open patching (1)
- Emerging options: Vonoprazan is a novel acid blocker that is noninferior to PPIs.

ADMISSION, INPATIENT, AND NURSING CONSIDERATIONS

- Discontinue ulcerogenic agents (e.g., NSAIDs).
- Bleeding peptic ulcers
  – Stable: Give PPI to reduce transfusion requirements, need for surgery, and duration of hospitalization (5).
  – Unstable: fluid/packed RBC resuscitation followed by emergent esophagogastroduodenoscopy (EGD) or surgery; use IV PPI.
  – Insufficient evidence for high-dose PPI treatment over lower doses in peptic ulcer bleeding (2)[A]
- Oral PPI equivalent to IV after endoscopic treatment (5)
- Perforated peptic ulcers are a surgical emergency (1).

ONGOING CARE

FOLLOW-UP RECOMMENDATIONS
Patient Monitoring

- *H. pylori* eradication: expected in >90% (with double antibiotic regimen): Confirm eradication with urea breath test or fecal antigen test.
- Acute duodenal ulcer: Monitor clinically.
- Acute gastric ulcer: Confirm healing via endoscopy after 12 weeks; biopsies (if not done initially) to confirm benign mucosa

PROGNOSIS

After *H. pylori* eradication (3):
- Low ulcer relapse rate; if relapse, consider use of NSAIDs or tobacco.
- Reinfection rates <1% per year
- Low risk of rebleeding
- Decreased NSAID ulcer recurrence (3)

COMPLICATIONS

- Hemorrhage: up to 25% of patients (initial presentation in 10%)
- Perforation: <5% of patients
- Gastric outlet obstruction: up to 5% of duodenal or pyloric channel ulcers; male predilection found
- Risk of gastric adenocarcinoma is increased in *H. pylori*–infected patients.
- Refractory peptic ulcer disease (5–10% after eradication of *H. pylori* or completion of 12 weeks of PPI)

REFERENCES

1. Lanas A, Chan FKL. Peptic ulcer disease. *Lancet.* 2017;390(10094):613–624.
2. Neumann I, Letelier LM, Rada G, et al. Comparison of different regimens of proton pump inhibitors for acute peptic ulcer bleeding. *Cochrane Database Syst Rev.* 2013;(6):CD007999.
3. Gisbert JP, Calvet X, Cosme A, et al; for *H. pylori* Study Group of the Asociación Española de Gastroenterología (Spanish Gastroenterology Association). Long-term follow-up of 1,000 patients cured of *Helicobacter pylori* infection following an episode of peptic ulcer bleeding. *Am J Gastroenterol.* 2012;107(8):1197–1204.
4. Laine L, Jensen DM. Management of patients with ulcer bleeding. *Am J Gastroenterol.* 2012;107(3):345–361.
5. Yen HH, Yang CW, Su WW, et al. Oral versus intravenous proton pump inhibitors in preventing re-bleeding for patients with peptic ulcer bleeding after successful endoscopic therapy. *BMC Gastroenterol.* 2012;12:66.

ADDITIONAL READING

Echizen H. The first-in-class potassium-competitive acid blocker, vonoprazan fumarate: pharmacokinetic and pharmacodynamic considerations. *Clin Pharmacokinet.* 2016;55(4):409–418.

CODES

ICD10
- K27.9 Peptic ulc, site unsp, unsp as ac or chr, w/o hemor or perf
- K26.9 Duodenal ulcer, unspecified as acute or chronic, without hemorrhage or perforation
- K25.9 Gastric ulcer, unspecified as acute or chronic, without hemorrhage or perforation

CLINICAL PEARLS

- PPIs have higher efficacy than H$_2$ blockers for healing duodenal ulcers.
- In patients with PUD, eradicate *H. pylori* to assist healing and reduce the risk of recurrence.
- Upper endoscopy is indicated for patients with suspected peptic ulcers and red flag symptoms and for those who do not respond to treatment.

PERICARDITIS
Veronica J. Ruston, DO

BASICS

DESCRIPTION
Inflammation of the pericardium, with or without associated pericardial effusion. Myopericarditis or perimyocarditis refers to cases that have myocardial involvement in addition to involvement of the pericardium.

EPIDEMIOLOGY
Incidence
- Epidemiologic studies are lacking. Exact incidence is unknown but occurs in up to 5% of patients evaluated in the emergency room (ER) for chest pain without myocardial infarction (MI), including children; appears to be a slightly increased prevalence in men ages 16–65 years old.
- After first episode of acute pericarditis, about 30% of patients will experience recurrence within next 18 months.

ETIOLOGY AND PATHOPHYSIOLOGY
- Inflammation of the pericardial sac can be *acute*, *chronic* (disease process lasting >3 months), or recurrent (subsequent episode after 4–6 weeks without symptoms). Chronic or recurrent inflammation may result in constrictive pericarditis.
- Can produce serous/purulent fluid/dense fibrinous material (depending on etiology), which may or may not lead to hemodynamic compromise
- Idiopathic: 85–90% of cases; likely related to viral infection, which may trigger immune-related process
- Infectious
  - Viral: coxsackievirus, echovirus, adenovirus, Epstein-Barr virus, cytomegalovirus, hepatitis viruses, influenza virus, HIV, measles, mumps, varicella
  - Bacterial: Mycobacterium tuberculosis (common in endemic countries), other bacterial causes rare
  - Fungal (more common in immunocompromised populations): *Blastomyces dermatitidis, Candida* sp., *Histoplasma capsulatum*
  - Parasites: *Echinococcus*
- Noninfectious causes
  - Acute MI (2 to 4 days after MI), Dressler syndrome (weeks to months after MI)
  - Aortic dissection
  - Renal failure, uremia, dialysis-associated
  - Malignancy (e.g., breast cancer, lung cancer, Hodgkin disease, leukemia, lymphoma)
  - Radiation therapy
  - Trauma
  - After cardiac procedures (e.g., catheterization, pacemaker placement, ablation, pericardiotomy)
  - Autoimmune disorders: connective tissue disorders, systemic lupus erythematosus (SLE), rheumatoid arthritis, scleroderma, hypothyroidism, inflammatory bowel disease, Wegener granulomatosis, spondyloarthropathies, sarcoidosis
- Medication-induced: dantrolene, doxorubicin, hydralazine, isoniazid, mesalamine, methysergide, penicillin, phenytoin, procainamide, rifampin

Genetics
No known factors

RISK FACTORS
Thoracic surgery, chronic kidney disease, pneumonia, autoimmune diseases, lung or breast cancer especially if treated with radiation therapy

GENERAL PREVENTION
Good hygiene including hand washing and use of masks

COMMONLY ASSOCIATED CONDITIONS
Depends on etiology

DIAGNOSIS

- Diagnostic clinical criteria
  - Acute pericarditis (at least two of four criteria)
    - Typical (pleuritic) chest pain
    - Pericardial friction rub (<33% of cases)
    - ECG changes with widespread (non-regional) ST-segment elevations (up to 60% of cases)
    - New/increasing pericardial effusion seen on imaging
  - Myopericarditis
    - 1. Definite pericarditis *and*
    - 2. Symptoms (dyspnea, chest pain, or palpitations) *and* ECG changes not previously documented (ST/T wave abnormalities, supraventricular/ventricular tachycardia) *or* focal/diffuse depressed left ventricular (LV) function documented on imaging study
    - 3. Absence of evidence of other cause
    - 4. One of the following: elevated cardiac enzymes (creatine kinase [CK]-MB, troponin I or T) *or* new focal/diffuse depressed LV function *or* abnormal imaging consistent with myocarditis (MRI with gadolinium, gallium-67 scanning, antimyosin antibody scanning)
  - Case definitions of myopericarditis using above criteria:
    - *Suspected myopericarditis*: criteria 1, 2, and 3
    - *Probable myopericarditis*: criteria 1, 2, 3, and 4
    - *Confirmed myopericarditis*: histopathologic evidence of myocarditis by endomyocardial biopsy (EMB) or autopsy (Note: In the clinical setting, for self-limited cases with predominantly pericarditis, EMB is rarely indicated.)

HISTORY
- Prodrome of fever, malaise, myalgias, viral upper respiratory
- Acute, sharp, stabbing chest pain, pathognomonic if pain radiates to trapezius
- Duration typically hours to days
- Pleuritic pain
- Pain reduced by leaning forward, worsened by lying supine
- Shortness of breath

PHYSICAL EXAM
- Heart rate is usually regular but may be rapid
- Pericardial friction rub: coarse, high-pitched sound best heard during end expiration at left lower sternal border with patient leaning forward. Highly specific for diagnosis (but not sensitive); may be transient and mono-, bi-, or triphasic
- New S_3 may suggest myopericarditis
- Cardiac tamponade

DIAGNOSTIC TESTS & INTERPRETATION
Initial Tests (lab, imaging)
- It is not necessary to order tests for uncomplicated cases or when the diagnosis is clear, especially in countries with low prevalence of tuberculosis. Following labs may be helpful:
  - CBC: typically shows leukocytosis
  - Inflammatory markers: elevated erythrocyte sedimentation rate (ESR), C-reactive protein (CRP), and lactate dehydrogenase (LDH)
  - Cardiac biomarkers: typically elevated CK, troponins
    - Elevated troponins associated with younger age, male sex, pericardial effusion at presentation, and ST segment elevation on ECG
    - Adverse outcomes are not predicted by elevated troponin.

- ECG: Findings include widespread upward concave ST segment elevation (in all or most leads, a diffuse, nonregional process) and PR segment depression that may evolve through four stages. ECG may be normal/show nonspecific abnormalities:
  - Stage 1: diffuse ST segment elevation and PR segment depression
  - Stage 2: Normalization of the ST and PR segments and T waves begin to flatten and invert.
  - Stage 3: widespread T wave inversions
  - Stage 4: normalization of T waves; may have persistent inversions if chronic pericarditis
- ECG may demonstrate low voltage and electrical alternans with large effusions and tamponade.
- Transthoracic echocardiogram is recommended to evaluate for the presence of pericardial effusion, tamponade, or myocardial disease (presence of effusion helps to confirm diagnosis of pericarditis). Effusions are readily diagnosed on echo.
- Chest x-ray (CXR) is performed to rule out pulmonary/mediastinal pathology. Enlarged cardiac silhouette suggests large pericardial effusion (at least 300 mL).
- CT and MRI allow visualization of pericardium to assess for complications or if initial workup is inconclusive.
- Additional testing (if clinically appropriate based on history or atypical presentation or course) may include tuberculin skin test, sputum cultures, rheumatoid factor, antinuclear antibody, and HIV serology.
- Viral cultures and antibody titers rarely clinically useful

Diagnostic Procedures/Other
- Pericardiocentesis indicated for cardiac tamponade; for suspected purulent, tuberculous, or neoplastic pericarditis; and for effusions >20 mm on echocardiography (1)[C]
- Surgical drainage with pericardial biopsy recommended if recurrent tamponade, ineffective pericardiocentesis, or hemodynamic instability (1)[C]

Test Interpretation
- Microscopic examination may reveal hyperemia, leukocyte accumulation, or fibrin deposition.
- Purulent fluid with neutrophilic predominance if bacterial etiology
- Lymphocytic predominance in viral, tuberculous, and neoplastic pericarditis

TREATMENT

- Goal of treatment is to relieve pain and reduce complications (e.g., recurrence, tamponade, chronic constrictive pericarditis).
- Outpatient therapy is reported to be successful in 85% patients with low-risk features.

GENERAL MEASURES
Specific therapy directed toward underlying disorder for patients with identified cause other than viral/idiopathic disease. Restrictions of physical activity are an important part of treatment for recurrences.

MEDICATION
First Line
- NSAIDs are considered the mainstay of therapy for acute pericarditis:
  - Ibuprofen 600 mg TID for 1 to 2 weeks (2 to 4 weeks for recurrence) then taper (2)[C]
  - Aspirin 750–1000 mg TID for 1 to 2 weeks (2 to 4 weeks for recurrence) then taper; preferable for patients with recent MI because other NSAIDs impair scar formation in animal studies (2)[C],(3)[C]

– Indomethacin 50 mg TID for 1 to 2 weeks (2 to 4 weeks for recurrence) then taper; should avoid in elderly due to flow restriction to coronaries (4)[C]

– Ketorolac 15 to 30 mg IV/IM q6h while inpatient; maximum duration of 5 days (4)[C]

– GI protection should be provided (4)[C].

– Tapering should be done only if the patient is asymptomatic and CRP/ESR are normal. Repeat CRP/ESR every 1 to 2 weeks (4)[C].

– Treatment duration using NSAIDs for initial attacks is 1 to 2 weeks, but for recurrences, consider 2 to 4 weeks of therapy (4)[C].

– Monitoring: NSAIDs: CBC and CRP at baseline and weekly until CRP normalizes

– Contraindications: hypersensitivity to aspirin or NSAIDs, active peptic ulcer/GI bleeding

– Precautions: Use with caution in patients with asthma, 3rd-trimester pregnancy, coagulopathy, and renal/hepatic dysfunction.

• Colchicine: common practice to use in combination with NSAIDs to decrease incidence of recurrence and for faster symptomatic response; 0.6 mg BID for up to 3 months (up to 6 months for recurrence); taper is not required. This is the only agent proven to prevent recurrences in RCTs. Adjunctive therapy can reduce rate of recurrence by 50% (1)[A]. Monitoring: Consider CBC, CRP, transaminases, CK, and creatinine at baseline and after 1 month at a minimum.

• Pregnant: <20 weeks' gestation: Aspirin is first choice, but NSAIDs and prednisone are also allowed; >20 weeks' gestation: Prednisone is allowed with avoidance of NSAIDs, aspirin, and colchicine.

Second Line

• Corticosteroid treatment is indicated in connective tissue disease, tuberculous pericarditis, or severe recurrent symptoms unresponsive to NSAIDs or colchicine; should be avoided in uncomplicated acute pericarditis or if infectious etiology is suspected. *Corticosteroid use alone has been found to be an independent risk factor for recurrence* (3)[C].

• If steroids are used, consider low dose (0.20 to 0.50 mg/kg/day until resolution of symptoms and normalization of CRP, then consider slow tapering (if >50 mg: 10 mg/day every 1 to 2 weeks; if 25 to 50 mg: 5 to 10 mg/day every 1 to 2 weeks; if 15 to 25 mg: 2.5 mg/day every 2 to 4 weeks; if <15 mg/day: 1.0 to 2.5 mg/day every 2 to 6 weeks). At threshold of 10–15 mg/day, decrease taper to 1.0–2.5 mg every 2–6 weeks to prevent recurrence (2)[C].

• Remember adequate prophylaxis treatment for osteoporosis prevention (3)[C].

• If recurrence while tapering, try to not increase dose or restart corticosteroids (2)[C].

• Intrapericardial administration of steroids may be effective and limits systemic side effects.

• Emerging alternative options include azathioprine, IV human immunoglobulins, and anakinra (3)[C].

ISSUES FOR REFERRAL

• Hospitalization and evaluation for etiology recommended for any patient with major medical comorbidities, for suspected or threatened tamponade, for poor prognostic factors (see next column), or for a presentation that suggests an underlying systemic inflammatory disease (2)[C].

• Refractory cases include those on unacceptably high long-term steroid doses (>25 mg/day).

• Consider trial of aspirin and/or NSAIDs plus steroid and colchicine.

• Uremic or dialysis-related cases require more frequent or urgent dialysis without significant benefit from pharmacologics.

SURGERY/OTHER PROCEDURES

• Pericardiocentesis is indicated in cases of cardiac tamponade, high likelihood of tuberculous/purulent/neoplastic pericarditis, and moderate-to-large symptomatic effusions refractory to medical therapy.

• Pericardial biopsy may be considered for diagnosis in those with persistent worsening pericarditis without a definite diagnosis.

• Pericardioscopy for targeted diagnostic imaging may be performed at experienced tertiary referral centers in refractory and difficult cases.

• Pericardial window may be performed in cases of recurrent cardiac tamponade with large pericardial effusion despite medical therapy and severe symptoms.

• Pericardiectomy is standard of care for chronic constrictive pericarditis with persistent symptoms, such as NYHA class III or IV. Mortality is high at 6–12% so is reserved only after careful evaluation by experienced surgeons at hospitals with specific interest in pericardial diseases (2)[C].

ADMISSION, INPATIENT, AND NURSING CONSIDERATIONS

• Inpatient therapy recommended for pericarditis associated with clinical predictors of poor prognosis:

– Major predictors: fever >38°C, subacute onset, large pericardial effusion, cardiac tamponade, lack of response to NSAID/aspirin therapy after at least 1 week (2)[C]

– Minor predictors: immunosuppressed state, trauma, oral anticoagulation therapy, myopericarditis (5)[C]

• IV fluids considered for hypotension or in the setting of pericardial tamponade

• Discharge criteria

– Response to therapy with symptom improvement

– Hemodynamic stability

 ONGOING CARE

FOLLOW-UP RECOMMENDATIONS

• 7 to 10 days to assess response to treatment

• 1 month to check CBC and CRP and thereafter if symptoms continue to be present

• Those with clinical predictors of poor prognosis may require closer follow-up based on lab data and echocardiographic findings.

Patient Monitoring

Myopericarditis

• Use lower doses of anti-inflammatory drugs to control symptoms for 1 to 2 weeks while minimizing deleterious effects on myocarditic process.

• Exercise restrictions for 4 to 6 weeks or until symptoms resolved and biomarkers normalized (1)[C]. For athletes, exercise restriction should be a minimum of 3 months after symptom onset (2)[C].

• Echocardiographic monitoring at 1, 6, and 12 months (especially in those with LV dysfunction)

DIET

Specific to underlying etiology only

PROGNOSIS

Overall good prognosis; disease usually benign and self-limiting; purulent and tuberculosis pericarditis with high mortality

COMPLICATIONS

• Recurrent pericarditis: occurs in ~30% of patients, with most instances resulting from idiopathic, viral, or autoimmune pericarditis; inadequate treatment of the initial attack; and, less commonly, neoplastic etiologies. Recurrence usually within 1st week following initial episode but may occur months to years later; rarely associated with tamponade/constriction

• About 5% of patients develop corticosteroid dependence and colchicine resistance.

• Cardiac tamponade: rare complication with increased incidence in neoplastic, purulent, and tuberculous pericarditis

• Effusive-constrictive pericarditis: reported in 24% of patients undergoing surgery for constrictive pericarditis and in 8% of patients undergoing pericardiocentesis and cardiac catheterization for cardiac tamponade. Failure of right atrial pressure to fall by 50% or to a level below 10 mm Hg after pericardiocentesis is diagnostic.

• Constrictive pericarditis: rare complication in which rigid pericardium produces abnormal diastolic filling with elevated filling pressures. Pericardiectomy remains definitive therapy.

REFERENCES

1. Imazio M, Brucato A, Belli R, et al. Colchicine for the prevention of pericarditis: what we know and what we do not know in 2014—systematic review and meta-analysis. *J Cardiovasc Med (Hagerstown)*. 2014;15(12):840–846.

2. Alder Y, Charron P, Imazio M, et al; for Task Force on the Diagnosis and Management of Pericardial Diseases of the European Society of Cardiology (ESC). Guidelines for the diagnosis and management of pericardial diseases executive summary. *Eur Heart J*. 2015;36(42):2921–2964.

3. Imazio M, Lazaros G, Brucato A, et al. Recurrent pericarditis: new and emerging therapeutic options. *Nat Rev Cardiol*. 2016;13(2):99–105.

4. Lilly LS. Treatment of acute and recurrent idiopathic pericarditis. *Circulation*. 2013;127(16):1723–1726.

5. Snyder MJ, Bepko J, White M. Acute pericarditis: diagnosis and management. *Am Fam Physician*. 2014;89(7):553–560.

ADDITIONAL READING

• Brucato A, Imazio M, Gattorno M, et al. Effect of anakinra on recurrent pericarditis among patients with colchicine resistance and corticosteroid dependence: the AIRTRIP randomized clinical trial. *JAMA*. 2016;316(18):1906–1912.

• Imazio M, Spodick DH, Brucato A, et al. Controversial issues in the management of pericardial diseases. *Circulation*. 2010;121(7):916–928.

• Khandaker MH, Espinosa RE, Nishimura RA, et al. Pericardial disease: diagnosis and management. *Mayo Clin Proc*. 2010;85(6):572–593.

CODES

ICD10

• I31.9 Disease of pericardium, unspecified

• I30.9 Acute pericarditis, unspecified

• I30.1 Infective pericarditis

CLINICAL PEARLS

• Therapy aimed at symptomatic relief and NSAIDs are first-line treatment. Colchicine is recommended as an adjunct to NSAIDs and has been shown to decrease risk of recurrence by 50%.

• Pericardiocentesis is recommended in the setting of cardiac tamponade or possible purulent pericarditis.

• Depending on risk factors and presentation, some patients should be hospitalized initially for treatment.

PERIODIC LIMB MOVEMENT DISORDER (PLMD)

Denise Sharon, MD, PhD, FAASM • Rochelle Zak, MD

BASICS

DESCRIPTION

Sleep-related movement disorder characterized by periodic limb movements of sleep (PLMS) with significant sleep disturbance and/or daytime functional impairment:

- Periodic limb movements of sleep (PLMS) demonstrated during polysomnography
- PLMS are repetitive contractions of tibialis anterior muscles occurring mainly in non–rapid eye movement (NREM) sleep.
- Movements consist of unilateral or bilateral, simultaneous or not, rhythmical extension of the big toe and ankle dorsiflexion.
- Sometimes, knee and hip flexion is noted.
- Arm movements or more generalized movements occur less commonly.
- Movements might be associated with cortical arousals from sleep unbeknownst to the patient (PLMs with arousals—PLMA).
- A clinical history of significant sleep disturbance and/or functional impairment is necessary for diagnosis.
- Complaints include insomnia, nonrestorative sleep, daytime fatigue, somnolence.
- Bed partner may complain of patient's movements.
- Other sleep disorders such as obstructive sleep apnea (OSA), narcolepsy, restless legs syndrome do not explain the PLMS.
- No associated restlessness or dysesthesia while awake
  - If there is an associated sensory perception or restlessness, the diagnosis is not PLMD but possibly restless leg syndrome (RLS).
- System(s) affected: musculoskeletal, nervous
- Synonym(s) referring to the PLMS: nocturnal myoclonus; sleep myoclonus

EPIDEMIOLOGY

Incidence

- PLMD is rare, affecting children and adults (1).
- PLMS occurs in >15% of insomnia patients.
- PLMS are frequent in narcolepsy, in OSA, and during initiation of CPAP.

Prevalence

- PLMS increases with age: 45% of patients >65 years exhibit PLMS >5/hr but not PLMD.
- PLMD is much less common: <5% of adults but also underdiagnosed (1)
- 85% of RLS patients have PLMS (2).

ETIOLOGY AND PATHOPHYSIOLOGY

- Understudied; most data reports on PLMS as it pertains to RLS:
  - CNS dopamine dysregulation supported by increased incidence of PLMS in untreated Parkinson disease (PD) and decreased incidence of PLMS in schizophrenia.
- Triggering and exacerbating factors:
  - Peripheral neuropathy
  - Arthritis
  - Renal failure
  - Spinal cord injury
  - Pregnancy

- Medication side effects:
  - Most antidepressants (except bupropion or desipramine) and lithium
  - Some antipsychotic and antidementia medications
  - Antiemetics (dopaminergic)
  - Sedating antihistamines

Genetics

BTBD9 on chromosome 6p associated with PLMS in patients with or without RLS but not in RLS patients without PLMS

RISK FACTORS

- Family history of RLS
- Iron deficiency and associated conditions
- History of prematurity

GENERAL PREVENTION

- Promoting adequate sleep
- Avoid PLMS triggers such as iron deficiency, frequently observed in children (3).

COMMONLY ASSOCIATED CONDITIONS

- Narcolepsy
- End-stage renal disease; cardiovascular disease; stroke
- Gastric surgery
- Pregnancy
- Arthritis
- Lumbar spine disease; spinal cord injury
- Peripheral neuropathy
- Insomnia, insufficient sleep, parasomnias
- ADHD, anxiety, oppositional behaviors

Pediatric Considerations

- PLMD may precede overt RLS by years (3).
- Association with RLS is more common.
- Association and differential diagnosis with restless sleep disorder, ADHD, oppositional behaviors, mood disorders, growing pains (3)

Pregnancy Considerations

- May be secondary to iron, folate deficiency
- Most severe in the 3rd trimester
- Usually resolves after delivery

Geriatric Considerations

- May cause or exacerbate circadian disruption and "sundowning"
- PLMS may increase risk of atrial fibrillation in elderly.

DIAGNOSIS

HISTORY

Sleep disturbance:

- Insomnia: difficulty maintaining sleep
- Nonrestorative sleep
- Daytime fatigue, tiredness, somnolence
- Oppositional behaviors
- Memory impairment
- Depression
- ADHD, particularly in children (3)

PHYSICAL EXAM

No specific findings

DIFFERENTIAL DIAGNOSIS

- PLMS occurring with RLS, RBD, narcolepsy, are secondary to the sleep disorder, not PLMD.
- PLMS occurring with OSA may be associated with respiratory events and is not PLMD.
- Sleep starts: nonperiodic, generalized, only at wake–sleep transition, <0.2" duration
- Sleep-related leg cramps: isolated, painful, muscle knots
- Fragmentary myoclonus: 75 to 150 ms of electromyographic (EMG) activity, minimal movement, no periodicity
- Nocturnal seizures: epileptiform EEG, motor pattern incongruent with PLMs
- Fasciculations, tremor: no sleep association
- Sleep-related rhythmic movement disorder: voluntary movement during wake–sleep transition; higher frequency than PLMs
- Restless sleep disorder—large body movements, no periodicity

DIAGNOSTIC TESTS & INTERPRETATION

Polysomnography (PSG) demonstrating PLMS:

- Tibialis ant EMG activation lasting 0.5" to 10.0"
- EMG amplitude increase >8 μV from baseline
- Movements occur in a sequence of ≥4 at intervals of 5 to 90 seconds.
- Associated with heart rate variability from autonomic-level arousals
- Most PLMs episodes occur in the first hours of NREM sleep.
- Night-to-night PLMS variability is common.

Initial Tests (lab, imaging)

Serum iron stores including ferritin, transferrin, iron-binding capacity, serum iron

Follow-Up Tests & Special Considerations

Repeat iron stores, at least ferritin if suspected change, or nonresponsive to treatment

Diagnostic Procedures/Other

EMG, nerve conduction studies for peripheral neuropathy/radiculopathy if indicated

Test Interpretation

On PSG: PLMSI >5/hr children, and >15/hr adults

TREATMENT

Treatment paradigm similar to that for RLS, except that all medications are off-label for PLMD (2),(4),(5)[B]

GENERAL MEASURES

- Assess for and correct iron insufficiency.
- Adequate nightly sleep
- Regular exercise, low impact in the evening
- Weighted blanket, warm the legs (long socks, leg warmers, electric blanket, etc.)
- Hot/leg baths, warm soaks before bedtime
- Avoid caffeine and alcohol.

MEDICATION
- Use minimum effective dose.
- Goals of medication:
  - Improve subjective sleep quality.
  - Control PLMS and their effect on sleep.
- Consider risks, side effects, interactions in different populations (e.g., benzodiazepines in elderly).
- Treatment should decrease daytime somnolence.

First Line
- Dopamine agonists reduce PLMS, increase sleep efficiency, but have no effect on sleep instability; start low, titrate slow to optimal dose (2),(4),(5)[C].
  - Pramipexole (Mirapex): 0.125 to 0.5 mg; titrate by 0.125 mg; take 2 hours HS
  - Ropinirole (Requip): 0.25 to 4.00 mg; titrate by 0.25 mg; take 1/2 to 1 hour HS; preferred in renal impairment
  - Transdermal rotigotine (Neupro): 1 to 3 mg/24 hr patch; initiate with 1 mg/24 hr; titrate up by 1 mg slowly to effectiveness.
- Avoid dopamine agonists in psychotic patients, especially if taking dopamine antagonists.
- Dopamine agonists may exert a stimulant effect, further disturbing sleep.

Second Line
- Voltage-gated calcium channel $\alpha 2\delta$ subunit ligands: useful for associated neuropathy; decrease PLMS and improve sleep architecture; caution with renal impairment (2)[C],(4)
  - Gabapentin enacarbil (Horizant): 600 mg early evening
  - Gabapentin (Neurontin): 300 to 600 mg HS
  - Pregabalin (Lyrica): 75 to 300 mg HS
- Benzodiazepines and agonists (2)[C],(4); most commonly used because of their effect on sleep; caution in the elderly
  - Clonazepam (Klonopin): 0.5 to 2.0 mg QHS
  - Zaleplon, zolpidem, temazepam, triazolam, alprazolam, diazepam

ISSUES FOR REFERRAL
To sleep medicine clinic, neurology and movement disorders clinic:
- High-dose medications
- Worsening of Sx while on medications
- Intractable iron deficiency
- Uncontrolled symptoms in adults and special populations

Pediatric Considerations
- First-line treatment: nonpharmacologic (3)[C]
- Assess/correct iron deficiency (6)[B].
- Consider low-dose clonidine 0.1 to 0.3 mg HS; caution: orthostatic hypotension (3)[C]

Pregnancy Considerations
- Initial approach: iron supplementation, nonpharmacologic therapies (5)
- In 2nd, 3rd trimester, can use clonazepam 0.25 to 1 mg QHS
- CarbiDOPA/levoDOPA 25/100 to 50/200 ER
- Refractory PLMD—may use oxycodone in 2nd, 3rd trimester: Discontinue 2 weeks prior delivery.

Geriatric Considerations
In weak or frail patients, avoid medications that may cause dizziness or unsteadiness.

ADDITIONAL THERAPIES
- If iron deficient, iron supplementation:
  - 325-mg ferrous sulfate with 200 mg vitamin C between meals BID or entire dose QD
  - Repletion may require months of treatment.
- Clonidine 0.05 to 0.30 mg/day
- Relaxis leg vibration device; limited data

SURGERY/OTHER PROCEDURES
Correction of orthopedic, neuropathic, or peripheral vascular problems

COMPLEMENTARY & ALTERNATIVE MEDICINE
Vitamin/mineral supplements, including calcium, magnesium, vitamin D, vitamin B_{12}, folate maybe helpful

 ONGOING CARE

FOLLOW-UP RECOMMENDATIONS
Patient Monitoring
- At monthly intervals until stable
- Assess symptom severity, medication side effects, augmentation.
- Annual and PRN follow-up thereafter
- Repeat iron blood work if previously low.

DIET
Avoid caffeine, alcohol, more so late in the day.

PATIENT EDUCATION
- National Sleep Foundation: http://sleepfoundation.org/
- American Academy of Sleep Medicine: http://www.sleepeducation.org/

PROGNOSIS
- Primary PLMD: lifelong, no current cure
- Secondary PLMD: may subside with resolution of cause(s) such as low iron stores
- Current therapies usually control symptoms.
- PLMD often precedes the emergence of RLS.

COMPLICATIONS
- Tolerance to meds requiring increased dose
- Augmentation (increased PLMs and sleep disturbance, emergence of RLS) from dopamine agonists:
  - Higher doses increase risk.
  - Iron deficiency increases augmentation risk.
  - Add alternative medication and then gradually discontinue dopaminergic agent.
- Iatrogenic PLMD (from antidepressants, etc.)

REFERENCES
1. Hornyak M, Feige B, Riemann D, et al. Periodic leg movements in sleep and periodic limb movement disorder: prevalence, clinical significance and treatment. *Sleep Med Rev*. 2006;10(3):169–177.
2. Fulda S. The role of periodic limb movements during sleep in restless legs syndrome: a selective update. *Sleep Med Clin*. 2015;10(3):241–248.
3. Sharon D, Walters AS, Simakajjornboon N. RLS and restless legs syndrome and periodic limb movement disorder in children. *J Child Sci*. 2019;9:e38–e49.
4. Aurora RN, Kristo DA, Bista SR, et al; for American Academy of Sleep Medicine. The treatment of restless legs syndrome and periodic limb movement disorder in adults—an update for 2012: practice parameters with an evidence-based systematic review and meta-analyses: an American Academy of Sleep Medicine clinical practice guideline. *Sleep*. 2012;35(8):1039–1062.
5. Garcia-Borreguero D, Silber MH, Winkelman JW, et al. Guidelines for the first-line treatment of restless legs syndrome/Willis–Ekbom disease, prevention and treatment of dopaminergic augmentation: a combined task force of the IRLSSG, EURLSSG, and the RLS-foundation. *Sleep Med*. 2016;21:1–11.
6. Gingras JL, Gaultney JF, Picchietti DL. Pediatric periodic limb movement disorder: sleep symptom and polysomnographic correlates compared to obstructive sleep apnea. *J Clin Sleep Med*. 2011;7(6):603A–609A.

ADDITIONAL READING
- American Academy of Sleep Medicine. Periodic limb movement disorder. In: *International Classification of Sleep Disorders*. 3rd ed. Darien, IL: American Academy of Sleep Medicine; 2014:292–299.
- Högl B, Comella C. Therapeutic advances in restless legs syndrome (RLS). *Mov Disord*. 2015;30(11):1574–1579.

 SEE ALSO

Restless Leg Syndrome

 CODES

ICD10
G47.61 Periodic limb movement disorder

CLINICAL PEARLS
- Many patients with PLMs may not require treatment; when sleep disturbance associated with PLMs causes insomnia and/or daytime consequences, PLMD should be treated.
- Assuring adequate iron stores, with a ferritin >75 is advised.
- Many antidepressants and some antihistamines cause or exacerbate PLMs.

PERIPHERAL ARTERIAL DISEASE

Mansi Katkar, MD • Joseph Francis Urbanik, DO

 BASICS

DESCRIPTION

Peripheral arterial disease (PAD) represents an atherosclerotic occlusive disease of the peripheral arteries, most commonly in the lower extremities. Following coronary artery disease and cerebrovascular disease, PAD is the third leading source of atherosclerotic vascular morbidity. PAD manifests as intermittent claudication (IC) or atypical leg pain and is commonly diagnosed with a resting ankle-brachial index (ABI) of <0.90 (1).

EPIDEMIOLOGY

- Age: ≥65 years, 50 to 64 years with atherosclerosis risk factors (e.g., diabetes mellitus [DM], hyperlipidemia [HLD], hypertension [HTN], history of smoking) or family history of PAD, or <50 years, with DM and one additional atherosclerosis risk factor
- Individuals with known atherosclerotic disease in another vascular bed (e.g., coronary, carotid, subclavian, renal, mesenteric artery stenosis, or AAA)
- Impacts at least 7.1 million people in the United States

Incidence

Incidence increases with age and the presence of cardiovascular risk factors.

Prevalence

- Data from the National Health and Nutrition Examination Survey (1999–2004) show that 5.9% of the U.S. population 40 years or older has a low ABI (<0.9) indicating the presence of PAD.
- However, the true prevalence of PAD is difficult to establish because more than half of persons with a low ABI are asymptomatic.

ETIOLOGY AND PATHOPHYSIOLOGY

- In PAD, arterial occlusion is most commonly a result of underlying atherosclerotic disease.
- The association between PAD and cardiovascular morbidity and mortality has been well established, with a lower ABI being an independent predictor.
- Other etiologies for PAD include phlebitis, trauma, or autoimmune/vasculitic diseases.
- Arterial narrowing results in insufficient oxygen delivery to the muscle during periods of increased demand (i.e., exercise), causing claudication and limiting exercise.
- Reperfusion at rest following ischemia can result in multiple subsequent physiologic changes, including inflammation, oxidant stress, endothelial dysfunction, and mitochondrial injury.

Genetics

Although several of the risk factors for PAD (as noted next) are heritable, genome-wide association studies isolating PAD-specific single nucleotide polymorphisms have not been as successful. This has been attributed to the increased clinical and genetic heterogeneity of PAD.

RISK FACTORS

- Older age, atherosclerotic disease of any vascular bed, current or history of smoking, diabetes mellitus, HTN, HLD, chronic kidney disease (CKD)
- Heritable conditions: chylomicronemia, hypercholesterolemia, hyperhomocysteinemia, and pseudoxanthoma elasticum

GENERAL PREVENTION

- Regular aerobic exercise program, smoking cessation, blood pressure (BP) and diabetes control
- Statin therapy is indicated in patients with clinical PAD for secondary prevention of atherosclerotic cardiovascular disease.

COMMONLY ASSOCIATED CONDITIONS

In addition to the aforementioned risk factors, PAD is associated with other forms of atherosclerotic disease including myocardial infarction (MI), transient ischemic attack (TIA), and cerebrovascular accident (CVA).

 DIAGNOSIS

HISTORY

- 20–40% of patients will be asymptomatic (2).
- 10–35% of patients present with classic IC (painful, aching, cramping, uncomfortable, or tired feeling in legs during walking, relieved by rest) (2).
- Atypical pain in 40–50% of patients
- 1–2% of patients will develop critical limb ischemia (threatened limb).
- Nonhealing wounds and ulceration
- Skin discoloration
- Erectile dysfunction (in conjunction with IC and absent or diminished femoral pulses constitutes Leriche syndrome, caused by severe atherosclerosis of the distal abdominal aorta, iliac arteries and femoral and popliteal arteries) (3)

PHYSICAL EXAM

- Pallor with leg elevation, dependent rubor
- Pale atrophic skin with hair thinning or loss (seen with chronic PAD)
- Brittle or hypertrophic nails
- Moderate to severe PAD can cause reduced/absent extremity pulses.
- Severe PAD may present nonhealing ulcers and wounds on distal toes or heels.
- Gangrene
- Distal lower extremities may feel cool.

DIFFERENTIAL DIAGNOSIS

- Arterial aneurysm or dissection
- Deep vein thrombosis (DVT)
- Thromboangiitis obliterans (Buerger disease) or other vasculopathies
- Arterial embolism
- Peripheral neuropathy
- Spinal stenosis or nerve root compression (pseudoclaudication)
- Popliteal entrapment syndrome

DIAGNOSTIC TESTS & INTERPRETATION

Screening

- Current AHA/ACC guidelines recommend resting ABI testing for symptomatic patients and also state that it could be reasonable to test asymptomatic patients with increased risk of PAD (patients with known atherosclerotic disease or risk factors of atherosclerosis including DM, HTN, HLD, smoking and age ≥65 years.
- Routine ABI screening for asymptomatic adults without PAD risk factors is not recommended by the AHA/ACC and is graded as having insufficient evidence (I) by the USPSTF.

Initial Tests (lab, imaging)

- Risk factor identification with fasting lipid profile and basic metabolic profile
- Exercise treadmill ABI is useful in patients who are symptomatic but have normal resting ABI.
- Imaging is reserved for patients who have lifestyle-limiting symptoms (IC) despite appropriate guideline-directed management and therapy.
  - Duplex ultrasound, magnetic resonance angiography (MRA), and computed tomography angiography (CTA) are recommended in symptomatic patients who are being considered for revascularization.
  - Invasive angiography is recommended in patients with critical limb ischemia and is reasonable in those with symptomatic PAD who are candidates for revascularization.

Diagnostic Procedures/Other

- Doppler ABI: ratio of systolic BP at the ankle and brachial artery
- Toe-brachial index (TBI) is recommended when ABI is ≥1.40, suggesting a noncompressible vessel.

Test Interpretation

- <0.90 abnormal, diagnostic for PAD, 0.91 to 0.99 borderline, correlated clinically, and consider additional testing
- 1.00 to 1.40 normal, >1.40 concern for incompressible arteries, association with diabetes mellitus

TREATMENT

GENERAL MEASURES

- The treatment of PAD is multifactorial and includes a supervised exercise program, guideline-based medical therapy, and risk factor modification (4). Recommendations below are based primarily on AHA/ACC Guideline (1)[C].
- Assess functional status via the Fontaine or Rutherford classification systems. Anatomic classification of complexity is determined by the Trans-Atlantic Inter-Society Consensus (TASC). This classification may be used to guide management (4),(5).
- Cardiovascular risk factor modification, especially in the setting of smoking cessation
  - High-intensity statin (lipid-lowering therapy) is recommended for all patients with PAD and has been shown to reduce all-cause mortality 1A.
  - Goal BP <140/90 mm Hg
  - ACE inhibitors are associated with a significant reduction in major adverse cardiovascular events in patients with PAD 1A.
  - Counselling on smoking cessation and offering pharmacologic agents (varenicline, bupropion, nicotine replacement syndrome) and behavioral counselling
- Supervised exercise training, which takes place in a hospital or outpatient facility, is the initial treatment modality recommended in patients with IC. Patients are instructed to walk for a minimum of 30 to 45 minutes (with rest when symptomatic) 3 times per week for a minimum of 12 weeks. A structured community or home-based exercise program can be beneficial and is recommended when a supervised program is not possible.
- An interdisciplinary approach is recommended for optimal treatment, including physicians (vascular specialists if indicated), nurses, exercise physiologists, podiatrists, nutritionists, and social workers.

MEDICATION

First Line

- Antiplatelet monotherapy is recommended in symptomatic PAD without bleeding risk contraindications (6)[A]. Aspirin (75 to 325 mg) or clopidogrel (75 mg) is acceptable first-line antiplatelet agent.
  - It is reasonable to prescribe antiplatelet monotherapy in asymptomatic patients who have an ABI diagnostic of PAD.
  - In asymptomatic patients with borderline ABIs (0.91 to 0.99), the utility of antiplatelet therapy is not well established.
- Dual antiplatelet therapy (DAPT; aspirin and clopidogrel) should be prescribed only following endovascular intervention; the data for efficacy is not well established, and bleeding risk is increased.
- Current professional society guidelines recommend statins for all individuals with symptomatic and asymptomatic PAD.

- Cilostazol (100 mg orally twice daily) has been shown to improve walking distance and should be considered in all patients with claudication that impacts daily living.
- The above medications can be prescribed concurrently with the initiation of an exercise program.

Second Line

Pentoxifylline (400 mg 3 times daily) was previously considered first line for symptomatic relief of claudication; however, evidence is of poor quality and benefit is uncertain (Cochrane, other reviews).

SURGERY/OTHER PROCEDURES

Percutaneous and surgical interventions should be considered in patients who had an inadequate response to less invasive modalities (i.e., exercise and pharmacotherapy) have significant disability from their claudication and have a favorable risk-benefit ratio.

- Percutaneous intervention involves accessing the artery with a wire or catheter and balloon angioplasty with possible stent placement to widen the stenosed arterial lumen. Balloons and stents may be drug eluting.
- Preferred for patients with aortoiliac disease and reasonable for femoropopliteal disease
- Current data are insufficient regarding infrapopliteal lesions, but ongoing studies are comparing efficacy between endovascular and surgical intervention.
- Surgical intervention involves using a bypass graft to revascularize the artery distal to the stenosis.

COMPLEMENTARY & ALTERNATIVE MEDICINE

- Chelation therapy and B-complex vitamins are not recommended in patients with PAD.
- Additional studies on Ginkgo biloba, L-arginine, propionyl-L-carnitine, omega-3 fatty acids, and vitamin E have been studied, and in general, their efficacy is uncertain. Thus, currently, they are not recommended for use in the primary care setting.

 ONGOING CARE

FOLLOW-UP RECOMMENDATIONS

- At follow-up, patients should undergo thorough history and physical examinations. They should be asked about their progress with risk-factor modification (i.e., smoking, glucose control, HTN), exercise endurance and compliance with training program, and effectiveness of pharmacotherapy.
- After endovascular or surgical intervention, patients should receive regular assessment of symptoms and occlusion via resting and exercise ABIs.

DIET

- A heart-healthy diet is recommended in all patients with PAD or atherosclerotic disease and risk factors.
- Balanced diets consisting of vegetables, fruit, nuts, protein, and healthy fats (such as the Mediterranean diet) are likely best.
- Consultation with a nutritionist can be used in patients when appropriate.

PROGNOSIS

- Limb ischemia and IC: 15–20% will have worsening claudication, 5–10% will require endovascular or surgical intervention, and 2–5% will undergo amputation (most commonly smokers and patients with diabetes).
- Considering cardiovascular outcomes, at 5 years, 20% of patients with PAD will experience a nonfatal cardiovascular event, and 15–20% will die, most commonly of cardiovascular disease.

REFERENCES

1. Gerhard-Herman MD, Gornik HL, Barrett C, et al. 2016 AHA/ACC guideline on the management of patients with lower extremity peripheral artery disease: executive summary. *Circulation.* 2017;135(12):e686–e725.
2. Firnhaber JM, Powell CS. Lower extremity peripheral artery disease: diagnosis and treatment [published correction appears in *Am Fam Physician.* 2019 Jul 15;100(2):74]. *Am Fam Physician.* 2019;99(6):362–369.
3. Frederick M, Newman J, Kohlwes J. Leriche syndrome. *J Gen Intern Med.* 2010;25(10):1102–1104.
4. Olin JW, White CJ, Armstrong EJ, et al. Peripheral artery disease: evolving role of exercise, medical therapy, and endovascular options. *J Am Coll Cardiol.* 2016;67(11):1338–1357.
5. Abu Dabrh AM, Steffen MW, Asi N, et al. Bypass surgery versus endovascular interventions in severe or critical limb ischemia. *J Vasc Surg.* 2016;63(1):244.e11–253.e11.
6. Wong PF, Chong LY, Mikhailidis DP, et al. Antiplatelet agents for intermittent claudication. *Cochrane Database Syst Rev.* 2011;(11):CD001272.

CODES

ICD10

- I73.9 Peripheral vascular disease, unspecified
- I70.209 Unsp athscl native arteries of extremities, unsp extremity
- I70.219 Athscl native arteries of extrm w intrmt claud, unsp extrm

CLINICAL PEARLS

- USPSTF (2018): Current evidence is insufficient to weigh harms and benefits of screening for PAD with ABI.
- Patients who fail noninvasive therapy with a supervised exercise training program and pharmacotherapy should be referred to vascular surgery. Patients with CLI (pain at rest, gangrene, ulceration) should be referred.
- Antiplatelet therapy (aspirin or clopidogrel) and cilostazol for symptomatic relief are at the cornerstone of pharmacotherapy. Additionally, appropriate BP control (BP <140/90 mm Hg) and HLD management with statin therapy are indicated in all patients.

PERITONITIS, ACUTE

Marie L. Borum, MD, EdD, MPH • Giancarlo Colón Rosa, MD

BASICS

DESCRIPTION
- Definition: inflammation of the peritoneum
- Classification:
  - Aseptic: chemical irritation or systemic inflammation of peritoneum
  - Bacterial: infection of peritoneal fluid
- Bacterial peritonitis types:
  - Primary/spontaneous bacterial peritonitis (SBP): infection of ascitic fluid in the absence of an intra-abdominal source
  - Secondary bacterial peritonitis: infection of ascitic fluid from a detectable intra-abdominal source
    - Secondary bacterial peritonitis can be further classified as either perforation peritonitis or nonperforation peritonitis.
  - Tertiary bacterial peritonitis: >48 hours of infection despite source control
  - Peritoneal dialysis–associated peritonitis
  - Perforated appendicitis and chronic peritoneal dialysis are the most common cause leading to acute peritonitis in children.

EPIDEMIOLOGY
Incidence
- In cirrhotic patients with ascites, the annual incidence of SBP is 10–25%.
- 25–75% of patients with secondary bacterial peritonitis progress to tertiary peritonitis.

Prevalence
- SBP: In asymptomatic patients with cirrhosis and ascites, the prevalence of SBP is <4% in outpatients. Nosocomial rates are 10%.
- In patients with cirrhosis and ascites, 5% of peritonitis is secondary.
- Secondary peritonitis is the most common cause of sepsis in surgical ICU patients.
- PD peritonitis is the primary reason for switching from PD to hemodialysis (HD).
- PD peritonitis in children is more common than in adults.

ETIOLOGY AND PATHOPHYSIOLOGY
- Mechanism
  - SBP:
    - Bacterial translocation via lymphatic spread through mesentery lymph nodes
    - Often develops in the setting of large-volume ascites in patients with advanced cirrhosis
    - Cirrhotic patients have:
      - Alterations to gut microbiota with higher prevalence of pathogenic organisms
      - Small intestinal bacterial overgrowth (SIBO) and increased intestinal mucosal permeability to bacteria
      - Decreased cellular and humoral immunity limiting peritoneal bacterial clearance
  - Secondary:
    - Translocation of bacteria from inflamed or perforated intraperitoneal (IP) organs or introduction of bacterial through instrumentation
  - Tertiary: evolves from secondary peritonitis
  - PD peritonitis:
    - Contamination with pathogenic skin flora during exchanges or exit-site infection
- Microbiology
  - SBP. Most cases (>90%) of SBP are monomicrobial.
    - Most common gram-negative pathogens are *Escherichia coli* (33%) and *Klebsiella* spp. (8%).

- Most common gram-positive pathogens are *Streptococcus* spp. (15%) and *Staphylococcus aureus* (13%).
  - Secondary: perforation of a viscus, small bowel strangulation, necrotizing pancreatitis. Organism depends on cause of peritonitis; gram-positive organisms more common with upper GI pathology, whereas gram-negative organisms more common with lower GI pathology. Common species include *E. coli*, *Klebsiella*, *Proteus*, *Streptococcus*, *Enterococcus*, *Bacteroides*, and *Clostridium*.
  - PD peritonitis is most commonly due to *Staphylococcus epidermidis* and *S. aureus*.

RISK FACTORS
- SBP: advanced cirrhosis with ascites, malnutrition, upper GI bleed, PPI usage, and prior SBP
  - Acid suppression (most commonly with PPIs) promotes gut bacterial growth and translocation.
  - 70% of SBP cases are in patients with Child-Pugh class C cirrhosis.
  - Low ascites protein (<1.0 g/dL) increases risk.
- Secondary:
  - *Helicobacter pylori* or NSAIDs-induced ulcers, vascular disease causing bowel ischemia, alcohol abuse causing pancreatitis, trauma, or IBD causing bowel perforation
- PD peritonitis:
  - Nonsterile technique
  - Recent instrumentation

GENERAL PREVENTION
- SBP prophylaxis decreases mortality in patients at high risk (e.g., ascitic fluid protein concentration <1.0 g/dL, esophageal varices, or history of previous SBP).
  - Antibiotics include norfloxacin, ciprofloxacin, TMP/SMZ PO, ceftriaxone IV.
  - Patients with cirrhotic ascites who have low ascitic fluid protein (<1.5 g/dL), renal impairment (creatinine ≥1.2 mg/dL, BUN ≥25 mg/dL, serum sodium [Na] ≤130 mEq/L), or liver failure (Child-Pugh score ≥9 and serum bilirubin ≥3 mg/dL) should also receive SBP prophylaxis.
- Limit use of PPIs.
- PD peritonitis:
  - Sterile techniques
  - Antibiotic prophylaxis prior to selected procedures

COMMONLY ASSOCIATED CONDITIONS
SBP almost always occurs in the setting of decompensated cirrhosis.

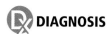**DIAGNOSIS**

HISTORY
- SBP: history of cirrhosis and/or ascites, fever, chills, mental status changes, abdominal pain (diffuse, continuous; may be subtle due to presence of ascites), nausea/vomiting, diarrhea, GI bleeding
- Secondary: may be clinically indistinguishable from SBP unless history of perforation, abscess, or other intra-abdominal pathology or recent surgical intervention is present
- Tertiary: persistent signs and symptoms despite initial treatment, or history of recurrent peritonitis
- PD peritonitis: presumptive diagnosis in PD patients with cloudy effluent

ALERT
Up to 30% of patients are asymptomatic.

PHYSICAL EXAM
- Tachycardia, tachypnea, altered mental status, hypotension, hyperthermia, or hypothermia
  - AMS may be subtle; Reitan trail test (connect-the-numbers test) helpful in detecting subtle changes in mental status. Suspect hepatic encephalopathy if the number of seconds it takes for patient to finish test is greater than their age.
- Abdominal pain and distention, ascites, abdominal wall guarding, rebound tenderness, hypoactive/absent bowel sounds, diarrhea
  - There is no rigidity because ascites separates parietal layer of peritoneum from visceral layer.

DIFFERENTIAL DIAGNOSIS
- Liver disease: hepatitis, decompensated cirrhosis
- Luminal disease: abscess formation, ileus, volvulus, intussusception, mesenteric adenitis, pancreatitis, cholecystitis, malignancy, peritoneal carcinomatosis, IBD
- Extraluminal disease: ruptured ectopic pregnancy, tubo-ovarian abscess, PID, UTI, pyelonephritis
- Systemic disease: tuberculosis, pneumonia, MI, porphyria, SLE

DIAGNOSTIC TESTS & INTERPRETATION

ALERT
Early diagnosis and immediate evaluation reduce mortality.

Initial Tests (lab, imaging)
- CBC: leukocytosis, anemia
  - Thrombocytopenia <100,000/mL predicts SBP (1)[B].
- BMP: metabolic acidosis, azotemia
- LFTs, coagulations often abnormal at baseline in cirrhotics
- CRP >60 mg/L + cirrhotic ascites is highly specific for SBP (96.5%) (1)[B].
- Secondary:
  - Abdominal x-rays or CT may show free air or source of infection (abscess, perforation, etc.).
  - Procalcitonin levels may predict severity; >10 ng/mL correlates with ICU admission.

Follow-Up Tests & Special Considerations
- Obtain ascites, blood, and urine cultures before antibiotics are given.
- If culture is monomicrobial but PMN <250, colonization generally resolves if patient asymptomatic but generally progresses to SBP if patient symptomatic.
- If culture is polymicrobial but PMN <250, cause is likely traumatic paracentesis.
- If culture negative but PMN >250, still likely to be SBP and requires broad-spectrum antibiotics
- Alcoholic hepatitis and SBP can occur concurrently.
- In hemorrhagic ascites, PMN count is corrected by subtracting 1 PMN per 250 RBCs.

Diagnostic Procedures/Other
- Ascitic fluid studies from diagnostic paracentesis: culture, Gram stain, cell count with differential, albumin; for secondary peritonitis, include LDH, total protein, glucose, alkaline phosphatase (ALP), and CEA.
- SBP: PMN >500 cells/mm³ is the best individual predictor of SBP (86% sensitivity; 98% specific). A cutoff of 250 cells/mm³ has a sensitivity of 93% and a specificity of 94%.
  - PMN >250 cells/mm³, a positive ascitic culture, and a lack of a cause of secondary peritonitis confirms the diagnosis of SBP.
  - Serum-ascites albumin gradient <1.1 g/dL rules out portal hypertension, making SBP unlikely.

- Secondary peritonitis: PMN >250 cells/mm³ on ascitic fluid analysis with polymicrobial culture and/or two of the following (Runyon criteria): ascitic fluid total protein >1 g/dL, glucose <50 mg/dL, and LDH > upper limit of normal for serum (67% sensitivity, 96% specific)
  - Perforation is likely with ALP >240 U/L or CEA >5 ng/mL (sensitivity 92%, specificity 88%)
  - Ascites-serum amylase ratio >6 suggests pancreatic source.
- PD peritonitis:
  - Two of the following: positive effluent culture, consistent clinical features, and peritoneal fluid WBC >100 mm³ with PMN >50%

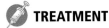 **TREATMENT**

GENERAL MEASURES
- Control ascites with salt restriction, spironolactone ±, furosemide, albumin infusion after large-volume paracentesis, and/or lactulose for encephalopathy.
- Discontinue β-blockers in SBP.
- Avoid nephrotoxic medications.

MEDICATION
- SBP
  - Community-acquired SBP without recent β-lactam antibiotic use: 3rd-generation cephalosporins, preferably cefotaxime 2 g IV q8h for 5 more days
  - SBP in absence of previous quinolone use/ prophylaxis, vomiting, shock, hepatic encephalopathy, or serum creatinine >3 mg/dL: can substitute ofloxacin 400 mg BID PO (must be renally dosed) for cefotaxime (2)[A]
  - Symptomatic bacterascites with PMN count <250 cells/mm³: cefotaxime 2 g IV q8h while awaiting sensitivities
  - Second-line antibiotics include fluoroquinolones (levofloxacin), piperacillin/tazobactam, or vancomycin.
    - Ciprofloxacin 200 mg IV BID can be used in patients for whom cephalosporins are contraindicated or poorly tolerated.
- SBP with renal or hepatic impairment (serum creatinine >1 mg/dL, BUN >30 mg/dL, or total bilirubin >4 mg/dL): Add albumin 1.5 g/kg within 6 hours and 1 g/kg on day 3.
- Most patients respond well to a 5-day course of parenteral antibiotics.
  - Longer therapy is considered for patients infected with:
    - Unusual or resistant organisms (e.g., *Pseudomonas*)
- Reassess patient after 5-day antibiotic course.
  - If asymptomatic, no further treatment is needed.
  - If fever or pain persists, repeat paracentesis.
- Secondary:
  - Empiric broad-spectrum antibiotic coverage for polymicrobial infection; IV cefotaxime or other 3rd- to 4th-generation cephalosporin plus metronidazole
- Tertiary:
  - If no unrepaired perforations or leaks, continue with medical management: broad-spectrum antibiotics (guided by susceptibilities), early enteral nutrition prevent atrophy.
  - Consider adding antifungal coverage.
  - Consider removing catheter if recurrent or persistent PD–associated infection.
- PD peritonitis:
  - IP route for antibiotics preferred over IV route unless patient is septic.
  - Gram-positive coverage: vancomycin or a 1st-generation cephalosporin (e.g., cefazolin)
  - Gram-negative coverage: 3rd-generation cephalosporin (e.g., ceftazidime, cefepime), an aminoglycoside, or a carbapenem

- Most patients usually improve within 48 hours of initiation of antibiotic therapy.
  - Clinical improvement, less cloudy efferent, and/ or lower cell count in peritoneal fluid all demonstrate infection is resolving.
  - PD does not have to be discontinued.
  - Remove catheter if:
    - Fungal or mycobacterial peritonitis
    - Culture-negative peritonitis with persistent symptoms and elevated WBC in peritoneal fluid
    - PD effluent is not clear after a 5-day course of antibiotics (refractory peritonitis).
    - Peritonitis recurring within 4 weeks of completion of antibiotic course
    - Laparotomy required
  - If catheter removed, can be replaced after 2 weeks if symptoms have resolved (3)[C]

SURGERY/OTHER PROCEDURES
- SBP:
  - Medical management only (80% mortality if patient with SBP receives exploratory laparotomy)
- Secondary:
  - Emergent surgical management, including source control with open laparotomy to repair any perforated viscus and eradicate infected material, is first-line treatment.
- Tertiary:
  - If there are no unrepaired perforations or leaks, additional surgery for severe abdominal infection correlates with deterioration and mortality.

ALERT
The mortality of secondary bacterial peritonitis approaches 100% if not treated surgically.

ADMISSION, INPATIENT, AND NURSING CONSIDERATIONS
- Acute peritonitis typically warrants hospitalization.
- In patients with cardiogenic or septic shock, use invasive monitoring with goal-directed fluid therapy.
- Patients who present with peritonitis can be severely hypovolemic, and volume resuscitation is critical.
- Cirrhotic patients are often on β-blockers. During an episode of SBP, β-blockers increase mortality, hepatorenal syndrome, and hospital stay.

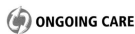 **ONGOING CARE**

FOLLOW-UP RECOMMENDATIONS
Patient Monitoring
Normalization of vital signs with resolution of leukocytosis is a sign of improvement.
- PMN decrease >25% is expected if repeat paracentesis is performed after 48 hours, although repeat paracentesis is not required in the setting of clinical improvement.

DIET
- NPO, total parental nutrition (TPN) as necessary, especially in secondary peritonitis
- Resume enteral feeding after return of bowel function.
- Na restriction can reduce future ascites.

PROGNOSIS
- SBP:
  - For inpatients with first episode of SBP, mortality is <5% with prompt diagnosis and treatment.
  - Prognosis improves if antibiotics are started early and prior to onset of shock or renal failure.
  - Renal insufficiency is the strongest negative prognostic indicator.
  - Patients with prior SBP have 1-year recurrence of 40–70% and 1-year mortality of 50–70%.

- Secondary:
  - In-hospital mortality of treated patients is 20%.
  - Prognosis is worse in perforation peritonitis (vs. nonperforation peritonitis) and mortality of perforation approaches 100% if not treated surgically.
- PD peritonitis
  - 2–6% mortality (highest in fungal, gram-negative, and *S. aureus* infection)
  - 5–20% switch to HD

COMPLICATIONS
- Renal and hepatic failure, encephalopathy, coagulopathy, secondary infection, iatrogenic infection, abscess, fistula formation, abdominal compartment syndrome
- Sepsis/septic shock, cardiovascular collapse, adrenal insufficiency, respiratory failure, ARDS

REFERENCES
1. MacIntosh T. Emergency management of spontaneous bacterial peritonitis—a clinical review. *Cureus*. 2018;10(3):e2253.
2. Dever JB, Sheikh MY. Review article: spontaneous bacterial peritonitis—bacteriology, diagnosis, treatment, risk factors and prevention. *Aliment Pharmacol Ther*. 2015;41(11):1116–1131.
3. Li PK, Szeto CC, Piraino B, et al. ISPD peritonitis recommendations: 2016 update on prevention and treatment. *Perit Dial Int*. 2016;36(5):481–508.

ADDITIONAL READING
- Aithal GP, Palaniyappan N, China L, et al. Guidelines on the management of ascites in cirrhosis. *Gut*. 2021;70(1):9–29.
- Popoiag RE, Fierbințeanu-Braticevici C. Spontaneous bacterial peritonitis: update on diagnosis and treatment. *Rom J Intern Med*. 2021;59(4):345–350.

 SEE ALSO

Appendicitis, Acute; Cirrhosis of the Liver; Diverticular Disease; Peptic Ulcer Disease

 CODES

ICD10
- K65.0 Generalized (acute) peritonitis
- K65.2 Spontaneous bacterial peritonitis
- K65.8 Other peritonitis

CLINICAL PEARLS
- Maintain a high index of suspicion for SBP in cirrhotic patients with ascites (up to 30% of cases may be asymptomatic) and start empiric therapy early.
- SBP is usually monomicrobial. Paracentesis is necessary to diagnose.
- *E. coli* is the most common bacterial isolate from cases of SBP. 3rd-generation cephalosporins are first-line treatment.
- Ascitic fluid analysis stratifies patients at risk for secondary peritonitis who need additional imaging.
- Renal function is an important prognostic indicator for SBP.

PERTUSSIS

Mary E. Cataletto, MD, FAAP, FCCP • Margaret J. McCormick, MS, RN, CNE

 BASICS

- Highly contagious among close contacts
- Synonyms: whooping cough, "100 day cough"

DESCRIPTION

- Host: humans
- Most common reservoir: adults
- Ages: all
- Distribution: worldwide
- Pattern: endemic or epidemic with outbreaks every 3 to 5 years (1)
- Seasonality: peaks late summer–autumn; can occur year-round
- Transmission: person to person via aerosolized droplets (1)
- Typical incubation period: 7 to 10 days (1)
- Effective vaccine: available
- Immunity: neither 100% nor lifelong immunity with either infection or vaccine (1)
- System(s) affected: respiratory

EPIDEMIOLOGY

Incidence
- United States (2012 most recent peak year): 48,277 cases reported (2)
- Worldwide: 24.1 million cases and about 160,700 deaths per year (2)

ETIOLOGY AND PATHOPHYSIOLOGY
- Toxin mediated
- Infectious process with predilection for ciliated respiratory epithelium
- Common organisms:
  - *Bordetella pertussis*
  - *Bordetella parapertussis*

Genetics
No known genetic predisposition

RISK FACTORS
- Exposure to a confirmed case
- Non- or underimmunized infants and children
- Premature birth
- Chronic lung disease
- Immunodeficiency (e.g., AIDS)
- Age <6 months (accounts for ~90% pediatric pertussis hospitalizations) (3)

GENERAL PREVENTION
- Public health measures
  - Surveillance
  - Outbreak management
  - Care of exposed individuals
- Prevention programs

- Immunizations (4)
  - Primary childhood immunization series against pertussis followed by boosters
  - Maternal immunization during each pregnancy
  - Adults, including health care providers in close contact with infants <1 year of age, should be immunized.

Pediatric Considerations
Strategies to reduce neonatal pertussis (1):
- Tdap with each pregnancy, ideally between 27 and 36 weeks' gestation
- Cocooning
- Tdap recommended for all persons in close contact with infants <1 year of age

Geriatric Considerations
Older adults are at increased risk for pertussis complications due to (5):
- Age-related changes in immunity
- Comorbid medical conditions

COMMONLY ASSOCIATED CONDITIONS
- Apnea in infants
- Secondary bacterial pneumonia
- Sinusitis
- Seizures
- Encephalopathy
- Urinary incontinence

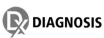 DIAGNOSIS

HISTORY
- Exposure to pertussis
- Insidious onset
- Incubation period 7 to 10 days (range 5 to 21 days)

PHYSICAL EXAM
- Classic pertussis has three phases, which occur over 6 to 10 weeks (6):
  - Catarrhal phase: rhinorrhea, mild cough, and low-grade fever
  - Paroxysmal phase: Cough occurs in bursts, with increased frequency and intensity, often followed by an inspiratory whoop and/or posttussive vomiting.
  - Convalescent phase: Coughing paroxysms decrease in frequency and intensity.
- Classic presentation is more common in adults and unvaccinated children.

ALERT
- In the absence of paroxysms or complications, the physical exam may be normal.
- Infants <6 months of age may have atypical presentations.

DIFFERENTIAL DIAGNOSIS
Sporadic, prolonged cough can also be caused by:
- *B. parapertussis*
- *Mycoplasma pneumoniae*
- *Chlamydia trachomatis*
- *Chlamydophila* pneumonia
- *Bordetella bronchiseptica*
- *Bordetella holmesii*
- Respiratory syncytial virus
- Adenovirus

DIAGNOSTIC TESTS & INTERPRETATION
Initial Tests (lab, imaging)
- Nasopharyngeal culture (gold standard): best results within 2 weeks of cough onset (6)[A]
- False results can occur in:
  - Previously immunized individuals
  - After initiation of appropriate antibiotic
  - After 2 weeks from cough onset
  - With incorrect collection or handling
- Polymerase chain reaction (PCR) assays: rapid turnaround time; good within first 3 weeks
- Serology:
  - Commercially available assay
  - Not FDA-approved for diagnosis

Follow-Up Tests & Special Considerations
- Evaluation and follow-up for associated conditions and complications
- Chest radiograph (two views) to evaluate for the presence of pneumonia
- EEG/neuroimaging may be considered in infant with seizure or apparent life-threatening events (ALTEs).
- Infants <1 month of age who are treated with macrolides should be monitored for the possible development of hypertrophic pyloric stenosis.

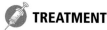 TREATMENT

GENERAL MEASURES
- Hospitalization with continuous cardiopulmonary monitoring is recommended for neonates with pertussis.
- Supplemental oxygen and/or mechanical ventilatory support may be needed.

MEDICATION
- Start empiric antibiotic therapy once diagnostic testing is performed in cases with strong clinical suspicion or in those at high risk for complications.
- Antibiotic therapy after cough is established may help to limit spread but is not expected to change clinical symptoms.

- Preferred antibiotics:
  - For patients >6 months:
    - Azithromycin, clarithromycin, or erythromycin
  - For infants <1 month of age, azithromycin is preferred but with caution (6)[A].

First Line
Azithromycin is the first line for treatment and for postexposure prophylaxis (5-day course) (6)[A].

ALERT
- Infantile hypertrophic pyloric stenosis has been associated with the use of macrolides in infants <1 month of age.
- Consultation and monitoring are recommended.

ALERT
- *Fatal cardiac dysrhythmias* have been reported with azithromycin.
- Caution is recommended in individuals with prolonged QT and proarrhythmic conditions.

Second Line
Trimethoprim/sulfamethoxazole (TMX/SMX) (for persons >2 months of age) if:
- Macrolide intolerance
- Macrolide resistance

ALERT
- TMP/SMX is *contraindicated* in infants <2 months of age.
- Clarithromycin is not recommended in infants <1 month of age.

ISSUES FOR REFERRAL
Evaluation and treatment of infants <6 months of age, especially those born prematurely, who are unimmunized and those who require hospitalization

ADDITIONAL THERAPIES
Symptomatic treatment of the cough in pertussis (e.g., corticosteroids, β_2-adrenergic agonists) has not shown consistent benefit (7).

ADMISSION, INPATIENT, AND NURSING CONSIDERATIONS
- Small, frequent meals may be necessary to ensure adequate nutrition.
- IV fluids indicated for dehydration and when oral fluids are either contraindicated or poorly tolerated
- In addition to standard precautions, hospitalized patients should be isolated with respiratory precautions for 5 days after the initiation of effective antibiotic treatment and for 3 weeks after the onset of paroxysms in older patients if antibiotics are not used.
- Gentle suctioning of nasal secretions
- Avoid stimuli that trigger paroxysms.
- Respiratory monitoring, including pulse oximetry
- Educate each family about the importance of immunization.
- Discuss chemoprophylaxis with each family.

ONGOING CARE
Supportive

FOLLOW-UP RECOMMENDATIONS
- Monitor infants who received EES or azithromycin for hypotrophic pyloric stenosis.
- Neurologic and/or pulmonary follow-up as necessary

Patient Monitoring
ICU care may be necessary for severely ill or compromised patients.

DIET
IV fluids/nutrition may be required to treat dehydration or supplement poor oral intake.

PATIENT EDUCATION
- American Academy of Pediatrics: http://www.aap.org
- Centers for Disease Control and Prevention: http://www.cdc.gov

PROGNOSIS
- Complete recovery in most cases
- Most severe morbidity and highest mortality in infants <6 months of age
- Worldwide overall mortality estimated at 160,799 deaths/year (2)

COMPLICATIONS
- Highest and most severe in infants; may include apnea, cyanosis, and sudden death
- In children: may include conjunctival hemorrhage, inguinal hernia, pneumonia, and seizures
- More frequent in adults than adolescents: may include sinusitis, otitis media, pneumonia, weight loss, fainting, rib fracture, urinary incontinence, seizures, and encephalopathy

REFERENCES
1. Daniels HL, Sabella C. *Bordetella pertussis* (Pertussis). *Pediatr Rev.* 2018;39(5):247–257.
2. Centers for Disease Control and Prevention. Pertussis fast facts. https://www.cdc.gov/pertussis/fast-facts.html. Accessed September 4, 2020.
3. Lopez MA, Cruz AT, Kowalkowski MA, et al. Trends in hospitalizations and resource utilization for pediatric pertussis. *Hosp Pediatr.* 2014;4(5):269–275.
4. Liang JL, Tiwari T, Moro P, et al. Prevention of pertussis, tetanus, and diphtheria with vaccines in the united states: recommendations of the Advisory Committee on Immunization Practices (ACIP). *MMWR Recomm Rep.* 2018;67(2):1–44.
5. Burke M, Rowe T. Vaccinations in older adults. *Clin Geriatr Med.* 2018;34(1):131–143.
6. Committee on Infectious Diseases. Pertussis (whooping cough). In: Kimberlin DW, Brady DW, Jackson MA, eds. *Red Book: 2018–2021 Report of the Committee on Infectious Diseases.* 31st ed. Itasca, IL: American Academy of Pediatrics; 2018:620–634.
7. Polinori I, Esposito S. Clinical findings and management of pertussis. *Adv Exp Med Biol.* 2019;1183:151–160.

CODES

ICD10
- A37.10 Whooping cough due to Bordetella parapertussis without pneumonia
- A37 Whooping cough
- A37.91 Whooping cough, unspecified species with pneumonia

CLINICAL PEARLS
- Hospitalizations for pertussis is highest in infants <6 months of age.
  - Maternal Tdap is effective in protecting young infants against pertussis, especially during first 2 months of life.
- Neither immunization nor active infection confers lifelong immunity.

PHARYNGITIS
Pratha Muthiah, MD, MPH

BASICS

DESCRIPTION
- Synonym(s): sore throat; tonsillitis; "strep throat"
- Acute or chronic inflammation of the pharyngeal mucosa and underlying structures of the throat
- Group A *Streptococcus* (GAS) pharyngitis is notable for preventable suppurative (e.g., retropharyngeal or peritonsillar abscess) and nonsuppurative (e.g., rheumatic sequelae) complications.

EPIDEMIOLOGY
- ~15 million cases are diagnosed yearly.
- Accounts for 1–2% of all outpatient visits and 6% of all pediatric visits to primary care physicians
- Most commonly viral (40–60% of cases)
- GAS is the most common bacterial cause of acute pharyngitis, accounting for 15–30% of pediatric and 5–15% of adult cases. The incubation period ranges from 24 to 72 hours.
- Rheumatic fever is a serious sequela, but is rare in the United States (<1 case per 100,000). Early antibiotic use has diminished occurrence.
- 3,000 to 4,000 patients with group A β-hemolytic streptococcal infection must be treated to prevent one case of acute rheumatic fever.
- Affects all age groups; some etiologies and sequelae occur more frequently in certain age groups.

Pediatric Considerations
The highest incidence of rheumatic fever is in children 5 to 18 years as a rare sequela of streptococcal pharyngitis.

ETIOLOGY AND PATHOPHYSIOLOGY
- Acute, viral (associated with lower grade fever)
  - Rhinovirus; adenovirus (associated with conjunctivitis); parainfluenza virus; coxsackievirus (hand-foot-mouth disease); coronavirus; echovirus
  - Herpes simplex virus (HSV) (vesicular lesions); Epstein-Barr virus (EBV/mononucleosis); cytomegalovirus (CMV)
  - HIV
- Acute, bacterial (associated with higher fevers)
  - Group A β-hemolytic streptococcus
  - *Neisseria gonorrhoeae*; *Corynebacterium diphtheriae* (diphtheria); *Haemophilus influenzae*
  - *Moraxella catarrhalis*; *Chlamydia pneumonia*
  - *Fusobacterium necrophorum* (20% young adult cases); Group C or G *Streptococcus*
  - *Arcanobacterium haemolyticum*; *Mycoplasma pneumoniae*; *Francisella tularensis* (tularemia)
- Acute, noninfectious
  - Various caustic, mechanical, or trauma-related (including endotracheal intubation)
- Chronic, more likely noninfectious
  - Chemical irritation (GERD)
  - Smoking
  - Neoplasms
  - Vasculitis
  - Radiation changes

Genetics
Patients with a family history of rheumatic fever have a higher risk of rheumatic sequelae following an untreated group A β-hemolytic streptococcal infection.

RISK FACTORS
- Epidemics of group A β-hemolytic streptococcal disease
- Cold and flu season (late fall through early spring)
- Age (rheumatic fever possible, especially in children/adolescents 5 to 15 years)
- Close contact with infected individuals (home, daycare, military barracks)
- Immunosuppression
- Smoking/secondhand smoke exposure
- Acid reflux
- Oral sex
- Diabetes mellitus
- Recent illness (secondary postviral bacterial infection)
- Chronic colonization of bacteria in tonsils/adenoids

GENERAL PREVENTION
- Avoid close contact with infectious patients.
- Wash hands frequently.
- Avoid first- or secondhand smoke.
- Manage preventable causes (e.g., GERD).

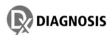

DIAGNOSIS

HISTORY
- Sore throat
- Difficulty swallowing (dysphagia) or pain on swallowing (odynophagia)
- Cough (uncommon in GAS pharyngitis)
- Hoarseness; "hot potato" voice
- Fever
- Anorexia
- Chills
- Malaise; fatigue
- Headache
- Dysuria and arthralgias (suggest gonococcal etiology)
- Sick contacts with similar symptoms or confirmed diagnosis

PHYSICAL EXAM
- Enlarged tonsils with or without exudate
- Pharyngeal erythema; palatal petechiae
- Unilateral tonsillar swelling ("frog's belly") or uvular deviation (concern for peritonsillar abscess)
- Trismus; stridor; drooling (concern for peritonsillar or retropharyngeal abscess)
- Cervical adenopathy (anterior suggestive of GAS, posterior most commonly associated with infectious mononucleosis)
- Fever (higher in bacterial infections)
- Pharyngeal ulcers (CMV, HIV, Crohn, other autoimmune vasculitides)
- Scarlet fever rash: Punctate erythematous macules with reddened flexor creases and circumoral pallor suggests streptococcal pharyngitis.
- Tonsillar/soft palate petechiae with hepatosplenomegaly suggest infectious mononucleosis (EBV/CMV).
- Gray oral pseudomembrane suggests diphtheria and occasionally infectious mononucleosis (EBV/CMV).
- Characteristic erythematous-based clear vesicles suggest HSV or coxsackie A virus infection (herpangina).
- Conjunctivitis suggests adenovirus.

DIFFERENTIAL DIAGNOSIS
- Viral infection
- Streptococcal infection
- Allergic rhinitis/postnasal drip
- GERD
- Malignancy (lymphoma or squamous cell carcinoma)
- Irritants/chemicals (detergent/caustic ingestion)
- Atypical bacterial (e.g., gonococcal, chlamydial, syphilis, pertussis, diphtheria)
- Oral candidiasis (Patients typically complain mostly of dysphagia.)
- Thyroiditis (can be painful or painless, possibly associated with hyperthyroid syndrome)
- Epiglottitis (associated with stridor, drooling, and progressive respiratory distress)

DIAGNOSTIC TESTS & INTERPRETATION
- Prediction rules determine need for further testing (see below).
- Additional testing generally not needed if viral-like clinical features (e.g., cough, rhinorrhea, hoarseness, oral ulcers, diarrhea, conjunctivitis, rash) (1)[A]
- Avoid testing for GAS pharyngitis in children <3 years as acute rheumatic flare is rare, unless there is a close sick contact who is GAS-positive (1)[B].
- Modified Centor clinical prediction rule for group A streptococcal infection (2)[A]:
  - +1 point: tonsillar exudates
  - +1 point: tender anterior chain cervical adenopathy
  - +1 point: absence of cough
  - +1 point: fever by history
  - +1 point: age <15 years
  - 0 point: age 15 to 45 years
  - −1 point: age >45 years
- Scoring:
  - If 4 points, positive predictive value of ~80%; treat empirically.
  - If 2 to 3 points, positive predictive value of ~50%, rapid strep antigen; treat if GAS-positive.
  - If 0 or 1 point, positive predictive value <20%; do not test; treat symptomatically with follow-up as needed.

Initial Tests (lab, imaging)
- Testing, if performed, is usually for GAS. Options include:
  - Rapid antigen streptococcus test (RAST); quick adjunct to throat culture with 96% specificity and 86% sensitivity (although sensitivity varies by modality kit) (3)[A]
  - Blood agar throat culture from swab; gold standard—90–95% sensitivity (3)[A]
    - Back up throat cultures are not needed for adults with negative RAST. They are recommended for children with negative RAST due to the higher likelihood of complications but can be omitted if a highly sensitive immunoassay or molecular test was used.
  - Antistreptolysin O (suspect carrier state if positive culture, and unchanged ASO titers)
- Special tests if history suggests a different diagnosis
  - Warm Thayer-Martin plate or antigen testing for *N. gonorrhoeae*
  - Viral cultures for HSV
  - Monospot for EBV
  - IgM serology for CMV

Follow-Up Tests & Special Considerations
Recurrent GAS infection may indicate β-lactamase production by host, may require antibiotic with anti-β-lactamase activity.

Test Interpretation
Bacitracin disk sensitivity of hemolytic colonies suggests group A β-hemolytic streptococcus.

TREATMENT

Treatment is largely for symptomatic relief, unless bacterial infection is confirmed or highly suspected.

GENERAL MEASURES
Conservative therapy recommended for most cases (unless bacterial etiology suspected):
- Salt water gargles
- Acetaminophen 10 to 15 mg/kg/dose q4h PRN pain or fever (pediatric). In adults, do not exceed >3 g/day.
- Nonsteroidal anti-inflammatory drugs (NSAIDs) for pain or fever (more effective than acetaminophen for GAS pharyngitis)
- Anesthetic lozenges
- Cool-mist humidifier
- Hydration (PO or IV if PO is not tolerated)
- Viscous lidocaine (2%) 5 to 10 mL PO q4h swish/spit (severe pain)

Pediatric Considerations
- Opioids not recommended due to black box warnings
- Lower threshold to start antibiotics due to higher risk of rheumatic fever
- Avoid aspirin for symptom relief in pediatric patients due to risk of Reye syndrome.

MEDICATION
- Antibiotics (particularly penicillin) are used primarily to prevent complications.
  - 60–70% primary care visits by children with pharyngitis result in antibiotic prescriptions (4). Empiric therapy results in antibiotic overuse.
  - Treatment duration generally 10 days (1)[A]
  - Antibiotics do not reduce risk of poststreptococcal glomerulonephritis.
  - Antibiotics shorten duration of symptoms by approximately 16 hours (5).
  - Antibiotics may prevent pharyngitis/fever by day 3 (NNT 4 if GAS-positive, 6.5 if GAS-negative, 14.4 if untested) (5)[A].
- Ulcers related to autoimmune diseases usually require systemic or intralesional injectable steroids.
- HIV-related ulcers are due to decreasing counts of CD4 and respond when patients' CD4 titers increase.
- Corticosteroids, when used concomitantly with antibiotics, may provide a small reduction in the duration of symptoms (24 hours). Routine use is not currently recommended (1)[B],(3)[B].

First Line
Recommended first-line therapies (1)[A]:
- Penicillin V: children (<27 kg): 250 mg PO TID (BID dosing sufficient if good compliance); adolescents and adults (>27 kg): 250 mg PO QID or 500 mg PO BID
- Penicillin G benzathine: children <60 lb (27 kg): 600,000 units IM 1 dose; children ≥60 lb and adults: 1.2 million units IM 1 dose
- Amoxicillin: 50 mg/kg PO once daily (max 1,000 mg/dose or 25 mg/kg PO BID (max = 500 mg/dose)

ALERT
Use with caution if diagnosis is unclear because using amoxicillin with EBV infection may induce rash.

Second Line
- If type IV hypersensitivity but no history of anaphylactic penicillin allergy:
  - Cephalexin 20 mg/kg PO BID or (children) 25 to 50 mg/kg/day divided BID or (adults) 1,000 mg PO QID (max = 4 g/day)
  - Cefadroxil 30 mg/kg PO once daily (max = 1 g/day)
- If history of anaphylactic penicillin allergy (type I hypersensitivity):
  - Azithromycin 12 mg/kg PO once daily for 5 days (max = 500 mg/dose)
  - Clarithromycin 7.5 mg/kg PO BID (max = 250 mg/dose) or (adults) 250 to 500 mg PO BID
  - Clindamycin 7 mg/kg PO TID (max = 300 mg/dose) or (children) 10 to 30 mg/kg/day PO divided TID–QID or (adults) 150 to 450 mg PO TID–QID
- Penicillin is most commonly used to prevent rheumatic sequelae; cephalosporins have a lower rate of antimicrobial failure for streptococcal pharyngitis.
- Newer macrolides are effective against streptococcal pharyngitis; they are also more expensive and unproven at preventing rheumatic complications.
- Macrolide-resistant strains of GAS are currently <10% in the United States but more prevalent worldwide.

ISSUES FOR REFERRAL
- Document each GAS-confirmed episode to support the need for future tonsillectomy and adenoidectomy.
- Tonsillectomy is recommended for patients who have had seven or more throat infections (viral or bacterial) in 1 year, five or more infections per year for the past 2 years, or three or more infections per year for the past 3 years. Tonsillectomy is also recommended in patients who are difficult to treat medically, including those who are allergic to multiple antibiotics.

ONGOING CARE

FOLLOW-UP RECOMMENDATIONS
- Complete the full course of antibiotic therapy, regardless of symptom response.
- Patients are generally noninfectious after 24 hours of antibiotics.
- Follow-up culture for GAS is not recommended (1)[A].

DIET
As tolerated. Encourage the consumption of fluids.

PROGNOSIS
- Streptococcal pharyngitis runs a 5- to 7-day course with peak fever at 2 to 3 days.
- Symptoms will resolve spontaneously without treatment, but rheumatic complications are still possible.

COMPLICATIONS
- Rheumatic fever (e.g., carditis, valve disease, arthritis)
- Poststreptococcal glomerulonephritis
- Peritonsillar abscess (a.k.a. quinsy tonsillitis): considered a clinical diagnosis and does not warrant ultrasound/computed tomography. Will generally require percutaneous/transoral drainage. Surgery may also involve a quinsy (acute) tonsillectomy. Most sources recommend resolution of the acute infection before surgery.

- Acute airway compromise (rare) can typically be bypassed with nasal trumpets. Consult anesthesiologist/otolaryngologist.
- Repeated episodes of GAS pharyngitis may represent recurrent viral infections in a chronic pharyngeal GAS carrier (1)[B]. IDSA recommends against repeated diagnostic efforts/antibiotic therapy in a known chronic pharyngeal GAS carrier, as they are seldom contagious or at risk for serious complications.

REFERENCES

1. Shulman ST, Bisno AL, Clegg HW, et al. Clinical practice guideline for the diagnosis and management of group A streptococcal pharyngitis: 2012 update by the Infectious Diseases Society of America. *Clin Infect Dis.* 2012;55(10):1279–1282.
2. Fine AM, Nizet V, Mandl KD. Large-scale validation of the Centor and McIsaac scores to predict group A streptococcal pharyngitis. *Arch Intern Med.* 2012;172(11):847–852.
3. Sauve L, Forrester AM, Top KA. Group A streptococcal pharyngitis: a practical guide to diagnosis and treatment. *Paediatr Child Health.* 2021;26(5):319–320.
4. Robinson JL. Paediatrics: how to manage pharyngitis in an era of increasing antimicrobial resistance. *Drugs Context.* 2021;10:2020-11-6.
5. Spinks A, Glasziou PP, Del Mar CB. Antibiotics for sore throat. *Cochrane Database Syst Rev.* 2013;2013(11):CD000023.

ADDITIONAL READING

Baugh RF, Archer SM, Mitchell RB, et al; American Academy of Otolaryngology-Head and Neck Surgery Foundation. Clinical practice guideline: tonsillectomy in children. *Otolaryngol Head Neck Surg.* 2011;144(1 Suppl):S1–S30.

 SEE ALSO

- Herpes Simplex; Infectious Mononucleosis, Epstein-Barr Virus Infections; Rheumatic Fever
- Algorithm: Pharyngitis

 CODES

ICD10
- J31.1 Chronic nasopharyngitis
- A54.5 Gonococcal pharyngitis
- B08.5 Enteroviral vesicular pharyngitis

CLINICAL PEARLS

- Most cases of pharyngitis are viral and do not require antibiotics.
- The risk associated with undiagnosed and untreated group A streptococcal infection is for rheumatic sequelae—a rare complication.
- Use of the Modified Centor Score helps to guide testing and treatment.
- Penicillin is the preferred first-line therapy for group A streptococcal infection.

PILONIDAL DISEASE

Tam T. Nguyen, MD

 BASICS

DESCRIPTION
- Pilonidal disease results from an abscess, or sinus tract, in the upper part of the natal (gluteal) cleft.
- Synonym(s): jeep disease

EPIDEMIOLOGY

Incidence
- 16 to 26/100,000 per year
- Predominant sex: male > female (3 to 4:1)
- Predominant age: 2nd to 3rd decade, rare >45 years
- Ethnic consideration: whites > blacks > Asians

Prevalence
Surgical procedures show male: female ratio of 4:1, yet incidence data are 10:1.

ETIOLOGY AND PATHOPHYSIOLOGY
Pilonidal means "nest of hair"; hair in the natal cleft allows hair to be drawn into the deeper tissues via negative pressure caused by movement of the buttocks (50%); follicular occlusion from stretching and blocking of pores with debris (50%) creating a pilonidal cyst
- Inflammation of SC gluteal tissues with secondary infection and sinus tract formation
- Polymicrobial, likely from enteric pathogens given proximity to anorectal contamination

Genetics
- Congenital dimple in the natal cleft/spina bifida occulta
- Follicular-occluding tetrad: acne conglobata, dissecting cellulitis, hidradenitis suppurativa, pilonidal

RISK FACTORS
- Sedentary/prolonged sitting
- Excessive body hair
- Obesity/increased sacrococcygeal fold thickness
- Congenital natal dimple
- Trauma to coccyx

GENERAL PREVENTION
- Weight loss
- Trim hair in/around gluteal cleft weekly.
- Hygiene
- Ingrown hair prevention/follicle unblocking

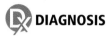 **DIAGNOSIS**

HISTORY
Three distinct clinical presentations
- Asymptomatic: painless cyst or sinus at the top of the gluteal cleft; fever is rare.
- Acute abscess: severe pain, swelling, discharge from the top of the gluteal cleft that may or may not have drained spontaneously
- Chronic abscess: persistent drainage from a sinus tract at the top of the gluteal cleft

PHYSICAL EXAM
- Common: inflamed cystic mass at the top of the gluteal cleft with limited surrounding erythema ± drainage or a sinus tract
- Inflamed sinus accompanied with one or more pits with or without hair debris
- Less common: significant cellulitis of the surrounding tissues near the gluteal cleft

DIFFERENTIAL DIAGNOSIS
- Furunculosis or folliculitis
- Hidradenitis suppurativa
- Anal fistula
- Perirectal abscess
- Crohn disease

DIAGNOSTIC TESTS & INTERPRETATION
Generally no tests are needed since can diagnose clinically.

Initial Tests (lab, imaging)
- Consider CBC and wound culture but generally not necessary for less severe infections.
- Ultrasound or MRI might be considered to differentiate between perirectal abscess and pilonidal disease.

Follow-Up Tests & Special Considerations
None

Diagnostic Procedures/Other
Wound culture if infection is suspected

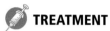 **TREATMENT**

GENERAL MEASURES
Shave area; remove hair from crypts weekly.

MEDICATION
- Antibiotics not indicated unless there is significant cellulitis (1)
- If antibiotics are needed, a culture to direct therapy might be useful.
- Cefazolin plus metronidazole or amoxicillin-clavulanate are often used empirically if cellulitis is suspected.

ISSUES FOR REFERRAL
- Patients who cannot comply with frequent dressing changes required after incision and drainage (I&D)
- Patients who have recurrence after I&D
- Patients who have complex disease with multiple sinus tracts

ADDITIONAL THERAPIES
- I&D with only enough packing to allow the cyst to drain; overpacking not indicated
- Antibiotics only if significant cellulitis; temporizing, not curative
- Negative pressure wound therapy

- Laser epilation of hair in the gluteal fold (2)[B]
- Phenol treatment can be used, especially for recurring disease.

SURGERY/OTHER PROCEDURES
- Several surgical techniques have proposed with limited data on superiority of one over another.
- Six levels of care based on severity or recurrence of disease; recent innovations in technique are aimed at expediting healing and minimizing recurrence.
  - I&D, remove hair, curette granulation tissue (3)[A]
  - Excision of midline "pits" allows drainage of lateral sinus tracts (pit picking).
  - Pilonidal cystotomy: Insert probe into sinus tract, excise overlying skin, and close wound (4)[B].
  - Marsupialization: Excise overlying skin and roof of cyst, and suture skin edges to cyst floor (3),(5)[B].
  - Excision: use of flap closure; no clear benefit for open healing over surgical closure
  - Off-midline surgical excision (cleft lift or modified Karydakis procedure): A systematic review showed a clear benefit in favor of off-midline rather than midline wound closure. When closure of pilonidal sinuses is the desired surgical option, off-midline closure should be the standard management (3)[A].
  - Endoscopic pilonidal sinus treatment (EPSiT): minimally invasive procedure (6)

ADMISSION, INPATIENT, AND NURSING CONSIDERATIONS
- Severe cellulitis
- Large area excision

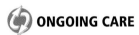 **ONGOING CARE**

FOLLOW-UP RECOMMENDATIONS
- Frequent dressing changes required after I&D
- Follow-up wound checks to assess for recurrence

Patient Monitoring
Monitor for fever; more extensive cellulitis

PATIENT EDUCATION
- Wash area briskly with washcloth daily.
- Shave the area weekly.
- Remove any embedded hair from the crypt.
- Avoid prolonged sitting.

PROGNOSIS
- Simple I&D has a 55% failure rate; median time to healing is 5 weeks.
- More extensive surgical excisions involve hospital stays and longer time to heal.

COMPLICATIONS
Malignant degeneration is a rare complication of untreated chronic pilonidal disease.

REFERENCES
1. Mavros MN, Mitsikostas PK, Alexiou VG, et al. Antimicrobials as an adjunct to pilonidal disease surgery: a systematic review of the literature. *Eur J Clin Microbiol Infect Dis*. 2013;32(7):851–858.
2. Loganathan A, Arsalani Zadeh R, Hartley J. Pilonidal disease: time to reevaluate a common pain in the rear! *Dis Colon Rectum*. 2012;55(4):491–493.
3. Humphries AE, Duncan JE. Evaluation and management of pilonidal disease. *Surg Clin North Am*. 2010;90(1):113–124.
4. da Silva JH. Pilonidal cyst: cause and treatment. *Dis Colon Rectum*. 2000;43(8):1146–1156.
5. Aydede H, Erhan Y, Sakarya A, et al. Comparison of three methods in surgical treatment of pilonidal disease. *ANZ J Surg*. 2001;71(6):362–364.
6. Meinero P, Stazi A, Carbone A, et al. Endoscopic pilonidal sinus treatment: a prospective multicentre trial. *Colorectal Dis*. 2016;18(5):O164–O170.

ADDITIONAL READING
- Aygen E, Arslan K, Dogru O, et al. Crystallized phenol in nonoperative treatment of previously operated, recurrent pilonidal disease. *Dis Colon Rectum*. 2010;53(6):932–935.
- Bradley L. Pilonidal sinus disease: a review. Part one. *J Wound Care*. 2010;19(11):504–508.
- Harlak A, Mentes O, Kilic S, et al. Sacrococcygeal pilonidal disease: analysis of previously proposed risk factors. *Clinics (Sao Paulo)*. 2010;65(2):125–131.
- Rao MM, Zawislak W, Kennedy R, et al. A prospective randomised study comparing two treatment modalities for chronic pilonidal sinus with a 5-year follow-up. *Int J Colorectal Dis*. 2010;25(3):395–400.
- Theodoropoulos GE, Vlahos K, Lazaris AC, et al. Modified Bascom's asymmetric midgluteal cleft closure technique for recurrent pilonidal disease: early experience in a military hospital. *Dis Colon Rectum*. 2003;46(9):1286–1291.

 CODES

ICD10
- L05.91 Pilonidal cyst without abscess
- L05.92 Pilonidal sinus without abscess
- L05.01 Pilonidal cyst with abscess

CLINICAL PEARLS
- Avoid prolonged sitting.
- Lose weight.
- Trim hair in gluteal cleft weekly.
- Refer recurring infections for more definitive surgical management.

PINWORMS

Jonathan Edward MacClements, MD, FAAFP

BASICS

DESCRIPTION
- Intestinal infection with *Enterobius vermicularis*
  - Characterized by perineal and perianal itching
  - Usually worse at night
- System(s) affected: gastrointestinal; skin/exocrine
- Synonym(s): enterobiasis

EPIDEMIOLOGY
Predominant age: 5 to 14 years

Prevalence
- Most common helminthic infection in the United States
  - 20 to 42 million people harbor the parasite.
- ~30% of children are infected worldwide.

Pediatric Considerations
More common in children, who are more likely to become reinfected

ETIOLOGY AND PATHOPHYSIOLOGY
- Small white worms (2 to 13 mm) inhabit the cecum, appendix, and adjacent portions of the ascending colon following ingestion.
- Female worms migrate to the perineal areas at night to deposit eggs; this causes local irritation and itching.
- Scratching leads to autoingestion of the eggs and continuation of pinworm's life cycle within the host. Eggs incubate 1 to 2 months in the host small intestine. When mature, female pinworms migrate to the colon where they lay eggs around the anus at night, and the lifecycle continues.
- Infestation by the intestinal nematode *E. vermicularis* (1)

RISK FACTORS
- Institutionalization (prevalence over 50%)
- Crowded living conditions
- Poor hygiene

- Warm climate
- Handling of infected children's clothing or bedding

GENERAL PREVENTION
- Hand hygiene, especially after bowel movements
- Clip and maintain short fingernails.
- Wash anus and genitals at least once a day, preferably during shower.
- Avoid scratching anus and putting fingers near nose (pinworm eggs can also be inhaled) or mouth.

COMMONLY ASSOCIATED CONDITIONS
Pruritus ani

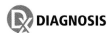

DIAGNOSIS

HISTORY
Many patients are asymptomatic. Common symptoms include the following:
- Perianal or perineal itching
- Vulvovaginitis
- Dysuria
- Abdominal pain (rare)
- Insomnia (typically due to pruritus)

PHYSICAL EXAM
Perineal and perianal exam; particularly in early morning to look for evidence of migrating worms

DIFFERENTIAL DIAGNOSIS
- Idiopathic pruritus ani
- Atopic dermatitis, contact dermatitis
- Psoriasis; lichen planus
- Human papillomavirus (HPV)
- Herpes simplex virus (HSV)
- Fungal infections; erythrasma
- Scabies
- Vaginitis; hemorrhoids
- Chron disease; ulcerative colitis

DIAGNOSTIC TESTS & INTERPRETATION
- Adhesive tape test
  - Place cellophane tape on the perianal skin in the early morning before bathing and affix to a microscope slide to look for pinworm eggs.
  - 90% sensitivity if performed on three consecutive mornings
  - Alternatively, use anal swabs or a pinworm paddle coated with adhesive material.
  - Scrapings from under fingernails of affected individuals can reveal pinworm eggs.
- Digital rectal exam with saline slide preparation of stool on gloved finger
- Stool samples are not helpful.
- *Routine stool examination for ova and parasites is positive in only 10–15% of infected patients.*

Initial Tests (lab, imaging)
Serologic tests are currently not available for diagnosing pinworm infections.

Test Interpretation
Identification of ova on low-power microscopy or direct visualization of the female worm (10 mm long); ova are asymmetric, flat on one side, and measure $56 \times 27\ \mu$m.

TREATMENT

MEDICATION
First Line
- Treatment options include:
  - Albendazole (Albenza): 400 mg PO as a single dose in adults and children >20 kg; may repeat in 2 weeks; 200 mg PO as a single dose repeated in 2 weeks in children ≤20 kg (1)[A]
  - Mebendazole (Emverm, Vermox): chewable 100-mg tablet as a single dose in adults and children >2 years of age; may repeat in 2 to 3 weeks; use with caution in children <2 years of age (1)[A].

– Pyrantel pamoate (Pin-X, Reese Pinworm Medicine): oral liquid or tablet 11 mg/kg as a single dose in adults and children >2 years of age; maximum dose 1 g. Use with caution in children <2 years of age (1)[A].

- Repeat treatment after 2 weeks is often recommended due to the high frequency of reinfection. Refractory cases may (rarely) require retreatment every 2 weeks for 4 to 6 cycles.
- All symptomatic family members should be treated.

Pregnancy Considerations
Avoid drug therapy in pregnancy as all three drugs are FDA pregnancy Category C. Treat after delivery but may consider treating in 3rd trimester if infection is compromising the pregnancy. Breastfeeding is allowed during mebendazole therapy (1)[A].

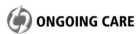 **ONGOING CARE**

FOLLOW-UP RECOMMENDATIONS
Unnecessary unless symptoms recur after initial therapy

PATIENT EDUCATION
- Take medicine with food.
- Practice good hygiene: hand washing and perianal hygiene; particularly after bowel movements
- Encourage frequent and careful hand washing.
- Clip fingernails.
- Wash clothing and bedding after diagnosis to prevent reinfection. Do not shake linen and clothing before laundering because this may spread the eggs.
- Do not share washcloths.
- Do not allow children to cobathe during treatment and for 2 weeks after treatment; showering is preferred.

PROGNOSIS
- Asymptomatic carriers are common.
- Drug therapy is 90% curative.
- Reinfection is common, especially among children.

COMPLICATIONS
- Perianal scratching may lead to bacterial superinfection.
- Females: vulvovaginitis, urethritis, endometritis, and salpingitis (2)[A]
- UTIs
- Rarely: ectopic disease with granulomas of the pelvis, genitourinary tract, and appendix; colonic intussusception (3)[A]

REFERENCES

1. The Medical Letter. *Enterobius vermicularis* (pinworm) infection. In: *Drugs for Parasitic Infection. Treatment Guidelines from the Medical Letter*. (vol 11). New Rochelle, NY: The Medical Letter; 2013:e7.
2. Dennie J, Grover SR. Distressing perineal and vaginal pain in prepubescent girls: an aetiology. *J Paediatr Child Health* (vol 11).
3. Adorisio O, De Peppo F, Rivosecchi M, et al. *Enterobius vermicularis* as a cause of intestinal occlusion: how to avoid unnecessary surgery. *Pediatr Emerg Care*. 2016;32(4):235–236.

ADDITIONAL READING

- Centers for Disease Control and Prevention. Parasites—enterobiasis (also known as pinworm infection). https://www.cdc.gov/parasites/pinworm/health_professionals/index.html. Accessed August 4, 2021.

- Kang WH, Jee SC. *Enterobius vermicularis* (pinworm) infection. *N Engl J Med*. 2019;381(1):e1.
- Schroeder JC, Jones D, Maranich A. Peripheral eosinophilia found in pediatric *Enterobius vermicularis* infections. *Clin Pediatr (Phila)*. 2019;58(1):13–16.
- von Höveling A, Carrasco L, Weitzel T, et al. Preschool girl with vaginal bleeding due to pinworm endometritis. *J Pediatr Adolesc Gynecol*. 2020;33(2):170–172.

 SEE ALSO

Pruritus Ani

 CODES

ICD10
B80 Enterobiasis

CLINICAL PEARLS
- Nocturnal or early morning perianal itch with restless sleep or insomnia (particularly in children) is the hallmark of symptomatic pinworm infection.
- Treatment includes of mebendazole, albendazole, or pyrantel pamoate.
- Treat close contacts.
- Retreatment after 2 weeks is generally recommended.

PITUITARY ADENOMA

Anup Sabharwal, MD, MBA, FACE, FASPC, FNLA

 BASICS

DESCRIPTION
Typically benign, slow-growing tumors that arise from cells in the pituitary gland
- Pituitary adenomas have been identified as the third most frequent intracranial tumor; accounts for 10–25%, at times identified incidentally on magnetic resonance imaging (MRI)
- Subtypes (hormonal): prolactinoma (PRL) 25–40%, nonfunctioning pituitary adenomas 30%, somatotroph adenoma (growth hormone [GH]) 15–20%, corticotroph adenoma (adrenocorticotropic hormone [ACTH]) 5–10%, thyrotroph adenoma (thyroid-stimulating hormone [TSH]) <1%, gonadotropinoma (luteinizing hormone/follicle-stimulating hormone [LH/FSH]), mixed (1)[A]
- Defined as microadenoma <10 mm and macroadenoma ≥10 mm
- May secrete hormones and/or cause mass effects, or visual changes

EPIDEMIOLOGY
- Predominant age: Age increases incidence.
- Predominant sex: female > male (3:2) for microadenomas (often delayed diagnosis in men)

Incidence
- Autopsy studies have found microadenomas in 3–27% and macroadenomas in <0.5% of people without any pituitary disorders.
- MRI scans illustrate abnormalities consistent with pituitary adenoma in 1/10 persons.
- Clinically apparent pituitary tumors are seen in 18/100,000 persons.

ETIOLOGY AND PATHOPHYSIOLOGY
- Monoclonal adenohypophysial cell growth
- Hormonal effects of functional microadenomas often prompt diagnosis before mass effect.
- PRL increased by functional prolactinomas or inhibited dopaminergic suppression by stalk effect

Genetics
- Carney complex
- Familial isolated pituitary adenomas: ~15% have mutations in the aryl hydrocarbon receptor–interacting protein gene (AIP); present at a younger age and are larger in size (2)
- McCune-Albright syndrome
- Multiple endocrine neoplasia type 1 (MEN1)
- MEN1-like phenotype (MEN4): germline mutation in the cyclin-dependent kinase inhibitor 1B (CDKN1B) (2)
- Gs-alpha ($G_s\alpha$): an activating mutation of the guanine nucleotide stimulatory protein ($G_s\alpha$) gene found in ~40% of somatotroph adenomas (3)

RISK FACTORS
Multiple endocrine neoplasias

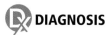 **DIAGNOSIS**

HISTORY
- Common
  - Hyperprolactinemia: infertility, amenorrhea, galactorrhea, gynecomastia, impotence
  - Headache (sellar expansion)
  - Visual disturbances: bitemporal hemianopsia

- Less common
  - Hypersomatotropinemia: acromegaly (coarse facial features, hand/foot swelling, carpal tunnel syndrome, hyperhidrosis, left ventricular hypertrophy)
  - Hyposomatotropinemia: failure to thrive (FTT) (children), asymptomatic (adults)
  - Intracranial pressure (ICP) elevation: headache, nausea, seizures
  - Hypercorticotropinemia: Cushing disease (supraclavicular/dorsocervical fat pad thickening, moon face, hirsutism, acne, plethora, abdominal striae, centripetal obesity with thin limbs, easy bruising and bleeding, hyperglycemia)
- Rare
  - Apoplexy: headache, sudden collapse
  - Secondary hyperthyroidism: palpitations, diaphoresis, heat intolerance, diarrhea
  - Secondary adrenal insufficiency: weakness, irritability, anorexia, nausea/vomiting
  - Hypothalamic compression: temperature, thirst/appetite disorders

PHYSICAL EXAM
- Common
  - Visual disturbances: bitemporal hemianopsia
  - Hyperprolactinemia: hypogonadism, galactorrhea, gynecomastia
  - Hypersomatotropinemia: acromegaly (coarse features, hand/foot swelling, diaphoresis)
  - Hyposomatotropinemia: FTT (children)
- Less common
  - ICP elevation: papilledema, dementia
  - Cushing disease: centripetal obesity, supraclavicular fat pad thickening, moon face, hirsutism, acne
- Rare
  - Apoplexy: hypotension, hypoglycemia, tachycardia, oliguria
  - Secondary hyperthyroidism: tachycardia, tachypnea, diaphoresis, warm/moist skin, tremor
  - Adrenal crisis: orthostatic hypotension
- Hypothalamic compression: temperature dysregulation, obesity, increased urination

DIFFERENTIAL DIAGNOSIS
Pituitary hyperplasia (e.g., pregnancy, primary hypothyroidism, menopause), Rathke cleft cyst, granulomatous disease (e.g., tuberculosis), lymphocytic hypophysitis, metastatic tumor, germinoma, craniopharyngioma

DIAGNOSTIC TESTS & INTERPRETATION
Select based on dysfunction(s) suspected
- Somatotrophic (GH secreting: 40 to 130/million)
  - Acromegaly/hypersomatotropinemia: serum IGF-1 elevated; oral glucose tolerance test with GH given at 0, 30, and 60 minutes (normally suppresses GH to <1 g/L)
  - Hyposomatotropinemia: low GH-releasing hormone response
  - Macimorelin is a noninvasive oral test to evaluate for adult GH deficiency (4)[A].
- Corticotropic
  - Cushing disease/hypercorticotropinemia
  - 24-hour urinary-free cortisol >50 μg
  - Overnight low-dose dexamethasone suppression test (DMST): normal free plasma cortisol (FPC) >1.8 μg/dL at 8 AM (after 1 mg given at 11 PM on night prior)
  - ACTH level assay (if DMST results abnormal): <20 pg/mL = adrenal tumor; ≥20 pg/mL = ectopic/pituitary source
  - Hypocorticotropinemia/secondary glucocorticoid deficiency: high-dose corticotropin stimulation test: FPC <10 g/dL at baseline, with an increase

of <25% 1 hour after 250 μg; metyrapone test: 11-deoxycortisol <150 ng/L after 2 g given (Prepare to give steroids because test may worsen insufficiency.)
- Gonadotrophic/hypogonadotropism: gonadotropin-releasing hormone stimulation of LH/FSH blunted in pituitary hypergonadism but increased in primary hypogonadism
- Lactotrophic (PRL secreting): hyperprolactinemia: serum PRL >20 ng/mL
- Thyrotrophic (TSH secreting): hyper-/hypothyroidism: TSH and free T_4 both increased for pituitary hyperthyroidism and both decreased for pituitary hypothyroidism.

Initial Tests (lab, imaging)
- A typical panel for asymptomatic tumors: PRL, GH, IGF-1, ACTH, 24-hour urinary-free cortisol or overnight DMST, β-HCG, FSH, LH, TSH, free T_4
- Maintain the same GH and IGF-1 through patient management (5)[C].
- Screening for AIP mutations may be offered to families of patients with pituitary adenoma, where available.
- MRI preferred (>90% sensitivity and specificity) after biochemically confirmed
- Octreotide scintigraphy is useful in identifying tumors with somatostatin receptors (5)[B].

Diagnostic Procedures/Other
Inferior petrosal sinus sampling: ACTH sampled from inferior petrosal sinuses to distinguish Cushing disease (pituitary source) from ectopic ACTH

Test Interpretation
- Cell types identified by immunohistochemistry
- Light microscope: eosinophilic (GH, PRL), basophilic (FSH/LH, TSH, ACTH), chromophobic

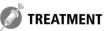 **TREATMENT**

Medical therapy is primary therapy for prolactinomas and adjunct for other tumors.

MEDICATION

First Line
- Hyperprolactinemia: Dopamine agonists increase dopaminergic suppression of PRL.
  - Cabergoline (Dostinex): D_2 receptor–specific
    - Initial dose: 0.25 mg PO once or twice weekly
    - Maintenance dose: Increase q4wk by 0.25 mg 2 times per week per PRL (max 2 mg/week).
    - Contraindications: hypersensitivity (ergots), uncontrolled hypertension (HTN), pregnancy
    - Precautions: caution with liver impairment
    - Interactions: may be inhibited by tricyclic antidepressants, phenothiazines, opiates
    - Adverse reactions: orthostatic hypotension, vertigo, dyspepsia, hot flashes
  - Bromocriptine (Parlodel): D_2 receptor–specific
    - Initial dose: 1.25 to 2.50 mg PO daily (give with food)
    - Maintenance dose: Increase by 2.5 mg/day q2–7d (max 15 mg/day).
    - Contraindications: hypersensitivity (ergots), uncontrolled HTN, pregnancy; preferred over cabergoline if required
    - Precautions: caution with liver impairment
    - Interactions: may be inhibited by tricyclic antidepressants, phenothiazines, opiates
    - Adverse reactions: orthostatic hypotension, seizures, hallucinations, stroke, myocardial infarction

- Somatotropinoma
  - Long-acting analogues of somatostatin (Sandostatin LAR and lanreotide Autogel)
    - Sandostatin LAR: 20 mg q28d (5)[A]; lanreotide Autogel 90 mg q28d; titrate per package insert.
    - Contraindication: hypersensitivity
    - Precautions: caution with biliary, thyroid, cardiac, liver, or kidney disease
    - Interactions: Pimozide increases risk of QT prolongation; variable effects with β-blockers, diuretics, oral glycemic agents
    - Adverse reactions: ascending cholangitis, arrhythmias, congestive heart failure, glycemic instability
    - More effective as adjuvant than as primary treatment for somatotropinomas
    - Consider use of somatostatin analogue or pegvisomant in patients with severe residual disease (5)[A].
    - Consider use of cabergoline in patients with mild residual disease (6)[B].
  - Pegvisomant (Somavert): GH receptor antagonist
    - Initial dose: 40 mg SC × 1, then 10 mg daily and titrate by 5 mg every 4 to 6 weeks based on IGF-1 levels (max 30 mg/day maintenance dose)
    - Contraindication: hypersensitivity
    - Precautions: caution if GH-secreting tumors, diabetes mellitus, impaired liver function
    - Interactions: NSAIDs, opiates, insulins, oral glycemic agents
    - Adverse reactions: hepatitis, tumor growth, GH secretion
- Corticotropinemia: peripheral inhibitors
  - Mitotane (Lysodren)
    - Initial dose: 2 to 6 g/day divided PO TID (max 19 g/day)
    - Maintenance dose: 2 to 16 g TID
    - Contraindication: hypersensitivity
    - Precautions: caution with liver dysfunction and brain damage
    - Interactions: contraindicated with rotavirus vaccine; caution with other vaccines
    - Adverse reactions: HTN, orthostatic hypotension, hemorrhagic cystitis, rash
  - Ketoconazole
    - Dosing: 200 mg PO TID (max 1,200 mg/day)
    - Contraindications: hypersensitivity, achlorhydria, fungal meningitis, impaired liver function
    - Precautions: caution with liver dysfunction
    - Interactions: contraindicated with dronedarone, methadone, statins, pimozide, sirolimus; caution with other antifungals
    - Adverse reactions: adrenal insufficiency, thrombocytopenia, hepatic failure, hepatotoxicity, anaphylaxis, leukopenia, hemolytic anemia
  - Pasireotide (Signifor)
    - Dosing: initially, 0.6 to 0.9 mg twice daily and then 0.3 to 0.9 mg twice daily
    - Contraindication: none
    - Precautions: hypocortisolism, hyperglycemia, bradycardia or QT prolongation, liver test elevations, cholelithiasis, and other pituitary hormone deficiencies
  - Mifepristone (Korlym)
    - Dosing: Administer PO once daily with a meal. The recommended starting dose is 300 mg once daily; not to exceed 600 mg daily in renal impairment
  - Contraindication: pregnancy, use of simvastatin or lovastatin and CYP3A substrates with narrow therapeutic range, concurrent long-term corticosteroid use, women with history of unexplained vaginal bleeding, women with endometrial hyperplasia with atypia or endometrial carcinoma
  - Precautions: adrenal insufficiency, hypokalemia, vaginal bleeding and endometrial changes, QT interval prolongation, use of strong CYP3A inhibitors

- Interactions: potential interactions with drugs metabolized by CYP3A, CYP2C8/9, CYP2B6, and hormonal contraceptives. Nursing mothers should discontinue drug or discontinue nursing.
- Adverse reactions: most common adverse reactions in Cushing syndrome (≥20%): nausea, fatigue, headache, decreased blood potassium, arthralgia, vomiting, peripheral edema, HTN, dizziness, decreased appetite, endometrial hypertrophy
- Gonadotropinemia
  - Bromocriptine: See earlier discussion.
- Thyrotropinemia
  - Somatostatin analogues: See earlier discussion.

Second Line
- Corticotropinemia: peripheral inhibitors
  - Metyrapone
    - Dose: 250 mg PO QID
    - Contraindication: porphyria
    - Precautions: caution in liver/thyroid disease
    - Interactions: Dilantin increases metabolism.
    - Adverse reactions: nausea, hypotension
- Gonadotropinemia
  - Octreotide: See earlier discussion.

ISSUES FOR REFERRAL
- Neurosurgery consultation for symptomatic tumors (except for prolactinoma)
- Ophthalmologist evaluation prior to surgery

ADDITIONAL THERAPIES
- Fractionated radiotherapy: often effective as adjunctive when surgery is inadequate (6)[B]
- Stereotactic radiosurgery: alternative to surgery in high-risk patients or as adjunct (6)[B]

SURGERY/OTHER PROCEDURES
- Most are now done endoscopically via translabial/transsphenoidal approach (7)[A].
- Indications: symptoms or treatment resistant
- Follow-up: serial neurologic/hormonal evaluations to evaluate complications (e.g., diabetes insipidus, CNS damage) and need for more treatment
- Remission rates: 72–87% for microadenoma but only 50–56% for macroadenomas

ADMISSION, INPATIENT, AND NURSING CONSIDERATIONS
- Outpatient management unless apoplexy or adrenal crisis
- Treat pituitary apoplexy immediately to prevent death (see "Complications") (7)[A].
- Consider stress-dose steroids in frail or hemodynamically unstable patients.
- Maintain BP with fluids and/or pressor agents.
- Check serum sodium, serum osmolality, and urine specific gravity if polyuric or electrolytes are imbalanced.
- Contact neurosurgery.
- Diabetes insipidus: hyperosmolar IV fluids
- Adrenal crisis: normal saline
- Pituitary apoplexy: Monitor inputs/outputs (I/Os), central venous pressure, and ICP and do frequent neurologic checks.
- Adrenal crisis: Monitor BP and I/Os.
- Keep as inpatient postoperatively until diabetes insipidus and/or adrenal insufficiency is managed.

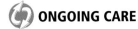 ONGOING CARE

FOLLOW-UP RECOMMENDATIONS
Patient Monitoring
- Follow-up MRIs at 6 and 12 months after discharge
- Involved hormone(s) are followed postoperatively, especially after radiation because

hypopituitarism may develop 10 to 15 years after treatment.

PROGNOSIS
Depends on type, size, symptoms, therapy

COMPLICATIONS
- Postoperative diabetes insipidus and/or hypogonadism (usually transient/common)
- Pituitary apoplexy (acute/uncommon): acute hemorrhagic pituitary infarction; adrenal crisis with severe headache; surgical decompression required to prevent shock, coma, and death
- Nelson syndrome (subacute/uncommon): rapid adenoma growth postadrenalectomy
- Pituitary hormone insufficiency (chronic/uncommon): often years after treatment
- Optic nerve neuropathy and brain necrosis after >60 Gy radiotherapy (chronic/rare)

REFERENCES
1. Dworakowska D, Grossman AB. The pathophysiology of pituitary adenomas. *Best Pract Res Clin Endocrinol Metab*. 2009;23(5):525–541.
2. Georgitsi M, Raitila A, Karhu A, et al. Molecular diagnosis of pituitary adenoma predisposition caused by aryl hydrocarbon receptor-interacting protein gene mutations. *Proc Natl Acad Sci U S A*. 2007;104(10):4101–4105.
3. Landis CA, Masters SB, Spada A, et al. GTPase inhibiting mutations activate the alpha chain of Gs and stimulate adenylyl cyclase in human pituitary tumours. *Nature*. 1989;340(6236):692–696.
4. Agrawal V, Garcia JM. The macimorelin-stimulated growth hormone test for adult growth hormone deficiency diagnosis. *Expert Rev Mol Diagn*. 2014;14(6):647–654.
5. Tichomirowa MA, Daly AF, Beckers A. Treatment of pituitary tumors: somatostatin. *Endocrine*. 2005;28(1):93–100.
6. Mondok A, Szeifert GT, Mayer A, et al. Treatment of pituitary tumors: radiation. *Endocrine*. 2005;28(1):77–85.
7. Buchfelder M. Treatment of pituitary tumors: surgery. *Endocrine*. 2005;28(1):67–75.

 SEE ALSO

Cushing Disease and Cushing Syndrome; Galactorrhea

 CODES

ICD10
D35.2 Benign neoplasm of pituitary gland

CLINICAL PEARLS
- An incidentaloma is an asymptomatic microadenoma found on imaging. General labs include PRL, GH, IGF-1, ACTH, 24-hour urinary-free cortisol/overnight DMST, β-subunit FSH, LH, TSH, and free T₄. Obtain follow-up MRIs at 6 and 12 months if normal, but consult endocrinology if not.
- Initial treatment selected for symptomatic pituitary adenoma includes a dopamine agonist for prolactinomas and surgical resection for all others.
- Pituitary apoplexy is a rapid hemorrhagic pituitary infarction due to compression of the blood supply. It is fatal within hours unless surgically decompressed.

PLANTAR FASCIITIS

Krystyna Guinevere Golden, MD • Blake R. Shaffer, MD, MBS • Brooke Organ, DO

BASICS

DESCRIPTION
- Degenerative change of plantar fascia at origin on medial tuberosity of calcaneus
- Pain on plantar surface, usually at calcaneal insertion of plantar fascia upon weight-bearing, especially in morning or on initiation of walking after prolonged rest
- Also referred to as: plantar fasciopathy, plantar heel pain syndrome, plantar fasciosis, painful heel syndrome

EPIDEMIOLOGY
Incidence
Estimated 1 million patient visits yearly in the United States

Prevalence
- Most common cause of plantar heel pain
- Lifetime: 10–15% of population
- Peak incidence between ages 40 and 60 years, earlier peak in runners

ETIOLOGY AND PATHOPHYSIOLOGY
- Repetitive microtrauma and collagen degeneration of plantar fascia
- Chronic degenerative change (-osis/-opathy rather than -itis) of plantar fascia generally at insertion on medial tuberosity of calcaneus

RISK FACTORS
- Intrinsic
  - Age (>40 to 60 years)
  - Female, pregnancy
  - Obesity (BMI >30)
  - Pes planus (flat feet), pes cavus (high arch), overpronation, leg length discrepancy
  - Hamstring, calf, and Achilles tightness
  - Calf and intrinsic foot muscle weakness
  - Decreased ankle range of motion with dorsiflexion (equinus or tight heel cord; <15 degrees of dorsiflexion)
  - Systemic connective tissue disorders
- Extrinsic
  - Dancers, runners, court sport athletes
  - Occupations with prolonged standing, especially on hard surfaces (nurses, letter carriers, warehouse/factory workers)
  - Overuse and rapid increase in activities involving repetitive loading

GENERAL PREVENTION
- Maintain normal body weight.
- Avoid training errors (increasing intensity, distance, duration, and frequency of high-impact activities too rapidly); avoid overtraining.
- Proper footwear (appropriate cushion/arch support)
- Runners should replace footwear every 250 to 500 miles.

COMMONLY ASSOCIATED CONDITIONS
- Usually isolated
- Heel spurs commonly seen but are not a marker of severity nor pathognomonic and surgical removal of unclear benefit
- Posterior tibial neuropathy

DIAGNOSIS

Typically made clinically

HISTORY
- Pain on plantar surface of foot, usually at fascial insertion at calcaneus (medial calcaneal tubercle), but can have pain anywhere along length of plantar fascia
- Pain is typically worse with first few steps in the morning or after prolonged rest or standing (poststatic dyskinesia).
- Pain typically improves after first few steps only to recur toward the end of the day or after prolonged ambulation.
- Pain commonly unilateral but can be bilateral in 1/3 of cases
- Pain can be dull and constant in chronic cases.
- Limp with excessive toe walking
- Numbness and burning of medial hindfoot is more suggestive of posterior tibial nerve compression.

PHYSICAL EXAM
- Point tenderness on medial tuberosity of calcaneus at insertion of plantar fascia
- Pain along plantar fascia with dorsiflexion of foot
- Windlass test: Extend MTP while allowing passive flexion of IP joint of hallux—pain indicates a positive test; high specificity, low sensitivity; sensitivity improves (13.5% → 31.8%) if performed while standing.
- Dorsiflexion-eversion test: pain with dorsiflexion plus eversion of the subtalar joint
- Decreased passive range of motion with dorsiflexion
- Evaluate for pes planus, pes cavus, and overpronation.
- Loss of heel fat pad suggests heel fat pad syndrome.
- Point tenderness on posterosuperior aspect of heel suggests Achilles tendinopathy.

DIFFERENTIAL DIAGNOSIS
- Calcaneal stress fracture
- Heel fat pad syndrome (painful or atrophic heel pad)
- Longitudinal arch strain
- Nerve entrapment (posterior tibial nerve—tarsal tunnel syndrome, medial calcaneal branch of posterior tibial nerve, abductor digiti quinti)
- Achilles tendinopathy
- Calcaneal contusion
- Plantar calcaneal bursitis
- Tendonitis of posterior tibialis
- Plantar fascia tear
- S1 radiculopathy
- Adolescents: calcaneal apophysitis (Sever disease)

DIAGNOSTIC TESTS & INTERPRETATION
- Usually not necessary; typically a clinical diagnosis
- Consider further imaging only to rule out other causes, uncertain diagnosis, or persistent heel pain after 4 to 6 months of conservative therapy.
- Radiographs: two views of foot to evaluate for fracture, tumor, cyst, periostitis, bony erosions; weight-bearing films preferred; calcaneal spurs common but not diagnostic

- Ultrasound: hypoechoic at insertion, thickened plantar fascia (≥4 mm); can improve delivery accuracy of injections and extracorporeal shock wave therapy (ESWT); can objectively evaluate change in plantar fascia thickness to monitor effects of an intervention
- MRI can evaluate for other soft tissue etiologies.
- CT or technetium-99m bone scan can rule out calcaneal stress fracture and evaluate for infection.
- Nerve conduction studies can rule out nerve entrapment.
- Inflammatory markers: can consider if bilateral heel pain or young patients

TREATMENT

Nonoperative management is mainstay of treatment.

GENERAL MEASURES
- Weight loss if overweight, pain reduction, improvement of intrinsic foot muscle strength
- Focus should be on intrinsic foot muscle strengthening to stabilize the arch.
- Strengthen calf and intrinsic foot muscles, using the towel drag/pickup exercise and barefoot single leg balance.
- Relative rest/activity modification with avoidance of high-impact causative activities
- Stretching: Plantar fascia stretches more effective than Achilles tendon/gastrocnemius-soleus stretches, and non–weight-bearing stretches may be preferable.
- Plantar fascia mobilization done in office and taught to patients is effective based on systematic review.
  - Plantar fascia mobilization: foot to inversion; compress tender point while moving foot to eversion; repeat along plantar fascia.
- Ice (frozen water bottle roll)
- Massage (golf or tennis ball roll) of tibialis anterior
- Weight reduction if BMI >25
- Supportive footwear with stable midfoot or orthoses may be helpful.
  - For relief of acute pain (2 to 3 weeks), not to be worn indefinitely as they can contribute to continued intrinsic muscle weakness
  - Options include: heel cup, soft heel pad, navicular pad, medial heel wedge, Thomas heel, and night splint (1)
  - Custom orthoses show no benefit over prefabricated orthoses and are more costly.
  - Improved effectiveness of night splints when used in association with orthotics
- Surgical treatment of "heel spurs" is not indicated.

MEDICATION
First Line
- NSAIDs scheduled for 2 to 3 weeks: naproxen 500 mg PO BID *or* ibuprofen 600 to 800 mg PO TID PRN for pain
- Acetaminophen 1,000 mg PO TID PRN for pain

Second Line
None

ISSUES FOR REFERRAL
- Physical therapy for patient instruction on proper stretching and strengthening techniques, manipulative treatments (joint and soft tissue mobilization), and massage. For chronic cases, consider analysis of gait and biomechanical factors.
- Podiatry: Consider if conservative measures fail after 3 to 6 months.
- Surgery: Consider if conservative measures fail after 6 to 12 months.

ADDITIONAL THERAPIES
- Corticosteroid injections (2)[B]
  – Short-term pain relief
  – Medial heel approach or points of maximal tenderness along plantar fascia
  – Recommend ultrasound guidance when possible.
  – Risk for plantar fascia rupture and calcaneal fat pad atrophy with resultant permanent heel pain
- Platelet-rich plasma (PRP) injections (3)[B]
  – May lead to greater improvement in pain and functional outcomes compared to CSI
- ESWT (4)[B]
  – Is an effective alternative to CSI in relieving pain and improving function
- Low-dye and calcaneal taping
- Short walking cast
- Promising therapies with inconsistent evidence
  – Radiofrequency nerve ablation (5)[B]
  – Plantar iontophoresis
  – Intralesional autologous blood injection
  – Low-level laser therapy
  – Acupuncture
  – Myofascial trigger point dry needling (6)[B]
  – Botulinum toxin (BT) A injection (7)[B]
  – Ozone injections
  – Polydeoxyribonucleotide (PDRN) injections

SURGERY/OTHER PROCEDURES
- Necessary in <10% of patients; more likely beneficial in severely obese
- Recommended if conservative treatment fails after 6 to 12 months and pain is unrelenting.
- Open/endoscopic plantar fasciotomy (less risk and complications with endoscopic technique but requires specialized equipment and skills; not widely used)
- Cryosurgery
- Calcaneal spur resection

COMPLEMENTARY & ALTERNATIVE MEDICINE
Acupuncture may reduce pain in short term, but further studies needed.

ONGOING CARE

FOLLOW-UP RECOMMENDATIONS
- Ensure patient adherence to proper stretching technique.
- Following 3 to 6 months of unsuccessful conservative treatment, consider additional therapies or referrals.

PATIENT EDUCATION
- Weight reduction if BMI >25
- Home plantar fascia mobilization exercises
- Strengthen foot muscles: Place a towel on the floor, pull toward yourself with ball of foot and toes without lifting the heel; progressive one-leg standing
- Proper footwear (adequate cushion and arch support)
- Stretch plantar fascia: Pull toes into dorsiflexion prior to walking after prolonged sitting or sleep.
- Ice the foot using a frozen water bottle: Roll foot over bottle for 10 minutes in the morning and after work.
- Massage plantar fascia: Roll foot over a golf ball.
- Decrease repetitive stress.

PROGNOSIS
- Generally good
- Self-limited (resolves within 12 months) in up to 80–90% of patients

COMPLICATIONS
- Rupture of plantar fascia (more common with repeated corticosteroid injections)
- Chronic pain
- Gait abnormality

REFERENCES

1. Choo YJ, Park CH, Chang MC. Rearfoot disorders and conservative treatment: a narrative review. *Ann Palliat Med*. 2020;9(5):3546–3552.
2. David JA, Sankarapandian V, Christopher PR, et al. Injected corticosteroids for treating plantar heel pain in adults. *Cochrane Database Syst Rev*. 2017;(6):CD009348.
3. Hurley ET, Shimozono Y, Hannon CP, et al. Platelet-rich plasma versus corticosteroids for plantar fasciitis: a systematic review of randomized controlled trials. *Orthop J Sports Med*. 2020;8(4):2325967120915704.
4. Hocaoglu S, Vurdem UE, Cebicci MA, et al. Comparative effectiveness of radial extracorporeal shockwave therapy and ultrasound-guided local corticosteroid injection treatment for plantar fasciitis. *J Am Podiatr Med Assoc*. 2017;107(3):192–199.
5. Landsman AS, Catanese DJ, Wiener SN, et al. A prospective, randomized, double-blinded study with crossover to determine the efficacy of radiofrequency nerve ablation for the treatment of heel pain. *J Am Podiatr Med Assoc*. 2013;103(1):8–15.
6. He C, Ma H. Effectiveness of trigger point dry needling for plantar heel pain: a meta-analysis of seven randomized controlled trials. *J Pain Res*. 2017;10:1933–1942.
7. Tsikopoulos K, Vasiliadis HS, Mavridis D. Injection therapies for plantar fasciopathy ('plantar fasciitis'): a systematic review and network meta-analysis of 22 randomised controlled trials. *Br J Sports Med*. 2016;50(22):1367–1375.

ADDITIONAL READING

- Al-Boloushi Z, Lopez-Royo MD, Arian M, et al. Minimally invasive non-surgical management of plantar fasciitis: a systematic review. *J Bodyw Mov Ther*. 2019;23(1):122–137.
- Bahrami MH, Raeissadat SA, Barchinejad M, et al. Local ozone versus corticosteroid injection efficacy in plantar fasciitis treatment: a double-blinded RCT. *J Pain Res*. 2019;12:2251–225.
- Berbrayer D, Fredericson M. Update on evidence-based treatments for plantar fasciopathy. *PM R*. 2014;6(2):159–169.
- Clark RJ, Tighe M. The effectiveness of acupuncture for plantar heel pain: a systematic review. *Acupunct Med*. 2012;30(4):298–306.
- Li Z, Yu A, Qi B, et al. Corticosteroid versus placebo injection for plantar fasciitis: a meta-analysis of randomized controlled trials. *Exp Ther Med*. 2015;9(6):2263–2268.
- Petraglia F, Ramazzina I, Costantino C. Plantar fasciitis in athletes: diagnostic and treatment strategies. A systematic review. *Muscles Ligaments Tendons J*. 2017;7(1):107–118.
- Sun J, Gao F, Wang Y, et al. Extracorporeal shock wave therapy is effective in treating chronic plantar fasciitis: a meta-analysis of RCTs. *Medicine (Baltimore)*. 2017;96(15):e6621.
- Yin MC, Ye J, Yao M, et al. Is extracorporeal shock wave therapy clinical efficacy for relief of chronic, recalcitrant plantar fasciitis? A systematic review and meta-analysis of randomized placebo or active-treatment controlled trials. *Arch Phys Med Rehabil*. 2014;95(8):1585–1593.

SEE ALSO

Algorithm: Heel Pain

CODES

ICD10
M72.2 Plantar fascial fibromatosis

CLINICAL PEARLS
- Plantar fasciitis occurs due to degeneration of plantar fascia at origin (medial calcaneal tuberosity) with characteristic pattern of pain.
- Plantar medial heel pain with weight-bearing (most noticeable with initial steps in the morning or after period of inactivity) is hallmark presentation.
- Generally, self-limited and conservative treatment is preferred. 85–90% of patients can be treated with conservative therapies.
- Strengthen intrinsic foot muscles, modify activity, stretch plantar fascia, ice (water bottle roll), and massage (golf ball roll).
- Weight loss helps control symptoms, particularly for BMI ≥25.

PLEURAL EFFUSION

Felix B. Chang, MD, DABMA, ABIHM, ABIM

 BASICS

Abnormal accumulation of fluid in the pleural space

DESCRIPTION
Types: transudate (low protein/low specific gravity) and exudate (high protein and cellular debris). Transudate: commonly caused by: congestive heart failure (CHF): 40%. Exudates: pneumonia 25%, malignancy 15%, and pulmonary embolism (PE) 10%

EPIDEMIOLOGY
Incidence
Estimated 1.5 million cases per year in the United States; CHF: 500,000; pneumonia: 300,000; malignancy: 150,000; PE: 150,000; cirrhosis: 150,000; tuberculosis (TB): 2,500; pancreatitis: 20,000; collagen vascular disease: 6,000

Prevalence
Estimated 320 cases per 100,000 people in industrialized countries; in hospitalized patients with AIDS, prevalence is 7–27%. No gender predilection: ~2/3 of malignant pleural effusions occur in women.

ETIOLOGY AND PATHOPHYSIOLOGY
- Pleural fluid formation exceeds pleural fluid absorption. Transudates result from imbalances in hydrostatic and oncotic forces. Increase in hydrostatic and/or low oncotic pressures; increase in pleural capillary permeability; lymphatic obstruction or impaired drainage; movement of fluid from the peritoneal or retroperitoneal space
- Transudates (1)[A]:CHF: 40% of transudative effusions; 80% bilateral; constrictive pericarditis, atelectasis; superior vena cava syndrome. Cirrhosis (hepatic hydrothorax), nephrotic syndrome, hypoalbuminemia; myxedema. Urinothorax, central line misplacement; peritoneal dialysis. Dressler syndrome (postmyocardial infarction syndrome). Yellow nail syndrome: yellow nails, lymphedema and pleural effusion; SARS-Cov-2
- Exudates (1)[A]: lung parenchyma infection, bacterial (parapneumonic, tuberculous pleurisy), fungal, viral, parasitic (amebiasis, *Echinococcus*). Cancer: lung cancer, metastases (breast, lymphoma, ovaries), mesothelioma. PE: 25% of PEs are transudate. Collagen vascular disease: rheumatoid arthritis, systemic lupus erythematosus (SLE), Wegener granulomatosis, sarcoidosis, Churg-Strauss, Sjogren syndrome, granulomatosis with polyangiitis. GI: pancreatitis, esophageal rupture, abdominal abscess, after liver transplant; chylothorax: thoracic duct tear, malignancy. Hemothorax: trauma, PE, malignancy, coagulopathy, aortic aneurysm. Others: after coronary artery bypass graft; uremia, asbestos exposure, radiation; drugs. Drugs: nitrofurantoin, bromocriptine, amiodarone, procarbazine, hydralazine, procainamide, quinidine, methotrexate, methysergide, interleukin-2, mitomycin, practolol, minoxidil, bleomycin, cyclophosphamide, procarbazine, imatinib, all-trans-retinoic acid, gemcitabine, dantrolene, valproic acid, sulfasalazine, minocy-

cline, acebutolol, phenytoin, practolol, minoxidil, methysergide, L-tryptophan, dasatinib, docetaxel, filgrastine, ergot alkaloids
  – Meigs syndrome; yellow nail syndrome; ovarian stimulation syndrome; lymphangiomatosis; acute respiratory distress syndrome (ARDS). Chylothorax: thoracic duct tear, malignancy, associated with lymphoma
  – PEEVO: pleural effusions of extravascular origin. Transudative PEEVO: hepatic hydrothorax, peritoneal dialysis, urinothorax, extravascular migration of central venous catheter, duropleural fistula, ventriculoperitoneal and ventriculopleural shunts, glycinothorax. Exudative PEEVO: esophageal or gastric perforation, misplaced enteral feeding tube, pancreaticopleural fistula and pancreatic pseudocyst, bilothorax

RISK FACTORS
Occupational exposures/drugs. PE, TB, bacterial pneumonias. Opportunistic infections (in HIV patients when CD4 count is <150 cells/μL)

COMMONLY ASSOCIATED CONDITIONS
Hypoproteinemia, heart failure, cirrhosis

 DIAGNOSIS

Presumptive diagnosis in 50% of cases. Small pleural effusions; radiographic area <2 intercostal spaces (<300 mL) are asymptomatic.

HISTORY
Dyspnea, fever, malaise, and weight loss; chest pain, cough, hemoptysis, and dull pain

PHYSICAL EXAM
Pleural effusion >300 mL: tachypnea, asymmetric expansion of the thoracic cage; decrease/absent tactile fremitus; dullness to percussion; decreased/inaudible breath sounds, egophony, pleural friction rub. Ascites suggest: hepatic hydrothorax, ovarian cancer, and Meigs syndrome. If associated with unilateral swelling in lower extremity, consider DVT with PE. Lymphadenopathy may suggest malignancy.

DIFFERENTIAL DIAGNOSIS
Pseudochylothorax: accumulation of cholesterol or lecithin-globulin complexes in pleural space

DIAGNOSTIC TESTS & INTERPRETATION
Initial Tests (lab, imaging)
- Thoracentesis: use of thoracic ultrasound (US) lowers rate of pneumothorax (4% vs. 9.5%) (2)[A]. US: detects as 5 to 50 mL of pleural fluid; identifies loculated effusions; site for thoracentesis, pleural biopsy, or pleural drainage. Chest CT scan with contrast for patients with undiagnosed pleural effusion; CT pulmonary angiography if PE is suspected. CT scan of the chest with contrast is recommended if the pleural fluid has complex ultrasonographic features such as septations and loculations.

- Pleural fluid: appearance, pH, WBC differential, total protein, lactate dehydrogenase (LDH), glucose, Gram stain and culture, and acid-fast bacilli (AFB) staining. Consider polymerase chain reaction (PCR) for *Mycobacterium tuberculosis* and *Streptococcus pneumoniae*. If comorbidities implying risk, consider amylase, triglycerides, cholesterol, LE cells, cytology, antinuclear antibodies (ANAs), adenosine deaminase, tumor markers, rheumatoid factor, cytology, creatinine (3)[C].
- Light criteria, transudate versus exudate (98% sensitivity; 80% specificity); fluid is considered an exudate if any of the following: ratio of pleural fluid-to-serum protein levels >0.5; ratio of pleural fluid-to-serum LDH levels >0.6; pleural fluid LDH level >2/3 the upper limit for serum LDH level; 99.5% sensitive for detecting exudative effusion
- Other exudate criteria: serum-effusion albumin gradient ≤1.2 (sensitivity 87%; specificity 92%), cholesterol effusion >45 mg/dL, and LDH effusion >200 mg/dL (sensitivity 90%; specificity 98%). Empyema: pus, putrid odor; culture. A putrid odor suggests an anaerobic empyema: LDH levels >1,000 IU/L (normal serum = 200 IU/L); glucose, <60 mg/dL; low pH. Malignancy: cytology, red, bloody; glucose, normal to low, depending on the tumor burden; RBCs >100,000/mm³
- Lupus pleuritis: LE cells present; pleural fluid-to-serum ANAs ratio >1; glucose <60 mg/dL; pleural fluid-to-serum glucose ratio <0.5. Fungal: positive KOH, culture; peritoneal dialysis: protein <1 g/dL; glucose 300 to 400 mg/dL. Urinothorax: creatinine: pleural/blood >0.5; high LDH pleural fluid, with low protein levels. Hemothorax: hematocrit: pleural/blood >0.5; benign asbestos effusion: unilateral, exudative; have elevated eosinophil count. Tuberculous pleuritis: lymphocytes >80% predominance effusion; elevated levels of adenosine deaminase >50 U/L and interferon-γ >140 pg/mL; positive AFB stain, culture; total protein >4 g/dL, nuclear acid amplification (NAA), LDH levels elevated in about 75% of patients (often >500 U/L). Chylothorax: milky; triglycerides >110 mg/dL; lipoprotein electrophoresis (chylomicrons). Pseudochylothorax: cholesterol level >200 mg/dL or presence of cholesterol crystals. Amebic liver abscess: anchovy paste effusion; Waldenström macroglobulinemia and multiple myeloma: protein >7 g/dL. Esophageal rupture: high salivary amylase; pleural fluid acidosis, pH <6; amylase rich: acute pancreatitis, chronic pancreatic pleural effusion, malignancy, esophageal rupture; rheumatoid pleurisy: glucose <60 mg/dL; pleural fluid/serum glucose <0.5
- Lymphocytosis: tuberculous pleurisy, lymphoma, sarcoidosis, chronic rheumatoid pleurisy, yellow nail syndrome, or chylothorax (80–95% of the nucleated cells); carcinomatosis in half of cases (50–70% are lymphocytes). Neutrophils >50% suggest parapneumonic effusion, empyema, PE, abdominal

disease, malignant pleural effusion, acute tuberculous pleurisy. COVID-19 5.88% of pleural effusion. Pleural fluid eosinophilia (>10% of total nucleated cells): pneumothorax, hemothorax, malignancy, drugs, pulmonary infarction, fungal (coccidioidomycosis, cryptococcosis, histoplasmosis), benign asbestos pleural effusion. Low glucose (<60 mg/dL): TB, malignancy, rheumatoid pleurisy, parapneumonic, empyema, hemothorax, paragonimiasis, Churg-Strauss syndrome. RBC count >100,000/mm³: trauma, malignancy, PE, injury after cardiac surgery, asbestos pleurisy, pancreatitis, TB. Pleural fluid LDH >1,000 IU/L: suggests empyema, malignant effusion, rheumatoid effusion, or pleural paragonimiasis. pH >7.3: rheumatoid pleurisy, empyema, malignant effusion, TB, esophageal rupture, or lupus nephritis .pH <7.2 necessitates fluid drainage in patient with parapneumonic effusion. Mesothelial cells in exudates: TB is unlikely if there are >5% of mesothelial cells. Adenosine deaminase >35 U/L suggests tuberculous pleurisy, empyema, complicated parapneumonic effusion, malignancy. ADA >250 U/L, consider empyema or lymphoma over TB. *S. pneumoniae* accounts for 50% of cases of parapneumonic effusions in AIDS patients, followed by *Staphylococcus aureus, Haemophilus influenzae, Mycoplasma pneumoniae, Legionella, Nocardia,* and *Bordetella bronchiseptica*; exudate with low count of nucleated cells. *Pneumocystis jiroveci* is an uncommon cause in HIV. Usually, it is a small effusion, unilateral or bilateral, and serous to bloody in appearance. Demonstration of the trophozoite or cyst is mandatory. Cancer-related HIV pleural effusion: Kaposi sarcoma, Castleman disease, and primary effusion lymphoma. Kaposi sarcoma: mononuclear predominance, exudate pH >7.4; LDH 111 to 330 IU/L; glucose >60 mg/dL
- Chest x-ray (CXR)—posteroanterior–anteroposterior views: Upright x-rays show a concave meniscus in the costophrenic angle that suggests >250 mL of pleural fluid; homogeneous opacity, with visibility of pulmonary vessels through diffuse haziness and absence of air bronchogram; 75 mL of fluid will obliterate the posterior costophrenic sulcus. Lateral x-rays show blunting of the posterior costophrenic angle and the posterior gutter; decubitus x-rays to exclude a loculated effusion and underlying pulmonary lesion or pulmonary thickening. Supine x-rays show costophrenic blunting, haziness, obliteration of the diaphragmatic silhouette, decreased visibility of the lower lobe vasculature, and widened minor fissure.

Follow-Up Tests & Special Considerations
75% of patients with exudative effusions have a non-CHF cause.

Diagnostic Procedures/Other
Diagnostic thoracentesis indicated for the following: clinically significant pleural effusion (>10 mm thick on US or lateral decubitus x-ray with no known cause)

 TREATMENT

MEDICATION
First Line
CHF: diuretics (75% clearing in 48 hours); parapneumonic effusion: antibiotics; rheumatologic conditions/inflammation: steroids and NSAID

ISSUES FOR REFERRAL
Uncertain etiology; malignant effusion; high-risk diagnostic thoracentesis; decortication

ADDITIONAL THERAPIES
- Pleurodesis for symptomatic patients whose pleural effusion reaccumulates too quickly for repeat therapeutic thoracentesis. Tunneled pleural catheter is the preferred treatment for patients with malignant pleural effusion and limited survival (2)[A],(3).
- Sclerosing agents for malignant effusions: Talc slurry (6, 95% credible interval [Cr-I] 3–10) may result in lesser pleurodesis failure in compare of bleomycin, doxycycline bleomycin versus talc slurry: odds ratio (OR) 2.24 95% Cr-I 1.10–4.68; low certainty; ranked 11, 95% Cr-I 7 to 15 (2)[A].
- There is little evidence of a difference between the pleurodesis failure rate of talc poudrage and talc slurry OR 0.50, 95% Cr-I 0.21–1.02 (2)[A].

SURGERY/OTHER PROCEDURES
- Percutaneous pleural biopsy if a cause is not clear after thoracentesis: closed pleural biopsy: Pleura is diffusely involved (Tuberculous pleuritis, noncaseating granuloma in rheumatoid pleuritis). CT-guided needle biopsy: pleural mass; video-assisted thoracoscopic pleural biopsy: Negative percutaneous biopsy, patchy disease, or CT scan does not show obvious mass.
- Parapneumonic effusion should be sampled if free-flowing, but layer is >10 mm on a lateral decubitus film; loculated, thickened pleura on a contrast-enhanced CT scan, clearly delineated by US open pleural biopsy by thoracotomy
- Contraindications for thoracentesis: anticoagulation, bleeding diathesis, thrombocytopenia <20,000/mm³, mechanical ventilation. Bronchoscopy: when malignancy is suspected (pulmonary infiltrate or mass on CXR or CT scan, hemoptysis, massive pleural effusion, or shift of the mediastinum toward the side of effusion). Thoracoscopy: No statistically significant difference in mortality between primary surgical and nonsurgical management of pleural empyema for all age groups. Video-assisted thoracoscopic surgery may reduce length of hospital stay compared to thoracostomy.

ADMISSION, INPATIENT, AND NURSING CONSIDERATIONS
Treat any underlying medical disorder.

 ONGOING CARE

FOLLOW-UP RECOMMENDATIONS
Patient Monitoring
Check for the amount and quality of fluid drained, air leak (bubbling), and oscillation. Repeat a CXR when drainage decreases to <100 mL/day to evaluate complete clearing.

DIET
Cardiac diet in heart failure; correct hypoproteinemia.

PROGNOSIS
- Low-pH malignant effusions have shorter survival and poorer response to chemical pleurodesis than those with pH >7.3. Low pleural fluid pH (≤7.15): high likelihood of pleural space drainage. Malignant pleural effusion has a poor prognosis with 84% reported 1-year mortality among patient with bilateral pleural effusion. Pleural fluid pH ≤7.28 associated with reduced survival (OR 4.42, 95% CI 2.39–8.46 for <1-month survival). Uncomplicated parapneumonic effusions and effusions from PE, tuberculous pleurisy, and postcardiac injury syndrome may persist for several weeks. Benign asbestos pleural effusion, rheumatoid pleurisy, and radiation pleuritis often persist for months to years.
- Reexpansion pulmonary edema carries a mortality rate of 20%.

COMPLICATIONS
Pleural effusion: constrictive fibrosis, pleurocutaneous fistula. 40% of pneumonia patients will develop up to 40% parapneumonic effusion and close to 10% will progress to empyema. Mortality approaches 20% and up to 30% in patients with comorbidites (1)[B]. Thoracentesis: pneumothorax (5–10%); hemothorax (~1%); empyema; spleen/liver laceration; reexpansion pulmonary edema (if >1.5 L is removed). Complications related to large-volume thoracentesis include reexpansion pulmonary edema and pneumothorax ex vacuo.

REFERENCES
1. Aboudara M, Maldonado F. Update in the management of pleural effusions. *Med Clin North Am.* 2019;103(3):475–485.
2. Gordon CE, Feller-Kopman D, Balk EM, et al. Pneumothorax following thoracentesis: a systematic review and meta-analysis. *Arch Intern Med.* 2010;170(4):332–339.
3. Dipper A, Jones HE, Bhatnagar R, et al. Interventions for the management of malignant pleural effusions: a network meta-analysis. *Cochrane Database Syst Rev.* 2020;4(4):CD010529.

 CODES

ICD10
- J86.9 Pyothorax without fistula
- J86.0 Pyothorax with fistula
- J91.0 Malignant pleural effusion

CLINICAL PEARLS
Rare causes of pleural exudates include constrictive pericarditis, urinothorax, Meigs syndrome. Most common pleural exudates include malignancy, parapneumonic effusions, TB, empyema.

PNEUMONIA, BACTERIAL

Jocelyn C. Young, DO, MSc • Rehan Azeem, MD

 BASICS

Bacterial pneumonia is an infection of the pulmonary parenchyma by a bacterial organism.

DESCRIPTION

Bacterial pneumonia can be classified as the following:

- Community-acquired pneumonia (CAP) is classified by severity:
  - CAP in an outpatient setting
  - Nonsevere CAP in an inpatient setting
  - CAP in an intensive care unit (ICU) OR severe CAP is based on validated illness severity criteria and is defined as the presence of one major criterion OR at least three minor criteria.
    - Major criteria: septic shock requiring vasopressors, respiratory failure requiring mechanical ventilation
    - Minor criteria: respiratory rate $\geq$30 breaths/min, PaO_2/FiO_2 ratio $\leq$250, multilobar infiltrates, confusion, BUN $\geq$20, WBC $\leq$4, platelets <100,000, hypothermia, and hypotension requiring aggressive fluid resuscitation
- Nosocomial pneumonia: acquired in health care settings
  - Hospital-acquired pneumonia (HAP): occurs $\geq$48 hours after admission and did not appear to be incubating at the time of admission
  - Ventilator-associated pneumonia (VAP): develops $\geq$ 48 hours after endotracheal intubation

EPIDEMIOLOGY

- In the United States as of 2018, CAP is the eighth most common cause of death (even higher in those >65 years).
- Rates of infection are 3 times higher in African Americans than in whites and are 5 to 10 times higher in Native American adults and 10 times higher in Native American children.
- Mortality rate in children is approximately 1.6 million a year. Respiratory viruses are the most commonly detected causes of pneumonia.

Incidence

- CAP: 5 to 6 cases per 1,000 persons with increased incidence occurring in the winter months
- HAP: 5 to 20 cases per 1,000 admissions; incidence increases 6- to 20-fold in ventilated patients.

ETIOLOGY AND PATHOPHYSIOLOGY

- Adults, outpatient CAP
  - Typical (85%): *Streptococcus pneumoniae, Haemophilus influenzae, Staphylococcus aureus,* group A *Streptococcus, Moraxella catarrhalis*
  - Atypical (15%): *Legionella* sp., *Mycoplasma pneumoniae, Chlamydophila pneumoniae*
- Adults, inpatient nonsevere or severe CAP, HAP, VAP
  - Aerobic gram-negative bacilli: *Pseudomonas aeruginosa, Escherichia coli, Klebsiella pneumoniae,* and *Acinetobacter* sp.
  - Gram-positive cocci: *Streptococcus* sp. and *S. aureus* (including MRSA)
- Pediatric
  - Birth to 3 weeks: *E. coli*, group B streptococci, *Listeria monocytogenes*
  - <3 months: *Chlamydia trachomatis, S. pneumoniae, H. influenzae*
  - 3 months to 18 years: typical: *S. pneumoniae;* atypical: *C. pneumoniae, M. pneumoniae*

RISK FACTORS

- Immunosuppression:
  - Chronic steroid use (>20 mg/day or >2 mg/kg/day of prednisone for >14 days)
  - HIV/immunoglobulin deficiencies/solid organ transplant/TNF-α inhibitor therapy
- Chronic health conditions: asthma, COPD, type 2 diabetes mellitus (DM), chronic renal failure, CHF, liver disease, tobacco use
- Other:
  - Age >65 years, antibiotic therapy in the past 6 months/resistance to antibiotics
  - Hospitalization for $\geq$2 days during past 90 days
  - Poor functional status

GENERAL PREVENTION

Vaccination recommendations:

- All children 2 to 59 months of age should be routinely vaccinated with pneumococcal conjugate (PCV13); given at 2, 4, and 6 months of age; a fourth dose at 12 to 15 months of age
- Adults $\geq$65 years who are vaccine naïve: should receive PPSV23 only. Adults >65 years in the high-risk group should receive PCV13 followed by pneumococcal polysaccharide (PPSV23) $\geq$1-year interval.
- For high-risk adults $\geq$65 years who have already received PPSV23, a dose of PCV13 is indicated after $\geq$1 year.
- Adults 19 to 64 years with tobacco use, chronic heart or lung disease, alcoholism, or chronic liver disease should receive a dose of PPSV23, followed by PCV13 at age 65 years and a subsequent PPSV23 $\geq$1 year after PCV13 and at least 5 years after the previous PPSV23 dose.
- High-risk adults $\geq$19 years old with immunocompromising conditions: Asplenia, CSF leaks, cochlear implants, HIV infection, immunodeficiencies require additional vaccinations as per the Centers for Disease Control.
- Annual influenza vaccine

DIAGNOSIS

HISTORY

- Fever, chills, rigors, malaise, fatigue, dyspnea, cough (with/without sputum), pleuritic chest pain, myalgias, GI symptoms
- Pediatric patients: lethargy, hypotonia, poor feeding, dry mucus membranes, vomiting

ALERT

- High fever (>104°F [40°C]), male sex, multilobar involvement, and GI and neurologic abnormalities have been associated with CAP caused by *Legionella*.
- History of advanced neurodegenerative disease or dementia who develop sudden high fever and cough should raise suspicion for aspiration pneumonia.

Geriatric Considerations

Older adults with pneumonia present with weakness, mental status change, agitation, or history of falls.

PHYSICAL EXAM

- Vitals: fever >100.4°F (38°C), tachypnea, tachycardia, hypoxemia
  - Severe cases may also present with hypothermia, bradycardia, or hypotension.
- Pulmonary exam: decreased breath sounds unilaterally with rales, rhonchi, egophony, increased fremitus, bronchial breath sounds, dullness to percussion, asymmetric breath sounds, abdominal tenderness
- Pediatric exam findings: grunting, retractions

DIFFERENTIAL DIAGNOSIS

Viral pneumonia, bronchitis, asthma or COPD exacerbation, pulmonary edema, lung cancer, pulmonary tuberculosis, pneumonitis, rheumatologic etiologies (i.e., sarcoidosis)

DIAGNOSTIC TESTS & INTERPRETATION

Initial Tests (lab, imaging)

- Outpatient setting:
  - No routine laboratory testing in outpatients is indicated.
  - CRP is the most useful and accurate biomarker for diagnosing outpatient CAP.
  - Clinical diagnosis with fever, tachypnea, and physical exam findings; chest x-ray not needed
  - A rapid influenza NAAT is preferred over a rapid influenza antigen test in all patients with CAP when influenza are in the community.
- Inpatient, noncritical care setting:
  - CBC, CRP, chest x-ray
  - Procalcitonin is no longer recommended.
  - Urine *Legionella* antigen testing if there is travel to a *Legionella* endemic area OR exposure to a *Legionella* outbreak
- Inpatient or critical care setting or severe CAP:
  - CBC, CRP, chest x-ray
  - Blood culture and sputum culture are recommended only for patients with severe CAP OR with a history of MRSA OR *P. aeruginosa* infections, OR being treated for MRSA/*P. aeruginosa* infections, OR hospitalized and treated with parental antibiotics within the previous 90 days.
  - Urine pneumococcal and *Legionella* antigen testing should be performed.
  - Procalcitonin is no longer recommended.
- Evidence of necrotizing/cavitary pneumonia should raise suspicion for MRSA pneumonia.

Follow-Up Tests & Special Considerations

- Viral testing including influenza as up to 80% of children <2 years old will have a viral cause.
- Obtain blood cultures only if no improvement on antibiotics or with severe CAP.

Diagnostic Procedures/Other

For HAP and VAP: By bronchoscopic or nonbronchoscopic means, obtain a lower respiratory tract sample for culture prior to initiation/change of therapy. Serial evaluations may be needed.

TREATMENT

GENERAL MEASURES

Use a risk calculator to determine need for hospitalization and efficacy of treatment:

- Pneumonia Severity Index: https://www.thecalculator.co/health/Pneumonia-Severity-Index-(PSI)-Calculator-977.html
- CURB-65: https://www.mdcalc.com/curb-65-score-pneumonia-severity

MEDICATION

First Line

- Adults (1)
  - CAP, outpatient empiric treatment: no risk factors for MRSA OR *P. aeruginosa* and no comorbidities
    - Amoxicillin 1,000 mg 3 times daily OR doxycycline 100 mg twice daily OR
    - If local macrolide resistance is <25%, then azithromycin 500 mg on day 1 and then 250 mg daily
  - CAP, outpatient empiric treatment: with comorbidities such as alcoholism, asplenia, DM, malignancy OR chronic heart/lung/liver/kidney disease but without risk factors for MRSA or *P. aeruginosa*
    - Combination therapy:
      - Amoxicillin/clavulanate 875 mg/125 BID, cefpodoxime 200 mg BID, or cefuroxime 500 mg BID PLUS
        □ Azithromycin 500 mg on the first day then 250 mg daily OR doxycycline 100 mg BID OR
    - Monotherapy with a respiratory fluoroquinolone: levofloxacin 750 mg daily or moxifloxacin 400 mg daily
  - Minimum duration of therapy is 5 days.
- CAP, inpatient: nonsevere pneumonia without risk factors for MRSA or *P. aeruginosa*
  - IV antibiotics initially, transition to PO with improvement
  - Minimum duration of therapy is 5 days.
  - Combination of:
    - Ampicillin/sulbactam (Unasyn), 1.5 to 3.0 g IV q6h OR cefotaxime, 1 to 2 g IV q8h OR ceftaroline, 600 mg IV q12h OR ceftriaxone, 1 to 2 g IV daily PLUS
      - Azithromycin 500 mg PO/IV daily OR clarithromycin 500 mg PO q12h OR
  - Monotherapy with a respiratory fluoroquinolone: levofloxacin 750 mg PO/IV daily OR moxifloxacin 400 mg PO/IV daily
- CAP, inpatient: severe pneumonia without risk factors for MRSA or *P. aeruginosa*
  - Combination of:
    - Ampicillin/sulbactam 1.5 to 3.0 g IV q6h OR cefotaxime 1 to 2 g IV q8h OR ceftriaxone 1 to 2 g IV daily PLUS
      - Azithromycin 500 mg PO/IV daily OR clarithromycin 500 mg PO q12h OR levofloxacin 750 mg PO/IV daily OR moxifloxacin 400 mg PO/IV daily

- CAP, inpatient: severe pneumonia with locally validated risk factors for MRSA or *P. aeruginosa*
  - For MRSA risk factors: linezolid, 600 mg PO/IV q12h OR vancomycin, 15 mg/kg IV q12h (adjust based on trough levels)
  - For *P. aeruginosa* risk factors: aztreonam, 2 g IV q8h OR cefepime, 2 g IV q8h OR meropenem, 1 g IV q8h OR piperacillin/tazobactam, 4.5 g IV q6h
- Routine use of corticosteroids is not recommended, including in severe CAP or HAP.
- HAP, inpatient (2)
  - Patients without MRSA risk factors and not at high risk of mortality, choose one of the following:
    - Piperacillin-tazobactam 4.5 mg IV q6h OR cefepime 2 g IV q8h OR levofloxacin 750 mg IV q24h OR imipenem 500 mg IV q6h OR meropenem 1 g IV q8h
  - Patients with MRSA risk factors add either vancomycin 15 mg/kg IV q8–12h based on trough OR linezolid 600 mg IV q12h
- VAP, inpatient (2)
  - Empirically cover *S. aureus*, *P. aeruginosa*, and other gram-negative bacilli
  - Cover MRSA if at risk for antimicrobial resistance or if prevalence of MRSA is not known.
  - Include double *Pseudomonas* coverage from two different classes only in patients at risk for antimicrobial resistance or in an ICU where susceptibility rates are not known.
- Pediatric, outpatient (≥3 months)
  - Antibiotic treatment in preschool-age children is not routinely required because viral pathogens are more common.
  - 10 days of therapy has been most studied; can consider shorter duration if treating mild pneumonia as an outpatient
  - Presumed typical bacterial pneumonia
    - Amoxicillin 90 mg/kg/day PO BID (max 4 g/day) OR amoxicillin-clavulanate 90 mg/kg/day PO BID (max 4 g/day)
  - Presumed atypical bacterial pneumonia
    - Azithromycin 10 mg/kg PO on day 1 (max 500 mg) and then 5 mg/kg/day (max 250 mg) on days 2 to 5
    - Clarithromycin 15 mg/kg/day PO BID (max 1 g/day) or erythromycin 40 mg/kg/day PO daily
    - Doxycycline 1 to 2 mg/kg/dose PO BID if >8 years old
- Pediatric, inpatient (≥3 months)
  - Presumed typical bacterial pneumonia
    - Fully immunized: ampicillin 200 mg/kg/day IV q6h
    - Not fully immunized: ceftriaxone 50 to 100 mg/kg/day IV q12–24h (max 2,000 mg)
    - Add vancomycin or clindamycin if suspecting community-acquired MRSA.
  - Presumed atypical bacterial pneumonia
    - Azithromycin 10 mg/kg IV daily on days 1 and 2 (max 500 mg) and then 5 mg/kg/day PO (max 250 mg) on days 3 to 5
    - Alternatives: clarithromycin, erythromycin, doxycycline (if >8 years old), levofloxacin (if reached growth maturity)

ADMISSION, INPATIENT, AND NURSING CONSIDERATIONS

- Patients with COPD or CHF are more likely to require ICU admission when suffering from CAP.
- Other considerations
  - Analgesia and antipyretics, chest physiotherapy, IV fluids (and conversely, diuretics) if indicated
  - Pulse oximetry and oxygen supplementation
  - Positioning minimize aspiration risk

Pediatric Considerations

- Inpatient treatment is recommended for infants ≤3 to 6 months, presence of respiratory distress (tachypnea, dyspnea, retractions, grunting, nasal flaring, apnea, altered mental status, O_2 sat <90%), or if known to have CAP as result of a virulent pathogen such as community-associated MRSA.
- Discharge criteria: clinical stability for 12 to 24 hours including temperature ≤100°F (37.8°C); HR ≤100 beats/min; RR ≤24 breaths/min; systolic BP ≤90 mm Hg; O_2 sat ≥90% on room air; maintain oral intake; normal mental status

 ## ONGOING CARE

PATIENT EDUCATION

Smoking cessation, vaccinations

COMPLICATIONS

Necrotizing pneumonia, respiratory failure, empyema, abscesses, cavitation, bronchopleural fistula, sepsis

REFERENCES

1. Metlay JP, Waterer GW, Long AC, et al. Diagnosis and treatment of adults with community-acquired pneumonia. An official clinical practice guideline of the American Thoracic Society and Infectious Diseases Society of America. *Am J Respir Crit Care Med*. 2019;200(7):e45–e67.
2. Kalil AC, Metersky ML, Klompas M, et al. Management of adults with hospital-acquired and ventilator-associated pneumonia: 2016 clinical practice guidelines by the Infectious Diseases Society of America and the American Thoracic Society. *Clin Infect Dis*. 2016;63(5):e61–e111.

 ## CODES

ICD10

- J15.9 Unspecified bacterial pneumonia
- J15.4 Pneumonia due to other streptococci
- J14 Pneumonia due to Hemophilus influenzae

CLINICAL PEARLS

- Bacterial pneumonia can usually be treated empirically based on its classification as outpatient CAP, inpatient nonsevere CAP, and inpatient severe CAP, or nosocomial pneumonia.
- A severity of illness score is helpful in determining the need for hospitalization of adult patients but does not replace a physician's clinical judgment.

PNEUMONIA, MYCOPLASMA

Kenneth A. Ballou, MD

BASICS

DESCRIPTION
- Bronchopulmonary infection caused by the *Mycoplasma* species, *Mycoplasma pneumoniae*
- Smallest free-living organism; fastidious and slow-growing; first isolated in cattle in 1898
- Most frequently affects children/young adults but can also occur in the elderly; often causes epidemics in closed communities (i.e., skilled nursing facilities)
- Infection may be asymptomatic, most often confined to the upper respiratory tract; however, may progress to pneumonia (5–10%)
- Course is usually acute with an incubation period of 1 to 4 weeks.
- Synonym(s): primary atypical pneumonia (PAP); Eaton agent pneumonia; cold agglutinin–positive pneumonia; walking pneumonia

Geriatric Considerations
The highest rate of ICU admissions for community-acquired pneumonia (CAP) secondary to *M. pneumoniae* occurs in seniors.

Pediatric Considerations
- Plays a significant role in pneumonias in children of all ages (Pneumonia <5 years, however, viral infection is far more common.)
- Increased incidence of asthma exacerbation in older children (1)[A]
- Infants 3 to 6 months with suspected bacterial pneumonia should be hospitalized.

EPIDEMIOLOGY
Incidence
- Estimated 1 million cases per year in the United States
- Responsible for 20% of CAP requiring hospitalizations annually
- Infection occurs most frequently in fall/winter seasons but may develop year round.

Prevalence
- Predominant sex: male = female
- Predominant age group affected: 5 to 20 years
  - May occur at any age
  - Rare in children <5 years of age
- Responsible for up to 15–20% of all cases of CAP yearly
  - Most common cause of pneumonia in school children and young adults who do not have a chronic underlying condition

ETIOLOGY AND PATHOPHYSIOLOGY
- *M. pneumoniae* is a short-rod mucosal pathogen, which lacks a cell wall and thus not visible on Gram stain.
- Can grow under both aerobic and anaerobic conditions
- Highly contagious, *M. pneumoniae* is transmitted primarily by aerosol droplets.
- Pathogenicity linked to its filamentous tips, which adhere selectively to respiratory epithelial cell membrane proteins with production of H_2O_2 and superoxide radicals, damaging cilia
- Many pathogenic features of infection are believed to be immune mediated, not directly induced.
- Decreased ciliary movement produces prolonged paroxysmal, hacking cough.
- Incubation period is 2 to 3 weeks.

RISK FACTORS
- Immunocompromised state (e.g., HIV, transplant recipients, chemotherapy)
- Smoking
- Close community living (e.g., military barracks, prisons, hospitals, dormitories, schools, household contacts, skilled nursing facilities)

GENERAL PREVENTION
Consider droplet isolation of active cases.

COMMONLY ASSOCIATED CONDITIONS
- Asthma exacerbations as a result of proinflammatory cytokine release (1)[A]
- Chronic obstructive pulmonary disease

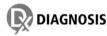DIAGNOSIS

HISTORY
- Infection may be asymptomatic.
- Gradual onset of headache, malaise, low-grade fevers, chills
- Symptoms of upper respiratory infection, including incessant, nonproductive cough, worsening cough (which may become mildly productive late in the disease) and pleurisy; rhinorrhea, pharyngitis, and sinusitis may occur subsequently (2).
- Pneumonia may occur with associated pleural effusion.
- The presence of pleuritic chest pain warrants a higher suspicion of *M. pneumoniae* (2).
- Extrapulmonary findings may develop in 5–10% of patients, including arthralgias, skin rashes, cervical adenopathy, hemolysis, congestive heart failure (CHF), and cardiac conduction abnormalities.
- Neurologic symptoms develop more commonly in children and may include encephalitis, aseptic meningitis, cranial nerve palsies, cerebellar ataxia, ascending paralysis, and coma (3).
- Persistent cough is common during convalescence; other sequelae are rare.

PHYSICAL EXAM
- Toxicity increases with advancing age or increased number of comorbidity factors.
- Hacking/pertussis-like cough may be present along with fever and lassitude.
- Normal lung findings with early infection, but rhonchi, rales, and/or wheezes may develop several days later (2).
- Mild pharyngeal injection without exudates
- Minimal/no cervical adenopathy
- Erythematous tympanic membranes or bullous myringitis in patients >2 years of age is an uncommon but unique sign.
- Some patients may develop an audible pleural friction rub.
- Various exanthems, including erythema multiforme and Stevens-Johnson syndrome

DIFFERENTIAL DIAGNOSIS
- Viral/bacterial/fungal pneumonia
- Tuberculosis

- Other atypical pneumonias, including *Chlamydia pneumoniae, Chlamydophila psittaci, Coxiella burnetii* (Q fever), *Francisella tularensis* (tularemia), *Pneumocystis jiroveci, Legionella pneumophila,* and other community-acquired pneumonias
- Must differentiate from COVID-19–related pulmonary infection; COVID-19 testing recommended

DIAGNOSTIC TESTS & INTERPRETATION
- *M. pneumoniae* is typically a clinical diagnosis and treated empirically; however, when specific pathogen testing is indicated, polymerase chain reaction (PCR) is the test of choice (4)[C].
- No clinical or radiographic findings can differentiate between *M. pneumoniae* and other atypical pneumonia pathogens (*Chlamydia/Legionella*).

Initial Tests (lab, imaging)
- WBC count may be normal or elevated.
- Hemolytic anemia has been described but is rare.
- Elevated erythrocyte sedimentation rate (ESR) may be present but is nonspecific.
- Use of procalcitonin levels is limited as the rise in levels is generally more modest for atypical etiologies and may be undetectable for *Mycoplasma* species.
- When available, PCR for *M. pneumoniae* DNA in nasopharyngeal and throat swabs as well as bronchoalveolar lavage respiratory secretions, CSF, and tissue samples may be the most sensitive and specific.
- CXR shows reticulonodular pattern with patchy areas of lower lobe consolidation, although this is not specific. Small pleural effusion may be present in 10–15% cases.

Follow-Up Tests & Special Considerations
- Sputum Gram stains are not helpful because *M. pneumoniae* lacks a cell wall and cannot be stained.
- *M. pneumoniae* is difficult to culture and requires 7 to 21 days to grow; culturing is successful in 40–90% of cases but does not provide information to guide treatment, thus infrequently performed.
- Complement fixation serologic assay shows 4-fold rise in IgM antibody titer at 2 to 4 weeks after symptom onset; this is an older technique.
- Positive cold agglutinins (titer of ≥1:128 or rising 4-fold) in 50% of infections but can take 1 to 2 weeks to develop; not sensitive/specific; not routinely recommended
- CT of chest may show a combination of patchy tree-in-bud opacities with segmental ground-glass opacities.

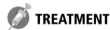TREATMENT

GENERAL MEASURES
- Avoid ill contacts.
- Supportive care indicated, especially for very ill patients who may require inpatient treatment
- Treatment is initially empiric and must be comprehensive to cover all likely pathogens in the context of the clinical setting.
- Calculation of pneumonia severity score (CAP score: http://www.mdcalc.com/psi-port-score-pneumonia-severity-index-adult-cap) may be helpful in determining inpatient versus outpatient treatment.

Pregnancy Considerations
- Azithromycin: pregnancy Category B (preferred treatment)
- Clarithromycin, levofloxacin, and moxifloxacin: pregnancy Category C

MEDICATION

First Line
- Azithromycin
  - <3 months of age: not established (5)[B]
  - >3 months of age: day 1, 10 mg/kg PO × 1 (not to exceed 500 mg); days 2 to 5, 5 mg/kg PO daily (not to exceed 250 mg/day)
  - Adults: 500 mg PO × 1 followed by 250 mg PO daily × 4 days
- Doxycycline
  - Children <8 years of age: not recommended
  - Children >8 years of age (≤45 kg): 2 to 4 mg/kg/day up to 200 mg/day PO divided BID for 10 to 14 days
  - Children >8 years of age (≥45 kg): Refer to adult dosing.
  - Adults: 100 mg PO BID × 7 to 14 days
  - Useful in macrolide-resistant strains of *M. pneumoniae*
- Clarithromycin
  - Children <6 months of age: not established
  - Patients >6 months of age: 15 mg/kg/day PO divided q12h for 10 to 14 days
  - Adults: 250 to 500 mg PO BID for 10 to 14 days
- Minocycline
  - 200 mg PO/IV × 1 dose and then 100 mg BID for 7 to 10 days
- Erythromycin
  - Children: 20 to 50 mg/kg/day (base) PO divided q6–8h for 10 to 14 days
  - Adults: 500 mg (base) PO q6h × 10 to 14 days

Second Line
- Levofloxacin
  - Children <18 years of age: not recommended
  - Adults: 750 mg PO daily × 5 days
- Moxifloxacin
  - Children <18 years of age: not recommended
  - Adults: 400 mg/day PO for 7 to 10 days
- Levofloxacin and moxifloxacin show good activity against *M. pneumoniae*. Consider use with comorbid conditions and other pneumonia pathogens; also useful if macrolide resistance is suspected

ADDITIONAL THERAPIES
- Albuterol inhaler: 2 puffs q4–6h as needed for wheezing
- Dexamethasone may downregulate cytokine release (6)[B].
- Acetaminophen/ibuprofen as needed for fever
- Supplemental oxygen as needed
- Up to 10.9% of hospitalized patients may require mechanical ventilation.
- Plasmapheresis in cases of severe hemolytic anemia

ADMISSION, INPATIENT, AND NURSING CONSIDERATIONS
- CAP score risk class IV/V
- Other scoring systems such as the CURB65 and Pneumonia Severity Index (PSI) may also be helpful in the inpatient versus outpatient treatment decision (6)[A].
- Advanced age with comorbidities
- Complicating neoplastic disease
- Significant cerebrovascular, cardiac, renal, liver, or GI symptoms
- Altered mental status
- Inability to maintain oxygen saturation
- Tachycardia/tachypnea
- Hypotension
- Neurologic symptoms
- Signs of Stevens-Johnson syndrome
- Significant hemolysis (autoimmune hemolytic anemia, cold agglutinin disease)
- Change from IV to PO antibiotic may be made when:
  - Respiratory distress and hypoxia have resolved.
  - Patients are tolerating oral hydration.
  - No significant complications are present.
  - Utilization of procalcitonin (PCT) may aid in this decision (4)[A].
- Generally, no need for 24-hour observation on PO antibiotics prior to discharge.

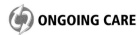 ## ONGOING CARE

FOLLOW-UP RECOMMENDATIONS
- Clearing of condition on CXR should be documented in patients >50 years of age.
- In smokers, document a clear CXR in 6 to 8 weeks.
- Worsening symptoms/development of rash or meningeal/neurologic signs should prompt immediate presentation to medical attention.
- Antibiotic prophylaxis for exposed contacts is not routinely recommended.
- For household contacts who may be predisposed to severe mycoplasmal infection, macrolide or doxycycline prophylaxis should be used.

DIET
- No special diet considerations
- Ensure adequate hydration.

PATIENT EDUCATION
- Smoking cessation
- Contact and droplet precautions
- Adequate hand washing techniques

PROGNOSIS
- Symptoms usually resolve in 2 weeks.
- Some constitutional symptoms may persist for several weeks.
- With correct therapy, even most severe cases can expect complete recovery.

COMPLICATIONS
- All complications are rare, except reactive airway disease, hemolytic anemia, and erythema multiforme.
- Reactive airway disease may persist indefinitely and can cause acute chest syndrome in patients with sickle cell anemia.
- Meningoencephalitis
- Aseptic meningitis
- Peripheral neuropathy
- Transverse myelitis/acute transverse myelitis
- Cerebellar ataxia
- Acute disseminated encephalomyelitis
- Guillain-Barré syndrome
- Encephalitis (especially in children)
- Polyneuritis/polyarthritis
- Stevens-Johnson syndrome
- Pericarditis/myocarditis
- Respiratory distress syndrome
- Cerebral ataxia
- Thromboembolic phenomena
- Pleural effusion
- Nephritis
- Occasional deaths occur primarily among the elderly and persons with sickle cell disease.

REFERENCES

1. Gao S, Wang L, Zhu W, et al. Mycoplasma pneumonia infection and asthma: a clinical study. *Pak J Med Sci.* 2015;31(3):548–551.
2. Marchello C, Dale AP, Thai TN, et al. Prevalence of atypical pathogens in patients with cough and community-acquired pneumonia: a meta-analysis. *Ann Fam Med.* 2016;14(6):552–566.
3. Wang K, Gill P, Perera R, et al. Clinical symptoms and signs for the diagnosis of *Mycoplasma pneumoniae* in children and adolescents with community-acquired pneumonia. *Cochrane Database Syst Rev.* 2012;(10):CD009175.
4. Sager R, Kutz A, Mueller B, et al. Procalcitonin-guided diagnosis and antibiotic stewardship revisited. *BMC Med.* 2017;15(1):15.
5. Gardiner S, Gavranich J, Chang A. Antibiotics for community-acquired lower respiratory tract infections secondary to *Mycoplasma pneumoniae* in children. *Cochrane Database Syst Rev.* 2015;(1):CD004875.
6. Sharma L, Losier A, Tolbert T, et al. Atypical pneumonia: updates on *Legionella*, *Chlamydophila*, and *Mycoplasma* pneumonia. *Clin Chest Med.* 2017;38(1):45–58.

ADDITIONAL READING

- Atkinson TP, Balish MF, Waites KB. Epidemiology, clinical manifestations, pathogenesis and laboratory detection of *Mycoplasma pneumoniae* infections. *FEMS Microbiol Rev.* 2008;32(6):956–973.
- Eliakim-Raz N, Robenshtok E, Shefet D, et al. Empiric antibiotic coverage of atypical pathogens for community-acquired pneumonia in hospitalized adults. *Cochrane Database Syst Rev.* 2012;(9):CD004418.
- Kashyap S, Sarkar M. Mycoplasma pneumonia: clinical features and management. *Lung India.* 2010;27(2):75–85.
- Kaysin A, Viera A. Community-acquired pneumonia in adults: diagnosis and management. *Am Fam Physician.* 2016;94(9):698–706.
- Khoury T, Sviri S, Rmeileh AA, et al. Increased rates of intensive care unit admission in patients with *Mycoplasma pneumoniae*: a retrospective study. *Clin Microbiol Infect.* 2016;22(8):711–714.
- Stuckey-Schrock K, Hayes B, George C. Community-acquired pneumonia in children. *Am Fam Physician.* 2012;86(7):661–667.
- Viasus D, Calatayud L, McBrown M, et al. Urinary antigen testing in community-acquired pneumonia in adults: an update. *Expert Rev Anti Infect Ther.* 2019;17(2):107–115.
- Waites KB, Xiao L, Liu Y, et al. *Mycoplasma pneumoniae* from the respiratory tract and beyond. *Clin Microbiol Rev.* 2017;30(3):747–809.

 ## CODES

ICD10
J15.7 Pneumonia due to Mycoplasma pneumoniae

CLINICAL PEARLS
- Most common atypical respiratory pathogens include *M. pneumoniae*, *C. pneumoniae*, and *L. pneumophila*.
- Atypical pneumonia is usually a clinical diagnosis.
- Watch closely for complicating symptoms that could indicate worsening disease.
- Atypical pneumonia with *M. pneumoniae* usually responds to empiric treatment.
- Outbreaks of *M. pneumoniae* can be seen in closed communities (i.e., dormitories).
- Presentation of infection is typically a gradual onset of symptoms.

PNEUMONIA, PNEUMOCYSTIS JIROVECI

Thomas J. Hansen, MD

 BASICS

DESCRIPTION
- *Pneumocystis jiroveci* causes pneumonia primarily in immunocompromised patients.
- The fungus that causes this pneumonia in humans was previously called *Pneumocystis carinii*.
- The name was formally changed to *Pneumocystis jiroveci* in 2001, following the discovery that the fungus that infects humans is unique and distinctive from the fungus that infects animals.
- *P. jiroveci* is extremely resistant to traditional antifungal agents, including both amphotericin and azole agents.
- To prevent confusion, the term PCP, which used to represent *P. carinii* pneumonia, now represents *Pneumocystis* pneumonia (1).

ALERT
No combination of symptoms, signs, blood chemistries, or radiographic findings is diagnostic of *P. jiroveci* pneumonia (2).

EPIDEMIOLOGY
- *P. jiroveci* has a worldwide distribution, and most children have been exposed to the fungus by 2 to 4 years (3).
- The reservoir and mode of transmission for *P. jiroveci* is still unclear.
  - Human studies favor an airborne transmission model, with person-to-person spread being the most likely mode of infection acquisition (2).

Incidence
- Infants with HIV infection have a peak incidence of PCP between 2 and 6 months (3).
- HIV-infected infants have a high mortality rate, with a median survival of only 1 month.

Prevalence
- The prevalence of *P. jiroveci* colonization among healthy adults is 0–20%.
- Recent studies have demonstrated the transient nature of *P. jiroveci* colonization in asymptomatic, immunocompetent patients (2).
- 50% of patients with PCP are coinfected with ≥2 strains of *P. jiroveci* (3).
- There is evidence that distinct strains are responsible for each episode in patients who develop multiple episodes of PCP (3).

ETIOLOGY AND PATHOPHYSIOLOGY
Mode of transmission is unknown; likely respiratory from infected host

RISK FACTORS
Individuals at risk (2)
- Patients with HIV infection, especially if not receiving prophylactic treatment for PCP
- Patients who are receiving high doses of glucocorticoids
- Patients who have an altered immune system not due to HIV
- Patients who are receiving chronic immunosuppressive medications
- Patients who have hematologic or solid malignancies resulting in malignancy-related immune depression

GENERAL PREVENTION
- Indications for prophylaxis
  - HIV-infected adults (3)
    - Should start when CD4 count is <200 cells/μL or if the patient develops oropharyngeal candidiasis
  - HIV-infected children (3)
    - Prophylaxis should be provided for children ≥6 years based on adult guidelines.
    - For children aged 1 to 5 years, start when CD4 count is <500 cells/μL.
    - For infants <12 months, start when the CD4 percentage is <15%.
  - Non–HIV-infected adults receiving immunosuppressive medications or with underlying immune system deficits should receive PCP prophylaxis, but currently, there are no specific guidelines on when to start this.
- Medication
  - Trimethoprim-sulfamethoxazole (TMP-SMX)
    - Adults: 1 double-strength tablet daily or 1 double-strength tablet 3 times per week
    - Children >2 months: TMP 150 mg/kg/day in divided doses q12h for 3 days/week
  - Atovaquone suspension
    - Adults: 1,500 mg PO once daily with food
    - Children: not to exceed 1,500 mg/day
      - 1 to 3 months: 30 mg/kg/day PO once daily
      - 4 to 24 months: 45 mg/kg/day PO once daily
      - >24 months: 30 mg/kg/day PO once daily
      - Adolescents ≥13 years: Refer to adult dosing.
  - Dapsone
    - Adults only: 50 mg BID or 100 mg once daily
  - Pentamidine
    - Adults only: 300 mg aerosolized every 4 weeks
- Discontinuation of prophylaxis
  - When CD4+ cell counts are >200 cells/μL for a period of 3 months in the adult population
  - There are no clear guidelines for discontinuation of prophylaxis in children.

COMMONLY ASSOCIATED CONDITIONS
- HIV Infection
- Chronic obstructive pulmonary disease (COPD)
- Interstitial lung disease
- Connective tissue diseases treated with corticosteroids
- Cancer and organ transplant patients on immunosuppressive medication

 DIAGNOSIS

HISTORY
- HIV-infected patients
  - Subacute onset over several weeks
    - Progressively worsening dyspnea
    - Tachypnea
    - Cough: nonproductive or productive of clear sputum
    - Low-grade fever, chills
    - Weakness, fatigue, malaise
- Non–HIV-infected immunocompromised patients
  - More acute onset with fulminant respiratory failure
    - Abrupt tachypnea, dyspnea
    - Fever
    - Dry cough

PHYSICAL EXAM
- Fever
- Tachypnea
- Tachycardia
- Lung exam is normal or near-normal.

DIFFERENTIAL DIAGNOSIS
- Tuberculosis
- Bacterial pneumonia
- Fungal pneumonia
- Viral pneumonia

DIAGNOSTIC TESTS & INTERPRETATION
P. jiroveci cannot be cultured. Therefore, a diagnosis relies on detection of the organism by colorimetric or immunofluorescent stains or by polymerase chain reaction (PCR) (3)[C].
- ABG: reveals hypoxemia and increased alveolar–arterial gradient that varies with severity of disease
- LDH: Serum lactate dehydrogenase is frequently increased (nonspecific; likely due to underlying lung inflammation and injury).
- CD4 cell count is generally <200 cells/μL in HIV-infected patients with PCP.
- S-adenosylmethionine levels are significantly lower in a patient with PCP. The levels increase with successful treatment (4)[B].
- Comprehensive metabolic profile
- Chest x-ray (CXR) (2)[C]
  - Bilateral, symmetric, fine, reticular interstitial infiltrates involving perihilar areas; becomes more homogeneous and diffuse as severity of infection progresses
  - Less common patterns include upper lobe involvement in patients receiving aerosolized pentamidine, solitary or multiple nodular opacities, lobar infiltrates, pneumatoceles, and pneumothoraces.
  - May be normal in up to 30% of patients with PCP (1)[C]
- High-resolution CT is more sensitive than CXR.

Diagnostic Procedures/Other
- Fiberoptic bronchoscopy with bronchoalveolar lavage (BAL) is the preferred diagnostic procedure to obtain samples for direct fluorescent antibody staining.
  - Sensitivities range from 89% to >98%.
- *Pneumocystis* trophic forms or cysts obtained from induced sputum, BAL fluid, or lung tissue, which can be visualized using conventional stains
- PCR can detect *Pneumocystis* from respiratory sources, but the potential remains for false positives (2)[C].

TREATMENT

The recommended duration of therapy differs in patients who are with/without AIDS:
- In patients with PCP who do not have AIDS, the typical duration of therapy is 14 days.
- Treatment of PCP in patients who have AIDS was increased to 21 days due to the risk for relapse after only 14 days of treatment (2)[C].

MEDICATION

First Line
- TMP-SMX (2)[C]
- Adult dosing
  - TMP: 15 to 20 mg/kg/day, PO or IV, divided into 4 doses
- Pediatric dosing (>2 months) (2)[C]
  - TMP: 15 to 20 mg/kg/day in divided doses q6–8h
- Reduce doses of TMP-SMX in patients with renal failure.
- Patients should receive 21 days of therapy.
- Treatment response to *Pneumocystis* therapy often requires at least 7 to 10 days before clinical improvement is documented.
- Pregnancy risk factor: category C (2)[C]
- Precautions
  - History of sulfa allergy
  - There is an emergence of drug-resistant PCP, especially against TMP-SMX.

Second Line
- Pentamidine (for moderate to severe cases)
  - Adults and children: 4 mg/kg IV or IM once daily
- Dapsone + trimethoprim (adults only)
  - Dapsone 100 mg PO once daily, *plus*
  - Trimethoprim 5 mg/kg PO TID
    - Check the glucose-6-phosphate dehydrogenase level before beginning dapsone because hemolysis may result.
- Clindamycin + primaquine (adults only)
  - Clindamycin 600 to 900 mg IV q8h or 300 to 450 mg PO QID *plus*
  - Primaquine 30 mg PO once daily
- Atovaquone
  - Adults: 750 mg PO BID (>13 years of age)
  - Children: 40 mg/kg/day PO divided BID (max 1,500 mg)
- Note: Pentamidine has greater toxicity than TMP-SMX: hypotension, hypoglycemia, pancreatitis (2)[C].

ADDITIONAL THERAPIES
Adjunctive corticosteroid (prednisone or methylprednisolone) (2)[C],(5)[A]

- Adjunctive corticosteroids are shown to provide benefits in patients who have HIV and symptoms of moderate to severe PCP.
- Corticosteroids provide the greatest benefit to HIV patients who have hypoxemia manifested as a partial pressure of arterial oxygen <70 mm Hg or an alveolar–arterial gradient >35 mm Hg on room air.
- Adults and children >13 years of age: prednisone, 40 mg PO BID on days 1 to 5; 40 mg daily on days 6 to 11; 20 mg daily on days 12 to 21

ADMISSION, INPATIENT, AND NURSING CONSIDERATIONS
- No set criteria for hospital admission
- Five predictors of mortality in HIV-associated *Pneumocystis* pneumonia (6)
  - Increased age of the patient
  - Recent IV drug use
  - Total bilirubin >0.6 mg/dL
  - Serum albumin <3 g/dL
  - Alveolar–arterial oxygen gradient ≥50 mm Hg (6)[C]

ONGOING CARE

FOLLOW-UP RECOMMENDATIONS
In patients with HIV/AIDS: Patients with previous episodes of PCP should receive lifelong secondary prophylaxis unless they respond well to highly active antiretroviral therapy (HAART) and have a CD4 count >200 cells/μL for at least 3 months.

Patient Monitoring
Serum lactate dehydrogenase levels, pulmonary function test results, and ABG measurements generally normalize with treatment.

DIET
No special diet needed

PATIENT EDUCATION
- Centers for Disease Control and Prevention: https://www.cdc.gov/dpdx/pneumocystis/index.html
- FamilyDoctor.org: http://familydoctor.org/familydoctor/en/diseases-conditions/hiv-and-aids/complications/pneumocystis-pneumonia-pcp-and-hiv.html

REFERENCES
1. D'Avignon LC, Schofield CM, Hospenthal DR. *Pneumocystis* pneumonia. *Semin Respir Crit Care Med.* 2008;29(2):132–140.
2. Krajicek BJ, Thomas CF Jr, Limper AH. *Pneumocystis* pneumonia: current concepts in pathogenesis, diagnosis, and treatment. *Clin Chest Med.* 2009;30(2):265–278.
3. Kovacs JA, Masur H. Evolving health effects of *Pneumocystis*: one hundred years of progress in diagnosis and treatment. *JAMA.* 2009;301(24):2578–2585.
4. Skelly MJ, Holzman RS, Merali S. S-adenosylmethionine levels in the diagnosis of *Pneumocystis carinii* pneumonia in patients with HIV infection. *Clin Infect Dis.* 2008;46(3):467–471.
5. Briel M, Bucher HC, Boscacci R, et al. Adjunctive corticosteroids for *Pneumocystis jiroveci* pneumonia in patients with HIV-infection. *Cochrane Database Syst Rev.* 2006;(3):CD006150.
6. Fei MW, Kim EJ, Sant CA, et al. Predicting mortality from HIV-associated *Pneumocystis* pneumonia at illness presentation: an observational cohort study. *Thorax.* 2009;64(12):1070–1076.

ADDITIONAL READING
- Benson CA, Kaplan JE, Masur H, et al; for Centers of Disease Control and Prevention, National Institutes of Health, Infectious Diseases Society of America. Treating opportunistic infections among HIV-infected adults and adolescents: recommendations from CDC, the National Institutes of Health, and the HIV Medicine Association/Infectious Diseases Society of America. *MMWR Recomm Rep.* 2004;53(RR-15):1–112.
- Catherinot E, Lanternier F, Bougnoux ME, et al. *Pneumocystis jirovecii* pneumonia. *Infect Dis Clin North Am.* 2010;24(1):107–138.

- Green H, Paul M, Vidal L, et al. Prophylaxis for *Pneumocystis* pneumonia (PCP) in non-HIV immunocompromised patients. *Cochrane Database Syst Rev.* 2007;(3):CD005590.
- Kaplan JE, Masur H, Holmes KK. Guidelines for preventing opportunistic infections among HIV-infected persons—2002. Recommendations of the U.S. Public Health Service and the Infectious Diseases Society of America. http://www.cdc.gov/mmwr/preview/mmwrhtml/rr5108a1.htm. Accessed October 3, 2016.
- Limper AH, Knox KS, Sarosi GA, et al; for American Thoracic Society Fungal Working Group. An official American Thoracic Society statement: treatment of fungal infections in adult pulmonary and critical care patients. *Am J Respir Crit Care Med.* 2011;183(1):96–128.
- Shankar SM, Nania JJ. Management of *Pneumocystis jiroveci* pneumonia in children receiving chemotherapy. *Paediatr Drugs.* 2007;9(5):301–309.
- Stringer JR, Beard CB, Miller RF, et al. A new name for *Pneumocystis* from humans and new perspectives on the host-pathogen relationship. *Emerg Infect Dis.* 2002;8(9):891–896.

SEE ALSO

HIV/AIDS

CODES

ICD10
B59 Pneumocystosis

CLINICAL PEARLS

- Colonization with *P. jiroveci* is common in the pediatric population.
- PCP only occurs in immunocompromised patients.
- Patients with HIV are at risk once their CD4 count is <200 cells/μL. At that time, TMP-SMX should be initiated as prophylaxis. Prophylaxis may end after HAART has been initiated and the CD4 count is >200 cells/μL for 3 months.
- Patients who are immunocompromised are also at risk. Currently, no clear clinical guidelines are available as to when to initiate or end prophylaxis.
- The first-line treatment is TMP-SMX. The typical duration of therapy is 14 days in non–HIV-infected patients and 21 days in HIV-infected patients.

POLYARTERITIS NODOSA

Ratnesh Chopra, MD • Yevgeniy Popov, DO, MPH

 BASICS

DESCRIPTION

- Polyarteritis nodosa (PAN) is an antineutrophil cytoplasmic antibody (ANCA)-negative necrotizing arteritis of medium-sized muscular arteries and (occasionally) small arteries. Arterioles, capillaries, and venules are spared (1).
- Involved systems include gastrointestinal (GI) tract, peripheral nervous system (sensory and motor), CNS, genitourinary, skin, and cardiovascular. Glomerulonephritis and pulmonary capillaritis are rare (1),(2).
- Features depend on location of vasculitis: for example, mesenteric ischemia–related symptoms, new onset or worsening hypertension (HTN), mononeuritis multiplex, purpuric or nodular skin lesions, or livedo reticularis (2).
- Renal disease in PAN usually manifests as HTN and mild proteinuria with/without azotemia. Renal infarction may also occur (2).
- PAN formerly encompassed several distinct entities (classic PAN, microscopic PAN, and cutaneous PAN). With ANCA testing, microscopic PAN appears pathophysiologically unrelated to the other two.
  - Idiopathic generalized PAN (classic PAN) is clinically variable, ranging from single organ involvement to polyvisceral failure (1).
  - HBV-associated PAN patients are positive for active hepatitis B infection and can present in similar fashion to idiopathic generalized PAN (1).
  - Microscopic PAN has ANCAs directed against myeloperoxidase (MPO) and involvement of small arterioles (microscopic polyangiitis [MPA]). This is now classified as ANCA-associated vasculitis.
  - Cutaneous (or limited) PAN is generally limited to the deep dermal and subcutaneous (SC) levels of the skin with characteristic histopathologic features of PAN. There are few systemic manifestations, although myalgias and peripheral motor neuropathy (mononeuritis multiplex) or sensory neuropathy may be present (2).
- Synonym(s): periarteritis; panarteritis; necrotizing arteritis

EPIDEMIOLOGY

Incidence
- Incidence of 0 to 1.6 cases per million
- Predominant age: peaks in 5th to 6th decade; incidence rises with age.
- Mean age at diagnosis is 50 years.
- Male predominance

Prevalence
Rare: up to 31 cases per 1 million adults (1)

ETIOLOGY AND PATHOPHYSIOLOGY
- Segmental, transmural, necrotizing inflammation of medium and small muscular arteries, with intimal proliferation, thrombosis, and ischemia of the end-organ/tissue supplied by the affected vessels; aneurysm formation at vessel bifurcations (2).
- Hepatitis B–related PAN results in direct vessel injury due to viral replication or deposition of immune complexes, with complement activation and subsequent inflammatory response (2).

- Most cases are idiopathic; 20% are related to hepatitis B or C infection.
- In patients with PAN and hepatitis B, HBsAg has been recovered from involved vessel walls.

Genetics
Mutations of adenosine deaminase 2 (ADA 2) have been identified in families with PAN (1).

RISK FACTORS
Hepatitis B > hepatitis C infection (cutaneous PAN)

COMMONLY ASSOCIATED CONDITIONS
- Hepatitis B (strong association with classic PAN)
- Hepatitis C (less strongly linked to cutaneous PAN)
- Hairy cell leukemia
- 27 cases of systemic PAN following hepatitis B vaccination
- Minocycline (Symptoms resolve on stopping drug, reoccur if rechallenged.)
- Case-based associations with CMV infection, amphetamines, and interferon

 DIAGNOSIS

- There are no formal diagnostic criteria for PAN (1),(2).
- Suspect PAN with:
  - Acute, sometimes fulminant multisystem disease with a relatively short prodrome (i.e., weeks to months)
  - Vasculitic skin rash with sensorimotor symptoms/findings
  - Recent-onset HTN with systemic symptoms
  - Unexplained sensory and/or motor neuropathy with systemic symptoms
  - Hepatitis B infection with multisystem disease

HISTORY
Symptoms reflect specific organ involvement (2).
- Constitutional symptoms (fever, weight loss, malaise)
- Organ-specific symptoms
  - Focal muscular weakness/extremity numbness
  - Myalgia and arthralgia
  - Rash (nodules, purpura, livedo)
  - Recurrent postprandial pain, intestinal angina, nausea, vomiting, and bleeding
  - Altered mental status, headaches, mononeuritis multiplex
  - Testicular/epididymal pain, neurogenic bladder (rare)

PHYSICAL EXAM
Findings/course reflect specific organ involvement (2).
- Peripheral nervous system: peripheral neuropathy, mononeuritis multiplex
- Renal: HTN
- Skin: purpura, urticaria, polymorphic rashes, SC nodules (uncommon but characteristic), livedo reticularis; deep skin ulcers, especially in lower extremities; Raynaud phenomenon (rare); single digit gangrene (rare)
- GI: acute abdomen; rebound, guarding, tenderness
- CNS: seizures, altered mental status, papillitis
- Lung: signs of pleural effusion—dullness to percussion; decreased breath sounds

- Cardiac: signs of congestive heart failure and/or myocardial infarction—S_3 gallop; pericarditis (Friction rub is rare.)
- Genitourinary: testicular/epididymal tenderness (can mimic testicular torsion)
- Musculoskeletal: arthritis (usually large joint in lower extremities)

DIFFERENTIAL DIAGNOSIS
- Other forms of vasculitis (ANCA-associated, such as granulomatosis with polyangiitis [GPA—formerly Wegener granulomatosis], Churg-Strauss syndrome, and MPA; Henoch-Schönlein purpura, drug-induced vasculitis, cryoglobulinemia, Goodpasture syndrome)
- Buerger disease
- Systemic lupus erythematosus (SLE)
- Embolic disease (atrial myxoma, cholesterol emboli)
- Thrombotic disease (antiphospholipid antibody syndrome)
- Dissecting aneurysm
- Ehlers-Danlos syndrome
- Multiple sclerosis, systemic amyloidosis
- Infection (subacute endocarditis, HIV infection, trichinosis, rickettsial diseases)
- Calciphylaxis lesions
- Fibromuscular dysplasia
- Ergotamine use
- Segmental arterial mediolysis

DIAGNOSTIC TESTS & INTERPRETATION
- No specific laboratory abnormalities. Confirm diagnosis with biopsy if possible (3)[A].
- Angiography (conventional, CT angiography, or MR angiography) may reveal microaneurysms and/or beading of bifurcating blood vessels.
- Avoid contrast in renal disease.
- Nonspecific laboratory abnormalities:
  - Elevated ESR and CRP
  - Mild proteinuria, elevated creatinine
  - Hepatitis B surface antigen positive in 10–50%
  - Hepatitis C antibody/hepatitis C virus RNA
  - ANCA, anti-proteinase 3 (PR3), and anti-MPO are negative. Positive ANCA argues against PAN.
  - Rheumatoid factor may be positive.
  - Anemia of chronic disease (2),(3)

Initial Tests (lab, imaging)
Look for evidence of systemic disease and rule out other causes (2),(3):
- CBC (thrombocytosis), ESR, and CRP (elevated) (3)[C]
- Chemistries: elevated creatinine/BUN (3)[C]
- Hepatitis B serology: often positive; hepatitis C less commonly positive
- LFTs: abnormal if associated hepatitis B, C, or involvement of hepatobiliary tract
- Urinalysis: proteinuria/hematuria, generally no cellular casts or active urinary sediment (3)[C]
- ANA, cryoglobulins (3)[C]
- ANCA, anti-MPO, and anti-PR3 (3)[A]
- Complement levels (C3, C4)
- Angiographic demonstration of aneurysmal changes/beading of small- and medium-sized arteries

Diagnostic Procedures/Other
- Electromyography and nerve conduction studies in patients with suspected mononeuritis multiplex. If abnormal, consider sural nerve biopsy.
- Arterial/tissue biopsy (least invasive approach preferable)
- Skin biopsy from edges of ulcers; include deep dermis and SC fat to assess small muscular artery involvement (excisional *not* punch biopsy) (2),(3).

Test Interpretation
- Necrotizing inflammation with fibrinoid necrosis of small- and medium-sized muscular arteries; segmental, often at bifurcations and branchings. Venules are not involved in classic PAN.
- Capillaritis/other lung parenchymal involvement by vasculitis *strongly suggests* another process (microscopic PAN, GPA, Churg-Strauss syndrome, or antiglomerular basement membrane disease).
- Acute lesions with infiltration of polymorphonuclear cells through vessel walls into perivascular area; necrosis, thrombosis, and infarction of involved tissue.
- Aneurysmal dilatations, including aortic dissection
- Peripheral nerves: 50–70% (vasa nervorum with necrotizing vasculitis)
- GI vessels: 50% (at autopsy) with bowel necrosis; gallbladder and appendix vasculature: 10%
- Muscle vessels: 50%
- Testicular vessels involved in symptomatic males
- *The key differences from other necrotizing vasculitides are lack of granuloma formation and sparing of veins and pulmonary arteries* (2).

TREATMENT

GENERAL MEASURES
Treat HTN aggressively to prevent complications (stroke, myocardial infarction, heart failure).

MEDICATION
First Line
- Severe (life-threatening) disease: corticosteroids (CS) (high-dose oral prednisone [1 mg/kg/day] or intravenous [IV] methylprednisolone [0.5 to 1.0 g/day] for 3 days, then transition to prednisone 1 mg/kg/day, and taper according to response) (3),(4)[A].
  - Only 50% of patients achieve and maintain remission with CS. Other patients require additional immunosuppressive therapy.
  - IV cyclophosphamide (0.6 g/m² every 2 weeks for 3 doses and then monthly for 4 to 12 months) in combination with CS: improves survival and spares use of chronic steroids in moderate/severe PAN (3),(4)[A]
    - Cyclophosphamide has risk of infertility and malignancy.
  - Plasma exchange for severe refractory disease, such as progressive renal disease (3)[A]
- Less severe disease: CS alone ± other immunosuppressive agents (azathioprine 2 mg/kg/day, methotrexate 20 to 25 mg/week, mycophenolate mofetil 2,000 to 3,000 mg daily). Hydroxychloroquine (5 mg/kg/day) use has been reported (3),(4)[A],(5)[C].
- Cutaneous PAN: Nonsteroidal anti-inflammatory drugs, dapsone, and colchicine are used (3)[C].
- HBV-associated PAN: antiviral agents, short-term CS, plasma exchange (1)
- Tocilizumab has been reported in treatment refractory, hepatitis B–negative PAN (6)[C].

Second Line
- There is no well-defined second-line therapy in PAN.
- Infliximab (3 to 5 mg/kg IV at 0, 2, and 6 weeks, and every 4 to 8 weeks thereafter) and rituximab (1,000 mg IV on days 0 and 14 and then every 6 months OR 375 mg/m² IV weekly for 4 weeks) anecdotally reported to be of benefit in refractory PAN (3)[C].

ADDITIONAL THERAPIES
- For patients receiving IV cyclophosphamide, mercaptoethanesulfonate reduces bladder exposure to carcinogenic metabolites (3).
- Prophylactically treat patients on cyclophosphamide for *Pneumocystis jiroveci (carinii)* pneumonia with trimethoprim-sulfamethoxazole (use dapsone 100 mg/day or atovaquone 1,500 mg/day in intolerant/allergic patients) (3).

ADMISSION, INPATIENT, AND NURSING CONSIDERATIONS
Depends on extent and involvement of specific organs

ONGOING CARE

FOLLOW-UP RECOMMENDATIONS
Patient Monitoring
- CBC, urinalysis, renal and hepatic function tests.
- Acute-phase reactants (e.g., ESR, CRP) may help monitor disease activity.
- The revised 2009 Five Factor Score (FFS) can predict mortality and guide treatment strategies. Four factors are used in the evaluation of patients with PAN, including age, renal insufficiency, cardiac involvement, and GI manifestations. The fifth factor, ENT manifestations, is only applied to patients with ANCA-associated vasculitis (1).
- Be alert for:
  - Side effects of immunosuppressant medications
  - Delayed appearance of neoplasms, especially bladder malignancy in patients treated with cyclophosphamide (Check annual urinalysis, urinary cytology with urologic evaluation if microscopic hematuria.) (1)
  - Steroid-induced osteoporosis

DIET
- Low-salt diet (HTN)
- Mediterranean diet for cardiovascular health
- Calcium and vitamin D–rich diets for patients on CS therapy

PATIENT EDUCATION
ACR Web site: https://www.rheumatology.org

PROGNOSIS
- Expected outcome of untreated PAN is poor.
- Steroid and cytotoxic treatment increases 5-year survival rate to 75–80% (2).
- Survival is greater for hepatitis B–related PAN as a result of the introduction of antiviral treatments.
- Patients presenting with proteinuria, renal insufficiency, GI tract involvement, cardiomyopathy, CNS involvement, or >65 years of age have a worse prognosis.

COMPLICATIONS
- End-organ damage from ischemia
- Complications from immunosuppressive agents

REFERENCES
1. De Virgilio A, Grego A, Magliulo G, et al. Polyarteritis nodosa: a contemporary overview. *Autoimmun Rev.* 2016;15(6):564–570.
2. Pagnoux C, Seror R, Henegar C, et al; for French Vasculitis Study Group. Clinical features and outcomes in 348 patients with polyarteritis nodosa: a systematic retrospective study of patients diagnosed between 1963 and 2005 and entered into the French Vasculitis Study Group Database. *Arthritis Rheum.* 2010;62(2):616–626.
3. Mukhtyar C, Guillevin L, Cid MC, et al; for European Vasculitis Study Group. EULAR recommendations for the management of primary small and medium vessel vasculitis. *Ann Rheum Dis.* 2009;68(3):310–317.
4. Ribi C, Cohen P, Pagnoux C, et al; for French Vasculitis Study Group. Treatment of polyarteritis nodosa and microscopic polyangiitis without poor-prognosis factors: a prospective randomized study of one hundred twenty-four patients. *Arthritis Rheum.* 2010;62(4):1186–1197.
5. Casian A, Sangle S, D'Cruz D. New use for an old treatment: hydroxychloroquine as a potential treatment for systemic vasculitis. *Autoimmun Rev.* 2018;17(7):660–664.
6. Krusche M, Ruffer N, Kötter I. Tocilizumab treatment in refractory polyarteritis nodosa: a case report and review of the literature. *Rheumatol Int.* 2019;39(2):337–344.

ADDITIONAL READING
Samson M, Puéchal X, Mouthon L, et al; for French Vasculitis Study Group. Microscopic polyangiitis and non-HBV polyarteritis nodosa with poor-prognosis factors: 10-year results of the prospective CHUSPAN trial. *Clin Exp Rheumatol.* 2017;35(1 Suppl 103):176–184.

SEE ALSO

Hepatitis B; Hepatitis C

CODES

ICD10
- M30.0 Polyarteritis nodosa
- M30.1 Polyarteritis with lung involvement [Churg-Strauss]
- M30.8 Other conditions related to polyarteritis nodosa

CLINICAL PEARLS
- PAN is a necrotizing vasculitis of small- to medium-sized muscular arteries with lack of granuloma formation that spares veins and pulmonary arteries.
- Clinical features of PAN depend on target organ.
- Skin biopsies at ulcer edges (include deep dermis and SC fat) improve diagnostic yield.
- Check hepatitis B and C serologies.
- ANCA is negative in classic PAN.
- At diagnosis, the revised FFS can determine prognosis and guide therapy.
- Treatment involves use of immunosuppressive drugs; choice depends on extent and severity of disease.

POLYCYSTIC KIDNEY DISEASE
Anila Khaliq, MD

BASICS

DESCRIPTION
- A group of monogenic disorders that results in renal cyst development
- The most frequent are two genetically distinct conditions: autosomal dominant polycystic kidney disease (ADPKD) and autosomal recessive polycystic kidney disease (ARPKD).
- ADPKD is one of the most common human genetic disorders.

EPIDEMIOLOGY
- ADPKD is generally late onset.
  - Mean age of end-stage kidney disease (ESKD) 57 to 69 years
  - More progressive disease in men than in women
  - Up to 90% of adults have cysts in the liver.
- ARPKD usually present in infants.
  - A minority in older children and young adults may manifest as liver disease.
  - Nonobstructive intrahepatic bile dilatation is sometimes seen.
  - Found on all continents and in all races

Incidence
- Mean age of ESKD: *PKD1* mutation, 54.3 years versus *PKD2* mutation, 74 years
- ARPKD affects 1/20,000 live births; carrier level is 1/70.
- ADPKD affects 1/400 to 1,000 live births.

Prevalence
As ESKD, ADPKD: 8.7/1 million in the United States; 7/1 million in Europe

ETIOLOGY AND PATHOPHYSIOLOGY
- ADPKD
  - *PKD1* and *PKD2* mutations, which encode for polycystin 1 (PC1) and polycystin 2 (PC2), disrupt the function of polycystins on the primary cilium, forming fluid-filled cysts that progressively increase in size, leading to gross enlargement of the kidney, and distortion of the renal architecture.
  - Glomerular hyperfiltration compensates for the progressive loss of healthy glomeruli, and therefore, by the time GFR decline becomes detectable, as much as ½ of the original functional glomeruli are irreversibly lost.
  - The majority of patients with ADPKD ultimately progress to ESKD (1).
- ARPKD
  - *PKHD1* product fibrocystin is also located in cilia.
- ADPKD: Cysts arise from only 1% of nephrons:
  - Autosomal dominant pattern of inheritance but a molecularly recessive disease with the 2-hit hypothesis
  - Requires genetic and environmental factors
- ARPKD: Mutations are scattered throughout the gene with genotype–phenotype correlation.

Genetics
- ADPKD
  - Autosomal dominant inheritance
  - 50% of children of an affected adult are affected.

- 100% penetrance; genetic imprinting and genetic anticipation are seen as well.
- Two genes isolated
  - *PKD1* on chromosome 16p13.3 (85% of patients) encodes polycystin 1.
  - *PKD2* on chromosome 4q21 (15% of patients) encodes polycystin 2.
- ARPKD
  - Autosomal recessive inheritance
  - Siblings have a 1:4 chance of being affected; gene *PKHD1* on chromosome 6p21.1–p12 encodes fibrocystin.

RISK FACTORS
A more rapidly progressive clinical course is predicted by onset of ESKD at <55 years, development of stage III CKD at <40 years old, onset of HTN at <18 years, total kidney volume greater than the expected for a given age, or presence of multiple complications (gross hematuria, microalbuminuria) (1).

GENERAL PREVENTION
Genetic counseling

COMMONLY ASSOCIATED CONDITIONS
- ADPKD
  - Cysts in other organs
    - Polycystic liver disease in 58% of young age group to 94% of 45-year-olds
    - Pancreatic (5%); seminal (40%); arachnoid (8%)
  - Vascular manifestations
    - Intracerebral aneurysms in 6% of patients without family history and in 16% with family history
    - Aortic root dilation, dissections
  - Cardiac manifestations
    - Mitral valve prolapse (25%); left ventricular hypertrophy
  - Diverticular disease
- ARPKD: liver involvement: affected in inverse proportion to renal disease; congenital hepatic fibrosis with portal HTN

DIAGNOSIS

HISTORY
- ADPKD
  - Positive family history (15% are de novo mutations.)
  - Flank pain: 60%
  - Hematuria
  - UTI
  - HTN: 50% aged 20 to 34 years; 100% with ESKD
  - Renal failure
  - Presymptomatic screening of ADPKD is not currently recommended for at-risk children (2).
- ARPKD
  - 30% of affected neonates die:
    - Enlarged echogenic kidneys and oligohydramnios are diagnosed in utero.
    - Later in childhood: HTN
  - Adolescents and adults present with complications of portal HTN: esophageal varices
  - Hypersplenism

PHYSICAL EXAM
- HTN
- Flank masses

DIFFERENTIAL DIAGNOSIS
- ADPKD and ARPKD
- Tuberous sclerosis: prevalence 1/6,000
- Von Hippel-Lindau syndrome: prevalence 1/36,000
- Nephronophthisis: accounts for 10–20% of cases of renal failure in children; medullary cystic kidney disease
- Renal cystic dysplasias: multicystic dysplastic kidneys: grossly deformed kidneys; most common type of bilateral cystic diseases in newborns (prevalence: 1/4,000)
- Simple cysts: most common cystic abnormality
  - Localized or unilateral renal cystic disease
  - Medullary sponge kidney
  - Acquired renal cystic disease
- Renal cystic neoplasms: benign multilocular cyst (cystic nephroma)

DIAGNOSTIC TESTS & INTERPRETATION
Electrolytes, BUN/creatinine, urine analysis plus urinary citrate

Initial Tests (lab, imaging)
- ADPKD
  - Renal dysfunction
    - Impaired renal concentration (3), hypocitraturia aciduria
    - Hyperfiltration
    - Elevated creatinine
  - Urinalysis: hematuria and mild proteinuria
- ARPKD
  - Electrolyte abnormalities and renal insufficiency
  - Anemia, thrombocytopenia, leukopenia
- ADPKD
  - US: It is the easiest diagnostic method; however, it is suboptimal for disease exclusion at age <40 years (2)[C].
    - Renal enlargement is universal.
    - In at-risk patients: By age 30 years, two renal cysts (bilateral or unilateral) are 100% diagnostic. In children, it sometimes appears similar to ARPKD; may be diagnosed in utero.
    - Presence of hepatic cysts in young adults is pathognomonic for ADPKD.
    - In the absence of family history, bilateral renal enlargement and cysts make the diagnosis.
  - CT scan/MRI ideally should be part of the initial evaluation (2)[C].
    - Kidney volume assessed by CT or MRI is a main predictor of progression.
    - Helpful in identifying cysts in other organs
    - In subjects <40 years, fewer than five cysts by MRI excludes the diagnosis (2)[B].
- ARPKD
  - US: Kidneys are enlarged, homogeneously hyperechogenic (cortex and medulla).
  - CT scan is more sensitive if diagnosis is in doubt.
  - Presence of hepatic fibrosis helps the diagnosis.

Follow-Up Tests & Special Considerations
- Diagnosis and prevention of secondary problems because of renal and liver abnormalities
- Follow-up of combined renal volume to assess disease severity
- Beyond age 2 years, renal size decreases in ARPKD but continues to grow in ADPKD at an average rate of 5.27% per year. Total kidney volume identifies patients with progressive disease (2).

Diagnostic Procedures/Other
- Genetic testing is available for *PKD1* and *PKD2* in ADPKD when imaging results are equivocal and for potential living related donors (4)[C].
- For *PKHD1* in ARPKD, a prenatal diagnosis is feasible in about 72% of patients.

Test Interpretation
- ADPKD
  - Kidneys are diffusely cystic and, although enlarged, retain their general shape.
  - Cysts range from a few millimeters to several centimeters and are distributed evenly throughout the cortex and medulla.
  - They arise in all segments of the nephron, although they arise initially from the collecting ducts.
  - One kidney may be larger than the other.
  - In patients without established family history, the detection of more than ten cysts per kidney by ultrasonography is usually considered diagnostic.
- ARPKD
  - Disease is a spectrum, ranging from severe renal disease with mild liver damage to mild renal disease with severe liver damage.
  - Renal enlargement is due to fusiform dilatation of the collecting ducts in the cortex and medulla in the newborn period.
  - Liver lesion is diffuse but limited to fibrotic portal areas.
  - Diagnosis is likely based on clinical imaging in severe neonatal or infantile cases on the basis of enlarged echogenic kidneys, a negative family history, and lack of additional features.
  - Molecular diagnostic analysis is the gold standard for diagnosing this disorder.

TREATMENT

GENERAL MEASURES
- HTN: moderate sodium restriction, weight control, and regular exercise
- Medications: ACE inhibitors; angiotensin receptor blockers (ARBs)
- Pain: narcotics and other analgesics; bed rest; limit NSAIDs (they worsen renal function).
- Urolithiasis: treated with alkalinization of urine and hydration therapy; surgery as needed
- UTIs/infections of cysts: lipid-soluble antibiotics more effective (e.g., trimethoprim-sulfamethoxazole and chloramphenicol); fluoroquinolones also useful
- Dialysis for ESKD patients
- Hematuria: Reduce physical activity.

MEDICATION
- Treatments that directly target cytogenic mechanisms such as decreasing cAMP levels in cystic tissues are now available. Tolvaptan slowed the rate of kidney growth and estimated GFR decline in patients with early ADPKD.
- HTN: should be very well controlled to prevent complications. ACE inhibitors are preferred if no contraindications are present.
- The use of antihypertensive medications has been found to decrease mortality (5)[B].
- Hyperlipidemia: statins preferred

ISSUES FOR REFERRAL
- Nephrologist primary management
- Urologic consultation for management of symptomatic/infected cysts
- Genetic counseling is critical.

SURGERY/OTHER PROCEDURES
- Indications for surgical intervention
  - Uncontrollable HTN
  - Severe back and loin pain, abdominal fullness
  - Renal deterioration due to enlarging cysts
  - Hematuria/hemorrhage or recurrent UTI
- Open and laparoscopic cyst unroofing: may decrease pain and narcotics requirements; has not been proven to prevent renal failure or to prolong current renal function
- Percutaneous cyst aspiration ± injection of sclerosing agent; not usually performed secondary to recurrent fluid accumulation
- Renal transplant for ESKD

ADMISSION, INPATIENT, AND NURSING CONSIDERATIONS
Severe pain, gross hematuria with clots

ONGOING CARE

FOLLOW-UP RECOMMENDATIONS
None in early stages of the disease; avoid vigorous activity if disease advances. Recurrent gross hematuria is secondary to trauma, associated with faster decline of renal function.

Patient Monitoring
- Monitor BP and renal function. Encourage hydration. Treat UTI and stone disease aggressively.
- Avoid nephrotoxic drugs.
- Creatinine and BP monitoring at least twice a year; more often as needed
- Screening for intracranial aneurysms (6)

DIET
- Low-protein diet may retard renal insufficiency.
- Limit caffeine because this might increase cyst growth.
- High water intake to decrease ADH >3 L/day (7)[C]

PROGNOSIS
- Renal failure in 2% by age 40 years; 23% by age 50 years; 48% by age 73 years
- ADPKD accounts for 10–15% of dialysis patients.
- No increased incidence of renal cell cancer

COMPLICATIONS
- Cyst rupture, infection, or hemorrhage
- Progression to renal failure
- Renal calculi

REFERENCES
1. Schrier RW, Brosnahan G, Cadnapaphornchai MA, et al. Predictors of autosomal dominant polycystic disease progression. *J Am Soc Nephrol*. 2014;25(11):2399–2418.
2. Chapman AB, Devuyst O, Eckardt KU, et al. Autosomal-dominant polycystic kidney disease (ADPKD): executive summary from a Kidney Disease: Improving Global Outcomes (KDIGO) controversies conference. *Kidney Int*. 2015;88(1):17–27. doi:10.1038/ki.2015.59.
3. Zittema D, Boertien WE, van Beek AP, et al. Vasopressin, copeptin, and renal concentrating capacity in patients with autosomal dominant polycystic kidney disease without renal impairment. *Clin J Am Soc Nephrol*. 2012;7(6):906–913.
4. Harris PC, Rossetti S. Molecular diagnostics for autosomal dominant polycystic kidney disease. *Nat Rev Nephrol*. 2010;6(4):197–206.
5. Patch C, Charlton J, Roderick PJ, et al. Use of antihypertensive medications and mortality of patients with autosomal dominant polycystic kidney disease: a population-based study. *Am J Kidney Dis*. 2011;57(6):856–862.
6. Rozenfeld MN, Ansari SA, Shaibani A, et al. Should patients with autosomal dominant polycystic kidney disease be screened for cerebral aneurysms? *AJNR Am J Neuroradiol*. 2014;35(1):3–9.
7. Mahnensmith RL. Novel treatments of autosomal dominant polycystic kidney disease. *Clin J Am Soc Nephrol*. 2014;9(5):831–836.

SEE ALSO

Chronic Kidney Disease

CODES

ICD10
- Q61.3 Polycystic kidney, unspecified
- Q61.2 Polycystic kidney, adult type
- Q61.1 Polycystic kidney, infantile type

CLINICAL PEARLS
- Most PKD patients eventually develop ESKD. No specific treatment has been proven to prevent ESKD, but hydration and control of BP are reasonable goals.
- Patients may benefit from a nephrology consultation after the initial diagnosis to counsel regarding disease progression prevention. Then, they can be followed by primary care if the disease was an incidental finding or no significant kidney dysfunction is present.

POLYCYSTIC OVARIAN SYNDROME (PCOS)

Melissa Dennis, MD, MHA • Akash Jani, MD

 BASICS

DESCRIPTION

- Polycystic ovarian syndrome (PCOS) is a common endocrine disorder with heterogeneous manifestations that affects 6–10% of the U.S. population.
- Characterized by hyperandrogenism, insulin resistance, and anovulation, typically presenting as amenorrhea or oligomenorrhea
- Diagnostic clinical characteristics include menstrual dysfunction, infertility, hirsutism, acne, obesity, and metabolic syndrome.
- The ovaries are often polycystic on imaging.
- The etiology of PCOS is unknown, but presentation and course can be modified by lifestyle factors.
- System(s) affected: reproductive, endocrine/metabolic, skin/exocrine
- Synonym(s): Stein-Leventhal syndrome; polycystic ovary disease

ALERT
- Condition may begin at puberty.
- Obesity may amplify PCOS, but it is not diagnostic.
- 20% of women with PCOS are not obese.
- Predisposes to and is associated with obesity, hypertension, diabetes, metabolic syndrome, hyperlipidemia, infertility, insulin-resistance syndrome, endometrial hyperplasia, and uterine cancer

EPIDEMIOLOGY

Incidence
Incidence and prevalence are still highly debated due to a wide spectrum of diagnostic features; the National Institutes of Health (NIH) criteria require chronic anovulation and hyperandrogenism.

Prevalence
- The prevalence based on NIH criteria is 7% of reproductive age women.
- Predominant age: reproductive age
- Predominant sex: females only

ETIOLOGY AND PATHOPHYSIOLOGY
- Recent evidence points to a primary role for insulin resistance with hyperinsulinemia.
- Increased GnRH pulsations in the hypothalamus lead to increased production of LH with limited production of FSH.
- Hyperandrogenism: Ovaries are the main source of excess androgens (75% of circulating testosterone originates in the ovary). Polycystic ovaries have thickened thecal layers and overexpressed LH receptors, which cause excess androgen secretion.
- Ovarian follicles: Abnormal androgen signaling may account for abnormal folliculogenesis causing polycystic ovaries.
- Obesity results in compensatory hyperinsulinemia: Women with PCOS have insulin resistance similar to that in type 2 diabetes. Elevated levels of insulin decrease sex hormone–binding globulin (SHBG), increasing bioavailability of testosterone. Insulin may also act directly on adrenal glands, ovaries, and hypothalamus to enhance androgen production.
- Insulin resistance causes elevated insulin levels and the frequently associated metabolic syndrome or frank diabetes mellitus.

Genetics
- Likely a combination of polygenic and environmental factors
- Implicated genes include *DENND1A* and *THADA*.

RISK FACTORS
See "Commonly Associated Conditions"; cause and effect are difficult to extricate in this disorder.

GENERAL PREVENTION
None known; focus on early diagnosis and treatment to prevent long-term complications.

COMMONLY ASSOCIATED CONDITIONS
- Infertility
- Obesity
- Obstructive sleep apnea
- Hypertension
- Diabetes mellitus
- Endometrial hyperplasia/carcinoma
- Fatty liver disease
- Mood disturbances and depression
- Hirsutism

℞ DIAGNOSIS

HISTORY
- A comprehensive history, including a family history of diabetes and premature onset of cardiovascular disease, is important in the differential diagnosis.
- Focus on the onset and duration of the various signs of androgen excess, menstrual history, and concomitant medications, including the use of exogenous androgens (1).
- Unpredictable, heavy, or absent menstrual cycles

PHYSICAL EXAM
- Vital signs: elevated body mass index (BMI), hypertension
- General appearance: central obesity, hirsutism, acne
- Skin: male hair pattern, balding, acne, seborrhea, acanthosis nigricans
- Pelvic: ovarian enlargement, clitoromegaly

ALERT
Look specifically for signs of virilization, such as hair pattern, deepened voice, and clitoromegaly because they indicate significant testosterone levels beyond that of PCOS.

DIFFERENTIAL DIAGNOSIS
- Cushing syndrome
- HAIR-AN syndrome
- Androgen-secreting ovarian or adrenal tumor
- Prolactin-producing pituitary adenoma
- Hyperthecosis
- Adult-onset adrenal hyperplasia
- Partial congenital adrenal hyperplasia (21-hydroxylase deficiency)
- 11β-Hydroxylase deficiency
- 17β-Hydroxysteroid dehydrogenase deficiency
- Acromegaly
- Drug-induced hirsutism, oligo-ovulation (e.g., danazol, steroids, valproic acid)
- Thyroid disease
- Idiopathic hirsutism
- Polycystic ovaries

DIAGNOSTIC TESTS & INTERPRETATION
- The value of measurement of circulating androgens to document PCOS is uncertain but should include calculating free testosterone concentration using mass spectrometry of total testosterone and measurement of SHBG (2)[C].

- Most commonly used diagnostic criteria is the Rotterdam criteria (need any 2 of 3):
  - Oligomenorrhea or amenorrhea
  - Clinical and/or biochemical signs of hyperandrogenism
  - Transvaginal ultrasonographic polycystic ovaries
- Must exclude other etiologies including Cushing disease, congenital adrenal hyperplasia, and androgen-secreting tumors
- Ultrasonographic polycystic ovaries are not necessary for the diagnosis of PCOS.
- More recent criteria also focus on similar criteria while acknowledging that there may be forms of PCOS without overt evidence of hyperandrogenism (3)[C].

Initial Tests (lab, imaging)
- Screening workup should rule out pregnancy, thyroid disease, hyperprolactinemia, congenital adrenal hyperplasia, and premature ovarian failure.
  - Serum testing includes human chorionic gonadotropin (hCG), TSH, prolactin, 17-OH progesterone, and FSH.
- Hirsute women should have a free testosterone determination (total testosterone minus SHBG) and a DHEA-S.
- Workup to rule out hypothalamic amenorrhea (LH and FSH), androgen-secreting tumors (FSH, estradiol, testosterone, DHEA-S), Cushing syndrome (24-hour urinary free cortisol), and acromegaly (IGF-1) should be considered based on clinical characteristics (4).
- Typical findings in PCOS include testosterone increased but <200 ng/dL (6.94 nmol/L), mild elevation in DHEA-S but <800 μg/dL (20.8 μmol/L), mild increase in 17-OH progesterone level, increased estrogen level, and decreased SHBG.
- Anovulation can be determined by a midluteal phase progesterone level (>3 ng/mL if the woman has ovulated).
- LH/FSH level ≥2.5 to 3.0 in ~50% of women with PCOS, but such testing is not generally necessary
- Drugs that may alter lab results:
  - Oral contraceptive pills (OCPs)
  - Steroids
  - Antidepressants
- Transvaginal ultrasound findings: one or both ovaries with ≥12 follicles measuring 2 to 9 mm or increased ovarian volume to 10 cm³

Follow-Up Tests & Special Considerations
- Consider fasting serum glucose, insulin level, and plasminogen activator inhibitor-1 determinations to establish presence of insulin resistance and glucose intolerance, especially if diagnosis is in doubt.
- Endometrial biopsy to rule out hyperplasia and/or carcinoma, if indicated
- If the syndrome is diagnosed, determination of fasting glucose and fasting lipid levels should be performed and formal glucose tolerance test is considered.

ALERT
Prolonged or heavy bleeding should prompt an endometrial biopsy for evaluation of endometrial hyperplasia and possible cancer.

Test Interpretation
- Ovary is usually enlarged with a smooth white glistening capsule.
- Ovarian cortex is lined with follicles in all stages of development but most atretic.
- Thecal cell proliferation with an increase in the stromal compartment

TREATMENT

GENERAL MEASURES
Lifestyle changes including appropriate nutrition and exercise to decrease body weight by as little as 5% can restore ovulation and increase insulin sensitivity (4)[A]. Treatment plan should be individualized based on patient needs and desires.

MEDICATION
- The goal of treatment in PCOS depends on symptoms and patient's goals for fertility.
- Treatment can be divided into four main categories: (i) restore menses, (ii) decrease insulin resistance, (iii) ameliorate androgen excess, and (iv) assist in fertility.

First Line
- Restore menses when pregnancy not desired:
  - OCPs and progestins provide improvement in menstrual irregularity and provide endometrial protection.
  - Low-dose OCPs (30 to 35 μg); newer formulations containing progestins with lower androgenicity (e.g., norethindrone, desogestrel, norgestimate, drospirenone) may be particularly beneficial, but all OCPs increase SHBG and decrease excess androgens. Discuss benefits and balance against slightly increased thrombotic potential of 3rd- and 4th-generation progestins as compared with older progestins.
  - Levonorgestrel IUD offers endometrial protection and pregnancy prevention but will not counteract hyperandrogenism (2).
  - If unable to tolerate OCPs, then intermittent medroxyprogesterone (Provera) 10 mg PO, or micronized progesterone (Crinone and Prometrium) 200 mg PO, for 10 to 14 days can be given every 1 to 3 months (2)[C]. These offer endometrial protection. However, these will not counteract hyperandrogenism or protect against pregnancy.
- Decrease insulin resistance:
  - Metformin may help to correct metabolic abnormalities in women who are insulin resistant. Initial dose is 500 mg daily for 1 week, increasing by 500 mg/week to a total of 1,500 to 2,000 mg/day divided BID; take with food.
    - Overall, data support the usefulness of metformin on both cardiometabolic risk and reproduction assistance in women with PCOS.
    - Thiazolidinediones may increase likelihood of ovulation and treat insulin resistance but do not increase live birth rate.
- If pregnancy is desired:
  - Previously, the first-line treatment for ovulation induction was clomiphene (Clomid, Serophene) and/or exogenous gonadotropins. Live birth rate with clomiphene (Clomid) is 10.1% (5).
  - More recent data shows that letrozole (an aromatase inhibitor) has increased ovulation rates, clinical pregnancy rates, and live birth rates compared to clomiphene (Clomid). Live birth rate with letrozole is 27.5%. Dosing starts on day 3, 4, or 5 with 2.5 mg daily for 5 days; can increase to 5 mg daily with max dose 7.5 mg daily for 5 days (5)
  - Counsel patients that letrozole is not approved by the FDA for ovulation induction.
  - Metformin: 500 to 2,000 mg PO divided BID has been shown to improve hyperandrogenism and restore ovulation. Some providers will choose to continue metformin throughout the 1st trimester or the entire pregnancy if there is a history of spontaneous abortion or glucose intolerance. It does improve ovulation rates and insulin resistance but does not improve live birth rates alone or in combination with clomiphene when used for ovulation induction.

- Metformin reduces the incidence of gestational diabetes.
- All ovulation induction drugs increase the risk of multiple births and obstetric complications, such as preterm birth and hypertensive disorders.

Second Line
- Acne:
  - OCPs with low-androgenicity progestins for example, norethindrone, desogestrel, norgestimate, drospirenone
  - Spironolactone: 50 to 200 mg daily in 1 to 2 divided doses for acne and hirsutism not addressed by OCP therapy. This medication is unsafe in pregnancy, and potassium levels must be followed closely when used.
- Hirsutism:
  - Eflornithine hydrochloride 13.9% cream BID
  - Finasteride 2.5 to 5.0 mg daily; must be on very reliable contraception as this medication is teratogenic

ISSUES FOR REFERRAL
- To reproductive endocrinologist for all women who cannot achieve pregnancy with clomiphene (Clomid) or letrozole
- To endocrinologist if Cushing syndrome, congenital adrenal hyperplasia, or adrenal or ovarian tumors are found during the workup

ADDITIONAL THERAPIES
If the excess hair is uncomfortable, mechanical means of hair removal, including laser, electrolysis, waxing, and depilatory, may improve cosmesis.

SURGERY/OTHER PROCEDURES
Ovarian wedge resection and laparoscopic laser drilling are controversial and rarely used today.

COMPLEMENTARY & ALTERNATIVE MEDICINE
Acupuncture may assist with cycle normalization and weight loss.

 ONGOING CARE

FOLLOW-UP RECOMMENDATIONS
6-month intervals to evaluate response to therapy and to monitor weight and medication side effects

Patient Monitoring
- Counsel patient about the risk of endometrial and breast carcinoma, insulin resistance, and diabetes as well as obesity and its role in infertility.
- See patient frequently throughout the menstrual cycle, depending on which drug combination is used to induce ovulation.
- All patients with PCOS who have not received medication or IUD for endometrial protection and have been amenorrheic for 1 year should undergo endometrial biopsy.

DIET
In overweight patients, weight loss is the most successful therapy because it improves cardiovascular risk, insulin sensitivity, menstrual patterns, and infertility: Counsel on lifestyle dietary changes; consider referral to nutritionist and weight center. No specific diet plan is proven to be better than another.

PATIENT EDUCATION
- Provide patient with information about PCOS, such as from http://www.acog.org/.
- Discuss the chronic nature of this condition and the risks and benefits and side effects of potential treatments.

- Review the importance of exercise and weight loss, if applicable. Modest weight loss of 5–10% of initial body weight has been demonstrated to improve many of the features of PCOS.

PROGNOSIS
- Fertility prognosis is good but may need assisted reproductive technologies.
- Proper follow-up and screening can prevent endometrial carcinoma.
- Early detection of diabetes may decrease morbidity and mortality associated with cardiovascular risk factor.

COMPLICATIONS
- Reproductive: infertility
- Metabolic: insulin resistance, diabetes mellitus, cardiovascular disease
- Psychosocial: increased anxiety, mood disorder, eating disorder, depression
- Predisposes to endometrial hyperplasia and as high as 9% lifetime risk of endometrial cancer
- Women with PCOS appear to be at increased risk for complications of pregnancy including gestational diabetes and hypertensive disorders.

REFERENCES
1. Azziz R, Carmina E, Dewailly D, et al; for Task Force on the Phenotype of the Polycystic Ovary Syndrome of the Androgen Excess and PCOS Society. The Androgen Excess and PCOS Society criteria for the polycystic ovary syndrome: the complete task force report. *Fertil Steril*. 2009;91(2):456–488.
2. McCartney CR, Marshall JC. Clinical practice. Polycystic ovary syndrome. *N Engl J Med*. 2016;375(1):54–64.
3. Carmina E, Oberfield SE, Lobo RA. The diagnosis of polycystic ovary syndrome in adolescents. *Am J Obstet Gynecol*. 2010;203(3):201.e1–201.e5.
4. Tang T, Lord JM, Norman RJ, et al. Insulin-sensitising drugs (metformin, rosiglitazone, pioglitazone, D-chiro-inositol) for women with polycystic ovary syndrome, oligo amenorrhoea and subfertility. *Cochrane Database Syst Rev*. 2010;(1):CD003053.
5. ACOG Practice Bulletin No. 194: polycystic ovary syndrome. *Obstet Gynecol*. 2018;131(6):e157–e171.

 SEE ALSO

Algorithm: Amenorrhea, Secondary

CODES

ICD10
- E28.2 Polycystic ovarian syndrome
- L68.0 Hirsutism

CLINICAL PEARLS
- Based on Rotterdam criteria, PCOS is diagnosed based on 2 of 3 of (i) oligo-ovulation, (ii) signs of hyperandrogenism, (iii) polycystic ovaries.
- Polycystic ovaries are not required for the diagnosis of PCOS.
- Chronic anovulation should be treated because chronic estrogen stimulation in absence of progesterone may lead to endometrial hyperplasia.
- Specific therapies must be individualized according to the needs and desires of each patient.
- Letrozole is the first-line medication for ovulation induction.

POLYCYTHEMIA VERA

Boris Calderon, DO

 BASICS

DESCRIPTION

- Polycythemia vera (PV) is a myeloproliferative clonal stem cell disorder marked by increased production of red blood cells (erythrocytosis) with excessive erythroid, myeloid, and megakaryocytic elements in the bone marrow.
- Morbidity and mortality are primarily related to complications from blood hyperviscosity leading to thrombosis development as well as malignant transformation. Untreated patients may survive 6 to 18 months. Adequate treatment may extend life to >10 years.
- Myelofibrosis (MF) can develop in the bone marrow, leading to progressive hepatosplenomegaly.
- Synonyms: primary polycythemia; maladie de Vaquez disease; primary PV; PV rubra; polycythemia, spleno-megalic; Vaquez-Osler disease

EPIDEMIOLOGY

Incidence

- Predominant age: 50 to 75 years; however, can occur in early adulthood and childhood
- Predominant sex: male > female (slightly)
- Incidence in the United States in 2012: 2.8/100,000 population of men and 1.3/100,000 population of women; highest for men 70 to 79 years at 23.5/100,000 persons per year

Prevalence

In the United States in 2010, estimates ranged from 45 to 57 cases per 100,000 patients.

ETIOLOGY AND PATHOPHYSIOLOGY

JAK2 V617F mutation associated with clonal prolifera-tive disorder

Genetics

JAK2 V617F (tyrosine kinase) mutation: >97% of patients with PV have an activating mutation; this is helpful in differentiating from secondary erythrocyto-sis. Homozygote carriers will have higher incidence of symptoms such as pruritus but will not have higher incidence of disease than heterozygotes.

RISK FACTORS

- PV may be slightly more prevalent among Jews of Eastern European descent than other Europeans or Asians.
- Familial history is rare.

COMMONLY ASSOCIATED CONDITIONS

- Budd-Chiari syndrome
- Ischemic digits
- Mesenteric artery thrombosis
- Myocardial infarction
- Cerebrovascular accident or transient ischemic attack
- Venous thromboembolism and pulmonary embolism

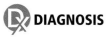 **DIAGNOSIS**

HISTORY

- Patients may be asymptomatic or present with nonspecific complaints, including fatigue, malaise, weight loss, sweating, and subjective weakness.

- Erythromelalgia (burning pain of feet/hands, occasionally with erythema, pallor, cyanosis, or paresthesias)
- Pruritus, especially after bathing (aquagenic pruritus)
- Arterial and venous occlusive events
- Headaches
- Blurred vision or blind spots
- Tinnitus, vertigo, dizziness
- Spontaneous bruising/bleeding
- Peptic ulcer disease (due to alterations in gastric mucosal blood flow)
- Early satiety due to enlarged spleen
- Bone pain (ribs and sternum)
- Gout
- Insomnia
- Depressed mood

PHYSICAL EXAM

- Hypertension (46%)
- Splenomegaly (75%), palpable spleen (36%)
- Hepatomegaly (30%)
- Facial plethora (ruddy cyanosis)
- Bone tenderness (especially ribs and sternum)
- Skin excoriations from significant pruritus
- Gouty tophi or arthritis
- Injection of the conjunctival small vessels and/or engorgement of the veins of the optic fundus

DIFFERENTIAL DIAGNOSIS

- Essential thrombocytopenia
- Secondary erythrocytosis:
  - Sleep apnea
  - Emphysema
  - Cigarette smoking
  - Renal artery stenosis
  - Carbon monoxide poisoning
  - Drugs: diuretics, testosterone replacement, erythropoietin (EPO)
- Hemoglobinopathy
- Ectopic EPO production
- Spurious polycythemia

DIAGNOSTIC TESTS & INTERPRETATION

- CBC; if suspicion is high, then obtain EPO level and gene testing for *JAK2 V617F*.
- If the only indication of PV is elevated hemoglobin (Hgb)/hematocrit (Hct), a CBC should be repeated. Further testing is unnecessary if the Hgb/Hct return to normal.

Initial Tests (lab, imaging)

- 2016 World Health Organization diagnostic criteria requires all three major criteria or the first two major criteria and the minor criterion* (1).
  - Major criteria:
    - Hgb >16.5 g/dL (men); Hgb >16.0 g/dL (women) or Hct >49% (men); Hct >48% (women) or increased cell mass (>25% above mean normal predictive value)
    - Bone marrow biopsy showing hypercellularity for age with trilineage growth (panmyelosis) including prominent erythroid, granulocytic, and megakaryocytic proliferation with pleomorphic, mature megakaryocytes (difference in sizes)
    - Presence of *JAK2 V617F* or similar mutation such as *JAK2* exon 12 mutation

  - Minor criteria:
    - Serum EPO level below normal *criterion number 2 (bone marrow biopsy) may not be required in cases with substantive absolute erythrocytosis: Hgb >18.5 g/dL in men (Hct, 55.5%) or >16.5 g/dL in women (Hct, 49.5%) if major criterion 3 and minor criterion are present. However, initial MF (present in up to 20% of points) can only be detected by perform-ing a bone marrow biopsy; this finding may predict a more rapid progression to overt MF (post-PV MF).
- Other lab findings that are common but not specific
  - Hyperuricemia
  - Hypercholesterolemia
  - Elevated serum vitamin B_{12} levels
  - Prolonged PT, aPTT due to low plasma volume
  - Thrombocytosis (>400,000 platelets/mm³)
  - Leukocytosis (>12,000/mm³)
  - Leukocyte alkaline phosphatase (100,000 U in the absence of fever or infection)
- CT or US to assess for splenomegaly, although not necessary for diagnosis
- Arterial oxygen saturation (<92% SaO_2) and carboxyhemoglobin (COHb)
- Bone marrow biopsy is not necessary. There is no staging system for this disease.

Diagnostic Procedures/Other

- Bone marrow aspiration if performed shows hypercellularity of erythroid, granulocytic and megakaryocytic lines, or MF.
- Cytogenetic testing (*JAK2 V617F*)

Test Interpretation

- If *JAK2 V617F* mutation testing is negative and the EPO level is normal or high, then PV is excluded; investigate causes of secondary erythrocytosis.
- *JAK2 V617* mutation in exon 14 is a distinguish-ing feature versus secondary polycythemia but not specific to PV as it can also be present in essential thrombocytopenia and primary MF (2).
- Other causes of erythrocytosis such as ectopic EPO production from a renal tumor, hypoxia from chronic lung, or cyanotic heart disease can be excluded with low or undetectable serum EPO level and normal oxygen saturation.

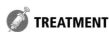 **TREATMENT**

GENERAL MEASURES

- Risk factors: Patients >60 years with history of thrombosis are high risk. Those who are <60 years with no history of thrombosis but with elevated platelets (>150,000) are intermediate risk. <60 years, with normal platelets, and no history of thrombosis are low risk.
- Phlebotomy and low-dose aspirin is first-line therapy for all patients.
- Although not curative, modern therapy for PV can relieve symptoms and prolong survival.
- If secondary PV, address etiology: aggressive treat-ment of obstructive sleep apnea, COPD (especially smoking cessation), renal disease; consider lowering dose in testosterone replacement.

- Phlebotomy reduces the blood hyperviscosity, improves platelet function, restores systemic pressures, and decreases risk of thrombosis.
- Phlebotomy:
  - Reduce Hct to <45%; will significantly lower rate of cardiovascular death and major thrombosis (3)[A]
  - Performed initially as often as every 2 to 3 days until normal Hct reached; phlebotomies of 250 to 500 mL (1 unit—500 mL—phlebotomy should reduce Hct by 3 percentage points). Reduce to 250 to 350 mL in elderly patients or patients with cerebrovascular disease.
  - Frail patients should have volume replaced with saline solution to avoid postural hypotension.
  - High risk for thrombosis or presence of elevated platelet count is indication for cytoreductive therapy.
  - Complications of phlebotomy: chronic iron deficiency (symptomatology: pica, angular stomatitis, and glossitis), possible muscle weakness, and dysphagia that is the result of esophageal webs (very rare)
- Other therapies:
  - Maintain hydration.
  - Pruritus therapy: H_1 and H_2 blockers, SSRIs, oatmeal baths, interferon α-2b
  - Uric acid reduction therapy

MEDICATION
First Line
- Primary therapies:
  - Low-dose aspirin 81 mg PO has been associated with a statistically nonsignificant reduction in the risk of fatal thrombotic events without increasing bleeding complications when used in conjunction with phlebotomy (4)[A]. Aspirin should not be used in those with acquired von Willebrand disease or those with other contraindications.
  - Hydroxyurea is recommended for patients at high risk for thrombosis (age >60 years or history of thrombotic event) and with splenomegaly and hepatomegaly. Common starting dose 500 to 1,500 mg PO daily, titrating to control Hct and platelet count. Be aware that hydroxyurea can lead to skin ulcer, myelosuppression, and higher risk of leukemic transformation (5)[A].
  - Ruxolitinib is approved for refractory PV or for patients who are intolerant to hydroxyurea.
  - Radioactive phosphorus (^{32}P) may control Hgb level and platelet count by destroying overactive marrow cells. May take up to 3 months before affecting cells. Consider for patients intolerant or nonadherent to hydroxyurea or short expected survival due to mutagenic potential.
  - Pegylated interferon α-2a is effective in controlling erythrocytosis, although dosing is generally limited secondary to intolerable side effects; usually recommended for younger patients (<40 years old) and those who might become pregnant (5)
  - Refer to hematologist/oncologist for further dosing and instructions.
- Symptomatic/adjunctive:
  - Allopurinol 300 mg/day PO for uric acid reduction
  - Cyproheptadine 4 to 16 mg PO daily as needed for pruritus

- H_2 receptor blockers or antacids for GI hyperacidity; cimetidine is also used for pruritus.
- Low-dose aspirin also used for pruritus/erythromelalgia
- SSRIs (paroxetine or fluoxetine) have shown some efficacy in controlling pruritus.
- Ultraviolet light therapy may help with pruritus.

Second Line
Myelosuppression: chlorambucil or busulfan; busulfan at 2 to 4 mg daily may be effective option for elderly patients with advanced PV refractory or intolerant to other agents such as hydroxyurea and interferon, but significant rate of transformation was observed.

ISSUES FOR REFERRAL
Referral to a hematologist to assist in diagnosis and management

COMPLEMENTARY & ALTERNATIVE MEDICINE
Osteopathic manipulative medicine to promote circulation

ADMISSION, INPATIENT, AND NURSING CONSIDERATIONS
DVT prophylaxis should be given.

 ONGOING CARE

FOLLOW-UP RECOMMENDATIONS
Patient Monitoring
Monitor Hct often and phlebotomize as needed to maintain target goal.

DIET
- Avoid high-sodium diet; can cause fluid retention
- Avoid iron supplement, a permissive chronic state of iron deficiency can help decrease blood production.

PATIENT EDUCATION
- Perform leg and ankle exercises to prevent clots.
- Continuous education regarding possible complications and seeking treatment early for any change or increase in symptoms

PROGNOSIS
- PV cannot be cured but can be controlled with treatment.
- Survival is >15 years with treatment.
- Patients are at risk for developing postpolycythemic MF (PPMF) and an increased risk of malignant transformation.

COMPLICATIONS
- Splenomegaly or hepatomegaly
- Budd-Chiari syndrome
- Vascular thrombosis (major cause of death) (20%)
- Transformation to acute leukemia (5%)
- Transformation to MF (10%)
- Hemorrhage
- Peptic ulcer
- Uric acid stones
- Secondary gout
- Increased risk for complications and mortality from surgical procedures. Assess risk/benefits and ensure optimal control of disorder before any elective surgery.

REFERENCES
1. Arber DA, Orazi A, Hasserjian R, et al. The 2016 revision to the World Health Organization classification of myeloid neoplasms and acute leukemia. *Blood*. 2016;127(20):2391–2405.
2. Tefferi A, Spivak JL. Polycythemia vera: scientific advances and current practice. *Semin Hematol*. 2005;42(4):206–220.
3. Marchioli R, Finazzi G, Specchia G, et al; for CYTO-PV Collaborative Group. Cardiovascular events and intensity of treatment in polycythemia vera. *N Engl J Med*. 2013;368(1):22–33.
4. Squizzato A, Romualdi E, Passamonti F, et al. Antiplatelet drugs for polycythaemia vera and essential thrombocythaemia. *Cochrane Database Syst Rev*. 2013;(4):CD006503.
5. Mascarenhas J, Mughal TI, Verstovsek S. Biology and clinical management of myeloproliferative neoplasms and development of the JAK inhibitor ruxolitinib. *Curr Med Chem*. 2012;19(26):4399–4413.

ADDITIONAL READING
- Passamonti F. How I treat polycythemia vera. *Blood*. 2012;120(2):275–284.
- Tefferi A, Fonseca R. Selective serotonin reuptake inhibitors are effective in the treatment of polycythemia vera–associated pruritus. *Blood*. 2002;99(7):2627.

 SEE ALSO

Myeloproliferative Neoplasms

CODES

ICD10
D45 Polycythemia vera

CLINICAL PEARLS
- Erythrocytosis: Hgb >16.5 g/dL in men, >16.0 g/dL in women
- *JAK2* mutations are an important component of myeloproliferative disorders.
- *Bone marrow biopsy can help in diagnosis showing hypercellularity and trilineage growth.*
- Common complications include thrombosis, malignant transformation, and MF.
- All patients should take low-dose aspirin unless there is major bleeding or GI intolerance.
- Phlebotomy is first-line treatment, and consultation with an experienced hematologist is recommended.

POLYMYALGIA RHEUMATICA

Juliana Chang, MD

BASICS

DESCRIPTION
- A clinical syndrome characterized by pain and stiffness of the shoulder, hip girdles, and neck; primarily impacts patients >50 years of age; associated with morning stiffness and elevated markers of inflammation
- System(s) affected: musculoskeletal; hematologic/lymphatic/immunologic
- Synonym(s): senile rheumatic disease; polymyalgia rheumatica (PMR) syndrome; pseudo-polyarthrite rhizomélique

Geriatric Considerations
- Incidence increases with age (age >50)
- Average age of onset ~70 years

Pediatric Considerations
Rare in patients <50 years of age. The peak incidence of PMR is between ages 70 and 80 years (1).

EPIDEMIOLOGY
Incidence
- Incidence increases after age 50 years. Incidence of PMR and giant cell arteritis (GCA) in the United States is 50 and 18 per 100,000 people, respectively.
- Predominant sex: female > male (2 to 3:1)
- Most common in Caucasians, especially those of northern European ancestry and in Scandinavian countries
- Peak incidence occurs between age 70 and 80.

Prevalence
Prevalence in those >50 years old: 700/100,000

ETIOLOGY AND PATHOPHYSIOLOGY
- Unknown. Symptoms relate to enhanced immune system and periarticular inflammatory activity.
- Pathogenesis
  - Polygenic; involves multiple environmental and genetic factors
  - Significant association between histologic evidence of GCA and parvovirus B19 DNA in temporal artery specimen

Genetics
Associated with human leukocyte antigen determinants (HLA-DRB1*04 and DRB1*01 alleles)

RISK FACTORS
- Age >50 years
- Presence of GCA

COMMONLY ASSOCIATED CONDITIONS
Concurrent GCA (temporal arteritis) in ~15–30% of patients; more commonly in females than males

DIAGNOSIS

HISTORY
- Suspect PMR in elderly patients with new onset of proximal limb pain and stiffness (neck, shoulder, hip). Patients may use the term stiffness and pain interchangeably (2). Shoulder pain is most typically present.
- Symptoms often have a rapid onset.
- Difficulty rising from chair or combing hair (proximal muscle involvement)
- Nighttime pain
- Can be unilateral however, soon becomes symmetrical
- Severe morning stiffness
- Systemic symptoms in ~25% (fatigue, weight loss, low-grade fever)
- Carpal tunnel syndrome can be seen in 10–15% of patients.

PHYSICAL EXAM
- Decreased range of motion (ROM) of shoulders, neck, and hips
- Muscle strength is usually normal—may be limited by pain and/or stiffness.
- Muscle tenderness
- Disuse atrophy
- Synovitis of the small joints and tenosynovitis; feet and ankles never affected
- Coexisting carpal tunnel syndrome

DIFFERENTIAL DIAGNOSIS
- Rheumatoid arthritis (RA)
- Palindromic rheumatism
- Late-onset seronegative spondyloarthropathies (e.g., psoriatic arthritis, ankylosing spondylitis)
- Systemic lupus erythematosus; Sjögren syndrome; fibromyalgia
- Polymyositis-dermatomyositis (Check creatine phosphokinase, aldolase.)
- Thyroid disease; hyperparathyroidism, hypoparathyroidism
- Hypovitaminosis D
- Osteoarthritis
- Rotator cuff syndrome; adhesive capsulitis
- RS3PE syndrome (remitting seronegative symmetrical synovitis with pitting edema)
- Occult infection or malignancy (e.g., lymphoma, leukemia, myeloma, solid tumor)
- Myopathy (e.g., steroid, alcohol, electrolyte depletion)
- Depression; fibromyalgia

DIAGNOSTIC TESTS & INTERPRETATION
ACR/EULAR classification criteria (3):
- Patients aged ≥50 years with bilateral shoulder aching and abnormal C-reactive protein concentrations or ESR, plus at least 4 points (without US) or 5 points or more (with US) from:
  - Morning stiffness for >45 minutes (2 points)
  - Hip pain or restricted range of motion (1 point)
  - Absence of rheumatoid factor (RF) or anti–citrullinated protein antibodies (ACPAs) (2 points)
  - Absence of other joint involvement (1 point)
  - If US is available, at least one shoulder with subdeltoid bursitis, biceps tenosynovitis or glenohumeral synovitis (either posterior or axillary), and at least one hip with synovitis or trochanteric bursitis (1 point)
  - If US is available, both shoulders with subdeltoid bursitis, biceps tenosynovitis, or glenohumeral synovitis (1 point)
- Temporal artery biopsy if symptoms of GCA present
- ESR (Westergren) elevation >40 mm/hr
  - ESR generally elevated, sometimes >100 mm/hr
  - ESR normal (<40 mm/hr) in 7–22% of patients
- Elevated C-reactive protein
- Normochromic/normocytic anemia
- Anti–cyclic citrullinated peptide (anti-CCP) antibodies usually negative (in contrast to elderly-onset RA)
- RF: negative (5–10% of patients >60 years have positive RF without RA.)
- Mild elevations in liver function tests, especially alkaline phosphatase
- Antibodies to ferritin peptide may be a useful diagnostic marker.
- Prednisone may alter lab results.
- Other disorders may cause elevation of ESR (e.g., infection, neoplasm, renal failure).
- Normal EMG
- Normal muscle histology
- CK is always normal.

Initial Tests (lab, imaging)
- ESR (usually >40 mm/hr); C-reactive protein; CBC
- MRI is not necessary for diagnosis but may show periarticular inflammation, tenosynovitis, and bursitis.
- US may show bursitis, tendinitis, and synovitis.
- MRI, PET, and temporal artery US may help in diagnosis of PMR.
- ACR/EULAR classification criteria help confirm the clinical diagnosis (4).
- ^{18}F-fluorodeoxyglucose PET scan prior to therapy improves diagnostic accuracy (5).

- A scoring algorithm (4) was devised consisting of the following: morning stiffness >45 minutes (2 points), hip pain/limited ROM (1 point), absence of RF and ACPA (2 points), and absence of peripheral joint pain (1 point).
- A score of >4 has 68% sensitivity and 78% specificity for PMR.

Diagnostic Procedures/Other
Temporal artery biopsy in patients with symptoms suggestive of GCA. Treat empirically pending results.

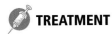

TREATMENT

GENERAL MEASURES
- Address risk of steroid-induced osteoporosis.
  - Obtain dual energy x-ray absorptiometry and check 25-OH vitamin D levels if necessary.
  - Consider antiresorptive therapies (bisphosphonates) for treatment of corticosteroid-induced osteoporosis.
- Encourage adequate calcium (1,500 mg/day) and vitamin D (800 to 1,000 U/day) supplementation.
- Physical therapy for ROM exercises, if needed

MEDICATION
First Line
- Prednisone: 10 to 20 mg/day PO initially; expect a dramatic (diagnostic) response within days. 15 mg/day is effective in almost all patients.
  - May increase to 20 mg/day if no immediate response
  - If no response to 10 to 20 mg/day within a week, reconsider diagnosis.
- Divided-dose steroids (BID or TID) may be useful initially (especially if symptoms recur in the afternoon).
- Consider using delayed-release prednisone taken at bedtime, which may help treat morning stiffness compared to immediate-release prednisone.
- Begin slow taper by 2.5 mg decrements every 2 to 4 weeks to a dose of 7.5 to 10.0 mg/day. Below this dose, taper by 1 mg/month to prevent relapse.
- Increase prednisone for symptom relapse (common).
- Corticosteroid treatment often lasts several years.
- May stop after 6 to 12 months if symptom free and ESR is normal
- Contraindications
  - Use steroids with caution in patients with chronic heart failure, diabetes mellitus (or other immunocompromised state), and systemic fungal or bacterial infection.
  - Treat any concurrent infections.
- Precautions
  - Long-term steroid use (>2 years) is associated with sodium and water retention, exacerbation of chronic heart failure, hypokalemia, increased susceptibility to infection, osteoporosis, fractures, hypertension, cataracts, glaucoma, avascular necrosis, depression, and weight gain.
  - Patients may develop temporal arteritis while on low-dose corticosteroid treatment for PMR. This requires an increase in prednisone dosing (up to 40–60 mg).
  - Alternate-day steroids are not effective.

Second Line
- Routine use of adjunctive therapy not recommended
- NSAIDs usually are not adequate for pain relief.
- Methotrexate modestly reduces relapse rate and lowers the cumulative dose of steroid therapy but has not been formally studied in PMR.
- Tocilizumab has been reported in case reports and small studies (6).
- There is conflicting evidence for anti–tumor necrosis factor (anti-TNF) agents (infliximab, etanercept).
- Corticosteroid injections (primarily for the shoulder) may help reduce pain and duration of morning stiffness, allowing for increased levels of activity.

ONGOING CARE

FOLLOW-UP RECOMMENDATIONS
Patient Monitoring
- Monthly evaluations initially and during medication taper; every 3 months otherwise
- Follow ESR as steroids are tapered; ESR and C-reactive protein should decline as symptoms improve.
- Follow up immediately for symptoms of GCA (e.g., headache, visual loss, and diplopia).
- Monitor side effects of corticosteroid therapy (osteoporosis, hypertension, and hyperglycemia).
- If patient is asymptomatic, do not treat elevated ESR (do not increase steroid dose to normalize ESR).

DIET
- Regular diet
- Adequate calcium and vitamin D

PATIENT EDUCATION
- Review adverse effects of corticosteroids.
- Discuss the symptoms of GCA (headache, visual loss, diplopia) and present immediately if any occur.
- Follow up if symptoms recur during steroid taper.
- Do not abruptly stop steroids.
- Ensure adequate calcium and vitamin D intake.
- Patient resources:
  - Arthritis Foundation: www.arthritis.org/
  - American College of Rheumatology: http://www.rheumatology.org/Practice/Clinical/Patients/Diseases_And_Conditions/Polymyalgia_Rheumatica/

PROGNOSIS
- Most patients require at least 2 years of corticosteroid treatment.
- Exacerbation or relapse is common if steroids are tapered too quickly.
- Prognosis is very good with proper treatment.
- Relapse is common (in 25–50% of patients).
- Higher age at diagnosis, female sex, high baseline ESR, increased levels of soluble IL-6 receptor, and high initial steroid dose have been associated with a prolonged disease course and more disease flares.

COMPLICATIONS
- Complications related to chronic steroid use
- Exacerbation of disease with taper of steroids; development of GCA (may occur when PMR is being treated adequately)

REFERENCES

1. El Chami S, Springer JM. Update on the treatment of giant cell arteritis and polymyalgia rheumatica. *Med Clin North Am.* 2021;105(2):311–324.
2. Lally L, Spiera R. Management of difficult polymyalgia rheumatica and giant cell arteritis: updates for clinical practice. *Best Pract Res Clin Rheumatol.* 2018;32(6):803–812.
3. Dasgupta B, Cimmino MA, Maradit-Kremers H, et al. 2012 Provisional classification criteria for polymyalgia rheumatica: a European League Against Rheumatism/American College of Rheumatology collaborative initiative. *Ann Rheum Dis.* 2012;71(4):484–492.
4. Macchioni P, Boiardi L, Catanoso M, et al. Performance of the new 2012 EULAR/ACR classification criteria for polymyalgia rheumatica: comparison with the previous criteria in a single-centre study. *Ann Rheum Dis.* 2014;73(6):1190–1193.
5. Henckaerts L, Gheysens O, Vanderschueren S, et al. Use of 18F-fluorodeoxyglucose positron emission tomography in the diagnosis of polymyalgia rheumatica—a prospective study of 99 patients. *Rheumatology (Oxford).* 2018;57(11):1908–1916.
6. Macchioni P, Boiardi L, Catanoso M, et al. Tocilizumab for polymyalgia rheumatica: report of two cases and review of the literature. *Semin Arthritis Rheum.* 2013;43(1):113–8.

ADDITIONAL READING
- Figus FA, Skoczyńska M, McConnell R, et al. Imaging in polymyalgia rheumatica: which technique to use? *Clin Exp Rheumatol.* 2021;39(4):883–888.
- Matteson EL, Deject C. Polymyalgia rheumatica. *Ann Int Med.* 2017;166(9):ITC65–ITC80.

 SEE ALSO

Arteritis, Temporal; Arthritis, Rheumatoid (RA); Depression; Fibromyalgia; Osteoarthritis; Polymyositis/Dermatomyositis

CODES

ICD10
- M35.3 Polymyalgia rheumatica
- M31.5 Giant cell arteritis with polymyalgia rheumatica

CLINICAL PEARLS
- Consider PMR in patients >50 years who present with hip, neck, and/or shoulder pain and stiffness.
- A normal ESR does not exclude PMR.
- Corticosteroids are the treatment of choice. If there is not a dramatic and rapid response, reconsider the diagnosis.
- Adjust steroids according to symptoms, not ESR.

POLYMYOSITIS/DERMATOMYOSITIS

Nehal R. Shah, MD • Christopher M. Wise, MD

BASICS

DESCRIPTION
- Systemic connective tissue disease characterized by inflammatory and degenerative changes in proximal muscles, sometimes accompanied by characteristic skin rash
  - If skin manifestations (Gottron sign [symmetric, scaly, violaceous, erythematous eruption over the extensor surfaces of the metacarpophalangeal and interphalangeal joints of the fingers]; heliotrope [reddish violaceous eruption on the upper eyelids]) are present, it is designated as dermatomyositis.
  - Different types of myositis include the following (1):
    ○ Idiopathic polymyositis
    ○ Idiopathic dermatomyositis
    ○ Polymyositis/dermatomyositis as an overlap (usually with lupus or systemic sclerosis or as part of mixed connective-tissue disease)
    ○ Myositis associated with malignancy
    ○ Necrotizing autoimmune myositis (often statin associated)
    ○ Inclusion body myositis (IBM), a variant with atypical patterns of weakness and biopsy findings
- System(s) affected: cardiovascular, musculoskeletal, pulmonary, skin/exocrine
- Synonym(s): myositis; inflammatory myopathy; antisynthetase syndrome (subset with certain antibodies)

EPIDEMIOLOGY
Incidence
- Estimated at 1.2 to 19 per million population per year
- Predominant age: 5 to 15 years, 40 to 60 years, peak incidence in mid-40s
- Predominant sex: female > male (2:1)

Prevalence
2.4 to 33.8 patients per 100,000 population

Geriatric Considerations
Elderly patients with myositis or dermatomyositis are at increased risk of neoplasm.

Pediatric Considerations
Childhood dermatomyositis is likely a separate entity associated with cutaneous vasculitis and muscle calcifications.

ETIOLOGY AND PATHOPHYSIOLOGY
- Inflammatory process, mediated by T cells and cytokine release, leading to damage to muscle cells (predominantly skeletal muscles)
- In patients with IBM, degenerative mechanisms may be important.
- Unknown; potential viral, genetic factors

Genetics
Mild association with human leukocyte antigen (HLA)-DR3, HLA-DRw52

RISK FACTORS
Family history of autoimmune disease (e.g., systemic lupus, myositis) or vasculitis

COMMONLY ASSOCIATED CONDITIONS
- Malignancy more common in dermatomyositis
- Progressive systemic sclerosis
- Vasculitis
- Systemic lupus erythematosus (SLE)
- Mixed connective tissue disease

DIAGNOSIS

HISTORY
- Symmetric proximal muscle weakness causing difficulty when
  - Arising from sitting or lying positions
  - Climbing stairs
  - Raising arms
- Joint pain/swelling
- Dysphagia
- Dyspnea
- Rash on face, eyelids, hands, arms

PHYSICAL EXAM
Proximal muscle weakness
- Shoulder muscles
- Hip girdle muscles (trouble standing from seated or squatting position, weak hip flexors in supine position)
- Muscle swelling, stiffness, induration
- Distal muscle weakness is seen only in patients with IBM.
- Rash over face (eyelids, nasolabial folds), upper chest, dorsal hands (especially knuckle pads), fingers ("mechanic's hands")
- Periorbital edema
- Calcinosis cutis (childhood cases)
- Mesenteric arterial insufficiency/infarction (childhood cases)
- Cardiac impairment; arrhythmia, failure

DIFFERENTIAL DIAGNOSIS
- Vasculitis
- Progressive systemic sclerosis
- SLE
- Rheumatoid arthritis
- Muscular dystrophy
- Lambert-Eaton syndrome
- Sarcoidosis
- Amyotrophic lateral sclerosis
- Endocrine disorders
  - Thyroid disease
  - Cushing syndrome
- Infectious myositis (viral, bacterial, parasitic)
- Drug-induced myopathies:
  - Cholesterol-lowering agents (statins)
  - Colchicine
  - Corticosteroids
  - Ethanol
  - Chloroquine
  - Zidovudine
- Electrolyte disorders (magnesium, calcium, potassium)
- Heritable metabolic myopathies
- Sleep apnea syndrome

DIAGNOSTIC TESTS & INTERPRETATION
- Diagnosis of muscle component (myositis) usually relies on four findings:
  - Weakness
  - Creatine kinase (CK) and/or aldolase elevation
  - Abnormal electromyogram (EMG)
  - Findings on muscle biopsy
- Presence of compatible skin rash of dermatomyositis
- There is an emerging role for myositis-specific antibody (MSA) profiles. MSAs can be used to guide the appropriate workup for malignancy and interstitial lung disease (ILD) (2).

Initial Tests (lab, imaging)
- Increased CK, aldolase
- Increased serum aspartate aminotransferase (AST)
- Increased lactate dehydrogenase (LDH)
- Myoglobinuria
- Increased ESR
- Positive rheumatoid factor (<50% of patients)
- Positive antinuclear antibody (ANA) (>50% of patients)
- Leukocytosis (<50% of patients)
- Anemia (<50% of patients)
- Hyperglobulinemia (<50% of patients)
- Anti-HMGCR (3-hydroxy-3-methylglutaryl-coenzyme A reductase) and anti-SRP antibodies seen in patient with necrotizing autoimmune myositis
- Antisynthetase antibodies (anti-Jo-1 and non–Jo-1 synthetases) present in antisynthetase syndrome
  - Associated with an increased incidence of ILD
- Anti–MDA-5 antibody seen in overlap myositis with atypical rashes and severe ILD
- Anti–U1 RNP, anti–PM-Scl, and anti-Ku antibodies seen in overlap myositis
- Chest radiograph as part of initial evaluation to assess for associated pulmonary involvement or malignancy

Follow-Up Tests & Special Considerations
- Changes in muscle enzymes (CK or aldolase) correlate with improvement and worsening.
- MRI to assess muscle edema and inflammation may be used in some patients to determine best biopsy site or response to therapy.

Diagnostic Procedures/Other
- EMG: muscle irritability, low-amplitude potentials, polyphasic action potentials, fibrillations
- Muscle biopsy (deltoid or quadriceps femoris)

Test Interpretation
- Microscopic findings:
  - Muscle fiber degeneration
  - Phagocytosis of muscle debris
  - Perifascicular muscle fiber atrophy
  - Inflammatory cell infiltrates in adult form
  - Via electron microscopy: inclusion bodies (IBM only)
  - Sarcoplasmic basophilia
- Muscle fiber increased in size
- Vasculopathy (childhood polymyositis/dermatomyositis)

TREATMENT

GENERAL MEASURES
Approach to treatment has varied by specialty involved (dermatology, rheumatology, neurology), but a consensus statement is available (3). Treatment approach should be informed by lesion type, degree of muscle involvement, presence of systemic symptoms, presence of MSAs, and patient age (2)[C].

MEDICATION
First Line
- Prednisone
  - 0.5 to 1.0 mg/kg/day PO in divided doses
  - IV pulse dose methylprednisolone 1,000 mg daily for 3 to 5 days in acute and severe cases
  - Consolidate doses and reduce prednisone slowly when enzyme levels are normal.
  - Probably need to continue 5 to 10 mg/day for maintenance in most patients

- Immunosuppressive maintenance therapy in parallel to steroids—recommended in most patients:
  – Azathioprine 1 mg/kg PO (arthritis dose) once daily or BID, or
  – Methotrexate 10 to 25 mg po weekly, or
  – Mycophenolate mofetil 2 to 3 mg daily
- Rash of dermatomyositis may require topical steroids or oral hydroxychloroquine.
- Patients with IBM have very poor response to steroids and other first- and second-line drugs in general.

Second Line
- Other immunosuppressant drugs (e.g., cyclophosphamide, chlorambucil, cyclosporin, tacrolimus) can be added to steroids in refractory cases. Adrenocorticotropic gel (ACTH gel) may have a role in refractory cases.
- Combination methotrexate and azathioprine also may be useful in refractory cases.
- IVIG and rituximab have been reported to be helpful in a small series of patients with refractory disease. Rituxan may be more effective in patients with autoantibodies positive myositis (especially anti–Jo-1 and anti–Mi-2). IVIG can be a reasonable alternative in patients whom steroids or other immunosuppressive drugs are contraindicated such as infection and neoplasm.
- Cyclophosphamide is usually reserved for severe cases with lung or heart involvement.
- Contraindications: Methotrexate is contraindicated with previous liver disease, alcohol use, pregnancy, and underlying renal disease (use with extreme caution in patients with serum creatinine >1.5 mg/dL in general).
- Precautions
  – Prednisone: Adverse effects associated with long-term steroid use include adrenal suppression, sodium and water retention, hypokalemia, osteoporosis, cataracts, and increased susceptibility to infection.
  – Azathioprine: Adverse effects include bone marrow suppression, increased liver function tests, and increased risk of infection.
  – Methotrexate: Adverse effects include stomatitis, bone marrow suppression, pneumonitis, and risk of liver fibrosis and cirrhosis with prolonged use.

ISSUES FOR REFERRAL
- Diagnostic uncertainty, usually related to elevated muscle enzymes without typical symptoms of findings of muscle weakness
- Poor response to initial steroid therapy
- Excessive steroid requirement (unable to taper prednisone to <20 mg/day after 4 to 6 months)

SURGERY/OTHER PROCEDURES
None indicated, other than initial biopsy

COMPLEMENTARY & ALTERNATIVE MEDICINE
Benefits and harms of physical therapy are not well-established, especially in active muscle disease (4)[A], although there is some suggestion of benefit in quiescent disease (5)[A]. Research is of low quality in this area.

ADMISSION, INPATIENT, AND NURSING CONSIDERATIONS
- Inability to stand, ambulate
- Respiratory difficulty
- Fever or other signs of infection
- Inpatient evaluation seldom needed

 ## ONGOING CARE

FOLLOW-UP RECOMMENDATIONS
Patient Monitoring
- Follow muscle enzymes along with muscle strength and functional capacity.
- Monitor for steroid-induced complications (e.g., hypokalemia, hypertension, and hyperglycemia).
- Bone densitometry and consideration of calcium, vitamin D, and bisphosphonate therapy
- If azathioprine, methotrexate, or other immunosuppressant is used, appropriate laboratory monitoring should be done periodically (e.g., hematology, liver enzymes, and creatinine).
- Attempt to decrease and/or discontinue steroid dose as patient responds to therapy.
- Maintain immunosuppression until patient's muscle strength stabilizes for prolonged period depending on individual patient parameters, risks of medication, risk of relapse; time period undefined (months, years)

DIET
Moderation of caloric and sodium intake to avoid weight gain from corticosteroid therapy

PATIENT EDUCATION
- Curtail excess physical activity in early phases when muscle enzymes are markedly elevated.
- Emphasize range of motion exercises.
- Gradually introduce muscle strengthening when muscle enzymes are normal or improved and stable (5).

PROGNOSIS
- Residual weakness: 30%
- Persistent active disease: 20%
- 5-year survival 65–75%, but mortality is 3- to 5-fold higher than general population. Most of the increase in mortality occurs in the 1st year after diagnosis.
- Survival is worse for women and African Americans and those with dermatomyositis, IBM, or cancer.
- Most patients improve with therapy.
- Patient with ILD have poor prognosis.
- Patients with IBM respond poorly to most therapies (6).
- 20–50% have full recovery.

COMPLICATIONS
- Pneumonia
- Infection
- Myocardial infarction
- Carcinoma (especially breast, lung)
- Severe dysphagia
- Respiratory impairment due to muscle weakness, ILD
- Aspiration pneumonitis
- Steroid myopathy
- Steroid-induced diabetes, hypertension, hypokalemia, osteoporosis

REFERENCES

1. Senécal JL, Raynauld JP, Troyanov Y. Editorial: a new classification of adult autoimmune myositis. *Arthritis Rheumatol.* 2017;69(5):878–884.
2. Waldman R, DeWane ME, Lu J. Dermatomyositis: diagnosis and treatment. *J Am Acad Dermatol.* 2020;82(2):283–296.
3. Kohsaka H, Mimori T, Kanda T, et al. Treatment consensus for management of polymyositis and dermatomyositis among rheumatologists, neurologists and dermatologists. *Mod Rheumatol.* 2019;29(1):1–19.
4. Voet NB, van der Kooi EL, van Engelen BG, et al. Strength training and aerobic exercise training for muscle disease. *Cochrane Database Syst Rev.* 2019;12(12):CD003907.
5. Van Thillo A, Vulsteke JB, Van Assche D, et al. Physical therapy in adult inflammatory myopathy patients: a systematic review. *Clin Rheumatol.* 2019;38(8):2039–2051.
6. Machado P, Brady S, Hanna MG. Update in inclusion body myositis. *Curr Opin Rheumatol.* 2013;25(6):763–771.

ADDITIONAL READING

- Anh-Tu Hoa S, Hudson M. Critical review of the role of intravenous immunoglobulins in idiopathic inflammatory myopathies. *Semin Arthritis Rheum.* 2017;46(4):488–508.
- Dobloug GC, Svensson J, Lundberg IE, et al. Mortality in idiopathic inflammatory myopathy: results from a Swedish nationwide population-based cohort study. *Ann Rheum Dis.* 2018;77(1):40–47.
- Fasano S, Gordon P, Hajji R, et al. Rituximab in the treatment of inflammatory myopathies: a review. *Rheumatology (Oxford).* 2017;56(1):26–36.
- Mammen AL. Statin-associated autoimmune myopathy. *N Engl J Med.* 2016;374(7):664–669

 ## CODES

ICD10
- M33.20 Polymyositis, organ involvement unspecified
- M33.90 Dermatopolymyositis, unspecified, organ involvement unspecified
- M33.92 Dermatopolymyositis, unspecified with myopathy

CLINICAL PEARLS

- Corticosteroids alone may be sufficient in patients who have rapid improvement in weakness and muscle enzymes. However, most patients require azathioprine, methotrexate, or other immunosuppressive medications.
- The risk of associated malignancy is higher in patients >50 years and in those with cutaneous manifestations.
- Elevated muscle enzymes (e.g., CK and aldolase) are seen frequently as transient phenomena in patients with febrile illness and injuries; may return to normal on repeat
- In patients with persistently elevated muscle enzymes and symptoms and findings of muscle weakness, EMG followed by muscle biopsy should be the initial studies considered.
- Suspect IBM in older patients with very slow onset and progression of symptoms, poor response to steroids and immunosuppressive therapy, and atypical patterns (asymmetric, sometimes distal) of muscle weakness.
- Suspect autoimmune necrotizing myositis in patients who develop myopathy while taking lipid-lowering drugs (statins) but fail to improve or who worsen after withdrawal of statin therapy.

POPLITEAL (BAKER) CYST
Shane L. Larson, MD • Christopher Morrow, PA-C

BASICS

DESCRIPTION
- A fluid-filled synovial sac arising in the popliteal fossa as a distention of (typically) the gastrocnemial-semimembranous bursa; not a true cyst
- Can be unilateral or bilateral
- Most frequent cystic mass around the knee
- Primary cysts are a distention of the bursa (arise independently without an intra-articular disorder).
- Secondary cysts occur if there is a communication between the bursa and knee joint, allowing articular fluid to fill the cyst.
- Associated with synovial inflammation

EPIDEMIOLOGY
Incidence
- Bimodal distribution
  - Children ages 4 to 7 years
  - Adults increasing with age
- Primary cysts usually seen in children <15 years
- Secondary cysts seen in adults

Prevalence
- Variable adult prevalence of 19–47% in symptomatic knees and 2–5% in asymptomatic knees
- In children: 6.3% in symptomatic knees; 2.4% in asymptomatic knees

ETIOLOGY AND PATHOPHYSIOLOGY
Associated intra-articular pathology includes
- Meniscal tears, mostly of the posterior horn
- Anterior cruciate ligament (ACL) insufficiency
- Degenerative articular cartilage lesions
- Rheumatoid arthritis (20%)
- Osteoarthritis (50%)
- Osteochondritis
- Gout (14%)
- Other potential factors
  - Infectious arthritis
  - Polyarthritis
  - Villonodular synovitis
  - Lymphoma
  - Sarcoidosis
  - Connective tissue diseases
- Extension or herniation of synovial membrane of the knee joint capsule or connection of normal bursa with the joint capsule
- May result from increased intra-articular pressure
- Commonly seen with knee effusions
- Direct trauma to the bursa is likely the primary cause in children because of no communication between the bursa and the joint.
- A valve-like mechanism allowing one-way passage of fluid from the joint to the bursal connection has been described.

RISK FACTORS
- Osteoarthritis of knee (most common)
- Rheumatoid arthritis
- Meniscal degeneration or tear
- Advancing age
- Ligamentous trauma
- Ligamentous insufficiency

COMMONLY ASSOCIATED CONDITIONS
Any condition causing knee joint effusion

DIAGNOSIS

HISTORY
- Painless mass arising in the popliteal fossa
- Most cysts are asymptomatic.
- Dull ache if cyst is large enough to impede joint motion—typically a restriction of flexion
- Painful if cyst ruptures
- Large cysts may cause entrapment neuropathy of the tibial nerve.
- Vascular compression, most commonly of the popliteal vein, may produce claudication or thrombophlebitis.
- Activity alters the cyst size.

PHYSICAL EXAM
- Examine in full extension and 90 degrees of flexion.
- Foucher sign: Mass increases with extension and disappears with flexion.
- Most commonly found in medial aspect of popliteal fossa lateral to the head of the gastrocnemius and medial to the neurovascular bundle
- Cyst is easiest to palpate when knee is slightly flexed and may occasionally be fluctuant or tender.
- Transillumination helps distinguish cyst from solid mass.
- Ruptured cysts are typically painful with associated swelling and bruising over the ipsilateral calf and ankle at the medial malleolus (crescent sign).
- Ruptured cysts also are associated with pseudothrombophlebitis, and rarely, compartment syndrome (1).

DIFFERENTIAL DIAGNOSIS
- Deep venous thrombosis
- Infection/abscess
- Ganglion cyst
- Hematoma
- Thrombophlebitis
- Lipoma, liposarcoma
- Fibroma, fibrosarcoma
- Vascular tumor
- Popliteal vein varices
- Xanthoma
- Aneurysm (rare)
- Muscular herniation (rare, related to trauma)

DIAGNOSTIC TESTS & INTERPRETATION
Initial Tests (lab, imaging)
- CBC, ESR (if septic arthritis suspected)
- Ensure not a popliteal aneurysm prior to aspiration. Send aspirate for cell count and culture to determine if fluid is infectious, inflammatory, or mechanical.
- Ultrasound confirms presence and size; Doppler can differentiate Baker cysts from popliteal vessel aneurysms, DVT, or soft tissue tumors (2).
- MRI helps assess derangements of internal joint structures and to identify cyst leakage.

Follow-Up Tests & Special Considerations
- Consider observation over invasive testing in children.
- Radiographs may show soft tissue density posteriorly.
- Arthrography may demonstrate communication with joint capsule or rupture.
- CT arthrography is superior for visualizing cystic details and can help distinguish lipomas, aneurysms, and malignancies from cysts.

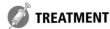 TREATMENT

GENERAL MEASURES
- No treatment if asymptomatic
- Treat any associated underlying conditions.
- Compressive wrap or sleeve for comfort

MEDICATION
If etiology is identified from cellular fluid examination, treat the underlying condition.

First Line
Analgesics and NSAIDs for symptomatic relief

ADDITIONAL THERAPIES
- Physical therapy improves knee ROM and strength, particularly with coexisting pathology.
- Temporary relief with needle aspiration; recurrence common
- Improvement in joint ROM, knee pain, swelling, accompanied reduction in bursa size after aspiration, and intra-articular/intracystic corticosteroid injection (3)[B]
- A combination of physical therapy and corticosteroid injection with or without aspiration leads to best improvements in pain, function, and reduction in cyst size (4)[A].
- Sclerotherapy injections of ethanol or dextrose/sodium morrhuate shown to have good results in small studies (5)[B].

SURGERY/OTHER PROCEDURES
- Consider excision when symptoms persist despite treatment or no etiology is found.
- Surgery usually not required in children
- Recurrence after standard surgery is common and is highest if chondral lesions are present.
- Arthroscopic surgery is highly successful if a valvular mechanism is identified and intra-articular pathology is treated (6)[B].
- Excision via arthroscopy or open procedure often requires concomitant treatment of underlying pathology.

 ONGOING CARE

PROGNOSIS
- Variable; many cysts remain asymptomatic.
- Some cysts resolve with treatment of underlying etiology (e.g., gout, rheumatoid arthritis).
- In children, most cysts resolve without treatment.

COMPLICATIONS
- Compartment syndrome in ruptured cyst
- Thrombophlebitis from compression of the popliteal vein
- Infection of popliteal cyst
- Hemorrhage into cyst if on anticoagulants

REFERENCES
1. Chatzopoulos D, Moralidis E, Markou P, et al. Baker's cysts in knees with chronic osteoarthritic pain: a clinical, ultrasonographic, radiographic and scintigraphic evaluation. *Rheumatol Int*. 2008;29(2):141–146.
2. Sanchez JE, Conkling N, Labropoulos N. Compression syndromes of the popliteal neurovascular bundle due to Baker cyst. *J Vasc Surg*. 2011;54(6):1821–1829.
3. Acebes JC, Sánchez-Pernaute O, Díaz-Oca A, et al. Ultrasonographic assessment of Baker's cysts after intra-articular corticosteroid injection in knee osteoarthritis. *J Clin Ultrasound*. 2006;34(3):113–117.
4. Di Sante L, Paoloni M, Dimaggio M, et al. Ultrasound-guided aspiration and corticosteroid injection compared to horizontal therapy for treatment of knee osteoarthritis complicated with Baker's cyst: a randomized, controlled trial. *Eur J Phys Rehabil Med*. 2012;48(4):561–567.
5. Centeno CJ, Schultz J, Freeman M. Sclerotherapy of Baker's cyst with imaging confirmation of resolution. *Pain Physician*. 2008;11(2):257–261.
6. Lie CW, Ng TP. Arthroscopic treatment of popliteal cyst. *Hong Kong Med J*. 2011;17(3):180–183.

ADDITIONAL READING
- Akagi R, Saisu T, Segawa Y, et al. Natural history of popliteal cysts in the pediatric population. *J Pediatr Orthop*. 2013;33(3):262–268.
- Akgul O, Guldeste Z, Ozgocmen S. The reliability of the clinical examination for detecting Baker's cyst in asymptomatic fossa. *Int J Rheum Dis*. 2014;17(2):204–209.
- Han JH, Bae JH, Nha KW, et al. Arthroscopic treatment of popliteal cysts with and without cystectomy: a systematic review and meta-analysis. *Knee Surg Relat Res*. 2019;31(2):103–112.
- Su C, Kuang S-D, Zhao X, et al. Clinical outcome of arthroscopic internal drainage of popliteal cysts with or without cyst wall resection. *BMC Musculoskelet Disord*. 2020;21(1):440.
- Van Nest DS, Tjoumakaris FP, Smith BJ, et al. Popliteal cysts: a systematic review of nonoperative and operative treatment. *JBJS Rev*. 2020;8(3):e0139.

 SEE ALSO

Algorithm: Knee Pain

 CODES

ICD10
- M71.20 Synovial cyst of popliteal space [Baker], unspecified knee
- M71.21 Synovial cyst of popliteal space [Baker], right knee
- M71.22 Synovial cyst of popliteal space [Baker], left knee

CLINICAL PEARLS
- Baker cyst: a fluid-filled synovial sac arising in the popliteal fossa as a distention of (typically) the gastrocnemial-semimembranous bursa; not a true cyst; often secondary to meniscal tear, osteoarthritis, etc.
- Conservative treatment of Baker cysts is preferred in children, as most will spontaneously resolve.
- In adults, treatment of underlying cause may resolve Baker cysts.
- Pain, bruising, and swelling over the medial malleolus (crescent sign) suggest cyst rupture.

PORTAL HYPERTENSION

Walter M. Kim, MD, PhD • Yu Sakai, MD

BASICS

DESCRIPTION
- Increased portal venous pressure >5 mm Hg that occurs in association with splanchnic vasodilatation, portosystemic collateral formation, and hyperdynamic circulation
- Most commonly secondary to elevated hepatic venous pressure gradient (HVPG; the gradient between portal and central venous pressures)
- Course is generally progressive, with risk of complications including acute variceal bleeding, ascites, hepatic encephalopathy, and hepatorenal syndrome.

EPIDEMIOLOGY
Incidence
The exact incidence of portal hypertension is unclear.

Prevalence
- Prevalence: <200,000 persons in the United States
- Predominant age: adult
- Predominant sex: male > female

ETIOLOGY AND PATHOPHYSIOLOGY
- Causes generally classified as follows:
  - Prehepatic (portal vein thrombosis or obstruction)
  - Intrahepatic (most commonly cirrhosis)
  - Posthepatic (hepatic vein thrombosis, Budd-Chiari syndrome, right-sided heart failure)
- 90% of intrahepatic cases are due to cirrhosis secondary to the following:
  - Virus (hepatitis B, hepatitis C, hepatitis D)
  - Alcoholism
  - Nonalcoholic fatty liver disease
  - Schistosomiasis
  - Wilson disease
  - Hemochromatosis
  - Primary biliary cirrhosis (PBC)
  - Sarcoidosis
- Increased HVPG results in venous collateral formation in the distal esophagus, proximal stomach, rectum, and umbilicus.
- Gastroesophageal variceal formation is found in 40% of patients with portal hypertension.
- Progression of portal hypertension results in splanchnic vasodilation and angiogenesis.

Genetics
No known genetic patterns except those associated with specific hepatic diseases that cause portal hypertension

RISK FACTORS
See "Etiology and Pathophysiology."

Pediatric Considerations
In children, portal vein thrombosis is the most common extrahepatic cause; intrahepatic causes are more likely to be biliary atresia, viral hepatitis, and metabolic liver disease.

GENERAL PREVENTION
Treatment of the underlying liver disease may reduce portal hypertension and prevent complications in patients with cirrhosis.

COMMONLY ASSOCIATED CONDITIONS
- Alcoholism
- Cirrhosis
- Nonalcoholic fatty liver disease
- Schistosomiasis
- Extrahepatic portal vein thrombosis

DIAGNOSIS

HISTORY
- Ascites; symptoms of heart failure including chest pain, shortness of breath, and/or edema
- Hematemesis
- Melena
- Oliguria
- Jaundice
- Weakness/fatigue
- History of chronic liver disease
- Alcoholic hepatitis
- Alcohol abuse

PHYSICAL EXAM
- Exam findings may be general or related to specific complications.
- General
  - Pallor
  - Icterus
  - Digital clubbing
  - Palmar erythema
  - Splenomegaly
  - Caput medusa
  - Spider angiomata
  - Umbilical bruit
  - Hemorrhoids
  - Gynecomastia
  - Testicular atrophy
- Gastroesophageal varices
  - Hypotension
  - Tachycardia
- Ascites
  - Distended abdomen
  - Fluid wave
  - Shifting dullness with percussion
- Hepatic encephalopathy
  - Confusion/coma
  - Asterixis
  - Hyperreflexia

DIFFERENTIAL DIAGNOSIS
Usually related to specific presentations
- Gastroesophageal varices with hemorrhage
  - Portal hypertensive gastropathy
  - Hemorrhagic gastritis
  - Peptic ulcer disease
  - Mallory-Weiss tear
- Ascites
  - Spontaneous bacterial peritonitis (SBP)
  - Pancreatic ascites
  - Peritoneal carcinomatosis
  - Tuberculous peritonitis
  - Hepatic malignancy
  - Fluid overload from heart failure
  - Nephrotic syndrome
- Hepatic encephalopathy
  - Delirium tremens
  - Intracranial hemorrhage
  - Sedative abuse
  - Uremia
- Hepatorenal syndrome
  - Drug nephrotoxicity
  - Renal tubular necrosis

DIAGNOSTIC TESTS & INTERPRETATION
Initial Tests (lab, imaging)
Direct calculation of HVPG (approximation of the gradient in pressure between portal vein and IVC) is the gold standard in diagnosing portal hypertension:

- HVPG = wedged hepatic venous pressure (WHVP) − free hepatic venous pressure (FHVP)
- WHVP is estimated by occlusion of the hepatic vein by a balloon catheter and measurement of the proximal static column of blood.
- FHVP is estimated by direct measurement of the patent hepatic vein, intra-abdominal inferior vena cava, or right atrium.
- Esophageal varices generally develop when HVPG >10 mm Hg in compensated cirrhosis and HVPG >16 mm Hg in decompensated cirrhosis.
- Nonspecific changes associated with underlying disease:
  - Hypersplenism: anemia (also may be due to malnutrition or bleeding), leukopenia, thrombocytopenia
  - Hepatic dysfunction
    ○ Hypoalbuminemia
    ○ Hyperbilirubinemia
    ○ Elevated alkaline phosphatase
    ○ Elevated liver enzymes (AST, ALT)
    ○ Abnormal clotting (prothrombin time, international normalized ratio, partial thromboplastin time)
  - GI bleeding
    ○ Iron deficiency anemia
    ○ Elevated serum ammonia
    ○ Fecal occult blood
    ○ Thrombocytopenia
  - Hepatorenal syndrome
    ○ Elevated serum creatinine (Cr), blood urea nitrogen (BUN)
    ○ Urine sodium <5 mEq/L (<20 mmol/L)
  - US and CT scan/MRI may detect cirrhosis, splenomegaly, ascites, and varices.
  - US/duplex Doppler
    ○ Can determine presence and direction of flow in portal and hepatic veins
    ○ Useful in diagnosing portal vein thrombosis, shunt thrombosis, or the presence of ascites
  - CT scan/MRI: angiographic measurement of hepatic venous wedge pressure via jugular or femoral vein
    ○ Correlates with portal pressure
    ○ Risk of variceal bleeding is increased if HVPG >12 mm Hg.
  - Upper GI series may outline varices in esophagus and stomach.
  - Transient elastography is a noninvasive method to determine hepatic fibrosis and to predict portal hypertension.

Follow-Up Tests & Special Considerations
- If portal hypertension is diagnosed in a patient with no risk factors, the patient should first be evaluated for cirrhosis.
- HVPG response to nonselective β-blockers is associated with a significant reduction in risk of variceal bleeding and decompensation.

Diagnostic Procedures/Other
- Diagnostic paracentesis and calculation of the serum-ascites albumin gradient (SAAG) can differentiate between portal hypertensive (SAAG >1.1 g/dL) from nonportal hypertensive (SAAG <1.1 g/dL) causes of ascites.
- Endoscopy can diagnose esophageal and gastric varices and portal hypertensive gastropathy.

Test Interpretation
Specific for underlying disease

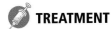 TREATMENT

GENERAL MEASURES
- Avoid sedatives that may precipitate encephalopathy.
- Limit sodium intake because cirrhotic patients avidly retain sodium (<2 g sodium per day).

MEDICATION
Therapy for encephalopathy: See "Hepatic Encephalopathy."

First Line
- Prophylaxis against variceal bleeding:
  - Nonselective β-blockade
    - Nadolol: 20 to 40 mg PO once-daily dosing
    - Propranolol: Start with 20 to 40 mg PO BID–TID.
  - May consider carvedilol: 6.25 mg PO once-daily dosing as an alternative β-blocker (1)[C]
  - Doses may be titrated up as tolerated to maximum recommended doses; goal resting heart rate of 55 to 60 bpm
- Therapy for acute variceal hemorrhage:
  - Octreotide: 50 μg IV bolus followed by 50 μg/hr continuous infusion; pediatric dose: 1 μg/kg bolus followed by 1 μg/kg/hr is used traditionally; treat for up to 5 days.
  - Vasopressin: Start with 0.2 to 0.4 U/min IV; increase to maximum dose 0.8 U/min as needed; pediatric dose: 0.002 to 0.005 U/kg/min; do not exceed 0.01 U/kg/min. After bleeding stops, continue at same dose for 12 hours and then taper off over 24 to 48 hours.
- For prevention of recurrence and for overall reduction in mortality:
  - Nadolol: 40 to 80 mg/day PO reduces portal venous blood inflow by blocking the adrenergic dilatation of the mesenteric arterioles.
  - Propranolol: 10 to 60 mg/day PO BID–QID; pediatric dose: 0.5 to 1.0 mg/kg/day PO divided q6–8h
  - Tetrandrine, a calcium channel blocker, also has been found to reduce the rate of rebleeding with fewer side effects.
- Initial treatment for ascites (along with salt and fluid restriction):
  - Furosemide: 20 to 40 mg/day PO; pediatric dose: 1 to 2 mg/kg/dose PO ± IV albumin infusion
  - Spironolactone: 50 to 100 mg/day PO; pediatric dose: 1 to 3 mg/kg/day PO

Second Line
- Terlipressin (2 mg IV q4h; titrate down to 1 mg IV q4h once hemorrhage is controlled; may be used for up to 48 hours) is a more selective splanchnic vasoconstrictor and may be associated with fewer complications. It is currently used when standard therapy with somatostatin or octreotide fails.
- Addition of nitrates, such as nitroglycerin or isosorbide mononitrate, reduces portal pressures and bleeding rates and has been shown to reduce mortality. Because the risk–benefit ratio is not clear, nitrates are not considered first-line treatment.
- Studies are ongoing for possible benefits of other agents including simvastatin, clonidine, verapamil, and losartan.

ISSUES FOR REFERRAL
Patients with portal hypertension should be managed longitudinally by both a primary care physician and a gastroenterologist.

SURGERY/OTHER PROCEDURES
- Treatments available for specific complications of portal hypertension (in addition to or if refractory to medications):
  - Gastroesophageal varices without hemorrhage
    - Endoscopic variceal ligation (EVL) is the preferred therapy for prevention of bleeding of large (grade III) varices and requires serial interventions every 2 to 8 weeks until the varices are eradicated.
  - Gastroesophageal varices with hemorrhage
    - EVL or sclerosis (the first-line treatment in many cases for acute hemorrhage) within 12 hours of presentation (2)[A]
    - Balloon tamponade (not used commonly when endoscopic treatment is available)
    - Transjugular intrahepatic portosystemic shunt (TIPS)
    - Portacaval shunting
  - Ascites refractory to medical management
    - Large-volume paracentesis
    - Peritoneovenous shunt
    - TIPS
- Liver transplantation should be considered for patients with advanced disease.

ADMISSION, INPATIENT, AND NURSING CONSIDERATIONS
- Acute GI bleeding should be managed in the inpatient setting, either on the regular medical floor if the patient is hemodynamically stable or in the ICU if the patient is unstable.
- Patients with mental status changes from encephalopathy need to be evaluated in the inpatient setting.
- Admission criteria/initial stabilization
  - Acute bleeding from the intestinal tract, either vomiting or per rectum
  - Acute confusional state/mental status changes
  - If acute variceal bleeding:
    - Type and cross patient's blood.
    - Initial resuscitation with isotonic fluid until packed RBCs are available
    - Correct coagulopathy with vitamin K and fresh frozen plasma (FFP).
    - Endoscopy as soon as the patient is stabilized (for diagnosis and treatment)
  - Avoid sedatives that may precipitate encephalopathy.
  - Limit sodium administration because cirrhotic patients avidly retain sodium.
  - Restrict protein only if encephalopathic.

ALERT
If the patient is an active alcohol drinker, assess for alcoholic hepatitis and watch for signs and symptoms of withdrawal. Follow inpatient protocols for alcohol withdrawal management.

- Use isotonic fluid for hydration.
- Discharge criteria
  - For GI bleeding:
    - No active bleeding in 24 hours
    - Stable hemoglobin and hematocrit
    - Hemodynamically stable (especially heart rate)
  - For encephalopathy: improvement in or resolution of mental status changes to baseline

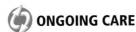 ONGOING CARE

FOLLOW-UP RECOMMENDATIONS
Patient Monitoring
- Treatment of the underlying etiology of chronic liver disease may improve both liver structure and function, which could translate into a reduction in portal pressure gradient.
- For patients without varices, there is currently no indication to use β-blockers as prophylaxis.

DIET
- In cirrhosis, patients retain sodium, so restrict sodium intake.
- Obesity can worsen cirrhosis, thus aggressively counsel on diet and exercise.
- Alcohol abstinence

PATIENT EDUCATION
Refrain from alcohol (refer to program if dependence), dietary sodium restriction.

PROGNOSIS
- Hepatic reserve defined by Child-Pugh classification: rating based on encephalopathy, ascites, bilirubin, albumin, prothrombin
- Variceal bleeding
  - 1/3 of patients with known varices will bleed eventually.
  - 50% rebleed, usually within 2 years, unless portal pressure is reduced by surgical or TIPS procedure.
  - 15–20% mortality rate
- Ascites and encephalopathy often recur.
- Prognosis of patients with ascites is poor: 50% 1-year survival without liver transplant (compared with 90% for patients with cirrhosis and no ascites).

COMPLICATIONS
- Acute gastroesophageal variceal bleed
- Ascites
- Hepatic encephalopathy
- Hepatic hydrothorax
- Hepatorenal syndrome
- Portal hypertensive gastropathy
- Portopulmonary hypertension
- Splenomegaly
- SBP

REFERENCES

1. Zacharias AP, Jeyaraj R, Hobolth L, et al. Carvedilol versus traditional, non-selective beta-blockers for adults with cirrhosis and gastroesophageal varices. *Cochrane Database Syst Rev*. 2018;(10):CD011510.
2. de Franchis R; for Baveno VI Faculty. Expanding consensus in portal hypertension: report of the Baveno VI Consensus Workshop: stratifying risk and individualizing care for portal hypertension. *J Hepatol*. 2015;63(3):743–752.

CODES

ICD10
K76.6 Portal hypertension

CLINICAL PEARLS
- Portal hypertension can be diagnosed based on physical examination in the setting of known risk factors, specifically cirrhosis.
- Endoscopic treatment is successful for acute variceal hemorrhage 85% of the time.
- Prognosis of patients with ascites is poor: 50% 1-year survival without liver transplant (compared with 90% for patients with cirrhosis and no ascites).

POSTCONCUSSION SYNDROME (MILD TRAUMATIC BRAIN INJURY)

Vicki R. Nelson, MD, PhD • Jose O. Malave, MD

 BASICS

DESCRIPTION

- Postconcussion syndrome (PCS) is a constellation of symptoms involving physical, cognitive, and/or behavioral symptoms persisting after a concussion (mild traumatic brain injury [mTBI]) that may continue for weeks to years (1).
- It is unclear when concussive symptoms transition to become postconcussive syndrome. A recent consensus defines this as persistent symptoms lasting >10 to 14 days in adults and 4 weeks in children (2).
- Symptoms of PCS may include (1)
  - Cognitive
    - Poor focus
    - Poor organization
    - Diminished academic/intellectual performance
    - Slowed response time
  - Physical
    - Headache
    - Nausea
    - Visual changes
    - Light and noise sensitivity
    - Tinnitus
    - Dizziness and balance problems
    - Fatigue and sleep disturbance
  - Behavioral
    - Depression
    - Irritability/emotional lability
    - Apathy
    - Increased sensitivity to alcohol
- Diagnosis is based on history and clinical symptoms.

EPIDEMIOLOGY

Incidence
The reported frequency of patients with mTBI who develop PCS varies widely between 5% and 80%.
- Largely due to difficulty differentiating postconcussion *symptoms* from PCS
- 80–90% of concussion victims recover from postconcussion *symptoms* within 7 to 10 days, slightly longer in children/adolescents (2). A diagnosis of PCS is made in patients with persistent concussive symptoms.

Prevalence
Predominant sex: Females are slightly more likely to experience prolonged symptoms following a concussive injury.

ETIOLOGY AND PATHOPHYSIOLOGY
- Controversial; exact mechanism(s) unknown
- Microscopic axonal injury from shearing forces leads to inflammation causing secondary brain injury.
- Conflicting data on structural brain damage and correlation of imaging with physical symptoms (1)
- Because the pathophysiology of PCS is not well understood and because of symptom overlap with other psychiatric conditions, PCS remains difficult to diagnose and to manage.
  - Only some individuals with mTBI develop PCS; it is unclear what causes postconcussion symptoms to persist leading to postconcussion syndrome.

- Behavioral factors are commonly associated with (and may play a role in) the development of PCS. It can be challenging to differentiate some behavioral disorders from PCS (1). Neuropsychiatry evaluation can be helpful.
  - Patients who reported high symptom burden following mTBI are at increased risk of PCS (3)[B].

RISK FACTORS
- Strongest predictor is severity of initial symptoms (2).
- Initial symptoms including retrograde amnesia, difficulty concentrating, disorientation, insomnia, loss of balance, sensitivity to noise, or visual disturbance (4)
- Preexisting psychiatric disease including depression, anxiety, personality disorder, and posttraumatic stress disorder (PTSD)
- Preexisting expectation of poor outcomes following mTBI (1)
- Nonsport concussion/mTBI
- Unclear if previous history of concussion(s) is a risk factor for PCS
- Low socioeconomic status
- Loss of consciousness is NOT predictive of PCS.

GENERAL PREVENTION
- Education of players, coaches, parents, and athletic trainers about concussion, PCS, and appropriate safety rules
- Head injury precautions are advised. Evidence is lacking that these decrease incidence of mTBI/PCS.
- Screening and intervention for anxiety and depression

COMMONLY ASSOCIATED CONDITIONS
- PTSD
- Anxiety
- Depression
- Fibromyalgia
- Personality disorders (namely, compulsive, histrionic, and narcissistic)
- ADHD

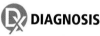 **DIAGNOSIS**

HISTORY
- Detailed history of recent impact and closed head injury, including:
  - Mechanism
  - Timing of injury related to symptoms
  - Previous head injuries, including concussion, and timing of those injuries
  - Previous medical, psychiatric, or social history
  - Thorough characterization of associated symptoms, intensity, and duration
- Report of neurologic, cognitive, or behavioral symptoms by patient/family

PHYSICAL EXAM
Complete neurologic exam, including the following:
- Glasgow Coma Scale (GCS)
- Anxiety/depression screening
  - Patient Health Questionnaire-9 (PHQ-9)
  - GAD-7

- Many additional screening and diagnostic tools are available (e.g., Sport Concussion Assessment Tool [SCAT], NFL Sideline Concussion Assessment Tool, or computerized neuropsychiatric testing) and may be utilized (2).

DIFFERENTIAL DIAGNOSIS
- Postconcussive symptoms
- PTSD
- Anxiety/depression
- Personality disorders
- Migraine headaches
- Chronic fatigue syndrome, fibromyalgia
- Evolving intracranial hemorrhage
- Exposure to toxins, including prescription and recreational drugs
- Endocrine/metabolic abnormality

DIAGNOSTIC TESTS & INTERPRETATION
Initial Tests (lab, imaging)
- Consider infection, intoxication, and endocrine or metabolic abnormality in appropriate clinical setting.
- Brain imaging both on initial evaluation of mTBI and PCS is not routinely indicated.
- Imaging to evaluate for bleeding is appropriate with comorbidities or anticoagulation therapy at the time of injury.
- Imaging indicated if cervical spine injury is suspected

Follow-Up Tests & Special Considerations
- Several computerized neuropsychiatric (CNP) tests are available to help guide return-to-play decisions; it is most useful to compare with baseline scores (if available).
- Formal neuropsychiatric evaluations are superior to CNP testing when available. None of these tests should be used in isolation for decision making, especially if a patient is still symptomatic (2)[C].
- Common neuropsychological testing programs
  - Immediate Post-Concussion Assessment and Cognitive Testing (ImPACT)
  - CNS Vital Signs
  - Balance Error Scoring System (BESS)
  - Axon Sports Computerized Cognitive Assessment Tool (CCAT)
  - Automated Neuropsychological Assessment Metrics (ANAM)

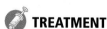 **TREATMENT**

GENERAL MEASURES
- Return to full activity should progress according to existing evidence-based recommendations, which include immediate cognitive rest in the acute period (24 to 48 hours) followed by gradual return to daily activities as tolerated (2)[C].
- When possible, controlling cognitive stress and providing extra school accommodations can be beneficial (2).

- Restrict individuals with concussion or PCS from sport activity until symptoms have resolved and patients have been weaned from any medications that might mask PCS symptoms (1),(2)[C].
- Physical therapy for coexisting cervical and vestibular injuries is beneficial. Cognitive-behavioral therapy helps with persistent mood disturbances (3).
- Limited evidence that pharmacotherapy is beneficial
- Subthreshold exercise helps resolve symptoms (5)[B].

MEDICATION
First Line
- Headache/neck pain
  - Nonopioid pain control (e.g., NSAIDs) preferred
    - With use of opioid medications, sedation obscures cognitive evaluation.
    - Possible association between the use of opiates and increased risk of anxiety/depression in PCS patients
    - Consider occipital nerve block.
  - Propranolol or amitriptyline alone or in combination
- Emotional dysregulation (irritability, sadness, anxiety, depression)
  - Anxiety/depression screening starting in the 1st week post-mTBI
    - Tricyclic antidepressants (e.g., amitriptyline 10 to 25 mg at night)
    - SSRIs (e.g., sertraline 25 mg daily titrated to effective dose with maximum 200 mg daily) for persistent depressive symptoms
  - Consider referral to behavioral health specialist(s).
- Sleep dysregulation
  - Sleep hygiene
  - Melatonin (up to 3 mg in older children and 5 mg in adolescents and adults)
  - Trazodone (25 to 50 mg at night)
- Cognitive disorders (poor concentration, fogginess, drowsiness)
  - Neuropsychological evaluation
  - Neurostimulants, such as amantadine (100 mg BID) (6), methylphenidate, atomoxetine
- Emotional disturbances

ISSUES FOR REFERRAL
- Neuropsychiatric therapy including comprehensive cognitive evaluation for potential TBI rehabilitation
- Cognitive-behavioral therapy for anxiety and depression symptoms
- Occupational therapy for vocational rehabilitation
- Physical therapy for vestibular rehabilitation
- Neurology referral if primary care interventions for seizures, headache, vertigo, or cognition are unsuccessful
- Substance abuse counseling, if needed

COMPLEMENTARY & ALTERNATIVE MEDICINE
- Massage therapy, osteopathic manipulative treatment, acupuncture for headache and neck pain
- Potential benefits shown with hyperbaric oxygen therapy in military veterans with concurrent PCS and PTSD (7)

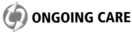 ## ONGOING CARE

FOLLOW-UP RECOMMENDATIONS
Schedule regular follow-up to evaluate for persistent symptoms, efficacy of and/or need for neuropsychiatric evaluation, and the efficacy of and/or need for pharmacologic therapy.

Patient Monitoring
- Consider serial neuropsychological testing.
- Follow return-to-play guidelines for resuming physical activity and sport (2)[C].

PATIENT EDUCATION
- Centers for Disease Control and Prevention: http://www.cdc.gov/headsup/
- Brain Injury Association of America: http://www.biausa.org/; (800) 444-6443

PROGNOSIS
- Prognosis generally is good. Most patients improve within 3 months.
- Adolescents may recover more slowly than adults.

COMPLICATIONS
- Repeat head injury or return to play before resolution of PCS can worsen/prolong symptoms.
- Case studies of second-impact syndrome, a rare but potentially fatal condition owing to a second head injury soon after the first, have been reported.

REFERENCES

1. Harmon KG, Clugston JR, Dec K, et al. American Medical Society for Sports Medicine position statement on concussion in sport. Br J Sports Med. 2019;53(4):213–225.
2. McCrory P, Meeuwisse W, Dvořák J, et al. Consensus statement on concussion in sport—the 5th International Conference on Concussion in Sport held in Berlin, October 2016. Br J Sports Med. 2017;51(11):838–847.
3. Meehan WP III, Mannix R, Monuteaux MC, et al. Early symptom burden predicts recovery after sport-related concussion. Neurology. 2014;83(24):2204–2210.
4. Kerr ZY, Zuckerman SL, Wasserman EB, et al. Factors associated with post-concussion syndrome in high school student-athletes. J Sci Med Sport. 2018;21(5):447–452.
5. Leddy JJ, Willer B. Use of graded exercise testing in concussion and return-to-activity management. Curr Sports Med Rep. 2013;12(6):370–376.
6. Reddy CC, Collins M, Lovell M, et al. Efficacy of amantadine on symptoms and neurocognitive performance among adolescents following sports-related concussion. J Head Trauma Rehabil. 2013;28:260–265.
7. Harch PG, Andrews SR, Fogarty EF, et al. Case control study: hyperbaric oxygen treatment of mild traumatic brain injury persistent post-concussion syndrome and post-traumatic stress disorder. Med Gas Res. 2017;7(3):156–174.

ADDITIONAL READING

- Morgan CD, Zuckerman SL, Lee YM, et al. Predictors of postconcussion syndrome after sports-related concussion in young athletes: a matched case-control study. J Neurosurg Pediatr. 2015;15(6):589–598.
- Schneider KJ, Leddy JJ, Guskiewicz KM, et al. Rest and treatment/rehabilitation following sport-related concussion: a systematic review. Br J Sports Med. 2017;51(12):930–934.

 ## SEE ALSO

Concussion (Mild Traumatic Brain Injury)

 ## CODES

ICD10
- F07.81 Postconcussional syndrome
- S06.9X0A Unsp intracranial injury w/o loss of consciousness, init
- S06.9X9A Unsp intracranial injury w LOC of unsp duration, init

CLINICAL PEARLS
- Imaging is rarely useful for postconcussion syndrome. If necessary, head CT is the test of choice for acute injury to exclude intracranial bleeding.
- Coordinate multidisciplinary treatment plans for patients with persistent symptoms.
- Return to sport/activity should not occur until the is fully asymptomatic (or has returned to preevent baseline).

POSTTRAUMATIC STRESS DISORDER (PTSD)

Siddhi Bhivandkar, MD • Saeed Ahmed, MD

 BASICS

Posttraumatic stress disorder (PTSD) is a psychiatric disorder that may occur in people who have experienced or witnessed a traumatic event or who have been threatened with death, sexual violence, or serious injury (1).

DESCRIPTION

- The disorder can appear at any age. In children >6 years of age, young adults, and adults, it presents with three cardinal characteristics:
  - Intrusion symptoms like flashbacks, nightmares, distressing recollections
  - Avoidance of anything related to the traumatic event and/or numbing of general responsiveness
  - Increased arousal
- Duration of PTSD can be:
  - Acute: symptoms lasting <3 months
  - Chronic: symptoms lasting ≥3 months
  - Delayed: onset 6 months after trauma exposure, <5% of cases
  - Symptoms of PTSD usually develop within 3 months after a trauma, although they can be delayed for years.

EPIDEMIOLOGY

- Probability of PTSD was assessed in about 29 types of traumatic experiences, divided into groups: sexual relationship violence, interpersonal violence, exposure to organized violence, participation in organized violence, and other life-threatening traumatic experiences.
- Unexpected death of loved one, rape, other sexual assault were associated with the highest rate of PTSD.
- 16% of children and adolescents exposed to trauma develop PTSD.

Incidence

~7.7 million American adults aged ≥18 years (3.5% of this age group) are diagnosed with PTSD each year.

Prevalence

Lifetime prevalence for PTSD ranges from 7% to 9% in the general population. More common in females than males.

ETIOLOGY AND PATHOPHYSIOLOGY

- Biologic dimensions: hypersensitivity of catecholamine pathways and overactivity of the central opioid pathways is seen; the amygdala and hippocampus dysfunction, with possible atrophy from overexposure to catecholamines, serotonergic dysregulation, glutamatergic dysregulation, and increased thyroid activity
- Learning theory: Life-threatening fear is classically conditioned by event exposure; any internal or external cue reminiscent of the event produces an intense "fight or flight" fear response.
- Cognitive theories: These models suggest that severe trauma becomes represented in complex memory structures. The activation of these memories triggers intense thoughts and emotions that cause discomfort and dysfunction.
- Psychodynamic theory: Traumatic memories overwhelm defense mechanisms. Repeated recall of the traumatic event with associated fear is an effort to understand the event in a less threatening way.

Genetics

Monozygotic twins exposed to combat in Vietnam were at increased risk of the cotwin having PTSD compared with dizygotic twins.

RISK FACTORS

- Pretrauma environment:
  - Female gender
  - Younger age
  - Psychiatric history
  - Sexual abuse
- Peritrauma environment:
  - Severity of the trauma
  - Peritrauma emotionality
  - Perception of threat to life
  - Perpetration of the trauma
- Posttrauma environment:
  - Perceived injury severity
  - Medical complications
  - Perceived social support
  - Persistent dissociation from traumatic event
- Subsequent exposure to trauma-related stimuli

GENERAL PREVENTION

Trauma-focused cognitive-behavioral therapy (CBT) and modified prolonged exposure delivered within weeks of a potentially traumatic event for people showing signs of distress have the most evidence in the prevention of PTSD.

COMMONLY ASSOCIATED CONDITIONS

- Major depressive disorder
- Alcohol/substance abuse
- Panic disorder/agoraphobia/social phobia
- Obsessive-compulsive disorder
- Traumatic brain injury
- Smoking (especially with assaultive trauma)
- Major neurocognitive disorders, dementia, or amnesia

Pediatric Considerations

Oppositional defiant disorder and separation anxiety are common comorbid conditions.

DIAGNOSIS

Diagnosis is based on *DSM-5* criteria (1):

- Criterion A: exposure to trauma (≥1 of the following):
  - Direct experience of a traumatic event
  - In-person witnessing of a traumatic event
  - Learning of a traumatic event involving a close friend or family member
  - Repeated exposure to details of a traumatic event
- Criterion B: intrusive symptoms associated with the traumatic event (≥1 of the following):
  - Recurrent, involuntary, and intrusive distressing memories of the event
  - Recurrent distressing dreams related to the event
  - Dissociative reactions that simulate a recurrence of the event
  - Intense or prolonged distress to stimuli that resemble an aspect of the event
- Criterion C: avoidance of stimuli associated with the trauma (≥1 of the following):
  - Avoidance of memories, thoughts, or feelings about the event
  - Avoidance of external reminders that trigger memories, thoughts, or feelings about the event

- Criterion D: negative cognitive and mood changes associated with the trauma (≥2 of the following):
  - Inability to remember aspects of event
  - Persistent and exaggerated negative opinion of self, others, or the world
  - Distorted beliefs about the cause or consequences of the event
  - Negative emotional state
  - Diminished interest in significant activities
  - Feeling detached from others
  - Inability to experience positive emotions
- Criterion E: hyperarousal (≥2 of the following):
  - Difficulty sleeping/falling asleep
  - Decreased concentration
  - Hypervigilance
  - Outbursts of anger/irritable mood
  - Exaggerated startle response
  - Self-destructive behavior
- Criterion F: Duration of the relevant criteria symptoms should be >1 month.
- Criterion G: clinically significant distress/impairment in functioning
- Criterion H: relevant criteria not attributed to substance effects or other medical conditions

Pediatric Considerations

- Reactions can include a fear of being separated from a parent, crying, whimpering, screaming, immobility and/or aimless motion, trembling, frightened facial expressions, excessive clinging, or regressive behavior.
- Older children may show extreme withdrawal, disruptive behavior, and/or an inability to pay attention. Regressive behaviors, nightmares, sleep problems, irrational fears, irritability, refusal to attend school, outbursts of anger, fighting, somatic complaints with no medical basis, and decline in schoolwork performance. Furthermore, depression, anxiety, feelings of guilt, and emotional numbing are often present.
- Parental posttraumatic stress has been shown to be a robust predictor of pediatric PTSD (2)[A].

HISTORY

Symptoms of intrusion, avoidance, alternations of mood and cognition, and hyperarousal must have lasted >1 month.

PHYSICAL EXAM

- Patients may present with physical injuries from the traumatic event.
- Mental status examination:
  - Thoughts and perceptions (e.g., hallucinations, delusions, suicidal ideation, phobias)
  - General appearance: disheveled, poor hygiene
  - Behavior: agitation; startle reaction extreme
  - Psychological numbness
  - Orientation may be affected.
  - Memory: forgetfulness, especially concerning the details of the traumatic event
  - Poor concentration
  - Poor impulse control
  - Altered speech rate and flow
  - Mood and affect may be changed: depression, anxiety, guilt, and/or fear.

Pediatric Considerations
Elevated heart rate immediately following trauma is associated with development of PTSD (2)[A].

DIFFERENTIAL DIAGNOSIS
- Generalized anxiety disorder/adjustment disorder
- Obsessive-compulsive disorder
- Schizophrenia
- Major depressive disorder/mood disorder with psychotic features
- Substance abuse
- Personality/dissociative/conversion disorders
- Factitious disorder, or malingering

DIAGNOSTIC TESTS & INTERPRETATION
- Diagnosis is based on *DSM-5* criteria (1)
- Primary Care PTSD Screen for *DSM-5* (PC-PTSD-5) (3)
- Trauma Screening Questionnaire (TSQ)

 TREATMENT

Combination psychotherapy and pharmacotherapy, initiated soon after the trauma, results in better prognosis.

MEDICATION
Both paroxetine and sertraline are FDA-approved drugs for the treatment of PTSD, but other SSRIs are also effective.

First Line
- Depression, panic attacks, startle response, sleep disruption: may improve with SSRIs (4)[A]:
  - Sertraline: 50 to 200 mg every day (FDA-approved)
  - Paroxetine: starting dose: 10-mg every day; may be increased in 10 mg increments at intervals ≥1 week (FDA-approved)
  - Fluoxetine: 20 mg every day/BID not to exceed 80 mg/day (demonstrates some efficacy for all three symptom clusters)
- Sleep disruption: Sleep disruption due to hyperarousal is ubiquitous in PTSD; standard sedatives, such as trazodone 50 to 300 mg at bedtime, mirtazapine 7.5 to 30.0 mg QHS, or amitriptyline 25 to 100 mg QHS
- Nightmares/nighttime hyperarousal: prazosin 2 to 15 mg QHS (5)[A], clonidine 0.1 to 0.2 mg QHS, amitriptyline 25 to 100 mg QHS

Second Line
Refractory/residual symptoms: Consider augmentation with:
- Depression: mirtazapine 15 to 45 mg/day; consider switch to a serotonin-norepinephrine reuptake inhibitor (SNRI), such as venlafaxine XR 37.5 to 300.0 mg/day, duloxetine 60 to 120 mg/day, or desvenlafaxine 50 to 100 mg/day. Nefazodone 300 to 600 mg/day in divided doses can be very effective but requires quarterly LFTs.
- Reexperiencing/intrusive thoughts: 1st-/2nd-generation antipsychotic medications: aripiprazole 5 to 15 mg/day, risperidone 0.5 to 2.0 mg/day, olanzapine 2.5 to 10.0 mg/day, quetiapine 50 to 400 mg/day (6)[A]. 2nd-generation Rx less prone to extrapyramidal symptoms (EPS): cognitive dulling

- Hyperarousal: clonidine, start 0.05 mg BID/TID; slowly titrate to as much as 0.45 mg/day divided doses; guanfacine 1 to 3 mg/day in divided doses (long-acting forms of both clonidine and guanfacine now available). Also consider 2nd-generation antipsychotics quetiapine, risperidone, and olanzapine as above; divided doses often more helpful
- Impulsivity/explosiveness: anticonvulsants: valproic acid 500 to 2,000 mg/day, carbamazepine 200 to 600 mg/day, topiramate 50 to 200 mg/day
- Anxiety: Benzodiazepines (especially short-acting) should be avoided given the risk of substance abuse and questionable benefit in PTSD (7)[A]. Consider hydroxyzine 25 to 50 mg TID/QID PRN or risperidone 0.25 to 0.50 mg TID PRN.

ADDITIONAL THERAPIES
- Exposure therapies have shown the highest effectiveness for treatment of PTSD (8)[A]:
  - Behavioral and CBT: Early CBT, including virtual exposure, has been shown to speed recovery. CBT is considered the standard of care for PTSD by the U.S. Department of Defense.
  - 1-week intensive CBT was as effective as 3 months weekly CBT in one study.
  - Prolonged exposure therapy: Reexperience distressing trauma-related memories and reminders to facilitate habituation and successful emotional processing of memory.
  - Eye movement desensitization and reprocessing (EMDR) has been shown to benefit patients with PTSD.
- Stress-reduction techniques:
  - Immediate symptom reduction (e.g., rebreathing in a bag for hyperventilation)
  - Early recognition and removal from a stress
  - Relaxation, meditation, and exercise techniques are also helpful in reducing the reaction to stressful events.
- Telemedicine-based collaborative care (nurse, case manager, pharmacy, psychology, psychiatry).

Pediatric Considerations
Little evidence to support use of pharmacologic interventions for pediatric PTSD.

 ONGOING CARE

- The initial stabilization phase can be prolonged.
- Ongoing exposure to trauma can undermine the improvement.
- Patients with a history of childhood sexual abuse (complex PTSD) are often challenging to treat; they have significant difficulties with affect regulation and trust (9).
- It can take years for patients of complex PTSD to build trust and develop a relationship with the therapist to manage the exploration of the trauma (9).

PATIENT EDUCATION
National Center for PTSD: http://www.ptsd.va.gov

PROGNOSIS
- In 50% of cases, the symptoms spontaneously remit after 3 months; however, symptoms may persist and cause long-term impairment in life functioning.

- Factors associated with a good prognosis include:
  - Rapid engagement of treatment
  - Early and ongoing social support
  - Avoidance of retraumatization
  - Absence of other psychiatric disorders/substance abuse

COMPLICATIONS
- Increased risk for panic disorder, agoraphobia, obsessive-compulsive disorder, social phobia, specific phobia, major depressive disorder, somatization disorder; impulsive behavior, suicide, and homicide
- Victims of sexual assault are at especially high risk for developing mental health problems and committing suicide.

REFERENCES
1. American Psychiatric Association. *Diagnostic and Statistical Manual of Mental Disorders*. 5th ed. Arlington, VA: American Psychiatric Association; 2013.
2. Brosbe MS, Hoefling K, Faust J. Predicting posttraumatic stress following pediatric injury: a systematic review. *J Pediatr Psychol*. 2011;36(6):718–729.
3. Prins A, Ouimette P, Kimerling R, et al. The Primary Care PTSD Screen (PC-PTSD): development and operating characteristics. *Primary Care Psychiatry*. 2003;9(1):9–14.
4. Stein DJ, Ipser JC, Seedat S. Pharmacotherapy for post traumatic stress disorder (PTSD). *Cochrane Database Syst Rev*. 2006;(1):CD002795.
5. Writer BW, Meyer EG, Schillerstrom JE. Prazosin for military combat-related PTSD nightmares: a critical review. *J Neuropsychiatry Clin Neurosci*. 2014;26(1):24–33.
6. Han C, Pae C-U, Wang S-M, et al. The potential role of atypical antipsychotics for the treatment of posttraumatic stress disorder. *J Psychiatr Res*. 2014;56:72–81.
7. Jeffreys M, Capehart B, Friedman MJ. Pharmacotherapy for posttraumatic stress disorder: review with clinical applications. *J Rehabil Res Dev*. 2012;49(5):703–715.
8. Kornør H, Winje D, Ekeberg Ø, et al. Early trauma-focused cognitive-behavioural therapy to prevent chronic post-traumatic stress disorder and related symptoms: a systematic review and meta-analysis. *BMC Psychiatry*. 2008;8:81.
9. Stern TA, Herman JB, eds. *Massachusetts General Hospital Psychiatry Update and Board Preparation*. 2nd ed. New York, NY: McGraw-Hill; 2004.

CODES

ICD10
- F43.10 Post-traumatic stress disorder, unspecified
- F43.11 Post-traumatic stress disorder, acute
- F43.12 Post-traumatic stress disorder, chronic

CLINICAL PEARLS

Treatment is often best accomplished with a combination of psychotherapy and pharmacotherapy.

PREECLAMPSIA AND ECLAMPSIA (TOXEMIA OF PREGNANCY)

Ann M. Aring, MD, FAAFP

 BASICS

DESCRIPTION
- Preeclampsia:
  - A disorder of pregnancy occurring after 20 weeks' gestation characterized by new-onset hypertension (HTN), new-onset proteinuria, ± impaired organ function:
    - May progress from mild to life-threatening in hours to days
    - Reversible by delivery
- Eclampsia:
  - New-onset grand mal seizure activity with no history of underlying neurologic disease
- Most postpartum cases of preeclampsia and eclampsia occur within 48 hours of delivery but can occur up to 4 weeks postpartum.
- System(s) affected: cardiovascular, renal, reproductive, fetoplacental, CNS, hepatic, pulmonary
- Synonym(s): toxemia of pregnancy

EPIDEMIOLOGY
Incidence
Preeclampsia occurs in 5–8% of all pregnancies.

Prevalence
- Predominant age
  - Most in younger women, primiparous women
  - Older (>40 years) patients with preeclampsia have 4 times the incidence of seizures compared with patients in their 20s.
- Eclampsia occurs:
  - 1.6 to 10 out of 10,000 deliveries in developed countries
  - 6 to 157 out of 10,000 deliveries in developing countries
- 40% of eclamptic seizures occur before delivery; 16% occur >48 hours after delivery.
- Eclampsia is a main cause of perinatal mortality and morbidity (2–8% of all pregnancies).

ETIOLOGY AND PATHOPHYSIOLOGY
- Cause of preeclampsia is becoming clearer.
  - Abnormal placental implantation
  - Angiogenic factors
  - Genetic predisposition
  - Immunologic phenomena
  - Vascular endothelial damage and oxidative stress
- Systemic derangements in eclampsia include the following:
  - Cardiovascular: generalized vasospasm
  - Hematologic: decreased plasma volume, increased blood viscosity, hemoconcentration, coagulopathy
  - Renal: decreased glomerular filtration rate
  - Hepatic: periportal necrosis, hepatocellular damage, subcapsular hematoma
  - CNS: cerebral vasospasm and ischemia, cerebral edema, cerebral hemorrhage

Genetics
2 to 4 times increased risk in pregnant women with family history of preeclampsia

RISK FACTORS
- Nulliparity
- Age >40 years
- Family history of preeclampsia
- High body mass index
- Diabetes
- Chronic HTN
- Chronic renal disease
- Multifetal pregnancy

- Previous pregnancy with preeclampsia
- Systemic lupus erythematosus
- In vitro fertilization

GENERAL PREVENTION
- Adequate prenatal care
- Inadequate prenatal care results in 7 times increase in mortality.
- Good control of preexisting HTN
- Low-dose aspirin (ASA) (60 to 80 mg):
  - ASA started early after 12 weeks' gestational age [GA] may lower the risk of developing preeclampsia and the rate of preterm delivery and neonatal death in moderate- to high-risk patients (1)[B] (see "Risk Factors" as mentioned earlier).
- Low-dose calcium supplementation has been shown to reduce the risk and severity of preeclampsia in calcium-deficient populations.
- Some evidence suggests vitamin C (1,000 mg/day) and vitamin E (400 IU/day) may reduce the risk for preeclampsia, but recent guidelines recommend against their use.

COMMONLY ASSOCIATED CONDITIONS
Abruptio placentae, placental insufficiency, fetal growth restriction, preterm delivery, fetal demise maternal seizures (eclampsia), maternal pulmonary edema, maternal liver/kidney failure, or maternal death

 DIAGNOSIS

- Preeclampsia diagnosis:
  - Blood pressure:
    - New-onset elevated blood pressure (BP): systolic BP (SBP) ≥140 mm Hg or diastolic BP (DBP) ≥90 mm Hg (on two occasions at least 4 hours apart) or ≥160/110 mm Hg after 20 weeks of gestation (within a shorter interval), *and either*
  - Proteinuria:
    - Proteinuria >300 mg/24 hr
    - Spot protein: creatinine ≥0.3
  - Or, without proteinuria and new onset of any of these features:
    - Platelets <100,000/μL
    - Liver transaminase levels >2 times normal
    - Creatinine >1.1 mg/dL or doubling of serum creatinine levels
    - Pulmonary edema
    - Cerebral or visual symptoms
  - Preeclampsia with severe features
    - Platelets <100,000/μL
    - Severe persistent right upper quadrant (RUQ)/epigastric pain, or both
    - Creatinine >1.1 mg/dL or doubling of serum creatinine levels
    - Visual disturbances
    - New-onset headache
    - Pulmonary edema
- Eclampsia diagnosis:
  - New-onset tonic clonic, focal, or multifocal seizures
  - No history of neurologic disease

HISTORY
- May be asymptomatic. In some cases, rapid excessive weight gain (>5 lb/week; >2.3 kg/week); more severe cases are associated with epigastric/RUQ pain, headache, altered mental status, and visual disturbance. Note: Headache, visual disturbance, and epigastric or RUQ pain often precede seizure.
- Seizures may occur once/repeatedly.

PHYSICAL EXAM
BP criteria:
- Preeclampsia *without* severe features: elevated BP ≥140/90 mm Hg
- Preeclampsia *with* severe features: elevated BP ≥160 systolic mm Hg or 110 mm Hg diastolic
- Eclampsia: tonic–clonic seizure activity (focal/generalized)
- Normal BP, even in response to treatment; does not rule out potential for seizures

DIFFERENTIAL DIAGNOSIS
- Chronic HTN: HTN before pregnancy; high BP before the 20th week
- Chronic HTN with superimposed preeclampsia
- Gestational HTN: Increased BP first discovered after 20 weeks, often close to term, with no proteinuria and without evidence of organ dysfunction. BP becomes normal by 12 weeks postpartum, or it is reclassified as chronic HTN.
- Seizures in pregnancy: epilepsy, cerebral tumors, meningitis/encephalitis, and ruptured cerebral aneurysm. Until other causes are proven; however, all pregnant women with convulsions should be considered to have eclampsia.

DIAGNOSTIC TESTS & INTERPRETATION
Initial Tests (lab, imaging)
- Routine spot urine testing or urinalysis for protein should be done at each prenatal visit in all hypertensive patients but is not indicated routinely for low-risk, nonhypertensive gravidas.
- Complete blood count (CBC), including platelets, creatinine, serum transaminase levels, and uric acid as baseline in hypertensive patients and if preeclampsia suspected or possible
- Coagulation profiles: Abnormalities suggest severe disease.
- 24-hour urine or spot protein/creatinine ratio if urine protein dips 1+ on more than one occasion or if preeclampsia is being considered
- Daily fetal movement monitoring by mother ("kick counts")
- US imaging is used to monitor growth and cord blood flow; perform, as indicated, based on clinical stability and laboratory findings.
- Nonstress test (NST) at diagnosis and then twice weekly until delivery
- Biophysical profile (BPP) if NST is nonreactive
- US imaging for growth progress every 3 weeks and amniotic fluid volume at least once weekly
- With seizures, CT scan and MRI should be considered if focal findings persist or uncharacteristic signs/symptoms are present.

Follow-Up Tests & Special Considerations
Disseminated intravascular coagulation, thrombocytopenia, liver dysfunction, and renal failure can complicate preeclampsia associated with HELLP syndrome.

Test Interpretation
CNS: cerebral edema, hyperemia, focal anemia, thrombosis, and hemorrhage. Cerebral lesions account for 40% of eclamptic deaths.

TREATMENT

GENERAL MEASURES

- Preeclampsia without severe features:
  - Outpatient care
  - Maternal: daily home BP monitoring; daily weights; weekly labs (CBC, creatinine, liver function test [LFT])
  - Fetal:
    - Patient-measured: daily "kick counts"
    - NST/BPP/US (see "Initial Tests (lab, imaging)" section above)
    - Delivery at 37 weeks (induction of labor) (2)[C]
    - Steroids for gestation <37 weeks
- Preeclampsia with severe features:
  - Inpatient care
  - Maternal:
    - Daily labs
    - IV magnesium sulfate (MgSO₄) as seizure prophylaxis
    - Antihypertensive therapy titrated to keep SBP <160 mm Hg and DBP <110 mm Hg (Some recommend <150/100 mm Hg postpartum.)
  - Fetal:
    - Continuous heart monitoring
    - Daily US with BPP
    - Check amniotic fluid levels and fetal growth.
  - Definitive management (delivery) depends on GA (2)[C].
  - <23 weeks:
    - Offer to terminate pregnancy.
  - At 23 to 34 weeks:
    - Antihypertensives
    - Evaluate maternal–fetal condition.
    - Steroids to enhance fetal lung maturity
    - Plan delivery at 34 weeks with magnesium sulfate prophylaxis.
    - If HELLP syndrome (full or partial), severe oligohydramnios, significant renal dysfunction, persistent symptoms, fetal growth restriction, onset of labor, OR PROM, proceed to delivery.
  - At ≥34 weeks: magnesium sulfate, steroids, and proceed to delivery; steroids indicated up to 37 weeks

ALERT

- Regardless of GA, emergent delivery is recommended if there are signs of maternal hypertensive crisis, abruptio placentae, uterine rupture, or fetal distress.
- Seizures: control of convulsions, correction of hypoxia and acidosis, lowering of BP, steps to effect delivery as soon as convulsions are controlled
- Administer betamethasone 12 mg IM daily × 2 doses or dexamethasone 6 mg every 12 hours × 4 doses if delivery <37 weeks possible.

MEDICATION

First Line

- Seizure prophylaxis for women with severe preeclampsia:
  - Magnesium sulfate: loading dose 4 g IV in 200 mL normal saline over 20 to 30 minutes; maintenance dose 1 to 2 g/hr IV continuous infusion (Although recent guidelines suggest it not be universally administered for seizure prophylaxis to prevent eclampsia, the quality of the evidence is low, and the strength of the recommendation is qualified.)
- BP control (3):
  - Antihypertensives are inadvisable for mildly elevated BP (without severe features).
  - Labetalol (IV): 20 mg over 2 minutes followed at 20- to 30-minute intervals with doses of 20 to 80 mg titrated to keep BP <160/110 mm Hg; max of 300 mg/24 hr (contraindicated in asthma, heart disease, congestive heart failure)

  - Hydralazine (IV): 5 to 10 mg over 2 minutes, followed at 20 minutes intervals with 5 to 10 mg IV boluses; titrated to keep BP <160/110 mm Hg; max of 25 mg/24 hr
  - Nifedipine immediate release 10 mg oral followed by 20 mg in 20 minutes if needed for severe range (4)[A]. Sustained release (PO) (used in the postpartum): 30 to 120 mg/day (caution with combination of nifedipine and magnesium sulfate resulting in hypotension and neuromuscular blockade)
- Eclampsia/seizures:
  - Magnesium sulfate for seizures
    - 4 to 6 g IV over 15 to 20 minutes followed by 1 to 2 g/hr infusion
    - Further boluses of magnesium may be given for recurrent convulsions with the amount given based on the neurologic examination and patellar reflexes.
    - Contraindications: myasthenia gravis, renal failure, pulmonary edema
  - Levels of 6 to 8 mEq/mL are considered therapeutic, but monitor clinical status of:
    - Patellar reflexes are present.
    - Respirations are not depressed.
    - Urine output is ≥25 mL/hr.
  - May be given safely, even in the presence of renal insufficiency
- Fluid therapy
  - Ringer lactated solution with 5% dextrose at 60 to 120 mL/hr, with careful attention to fluid volume status
- Calcium gluconate or chloride (1 g, administered slowly IV) may reverse magnesium-induced respiratory depression (2).

Second Line

- In randomized trials, magnesium sulfate was found to be superior to phenytoin in treatment and prevention of eclampsia and probably more effective and safer than diazepam.
- Diazepam 2 mg/min until resolution or 20 mg given or
- Lorazepam 1 to 2 mg/min up to total of 10 mg or
- Phenytoin 15 to 20 mg/kg at a maximum rate of 50 mg/min or
- Levetiracetam 500 mg IV or oral may be repeated in 12 hours (dose needs to be adjusted in renal impairment) or
- Phenobarbital 20 mg/kg infused at 50 mg/min; may repeat with additional 5 to 10 mg/kg after 15 minutes

 ONGOING CARE

FOLLOW-UP RECOMMENDATIONS

- Without severe features: restricted activity and close monitoring; with severe features: restricted activity, in hospital
- Women with a history of preeclampsia should report this to physicians caring for them in later life. It is a potent cardiovascular disease risk factor.

DIET

- Salt restriction is inadvisable because the patient often is experiencing intravascular hypovolemia.
- Calcium supplementation may be recommended for women who have low calcium intake (<600 mg/day).

PATIENT EDUCATION

American College of Obstetricians and Gynecologists, 409 12th St. SW, Washington, DC 20024-2188; (800) 762-ACOG; http://www.acog.org/

PROGNOSIS

- For nulliparous women with preeclampsia before 30 weeks of gestation, the recurrence rate for the disorder may be as high as 40% in future pregnancies.

- 25% of eclamptic women will have HTN during subsequent pregnancies, but only 5% of these will be severe and only 2% will be eclamptic again.
- Preeclamptic, multiparous women may be at higher risk for subsequent essential HTN; they also have higher mortality during subsequent pregnancies than do primiparous women.

COMPLICATIONS

- Most women do not have long-term sequelae from eclampsia, although many may have transient neurologic deficits.
- A history of preeclampsia is equivalent to traditional risk factors for cardiovascular disease. Women with a history of preeclampsia should be strongly advised to avoid obesity and smoking. Other signs of metabolic syndrome should be closely monitored as well.
- Intrauterine growth restriction (IUGR)
- Maternal and/or fetal death

REFERENCES

1. Rolnik DL, Wright D, Poon LC, et al. Aspirin versus placebo in pregnancies at high risk for preterm preeclampsia. *N Engl J Med*. 2017;377:613–622.
2. Leeman L, Dresang LT, Fontaine P. Hypertensive disorders of pregnancy. *Am Fam Physician*. 2016;93(2):121–127.
3. ACOG Committee Opinion No. 767: emergent therapy for acute-onset, severe hypertension during pregnancy and the postpartum period. *Obstet Gynecol*. 2019;133(2):e174–e180.
4. Duley L, Meher S, Jones L. Drugs for treatment of very high blood pressure during pregnancy. *Cochrane Database Syst Rev*. 2013;(7):CD001449.

ADDITIONAL READING

- Abalos E, Duley L, Steyn DW. Antihypertensive drug therapy for mild to moderate hypertension during pregnancy. *Cochrane Database Syst Rev*. 2014;(2):CD002252.
- ACOG Committee Opinion No. 764: medically indicated late-preterm and early-term deliveries. *Obstet Gynecol*. 2019;133(2):e151–e155.
- Gestational hypertension and preeclampsia: ACOG Practice Bulletin, Number 222. *Obstet Gynecol*. 2020;135(6):e237–e260.
- Phipps E, Prasanna D, Brima W, et al. Preeclampsia: updates in pathogenesis, definitions, and guidelines. *Clin J Am Soc Nephrol*. 2016;11(6):1102–1113.

CODES

ICD10

- O14.90 Unspecified pre-eclampsia, unspecified trimester
- O15.00 Eclampsia in pregnancy, unspecified trimester
- O14.00 Mild to moderate pre-eclampsia, unspecified trimester

CLINICAL PEARLS

- Management of preeclampsia depends on both the severity of the condition and the GA of the fetus.
- Magnesium sulfate is the treatment of choice for women demonstrating preeclampsia with severe features.
- Low-dose ASA starting in early pregnancy in high-risk patients may lower rate of preeclampsia.
- Continue to monitor maternal BP postpartum—still at risk for developing preeclampsia.
- History of preeclampsia is a cardiovascular risk factor later in life.

PREMENSTRUAL SYNDROME (PMS) AND PREMENSTRUAL DYSPHORIC DISORDER (PMDD)

Andrew Lutzkanin, MD • Madie D. Hartman, DO

 BASICS

DESCRIPTION
- Premenstrual syndrome (PMS), a complex of physical and emotional symptoms sufficiently severe to interfere with everyday life, occurs cyclically during the luteal phase of menses.
- Premenstrual dysphoric disorder (PMDD) is a severe form of PMS characterized by severe recurrent depressive and anxiety symptoms, with premenstrual (luteal phase) onset, that remits a few days after the start of menses as defined in the *Diagnostic and Statistical Manual of Mental Disorders*, 5th edition (*DSM-5*).
- System(s) affected: endocrine/metabolic, nervous, reproductive

EPIDEMIOLOGY
Prevalence
- Many women have some physical and psychological symptoms before menses that can encompass a spectrum from mild molimina to severe and disabling symptoms.
- The prevalence of PMS is reported anywhere between 20% and 30% of menstruating women. 1.2% to 6.4% of women have PMDD based on *DSM-5* criteria (1) with upward of 18% of menstruating women meeting partial *DSM* criteria (2).

ETIOLOGY AND PATHOPHYSIOLOGY
While not yet fully understood, there are two main views on the pathophysiology (1):
- Changing levels of the progesterone metabolite allopregnanolone interacts with serotonin and γ-aminobutyric acid (GABA) receptors, provoking downstream effects of decreased GABA-mediated inhibition and decreased serotonin levels.
- Decreased function of the serotonin system (in particular the serotonin transporter) serves as the primary abnormality and thus when modulated by sex hormones leads to decreased serotonin levels in patients with PMS/PMDD.

Genetics
- The role of genetic predisposition is controversial; however, twin studies do suggest a genetic component.
- Involvement of gene coding for the serotonergic *5HT1A* receptor and allelic variants of the estrogen receptor-α gene (*ESR1*) is suggested.

RISK FACTORS
- Age: usually presents in the late 20s to mid-30s
- History of mood disorder (major depression, bipolar disorder), anxiety disorder, personality disorder, or substance abuse
- Family history
- Low parity
- Cigarette smoking and other nicotine-containing products
- Psychosocial stressors/history of trauma
- High BMI (>27.5)

COMMONLY ASSOCIATED CONDITIONS
There is a high prevalence of comorbid mood disorders and/or anxiety disorders in patients with PMS/PMDD.

 DIAGNOSIS

HISTORY
- Criteria for the diagnosis of PMS has been established by the International Society for Premenstrual Disorders (ISPMD) and include:
  - Physical or emotional symptoms
  - Symptoms are present during the luteal phase and abate as menstruation begins
  - A symptom-free week
  - Symptoms are associated with significant impairment during the luteal phase
- Criteria for the diagnosis of PMDD was established by the American Psychiatric Association in 2013 and included in the *DSM-5*.
- Symptoms occur 1 week before menses, improve in the first few days after menses begin, and are minimal/absent in the week following menses (over most menstrual cycles during the past year).
- ≥5 of the following (1 must be among the first 4):
  - Marked depressed mood, feelings of hopelessness, or self-deprecating thoughts
  - Marked anxiety, tension, and/or feelings of being keyed up or on edge
  - Marked affective lability (mood swings)
  - Marked irritability or anger or increased interpersonal conflicts
  - Decreased interest in usual activities and social withdrawal
  - Lethargy, easy fatigability, or lack of energy
  - Appetite change, overeating, food cravings
  - Hypersomnia or insomnia
  - Feeling out of control or overwhelmed
  - Subjective difficulty concentrating
  - Physical symptoms, such as abdominal bloating, breast tenderness, headaches, weight gain, and joint/muscle pain
- Emotional symptoms must be sufficiently severe to interfere with work, school, usual social activities, or relationships with others.
- Symptoms may be superimposed on an underlying psychiatric disorder but may not be an exacerbation of another condition, such as panic disorder/major depression.
- Criteria should be confirmed by prospective patient record of symptoms for a minimum of two consecutive menstrual cycles (without confirmation, "provisional" should be noted with diagnosis).
- Symptoms should not be attributable to drug abuse, medications, or other medical conditions.
- Diagnosis can be established through the use of a validated tool such as the Daily Record of Severity of Problems (available online at http://www.aafp.org/afp/2011/1015/p918-fig1.pdf) or similar inventory.

PHYSICAL EXAM
No specific physical exam is required; may consider thyroid and pelvic exams if indicated by additional patient symptoms

DIFFERENTIAL DIAGNOSIS
- Premenstrual exacerbation of underlying psychiatric disorder
- Psychiatric disorders (especially bipolar disorder, major depression, anxiety)
- Thyroid disorders
- Perimenopause
- Premenstrual migraine
- Chronic fatigue syndrome
- Irritable bowel syndrome (painful symptoms)
- Seizures
- Anemia
- Endometriosis (painful symptoms)
- Drug/alcohol abuse

DIAGNOSTIC TESTS & INTERPRETATION
- The repetitive nature of symptoms precludes the need for labs if a classic history is present.
- Consider
  - Hemoglobin to rule out anemia
  - Serum thyroid-stimulating hormone (TSH) to rule out hypothyroidism
- Imaging with pelvic ultrasound to diagnose causes of pelvic pain and dysmenorrhea may be needed.

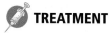 **TREATMENT**

GENERAL MEASURES
Exercise increases beta-endorphins in the brain, but the role of physical activity in the treatment of premenstrual disorders remains unclear (3).

MEDICATION
First Line
- SSRIs are recommended as the first-line therapy in the treatment of physical, functional, and behavioral symptoms of PMS and PMDD compared to placebo (4)[A]:
  - Both intermittent luteal phase dosing and continuous full-cycle dosing are effective with no clear evidence of a difference between modes of administration (4)[A].
  - All SSRIs tested appeared effective (4)[A].
  - SSRIs are effective at low doses but may require titration of the dose for the desired response in certain patients. Higher doses have increased effect but are accompanied by increased side effects (4)[A].
- Fluoxetine (Prozac, Sarafem) 20 mg/day every day or 20 mg/day only during the luteal phase, or 90 mg once a week for 2 weeks in the luteal phase
- Sertraline (Zoloft) 50 to 150 mg/day every day or 50 to 150 mg/day only during the luteal phase
- Citalopram (Celexa) 10 to 30 mg/day every day or 10 to 30 mg/day only during the luteal phase
- Adverse effects (number needed to harm [NNH] with moderate-dose SSRI): nausea (NNH = 7), asthenia (NNH = 9), somnolence (NNH = 13), fatigue (NNH = 14), decreased libido (NNH = 14), and sweating (NNH = 14) (4)[A]
- Contraindications: patients taking monoamine oxidase inhibitors (MAOIs)
- Precautions
  - Increased risk of suicidal thinking and behavior in children and adolescents with depressive disorders; uncertain if this risk applies to those taking SSRIs for PMDD
  - Bipolar disorder
  - Seizure disorder
  - QTc prolongation (with citalopram)

– Hepatic dysfunction
– Renal dysfunction

Second Line
Alternative therapies should be considered if no response to SSRIs:

- Spironolactone (Aldactone) 50 to 100 mg/day for 7 to 10 days during the luteal phase; helpful for fluid retention.
  - Adverse reactions: lethargy, headache, irregular menses, hyperkalemia
  - Regular monitoring of electrolytes is recommended due to the risk of hyperkalemia.
- Oral contraceptive pills (OCPs)
  - OCPs can cause adverse effects similar to PMDD symptoms.
  - Extended-cycle use of OCPs (e.g., 12 weeks on and 1 week off) or a shorter placebo interval (e.g., 24 active pills with 4 placebo days [24/4] compared with 21/7 preparations) may be beneficial.
  - OCPs containing the progestin drospirenone (structurally similar to spironolactone) may improve physical symptoms and mood changes associated with PMDD (5)[A]. Caution: The risk of venous thromboembolism may be modestly higher than with other OCPs.
  - Continuous administration of levonorgestrel/ethinyl estradiol may improve patient symptoms in PMDD.
    - Suggested OCP formulations:
      - Ethinyl estradiol 0.02 to 0.03 mg/drospirenone 3 mg (Gianvi/Loryna/Nikki/Ocella/Syeda/Vestura/Yasmin/Yaz Zarah): 1 tablet/day
      - Ethinyl estradiol 0.02 to 0.03 mg/drospirenone 3 mg/levomefolate 0.451 mg (Beyaz/Safyral): 1 tablet/day
      - Levonorgestrel 90 μg/ethinyl estradiol 20 μg (Amethyst/Lybrel): 1 tablet/day
- Anxiolytics
  - Alprazolam (Xanax) 0.25 mg TID–QID only during luteal phase; taper at the onset of menses (other benzodiazepines not studied for PMDD); caution: addictive potential
  - Buspirone (BuSpar) 10 to 30 mg/day divided BID–TID in the luteal phase
- Ovulation inhibitors
  - Gonadotropin-releasing hormone (GnRH) agonists: leuprolide (Lupron) depot 3.75 mg/month IM
    - Precautions: Menopause-like side effects (e.g., osteoporosis, hot flashes, headaches, muscle aches, vaginal dryness, irritability) limit treatment to 6 months; may be the first step if considering bilateral oophorectomy for severe, refractory PMDD
  - Danazol (Danocrine) 300 to 400 mg BID; adverse reactions: androgenic and antiestrogenic effects (e.g., amenorrhea, weight gain, acne, fluid retention, hirsutism, hot flashes, vaginal dryness, emotional lability)
  - Estrogen, transdermal preferred, 100 to 200 μg:
    - Precautions: increased risk of blood clots, stroke, heart attack, and breast cancer
    - Requires concomitant progesterone add-back therapy to protect against uterine hyperplasia and endometrial cancer
- Progesterone: insufficient evidence to support use

ISSUES FOR REFERRAL
Short-term follow-up (within 1–3 months) can assess if the patient has an adequate response to treatment. If not, referral to a psychiatrist may be indicated for further evaluation.

ADDITIONAL THERAPIES
Cognitive-behavioral therapy (CBT) is theoretically helpful for PMS/PMDD given its application for symptom reduction in other mood disorders, but direct evidence is lacking.

SURGERY/OTHER PROCEDURES
Bilateral oophorectomy, usually with concomitant hysterectomy, is an option for rare, refractory cases with severe, disabling symptoms.

COMPLEMENTARY & ALTERNATIVE MEDICINE
Acupuncture demonstrated superiority to progestins, anxiolytics, and sham acupuncture with no evidence of harm (6)[A].

- Some data support the use of the following:
  - Calcium: 600 mg BID
  - Vitamin B_6: 50 to 100 mg/day
  - Chasteberry (*Vitex agnus-castus*): 4 mg/day of extract containing 6% of agnuside (or 20 to 40 mg/day of fruit extract)
  - Omega-3 fatty acids 2 g/day
- Data insufficient regarding the following:
  - Magnesium: 200 to 400 mg/day
  - Vitamin D: 2,000 IU/day
  - Vitamin E: 400 IU/day
  - Manganese: 1.8 mg/day
  - St. John's wort: 900 mg/day
  - Soy: 68 mg/day isoflavones
  - Ginkgo: 160 to 320 mg/day
  - Saffron: 30 mg/day
- Evidence supporting efficacy and/or safety of herbal products is lacking; the following products/interventions have not been found useful for PMS/PMDD, although not all studies are of high quality and able to eliminate the possibility of benefit completely:
  - Evening primrose oil
  - Black currant oil
  - Black cohosh
  - Wild yam root
  - Dong quai
  - Kava kava
  - Light-based therapy

ONGOING CARE

FOLLOW-UP RECOMMENDATIONS
Patient Monitoring
Increased risk of suicidal thinking and behavior in children and adolescents with depressive disorders on initiation of SSRIs; uncertain if this risk applies to those taking SSRIs for PMDD

DIET
- Reduce consumption of salt, sugar, caffeine, dairy products, and alcohol (anecdotal reports).
- Eat small, frequent portions of food high in complex carbohydrates (limited data).

PATIENT EDUCATION
- Counsel patients to eat a balanced diet rich in calcium, vitamin D, and omega-3 fatty acids and low in saturated fat and caffeine.
- Counsel patients to quit tobacco and other nicotine use (more research is needed on the benefit of smoking cessation in PMS and PMDD).
- Counsel women that they are not "crazy." PMDD is a real disorder with a physiologic basis.
- Although incompletely understood, successful treatment is often possible.

PROGNOSIS
- Many patients can have their symptoms adequately controlled. PMS disappears at menopause.
- PMS can continue after hysterectomy if ovaries are left in place.

REFERENCES
1. Yonkers KA, Simoni MK. Premenstrual disorders. *Am J Obstet Gynecol*. 2018;218(1):68–74.
2. Carlini SV, Deligiannidis KM. Evidence-based treatment of premenstrual dysphoric disorder: a concise review. *J Clin Psychiatry*. 2020;81(2):19ac13071.
3. Lanza di Scalea T, Pearlstein T. Premenstrual dysphoric disorder. *Med Clin North Am*. 2019;103(4):613–628.
4. Marjoribanks J, Brown J, O'Brien PM, et al. Selective serotonin reuptake inhibitors for premenstrual syndrome. *Cochrane Database Syst Rev*. 2013;2013(6):CD001396.
5. Lopez LM, Kaptein AA, Helmerhorst FM. Oral contraceptives containing drospirenone for premenstrual syndrome. *Cochrane Database Syst Rev*. 2012;(2):CD006586.
6. Kim S-Y, Park H-J, Lee H, et al. Acupuncture for premenstrual syndrome: a systematic review and meta-analysis of randomised controlled trials. *BJOG*. 2011;118(8):899–915.

CODES

ICD10
N94.3 Premenstrual tension syndrome

CLINICAL PEARLS
- Have the patient keep a daily log of her symptoms and menses. Symptoms beginning in the week before menses and abating before the end of menses, occurring over at least 2 months, and sufficiently severe to interfere with daily functioning are diagnostic of PMS.
- Treatment only during the luteal phase is likely as effective as continuous-cycle treatment with SSRIs but has fewer adverse effects.

PRENATAL CARE AND TESTING
Anna K. Zheng, MD • Henry Del Rosario, MD

BASICS

The goal of prenatal care is to ensure the well-being of mother and baby using the best available evidence and a patient-centered approach. General concepts include: estimating the gestational age (GA) accurately; identifying risk for complications; encouraging and empowering the patient for motherhood, newborn care, and breastfeeding; intervening when fetal abnormalities are present to prevent morbidity and mortality.

GENERAL PREVENTION
In the United States, the typical prenatal visit schedule consists of monthly visits for weeks 4 to 28 of pregnancy, visits twice monthly from 28 to 36 weeks, weekly after week 36 (until delivery, typically at weeks 38 to 41).

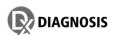

DIAGNOSIS

HISTORY
Collect the following histories in the initial prenatal visit and continually update throughout the pregnancy (1),(2):

- Medical history, with an emphasis on the following but not limited to:
  - Prediabetes/DM, obesity/overweight
  - Thyroid disorders
  - Pregestational hypertension or history of hypertensive disease in pregnancy (e.g., chronic HTN, gestational HTN, preeclampsia with or without severe features, HELLP syndrome)
  - Maternal age at delivery
  - Previous DVT/PE
  - Known uterine anomaly
  - Autoimmune disease (e.g., systemic lupus erythematosus, rheumatoid arthritis, Sjögren)
  - Strong family history of diseases in pregnancy or congenital/inheritable conditions
- Obstetrical history, including but not limited to:
  - History of preterm delivery or PTL
  - History of hypertensive disease in pregnancy
  - History of gestational diabetes (GDM) or early onset GDM
  - Other medical conditions raising maternal risk: HIV/AIDS or other STIs in the past, sickle cell disease, intrahepatic cholestasis of pregnancy
  - Personal history of delivering a newborn with birth defects/trisomies or congenital/inheritable condition
- Psychosocial history, including but not limited to:
  - Depression screening (use EPDS or PHQ-9), intimate partner violence (ACOG guidelines: Screen *all* pregnant patients at the first prenatal visit, 1x/trimester, and at postpartum checkup.)
  - Tobacco, alcohol, and drug use
  - Lifestyle, nutrition, toxin exposures, travel to areas with endemic diseases, stressors/supports; potential barriers to care (preferred language, housing, transportation, child care issues, economic constraints, work schedule)

PHYSICAL EXAM
- A full physical exam on intake (1),(2).
- At each subsequent prenatal visit, the following should be recorded (1),(2):
  - Weight gain recommendations (2009 IOM)
    - BMI <18.5 kg/m² (underweight): 28 to 40 lb (12.5 to 18.0 kg)
    - BMI 18.5 to 24.9 kg/m² (normal weight): 25 to 35 lb (11.5 to 16.0 kg)
    - BMI 25.0 to 29.9 kg/m² (overweight): 15 to 25 lb (7.0 to 11.5 kg)
    - BMI ≥30.0 kg/m² (obese): 11 to 20 lb (5 to 9.0 kg)
  - BP (mm Hg): Assess for mild (≥140/≥90 to <160 <110) or severe range (≥160/≥110) BP if not normal.
  - Fundal height: Start after week 20–24 week.
  - Fetal heart rate: usually audible by 8 weeks' GA with a Doppler device
  - Pelvic/cervical exam if indicated
  - Fetal position by Leopold maneuver at weeks 32 to 36; confirm by ultrasound if available.

DIAGNOSTIC TESTS & INTERPRETATION
- First prenatal visit (1):
  - Lab tests
    - Hematocrit or hemoglobin, blood type, Rhesus type, and antibody screen
    - Hemoglobin electrophoresis: Screen for sickle cell disease, SCT, or thalassemia.
    - Urine culture
    - Ab titers for Rubella and Varicella
    - STI screen: RPR/VDRL, GC/C, Hep B, HIV
    - Not recommended: routine screening for bacterial vaginosis, toxoplasmosis, CMV, and parvovirus; thyroid and vitamin D deficiency
  - Carrier screening (including, but not limited to):
    - Cystic fibrosis screening: Counseling needed first, and screening should be offered when one partner is of Caucasian, European, or Ashkenazi Jewish descent.
    - Spinal muscular atrophy
    - Hemoglobinopathies (i.e., risk for sickle cell disease, thalassemia)
  - Screening for fetal aneuploidy:
    - Counseling should be provided before any shared decision-making on testing.
    - All women should be offered screening or diagnostic testing, regardless of maternal age.
    - Ultrasound (US) nuchal translucency (NT): measures thickness at the back of the neck of the fetus
    - Blood screens: human chorionic gonadotropin (hCG), pregnancy-associated plasma protein A (PAPP-A), quadruple test: α-fetoprotein (AFP), unconjugated estriol (UE3), hCG, dimeric inhibin-A (DIA)
    - Cell-free DNA testing: should not be used as a substitute for diagnostic testing due to potential for false-positive or false-negative results; all women with positive screening test should have a diagnostic procedure before any irreversible action is taken.

- 1st-trimester "combined test" between 11 and 13 weeks' GA using both NT and hCG/PAPP-A blood testing is an effective protocol; may be performed either as a single combined stand-alone test (US NT 1 blood [HCG and PAPP-A]) or as part of a sequential "step-by-step" 1st- and 2nd-trimester screening process (see the following discussion)
- Women who undergo 1st-trimester screening should be offered 2nd-trimester assessment for open fetal defects and US screening for other fetal structural defects.
- 2nd-trimester screening: Obtain quadruple test ideally at weeks 15–18 but can be done as late as week 22.
- If risk found, all pregnant women should be offered invasive prenatal diagnostic testing regardless of maternal age or other risk factors (3). Diagnostic tests for genetic disorders:
  - CVS: 1st trimester: usually done weeks 10 to 12. Small sample of the placenta; chorionic tissue sample obtained either transcervical (TC) or transabdominal (TA)
  - Amniocentesis: usually done weeks 15 to 18. Small sample of amniotic fluid from the amniotic sac surrounding the developing fetus is obtained by an US-guided TA approach.
  - The rate of procedure-related pregnancy loss that is attributable to a prenatal diagnostic procedure is 0.1–0.3% when performed by experienced health care providers (3).
  - Chromosomal microarray analysis: can detect a pathogenic copy number variant in about 1.7% of patients with normal US and normal karyotype; make available to any patient choosing to undergo invasive diagnostic testing; primary test for patients undergoing diagnostic testing for indication of a fetal structural abnormality detected by US examination (3)
  - Cervical cancer screening:
    - A Pap smear or approved high-risk HPV screen should be obtained when indicated by standard Pap screening guidelines, regardless of gestation, to start at age 21.
    - Squamous intraepithelial lesions can progress during pregnancy but often regress postpartum.
    - LSIL/CIN1 in pregnancy: colposcopy preferred, but it is acceptable to defer colposcopy to 6 weeks postpartum
    - CIN 2 or CIN 3 in pregnancy: In the absence of invasive disease or advanced pregnancy, additional colposcopic and cytologic examinations are acceptable; repeat biopsy is recommended only if appearance of lesion worsens or if cytology suggests invasive cancer; it is acceptable to defer reevaluation until 6 weeks postpartum.
    - Endocervical sampling is contraindicated in pregnancy.
- Subsequent prenatal visits (1),(2):
  - Urinalysis for glucose and protein: limited evidence for benefit or harm. Baseline during initial intake may be useful for high-risk patients (e.g., chronic HTN).

- 24- to 28-week prenatal visits (1),(2):
  - Obtain diabetes screen.
  - Repeat hematocrit or hemoglobin and repeat antibody screen in Rh-negative mother prior to receiving prophylactic Rh immunoglobulin. Repeat syphilis testing in the 3rd trimester around 28 weeks in all cases (2018 CDC, ACOG and AAP guidelines due to rising cases of congenital syphilis). Retest for HIV at 28 weeks in high-risk cases. Retest for syphilis and HIV at delivery in high-risk cases.
  - GDM screening (2)
    - The ADA and ACOG define increased risk of diabetes in pregnancy who need earlier screening based on BMI≥25 kg/m² (≥23 kg/m² in Asian Americans) plus one or more of the following:
      - Previous pregnancy history of GDM, fetal macrosomia (≥4,000 g BW prior delivery), or stillbirth
      - Hypertension (140/90 mm Hg or being treated for hypertension)
      - HDL cholesterol ≤35 mg/dL (0.90 mmol/L)
      - Fasting triglyceride ≥250 mg/dL (2.82 mmol/L)
      - Hemoglobin A1C ≥5.7%, impaired glucose tolerance or impaired fasting glucose
      - PCOS, acanthosis nigricans, nonalcoholic steatohepatitis, morbid obesity pre-pregnancy BMI ≥40, and other conditions associated with insulin resistance
      - Current or past history of cardiovascular disease
      - Family history of diabetes—first-degree relative (parent or sibling)
      - High-risk ethnicity or communities
    - Early-onset diagnosis is made via 2-step testing (see below) ideally between weeks 12 to 16 of pregnancy for at-risk cases.
    - For typical low-risk cases, employ 2-step testing starting week 24 to 28: screen using a 1-hour glucola test and, if needed and appropriate (see below*), a 3-hour diagnostic test.
    - The risk of developing type 2 diabetes with the personal history of GDM is up to 50% in the next 20 years after delivery. Therefore, a fasting 75-g 2-hour oral glucose tolerance test (OGTT) since it is only 1 step may be helpful in diagnosing postpartum diabetes or glucose intolerance. It is unclear if the 75-g 2-hour GTT is comparable to the 2-step approach in diagnosing GDM*.
    - Assess for readiness for change in diet +/− exercise. Provide counseling, nutrition, and other support upon diagnosis of GDM. Continue to support during the postpartum period and beyond.
    - Diagnosing GDM (ACOG and AAFP guidelines):
      - Setting cutoff for "elevated 1-hour GCT": Setting the cutoff at 130 or 135 may be prudent for a practice with higher local prevalence of GDM. Setting the cutoff at 140 may be prudent for a practice with low local prevalence of GDM.
      - Routine screening for GDM (~week 24 to 28): 50 g PO nonfasting glucose load with blood glucose testing 1 hour later. If elevated, then proceed to 3-hour testing for diagnosis.
        - *Each practice or institution may have internal guidelines for 1-hour results if ≥180 to 185 and proceed with fasting BG monitoring instead of proceeding with 3-hour GTT.

- Diagnostic test: 3-hour GTT is achieved, on a separate day from 1-hour GCT, by 100 g PO glucose load after fasting for ≥ 8 hours with blood drawn: fasting, 1, 2, and 3 hours after ingestion of glucose
  - *A positive diagnosis of GDM requires that ≥2 positive thresholds by either criteria below.
    - Carpenter and Coustan standard: ≥95 (fasting), ≥180 (1-hour), ≥155 (2-hour), ≥140 (3-hour)
    - NDDG standard: ≥105 (fasting), ≥190 (1-hour), ≥165 (2-hour), ≥145 (3-hour)
  - ACOG states, due to known adverse events, one elevated value from the 3-hour GTT may be sufficient to demonstrate evidence of glucose intolerance.
  - 1-step approach (75-g OGTT) on all women will increase the diagnosis of GDM, but sufficient prospective studies demonstrating improved outcomes still lacking and needs further research. ACOG does acknowledge that some centers may opt for "1 step" if warranted based on their population.

- 35 to 37 week prenatal visits (1):
  - Group B *Streptococcus* (GBS) culture: Screen all low-risk cases at 35 to 37 weeks' GA to identify women colonized with GBS. For cases requiring induction at 37 weeks or earlier, screen as soon as possible.
  - High-risk patients: High-risk patients should be screened again for gonorrhea, chlamydia, syphilis, and HIV.

- Postterm pregnancy:
  - Rate of stillbirth increases with GA by 1/3,000 per week at 41 weeks, 3/3,000 per week at 42 weeks, and 6/3,000 at 43 weeks. In one meta-analysis, routine induction of labor at 41 weeks' GA reduced rates of perinatal death without increased rates of cesarean delivery.
  - For prenatal care beyond 41 to 42 weeks, fetal well-being should be assessed with nonstress testing and US assessment of amniotic fluid volume.

 TREATMENT

ISSUES FOR REFERRAL
Abnormal screening labs or imaging may prompt referral to maternal–fetal medicine specialist or other medical specialists as indicated.

 ONGOING CARE

PATIENT EDUCATION
- Immunizations during pregnancy per CDC:
  - Tdap during each pregnancy (should be given between 27 and 36 weeks' GA); hepatitis B and influenza. Likely safe include meningococcal, rabies. Contraindicated or safety not established: live vaccines including BCG, MMR, and varicella
  - Vaccination against COVID-19 is recommended in pregnancy. COVID-19 increases risk for patient and fetus (4).

- Recommendations for use of dietary supplements in pregnancy (1),(2)
  - Folic acid 0.4 mg daily beginning at least 1 month prior to attempting conception and continuing throughout pregnancy; 1 to 4 mg for women at higher risk of having child with neural tube defect beginning 1 to 3 months before conception, continued through first 12 weeks of gestation, and then reduced to 0.4 mg daily
  - Calcium: 1,000 to 1,300 mg/day; supplement may be beneficial for women with high risk for gestational hypertension or communities with low dietary calcium intake.
  - Caffeine: Limit to <200 mg/day. More research needed
  - Iron: Screen for anemia (hemoglobin/hematocrit) and order extra iron supplementation if necessary.
  - Vitamin A: Pregnant women in industrialized countries should limit to <5,000 IU/day.
  - Vitamin D: 200 to 1,200 IU (dose in standard prenatal vitamin) is recommended until more evidence is available to support different dose.
- Other important counseling topics during pregnancy (2):
  - Airline travel: generally safe until up to week 35; >2 hours without ambulation increases risk of thrombosis
  - Exercise: Healthy women with uncomplicated pregnancies should continue to exercise.
  - Seat belts/air bags: Wear lap and shoulder seatbelts. Working air bags (ACOG and AAFP)
  - Sexual activity: Intercourse while pregnant is not associated with adverse outcomes. Avoiding sex may be necessary in cases of low lying placenta, placenta previa, or vasa previa.
  - Alcohol, cigarettes, and illicit drugs are injurious to fetal and maternal health.
  - Pregnancy-safe medications (teratogenicity)
  - Avoid large fish such as shark, tuna, swordfish and mackerel (high levels of mercury).
  - Preconception counseling offers the opportunity to discuss individualized risks.

REFERENCES

1. Zolotor AJ, Carlough MC. Update on prenatal care. *Am Fam Physician*. 2014;89(3):199–208.
2. Kilpatrick SJ, Papile L, Macones GA, eds. *Guidelines for Perinatal Care*. 8th ed. Itasca, IL: American Academy of Pediatrics; 2017.
3. American College of Obstetricians and Gynecologists' Committee on Practice Bulletins—Obstetrics, Committee on Genetics, Society for Maternal-Fetal Medicine. Practice Bulletin No. 162: prenatal diagnostic testing for genetic disorders. *Obstet Gynecol*. 2016;127(5):e108–e122.
4. Shimabukuro TT, Kim SY, Myers TR, et al. Preliminary findings of mRNA Covid-19 vaccine safety in pregnant persons. *N Engl J Med*. 2021;384(24):2273–2282.

 CODES

ICD10
- Z34.90 Encntr for suprvsn of normal pregnancy, unsp, unsp trimester
- Z36 Encounter for antenatal screening of mother
- Z34.00 Encntr for suprvsn of normal first pregnancy, unsp trimester

PREOPERATIVE EVALUATION OF THE NONCARDIAC SURGICAL PATIENT

Andrew Grimes, MD

 BASICS

DESCRIPTION

- Preoperative medical evaluation should determine the presence of established or unrecognized disease or other factors that may increase the risk of perioperative morbidity and mortality in patients undergoing surgery.
- Specific assessment goals include the following:
  - Conducting a thorough medical history and physical exam to assess the need for further testing and/or consultation
  - Recommending strategies to reduce risk and optimize patient condition prior to surgery
  - Encouraging patients to optimize their health for possible improvement of both perioperative and long-term outcomes
- Synonym(s): preoperative diagnostic workup; preoperative preparation; preoperative general health assessment

EPIDEMIOLOGY

Overall patient morbidity and mortality related to surgery is low. One large study of inpatients in the United States showed a 30-day mortality rate of 1.32%. Another study found that perioperative acute myocardial infarction (MI) and death decreased from 2004 to 2013, but the rate of ischemic stroke has increased. Preoperative patient evaluation and subsequent optimization of perioperative care can reduce both postoperative morbidity and mortality.

RISK FACTORS

- Functional capacity (1): Exercise tolerance is one of the most important determinants of cardiac risk:
  - Self-reported exercise tolerance may be an extremely useful predictive tool when assessing risk. Patients unable to meet a 4–metabolic equivalents (METs) demand (defined in the "Diagnosis" section) during daily activities have increased perioperative cardiac and long-term risks. A study compared physicians' subjective assessment of functional capacity to objective measures of functional capacity. It found that the subjective assessment tended to misclassify high-risk patients as low risk. Structured questionnaires such as the Duke Activity Status Index had much better prognostic accuracy to assess functional status (2).
  - Patients who report good exercise tolerance require minimal, if any, additional testing.
- Levels of surgical risk
  - An increased risk for major adverse cardiac events (MACE) is associated with procedures that are intrathoracic, intra-abdominal, or vascular procedures that are suprainguinal in nature.
- Clinical risk factors: history of ischemic heart disease, the presence of compensated heart failure or a history of prior congestive heart failure (CHF), cerebrovascular disease, diabetes mellitus (DM), and renal insufficiency; these risk factors plus surgical risk can dictate the need for further cardiac testing.
- Age: Patients >70 years of age are at higher risk for perioperative complications and mortality and have a longer length of stay in the hospital postoperatively (likely attributed to increasing medical comorbidities with increasing age). Age alone should not be a deciding factor in the decision to proceed or not to proceed with surgery.

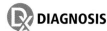 **DIAGNOSIS**

HISTORY

- Evaluate pertinent medical records and interview the patient. Many institutions provide standard patient questionnaires that screen for preoperative risk factors:
  - History of present illness and treatments
  - Past medical and surgical history
  - Patient and family anesthetic history and associated complications
  - Current medications (including over-the-counter [OTC] medications, vitamins, supplements, and herbals) as well as reasons for use
  - Allergies (including specific reactions)
  - Social history: tobacco, alcohol, drug use, and cessation
- Systems (both history and current status)
  - Cardiovascular: Inquire about exercise capacity.
    - 1 MET: can take care of self, eat, dress, and use toilet; walk around house indoors; walk a block or two on level ground at 2 to 3 mph
    - 4 METs: can climb 2 flights of stairs or walk uphill, walk on level ground at 4 mph, run a short distance, do heavy work around house, participate in moderate recreational activities
    - 10 METs: can participate in strenuous sports such as swimming, singles tennis, football, basketball, or skiing
  - Note presence of CHF, cardiomyopathy, ischemic heart disease (stable vs. unstable), valvular disease, hypertension (HTN), arrhythmias, murmurs, pericarditis, history of pacemaker or implantable cardioverter defibrillator (ICD):
    - Rhythm management devices (pacemakers and automatic ICDs [AICDs]) affect the perioperative course. Most importantly, the following information needs to be available for proper management: name of cardiologist who manages the device, type of device, manufacturer, last interrogation, and any problems that have occurred recently. Based on this information and the location and type of surgery, a perioperative plan of management will be made.
    - Stents: Patients with coronary stents are maintained on duel antiplatelet therapy (DAPT) for a prescribed period of time. This is typically done with a thienopyridine, such as clopidogrel, in combination with aspirin. The perioperative period is associated with a prothrombotic state. Premature discontinuation of DAPT markedly increases the risk of acute stent thrombosis, MI, and death. Elective surgery should be delayed and DAPT continued for a minimum of 30 days after bare metal stent placement. Duration of dual antiplatelet therapy following drug-eluting stent (DES) placement depends on the type of stent and risk of thrombosis. DAPT has been advised for 6 to 12 months following DES, but shorter durations may be possible for newer stents (3). Several caveats to these recommendations exist. Any perioperative disruption in the patient's DAPT regimen needs to be discussed with the patient's cardiologist and surgeon. The risk of perioperative bleeding must be weighed against the risks of discontinuation of DAPT prior to surgery.
  - Pulmonary: Chronic and active disease processes should be addressed: chronic infections, bronchitis, emphysema, asthma, wheezing, shortness of breath, cough (productive or otherwise):
    - Sleep apnea: Patients with obstructive sleep apnea (OSA) are at increased risk for perioperative adverse events. Screening tools (such as the STOP-Bang) can help risk stratify patients. Additional evaluation should be considered if a patient has associated significant systemic disease, hypoventilation syndrome, severe pulmonary HTN, or resting hypoxemia (4).
    - Often, patients with an existing diagnosis of OSA who use positive airway pressure (PAP) at night are asked to bring their PAP machine to the hospital or surgery center when they are admitted for surgery. For patients with suspected but previously undiagnosed OSA, PAP therapy should be considered on a case-by-case basis.
    - Some studies suggest that even short periods (3 weeks) of treatment with PAP can improve some indices of ventilation and therefore may reduce postoperative morbidity.
  - GI: hepatic disease, gastric ulcer, inflammatory bowel disease, hernias (especially hiatal), significant weight loss, nausea, vomiting, history of postoperative nausea, and vomiting: Any symptoms consistent with gastroesophageal reflux disease (GERD) should be optimally treated.
  - Hematologic: anemia, serious bleeding, clotting problems, blood transfusions, hereditary disorders
  - Renal: kidney failure, dialysis, infections, stones, changes in bladder function
  - Endocrine: nocturia, parathyroid, pituitary, adrenal disease, thyroid disease
    - Diabetes: Evidence that hyperglycemia in the perioperative period is associated with increased perioperative complications. Although recommendations vary, most experts recommend keeping perioperative blood glucose levels <180 mg/dL.
  - Neurologic/psychiatric: seizures, stroke, paralysis, tremor, migraine headaches, nerve injury, multiple sclerosis, extremity numbness, psychiatric disorders (e.g., anxiety, depression)
  - Musculoskeletal: arthritis, lower back pain
  - Frailty is increasingly recognized as a perioperative risk factor. Research is being done on various screening tools and interventions that can decrease perioperative mortality and morbidity in the frail population (5).
  - Reproductive: possibility of pregnancy in women of childbearing potential
- Mouth/upper airway: dentures, crowns, partials, bridges, teeth (loose, chipped, cracked, capped)

PHYSICAL EXAM

- Assess vital signs, including arterial BP bilaterally.
- Check carotid pulses; auscultate for bruits.
- Examine lungs by auscultating all lung fields and listening for rales, rhonchi, wheezes, or other sounds indicating disease.
- Examine cardiovascular system by auscultating heart and noting any irregular rhythms or murmurs; precordial palpation
- If a regional anesthesia technique is being contemplated, perform a relevant, focused neurologic exam.

DIAGNOSTIC TESTS & INTERPRETATION
Initial Tests (lab, imaging)

- Laboratory testing should never be "routine" prior to surgery. Tests should be obtained only when indicated by specific conditions or risk factors. "Routine" testing results in unnecessary delays and disruptions to planned surgery. Specific tests should be requested if the evaluator suspects findings from the clinical evaluation that may influence perioperative patient management.
- Labs performed within the past 4 months prior to evaluation are reliable, unless the patient has had an interim change in clinical presentation or is taking medications that require monitoring of plasma level or effect.
- CBC
  - Hemoglobin: if a patient has symptoms of anemia or is undergoing a procedure with major blood loss; extremes of age; liver or kidney disease
  - WBC count: if symptoms suggest infection or myeloproliferative disorder or the patient is at risk for chemotherapy-induced leukopenia
  - Platelet count: if history of bleeding, myeloproliferative disorder, liver or renal disease, or the patient is at risk for chemotherapy-induced thrombocytopenia
- Serum chemistries (electrolytes, glucose, renal and liver function tests): should be obtained for extremes of age; in known renal insufficiency, CHF, liver dysfunction, or endocrine abnormalities; or the patient is on medications that alter electrolyte levels, such as diuretics
- PT/PTT: if history of a bleeding disorder, chronic liver disease, or malnutrition, or those with recent or chronic antibiotic or anticoagulant use
- Urinalysis: Routine urinalysis is not recommended preoperatively.
- Pregnancy test: controversial; should be *considered* for all female patients of childbearing age
- CXR is not generally indicated unless there is a history of significant heart or lung disease or there is a recent change of symptoms.

Diagnostic Procedures/Other

- ECG
  - Preoperative resting 12-lead ECG is reasonable for patients with known coronary disease, known peripheral vascular disease, significant arrhythmia, or known significant structural heart disease.
  - ECGs are not indicated for asymptomatic patients undergoing low-risk procedures.
- The American Heart Association (AHA) guidelines recommend using the Revised Cardiac Risk Index or the ACS NSQIP online risk calculator to make an estimate of risk of MACE in the perioperative period. If the risk of MACE is low (<1%), then proceed with surgery. If the risk is >1%, the functional capacity needs to be considered. For patients with a functional capacity of >4 METs, then proceed with surgery. If the functional capacity is <4 METs or unknown, consider pharmacologic stress testing if it will change management.
- PFTs: Definitive data regarding the efficacy of preoperative testing are lacking. The most important factor is preoperative optimization of patients with chronic obstructive pulmonary disease (COPD) or reactive airways disease with indicated use of antibiotics, bronchodilators, and inhaled corticosteroids. Spirometry can help guide therapy. Upper abdominal and thoracic surgery has a higher risk of postoperative pulmonary complications.

 TREATMENT

MEDICATION

- Reducing cardiac risk
  - Elective surgery should be delayed or cancelled if the patient has any of the following: unstable coronary syndromes (unstable or severe angina), recent MI (<30 days), decompensated heart failure, significant arrhythmias, or severe valvular disease.
  - Timing of elective noncardiac surgery after ischemic stroke or MI can have a significant effect on perioperative morbidity and mortality. The AHA/ACC guidelines recommend waiting at least 60 days after an MI if the patient did not require a coronary intervention. There is a significant increase in both risk of MACE and mortality associated with elective surgery within 3 months of an ischemic stroke.
  - Perioperative β-blockade has been shown to reduce mortality and the incidence of perioperative MIs in high-risk patients. Studies conflict, however, in which patients need to be treated, the dosage and timing of treatment, and for what surgeries. *Patients chronically on β-blockers* should have the medication continued in the perioperative period. When β-blockers are discontinued in the perioperative period, 30-day mortality increases. It is not recommended to start β-blockers on the day of surgery in β-blocker–naive patients.
  - A recent review examined prophylactic use of aspirin in the perioperative period and did not find a significant effect on perioperative mortality or risk for MI in patients undergoing noncardiac surgery and may be associated with an increased risk of perioperative bleeding. There were important exclusion criteria, including patients with recent stent placement.
- Reducing pulmonary risk
  - Recommend cigarette cessation for at least 8 weeks prior to elective surgery.
  - Patients with asthma should not be wheezing and should have a peak flow of at least 80% of their predicted or personal-best value.
  - Treatment of COPD and asthma should focus on maximally reducing airflow obstruction and is identical to treatment of nonsurgical patients.

REFERENCES

1. Fleisher LA, Fleischmann KE, Auerbach AD, et al. 2014 ACC/AHA guideline on perioperative cardiovascular evaluation and management of patients undergoing noncardiac surgery: executive summary: a report of the American College of Cardiology/American Heart Association Task Force on practice guidelines. Developed in collaboration with the American College of Surgeons, American Society of Anesthesiologists, American Society of Echocardiography, American Society of Nuclear Cardiology, Heart Rhythm Society, Society for Cardiovascular Angiography and Interventions, Society of Cardiovascular Anesthesiologists, and Society of Vascular Medicine Endorsed by the Society of Hospital Medicine. *J Nucl Cardiol.* 2015;22(1):162–215.
2. Wijeysundera DN, Pearse RM, Shulman MA, et al. Assessment of functional capacity before major noncardiac surgery: an international, prospective cohort study. *Lancet.* 2018;391(10140):2631–2640.
3. Watanabe H, Domei T, Moriomoto T, et al. Effect of 1-month dual antiplatelet therapy followed by clopidogrel vs 12-month dual antiplatelet therapy on cardiovascular and bleeding events in patients receiving PCI: the STOPDAPT-2 randomized clinical trial. *JAMA.* 2019;321(24):2414–2427.
4. Chan MT, Wang CY, Seet E, et al. Association of unrecognized obstructive sleep apnea with postoperative cardiovascular events in patients undergoing major noncardiac surgery. *JAMA.* 2019;321(18):1788–1798.
5. Nidadavolu LS, Ehrlich AL, Sieber FE, et al. Preoperative evaluation of the frail patient. *Anesth Analg.* 2020;130(6):1493–1503.

 SEE ALSO

Algorithm: Preoperative Evaluation of Noncardiac Surgical Patient

CODES

ICD10

- Z01.818 Encounter for other preprocedural examination
- Z01.811 Encounter for preprocedural respiratory examination
- Z01.812 Encounter for preprocedural laboratory examination

CLINICAL PEARLS

- The preoperative evaluation should include medical record evaluation, patient interview, and physical exam.
- Functional capacity, the level of surgical risk, and clinical risk factors determine if further cardiac testing is needed.
- No preoperative tests are or should be routine.
- Active cardiac conditions should lead to delay or cancellation of nonemergent surgery.

PRESBYCUSIS

Ronald L. Cook, DO, MBA • Joshua McGuire, MD

BASICS

DESCRIPTION

- Presbycusis is an age-related hearing loss (HL), showing increased incidence with age. It often presents as difficulty communicating in noisy conditions.
- May be divided into central and peripheral causes:
  - Central presbycusis: age-related change in the auditory portions of the central nervous system negatively impacting auditory perception, speech-communication performance, or both
  - Peripheral presbycusis: age-related, bilateral sensorineural HL (SNHL) typically symmetric
- Represents a lifetime of insults to the auditory system from toxic noise exposure and natural decline
- Initially presents as high-frequency SNHL with tinnitus (ringing)
- Impacts the "clarity" of sounds (i.e., ability to detect, identify, and localize sounds)
- Due to mild and progressive nature, presbycusis is often treated with amplification alone.
- Can lead to adverse effects on physical, cognitive, emotional, behavioral, and social function in the elderly (e.g., depression, social isolation) and is a contributor to all cause dementia (1)

EPIDEMIOLOGY

Incidence
According to an ongoing community-based epidemiologic study, the 10-year cumulative incidence rates of HL are as follows, approximately:

- Age 48 to 59 years: M (31.7%), F (15.6%); all (21.8%)
- Age 60 to 69 years: M (56.8%), F (40.7%); all (45.5%)
- Age 70 to 79 years: M (87.1%), F (70.6%); all (73.7%)
- Age 80 to 92 years: M (100%), F (100%); all (100%)

Prevalence
- 10% of the population develops SNHL severe enough to impair communication.
- Increases to 40% in the population >65 years of age
- 80% of HL cases occur in elderly patients.
- Only 10–20% of older adults with HL have ever used hearing aids (HAs).
- Predominant sex: male > female
- Hearing levels are poorer in industrialized societies than in isolated or agrarian societies.

ETIOLOGY AND PATHOPHYSIOLOGY

- The external ear transmits sound energy to the tympanic membrane. The middle ear ossicles amplify and conduct the sound waves into the inner ear (cochlea) via the oval window. The organ of Corti, located in the cochlea, contains hair cells that detect these vibrations and depolarize, producing electrical signals that travel through the auditory nerve to the brain. Toxic noise exposure traumatizes the hair cells and leads to cell death and HL. Research also suggests that overexcitation of the neuro synapses causes increased glutamate, which is also neurotoxic (2).
  - Sensory presbycusis: primary loss of the hair cells in the basal end of the cochlea (high-frequency HL)
  - Neural presbycusis: loss of spiral ganglion cells (nerve cells induced by hair cells to produce action potentials to travel to the brainstem)
  - Strial (metabolic) presbycusis: atrophy of the stria vascularis (cochlear tissue that generates the endocochlear electrical potential)
  - Cochlear conductive (mechanical) presbycusis: no morphologic findings (presumed stiffening of the basilar membrane)
  - Mixed presbycusis: combinations of hair cell, ganglion cell, and stria vascularis loss
  - Indeterminate presbycusis: no morphologic findings (presumed impaired cellular function)
- Presbycusis is caused by the accumulated effects of noise exposure, systemic disease, oxidative damage, ototoxic drugs, and genetic susceptibility.

Genetics
Presbycusis has a clear familial aggregation:

- Heritability estimates show 35–55% of the variance of sensory presbycusis is from genetic factors; even greater percentage in strial presbycusis
- Heritability is stronger among women than men.

RISK FACTORS

- Noise exposure (military, industrial, etc.)
- Ototoxic substances
  - Organic solvents
  - Heavy metals
  - Carbon monoxide
- Drugs
  - Aminoglycosides
  - Cisplatin (dose dependent)
  - Salicylates
  - Diuretics
- Tobacco smoking
- Alcohol abuse
- Lower socioeconomic status
- Family history of presbycusis
- Head trauma (temporal bone fractures)
- Cardiovascular disease (hypertension, atherosclerosis, hyperlipidemia); labyrinthine artery is terminal artery to the cochlea.
- Diabetes mellitus
- Obesity
- Autoimmune disease (auto cochleitis/labyrinthitis)
- Metabolic bone disease
- Endocrine medical conditions: levels of aldosterone
- Alzheimer disease
- Otologic conditions (e.g., Ménière disease or otosclerosis)

GENERAL PREVENTION

- Avoid hazardous noise exposure.
- Use hearing protection.
- Maintain healthy diet and exercise.
- Screening
  - Patient self-screening tools that are available online and through mobile apps
  - Hearing Handicap Inventory for the Elderly Screening (3)
  - RCT published in 2010 on screening for HL, HA use was significantly higher in three screened groups (4.1% in those using a questionnaire, 6.3% using handheld audiometry, and 7.4% using both modalities) versus unscreened control participants (3.3%) at 1-year follow-up (4)[B].
  - Based on a 2021 review, according to the USPSTF, there is insufficient evidence to assess the relative benefits and harms of HL screening in adults ≥50 years (5)[B].

COMMONLY ASSOCIATED CONDITIONS

- A 2018 meta-analysis showed that ARHL had significant associations with accelerated multidomain cognitive decline, cognitive impairment, and dementia (6)[A].
- Depression, social isolation (3)

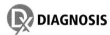

DIAGNOSIS

HISTORY

- Reduced hearing sensitivity and speech understanding in noisy/public environments
- Impaired localization of sound sources
- Increased difficulty understanding conversations, especially with women, due to higher frequency of spoken voice
- Presents bilaterally and symmetrically
- If unilateral HL, alternative diagnosis should be pursued.
- Additional history if HL is suspected or detected (7)[B]:
  - Time course of HL
  - Symptoms of tinnitus, otalgia, otorrhea, or vertigo
  - History of noise exposure, ear trauma, or head trauma
  - Presence of any neurologic deficit
- Reports from patient/family/caregiver (7)[B]
  - Confusion in social situations
  - Excessive volume of television/radio/computer
  - Social withdrawal
  - Anxiety in group settings

PHYSICAL EXAM

- Rinne and Weber tests are helpful for determining conductive versus SNHL but not recommended for general screening.
- Pneumatic otoscopy to evaluate for simple middle ear effusion as cause of conductive HL

DIFFERENTIAL DIAGNOSIS

- Complete canal occlusion (cerumen, foreign body)
- Large external ear tumors (e.g., polyp, exostosis, squamous cell)
- Otitis externa
- Chronic otitis media or effusion
- Cholesteatoma
- Otosclerosis
- Osteogenesis imperfecta
- Large middle ear tumors (e.g., facial nerve schwannomas, paragangliomas)
- Perilymph fistula (trauma/iatrogenic)
- Ménière disease
- Acoustic neuroma (usually unilateral)
- Vascular anomaly
- Acute noise-induced traumatic loss (explosion)
- Autoimmune HL

DIAGNOSTIC TESTS & INTERPRETATION

- Central: synthetic sentence identification test with ipsilateral competing message and the dichotic sentence identification test (3)[C]
- Peripheral: handheld audiometry; insert probe in ear (sealing canal) and have patient indicate if tones can be heard.
  - Positive likelihood ratio (LR) range, 3.1 to 5.8; negative LR range, 0.03 to 0.40

- Screening audiometry
  - Symmetric high-frequency HL in descending slope pattern
  - SNHL frequencies >2 KHz initially
  - Essential to determine global clinical hearing status and if etiology is conductive HL versus SNHL or pseudohypacusis (conversion)

TREATMENT

- Analog HA: picks up sound waves through a microphone; converts them into electrical signals; amplifies and sends them through the ear canal to the tympanic membrane
- Digital HA: programmable; may reduce acoustic feedback, reduce background noise, detect and automatically accommodate different listening environments, control multiple microphones
  - HAs have an average decibel gain of 16.3 dB.
  - Associated with hypersensitivity to loud sounds ("loudness recruitment")
- Hearing-assistive technologies (HATs) (3)
  - Can be used alone or in combination with HAs (for difficult listening conditions)
  - Addresses face-to-face communication, broadcast or other electronic media (radio, TV), telephone conversation, sensitivity to alerting signals and environment stimuli (doorbell, baby's cry, alarm clock, etc.)
  - Includes personal FM systems, infrared systems, induction loop systems, hardwired systems, telephone amplifier, telecoil, TDD (telecommunication device for the deaf), situation-specific devices (e.g., television), alerting devices
- Aural rehabilitation (also known as audiologic orientation or auditory training) (7)[A]
  - Adjunct to HA or HATs
  - Involves education regarding proper use of amplification devices, coaching on how to manage the auditory environment, training in speech perception and communication, and counseling for coping strategies to deal with the difficulties of HAs or HATs

ISSUES FOR REFERRAL
Refer to audiologist for formal evaluation and optimal fitting of HAs and/or HATs.
- Individuals receiving post fitting orientation/education have significantly fewer HA returns.
- Individuals receiving >2 hours of education and counseling report higher levels of satisfaction.

ADDITIONAL THERAPIES
- Gene therapy: Ongoing research targets includes investigation of various transcription factors, cell cycle modulators, and cyclin-dependent kinase inhibitors, which are all associated with various aspects of formation and regeneration of hair cells, and maintenance of supporting cells.
- Pharmacotherapy: Ongoing research includes cellular signaling pathways and molecules as the most investigated targets for pharmacotherapy. Wnt and Notch signaling cascades are highly studied and both implicated in proliferation of supporting cells but so far are associated with limited hair cell growth.
- Stem cell therapy: Ongoing research has been focused predominantly on hair cell-like cells from mouse embryonic stem cells or induced pluripotent stem cells as well as the neural component of the inner ear system. Mesenchymal stem cells have also shown success in regenerating cochlear spiral ganglion neurons. Endogenous stem cells show the most promising results (3).

SURGERY/OTHER PROCEDURES
- Cochlear implants (CIs)
  - Works by bypassing the ear canal, middle ear, and hair cells in the cochlea to provide electric stimulation directly to the auditory nerve
  - Indications include hearing no better than identifying ≤50% of key words in test sentences in the best aided condition in the worst ear and 60% in the better ear.
  - Incoming sounds are received through the microphone in the audio processor component (resembles a small HA), which converts them into electrical impulses and sends them to the magnetic coil (located on the skin). The impulses transmit these across intact skin via radio waves to the implanted component (directly subjacent to the coil). The pulses travel to the electrodes in the cochlea and stimulate the cochlea at high rates.
  - Receiving a unilateral CI is most common; some may receive bilateral CIs (either sequentially or in the same surgery). Others may wear a CI in one ear and an HA in the contralateral ear (bimodal fit).
  - Younger age at CI placement derives greatest benefit.
- Active middle ear implants (AMEIs)
  - Suitable for elderly adults who cannot wear conventional HAs for medical or personal (cosmetic) reasons and whose HL is not severe enough for a CI
  - Different models available and may include components that are implantable under the skin
- Electric acoustic stimulation: use of CI and HA together in one ear
  - Addresses the specific needs of patients presenting with good low-frequency hearing (a mild to moderate sensorineural HL in frequencies up to 1,000 Hz) but poorer hearing in the high frequencies (sloping to 60 dB or worse HL >1,000 Hz)
    - Contraindications: progressive HL, autoimmune disease; HL related to meningitis, otosclerosis, or ossification; malformation of the cochlea; a gap in air conduction and bone conduction thresholds of >15 dB; external ear contraindications, active infection, or unwillingness to use amplification device (3)

ONGOING CARE

FOLLOW-UP RECOMMENDATIONS
Patient Monitoring
- During follow-up visits, check for compliance of HA use as 25–40% of adults will either stop wearing them or use them only occasionally.
- Assess perceived benefit of HA and, if ineffective, for indications for possible surgical treatments.
- Annual audiograms
- Can follow up with audiologists for HA fittings if HA becomes uncomfortable
- Asymmetric HL should have evaluation via MRI for acoustic neuroma.
- Sudden SNHL is atypical and warrants urgent otolaryngologic evaluation/audiometry. The most recent recommendations by the American Academy of Otolaryngology recommend steroids empirically.

PATIENT EDUCATION
- Should be face-to-face; spoken clearly and unhurriedly, without competing background noise (e.g., radio, TV); and include a confirmation that the message is received
- Formal speech reading classes may be beneficial; however, availability may be limited.

REFERENCES
1. Deal JA, Sharrett AR, Albert MS, et al. Hearing impairment and cognitive decline: a pilot study conducted within the atherosclerosis risk in communities neurocognitive study. *Am J Epidemiol*. 2015;181(9):680–690.
2. Yamasoba T, Lin FR, Someya S, et al. Current concepts in age-related hearing loss: epidemiology and mechanistic pathways. *Hear Res*. 2013;303:30–38.
3. Vaisbuch Y, Santa Maria PL. Age-related hearing loss: innovations in hearing augmentation. *Otolaryngol Clin North Am*. 2018;51(4):705–723.
4. Yueh B, Collins MP, Souza PE, et al. Long-term effectiveness of screening for hearing loss: the Screening for Auditory Impairment—Which Hearing Assessment Test (SAI-WHAT) randomized trial. *J Am Geriatr Soc*. 2010;58(3):427–434.
5. Feltner C, Wallace IF, Kistler CE, et al. *Screening for Hearing Loss in Older Adults, an Evidence Review for the U.S. Preventative Task Force* (Evidence Synthesis No. 200). Rockville, MD: Agency for Healthcare Research and Quality; 2021.
6. Loughrey DG, Kelly ME, Kelley GA, et al. Association of Age-Related Hearing Loss With Cognitive Function, Cognitive Impairment, and Dementia: A Systematic Review and Meta-analysis. *JAMA Otolaryngol Head Neck Surg*. 2018;144(2):115–126.
7. Pacala JT, Yueh B. Hearing deficits in the older patient: "I didn't notice anything." *JAMA*. 2012;307(11):1185–1194.

CODES

ICD10
- H91.10 Presbycusis, unspecified ear
- H91.13 Presbycusis, bilateral
- H91.11 Presbycusis, right ear

CLINICAL PEARLS
- Presbycusis is an age-related HL, showing increased incidence with age. It is often bilateral and initially begins as high-frequency HL It presents as difficulty communicating in noisy conditions.
- HL is significantly associated with social isolation, depression, and progressive cognitive impairment leading to dementia.
- Early audiology referral for individuals with suspected HL may improve treatment efficacy.
- Use of auditory assistive devices, HAs, CIs, and AMEIs is associated with improvement in cognitive function, social isolation, and depression.

PRESSURE ULCER

Ramanpreet Grewal, MD • Moiz A. Suhail, MD • Ghulam Abbas Harrie, MD

BASICS

DESCRIPTION
- A localized area of skin or underlying tissue injury resulting from pressure and/or shear
- Usually over a bony prominence (e.g., sacrum, calcaneus, ischium)
- Classified in stages according to the National Pressure Injury Advisory Panel (NPIAP):
  - Stage I: nonblanchable erythema—intact skin with nonblanchable redness; darkly pigmented skin may not have visible blanching.
  - Stage II: partial-thickness skin loss—shallow open ulcer with a viable red-pink, moist wound bed, without slough; or intact or open/ruptured serum-filled blister
  - Stage III: full-thickness skin loss—subcutaneous fat may be visible, but bone, tendon, or muscle is not exposed; slough, if present, does not obscure depth of tissue loss.
  - Stage IV: full-thickness tissue loss—exposed bone, tendon, or joint; slough or eschar may be present but does not completely obscure wound base.
  - Unstageable: depth unknown—base of the ulcer is covered by slough and/or eschar in the wound bed.
  - Suspected deep tissue injury: depth unknown—purple or maroon area of intact skin or blood-filled blister. Pain and temperature change precede skin color changes.
- Synonyms: decubitus ulcer; bedsore; pressure injury, pressure sore

EPIDEMIOLOGY
Incidence
Dependant on setting and population: 0–53.4% (1),(2)

Prevalence
Dependant on setting and population: 0–72.5% (1),(2)

ETIOLOGY AND PATHOPHYSIOLOGY
Complex process of risk factors interacting with external forces (pressure and/or shear, friction, and moisture) (3)

RISK FACTORS
- Mobility impairment
- Malnutrition
- Reduced skin perfusion
- Sensory impairment
- Medical devices

GENERAL PREVENTION
- Structured risk assessment (1)
- Skin and tissue assessment (1)
- Preventive skin care (1)
- Nutrition screening (1)
- Repositioning (1)
- Early mobilization (1)
- Support surfaces (1)
- Microclimate control (1)
- Prophylactic dressings (1)
- Electrical stimulation of the muscles (1)

COMMONLY ASSOCIATED CONDITIONS
- Advanced age
- Immobility
- Trauma
- Hip fractures
- Diabetes
- Cerebrovascular and cardiovascular disease
- Incontinence

DIAGNOSIS

HISTORY
- Risk factors
- Nutritional assessment (1)
- Pain assessment (1)
- Date of ulcer diagnosis
- Treatment course

PHYSICAL EXAM
- Full skin examination on initial contact and repeatedly throughout visits
- Assess location, stage, size (length, width, depth), identify the presence of sinus tracts, undermining, tunneling, exudate, necrosis, odor, and signs of healing (e.g., granulation tissue) (1).
- Identify factors that may affect healing (impaired perfusion, sensation, presence of infection).

DIFFERENTIAL DIAGNOSIS
- Venous ulcers
- Arterial ulcers
- Diabetic foot ulcer
- Cellulitis and erysipelas
- Incontinence associated dermatitis
- Skin tears
- Intertrigo
- Neuropathic ulcers
- Cutaneous squamous cell carcinomas
- Hypertensive ulcers
- Pyoderma gangrenosum, cancers, vasculitides, and other dermatologic conditions

DIAGNOSTIC TESTS & INTERPRETATION
Initial Tests (lab, imaging)
- Wound culture: Do not culture surface drainage. If culture is necessary, do deep tissue culture/bone biopsy.
- If systemic infection or that of bone, muscle is suspected add infectious workup, including inflammatory markers, CBC, blood cultures, x-ray. MRI may be necessary to confirm osteomyelitis.
- Ankle-brachial index and Doppler ultrasound (for lower extremity wounds)

Follow-Up Tests & Special Considerations
Additional tests may be indicated when additional medical illness complicates assessment. This may include testing for diabetes (i.e., A1c), thyroid disease (i.e., TSH), vascular disease, and other dermatologic diagnoses.

TREATMENT

GENERAL MEASURES
- Comprehensive initial assessment of the patient
- Pressure reduction/redistribution (4)[A]
- Nutritional support (e.g., protein-containing supplements) (5)[B]
- Wound assessment and treatment
  - Wound bed preparation (tissue management, infection and inflammation control, moisture balance, epithelial edge advancement) (1)
  - Wound cleansing (1)[C]
  - Débridement (1)[C]
- Address immobility.
- Manage incontinence.
- Address pain.
- Assess goals of care and advance directives.

MEDICATION
First Line
- Wound dressings as appropriate for the category of ulcer (transparent film, hydrocolloid, hydrogel, alginate, foam, silver-impregnated, honey impregnated, cadexomer iodine, gauze, silicone, collagen matrix, composite) (1)[C].
- Systematic reviews find evidence of superiority of one dressing compared to another is of poor quality. Therefore, it is impossible to recommend one dressing over another (6)[A].
- Enzymatic débriding agents

Second Line
- Activated charcoal
- Topical antiseptics (hydrogen peroxide, Dakin solution, povidone-iodine)

ISSUES FOR REFERRAL
- Consider referral to a wound care specialist (if available) for complex or nonhealing wounds.
- Consider vascular surgery for improvement of blood flow to wound via vascular bypass if appropriate.
- Consider a surgical consultation for possible urgent drainage and/or débridement if advancing cellulitis; suspected source of sepsis; undermining, tunneling, sinus tracts, and/or extensive necrotic tissue that cannot otherwise be removed by nonsurgical débridement methods; or for stage III or IV that are not closing with conservative management (1)[C].
- Consider plastic surgery for skin graft/flap if appropriate.
- Consider dermatology referral if suspected pyoderma gangrenosum, cancer, vasculitis, or other dermatologic conditions.

ADDITIONAL THERAPIES
- Direct contact electrical stimulation for recalcitrant stage II and any category/stage III and IV (1)[A]
- Electromagnetic field for recalcitrant category/stage II and any stage III and IV (1)[C]
- Pulsed radio frequency energy for recalcitrant stage II and any stage III and IV (1)[C]

COMPLEMENTARY & ALTERNATIVE MEDICINE
- Low-frequency ultrasound for débridement of necrotic soft tissue (not eschar) (1)[C]
- High-frequency ultrasound as adjunct for infected pressure ulcers (1)[C]
- Negative pressure wound therapy as an early adjuvant treatment for deep, stage III and IV (1)[C]
- Consider course of hydrotherapy with pulsed lavage with suction for wound cleansing and débridement (1)[C].
- Phototherapy: short-term UVC light if traditional therapies fail (1)[C]; laser not recommended (1)[C]; infrared is not recommended (1)[C].
- Hyperbaric and topical oxygen therapy not recommended for routine use (1)[C]
- Hydrotherapy with whirlpool should not be considered for routine use (1)[C].
- Vibration therapy not recommended (1)[C]
- Consider maggot débridement therapy.

ADMISSION, INPATIENT, AND NURSING CONSIDERATIONS
- Admission criteria/initial stabilization: refractory cellulitis, osteomyelitis, systemic infection, advanced nutritional decline, suspected patient mistreatment, inability to care for self
- Dressing changes 1 to 3 times daily based on wound assessment and plan of care
- Assess risk factors according to scales.
- Assess for changing or new wounds.
- Discharge criteria: clinical improvement in wound and systemic illness; when applicable, safe, and appropriate location for discharge

ONGOING CARE

FOLLOW-UP RECOMMENDATIONS
Weekly assessment by nurse with wound experience; biweekly assessment by a physician

Patient Monitoring
- Home health nursing
- Change plan of care if no improvement in 2 to 3 weeks.

DIET
- Approximately 1.0 to 1.5 kg/day of protein
- Strict glycemic control
- Include micronutrients in diet or as supplements (vitamin C and zinc).

PATIENT EDUCATION
- Check skin regularly.
- Signs and symptoms of infection
- Report new or increased pain.
- Prevention of new wound where old wound healed
- Skin care, moisture prevention
- Smoking cessation

PROGNOSIS
Variable, depending on the following:
- Removal of pressure
- Nutrition
- Wound care

COMPLICATIONS
- Infection
- Amputation
- Increased mortality

REFERENCES

1. Haesler E, ed. *Prevention and Treatment of Pressure Ulcers: Clinical Practice Guideline*. Osborne Park, Western Australia: Cambridge Media; 2014.
2. Pieper B, ed. *Pressure Ulcers: Prevalence, Incidence, and Implications for the Future.* Washington, DC: National Pressure Ulcer Advisory Panel; 2012.
3. Sibbald RG, Krasner DL, Woo KY. Pressure ulcer staging revisited: superficial skin changes & Deep Pressure Ulcer Framework. *Adv Skin Wound Care*. 2011;24(12):571–580; quiz 581–582.
4. Bergstrom N, Horn SD, Rapp MP, et al. Turning for ulcer reduction: a multisite randomized clinical trial in nursing homes. *J Am Geriatr Soc*. 2013;61(10):1705–1713.
5. Smith ME, Totten A, Hickam DH, et al. Pressure ulcer treatment strategies: a systematic comparative effectiveness review. *Ann Intern Med*. 2013;159(1):39–50.
6. Westby MJ, Dumville JC, Soares MO, et al. Dressings and topical agents for treating pressure ulcers. *Cochrane Database Syst Rev*. 2017;6(6):CD011947.

ADDITIONAL READING

- Qaseem A, Humphrey LL, Forciea MA, et al; for Clinical Guidelines Committee of the American College of Physicians. Treatment of pressure ulcers: a clinical practice guideline from the American College of Physicians. *Ann Intern Med*. 2015;162(5):370–379.
- Reddy M, Gill SS, Rochon PA. Preventing pressure ulcers: a systematic review. *JAMA*. 2006;296(8):974–984.
- Stansby G, Avital L, Jones K, et al. Prevention and management of pressure ulcers in primary and secondary care: summary of NICE guidance. *BMJ*. 2014;348:g2592.

CODES

ICD10
- L89.95 Pressure ulcer of unspecified site, unstageable
- L89.91 Pressure ulcer of unspecified site, stage 1
- L89.92 Pressure ulcer of unspecified site, stage 2

CLINICAL PEARLS
- Create assessment and prevention protocols for all patients.
- Identify risk factors, reduce/redistribute pressure, maximize nutrition, regular skin checks, and assess and treat wounds appropriately.
- All care needs to be done in a time-sensitive, patient-centered fashion.

PRETERM LABOR

Brooke Ersland, MD

BASICS

DESCRIPTION
Regular contractions occurring between 20 and 36 weeks and 6 days with either a change in effacement and cervical dilation or cervical dilation of ≥2cm on presentation.

EPIDEMIOLOGY
Preterm birth is the leading cause of perinatal morbidity and mortality in the United States.

Incidence
10–15% of pregnancies experienced at least one episode of preterm labor.

Prevalence
10.23% of all births in the United States in 2019 were preterm (1). Non-Hispanic blacks are 50% more likely to have a preterm birth than Hispanic or white patients (1).

ETIOLOGY AND PATHOPHYSIOLOGY
- Premature formation and activation of myometrial gap junctions
- Abnormal placental implantation
- Systemic inflammation/infections (e.g., UTI)
- Local inflammation/infections (e.g., intra-amniotic infections)
- Uterine abnormalities
- Overdistension (by multiple gestation or polyhydramnios)
- Preterm premature rupture of membranes
- Trauma
- Placental abruption
- Immunopathology (e.g., antiphospholipid antibodies)
- Placental ischemic disease (preeclampsia and fetal growth restriction)

Genetics
Familial predisposition. Numerous gene candidates mediating various pathways have been identified, but causality and gene-environment interactions are not well-defined.

RISK FACTORS
- Prior preterm delivery (most significant risk factor)
- Demographic factors, including social and economic disadvantages and black race with concern for chronic stress from structural racism
- Short interpregnancy interval (<18 months)
- Prepregnancy weight <45 kg (100 lb), body mass index <18.5
- Substance abuse (e.g., cocaine, tobacco)
- Unintended pregnancy
- History of dilation and curettage
- Cervical insufficiency
- Short cervical length of <25 mm
- Abdominal surgery/trauma during pregnancy
- Uterine structural abnormalities, such as large fibroids or müllerian abnormalities
- Serious maternal infections/diseases

- Bacterial vaginosis
- Bacteriuria
- Multiple gestation
- Intrauterine growth restriction
- Placenta previa
- Premature placental separation (abruption)
- Polyhydramnios

GENERAL PREVENTION
- Patient education at each visit in 2nd and 3rd trimesters for those at risk and periodically in the last 2 trimesters for the general population
- For women with a singleton pregnancy and no history of spontaneous preterm births, visualization of the cervix on routine fetal anatomical scan at 18 0/7 and 22 6/7 should be performed. If found to be shortened, a transvaginal ultrasound should be done for further evaluation (2)[C]. This recommendation is the same for multiple gestation and women with a history of medically induced preterm birth. Twin pregnancies are more likely to have a shortened cervix during the 2nd trimester, and women with a history of medically induced preterm birth are more likely to have a subsequent preterm birth (2).
- For women with history of spontaneous preterm birth and singleton pregnancy, a screening transvaginal ultrasound to evaluate cervix length should be done at 16 0/7 weeks and repeated until 24 0/7 weeks. Many protocols will repeat every 1 to 4 weeks during this time (2).
- Primary prevention:
  - Interval contraception to optimize pregnancy spacing
  - Smoking cessation
  - If previous preterm birth, evaluate if etiology is likely to recur and target intervention to specific condition.
  - Women with history of spontaneous preterm birth and singleton pregnancy should be offered vaginal or intramuscular progesterone to prevent preterm birth with a shared decision model (2).
- Secondary prevention:
  - For patients with a cervix of <25 mm with or without a history of previous spontaneous preterm delivery and singleton pregnancy, it is recommended to give vaginal progesterone if not already on progesterone. Most protocols give 200 mg daily at diagnosis at 18 0/7 to 25 6/7 to continue until 36 to 37 weeks (2).
  - Women with a singleton pregnancy and history of spontaneous preterm birth with shortened cervix should be considered for a cerclage (2).
  - Data is insufficient to recommend vaginal progesterone for multiple gestation (2).
  - Cerclage can be considered for any patient who is noted to have cervical insufficiency on physical exam (2).
  - It is not recommended to do a cervical pessary in any patient with shortened cervix (2).
- Tocolysis

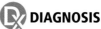

DIAGNOSIS

Diagnosis is generally based on a combination of significant cervical changes (such as dilation, effacement) with regular contractions. However, there is no single test that will reliably diagnose or predict true preterm labor. The diagnosis is based on a combination of physical findings and diagnostic tests that are interpreted in the context of the degree of risk to the patient.

HISTORY
- Address risk factors.
- Regular uterine contractions or cramping
- Dull, low backache or pain
- Intermittent lower abdominal pain
- Increased low pelvic pressure
- Change in vaginal discharge
- Vaginal bleeding
- Fluid leakage

PHYSICAL EXAM
- Sterile speculum exam for membrane rupture evaluation, cultures, and cervical inspection
- Bimanual cervical exam if intact membranes.

> **ALERT**
> Avoid bimanual examination when possible if rupture of the membranes is suspected.

DIFFERENTIAL DIAGNOSIS
- Braxton-Hicks contractions/false labor
- Round ligament pain
- Lumbosacral muscular back pain
- UTI or vaginal infections
- Adnexal torsion
- Appendicitis
- Nephrolithiasis

DIAGNOSTIC TESTS & INTERPRETATION
Initial Tests (lab, imaging)
- There are no specific tests that completely accurately predict preterm birth, although several can help with risk stratification.
- In symptomatic women from 22 to 34 weeks' gestation with intact membranes and no intercourse or bleeding in past 24 hours, obtain a fetal fibronectin (FFN) swab from the posterior vaginal fornix. FFN must be obtained prior to digital cervical exam.
  - If results are positive (≥50 ng/mL), patient is at a modest increased risk for preterm birth (positive predictive value [PPV] 13–30% for delivery within 2 weeks).
  - If results are negative, >97% of patients will not deliver in 14 days, so can consider avoiding complicated or high-risk interventions.
  - Fetal fibronectin and shortened cervix alone has low predictive value, so other data should be used as well in acute management of patient (3).
- Urinalysis and urine culture
- Cultures for gonorrhea, chlamydia, and wet prep

- Vaginal introitus and rectal culture for group B *Streptococcus* if indicated
- pH and ferning test of vaginal fluid to evaluate for rupture of membranes
- CBC with differential and Kleihauer-Betke test if abruption suspected
- US to identify number of fetuses and fetal position, confirm gestational age, estimate fetal weight, quantify amniotic fluid, and look for conditions making tocolysis contraindicated
- Transvaginal US to evaluate CL, funneling, and dynamic changes after obtaining FFN (if clinical assessment of the cervix is uncertain or if the cervix is closed on digital exam)

Follow-Up Tests & Special Considerations
- Repeat FFN as indicated by symptoms.
- After successful treatment, progressive changes of the cervix on repeat examination or US (in 1 to 2 weeks) may indicate need for hospitalization.

Diagnostic Procedures/Other
- Monitor contractions with external tocodynamometer.
- Consider amniocentesis at any preterm gestational age to evaluate for intra-amniotic infection.

 ## TREATMENT

GENERAL MEASURES
- Treat underlying risk factors.
- Hospitalization is necessary if the patient needs IV tocolysis.

MEDICATION
Tocolysis may allow time for interventions such as transfer to tertiary care facility and administration of corticosteroids but may not prolong pregnancy significantly (3).

First Line
- Corticosteroids (3):
  – Give if the mother is at 24 to 34 weeks' gestation and is at risk for delivery in the next 7 days (3); can consider if mother is 23 weeks to 23 weeks and 6 days and at risk for delivery in the next 7 days
  – Corticosteroids decrease neonatal respiratory distress, intraventricular hemorrhage, necrotizing enterocolitis, and overall perinatal mortality.
  – Betamethasone 12 mg IM × 2 doses 24 hours apart *or* dexamethasone 6 mg IM q12h for 4 doses (3).
  – Steroids may reduce the risk of respiratory morbidities in singleton infants born to nondiabetic mothers in the late preterm period (34 + 0 to 36 + 6 weeks' gestation). If delivery is likely during this time period, administration of steroids may be considered as above. Tocolysis is not recommended.
- Tocolysis:
  – Should be reserved for women who benefit from a 48-hour delay to receive corticosteroids as there is no evidence showing tocolysis causes improvement in neonatal outcomes (3)
  – Nifedipine: 20 mg PO loading dose, then 10 to 20 mg q4–6h for 48 hours (do not use sublingual route); check BP often and avoid hypotension. Concurrent use with magnesium sulfate is discouraged due to the theoretical risk of neuromuscular blockade (4).

  – Indomethacin: 50 to 100 mg PO initial dose and then 25 to 50 mg q6–8h. Use for longer than 72 hours is not recommended due to risk of premature closure of ductus arteriosus, oligohydramnios, and possibly neonatal necrotizing enterocolitis. Best to use in combination with magnesium if it is being used for neuroprotection (3),(4).
  – Contraindications to tocolysis: severe preeclampsia, hemorrhage, chorioamnionitis, advanced labor, intrauterine growth restriction, fetal distress, or lethal fetal abnormalities
- Antibiotics: antibiotics for group B *Streptococcus* prophylaxis if culture is indicated
- Magnesium sulfate is recommended for imminent delivery prior to 32 weeks for neuroprotection as it reduces the risk of cerebral palsy (3).

Second Line
Tocolysis
- Magnesium sulfate by IV infusion has not been shown to be superior to placebo in prolonging pregnancy beyond 48 hours. The side effects are generally greater than those with calcium channel blockers or NSAIDs. Therefore, this agent should be used cautiously.
- Terbutaline given via SC administration. If contractions persist or pulse >120 beats/min, change to another tocolytic agent (4). Due to reports of serious cardiovascular events and maternal deaths, PO or long-term SC administration of terbutaline should not be given (4).
- Significant possible interactions include pulmonary edema from crystalloid fluids and tocolytic agents, especially magnesium sulfate.
- Antibiotics should not be used as tocolysis or to improve neonatal outcomes for preterm labor with intact membranes and may be associated with harm. This is separate from recommendation for GBS and ruptured membranes.

ISSUES FOR REFERRAL
- If delivery is inevitable but not immediate, consider transport to a tertiary care center or hospital equipped with a neonatal ICU.
- Consider consultation with maternal–fetal medicine specialist.

ADDITIONAL THERAPIES
- Data to prove efficacy of pelvic rest (e.g., no douching or intercourse) is lacking.
- Bed rest and hydration have not been shown to be effective in the prevention of preterm delivery and are not recommended (3).

SURGERY/OTHER PROCEDURES
- For malpresentation or fetal compromise, consider cesarean delivery if labor is progressing.
- Consider cerclage for cervical insufficiency (until 24 weeks' gestation).

ADMISSION, INPATIENT, AND NURSING CONSIDERATIONS
Suspected/threatened preterm labor
- IV access
- Continuous fetal and contraction monitoring
- Assess cervix for dilatation and effacement.
- IV hydration
- Monitor for fluid overload.

 ## ONGOING CARE

FOLLOW-UP RECOMMENDATIONS
Patient Monitoring
- Weekly office visits with contraction monitoring, cervical checks, or cervical US if at high risk for recurrence
- Routine use of maintenance tocolysis is ineffective in preventing recurrent preterm labor or preterm birth.

PATIENT EDUCATION
Call physician or proceed to hospital whenever regular contractions last >1 hour, bleeding, increased vaginal discharge or fluid, decreased fetal movement.

PROGNOSIS
- If membranes are ruptured and no infection is confirmed, delivery often occurs within 3 to 7 days.
- If membranes are intact, 20–50% deliver preterm.

COMPLICATIONS
Labor resistant to tocolysis, pulmonary edema, intra-amniotic infection

REFERENCES

1. Martin JA, Hamilton BE, Osterman MJK. Births in the United States, 2019. *NCHS Data Brief*. 2020;(387):1–8.
2. American College of Obstetricians and Gynecologists Committee on Practice Bulletins—Obstetrics. Prediction and prevention of spontaneous preterm birth: ACOG Practice Bulletin, Number 234. *Obstet Gynecol*. 2021;138(2):e65–e90.
3. Practice Bulletin No. 171 summary: management of preterm labor. *Obstet Gynecol*. 2016;128(4):931–933.
4. Rundell K, Panchal B. Preterm labor: prevention and management. *Am Fam Physician*. 2017;95(6):366–372.

ADDITIONAL READING

Purisch SE, Gyamfi-Bannerman C. Epidemiology of preterm birth. *Semin Perinatol*. 2017;41(7):387–391.

 ## CODES

ICD10
- O60.03 Preterm labor without delivery, third trimester
- O60.0 Preterm labor without delivery
- O60.02 Preterm labor without delivery, second trimester

CLINICAL PEARLS
- Treatment of preterm labor may delay delivery to facilitate short-term interventions.
- Steroids improve neonatal outcomes.
- Magnesium sulfate is recommended for neuroprotection for imminent deliveries prior to 32 weeks.

PRIAPISM

Dongsheng Jiang, MD, MSc • Joanna Jiang, MD

 BASICS

DESCRIPTION
- Penile (or less common clitoral) erection lasting for >4 hours and unrelated to sexual stimulation or arousal
- Classification:
  - Ischemic (low-flow, veno-occlusive): 95% of cases. It is associated with ischemia of the corpora cavernosa.
  - Nonischemic (high-flow, arterial): less common and often painless, may be related to prior trauma, and does not require urgent treatment
  - Recurrent ischemic ("stuttering") priapism: episodic, short-lived, and may not require intervention
- Malignant priapism: rare, resulting most commonly from penile metastases related to primary bladder, prostatic, rectosigmoid, and renal tumors
- System(s) affected: reproductive and vascular
- Functional impairment: neurophysiologic, sexual, psychosocial

Pediatric Considerations
In children, the most common etiology is sickle cell disease (SCD) (63% of cases). Less common etiologies, occurring more typically in the adolescent years, are leukemia, idiopathic, penile trauma (e.g., post circumcision), or illicit drugs (up to 35% of cases).

EPIDEMIOLOGY
Incidence
- About 5.3 per 100,000 men per year
- Age: There has been an age shift since 2008 toward men in their 40s. The incidence doubles in men aged >40 years (2.9 vs. 1.5/100,000 person-years).
- Race: 61.1% African American (correlated with incidence of SCD), 30% Caucasian, 6.3% Hispanic

ETIOLOGY AND PATHOPHYSIOLOGY
- Anatomy and physiology:
  - The penis consists of three longitudinally oriented corpora: two dorsolaterally paired corpora cavernosa that are responsible for penile erection and a single ventral corpus spongiosum that surrounds the glans penis and extends distally to form the glans penis.
  - In general, the penile artery (a branch of the internal pudendal artery that, in turn, is a branch from the internal iliac artery) supplies the penis. It divides into three branches: dorsal artery, bulbar artery (supplies the corpus spongiosum), and cavernosal artery (the main blood supply to the erectile tissue).
  - During an erection, smooth muscle relaxation of the cavernosal arterioles results in high-volume inflow to the sinusoids, resulting in compression of the exiting venules. This leads to significant volume expansion of the corpora cavernosa.
  - During the flaccid resting state, the sympathetic nervous system is predominantly in control. Penile tumescence and erection are driven by the parasympathetic nervous system through the generation of nitric oxide.
- Smooth muscle relaxation occurs via usage of the phosphodiesterase type 5A (PDE5A) pathway, which generates cyclic guanosine monophosphate (cGMP).
  - In ischemic priapism, decreased venous outflow results in increased intracavernosal pressure. This leads to erection, decreased arterial inflow, blood stasis, local hypoxia, and acidosis (a compartment syndrome). Penile tissue necrosis and fibrosis may occur if priapism persists >24 hours. Pathophysiology mechanisms thought to contribute to impaired smooth muscle relaxation and decreased venous outflow include dysregulation of the NO/cGMP, RhoA/Rho kinase, and opiorphin signaling pathways as well as excessive adenosine signaling (1).
- In nonischemic priapism, increased arterial flow without decreased venous outflow results in a sustained, nonpainful, partially rigid erection.
- Causes:
  - Ischemic priapism (2):
    - Idiopathic: about 50% cases
    - Hematologic dyscrasias: SCD, thalassemia, leukemia, multiple myeloma, fat emboli during hyperalimentation, hemodialysis, glucose-6-phosphate dehydrogenase deficiency, factor V Leiden mutation
    - Infections (toxin mediated): urinary tract infections, scorpion sting, spider bite, rabies, malaria
    - Metabolic disorders: nephrolithiasis, amyloidosis, Fabry disease, gout
    - Neurogenic disorders: syphilis, spinal cord injury, cauda equina syndrome, autonomic neuropathy, lumbar disc herniation, spinal stenosis, cerebrovascular accident, brain tumour, spinal anesthesia
    - Neoplasms: penis, urethra, bladder, prostate, kidney and rectum
    - Medications:
      - Vasoactive erectile agents (i.e., papaverine, phentolamine, prostaglandin E1/alprostadil)
      - α-Adrenergic receptor antagonists (i.e., prazosin, terazosin, doxazosin, tamsulosin)
      - Antidepressants and antipsychotics (i.e., trazodone, bupropion, fluoxetine, sertraline, lithium, clozapine, risperidone, olanzapine, chlorpromazine, thioridazine, phenothiazines)
      - Antihypertensives (i.e., hydralazine, guanethidine, propranolol)
      - Hormones (i.e., gonadotropin-releasing hormone, testosterone)
      - Anxiolytics (hydroxyzine)
      - Anticoagulants (heparin, warfarin)
      - Recreational drugs (i.e., alcohol, marijuana, cocaine)
  - Nonischemic priapism (2):
    - Penile or perineal trauma resulting in a fistula between the cavernous artery and the corpus cavernosum.
    - Acute spinal cord injury
    - Treatment of ischemic priapism

RISK FACTORS
- SCD has a lifetime risk of ischemic priapism 29–42%.
- Dehydration correlated with SCD or trait
- Prior history of priapismic episodes

GENERAL PREVENTION
- Avoid dehydration (SCD cases).
- Avoid excessive sexual stimulation.
- Avoid or limit causative drugs.
- Avoid trauma to the genital area

COMMONLY ASSOCIATED CONDITIONS
- SCD (42.9%) or sickle cell trait (2.5%)
- Drug abuse (7.9%)
- G6PD deficiency
- Leukemia
- Neoplasm

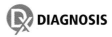 **DIAGNOSIS**

HISTORY
- Prior priapism episodes or prolonged erections after waking and degree of pain
- Duration of erection
- Perineal or penile trauma (blunt force or needle injury)
- Urination difficult during erection
- History of any hematologic abnormalities (e.g., SCD or trait)
- Cardiovascular disease
- Medications
- Recreational drug use

PHYSICAL EXAM
- In general, physical examination should include the following:
  - A complete penile, scrotal, and perineal exam to identify the presence of trauma, gangrene (rare), or prosthesis
  - An abdominal and lymph noted exam to rule out underlying conditions
- Observations on examination should include the following:
  - Ischemic (or stuttering) priapism: Penis is fully erect, painful, or tender; corpora cavernosa are rigid; and corpora spongiosum and glans are flaccid.
  - Nonischemic priapism: Penis is partially erect (not tender or painful), and the corpora cavernosa are semirigid and nontender, with the glans and corpora spongiosum flaccid.

DIAGNOSTIC TESTS & INTERPRETATION
- CBC with reticulocyte count
- Sickling hemoglobin (Hgb) solubility test and Hgb electrophoresis
- Coagulation profile
- Urinalysis/urine toxicology

824

- Corporal blood gas (CBG) should be obtained to distinguish ischemic from nonischemic priapism. Nonischemic blood gas analysis is identical to normal arterial blood, whereas the following is concerning for ischemic priapism: pH <7.25, pO_2 <30 mm Hg, and pCO_2 >60 mm Hg.
- A color Doppler ultrasound (CDUS) may be necessary to differentiate ischemic (no blood flow in the cavernosal arteries) from nonischemic (high blood flow) priapism.
- Penile arteriography can be used to identify the presence and arterial cavernous fistula or pseudoaneurysms (nonischemic) (3).
- Penile MRI can be used for cases >48–72 hour duration to evaluate for corporal smooth muscle necrosis and candidacy for immediate penile prosthesis implantation.

 TREATMENT

- Based on the type:
  – Ischemic priapism: requires immediate treatment and urology consultation
    ◦ Between 4 and 24 hours, initial conservative management should include pain control, encouraging ejaculation, vigorous physical exercise, and icing (4).
    ◦ Cavernosal aspiration with a large-bore needle (success rate ~30%)
    ◦ Cavernosal injection of phenylephrine 200 μg repeated to a maximum of 1,500 μg (with BP monitoring)
    ◦ If this fails, shunt procedures are considered.
  – Nonischemic priapism
    ◦ Observation, icing, site specific compression; causative fistula may close spontaneously.
    ◦ If nonischemic priapism does not resolve arteriography and selective embolization
  – Stuttering priapism
    ◦ The initial goal is to prevent recurrence. But, if the episode is prolonged, there is a risk of conversion to ischemic priapism.
    ◦ Initial conservative treatment including ejaculation, physical exercise, icing, and/or cold shower.
    ◦ Manage acute episodes as ischemic cases— aspiration then intracavernous injections of:
      ▪ Phenylephrine: 200 μg every 3 to 5 minutes to a maximum of 1 mg within 1 hour;
      ▪ Etilefrine: 2.5 mg diluted in 1- to 2-mL saline;
      ▪ Adrenaline: 2 mL of 1/100,000 solution given up to 5 times in a 20-minute period;
      ▪ Methylene blue: 50 to 100 mg
- In all cases, particularly SCD cases, treat the underlying condition (e.g., SCD does not delay intracavernous treatment).
- Although blood transfusion is an option, particularly in SCD cases, other interventions should be explored and exhausted first.

GENERAL MEASURES
- Treat any underlying cause or disease process.
- In SCD cases: IV hydration; supplemental oxygen; partial exchange or repeated transfusions to reduce percentage of sickle cells to <50%

MEDICATION
- Analgesics (e.g., opioids) for pain, if needed
- May try oral pseudoephedrine or terbutaline while awaiting for intracavernous injection

First Line
Intracavernous injection of phenylephrine is considered to be first line.

Second Line
- Ischemic priapism:
  – Etilefrine (intracavernous) is a the second most used sympathomimetic.
  – Methylene blue (intracavernous) can be used for pharmacologically induced priapism (cGMP inhibitor).
  – Epinephrine (intracavernous) has a higher success rate than phenylephrine, but greater cardiovascular side effects.
- Stuttering priapism:
  – Prevention of recurrence with daily oral medications:
    ◦ Adrenergic agonists: pseudoephedrine and etilefrine
    ◦ Androgen suppression: antiandrogens, 5α-reductase inhibitors, and ketoconazole
    ◦ PDE5 inhibitors: sildenafil
    ◦ Smooth muscle regulation: digoxin or terbutaline
    ◦ Others: gabapentin, baclofen, hydroxyurea

ISSUES FOR REFERRAL
A urologist should be consulted in all cases of suspected priapism.

SURGERY/OTHER PROCEDURES
- For ischemic priapism, surgical options after medical therapy include the following:
  – Distal cavernoglandular shunts
    ◦ Percutaneous: Ebbehoj, Winter, or T shunt
    ◦ Open: Al-Ghorab or Burnett
  – Proximal cavernoglandular shunts
    ◦ Open: Quackles or Sacher
  – Venous shunts
    ◦ Grayhack (saphenous vein shunt)
    ◦ Barry (deep dorsal vein shunt)
  – Immediate penile prothesis placement: relative indications include failure of intracavernous therapies or corporal smooth muscle necrosis or MRI/biopsy; early surgery avoids cavernous fibrosis, which offers the opportunity to maintain penile size and prevent penile curvature due to cavernosal fibrosis.
- For nonischemic priapism, surgical options include the following:
  – Selective embolization with autologous blood clot, absorbable (gel foam or sponge) or nonabsorbable materials (coils or acrylic glue), or surgical ligation as a last resort

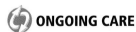 ONGOING CARE

FOLLOW-UP RECOMMENDATIONS
Patient Monitoring
Close follow-up with a urologist is mandatory.

PROGNOSIS
- Even with excellent treatment for a prolonged priapism, complete detumescence may require several weeks secondary to edema.
- Impotence due to irreversible corporal fibrosis is likely in ischemic priapism and is up to 90% if the priapism lasts >24 hours (2).

COMPLICATIONS
Erectile dysfunction

REFERENCES
1. Anele UA, Morrison BF, Burnett AL. Molecular pathophysiology of priapism: emerging targets. *Curr Drug Targets*. 2015;16(5):474–483.
2. Huang Y-C, Harraz AM, Shindel AW, et al. Evaluation and management of priapism: 2009 update. *Nat Rev Urol*. 2009;6(5):262–271.
3. Montague DK, Jarow J, Broderick GA, et al; for Members of the Erectile Dysfunction Guideline Update Panel, American Urological Association. American Urological Association guideline on the management of priapism. *J Urol*. 2003;170(4, Pt 1):1318–1324.
4. Muneer A, Alnajjar HM, Ralph D. Recent advances in the management of priapism. *F1000Res*. 2018;7:37.

 SEE ALSO

Anemia, Sickle Cell; Erectile Dysfunction

 CODES

ICD10
- N48.30 Priapism, unspecified
- N48.39 Other priapism
- N48.31 Priapism due to trauma

CLINICAL PEARLS
- Priapism is a prolonged penile erection that lasts >4 hours and is unrelated to sexual stimulation. If priapism lasts >24 hours, it likely results in permanent sexual impairment.
- Priapism can occur in children, particularly in SCD. Treatment should address both the underlying disease as well as developmental needs.
- In evaluating priapism, the clinician must distinguish ischemic from nonischemic priapism by history and physical exam as well as cavernosal blood gas and possibly ultrasound or MRI, if indicated.
- Ischemic priapism is an emergent condition that requires immediate urologic evaluation and treatment.

PROSTATE CANCER

Dylan Buller, MD • Joseph R. Wagner, MD

 BASICS

DESCRIPTION

- The prostate is a male reproductive organ that contributes seminal fluid to the ejaculate.
- The prostate gland is about the size of a walnut, averaging 20 to 25 g in volume in an adult male; tends to enlarge after age 50
- Three distinct zones delineate the functional anatomy of the prostate: peripheral zone (largest, neighbors rectal wall, palpable on digital rectal exam [DRE], most common location for prostate cancer), central zone (contains the ejaculatory ducts), and transition zone (located centrally, adjacent to the urethra).
- Prostatic epithelial cells produce prostate-specific antigen (PSA), which is used as a tumor marker and in screening.

EPIDEMIOLOGY

Incidence
An estimated 248,530 men in the United States will be newly diagnosed with carcinoma of the prostate (CaP) in 2021, representing 13.1% of all new cancer diagnoses.

Prevalence
- An estimated 34,130 men in the United States will die of CaP in 2021, representing 5.6% of all cancer deaths.
- Median age at diagnosis is 67 years; probability of CaP 10.9% (1 in 9) ≥70 years
- PCa most commonly diagnosed nonskin cancer in men in the United States (~12.1% lifetime risk) and second leading cause of cancer death in men (only ~3% of all CaP results in CaP-related death.)
- Autopsy studies find foci of latent CaP in 50% of men in their 8th decade of life.

ETIOLOGY AND PATHOPHYSIOLOGY
- Adenocarcinoma: >95%; nonadenocarcinoma: <5% (most common transitional cell carcinoma)
- Location of CaP: 70% peripheral zone, 20% transitional zone, 5–10% central zone

RISK FACTORS
Age >50 years, African American race, positive family history

GENERAL PREVENTION
There are no FDA-approved drugs or diet modifications to prevent CaP.

- Finasteride use associated with moderate risk reduction in CaP but associated with an increased risk of high-grade disease.

ALERT
Screening for prostate cancer is controversial:

- U.S. Preventive Services Task Force (USPSTF): "for men aged 55 to 69 years, the decision to undergo periodic PSA-based screening for prostate cancer should be an individual one and should include discussion of the potential benefits and harms of screening with their clinician. Screening offers a small potential benefit of reducing the chance of death from prostate cancer in some men. However, many men will experience potential harms of screening" (1)[A]. USPSTF recommends against PSA screening for men ≥70 years old (1)[A].

- The American Urological Association (AUA) panel recommends for men 55 to 69 shared decision-making between physician and patient regarding PSA screening.
- PSA screening is not recommended in men age <40 years or any man with <10 years of estimated life expectancy.
- When providing informed consent, data shows if you screen 1,000 men between 55 and 69 years:
  – 240 will have a positive result; only ~100 will truly have PCa; of the 100 with cancer, 80 will agree to treatment.
  – Treatment will result in one less person dying, but 50 will develop erectile dysfunction (ED); 15 permanent incontinence

 DIAGNOSIS

HISTORY
Inquire about family history of CaP, symptoms of bladder outlet obstruction, and other voiding symptoms.

PHYSICAL EXAM
- DRE to assess for prostatic masses, firmness, or asymmetry
- Evaluate lumbar spine and lymph nodes for evidence of metastasis.

DIFFERENTIAL DIAGNOSIS
Benign prostatic hyperplasia, prostatitis, prostatic intraepithelial neoplasia (PIN), prostate stones, atypical small acinar proliferation (ASAP)

DIAGNOSTIC TESTS & INTERPRETATION
Initial Tests (lab, imaging)
- In general, total PSA ≥4 ng/mL is concerning for CaP (sensitivity 21%, specificity 91%).
  – Other benign conditions can elevate PSA (infection, inflammation, normal growth, natural PSA fluctuations, normally high variants).
  – Rectal manipulation will not significantly elevate PSA.
  – 5-α-Reductase inhibitors decrease PSA by ~50%.
- Other PSA metrics used to aid in CaP diagnosis:
  – Total PSA velocity: ≥0.75 ng/mL/year or >20% baseline for higher values increases CaP risk.
  – Free PSA and age-/race-adjusted PSA helpful in evaluating risk. For patients with PSA between 4 and 10 ng/mL, a low percent free PSA is associated with higher risk of CaP.
  – PSAD ≥0.15 associated with higher prevalence of CaP
- Prostate biopsy
  – Decision to biopsy involves PSA, DRE findings, MRI, and overall clinical suspicion of CaP with consideration of comorbidities and life expectancy
  – Standard biopsy: systematic random cores from peripheral zone base, mid-gland, and apex, 8 to 12 cores
  – Prebiopsy MRI used to identify suspicious prostate lesions to be targeted at biopsy
  – The Gleason grade is the standard pathologic grading system but is being replaced by grade groups 1 to 5.
    ◦ Gleason grade ranks specimens from 1 (most differentiated) to 5 (least differentiated).

- Primary and secondary patterns are identified and reported, and the sum is the Gleason score (e.g., 3 + 4 = 7).
- Most prostate cancer are scored 6 to 10, with 10 having the worst prognosis.
- Grade group 1 = Gleason 6; grade group 2 = Gleason 3 + 4 = 7; grade group 3 = Gleason 4 + 3 = 7; grade group 4 = Gleason 8; grade group 5 = Gleason 9 and 10
- Staging
  – TNM (tumor, node, and metastasis) staging used to generate a clinical and pathologic stage, which directs treatment. Clinical staging is as follows:
    ◦ T1: cancer found incidentally on TURP or found on biopsy for elevated PSA
    ◦ T2: cancer found on DRE but confined to the prostate
    ◦ T3: cancer found to be extended locally outside of the prostate and/or the seminal vesicle
    ◦ T4: cancer invading adjacent organs
    ◦ N1: denotes local lymph node spread
    ◦ M1: distant metastasis

Follow-Up Tests & Special Considerations
Some combination of bone scan, MRI, CT, or PET scan may be indicated for high-risk cancers.

TREATMENT

- Use Prostate Predict Calculator to help patient consider treatment options: https://prostate.predict.nhs.uk/.
- Treatment options include:
  – Watchful waiting: monitoring with expectation to provide palliation with symptoms
    ◦ ProtecT trial (2016) found watchful waiting had equal cancer-specific and all-cause mortality compared to surgery or radiotherapy. In the treatment arms, there was less disease progression (including metastatic disease) but resulted in significantly more morbidity (urinary and bowel dysfunction, ED).
  – Active surveillance: close monitoring of PSA, DRE, and repeat biopsy at regular intervals
  – Radical prostatectomy: ± pelvic lymph node dissection (PLND)
  – Radiation therapy: external beam (EBRT)
  – Brachytherapy: radioactive implants placed in prostate; option for early clinical stage localized to the prostate
  – Antiandrogen therapy
    ◦ Bilateral orchiectomy (surgical castration)
    ◦ Gonadotropin-releasing hormone (GnRH) agonist, antagonist, or antiandrogen (medical castration)
    ◦ Abiraterone: 17α-hydroxylase inhibitor (CYP17A adrenal androgen production)
    ◦ Bicalutamide/nilutamide/flutamide/enzalutamide/apalutamide: androgen receptor antagonists
  – Chemotherapy: includes multiple chemotherapeutic agents used to treat castrate-resistant prostate cancer (CRPC)
  – Risk factors
    ◦ Treatment options based on risk: very low-, low-, favorable intermediate-, unfavorable intermediate-, high-, and very high-risk categories; this is based on risk of recurrence after definitive treatment.

○ Must meet all three criteria to be low risk; any one criterion moves patient to a higher risk group: risk category clinical stage/serum PSA (ng/mL)/grade group: low T1–T2a/<10/1; intermediate T2b–T2c/10–20/2–3; high T3a/>20/4–5

○ Very low and very high-risk categories, as well as differentiating favorable versus unfavorable intermediate risk, are based on additional clinical/pathologic criteria.

○ Updated risk stratification algorithms include additional groups of very low risk, favorable and unfavorable intermediate risk, and very high risk.

○ Localized CaP
  ▪ Very low and low risk:
    □ Mainstay of therapy is active surveillance.
    □ Radical prostatectomy and radiation therapy may be offered.
  ▪ Intermediate risk:
    □ Mainstay of therapy is radical prostatectomy or radiation therapy.
    □ Radical prostatectomy has shown a possible survival benefit in intermediate prostate cancer.
    □ Active surveillance may be offered to patients in the favorable intermediate risk group
  ▪ High and very high risk:
    □ Mainstay of therapy is radical prostatectomy or radiation therapy.
    □ Adjuvant radiation may be considered based on adverse pathologic findings after prostatectomy.

ALERT

Life expectancy determination, as well as educating the patient of the risks and benefits of surveillance and treatment options, is critical.

• Locally advanced CaP:
  – Mainstay of therapy is androgen deprivation therapy (ADT) and radiation; surgery and adjuvant radiation also used
  – Adding abiraterone + prednisone in patients commencing long-term ADT for high risk (T3–T4, Gleason 8 to 10, PSA >40), locally advanced prostate cancer has been shown to significantly increase overall survival.
• Metastatic CaP:
  – Mainstay of therapy is RT and ADT.
  – Early chemotherapy (docetaxel) with ADT may be considered for high-volume disease; ADT with abiraterone + prednisone for lower volume disease
  – ADT specifics:
    ○ GnRH agonists include leuprolide, goserelin, histrelin, or triptorelin.
    ○ GnRH antagonists include degarelix: an alternative to GnRH agonists; suppresses testosterone production and avoids flare phenomenon observed with GnRH agonists
    ○ Side effects of ADT: osteoporosis, gynecomastia, ED, decreased libido, obesity, lipid alterations, diabetes, and cardiovascular disease

○ Flare phenomenon (disease flare: hot flashes, fatigue) can occur owing to transient increase in testosterone levels on initiation of GnRH agonist therapy.
○ If spinal cord metastases are present, the concern for cord compression with a testosterone flare can be avoided by starting antiandrogen therapy prior to initiation of a GnRH agonist.
○ Combined androgen blockade with GnRH agonist and antiandrogen (e.g., bicalutamide, nilutamide, or flutamide) may be used to prevent flare.

• CRPC
  – CRPC is defined as progression of disease following ADT. Treatment includes the following:
    ○ Nonmetastatic
      ▪ Continue ADT.
      ▪ Add antiandrogen (apalutamide, darolutamide, or enzalutamide).
    ○ Metastatic: tumor and germline testing recommended. First-line treatment:
      ▪ Abiraterone: inhibitor of CYP17A (adrenal androgen production), used with prednisone
      ▪ Enzalutamide: androgen receptor inhibitor
      ▪ Docetaxel: chemotherapeutic that inhibits microtubules
      ▪ Sipuleucel-T: immunotherapy
      ▪ Radium-223 (radiopharmaceutical) for patients with symptomatic bony metastases
      ▪ Mitoxantrone for patients with symptomatic visceral metastases intolerant of other therapies
    ○ Second line (if first-line abiraterone/enzalutamide):
      ▪ Docetaxel or sipuleucel-T preferred
      ▪ Olaparib, pembrolizumab, radium-223, or rucaparib in specific patient populations
      ▪ Abiraterone, cabazitaxel, enzalutamide, fine-particle abiraterone also recommended
    ○ Second line (if first-line docetaxel):
      ▪ Abiraterone, cabazitaxel, or enzalutamide preferred
      ▪ Mitoxantrone, olaparib, pembrolizumab, radium-223, or rucaparib in specific patient populations
      ▪ Docetaxel rechallenge, fine-particle abiraterone, sipuleucel-T also recommended
    ○ 177Lu-PSMA-617 granted FDA Breakthrough Therapy designation and may represent new treatment modality for patients with metastatic CRPC.
• Bone health
  – Men with prostate cancer, especially on ADT, are at elevated risk of pathologic fractures
    ○ Offer bone density and vitamin D supplementation.
    ○ Denosumab (RANK-ligand inhibitor—prevents osteoclast activation) and zoledronic acid (bisphosphonate) can be offered for prevention.

 ONGOING CARE

FOLLOW-UP RECOMMENDATIONS
• Prostatectomy: PSA and DRE at regular intervals. Some combination of CT/MRI/PET/bone scan obtained at recurrence. If the PSA recurrence is due to local disease, salvage radiation +/− ADT is considered. For metastatic disease, androgen deprivation.
• XRT: PSA and DRE are recommended at regular intervals. Biochemical recurrence is defined as PSA increase ≥2 ng/mL above nadir; some combination of CT/MRI/PET/bone scan is usually obtained. If the PSA recurrence is thought to be from local disease, salvage prostatectomy, cryosurgery, brachytherapy, or high-intensity focused ultrasound (HIFU) are considered. For metastatic disease, androgen deprivation is considered.

PROGNOSIS
• Localized disease is frequently curable; advanced disease has a favorable prognosis if lesions are hormone sensitive.
• 5-year CaP survival by stage: local 100%, regional 100%, distant 30.2%
• Recurrence risk increased if: extraprostatic extension, seminal vesicle invasion, positive surgical margins

COMPLICATIONS
• Prostatectomy: Urinary incontinence and ED are the most common long-term issues.
• Radiation therapy: urinary incontinence, ED, radiation cystitis, and radiation proctitis
• Treatment options for ED: PDE5 inhibitors, intracavernosal injections, intraurethral suppositories, vacuum pump, penile prosthesis
• Treatment options for incontinence: oral medications, urethral sling, artificial sphincter

REFERENCES

1. Grossman DC, Curry SJ, Owens DK, et al; and US Preventive Services Task Force. Screening for prostate cancer: US Preventive Services Task Force recommendation statement. *JAMA.* 2018;319(18):1901–1913.

 CODES

ICD10
• C61 Malignant neoplasm of prostate
• Z80.42 Family history of malignant neoplasm of prostate
• D07.5 Carcinoma in situ of prostate

CLINICAL PEARLS
• The use of PSA for CaP screening is controversial; shared decision-making is recommended.
• Care must be taken when interpreting PSA levels in patients taking 5-α-reductase inhibitors.

PROSTATIC HYPERPLASIA, BENIGN (BPH)

Michael T. Partin, MD • Sahel Uddin, DO

BASICS

- Benign prostatic hyperplasia (BPH) is due to proliferation of both smooth muscle and epithelial cell lines of the prostate which causes increased prostate volume and may lead to compression of the urethra and obstructive symptoms.
- BPH presents clinically with storage and/or voiding symptoms known collectively as lower urinary tract symptoms (LUTS). These include difficulty initiating a urinary stream, frequency, urgency, nocturia, and/or dysuria.
- Symptoms do not directly correlate to prostate volume. It is estimated that only half of all men with histologic evidence of BPH experience moderate to severe LUTS.
- Progression may result in upper and lower urinary tract infections and may progress to direct bladder outlet obstruction and acute renal failure (ARF).

EPIDEMIOLOGY
Age related with nearly universal development in men

Incidence
Incidence increases with age with an estimated prevalence varying from 70% to 90% by the age of 80 years (estimated at 8–20% by age 40 years).

ETIOLOGY AND PATHOPHYSIOLOGY
- Unknown etiology
- Develops in prostatic periurethral or transition zone
- Hyperplastic nodules of stromal and epithelial components increase glandular components.

RISK FACTORS
- Increasing age
- Higher free prostate-specific antigen (PSA) levels, heart disease, and use of β-blockers
- Low androgen levels from cirrhosis/chronic alcoholism reduces the risk of BPH
- Obesity and sedentary lifestyle can worsen LUTS
- No evidence of increased or decreased risk with smoking, alcohol, or any dietary factors

GENERAL PREVENTION
Symptoms can be managed through weight loss, regulation of fluid intake (especially in the evening), decreased intake of caffeine, and increased physical activity.

COMMONLY ASSOCIATED CONDITIONS
- LUTS can be divided into two groups:
  - Filling/storage symptoms: frequency, nocturia, urgency, and urge incontinence
  - Voiding symptoms: difficulty initiating urinary stream, incomplete voiding, or weak stream
- Sexual dysfunction, including erectile dysfunction and ejaculatory disorders
- LUTS can also be secondary to cardiovascular, respiratory, or renal disease (1).

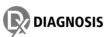

DIAGNOSIS

HISTORY
- Evaluate symptom severity with the American Urological Society Symptom Index (AUA-SI) or the International Prostate Symptom Score (IPSS)
- Screen for other causes such as infection, procedural history, or neurogenic causes.

- Evaluate for comorbid conditions such as diabetes, congestive heart failure (CHF), or Parkinson disease.
- Review medication list and family history of BPH/prostate cancer.
- Screen for gross hematuria.
- Nocturia >2 times per night warrants a frequency/volume chart for 2 to 3 days to detect urinary patterns

PHYSICAL EXAM
- Digital rectal exam (DRE): symmetrically enlarged prostate (*Size does not always correlate with symptoms.*)
- Signs of renal failure due to obstructive uropathy (edema, pallor, pruritus, ecchymosis, nutritional deficiencies)
- If DRE is suggestive of prostate cancer, or if there is hematuria, recurrent infections, concern for stricture, or evidence of neurologic disease, the patient should be referred to urology.

DIFFERENTIAL DIAGNOSIS
- Obstructive
  - Prostate cancer
  - Urethral stricture or valves
  - Bladder neck contracture (usually secondary to prostate surgery)
  - Inability of bladder neck or external sphincter to relax appropriately during voiding
- Neurogenic
  - Spinal cord injury or stroke
  - Parkinsonism
  - Multiple sclerosis
- Medical
  - Poorly controlled diabetes mellitus
  - CHF
- Pharmacologic
  - Diuretics (increased urine production)
  - Decongestants (increased sphincter tone)
  - Opioids (impaired autonomic function)
  - Tricyclic antidepressants (anticholinergic)
- Other
  - Bladder carcinoma
  - Overactive bladder
  - Nocturnal polyuria
  - Bladder calculi
  - UTI and prostatitis
  - Urethritis/sexually transmitted infections
  - Obstructive sleep apnea (OSA) (nocturia)
  - Caffeine

DIAGNOSTIC TESTS & INTERPRETATION

Initial Tests (lab, imaging)
- Urinalysis (UA) in all patients presenting with LUTS can help rule out other etiologies such as bladder/kidney stones, cancer, UTI, or urethral strictures.
- PSA (especially for men with a life expectancy of 10 years or more who would be surgical candidates if prostate cancer was identified)
- PSA levels correlate with prostate volume which can help guide treatment choice.
- With bladder cancer risk factors (smoking history or hematuria), obtain urine cytology and/or cystoscopy.
- If nocturia is the main concern, consider using a frequency volume chart for urine output.

- Uroflow: volume voided per unit time (Peak flow <10 mL/sec is abnormal.)
- Postvoid residual (PVR): either with catheterization or bladder ultrasound (>100 mL = incomplete emptying)
- Sleep study if OSA or primary nocturnal polyuria is suspected

Follow-Up Tests & Special Considerations
- No additional testing is recommended in uncomplicated LUTS.
- Further testing if symptoms do not respond to medical management or if initial evaluation suggests underlying disease
- Transrectal ultrasound or cross-sectional imaging (MRI/CT): assessment of prostate gland size; not necessary in the routine evaluation
- Abdominal ultrasound: can demonstrate increased PVR or hydronephrosis; not necessary in the routine evaluation

Diagnostic Procedures/Other
- Pressure-flow studies (urine flow vs. voiding pressures) to determine etiology of symptoms
  - Obstructive pattern shows high voiding pressures with low-flow rate.
- Cystoscopy
  - Demonstrates presence, configuration, cause (stricture, stone), and site of obstructive tissue
  - Not recommended in routine evaluation unless other factors, such as hematuria, are present

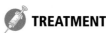

TREATMENT

GENERAL MEASURES
- Treatment ranges from watchful waiting to lifestyle modifications, medications, or surgical management.
- Mild symptoms (score of <7) or moderate symptoms (score 8 to 15) on IPSS that are nonbothersome require no treatment with repeat evaluation performed annually.
- For moderate-severe symptoms, attempt lifestyle interventions including regulation of fluid intake, avoidance of alcohol and caffeine, exercise, diet, and eliminating/reducing contributing medications.

MEDICATION
- α-Adrenergic antagonists
  - First-line option for moderate/severe and bothersome LUTS (2)
  - Affects contraction of smooth muscle in the prostatic urethra and bladder neck
  - Clinical improvement typically takes 2 to 4 weeks
  - May affect blood pressure and lead to orthostatic hypotension
  - AUA recommends alfuzosin (Uroxatral), doxazosin (Cardura), and tamsulosin (Flomax) because they are thought to be more selective and have less effect on blood pressure. Prazosin (Minipress) and phenoxybenzamine (Dibenzyline) have insufficient evidence and are not recommended.
    ○ Doxazosin (Cardura): 1 to 8 mg/day PO
    ○ Tamsulosin (Flomax): 0.4 to 0.8 mg/day PO
    ○ Alfuzosin (Uroxatral): 10 mg/day PO
    ○ Terazosin (Hytrin): Start at 1 mg PO daily at bedtime, max 20 mg daily.

- **Contraindications**
  - Use caution in patients who are also using phosphodiesterase type 5 inhibitors for erectile dysfunction.
  - Do not use in men pursuing cataract surgery until they are postoperative due to the risk for perioperative floppy iris syndrome.
- **5-α-Reductase inhibitors**
  - Blocks conversion of testosterone to dihydrotestosterone to gradually reduce prostatic volume
  - Greatest clinical benefit when prostate volume exceeds 40 mL and thus recommended to avoid use without evidence of enlarged prostate
  - Generally requires 6 months to show clinical benefits
    - Finasteride (Proscar): 5 mg/day PO
    - Dutasteride (Avodart): 0.5 mg/day PO
  - Shows reduced risk of acute urinary retention and less need for surgical intervention
  - Used in patients with refractory hematuria after other causes have been ruled out
  - Side effects include decreased libido and erectile dysfunction; low risk of prostate cancer (3)[C].

ALERT
A PSA value in a patient taking a **5-α-reductase inhibitors will be artificially low by up to 50%.** Test before and after initiating treatment.

- Combination therapy of α-blocker plus 5-α-reductase inhibitor is superior to monotherapy with an α-blocker only in men with evidence of enlarged prostates.
- Anticholinergic agents are appropriate for moderate to severe predominant storage LUTS without an elevated PVR. Options include solifenacin (VESIcare), tolterodine (Detrol LA), or oxybutynin (Ditropan XL); should be avoided in patients with PVR >250 mL
- β3 adrenergic agonists in combination with an α-blocker can be offered for patients with moderate to severe storage LUTS (3)[C].
- Phosphodiesterase-5 inhibitors lead to mild improvement of LUTS; can use tadalafil (Cialis): 5 mg/day PO but avoid use in combination with α-blockers or in those with CrCl <30 mL/min irrespective of comorbid erectile dysfunction (3)[B].

Geriatric Considerations
Use caution with anticholinergics, antihistamines, sympathomimetics, tricyclic antidepressants, and opioids.

ISSUES FOR REFERRAL
- Moderate or severe LUTS that do not respond to medical management
- BPH-related complications such as recurrent UTIs or hematuria, renal insufficiency, and urinary retention
- Abnormal PSA or prostate exam
- Any history of urethral trauma or stricture, or neurologic disease of the bladder/urinary system

SURGERY/OTHER PROCEDURES
- Indications for surgery
  - Urinary retention due to prostatic obstruction, recurrent, no improvement with medications
  - Intractable symptoms due to prostatic obstruction AUA score >8 and symptoms

- Obstructive uropathy (renal insufficiency)
  - Recurrent or persistent UTIs due to prostatic obstruction
  - Recurrent gross hematuria due to enlarged prostate
  - Bladder calculi
- Surgical procedures: TURP remains the gold standard of surgical procedures; however, for selected patient populations, there are other options available.
- Common complications of TURP:
  - Bleeding, retrograde ejaculation, urinary incontinence
  - TURP syndrome: hyponatremia secondary to absorption of hypotonic irrigation fluid
- Other options include transurethral vaporization of the prostate (TUVP), transurethral microwave thermotherapy (TUMT), transurethral incision of the prostate (TUIP), photoselective vaporization of the prostate (PVP), prostatic urethral lift (PUL), water vapor thermal therapy (WVTT), laser enucleation, and robotic waterjet treatment (RWT).
- Holmium laser enucleation (HoLEP), thulium laser enucleation of the prostate (ThuLEP), and PVP are options for patients on anticoagulation (4).
- PUL and WVTT can be offered as a treatment option for patients who prefer conservation of erectile and ejaculatory function (4)[C].
- Transurethral needle ablation and prostate artery embolization are not supported by current data (4)[C].

COMPLEMENTARY & ALTERNATIVE MEDICINE
- There are no recommended complementary or alternative treatments for BPH (2).
- Saw palmetto (*Serenoa repens*) has been thoroughly studied in a Cochrane review and did not improve LUTS.

 ONGOING CARE

FOLLOW-UP RECOMMENDATIONS
Patient Monitoring
- DRE yearly in patients who choose watchful waiting
- PSA yearly in patients who choose watchful waiting: should not be checked while patient is in retention, recently catheterized, or within a week of any surgical procedure to the prostate
- Consider monitoring PVR, if elevated.

DIET
Large boluses of oral/IV fluids, alcohol, or caffeine may exacerbate LUTS.

PATIENT EDUCATION
National Kidney and Urologic Diseases Information Clearinghouse, Box NKUDIC, Bethesda, MD 20893; 301-468-6345

PROGNOSIS
- Symptoms improve or stabilize in 70–80% of patients.
- 25% of men with LUTS will have persistent storage symptoms after prostatectomy.
- Of men with BPH, 11–33% have occult prostate cancer.

COMPLICATIONS
- Urinary retention (acute or chronic)
- Bladder stones, prostatitis, hematuria

REFERENCES

1. McVary KT, Roehrborn CG, Avins AL, et al. Update on AUA guideline on the management of benign prostatic hyperplasia. *J Urol.* 2011;185(5): 1793–1803.
2. Pearson R, Williams PM. Common questions about the diagnosis and management of benign prostatic hyperplasia. *Am Fam Physician.* 2014;90(11): 769–774.
3. Lerner LB, McVary KT, Barry MJ, et al. Management of lower urinary tract symptoms attributed to benign prostatic hyperplasia: AUA GUIDELINE PART I—initial work-up and medical management. *J Urol.* 2021;206(4):806–817.
4. Lerner LB, McVary KT, Barry MJ, et al. Management of lower urinary tract symptoms attributed to benign prostatic hyperplasia: AUA GUIDELINE PART II—surgical evaluation and treatment. *J Urol.* 2021;206(4):818–826.

ADDITIONAL READING
- American Urological Association. Management of benign prostatic hyperplasia/lower urinary tract symptoms: AUA Guideline 2021. https://www.auanet.org/guidelines/guidelines/benign-prostatic-hyperplasia-(bph)-guideline. Accessed October 20, 2021.
- Edwards JL. Diagnosis and management of benign prostatic hyperplasia. *Am Fam Physician.* 2008;77(10):1403–1410.

CODES

ICD10
- N40.0 Enlarged prostate without lower urinary tract symptoms
- N40.1 Enlarged prostate with lower urinary tract symptoms

CLINICAL PEARLS
- Although medical therapy has changed the management of BPH, it has only delayed the need for TURP by 10 to 15 years, not eliminated it.
- Urinary retention, obstructive uropathy, recurrent UTIs, elevated PSA, bladder calculi, hematuria, and failure of medical therapy are indications for surgical management of BPH.

PROSTATITIS

Robert Bonanno, MD • Mark Micolucci, MD

 BASICS

DESCRIPTION

- Painful or inflammatory condition affecting the prostate gland with or without bacterial etiology, often characterized by urogenital pain, voiding symptoms, and/or sexual dysfunction
- Significant impact on quality of life
- <10% bacteria-proven infection
- National Institutes of Health's (NIH) classification
  - *Class I: acute bacterial prostatitis*: symptomatic with fever, perineal pain, dysuria, and obstructive symptoms; polymorphonuclear leukocytes (PMNL) and bacteria in urine
  - *Class II: chronic bacterial prostatitis*: symptomatic chronic or recurrent bacterial infection with pain and voiding disturbances; PMNL and bacteria in expressed prostatic secretions (EPS), or urine after prostate massage, or in semen
  - *Class III: chronic prostatitis/chronic pelvic pain syndrome* (CP/CPPS)
    - Inflammatory (subtype IIIA): chronic symptoms with PMNL in EPS/urine after prostate massage or in semen
    - Noninflammatory (subtype IIIB): chronic symptoms without presence of PMNL in EPS/urine after prostate massage or in semen
  - *Class IV*: asymptomatic *inflammatory prostatitis*: incidental finding during prostate biopsy; presence of PMNL and/or bacteria in EPS/urine after prostatic massage or in semen
- System(s) affected: genitourinary, renal, reproductive

EPIDEMIOLOGY

Incidence
- 2 million cases annually in the United States
- Bimodal peak 20 to 40 and >60 years old
- Chronic is more common in those >50 years.
- Bacterial prostatitis more frequently in HIV.

Prevalence
- Affects approximately 8.2% of males
- Lifetime probability of diagnosis >25%
- Accounts for 8% of visits to urologists and 1% of visits to primary care physicians
- Percentage of cases by class: class I: <1%, class II: 5–10%, class III: 80–90%, class IV: 10%

ETIOLOGY AND PATHOPHYSIOLOGY

- Acute bacterial prostatitis (NIH class I)
  - Likely, etiology from ascending urethral infection with intraprostatic reflux of infected urine into prostatic ducts, often associated with cystitis
  - Can occur after instrumentation of prostate
  - Usually, gram-negative bacteria (*Escherichia coli* [most common]; *Proteus, Klebsiella, Serratia,* and *Enterobacter* species; *Pseudomonas aeruginosa*)
  - Rarely, gram-positive bacteria (*Staphylococcus aureus, Streptococcus,* and *Enterococcus* species)
  - Confirmed staphylococcal prostatitis should warrant evaluation for hematogenous spread, including endovascular source.
  - Atypical bacteria include *Chlamydia trachomatis, Trichomonas vaginalis, Ureaplasma urealyticum, Mycobacterium tuberculosis,* and fungal etiologies in immunocompromised hosts.
  - Consider *Neisseria gonorrhoeae* or *C. trachomatis* in sexually active men <35 years.
- Chronic bacterial prostatitis (NIH class II)
  - Similar pathogens possibly higher rate of gram-positive bacteria than in acute prostatitis
  - Often as recurrent episodes of same organism

- Progression from acute to CP is poorly understood but could result from inadequate treatment of acute prostatitis.
- CP/CPPS (NIH class III)
  - Unclear etiology with no current data to support an infectious cause
  - Inciting agent may cause inflammation or neurologic damage around prostate and leads to pelvic floor neuromuscular and/or neuropathic pain.
  - No correlation between histologic inflammation of prostate and presence or absence of symptoms
  - Patients with chronic inflammation on histology have shorter time to symptomatic progression.

RISK FACTORS
- Urinary tract infections (including sexually transmitted infections [STIs])
- HIV infection
- Prostatic calculi
- Urethral stricture
- Urinary catheterization: indwelling, intermittent
- Genitourinary instrumentation, including prostate biopsy (especially in patients with prior quinolone intake), transurethral resection of the prostate (TURP), cystoscopy
- Urinary retention
- Benign prostatic hypertrophy
- Unprotected sexual intercourse
- Prostate cancer

GENERAL PREVENTION
Antibiotic prophylaxis for genitourinary instrumentation and prostatic biopsy

COMMONLY ASSOCIATED CONDITIONS
- Benign prostatic hypertrophy
- Cystitis
- Urethritis
- Sexual dysfunction, including erectile dysfunction and premature ejaculation

 DIAGNOSIS

HISTORY
- Acute prostatitis (class I):
  - Acutely ill with fever, chills, malaise
  - Low back pain, myalgias
  - Nausea, vomiting
  - Frequency, urgency, dysuria, nocturia
  - Prostatodynia, pelvic pain, perineal pain
  - Cloudy urine
  - Obstructive voiding symptoms: poor stream, hesitancy, retention, urge incontinence
  - Recent prostate instrumentation
- CP (classes II and III) (symptoms vary from patient to patient and may include the following):
  - More insidious presentation than class I
  - Symptoms for 3 of 6 previous months
  - High caffeine and alcohol intake
  - Low-grade fever (class II only)
  - Prostatodynia, perineal pain
  - Dysuria, frequency, urgency
  - Lower abdominal pain
  - Low back, testicular, and/or penile pain
  - Hematospermia
  - Sexual dysfunction/painful ejaculation

PHYSICAL EXAM
- Vital signs (Unstable vitals suggest sepsis.)
- Back exam (CVA tenderness)
- Abdominal exam (bladder distension)

- Prostate exam
  - NIH class I: acute bacterial prostatitis: Prostate is very tender, warm, firm, and edematous.
  - NIH class II: chronic bacterial prostatitis: Prostate is often normal but enlarged, tender, edematous, nodular prostate also encountered.
  - NIH class III: CP/CPPS: often normal prostate

ALERT
Avoid vigorous massage of the prostate in acute bacterial prostatitis; may induce iatrogenic bacteremia; safe if done gently

DIFFERENTIAL DIAGNOSIS
- Lower urinary tract infection
- Pyelonephritis
- Cystitis (bacterial, interstitial)
- Urethritis
- Epididymitis
- Proctitis
- Prostatic abscess
- Acute/chronic urinary retention
- Benign prostatic hypertrophy or malignancy (prostate, bladder)
- Obstructive calculi
- Foreign body

DIAGNOSTIC TESTS & INTERPRETATION

Initial Tests (lab, imaging)
- Suspected acute prostatitis (NIH class I)
  - Urinalysis, urine culture and sensitivity (1)[A]
  - Complete blood count with differential, blood culture if immunocompromised or signs of SIRS/sepsis are present
  - Prostate-specific antigen (PSA) is not recommended unless specific indications.
  - Imaging is optional (1)[A] and used as indicated to rule out complications, for example, transrectal prostatic ultrasound [TRUS] or CT scan of abdomen to rule out abscess, pelvic ultrasound (US)/ bladder scan if symptoms of urinary retention. Initial imaging of prostate is not recommended.
  - STI testing (higher risk in men <35 or >35 years old with risky risk sexual behavior)
- Suspected chronic bacterial prostatitis (NIH class II)
  - Microbiologic localization cultures of lower urinary tract 4- or 2-glass test (pre- and postmassage urine culture)
  - Semen cultures are not recommended.
  - TRUS is not recommended.
  - Urodynamics studies are optional and could help to document obstruction/bladder problems.
- Suspected CP/CPPS (NIH class III)
  - Diagnosis of exclusion (especially to rule out urinary tract infection/STI with history/physical exam and appropriate laboratory investigation if indicated)
  - Administration of NIH Chronic Prostatitis Symptom Index (NIH-CPSI): nine-question symptom survey (http://www.prostatitis.org/symptomindex.html) is useful for symptom evaluation (not diagnosis) at diagnosis and with ongoing treatment.
  - 4- or 2-glass test pre- and postmassage test with urine microscopy considered optional (prostatic massage rarely and anecdotally associated with sepsis; proceed with caution.)
  - Urodynamic studies are optional and could be helpful to investigate obstructive symptoms.
  - Semen cultures are not recommended.
  - Cystoscopy may be indicated for select patients (i.e., with hematuria or obstructive symptoms refractory to treatment).

– TRUS is not recommended.
– Serum PSA levels not recommended unless specific indications (e.g., abnormal DRE, >45 years, family history of prostate cancer or risk factors)
– Psychological assessment
– If hematuria present: urine cytology, cystoscopy, CT urography with or without contrast
– Urethral symptoms (dysuria, discharge, penile pain): urethral swab
– Concomitant abdominal pain: CT scan
– Testicular pain: scrotal US
– Lumbar radiculopathy: MRI of spine

Follow-Up Tests & Special Considerations
- Failure to respond to initial antibiotic therapy: US, CT scan, or MRI to image prostate and urology referral
- TRUS, CT scan, or MRI if prostatic calculi, malignancy, or abscess is suspected.
- Acute bacterial: Repeat urinalysis and/or culture if symptoms persist after appropriate course of treatment. Consider repeating urine culture 7 days after antibiotic therapy to ensure resolution of infection.

Diagnostic Procedures/Other
- Needle biopsy or aspiration for culture
- Urodynamic testing if obstructive symptoms present
- Cystoscopy (to investigate for bladder cancer, interstitial cystitis if hematuria, or obstructive symptoms refractory to treatment present)

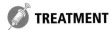

TREATMENT

GENERAL MEASURES
- NSAIDs for analgesia
- α_1-Blockers for lower urinary tract symptoms (obstructive/voiding symptoms)
- Antipyretics/stool softeners
- Hydration
- Sitz baths to relieve pain and spasm
- Urinary drainage for urine retention
- Anxiolytics, antidepressants if indicated

MEDICATION

First Line
- Acute bacterial NIH class I (outpatient)
  – Antimicrobial therapy is recommended (1).
  – Fluoroquinolones are preferred first-line agents.
    ○ Fluoroquinolones: ciprofloxacin 500 mg PO q12h or levofloxacin 500 to 750 mg PO once daily
      ▪ No clinically significant difference between different fluoroquinolones
    ○ Trimethoprim-sulfamethoxazole 160/800 mg PO q12h (Consider local *E. Coli* resistance rates.)
  – Duration of therapy is 2 to 4 weeks (up to 4 to 6 weeks recommended by some authorities).
  – If at risk for STI ceftriaxone 250 mg IM for 1 dose (or cefixime 400 mg PO 1 dose) plus azithromycin 1 g PO for 1 dose or doxycycline 100 mg PO q12h for 10 days
  – α_1-Blockers for symptomatic relief of lower urinary tract symptoms and NSAIDs for analgesia
- Acute bacterial NIH class I (inpatient) (1)
  – Urinary drainage (indwelling, intermittent, or suprapubic catheterization)
  – Obtain both blood and urine cultures.
  – Initial broad-spectrum IV antibiotic therapy in acutely ill patients:
    ○ IV fluoroquinolone + aminoglycoside (ciprofloxacin 400 mg IV q12h or levofloxacin 500 to 750 mg IV q24h + gentamycin 5 mg/kg IV daily) with or without a broad penicillin

(ampicillin 1 to 2 g q4–6h) or 2nd-/3rd-generation cephalosporin (cefuroxime IV 1.5 g q8h ceftriaxone 1 to 2 g IV q24h
    – De-escalate to oral regimen pending blood/urine culture results and with clinical improvement for additional 2 to 4 weeks of therapy.
- Chronic bacterial NIH class II (1)
  – Antimicrobial therapy (1)[A]
  – Fluoroquinolones are preferred first-line agents (ciprofloxacin 500 mg PO q12h or levofloxacin 500 to 750 mg PO daily for 4 to 6 weeks) or trimethoprim-sulfamethoxazole (160/800 mg PO q12h for 8 to 12 weeks).
    ○ No clinically significant difference between different fluoroquinolones
  – If gram-positive bacteria (*Enterococcus faecalis*) and failed ciprofloxacin or levofloxacin, consider moxifloxacin 400 mg PO once daily or linezolid 600 mg PO q12h.
  – Therapy with macrolide (azithromycin) has higher clinical improvement and eradication rates than ciprofloxacin for chlamydial prostatitis.
  – Refractory cases: can consider intermittent antimicrobial treatment of acute symptomatic episodes (cystitis), low-dose antimicrobial suppression, radical TURP, or open prostatectomy if all options failed
  – α-Blockers combined with antimicrobial therapy reduce the high recurrence rate and are optimal for patients with obstructive symptoms.
- CP/CPPS NIH class III
  – Unclear source of disease so limited evidence on effective treatment
  – Treatment choice is patient-centered, focusing on symptoms relief of four domains: pain, lower urinary tract symptoms, psychological stress, and sexual dysfunction.
  – Empiric trial of eliminating caffeine and alcohol
  – α_1-Blockers (tamsulosin 0.4 mg PO daily) can be beneficial, especially in men with lower urinary tract symptoms; however, studies do not show statistically significant differences.
  – Fluoroquinolones (ciprofloxacin 500 mg PO BID) may help for symptoms in patients but studies do not show it is statistically significant.
  – NSAIDs can help with symptoms.

ISSUES FOR REFERRAL
Urology referral if antibiotic treatment fails, symptoms persist (especially obstructive voiding symptoms), hematuria, elevated PSA; or for surgical drainage if an abscess persists after ≥1 week of therapy

ADDITIONAL THERAPIES
- Psychotherapy (ideally including cognitive-behavioral therapy [CBT]) in cases of psychosocial stressors or sexual dysfunction
- Pudendal nerve block or neurolysis beneficial if secondary to pudendal nerve entrapment.

SURGERY/OTHER PROCEDURES
Surgical resection may be considered for refractory cases of recurrent bacterial prostatitis or to drain an abscess. For CP/CPPS class III, procedures such as balloon dilation, neodymium: YAG laser, transurethral needle ablation, microwave hyperthermia, thermotherapy are not recommended at this time (1)[A]. For CP/CPPS class III, radical transurethral resection or total prostatectomy is not recommended.

COMPLEMENTARY & ALTERNATIVE MEDICINE
CP/CPPS class III: Acupuncture and extracorporeal shockwave therapy have best evidence of decrease in prostatitis symptoms without adverse effects.

ADMISSION, INPATIENT, AND NURSING CONSIDERATIONS
- Sepsis
- PO intolerance
- Urinary retention
- Proven or suspected abscess
- Risk factors for resistance (recent prostatic instrumentation or recent fluoroquinolone use)
- Immunocompromised

 ## ONGOING CARE

FOLLOW-UP RECOMMENDATIONS
- Negative urine culture at 7 days predictive of cure after completion of treatment course
- Consider prostatic abscess in patients who do not respond well to therapy.

Patient Monitoring
NIH-CPSI: nine questions, which can be used to evaluate severity of patient symptoms and response to treatment within three domains:
- Pain
- Urinary symptoms
- Quality of life

PROGNOSIS
- Fever and dysuria usually resolve in 2 to 6 days.
- Acute infection usually improves in 3 to 4 weeks.
- Course of CP is often prolonged; 55–97% cure rate depending on population and drug used
- 20% have reinfection or persistent infection.
- 10% with acute bacterial prostatitis may progress to CP.

COMPLICATIONS
- Prostatic abscess (common in HIV infected)
- Pyelonephritis
- Gram-negative sepsis, bacteremia
- Urinary retention
- Epididymitis
- Infertility
- Chronic bacterial prostatitis (following acute prostatitis)
- Metastatic infection (spinal, sacroiliac)
- Erectile dysfunction

REFERENCE
1. Gill BC, Shoskes DA. Bacterial prostatitis. *Curr Opin Infect Dis*. 2016;29(1):86–91.

 ## SEE ALSO

- Prostate Cancer; Prostatic Hyperplasia, Benign (BPH); Urinary Tract Infection (UTI) in Males
- Algorithm: Hematuria

 ## CODES

ICD10
- N41.8 Other inflammatory diseases of prostate
- N41 Inflammatory diseases of prostate
- N41.4 Granulomatous prostatitis

CLINICAL PEARLS
- Prostatic massage is contraindicated in acute prostatitis.
- Fluoroquinolones are recommended first-line antibiotic for bacterial prostatitis.
- At least 14 to 30 days of antibiotic therapy is required for acute prostatitis; longer for chronic bacterial prostatitis

PROTEIN C DEFICIENCY

Shilpa Das, DO, MS • Kyle J. Fletke, MD

 BASICS

A rare heritable disorder or acquired risk factor causing increased risk of blood clots due to decreased anticoagulation. Symptoms range from asymptomatic presentation to recurrent venous thromboembolism (VTE), life-threatening neonatal purpura fulminans, or severe disseminated intravascular coagulation (DIC).

DESCRIPTION
- Protein C is a vitamin K–dependent anticoagulant protein synthesized, in an inactive form, by the liver.
- Activated protein C (APC) inhibits generation of thrombin by inactivating factors Va and VIIIa, using protein S as a cofactor.
- Deficiency in protein C activity therefore leads to a prothrombotic state.
- System(s) affected: cardiovascular, pulmonary, integumentary, hematologic, and immunologic

EPIDEMIOLOGY
Incidence
The estimated incidence is between 1 in 200 and 1 in 500. Clinically substantial protein C deficiency (PCD) estimated to be 1 in 20,000. Severe PCD is rare, predicted in 1 in 4 million infants.

Prevalence
- 0.3% of the general population
- 3–5% of persons with VTE
- Mean age of first thrombosis is 45 years.
- There is no known gender predominance.

ETIOLOGY AND PATHOPHYSIOLOGY
- PCD can be inherited or acquired.
- Genetic mutations can lead to two types of PCD; however, the distinction between the two is clinically irrelevant.
  - Type I (most common) results in the reduction of protein C levels.
  - Type II results in a decreased functionality, despite having normal levels of protein C.
- Acquired PCD is more common and can occur in many disease states such as:
  - Liver disease
  - DIC
  - Severe infections (especially meningococcemia)
  - Autoantibody inhibitors directed toward protein C
  - Cancer and chemotherapy (i.e., L-asparaginase, 5-FU, methotrexate, and cyclophosphamide)
  - Initial use of vitamin K antagonists (warfarin)
  - Vitamin K deficiency (malnutrition or malabsorption of fat-soluble vitamins)
- Heterozygous PCD and mild deficiency can cause a wide range of symptom severity from asymptomatic to recurrent thromboses.
  - There is an increased risk of DVT, PE, and sequelae such as ischemic arterial stroke and pregnancy-associated thrombosis.

Genetics
- Autosomal dominant inheritance pattern with incomplete penetrance
- At least 270 genetic mutations have been described in the protein C (PROC) gene that can lead to a functional deficiency.
- Heterozygous patients often have mild or asymptomatic disease.

- Homozygous patients, or those with another coexisting genetic thrombophilia, often have more severe disease.
- Additionally, mutations in other genes (GCKR, EDEM2, BAZ1B, etc.) are associated with variability in the levels of protein C expression in the general population, although their clinical significance is currently unknown.
- Patients with PCD who start warfarin without concomitant heparin are at increased risk of developing warfarin-induced skin necrosis (WISN). This is thought to be due to the shorter half-life of protein C (5 to 8 hours) compared to other vitamin K–dependent clotting factors. However, not all patients who develop WISN have PCD.

ALERT
The prevention of warfarin necrosis has been achieved by avoiding loading doses of warfarin and the use of heparin bridging. Screening all patients for inherited or acquired forms of PCD prior to initiating warfarin is not cost-effective nor prognostic because many patients with documented deficiency do not progress to WISN.

RISK FACTORS
Acquired conditions such as heart failure, severe liver disease, DIC and vitamin K antagonists.

GENERAL PREVENTION
Because PCD is usually a congenital disease, there are no preventive measures.

COMMONLY ASSOCIATED CONDITIONS
- VTE at any site, often spontaneous
- Arterial thrombosis is rare, and a causative relationship has not been clearly demonstrated.
- Homozygosity can be associated with catastrophic thrombotic complications at birth (e.g., *purpura fulminans*).
- Recurrent pregnancy losses

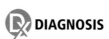 **DIAGNOSIS**

Can be suspected with increased history as noted below

HISTORY
- Recurrent VTE
- VTE at <40 years of age
- Thrombosis in unusual locations (e.g., mesentery, sagittal sinus, portal vein)
- Thrombosis at a young age (<50 years)
- Family history of thrombosis, spontaneous abortion, or WISN

PHYSICAL EXAM
Normal

DIFFERENTIAL DIAGNOSIS
- Factor V Leiden
- Protein S deficiency
- Antithrombin deficiency

- Dysfibrinogenemia
- Dysplasminogenemia
- Hyperhomocysteinemia
- Prothrombin 20210 mutation
- Elevated factor VIII, IX, or XI levels
- Antiphospholipid antibody syndrome
- DIC
- Heparin-induced thrombocytopenia (HIT)

DIAGNOSTIC TESTS & INTERPRETATION
PCD can be diagnosed using clotting assays, ELISA, and chromogenic tests to assess protein C levels. PROC gene mutational analysis is also available.

Initial Tests (lab, imaging)
- Initial evaluation of a new clot in patients should include a CBC with peripheral smear, INR, aPTT, hepatic and renal function tests, as well as appropriate imaging.
- Testing for heritable causes of thrombophilia in unselected patients presenting with a first-time VTE (provoked or unprovoked) is not indicated (1).
- Consider screening for antiphospholipid syndrome rather than other thrombophilia (PCD) for women with recurrent early pregnancy loss (three loses prior to 10 weeks' gestation) (2)[B].

Follow-Up Tests & Special Considerations
- Testing for heritable or acquired thrombophilia is suggested in the following circumstances:
  - First episode of VTE and patient age <40 years
  - Recurrent VTE regardless of the presence of risk factors
  - Patients with VTE at unusual sites
- Testing for PCD should be considered in patients with history of WISN.
- Testing for protein C and S deficiencies should be done urgently in neonates and children suspected to have purpura fulminans (1).
- Testing for hereditary thrombophilia should only be considered in asymptomatic first-degree relatives of those with proven hereditary thrombophilia if they are female, of childbearing age, and have no history of prior pregnancy complications (2)[C].
- When ordering additional testing for hereditary or acquired thrombophilia, the following conditions should be considered:
  - Antiphospholipid antibody syndrome
  - Antithrombin III deficiency
  - Factor V Leiden
  - PCD
  - Protein S deficiency
  - Prothrombin G20210A

Diagnostic Procedures/Other
Testing for PCD is done using two separate lab tests:
- An immunoassay for a quantitative assessment of protein C levels
- A functional activity assay using a snake venom protease to activate protein C

Test Interpretation
- Drugs that may alter lab results
  - Oral contraceptives can raise protein C levels.
  - Warfarin reduces protein C levels and should be discontinued 2 to 3 weeks before reliable testing.
- Disorders that may alter lab results
  - Liver disease reduces protein C levels.

ALERT
Acute thrombosis can lower protein C levels. Repeat confirmatory test of low protein C level at a separate time is advisable. If a normal level of protein C is obtained at presentation, then deficiency can be excluded.

 TREATMENT

Treat active thrombosis; follow-up

GENERAL MEASURES
- Individuals with PCD should be educated regarding signs and symptoms of VTE.
- Women with any of the following history should avoid estradiol-containing contraceptives and hormone replacement therapy during menopause:
  - Diagnoses of PCD
  - First-degree relative with PCD
  - First-degree relative with VTE at age <50 years
- Women may use progestin-only hormonal contraception options.
- Routine anticoagulation for asymptomatic patients with PCD is not recommended (2)[C].
- Anticoagulation is recommended for at least 3 months in patients with inherited thrombophilia following their first VTE (1).
  - There is some argument for indefinite anticoagulation; however, data are limited.
  - Shared decision-making should be used to discuss duration of therapy beyond 3 months.
- Indefinite anticoagulation is indicated for patients with recurrent VTE (2)[A].
- Treat VTE as an outpatient when possible if clinically stable (2)[B].
- Severe congenital PCD may be treated with protein C concentrates.

Pregnancy Considerations
- Heparin-based products should be used during pregnancy when therapeutic or prophylactic treatment of VTE is needed.
- For pregnant women with known PCD but no personal history of VTE or additional thrombotic risk factors (i.e., family history of VTE in first-degree relative <50 years of age, obesity, prolonged immobility), antepartum and postpartum clinical monitoring is recommended over prophylactic therapy.
- For pregnant women with known PCD, no personal history of VTE but with an additional thrombotic risk factor, antepartum surveillance is recommended with postpartum prophylactic therapy for 6 weeks of either prophylactic or intermediate dose.
- For pregnant women with known PCD and previous VTE, it is recommended to give postpartum preventative therapy with either prophylactic or intermediate-dose LMWH. This could also be given antepartum versus surveillance at the provider's discretion.

MEDICATION
First Line
- LMWH (2)[A]: initially started with warfarin for a minimum of 5 days and two consecutive INRs between 2 and 3 to bridge. Additionally, LMWH may be started 5 to 10 days prior to starting dabigatran or edoxaban.
  - Enoxaparin (Lovenox) 1 mg/kg SC BID or 1.5 mg/kg/day SC
  - Tinzaparin (Innohep): 175 anti-Xa IU/kg/day SC
  - Dalteparin (Fragmin) 200 U/kg/day
- Novel oral anticoagulants (NOACs):
  - Rivaroxaban (Xarelto) 15 mg PO BID with food for 21 days and then 20 mg PO QD with food
  - Apixaban (Eliquis) 10 mg PO BID for 7 days and then 5 mg PO BID
  - Dabigatran (Pradaxa) 150 mg PO BID (after 5 to 10 days of parenteral anticoagulation)
  - Edoxaban (Savaysa) 60 mg PO QD (after 5 to 10 days of parenteral anticoagulation)
- Oral vitamin K antagonist:
  - Warfarin (Coumadin) titrated to an INR of 2 to 3 (2)[A]
- Factor Xa inhibitors:
  - Fondaparinux (Arixtra) <50 kg: 5 mg/day SC; 50 to 100 kg: 7.5 mg/day SC; >100 kg: 10 mg/day SC; contraindicated if CrCl <30 mL/min
- Contraindications
  - Active bleeding
  - Risk of bleeding is a relative contraindication to long-term anticoagulation
- Precautions
  - Observe patient for signs of embolization, further thrombosis, or bleeding.
  - Monitor kidney function, drug–drug interactions, and CBC, including platelets (concern for HIT).

Second Line
- Heparin 80 U/kg IV bolus followed by 18 U/kg/hr; adjust dose depending on PPT.
- In patients requiring large daily doses of heparin, measure an anti-Xa level for dose guidance.
- Alternatively, and for outpatients, unfractionated heparin can be given at 333 U/kg and then 250 U/kg SC, without monitoring (2)[C].
- May be treatable with replacement protein C concentrate. Neonatal purpura fulminans can be controlled with protein C replacement from fresh frozen plasma (FFP).

ISSUES FOR REFERRAL
Patients with suspected PCD should be referred to a hematologist.

SURGERY/OTHER PROCEDURES
- Anticoagulation may be held for surgical interventions.
- In patients with acute proximal DVT of the lower extremity *and* an absolute contraindication to anticoagulation, inferior vena cava (IVC) filters are recommended; otherwise, the use of an IVC filter in addition to anticoagulants is not recommended (2)[B].

ADMISSION, INPATIENT, AND NURSING CONSIDERATIONS
- Life-threatening VTE
- Significant bleeding while on anticoagulant therapy

 ONGOING CARE

FOLLOW-UP RECOMMENDATIONS
Patient Monitoring
- Warfarin requires periodic monitoring of the INR to maintain a range of 2 to 3 (monthly, after initial stabilization).
- LMWH is the treatment of choice in pregnancy. Periodic monitoring with anti-Xa levels is recommended in these patients.

DIET
Unrestricted (except if on warfarin—avoid varying diet with foods that have significant amounts of vitamin K)

PATIENT EDUCATION
- Patients should be educated about signs and symptoms of VTE as well as the use of oral anticoagulant therapy if taking such.
- Avoid NSAIDs while on warfarin.
- Avoid OCPs because of increased risk of thrombosis.

PROGNOSIS
When compared with normal individuals, persons with PCD have normal life spans.

COMPLICATIONS
Primary or recurrent VTE

REFERENCES
1. Baglin T, Gray E, Greaves M, et al; and British Committee for Standards in Haematology. Clinical guidelines for testing for heritable thrombophilia. *Br J Haematol*. 2010;149(2):209–220.
2. Guyatt GH, Akl EA, Crowther M, et al; for American College of Chest Physicians Antithrombotic Therapy and Prevention of Thrombosis Panel. Executive summary: Antithrombotic Therapy and Prevention of Thrombosis, 9th ed: American College of Chest Physicians evidence-based clinical practice guidelines. *Chest*. 2012;141(Suppl 2):7S–47S.

 CODES

ICD10
D68.59 Other primary thrombophilia

CLINICAL PEARLS
- Screening of asymptomatic family members is not justified with the possible exception of females of childbearing age with no previous history of pregnancy complications.
- Asymptomatic patients with PCD do not need prophylactic anticoagulation because the risk of thrombosis is low.
- Patients with PCD presenting with first-time VTE should be anticoagulated for at least 3 months. Other risk factors and shared decision-making should be used to determine if anticoagulation should be used for a longer duration.
- Recurrent VTE is an indication for indefinite anticoagulation.

PROTEIN S DEFICIENCY

Boris Calderon, DO

BASICS

DESCRIPTION

- Protein S is a vitamin K–dependent glycoprotein, produced mainly in the liver that acts as a cofactor for protein C. It is also produced by megakaryocytes and endothelial cells.
- Protein C becomes activated when thrombin binds to the endothelial receptor, thrombomodulin.
- Activated protein C, with protein S (a cofactor), inactivates clotting factors Va and VIIIa enhancing fibrinolysis.
- Protein S is also able to directly inhibit factors Va, VIIa, and Xa independently of activated protein C.
- Protein S deficiency is a congenital thrombophilia, which increases the risk of thromboembolism.
- It primarily affects the venous system.
- System(s) affected: cardiovascular; hematologic/immunologic; pulmonary

EPIDEMIOLOGY

Incidence
- Mean age of first thrombosis: 2nd decade
- Predominant sex: male = female

Prevalence
- ~0.2% of general population
- Found in ~1% of persons with venous thrombosis embolism (VTE)

ETIOLOGY AND PATHOPHYSIOLOGY

- It is an autosomal dominant disease.
- Only the free form of protein S (30–40%) acts as a cofactor for activated protein C. Protein S reversibly binds to the C4b protein, which leads to conditions in which free protein S is low but total protein S is normal. These individuals are prone to thrombosis.
- Conditions with reduced protein S: pregnancy, disseminated intravascular coagulation (DIC), liver disease, nephrotic syndrome, HIV, acute thrombosis, and acute varicella-zoster virus infection
- Drugs: oral contraceptives, warfarin, and L-asparaginase chemotherapy

Genetics
- Is due to mutations in the PROS1 gene on chromosome 3. Most individuals are heterozygous.
- Heterozygotes have an odds ratio (OR) of VTE of 1.6 to 11.5.
- Homozygosity or compound heterozygosity, if untreated, is usually incompatible with adult life.
- Homozygotes can have a fulminant thrombotic event in infancy, termed *neonatal purpura fulminans*.

RISK FACTORS

- Oral contraceptives, pregnancy, and the use of hormone replacement therapy (HRT) increase the risk of VTE in patients with protein S deficiency (1)[A].
- Patients with protein S deficiency and other prothrombotic states have further increased rate of thrombosis (1)[A].
- Arterial thrombosis is more frequent in patients with protein S deficiency who smoke.

- Patients heterozygous for protein S deficiency who are initiated on warfarin without concomitant heparin can develop warfarin-induced skin necrosis because the half-life of other vitamin K–dependent clotting factors (e.g., prothrombin, factor IX, and factor X) is much longer than the anticoagulant protein S (4 to 8 hours), leading to a transient hypercoagulable state when protein S becomes depleted. These patients develop extremely low levels of protein S and develop necrosis of the skin over central areas of the body such as the breast, abdomen, buttocks, and genitalia (1)[A].

Pregnancy Considerations
Increased thrombotic risk and pregnancy losses

GENERAL PREVENTION
There are no preventive measures.

COMMONLY ASSOCIATED CONDITIONS

- Deep and superficial VTE, often unprovoked
- Up to 50% of homozygotes will have thrombosis.
- Homozygosity is associated with catastrophic thrombotic complications at birth: *neonatal purpura fulminans*.
- Sites of thrombosis can be unusual, including the mesentery, cerebral veins, and axillary veins.
- Arterial thrombosis is rare but reported in several case reports.
- Skin necrosis in patients treated with warfarin
- Recurrent pregnancy losses (2)

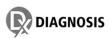

DIAGNOSIS

HISTORY
Inherited thrombophilias should be suspected in:

- Unprovoked VTE at age <50 years
- VTE with a strong family history of VTE or known familial protein S deficiency
- VTE in unusual sites as mesenteric or cerebral vein
- Recurrent VTE

PHYSICAL EXAM
Normal

DIFFERENTIAL DIAGNOSIS
Other inherited thrombophilias:

- Factor V Leiden (most common; usually in Caucasians)
- Protein C deficiency (in Caucasians)
- Antithrombin deficiency
- Dysfibrinogenemia
- Dysplasminogenemia
- Homocystinemia
- Prothrombin G20210A mutation
- Elevated factor VIII levels
- Acquired VTE risk factors: surgery, immobility, cancer, myeloproliferative neoplasms, trauma, antiphospholipid syndrome, paroxysmal nocturnal hemoglobinuria, pregnancy, HRT, postpartum, DIC

DIAGNOSTIC TESTS & INTERPRETATION
Initial Tests (lab, imaging)

- For evaluation of new clot in a patient at risk: CBC with peripheral smear, PT/INR, aPTT, thrombin time, lupus anticoagulant, antiphospholipid antibodies, anticardiolipin antibody, anti-β_2-glycoprotein I antibody, activated protein C resistance, protein S antigen and resistance, antithrombin III assay, fibrinogen, factor V Leiden, prothrombin G20210A
- Immunoassay for quantitative assessment of total and free protein S levels
- Protein S activity assay (mainly after obtaining activated protein C resistance)
- Disorders that may alter lab results: acute thrombosis, vitamin K antagonists (VKA), any acute illness response, liver disease, and pregnancy-reduce protein S levels. Direct oral anticoagulants affect protein S activity assay.
- Heparin and low-weight heparin do not alter lab results.
- Total protein S levels are markedly decreased in newborns and young infants; use age-adjusted norms.

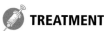

TREATMENT

GENERAL MEASURES

- Routine anticoagulation for asymptomatic patients with protein S deficiency is not recommended.
- Antithrombotic therapy recommendations for patients with protein S deficiency can be guided by antithrombotic therapy for VTE disease guidelines.
- Patients with unprovoked VTE and who have a low or moderate bleeding risk are suggested to receive extended anticoagulant therapy (no scheduled stop date) over 3 months of therapy (1)[B],(3), and those who have a high bleeding risk are recommended to receive 3 months of anticoagulant therapy (3),(4)[B].
- Patients with a second unprovoked VTE and who have a low to moderate bleeding risk are recommended to receive extended anticoagulant therapy over 3 months (3),(4)[B]; those who have high bleeding risk are suggested to receive 3 months of anticoagulant therapy (1)[B],(3).
- Patients with VTE and no history of cancer are suggested to receive dabigatran, rivaroxaban, apixaban, or edoxaban over VKA therapy as long-term (first 3 months) anticoagulant therapy; VKA therapy over low-molecular-weight heparin (LMWH) (3)
- Patients with VTE and active cancer are suggested to receive LMWH, rivaroxaban, or edoxaban for long-term anticoagulation (5). It is recommended that these patients receive extended anticoagulant therapy (3).
- Treatment of thrombosis with LMWH is recommended over unfractionated heparin, unless the patient has severe renal failure.
- Treat as outpatient, if possible.
- Prophylaxis should be considered in risk situations such us surgery, immobility or postpartum, especially in patients with family history.

- The role of family screening for protein S deficiency is unclear because most patients with this mutation do not have thrombosis. Screening should be considered for women considering oral contraceptives or pregnancy and who have a family history of protein S deficiency (6)[B].

MEDICATION
- LMWH
  - Enoxaparin (Lovenox) 1 mg/kg SC BID
    ○ Alternatively, 1.5 mg/kg/day SC
  - Tinzaparin (Innohep) 175 anti-Xa U/kg/day SC
  - Dalteparin (Fragmin) 200 U/kg/day SC divided QD–BID
- Factor Xa inhibitor
  - Fondaparinux (Arixtra) <50 kg: 5 mg/day SC; 50 to 100 kg: 7.5 mg/day SC; >100 kg: 10 mg/day SC; contraindicated if CrCl <30 mL/min
- Dual oral anticoagulants (DOACs)
  - Dabigatran 150 mg PO BID (after 5 to 10 days of parenteral anticoagulation)
  - Rivaroxaban 15 mg PO BID for 21 days and then 20 mg PO QD
  - Apixaban 10 mg PO BID for 7 days and then 5 mg PO BID
  - Edoxaban: person weighs ≤60 kg: 30 mg PO QD OR >60 kg: 60 mg PO QD (after 5 to 10 days of parenteral anticoagulation)
- Oral anticoagulant: warfarin (Coumadin): 2 to 5 mg PO QD then adjusted to an INR of 2 to 3. LMWH initially for a minimum of 5 days and two consecutive INRs between 2 and 3, at which time it can be stopped; contraindications
  - Active bleeding precludes anticoagulation; risk of bleeding is a relative contraindication to long-term anticoagulation.
  - Warfarin is contraindicated in patients with a prior history of warfarin-induced skin necrosis.
- Precautions
  - Observe patient for signs of embolization, further thrombosis, or bleeding.
  - Avoid IM injections.
  - Periodically, check stool and urine for occult blood; monitor CBC, including platelets.
  - Heparin: thrombocytopenia and/or paradoxical thrombosis with thrombocytopenia
  - Warfarin: necrotic skin lesions (typically breasts, thighs, and buttocks)
  - LMWH: Adjust dose in renal insufficiency.
- Significant possible interactions
  - Agents that intensify the response to oral anticoagulants: ethanol, allopurinol, amiodarone, anabolic steroids, androgens, many antimicrobials, cimetidine, chloral hydrate, disulfiram, NSAIDs, sulfinpyrazone, tamoxifen, levothyroxine, vitamin E, ranitidine, salicylates, and acetaminophen
  - Agents that diminish the response to oral anticoagulants: aminoglutethimide, antacids, barbiturates, carbamazepine, cholestyramine, diuretics, griseofulvin, rifampin, and oral contraceptives

ISSUES FOR REFERRAL
- Patients with suspected protein S deficiency should be seen by a hematologist.
- Screening and prophylactic treatment of asymptomatic family members is not justified (7).

SURGERY/OTHER PROCEDURES
- Anticoagulation must be held for surgical interventions.
- For most patients with DVT, recommendations are against routine use of vena cava filter in addition to anticoagulation. IVC filter is only recommended in case of contraindication to anticoagulation (3)[A].

COMPLEMENTARY & ALTERNATIVE MEDICINE
Diet modifications if taking VKA

ADMISSION, INPATIENT, AND NURSING CONSIDERATIONS
- Life-threatening VTE
- Significant bleeding while on anticoagulant therapy
- Look for signs of bleeding while on anticoagulation therapy.

 ONGOING CARE

FOLLOW-UP RECOMMENDATIONS
Patient Monitoring
- Warfarin requires periodic (monthly after initial stabilization) monitoring of the INR.
- Periodic measurement of INR to maintain a range of 2 to 3
- LMWH is the treatment of choice in pregnancy. Periodic monitoring with anti-Xa levels is recommended in some cases, such as overweight and borderline renal failure.

DIET
Unrestricted, unless taking VKA

PATIENT EDUCATION
- Patients should be educated about use of oral anticoagulant therapy if taking such.
- Patients undergoing warfarin therapy should avoid drinking alcohol on a daily basis.
- Avoid NSAIDs while on warfarin.

PROGNOSIS
- Persons with protein S deficiency have normal lifespan.
- By age 45 years, 50% of the people heterozygous for protein S deficiency will have VT; half will be spontaneous.

COMPLICATIONS
Recurrent thrombosis (requires indefinite anticoagulation)

REFERENCES
1. Bick RL. Prothrombin G20210A mutation, antithrombin, heparin cofactor II, protein C, and protein S defects. *Hematol Oncol Clin North Am*. 2003;17(1):9–36.
2. Parand A, Zolghadri J, Nezam M, et al. Inherited thrombophilia and recurrent pregnancy loss. *Iran Red Crescent Med J*. 2013;15(12):e13708.
3. Kearon C, Akl EA, Ornelas J, et al. Antithrombotic therapy for VTE disease: CHEST Guideline and Expert Panel Report. *Chest*. 2016;149(2):315–352.
4. Moll S. Thrombophilias—practical implications and testing caveats. *J Thromb Thrombolysis*. 2006;21(1):7–15.
5. Key NS, Khorana AA, Kuderer NM, et al. Venous thromboembolism prophylaxis and treatment in patients with cancer: ASCO clinical practice guideline update. *J Clin Oncol*. 2020;38(5):496–520.
6. Langlois NJ, Wells PS. Risk of venous thromboembolism in relatives of symptomatic probands with thrombophilia: a systematic review. *Thromb Haemost*. 2003;90(1):17–26.
7. Hornsby LB, Armstrong EM, Bellone JM, et al. Thrombophilia screening. *J Pharm Pract*. 2014;27(3):253–259.

ADDITIONAL READING
Ameku K, Higa M. Rivaroxaban treatment for warfarin-refractory thrombosis in a patient with hereditary protein S deficiency. *Case Rep Hematol*. 2018;2018:5217301.

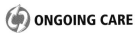 **CODES**

ICD10
D68.59 Other primary thrombophilia

CLINICAL PEARLS
- Asymptomatic patients with protein S deficiency do not require prophylactic anticoagulation because the risk of thrombosis is low; asymptomatic patients do not require anticoagulation.
- Patients with protein S deficiency and DVT should be anticoagulated for at least 6 months, especially if first episode.

PROTEINURIA

Marvin H. Sineath Jr., MD, FAAFP, CAQSM • Algimantas Simpson, MD

BASICS

DESCRIPTION
Urinary protein excretion of >150 mg/day
- Nephrotic-range proteinuria: urinary protein excretion of >3.5 g/day; also called *heavy proteinuria*
- Three pathologic types:
  – Glomerular proteinuria: increased permeability of proteins across glomerular capillary membrane
  – Tubular proteinuria: decreased proximal tubular reabsorption of proteins
  – Overflow proteinuria: increased production of low-molecular-weight proteins

Pediatric Considerations
- Proteinuria: Normal is daily excretion of up to 100 mg/m^2 (body surface area).
- Nephrotic-range proteinuria: daily excretion of >1,000 mg/m^2 (body surface area)

Pregnancy Considerations
- Proteinuria in pregnancy beyond 20 weeks' gestation is a hallmark of preeclampsia/eclampsia and demands further workup.
- Proteinuria in pregnancy before 20 weeks' gestation is suggestive of underlying renal disease.

ETIOLOGY AND PATHOPHYSIOLOGY
- Glomerular proteinuria: increased filtration/larger proteins (albumin) due to the following:
  – Increased size of glomerular basement membrane pores and
  – Loss of proteoglycan negative charge barrier
- Tubular proteinuria: Tubulointerstitial disease prevents proximal tubular reabsorption of smaller proteins (β_2-microglobulin, immunoglobulin [Ig] light chains, retinol-binding protein, amino acids).
- Overflow proteinuria: proximal tubular reabsorption overwhelmed by increased production of smaller proteins
- Glomerular proteinuria
  – Primary glomerulonephropathy
    ○ Minimal change disease
    ○ Idiopathic/primary membranous glomerulonephritis
    ○ Focal segmental glomerulonephritis
    ○ Membranoproliferative glomerulonephritis
    ○ IgA nephropathy
  – Secondary glomerulonephropathy
    ○ Diabetic nephropathy
    ○ Autoimmune/collagen vascular disorders (e.g., lupus nephritis, Goodpasture syndrome)
    ○ Amyloidosis
    ○ Preeclampsia
    ○ Infection (HIV, hepatitis B and C, poststreptococcal, endocarditis, syphilis, malaria)
    ○ Malignancy (GI, lung, lymphoma)
    ○ Renal transplant rejection
    ○ Structural (reflux nephropathy, polycystic kidney disease)
    ○ Drug induced (NSAIDs, penicillamine, lithium, heavy metals, gold, heroin)
- Tubular proteinuria
  – Hypertensive nephrosclerosis
  – Tubulointerstitial disease (uric acid nephropathy, hypersensitivity, interstitial nephritis, Fanconi syndrome, heavy metals, sickle cell disease, NSAIDs, antibiotics)
  – Acute tubular necrosis

- Overflow proteinuria
  – Multiple myeloma (light chains; also tubulotoxic)
  – Hemoglobinuria
  – Myoglobinuria (in rhabdomyolysis)
  – Lysozyme (in acute monocytic leukemia)
- Benign proteinuria
  – Functional (fever, exercise, cold exposure, stress, CHF)
  – Idiopathic transient
  – Orthostasis (postural)

Genetics
No known genetic pattern

RISK FACTORS
- Hypertension
- Diabetes
- Obesity
- Strenuous exercise
- CHF
- UTI
- Fever

GENERAL PREVENTION
Control of weight, BP, and blood glucose reduces the risk of proteinuria.

COMMONLY ASSOCIATED CONDITIONS
- Hypertension (common)
- Diabetes mellitus (DM) (common)
- Preeclampsia (common)
- Multiple myeloma (rare)

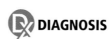

DIAGNOSIS

HISTORY
- Frothy/foamy urine
- Change in urine output
- Blood- or cola-colored urine
- Recent weight change
- Swelling
- Rule out systemic illness: diabetes, heart failure, autoimmune, poststreptococcal infection.

PHYSICAL EXAM
- BP
- Weight
- Peripheral edema
- Periorbital/facial edema
- Ascites
- Palpation of kidneys
- Check lungs, heart for signs of CHF.

DIFFERENTIAL DIAGNOSIS
Includes all causes listed under "Etiology and Pathophysiology"

DIAGNOSTIC TESTS & INTERPRETATION
All adults with CKD risk factors should be screened via serum creatine determination for GFR estimation and analysis of random urine sample for proteinuria (1)[C].

Initial Tests (lab, imaging)
- Urinalysis (UA) quantitatively estimates proteinuria:
  – Only sensitive to albumin; will not detect smaller proteins of overflow/tubular etiologies
  – False-positive finding if urine pH >7, highly concentrated (specific gravity [SG] >1.015), gross hematuria, mucus, semen, leukocytes, iodinated contrast agents, penicillin analogues, sulfonamide metabolites

  – False-negative finding if urine is dilute (SG 1.005), albumin excretion <20 to 30 mg/dL, protein is nonalbumin
  – Sensitivity, 32–46%; specificity, 97–100%
  – Also can perform sulfosalicylic acid test to detect nonalbumin protein
  – Initial timed 24-hour urine test not recommended due to faulty collection and inconvenience to patients (1).
  – Sensitive for heavy proteinuria >300 mg/24 hr (might not detect 30 to 300 mg) (1)
- If UA positive, perform urine microscopy. Refer to nephrologist if positive for signs of glomerular disease.
- If UA shows trace to 2+ protein, rule out transient proteinuria with repeat UA at another visit:
  – More common than persistent proteinuria
  – Causes include exercise, fever, CHF, UTI, and cold exposure.
  – Reassure patient that transient proteinuria is benign and requires no further workup.
- Spot urine protein-to-creatine ratio should be used instead of 24-hour urine collection to confirm nephrotic-range proteinuria (2).
- If initial UA shows 3+ to 4+ protein or repeat UA is positive, measure creatinine clearance and quantify proteinuria with 24-hour urine collection (gold standard) or spot urine protein-to-creatinine (P/C) ratio (acceptable practice) (3)[A]:
  – Numerical P/C ratios correlate with total protein excreted in grams per day (i.e., ratio of 0.2 correlates with 0.2 g during a 24-hour collection).
  – Patients age <30 years with 24-hour urine excretion of <2 g/day and normal creatinine clearance should be tested for orthostatic proteinuria:
    ○ Benign condition is present in 2–5% of adolescents.
    ○ Diagnosed with a normal urine P/C ratio in first morning void and an elevated urine P/C ratio in a second specimen taken after standing for several hours
- If protein excretion >2 g/day, consider nephrology referral and begin workup for systemic/renal disease.
- Patients with persistent proteinuria not explained by orthostatic changes should undergo renal ultrasound to rule out structural abnormalities (e.g., reflux nephropathy, polycystic kidney).

Follow-Up Tests & Special Considerations
Renal/systemic disease workup can include the following:
- CBC, ferritin, ESR, serum iron
- Electrolytes, LFTs
- Lipid profile (ideally, fasting)
- Prothrombin time/international normalized ratio
- Antiphospholipase A2 receptor antibody: positive in ~70% of primary membranous nephropathy
- Antinuclear antibodies: elevated in lupus
- Antistreptolysin O titer: elevated after streptococcal glomerulonephritis
- Complement C3/C4: low in most glomerulonephritis
- HIV, syphilis, and hepatitis serologies: all associated with glomerular proteinuria
- Serum and urine protein electrophoresis: abnormal in multiple myeloma

- Patients with nephrotic-range proteinuria are at increased risk for hypercholesterolemia and thromboembolic events (~25% of adult patients) with highest risk in membranous nephropathy. Optimal duration of prophylactic anticoagulation is unknown but may extend for the duration of the nephrotic state (4).
- Proteinuric pregnant patients beyond 20 weeks' gestation should be examined for other signs/symptoms of preeclampsia (e.g., hypertension, thrombocytopenia, elevated liver transaminases).

 TREATMENT

- BP goal for both diabetic and nondiabetic adults is ≤140/90 mm Hg (5)[C].
- Proteinuria goal is <0.5 g/day (6)[A].
- BP goal of 130/80 mm Hg for patients with normal urinary albumin concentration (1).
- BP goal of 125/75 mm Hg for patients with greater or equal to 1 g/24 hr proteinuria (1).

GENERAL MEASURES
- Limit protein intake to 0.8 g/kg/day in adults with DM or without DM and glomerular filtration rate (GFR) <30 mL/min/1.73 m^2. Soy protein may be renoprotective. Monitor protein intake with 24-hour urine urea excretion (6)[A].
- Limit sodium chloride intake to <2 g/day to optimize antiproteinuric medications (5)[B].
- Effect on BP is further protective (6)[A].
- Limit fluid intake for urine output goal of <2 L/day. Larger urine volumes are associated with increased proteinuria and later GFR decline (6)[B],(7).
- Smoking cessation: Smoking is associated with increased proteinuria and faster kidney disease progression (6)[B].
- Encourage supine posture (up to 50% reduction vs. upright) (6)[B].
- Discourage severe exertion (6)[B].
- Encourage weight loss (6)[B].

MEDICATION
First Line
- Loop diuretics, ACE inhibitors, or ARB use is a conservative management approach with nephrotic syndrome.
- ACE inhibitors: first choice; use maximally tolerated doses; use even if normotensive (6)[A].
- Angiotensin receptor blockers (ARBs): proven antiproteinuric and renoprotective; ARBs are first choice if ACE inhibitors are not tolerated (6)[A].
- Combination ACE inhibitor and ARB should not be used. Although shown to reduce proteinuria, combination does not reduce poor CV outcomes and does increase risk of adverse drug reactions (7),(8)[A],(9)[A].

Second Line
- β-Blockers: antiproteinuric and cardioprotective (6)[A]
- Dihydropyridine calcium channel blockers (DHCCBs): should be avoided unless needed for BP control; not antiproteinuric (6)[A]
- Non-DHCCB: antiproteinuric; may be renoprotective (6)[B]
- Aldosterone antagonists: antiproteinuric independent of BP control (6)[B]
- NSAIDs: antiproteinuric but also nephrotoxic; generally should be avoided (6)[C]

ISSUES FOR REFERRAL
Consider nephrology referral for possible renal biopsy if
- Impaired creatinine clearance
- Nephrotic-range proteinuria
- Unclear etiology

COMPLEMENTARY & ALTERNATIVE MEDICINE
- Corticosteroids: No proven benefit in mortality or need for renal replacement in adults with nephrotic syndrome, although steroids are recommended in some patients who do not respond to conservative treatment. Classically, children with nephrotic syndrome respond better than adults, especially those with minimal change disease (7),(9)[A].
- Corticosteroids and other immunosuppressant drugs: Some benefit with NS. Have significant potential risks. No evidence or guideline that recommends use of these drugs in all patients with nephrotic syndrome (10).
- Estrogen/progesterone replacement: may be renoprotective in premenopausal women but should be avoided in postmenopausal women (6)[B]
- Antioxidant therapy: may be antiproteinuric in diabetic nephropathy (6)[C]
- Sodium bicarbonate: not antiproteinuric but may block tubular injury caused by proteinuria; correcting metabolic acidosis may decrease protein catabolism (6)[C].
- Avoid excessive caffeine consumption: antiproteinuric in diabetic rat models (6)[C].
- Avoid iron overload (6)[C].
- Pentoxifylline: prevents progression of renal disease by unclear mechanisms (6)[C]
- Mycophenolate mofetil: antiproteinuric and renoprotective in animal models (6)[C]

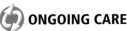 **ONGOING CARE**

FOLLOW-UP RECOMMENDATIONS
Patient Monitoring
All patients with persistent proteinuria should be followed with serial BP checks, UA, and renal function tests in the outpatient setting. Intervals depend on underlying etiology.

PROGNOSIS
- Transient and orthostatic proteinuria are benign conditions that do not convey a poor prognosis.
- Clinical significance of persistent proteinuria varies greatly and depends on underlying etiology.
- Degree of proteinuria is associated with disease progression in chronic kidney disease.
- Independent of GFR, higher levels of proteinuria likely convey an increased risk of mortality, myocardial infarction, and progression to kidney failure.

COMPLICATIONS
- Progression to chronic renal failure and the need for dialysis/renal transplant
- Hypercholesterolemia
- Hypercoagulable state
- Increased risk for infection for patient with nephrotic syndrome
- In nephrotic syndrome, ACIP recommends first dose of PCV13, followed by first dose of PPSV23 ≥8 weeks and then second dose of PPSV23 5 years after the first PPSV.

REFERENCES
1. Gaitonde DY, Cook DL, Rivera IM. Chronic kidney disease: detection and evaluation. *Am Fam Physician*. 2017;96(12):776–783.
2. Hull RP, Goldsmith DJ. Nephrotic syndrome in adults. *BMJ*. 2008;336(7654):1185–1189.
3. National Kidney Foundation. K/DOQI clinical practice guidelines for chronic kidney disease: evaluation classification, and stratification: guideline 5. Assessment of proteinuria. http://www2.kidney.org/professionals/KDOQI/guidelines_ckd/toc.htm. Accessed November 16, 2017.
4. Kerlin BA, Ayoob R, Smoyer WE. Epidemiology and pathophysiology of nephrotic syndrome-associated thromboembolic disease. *Clin J Am Soc Nephrol*. 2012;7(3):513–520.
5. James PA, Oparil S, Carter BL, et al. 2014 Evidence-based guideline for the management of high blood pressure in adults: report from the panel members appointed to the Eighth Joint National Committee (JNC 8). *JAMA*. 2014;311(5):507–520.
6. Wilmer WA, Rovin BH, Hebert CJ, et al. Management of glomerular proteinuria: a commentary. *J Am Soc Nephrol*. 2003;14(12):3217–3232.
7. Kodner C. Diagnosis and management of nephrotic syndrome in adults. *Am Fam Physician*. 2016;93(6):479–485.
8. Fried LF, Emanuele N, Zhang JH, et al; for VA NEPHRON-D Investigators. Combined angiotensin inhibition for the treatment of diabetic nephropathy. *N Engl J Med*. 2013;369(20):1892–1903.
9. Kodner C. Nephrotic syndrome in adults: diagnosis and management. *Am Fam Physician*. 2009;80(10):1129–1134.
10. Chen Y, Schieppati A, Chen X, et al. Immunosuppressive treatment for idiopathic membranous nephropathy in adults with nephrotic syndrome. *Cochrane Database Syst Rev*. 2014;(10):CD004293.

 CODES

ICD10
- R80.9 Proteinuria, unspecified
- R80.2 Orthostatic proteinuria, unspecified
- R80.1 Persistent proteinuria, unspecified

CLINICAL PEARLS
- Transient and orthostatic proteinuria are benign conditions that do not convey a poor prognosis.
- Proteinuria >2 g/day likely represents glomerular malfunction and warrants a nephrology consultation.
- Clinical course varies greatly, but, in general, the degree of proteinuria correlates with kidney disease progression.
- First-line therapy for persistent proteinuric patients is a high-dose ACE inhibitor.

PROTHROMBIN 20210 (MUTATION)

Katyayini Aribindi, MD • Adrian DaSilva-DeAbreu, MD • Raymundo A. Quintana, MD

 BASICS

DESCRIPTION

- The G20210A is a gain of function mutation where adenine is substituted for a guanine at the 20210 noncoding position of the prothrombin (a.k.a. factor II) gene.
- Prothrombin 20210 mutation is the second most common venous thrombophilia after the factor V Leiden mutation.
- The mechanism of increasing the risk of thrombosis is incompletely understood but has been attributed to increased prothrombin or factor II levels in circulation by increased prothrombin protein translation without changing the levels of prothrombin mRNA transcription.
- Autosomal dominant condition, where heterozygotes have a 30% higher prothrombin level and a 3- to 4-fold increased risk of venous thromboembolism (VTE)
- System(s) affected: cardiovascular, hematologic/lymphatic/immunologic, nervous, pulmonary, reproductive, and hepatic
- Synonym(s): prothrombin G20210A mutation; prothrombin G20210A gene polymorphism; prothrombin gene mutation; and FII A^{20210} mutation

EPIDEMIOLOGY

- Found largely in Caucasian population with a prevalence ranging between 1% and 6%, but overall, it is about 2%
- In patients presenting with a VTE, prothrombin 20210 mutation has a prevalence that ranges from 4.6% to 18% with increased prevalence attributed to highly thrombophilic families.
- Mean age of first thrombosis is in the 2nd decade of life.
- Inheritance is similar between both genders (autosomal).

ETIOLOGY AND PATHOPHYSIOLOGY

- Noncoding substitution of adenine for guanine at the 20210 position at the terminal nucleotide of the 3′ resulting in a gain of function of prothrombin gene, leading to increased levels of prothrombin (factor II), by increased translation of prothrombin mRNA but not transcription
- The base change location is in the 3′ terminal nucleotide of the untranslated region associated with the mRNA sequence for polyadenylation. The gain of function is possible due to increased rate of processing, alteration of the site of cleavage, or increased mRNA stability.
- In the coagulation cascade, prothrombin (factor II) is the precursor of thrombin, which cleaves fibrinogen to fibrin. Elevated prothrombin activity leads to elevated thrombin levels and subsequent clot formation.
- The majority of thrombus formation occurs in the venous circulation: deep venous thrombosis (DVT)/PE, mesenteric, and cerebral. Recent studies have shown that prothrombin 20210 mutation did not correlate with Budd-Chiari syndrome or a portal or hepatic vein thrombosis.
- G20210A mutation is not known to be a risk factor for some arterial thrombotic events (myocardial infarction or acute ischemic stroke); however, studies have shown an increased prevalence of the mutation in patients with critical limb ischemia (1).

Genetics

- Caused by the G20210A mutation of the *F2* gene (prothrombin gene) located in the short (p) arm of chromosome 11 that causes a gain of function
- Heterozygotes have a 30% increased levels of prothrombin levels, with a 3- to 4-fold increase of VTE events. Homozygotes are at an even greater risk.
- There are three other prothrombin mutations not related to the G20210A area:
  – Yukuhashi: missense mutation G1787T, arginine for leucine at amino acid 596, leading to prolonged procoagulant activity
  – C20209T: adjacent to G20210A mutation, primarily found in African individuals; newer studies have suggested a possible relationship between this mutation and recurrent pregnancy loss, although it is not fully understood.
  – A19911G: located in the intron of the prothrombin gene; may affect the G20210A mutation by increasing the odds ratio of the venous thromboembolic event. Mechanism is still unknown.

RISK FACTORS

- Being a hereditary condition, the presence of such mutation in the parents poses risk of transmission to offspring.
- Regarding the risk of developing VTE:
  – Patients with both the prothrombin 20210 mutation and factor V Leiden mutation increases the odds ratio of VTE by 20-fold.
  – Virchow triad of thrombogenesis consists of stasis, endothelial injury, and thrombophilia. Any condition that promotes stasis and endothelial injury will consequently increase the risk of VTE, for example, oral contraceptive, pregnancy, malignancy, orthopedic surgery, congestive heart failure, cerebrovascular accident in the past 3 months, air travel, obesity, and smoking.

Pregnancy Considerations

- Increased thrombotic risk in patients with prothrombin 20210 mutation during pregnancy and in the postpartum state is attributed to relative stasis.
- Anticoagulation should begin in the 1st trimester because the risk of VTE increases early in pregnancy and should be discontinued at onset of labor or before scheduled induction/cesarean delivery. Postpartum risk of VTE is usually greater, and anticoagulation can resume 4 to 6 hours after a vaginal delivery or 6 to 12 hours after surgery. Warfarin may begin immediately due to slow onset of action.
- C20209T mutation may have some relation with recurrent pregnancy loss; however, it is not well studied (2).

GENERAL PREVENTION

Asymptomatic individuals with the mutation do not require any prophylactic anticoagulation. Exceptions are generally made for pregnant women with very high-risk thrombophilic mutations (usually factor V Leiden) with a strong family history. After the first VTE, lifelong prophylaxis may be warranted if some features are present: unprovoked or in a nontraditional area like hepatic, portal, mesenteric, or cerebral.

COMMONLY ASSOCIATED CONDITIONS

- VTE
- Factor V Leiden

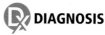 **DIAGNOSIS**

HISTORY

- Previous VTE
- Family history of VTE
- Family history of prothrombin 20210 mutation

PHYSICAL EXAM

- Unilateral swollen, erythematous, and tender calf is significant for a possible DVT.
- Positive Homans sign, sensitivity of 10–54%, specificity of 39–89% for DVT
- Tachycardia is the most common sign of a pulmonary embolism; however, patients may have chest pain and hypotension depending on the severity of the pulmonary embolus.
- A tender abdomen may be indicative of mesenteric veins thrombosis; however, other causes of an acute abdomen should be worked up as appropriate.

DIFFERENTIAL DIAGNOSIS

- Factor V Leiden mutation
- Protein C deficiency
- Protein S deficiency
- Antithrombin deficiency
- Other causes of activated protein C resistance (e.g., antiphospholipid antibodies)
- Dysfibrinogenemia
- Dysplasminogenemia
- Homocystinemia
- Elevated factor VIII levels

DIAGNOSTIC TESTS & INTERPRETATION

Screening for prothrombin G20210A mutation in asymptomatic individuals is not recommended; except for those with very strong family history (3)[B]. Testing can take place in patients with thrombosis at a very early age, recurrent unprovoked VTE, or those with thrombosis in unusual locations.

Initial Tests (lab, imaging)

- This mutation can be diagnosed using PCR with electrophoresis or immunoassays.
- Imaging should be obtained as appropriate for the suspected site of thrombosis: ultrasound with Doppler, computed tomography scan with contrast to evaluate venous phase, and V/Q scan.
- Testing for an inherited thrombophilic condition is reliable during an acute embolic event or with anticoagulation use (4)[A].

Follow-Up Tests & Special Considerations

Although prothrombin levels are elevated, this is not a sensitive test to make the diagnosis.

Diagnostic Procedures/Other

MR angiography (MRA), venography, or arteriography to detect thrombosis

Test Interpretation

Imaging is likely to show presence of arterial or venous thrombus.

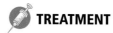 **TREATMENT**

GENERAL MEASURES

Management of patients with a first-time VTE with or without an acquired thrombophilic condition remains overall very similar.

MEDICATION

Is directed to treat those patients with VTE (prophylactic doses may vary). We recommend the reader to check the most updated doses, dose adjustments, and contraindications for the medications listed below. The doses listed apply to most adults.

First Line

In adult patients without cancer, the following oral anticoagulants are preferred over warfarin and low-molecular-weight heparin (LMWH): dabigatran, rivaroxaban, apixaban, or edoxaban are preferred over warfarin (5)[A].

- Apixaban (Eliquis): Initial dose is 10 mg BID for 7 days, followed by 5 mg BID.
- Dabigatran (Pradaxa): requires initial parenteral anticoagulation for 5 to 10 days, followed by 150 mg BID
- Edoxaban (Savaysa): requires initial parenteral anticoagulation for 5 to 10 days, followed by 60 mg daily
- Rivaroxaban (Xarelto): Initial dose is 15 mg BID with food for 21 days, followed by a daily dose of 20 mg with food.

Second Line

For patients without cancer that cannot be treated with DOAC, warfarin is preferred over LMWH (5)[A].

- Warfarin (Coumadin): Initial dose may range from 2 to 10 mg PO daily and then adjusted to an INR of 2 to 3.
- Enoxaparin (Lovenox): 1 mg/kg subcutaneous injection every 12 hours

MEDICATION CONSIDERATIONS

- Contraindications
  - Absolute contraindications: active bleeding, severe bleeding diathesis, planned or recent high bleeding risk surgery or procedure, major trauma, recent or history of intracranial hemorrhage
  - Relative contraindications: recurrent gastrointestinal bleeding, intracranial or spinal tumors, thrombocytopenia with platelets <50,000 (enoxaparin can be dose adjusted depending on severity of thrombocytopenia), large AAA with severe hypertension, recent or emergent low bleeding risk surgery
  - Warfarin: history of warfarin skin necrosis
  - Doses of LMWH and new oral anticoagulants need to be adjusted in patients with renal dysfunction. Rivaroxaban should be avoided in patients with severe renal dysfunction. Apixaban may be relatively safer to use in patients with CKD and has a significantly lower risk of major bleeding or clinically relevant nonmajor bleeding than rivaroxaban or dabigatran (6)[A].
  - Apixaban can be given for DVT prophylaxis as well as at a reduced dose of 2.5 mg PO BID.
- Precautions
  - Observe patient for signs of embolization, further thrombosis, or bleeding.
  - Periodically monitor CBCs.
  - Oral contraceptives are generally avoided in women already known to have the mutation; however, it is not recommended to check for the mutation before starting oral contraceptives in asymptomatic women.
- Complications of medications
  - Heparins: heparin-induced thrombocytopenia
  - Warfarin may cause necrotic skin lesions (typically breasts, thighs, or buttocks).

- Significant possible interactions
  - Agents that increase the effect of some anticoagulants: alcohol, allopurinol, amiodarone, anabolic steroids, androgens, many antimicrobials, cimetidine, chloral hydrate, disulfiram, all NSAIDs, sulfinpyrazone, tamoxifen, thyroid hormone, vitamin E, ranitidine, salicylates, acetaminophen
  - Agents that decrease the effect of some anticoagulants: aminoglutethimide, antacids, barbiturates, carbamazepine, cholestyramine, diuretics, griseofulvin, rifampin, oral contraceptives

ISSUES FOR REFERRAL

- Recurrent thrombosis on anticoagulation
- Difficulty anticoagulating
- Genetic counseling

SURGERY/OTHER PROCEDURES

- Anticoagulation must be held for surgical interventions.
- For most patients with DVT, recommendations are against routine use of vena cava filter in addition to anticoagulation, except in case with contraindication to anticoagulation (5)[A].
- Thrombectomy may be necessary in some cases.

ADMISSION, INPATIENT, AND NURSING CONSIDERATIONS

- Admission criteria/initial stabilization: complicated thrombosis, such as pulmonary embolus; required heparin drip
- Patient can be safely discharged if patient is stable on anticoagulation.

 ONGOING CARE

- Compression stockings for prevention
- DVT prophylaxis as appropriate if patient admitted to hospital

FOLLOW-UP RECOMMENDATIONS

Patient Monitoring

- Warfarin use requires periodic (weekly and then monthly after initial stabilization) INR measurements, with a goal of 2 to 3 (5)[A].
- Heterozygosity for the prothrombin 20210 mutation increases the risk for recurrent VTE only slightly, thus its presence does not alter the length of anticoagulation treatment decision.

DIET

- No restrictions; unless taking warfarin
- Food rich in vitamin K may interfere with warfarin anticoagulation.
- Grapefruit and St. John's wort interfere with the cytochrome P450 and can alter the levels and clearance of anticoagulant therapy.

PATIENT EDUCATION

Patients should be educated about:

- Use of oral anticoagulant therapy
- Signs and symptoms of acute blood loss
- Avoidance of NSAIDs while on warfarin

PROGNOSIS

When compared with normal individuals, persons with prothrombin 20210 have normal lifespans.

COMPLICATIONS

- Recurrent thrombosis on anticoagulation
- Bleeding on anticoagulation
- Complications are usually location dependent and can lead to death, possibly from a massive pulmonary embolism.
- Venous stasis ulcers

REFERENCES

1. Vazquez F, Rodger M, Carrier M, et al. Prothrombin G20210A mutation and lower extremity peripheral arterial disease: a systematic review and meta-analysis. Eur J Vasc Endovasc Surg. 2015;50(2):232–240.
2. Prat M, Morales-Indiano C, Jimenez C, et al. "20209C-T" a variant mutation of prothrombin gene mutation in a patient with recurrent pregnancy loss. Ann Clin Lab Sci. 2014;44(3):334–336.
3. Bucciarelli P, De Stefano V, Passamonti SM, et al. Influence of proband's characteristics on the risk for venous thromboembolism in relatives with factor V Leiden or prothrombin G20210A polymorphisms. Blood. 2013;122(15):2555–2561.
4. Cooper PC, Rezende SM. An overview of methods for detection of factor V Leiden and the prothrombin G20210A mutations. Int J Lab Hematol. 2007;29(3):153–162.
5. Kearon C, Akl EA, Ornelas J, et al. Antithrombotic therapy for VTE disease: CHEST guideline and expert panel report. Chest. 2016;149(2):315–352.
6. Cohen AT, Hamilton M, Mitchell SA, et al. Comparison of the novel oral anticoagulants apixaban, dabigatran, edoxaban, and rivaroxaban in the initial and long-term treatment and prevention of venous thromboembolism: systematic review and network meta-analysis. PLoS One. 2015;10(12):e0144856.

ADDITIONAL READING

- Kearon C, Akl EA. Duration of anticoagulant therapy for deep vein thrombosis and pulmonary embolism. Blood. 2014;123(12):1794–1801.
- Moll S. Thrombophilias—practical implications and testing caveats. J Thromb Thrombolysis. 2006;21(1):7–15.
- Seligsohn U, Lubetsky A. Genetic susceptibility to venous thrombosis. N Engl J Med. 2001;344(16):1222–1231.
- Wells PS, Forgie MA, Rodger MA. Treatment of venous thromboembolism. JAMA. 2014;311(7): 717–728.

 SEE ALSO

Antithrombin Deficiency; Deep Vein Thrombophlebitis; Factor V Leiden; Protein C Deficiency; Protein S Deficiency

 CODES

ICD10

D68.52 Prothrombin gene mutation

CLINICAL PEARLS

- Prothrombin 20210 mutation is the second most common inherited risk factor for VTE after factor V Leiden mutation.
- Asymptomatic patients with prothrombin 20210 mutation do not need anticoagulation or screening.
- Management of VTE is no different with or without the prothrombin G20210A mutation. However, indefinite anticoagulation may be considered in people with an unprovoked VTE or thrombus in a nontraditional area (mesenteric or cerebral).

PRURITUS ANI

Marie L. Borum, MD, EdD, MPH • Faraz A. Sohail, MD

BASICS

DESCRIPTION
- Intense anal/perianal itching and/or burning
- Usually acute (defined as <6 weeks of symptoms)
- Classified as primary (idiopathic) or secondary (25–75% of cases) to anorectal pathology (1)

EPIDEMIOLOGY
Incidence
- 1–5% of the general population (1)
- Predominant age: 30 to 50 years; although seen in all ages groups (1)
- Predominant sex: male > female (4:1) (1)

Prevalence
Difficult to estimate because many patients do not report symptoms; affects 1–5% of the population

ETIOLOGY AND PATHOPHYSIOLOGY
- Multiple etiologies categorized by inflammatory, infectious, systemic, neoplastic, neuropathic, neurogenic, and psychogenic causes (1),(2),(3)
- Most cases are idiopathic (25–90%), which are likely due to trauma from wiping or scratching and perianal fecal contamination (1).
- Pruritus may create an irresistible desire to scratch, leading to a self-perpetuating "itch–scratch–itch" cycle.
- Depending on underlying etiology, itch pathway may be histamine mediated or nonhistamine mediated (2).
- Pruritus ani is typically intensely perceived by the patient due to dense innervation.
- Consider primary pruritus ani when no other demonstrable causes can be found, including:
  – Poor anal hygiene
  – Loose or leaking stool that makes hygiene difficult. Patients with abdominal ostomy bags typically do not complain of pruritus.
  – Internal sphincter laxity
- Etiologies of secondary pruritus ani:
  – Inflammatory dermatologic diseases:
    ○ Allergic contact dermatitis (soaps, perfumes, or dyes in toilet paper, topical anesthetics, oral antibiotics)
    ○ Atopic dermatitis ± lichen simplex chronicus (Patients also have asthma and/or eczema.)
    ○ Psoriasis (Lesions tend to be poorly demarcated, pale, and nonscaling.)
    ○ Seborrheic dermatitis
    ○ Scleroderma
    ○ Lichen planus (may be seen in patients with ulcerative colitis and myasthenia gravis)
    ○ Hidradenitis suppurativa
    ○ Radiation dermatitis (3)
  – Colorectal/anorectal diseases: rectal prolapse, hemorrhoids, fissures or fistulas, proctitis, chronic diarrhea/constipation, polyps
  – Infectious etiologies may be sexually transmitted: bacteria (gonorrhea, chlamydia, syphilis), viruses (herpes simplex virus [HSV], condyloma acuminate from human papillomavirus [HPV], molluscum), parasites (pinworms, lice, scabies, or bed bugs), fungal (*Candida*, or dermatophytes like tinea); other bacteria (*Staphylococcus aureus*, β-hemolytic *Streptococcus*, *Corynebacterium minutissimum* [erythrasma]) (3).
  – Malignancies: melanoma, basal cell/squamous cell carcinoma, colorectal cancer, leukemia, lymphoma, or (uncommon) the presenting symptom of Bowen or Paget disease
  – Mechanical factors: vigorous cleaning and scrubbing, tight-fitting clothes, synthetic undergarments
  – Systemic diseases (often presents as generalized pruritus): diabetes mellitus (most common), cholestasis, chronic liver disease, renal failure, hyperthyroidism, anemia, HIV, vitamin or iron deficiencies, lumbosacral radiculopathy (particularly in the elderly).
  – Chemical irritants: local anesthetics, chemotherapy, diarrhea (often from antibiotic use)
  – Dietary elements (citrus, milk products, coffee, tea, cola, chocolate, beer, wine, tomatoes, nuts)
  – Psychogenic factors: anxiety–itch–anxiety cycle

RISK FACTORS
- Obesity
- Excess perianal hair growth and/or perspiration
- Underlying anorectal pathology
- Atopic disease
- Underlying anxiety disorder
- Caffeine intake has been correlated with symptoms.

GENERAL PREVENTION
- Good perianal hygiene; avoid overzealous hygiene.
- Avoid mechanical irritation of skin (vigorous cleaning or rubbing with dry toilet paper or baby wipes, harsh soaps or perfumed products, excessive scratching with fingernails, or tight/synthetic undergarments).
- Minimize moisture in perianal area (absorbent cotton in anal cleft may help keep area dry).
- Avoid laxative use (loose stool is an irritant).

COMMONLY ASSOCIATED CONDITIONS
- Psoriasis is seen in 5–55% of patients with pruritus ani (1).
- Coexisting anorectal disease, such as hemorrhoids, can be seen in up to 52% of patients with pruritus ani (1).

DIAGNOSIS

HISTORY
- Patients present with complaints of anal and/or perianal itching, burning, or excoriation.
- Inquire about:
  – Timing (when it started, when it is worse)
  – Perianal hygiene (frequency of cleansing and products used)
  – Change in bowel habits
  – Bleeding (spotting of toilet paper, melena, hematochezia)
  – Recent antibiotic use
  – Skin disorders (psoriasis, eczema)
  – Rectal or vaginal discharge, menstrual cycle
  – Dietary history: Focus on the "C"s: caffeine, coffee, cola, chocolate, citrus, calcium (dairy) (3).
  – Medical history (hepatitis, iron deficiency anemia, and diabetes in particular)
  – Family history of colorectal cancer
  – Anal receptive intercourse
  – Change in toiletry products
  – Household members (particularly children) with itching (possible pinworms)
  – Pets
  – Clothing preference (tight, synthetic) (4)

PHYSICAL EXAM
- Perianal visual inspection for erythema, hemorrhoids, anal fissures, maceration, lichenification, warts, polyps, excoriations, neoplasia, stool seepage
- Classification based on gross appearance
  – Stage 1: erythema, inflamed appearance
  – Stage 2: lichenification
  – Stage 3: lichenification, coarse skin, potential fissures or ulcerations (4)
- Digital rectal exam to evaluate for masses, internal sphincter tone, pain
- Valsalva to evaluate for prolapse
- Anoscopy to evaluate for hemorrhoids, fissures, other internal lesions

DIFFERENTIAL DIAGNOSIS
"ITCHeS" acronym (5)
- **I**nfection: *Candida*, parasites (scabies, pinworms), HPV, HSV, bacterial (gram-positive bacteria, gonorrhea, chlamydia, syphilis)
- **T**opical irritants: soaps/detergents, garments, deodorants, perfumes, stool leakage
- **C**utaneous/**C**ancer/**C**olorectal: eczema, psoriasis, lichen planus, lichen sclerosus, seborrhea, skin cancer, extramammary Paget disease, Bowen disease, fistula, fissure, prolapse, hemorrhoids, colorectal cancer
- **H**ypersensitivity: foods, medications (colchicine, quinidine, mineral oil)
- **eS**ystemic: diabetes, iron deficiency anemia, uremia, cholestasis, hematologic malignancy

DIAGNOSTIC TESTS & INTERPRETATION
Initial Tests (lab, imaging)
Use history and exam to suggest a specific etiology, and guide testing:
- Pinworm tape test; stool for ova and parasites
- CBC, comprehensive metabolic panel, A1c, thyroid studies to identify underlying systemic disease
- Wood lamp examination will show coral-red fluorescence in erythrasma (3).
- Skin scraping with potassium hydroxide (KOH) prep for dermatophytes or candidiasis (as etiology or as superinfection) and mineral oil prep for scabies
- Perianal skin culture (bacterial superinfection)
- Hemoccult testing of stool

Pediatric Considerations
Pinworms common in children. Consider perianal Crohn disease.

Follow-Up Tests & Special Considerations
Anal DNA polymerase chain reaction (PCR) probe for gonorrhea and chlamydia. Test for anal HPV if receptive anal intercourse. HIV testing in patients with HIV risk factors.

Diagnostic Procedures/Other
- Biopsy suspicious lesions (e.g., lichenification, ulcerated epithelium, refractory cases) to exclude neoplasia; evaluate etiology.
- Consider colonoscopy if history, exam, or testing suggests colorectal pathology (family history of colorectal disease, especially if age >40 years, weight loss, rectal bleeding, change in bowel habits).

Geriatric Considerations
- Stool incontinence may be a predisposing factor.
- Consider systemic disease.
- Higher likelihood of colorectal pathology

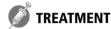 **TREATMENT**

GENERAL MEASURES

- Proper anal/perianal hygiene. Avoid vigorous rubbing while cleansing after bowel movement. Use cotton swabs moistened with warm water instead of tissue paper. Avoid chemical and mechanical irritants and wear proper undergarments (1)[A].
- High-fiber diet and/or bowel regimen to maintain regular bowel movements (1)[A]
- Avoid tight-fitting clothing. Use cotton undergarments.
- Avoiding moisture; absorbent cotton, talcum powder, or cornstarch if excess moisture. Can use hair dryer on cool setting to dry anal area (4)[C]
- Cotton gloves at night to control nocturnal scratching

MEDICATION

First Line

- Treat underlying infections: fungal or dermatophyte infection with topical imidazoles, bacterial infection with topical antibacterials (1)[A].
- Treat underlying anorectal anatomic pathology: banding of prolapsing internal hemorrhoids, treat fistulas, or fissures (1)[A].
- Break itch–scratch cycle with low-potency steroid cream such as hydrocortisone 1% ointment applied sparingly up to 4 times daily (1)[A],(4)[C]. Discontinue when itching subsides. Avoid use >2 weeks due to risk of skin atrophy.
- If no response with low-potency steroid, consider high-potency steroid cream.
- Antihistamines, particularly sedating antihistamines, may be useful in reducing nighttime itching until local measures take effect (1)[A]. Avoid in elderly patients due to anticholinergic properties.
- Tricyclic antidepressants may reduce nighttime scratching. SSRIs or gabapentin may be used in resistant cases (2)[C].
- Zinc oxide can be used after steroid course for barrier protection (3)[C]; petroleum jelly is another barrier. Avoid mineral oil as it can worsen pruritus.
- Albendazole for pinworm.

Second Line

- Low-dose topical capsaicin cream in combination with steroid cream if refractory symptoms (1)[A],(4)[C]
- 0.03% tacrolimus ointment can be considered in cases not responsive to high potency steroids (4)[C].
- Intradermal methylene blue injections, sometimes known as anal tattooing, may be used to destroy nerve endings and create permanent anesthesia in cases not responsive to medical management (1)[A],(4)[C].
- Biologics, such as the IL-4 inhibitor dupilumab, show promise for recalcitrant cases, though there is limited data currently.

ISSUES FOR REFERRAL

- Intractable pruritus: Consider referral to gastroenterology (for colonoscopy) or dermatology (for additional treatment, possibly injections, or biopsies). Refractory or persistent symptoms should signal the possibility of underlying neoplasia because pruritus ani of long duration is associated with a greater likelihood of colorectal pathology.
- Refer for colonoscopy if at risk for colon cancer.

SURGERY/OTHER PROCEDURES

As above, especially if concern for malignancy identified

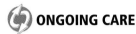 **ONGOING CARE**

FOLLOW-UP RECOMMENDATIONS

- See patient every 2 weeks if not improving.
- Ensure proper hygiene and avoidance of irritants.
- Work up for systemic disease and check for persistent lichenification. If refractory pruritus or lichenification does not resolve, consider underlying malignancy.

DIET

- Eliminate foods and beverages known or suspected to exacerbate symptoms: coffee, tea, chocolate, beer, cola, vitamin C tablets in excessive doses, citrus fruits, tomatoes, or spices.
- Eliminate foods or drugs contributing to loose bowel movements or dermatitis.
- Add fiber supplementation to bulk stools and prevent fecal leakage in patients who have fecal incontinence or partially formed stools.

PATIENT EDUCATION

- Review proper anal hygiene:
  – Resist overuse of soap and rubbing.
  – Avoid products with irritating perfumes and dyes.
  – Avoid use of ointments and mineral oil.
  – Wear loose, light cotton clothing.
  – If moisture is a problem, use cotton, unmedicated talcum powder, or cornstarch to keep the area dry.
  – Cleanse perianal area after bowel movements with water-moistened cotton.
  – Dry area after bathing by patting with a soft towel or by using a hair dryer on cool setting (4)[C].
- Avoid medications that cause diarrhea or constipation.
- Avoid caffeine, cola, chocolate, citrus, tomatoes, tea, alcohol, nuts, and milk products (3)[C].
- Use barrier protection if engaging in anal intercourse.
- If unable to completely empty rectum with defecation, use small plain-water enema (infant bulb syringe) after each bowel movement to prevent soiling and irritation.
- If persists, consider underlying medical disease.

PROGNOSIS

- Conservative treatment successful in ~90% of cases
- Idiopathic pruritus ani is often chronic—waxes and wanes.

COMPLICATIONS

- Bacterial superinfection at site of excoriations and potential abscess formation or penetrating infection via self-inoculation with colonic pathogens
- Lichenification
- Significant effect on quality of life

REFERENCES

1. Siddiqi S, Vijay V, Ward M, et al. Pruritus ani. *Ann R Coll Surg Engl.* 2008;90(6):457–463.
2. Swamiappan M. Anogenital pruritus—an overview. *J Clin Diagn Res.* 2016;10(4):WE01–WE03.
3. Nasseri YY, Osborne MC. Pruritus ani: diagnosis and treatment. *Gastroenterol Clin North Am.* 2013;42(4):801–813.
4. Ortega AE, Delgadillo X. Idiopathic pruritus ani and acute perianal dermatitis. *Clin Colon Rectal Surg.* 2019;32(5):327–332.
5. Henderson PK, Cash BD. Common anorectal conditions: evaluation and treatment. *Curr Gastroenterol Rep.* 2014;16(10):408.

ADDITIONAL READING

- Davies D, Bailey J. Diagnosis and management of anorectal disorders in the primary care setting. *Prim Care.* 2017;44(4):709–720.
- Misery L. Itch in special skin locations management. *Curr Probl Dermatol.* 2016;50:111–115.
- Ucak H, Demir B, Cicek D, et al. Efficacy of topical tacrolimus for the treatment of persistent pruritus ani in patients with atopic dermatitis. *J Dermatolog Treat.* 2013;24(6):454–457.

 SEE ALSO

Pinworms; Pruritus Vulvae

 CODES

ICD10
L29.0 Pruritus ani

CLINICAL PEARLS

- Pruritus ani is characterized by anal/perianal itching and/or burning. It is a skin irritation with itch–scratch–itch cycle.
- Conservative treatment with perianal hygiene and reassurance is successful in 90% of patients.
- Consider trial of dietary elimination of "C"s—citrus, vitamin C supplements, calcium products, caffeine, coffee, cola, chocolate.
- Rule out infection (viral, bacterial, parasitic) in immunosuppressed patients.
- Consider underlying malignancy if refractory.

PRURITUS VULVAE

Maeve K. Hopkins, MD, MA • Michael P. Hopkins, MD, MEd

 BASICS

DESCRIPTION
- Pruritus vulvae is a symptom or can be a primary diagnosis.
- If a primary diagnosis, other etiologies must be excluded.
- Pruritus vulvae as a primary diagnosis may also be more appropriately documented as vulvodynia (see "Vulvodynia" topic) or burning vulva syndrome.

EPIDEMIOLOGY
Symptoms may occur at any age during a woman's lifetime.
- Young girls most commonly have infectious or hygiene etiology.
- The primary diagnosis is more common in post-menopausal women.

Incidence
The exact incidence is unknown, although most women complain of vulvar pruritus at some point in their lifetime.

ETIOLOGY AND PATHOPHYSIOLOGY
Vulvar tissue is more permeable than exposed skin due to differences in structure, occlusion, hydration, and susceptibility to friction. It is particularly vulnerable to irritants such as (1)
- Perfumes
- Soaps
- Vaginal hygiene products
- Topical medications
- Dyes
- Body fluids

RISK FACTORS
- High-risk sexual behavior
- Immunosuppression
- Obesity

GENERAL PREVENTION
- Avoid irritants.
- Tight-fitting clothing should be avoided.
- Only cotton underwear should be worn.

COMMONLY ASSOCIATED CONDITIONS
- Infectious etiology
  - Vaginal or vulvar candida
  - *Gardnerella vaginalis*
  - *Trichomonas*
  - Human papillomavirus
  - Herpes simplex virus
- Vulvar vestibulitis
- Lichen sclerosus
- Lichen planus
- Lichen simplex chronicus (squamous cell hyperplasia)
- Malignant or premalignant conditions
- Psoriasis
- Fecal or urinary incontinence
- Dermatophytosis
- Parasites: scabies, *Pthirus pubis*
- Extramammary Paget
- Dietary: methylxanthines (e.g., coffee, cola), tomatoes, peanuts
- Autoimmune progesterone dermatitis: perimenstrual eruptions
- Irritant or allergic contact dermatitis
- Atopic dermatitis

 DIAGNOSIS

Pruritus vulvae is a diagnosis of exclusion. Delay in diagnosis is common due to patient hesitancy to seek treatment or provider delay in biopsy. Delayed diagnosis can have profound negative effect on women's sexual comfort and quality of life (2).

HISTORY
- Persistent itching
- Persistent burning sensation over the vulva or perineum
- Change in vaginal discharge
- Postcoital bleeding
- Dyspareunia

PHYSICAL EXAM
- Visual inspection of the vulva, vagina, perineum, and anus
  - Superior surfaces of the labia majora—extending from mons to the anal orifice—are most involved.
  - Vulvar skin is leathery or lichenified in appearance.
  - Papillomatosis may be a sign of chronic inflammation.
- Cotton swab–applied pressure to area of pain and to vestibular glands
- Musculoskeletal evaluation to confirm not contributing if persistent vulvar pain

DIAGNOSTIC TESTS & INTERPRETATION
- Sodium chloride: *Gardnerella* or *Trichomonas*
- 10% potassium hydroxide: *Candida*
- Viral culture or polymerase chain reaction: herpes simplex virus
- Directed biopsy recommended (3)[B]: human papillomavirus, lichen, malignancy, chronic inflammation
- Colposcopy with acetic acid or Lugol solution of vagina and vulva

Follow-Up Tests & Special Considerations
- A patch test may be performed by a dermatologist to assist in identifying a causative agent if contact dermatitis is suspected or if topical products are suspected as source of dermatitis (4)[A].
- Exam-directed tissue biopsies are essential in the postmenopausal population to rule out malignancy.

Diagnostic Procedures/Other
Biopsies should be collected from any ulceration, discoloration, raised areas, macerated areas, and the area of most intense pruritus.

Test Interpretation
- Only in the absence of pathologic findings can the primary diagnosis of pruritus vulvae be made.
- Biopsies of visible lesions most commonly show lichen simplex chronicus (25%), lichen sclerosus (20%), or chronic inflammation (15%) (3).

TREATMENT

Identify the underlying cause or disease to target treatment.

- Stop all potential irritants.
- Eliminate bacterial and fungal infection.
- Cool the affected area: Use cool gel packs (not ice packs, which may cause further injury).
- Sitz baths and bland emollients to soothe fissured or eroded skin

MEDICATION

First Line
- Topical steroids (1),(5)
  - Triamcinolone 0.1% applied daily for 2 to 4 weeks and then twice weekly
  - Hydrocortisone 1–2.5% cream applied 2 to 4 times daily
  - Avoid long-term use due to risk of atrophy.
- 1st-generation antihistamines
  - Hydroxyzine: Initiate with 10 mg before bedtime (slowly increase up to 100 mg).
  - Doxepin: Initiate with 10 mg before bedtime.
  - 2nd-generation antihistamines are of little benefit.

Second Line
- *SSRI such as* citalopram 20 to 40 mg for resistant cases (6)
- Calcineurin inhibitors such as 1% pimecrolimus (5)[A]

ISSUES FOR REFERRAL
- Persistent symptoms should prompt additional investigation and referral to a gynecologist or gynecologic oncologist.
- Gynecologic oncology referral for proven or suspected malignancy
- Dermatology referral for patch testing to evaluate for contact dermatitis

ADDITIONAL THERAPIES
- Sacral neuromodulation device
- Laser therapy
- GnRH analogues
- Naltrexone

 ONGOING CARE

- Frequent evaluation, repeat cultures, and biopsies are necessary for cases resistant to treatment.
- Refractory cases may require referral to gynecologist or gynecologic oncology for further management.

DIET
Dietary alterations include avoidance of the following:
- Coffee and other caffeine-containing beverages
- Tomatoes
- Peanuts

PATIENT EDUCATION
- American College of Obstetricians and Gynecologists: https://www.acog.org
- National Vulvodynia Association: https://www.nva.org

PROGNOSIS
Conservative measures and short-term topical steroids control most patients' symptoms.

COMPLICATIONS
Malignancy

REFERENCES

1. Stockdale CK, Boardman L. Diagnosis and treatment of vulvar dermatoses. *Obstet Gynecol*. 2018;131(2):371–386.
2. Kellogg Spadt S, Kusturiss E. Vulvar dermatoses: a primer for the sexual medicine clinician. *Sex Med Rev*. 2015;3(3):126–136.
3. Ozalp SS, Telli E, Yalcin OT, et al. Vulval pruritus: the experience of gynaecologists revealed by biopsy. *J Obstet Gynaecol*. 2015;35(1):53–56.
4. Corazza M, Virgili A, Toni G, et al. Level of use and safety of botanical products for itching vulvar dermatoses. Are patch tests useful? *Contact Dermatitis*. 2016;74(5):289–294.
5. Chi CC, Kirtschig G, Baldo M, et al. Systematic review and meta-analysis of randomized controlled trials on topical interventions for genital lichen sclerosus. *J Am Acad Dermatol*. 2012;67(2):305–312.
6. Swamiappan M. Anogenital pruritus—an overview. *J Clin Diagn Res*. 2016;10(4):WE01–WE03.

ADDITIONAL READING

- Böttcher B, Wildt L. Treatment of refractory vulvo-vaginal pruritus with naltrexone, a specific opiate antagonist. *Eur J Obstet Gynecol Reprod Biol*. 2014;174:115–116.
- Caro-Bruce E, Flaxman G. Vulvar pruritus in a post-menopausal woman. *CMAJ*. 2014;186(9):688–699.
- Hill A, Paraiso M. Resolution of chronic vulvar pruritus with replacement of a neuromodulation device. *J Minim Invasive Gynecol*. 2015;22(5):889–891.
- Pichardo-Geisinger R. Atopic and contact dermatitis of the vulva. *Obstet Gynecol Clin North Am*. 2017;44(3):371–378.

CODES

ICD10
- L29.2 Pruritus vulvae
- N94.819 Vulvodynia, unspecified

CLINICAL PEARLS

- Pruritus vulvae is a common complaint.
- Pruritus vulvae is a diagnosis of exclusion once other causes of itching have been ruled out.
- Exam-directed biopsies from any ulceration, discoloration, raised areas, macerated areas, and the area of most intense pruritus are essential to rule out malignancy.
- Initial treatment is conservative.

PSEUDOFOLLICULITIS BARBAE

Maurice Duggins, MD, FAAFP

BASICS

DESCRIPTION

- Foreign body inflammatory reaction from an ingrown hair resulting in the appearance of papules and pustules. This is found mainly in the bearded area (barbae) but may occur in other hairy locations such as the scalp, axilla, or pubic areas where shaving is done (1).
- A mechanical problem: extrafollicular and transfollicular hair penetration
- System(s) affected: skin/exocrine
- Synonym(s): chronic sycosis barbae; pili incarnati; folliculitis barbae traumatica; razor bumps; shaving bumps; tinea barbae; pseudofolliculitis barbae (PFB)

EPIDEMIOLOGY

- Predominant age: postpubertal, middle age (14 to 25 years)
- Predominant sex: male > female (can be seen in females of all races who wax/shave)

Incidence

- Adult male African Americans: unknown
- Adult male whites: unknown

Prevalence

- Widespread in Fitzpatrick skin types IV to VI (darker complexions) who shave
- 45–83% of African American soldiers who shave (1)

ETIOLOGY AND PATHOPHYSIOLOGY

- Transfollicular escape of the low-cut hair shaft as it tries to exit the skin is accompanied by inflammation and often an intraepidermal abscess.
- As the hair enters the dermis, more severe inflammation occurs, with downgrowth of the epidermis in an attempt to sheath the hair.
- A foreign body reaction forms at the tip of the invading hair, followed by abscess formation.
- Shaving too close
- Plucking/tweezing or wax depilation of hair may cause abnormal hair growth in injured follicles.

Genetics

- People with curly hair have an asymmetric accumulation of acidic keratin hHa8 on hair shaft.
- Single-nucleotide polymorphism (disruption Ala12Thr substitution) affects keratin of hair follicle.

RISK FACTORS

- Curly hair
- Shaving too close or shaving with multiple razor strokes
- Plucking/tweezing hairs
- South Mediterranean/American, Middle Eastern, Asian, or African descent (skin types IV to VI)

GENERAL PREVENTION

- Prior to shaving, rinse face with warm water to hydrate and soften hairs.
- Use adjustable hair clippers that leave very low hair length above skin.
- Shave with either a manual adjustable razor at coarsest setting (avoids close shaves), a single-edge blade razor (e.g., Bump Fighter), a foil-guarded razor (e.g., PFB razor), or electric triple "O-head" razor.
- Empty razor of hair frequently.
- Shave in the direction of hair growth. Do not overstretch skin when shaving.
- Use a generous amount of the correct shaving cream/gel (e.g., Ef-Kay shaving gel, Edge shaving gel, Aveeno therapeutic shave gel, Easy Shave medicated shaving cream).
- Daily shaving reduces papules/pruritus.
- Regular use of depilatories

COMMONLY ASSOCIATED CONDITIONS

- Keloidal folliculitis
- Pseudofolliculitis nuchae

DIAGNOSIS

HISTORY

Pain on shaving; pruritus of shaved areas, irritated "razor bumps"

PHYSICAL EXAM

- Tender, exudative, erythematous follicular papules or pustules in beard area (less commonly in scalp, axilla, and pubic areas); range from 2 to 4 mm
- Hyperpigmented "razor or shave bumps"
- Alopecia
- Lusterless, brittle hair

DIFFERENTIAL DIAGNOSIS

- Bacterial folliculitis
- Impetigo
- Acne vulgaris
- Tinea barbae
- Sarcoidal papules

DIAGNOSTIC TESTS & INTERPRETATION

Initial Tests (lab, imaging)

- Clinical diagnosis
- Culture of pustules: usually sterile; may show coagulase-negative *Staphylococcus epidermidis* (normal skin flora)
- Additional hormonal testing may be indicated in females with hirsutism and/or polycystic ovary syndrome: dehydroepiandrosterone sulfate, luteinizing hormone (LH)/follicle-stimulating hormone (FSH), and free and total testosterone (2)[C].

Test Interpretation

Follicular papules and pustules

TREATMENT

- Mild cases
  - Stop shaving or avoid close shaving for 30 days while keeping beard groomed and clean (1),(3).
  - Consider 5% benzoyl peroxide after shaving and application of 1% hydrocortisone cream at bedtime (or LactiCare-HC lotion after shaving).
  - Tretinoin 0.025% cream; apply daily (1)[C].
- Moderate cases
  - Chemical depilatories (barium sulfide; Magic shaving powder); first test on forearm for 48 hours (for irritation) (1),(2)[B]
  - Consider eflornithine HCl cream (Vaniqa) to reduce hair growth and stiffness in combination with other therapies (1),(4)[B].
- Severe cases
  - Laser therapy: Longer wavelength laser (e.g., neodymium [Nd]:YAG) is safer for dark skin (5)[B].
  - Avoid shaving altogether; grow beard (1),(2)[C].

GENERAL MEASURES

Acute treatment

- Dislodge embedded hair with sterile needle/tweezers.
- Discontinue shaving until red papules have resolved (minimum 3 to 4 weeks; longer if moderate or severe); can trim to length >0.5 cm during this time
- Massage beard area with washcloth, coarse sponge, or a soft brush several times daily.
- Hydrocortisone 1–2.5% cream to relieve inflammation
- Selenium sulfide if seborrhea is present and to help reduce pruritus
- Systemic antibiotics if secondary infection is present

Pregnancy Considerations

Do not use tretinoin (Retin-A), tetracycline, or benzoyl peroxide.

MEDICATION

First Line

- Topical or systemic antibiotic for secondary infection
  - Application of clindamycin (Cleocin T) solution BID or topical erythromycin
  - Low-dose erythromycin or tetracycline 250 to 500 mg PO BID for more severe inflammation
  - Benzoyl peroxide 5%–clindamycin 1% gel BID: Administer until papule/pustule resolves.
- Mild cases: tretinoin 0.025% cream at bedtime; combination of the above therapies

- Moderate disease/chemical depilatories
  - Disrupt cross-linking of disulfide bonds of hair to produce blunt (less sharp) hair tip.
  - Apply no more frequently than every 3rd day: 2% barium sulfide (Magic Shave) or calcium thioglycolate (Surgex); calcium hydroxide (Nair)
- Contraindications
  - Clindamycin: hypersensitivity history; history of regional enteritis or ulcerative colitis; history of antibiotic-associated colitis
  - Erythromycin, tetracycline, tretinoin: hypersensitivity history
- Precautions
  - Clindamycin: colitis, eye burning and irritation, skin dryness; pregnancy Category B
  - Erythromycin: Use cautiously in patients with impaired hepatic function; GI side effects, especially abdominal cramping; pregnancy Category B (erythromycin base formulation)
  - Chemical depilatories: Use cautiously; frequent use and prolonged application may lead to irritant contact dermatitis and chemical burns.
  - Tetracycline: Avoid in pregnancy.
  - Tretinoin: severe skin irritation; avoid in pregnancy.
  - Benzoyl peroxide: skin irritation and dryness, allergic contact dermatitis
  - Hydrocortisone cream: local skin irritation, skin atrophy with prolonged use, lightening of skin color
- Significant possible interactions
  - Erythromycin: increases theophylline and carbamazepine levels; decreases clearance of warfarin
  - Tetracycline: depresses plasma prothrombin activity

Second Line
Chemical peels with either glycolic acid or salicylic acid

ISSUES FOR REFERRAL
- Worsening or poor response to the above therapies after 4 to 6 weeks should prompt dermatology consultation.
- Occupational demands may also prompt earlier referral to dermatology for more aggressive therapy.

SURGERY/OTHER PROCEDURES
Laser treatment with long-pulsed Nd:YAG is helpful for severe cases.

ONGOING CARE

FOLLOW-UP RECOMMENDATIONS
Patient Monitoring
- As needed
- Educate patient on curative and preventive treatment.

DIET
- No restrictions
- No dietary studies available

PATIENT EDUCATION
https://medlineplus.com

PROGNOSIS
- Good, with preventive methods
- Prognosis is poor in the presence of progressive scarring and foreign body granuloma formation.

COMPLICATIONS
- Scarring (occasionally keloidal)
- Foreign body granuloma formation
- Disfiguring postinflammatory hyperpigmentation (use sunscreens; can treat with hydroquinone 4% cream, Retin-A, clinical peels)
- Impetiginization of inflamed skin
- Epidermal (erythema, crusting, burns with scarring) and pigmentary changes with laser

REFERENCES

1. Bridgeman-Shah S. The medical and surgical therapy of pseudofolliculitis barbae. *Dermatol Ther*. 2004;17(2):158–163.
2. Quarles FN, Brody H, Johnson BA, et al. Pseudofolliculitis barbae. *Dermatol Ther*. 2007;20(3):133–136.
3. Nussbaum D, Friedman A. Pseudofolliculitis barbae: a review of current treatment options. *J Drugs Dermatol*. 2019;18(3):246–250.
4. Xia Y, Cho S, Howard RS, et al. Topical eflornithine hydrochloride improves the effectiveness of standard laser hair removal for treating pseudofolliculitis barbae: a randomized, double-blinded, placebo-controlled trial. *J Am Acad Dermatol*. 2012;67(4):694–699.
5. Weaver SM III, Sagaral EC. Treatment of pseudofolliculitis barbae using the long-pulse Nd:YAG laser on skin types V and VI. *Dermatol Surg*. 2003;29(12):1187–1191.

ADDITIONAL READING

- Daniel A, Gustafson CJ, Zupkosky PJ, et al. Shave frequency and regimen variation effects on the management of pseudofolliculitis barbae. *J Drugs Dermatol*. 2013;12(4):410–418.
- Kindred C, Oresajo CO, Yatskayer M, et al. Comparative evaluation of men's depilatory composition versus razor in black men. *Cutis*. 2011;88(2):98–103.
- Kundu RV, Patterson S. Dermatologic conditions in skin of color: part II. Disorders occurring predominately in skin of color. *Am Fam Physician*. 2013;87(12):859–865.
- Taylor SC, Barbosa V, Burgess C, et al. Hair and scalp disorders in adult and pediatric patients with skin of color. *Cutis*. 2017;100(1):31–35.

SEE ALSO

Folliculitis; Impetigo

CODES

ICD10
- L73.1 Pseudofolliculitis barbae
- B35.0 Tinea barbae and tinea capitis
- L73.8 Other specified follicular disorders

CLINICAL PEARLS
- Electrolysis is not recommended as a treatment. It is expensive, painful, and often unsuccessful.
- Combination of laser therapy with eflornithine is more effective than laser alone.
- The unpleasant smell of sulfur could be a problem with some depilatory products.
- Have patient test for skin sensitivity with a small (coin sized) amount of the depilatory on the bearded area or forearm.

PSEUDOGOUT (CALCIUM PYROPHOSPHATE DIHYDRATE)

Juliana Chang, MD

BASICS

DESCRIPTION
- Autoinflammatory disease triggered by calcium pyrophosphate dihydrate (CPPD) crystal deposition within joints
- One of many diseases associated with pathologic deposition of crystal; mineralization and ossification
  - CPPD crystal deposition = chondrocalcinosis (calcification of hyaline or fibrocartilage), pseudogout, and pyrophosphate arthropathy
  - Monosodium urate crystal deposition = gout
  - Hydroxyapatite deposition = ankylosing spondylitis, osteoarthritis, and vascular calcification
- Suspect pseudogout with arthritis and a pattern of joint involvement inconsistent with degenerative joint disease (e.g., metacarpophalangeal joints, wrists).
- Clinical presentation is broad:
  - Asymptomatic CPPD (incidentally identified on radiograph with or without additional findings of osteoarthritis)
  - Acute CPPD arthritis (acute onset, self-limiting, synovitis)
    ○ Knee is affected in >50% of all acute attacks versus MTP in gout.
    ○ Can be brought on my trauma, medical illness, or surgery (after parathyroidectomy) (1)
  - Chronic CPPD crystal inflammatory arthritis (2)[C]
- Chronic CPPD crystal deposition may cause a progressive degenerative arthritis in numerous joints; usually large joints; primarily in elderly patients
- Symptom onset is usually insidious.
- Definitive diagnosis requires the identification of CPPD crystals in synovial fluid.
- System(s) affected: endocrine/metabolic; musculoskeletal
- Synonyms: pseudogout; CPPD; pyrophosphate arthropathy; chondrocalcinosis

EPIDEMIOLOGY
Prevalence
- Thought to affect 4–7% of adults in Europe and United States; 80% of patients >60 years
- No gender predominance. Men more likely to present acutely; women more likely to present atypically
- Chondrocalcinosis present in 1:10 adults age 60 to 75 years, 1:3 age >80 years; only a small percentage develop arthropathy.

ETIOLOGY AND PATHOPHYSIOLOGY
- Arthropathy results from an acute autoinflammatory reaction to CPPD crystals in the synovial cavity.
- CPPD crystal deposition occurs in three stages:
  - Overproduction of anionic pyrophosphate (PPi) in articular cartilage
  - PPi binds calcium to form CCPD crystals, eliciting an inflammatory response. Neutrophils engulf CPPD crystals, inducing extracellular trap formation.
  - Increased CPPD crystal deposition causes inflammation and damage (3)[C].

Genetics
Most cases are sporadic; rare familial pattern with autosomal dominant inheritance (<1% of patients). Mutation in *ANKH* gene increases risk for calcium crystal formation.

RISK FACTORS
Advanced age; joint trauma

GENERAL PREVENTION
Colchicine 0.6 mg BID may be used prophylactically to reduce frequency of episodes in recurrent CPPD.

COMMONLY ASSOCIATED CONDITIONS
- Gout
- Hyperparathyroidism
- Amyloidosis
- Hemochromatosis; ochronosis
- Hypothyroidism
- Wilson disease
- Hypomagnesemia
- Familial hypocalciuric hypercalcemia
- X-linked hypophosphatemic rickets
- Acromegaly

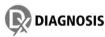

DIAGNOSIS

HISTORY
- Presentation often mimics gout ("pseudogout").
- Acute CPPD: pain and swelling of ≥1 or more joints; knee involved 50% of the time; ankle, wrist, toe, and shoulder are also common.
- Proximal joint involvement (mimicking polymyalgia rheumatica), often with tibiofemoral and ankle arthritis and tendinous calcifications
- Multiple symmetric joint involvement (mimicking RA) in <5% of cases
- May develop after intra-articular injection of hyaluronic acid (Hyalgan, Synvisc)
- Chronic CPPD: progressive degenerative arthritis with superimposed acute inflammatory attacks

PHYSICAL EXAM
- Inflammation (erythema, warmth, tender to touch), joint effusion, decreased range of motion (ROM)
- 50% associated with fever

DIFFERENTIAL DIAGNOSIS
- Illnesses that may cause acute inflammatory arthritis in a single or multiple joint(s): gout, septic arthritis, trauma
- Other acute inflammatory arthritides: Reiter syndrome, Lyme disease, acute RA

DIAGNOSTIC TESTS & INTERPRETATION
Initial Tests (lab, imaging)
Synovial fluid analysis shows an inflammatory effusion:
- Cell count 2,000 to 100,000 WBCs/mL
- Neutrophil predominance (80–90%)

- >50,000 WBC count increases likelihood of septic arthritis; >100,000 WBCs/mL
- Polarized microscopy shows small number of positively birefringent crystals; high false-negative rate
- Consider the following to exclude underlying disease:
  - Serum calcium, phosphorus, and magnesium
  - Serum alkaline phosphatase
  - Serum parathormone (i-PTH)
  - Serum iron, total iron-binding capacity, and serum ferritin
  - Serum thyroid-stimulating hormone (TSH) level
- Plain radiograph:
  - Radiographic findings in pseudogout are neither sensitive nor specific.
  - Punctate and linear calcifications in fibrocartilage, particularly of knees, hips, symphysis pubis, and wrists
  - Chronic CPPD: subchondral cysts and loose bodies in joints not typically affected by degenerative joint disease
- Ultrasound: joint effusion, synovial thickening, and hyperechoic deposits
  - May be more useful than plain radiography for the diagnosis of pseudogout in peripheral joints, with a positive predictive value of 92% and negative predictive value of 93% (4)[C]
- MRI: chondrocalcinosis evident as hypointense lesions, particularly of knee menisci

Diagnostic Procedures/Other

> **ALERT**
> Synovial fluid analysis with demonstration of CPPD crystals is required for diagnosis; aspiration may help relieve symptoms and speed resolution.

Test Interpretation
CPPD crystal deposition in articular cartilage, synovium, ligaments, and tendons

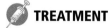

TREATMENT

GENERAL MEASURES
Target symptom relief (reduce inflammation):
- Rest and elevate affected joint(s).
- Apply ice/cool compresses to affected joints.
- Non–weight-bearing on affected joint while painful; use crutches or a walker.

MEDICATION
First Line
- Acute attacks: ice packs, rest, and joint aspiration with or without steroid injection
- Chronic CPPD: prophylactic management with oral NSAIDs and/or colchicine (4)[C]

- Oral NSAIDs
  - Ibuprofen 600 to 800 mg PO TID–QID with food; maximum 3.2 g/day
  - Naproxen 500 mg PO BID with food
  - Other NSAIDs are effective, although indomethacin has higher complication rates (relative risk [RR] = 2.2) compared with ibuprofen (RR = 1.2).
- Contraindications:
  - History of hypersensitivity to NSAIDs or aspirin
  - Active peptic ulcer disease or history of recurrent upper GI lesions
  - Avoid in renal insufficiency.
  - Serious GI bleeding can occur without warning; patient should be instructed on signs/symptoms. Administer proton pump inhibitor (PPI) or misoprostol 200 μg PO QID in patients at risk for NSAID-induced gastric ulcers.
  - Caution in cardiovascular disease, particularly heart failure or difficult to control hypertension
  - Avoid in concomitant aspirin and anticoagulant use.
- Oral colchicine: 0.5 mg up to 3 to 4 times daily, with or without 1 mg initial dose; 1.2 mg at the first sign of flare, followed in 1 hour
- Intra-articular steroid injection: prednisolone sodium phosphate 4 to 20 mg or triamcinolone diacetate 2 to 40 mg with local anesthetic
- Supportive measures for symptomatic relief (application of ice or cool packs) and immobilization

Second Line
- Oral prednisone: 30 to 50 mg/day for 7 to 10 days
- IM triamcinolone acetonide 40 mg; if necessary, may repeat in 1 to 4 days
- Consider referring patients with large space-occupying tophaceous lesions for surgical removal.
- Alternative therapies for chronic CPPD
  - ACTH, anakinra (anti–IL-1), hydroxychloroquine, infliximab, probenecid, magnesium, ethylenediaminetetraacetic acid (EDTA) have all been suggested. Large-scale studies are needed to evaluate effectiveness (5)[C].

> **ALERT**
> Recent randomized trial showed no significant effect of methotrexate in chronic-recurrent CPPD (6)[B].

ISSUES FOR REFERRAL
Consider consultation with orthopedist or rheumatologist if septic joint or patient is not responding.

ADDITIONAL THERAPIES
Physical therapy
- Isometric exercises to maintain muscle strength during the acute stage
- Begin joint ROM exercises as inflammation and pain subside.
- Resume weight bearing when pain subsides.

SURGERY/OTHER PROCEDURES
Perform arthrocentesis and joint fluid analysis.

ADMISSION, INPATIENT, AND NURSING CONSIDERATIONS
Consider admission for septic arthritis if:
- Synovial fluid WBC count >50,000/mL
- Treat with appropriate antibiotics pending culture results.

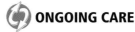 ONGOING CARE

FOLLOW-UP RECOMMENDATIONS
Patient Monitoring
Reevaluate response to therapy 48 to 72 hours after beginning treatment; reexamine in 1 week then as needed.

DIET
No known relationship to diet

PATIENT EDUCATION
- Rest affected joint.
- Symptoms usually resolve in 7 to 10 days.

PROGNOSIS
- Acute attack usually resolves in 10 days; prognosis for resolution of acute attack is excellent.
- Patients may experience progressive joint damage and functional limitation with recurrent attacks.

COMPLICATIONS
- Recurrent acute attacks
- Osteoarthritis

Geriatric Considerations
Elderly patients treated with NSAIDs require careful monitoring and are at higher risk for GI bleeding and acute renal insufficiency; no loading dose for colchicine due to high rates of renal insufficiency in elderly patients

REFERENCES
1. Bilezikian JP, Connor TB, Aptekar R, et al. Pseudogout after parathyroidectomy. *Lancet.* 1973;1(7801):445–446.
2. Zhang W, Doherty M, Bardin T, et al. European League Against Rheumatism recommendations for calcium pyrophosphate deposition. Part I: terminology and diagnosis. *Ann Rheum Dis.* 2011;70(4):563–570.
3. Rosenthal AK, Ryan LM. Nonpharmacologic and pharmacologic management of CPP crystal arthritis and BCP arthropathy and periarticular syndromes. *Rheum Dis Clin North Am.* 2014;40(2):343–356.
4. Zhang W, Doherty M, Pascual E, et al. EULAR recommendations for calcium pyrophosphate deposition. Part II: management. *Ann Rheum Dis.* 2011;70(4):571–575.
5. Pascart T, Richette P, Flipo RM. Treatment of nongout joint deposition diseases: an update. *Arthritis.* 2014;2014:375202.
6. Finckh A, Mc Carthy GM, Madigan A, et al. Methotrexate in chronic-recurrent calcium pyrophosphate deposition disease: no significant effect in a randomized crossover trial. *Arthritis Res Ther.* 2014;16(5):458.

ADDITIONAL READING
- Bruges-Armas J, Bettencourt BF, Couto AR, et al. Effectiveness and safety of infliximab in two cases of severe chondrocalcinosis: nine years of follow-up. *Case Rep Rheumatol.* 2014;2014:536856.
- Daoussis D, Antonopoulos I, Andonopoulos AP. ACTH as a treatment for acute crystal-induced arthritis: update on clinical evidence and mechanisms of action. *Semin Arthritis Rheum.* 2014;43(5):648–653.
- Demertzis JL, Rubin DA. MR imaging assessment of inflammatory, crystalline-induced, and infectious arthritides. *Magn Reson Imaging Clin N Am.* 2011;19(2):339–363.
- Macmullan P, McCarthy G. Treatment and management of pseudogout: insights for the clinician. *Ther Adv Musculoskelet Dis.* 2012;4(2):121–131.
- Sattui SE, Singh JA, Gaffo AL. Comorbidities in patients with crystal diseases and hyperuricemia. *Rheum Dis Clin North Am.* 2014;40(2):251–278.

 CODES

ICD10
- M11.20 Other chondrocalcinosis, unspecified site
- M11.269 Other chondrocalcinosis, unspecified knee
- M11.29 Other chondrocalcinosis, multiple sites

CLINICAL PEARLS
- Suspect CPPD in arthritis cases that do not follow a pattern typical of degenerative joint disease
- Perform arthrocentesis to confirm diagnosis.
- If septic arthritis is suspected, treat empirically with antibiotics while awaiting culture.
- NSAIDs are preferred pharmacologic treatment for acute flare.
- Oral steroids are useful if NSAIDs are contraindicated.
- Intra-articular steroids can be used *if* septic arthritis has been excluded.

PSORIASIS

Karl T. Clebak, MD, MHA, FAAFP • Roland W. Newman II, DO

BASICS

DESCRIPTION

- A chronic, inflammatory disorder commonly characterized by cutaneous erythematous plaques with silvery scale with varying phenotypes and severity
- Clinical phenotypes
  - Plaque (vulgaris): most common variant (~80% of cases); well-demarcated, red plaques with silvery scale; symmetrically distributed commonly on the scalp, extensor surfaces, and trunk.
  - Guttate: <2% of psoriasis patients, usually in patients <30 years of age; presents abruptly with 1- to 10-mm droplet-shaped erythematous papules with fine scale over trunk and extremities; often preceded by group A β-hemolytic streptococcal infection 2 to 3 weeks prior. Most cases resolve spontaneously.
  - Inverse: affects intertriginous areas and flexural surfaces; pink-to-red plaques with minimal scale; absence of satellite pustules distinguishes it from candidiasis.
  - Erythrodermic: generalized erythema and scaling, affecting 90% of body surface area (BSA) or more; associated with desquamation; hair loss; nail dystrophy; and systemic symptoms such as fever, chills, malaise, lymphadenopathy, and/or high-output cardiac failure
  - Pustular: sterile pustules; several forms including generalized pustular psoriasis, localized pustular psoriasis, and impetigo herpetiformis (in pregnancy); generalized type can result in life-threatening bacterial superinfections
  - Nail disease: pitting, oil spots, and onycholysis; nails involved in up to 50% of patients with psoriasis with lifetime incidence of 80–90%; increased association with psoriatic arthritis

EPIDEMIOLOGY

Incidence
Predominant sex: female > male; predominant age: two peaks of incidence between the ages of 20 to 30 years and 50 to 60 years

Prevalence
- 2–4% prevalence in the United States
- In the United States, the most commonly affected demographic group is non-Hispanic Caucasian.

ETIOLOGY AND PATHOPHYSIOLOGY
Psoriasis is a complex immune-mediated disorder with interactions between dendritic cells, T lymphocytes, neutrophils, and keratinocytes that results from a polygenic predisposition in the setting of environmental triggers; associated with relapsing flares related to systemic, psychological, infectious, and environmental factors

Genetics
- Genetic predisposition (polygenic)
- 40% have psoriasis in a first-degree relative.
- Multiple susceptibility loci contain genes involved in immune system regulation.
- HLA-C*06 is most strongly correlated with early-onset psoriasis.

RISK FACTORS
- Family history
- Obesity
- Local trauma; local irritation (Koebner phenomenon)
- HIV
- Streptococcal infection

- Stress (may contribute to exacerbation)
- Medications (lithium, antimalarials, β-blockers, interferon, TNF-α inhibitors, withdrawal of steroids)
- Smoking
- Alcohol abuse

GENERAL PREVENTION
Control cardiovascular risk factors. Avoidance of triggers including trauma, sunburns, smoking, and exposure to certain medications, alcohol, and stress.

COMMONLY ASSOCIATED CONDITIONS
- Psoriatic arthritis
- Seborrheic dermatitis
- Obesity, metabolic syndrome, diabetes, chronic kidney disease
- Cardiovascular disease, atherosclerotic disease
- Nonalcoholic fatty liver disease (NAFLD)
- Other autoimmune conditions: Crohn disease, ulcerative colitis, ankylosing spondylitis
- Psychiatric/psychological conditions: depression, anxiety, suicidal ideation, poor self-esteem, emotional burden/anxiety, alcohol abuse, sexual dysfunction
- Myopathy

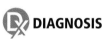

DIAGNOSIS

HISTORY
- May include: sudden onset of clearly demarcated, erythematous plaques with overlying silvery scales or exacerbation of chronic plaques, especially on extensor surfaces and scalp. Typically no or mild pruritus. Triggers may include recent streptococcal infection or trauma.
- Family history of similar condition

PHYSICAL EXAM
- Well-demarcated salmon pink-to-red erythematous papules and plaques with silvery scale
- Distribution favors scalp, auricular conchal bowls and postauricular area, extensor surface of extremities, especially knees and elbows, umbilicus, lower back, intergluteal cleft, and nails.
- Nail findings: pitting, oil spots, onycholysis
- Auspitz sign: pinpoint bleeding with removal of scale
- Koebner phenomenon: new psoriatic lesions arising at sites of skin injury/trauma
- Woronoff ring is a pale blanching ring that may be seen around a psoriatic lesion.
- Sebopsoriasis: Psoriasis can overlap with seborrheic dermatitis as greasy scales on the scalp, eyebrows, nasolabial folds, postauricular, and presternal areas.

DIFFERENTIAL DIAGNOSIS
- Plaque: seborrheic dermatitis (may coexist), nummular eczema, atopic dermatitis, contact dermatitis, lichen simplex chronicus (may coexist), tinea, pityriasis rubra pilaris, dermatomyositis, squamous cell carcinoma in situ, reactive arthritis, pityriasis rosea, lichen planus, lichen sclerosus et atrophicus
- Guttate: pityriasis rosea, pityriasis lichenoides chronica, secondary syphilis, small plaque parapsoriasis
- Inverse: cutaneous candidiasis, tinea, seborrheic dermatitis, contact dermatitis
- Pustular: subcorneal pustulosis, acute generalized exanthematous pustulosis, folliculitis
- Erythrodermic: cutaneous T-cell lymphoma, drug-induced erythroderma, pityriasis rubra pilaris

DIAGNOSTIC TESTS & INTERPRETATION

Initial Tests (lab, imaging)
- Clinical diagnosis based on history and physical exam.
- Labs generally not needed, although KOH to rule out tinea helpful, especially in inverse psoriasis.
- Consider skin biopsy if diagnosis unclear.
- Consider x-rays if complaints of joint pain to evaluate for psoriatic arthritis.

Diagnostic Procedures/Other
- Psoriasis Area and Severity Index (PASI) evaluates overall severity and BSA involvement.
- Dermatology Life Quality Index (DLQI)

Test Interpretation
Biopsy findings: thickening of the stratum corneum (hyperkeratosis) with retention of nuclei (parakeratosis); elongation, thickening, and clubbing of rete ridges; dilated tortuous capillary loops in the dermal papillae; perivascular lymphocytic infiltrate, Munro microabscesses: neutrophils in stratum corneum

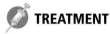

TREATMENT

GENERAL MEASURES
Adequate topical hydration (emollients); avoidance of triggers; weight loss

MEDICATION

First Line
- Assess for concurrent psoriatic arthritis, if present start with therapies with dual approval for psoriasis and psoriatic arthritis, even if skin manifestations are mild due to risk of joint destruction secondary to psoriatic arthritis (1)[C].
- Mild-to-moderate disease
  - Emollients: petrolatum/ointments to maintain skin hydration and minimize pruritus and risk of koebnerization
  - Topical corticosteroids
    ○ Anti-inflammatory, antiproliferative, immunosuppressive, and vasoconstrictive effects
    ○ Local side effects: skin atrophy, hypopigmentation, striae, acne, folliculitis, and purpura. Systemic side effects: Risk is higher, with higher potency formulations used over a large surface for a prolonged period; pregnancy Category C
    ○ Applications are typically twice daily until lesions flatten/resolve and then taper to PRN use for maintenance.
    ○ Scalp: high potency in solution/foam vehicle; shampoos and sprays also available
    ○ Face, intertriginous areas, infants: low-potency corticosteroids: 1% hydrocortisone
    ○ Adult initial therapy: medium-potency corticosteroids daily: 0.1% mometasone or triamcinolone; strong-potency corticosteroids: 0.05% betamethasone or fluocinonide daily; superpotent corticosteroids: clobetasol, halobetasol; caution with use over 2 to 4 weeks; avoid occlusive dressings; reserved for recalcitrant plaques
  - Vitamin D analogues: calcipotriene 0.005% cream daily to BID; may be used in combination with a superpotent corticosteroid; should not be used with products that can alter pH (e.g., topical lactic acid) local side effects: burning, pruritus, edema, peeling, dryness, and erythema; pregnancy Category C

- Topical retinoids: tazarotene 0.05% or 0.1% (Tazorac) daily; may be combined with corticosteroids; side effects: local irritation, photosensitivity; pregnancy Category X
- Topical calcineurin inhibitors: Tacrolimus 0.1% or pimecrolimus 1% may be used as steroid-sparing agents, especially in facial and intertriginous areas.
- Comparison of topical therapies: Vitamin D analogues have slower onset of action than topical corticosteroids but longer disease-free periods for body plaques; for scalp, potent and superpotent steroids are more effective (2)[A].
- Combination of superpotent steroids and vitamin D analogues has better efficacy than either as monotherapy (3)[A].
- Severe disease: may need combination therapy
  - Light therapy: UVB (broad/narrow band [BB, NB]) or PUVA: Treatment protocols are skin type dependent. PUVA with GI SE, photosensitivity, and increased risk of nonmelanoma skin cancers; can be used as adjunct therapy
  - Oral systemic therapies
    o Methotrexate: Start with 5-mg test dose, then increase to 7.5 to 15.0 mg/week IV, PO, IM, or SC, and then increase 2.5 mg every 2 to 3 weeks, up to 25 mg; contraindicated in pregnancy and use caution in women of childbearing age; supplement with folic acid 1 mg/day baseline chest x-ray, monitor LFTs, renal function, CBC, testing for latent tuberculosis (TB); consider liver biopsy when cumulative dose reaches 3.5 to 4.0 g; avoid alcohol and medications that interfere with folic acid metabolism including trimethoprim—sulfamethoxazole (Bactrim), NSAIDs, sulfamethoxazole, or hepatotoxic agents (e.g., retinoids).
    o Cyclosporine: Start 2.5 mg/kg/day; if insufficient response after 4 weeks, increase by 0.5 mg/kg/day; additional dosage increases every 2 weeks (max dose: 5 mg/kg/day); pregnancy Category C; side effects: renal toxicity and hypertension, limit use to 6 months to 1 year: Monitor renal function and electrolytes with Mg^{2+}, CBC, lipids, and blood pressure.
    o Acitretin (Soriatane): Start at 10 to 25 mg/day; effective for pustular psoriasis and as a maintenance therapy after stabilization with other agents; pregnancy Category X: pregnancy test before starting; two forms of contraception 1 month before, during, and for at least 3 years after treatment; avoid alcohol ; side effects: alopecia, xerosis, cheilitis, hepatotoxicity, hyperlipidemia, cataracts; monitor LFTs, renal function, lipid profile, CBC, regular eye exams.
    o Phosphodiesterase-4 enzyme inhibitor: Apremilast (Otezla): 10 mg PO, titrate up by 10 mg/day on days 2 to 5 maintenance dose of 30 mg BID starting on day 6. Routine lab monitoring not required. Most common SE are GI symptoms, depression; pregnancy Category C

- Biologics—Achieve remission for patients with moderate to severe disease. Expensive and long-term outcomes and safety data not available (4)[A].
  o General guidelines: Screen for latent TB at baseline and yearly, hepatitis panel at baseline, avoid live vaccines; monitor CBC with differential, signs/symptoms of infections, heart failure, malignancy, drug-induced lupus, demyelinating disorder. All should be considered effective first-line treatments; pregnancy Category B
    ▪ TNF-α inhibitors: also approved for treatment of psoriatic arthritis. Options include etanercept (Enbrel), adalimumab (Humira), and infliximab (Remicade).
    ▪ IL-12/IL-23 antagonist: ustekinumab (Stelara); also approved for treatment of psoriatic arthritis
    ▪ IL-17 antagonists: secukinumab (Cosentyx), brodalumab (Siliq). Also approved for the treatment of psoriatic arthritis. Avoid in patients with inflammatory bowel disease.

Second Line
- Immunosuppressives: azathioprine, hydroxyurea, 6-thioguanine, fumaric acid esters
- Topicals: salicylic acid, anthralin, coal tar

ISSUES FOR REFERRAL
Refer patients with psoriasis >20% of BSA, psoriatic arthritis, pustular psoriasis, severe extremity involvement, or disease not responding to topical therapy.

SURGERY/OTHER PROCEDURES
Psoriasis and psoriatic medications can affect wound healing postoperatively.

COMPLEMENTARY & ALTERNATIVE MEDICINE
Balneotherapy, climatotherapy, and stress management interventions

ADMISSION, INPATIENT, AND NURSING CONSIDERATIONS
Rule out sepsis; restoration of barrier function of skin with cleaning and bandaging; intensive topical corticosteroid therapy, initiate systemic therapy; management of electrolytes

 ONGOING CARE

FOLLOW-UP RECOMMENDATIONS
Measure BSA involvement to determine if therapy is working; change therapy or add agent if no improvement is seen.

DIET
Well-balanced diet and exercise to limit cardiovascular risk factors

PATIENT EDUCATION
National Psoriasis Foundation: https://www.psoriasis.org; (800) 723-9166

PROGNOSIS
Guttate form may be self-limited and remit after months; chronic plaque type is lifelong, with intermittent spontaneous remissions and exacerbations; erythrodermic and generalized pustular forms may be severe and persistent.

COMPLICATIONS
- Psoriatic arthritis, generalized pustular psoriasis, erythrodermic psoriasis
- Cardiovascular disease

REFERENCES
1. Armstrong AW, Read C. Pathophysiology, clinical presentation, and treatment of psoriasis. *JAMA.* 2020;323(19):1945–1960.
2. Mason AR, Mason J, Cork M, et al. Topical treatments for chronic plaque psoriasis. *Cochrane Database Syst Rev.* 2013;(3):CD005028.
3. Hendriks AG, Keijsers RR, de Jong EM, et al. Efficacy and safety of combinations of first-line topical treatments in chronic plaque psoriasis: a systematic literature review. *J Eur Acad Dermatol Venereol.* 2013;27(8):931–951.
4. Sbidian E, Chaimani A, Garcia-Doval I, et al. Systemic pharmacological treatments for chronic plaque psoriasis: a network meta-analysis. *Cochrane Database Syst Rev.* 2020;(1):CD011535. doi:10.1002/14651858.CD011535.pub3.

ADDITIONAL READING
- Clebak KT, Helm L, Helm MF, et al. The many variants of psoriasis. *J Fam Pract.* 2020;69(4):192–200.
- Sendur N, Buyukpapuscu O, Karaman G, et al. Biologics in psoriasis. *J Am Acad Dermatol.* 2016;74(5):AB238.
- Weigle N, McBane S. Psoriasis. *Am Fam Physician.* 2013;87(9):626–633.

 SEE ALSO

Arthritis, Psoriatic

CODES

ICD10
- L40.2 Acrodermatitis continua
- L40.5 Arthropathic psoriasis
- L40.59 Other psoriatic arthropathy

CLINICAL PEARLS
Chronic lifelong inflammatory skin condition with remissions and exacerbations; set realistic expectations with patient. Disease burden not limited to skin. If one medication does not work, use/combine with another agent. Control cardiovascular risk factors; patients with psoriasis have a higher risk of cardiovascular disease.

PSYCHOSIS

Matthew J. Filippo, DO • Ashley F. Chin, MD

 BASICS

DESCRIPTION
A disorder where thoughts and emotions are disrupted; seen in schizophrenia, mood disorders, substance use, medical problems, delirium, and dementia

- Positive symptoms: hallucinations and delusions (fixed false beliefs not typical of cultural background)
- Negative symptoms: anhedonia, poverty of speech, lack of motivation, social withdrawal, affective blunting
- Cognition: poor working memory, information processing, inattention, disorganized speech and/or behavior

EPIDEMIOLOGY
Incidence
The incidence of schizophrenia is 1.5 per 10,000 people.

Prevalence
- Schizophrenia: peak onset: males: 18 to 25 years; females: 25 to 35 years
- 1% of the U.S. population; similar percentage worldwide
- Seen in ~50% of bipolar cases and 20% of unipolar depression cases

ETIOLOGY AND PATHOPHYSIOLOGY
- Many causes including psychiatric, medical, and/or substance use
- Positive symptoms: excessive dopaminergic activity in the mesolimbic pathway
- Negative symptoms: diminished dopaminergic activity in mesocortical pathway

Genetics
Schizophrenia: 50% concordance in monozygotic twins, little shared environmental effect; many genes involved

RISK FACTORS
Substance use (particularly stimulants and THC), family history of psychosis, lower socioeconomic status

GENERAL PREVENTION
Community interventions for early detection and treatment of prodromal symptoms

COMMONLY ASSOCIATED CONDITIONS
- Associated with metabolic syndrome, autonomic dysfunction, sudden cardiac death, and breast and lung cancer
- Substance use, including nicotine dependence

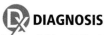 **DIAGNOSIS**

Rule out delirium: Unlike delirium, psychosis should not have fluctuating mentation.

HISTORY
- Delusions: persecutory, bizarre, somatic, referential, or grandiose
- Hallucinations: auditory, visual, tactile, gustatory, olfactory
- Bipolar, unipolar depression, and dementia are associated with psychosis.

- Screen for drugs of abuse and history of epileptiform activity.
- Suicidality: higher risk with comorbid depression/mania, previous attempts, drug use, agitation/akathisia, poor adherence

PHYSICAL EXAM
- Mental status exam: disorganized speech, behavior, and/or thought process; thought blocking; response latency; blunted affect; social withdrawal; lack of initiative; poverty of thought/speech; hallucinations
- Pay attention to focal neurologic signs, parkinsonism, tardive dyskinesia, and akathisia.
- May present with catatonia: lack of movement or extreme excitement, posturing, mutism, grimacing, waxy flexibility

DIFFERENTIAL DIAGNOSIS
- Schizophrenia: positive symptoms and negative symptoms, prodrome of social withdrawal, cognitive impairment. Schizophreniform: psychotic/prodromal symptoms <6 months. Schizoaffective: manic/depressive mood disorder with psychosis that persists when euthymic. Schizotypal personality disorder: distance in relationships and odd beliefs. Delusional disorder: nonbizarre delusion (e.g., erotomanic, grandiose, jealous, persecutory, somatic)
- Mood disorder with psychotic features: occur in mania and depression. Mood congruent; psychosis remits as mood improves.
- Substance-induced: alcohol and benzodiazepine withdrawal, intoxication with cocaine, bath salts, PCP, THC, amphetamines, hallucinogens, and alcohol; may persist beyond acute intoxication
- Posttraumatic stress disorder: psychosis associated with traumatic recollections; often visual hallucinations
- Psychosis due to general medical condition: delirium, stroke, infection, collagen vascular disease, head injury, tumor, interictal, porphyria, syphilis, autoimmune encephalitis, etc.
- Medication-induced psychosis: steroids especially >40 mg prednisone equivalent, L-dopa, anticholinergics, antidepressants in bipolar patients, interferon, digoxin, stimulants

DIAGNOSTIC TESTS & INTERPRETATION
Labs: CBC, CMP, LFTs, thyroid-stimulating hormone (TSH), rapid plasma reagin (RPR), HIV, ANA, ESR, vitamin B_{12}, vitamin D, urinalysis, tox screen

Initial Tests (lab, imaging)
- Imaging: not necessary for diagnosis. Consider CT or MRI if focal neurologic signs, first break, or new onset in elderly.
- Consider MRI if sudden onset of symptoms, especially with comorbid fever or headache.
- Consider ECG to assess QTc interval if patient has a cardiac history, age >50.

Follow-Up Tests & Special Considerations
- Consider Wilson disease, porphyria, metachromatic leukodystrophy, and inflammatory conditions.
- Consider lumbar puncture if unable to distinguish from delirium and/or rapid-onset psychosis.
- Consider electroencephalogram (EEG) for seizures and psychosis associated with ictal events.
- Consider anti-NMDA receptor antibodies in suspected autoimmune encephalitis.

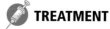 **TREATMENT**

GENERAL MEASURES
Ensure safety of person and environment and rule out medical causes particularly delirium.

MEDICATION
- Antipsychotics are mainstay of treatment (1)[B].
- Classified as typical versus atypical. Dopamine-2 (D_2) antagonists with varied affinity for the receptor. Atypicals also block serotonin 5-HT$_{2A}$ receptors. They treat positive symptoms > negative. Effect on agitation begins early; antipsychotic effect may take 1 week.
- For mania with psychotic features, a mood stabilizer may be used with an antipsychotic.
- For depression with psychotic features, antidepressant and antipsychotic combination improves response more than either alone. In delirium, must treat underlying cause; may not require antipsychotic therapy
- Side effects
  - Acute dystonia: benztropine 1 to 3 mg IM/IV then 0.5 to 2.0 mg BID–TID or diphenhydramine 50 to 100 mg IM/IV BID–TID max 400 mg/day
  - Parkinsonism: Lower antipsychotic dose; switch to atypical (particularly, quetiapine or clozapine) and/or add benztropine 0.5 to 2.0 mg PO BID–TID
  - Akathisia (intense restlessness): Lower antipsychotic dose; treat with β-blocker or benzodiazepine; may switch to antipsychotic with lower akathisia risk such as quetiapine or clozapine
  - Tardive dyskinesia: seen in ~1/3 of those treated long term with typicals, ~1/8 with atypicals. Switch to clozapine or quetiapine. Otherwise minimize dose. Symptomatic treatment has been tried with low-dose benzodiazepines, botulinum toxin, and VMAT2 inhibitors such as valbenazine and deutetrabenazine.
  - Neuroleptic malignant syndrome: potentially fatal; rigidity, tremor, fever, autonomic instability, mental status changes; discontinue neuroleptic; ICU; volume resuscitation; cooling blankets; no anticholinergics/antihistamines; consider dantrolene, amantadine, bromocriptine, and electroconvulsive therapy (ECT).
  - Metabolic syndrome, sudden cardiac death (risk higher IM/IV droperidol, IV haloperidol), stroke, heart failure, PNA (elderly), pulmonary embolus; can minimize metabolic risk by using anorexigenics and behavioral counseling

First Line
- Atypical versus typical antipsychotics lower risk of extrapyramidal symptoms and dyskinesias (clozapine, quetiapine)
- Greater risk of weight gain, diabetes, and hyperlipidemia especially with olanzapine and clozapine
- Acute psychotic agitation: olanzapine 5 to 10 mg IM NTE 30 mg/day; do not administer with IM benzodiazepine; ziprasidone 10 mg IM q2h or 20 mg q4h; NTE 40 mg/day; haloperidol 2 to 5 mg +/− lorazepam 2 mg IM, can be given with 1 mg IM benztropine, NTE 20 mg haloperidol and 8 mg lorazepam per day

Medications

Haloperidol	Haldol Decanoate: 50 mg, 50–200 mg, q3–4wk
Fluphenazine	Haldol Decanoate: 12.5 mg, 12.5–50 mg, q2–3wk
Aripiprazole	Abilify Maintena: 400 mg monthly (2-week PO overlap), 300–400 mg monthly
	Lauroxil: 441–1,064 mg, 3-week PO overlap. 15 mg/day PO: 662 mg IM monthly
	OR 30 mg PO and Aristada Initio + lauroxil or 882 mg IM q6wk or 1,064 mg IM q2mo
Paliperidone	Invega Sustenna: 234 mg then 156 mg in 1 week, 39–234 mg monthly
	Invega Trinza: 273–819 mg q3mo, needs 4 months of Sustenna
	Invega Hayfera: 1,092–1,560 mg q6mo; needs 4 months of Sustenna or one Trinza cycle
Olanzapine	Pamoate: 210–405 mg
Risperidone	Risperdal Consta: 12.5–50.0 mg q2wk (PO overlap), 12.5–50.0 mg q2wk
	Perseris: 90 or 120 mg monthly (no PO overlap), 90 mg = 3 mg QD, 120 = 4 mg QD

- Psychosis in schizophrenia
  - Risperidone: Start 1 to 2 mg QD; target dose of 2 to 8 mg/day reached over 1 to 2 weeks; >6 mg rarely more effective and higher risk of parkinsonism; higher risk of prolactinemia/parkinsonism due to D_2 blockade
  - Ziprasidone: Start 20 to 40 mg PO BID with at least 500 calories. Target dose 100 to 160 mg/day in divided doses over 2 weeks; prolongs QTc; less likely to cause weight gain than other atypicals; higher risk of akathisia/parkinsonism
  - Aripiprazole: Start 10 to 15 mg QD, may increase to 30 mg/day over 1 to 2 weeks; less weight gain but high rates of akathisia; lowers QTc
  - Lurasidone: Start 20 to 40 mg QD with at least 350 calories, increase up to 160 mg QHS over 2 to 4 weeks; less weight gain but high rates of akathisia/parkinsonism

Second Line
- Olanzapine: Start 5 to 10 mg QHS; target dose 5 to 20 mg/day within 2 days. More likely weight gain, hyperlipidemia, and hyperglycemia than other atypicals except clozapine; sedating; drug metabolism increased 50% by tobacco use
- Quetiapine: Start 25 mg BID, increase 25 to 50 mg q8–12h days 2 and 3, up to 3 to 400 mg by day 4. Can then increase 50 to 100 mg/day, NTE 800 mg/day divided BID–TID; less risk of parkinsonism but more weight gain; sedation, restless legs syndrome; gradual titration better tolerated; prolongs QTc
- Paliperidone: Start 3 to 6 mg QD; target dose 6 to 12 mg QD; titrate over 1 to 2 weeks. Higher risk of prolactinemia/parkinsonism than others; minimal hepatic metabolism, ideal for hepatic impairment
- Asenapine: Start 5 mg QHS or BID sublingually, increase to 10 mg BID if needed over 1 to 2 weeks; less weight gain than some, high rates of akathisia/parkinsonism; sedation, orthostatic hypotension; transdermal patch available
- Iloperidone: Start 1 mg BID, may increase by 2 mg daily, but slower can be better due to significant orthostasis (max 12 mg BID); little akathisia/parkinsonism, less weight gain but long titration, orthostasis, sedation; prolongs QTc
- Brexpiprazole: Start 1 mg QD for first 4 days, 2 mg QD days 5 to 7, can increase dose up to 4 mg/day based on response. Lower rates of akathisia than aripiprazole but higher rates than others; less weight gain than others

- Cariprazine: Start at 1.5 mg QD, can be increased to 3 mg QD on day 2, dosed up to 6 mg QD based on response; in 6-week study, fasting glucose, cholesterol, triglycerides, and weight were similar to placebo
- Lumateperone: 42 mg daily. No titration required. Mild average weight loss; moderate sedation and dry mouth
- First-generation antipsychotics such as haloperidol which can be started at 0.5 to 2.0 mg q8–12h. Target dose of 10 mg QD or less divided doses. High rates of tardive dyskinesia; decreased rates of metabolic syndrome
- Olanzapine/samidorphan: Start at 5 mg/10 mg QD. Increase olanzapine at weekly intervals of 5 mg pending response, up to 20 mg/10 mg QD. Less weight gain risk attributed to samidorphan—a novel opioid-system modulator, similar to naltrexone

Geriatric Considerations
Antipsychotics increase risk of death compared to placebo when used in the elderly with dementia. Pimavanserin is approved for Parkinson disease psychosis.

ADDITIONAL THERAPIES
Psychotherapy, vocational, art, and group are effective adjuvants to antipsychotics (1)[B].

COMPLEMENTARY & ALTERNATIVE MEDICINE
- Vitamin treatments if there is a deficiency (common with folic acid, B_6, B_{12}, D), omega 3 supplements, glycine
- CBD proposed as an adjunctive treatment. Do not confuse with THC, which can precipitate psychosis.

ADMISSION, INPATIENT, AND NURSING CONSIDERATIONS
Admission if at risk for harm to self or others; extreme functional impairment; new-onset psychosis

 ONGOING CARE

Medication management, psychotherapy. Cognitive-behavioral therapies can be very effective.

FOLLOW-UP RECOMMENDATIONS
Close follow-up for inpatient discharge (high risk for suicide); use therapy, exercise, smoking cessation, AIMS testing.

Patient Monitoring
- For patients treated with antipsychotics, screen initially for metabolic syndrome (lipid panel, glucose, HgbA1c, CBC, CMP, LFTs, weight, waist circumference) and AIMS testing. Continue monitoring with long-term use.
- EPS: Evaluate every week until dose is stable for 2 weeks. Once stabilized, assess EPS and TD at least q6–12mo.

DIET
- Omega-3, which may be found in fish, fruits, vegetables, nuts, and seeds
- Avoid alcohol and sugar-sweetened beverages.

PATIENT EDUCATION
National Alliance on Mental Illness:
https://www.nami.org/

PROGNOSIS
- Schizophrenia: fluctuating course; 70% first-episode psychosis patients improve in 3 to 4 months, 20–40% attempt suicide. 7% die of suicide.
- Medications are a mainstay of treatment but are only one component; others include psychosocial interventions, cognitive-behavioral therapy, self-help–based interventions, and motivational enhancement techniques.

COMPLICATIONS
- Metabolic disturbances secondary to antipsychotic medications, sedentary lifestyle, and smoking
- Life expectancy reduced over a decade compared to general population (largely mediated by heart disease)

REFERENCE
1. National Institute for Health and Care Excellence. Psychosis and schizophrenia in adults: prevention and management. http://www.nice.org.uk/guidance/cg178. Accessed October 16, 2018.

ADDITIONAL READING
American Psychiatric Association. Clinical practice guidelines. https://www.psychiatry.org/psychiatrists/practice/clinical-practice-guidelines. Accessed November 24, 2021.

 SEE ALSO

Delirium; Schizophrenia

CODE
ICD
60
CODES

ICD10
- F29 Unsp psychosis not due to a substance or known physiol cond
- F20.9 Schizophrenia, unspecified
- F39 Unspecified mood [affective] disorder

CLINICAL PEARLS
- Antipsychotics are the mainstay of treatment; decrease all-cause mortality and increase quality of life
- Aripiprazole shortens QTc.
- Clozapine and long-acting injectables may increase adherence.

PULMONARY ARTERIAL HYPERTENSION

Nasheena Jiwa, MD

 BASICS

DESCRIPTION

- Pulmonary arterial hypertension (PAH) is a category of pulmonary hypertension (PH) characterized by abnormalities in the small pulmonary arteries (precapillary PH) that produce increased pulmonary arterial pressure (PAP) and vascular resistance, eventually resulting in right-sided heart failure. PAH is a progressive disorder associated with increased mortality.
  - Previously, PH was classified as primary PH (without cause, now idiopathic IPAH) or secondary PH (with cause or associated condition); now, it is clear that some types of secondary PH closely match primary PH (IPAH) in their histology, natural history, and response to treatment. Therefore, WHO classifies PH into five groups based on mechanism, with PAH as group 1 in this classification.
  - PAH is diagnosed by right-heart catheterization and defined by a mean PAP ≥20 mm Hg at rest and a pulmonary vascular resistance (PVR) of ≥3 Wood units, when other groups of PH are ruled out; pulmonary capillary wedge pressure ≤15 mm Hg (excludes PH owing to left heart disease; i.e., group 2 PH).
  - Mild or absent chronic lung disease or other causes of hypoxemia (excludes PH owing to lung disease or hypoxemia; i.e., group 3 PH)
  - Absent venous thromboembolic disease (excludes chronic thromboembolic PH [CTEPH]; i.e., group 4 PH)
  - Absent systemic disorder (like sarcoidosis), hematologic disorders (like myeloproliferative disease), and metabolic disorders (like glycogen storage disease) (excludes group 5 PH)
- PAH is divided into following main categories:
  - Idiopathic: sporadic, with no family history or risk factors
  - Heritable: IPAH with mutations or familial cases with or without mutations
  - Drug or toxin induced: mostly associated with anorectics (e.g., fenfluramine), rapeseed oil, L-tryptophan, dasatinib (Bcr-Abl tyrosine kinase inhibitor), and illicit drugs such as methamphetamine and cocaine
  - Associated: connective tissue diseases (e.g., systemic lupus erythematosus, rheumatoid arthritis, scleroderma), HIV infection, portal hypertension (HTN), congenital heart disease, schistosomiasis (chronic hemolytic anemia added to group 5 PH—unclear/multifactorial mechanisms) (1)
  - Pulmonary veno-occlusive disease (PVOD) and/or pulmonary capillary hemangiomatosis (PCH) and persistent PH of the newborn (PPHN) are classified as separate categories due to more differences than similarities with PAH.
    - PVOD and/or PCH: rare cause of PH characterized by extensive diffuse occlusion of the pulmonary veins (unlike PAH which involves the small muscular pulmonary arterioles)

EPIDEMIOLOGY

- Age: can occur at any age; mean age 37 years
- Sex (IPAH): female > male (female:male ratio ranges from 1.7 to 4.8:1.0)

Incidence

- Overall PAH: 5 to 52 cases per million
- IPAH: low, ~2 to 6 per million
- Drug-induced PAH: 1/25,000 with >3 months of anorectic use
- HIV associated: 0.5/100

- Portal HTN associated: 1 to 6/100
- Scleroderma associated: 6–60%

Prevalence

- PAH: ~15 to 50 cases per million
- IPAH: ~6 cases per million

ETIOLOGY AND PATHOPHYSIOLOGY

- Pulmonary: Inflammation, vasoconstriction, endothelial dysfunction, and intimal proliferation causing remodeling of pulmonary arteries produced by increased cell proliferation and reduced rates of apoptosis lead to obstruction.
- Cardiovascular: Right ventricular hypertrophy (RVH), eventually leading to right-sided heart failure and right ventricular (RV) ischemia due to reduced right coronary artery flow, causes RV remodeling associated with PAH.
- IPAH: by definition, unknown. True IPAH is mostly sporadic or sometimes familial in nature.
- Pulmonary arteriolar hyperactivity and vasoconstriction, occult thromboembolism, or autoimmune (high frequency of antinuclear antibodies)

Genetics

- 75% of heritable PAH (HPAH) cases and 25% of IPAH cases have mutations in *BMPR2* (autosomal dominant).
- Mutations in *ALK1* and endoglin (autosomal dominant) also are associated with PAH.

RISK FACTORS

- Female sex
- Previous anorectic drug use
- Recent acute pulmonary embolism
- First-degree relatives of patient with familial PAH

COMMONLY ASSOCIATED CONDITIONS

See associated PAH, discussed earlier.

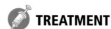 **DIAGNOSIS**

Symptoms of PAH are nonspecific, which can lead to missed or delayed diagnosis of this serious disease.

HISTORY

Dyspnea, weakness, syncope, dizziness, chest pain, palpitations, lower extremity edema

PHYSICAL EXAM

- Pulmonary component of S_2 (at apex in >90% of patients)
- RV lift
- Early systolic click of pulmonary valve
- Pansystolic murmur of tricuspid regurgitation
- Diastolic murmur of pulmonic insufficiency (Graham Steell murmur)
- RV S_3 or S_4
- Edema as jugular vein distention, ascites, hepatomegaly, or peripheral edema

DIFFERENTIAL DIAGNOSIS

Other causes of dyspnea:

- Pulmonary parenchymal disease such as chronic obstructive pulmonary disease, interstitial lung disease, or restrictive lung disease
- Pulmonary vascular disease such as pulmonary thromboembolism
- Cardiac disease such as cardiomyopathy
- Other disorders of respiratory function such as sleep apnea

DIAGNOSTIC TESTS & INTERPRETATION

- Echocardiography (ECG): RVH and right axis deviation, or RV strain (increased P wave amplitude, incomplete right bundle branch block pattern, an R-to-S ratio >1 in lead V_1)
- Pulmonary function testing: reduced diffusion capacity
- Arterial blood gas: arterial hypoxemia, hypocapnia
- Ventilation/perfusion (V/Q) scan: Look for proximal pulmonary artery emboli and CTEPH; rule out group 4 PH.
- Exercise test: reduced maximal O_2 consumption, high-minute ventilation, low anaerobic threshold, increased PO_2 alveolar–arterial gradient; correlation to severity of disease with 6-minute walk distance (6MWD) test
- Antinuclear antibody positive (up to 40% of patients)
- LFTs: Evaluate for portopulmonary HTN as a complication of chronic liver disease.
- HIV test, thyroid function tests, sickle cell disease screening
- Elevated brain natriuretic peptide (BNP) and N-terminal-proBNP may be useful for early detection of PAH in young, otherwise healthy patients with mild symptoms. It can also be used to assess disease severity and prognosis.
- Chest radiograph
  - Prominent central pulmonary arteries with peripheral hypovascularity of pulmonary arterial branches
  - RV enlargement is a late finding.
- Echo Doppler
  - Should be performed with suspicion of PAH; echo suggests, but does not diagnose, PAH; most commonly used screening tool
    - Estimates mean PAP and assesses cardiac structure and function, excludes congenital anomalies
    - Right atrial and ventricular enlargement; tricuspid regurgitation
    - Important to rule out underlying cardiac disease such as atrial septal defect with secondary PH or mitral stenosis
- In patients at risk for HPAH, screen for gene mutations *BMPR2*.
- Polysomnography: for suspected symptoms of obstructive sleep apnea

Diagnostic Procedures/Other

- Pulmonary angiography
  - Should be done if V/Q scan suggests CTEPH
  - Use caution; can lead to hemodynamic collapse; use low osmolar agents, subselective angiograms.
- Right-sided cardiac catheterization (gold standard for diagnosis of PAH)
- Essential to confirm diagnosis and determine severity and prognosis by measuring PAPs and hemodynamics
  - Rule out underlying cardiac disease (e.g., left-sided heart disease) and assess response to vasodilator therapy.
- Lung biopsy: not recommended unless primary pulmonary parenchymal disease exists
- 6MWD: classifies severity of PAH and estimates prognosis

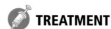 **TREATMENT**

- Treat underlying diseases/conditions that may cause PAH to relieve symptoms and improve quality of life and survival.
- Reasonable goals of therapy include the following:
  - Modified NYHA FC I or II
  - ECG/CMR of normal/near-normal RV size and function

– Hemodynamic parameters showing normalization of the RV function (RAP <8 mm Hg and cardiac index [CI] >2.5 to 3.0 L/min/m²)
– 6MWD of >380 to 440 m
– Cardiopulmonary exercise testing, including peak oxygen consumption of >15 mL/min/kg and EqCO2 <45 L/min
– Normal BNP levels (2)[C]

GENERAL MEASURES
- Supervised exercise training (3)[A]
- Psychosocial support (3)[C]
- Avoid strenuous physical activity (3)[C].
- Avoid pregnancy (3)[C].
- Influenza and pneumococcal immunization (3)[C]
- Oxygen—maintain arterial blood O_2 pressure >60 mm Hg (3)[C]

MEDICATION
- Acute vasodilator test during heart catheterization for all patients who are potential candidates for long-term oral calcium channel blocker (CCB) therapy (3)[C]
  – Screens for pulmonary vasoreactivity/responsiveness using inhaled nitrous oxide; epoprostenol (IV) or adenosine (IV): Positive response may be a prognostic indicator.
  – Contraindicated in right-sided heart failure or hemodynamic instability
- Chronic vasodilator therapy
  – If IPAH with positive response to acute vasodilator test (a fall in mean PAP of ≥10 mm Hg and to a value <40 mm Hg, with unchanged/increased cardiac output), use CCBs.
    o Adequate response confirmed after 3 to 4 months of treatment
    o ~13% will initially respond. Long-term clinical response to CCB therapy is small (~7%) (3)[C].
    o CCBs include nifedipine (long acting), diltiazem, and amlodipine.
    o Avoid verapamil due to its significant negative inotropic effect.
  – CCBs are contraindicated in patients with a cardiac index of <2 L/min/m² or a right atrial pressure >15 mm Hg if PAH with negative response to acute vasodilator test or worsening on therapy; specific vasodilator choice based on risk stratification (3)[C].
    o Nonresponders to acute vasoreactivity who are in WHO-FC II should be treated with an oral compound (3)[B].
    o Nonresponders who remain or progress to WHO-FC III should be considered for treatment with any approved PAH drugs (3)[B].
    o Continuous IV epoprostenol is recommended as first-line therapy for WHO-FC IV PAH due to survival benefit (NNT = 5) (3)[A].
    o In case of inadequate clinical response, sequential combination therapy should be considered. Therapy includes ERA plus a phosphodiesterase type 5 (PDE5) inhibitor or a prostanoid plus ERA or a prostanoid plus a PDE5 inhibitor (3)[A].
    o WHO-FC II PAH—approved drugs: ambrisentan, bosentan, macitentan, riociguat, sildenafil, tadalafil (3)[B]
    o WHO-FC III PAH—approved drugs: ambrisentan, bosentan, epoprostenol (IV), macitentan, riociguat, sildenafil, tadalafil, treprostinil (SC, inhaled) (3)[B]
    o WHO-FC IV PAH—approved drugs: epoprostenol (IV) (3)[A]

– Drug classes:
  o Prostacyclins: improve exercise capacity, cardiopulmonary hemodynamics: epoprostenol (IV), treprostinil (IV, SC, or inhaled), iloprost, beraprost
  o Prostacyclin IP: receptor agonist—selexipag
  o Endothelin receptor antagonists: improve exercise capacity; reducing mortality has been noted (4)[A]: bosentan (PO), ambrisentan (PO), macitentan. Pregnancy Category X; monitor LFTs monthly.
  o PDE5 inhibitor: suggested improvement in exercise capacity, cardiopulmonary hemodynamics, and symptoms (3)[C]: sildenafil (PO), tadalafil (PO), vardenafil
  o Guanylate cyclase stimulant: stimulators of the nitric oxide receptor, improves exercise capacity: riociguat (PO)
- Anticoagulation
  – Improved survival originally suggested in patients with IPAH only. Newer studies show some evidence for favorable effects of anticoagulation on survival in IPAH, HPAH, or PAH associated with anorexigens (3)[C].
  – Warfarin with international normalized ratio of 1.5 to 2.5 shows survival advantage in patients in multiple observational studies.
    o Contraindications: Avoid in patients with syncope or significant hemoptysis; consider drug interactions.
- Diuretics indicated in patients with RV volume overload (e.g., peripheral edema or ascites) (3)[B]
- Digoxin has little long-term data in PAH: used in RV failure and/or atrial dysrhythmias, increases cardiac output, and preserves RV contractility

ISSUES FOR REFERRAL
Refer to a pulmonologist and/or a cardiologist for further evaluation/treatment if PAH is suspected.

SURGERY/OTHER PROCEDURES
- Patients with documented large-vessel thromboembolic disease should be considered for pulmonary thrombectomy.
- Balloon atrial septostomy for severe PAH with right-sided heart failure despite optimized medical therapy to relieve symptoms prior to lung transplant or as a treatment on its own
- Heart–lung or lung transplantation

ADMISSION, INPATIENT, AND NURSING CONSIDERATIONS
- Medical therapy is primarily palliative.
- Hospitalization with invasive monitoring is needed to screen vasodilator responsiveness and initiate vasodilator therapy.
- National registry has been established by the National Heart, Lung, and Blood Institute.

ONGOING CARE

FOLLOW-UP RECOMMENDATIONS
- Pneumococcal and influenza vaccines
- Exercise: walking or low-level aerobic activity, as tolerated, once stable; respiratory training

Patient Monitoring
Frequently evaluate disease progression and therapeutic efficacy. Tests to measure treatment response include 6-minute walk test and cardiopulmonary exercise test.

DIET
Fluid and salt restrictions, especially with RV failure

PATIENT EDUCATION
Discuss prognosis, lifestyle changes, and all therapeutic options (including transplant).

PROGNOSIS
- Median survival is 2 to 3 years from diagnosis; 5-year survival rate is 34% (NIH registry); newer data show 5-year survival ~70% with new treatment.
- Mode of death: right-sided heart failure (most common), pneumonia, sudden death, cardiac death
- Poor prognostic factors
  – Rapid symptom progression
  – Clinical evidence of RV failure
  – WHO functional PAH class IV (or NYHA functional class III or IV)
  – 6MWD <300 m
  – Peak VO_2 during cardiopulmonary exercise testing <10.4 mL/kg/min
  – ECG with pericardial effusion, significant RV enlargement/dysfunction, right atrial enlargement
  – Mean right atrial pressure >20 mm Hg
  – Cardiac index <2 L/min/m²
  – Elevated mean PAP
  – Significantly elevated BNP and NT-proBNP; other markers also show promise in predicting survival: RDW, GDF-15, interleukin-6, creatinine.
  – Scleroderma spectrum of diseases

COMPLICATIONS
- Thromboembolism, heart failure, pleural effusion, and sudden death
- Pregnancy should be avoided due to high maternal mortality (30–50%) and fetal wastage.

REFERENCES
1. Simonneau G, Gatzoulis MA, Adatia I, et al. Updated clinical classification of pulmonary hypertension. *J Am Coll Cardiol*. 2013;62(Suppl 25):D34–D41.
2. McLaughlin VV, Gaine SP, Howard LS, et al. Treatment goals of pulmonary hypertension. *J Am Coll Cardiol*. 2013;62(Suppl 25):D73–D81.
3. Galiè N, Corris PA, Frost A, et al. Updated treatment algorithm of pulmonary arterial hypertension. *J Am Coll Cardiol*. 2013;62(Suppl 25):D60–D72.
4. Liu C, Chen J, Gao Y, et al. Endothelin receptor antagonists for pulmonary arterial hypertension. *Cochrane Database Syst Rev*. 2009;(3):CD004434.

ADDITIONAL READING
Taichman DB, Ornelas J, Chung L, et al. Pharmacologic therapy for pulmonary arterial hypertension in adults: CHEST guideline and expert panel report. *Chest*. 2014;146(2):449–475.

 CODES

ICD10
- I27.0 Primary pulmonary hypertension
- I27.2 Other secondary pulmonary hypertension

CLINICAL PEARLS
- PAH involves abnormalities in the small pulmonary arteries (precapillary PH) which increase PAP and vascular resistance leading to right heart failure. Diagnosis is made by right heart catheterization.
- For positive vasodilator test, CCBs are the first-line agents to manage IPAH.
- For nonresponders, treatment depends on WHO-FC.

Umair Usman Khan, MD • Naureen Bashir Rafiq, MD

 BASICS

Pulmonary embolism (PE) is an acute cardiovascular disorder that requires emergent medical attention due to its high early mortality rates. PE causes pulmonary vascular bed obstruction, which results in acute right ventricular failure, a life-threatening condition.

DESCRIPTION
- PE is the most serious presentation of venous thromboembolism (VTE).
- Classified based on severity:
  - Low-risk PE: acute and absence of clinical markers of adverse prognosis
  - Submassive PE: no systemic hypotension, but there is either myocardial necrosis (elevated troponin) or right ventricle (RV) dysfunction (RV dilation or systolic dysfunction on echocardiography [echo], RV/LV ratio >1 on computed tomography [CT], elevation of B-type natriuretic peptide [BNP] or N-terminal pro-BNP, or consistent electrocardiogram [ECG] changes)
  - Massive PE: hemodynamic instability with sustained hypotension; pulselessness; or persistent bradycardia, cardiogenic shock, acute manifesting RV failure

EPIDEMIOLOGY
Case fatality rates vary widely (1–60%); case fatality rate is approximately 11% at 2 weeks.

Incidence
- Approximately 30 to 80/100,000, with higher incidence in African Americans and lower in Asians; >100,000 cases annually in the United States
- Incidence increases with age, most occurring at 60 to 70 years of age.
- 250,000 hospitalizations per year in the United States, 10–60% in hospitalized patients
  - Highest risk for orthopedic and cancer patients
  - 1:1,000 pregnancies (including postpartum)

Prevalence
- Epidemiology is difficult to determine outside of the hospital setting because some patients with PE may remain asymptomatic, the first presentation of PE can be sudden death, or diagnosis of PE is incidental.
- Within hospitalized patients:
  - 17.3% prevalence of PE in hospitalized adults who were admitted for first episode of syncope (between 2012 and 2014)
  - 2.5 to 23 per 10,000 patient prevalence of PE in Asian countries (China, India, Japan, Korea, Singapore) (1)

ETIOLOGY AND PATHOPHYSIOLOGY
- Venous stasis, endothelial damage, and changes in coagulation properties trigger thrombus.
- Causes increased pulmonary vascular resistance, impaired gas exchange, and decreased pulmonary compliance. RV failure due to pressure overload is usually the primary cause of death.
- The most common source (85%) of PE is proximal lower extremity deep vein thrombosis (DVT).

Genetics
- Factor V Leiden: most common thrombophilia. +5.5% in Caucasian, 2.2% in Hispanics, 1.2% in African American, 0.5% in Asian; associated with 20% of VTE
- Prothrombin G20210A: 3% of Caucasians; rare in African American, Asian, and Native American; 6% in patients with VTE
- Rarely, deficiencies in protein C, S, and antithrombin

RISK FACTORS
- Older age, obesity, prolonged immobilization, surgery, major trauma, joint replacement, spinal cord injury, cancer, hormonal replacement therapy, pregnancy/puerperium, previous thrombosis, antiphospholipid syndrome, genetics
- Oral contraceptive most frequent risk factor in women

GENERAL PREVENTION
- Low VTE risk: early ambulation after surgery, compression stockings, and intermittent pneumatic compression
- Use of thromboprophylaxis in COVID-19 infection is not commonly done but may be considered in those at high risk (prior VTE, recent surgery, limb immobilization, recent trauma, etc.).
- Hip or knee arthroplasty (high VTE risk): 10 or more days prophylaxis with low-molecular-weight heparin (LMWH), fondaparinux, apixaban, dabigatran, rivaroxaban, or low-dose unfractionated heparin (UFH)
- Spinal cord injury, hip fracture surgery, and trauma surgery (high VTE risk): 28 to 35 days with LMWH, fondaparinux, UFH, or vitamin K antagonists (VKA)
- Long-distance travel (>8 hours): hydration, walking, avoidance of constrictive clothing and frequent calf exercises, compression stockings below knee
- Patients with factor V Leiden, prothrombin *G20210A* with no previous thrombosis do not need prophylaxis.

COMMONLY ASSOCIATED CONDITIONS
COVID-19 infection

 DIAGNOSIS

- Establish a pretest probability based on clinical criteria.
  - Wells score
    - Clinical signs and symptoms of DVT +3
    - Alternative diagnosis is less likely than PE +3.
    - Heart rate >100 +1.5
    - Immobilization previous 4 weeks +1.5
    - Previous DVT/PE +1.5
    - Hemoptysis +1
    - Malignancy +1
    - D-dimer has very high negative predictive value (NPV), so if <500 ng/mL, PE is ruled out
    - Interpretation:
      - <2 points, low probability (obtain D-dimer)
      - 2 to 4 points, moderate probability (Obtain D-dimer but consider initiating anticoagulation.)
      - >4 points, high probability (Obtain spiral CT angiogram if patient is stable, and initiate anticoagulation if no contraindications.)
- Wells and revised Geneva score were simplified.
  - Wells score: Each predictor is +1; PE unlikely if 0 to 1, PE likely if >2
  - Geneva score: Each predictor is +1 except for heart rate >95 beats/min, which is +2; PE unlikely if 0 to 2 and PE likely if >3

HISTORY
- Determine if the presentation is provoked or idiopathic. Approximately 30% of cases develop without identifiable risk factor.
- Bleeding risk (previous anticoagulation, history of bleeding, recent interventions/surgeries, liver disease, kidney disease)
- Sudden onset dyspnea (>85%), chest pain (>50%), cough (20%), syncope (14%), hemoptysis (7%)

PHYSICAL EXAM
- Dyspnea, syncope, hemoptysis, tachycardia, tachypnea, accentuated S_2; pleuritic chest pain, pleural friction rub, rales
- Signs of DVT: leg swelling, tenderness, visible collateral veins
- Signs of RV failure: jugular vein distention, S_3 or S_4, systolic murmur at left sternal edge, hepatomegaly

DIFFERENTIAL DIAGNOSIS
- Pulmonary: pneumonia, bronchitis, pneumothorax, pneumonitis, chronic obstructive pulmonary disease exacerbation, pulmonary edema
- Cardiac/vascular: myocardial infarction, pericarditis, congestive heart failure, aortic dissection
- Musculoskeletal: rib fracture(s), chest wall pain

DIAGNOSTIC TESTS & INTERPRETATION
- D-dimer ELISA: In patients with low pretest probability, it can rule out PE if it is negative (high NPV). It is not diagnostic if positive (low positive predictive value [PPV]), and it is not helpful if pretest probability is intermediate or high.
- CBC, creatinine, aPTT and PT, ABG: In young patients with idiopathic, recurrent, or significant family history of VTE, consider hypercoagulable tests.
  - Do not test for protein C, S, factor VIII, or antithrombin in the acute setting.
  - Patients with intermediate or high pretest probability and low probability with elevated D-dimer need further diagnostic testing.
- Chest x-ray (CXR): Westermark sign (lack of vessels in an area distal to the embolus), Hampton hump (wedge-shaped opacity with base in pleura), Fleischner sign (enlarged pulmonary arteries), pleural effusion, hemidiaphragm elevation
- ECG: right heart strain, S1Q3T3
- CT pulmonary angiography: sensitivity 96–100%, specificity 86–89%; NPV 99.8%. If normal, it excludes PE if low or intermediate clinical probability.
- Ventilation/perfusion scintigraphy (V/Q scan): use if CT angiography is not available or contraindicated. A high-probability V/Q scan makes the diagnosis of PE; normal V/Q scan excludes PE.
- Pulmonary angiography: gold standard invasive and technically difficult: 2% morbidity and <0.01 mortality risk
- Echo: assesses RV function and thrombus in transit
- Magnetic resonance (MR) angiography: lower sensitivity and specificity than CT angiography
- Compression venous ultrasound (CUS): noninvasive. Sensitivity >90%, specificity ~95%. It confirms the diagnosis of PE in patients with clinical suspicion.
- CT venography: can be done at the same time as CT angiography; increases diagnostic yield

ALERT
If preclinical probability is intermediate or high and patient has low bleeding risk, start treatment while waiting for results.

Initial Tests (lab, imaging)
- Labs:
  - CBC: for anemia, thrombocytosis, leukocytosis
  - CMP: to check electrolyte abnormalities
  - D-dimer: *used to rule out DVT/PE when clinical suspicion for PE is low to moderate
  - BNP: to rule-out congestive heart failure as cause
  - Troponins: Rule out myocardial causes.
- Imaging:
  - CXR: If normal with hypoxemia, suspect PE.
  - Venous Doppler: initial test for DVT; positive venous Doppler with SOB and tachypnea can begin treatment for PE.

Follow-Up Tests & Special Considerations

- Spiral CTA: test of choice to diagnose PE, performed when clinical suspicion for PE is high
  - *Contraindication: renal failure or contrast allergy
- Lung V/Q scan: can rule out PE if low clinical suspicion/Wells score

Diagnostic Procedures/Other

Pulmonary angiography—definitive test

Test Interpretation

- D-dimer (performed if Wells criteria for PE is less than or equal to 4)
  - Normal: PE is ruled-out.
  - High: Move on to imaging (spiral CTA).
- Spiral CTA (performed if Wells is >4 or D-dimer is high)
  - Diagnostic/positive: Treat for PE.
  - Nondiagnostic/contraindicated: Perform V/Q scan, CUS.
- V/Q scan, CUS
  - Negative: TEE or MR or pulmonary angiography
  - Positive: Treat for PE.

 ## TREATMENT

Treatment is based on risk stratification.

- Low-risk PE → use anticoagulation or inferior vena cava (IVC) filter.
- Submassive PE → anticoagulation + possible INR-guided thrombolysis
- Massive PE → anticoagulation + definite INR consult for thrombolysis/embolectomy catheter/surgery

GENERAL MEASURES

Goal to maintain SaO_2 at >92%

MEDICATION

- Start LMWH, fondaparinux, UFH, as initial therapy for first 5 to 10 days. VKA can be started the 1st day and must overlap with parenteral treatment for minimum of 5 days, until INR is 2 to 3 for 24 hours.
- Following 5 to 10 days of parenteral therapy, dabigatran or edoxaban is also approved.
- An oral option for initial and long-term treatment is rivaroxaban or apixaban.
- Patients with massive PE with low bleeding risk: Consider systemic thrombolytics if no contraindications.

First Line

- UFH:
  - IV bolus of 80 U/kg or 5,000 U followed by continuous infusion (initially 18 U/kg/hr or 1,300 U/hr) with dose adjustments to maintain aPTT that corresponds to anti-Xa levels of 0.3 to 0.7
  - SC injection: two options:
    - Monitored: 17,500 U or 250 U/kg BID with dose adjustments to maintain an aPTT that corresponds to anti-Xa levels of 0.3 to 0.7 measured 6 hours after a dose
    - Fixed dose: 333 U/kg initial dose, followed by 250 U/kg BID
- LMWH: preferred due to lower risk of major bleeding and heparin-induced thrombocytopenia (HIT)
  - Enoxaparin (Lovenox) 1 mg/kg/dose SC q12h
  - Dalteparin (Fragmin) 200 U/kg SC q24h
  - Fondaparinux (Arixtra) 5 mg (body weight <50 kg), 7.5 mg (body weight 50 to 100 kg), or 10 mg (body weight >100 kg) SC q24h
- Maintenance therapy: warfarin on day 1, if possible; 5 mg/day for 3 days in hospitalized or older patients and at a dose of 10 mg in <60 years of aged patients; adjust dose to maintain an INR of 2 to 3; needs to overlap with UFH, LMWH, or fondaparinux: 5 to 7 days, until 2 consecutive days of therapeutic INR

- Rivaroxaban: 15 mg BID × 3 weeks and then 20 mg once daily to complete treatment. Compared to warfarin, it has less major bleeding side effects while having same efficacy; ok to use in HIT
- Edoxaban: 60 mg once daily (reduced to 30 mg once daily if CrCl 30 to 50 mL/min or body weight <60 kg). Patients require initial treatment with LMWH at least 5 days before starting edoxaban. Compared to warfarin, less bleeding and lower rate of recurrence in PE with RV dysfunction; increased bleeding risk in cancer-associated thrombosis compared to dalteparin
- Apixaban: 10 mg BID for 7 days, then 5 mg once daily; less major bleeding episodes; ok to use in HIT
- Dabigatran: requires initial treatment with LMWH; ok to use in HIT

ALERT

- Contraindications:
  - Active bleeding
  - Heparin: HIT
  - LMWH: HIT, renal failure
  - Warfarin: pregnancy
  - Rivaroxaban and fondaparinux: renal failure
  - Edoxaban: severe kidney or liver failure
  - Apixaban: renal impairment and nonvalvular atrial fibrillation
  - Dabigatran: severe kidney problems. Use of dronedarone or ketoconazole increases risk.
- No dose reduction strategy needed to treat acute PE with dabigatran, apixaban, or rivaroxaban

Pregnancy Considerations

- Warfarin: teratogenic; safe while breastfeeding
- LMWH: Dalteparin, enoxaparin, and fondaparinux are Category B; heparin is Category C: Use if the benefit outweighs risks.
- UFH: requires aPTT monitoring; can cause osteoporosis if used for prolonged period
- Rivaroxaban is Category C.
- Edoxaban and apixaban: Category B; increase risk of hemorrhage
- Dabigatran: Category C; only if benefit > risk

Second Line

Massive PE: thrombolytics if hemodynamic compromise and low bleeding risk, intracranial hemorrhage risk: 0.7–6.4%:

- Tissue plasminogen activator (tPA) 100 mg infused over 2 hours
- Absolute contraindications:
  - Intracranial hemorrhage, intracranial cerebrovascular or malignancy, ischemic stroke <3 months, possible aortic dissection, bleeding diathesis, active bleeding, recent neurosurgery, or major trauma

SURGERY/OTHER PROCEDURES

- IVC filter placement if absolute contraindication for anticoagulation or recurrent PE despite adequate anticoagulation treatment
- Emergency embolectomy can be considered in patients with massive PE with contraindications for thrombolysis.
- Consider US-assisted catheter-directed thrombolysis with intermediate risk of death or submassive PE.

ADMISSION, INPATIENT, AND NURSING CONSIDERATIONS

- In selected, low-risk acute PE population (Pulmonary Embolism Severity Index [PESI] score class I or II), patients could be managed safely and effectively in the outpatient setting with close follow-up.
- ICU-level care if hemodynamically unstable

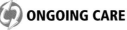 ## ONGOING CARE

Duration of anticoagulation

- Provoked PE (trigger no longer present): 3 months

- Unprovoked PE: >3 months; consider long-term or prolonged secondary prophylaxis if bleeding risk is low. HERDOO2 Score provides guidance to determine duration of therapy in women with first unprovoked VTE. Low risk (0 to 1 criteria) can safely stop treatment after 6 months.
- Cancer-related PE: LMWH first 3 to 6 months. Consider secondary prophylaxis as long as the patient has active cancer.
- Recurrent unprovoked PE: long-term anticoagulation

FOLLOW-UP RECOMMENDATIONS

If concomant DVT, consider 30 to 40 mm Hg knee-high compression stockings.

Patient Monitoring

- INR should be checked regularly; target is 2 to 3.
- aPTT needs to be monitored in SC UFH.
- Anti-Xa can be checked in special circumstances if treated with LMWH, including pregnancy, younger patients, renal disease.

PATIENT EDUCATION

Patients at risk for clots (i.e,. sedentary, postsurgical, hypercoagulable states pregnancy or cancer) should be counseled on preventive measures.

PROGNOSIS

- Mortality: submassive 6–14%; massive PE 15–60%
- PESI score predicts 30-day mortality. Stratified by risk classes depending on number of risk factors: class I (very low mortality risk; 0–1.6%), class II (low mortality risk; 1.7–3.5%), class III (moderate mortality risk; 3.2–7.1%), class IV (high mortality risk; 4–11.4%), and class V (very high mortality risk; 10–24.5%)
- Any one of the following defines high risk: age >80 years, cancer, chronic cardiopulmonary disease, heart rate 110 beats/min, systolic blood pressure <100 mm Hg, O_2 saturation <90%.
- High early mortality risk: shock or hypotension, + sPESI >1 + RV dysfunction signs
- Intermediate high early mortality risk: no shock or hypotension + sPESI >1 + RV dysfunction signs
- Intermediate low early mortality risk: no shock or hypotension + sPESI >1 + either RV dysfunction by imaging or cardiac laboratory biomarkers
- Low early mortality risk: no shock or hypotension, no sPESI; imaging is optional.
- PE mortality rate is significantly higher in patients with active cancer (up to 47-fold higher).

COMPLICATIONS

Post-PE syndrome: permanent pulmonary vasculature changes, dyspnea, reduced exercise capacity

REFERENCE

1. Lee LH, Gallus A, Jindal R, et al. Incidence of venous thromboembolism in Asian populations: a systemic review. *Thromb Haemost*. 2017;117(12):2243–2260.

 ## CODES

ICD10

- I26.02 Saddle embolus of pulmonary artery with acute cor pulmonale
- I26.92 Saddle embolus of pulmonary artery without acute cor pulmonale
- I26.01 Septic pulmonary embolism with acute cor pulmonale

CLINICAL PEARLS

Use Wells criteria; obtain D-dimer for low and intermediate risk; spiral CT angiography for high risk

PULMONARY FIBROSIS

Avignat S. Patel, MD

BASICS

DESCRIPTION
- Pulmonary fibrosis (PF) is an interstitial lung diseases (ILDs), a family of >200 different lung diseases, characterized by inflammation, cellular proliferation, and/or fibrosis within lung interstitium and bronchial walls. If no cause identified, ILD is called idiopathic interstitial pneumonia.
- The most common idiopathic interstitial pneumonia is idiopathic PF (IPF).
- IPF is defined as a form of chronic fibrosing ILD associated with the histologic and/or radiologic appearance of usual interstitial pneumonia (UIP) when other causes have been excluded.

EPIDEMIOLOGY
- Most common ILD prevalent worldwide (25–30% of all ILD)
- Most common in men >60 years of age

Incidence
Higher in North America and Europe (3 to 9 cases per 100,000 person-years) than in South America and East Asia (fewer than 4 cases per 100,000 person-years)

Prevalence
In the United States, the prevalence has been reported to range from 10 to 60 cases per 100,000.

ETIOLOGY AND PATHOPHYSIOLOGY
- A favored model for the pathogenesis of IPF is that recurrent, alveolar epithelial damage with accelerated cell senescence leads to abnormal cellular repair and deposition of interstitial fibrosis by myofibroblasts.
- Causes of nonidiopathic PF include occupational and environmental exposures, drugs, and connective tissue diseases.

Genetics
- The role of host genetic factors and their interactions with environmental factors is unknown.
- Mutations in genes involved in maintenance of telomere length are associated with increased risk of IPF.
- An SNP in the MUC5B promoter leads to gene overexpression and is associated with increased risk of IPF. However, the mechanism linking MUC5B and IPF is not clear.

RISK FACTORS
- Family history of IPF
- Smoking—most significant association
- GERD, OSA
- Occupational and environmental exposures: wood (pine), metal dusts (lead, brass, steel), farming, birds, hairdressing, stone cutting, exposure to livestock, vegetable and animal dust, air pollution, mold

GENERAL PREVENTION
Avoidance of above risk factors

COMMONLY ASSOCIATED CONDITIONS
- Pulmonary hypertension: 30–80% of patients with IPF
- GERD
- Nonidiopathic PF may be related to connective tissue diseases (RA and scleroderma).

DIAGNOSIS

HISTORY
- Gradual onset
- Exertional breathlessness and nonproductive cough
- Constitutional symptoms (weight loss, fever, fatigue, myalgias, arthralgias) are uncommon.
- History of exposure (see "Risk Factors" above)

PHYSICAL EXAM
- Lung auscultation: bibasilar fine, late inspiratory crackles: "Velcro" crackles
- Clubbing in late stages, cyanosis (rare)
- Findings of pulmonary hypertension and RV failure (elevated JVP, right ventricular (RV) parasternal heave, loud P_2, LE edema)
- Signs of connective tissue disorders (skin/nail fold changes, arthritis)

DIFFERENTIAL DIAGNOSIS
- Other ILDs such as chronic hypersensitivity pneumonitis, nonspecific interstitial pneumonia, occupational lung disease, connective tissue disease-ILD (CTD-ILD)
- See below for histologic differential diagnosis of UIP.

DIAGNOSTIC TESTS & INTERPRETATION

Initial Tests (lab, imaging)
- Blood tests: Most labs are normal.
- Chest radiograph:
  - Reduced lung volumes and reticular opacities mostly at lung bases
  - Coarse reticular pattern and honeycombed cysts in advanced stages
- Pleural abnormalities (such as pleural plaques, effusions) are uncommon.

Follow-Up Tests & Special Considerations
- Chest CT scan:
  - Once diagnosis of IPF is suspected, obtain high-resolution CT (HRCT) chest, including inspiratory and expiratory images with thin <1.25 mm slices and prone images if subtle subpleural basal changes present.
  - In diagnosing IPF, HRCT is categorized into one of four patterns: UIP, probable UIP, indeterminate, and alternative diagnosis.
  - UIP pattern requires bilateral, primary peripheral, lower lobe reticulation, and honeycombing with or without traction bronchiectasis. UIP pattern on HRCT is diagnostic of IPF without need for surgical lung biopsy.
  - Similar changes (as described above) with traction bronchiectasis but in the absence of honeycombing are categorized as probable UIP.
  - Atypical features on HRCT include upper- or mid-lung predominance, predominant consolidation, ground-glass opacities, and diffuse nodules or cysts; these increase the likelihood of an ILD other than IPF.
- Serologic testing for connective tissue diseases to exclude nonidiopathic causes: ANA; RF; anti–CCP antibodies; Scl-70, Ro, La, U1-RNP, and Jo-1; creatine kinase; and myoglobin, and antisynthetase antibodies
- Echocardiogram to assess cardiac function, RV function, and pulmonary hypertension

Diagnostic Procedures/Other
- Pulmonary function testing (PFT):
  - PFTs in all patients undergoing evaluation and treatment of IPF/ILD
  - Findings include:
    - Decreased diffusion capacity for carbon monoxide (DLCO)
    - Decreased lung volumes (TLC, RV, FRC)
    - Decreased spirometric values: FVC and FEV_1 due to the reduction in lung volume with preserved FEV_1/FVC ratio
- ABG may show hypoxemia and respiratory alkalosis.
- 6-minute walk distance (6MWD): reduced distance and exertional hypoxemia
- Sleep study:
  - Sleep disturbances with reduced REM sleep, lighter and more fragmented sleep, and hypoxemia during REM sleep
  - Tachypnea persists during sleep.
- Bronchoscopy:
  - Bronchoalveolar lavage (BAL):
    - Can be helpful in excluding other diagnoses like infection, malignancy, etc.
    - ATS/ERS does not recommend routine use of BAL for diagnosis of IPF.
  - Bronchoscopic transbronchial biopsy:
    - Not recommended for diagnosis of IPF as sensitivity and specificity is poor
    - May help exclude other ILDs
    - Transbronchial lung cryobiopsy is a potential replacement for thoracoscopic biopsy, but data is limited at this point.
    - A genomic classifier that can be run on transbronchial biopsy specimens can assist in diagnosing patients whose CT is not definite for IPF.
- Surgical lung biopsy:
  - Gold standard for diagnosis of ILDs
  - When the combination of clinical and imaging data is not diagnostic, a thoracoscopic lung biopsy can be considered.
  - Biopsy samples should be taken from multiple lobes avoiding the most severely affected areas as they will show nondiagnostic fibrosis.
  - Procedure should not be performed in high-risk patients, including:
    - High oxygen requirements (>2 L/min)
    - Significant pulmonary hypertension
    - Rapid disease progression
    - Severely reduced FVC or DLCO
  - Several studies have compared video-assisted thoracoscopic biopsy (VATS) with open thoracotomy biopsy and noted that diagnostic yield is similar but morbidity less with VATS.

Test Interpretation
- Histopathology
  - Gross pathology distinctive nodular pleural surface
  - Histopathologic pattern in IPF is UIP.
    - UIP pattern requires dense fibrosis with architectural distortion, subpleural, and basal distribution, spatial and temporal heterogeneity, fibroblastic foci, and honeycomb changes plus absence of features suggestive of alternate diagnosis.
    - Differential diagnosis of UIP histologic pattern includes IPF, CTD-ILD, chronic hypersensitivity pneumonitis, asbestosis, chronic radiation pneumonitis, Hermansky-Pudlak syndrome and neurofibromatosis.

- Diagnostic strategies:
  - As per ATS/ERS statement of IPF in 2018, diagnosis of IPF requires (1):
    - Exclusion of other known causes of ILD and either of the following:
      - UIP pattern on HRCT
      - Specific combinations of HRCT patterns and histopathology patterns
  - UIP pattern on HRCT would be diagnostic with all histology patterns except alternate diagnosis findings.
  - UIP pattern on histology would be diagnostic with all HRCT patterns except alternate diagnosis findings.
  - Per ATS/ERS, for patients suspected of having IPF, a multidisciplinary discussion (pulmonologists, radiologists, pathologists, rheumatologists) is recommended for diagnostic decision-making.

 TREATMENT

GENERAL MEASURES
- Smoking cessation
- Vaccinations: pneumococcus, influenza, SARS-CoV-2
- Pulmonary rehabilitation
- Referral to a transplant center
- Supplemental oxygen:
  - Clinical practice guidelines strongly recommend supplemental oxygen if SpO_2 <88%.
  - The oxygen prescription should be informed by 6-minute walk tests or treadmill testing of oxygen saturation as well as by nocturnal oximetry or polysomnography when indicated.

MEDICATION
Two medications, nintedanib and pirfenidone, have been shown to be safe, effective, and are recommended in the treatment of IPF.
- In placebo-controlled, randomized trials, each drug has been shown to slow the rate of FVC decline by approximately 50% over the course of 1 year.
- Both have shown some efficacy in reducing severe respiratory events, such as acute exacerbations and hospitalization.
- Pooled data and meta-analyses also suggest reduced mortality.
- The cost of each medication is estimated to exceed $100,000 annually.

First Line
- Nintedanib:
  - Mechanism of action: tyrosine kinase inhibitor that targets growth factor pathways including VEGF, FGF, and PDGF receptors
  - Most common side effect is diarrhea. It is also associated with a small risk of bleeding and should be used cautiously, if at all, in patients on therapeutic anticoagulation.
  - Liver function should be monitored as liver toxicity has been reported.
- Pirfenidone:
  - Mechanism of action: anti-inflammatory and antifibrotic effects, including inhibition of collagen synthesis, down regulation of TGF-β and TNF-α, and reduction in fibroblast proliferation
  - Common side effects: anorexia, nausea, vomiting, photosensitive rash, abnormal liver function

- Cannot recommend one agent over the other because there have been no head-to-head comparisons and efficacy is similar
- Reflux management:
  - Some data suggested worsening of IPF with ongoing/untreated GERD. However, there is no data from clinical trials to support routine treatment.

Second Line
- No second-line agents available.
- Treatment guidelines for IPF by ATS/ERS include:
  - Strong recommendations against use of:
    - Anticoagulation (warfarin)
    - Combination prednisone + azathioprine + N-acetylcysteine (NAC)
    - Selective endothelin receptor antagonist (ambrisentan)
    - Imatinib, a tyrosine kinase inhibitor with one target
  - Conditional recommendations against:
    - Dual endothelin receptor antagonists (macitentan, bosentan)
    - Phosphodiesterase-5 inhibitor (sildenafil)
    - NAC monotherapy

ISSUES FOR REFERRAL
- Referral to pulmonologist for diagnosis and management
- Thoracic surgeon referral is indicated if patient cannot be diagnosed by ATS clinical and radiographic criteria.
- Referral to lung transplant center is indicated early on for patients showing progressive worsening of the disease.

ADDITIONAL THERAPIES
Several investigational therapies are being studied in randomized controlled trials.

SURGERY/OTHER PROCEDURES
Lung transplant:
- Can prolong survival and improve quality of life for highly selected candidates
- Only a minority of patients with IPF receive lung transplants.
- Only 66% of lung transplant recipients survive for >3 years after transplant and only 53% survive for >5 years.
- Common complications include primary graft dysfunction, acute and chronic allograft rejection, opportunistic infections, and cancer.

COMPLEMENTARY & ALTERNATIVE MEDICINE
No proven benefit of any of the complementary and alternative medications

ADMISSION, INPATIENT, AND NURSING CONSIDERATIONS
- Patient with acute exacerbation of IPF should be admitted to the hospital for management with corticosteroids.
- Need for mechanical ventilation portends a poor prognosis and should be avoided if possible.
- Palliative care consult is appropriate for all patients diagnosed with IPF.

 ONGOING CARE

FOLLOW-UP RECOMMENDATIONS
- Pulmonary clinic and, if possible, at an ILD clinic
- Monitoring with serial HRCT, PFT along with 6MWD
- If on antifibrotic medications, monitor LFTs.

PROGNOSIS
IPF carries a poor prognosis with a median survival of 3.8 years among adults ≥65 years in the United States.

COMPLICATIONS
- Acute exacerbation of IPF
  - 10–20% per patient per year
  - It is characterized by worsening hypoxemia, new bilateral ground-glass opacities, consolidation, or both on HRCT imaging that are not fully explained by volume overload or infection.
  - Triggers: infection, aspiration, drug toxicity, or idiopathic
  - Treatment: Available guidelines make weak recommendations for the use of glucocorticoids (no definitive benefit based on available data) and do not recommend the use of mechanical ventilation. Consider palliative care referral.
- Increased risk for VTE, lung cancer, and pulmonary hypertension
  - Management of pulmonary hypertension in the outpatient setting should consist of supplemental oxygen. A recent study of inhaled treprostinil in ILD, including IPF, demonstrated a clinical benefit but, in general, pulmonary vasodilator therapy has not proven beneficial in IPF. IPF patients with significant pulmonary hypertension should be referred to a pulmonary hypertension specialist.

REFERENCE
1. Raghu G, Remy-Jardin M, Myers JL, et al; for American Thoracic Society, European Respiratory Society, Japanese Respiratory Society, Latin American Thoracic Society. Diagnosis of idiopathic pulmonary fibrosis. An official ATS/ERS/JRS/ALAT clinical practice guideline. *Am J Respir Crit Care Med.* 2018;198(5):e44–e68.

 CODES

ICD10
- J84.10 Pulmonary fibrosis, unspecified
- J84.112 Idiopathic pulmonary fibrosis

CLINICAL PEARLS
- IPF is the most common idiopathic ILD and frequently misdiagnosed or has delayed diagnosis.
- HRCT scan is the cornerstone for diagnosis.
- Two antifibrotic drugs are the only approved therapy for IPF.
- Oxygen supplementation, pulmonary rehab, anti-reflux treatment, vaccinations against pneumococcus and influenza should be considered in all patients.
- Referral to pulmonary clinic, ILD clinic, and lung transplant center should be considered very early in course.

PYELONEPHRITIS

Katelin M. Lisenby, PharmD, BCPS • Connie Leeper, MD, MPH •
Dana G. Carroll, PharmD, BCPS, CDCES, BCGP

 BASICS

DESCRIPTION
- A syndrome caused by infection of the renal parenchyma and/or renal pelvis, often producing localized flank/back pain combined with systemic symptoms, such as fever, chills, nausea and vomiting; there is a wide spectrum of illness ranging from mild symptoms to septic shock.
- Chronic pyelonephritis is the result of progressive inflammation of the renal interstitium and tubules, due to recurrent infection, vesicoureteral reflux, or both.
- Pyelonephritis is considered uncomplicated if the infection is caused by a typical pathogen in an immunocompetent patient with normal urinary tract anatomy and renal function.
- System(s) affected: renal; urologic
- Synonym: acute upper urinary tract infection (UTI)

Geriatric Considerations
- May present as altered mental status; absence of fever is common in the elderly.
- Older patients with diabetes and pyelonephritis are at higher risk for bacteremia, prolonged hospitalization, and mortality.
- The high prevalence of asymptomatic bacteriuria in the elderly makes the use of urine dipstick less reliable for diagnosing UTI in this population.

Pregnancy Considerations
- Most common medical complication requiring hospitalization. Pregnant women with asymptomatic bacteriuria (ABU) have 20–30% risk to develop acute pyelonephritis if ABU is not treated.
- Affects 1–2% of all pregnancies. Morbidity does not differ between trimesters.
- Urine culture for test of cure 1 to 2 weeks after therapy.
- Consider low-dose suppressive antibiotics for the remainder of pregnancy following treatment for pyelonephritis or recurrent cystitis in pregnancy.

Pediatric Considerations
- UTI is present in ~5% of patients age 2 months to 2 years with fever and no apparent source on history and physical exam.
- Treatment (PO or IV; inpatient or outpatient) should be based on the clinical situation and patient toxicity.

EPIDEMIOLOGY
Incidence
Community-acquired acute pyelonephritis: 3 to 4 cases per 10,000 males; 15 to 17 cases per 10,000 females; 28 cases per 10,000 women ages 18 to 49 years.

Prevalence
Adult cases: 250,000/year, with 200,000 hospitalizations

ETIOLOGY AND PATHOPHYSIOLOGY
- *Escherichia coli* (>80%)
- Other gram-negative pathogens: *Proteus, Klebsiella, Serratia, Clostridium, Pseudomonas,* and *Enterobacter* spp.
- *Enterococcus* spp.
- *Staphylococcus: Staphylococcus epidermidis, Staphylococcus saprophyticus* (number 2 cause in young women), and *Staphylococcus aureus*
- *Candida* spp.

RISK FACTORS
- Underlying urinary tract abnormalities
- Indwelling catheter/recent urinary tract instrumentation
- Nephrolithiasis
- Immunocompromised, including diabetes
- Elderly, institutionalized patients (particularly women)
- Prostatic enlargement, stress incontinence
- Childhood UTI
- Acute pyelonephritis within the prior year
- Recent sexual intercourse; spermicide use; new sex partner within the prior year
- Pregnancy
- Hospital-acquired infection
- Symptoms >7 days at time of presentation

COMMONLY ASSOCIATED CONDITIONS
- Indwelling catheters, renal calculi
- Benign prostatic hyperplasia

 DIAGNOSIS

HISTORY
- In adults
  - Fever; flank pain; nausea ± vomiting
  - Malaise, anorexia, myalgia
  - Dysuria, urinary frequency, urgency
  - Suprapubic discomfort
  - Mental status changes (elderly)
- In infants and children
  - Fever, irritability and poor feeding
  - GI symptoms

PHYSICAL EXAM
- In adults
  - Fever: ≥38°C (100.4°F)
  - Costovertebral angle tenderness
  - Presentation ranges from no physical findings to septic shock.
  - Mental status changes common in the elderly
  - Depending on presentation, consider a pelvic exam in women to exclude pelvic inflammatory disease.
- In infants and children
  - Lethargy, fever, poor skin perfusion
  - Inadequate weight gain/weight loss
  - Jaundice; pallor; gray skin color

DIFFERENTIAL DIAGNOSIS
- Obstructive uropathy
- Acute bacterial pneumonia (lower lobe)
- Cholecystitis, acute pancreatitis, appendicitis
- Perforated viscus; aortic dissection
- Pelvic inflammatory disease; ectopic pregnancy
- Kidney stone, diverticulitis

DIAGNOSTIC TESTS & INTERPRETATION
Initial Tests (lab, imaging)
- Urinalysis: pyuria (>5 WBC/HPF) ± leukocyte casts, hematuria, nitrites (sensitivity 35–85%; specificity 92–100%), and mild proteinuria
- Urine leukocyte esterase positive (sensitivity 74–96%; specificity 94–98%)
- Urine Gram stain; urine culture (>100,000 colony forming units/mL or >100 colony forming units/mL + symptoms) and sensitivities

- Complete blood count, blood urea nitrogen, creatinine, glomerular filtration rate (GFR), and pregnancy test (if indicated)
- C-reactive protein levels correlate with prolonged hospitalization and recurrence; serum albumin <3.3 g/dL also associated with increased risk for hospital admission
- Imaging not necessary in routine cases. Imaging is primarily used to diagnose complications (emphysematous pyelonephritis or renal abscess).
- Pediatrics: Guidelines recommend renal/bladder US (not voiding cystourethrogram) after first febrile UTI between age 2 and 24 months.

Follow-Up Tests & Special Considerations
- Catheterization/suprapubic aspirate to obtain samples from non–toilet-trained children
- Blood culture(s): if hospitalized, diagnosis uncertain, suspected hematogenous source or immunosuppression
- Recent antibiotic use may alter lab results.
- If patient's condition does not improve within 72 hours, if obstruction/anatomic abnormality suspected, in patients with immunosuppression or multiple comorbidities, and/or if certain lab abnormalities are present (urine pH >7, GFR <40, 50% decline in renal function), consider:
  - CT scan of abdomen and pelvis ± contrast. Contrast-enhanced computed tomography (CECT) is typically the image of choice for children and adults with acute pyelonephritis.
  - US of kidneys, ureter, bladder is not as sensitive as CT but is cheaper and more readily available.
  - Cystoscopy with ureteral catheterization

Test Interpretation
- Acute: abscess formation with neutrophil response
- Chronic: fibrosis with reduction in renal tissue

 TREATMENT

- ≤7 days of treatment is equivalent to longer regimens in adults (including those with bacteremia) without urogenital abnormalities (1),(2)[A].
- IV antibiotics for inpatients who are toxic appearing or unable to tolerate oral antibiotics

GENERAL MEASURES
- Broad-spectrum antibiotics initially based on severity of illness, health status, and risk factors for resistant pathogens; tailor to culture and sensitivity results.
  - Risk factors for a multidrug-resistant (MDR) pathogens/infections if present within last 3 months:
    ○ History of urinary MDR pathogen
    ○ Inpatient stay at a health care facility (hospital, nursing home, etc.)
    ○ Use of fluoroquinolone, trimethoprim-sulfamethoxazole (TMP-SMX), or broad-spectrum β-lactam
    ○ Travel to geographic regions with significant incidence of MDR pathogens (e.g., India, Middle East, Central America)
- Analgesics and antipyretics
- Consider urinary analgesics (e.g., phenazopyridine 200 mg q8h) for dysuria

MEDICATION

- For empiric oral therapy, a fluoroquinolone is recommended. Should fluoroquinolone resistance exceed 10% or the patient has nausea/vomiting, a single initial IV dose of a long-acting antibiotic such as ceftriaxone 1 g is recommended.
- For parenteral therapy, fluoroquinolone, an aminoglycoside with or without ampicillin, an extended-spectrum cephalosporin with or without a β-lactamase inhibitor, an extended-spectrum penicillin with or without an aminoglycoside, or a carbapenem are recommended.
- Contraindications:
  - Known drug allergy
  - Fluoroquinolones are not recommended in children, adolescents, and pregnant women unless other alternatives are not available.
  - Nitrofurantoin does not achieve reliable tissue levels to treat pyelonephritis.
- Precautions
  - Adjust antibiotic dosages in patients with renal insufficiency.
  - Monitor aminoglycoside levels and renal function.
  - If *Enterococcus* is suspected based on Gram stain, ampicillin ± gentamicin or piperacillin-tazobactam are good empiric choices; unless patient is penicillin allergic, then use vancomycin. If outpatient, add amoxicillin to fluoroquinolone, pending culture results and sensitivity. Do not use a 3rd-generation cephalosporin for suspected/proven enterococcal infections.
  - >20% *E. coli* strains are resistant to ampicillin and TMP-SMX in community-acquired infections.
  - Extended-spectrum β-lactamase (ESBL)-producing strains should be treated with a carbapenem ± β-lactamase inhibitor or ceftolozane-tazobactam or plazomicin (3)[A],(4)[A].

First Line

- Adults
  - Oral (initial outpatient treatment)
    - Ciprofloxacin: 500 mg q12h for 7 days
    - Ciprofloxacin XR: 1,000 mg/day for 7 days
    - Levofloxacin: 750 mg/day for 5 days
    - TMP-SMX (160/800 mg): 1 tablet q12h for 14 days provided uropathogen known to be susceptible ± ceftriaxone 1 g initial IM/IV dose
  - IV (initial inpatient treatment for patients with no risk factors for MDR organisms)
    - Ciprofloxacin: 400 mg q12h
    - Levofloxacin: 750 mg/day
    - Cefotaxime: 1 g q8–12h up to 2 g q4h
    - Ceftriaxone: 1 to 2 g/day
    - Cefepime: 1 to 2 g q12h
    - Gentamicin: 5 to 7 mg/kg body weight daily
    - Piperacillin-tazobactam: 3.375 g q6–8h
    - Ampicillin: 2 g q6h ± gentamicin for *Enterococcus*
  - IV (initial inpatient treatment for patients with at least one risk factor for MDR organisms)
    - Antipseudomonal carbapenem
      - Meropenem: 1 g q8h
      - Imipenem: 500 mg q6h
      - Doripenem: 500 mg q8h
    - Add vancomycin for methicillin-resistant *S. aureus* (MRSA) or daptomycin or linezolid for vancomycin-resistant *Enterococcus* (VRE).
  - Severe illness: IV therapy until afebrile for 24 to 48 hours and tolerating PO intake. Switch to oral agents to complete up to a 2-week course.
- Pediatric
  - Oral: cefdinir: 14 mg/kg/day for 10 to 14 days; ceftibuten 9 mg/kg/day for 10 to 14 days; cefixime 8 mg/kg/day for 10 to 14 days

- IV (General indication for IV therapy is age <2 months or clinical concern in other ages.)
  - Ceftriaxone: 75 mg/kg/day (IM use acceptable in outpatient setting)
  - Cefotaxime: 150 mg/kg/day divided in 3 to 4 doses
  - Ampicillin: 100 mg/kg/day divided in 4 doses + gentamicin 7.5 mg/kg/day divided in 3 doses

Second Line

Adults

- Oral
  - Use oral β-lactams with caution; if used, provide an initial IV dose of ceftriaxone or a consolidated 24-hour dose of an aminoglycoside; longer courses of therapy (10 to 14 days) recommended
  - Cefpodoxime (Proxetil): 200 mg q12h
  - Amoxicillin-clavulanate: 875/125 mg q12h or 500/125 mg q8h
- IV
  - Ticarcillin-clavulanate: 3.1 g q4–6h
  - Targeted therapy for MDR organisms
    - Ertapenem: 1 g q24h
    - Ceftazidime-avibactam: 2.5 g q8h
    - Ceftolozane-tazobactam: 1.5 g q8h
    - Meropenem-vaborbactam: 4 g q8h (3)[A]
    - Plazomicin: 15 mg/kg/day (4)[A]
    - Cefiderocol: 2 g q8h (5)[A]

Pediatric Considerations

- Treat children <2 years of age and children with febrile or recurrent UTI for 10 to 14 days.
- Initial empiric antibiotic choice should cover *E. coli*. Add ampicillin if *Enterococcus* is suspected.
  - Oral antibiotics (ceftibuten, cefixime, and amoxicillin/clavulanic acid) may be used alone, *or*
  - IV antibiotics (single daily dosing if an aminoglycoside is chosen) for 2 to 4 days, followed by oral antibiotics for a total of 10 to 14 days
- Complete outpatient antibiotic course in entirety.

ISSUES FOR REFERRAL

- Acute pyelonephritis unresponsive to therapy
- Chronic pyelonephritis, abnormal urogenital anatomy

SURGERY/OTHER PROCEDURES

Perinephric abscess may require surgical drainage.

ADMISSION, INPATIENT, AND NURSING CONSIDERATIONS

- Inpatient therapy for severe illness (e.g., high fevers, severe pain, marked debility, intractable vomiting, inability to tolerate oral intake, possible sepsis), risk factors for complicated pyelonephritis, pregnancy, or extremes of age
- Outpatient therapy if mild to moderate illness, uncomplicated course, and tolerating oral intake.
- IV fluids for dehydration; blood cultures for patients admitted with pyelonephritis
- Discharge on oral agent after patient is afebrile 24 to 48 hours to complete up to 2 weeks of therapy.

 ONGOING CARE

FOLLOW-UP RECOMMENDATIONS

- Women: routine follow-up cultures not recommended unless symptoms recur after 2 weeks and then urologic evaluation is necessary
- Men, children, adolescents, patients with recurrent infections, patients with risk factors: Repeat cultures 1 to 2 weeks after completing therapy; urologic evaluation after first episode of pyelonephritis and with recurrences

Patient Monitoring

- If no response within 48 hours (5% of patients): Reevaluate and review cultures, CT scan, or US to review anatomy; adjust therapy as needed; urologic or infectious disease consult. The two most common causes of failure to respond are a resistant organism and nephrolithiasis.
- Work with parents to monitor response in children.

DIET

Encourage fluid intake.

PROGNOSIS

95% of treated patients respond within 48 hours.

COMPLICATIONS

- Renal abscess; perinephric abscess
- Metastatic infection: skeletal system, endocardium, eye, meningitis with subsequent seizures
- Septic shock and death
- Acute/chronic renal failure

REFERENCES

1. Eliakim-Raz N, Yahav D, Paul M, et al. Duration of antibiotic treatment for acute pyelonephritis and septic urinary tract infection—7 days or less versus longer treatment: systematic review and meta-analysis of randomized controlled trials. *J Antimicrob Chemother*. 2013;68(10):2183–2191.
2. Ren H, Li X, Ni ZH, et al. Treatment of complicated urinary tract infection and acute pyelonephritis by short-course intravenous levofloxacin (750 mg/day) or conventional intravenous/oral levofloxacin (500 mg/day): prospective, open-label, randomized, controlled, multicenter, non-inferiority clinical trial. *Int Urol Nephrol*. 2017;49(3):499–507.
3. Wunderink RG, Giamarellos-Bourboulis EJ, Rahav G, et al. Effect and safety of meropenem-vaborbactam versus best-available therapy in patients with carbapenem-resistant Enterobacteriaceae infections: the TANGO II randomized clinical trial. *Infect Dis Ther*. 2018;7(4):439–455.
4. Wagenlehner FME, Cloutier DJ, Komirenko AS, et al. Once-daily plazomicin for complicated urinary tract infections. *N Engl J Med*. 2019;380(8):729–740.
5. Portsmouth S, van Veenhuyzen D, Echols R, et al. Cefiderocol verses imipenem-cilastin for the treatment of complicated urinary tract infections caused by gram-negative uropathogens: a phase 2, randomised, double-blind, non-inferiority trial. *Lancet Infect Dis*. 2018;18(12):1319–1328.

CODES

ICD10

- N12 Tubulo-interstitial nephritis, not spcf as acute or chronic
- N10 Acute tubulo-interstitial nephritis
- N11.9 Chronic tubulo-interstitial nephritis, unspecified

CLINICAL PEARLS

- Pyelonephritis can present with isolated confusion or mental status changes (no fever) in the elderly.
- The most common causes of poor response to treatment are antibiotic resistance and coexisting nephrolithiasis.
- Fluoroquinolones are generally the initial antibiotic of choice for pyelonephritis. Oral β-lactams are less effective. Parenteral β-lactams may be used in cases of complicated UTIs.

PYLORIC STENOSIS
Blake Leeds, DO • Laura B. Bishop, MD

BASICS

DESCRIPTION
- Acquired narrowing of the pyloric canal due to progressive hypertrophy of pyloric muscle leading to obstruction, usually occurs in the first 2 to 12 weeks of life
- Synonym(s): infantile hypertrophic pyloric stenosis (IHPS)

EPIDEMIOLOGY
- Onset almost always between 2 and 12 weeks of age
- Highest incidence found in first-born infants.
- May be more common in bottle-fed infants
- The most common condition requiring surgical intervention in the 1st year of life
- A recent decline in incidence has been reported in a number of countries.
- Predominant sex: male > female (4 to 5:1)

Incidence
In Caucasian infants, 2 to 5:1,000 babies; less common in African American and Asian babies

Prevalence
National prevalence level is 1 to 2:1,000 infants, ranging from 0.5 to 4.21:1,000 live births.

ETIOLOGY AND PATHOPHYSIOLOGY
- Abnormal relaxation of the pyloric muscles leads to hypertrophy.
- Redundant mucosa fills the pyloric canal.
- Gastric outflow is obstructed, leading to gastric distension and forceful projectile postprandial vomiting.
- The exact cause remains unknown, but multiple genetic and environmental factors have been implicated.
- Increased vasoactive intestinal peptide in breast milk may mediate pyloric relaxation and increase gastric emptying, protecting from pyloric stenosis.
- Formula feeding may cause higher serum levels associated with pylorospasm, increasing rates of pyloric stenosis (1)[C].

Genetics
Recent studies have identified linkage to chromosomes 3, 5, 11, and 19.

RISK FACTORS
- 5 times increased risk with affected first-degree relative
- Strong familial aggregation and >80% heritability
- Premature birth is NOT a risk factor.

- Multiple gestation
  - 200-fold increased risk if monozygotic twin affected
  - 20-fold increased risk if dizygotic twin affected
- Maternal white ethnicity
- Maternal alcohol and cigarette use perinatally
- Perinatal risk factors include C-section and first born.
- Postnatal macrolide antibiotics, especially erythromycin, could potentially cause sustained contraction of pyloric muscle.
- Formula feeding increases risk.

GENERAL PREVENTION
Breastfeeding appears to be protective.

COMMONLY ASSOCIATED CONDITIONS
Associated anomalies present in ~4–7% of infants with pyloric stenosis.
- Hiatal and inguinal hernias (most common)
- Rare associated anomalies include the following:
  - Congenital heart disease
  - Esophageal atresia
  - Tracheoesophageal fistula
  - Renal abnormalities
  - Turner syndrome and trisomy 18
  - Cornelia de Lange syndrome
  - Smith-Lemli-Opitz syndrome

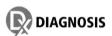

DIAGNOSIS

HISTORY
- Nonbilious projectile vomiting after feeding, increasing in frequency and severity
- Emesis may become blood-tinged from gastric irritation.
- Hunger due to inadequate nutrition
- Excessive crying
- Decrease in bowel movements
- Weight loss
- Median duration of symptoms is 10 days.

PHYSICAL EXAM
- Firm, mobile ("olive-like") mass palpable in the right upper quadrant (historically 70–90% of the time)
- Use of ultrasound (US) has led to earlier diagnosis, decreasing "olive-like" mass finding to 14% present with classic triad of nonbilious vomiting, visible peristalsis, and a palpable olive (1)[C].
- Epigastric distention
- Visible gastric peristalsis after feeding
- Late signs: dehydration, weight loss
- Rarely, jaundice when starvation leads to decreased glucuronyl transferase activity resulting in indirect hyperbilirubinemia.

DIFFERENTIAL DIAGNOSIS
- Inexperienced or inappropriate feeding
- GERD
- Gastritis
- Congenital adrenal hyperplasia, salt-wasting
- Pylorospasm
- Gastric volvulus
- Antral or gastric web
- Neonatal intestinal obstruction
- Hiatal hernia

DIAGNOSTIC TESTS & INTERPRETATION
Metabolic disturbances are late findings and uncommon due to early diagnosis and intervention.
- If prolonged vomiting, check electrolytes: hypokalemia, hypochloremia, metabolic alkalosis
- Elevated unconjugated bilirubin level (rare)
- Paradoxical aciduria: The kidney tubules excrete hydrogen to preserve potassium in face of hypokalemic alkalosis.

Initial Tests (lab, imaging)
- Pyloric US is the study of choice.
  - US shows thickened and elongated pyloric muscle and redundant mucosa.
  - Pathologic limits are 3-mm pyloric muscle thickness, 15-mm pyloric length, 11-mm pyloric diameter, and 12-mL pyloric volume with muscle thickness being the key factor. Although these measurements remain diagnostic, they may exclude younger (<3 weeks old), smaller infants who can be clinically diagnosed (2)[B].
- Upper GI series: rarely indicated; may be used if history, exam, and US are not conclusive
  - Strong gastric contractions; pyloric canal outlined by string of contrast material (string sign); and parallel lines of barium in the narrow channel separated by mucosa (double-tract sign or railroad track sign)

Test Interpretation
Concentric hypertrophy of pyloric muscle

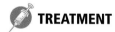

TREATMENT

GENERAL MEASURES
- Treat dehydration and alkalosis before surgery.
- Preoperative antibiotics (cefazolin 30 mg/kg or clindamycin 10 mg/kg IV) for infection prophylaxis
- Usually no need for preoperative NG tube

MEDICATION

First Line

Medical treatment with oral or IV atropine is an alternative to surgical treatment (3)[A].

- Oral atropine: initial dose of 0.05 mg/kg/day and increased to max of 0.1 mg/kg/day
- IV atropine: initial dose of 0.1 mg/kg/day and increased by 0.01 mg/kg/day until vomiting ceases then change to oral atropine at twice the effective IV dose
- Recommended for use in patients when anesthesia or surgery is not possible
- Takes 5 to 15 months for pyloric muscle to normalize on medical therapy, although vomiting will usually cease within 7 days
- Associated with lower success rates and longer stays as compared to surgery

SURGERY/OTHER PROCEDURES

- Ramstedt pyloromyotomy is curative. The entire length of hypertrophied muscle is divided, with preservation of the underlying mucosa.
- Surgical approaches include traditional right upper quadrant transverse incision, more contemporary circumumbilical incision, and laparoscopic techniques.
- Laparoscopic approach results in less postoperative pain, shorter hospital stays, shorter postoperative recovery, lower complication rates, improved cosmesis, and can be performed with no increase in operative time or complications (3),(4)[A],(5)[B].

ADMISSION, INPATIENT, AND NURSING CONSIDERATIONS

- Prompt treatment to avoid dehydration and malnutrition
- Correct acid–base and electrolyte disturbances. Surgery should be delayed until metabolic derangements are corrected.
- Patients need pre- and postoperative apnea monitoring due to a tendency to compensate with respiratory acidosis (apnea) for their metabolic alkalosis.
- IV fluids to correct dehydration and metabolic abnormalities. For optimal resuscitation in infants, use D5 1/2NS with 20 mEq of KCl (1)[C].

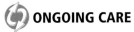 **ONGOING CARE**

FOLLOW-UP RECOMMENDATIONS

Discharge following surgery when tolerating 2 to 3 full feeds (1)[C].

Patient Monitoring

- Routine pediatric health maintenance
- Postoperative monitoring, including monitoring for pain, emesis, apnea
- If significant emesis present after 1 to 2 weeks, then upper GI studies needed to rule out incomplete pyloromyotomy or duodenal leak (1)[C]

DIET

- Adlib feedings are recommended after pyloromyotomy as they decrease length of stay.
- Timing of first feed is not significant, but early feeding is associated with increased potential for emesis without impacting length of stay (6)[A].

PATIENT EDUCATION

Counsel caregivers on postoperative emesis, signs and symptoms of infection, and assessment of hydration status.

PROGNOSIS

Surgery is curative.

COMPLICATIONS

- Dehydration
- Failure to thrive
- Jaundice
- Chronic abdominal pain and pain-associated functional GI disorders following surgery
- Incomplete pyloromyotomy
- Mucosal perforation
- Wound infections
- Delayed feeding due to postoperative vomiting
- Serosal tear
- Subcutaneous emphysema
- 4.6–12% complication rate (2)[C]

REFERENCES

1. Peters B, Oomen MWN, Bakx R, et al. Advances in infantile hypertrophic pyloric stenosis. *Expert Rev Gastroenterol Hepatol.* 2014;8(5):533–541.
2. Said M, Shaul DB, Fujimoto M, et al. Ultrasound measurements in hypertrophic pyloric stenosis: don't let the numbers fool you. *Perm J.* 2012;16(3):25–27.
3. Wu SF, Lin HY, Huang FK, et al. Efficacy of medical treatment for infantile hypertrophic pyloric stenosis: a meta-analysis. *Pediatr Neonatol.* 2016;57(6):515–521.
4. Oomen MWN, Hoekstra LT, Bakx R, et al. Open versus laparoscopic pyloromyotomy for hypertrophic pyloric stenosis: a systematic review and meta-analysis focusing on major complications. *Surg Endosc.* 2012;26(8):2104–2110.
5. Mahida JB, Asti L, Deans KJ, et al. Laparoscopic pyloromyotomy decreases postoperative length of stay in children with hypertrophic pyloric stenosis. *J Pediatr Surg.* 2016;51(9):1436–1439.
6. Sullivan KJ, Chan E, Vincent J, et al; for the Canadian Association of Paediatric Surgeons Evidence-Based Resource. Feeding post-pyloromyotomy: a meta-analysis. *Pediatrics.* 2016;137(1):1–11.

ADDITIONAL READING

- Ein SH, Masiakos PT, Ein A. The ins and outs of pyloromyotomy: what we have learned in 35 years. *Pediatr Surg Int.* 2014;30(5):467–480.
- Graham KA, Laituri CA, Markel TA, et al. A review of postoperative feeding regimens in infantile hypertrophic pyloric stenosis. *J Pediatr Surg.* 2013;48(10):2175–2179.
- Krogh C, Fischer TK, Skotte L, et al. Familial aggregation and heritability of pyloric stenosis. *JAMA.* 2010;303(23):2393–2399.
- Murchison L, De Coppi P, Eaton S. Post-natal erythromycin exposure and risk of infantile hypertrophic pyloric stenosis: a systematic review and meta-analysis. *Pediatr Surg Int.* 2016;32(12):1147–1152.
- Owen RP, Almond SL, Humphrey GM. Atropine sulphate: rescue therapy for pyloric stenosis. *BMJ Case Rep.* 2012;2012:bcr2012006489.
- Wyrick DL, Smith SD, Dassinger MS. Surgeon as educator: bedside ultrasound in hypertrophic pyloric stenosis. *J Surg Educ.* 2014;71(6):896–898.
- Zhu J, Zhu T, Lin Z, et al. Perinatal risk factors for infantile hypertrophic pyloric stenosis: a meta-analysis. *J Pediatr Surg.* 2017;52(9):1389–1397.

 CODES

ICD10

Q40.0 Congenital hypertrophic pyloric stenosis

CLINICAL PEARLS

- Pyloric stenosis is the most common condition requiring surgical intervention in the 1st year of life.
- The condition classically presents between 1 and 5 months of life, with projectile vomiting after feeds and a firm, mobile mass in the right upper quadrant.
- Abdominal US is the study of choice.
- Surgery (laparoscopic Ramstedt pyloromyotomy is the preferred method) is curative, but conservative medical management with atropine can be safe and effective as well.

RABIES

Mallory Zaino, MD • Laura B. Bishop, MD

 BASICS

DESCRIPTION

- A rapidly progressive central nervous system (CNS) infection caused by RNA rhabdovirus affecting humans and mammals
- May present with symptoms of encephalitis or paralysis
- Generally considered 100% fatal after symptoms onset
- Vaccine-preventable
- System(s) affected: CNS
- Synonym(s): hydrophobia (inability to swallow water)

EPIDEMIOLOGY

- Present on all continents except Australia and Antarctica
- >95% of human deaths related to rabies occur in Asia and Africa.
- Bats are the most common reservoir in the United States.
- Dogs are the most common reservoir worldwide.

Incidence

- Estimated 55,000 deaths worldwide per year
- Typically only 1 to 3 cases per year in the United States: 1/3 of those exposures occur outside of the United States

ETIOLOGY AND PATHOPHYSIOLOGY

- Family Rhabdoviridae; genus Lyssavirus: bullet-shaped enveloped, negative-sense single-stranded RNA, neurotropic virus
- Transmission occurs from a bite by an infected animal or when the saliva of an infected animal comes into contact with an open wound or mucous membrane.
  - 60% of human cases of bat-variant virus in North America report no history of bat bite or scratch and 33% report no history of bat contact.
  - Although rare, there are reported cases of laboratory aerosolization and infection from transplanted organs.
- Following transmission, the virus replicates within the muscle and binds to acetylcholine receptors located at the neuromuscular junction.
  - The virus travels retrograde through nerves to the CNS where infection of the dorsal ganglia leads to pain. Viral replication in the brain can disseminate to other organs, including the salivary glands where it can be shed.

RISK FACTORS

- Professions or activities with exposure to infected animals (e.g., animal handlers, lab workers, veterinarians, cave explorers)
- Travel to countries where canine rabies is endemic.
- In the United States, most cases are associated with bat exposure.
- Internationally, exposure occurs through both domestic and feral dogs.
- There are reports of human-to-human transmission through cornea, solid organ, and other tissue transplants.

GENERAL PREVENTION

- Preexposure vaccination
  - For high-risk groups (veterinarians, animal handlers, wildlife rangers, and certain laboratory workers)
  - Consider preexposure vaccination for travelers to parts of the world with increased risk of rabies from domestic animals (i.e., North Africa).
- Source control and avoidance
  - Immunization of dogs and cats has led to a dramatic decrease in U.S. cases since the 1950s.
  - Contact animal control and avoid approaching or handling wild (or domestic) animals exhibiting strange behaviors.
- Postexposure prophylaxis
  - Seek treatment promptly if bitten, scratched, or in contact with saliva from potentially infected animal.
  - Prevent infection by prompt postexposure treatment.
  - Consider postexposure prophylaxis for individuals in direct contact with bats.
  - Hospital contacts of patients infected with rabies do not require postexposure prophylaxis unless there has been exposure through mucous membranes or an open wound (including a bite) to saliva, cerebrospinal fluid (CSF), or brain tissue from the infected patient.
  - Hospitalized patients should be placed in contact isolation with gowns, gloves, goggles, and masks.

 DIAGNOSIS

Diagnosis can be made antemortem through isolation of the virus or antibodies in the serum, saliva, CSF, or nuchal biopsy and postmortem by brain biopsy.

HISTORY

- History of animal exposure; however, most patients do not recall exposure.
- Five stages (may overlap):
  - Incubation period: the time between bite and symptom onset ranges: <1 week to 1 year
  - Prodrome: lasts days to weeks and include nonspecific symptoms of fever, malaise, and anorexia +/− pain and paresthesia at site of infection
  - Acute neurologic period: lasts 2 to 10 days. CNS symptoms dominate; generally 1 of 2 forms:
    ○ Encephalitic (furious) rabies: (80% of cases) hyperactivity with hydrophobia, aerophobia, hyperventilation, hypersalivation, and autonomic instability; progresses to hallucinations, paralysis, stupor
    ○ Paralytic (dumb) rabies: (20% of cases) symmetric or asymmetric paresis, often starting at the site of infection
      ■ Misdiagnosis of paralytic rabies contributes to underreporting of the disease
  - Coma: lasts hours to days; may evolve over several days following acute neurologic period; may be sudden, with respiratory arrest
  - Death: occurs in days to weeks due to diaphragmatic paralysis

PHYSICAL EXAM

Findings range from normal exam to severe neurologic findings, including paralysis and coma, depending on the stage of rabies at the time of presentation

- Assess bite site for excoriation and swelling.
- Encephalitis— fluctuating consciousness with hyperarousal alternating with lucid periods
- Hydrophobia—asking the patient to swallow water or offering a glass of water causes spasms of the accessory muscles of the neck, pharyngeal muscles, and diaphragm
- Aerophobia—blowing or fanning air on the face causes spasms of the accessory muscles of the neck, pharyngeal muscles, and diaphragm.
  - May exhibit fearful facial expression during these episodes
- Signs of autonomic dysfunction—hypersalivation, hyperhidrosis, anisocoria, mydriasis, piloerection, and priapism
- Limb weakness may be the presenting symptom with paralytic rabies.
- Neuropathic and/or radicular pain, sensory deficits, and seizures may be presenting symptoms with bat-variant rabies.
- Nonspecific prodrome of fever, malaise, anorexia, and headache often occur.

DIFFERENTIAL DIAGNOSIS

- Any rapidly progressive encephalitis; important to exclude treatable causes of encephalitis
  - HSV encephalitis, Japanese encephalitis, West Nile virus, Eastern equine encephalitis, enterovirus, Nipah virus
- Tetanus
- Botulism
- Substance use disorder with intoxication
- Transverse myelitis
- Guillain-Barré Syndrome

DIAGNOSTIC TESTS & INTERPRETATION

- Negative predictive value of laboratory tests are low due to multiple factors including intermittent shedding, antibody production, and phase of disease.
- Therefore, multiple types of samples are tested to increase chances of a positive test: serum, saliva, CSF, skin biopsy.

ALERT

Contact state or local health department in suspected rabies testing so that collection and transportation of labs (skin biopsy, saliva, serum and CSF) to the Centers for Disease Control and Prevention (CDC) can be safely arranged.

Initial Tests (lab, imaging)

- Lumbar puncture
  - White blood cell count is normal or shows moderate pleocytosis; protein normal or moderately elevated
  - Rabies antibody titer
- Serum
  - Rabies antibody titer
- Saliva
  - Reverse transcriptase and polymerase chain reaction (RT-PCR) or isolation of the virus by immunofluorescence

- Skin biopsy from nape of neck
  - To detect rabies through RT-PCR and/or direct fluorescent antigen (DFA), needs to include hair follicles
- Corneal smear stains are positive by immunofluorescence in 50% of patients.
- Hyponatremia is common.
- Head CT shows normal or nonspecific findings consistent with encephalitis.
- MRI can help rule out other forms of encephalitis.
- Postmortem diagnoses can be confirmed by brain tissue analysis with DFA or RT-PCR.

Follow-Up Tests & Special Considerations

Testing/observing the suspected rapid animal:

- No case of human rabies in the United States has been attributed to a dog, cat, or ferret that has remained healthy throughout the standard 10-day period of confinement after an exposure.
- Submit the brain tissue from at least two different locations, preferably the brainstem and the cerebellum of the suspected rabid animal for direct fluorescent antibody testing if possible.

Test Interpretation

- Encephalitis may be found on brain biopsy. Other abnormal findings (e.g., brainstem, midbrain, cerebellum) often found only postmortem.
- Negri bodies—round or oval eosinophilic inclusions found in the cytoplasm of the pyramidal cells of Ammon horn, and the Purkinje cells of the cerebellum

 TREATMENT

After symptoms have developed, treatment is palliative (analgesia and sedation). Postexposure prophylaxis is used for patients following exposure to rabies, but before the onset of symptoms. Preexposure prophylaxis is used for individuals at risk for infection.

GENERAL MEASURES

Thorough wound cleansing with soap and water is first line of treatment. Irrigate wound with virucidal agent, such as povidone-iodine, if available.

MEDICATION

ALERT

- Assess need for postexposure prophylaxis with local wound care, rabies vaccination and rabies immunoglobulin (RIG) based on circumstances of possible exposure, consulting public health officials for recommendations.
- Increased risk:
  - Bites involving skin puncture are at higher risk than a scratch; saliva exposure is a risk only if it comes in contact with an open wound or mucous membranes.
  - Wild or domestic animals unavailable for quarantine
  - Bat exposure
  - Hybrid animals of wild and domestic species (e.g., wolf-dog)
  - Unprovoked attack (Feeding a wild animal is considered a provoked attack.)

- Management:
  - Bites from cats, dogs, and ferrets that can be watched for 10 days do not require prophylaxis unless animal shows signs of illness.
  - Skunks, foxes, bats, raccoons, and most carnivores are high risk, and prophylaxis should begin promptly unless animal can be captured and euthanized for pathologic evaluation.
  - For rodents or livestock, consult local public health authorities before initiating prophylaxis.
- Postexposure prophylaxis
  - Passive vaccination: RIG (HyperRAB) 20 IU/kg administered once. Infiltrate RIG around the wound if possible. Administer remaining RIG IM. Do not administer RIG using the same syringe or into the same anatomic site as vaccine.
  - Active vaccination: rabies vaccine, human diploid cell vaccine (HDCV), or rabies vaccine adsorbed (RVA) or purified chick embryo cell vaccine IM in the deltoid. Give the first dose, 1 mL, as soon as possible after exposure. The day of the first dose is designated day 0. Give additional 1-mL doses on days 3, 7, 14, and 28. For children, use the anterolateral aspect of the thigh and avoid the gluteal area (1).
  - Immunosuppression alters immunity after vaccination. Immunosuppressive drugs should be avoided during postexposure prophylaxis if possible. If postexposure prophylaxis is given to an immunosuppressed patient, check serum samples for the presence of rabies virus–neutralizing antibody to assess response to vaccination.
- Previously vaccinated patients: Administer an initial 1-mL IM dose of vaccine immediately and an additional 1-mL dose 3 days later. RIG is not necessary in these patients.
- Preexposure vaccination: for people in high-risk groups, such as veterinarians, animal handlers, wildlife rangers, certain laboratory workers, and those spending time in foreign countries where rabies is enzootic:
  - Primary preexposure: 3 IM 1-mL injections of HDCV or RVA in deltoid area on days 0, 7, and 21, or 28
  - Preexposure boosters: For people at risk of exposure to rabies, test serum every 2 years. Administer preexposure booster of 1-mL IM if immunity is waning. If titer cannot be obtained, a booster can be administered instead.
- Adverse effects: 0.6% of people develop mild serum sickness reaction following HDCV boosters.

ADDITIONAL THERAPIES

- Symptomatic rabies necessitates a palliative approach and should be focused on analgesia, sedation, and seizure control.
- Milwaukee protocol: experimental treatment using ketamine, midazolam, and amantadine (originally included ribavirin but no longer recommended) (2)[C]. One patient who did not receive pre- or postexposure prophylaxis recovered from clinical rabies in 2004 after being treated with medically induced coma and amantadine.
- Control cerebral artery vasospasm (with an agent such as nimodipine) (2)[C].
- Fludrocortisone and hypertonic saline if needed to maintain normal sodium level

 ONGOING CARE

PROGNOSIS

- If untreated, rabies has the highest case fatality rate of any infectious disease; generally considered to be 100% fatal once symptoms develop.
- To date, fewer than 20 cases of survival from clinical rabies. Almost all received some form of pre- or postexposure immunization.

COMPLICATIONS

- During latter stages of disease, multiorgan failure ensues:
  - Cardiac arrhythmias, heart failure, cardiac arrest, myocarditis
  - Hyperventilation, hypoxemia, respiratory depression, aspiration pneumonia, neurogenic pulmonary edema
  - Gastrointestinal hemorrhage
- In the very rare cases where patients survive, there are varying reports of neurologic impairment.

REFERENCES

1. Jackson AC. Rabies. *Handb Clin Neurol*. 2014;123:601–618.
2. Aramburo A, Willoughby RE, Bollen AW, et al. Failure of the Milwaukee protocol in a child with rabies. *Clin Infect Dis*. 2011;53(6):572–574.

ADDITIONAL READING

- Centers for Disease Control and Prevention. Rabies. http://www.cdc.gov/rabies.
- Moore SM. Challenges of rabies serology: defining context of interpretation. *Viruses*. 2021;13(8):1516.
- World Health Organization. Fact sheets: rabies. https://www.who.int/news-room/fact-sheets/detail/rabies. Accessed November 17, 2021.

 CODES

ICD10

- A82.9 Rabies, unspecified
- Z20.3 Contact with and (suspected) exposure to rabies

CLINICAL PEARLS

- Caused by RNA virus and transmitted by infected animal saliva
- Rabies is a vaccine-preventable virus.
- Seek immediate treatment if exposed to scratch, bite, or saliva of potentially infected animal (e.g., feral dog, bat, fox, raccoon, or other wild mammals).
- Postexposure prophylaxis consists of three steps: local wound cleansing, passive immunization with RIG, and active immunization with HDCV.
- Contact local health department for all suspected cases and particularly if sending antemortem samples to the CDC.

RAPE CRISIS SYNDROME

Elizabeth Ashley Suniega, MD

BASICS

DESCRIPTION

Definitions (vary by jurisdiction on local, state, and national levels):

- Rape (a legal term), sexual assault (a medical term), or sexual violence (a general term): any form of sexual activity that occurs without consent between a victim and perpetrator(s)/suspect(s)
- Rape/sexual assault/sexual violence: may be associated with the use of force and/or threats, alcohol, and/or illicit and/or prescription drugs
- Rape crisis syndrome is historical term that has previously been utilized to define what is now known as an acute stress reaction (ASR), acute stress disorder (ASD), and/or a posttraumatic stress disorder (PTSD) in persons exposed to sexual violence.
  - Psychological responses to sexual violence range from transient to chronic and debilitating.
  - The neurobiology and traumatic impact of sexual violence on victims is complex. It is associated with a profound flight, fight, and/or freeze-related fear response as well as a hormonal cascade (involving catecholamines, cortisol, opiates, and oxytocin), and the use of primitive brain structures (e.g., the prefrontal cortex, amygdala, and hippocampus) and can trigger the development of numerous posttraumatic psychological, emotional, physical, and social effects.

EPIDEMIOLOGY

- In the United States, 33% of women and 25% of men have reported experiencing sexual violence during their lifetime.
- Around 1.5 million women and 834,700 men are victims of sexual violence annually in the United States.
- The following populations are especially vulnerable to sexual violence:
  - Adolescents and young children
  - Persons with disabilities
  - Elderly adults
  - Those with a low socioeconomic status and/or that are homeless
  - Sex workers and persons being trafficked
  - People living in institutions/areas of conflict/training environments
- The incidence of sexual violence peaks in those 11 to 24 years of age.
- 33% of female victims first experienced sexual violence before age 18; 13% first experienced it before age 10
- 25% of male victims first experienced sexual violence before age 18; 25% first experienced it before age 10
- Only 16–38% of victims of sexual violence report to law enforcement, and 17–43% of victims obtain a medical evaluation.
- 33% of victims of sexual violence never report it to their primary care providers.

RISK FACTORS

- History of sexual violence, psychological aggression, physical violence, trafficking, and/or stalking
- Early initiation of sexual activity
- Engagement in high-risk sexual behavior
- Exposure to familial and/or environmental violence
- Consumption of alcohol/use of illicit drugs
- Belief in traditional gender roles

GENERAL PREVENTION

- Primary prevention: Promoting gender equality, teaching skills to prevent sexual violence, empowering and supporting females, and creating protective environments decrease the occurrence of sexual violence perpetration.
- Secondary prevention: The United States Preventive Services Task Force recommends screening all women of childbearing age for intimate partner violence (IPV) and referring women who screen positive for interventional services.
  - The HARK screening tool, which includes questions that assess if a patient has felt humiliated (H) and/or afraid (A) and been raped (R) and/or kicked (K) within the past year, is 81% sensitive and 95% specific for IPV, as well as clinically useful (1).

DIAGNOSIS

- History and/or objective physical exam findings concerning for sexual violence
- The PTSD Checklist for *DSM-5* (PCL-5) is a clinically useful screening tool for PTSD and 86% sensitive and 63% specific.

HISTORY

- Medical and forensic histories and exams should ideally be performed by providers with specialized training in providing medical and forensic care (e.g., Sexual Assault Nurse Examiners [SANEs]).
  - These providers should be willing and able to testify in court on behalf of the patient, if indicated.
- States usually require the completion of specific forms for documenting the history of a victim and/or suspect/perpetrator of sexual violence.
- Utilize a trauma-informed approach to patient care in order to help prevent retraumatization by incorporating the "four Rs" (1): (i) realizing the widespread impact of trauma; (ii) recognizing signs and symptoms of trauma; (iii) responding by integrating knowledge about trauma into practices, procedures, and policies; and (iv) resisting retraumatization (2).
- Avoid questioning that may imply that a patient is at fault or be interpreted as investigative.
- Inquire about patient safety.
- Record answers in the patient's own words, and request clarification on unclear terminology.
- Describe all types of physical trauma and sexual contact and whether it was actual/attempted and with/without use of force.

- Inquire about any alcohol and/or illicit drug use before and/or after the episode of sexual violence.
- Document the time of occurrence of activities that could potentially alter biologic specimens (e.g., taking a bath or shower, using a douche or mouthwash, brushing teeth, eating/drinking, and/or changing clothes).
- Obtain a thorough gynecologic history, including the LMP, last consenting sexual contact, last use of contraception, and prior surgeries.
- Inquire about a recent history of strangulation.
  - If positive, advise obtaining angiographic neck imaging (e.g., a CT angiogram [CTA]) to assess for a potential carotid artery dissection, embolus, hematoma, and/or edema around the larynx and/or trachea.

PHYSICAL EXAM

- Request for exams to be performed by SANEs, if available.
- Document all atypical physical findings and/or signs concerning for sexual and/or physical trauma.
- Document the patient's mental status and emotional state during the exam.
- In patients with a recent history of strangulation, examine the patient's scalp, eyes, eyelids, ears, face, oropharynx, neck, and chest and assess for any neurologic, respiratory, voice, and throat-related changes.
- Obtain the patient's consent prior to each step of the examination, as it is both mandatory and empowering to patients.
- Pending the patient's preferences, may obtain confidential medical photographs (i.e., on a secure digital camera that is reserved solely for use on this unique patient population) prior to swabbing and physically examining the patient
- May use a UV light (Wood lamp) and orange-tinted forensic goggles to detect biologic specimens on clothing and/or skin prior to swabbing and physically examining the patient

ALERT

- A medical and forensic SAFE Kit (previously referred to as a "rape kit") contains sterile cotton swabs that can be used to collect biologic specimens from the oropharyngeal cavity, anogenital regions, and other bodily sites as clinically indicated. Detailed instructions are provided within the kit.
- Perform a complete oropharyngeal, genital, and rectal exam and assess for physical signs concerning for physical and sexual trauma, blood and/or other biologic fluids, and/or foreign objects.
  - Use a nonlubricated, water-moistened speculum for female patients.
  - Perform testing and/or collect biologic specimens as indicated based on the patient's history and physical exam.

DIAGNOSTIC TESTS & INTERPRETATION
- Pregnancy test
- Drug and/or alcohol testing as clinically indicated
- Diagnostic testing for sexually transmitted infections (STIs) is medically indicated but not required prior to prescribing treatment; recommend screening for chlamydia, gonorrhea, bacterial vaginosis, trichomoniasis, HIV, hepatitis B, and syphilis.

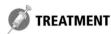 **TREATMENT**

GENERAL MEASURES
- Employ enhanced sensitivity and privacy measures, as well as a trauma-informed care approach.
- All cases of sexual violence must be reported immediately to the appropriate law enforcement agency.
- With a victim's permission, enlist the help of personnel from local support agencies (e.g., sexual violence/"rape crisis" support centers) and in-house social services (e.g., SANEs, victim advocates, sexual assault response and care coordinators, sexual assault care providers, behavioral health specialists, and chaplains).
- Administer tetanus prophylaxis, if clinically indicated.
- Discuss risks of STI exposure and test/treat as indicated.
- Evaluate for psychological sequelae, and refer for further evaluation and treatment by behavioral health specialists.

MEDICATION
First Line
- The Centers for Disease Control and Prevention (CDC) 2021 Sexually Transmitted Diseases Treatment Guidelines recommend empirically and prophylactically treating STIs (especially gonorrhea, chlamydia, trichomoniasis, bacterial vaginosis, hepatitis B, and human papilloma virus [HPV]), as well as considering treatment for HIV and syphilis, depending on a patient's level of risk (3).
- Cultures are not required before treatment.
- Gonorrhea: (adult dosing) (i) weight <150 kg: ceftriaxone 500 mg IM single dose, (ii) weight ≥150 kg: ceftriaxone 1 g IM single dose; (pediatric dosing) (i) weight ≤45 kg: ceftriaxone 25 to 50 mg/kg IV or IM single dose (not to exceed 250 mg), (ii) weight >45 kg: refer to adult dosing.
- Chlamydia: (adult dosing) azithromycin 1 g PO single dose, or doxycycline 100 mg PO BID for 7 days, or levofloxacin 500 mg PO daily for 7 days; (pediatric dosing) (i) age ≥8 years: azithromycin 1 g PO single dose or doxycycline 100 mg PO BID for 7 days, (ii) age <8 years with weight ≥45 kg: azithromycin 1 g PO single dose, (iii) age <8 years with weight <45 kg: erythromycin base or ethylsuccinate 50 mg/kg/day PO divided into 4 doses daily for 14 days
- Trichomoniasis: (adult and pediatric dosing) (i) men: metronidazole or tinidazole 2 g PO single dose, (ii) women: metronidazole 500 mg BID for 7 days or tinidazole 2 g PO single dose
- Bacterial vaginosis: (adult and pediatric dosing) metronidazole 500 mg PO BID for 7 days, or metronidazole gel 0.75% 5 g (one full applicator) intravaginally daily for 5 days, or clindamycin cream 2% 5 g (one full applicator) intravaginally nightly for 7 days

- HIV: although there is usually a low likelihood of HIV transmittance during most episodes of sexual violence, prescribing nonoccupational postexposure prophylaxis (nPEP) for victims with a high-risk of HIV exposure (e.g., the suspect/perpetrator's HIV status is positive and/or history is positive for IV drug use)
  - nPEP options (4):
    - Tenofovir disoproxil fumarate (Viread) 300 mg PO daily with emtricitabine (Truvada) 200 mg PO daily for 28 days plus
    - Raltegravir (Isentress) 400 mg PO BID or dolutegravir (Tivicay) 50 mg PO daily for 28 days
    - Pregnant: Dolutegravir should be cautiously prescribed, especially during the first 28 days, given the potential risk of congenital neural tube defects; recommend consulting an infectious disease (ID) provider.
    - Nonpregnant women: nPEP should be cautiously prescribed in nonpregnant women of childbearing age who are effectively using birth control.
    - Children (age ≤12 years): Recommend consulting an ID provider.
  - Treatment is most effective if started within 4 hours of an episode of sexual assault and can reduce HIV transmission by ~80%; it is unlikely to be beneficial if started after 72 hours.
- Hepatitis B: hepatitis B immunoglobulin 0.06 mL/kg IM single dose and initiate a 3-dose total hepatitis B virus immunization series (1st dose administered at initial exam)
  - No treatment is indicated if the victim has received a complete hepatitis B vaccine series and has documented levels of immunity.
- HPV: HPV vaccination is recommended for all victims of sexual violence between 9 and 26 years of age and may be considered after shared clinical decision-making in victims between 27 and 45 years of age. Administer 1st dose at initial exam, 2nd dose 1 to 2 months after 1st dose, and 3rd dose 6 months after 1st dose.
- Syphilis: Evidence does not currently support the empiric and prophylactic treatment of patients with a low risk of developing syphilis. However, patients with a high risk of contracting syphilis may be treated with benzathine penicillin G 2.4 million units IM single dose.

Pregnancy Considerations
- Perform a screening pregnancy test in all female victims.
- Discuss unplanned pregnancy prevention and termination-related options, which are listed in order of increasing effectiveness (5).
  - Levonorgestrel (Plan B) 0.75 mg PO q12h × 2 doses or 1.5 mg PO single dose (Plan B One-Step) has a low incidence of GI side effects; effective up to 72 hours but with a decreased efficacy in overweight and obese females
  - Ulipristal acetate (Ella) 30 mg PO single dose. Lacks a hormonal component. Effective up to 120 hours; preferred for use in overweight and obese females
  - Copper IUD (ParaGard) 313.4 mg IU single device. Lacks a hormonal component. Effective up to 120 hours; most effective emergency contraceptive method

 ONGOING CARE

FOLLOW-UP RECOMMENDATIONS
Patient Monitoring
Patients should be frequently evaluated for follow-up medical care: (i) 1 to 2 weeks: pregnancy retesting and counseling, gonorrhea and chlamydia retesting, and vaginitis and/or UTI assessment; (ii) 6, 12, and 24 weeks: syphilis and HIV retesting; and (iii) 4 to 8 weeks: HPV anogenital wart assessment.

REFERENCES
1. Nelson HD, Bougatsos C, Blazina I. *Screening Women for Intimate Partner Violence and Elderly and Vulnerable Adults for Abuse: Systematic Review to Update the 2004 U.S. Preventive Services Task Force Recommendation.* Rockville, MD: Agency for Healthcare Research and Quality; 2012. Evidence synthesis no. 92. AHRQ publication no. 12-05167-EF-1.
2. Ravi A, Little V. Providing trauma-informed care. *Am Fam Physician.* 2017;95(10):655–657.
3. Meehan PJ, Rosenstein NE, Gillen M, et al. Responding to detection of aerosolized *Bacillus anthracis* by autonomous detection systems in the workplace. *MMWR Recomm Rep.* 2004;53(RR-7):1–12.
4. Centers for Disease Control and Prevention, U.S. Department of Health and Human Services. *Updated Guidelines for Antiretroviral Postexposure Prophylaxis After Sexual, Injection Drug Use, or Other Nonoccupational Exposure to HIV—United States, 2016.* Atlanta, GA: U.S. Department of Health and Human Services; 2016.
5. Cheng L, Che Y, Gülmezoglu AM. Interventions for emergency contraception. *Cochrane Database Syst Rev.* 2012;(8):CD001324.

 CODES

ICD10
- T74.21XA Adult sexual abuse, confirmed, initial encounter
- T74.22XA Child sexual abuse, confirmed, initial encounter
- Z04.41 Encounter for exam and obs following alleged adult rape

CLINICAL PEARLS
- Employ enhanced sensitivity and privacy measures, as well as a trauma-informed care approach, when providing care.
- All cases of sexual violence must be reported immediately to the appropriate law enforcement agency.

R

RAYNAUD PHENOMENON

Kelsey E. Phelps, MD

 BASICS

DESCRIPTION

- Idiopathic intermittent episodes of vasoconstriction of digital arteries, precapillary arterioles, and cutaneous arteriovenous shunts in response to cold, emotional stress, or blunt trauma
  - A triphasic color change of the fingers (occasionally the toes, rarely nipples) is the principal physical manifestation.
    - The initial color is *white* from extreme pallor, then *blue* from cyanosis, and finally with warming/vasodilatation, the skin appears *red*.
    - Thumbs are rarely involved.
  - Swelling, throbbing, and paresthesias are associated symptoms.
  - Primary
    - 80% of patients have primary disease.
    - Episodes are bilateral and nonprogressive.
    - Diagnosis confirmed if after 2 years of symptoms no underlying connective tissue disease develops
  - Secondary
    - Progressive and asymmetric
    - Vascular spasm is more frequent and more severe over time. Ulceration is rare; gangrene does not develop; 13% progress to digital fat pad atrophy and ischemic fingertip changes.
    - Typically associated with an underlying connective tissue disorder
- System(s) affected: hematologic, lymphatic, immunologic, musculoskeletal, dermatologic, exocrine

Pregnancy Considerations
- Raynaud phenomenon can appear as breast pain in lactating women.
- Positive breast milk bacterial culture distinguishes mastitis from Raynaud phenomenon.

Geriatric Considerations
Initial appearance of Raynaud phenomenon after age 40 years suggests underlying connective tissue disease.

Pediatric Considerations
Associated with systemic lupus erythematosus (SLE) and scleroderma

EPIDEMIOLOGY

Incidence
- Primary
  - Predominant age: 14 years; ~1/4 begin >40 years
  - Predominant sex: female > male (4:1)
- Secondary
  - Predominant age: >40 years
  - Predominant sex: no gender predilection

Prevalence
- Primary: 3–12% of men; 6–20% of women (based on clinical history)
- Secondary: ~1% of population

ETIOLOGY AND PATHOPHYSIOLOGY
Unknown. Dysregulation of vascular control mechanisms leads to imbalance between vasodilation and vasoconstriction. There is a reduced endothelin-dependent vasodilation activity and an increased vasoconstriction in peripheral vessels by overproduction of endothelin-1. 5-HT$_2$ serotonin receptors may be involved in secondary Raynaud phenomenon. Platelet and blood viscosity abnormalities in secondary disease contribute to ischemic pathology.

Genetics
Some studies suggest dominant inheritance pattern. ~1/4 of patients with primary condition also have a first-degree relative with Raynaud phenomenon.

RISK FACTORS
- Existing autoimmune or connective tissue disorder
- End-stage renal disease with hemodialysis may increase risk if a steal phenomenon develops in association with the arterial-venous shunt.
- Primary and secondary disease associated with elevated homocysteine levels
- Smoking is not associated with increased risk of Raynaud phenomenon but may worsen symptoms.

GENERAL PREVENTION
- Avoid cold exposure.
- Tobacco cessation
- No relationship has been established between Raynaud phenomenon and vibratory tool use.
- Stress and anxiety can trigger attacks.

COMMONLY ASSOCIATED CONDITIONS
Secondary Raynaud
- Scleroderma; SLE; polymyositis
- Sjögren syndrome; occlusive vascular disease
- Cryoglobulinemia

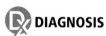 **DIAGNOSIS**

HISTORY
- Primary
  - Symmetric attacks involving fingers
  - Family history of connective tissue disorder
  - Absence of tissue necrosis, ulceration, or gangrene
  - If after ≥2 years of symptoms, no abnormal clinical or laboratory signs have developed, secondary disease is unlikely.
- Secondary
  - Onset typically after 40 years of age
  - Asymmetric episodes more intense and painful
  - Arthritis, myalgias, fever, dry eyes and/or mouth, rash, or cardiopulmonary symptoms
  - History of medication and/or recreational drug use
  - Exposure to toxic agents
  - Repetitive trauma

PHYSICAL EXAM
Pallor (whiteness) of fingertips with cold exposure, then cyanosis (blue), and then redness and pain with warming
- Ischemic attacks evidenced by demarcated or cyanotic skin limited to digits; usually starts on one digit and spreads symmetrically to remaining fingers of both hands. The thumb is typically spared.
- Rarely involves other tissues (e.g., tongue) (1),(2)
- Beau lines: transverse linear depressions in nail plate on most or all fingernails that occurs after exposure to cold or any insult that disrupts normal nail growth
- Livedo reticularis: mottling of the skin of the arms and legs; benign and reverses with warming
- Primary
  - Normal physical exam
  - Nail bed capillaries have normal appearance: Place 1 drop of grade B immersion oil on skin at base of fingernail and view capillaries with hand-held ophthalmoscope at 10 to 40 diopters.
- Secondary
  - Skin changes, arthritis, and abnormal lung findings suggest connective tissue disease.
  - Ischemic skin lesions: ulceration of finger pads (autoamputation in severe, prolonged cases)
  - Nail bed capillary distortion including giant loops, avascular areas, and increased tortuosity
  - Abnormal Allen test (Have patient open and close hand several times and then tightly into a fist. Sequentially occlude the ulnar and radial arteries while the patient opens hand to reveal the return of color as a measure of circulation.)

DIFFERENTIAL DIAGNOSIS
- Thromboangiitis obliterans (Buerger disease): primarily affects men; smoking related
- Rheumatoid arthritis (RA)
- Progressive systemic sclerosis (scleroderma): Raynaud phenomenon precedes other symptoms.
- SLE
- Carpal tunnel syndrome; thoracic outlet syndrome
- Hypothyroidism
- CREST syndrome (calcinosis cutis, Raynaud phenomenon, esophageal dysmotility, sclerodactyly, and telangiectasias)
- Cryoglobulinemia; Waldenström macroglobulinemia
- Acrocyanosis
- Polycythemia
- Occupational (e.g., especially from vibrating tools, masonry work, exposure to polyvinyl chloride)
- Drug induced (e.g., clonidine, ergotamine, methysergide, amphetamines, bromocriptine, bleomycin, vinblastine, cisplatin, cyclosporine)

DIAGNOSTIC TESTS & INTERPRETATION
Provocative test (e.g., ice water immersion) unnecessary
- Primary
  - Antinuclear antibody: negative
  - ESR: normal
- Secondary
  - Tests for secondary causes (e.g., CBC, ESR)
  - Positive autoantibody has low positive predictive value for connective tissue disease (30%).
  - Antibodies to specific autoantigens (e.g., scleroderma with anticentromere or anti-topoisomerase antibodies)
  - Videocapillaroscopy is gold standard (200 times magnification).

Follow-Up Tests & Special Considerations
Periodic assessments for a connective tissue disorder

Diagnostic Procedures/Other
Diagnosis is determined by history and physical exam.

TREATMENT

Assess using a Raynaud Condition Score.

GENERAL MEASURES
- Dress warmly, wear gloves, avoid cold temperatures.
- During attacks, rotate the arms in a windmill pattern or place the hands under warm water or in a warm body fold to alleviate symptoms.
- Tobacco cessation
- Avoid β-blockers, amphetamines, ergot alkaloids, OTC medications containing pseudoephedrine, and sumatriptan.
- Temperature-related biofeedback may help patients increase hand temperature. 1-year follow-up is no better than control.
- Finger guards to protect ulcerated fingertips
- Recognition and avoidance of stressful situations

MEDICATION
First Line
- Calcium channel blockers (CCBs). Nifedipine is the best studied and most frequently used.
- Nifedipine: 30 to 180 mg/day (sustained-release form); seasonal (winter) use is effective with up to 75% of patients experiencing improvement.
- Compatible with breastfeeding
- Contraindications: allergy to drug, pregnancy, CHF
- Precautions: may cause headache, dizziness, light-headedness, edema, or hypotension
- Significant possible interactions
  – Increases serum level of digoxin

Second Line
- Amlodipine (5 to 10 mg/day) and nicardipine are effective and may have fewer adverse effects.
- No data exist to support switching CCB if initial drug is ineffective.
- Small studies support benefit from losartan and fluoxetine.
- Phosphodiesterase type-5 inhibitors (sildenafil, vardenafil) may reduce symptoms without increasing blood flow.
- Parenteral iloprost, a prostacyclin, in low doses (0.5 ng/kg/min over 6 hours), has improved ulcerations with severe Raynaud phenomenon when CCBs failed. Oral prostacyclin has not proven useful.
- Nitroglycerin patches may be helpful, but use is limited by the incidence of severe headache. Nitroglycerin gel has shown promise as a topical therapy.
- Topical sildenafil cream may also improve digital arterial blood flow in patients with secondary Raynaud phenomenon (3).
- Prazosin (1 to 2 mg TID) is the only well-studied α_1-adrenergic receptor blocker with modest effect; adverse effects may outweigh any benefit.
- ACE inhibitors are no longer recommended.

ISSUES FOR REFERRAL
If an underlying disease is suspected, consider rheumatology consultation for evaluation and treatment.

ADDITIONAL THERAPIES
- Botulinum toxin somewhat effective in reducing vasospastic episodes, frequency of attacks, rest pain, and helping to promote digital ulcer healing (4)[C]
- Aspirin
- Digital or wrist block with lidocaine or bupivacaine (without epinephrine) for pain control
- Short-term anticoagulation with heparin if persistent critical ischemia, evidence of large-artery occlusive disease, or both

SURGERY/OTHER PROCEDURES
Surgical intervention is rare in Raynaud phenomenon. Effect of cervical sympathectomy is transient; symptoms return in 1 to 2 years. Digital fat grafting is a novel modality that has shown improved symptomatology and evidence of measurably increased perfusion in several cases (5)[C].

COMPLEMENTARY & ALTERNATIVE MEDICINE
- *Ginkgo biloba* with unclear benefit
- Fish oil supplements may increase digital systolic pressure and time to onset of symptoms after exposure to cold; not proven in controlled trials
- Vitamin D supplementation led to improvement in self-reported symptoms in vitamin D–deficient patients with Raynaud phenomenon (6)[B].
- Evening primrose oil reduced severity of attacks in one study.
- Oral arginine is no better than placebo.
- Acupuncture and accupressure found to be helpful in symptom reduction, but studies have been small and evidence is not statistically significant (7).
- Biofeedback is not likely helpful.

ONGOING CARE

FOLLOW-UP RECOMMENDATIONS
Avoid exposure to cold; reassess for secondary causes.

Patient Monitoring
Manage fingertip ulcers and rapidly treat infection.

DIET
No special diet

PATIENT EDUCATION
- Tobacco cessation
- Avoid triggers (e.g., trauma, vibration, cold).
- Dress warmly; wear gloves.
- Warm hands when experiencing vasospasm.

PROGNOSIS
- Attacks may last from several minutes to a few hours.
- 2/3 of attacks resolve spontaneously.
- ~13% of Raynaud patients develop a secondary disorder, typically connective tissue diseases.

COMPLICATIONS
- Primary: very rare
- Secondary: gangrene, autoamputation of fingertips

REFERENCES
1. Wigley FM, Flavahan NA. Raynaud's phenomenon. *N Engl J Med*. 2016;375(6):556–565.
2. Devgire V, Hughes M. Raynaud's phenomenon. *Br J Hosp Med (Lond)*. 2019;80(11):658–664.
3. Wortsman X, Del Barrio-Díaz P, Meza-Romero R, et al. Nifedipine cream versus sildenafil cream for patients with secondary Raynaud phenomenon: a randomized, double-blind, controlled pilot study. *J Am Acad Dermatol*. 2018;78(1):189–190.
4. Neumeister MW, Webb KN, Romanelli M. Minimally invasive treatment of Raynaud phenomenon: the role of botulinum type A. *Hand Clin*. 2014;30(1):17–24.
5. Bank J, Fuller SM, Henry GI, et al. Fat grafting to the hand in patients with Raynaud phenomenon: a novel therapeutic modality. *Plast Reconstr Surg*. 2014;133(5):1109–1118.
6. Hélou J, Moutran R, Maatouk I, et al. Raynaud's phenomenon and vitamin D. *Rheumatol Int*. 2013;33(3):751–755.
7. Gladue H, Berrocal V, Harris R, et al. A randomized controlled trial of acupressure for the treatment of Raynaud's phenomenon: the difficulty of conducting a trial in Raynaud's phenomenon. *J Scleroderma Relat Disord*. 2016;1(2):226–233.

ADDITIONAL READING
Herrick AL. Evidence-based management of Raynaud's phenomenon. *Ther Adv Musculoskelet Dis*. 2017;9(12):317–329.

SEE ALSO

Algorithm: Raynaud Phenomenon

CODES

ICD10
- I73.00 Raynaud's syndrome without gangrene
- I73.01 Raynaud's syndrome with gangrene

CLINICAL PEARLS
- Raynaud phenomenon is a clinical diagnosis.
- Provocative testing is not recommended.
- Initial presentation of Raynaud phenomenon after age 40 years suggests underlying (secondary) disease.
- Cold avoidance and stress reduction are foundational in treating Raynaud phenomenon.
- Digital ulcers are not normal and always merit a workup for secondary disease.
- Acute digital ischemia is a medical emergency.

R

REACTIVE ARTHRITIS (REITER SYNDROME)

Douglas William MacPherson, MD, MSc(CTM), FRCPC

 BASICS

Reiter syndrome is a seronegative, multisystem, inflammatory disorder classically involving joints, the eye, and the lower genitourinary (GU) tract, and skin. It is a postinfectious autoimmune process. Axial joint (e.g., spine, sacroiliac joints) and dermatologic manifestations are common (1)[C],(2)[C].

DESCRIPTION
The classic triad includes arthritis, conjunctivitis/iritis, and either urethritis or cervicitis ("can't see; can't pee; can't bend my knee").

- The epidemiology is similar to other reactive arthritides, characterized by sterile joint inflammation associated with infections originating at nonarticular sites. A fourth feature (dermatologic involvement) may include buccal ulceration, balanitis, or a psoriasiform skin eruption. (Having only two features does not rule out the diagnosis.)
- Two forms of Reiter syndrome:
  - Sexually transmitted: Symptoms emerge 7 to 14 days after exposure to *Chlamydia trachomatis* and other sexually acquired pathogens.
  - Postenteric infection (including traveler's diarrhea)
- In individuals with new or frequent sexual partners, the triggering infection is likely sexually transmitted (rather than enteric).
- In individuals with a history of recent enteric illness, the triggering event is more likely to be a bacterial enteric infection than sexual transmission.
- System(s) affected: musculoskeletal, renal/urologic, dermatologic/exocrine
- Synonym(s): idiopathic blennorrheal arthritis; arthritis urethritica; urethro-oculo-synovial syndrome; Fiessinger-Leroy-Reiter disease; reactive arthritis

Pediatric Considerations
Juvenile rheumatoid arthritis (RA) has many of the same clinical features as Reiter syndrome.

Pregnancy Considerations
No special considerations; usual drug precautions

EPIDEMIOLOGY
Incidence
- Predominant age: 20 to 40 years
- Predominant sex: male > female
- 0.2–1% incidence after bacterial dysentery outbreaks
- Complicates 1–2% of nongonococcal urethritis cases
- ~3 to 5 cases per 100,000 individuals per year

ETIOLOGY AND PATHOPHYSIOLOGY
- The pathophysiology of all the seronegative reactive arthritis syndromes and the immunologic role of infectious diseases as precipitants for clinical illness are incompletely understood. Proinflammatory cytokines lead to synovitis. Toll-like receptors (TLR) have been implicated in the recognition of gram-negative lipopolysaccharide as part of the disease cascade.
- Avoiding precipitant infections and early management of multiorgan inflammation is important. Antibiotic treatment following onset of syndrome does not appear to benefit inflammatory joint, eye, or urinary tract symptoms.

- *C. trachomatis* is the most common sexually transmitted infection associated with Reiter syndrome.
- Dysentery-associated Reiter syndrome follows infection with *Shigella*, *Salmonella*, *Yersinia*, and *Campylobacter* spp. Enteric-associated Reiter syndrome is more common in women, children, and the elderly than the postvenereal form.

Genetics
HLA-B27 tissue antigen present in 60–80% of patients, suggesting a genetic predisposition

RISK FACTORS
- New or high-risk sexual contacts 1 to 4 weeks before the onset of clinical presentation; the primary infection may be subclinical and undiagnosed.
- Food poisoning or bacterial dysentery

GENERAL PREVENTION
- The immune-response characteristics of this syndrome make avoidance of infectious precipitants the most important general precaution (and potentially the most difficult to achieve).
- Safe sexual practices; proper food and water hygiene

COMMONLY ASSOCIATED CONDITIONS
- Enteric disease
  - Shigellosis; Salmonellosis; Campylobacteriosis
  - Enteric infection with *Yersinia* spp.
- Urogenital infection
  - *Chlamydia* urethritis/cervicitis (3)[C]
  - *Mycoplasma* or *Ureaplasma* spp.
- HIV/AIDS

DIAGNOSIS

- Clinical presentation with joint, eye, and GU inflammation ("classic triad") and negative serologic testing for rheumatoid factor
- Classic symptoms not always present
- HLA-B27 testing is not required for diagnosis.

HISTORY
The presence of the clinical syndrome plus
- Diarrhea, dysentery, urethritis, or genital discharge and appropriate exposure history
- Exposure risks, including travel or migration history and potential infectious exposure
- Arthritis associated with urethritis for >1 month (84% sensitive; 98% specific for diagnosis)
- Urethritis occurs 1 to 15 days after sexual exposure.
- Reiter syndrome onset within 10 to 30 days of either enteric infection or STI
- Mean duration of symptoms is 19 weeks.

PHYSICAL EXAM
- Musculoskeletal
  - Asymmetric arthritis (especially knees, ankles, and metatarsophalangeal joints)
  - Enthesopathy (inflammation at tendinous insertion into bone, such as plantar fasciitis, digital periostitis, polydactylitis, and Achilles tendinitis)
  - Spondyloarthropathy (spine and sacroiliac joint involvement)

- Urogenital tract
  - Urethritis; prostatitis; cystitis (rare)
  - Balanitis
  - Cervicitis: usually asymptomatic
- Eye
  - Conjunctivitis of one or both eyes
  - Occasionally, scleritis, keratitis, and corneal ulceration
  - Rarely, uveitis and iritis
- Skin
  - Mucocutaneous lesions (small, painless superficial ulcers on oral mucosa, tongue, or glans penis)
  - Keratoderma blennorrhagica (hyperkeratotic skin lesions of palms and soles and around nails—can be mistaken for psoriasis)
- Cardiovascular: occasionally, pericarditis, murmur, conduction defects, and aortic incompetence
- Nervous system: rarely, peripheral neuropathy, cranial neuropathy, meningoencephalitis, and neuropsychiatric changes
- Constitutional
  - Fever, malaise, anorexia, and weight loss
  - Patient can appear seriously ill (e.g., fever, rigors, tachycardia, and exquisitely tender joints).

DIFFERENTIAL DIAGNOSIS
- Seropositive arthritides: rheumatoid arthritis and others
- Ankylosing spondylitis
- Arthritis associated with inflammatory bowel disease
- Psoriatic arthritis
- Juvenile RA
- Bacterial arthritis, including gonococcal
- Rheumatic fever

DIAGNOSTIC TESTS & INTERPRETATION
- Blood
  - Negative rheumatoid factor
  - Leukocyte count: 10,000 to 20,000 cells/mm^3
  - Neutrophil predominance
  - Elevated ESR and/or CRP
  - Moderate normochromic, normocytic anemia
  - Hypergammaglobulinemia
- Synovial fluid
  - Leukocyte count: 1,000 to 8,000 cells/mm^3
  - Bacterial culture negative
- Supportive tests
  - Cultures, antigens, or PCR positive for *C. trachomatis* or stool test positive for *Salmonella*, *Shigella*, *Yersinia*, or *Campylobacter* spp.
  - HIV serology positive (acute retroviral syndrome)
  - HLA-B27-positive (*not required for diagnosis*)
  - Drugs that may alter lab results: Antibiotics may affect isolation of the bacterial pathogens.
  - Rheumatoid factor is negative.
- X-ray
  - Periosteal proliferation, thickening
  - Articular bony spurs; erosions at articular margins
  - Residual joint destruction
  - Syndesmophytes (spine); sacroiliitis

Diagnostic Procedures/Other
HLA-B27 histocompatibility antigen: positive in 60–80% of cases in non–HIV-related Reiter syndrome; HLA testing is not required or recommended for diagnosis.
- Screen for STI if clinically indicated.
- Screening for enteric infections is rarely useful and generally not indicated.

Test Interpretation
- Seronegative spondyloarthropathy (similar to ankylosing spondylitis, enteric arthritis, and psoriatic arthritis)
- Villous formation within joints; hyperemia, and inflammation
- Prostatitis and seminal vesiculitis
- Skin biopsy similar to psoriasis

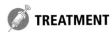

TREATMENT

GENERAL MEASURES
Treatment is determined by symptoms.
- Conjunctivitis does not require specific treatment.
- Iritis requires treatment.
- Mucocutaneous lesions do not require treatment.
- Physical therapy (PT) aids recovery.
- Arthritis may become prominent and disabling during the acute phase.

MEDICATION
First Line
- Symptomatic management: NSAIDs, including indomethacin, naproxen, and others; intra-articular or systemic corticosteroids for refractory arthritis and enteritis
  - Contraindications
    - GI bleeding
    - Peptic ulcer, gastritis, or ulcerative colitis
    - Renal insufficiency
- Specific treatment of isolated microorganism (4)[A]:
  - *C. trachomatis*: doxycycline 100 mg PO BID for 7 to 14 days (*Note*: All STIs should be treated whether associated with Reiter syndrome or not.)
  - *Salmonella, Shigella, Yersinia,* and *Campylobacter* infections: ciprofloxacin 500 mg PO BID for 5 to 10 days (*Note*: Emerging antimicrobial resistance will limit the utility of ciprofloxacin. Antibiotic treatment does not reduce GI symptoms or duration of infection or prevent carrier state [Salmonella only].)
  - Trials of antibiotic treatment for reactive arthritis have produced mixed results, rendering the efficacy of antibiotics uncertain.
- GI upset: antacids
- Iritis: intraocular steroids
- Keratitis: topical steroids

Second Line
- Aspirin or other NSAIDs
- Sulfasalazine is promising but not FDA-approved.
- Methotrexate or azathioprine in severe cases (experimental, not approved or known to be effective); immunosuppressive therapy is relatively contraindicated in HIV-related Reiter syndrome.

- Specialty consultation is recommended, particularly if considering immunomodulatory agents such as sulfasalazine, methotrexate, or azathioprine or for treatment with anti-TNF medications (etanercept and infliximab), which have shown benefit in isolated case reports.
- Role of antibiotics under investigation—currently unproven effectiveness in seronegative arthritides
- No published evidence supports the beneficial effect of antibiotics on the long-term outcome in patients with Reiter syndrome.

ISSUES FOR REFERRAL
Joint and eye complications; complex cases—consider consultation with rheumatology; ophthalmology

ADMISSION, INPATIENT, AND NURSING CONSIDERATIONS
- Based on severity of disease and associated complications
- Inpatient care may be needed during acute phase.

 ## ONGOING CARE

FOLLOW-UP RECOMMENDATIONS
Activity modification until joint inflammation subsides

Patient Monitoring
Monitor clinical response to anti-inflammatory drugs. Observe for complications, particularly with sulfasalazine and immunosuppressive drugs.

PATIENT EDUCATION
- Educate on risk factors for exposure and recurrence.
- Home PT
- National Institute of Arthritis and Musculoskeletal and Skin Diseases: http://www.niams.nih.gov/

PROGNOSIS
Prognosis is poor in cases involving the heel, eye, or heart.

COMPLICATIONS
- Chronic or recurrent disease in 5–50% of patients
- Ankylosing spondylitis develops in 30–50% of patients who test positive for HLA-B27 antigen.
- Urethral strictures
- Cataracts and blindness
- Aortic root necrosis

REFERENCES
1. Schmitt SK. Reactive arthritis. *Infect Dis Clin North Am*. 2017;31(2):265–277.
2. Padhan P, Danda D. Clinical spectrum of post-streptococcal reactive arthritis (PSRA) revisited: juvenile versus adult-onset disease. *Int J Rheum Dis*. 2019;22(4):750–751.
3. Zeidler H, Hudson AP. New insights into *Chlamydia* and arthritis. Promise of a cure? *Ann Rheum Dis*. 2014;73(4):637–644.
4. Barber CE, Kim J, Inman RD, et al. Antibiotics for treatment of reactive arthritis: a systematic review and metaanalysis. *J Rheumatol*. 2013;40(6):916–928.

ADDITIONAL READING
- Boring MA, Hootman JM, Liu Y, et al. Prevalence of arthritis and arthritis-attributable activity limitation by urban-rural county classification—United States, 2015. *MMWR Morb Mortal Wkly Rep*. 2017;66(20):527–532.
- García-Kutzbach A, Chacón-Súchite J, García-Ferrer H, et al. Reactive arthritis: update 2018. *Clin Rheumatol*. 2018;37(4):869–874.
- Lucchino B, Spinelli FR, Pericone C, et al. Reactive arthritis: current treatment challenges and future perspectives. *Clin Exp Rheumatol*. 2019;37(6):1065–1076.
- Mathew AJ, Ravindran V. Infections and arthritis. *Best Pract Res Clin Rheumatol*. 2014;28(6):935–959.

 ### SEE ALSO

Ankylosing Spondylitis; Arthritis, Psoriatic; Behçet Syndrome

 ### CODES

ICD10
- M02.30 Reiter's disease, unspecified site
- M02.39 Reiter's disease, multiple sites

CLINICAL PEARLS
- Diagnosis of reactive arthritis is based on the clinical presentation of the classic triad of joint, eye, and GU inflammation and negative serologic testing for rheumatoid factor (signs and symptoms may not all be present at the same time).
- Screen for STI (including HIV) if sexually acquired. Enteric studies are rarely clinically indicated.
- Refer patients with a chronic or recurrent course and those who have clinical complications.
- Treatment focuses on symptom relief and treating any underlying infection.

RENAL TUBULAR ACIDOSIS

Ryan M. Song, MD • Venkata Raju Behara, MD

 BASICS

DESCRIPTION

- Renal tubular acidosis (RTA) is a group of disorders characterized by an inability of the kidney to resorb bicarbonate (HCO_3)/secrete hydrogen ions, resulting in normal anion gap metabolic acidosis. Renal function must be normal or near normal.
- Several types have been identified:
  - Type I (distal) RTA: inability of the distal tubule to acidify the urine due to impaired hydrogen ion secretion, increased back leak of secreted hydrogen ions, or impaired sodium reabsorption; urine pH >5.5.
  - Type II (proximal) RTA: defect of the proximal tubule in HCO_3 reabsorption. Proximal tubular HCO_3 reabsorption is absent; plasma HCO_3 concentration stabilizes at 12 to 18 mEq/L due to compensatory distal HCO_3 reabsorption; urine pH <5.5
  - Type III RTA: extremely rare autosomal recessive syndrome with associated osteopetrosis, cerebral calcification, intellectual disability.
  - Type IV RTA (hypoaldosteronism): due to aldosterone resistance/deficiency that results in hyperkalemia. Urine pH usually is <5.5.

EPIDEMIOLOGY

Incidence

Predominant sex: male > female (with regard to type II RTA with isolated defect in HCO_3 reabsorption)

ETIOLOGY AND PATHOPHYSIOLOGY

- Type I RTA—caused by conditions and medications that impair adequate urine acidification at the distal tubule:
  - Autoimmune diseases: Sjögren syndrome, rheumatoid arthritis (RA), systemic lupus erythematosus (SLE), thyroiditis (1)
  - Medications: amphotericin B, lithium, ifosfamide, foscarnet, triamterene, trimethoprim, pentamidine
  - Obstructive uropathy (hyperkalemic)
  - Other familial disorders: Ehlers-Danlos syndrome, glycogenosis type III, Fabry disease, Wilson disease
  - Hematologic diseases: sickle cell disease (hyperkalemic), hereditary elliptocytosis
  - Toxins: toluene, glue
  - Hypercalciuria, diseases causing nephrocalcinosis
  - Vitamin D intoxication
  - Medullary cystic disease
  - Hypergammaglobulinemic syndrome
  - Chronic pyelonephritis
  - Chronic active hepatitis, primary biliary cirrhosis
  - Malnutrition
  - Incomplete distal RTA—a form in which patients are unable to appropriately acidify their urine, however are able to excrete sufficient acid to maintain normal serum HCO_3 and pH (2). Cause and pathophysiology is poorly understood.
  - Voltage-dependent RTA—a form of distal RTA in which the impairment in urine acidification is due to poor delivery of Na^+ to the distal tube, leading to disruption of favorable transepithelial voltage gradient, and retention of K^+ and H^+. This form will lead to hyperkalemia, as opposed to hypokalemia in classic distal RTA (3).
    - Amiloride causes voltage-dependent RTA rather than classic distal RTA (3).
- Type II RTA—caused by conditions and medications that impair adequate $HCO3$ reabsorption in the proximal convoluted tubule (4):
  - Genetic inheritance (see below)
  - Primary Fanconi syndrome

- Systemic diseases causing Fanconi syndrome: multiple myeloma and other dysproteinemic states, amyloidosis, paroxysmal nocturnal hemoglobinuria, tubulointerstitial nephritis
  - Medications
    - Carbonic anhydrase inhibitors: acetazolamide, methazolamide and dichlorphenamide
    - Chemotherapy agents: ifosfamide, oxaliplatin, cisplatin
    - Antiretroviral medications: tenofovir, didanosine
    - Anticonvulsant medications: topiramate, valproic acid
    - Antibiotics: sulfanilamide, outdated tetracycline, aminoglycosides
    - Other miscellaneous medications: deferasirox, apremilast, heavy metals
  - Familial (cystinosis, tyrosinemia, hereditary fructose intolerance, galactosemia, glycogen storage disease type I, Wilson disease, Lowe syndrome, inherited carbonic anhydrase deficiency)
  - Defects in calcium metabolism (hyperparathyroidism)
- Type IV RTA (5)
  - Medications: NSAIDs, ACE inhibitors, ARBs, heparin/low-molecular-weight (LMW) heparin (hyperkalemia in 5–10% of patients), ketoconazole, tacrolimus, cyclosporine, spironolactone, eplerenone
  - Diabetic nephropathy
  - Tubulointerstitial nephropathies
  - Primary adrenal insufficiency
  - Markedly decreased distal Na^+ delivery
  - Pseudohypoaldosteronism (PHA) (end-organ resistance to aldosterone)
    - PHA type 1
    - PHA type 2 (Gordon syndrome)

Genetics

- Type I RTA: hereditary forms due to mutations affecting intercalated cells in collecting tubules. Loss of function mutations of a chloride-bicarbonate exchanger (AE1) found in the kidney and red blood cell are inherited in autosomal dominant and recessive manners and may be associated with hemolytic anemia, spherocytosis, or ovalocytosis. Loss of function mutations of a vacuolar-type H^+ ATPase (V-ATPase) found in the kidney and inner ear are autosomal recessive, and are associated with enlarged vestibular aqueducts, dizziness, and sensorineural deafness (2). More recently, whole exome genomic sequencing has implicated mutations in a protein transcription factor FOXI1, which regulates both AE1 and V-ATPase, as another cause of distal RTA with early-onset sensorineural deafness.
- Type II RTA: Autosomal dominant form is extremely rare. Autosomal recessive form is associated with mutation in a basolateral electrogenic sodium-bicarbonate cotransporter (NBCe1) and can be seen with severe growth retardation, ophthalmologic abnormalities, and intellectual disability. Fanconi syndrome, which is associated with several genetic diseases (e.g., cystinosis, Wilson disease, tyrosinemia, hereditary fructose intolerance, Lowe syndrome, galactosemia, glycogen storage disease, metachromatic leukodystrophy), can also be inherited by sporadic missense mutation in a sodium phosphate cotransporter. More recent studies identified other causes of inherited Fanconi syndrome, including mutation of EHHADH, a gene involved in peroxisomal fatty acid oxidation, and HNF4A, a gene that encodes a nuclear transcription factor (4).
- Type IV RTA: Some cases are familial, such as PHA type I (autosomal dominant).

GENERAL PREVENTION

Careful use/avoidance of causative agents

COMMONLY ASSOCIATED CONDITIONS

- Type I RTA in children: hypercalciuria leading to rickets, nephrocalcinosis
- Type I RTA in adults: autoimmune diseases (Sjögren syndrome, RA, SLE), obstructive uropathy, hypercalciuria
- Type II RTA: Fanconi syndrome (generalized proximal tubular dysfunction resulting in glycosuria, aminoaciduria, hyperuricosuria, phosphaturia, bicarbonaturia)
- Type II RTA in adults: multiple myeloma, carbonic anhydrase inhibitors, aminoglycosides
- Type IV RTA: diabetic nephropathy, solid-organ transplant (due to calcineurin inhibitors)

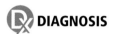 **DIAGNOSIS**

HISTORY

- Often asymptomatic (particularly type IV)
- In children: failure to thrive, rickets
- Anorexia, nausea/vomiting, constipation
- Weakness or polyuria (due to hypokalemia or hypercalciuria)
- Polydipsia
- Osteomalacia in adults

DIFFERENTIAL DIAGNOSIS

- Plasma anion gap should be normal, if not, evaluate for causes of anion-gap metabolic acidosis: ketoacidosis, ingestions (ASA, methanol, ethylene glycol, propylene glycol), lactic acidosis, D-lactic acidosis, uremia.
- Extrarenal HCO_3 losses
  - Chronic diarrhea
  - Small bowel, pancreatic, or biliary fistulas
  - Urinary diversion (e.g., ureterosigmoidostomy, ileal conduit)
- Acidosis of chronic renal failure (develops when GFR ≤20 to 30 mL/min).
- Excessive administration of acid load via chloride salts, including dilutional acidosis via normal saline (NaCl, HCl, NH_4Cl, lysine HCl, $CaCl_2$, $MgCl_2$)

DIAGNOSTIC TESTS & INTERPRETATION

Initial Tests (lab, imaging)

- Serum chemistries and electrolytes
  - Hyperchloremic metabolic acidosis with a normal anion gap (anion gap = $Na^+ - [Cl^- + HCO_3]$)
  - Plasma potassium:
    - Low: in type I RTA (due to impaired distal H^+ secretion/increased H^+ back leak) and type II RTA
    - High: in type IV RTA and type I (if due to voltage-dependent RTA)
  - BUN and Cr should be normal/near baseline to rule out renal failure as a cause of acidosis.
  - Electrolyte abnormalities of Fanconi syndrome (hypophosphatemia, hyponatremia, hypoglycemia, hypoproteinemia) may be seen in type II RTA (3).
- Urine studies (3)
  - Urine pH >5.5 in the presence of hyperchloremic metabolic acidosis is strongly suggestive of type I and II RTA if serum HCO_3^- is above resorptive threshold of distal tubules (12 to 18 mEq/L). Urine pH is typically <5.5 in type IV RTA.
    - Urine pH can be altered in intravascular volume depletion and the presence of urea-splitting organisms, which can mimic RTA nonanion gap metabolic acidosis.

- Urine calcium is typically high in type I RTA (3). Increased fractional excretion of phosphate, uric acid, glucose, amino acids, LMW proteins, and presence of urinary retinol-binding protein 4 (not readily available in most places) are sensitive for type II RTA (4).
- Urine anion gap (UAG; $U_{Na} + U_K - U_{Cl}$) is inversely related to urine NH_4^+ excretion (NH_4^+ cannot be directly measured in urine). Positive UAG in acidemic patient indicates impaired urine acid excretion and is a sign of type I and type IV RTA.
  - Accurate UAG requires $U_{Na} > 25$ mEq/L. UAG will also be positive in renal failure, in which acid excretion is impaired.
  - There is limited utility of UAG in type II RTA, as patients may not have maximal ammonium excretion during acidosis, and UAG may not be appropriately negative (4).

Pediatric Considerations
Audiogram to evaluate hearing loss or MRI/CT to evaluate presence of enlarged vestibular aqueducts in type I RTA (2).

Pregnancy Considerations
Studies have identified severe acid–base disturbances in pregnant women with inherited type I RTA, who presented with severe hypokalemia and metabolic acidosis. Other issues that may complicate pregnancy include recurrent UTIs and nephrolithiasis due to nephrocalcinosis as well as issues with alkali supplementation in patients with hyperemesis gravidarum (2).

Diagnostic Procedures/Other
- Helpful to measure urine pH on fresh sample with pH meter for increased accuracy instead of dipstick. Pour film of oil over urine to avoid loss of CO_2 if pH cannot be measured quickly.
- Ammonium chloride loading test can provide definitive diagnosis of type I RTA—presence of non-acidified urine (pH >5.3) or positive UAG 6 hours after 100 mg/kg of NH_4Cl is diagnostic. Urine pH <5.3 excludes type I RTA (3).
  - Study is limited by long duration of the test and gastrointestinal upset from the side effects of ammonium chloride. A reasonable and safe alternative is the simultaneous 40 mg furosemide and 1 mg fludrocortisone test (f+f test); patients with type I RTA unable to reduce urine pH to <5.3 (2)
- HCO_3 loading test is gold standard for diagnosis for type II RTA. Fractional excretion of HCO_3 >15% during 1 mEq/kg/hr HCO_3 infusion is diagnostic of type II RTA (1). <5% excludes type II RTA (3).

Test Interpretation
- Nephrocalcinosis
- Nephrolithiasis
- Rickets
- Osteomalacia, osteopenia
- Findings of an underlying disease causing RTA

 TREATMENT

MEDICATION
First Line
- Provide oral alkali to raise serum HCO_3 to normal. Start at a low dose and increase until HCO_3 is normal. Give as sodium bicarbonate ($NaHCO_3$) (7.7 mEq $NaHCO_3$/650 mg tab), sodium citrate (oral solution, 1 mEq HCO_3 equivalent/mL), sodium/potassium citrate (oral solution), or potassium citrate (tablet, powder, or oral solution: 2 mEq K/mL, 2 mEq HCO_3/mL), depending on need for potassium.

- Type I RTA: typical doses 1 to 2 mEq/kg/day (in adults), 3 to 4 mEq/kg/day (in children) HCO_3 equivalent divided 3 to 4 times per day (require much higher doses if HCO_3 wasting is present); may require K^+ supplementation (1)[C]
- Type II RTA: typical doses 10 to 15 mEq/kg/day HCO_3 equivalent, divided 4 to 6 times per day. Very difficult to restore plasma HCO_3 to normal, as renal HCO_3 losses increase once plasma HCO_3 is corrected above resorptive threshold. Exogenous HCO_3 increases K^+ losses, requiring supplemental K^+; often need supplemental PO_4 and vitamin D due to proximal PO_4 losses
- Type IV RTA: Avoid inciting medications and treat the underlying cause of hypoaldosteronism; restrict dietary K^+. May augment K^+ excretion with loop diuretic, thiazide diuretic, or polystyrene sulfonate (Kayexalate). Correcting hyperkalemia increases activity of the urea cycle, augmenting renal ammoniagenesis and adding substrate for renal acid excretion (1)[C]. If necessary, 1 to 5 mEq/kg/day alkali divided 2 to 3 times per day. If mineralocorticoid deficiency, fludrocortisone: 0.1 to 0.3 mg/day.
- Precautions
  - Sodium-containing compounds will increase urinary calcium excretion, potentially increasing the risk of nephrolithiasis.
  - Mineralocorticoids and sodium-based alkali may lead to hypertension and/or edema.
  - Aluminum-containing medications (antacids, sucralfate) should be avoided if solutions containing citric acid are prescribed because citric acid increases aluminum absorption.
  - $NaHCO_3$ may cause flatulence because CO_2 is formed, whereas citrate is metabolized to HCO_3 in the liver, avoiding gas production.

Second Line
- Thiazide diuretics may be used as adjunctive therapy in type II RTA (after maximal alkali replacement) to induce mild hypovolemia, which increases proximal Na^+/HCO_3^- reabsorption and reduces amount of alkali replacement needed but are likely to further increase urinary K^+ losses (4). They can also be considered in type I RTA to reduce calcium excretion; however, they carry the same risk of hypokalemia (2).
- Indomethacin can also be considered to reduce severity of polyuria and hypokalemia in type I RTA (2).
- Recent case reports and case studies have described the safety and efficacy of low-dose fludrocortisone in normalizing recurrent hyperkalemia in type IV RTA in the context of diabetes, amyloidosis, and patients undergoing renal transplant or newly entering dialysis (6).

SURGERY/OTHER PROCEDURES
If distal RTA is due to obstructive uropathy.

ADMISSION, INPATIENT, AND NURSING CONSIDERATIONS
Admit if severe acidosis patient unreliable, emesis persistent, or infant with severe failure to thrive

 ONGOING CARE

FOLLOW-UP RECOMMENDATIONS
Patient Monitoring
- Electrolytes 1 to 2 weeks following initiation of therapy, monthly until serum HCO_3 corrected to desired range, and then as clinically indicated
- Poor compliance common due to 3 to 6 times per day alkali dosing schedule

DIET
Varies based on serum K^+ level and volume status

PATIENT EDUCATION
National Kidney Foundation: https://www.kidney.org/

PROGNOSIS
- Depends on associated disease:
  - Type I RTA: Amount of alkali supplementation decreases with age due to increased release of H^+ from bone during skeletal growth. Primary disease is permanent and will require lifelong alkali replacement. Compliance with therapy will restore growth in children and prevent nephrocalcinosis.
  - Type II RTA: Long term compliance to therapy is poor due to large amounts of supplementation required. Prognosis depends on cause; sporadic cases can improve over and therapy stopped.
  - Type IV RTA: Treatment and prognosis depends on underlying cause.
- Transient forms of all types of RTA may occur.

COMPLICATIONS
- Nephrocalcinosis, nephrolithiasis (type I)
- Hypercalciuria (type I)
- Hypokalemia (type I, type II if given HCO_3)
- Hyperkalemia (type IV, some causes of type I)
- Osteomalacia (type II due to phosphate wasting), osteopenia (due to buffering of acid in bone)

REFERENCES

1. Reddy P. Clinical approach to renal tubular acidosis in adult patients. *Int J Clin Pract.* 2011;65(3):350–360.
2. Mohebbi N, Wagner CA. Pathophysiology, diagnosis and treatment of inherited distal renal tubular acidosis. *J Nephrol.* 2018;31(4):511–522.
3. Yaxley J, Pirrone C. Review of the diagnostic evaluation of renal tubular acidosis. *Ochsner J.* 2016;16(4):525–530.
4. Kashoor I, Batlle D. Proximal renal tubular acidosis with and without Fanconi syndrome. *Kidney Res Clin Pract.* 2019;38(3):267–281.
5. Karet FE. Mechanisms in hyperkalemic renal tubular acidosis. *J Am Soc Nephrol.* 2009;20(2):251–254.
6. Dobbin SJH, Petrie JR, Lean MEJ, et al. Fludrocortisone therapy for persistent hyperkalaemia. *Diabet Med.* 2017;34(7):1005–1008.

CODES

ICD10
N25.89 Oth disorders resulting from impaired renal tubular function

CLINICAL PEARLS
- Consider RTA in cases of normal anion gap metabolic acidosis with normal renal function.
- Type I RTA: urine pH >5.5 in setting of acidemia; positive UAG; acidemia can be severe.
- Type II RTA: urine pH <5.5 unless HCO_3 raised above reabsorptive threshold (12 to 18 mEq/L)
- Type IV RTA: most common subtype; hyperkalemia; urine pH <5.5; acidemia usually mild
- Treatment includes avoidance of inciting causes, provision of oral alkali (HCO_3 or citrate), and measures to supplement (type II, many type I) or restrict (type IV) potassium.

RESPIRATORY DISTRESS SYNDROME, ACUTE (ARDS)

Marianna G. Weaver, MA, DO • Sally Suliman, MD

 BASICS

DESCRIPTION

- Acute respiratory distress syndrome (ARDS) is defined as the onset of acute hypoxemia within 7 days of a known clinical insult or new or worsening respiratory symptoms with bilateral opacities (patchy, diffuse, or homogenous) consistent with pulmonary edema on imaging.
- Severity of ARDS is measured with a ratio of partial pressure of arterial oxygen (PaO_2) to fraction of inspired oxygen (FiO_2) at a positive end-expiratory pressure (PEEP) or continuous positive airway pressure (CPAP) of at least 5 cm H_2O.
  - Mild—200 mm Hg $< PaO_2/FiO_2 \leq 300$ mm Hg
  - Moderate—100 mm Hg $< PaO_2/FiO_2 \leq 200$ mm Hg
  - Severe—$PaO_2/FiO_2 \leq 100$ mm Hg
- Synonym(s): acute lung injury; increased permeability pulmonary edema; noncardiac pulmonary edema
- Systems affected: pulmonary, cardiovascular

EPIDEMIOLOGY

Incidence

- Incidence of ARDS is highly variable and underrecognized.
- Incidence rate varies from 10 to 86 cases per 100,000 persons.

ETIOLOGY AND PATHOPHYSIOLOGY

- ARDS is a response to direct or indirect alveolar injury leading to diffuse alveolar damage.
  - Direct
    - Pneumonia (bacterial, viral, fungal, or opportunistic)
    - Aspiration of gastric contents
    - Near drowning
    - Pulmonary contusion
    - Inhalation injury
  - Indirect
    - Sepsis (nonpulmonary)
    - Shock
    - Transfusion of blood products
    - Major burn injury
    - Nonthoracic trauma
    - Drug overdose
    - Cardiopulmonary bypass
    - Reperfusion edema after lung transplant or embolectomy
- Progression of the diffuse alveolar damage in ARDS is divided into three phases.
  - Exudative phase—The initial highly inflammatory phase when alveolar macrophages are activated due to lung injury, leading to complement activation, release of proinflammatory mediators, and activation of neutrophils. This causes epithelial–endothelial barrier disruption, leading to intra-alveolar and extra-alveolar flooding with fluid. This is followed by hyaline membrane formation leading to alveolar collapse.

  - Proliferative phase—The second phase characterized by fibroblasts, myofibroblasts, and alveolar epithelial cell (ACE) II mediated repair. Formation of new matrix, differentiation into ACE I, and formation of cellular junctions begins which leads to expression of aquaporin and ion channels, aiding in the reabsorption of fluid.
  - Fibrotic phase—The final phase, not experience by every patient, is characterized by prolonged mechanical ventilation and associated with increased mortality.

Genetics

No single gene has been identified for clinical use.

RISK FACTORS

Increased levels of markers of systemic inflammation have been associated with adverse outcomes.

GENERAL PREVENTION

Early identification of sepsis with appropriate resuscitation and antibiotic use

COMMONLY ASSOCIATED CONDITIONS

- Pneumonia, sepsis, and aspiration of gastric contents cause 85% of ARDS cases.
- Other causes can include:
  - Trauma
  - Burns
  - Cardiothoracic surgery
  - Pancreatitis
  - Inhalational injuries and near drownings
  - Transfusion-related acute lung injury (TRALI)
  - Shock
  - Medication toxicity

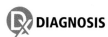 **DIAGNOSIS**

HISTORY

Precipitating event (see "Etiology and Pathophysiology") followed by abrupt onset of respiratory distress and hypoxemia

PHYSICAL EXAM

- Tachypnea and tachycardia during the first 12 to 24 hours
- Increased oxygen requirements
- Decreased breath sounds with or without rales

DIFFERENTIAL DIAGNOSIS

- Bilateral pneumonia (including COVID-19)
- Congestive heart failure
- Interstitial and airway diseases
- Hypersensitivity pneumonitis
- Endobronchial tuberculosis
- Diffuse alveolar hemorrhage
- Veno-occlusive disease
- Mitral stenosis: intravascular volume overload
- Drug-induced lung disease especially vascular leak syndrome with immunotherapy

DIAGNOSTIC TESTS & INTERPRETATION

Initial Tests (lab, imaging)

- Initial labs should include a CBC, CMP, and ABG with evidence of hypoxemia.
- ECG: can show sinus tachycardia; nonspecific ST–T wave changes
- Chest x-ray (CXR): bilateral opacities; air bronchograms can be common.
- Chest CT scan: diffuse interstitial opacities

Follow-Up Tests & Special Considerations

- Blood cultures, sputum cultures, COVID-19 PCR
- Consider transthoracic echocardiography (TTE) in patients when the diagnosis of cardiac failure cannot be excluded.
- Consider bronchoscopy when the cause of ARDS cannot be clearly identified.

Diagnostic Procedures/Other

- Old approach: Invasive monitoring of pulmonary artery wedge pressure (PAWP) has fallen out of favor after clinical trials have shown no increased benefit and an increase in catheter-related complications.
- New approach: Measuring esophageal pressure with a manometer to estimate pleural pressure allows for adjustment of PEEP to achieve a positive end-expiratory transpulmonary pressure gradient, an approach that is increasingly used in clinical care and especially useful in the morbidly obese (1)[C].

Test Interpretation

- With introduction of the Berlin criteria, a diagnosis of ARDS can be made with a calculated PaO_2/FiO_2 of ≤ 300 mm Hg along with radiologic evidence of new bilateral infiltrates. If an ABG is not available, the oxygen saturation can be used as a surrogate for the PaO_2.
- Severity based on the Berlin criteria:
  - Mild—200 mm Hg $< PaO_2/FiO_2 \leq 300$ mm Hg
  - Moderate—100 mm Hg $< PaO_2/FiO_2 \leq 200$ mm Hg
  - Severe—$PaO_2/FiO_2 \leq 100$ mm Hg

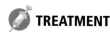 **TREATMENT**

GENERAL MEASURES

- Identify and treat the cause of ARDS.
- Lung protective ventilation and conservative fluid therapy
- Using tidal volumes of 6 mL/kg of predicted body weight with a plateau pressure goal of ≤ 30 cm H_2O has shown a decrease in mortality in comparison to higher volumes.
- Tidal volumes can be reduced to 4 mL/kg if plateau pressures exceed 30 cm H_2O (1)[A].
- Respiratory rate can be set to maintain adequate minute ventilation. Permissive hypercapnia is allowed as long as pH > 7.30. Recent data supports lower respiratory rates (1)[C].

- No clear guideline for PEEP has been established. No clinical trial has shown consistent benefit of high PEEP. There is a possible benefit of reduced mortality in patients with moderate to severe ARDS with high PEEP (1)[C].
- In patients with early moderate to severe ARDS (PaO_2/FiO_2 <150 mm Hg), use of neuromuscular blockade with sedation compared with placebo resulted in a mortality benefit. Proposed mechanisms include prevention of breath stacking and limiting patient-ventilator dyssynchrony along with increased efficacy of lung protective ventilation.
- Prone positioning has shown a decrease in mortality and has led to early extubation in patients with moderate to severe ARDS (PaO_2/FiO_2 <150 mm Hg and PEEP >5 cm H_2O) who have been intubated for <36 hours. Patients are placed in a prone position for 16 consecutive hours a day for up to 28 days or until a PaO_2/FiO_2 ratio is ≥150 mm Hg. While in the supine position, patients need a PEEP of ≤10 cm H_2O and an FiO_2 of ≤0.6 for >4 hours. The benefit of prone positioning is reduction in deleterious effects of positive pressure ventilation on nondependent and less injured airspaces.
- Extracorporeal membrane oxygenation (ECMO) is reserved for severe ARDS after standard supportive measures have failed. One randomized controlled trial suggested improved mortality in select individuals with ARDS referred to an ECMO center (1)[C].
- In patients with very severe ARDS (PaO_2/FiO_2 <80 mm Hg), the use of early ECMO versus conventional mechanical ventilation that included ECMO as a rescue therapy had no difference in 60-day mortality (2)[A].

MEDICATION

No single medication or combination of medications prevents or improves clinical outcomes in ARDS. Treatment is aimed at addressing the underlying cause and is mostly supportive.

ADDITIONAL THERAPIES

- For fluid management, central venous pressure (CVP) can be used to estimate fluid status. Liberal fluid management strategy targeting CVP of 10 to 14 cm H_2O was compared to conservative fluid management strategy targeting CVP of 4 cm H_2O. The conservative approach led to increased ventilator-free days and a decreased stay in the ICU with no change in mortality.
- High-frequency oscillation ventilation showed increased mortality in a clinical trial, although a meta-analysis suggested some benefit when patients with PaO_2/FiO_2 <60 mm Hg (1)[C].
- Airway pressure release ventilation may improve oxygenation, but studies have shown no mortality benefit (1)[C].
- Noninvasive ventilation in patients with severe hypoxemia may increase the risk of ventilation-induced lung injury in ARDS (1)[C].
- Corticosteroids may improve airway pressures and oxygenation, but there is not a consensus on mortality benefit in ARDS. There is potential harm when started after 14 days in the disease course (1)[C].

- Inhaled nitric oxide, surfactant, statins, nonsteroidal anti-inflammatory agents, antioxidants, albuterol, and neutrophil elastase inhibitor have not shown any benefit in clinical trials (1)[C].
- Clinical trials for additional therapies such as dexamethasone, vitamin D, aspirin, mesenchymal stem cells, and others are underway.

Pregnancy Considerations

Supportive care while identifying the underlying cause of ARDS continues to be important in the management of pregnant women with ARDS. However, fetal well-being, possible need for delivery, and physiologic changes associated with pregnancy must be considered. All pregnant patient should be followed by an obstetrician.

ADMISSION, INPATIENT, AND NURSING CONSIDERATIONS

All patients with ARDS should be managed in an ICU setting.

- Use lung protective ventilation while providing adequate PEEP.
- Consider prone positioning and paralysis if PaO_2/FiO_2 <120 to 150 mm Hg.
- If failing initial supportive measures, consider early referral to an ECMO center.
- If perfusion is inadequate after restoration of intravascular volume (e.g., septic shock), vasopressor therapy is indicated.
- Early physical therapy
- Nursing care may include any or all of the following:
  - Skin, eye, and mouth care
  - Deep vein thrombosis (DVT) prophylaxis
  - Stress ulcer prophylaxis
  - Suctioning of endotracheal tube
  - Adequate care while changing position of patient from supine to prone and vice versa
  - Ensure adequate level of sedation and/or paralysis while on mechanical ventilation.
  - Tracheostomy care
- Discharge criteria
  - Resolution or improvement of underlying cause, improving respiratory status, and return to baseline oxygen status

 ## ONGOING CARE

FOLLOW-UP RECOMMENDATIONS

Patient Monitoring

- Driving pressure and static lung compliance are important measures of lung mechanics.
- Daily labs are needed until the patient is no longer critical.
- Daily CXRs are not needed but should be ordered when evaluating for endotracheal tube placement, the presence of progressing infiltrates, catheter placement, worsening hypoxia, or complications of mechanical ventilation (e.g., air leaks).

DIET

Trophic and full-calorie enteral nutrition has shown no difference in mortality, whereas early parenteral nutrition might be harmful (1)[C].

PATIENT EDUCATION

https://www.thoracic.org/patients/patient-resources/resources/acute-respiratory-distress-syndrome.pdf

PROGNOSIS

- Mortality rate is up to 45% with a significant increase across the severity categories.
- Mortality is 34.9% in mild ARDS, 40.3% in moderate, and 46.1% in severe ARDS.

COMPLICATIONS

- Short-term complications include:
  - Barotrauma
  - Nosocomial infection
  - Delirium
  - Catheter-related infection
  - DVT
  - Gastrointestinal bleeding due to stress ulcer
  - Poor nutrition
  - Multiple organ dysfunction syndrome
  - Death
- Long-term complications are related to the age and comorbidities of the patient.
  - Pulmonary dysfunction
  - Reduced health-related quality of life
  - Persistent reticular pattern/ground glass opacities on radiographic imaging
  - Neuropsychological disability, such as depression and PTSD

REFERENCES

1. Thompson BT, Chambers RC, Liu KD. Acute respiratory distress syndrome. *N Engl J Med*. 2017;377(6): 562–572. doi:10.1056/NEJMra1608077.
2. Combes A, Hajage D, Capellier G, et al; for EOLIA Trial Group, REVA, ECMONet. Extracorporeal membrane oxygenation for severe acute respiratory distress syndrome. *N Engl J Med*. 2018;378(21):1965–1975.

ADDITIONAL READING

Matthay MA, McAuley DF, Ware LB. Clinical trials in acute respiratory distress syndrome: challenges and opportunities. *Lancet Respir Med*. 2017;5(6):524–534.

 ## SEE ALSO

http://www.ardsnet.org/

CODES

ICD10

J80 Acute respiratory distress syndrome

CLINICAL PEARLS

- ARDS is the acute onset of hypoxemia secondary to alveolar injury with a PaO_2/FiO_2 ≤300 mm Hg and bilateral infiltrates on CXR.
- Treatment includes identifying and treating the underlying cause.
- Lung protective mechanical ventilation can improve morbidity and mortality.
- Prone positioning and paralytics can be considered in PaO_2/FiO_2 <150 mm Hg.

R

RESPIRATORY DISTRESS SYNDROME, NEONATAL

Tauhid Mahmud, MD, MPH • Amoreena Ranck Howell, MD, MSPH

BASICS

DESCRIPTION
- Neonatal respiratory distress syndrome (NRDS) is a disorder primarily of prematurity manifest by respiratory distress.
- System(s) affected: respiratory
- Synonym(s): hyaline membrane disease; surfactant deficiency

ALERT
A disorder of the neonatal period

EPIDEMIOLOGY
Incidence
- >90% incidence in infants born ≤28 weeks' gestation
- 1% all newborns, 10% of preterm infants
- Inversely proportional to gestational age
- Gender: slight male predominance
- Eighth leading cause of infant death in United States in 2019: 11.3 infant deaths per 100,000 live births (1)

ETIOLOGY AND PATHOPHYSIOLOGY
- Impaired surfactant synthesis and secretion
  - Usually secondary to deficient surfactant (dipalmitoyl lecithin) production in immature lungs
  - Leads to low lung compliance, low lung volume, and increased lung resistance
- High oxygen exposure and barotrauma during treatment can cause further damage to alveolar epithelium.

Genetics
No known genetic pattern

RISK FACTORS
- Premature birth
- Infants of diabetic mothers
- Perinatal asphyxia
- History of RDS in a sibling
- Cesarean delivery

GENERAL PREVENTION
- Prevention of premature birth:
  - Education
  - Regular prenatal care
  - Management of maternal medical conditions
- Promote healthy behaviors during pregnancy focusing on:
  - Diet
  - Exercise
  - Avoidance of exposure to tobacco smoke, alcohol, and illegal drugs

- Antenatal corticosteroids: for women at risk for preterm delivery within 7 days and are between 24 0/7 and 33 6/7 weeks' gestation, including those with ruptured membranes and multiple gestations (2)

COMMONLY ASSOCIATED CONDITIONS
- Patent ductus arteriosus
- Bronchopulmonary dysplasia (BPD)
- Pneumothorax

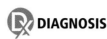

DIAGNOSIS

HISTORY
- Preterm neonates with worsening respiratory distress beginning at or shortly after birth and progressing over first few hours of life
- Early interventions can modify classic course.

PHYSICAL EXAM
- Tachypnea
- Grunting
- Nasal flaring
- Subcostal and intercostal retractions
- Cyanosis
- Decreased breath sounds
- Pallor
- Diminished pulses
- Peripheral edema
- Decreased urine output

DIFFERENTIAL DIAGNOSIS
- Bacterial pneumonia
- Transient tachypnea of newborn
- Interstitial lung disease
- Persistent pulmonary hypertension
- Cyanotic congenital heart disease

DIAGNOSTIC TESTS & INTERPRETATION
Initial Tests (lab, imaging)
- Arterial blood gases (ABGs)
  - Evaluate for evidence of acid–base abnormalities (respiratory acidosis, metabolic acidosis), hypoxemia, and hypercarbia.
- Chest x-ray (CXR):
  - Diffuse reticulogranular pattern (ground-glass appearance)
  - Air bronchograms
  - Low lung volumes

Follow-Up Tests & Special Considerations
- Complete blood count
- Blood culture
- Blood glucose

Diagnostic Procedures/Other
- Echocardiogram: Consider if murmur is present to evaluate for patent ductus arteriosus (PDA) and contribution to lung disease due to L → R shunting.
- Lung pathology (autopsy findings)
  - Macroscopically: uniformly ruddy, airless appearance of lungs
  - Microscopically: diffuse atelectasis and hyaline membranes (eosinophilic and fibrinous membrane lining air spaces)

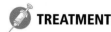

TREATMENT

GENERAL MEASURES
- Respiratory support (3)[C]
  - If no respiratory failure: early initiation of continuous positive airway pressure (CPAP)
  - If respiratory failure: Intubate, ventilate as needed, and administer pulmonary surfactant.
- Respiratory monitoring options
  - Noninvasive
    - Transcutaneous monitor or end-tidal CO_2 monitor
    - Pulse oximetry: target >90% to <95% O_2 saturation
  - Invasive
    - Umbilical artery catheter placement
      - Direct sampling of ABGs
- Empiric antibiotic therapy with ampicillin and gentamicin pending evaluation of blood cultures
- Supportive care:
  - Thermoneutral environment
  - Maintain adequate perfusion.
  - Optimize fluid and electrolyte balance (avoid overhydration).
  - Routine use of diuretics is not indicated.
  - Provide for nutritional needs

MEDICATION
- Pulmonary surfactant (4)[A]
  - Poractant alfa (Curosurf)—porcine lung minced extract
  - Calfactant (Infasurf)—bovine lung lavage extract
  - Beractant (Survanta)—bovine lung minced extract
  - Each surfactant has specific protocols for delivery; consult local standards.

– Administer within first 30–60 minutes of life; should be balanced with less invasive forms of respiratory support
– Strong evidence for use with gestational age <30 weeks
– Side effects
  ○ Bradycardia
  ○ Hypotension
  ○ Airway obstruction/endotracheal tube blockage with administration
  ○ Rapid changes in tidal volume (due to increased compliance) can cause a pneumothorax and small risk of pulmonary hemorrhage.
  ○ Transient adverse effects indicates surfactant administration should be temporarily stopped until neonate is stable and dosing can be continued.
– Contraindications: presence of congenital anomalies incompatible with life beyond neonatal period; infant with laboratory evidence of lung maturity
• Caffeine: increases respiratory drive
• No indication for inhaled nitrous oxide
• No current data to support routine diuretic use

ISSUES FOR REFERRAL
Comorbid conditions associated with prematurity
• PDA (cardiology consult)
• Necrotizing enterocolitis (NEC) (gastroenterology)
• Retinopathy of prematurity (ROP) (ophthalmology)

ADDITIONAL THERAPIES
Treat associated problems of prematurity.

ADMISSION, INPATIENT, AND NURSING CONSIDERATIONS
• All neonates with respiratory distress require immediate evaluation, monitoring, and treatment in the delivery room with transfer to a NICU.
• Supportive care
  – Thermoneutral environment
  – Respiratory monitoring
  – Establish relationship with family to provide education and emotional support.
• Discharge criteria
  – Should have stable vital signs and pulse oximetry before discharge
  – Medical home and support services should be in place.

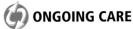 ONGOING CARE

FOLLOW-UP RECOMMENDATIONS
Following discharge, infants should be followed closely by their physicians to monitor growth and respiratory symptomatology.

DIET
As clinically indicated

PATIENT EDUCATION
• Educate parents regarding the risks in subsequent pregnancies.
• Advise parents regarding potential issues with chronic lung disease.

PROGNOSIS
• Progressive worsening of clinical picture during first 2 days of life (5)
• Prognosis and outcome are highly dependent on gestational age; significant neurodevelopmental delays in almost half infants ≤25 weeks' gestation (6)
• Survival rare in infants <25 weeks' gestation (7)

COMPLICATIONS
• Complications specific to NRDS
  – Pneumothorax
  – Chronic lung disease, BPD
  – Pulmonary interstitial edema (PIE)
• Additional complications may occur related to therapeutic interventions and comorbid conditions.

REFERENCES

1. Kochanek KD, Murphy SL, Xu J, et al. Mortality in the United States, 2019 (National Center for Health Statistics Data Brief No. 395). http://www.cdc.gov/nchs/data/databriefs/db395-H.pdf. Accessed October 13, 2016.
2. American College of Obstetricians and Gynecologists' Committee on Obstetric Practice, Society for Maternal–Fetal Medicine. Committee Opinion No. 713: antenatal corticosteroid therapy for fetal maturation. *Obstet Gynecol*. 2017;130(2):e102–e109.
3. Committee on Fetus and Newborn, American Academy of Pediatrics. Respiratory support in preterm infants at birth. *Pediatrics*. 2014;133(1):171–174.
4. Polin RA, Carlo WA; for Committee on Fetus and Newborn, American Academy of Pediatrics. Surfactant replacement therapy for preterm and term neonates with respiratory distress. *Pediatrics*. 2014;133(1):156–163.
5. Sweet DG, Carnielli V, Greisen G, et al. European consensus guidelines on the management of neonatal respiratory distress syndrome in preterm infants—2013 update. *Neonatology*. 2013;103(4):353–368.
6. Jarjour IT. Neurodevelopmental outcome after extreme prematurity: a review of the literature. *Pediatr Neurol*. 2015;52(2):143–152.
7. Ancel PY, Goffinet F, Kuhn P, et al. Survival and morbidity of preterm children born at 22 through 34 weeks' gestation in France in 2011: results of the EPIPAGE-2 cohort study. *JAMA Pediatr*. 2015;169(3):230–238.

ADDITIONAL READING

• Bell EF, Acarregui M. Restricted versus liberal water intake for preventing morbidity and mortality in preterm infants. *Cochrane Database Syst Rev*. 2014;(12):CD000503.
• Keszler M. Mechanical ventilation strategies. *Semin Fetal Neonatal Med*. 2017;22(4):267–274.
• Lemyre B, Laughon M, Bose C, et al. Early nasal intermittent positive pressure ventilation (NIPPV) versus early nasal continuous positive airway pressure (NCPAP) for preterm infants. *Cochrane Database Syst Rev*. 2016;(12):CD005384.
• Reiterer F, Schwaberger B, Freidl T, et al. Lung-protective ventilatory strategies in intubated preterm neonates with RDS. *Paediatr Respir Rev*. 2017;23:89–96.
• Roberts D, Brown J, Medley N, et al. Antenatal corticosteroids for accelerating fetal lung maturation for women at risk of preterm birth. *Cochrane Database Syst Rev*. 2017;(3):CD004454.

CODES

ICD10
P22.0 Respiratory distress syndrome of newborn

CLINICAL PEARLS
• NRDS is a disorder primarily of prematurity manifest by respiratory distress.
• Early treatment with CPAP or pulmonary surfactant can modify clinical course.
• Prognosis and outcome are highly dependent on gestational age.

RESPIRATORY SYNCYTIAL VIRUS (RSV) INFECTION

Sahil Mullick, MD • Sakshi Duggal, MBBS

BASICS

Respiratory syncytial virus (RSV) is a medium-sized, membrane-bound RNA virus that causes acute respiratory tract illness in patients of all ages.

DESCRIPTION
- In adults, RSV causes upper respiratory tract infection (URTI).
- In infants and children, RSV commonly presents as lower respiratory tract infection (LRTI) that manifests as bronchiolitis and rarely pneumonia, respiratory failure, and death.

Pediatric Considerations
- 90–95% of children are infected by 24 months.
- Leading cause of pediatric bronchiolitis (50–90%)
- Premature infants and infants under the age of 6 months are at increased risk.

EPIDEMIOLOGY
- Seasonality:
  - Outbreaks of RSV disease occur each winter (October to late January).
- Morbidity and mortality:
  - RSV infection leads to >100,000 annual hospitalizations.
  - In the United States, 2.1 million outpatient visits for RSV in children <5 years.

Incidence
- Worldwide, RSV is responsible for approximately 33 million LRTI/year and up to 199,000 childhood deaths.
- RSV is the most common etiology of pneumonia in children (29%).
- 177,000 hospitalizations, 14,000 annual deaths are attributable to RSV in the elderly.
- The COVID-19 pandemic significantly impacted RSV presentations to clinical care.

Prevalence
Difficult to conclude accurately

ETIOLOGY AND PATHOPHYSIOLOGY
- RSV is a single-stranded, negative-sense RNA virus belonging to the Paramyxoviridae family.
- Two subtypes, A and B, are simultaneously present in most outbreaks with A subtypes causing more severe disease.
- RSV is spread via direct contact or droplet aerosols. Incubation period ranges from 2 to 8 days, mean 4 to 6.
- Natural RSV infections result in incomplete immunity; recurrent infections are common.
  - RSV causes a neutrophil-intensive inflammation of the airway.
  - RSV develops in the cytoplasm of infected cells and matures by budding from the plasma membrane.
  - RSV is a major cause of exacerbation of asthma and chronic obstructive pulmonary disease (COPD).

Genetics
- Severe RSV infections may be associated with polymorphisms in cytokine-related genes, including *CCR5*; *IL4*; *IL8, IL10*, and *IL13*.
- RSV replicates in apical ciliated bronchial epithelial cells. The airway epithelium produces chemokines, which recruit neutrophils.

RISK FACTORS
- Significant association with RSV-associated acute LRTI
  - Infants born before the 35 weeks' gestation
  - Low birth weight, male gender
  - Underlying cardiopulmonary disease
  - HIV
  - Down syndrome
  - Any age group with persistent asthma
  - Children <5 years with socioeconomic vulnerability
  - Immunodeficiency
  - Siblings with asymptomatic RSV infection
  - Secondhand smoke
  - History of atopy, no breastfeeding
  - Adult patients with COPD or functional disability
  - Other risk factors
    ○ Daycare center attendance
    ○ Exposure to indoor and environmental air pollutants
    ○ Multiple births, malnutrition, higher altitude

GENERAL PREVENTION
- Hand hygiene is the most important step to prevent the spread of RSV (1)[B].
  - Use alcohol-based rubs for hand decontamination when caring for children with bronchiolitis. When alcohol-based rubs are not available, wash hands with soap and water (1)[B].
- Avoid passive smoke exposure (1)[B].
- Isolate patients with proven or suspected RSV.
- Palivizumab is a humanized monoclonal antibody for the prevention of severe RSV in high-risk children (2)[A]:
  - Preterm infants born ≤28 weeks, 6 days of gestation, or who are <12 months at start of RSV season
  - Infants with bronchopulmonary dysplasia who are <1 year or <23 months and requiring treatment
  - Infants ≤12 months of age who are being medically treated for acyanotic heart disease or have moderate to severe pulmonary hypertension
- Prophylactic use is indicated for infants and children <24 months of age with:
  - Chronic lung disease (CLD) of prematurity
  - Hemodynamically significant congenital heart disease
    ○ Congenital abnormalities of the airway or neuromuscular disease
- AAP guidelines (2)[A]:
  - Preterm infants born <29 weeks' gestational age (wGA) and <1 year at the RSV season start date
  - Infants in the 1st year of life with CLD of prematurity
  - Infants with HS-CHD <1 year at the season start date

- Dosage: maximum of 5 monthly doses beginning in November or December at 15 mg/kg per dose IM
- Breastfeeding can significantly reduce hospitalizations due to respiratory infections (3)[A].

COMMONLY ASSOCIATED CONDITIONS
In hospitalized infants:
- Pulmonary infiltrates/atelectasis (42.8%)
- Otitis media (25.3%)
- Hyperinflation (20.8%); respiratory failure (14%)
- Hyperkalemia (10.1%, defined as K^+ >6.0)
- Apnea (8.8%); bacterial pneumonia (7.6%)

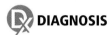

DIAGNOSIS

HISTORY
- History of prematurity, secondhand tobacco smoke exposure, daycare, number and age of siblings
- Immunization history
- Family history of respiratory disease
- Children
  - Nasal congestion, cough, and coryza
  - Low-grade fever, wheezing
  - Nasal flaring, chest wall retraction
- Adults
  - Young adults present with URI symptoms.
  - Mild fever, cough in 90%, wheeze in 40%

PHYSICAL EXAM
- Vital signs: fever, signs of increased work of breathing (tachypnea, grunting, flaring, retracting), apnea, pulse rate; pulse oximetry
- Dry mucous membranes; skin turgor (dehydration)
- Serous otitis or acute otitis
- Upper respiratory findings: rhinorrhea, nasal congestion, cough, sneezing, and sometimes fever and myalgia
- Lower respiratory tract involvement with various permutations of the classic findings of bronchiolitis:
  - Rhonchus breath sounds, tachypnea
  - Accessory muscle use, wheezes and crackles
  - Prolonged expiration

Pediatric Considerations
- Young infants with bronchiolitis may develop apnea.
- Hospital admission based on apnea, hypoxia, respiratory failure, reduced oral intake, and hydration status

DIFFERENTIAL DIAGNOSIS
- Mild illness/URTI
  - Other respiratory viral infections: parainfluenza virus, metapneumovirus, influenza virus, rhinovirus, coronavirus, human bocavirus, and adenovirus.
  - Coinfection with other viruses (e.g., adenovirus, influenza), mycoplasma, or bacteria, including Bordetella pertussis, should be considered.
  - Allergic rhinitis, sinusitis
  - Asthma exacerbation, croup
- Severe illness/LRTI
  - Bronchiolitis, asthma
  - Pneumonia, foreign body aspiration

DIAGNOSTIC TESTS & INTERPRETATION

Initial Tests (lab, imaging)
- The diagnosis of RSV is clinical and does not require confirmatory testing or imaging (4)[B]. However, it is recommended in hospitalized patients being treated prophylactically with palivizumab.
  - If obtained, WBC count normal or elevated
  - Virologic tests for RSV rarely change management decisions or outcomes.
- Septic workups are not necessary, unless the child is toxic in appearance.
- When obtained, typical CXR findings include:
  - Hyperinflation and peribronchiolar thickening
  - Atelectasis, interstitial infiltrates
  - Segmental or lobar consolidation

Follow-Up Tests & Special Considerations
Real-time PCR have superior sensitivity and specificity compared with antigen detection assays and tissue culture.

Diagnostic Procedures/Other
Evidence of inadequate feeding or fluid intake, history of apnea, lethargy, or moderate to severe respiratory distress (nasal flaring, tachypnea, grunting, retractions or cyanosis), and / or an SpO_2 ≤92% in room air (cutoffs for acceptable SpO_2 vary per country), warrant hospitalization, ideally in a secondary care level hospital (3)[A]

Test Interpretation
Antigen test for RSV: Sensitivity ranges from 72% to 94% and specificity 95–100%, in children up to 32 months of age, but sensitivity is 0–25% in older children and adults.

TREATMENT

GENERAL MEASURES
- Treatment for patients with RSV is supportive (4)[A].
- Nasal suction and lubrication
- Antipyretics for fever
- Treat dehydration (oral or intravenous/nasogastric)—particularly in infants.
- Oxygen for hypoxia, with an SpO_2 of 92% as the cutoff for supplementation (3),(5)[C]

MEDICATION

First Line
Treatment is supportive; oxygen as needed

Second Line
- Do not administer albuterol (or salbutamol) to infants and children with a diagnosis of bronchiolitis (1)[B].
- Do not administer epinephrine to infants and children with a diagnosis of bronchiolitis (1)[B].
- Do not administer systemic corticosteroids to infants with a diagnosis of bronchiolitis in any setting (1)[A].
- Nebulized hypertonic saline should not be administered to infants with a diagnosis of bronchiolitis in the emergency department (1)[B].
- May choose not to administer supplemental oxygen if the oxyhemoglobin saturation exceeds 90% in infants and children with a diagnosis of bronchiolitis (1)[C]
- Do not use chest physiotherapy for infants and children with a diagnosis of bronchiolitis (1)[B].

- Do not administer antibacterial medications to infants and children with bronchiolitis, unless there is a concomitant bacterial infection or a strong suspicion of one (1)[B].
- Clinicians should administer nasogastric or intravenous fluids for infants with a diagnosis of bronchiolitis who cannot maintain hydration orally (1)[A].
- Routine use of ribavirin is discouraged but can be considered on case-by-case basis (4)[A].
- Suctioning is often used to reduce secretions in nasopharynx. However, studies have shown that it prolongs duration of hospitalization particularly in infant aged 2–12 months (6).

ADDITIONAL THERAPIES
Bulb suctioning of the nares

Pediatric Considerations
- Over-the-counter (OTC) cough and cold medications should not be used in children <6 years.
- If a hospitalized infant cannot receive oral feedings, use a nasogastric tube to restore adequate feeding and hydration (3)[A].

COMPLEMENTARY & ALTERNATIVE MEDICINE
No complementary, alternative, or integrative therapies are of proven benefit.

ADMISSION, INPATIENT, AND NURSING CONSIDERATIONS
- The main goal is to achieve an adequate fluid balance and normal oxygen saturation levels.
- Patients with worsening despite oxygen supplementation may benefit from CPAP (3)[B].
- Mechanical ventilation is required in about 5% of infants hospitalized with RSV.
- Nursing considerations/education:
  - Educate the family on hand washing (4)[A].
  - Cleaning of environmental surfaces
  - Universal precautions
- No set criteria for discharge; patients should be recovering and demonstrate:
  - Stable respiratory status with no oxygen requirement
  - Ability to maintain oral intake and hydration status
  - Adequate follow-up and patient education

ONGOING CARE

FOLLOW-UP RECOMMENDATIONS

Patient Monitoring
- Adequate fluid intake
- Maintaining oxygen saturation

PATIENT EDUCATION
- Bronchiolitis and Your Child: http://familydoctor.org/familydoctor/en/diseases-conditions/bronchiolitis.html
- Parent education—emphasize use of alcohol-based hand gels/wash and/or to wash hands with soap and water. Clean surfaces with gloves and avoid daycare/kindergarten during recovery.

PROGNOSIS
Most patients recover fully within 7 to 10 days. Reinfection is common.

COMPLICATIONS
- The overall mortality for RSV is <1% with <400 deaths attributed to RSV each year.
- Infants hospitalized for RSV may be at increased risk for recurrent wheezing, allergic sensitization, and reduced pulmonary function, particularly during the 1st decade of life.

REFERENCES
1. Ralston SL, Lieberthal AS, Meissner HC, et al. Clinical practice guideline: the diagnosis, management, and prevention of bronchiolitis [published correction appears in *Pediatrics*. 2015;136(4):782]. *Pediatrics*. 2014;134(5):e1474–e1502.
2. Simões EAF, Bont L, Manzoni P, et al. Past, present and future approaches to the prevention and treatment of respiratory syncytial virus infection in children. *Infect Dis Ther*. 2018;7(1):87–120.
3. Caballero MT, Polack FP, Stein RT. Viral bronchiolitis in young infants: new perspectives for management and treatment. *J Pediatr (Rio J)*. 2017;93 (Suppl 1):75–83.
4. Taveras J, Ramilo O, Mejias A. Preventive strategies for respiratory syncytial virus infection in young infants. *Neoreviews*. 2020;21(8):e535–e545.
5. Bianchi S, Silvestri E, Argentiero A, et al. Role of respiratory syncytial virus in pediatric pneumonia. *Microorganisms*. 2020;8(12):2048.
6. Behzadi MA, Leyva-Grado VH. Overview of current therapeutics and novel candidates against influenza, respiratory syncytial virus, and middle east respiratory syndrome coronavirus infections. *Front Microbiol*. 2019;10:1327.

ADDITIONAL READING
Binns E, Koenraads M, Hristeva L, et al. Influenza and respiratory syncytial virus during the COVID-19 pandemic: time for a new paradigm? [published online ahead of print October 13, 2021]. *Pediatr Pulmonol*. doi:10.1002/ppul.25719.

CODES

ICD10
- B97.4 Respiratory syncytial virus causing diseases classd elswhr
- J06.9 Acute upper respiratory infection, unspecified
- J21.0 Acute bronchiolitis due to respiratory syncytial virus

CLINICAL PEARLS
- RSV causes 50–90% of pediatric bronchiolitis.
- Hand sanitation (alcohol-based rubs are preferred) is the key to RSV prevention.
- The diagnosis of RSV is typically clinical. Routine laboratory or radiology studies are not necessary.
- Treatment of RSV is usually supportive.
- Palivizumab should be used to prevent RSV in high-risk patients.

RESTLESS LEGS SYNDROME

Denise Sharon, MD, PhD, FAASM • Rochelle Zak, MD

 BASICS

DESCRIPTION

- Sensorimotor disorder consisting of a strong, nearly irresistible urge to move the limbs. Legs are usually affected initially but may involve arms or other body parts.
- The symptoms (Sx):
  - Begin or worsen during rest or inactivity
  - Are relieved by movement but recur with inactivity. If not current, previous relief by movement
  - Occur preferentially in the evening/night. If not current, previously reported circadian aspect
- Involuntary leg jerks reported during wake/sleep.
- Early (<45 years) versus late (>45 years) onset
  - Early onset phenotype: 40–92% familial, stable, slow progression of Sx
  - Late onset phenotype: more aggravating factors; rapid progression is common.
- Synonym(s): Willis-Ekbom disease

EPIDEMIOLOGY

Incidence
- 0.8–2.2% annually
- Onset at any age
- Parous females have twice the prevalence of males.
- Temperature (cold weather, other environmental factors may increase incidence/trigger Sx)

Prevalence
- 1–3% of Caucasians (likely underdiagnosed)
- Increases with age
- Lower in non-Caucasians (except Koreans)

Pregnancy Considerations
- 10–30% prevalence; triggers/exacerbates RLS
- Predictors: past history (Hx), family Hx , iron deficiency (ID), Hgb ≤11 g/dL (1)[C]
- Peaks in 3rd trimester
- Most are relieved by 1-month postpartum.

ETIOLOGY AND PATHOPHYSIOLOGY

- Brain iron deficiency (BID), from either low serum iron or impaired transport of iron into the brain, leading to CNS dopamine dysregulation:
  - Higher than normal dopamine (DA) levels in the morning and lower than normal DA at night leading to downregulation of DA D_2 receptors
  - Increased glutamate and decreased adenosine leading to hyperarousal and insomnia
- Sensorimotor pathways abnormalities and increased motor excitability
- Triggered by prolonged immobility, such hospitalizations
- Medication induced:
  - Most antidepressants (except bupropion)
  - DA-blocking antiemetics (e.g., metoclopramide, prochlorperazine)
  - Phenothiazine antipsychotics (risperidone, clozapine, olanzapine quetiapine, etc.). Possible exception: aripiprazole (partial D_2 agonist)
  - Cognition-enhancing meds: memantine
  - Theophylline and other xanthines
  - Sedating antihistamines, OTC cold preparations

Genetics
- Susceptibility loci: 2p14, 2q, 6p21.2, 9p, 12q, 14q, 15q23, and 20p
- Genes: MEIS1, MAP2K5/LBXCOR1, BTBD9, PRPRD, TOX3

RISK FACTORS
- ID: ferritin <75 ng/mL or transferrin saturation (TSAT) <16
- Family history
- Chronic renal failure
- Sleep deprivation
- Alcohol, caffeine (limited data)

GENERAL PREVENTION
- Regular physical activity/exercise during the day, low-impact activity at night such as stretches, walks
- Adequate sleep; delay wake time if possible.
- Avoid caffeine, alcohol, nicotine mainly in the evening.
- Avoid use of medications that may trigger RLS (2)[C].

COMMONLY ASSOCIATED CONDITIONS
- Insomnia, sleep walking, delayed sleep phase
- Iron deficiency, renal disease/uremia/dialysis, gastric surgery, IBS, liver disease
- Parkinson disease, multiple sclerosis, peripheral neuropathy, Machado-Joseph disease, migraine
- Anxiety, depression, ADHD
- Cardiovascular disease, coronary artery disease and stroke
- Venous insufficiency/peripheral vascular disease
- Pulmonary hypertension, lung transplantation, chronic obstructive pulmonary disease (COPD)
- Orthopedic problems, arthritis, fibromyalgia

 DIAGNOSIS

- Clinical, based on Hx, "difficult to describe"
- All criteria must be met for RLS diagnosis (3)[C]:
  - An urge to move the legs, usually accompanied by or thought to be caused by uncomfortable and unpleasant sensations in the legs. The urge must:
    - Begin or worsen during periods of rest or inactivity such as lying down or sitting
    - Be partially or totally relieved by movement such as walking or stretching at least as long as the activity continues. Relief by movement may not be noticeable but must have been previously reported.
    - Occur exclusively or predominantly in the evening or night rather than during the day. Circadian aspect may not be noticeable but must have been previously reported.
  - The above features are not solely accounted for by "mimics" or another sleep, medical or behavioral condition. (Mimics include leg cramps, positional discomfort, habitual foot tapping, arthralgias/arthritis, myalgias, leg edema, peripheral neuropathy, radiculopathy; even though some may coexist.)
  - The symptoms of RLS cause concern/distress; sleep disturbance; or impairment in mental, physical, social, occupational, educational, behavioral, or other area of functioning.

HISTORY
- Signs/symptoms (see also "Description") (4)[A]
  - Painful in ~35% of patients
  - Example descriptions: antsy, burning, achy, itching, "can't get comfortable"
  - Urge to move may be the only "discomfort."
  - Some patients must get up and walk.
  - PLMS in ~80% of patients
  - Insomnia, fatigue, anxiety, depression
- Severity range: from rare, minor problem to daily, mild to moderate, to severe impact on quality of life

Pediatric Considerations
Additional supportive findings (3)[A],(4):
- Insomnia or sleep disturbance
- RLS in immediate biologic relative
- PLMS

PHYSICAL EXAM
Usually normal

DIFFERENTIAL DIAGNOSIS
- Vascular compression: Single position change eliminates discomfort without requiring repetitive movements.
- Claudication: Movement doesn't relieve pain.
- Motor neuron disease fasciculation/tremor: no discomfort or circadian pattern
- Peripheral neuropathy: prominent daytime component unresponsive to dopamine agonists (DAs)
- Dermatitis/pruritus: movement only to scratch; no circadian pattern
- Sleep-related leg cramps: presence of muscle knot
- PLMD: no waketime urge to move
- Growing pains: no urge to move or relief by movement

DIAGNOSTIC TESTS & INTERPRETATION
Assessment of serum iron stores: ferritin, TSAT, iron-binding capacity, serum iron (see also "General Measures") (5)[C]

Diagnostic Procedures/Other
- Sleep study (PSG) helpful but not required
  - Frequent, PLM during wake, prior to sleep and
  - Frequent PLMS on PSG support diagnosis
- Suggested immobilization test (SIT) or multiple SIT (m-SIT)
  - Conducted before or without nocturnal PSG
  - Patient attempts to sit still in bed for 1 hour (SIT) or four 1-hour periods, every 2 hours (m-SIT) while completing every 10 minutes a visual analogue scale (VAS) or m-SIT disturbance scale.
  - SIT >40 movements per hour suggest RLS.

 TREATMENT

GENERAL MEASURES
- If iron insufficient, supplement (2)[C]:
  - 325 mg $FeSO_4$ in the eve + 100 mg vit C
  - Repletion requires months till serum ferritin >75 ng/mL and TSAT >16%.
- Daily exercise; avoid activities that exacerbate RLS.
- Avoid exacerbating factors; maintain regular sleep.
- Treat obstructive sleep apnea (OSA) if present

- Hot baths, warm soaks, leg massage (6)[C]
- In bed: long socks, electric blanket, weighted blanket
- Intense mental activity (games, puzzles, etc.)

MEDICATION
- Consider not initiating medications in mild to moderate cases until general measures have failed. Use minimum dose necessary to control Sx, including sleep disturbance.
- Assess Sx severity every encounter using a scale such as John Hopkins' (JHRLSS), IRLS, sIRLS.
- Opt for longer acting/extended-release options (2),(5),(6)[C].
- Refractory RLS may require combination therapy Tx.

First Line
- Anticonvulsants—less risk for augmentation and more effective in DA-naive patients (2),(5),(6)[C]:
  – Gabapentin enacarbil (Horizant): 300 to 1,200 mg every day ~5:00 PM (2),(5)[C]
  – Pregabalin (Lyrica): 50 to 450 mg/day (off-label)
  – Gabapentin (Neurontin): 100 to 2,400 mg/day (off-label)
- DA—every encounter: Assess for augmentation, impulse-control disorders (ICD) (2),(5),(6)[C].
  – Pramipexole (Mirapex): 0.125 to 0.5 mg 1 to 2 hours before Sx; titrate by 0.125 mg every 4 days.
  – Pramipexole ER 0.375 mg tablet
  – Ropinirole (Requip): 0.25 to 4.0 mg 30 minutes to 1 hour before Sx; titrate by 0.25 mg every 4 days.
  – Ropinirole XL 2 mg
  – Transdermal rotigotine (Neupro): 1 to 3 mg/24 hr patch; start at 1 mg/d; titrate by 1 mg/wk.
- Avoid DAs in psychotic patients, particularly if taking dopamine antagonists.
- Avoid exceeding DA-recommended dose.

Second Line
- Off-label (2),(5),(6)[C]
  – Buprenorphine naloxone 20/0.5 QD–BID
- Benzodiazepines and agonists—insomnia/anxiety
  – Clonazepam (Klonopin): 0.5 to 3.0 mg/day
  – Temazepam, triazolam, alprazolam, zaleplon, zolpidem, and diazepam
- Short-acting DAs for occasional symptoms
  – Carbidopa/levodopa (Sinemet or Sinemet CR): 10/100 to 25/250; PRN up to twice per week

Pregnancy Considerations
- Initial approach: nonpharmacologic therapies, assess/correct ID
- Avoid medications class C or D.
- In 3rd trimester, if severe and failed above, may consider low-dose clonazepam, clonidine, carbidopa/levodopa, or opioids (1)[B]

Pediatric Considerations
- First-line treatment: nonpharmacologic therapies, healthy sleep habits, assess/correct iron deficiency
- Consider low-dose, age-adjusted gabapentin, clonidine, melatonin for sleep.

Geriatric Considerations
- Avoid medications causing dizziness/unsteadiness.
- Many medications trigger/worsen RLS in the elderly.

ISSUES FOR REFERRAL
Severe, intractable symptoms

ADDITIONAL THERAPIES
- Vitamin, mineral suppl: Ca, Mg, D, B_{12}, folate
- Clonidine: 0.05 to 0.10 mg/day
- Baclofen: 20 to 80 mg/day

SURGERY/OTHER PROCEDURES
For orthopedic, neuropathic, or lower extremities vein disease (laser ablation, sclerotherapy)

COMPLEMENTARY & ALTERNATIVE MEDICINE
- Pneumatic compression devices for the legs
- Relaxis leg vibration device (FDA-approved)
- Enhanced external counterpulsation
- Compression stockings
- Acupuncture, yoga
- MicroVas therapy

ADMISSION, INPATIENT, AND NURSING CONSIDERATIONS
Prolonged hospitalization can trigger/worsen RLS.

 ## ONGOING CARE

FOLLOW-UP RECOMMENDATIONS
Patient Monitoring
- At 1- to 4-week intervals until stable and then annually
- If taking iron, reassess iron stores, at least ferritin.
- If status changes, assess for augmentation, ICD, associated conditions, and medications.

DIET
Avoid caffeine and alcohol, mainly in the evening.

PATIENT EDUCATION
- RLS Foundation: www.rls.org
- National Sleep Foundation: https://www.sleepfoundation.org/
- American Academy of Sleep Medicine: http://sleepeducation.org/

PROGNOSIS
- Early onset: lifelong condition with no current cure
- Late onset/secondary: may subside with resolution of precipitating factors, otherwise chronic, progressive
- Current therapies usually control symptoms.

COMPLICATIONS
- Augmentation of symptoms following DA therapy to be assessed at every visit (5)[C]:
  – 4-hour time advance of Sx or 2 to 4 hours advance of Sx together with shorter latency at rest; Sx spread to other body parts or have greater intensity.
  – Higher doses increase risk, and increasing the dose makes Sx worse.
  – Greater risk with meds with shorter half-lives
  – Iron deficiency increases risk.
  – Down-titrate and discontinue DAs for at least 10 days, may add alternative medication then or to continue treatment
- The potential for ICD/Sx needs to be assessed at every visit in patients receiving DA (5)[C].
- Iatrogenic RLS (following blood loss or donation)

REFERENCES
1. Picchietti DL, Hensley JG, Bainbridge JL, et al; for International Restless Legs Syndrome Study Group. Consensus clinical practice guidelines for the diagnosis and treatment of restless legs syndrome/Willis-Ekbom disease during pregnancy and lactation. *Sleep Med Rev*. 2015;22:64–77.
2. Garcia-Borreguero D, Silber MH, Winkelman JW, et al. Guidelines for the first-line treatment of restless legs syndrome/Willis-Ekbom disease, prevention and treatment of dopaminergic augmentation: a combined task force of the IRLSSG, EURLSSG, and the RLS-foundation. *Sleep Med*. 2016;21:1–11.
3. American Academy of Sleep Medicine. Restless legs syndrome. In: *International Classification of Sleep Disorders*. 3rd ed. Darien, IL: American Academy of Sleep Medicine; 2014:281–291.
4. Allen RP, Picchietti DL, Garcia-Borreguero D, et al. Restless legs syndrome/Willis-Ekbom disease diagnostic criteria: updated International Restless Legs Syndrome Study Group (IRLSSG) consensus criteria—history, rationale, description, and significance. *Sleep Med*. 2014;15(8):860–873.
5. Trotti LM, Goldstein CA, Harrod CG, et al. Quality measures for the care of adult patients with restless legs syndrome. *J Clin Sleep Med*. 2015;11(3):293–310.
6. Sharon D. Nonpharmacologic management of restless legs syndrome (Willis-Ekbom disease): myths or science. *Sleep Med Clin*. 2015;10(3):263–278.

ADDITIONAL READING
- Garcia-Borreguero D, Cano-Pumarega I. New concepts in the management of restless legs syndrome. *BMJ*. 2017;356:j104.
- Silber MH, Buchfuhrer MJ, Earley CJ, et al; for Scientific and Medical Advisory Board of the Restless Legs Syndrome Foundation. The management of RLS: an updated algorithm. *Mayo Clin Proc*. 2021;96(7):1921–1937.

 ## SEE ALSO
- Periodic Limb Movement Disorder (PLMD)
- International Restless Legs Syndrome Study Group: irlssg.org

 ## CODES

ICD10
G25.81 Restless legs syndrome

CLINICAL PEARLS
- Insomnia is often a symptom of RLS.
- Antidepressants, antipsychotics, antiemetics, and sedating antihistamines can trigger or worsen RLS.
- Severity and change in Sx can be monitored using a severity scale such as sIRLS, IRLS, or JHRLSS.
- Iron supplement is an often well-tolerated, easily available treatment for RLS.
- Anticonvulsants (e.g., gabapentins) should be considered as initial therapy.
- To avoid augmentation, titrate DAs only up to the minimum dose necessary to control Sx.

RETINAL DETACHMENT

Richard W. Allinson, MD • Alyce D. Alven, OD, MS

 BASICS

DESCRIPTION

- Separation of the sensory retina from the underlying retinal pigment epithelium
- Rhegmatogenous retinal detachment (RRD): most common type; occurs when the fluid vitreous gains access to the subretinal space through a break in the retina (Greek *rhegma*, "rent")
- Exudative or serous detachment: occurs in the absence of a retinal break, usually in association with inflammation or a tumor
- Traction detachment: Vitreoretinal adhesions mechanically pull the retina from the retinal pigment epithelium. The most common cause is proliferative diabetic retinopathy.
- System(s) affected: nervous

EPIDEMIOLOGY

Incidence
- Predominant age: Incidence increases with age.
- Predominant sex: male > female (3:2)
- Per year: 1/10,000 in patients who have not had cataract surgery

Prevalence
After cataract surgery, 1–3% of patients will develop a retinal detachment.

ETIOLOGY AND PATHOPHYSIOLOGY

- Traction from a posterior vitreous detachment (PVD) causes most retinal tears. With aging, vitreous gel liquefies, leading to separation of the vitreous from the retina. Vitreoschisis (lamellar separation of the posterior vitreous cortex) commonly precedes a complete PVD. The vitreous gel remains attached at the vitreous base, in the retinal periphery, resulting in vitreous traction that produces tears in the retinal periphery. There is an ~15% chance of developing a retinal tear from a PVD.
- PVD associated with vitreous hemorrhage has a high incidence of retinal tears.
- Exudative detachment
  - Tumors
  - Inflammatory diseases (Vogt-Koyanagi-Harada disease, systemic lupus erythematosus, posterior scleritis, sympathetic ophthalmia)
  - Miscellaneous (central serous retinopathy, uveal effusion syndrome, malignant hypertension, drugs—ipilimumab, topiramate)
- Traction detachment
  - Proliferative diabetic retinopathy
  - Cicatricial retinopathy of prematurity
  - Proliferative sickle-cell retinopathy
  - Proliferative vitreoretinopathy (PVR)
  - Pars planitis
- Penetrating trauma

Genetics
- Most cases are sporadic.
- There is an increased risk of RRD if a sibling has been affected by this condition. The risk increases with higher levels of myopia in the family history.

RISK FACTORS
- Myopia (>5 diopters)
- Aphakia or pseudophakia
  - In patients undergoing small-incision coaxial phacoemulsification with high myopia (axial length ≥26 mm), the incidence of retinal detachment is 2.7%.
- PVD
- Trauma

- Retinal detachment in fellow eye
- Lattice degeneration: a vitreoretinal abnormality found in 6–10% of the general population
- Glaucoma: 4–7% of patients with retinal detachment have chronic open-angle glaucoma
- Vitreoretinal tufts: Peripheral retinal tufts are caused by focal areas of vitreous traction.
- Meridional folds: Redundant retina usually is found in the supranasal quadrant.
- The risk of retinal detachment after intravitreal injection for age-related macular degeneration or retinal vein occlusion is low with a rate of approximately 1 in 7,500 injections (1)[B].

GENERAL PREVENTION
Patients at risk for retinal detachment should have regular ophthalmologic exams.

Geriatric Considerations
- PVD
- Cataract surgery

Pediatric Considerations
Usually associated with underlying vitreoretinal disorders and/or retinopathy of prematurity

COMMONLY ASSOCIATED CONDITIONS
- Lattice degeneration
- High myopia
- Cataract surgery
- Glaucoma
- History of retinal detachment in the fellow eye
- Trauma

Pregnancy Considerations
Preeclampsia/eclampsia may be associated with exudative retinal detachment. No intervention is indicated, provided hypertension is controlled. Prognosis is usually good.

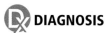 **DIAGNOSIS**

HISTORY
- Sudden flashes of light (photopsia)
- Shower of floaters
- Visual field loss: "curtain coming across vision"
- Central vision will be preserved if the macula is not detached.
- Poor visual acuity (20/200 or worse), with loss of central vision when macula is detached

PHYSICAL EXAM
- Elevation of the neurosensory retina from the underlying retinal pigment epithelium
- Elevation of retina associated with ≥1 retinal tears in RRD or elevation of the retina without tears in exudative detachment
- In 3–10% of patients with presumed RRD, no definite retinal break is found.
- Tenting of the retina without retinal tears in traction detachment
- Pigmented cells within the vitreous ("tobacco dust")

DIFFERENTIAL DIAGNOSIS
Retinoschisis (splitting of the retina)
- Vitreous cells and vitreous hemorrhage are found rarely in the vitreous with retinoschisis, whereas they are seen commonly in RRD.
- Retinoschisis usually has a smooth surface and is dome shaped, whereas RRD often has a corrugated, irregular surface.

DIAGNOSTIC TESTS & INTERPRETATION
Visual field testing: differentiates RRD from retinoschisis. An absolute scotoma is seen in retinoschisis, whereas RRD causes a relative scotoma.

Initial Tests (lab, imaging)
- Ultrasound (US) can demonstrate a detached retina and may be helpful when the retina cannot be visualized directly (e.g., with cataracts or vitreous hemorrhage).
- Fluorescein dye leakage can be seen in exudative retinal detachment; caused by central serous retinopathy and other inflammatory conditions
- Optical coherence tomography (OCT) (2)

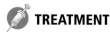 **TREATMENT**

GENERAL MEASURES
- Not all retinal tears or breaks need to be treated:
  - Flap or horseshoe tears in symptomatic patients (e.g., patients with flashes or floaters) are treated frequently.
  - Operculated holes in symptomatic patients are treated sometimes.
  - Asymptomatic atrophic round holes are rarely treated.
- Lattice degeneration with or without holes within the lattice in an asymptomatic patient with prior retinal detachment in the fellow eye may be treated prophylactically.
- Flap retinal tears in asymptomatic patients frequently are treated prophylactically.
- Exudative detachments usually are managed by treating underlying disorder.
- Traction detachments usually are managed by observation. If the fovea is involved, a vitrectomy is needed.

MEDICATION

First Line
The following may be used at the time of surgery to facilitate repair of the RRD:
- Intraocular gases (air, perfluoropropane, sulfur hexafluoride)
- Perfluorocarbon liquids
- Silicone oil (SO)
- Contraindications to intraocular gas: patients with poorly controlled glaucoma
- Precautions with intraocular gas: Expanding intraocular gas bubble increases intraocular pressure; therefore, avoid higher altitudes.
- Significant possible interactions with intraocular gas: Nitrous oxide used in general anesthesia can expand an intraocular gas bubble.

Second Line
Steroids can treat some causes of exudative retinal detachment. Steroids may cause worsening of central serous retinopathy.

SURGERY/OTHER PROCEDURES
- Timing of repairs
  - Macula attached: within 24 hours if possible. If the detachment is peripheral and does not have features suggestive of rapid progression (e.g., large and/or superior tears), repair can be performed within a few days.
    - Preoperative posturing consisting of bed rest and positioning is frequently prescribed to patients with macula-on retinal detachment. Preoperative posturing can reduce the progression of macula-on retinal detachments.

- Macula recently detached: within 10 days of development of a macula-off retinal detachment (3)[B]
  - Old macular detachment: elective repair within 2 weeks
- If a retinal break has led to the development of a retinal detachment, surgery is needed. Surgical options (and combinations) include the following:
  - Demarcation laser treatment
  - Pneumatic retinopexy (PR) is when air or gas is injected intraocularly in the office: Head positioning is required postoperatively.
  - Scleral buckle (SB)
  - Pars plana vitrectomy (PPV)
  - Perfluorocarbon liquids, especially for giant tears (circumferential tears ≥90 degrees)
  - SO for complex repairs
- RRD may have >1 break. If any retinal break is not closed at the time of surgery, the surgery will fail.
- In patients 50 years of age or greater, there is a higher incidence of inferior retinal breaks and inferior retinal detachments in pseudophakic eyes compared to phakic eyes (4)[A].
- Additional surgery may be required if the retina redetaches secondary to a new retinal break or because of PVR.
- If a vitreous hemorrhage is present, presumably from a retinal tear and the fundus cannot be well visualized, consideration can be given for early vitrectomy.
  - Patients who underwent PPV within the 1st week of presentation had a significantly lower risk of having a macula-off RD.
  - Both phakic and pseudophakic patients had a similar chance of developing a retinal detachment. Phakic patients who underwent PPV had a higher chance of requiring subsequent cataract surgery.
- There is a trend toward primary vitrectomy in the management of RRD. Eyes undergoing PPV for primary RRD repair may not need the addition of a scleral buckle.
- Patients with RRD who are at high risk for PVR (retinal detachment in two or more quadrants, retinal tears >1 clock hour, preoperative PVR, or vitreous hemorrhage), PPV + SB were associated with higher rates of anatomical success compared to PPV alone.
- The single-procedure anatomic success rate of PPV, retinectomy, and SO tamponade without SB for PVR-related recurrent RRD is comparable to similar surgery incorporating a SB (5)[C].

ADMISSION, INPATIENT, AND NURSING CONSIDERATIONS
- Recognition of condition is key (see "Diagnosis").
- Refer to an ophthalmologist for exam and treatment, if indicated.

ONGOING CARE

FOLLOW-UP RECOMMENDATIONS
- Bed rest prior to surgery in macula-on cases
- Postoperatively, if intraocular gas has been used, the patient may need specific head positioning and should not travel to high altitudes to avoid expanding the intraocular gas bubble.

Patient Monitoring
- Alert ophthalmologist if there is new onset of floaters or flashes, increase in floaters or flashes, sudden shower of floaters, curtain or shadow in the peripheral visual field, or reduced vision.
- Patients with acute symptomatic PVD should be reexamined by the ophthalmologist in 3 to 4 weeks. Delayed retinal breaks and RRDs can occur for several months after an acute PVD, so the patient should be monitored and be given the warning signs of a RRD (6)[B].

- If acute symptomatic PVD is associated with gross vitreous hemorrhage that interferes with complete visualization of the retinal periphery by indirect ophthalmoscopy, the patient should be reexamined at shorter intervals with indirect ophthalmoscopy until the entire retinal periphery can be observed. Early PPV can be considered.
- If the examiner is not certain whether the retina is detached in the presence of opaque medium, US should be performed.

DIET
NPO if surgery is imminent

PROGNOSIS
- RRD
  - 90% of retinal detachments can be reattached successfully after 1 or more surgical procedures. Postoperative visual acuity depends primarily on the status of the macula preoperatively. Also important is the length of time between the detachment and the repair (75% of eyes with macular detachments of <1 week will obtain a final visual acuity of 20/70 or better).
  - 87% of eyes with a retinal detachment not involving the macula attain a visual acuity of 20/50 or better postoperatively. 37% of eyes with a detached macula preoperatively attain 20/50 or better vision postoperatively.
  - In 10–15% of successfully repaired retinal detachments not involving the macula preoperatively, visual acuity does not return to the preoperative level. This decrease is secondary to complications such as macular edema and macular pucker.
  - Failed primary pneumatic retinopexy selects for RDs that are inherently more difficult to reattach.
- Risk factors associated with primary RRD repair failure include choroidal detachment, significant hypotony, grade C-1 PVR or worse, four detached quadrants, and large or giant retinal breaks. Additional risk factors associated with primary RRD repair failure include increased number of breaks and inferior location of retinal breaks.
- 18% of patients undergoing primary RRD repair by either laser barricade, PR, PPV, or SB required a secondary procedure within 90 days. PR was associated with the highest rate of reoperation of 29%. Most secondary repairs were performed by PPV (7)[A].
- Tractional retinal detachment
  - When not involving the fovea, the patient usually can be observed because it is uncommon for these to extend into the fovea.
- Exudative retinal detachment
  - Management is usually nonsurgical.
  - The presence of shifting fluid is highly suggestive of an exudative retinal detachment. Fixed retinal folds, which are indicative of PVR, are seen rarely in exudative retinal detachment. If the underlying condition is treated, the prognosis generally is good.

COMPLICATIONS
- PVR is the most common cause of failed retinal detachment repair; 10–15% of retinas that reattach initially after retinal surgery will redetach subsequently, usually within 6 weeks, as a result of cellular proliferation and contraction on the retinal surface.
- Partial or total loss of vision due to macular detachment and/or PVR.
- Moderate to severe forms of PVR usually are treated with PPV and fluid–gas exchange. If a segmental scleral buckle was placed at the initial procedure, it may need to be revised.

- Primary retinectomy can be used in cases of PVR without a SB.
- Scleral buckles may erode the overlying conjunctiva and lead to an infection.
- Optic neuropathy after PPV for macula-sparing primary RRD.

REFERENCES

1. Storey PP, Pancholy M, Wibbelsman TD, et al. Rhegmatogenous retinal detachment after intravitreal injection of anti-vascular endothelial growth factor. *Ophthalmology*. 2019;126(10):1424–1431.
2. Tsukaahara M, Mori K, Gehlbach PL, et al. Posterior vitreous detachment as observed by wide-angle OCT imaging. *Ophthalmology*. 2018;125(9):1372–1383.
3. Hassan TS, Sarrafizadeh R, Ruby AJ, et al. The effect of duration of macular detachment on results after the scleral buckle repair of primary, macula-off retinal detachments. *Ophthalmology*. 2002;109(1):146–152.
4. Ferrar M, Mehta A, Qureshe H, et al. Phenotype and outcomes of phakic versus pseudophakic primary rhegmatogenous retinal detachments: Cataract or cataract surgery related? *Am J Ophthalmol*. 2021;222:318–327.
5. Deaner JD, Aderman CM, Bonafede KM, et al. PPV, retinectomy, and silicone oil without scleral buckle for recurrent RRD from proliferatiave vitreoretinopathy. *Ophthalmic Surg Lasers Imaging Retina*. 2019;50(11):e278–e287.
6. Uhr JH, Obeid A, Wibbelsman TD, et al. Delayed retinal breaks and detachments after acute posterior vitreous detachment. *Ophthalmology*. 2020;127(4):516–522.
7. Reeves M-G, Afshar AR, Pershing S. Need for retinal detachment reoperation based on primary repair method among commercially insured patients, 2003–2016. *Am J Ophthalmol*. 2021;229:71–81.

 SEE ALSO

Retinopathy, Diabetic

 CODES

ICD10
- H33.059 Total retinal detachment, unspecified eye
- H33.20 Serous retinal detachment, unspecified eye
- H33.0 Retinal detachment with retinal break

CLINICAL PEARLS

- If a patient complains of the new onset of floaters or flashes of light, the patient should undergo a dilated eye exam to rule out a retinal tear or retinal detachment.
- There is an increased risk of retinal detachment after cataract surgery.

RETINOPATHY, DIABETIC

Richard W. Allinson, MD • Alyce D. Alven, OD, MS

 BASICS

DESCRIPTION
- Noninflammatory retinal disorder characterized by retinal capillary closure and microaneurysms. Retinal ischemia leads to release of a vasoproliferative factor, stimulating neovascularization (NV) on retina, optic nerve, or iris.
- Most patients with diabetes mellitus (DM) will develop diabetic retinopathy (DR). It is the leading cause of new cases of legal blindness among residents in the United States between the ages of 20 and 64 years.
- DR can be divided into three stages:
  - Nonproliferative (NPDR) (background)
  - Severe NPDR (preproliferative)
  - Proliferative (PDR)

Pregnancy Considerations
- Pregnancy can exacerbate condition.
- Pregnant diabetic women should be examined in 1st trimester and then every 3 months until delivery.

EPIDEMIOLOGY
Incidence
- Peak incidence of type 1, juvenile-onset DM is between the ages of 12 and 15 years. In type 1 DM (T1DM), there is β-cell destruction, leading to insulin deficiency.
- Peak incidence of type 2, adult-onset DM is between the ages of 50 and 70 years. Type 2 DM (T2DM) ranges from a condition characterized by insulin resistance with relative insulin deficiency to one that is predominantly an insulin secretory defect with insulin resistance.
- Incidence of DR is directly related to the duration of diabetes.
- <10 years of age, it is unusual to see DR, regardless of DM duration.

Prevalence
- 13.0% of all U.S. adults, 18 years or older, have DM. Prevalence increases with age, reaching 26.8% of U.S. adults aged >65.
- Worldwide, DR affects 1 out of 3 persons with DM.
- Predominant age:
  - Risk increases after puberty.
  - 2/3 of T1DM patients who have had DM for at least 35 years will develop PDR, and 1/3 will develop diabetic macular edema (DME). Proportions are reversed for T2DM.
- Predominant sex: male = female (T1DM); female > male (T2DM).

ETIOLOGY AND PATHOPHYSIOLOGY
- Related to development of diabetic microaneurysms and microvascular abnormalities
- Reduction in perifoveal capillary blood flow velocity, perifoveal capillary occlusion, and increased retinal thickness at the central fovea in diabetic patients are associated with visual impairment in patients with DME.
- Vascular endothelial growth factor (VEGF) is elevated in patients with hypoxic retina. Intraocular levels of VEGF are elevated in patients with retinal or iris NV. Retinal hypoxia also contributes to DME, and VEGF is a major contributor to DME.

RISK FACTORS
- Duration of DM (usually >10 years)
- Poor glycemic control
- Pregnancy
- Renal disease
- Systemic hypertension (HTN)
- Smoking
- Elevated lipid levels
- Myopic eyes (eyes with longer axial length) have a lower risk of developing DR and of its progression.

GENERAL PREVENTION
- Monitor and control of blood glucose.
- Schedule yearly ophthalmologic eye exams.

COMMONLY ASSOCIATED CONDITIONS
- Glaucoma
- Cataracts
- Retinal detachment
- Vitreous hemorrhage (VH)
- Disc edema (diabetic papillopathy); may occur in T1DM and T2DM

 DIAGNOSIS

PHYSICAL EXAM
- Eye exam: measurement of visual acuity and documentation of the status of the iris, lens, vitreous, and fundus
- NPDR (background)
  - Microaneurysms
  - Intraretinal hemorrhage
  - Lipid deposits
- Severe NPDR (preproliferative)
  - Nerve fiber layer infarctions ("cotton wool spots")
  - Venous beading
  - Venous dilatation
  - Intraretinal microvascular abnormalities (IRMA)
  - Extensive retinal hemorrhage
  - The Early Treatment Diabetic Retinopathy Study (ETDRS) developed the 4:2:1 rule for severe nonproliferative diabetic retinopathy (NPDR). Severe NPDR was defined as having any one of the following features:
    ○ Severe intraretinal hemorrhages and microaneurysms in four quadrants
    ○ Venous beading in two or more quadrants
    ○ IRMAs in one or more quadrants
- PDR
  - New blood vessel proliferation: NV can be found on the retinal surface, optic nerve, and iris.
  - Visual loss caused by VH, traction retinal detachment. Contraction of fibrovascular tissue on a vitreous scaffold can lead to VH and traction retinal detachment.

DIFFERENTIAL DIAGNOSIS
Other causes of retinopathy (e.g., radiation, retinal venous obstruction, HTN)

DIAGNOSTIC TESTS & INTERPRETATION
Diagnostic Procedures/Other
- Fluorescein angiography demonstrates retinal nonperfusion, retinal leakage, and PDR.
- Optical coherence tomography (OCT) can be used to help detect DME by measuring retinal thickness.
- Swept-source optical coherence tomography angiography (SS-OCTA) can detect diabetic NV.

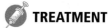 **TREATMENT**

GENERAL MEASURES
- The Diabetes Control and Complications Trial (DCCT) recommended that for most patients with T1DM with insulin-dependent DM, blood glucose levels should be as close to the nondiabetic range as is safe to reduce the risk and rate of progression of DR.
  - In the DCCT, insulin-dependent T1DM patients were randomly assigned into either conventional or intensive insulin treatment. The DCCT demonstrated that intensive insulin therapy reduced the risk of DME and retinal NV. The benefit of intensive insulin therapy with the reduced risk of DR-associated microvascular complications persists for at least 10 years.
  - In the DCCT, intensive insulin therapy was more effective in reducing the risk of progression of DR in the less advanced stages. However, advanced DR also benefited from the intensive insulin therapy.
- The United Kingdom Prospective Diabetes Study (UKPDS) demonstrated patients with T2DM had slower progression of DR with intensive blood glucose control. It also showed that intensive control of blood pressure slowed progression of DR (1).
- Microvascular complications, including PDR, are increased when blood sugar levels are ≥200 mg/dL.
- Cataracts are more common among those with DM. Cataract surgery can cause retinopathy to worsen and increase the risk for development of DME.
- HTN has a detrimental effect on DR and must be controlled.
- Severe obstructive sleep apnea (OSA) is a risk factor for DME in patients with T2DM. Refractory DME is more frequent in patients with severe OSA. Continuous positive airway pressure (CPAP) may help prevent refractory DME in patients with OSA (2)[B].

MEDICATION
- Treatment of HTN with the angiotensin receptor blocker candesartan has been shown to result in regression of DR in some patients.
- Statin therapy in patients with T2DM is associated with a decreased risk of DR:
  - T2DM patients on lipid-lowering medications are less likely to develop NPDR, PDR, or DME (3)[A].
- Aspirin
  - Does not alter progression of DR
  - Does not increase the risk of VH

SURGERY/OTHER PROCEDURES
- Preventive treatment of moderate to severe NPDR without centered-involved diabetic macular edema (CI-DME) with intravitreal aflibercept injection (IAI) reduced the development of PDR or vision-reducing CI-DME. After 2 years of follow-up, preventive treatment with IAI did not confer VA benefit compared with observation plus IAI only after development of PDR or vision-reducing CI-DME (4)[A].
- Treatment for DME
  - Intravitreal anti-VEGF is first-line treatment for DME:
    ○ Ranibizumab, an antibody fragment that binds VEGF, can be used to treat DME when injected intravitreally. Ranibizumab 0.3 mg (0.05 mL) injected intravitreally monthly resulted in improved vision and reduced central foveal thickness.
    ■ Anti-VEGF treatment by intravitreal injection (IVI) results in superior clinical outcomes compared to laser photocoagulation for DME.

- Intravitreal ranibizumab injections (IRIs) are beneficial for patients with DME and concurrent macular nonperfusion.
- IRI for DME may also improve DR severity and reduce the risk of DR progression.
- Treat and extend dosing for IRI decreased the number of injections while giving similar visual and anatomic outcomes compared with monthly dosing at 1 year.
- As-needed treatment after a loading dose of 3 monthly injections has been shown to result in comparable results to more frequent treatments.
- Topical povidone-iodine prophylaxis is important to help prevent endophthalmitis from IVIs from anti-VEGF treatment.
  - Bevacizumab, a full-length antibody that binds VEGF, can be used to treat DME when injected intravitreally. Intravitreal bevacizumab injection (IBI) is an off-label use.
  - Aflibercept, a decoy receptor for VEGF that inhibits all isoforms of VEGF-A and placental growth factor. Aflibercept 2 mg (0.05 mL) injected intravitreally every 4 weeks for the first 5 injections followed by 2 mg (0.05 mL) intravitreally once every 8 weeks. It is indicated for patients with DME and for DR in patients without DME.
    - Intravitreal aflibercept injection (IAI) has demonstrated significant superiority in functional and anatomic end points over macular laser photocoagulation.
    - At worse levels of initial visual acuity (VA) (20/50 or worse) in patients with DME, IAI was more effective in improving vision than ranibizumab or bevacizumab with 1-year follow-up. When the initial vision loss was mild (20/32 to 20/40) in patients with DME, there was no significant difference between aflibercept, ranibizumab, and bevacizumab.
      □ Aflibercept had superior 2-year VA outcomes compared with bevacizumab. The superiority of aflibercept over ranibizumab, noted at 1 year, was no longer seen at 2 years of follow-up.
    - Among eyes with CI-DME and good VA (20/25 or better), there was no significant difference in vision loss whether eyes were initially managed with observation plus IAI only if VA decreased, or with initial focal laser treatment plus IAI only if VA decreased, or prompt IAI. Observation without treatment unless VA worsens may be a reasonable plan of action for CI-DME (5)[A].
    - As-needed IAI has been shown to maintain vision and reduce treatment frequency.
  - Faricimab inhibits both angiopoietin-2 and VEGF-A. It is being studied for the treatment of DME at a dosing of every 4 months.
- Focal laser treatment.
- Vitrectomy may benefit some with diffuse macular edema. This may apply especially to eyes with vitreomacular traction found on OCT and with persistent DME.
- Intravitreal triamcinolone may be used for DM-related macular edema that fails laser treatment; no long-term benefit of intravitreal triamcinolone relative to focal/grid photocoagulation in patients with DME.
- Intraocular steroid implants for DME. Either a dexamethasone implant or a fluocinolone acetonide implant. Complications of these implants include cataract and glaucoma.

- Treatment for PDR:
  - Thermal laser photocoagulation in a panretinal pattern is a common form of treatment for PDR. The goal of panretinal photocoagulation (PRP) is regression or involution of NV. PRP destroys ischemic retina and decreases the neovascular stimulus.
    - The Diabetic Retinopathy Study demonstrated that when PRP was used to treat PDR or severe NPDR, eyes treated with PRP had a reduction of 50% or more in the rates of severe vision loss compared with untreated control eyes. In certain subgroups, the incidence of severe visual loss in untreated eyes was as high as 36.9% at 2 years.
    - Patients with DME and high-risk proliferative disease can have simultaneous focal and PRP without adversely affecting the visual outcome.
  - Both IRI and IAI are alternative therapies to PRP for PDR. They can be used in conjunction with PRP to treat PDR.
  - Inital IAI or pars plana vitrectomy (PPV) with PRP can be used to treat PDR-related VH (6)[A].
  - IVI of anti-VEGF therapy for PDR does not increase the risk for TRD (7)[B].
  - PPV recommended for patients with severe PDR, traction retinal detachment involving the macula, and nonclearing VH.
    - The Diabetic Retinopathy Vitrectomy Study (DRVS) demonstrated the benefits of early PPV (1 to 6 months after onset of VH) in T1DM and for eyes with very severe PDR.
    - Immediate PPV with endolaser may be considered for PDR-associated VH (<30 days).
    - Preoperative IBI can be used as an adjuvant to vitrectomy for complications of PDR. This is an off-label use.

COMPLEMENTARY & ALTERNATIVE MEDICINE
Nutritional antioxidant intake of vitamins C and E and of β-carotene has no protective effect on DR.

 ONGOING CARE

FOLLOW-UP RECOMMENDATIONS
Patient Monitoring
Scheduled ophthalmologic eye exams
- Yearly follow-up if no retinopathy
- Every 6 months with background DR
- At least every 3 to 4 months with pre-PDR
- Every 2 to 3 months with active PDR
- Patients with DME should be followed every 4 to 6 weeks.

DIET
In middle-aged and older individuals with T2DM, intake of at least 500 mg/day of dietary long-chain omega-3 polyunsaturated fatty acids, achievable with 2 weekly servings of oily fish, is associated with a decreased risk of visual loss from DR.

PATIENT EDUCATION
- Advise regular ophthalmic exams.
- Stress importance of glucose control through diet, exercise, drugs/insulin.

PROGNOSIS
If the condition is diagnosed and treated early in development, outlook is good. If treatment is delayed, blindness may result.

COMPLICATIONS
- Repeated intravitreal injection of anti-VEGF therapy may increase the risk of sustained intraocular pressure elevation and the possible need for ocular hypotensive treatment.
- Blindness

REFERENCES
1. UK Prospective Diabetes Study Group. Tight blood pressure control and risk of macrovascular and microvascular complications in type 2 diabetes: UKPDS 38. BMJ. 1998;317(7160):703–713.
2. Chiang J-F, Sun M-H, Chen K-J, et al. Association between obstructive sleep apnea and diabetic macular edema in patients with type 2 diabetes. Am J Ophthalmol. 2021;226:217–225.
3. Vail D, Callaway NF, Ludwig CA, et al. Lipid-lowering mediations are associated with lower risk of retinopathy and ophthalmic interventions among U.S. patients with diabetes. Am J Ophthalmol. 2019;207:378–384.
4. Maturi RK, Glassman AR, Josic K, et al. Effect of intravitreous anti-vascular endothelial growth factor vs sham treatment for prevention of vision-threatening complications of diabetic retinopathy: the Protocol W randomized clinical trial. JAMA Ophthalmol. 2021;139(7):701–712.
5. Glassman AR, Baker CW, Beaulieu WT, et al. Assessment of the DRCR Retina Network approach to management with initial observation for eyes with center-involved diabetic macular edema and good visual acuity: a secondary analysis of a randomized clinical trial. JAMA Ophthalmol. 2020;138(4):341–349.
6. Glassman AR, Beaulieu WT, Maguire MG, et al. Visual acuity, vitreous hemorrhage, and other ocular outcomes after vitrectomy vs aflibercept for vitreous hemorrhage due to diabetic retinopathy: a secondary analysis of a randomized clinical trial. JAMA Ophthalmol. 2021;139(7):725–733.
7. Bressler NM, Beaulieu WT, Bressler SB, et al. Anti-vascular endothelial growth factor therapy and risk of traction retinal detachment in eyes with proliferative diabetic retinopathy: pooled analysis of five DRCR Retina Network randomized clinical trials. Retina. 2020;40(6):1021–1028.

ADDITIONAL READING

Wells JA, Glassman AR, Ayala AR, et al; for Diabetic Retinopathy Clinical Research Network. Aflibercept, bevacizumab, or ranibizumab for diabetic macular edema: two-year results from a comparative effectiveness randomized clinical trial. Ophthalmology. 2016;123(6):1351–1359.

CODES

ICD10
- E11.319 Type 2 diabetes mellitus with unspecified diabetic retinopathy without macular edema
- E10.319 Type 1 diabetes mellitus with unspecified diabetic retinopathy without macular edema
- E10.329 Type 1 diab w mild nonprlf diabetic rtnop w/o macular edema

CLINICAL PEARLS
- Schedule yearly ophthalmologic eye exams.
- Options for the treatment of diabetic macular edema include focal laser treatment, intravitreal triamcinolone, intravitreal ranibizumab, intravitreal bevacizumab (off-label), intravitreal aflibercept, intraocular steroid implants, and vitrectomy.

RH INCOMPATIBILITY
Jennifer G. Chang, MD

BASICS

DESCRIPTION
- Antibody-mediated destruction of red blood cells (RBCs) that bear Rh surface antigens in individuals who lack the antigens and have become isoimmunized (sensitized) to them
- System(s) affected: hematologic/lymphatic/immunologic
- Synonym(s): Rh isoimmunization; Rh alloimmunization; Rh sensitization

EPIDEMIOLOGY
Incidence
- Predominantly affects fetuses/neonates of isoimmunized, childbearing females; varies by race and ethnicity
- ~15% of the white population and smaller fractions of other races are Rh-negative and thus may be susceptible to sensitization.

ETIOLOGY AND PATHOPHYSIOLOGY
- Circulating antibodies to Rh antigens (transplacentally transferred antibodies in the case of a fetus/newborn) attach to Rh antigens on RBCs.
- Immune-mediated destruction of RBCs leads to hemolysis, anemia, and increased bilirubin production.
- Transplacental fetomaternal hemorrhage may occur during pregnancy but is more common at delivery.
- Most cases of alloimmunization involve small volume fetomaternal hemorrhage (0.1 mL or less) during uncomplicated vaginal delivery.
- Other causes: transfusion of Rh-positive blood to Rh-negative recipient; exposure to needles contaminated with Rh-positive blood

Genetics
- Complex autosomal inheritance of polypeptide Rh antigens; three genetic loci with closely related genes carry an assortment of alleles: Dd, Cc, and Ee.
- Individuals who express the D antigen (also called *Rho* or *Rho[D]*) are considered Rh-positive. Individuals lacking the D antigen are Rh-negative.
- Variant D alleles (weak D and partial D) are heterogeneous, altered forms of the D antigen. Some D variants are at risk for formation of anti-D antibodies, whereas others are not. With current blood typing procedures, certain D variants likely to produce alloimmunization are typed as D-negative, although this does not include all genetic subtypes at risk for isoimmunization.
- Another variant D antigen, DEL, has been identified in some individuals (predominantly Asians). Those with partial DEL expression are at risk for alloimmunization and should be considered clinically Rh-negative. Women with complete DEL are not likely to be sensitized by exposure to Rh-D antigens through pregnancy or transfusion and should be considered clinically Rh-positive and do not need RhD prophylaxis.

- Antibodies may be produced to C, c, D, E, or e in individuals lacking the specific antigen; only D is strongly immunogenic.
- Isoimmunization to Rh antigens in susceptible individuals is acquired, not inherited.

RISK FACTORS
- Any Rh-positive fetus in an Rh-negative pregnant woman can result in sensitization.
- Weak D and partial D women are a heterogeneous group. Although previously reported to be Rh-positive and treated as such, alloimmunization has been reported (though is rare) and can result in hemolytic disease of the fetus and newborn (HDFN).
- Native risk of isoimmunization after Rh-positive pregnancy had been estimated at ≤15% but seems to be decreasing.
- 1–2% of Rh isoimmunization occurs antepartum.
- The risk of isoimmunization is 1–2% after spontaneous abortion and 4–5% after induced abortion. It is unclear what the risk is with early medication-induced abortion but is likely very low due to the small volume of embryonic red cells.
- Increased volume of fetomaternal hemorrhage may occur in cesarean delivery, multifetal gestation, placenta previa or abruption, manual removal of the placenta and during antenatal procedures such as chorionic villus sampling, amniocentesis, and external cephalic version.
- Use of Rho(D) immunoglobulin prophylaxis has reduced incidence of isoimmunization to <1% in susceptible pregnancies (1)[C].

GENERAL PREVENTION
- Blood typing (ABO and Rh) on all pregnant women and prior to blood transfusions
- Antibody screening early in pregnancy
- Rh immunoglobulin prevents only sensitization to the D antigen.
- Cell-free fetal (Cff) DNA testing with selective administration of Rh immunoglobulin when the fetus tests Rh-positive has been shown to be as effective at preventing new Rh sensitization when compared to routine administration of Rh-immunoglobulin to all Rh-negative women. Such an approach avoids unnecessary use of Rh immunoglobulin (2)[B].
- Currently, routine administration of Rh immune globulin is more cost-effective than use of Cff DNA testing in the United States (1)[C].
- For prophylaxis, Rho(D) immunoglobulin (RhIG, RhoGAM, HyperRHO, Rhophylac) given to unsensitized, Rh-negative women after the following:
  - Threatened miscarriage or miscarriage (controversial before 12 weeks gestation)
  - Therapeutic pregnancy termination (no evidence for or against prophylaxis before 6 to 7 weeks in medication-induced abortion)
  - Ectopic pregnancy
  - Evacuation of molar pregnancy
  - Intrauterine fetal death
  - Antepartum hemorrhage
  - Trauma to abdomen

- Amniocentesis or cordocentesis
- Chorionic villus sampling
- External cephalic version
- Within 72 hours of delivery of an Rh-positive infant
- Given routinely at 28 weeks' gestation
- Prophylaxis prevents sensitization that could affect a subsequent pregnancy and has little effect on the current pregnancy.
- Dose for prophylaxis
  - 50-μg (up to 120-μg) dose for events up to 12 weeks' gestation
  - 300-μg dose for events after 12 weeks' gestation
  - Higher doses may be required in the event of a large fetal–maternal hemorrhage (>30 mL of whole blood).

COMMONLY ASSOCIATED CONDITIONS
- Neonatal jaundice (common)
- Hemolytic disease of the fetus and newborn (HDFN) (less common)
- Hydrops fetalis (rare)
- Kernicterus (rare)
- See "Erythroblastosis Fetalis."

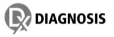

DIAGNOSIS

PHYSICAL EXAM
- Jaundice of newborn
- Kernicterus signs/symptoms (choreoathetoid movements, gaze abnormalities, dental enamel dysplasia)
- Fetal hydrops or fetal death in utero if severe (see "Erythroblastosis Fetalis" topic)

DIFFERENTIAL DIAGNOSIS
- ABO incompatibility
- Other blood group (non-Rh) isoimmunization
- Nonimmune fetal hydrops
- Hereditary spherocytosis
- RBC enzyme defects

DIAGNOSTIC TESTS & INTERPRETATION
Initial Tests (lab, imaging)
- Positive indirect Coombs test (antibody screen) during pregnancy
- Paternal blood type; if unknown or heterozygous, amniocentesis for fetal antigen type using PCR is highly sensitive (98.7%) and specific (100%); current standard practice in United States (1)[C].
- Cell-free fetal DNA (Cff DNA) test: standard practice in many European countries; available in the United States but is not currently a widely covered benefit. It allows detection of fetal Rh genotype with accuracy of 97.1%, sensitivity of 97.2%, and specificity of 96.8%.
- Rosette test (qualitative detection of fetomaternal bleeding); if positive, perform Kleihauer-Betke test (fetal hemoglobin acid elution, Hb F slide elution) or flow cytometry (more sensitive but not widely available) to quantify an acute fetal–maternal bleed.
- Assess degree of fetal anemia.
- Blood type and direct Coombs test in newborn

Follow-Up Tests & Special Considerations

Prior administration of Rho(D) may lead to weakly (false-) positive anti-D (indirect Coombs test) in mother and direct Coombs test in infant.

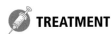

TREATMENT

GENERAL MEASURES

- Depending on severity of involvement, treatment of fetus may include the following:
  - Intrauterine transfusion (3)[B],(4)[A]
  - Early delivery—typically no later than 37 to 38 weeks' gestation (1)[C],(4)[A]
- Treatment of newborn may include the following:
  - Exchange transfusion
  - Transfusion after delivery
  - Phototherapy
- Inconclusive evidence on efficacy of IVIG to reduce need for exchange transfusion (5)[A].

ISSUES FOR REFERRAL

Because of the specialized, somewhat hazardous, treatment measures involved, pregnancies in Rh-sensitized women are usually managed at tertiary care facilities with maternal–fetal medicine specialists.

ADMISSION, INPATIENT, AND NURSING CONSIDERATIONS

Initial monitoring of the newborn as inpatient or in special care nursery if treatment interventions are needed.

ONGOING CARE

FOLLOW-UP RECOMMENDATIONS

Patient Monitoring

- In most cases, outpatient ambulatory management is appropriate during the antepartum period.
- Antibody titer measured monthly in isoimmunized women until 24 weeks and every 2 weeks thereafter during first affected pregnancy; a titer of ≥1:16 indicates the need for further testing (4)[A].
- If the patient had a previously affected infant, an Rh-positive fetus in the current pregnancy should be considered at risk regardless of antibody titers (4)[A].
  - Fetal heart rate testing/US to assess fetal status
  - Doppler US measurement of cerebral blood flow (should be performed only by adequately trained providers). If peak MCA systolic velocity >1.5 multiples of the median for gestational age, further testing is needed (cordocentesis) for diagnosing fetal anemia (4)[A].
  - Umbilical blood sampling (cordocentesis) for fetal blood type, hematocrit, reticulocyte count, and presence of erythroblasts (4)[A]
  - Amniocentesis for amniotic fluid bilirubin levels (4)[A]
  - Amniocentesis for fetal lung maturity if early delivery is a treatment option (1)[C],(4)[A]

PROGNOSIS

- With appropriate monitoring and treatment, infants born of severely affected pregnancies have a survival rate of >80% (4)[A].
- Even with severe disease, the neurologic outcome of survivors is generally good.
- Fetuses with hydrops have a higher mortality rate and higher risk of neurologic impairment.
- Disease is likely to be more severe in affected subsequent pregnancies.

COMPLICATIONS

- Pregnancy loss from umbilical blood sampling
- Pregnancy loss from intrauterine transfusion
- Fetal distress requiring emergent delivery

REFERENCES

1. ACOG Practice Bulletin No. 192: management of alloimmunization during pregnancy. *Obstet Gynecol*. 2018;131(3):e82–e90.
2. Tiblad E, Tuane Wikman A, Ajne G, et al. Targeted routine antenatal anti-D prophylaxis in the prevention of RhD immunization—outcome of a new antenatal screening and prevention program. *PloS One*. 2013;8(8):e70984.
3. Lindenburg IT, Smits-Wintjens VE, van Klink JM, et al. Long-term neurodevelopmental outcome after intrauterine transfusion for hemolytic disease of the fetus/newborn: the LOTUS study. *Am J Obstet Gynecol*. 2012;206(2):141.e1–141.e8.
4. Moise KJ Jr, Argoti PS. Management and prevention of red cell alloimmunization in pregnancy: a systematic review. *Obstet Gynecol*. 2012;120(5):1132–1139.
5. Louis D, More K, Oberoi S, et al. Intravenous immunoglobulin in isoimmune haemolytic disease of newborn: an updated systematic review and meta-analysis. *Arch Dis Child Fetal Neonatal Ed*. 2014;99(4):F325–F331.

ADDITIONAL READING

- Agre P, Cartron JP. Molecular biology of the Rh antigens. *Blood*. 1991;78(3):551–563.
- Bowman J. Thirty-five years of Rh prophylaxis. *Transfusion*. 2003;43(12):1661–1666.
- Delaney M, Matthews DC. Hemolytic disease of the fetus and newborn: managing the mother, fetus, and newborn. *Hematology Am Soc Hematol Educ Program*. 2015;2015:146–151.
- Flegel WA. Molecular genetics and clinical applications for RH. *Transfus Apher Sci*. 2011;44(1):81–91.
- Hawk AF, Chang EY, Shields SM, et al. Costs and clinical outcomes of noninvasive fetal RhD typing for targeted prophylaxis. *Obstet Gynecol*. 2013;122(3):579–585.

- McBain RD, Crowther CA, Middleton P. Anti-D administration in pregnancy for preventing Rhesus alloimmunisation. *Cochrane Database Syst Rev*. 2015;(9):CD000020.
- Wang M, Wang BL, Xu W, et al. Anti-D alloimmunisation in pregnant women with DEL phenotype in China. *Transfus Med*. 2015;25(3):163–169.

 SEE ALSO

- Anemia, Autoimmune Hemolytic; Erythroblastosis Fetalis
- Algorithm: Jaundice

 CODES

ICD10

- P55.0 Rh isoimmunization of newborn
- O36.0990 Maternal care for other rhesus isoimmunization, unspecified trimester, not applicable or unspecified
- T80.40XA Rh incompat react due to tranfs of bld/bld prod, unsp, init

CLINICAL PEARLS

- If paternity is certain, determining that the father does not carry the Rh(D) blood group antigen eliminates the need to give RhIG prophylaxis during pregnancy or the need for special fetal surveillance if the mother is already sensitized.
- The dose of RhIG for prophylaxis is affected by gestational age. The fetal blood volume is only a few milliliters at 12 weeks' gestation. Therefore, a 50-μg dose of RhIG may be used for threatened, spontaneous, or induced abortions up to 12 weeks' gestation, instead of the standard 300-μg dose.
- Diagnosis is made by antibody screen and titer. Affected pregnancies will require maternal–fetal medicine consultations and monitoring of antibody levels; if titer >1:16, will also require serial monitoring of MCA peak velocity. This will determine the need for invasive testing and transfusions.
- If the patient had a previously affected infant, an Rh-positive fetus in the current pregnancy should be considered at risk regardless of antibody titers—proceed to MCA peak velocity monitoring.
- The current standard in the United States is to provide prophylaxis to all unsensitized Rh-negative mothers; however, determination of the fetal Rh status by Cff DNA testing is reliable and could allow for targeted, rather than universal prophylaxis. Currently, routine prophylaxis is more cost-effective in the United States.

R

RHABDOMYOLYSIS

Chirag N. Shah, MD

BASICS

DESCRIPTION
- Breakdown of skeletal muscle with systemic release of intracellular contents
- Rhabdomyolysis typically presents with muscle pain, weakness, and reddish brown (tea-colored) urine. Up to 50% of patients are asymptomatic.

EPIDEMIOLOGY
Incidence
26,000 hospitalizations annually in United States

ETIOLOGY AND PATHOPHYSIOLOGY
Risk factors
- Direct muscle trauma (most common cause)
  - Crush injuries
  - Extended periods of muscle pressure (during surgery, unconscious from alcohol ingestion)
  - Burns, electrocution, lightning strike
- Muscle exertion
  - Intense and/or prolonged physical exercise (marathon runners, athletes, contact sports)
  - Seizures
  - Delirium tremens
- Drugs and toxins
  - Alcohol
  - Cocaine (most common recreational drug), methamphetamine, phencyclidine, heroin, bath salts (1)[B]; synthetic marijuana has been associated with severe rhabdomyolysis.
  - Antipsychotics (due to neuroleptic malignant syndrome, malignant hyperthermia, and dystonia)
  - Zidovudine
  - Antimalarials
  - HMG-CoA reductase inhibitors (statins) (risk <0.01%—elevated with higher doses and in combination with fibrates)
  - Colchicine
  - Corticosteroids
  - Carbon monoxide
  - Snake envenomation
- Muscle ischemia
  - Thrombosis, embolism, sickle cell disease
  - Compartment syndrome
  - Tourniquets
- Infections
  - Viral: influenza A and B, coxsackievirus, HIV, varicella
  - Bacterial: *Streptococcus* or *Staphylococcus* sepsis, gas gangrene, necrotizing fasciitis, *Salmonella*, *Legionella*
  - Malaria
- Hypothermia
- Hyperthermia
- Autoimmune disorders
  - Polymyositis, dermatomyositis
- Metabolic and endocrinologic
  - Hypothyroidism or thyrotoxicosis
  - Electrolyte imbalances (e.g., hyponatremia, hypernatremia, hypokalemia, hypocalcemia, hypophosphatemia)
  - Diabetic ketoacidosis
  - Hyperosmolar state

Genetics
Hereditary causes of rhabdomyolysis are rare but should be suspected in children; patients with recurrent attacks; or patients who have attacks after minimal exertion, mild illness, or starvation.
- Genetic disorders (1)[C]
  - Muscular dystrophies
  - Disorders of lipid metabolism (e.g., carnitine palmitoyltransferase deficiency)
  - Disorders of carbohydrate metabolism (i.e., phosphofructokinase deficiency, phosphoglycerate mutase, myophosphorylase deficiency, a.k.a. McArdle disease/deficiency)
  - Glycogen storage diseases (e.g., phosphorylase B kinase deficiency) and others (e.g., lactate dehydrogenase A deficiency)
  - Mitochondrial disorders

GENERAL PREVENTION
- Avoid excessive exertion; ensure adequate hydration.
- Avoid precipitating drugs, metabolic and electrolyte abnormalities.

DIAGNOSIS

HISTORY
- Crush injury: direct trauma, prolonged compression/immobility. Causes include motor vehicle accidents (MVA) and entrapment in collapsed buildings. The elderly are more susceptible to crush injury due to immobility and falls. Rhabdomyolysis usually occurs after 1 hour of immobilization, but cases reported with compression lasting <20 minutes.
- Possible history of overexertion or use of drug/toxin (e.g., cocaine, amphetamine, statins), particularly in warm environments
- Patient may complain of fever, malaise, muscle aches, weakness, cramps, or fatigue.
- Nausea, vomiting, diarrhea
- Dark urine
- Agitation while patients are in restraints
- Prolonged periods of lying on a hard surface (e.g., intoxicated or obtunded individuals)

PHYSICAL EXAM
- Vital signs—temperature, pulse, respirations, blood pressure, and oxygenation status
- May have obvious muscle tenderness, evidence of crush injury, weakness, and/or swelling on exam. The muscle exam may also be completely normal.
- Tea-colored urine is indicative of myoglobinuria.
- Decreased urine output may indicate renal failure.

DIFFERENTIAL DIAGNOSIS
- Any disease that causes acute tubular necrosis may be confused with rhabdomyolysis.
- Inflammatory myopathies
- Infection (bacterial or viral)
- Phosphorylase, phosphofructokinase, carnitine palmityl transferase, phosphoglycerate mutase deficiency
- Guillain-Barré syndrome
- Myocardial infarction

DIAGNOSTIC TESTS & INTERPRETATION
Initial Tests (lab, imaging)
- Creatine kinase (CK) is the most important diagnostic test: elevated >5 times the upper limit of normal or >1,000 U/L. CK levels >5,000 U/L are causally related to acute renal failure (ARF) (2)[B],(3)[A] and should prompt aggressive fluid resuscitation.
- CK levels peak at ~24 hours and return to normal after 3 to 5 days, making CK a more sensitive marker than myoglobin. Myoglobin is responsible for renal damage (2)[B],(3)[C].
- Serum myoglobin levels peak within a few hours and return to normal after ~24 hours. Normal myoglobin levels do not rule out rhabdomyolysis (due to rapid clearance).
- Urinalysis: Dipstick test positive for blood without erythrocytes in sediment suggests injury from either hemoglobin or myoglobin.
- Elevations of serum potassium from muscle injury can be compounded by ARF.
- Initial hypocalcemia: Calcium enters the injured muscle cells and precipitates as calcium phosphate, leading to calcification of ischemic muscle cells. Only correct initial hypocalcemia if patient is symptomatic or has ECG changes; resolves during the renal recovery phase
- Hypercalcemia during renal recovery phase: unique to rhabdomyolysis-induced ARF for 20–30% of patients (3)[A]. As renal function improves, there is mobilization of the precipitated calcium, increase in calcitriol, and hyperphosphatemia resolves.
- Extreme hyperuricemia may be present and can cause acute uric acid nephropathy.
- Elevations in BUN and creatinine suggest ARF.
- Reversible hepatic dysfunction can occur. However, elevations in alanine aminotransferase (ALT), aspartate aminotransferase (AST), and lactic dehydrogenase may be due to muscle injury rather than hepatic injury.
- Disseminated intravascular coagulation (DIC) suggested by increase in coagulation times, fibrin degradation products, and D-dimer with decreases in platelets and fibrinogen
- 12-lead ECG because hyperkalemia can induce fatal arrhythmias

Follow-Up Tests & Special Considerations
- Delayed renal failure/electrolyte abnormalities despite normal initial levels
- Ongoing muscle injury is manifested by rising creatine phosphokinase (CPK).
- Renal imaging shows findings similar to other mechanisms of ARF.

Diagnostic Procedures/Other
Muscle compartment pressures if compartment syndrome is suspected

Test Interpretation
- Muscle necrosis
- Myoglobin-related renal injury may resemble acute tubular necrosis from other causes.

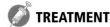 TREATMENT

GENERAL MEASURES
- Address underlying cause (e.g., medications cessation, temperature control, trauma, infection).
- Aggressive hydration is often necessary. With severe muscle trauma (crush injuries), up to 12 L of fluid may be sequestered in the muscles.
- Monitor CK levels, renal function, and electrolytes.
- Follow potassium levels due to potential for arrhythmias.
- Treat DIC or hepatic dysfunction appropriately.
- Recognize and treat compartment syndrome promptly.

MEDICATION
First Line
- Aggressive fluid resuscitation is the most important intervention: normal saline (NS) and 5% glucose solution with a target urine output of 200 to 300 mL/hr. Alternating NS and 5% glucose is recommended to prevent volume overload. Infusion rate should be 500 mL/hr (4)[A],(5)[A].
- Alkalinization of the urine may decrease myoglobin-induced nephrotoxicity in the tubules (sodium bicarbonate to increase urine pH >6.5):
  – Use is controversial.
  – Side effects include worsening hypocalcemia.
  – Sodium bicarbonate may be of use in patients with very high CK levels, acidosis, or coexisting hyperkalemia.
  – Place 150 mEq (3 ampules) NaHCO₃ in 1 L of D5W and infuse at 200 mL/hr.

Second Line
- IV mannitol as a bolus if urine output remains low, 1 to 2 g/kg, not to exceed 200 g in 24 hours with a cumulative dose of 800 g. It is used to prevent ARF only if diuresis is not adequate (<200 mL/hr) despite fluid therapy (4)[A],(5)[A].
  – Increases prostaglandin production leading to renal vasodilation and diuresis, reducing susceptibility to myoglobin injury. As an osmotic agent, filtered but not reabsorbed by the tubules, mannitol increases sodium delivery and diuresis. This may remove necrotic cell debris and prevent rise in compartment pressures.
  – Use of mannitol is controversial. No good evidence that it improves outcomes more than aggressive IV hydration. As a free-radical scavenger, mannitol has renal protective effects if used before tubular occlusion.
  – Consider adding furosemide to force diuresis if necessary (40 to 120 mg/day).
  – Do not diurese in anuric renal failure; caution also in the elderly and patients with heart disease
- Hyperkalemia can result from massive release of intracellular potassium stores or ARF. Severe hyperkalemia may be life-threatening; treatment when ECG changes are present (tall, thin T waves; PR prolongation; QRS widening; P wave flattening)
  – Calcium gluconate: to stabilize the cardiac membrane; IV 1 to 2 ampules (0.5 mL 10% calcium gluconate = 4 mg elemental calcium; give 4 mg/kg/hr for 4 hours.)

– If acidosis is present: 1 to 2 ampules (2 to 3 mL/kg) sodium bicarbonate IV. Sodium bicarbonate can worsen hypocalcemia.
– If tolerated: Oral sodium polystyrene sulfonate (Kayexalate) as much as 20 g (1 g/kg) can be given via enema.
– Insulin and albuterol transiently drive potassium into the cells. Administration of glucose can prevent the hypoglycemic effects of insulin.
– Precautions: continuous monitoring of potassium levels to prevent overcorrecting with potential hypokalemia and arrhythmias
– Indications for dialysis include resistant and symptomatic hyperkalemia (ECG), oliguria (<0.5 mL/kg over 12-hour period), anuria, volume overload, or persistent acidosis (pH <7.1).

ISSUES FOR REFERRAL
- Usually managed as an inpatient
- Diagnosis of compartment syndrome merits surgical consultation for consideration of fasciotomy.
- Renal dialysis may be indicated in ARF.

ADDITIONAL THERAPIES
During the oliguric phase, symptomatic hypocalcemia (rare) may benefit from IV calcium gluconate.

SURGERY/OTHER PROCEDURES
For muscle entrapment/compartment syndrome

ADMISSION, INPATIENT, AND NURSING CONSIDERATIONS
- Patients with significant elevations of CK should be admitted for IV hydration and clinical monitoring.
- Volume expansion with NS to increase urine output to at least 150 mL/hr
- CK usually peaks 24 to 36 hours after muscle injury, so monitoring should confirm that the CK is trending down. Renal function should be stable/improving. Electrolytes should be normal.
- Patients with mild CK elevation and normal renal function may be discharged after observation phase if CK is trending down.

 ONGOING CARE

FOLLOW-UP RECOMMENDATIONS
Follow up within a few days to recheck CK, electrolytes, and renal function.

Patient Monitoring
- Contingent on disease: essential for metabolic myopathies
- Myotoxic drugs should be discontinued/monitored closely.

DIET
- With renal failure, restrict protein intake to lower BUN level.
- Limit potassium intake.
- With anuria, essential to restrict volume intake

PROGNOSIS
Contingent on primary cause of rhabdomyolysis and on recovery from ARF without complications

COMPLICATIONS
- Death, especially from hyperkalemia/renal failure
- With dialysis and supportive care, the prognosis is very good.

REFERENCES
1. Scalco RS, Gardiner AR, Pitceathly RD, et al. Rhabdomyolysis: a genetic perspective. *Orphanet J Rare Dis*. 2015;10:51.
2. Cervellin G, Comelli I, Benatti M, et al. Non-traumatic rhabdomyolysis: background, laboratory features, and acute clinical management. *Clin Biochem*. 2017;50(12):656–662.
3. Long B, Koyfman A, Gottlieb M. An evidence-based narrative review of the ermegency department evaluation and management of rhabdomyolysis. *Am J Emerg Med*. 2019;37(3):518–523.
4. Chavez LO, Leon M, Elinav S, et al. Beyond muscle destruction: a systematic review of rhabdomyolysis for clinical practice. *Crit Care*. 2016;20(1):135.
5. Petejova N, Martinek A. Acute kidney injury due to rhabdomyolysis and renal replacement therapy: a critical review. *Crit Care*. 2014;18(3):224.

ADDITIONAL READING
- Cabral BMI, Edding SN, Portocarrero JP, et al. Rhabdomyolysis. *Dis Mon*. 2020;66(8):101015.
- Durand D, Delgado LL, de la Parra-Pellot DM, et al. Psychosis and severe rhabdomyolysis associated with synthetic cannabinoid use: a case report. *Clin Schizophr Relat Psychoses*. 2015;8(4):205–208.
- Knafl EG, Hughes JA, Dimeski G, et al. Rhabdomyolysis: patterns, circumstances, and outcomes of patients presenting to the emergency department. *Ochsner J*. 2018;18(3):215–221.
- Shawkat H, Westwood MM, Mortimer A. Mannitol: a review of its clinical uses. *Contin Educ Anaesth Crit Care Pain*. 2012;12(2):82–85.

 SEE ALSO

Algorithm: Acute Kidney Injury (Acute Renal Failure)

 CODES

ICD10
- M62.82 Rhabdomyolysis
- T79.6 Traumatic ischemia of muscle
- T79.6xxS Traumatic ischemia of muscle, sequela

CLINICAL PEARLS
- Elevation of CK is the diagnostic hallmark of rhabdomyolysis.
- The cornerstone of treatment of rhabdomyolysis is aggressive fluid administration.
- Electrolyte abnormalities, acute kidney injury, hepatic injury, compartment syndrome, and (rarely) DIC are the most worrisome complications of rhabdomyolysis.

R

RHABDOMYOSARCOMA
Vincent L. Shaw Jr., MD, CAQ-SM

BASICS

DESCRIPTION
Rhabdomyosarcoma (RMS) is a malignant tumor of soft tissue assumed to originate from the same pluripotent mesenchyme cell as striated skeletal muscle. It occurs mainly as primary malignancy but can also be a component of heterogeneous neoplasias, like malignant teratoma.

- Common primary sites:
  - Head and neck 25% presentation (common in young children, almost always embryonal type)
  - Genitourinary 31% of cases (mostly embryonal type)
  - Musculoskeletal 13% of cases (most common in extremities primary sites in adolescents and adults, alveolar subtype)
- The 4th edition of the *WHO Classification of Tumours of Soft Tissue and Bone* of RMS describes four major subtypes:
  - Embryonal RMS (ERMS): represents 60–70% among all RMS. Has early onset and is the most common subtype in children. Commonly presents in the head, neck, and genitourinary areas. ERMS is subdivided into:
    ○ Classic
    ○ Botryoid (6% overall embryonal): seen in infants, although can happen <4-year-old patients
    ○ Spindle cell: 3% of cases and affects young children
      ■ Both botryoid and spindle cell variants have better prognosis than the classical one.
  - Alveolar RMS (ARMS): represents 30% of pediatric cases, very aggressive subtype; more common in the trunk, perineum/perianal area, and extremities
  - Spindle cell/sclerosing: most frequently seen at the paratesticular site
  - Anaplastic (children)/pleomorphic (adults) seen in patients aged 30 to 50 years, rarely in children, represents 1% of all RMS, mostly associated with Li-Fraumeni symptoms
- Clinicopathologic and molecular studies have now delineated five to six distinct subfamilies of RMSs (1).

EPIDEMIOLOGY
It presents most commonly in children and young adults rather than adults. Male sex was directly associated with RMS. When diagnosed in adults, it is often found in more unfavorable sites and is associated with a more aggressive course.

Incidence
- 4.5 cases of RMS per 1 million children per year, in children, adolescents, and young adults.
- RMS accounts for 60% of sarcomas in children and adolescents. 50% of pediatric cases occur before the age of 10 years.
- In adults, RMS represents 3% of all soft tissue sarcomas in adults.
- More common in the black population

Prevalence
- RMS comprises 3.5% of childhood cancers overall.
- The more frequent in males (male:female ratio, 1:5)

ETIOLOGY AND PATHOPHYSIOLOGY
Genetics
Genetic characteristics vary according to the RMS subtype:
- Alveolar:
  - Associated with recurrent Forkhead box O1 (FOXO1) fusions, (found in 90% of cases)
  - t(2;13)(q35;q14); causing *PAX3-FOXO1* fusion
  - t(1;13)(p36;q14); causing *PAX7-FOXO1* fusion
  - t(X;2)(q13;q35); causing *PAX3-FOXO4* fusion
  - t(2;2)(q35;p23); causing *PAX3-NCOA1* fusion
  - t(2;8)(q35;q13); causing *PAX3-NCOA2* fusion
  - t(8;13)(p12;q13); causing *FOXO1-FGFR1* fusion
- Embryonal:
  - Multiple complex genetic aberrations, including *MYOD1* mutations
  - Loss or uniparental disomy of 11p15.5 +2, +8, +11, +12, +13, +20 affecting the genes *IGF-2, H19, CDKN1C,* and/or *HOTS*
- Spindle cell/sclerosing RMS:
  - 8q13 rearrangements involving *SRF-NCOA2* and *TEAD1-NCOA2*

RISK FACTORS
Although not yet proven, RMS has been associated with high birth weight, large gestational size for age, exposure to recreational drugs and/or radiation while in utero, low socioeconomic status, and the genetic conditions as described below.

COMMONLY ASSOCIATED CONDITIONS
- Beckwith-Wiedemann syndrome (11p15 mutations) presents as fetal overgrowth.
- Costello syndrome (germline *HRAS* mutations) presents as postnatal growth delay and morphologic abnormalities (including macrocephaly).
- Li-Fraumeni (germline *TP53*; known as *p53* mutations)
- Neurofibromatosis type I (*NF1* mutations)
- Noonan syndrome (*PTPN11* mutations)
- Pleuropulmonary blastoma (*DICER1* mutations)

DIAGNOSIS

HISTORY
- Presents as a progressive nontender palpable mass
- When presents in the head/neck, patients report diplopia (due to ophthalmoplegia), recurrent sinusitis, or persistent nasal discharge.
- RMS of genitourinary tissue may present as hematuria, polyuria, vaginal bleeding in females
- Other symptoms may be noted due to the mass effect of the primary or metastatic lesions.
- Personal or family history of genetic syndromes (i.e., NF1, Li-Fraumeni, etc.)

PHYSICAL EXAM
- Painless, enlarging mass
- Polypoid mass protruding from the vagina (botryoid)
- Exophthalmos and chemosis (orbital involvement)
- Abdominal pain and compression symptoms (i.e., seizures, visual field defects, nerve palsy, headaches)

DIAGNOSTIC TESTS & INTERPRETATION
Initial Tests (lab, imaging)
- Standard blood tests, including complete blood count, serum chemistry, liver function test, and coagulation profile, should be obtained for clinical optimization prior to treatment.
- MRI with/without contrast or CT with contrast of the primary tumor (to define anatomy)
- Staging workup:
  - Chest x-ray or CT chest without contrast (preferred). The most common site of metastasis is the lungs. PET/CT scans for lymph node or distant metastases detection that are not readily evident on other imaging. It is also helpful in monitoring the response to treatment for deep, firm lesions >3 cm.
  - Lymph node biopsy

Diagnostic Procedures/Other
- For pathology diagnosis:
  - Core needle biopsy, incisional biopsy, or excisional biopsy (based on the size of the mass). The histologic characteristics are similar to others and comprise small, blue, round-cell, which raises the need for advanced immunohistochemical (IHC) and genetic tests.
  - Histologic classification:
    ○ Alveolar: rhabdomyoblasts grossly mimicking pulmonary alveoli. The alveolar component must be ≥ 50%; has high levels of myogenin when compared to other subtypes
    ○ Embryonal:
      ■ Classic: rhabdomyoblasts configured in sheets, large nest, eosinophilic cytoplasm; no alveolar pattern, instead of poor myofilaments arrangement
      ■ Botryoid: "grape-like" appearance of rhabdomyoblasts with notable clustering in the subepithelium forming the cambium layer; seen within the vagina and bladder
      ■ Spindle cell: rhabdomyoblasts with spindle-like appearance
    ○ Anaplastic (children)/pleomorphic (adults): rhabdomyoblast with large hyperchromatic nuclei and strange mitotic morphologies
- IHC markers:
  - Muscle-specific actin, myosin, desmin (in 99% of RMS), myoglobin, Z-band protein, and MyoD1
- Molecular testing for PAX/FOXO1 fusion, which is tested by PCR and fluorescence in situ hybridization (FISH) with good concordance (94.9%). Although both have similar sensitivity (85.7% vs. 83.3%), PCR seems to have a slightly higher specificity (100% vs. 96%).
- Although not established yet, genetic profiling will become the gold standard for diagnosis and prognosis.
  - The Children's Oncology Group (COG) has incorporated fusion status into their risk stratification system.
- Staging is based on the site, size, regional nodal involvement, and distance spread (Table 1).

Table 1. TNM Staging System for Rhabdomyosarcoma

Stage	Site	T	Tumor diameter	N	M
1	Orbit; head and neck (excluding parameningeal), genitourinary—nonbladder and nonprostate, biliary tract	T1 or T2	a or b	Any N	M0
2	Bladder or prostate, extremity, cranial parameningeal, other	T1 or T2	a	N0 or NX	M0
3a	Bladder or prostate, extremity, cranial parameningeal, other	T1 or T2	a	N1	M0
3b	Bladder or prostate, extremity, cranial parameningeal, other	T1 or T2	b	Any N	M0
4	All sites	T1 or T2	a or b	N0 or N1	M1

T1, confined to organ of origin; T2, extends outside the organ of origin; a, ≤5 cm in diameter; b, >5 cm in diameter; M0, no distant metastasis; N0, regional nodes not clinically involved; NX, clinical status of regional nodes unknown; N1, regional nodes clinically involved by neoplasm; M1, distant metastasis.

TREATMENT

Encompasses surgical resection, radiation, chemotherapy. Patients should always be referred to a multidisciplinary team with expertise in oncology for definitive treatment.

SURGERY/OTHER PROCEDURES
- Surgery:
  - Local resection of tumor along with metastasis and nodal resection. Lymph node sampling is intended to identify unknown metastasis and guide decision for postop radiation. However, wide resection may not be feasible in cases where grossly impaired functionality results (i.e., head/neck).
- Radiation therapy (RT): is widely recommended to enhance local control, except in patients with embryonal type and fusion negative ICH. Emergent RT is only considered in patients with compression symptoms. Proton beam over photon beam due to safety profile. Brachytherapy can be considered in patients with difficult to treat tumors due to location (head/neck and parameningeal).
- Chemotherapy:
  - Selected based on prognosis risk stratification assessment (i.e., low, intermediate, high). For nonmetastatic RMS, stratification is made based on the TNM staging as well as the surgical/pathologic clinical grouping system. The latter is determined after the surgical resection based on histopathologic features and the extent of residual tumor. In other words, nonmetastatic RMS, risk stratification cannot be fully determined until surgery is performed.
    - Gold standard is VAC (vincristine, dactinomycin [also known as actinomycin D], and cyclophosphamide) (2)[A]. Low-risk patients may be prescribed VA instead (2)[A].
    - Most common adverse reactions are:
      - Vincristine: peripheral neuropathy
      - Dactinomycin: myelosuppression and hepatotoxicity
      - Cyclophosphamide: hemorrhagic cystitis (mesna is used for prophylaxis), transitional cell carcinoma, myelosuppression with leukopenia, and infertility
- In addition, ifosfamide, topotecan, doxorubicin, etoposide, and irinotecan may also be used in alternative regimens.
- Duration also depends on risk stratification but in general ranges from 12 to 24 months given in separate cycles (usually 14 to 15 cycles).

- European Paediatric Soft Tissue Sarcoma Study Group (EPSTSSG) recently demonstrated improvement in 3 years survival with maintenance chemotherapy, with vinorelbine and cyclophosphamide. Although according to COG guidelines, these recommendations cannot yet be established as standard therapy.
- Immune-mediated thru natural killer cells are being studied with great potential, although remains in vitro experiment.
- Given the low frequency of RMS in adults, there are no large trials to set appropriate regimen; therefore, standard VAC is used empirically; although this practice showed low efficacy in some case series, has allowed recommending alternative regimen (doxorubicin, ifosfamide, and vincristine), which demonstrated improvement in short-term (2 years) overall survival and disease-free survival

ONGOING CARE

FOLLOW-UP RECOMMENDATIONS
All patients should follow up with their multidisciplinary team. This allows monitoring of treatment response, early detection of locoregional relapse, metastatic disease, or development of secondary malignancies. For this effort, physical exam and imaging surveillance for the first 5 years are paramount (CT/MRI/x-ray). Imaging should be done every 3 months for the 1st year, then every 4 months for the following 2 years, finally every 6 months for the next 2 years. After the first 5 years, no more imaging surveillance is recommended as it has not shown further benefits. Other imaging techniques such as bone scan/PET scan should be considered based on clinical decisions, and echocardiograms are recommended if the patient received anthracycline therapy.

PROGNOSIS
- RMS (overall): 70% 5-year survival
- The survival rate has increased from 30% to 51% in adolescents 15 to 19 years old.
- In orbital RMS, survival can be as high as 95%.
- Prognosis as in other tumors depends on size, presence or not of metastasis, and location of the tumor, which help to risk-stratify patients into low, intermediate, and high risk. Favorable sites include orbit/eyelid, head and neck (with no parameningeal involvement), genitourinary (without bladder or prostate involvement), and biliary tract. Unfavorable site: bladder, prostate, extremity, parameningeal, trunk, retroperitoneal, pelvis

- 5-year survival based on *PAX/FOXO1* fusion status and risk stratification: low risk + fusion negative 90%; intermediate risk + fusion negative 78%; intermediate risk + fusion positive 56%; high risk + fusion negative 41%; high risk + fusion positive 11%
- In terms of histologic classification, botryoid and spindle cell RMS have a favorable prognosis, embryonal subtype has intermediate; sclerosing, spindle cell RMS and alveolar subtype being the poorest, with alveolar RMS being the poorest.
- Adults have a worse prognosis when compared to children not only due to lower rates of treatment adherence and lack of clinical trials identifying best treatment but also due to less favorable location and histopathology and metastasis at the time of diagnosis.
- The alveolar subtype has the poorest prognosis; however, any subtype metastatic presentation has a bad prognosis. Risk factors associated with the poorest outcome: metastatic disease at relapse, prior RT treatment, initial tumor size >5 cm, and relapse within 18 months

COMPLICATIONS
- Relapse
- Secondary neoplasm
- Growth abnormalities
- Treatment side effects

REFERENCES
1. Leiner J, Le Loarer F. The current landscape of rhabdomyosarcomas: an update. *Virchows Arch.* 2020;476(1):97–108.
2. National Comprehensive Cancer Network. Soft tissue sarcoma. Version 2.2017. https://www.nccn.org/professionals/physician_gls/pdf/sarcoma.pdf. Updated August 9, 2018. Accessed August 14, 2018.

 ## CODES

ICD10
- C49.9 Malignant neoplasm of connective and soft tissue, unsp
- C49.0 Malignant neoplasm of connective and soft tissue of head, face and neck
- C49.5 Malignant neoplasm of connective and soft tissue of pelvis

CLINICAL PEARLS
- RMS is more common in children but can develop in adults, the latest having the highest mortality.
- Genetic disorders and congenital syndromes are associated with a higher risk of developing RMS.
- If a localized tumor is identified with concurrent lymph node involvement, implement more aggressive therapy.
- The most common site of metastasis is the lung, followed by bone marrow/bone and peritoneum.
- High-dose chemotherapy followed by autologous stem cell transplant remains a promising therapy for patients who can tolerate side effects and toxicity but still needs further investigation prior to standardization.

RHEUMATIC FEVER

Stuart H. Batten, MD • Hillary J. Darrow, MD • Reggie Taylor, DO, MA

BASICS

DESCRIPTION
- Acute rheumatic fever (ARF) is an autoimmune, inflammatory response to infection with group A *Streptococcus* (GAS) that affects multiple organ systems.
- Untreated acute disease can lead to chronic rheumatic heart disease (RHD).
- Recurrence is common without adequate antibiotic treatment.

Pediatric Considerations
Most cases occur in children aged 5 to 15 years; rare in children <5 years (1)

EPIDEMIOLOGY
- ARF and RHD are largely restricted to low-income countries and marginalized sections of wealthy countries.
- Male = female; females more likely to develop chorea and RHD.
- Endemic regions include South Pacific, indigenous populations of Australia and New Zealand, Africa, and Asia (2).

Incidence
- Worldwide, incidence has been declining for 25 years. The large majority of new cases are in developing countries (2).
- Mean worldwide incidence ranges from 8 to 51/100,000 school-aged children (1); in endemic regions, prevalence can be >1,000 cases per 100,000 people (2).
- Incidence of ARF in the United States is approximately 0.6–3.4/100,000 school-aged children (2).

Prevalence
- In developing areas, RHD affects >33 million people and is the leading cause of cardiovascular death during the first 5 decades of life.
- Prevalence has been rising due to improved medical care and longer survival.

ETIOLOGY AND PATHOPHYSIOLOGY
- ARF most commonly occurs 2 to 3 weeks after GAS pharyngitis infection, but GAS impetigo may also be a preceding infection.
- Although pathogenicity is not completely understood, expert consensus implicates genetic and molecular mimicry leading to an inflammatory cascade as key to disease development.
- Joint involvement is a likely result of immune complex accumulation.

Genetics
- Susceptibility is associated with certain indigenous populations.
- ARF is heritable, polygenic, and displays variable and incomplete penetrance.

RISK FACTORS
Poverty, household crowding, genetic susceptibility, ethnic predisposition, and social disadvantage are the strongest risk factors.

GENERAL PREVENTION
- Primary prevention: Appropriate treatment of streptococcal infection prevents ARF in most cases (1).
- Secondary prevention: long-term antibiotic prophylaxis (up to 5 to 10 years) to prevent recurrence (2)

DIAGNOSIS

- 2015 Revised Jones Criteria and lab evidence of preceding GAS infection are used for diagnosis.
- Initial ARF: 2 major OR 1 major + 2 minor
- Recurrent ARF: 2 major OR 1 major + 2 minor OR 3 minor
- Sydenham chorea is independently sufficient to diagnosis ARF, even without lab evidence of preceding infection (1)[C].

Low-Risk Population	Moderate- and High-Risk Population
Major criteria:	Major criteria:
• Carditis: clinical or subclinical (echocardiogram)	• Carditis: clinical or subclinical (echocardiogram)
• Polyarthritis ONLY	• Polyarthritis OR monoarthritis
• Chorea	• Chorea
• Erythema marginatum	• Erythema marginatum
• Subcutaneous nodules	• Subcutaneous nodules
Minor criteria:	Minor criteria:
• Polyarthralgia	• Monoarthralgia
• Fever ≥38.5°C	• Fever ≥38.0°C
• ESR ≥60 mm/hr	• ESR ≥30 mm/hr
• CRP ≥3 mg/dL	• CRP ≥3 mg/dL
• ↑PR interval	• ↑PR interval

- The revised criteria distinguish between low-risk and moderate- to high-risk patient populations. Patients can be considered low risk if they are from and among a low-incidence group.
- Subclinical carditis can be diagnosed with echocardiographic evidence of mitral or aortic valve regurgitation and can be supported by chest x-ray demonstrating cardiomegaly or left atrial enlargement (1)[C].

HISTORY
- ARF typically presents 2 to 3 weeks following GAS pharyngitis or impetigo.
- Polyarthritis (knees, ankles, elbows, wrists) (35–66%) is self-limited and often the first symptom; each resolves in days, thus seems to "migrate." Rapid improvement occurs with aspirin or NSAIDs, which may mask initial symptoms. Moderate- and high-risk patients may only have monoarthritis.
- Fever
- Erythema marginatum rash
- Pancarditis or valvulitis (50–70%) can be subclinical (asymptomatic without auscultatory findings) or clinically apparent.
- Sydenham chorea (late manifestation [1 to 6 months after infection] in 10–30%): purposeless, involuntary, nonstereotypical movements, most commonly involving the face and hands
  - More common in 5 to 15 years old females
  - Improves or ceases during sleep
  - Can have associated muscular weakness, may manifest as deteriorating handwriting
  - Psychiatric symptoms may have onset prior to chorea, with emotional lability and obsessive-compulsive symptoms.
  - Self-resolves over several months and can relapse

PHYSICAL EXAM
- Neuro: Sydenham chorea: Involuntary movements may be general or unilateral and involve the face. "Milkmaid grip" is intermittent hypotonia on test of grip strength.
- Cardiac: pericardial friction rub, holosystolic murmur of mitral/aortic regurgitation, rarely diastolic; rarely evidence of heart failure
- Skin
  - Subcutaneous nodules (<10%): firm, painless protuberances on extensor surfaces involving knees, elbows, wrists, occiput, and spinous process of thoracic and lumbar vertebrae; more common in severe ARF, persists several weeks
  - Erythema marginatum (5–13%): evanescent, pink rash with pale centers and rounded/serpiginous margins found on trunk and proximal extremities. Rare to be found on face; typically nonpruritic; blanches with pressure and can be induced with heat

DIFFERENTIAL DIAGNOSIS
- Systemic lupus erythematosus
- Poststreptococcal reactive arthritis
- Juvenile rheumatoid arthritis
- Infectious arthritis
- Myocarditis (viral or idiopathic)
- Innocent cardiac murmur
- Cardiomyopathy
- Tourette syndrome
- Kawasaki syndrome
- Pediatric autoimmune neuropsychiatric disorders associated with streptococcal infections (PANDAS)
- Lyme disease
- Henoch-Schönlein purpura
- Wilson disease
- Substance abuse
- Tic disorder
- Encephalitis
- Huntington chorea
- Drug reaction

DIAGNOSTIC TESTS & INTERPRETATION
Initial Tests (lab, imaging)
- Serologic evidence of GAS infection is needed whenever possible, and diagnosis is in question when it cannot be obtained (chorea and chronic indolent rheumatic carditis being the exception due to delayed onset).
  - Rapid streptococcal antigen test with high pretest probability
  - Positive GAS throat culture
  - Elevated or rising antistreptococcal antibody titer (ASO or ADB); ASO peaks 3 to 5 weeks postinfection, ADB 6 to 8 weeks. A rise in titer is better than a single titer result.
- ESR and CRP are acute-phase reactants; almost always increased in ARF
- CBC with differential: leukocytosis, normocytic anemia
- ECG: PR prolongation, AV block, signs of pericarditis
- Joint aspiration and synovial fluid evaluation is indicated if significant effusion or septic arthritis is suspected.

- Echocardiogram: chamber size and function, pericardial effusion, and valve disease
- All cases of confirmed OR suspected ARF should have an echocardiogram within 12 weeks due to 18% prevalence of subclinical carditis.

Follow-Up Tests & Special Considerations

- CRP is useful to monitor the acute disease process and can initially be trended twice weekly, followed by every 1 to 2 weeks until normalized.
- Due to morbidity associate with untreated cardiac disease, all confirmed cases of ARF should have serial echocardiograms, even if the initial screen was negative for carditis (2)[C].
- All household contacts should be screened with GAS throat cultures. Positive results should be treated with antibiotics, even if asymptomatic.

Test Interpretation

Prior treatment with aspirin or steroids may lead to falsely negative lab results.

 TREATMENT

GENERAL MEASURES

- Antibiotic
- Anti-inflammatory agent (aspirin or naproxen)
- Manage other manifestations as indicated (e.g., chorea, dysrhythmia, carditis, or heart failure).

MEDICATION

First Line

- Eradication: GAS infection treatment should begin within 9 days of illness to prevent ARF. If confirmed diagnosis, begin secondary prophylaxis.
- If no penicillin allergy:
  – Penicillin VK 250 mg PO BID for 10 days, benzathine penicillin G IM for 1 day, or amoxicillin 50 mg/kg PO for 10 days (preferred in children)
- If penicillin allergy:
  – 1st-generation cephalosporin PO for 10 days, azithromycin 12 mg/kg PO for 5 days, clindamycin 7 mg/kg/dose PO for 10 days, or clarithromycin 7.5 mg/kg/dose PO for 10 days
- Arthritis: naproxen 10 to 20 mg/kg/day divided BID is now recommended over aspirin, given superior side effect profile and less risk of Reye syndrome.
- Carditis: If heart failure, 3rd-degree AV block, or other severe manifestations, appropriate traditional management should be initiated as indicated.
- NSAIDs, glucocorticoids, and IVIG are not recommended for carditis, although glucocorticoids can be considered in severe carditis with acute cardiac failure.
- Chorea: generally self-limited, not requiring treatment. Valproic acid or carbamazepine may be used for severe cases. IVIG and glucocorticoids are restricted to failure of initial management. Antipsychotics are not routinely used due to extrapyramidal side effects.

Second Line

If penicillin allergy is present, erythromycin is preferred by the New Zealand Guidelines Group but not by the Infectious Diseases Society of America.

ISSUES FOR REFERRAL

- A cardiologist should be involved in management of ARF.
- Pediatric neurologist or movement specialist can help guide therapy with severe chorea.

SURGERY/OTHER PROCEDURES

Valve stenosis is a late sequela resulting from fibrosis and calcification; mainstay of therapy is surgical correction (2).

ADMISSION, INPATIENT, AND NURSING CONSIDERATIONS

- Initial hospitalization may be helpful for diagnosis and to ensure stability.
- Heart failure requires prompt hospitalization.
- IV fluids
  – Only if signs of dehydration or hypotension; use caution in heart failure.
- Nursing
  – Activity as tolerated

 ONGOING CARE

FOLLOW-UP RECOMMENDATIONS

- Secondary prophylaxis: antibiotic therapy from time of diagnosis until at least age 21 years, or 5 years after diagnosis (whichever comes later)
- Indefinite prophylactic antibiotics can be indicated based on cardiac damage, as recurrence of disease can worsen severity of carditis.
  – First-line prophylaxis is long-acting benzathine penicillin G monthly IM injections.
  – Penicillin V PO 250 mg BID is an alternative.
  – If penicillin allergy, sulfadiazine 0.5 to 1.0 g daily
  – If penicillin and sulfa drug allergy, azithromycin
  – Patients on penicillin prophylaxis who develop GAS pharyngitis while on penicillin should be treated with clindamycin.
- If ARF is possible, but uncertain, treat with 1 year of secondary antibiotic prophylaxis until repeat echocardiogram (2)[C].
- Prophylaxis duration is the same in patients that have ARF but no evidence of carditis.
- Routine antibiotic prophylaxis for dental procedures is no longer recommended for patients with RHD.

Patient Monitoring

Weekly monitoring after the initial diagnosis; every 6 months thereafter, based on clinical stability.

Pediatric Considerations

Use aspirin with caution in children given the risk of Reye syndrome.

Pregnancy Considerations

May exacerbate valve disease, particularly mitral stenosis in RHD. Refer pregnant patients to a cardiologist.

DIET

No dietary restrictions; low-sodium if heart failure present

PATIENT EDUCATION

American Heart Association: http://www.heart.org

PROGNOSIS

Long-term sequelae are generally limited to the heart and depend on the severity of carditis during an acute attack. Recurrence is most common in the 1st year after diagnosis (2).

COMPLICATIONS

- Recurrence of ARF due to GAS reinfection
- RHD can occur 10 to 20 years after ARF, with mitral more common than aortic regurgitation, can lead to mitral stenosis. Heart failure is the worst complication.
- Jaccoud arthropathy is chronic and involves painless deformities of hands/feet.
- Patients with a history of ARF have a higher incidence of infective endocarditis in the future.

REFERENCES

1. Lahiri S, Sanyahumbi A. Acute rheumatic fever. *Pediatr Rev.* 2021;42(5):221–232.
2. Kumar RK, Antunes MJ, Beaton A, et al. Contemporary diagnosis and management of rheumatic heart disease: implications for closing the gap: a scientific statement from the American Heart Association. *Circulation.* 2020;142(20):e337–e357.

ADDITIONAL READING

Ralph AP, Noonan S, Wade V, et al. The 2020 Australian guideline for prevention, diagnosis, and management of acute rheumatic fever and rheumatic heart disease. *Med J Aust.* 2021;214(5):220–227.

 CODES

ICD10

- I00 Rheumatic fever without heart involvement
- I01.9 Acute rheumatic heart disease, unspecified
- I01.0 Acute rheumatic pericarditis

CLINICAL PEARLS

- ARF is an autoimmune, inflammatory disease that follows GAS pharyngitis or impetigo and affects multiple organ systems, including the heart.
- Modified Jones criteria delineate between low-risk and moderate-/high-risk patients. Diagnosis requires 2 major or 1 major plus 2 minor manifestations in the context of a preceding documented GAS infection.
- Early echocardiogram evaluation for subclinical carditis can expedite initial diagnosis and improve clinical outcomes.
- Treatment involves acute antibiotic eradication followed immediately by long-term antibiotic prophylaxis to prevent chronic RHD.

RHINITIS, ALLERGIC
Madhavi Singh, MD • Daniel Abelev, MD

BASICS

Allergic rhinitis is the collection of symptoms involving mucous membranes of nose, eyes, ears, and throat after an exposure to allergens such as pollen, dust, or dander.

DESCRIPTION
- IgE-mediated inflammation of the nasal mucosa following exposure to an extrinsic protein; an immediate symptomatic response is characterized by sneezing, congestion, and rhinorrhea followed by a persistent late phase dominated by congestion and mucosal hyperreactivity.
- Allergic rhinitis can be classified into seasonal or perennial and can be intermittent or persistent.
- Seasonal responses are usually due to outdoor allergens such as tree pollen, flowering shrubs in spring, grasses and flowering plants in summer, and ragweed and mold in fall.
- Perennial responses, or year-round symptoms, are usually associated with indoor allergens like dust mites, mold, and animal dander.
- Occupational allergic rhinitis is caused by allergens at the workplace and can be sporadic or year-round.
- Nonallergic rhinitis (e.g., vasomotor, rhinitis of pregnancy, and rhinitis medicamentosa) can occur.

Pediatric Considerations
Chronic nasal obstruction can result in facial deformities, dental malocclusions, and sleep disorders.

Pregnancy Considerations
Physiologic changes during pregnancy may aggravate all types of rhinitis, frequently in the 2nd trimester.

EPIDEMIOLOGY
- Onset usually in first 2 decades, rarely before 6 months of age, with tendency declining with advancing age
- The mean age of onset is 8 to 11 years, and about 80% of cases have established allergic rhinitis by age 20 years.

Prevalence
- ~10–25% of the U.S. adult population and 9–42% of the U.S. pediatric population are affected.
- 44–87% of patients with allergic rhinitis have mixed allergic and nonallergic rhinitis, which is more common than either pure form (1).
- Scandinavian studies have demonstrated cumulative prevalence rate of 14% in men and 15% in women.

ETIOLOGY AND PATHOPHYSIOLOGY
- Aeroallergen-driven mucosal inflammation due to resident and infiltrating inflammatory cells as well as vasoactive and proinflammatory mediators (e.g., cytokines)
- Inhalant allergens:
  - Perennial: house dust mites, indoor molds, animal dander, cockroach/insect detritus
  - Seasonal: tree, grass, and weed pollens; outdoor molds
  - Occupational: latex, plant products (e.g., baking flour), sensitizing chemicals, and certain animals for people working in farms and vet clinics

Genetics
Complex but strong genetic predilection present (80% have family history of allergic disorders.)

RISK FACTORS
- Family history of atopy, with a greater risk if both parents have atopy
- Higher socioeconomic status
- Tobacco smoke can exacerbate symptoms and increase risk of developing asthma in patients with allergic rhinitis.
- Having other allergies such as asthma
- Unclear evidence regarding risk due to early, repeated exposure to offending allergen and early introduction of solid food
- Pets in house and houses infested with cockroaches can cause perennial allergic rhinitis.
- Male sex

GENERAL PREVENTION
- Primary prevention of atopic disease has not been proven effective by maternal diet or maternal allergen avoidance (2).
- Exclusive breastfeeding to 6 months of age lowers risk of some atopic disorders.
- Symptomatic control by environmental avoidance is the "first-line treatment."
- No evidence to support use of acaricides with mite-proof mattress and pillow covers, carpet and drape removal, removal of plants in the home, and pet control (2),(3)[B]
- Air conditioning and limited outside exposure during allergy season (1)[B]
- HEPA air cleaners and vacuum bags of unclear efficacy
- Close doors and windows during allergy season.
- Use a dehumidifier to reduce indoor humidity.

COMMONLY ASSOCIATED CONDITIONS
Other IgE-mediated conditions: asthma, atopic dermatitis, allergic conjunctivitis, food allergy

DIAGNOSIS

Diagnosis is made primarily by history and physical exam.

HISTORY
- Evaluation of nature, duration, and time course of symptoms
- History of atopic dermatitis and/or food allergies
- History of nasal congestion; rhinorrhea; pruritus of nose, eyes, ears, and/or palate; sneezing; itching; and watering eyes
- Family history of allergic diseases
- History of environmental and occupational exposure and various nasal stimuli can help differentiate between allergic and vasomotor rhinitis.

PHYSICAL EXAM
Many findings are suggestive of but not specific for allergic rhinitis:
- Dark circles under eyes, "allergic shiners" (infraorbital venous congestion)
- Transverse nasal crease from rubbing nose upward; typically seen in children

- Rhinorrhea, usually with clear discharge
- Pale, boggy, blue-gray nasal mucosa
- Postnasal mucus discharge
- Oropharyngeal lymphoid tissue hypertrophy

DIFFERENTIAL DIAGNOSIS
- Infectious rhinitis: usually viral, commonly with secondary bacterial infection
  - Usually associated with sinusitis and is known as rhinosinusitis
  - Viral rhinitis averages six episodes per year from ages 2 to 6 years.
  - IgA deficiency with recurrent sinusitis
  - Rhinitis medicamentosa (RM):
    ○ Rebound effect associated with continued use of certain medications; topical decongestant drops and sprays are most common
    ○ Other medications that may indue RM include: ACE inhibitors, reserpine, β-blockers, oral contraceptive pills (OCPs), guanethidine, methyldopa, Aspirin, NSAIDs
  - Vasomotor (idiopathic) rhinitis caused by numerous nasal stimuli such as warm or cold air, scents and odors, light or particulate matter
  - Hormonal: pregnancy, thyroid, OCPs
  - Nonallergic rhinitis with eosinophilia syndrome (NARES)
  - Gustatory: watery rhinorrhea in response to alcohol or food
  - "Skier's nose": watery rhinorrhea in response to cold air
- Conditions associated with rhinitis:
  - Nasal polyps, tumor
  - Septal/anatomic obstruction
    ○ Adenoidal hypertrophy, particularly in children
    ○ Septal abnormality or deflected nasal septum (DNS) in adults

DIAGNOSTIC TESTS & INTERPRETATION
- Lab tests rarely needed
- Skin testing is done to identify the allergen for immunotherapy.

Initial Tests (lab, imaging)
- Testing is rarely indicated.
- If diagnosis implies other causes, consider the following:
  - CBC with differential may show elevated eosinophils.
  - Increased total serum IgE level
  - Nasal probe smear may show elevated eosinophils.
- Medications that may alter lab results
  - Corticosteroids may decrease eosinophilia.
  - Antihistamines suppress reactivity to skin tests; stop antihistamines 7 days before testing.
- CT scan of sinuses is not routinely done but can be used to check for complete opacity, fluid level, and mucosal thickening.

Diagnostic Procedures/Other
- Consider testing in only those cases where allergic symptoms do not respond to treatment and/or considering immunotherapy.
- Specific allergen sensitivity with allergen skin testing or radioallergosorbent test (RAST); clinical correlation based on history is essential in interpreting results.

- Diagnostic allergen prick tests are used to select agent to determine appropriate environmental control measures as well as to direct immunotherapy:
  - Prick or puncture: superficial injury to epidermis with application of test antigen
  - Intradermal
- RAST: more expensive and less sensitive than skin testing; typically used in patients in whom skin testing is not practical or a severe reaction is possible
- Rhinoscopy: useful to visualize intranasal anatomy and posterior pharyngeal structures, including adenoids, polyps, and larynx

Test Interpretation
- Nasal washing/scraping: Eosinophils predominate but may see basophils, mast cells.
- Nasal mucosa: submucosal edema but without destruction; eosinophilic infiltration; congested mucous glands and goblet cells

TREATMENT

There are three mainstays of treatment of allergic rhinitis:
- Allergen avoidance
- Medication
- Allergy immunotherapy

GENERAL MEASURES
Limit exposure to offending allergen.

MEDICATION
Oral medication and intranasal sprays are commonly used.

First Line
- Mild symptoms: 2nd-generation nonsedating antihistamines are the first-line therapy for mild to moderate allergic rhinitis (1).
- Adverse effects: mild sedation, mild anticholinergic effects
- Generic (cetirizine, fexofenadine, loratadine; most to least effective)
  - Levocetirizine is a 2nd-generation nonsedating antihistamine that is effective but costly.
- Moderate to severe symptoms: Intranasal corticosteroids are first-line therapy for moderate to severe allergic rhinitis (1):
  - Most effective drug class for symptoms of allergic rhinitis
  - Use nasal sprays after showering and direct spray away from septum to improve deposition on mucosal surface.
  - May be used as needed; however, more effective with daily use (1)
  - Adverse effects: nosebleed, nasal septal perforation, and systemic corticosteroid effects
  - Ciclesonide is a new-generation corticosteroid with previously demonstrated efficacy in the treatment of asthma when delivered through a metered-dose inhaler. Ciclesonide is also currently in clinical development as an intranasal formulation for use in the treatment of AR.
- Systemic steroids should be considered only in urgent cases and only for short-term use.

Second Line
Nasal antihistamines effective but may be systemically absorbed and may cause sedation: azelastine, olopatadine
- Decongestants
  - Phenylephrine: 10 mg PO q4h PRN
  - Pseudoephedrine: 60 mg PO q4–6h PRN
  - Oxymetazoline nasal spray (Afrin): 2 to 3 sprays per nostril q10–12h PRN (max 3 days). Intranasal agents should not be used for >3 days due to rebound rhinitis. Discourage use in patients with hypertension (HTN) or cardiac arrhythmia.
- Intranasal anticholinergics such as ipratropium nasal spray 2 sprays per nostril BID–TID
  - Intranasal anticholinergics can increase efficacy in combination with steroid use.
- Leukotriene antagonists such as montelukast 10 mg/day PO
  - Should generally be used as an adjunct, not monotherapy
  - May be first line in those with concomitant asthma
- Mast cell stabilizers such as cromolyn nasal spray 1 spray per nostril TID–QID
  - May take 2 to 4 weeks of therapy for optimal efficacy
  - May be ineffective in patients with nonallergic rhinitis and nasal polyps
- 3rd-generation antihistamines, such as the following:
  - Brompheniramine: 12 to 24 mg PO BID
  - Chlorpheniramine: 4 mg PO q4–6h PRN
  - Clemastine: 1 to 2 mg PO BID PRN
  - Diphenhydramine: 25 to 50 mg PO q4–6h PRN:
    ○ May precipitate urinary retention in men with prostatism and/or hypertrophy
    ○ Adverse effects: sedation, prolonged QT interval, performance impairment, and anticholinergic effect

ISSUES FOR REFERRAL
Refer to allergist for consideration of immunotherapy.

ADDITIONAL THERAPIES
- Nasal saline use has evidence of efficacy as sole agent or as adjunctive treatment (1).
- Other treatment strategies
  - When initiating intranasal steroids, consider starting with a "burst," using 2 sprays in each nostril daily for 2 weeks and then decreasing to 1 spray in each nostril daily thereafter.
  - To mitigate long-term side effects of intranasal steroids, consider a "5 days on, 2 days off" strategy, with the days off being the days of lowest exposure to allergens.
  - Allergen immunotherapy (desensitization)
    ○ Reserved when symptoms are uncontrollable with medical therapy or have a comorbidity (e.g., asthma)
    ○ Specific allergen extract is injected SC in increasing doses to induce patient tolerance.

 ONGOING CARE

FOLLOW-UP RECOMMENDATIONS
Patient Monitoring
Initiation of patient education is critical.

DIET
Some patients with severe sensitivity to seasonal pollens may have oral allergy syndrome, which is associated with itching in the mouth with the ingestion of fresh fruits that may cross-react with the allergens.

PATIENT EDUCATION
- Asthma and Allergy Foundation of America, 1235 South Clark St., Suite 305, Arlington, VA 22202; (800) 7-ASTHMA: http://www.aafa.org/
- Other helpful information available at http://www.acaai.org/ and http://www.aaaai.org/home.aspx

PROGNOSIS
- Acceptable control of symptoms is the goal.
- Treatment is helpful to reduce the risk of comorbidities, such as sinusitis and asthma.

COMPLICATIONS
- Secondary infection such as otitis media or sinusitis
- Epistaxis
- Nasopharyngeal lymphoid hyperplasia
- Airway hyperreactivity with allergen exposure
- Asthma
- Facial changes, especially in children who are mouth breathers
- Sleep disturbance

REFERENCES

1. Wallace DV, Dykewicz MS, Bernstein DI, et al; for Joint Task Force on Practice Parameter for Allergy and Immunology. The diagnosis and management of rhinitis: an updated practice parameter. *J Allergy Clin Immunol*. 2008;122(Suppl 2):S1–S84.
2. Kramer MS, Kakuma R. Maternal dietary antigen avoidance during pregnancy or lactation, or both, for preventing or treating atopic disease in the child. *Cochrane Database Syst Rev*. 2012;(9):CD000133.
3. Sheikh A, Hurwitz B, Nurmatov U, et al. House dust mite avoidance measures for perennial allergic rhinitis. *Cochrane Database Syst Rev*. 2010;(7):CD001563.

 SEE ALSO

Conjunctivitis, Acute

CODES

ICD10
- J30.89 Other allergic rhinitis
- J30.81 Allergic rhinitis due to animal (cat) (dog) hair and dander
- J30.2 Other seasonal allergic rhinitis

CLINICAL PEARLS
- Nasal saline irrigation (flushing 6 to 8 oz) may be very helpful in clearing upper airway of secretions and may precede the use of nasal corticosteroids.
- 2nd-generation antihistamines and intranasal corticosteroids are first-line therapies for allergic rhinitis.

R

ROCKY MOUNTAIN SPOTTED FEVER

Christopher A. Zagar, MD, FAAFP • Kimberly M. Chekan, DO, MPH

BASICS

Rocky Mountain spotted fever (RMSF) is the most common spotted fever rickettsiosis (SFR) in North America. It is associated with the highest rates of severe and fatal outcomes of all reportable rickettsial diseases in the United States (1)[A],(2)[C].

DESCRIPTION
- RMSF is a tick-borne systemic small and medium vessel vasculitis caused by the bacterium *Rickettsia rickettsii* (2)[C].
- Symptoms include fever, headache, and myalgia followed by a macular rash; begins at wrists and ankles, spreading toward palms, soles, and the trunk
- System(s) affected: cardiovascular, musculoskeletal, skin, central nervous system (CNS), renal, hepatic, and pulmonary

EPIDEMIOLOGY
In the United States, ticks are both vectors and main reservoirs. Important species in the United States include the American dog tick, *Dermacentor variabilis*, in the eastern two-thirds of the United States; the Rocky Mountain wood tick, *Dermacentor andersoni*, in the western United States; and the brown dog tick, *Rhipicephalus sanguineus*, distributed throughout all states (1)[A],(3)[C].

Incidence
- In the United States, the annual incidence of SFR increased from 1.7 cases per million persons in 2000 to 13.2 in 2016. Cases have been reported in all states except Hawaii and Alaska. RMSF also seen in Canada, Mexico, and throughout Central and South America (4)[B].
- Arkansas, Missouri, North Carolina, Tennessee, and Virginia account for over 50% of SFR cases. Cases have also been identified in Arizona where they had not previously (5).
- Cases occur year round. Most cases are reported from May through August during the peak of outdoor activity (5).
- Highest incidence occurs in age 60 to 64 years. Highest number of reported deaths is in children <10 years (5).

Prevalence
In the United States, 4,470 cases were reported in 2012. <0.1% of ticks carry virulent rickettsial species.

ETIOLOGY AND PATHOPHYSIOLOGY
- An adult tick releases *R. rickettsii*, from its salivary glands after 6 to 10 hours of feeding.
- Pathogens infect vascular endothelial cells, causing small and medium vessel injury throughout the body leading to disseminated inflammation. Subsequent vascular permeability can cause pulmonary and cerebral edema. Local consumption of platelets results in characteristic petechial rash.
- Subsequent end-organ injury may also result in meningoencephalitis, ARF, acute respiratory distress syndrome, shock, arrhythmia, and seizure (1).
- Symptoms appear 3 to 12 days after bite or between 4 and 8 days after discovery of an attached tick.
- It is unknown whether *R. rickettsii* crosses the placenta and causes in utero infection.
- RMSF can rarely be caused by direct inoculation of tick blood into open wounds or conjunctivae.

RISK FACTORS
- Known tick bite, engorged tick, or presence of tick for >20 hours
- Tick crushed during removal
- Accumulated outdoor exposure or residence in wooded areas; contact with outdoor pets or wild animals

GENERAL PREVENTION
- Limit tick exposure; highest tick exposure is in tall grasses, open areas of low bushy vegetation or wooded areas.
- Wear light-colored clothing, long sleeves, pants, socks, and closed-toe shoes. Use DEET-containing insect repellents.
- Permethrin spray on clothing
- Regular tick checks, prompt and proper tick removal; do not use bare hands to remove ticks.
- Wash hands and site of bite with soap and water after tick removal to avoid potential mucosal inoculation.
- Protect pets through ectoparasite control (1)[A].

DIAGNOSIS

- Maintain high incidence of suspicion for rickettsial infections when patients present with "influenza-like" symptoms during summer months regardless of a known history of tick exposure (2)[C].
- Delay of empirical therapy increases risk of long-term sequelae and mortality.

HISTORY
Consider RMSF in acute febrile illness and rash, particularly with a history of potential tick exposure within previous 14 days; outdoor activities or travels to an endemic area, during late spring or summer months. *The tick bite goes unnoticed 30–50% of the time.*

- Typically presents like a viral illness in the first 1 to 4 days with sudden onset of fever, severe frontal headache, malaise, myalgia, anorexia, nausea, vomiting, and photophobia (1)
- Rash typically appears 2 to 4 days after onset of fever; starts as a small blanching, pink macules on wrist and ankles before spreading to the trunk where rash may become maculopapular in appearance
- Involvement of palms and soles usually present by 5th to 6th day, along with generalized petechial rash; a sign of advanced disease. Rash generally spares the face.
- Although children <15 years more frequently (>90%) have a rash, the classic triad of fever, rash, and tick bite occurs in <60% of children with RMSF. 10% of patients never develop a rash and decision to treat should not be based on presence of rash (1)[A].
- Other symptoms include conjunctival injection, mental status impairments, restlessness, arthralgia, peripheral or periorbital edema, calf pain, and hearing loss (1)[A].

PHYSICAL EXAM
- Fever is typically >102°F.
- The rash typically starts as an erythematous, macular, or maculopapular exanthema (1 to 5 mm in diameter); 50% become petechial or purpuric.
- Rash can be difficult to visualize on dark skin.
- In severe cases, the rash can involve the entire body (including mucous membranes) and may progress to necrotic or gangrenous lesions.
- The rash is not associated with pruritus or urticaria.
- AMS, lymphadenopathy, diffuse right upper quadrant pain, hepatosplenomegaly, and edema of dorsum of hands or feet

DIFFERENTIAL DIAGNOSIS
- Viral exanthema (e.g., hand-foot-mouth disease, measles, rubella, roseola)
- Viral gastroenteritis, mononucleosis, pharyngitis
- Upper respiratory infection, urinary tract infection, TTP/ITP, idiopathic vasculitides, toxic shock syndrome
- Meningoencephalitis, meningococcemia
- Other tick-borne infections: typhus, ehrlichiosis, Lyme disease, babesiosis, boutonneuse fever, leptospirosis
- Drug reaction or serum sickness
- Kawasaki disease, infective endocarditis

DIAGNOSTIC TESTS & INTERPRETATION
Most cases of RMSF are diagnosed based on IgM and IgG serologic response to *R. rickettsii*, in conjunction with a high degree of clinical suspicion. Do not delay therapy awaiting results (2)[C].

Initial Tests (lab, imaging)
- Specific laboratory diagnosis
  - Indirect fluorescent antibody (IFA) testing is the gold standard for serology.
  - Sensitivity of IFA 2 weeks after onset of illness is 94–100% but cannot distinguish between *R. rickettsii* and other spotted fever–group rickettsii (3)[C].
  - Due to seroprevalence, it is impossible to differentiate a single elevated IgG titer associated with acute illness from previous infections (4)[B].
  - Testing two sequential serum or plasma samples allows demonstrating rising IgG or IgM antibody levels, which is essential to confirm acute infection (4)[B].
  - Typically, these specimens should be taken at least 2 to 3 weeks apart to examine for a 4-fold or greater increase in antibody titer to confirm diagnosis (3)[C].
  - Optimal time for testing is 14 to 21 days after symptom onset.
- Nonspecific laboratory tests
  - WBC count: variable, frequently normal
  - Platelet: thrombocytopenia (<150,000 cells/μL) in 60% of kids
  - Hyponatremia <135 mEq/dL, and elevated hepatic transaminases in 50% of patients
  - Anemia, increase in blood urea nitrogen/creatinine, PT/PTT, hyperbilirubinemia, and hypoalbuminemia may also be present.
  - CSF may have mononuclear pleocytosis and elevated protein, and normal glucose (1)[A],(3)[C].
- Imaging procedures are rarely helpful.

Diagnostic Procedures/Other
- Skin biopsy can offer definitive diagnosis; a 3-mm punch biopsy to perform a rapid direct fluorescent antibody (DFA) test (sensitivity 70%, specificity 100%)
- Rickettsial DNA detection using PCR of skin biopsy samples is a new approach to diagnosis of suspected rickettsial infections during the acute phase of illness (2)[C].
- Qualitative enzyme-linked immunosorbent assay

Test Interpretation
- Test acute and convalescent phase sera in tandem.
- Early treatment may limit antibody formation.
- Seropositivity increases with age in endemic states. Positive spotted fever-group *Rickettsia* antibody does not necessarily signify an acute infection.

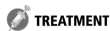 **TREATMENT**

MEDICATION
First Line
Doxycycline is the treatment of choice in both adults and children (1)[A],(2)[C],(3)[C].
- Untreated rickettsial infections have a high rate of morbidity and mortality (20–30% without prompt antibiotic treatment). Other antibiotics are considerably less effective (2)[C].
- Adults and children <18 years who are >45 kg: doxycycline 100 mg PO or IV q12h until 3 days after the fever subsides (1)[A],(3)[C]
- Children <45 kg: doxycycline 2.2 mg/kg PO or IV q12h until 3 days after fever subsides (1)[A].
- Pregnancy: Doxycycline 100 mg PO or IV q12h until 3 days after fever subsides is the first-line therapy and chloramphenicol 50 to 75 mg/kg IV divided into 4 doses daily for 7 days is the second-line therapy. Current evidence, while limited, suggests no increased risk of teratogenicity (3)[C].
- Total course of treatment is typically 5 to 7 days, at a minimum, possibly longer if severe or complicated disease (1)[A].
- Fever typically subsides within 24 to 48 hours with early treatment; longer if patient is severely ill. If promptly treated, and patient lack response to doxycycline in 48 hours, consider an alternate diagnosis.
- RMSF resistance to doxycycline has not been documented.
- Adverse effects may include the following:
  - Dyspepsia. Take medication with food and water. Avoid dairy, iron, or antacids, as they may inhibit drug absorption.
  - Photosensitivity may occur. Minimize sun exposure and use sunscreen.
  - No risk of dental staining in children <8 years old (1)[A],(2)[C]
- Severe allergy is a contraindication to doxycycline; rapid desensitization may be considered for life-threatening disease in severe illness.

Second Line
Chloramphenicol is the alternative to treat RMSF; associated with adverse hematologic effects (e.g., aplastic anemia) and increased case mortality (1)[A]

Pregnancy Considerations
- Doxycycline is appropriate for this life-threatening infection in pregnancy if suspicion is high, despite the potential risk to fetal bones/teeth along with maternal hepatotoxicity and pancreatitis (1)[A],(3)[C].
- Short-term doxycycline is compatible with breastfeeding (1)[A].
- Chloramphenicol may be considered but should be avoided in the 3rd trimester due to risk for gray baby syndrome.

ISSUES FOR REFERRAL
- Consider infectious disease consult along with immunology/allergist if patient is severely allergic to doxycycline.
- Report cases of RMSF to public health authorities.

ADDITIONAL THERAPIES
Patients with neurologic injury may require prolonged physical and cognitive therapy.

ADMISSION, INPATIENT, AND NURSING CONSIDERATIONS
- Admission criteria/initial stabilization
  - CNS dysfunction
  - Nausea/vomiting preventing oral antibiotic therapy
  - Immunocompromised patients
  - Specific acute organ failure
  - Failure of oral pain management
  - ICU for patients with shock
- Discharge criteria
  - Resolution of fever
  - Ability to take oral therapy and nutrition

 ONGOING CARE

FOLLOW-UP RECOMMENDATIONS
- Patients with mild disease may be treated as outpatients if close follow-up is available.
- Hospitalize patients with moderate to severe disease.
- Infection does not confer lifelong immunity.

Patient Monitoring
- Follow patients treated as outpatients every 2 to 3 days until symptoms resolve.
- Follow-up CBC, electrolytes, LFTs if clinically indicated

DIET
Consider nutritional supplementation if intake is poor.

PATIENT EDUCATION
General prevention and caution regarding tick avoidance during outside activities in endemic areas

PROGNOSIS
- Prognosis is closely related to timely administration of appropriate antibiotics.
- Delay in treatment may increase mortality by 3-fold if delayed to 5th day of illness (1)[A].
- When treated promptly, prognosis is excellent with resolution of symptoms and no sequelae.
- Children aged <10 years and elderly >70 years are at higher risk of morbidity and/or mortality.
- Patients with G6PD deficiency are at highest risk for fulminant RMSF, in which death can occur ≤5 days.

COMPLICATIONS
- Encephalopathy, most commonly transient impaired level of consciousness or meningismus
- Seizures, focal neurologic deficit
- Renal injury leading to acute renal failure
- Hepatitis, congestive heart failure (CHF), respiratory failure
- Proximal muscle weakness, changes in personality, paresthesias, deafness, secondary thromboses, and tissue necrosis may also be seen.

REFERENCES
1. Biggs HM, Behravesh CB, Bradley KK, et al. Diagnosis and management of tickborne rickettsial diseases: Rocky Mountain spotted fever and other spotted fever group rickettsioses, ehrlichioses, and anaplasmosis—United States. *MMWR Recomm Rep*. 2016;65(2):1–44.
2. Snowden J, Simonsen KA. *Rickettsia Rickettsiae (Rocky Mountain Spotted Fever)*. Treasure Island, FL: StatPearls; 2020.
3. Gottlieb M, Long B, Koyfman A. The evaluation and management of Rocky Mountain spotted fever in the emergency department: a review of the literature. *J Emerg Med*. 2018;55(1):42–50.
4. Binder AM, Nichols Heitman K, Drexler NA. Diagnostic methods used to classify confirmed and probable cases of spotted fever rickettsioses—United states, 2010-2015. *MMWR Morb Mortal Wkly Rep*. 2019;68(10):243–246.
5. Centers for Disease Control and Prevention. National Center for Emerging and Zoonotic Infectious Diseases (NCEZID), Division of Vector-Borne Diseases (DVBD). CDC > Rocky Mountain Spotted Fever [Internet]. 2020. https://www.cdc.gov/ticks/tickbornediseases/rmsf.html.

ADDITIONAL READING
Blanton LS. The rickettsioses: a practical update. *Infect Dis Clin North Am*. 2019;33(1):213–229.

 CODES

ICD10
A77.0 Spotted fever due to Rickettsia rickettsii

CLINICAL PEARLS
- Diagnosis of RMSF requires a high index of clinical suspicion.
- Tick bites are often unnoticed, and some patients may never develop a rash.
- Begin treatment immediately without waiting for confirmatory testing in suspected cases. Doxycycline is drug of choice for RMSF in both adults and children. The only absolute contraindication is severe allergy to the drug.
- There is no evidence to support prophylaxis against RMSF in patients with known tick bite (2)[C].

R

ROSEOLA

Jeffrey D. Quinlan, MD, FAAFP

 BASICS

Omnipresent infection occurring in infancy and childhood. Majority of cases are caused by human herpesvirus 6 (HHV-6); may be associated with other diseases including encephalitis

DESCRIPTION

- Acute infection of infants or very young children (1)
- Causes a high fever followed by a skin eruption as the fever resolves (1)
- Transmission via contact with salivary secretions or respiratory droplet (1)
- Incubation period of 9 to 10 days (1)
- System(s) affected: skin/exocrine, metabolic, gastrointestinal, respiratory, neurologic
- Synonym(s): roseola infantum, exanthem subitum; pseudorubella; sixth disease; 3-day fever (1)

Pediatric Considerations
A disease of infants and very young children (2)

EPIDEMIOLOGY

- Predominant age
  - HHV-6
    - Infants and very young children (<2 years old) (3)
    - Peak age infection 6 to 9 months, rarely congenital or perinatal infection (1)
    - 95% of children have been infected with HHV-6 by 2 years of life.
  - HHV-7
    - Later childhood
    - Mean age of infection 26 months
    - >90% population with HHV-7 by 10 years (1)
- Predominant sex: male = female (1)
- No seasonal variance

Incidence
Common—accounts for 20% ED visits for febrile illness among children 6 to 8 months (4)

Prevalence
- Peak prevalence is between 9 and 21 months (3).
- Nearly 100% population carrying HHV-6 by 3 years (1)
- Approximately 20% patients with primary HHV-6 have roseola (4).

ETIOLOGY AND PATHOPHYSIOLOGY

- HHV-6 and HHV-7 (2)
- Majority of cases (60–74%) due to HHV-6
  - HHV-6B > HHV-6A (2)
  - HHV-6A seen in children in Africa
  - HHV-6 binds to CD46 receptors on all nucleated cells (2).
- Primary infection typically through respiratory droplets or saliva

- Congenital infection/vertical transmission occurs in 1% of cases (1).
  - Transplacental transmission
  - Chromosomal integration (clinical significance unknown)
- Lifelong latent or persistent asymptomatic infection occurs after primary infection (1).
  - 80–90% of population intermittently sheds HHV-6/HHV-7 in saliva (2).
  - Patients are viremic from 2 days prior to fever until defervescence and onset of rash.
  - HHV-6 latency is also implicated in CSF (4).

Genetics
HHV-6 is integrated into the chromosomes of 0.2–3.0% of the population. This leads to vertical transmission of the virus. Clinical significance of this is unknown (1).

RISK FACTORS

- Female gender (3)
- Having older siblings (3)
- At-risk adults: immunocompromised (5)
  - Renal, liver, other solid organ, and bone marrow transplant (BMT) (3)
  - HHV-6 reactivation can occur in 1st week post-transplant (5). HHV-6 viremia occurs in 30–45% of BMT within the first several weeks after transplantation (4).
    - Usually asymptomatic (4)
    - Up to 82% of HHV-6 reactivation/reinfection in solid organ transplant (5)
- Nonrisk factors (3)
  - Child care attendance
  - Method of delivery
  - Breastfeeding (HHV does not appear to pass through breast milk.)
  - Maternal age
  - Season

 DIAGNOSIS

HISTORY

- 3 to 5 days abrupt fever 102.2–104.0°F (39–40°C) not associated with a rash (1)
- The child may be fussy during this prodrome (1),(6).
- Sudden drop of fever associated with appearance of rash (1)
  - Rash on trunk then spreads centrifugally mainly to neck, possibly also to peripheral extremities, and face
- Diarrhea (3)
- Mild upper respiratory symptoms (3)
- Rhinorrhea (3)
- Febrile seizure occurs in 13% of cases (1).

PHYSICAL EXAM

- Rash (exanthem subitum) (1)
  - Rose-pink macules and/or papules that blanch
  - First appears on the trunk then peripherally
  - May occur up to 3 days after fever resolves (1)
  - Fades within 2 days
  - Occurs in approximately 20% of patients in the United States (1)
- Mild inflammation of tympanic membrane, pharynx, and/or conjunctiva (1),(6)
- Ulcers on soft palate and uvula (Nagayama spots) (1)
- Cervical lymphadenopathy (1)
- Periorbital edema (2)

DIFFERENTIAL DIAGNOSIS

- Enterovirus infection
- Adenovirus infection (1)
- Epstein-Barr virus
- Fifth disease—parvovirus B19
- Rubella (1)
- Scarlet fever (1)
- Drug eruption (1)
- Measles (1)

DIAGNOSTIC TESTS & INTERPRETATION

- Primarily a clinical diagnosis not requiring laboratory or radiologic testing (1)[C]
- Tests often cannot differentiate latent or active disease (1)[C].
- Specific diagnosis only necessary in severe cases, unclear diagnosis where more serious disease needs to be ruled out, or if considering antiviral therapy (1)[C]

Initial Tests (lab, imaging)
- If necessary, HHV-6 and HHV-7 by PCR (1),(5)[C]
  - Serum, whole blood, CSF, or saliva
  - Becoming more widely available
  - Not required in nonimmunocompromised individuals
- HHV-6 IgM immunofluorescence (1)
- Diagnostic for acute infection
  - Spike seen in 1st week of illness
- HHV-6 IgG immunofluorescence (1)
  - Check at diagnosis and then 2 weeks later.
  - Use with IgM to show primary infection.
  - Negative initial test and rise on follow-up suggest primary infection.
- Viral culture (5)
  - Rarely done
  - No clinical use (very time-consuming)
- Other laboratory findings (1)
  - Decreased total leukocytes, lymphocytes, and neutrophils
  - Elevated transaminases
  - Thrombocytopenia

Diagnostic Procedures/Other
- Urine culture: to rule out UTI as source of fever (2)
- Chest x-ray (CXR): if a child has respiratory symptoms

TREATMENT
No treatment necessary, resolves without sequelae (1)[C]

GENERAL MEASURES
- Symptomatic relief including antipyretics (1)[C]
- Hydration (1)[C]

MEDICATION
First Line
- No specific first-line treatment in immunocompetent hosts beyond supportive measures (2)[C]
  - Antivirals are not recommended in immunocompetent.
- No approved antiviral treatment in immunocompromised (2)[C]
- Second-line IV ganciclovir, cidofovir, foscarnet tested in vitro studies in stem cell transplant patients
  - HHV-6B susceptible: ganciclovir and foscarnet (5)[C]
  - HHV-6A and HHV-7 are more resistant to ganciclovir (5).
- Antivirals suggested in individual cases of encephalitis (associated with reactivation of HHV-6) (5)
- In bone marrow and stem cell transplant recipients receiving immunosuppression, ganciclovir prophylaxis is effective in preventing reactivation of HHV-6 (6)[B].

ONGOING CARE

FOLLOW-UP RECOMMENDATIONS
Patient Monitoring
- During febrile prodrome, monitor for dehydration.
- None after typical rash appears and fever resolves
- Mean duration of illness is 6 days (4).
- If febrile seizures occur, they will cease after fever subsides and will not likely recur (4).
- Symptomatic reactivation in immunocompromised (1)

DIET
Encourage fluids.

PATIENT EDUCATION
- Parental reassurance that this is usually a benign, self-limited disease (1)
- There is no specific recommended period of exclusion from out-of-home care for affected children.
- Patient is viremic a few days prior to fever until time of defervescence and rash onset.

PROGNOSIS
- Course: acute, complete recovery without sequelae (1)
- Reactivation in immunocompromised patients is common (4).

COMPLICATIONS
- Febrile seizures
  - 13% patients with roseola (1),(6)
  - Accounts for 1/3 of primary seizures in children <2 years old (1)
- Medication hypersensitivity syndromes (drug reaction with eosinophilia and systemic symptoms) (2)
- Reactivation can occur in transplant patients, HIV-1 infection, and other immunocompromised individuals (4).
- Meningoencephalitis occurs in immunocompetent and in immunosuppressed patients (4); poor association with multiple sclerosis (4)
- Pityriasis rosea (1)
- Possible association with progressive multifocal leukoencephalopathy (4)

REFERENCES
1. Stone RC, Micali GA, Schwartz RA. Roseola infantum and its causal human herpesviruses. *Int J Dermatol*. 2014;53(4):397–403.
2. Wolz MM, Sciallis GF, Pittelkow MR. Human herpesviruses 6, 7, and 8 from a dermatologic perspective. *Mayo Clin Proc*. 2012;87(10):1004–1014.
3. Zerr DM, Meier AS, Selke SS, et al. A population-based study of primary human herpesvirus 6 infection. *N Engl J Med*. 2005;352(8):768–776.
4. Caserta MT, Mock DJ, Dewhurst S. Human herpesvirus 6. *Clin Infect Dis*. 2001;33(6):829–833.
5. Le J, Gantt S; for AST Infectious Diseases Community of Practice. Human herpesvirus 6, 7 and 8 in solid organ transplantation. *Am J Transplant*. 2013;13(Suppl 4):128–137.
6. Tokimasa S, Hara J, Osugi Y, et al. Ganciclovir is effective for prophylaxis and treatment of human herpesvirus-6 in allogeneic stem cell transplantation. *Bone Marrow Transplant*. 2002;29(7):595–598.

ADDITIONAL READING
- Ablashi DV, Devin CL, Yoshikawa T, et al. Review part 3: human herpesvirus-6 in multiple non-neurological diseases. *J Med Virol*. 2010;82(11):1903–1910.
- Caselli E, Di Luca D. Molecular biology and clinical associations of roseoloviruses human herpesvirus 6 and human herpesvirus 7. *New Microbiol*. 2007;30(3):173–187.
- Dockrell DH, Smith TF, Paya CV. Human herpesvirus 6. *Mayo Clin Proc*. 1999;74(2):163–170.
- Dyer JA. Childhood viral exanthems. *Pediatr Ann*. 2007;36(1):21–29.
- Evans CM, Kudesia G, McKendrick M. Management of herpesvirus infections. *Int J Antimicrob Agents*. 2013;42(2):119–128.
- Fölster-Holst R, Kreth HW. Viral exanthems in childhood—infectious (direct) exanthems. Part 1: classic exanthems. *J Dtsch Dermatol Ges*. 2009;7(4):309–316.
- Huang CT, Lin LH. Differentiating roseola infantum with pyuria from urinary tract infection. *Pediatr Int*. 2013;55(2):214–218.
- Leach CT. Human herpesvirus-6 and -7 infections in children: agents of roseola and other syndromes. *Curr Opin Pediatr*. 2000;12(3):269–274.
- Lowry M. Roseola infantum. *Pract Nurse*. 2013;43:40–42.
- Stoeckle MY. The spectrum of human herpesvirus 6 infection: from roseola infantum to adult disease. *Annu Rev Med*. 2000;51:423–430.
- Vianna RA, de Oliveira SA, Camacho LA, et al. Role of human herpesvirus 6 infection in young Brazilian children with rash illnesses. *Pediatr Infect Dis J*. 2008;27(6):533–537.

 CODES

ICD10
- B08.20 Exanthema subitum [sixth disease], unspecified
- B08.21 Exanthema subitum [sixth disease] due to human herpesvirus 6
- B08.22 Exanthema subitum [sixth disease] due to human herpesvirus 7

CLINICAL PEARLS
- Roseola infection should be suspected if an infant or young child presents with a high temperature without other clinical findings.
- As the fever abates, a macular rash will be seen on the trunk, with eventual spread to the face and extremities in 20% of patients.
- Roseola is a clinical diagnosis, and laboratory testing is not necessary for most children with classic presentation.
- For atypical presentations, complications, and immunocompromised hosts, several laboratory tools are available, including serologic testing for antibody, viral PCR testing, and viral culture.
- Infection is typically self-limiting and without sequelae.
- Usually, only symptomatic treatment is needed.
- Consider prophylaxis in patients undergoing bone marrow or stem cell transplant and receiving immunosuppressive therapy.

R

ROTATOR CUFF IMPINGEMENT SYNDROME

Faren H. Williams, MD, MS • Minjin Fromm, MD

BASICS

DESCRIPTION

- Compression of rotator cuff tendons and subacromial bursa between the humeral head and the structures comprising the coracoacromial arch and proximal humerus
- Most common cause of atraumatic shoulder pain in patients >25 years of age
- Primary symptom is pain that is most severe when the arm is abducted between 60 and 120 degrees (the "painful arc").
- Classically divided into three stages:
  - Stage I: acute inflammation, edema, or hemorrhage of the underlying tendons due to overuse (typically in those age <25 years)
  - Stage II: progressive tendinosis that leads to partial rotator cuff tear along with underlying thickening or fibrosis of surrounding structures (commonly, ages 25 to 40 years)
  - Stage III: full-thickness tear (typically in patients age >40 years)

EPIDEMIOLOGY

Incidence

- Shoulder pain accounts for 1% of all primary care visits.
- Peak incidence of 25/1,000 patients per year occurs in patients aged 42 to 46 years.
- Impingement responsible for 18–74% of shoulder pain diagnoses

Prevalence

Prevalence of shoulder pain in general population ranges from ~7% to 30%.

RISK FACTORS

- Repetitive overhead motions (throwing, swimming)
- Glenohumeral joint instability or muscle imbalance
- Acromioclavicular arthritis or osteophytes
- Thickened coracoacromial ligament
- Shoulder trauma
- Increasing age
- Smoking

GENERAL PREVENTION

- Proper throwing and lifting techniques
- Proper strengthening to balance rotator cuff and scapula stabilizer muscles

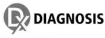

DIAGNOSIS

HISTORY

- Gradual increase in shoulder pain with overhead activities (Sudden onset of sharp pain suggests a tear.)
- Night pain is common, exacerbated by lying on the affected shoulder or sleeping with the affected arm above the head.
- Anterolateral shoulder pain with overhead activities
- May progress to weakness and decreased range of motion if shoulder is not used through full range of motion

PHYSICAL EXAM

- Examine patient for atrophy/asymmetry. Observe how the patient takes off his or her shirt during exam.
- Neer impingement test: Examiner stabilizes the scapula and moves the affected upper extremity through a flexion arc. Positive is pain with flexion of the shoulder. Sensitivity: 78%. Specificity: 58% (1)[A]
- Hawkins-Kennedy impingement test: Examiner places the arm in 90 degrees of forward flexion and then gently internally rotates the arm. End point for internal rotation is when the patient feels pain or when the rotation of the scapula is felt or observed by the examiner. Test is positive when patient experiences pain during the maneuver. Sensitivity: 74%. Specificity: 57% (1)[A]
- Empty can test (supraspinatus): Examiner asks the patient to elevate and internally rotate the arm with thumbs pointing downward in the scapular plane. Elbow should be fully extended. Examiner applies downward pressure on upper surface of the arm. Test is positive when patient complains of pain with resistance. Sensitivity: 69%. Specificity: 62% (1)[A]
- Lift-off test (subscapularis): Patient internally rotates the shoulder, placing the back of the hand on ipsilateral buttock, then lifts hand off buttock against resistance. A tear in the subscapularis muscle produces weakness of this action. Sensitivity: 42%. Specificity: 97% (1)[A]
- Drop-arm test: Patient fully elevates arm and then slowly reverses the motion. If the arm is dropped suddenly or the patient has extreme pain, the test is positive for a possible rotator cuff tear. Sensitivity: 21%. Specificity: 92% (1)[A]
- Resisted external rotation: weakness suggestive of infraspinatus and/or teres minor tendon involvement
- Apprehension-relocation test for anterior glenohumeral joint instability: Have the patient supine or sitting; abduct the arm to 90 degrees and flex the patient's elbow to 90 degrees; examiner slowly rotates the humerus (pushes hand posteriorly while patient resists then anteriorly while the patient resists). If the patient becomes anxious or has apprehension from this maneuver, test is positive implying instability and risk for dislocation. If pain is present, rather than instability, consider labral tear and/or impingement syndrome.
- Examine cervical spine to rule out cervical pathology as source of shoulder pain.
- Neurovascular exam of the upper extremity

DIFFERENTIAL DIAGNOSIS

- Labral injury
- Acromioclavicular arthritis (more common in older patients; positive cross-arm test—pain when affected arm is fully adducted across the chest in the horizontal plane)
- Adhesive capsulitis (rotator cuff tendonitis leads to decreased use and atrophy of rotator cuff muscles, followed by contracture; linked to diabetes and potentially prior trauma)
- Anterior shoulder instability (prior trauma; more common in patients <25 years old)
- Multidirectional instability
- Biceps tendonitis or rupture (Perform Speed and Yergason tests and look for visible or palpable defect of biceps—"Popeye sign.")
- Calcific tendonitis
- Cervical radiculopathy (spinal or foraminal stenosis, can test with Spurling maneuver)
- Glenohumeral arthritis (Evaluate with plain films.)
- Suprascapular nerve entrapment (Look for focal muscle atrophy of supra- or infraspinatus.)
- Traumatic rotator cuff tear

DIAGNOSTIC TESTS & INTERPRETATION

Initial Tests (lab, imaging)

- Plain-film radiographs of the shoulder (three views): anteroposterior, axillary, scapular Y views
- Plain films may reveal:
  - Osteoarthritis of the acromioclavicular and glenohumeral joints
  - Superior migration of the humeral head (indicative of a large rotator cuff tear)
  - Cystic change of the humeral head and sclerosis of the inferior acromion (indicative of chronic rotator cuff disease)
  - Calcific tendonitis
- MRI is used to definitively assess rotator cuff tendinopathy, partial tears, and complete tears.
- MR arthrogram is preferred for labral pathology.
- Ultrasound is sensitive and specific for rotator cuff tears but is highly operator dependent.
- CT scan is preferred for bony pathology or for those unable to undergo MRI.

Diagnostic Procedures/Other

- Lidocaine injection test
  - Inject lidocaine into the subacromial space:
    - Repeat impingement tests; if pain is completely relieved and range of motion is improved, likely impingement syndrome (rather than cuff tear)
  - Allows for more accurate strength testing on physical examination:
    - If strength is intact, rule out rotator cuff tear.
    - If range of motion does not improve in any plane, more likely adhesive capsulitis
  - Some pain relief and improved range of motion occurs after lidocaine injection with
    - Glenoid labral tear
    - Capsular strain
    - Glenohumeral osteoarthritis
    - Glenohumeral instability
- A lack of any pain relief suggests other sources (i.e., cervical radiculopathy) or inappropriate placement of injection.

Test Interpretation

May have tendinosis, tendonitis, or muscle/tendon tear

TREATMENT

Pain control in combination with aggressive rehabilitation improves and fully resolves rotator cuff tendonitis in most patients.

GENERAL MEASURES
- Rest initial, then mandatory supervised physical therapy for 6 to 8 weeks
- Ice or heat for symptom relief
- Activity modification, with avoidance of aggravating activities, particularly overhead motions
- Range of motion exercises
- Rotator cuff and adjacent muscle strengthening to enhance stability and prevent further injuries

MEDICATION
First Line
NSAIDs or other analgesic, often for 6 to 12 weeks

ISSUES FOR REFERRAL
Failure of conservative treatment, persistent pain, weakness, or complete tear of rotator cuff

ADDITIONAL THERAPIES
- Supervised- or home-exercise regimens provide significant pain reduction and improve function (2)[A].
- Physical therapy is effective for short-term and long-term recovery of function (3)[A]:
  – Initial goal is to restore range of motion.
  – After pain resolves, gradually strengthen rotator cuff muscles in internal rotation, external rotation, and abduction.

SURGERY/OTHER PROCEDURES
- Steroid injections may have a significant benefit on pain and function in the short term but do not appear to have a significant long-term effect (4)[A].
- No evidence that surgery is superior to conservative management or that one surgical technique is superior to another for impingement syndrome (5)[A]
- Platelet-rich therapies for musculoskeletal soft tissue injuries are increasingly common.
  – No apparent effect of platelet-rich plasma injection during arthroscopic rotator cuff repair on overall retear rates or shoulder-specific outcomes
- Extracorporeal shock wave therapy is currently under study as an emerging treatment for calcific tendonitis.

COMPLEMENTARY & ALTERNATIVE MEDICINE
Acupuncture is potentially beneficial for reducing pain and improving function, particularly when used with physical therapy (6)[A].

 ONGOING CARE

PATIENT EDUCATION
- Physical rehabilitation is necessary, both in conservative course of treatment (i.e., NSAIDs, physical therapy, home exercises) and in surgical intervention.
- An aggressive trial of rehabilitation should be encouraged prior to extensive testing or surgical intervention. Providing pain relief prior to beginning a program of physical therapy improves adherence and outcomes.
- Symptoms often recur if not fully addressed.

PROGNOSIS
- Variable, depends on underlying pathology
- Most patients improve with conservative management. Recovery can be slow.
- Patients with more severe symptoms—those with symptoms for >1 year—are less likely to respond well with conservative therapies.

COMPLICATIONS
- Progression of injury
- Tendon retraction in complete rotator cuff tear

REFERENCES

1. Alqunaee M, Galvin R, Fahey T. Diagnostic accuracy of clinical tests for subacromial impingement syndrome: a systematic review and meta-analysis. *Arch Phys Med Rehabil*. 2012;93(2):229–236.
2. Kuhn JE. Exercise in the treatment of rotator cuff impingement: a systematic review and a synthesized evidence-based rehabilitation protocol. *J Shoulder Elbow Surg*. 2009;18(1):138–160.
3. Green S, Buchbinder R, Hetrick S. Physiotherapy interventions for shoulder pain. *Cochrane Database Syst Rev*. 2003;(2):CD004258.
4. Gaujoux-Viala C, Dougados M, Gossec L. Efficacy and safety of steroid injections for shoulder and elbow tendonitis: a meta-analysis of randomised controlled trials. *Ann Rheum Dis*. 2009;68(12):1843–1849.
5. Gebremariam L, Hay EM, Koes BW, et al. Effectiveness of surgical and postsurgical interventions for the subacromial impingement syndrome: a systematic review. *Arch Phys Med Rehabil*. 2011;92(11):1900–1913.
6. Vas J, Ortega C, Olmo V, et al. Single-point acupuncture and physiotherapy for the treatment of painful shoulder: a multicentre randomized controlled trial. *Rheumatology (Oxford)*. 2008;47(6):887–893.

ADDITIONAL READING

- Baumgarten KM, Gerlach D, Galatz LM, et al. Cigarette smoking increases the risk for rotator cuff tears. *Clin Orthop Relat Res*. 2010;468(6):1534–1541.
- Burbank KM, Stevenson JH, Czarnecki GR, et al. Chronic shoulder pain: part I. Evaluation and diagnosis. *Am Fam Physician*. 2008;77(4):453–460.
- Burbank KM, Stevenson JH, Czarnecki GR, et al. Chronic shoulder pain: part II. Treatment. *Am Fam Physician*. 2008;77(4):493–497.
- Hanchard NC, Lenza M, Handoll HH, et al. Physical tests for shoulder impingements and local lesions of bursa, tendon or labrum that may accompany impingement. *Cochrane Database Syst Rev*. 2013;(4):CD007427.

 CODES

ICD10
- M75.40 Impingement syndrome of unspecified shoulder
- M75.110 Incmpl rotatr-cuff tear/ruptr of unsp shoulder, not trauma
- M75.120 Complete rotatr-cuff tear/ruptr of unsp shoulder, not trauma

CLINICAL PEARLS

- Consider impingement syndrome in patients who engage in activities with repetitive overhead motions (e.g., swimming, throwing) who present with shoulder pain.
- Atraumatic shoulder pain in middle age often represents rotator cuff tendonitis.
- The supraspinatus tendon is most commonly affected in impingement syndrome.
- Neer and Hawkins tests specifically check for shoulder impingement.
- The empty can maneuver tests for weakness of supraspinatus muscle.
- The drop-arm test is specific for rotator cuff tear.
- Physical therapy over 6 to 12 weeks promotes return to function.
- Most patients with shoulder impingement respond well to conservative management.

R

SALIVARY GLAND CALCULI/SIALADENITIS

Sahil Mullick, MD • Sudeshna Dutta, MD

BASICS

DESCRIPTION

- Inflammation of one or more salivary glands
- Infectious, obstructive, or autoimmune.
- "Sialolithiasis" is characterized by a painful swelling of the affected gland when eating due to an obstructing stones within the salivary glands or ducts.
- "Sialadenitis" is inflammation of the salivary gland classified as acute or chronic sialadenitis.
  - Acute can be caused by a primary infection (viral/bacterial) or secondary infection.
  - Chronic sialadenitis is due to repeated episodes of inflammation resulting in progressive loss of salivary gland function.
- Parotid gland and submandibular glands are commonly affected by sialadenitis. However, parotid gland is affected mostly by acute suppurative sialadenitis. The submandibular gland is more commonly affected (80–90% of cases) by stones than the parotid gland due to higher mucinous content of saliva, longer course of Wharton duct, and slow salivary flow against gravity.

EPIDEMIOLOGY

Incidence

- Peak incidence is 30 to 60 years; rarely in children
- Most common in debilitated and dehydrated patients
- 70% of the stones are single; 30% bilateral

ETIOLOGY AND PATHOPHYSIOLOGY

- Stagnation of salivary flow and elevated calcium concentrations are thought to be important.
- Decreased salivary outflow from anticholinergics, dehydration, or radiation
- Salivary calculi are composed of calcium phosphate and hydroxyapatite with smaller amounts of magnesium, potassium, and ammonium.
- Predisposing factors include inflammation of the salivary gland or duct, salivary stasis, retrograde bacterial contamination from the oral cavity, increased alkalinity of saliva, and physical trauma to salivary duct or gland.
- Gout associated with salivary stone development. In gout, sialoliths are composed of uric acid.
- Bacterial sialadenitis tends to be unifocal caused by *Staphylococcus aureus*, *Streptococcus viridans*, *Streptococcus pyogenes*, *Haemophilus influenzae*, *Escherichia coli*, *Pseudomonas aeruginosa*, and group B streptococci (neonates and children).
- Viral sialadenitis tends to be multifocal caused by mumps, cytomegalovirus, Epstein-Barr virus, HIV, and enteroviruses.
- Other common causes include radioiodine use, positive pressure ventilation use with anesthesia, Sjögren syndrome, and sarcoidosis (1).

Pediatric Considerations

Common causes of sialadenitis in children are mumps and idiopathic juvenile recurrent parotitis.

RISK FACTORS

- Anticholinergic use
- Poor oral hygiene, malnutrition, smoking, dehydration
- Head/neck radiation

GENERAL PREVENTION

- Maintain proper oral care and hygiene.
- Avoid anticholinergics and other causes of xerostomia.

COMMONLY ASSOCIATED CONDITIONS

- Radiation or drug-induced xerostomia
- Sjögren syndrome, Mikulicz syndrome
- Hypercalcemia

DIAGNOSIS

Most (~80%) salivary gland stones occur in the submandibular glands, 6–20% occur in the parotid gland and 1–2% occur in the sublingual or minor salivary glands. Submandibular stones are more often located in the duct. Parotid stones tend to be smaller than mandibular stones, are more often multiple, and located within the gland itself (1).

HISTORY

- Review history for
  - Alcoholism, bulimia, malnutrition; radiation therapy, past malignancy; TB or HIV exposure
- Acute onset of pain and swelling over the affected salivary gland, especially postprandial or following the anticipation of eating
- Dental pain, discharge, foul breath (halitosis) hypersalivation, and pain with chewing
- Xerostomia
- 33% of the patients with submandibular sialolithiasis present with painless swelling and 10% with pain but not swelling.
- Worsening pain, erythema and/or fever may indicate secondary infection.
- Pus drainage through the gland duct into the mouth

PHYSICAL EXAM

- Visual inspection of the glands and ducts; for submandibular gland a stone may be felt within the Wharton duct or seen near the frenulum of the tongue. For parotid glands, a stone may be felt within Stensen duct or seen at the orifice.
- Bimanual exam of oral cavity palpating all salivary glands, floor of mouth, tongue, and neck to assess symmetry, tenderness, induration, edema, presence of stones, lymphadenopathy, and the number of glands involved. A functioning gland is usually spongy and elastic.

- Examine duct openings for purulent discharge and presence of saliva. Purulent discharge at the orifice raises concern for acute bacterial sialadenitis.
- Gently palpate gland to express normal, thin absent or reduced amounts of saliva, assess for bubbling appearance or purulent drainage.
- Examine eyes for interstitial keratitis.
- Evaluation of facial nerve (CN VII) function, which is at risk for compromise if parotid gland is involved

Pediatric Considerations

Stones in children are often within the distal duct. Ultrasound with sialendoscopy is diagnostic and therapeutic.

DIFFERENTIAL DIAGNOSIS

- Bacterial parotitis
- Idiopathic juvenile recurrent parotitis; cystic fibrosis
- Mumps; tularemia
- Collagen vascular disease
- Metal poisoning
- Salivary gland tumors; lymphoma

DIAGNOSTIC TESTS & INTERPRETATION

Sialolithiasis is a clinical diagnosis based on a characteristic history and physical examination. There is typically sudden onset of swelling and pain in the affected gland associated with eating or anticipation of eating. A stone may be seen at the opening of the affected salivary duct or palpated along the course of the duct.

Initial Tests (lab, imaging)

- Consider CBC.
- Culture and sensitivity of any expressed pus
- Ultrasound is able to detect up to 90% of stones 2 mm or larger (2)[C].
- CT scan with IV contrast is more sensitive but has radiation exposure (3)[C].
- MR sialography for patients with an inconclusive ultrasound and persistent symptoms without the use of intraductal contrast.
- Sonopalpation (concurrent ultrasound with transoral palpation) proved to have a sensitivity and specificity of 96.6% and 90% in finding a calculus (3)[B].

Follow-Up Tests & Special Considerations

- If autoimmune process is suspected, order rheumatoid factor (RF) and antinuclear antibodies (ANAs) (4)[C].
- Salivary gland biopsy

Diagnostic Procedures/Other

- Sialography to evaluate sialolithiasis and other obstructive lesions
- Sialendoscopy to find and remove sialoliths. In one study, sialendoscopy confirmed 221 (79%) parotid and 812 (93%) submandibular stones (5)[A].

- One study revealed that sonography, cone beam CT, and sialendoscopy all had excellent specificity and positive predictive value in diagnosing stones (3)[B].
- When sialendoscopy fails, a novel ultrasound-guided needle localization approach has been proposed.
- Technetium-99m pertechnetate scintigraphy showed decreased gland excretion and decreased uptake in patients with sialolithiasis.

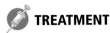 **TREATMENT**

GENERAL MEASURES
- Maintain hydration.
- Apply warm compresses.
- Massage the gland and milk the duct.
- Sialagogues (agents that promote salivary flow) like tart, lemon juice, and hard candies (lemon drops) may be helpful. Use throughout the day as tolerated.
- Maintain good oral hygiene.
- Chlorhexidine 0.12% mouth rinses 3 times a day will help to reduce the bacterial burden in oral cavity and will promote oral hygiene.
- Discontinue medications with anticholinergic effects that reduce salivary flow.

MEDICATION
- Pain management with NSAIDs
- Antibiotics for suspected secondary infection (fever, purulent discharge)

First Line
- Antistaphylococcal antibiotics such as dicloxacillin 500 mg or cephalexin 500 mg QID for 7 to 10 days
- If no improvement within 5 to 7 days, a culture of the duct discharge should be obtained and the antibiotic coverage broadened by substituting amoxicillin/clavulanate or clindamycin.
- Penicillin-allergic: Use clindamycin 300 mg PO q8h.
- Gram negative: 3rd-generation cephalosporin or fluoroquinolone
- Anaerobic: metronidazole or clindamycin

Second Line
- 1st-generation cephalosporin (cephalexin or cefazolin) or clindamycin is also indicated for empiric coverage.
- If MRSA, then vancomycin

ISSUES FOR REFERRAL
- Dentist if poor dentition/dental abscess.
- ENT if failure to improve with conservative management, recurrent symptoms (6)

ADDITIONAL THERAPIES
In the case of chronic sialadenitis with strictures, consider sialostent placement.

SURGERY/OTHER PROCEDURES
- Submandibular stones found in the anterior floor of the mouth can be excised intraorally (sialodochoplasty), whereas those in the hilum require gland excision. Parotid stones usually require parotidectomy (4)[A].
- Good results in patient symptom relief, quality of life, and safety have been reported in sialadenitis and sialolithiasis using sialendoscopy (4),(5). Complications include strictures, ranulas, and lingual nerve injury. However, sialendoscopy is contraindicated in acute sialadenitis.
- A combined approach using limited intraoral incision with sialendoscopy has shown an 86% success rate.
- Incision and drainage of parotid abscess is indicated after failing 3 to 5 days of medical management (7).
- Sialoliths larger than 4 mm and stenoses can be successfully treated by radiologically or fluoroscopically controlled or sialendoscopically based methods in ~80% of cases. Extracorporeal shock wave lithotripsy (ESWL) is successful in up to 50% of cases.
- Transoral duct slitting for extraparenchymal submandibular stones; 90% success rate

COMPLEMENTARY & ALTERNATIVE MEDICINE
Consider lemon drops or other sialogogues to promote salivation. In one study, postoperative use of sialogogues nearly halved rates of sialadenitis (4)[C].

ADMISSION, INPATIENT, AND NURSING CONSIDERATIONS
- Parotid abscess
- Inability to tolerate PO intake

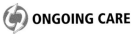 **ONGOING CARE**

FOLLOW-UP RECOMMENDATIONS
Avoid prescribing medications that cause xerostomia.

Patient Monitoring
Monitor patients with chronic sialadenitis because decreased salivary gland function due to fibrosis and loss of acini can lead to acute exacerbations.

DIET
- Avoid sialogogues during acute attacks.
- Maintain adequate hydration.

PATIENT EDUCATION
Maintaining excellent oral hygiene/hydration

PROGNOSIS
- Acute symptoms usually resolving in about a week with appropriate treatment. Complete resolution is expected after conservative outpatient treatment.
- Patients with autoimmune etiology may have prolonged course due to systemic involvement.
- In patients who undergo transoral surgical stone removal, recurrence has been reported in 18%.

COMPLICATIONS
- Local spreading of infection, causing cellulitis or Ludwig's angina
- Facial nerve impingement, hypoglossal and lingual nerve injuries
- Dental decay: Hypofunction of salivary gland causes decrease protection from acid erosion, promoting dental decay.

REFERENCES
1. Kao WK, Chole RA, Ogden MA. Evidence of a microbial etiology for sialoliths. *Laryngoscope.* 2020;130(1):69–74.
2. Goncalves M, Mantsopoulos K, Schapher M, et al. Ultrasound supplemented by sialendoscopy: diagnostic value in sialolithiasis. *Am Academy of Otolaryngol Head Neck Surg.* 2018;159(3):449–455.
3. Schwarz D, Kabbasch C, Scheer M, et al. Comparative analysis of sialendoscopy, sonography, and CBCT in the detection of sialolithiasis. *Laryngoscope.* 2015;125(5):1098–1101.
4. Wilson KF, Meier JD, Ward PD. Salivary gland disorders. *Am Fam Physician.* 2014;89(11):882–888.
5. Atienza G, López-Cedrún JL. Management of obstructive salivary disorders by sialendoscopy: a systematic review. *Br J Oral Maxillofac Surg.* 2015;53(6):507–519.
6. Wallace E, Tauzin M, Hagan J, et al. Management of giant sialoliths: review of the literature and preliminary experience with interventional sialendoscopy. *Laryngoscope.* 2010;120(10):1974–1978.
7. Capaccio P, Torretta S, Pignataro L, et al. Salivary lithotripsy in the era of sialendoscopy. *Acta Otorhinolaryngol Ital.* 2017;37(2):113–121.

 CODES

ICD10
- K11.5 Sialolithiasis
- K11.20 Sialoadenitis, unspecified
- K11.21 Acute sialoadenitis

CLINICAL PEARLS
- Mainstay of treatment is hydration, good oral hygiene, sialogogues, and possible surgical excision.
- Nonpharmacologic agents that promote salivary flow like tart and hard candies such as lemon drops may be helpful and should be used throughout the day.

S

SALMONELLA INFECTION

Marie L. Borum, MD, EdD, MPH • Matthew Houle, BS

BASICS

DESCRIPTION
- Infection caused by any serotype of the bacterial genus *Salmonella*, a gram-negative facultatively anaerobic bacillus
- Nontyphoidal *Salmonella* typically causes gastroenteritis via foodborne infection and sporadic outbreaks; less commonly causes infection outside the gastrointestinal (GI) tract
- Clinical syndromes
  – Enteric fever (see "Typhoid Fever")
  – Nontyphoidal gastroenteritis
    ○ Chronic carrier state (>1 year)
  – Nontyphoidal invasive disease
    ○ Bacteremia
      ▪ Endovascular complications
      ▪ Localized infection outside GI tract (i.e., osteomyelitis, abscess)

Geriatric Considerations
Patients >65 years old have increased risk of invasive disease with bacteremia and endovascular complications due to comorbidities (atherosclerotic endovascular lesions, prostheses, etc.) that increase risk of bacterial seeding.

Pediatric Considerations
Neonates (<3 months) are more susceptible to invasive disease and complications.

EPIDEMIOLOGY
Incidence
- Global incidence of nontyphoidal *Salmonella enteritidis* estimated to be ~94 million per year (mostly foodborne)
  – Wide variation by region from 40 to 3,980 estimated cases per 100,000
- Global incidence of invasive nontyphoidal *Salmonella* infection estimated to be 535,000 cases in 2017
- Most commonly identified foodborne bacterial illness in the United States and a common cause of traveler's diarrhea.
  – Estimated 1.4 million cases per year in the United States, with annual incidence of 15 illnesses per 100,000
- Second most common bacteria isolated from stool cultures in diarrheal illness (following *Campylobacter*) in the United States
- Highest incidence of bacteremia in children <5 years old
- Hospitalization rates higher in patients >50 years old
- Peak frequency: July to November

ETIOLOGY AND PATHOPHYSIOLOGY
- *Salmonella enterica*
  – Most pathogenic species in humans
  – 2,500 different serotypes
- Etiology
  – ~95% of cases are foodborne
  – Other cases (5%) are due to direct or indirect fecal–oral contact with animals or human carriers.
  – Iatrogenic contamination (e.g., blood transfusion, endoscopy) is rare.
- Pathophysiology
  – Typical infectious dose in immunocompetent patients is ingestion of 1 million bacteria but can be lower in patients taking antibiotics or in the setting of gastric acid reduction.
  – Bacteria ingested invade the distal ileal and proximal colonic mucosa to produce an inflammatory and cytotoxic response.
  – Bacteria can enter the mesenteric lymphatic system and then the systemic circulation to cause disseminated/invasive disease.

RISK FACTORS
- Recent travel to underdeveloped nations
- Consumption of undercooked meat, egg, or unpasteurized dairy products. Nonanimal products have also been implicated in outbreaks.
- Contact with live reptiles or poultry
- Contact with human carrier (*Salmonella* fecal shedding)
- Impaired gastric acidity: H_2 receptor blockers, antacids, proton pump inhibitors (PPIs), gastrectomy, achlorhydria, pernicious anemia, infants
- Recent antibiotic use
- Reticuloendothelial blockade: sickle cell disease, malaria, bartonellosis
- Immunosuppression: HIV, diabetes, corticosteroid or other immunosuppressant use, chemotherapy
- Impaired phagocytic function: chronic granulomatous disease, hemoglobinopathies, malaria
- Age <5 years or >50 years

GENERAL PREVENTION
- Proper hygiene in production, transport, and storage of food (e.g., refrigeration during food storage and thoroughly cooking food prior to consumption)
- Control of animal reservoirs: Avoid contact with high-risk animals, feces, and polluted waters.
- Hand hygiene
- CDC tracks outbreaks (http://www.cdc.gov/salmonella/).

COMMONLY ASSOCIATED CONDITIONS
- Gastroenteritis
- Bacteremia: immunocompromised or patients with underlying disease (e.g., cholelithiasis, prostheses)
- Osteomyelitis: higher incidence in sickle cell disease
- Abscesses: higher incidence with malignant tumors
- Reactive arthritis

DIAGNOSIS

HISTORY
- *Salmonella* infections are typically asymptomatic or result in mild, self-limited gastroenteritis
- Exposure history: travel; contact with infected human, reptile, or poultry; improper food preparation
- Local outbreaks
- Host factors: age, immune status, other risk factors
- Symptoms typically begin 8 to 72 hours after ingestion and resolve within 4 to 10 days.
- Acute uncomplicated illness
  – Sudden onset of diarrhea
    ○ Not typically grossly bloody but can be bloody especially among pediatric patients
  – Vomiting is infrequent.
  – Abdominal cramping
  – Headache
  – Myalgias
  – Fever

PHYSICAL EXAM
- Fever
- Evidence of hypovolemia
- Abdominal tenderness
- Heme-positive stool in some patients
- Hepatosplenomegaly in some patients

DIFFERENTIAL DIAGNOSIS
- Viral gastroenteritis
- Bacterial enteritis due to other organisms
- Pseudomembranous colitis
- Inflammatory bowel disease

DIAGNOSTIC TESTS & INTERPRETATION
Initial Tests (lab, imaging)
- Gastroenteritis
  – Stool culture for *Salmonella*, *Escherichia coli*, *Shigella*, and *Campylobacter* (1)[C] (Optimal specimen is a diarrheal stool sample.)
  – Indications for stool culture include the following:
    ○ Severe diarrhea (≥6 loose stools daily) (1)[C]
    ○ Diarrhea >1 week in duration (2)[C]
    ○ Fever (1)[C]
    ○ Diarrhea containing blood or mucous (1)[C]
    ○ Multiple cases suggesting an outbreak (1)[C]
  – Fecal leukocytes: positive
  – Blood cultures are warranted in:
    ○ Infants <3 months
    ○ People of any age with signs of septicemia or other systemic manifestations of infection
    ○ Cases where enteric fever is suspected
    ○ Immunocompromised patients
- Bacteremia
  – Blood cultures if febrile (1)[C]
  – Stool cultures: may also be positive (1)[C]
  – Culture CSF if patient is <3 months of age with positive blood culture.
- Endovascular infection
  – Consider angiography in bacteremic patients >50 years of age if aortic or vascular source is suspected (3)[A].
- Local infections
  – Wound culture
  – Consider CT or MRI for soft tissue or bone infections (1)[C].
- Chronic carrier state
  – Stool culture positive for >1 year (1)[C]
  – Urine culture may be positive in chronic carriers.

Follow-Up Tests & Special Considerations
- Look for other causes in diarrhea lasting >14 days.
- Asymptomatic excretion of *Salmonella* may occur for weeks after infection; follow-up fecal cultures are routinely not indicated for patients with uncomplicated gastroenteritis (1),(3)[C].
- Follow-up blood cultures suggested for patients with bacteremia (1)[C]

Test Interpretation
Intestinal biopsies (if taken) may show mucosal ulceration, hemorrhage, and necrosis seen on along with reticuloendothelial hypertrophy/hyperplasia.

TREATMENT

- Treatment is supportive for nonsevere nontyphoidal *Salmonella* gastroenteritis in immunocompetent patients between 12 months and 50 years of age. The illness is typically self-limited. There is no proven benefit for treatment of mild disease. Treatment can suppress the host immunologic response. Higher rates of relapse have also been reported and there is the potential to extend asymptomatic carriage (1),(2)[C].
- Consider antibiotics in immunocompetent hosts with severe diarrhea, high fever, or those requiring hospitalization (1)[C].

- Patients at increased risk of bacteremia benefit from antibiotics:
  - Infants <3 months of age (1)[C]
  - Patients >50 years old (Risk particularly increases after age 65 years.) (1)[C]
  - HIV-infected patients
  - Patients with hemoglobinopathies, atherosclerotic lesions, and prosthetic valves, grafts, or joints or any immunosuppressed state (1)[C],(3)[A]
- Chronic carriage of nontyphoidal *Salmonella*
  - 4 to 6 weeks of antimicrobial therapy
  - Prophylactic therapy in immunocompromised patients (3)[A]

GENERAL MEASURES

- Hydration and electrolyte replacement
- Hand washing and barrier precautions for inpatients
- Avoid antimotility drugs in patients with fever or dysentery. Antimotility drugs may increase contact time of the enteropathogen in the gut mucosa (1)[C].

MEDICATION

First Line

- Gastroenteritis, uncomplicated: No specific medications are necessary; supportive care (2)[A]
- Gastroenteritis, complicated (due to illness severity or host risk factors such as immunocompromised)
  - Adults (Treat for 14 days if immunocompromised.)
    - Levofloxacin: 500 mg/day PO for 1 to 3 days (2)[C] *or*
    - Ciprofloxacin: 750 mg/day PO for 1 day or 500 mg/day PO for 3 days (2)[C] or
    - Ofloxacin: 400 mg/day PO for 1 to 3 days (2)[C] or
    - Azithromycin: 500 mg/day PO for 3 days or 1 g followed by 500 mg daily for 3 days (2)[C]
      - Preferred agent for febrile diarrhea or dysentery
  - Children
    - Ceftriaxone: 100 mg/kg/day IV or IM in 2 equally divided doses for 7 to 10 days (3)[C] or
    - Azithromycin: 20 mg/kg PO for first dose and then 10 mg/kg/day for subsequent doses daily for 7 days (3)[C]
  - HIV patients
    - Increased duration (range of 2 to 6 weeks) of antimicrobial therapy and/or zidovudine may decrease relapse (3)[C].
- Bacteremia: Due to resistance trends, treat life-threatening infections in adults with a fluoroquinolone *or* a 3rd-generation cephalosporin until susceptibilities are determined (3)[A].
  - Adults
    - Ciprofloxacin (or other fluoroquinolone): 400 mg IV BID for 10 to 14 days *plus*
    - Ceftriaxone: 1 to 2 g/day IV for 10 to 14 days *or*
    - Cefotaxime: 2 g IV q8h for 10 to 14 days
  - Children
    - Amoxicillin: 30 mg/kg/dose TID for 10 to 14 days
    - Trimethoprim-sulfamethoxazole: 8 to 12 mg/kg/day of trimethoprim component in 2 divided doses for 10 to 14 days *or*
    - Ceftriaxone: 50 mg/kg/day (max 1 g) BID for 10 to 14 days
- Localized infection (e.g., septic arthritis, osteomyelitis, cholangitis, and pneumonia); surgical drainage or débridement in addition to a minimum of 3 weeks of antimicrobial therapy
  - In sustained bacteremia, prolonged local infection, or immunocompromised patients, give antibiotics PO for 4 to 6 weeks (3)[A].
- Chronic carrier state (shedding >1 year duration)
  - Amoxicillin: 1 g PO TID for 12 weeks *or*
  - Trimethoprim-sulfamethoxazole 160 mg/800 mg PO BID for 12 weeks *or*

- Ciprofloxacin: 500 mg PO BID for 4 weeks *or*
- Levofloxacin 500 mg/day for 4 weeks *or*
- Norfloxacin 400 mg PO BID for 4 weeks if gallstones are present

ALERT
Antimicrobial resistance

- Strains resistant to ampicillin, chloramphenicol, and trimethoprim-sulfamethoxazole have been reported.
- Fluoroquinolone resistance is increasing, perhaps due to increasing use in livestock.
- Extended-spectrum cephalosporin resistance has been reported with increasing frequency.

Second Line

- Aztreonam is an alternative agent that may be useful in patients with multiple allergies or if the organism demonstrates an unusual resistance pattern (3)[A].
- Fluoroquinolones are now routinely given to children for 5 to 7 days in areas of the world where multidrug-resistant *Salmonella typhi* is common (3)[A].

SURGERY/OTHER PROCEDURES

- Surgical excision and drainage for infected tissue sites, followed by a minimum of 3 weeks of antibiotic therapy
- If biliary tract disease is present, a preoperative 10- to 14-day course of parenteral antibiotics is recommended prior to cholecystectomy.

 ONGOING CARE

FOLLOW-UP RECOMMENDATIONS

Patient Monitoring

- Asymptomatic shedding of *Salmonella* may occur for weeks after infection. Follow-up fecal cultures are generally not indicated for patients with uncomplicated gastroenteritis. Requirements may differ during a *Salmonella* outbreak.
- Criteria may vary by state and local regulations. Some public health departments require negative stool cultures for health workers and food handlers prior to returning to work. Shedding may last 4 to 8 weeks.
- Serotyping of isolates can be performed at public health laboratories.

DIET
Easily digestible foods

PATIENT EDUCATION

- Meticulous hand hygiene; caution handling raw meat, poultry, and eggs
- Fruits and vegetables should be thoroughly washed prior to consumption.
- Thoroughly cooking meats eliminates *Salmonella*.
- Caution when handling animals with high fecal carriage rates
- www.cdc.gov/salmonella/general/prevention.html

PROGNOSIS

- Most cases of *Salmonella* gastroenteritis are self-limited and have an excellent prognosis.
- Increased mortality is seen in the young (<3 months), elderly (>65 years), and immunocompromised.
- Increased mortality is seen with bacteremia and other invasive infections.
- Mortality is increased in multidrug-resistant strains.

COMPLICATIONS
Toxic megacolon, hypovolemic shock, metastatic abscess formation, endocarditis, infectious endarteritis, meningitis, septic arthritis, reactive arthritis, osteomyelitis, pneumonia, appendicitis, cholecystitis

REFERENCES

1. Shane AL, Mody RK, Crump JA, et al. 2017 Infectious Diseases Society of America clinical practice guidelines for the diagnosis and management of infectious diarrhea. *Clin Infect Dis*. 2017;65(12):e45–e80
2. Riddle MS, Dupont HL, Connor BA. ACG clinical guideline: diagnosis, treatment, and prevention of acute diarrheal infections in adults. *Am J Gastroenterol*. 2016;111(5):602–622
3. Wen SC, Best E, Nourse C. Non-typhoidal *Salmonella* infections in children: review of literature and recommendations for management. *J Paediatr Child Health*. 2017;53(10):936–941.

ADDITIONAL READING

- Chen HM, Wang Y, Su LH, et al. Nontyphoid *Salmonella* infection: microbiology, clinical features, and antimicrobial therapy. *Pediatr Neonatol*. 2013;54(3):147–152.
- Hurley D, McCusker MP, Fanning S, et al. *Salmonella*–host interactions—modulation of the host innate immune system. *Front Immunol*. 2014;5:481.
- Lee MB, Greig JD. A review of nosocomial *Salmonella* outbreaks: infection control interventions found effective. *Public Health*. 2013;127(3):199–206.
- Odey F, Okomo U, Oyo-Ita A. Vaccines for preventing invasive salmonella infections in people with sickle cell disease. *Cochrane Database Syst Rev*. 2015;(6):CD006975.
- Onwuezobe IA, Oshun PO, Odigwe CC. Antimicrobials for treating symptomatic non-typhoidal *Salmonella* infection. *Cochrane Database Syst Rev*. 2012;(11):CD001167.

 SEE ALSO

Gastroenteritis; Typhoid Fever

 CODES

ICD10
- A02.25 Salmonella pyelonephritis
- A01.02 Typhoid fever with heart involvement
- A01.3 Paratyphoid fever C

CLINICAL PEARLS

- Nontyphoidal *Salmonella* infection is typically a foodborne infection associated with a self-limited gastroenteritis.
- Clinical syndromes include gastroenteritis, bacteremia, endovascular infection, localized infection outside the GI tract, and a chronic carrier state.
- Those at greatest risk of complications from *Salmonella* infection include the young, the elderly, and immunocompromised patients.
- Uncomplicated gastroenteritis in healthy patients can be treated with supportive care.
- Antibiotics should be used in infants, the elderly, immunocompromised patients, and for invasive infections such as bacteremia outside the GI tract.

S

SARCOIDOSIS

Donnah Mathews, MD, FACP

 BASICS

DESCRIPTION

- Sarcoidosis is a noninfectious, multisystem, granulomatous disease of unknown cause, affecting young and middle-aged adults.
  - Frequently presents with bilateral hilar adenopathy, pulmonary infiltrates, ocular or skin lesions
  - In ~50% of cases, it is diagnosed in asymptomatic patients with abnormal chest x-rays (CXRs).
  - Almost any organ may be involved.
- System(s) affected: primarily pulmonary but also cardiovascular, gastrointestinal, hematologic, endocrine, renal, neurologic, dermatologic, ophthalmologic, musculoskeletal
- Synonym(s): Löfgren syndrome (erythema nodosum [EN], hilar adenopathy, fever, arthralgias); Heerfordt syndrome (uveitis, parotid enlargement, facial palsy, fever); Besnier-Boeck disease; Boeck sarcoid; Scheuermann disease (1),(2)

EPIDEMIOLOGY

Incidence
Estimated 6/100 person-years (1)

Prevalence
- Estimated 10 to 20/100,000 persons
- 11/100,000 annual incidence rate for women (2)
- Usually occurs in younger persons, with the peak age of incidence for women 50 to 69 years and for men 40 to 59 years. Rare in children

ETIOLOGY AND PATHOPHYSIOLOGY
- Despite extensive research, etiology unknown. Thought to be due to exaggerated cell-mediated immune response to unknown antigen(s)
- In the lungs, the initial lesion is CD4+ T-cell alveolitis, causing noncaseating granulomata, which may resolve or may undergo fibrosis. "Immune paradox" with affected organs showing an intense immune response and yet anergy exists elsewhere

Genetics
- Reports of familial clustering, with genetic linkage to a section within MHC on short arm of chromosome 6
- Although worldwide in distribution, increased prevalence in Scandinavians, Japanese, Black Americans, and women
- In Northern Europe, 5 to 40 cases per 100,000 persons. In Black Americans, 35 cases per 100,000 persons; in Caucasian Americans, 11 cases per 100,000 persons (1)

RISK FACTORS
Exact etiology and pathogenesis remain unknown.

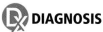 **DIAGNOSIS**

A comprehensive exam should be done in all patients with suspected sarcoidosis.

HISTORY
- Patients may be asymptomatic.
- Patients may have nonspecific complaints, such as the following:
  - Nonproductive cough or shortness of breath
  - Fever or night sweats
  - Weight loss
  - General fatigue
  - Eye pain
  - Chest pain/palpitations
  - Skin lesions
  - Polyarthritis
  - Encephalopathy, seizures, hydrocephalus (rare)
  - Patients >70 years old more likely to have systemic symptoms

PHYSICAL EXAM
- Many patients have a normal physical exam.
- Lungs may reveal wheezing/fine interstitial crackles
- ~30% of patients have extrapulmonary manifestations, including the following:
  - Uveitis or other eye findings: conjunctival nodules, lacrimal gland enlargement, cataracts, glaucoma, papilledema
  - Cranial nerve palsies
  - Salivary gland swelling or lymphadenopathy
  - Arrhythmias
  - Hepatosplenomegaly
  - Polyarthritis
  - Rashes
    ○ Maculopapular of nares, eyelids, forehead, base of neck at hairline, and previous trauma sites
    ○ Waxy nodular of face, trunk, and extensor surfaces of extremities
    ○ Plaques (lupus pernio) of nose, cheeks, chin, and ears
    ○ EN (component of Löfgren syndrome)

DIFFERENTIAL DIAGNOSIS
- Sarcoidosis is a diagnosis of exclusion.
- Infectious granulomatous disease, such as tuberculosis and fungal infections
- Hypersensitivity pneumonitis
- Lymphoma or other malignancies
- Berylliosis

DIAGNOSTIC TESTS & INTERPRETATION
No definitive test for diagnosis, but diagnosis is suggested by the following:
- Clinical and radiographic manifestations
- Exclusion of other diagnoses
- Histopathologic detection of noncaseating granulomas

Initial Tests (lab, imaging)
- CBC: anemia/leukopenia ± eosinophilia
- Hypergammaglobulinemia
- Abnormal liver function and increased alkaline phosphatase with hepatic involvement.

- Hypercalciuria occurs in up to 10% of patients, with hypercalcemia less frequent.
- Serum ACE elevated in >75% of patients but is not diagnostic or exclusionary
  - Drugs may alter lab results: Prednisone will lower serum ACE and normalize gallium scan. ACE inhibitors will lower serum ACE level.
  - Disorders may alter lab results: Hyperthyroidism, diabetes, tuberculosis, other cancers may also increase serum ACE level.
- CXR or CT scan may reveal granulomas/hilar adenopathy. CXRs are staged using Scadding classification.
  - Stage 0 = normal
  - Stage 1 = bilateral hilar adenopathy alone
  - Stage 2 = bilateral hilar adenopathy + parenchymal infiltrates (primarily upper lobes)
  - Stage 3 = parenchymal infiltrates with shrinking hilar adenopathy
  - Stage 4 = parenchymal infiltrates with volume loss, bronchiectasis, calcification, or cyst formation
- High-resolution chest CT scan may reveal peribronchial disease.
- Positron emission tomography (PET) scan can indicate areas of disease activity in lungs, lymph nodes, and other areas of the body but does not differentiate between malignancy and sarcoidosis. Cardiac PET scan may detect cardiac sarcoidosis (1)[C].
- Serum amyloid A and adenosine deaminase has been found to be elevated with sarcoidosis but are not clinically used due to low sensitivity and specificity.

Diagnostic Procedures/Other
- Pulmonary function tests (PFTs) may reveal restrictive pattern with decreased carbon monoxide diffusing capacity (DLCO).
- In active disease, bronchoalveolar lavage fluid has an increased CD4-to-CD8 ratio. Ongoing research on whether the presence of D-dimer in BAL supports diagnosis of sarcoidosis.
- Ophthalmologic examination may reveal uveitis, retinal vasculitis, or conjunctivitis.
- ECG
- Tuberculin skin test
- Biopsy of lesions should reveal noncaseating granulomas.
- If lungs are affected, bronchoscopy with biopsy of central and peripheral airways is helpful. Endobronchial US (EBUS)—guided transbronchial needle aspiration may have a better diagnostic yield.
- Kveim test (ongoing research): Suspension of sterilized splenic cells from a patient with sarcoidosis is injected in an intradermal skin test to evoke a sarcoid granulomatous response over 3 weeks, similar to a tuberculin skin test.

Test Interpretation

Noncaseating epithelioid granulomas without evidence of fungal/mycobacterial infection

 TREATMENT

- Many patients undergo spontaneous remission.
- No treatment may be necessary in asymptomatic individuals, but treatment may be required for cardiac, CNS, renal, or ocular involvement.
- No treatment indicated for asymptomatic patients with stage I to III radiographic changes with normal/mildly abnormal lung function, although close follow-up recommended.
- Treatment of pulmonary manifestations is done on the basis of impairment.
  - Worsening pulmonary symptoms and deteriorating lung function
  - Worsening radiographic findings

MEDICATION

Systemic therapy is indicated for hypercalcemia or cardiac, neurologic, or eye disease. Most patients with pulmonary sarcoidosis do not require treatment with medications as many are asymptomatic or have a spontaneous remission.

First Line

- No FDA-approved treatment for sarcoidosis.
- Systemic corticosteroids in the symptomatic individual or with worsening lung function or radiographic findings
  - Optimal dose of glucocorticoids is not known. Prior to initiating glucocorticoids, must exclude tuberculosis.
  - Usually prednisone, 0.3 to 0.6 mg/kg ideal body weight (20 to 40 mg/day) for 4 to 6 weeks
  - If stable, taper by 5 mg/week to 10 to 20 mg/day over the next 6 weeks.
  - If no relapse, 10 to 20 mg/day for 8 to 12 months. Relapse is common.
  - Higher doses (80 to 100 mg/day) may be warranted in patients with acute respiratory failure and cardiac, neurologic, or ocular disease.
- In patients with skin disease, topical steroids may be effective.
- Inhaled steroids (budesonide 800 to 1,600 μg BID) may be of some clinical benefit in early disease with mild pulmonary symptoms.
  - Contraindications and significant possible interactions: Refer to the manufacturer's profile of each drug (1),(3).

Second Line

- All alternative agents to glucocorticoids carry substantial risk for toxicity, including myelosuppression, hepatotoxicity, and opportunistic infection. Prior to utilizing these medications, assess for steroid compliance, comorbid disease, or other complicating factors contributing to steroid failure. Referral to specialist is recommended.
- Methotrexate: initially 7.5 mg/week, increasing gradually to 10 to 15 mg/week. Cannot be used with underlying liver disease
- Azathioprine: generally a supplement to prednisone in an attempt to lower steroid doses
- Use of immunosuppressants, such as methotrexate or azathioprine, will require regular monitoring of CBC and LFTs.
- Antimalarial agents have been trialed without clear benefit, such as chloroquine or hydroxychloroquine.
- Tumor necrosis factor antagonists, such as infliximab, have been useful in refractory cases (1).

ISSUES FOR REFERRAL

May be followed by a pulmonologist, with referrals to other specialists as dictated by involvement of other organ systems; if requiring a second-line therapy, should be followed by a specialist.

SURGERY/OTHER PROCEDURES

Lung transplantation in severe, refractory cases; long-term outcomes are unknown.

 ONGOING CARE

FOLLOW-UP RECOMMENDATIONS

There is limited data on indications for the specific tests and optimal frequency of monitoring of disease activity. Suggestions follow.

Patient Monitoring

- Patients on prednisone for symptoms should be seen q1–2mo while on therapy.
- Patients not requiring therapy should be seen q3mo for at least the first 2 years after diagnosis, obtaining a history and physical exam, laboratory testing tailored to sites of disease activity, PFTs, and ambulatory pulse oximetry.
- If active disease
  - Every 6 to 12 months, obtain ophthalmologic exam if on hydroxychloroquine.
  - Annually, CBC, creatinine, calcium, LFTs, ECG, 25-hydroxy vitamin D and 1,25 dihydroxyvitamin D, CXR, ophthalmologic examination
- Other testing per individual patient's symptoms, including HRCT, echocardiogram, Holter monitoring, urinalysis (UA), thyroid-stimulating hormone (TSH), bone density, MRI of brain

- The serum ACE level is used by some physicians to follow the disease activity. In patients with an initially elevated ACE level, it should fall toward normal while on the therapy or when the disease resolves.
- If inactive disease, follow annually with history and physical exam, PFTs, ambulatory pulse oximetry, CBC, creatinine, calcium, liver enzymes, 1,25 dihydroxy vitamin D, ECG, and ophthalmologic exam.

PATIENT EDUCATION

- The American Lung Association: https://www.lung.org/lung-health-diseases/lung-disease-lookup/sarcoidosis
- Sarcoidosis by MedlinePlus: www.nlm.nih.gov/medlineplus/sarcoidosis.html

PROGNOSIS

- 50% of patients will have spontaneous resolution within 2 years.
- 25% of patients will have significant fibrosis, but no further worsening of the disease after 2 years.
- 25% of patients (higher in some populations, including Black Americans) will have chronic disease.
- Patients on corticosteroids for >6 months have a greater chance of having chronic disease.
- Overall death rate: <5%

COMPLICATIONS

- Patients may develop significant respiratory involvement, including cor pulmonale. Pulmonary hemorrhage from infection with aspergillosis in the damaged lung is possible.
- Other organs, especially the heart (congestive heart failure, arrhythmias), eyes (rarely blindness), and CNS, can be involved with serious consequences.

REFERENCES

1. Iannuzzi MC, Rybicki BA, Teirstein AS. Sarcoidosis. *N Engl J Med*. 2007;357(21):2153–2165.
2. Dumas O, Abramovitz L, Wiley AS, et al. Epidemiology of sarcoidosis in a prospective cohort study of U.S. women. *Ann Am Thorac Soc*. 2016;13(1):67–71.
3. Melani AS, Bigliazzi C, Cimmino FA. A comprehensive review of sarcoidosis treatment for pulmonologists. *Pulm Ther*. 2021;7(2):325–344.

CODES

ICD10

- D86.89 Sarcoidosis of other sites
- D86.81 Sarcoid meningitis
- D86.2 Sarcoidosis of lung with sarcoidosis of lymph nodes

CLINICAL PEARLS

- Sarcoidosis is a noninfectious, multisystem, granulomatous disease of unknown cause, typically affecting young and middle-aged adults.
- Diagnosis is based on clinical findings, exclusion of other disorders, and pathologic detection of noncaseating granulomas.

S

SCABIES
Roland W. Newman II, DO • Matthew J. Kor, MD

BASICS

DESCRIPTION
- A contagious parasitic infection of the skin caused by the mite *Sarcoptes scabiei*, var. *hominis*
- Typically, a clinical diagnosis based on history and physical exam
- System(s) affected: skin/exocrine

EPIDEMIOLOGY
Incidence
- Predominant age: children, sexually active young adults, and the elderly
- Male children from lower income quartiles were more likely to visit the ED in a retrospective analysis of nationally representative National Emergency Department Sample for 2013 to 2015, whereas older male patients, insured by Medicare, from the highest income quartile in the Midwest/West were most likely to be admitted to the hospital (1).

Prevalence
Prevalence varies substantially worldwide but is more common in resource-poor settings.
- More prevalent in areas of overcrowding and in developing countries, particularly tropical climates
- Added to World Health Organization's list of neglected tropical diseases in 2017

ETIOLOGY AND PATHOPHYSIOLOGY
- *S. scabiei*, var. *hominis*
  - An obligate human parasite
  - Primarily transmitted by prolonged human-to-human direct skin contact
  - Infrequently transmitted via fomites (e.g., bedding, clothing, or furnishings)
- Female mite lays eggs in burrows in the stratum corneum and epidermis.
- Itching is caused by a delayed type IV hypersensitivity reaction to the mite saliva, eggs, or excrement.

RISK FACTORS
- Prolonged skin-to-skin contact (e.g., sexual, overcrowding, nosocomial infection)
- Poor nutritional status, poverty, and homelessness
- Hot, tropical climates
- Seasonal variation: Incidence may be higher in the winter than in the summer (due to overcrowding).
- Immunocompromised patients, including those with HIV/AIDS, are at increased risk of developing severe (crusted/Norwegian) scabies.

GENERAL PREVENTION
Prevent outbreaks by prompt treatment and cleansing of fomites (see "General Measures").

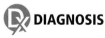 DIAGNOSIS

HISTORY
- Generalized itching is often severe and worse at night.
- Identify potential contact with infected individuals.
- Initial/primary infection usually asymptomatic for the first 3 to 4 weeks (until sensitivity occurs)
- Subsequent reinfection typically develops symptoms after only 1 to 3 days.

PHYSICAL EXAM
- Lesions (inflammatory, erythematous, pruritic papules) most commonly located in the finger webs, flexor surfaces of the wrists, elbows, axillae, buttocks, genitalia, feet, and ankles; often spares the head/neck in adults

- Burrows (thin, curvy lines in the upper epidermis that measure 1 to 10 mm in length)—a pathognomonic sign of scabies most common in hands and wrists
- Secondary erosions and excoriations from scratching
- Pustules (if secondarily infected)
- Pruritic papular or nodular lesions in covered areas (buttocks, groin, axillae) resulting from an exaggerated hypersensitivity reaction
- Crusted scabies (or Norwegian scabies) is a psoriasiform dermatosis occurring with hyperinfestation with thousands/millions of mites (more common in immunosuppressed patients).

Geriatric Considerations
The elderly often itch more severely despite fewer cutaneous lesions and are at risk for extensive infestations, perhaps related to a decline in cell-mediated immunity. There may be back involvement in those who are bedridden.

Pediatric Considerations
Infants and very young children often present with vesicles, papules, and pustules and have more widespread involvement, including the hands, palms, feet, soles, body folds, and head (rare for adults).

DIFFERENTIAL DIAGNOSIS
- Atopic dermatitis
- Contact dermatitis
- Dermatitis herpetiformis
- Eczema
- Folliculitis/impetigo
- Insect bites
- Papular urticaria
- Pediculosis corporis
- Psoriasis (crusted scabies)
- Pyoderma
- Seborrheic dermatitis
- Syphilis
- Tinea corporis

DIAGNOSTIC TESTS & INTERPRETATION
- Based on 2018 IACS (International Alliance Control for Scabies) Criteria for the Diagnosis of Scabies:
  - Confirmed scabies diagnosis: based on microscopic identification of mites, eggs, or fecal pellets (scybala) OR visualization of mite with dermoscopy
  - Clinical scabies diagnosis: detection of burrows, OR typical lesions on male genitalia, OR typical lesions in a typical distribution with two history features of itch and known infectious contact
  - Suspected scabies diagnosis: typical lesions in a typical distribution with one history feature of itch or known infectious contact, OR atypical lesions or atypical distribution with two history features of itch and known infectious contact
- A failure to find mites does not rule out scabies.

Initial Tests (lab, imaging)
CBC is rarely needed but may show eosinophilia.

Diagnostic Procedures/Other
- Examination of skin with dermoscopy
  - Look for typical burrows in finger webs, on flexor aspect of the wrists, and on the penis.
  - Look for a dark point at the end of the burrow (the mite, also known as "delta wing sign").
- Skin scraping
  - Place a drop of mineral oil over a nonexcoriated lesion or burrow.
  - Scrape the lesion with a surgical blade (no. 15).
  - Examine scrapings under a microscope for mites, eggs, egg casings, or feces.

- Scraping under fingernails may be positive.
  - When mite is not found with scraping, biopsy may reveal mite, eggs, or feces (2).
- Potassium hydroxide (KOH) wet mount NOT recommended because it can dissolve mite pellets
- Burrow ink test
  - If burrows are not obvious, apply gentian violet or India ink to an area of rash. Wash off the ink with alcohol. A burrow should remain stained and become more evident. Then apply mineral oil, scrape, and observe microscopically, as noted previously.

Test Interpretation
Skin biopsy of a nodule (although performed rarely) will reveal portions of the mite in the corneal layer.

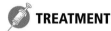 TREATMENT

GENERAL MEASURES
- Treat all intimate contacts (including close household and family members).
- Treat items in contact with skin. Wash all clothing, bed linens, and towels in hot (60°C) water and dry in hot dryer. Personal items that cannot be washed should be sealed in a plastic bag for at least 7 days.
- Itching and dermatitis can persist for up to 4 weeks despite appropriate treatment and can be treated with oral antihistamines and/or topical/oral corticosteroids. It is important to educate patients this is likely not a sign of treatment failure. However, persistent symptoms greater than 4 weeks posttreatment may need further workup for an alternative diagnosis, failure of initial treatment, or irritation secondary to treatment (2).

MEDICATION
First Line
- Permethrin 5% cream (Elimite) is generally accepted as first-line therapy (3)[A].
  - After bathing or showering, apply cream from the neck to the soles of the feet, paying particular attention to areas that are most involved and then wash off after 8 to 14 hours.
  - It is recommended to repeat treatment 1 to 2 weeks later.
  - The adult dose is usually 30 g per treatment.
  - Side effects include itching, stinging, erythema, and burning (minimal absorption).
- Ivermectin (Stromectol) (3)[A]
  - Not FDA-approved for scabies
  - 200 μg/kg PO as a single dose, which may be repeated in 2 weeks, is an option according to the CDC. Failure of a second dose of ivermectin has been shown to be a predictor of unsuccessful treatment (4).
  - Take with food to improve bioavailability and enhance penetration into the epidermis.
  - May need higher doses or may need to use in combination with topical scabicide for HIV-positive patients
  - Side effects may include headache and nausea (5).
- Both permethrin and ivermectin are associated with high clearance rates in the treatment of scabies without highly significant differences between the two (5).
- Choice between either permethrin or ivermectin can be based on availability, practicality, and associated cost depending on the individual situation (5).
  Crusted scabies often require more frequent application of permethrin (q2–3d for 1 to 2 weeks) in combination with repeated doses of PO ivermectin on days 1, 2, 8, 9, and 15. Severe cases may need further dosing of ivermectin on days 22 and 29.

Pediatric Considerations
- Permethrin may be used on infants >2 months of age. In children <5 years of age, the cream should be applied to the head and neck as well as to the entire body.
- PO ivermectin should be avoided in children <5 years and in those weighing <15 kg.

Second Line
- Crotamiton (Eurax) 10% cream may be used on infants >3 months of age.
  - Apply from the neck down for 24 hours, rinse off, reapply for an additional 24 to 48 hours, and then thoroughly wash off.
  - Nodular scabies: Apply to nodules for 24 hours, rinse off, reapply for an additional 24 hours, and then thoroughly wash off.
- Precipitated sulfur 2–10% in petrolatum
  - Not FDA-approved for scabies
  - Apply to the entire body from the neck down for 24 hours, rinse by bathing and then repeat for 2 more days (3 days total). It is malodorous and messy but is thought to be safer than lindane, especially in infants <6 months of age and safer than permethrin in infants <2 months of age.
- Lindane (γ-benzene hexachloride, Kwell) 1% lotion
  - Apply a thin layer to all skin surfaces from the neck down and wash off 6 to 8 hours later.
  - Two applications 1 week apart are recommended but may increase the risk of toxicity.
  - 2 oz is usually adequate for an adult.
  - Side effects: neurotoxicity (seizures, muscle spasms), aplastic anemia
  - Contraindications: uncontrolled seizure disorder, premature infants
  - Precautions: Do not use on excoriated skin, on immunocompromised patients, in conditions that may increase risk of seizures, or with medications that decrease seizure threshold.
  - Possible interactions: concomitant use with medications that lower the seizure threshold.
  - Some instances of lindane-resistant scabies have been reported. These cases do respond to permethrin.

ALERT
Lindane: FDA black box warning of severe neurologic toxicity; use only when all other agents have failed.

Pediatric Considerations
- The FDA recommends caution when using lindane in patients who weigh <50 kg. It is not recommended for infants and is contraindicated in premature infants.
- Infants <2 months should be treated with crotamiton or sulfur preparation.

Pregnancy Considerations
- Permethrin is pregnancy Category B, and lindane, ivermectin, and crotamiton are Category C.
- Permethrin is considered compatible with lactation, but if permethrin is used while breastfeeding, the infant should be bottle-fed until the cream has been thoroughly washed off.

ISSUES FOR REFERRAL
Consider referral to dermatology if unable to confirm diagnosis and/or resistant to repeated treatments.

ADDITIONAL THERAPIES
- Crusted scabies may require use of keratolytics to improve penetration of permethrin.
- Nodular scabies may require intralesional steroids for complete resolution, if they persist for several weeks after treatment.

- Benzyl benzoate lotion (not available in the United States but used widely in developing countries)
  - Not FDA-approved for scabies
  - Dose for adults is 25–28%; dilute to 12.5% for children and 6.25% for infants.
  - After bathing, apply lotion from the neck to soles of feet for 24 hours.
- Topical ivermectin 1% lotion (investigational, moderate level of certainty)
  - Not FDA-approved for scabies
  - Apply to affected sites and wash off 8 hours later (3)[A].

COMPLEMENTARY & ALTERNATIVE MEDICINE
Tea tree oil (TTO) derived from the plant Melaleuca alternifolia is a safe, effective, and generally well tolerated alternative option as a treatment for scabies.
- 5% TTO has proven efficacy as a scabicidal agent in vitro.
- Topical application of TTO is generally associated with a low incidence of adverse effects (irritant or localized reactions to the oil) (6).
  - Most irritant skin reactions can be avoided by use of TTO concentrations of less than 20% (6).

 ## ONGOING CARE

FOLLOW-UP RECOMMENDATIONS
Patient Monitoring
Recheck patient at weekly intervals only if rash or itching persists. Scrape new lesions and retreat if mites or products are found.

PATIENT EDUCATION
- Patients should be instructed on proper application and cautioned not to overuse the medication when applying it to the skin.
- A patient fact sheet is available from the CDC: http://www.cdc.gov/parasites/scabies/

PROGNOSIS
Lesions begin to regress in 1 to 2 days, but eczema and itching may persist for up to 4 weeks after treatment.

COMPLICATIONS
- Eczema
- Nodules (nodular scabies) may persist for weeks to months after treatment.
- Postscabetic pruritus
- Poor sleep due to pruritus
- Pyoderma
- Secondary bacterial infection (more common in developing countries). Impetigo due to Group A Streptococci and Staphylococcus aureus may lead to sepsis, poststreptococcal glomerulonephritis, and rheumatic heart disease.
- Social stigma

REFERENCES
1. Tripathi R, Knusel KD, Ezaldein HH, et al. Emergency department visits due to scabies in the United States: a retrospective analysis of a nationally representative emergency department sample. Clin Infect Dis. 2020;70(3):509–517.
2. Gunning K, Pippitt K, Kiraly B, et al. Lice and scabies: treatment update. Am Fam Physician. 2019;99(10):635–642.
3. Rosumeck S, Nast A, Dressler C. Ivermectin and permethrin for treating scabies. Cochrane Database Syst Rev. 2018;(4):CD012994.
4. Aussy A, Houivet E, Hebert V, et al. Risk factors for treatment failure in scabies. Br J Dermatol. 2019;180(4):e121–e121.
5. Rosumeck S, Nast A, Dressler C. Evaluation of ivermectin vs permethrin for treating scabies—summary of a Cochrane review. JAMA Dermatol. 2019;155(6):730–732. doi:10.1001/jamadermatol .2019.0279.
6. Thomas J, Carson CF, Peterson GM, et al. Therapeutic potential of tea tree oil for scabies. Am J of Trop Med Hyg. 2016;94(2):258–266.

ADDITIONAL READING
- Chosidow O, Roderick J. Control of scabies and secondary impetigo: optimising treatment effectiveness in endemic settings. Lancet Infect Dis. 2019;19(5):454–456.
- Engelman D, Fuller LC, Steer AC; for International Alliance for the Control of Scabies Delphi Panel. Consensus criteria for the diagnosis of scabies: a Delphi study of international experts. PLoS Negl Trop Dis. 2018;12(5):e0006549.
- Gopinath H, Aishwarya M, Karthikeyan K. Tackling scabies: novel agents for a neglected disease. Intl J Dermatol. 2018;57(11):1293–1298. doi:10.1111/ijd.13999.
- Romani L, Steer AC, Whitfeld MJ, et al. Prevalence of scabies and impetigo worldwide: a systematic review. Lancet Infect Dis. 2015;15(8):960–967.
- Strong M, Johnstone P. Interventions for treating scabies. Cochrane Database Syst Rev. 2007;(3):CD000320.
- Yeoh D, Asha B, Carapetis JR. Impetigo and scabies–disease burden and modern treatment strategies. J Infect. 2016;72:S61–S67.

 ## SEE ALSO

Arthropod Bites and Stings; Pediculosis (Lice)

 ## CODES

ICD10
B86 Scabies

CLINICAL PEARLS
- Prior to diagnosis, use of a topical steroid to treat pruritic symptoms may mask symptoms and is termed scabies incognito.
- Environmental control is recommended. All linens, towels, and clothing used in the previous 4 days should be washed in hot water or dry-cleaned. Personal items that cannot be washed or dry-cleaned should be sealed in a plastic bag for 7 days.
- All intimate contacts should receive treatment.
- Close contacts (those sharing the same bed or who have intimate contact) may not show signs and symptoms immediately but should be treated simultaneously to avoid reinfestation.
- Eczema and itching may persist for up to 4 weeks after treatment, causing many patients to falsely believe that they have failed treatment or are being reinfected.
- In patients with actual reinfection, it is possible the patient has not applied the medication properly or, more likely, the index patient has not been identified and treated.

SCARLET FEVER

Christina Scartozzi, DO • Leesha A. Helm, MD, MPH

BASICS

DESCRIPTION
- A disease (typically in childhood) characterized by fever, pharyngitis, and rash caused by group A β-hemolytic *Streptococcus pyogenes* (GAS) that produces erythrogenic toxin
- Incubation period: 1 to 7 days
- Duration of illness: 4 to 10 days
- Rash usually appears within 24 to 48 hours after symptom onset.
- Rash first appears in the groin, trunk, and axillae accompanied by strawberry tongue and circumoral pallor and then rapidly spreads outward all over the body.
- Rash clears at the end of the 1st week and is followed by several weeks of desquamation.
- Rash is not dangerous but is a marker for GAS infection with suppurative and nonsuppurative complications.
- System(s) affected: head, eyes, ears, nose, throat, skin/exocrine
- Synonym(s): scarlatina

EPIDEMIOLOGY
Incidence
- In developed countries, 15% of school age children and 4–10% of adults have an episode of GAS pharyngitis each year.
- Scarlet fever is rare in infancy because of maternal antitoxin antibodies.
- Predominant age: 6 to 12 years
- Peak age: 4 to 8 years
- Predominant sex: male = female
- Rare in the United States in persons >12 years because of high rates (>80%) of lifelong protective antibodies to erythrogenic toxins

Prevalence
- 15–30% of cases of pharyngitis in children are due to GAS; 5–15% in adults
- <10% of children with streptococcal pharyngitis develop scarlet fever.

ETIOLOGY AND PATHOPHYSIOLOGY
- Erythrogenic toxin production is necessary to develop scarlet fever.
- Three toxin types: A, B, C
- Toxins damage capillaries (producing rash) and act as superantigens, stimulating cytokine release.
- Antibodies to toxins prevent development of rash but do not protect against underlying infection.
- Primary site of streptococcal infection is usually within the tonsils, but scarlet fever may also occur with infection of skin, surgical wounds, or uterus (puerperal scarlet fever).

RISK FACTORS
- Winter/early spring seasonal increase
- More common in school-aged children
- Contact with infected individual(s)
- Crowded living conditions (e.g., lower socioeconomic status, barracks, child care, schools)

GENERAL PREVENTION
- Spread by contact with airborne respiratory droplets, saliva, and nasal secretions
- Foodborne outbreaks have been reported, but are rare.
- Asymptomatic contacts do not require cultures/prophylaxis.

- Symptomatic contacts of a child with documented GAS infection who have recent or current clinical evidence of a GAS infection should undergo appropriate laboratory tests and should be treated if test results are positive.
- Children should not return to school/daycare until they are afebrile and have received 24 hours of antibiotic therapy.

COMMONLY ASSOCIATED CONDITIONS
- Pharyngitis
- Impetigo
- Rheumatic fever
- Glomerulonephritis

DIAGNOSIS

HISTORY
Prodrome 1 to 2 days
- Sore throat
- Headache
- Myalgias
- Malaise
- Fever (>38°C [100.4°F])
- Vomiting
- Abdominal pain (may mimic acute abdomen)
- Rash—scarlatiniform erythematous punctate eruption
- Cough, conjunctivitis, hoarseness, diarrhea, coryza, oral ulceration, and rhinorrhea are more commonly associated with viral infections.

PHYSICAL EXAM
- Oral exam
  - Beefy red tonsils and pharynx with/without exudate
  - Petechiae on palate
  - White coating on tongue: White strawberry tongue appears on days 1 to 2. This sheds by days 4 to 5, leaving a red strawberry tongue, which is shiny and erythematous with prominent papillae.
- Exanthem (appears within 1 to 5 days)
  - Scarlet, nonconfluent, 1 to 2 mm papules with generalized erythema; blanches when pressed
  - Orange-red punctate skin eruption with sandpaper-like texture, "sunburn with goose pimples"
  - Coarse "sand paper" rash, initially appearing in groin, upper trunk, and axillae and then spreading outward to extremities; prominent in skin folds, flexural surfaces (e.g., axillae, groin, buttocks), with sparing of palms and soles
  - Flushed face with circumoral pallor, red lips
  - Pastia lines: transverse red streaks in skin folds of abdomen, antecubital space, and axillae
  - Desquamation begins on face after 7 to 10 days and proceeds over trunk to hands and feet; may persist for 6 weeks
  - In severe cases, small vesicular lesions (miliary sudamina) may appear on abdomen, hands, and feet.

DIFFERENTIAL DIAGNOSIS
- Viral exanthem: measles; rubella; roseola; erythema infectiosum (fifth disease)
- Infectious mononucleosis
- *Mycoplasma* pneumonia
- Secondary syphilis
- Toxic shock syndrome
- Staphylococcal scalded-skin syndrome
- Kawasaki disease
- Acute systemic lupus erythematosus
- Juvenile arthritis

- Drug hypersensitivity
- Severe sunburn

DIAGNOSTIC TESTS & INTERPRETATION
- The signs and symptoms of streptococcal and nonstreptococcal pharyngitis overlap too broadly for diagnosis to be made with precision on clinical grounds alone. Even patients with all clinical features are confirmed to have streptococcal pharyngitis only about 35–50% of the time, particularly in children.
- Use results from rapid antigen detection testing (RADT) or polymerase chain reaction (PCR)-based rapid testing.
- Modified Centor clinical decision rule
  - Absence of cough — 1 point
  - Swollen, tender anterior cervical nodes — 1 point
  - Temperature 100.4°F (38°C) — 1 point
  - Tonsillar exudate or swelling — 1 point
  - Age:
    - 3 to 14 years — 1 point
    - 15 to 44 years — 0 point
    - >45 years — −1 point
- Cumulative score
  - 0: Risk of GAS pharyngitis 1–2.5%—no further testing or antibiotics indicated
  - 1: Risk of GAS pharyngitis 5–10%—no further testing or antibiotics indicated—option to perform throat culture or RADT—treat if positive
  - 2: Risk of GAS pharyngitis 11–17%—perform throat culture or RADT—treat if positive
  - 3: Risk of GAS pharyngitis 28–35%—perform throat culture or RADT—treat if positive
  - 4+: Risk of GAS pharyngitis 51–53%—consider empiric treatment with antibiotics
- Testing for GAS pharyngitis is *not recommended* for patients with symptoms suggesting a viral etiology (e.g., cough, coryza, diarrhea, conjunctivitis, rhinorrhea, hoarseness, oral ulcers).

Initial Tests (lab, imaging)
- RADT: diagnostic if positive, sensitivity approaches that of culture, 95% specific. In children, negative RADT should be confirmed by throat culture (not necessary in adults). Positive RADT does not require confirmatory culture (1)[C].
- PCR: diagnostic if positive, 100% sensitive, 94.1% specific, 84.1% positive predictive value, 100% negative predictive value. Positive PCR does not require confirmatory culture.
- Throat culture is the gold standard to confirm streptococcal infection (99% specific, 90–97% sensitive; 5–10% of healthy individuals are carriers) (1).
- Serologic tests (antistreptolysin O titer and streptozyme tests, antihyaluronidase): Confirm recent GAS infection; not helpful or recommended for diagnosis of acute disease
- Gram stain: gram-positive cocci in chains
- CBC may show elevated WBC count (12,000 to 16,000/mm^3); eosinophilia later (second week)
- Follow-up (posttreatment) throat cultures or RADT/PCR not routinely recommended
- Diagnostic testing and empiric treatment of asymptomatic household contacts of patients with acute streptococcal pharyngitis is not routinely recommended (2)[B].

Follow-Up Tests & Special Considerations
- Recent antibiotic therapy may impact culture results.
- Within 5 days of symptoms, antibiotics can delay/abolish antistreptolysin O response.

Test Interpretation
Skin lesions reveal characteristic inflammatory reaction, specifically hyperemia, edema, and polymorphonuclear cell infiltration.

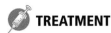 **TREATMENT**

GENERAL MEASURES
Supportive care; analgesic/antipyretic such as acetaminophen or NSAID, for moderate to severe symptoms or to control fever. Symptomatic treatment can include medicated throat lozenges and topical anesthetics.

MEDICATION
First Line
The primary reason for treating GAS is to decrease the risk of acute rheumatic fever. Early treatment decreases duration of symptoms by 1 to 2 days and decreases the period of contagiousness. Penicillin is the drug of choice for GAS pharyngitis given its proven efficacy, safety, narrow spectrum, and low cost.

- Penicillin (PO; penicillin V and others) for 10 days
  - 250 mg PO BID or TID for <27 kg (60 lb); 250 mg QID or 500 mg BID for >27 kg (60 lb) adolescents and adults (1)[A],(3)[A],(4)
  - If compliance is questionable, use penicillin G benzathine: single IM dose 600,000 U for <27 kg (60 lb); 1.2 mU for those >27 kg
- Amoxicillin (PO) 50 mg/kg (max dose 1,000 mg) once daily or 25 mg/kg (max dose 500 mg) twice daily for 10 days (use only for definitive GAS because it can induce rash with some viral infections)
  - Contraindications: penicillin allergy
  - Amoxicillin has similar efficacy to penicillin and is more palatable for children (5).
- Precautions: Avoid in patients with penicillin allergy (anaphylaxis).

Second Line
For patients allergic to penicillin
- Type IV hypersensitivity to penicillin:
  - Oral cephalosporins: Many are effective, but 1st-generation cephalosporins are less expensive:
    ○ Cephalexin 20 mg/kg dose twice daily for 10 days; max 500 mg every 12 hours (1)[A]
    ○ Cefadroxil 30 mg/kg once daily; max 1,000 mg for 10 days (1)
- Type I hypersensitivity to penicillin:
  - Azithromycin (Zithromax, Z pack): 12 mg/kg/day (max 500 mg) for 5 days (3)[A]
  - Clarithromycin (Biaxin): children >6 months: 7.5 mg/kg BID for 10 days; adults: 250 mg BID for 10 days
  - Clindamycin 7 mg/kg (max 300 mg/dose) TID for 10 days (3)[B]
- Tetracyclines and sulfonamides should not be used.

ALERT
Avoid aspirin in children due to risk of Reye syndrome.

ISSUES FOR REFERRAL
Peritonsillar abscess/retropharyngeal abscess; shock symptoms: hypotension, disseminated intravascular coagulation (DIC), cardiac, liver, renal dysfunction

SURGERY/OTHER PROCEDURES
- Tonsillectomy is recommended with recurrent bouts of pharyngitis (≥6 positive strep cultures in 1 year).
- Although children still may get streptococcal pharyngitis ("strep throat") after a tonsillectomy, the procedure reduces the frequency and severity of infections.

 ONGOING CARE

FOLLOW-UP RECOMMENDATIONS
Follow-up throat culture not needed unless symptomatic

Patient Monitoring
GAS is uniformly susceptible to penicillin, treatment failures are typically due to:
- Poor adherence to recommended antibiotic therapy
- β-Lactamase oral flora hydrolyzing penicillin
- GAS carrier state and concurrent viral rash (requires no treatment)
- Repeat exposure to carriers in family: Streptococci persist on unrinsed toothbrushes and orthodontic appliances for up to 15 days.
- Retreat recurrent GAS pharyngitis with the same agent, an alternative oral agent, or IM penicillin G.

DIET
No special diet

PATIENT EDUCATION
- Delay in treatment awaiting culture results does not increase the risk of rheumatic fever.
- Complete the entire course of antibiotics.
- Children should not return to school/daycare until they have received >24 hours of antibiotic therapy.
- Can spread person to person. Personal hygiene is important (wash hands, don't share utensils).
- "Recurring strep throat: When is tonsillectomy useful?": http://www.mayoclinic.org/diseasesconditions/strep-throat/expert-answers/recurringstrep-throat/faq-20058360

PROGNOSIS
- Treatment shortens symptoms by 12 to 24 hours.
- Recurrent attacks are possible (different erythrogenic toxins).

COMPLICATIONS
- Suppurative
  - Sinusitis
  - Otitis media/mastoiditis
  - Cervical lymphadenitis
  - Peritonsillar abscess/retropharyngeal abscess
  - Pneumonia
  - Bacteremia with metastatic infectious foci: meningitis, brain abscess, osteomyelitis, septic arthritis, endocarditis, intracranial venous sinus thrombosis, necrotizing fasciitis
- Nonsuppurative
  - Rheumatic fever: Therapy prevents rheumatic fever when started as long as 10 days after onset of acute GAS infection.
  - Glomerulonephritis: due to nephritogenic strain of *Streptococcus*; prevention even after adequate treatment of GAS is less certain.
  - Streptococcal toxic shock syndrome: fever; hypotension; DIC; and cardiac, liver, and/or kidney dysfunction due to other toxin-mediated sequelae
  - Poststreptococcal reactive arthritis—a reactive arthritis following a pharyngeal streptococcal infection with a symptom-free interval and subsequent aseptic inflammation of one or more joints typically without cardiac involvement
  - Cellulitis
  - Weeks to months later, may develop transverse grooves in nail plates and hair loss (telogen effluvium)
  - Pediatric autoimmune neuropsychiatric disorder associated with GAS (PANDAS). A subset of children has been recognized whose symptoms of obsessive-compulsive disorder (OCD) or tic disorders are exacerbated by GAS infection.

REFERENCES
1. Kalra MG, Higgins KE, Perez ED. Common questions about streptococcal pharyngitis. *Am Fam Physician*. 2016;94(1):24–31.
2. Shulman ST, Bisno AL, Clegg HW, et al. Clinical practice guideline for the diagnosis and management of group A streptococcal pharyngitis: 2012 update by the Infectious Diseases Society of America. *Clin Infect Dis*. 2012;55(10):1279–1282.
3. Gerber MA, Baltimore RS, Eaton CB, et al. Prevention of rheumatic fever and diagnosis and treatment of acute streptococcal pharyngitis: a scientific statement from the American Heart Association Rheumatic Fever, Endocarditis, and Kawasaki Disease Committee of the Council on Cardiovascular Disease in the Young, the Interdisciplinary Council on Functional Genomics and Translational Biology, and the Interdisciplinary Council on Quality of Care and Outcomes Research: endorsed by the American Academy of Pediatrics. *Circulation*. 2009;119(11):1541–1551.
4. van Driel ML, De Sutter AI, Thorning S, et al. Different antibiotic treatments for group A streptococcal pharyngitis. *Cochrane Database Syst Rev*. 2021;(3):CD004406.
5. Choby BA. Diagnosis and treatment of Streptococcal Pharyngitis. *Am Fam Physician*. 2009;79(5):383–390.

ADDITIONAL READING
- Basetti S, Hodgson J, Rawson TM, et al. Scarlet fever: a guide for general practitioners. *London J Prim Care (Abingdon)*. 2017;9(5):77–79.
- Dietrich ML, Steele RW. Group A *Streptococcus*. *Pediatr Rev*. 2018;39(8):379–391.
- Committee on Infectious Diseases. Group A streptococcal infections. In: Kimberlin DW, Brady MT, Jackson MA, eds. *Red Book: 2018 Report of the Committee on Infectious Diseases*. 31st ed. Elk Grove Village, IL: American Academy of Pediatrics; 2018:748–762.

 SEE ALSO

- Pharyngitis
- Algorithm: Pharyngitis

CODES

ICD10
- A38.9 Scarlet fever, uncomplicated
- J02.0 Streptococcal pharyngitis
- A38.0 Scarlet fever with otitis media

CLINICAL PEARLS
- Consider scarlet fever in the differential diagnosis of children with fever and an exanthematous rash.
- Key clinical findings include strawberry tongue, circumoral pallor, and a coarse sandpaper rash.
- Desquamation (7 to 10 days after symptom onset) may last for several weeks following scarlet fever.
- Diagnose GAS pharyngitis using a validated clinical decision rule (modified Centor score) and selective use of RADT.
- Penicillin remains the drug of choice; however, amoxicillin is as effective and is more palatable for children.

S

SCHIZOPHRENIA

Lauren Elizabeth Kwan, MD • Jeffrey Stovall, MD

BASICS

A severe and persistent mental illness characterized by delusions, hallucinations, disorganization of thought and behavior, cognitive dysfunction, and impairment in reality testing

DESCRIPTION
- Major psychiatric disorder with a variable course, typically involving prodromal, active, and residual psychotic symptoms with disturbances in thought, speech, affect, behavior, and perception
- *DSM-5* eliminated subcategories of schizophrenia (paranoid, disorganized, catatonic, etc.).
- System(s) affected: central nervous system (CNS)

EPIDEMIOLOGY
Incidence
- 7.7 to 43/100,000
- Predominant sex: male-to-female ratio = 1.4:1.0
- Age of onset: typically <30 years, earlier in males (late teens to mid-20s) than in females (early 20s to early 30s), with a smaller peak that occurs in women >45 years; more subtle changes in cognition and functioning can precede the diagnosis (prodromal period) by several years.

Prevalence
- Lifetime (1%): highest prevalence in lower socioeconomic classes and urban settings (2-fold higher risk)
- 1.1% of the population >18 years old; similar rates in all countries

ETIOLOGY AND PATHOPHYSIOLOGY
- Stems from a complex interaction between genetic and environmental factors; higher incidence if prenatal infection or hypoxia, winter births, first-generation immigrants, advanced paternal age, drug use, and genetic (velocardiofacial) syndromes
- Overstimulation of mesolimbic dopamine D_2 receptors, deficient prefrontal dopamine, and aberrant prefrontal glutamate (NMDA) activity results in perceptual disturbances, disordered thought process, and cognitive impairments

Genetics
If first-degree biologic relative has schizophrenia, risk is 8–10% (a 10-fold increase).

GENERAL PREVENTION
Educate all patients on the risks around marijuana use, especially those in a potential prodromal period or those with a family history of psychosis.

COMMONLY ASSOCIATED CONDITIONS
- Nicotine dependence (>50%) and substance use disorders
- Metabolic syndrome, diabetes mellitus, obesity, and infectious diseases, including HIV, hepatitis B, and hepatitis C all occur in higher-than-expected rates.

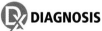

DIAGNOSIS

Focus on identifying an insidious social and functional decline over a ≥ 6-month period (differentiates schizophrenia from brief psychotic and schizophreniform disorders). At least 2 of the following core symptoms must be present for ≥1 month:
- Delusions (fixed, false beliefs)
- Hallucinations (auditory > visual disturbances)

- Disorganized thought (derailed or incoherent speech)
- Grossly disorganized/catatonic behavior (hyper- or hypoactive movements that are often repetitive)
- Negative symptoms (diminished emotional expression, poverty of speech and thought, amotivation, lack of social interest)

PHYSICAL EXAM
No physical findings characterize the illness; however, chronic treatment with neuroleptic agents may result in extrapyramidal symptoms, including dystonia (sustained muscle contractions), akathisia (restlessness), parkinsonism (tremor, shuffling gait), or tardive dyskinesia (repetitive, involuntary movements).

DIFFERENTIAL DIAGNOSIS
- Brief psychotic disorder (symptom duration <1 month)
- Schizophreniform disorder (symptom duration 1 to 6 months)
- Psychotic disorder due to another medical condition
- Disorientation and altered level of arousal raise concern for delirium.
- Substance-induced psychosis: secondary to substance use/abuse, such as cocaine, hallucinogens (amphetamines, LSD, phencyclidine), cannabis (including synthetic), bath salts, alcohol, or prescribed medications including steroids, anticholinergics, and opiates
  - About 25% of patients with substance-induced psychosis will transition to schizophrenia. Highest transition rates are associated with cannabis use (1)[A].
- Personality disorders: paranoid, schizotypal, schizoid, borderline personality disorders
- Mood disorders: bipolar disorder, major depressive disorders with psychotic features or catatonia
- Posttraumatic stress disorder
- Autism spectrum disorder or neurodevelopmental disorders

DIAGNOSTIC TESTS & INTERPRETATION
- No tests are available to diagnose schizophrenia.
- Imaging (MRI), EEG, LP, and laboratory tests may be indicated to rule out other causes and may be used as clinical presentation warrants.

Initial Tests (lab, imaging)
- The following labs are often used to rule out a medical etiology of psychotic symptoms (2):
  - Thyroid-stimulating hormone (TSH), complete blood count (CBC), blood chemistries
  - Vitamin levels (thiamine, vitamin D, methylmalonic acid/vitamin B_{12}, folate)
  - Drug/alcohol screen of blood and urine, urinalysis
  - Syphilis screen, HIV
  - Heavy-metal exposure: lead, mercury
  - Ceruloplasmin, urine porphobilinogen as indicated
  - Erythrocyte sedimentation rate, antinuclear antibody
  - Hepatitis C, hepatitis B
- The following labs are used to assess for comorbidities and baseline values prior to antipsychotic initiation:
  - Electrocardiogram (ECG) for baseline QTc
  - CBC, blood chemistries, TSH, hemoglobin A1C
  - Lipid panel
  - Pregnancy test, if indicated

Follow-Up Tests & Special Considerations
Clinical and laboratory tests for routine monitoring, at least yearly, if using antipsychotic medications:
- Weight, waist circumference, and blood pressure
- CBC, hemoglobin A1C, lipid panel
- Pregnancy test and prolactin level, if indicated
- ECG, monitoring for QTc prolongation
- Clinical assessment of extrapyramidal symptoms using a standardized test such as the Abnormal Involuntary Movement Scale (AIMS)

Diagnostic Procedures/Other
Neuropsychological testing: not a routine part of assessment but can help assess cognitive level to predict functioning and need for assistance

Test Interpretation
No diagnostic pathologic findings; however, ventriculomegaly is frequently seen on MRI with whole brain gray matter loss and white matter loss in medial temporal lobe structures preferentially.

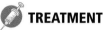

TREATMENT

MEDICATION
First Line
- Two classes of antipsychotic medications: typical and atypical. First-line treatment is with an atypical antipsychotic given lower potential for extrapyramidal side effects.
  - Atypical (2nd generation)
    - Risperidone, olanzapine, ziprasidone, aripiprazole, quetiapine, paliperidone, iloperidone, asenapine, lurasidone, clozapine, brexpiprazole, cariprazine, pimavanserin (Parkinson disease–related psychosis)
  - Typical (1st generation)
    - Haloperidol, chlorpromazine, fluphenazine, trifluoperazine, perphenazine, thioridazine, thiothixene, loxapine
- Medication choice is based on clinical and subjective response and side-effect profile (3)
  - Sensitivity to extrapyramidal adverse effects: atypical
  - For least risk of tardive dyskinesia: quetiapine, clozapine
  - For least risk of metabolic syndrome: aripiprazole, ziprasidone, lurasidone, perphenazine, brexpiprazole
  - For least risk of QTc prolongation: aripiprazole
    - Avoid use of thioridazine and ziprasidone in patients with a prolonged QT interval.
- For poor compliance/high risk of relapse: Injectable form of long-acting antipsychotic may be used.
  - Haloperidol, fluphenazine, risperidone, olanzapine, aripiprazole, and paliperidone
- Usual maintenance daily range (Initiation is commonly at a lower dose.)
  - Chlorpromazine: 200 to 800 mg/day divided BID/TID/QID
  - Aripiprazole: 10 to 30 mg/day
  - Asenapine: 5 to 10 mg BID (sublingual), once daily patch (FDA approved in October 2019)
  - Fluphenazine: 5 to 20 mg/day
  - Haloperidol: 5 to 20 mg/day

- Lurasidone: 40 to 80 mg/day (with meal)
- Olanzapine: 10 to 30 mg/day
- Paliperidone: 3 to 12 mg/day
- Perphenazine: 24 mg/day divided BID/TID
- Quetiapine: 200 to 400 mg BID
- Risperidone: 2 to 8 mg/day
- Ziprasidone: 20 to 80 mg BID (with meal)
- Cariprazine: 1.5 to 6.0 mg/day
- Brexpiprazole: 2 to 4 mg/day
- Pimavanserin (for Parkinson disease–related psychosis): 34 mg/day
- Clozapine: 200 mg BID
  ○ Typical dosage range is 300 to 600 mg/day split into BID dosing.
  ○ The gold standard treatment for refractory schizophrenia
  ○ Effective in treatment of suicidal patients
  ○ Serious risk of agranulocytosis mandates registration with National Clozapine Registry and weekly to monthly monitoring of CBC with differential
  ○ Significant risk of seizure at higher doses
  ○ SE can include myocarditis, DVT, sialorrhea, tachycardia, and weight gain.

ALERT
All antipsychotics are associated with weight gain and carry the risk of metabolic syndrome and tardive dyskinesia.

- Managing adverse effects of antipsychotics
  - Dystonic reaction (especially of head and neck): diphenhydramine 25 to 50 mg IM or benztropine 1 to 2 mg IM
  - Akathisia (restlessness): propranolol 20 to 30 mg BID or lorazepam 0.5 to 1.0 mg BID
  - Parkinsonism: trihexyphenidyl 2 mg BID (up to 15 mg daily) or benztropine 0.5 BID (1 to 4 mg/day); amantadine 100 mg daily (up to 300 mg daily)
  - Tardive dyskinesia: valbenazine (80 mg daily), tetrabenazine (25 to 50 mg TID), or deutetrabenazine (6 to 24 mg BID)
  - Neuroleptic malignant syndrome: hyperthermia, autonomic dysfunction, and extrapyramidal symptoms; requires hospitalization and supportive management (IVF and cessation of offending neuroleptic)
  - Metabolic syndrome: metformin, topiramate (4)
  - Geriatric considerations: All antipsychotics carry a black box warning for increased mortality risk in elderly patients with dementia.
- Adjunctive treatments
  - Benzodiazepines
    ○ May be effective adjuncts to antipsychotics during acute phase of illness, especially when anxiety is prominent
    ○ First-line for the treatment of catatonia
    ○ Withdrawal reactions with psychosis or seizures; risk for dependence and cognitive impairment
    ○ Best when used only in the short term; high cumulative exposure to benzodiazepines is associated with a significantly increased risk of death in patients with schizophrenia.
  - Mood stabilizers
    ○ Valproic acid may be effective adjunct for those with agitated/violent behavior (3).
    ○ Lithium may be effective adjunct for patients with prominent affective symptoms or suicidal ideation (3).

- Antidepressants:
  ○ Useful if comorbid depression and/or anxiety are present
  ○ Associated with a lower risk of psychiatric hospitalization when added to antipsychotic monotherapy compared to adding a second antipsychotic (5)[B]

ISSUES FOR REFERRAL
- Consider referral in cases of suicidality, coexistence of a substance use disorder, difficulty in engagement, or poor self-care.
- Multidisciplinary care from both a primary care clinician and a psychiatrist is recommended.
- Family members often benefit from referral to family advocacy organizations such as NAMI.

ADDITIONAL THERAPIES
- Psychoeducation and psychotherapy for patient and family: These include specific treatments to reduce the impact of psychotic symptoms, enhance social functioning, and reduce risk of symptom exacerbation. Cognitive-behavioral therapy has been shown to be effective for specific symptoms of schizophrenia (3).
- Cognitive remediation is a new approach for cognitive retraining and psychosocial recovery.
- Vocational support programs have shown success in returning individuals to work.
- Negative symptoms typically respond better to these nonpharmacologic interventions than they do to medications

SURGERY/OTHER PROCEDURES
Electroconvulsive therapy (ECT) should be considered for patients presenting with catatonic features, severe depression, or aggression and suicidality.

ADMISSION, INPATIENT, AND NURSING CONSIDERATIONS
The decision to admit is based on the risk of self-harm or harm to others and the inability to care for self.

 ## ONGOING CARE

FOLLOW-UP RECOMMENDATIONS
- Long-term symptom management and rehabilitation depend on engagement in ongoing pharmacologic and psychosocial treatment.
- Monitoring is based on evaluation of symptoms (including safety and psychotic symptoms), looking for the emergence of comorbidities, medication side effects, and prevention of complications.

DIET
Antipsychotics confer a higher risk of metabolic side effects such as diabetes, hypercholesterolemia, and weight gain.

PATIENT EDUCATION
- *Helping a Family Member with Schizophrenia*: https://www.aafp.org/afp/2007/0615/p1830.html
- National Alliance on Mental Illness: www.NAMI.org

PROGNOSIS
- Typical course is one of remissions and exacerbations; although uncommon, there are known cases of complete remission and of refractory illness.
- Negative symptoms are often most difficult to treat; antipsychotics are better at treating positive symptoms.

- About 20% attempt and 5–6% die of suicide.
- Decreased life span related to comorbidities

COMPLICATIONS
- Medication side effects (tardive dyskinesia, orthostatic hypotension, QTc prolongation, metabolic syndrome)
- Combative behavior toward others (Note that only 5% of crimes are caused by those with mental illness including psychosis, and the mentally ill are more likely to be victims of violence.)
- Comorbid substance use disorders

REFERENCES
1. Murrie B, Lappin J, Large M. Transition of substance-induced, brief, and atypical psychoses to schizophrenia: a systematic review and meta-analysis. *Schizophr Bull*. 2020;46(3):505–516.
2. Skikic M, Arriola JA. First episode psychosis medical workup: evidence-informed recommendations and introduction to a clinically guided approach. *Child Adolesc Psychiatr Clin N Am*. 2020;29(1):15–28.
3. Hasan A, Falkai P, Wobrock T, et al; WFSBP Task Force on Treatment and Guidelines for Schizophrenia. World Federation of Societies of Biological Psychiatry (WFSBP) guidelines for biological treatment of schizophrenia—a short version for primary care. *Int J Psychiatry Clin Pract*. 2017;21(2):82–90.
4. Gracious BL, Meyer AE. Psychotropic-induced weight gain and potential pharmacologic treatment strategies. *Psychiatry (Edgmont)*. 2005;2(1):36–42.
5. Stroup TS, Gerhard T, Crystal S, et al. Comparative effectiveness of adjunctive psychotropic medications in patients with schizophrenia. *JAMA Psychiatry*. 2019;76(5):508–515.

 ## SEE ALSO

Algorithm: Delirium

CODES

ICD10
- F20.3 Undifferentiated schizophrenia
- F20.5 Residual schizophrenia
- F20.2 Catatonic schizophrenia

CLINICAL PEARLS
- Schizophrenia is a severe and persistent mental illness that impacts cognition and functioning and requires a multidisciplinary team approach to assist with coping, treatment, and to promote recovery.
- Schizophrenia is characterized by positive symptoms, including hallucinations and delusions, and negative symptoms, including flattened affect, anhedonia, amotivation, and social withdrawal.
- Substance use disorders are the most common psychiatric comorbidities and should be monitored and treated appropriately.

SCLERITIS
Matthew J. Schear, DO, MS

BASICS

DESCRIPTION
- Scleritis is a painful, inflammatory process of the sclera, part of the eye's outer coat.
  - Categorized into anterior or posterior and diffuse, nodular, or necrotizing
  - Commonly associated with systemic disorders
  - Potentially vision threatening
- In contrast, episcleritis is a self-limited inflammation of the superficial episclera with only mild discomfort.
- System(s) affected: ocular

EPIDEMIOLOGY
- Mean age is 54 years (range 12 to 96).
- Predominant sex: female > male (1.6:1)

Incidence
Estimated to be 6 cases per 100,000 people in the general population

Prevalence
- Anterior scleritis, about 94% of cases (1)
  - Diffuse anterior scleritis, about 75% (most common)
- Remaining 6% have posterior scleritis.

ETIOLOGY AND PATHOPHYSIOLOGY
- Frequently associated with a systemic illness (1)[B]
  - Most commonly associated with rheumatoid arthritis
  - In about 38% of cases, scleritis is the presenting manifestation of an underlying systemic disorder.
  - Necrotizing scleritis has the highest association with systemic disease.
- Other etiologies
  - Proposed pathogenesis is dependent on type of scleritis. In necrotizing scleritis, the predominant mechanism is likely due to the activity of matrix metalloproteinases.
  - Drug-induced scleritis has been reported in patients on bisphosphonate therapy.
  - Surgically induced necrotizing scleritis is exceedingly rare and occurs after multiple surgeries.
  - Infectious scleritis occurs most commonly after surgical trauma, and *Pseudomonas aeruginosa* in poorly controlled diabetic patients is the most common causative organism (2)[B].

RISK FACTORS
Individuals with autoimmune disorders are most at risk.

COMMONLY ASSOCIATED CONDITIONS
- Rheumatoid arthritis (most common)
- Sjögren syndrome
- Granulomatosis with polyangiitis
- HLA-B27–associated ankylosing spondylitis
- Systemic lupus erythematosus
- Behçet disease
- Juvenile idiopathic arthritis
- Cogan disease
- Relapsing polychondritis
- Polyarteritis nodosa
- Sarcoidosis
- Inflammatory bowel disease
- Herpes zoster, herpes simplex
- HIV, syphilis, Lyme disease, tuberculosis

DIAGNOSIS

HISTORY
- Redness and inflammation of the sclera
  - Can be bilateral in about 40% of cases (1)
- Photophobia and tearing
- Pain ranging from mild discomfort to extreme localized tenderness
  - May be described as constant, deep, boring, or pulsating
  - Pain may be referred to the eyebrow, temple, or jaw.
  - Pain may awaken patient from sleep in early hours of morning.
  - Severe pain is most commonly associated with necrotizing scleritis (1)[B].

PHYSICAL EXAM
- Examine sclera in all directions of gaze by gross inspection.
  - A bluish hue may suggest thinning of sclera.
  - Inspect for degree of injection and extent of thinning.
- Check visual acuity.
  - Decrease in visual acuity of two or more Snellen lines occurs in about 16% of patients (1)[B].
- Slit-lamp exam
  - Episcleritis: conjunctival and superficial vascular plexuses displaced anteriorly; blanches with phenylephrine
  - Scleritis: Deep episcleral plexus is the maximum site of vascular congestion, displaced anteriorly d/t edema of underlying sclera; characteristic blue or violet color, absent in patients with episcleritis

- Dilated fundus exam to rule out posterior involvement
- A complete physical exam, particularly of the skin, joints, heart, and lungs, should be done to evaluate for associated conditions.

DIFFERENTIAL DIAGNOSIS
- Conjunctivitis
- Episcleritis
- Iritis (anterior uveitis)
- Posterior uveitis
- Blepharitis
- Ocular rosacea

DIAGNOSTIC TESTS & INTERPRETATION
- Routine tests to exclude systemic disease: CBC; serum chemistry; urinalysis; ESR; and/or C-reactive protein, blood, and urine cultures
- Specific tests for underlying systemic illness: Rheumatoid factor, anticyclic citrullinated peptide antibodies, ACE level, HLA-B27, antineutrophil cytoplasmic antibodies, PPD or QuantiFERON-TB level, fluorescent treponemal antibody absorption (FTA-ABS), rapid plasma regain (RPR), Lyme titers, and antinuclear antibody may aid in the diagnosis.
- Further imaging studies, such as a chest x-ray, sacroiliac joint films, colonoscopy, may be useful if a specific systemic illness is suspected.
- B-scan US to detect posterior scleritis. Look at thickness of sclera and for T-sign (fluid in Tenon's space at interface between the optic nerve and sclera).
- MRI/CT scan may provide additional diagnostic benefit and detect orbital disease (3)[C].
- Different subtypes of scleritis are associated with varying presentations and distinct findings:
  - Diffuse anterior scleritis: widespread inflammation
  - Nodular anterior scleritis: immovable, inflamed nodule
  - Necrotizing anterior scleritis: "with inflammation": Sclera becomes transparent. Scleromalacia perforans without inflammation: painless and often associated with rheumatoid arthritis
  - Posterior scleritis: associated with retinal and choroidal complications; adjacent swelling of orbital tissues may occur.

Diagnostic Procedures/Other
Biopsy is not routinely required unless diagnosis remains uncertain after above investigations. Culture if suspecting infectious etiology.

TREATMENT

GENERAL MEASURES

If scleral thinning, glasses/eye shield should be worn to prevent perforation; should be managed by an appropriate eye care professional

MEDICATION

- First-line therapies for noninfectious scleritis (4)[C]
  - Oral NSAID therapy, choice based on availability, example is ibuprofen 600 to 800 mg PO TID–QID or indomethacin 50 mg PO TID provided no contraindications exists; about 37% successful (5)[B]
  - Systemic steroids (initial if necrotizing scleritis and preferentially IV if vision threatening, otherwise use if failure of NSAIDs), prednisone 40 to 60 mg PO QD or 1 mg/kg/day, taper over 4 to 6 weeks. Use caution if suspect infectious etiology.
  - Antimetabolites including methotrexate, azathioprine, mycophenolate mofetil, cyclophosphamide, and cyclosporine may be used as steroid-sparing agents. They are generally recommended if steroids cannot be tapered below 10 mg PO QD (5)[C].
- Second-line therapies (5)[C],(6)[A],(7)[C]
  - Immunomodulatory agents, infliximab, rituximab, and adalimumab can be used if patient has failed or is not a candidate for antimetabolites or calcineurin inhibitors. These agents are preferred over etanercept due to higher treatment success and its potential paradoxic effect on ocular inflammation.
- Adjunct therapy considerations
  - Topical steroids: prednisolone acetate 1% or difluprednate 0.05% under ophthalmologist care
  - Subconjunctival triamcinolone acetonide injection only for nonnecrotizing, 40 mg/mL, 97% improvement after one injection; increased risk of ocular HTN, cataract, and globe perforation
- Necrotizing anterior scleritis and posterior scleritis
  - May require immunosuppressive therapy in addition to systemic steroids
  - Treat aggressively due to possible complications if left untreated; may need patch grafting to maintain globe integrity
- Infectious
  - Antibiotic therapy resolves about 18% of cases, whereas the remaining often requires surgical intervention such as débridement (2)[B].

ISSUES FOR REFERRAL

- All patients with scleritis should be managed by an ophthalmologist familiar with this condition.
- Rheumatology referral for coexistent systemic disease is helpful for long-term success.

ADDITIONAL THERAPIES

Immunosuppressants used for autoimmune and collagen vascular disorders may be of help in active scleritis.

SURGERY/OTHER PROCEDURES

- In rare cases, scleral biopsy may be indicated to confirm infection or other etiology.
- Ocular perforation requires scleral grafting.

 ONGOING CARE

FOLLOW-UP RECOMMENDATIONS

Avoid contact lenses—wear only if there is corneal involvement, which is rare.

Patient Monitoring

- Patient in the active stage of inflammation should be followed very closely by an ophthalmologist to assess the effectiveness of therapy.
- Medication use mandates close surveillance for adverse effects.

PATIENT EDUCATION

Scleritis at The Ocular Immunology and Uveitis Foundation: http://www.uveitis.org/patient_articles/scleritis/

PROGNOSIS

Scleritis is indolent, chronic, and often progressive.

- Diffuse anterior scleritis (best prognosis)
- Necrotizing anterior scleritis (worst prognosis)
- Recurrent bouts of inflammation may occur.
- Scleromalacia perforans has the highest risk of perforation of the globe.

COMPLICATIONS

- Decrease in vision, anterior uveitis, ocular HTN, and peripheral keratitis
- Cataract and glaucoma can result from disease or treatment with steroids.
- Ocular perforation can occur in severe stages.

REFERENCES

1. Sainz de la Maza M, Molina N, Gonzalez-Gonzalez LA, et al. Clinical characteristics of a large cohort of patients with scleritis and episcleritis. *Ophthalmology.* 2012;119(1):43–50.
2. Hodson KL, Galor A, Karp CL, et al. Epidemiology and visual outcomes in patients with infectious scleritis. *Cornea.* 2013;32(4):466–472.
3. Diogo MC, Jager MJ, Ferreira TA. CT and MR imaging in the diagnosis of scleritis. *AJNR Am J Neuroradiol.* 2016;37(12):2334–2339.
4. Beardsley RM, Suhler EB, Rosenbaum JT, et al. Pharmacotherapy of scleritis: current paradigms and future directions. *Expert Opin Pharmacother.* 2013;14(4):411–424.
5. Sainz de la Maza M, Molina N, Gonzalez-Gonzalez LA, et al. Scleritis therapy. *Ophthalmology.* 2012;119(1):51–58.
6. Levy-Clarke G, Jabs DA, Read RW, et al. Expert panel recommendations for the use of anti-tumor necrosis factor biologic agents in patients with ocular inflammatory disorders. *Ophthalmology.* 2014;121(3):785–796.e3.
7. Cao JH, Oray M, Cocho L, et al. Rituximab in the treatment of refractory noninfectious scleritis. *Am J Ophthalmol.* 2016;164:22–28.

CODES

ICD10

- H15.009 Unspecified scleritis, unspecified eye
- H15.019 Anterior scleritis, unspecified eye
- H15.039 Posterior scleritis, unspecified eye

CLINICAL PEARLS

- Episcleritis is a self-limited inflammation of the eye with mild discomfort.
- Scleritis is a painful, severe, and potentially vision-threatening condition.
- While both conditions can be associated with underlying inflammatory diseases, 35% of scleritis cases are associated with a systemic disease such as rheumatoid arthritis. Necrotizing scleritis has the highest association.

SCLERODERMA
Ann M. Lynch, PharmD, RPh, AE-C • Jeremy Golding, MD, FAAFP

BASICS

DESCRIPTION
- Scleroderma (systemic sclerosis [SSc]) is a chronic disease of unknown cause involving connective tissue, characterized by diffuse fibrosis of skin and visceral organs and vascular abnormalities.
- Most manifestations have vascular features (e.g., Raynaud phenomenon), but frank vasculitis is rarely seen.
- Can range from a mild disease, affecting the skin, to a systemic disease that can cause death in a few months
- The disease is categorized into two major clinical variants (1).
  - Diffuse: distal and proximal extremity and truncal skin thickening
  - Limited
    - Restricted to the fingers, hands, and face
    - CREST syndrome (calcinosis, Raynaud phenomenon, esophageal dysmotility, sclerodactyly, telangiectasia)
- System(s) affected: include, but not limited to skin, renal, cardiovascular, pulmonary, musculoskeletal, gastrointestinal (GI)

Geriatric Considerations
Uncommon >75 years of age

Pediatric Considerations
Rare in this age group

Pregnancy Considerations
- Safe and healthy pregnancies are common and possible despite higher frequency of premature births.
- High-risk management must be standard care to avoid complications, specifically renal crisis.
- Diffuse scleroderma causes greater risk for developing serious cardiopulmonary and renal problems. Pregnancy should be delayed until disease stabilizes.

EPIDEMIOLOGY
Incidence
- In the United States: 1 to 5/100,000 per year
- Predominant age
  - Young adult (16 to 40 years); middle-aged (40 to 75 years); peak onset 30 to 50 years
  - Symptoms usually appear in the 3rd to 5th decades.
- Predominant sex: female > male (4:1)

Prevalence
In the United States: 1 to 25/100,000

ETIOLOGY AND PATHOPHYSIOLOGY
Pathophysiology involves both a vascular component and a fibrotic component. Both occur simultaneously. The inciting event is unknown, but there is an increase in certain cytokines after endothelial cell activation that are profibrotic (TGF-β and PDGF).
- Unknown
- Possible alterations in immune response
- Possibly some association with exposure to quartz mining, quarrying, vinyl chloride, hydrocarbons, toxin exposure
- Treatment with bleomycin has caused a scleroderma-like syndrome, as has exposure to rapeseed oil.

Genetics
Familial clustering is rare but has been seen.

RISK FACTORS
Unknown

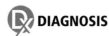

DIAGNOSIS

HISTORY
- Raynaud phenomenon is generally the presenting complaint (differentiated from Raynaud disease, generally affecting younger individuals and without digital ulcers).
- Skin thickening, "puffy hands," pruritus, and gastroesophageal reflux disease (GERD) are often noted early in the disease process.

PHYSICAL EXAM
- Skin
  - Digital ulcerations
  - Digital pitting
  - Tightness, swelling, thickening of digits
  - Hyperpigmentation/hypopigmentation
  - Narrowed oral aperture
  - SC calcinosis
- Peripheral vascular system
  - Telangiectasia
- Joints, tendons, and bones
  - Flexion contractures
  - Friction rub on tendon movement
  - Hand swelling
  - Joint stiffness
  - Polyarthralgia
  - Sclerodactyly
- Muscle
  - Proximal muscle weakness
- GI tract
  - Dysphagia
  - Esophageal reflux due to dysmotility (most common systemic sign in diffuse disease)
  - Malabsorptive diarrhea
  - Nausea and vomiting
  - Weight loss
  - Xerostomia
- Kidney
  - Hypertension
  - May develop scleroderma renal crisis: acute renal failure (ARF)
- Pulmonary
  - Dry crackles at lung bases
  - Dyspnea
- Nervous system
  - Peripheral neuropathy
  - Trigeminal neuropathy
- Cardiac (progressive disease)
  - Conduction abnormalities
  - Cardiomyopathy
  - Pericarditis
  - Secondary cor pulmonale

DIFFERENTIAL DIAGNOSIS
- Mixed connective tissue disease/overlap syndromes
- Scleredema
- Nephrogenic systemic fibrosis
- Toxic oil syndrome (Madrid, 1981, affecting 20,000 people)
- Eosinophilia-myalgia syndrome
- Diffuse fasciitis with eosinophilia
- Scleredema of Buschke

DIAGNOSTIC TESTS & INTERPRETATION
Initial Tests (lab, imaging)
- Nail fold capillary microscopy—drop out is most significant finding
- CBC
- Creatinine
- Urinalysis (albuminuria, microscopic hematuria)
- Antinuclear antibodies (ANA): positive in >90% of patients
- Anti-Scl-70 (anti-topoisomerase [ATA]) antibody is highly specific for systemic disease and confers a higher risk of interstitial lung disease (ILD).
- Anticentromere antibody usually associated with CREST variant
- Chest radiograph
  - Diffuse reticular pattern
  - Bilateral basilar pulmonary fibrosis
- Hand radiograph
  - Soft tissue atrophy and acroosteolysis
  - Can see overlap syndromes such as rheumatoid arthritis
  - SC calcinosis

Follow-Up Tests & Special Considerations
- Pulmonary function tests (PFTs)
  - Decreased maximum breathing capacity
  - Increased residual volume
  - Diffusion defect
- Antibodies to U3-RNP—higher risk for scleroderma-associated pulmonary hypertension
- Anti–PM-Scl antibodies (for myositis) (2)[B]
- Anti-RNA polymerase III—higher risk for diffuse cutaneous involvement and renal crisis (3)[A]
- ECG (low voltage): possible nonspecific abnormalities, arrhythmia, and conduction defects
- Echocardiography: pulmonary hypertension or cardiomyopathy
- Nail fold capillary loop abnormalities
- Upper GI
  - Distal esophageal dilatation
  - Atonic esophagus
  - Esophageal dysmotility
  - Duodenal diverticula
- Barium enema
  - Colonic diverticula
  - Megacolon
- High-resolution CT scan for detecting alveolitis, which has a ground-glass appearance or fibrosis predominant in bilateral lower lobes

Diagnostic Procedures/Other
- Skin biopsy
  - Compact collagen fibers in the reticular dermis and hyalinization and fibrosis of arterioles
  - Thinning of epidermis, with loss of rete pegs, and atrophy of dermal appendages
  - Accumulation of mononuclear cells is also seen.
- Right-sided heart catheterization: Pulmonary hypertension is an ominous prognostic feature.

Test Interpretation
- Skin
  - Edema, fibrosis, or atrophy (late stage)
  - Lymphocytic infiltrate around sweat glands
  - Loss of capillaries
  - Endothelial proliferation
  - Hair follicle atrophy

- Synovium
  - Pannus formation
  - Fibrin deposits in tendons
- Kidney
  - Small kidneys
  - Intimal proliferation in interlobular arteries
- Heart
  - Endocardial thickening
  - Myocardial interstitial fibrosis
  - Ischemic band necrosis
  - Enlarged heart
  - Cardiac hypertrophy
  - Pulmonary hypertension
- Lung
  - Interstitial pneumonitis
  - Cyst formation
  - Interstitial fibrosis
  - Bronchiectasis
- Esophagus
  - Esophageal atrophy
  - Fibrosis

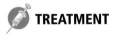 TREATMENT

GENERAL MEASURES

- Treatment is symptomatic and supportive.
- Esophageal dilation may be used for strictures.
- Avoid cold; dress appropriately in layers for the weather; be wary of air conditioning.
- Avoid smoking (crucial).
- Avoid fingersticks (e.g., blood tests).
- Elevate the head of the bed during sleep to help relieve GI symptoms.
- Use softening lotions, ointments, and bath oils to help prevent dryness and cracking of skin.
- Dialysis may be necessary in renal crisis.

MEDICATION

First Line

- ACE inhibitors (ACEIs): for preservation of renal blood flow and for treatment of hypertensive renal crisis
- Dihydropyridine calcium channel blockers (e.g., nifedipine, amlodipine) for Raynaud phenomenon
- Corticosteroids: for disabling myositis, pulmonary alveolitis, or mixed connective tissue disease (not recommended in high doses due to increased incidence of renal failure)
- NSAIDs: for joint or tendon symptoms; caution with long-term concurrent use with ACEIs (potential renal complications)
- Antibiotics: for secondary infections in bowel and active skin infections
- Antacids, proton pump inhibitors: for gastric reflux
- Metoclopramide: for intestinal dysfunction
- Hydrophilic skin ointments: for skin therapy
- Topical clindamycin, erythromycin, or silver sulfadiazine, and PDE5 inhibitors for prevention of recurrent infectious cutaneous ulcers
- Consider immunosuppressives for treatment of life-threatening or potentially crippling scleroderma or interstitial pneumonitis such as cyclophosphamide for ILD (4)[B].
- Nitrates, dihydropyridine calcium-channel blockers, PDE5 antagonists, and fluoxetine for Raynaud phenomenon (5)[A]
- Avoidance of caffeine, nicotine, and sympathomimetics may ease Raynaud symptoms.

- PDE5 antagonists (e.g., sildenafil), prostanoids, and endothelin-1 antagonists are changing the management of pulmonary hypertension (6).
- Alveolitis: immunosuppressants and alkylating agents (e.g., cyclophosphamide)

ADDITIONAL THERAPIES

- Anti–TNF-α therapy: Preliminary suggestion is that this may reduce joint symptoms and disability in inflammatory arthritis, but small sample sizes and observational biases lend to the need for further well-designed, adequately powered, longitudinal clinical trials.
- Physical therapy to maintain function and promote strength
- Heat therapy to relieve joint stiffness

SURGERY/OTHER PROCEDURES

- Some success with gastroplasty for correction of GERD
- Limited role for sympathectomy for Raynaud phenomenon
- Lung transplantation for pulmonary hypertension and ILD
- Hematopoietic stem cell transplantation for selected patients with rapidly progressive SSc (5)

 ONGOING CARE

FOLLOW-UP RECOMMENDATIONS

Patient Monitoring

- Monitor every 3 to 6 months for end organ and skin involvement and medications. Provide encouragement.
- Echocardiology and PFTs yearly

DIET

- Drink plenty of fluids with meals.
- Adjust eating habits if GI symptoms are present.

PATIENT EDUCATION

- Stay as active as possible, but avoid fatigue.
- Printed patient information available from the Scleroderma Federation, 1725 York Avenue, No. 29F, New York, NY 10128; (212) 427-7040; www.scleroderma.org
- Advise the patient to report any abnormal bruising or nonhealing abrasions.
- Assist the patient about smoking cessation, if needed.

PROGNOSIS

- Possible improvement but incurable
- Prognosis is poor if cardiac, pulmonary, or renal manifestations present early.

COMPLICATIONS

- Renal failure
- Respiratory failure
- Flexion contractures
- Disability
- Esophageal dysmotility
- Reflux esophagitis
- Arrhythmia
- Megacolon
- Pneumatosis intestinalis
- Obstructive bowel
- Cardiomyopathy
- Pulmonary hypertension
- Possible association with lung and other cancers
- Death

REFERENCES

1. van den Hoogen F, Khanna D, Fransen J, et al. 2013 Classification criteria for systemic sclerosis: an American College of Rheumatology/European League Against Rheumatism collaborative initiative. *Arthritis Rheum.* 2013;65(11):2737–2747.
2. D'Aoust J, Hudson M, Tatibouet S, et al; for Canadian Scleroderma Research Group. Clinical and serologic correlates of anti-PM/Scl antibodies in systemic sclerosis: a multicenter study of 763 patients. *Arthritis Rheumatol.* 2014;66(6): 1608–1615.
3. Sobanski V, Dauchet L, Lefèvre G, et al. Prevalence of anti-RNA polymerase III antibodies in systemic sclerosis: new data from a French cohort and a systematic review and meta-analysis. *Arthritis Rheumatol.* 2014;66(2):407–417.
4. Roth MD, Tseng CH, Clements PJ, et al; and Scleroderma Lung Study Research Group. Predicting treatment outcomes and responder subsets in scleroderma-related interstitial lung disease. *Arthritis Rheum.* 2011;63(9):2797–2808.
5. Kowal-Bielecka O, Fransen J, Avouac J, et al; for EUSTAR Coauthors. Update of EULAR recommendations for the treatment of systemic sclerosis. *Ann Rheum Dis.* 2017;76(8):1327–1339.
6. Volkmann ER, Saggar R, Khanna D, et al. Improved transplant-free survival in patients with systemic sclerosis-associated pulmonary hypertension and interstitial lung disease. *Arthritis Rheumatol.* 2014;66(7):1900–1908.

ADDITIONAL READING

- Curtiss P, Schwager Z, Cobos G, et al. A systematic review and meta-analysis of the effects of topical nitrates in the treatment of primary and secondary Raynaud's phenomenon. *J Am Acad Dermatol.* 2018;78(6):1110–1118.e3.
- Steen VD. Pregnancy in scleroderma. *Rheum Dis Clin North Am.* 2007;33(2):345–358.
- Valerio CJ, Schreiber BE, Handler CE, et al. Borderline mean pulmonary artery pressure in patients with systemic sclerosis: transpulmonary gradient predicts risk of developing pulmonary hypertension. *Arthritis Rheum.* 2013;65(4):1074–1084.

 SEE ALSO

Morphea

 CODES

ICD10

- M34.2 Systemic sclerosis induced by drug and chemical
- M34.9 Systemic sclerosis, unspecified
- M34.0 Progressive systemic sclerosis

CLINICAL PEARLS

- Raynaud phenomenon is frequently the initial complaint.
- Skin thickening, "puffy hands," and GERD are often noted early in disease.
- Patients must be followed proactively for development of pulmonary hypertension or ILD.

SEASONAL AFFECTIVE DISORDER

Matthew J. Filippo, DO • Greer Park, DO

BASICS

DESCRIPTION
- Seasonal affective disorder (SAD) describes mood episodes that occur as a part of major depressive or bipolar disorder in a seasonal pattern. Patients may experience depressive, hypomanic, or manic episodes, although depression is more common.
- Depressive episodes typically occur during winter months (fall-winter onset), with full remission in the spring and summer. Less commonly, patients may experience a spring-summer onset with remission in the fall-winter months.
- Ranges from a milder form (winter blues) to a seriously disabling illness

EPIDEMIOLOGY
Incidence
- Affects up to 500,000 Americans every winter
- Up to 30% of patients visiting a primary care physician (PCP) during winter may report winter depressive symptoms.
- Predominant age: occurs at any age; peaks in 20s and 30s
- Predominant sex: female > male (3:1)
Prevalence
- Lifetime prevalence of the general population is 0.5–3%.
- Point prevalence in primary care patients is 5–10%, while in depressed patients, this is 15%.

ETIOLOGY AND PATHOPHYSIOLOGY
- The major theories currently involve the interplay of phase-shifted circadian rhythms, genetic vulnerability, and serotonin dysregulation.
- Photoperiod and Phase Shift Hypotheses:
  - During the winter months, the period of natural daylight is shorter. When there is less sunlight, the pineal gland increases melatonin secretion, which can lead to a phase shift in circadian rhythm. This process has been linked to symptoms of depression. Light therapy in the morning or evening can suppress melatonin secretion to correct the phase shift and improve symptoms of depression. Reduced sunlight may also decrease vitamin D levels, which may contribute to symptoms of depression.
- Serotonin Dysregulation Hypothesis:
  - It is suspected that dysregulation of serotonin, particularly increased clearance from the synaptic cleft and reduced secretion, contributes to SAD pathophysiology. Central acting serotonergic agents such as SSRIs appear to reverse SAD symptoms.
Genetics
- Twin studies and a preliminary study on GPR50 melatonin receptor variants suggest a genetic component.
- Studies also indicate an association with melanopsin gene (OPN4) variants.
- Increased incidence of depression, ADHD, and alcoholism in close relatives, or first-degree relatives with SAD increase the chance an individual will develop SAD.

RISK FACTORS
- Most common during months of January and February: Patients frequently visit their PCP during winter months complaining of recurrent flu, chronic fatigue, and unexplained weight gain.
- Working in a building without windows or other environments without significant exposure to sunlight

GENERAL PREVENTION
- Consider use of light therapy at the start of winter (if prior episodes begin in October), increase time outside during daylight hours, or move to a more southern location.
- Bupropion (Wellbutrin) is the only FDA-approved antidepressant for the prevention of SAD.
- While studies show mixed results, low-dose melatonin in the evening may help prevent symptoms of depression from occurring if taken before and during winter months.

COMMONLY ASSOCIATED CONDITIONS
Patients with SAD often have other comorbid psychiatric disorders including alcohol use disorder, ADHD, and binge eating disorder, among others. Some individuals with SAD have a weakened immune system and may be more vulnerable to infections.

DIAGNOSIS

Under *DSM-5*, SAD is denoted by adding the "with seasonal pattern" specifier to a diagnosis of major depressive disorder, bipolar 1 disorder, or bipolar 2 disorder.
- Remission of symptoms during nonseasonal months (usually spring and summer)
- Symptoms have occurred for the past 2 years.
- Seasonal episodes substantially outnumber any nonseasonal depressive episodes in the patient's lifetime.
- Carefully document the presence or absence of prior manic episodes.
- Screen for the existence of any suicidal ideation and safety risk factors.

HISTORY
- Symptoms of depression meeting the criteria for major depressive disorder are the following:
  - Sleep disturbance: either too much or too little
  - Lack of interest in life and absence of pleasure from hobbies/activities
  - Guilt: feelings of guilt or worthlessness
  - Energy: fatigue or constantly feeling tired
  - Concentration: difficulty with concentration and memory
  - Appetite: changes in appetite and weight
  - Psychomotor retardation: Patients feel slowed down with decreased activity.
  - Suicidal thoughts: Patients report thoughts of suicide.
- In SAD episodes with fall-winter onset, hypersomnia, hyperphagia (craving for carbohydrates and sweets), and weight gain usually predominate. Despite sleeping more, patients report daytime sleepiness and fatigue. Cravings may lead to binge eating and weight gains >20 lb.

- In SAD episodes with spring-summer onset, depression symptoms of insomnia and loss of appetite are more common.
- Obtain collateral history if patient is unable to provide insight into the seasonal component.

PHYSICAL EXAM
Use exam to exclude other organic causes for symptoms. Neurologic deficits, signs of endocrine dysfunction, or stigmata of substance abuse should prompt further testing.

DIFFERENTIAL DIAGNOSIS
- Organic causes of low energy and fatigue, such as hypothyroidism, anemia, and mononucleosis (or other viral syndromes), need to be considered.
- Symptoms should not be better accounted for by seasonal psychosocial stressors, which often accompany the winter or holiday seasons.
- Substance use disorders

DIAGNOSTIC TESTS & INTERPRETATION
- Thyroid-stimulating hormone to rule out hypothyroidism
- CBC to rule out anemia
- Rule out electrolyte and glucose dysregulation.
- 25-OH vitamin D level
- Pregnancy test for women of childbearing potential
- Urine toxicology screen if substance use is a concern
- Imaging is not useful unless focal neurologic finding or looking to exclude an organic cause.

TREATMENT

MEDICATION
There is a lack of evidence to determine whether light therapy or medication should be the first-line agent. Both are strongly supported by the literature and may have equal efficacy. The combination of medication and light therapy has been shown to be more efficacious than monotherapy. Medications may have more side effects. Adherence to both remains a critical issue. The ultimate choice depends on the acuity of the patient and the comfort level of the prescribing clinician with each treatment modality (1)[B].

First Line
- SSRIs such as sertraline (Zoloft), paroxetine (Paxil), fluoxetine (Prozac), citalopram (Celexa), and escitalopram (Lexapro) can be used at typical antidepressant doses (2)[B]. It may be reasonable to decrease a patient's dose during nonseasonal months when patients do not experience symptoms of depression.
- Bupropion (Wellbutrin) is the only antidepressant currently approved by the FDA for the prevention of SAD (3)[B].
- There is evidence that suggests low-dose melatonin given in the early evening (not at nighttime) paired with early morning light therapy helps shift one's circadian rhythm and reduces SAD symptoms.

Second Line
Short-acting β-blockers in the early morning given before sunrise suppress melatonin release and can be helpful in reducing SAD symptoms in treatment-resistant cases (4)[B].

ISSUES FOR REFERRAL

- Patients with a history of ocular disease should be referred for an ophthalmologic exam before phototherapy and for serial monitoring.
- Patients who fail to respond or who develop manic symptoms or suicidal ideation once treatment is initiated should be considered for psychiatric referral.

ADDITIONAL THERAPIES

- Phototherapy using special light sources has been shown to be effective in 60–90% of patients and can be considered a first-line treatment, often providing relief with a few sessions (2),(5),(6). This has been shown to be effective for both unipolar and bipolar depression.
- Variables that can regulate effect of bright light therapy are the following:
  - Light intensity: Although the minimum light source intensity is under investigation, at least 2,500 lux is suggested (domestic lights emit, on average, 200 to 500 lux). There is stronger evidence using 7,000 to 10,000 lux (2)[B].
  - Treatment duration: Exposure time varies based on intensity of light source, with daily sessions of 30 minutes to a few hours. Treatment should continue into the season of remission until symptoms improve.
  - Time of treatment: Most patients respond better by using the light therapy early in the morning.
  - Color of light source: Emerging data suggest that shorter sessions of lower intensity light-emitting diodes enriched in the blue spectrum have equal efficacy to the traditional white light treatment (7)[B].
- Light box is placed on table several feet away, and the light is allowed to shine onto the patient's retinas (sunglasses should be avoided). Ensure that the light box has an ultraviolet filter.
- Most common side effects are eye strain and headache. Insomnia can result if the light box is used too late in the evening. Light boxes can rarely precipitate mania in some patients but can still be used in patients with bipolar disorder.
- Dawn simulation machines gradually increase illumination while the patient sleeps, simulating sunrise while using a significantly less intense light source. These devices have been shown in studies to improve SAD symptoms similar to bright light therapy, and more effectively than placebo.
- In addition to action through circadian rhythms, light therapy may alter mood more directly through stimulation of the retina, which connects to areas of the brain responsible for mood regulation.
- Separately from mood symptoms, light therapy may also improve alertness when utilizing high Kelvin white lights.

COMPLEMENTARY & ALTERNATIVE MEDICINE

- Work to reduce stress levels through meditation, progressive relaxation exercises, and/or lifestyle modification.
- The potential role of vitamin D supplementation is under investigation. Currently, there is a lack of consistent research to satisfactorily demonstrate this treatment improves SAD symptoms. Reported doses vary widely, but typically, maintenance doses are between 400 and 800 IU/day (8)[C].

ADMISSION, INPATIENT, AND NURSING CONSIDERATIONS

If the patient develops suicidal ideation as part of his or her depression or mania after treatment is initiated, inpatient admission should be considered.

 ONGOING CARE

FOLLOW-UP RECOMMENDATIONS

Regular monitoring by PCP or psychiatrist for response to treatment; rarely, patients may become manic when treated with SSRIs or light therapy.

Patient Monitoring

Patients should be seen monitored weekly to biweekly when initiating light or pharmacotherapy to monitor treatment results, side effects, and any increased suicidal thoughts if using SSRIs.

DIET

No specific diet modification needed

PATIENT EDUCATION

- Increase time outdoors during daylight.
- Rearrange home or work environment to get more direct sunlight through windows.

PROGNOSIS

Symptoms, if untreated, generally remit within 5 months with exposure to spring light, only to return in subsequent winters. If treated, patients usually respond within 3 to 6 weeks.

COMPLICATIONS

Development of suicidal ideation and mania are two outcomes the clinician needs to monitor.

REFERENCES

1. Lam RW, Levitt AJ, Levitan RD, et al. The Can-SAD study: a randomized controlled trial of the effectiveness of light therapy and fluoxetine in patients with winter seasonal affective disorder. *Am J Psychiatry*. 2006;163(5):805–812.
2. Kurlansik SL, Ibay AD. Seasonal affective disorder. *Am Fam Physician*. 2012;86(11):1037–1041.
3. Magovern M, Crawford-Faucher A. Extended-release bupropion for preventing seasonal affective disorder in adults. *Am Fam Physician*. 2017;95(1):10–11.
4. Schlager D. Early-morning administration of short-acting beta blockers for treatment of winter depression. *Am J Psychiatry*. 1994;151(9):1383–1385.
5. Terman M, Terman JS. Light therapy for seasonal and nonseasonal depression: efficacy, protocol, safety, and side effects. *CNS Spectr*. 2005;10(8):647–663.
6. Golden R, Gaynes B, Ekstron R, et al. The efficacy of light therapy in the treatment of mood disorders: a review and meta-analysis of the evidence. *Am J of Psychiatry*. 2005;162(4):656–662.
7. Meesters Y, Duijzer W, Hommes V. The effects of low-intensity narrow-band blue-light treatment compared to bright white-light treatment in seasonal affective disorder. *J Affect Disord*. 2018;232:48–51.
8. Frandsen TB, Pareek M, Hansen JP, et al. Vitamin D supplementation for treatment of seasonal affective symptoms in healthcare professionals: a double-blind randomised placebo-controlled trial. *BMC Res Notes*. 2014;7:528.

ADDITIONAL READING

Cools O, Hebbrecht K, Coppens V, et al. Pharmacotherapy and nutritional supplements for seasonal affective disorders: a systematic review. *Expert Opin Pharmacother*. 2018;19(11):1221–1233.

 SEE ALSO

- Bipolar I Disorder; Bipolar II Disorder; Depression
- Algorithm: Depressive Episode, Major

CODES

ICD10

- F33.9 Major depressive disorder, recurrent, unspecified
- F33.0 Major depressive disorder, recurrent, mild
- F33.1 Major depressive disorder, recurrent, moderate

CLINICAL PEARLS

- SAD is a subtype of both major depressive disorder and bipolar disorder, with seasonal pattern. Once the patient has a diagnosed mood disorder, ask whether the symptoms vary in a seasonal pattern to qualify for the diagnosis of SAD. Generally, these patients will report sleeping too much, eating too much (especially carbs and sweets), and gaining weight during winter months.
- Ensure that symptoms are not due to an organic process or better explained by substance use.
- Guidelines suggest using SSRIs first if the patient is more acute or has contraindications to light therapy or the clinician is not comfortable with light therapy.
- Light therapy boxes are available from numerous online suppliers but are not extensively regulated; practitioners should take care to ensure that patients are using devices from reputable suppliers. Dawn simulation therapy can be utilized as an alternative if bright light therapy is less tolerable.
- If using SSRIs, recent studies indicate some patients may experience increased suicidal thoughts after starting therapy; these patients need to be monitored closely as outpatients every 1 to 2 weeks.

SEIZURE DISORDER, ABSENCE

Christine Young, MD • Vaidehi Joshi, MD, MHA • Brittany E. Zeller, DO

BASICS

DESCRIPTION
- A type of generalized nonmotor seizure characterized by a brief lapse of awareness
- Classified by the International League Against Epilepsy (ILAE) (1):
  - Typical have an abrupt onset and offset of behavioral arrest, loss of awareness, and blank staring, sometimes with eyelid movements, eye opening, or oral automatisms (e.g., lip smacking).
    - Typically occurs at 3 Hz
    - Lasts 5 to 30 seconds, with immediate return to normal consciousness with no aura or postictal phase
    - Commonly associated with epilepsy disorders such as childhood absence epilepsy, juvenile absence epilepsy, juvenile myoclonic epilepsy, and epilepsy with myoclonic absences
  - Atypical have a less abrupt onset and offset and often associated with loss of muscle tone or subtle myoclonic jerks.
    - Typically occurs at <2.5 Hz
    - Lasts 10 to 45 seconds with often incomplete impairment of consciousness with continued purposeful activity, albeit done more slowly.
    - Brief postictal confusion can sometimes occur.
    - Associated with Lennox-Gastaut syndrome and Dravet syndrome
  - Myoclonic have an abrupt onset and offset of staring and loss of awareness with continuous rhythmic jerks of shoulders, arms, legs, head, or perioral muscles.
    - Typically occurs at 2.5 to 4.5 Hz
    - Lasts 10 to 60 seconds with impairment of consciousness varying from complete loss of awareness to retained awareness
    - Associated with epilepsy with myoclonic absences, learning disability, and behavioral problems
  - Eyelid myoclonia have an abrupt onset and offset of repetitive, rhythmic jerks of the eyelids with simultaneous upward deviation of the eyeballs and extension of the head.
    - Typically occurs at 4 to 6 Hz
    - Lasts <6 seconds with incomplete impairment of consciousness and often with awareness mostly retained
    - Associated with epilepsy with eyelid myoclonus

EPIDEMIOLOGY
- Predominant age of onset: between 4 and 10 years, with peak onset between 5 and 7
- Predominant gender: female > male (2:1) with male predominance in myoclonic absence seizure

Incidence
- 0.7 to 4.6 /100,000 in general population (2)
- 6 to 8/100,000 per year in children up to 15 years of age (2)

Prevalence
Prevalence: 5 to 50/10,000 (3)

ETIOLOGY AND PATHOPHYSIOLOGY
- Etiology is mainly genetic with complex, multifactorial inheritance; however, may be secondary to a variety of congenital or acquired brain disorders such as hypoxia–ischemia, trauma, CNS infection, cortical malformations, or inborn errors of metabolism.
- Absences are triggered in the cortico-thalamic-cortical system when γ-aminobutyric acid (GABA)-mediated activity induces prolonged hyperpolarization and activates T-type ("low-threshold") calcium channels, resulting in sustained-burst firing of these neurons, causing absence seizures.

Genetics
- 75% concordance occurs in monozygotic twins; 84% share EEG features (4).
- 15–44% of patients with CAE have a family history of epilepsy.
- Mutations of GABA-A/B receptors—involved in spike-wave discharges
- Mutations in calcium channels (CACNA1 A, CACNA1 H, CACNA1 I, CACNG3)—thalamocortical dysrhythmia
- Mutations of SLC21A, which encodes GLUT1—associated with worse prognosis

> **ALERT**
> Onset of absence seizures <4 years; consider GLUT1 deficiency syndrome.

RISK FACTORS
Seizures of any kind can be triggered by:
- Lack of compliance with medications
- Lack of sleep
- Alcohol use
- Use of medications that lower seizure threshold
- Hyperventilation

COMMONLY ASSOCIATED CONDITIONS
Approximately 60% of children have neuropsychiatric comorbidities including attention deficit and mood disorders (5).
- Includes difficulties in visual attention and visuospatial skills, verbal learning and memory, fine motor skills, executive functions, reduced language abilities, ADHD, anxiety, depression, social isolation, and low esteem

DIAGNOSIS

HISTORY
- Detailed description of episode, including activity at onset, any automatisms, duration of episode, frequency of episodes, aura or postictal state, age of onset, and birth and developmental history.
- Teachers report that child seems to daydream or zone out frequently and during episodes become unresponsive and unaware with a blank stare.
- Pallor is frequently reported.
- Child will forget portions of conversations.
- Child with normal IQ underperforms in school.

> **ALERT**
> Seizures are often so brief that untrained observers are not aware of the occurrence.

PHYSICAL EXAM
- Unless a child has another genetic or acquired abnormality, a neurologic exam usually is normal. Abnormal physical exam indicates the need for further diagnostic workup (e.g., MRI, metabolic, or genetic testing).
- Seizures may be induced by hyperventilation:
  - Have the child blow on a pinwheel or similar exercise for 3 to 5 minutes to provoke seizure.
  - Alternatively, ask the patient to perform hyperventilation with eyes closed and count. Patient will open eyes at onset of seizure and stop counting.

> **ALERT**
> Absence seizures are not associated with sensitivity to light or other photic stimuli (e.g., strobe lights).

DIFFERENTIAL DIAGNOSIS
- CAE
- JAE
- Juvenile myoclonic epilepsy (JME)
- GLUT1 deficiency syndrome
- Complex partial seizures
- Psychogenic nonepileptic seizures
- ADHD
- Confusional states and acute memory disorders
- Migraine variants
- Panic/anxiety attacks
- Breath-holding spells
- Nonepileptic staring spells
- Febrile seizures
- Status epilepticus

DIAGNOSTIC TESTS & INTERPRETATION

Initial Tests (lab, imaging)
- Video-EEG, including sleep and awake with hyperventilation resulting in spike-wave complexes from <2.5 to 6.0 Hz, depending on type of absence seizure, is standard for diagnosis (6)[B].
- Imaging is not routinely indicated in children with typical absence and normal neurologic exam and cognition. If imaging is performed, MRI is preferable to CT scan due to higher sensitivity for anatomic abnormalities (6)[B].
- Presently, no laboratory values can definitively prove or rule out the diagnosis of an absence seizure. However, labs such as electrolytes, creatinine, liver and renal function tests, TSH, CBC, and toxicology screen can rule out endocrine, metabolic, toxic, or infectious etiologies (7)[C].

Follow-Up Tests & Special Considerations
- Drug levels are useful in evaluating symptoms of toxicity or for breakthrough seizures.
- Follow blood chemistry, hepatic function, blood counts, etc., specific to drug regimen.

TREATMENT

GENERAL MEASURES

> **ALERT**
> Review seizure precautions with every patient diagnosed with or suspected to have epilepsy. Seizure precautions are to prevent injury. Patients should refrain from activities that would put them at risk if a seizure occurred (e.g., climbing heights, swimming unsupervised, cycling on busy roads, driving). Providers should be familiar with state laws concerning driving with epilepsy.

MEDICATION

ALERT
- Certain common anticonvulsants may exacerbate absence including carbamazepine, oxcarbazepine, phenytoin, phenobarbital, tiagabine, vigabatrin, pregabalin, and gabapentin.
- 30% of children are pharmacoresistant (4).

First Line
- Ethosuximide blocks T-type calcium channels:
  - First line, high efficacy (8)[A], fastest onset of efficacy (9)[B], and fewer adverse attentional effects compared to valproic acid (8)[A]; however, is only effective against absence seizures
  - Side effects: vomiting, diarrhea, abdominal discomfort, hiccups, headache, sedation
  - Adverse effects: aplastic anemia, skin reactions, and renal/hepatic impairment. Monitor CBC and CMP (3)[C].
- Valproic acid has multiple mechanisms:
  - Alternative first line
    - Very effective but has highest rate of adverse events leading to treatment discontinuation, including negative attentional effects and weight gain (8)[A]; is considered broad spectrum due to effective against absence and comorbid seizure types such as myoclonic, tonic–clonic, and partial
    - Side effects: tremor, drowsiness, dizziness, weight gain, alopecia, sedation, vomiting
    - Adverse effects: teratogenicity, behavior/cognitive abnormalities, hepatotoxicity, pancreatitis. Monitor CMP, amylase, and lipase (3)[C]; reduced bone mineral density and increased risk of osteoporosis and fractures
    - Attention deficits persist more frequently with valproic acid monotherapy compared to ethosuximide or lamotrigine.

Second Line
Lamotrigine affects sodium channels:
- Controls seizures but may be less efficacious than ethosuximide or valproic acid (8)[A]
- Side effects: rash, diplopia, headache, insomnia, dizziness, nausea, vomiting, diarrhea
- Adverse effects: rare Stevens-Johnson rash, more often when coadministered with valproic acid

ISSUES FOR REFERRAL
Failure to gain seizure control for at least 1 year with two AEDs (whether as monotherapy or in combination) should prompt referral to neurologist for confirmation of the diagnosis for seizure and/or syndrome classification and, if appropriate, for consideration of epilepsy surgery (9)[B].

Pediatric Considerations
- Prescribe vitamin D supplementation (usual dose 400 to 1,000 IU/day) in children taking valproic acid due to AE of reduced bone mineral density (10)[A].
- Fatal hepatotoxicity with valproic acid risk is greatest in <2 years old (3)[C].

Pregnancy Considerations
- Anticonvulsants, especially valproic acid, are associated with an increase in fetal malformations. Use of valproic acid in women of childbearing age, who are not using adequate birth control, is contraindicated.
- Pregnant women with epilepsy can enroll in The North American AED Pregnancy Registry: http://www.aedpregnancyregistry.org.

ADDITIONAL THERAPIES
Vagal nerve stimulator (VNS) may be considered as an option for medically refractory absence epilepsy (11)[C].

SURGERY/OTHER PROCEDURES
Epilepsy surgery including ablation and resection for medically refractive absence epilepsy.

COMPLEMENTARY & ALTERNATIVE MEDICINE
According to a 2020 Cochrane review, a ketogenic diet can reduce seizure frequency by 50% in children with drug-resistant epilepsy (12).

ADMISSION, INPATIENT, AND NURSING CONSIDERATIONS
Status epilepticus requires inpatient management.

 ONGOING CARE

FOLLOW-UP RECOMMENDATIONS
Patients should be monitored periodically by a neurologist for evolution of absence epilepsy into other seizure types.

PATIENT EDUCATION
- Caregivers should be informed that tonic–clonic seizures are rare in absence seizures but should be taught how to manage a generalized tonic–clonic seizure.
- Caregivers who question the need to treat these seizures should be informed that though brief, these can interfere with learning and daily activities and can increase the risk of accidents.
- Sarah Jayne Has Staring Moments: a fictional children's book for child absence seizure epilepsy by Kate Lambert

PROGNOSIS
- Prognosis for CAE is excellent with 56–84% remission rate (2).
- Successful control with initial AED is a good prognostic sign.
- Remission is less common in JAE, JME, and those who progress to generalized tonic–clonic seizures or myoclonic seizures.
- Patients whose shortest pretreatment EEG seizures are >20 seconds in duration are more likely to achieve seizure freedom, regardless of treatment.
- Typical absence seizures generally cease spontaneously by age 12 years or sooner.

COMPLICATIONS
- Reported frequencies of typical absence status epilepticus range from 5.8% to 9.4%.
- <10% develop generalized tonic–clonic seizures.

REFERENCES

1. Fisher RS, Cross JH, D'Souza C, et al. Instruction manual for the ILAE 2017 operational classification of seizure types. *Epilepsia*. 2017;58(4):531–542.
2. Guilhoto LM. Absence epilepsy: continuum of clinical presentation and epigenetics? *Seizure*. 2017;44:53–57.
3. Posner E. Absence seizures in children. *Am Fam Physician*. 2015;91(2):114–115.
4. Matricardi S, Verrotti A, Chiarelli F, et al. Current advances in childhood absence epilepsy. *Pediatr Neurol*. 2014;50(3):205–212.
5. Crunelli V, Lőrincz ML, McCafferty C, et al. Clinical and experimental insight into pathophysiology, comorbidity and therapy of absence seizures. *Brain*. 2020;143(8):2341–2368.
6. Uysal-Soyer O, Yalnizoğlu D, Turanli G. The classification and differential diagnosis of absence seizures with short-term video-EEG monitoring during childhood. *Turk J Pediatr*. 2012;54(1):7–14.
7. Nass RD, Sassen R, Elger CE, et al. The role of postictal laboratory blood analyses in the diagnosis and prognosis of seizures. *Seizure*. 2017;47:51–65.
8. Glauser TA, Cnaan A, Shinnar S, et al; for Childhood Absence Epilepsy Study Team. Ethosuximide, valproic acid and lamotrigine in childhood absence epilepsy: initial monotherapy outcomes at 12 months. *Epilepsia*. 2013;54(1):141–155.
9. Mohanraj R, Brodie M. Early predictors of outcome in newly diagnosed epilepsy. *Seizure*. 2013;22(5):333–344.
10. Crepeau A, Moseley B, Wirrell E. Specific safety and tolerability considerations in the use of anticonvulsant medications in children. *Drug Healthc Patient Saf*. 2012;4:39–54.
11. Arya R, Greiner HM, Lewis A, et al. Vagus nerve stimulation for medically refractory absence epilepsy. *Seizure*. 2013;22(4):267–270.
12. Covey C. Ketogenic diets for drug-resistant epilepsy. *Am Fam Physician*. 2021;103(9):524–525.

CODES

ICD10
- G40.409 Other generalized epilepsy and epileptic syndromes, not intractable, without status epilepticus
- G40.419 Oth generalized epilepsy, intractable, w/o stat epi
- G40.401 Oth generalized epilepsy, not intractable, w stat epi

CLINICAL PEARLS
- Children with CAE can exhibit cognitive, behavioral, and psychosocial comorbidities. For these children, attentional deficits are the most important marker of cognitive dysfunction and often associated with reduced academic performance, anxiety, depression, and behavioral disorders.
- If parents are unable to determine the cause of a staring spell, try suggesting that parents mention something exciting or unexpected like "ice cream" during a spell to get the child's attention rather than calling his or her name.
- Ethosuximide and valproic acid are first-line agents in treatment of absence seizures.
- If failure to gain seizure control for at least 1 year with two AEDs, consider referral to neurologist for confirmation of seizure disorder and/or additional/alternative therapies including ketogenic diet, VNS, and surgery.
- Maintain a seizure diary to help identify type and cause of seizures (https://diary.epilepsy.com/login).
- Review seizure precautions and create a seizure response plan: https://www.epilepsy.com/sites/core/files/atoms/files/GENERAL%20Seizure%20Action%20Plan%202020-April7_FILLABLE.pdf.

S

SEIZURE DISORDER, FOCAL

Noel Dunn, MD • Molly E. Chandler, MD

 BASICS

DESCRIPTION
- Seizures occur when abnormal synchronous neuronal discharges in the brain cause transient cortical dysfunction.
- Focal or localization-related seizures have previously been referred to as partial seizures and originate from a discrete focus limited to one cerebral hemisphere.
- Focal seizures are further divided into aware versus unaware and motor versus nonmotor.
- Presence of impaired awareness is defined as the inability to respond normally to exogenous stimuli due to altered awareness and/or responsiveness:
  - Focal seizures with impairment of awareness (formerly "complex partial seizures")
  - Focal seizures without impairment of awareness (formerly "simple partial seizures")

EPIDEMIOLOGY
Prevalence
Focal seizures occur in 20/100,000 persons in the United States.

ETIOLOGY AND PATHOPHYSIOLOGY
- Focal seizures begin when a localized seizure focus produces an abnormal, synchronized depolarization within a neuronal network limited to one cerebral hemisphere; it may stay discretely localized or be widely distributed throughout that hemisphere.
- The area of cortex involved in the seizure determines the symptoms; for example, an epileptogenic focus in motor cortex produces contralateral motor symptoms.
- Most common etiologies vary by life stage:
  - Early childhood: developmental/congenital malformation, trauma
  - Young adults: developmental, infection, trauma
  - Adults 40 to 60 years of age: cerebrovascular insult, infection, trauma
  - Adults >60 years of age: cerebrovascular insult, trauma, neoplasm

Genetics
Benign rolandic epilepsy; has an autosomal dominant inheritance pattern

RISK FACTORS
- History of traumatic brain injury (TBI)
- Thiamine-deficient formula

COMMONLY ASSOCIATED CONDITIONS
Depression

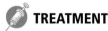 **DIAGNOSIS**

- Duration: seconds to minutes, unless status epilepticus develops; status epilepticus may present as focal/generalized convulsions/altered mental status without convulsions.
- Focal seizures without impairment of awareness (simple partial seizures)
  - Motor onset: Seizure activity in motor strip causes contraction (tonic) or rhythmic jerking (clonic) movements that may involve one entire side of body or may be more localized (i.e., hands, feet, or face).
    ○ Jacksonian march: As discharge spreads through motor cortex, tonic–clonic activity spreads in predictable fashion (i.e., beginning in hand and progressing up arm and to the face).
  - Nonmotor onset:
    ○ Todd paralysis: after motor seizure, residual, temporary weakness in the affected area
    ○ Parietal lobe: sensory loss/paresthesias, dizziness
    ○ Temporal lobe: déjà vu, rising sensation in epigastrium, auditory hallucinations/forced memories, unpleasant smell/taste
    ○ Occipital: visual hallucinations
- Focal seizures with impairment of awareness (complex partial seizures):
  - May have aura; indicates the onset of the seizure
  - Amnesia for the event, postictal confusion
  - Most often, focus is temporal/frontal.
  - Motor manifestations may include dystonic posturing/automatisms (i.e., simple, repetitive movements of face and hands such as lip smacking, picking, or more complex actions such as purposeless walking).
  - Frontal lobe seizure is characterized by brief, bilateral complex movements, vocalizations, often with onset during sleep.

HISTORY
- A detailed description of the seizure should be obtained from an observer.
- Review medication list for drugs that lower seizure threshold (e.g., tramadol, bupropion, theophylline).
- Obtain history of drugs of abuse (e.g., cocaine) that may lower seizure threshold.
- Review history of prior TBI.

PHYSICAL EXAM
Include neurologic exam, with attention to lateralizing signs suggestive of structural lesion.

DIFFERENTIAL DIAGNOSIS
- Syncope/postanoxic myoclonus
- Hypoglycemia
- Psychogenic nonepileptic seizure
- For hemiparesis following event: TIA, hemiplegic migraine

DIAGNOSTIC TESTS & INTERPRETATION
- CBC; complete metabolic panel; urinalysis; urine drug screen; levels of antiepileptic drugs; chest x-ray
- Elevated prolactin, if measured within 10 to 20 minutes of suspected seizure, or elevated creatine phosphokinase; if measured within 6 to 24 hours, may help to differentiate generalized/focal seizure from psychogenic nonepileptic seizure (1)[B]
- Emergency evaluation of new seizure: CT scan to screen for hemorrhage and stroke
- CSF exam if infection is suspected
- EEG should be considered in patients with first time unprovoked seizure (2)[B].
- Yield of EEG is increased by being obtained in the first 24 hours following seizure and by sleep deprivation.
- If difficulty with diagnosis, continuous video–EEG monitoring may be appropriate.
- In patients without recent neuroimaging, consider CT or MRI (2)[B].

TREATMENT

GENERAL MEASURES
Maintain a seizure diary, noting potential triggers, such as stress, sleep deprivation, drug use, discontinuation of alcohol/benzodiazepines, menses.

MEDICATION
- Current guidelines do not recommend for or against starting an AED after a single unprovoked seizure. Patients should be counseled that AEDs will reduce risk of repeat seizure over 2 years but have no effect on long-term remission (3)[C].
- AEDs act on voltage-gated ion channels, affect neuronal inhibition via enhancement of γ-aminobutyric acid (GABA, an inhibitory neurotransmitter), or decrease neuronal excitation. End result is to decrease the abnormal synchronized firing and to prevent seizure propagation.
- 50% of those with newly diagnosed focal seizures respond to, and tolerate, first AED trial. Up to 50% of those who fail the first AED trial will also fail a second AED trial (4)[B].
- Choose AED based on seizure type, side effect profile, and patient characteristics. Increase dose until seizure control is obtained/side effects become unacceptable.
- Attempt monotherapy, but many patients will require adjunctive agents.
- AEDs may prevent seizures after a TBI in the short term, although they provide no efficacy in long-term prevention (5)[B].
- Several AEDs induce/inhibit cytochrome P450 enzymes (watch for drug interactions).

First Line
- Carbamazepine: affects sodium channels; side effects include GI distress, hyponatremia, diplopia, dizziness, rare pancytopenia/marrow suppression, and exfoliative rash.
- Oxcarbazepine: affects sodium channels; side effects include dizziness, diplopia, hyponatremia, and headache.
- Lamotrigine: affects sodium channels
  - Side effects include insomnia, dizziness, and ataxia.
  - Risk of Stevens-Johnson reaction (potentially fatal exfoliative rash), especially when given with valproate, requires slow titration
- Levetiracetam: multiple mechanisms; side effects include sedation, ataxia, and irritability.

Second Line
- Phenytoin: affects sodium channels; side effects include ataxia, dizziness, diplopia, tremor, GI upset, gingival hyperplasia, and fever.
- Phenobarbital: multiple mechanisms; side effects include sedation and withdrawal seizures.
- Valproate: multiple mechanisms; side effects include GI upset, weight gain, alopecia, and tremor; less common, thrombocytopenia, hepatitis, pancreatitis
- Topiramate: multiple mechanisms; side effects include anorexia, cognitive slowing, sedation, nephrolithiasis, and anhidrosis.
- Gabapentin: multiple mechanisms; side effects include sedation, dizziness, and ataxia.
- Pregabalin: affects calcium channels; side effects include sedation, dizziness, and weight gain.
- Zonisamide: affects sodium channels
  - Side effects include sedation, anorexia, nausea, dizziness, ataxia, anhidrosis, and nephrolithiasis.
  - Cross-reaction with sulfa allergy

Pregnancy Considerations
- Folate should be prescribed for all women of childbearing age who are taking AEDs. AED therapy during the 1st trimester is associated with doubled risk for major fetal malformations (6% vs. 3%).
- Phenytoin in pregnancy may result in fetal hydantoin syndrome.
- Valproate is associated with neural tube defects and should be avoided in pregnancy when possible.
- Fetal insult from seizures following withdrawal of therapy also may be severe. Risk-to-benefit balance should be evaluated with high-risk pregnancy and neurology consultations. Most patients remain on anticonvulsants.
- AED levels should be monitored at least every trimester.

ISSUES FOR REFERRAL
Epilepsy specialist for refractory seizures

ADDITIONAL THERAPIES
- Vagal nerve stimulator provides periodic stimulation to vagus nerve. High-frequency stimulation in adults provides greater reduction in seizure frequency than low-frequency stimulation but also has greater rates of side effects (6)[B].
- Deep brain stimulation may decrease seizure frequency in medically refractive epilepsy.
- Repetitive magnetic transcranial stimulation may reduce seizures with refractory focal seizures.

SURGERY/OTHER PROCEDURES
- For refractory focal seizures with identifiable focus
- Preoperative testing, such as Wada test, should be done to decrease likelihood of inducing aphasia and memory loss.
- 34–74% will be seizure free after temporal lobe surgery. Prognosis varies for surgical resection of extratemporal foci.
- Goal of surgical intervention is to reduce reliance on medications; most patients remain on anticonvulsants postoperatively.

ADMISSION, INPATIENT, AND NURSING CONSIDERATIONS
Admit for unremitting seizure (status epilepticus).

ONGOING CARE

FOLLOW-UP RECOMMENDATIONS
- Most states have restrictions on driving for those with seizure disorders.
- Depending on seizure manifestation, may also recommend against activities such as swimming, climbing to heights, or operating heavy machinery

Patient Monitoring
AED levels if concern over toxicity, noncompliance, or for breakthrough seizures

DIET
Ketogenic or low-glycemic index diet may improve seizure control in some patients.

PATIENT EDUCATION
Avoid potential triggers such as alcohol or drug use and sleep deprivation.

PROGNOSIS
- Risk of seizure recurrence: ~30% after first seizure; of these, 50% will occur in the first 6 months, 90% in the first 2 years.
- Depends on seizure type; rolandic epilepsy has a good prognosis; temporal lobe epilepsy is more likely to be persistent.
- ~25–30% of all seizures are refractory to current medications.
- AEDs initiated after an initial seizure have been shown to decrease the risk of seizure over the first 5 years but are not demonstrated to reduce long-term risk of recurrence or mortality.
- The risk of developing seizure after mild TBI remains high for a long period (>10 years).

COMPLICATIONS
- Risk of accidental injury
- Depression and anxiety
- Memory impairment

REFERENCES
1. Brigo F, Igwe SC, Erro R, et al. Postictal serum creatine kinase for the differential diagnosis of epileptic seizures and psychogenic non-epileptic seizures: a systematic review. *J Neurol.* 2015;262(2):251–257.
2. Krumholz A, Wiebe S, Gronseth G, et al. Practice parameter: evaluating an apparent unprovoked first seizure in adults (an evidence-based review): report of the Quality Standards Subcommittee of the American Academy of Neurology and the American Epilepsy Society. *Neurology.* 2007;69(21):1996–2007.
3. Krumholz A, Wiebe S, Gronseth GS, et al. Evidence-based guideline: management of an unprovoked first seizure in adults: report of the Guideline Development Subcommittee of the American Academy of Neurology and the American Epilepsy Society. *Neurology.* 2015;84(16):1705–1713.
4. Bonnett LJ, Tudur Smith C, Donegan S, et al. Treatment outcome after failure of a first antiepileptic drug. *Neurology.* 2014;83(6):552–560.
5. Thompson K, Pohlmann-Eden B, Campbell LA, et al. Pharmacological treatments for preventing epilepsy following traumatic head injury. *Cochrane Database Syst Rev.* 2015;(8):CD009900.
6. Panebianco M, Rigby A, Weston J, et al. Vagus nerve stimulation for partial seizures. *Cochrane Database Syst Rev.* 2015;(4):CD002896.

ADDITIONAL READING
- Gavvala JR, Schuele SU. New-onset seizure in adults and adolescents: a review. *JAMA.* 2016;316(24):2657–2668.
- Pack AM. Epilepsy overview and revised classification of seizures and epilepsies. *Continuum (Minneap Minn).* 2019;25(2):306–321.

CODES

ICD10
- G40.109 Local-rel symptc epi w simp prt seiz, not ntrct, w/o stat epi
- G40.209 Local-rel symptc epi w cmplx prt seiz, not ntrct, w/o stat epi
- G40.119 Local-rel symptc epi w simple part seiz, ntrct, w/o stat epi

CLINICAL PEARLS
- Focal seizures originate from a discrete focus limited to one hemisphere in the cerebral cortex and are further divided into aware versus unaware and motor versus nonmotor, depending on patient presentation.
- It is controversial whether AED treatment is indicated after a first seizure. Treatment should be strongly considered when a clear structural cause is identified/risk of injury from seizure is high (e.g., osteoporosis, anticoagulation).
- An EEG and neuroimaging (CT or MRI) should be considered in evaluating a first unprovoked seizure.
- Postictal elevation in prolactin and CPK levels can help distinguish physiologic from psychogenic nonepileptic seizures.

SEIZURE DISORDERS

Sahil Mullick, MD • Joseph Braddock, MD

 BASICS

DESCRIPTION

- Seizure: sudden and transient symptoms (altered level of consciousness, motor manifestations) due to abnormal neuronal electrical activity
- Epilepsy: two or more unprovoked seizures apart in a >24-hour period or one unprovoked seizure with a risk of further seizures that is similar to the risk after two unprovoked seizures (at least 60%)
- Status epilepticus: epileptic seizure that lasts >5 minutes or multiple seizures without returning to normal between them. Classification: generalized, simple and complex partial, absence, nonconvulsive; based on three key features:
  – Seizure origin: focal (previously partial), focal to bilateral, generalized
  – Awareness: aware, focal impaired or generalized
  – Clinical features: motor, nonmotor (absence, behavior, cognitive, autonomic)
- System(s) affected: nervous
- Synonym(s): convulsion; attacks; spells

Pregnancy Considerations
- Pregnancy: Avoid valproate as possible. Monitor AED levels every trimester for dose adjustment, continue folic acid supplementation, and screen for congenital abnormalities.
- Levetiracetam, topiramate, lamotrigine are alternatives for women of childbearing potential (1).

EPIDEMIOLOGY

Incidence
200,000 new cases of epilepsy are diagnosed in United States annually, with 45,000 new cases in children <15 years of age.

ETIOLOGY AND PATHOPHYSIOLOGY
- Synchronous and excessive firing of neurons, resulting in an imbalance of regulatory mechanisms in favor of excitatory activity
- Acute symptomatic seizures: triggered by acute insult to the brain, medical illness, metabolic disturbance, substance/medication ingestion or withdrawal (such seizures do not necessarily define the presence of epilepsy)
  – Stroke, subdural hematoma, subarachnoid bleed, traumatic brain injury, hypoxic-ischemic injury, acute infection
  – Metabolic and endocrine disorders, drug intoxication/poisoning/overdose
  – Medications: opioids, anticancer drugs, various antibiotics, hypoglycemic agents, immunosuppressants, psychotropic medications, and decongestants
- Vascular malformations
- Familial/genetic seizure syndromes
- Benign neonatal seizures, benign familial neonatal epilepsy, EME, Ohtahara syndrome
- Infancy (<2 years): febrile seizures, metabolic causes (e.g., hypoglycemia, B_6 deficiency)

- Childhood (2 to 10 years): absence or febrile seizure
- Adolescent (10 to 18 years): AV malformation
- Late adulthood (>60 years): stroke, metabolic disturbances (hypoglycemia, uremia, hepatic failure, electrolyte abnormality), and drugs

Genetics
Family history increases risk 3-fold.

RISK FACTORS
History of congenital brain malformations, CNS infections, head trauma, stroke, tumors

GENERAL PREVENTION
Prevent head injuries. Avoid sleep deprivation and excessive alcohol intake.

COMMONLY ASSOCIATED CONDITIONS
Genetic syndromes (Angelman, tuberous sclerosis, Sturge-Weber), infections, tumors, drug abuse, alcohol and drug withdrawal, trauma, metabolic disorders

 DIAGNOSIS

Conventional classification of seizures
- Generalized seizures
  – Tonic–clonic: tonic phase: sudden loss of consciousness; clonic phase: sustained contraction followed by rhythmic contractions of all four extremities; postictal phase: headache, confusion, fatigue; clinically hypertensive, tachycardic, and otherwise hypersympathetic
  – Absence: impaired awareness and responsiveness
  – Atonic: abrupt loss of muscle tone
  – Myoclonic: repetitive muscle contractions
- Febrile seizures
  – Usually ≤6 years; fever without evidence of any other defined cause of seizures
  – Recurrent febrile seizures probably do not increase the risk of epilepsy.
- Focal seizures with retained awareness (previously called simple partial seizures): Symptoms vary depending entirely on the part of the cortex involved; can present with auras and postictal phase
- Focal seizures with impaired awareness (previously called complex partial seizures): most common type of seizure in adults with epilepsy; can stare into space, motionless, or engage in automatisms and then enters postictal phase
- Both focal seizures may propagate diffusely to cause bilateral tonic–clonic seizures.
- Nonconvulsive status epilepticus: most commonly seen in ICU patients; no tonic–clonic activity seen so must diagnose with bedside EEG
- Status epilepticus: repetitive generalized seizures without recovery between seizures; considered a neurologic emergency
- PNES: nonrhythmic pattern of movement, eye closure during event, anterior tongue biting, history of psychiatric disorders. Patients can also have coexisting epilepsy.

HISTORY
- Eyewitness descriptions of event; patient impressions of what occurred before, during, and after the event
- Screen for etiologies, including provoking/ameliorating factors for the event, such as sleep deprivation.
- Ask about bowel/bladder incontinence, tongue biting, other injury, automatisms, or prior seizure activity.
- Ictal behaviors are useful for localization.
- Evaluate for medication or substance use.

PHYSICAL EXAM
Thorough neurologic exam; lateral tongue biting suggestive of generalized seizure, whereas tip of tongue more suggestive of nonepileptic event. Tongue biting lacks sensitivity but has high specificity to differentiate from PNES and syncope. Urinary incontinence has low specificity and sensitivity.

DIFFERENTIAL DIAGNOSIS
- Syncope, orthostatic hypotension, convulsive syncope
- Transient ischemic attack, stroke
- Complicated migraine
- Sleep disorders: cataplexy, narcolepsy
- Psychiatric disorders: conversion, malingering, panic

DIAGNOSTIC TESTS & INTERPRETATION
A negative EEG does not rule out a seizure disorder. Interictal EEG sensitivity may be as low as 20%; multiple EEGs (at least three) may increase sensitivity to 80% (2)[C].
- Sleep deprivation may be helpful prior to EEG, and hyperventilation and photic stimulation during recording may increase sensitivity.
- Video EEG monitoring is used to differentiate PNES from true cortical events.
- EEG is necessary for diagnosis of nonconvulsive status epilepticus.

Initial Tests (lab, imaging)
- Glucose, sodium, potassium, calcium, phosphorus, magnesium, BUN, ammonia; drug and toxin screens
- AED levels (if patient is taking antiepileptic medication)
- CBC, UA, ECG, lumbar puncture if needed: Rule out infection.
- Serum prolactin has limited utility; may be useful in differentiating generalized tonic–clonic and focal seizure from PNES
- Imaging is recommended for new-onset seizures. MRI is preferred to CT.
  – CT scan of brain: indicated routinely as initial evaluation, especially in the ER
  – Brain MRI: superior in evaluation of the temporal lobes (e.g., mesial temporal sclerosis), stroke, and other structural abnormalities

Diagnostic Procedures/Other
Lumbar puncture for spinal fluid analysis may be necessary to rule out meningitis.

TREATMENT

- Older adults are more sensitive to side effects from AEDs; use lower initial dosing (3).
- After an initial unprovoked seizure, 21–45% will have a recurrence within 2 years (4).
- Starting antiepileptic medications is likely to reduce recurrences of seizures but does not alter long-term outcomes or improve quality of life (4).
- Patients with a single unprovoked seizure and associated risk factors that increase recurrence risk up to 60% (abnormal EEG, neurologic exam, or neuroimaging) can potentially benefit from starting therapy.

GENERAL MEASURES

- Most seizures remit spontaneously within 2 minutes.
- Treat metabolic and infectious etiologies.
- Main goals: Control seizures, avoid side effects, and restore quality of life.

MEDICATION

- AED: Select based on type of seizure, potential adverse effects/drug interactions, comorbid medical conditions.
- Treatment should begin with a single agent, and the dose titrated until seizures are controlled or side effects become problematic. Consider switching to a different agent versus adding a second agent.
- Patients treated with loading doses of AED in status epilepticus can be started on maintenance dose of a different AED afterward.

First Line

Treatment options include the following:

- Levetiracetam (Keppra): 1,000 to 4,000 mg/day in 2 doses
- Carbamazepine (Tegretol): 100 to 200 mg/day, 2 to 4 doses; therapeutic range 4 to 12 mg/L
- Lamotrigine (Lamictal): 25 mg/day, titrate by 50 mg/day every 1 to 2 weeks to 225 to 375 mg/day in 2 doses for immediate release or 300 to 400 mg/day for extended release
- Oxcarbazepine (Trileptal): 900 to 2,400 mg/day in 2 to 3 doses
- Lacosamide (Vimpat): 200 to 400 mg/day in 2 doses
- Ethosuximide (Zarontin): 20 to 40 mg/kg/day in 1 to 3 doses, therapeutic concentration 40 to 100 μg/mL
- Generalized status epilepticus:
  - Lorazepam 4 mg, fosphenytoin 20 mg/kg load, valproic acid 30 mg/kg load, levetiracetam 60 mg/kg load, lacosamide 300 mg load

Second Line

- Phenytoin (Dilantin): 300 to 400 mg/day in 1 to 3 doses; therapeutic range 10 to 20 mg/L
- Valproic acid (Depakene): 750 to 3,000 mg/day in 1 to 3 doses to begin at 15 mg/kg/day; therapeutic range 50 to 125 μg/mL
- Topiramate (Topamax): 50 mg/day; adjust weekly to effect; 400 mg/day in 2 doses, max 1,600 mg/day
- Gabapentin (Neurontin): 1,800 to 3,600 mg in 3 doses for adjunct therapy
- Pregabalin (Lyrica): 150 to 300 mg/day in 2 to 3 doses

- Zonisamide (Zonegran): 100 to 600 mg/day in 1 to 2 doses
- Perampanel (Fycompa): 4 to 12 mg daily
- Clonazepam (Klonopin): 1.5 to 8.0 mg in 2 to 3 doses (maximum 20 mg daily)
- Clobazam (Onfi): 20 to 40 mg in 1 to 2 doses
- Rufinamide (Banzel): 3,200 mg in 2 doses
- Brivaracetam (Briviact) (an analog of levetiracetam): 50 to 200 mg/day in 2 doses
- Consider cautioning about increased risk of suicide, but risk of untreated seizures is far greater.
- Patients are susceptible to sudden unexpected death in epilepsy, possibly due to cardiac arrhythmia.

ISSUES FOR REFERRAL

- Psychological therapies may be used in conjunction with AED therapy. Cognitive-behavioral therapy, relaxation, biofeedback, and yoga all may be helpful as adjunctive therapy.
- Neurology referral for first time seizure patients, unless clearly provoked and initial studies unremarkable

SURGERY/OTHER PROCEDURES

For patients that fail traditional therapy: lobectomy, resection, laser ablation, and vagus nerve stimulation

COMPLEMENTARY & ALTERNATIVE MEDICINE

Complimentary supplements may induce drug interactions with prescribed AEDs.

ADMISSION, INPATIENT, AND NURSING CONSIDERATIONS

- Admit for status epilepticus, prolonged postictal state, or serious seizure related injury.
- Admissions to epilepsy monitoring units for video EEG monitoring may benefit patients with events that pose a diagnostic challenge or patients with intractable seizures already on two AED.

 ONGOING CARE

FOLLOW-UP RECOMMENDATIONS

Maintain adequate drug therapy; ensure compliance and/or access to medication. Drug therapy withdrawal and tapering of doses may be considered after a seizure-free 2-year period. Expect a 33% relapse rate in the following 3 years.

Patient Monitoring

- Monitor drug levels and seizure frequency.
- CBC and lab values (e.g., calcium, vitamin D) as indicated; BMD
- Monitor for side effects and adverse reactions.
- All patients currently taking any AED should be monitored closely for notable changes in behavior that could indicate the emergence/worsening of suicidal thoughts/behavior/depression.

DIET

Ketogenic diet may be beneficial in children in conjunction with AED therapy and refractory seizures.

PATIENT EDUCATION

- Seizure precautions: Be aware of common triggers or precipitating factors and avoid them.
- Caution with unsupervised activities that can be dangerous with a sudden loss of consciousness.
- Emphasize the danger of driving unless seizure free for a certain period. Laws vary by state: http://www.epilepsy.org.

PROGNOSIS

- Depends on type of seizure disorder: ~70% will become seizure free with treatment. The number of seizures within 6 months after first presentation is a prognostic factor for remission.
- ~90% with an unprovoked seizure attain a 1- to 2-year remission within 4 or 5 years of the initial event.
- Life expectancy is shortened in persons with epilepsy.
- The case fatality rate for status epilepticus: 20%

REFERENCES

1. Perucca E, Tomson T. The pharmacological treatment of epilepsy in adults. *Lancet Neurol*. 2011;10(5):446–456.
2. Fisher RS, Acevedo C, Arzimanoglou A, et al. ILAE official report: a practical clinical definition of epilepsy. *Epilepsia*. 2014;55(4):475–482.
3. Lee SK. Epilepsy in the elderly: treatment and consideration of comorbid diseases. *J Epilepsy Res*. 2019;9(1):27–35.
4. Rizvi S, Ladino LD, Hernandez-Ranquillo L, et al. Epidemiology of early stages of epilepsy: risk of seizure recurrence after a first seizure. *Seizure*. 2017;49:46–53.

 SEE ALSO

Seizures, Febrile; Status Epilepticus

 CODES

ICD10

- G40.B1 Juvenile myoclonic epilepsy, intractable
- G40.804 Other epilepsy, intractable, without status epilepticus
- G40.A0 Absence epileptic syndrome, not intractable

CLINICAL PEARLS

- Initiation of treatment depends on multiple variables, including type of seizure, underlying risk factors, risk of recurrence.
- Semiology of event is very important for diagnosis of seizures versus PNES. Patients with PNES can have concomitant epileptic seizures.
- Patients in status epilepticus who receive a loading dose of one AED do not require to be continued on the same medication.

S

SEIZURES, FEBRILE

Joo Hyun Lee, MD • Swati B. Avashia, MD, FAAP, FACP

 BASICS

DESCRIPTION

Febrile seizures (FS) occur in children aged 6 months to 5 years with fever ≥100.4°F (38°C) in the absence of an underlying neurologic abnormality, metabolic condition, or intracranial infection. There are three distinct categories (1),(2):

- Simple febrile seizure (SFS) (70–75%; must meet all criteria)
  - Generalized clonic or tonic–clonic seizure activity without focal features
  - Duration <15 minutes
  - Does not recur within 24 hours
  - Resolves spontaneously
  - No history of previous afebrile seizure, seizure disorder, or other neurologic problem
- Complex febrile seizure (CFS) (20–25%; only one criterion must be met)
  - Partial seizure, focal activity
  - Duration >15 minutes but <30 minutes
  - Recurrence within 24 hours
  - Postictal focal neurologic abnormalities (e.g., Todd paralysis)
- Febrile status epilepticus (FSE) (5%)
  - Lasts >30 minutes

EPIDEMIOLOGY

Incidence
- About 500,000 FS in the United States annually.
- Occurs in 2–4% of children 6 months to 5 years of age. Peak incidence is 18 months of age with 90% of children having their first FS before age 3. Only 6% of FS occur before age 6 months (3).
- Bimodal seasonal pattern that mirrors peaks of febrile respiratory (November to January) and gastrointestinal infections (June to August) (4)

Prevalence
Children of any ethnic group can develop FS, but there is higher prevalence in Asian population, specifically the Japanese (3.4–9.3%), Indians (5–10%), and Guamanians (14%). Children in United States and Western Europe have a prevalence of 2–5%.

ETIOLOGY AND PATHOPHYSIOLOGY
The pathophysiology of FS remains unclear but current research suggests the following mechanisms that lower seizure threshold:
- Age-dependent vulnerability of developing nervous system (2)
- Increased neuronal activity (i.e., seizures) secondary to temperature-sensitive ion channels and secretion of cytokines from inflammatory processes such as fever-promoting pyrogen interleukin-1β
  - Interleukin-1β can increase neuronal activity by modulating glutamate and GABA.
- Hyperthermia-induced hyperventilation and alkalosis, which provokes neuronal excitability

Genetics
- FEB1 and FEB2 are known to increase susceptibility to FS.
  - Sodium channel 1alpha (SCN1A) mutation is also known to increase susceptibility to FS; however, epileptic syndromes can also carry the same mutation:
    - Dravet syndrome: most severe form of epileptic encelphalopathy that presents with FS and is commonly caused by a de novo mutation of SCN1A
- Mode of inheritance thought to be through polygenic multifactorial transmission (several different pairs of genes that are contributory and additive to the phenotype) or autosomal dominant pattern with reduced penetrance

RISK FACTORS
- Most common risk factors for developing first FS (1),(5):
  - Height of fever, more so than rate of rise
  - Viral infection (80% of FS caused by virus)—HHV6, influenza A, adenovirus, and parainfluenza are commonly associated viruses
  - Recently immunized, particularly with MMR and DTwP
  - Family history of FS
    - As many as 25–40% of cases have a positive family history of FS. Risk increases with number of affected first-degree (OR = 4.5%) and second-degree relatives (OR = 3.6%); greater concordance rate in monozygotic than dizygotic twins (1)
- Other general risk factors for FS: nicotine exposure in utero, NICU stay >28 days, developmental delay or day care attendance
- Risk is slightly increased for males (2).
- Recent vaccination (6)
  - Certain vaccines (e.g., MMR, DTP, PCV13), method of preparation, vaccine coadministration, and associated age of administration have shown to increase risk of FS.
  - No evidence of increased risk with isolated influenza vaccination
- Perhaps increased risk with iron deficiency anemia and low zinc levels (1),(4)

GENERAL PREVENTION
Choose vaccines with lower risk of developing FS and ask if the child has ever had a history of FS after vaccine administration (5).
- Increased risk of FS if vaccine administrations are delayed
- Separate MMR and varicella vaccine and administer between 12 and 15 months of age.
- Administer DTaP (acellular) rather than DTwP (whole cell) vaccine.

COMMONLY ASSOCIATED CONDITIONS
- Viral infections are the cause of fever in nearly 80% of FS cases, particularly human herpesvirus 6 (HHV-6), influenza, parainfluenza, adenovirus, and respiratory syncytial virus (RSV) (4).
- Bacterial infections: otitis media, pharyngitis, urinary tract infection (UTI), pneumonia, and gastroenteritis (specifically with *Shigella*)

- Vaccinations (6):
  - MMRV vaccination had 2-fold increase in risk of FS compared to separation of MMR and varicella vaccine.
  - DTwP vaccine had roughly 15% greater chance of causing FS compared to DTaP (1 per 2,835 vaccines and 1 per 19,496 vaccines, respectively).
  - There is a small increased risk for FS when activated influenza vaccine (flu shot) is given at the same time as either the PCV13 (pneumococcal) vaccine or the DTaP vaccine (7).
    - Also small increased risk with PCV13 given alone (7)
    - No increased risk if influenza or DTaP given alone (7)

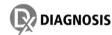 **DIAGNOSIS**

HISTORY
- Symptoms of underlying infection or neurologic deficits
- Onset, duration, type, and number of seizure (4)
  - A SFS is generalized and associated with tonic–clonic movements of the limb and rolling back of the eyes. It may last a few seconds to 15 minutes, although generally <5 minutes, and does not recur within 24 hours.
- Presence of postictal state (such as weakness or paralysis)
  - Postictal drowsiness should resolve within 5 to 10 minutes. Encephalopathy beyond this range raises suspicion of CNS or systemic infection.
- Any interventions made to stop seizure
- Past medical history:
  - Immunization status, recent vaccines
  - Preexisting conditions: developmental delay, cerebral palsy, metabolic disorders, injury
  - Recent antibiotic course
- Family history: FS, afebrile seizures, epilepsy, metabolic disorders, and other neurologic conditions
- Factors concerning for child abuse or trauma

PHYSICAL EXAM
- Monitoring vital signs and close observation of neurologic status/change are essential in all children (1)[A].
  - Unstable vital signs or toxic appearance warrants further evaluation.
  - Look for tachypnea, hypoxemia, lesions in oropharynx, or viral exanthem.
    - Observe for presence of closed eyes and a deep breath to indicate cessation of seizure. Children with persistently open and deviated eyes may still be seizing in absence of convulsive motor activities.
    - Average duration of FSE is 67 minutes.
  - Assess mental status and signs of meningitis—obtunded or comatose mental state, nuchal rigidity, prolonged focal seizure or petechial rash, and multiple seizures.
  - Duration of seizures greater than 30 minutes, presence of postictal drowsiness and neurologic deficits were predictive factors for meningitis.
- A thorough physical exam should not be deferred until postictal state has resolved. Although exam may be limited, prompt evaluation may reveal focal neurologic deficits or Todd paresis (2)[A].
- Assess for nonaccidental trauma with skin inspection, palpation for occult trauma, and retinal exam.

DIFFERENTIAL DIAGNOSIS

- Seizures due to other etiology: meningitis, encephalitis, primary epilepsy, intracranial mass, trauma, electrolyte abnormality, hypoglycemia, metabolic disorder
- Seizure mimics: rigors, crying, breath-holding spell, choking episode, tic disorder, parasomnia, dystonic reaction, shaking chills (shivering)

DIAGNOSTIC TESTS & INTERPRETATION

Initial Tests (lab, imaging)

- Routine laboratory tests not routinely recommended if the child is well appearing (5)[B].
  - Blood workup if other symptoms, such as vomiting, diarrhea, and poor fluid intake that points toward another etiology for seizure.
  - Urinalysis only if indicated by current UTI rates in children with SFS are comparable to febrile children without seizure.
- Lumbar puncture (LP) not necessary well-appearing children who quickly return to baseline.
  - Following situations may warrant LP:
    o Meningeal signs and symptoms (5)[B]. Infant 6 to 12 months of age without known *Haemophilus influenzae* type b (Hib) or
    o *Streptococcus pneumoniae* immunization (5)[C]. Child was treated with antibiotics as it can mask the signs and symptoms of meningitis (5)[C]
- Neuroimaging is not routinely recommended to identify the cause of an FS (2)[A],(5)[A].
  - Studies demonstrate limited utility of emergent imaging in most patients with FS; no advantage of MRI versus CT for management of FS in ED
  - Warranted if strong indication of acute/subacute bleeding or structural lesion
  - Nonurgent, outpatient MRI brain is recommended for patients with focal CFS especially with postictal neurologic deficits.
    o No evidence to support routine use of neuroimaging in absence of interictal or postictal focality
- Check for anemia if iron deficiency is suspected.

Follow-Up Tests & Special Considerations

If there is a need to perform both EEG and MRI for a child presenting with FS, do EEG first. MRI in children will most often require complete sedation, which may alter the results of an EEG.

Test Interpretation

If the CSF show any pleocytosis, even in the absence of any glucose or protein abnormalities, this should be considered as a sign of meningitis rather than consequence of FS (3)[A].

 TREATMENT

Most FS are self-limited, however, if health care professionals are able to witness the FS, acute abortive treatment should be no different than any other seizure treatment. FSE rarely stops spontaneously and often required more than one medication to control. Early intervention with AEDs is important for duration of FSE and outcome (2)[A].

GENERAL MEASURES

During an acute seizure management, continue to monitor patient's ABCs (1).

- Airway: Position the patient laterally, suction secretions, and place a nasopharyngeal airway
- Breathing: Administer oxygen for cyanosis; consider bag-mask ventilation or intubation for inadequate ventilation.
- Circulation: Establish IV access for any medication and fluid bolus.

MEDICATION

First Line

- Treat seizures of ≥5 minutes duration with anticonvulsants. If seizures continue 5 minutes after administration of medication, can repeat dose (2)[A]:
  - Out of hospital (e.g., home or paramedics on route): rectal diazepam 0.5 mg/kg, buccal midazolam (0.2 to 0.4 mg/kg), or nasal midazolam (0.2 mg/kg)
  - In hospital: IV or IM lorazepam 0.05 to 0.10 mg/kg or IV diazepam 0.1 to 0.2 mg/kg; "out of hospital" options can also be used if IV option is not available.
- If seizures are prolonged or recurrent, administer IV fosphenytoin (20 mg PE/kg); if seizures persist after 10 minutes of loading dose, can give additional dose (5 to 10 mg phenytoin equivalent/kg) (2)[A]
  - There is some evidence that fosphenytoin should be avoided due to risk of worsening seizures in patients with SCN1A mutations (2)[C].
- Antipyretics should be used to reduce fever as it often helps with overall comfort level of patients (1)[A].
  - In one study, rectal acetaminophen (10 mg/kg, every 6 hours for 24 hours) showed potential to prevent FS recurrence during same fever episode (1)[B].
  - Prophylactic antipyretics before vaccination is not recommended as not effective and could decrease immune response to certain vaccines (4)[B].

Second Line

IV phenobarbital (15 to 20 mg/kg), valproic acid (20 to 40 mg/kg), or levetiracetam (20 to 60 mg/kg)

ISSUES FOR REFERRAL

Neurology consultation if persistent neurologic deficits, recurrent FS, or abnormal exam on evaluation (2).

ADMISSION, INPATIENT, AND NURSING CONSIDERATIONS

Abnormal or concerning findings on history or physical exam or prolonged/delayed recovery

 ONGOING CARE

FOLLOW-UP RECOMMENDATIONS

Anticonvulsant prophylaxis during subsequent febrile episodes is not recommended (5).

PATIENT EDUCATION

Guidance for parents should focus on reassurance, emphasizing the benign nature of FS, overall excellent prognosis of the disease, and basic guidelines on interventions of FS were to reoccur (1).

- FS often do not cause brain damage, have a low risk for sequelae, and do not have a negative impact on intellect, behavior, or risk of death (3).
- The benefits of vaccinations greatly outweigh the side effects. The vaccine-induced FS risk is more affected by personal and family history rather than the sole act of receiving the vaccination (4).

PROGNOSIS

Favorable for children with normal neurodevelopmental status.

- A second FS occurs in about 1/3 of the patients; a third FS in 15% of patients
- Risk factors for recurrent FS (1),(2),(4):
  - Age of onset: younger the age, higher the risk (3)
  - Relatively low temp (<104°F) at time of first FS
  - Shorter interval (<1 hr) between onset of fever and seizure
  - First-degree relative with history of FS or epilepsy
  - First FS has complex FS features, particularly focal or prolonged CFS (continued topic of debate)
- Risk of FS developing into epilepsy (1),(3):
  - Age >3 years at time of first FS
  - Developmental delay or abnormal neurologic exam prior to onset of first FS
  - Complex FS
  - Family history of epilepsy
  - Fever duration of <1 hour before seizure onset
- An unprovoked, afebrile seizure (epilepsy) after FS is estimated to be 1% for simple FS and 4–6% for complex FS.

REFERENCES

1. Smith DK, Sadler KP, Benedum M. Febrile seizures: risks, evaluation, and prognosis. *Am Fam Physician*. 2019;99(7):445–450.
2. Whelan H, Harmelink M, Chou E, et al. Complex febrile seizures—a systematic review. *Dis Mon*. 2017;63(1):5–23.
3. Gupta A. Febrile seizures. *Continuum (Minneap Minn)*. 2016;22(1 Epilepsy):51–59.
4. Leung AK, Hon KL, Leung TN. Febrile seizures: an overview. *Drugs Context*. 2018;7:212536.
5. Subcommittee on Febrile Seizures, American Academy of Pediatrics. Neurodiagnostic evaluation of the child with a simple febrile seizure. *Pediatrics*. 2011;127(2):389–394.
6. Li X, Lin Y, Yao G, et al. The influence of vaccine on febrile seizure. *Curr Neuropharmacol*. 2018;16(01):59–65.
7. Centers for Disease Control and Prevention. Febrile seizures and childhood vaccines. https://www.cdc.gov/vaccinesafety/concerns/febrile-seizures.html. Accessed February 6, 2021.

CODES

ICD10

- R56.00 Simple febrile convulsions
- R56.01 Complex febrile convulsions
- G40.901 Epilepsy, unsp, not intractable, with status epilepticus

CLINICAL PEARLS

- FS are generally benign and without sequelae if the underlying causes are ruled out.
- Labs, LP, neuroimaging, and EEG not routinely recommended in an acute setting in the absence of suspicion for underlying pathology.
- Prophylaxis with anticonvulsants or antipyretics during subsequent febrile episodes is not recommended.

SEROTONIN SYNDROME

Michael T. Partin, MD • Karl T. Clebak, MD, MHA, FAAFP • Munima Nasir, MD

 BASICS

DESCRIPTION

- A potentially life-threatening drug-induced syndrome that results from synaptic increase in serotonin (5-hydroxytryptamine [5-HT]) concentrations and stimulation of peripheral and CNS serotonergic receptors
- Classically characterized by a triad of symptoms that include mental status changes, neuromuscular hyperactivity, and autonomic instability.
- Onset is usually within 24 hours with the majority occurring within 6 hours of exposure to, or change in, dosing of a serotonergic agent. Rarely, reported weeks after discontinuation of serotonergic agents
- It is a concentration-dependent toxicity that can develop in any individual who has ingested drug combinations that synergistically increase synaptic 5-HT.
- Serotonin toxicity occurs in three main settings: (i) therapeutic drug use, which often results in mild to moderate symptoms; (ii) intentional overdose of a single serotonergic agent, which typically leads to moderate symptoms; and (iii) as the result of a drug interaction between numerous serotonergic agents (most commonly, selective serotonin reuptake inhibitors [SSRIs], serotonin noradrenergic reuptake inhibitors [SNRIs], and monoamine oxidase inhibitors [MAOIs]), most often associated with severe serotonin toxicity.

Geriatric Considerations
Increased risk through polypharmacy given frequent use of serotonergic analgesics, antibiotics, and antidepressants.

Pediatric Considerations
- Similar manifestations in children and adults.
- Aside from altering medication dosing, general management is unchanged in pediatric patients.
- Consider toxic ingestion of serotonergic agents prescribed to caregivers of pediatric patients.
- Symptoms in neonates may include tremors, increased muscle tone, jitteriness, shivering, feeding/digestive disturbances, irritability, agitation, sleep disturbances, increased reflexes, excessive crying, and respiratory disturbances.

Pregnancy Considerations
- Serotonin levels are increased from baseline during an uncomplicated pregnancy with preeclamptic patients demonstrating a 10-fold increase in serotonin levels.
- Third-trimester exposure to SSRIs has been associated with transient neonatal complications that may reflect either acute drug withdrawal or serotonergic toxicity.

EPIDEMIOLOGY
Seen in about 14–16% of SSRI overdose patients

Incidence
- In a 2008 study, SSRIs were responsible for adverse events in 18.8% of cases, with 55.7% due to intentional causes, 39.5% unintentional, and remainder of causes unknown. 46.6% had symptoms requiring hospitalization, and significant toxic effects occurred in 90 patients with two resultant deaths (1)[A].
- The incidence of serotonin syndrome is rising because serotonergic agents are increasingly prescribed and often in combination with other serotonergic agents. However, the true incidence is unclear due to potential misdiagnosis and unreported mild cases.

- Affects all age groups
- Predominant sex: male = female

ETIOLOGY AND PATHOPHYSIOLOGY
- Increased synaptic 5-HT or agonist concentration as a result of one or more of the following mechanisms: (i) decreased 5-HT breakdown (e.g., MAOI), (ii) decreased 5-HT reuptake (e.g., SSRI), (iii) increased 5-HT agonists (e.g., tryptophan), (iv) increased 5-HT release (e.g., amphetamines), and (v) CYP2D6 and CYP3A4 inhibitors (e.g., erythromycin)
- Risk is mediated in a dose-related manner by the action of 5-HT/5-HT agonists on 5-HT_{1A} and/or 5-HT_{2A} receptors.
- A number of drugs are associated with serotonin syndrome, which usually involves combination with an SSRI. These include SSRIs (e.g., citalopram, escitalopram, fluoxetine, fluvoxamine, paroxetine, sertraline); MAOIs; SNRIs (duloxetine, venlafaxine, desvenlafaxine); tricyclic antidepressants (e.g., amitriptyline); other antidepressants (nefazodone, trazodone); anxiolytic (buspirone); lithium; triptans; anticonvulsants (Depakote); analgesics (fentanyl, meperidine, pentazocine, tramadol); antibiotics/antivirals (linezolid, tedizolid [weak MAOI], ritonavir); over-the-counter (OTC) cough medications (dextromethorphan); some antipsychotics (risperidone, olanzapine); antiemetics (ondansetron, granisetron); other medications, such as metoclopramide, cyclobenzaprine, L-dopa; dietary supplements (tryptophan); herbal supplements (St. John's wort, nutmeg); methylene blue; and drugs of abuse (e.g., methylenedioxymethamphetamine [MDMA], cocaine, D-lysergic acid diethylamide [LSD], and amphetamine) (2)[A].

Genetics
Unknown

RISK FACTORS
- Recent dose change or overdose of drugs associated with serotonin syndrome
- Comorbid conditions leading to polypharmacy
- The greatest number of adverse events has been shown to be associated with SSRIs in combination with other substances, and the combination of SSRIs and MAOIs carries the greatest risk of developing serotonin toxicity.

GENERAL PREVENTION
- Consider drug–drug interactions when a multidrug regimen is required and avoid if possible.
- Caution patients about taking SSRIs with OTC medications (e.g., dextromethorphan) or herbal supplements (e.g., St. John's wort) prior to consulting a physician.
- Avoid serotonergic agents for nonpsychiatric disorders (e.g., tramadol for pain relief).

COMMONLY ASSOCIATED CONDITIONS
Intentional ingestions/overdose, illicit drug use

DIAGNOSIS

- Serotonin syndrome is a clinical diagnosis.
- *Hunter Toxicity Criteria Decision Rules* (3) aid in the diagnosis of clinically significant serotonin toxicity (sensitivity, 84%; specificity, 97%). A patient who took a serotonergic agent must have one of the following:
  – Spontaneous clonus
  – Inducible clonus with agitation or diaphoresis

  – Ocular clonus with agitation or diaphoresis
  – Hypertonia and hyperthermia (temperature >38°C) with inducible clonus or ocular clonus (3)[A]
  – Tremor and hyperreflexia

HISTORY
- Obtain a thorough drug history including prescriptions, OTC remedies, dietary and herbal supplements, and illicit drugs. Ask about dose, formulation, and recent changes.
- Review comorbidities (e.g., depression and chronic pain).
- Address possibility of drug overdose and obtain collateral information if intentional overdose is suspected.
- Elicit description of symptoms, including onset and progression.

PHYSICAL EXAM
Neuromuscular findings are seen in over half of patients with serotonin syndrome. Initially, patients can develop a peripheral tremor, confusion, and ataxia; systemic signs follow (e.g., agitation, diaphoresis, hyperreflexia, and shivering). Severe signs include fever, jerking, and diarrhea.

- Tachycardia, hypertension, and hyperthermia (≥40°C in severe cases)
- Neuromuscular abnormalities
  – Mild: hyperreflexia, myoclonus, and tremor all greater in lower extremities; bilateral Babinski sign
  – Moderate: opsoclonus, spontaneous or inducible clonus (involuntary muscle contractions, most commonly tested by rapid dorsiflexion of foot)
  – Severe: rigidity, respiratory failure, tonic–clonic seizure
- Autonomic dysfunction:
  – Mild: diaphoresis, mydriasis, tachycardia
  – Moderate: hyperactive bowel sounds, diarrhea, nausea, vomiting, hyperthermia (<40°C)
  – Severe: hyperthermia (≥40°C), rapidly changing blood pressure (BP)
- Mental status changes:
  – Mild: anxiety, akathisia (restlessness), insomnia
  – Moderate: agitation
  – Severe: coma, delirium, confusion (4)[B]
- Severe cases have led to altered level of consciousness, rhabdomyolysis, metabolic acidosis, and disseminated intravascular coagulation (DIC).

DIFFERENTIAL DIAGNOSIS
- Neuroleptic malignant syndrome (NMS): lead pipe rigidity and extrapyramidal features without clonus or hyperreflexia
- Anticholinergic fever (e.g., benztropine, diphenhydramine, oxybutynin, nifedipine, famotidine, atropine, scopolamine; plant poisoning from belladonna/"deadly nightshade," datura, henbane, mandrake, brugmansia): urinary retention, decreased bowel sounds, normal reflexes
- Malignant hyperthermia: generally following administration of anesthetics or depolarizing muscle relaxants
- Heat stroke
- CNS infection (e.g., meningitis, encephalitis)
- Sympathomimetic toxicity (cocaine, methamphetamine, PCP)
- Nonconvulsive seizures
- Hyperthyroidism (thyroid storm)
- Tetanus
- Rabies
- Acute baclofen withdrawal

DIAGNOSTIC TESTS & INTERPRETATION

- No single test confirms diagnosis of serotonin syndrome.
- Serum serotonin levels do not correlate with clinical findings.
- Nonspecific lab findings may include:
  - Elevated WBC count
  - Elevated creatine phosphokinase (CK or CPK)
  - Decreased serum bicarbonate
  - Elevated hepatic transaminases
- In severe cases, the following complications may develop:
  - DIC
  - Metabolic acidosis
  - Rhabdomyolysis
  - Renal failure
  - Myoglobinuria
  - Acute respiratory distress syndrome (ARDS) (3)[A]
- Consider urine toxicology screening for illicit drugs.

 TREATMENT

- Discontinuation of all serotonergic agents regardless of severity.
- Supportive care is the mainstay of therapy: administrating oxygen and aggressive IV fluids, continuous cardiac monitoring, monitoring urine output, and stabilizing vital signs.
  - Benzodiazepines may be effective for the management of agitation.
  - Administration of serotonin antagonists: Cyproheptadine may be useful if supportive measures and sedation (benzodiazepines) are unable to control agitation and correct vital signs. This agent does not reduce the duration of serotonin syndrome.
- Mild cases (afebrile, tachycardia, shivering, diaphoresis, mydriasis, hyperreflexia, intermittent tremor or myoclonus)
  - Discontinue precipitating agent(s).
  - Supportive care
  - Sedation
  - Observe for 12 to 24 hours.
- Moderate cases (temperature >38°C, autonomic instability, hyperactive bowel sounds, diarrhea, diaphoresis, ocular clonus, hyperreflexia, tremor, mild agitation, or hypervigilance)
  - Discontinue precipitating agent(s).
  - Supportive care
  - Sedation
  - Aggressive treatment of autonomic instability
  - Treatment with cyproheptadine should be initiated if agitation and vital sign abnormalities are unimproved with benzodiazepines and supportive care.
  - Hypotension from MAOI interactions should be treated with low doses of direct-acting sympathomimetics (e.g., norepinephrine, phenylephrine, epinephrine); indirect serotonin agonists, such as dopamine, should be avoided.
  - Severe hypertension and tachycardia should be treated with short-acting agents, such as nitroprusside or esmolol.
  - Avoid use of longer acting agents, such as propranolol, to prevent hypotension and falsely lowering heart rate, which can be used to monitor treatment response.
  - Observe for 12 to 24 hours.

- Severe cases (temperature >41.1°C, autonomic instability, delirium, muscular rigidity, and hypertonicity)
  - Discontinue precipitating agent(s).
  - Immediate sedation
  - Endotracheal intubation as clinically indicated
  - Paralysis as clinically indicated (maintained with nondepolarizing continuous paralytic agents such as vecuronium, cisatracurium, rocuronium)
  - Succinylcholine should not be used in cases of rhabdomyolysis to avoid exacerbation of hyperkalemia (5)[A].
  - Antipyretic medications are not effective (4)[A]; the increased body temperature is due to muscle activity, not an alteration in the hypothalamic set point.
  - Avoid physical restraints because it can worsen hyperthermia and lactic acidosis in agitated patients (5)[A].

MEDICATION

- Benzodiazepines: may be used to manage agitation in serotonin syndrome and also may correct mild increases in BP and heart rate. Use with caution in patients with delirium, given the known paradoxical effect of exacerbating delirium.
- Cyproheptadine (Periactin): Consider use if benzodiazepines and supportive measures are unable to control agitation and correct vital signs:
  - Adults: initial dose 12 mg PO (can also be crushed and given via nasogastric [NG] tube) followed by 2 mg q2h until clinical response observed; 12 to 32 mg of drug may be required in a 24-hour period.
  - Children:
    - <2 years: 0.06 mg/kg q6h
    - 2 to 6 years: 2 mg q6h
    - 7 to 14 years: 4 mg q6h
  - Unlikely to be effective in patients who have received activated charcoal
  - Pregnancy Category B
- Use of antipsychotics with 5-HT$_{2A}$ antagonist activity, such as olanzapine and chlorpromazine, is not recommended (4)[B].

ISSUES FOR REFERRAL

- Psychiatry: for assistance with medication management and follow-up care (inpatient psychiatric care vs. outpatient psychiatric follow-up)
- Toxicology/clinical pharmacology service
- Poison control center

ADMISSION, INPATIENT, AND NURSING CONSIDERATIONS

- Patients with known/suspected serotonin syndrome should be admitted to a medical inpatient unit for observation.
- ICU admission is often indicated in severe cases.
- Discharge when
  - Mental status has returned to baseline, with stable vital and neurologic (e.g., clonus) signs. Ensure close patient follow-up.

 ONGOING CARE

FOLLOW-UP RECOMMENDATIONS

- In mild cases address risks and benefits of restarting offending agents. Serotonergic medications need to be titrated slowly, and patients must have close outpatient follow-up.

- In severe cases, the offending agent should likely not be resumed unless precipitant for serotonin syndrome is found (e.g., combination with another serotonin agonist); the patient can be carefully monitored, or there is clear benefit versus risk of restarting the medication.

PROGNOSIS

- Generally favorable with early recognition of the syndrome and prompt initiation of treatment
- Most cases resolve within 24 hours of discontinuation of serotonergic agents; this can be longer depending on the drug's half-life:
  - MAOIs can result in toxicity for several days.
  - SSRIs can result in toxicity for up to several weeks after discontinuation.

COMPLICATIONS

- Adverse outcomes, including death, are usually the consequence of poorly treated hyperthermia and may include acute renal failure, acute respiratory distress syndrome, arrhythmia, coma, disseminated intravascular coagulation, seizure, metabolic acidosis, multiorgan failure, myoglobinuria, respiratory arrest, and rhabdomyolysis.
- Nonhyperthermic patients who survive typically do not have long-term sequelae.

REFERENCES

1. Bronstein AC, Spyker DA, Cantilena LR Jr, et al. 2008 Annual report of the American Association of Poison Control Centers' National Poison Data System (NPDS): 26th annual report. *Clin Toxicol (Phila)*. 2009;47(10):911–1084.
2. Moss MJ, Hendrickson RG; and Toxicology Investigators Consortium (ToxIC). Serotonin toxicity: associated agents and clinical characteristics. *J Clin Psychopharmacol*. 2019;39(6):628–633.
3. Dunkley EJ, Isbister GK, Sibbritt D, et al. The Hunter Serotonin Toxicity Criteria: simple and accurate diagnostic decision rules for serotonin toxicity. *QJM*. 2003;96(9):635–642.
4. Buckley NA, Dawson AH, Isbister GK. Serotonin syndrome. *BMJ*. 2014;348:g1626.
5. Heitmiller DR. Serotonin syndrome: a concise review of a toxic state. *R I Med J (2013)*. 2014;97(6):33–35.

ADDITIONAL READING

- Mas Serrano M, Pérez-Sánchez JR, Portela Sánchez S, et al. Serotonin syndrome in two COVID-19 patients treated with lopinavir/ritonavir. *J Neurol Sci*. 2020; 415:116944.
- Nordstrom K, Vilke GM, Wilson MP. Psychiatric emergencies for clinicians: emergency department management of serotonin syndrome. *J Emerg Med*. 2016;50(1):89–91.

 CODES

ICD10
G25.79 Other drug induced movement disorders

CLINICAL PEARLS

Consider serotonin syndrome in patients with recent use of a serotonergic agent (particularly if multiple proserotonergic agents are involved) presenting with unexplained tachycardia, hypertension, hyperthermia, clonus, hyperreflexia, and change in mental status.

SEXUAL DYSFUNCTION IN WOMEN

Fehima C. Dawy, MD • Miguel A. Palacios, MD

 BASICS

- Very common: ~40% of women surveyed in the United States have sexual concerns.
- May present as a lack of sexual desire, impaired arousal, inability to achieve orgasm or pain with sexual activity, and may be lifelong or acquired

DESCRIPTION

- Female sexual interest or arousal disorder—lack of or significantly reduced sexual interest or arousal as manifested by three of the following:
  - Absent or reduced interest in sexual activity
  - Absent or reduced sexual or erotic thoughts or fantasies
  - No or reduced initiation of sexual activity and unreceptive to partner's attempts to initiate
  - Absent or reduced sexual excitement or pleasure during sexual activity in almost all (75–100%) of sexual encounters
  - Absent or reduced sexual interest or arousal in response to any internal or external sexual or erotic cues
  - Absent or reduced genital or nongenital sensation during sexual activity in almost all (75–100%) of sexual encounters
- Subjective sexual arousal disorder—absent or diminished feelings of sexual arousal from sexual stimulation, but physical responses, such as vaginal lubrication, occur
- Genital sexual arousal disorder—subjective sexual excitement occurs with nongenital sexual stimuli; however, there is notable impaired genital sexual arousal, that is, minimal vulvar swelling or vaginal lubrication from genital stimulation
- Female orgasmic disorder—presence of either of the following in almost all (75–100%) occasions of sexual activity:
  - Marked delay in, marked infrequency of, or absence of orgasm
  - Markedly reduced intensity of orgasmic sensations
- Genito-pelvic pain or penetration disorder, which can include dyspareunia, vaginismus and sexual aversion disorder—persistent or recurrent difficulties with one or more of the following:
  - Vaginal penetration during intercourse
  - Marked vulvovaginal or pelvic pain during intercourse or penetration attempts
  - Marked fear or anxiety about vulvovaginal or pelvic pain in anticipation of, during, or because of vaginal penetration
  - Marked tensing or tightening of pelvic floor muscles during attempted vaginal penetration

ALERT
Symptoms must be present for ≥6 months; cause clinically significant distress or impairment; and not be better explained by a nonsexual mental disorder, a consequence of severe relationship distress, or other significant stressors

- System(s) affected: nervous; reproductive; genitourinary; psychiatric
- Synonym(s): hypoactive sexual desire disorder; sexual aversion disorder; female sexual arousal disorder; inhibited female orgasm

EPIDEMIOLOGY
In two large studies, approximately 40% of women reported sexual problems.

Incidence
Sexual problems are highest in women aged 45 to 64 years and then decline secondary to changes in sexual-related personal distress.

Prevalence
- Low sexual desire is the most common manifestation, followed by difficulty with orgasm, difficulty with arousal, and sexual pain.
- Lack of interest in sexual activity is notably greater than the normal decrease experienced with increasing age and relationship duration.

ETIOLOGY AND PATHOPHYSIOLOGY
- The pathophysiology of sexual dysfunction is complex and multifactorial because it can be the result of any etiology that interferes with the female sexual response cycle (desire, arousal, orgasm, and resolution). The etiology of female sexual dysfunction may encompass biologic, psychological, relational, and sociocultural factors. Phases can vary in sequence, overlap, or be absent during all or some sexual encounters.
  - Biologic
    - Disorders of the hypothalamic-pituitary-adrenal system, hormonal imbalance/disorders of ovarian function, menopause (surgical or natural), chronic illness (vascular disease, diabetes mellitus, and malignancy)
    - Prescription medications (SSRIs, MAOIs, TCAs, β-blockers)
    - Thyroid disease
    - Neuromuscular disease (multiple sclerosis, spinal cord damage, disorders of central or peripheral nervous system)
    - Musculogenic disorders causing hyper- or hypotonicity of pelvic floor muscles
    - Malignancy
  - Psychological
    - Anxiety/depression
    - Maladaptive thoughts/behaviors
    - Interrelational difficulties
    - Body image issues
    - Drug and alcohol abuse
    - Sexual abuse
- There are a multitude of sex hormones and neurotransmitters involved in sexual functioning with different effects:
  - Positive effects on desire, arousal: dopamine, estrogen, norepinephrine, serotonin, testosterone
  - Negative effect on desire, arousal: prolactin, serotonin
  - Vasocongestion of clitoral tissue: nitric oxide, vasoactive intestinal peptide
  - Receptivity, orgasm: oxytocin, progesterone

Genetics
Sexual dysfunction in women is a multifactorial issue, often including a combination of biologic and psychosocial causes. However, genetics can affect certain medication responses and medical conditions. As psychoactive medications can affect sexual desire, the genetic differences of neurotransmitter receptor profiles can affect how SSRIs influence levels of sexual desire. Other medical conditions affected by genetics may also result in sexual dysfunction in women.

RISK FACTORS
- Advancing age/menopause
- Previous sexual trauma
- Lack of knowledge about sexual stimulation and response

- Chronic medical problems
  - Depression, anxiety, chronic pain syndromes, and other psychiatric disorders
  - Cardiovascular disease
  - Endocrine disorders
  - Dermatologic disorders
  - Neurologic disorders
  - Cancer
- Gynecologic issues
  - Childbirth
  - Pelvic floor or bladder dysfunction
  - Endometriosis
  - Uterine fibroids
  - Chronic vulvovaginal candidiasis/vaginal infections
  - Female genital mutilation
- Relationship factors such as couple discrepancies in expectations and/or cultural backgrounds and attitudes toward sexuality in family of origin
- Medications or substance abuse

GENERAL PREVENTION
- Typically, sexual health is usually not discussed until or unless a problem arises. Effective sexual health care, through thorough sexual history can not only assist with control of fertility and prevention of sexually transmitted diseases but also with detection of psychosocial problems associated with sexual dysfunction. Additionally, eliciting a sexual history may aid in the early diagnosis of chronic disorders such as diabetes or depression.
- To take a detailed sexual history, consider using the 5 P's model to shape the interview:
  - Partners: How do partners identify, how many, how satisfied, any changes in sexual desire or frequency of sexual activity?
  - Practices: What types of sexual activities?
  - Past history/protection from sexually transmitted diseases/infections
  - Pregnancy plans: interest in pregnancy, contraception
  - Pleasure: any pain with intercourse, difficulty with orgasm, difficulty with lubrication, asking about concerns or questions about sexual function

COMMONLY ASSOCIATED CONDITIONS
- Marital/relationship discord
- Depression
- Anxiety

 DIAGNOSIS

- Female sexual dysfunction is diagnosed by utilizing a validated sexual function screening instrument and a structured interview, including detailed medical and sexual history, to confirm diagnosis.
  - Female Sexual Function Index
  - Brief Index of Sexual Functioning for Women
  - Brief Sexual Symptom Checklist
  - Decreased Sexual Desire Screener
- The diagnosis requires that the sexual problem be recurrent or persistent and causes personal distress rather than be due solely to partner or relationship issues.

HISTORY
- Detailed sexual history
  - Degree of personal distress
  - Lifelong versus acquired problem
  - Situational versus generalized problem
  - Cultural/societal beliefs regarding sexuality

- History of sexual trauma
- Concerns about safety, pregnancy, or STIs
- Concerns regarding privacy
- Interpersonal relationship factors
  - Current relationship status
  - Family dysfunction
- Physiologic/biologic history
  - Urinary/anal incontinence
  - Medications (including herbal and OTC)
  - Pregnancy/childbirth history
  - Infertility
  - Menopausal status (natural, surgical, or postchemotherapy)
  - STIs and vaginitis
  - Pelvic surgery, injury, or cancer
  - Chronic pelvic pain
  - Abnormal genital tract bleeding
- Psychological history
  - Low self-image
  - Anxiety
  - Depression
  - Negative past sexual experiences
  - Substance misuse/abuse

PHYSICAL EXAM
- Most commonly, patients have a normal physical exam.
  - Assess for anatomic abnormalities.
  - Assess for scars or evidence of trauma.
  - Assess for vaginal atrophy, adequate estrogenization.
  - Assess for infection.
  - Recognize signs of anxiety, apprehension, and pain during the speculum and pelvic exam.
- General physical exam, signs of chronic disease

DIFFERENTIAL DIAGNOSIS
- Medication side effects
- Vaginitis
- Decreased vaginal lubrication secondary to hormonal imbalance
- Decreased sensation secondary to nerve injury
- Multiple sclerosis
- Anatomic abnormalities
- Abdominal surgery (which can interfere with pelvic innervation)
- Depression
- Marital dysfunction, including domestic violence
- Pregnancy
- Pseudodyspareunia (use of complaint of pain to distance self from partner)

DIAGNOSTIC TESTS & INTERPRETATION
Laboratory studies are rarely helpful. There are no reliable correlations between serum hormone levels and sexual dysfunction. Assessment of sexual dysfunction in women is best approached with biopsychosocial model that includes a sexual history and physical examination.

Initial Tests (lab, imaging)
As needed to identify infections and other medical causes, including blood glucose levels, cholesterol, lipids, hormonal profile

Follow-Up Tests & Special Considerations
- Foundation of treatment is most notably patient education and therapy.
- Currently, limited research for benefit of pharmacotherapy
- If an infective etiology of dyspareunia is noted, further studies of vaginal/cervical microscopy and cultures should be performed.

Diagnostic Procedures/Other
As noted above, speculum and pelvic exam provides an opportunity to recognize signs of anxiety, apprehension, or pain that may provide insight to sexual dysfunction.

TREATMENT
- Set realistic goals and expectations (1)[C].
- Address underlying medical and psychiatric conditions.
- If SSRIs, consider switching to an antidepressant with fewer sexual adverse effects or adding bupropion.
- Review sexual response, heterogeneity of normal response, and sexual activity other than intercourse (1)[C].
- Education on communication
- Educate on healthy lifestyle, diet, exercise, sleep, avoidance of tobacco, and reduced alcohol (1)[C].
- Vaginal moisturizers and lubricants
- Cognitive-behavioral therapy (CBT) (individual or couples) to target maladaptive thoughts and behaviors and to disrupt the dysfunctional cycle
- Mindfulness-based CBT (1)[C]
- Sex therapy: sensate focus, systematic desensitization exercises, homework exchanging physical touch with partner, scheduled attempt of sexual activity 3 times per week, or directed masturbation alone
- Physical therapy/biofeedback
- Pelvic muscle exercises to help muscles surrounding the vagina

GENERAL MEASURES
Ensure a sexual history is performed for patients to identify sexual dysfunction early to educate and assist.

MEDICATION
Sexual dysfunction is often a multifactorial psychosocial condition. Using medications does not usually address the cause of the problem and can, in some cases, make the condition worse.
- Bupropion (1)[C]: adjunct for SSRI-induced sexual dysfunction. Improves sexual arousal and orgasm but not desire. Dose: bupropion SR 150 mg orally once or twice daily
- Flibanserin: possible improvement in sexual desire. Clinical improvement versus placebo is minimal, and side effects are common. Mechanism of action: 5-HT$_{1A}$ agonist and 5-HT$_{2A}$ antagonist. Dose: 100 mg at bedtime; FDA-approved for premenopausal women with hypoactive sexual desire
- Estrogen replacement with or without progestins (1): may improve sexual desire, vaginal atrophy, and clitoral sensitivity. Vaginal estrogen therapy (preferred route of administration) is available in cream, vaginal tablet, or ring form.
- Ospemifene (1): selective estrogen receptor modulator FDA-approved for dyspareunia due to vulvo- or vaginal atrophy in postmenopausal women. Dose: ospemifene 60 mg orally once daily
- Testosterone (1)
  - Use in premenopausal women not supported
  - In postmenopausal women, adding <6 months of testosterone to hormone replacement may increase desire
  - Side effects: hirsutism, androgenic alopecia, acne, decreased HDL, liver dysfunction; not FDA-approved for sexual dysfunction in women

  - Contraindicated in breast or endometrial cancer, thromboembolic disease, or coronary artery disease
  - Dose: oral methyltestosterone 1.25 to 2.50 mg/day (1/10 of men's dose) or topical (patch, gel)
- Dehydroepiandrosterone (DHEA): vaginal formulation 6.5 mg FDA-approved for dyspareunia due to vaginal atrophy in postmenopausal women
- Phosphodiesterase type 5 (PDE5) inhibitors: adjunct for SSRI- or SNRI-induced sexual dysfunction

ISSUES FOR REFERRAL
Consider referral for CBT, marriage/couples counseling, pelvic floor therapy, or sex therapy.

ADDITIONAL THERAPIES
- Smoking cessation and reduction of alcohol intake
- For childhood trauma: scripting, psychotherapy, cognitive restructuring

COMPLEMENTARY & ALTERNATIVE MEDICINE
- Yohimbine: not recommended, potentially dangerous
- Ginseng and St. John's wort: no evidence to support

ONGOING CARE

FOLLOW-UP RECOMMENDATIONS
Lifestyle modifications and medication changes.

DIET
Weight reduction if overweight or obese

PATIENT EDUCATION
- American Association of Sexuality Educators, Counselors, and Therapists: www.aasect.org
- National Women's Health Resource Center: www.healthywomen.org

PROGNOSIS
Lack of desire is most difficult type to treat with <50% success. Treatment is most successful with multidisciplinary approach.

REFERENCE
1. Kingsberg SA, Woodard T. Female sexual dysfunction: focus on low desire. *Obstet Gynecol.* 2015;125(2):477–486.

CODES

ICD10
- R37 Sexual dysfunction, unspecified
- F52.0 Hypoactive sexual desire disorder
- N94.1 Dyspareunia

CLINICAL PEARLS
- Female sexual dysfunction is a common, complex, multifactorial problem.
- Usually, patients with sexual dysfunction have a normal physical exam.
- Symptoms of sexual dysfunction peak during perimenopause between the ages of 45 and 64 years.
- Combination of behavioral, physical, and medical therapy leads to greater treatment success. There is rarely a simple "fix" with a medication.

S

SHOULDER PAIN

Lee A. Mancini, MD, CSCS*D, CSN • Nicholas R. Martin, MD • Michael J. Maddaleni, MD

 BASICS

DESCRIPTION
- Shoulder pain commonly affects patients of all ages.
- Causes include acute trauma, overuse during sports, infection, and activities of everyday living.
- Age plays an important role in determining the etiology of shoulder pain.
- Onset and characteristics of pain, mechanism of injury, and limitation narrow the differential diagnosis.

EPIDEMIOLOGY
- Shoulder pain accounts for 16% of all musculoskeletal (MSK) complaints.
- The lifetime prevalence of shoulder pain is ~70%.
- Predominant etiology varies with age:
  - <30 years: shoulder instability
  - 30 to 60 years: rotator cuff (RTC) disorder, impingement syndrome, partial tears
  - >60 years: full-thickness tear, glenohumeral OA

Incidence
The incidence of shoulder pain is 7 to 25 cases per 1,000 patients, with a peak incidence in the 4th to 6th decades.

ETIOLOGY AND PATHOPHYSIOLOGY
Pathology varies with cause:
- Trauma—fracture, dislocation, ligament/tendon tear, acromioclavicular (AC) separation
- Overuse—RTC pathology, biceps tenosynovitis, bursitis, muscle strain, apophyseal injuries
- RTC disorders most commonly result from repetitive overhead activity, leading to RTC impingement with a three-stage progression:
  - Stage I: tendinopathy
  - Stage II: partial RTC tear
  - Stage III: full-thickness RTC tear
- Subacromial bursitis can occur with RTC disorders but is rarely an isolated diagnosis.
- Age related: In pediatric athletes, instability and physeal injuries are more common. With increasing age, the incidence of AC and glenohumeral joint OA, adhesive capsulitis, and RTC tear rises.
- Rheumatologic: rheumatoid arthritis, polymyalgia rheumatica, fibromyalgia
- Infectious: septic arthritis
- Referred pain: neck, gallbladder, diaphragm

RISK FACTORS
- Repetitive overhead activity
- Overhead and upper extremity weight-bearing sports (baseball, softball, swimming, tennis, volleyball)
- Weight lifting: AC joint disorders
- Rapid increases in training frequency or load (often associated with improper technique)
- Muscle weakness or imbalance
- Trauma or fall onto the shoulder
- Diabetes, thyroid disorders and other autoimmune diseases, female gender, and age 40 to 60 years are risk factors for adhesive capsulitis.

GENERAL PREVENTION
- Maintain strength and range of motion (ROM).
- Avoid repetitive overhead activities (pitch counts).
- Proper technique (pitching, weight lifting)

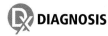 **DIAGNOSIS**

HISTORY
- Pain characteristics location
  - Superior: AC pathology, trapezius strain
  - Lateral: RTC pathology
  - Anterior: proximal biceps tendinosis
  - Diffuse pain: RTC pathology, adhesive capsulitis, glenohumeral OA
- Descriptors
  - Night pain, worse lying on affected side: RTC pathology, adhesive capsulitis, glenohumeral OA
  - Stiff shoulder, limited ROM: adhesive capsulitis, glenohumeral OA
- Aggravating movements
  - Cross-body adduction, "scarf test": AC pathology
  - Abduction/external rotation (reaching behind): instability, RTC pathology, glenohumeral OA
  - Overhead activity: RTC pathology, AC pathology, labrum pathology, glenohumeral OA
  - Turning neck, pain past elbow: cervical pathology
- Mechanism of injury
  - Forceful abduction and external rotation: traumatic shoulder instability/dislocation
  - Fall directly onto lateral shoulder: AC joint sprain or separation, clavicular fracture
  - Repetitive overhead activity: RTC pathology
  - Fall on outstretched hand (FOOSH): shoulder separation; forearm/wrist fracture
- Age
  - Shoulder instability (subluxation, dislocation, multi-directional instability) is the most common cause of shoulder pain in young athletes (<30 years old).
  - RTC disorders are the most common cause of shoulder pain in patients >30 years old. Severity of RTC disorder increases with age.
  - Older patients (>60 years old) commonly have OA.
  - Trauma in a young person <40 years is more commonly associated with dislocation/subluxation. In patients >40 years, trauma is more commonly associated with RTC tear.

PHYSICAL EXAM
- Three main joints combine to create the shoulder: glenohumeral, AC, sternoclavicular.
- Four RTC muscles/tendons (SITS): supraspinatus (abduction), infraspinatus (external rotation), teres minor (external rotation, adduction), and subscapularis (adduction, internal rotation)
- Observe face and shoulder movements as patient disrobes, moves arm, and shakes hand.
- Inspect for malalignment, muscle atrophy, asymmetry, erythema, ecchymosis, and swelling. Scapular winging suggests long thoracic nerve or muscular (trapezius, serratus anterior) dysfunction. Prominent scapular spine with scalloped infraspinatus fossa suggests infraspinatus atrophy.
- Palpate SC joint, AC joint, acromion, biceps tendon for tenderness, warmth, bony step-offs.
- Evaluate active AND passive ROM and flexibility.
- Decreased active AND passive ROM is more common with adhesive capsulitis. Normal abduction is to 180 degrees.
- Pain from 60 to 180 degrees suggests subacromial impingement; 120 to 180 degrees suggests AC joint pathology (1).
- Mildly decreased active and/or passive ROM may also indicate glenohumeral OA.
- Decreased active ROM with full passive ROM: RTC pathology
- Evaluate for muscle strength, including grip, biceps, triceps, and deltoid.
- Test RTC strength: supraspinatus (empty can test), infraspinatus/teres minor (resisted external rotation, external lag test), subscapularis (lift-off test, belly press, resisted internal rotation).
- Pain with RTC strength testing indicates RTC pathology. Weakness could suggest tear.
- Special diagnostic tests
  - Neer RTC impingement test: Examiner stabilizes the scapula and internally rotates the patient's arm and flexes the shoulder through the full ROM or until the patient reports pain.
  - Hawkins RTC impingement test: Examiner internally rotates the shoulder with the elbow, and shoulder flexed to 90 degrees to the end of ROM or until the patient reports pain.
  - Drop-arm test for RTC tear: positive if patient is unable to smoothly control the lowering of their arm or to hold the arm in 90 degrees of abduction
  - Cross-arm adduction is painful in AC joint arthritis or sprain.
  - Speed test for biceps tendinopathy: With arm 30 degrees of flexion and palm supinated, patient attempts to flex the elbow against resistance. Pain over biceps is positive.
  - Yergason test for biceps tendinopathy: With the elbow stabilized to the patient's side and flexed to 90 degrees, place the patient's forearm in pronation and resist against supination.
  - Apprehension, relocation test for anterior glenohumeral joint instability: Examiner supports the elbow of the patient and with the other hand holding the wrist, slowly externally rotates the humerus with the shoulder at 90 degrees abduction, patient apprehensive with maneuver.
  - Sulcus sign for inferior glenohumeral joint instability: Examiner pulls down with the hand grasping the subject's elbow, positive if significant inferior movement of the arm, relative to shoulder.
  - O'Brien, clunk test for labral pathology: move arm at 90 degrees of flexion, 10 degrees of adduction, thumb pointed down (arm in internal rotation), examiner resists flexion distally. Maintain same position and have the patient turn thumb up. Pain with thumb down and no pain with thumb up is positive.
  - Spurling test for cervical pathology: rotation of head toward side of symptoms along with neck extension with applied downward force to reproduce radicular symptoms

DIFFERENTIAL DIAGNOSIS

- Fracture (clavicle, humerus, scapula), contusion
- RTC disorder: impingement, tear, calcific tendonitis
- Subacromial bursitis
- Scapulothoracic dyskinesis
- AC joint pathology (AC separation/OA, osteolysis)
- Biceps tenosynovitis or tear
- Acromial apophysitis or os acromiale
- Glenohumeral joint OA
- Glenohumeral joint instability (acute dislocation or chronic multidirectional instability)
- Adhesive capsulitis
- Labral tear or associated bony pathology
- Muscle strain (trapezius, deltoid, biceps)
- Cervical radiculopathy
- Other: autoimmune, rheumatologic, referred pain, septic joint (biliary/splenic, cardiac, pneumonia/lung mass)

DIAGNOSTIC TESTS & INTERPRETATION

Initial Tests (lab, imaging)

- A history of significant trauma, prolonged symptoms, or red flags (older age, fever, rest pain) suggests a need for imaging.
- Adults with nontraumatic shoulder pain of <4 weeks duration may not require initial imaging.
- Plain radiographs anteroposterior, scapular Y, axillary views
- EMG study of the upper extremity may help differentiate referred cervical pain and brachial plexopathy from a primary shoulder disorder.
- Obtain ECG if any suspicion for cardiac etiology.
- Serologic tests if autoimmune etiology is suspected.

Follow-Up Tests & Special Considerations

- CT or MRI can rule out an occult fracture.
- MRI is gold standard for noninvasive soft tissue imaging, including RTC, biceps tendon.
- MR arthrogram may be necessary to assess for labral tears.
- Ultrasound (US) can assess for RTC tears, biceps tendinopathy, and AC joint pathology.
- US is operator dependent but in the hands of a good technician can be equivalent to MRI in detecting full-thickness tears (sensitivity 92%, specificity 94%) and partial-thickness tears (sensitivity 67%, specificity 94%) (1).

Diagnostic Procedures/Other

Consider diagnostic arthroscopy after failing conservative management if structural injury is suspected.

Test Interpretation

- Tendinosis rather than tendonitis is common with stage I impingement.
- Capsular scarring is the hallmark of adhesive capsulitis.
- RTC enthesophytes visualized with calcific tendonitis
- Tear enlargement and pain development in asymptomatic tears are more common with involvement of the dominant shoulder.

TREATMENT

- Treatment is based on underlying diagnosis.
- In general, conservative therapy includes activity modification, analgesics, and/or anti-inflammatory medicines in association with appropriate rehabilitative programs.
- Physical therapy almost always required for full resolution

MEDICATION

First Line

- Analgesics and anti-inflammatory medications for symptomatic relief include NSAIDs, such as ibuprofen, naproxen, and meloxicam. Acetaminophen may also be used especially if the patient has a history of a GI bleed.
- Corticosteroid injections (subacromial, glenohumeral, AC, subscapular bursa) can be used to acutely relieve pain due to RTC pathology, adhesive capsulitis, OA, or scapulothoracic dyskinesis.
- Steroid injections can improve ability to engage in rehabilitative activities.
- US guidance improves accuracy of anatomic placement of corticosteroid injections; long-term outcomes similar between US-guided versus nonguided versus NSAID; use after 6 to 8 weeks.

ISSUES FOR REFERRAL

- If etiology remains unclear, patient is not responsive to conservative care, for complicated or displaced fractures.
- Full-thickness RTC tears >1 cm (acute or chronic) in patients <65 years old or any tear with significant changes in functional status require surgical referral. These tears have a high rate of progression, fatty infiltration, or retraction with nonoperative care.

ADDITIONAL THERAPIES

- Physical therapy can benefit persistent RTC disorders, adhesive capsulitis, and shoulder instability.
- Manual therapy and exercises may improve pain and increase function in RTC disease.
- Manual manipulative therapy (MMT) by chiropractors, osteopathic physicians, or physical therapists improves pain with adhesive capsulitis, RTC, and soft tissue disorders. In adhesive capsulitis, MMT is generally less effective than glucocorticoid injections at 6-week mark, but both have similar long-term outcomes. Acupuncture may improve short-term pain and function in RTC impingement.

SURGERY/OTHER PROCEDURES

- Surgery is recommended for shoulder pain caused by acute displaced fractures, large RTC tears (criteria as above). It may also be recommended for multiple shoulder dislocation in patients <20 years of age.
- Surgery can be considered for shoulder pain unresponsive to conservative measures >3 to 6 months. Surgery is not more effective than active nonsurgical treatment in impingement syndrome (2)[A].

- Platelet-rich therapies need more conclusive evidence before routine use in treatment of MSK soft tissue injuries.

COMPLEMENTARY & ALTERNATIVE MEDICINE

Acupuncture may help with acute shoulder pain. There is no conclusive evidence for the effectiveness of acupuncture.

ONGOING CARE

FOLLOW-UP RECOMMENDATIONS

Limit overhead activity to reduce impingement symptoms.

PATIENT EDUCATION

Refer to specific diagnosis for shoulder pain.

PROGNOSIS

Shoulder pain generally has a favorable outcome with conservative care, but recovery can be slow, with 40–50% of patients complaining of persistent pain or recurrence at 12 months.

REFERENCES

1. Greenberg DL. Evaluation and treatment of shoulder pain. *Med Clin North Am*. 2014;98(3): 487–504.
2. Coghlan JA, Buchbinder R, Green S, et al. Surgery for rotator cuff disease. *Cochrane Database Syst Rev*. 2008;(1):CD005619.

ADDITIONAL READING

Littlewood C, Ashton J, Chance-Larsen K, et al. Exercise for rotator cuff tendinopathy: a systematic review. *Physiotherapy*. 2012;98(2):101–109.

CODES

ICD10

M25.519 Pain in unspecified shoulder

CLINICAL PEARLS

- RTC disorders (tendinopathy, tears) are the most common cause of shoulder pain in individuals >30 years of age.
- Shoulder instability (acute dislocation/subluxation or chronic instability) is the most common source of shoulder pain in individuals <30 years of age.
- Patients with diabetes are at increased risk for adhesive capsulitis.
- Most patients do well with a structured program of pain control and rehabilitation.

S

SINUSITIS

Chirag N. Shah, MD • Grant Wei, MD, FACEP

BASICS

DESCRIPTION
- Acute sinusitis is a symptomatic inflammation of ≥1 paranasal sinuses of <4 weeks duration resulting from impaired drainage and retained secretions accompanied by obstruction, facial pain/pressure/fullness, or both. Because rhinitis and sinusitis usually coexist, "rhinosinusitis" is the preferred term.
- Disease is subacute when symptomatic for 4 to 12 weeks, recurrent acute when ≥4 annual episodes without persistent symptoms in between, and chronic when symptomatic for >12 weeks.
- Uncomplicated rhinosinusitis has no extension of inflammation beyond paranasal sinuses and nasal cavity.
- System(s) affected: head/eyes/ears/nose/throat (HEENT), pulmonary

EPIDEMIOLOGY
- Affects 1 in 8 adults accounting for >30 million individuals in the United States each year diagnosed with rhinosinusitis
- Diagnosis of acute bacterial rhinosinusitis remains the fifth leading reason for prescribing antibiotics.
- Viral cause in 90–98% of cases
  - 0.5–2% of viral rhinosinusitis episodes have a bacterial superinfection.

Incidence
Incidence is highest in early fall through early spring (related to incidence of viral upper respiratory infection [URI]). Adults have two to three viral URIs per year; 90% of these colds are accompanied by viral rhinosinusitis. It is the fifth most common diagnosis made during family physician visits.

ETIOLOGY AND PATHOPHYSIOLOGY
- Important features
  - Inflammation and edema of the sinus mucosa
  - Obstruction of the sinus ostia
  - Impaired mucociliary clearance
- Secretions that are not cleared become hospitable to bacterial growth.
- Inflammatory response (neutrophil influx and release of cytokines) damages mucosal surfaces.
- Viral: vast majority of cases (rhinovirus; influenza A and B; parainfluenza virus; respiratory syncytial, adeno-, corona-, and enteroviruses)
- Bacterial (complicates 0.5–2% of viral cases)
  - More likely if symptoms worsen within 5 to 6 days after initial improvement
  - No improvement within 10 days of symptom onset
  - >3 to 4 days of fever >102°F and facial pain and purulent nasal discharge
  - *Streptococcus pneumoniae, Haemophilus influenzae,* and *Moraxella catarrhalis* are the most common bacterial pathogens.
  - Often overdiagnosed, which leads to overuse of and increasing resistance to antibiotics
  - Methicillin-resistant *Staphylococcus aureus* present in 0–15.9% of patients
- Fungal: seen in immunocompromised hosts (uncontrolled diabetes, neutropenia, use of corticosteroids) or as a nosocomial infection

RISK FACTORS
- Viral URI
- Allergic rhinitis
- Asthma
- Cigarette smoking
- Dental infections and procedures
- Anatomic variations
  - Tonsillar and adenoid hypertrophy
  - Turbinate hypertrophy, nasal polyps
  - Cleft palate
- Immunodeficiency (e.g., HIV)
- Cystic fibrosis (CF)

GENERAL PREVENTION
- Hand washing to prevent transmission of viral infection
- Childhood vaccinations up to date
- Avoid close contacts with symptomatic individuals.
- Avoid smoking and exposure to secondhand smoke.

DIAGNOSIS

- History and physical exam suggest and establish the diagnosis but are rarely helpful in distinguishing bacterial from viral causes.
- Use a constellation of symptoms rather than a particular sign or symptom in diagnosis.

HISTORY
- Symptoms somewhat predictive of bacterial sinusitis (1)[C]
  - Worsening of symptoms >5 to 6 days after initial improvement
  - Persistent symptoms for ≥10 days
  - Persistent purulent nasal discharge
  - Unilateral upper tooth or facial pain
  - Unilateral maxillary sinus tenderness
  - Fever
- Associated symptoms
  - Headache
  - Nasal congestion
  - Retro-orbital pain
  - Otalgia
  - Hyposomia
  - Halitosis
  - Chronic cough
- Symptoms requiring urgent attention
  - Visual disturbances, especially diplopia
  - Periorbital swelling or erythema
  - Altered mental status

PHYSICAL EXAM
- Fever
- Edema and erythema of nasal mucosa
- Purulent discharge
- Tenderness to palpation over sinus(es)
- Pain localized to sinuses when bending forward
- Transillumination of the sinuses may confirm fluid in sinuses (helpful if asymmetric; not helpful if symmetric exam).

Pediatric Considerations
- Sinuses are not fully developed until age 20 years. Maxillary and ethmoid sinuses, although small, are present from birth.
- Because children have an average of six to eight colds per year, they are at risk for developing sinusitis.
- Diagnosis can be more difficult than in adults because symptoms are often more subtle.

DIFFERENTIAL DIAGNOSIS
- Dental disease
- CF
- Wegener granulomatosis
- HIV infection
- Kartagener syndrome
- Neoplasm
- Headache, tension, or migraine

DIAGNOSTIC TESTS & INTERPRETATION
Diagnostic tests are not routinely recommended; no diagnostic tests can adequately differentiate between viral and bacterial rhinosinusitis (2)[C].
- None indicated in routine evaluation
- Routine use of sinus radiography discouraged because of the following:
  - ≥3 clinical findings have similar diagnostic accuracy as imaging.
  - Imaging does not distinguish viral from bacterial etiology.
- Limited coronal CT scan can be useful in recurrent infection or failure to respond to medical therapy.

Diagnostic Procedures/Other
Sinus CT if signs suggest extra sinus involvement or to evaluate chronic rhinosinusitis

Test Interpretation
- Inflammation, edema, thickened mucosa
- Impaired ciliary function
- Metaplasia of ciliated columnar cells
- Relative acidosis and hypoxia within sinuses
- Polyps

TREATMENT

Most cases resolve with supportive care (treating pain, nasal symptoms). Antibiotics should be reserved for symptoms that persist >10 days, onset with severe symptoms (high fever, purulent nasal discharge, facial pain) for at least 3 to 4 consecutive days, or worsening signs/symptoms that were initially improving (1)[C],(2).

GENERAL MEASURES
- Hydration
- Steam inhalation 20 to 30 minutes TID
- Saline irrigation (Neti pot) or nose drops
- Sleep with head of bed elevated.
- Avoid exposure to cigarette smoke or fumes.
- Avoid caffeine and alcohol.
- Antibiotics are indicated only when findings suggest bacterial infection.
- Analgesics, NSAIDs
- Acute viral sinusitis is self-limiting; antibiotics should not be used.

MEDICATION

First Line
- Decongestants
  - Pseudoephedrine HCl
  - Phenylephrine nasal spray (limited use)
  - Oxymetazoline nasal spray (e.g., Afrin) (not to be used >3 days)
- Analgesics
  - Acetaminophen
  - Aspirin
  - NSAIDs

- Antibiotics
  - Antibiotics can shorten time to cure but only in 5 to 11 people per 100 (3)[A]; most improve without antimicrobial therapy.
  - Reserve antibiotic use for patients with moderate to severe disease.
  - Choice should be based on understanding of antibiotic resistance in the community.
  - Infectious Disease Society of America (IDSA) recommends the following (1)[C]:
    - Start antibiotics as soon as clinical diagnosis of acute bacterial sinusitis is made.
    - Use amoxicillin-clavulanate rather than amoxicillin alone.
    - Amoxicillin-clavulanate 875/125 mg q12h; 2 g PO BID in geographic regions with high rates of resistant *S. pneumoniae*
    - Doxycycline: 100 mg PO BID an alternative to amoxicillin-clavulanate for initial therapy (adults only)
    - Trimethoprim-sulfamethoxazole (TMP/SMX) and 3rd-generation cephalosporins not recommended due to high rate of resistance (1)[C]
    - Treat for 5 to 7 days in adults if uncomplicated bacterial rhinosinusitis (IDSA low- to moderate-quality evidence). Treat for 10 to 14 days in children if uncomplicated bacterial rhinosinusitis (IDSA low- to moderate-quality evidence).
  - American Academy of Pediatrics recommends the following (4)[C]:
    - Amoxicillin: 45 to 90 mg/kg/day in 2 divided doses if uncomplicated acute bacterial sinusitis in children
    - Amoxicillin-clavulanate: 80 to 90 mg/6.4 mg/kg/day in 2 divided doses for children with severe illness, recent antibiotics, or attending daycare
    - Levofloxacin: 10 to 20 mg/kg/day max 750 mg/day if history of type 1 hypersensitivity to PCN (1)[C]
    - Clindamycin (30 to 40 mg/kg/day) + cefixime (8 mg/kg/day in 2 divided doses) or cefpodoxime (10 mg/kg/day in 2 divided doses) (1)[C] for non–type 1 PCN allergy
    - Ceftriaxone: 50 mg/kg IM single dose if not able to tolerate oral meds
- Because allergies may be a predisposing factor, some patients may benefit from use of the following agents:
  - Oral antihistamines
    - Loratidine (Claritin), fexofenadine (Allegra), cetirizine (Zyrtec), desloratadine (Clarinex), or levocetirizine (Xyzal)
    - Chlorpheniramine (Chlor-Trimeton)
    - Diphenhydramine (Benadryl)
  - Leukotriene inhibitors (Singulair, Accolade), especially in patients with asthma
  - Nasal steroids (i.e., fluticasone [Flonase])

Second Line
- Levofloxacin (Levaquin): 750 mg/day for 5 days or moxifloxacin 400 mg/day for 5 to 7 days (adults only) (1)[C]
- If no response to first-line therapy after 72 hours
  - Broaden antibiotic coverage or switch to a different class; evaluate for resistant pathogens or other causes for treatment failure (i.e., noninfectious etiology); fluoroquinolones as above
- *Note*: Bacteriologic failure rates of up to 20–25% are possible with use of azithromycin and clarithromycin.

- If lack of response to 3 weeks of antibiotics, consider the following:
  - CT scan of sinuses
  - Ear/nose/throat (ENT) referral

ISSUES FOR REFERRAL
Complications or failure of treatment

ALERT
- Meta-analyses have demonstrated no benefit of newer antibiotics over amoxicillin or doxycycline.
- Antibiotics recommendations vary with different guidelines. Patients seen by specialists are different from those in a primary care setting. Patients usually do not have complicated sinusitis in primary care setting.
  - American Academy of Otolaryngology—Head and Neck Surgery Foundation (2)[C] recommends the following:
    - Consider watchful waiting without antibiotics in patients with uncomplicated mild illness (mild pain and temperature <101°F) with assurance of follow-up within 7 days.
- PCV-13 pneumococcal vaccine can be helpful in reducing chronic sinusitis in children (5)[B].
- Use of intranasal steroids small but significant improvement in symptoms when used alone or in combination with antibiotics (6)[A]
- Precautions
  - Decongestants can exacerbate hypertension.
  - Intranasal decongestants should be limited to 3 days to avoid rebound nasal congestion.

Pregnancy Considerations
- Nasal irrigation with saline, pseudoephedrine, most antihistamines, and some nasal steroids are safe during pregnancy and lactation.
- Antibiotics safe in pregnancy and lactation
  - Amoxicillin, amoxicillin-clavulanate, cephalosporins
- Antibiotic contraindicated: doxycycline, fluoroquinolones
- Antibiotic safe in lactation but not pregnancy: levofloxacin

SURGERY/OTHER PROCEDURES
- If medical therapy fails, consider sinus irrigation.
- Functional endoscopic sinus surgery is the preferred treatment for medically recalcitrant cases.
- Absolute surgical indications
  - Massive nasal polyposis
  - Acute complications: subperiosteal or orbital abscess, frontal soft tissue spread of infection
  - Mucocele or mucopyocele
  - Invasive or allergic fungal sinusitis
  - Suspected obstructing tumor
  - CSF rhinorrhea

ADMISSION, INPATIENT, AND NURSING CONSIDERATIONS
Hospitalization for complications (e.g., meningitis, orbital cellulitis or abscess, brain abscess)

ONGOING CARE

FOLLOW-UP RECOMMENDATIONS
Return if no improvement after 72 hours or no resolution of symptoms after 10 days of antibiotics.

PATIENT EDUCATION
http://familydoctor.org

PROGNOSIS
Alleviation of symptoms within 72 hours with complete resolution within 10 to 14 days

COMPLICATIONS
- Serious complications are rare.
- Meningitis, orbital cellulitis, brain abscess
- Cavernous sinus thrombosis
- Osteomyelitis, subdural empyema

REFERENCES
1. Chow AW, Benninger MS, Brook I, et al; for Infectious Diseases Society of America. IDSA clinical practice guideline for acute bacterial rhinosinusitis in children and adults. *Clin Infect Dis*. 2012;54(8):e72–e112.
2. Rosenfeld RM, Piccirillo JF, Chandrasekhar SS, et al. Clinical practice guideline (update): adult sinusitis. *Otolaryngol Head Neck Surg*. 2015;152(Suppl 2): S1–S39.
3. Lemiengre MB, van Driel ML, Merenstein D, et al. Antibiotics for acute rhinosinusitis in adults. *Cochrane Database Syst Rev*. 2018;(9):CD006089.
4. Wald ER, Applegate KE, Bordley C, et al; for American Academy of Pediatrics. Clinical practice guideline for the diagnosis and management of acute bacterial sinusitis in children aged 1 to 18 years. *Pediatrics*. 2013;132(1):e262–e280.
5. Olarte L, Hulten KG, Lamberth L, et al. Impact of the 13-valent pneumococcal conjugate vaccine on chronic sinusitis associated with *Streptococcus pneumoniae* in children. *Pediatr Infect Dis J*. 2014;33(10):1033–1036.
6. Hayward G, Heneghan C, Perera R, et al. Intranasal corticosteroids in management of acute sinusitis: a systematic review and meta-analysis. *Ann Fam Med*. 2012;10(3):241–249.

ADDITIONAL READING
Aring AM, Chan MM. Acute rhinosinusitis in adults. *Am Fam Physician*. 2011;83(9):1057–1063.

CODES

ICD10
- J01.41 Acute recurrent pansinusitis
- J01.0 Acute maxillary sinusitis
- J01.80 Other acute sinusitis

CLINICAL PEARLS
- Most cases resolve with supportive care (treating pain, nasal symptoms).
- Reserve antibiotics for symptoms that persist >10 days or if presenting with 3 to 4 consecutive days of severe symptoms (high fever, purulent nasal discharge, facial pain).
- Multiple meta-analyses have demonstrated *no* benefit of newer antibiotics over amoxicillin or doxycycline.
- Antibiotic NNT is 10 to 19 for shortening time course, whereas NNH is 8 from medication side effects.
- Significant patient symptom relief with nasal saline spray or drops or irrigation (Neti pot)

SJÖGREN SYNDROME
Mariya Milko, DO, MS

BASICS

- Chronic inflammatory disorder characterized by lymphocytic infiltrates in exocrine organs
- Typically presents with diminished salivary and lacrimal gland function, resulting in sicca symptoms such as dry eyes (xerophthalmia), dry mouth (xerostomia), and parotid enlargement
- Extraglandular manifestations: arthralgia, myalgia, Raynaud phenomenon, pulmonary disease, GI disease, leukopenia, anemia, lymphadenopathy, vasculitis, renal tubular acidosis, lymphoma, CNS involvement with longitudinal transverse myelitis (>4 vertebral segments), and optic neuritis associated with anti–aquaporin-4 antibodies, PNS involvement with small fiber neuropathy
- Primary Sjögren: not associated with other diseases; *HLA-DRB1*0301* and *HLA-DRB1*1501* are the most common.
- Secondary Sjögren: complication of other rheumatologic conditions, most commonly rheumatoid arthritis; associated with HLA-DR4
- First described by Swedish ophthalmologist Henrik Sjögren

EPIDEMIOLOGY
Incidence
Annual incidence: ~4/100,000. Primary Sjögren syndrome (SS) is one of the most common autoimmune diseases, affecting 1–4% of population.
- All races are affected.
- Predominant sex: female > male (9:1)
- Predominant age: can affect patients of any age but is most common in the elderly; onset typically in the 4th to 5th decades of life

Prevalence
SS affects 1 to 4 million people in the United States.

ETIOLOGY AND PATHOPHYSIOLOGY
- Multifactorial systemic autoimmune process characterized by infiltration of glandular tissue by CD4 T lymphocytes
- Theorized that glandular epithelial cells present antigen to the T cells inducing cytokine production. There is also evidence for B-cell activation, resulting in autoantibody production and an increased incidence of B-cell malignancies.
- Etiology is unknown. Estrogen may play a role because SS is more common in women. Exogenous factors such as viral proteins (EBV, HCV, HTLV-1) have also been implicated.

Genetics
- A familial tendency suggests a genetic predisposition.
- Associations in the HLA regions *HLA-DQA1*0501*, *HLA-DQB1*0201*, and *HLA-DRB*0301* are the strongest genetic risk factors for SS.

RISK FACTORS
There are no known modifiable risk factors.

GENERAL PREVENTION
- No known prevention. Complications can be prevented by early diagnosis and treatment.
- Oral health providers play a key role in early detection and management of salivary dysfunction (1)[C].

COMMONLY ASSOCIATED CONDITIONS
Secondary SS associated with rheumatoid arthritis, scleroderma, systemic lupus erythematosus (SLE), polymyositis, HIV, hepatitis C, MCTD, PBC, hypergammaglobulinemic purpura, necrotizing vasculitis, autoimmune thyroiditis, chronic active hepatitis, mixed cryoglobulinemia

Pregnancy Considerations
Pregnant SS patients with anti-SSA Abs have increased risk of delivering fetus with skin rash and 3rd-degree heart block.

DIAGNOSIS

- 2016 ACR/EULAR classification criteria (2)[A]:
  - Based on five objective tests/items
  - Inclusion criteria applicable if the patient is positive for one ocular/oral dryness symptom based on the AECG questions or at least one positive domain from the EULAR SS disease activity index questionnaire and a total score of ≥4 from the following:
    - Positive serum anti-SSA/Ro antibody—3 points
    - Focal lymphocytic sialadenitis with a focus score ≥1 foci/4 mm² from labial salivary gland biopsy—3 points
    - Abnormal ocular staining score of ≥5 or van Bijsterveld score of ≥4—1 point
    - Schirmer test result of ≤5 mm/5 min—1 point
    - An unstimulated salivary flow rate of ≤0.1 mL/min—1 point
- Ocular signs and symptoms
  - Troublesome dry eyes daily for ≥3 months
  - Recurrent sandy/gritty ocular sensation
  - Use of tear substitute ≥3 times per day
- Oral signs and symptoms
  - Daily symptoms of dry mouth for ≥3 months
  - Recurrent feeling of swollen salivary glands
  - Need to drink liquid to help swallow dry foods
- Other manifestations: chronic arthritis, type 1 RTA, tubular interstitial nephritis, rheumatoid arthritis, vasculitis, vaginal dryness, pleuritis, pancreatitis

HISTORY
- Decreased tear production; burning, scratchy sensation in eyes
- Difficulty speaking/swallowing, dental caries, xerotrachea
- Enlarged or intermittent swelling of parotid glands (bilateral)
- Dyspareunia; vaginal dryness
- From consensus criteria and EULAR questionnaire:
  - (1) Have you had daily, persistent, troublesome dry eyes for >3 months?
  - (2) Do you have a recurrent sensation of sand or gravel in the eyes?
  - (3) Do you use tear substitutes >3 times a day?
  - (4) Have you had a daily feeling of dry mouth for >3 months?
  - (5) Do you frequently drink liquids to aid in swallowing dry food?

PHYSICAL EXAM
- Eye exam: dry eyes (keratoconjunctivitis sicca), decreased tear pool in the lower conjunctiva, dilated conjunctival vessels, mucinous threads, and filamentary keratosis (slit-lamp examination)
- Mouth exam: dry mouth (xerostomia); decreased sublingual salivary pool (tongue may stick to the tongue depressor); frequent oral caries (sometimes in unusual locations such as the incisor surface and along the gum line); dark red tongue from prolonged xerostomia
- Ear, nose, and throat exam: parotid enlargement, submandibular enlargement
- Skin exam: nonpalpable or palpable vasculitic purpura (typically 2 to 3 mm in diameter and on the lower extremities)

DIFFERENTIAL DIAGNOSIS
- Causes of ocular dryness: hypovitaminosis A, decreased tear production unrelated to autoimmune process, chronic blepharitis or conjunctivitis, impaired blinking (i.e., due to Parkinson disease or Bell palsy), infiltration of lacrimal glands (i.e., amyloidosis, lymphoma, sarcoidosis), low estrogen levels
- Causes of oral dryness: anticholinergic medications, sialadenitis due to chronic obstruction, chronic viral infections (e.g., hepatitis C or HIV), radiation of head/neck
- Causes of salivary gland swelling: unilateral: obstruction, chronic sialadenitis, bacterial infection, neoplasm; bilateral (asymmetric): IgG4-related disease, HIV; bilateral (symmetric): hepatic cirrhosis, DM, anorexia/bulimia, acromegaly, alcoholism, hypolipoproteinemia, chronic pancreatitis, acute or chronic viral infection (i.e., mumps, Epstein-Barr virus [EBV]), coxsackievirus, echovirus, granulomatous diseases (i.e., tuberculosis, sarcoidosis)

DIAGNOSTIC TESTS & INTERPRETATION
- Schirmer test (<5-mm wetness after 5 minutes)
- Rose Bengal test (slit lamp)
- Minor salivary gland biopsy (gold standard)
- Auto antibodies: +ANAs (95%), +RF (75%)
- In primary SS: +anti-Ro (anti-SSA, 56%) and +anti-La (anti-SSB, 30%)

Initial Tests (lab, imaging)
Preliminary lab workup
- Basic labs: CBC with differential, BUN/creatinine (Cr), AST/ALT, ESR, C-reactive protein (CRP), urinalysis
- Special labs: ANA, rheumatoid factor (RF), anti-Ro/SSA, anti-La/SSB, ESR, CRP
- Anti-SSA and anti-SSB antibodies present in 33–74% and 23–52% of SS patients, respectively
- Other autoantibodies-muscarinic type 3 receptor (M3R) and anti-α-fodrin are being explored with good specificity (3)[A].
- Imaging may include:
  - Imaging for xerostomia: salivary gland scintigraphy (insensitive but highly specific)
  - Parotid gland sialography (should not be used in acute parotitis)
  - MRI (correlates well with salivary gland biopsy)
- A novel diagnostic tool is salivary gland US (SGUS), which is noninvasive and highly specific for salivary gland involvement in SS (4)[A].

Diagnostic Procedures/Other
- Salivary gland biopsy: used to confirm suspected diagnosis of SS or to exclude other causes of xerostomia and bilateral glandular enlargement
- Parotid biopsy if malignancy is suspected
- Lymph node biopsy to rule out pseudolymphoma or lymphoma if suspected

Test Interpretation
- Salivary gland histology shows focal collections of lymphocytes; immunocytology shows CD4+ T-cell lymphocyte predominance.
- SGUS parameters include:
  – Parenchymal nonhomogeneity—the most useful diagnostic marker (4)[A]
  – US inflammatory findings include hypoechoic and hyperechoic bands (4)[A].
  – Real-time sonoelastography (RTS) to quantify tissue rigidity and assess glandular damage (4)[A]

TREATMENT
- Treatment is primarily supportive.
- Treat sicca symptoms—dry eyes, dry mouth.
- Avoid medications that may worsen oral dryness (i.e., anticholinergics).
- Promote good oral hygiene.
- Treat systemic manifestations.
- Address fatigue and pain.

MEDICATION
- Therapy for sicca symptoms: artificial tears and ocular lubricants (5)[C]
- Topical therapy for dry mouth: liberal sips of water, sugar-free lemon drops, or artificial saliva preparations such as Salivart, Saliment, Xero-Lube, MouthKote
- Immunosuppressive therapy such as hydroxychloroquine can be used for systemic symptoms; however, it has not shown any benefit in relieving refractory sicca symptoms.
- Cevimeline (Evoxac) works by stimulating muscarinic cholinergic receptors to increase salivary gland secretion and may be prescribed for SS-associated xerostomia.
- Dry eyes are graded by severity of symptoms, conjunctival injection and staining, corneal damage, tear quality, and lid involvement. Artificial tears may be used; however, artificial tears with hydroxyethylcellulose or dextran are more viscous and can last longer.
- Acetaminophen or NSAIDs for arthralgias

First Line
- Xerostomia: sugar-free lozenges, especially malic acid, artificial saliva; pilocarpine 5 mg PO QID or cevimeline 30 mg PO TID
- Keratoconjunctivitis sicca: artificial tears and ocular lubricants for symptomatic relief, topical cyclosporine (Restasis), or autologous tears

Second Line
- Xerostomia: Interferon-α lozenges may enhance salivary gland flow.
- Keratoconjunctivitis sicca: topical glucocorticoids or topical NSAIDs (Use with caution.)

- Immunosuppressive therapy: antimalarials (e.g., hydroxychloroquine) for arthralgias, lymphadenopathies, and skin manifestations; may then consider methotrexate or cyclosporine, which showed subjective improvement but no significant objective improvement
- Early studies show improvement in fatigue with rituximab (6)[B].
- For life-threatening extraglandular manifestations, cyclophosphamide (PO or IV), mycophenolate mofetil, and azathioprine are often used.

ISSUES FOR REFERRAL
- Rheumatology to help manage systemic manifestations or resistant symptoms
- Oral health
- Ophthalmology for grading of severity and management of xerophthalmia

ADDITIONAL THERAPIES
- Patients should use vaginal lubricants (e.g., Replens) for vaginal dryness. Vaginal estrogen creams can help in postmenopausal women. Be alert for and treat vaginal yeast infections.
- Xerostomia: small sips of water, good dental care
- Keratoconjunctivitis sicca: Conserve tears with side shields or ski/swim goggles, humidifiers, and moist washcloths.
- Dehydroepiandrosterone (DHEA) does not offer improvement in fatigue and well-being above placebo.

SURGERY/OTHER PROCEDURES
Keratoconjunctivitis sicca: If refractory to artificial tears, punctal occlusion is the treatment of choice.

COMPLEMENTARY & ALTERNATIVE MEDICINE
- Some studies show acupuncture benefits saliva production and symptoms of xerostomia.
- There is insufficient evidence to determine the effects of electrostimulation devices on dry mouth symptoms or saliva production in patients with SS.

ADMISSION, INPATIENT, AND NURSING CONSIDERATIONS
May be required for extraglandular manifestations, such as cardiopulmonary disease, renal involvement, and CNS manifestations (e.g., optic neuritis, transverse myelitis, vasculitis, or ischemic stroke)

ONGOING CARE

FOLLOW-UP RECOMMENDATIONS
Frequency of follow-up depends on severity.

Patient Monitoring
- Monitor for complications, systemic manifestations, and relief of symptoms.
- Medicolegal pitfalls: Monitor for parotid tumor or lymphoma.

PATIENT EDUCATION
In most cases, simple measures are adequate: humidifiers, sips of water, chewing gum, artificial tears.

PROGNOSIS
- Hypocomplementemia is an independent risk factor for premature death.
- Primary SS is associated with increased risks of malignancy, non-Hodgkin lymphoma, and thyroid cancer.

COMPLICATIONS
Complications include dental caries, gum disease, dysphagia, salivary gland calculi, keratitis, conjunctivitis, and scarring of the ocular surface.

REFERENCES
1. Mays JW, Sarmadi M, Moutsopoulos NM. Oral manifestations of systemic autoimmune and inflammatory diseases: diagnosis and clinical management. J Evid Based Dent Pract. 2012;12(Suppl 3):265–282.
2. Shiboski CH, Shiboski SC, Seror R, et al; and International Sjögren's Syndrome Criteria Working Group. 2016 American College of Rheumatology/European League Against Rheumatism classification criteria for primary Sjögren's syndrome: a consensus and data-driven methodology involving three international patient cohorts. Arthritis Rheumatol. 2017;69(1):35–45.
3. Deng C, Hu C, Chen S, et al. Meta-analysis of anti-muscarinic receptor type 3 antibodies for the diagnosis of Sjögren syndrome. PLoS One. 2015;10(1):e0116744.
4. Ferro F, Marcucci E, Orlandi M, et al. One year in review 2017: primary Sjogren's syndrome. Clin Exp Rheumatol. 2017;35(2):179–191.
5. Aragona P, Spinella R, Rania L, et al. Safety and efficacy of 0.1% clobetasone butyrate eyedrops in the treatment of dry eye in Sjögren syndrome. Eur J Ophthalmol. 2013;23(3):368–376.
6. Meijer JM, Meiners PM, Vissink A, et al. Effectiveness of rituximab treatment in primary Sjögren's syndrome: a randomized, double-blind, placebo-controlled trial. Arthritis Rheum. 2010;62(4):960–968.

CODES

ICD10
- M35.00 Sicca syndrome, unspecified
- M35.02 Sicca syndrome with lung involvement
- M35.09 Sicca syndrome with other organ involvement

CLINICAL PEARLS
- Many symptoms of SS can be treated with simple interventions such as artificial tears and sugar-free lozenges.
- Consider lacrimal duct plugs for dry eyes.
- Consider SS in patients with unexplained lung disease and +ANA.
- Patients with primary SS may have an increased incidence of celiac disease.

S

SLEEP APNEA, OBSTRUCTIVE

Thomas J. Hansen, MD

BASICS

DESCRIPTION

- Obstructive sleep apnea (OSA) is defined as repetitive episodes of cessation of airflow (apnea) through the nose and mouth during sleep due to obstruction at the level of the pharynx.
  - Apneas often terminate with a snort/gasp.
  - Repetitive apneas produce sleep disruption, leading to excessive daytime sleepiness (EDS).
  - Associated with oxygen desaturation and nocturnal hypoxemia
  - Usual course is chronic.
- System(s) affected: cardiovascular; nervous; pulmonary
- Synonym(s): sleep apnea syndrome; nocturnal upper airway occlusion

EPIDEMIOLOGY

Incidence

- Predominant age: middle-aged men and women
- Predominant sex: male > female (2:1)

Prevalence

- Up to 15% in men; 5% in women
- Prevalence is higher in obese/hypertensive patients.

ETIOLOGY AND PATHOPHYSIOLOGY

OSA occurs when the naso- or oropharynx collapses passively during inspiration. Anatomic and neuromuscular factors contribute to pharyngeal collapse, which leads to hypoxic arousal.

- Anatomic abnormalities, such as increased soft tissue in the palate, tonsillar hypertrophy, macroglossia, and craniofacial abnormalities, predispose the airway to collapse by decreasing the area of the upper airway or increasing the pressure surrounding the airway.
- During sleep, decreased muscle tone in the naso- or oropharynx contributes to airway obstruction and collapse.
- Upper airway narrowing may be due to the following:
  - Obesity, redundant tissue in the soft palate
  - Enlarged tonsils/uvula or a low soft palate
  - Large/posteriorly located tongue
  - Craniofacial abnormalities or neuromuscular disorders
  - Alcohol/sedative use before bedtime

RISK FACTORS

- Obesity (strongest risk factor)
- Age >40 years
- Alcohol/sedative intake before bedtime
- Smoking
- Nasal obstruction (due to polyps, rhinitis, or deviated septum)
- Anatomic narrowing of nasopharynx (e.g., tonsillar hypertrophy, macroglossia, micrognathia, retrognathia, craniofacial abnormalities)
- Acromegaly
- Hypothyroidism
- Neurologic syndromes (e.g., muscular dystrophy, cerebral palsy)

GENERAL PREVENTION

Weight control and avoidance of alcohol and sedatives at night can help to prevent airway collapse.

COMMONLY ASSOCIATED CONDITIONS

- Common
  - Hypertension
  - Obesity
  - Daytime sleepiness
  - Metabolic syndrome
- Rare
  - Cardiac arrhythmias
  - Cardiovascular disease
  - Congestive heart failure
  - Pulmonary hypertension
  - Nasal obstructive problems

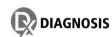

DIAGNOSIS

HISTORY

- Elicit a complete history of daytime and nighttime symptoms. Symptoms can be insidious and may have been present for years.
- Daytime symptoms
  - Excessive daytime sleepiness (EDS) or fatigue (cardinal symptom) (1)
    - Mild symptoms are those that occur during quiet activities (e.g., reading, watching television).
    - More severe symptoms are those that occur during dynamic activities (e.g., work, driving).
  - Tired on morning awakening "nonrestorative sleep"
  - Sore/dry throat
  - Poor concentration, memory problems, irritability, mood changes, behavior problems (in children)
  - Morning headaches
  - Decreased libido
  - Depression
- Nighttime symptoms
  - Loud snoring (present in 60% of people with OSA)
  - Snort/gasp that arouses patient from sleep but not usually to full consciousness
  - Disrupted sleep
  - Witnessed apneic episodes at night
- Screening—the USPSTF found that there is insufficient evidence to screen for OSA in asymptomatic adults or in adults with unrecognized symptoms (2)[A].

PHYSICAL EXAM

- OSA is commonly associated with obesity. It is unlikely to be found in those with normal body weight who do not snore (1).
- Focused head and neck exam
  - Short neck with large circumference
  - Oropharynx
    - Narrowing of the lateral airway wall
    - Tonsillar hypertrophy
    - Macroglossia
    - Micrognathia/retrognathia
    - Soft palate edema
    - Long/thick uvula
    - High, arched hard palate
  - Nasopharynx
    - Deviated nasal septum
    - Poor nasal airflow

DIFFERENTIAL DIAGNOSIS

- Other causes of EDS such as the following:
  - Narcolepsy
  - Idiopathic daytime hypersomnolence
  - Inadequate sleep time
  - Depressive episodes with EDS
  - Periodic limb movements disorder
- Respiratory disorders with nocturnal awakenings such as the following:
  - Asthma
  - Chronic obstructive pulmonary disease
  - Congestive heart failure
- Central sleep apnea (Respiratory effort is absent as compared to OSA where effort is present.)
- Sleep-related choking/laryngospasm
- Gastroesophageal reflux
- Sleep-associated seizures (temporal lobe epilepsy)

DIAGNOSTIC TESTS & INTERPRETATION

Initial Tests (lab, imaging)

When clinically indicated

- Thyroid-stimulating hormone to evaluate hypothyroidism
- CBC to evaluate anemia and polycythemia, which can indicate nocturnal hypoxemia
- Fasting glucose in obesity to evaluate for diabetes
- Rare: arterial blood gases to evaluate daytime hypercapnia
- Cephalometric measurements from lateral head and neck radiographs aid in surgical treatment.

Diagnostic Procedures/Other

- The gold standard for OSA is a full-night, in-laboratory polysomnography (PSG), a nighttime sleep study (1)[A],(3)[B].
  - Demonstrates severity of hypoxemia, sleep disruption, and cardiac arrhythmias associated with OSA and elevated end-tidal CO_2
  - Shows repetitive episodes of cessation/marked reduction in airflow despite continued respiratory efforts
  - Apneic episodes must last at least 10 seconds and occur 10 to 15 times per hour and cause decreased oxygen saturation to be considered clinically significant.
  - Complete PSG is expensive, and health insurance may not cover the cost.
- Multiple sleep latency testing is a diagnostic tool used to measure the time it takes from the start of a daytime nap period to the first signs of sleep (sleep latency). It provides an objective measurement of daytime sleepiness.
- The Apnea-Hypopnea Index (AHI) is defined as the total number of apneas and hypopneas divided by the total sleep time in hours.
  - Mild OSA: AHI = 5 to 15
  - Moderate OSA: AHI = 15 to 30
  - Severe OSA: AHI >30
- Split-night PSG (as compared to a full-night PSG) occurs when patients are diagnosed with OSA within the first part of the night, and then they can initiate positive pressure device titration during the second half of the night.
- Drugs that may alter the test results include benzodiazepines and other sedatives that can amplify the severity of apnea seen during the sleep study.
- Early data suggest that home-based diagnosis using portable monitoring devices may be an alternative to laboratory-based PSG if the test is of sufficient duration (4)[B].

TREATMENT

- Lifestyle modification is the most frequently recommended treatment for mild to moderate OSA. This includes weight loss; exercise; and avoidance of alcohol, smoking, and sedatives, especially before bedtime.
- Weight loss—shown to decrease the severity of symptoms in obese patients. Lifestyle modifications should be seen as adjunctive rather than curative therapy (5)[A], and a lack of improvement of symptoms with lifestyle modification should not preclude patients from receiving other therapy such as continuous positive airway pressure (CPAP).
- Position changes—if OSA is present only when supine, keep the patient off his or her back when sleeping (e.g., tennis ball worn on back of nightshirt or using a sleep position trainer).
- Positive airway pressure—the most effective therapy for mild, moderate, or severe OSA is CPAP (6)[A]. Treatment with CPAP uses a mask interface and a flow generator to prevent airway collapse, thus helping to prevent apnea, hypoxia, and sleep disturbance. Compared with inactive controls, CPAP significantly improves both objective (24-hour systolic and diastolic blood pressures) and subjective measures (Epworth Sleepiness Scale) in OSA patients with symptoms of daytime sleepiness. CPAP may also decrease the risk for atherosclerosis as well as improves insulin resistance in nondiabetic patients. Early data show that these benefits may not be seen in patients who do not have symptoms of daytime sleepiness.
- Several types of mask interfaces, including nasal masks, oral masks, and nasal pillows exist for CPAP therapy. Short-term data suggest that nasal pillows are the preferred interface in almost all patients. In patients with compliance difficulty, a different choice of interface may be appropriate.
- Oral appliances to treat OSA are available and often subjectively preferred by patients (mandibular advancement devices vs. tongue retaining devices). Although oral appliances have been shown to improve symptoms compared with inactive controls, they are not as effective for reduction of respiratory disturbances as CPAP over short-term data. Treatment with oral appliances may be considered in patients who fail to comply with CPAP therapy.

MEDICATION
Medications are yet to be proven effective in treating OSA. Further studies in this area are needed (7).

First Line
Some short-term data found fluticasone nasal spray, mirtazapine, physostigmine, and nasal lubricant of some benefit; longer term studies needed

ISSUES FOR REFERRAL
If sleep apnea is suspected, patient should be referred for a sleep study evaluation.

SURGERY/OTHER PROCEDURES
Surgical corrections of the upper airway include alteration of the uvula and/or palate such as uvulopalato-pharyngoplasty (UPPP), tracheostomy, and craniofacial surgery. Currently, no evidence supports the use of surgery for the treatment of OSA (8)[A].

ADMISSION, INPATIENT, AND NURSING CONSIDERATIONS
On admission, patients should bring in their own appliance and know their CPAP settings to continue to use CPAP/dental devices as they do so at home.

 ONGOING CARE

Lifelong compliance with weight loss or CPAP is necessary for successful OSA treatment.

DIET
Overweight and obese patients should be encouraged to lose weight, and all patients must avoid weight gain. Weight loss alone could reduce symptoms of OSA.

PATIENT EDUCATION
- Weight loss and avoidance of alcohol and sedatives may reduce OSA symptoms particularly in severe cases.
- Significantly sleepy patients should not drive a motor vehicle/operate dangerous equipment.

PROGNOSIS
- EDS is reduced dramatically with appropriate apnea control.
- Lifelong compliance with weight loss or CPAP is necessary for effective treatment of OSA, but long-term adherence is poor.
- If untreated, OSA is progressive.
- Significant morbidity and mortality with OSA usually due to motor vehicle accidents or are secondary to cardiac complications, including arrhythmias, cardiac ischemia, and hypertension; data insufficient on whether identification and treatment changes outcomes.

COMPLICATIONS
Untreated OSA may increase the risk for development of hypertension, stroke, myocardial infarction, diabetes, cardiovascular disease, and work-related and driving accidents, but it is unclear that treatment reduces or prevents any of these problems.

Pediatric Considerations
- The prevalence of pediatric OSA is 1–2% in children 4 to 5 years of age, and the peak incidence is between 3 and 6 years of age (9).
- Etiology: The most common cause is tonsillar hypertrophy. Additional causes are obesity and craniofacial abnormalities. OSA is also seen in children with neuromuscular diseases, such as cerebral palsy and spinal muscular atrophy, due to abnormal pharyngeal muscle control.
- Signs and symptoms
  - Nighttime: loud snoring, restlessness, and sweating
  - Daytime: hyperactivity and decreased school performance
  - EDS is not a significant symptom.
- Diagnosis: Gold standard is PSG. (PSG may be an even better tool in children due to lessened night-to-night variation. There is a lack of studies showing efficacy of home-based diagnostic studies vs. PSG in children.) Abnormal AHI is different in children: >1 to 2 per hour is abnormal.

- Treatment: Surgery is the first-line treatment in cases due to tonsillar enlargement (reduces symptoms in 70%). Some data suggest improved academic performance if tonsillectomy is performed for OSA. For cases due to obesity/craniofacial abnormalities, patients can use CPAP treatment.

Geriatric Considerations
The presence of sleep apnea in the geriatric population may be associated with earlier onset of mild cognitive impairment as well as Alzheimer dementia at an earlier age. The rate of decline of cognitive function may be slowed by the usage of CPAP.

REFERENCES
1. Myers KA, Mrkobrada M, Simel DL. Does this patient have obstructive sleep apnea? The rational clinical examination systematic review. *JAMA.* 2013;310(7):731–741.
2. Bibbins-Domingo K, Grossman DC, Curry SJ, et al; and US Preventive Services Task Force. Screening for obstructive sleep apnea in adults: US Preventive Services Task Force recommendation statement. *JAMA.* 2017;317(4):407–414.
3. Kapur VK, Auckley DH, Chowdhuri S, et al. Clinical practice guideline for diagnostic testing for adult obstructive sleep apnea: an American Academy of Sleep Medicine clinical practice guideline. *J Clin Sleep Med.* 2017;13(3):479–504.
4. Wittine LM, Olson EJ, Morgenthaler TI. Effect of recording duration on the diagnostic accuracy of out-of-center sleep testing for obstructive sleep apnea. *Sleep.* 2014;37(5):969–975.
5. Anandam A, Akinnusi M, Kufel T, et al. Effects of dietary weight loss on obstructive sleep apnea: a meta-analysis. *Sleep Breath.* 2013;17(1):227–234.
6. Giles TL, Lasserson TJ, Smith BH, et al. Continuous positive airways pressure for obstructive sleep apnoea in adults. *Cochrane Database Syst Rev.* 2006;(3):CD001106.
7. Mason M, Welsh EJ, Smith I. Drug therapy for obstructive sleep apnoea in adults. *Cochrane Database Syst Rev.* 2013;(5):CD003002.
8. Sundaram S, Bridgman SA, Lim J, et al. Surgery for obstructive sleep apnoea. *Cochrane Database Syst Rev.* 2005;(4):CD001004.
9. Marcus CL, Brooks LJ, Draper KA, et al; for American Academy of Pediatrics. Diagnosis and management of childhood obstructive sleep apnea syndrome. *Pediatrics.* 2012;130(3):576–584.

 CODES

ICD10
- G47.33 Obstructive sleep apnea (adult) (pediatric)
- G47.30 Sleep apnea, unspecified

CLINICAL PEARLS
- OSA is characterized by repetitive episodes of apnea often terminating in a snort/gasp.
- Laboratory PSG is the key to diagnosis.
- CPAP is the most effective form of treatment for both mild to moderate and moderate to severe OSA.
- Central sleep apnea may mimic OSA.

SLEEP DISORDER, SHIFT WORK

Michael McShane, MD, EdM

 BASICS

DESCRIPTION

Shift work disorder (SWD), classified as a circadian rhythm sleep-wake disorder, is characterized by symptoms of insomnia and/or excessive sleepiness when required to work during usual sleep times (1). SWD is caused by a misalignment between the internal circadian rhythm and the required sleep-wake schedule defined by nontraditional work shifts including night shifts, afternoon or evening shifts, early morning shifts, irregular shifts, and rotating shifts (2).

EPIDEMIOLOGY

Prevalence

- In the United States, approximately 20% of employed adults are shift workers, particularly in service-related occupations such as health care, protective services, transportation, and food services (2).
- SWD has an estimated prevalence of approximately 2–5% in the general population of the United States (2).
- Prevalence of SWD rises with age, particularly for adults age >50 years (1).

ETIOLOGY AND PATHOPHYSIOLOGY

- Sleep disturbances in shift workers are explained by disruptions in two biologic processes. The homeostatic sleep drive and circadian rhythm of alertness interact with each other to regulate sleep. The homeostatic sleep drive increases with wakefulness and decreases with sleep. Alertness is regulated by the suprachiasmatic nucleus (SCN) of the anterior hypothalamus and promotes wakefulness during the daytime and sleep at night. As homeostatic sleep drive increases during the day, the circadian rhythm of alertness increases and vice versa (2),(3).
- Circadian rhythms play a role multiple biologic functions, including regulation of body temperature, hormone levels, blood pressure, metabolism, cellular regeneration, sleep-wake cycles, and DNA transcription and translation (4). This internal biologic clock fluctuates with 24-hour cycles and is primarily regulated by external and environmental cues (3).
- The strongest influence on circadian rhythm is light. Light entering the eyes stimulates the retinohypothalamic and retino-geniculo-hypothalamic pathways to the SCN of the hypothalamus, subsequently suppressing melatonin from the pineal gland. During the day, melatonin levels are low, and the circadian rhythm of alertness is high (2).
- Periods of darkness cause the SCN to induce melatonin release from the pineal gland, which can also help to reset the molecular clock (4).
- In shift workers, there is a misalignment between one's endogenous circadian rhythm of sleep and wakefulness and a sleep-wake schedule based on nontraditional shift work. Dyssynchrony results in excessive sleepiness during the work shift and/or insomnia during desired sleep time (2),(3),(4).

Genetics

Not all shift workers experience SWD and there is variability in symptoms occurring among shifts workers with SWD. One possibly genetically linked trait is a person's preference for the morning versus the evening. This is partially linked to the polymorphism of the PER3 "clock" gene involved in sleep-wake regulation (2).

RISK FACTORS

- Age >50 years (2)
- Strong competing social and domestic needs (1)

GENERAL PREVENTION

- Reduce or eliminate shift work.
- Try to rotate shifts forward if shifts must be rotated.
- Use bright light during shifts.
- Improve sleep hygiene.
- Schedule regular sleep including naps (<1 hour) just before a shift or, if possible, during a shift.

COMMONLY ASSOCIATED CONDITIONS

- SWD has been associated with functional consequences including impaired immediate free recall, decreased processing speed, and selective attention impairments (4).
- SWD has been associated with higher risk of vehicular accidents, job-related injuries (4).
- SWD has been associated with poor physical health (including increased incidence of gastrointestinal [GI] disorders, cardiovascular disease [CVD], diabetes, and possible increase risk of cancers), as well as poor mental health (including increased incidence of substance use disorders and mood disorders) (4),(5).

 DIAGNOSIS

- This is a clinical diagnosis. Criteria for circadian rhythm disorder per *DSM-5* include all three of the following (1):
  - A persistent or recurrent pattern of sleep disruption that is primarily due to an alteration of the circadian system or to a misalignment between the endogenous circadian rhythm and sleep-wake schedule required by an individual's physical environment or social or professional schedule
  - The sleep disruption leads to excessive sleepiness or insomnia, or both.
  - The sleep disturbance causes clinically significant distress or impairment in social, occupational, and other important areas of functioning.
- Additional specification per *DSM-5* for SWD includes (1):
  - Insomnia during the major sleep period and/or excessive sleepiness (including inadvertent sleep) during the major awake period associated with a shift work schedule (i.e., requiring unconventional work hours).
  - The disorder is classified as to whether it is episodic (symptoms at least 1 month but <3 months), persistent (symptoms at least 3 months or longer) or recurrent (two or more episodes occurring within 1 year).

HISTORY

- A careful history is critical. Assess work history, detailed sleep history, level of sleepiness, safety risk, and performance impairments during work shifts.
- Note the following in particular (3),(6)[C]:
  - Sleep-wake habits, sleep environment
  - Degree of alertness or sleepiness
  - Light exposure before, during, and after the shift
  - Job-related factors: occupation, work schedule, years of shift work, length of shift, number of consecutive shifts, and commute after shift
  - Sedating or stimulating medications or substance use
  - Impact on social and domestic responsibilities (including drowsy driving)

- Evaluate for symptoms of other sleep disorders, which often coexist and can exacerbate SWD such as the following (3):
  - Loud snoring and pauses in breathing during sleep (obstructive sleep apnea [OSA])
  - Sudden sleep attacks and leg symptoms (restless legs syndrome [RLS])
  - Falling asleep at inappropriate times, drop attacks, and daytime fatigue (narcolepsy)

PHYSICAL EXAM

Evaluate for findings suggestive of mood disorders, GI disease, diabetes, CVD, cancer signs of OSA such as obesity, and large neck (3),(6)[C].

DIFFERENTIAL DIAGNOSIS

- Other primary sleep disorders: insomnia, sleep-related breathing disorders, central disorders of hypersomnolence, parasomnias, sleep-related movement disorders (3)
- Other circadian rhythm sleep disorders such as delayed sleep phase type or irregular sleep-wake type. Distinguishing among these can be challenging.

DIAGNOSTIC TESTS & INTERPRETATION

No diagnostic testing required for the diagnosis. If concern for another sleep disorder, consider polysomnography or multiple sleep latency testing (testing for narcolepsy). Given possible increased risk, consider screen for potential medical comorbidities as discussed above including mood disorders and metabolic disorders among shift workers (2),(3).

Diagnostic Procedures/Other

- Sleep diaries can help identify sleep-wake disturbances related to shift work and should be recorded for 2 weeks. Sleep diaries can provide useful information on sleep-wake patterns on work days, nonwork days, transitional periods, sleep efficiency, sleep onset latency, duration of wakefulness after sleep onset, and sleep quality. Two types of sleep diary include the 24-hour sleep diary which is more commonly used to evaluate sleep-wake patterns across multiple days, and the consensus sleep diary which is the preferred form for evaluation of insomnia (3).
- Standardized measures of sleepiness can be obtained using several tools including the Insomnia Severity Index (ISI) and Epworth Sleepiness Scale (ESS). ISI assesses for sleep disturbances with a score ≥10 being clinically significant for insomnia. ESS assesses for sleepiness during wake periods with a score ≥10 indicating excessive sleepiness (3).

Test Interpretation

Sleep diaries often reveal:

- Increased sleep latency
- Decreased total sleep time
- Frequent awakenings
- Most people revert to nocturnal sleeping on their days off. Every work week, they must "start over" to shift circadian rhythms to align with work schedules.

 TREATMENT

- The only standard recommendation by the American Academy of Sleep Medicine (AASM) is planned (prescribed) sleep schedules (7)[C].
- Other commonly used strategies include promoting wakefulness while at work with bright light exposure, caffeine or rarely other stimulants, and/or promoting sleep with sleep hygiene optimization, melatonin, and hypnotics.

GENERAL MEASURES

- Sleep hygiene: An important first step in approaching the treatment of sleep disorders is proper sleep hygiene. This includes minimizing exposure to bright light before and during scheduled sleep periods (maintain a dark sleeping space, wear dark sunglasses following work shift, wear an eye mask to sleep), maintain a quiet sleep environment (wear ear plugs to sleep, disconnect phone/doorbell, use a white noise generator), maintain cool sleeping quarters to help retrain core body temperature to align with modified sleep-wake cycle, and avoid use of stimulants during second half of work shift (4)[C].
- Sleep time: protected time for sleep prior to and following work shifts with strategic naps where possible (6)[C]. Shift workers, particularly night shift workers, should be aware of postnap sleep inertia and avoid driving when drowsy (2).
- Anchor sleep: Even if circadian rhythm can be retrained, these efforts are often unraveled due to workers attempting to resume a normal circadian rhythm on their days off. This process can be mitigated by scheduling sleep periods so that at least 1 to 2 hours of designated sleep time overlap on work days and nonwork days. Anchor sleep can help increase sleep duration as well as allow workers to maintain time for socialization and recreation.
- Work/social/domestic factors: Treat psychosocial stress, depression; encourage healthy eating habits; limit substance use; increase exercise to at least 30 minutes 5 times per week (not within 2 to 4 hours of bedtime) (6)[C]. Seek family member and social support for protected sleep time (2).
- Work-related interventions: If possible, reduce number of consecutive shifts (<4) or reduce shift duration (<12 hours), allow adequate time between shifts (>11 hours), move heavy workload outside circadian nadir (04:00 to 07:00) (6)[C].
- Light exposure: Timed bright light exposure can delay the physiologic nadir of alertness and thus, promote alertness during the night/early shift and possibly reduce circadian misalignment. Light avoidance during the day may also help with circadian adaption and improve sleep (2),(3).

MEDICATION

- Sleep-promoting medications:
  - Melatonin may help shift circadian rhythms and can increase the quality and duration of sleep as well as increase alertness during the work shift. AASM recommends 3 mg of melatonin for daytime sleep for shift workers (2); clinical effectiveness of melatonin is unclear.
  - Ramelteon (Rozerem), a melatonin receptor agonist, is FDA approved to treat insomnia, and may also provide benefit in SWD (4)[C].
  - Doxepin (tricyclic antidepressant) given at low doses may improve sleep without residual daytime impairment (4)[C]. Trazodone is a non–first-line agent for treatment of insomnia; it may also provide some benefit in SWD.
  - Intermediate-acting hypnotics such as zolpidem (Ambien) or eszopiclone (Lunesta) can cause postsleep sedation (4)[C]. Long-term use is discouraged due to potential dependence. Additionally, side effects such as anxiety or irritability may affect sleep (2).
- Wakefulness-promoting medications:
  - Modafinil (Provigil) and armodafinil (Nuvigil) are FDA approved for excessive sleepiness in patients with SWD and can reduce daytime sleepiness and improve cognitive performance (4). Notably, modafinil has been tied to rare instances of Stevens-Johnson syndrome (3).
  - Prophylactic caffeine use immediately prior to work shift and during work shift (6)[C]. Limiting caffeine to the first half of the night shift is recommended to limit disruption of daytime sleep (3).

First Line

Circadian shift/sleep promoting: melatonin 3 mg PO or sublingual, 30 minutes before daytime sleep period. Take only when the patient is home and able to go to bed (4)[C].

Second Line

- Wakefulness promoting:
  - Modafinil initially 200 mg PO 1 hour prior to work shift
  - Armodafinil 150 mg PO 1 hour prior to work shift; long-acting (12 to 16 hours, depending on food intake) use judiciously in SWD to impede a patient's ability to sleep after the shift
- Sleep promoting:
  - Nonbenzodiazepine hypnotics:
    - Zolpidem 5 to 10 mg or eszopiclone 1 to 3 mg immediately prior to bed; suvorexant 10 to 20 mg PO 30 minutes prior to bed
  - Antidepressants
    - Doxepin (3 to 6 mg) and trazodone (25 to 150 mg), 1 to 2 hours prior to bed (4)[C]
  - Benzodiazepines: Estazolam, flurazepam, quazepam, temazepam, and triazolam are FDA approved for the treatment of insomnia. Due to high risk of tolerance/withdrawal, use cautiously for short-term treatment of insomnia (4)[C].
  - In general, hypnotics may improve daytime sleep but does not appear to improve sleep maintenance or nighttime alertness. They may also cause residual sedation during work hours. This may worsen SWD symptoms (4)[C].

ISSUES FOR REFERRAL

Refer to a sleep specialist for suspicion of other primary sleep disorders or dependence on hypnotics, alcohol, or stimulants.

ADDITIONAL THERAPIES

- Bright light therapy: Multiple studies have demonstrated that bright light prior to or early in night shift can increase alertness. There is less consensus as to the appropriate duration of bright light exposure (20 minutes is generally the recommended minimum); however, there is consensus that blue wavelengths are more effective and higher intensities (>2,000 lux) are recommended (2),(3).
- On the other hand, bright light can be detrimental to daytime sleeping schedule. Patients exposed to bright light on their drive home, or otherwise prior to initiating day sleep have been shown to have longer sleep latency. There is some low-quality evidence that wearing sun glasses or blue wave blocking glasses during the early morning hours can help shield workers from these effects (3).
- Cognitive-behavioral therapy for insomnia (CBT-I): It has been shown to have positive effects on sleep latency and total sleep time in small studies but has not been evaluated in large, high-powered randomized control trials as of yet (3).
- Notably, there have been no high-powered, long-term studies to evaluate what effect these therapies have on comorbidities associated with SWD. For example, there is no strong longitudinal data to access what effect bright light therapy has on stroke risk.

 ONGOING CARE

PATIENT EDUCATION

- Discuss sleep hygiene and optimizing the sleep environment.
- Shift workers who sleep in the daytime should ensure a cool, dark, quiet sleep environment.
- Reserve bedroom for sleeping and intimacy only. Remove televisions, cell phones, tablets, and laptop computers from the bedroom.
- When going to sleep, turn clock away from bed and discourage prolonged reading in bed.
- Blackout shades help achieve the proper darkness.
- Symptoms are associated with shift work and should resolve if shift work is eliminated, this may not be feasible for patients.

REFERENCES

1. American Psychiatric Association. *Diagnostic and Statistical Manual of Mental Disorders: DSM-5*. Arlington, VA: American Psychiatric Association; 2013.
2. Wickwire EM, Geiger-Brown J, Scharf SM, et al. Shift work and shift work sleep disorder: clinical and organizational perspectives. *Chest*. 2017;151(5):1156–1172.
3. Cheng P, Drake C. Shift work disorder. *Neurol Clin*. 2019;37(3):563–577.
4. Morrissette DA. Twisting the night away: a review of the neurobiology, genetics, diagnosis, and treatment of shift work disorder. *CNS Spectr*. 2013;18(Suppl 1):45–54.
5. Vyas MV, Garg AX, Iansavichus AV, et al. Shift work and vascular events: systematic review and meta-analysis. *BMJ*. 2012;345:e4800.
6. Wright KP Jr, Bogan RK, Wyatt JK. Shift work and the assessment and management of shift work disorder (SWD). *Sleep Med Rev*. 2013;17(1):41–54.
7. American Academy of Sleep Medicine. *International Classification of Sleep Disorders*. 3rd ed. Darien, IL: American Academy of Sleep Medicine; 2014.

ADDITIONAL READING

HelpGuide. Weekly sleep diary. https://www.helpguide.org/wp-content/uploads/2018/12/sleep-diary.pdf. Accessed November 17, 2021.

 CODES

ICD10

G47.26 Circadian rhythm sleep disorder, shift work type

CLINICAL PEARLS

- SWD has been associated with increased risk for metabolic disorders and mood disorders.
- The first diagnostic step in SWD is to obtain a comprehensive sleep history and work history. Sleep diaries are helpful tools to assess sleep-wake patterns.
- Shift workers are at greater risk for accidents during night and early morning shifts.

S

SMELL AND TASTE DISORDERS
Beth K. Mazyck, MD • Daniel B. Kurtz, PhD, BS

BASICS

DESCRIPTION
- Physiologically, the senses of smell and taste aid in normal digestion by triggering GI secretions.
- Loss of smell occurs more frequently than loss of taste, and patients frequently confuse the concepts of flavor loss (as a result of smell impairment) with taste loss (an impaired ability to sense sweet, sour, salty, or bitter).
- Smell depends on the functioning of CN I (olfactory nerve) and CN V (trigeminal nerve).
- Taste depends on the functioning of CNs VII, IX, and X. Because of these multiple pathways, total loss of taste (ageusia) is rare.
- Systems affected: nervous, upper respiratory

EPIDEMIOLOGY
Incidence
There are ~200,000 patient visits a year for smell and taste disturbances.

Prevalence
- Predominant sex: male > female. Men begin to lose their ability to smell earlier in life than women.
- Predominant age:
  – Age >80 years: 80% have major olfactory impairment; nearly 50% are anosmic.
  – Ages 65 to 80 years: 60% have major olfactory impairment; nearly 25% are anosmic.
  – Age <65 years: 1–2% have smell impairment.
- Estimated >2 million affected in the United States

ETIOLOGY AND PATHOPHYSIOLOGY
- Smell and/or taste disturbances:
  – COVID-19—common in mildly symptomatic patients (~65%) but even more common in patients needing hospitalization (85%) (1),(2),(3). While most recovery occurs within a few weeks, 7% of chemosensory disorders persist beyond 60 days (3). Unexplained chemosensory loss is a good predictor of COVID-19 (4),(5)[B].
  – Nutritional factors (e.g., malnutrition, vitamin deficiencies, liver disease, pernicious anemia)
  – Endocrine disorders (e.g., thyroid disease, diabetes mellitus, renal disease)
  – Migraine headache (e.g., gustatory aura, olfactory aura)
  – Sjögren syndrome
  – Toxic exposures
  – Neurodegenerative diseases (e.g., multiple sclerosis, Alzheimer disease, cerebrovascular accident, Parkinson disease)
  – Infections

- Smell-specific disturbance:
  – Nasal and sinus disease (e.g., allergies, rhinitis, rhinorrhea, URI)
  – Cigarette smoking
  – Cocaine abuse (intranasal)
  – Hemodialysis
  – Neoplasm (e.g., brain tumor, nasal polyps, intranasal tumor)
  – Systemic lupus erythematosus (SLE)
  – Bell palsy
- Taste-specific loss:
  – Oral appliances, procedures
  – Intraoral abscess, gingivitis
  – Damage to CN VI, IX, or X
  – Stroke (especially frontal lobe)
- Selected medications:
  – Antibiotics: amikacin, ampicillin, azithromycin, ciprofloxacin, clarithromycin, doxycycline, griseofulvin, metronidazole, ofloxacin, tetracycline, terbinafine, β-lactamase inhibitors
  – Anticonvulsants: carbamazepine, phenytoin
  – Antidepressants: amitriptyline, doxepin, imipramine, nortriptyline
  – Antihistamines and decongestants: zinc-based cold remedies (Zicam)
  – Antihypertensives and cardiac medications: acetazolamide, amiloride, captopril, diltiazem, hydrochlorothiazide, nifedipine, propranolol, spironolactone
  – Anti-inflammatory agents: auranofin, gold, penicillamine
  – Antimanic drugs: lithium
  – Antineoplastics: cisplatin, doxorubicin, methotrexate, vincristine
  – Antiparkinsonian agents: levodopa, carbidopa
  – Antiseptic: chlorhexidine
  – Antithyroid agents: methimazole, propylthiouracil
  – Lipid-lowering agents: statins

Genetics
Unknown

RISK FACTORS
- Poor nutritional status
- Smoking

GENERAL PREVENTION
- Well-balanced diet
- Maintain good oral and nasal health.
- Avoid tobacco products, chemical exposures.

Geriatric Considerations
Anosmia also may be an early sign of degenerative disorders and has been shown to predict increased 5-year mortality (6)[B].

Pediatric Considerations
- In developing countries with poor nutrition (particularly zinc depletion), smell and taste disorders may occur.
- Delayed puberty in association with anosmia (± midline craniofacial abnormalities, deafness, or renal abnormalities) suggests the possibility of Kallmann syndrome (hypogonadotropic hypogonadism).

Pregnancy Considerations
Many women report increased sensitivity to odors during pregnancy as well as an increased dislike for bitterness and a preference for salty substances.

COMMONLY ASSOCIATED CONDITIONS
URI, allergic rhinitis, dental abscesses

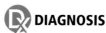**DIAGNOSIS**

Smell and taste disturbances are symptoms; it is essential to look for possible underlying causes.

HISTORY
- Symptoms of URI, environmental allergies
- Fever, cough, sore throat suggestive of COVID-19 infection
- Oral pain, other dental problems
- Cognitive/memory difficulties
- Current medications
- Nutritional status, ovolactovegetarian
- Weight loss or gain
- Frequent infections (impaired immunity)
- Worsening of underlying medical illness
- Increased use of salt and/or sugar to increase taste of food
- Neurodegenerative disease

PHYSICAL EXAM
Thorough HEENT exam

DIFFERENTIAL DIAGNOSIS
- Epilepsy (gustatory or olfactory aura)
- Memory impairment
- Psychiatric conditions

DIAGNOSTIC TESTS & INTERPRETATION
Initial Tests (lab, imaging)
Consider (Not all patients require all tests.)
- SARS-CoV-2
- CBC, chemistry panel
- Liver function tests
- Vitamin B_{12} level
- Thyroid-stimulating hormone (TSH)
- Serum IgE
- CT scanning is the most useful and cost-effective technique for assessing sinonasal disorders and is superior to an MRI in evaluating bony structures and airway patency. Coronal CT scans are particularly valuable in assessing paranasal anatomy (7)[B].

Follow-Up Tests & Special Considerations

Diagnosis of smell and taste disturbances is usually possible through history; however, the following tests can be used to confirm:

- Olfactory tests
  - Smell identification test: evaluates the ability to identify 40 microencapsulated scratch-and-sniff odorants (8)[B]
  - Brief smell identification test (9)[B]
  - Taste tests (more difficult because no convenient standardized tests are presently available): Solutions containing sucrose (sweet), sodium chloride (salty), quinine (bitter), and citric acid (sour) are helpful.
  - An MRI is useful in defining soft tissue disease; therefore, a coronal MRI is the technique of choice to image the olfactory bulbs, tracts, and cortical parenchyma; possible placement of an accessory coil (TMJ) over the nose to assist in imaging

 TREATMENT

GENERAL MEASURES
- Appropriate treatment for underlying cause
- Quit smoking.
- Treatment of underlying nasal congestion with nasal decongestants and/or nasal/oral steroids (10)[B]
- Surgical correction of nasal blockage/nasal polyps
- Drug-related smell or taste loss can be reversed with cessation of the offending medication, but it may take many months.
- Proper nutritional and dietary assessment (7)[C]
- Formal dental evaluation

MEDICATION
- Treat underlying causes as appropriate. Idiopathic cases will often resolve spontaneously.
- Consider trial of corticosteroids topically (e.g., fluticasone nasal spray daily to qBID) and/or systemically (e.g., oral prednisone 60 mg daily for 5 to 7 days) (10)[B].
- Zinc and vitamins (A, B complex) when deficiency is suspected

ISSUES FOR REFERRAL
Consider referral to an otolaryngologist or neurologist for persistent cases.

 ONGOING CARE

DIET
- Weight gain/loss is possible because the patient may reject food or may switch to calorie-rich foods that are still palatable.
- Ensure a nutritionally balanced diet with appropriate levels of nutrients, vitamins, and essential minerals.

PATIENT EDUCATION
- Caution patients not to overindulge as compensation for the bland taste of food. For example, patients with diabetes may need help in avoiding excessive sugar intake as an inappropriate way of improving food taste.
- Patients with chemosensory impairments should use measuring devices when cooking and should not cook by taste.
- Optimizing food texture, aroma, temperature, and color may improve the overall food experience when taste is limited.
- Patients with permanent smell dysfunction must develop adaptive strategies for dealing with hygiene, appetite, safety, and health.
- Natural gas and smoke detectors are essential; check for proper function frequently.
- Check food expiration dates frequently; discard old food.

PROGNOSIS
- If smell loss is associated with a COVID-19 infection, the loss lasts on average 3 weeks, and 90% has resolved within 4 weeks. A small number will experience long-term loss. Additionally, a small number will experience phantosmia or parosmia (phantom smells, or previously pleasant smells become foul).
- In general, the olfactory system regenerates poorly after a head injury. Most patients who recover smell function following head trauma do so within 12 weeks of injury.
- Patients who quit smoking typically recover improved olfactory function and flavor sensation.
- Many taste disorders (dysgeusias) resolve spontaneously within a few years of onset.
- Phantosmias that are flow dependent may respond to surgical ablation of olfactory mucosa.
- Conditions such as radiation-induced xerostomia and Bell palsy generally improve over time.

COMPLICATIONS
- Permanent loss of ability to smell/taste
- Psychiatric issues with dysgeusias and phantosmia

REFERENCES
1. Spinato G, Fabbris C, Polesel J, et al. Alterations in smell or taste in mildly symptomatic outpatients with SARS-CoV-2 infection. *JAMA*. 2020;323(20):2089–2090.
2. Menni C, Valdes AM, Freidin MB, et al. Real-time tracking of self-reported symptoms to predict potential COVID-19. *Nat Med*. 2020;26(7):1037–1040.
3. Vaira LA, Hopkins C, Petrocelli M, et al. Smell and taste recovery in coronavirus disease 2019 patients: a 60-day objective and prospective study. *J Laryngol Otol*. 2020;134(8):703–709.
4. Parma V, Ohla K, Veldhuizen MG, et al. More than smell-COVID-19 is associated with severe impairment of smell, taste, and chemesthesis. *Chem Senses*. 2020;45(7):609–622.
5. Gerkin RC, Ohla K, Veldhuizen MG, et al. The best COVID-19 predictor is recent smell loss: a cross-sectional study. *medRxiv*. 2020. doi:10.1101/2020.07.22.20157263.
6. Pinto JM, Wroblewski KE, Kern DW, et al. Olfactory dysfunction predicts 5-year mortality in older adults. *PLoS One*. 2014;9(10):e107541.
7. Malaty J, Malaty IAC. Smell and taste disorders in primary care. *Am Fam Physician*. 2013;88(12):852–859.
8. Doty RL, Shaman P, Dann M. Development of the University of Pennsylvania Smell Identification Test: a standardized microencapsulated test of olfactory function. *Physiol Behav*. 1984;32(3):489–502.
9. Jackman AH, Doty RL. Utility of a three-item smell identification test in detecting olfactory dysfunction. *Laryngoscope*. 2005;115(12):2209–2212.
10. Seiden AM, Duncan HJ. The diagnosis of a conductive olfactory loss. *Laryngoscope*. 2001;111(1):9–14.

 CODES

ICD10
- R43.9 Unspecified disturbances of smell and taste
- R43.1 Parosmia
- R43.2 Parageusia

CLINICAL PEARLS
- Smell loss is often the first and only symptom of mild cases of COVID-19.
- Smell disorders are often mistaken as decreased taste by patients.
- Most temporary smell loss is due to nasal passage obstruction.
- Actual taste disorders are often related to dental problems or medication side effects.
- Gradual smell loss is very common in the elderly; extensive workup in this population may not be indicated if no associated signs/symptoms are present but may be predictive of 5- to 13-year mortality.
- Sudden unexplained smell loss may be a predictor of COVID-19.

S

SOMATIC SYMPTOM (SOMATIZATION) DISORDER

William G. Elder, PhD

 BASICS

DESCRIPTION

- Somatic symptom disorders (SSD) are a pattern of one or more somatic symptoms recurring or persisting for >6 months that are distressing or result in significant disruption of daily life.
- Designation of a symptom as somatic means that it appears to be physical problem or complaint yet is medically unexplained.
- Conceptualization and diagnostic criteria for somatic symptom presentations were significantly modified with the advent of *DSM-5*. SSD is similar in many aspects to the former somatization disorder, which required presentation with multiple physical complaints. No longer based on symptoms counts; current diagnosis is based on the way the patient presents and perceives his or her symptoms.
- SSD now includes most presentations that would formerly be considered hypochondriasis. Hypochondriasis has been replaced by illness anxiety disorder, which is diagnosed when the patient presents with significant preoccupation with having a serious illness in the absence of illness-related somatic complaints.
- Somatization increases disability independent of comorbidity, and individuals with SSD have health-related functioning that is 2 standard deviations below the mean.
- Symptoms may be specific (e.g., localized pain) or relatively nonspecific (e.g., fatigue).
- Symptoms sometimes may represent normal bodily sensations or discomfort that does not signify serious disease.
- Suffering is authentic. Symptoms are not intentionally produced or feigned.
- SSDs are sometimes referred to as "functional disorders" to denote their nonphysical basis and with the assumption that the illness behavior is a function of the environment.

EPIDEMIOLOGY

Incidence
- Usually, first symptoms appear in adolescence.
- Predominant sex: female > male (10:1)
- Type and frequency of somatic complaints may differ among cultures, so symptom reviews should be adjusted based on culture; more frequent in cultures without Western/empirical explanatory models

Prevalence
- Expected 2% among women and <0.2% among men
- Somatization seen in up to 29% of patients presenting to primary care offices
- Somatic concerns may increase, but other features of the presentation decrease such that prevalence declines after age 65 years.

ETIOLOGY AND PATHOPHYSIOLOGY
Patients with SSD demonstrate different patterns of heart rate variability. Although this cannot be used to clinically differentiate, it does point to the differences in psychophysiology of SSD. Also, not to be used clinically, patients with SSD display differences in brain functional connectivity, with the possibility that deficits in attention distort perception of external stimuli, affecting regulation of externally responsive body functioning (1)[C].

Genetics
Consanguinity studies and single nucleotide polymorphism genotyping indicate that both genetic and environmental factors contribute to the risk of SSD.

RISK FACTORS
- Child abuse, particularly sexual abuse, has been shown to be a risk factor for somatization.
- Symptoms begin or worsen after losses (e.g., job, close relative, or friend).
- Greater intensity of symptoms often occurs with stress.

COMMONLY ASSOCIATED CONDITIONS
Comorbid with other psychiatric conditions is yet to be determined but is likely to be 20–50% with anxiety, depression, or personality disorders.

DIAGNOSIS

- Determining that a somatic symptom is medically unexplained is unreliable, and it is inappropriate to diagnose a mental disorder solely because a medical diagnosis is not demonstrated. Rely on symptoms and presentation rather than ruling out medical causes in making the SSD diagnosis.
- Among studies reviewing accuracy of SSD under *DSM-IV* and *DSM-5* criteria, 0.5–8% of diagnoses had to be revised based on subsequent findings of underlying organic pathology (2)[B].
- Illness anxiety and somatic distress are independent but often co-occur.

HISTORY
- One or more somatic complaints, with sometimes a grossly positive review of symptoms
- SSD involves patient unrealistic thoughts, feelings, or behaviors associated with symptoms or associated health concerns manifested by at least one of the following:
  - Disproportionate and persistent thoughts about the seriousness of the symptoms
  - Persistent high level of anxiety about health or symptoms
  - Excessive time or energy devoted to symptoms or health concerns

- Diagnoses no longer rely on symptom counts, but common symptoms include:
  - Pain symptoms related to different sites such as head, abdomen, back, joints, extremities, chest, or rectum or related to body functions such as menstruation, sexual intercourse, or urination
  - GI symptoms such as nausea, bloating, vomiting (not during pregnancy), diarrhea, intolerance of several foods
  - Sexual symptoms such as indifference to sex, difficulties with erection or ejaculation, irregular menses, excessive menstrual bleeding, or vomiting throughout all 9 months of pregnancy
  - Pseudoneurologic symptoms such as impaired balance or coordination, weak or paralyzed muscles, lump in throat or trouble swallowing, loss of voice, retention of urine, hallucinations, numbness (to touch or pain), double vision, blindness, deafness, seizures, amnesia or other dissociative symptoms, loss of consciousness (other than with fainting); none of these is limited to pain.
- Patients with SSD frequently use alternative treatments, which should be explored for their effects on health and physical functioning.

PHYSICAL EXAM
Physical exam remarkable for absence of objective findings to explain the many subjective complaints

DIFFERENTIAL DIAGNOSIS
- Other psychiatric illnesses must be ruled out:
  - Depressive disorders
  - Anxiety disorders
  - Schizophrenia
  - Other somatic disorders: illness anxiety disorder, conversion disorder
  - Factitious disorder
  - Body dysmorphic disorder
- Malingering
- General medical conditions, with vague, multiple, confusing symptoms, must be ruled out.
  - Systemic lupus erythematosus
  - Hyperparathyroidism
  - Hyper- or hypothyroidism
  - Lyme disease
  - Porphyria

DIAGNOSTIC TESTS & INTERPRETATION
Several screening tools are available that help to identify symptoms as somatic:
- Patient Health Questionnaire (PHQ)-15 (screens and monitors symptoms)
- Minnesota Multiphasic Personality Inventory (MMPI) (identifies somatization)

Initial Tests (lab, imaging)
- Laboratory test results do not support the subjective complaints.
- Imaging studies do not support the subjective complaints.

Test Interpretation
None are identified.

TREATMENT

GENERAL MEASURES

- The goal of treatment is to help the person learn to control the symptoms.
- It is not helpful to tell patients that their symptoms are imaginary. Enhanced or structured care as follows can be as effective as psychological interventions in adults (3)[A].
- The involvement of a single provider is important because a history of seeking medical attention and "doctor shopping" is common.
- Patients usually receive the most benefit from primary care providers who accept the limitations of treatment, listen to their patient's concerns, and provide reassurance.
- A supportive relationship with a sympathetic health care provider is the most important aspect of treatment:
  – Regular scheduled appointments should be maintained to review symptoms and the person's coping mechanisms (at least 15 minutes once a month).
  – Acknowledge and explain test results.
- Antidepressant or antianxiety medication and referral to a support group or mental health provider can help patients who are willing to participate in their treatment.

MEDICATION

- Fluoxetine has been shown to have efficacy with illness anxiety disorder (formerly hypochondriasis), although >50% of those patients did not respond to the medication (4)[B].
- Antidepressants (e.g., SSRIs) help to treat comorbid depression and anxiety (5)[C].

ISSUES FOR REFERRAL

- Discourage referrals to specialists for further investigation of somatic complaints.
- Referrals to support groups or to a mental health provider may be helpful.

ADDITIONAL THERAPIES

- Treatments have not been evaluated for this recently reformulated disorder. However, there are numerous studies with positive outcomes for child and adult patients with various forms of somatization or medically unexplained symptoms.
- Treatment typically includes long-term therapy, which has been shown to decrease the severity of symptoms.
- Individual or group cognitive-behavioral therapy addressing health anxiety, health beliefs, and health behaviors has been shown to be the most efficacious treatment for somatoform disorders. Cognitive processes modified in therapy include patient tendencies to ruminate and catastrophize (6)[A].

- For children, psychological interventions reduce symptom numbers and severity, disability, and school absence (7)[A].
- Consideration should be given to providing integrated multidisciplinary care. For example, for patients with a functional gastrointestinal disorder, inclusion of dietitians, gut-focused hypnotherapists, psychiatrists, and behavioral (biofeedback) physiotherapists, has been shown to improved symptoms, specific functional disorders, psychological state, quality of life, and cost of care for the treatment of functional gastrointestinal disorders (8).

 ONGOING CARE

FOLLOW-UP RECOMMENDATIONS

Patients should have regularly scheduled follow-up with a primary care doctor, psychiatrist, and/or therapist.

PATIENT EDUCATION

Encourage interventions that decrease stressful elements of the patient's life:
- Psychoeducational advice
- Increase in exercise
- Pleasurable private time

PROGNOSIS

- Chronic course, fluctuating in severity
- Full remission is rare.
- Individuals with this disorder do not experience any significant difference in mortality rate or significant physical illness.
- Patients with this diagnosis do experience substantially greater functional disability and role impairment than nonsomatizing patients.

COMPLICATIONS

- May result from invasive testing and from multiple evaluations that are performed while looking for the cause of the symptoms
- A dependency on pain relievers or sedatives may develop.

REFERENCES

1. Kim S, Hong J, Min K, et al. Brain functional connectivity in patients with somatic symptom disorder. *Psychosom Med*. 2019;81(3):313–318.
2. Henningsen P. Management of somatic symptom disorder. *Dialogues Clin Neurosci*. 2018;20(1):23–31.
3. van Dessel N, den Boeft M, van der Wouden JC, et al. Non-pharmacological interventions for somatoform disorders and medically unexplained physical symptoms (MUPS) in adults. *Cochrane Database Syst Rev*. 2014;(11):CD011142.
4. Fallon BA, Ahern DK, Pavlicova M, et al. A randomized controlled trial of medication and cognitive-behavioral therapy for hypochondriasis. *Am J Psychiatry*. 2017;174(8):756–764.
5. Somashekar B, Jainer A, Wuntakal B. Psychopharmacotherapy of somatic symptoms disorders. *Int Rev Psychiatry*. 2013;25(1):107–115.
6. Moreno S, Gili M, Magallón R, et al. Effectiveness of group versus individual cognitive-behavioral therapy in patients with abridged somatization disorder: a randomized controlled trial. *Psychosom Med*. 2013;75(6):600–608.
7. Bonvanie I, Kallesøe K, Janssens K, et al. Psychological interventions for children with functional somatic symptoms: a systematic review and meta-analysis. *J Pediatr*. 2017;187:272–281.e17.
8. Basnayake C, Kamm MA, Stanley A, et al. Standard gastroenterologist versus multidisciplinary treatment for functional gastrointestinal disorders (MANTRA): an open-label, single-centre, randomised controlled trial. *Lancet Gastroenterol Hepatol*. 2020;5(10):890–899.

ADDITIONAL READING

- Elder WG, King M, Dassow P, et al. Managing lower back pain: you may be doing too much. *J Fam Pract*. 2009;58(4):180–186.
- Sharma MP, Manjula M. Behavioural and psychological management of somatic symptom disorders: an overview. *Int Rev Psychiatry*. 2013;25(1):116–124.

CODES

ICD10
- F45.9 Somatoform disorder, unspecified
- F45.20 Hypochondriacal disorder, unspecified
- F45.22 Body dysmorphic disorder

CLINICAL PEARLS

- Diagnosis is based on a pattern of symptoms rather than an absence of medical explanation.
- A clue is accumulation of several diagnoses with >13 letters (e.g., chronic fatigue syndrome, fibromyalgia syndrome, reflex sympathetic dystrophy, temporomandibular joint syndrome, carpal tunnel syndrome, mitral valve prolapse).
- Inability of more than three physicians to make a meaningful diagnosis suggests somatization.
- Acknowledge the patient's pain, suffering, and disability.
- Do not tell patients the symptoms are "all in their head."
- Emphasize that this is not a rare disorder.
- Discuss the limitations of treatment while providing reassurance that there are interventions that will lessen suffering and reduce symptoms.

S

SPINAL STENOSIS

Birju B. Patel, MD, FACP • N. Wilson Holland, MD, FACP

 BASICS

DESCRIPTION

Narrowing of the spinal canal and foramen:

- Spondylosis or degenerative arthritis is the most common cause of spinal stenosis, resulting from compression of the spinal cord by disc degeneration, facet arthropathy, osteophyte formation, and ligamentum flavum hypertrophy.
- The L4–L5 level is most commonly involved.

EPIDEMIOLOGY

The prevalence of spinal stenosis increases with age.

Incidence

Symptomatic spinal stenosis affects up to 8% of the general population.

Prevalence

- The prevalence of spinal stenosis is high if assessed solely by imaging in elderly patients. Not all patients with radiographic spinal stenosis are symptomatic. The degree of radiographic stenosis does not always correlate with patient symptoms. Lumbar MRI shows significant abnormalities in 57% of patients >60 years.
- Predominant age: Symptoms develop in 5th to 6th decades (congenital stenosis is symptomatic earlier).

ETIOLOGY AND PATHOPHYSIOLOGY

- Spinal stenosis can result from congenital or acquired causes. Degenerative spondylosis is most common.
- Disc dehydration leads to loss of height with bulging of the disc annulus and ligamentum flavum into the spinal canal, increasing facet joint loading.
- Facet loading leads to reactive sclerosis and osteophytic bone growth, further compressing spinal canal, and foraminal elements.
- Other causes of acquired spinal stenosis include:
  - Trauma
  - Neoplasms
  - Neural cysts and lipomas
  - Postoperative changes
  - Rheumatoid arthritis
  - Diffuse idiopathic skeletal hyperostosis
  - Ankylosing spondylitis
  - Metabolic/endocrine causes: osteoporosis, renal osteodystrophy, and Paget disease

Genetics

No definitive genetic links

RISK FACTORS

Increasing age and degenerative spinal disease

GENERAL PREVENTION

There is no proven prevention for spinal stenosis.

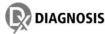 **DIAGNOSIS**

HISTORY

- Helps distinguish spinal stenosis from other causes of back pain and peripheral vascular disease
  - Insidious onset and slow progression are typical; discomfort with standing, paresthesias, and weakness (often bilateral) (1)
  - Symptoms *worsen with extension* (prolonged standing, walking downhill or downstairs).
  - Symptoms *improve with flexion* (sitting, leaning forward while walking, walking uphill or upstairs, lying in a flexed position). Symptoms can be alleviated with flexion at the waist: leaning forward while walking, pushing a shopping cart, lying in flexed position, sitting, avoiding provocative maneuvers (back extension, ambulating long distances without resting).
- Neurogenic claudication (i.e., pain, tightness, numbness, and subjective weakness of lower extremities) may mimic vascular claudication.
- The Zurich Claudication Questionnaire (ZCQ) is a self-administered measure to evaluate symptom severity, physical function, and surgery satisfaction.

PHYSICAL EXAM

Neurologic exam may be normal. Key exam areas:

- Examine gait (rule out cervical myelopathy or intracranial pathology).
  - Measurement of free walking can be used as a functional assessment (2).
- Loss of lumbar lordosis
- Evaluate range of motion of lumbar spine.
- Pain with extension of the lumbar spine is typical.
- Straight leg raise test may be positive if nerve root entrapment is present.
- Muscle weakness when apparent usually involves L4–L5 nerve roots (demonstrated by weakness in great toe extension and hip abduction) and less commonly S1 nerve roots (demonstrated by hip extension weakness).
- About half of patients with symptomatic stenosis have a reduced or absent Achilles reflex. Some have reduced or absent patellar reflex.

DIFFERENTIAL DIAGNOSIS

- Vascular claudication. Symptoms of vascular claudication do not improve with leaning forward and usually abate with standing or rest.
- Disc herniation
- Cervical myelopathy

DIAGNOSTIC TESTS & INTERPRETATION

Generally, a clinical diagnosis. Imaging (MRI is best) is used to stage severity and plan treatment.

Initial Tests (lab, imaging)

- CBC, ESR, C-reactive protein (if considering infection or malignancy)
- New back pain lasting >2 weeks or back pain accompanied by neurologic findings in patients >50 years generally warrants further evaluation, including evaluation for potential metastatic disease.
- MRI is the modality of choice.
- CT myelography is an alternative to MRI but is invasive and has higher risk of complications.
- Plain radiography helps exclude other causes of new back pain (e.g., malignant lytic lesions, vertebral compression fractures) but does not reveal the underlying pathology.
- Radiologic abnormalities in general do not correlate with the clinical severity.

Test Interpretation

Common radiographic findings include decreased disc height, facet hypertrophy, and spinal canal and/or foraminal narrowing.

 TREATMENT

- In general, nonoperative interventions are preferred in the absence of progressive or debilitating neurologic symptoms:
  - Physical therapy, exercise, weight management, medications, followed by epidural steroid injections are options.
  - Patients should understand that the benefits of surgery may diminish over time.
  - Rule out other neuropathies and peripheral vascular disease.
- When medications and physical therapy have failed, other treatments can be considered such as: intra-articular facet injections and medial branch radiofrequency thermal ablation of lumbar facet joint nerve.

MEDICATION

First Line

NSAIDs: Consider potential for GI side effects, fluid retention, and renal failure.

Second Line

- The available evidence does not support the routine use of epidural steroid injections. A randomized study comparing injections of glucocorticoids plus lidocaine versus lidocaine alone showed no significance in symptoms at 6 weeks in these two groups (3)[B].
- Use opioids sparingly and only when other treatments have failed to control severe pain.

Geriatric Considerations

- Anti-inflammatory medications should be used with caution in the elderly due to the risks of GI bleeding, fluid retention, renal failure, and cardiovascular risks.
- Side effects of opioids include constipation, confusion, urinary retention, drowsiness, nausea, vomiting, and the potential for dependence and abuse.
- >10% of elderly lack Achilles reflexes.

ISSUES FOR REFERRAL

Patients in unremitting pain or with a neurologic deficit should see a neurosurgeon.

ADDITIONAL THERAPIES

- Patients with spinal stenosis are typically able to ride a bicycle (leaning forward tends to relieve symptoms).
- Aquatic therapy (helpful for muscle training and general conditioning)
- Strengthening of abdominal and back muscles
- Gait training
- Although a brace may help in the short term, use is not recommended for prolonged periods due to development of paraspinal muscle weakness.
- Encourage physical activity to prevent deconditioning.

SURGERY/OTHER PROCEDURES

- Surgery is indicated when symptoms persist despite conservative measures.
  - Surgical decompression is definitive for patients who are symptomatic after nonoperative treatment:
    - ○ Spinal stenosis generally does not lead to neurologic damage.
    - ○ Surgery may be required for pain relief to increase mobility and improve quality of life.
- Age alone should not be an exclusion factor for surgical intervention. Cognitive impairment, multiple comorbidities, and osteoporosis may increase the risk of perioperative complications in the elderly.
- Interspinous process spacers (IPS) maybe used for moderate disease. Advantages of this procedure include being less invasive and preserving more spinal mobility as compared to laminectomy (4)[B].
  - Spacers should not be used for patients with unstable spondylolisthesis.

- Minimally invasive lumbar decompression (MILD) is an option for decompression for central stenosis.
- Invasive decompression surgery can be considered in a stepwise manner from limited open decompression to extensive decompression and fusion (5).

ADMISSION, INPATIENT, AND NURSING CONSIDERATIONS

- Admission criteria/initial stabilization: acute or progressive neurologic deficit
- Discharge criteria: improved pain or after neurologic deficit has been addressed

 ONGOING CARE

FOLLOW-UP RECOMMENDATIONS

- Follow up based on progression of symptoms.
- No limitations to activity; patients may be as active as tolerated. Exercise should be encouraged.

Patient Monitoring

Patients are monitored for improvement of symptoms and development of any complications.

DIET

Optimize nutrition for weight management.

PATIENT EDUCATION

- Activity as tolerated, if no other pathology is present (e.g., fractures)
- Patients should present for care if they develop progressive motor weakness and/or bladder/bowel dysfunction.
- Patients should know the natural history of the condition and how best to relieve symptoms.

PROGNOSIS

- Spinal stenosis can usually be managed conservatively, but the pain can lead to limitation in ADLs and progressive disability.
- Surgery usually improves pain and symptoms in patients who fail nonoperative treatment.
- Surgical outcomes are similar in terms of pain relief and functional improvement for patients of all ages.

COMPLICATIONS

- Severe spinal stenosis can lead to bowel and/or bladder dysfunction.
- Surgical complications include infection, neurologic injury, chronic pain, and disability.

REFERENCES

1. Suri P, Rainville J, Kalichman L, et al. Does this older adult with lower extremity pain have the clinical syndrome of lumbar spinal stenosis? *JAMA.* 2010;304(23):2628–2636.
2. Grelat M, Gouteron A, Cassilas JM, et al. Walking speed as an alternative measure of functional status in patients with lumbar spinal stenosis. *World Neurosurg.* 2019;122:e591–e597.
3. Friedly JL, Comstock BA, Turner JA, et al. A randomized trial of epidural glucocorticoid injections for spinal stenosis. *N Engl J Med.* 2014;371(1):11–21.
4. Gala RJ, Russo GS, Whang PG, et al. Interspinous implants to treat spinal stenosis. *Curr Rev Musculoskelet Med.* 2017;10(2):182–188.
5. Diwan S, Sayed D, Deer TR, et al. An algorithmic approach to treating lumbar spinal stenosis: an evidence-based approach. *Pain Med.* 2019;20(Suppl 2):S23–S31.

 SEE ALSO

Algorithm: Low Back Pain, Acute

CODES

ICD10

- M48.00 Spinal stenosis, site unspecified
- M48.06 Spinal stenosis, lumbar region
- M48.04 Spinal stenosis, thoracic region

CLINICAL PEARLS

- Spinal stenosis typically presents as neurogenic claudication (pain, tightness, numbness, and subjective weakness of lower extremities), which can mimic vascular claudication.
- Flexion of the spine generally relieves symptoms associated with spinal stenosis.
- Spinal extension (prolonged standing, walking downhill, and walking downstairs) can worsen symptoms of spinal stenosis.
- Consider urgent surgery for patients with cauda equina/conus medullaris syndrome or progressive bladder dysfunction. Other patients with lumbar spinal stenosis typically do well with initial conservative management.
- For patients with lumbar spinal stenosis who do not have fixed or progressive neurologic deficits should be managed with conservative treatment. Physical therapy and/or oral pain medication are often used, although their efficacy has not well evaluated.

SPRAIN, ANKLE
Shane L. Larson, MD • Brandon J. Moore, PA-C, MPAS

BASICS

DESCRIPTION
The most common cause of ankle injury comprising a significant proportion of sports injuries:
- Types of ankle sprains: lateral, medial, and syndesmotic (or high ankle sprain)
  - Lateral ankle sprains are the most common, accounting for up to 89% of all ankle sprains (1):
    - In lateral ankle sprains, the anterior talofibular ligament (ATFL) is most likely to be injured.
    - The calcaneofibular ligament (CFL) is the second most likely ligament to be injured.
    - The posterior talofibular ligament (PTFL) is the least likely to be injured.
  - Medial ankle sprains (5–10%) result from an injury to the deltoid ligament.
  - Syndesmotic ("high ankle sprain") injuries account for 5–10% of ankle sprains.
    - The syndesmosis between the distal tibia and distal fibula bones consists of the anterior, posterior, and transverse tibiofibular ligaments; the interosseous ligament; and interosseous membrane.
- Ankle sprains are classified according to the degree of ligamentous disruption:
  - Grade I: mild stretching of a ligament with possible microscopic tears
  - Grade II: incomplete tear of a ligament
  - Grade III: complete ligament tear

Geriatric Considerations
Increased risk of fracture in patients with preexisting bone weakness (osteoporosis/osteopenia)

Pediatric Considerations
- Increased risk of physeal injuries instead of ligament sprain because ligaments have greater tensile strength than physes
- Inversion ankle injuries in children may have a concomitant fibular physeal injury (Salter-Harris type I or higher fracture).
- Consider tarsal coalition with recurrent ankle sprains.

EPIDEMIOLOGY
Incidence
- Ankle sprains are more common in childhood and adolescents, particularly in active individuals (2).
- 1/2 of all ankle sprains are sports related; highest incidence in indoor/court sports (basketball, volleyball, tennis), followed by football and soccer (3)
- Most common sports injury
- More common in males age <30 years and females >30 years old

Prevalence
- 25% of sports injuries in the United States
- 75% of all ankle injuries are sprains.

ETIOLOGY AND PATHOPHYSIOLOGY
- Lateral ankle sprains result from an inversion force with the ankle in plantar flexion.
- Medial ankle sprains are due to forced eversion while the foot is in dorsiflexion.
- Syndesmotic sprains result from eversion stress/extreme dorsiflexion along with internal rotation of tibia.

RISK FACTORS
- The greatest risk factor is a prior history of an ankle sprain (3–34% recurrence rate).
- Postural instability, gait alterations
- Joint laxity and decreased proprioception are not risk factors.

GENERAL PREVENTION
- Improve overall physical conditioning:
  - Training in agility and flexibility
  - Single-leg balancing
  - Proprioceptive training
- Taping and bracing may help prevent primary injury in selected sports (i.e., volleyball, basketball, football) or reinjury (4). Taping and bracing do not reduce sprain severity.
- Weight loss may help in overweight patients (4)[A].

COMMONLY ASSOCIATED CONDITIONS
- Contusions
- Fractures
  - Fibular head fracture/dislocation (Maisonneuve)
  - Fracture of the base of the 5th metatarsal
  - Distal fibula physeal fracture (includes Salter-Harris fractures in pediatric patients; most common type of pediatric ankle fracture)

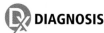

DIAGNOSIS

HISTORY
- Elicit specific mechanism of injury (inversion vs. eversion)
- Popping/snapping sensation during the injury
- Previous history of ankle injuries
- Ability to ambulate immediately after the injury
- Rapid onset of pain, swelling, or ecchymosis
- Location of pain (lateral/medial)
- Difficulty bearing weight
- Past medical history of systemic disorders

PHYSICAL EXAM
- Timing: Initial assessment for laxity may be difficult due to pain, swelling, and muscle spasm. Repeating exam ~5 days after injury often improves sensitivity.
- Compare to uninjured ankle for swelling, ecchymosis, weakness, and laxity.
- Neurovascular exam
- Palpate ATFL, CFL, PTFL, and deltoid ligament for tenderness.
- Palpate lateral and medial malleolus, base of 5th metatarsal, navicular, and entire fibula.
  - High ankle sprain associated with fracture of proximal fibula
- Grade I sprain: mild swelling and pain; no laxity; able to bear weight/ambulate without pain
- Grade II sprain: moderate swelling and pain; mild laxity with firm end point noted; weight-bearing/ambulation painful
- Grade III sprain: severe swelling, pain, and bruising; laxity with no end point; significant instability and loss of function/motion; unable to bear weight/ambulate
  - Swelling less sensitive for grade of tear in pediatric patient

- Special tests:
  - Anterior drawer test to check for ATFL laxity
  - Talar tilt test to check laxity in CFL (with inversion) or deltoid ligament (eversion)
  - Squeeze test: Compress tibia and fibula midcalf to check for syndesmotic injury; sensitivity 30%, specificity 93.5%
  - Dorsiflexion/external rotation test: Positive test is pain at syndesmosis with rotation; sensitivity 20%, specificity 85%

DIFFERENTIAL DIAGNOSIS
- Tendon injury
  - Tendinopathy/tendon tear
- Fracture and/or dislocation of the ankle/foot
- Hindfoot/midfoot injuries
- Nerve injury
- Contusion

DIAGNOSTIC TESTS & INTERPRETATION
Initial Tests (lab, imaging)
- Ottawa Ankle Rules (nearly 100% sensitive, 30–50% specific) determine need for radiographs to rule out ankle fractures (patient must be 18 to 55 years; certain patients, e.g., diabetics with diminished sensation, may still need radiographs):
  - Pain in malleolar zone
  - Inability to bear weight (walk ≥4 steps) immediately and in the exam room
  - Bony tenderness at tip/posterior edge of the lateral and/or medial malleolus
  - Reported pain in the midfoot zone AND pain with palpation of navicular
  - Pain on palpation at the base of 5th metatarsal
  - Although Ottawa rules are highly sensitive, they should not overrule clinical judgment.
- If radiographs are indicated, obtain anteroposterior, lateral, and mortise views of the ankle.
  - Small avulsion fractures are associated with grade III sprains.
- Consider CT if radiographs are negative but occult fracture is suspected clinically.
- MRI is the gold standard for soft tissue imaging but is expensive and rarely necessary.
  - Syndesmotic ankle sprains: MRI is more sensitive.
- US is a good second-line imaging option with sensitivity comparable to MRI with experienced sonographers and providers.

Follow-Up Tests & Special Considerations
If patient's condition does not improve in 6 to 8 weeks, consider CT, MRI, or US. Failure to resolve could indicate an injury such as a fracture or osteochondral lesion of the talus.

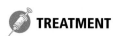

TREATMENT

GENERAL MEASURES
- Most grade I, II, and III lateral ankle sprains can be managed conservatively.
- Conservative therapy: PRICE (protection, relative rest, ice, compression, elevation) (4)[A]

- Protection/compression: For grade I/II sprains, lace-up bracing is superior to air-filled/gel-filled ankle brace, which is superior to elastic bandage/taping to provide support and decrease swelling.
  - Note: The combination of air-filled brace and compression wrap is superior to each individual modality for return to preinjury joint function at 10 days and 1 month following grade I and II sprains.
  - Grade III sprains should have short-term immobilization (10 days) with below-the-knee cast, followed by a semirigid brace (air cast). If a patient refuses casting, a 10-day period of strict non–weight-bearing with air cast splint and elastic bandage is a comparable alternative if non–weight-bearing is maintained.
- Rest: initially, activity as tolerated. Early mobilization and physical therapy speed recovery/reduce pain:
  - Weight-bearing, as tolerated
  - Consider crutches if unable to bear weight.
  - Initiate exercises as early as tolerated. Limit to pain-free range of motion.
  - Start mobilization by tracing the alphabet with the foot or toes.
  - Resistance exercises with an elastic band
- Ice: Ice for first 3 to 7 days reduces pain and decreases recovery time.
- Elevation: Elevate ankle to decrease swelling.

MEDICATION
- NSAIDs: preferably oral; topical forms (e.g., diclofenac 1% gel) may be used to minimize GI side effects. PRN NSAID dosing has similar outcomes to scheduled dosing with improved safety profile.
  - Example: naproxen 500 mg BID PRN
- Acetaminophen 650 mg q4–6h (max outpatient therapy dose: 3,250 mg/day) (may be combined with NSAIDs without risk of adverse drug interaction)
- Opioids (<5 days) if severe pain (rarely needed)

ISSUES FOR REFERRAL
- Malleolar/talar dome fracture
- Syndesmotic sprain
- Dislocation/subluxation
- Tendon rupture
- Ongoing instability
- Uncertain diagnosis

ADDITIONAL THERAPIES
Physical therapy:
- After the acute phase of the injury, patients with grade II or III sprain should start physical therapy as soon as possible to increase range of motion, strength, flexibility, and improve proprioceptive balance (wobble board/ankle disk).
- Functional rehabilitation prevents chronic instability and speeds healing.
- Athletes should undergo sport-specific rehabilitation before returning to play.

SURGERY/OTHER PROCEDURES
- Surgery is typically reserved for treatment of complicated recurrent sprains and certain syndesmotic sprains.
- Patients with chronic ankle instability who fail functional rehabilitation or with poor tissue quality may need anatomic repair/reconstructive surgery.

ONGOING CARE

FOLLOW-UP RECOMMENDATIONS
- After an ankle sprain, consider ankle-stabilizing orthoses (air stirrup braces, lace-up supports, athletic taping, etc.) for athletes participating in high-risk sports to prevent future ankle sprains.
- Moderate and severe sprains require ankle orthoses for ≥6 months during sports participation.
- Gradual return to play for athletes with a grade I lateral ankle sprain can generally be accomplished in 1 to 2 weeks; grade II sprain return to play time is 2 to 3 weeks; grade III sprain is approximately 4 weeks.
- Syndesmotic sprains take longer (~8 to 9 weeks) to heal than lateral ankle sprains.

Patient Monitoring
If athletes continue to have symptoms when they return to play or if a patient has pain for 6 to 8 weeks after injury, repeat examination and imaging.

PATIENT EDUCATION
- Crutch training
- Provide training on proper use of elastic bandages, brace, and/or orthoses.
- Demonstrate mobilization exercises (alphabet trace, towel grab).

PROGNOSIS
- Earlier physical therapy and mobilization with bracing allows for faster return to daily living and/or sports.
- Higher grade sprains, older patient age, and initial non–weight-bearing status have poorer prognosis and longer recovery.
- Ligamentous strength does not return for months after the injury.

COMPLICATIONS
- Joint instability
- Intermittent swelling/pain if not properly treated
- 5–33% continue to have pain 1 year postinjury.
- Accumulation of cartilage damage, leading to degenerative changes

REFERENCES

1. Feger MA, Glaviano NR, Donovan L, et al. Current trends in the management of lateral ankle sprain in the United States. *Clin J Sport Med*. 2017;27(2):145–152.
2. Doherty C, Delahunt E, Caulfield B, et al. The incidence and prevalence of ankle sprain injury: a systematic review and meta-analysis of prospective epidemiological studies. *Sports Med*. 2014;44(1):123–140.
3. Waterman BR, Owens BD, Davey S, et al. The epidemiology of ankle sprains in the United States. *J Bone Joint Surg Am*. 2010;92(13):2279–2284.
4. McCriskin BJ, Cameron KL, Orr JD, et al. Management and prevention of acute and chronic lateral ankle instability in athletic patient populations. *World J Orthop*. 2015;6(2):161–171.

ADDITIONAL READING

- Caldemeyer LE, Brown SM, Mulcahey MK. Neuromuscular training for the prevention of ankle sprains in female athletes: a systematic review. *Phys Sportsmed*. 2020;48(4):363–369.
- Camacho LD, Roward ZT, Deng Y, et al. Surgical management of lateral ankle instability in athletes. *J Athl Train*. 2019;54(6):639–649.
- D'Hooghe P, Cruz F, Alkhelaifi K. Return to play after a lateral ligament ankle sprain. *Curr Review Musculoskelet Med*. 2020;13(3):281–288.
- Farwell KE, Powden CJ, Powell MR, et al. The effectiveness of prophylactic ankle braces in reducing the incidence of acute ankle injuries in adolescent athletes: a critically appraised topic. *J Sport Rehabil*. 2013;22(2):137–142.
- Ortega-Avila AB, Cervera-Garvi P, Marchena-Rodriguez A, et al. Conservative treatment for acute ankle sprain: a systematic review. *J Clin Med*. 2020;9(10):3128.
- Richie DH, Izadi FE. Return to play after an ankle sprain: guidelines for the podiatric physician. *Clin Podiatr Med Surg*. 2015;32(2):195–215.

CODES

ICD10
- S96.919A Strain of unsp msl/tnd at ank/ft level, unsp foot, init
- S93.499A Sprain of other ligament of unspecified ankle, init encntr
- S93.419A Sprain of calcaneofibular ligament of unsp ankle, init

CLINICAL PEARLS
- Children are at an increased risk for physeal injuries because ligaments are stronger than physes.
- Conditioning, including proprioceptive training, before participating in sports and throughout the season helps to prevent ankle sprains.
- Functional rehabilitation, rather than total immobilization, is recommended for quicker return to sport and work.
- Patients who do not adequately rehabilitate an ankle sprain are at increased risk for recurrence and chronic ankle instability.
- If patient's condition is not improving in 6 to 8 weeks, consider advanced imaging with CT, MRI, or US.

S

SPRAINS AND STRAINS

Lee A. Mancini, MD, CSCS*D, CSN • Alec L. Tributino, DO • Grant Pierre, MD, CAQSM

 BASICS

DESCRIPTION

- *Sprains* are complete or partial ligamentous injuries either within the body of the ligament or at the site of attachment to bone.
  - Classified as grade 1, 2, or 3 (AMA Ligament Injury Classification)
    - Grade 1: stretch injury without ligamentous laxity
    - Grade 2: partial tear with increased ligamentous laxity but firm end point on exam
    - Grade 3: complete tear with increased ligamentous laxity and no firm end point on exam
  - Usually secondary to trauma (e.g., falls, twisting injuries, motor vehicle accidents)
  - Physical exam is the key to accurate diagnosis.
- *Strains* are partial or complete disruptions of the muscle, muscle–tendon junction, or tendon.
  - Classified as
    - First degree: minimal damage to muscle, tendon, or musculotendinous unit
    - Second degree: partial tear to the muscle, tendon, or musculotendinous unit
    - Third degree: complete disruption of the muscle, tendon, or musculotendinous unit
  - Often associated with overuse injuries

Geriatric Considerations
More likely to see associated bony injuries due to decreased joint flexibility and increased prevalence of osteoporosis and osteopenia

Pediatric Considerations
- Sprains and strains account for 24% of pediatric injuries.
- 3 million pediatric sports injuries occur annually.
- Consider physeal/apophyseal injuries in the skeletally immature patient.

EPIDEMIOLOGY

Incidence
~80% of all U.S. athletes experience a sprain or strain at some point.

Prevalence
- Ankle sprains are among the most common injuries in primary care, accounting for ~30% of sports medicine clinic visits. Most ankle sprains are due to inversion injuries (lateral sprains) involving the anterior talofibular ligament; account for 650,000 annual ER visits in the United States
- Predominant age
  - Sprains: any age in physically active patient
  - Strains: usually 15 to 40 years of age
- Predominant sex: male > female for most; female > male for sprain of anterior cruciate ligament (ACL)

ETIOLOGY AND PATHOPHYSIOLOGY
- Trauma, falls, motor vehicle accidents
- Excessive exercise; poor conditioning
- Improper footwear
- Inadequate warm-up and stretching before activity
- Prior sprain or strain

RISK FACTORS
- Prior history of sprain or strain is greatest risk factor for future sprain/strain.
- Change in or improper footwear, protective gear, or environment (e.g., surface)
- Sudden increase in training schedule or volume
- Tobacco use, medication adverse effects

GENERAL PREVENTION
- Appropriate warm-up and cooldown exercises
- Use proper equipment and footwear.
- Balance training programs improve proprioception and reduce the risk of ankle sprains.
- Semirigid orthoses may prevent ankle sprains during high-risk sports, especially in athletes with history of sprain.
- Proprioception and strength training decrease injury risk; stretching does not

COMMONLY ASSOCIATED CONDITIONS
- Effusions, ecchymosis, hemarthrosis
- Stress, avulsion, and/or other fractures
- Syndesmotic injuries
- Contusions
- Dislocations/subluxations

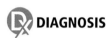 **DIAGNOSIS**

HISTORY
- Obtain thorough description of mechanism of injury including activity, trauma, baseline conditioning, and prior musculoskeletal injuries.
- May describe feeling or hearing pop or snap

PHYSICAL EXAM
- Inspect for swelling, asymmetry, ecchymosis, and gait disturbance.
- Evaluate for neurovascular compromise.
- Palpate for tenderness.
- Evaluate for decreased range of motion (ROM) of joint and joint instability/laxity.
- Evaluate for strength.
- Sprains
  - Grade 1: tenderness without laxity; minimal pain, swelling; little ecchymosis; can bear weight
  - Grade 2: tenderness with increased laxity on exam but firm end point; more pain, swelling; often ecchymosis; some difficulty bearing weight
  - Grade 3: tenderness with increased laxity on exam and no firm end point; severe pain, swelling; obvious ecchymosis; difficulty bearing weight

DIFFERENTIAL DIAGNOSIS
- Tendonitis
- Bursitis
- Contusion
- Hematoma
- Fracture
- Osteochondral lesion
- Rheumatologic process

DIAGNOSTIC TESTS & INTERPRETATION
- Ankle
  - Anterior drawer test assesses integrity of anterior talofibular ligament.
  - Talar tilt test assesses integrity of calcaneofibular ligament.
  - Squeeze test assesses for syndesmotic injury.
  - Palpate lateral and medial malleoli.
- Knee
  - Lachman and anterior drawer tests assess integrity of ACL. Posterior drawer and sag tests assess integrity of posterior cruciate ligament.
  - Valgus/varus stress tests assess integrity of medial and lateral collateral ligaments, respectively.
- Shoulder
  - Load and shift test; sulcus sign; and the apprehension, relocation, surprise test assess for instability of the glenohumeral joint.
- Radiographs help rule out bony injury; stress views may be necessary. Obtain bilateral radiographs in children to rule out growth plate injuries.
- Use Ottawa Foot and Ankle Rules (age 18 to 55 years) to determine if radiographs are necessary.
- Ottawa Ankle Rules: x-ray required if pain in the malleolar zone *and*
  - Bone tenderness in posterior aspect distal 6 cm of tibia or fibula *or*
  - Unable to bear weight immediately or in emergency department
- Ottawa Foot Rules: x-ray required if midfoot zone pain is present *and*
  - Bone tenderness at base of 5th metatarsal *or*
  - Bone tenderness at navicular *or*
  - Inability to bear weight immediately or in emergency department

Follow-Up Tests & Special Considerations
- Can consider repeat x-rays in 1 to 2 weeks if symptoms not improved to rule out occult fracture
- CT scan can be considered if occult fracture is suspected.
- MRI is the gold standard for imaging soft tissue structures, including muscle, ligaments, and intra-articular structures. If tibiofibular syndesmotic disruption is suspected, MRI is highly accurate for diagnosis. Contrast is usually not necessary for diagnosis of most ligamentous and labral injuries.
- Ultrasound evaluation of a variety of muscles, tendons, and ligaments by a skilled operator allows for dynamic evaluation of potential sprain/strain that can add to traditional diagnostic imaging.

Diagnostic Procedures/Other
Surgery may be required for some partial and complete sprains depending on location, mechanism, and chronicity.

TREATMENT

GENERAL MEASURES
- Acute: *protection*, relative *rest* (activity modification), *ice*, *compression*, *elevation*, *medications*, *modalities* (PRICEMM) therapy
- Ankle sprains: should consist of functional support, possibly augmented by nonsteroidal anti-inflammatory drugs in the early phases after injury
- Grade 1 and 2 ankle sprain: functional treatment with brace, orthosis, taping, elastic bandage wrap
  - Ankle braces (lace-up, stirrup-type, air cast) are a more effective functional treatment than elastic bandages or taping (1)[A].
- Grade 3 ankle sprain: Short period of immobilization may be needed. Consider short walking boot and/or crutches.
- Refer for early physical therapy.
- For high-level athletes with more extensive damage (e.g., biceps or pectoralis disruption), consider surgical referral.

MEDICATION
First Line
- Acetaminophen: not to exceed 3 g/day
- NSAIDs
  - Ibuprofen: 200 to 800 mg TID
  - Naproxen: 250 to 500 mg BID
  - Diclofenac: 50 to 75 mg BID
- Acetaminophen and NSAIDs have similar efficacy in reducing pain after soft tissue injuries with less GI side effects; NSAIDs are better than narcotics.
- Topical diclofenac, ibuprofen, and ketoprofen are effective for pain related to strains and sprains, especially in gel form or patch (2)[A].

Second Line
- Platelet-rich plasma injections may aid recovery in treatment of muscle strains, but more studies are needed.
- Opioids should rarely be considered acutely for severe pain, but discretion is advised.

ISSUES FOR REFERRAL
- ACL sprain in athletes/physically active
- Salter-Harris physeal fractures
- Joint instability especially if chronic
- Tendon disruption (i.e., Achilles, biceps, ACL)
- Lack of improvement with conservative measures

ADDITIONAL THERAPIES
- Physical therapy is a useful adjunct after a sprain, particularly if early mobilization is crucial.
  - Proprioception retraining
  - Core strengthening
  - Eccentric exercises
  - Thera-Band exercises
- After hamstring strain, frequent daily stretching and progressive agility and trunk stabilization exercises may speed recovery and reduce risk of reinjury (3)[A]. Rehab protocols emphasizing eccentric/lengthening exercises are more effective than conventional exercises (4)[B].

SURGERY/OTHER PROCEDURES
- Casting and surgery are reserved for select partial and complete sprains. Need for surgery depends on the neurovascular supply to the injured area as well as the ability to attain full ROM and stability of the affected joint. The need for surgery also depends on activity level and patient preference.
- For primary management of acute lateral ankle sprains, there is no difference between surgical versus conservative therapy. Risks are increased with surgical intervention.
- Chronic ankle instability affects 10–20% of people who sustain an acute sprain. If conservative management fails and laxity is present, surgery is considered (5)[A].
- Percutaneous needle tenotomy versus surgical tenotomy are available as options for chronic tendinosis (chronic, recurrent strains).

 ## ONGOING CARE

FOLLOW-UP RECOMMENDATIONS
If the affected joint has full strength and ROM, the patient can advance activity as tolerated using pain as a guide for return to activity.

Patient Monitoring
After initial treatment, consider early rehabilitation. Limit swelling and work on increasing ROM.

DIET
Weight loss if overweight

PATIENT EDUCATION
- Injury prevention through proprioceptive training and physical therapy
- ROM and strengthening exercises to restore functional capacity

PROGNOSIS
Favorable with appropriate treatment and rest. Duration of recovery depends on the severity and location of injury.

COMPLICATIONS
- Chronic joint instability
- Arthritis
- Muscle contracture
- Chronic tendinopathy

REFERENCES

1. Petersen W, Rembitzki IV, Koppenburg AG, et al. Treatment of acute ankle ligament injuries: a systematic review. *Arch Orthop Trauma Surg*. 2013;133(8):1129–1141.
2. Derry S, Moore RA, Gaskell H, et al. Topical NSAIDs for acute musculoskeletal pain in adults. *Cochrane Database Syst Rev*. 2015;(6):CD007402.
3. Pas HI, Reurink G, Tol JL, et al. Efficacy of rehabilitation (lengthening) exercises, platelet-rich plasma injections, and other conservative interventions in acute hamstring injuries: an updated systematic review and meta-analysis. *Br J Sports Med*. 2015;49(18):1197–1205.
4. Askling CM, Tengvar M, Tarassova O, et al. Acute hamstring injuries in Swedish elite sprinters and jumpers: a prospective randomised controlled clinical trial comparing two rehabilitation protocols. *Br J Sports Med*. 2014;48(7):532–539.
5. McCriskin BJ, Cameron KL, Orr JD, et al. Management and prevention of acute and chronic lateral ankle instability in athletic patient populations. *World J Orthop*. 2015;6(2):161–171.

ADDITIONAL READING

- Hamilton BH, Best TM. Platelet-enriched plasma and muscle strain injuries: challenges imposed by the burden of proof. *Clin J Sport Med*. 2011;21(1):31–36.
- Kim T, Lee M, Kim K, et al. Acupuncture for treating acute ankle sprains in adults. *Cochrane Database Syst Rev*. 2014;(6):CD009065.
- Monk AP, Davies LJ, Hopewell S, et al. Surgical versus conservative interventions for treating anterior cruciate ligament injuries. *Cochrane Database Syst Rev*. 2016;(4):CD011166.
- Seah R, Mani-Babu S. Managing ankle sprains in primary care: what is best practice? A systematic review of the last 10 years of evidence. *Br Med Bull*. 2011;97:105–135.

 ## SEE ALSO

Tendinopathy

CODES

ICD10
- S93.6 Sprain of foot
- S93.4 Sprain of ankle
- S93.5 Sprain of toe

CLINICAL PEARLS

For acute injury, remember PRICEMM:
- Protection of the joint
- Relative rest (activity modification)
- Apply ice.
- Apply compression.
- Elevate joint.
- Medications/ice for pain
- Other modalities as needed
- Wean out of brace as tolerated to limit atrophy of stabilizing muscles.

SQUAMOUS CELL CARCINOMA, CUTANEOUS

Sujitha Yadlapati, MD • Faraz Yousefian, DO

BASICS

DESCRIPTION
Cutaneous squamous cell cancer is the second most common nonmelanoma skin cancer after basal cell carcinoma (1).

EPIDEMIOLOGY
Nonmelanoma skin cancer is the most common malignancy worldwide. Historically, squamous cell carcinoma (SCC) has been thought to account for 20% of nonmelanoma skin cancers, thus being the second most common malignancy after basal cell carcinoma (2),(3). However, recent data indicate that the ratio of basal cell carcinoma to SCC is 1.0 in the U.S. Medicare population (1). An accurate incidence of cutaneous SCC is not known since this is not required to be reported to national cancer registries.

Incidence
- The average age for incidence is around 60 years, more common in men (4).
- Incidence increases the closer the person gets to the equator or higher altitude (4).

ETIOLOGY AND PATHOPHYSIOLOGY
Genetics
Some of the hereditary disorders have genes that are associated with cutaneous squamous cell cancer (5). They include:
- Xeroderma pigmentosum (5)
- Oculocutaneous albinism (5)
- Epidermodysplasia verruciformis (5)
- Genes mutated include: TP53, CDKN2A, NOTCH1, Ras, TP53 (most common gene involved in cutaneous SCC) (5)

RISK FACTORS
- Most SCCs arise in:
  - Sun-damaged skin of elderly white individuals of European ancestry
  - Gender (more common in men)
  - Increasing age (average age of onset is the mid-60s)
  - Background of preexisting lesions of actinic keratosis (AK) (2)
  - UV radiation exposure (5),(6)
  - Preexisting conditions
  - Immunosuppression (5)
    - Solid organ transplantation (5)
    - HIV/AIDS, non-Hodgkin lymphoma, chronic lymphocytic leukemia have increasing rates of developing cutaneous squamous cell cancer (5).
- Chronic skin conditions (5)
  - Burn scars, hidradenitis suppurativa, chronic osteomyelitis, discoid lupus erythematosus, lichen planus, lichen sclerosus et atrophicus
- Inherited genetic conditions (5)
  - Albinism, epidermolysis bullosa, xeroderma pigmentosum
- Ionizing radiation exposure (6)
- Arsenic exposure (5),(6)

- Ulcers (6)
- Bowen disease (SCC in situ) (6)
- Erythroplasia of Queyrat (SCC in situ of penis) (6)
- HPV infection (6, 11, 16, 18) (6)
- Treatment with BRAF inhibitors (vemurafenib and dabrafenib) (7)

GENERAL PREVENTION
- Protect skin from sun exposure (5).
- Wear sunscreen, hats, and UV protective clothing.
- Vitamin B_3 (nicotinamide) can repair DNA by preventing UVR-induced adenosine triphosphate depletion (5).

COMMONLY ASSOCIATED CONDITIONS
Actinic keratosis is the precursor of cutaneous squamous cell cancer, Bowen disease, erythroplasia of Queyrat (4).

DIAGNOSIS

- Histopathology remains the gold standard for the diagnosis of SCC. A punch or shave biopsy can be used to obtain a sample (8).
- Dermoscopy is a noninvasive technique that can help improve diagnostic accuracy (8).

PHYSICAL EXAM
- Lesions occur mainly in chronically exposed areas:
  - Face (especially lips, ear, nose, cheek, and eyelid) (4)
- Lesions occur chiefly in chronically sun-exposed areas:
  - Face and backs of the forearms and hands
  - Bald areas of the scalp and top of ears in men
  - The sun-exposed "V" of the neck as well as the posterior neck below the occipital hairline
  - In elderly females, lesions tend to occur on the legs and other sun-exposed locations.
  - In African Americans, equal frequency in sun-exposed and unexposed areas
- Clinical appearance
  - Generally slow-growing, firm, hyperkeratotic papules, nodules, or plaques
  - Most SCCs are asymptomatic, although bleeding, pain, and tenderness may be noted.
  - Lesions may have a smooth, verrucous, or papillomatous surface.
  - Varying degrees of ulceration, erosion, crust, or scale
  - Color is often red to brown, tan, or pearly (indistinguishable from basal cell carcinoma).
- Clinical variants of SCC
  - Bowen disease (SCC in situ): a solitary lesion that resembles a scaly psoriatic plaque
  - Invasive SCC: often a raised, firm papule, nodule, or plaque. Lesions may be smooth, verrucous, or papillomatous, with varying degrees of ulceration, erosion, crust, or scale.

- Cutaneous horn: SCC with an overlying cutaneous horn. A cutaneous horn represents a thick, hard, fingernail-like keratinization produced by the SCC. Bowen disease may also have a cutaneous horn on its surface.
- Erythroplasia of Queyrat refers to Bowen disease of the glans penis, which manifests as one or more velvety red plaques.
- Subungual SCC appears as hyperkeratotic lesions under the nail plate or surrounding periungual skin, often mimicking warts.
- Marjolin ulcer: an SCC evolving from a new area of ulceration or elevation at the site of a scar or ulcer
- HPV-associated SCC: virally induced; an SCC most commonly seen as a new or enlarging warty growth on penis, vulva, perianal area, or periungual region
- Verrucous carcinoma: a subtype of SCC that is extremely well-differentiated, can be locally destructive, but rarely metastasizes. Lesions are "cauliflower-like" verrucous nodules or plaques.
- Basaloid SCC: less common than typical SCC; seen more often in men aged 40 to 70 years

DIFFERENTIAL DIAGNOSIS
- Actinic keratosis
- Basal cell carcinoma

DIAGNOSTIC TESTS & INTERPRETATION
- Biopsy of the lesion will demonstrate characteristic histologic findings. Shave biopsy, punch biopsy, or excisional biopsy can be utilized (8).
- Histopathologic findings are as follows (8):
  - Pleomorphic, hyperchromatic squamous cells with nuclear pleomorphism (8)
  - Aggregates of glassy, eosinophilic keratinocytes (8)
  - Full-thickness atypia of the epidermis (8)
  - Keratinocyte mitoses (8)
  - Squamous pearls (8)
  - Inflammatory infiltrate of lymphocytes and plasma cells may be seen (8).

Follow-Up Tests & Special Considerations
- For high-risk cutaneous squamous cell cancer: These are the follow-up recommendations (9):
  - Complete skin exam and lymph node exam required every 2 to 6 months (9)
  - Every 6 to 12 months for the next 3 years
  - Annually after 5 years (9)
- For high-risk cutaneous squamous cell cancer with regional disease: These are the follow-up recommendations (9):
  - Complete skin exam and lymph node exam every 1 to 3 months (9)
  - Every 2 to 4 months for the next year (9)
  - Every 4 to 6 months until the 5th year (9)
  - Every 6 to 12 months for the patient's lifetime (9)

TREATMENT

Selecting the most appropriate treatment options should involve consideration of:

- Tumor location and characteristics
- High-risk areas
- Recurrence rate
- Patient expectations
- Patient's functional status and life expectancy

MEDICATION

First Line

- First-line treatment for cutaneous SCC is complete surgical excision with histopathologic control of excision margins.
- Surgical excision provides these benefits (9):
  – Shorter healing time
  – Cure rate as high as 95%
- Mohs micrographic surgery (MMS) is the treatment for high-risk tumors instead of surgical excision (9).
  – MMS is the gold standard for surgical removal of high-risk SCCs (9).
  – SCCs with a low risk of metastasis can be eliminated by excision, electrodesiccation, curettage, or cryosurgery.
  – For high-risk cancer, surgical resection and MMS provide decreased recurrence and metastasis.
  – Cryotherapy is used to treat small squamous cell cancers.
  – Cryotherapy or radiation can be used to treat patients who have bleeding disorders or contraindications to surgery.
  – MMS offers the highest cure for patients who have recurrent or high-risk primary squamous cell cancer.

Second Line

Advances in the management of cutaneous SCC

- Monoclonal antibodies (cetuximab, panitumumab) (9)
- Tyrosine kinase inhibitors (erlotinib) (9)
- Chemotherapy—used in locally advanced or metastatic skin squamous cell cancer (9)
- Chemotherapeutic drugs used are methotrexate, bleomycin, doxorubicin, cisplatin (9).
- Oral retinoids decrease the incidence of actinic keratosis and cutaneous squamous cell cancer (9).

SURGERY/OTHER PROCEDURES

- For high-risk cutaneous squamous cell cancer patients, who have tumors in inoperable locations and are poor candidates for surgery, they have the option for radiation therapy (9).
- Radiation therapy side effects include (9):
  – Malaise
  – Nausea
  – Radiation-induced erythema
  – Telangiectasia
  – Hypopigmentation
  – Epidermal atrophy
  – Soft tissue necrosis
  – Radiation-induced malignancy

ADMISSION, INPATIENT, AND NURSING CONSIDERATIONS

Examine sentinel lymph nodes for early detection of metastasis. This can decrease disease-related morbidity and mortality (9).

 ONGOING CARE

PROGNOSIS

- Patients with high-risk cutaneous squamous cell cancer have an increased risk of recurrence, lymph node, or distant metastases (9).
- From the lesions at risk, 7–80% will locally recur or metastasize within the first 2 years and 95% within the first 5 years of initial diagnosis (9).
- 30–50% of high-risk cutaneous squamous cell cancer patients will develop second skin cancer within 5 years (9).
- Cutaneous squamous cell cancer has an increased risk of metastasis if these characteristics below are present (9):
  – Tumor recurrence
  – Diameter ≥2 cm
  – Thickness >2 mm
  – Poorly differentiated histology
  – Invasion of subcutaneous tissue or structures such as perineural, vascular, or lymphatic
  – If the tumor is located on
    ○ Eye
    ○ Vermilion lip
    ○ "Mask areas" of face
    ○ Hands
    ○ Feet
    ○ Genitalia
- MMS provides cure rates of 97% for primary cutaneous squamous cell cancer and 94% for recurrent cutaneous squamous cell cancer.
- MMS is very beneficial for treating specifically high-risk cutaneous squamous cell cancers and preventing local recurrence (9).
- Staging is essential for treating high-risk cutaneous SCC (9).
- High-risk factors include (9):
  – Diameter ≥0.1 mm
  – Poorly differentiated histology
  – Tumor invasion beyond fat
  – Perineural invasion ≥0.1 mm
- Excellent prognosis
- After recurrence, the prognosis is inferior. There is a risk of distant metastasis and metastasis to regional lymph nodes.
- After resection of cancer, recurrent cancers have twice the risk of recurrence.
- For patients with metastatic disease, the long-term prognosis is poor.
  – For patients having distant metastasis, 10-year survival rates are <10%.
  – For patients having regional lymph node involvement, 10-year survival rates are <20%.

- Distant metastasis occurs in 15% of cases and involves these sites:
  – Brain
  – Lungs
  – Liver
  – Skin
  – Bone

COMPLICATIONS

- Local recurrence
- Metastasis

REFERENCES

1. Rogers HW, Weinstock MA, Feldman SR, et al. Incidence estimate of nonmelanoma skin cancer (keratinocyte carcinomas) in the U.S. population, 2012. *JAMA Dermatol*. 2015;151(10):1081–1086.
2. Elder DE. *Lever's Histopathology of the Skin*. 10th ed. Philadelphia, PA: Wolters Kluwer; 2008.
3. Miller DL, Weinstock MA. Nonmelanoma skin cancer in the United States: incidence. *J Am Acad Dermatol*. 1994;30(5 Pt 1):774–778.
4. Simonacci F, Bertozzi N, Grieco MP, et al. Surgical therapy of cutaneous squamous cell carcinoma: our experience. *Acta Biomed*. 2018;89(2):242–248.
5. Green AC, Olsen CM. Cutaneous squamous cell carcinoma: an epidemiological review. *Br J Dermatol*. 2017;177(2):373–381.
6. Alam M, Ratner D. Cutaneous squamous-cell carcinoma. *N Engl J Med*. 2001;344(13):975–983.
7. Su F, Viros A, Milagre C, et al. RAS mutations in cutaneous squamous-cell carcinomas in patients treated with BRAF inhibitors. *N Engl J Med*. 2012;366(3):207–215.
8. Combalia A, Carrera C. Squamous cell carcinoma: an update on diagnosis and treatment. *Dermatol Pract Concept*. 2020;10(3):e2020066.
9. Parikh SA, Patel VA, Ratner D. Advances in the management of cutaneous squamous cell carcinoma. *F1000Prime Rep*. 2014;6:70.

CODES

ICD10

- C44.92 Squamous cell carcinoma of skin, unspecified
- C44.320 Squamous cell carcinoma of skin of unspecified parts of face
- C44.42 Squamous cell carcinoma of skin of scalp and neck

CLINICAL PEARLS

- Cutaneous SCC associated with UV light exposure and immunosuppression
- The head and neck are the most common regions for invasive cutaneous SCC.
- MMS provides cure rates of 97% for primary cutaneous SCC.

STRESS FRACTURE
Dongsheng Jiang, MD, MSc • Joanna Jiang, MD

 BASICS

DESCRIPTION
- Stress fractures are overuse injuries caused by cumulative microdamage from repetitive bone loading.
- Stress fractures occur in different situations:
  - Fatigue fracture: abnormal repetitive stress applied to normal bone (e.g., young college athletes or new military recruits with increased physical activity demands and inadequate conditioning). Common sites include tibia, fibula, metatarsals, femoral neck, and navicular.
  - Insufficiency fracture: normal stress applied to structurally abnormal bone (e.g., femoral neck fracture in osteopenic bone, metabolic bone disease). Common sites include spine, sacrum, femoral neck, and medial femoral condyle.
  - Combination fracture: abnormal stress applied to abnormal bone (e.g., female long-distance runners with premature osteoporosis from athletic triad)
- Weight-bearing bones of the lower extremity are most commonly affected at the following sites:
  - Tibia/fibula (most common)
  - Metatarsals (second most)
  - Navicular
  - Femoral neck
  - Pars interarticularis
- High-risk stress fractures occur in zones of tension or areas with poor blood supply and are more likely to result in fracture displacement and/or nonunion. High-risk sites include the following:
  - Femoral neck
  - Anterior tibial diaphysis
  - Sesamoids
  - Pars interarticularis of lumbar spine (L4, L5)
  - 5th metatarsal at metaphyseal–diaphyseal junction
  - Proximal 2nd metatarsal
  - Medial malleolus
  - Tarsal navicular
  - Patella
  - Talar neck
- Synonym(s): march fracture; fatigue fracture

EPIDEMIOLOGY
Incidence
- Greatest incidence in 15- to 27-year-olds
- Females > males
- Accounts for up to 20% of visits to sports medicine and orthopedic clinics
Prevalence
- Lifetime athletic stress fracture is 10% (1).
- Affects up to 6.9% of male and 21.0% of female military members

ETIOLOGY AND PATHOPHYSIOLOGY
- Bone is dynamic and constantly remodeling in response to applied physiologic stress.
- Repetitive loading or overuse causes microfractures that fail to heal due to imbalance between bone resorption and bone formation.
- If microdamage accumulates in excess of reparation, bony fatigue leads to stress fracture.

RISK FACTORS
- Intrinsic
  - Females are at 2.3 times higher risk than males
  - Female athlete triad
  - Small tibial width
  - Later menarche, amenorrhea, or irregular menses
  - History of stress fracture
  - History of osteoporosis, osteomalacia, rheumatoid arthritis, prolonged corticosteroid therapy
  - BMI <19
  - Skeletal malalignment: pes cavus/planus, leg length discrepancies, excessive forefoot varus, tarsal coalitions, prominent posterior calcaneal process, tight heel cords
  - Biomechanical factors such as increased vertical loading rate (e.g., heel-to-toe running instead of forefoot striking)
- Extrinsic
  - High-risk exercises—track and field, cross country
  - Training regimen—running >20 miles/week or training >5 hr/day
  - Nutritional—inadequate caloric intake or history of eating disorder
  - Chronic low vitamin D
  - Rapid increase in mileage, running pace, or training volume
  - Inappropriate footwear
  - Hard training/running surface
  - Inadequate recovery or rest and training with fatigued muscle
  - Meds: glucocorticoids, anticonvulsants, antidepressants, medroxyprogesterone (DMPA), methotrexate, antiretrovirals, chronic cannabis use, >5 years of bisphosphonate use

GENERAL PREVENTION
- Prevention is key especially in adolescent athletes (1).
- Graduated increments in training load intensity: no more than 10% per week
- Optimize energy balance.
- Diversify sports participation (minimizing sports specialization).
- Reduce intensity and duration of activity if new-onset pain.
- Proper footwear (Athletes should have a gait analysis prior to training.)
- Increasing dynamic physical activity (jumping; plyometric training) increases bone density and resistance to mechanical stress.
- Decrease vertical loading rate either by switching to forefoot strike running or (if continuing with heel-to-toe strike) by using a heel pad insert.
- Vitamin D supplementation (800 IU/day) in combination with calcium (2,000 mg/day)

COMMONLY ASSOCIATED CONDITIONS
- Osteoporosis/osteopenia
- Female athlete triad
- Metabolic bone disorders

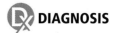 **DIAGNOSIS**

HISTORY
- Insidious onset of vague bony pain over period of weeks. Pain is typically worse with physical activity.
- Initially relieved by rest, then pain persists with rest or slight activity
- If untreated, pain progresses and may occur earlier during training sessions. With time and repetitive loading, the pain also becomes more localized.
- History of recent change in training intensity, alteration in training terrain, and/or footwear
- Assess dietary practices: energy availability, disordered eating, weight fluctuations, and calcium and vitamin D intake.
- In female athletes, assess menstrual history: menarche, oligomenorrhea, or amenorrhea.

PHYSICAL EXAM
- Height, weight, BMI, and any stigmata of disordered eating (cold extremities, hypercarotenemia, lanugo hair, calluses on back of fingers, poor oral hygiene, parotid gland hypertrophy, or orthostatic hypotension)
- Antalgic gait (limp; limiting weight on affected leg)
- Point or percussion tenderness over injury site: A vibrating tuning fork over the fracture site may intensify pain.
- Swelling may be present.
- Specific tests:
  - Hop test for tibial stress fracture: With a stress fracture, the patient cannot hop on one leg 10 times; if able to perform test, consider shin splints (medial tibial stress syndrome).
  - Fulcrum test for femoral stress fracture: With patient seated, provoke pain by applying downward force on the distal femur while other hand is under the midthigh on femoral shaft (if clinical suspicion is high, defer or use only with extreme caution to avoid completing a femoral neck stress fracture).
  - Single-leg hyperextension (Stork) test for pars interarticularis fracture of lumbar spine: Stand on one leg and extend lumbar spine; positive if painful on symptomatic side
- Anatomic malalignment may be present (leg length discrepancy, scoliosis, pes planus/cavus).

DIFFERENTIAL DIAGNOSIS
- Shin splints (medial tibial stress syndrome—pain resolves with rest; stress fracture pain does not)
- Infection (osteomyelitis)
- Soft tissue injury (sprain, tendonitis, and periostitis)
- Exertional compartment syndrome
- Bony fracture, pathologic fracture, insufficiency fracture
- Neoplasm (osteoid osteoma)
- Nerve entrapment syndromes
- Intermittent claudication

DIAGNOSTIC TESTS & INTERPRETATION
Initial Tests (lab, imaging)
- Laboratory tests are not required unless clinically indicated for suspected disease (e.g., female athlete triad, hyperparathyroidism, and vitamin D deficiency)
- May consider CBC, CMP, TSH, 25-hydroxyvitamin D, FSH, LH plus 24-hour urine calcium and PTH.
- Plain films (x-ray):
  - First line in suspected stress fracture
  - Findings typically seen 2 to 8 weeks after pain onset
  - High false-negative rate during early stages (1 to 2 weeks)
  - May see periosteal callus, "gray cortex sign" (region of decreased cortical intensity), osteopenia, endosteal reaction, or ill-defined cortical margin
  - Severe cases may show discrete fracture.

Follow-Up Tests & Special Considerations
- MRI:
  - Gold standard for imaging stress fractures
  - Early signs (edema of bone and surrounding soft tissue) can be identified as early as 1 or 2 days after the onset of symptoms.
  - Sensitivity is up to 88%; specificity up to 100%, accuracy 90% (1)
- Bone scan:
  - Sensitive but has potential for false positives
  - Can show signs of stress fracture as early as 3 to 5 days after onset of symptoms
  - Useful for suspected rib or spine stress fractures
  - Should not be used to assess healing
- CT scan:
  - Less sensitive than MRI or bone scan for early stress fractures but has an important role in evaluating longitudinal fracture lines and occult fractures of foot, tibia, carpal scaphoid, and pars interarticularis
  - Can distinguish conditions (osteoid osteoma, malignancy, and osteomyelitis) that mimic stress fracture on bone scan; useful when fractures are chronic and are associated with low bone turnover.
  - Bony detail provided by CT scan allows differentiation of complete versus incomplete fracture, especially if MRI is equivocal.
- US: not routinely used but beneficial for superficial stress fracture
- Classification by radiographic findings (CT, MRI, bone scan, or x-ray)
  - Grade I: asymptomatic stress reaction; no pain, periosteal edema only, no fracture line
  - Grade II: symptomatic stress reaction; pain on exam, bone marrow edema, no fracture line seen on imaging
  - Grade III: nondisplaced fracture; pain on exam, nondisplaced fracture line seen on imaging
  - Grade IV: displaced fracture; pain on exam, displaced fracture >2 mm seen on imaging
  - Grade V: nonunion; pain on exam, nonunion characteristics on imaging, long-standing symptoms

TREATMENT
- Low-risk stress fractures are generally treated nonoperatively.
- Protection, rest, ice, compression, and elevation (PRICE) for acute pain and edema
- Activity modification: Decrease activity to the level of pain-free functioning.
- Consider temporarily immobilizing patients who have pain at rest or with gentle range of motion.
- If patients have pain with ambulation, use crutches with periodic walking trial to monitor readiness for nonaided (pain free) ambulation.
- Pneumatic leg brace is effective in decreasing the return-to-play time for tibial shaft stress fracture.
- Adequate recovery time is important to ensure proper healing of all stress fractures. The patient should be pain free before starting rehabilitation. Return to sports should start 10 to 14 days after the patient is pain free.
- High-risk fractures typically require immediate immobilization and a period of non–weight-bearing. May require early surgical intervention to avoid nonunion and facilitate earlier return to sport
- A low-grade stress fracture at a high-risk location must heal fully prior to returning to full activity versus a low-grade fracture at a low-risk location.
- Criteria for allowing an athlete to return should include complete resolution of symptoms with activities of daily living; radiographic evidence of healing; no tenderness to palpation at the injury site; and optimization of the athlete's nutritional, biomechanical, hormonal, and psychological status.

MEDICATION
First Line
- Calcium (up to 2 g/day through diet sources) and vitamin D (800 to 4,000 IU/day)
- Acetaminophen is useful for pain.
- NSAIDs are beneficial for pain and inflammation but may adversely affect fracture healing.

Second Line
- Some have tried PTH (1–34) 20 μg subcutaneous daily for 8 weeks.
- Oral contraceptives do not restore bone density in athletes (1).

ISSUES FOR REFERRAL
Orthopedic consultation for high-risk fractures, failure to improve with standard treatment, evidence of nonunion within 3 to 4 weeks, or inability to tolerate rehabilitation

ADDITIONAL THERAPIES
- Electrical stimulation may be an adjunct for delayed union and nonunion.
- Extracorporeal shock wave therapy (ESWT) and pulsed US require additional study.
- Physical therapy
- May consider other exercises such as stationary cycling, hydrotherapy and swimming, antigravity treadmills, Pilates, and seated exercise (1)

ONGOING CARE
FOLLOW-UP RECOMMENDATIONS
Once the patient is pain free, low-impact training can start and be advanced gently as tolerated.

Patient Monitoring
Imaging every 4 to 6 weeks to assess healing

DIET
- Adequate caloric intake
- Adequate calcium and vitamin D

PATIENT EDUCATION
Correct training errors with gait retraining.

COMPLICATIONS
- Delayed union
- Nonunion

REFERENCE
1. Beck B, Drysdale L. Risk factors, diagnosis and management of bone stress injuries in adolescent athletes: a narrative review. *Sports (Basel)*. 2021;9(4):52.

SEE ALSO

Algorithm: Foot Pain

CODES
ICD10
- M84.38XA Stress fracture, other site, initial encounter for fracture
- M84.369A Stress fracture, unsp tibia and fibula, init for fx
- M84.376A Stress fracture, unspecified foot, init encntr for fracture

CLINICAL PEARLS
- The diagnosis of stress fractures requires a high index of suspicion. X-rays are often negative initially.
- Identify and treat female athletic triad or underlying metabolic conditions.
- To help prevent stress fractures, gradually increase training volume and avoid sudden increases in high-impact activity or running mileage. Ensure adequate nutrition intake including calcium, vitamin D.
- High-risk fractures require immediate immobilization and non–weight-bearing.
- Ensure gradual return to training with proper rehabilitation protocol for all stress fractures. Treat any underlying metabolic causes and mitigate risk factors.

S

STROKE, ACUTE (CEREBROVASCULAR ACCIDENT [CVA])

Audrey Dong, DO • Kiyomi K. Goto, DO

 BASICS

DESCRIPTION
The sudden onset of a focal neurologic deficit(s) resulting from either infarction or hemorrhage within the brain

- Two broad categories: ischemic (thrombotic or embolic) (87%) and hemorrhagic (13%)
- Hemorrhage: intracerebral or subarachnoid
- Synonym(s): CVA; cerebral infarct
- Related terms: transient ischemic attack (TIA), a transient episode of neurologic dysfunction due to focal ischemia without permanent infarction on imaging (See "Transient Ischemic Attack (TIA).")

Pediatric Considerations
- Incidence: 2 to 13/100,000
- Frequent risk factors: arteriopathies (53%), cardiac disorders (31%), and infection (24%) (1)

EPIDEMIOLOGY
Incidence
Annual incidence in the United States is ~795,000.

Prevalence
- Prevalence in the United States: 550/100,000
- Predominant age: Risk increases >45 years of age; highest during the 7th and 8th decades
- Predominant sex: male > female at younger age but higher incidence in women with age ≥75 years

ETIOLOGY AND PATHOPHYSIOLOGY
- 87% of strokes are ischemic, three main subtypes: thrombosis, embolism, and systemic hypoperfusion. Large vessel atherothrombotic strokes often involve the origin of the internal carotid artery. Small vessel lacunar strokes are commonly due to lipohyalinosis occlusion. Embolic strokes are largely from a cardiac source (due to left atrial thrombus, atrial fibrillation, recent MI, valve disease, or mechanical valves) or ascending aortic atheromatous disease (>4 mm) (2).
- 13% of strokes are hemorrhagic; most commonly due to hypertension (HTN). Other causes include intracranial vascular malformations (cavernous angiomas, AVMs), cerebral amyloid angiopathy (lobar hemorrhages in elderly), and anticoagulation (2).
- Fibromuscular dysplasia (rare), vasculitis, or drug use (cocaine, amphetamines) are other causes of stroke.

Genetics
Stroke is a polygenic multifactorial disease.

RISK FACTORS
- Uncontrollable: age, gender, race, family history/genetics, prior stroke or TIA
- Controllable/modifiable/treatable
  - Metabolic: diabetes, dyslipidemia
  - Lifestyle: smoking, alcohol, cocaine/amphetamine use, physical inactivity
  - Cardiovascular: HTN, atrial fibrillation, valvular heart disease, endocarditis, recent MI, severe carotid artery stenosis, hypercoagulable states, patent foramen ovale (2)

GENERAL PREVENTION
Smoking cessation, regular exercise, avoid prolonged physical inactivity (3), weight control to maintain BMI<30 and maximize glucose control, low-salt diet, moderate alcohol use; control BP; manage hyperlipidemia; antiplatelet therapy (e.g., aspirin) in high-risk persons; treat anticoagulation therapy for nonvalvular atrial fibrillation.

COMMONLY ASSOCIATED CONDITIONS
Coronary artery disease is the major cause of death in the first 5 years after a stroke.

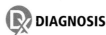 **DIAGNOSIS**

HISTORY
- Determining time course is critical: Assess onset of symptoms. History from witnesses may be helpful.
- Acute onset of focal arm/leg weakness, facial weakness, difficulty with speech or swallowing, vertigo, visual disturbances, diminished consciousness
- Assess risk factors.
- Vomiting and severe headache favor hemorrhagic stroke (2).

PHYSICAL EXAM
- Assess airway, breathing, and circulation (ABC).
- Vital signs—pulse (character and rate) and BP
- Cardiovascular exam: bruits, pulses (regularity); murmurs; gallops; peripheral stigmata
- Pulmonary exam: signs of fluid overload or bronchospasm
- Neurologic exam:
  - Anterior cerebral artery: motor/sensory deficit: (leg > face/arm), gait apraxia; abulia (inability to act willfully)
  - Middle cerebral artery (MCA):
    ○ Dominant: aphasia (inability to speak); motor/sensory deficit (face > arm > leg > foot); homonymous hemianopia
    ○ Nondominant: neglect, motor/sensory deficit (face/arm > leg > foot), homonymous hemianopia
  - Posterior cerebral artery: homonymous hemianopia; visual hallucinations; visual palsies; motor/sensory deficits; alexia (inability to read—"word blindness") without agraphia (inability to write)
  - Posterior (vertebrobasilar) circulation: diplopia, vertigo, gait and limb ataxia, facial paresis, Horner syndrome, dysphagia, dysarthria, alternating sensory loss
- The three most predictive findings for stroke on physical examination are: (i) facial paresis, (ii) arm weakness or drift, and (iii) abnormal speech.
- National Institutes of Health Stroke Scale (NIHSS): stroke.nih.gov/documents/NIH_Stroke_Scale_508C.pdf

DIFFERENTIAL DIAGNOSIS
- Migraine (complicated)
- Postictal state (Todd paralysis)
- Systemic infection, including meningitis or encephalitis (Infection may uncover or enhance previous deficits.)
- Toxic or metabolic disturbance (hypoglycemia, acute renal failure, liver failure, drug intoxication)
- Brain tumor, primary or metastases
- Head trauma, encephalopathy, septic emboli (2)
- Other types of intracranial hemorrhage (epidural, subdural, subarachnoid)

DIAGNOSTIC TESTS & INTERPRETATION
Used to narrow differential and identify etiology of stroke

Initial Tests (lab, imaging)
- Serum glucose (REQUIRED to exclude hypo-/hyperglycemia prior to IV alteplase)
- Electrocardiogram (ECG)
- CBC; electrolyte panel; baseline troponin
- Coagulation studies: PT, PTT, INR
- Emergent noncontrast head CT, within 20 minutes of arrival to the emergency department (ED)
- Subsequent multimodal CT (perfusion CT, CTA, unenhanced CT) or MRI improves diagnosis of acute ischemic stroke (AIS).

Follow-Up Tests & Special Considerations
Consider LFT, toxicology screen, blood alcohol, ABG, lumbar puncture if suspected subarachnoid hemorrhage (SAH); EEG if suspect seizures, blood type and cross
- Diffusion-weighted MRI (DW-MRI) is more sensitive than CT for AIS.
- MRI is better than CT for posterior fossa lesions.
- Prior to IV tissue plasminogen activator (tPA), a noncontrast head CT (rule out ICH) and glucose are the only required tests unless contraindications exist. MRI is not required.
- Multimodal imaging studies should not delay IV tPA.
- For patients who meet criteria for thrombectomy, multimodal CT and MRI to rule out large vessel occlusion is recommended. Selected patients may be treated up to 16 to 24 hours after onset of symptoms.

Diagnostic Procedures/Other
Echocardiogram (transthoracic and/or transesophageal) if there is suspicion for cardioembolic source. In cryptogenic stroke patients, perform prolonged ECG monitoring with a 30-day event monitor.

Test Interpretation
Early CT findings of ischemia: hyperdense MCA sign (increased attenuation of proximal portion of the MCA; associated with MCA thrombosis), loss of gray-white matter differentiation, sulcal effacement

 TREATMENT

- Monitor BP closely in the first 24 hours.
  - Withhold antihypertensives unless systolic BP >220 mm Hg or diastolic BP >120 mm Hg. Goal is to lower BP ~15% in the first 24 hours if treatment is undertaken. If thrombolytic therapy is planned, BP must be <185/110 mm Hg prior to administration of thrombolytics (4).
  - In acute spontaneous intracranial hemorrhagic stroke, goal BP is 160/90 mm Hg or MAP of 110.
  - If there is suspicion of elevated ICP, reduce BP to a target cerebral perfusion pressure of between 61 mm Hg and 80 mm Hg.
  - Start/restart antihypertensive medications 24 hours after stroke onset for patients with BP >140/90 mm Hg who are neurologically stable.

ALERT
Thrombolysis: Individualize discussion about the use of IV thrombolysis with eligible patients who have measurable neurologic deficits that do not clear spontaneously and present within 3.0 to 4.5 hours of symptom onset.

- Exclusion criteria for thrombolysis within 3 hours of onset include the following:
  - History of ICH/ symptoms suggestive of ICH
  - Head trauma, MI or prior stroke within 3 months
  - GI malignancy or bleed within 21 days
  - Major surgery within 14 days
  - Arterial puncture at noncompressible site within 7 days

– Elevated BP (systolic >185 mm Hg and diastolic >110 mm Hg)

– Active bleeding or evidence of acute trauma

– Taking anticoagulant and INR ≥1.7

– Low-molecular-weight heparin received during previous 24 hours; platelet count <100,000 mm^3

– Blood glucose concentration <50 mg/dL

– Seizure with postictal neurologic impairment

– Multilobar infarction on CT (hypodensity >1/3 cerebral hemisphere)

– Patient/family members unable to provide input and understand potential risk/benefits of treatment

• Extended AHA/ASA exclusion criteria for thrombolysis within 4.5 hours include:

– Age >80 years

– All patients taking oral anticoagulants

– NIHSS >25

– History of stroke and diabetes

MEDICATION

First Line

• Thrombolysis, IV administration of rtPA: Infuse 0.9 mg/kg, maximum dose 90 mg over 60 minutes with 10% of dose given as bolus over 1 minute. There is no benefit for patients with mild, nondisabling stroke symptoms (NIHSS score 0 to 5) (4).

– Door-to-needle time of <60 minutes

– Admit to ICU or stroke unit, with neurologic exams every 15 minutes during infusion, every 30 minutes for next 6 hours, and then hourly until 24 hours after treatment.

– Discontinue infusion and obtain emergent CT scan if severe headache, angioedema, acute HTN, or nausea and vomiting develop.

– Measure BP every 15 minutes for first 2 hours, every 30 minutes for next 6 hours, and then every hour until 24 hours after treatment. Maintain BP <185/105 mm Hg; follow-up CT before starting anticoagulants or antiplatelet agents

• Antiplatelet: aspirin 160 to 300 mg/day within 24 to 48 hours after AIS (4)

• BP management options include:

– Labetalol 10 to 20 mg IV over 1 to 2 minutes, may be repeated once

– Nicardipine infusion 5 mg/hr, titrate 2.5 mg/hr at 5 to 15 minutes intervals to maximum of 15 mg/hr; reduce to 3 mg/hr when target BP is reached.

Second Line

Carotid endarterectomy (CEA) is indicated for >70% ipsilateral stenosis; may be indicated for 50–69% stenosis in carefully selected patients, depending on risk factors, and skill and experience of surgeons

ISSUES FOR REFERRAL

Follow-up with neurologist 1 week after discharge

ADDITIONAL THERAPIES

• If no contraindications, consider a trial of fluoxetine to improve motor outcomes (5)[A].

• Deep vein thrombosis (DVT) prophylaxis

• Corticosteroids are *not* recommended for cerebral brain edema.

• Continued statin following acute stroke

• Refer to PT, OT, and speech therapy as necessary.

SURGERY/OTHER PROCEDURES

• Ventricular drain for patients with acute hydrocephalus secondary to stroke

• Decompressive surgery is recommended for major cerebellar infarction.

• Endovascular thrombectomy (EVT) is an effective treatment for AIS patients up to 16 to 24 hours after the event (6).

COMPLEMENTARY & ALTERNATIVE MEDICINE

Acupuncture within 30 days of stroke onset may improve neurologic functioning.

ADMISSION, INPATIENT, AND NURSING CONSIDERATIONS

• Observe closely with frequent neurologic exams in first 24 hours for neurologic decline, particularly due to cerebral edema.

• Elevate bed to at least 30 degrees if elevated ICP is suspected. Patients with ischemic stroke may benefit from a horizontal bed position during the acute phase.

• Monitor cardiac rhythm for at least 24 hours to identify arrhythmias.

• Airway support and ventilatory assistance may be necessary due to diminished consciousness or bulbar involvement; reserve supplemental oxygen for hypoxic patients. Consider elective intubation for patients with malignant edema.

• Maintain oxygen saturation >94%.

• Correct hypovolemia with normal saline.

• Keep patients NPO until a formal swallow evaluation has been performed; to reduce risk of aspiration pneumonia, elevate head of bed to 30 degrees.

• Maintenance IV hydration with normal saline until swallowing status is assessed

• Hypoglycemia (especially <60 mg/dL) can cause neurologic dysfunction; correct initially.

• Hyperglycemia within first 24 hours of stroke is associated with poor outcomes: insulin recommended to maintain glucose levels 140 to 180 mg/dL.

• In patients with ICH secondary to anticoagulant use, correct an elevated INR with IV vitamin K and fresh frozen plasma or prothrombin concentrate complex.

• DVT prophylaxis

• Early PT and discharge planning for rehabilitation and placement

• Fall precautions; frequent repositioning to prevent skin breakdown

• Discharge criteria: medically stable, adequate nutritional support, neurologic status stable

• COVID-19 has been linked with hypercoagulability, with elevated D-dimer and fibrinogen levels that may explain a rise in stroke, although patients with severe disease are often older with other comorbidities that increase their risk as well.

• Admissions for mild and severe strokes have decreased since the COVID-19 pandemic, likely multifactorial, may be related to improved hygiene preventing against other infections linked to stroke or patient reluctance to visit the ED due to fear of exposure to SARS-CoV-2 virus.

ONGOING CARE

FOLLOW-UP RECOMMENDATIONS

• Secondary prevention of stroke with aggressive management of risk factors

• Platelet inhibition using aspirin, clopidogrel, or aspirin plus extended-release dipyridamole (Aggrenox) based on physician and patient preference

• Stroke-like symptoms within 2 weeks of the initial event have a high chance of being recurrent stroke and should be followed up within 24 hours (6).

Patient Monitoring

Follow-up every 3 months for 1st year and then annually

DIET

Patients with impaired swallowing should receive nasogastric or percutaneous endoscopic gastrostomy feedings to maintain nutrition and hydration.

PATIENT EDUCATION

National Stroke Association (800-STROKES or http://www.stroke.org)

PROGNOSIS

Variable depends on subtype and severity of stroke; NIHSS may be used for prognosis.

COMPLICATIONS

• Acute: brain herniation, hemorrhagic transformation, MI, CHF, dysphagia, aspiration pneumonia, UTI, DVT, pulmonary embolism, malnutrition, pressure sores

• Chronic: falls, depression, dementia, orthopedic complications, contractures, OSA

REFERENCES

1. Hankey GJ. Stroke. *Lancet*. 2017;389(10069): 641–654.
2. Yew KS, Cheng EM. Diagnosis of acute stroke. *Am Fam Physician*. 2015;91(8):528–536.
3. Kleindorfer DO, Towfighi A, Chaturvedi S, et al. 2021 Guideline for the prevention of stroke in patients with stroke and transient ischemic attack: a guideline from the American Heart Association/American Stroke Association. *Stroke*. 2021;52(7):e364–e467.
4. Powers WJ, Rabinstein AA, Ackerson T, et al; for American Heart Association. Guidelines for the early management of patients with acute ischemic stroke: 2019 update to the 2018 guidelines for the early management of acute ischemic stroke: a guideline for healthcare professionals from the American Heart Association/American Stroke Association. *Stroke*. 2019;50(12):e344–418.
5. Chollet F, Tardy J, Albucher JF, et al. Fluoxetine for motor recovery after acute ischaemic stroke (FLAME): a randomised placebo-controlled trial. *Lancet Neurol*. 2011;10(2):123–130.
6. Boulanger JM, Lindsay MP, Gubitz G, et al. Canadian stroke best practice recommendations for acute stroke management: Prehospital, Emergency Department, and Acute Inpatient Stroke Care, 6th Edition, Update 2018. *Int J Stroke*. 2018;13(9):949–984.

CODES

ICD10

• I63.9 Cerebral infarction, unspecified

• I61.9 Nontraumatic intracerebral hemorrhage, unspecified

• I63.50 Cereb infrc due to unsp occls or stenos of unsp cereb artery

CLINICAL PEARLS

• Unless stroke is hemorrhagic or patient is undergoing thrombolysis, do not lower BP acutely. This helps to maintain perfusion of penumbra region.

• Consider IV thrombolysis in eligible patients with neurologic deficits that do not clear spontaneously within 3.0 to 4.5 hours of symptom onset.

• DW-MRI is more sensitive than conventional CT for the diagnosis of AIS. MRI is also superior for diagnosing posterior fossa lesions.

S

SUBCONJUNCTIVAL HEMORRHAGE

Nisarg Joshi, MD, BS • Ankur Sudhir Gupta, MD, MS

 BASICS

DESCRIPTION

- Subconjunctival hemorrhage (SCH) is bleeding from small blood vessels underneath the conjunctiva, the thin clear skin covering the sclera (white part) of the eye.
- SCH is diagnosed clinically:
  - Well-demarcated areas of extravasated blood can be seen just under the surface of the conjunctiva of the eye.
  - Lesions can be flat, elevated, or bullous.
- Typically, SCH self-resolves in 1 to 3 weeks depending on the severity.

EPIDEMIOLOGY

- Male = female; no gender predilection
- Common; 3% rate of diagnosis in ophthalmology clinics (1)

Incidence

Incidence increases
- With increasing age
- In contact lenses wearers (5% of cases) (2)
- With systemic diseases such as diabetes, hypertension (HTN), and coagulation disorders
- With trauma
- During summer months, possibly due to trauma (1)

ETIOLOGY AND PATHOPHYSIOLOGY

- SCH results from damage to conjunctival and episcleral vessels from direct or indirect injury.
- Anti-thrombogenic and anti-coagulated states (blood dyscrasias, thrombocytopenia, anemia, anti-platelet use, anti-coagulant use) increase the risk and severity of SCH.
- Causes include the following:
  - Idiopathic (most common cause)
  - Direct trauma from
    - Blunt or penetrating injury to the eye
    - Contact lenses placement or removal; improper contact lenses wear
    - Rubbing eyes
    - Foreign body in eye
    - Ocular surgery, injection, or other procedure

- Valsalva maneuvers causing sudden severe venous congestion such as coughing, sneezing, vomiting, straining, severe asthma or COPD exacerbation, weightlifting, or childbirth/labor
  - Damaged vessels from atherosclerotic disease or diabetes (which is a cause of recurrent SCH without trauma)
- In patients age >60 years, HTN is the most common etiology.
- In patients age <40 years, trauma, Valsalva, and contact lenses use are the most common etiologies.
- In patients age >40 years, conjunctivochalasis (redundant conjunctival folds) and presence of pinguecula are strongly associated (2).

RISK FACTORS

- Trauma
- Age
- Contact lenses wearer
- Systemic diseases (HTN, diabetes)
- Bleeding disorders (1)
- Recent ocular surgery (cataract, laser-assisted in situ keratomileusis [LASIK])

GENERAL PREVENTION

- Avoid rubbing eyes.
- Proper cleaning and maintenance of contact lenses
- Protective eyewear in sports and hobbies
- Optimizing control of systemic diseases such as HTN, diabetes, atherosclerotic disease, and thrombocytopenia
- Control of PT/INR in patients on warfarin therapy (3)

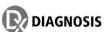 **DIAGNOSIS**

HISTORY

- Usually, the patient notices redness in the mirror or another person mentions it to the patient.
- Generally, patients do not have ocular symptoms.
- May complain of mild irritation or foreign body sensation

- Obtain history of trauma, recent ocular surgery, rubbing eyes, contact lenses use, heavy Valsalva maneuvers (coughing, straining going to the bathroom, lifting heavy objects, etc.) (1). SCH can occur 12 to 24 hours after orbital fracture (4).
- Evaluate medical history of systemic disease like diabetes mellitus, HTN, and coagulopathy.
- Ask about medications that may increase risk: aspirin, clopidogrel, other anti-platelets, anti-coagulants.
- Obtain history of other systemic symptomatology.

PHYSICAL EXAM

- Visual acuity, intra-ocular pressure, and pupils should be unaffected (3).
- Slit lamp exam shows bright red well-demarcated spots or patches. They are more often inferior due to gravity (2).
- Lesions can be flat, elevated, or bullous.
- The color of the conjunctiva changes over time. When the blood newly accumulates, the color is bright red. Older blood has a darker red color. The conjunctiva may have a yellow hue from blood-breakdown products as the hemorrhage dissipates.
- Fluorescein can be applied to assess for conjunctival and cornea abrasions/lacerations. Under cobalt blue light, there should be no stain uptake with a simple SCH.
- If the conjunctiva was lacerated, drops of blood can extrude from the conjunctiva onto the eyelid and periorbital skin.
- If a foreign body was involved, it could be hidden by the SCH.
- If there is concern for penetrating or perforating ocular trauma, a shield should be placed over the eye and the patient should be evaluated emergently by an ophthalmologist and/or trauma team.
- Measure blood pressure to evaluate for uncontrolled HTN (1).

Geriatric Considerations

In older adults, the area of SCH will be more widespread across the sclera (2). Elastic and connective tissues are more fragile with age, and underlying conditions such as HTN and diabetes may contribute.

DIFFERENTIAL DIAGNOSIS
- Viral, bacterial, allergic, or chemical conjunctivitis (enterovirus and coxsackievirus most common) (4)[B]
- Foreign body in/on the conjunctiva
- Penetrating or perforating trauma
- Recent ocular surgery/injection
- Contact lenses-induced
- Child abuse (particularly if bilateral in an infant or toddler) (4)
- Occasionally found in newborns following vaginal delivery

DIAGNOSTIC TESTS & INTERPRETATION
- Typically no testing is indicated; SCH is a clinical diagnosis. If a foreign body is suspected, perform a fluorescein exam.
- Fluorescein exam of a patient with an SCH should show no uptake of fluorescein (3)[C].
- If an orbital fracture is suspected, an orbital/maxillofacial CT may be obtained (5)[C].

Follow-Up Tests & Special Considerations
If history and physical exam suggest a bleeding disorder (3)[C]
- CBC
- PT/INR

ALERT
- If a penetrating injury is suspected, may obtain a CT scan of the orbits
- Do not perform MRI because the foreign object may be metallic (5)[C].

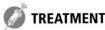 **TREATMENT**
- Reassurance is important.
- SCH self-resolves with time.
- Artificial tears can be used four times a day as needed for eye irritation (3)[C].

GENERAL MEASURES
- Control BP.
- Control blood glucose.
- Control INR.
- Wear protective eyewear.

ISSUES FOR REFERRAL
- If there is a history of any significant trauma, even blunt trauma, seek emergent ophthalmology consultation.
- If the patient complains of any decreased visual acuity or visual disturbances (i.e., new floaters), refer to an ophthalmologist as soon as possible.
- If there is no resolution of SCH within 2 weeks or if SCH is recurrent, patient may need referral to an ophthalmologist.

 ONGOING CARE

FOLLOW-UP RECOMMENDATIONS
- Follow up only if the area does not resolve in about 2 weeks.
- If SCH recurs, then work up patient for systemic sources such as bleeding disorders (3)[C] or diabetes.

PATIENT EDUCATION
- Reassurance of the self-limited nature of the problem and typical time frame for resolution
- Education to return to clinic if the area does not heal or recurs
- Correct cleaning and maintenance of contact lenses
- Eye lubricants for ocular irritation

PROGNOSIS
Excellent

COMPLICATIONS
Rare

REFERENCES
1. Mimura T, Usui T, Yamagami S, et al. Recent causes of subconjunctival hemorrhage. *Ophthalmologica.* 2010;224(3):133–137.
2. Mimura T, Yamagami S, Mori M, et al. Contact lens-induced subconjunctival hemorrhage. *Am J Ophthalmol.* 2010;150(5):656.e1–665.e1.
3. Cronau H, Kankanala RR, Mauger T. Diagnosis and management of red eye in primary care. *Am Fam Physician.* 2010;81(2):137–144.
4. Tarlan B, Kiratli H. Subconjunctival hemorrhage: risk factors and potential indicators. *Clin Ophthalmol.* 2013;7:1163–1170.
5. Wirbelauer C. Management of the red eye for the primary care physician. *Am J Med.* 2006;119(4):302–306.

 CODES

ICD10
- H11.30 Conjunctival hemorrhage, unspecified eye
- H11.31 Conjunctival hemorrhage, right eye
- H11.32 Conjunctival hemorrhage, left eye

CLINICAL PEARLS
- SCH is a clinical diagnosis. The condition is typically asymptomatic and will self-resolve within 2 weeks.
- Risk factors include trauma, intense Valsalva, HTN, and diabetes.
- Indications for immediate referral to an ophthalmologist include eye pain, changes in vision, lack of pupil reactivity, and/or suspected penetrating eye injury.
- Reassurance and comfort measures (i.e., ocular lubrication) are mainstays of treatment.

S

SUBSTANCE USE DISORDERS

S. Lindsey Clarke, MD, FAAFP • Benjamin J. Velky, MD

 BASICS

DESCRIPTION

Any pattern of substance use causing significant physical, mental, or social dysfunction

- Substances of abuse include:
  - Alcohol
  - Tobacco
  - Prescription medications
    - Opioids and morphine derivatives (buprenorphine, codeine, fentanyl, hydrocodone, hydromorphone, meperidine, methadone, morphine, oxycodone, oxymorphone)
    - CNS depressants (barbiturates, benzodiazepines, hypnotics)
    - Stimulants (amphetamines, methylphenidate)
    - Dextromethorphan ("Robo-tripping")
  - Cannabis (marijuana, hashish, cannabis oil, and extracts); also sold as highly concentrated extracts (up to 90% THC) for use in vaporizers
  - Synthetic cannabinoids (Spice, K2, fake weed); often much more potent than marijuana; may be smoked, brewed in tea, or vaporized
  - Stimulants (cocaine, amphetamines, methamphetamines, Khat)
  - "Club drugs" (MDMA [ecstasy, Molly], PMMA [Superman], flunitrazepam, γ-hydroxybutyrate [GHB])
  - Opioids (heroin, opium, kratom, carfentanil, desomorphine [Krokodil], U-47700 [Pink])
  - Dissociative drugs (ketamine, phencyclidine [PCP], tenocyclidine [TCP])
  - Hallucinogens (lysergic acid diethylamide [LSD], salvia, ayahuasca, N,N-dimethyltryptamine [DMT])
  - Synthetic cathinones (bath salts, α-PVP [Flakka])
  - Inhalants (glue, paint thinners, nitrous oxide)
- Synonym(s): drug abuse; drug dependence; substance abuse

Geriatric Considerations
- Alcohol is the most commonly abused substance, and abuse often goes unrecognized.
- Higher potential for drug interactions

Pregnancy Considerations
Substance abuse may cause fetal abnormalities, morbidity, and fetal or maternal death.

ALERT
The prevalence of opioid use in pregnancy and associated neonatal abstinence syndrome have increased significantly in recent years. Screen for substance use at the first prenatal visit with a brief intervention and refer for treatment to improve maternal and neonatal outcomes (1)[C].

EPIDEMIOLOGY

Incidence
- Predominant age: 18 to 25 years
- Predominant sex: male > female

Prevalence
- 57.2 million Americans (20.8%) reported illicit drug use in the past year in 2019.
- 17.2% of 12- to 17-year-olds; 39.1% of 18- to 25-year-olds
- 1 in 3 (35.4%) young adults were past year users of marijuana.
- 70.6% of drug overdose deaths in 2019 were opioid related.

ETIOLOGY AND PATHOPHYSIOLOGY
Multifactorial, including genetic, environmental

Genetics
Substances of abuse affect dopamine, acetylcholine, γ-aminobutyric acid, norepinephrine, opioid, and serotonin receptors. Variant alleles may account for differences in susceptibility to misuse of different substances.

RISK FACTORS
- Male gender, young adult
- Depression, anxiety
- Family history
- Peer or family use or approval; family dysfunction or trauma
- Low socioeconomic status; unemployment
- Accessibility of substances of abuse
- Antisocial personality disorder
- Academic problems, school dropout
- Criminal involvement

GENERAL PREVENTION
- Early identification and aggressive early intervention improve outcomes.
- Universal school-based interventions are modestly effective for preventing drug use among adolescents.

COMMONLY ASSOCIATED CONDITIONS
- Depression; bipolar affective disorder
- Personality disorders

ALERT
Prescription narcotic overdose is the leading cause of accidental death in patients between the ages of 23 and 45 years in the United States.

- Many states require naloxone to be prescribed or offered when issuing a prescription of opioids to patients at increased risk of overdose, such as those receiving ≥50 morphine milligram equivalents per day of an opioid, those taking both opioids and benzodiazepines, and those with a history of substance abuse.

DIAGNOSIS

Substance use disorder (*DSM-5* criteria): ≥2 of the following in past year severity based on number of criteria present:

- Missed work or school
- Use in hazardous situations
- Continued use despite social or personal problems
- Craving
- Tolerance (decreased response to effects of drug due to constant exposure)
- Withdrawal on discontinuation
- Using more than intended
- Failed attempts to quit
- Increased time spent obtaining, using, or recovering from the substance
- Interference with important activities
- Continued use despite health problems

HISTORY
- History of infections (e.g., endocarditis, hepatitis B or C, HIV, TB, HIV, STI, or recurrent pneumonia)
- Social or behavioral problems, including chaotic relationships and/or employment difficulties
- Frequent visits to emergency department
- Criminal incarceration
- History of blackouts, insomnia, mood swings, chronic pain, repetitive trauma
- Anxiety, fatigue, depression, psychosis

PHYSICAL EXAM
- Vital sign abnormalities (changes in HR, RR, BP, and temperature all manifest with substance misuse)
- Abnormally dilated or constricted pupils
- Cutaneous needle marks
- Nasal septum perforation (with cocaine use)
- Cardiac dysrhythmias, pathologic murmurs
- Malnutrition with severe dependence
- Mental status examination

DIFFERENTIAL DIAGNOSIS
- Depression, anxiety, or other behavioral conditions
- Metabolic delirium (hypoxia, hypoglycemia, infection, thiamine deficiency, hypothyroidism, thyrotoxicosis)
- ADHD
- Medication toxicity

DIAGNOSTIC TESTS & INTERPRETATION

ALERT
USPSTF recommends screening adults ≥18 years for unhealthy drug use when appropriate diagnosis and treatment services can be provided. USPSTF found insufficient evidence for or against such screening in adolescents (2)[A].

- Substance Use Brief Screen and single-question screening tools (e.g., "How many times in the past year have you used an illegal drug or used a prescription medication for nonmedical reasons?") have high sensitivity (71–100%) and specificity (61–96%) for identifying problem use in hospital and primary care settings (3)[A].
- CRAFFT questionnaire (sensitivity 94% with ≥2 "yes" answers):
  - C: Have you ever ridden in a CAR driven by someone (including yourself) who was "high" or who had been using alcohol or drugs?
  - R: Do you ever use alcohol or drugs to RELAX, feel better about yourself, or fit in?
  - A: Do you ever use alcohol or drugs while you are ALONE?
  - F: Do you ever FORGET things you did while using alcohol or drugs?
  - F: Do your FAMILY or FRIENDS ever tell you that you should cut down on your drinking or drug use?
  - T: Have you gotten into TROUBLE while you were using alcohol or drugs?
- American Academy of Pediatrics also recommends the following brief screening tools for adolescents:
  - Screening to Brief Intervention (S2B1)
  - Brief Screener for Tobacco, Alcohol, and Other Drugs (BSTAD)

Initial Tests (lab, imaging)
- Blood alcohol concentration
- Urine drug screen (UDS) (Order qualitative UDS and, if specific drug is in question, a quantitative analysis for specific drug; order confirmatory serum tests if false positive suspected)
- Standard screening immunoassays may miss synthetic cannabinoids and opioids.
- Approximate detection limits
  - Alcohol: 6 to 10 hours
  - Amphetamines and variants: 2 to 3 days
  - Barbiturates: 2 to 10 days
  - Benzodiazepines: 1 to 6 weeks
  - Cocaine: 2 to 3 days
  - Heroin: 1 to 1.5 days
  - LSD, psilocybin: 8 hours
  - Marijuana: 1 to 7 days; up to 1 month with chronic/heavy use

– Methadone: 1 day to 1 week
– Opioids: 1 to 3 days
– PCP: 7 to 14 days
– Anabolic steroids: oral, 3 weeks; injectable, 3 months; nandrolone, 9 months
- Liver transaminases
- HIV, hepatitis B and C screens

Follow-Up Tests & Special Considerations
- Blood cultures, echocardiogram for endocarditis
- Head CT scan for seizure, delirium, trauma
- Right upper quadrant abdominal ultrasound for cirrhosis

 ## TREATMENT

Determine substances abused early (may influence disposition).

GENERAL MEASURES
- Treatment should combine pharmacotherapy and cognitive-behavioral therapy or another evidence-based modality such as motivational enhancement therapy or contingency management when applicable (4)[A].
- Nonjudgmental, medically oriented attitude
- Motivational interviewing and brief interventions can overcome denial and promote change.
- Community reinforcement
- Interventional counseling
- Self-help groups to aid recovery (Alcoholics Anonymous, other 12-step programs)
- Support groups for family (Al-Anon/Alateen)

MEDICATION
- Alcohol withdrawal: See "Alcohol Use Disorder (AUD)" and "Alcohol Withdrawal."
- Benzodiazepine or barbiturate withdrawal
  – Gradual taper preferable to abrupt discontinuation
  – Substitution of long-acting benzodiazepine (e.g., clonazepam) or phenobarbital
- Nicotine withdrawal: See "Tobacco Use and Smoking Cessation."
- Opioid dependence
  – Buprenorphine: 8 to 24 mg SL daily, 100 to 300 mg SC monthly or as 6-month subdermal implant; may precipitate a more severe withdrawal if initiated too soon; use restricted to licensed clinics and certified physicians (5)[A],(6)[A]
  – Buprenorphine/naloxone: 2/0.5 to 16/4 mg SL daily; available as SL tabs and films and buccal films; combination limits abuse potential compared with buprenorphine alone.
  – Methadone: 10 to 40 mg/day PO; use restricted to inpatient settings and especially licensed clinics (5)[A],(6)[A]
  – Naltrexone: 50 mg PO daily, 100 mg PO every 2 days, 150 mg PO every 3 days, or 380 mg IM every 4 weeks; must be opioid-free for 7 to 10 days prior to treatment to avoid precipitating withdrawal
  – Naloxone: For opioid overdose 0.4 to 2.0 mg IV/IM/SC, repeat every 2 to 3 minutes as needed; intranasal 4 to 8 mg, repeat every 2 to 3 minutes as needed. Refer to state mandates for co-prescribing with opioid medications.
- Opioid withdrawal
  – Clonidine: 0.1 to 0.2 mg PO BID or TID for autonomic hyperactivity (5)[A]
  – Tramadol ER: 100 to 300 mg PO daily, then taper (off label) (5)[B]
- Stimulant withdrawal
  – No agent with clear benefit for withdrawal

– Methylphenidate ER: titrated up to 54 mg/day PO might enhance abstinence in amphetamine-dependent patients
- Adjuncts to therapy
  – Use all medications in conjunction with psychosocial behavioral interventions.
  – Antiemetics, nonaddictive analgesics for opioid withdrawal
  – Nonhabituating antidepressants, mood stabilizers, anxiolytics, and hypnotics for comorbid mood, anxiety, and sleep disorders that persist after detoxification
- Contraindications
  – Buprenorphine in breastfeeding, hepatic impairment
  – Methadone in hepatic impairment
  – Naltrexone in pregnancy, breastfeeding, hepatic impairment
- Precautions: Clonidine can cause hypotension.
- Significant possible interactions
  – Buprenorphine and opioids, CNS depressants, or HIV protease inhibitors
  – Methadone and opioids, CNS depressants, or strong inhibitors of CYP3A4 (clarithromycin, ketoconazole, HIV protease inhibitors)
  – Naltrexone and opioid medications (may induce or exacerbate withdrawal)

ISSUES FOR REFERRAL
- Consider addiction specialist, especially for opioid and polysubstance abuse.
- Psychiatrist for comorbid psychiatric disorders
- Social services

ADMISSION, INPATIENT, AND NURSING CONSIDERATIONS
- Indications for inpatient detoxification
  – History of severe withdrawal (e.g., seizures)
  – Mental status changes; hallucinations or psychotic features
  – Threat of harm to self or others
  – Obstacles to close monitoring/follow-up
  – Comorbid medical illness
  – Pregnancy
- Look for signs of infection (e.g., bacterial endocarditis).

 ## ONGOING CARE

FOLLOW-UP RECOMMENDATIONS
Initially frequent visits to monitor for medical stability and adherence and then progressive follow-up intervals

Patient Monitoring
Verify patient's adherence with the substance abuse treatment program.

DIET
Patients often are malnourished.

PATIENT EDUCATION
- Substance Abuse and Mental Health Services Administration: https://www.samhsa.gov or 800-662-HELP (4357) for information, treatment facility locator
- National Institute on Drug Abuse: http://www.drugabuse.gov/patients-families
- Alcoholics Anonymous: http://www.aa.org
- Narcotics Anonymous: http://www.na.org

PROGNOSIS
- Patients in treatment for longer periods have higher success rates.
- Behavioral therapy and pharmacotherapy are most successful when used in combination.

COMPLICATIONS
- Serious harm to self and others: accidents, violence
- Overdoses resulting in seizures, arrhythmias, cardiac and respiratory arrest, coma, death
- Cirrhosis, hepatic malignancy, hepatitis, HIV, tuberculosis, syphilis
- Subacute bacterial endocarditis
- Malnutrition
- Social problems, including arrest, poor marital adjustment and violence
- Depression, schizophrenia
- Sexual assault (alcohol, flunitrazepam, GHB)

REFERENCES

1. Committee on Obstetric Practice. Committee Opinion No. 711: opioid use and opioid use disorder in pregnancy. *Obstet Gynecol*. 2017;130(2):e81–e94.
2. Krist AH, Davidson KW, Mangione CM, et al; for U.S. Preventive Services Task Force. Screening for unhealthy drug use: US Preventive Services Task Force recommendation statement. *JAMA*. 2020;323(22):2301–2309.
3. Han BH, Sherman SE, Link AR, et al. Comparison of the Substance Use Brief Screen (SUBS) to the AUDIT-C and ASSIST for detecting unhealthy alcohol and drug use in a population of hospitalized smokers. *J Subst Abuse Treat*. 2017;79:67–74.
4. Ray LA, Meredith LR, Kiluk BD, et al. Combined pharmacotherapy and cognitive behavioral therapy for adults with alcohol or substance use disorders: a systematic review and meta-analysis. *JAMA Netw Open*. 2020;3(6):e208279.
5. Srivastava AB, Mariani JJ, Levin FR. New directions in the treatment of opioid withdrawal. *Lancet*. 2020;395(10241):1938–1948.
6. Gowing L, Ali R, White JM, et al. Buprenorphine for managing opioid withdrawal. *Cochrane Database Syst Rev*. 2017;(2):CD002025.

 ## SEE ALSO

Alcohol Use Disorder (AUD); Alcohol Withdrawal; Tobacco Use and Smoking Cessation

 ## CODES

ICD10
- F18.951 Inhalant use, unspecified with inhalant-induced psychotic disorder with hallucinations
- F11.120 Opioid abuse with intoxication, uncomplicated
- F17.201 Nicotine dependence, unspecified, in remission

CLINICAL PEARLS
- Substance use disorders are prevalent, serious, and often unrecognized in clinical practice. Comorbid psychiatric disorders are common.
- Substance abuse is distinguished by family, social, occupational, legal, or physical dysfunction that is caused by persistent use of the substance.
- Dependence is characterized by tolerance, withdrawal, compulsive use, and repeated overindulgence.
- Treatment should combine pharmacotherapy and cognitive-behavioral therapy or another evidence-based modality when applicable.
- Consider referring patients with alcohol or opioid dependence to an addiction specialist or treatment program.

S

SUICIDE

Harold J. Bursztajn, MD • Irene Coletsos, MD

BASICS

DESCRIPTION
Suicide and attempted suicide are significant causes of morbidity and mortality.

EPIDEMIOLOGY
- Predominant sex
  - Women *attempt* suicide 1.5 times more often than men. Men *complete* suicide 3 times more often than women. Men are more likely to choose a means with high lethality, such as firearms.
- In the United States: predominant age: adolescence through age 34 (2nd leading cause of death), 11th leading cause of death overall, per 2019 Centers for Disease Control and Prevention (CDC) (latest available)
- Worldwide, suicide is the 4th leading cause of death among youths (age 15 to 29), 17th leading cause of death per World Health Organization (WHO) reports from 2019.

Incidence
The COVID-19 pandemic—with its lockdowns, school closures, excess deaths (3rd leading cause in the United States) in 2020—led to concerns for a possible "tidal wave" of suicides. While initial data from WHO and CDC for 2020 showed an overall decrease in completed suicides, several early U.S. studies showed 27% to a doubling of suicides in non-whites during this period (1).

RISK FACTORS
- "Human understanding is the most effective weapon against suicide. The greatest need is to deepen the awareness and sensitivity of people to their fellow man" (Shneidman; American Association of Suicidology [AAS]).
- Be alert to a combination of increased emotional disturbance and access to the potential tools to cause death).
- 80% who complete suicide had a previous attempt.
- 90% who complete suicide meet *Diagnostic and Statistical Manual* criteria for major depression, bipolar disorder, anorexia, panic, personality disorders. Schizophrenia or acute onset of psychosis are also risk factors due to command hallucinations and hopelessness that can accompany these states.
- Substance use and withdrawal
- Family history of suicide
- Physical illness, including head injury (associated with 20% increased risk of death by suicide) (2)
- Despair: emotional pain *and* without hope; feeling unworthy of help
- For teenagers: not feeling "connected" to their peers or family; being bullied; gender identity issues; poor grades
- Among veterans: childhood abuse; major depression; multiple psychiatric hospitalizations are the best predictors of suicide risk (3).

- Psychosocial: recent loss. What may seem to be a small loss may be a devastating for the patient. *Patient-specific* factors need to be taken into account including anniversaries and holidays. Providers should inquire how COVID-19 has affected them: isolation; deaths of loved ones; job loss; infection (leading to risk of "long COVID," with physical and mental health disability). Screen for impaired decision-making skills: lack of risk awareness and increased impulsivity are more common in patients who have attempted suicide (4).
- If a patient is incompetent (e.g., too delusional, too psychotic) to alert providers about the potential for suicide and appears to be at increased risk for self-harm, providers should consider hospitalizing the patient.
- Access to lethal means: firearms, poisons; including prescription and nonprescription drugs; pesticides

GENERAL PREVENTION
- Educate patients about 24/7 resources.
- Screen for risk: Use screening instruments BUT providers need to keep in mind: (i) risks particular to each patient, and might not be captured in some screening tools (see "Risk Factors" above) and (ii) providers own biases in assessing risk (e.g., in wheelchair mobile patients, assuming a lower quality of life and underestimating resilience) (5). Screening instruments include the Patient Health Questionnaire-2 (PHQ-2), the PHQ-9, the Columbia Suicide Severity Rating Scale, Beck Scale for Suicide Ideation, Linehan Reasons for Living Inventory, and Risk Estimator for Suicide.
- Treat underlying mental and medical illnesses and substance abuse.
- Screen for possession of means of harm, including prescribed/unprescribed drugs, poisons, and firearms (encourage the removal of guns from the home and the relinquishment of gun licenses).
- Create a safety plan for patients at risk and their families, including how to access 24/7 emergency care.
- Public education about how to help others access emergency psychiatric care. Suicidal people may initially confide in those they trust outside health care.
- Law enforcement education through the FBI's National Center for Analysis of Violent Crime in recognizing and triaging potential "suicide by cop" events (deliberate attempt to trigger lethal force); thought to be responsible for approximately 20% of fatal police shootings in the United States between 1998 and 2006 (2)
- For the military: multiple resources: www.realwarriors.net. Suggested treatments include cognitive restructuring techniques (that their experience with adversity can be a source of strength) and help with problem solving (so the service member does not feel like a "burden"), therapeutic martial arts training, focus on Vets' helping others: "power of 1" initiative (any "one" helpful contact could save a life).

- For teens, their families, and their educators: http://www.cdc.gov/healthyyouth; http://www.stopbullying.gov
- In developing world countries, pesticide ingestion is a common method of suicide. Limiting free access has led to reduced suicide rates.

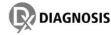

DIAGNOSIS

HISTORY
- Depressed patients should be asked about suicidal ideation and a potential plan:
  - "Have you ever felt that life isn't worth living? Do you ever wish you could go to sleep and not wake up? Are you having thoughts about killing yourself?"
- Use psychodynamic formulation: mental-state exam (including judgment, if the patient is able to able to make decisions or affected by prescribed or nonprescribed drugs/drug withdrawal), history. If the patient is experiencing a loss, or is under stress, and does not have access to a previously sustaining resource (e.g., a significant other, a pet, sports ability, a job), that patient is under increased risk for suicide.
- Prior attempts: precipitants, lethality, intent to die, precautions taken to avoid being rescued, reaction to survival (A patient who is upset that the suicide was not completed is at increased risk for a subsequent attempt.)
- History of psychiatric symptoms, substance abuse
- Also note strengths, such as reasons to live, hopes for future, social supports. A patient without these is at increased risk.
- Gather collateral history (from friends, family, physicians). Break confidentiality if patient is at imminent risk.

PHYSICAL EXAM
- Medical conditions: delirium, intoxication, withdrawal, medication side effects
- Psychosis
- In adults: See "Risk Factors."
- In teens: may not appear to be depressed; therefore, screen for risk factors: substance abuse, bullying and social isolation (commonly through electronic media), poor grades

DIFFERENTIAL DIAGNOSIS
Suicidal threats and gestures need to be immediately triaged to assess patient safety, although in some cases, the threat could be an attempt to manipulate others, such as in the case of personality disorders.

DIAGNOSTIC TESTS & INTERPRETATION

Diagnostic Procedures/Other

During any assessment:

- PHQ-9: www.med.umich.edu/1info/FHP/practiceguides/depress/score.pdf
- Columbia Suicide Severity Rating Scale (clinical instructions): https://cssrs.columbia.edu/wp-content/uploads/C-SSRS_Pediatric-SLC_11.14.16.pdf
- Suicide Trigger Scale Version 3 (STS-3), which measures a patient's "ruminative flooding" (self-critical, repetitive thoughts) and "frantic hopelessness" (feeling suicide is the only choice): www.ncbi.nlm.nih.gov/pmc/articles/PMC3443232/

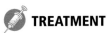 TREATMENT

GENERAL MEASURES

- Patients expressing active suicidal thoughts or who made an attempt require immediate evaluation for risk factors and a formal psychiatric consultation.
- Cognitive therapy decreased reattempt rate in prior suicide attempters by half (6),(7).
- Psychotherapy with suicidal patients is a challenge even for experienced clinicians. The countertransference, a clinician's feelings toward a patient, can evolve into wanting to be rid of the patient. If the patient detects this, the risk of suicide increases. Clinicians should be on the lookout for countertransference and get counseling if needed (8).
- Among military personnel: ACE campaign: Ask about suicidal thoughts; Care for the person, including removing access to lethal weapons; "Escort" the soldier/vet to help: an emergency room, a 911 call; call to a support hotline such as (800) 273-TALK (8255); text: 838255.

MEDICATION

- Psychopharmacology "is not a substitute for getting to know the patient" (9).
- Patients are at increased risk for suicide at the outset of antidepressant treatment and when it is discontinued. Consider tapering/switching medicines rather than sudden discontinuation. Monitor carefully.
- Anxiety, agitation, and delusions increasing in intensity should be treated aggressively.
- In the inpatient/emergency room setting, agitated or combative patients may require sedation with IV or IM benzodiazepines and/or antipsychotics.

Pediatric Considerations

FDA posted black box warning for antidepressant use in the pediatric population after increased suicidality was noted. Weigh risks vs. benefits of starting an antidepressant and closely monitor.

First Line

ECGs before prescribing or continuing antidepressants or antipsychotics to look for QT prolongation

ISSUES FOR REFERRAL

Consider a psychiatric consult. All decisions regarding treatment must be carefully documented and communicated to all involved health care providers.

ADMISSION, INPATIENT, AND NURSING CONSIDERATIONS

- Inpatient hospitalization if patient is suicidal with a plan, or otherwise at high risk; involuntary if at immediate risk
- Immediately after a suicide attempt, treat the medical problems resulting from the self-harm before initiating psychiatric care.
- Order lab work (e.g., solvent screen, blood and urine toxicology screen, aspirin and acetaminophen levels). Patients may not disclose ingestions.
- Risk for self-harm continues while inpatient: upon arrival, patients should be searched for potentially dangerous items; be on one-to-one observation; offered medication to ease symptoms. Use restraints only if necessary for patient safety.
- The period after transfer (involuntary to voluntary hospitalization; postdischarge) are times of high risk.
- Discharge criteria
  - No longer considered a danger to self/others
  - However, a patient may *claim* that he or she is no longer suicidal in order to be discharged—and complete the act. Look for signs that the patient is truly at reduced risk, such as improved appetite, sleep, engagement with staff and group therapy.
  - Provide information about 24/7 resources.

 ONGOING CARE

FOLLOW-UP RECOMMENDATIONS

Patient Monitoring

- Increase monitoring at the beginning of treatment, when changing medications, and after hospital discharge.
- Educate family and other close contact to the warning signs of suicidality (see above).
- Make sure that the patient is willing to accept recommended follow-up.
- Curtail access to firearms.
- Limit the number of pills to impulsive patients, but it might not prevent further attempts.

PATIENT EDUCATION

Patients who feel they are in danger of hurting themselves should consider one or several of these options:

- Call 911 or go directly to an emergency room.
- Contact treating therapist immediately.
- Call the National Suicide Prevention Hotline at (800) 273-TALK (8255).
- Service members and their families: Call (800) 796-9699 or call (800) 273-TALK (8255); text 838255.

PROGNOSIS

The key to a favorable prognosis is early recognition of risks, early treatment of disorders that had led to distress.

COMPLICATIONS

According to the AAS, the significant others of suicide victims may not seek help due to guilt or shame. It recommends counseling, including focus on the survivors' relationships. They may often seek out life partners to replace those they lost—interferring with mourning (W. J. Massicotte, National Scientific Program Committee, written communication, April 24, 2009).

- Sympathetic listening
- Support during holidays
- More self-help strategies: https://www.survivorsofsuicide.com

REFERENCES

1. Rabin CR. U.S. suicides reduced overall in 2020 but may have risen among people of color. http://www.NYTimes.com/2021/04/15/health/coronavirus.suicide-cdc.html. Updated September 10, 2021. Accessed September 11, 2021.
2. American Association of Suicidology: http://www.suicidology.org.
3. Koola MM, Ahmed AO, Sebastian J, et al. Childhood physical and sexual abuse predicts suicide risk in a large cohort of veterans. *Prim Care Companion CNS Disord.* 2018;20(4):18m02317.
4. Jollant F, Bellivier F, Leboyer M, et al. Impaired decision making in suicide attempters. *Am J Psychiatry.* 2005;162(2):304–310.
5. Budd MA, Haque OS, Stein MA. Biases in the evaluation of self-harm in patients with disability due to spinal cord injury. *Spinal Cord Ser Cases.* 2020;6(1):43.
6. Brown GK, Ten Have T, Henriques GR, et al. Cognitive therapy for the prevention of suicide attempts: a randomized controlled trial. *JAMA.* 2005;294(5):563–570.
7. Ghahramanlou-Holloway M, Neely L, Tucker J. A cognitive-behavioral strategy for preventing suicide. *Current Psychiatry.* 2014;13(8):18–28.
8. Maltsberger JT, Buie DH. Countertransference hate in the treatment of suicidal patients. *Arch Gen Psychiatry.* 1974;30(5):625–633.
9. Cipriani A, Pretty H, Hawton K, et al. Lithium in the prevention of suicidal behavior and all-cause mortality in patients with mood disorders: a systematic review of randomized trials. *Am J Psychiatry.* 2005;162(10):1805–1819.

ADDITIONAL READING

Gutheil TG, Bursztajn H, Brodsky A. The multidimensional assessment of dangerousness: competence assessment in patient care and liability prevention. *Bull Am Acad Psychiatry Law.* 1986;14(2):123–129.

 CODES

ICD10

- R45.851 Suicidal ideations
- T14.91 Suicide attempt
- Z91.5 Personal history of self-harm

CLINICAL PEARLS

- Key preventative measure is to listen to patients and take steps to keep them safe. This could include immediate hospitalization.
- Clozapine lithium and CBT are associated with a reduction in the risk of suicide.
- Family and contacts of people who have attempted or committed suicide suffer from reactions ranging from rage to despair. Encourage counseling.
- Resources for clinicians: https://www.suicidology.org; https://www.suicideassessment.com

SUPERFICIAL THROMBOPHLEBITIS
Jarrett Keller Sell, MD, FAAFP, AAHIVS • Jared M. Roberts

 BASICS

DESCRIPTION
- Superficial thrombophlebitis is venous inflammation with secondary thrombosis of a superficial vein.
- Most common in the lower extremities (60–80%), but can occur in the upper extremities/neck
- Generally a benign and self-limiting process but can be painful
- Traumatic thrombophlebitis types:
  - Injury
  - IV catheter related
  - Intentional (i.e., sclerotherapy)
- Aseptic thrombophlebitis types:
  - Primary hypercoagulable states: disorders with measurable defects in the proteins of the coagulation and/or fibrinolytic systems
  - Secondary hypercoagulable states: clinical conditions with a risk of thrombosis (venous stasis, pregnancy)
- Septic (suppurative) thrombophlebitis types:
  - Iatrogenic, long-term IV catheter use
  - Infectious, mainly syphilis and psittacosis
- Mondor disease
  - Rare presentation of groin, penis, or anterior chest/breast veins
- System(s) affected: cardiovascular
- Synonym(s): phlebitis; phlebothrombosis, superficial vein thrombosis (SVT)

Geriatric Considerations
Septic thrombophlebitis is more common; prognosis is poorer.

Pediatric Considerations
Subperiosteal abscesses of adjacent long bone may complicate the disorder.

Pregnancy Considerations
- Associated with increased risk of aseptic superficial thrombophlebitis, especially during postpartum
- As NSAIDs are contraindicated during pregnancy, alternative therapeutic approaches are advised.

EPIDEMIOLOGY
- Predominant age
  - Traumatic/IV related has no predominant age/sex.
  - Aseptic primary hypercoagulable state
    - Childhood to young adult
- Aseptic secondary hypercoagulable state
  - Mondor disease: women, ages 21 to 55 years
  - Thromboangiitis obliterans onset: ages 20 to 50 years
- Predominant sex
  - Suppurative: male = female
  - Aseptic
    - Spontaneous formation: female (55–70%)
    - Mondor: female > male (2:1)

Incidence
- Septic
  - Incidence of catheter-related thrombophlebitis is 88/100,000 persons per year.
  - Develops in 4–8% if cutdown is performed

- Aseptic primary hypercoagulable state: Antithrombin III and heparin cofactor II deficiency incidence is 50/100,000 persons.
- Aseptic secondary hypercoagulable state
  - In pregnancy, 49-fold increased incidence of phlebitis
  - Superficial migratory thrombophlebitis in 27% of patients with thromboangiitis obliterans

Prevalence
- Superficial thrombophlebitis is common.
- 1/3 of patients in a medical ICU develop thrombophlebitis that eventually progresses to the deep veins.

ETIOLOGY AND PATHOPHYSIOLOGY
- Similar to deep venous thrombosis; Virchow triad of vessel trauma, stasis, and hypercoagulability (genetic, iatrogenic, or idiopathic)
- Varicose veins play a primary role in etiology of lower extremity phlebitis.
- Mondor disease pathophysiology not completely understood
- Less commonly due to infection (i.e., septic)
  - *Staphylococcus aureus, Pseudomonas, Klebsiella, Peptostreptococcus* sp.
  - *Candida* sp.
- Aseptic primary hypercoagulable state
  - Due to inherited disorders of hypercoagulability
- Aseptic secondary hypercoagulable states
  - Malignancy (Trousseau syndrome: recurrent migratory thrombophlebitis): most commonly seen in metastatic mucin or adenocarcinomas of the GI tract (pancreas, stomach, colon, and gallbladder), lung, prostate, and ovary
  - Pregnancy
  - Estrogen-based oral contraceptives
  - Behçet, Buerger, or Mondor disease

Genetics
Not applicable other than hypercoagulable states

RISK FACTORS
- Nonspecific
  - Varicose veins
  - Immobilization
  - Obesity
  - Advanced age
  - Postoperative states
  - History of previous venous thromboembolic event (VTE)
- Traumatic/septic
  - IV catheter (plastic > coated)
  - Lower extremity IV catheter
  - Cutdowns
  - Burn patients
  - AIDS
  - IV drug use
- Aseptic
  - Pregnancy
  - Cancer, debilitating diseases
  - Estrogen-based oral contraceptives
  - Surgery, trauma, infection
  - Hypercoagulable state (i.e., factor V, protein C, or S deficiency, others)

- Thromboangiitis obliterans: persistent smoking
- Mondor disease
  - Breast cancer or breast surgery

GENERAL PREVENTION
- Avoid lower extremity cannulations or IVs.
- Insert catheters under aseptic conditions, secure cannulas, and replace every 3 days.
- Avoid stasis and use usual deep vein thrombosis (DVT) prophylaxis in high-risk patients (i.e., ICU, immobilized).

COMMONLY ASSOCIATED CONDITIONS
- Frequently seen with concurrent DVT (6–53%)
- Symptomatic pulmonary embolism can also be seen concurrently (0–10%).
- Both DVT/PE can occur up to 3 months after onset of superficial thrombophlebitis.

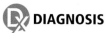 DIAGNOSIS

HISTORY
Pain along the course of a vein

PHYSICAL EXAM
- Swelling, tenderness, redness along the course of a vein or veins
- May have a palpable cord along the course of the vein
- Fever in 70% of patients in septic phlebitis
- Sign of systemic sepsis in 84% of suppurative cases

DIFFERENTIAL DIAGNOSIS
- Cellulitis
- DVT
- Erythema nodosum
- Cutaneous polyarteritis nodosa
- Lymphangitis

DIAGNOSTIC TESTS & INTERPRETATION
Initial Tests (lab, imaging)
Often none necessary if afebrile, otherwise healthy
- Small or distal veins (i.e., forearms or below the knee): no recommended imaging
- If concern for more proximal extension: venous Doppler US to assess extent of thrombosis and rule out DVT

Follow-Up Tests & Special Considerations
- If suspicious for sepsis
  - Blood cultures (bacteremia in 80–90%)
  - Consider culture of the IV fluids being infused.
  - CBC demonstrates leukocytosis.
- Aseptic: evaluation for coagulopathy if recurrent or without another identifiable cause (e.g., protein C and S, lupus anticoagulant, anticardiolipin antibody, factor V and VIII, homocysteine)
- In migratory thrombophlebitis, have a high index of suspicion for malignancy.
- Consider repeat venous ultrasound to assess effectiveness of therapy.
  - If thrombosis is extending, more aggressive therapy required

Test Interpretation

The affected vein is enlarged, tortuous, and thickened with endothelial damage and necrosis.

TREATMENT

GENERAL MEASURES

- Suppurative: consultation for urgent surgical venous excision
- Local, mild (1)[C]
  - Conservative management; antibiotics not useful
  - For varicosities
    - Compression stockings; maintain activities.
  - Catheter/trauma associated
    - Immediately remove IV and culture tip.
    - Elevate with application of warm compresses.
    - If slow to resolve, consider LMWH.
- Large, severe, or septic thrombophlebitis
  - Inpatient care or bed rest with elevation and local warm compress
  - When the patient is ambulating, then start compression stockings or Ace bandages.

MEDICATION

First Line

- Best medication(s) and duration of treatment are not well-defined, as 2018 Cochrane review found that most trials were small and of poor quality (2)[A].
- Localized, mild thrombophlebitis (usually self-limited)
  - NSAIDs and ASA for inflammation/pain to reduce symptoms and local progression
  - Use of compression stockings can also provide symptomatic relief (3).

Second Line

- Septic/suppurative
  - May present or be complicated by sepsis
  - Requires IV antibiotics (broad spectrum initially) and anticoagulation
- Increasing evidence shows that LMWH/fondaparinux treatment can prevent extension of superficial venous thrombosis in addition to venous thromboembolism (VTE) prevention.
  - Consider if thrombus is large, close to the junction with deep veins, or involves the long saphenous vein
    - To prevent VTE, 4 weeks of LMWH, such as enoxaparin
    - 45 days of fondaparinux was found to reduce DVT and VTE by 85% (relative risk reduction) in one large study (4)[B].
- Superficial thrombophlebitis related to inherited or acquired hypercoagulable states is addressed by treating the related disease.

ISSUES FOR REFERRAL

Severely inflamed or very large superficial thrombophlebitis should be evaluated for excision.

SURGERY/OTHER PROCEDURES

- Septic
  - Surgical consultation for excision of the involved vein segment and involved tributaries
  - Drain contiguous abscesses.
  - Remove all associated cannula and culture tips.
- Aseptic: Manage underlying conditions.
  - Evaluate for saphenous vein ligation to prevent deep vein extension after acute phase resolved.
  - Consider referral for varicosity excision.

ADMISSION, INPATIENT, AND NURSING CONSIDERATIONS

- Septic: inpatient
- Aseptic: outpatient

ONGOING CARE

FOLLOW-UP RECOMMENDATIONS

Patient Monitoring

- Septic: routine WBC count and differential. Target treatment based on culture results.
- Severe aseptic
  - Repeat venous Doppler US in 1 to 2 weeks to ensure no DVT and assess treatment effectiveness: Do not expect resolution, just no progression.
  - Repeat clotting studies.
- Local, mild thrombophlebitis typically resolves with conservative therapy and does not require specific monitoring unless there is a failure to resolve.

DIET

No restrictions

PATIENT EDUCATION

Review local care, elevation, and use of compression hose for acute treatment and prevention of recurrence.

PROGNOSIS

- Septic/suppurative
  - High mortality (50%) if untreated
  - Depends on treatment delay or need for surgery
- Aseptic
  - Usually benign course; recovery in 2 to 3 weeks
  - Depends on development of DVT and early detection of complications
  - Aseptic thrombophlebitis can be isolated, recurrent, or migratory.
  - Recurrence likely if related to varicosity or if severely affected vein not removed

COMPLICATIONS

- Septic: systemic sepsis, bacteremia (84%), septic pulmonary emboli (44%), metastatic abscess formation, pneumonia (44%), subperiosteal abscess of adjacent long bones in children
- Aseptic: DVT (6–53%), VTE (up to 10%), thromboembolic phenomena

REFERENCES

1. Nasr H, Scriven JM. Superficial thrombophlebitis (superficial venous thrombosis). *BMJ*. 2015;350:h2039.
2. Di Nisio M, Wichers IM, Middeldorp S. Treatment for superficial thrombophlebitis of the leg. *Cochrane Database Syst Rev*. 2018;2(2):CD004982.
3. Decousus H, Epinat M, Guillot K, et al. Superficial vein thrombosis: risk factors, diagnosis, and treatment. *Curr Opin Pulm Med*. 2003;9(5):393–397.
4. Decousus H, Prandoni P, Mismetti P, et al; for CALISTO Study Group. Fondaparinux for the treatment of superficial-vein thrombosis in the legs. *N Engl J Med*. 2010;363(13):1222–1232.

ADDITIONAL READING

- Decousus H, Quéré I, Presles E, et al; for POST Study Group. Superficial venous thrombosis and venous thromboembolism: a large, prospective epidemiologic study. *Ann Intern Med*. 2010;152(4):218–224.
- Di Nisio M, Middeldorp S. Treatment of lower extremity superficial thrombophlebitis. *JAMA*. 2014;311(7):729–730.
- Wichers IM, Di Nisio M, Büller HR, et al. Treatment of superficial vein thrombosis to prevent deep vein thrombosis and pulmonary embolism: a systematic review. *Haematologica*. 2005;90(5):672–677.

SEE ALSO

Deep Vein Thrombophlebitis

CODES

ICD10

- I80.9 Phlebitis and thrombophlebitis of unspecified site
- I80.00 Phlbts and thombophlb of superfic vessels of unsp low extrm
- I80.8 Phlebitis and thrombophlebitis of other sites

CLINICAL PEARLS

- Mild superficial thrombophlebitis is typically self-limiting and responds well to conservative care.
- Lower extremity disease involving large veins or proximal saphenous vein likely benefits from anticoagulation to prevent DVT.
- Septic thrombophlebitis requires admission for antibiotics and anticoagulation. If severe, consider surgical consultation for venous excision.

SYNCOPE

Santiago O. Valdes, MD, FAAP • Michael Bruno, MD • Patrick Sean Connell, MD, PhD

 BASICS

EPIDEMIOLOGY

Incidence
- Accounts for 1–3% of emergency room visits and 1% of hospital admissions
- Increased incidence after the age of 70 years, and annual incidence in institutionalized elderly (>75 years of age) is 7%.

Prevalence
- Approximately 20–35% of adults report ≥1 episode during their lifetime; 15% of children <18 years of age
- The prevalence in institutionalized elderly (>75 years of age) is 23%.

ETIOLOGY AND PATHOPHYSIOLOGY
- Systemic hypotension secondary to decreased cardiac output and/or systemic vasodilation leads to a drop in cerebral perfusion and resultant loss of consciousness.
- Cardiac
  - Obstructions to outflow
    - Aortic stenosis
    - Hypertrophic cardiomyopathy: most common cause of sudden cardiac death during exercise in young athletes
    - Pulmonary embolus (PE)
    - Pulmonary hypertension
  - Cardiac arrhythmias
    - Sustained ventricular tachycardia (VT)
    - Supraventricular tachycardia (SVT) (atrial fibrillation, atrial flutter, reentrant SVT)
    - Torsades de pointes (TdP)
    - Bradyarrhythmia
      - 2nd- and 3rd-degree AV block
      - Sick sinus syndrome
- Noncardiac
  - Reflex-mediated vasovagal (neurally mediated syncope [NMS]/neurocardiogenic): inappropriate vasodilation leading to neurally mediated systemic hypotension and decreased cerebral blood flow; situational (micturition, defecation, cough, pain, emotions, hair combing)
  - Orthostatic hypotension (OHT): Consider volume depletion, pregnancy, anemia, medications.
  - Drug/alcohol induced
  - Primary autonomic failure: pure autonomic failure, Parkinson
  - Secondary autonomic failure: diabetes, amyloidosis
  - Carotid sinus hypersensitivity
  - Unexplained
- NMS is most common cause in adult cases.
- Vast majority of pediatric cases represent benign alterations in vasomotor tone.
- Strokes, seizures, and psychogenic nonepileptic seizures may mimic syncope but are a distinct diagnosis.

Genetics
Specific cardiomyopathies and arrhythmias may be inherited (e.g., long QT syndrome, catecholaminergic polymorphic VT, Brugada syndrome, hypertrophic cardiomyopathy). Primary and secondary autonomic failure syndromes and NMS may also have genetic links.

RISK FACTORS
- Heart disease (acquired or structural)
- Dehydration

- Drugs
  - Antihypertensives
  - Vasodilators (including calcium channel blockers, ACE inhibitors, and nitrates)
  - Phenothiazines
  - Antidepressants
  - Antiarrhythmics
  - Diuretics

GENERAL PREVENTION
See "Risk Factors."

COMMONLY ASSOCIATED CONDITIONS
See "Etiology and Pathophysiology."

DIAGNOSIS

HISTORY
- Careful history, physical exam, and an ECG are more important than other investigations in determining the diagnosis (1).
- Make sure that the patient or witness (if present) is not referring to vertigo (i.e., sense of rotary motion, spinning, and whirling), seizure, or causes of fall without loss of consciousness. Onset of syncope is usually rapid, and recovery is spontaneous, rapid, and complete. Duration of episodes are typically brief (<60 seconds).
- Circumstances: Prolonged standing, urination, coughing, defecation, postprandial, and intense emotions are more likely to be associated with NMS. Consider carotid sinus hypersensitivity with abrupt neck movements. Consider cardiac cause with exertional syncope.
- Number of previous episodes (benign causes of syncope tend to be associated with a single episode)
- Presence of prodromal symptoms: Consider NMS.
  - Elderly patients less likely to experience a prodrome.
- Palpitations, chest pain or dyspnea: Consider cardiac.
- Position (supine: arrhythmia; erect: NMS; supine → erect: orthostatic hypotension)
- Prolonged syncope: Consider psychiatric or neurologic.
- Delayed recovery: Consider neurologic (postictal).
- Ask for family history of long QT syndrome, catecholaminergic polymorphic VT, Brugada syndrome, implantable cardioverter-defibrillator (ICD), hypertrophic cardiomyopathy, or unexplained sudden cardiac death in young family members (<50 years).
- High-risk findings: new-onset chest discomfort, breathlessness, abdominal pain, headache, syncope during exertion or when supine, or sudden palpitations immediately followed by syncope
- Even after careful evaluation, including diagnostic procedures and special tests, the cause will be found in only 50–60% of patients.

PHYSICAL EXAM
Check for orthostasis:
- Measure the BP and pulse after the patient is supine for 5 minutes, then have the patient stand and repeat BP and pulse immediately, after standing 1 and 3 minutes.
  - A drop in systolic BP of ≥20 mm Hg, or diastolic BP of ≥10 mm Hg, or experiencing light-headedness or dizziness is considered abnormal.

- Check for cardiac murmur or focal neurologic abnormality.
- High-risk findings: unexplained systolic BP <90 mm Hg, suggestion of GI bleed on rectal exam, persistent bradycardia (<40 beats/min) in absence of physical training, or undiagnosed systolic murmur

DIFFERENTIAL DIAGNOSIS
- Drop attacks
- Vertigo
- Seizure disorder
- Stroke/transient ischemic attacks (TIAs)
- Psychiatric (conversion, somatization): lack hemodynamic and/or autonomic changes

DIAGNOSTIC TESTS & INTERPRETATION
- Goal is to identify life-threatening conditions or those associated with significant risk of injury (2)[C].
- Comprehensive medical and family history, physical examination, and ECG should guide future testing.
- Evaluation of Guidelines in Syncope Study (EGSYS) Score may be used, as other algorithms to suspect cardiac syncope (3)[C].
- No one single test defines the cause of syncope (2).

Initial Tests (lab, imaging)
- ECG should be obtained in most patients.
  - Consider cardiac if there are ischemic changes, bifascicular block, AV block, sinus bradycardia <40 beats/min or sinus pause >3 seconds, prolonged QTc, preexcitation, and alternating BBB.
- Other testing should be guided by history and physical:
  - CBC, electrolytes, BUN, creatinine
  - Glucose (rarely helpful if asymptomatic or presenting hours later)
  - BNP
  - Cardiac enzymes (only if history suggestive of MI)
  - D-dimer (for pulmonary embolism workup)
  - Urine pregnancy and urine drug screen
  - Initial cardiac or neuroimaging only if indicated
  - Lung scan or helical CT scan of chest if concern for PE

Follow-Up Tests & Special Considerations
- If history and physical suggest ischemic, valvular, or congenital heart disease (1),(2)[B]
  - Exercise stress test (if syncope with exertion) (1),(2)[C]
  - Echocardiogram (1),(2)[B]
- ECG monitoring, either in hospital or ambulatory (1)[B]
  - Consider when concerned for cardiac cause.
  - Choice of outpatient device (e.g., Holter, external loop recorder, implantable loop recorder) should be determined by frequency of symptoms.
- Electrophysiologic studies (1),(2)[B]
  - Consider when concerned for cardiac cause.
  - Positive results seen in 22–82% of patients with preexisting heart disease and/or abnormal ECG
- Head imaging, carotid US, and EEG are not recommended in routine evaluation of syncope but may be useful if history and physical is concerning for neurologic issues (1)[C].
- Carotid hypersensitivity evaluation (2)[B]
  - Carotid hypersensitivity should be considered in patients >40 years old or with syncope during head turning, especially while wearing tight collars, and with neck tumors or scars.

– The technique is not standardized; one side at a time is massaged gently for 5–10 seconds with constant monitoring of pulse and BP/ECG. Generally, reproduction of symptoms with ventricular pause ≥3 seconds and/or fall in systolic BP ≥50 mm Hg is considered positive. Avoid in patients with history of TIA or stroke.

– Atropine should be readily available.

- Tilt-table testing (1),(2)[B]
  – Provocative test for vasovagal syncope
  – Often, results are not reproducible.
  – High false-positive rate
- Psychiatric evaluation (2)[C]: indicated when syncope is thought to be psychogenic. Psychiatric disease and substance abuse may be associated with syncope.

Diagnostic Procedures/Other
External or implantable loop recorders may be more helpful than short-term ambulatory monitoring; helpful in selective patients with recurrent syncope, with yield of ~55% (1)[B]

Test Interpretation
Depends on etiology and presence of underlying cardiac or neurologic conditions

 ## TREATMENT

- Maintaining good hydration status and normal salt intake are initial therapy. Educate patients of the premonitory signs of syncope (1).
- Majority of pediatric patients improve with nonpharmacologic measures.

GENERAL MEASURES
- NMS: reassurance, education, behavior modification
- Elderly patients without previously recognized heart disease should be admitted if the physician thinks that the cause of syncope is likely cardiac.
- Patients without heart disease, especially young patients (age <60 years), can be worked up safely as outpatients.
- Prescribe antiarrhythmics for documented arrhythmias occurring simultaneously with syncope or symptoms of presyncope. Asymptomatic arrhythmias do not necessarily require treatment.
- The EGSYS Score may be used to help distinguish a cardiac from noncardiac syncope using basic history findings. These include palpitations, syncope during effort or supine position, neurovegetative prodromes and specific precipitating events. An abnormal ECG is also taken into consideration for this score (3)[C].

MEDICATION
First Line
- Geared toward specific underlying cardiac or neurologic abnormalities
- In cases of recurrent NMS and OHT (1)[B],(4)
  – Mineralocorticoids (fludrocortisone)
  – α-Adrenergic agonists (midodrine)
  – Norepinephrine precursor (droxidopa)

Second Line
- SSRIs (paroxetine, sertraline, fluoxetine) (1)[C]
- Vagolytics (disopyramide)

ISSUES FOR REFERRAL
When cardiac or neurologic etiologies are suspected, obtain appropriate consultation, as indicated.

ADDITIONAL THERAPIES
For vasovagal/neurocardiogenic/NMS
- Counterpressure maneuvers and exercise improve vasovagal symptoms and recurrence (1).
- Head-up tilt sleeping (2)[C]

- Abdominal binders and/or support stockings (1),(2)[C]
- Increased fluid and salt intake to maintain intravascular volume in cases of recurrent NMS

SURGERY/OTHER PROCEDURES
- ICD placement for patients with cardiac conditions with high risk of sudden death and/or recurrent syncope on medications (e.g., long QT syndrome, Brugada, catecholaminergic polymorphic VT, hypertrophic cardiomyopathy) (1),(2)[B]
- Many recommend pacemaker implantation in patients with the following:
  – 2nd- (Mobitz type II) and 3rd-degree heart block
  – High risk of developing 3rd-degree heart block (bifascicular block, HV interval >100 ms by EPS)
  – Pacing-induced infranodal block
  – Sinus node recovery time ≥3 seconds

ADMISSION, INPATIENT, AND NURSING CONSIDERATIONS
- Patients with benign etiologies of syncope with negative ED workups are associated with benign outcomes, even with other risk factors (5)[B].
- ROSE rule recommends hospital admission if any of the following is present: BNP level ≥300 pg/mL, bradycardia HR ≤50, + fecal occult blood, anemia with hemoglobin ≤9 g/dL, chest pain associated with syncope, ECG showing Q wave (not in lead III), or oxygen saturation ≤94% on room air (6).
- Discharge after
  – Attainment of hemodynamic stability with
  – Adequate control of arrhythmia or seizure, if present

 ## ONGOING CARE

FOLLOW-UP RECOMMENDATIONS
Patient Monitoring
- Frequent follow-up visits for patients with cardiac causes of syncope, especially if on antiarrhythmics
- Patients with an unknown cause of syncope rarely (5%) are diagnosed during the follow-up.
- Home video recording with smartphone technology is recommended for recurrent episodes.

DIET
No specific diet unless the patient has heart disease or NMS (see "Additional Therapies")

PATIENT EDUCATION
- Reassurance that most cardiac causes can be treated, and those with noncardiac causes do well, even if the cause is never discovered.
- Physical counterpressure maneuvers can prevent recurrences of vasovagal syncope.
- Carefully consider whether the patient should drive while syncope is being evaluated. Physicians should be aware of pertinent laws in their own states.

PROGNOSIS
- The majority of patients (80%) have no recurrence of syncope.
- Cumulative mortality at 2 years
  – Low: young patients (<60 years of age) with noncardiac or unknown cause of syncope
  – Intermediate: older patients (>60 years of age) with noncardiac or unknown cause of syncope
  – High: patients with cardiac cause of syncope
- Independent predictors of poor short-term outcomes (5),(6)[B]
  – BNP ≥300 pg/ml
  – Abnormal ECG
  – Shortness of breath or chest pain

– Systolic BP <90 mm Hg
– Hematocrit <30%
– Congestive heart failure

COMPLICATIONS
Trauma from falling

REFERENCES

1. Shen WK, Sheldon RS, Benditt DG, et al. 2017 ACC/AHA/HRS guideline for the evaluation and management of patients with syncope: a report of the American College of Cardiology/American Heart Association Task Force on Clinical Practice Guidelines and the Heart Rhythm Society. Circulation. 2017;136(5):e60–e122.
2. Brignole M, Moya A, de Lange FJ, et al; for ESC Scientific Document Group. 2018 ESC guidelines for the diagnosis and management of syncope. Eur Heart J. 2018;39(21):1883–1948.
3. Albassam OT, Redelmeier RJ, Shadowitz S, et al. Did this patient have cardiac syncope? The rational clinical examination systematic review. JAMA. 2019;321(24):2448–2457.
4. Eschlböck S, Wenning G, Fanciulli A. Evidence-based treatment of neurogenic orthostatic hypotension and related symptoms. J Neural Transm. 2017;124(12):1567–1605.
5. Saccilotto RT, Nickel CH, Bucher HC, et al. San Francisco Syncope Rule to predict short-term serious outcomes: a systematic review. CMAJ. 2011;183(15):E1116–E1126.
6. Reed MJ, Newby DE, Coull AJ, et al. The ROSE (Risk stratification Of Syncope in the Emergency department) study. J Am Coll Cardiol. 2010;55(8):713–721.

ADDITIONAL READING
Anderson JB, Willis M, Lancaster H, et al. The evaluation and management of pediatric syncope. Pediatr Neurol. 2016;55:6–13.

 ## SEE ALSO

- Aortic Valvular Stenosis; Atrial Septal Defect; Carotid Sinus Hypersensitivity; Patent Ductus Arteriosus; Pulmonary Arterial Hypertension; Pulmonary Embolism; Seizure Disorders; Stokes-Adams Attacks
- Algorithms: Syncope; Transient Ischemic Attack and Transient Neurologic Defects

CODES

ICD10
R55 Syncope and collapse

CLINICAL PEARLS
- Careful history and physical exam are keys to a diagnosis.
- Use the ECG/event-recorder to evaluate for arrhythmias.
- Reflex-mediated vasovagal (neurally mediated syncope [NMS]/neurocardiogenic) is the most common cause in children and adults.
- True neurologic causes of syncope are rare.

SYNCOPE, REFLEX (VASOVAGAL SYNCOPE)

Melinda Kwan, DO, MPH • Norton Winer, MD

 BASICS

A reversible loss of consciousness and postural tone secondary to systemic hypotension and cerebral hypoperfusion due to vasodilation and/or bradycardia (rarely, tachycardia) with spontaneous recovery and no neurologic sequelae. The term syncope excludes seizures, coma, shock, or other states of altered consciousness.

DESCRIPTION
- Derived from the Greek *syncopa*, "to cut short"
- Sudden, transient loss of consciousness characterized by unresponsiveness, falling, and spontaneous recovery
- Common cause of syncope in all age groups, especially in patients with no evidence of neurologic or cardiac disease
- Five main types of syncope: vasovagal or neurocardiogenic syncope, situational syncope, orthostatic hypotension, carotid sinus hypersensitivity, and glossopharyngeal/trigeminal neuralgia syncope (uncommon) (1)

EPIDEMIOLOGY
- Mortality: cardiac-related syncope 20–30% and 5% in idiopathic syncope
- Age: any age

Incidence
- Ranges from 7% in children aged <18 years and 15% in adults aged >70 years
- 36–62% of all syncopal episodes
- 30% recurrence rate

Prevalence
22% in the general population

ETIOLOGY AND PATHOPHYSIOLOGY
Cause: an abnormal response of the normal mechanisms that maintain BP in an upright posture
- In normal individuals, upright posture results in venous pooling and transient decrease in BP.
- Neurally induced syncope may result from a cardioinhibitory response, a vasodepressor response, or a combination of the two.
- Increased cardiovagal tone leads to bradycardia or asystole, and decreased peripheral sympathetic activity leads to venodilation and hypotension (2).
- Vasovagal syncope usually has a precipitating event, often related to fright, pain, panic, exercise, noxious stimuli, or heat exposure (2).
- Carotid sinus syncope is precipitated by position change, turning head, or wearing a tight collar (possible neck tumors or surgical scarring).
- Situational syncope is related to micturition, defecation, postexercise, cough, or swallow (3).
- Glossopharyngeal syncope is related to throat or facial pain.

Genetics
Vasovagal syncope is associated with certain genetic markers, particularly involving serotonin and dopamine signaling (4).

RISK FACTORS
- Low-resting BP
- Age: older age
- Prolonged supine position with resulting deconditioning of autonomic control

GENERAL PREVENTION
Avoid precipitating events or situations. Optimize diabetes control, use of elastic stockings, adequate hydration.

COMMONLY ASSOCIATED CONDITIONS
- Cardiopulmonary disorders: CHF, MI, arrhythmias, hypertrophic obstructive cardiomyopathy, HTN, pulmonary embolism (PE)
- Neurologic disorders: autonomic dysfunction, Shy-Drager syndrome, Parkinson disease, multiple system atrophy, transient ischemic attack, vertebrobasilar insufficiency, peripheral neuropathy
- Psychiatric disorders:
  – Generalized anxiety disorder
  – Panic disorder
  – Major depression
  – Alcohol dependence

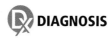 **DIAGNOSIS**

HISTORY
- History of syncope during or immediately after exertion is concerning for cardiac syncope.
- Neurally mediated syncope is preceded by blurred vision, palpitations, nausea, warmth, diaphoresis, or light-headedness, or there may be history of nausea, warmth, diaphoresis, or fatigue *after* syncope.
- Vasovagal syncope
  – Three phases: prodrome, loss of consciousness, and postsyncope
  – Precipitating event or stimulus is usually identified, such as panic, fright, pain, or exercise.
  – May be postexertional in athletes (diagnosis of exclusion)
  – Position: *can be preceded by prolonged standing but can occur from any position; generally resolves when the patient becomes supine*
    ○ Preceding events: as discussed above
    ○ Prodrome: as listed above for neurally mediated syncope
  – Duration: generally brief (seconds to minutes)
  – Recovery: may be prolonged with persistent nausea, pallor, and diaphoresis but without neurologic change or confusion
- Carotid sinus syncope is precipitated by position change, after turning head, or wearing a tight collar.
- Situational syncope is related to micturition, defecation, or coughing.
- Glossopharyngeal syncope (less common) is related to throat or facial pain.
  – Precipitating events or situations may include panic, pain, exercise, micturition, defecation, coughing, or swallowing.
- Pregnant women can have reflex syncope when moving from supine to lateral decubitus or upright positions.

PHYSICAL EXAM
- Vital signs, including orthostatic and bilateral BP
- Cardiac exam: volume status, murmurs, rhythm, carotid bruits
- Neurologic exam: signs of focal deficit
- Assess for occult blood loss.
- Dix-Hallpike if benign paroxysmal vertigo is suspected

DIFFERENTIAL DIAGNOSIS
- Seizure
- Arrhythmia
- Hypoglycemia
- Cardiac syncope
- Cerebrovascular syncope
- Orthostatic hypotension
- Drop attacks
- Psychiatric illness

DIAGNOSTIC TESTS & INTERPRETATION
Guided by history and physical, includes basic tests to rule out three primary causes of syncope: hypoglycemia, arrhythmia, and anemia

Initial Tests (lab, imaging)
- Blood glucose (hypoglycemia)
- ECG should be ordered for all patients. Abnormal ECG findings are common in patients with cardiac syncope (arrhythmia).
- CBC (rule out anemia)
- Head CT, MRI/MRA, carotid ultrasound only if history or physical exam suggests a neurologic cause
  – Radiology studies are not indicated for insignificant trauma in the presence of a normal neurologic exam (5).

Follow-Up Tests & Special Considerations
- 24-hour Holter monitoring only if a high probability of cardiac cause and/or abnormal ECG findings is present
- A low hemoglobin without obvious cause of bleed warrants stool guaiac, head CT (rule out subarachnoid hemorrhage), abdominal CT (rule out retroperitoneal bleed)
- Negative imaging prompts workup for alternative causes.
- Stroke, bleed, or carotid stenosis require appropriate disease-oriented management.
- EEG only if history or physical exam suggests seizure
- Implantable loop recorder

Diagnostic Procedures/Other
- Head-up tilt table testing:
  – Contraindicated in patients with known cardiac or neurovascular disease or in pregnancy
  – Indicated for recurrent syncope or single episode accompanied by injury or risk to others (e.g., pilots, surgeons)
  – Uses positional changes to reproduce symptoms
  – Positive test diagnostic for vasovagal syncope

- Carotid sinus massage, only in a monitored setting (i.e., BP and HR monitoring, IV access):
  - Contraindicated in patients with carotid disease (Careful auscultation prior to massage is essential.)
  - Pressure at the angle of the jaw for 5 seconds with simultaneous ECG monitoring
  - Positive tests (causing syncope or cardiac pause >3 seconds) are diagnostic of carotid sinus syncope.
- Psychiatric evaluation: to rule out anxiety, depression, and alcohol abuse

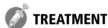 **TREATMENT**

Therapy is primarily for recurrent syncope. Situational syncope does not warrant specific treatment.

GENERAL MEASURES
Identify and avoid precipitating events or situations.

MEDICATION
First Line
Nonpharmacologic treatment
- Patient counseling
  - Development of coping skills
  - Increased salt and fluid intake
- Moderate exercise training
  - Isometric muscle contractions
    - Leg crossing and buttocks clenching
    - Intense gripping of the hands and tensing of the arms
    - These maneuvers increase cardiac output and arterial blood pressure (6).
- Tilt-table training
  - Progressively prolonged periods of enforced upright posture

Second Line
- α-Agonists mainly used for orthostatic hypotension
  - Midodrine is commonly used, particularly in younger, healthy patients with a high "syncope burden" (7). It increases peripheral vascular resistance and venous return. Side effects include HTN, paresthesia, urinary retention, "goose bumps," hyperactivity, dizziness, tremor, and nervousness.
- SSRIs: Paroxetine and fluoxetine are useful in treating neurocardiogenic/vasovagal syncope.
  - Serotonin affects BP and HR via the central nervous system. Serotonin decreases a sympathetic withdrawal response to rapid increases in serotonin levels.
  - Side effects include weight gain, nausea, anxiety, sexual dysfunction, and insomnia.
- Mineralocorticoids: Fludrocortisone has been found helpful mainly in orthostatic hypotension.
  - Helpful in renal sodium absorption and increasing the vasoconstrictive peripheral vascular response
  - Adverse reactions include fluid retention, HTN, CHF, peripheral edema, and hypokalemia.
- β-Blockers: metoprolol, atenolol, or pindolol mainly for postural orthostatic tachycardia syndrome (POTS)
  - Block peripheral vasodilators and ventricular mechanoreceptor stimulation
  - Stabilization of HR and BP
  - Side effects: hypotension and bradycardia (with worsening of syncope), fatigue, depression, and sexual dysfunction
  - Contraindicated in asthma

ISSUES FOR REFERRAL
Neurology or cardiology, as needed

ADDITIONAL THERAPIES
Use of support/pressure stockings

SURGERY/OTHER PROCEDURES
Pacemaker placement may be of use in patients with frequent neurocardiogenic/vasovagal syncope that is refractory to other therapies (3)[C].
- Prevents prolonged bradycardia or asystole during syncopal episodes
- Long-term effect
- Invasive placement procedure

COMPLEMENTARY & ALTERNATIVE MEDICINE
Treatments for underlying heart disease or precipitating factors (e.g., anxiety); none are proven therapies.
- Nutrition and supplements: omega-3 fatty acids, multivitamin, CoQ10, acetyl-L-carnitine, α-lipoic acid, and L-arginine
- Herbs: green tea (*Camellia sinensis*), bilberry (*Vaccinium myrtillus*), ginkgo (*Ginkgo biloba*)
- Homeopathy: carbo vegetabilis, opium, sepia
- Acupuncture: It may precipitate fainting.

ADMISSION, INPATIENT, AND NURSING CONSIDERATIONS
Hospital admission or intense evaluation for (8):
- Severe coronary artery disease or structural heart disease (severe CHF, low ejection fraction or previous myocardial infarction, aortic stenosis)
- Arrhythmic syncope:
  - ECG may show bifascicular block, sinus bradycardia <40 without SA block or β-blockers, Brugada syndrome, abnormal QT interval, etc.
- Severe anemia or electrolyte abnormalities
- Family history of sudden death
- Isotonic crystalloids, as needed
- Vital sign monitoring
- Discharge when hemodynamically stable and workup satisfactory.

 ONGOING CARE

DIET
- Increased salt intake may help if not otherwise contraindicated (2)[C].
- Maintain fluid intake.

PATIENT EDUCATION
- Identify and avoid precipitating events or situations.
- Avoid dehydration, alcohol consumption, warm environments, tight clothing, and long periods of standing motionless.
- Recognize presyncopal symptoms.
- Use behaviors, such as lying down, to avoid syncope.

PROGNOSIS
May be recurrent but not life-threatening

COMPLICATIONS
May result in injury from fall

REFERENCES
1. Zou R, Wang S, Lin P, et al. The clinical characteristics of situational syncope in children and adults undergoing head-up tilt testing. *Am J Emerg Med*. 2020;38(7):1419–1423.
2. Rocha BML, Gomes RV, Cunha GJL, et al. Diagnostic and therapeutic approach to cardioinhibitory reflex syncope: a complex and controversial issue. *Rev Port Cardiol (Engl Ed)*. 2019;38(9):661–673.
3. Walsh K, Hoffmayer K, Hamdan MH. Syncope: diagnosis and management. *Curr Probl Cardiol*. 2015;40(2):51–86.
4. Sheldon RS, Gerull B. Genetic markers of vasovagal syncope. *Auton Neurosci*. 2021;235:102871.
5. Runser LA, Gauer RL, Houser A. Syncope: evaluation and differential diagnosis. *Am Fam Physician*. 2017;95(5):303–312.
6. Kenny RA, McNicholas T. The management of vasovagal syncope. *QJM*. 2016;109(12):767–773.
7. Sheldon R, Faris P, Tang A, et al. Midodrine for the prevention of vasovagal syncope: a randomized clinical trial. *Ann Intern Med*. 2021;174(10):1349–1356.
8. Moya A, Sutton R, Ammirati F, et al; for Task Force for the Diagnosis and Management of Syncope, European Society of Cardiology, European Heart Rhythm Association, et al. Guidelines for the diagnosis and management of syncope (version 2009). *Eur Heart J*. 2009;30(21):2631–2671.

ADDITIONAL READING
Romano S, Branz L, Fondrieschi L, et al. Does a therapy for reflex vasovagal syncope really exist? *High Blood Press Cardiovasc Prev*. 2019;26(4):273–281.

 SEE ALSO

Algorithms: Syncope; Transient Ischemic Attack and Transient Neurologic Defects

CODES

ICD10
R55 Syncope and collapse

CLINICAL PEARLS
- A careful history of the events preceding the syncopal episode helps guide evaluation and management.
- Rule out cardiac or neurogenic syncope.
- Prodrome is common with reflex syncope.
- Recovery may be prolonged, with persistent symptoms, but there is no residual neurologic deficit or confusion.
- Patients should avoid precipitating situations or events.

S

SYNDROME OF INAPPROPRIATE ANTIDIURETIC HORMONE SECRETION (SIADH)

Elise Joyce Barney, DO

BASICS

Syndrome of inappropriate secretion of antidiuretic hormone (SIADH) is a common cause of hyponatremia in hospitalized patients.

DESCRIPTION

- The syndrome of inappropriate secretion of antidiuretic hormone (SIADH) is a disorder with impaired water excretion (concentrated urine), caused by abnormal production of antidiuretic hormone (ADH) despite low serum osmolality.
  - Decreased urinary electrolyte-free water excretion leads to dilutional hyponatremia (total body sodium [Na] levels may be normal or near-normal, but the patient's total body water is increased).
  - Often secondary to medications but may be associated with an underlying disorder, such as neoplasm, a pulmonary disorder, or CNS disease
- Synonym(s): syndrome of inappropriate secretion of ADH; syndrome of inappropriate antidiuresis

EPIDEMIOLOGY

Incidence

- Often found in the hospital setting, where incidence can be as high as 35%
- Predominant age: elderly
- Predominate sex: females > males

Prevalence

It is also prevalent in hospitalized perioperative patients in response to stress, hypotonic fluids, and drugs.

ETIOLOGY AND PATHOPHYSIOLOGY

- Drugs:
  - Antidepressants (e.g., SSRIs, tricyclics, monoamine oxidase inhibitors [MAOIs])
  - Antineoplastic drugs (e.g., vincristine, vinblastine, cisplatin, cyclophosphamide)
  - Antipsychotic agents (e.g., risperidone, quetiapine, phenothiazines, haloperidol)
  - Analgesics (e.g., duloxetine, pregabalin, tramadol, NSAIDs)
  - Anticonvulsants (e.g., carbamazepine, oxcarbazepine, valproic acid, phenytoin)
  - Others (e.g., vasopressin, DDAVP, oxytocin, ciprofloxacin, α-interferon, ecstasy)
- Malignancies (ectopic ADH production):
  - Bronchogenic carcinoma
  - Lymphoma
  - Mesothelioma
  - Small cell carcinoma of the lung
  - Pancreatic carcinoma
  - Thymoma
- Pulmonary conditions:
  - Asthma/COPD/pneumothorax
  - Atelectasis
  - Cystic fibrosis
  - Positive pressure mechanical ventilation
  - Pneumonia (viral, bacterial)

- Pulmonary tuberculosis (TB)
- Sarcoidosis
- Neurologic causes:
  - Brain tumor
  - CNS injury (i.e., subarachnoid hemorrhage, trauma, stroke)
  - CNS lupus
  - Encephalitis
  - Epilepsy
  - Guillain-Barré syndrome
  - Intracranial surgery
  - Meningitis
  - Multiple sclerosis
- Nephrogenic/hereditary:
  - A gain of function mutation in the gene for vasopressin 2 receptors (V2R)
- Other:
  - Acute intermittent porphyria
  - Delirium tremens
  - HIV infection/AIDS
  - Rocky Mountain spotted fever

Genetics

- 10% of patients have an X-linked mutation of V2R.
- Polymorphisms in TRPV4 gene

RISK FACTORS

- Advanced age
- Postoperative status
- Institutionalization
- Use of predisposing drugs

GENERAL PREVENTION

- Search for the cause, if unknown.
- Reduce/change medications, if drug-induced.
- Lifelong restriction of fluid intake

COMMONLY ASSOCIATED CONDITIONS

See "Etiology and Pathophysiology."

DIAGNOSIS

- Bartter and Schwartz criteria for SIADH:
  - Decreased osmolality (<275 mosm/kg) with inappropriately concentrated urine (>100 mosm/kg) and euvolemia
- Signs and symptoms depend on the rate and severity of hyponatremia and the degree of cerebral edema.

HISTORY

Symptoms:

- Fatigue, lethargy
- Anorexia
- Nausea, vomiting
- Increased thirst
- Headaches
- Dizziness, changes in vision
- Unsteady gait, falls

- Myalgias/weakness
- Confusion
- Seizures, coma

PHYSICAL EXAM

- Euvolemic state
- Mild hyponatremia (serum Na 125 to 135 mEq/L)
  - Slow cognition and reaction times
  - Hyporeflexia
  - Ataxia
- Moderate to severe hyponatremia (serum Na <125 mEq/L)
  - Altered mental status
  - Lethargy
  - Seizures
  - Psychosis
  - Coma
  - Death

DIFFERENTIAL DIAGNOSIS

- Intravascular volume depletion and thiazide-diuretic induced
- Appropriate ADH secretion secondary to decreased effective arterial blood volume (e.g., congestive heart failure [CHF], nephrotic syndrome, liver cirrhosis)
- Low solute intake hyponatremia
  - "Tea and toast" diet
  - Beer potomania
- Psychogenic polydipsia
  - Intake water usually >10 L/day
  - Diuresis occurs when intake is stopped.
- Endocrinopathies
  - Adrenal insufficiency
  - Hypothyroidism
- Translocational hyponatremia: caused by hyperglycemia, mannitol, sucrose, glycine
- Pseudohyponatremia
  - Lab artifact caused by hyperlipidemia, paraproteinemias, administration of IVIG
  - Labs using flame photometry or indirect potentiometry susceptible
- Postoperative complications:
  - Caused by nonosmotic release of ADH, probably mediated by pain afferents
  - ADH stimulated by pain, nausea, vomiting, and hypotension
- Cerebral salt-wasting syndrome (hyponatremia, extracellular fluid depletion, CNS insult)

DIAGNOSTIC TESTS & INTERPRETATION

- Serum Na level: low
- Serum urea level: normal to low
- Serum osmolality: low
- Urine osmolality: high; urine osmolality >100 mOsm/kg H_2O (1)
- Urine Na concentration: high; urine Na >30 mEq/L (1)
- Fractional excretion of Na >0.5% (1)
- Serum ADH level: high (not clinically useful)

- Not usually required for diagnosis but to assist in the diagnosis and assess for other causes:
  – Serum uric acid
  – Serum glucose; creatinine
  – Thyroid function
  – Morning cortisol

Initial Tests (lab, imaging)
- Serum osmolality
- Urine electrolytes (urine Na and urine potassium) and urine osmolality

Follow-Up Tests & Special Considerations
- Consider chest X-ray as part of SIADH workup to evaluate for pulmonary disease.
- Patients with nausea, vomiting, headache, vision changes, and confusion should have a CT scan of the head to look for signs of trauma or space-occupying lesions.

 TREATMENT

GENERAL MEASURES
- Treatment of the underlying cause is essential.
- Fluid restriction (usually <1,000 mL/day) is the main treatment (2)[B].
- Avoid isotonic saline because this can worsen the hyponatremia.
- Correct hypokalemia.
- Mild asymptomatic hyponatremia (serum Na >125 mEq/L [>125 mmol/L]): Restrict fluid and treat the underlying cause.
- Moderate hyponatremia (serum Na 120 to 125 mEq/L):
  – Restrict free water intake.
  – Increase oral solute intake.
  – Calculate urine/plasma electrolyte ratio ([urine Na + K] / [serum Na + serum K]) to determine efficacy of fluid restriction; ineffective if ratio >1 (3) and may need pharmacologic therapy
  – Treat underlying cause/remove the offending agent.
- Severe or with neurologic manifestations
  – Hypertonic saline (3% sodium chloride [NaCl] IV bolus)
  – Increase serum Na slowly with hypertonic saline by 4 to 6 mEq/L over 4 to 6 hours (not to exceed 8 mEq/L in a 24-hour period) (1),(4)[C].
- Acute (<48 hours duration)
  – Can initially correct rapidly but the 24-hour goal is the same as in chronic hyponatremia (4)[C]

MEDICATION
- If severe or neurologic symptoms: IV 3% NaCl to increase serum Na cautiously (5)[B]:
  – If serum Na <120 mEq/L or severe neurologic symptoms, consider bolus of hypertonic saline to increase serum Na by 4 to 6 mEq/L over the first 4 to 6 hours.
- NaCl oral tablets
- Oral urea is an option but limited due to bitter taste.
- Loop diuretics: furosemide + potassium replacement

- Vasopressin-2 receptor antagonist (the vaptans: tolvaptan, conivaptan) (5)[B]
  – Good efficacy and safety profiles in the treatment of moderate hyponatremia due to SIADH
  – Liberal fluid intake encouraged
  – Must be initiated in the hospital setting
  – Avoid tolvaptan in patients with liver disease.
- Demeclocycline (limited use)
  – Blocks ADH at renal tubule; produces nephrogenic diabetes insipidus
  – Dosage for long-term management: 300 to 600 mg PO BID
  – Onset of action within 1 week; therefore, not best for acute management
  – Adverse effects of GI intolerance and nephrotoxicity limit its use.
  – Paucity of evidence for efficacy
- Contraindications: Avoid fluids in HF, nephrotic syndrome, or cirrhosis. Avoid tolvaptan in patients with cirrhosis due to possible liver injury.
- Precautions: Overly rapid correction (>10 mEq/L/day) can increase the risk for osmotic demyelination syndrome (ODS):
  – Permanent CNS damage in pons leading to quadriplegia and pseudobulbar palsy
  – Increased risk in women, alcoholics, malnutrition, hypoxia, chronic hyponatremia of <110 mEq/L, and hypokalemia

ALERT
Increase Na levels slowly, not >8 mEq/L/24 hr, to prevent ODS (1)[C].

 ONGOING CARE

FOLLOW-UP RECOMMENDATIONS
Patient Monitoring
- Careful continuous clinical and laboratory monitoring of hyponatremic state during the acute phase:
  – Hourly urine output
  – Urine Na, urine potassium, urine osmolality
  – Goal Na increase is <8 mEq/L/24 hr until Na reaches 130 mEq/L (1),(4)[C].
  – If moderate/severe, check serial serum chemistry every 4 to 8 hours to ensure an appropriate rate of correction.
- Chronic management: Treat underlying cause; continue fluid restriction and NaCl tablets as needed; referral to nephrologist

DIET
Increase protein/solute intake and decrease water intake.

PATIENT EDUCATION
Diet and fluid restrictions

PROGNOSIS
- Higher morbidity and mortality in hospitalized patients with hyponatremia (6)
- Higher risk of ICU admission and increased risk of 30-day hospital readmission in hyponatremic patients (6)
- If symptomatic (seizure, coma): high mortality due to cerebral edema if serum Na <120 mEq/L

COMPLICATIONS
- Falls and hip fractures
- Cerebral edema (see "Prognosis")
- Osmotic demyelination with overcorrection (see "Treatment" precautions): central pontine and extrapontine irreversible myelinolysis (4)
- Chronic hyponatremia
- Chronic hyponatremia is associated with osteoporosis (6)[C].

REFERENCES

1. Decaux G, Musch W. Clinical laboratory evaluation of the syndrome of inappropriate secretion of antidiuretic hormone. *Clin J Am Soc Nephrol.* 2008;3(4):1175–1184.
2. Ellison DH, Berl T. Clinical practice. The syndrome of inappropriate antidiuresis. *N Engl J Med.* 2007;356(20):2064–2072.
3. Furst H, Hallows KR, Post J, et al. The urine/plasma electrolyte ratio: a predictive guide to water restriction. *Am J Med Sci.* 2000;319(4):240–244.
4. Adrogué HJ, Madias NE. The challenge of hyponatremia. *J Am Soc Nephrol.* 2012;23(7):1140–1148.
5. Esposito P, Piotti G, Bianzina S, et al. The syndrome of inappropriate antidiuresis: pathophysiology, clinical management and new therapeutic options. *Nephron Clin Pract.* 2011;119(1):c62–c73.
6. Usala RL, Fernandez SJ, Mete M, et al. Hyponatremia is associated with increased osteoporosis and bone fractures in a large US health system population. *J Clin Endocrinol Metab.* 2015;100(8):3021–3031.

 SEE ALSO

Hyponatremia

 CODES

ICD10
E22.2 Syndrome of inappropriate secretion of antidiuretic hormone

CLINICAL PEARLS
- Treatment of the underlying cause is key. Review all medications for potential culprits.
- Fluid restriction is the mainstay of treatment in SIADH. Fluid restriction fails to correct hyponatremia and Na wasting in salt-losing renal disease.
- ODS is a cerebral demyelination syndrome that causes quadriplegia, pseudobulbar palsy, seizures, coma, and death. It is caused by an overly rapid rate of Na correction. Increase Na levels slowly, not >8 mEq/L/24 hr, to prevent ODS.
- Safe correction of hyponatremia is important. Online calculators are available: http://www.medcalc.com/sodium.html.

S

SYPHILIS

Melissa E. Badowski, PharmD, MPH • Mahesh C. Patel, MD

 BASICS

DESCRIPTION

- A chronic, systemic infectious disease caused by the spirochete *Treponema pallidum*
- Transmitted sexually by direct contact with an active lesion; also transmitted vertically (maternal–fetal) and via blood transfusions
- Untreated disease includes four overlapping stages.
  - Primary: single (usually) painless chancre at point of entry; appears in 10 to 90 days; chancre heals without treatment in 3 to 6 weeks.
  - Secondary: appears 2 to 8 weeks after primary chancre; nonpruritic rash on palms or soles of feet, mucous membrane lesions, headache, fever, lymphadenopathy, alopecia
  - Latent: seroreactive without evidence of disease
    - Early latent: acquired within the last year
    - Late latent: exposure >12 months prior to diagnosis
  - Tertiary (late): Serology may be negative (fluorescent treponemal antibody absorption [FTA-ABS] test typically positive).
    - Gumma, cardiovascular, and late neurosyphilis; may be fatal
  - Neurosyphilis: *any* type of CNS involvement; can occur at *any* stage
    - Psychosis, delirium, dementia
- Syphilis can affect nearly every organ/tissue.

Pediatric Considerations
In noncongenital cases, consider child abuse.

Pregnancy Considerations
- Screen all pregnant patients with venereal disease research laboratory (VDRL) test or rapid plasma reagin (RPR) test early in pregnancy, (i.e., first prenatal visit). If high risk, repeat at 28 weeks and at delivery (1),(2)[A].
- Use the same nontreponemal test for initial screening and for follow-up (1),(2)[A].

EPIDEMIOLOGY

Incidence
- Syphilis rate decreased through 2000 and have since increased (primarily in men who have sex with men [MSM]) (3).
  - All stages: 40 per 100,000
- Congenital: 49/100,000 live births (3)
- Primary and secondary syphilis statistics (3)
  - HIV coinfection
    - MSM: 44.2%
    - Men who have sex with women only (MSW): 7.6%
    - Women: 4.3%
  - Male (per 100,000 population)
    - Overall: 20.1 (highest for males ages 25 to 29 years)
    - Whites, non-Hispanic: 11.0; blacks, non-Hispanic: 53.5
    - Hispanics: 23.4; Asians: 8.9
    - American Indians/Alaska natives: 27.1
    - Native Hawaiians/Pacific Islanders: 35.9
    - Multirace: 18.1
  - Female (per 100,000 population)
    - Overall: 3.9 (highest for females ages 25 to 29 years)
    - Whites, non-Hispanic: 2.3; blacks, non-Hispanic: 10.2
    - Hispanics: 3.8; Asians: 0.6
    - American Indians/Alaska natives: 15.4
    - Native Hawaiians/Pacific Islanders: 9.6
    - Multirace: 3.3

Prevalence
- Predominant sex: male (83%) > female (17%) (3)
- Highest prevalence in MSM (3)

ETIOLOGY AND PATHOPHYSIOLOGY
T. pallidum enters through intact mucous membranes or breaks in skin. The organism quickly enters the lymphatics to cause systemic disease. Highly infectious; exposure to as few as 60 spirochetes is associated with ~50% chance of infection.

RISK FACTORS
MSM, multiple sexual partners, exposure to infected body fluids, injection drug use, transplacental transmission, adult inmates, high-risk sexual behavior, people living with HIV (PLWH)

GENERAL PREVENTION
Education regarding safe sex; condoms reduce but do not eliminate transmission (4)[A].

COMMONLY ASSOCIATED CONDITIONS
HIV infection, hepatitis B, other sexually transmitted infections (STIs)

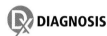 **DIAGNOSIS**

HISTORY
- As a "great imitator," a high index of suspicion is often required for accurate diagnosis.
- Previous sexual contact with partner with known infection or high-risk sexual behavior
- Genital lesions (chancre—primary syphilis)
- Rash, alopecia, malaise, headache, anorexia, nausea, fatigue (secondary syphilis)
- Mental status changes (tertiary syphilis)

PHYSICAL EXAM
Signs/symptoms depend on stage.
- Primary: single (occasionally multiple), usually painless ulcer (chancre) in groin or at other point of entry; regional adenopathy
- Chancres begin as solitary firm, raised painless papules that erode and ulcerate. Spontaneous healing occurs in 4 to 8 weeks regardless of treatment
- Secondary
  - Rash: skin/mucous membranes
    - Rough, red-brown macules, usually on palms and soles
    - May appear with chancre or after it has healed
    - Condylomata lata
    - Alopecia
  - Nonspecific symptoms: fever, adenopathy, malaise, headache, hair loss
- Tertiary (late) syphilis
  - Focal neurologic findings (hearing loss, vision loss; meningeal findings; loss of pain, temperature; proprioception)
  - Gummas (skin, mucous membranes, other organ systems)

DIFFERENTIAL DIAGNOSIS
- Primary: chancroid, lymphogranuloma venereum, granuloma inguinale, condylomata acuminata, herpes simplex, Behçet syndrome, trauma, carcinoma, mycotic infection, lichen planus, psoriasis, fungal infection
- Secondary: pityriasis rosea, drug eruption, psoriasis, lichen planus, viral exanthema, Stevens-Johnson syndrome
- Positive serology, asymptomatic: previously treated syphilis/other spirochetal disease (yaws, pinta)

DIAGNOSTIC TESTS & INTERPRETATION

Initial Tests (lab, imaging)
- Dark-field microscopy demonstrating *T. pallidum* spirochetes in lesion exudate/tissue biopsy is gold standard but difficult and not very sensitive (5)[A].
- Nontreponemal tests (VDRL/RPR) (3),(5)[A]
  - Primary screening test: positive within 7 days of exposure
  - Nonspecific false-positive results are common; must confirm diagnosis with treponemal tests
  - Positive test should be quantified and titers followed regularly after treatment.
    - Titers usually correlate with disease activity; 4-fold change is clinically significant.
    - Titers decrease with time/treatment; following adequate treatment for primary/secondary disease, a 4-fold decline is typical in 6 to 12 months.
    - Absence of a 4-fold decline suggests potential treatment failure.
    - ~15% of appropriately treated patients do not have a 4-fold decline in titer 12 months after treatment. Management is unclear; repeat HIV testing and/or CSF examination and continue to follow titers.
    - With appropriate treatment, titers should become negative (see serofast reaction).
    - Titers of patients treated in latent stages decline more gradually.
  - Prozone phenomenon: negative results from high titers of antibody; test with diluted serum.
  - Serofast reaction: persistently positive results years after successful treatment; new infection diagnosed by 4-fold rise in titer
  - Conditions that may alter treponemal testing (All stages of syphilis can have a false-negative RPR result, especially in primary syphilis.)
    - Pregnancy, autoimmune disease, mononucleosis, malaria, leprosy, viral pneumonia, cardiolipin antigens, injection drug use, acute febrile illness, HIV infection; elderly can have false-positive results.
- TP-PA (*T. pallidum* particle agglutination) increasingly used for primary testing as high sensitivity overcomes challenges of nontreponemal tests
- Treponemal tests (*confirmatory test after positive nontreponemal screening test*): for example, FTA-ABS, TP-PA (*T. pallidum particle agglutination*), others (5)[A]:
  - Confirmatory test
  - Usually positive for life after treatment
  - Titers of no benefit
  - 15–25% of patients treated during primary stage revert to serologic nonreactivity after 2 to 3 years.
- Lumbar puncture (LP) indicated for (5)[A]:
  - Neurologic, ocular, or auditory manifestations
  - Some advise LP in all secondary and early latent cases—even without neurologic symptoms.
  - PLWH with late latent/latent disease of unknown duration
  - Patients with late latent/latent disease of unknown duration if nonpenicillin therapy planned
  - Treatment failures
  - Evidence of active tertiary syphilis (e.g., aortitis, gumma, iritis)
  - Children to rule out neurosyphilis
  - VDRL, not RPR, used on CSF; may be negative in neurosyphilis; highly specific but insensitive
  - Send CSF for protein, glucose, and cell count.
  - Monitor resolution with cell count at 6 months along with serologies (see "Patient Monitoring").

– Negative FTA-ABS or microhemagglutination (MHA)-TP on CSF excludes neurosyphilis (highly sensitive).
– Positive FTA-ABS or MHA-TP on CSF is not diagnostic because of high false-positive rate.
– Traumatic tap, tuberculosis (TB), pyogenic/aseptic meningitis can all result in false-positive VDRL.

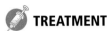 TREATMENT

GENERAL MEASURES

• Advise patients to notify partner(s) and to avoid intercourse until treatment is complete (5)[A].
• Test for HIV infection.
• Management of sexual contacts (3),(5)[A]
  – Presumptively treat partners exposed within 90 days of diagnosis.
  – Presumptively treat partners exposed >90 days before diagnosis if serologic results are not available immediately and follow-up is uncertain.
  – Presumptively treat those exposed to a patient diagnosed with syphilis of unknown duration who has high treponemal titers (>1:32).
  – Long-term sex partners of patients with latent infection should be evaluated clinically (including serologies) and treated accordingly.

MEDICATION

ALERT
Use Bicillin L-A instead of Bicillin C-R (combination benzathine–procaine penicillin).

First Line
Parenteral penicillin G is the drug of choice. The formulation is determined by the disease stage and clinical presentation.

• Primary, secondary, and early latent <1 year (5)[A]
  – Penicillin G benzathine 2.4 million U IM × 1 dose
  – Penicillin-allergic patients: doxycycline 100 mg PO BID for 2 weeks or ceftriaxone 1 to 2 g IM or IV daily for 10 to 14 days
    ○ Azithromycin 2 g PO for 1 dose (early syphilis only; should not be used in HIV, MSM, or pregnancy)
    ○ Resistance and treatment failures have been noted in several U.S. regions.
• Late latent/latent of unknown duration and tertiary without evidence of neurosyphilis (5)[A]
  – Penicillin G benzathine 2.4 million U IM weekly × 3 doses
  – Penicillin-allergic patients: Attempt desensitization and treatment with penicillin or doxycycline 100 mg PO BID for 28 days; adherence may be an issue.
• Ocular or neurosyphilis (5)[A]
  – Aqueous crystalline penicillin G 3 to 4 million U IV q4h as a continuous infusion for 10 to 14 days
  – Alternative: penicillin G procaine 2.4 million U IM daily in conjunction with probenecid 500 mg PO QID for 10 to 14 days (if compliance can be ensured)
  – Penicillin-allergic patients: Attempt desensitization and treat with penicillin; ceftriaxone 2 g/day IM or IV for 10 to 14 days
  – If late latent, latent of unknown duration, or tertiary in addition to neurosyphilis, consider treating as late latent after completion of neurosyphilis treatment regimen.

• Congenital (5)[A]
  – Aqueous crystalline penicillin G 50,000 U/kg/dose IV q12h for the first 7 days of life and q8h thereafter for a total of 10 days, or penicillin G procaine 50,000 U/kg/dose IM daily for 10 days
  – If negative CSF serologies, normal physical exam, and maternal titer, then give 50,000 U/kg penicillin G benzathine IM in single dose
  – If >1 day of drug is missed, restart course.
  – Children (after newborn period): aqueous crystalline penicillin G 50,000 U/kg/dose IV q4–6h for 10 days; late latent, 50,000 U/kg IM as 3 doses at 1-week intervals
  – For contacts without symptoms: Treat as primary disease after serologies are obtained.
  – PLWH and pregnant patients may show poor response to recommended IM doses. Use IV therapy for all treatment failures in these patients.
  – Do not give benzathine or procaine penicillins IV.
• Children (after newborn period) (5)[A]: aqueous crystalline penicillin G 50,000 U/kg/dose IV q4–6h for 10 days; late latent, 50,000 U/kg IM as 3 doses at 1-week intervals
• Pregnancy (5)[A]
  – Treatment is same as for nonpregnant patients.
  – Some recommend second dose of penicillin G benzathine 2.4 million U IM 1 week after initial dose in 3rd trimester or with primary, secondary, or early latent syphilis.
  – Penicillin sensitivity: no proven alternatives to penicillin available for treatment during pregnancy
  – Penicillin-allergic patients: Desensitize and treat with penicillin.
  – Pregnant PLWH may show poor response to recommended IM doses. Use IV therapy for all treatment failures in these patients.
• Treat contacts without symptoms as primary disease after obtaining serologies.
• History of penicillin allergy:
  – Confirmed IgE-mediated reaction: desensitization
  – Questionable history of IgE-mediated hypersensitivity: penicillin skin testing if major and minor penicillin determinants available
• Precautions (5)[A]
  – PLWH and pregnant patients may show poor response to recommended IM doses. Use IV therapy for all treatment failures in these patients.
  – Do not give benzathine or procaine penicillins IV.

 ONGOING CARE

FOLLOW-UP RECOMMENDATIONS

• Clinical and serologic evaluation 6 to 12 months after treatment; if >1 year duration, check at 24 months (5)[A].
• In PLWH, clinical and serologic evaluation at 3, 6, 9, 12, and 24 months after therapy (5)[A]

Patient Monitoring

• Use VDRL or RPR test to monitor therapy: 4-fold rise (two dilutions) in titer indicates new infection, whereas failure to decrease 4-fold (two dilutions) in 6 to 12 months may indicate treatment failure (although definitive criteria for cure not established); always use same test (preferably same lab) (5)[A].
• Retreatment for persistent clinical signs or recurrence, 4-fold rise in titers, or failure of initially high titer to decrease 4-fold by 6 to 12 months
• Neurosyphilis: Repeat LP every 6 months to check for normalization of CSF cell count (± CSF-VDRL and protein evaluation) (5)[A].

PATIENT EDUCATION
No intimate contacts until 4-fold titer drop

PROGNOSIS

• Excellent in all cases except patients with late syphilis complications and with HIV infection
• Syphilis in PLWH
  – Treatment same as for HIV-negative patients
  – More often false-negative treponemal and nontreponemal tests or unusually high titers
  – Response to therapy less predictable
  – Early syphilis: increased risk of neurosyphilis and higher rates of treatment failure
  – Late neurosyphilis: harder to treat; can occur up to 20 years or more after infection

COMPLICATIONS

• Membranous glomerulonephritis
• Paroxysmal cold hemoglobinemia
• Meningitis and tabes dorsalis
• Cardiovascular aneurysms; valvular damage
• Irreversible organ damage
• Jarisch-Herxheimer reaction
  – Fever, chills, headache, myalgias, new rash
  – Common when starting treatment (of primary/secondary disease; less common with tertiary) owing to treponemal lysis
  – Should not be confused with drug reaction
  – Managed with analgesics and antipyretics

REFERENCES

1. Gomez GB, Kamb ML, Newman LM, et al. Untreated maternal syphilis and adverse outcomes of pregnancy: a systematic review and meta-analysis. *Bull World Health Organ*. 2013;91(3):217–226.
2. Ghanem KG, Ram S, Rice PA. The modern epidemic of syphilis. *N Engl J Med*. 2020;382(9):845–854.
3. Centers for Disease Control and Prevention. *Sexually transmitted disease surveillance 2019*. Atlanta, GA: U.S. Department of Health and Human Services; 2021.
4. Stamm LV. Syphilis: antibiotic treatment and resistance. *Epidemiol Infect*. 2015;143(8):1567–1574.
5. Workowski KA, Bachmann LH, Chan PA, et al; for Centers for Disease Control and Prevention. Sexually transmitted infections treatment guidelines, 2021. *MMWR Recomm Rep*. 2021;70(4):1–192.

 SEE ALSO

Chlamydia Infection (Sexually Transmitted); Gonococcal Infections

CODES

ICD10
• A52.71 Late syphilitic oculopathy
• A51.0 Primary genital syphilis
• A52.74 Syphilis of liver and other viscera

CLINICAL PEARLS

• Screen all people living with HIV and all individuals with high-risk sexual behaviors for syphilis.
• Penicillin is the treatment of choice for syphilis.
• Syphilis rates are rising—prevalence is highest among MSM.

TARSAL TUNNEL SYNDROME

Terrence Tsui, DO • J. Herbert Stevenson, MD

 BASICS

DESCRIPTION

Tarsal tunnel syndrome refers to a compression or entrapment neuropathy of the posterior tibial nerve as it passes through a fibro-osseous tunnel (tarsal tunnel) located posterior and inferior to the medial malleolus and deep to the flexor retinaculum (laciniate ligament) in the medial ankle.

EPIDEMIOLOGY

- Women are slightly more affected than men (56%).
- All postpubescent ages are affected.

ETIOLOGY AND PATHOPHYSIOLOGY

- Contents within the tarsal tunnel from the anterior medial to the posterior lateral side include the following: the posterior tibial tendon, the flexor digitorum longus tendon, the posterior tibial artery and veins, the posterior tibial nerve, and the flexor hallucis tendon.
- The posterior tibial nerve passes through the tarsal tunnel, which is formed by three osseus structures—sustentaculum tali, medial calcaneus, and medial malleolus—covered by the laciniate ligament.
- Compression of the posterior tibial nerve within the tarsal tunnel results in decreased blood flow, ischemic damage, and resultant symptoms (1).
- Chronic compression can destroy endoneurial microvasculature, leading to edema and (eventually) fibrosis and demyelination (2).
- Increased pressure in the tarsal tunnel is caused by a variety of mechanical and biochemical mechanisms. The specific cause for compression is identifiable in only 60–80% of cases (1).
- Three general categories: trauma, space-occupying lesions, deformity (1)
  - Trauma including displaced fractures, deltoid ligament sprains, or tenosynovitis
  - Varicosities
  - Hindfoot varus or valgus
  - Fibrosis of the perineurium
- Other causes:
  - Osseous prominences; osteophytes
  - Ganglia; lipoma; neurilemmoma
  - Inflammatory synovitis
  - Pigmented villonodular synovitis
  - Tarsal coalition
  - Accessory musculature
- In patients with systemic disease (e.g., diabetes), the "double crush" syndrome refers to the development of a second compression along the same nerve at a site of anatomic narrowing in patients with previous proximal nerve damage (3).

RISK FACTORS

- Tarsal tunnel syndrome is associated with certain occupations and activities involving repetitive and prolonged weight-bearing on the foot and ankle (walking, running, dancing).
- Other possible risk factors include (4):
  - Diabetes
  - Systemic inflammatory arthritis
  - Connective tissue disorders

- Obesity
- Varicosities
- Heel varus or valgus
- Bifurcation of the posterior tibial nerve into medial and lateral plantar nerves proximal to the tarsal tunnel

 DIAGNOSIS

Tarsal tunnel syndrome is largely a clinical diagnosis, characterized by pain and paresthesias in a predictable distribution along the medial aspect of the ankle and plantar surface of the foot (1).

HISTORY

- History of trauma (which may be trivial) to the foot precipitating pain
- Pain, tightness, burning, tingling, and/or numbness behind medial malleolus radiating to the longitudinal arch and plantar aspect of foot including the heel (1)
- Pain usually worsens during standing or activity.
- Pain radiates proximally up the medial leg (Valleix phenomenon) in 33% of patients with severe compression.
- Some patients have substantial night pain (may be related to venostasis).
- Symptoms improve with rest, wearing loose footwear, and elevation.
- In advanced nerve compression, motor involvement may cause weakness, atrophy, and digital contractures of the intrinsic foot muscles (4).

ALERT

Other systemic neuropathies (diabetes, alcoholism, HIV, drug reactions) present with similar symptoms.

PHYSICAL EXAM

- Inspect: foot alignment
  - Examine for excessive foot pronation during standing or walking.
  - Examine for hindfoot varus or valgus deformity while standing.
- Palpate the tarsal tunnel and the course of the tibial nerve for tenderness and swelling.
- Tinel sign: Percussion over the tibial nerve may reproduce paresthesias that radiate distally.
- Valleix sign: Percussion over the tibial nerve may produce paresthesias that radiate proximally.
- Compression test: Applying pressure to the tarsal tunnel for 60 seconds may reproduce symptoms.
- Provocative testing: reproduction of symptoms with stretching of the nerve with exaggerated dorsiflexion and eversion of the foot/ankle or compression of the nerve with plantar flexion and inversion of the foot/ankle
- Sensory examination
  - The medial calcaneal nerve usually is spared, but numbness and altered sensation may be present in the distribution of the medial or lateral plantar nerves.
  - Vibratory sensation and two-point discrimination are decreased early in the disease process.

- Motor examination
  - Intrinsic foot muscle weakness (difficult to assess)
  - Rarely, weakness of toe plantar flexion may be present.
  - Toe contractures in flexion and atrophy of the abductor hallucis or abductor digiti minimi may be seen late in the disease process.

DIFFERENTIAL DIAGNOSIS

- Peripheral neuropathies (diabetes, alcoholism, HIV, or drug related)
- Inflammatory arthritis (rheumatoid arthritis)
- Morton neuroma
- Metatarsalgia
- Subtalar joint arthritis
- Tibialis posterior tendinopathy
- Plantar fasciitis
- Plantar callosities
- Peripheral vascular disease
- Lumbar radiculopathy
- Proximal injury or compression of the tibial branch of the sciatic nerve

DIAGNOSTIC TESTS & INTERPRETATION

Initial Tests (lab, imaging)

Routine lab tests help rule out other conditions that may mimic tarsal tunnel syndrome, including diabetic neuropathy, rheumatoid arthritis, thyroid dysfunction, or other systemic illnesses (5).

- Routine weight-bearing radiographs, followed by CT (if necessary) to assess for fracture or structural abnormality
- Consider evaluation of lumbar spine x-ray if double crush (injury to lumbar nerve results in compensatory injury to posterior tibial nerve) is suspected (5).
- MRI: helps assess the tarsal tunnel for soft tissue masses or other sources of nerve compression before surgery (1)
- Ultrasound (US): gaining importance and with several advantages over MRI; dynamic testing in positions where the nerve may be stretched or compressed; can assess for space-occupying lesions (ganglia, varicose veins, lipomas, etc.) and tenosynovitis (1)

Pregnancy Considerations

- Tarsal tunnel syndrome can occur during pregnancy, typically secondary to local compression caused by fluid retention and volume changes (1).
- Care is supportive. Most cases resolve after pregnancy.

Pediatric Considerations

MRI is recommended for evaluating pediatric tarsal tunnel syndrome to exclude neoplastic mass.

Diagnostic Procedures/Other

Electrodiagnostic studies

- Electromyography (EMG) of the intrinsic muscles of the foot can confirm the diagnosis of tarsal tunnel syndrome. A normal EMG does not exclude the diagnosis (false-negative rate is ~10%) (1).
- Nerve conduction studies may reveal slowed conduction of the tibial nerve.
- Evaluate for proximal nerve compression, including a lumbar radiculopathy or a double crush phenomenon.

TREATMENT

- Conservative management is recommended, except for acute onset tarsal tunnel syndrome or in the setting of a known space-occupying lesion (excluding synovitis).
- Tarsal tunnel decompression may improve sensory impairment and restore protective sensation in diabetic peripheral neuropathies if there is nerve entrapment at the tarsal tunnel.

MEDICATION
First Line
- Analgesics and anti-inflammatory medications
- Local corticosteroid injection into the tarsal tunnel
- Medications that alter neurogenic pain (tricyclic antidepressants, antiepileptic drugs, nerve blockers)

ADDITIONAL THERAPIES
- Rest and elevation
- Immobilization with a night splint or cam walker boot
- Taping and bracing
- Orthotics or shoe modification
- Physical therapy to strengthen the intrinsic and extrinsic muscles of the foot, nerve mobilization exercises, and to restore the medial longitudinal arch of the foot
- Other modalities (stretching, US, massage, icing)
- Compression stockings to decrease swelling
- Weight loss for obese patients

SURGERY/OTHER PROCEDURES
- Surgery is indicated (1),(2):
  - If nonoperative measures fail following a 6-month trial
  - In the setting of acute tarsal tunnel syndrome
  - If there are signs of motor involvement/weakness or muscle atrophy
  - If a space-occupying lesion is identified
- The surgical outcome is dependent on technique and postoperative management. 50–95% of cases have good to excellent outcomes.
- At the time of surgery, assess focal swelling, scarring, or nerve abnormalities and look for a pathologic source of compression.
- Postoperative management includes:
  - Non–weight-bearing splint until incision heals (2 to 3 weeks), followed by progressively increased weight-bearing and range of motion exercises
  - Rest, ice, compression, elevation to limit swelling

 ONGOING CARE

PATIENT EDUCATION
- Discuss conservative and surgical options based on individual patient circumstance and preference.
- A decision about surgical intervention should be made with a clear understanding of risks, benefits, and potential adverse outcomes.

PROGNOSIS
Surgery is most helpful for:
- Patients with a positive Tinel sign (3)[B]
- Young patients
- Short period between occurrence of symptoms and surgery <1 year
- Localized space-occupying lesion (1)
- No motor neuron involvement

COMPLICATIONS
- The main adverse outcome is an unsuccessful surgical intervention characterized by lack of improvement or recurrence of symptoms (1).
- Causes for a failed tarsal tunnel release include:
  - Incorrect diagnosis
  - Incomplete release
  - Adhesive neuritis (external scar formation)
  - Intraneural damage (systemic disease, direct nerve injury)
  - Failure to treat all sources of nerve compression in a double crush phenomenon
- Electrodiagnostic studies are rarely helpful in determining the cause of a failed tarsal tunnel release.
- Results with surgical revision are poorer than those for the primary surgical release.

REFERENCES

1. Ahmad M, Tsang K, Mackenney PJ, et al. Tarsal tunnel syndrome: a literature review. *Foot Ankle Surg*. 2012;18(3):149–152.
2. Dellon AL. The four medial ankle tunnels: a critical review of perceptions of tarsal tunnel syndrome and neuropathy. *Neurosurg Clin N Am*. 2008;19(4):629–648.
3. Dellon AL, Muse VL, Scott ND, et al. A positive Tinel sign as predictor of pain relief or sensory recovery after decompression of chronic tibial nerve compression in patients with diabetic neuropathy. *J Reconstr Microsurg*. 2012;28(4):235–240.
4. Franson J, Baravarian B. Tarsal tunnel syndrome: a compression neuropathy involving four distinct tunnels. *Clin Podiatr Med Surg*. 2006;23(3):597–609.
5. Fantino O. Role of ultrasound in posteromedial tarsal tunnel syndrome: 81 cases. *J Ultrasound*. 2014;17(2):99–112.

ADDITIONAL READING

- Abouelela AA, Zohiery AK. The triple compression stress test for diagnosis of tarsal tunnel syndrome. *Foot (Edinb)*. 2012;22(3):146–149.
- Allen JM, Greer BJ, Sorge DG, et al. MR imaging of neuropathies of the leg, ankle, and foot. *Magn Reson Imaging Clin N Am*. 2008;16(1):117–131.
- Gondring WH, Tarun PK, Trepman E. Touch pressure and sensory density after tarsal tunnel release in diabetic neuropathy. *Foot Ankle Surg*. 2012;18(4):241–246.
- Gould JS. Recurrent tarsal tunnel syndrome. *Foot Ankle Clin*. 2014;19(3):451–467.

- Imai K, Ikoma K, Imai R, et al. Tarsal tunnel syndrome in hemodialysis patients: a case series. *Foot Ankle Int*. 2013;34(3):439–444.
- Lui TH. Endoscopic resection of the tarsal tunnel ganglion. *Arthrosc Tech*. 2016;5(5):e1173–e1177.
- Patel AT, Gaines K, Malamut R, et al; for American Association of Neuromuscular and Electrodiagnostic Medicine. Usefulness of electrodiagnostic techniques in the evaluation of suspected tarsal tunnel syndrome: an evidence-based review. *Muscle Nerve*. 2005;32(2):236–240.
- Reichert P, Zimmer K, Wnukiewicz W, et al. Results of surgical treatment of tarsal tunnel syndrome. *Foot Ankle Surg*. 2015;21(1):26–29.
- Sung KS, Park SJ. Short-term operative outcome of tarsal tunnel syndrome due to benign space-occupying lesions. *Foot Ankle Int*. 2009;30(8):741–745.
- Yang Y, Du ML, Fu YS, et al. Fine dissection of the tarsal tunnel in 60 cases. *Sci Rep*. 2017;7:46351.

 SEE ALSO

Algorithm: Foot Pain

CODES

ICD10
- G57.50 Tarsal tunnel syndrome, unspecified lower limb
- G57.51 Tarsal tunnel syndrome, right lower limb
- G57.52 Tarsal tunnel syndrome, left lower limb

CLINICAL PEARLS
- Tarsal tunnel syndrome typically presents with pain and numbness/tingling/burning/paresthesias of the medial ankle and plantar foot.
- Tinel sign is the most sensitive and specific physical examination test for diagnosing tarsal tunnel.
- Tarsal tunnel syndrome is a clinical diagnosis, which can be supported with imaging and electrodiagnostic studies.
- Conservative management is recommended, except for patients with an acute onset tarsal tunnel syndrome or known space-occupying lesion.

TELOGEN EFFLUVIUM

Bonnie A. Buechel, MD, MS • Shawn Phillips, MD

BASICS

Acute, self-limited diffuse hair loss or hair thinning

DESCRIPTION

Telogen effluvium (TE) is a transient condition in which there is a premature conversion of a significant proportion of anagen (growth phase) hairs into telogen (resting phase) hairs resulting in subsequent increased shedding of these resting hair follicles when the follicles re-enter anagen, and the clinical appearance of moderate to severe hair thinning. Normally, each hair follicle cycles independently of others through anagen, catagen (end-of-growth transformation), and telogen, with the large majority of hair follicles in anagen at any given time.

- Five proposed types of TE:
  - Immediate anagen release: a highly common form, lasting 3 to 4 weeks, in which follicles meant to remain in anagen phase enter telogen prematurely due to a signal, including high fever, drug induced, or stress.
  - Delayed anagen release: large group of hair follicles that have remained in the anagen phase for an extended period all together enter the telogen phase, resulting in hair loss. Common postpartum.
  - Short anagen: a speculative type in which at least 50% of the hair follicles have an idiopathic shortening of the anagen phase. Results in a doubling of the follicles in the telogen phase.
  - Immediate telogen release: normal resting club hairs remain within the hair follicle until an unknown signal causes their release, initiating the anagen stage to begin. In this type, the resting club hairs are prematurely released, ending the telogen phase abruptly and causing diffuse shedding.
  - Delayed telogen release: the presence of increased visible light, whether it be a seasonal or environmental change, is thought to end a prolonged telogen phase and initiate the anagen phase; results in diffuse shedding of hair follicles

EPIDEMIOLOGY

Incidence
Second most common cause of alopecia

Prevalence
Unknown

ETIOLOGY AND PATHOPHYSIOLOGY

- The hair cycle consists of two predominant phases: the anagen (growth phase) and the telogen (resting phase), which last ~3 years and 3 months, respectively. In a normal scalp, ~10–15% of hairs are in the telogen phase. Due to the presence of some types of external/internal stress, there may be an increase in the percentage of telogen hairs. As new anagen hairs emerge, these telogen hair follicles are forced out. The preceding event usually occurs 2 to 3 months prior to the appearance of hair loss.
- It is hypothesized that substance P plays a key role in the pathogenesis of TE through various mechanisms (1). Studies have been conducted on human hair follicles in vitro and mice hair follicles in vivo, which support this theory.
- Role of substance P includes the following (2):
  - Upregulation of substance P receptor, NK1, at the gene and protein level, leading to premature catagen development and hair growth inhibition
  - Upregulation of nerve growth factor (NGF) and subsequently its hair apoptosis–producing receptor, p75NTR
  - Downregulation of hair growth–promoting receptor, TrkA
  - Upregulation of major histocompatibility class (MHC) I and β_2-microglobulin resulting in loss of hair follicle immune-privilege
  - Increase in tumor necrosis factor-α release by mast cells resulting in hair keratinocyte apoptosis
- Decreased cortisol levels in chronic stress states may also enhance the effects of substance P.

RISK FACTORS
- Infection
- Trauma
- Major surgery
- Thyroid disorder
- Febrile illness
- Malignancy
- Allergic contact dermatitis
- Iron deficiency anemia

- Excess vitamin A
- Protein-calorie restriction
- End-stage liver or renal disease
- Hormonal changes (including pregnancy, delivery, and estrogen-containing medications)
- Chronic stress
- Drug induced (e.g., β-blockers, anticonvulsants, antidepressants, anticoagulants, retinoids, ACE-inhibitors)
- Immunizations

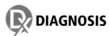
DIAGNOSIS

HISTORY
- Commonly, an inciting event 2 to 6 months previous to noted hair loss
- Fear of becoming bald
- Patients often present with evidence of hair loss with collections of hair or photographs

PHYSICAL EXAM
- Decreased density of hair on the scalp, most commonly involving the crown and temples.
- In rare cases of chronic TE, there is hair loss at the eyebrows and pubic region.
- May have diffuse shedding of hair when fingers are run through the scalp.
- Shed hairs are telogen hairs, which have a small bulb of unpigmented or pigmented keratin on the root end (so-called 'club' hairs).
- May affect nail growth, resulting in the appearance of Beau lines, which are transverse grooves on the nails of the hands and feet.

DIFFERENTIAL DIAGNOSIS
- Hypothyroidism
- Hyperthyroidism
- Alopecia areata (diffuse pattern)
- Androgenetic alopecia
- Drug-induced alopecia
- Systemic lupus erythematosus
- Secondary syphilis
- Trichotillomania

DIAGNOSTIC TESTS & INTERPRETATION

Most often, TE is a clinical diagnosis based on typical history and exclusion of other scalp pathology and medical conditions. Blood work may be collected primarily to rule out other possible causes of hair loss. Nutritional deficiencies in iron and zinc have been associated with TE.

Initial Tests (lab, imaging)

If indicated:
- Complete blood count, ferritin
- Thyroid-stimulating hormone
- Creatinine
- Consider iron profile, zinc
- Consider hepatic enzymes
- Consider rapid plasma reagin/venereal disease research laboratory

Diagnostic Procedures/Other

- Hair pull test: unreliable; performed by gently pulling 25 to 30 hairs from various sites on a patient's scalp. Each pull should elicit <5 normal club hairs; increased quantity may indicate possibility of TE.
- Hair clip test: performed by cutting 25 to 30 hairs from the patient's scalp and examining them under a microscope. A negative test (not indicative of TE) will demonstrate <10% of hair shafts of small diameter. A positive test will demonstrate >10% of hair shafts of small diameter.
- Trichogram: ~50 hairs are plucked using a hemostat from the patient's scalp, and the number of telogen and anagen hairs present are counted. In TE, there will be >10% of hairs in the telogen phase.
- Scalp biopsy: rarely needed; it is recommended that several 4-mm punch biopsies be obtained, all horizontally embedded to determine an accurate anagen-to-telogen ratio. Histologically, catagen-to-telogen hairs have numerous apoptotic cells in the outer sheath epithelium. >12–15% of hair follicles in telogen phase is consistent with TE.

 TREATMENT

TE is a benign, self-limited process. Identify and correct underlying cause. Patient should be reassured that hair growth will resume in 3–6 months, with full growth to return in 12–18 months (3). No treatment is required; however, when a nutritional deficiency is identified, there may be some benefit to taking a specific supplement.

MEDICATION

- Minoxidil stimulates hair regrowth via arteriolar smooth muscle vasodilation; not effective in TE
- Oral zinc therapy: new medication that may have benefits for patients with TE through various mechanisms all essential to hair growth, including the following (4)[C]:
  – Cofactor for enzymes needed in nucleic acid and protein synthesis and cell division
  – Inhibition of the catagen phase by blocking certain enzymes involved in hair apoptosis
  – Involved in hair growth regulation via hedgehog signaling
- An extract from millet mixed with polar lipids has been found to enhance the cell proliferation in the hair bulb, reduce hair density in the telogen phase, improve scalp dryness, and improve hair brightness.

COMPLEMENTARY & ALTERNATIVE MEDICINE

- Combination oral vitamin therapy: A formulation of zinc; biotin; iron; vitamins A, C, E, and B complex; folic acid; magnesium; and amino acids of keratin and collagen was associated with statistically significant improvement compared to a formulation of calcium pantothenate cystine, thiamine nitrate, medicinal yeast, keratin, and aminobenzoic acid in the following measures after 180 days of use: hair loss, hair volume, scalp hair density, hair shine, and hair strength (5)[C].
- An extract from millet mixed with polar lipids has been found to enhance the cell proliferation in the hair bulb, reduce hair density in the telogen phase, improve scalp dryness, and improve hair brightness.

REFERENCES

1. Grover C, Khurana A. Telogen effluvium. *Indian J Dermatol Venereol Leprol*. 2013;79(5):591–603.
2. Peters EMJ, Liotiri S, Bodó E, et al. Probing the effects of stress mediators on the human hair follicle: substance P holds central position. *Am J Pathol*. 2007;171(6):1872–1886.
3. Malkud S. Telogen effluvium: a review. *J Clin Diagn Res*. 2015;9(9):WE01–WE03.
4. Karashima T, Tsuruta D, Hamada T, et al. Oral zinc therapy for zinc deficiency-related telogen effluvium. *Dermatol Ther*. 2012;25(2):210–213.
5. Sant'Anna Addor F, Donato L, Melo C. Comparative evaluation between two nutritional supplements in the improvement of telogen effluvium. *Clin Cosmet Investig Dermatol*. 2018;11:431–436.

ADDITIONAL READING

- Headington JT. Telogen effluvium. New concepts and review. *Arch Dermatol*. 1993;129(3):356–563.
- Mounsey AL, Reed SW. Diagnosing and treating hair loss. *Am Fam Physician*. 2009;80(4):356–362.

 CODES

ICD10
L65.0 Telogen effluvium

CLINICAL PEARLS

- TE is a self-limited form of nonscarring alopecia, most often acute.
- TE is due to a premature conversion of a significant proportion of anagen (growth phase) hairs into telogen (resting phase) hairs, resulting in increased shedding of these resting hair follicles and the clinical appearance of moderate to severe hair thinning and loss when growth resumes.
- There are many potential causes of TE, both emotional and physiologic. Often it is hard to determine the etiology, but eliminating the stressor is the key to resolving TE and stimulating new hair growth.
- No treatment is needed. Patient should be reassured that complete hair regrowth will occur in 12 to 18 months.

T

TEMPOROMANDIBULAR JOINT DISORDER (TMD)

Rita M. Lahlou, MD, MPH • Jaimei Zhang, MD, MPH

 BASICS

DESCRIPTION
- Syndrome characterized by
  - Pain and tenderness involving the muscles of mastication and surrounding tissues
  - Sound, pain, stiffness, or grating in the temporomandibular joint (TMJ) with movement
  - Limitation of mandibular movement with possible locking or dislocation
  - Recent research suggests that TMD is a complex disorder with multiple causes consistent with a biopsychosocial model of illness (1).
- System(s) affected: musculoskeletal
- Synonym(s): TMJ syndrome; TMJ dysfunction; myofascial pain–dysfunction syndrome; bruxism; orofacial pain

EPIDEMIOLOGY
Incidence
- Annual first-onset incidence is 3.9%.
- Peak incidence in ages 30 to 50 years

Prevalence
- 6–12% in both adults and older children
- Twice as common in female patients
- Up to 1/2 the population may have at least one sign or symptom of TMD, but most are not limited by symptoms, and <1:4 seek medical or dental treatment.

ETIOLOGY AND PATHOPHYSIOLOGY
- Pathophysiology is multifactorial, involving anatomic, behavioral, emotional, and cognitive factors.
- The American Academy of Orofacial Pain categorizes TMD according to three anatomic origins of pain. The change in name from TMJ to TMD emphasizes that many do not suffer from true articular pain.
- Muscle disorders involving the muscles of mastication
  - Occlusomuscular dysfunction (bruxism)
  - Masticatory muscle spasm
  - Myositis
  - Myofibrosis
  - Poorly fitting oral devices (dentures, splints, etc.)
  - Contracture
  - Neoplasia
- Articular disorders of the joint
  - Congenital disorders
  - Inflammatory disorders: synovitis, arthritides, capsulitis, ankyloses
  - Avascular necrosis (rare)
  - TMJ disk derangement, osteoarthritis
  - Hyper- or hypomobile TMJ
  - TMJ trauma: condylar fractures, dislocation
- Cranial bone disorder including the mandible
  - Congenital and developmental disorders
  - Acquired disorders (fracture, neoplasm)

- Current consensus is that TMD is not only a local condition, so much as a family of complex disorders that can lead to chronic pain, and often overlap with other chronic pain conditions that reflect CNS sensitization.
- OPPERA study (Orofacial Pain: Prospective Evaluation and Risk Assessment) is assessing the heterogeneity in these disorders.

Genetics
Research is ongoing in gene polymorphisms associated with TMD and other pain disorders. These include the catechol O-methyltransferase (COMT) gene, which is thought to be associated with changes in pain responsiveness.

RISK FACTORS
- Macrotrauma to the face, jaw, and neck, including cervical whiplash injuries and hyperextension of jaw
- Rheumatologic and degenerative conditions involving the TMJ
- Psychosocial stress and poor adaptive capabilities
- Repetitive microtrauma from dental malocclusion, including inappropriate dental treatment
- Inconsistent association with bruxism and jaw/teeth clenching
- Hormonal contraceptive use

GENERAL PREVENTION
- Elimination of tension-causing oral habits
- Reduction in overall muscle tension

COMMONLY ASSOCIATED CONDITIONS
Craniomandibular disorders, somatization disorder, somatoform pain disorder, other chronic pain syndromes, fibromyalgia, juvenile idiopathic arthritis, tension headache, irritable bowel syndrome, sleep disturbance, tobacco use

 DIAGNOSIS

- TMD is a clinical diagnosis, and localized pain is the unifying feature.
- Several research classification systems exist. Most share several of the history and physical findings listed below.

HISTORY
- Facial and/or TMJ pain
- Locking/catching of jaw; decreased range of motion
- TMJ noises: clicking, grinding, popping
- Headache, earache, neck pain

PHYSICAL EXAM
- Muscle tenderness and restricted pain-free jaw opening are most consistent distinguishing signs.
- Check facial symmetry, muscle hypertrophy, and intraoral exam including tooth wear.
- Palpation of muscles of mastication may reproduce pain.
- There may be tenderness over the TMJ.

- Test jaw range of motion (opening, closing, lateral, protrusive) and masticatory muscle strength.
  - Maximal (pain free) jaw opening with interincisal distance <40 mm is suggestive of joint rather than muscle pathology if accompanied by other signs and symptoms (normal 35 to 55 mm).
  - Deviation to the affected side is common.
- Clicking or crepitus of jaw with opening

DIFFERENTIAL DIAGNOSIS
- Condylar fracture/dislocation
- Trigeminal neuralgia
- Dental or periodontal conditions
- Neoplasm of the jaw, orofacial muscles, or salivary glands
- Acute, nondental infection: parotitis, sialadenitis, otitis, mastoiditis
- Jaw claudication: giant cell arteritis
- Migraine or tension-type headache
- Ramsay Hunt syndrome (zoster auricular syndrome)

DIAGNOSTIC TESTS & INTERPRETATION
Blood work may be useful to rule out other conditions (CBC, CMP, ESR, CRP).

Initial Tests (lab, imaging)
- TMD is a clinical diagnosis based primarily on history and physical exam.
- Often, a poor correlation is found between pain severity and pathologic changes seen in joint or muscle tissues. Consider the following for traumatic, infectious, severe, or treatment-resistant cases, with MR or CT more useful as part of surgical workup:
  - Panoramic dental radiographs are a good first-line screen.
  - CT scan allows fine detail of bony structures, preferred for trauma.
  - US: Effusion and findings correlate with MRI and subjective pain.
  - MRI: noninvasive study for disc position; more sensitive than US; can help determine need for surgical management

Diagnostic Procedures/Other
- Local anesthetic nerve block can differentiate orofacial pain of articular versus muscular origin.
- Arthroscopy can be diagnostic for cartilage and bony pathology.

Test Interpretation
Positive findings include:
- Condylar head displacement
- Anterior disc displacement
- Posterior capsulitis
- Loosening of disc and capsular attachments
- Chondroid metaplasia of disc leading to disc perforation and degeneration

TREATMENT

Signs and symptoms will abate without any interventions in most patients. 50% report improvement at 1 year and 85% by 3 years. With conservative therapy, symptoms resolve in 75% of cases within 3 months. Only 5–10% will require surgical intervention.

- Patient education and setting expectations are important because there is no "cure" for TMD; yet, most patients will improve with limited interventions.
- Psychosocial interventions, including cognitive-behavioral therapy with or without biofeedback (2)[A]
- Behavior modification to eliminate tension-relieving oral habits including heavy chewing of food and nonfood items as well as potential strain from playing musical instruments that stress or strain the jaw (wind, brass, or string) (2)[A]
- Therapeutic exercises, especially if displacement is present, including formal physical therapy
- Occlusal adjustment cannot be recommended for the management or prevention of TMD because there is an absence of evidence from RCTs that occlusal adjustment treats or prevents TMD (3)[A],(4).
- Insufficient evidence exists either for or against the use of stabilization splint therapy for the treatment of TMD.
- The American Dental Association recommends a "less is often best" stepwise approach and offers the following stepwise progression for therapy:
  – Eating softer foods
  – Avoiding chewing gum and nail biting
  – Modifying pain with heat or ice
  – Relaxation techniques including meditation and biofeedback
  – Exercises to strengthen jaw muscles
  – Medications
  – Night guards and orthotics

MEDICATION

First Line
- NSAIDs:
  – Naproxen: 500 mg BID stronger evidence than for other NSAIDs [B]
  – Ibuprofen, if osteoarthritis is suspected [B]
  – Topical diclofenac if oral medication is contraindicated
- Gabapentin: Titrate up to 1,800 mg/day divided.
- Acetaminophen

Second Line
- Cyclobenzaprine 10 mg nightly more effective than placebo for pain reduction (5)[B]
- Tricyclic antidepressants: nortriptyline or amitriptyline
- Acupuncture and dry needling can reduce pain (4).
- Opiates should be reserved for perioperative or severe or recalcitrant cases (6)[B].
- DMARDs may benefit inflammatory arthropathies such as rheumatoid or psoriatic arthritis.
- Ineffective medications (6)[B]
  – The following medications when compared with placebo in RCTs were shown to be ineffective in improving pain and should not be used for the treatment of TMD:
    ○ Benzodiazepines
    ○ Topical capsaicin
    ○ Celecoxib

ADDITIONAL THERAPIES
Joint and muscle injections
- A systematic review of arthrocentesis with injection of hyaluronic acid and platelet-rich plasma showed no clinical improvement (7).
- Steroids given >3 times annually may accelerate degenerative changes.
- Injections into inferior space or double spaces have better effect than superior space injections alone.
- A systematic review of studies evaluating botulinum toxin type A (Botox) injections revealed mixed results (4).
- For advanced structural abnormalities, referral for discectomy, arthroplasty, or joint replacement can be considered; however, strong evidence is lacking for lavage or surgical treatments over conservative management (4).

COMPLEMENTARY & ALTERNATIVE MEDICINE
- Glucosamine may be effective if pain is secondary to osteoarthritis of the TMJ (6)[B].
- Multiple electronic diagnostic and treatment modalities are currently marketed to patients; however, the scientific literature does not support the use of electronic diagnostic and treatment devices for TMD at this time.

 ONGOING CARE

FOLLOW-UP RECOMMENDATIONS
- Relax jaw by disengaging teeth.
- Avoid wide, uncontrolled opening, such as yawning.
- Trial of soft diet
- Stress management and behavior modification counseling may be helpful.
- Be aware of any teeth-clenching or grinding habits.

Patient Monitoring
- Ongoing assessment of clinical response to conservative therapies (NSAIDs, behavior modification, occlusal splints) is necessary.
- Surgical procedure (arthroplasty, joint replacement) to correct disc displacement or replace a damaged disc may be indicated only if the patient has not responded to conservative treatment.

DIET
Soft diet to reduce chewing

PROGNOSIS
- With conservative therapy, symptoms resolve in 75% of cases within 3 months.
- Patients benefit most from a comprehensive treatment approach including the following (5):
  – Restoration of normal muscle function
  – Pain control
  – Stress management
  – Behavior modification

COMPLICATIONS
- Secondary degenerative joint disease
- Chronic TMJ dislocation
- Loss of joint range of motion
- Depression and chronic pain syndromes
- Secondary headache disorder

REFERENCES

1. Slade GD, Fillingim RB, Sanders AE, et al. Summary of findings from the OPPERA prospective cohort study of incidence of first-onset temporomandibular disorder: implications and future directions. *J Pain*. 2013;14(Suppl 12):T116–T124.
2. Aggarwal VR, Lovell K, Peters S, et al. Psychosocial interventions for the management of chronic orofacial pain. *Cochrane Database Syst Rev*. 2011;(11):CD008456.
3. Koh H, Robinson PG. Occlusal adjustment for treating and preventing temporomandibular joint disorders. *Cochrane Database Syst Rev*. 2003;(1):CD003812.
4. Gil-Martínez A, Paris-Alemany A, López-de-Uralde-Villanueva I, et al. Management of pain in patients with temporomandibular disorder (TMD): challenges and solutions. *J Pain Res*. 2018;11:571–587.
5. Gauer RL, Semidey MJ. Diagnosis and treatment of temporomandibular disorders. *Am Fam Physician*. 2015;91(6):378–386.
6. Mujakperuo HR, Watson M, Morrison R, et al. Pharmacological interventions for pain in patients with temporomandibular disorders. *Cochrane Database Syst Rev*. 2010;(10):CD004715.
7. Derwich M, Mitus-Kenig M, Pawlowska E. Mechanisms of action and efficacy of hyaluronic acid, corticosteroids and platelet-rich plasma in the treatment of temporomandibular joint osteoarthritis—a systematic review. *Int J Mol Sci*. 2021;22(14):7405.

 SEE ALSO

Headache, Tension

 CODES

ICD10
- M26.60 Temporomandibular joint disorder, unspecified
- M26.62 Arthralgia of temporomandibular joint
- M26.63 Articular disc disorder of temporomandibular joint

CLINICAL PEARLS

- TMD refers to a number of potential underlying joint and muscle conditions involving the jaw. Characteristics of all conditions are pain and functional limitation.
- TMD is a clinical diagnosis; imaging and labs are often of limited utility.
- Cognitive-behavioral therapy reduces pain, depression, and limitation of function.
- Exercises may improve function and pain.
- Evidence is lacking to support occlusion correction or splinting.
- Naproxen, gabapentin, topical methyl salicylate, glucosamine, amitriptyline, acupuncture, and botulinum toxin injections have some evidence of efficacy.

T

TESTICULAR MALIGNANCIES

Huy T. Tran, MD

BASICS

DESCRIPTION
- Testicular cancer accounts for <1% of all cancers in men; it is the most common solid malignancy in men aged 20 to 34 years (1).
- An estimated 9,610 new cases were diagnosed, and an estimated 440 deaths occurred in the United States in 2020 (2).
- Rates for new cases have been rising 0.8% each year over the last 10 years, but death rates have been stable.
- The median age at diagnosis is 33 years. The median age at death is 41 years (2).
- Treatment produces an overall 5-year survival of 95%; for African American patients, this 5-year survival rate is alarmingly lower but has improved from 86% to 92.3% (2).

EPIDEMIOLOGY
Incidence
The number of new cases of testicular cancer was 5.9 per 100,000 men per year with the number of deaths at 0.3 per 100,000 men per year (2).

Prevalence
In 2017, there were an estimated 269,769 men living with testicular cancer in the United States (2).

ETIOLOGY AND PATHOPHYSIOLOGY
95% of all malignant tumors arising in the testes are germ cell tumors (GCTs), which are subclassified as follows:
- Seminomatous GCTs: most common type overall
- Nonseminomatous GCTs (NSGCTs): These include embryonal cell carcinoma, choriocarcinoma, yolk sac tumor, teratomas, or often multiple cell types; these are more clinically aggressive tumors.

Genetics
Approximately 48.9% of the risk of getting testicular cancer is explained by heritable factors (3).

RISK FACTORS
- Cryptorchidism is the most firmly established risk factor: Relative risk of testicular cancer in all patients with cryptorchidism is 3 to 8, with a lower relative risk of 2 to 3 in those undergoing orchiopexy by age 12 years; in patients with unilateral cryptorchidism, the relative risk of testicular cancer in the contralateral normally descended testis is negligible (4).
- Personal history of testicular cancer
- Use of muscle building supplements
- Positive family history for testicular cancer
- Testicular dysgenesis
- Klinefelter syndrome
- Caucasian race
- HIV infection

GENERAL PREVENTION
No evidence that screening for testicular cancer is effective (5).

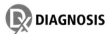

DIAGNOSIS

HISTORY
- A painless solid testicular mass is pathognomonic for testicular cancer.
- Clinical symptoms of epididymitis or orchitis that do not respond to treatment warrant further evaluation.
- Gynecomastia can be a rare systemic endocrine manifestation of testicular neoplasm.

PHYSICAL EXAM
- Testicular exam: Palpate for size, consistency, and nodules; masses do not transilluminate; a firm, hard, or fixed area should be considered suspicious.
- Lymph node and abdominal exam
- Gynecomastia

DIFFERENTIAL DIAGNOSIS
Epidermoid cyst, epididymitis, hernia, hydrocele, hematoma, lymphoma, orchitis, spermatocele, testicular torsion, varicocele

DIAGNOSTIC TESTS & INTERPRETATION
Initial Tests (lab, imaging)
- Testicular US is the initial study.
- If an intratesticular mass is identified, measure serum α-fetoprotein AFP, LDH, and β-human chorionic gonadotropin (β-hCG) and order a CXR.
- AFP, β-hCG, lactate dehydrogenase (LDH), creatinine, chemistry profile, complete blood count, liver enzymes, chest x-ray (CXR), and testicular ultrasound (US)
- Tumor markers AFP, β-hCG, and LDH are used to assist with diagnosis, prognosis, assessing treatment outcome, and monitoring for relapse:
  – AFP
    ○ Produced by nonseminomatous testicular cancer and is therefore associated with this histologic type
    ○ Those with a histologically "pure" testicular seminoma and an elevated AFP are assumed to possess an undetected focus of nonseminoma tumor.
  – β-hCG
    ○ May be associated with both seminomatous or nonseminomatous tumors
    ○ Hypogonadism and marijuana use may cause benign elevations of β-hCG.

Follow-Up Tests & Special Considerations
- CT scan of the abdomen/pelvis, positron emission tomography (PET) scan, MRI of the brain, and bone scan are used for staging and metastases evaluation as clinically indicated.
- LDH is less specific than AFP.

Diagnostic Procedures/Other
- Radical inguinal orchiectomy is the primary procedure for diagnosis and treatment.
- Testicular biopsy may be rarely considered if a suspicious intratesticular abnormality is identified on US; however, testicular microcalcification on US without any other abnormality can simply be observed and does not demand a biopsy.
- For those with unilateral testicular cancer, contralateral testicular biopsy is not routinely performed but should be considered when there is a cryptorchid testis, marked testicular atrophy, or a suspicious US for intratesticular abnormalities.

Test Interpretation
Clinical staging (6):
- Stage 0: carcinoma in situ
- Stage IA: tumor limited to testis and epididymis without vascular/lymphatic invasion; tumor may invade into the tunica albuginea but not the tunica vaginalis; normal serum tumor markers
- Stage IB: tumor limited to testis and epididymis with vascular/lymphatic invasion or tumor extending through tunica albuginea with involvement of tunica vaginalis; tumor invades the spermatic cord with or without vascular/lymphatic invasion; tumor invades the scrotum with or without vascular/lymphatic invasion; no lymph node involvement or distant metastasis; normal serum tumor markers

- Stage IS: any tumor with elevated serum tumor markers but no nodal involvement or metastasis
- Stage IIA: any tumor with lymph node mass/masses <2 cm
- Stage IIB: any tumor with lymph node mass/masses 2 to 5 cm
- Stage IIC: any tumor with lymph node mass >5 cm
- Stage IIIA: any tumor/lymph node presence; with nonregional nodal or pulmonary metastasis; either serum tumor markers normal or with mild elevation
- Stage IIIB: any tumor/lymph node presence; no distant metastasis or nonregional nodal involvement or pulmonary metastasis; with moderately elevated serum tumor markers
- Stage IIIC: any tumor/lymph node presence; with or without any metastasis; with greatly elevated serum tumor markers

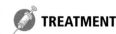

TREATMENT

GENERAL MEASURES
- Seminoma: Specifics are noted in the National Comprehensive Cancer Network guidelines (1):
  – Stages IA, IB: Options may include surveillance (preferred) (for low tumor load malignancy, i.e., pT1–pT3), single-agent carboplatin, or radiotherapy.
  – Stage IS: Repeat elevated serum tumor marker and abdominal/pelvic CT scan.
  – Stage IIA: radiotherapy to include para-aortic and ipsilateral iliac lymph nodes (preferred) or primary chemotherapy
  – Stage IIB: primary chemotherapy (preferred) or radiotherapy in select nonbulky cases to include para-aortic and ipsilateral iliac lymph nodes
  – Stages IIC, III
    ○ Good risk (any primary site and no nonpulmonary visceral metastases and normal AFP with any β-hCG or LDH): primary etoposide and cisplatin (EP) or bleomycin, etoposide, and cisplatin (BEP) chemotherapy (1)
    ○ Intermediate risk (any primary site and nonpulmonary visceral metastases and normal AFP with any β-hCG or LDH): primary BEP chemotherapy (1)
- Nonseminoma: Tumors with both seminomatous and nonseminomatous histology are managed as nonseminomatous. See "National Comprehensive Cancer Network guidelines" (1):
  – Stage IA: nonseminomatous surveillance protocol (preferred) or nerve-sparing retroperitoneal lymph node dissection (RPLND)
  – Stage IB: nerve-sparing RPLND or primary BEP chemotherapy; for T2 only can enter nonseminomatous surveillance protocol
  – Stage IS: primary chemotherapy followed by response evaluation:
    ○ Complete response, negative tumor markers: nonseminomatous surveillance protocol
    ○ Partial response, negative tumor markers: surgical resection of all residual masses
    ○ Incomplete response: Consider second-line therapy.
  – Stage IIA
    ○ Negative tumor markers: nerve-sparing RPLND or primary chemotherapy
    ○ Persistent marker elevation: primary chemotherapy followed by response evaluation

- ○ Complete response, negative tumor markers: nonseminomatous surveillance protocol or bilateral RPLND +/− nerve-sparing in select cases
- ○ Partial response, negative tumor markers: surgical resection of all residual masses
- ○ Incomplete response: Consider second-line therapy.
- – Stage IIB
  - ○ Negative tumor markers: primary chemotherapy or nerve-sparing RPLND in highly selected cases
  - ○ Persistent marker elevation: primary chemotherapy followed by response evaluation
    - ▪ Complete response, negative tumor markers: nonseminomatous surveillance protocol or bilateral RPLND +/− nerve-sparing in selected cases
    - ▪ Partial response, negative tumor markers: surgical resection of all residual masses
    - ▪ Incomplete response: Consider second-line therapy.
- – Stage IIC: primary chemotherapy followed by response evaluation as per stages IIA and IIB
- – Stages IIIA, IIIB, and IIIC: primary chemotherapy depending on risk profile, which is based on tumor, metastases, and postorchiectomy serum tumor markers
- Brain metastases: primary chemotherapy +/− radiotherapy, +/− surgery, as clinically indicated

MEDICATION

First Line
Primary chemotherapy regimens for GCTs:

- EP: etoposide 100 mg/m^2/day IV on days 1 to 5, cisplatin 20 mg/m^2/day IV on days 1 to 5; repeat every 21 days (1)[A].
- BEP: etoposide 100 mg/m^2/day IV on days 1 to 5, cisplatin 20 mg/m^2/day IV on days 1 to 5; bleomycin 30 U/dose IV weekly on days 1, 8, and 15 or days 2, 9, and 16; repeat every 21 days (1)[A].
- VIP: etoposide 75 mg/m^2/day IV on days 1 to 5; mesna 120 mg/m^2 slow IV push before ifosfamide on day 1 and then mesna 1,200 mg/m^2 IV continuous infusion on days 1 to 5; ifosfamide 1,200 mg/m^2/day on days 1 to 5; cisplatin 20 mg/m^2/day IV on days 1 to 5, repeat every 21 days (1)[A].

Second Line
- These agents are considered in patients who do not respond to first-line therapy or those who experience a recurrence: carboplatin, cisplatin, etoposide, ifosfamide, mesna, paclitaxel, and vinblastine (1)[A].
- Gemcitabine, oxaliplatin, and paclitaxel are used in palliative chemotherapy regimens (1)[A].

ISSUES FOR REFERRAL
Recurrent cancers should be treated at centers with extensive experience in treating relapsed testicular cancer.

ADDITIONAL THERAPIES
Consider sperm banking before treatment that may compromise fertility; rarely covered by insurance

SURGERY/OTHER PROCEDURES
- Radical inguinal orchiectomy: primary treatment for testicular cancer for all patients; prosthesis can be inserted at this time.
- RPLND identifies nodal metastases and provides accurate pathologic staging of the retroperitoneum.

⚡ ONGOING CARE

FOLLOW-UP RECOMMENDATIONS
- Pure seminoma: Specifics are noted in the National Comprehensive Cancer Network guidelines (1)[A]:
  - – Stages IA, IB: in general, H&P, optional tumor markers every 3 to 6 months for 1 year, every 6 to 12 months for years 2 to 3, and then annually for years 4 to 5; abdominal/pelvic CT at 3, 6, and 12 months and then every 6 to 12 months for years 2 to 3, every 12 to 24 months for years 4 to 5; CXR, as clinically indicated; less frequent if adjuvant therapy is given
  - – Stage IS: Repeat elevated serum tumor marker and assess with abdominal/pelvic CT scan for evaluable disease.
  - – Stages IIA, IIB (select): in general, H&P, optional tumor markers every 3 months for year 1, every 6 months for years 2 to 5; abdominal/pelvic CT at 3 and 6 to 12 months, then annually for years 2 to 3, and then as clinically indicated; CXR every 6 months for years 1 to 2
  - – Stages IIB (select), IIC, and III: Check all serum tumor markers along with chest, abdominal, and pelvic CT:
    - ○ Residual mass 0 to 3 cm and normal serum tumor markers: H&P, AFP, β-hCG, LDH, CXR every 2 months for year 1, every 3 months for year 2, every 6 months for years 3 to 4, and then annually; abdominal/pelvic CT scan at 3 to 6 months and then as clinically indicated, PET scans as clinically indicated
    - ○ Residual mass >3 cm and normal serum tumor markers: PET scan 6 weeks after chemotherapy:
      - ▪ Negative PET scan: abdominal/pelvic CT scans every 6 months for year 1 and then annually for 5 years
      - ▪ Positive PET scan: Consider RPLND or second-line chemotherapy or radiotherapy.
  - – Any recurrence: Treat according to extent of disease at relapse.
- Nonseminoma: Specifics are noted in the National Comprehensive Cancer Network guidelines (1):
  - – Stages IA and IB on surveillance only: H&P, AFP, β-hCG, LDH every 2 months for year 1, every 3 months for year 2, every 4 to 6 months for year 3, every 6 months for year 4, annually thereafter; CXR and abdominal/pelvic CT depending on stage IA or stage IB
  - – Follow-up after complete response to chemotherapy and RPLND in general: H&P, AFP, β-hCG, LDH every 2 to 3 months for years 1 to 2, every 6 months for years 3 to 5, annually thereafter; abdominal/pelvic CT every 6 months for year 1, annually for year 2, as clinically indicated thereafter
  - – Follow-up after RPLND only: H&P, AFP, β-hCG, LDH, CXR every 2 months for year 1, every 3 months for year 2, every 4 months for year 3, every 6 months for year 4, annually thereafter; abdominal/pelvic CT at 3 to 4 months and, as clinically indicated, thereafter; CXR every 2 to 4 months for year 1, 3 to 6 months for year 2, annually thereafter

Patient Monitoring
- No single follow-up plan is appropriate for all patients and should be modified for the individual patient based on sites of disease, biology of disease, and length of time on treatment.
- Monitoring may extend beyond 5 years at the discretion of the physician.

PROGNOSIS
>90% of patients diagnosed are cured, including 70–80% with advanced tumors (1).

COMPLICATIONS
- Surgical: hematoma, hemorrhage, infection, and infertility
- Radiotherapy: radiation enteritis and infertility
- Late complications (7):
  - – Cardiovascular toxicity and second malignancies each have a 25-year risk of about 16% in those treated with chemotherapy and/or radiotherapy.
  - – Risk for secondary malignancies remains increased for at least 35 years after treatment.
  - – Increased incidence of metabolic syndrome occurs and is likely associated with lower testosterone levels.
  - – Other late complications associated with chemotherapy, depending on the regimen, include chronic neurotoxicity, ototoxicity, renal function impairment, and pulmonary fibrosis.
- The incidence of late relapse in treated testicular cancer is now estimated to be 2–6%; the time to late relapse ranges from 2 to 32 years, with a median of 6 years (7).

REFERENCES

1. Gilligan T, Lin DW, Aggarwal R, et al. Testicular cancer, Version 3.2020. https://www.nccn.org/about/news/ebulletin/ebulletindetail.aspx?ebulletinid=1537. Accessed September 15, 2020.
2. Howlader N, Noone AM, Krapcho M, et al. *SEER Cancer Statistics Review, 1975-2017*. Bethesda, MD: National Cancer Institute. https://seer.cancer.gov/csr/1975_2017/. Published April 2020. Accessed January 25, 2021.
3. Litchfield K, Thomsen H, Mitchell J, et al. Quantifying the heritability of testicular germ cell tumour using both population-based and genomic approaches. *Sci Rep*. 2015;5:13889. doi:10.1038/srep13889.
4. Lip SZ, Murchison LE, Cullis PS, et al. A meta-analysis of the risk of boys with isolated cryptorchidism developing testicular cancer in later life. *Arch Dis Child*. 2013;98(1):20–26.
5. Ilic D, Misso ML. Screening for testicular cancer. *Cochrane Database Syst Rev*. 2011;(2):CD007853.
6. Edge SB, Byrd DR, Compton CC, et al., eds. Testis. In: *AJCC Cancer Staging Manual*. 7th ed. New York, NY: Springer; 2010:469–478.
7. Efstathiou E, Logothetis CJ. Review of late complications of treatment and late relapse in testicular cancer. *J Natl Compr Canc Netw*. 2006;4(10):1059–1070.

CODES

ICD10
- C62.90 Malig neoplasm of unsp testis, unsp descended or undescended
- C62.00 Malignant neoplasm of unspecified undescended testis
- C62.10 Malignant neoplasm of unspecified descended testis

CLINICAL PEARLS
- Testicular cancer is the most common solid organ tumor in men aged 20 to 34 years.
- Testicular US is the initial imaging of choice for testicular pathology.
- Radical inguinal orchiectomy is used for both diagnosis and treatment, with possible radiotherapy or chemotherapy as adjuvant treatment.
- 96% overall survival at 10 years after diagnosis and treatment

TESTICULAR TORSION
Adedamola Ayo Omole, MD • Jyothi R. Patri, MD, MHA, FAAFP, HMDC

BASICS

DESCRIPTION
- Twisting of testis and spermatic cord, resulting in acute ischemia and loss of testis if unrecognized:
  - Intravaginal torsion: occurs within tunica vaginalis, only involves testis and spermatic cord
  - Extravaginal torsion: involves twisting of testis, cord, and processus vaginalis as a unit; typically seen in neonates
- System(s) affected: reproductive

Geriatric Considerations
Rare in this age group

Pediatric Considerations
Peak incidence at age 14 years (1)[B]

EPIDEMIOLOGY
Incidence
- ~1/4,000 males before age 25 years
- Predominant age:
  - Occurs from newborn period to 7th decade
  - 65% of cases occur in 2nd decade, with peak at age 14 years (1).
  - Second peak in neonates (in utero torsion usually occurs around week 32 of gestation) (1)

ETIOLOGY AND PATHOPHYSIOLOGY
- Initial incomplete twisting of spermatic cord causes venous obstruction, edema of testis, leading to ischemia.
- Complete twisting of the spermatic cord causes arterial occlusion, in addition to the above, leading to rapid ischemia.
- Congenital bell clapper deformity, which is bilateral in at least 2/5 of cases: A high mesorchium (the posterior lateral attachment of the testis to the tunica vaginalis) allows more room for the testis to twist within the tunica vaginalis and is associated intravaginal testicular torsion (2).
- No clear anatomic defect is associated with extravaginal testicular torsion:
  - In neonates, the tunica vaginalis is not yet well attached to scrotal wall, allowing torsion of entire testis including tunica vaginalis (1)[B].
- Usually spontaneous and idiopathic (1)[B]
- 20% of patients have a history of trauma.
- 1/3 have had prior episodic testicular pain.
- Contraction of cremaster muscle or dartos may play a role and is stimulated by trauma, exercise, cold, and sexual stimulation.
- Increased incidence may be due to increasing weight and size of testis during pubertal development.
- Possible alterations in testosterone levels during nocturnal sex response cycle; possible elevated testosterone levels in neonates (1)[B]

- Testis must have inadequate, incomplete, or absent fixation within scrotum (1)[B].
- Torsion may occur in either clockwise or counter-clockwise direction.

Genetics
- Unknown
- Familial testicular torsion, although previously rarely reported, may involve as many as 10% of patients.

RISK FACTORS
- May be more common in colder months
- Paraplegia
- Previous contralateral testicular torsion

DIAGNOSIS

Testicular torsion is a clinical diagnosis. A good history and physicals are the most important and helpful tools in evaluating and managing testicular torsion. If H&P are highly suggestive of testicular torsion, imaging studies may be skipped and immediate urologic consult should be done, as time is of the utmost essence (3).

HISTORY
- Acute onset of unrelenting pain, often during period of inactivity
- Onset of pain usually sudden but may start gradually with subsequent increase in severity
- Nausea and vomiting are common:
  - Presence may increase the likelihood of testicular torsion versus other differential diagnoses.
- Prior history of multiple episodes of testicular pain with spontaneous resolution in an episodic crescendo pattern may indicate intermittent testicular torsion.

PHYSICAL EXAM
- Scrotum is enlarged, red, edematous, and painful unilaterally.
- Testicle is swollen and exquisitely tender.
- "Bell clapper" deformity: an asymmetrically high-riding testis oriented transversely instead of longitudinally occurring due to shortening spermatic cord from the torsion (4)
- Testis may be high in scrotum with a transverse lie; this is called Brunzel sign.
- Prehn sign: when elevation of the testis does not decrease pain in the affected testicle.
- Absent cremasteric reflex. Elicit cremasteric reflex by lightly stroking the inner thigh of the suspected side.

DIFFERENTIAL DIAGNOSIS
- Torsion appendix testis (This may account for 35–67% of acute scrotal pain cases in children.)
- Epididymitis (8–18% of acute scrotal pain cases)
- Orchitis
- Incarcerated or strangulated inguinal hernia
- Acute hydrocele
- Traumatic hematoma

- Testicle rupture
- Idiopathic scrotal edema
- Acute varicocele
- Epididymal hypertension (venous congestion of testicle or prostate due to sexual arousal that does not end in orgasm)
- Testis tumor
- Henoch-Schönlein purpura
- Scrotal abscess
- Leukemic infiltrate

DIAGNOSTIC TESTS & INTERPRETATION
- Doppler US may confirm testicular swelling but is diagnostic by demonstrating lack of blood flow to the testicle; PPV of 89.4% (5),(6)[B]. A normal testicular US does not rule out testicular torsion.
- In boys with intermittent, recurrent testicular torsion, both Doppler US and radionuclide scintigraphy findings will be normal (6)[B].

Initial Tests (lab, imaging)
Urinalysis to rule out any infection such as epididymitis, orchitis, UTI

Diagnostic Procedures/Other
- Doppler US flow detection demonstrates absent or reduced blood flow with torsion and increased flow with inflammatory process (reliable only in first 12 hours) (6)[B].
- Radionuclide testicular scintigraphy with technetium-99m pertechnetate demonstrates absent/decreased vascularity in torsion and increased vascularity with inflammatory processes (including torsion of appendix testes) (7)[C].

Test Interpretation
- Venous thrombosis
- Tissue edema and necrosis
- Arterial thrombosis
- Decreased Doppler flow also seen in hydrocele, abscess, hematoma, or scrotal hernia (6)[B]
- Sensitivity of radionuclide testicular scintigraphy is decreased relative to US because hyperemia in the torsed testicle can mimic flow (7)[C].

TREATMENT

- Manual reduction/detorsion: best performed by experienced physician, especially if a surgeon is not available; may be successful, facilitated by lidocaine 1% (plain) injection at level of external ring:
  - Performed by rotating the affected testicle in a medial to lateral direction; described as the "open book." 1/3 of torsion, however, is medial to lateral on presentation.
  - If successful will usually provide immediate relief; may need to rotate anywhere from 180 to 1,080 degrees, resulting in possible partial untwisting (8)

– Difficult to determine success of manual reduction, especially after giving local anesthesia
– Manual reduction might require sedation, and the entire process may delay definitive treatment.
– Even if successful, must always be followed by surgical exploration, urgently but not emergently (9)[C]
- Surgical exploration via scrotal approach with detorsion, evaluation of testicular viability, orchidopexy of viable testicle, orchiectomy of nonviable testicle (5)[B]
- In boys with a history of intermittent episodes of testicular pain, scrotal exploration is warranted with testicular fixation if abnormal testicular attachments are confirmed (5)[B].

GENERAL MEASURES
Early exam is crucial because necrosis of the testicle can occur after 6 to 8 hours (10)[C].

MEDICATION
Studies are ongoing on medications used to prevent reperfusion injury and increase blood flow.

SURGERY/OTHER PROCEDURES
Operative testicular fixation of the torsed testicle after detorsion and confirmation of viability:
- At least 3- or 4-point fixation with nonabsorbable sutures between the tunica albuginea and the tunica vaginalis (5)[B]
- Excision of window of tunica albuginea with suture to dartos fascia (5)[B]
- Any testis that is not clearly viable should be removed (1)[B].
- Testes of questionable viability that are preserved and pexed invariably atrophy (5)[B]
- Bilateral testicular fixation is recommended by many surgeons (5)[B].
- Contralateral testicle frequently has similar abnormal fixation and should be explored (5)[B],(9)[C].

ADMISSION, INPATIENT, AND NURSING CONSIDERATIONS
Patients can usually be discharged from recovery.

 ## ONGOING CARE

FOLLOW-UP RECOMMENDATIONS
Patient Monitoring
- Postoperative visit at 1 to 2 weeks
- Yearly visits until puberty may be needed to evaluate for atrophy.
- Counsel high-risk patients during primary care visits on emergency room return precautions.

DIET
Regular

PATIENT EDUCATION
Possibility of testicular atrophy in salvaged testis with depressed sperm counts. Importantly, fertility rates in patients with one testicle remain excellent.

PROGNOSIS
- Testicular salvage:
  – Salvage is related directly to duration of torsion (85–97% if within 6 hours, 20% after 12 hours, <10% if >24 hours) (10)[C].
  – The degree of torsion is related to testicular salvage:
    ○ The median degree of torsion is <360 in patients who are explored and orchidopexy performed.
- 80–94% may have depressed spermatogenesis related to duration of ischemic injury (possibly related to autoimmune-mediated injury) (10)[C].
- Up to 45% of patients undergoing orchidopexy for testicular torsion will develop atrophy of testicle.

COMPLICATIONS
- Possible testicular atrophy
- Abnormal spermatogenesis
- Infertility:
  – Fertility rates with one testicle remain excellent.
  – Nearly 36% of patients who experience torsion have sperm counts <20 million/mL (7)[C].

REFERENCES
1. Boettcher M, Bergholz R, Krebs TF, et al. Clinical predictors of testicular torsion in children. *Urology*. 2012;79(3):670–674.
2. Schick MA, Sternard BT. *Testicular Torsion*. In: StatPearls [Internet]. Treasure Island, FL: StatPearls Publishing; 2021. Available from: https://www.ncbi.nlm.nih.gov/books/NBK448199/. Updated August 2, 2021.
3. Sharp VJ, Kieran K, Arlen AM. Testicular torsion: diagnosis, evaluation, and management. *Am Fam Physician*. 2013;88(12):835–840.
4. Schmitz D, Safranek S. Clinical inquiries. How useful is a physical exam in diagnosing testicular torsion? *J Fam Pract*. 2009;58(8):433–434.
5. Van Glabeke E, Khairouni A, Larroquet M, et al. Acute scrotal pain in children: results of 543 surgical explorations. *Pediatr Surg Int*. 1999;15(5–6):353–357.
6. Yagil Y, Naroditsky I, Milhem J, et al. Role of Doppler ultrasonography in the triage of acute scrotum in the emergency department. *J Ultrasound Med*. 2010;29(1):11–21.
7. Saleh O, El-Sharkawi MS, Imran MB. Scrotal scintigraphy in testicular torsion: an experience at a tertiary care centre. *Int Med J Malaysia*. 2012;11(1):9–14.
8. Bowlin PR, Gatti JM, Murphy JP. Pediatric testicular torsion. *Surg Clin North Am*. 2017;97(1):161–172.
9. Eaton SH, Cendron MA, Estrada CR, et al. Intermittent testicular torsion: diagnostic features and management outcomes. *J Urol*. 2005;174(4, Pt 2):1532–1535.
10. Kapoor S. Testicular torsion: a race against time. *Int J Clin Pract*. 2008;62(5):821–827.

ADDITIONAL READING
- Fehér AM, Bajory Z. A review of main controversial aspects of acute testicular torsion. *J Acute Dis*. 2016;5(1):1–8.
- Jacobsen FM, Rudlang TM, Fode M, et al. The impact of testicular torsion on testicular function. *World J Mens Health*. 2020;38(3):298–307.
- Kühn AL, Scortegagna E, Nowitzki KM, et al. Ultrasonography of the scrotum in adults. *Ultrasonography*. 2016;35(3):180–97.

 ## CODES

ICD10
- N44.03 Torsion of appendix testis
- N44.0 Torsion of testis
- N44.02 Intravaginal torsion of spermatic cord

CLINICAL PEARLS
- The diagnosis of testicular torsion is usually made by physical exam. Patients with suspected torsion should be taken to the OR without delay. If the diagnosis is in question, a testicular Doppler US may be done to evaluate blood flow.
- Although testicular necrosis may be present within 6 to 8 hours of torsion, this is highly variable.
- Infertility can be a problem even if the testicle is viable. Autoimmune antisperm antibodies may be produced, and they may affect subsequent fertility.

T

TESTOSTERONE DEFICIENCY

Stanton C. Honig, MD • Dylan Buller, MD

 BASICS

DESCRIPTION

- Testosterone (T) is the principal circulating androgen in males. Testosterone deficiency (TD) is characterized by low levels of T in addition to signs and symptoms.
- No universally accepted threshold of T concentration to distinguish eugonadal from hypogonadal men, but the U.S. Food and Drug Administration (FDA) definition is T <300 ng/dL.
- T levels correlate with overall health and may be associated with sexual dysfunction.
- Synonym(s): hypogonadism; hypoandrogenism; androgen deficiency; low T

EPIDEMIOLOGY

Incidence
Overall incidence increases with age. T levels decline by 1% per year after age 40 years.

Prevalence
- Estimates of TD vary; typically 20% of men >60 years, 30% >70 years, and 50% >80 years of age
- Symptomatic TD in United States ages 40 to 69 years is 6–12.3%.
- 2.4 million men in United States ages 40 to 69 years

ETIOLOGY AND PATHOPHYSIOLOGY
Hypothalamus produces GnRH, which stimulates pituitary to produce follicle-stimulating hormone (FSH) and luteinizing hormone (LH). LH stimulates Leydig cells to produce T. Leydig cells are responsible for 90% of the body's T.

- Primary hypogonadism: testes produce insufficient amount of T; FSH/LH levels are elevated.
- Secondary hypogonadism: low T from inadequate production of LH
- Congenital syndromes: cryptorchidism, Klinefelter, hypogonadotropic hypogonadism (Kallmann)
- Acquired: cancer, trauma, orchiectomy, steroids
- Infectious: mumps orchitis, HIV, tuberculosis
- Systemic: Cushing, hemochromatosis, autoimmune, severe illness (e.g., renal and liver disease), metabolic syndrome, obesity, obstructive sleep apnea
- Medications and drugs: LHRH agonists, corticosteroids, ethanol, marijuana, opioids, SSRIs
- Elevated prolactin: prolactinoma, dopamine antagonists (neuroleptics and metoclopramide)

Genetics
- Klinefelter: XXY karyotype
- Kallmann syndrome: abnormal GnRH secretion due to abnormal hypothalamic development

RISK FACTORS
- Obesity, diabetes, COPD, depression, thyroid disorders, malnutrition, alcohol, stress
- Chronic infections, inflammatory states, narcotic use
- Undescended testicles, varicocele
- Trauma, cancer, testicular radiation, chemotherapy, disorders of the pituitary and/or hypothalamus

GENERAL PREVENTION
General health maintenance and treatment of obesity

COMMONLY ASSOCIATED CONDITIONS
- Infertility, erectile dysfunction, low libido
- Osteopenia/osteoporosis
- Diabetes, insulin resistance, metabolic syndrome, adiposity
- Depressed mood, poor concentration, irritability

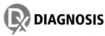 **DIAGNOSIS**

HISTORY
- Congenital and developmental abnormalities
- Infertility, loss of libido, erectile dysfunction
- Depression, fatigue, difficulty with concentration
- Decreased muscle strength, energy level
- Increase in body fat, development of diabetes
- Bone fractures from relatively minor trauma
- Testicular trauma, infection, radio- or chemotherapy
- Decrease in testicle size or consistency
- Headaches or vision changes
- Medications, narcotic use

PHYSICAL EXAM
- Infancy: ambiguous genitalia
- Puberty
  - Impaired growth of penis, testicles
  - Lack of secondary male characteristics
  - Gynecomastia, eunuchoid habitus
- Adulthood
  - Decreased muscular development, visceral fat distribution
  - Presence of gynecomastia
  - Small and/or soft testicles
  - Digital rectal exam, and International Prostate Symptom Score (IPSS)

DIFFERENTIAL DIAGNOSIS
- Delayed puberty
- Obesity, depression, chronic illness, hypothyroidism
- Normal aging
- Prior anabolic steroid abuse

DIAGNOSTIC TESTS & INTERPRETATION
- T levels vary widely and are subject to diurnal, seasonal, and age-related variations.
- Measurement should be obtained between 6 and 10 AM. Confirmation with a second measurement may be necessary. Free T with total T may be preferred in some cases. Measurements should not be obtained during acute illness. T circulates in blood primarily bound to SHBG or albumin. Only 2–3% of total T is found free. Free and albumin-bound T is considered bioavailable. Laboratory findings must be interpreted in the appropriate clinical setting.

Initial Tests (lab, imaging)
Morning T level is the initial test. If initial morning T is low and confirmed on repeat test, further evaluation is appropriate (1).

- Evaluation should include LH and FSH to differentiate between primary versus secondary hypogonadism.
- Consider estradiol and prolactin, especially if LH is low, or if breast symptoms and gynecomastia.
- If primary hypogonadism of unknown origin and physical exam reveals severe testis atrophy, consider obtaining karyotype (Klinefelter 1:500 to 1,000 risk).
- If secondary hypogonadism, consider prolactin, iron saturation, pituitary function testing, and/or MRI.

Follow-Up Tests & Special Considerations
- Prior to initiating therapy:
  - Hemoglobin and hematocrit (to determine risk of polycythemia)
  - Prostate-specific antigen (PSA) in men over 40 years of age (to exclude prostate cancer diagnosis)
  - Estradiol in men with breast symptoms or gynecomastia
- Dual energy x-ray absorptiometry (DEXA) in men with severe TD or fracture from minimal trauma
- Pituitary MRI: if there is elevation of prolactin more than twice the upper limit of normal or LH/FSH below normal range

 TREATMENT

Testosterone therapy (TT) recommended for symptomatic men (e.g., low libido and/or erectile dysfunction, low energy level, constitutional symptoms) with low T levels ≤300 ng/dL obtained in the morning; not recommended for older men with low T levels in absence of signs or symptom (2)[C]

- Recent data suggest T replacement can significantly increase hemoglobin levels in men with low T and unexplained anemia.
- Recent data suggest men with low bone mineral density and low T can increase bone density and bone strength with T replacement (3)[A].
- In older men with low T and age-associated memory impairment, T replacement was not seen as beneficial.

GENERAL MEASURES

- Future fertility? Impact of exogenous T should be discussed because it relates to fertility.
- Prostate cancer? Safety of TT is uncertain and a contraindication (4)[B].
  - 2018 American Urological Association AUA) guidelines: Patients with TD and history of prostate cancer should be informed that there is inadequate evidence to quantify the risk–benefit ratio of TT (2)[B].
  - 2018 endocrine guidelines: Patients with organ-confined prostate cancer who have undergone radical prostatectomy and disease free for ≥2 years with undetectable PSA may be considered for TT on an individualized basis.
  - TT should be avoided in men with PSA >4 or PSA >3 and increased risk of prostate cancer (African Americans, men with first-degree relative with prostate cancer).
- TT should not be used in men with metastatic prostate cancer, breast cancer, hematocrit >54%, untreated obstructive sleep apnea, uncontrolled congestive heart failure (CHF), severe lower urinary tract symptoms with an IPSS >19 (2).
- TT is not recommended for mood or strength improvement in otherwise healthy men or asymptomatic men with low T (2).
- Cardiovascular disease (CVD) risk?
  - Cannot state definitively if TT increases risk of cardiovascular events. However, TD is also a risk factor for CVD (2).
  - No definitive evidence linking TT to a higher incidence of venothrombotic events (2)[A]
- Consider short-term TT as an adjunctive in men with HIV and low T to promote weight maintenance and gains in lean body mass and strength.

MEDICATION

ALERT
Avoid contact with females or children.

- Oral therapy with methyltestosterone is not recommended due to association with significant hepatotoxicity.
  - Oral T undecanoate (Jatenzo) was FDA approved in March 2019.
- FDA cautions that TT is approved for men with confirmed low T by blood work with signs and symptoms, not solely due to aging.
- TT should NOT be started for a period of 3 to 6 months in patients with acute cardiovascular event.
- Topical gels/solutions: most common
  - Mimics normal daily circadian rhythm
  - Good absorption, 15–20% are nonresponders
- T pellets (Testopel)
  - Minor office procedure
  - Long-acting formulation, 3 to 4 months
  - 1–2% risk of infection or pellet extrusion
- Transdermal patch (Androderm)
  - Achieves less robust levels
  - High incidence of skin irritation

- T enanthate (Xyosted) SC weekly injection
  - Boxed warning for increased blood pressure
- T cypionate (IM every 1 to 3 weeks)
  - Starting dose: 100 mg/week or 200 mg/2 weeks
- T undecanoate (IM every 8 to 12 weeks)
  - Small risk of oil embolism, needs observation in office for 30 minutes postinjection
- Buccal application (Striant) BID dosing
  - Adheres to gum line, irritation in 16.3%
- Nasal gel (Natesto) TID dosing
  - Nasal irritation
  - May be protective of fertility
- Oral T undecanoate (Jatenzo) BID dosing
  - FDA warning for blood pressure elevation
  - Titration required to determine appropriate dose

ISSUES FOR REFERRAL
PSA elevation, abnormal prostate exam, worsening BPH (IPSS >19), refractory to replacement therapy should be referred to urology.

 ONGOING CARE

FOLLOW-UP RECOMMENDATIONS
Patient Monitoring
- 3 to 6 months after treatment initiation and then every 6 to 12 months
- Adjust dosing to achieve a total T in the middle tertile of the normal reference range.
- Measure hematocrit at baseline, at 3 to 6 months, and then annually.
- Stop treatment 3 to 6 months after starting in patients who experience normalization of T but fail to achieve symptom improvement.
- Bone mineral density after 1 to 2 years of therapy in men with osteoporosis
- Prostate exam every 6 to 12 months

DIET
Lifestyle changes and weight loss may raise T levels without need for T replacement (5).

PATIENT EDUCATION
- TD can be chronic and may need lifelong therapy.
- T replacement comes with many risks, and it is very important to regularly monitor outcomes.
- Women and children must not be allowed to come in contact with TT gel products.

PROGNOSIS
There is evolving evidence that TT may improve metabolic functions such as glycosylated hemoglobin, blood sugar, total cholesterol, and visceral fat in patients with diabetes; bone mineral density, and also unexplained anemia.

COMPLICATIONS
Complications of T replacement
- Decreased testicular volume, azoospermia in 40% of patients on TT, infertility
- Fluctuations in mood or libido

- Gynecomastia and growth of breast cancer
- Acne and oily skin
- Erythrocytosis (increased hematocrit)
- Exacerbation of sleep apnea
- Hepatotoxicity with prolonged oral use
- Possible prostate enlargement with or without worsening symptoms of BPH

REFERENCES

1. Paduch DA, Brannigan RE, Fuchs EF, et al. The laboratory diagnosis of testosterone deficiency. *Urology.* 2014;83(5):980–988.
2. Mulhall JP, Trost LW, Brannigan RE, et al. Evaluation and management of testosterone deficiency: AUA guideline. *J Urol.* 2018;200(2):423–432.
3. Roy CN, Snyder PJ, Stephens-Shields AJ, et al. Association of testosterone levels with anemia in older men: a controlled clinical trial. *JAMA Intern Med.* 2017;177(4):480–490.
4. Debruyne FM, Behre HM, Roehrborn CG, et al; for RHYME Investigators. Testosterone treatment is not associated with increased risk of prostate cancer or worsening of lower urinary tract symptoms: prostate health outcomes in the Registry of Hypogonadism in Men. *BJU Int.* 2017;119(2):216–224.
5. Kumagai H, Zempo-Miyaki A, Yoshikawa T, et al. Lifestyle modification increases serum testosterone level and decrease central blood pressure in overweight and obese men. *Endocr J.* 2015;62(5):423–430.

 CODES

ICD10
- E29.1 Testicular hypofunction
- E89.5 Postprocedural testicular hypofunction

CLINICAL PEARLS

- TD is common, and prevalence increases with age.
- Men with sexual dysfunction, obesity, unexplained anemia, bone density loss, chronic steroid or narcotic use, and metabolic diseases should be tested for TD.
- Initial test of choice is a morning total and free T; if low, repeat measurements.
- TT in the appropriately selected population can increase lean mass, reduce fat mass, increase bone mineral density, improve libido, improve unexplained anemia, and improve erections. However, it has not been shown to improve cognition or memory impairment in the elderly.
- Lifestyle changes such as diet and exercise may restore T levels.

T

THALASSEMIA
Garland E. Anderson II, MD

BASICS

DESCRIPTION
- A group of inherited hematologic disorders that affect the synthesis of adult hemoglobin tetramer (HbA) (1),(2)[C]
- α-Thalassemia is due to a deficient synthesis of α-globin chain, whereas β-thalassemia is due to a deficient synthesis of β-globin chain:
  - The synthesis of the unaffected globin chain proceeds normally.
  - This unbalanced globin chain production causes unstable hemoglobin tetramers, which leads to hypochromic, microcytic red blood cells (RBCs), and hemolytic anemia.
- α-Thalassemia is more common in persons of Mediterranean, African, and Southeast Asian descent, whereas β-thalassemia is more common in patients of African and Southeast Asian descent.
- Types
  - Thalassemia (minor) trait (α or β): absent or mild anemia with microcytosis and hypochromia
  - α-Thalassemia major with hemoglobin Bart usually results in fatal hydrops fetalis (fluid in ≥2 fetal compartments secondary to anemia and fetal heart failure).
  - α-Thalassemia intermedia with hemoglobin H (hemoglobin H disease): results in moderate hemolytic anemia and splenomegaly
  - β-Thalassemia major: results in severe anemia, growth retardation, hepatosplenomegaly, bone marrow expansion, and bone deformities. Transfusion therapy is necessary to sustain life.
  - β-Thalassemia intermedia: milder disease; transfusion therapy may not be needed or may be needed later in life.
- Other variants include hemoglobin E/β-thalassemia in Southeast Asians, which often mimics the severity of α-thalassemia major; δ-thalassemia; hemoglobin H Constant Spring
- System(s) affected: hematologic/lymphatic/immunologic, cardiac, hepatic
- Synonym(s): Mediterranean anemia; hereditary leptocytosis; Cooley anemia

Pediatric Considerations
- β-Thalassemia major causes symptoms during early childhood, usually starting at 6 months of age, and requires periodic transfusions to sustain life.
- Newborn's cord blood or heel stick should be screened for hemoglobinopathies with hemoglobin electrophoresis or comparably accurate test, although this primarily detects sickle cell disease.

Pregnancy Considerations
- Preconception genetic counseling is advised for couples at risk for having a child with thalassemia and for parents or other relatives of a child with thalassemia (3)[A].
- Once pregnant, a chorionic villus sample at 10 to 11 weeks' gestation or an amniocentesis at 15 weeks' gestation can be done to detect point mutations or deletions with polymerase chain reaction (PCR) technology.

EPIDEMIOLOGY
Incidence
- Occurs in ~4.4/10,000 live births
- Predominant age: Symptoms start to appear 6 months after birth with β-thalassemia major.
- Predominant sex: male = female

Prevalence
- Worldwide, ~200,000 people are alive with β-thalassemia major and <1,000 patients are in the United States.
- In the worldwide population, an estimated 1.5% are β-thalassemia carriers and 5% α-thalassemia carriers (4).

ETIOLOGY AND PATHOPHYSIOLOGY
Unknown; it is unclear how the imbalance of β-globulin in α-thalassemia and α-globin in β-thalassemia results in ineffective RBC genesis and hemolysis.

Genetics
- Inherited in an autosomal recessive pattern
- α-Thalassemia results from a deletion of ≥1 of the 4 genes, 2 on each chromosome 16, responsible for α-globin synthesis. 1-gene deletion is a silent carrier state, 2-gene deletion is the trait, 3-gene deletion results in hemoglobin H, and 4-gene deletion results in hemoglobin Bart, causing fatal hydrops fetalis.
- Nondeletional forms do occur rarely. Hemoglobin H Constant Spring is the most common nondeletional form.
- β-Thalassemia is caused by any of >200-point mutations and, very rarely, deletions on chromosome 11; 20 alleles account for >80% of the mutations.
- Significantly disparate phenotype with the same genotype occurs because β-globin chain production can range from near-normal to absent.

RISK FACTORS
Family history of thalassemia

GENERAL PREVENTION
- Prenatal information: genetic counseling regarding partner selection and information on the availability of diagnostic tests during the pregnancy
- Complication prevention
  - For offspring of adult thalassemia patients, an evaluation for thalassemia by 1 year of age
  - Severe forms
    - Avoid exposure to sick contacts.
    - Keep immunizations up to date.
  - Promptly treat bacterial infections. (After splenectomy, patients should maintain a supply of an appropriate antibiotic to take at the onset of symptoms of a bacterial infection.)
  - Dental checkups every 6 months
  - Avoid activities that could increase the risk of bone fractures.

COMMONLY ASSOCIATED CONDITIONS
See "Complications."

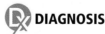

DIAGNOSIS
Thalassemia (minor) trait has no signs or symptoms.

HISTORY
- Poor growth
- Excessive fatigue
- Cholelithiasis
- Pathologic fractures
- Shortness of breath

PHYSICAL EXAM
- Pallor
- Splenomegaly
- Jaundice

- Maxillary hyperplasia/frontal bossing due to massive bone marrow expansion
- Dental malocclusion

DIFFERENTIAL DIAGNOSIS
- Iron deficiency anemia
- Other microcytic anemias: lead toxicity, sideroblastic
- Other hemolytic anemias
- Other hemoglobinopathies

DIAGNOSTIC TESTS & INTERPRETATION
Special tests
- Bone marrow aspiration to evaluate for causes of microcytic anemia is rarely needed.
- Multiple indices have been evaluated to discriminate β-thalassemia trait from iron deficiency anemia, yet none is sensitive enough to exclude β-thalassemia.
- Hemoglobin: usual range 10 to 12 g/dL with thalassemia trait and 3 to 8 g/dL with β-thalassemia major before transfusions
- Hematocrit
  - 28–40% in thalassemia trait
  - May fall to <10% in β-thalassemia major
- Peripheral blood
  - Microcytosis (MCV <70 fL)
  - Hypochromia (MCH <20 pg)
  - High percentage of target cells
  - Reticulocyte count is elevated.
- Red cell distribution width (RDW)
  - A normal RDW with a microcytic hypochromic anemia is almost always thalassemia trait.
  - The RDW can be elevated in ~50% of thalassemia trait patients. This is in contrast to iron deficiency anemia, where the RDW is almost always elevated (90%).
- Hemoglobin electrophoresis
  - In α-thalassemia trait, no recognizable electrophoretic pattern occurs in adults.
  - However, in the neonatal period, 3–10% of trait patients will have hemoglobin H or hemoglobin Bart at birth, which would confirm α-thalassemia.
  - If HbA_2 is below normal (<2.5%) with a normal HbF level, the diagnosis is α-thalassemia intermedia (HbH disease).
  - In the neonatal period with β-thalassemia trait, the electrophoresis is normal. However, in adults, elevated HbA_2 levels (>4%) may be present but are usually normal (5)[C].
  - β-Thalassemia major or intermedia has elevated HbA_2, elevated HbF, and reduced or absent HbA.
- DNA analysis
  - α-Thalassemia can definitively be diagnosed with genetic testing of hemoglobin A1 and A2 (for deletions and point mutations), but this is not routinely done due to the high cost.
  - High-performance liquid chromatography
  - Cost-effective primary screening tool for children and adolescents
  - Equivocal results should be confirmed with DNA analysis.

Pediatric Considerations
For children, calculate Mentzer index (mean corpuscular volume/RBC count).
- <13: suggests thalassemia
- >13: suggests iron deficiency anemia
- Liver iron concentrations can be assessed with MRI (FerriScan).

TREATMENT

- Outpatient for mild cases
- Inpatient for transfusion therapy

GENERAL MEASURES

- Mild cases (trait or minor) require no therapy.
- Thalassemia intermedia: No therapy is necessary unless hemoglobin falls to a level that causes symptoms; then, transfusion therapy is needed. Decision is based on patient's quality of life.
- Iron supplements should not be given unless iron deficiency occurs and is confirmed with low ferritin. Supplements increase the risk of iron overload (1)[C].
- Thalassemia major
  - A regular transfusion schedule to increase post-transfusion hemoglobin to 13.0 to 14.0 g/L and maintain a mean hemoglobin level of at least 9.3 g/dL (1.4 mmol/L) (1)[B]
  - Patients require >8 transfusion events per year. An event may be multiple transfused units.
  - Iron overload (6)[C]
    - Patients receiving transfusion therapy increase total body iron 4 times the normal amount.
    - Therapy is iron chelation. (See "Medication.")

MEDICATION

Thalassemia intermedia and major: folic acid supplements (1 mg/day)

First Line

β-Thalassemia major

- Iron chelation with deferoxamine (Desferal)
  - Usually continuous SC or IV infusion
  - Acute toxicity: initial—1,000 mg IV, may be followed by 500 mg every 4 hours for 2 doses; subsequent doses of 500 mg every 4 to 12 hours based on response (max 6,000 mg/day)
  - Chronic: 20 to 40 mg/kg over 8 to 12 hours daily
  - Usually started by 5 to 8 years of age
  - Treatment lasts 3 to 5 years to reach serum ferritin <1,000 ng/mL.
- Deferasirox (Exjade): 20 to 30 mg/kg/day PO acceptable alternative; approved for transfusion and non–transfusion-dependent patients with hepatic iron concentrations ≥5 mg/g of dry weight and serum ferritin >300 μg/L; renal and hepatic monitoring is recommended.

Second Line

Chelation with deferiprone (Ferriprox) 25 mg/kg TID PO initially is an acceptable alternative for patients who have not responded to deferoxamine; may provide more cardioprotection. A drawback is weekly CBC because ~1% of patients develop agranulocytosis.

ISSUES FOR REFERRAL

Thalassemia major usually requires hematology consult.

ADDITIONAL THERAPIES

β-Thalassemia intermedia

- Hydroxyurea may improve hemoglobin 1 to 2 g/dL.
- Psychological support seems appropriate for this chronic disease. However, no conclusions can be made regarding specific psychological therapies.

SURGERY/OTHER PROCEDURES

- Splenectomy
  - May be needed if hypersplenism causes an increase in the transfusion requirements (>180 to 200 mL/kg/year)
  - Defer surgery until patient is at least 4 years of age (due to increased infection risk).
  - Administer pneumococcal polyvalent-23 vaccine 1 month before splenectomy. Children should complete their pneumococcal conjugate vaccine series before surgery.
  - Daily penicillin prophylaxis, 250 mg BID, after splenectomy for 2 years for all patients and for children until age 16 years
- Bone marrow transplantation with HLA-identical related donor stem cells in children before developing hepatitis or iron overload has high likelihood of remission but may impair fertility.

 ONGOING CARE

FOLLOW-UP RECOMMENDATIONS

- Thalassemia trait requires no restrictions.
- β-Thalassemia major
  - Avoid strenuous activities (e.g., football, soccer).
  - Acceptable activity levels will be determined on an individual basis depending on the severity of the disorder.

Patient Monitoring

- Thalassemia-trait patients require no special follow-up.
- For β-thalassemia major, lifelong monitoring is necessary because the therapy and disease progression have numerous potential complications.

DIET

- Thalassemia trait requires no restrictions.
- β-Thalassemia major
  - Limit intake of iron-rich foods (e.g., red meats such as liver and some cereals).

PATIENT EDUCATION

Printed patient information available from Cooley's Anemia Foundation, 330 7th Ave. Suite 900, New York, NY 10001; http://www.thalassemia.org or http://www.cooleysanemia.org

PROGNOSIS

- Outlook varies depending on type.
- Thalassemia-trait patients live a normal lifespan.
- β-Thalassemia major patients live an average of 17 years and usually die by age 30 years.
- Iron overload causes most of the morbidity and mortality:
  - Cardiac events are the primary cause of death.
  - Myocardial iron deposition is best assessed with MRI T2.
  - Effective iron chelation improves longevity.

COMPLICATIONS

- Chronic hemolysis
- Susceptibility to infections after splenectomy
- Infections from blood transfusion
- Jaundice
- Leg ulcers
- Cholelithiasis
- Osteoporosis and low-trauma fractures
- Impaired growth rate
- Delayed or absent puberty
- Hypogonadism
- Hepatic siderosis
- Splenomegaly
- Cardiac disease from iron overload
- Thromboembolic phenomenon
- Aplastic and megaloblastic crises
- Increased risk of hematologic and abdominal cancer
- Increased risk of dementia

REFERENCES

1. Muncie HL Jr, Campbell J. Alpha and beta thalassemia. *Am Fam Physician*. 2009;80(4):339–344.
2. Higgs DR, Engel JD, Stamatoyannopoulos G. Thalassaemia. *Lancet*. 2012;379(9813):373–383.
3. Tamhankar PM, Agarwal S, Arya V, et al. Prevention of homozygous beta thalassemia by premarital screening and prenatal diagnosis in India. *Prenat Diagn*. 2009;29(1):83–88.
4. Peters M, Heijboer H, Smiers F, et al. Diagnosis and management of thalassaemia. *BMJ*. 2012;344:e228.
5. Mosca A, Paleari R, Ivaldi G, et al. The role of haemoglobin A(2) testing in the diagnosis of thalassaemias and related haemoglobinopathies. *J Clin Pathol*. 2009;62(1):13–17.
6. Fleming RE, Ponka P. Iron overload in human disease. *N Engl J Med*. 2012;366(4):348–359.

ADDITIONAL READING

- Paulson RF. Targeting a new regulator of erythropoiesis to alleviate anemia. *Nat Med*. 2014;20(4): 334–335.
- Piel FB, Weatherall DJ. The α-thalassemias. *N Engl J Med*. 2014;371(20):1908–1916.

CODES

ICD10

- D56.5 Hemoglobin E-beta thalassemia
- D56.3 Thalassemia minor
- D56.0 Alpha thalassemia

CLINICAL PEARLS

- Thalassemia (group of inherited hematologic disorders that affect the synthesis of adult hemoglobin tetramer) is a genetic condition; hemoglobin will not improve over time.
- α-Thalassemia is due to a deficient synthesis of the α-globin chain, whereas β-thalassemia is due to a deficient synthesis of the β-globin chain.
- Hemoglobin electrophoresis is needed for genetic counseling but not to make the diagnosis of thalassemia minor when evaluating a patient with mild hypochromic, microcytic anemia, and normal serum ferritin.
- Anemia from thalassemia minor is not due to inadequate iron availability or iron storage. Therefore, iron supplements will not improve the anemia and could be harmful due to GI distress and iron overload. If coexisting iron deficiency is proven, then iron therapy is appropriate.

THORACIC OUTLET SYNDROME

Ashley Nicole Koontz, DO • Jayson R. Loeffert, DO

BASICS

DESCRIPTION
- This syndrome consists of a constellation of symptoms that affect the head, neck, shoulders, and upper extremities caused by compression of the neurovascular structures (brachial plexus and subclavian vessels) at the thoracic outlet, specifically in the area superior to the 1st rib and posterior to the clavicle.
- Three forms of thoracic outlet syndrome (TOS) have been described: neurogenic (nTOS), venous (vTOS), and arterial (aTOS).
- Synonym(s): scalenus anticus syndrome; cervical rib syndrome; costoclavicular syndrome

Pregnancy Considerations
Generalized tissue fluid accumulations and postural changes may aggravate symptoms.

EPIDEMIOLOGY
- There are no universal diagnostic criteria to accurately determine epidemiology.
- Estimated 3 to 80 cases per 1,000 people (1)
- nTOS
  - Approximately 95% of all TOS cases
  - Predominant in 20- to 50-year-old females
- vTOS
  - Approximately 4% of all TOS cases
  - Predominant in 20- to 35-year-old physically active males
- aTOS
  - Approximately 1% of all TOS cases
  - No gender preference
  - Typically seen in young adults and associated with congenital anomalies

ETIOLOGY AND PATHOPHYSIOLOGY
- TOS primarily impacts 3 anatomic spaces within the thoracic outlet:
  - Scalene triangle
    - Bordered by the anterior scalene, middle scalene and 1st rib
    - Contains trunks of the brachial plexus and subclavian artery
  - Costoclavicular space
    - Bordered by the clavicle, 1st rib and upper portion of the scapula
    - Contains divisions of the brachial plexus, subclavian artery and vein
  - Subcoracoid space
    - Bordered by the pectoralis muscle, 2nd to 4th ribs, and coracoid process
    - Contains cords of the brachial plexus, axillary artery and vein
- 70% of cases are soft tissue in nature, causing compression of neurovascular structures (local tumor, muscle hypertrophy, variant anatomy). The remainder are bony in nature (cervical rib, malunion) (1).
- Cases are also divided into traumatic and non-traumatic etiologies. Trauma is most common, particularly for nTOS.
- Prolonged or repetitive motion of the shoulder in abduction or extension can provoke symptoms

RISK FACTORS
- Trauma, especially to the shoulder girdle
- Presence of a cervical rib
- Posttraumatic, exostosis of clavicle or 1st rib, postural abnormalities (e.g., drooping of shoulders, scoliosis), body building with increased muscular bulk in thoracic outlet area, rapid weight loss with vigorous physical exertion and/or exercise, pendulous breasts
- Occupational exposure via repetitive activity: computer users; musicians; repetitive work involving shoulders, arms, hands
- Young, thin females with long necks and drooping shoulders

GENERAL PREVENTION
Consider workplace evaluation for proper occupational ergonomics, including proper posture.

COMMONLY ASSOCIATED CONDITIONS
- Paget–Schrötter syndrome: thrombosis of subclavian vein
- Gilliatt-Sumner hand: neurogenic atrophy of abductor pollicis brevis
- Pancoast tumor

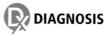

DIAGNOSIS

HISTORY
- nTOS
  - High index of suspicion for history of MVA trauma and overhead lifting athletes
  - 76% of patients will have occipital headache (2).
  - Symptoms of the upper plexus (C5 to C7)
    - Occipital and orbital headache
    - Pain and paresthesias in head, neck, mandible, face, temporal area, upper back/chest, outer arm, and hand in a radial nerve distribution
  - Symptoms of the lower plexus (C7 to T1)
    - Pain and paresthesias in axilla, inner arm, and hand in an ulnar nerve distribution, often nocturnal
    - Hypothenar and interosseous muscle atrophy
- vTOS
  - High index of suspicion if symptoms worsen with shoulder abduction particularly in overhead lifting athletes
  - Common symptoms: unilateral arm claudication, cyanosis, swelling, pain, venous enlargement
- aTOS
  - 85% of cases estimated to be related to cervical rib (3)
  - Highest morbidity of all types due to risk for limb ischemia
  - Common symptoms: unilateral arm weakness, pallor, paresthesia, pain, weak or absent pulse, blood pressure asymmetry

PHYSICAL EXAM
- Initial considerations
  - Posture (1)
  - Cervical alignment (1)
  - Scapular stability (1)
  - Inspection and palpation of thoracic outlet anatomy
  - Upper extremity and cranial nerve neurologic examination
- Have a high suspicion for TOS if there is loss of vibratory sensation along the distribution of brachial plexus nerves (1).
- Specialized testing
  - Adson maneuver (aTOS)
    - Head rotation to the affected side with cervical extension and then deep inhalation
    - Positive if paresthesias occur or if radial pulse is not palpable during maneuver
  - Morley test (vTOS)
    - Positive with reproduction of an aching sensation and typical localized paresthesia
    - Manual compression of brachial plexus for 30 seconds in the supraclavicular area of the scalene triangle
  - Hyperabduction test (aTOS)
    - Elevation of arm above the head
    - Positive if diminished of radial pulse
  - Military maneuver (i.e., costoclavicular bracing)
    - Patient elevates chin and pushes shoulders posteriorly in an extreme "at-attention" position.
    - Positive test reproduces symptoms
  - 1-minute Roos test
    - Shoulders and arms are braced in a 90-degree abducted and externally rotated position; patient is required to clench and relax fists repetitively for 1 minute.
    - Positive test reproduces symptoms.

DIFFERENTIAL DIAGNOSIS
- Cervical disc or carpal tunnel syndrome
- Orthopedic shoulder problems (shoulder strain, rotator cuff injury, tendonitis)
- Cervical spondylitis
- Ulnar nerve compression at elbow and hand
- Multiple sclerosis
- Spinal cord tumor/disease
- Angina pectoris
- Migraine
- Complex regional pain syndromes
- C3 to C5 and C8 radiculopathies
- Pancoast tumor

DIAGNOSTIC TESTS & INTERPRETATION
Initial Tests (lab, imaging)
- History and physical are the strongest clinical indicators for TOS. However, additional imaging helps to confirm subtype to guide proper treatment.
- Chest x-ray is often the best initial imaging modality for all subtypes (1).

- American College of Radiology recommends MR angiography and venography for diagnosis of aTOS and vTOS (4). However, duplex ultrasound can be beneficial as initial and easily accessible imaging modality (1).
- Laboratory testing is typically not considered in the initial workup.

Follow-Up Tests & Special Considerations
MRI and CT assist with definitive subtype diagnosis after initial workup (5)[C]

Diagnostic Procedures/Other
No indicated procedures; anesthetic anterior scalene block may relieve pressure by scalene muscles on the brachial plexus, making this type of block diagnostic and potentially therapeutic, but it poses the risk of procedural damage to the brachial plexus.

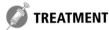 TREATMENT

GENERAL MEASURES
- Conservative management usually involves approaches to reduce and redistribute pressure and traction on the thoracic outlet.
- Physical therapy is first-line treatment along with activity modification, rest, and NSAIDs (6)[B].
- Interscalene injections of botulinum toxin have been shown to decrease symptoms of nTOS (7)[C]. A single, CT-guided Botox injection into the anterior scalene muscle may offer an effective, minimally invasive treatment (8)[A].
- Severe cases may use taping, adhesive elastic bandages, moist heat, TENS, or US but should not substitute active exercise and correction of posture and muscle imbalance (6)[B].

MEDICATION
No firm evidence exists for any specific pharmacologic approach to the four types of TOS.
- Anti-inflammatory (ibuprofen)
  - Adult dose: 400 to 800 mg PO q8h; not to exceed 3,200 mg/day
  - Pediatric dose:
    ○ <12 years: 10 mg/kg/dose q6–8h
  - Contraindications: documented hypersensitivity, active PUD, renal or hepatic impairment, recent use of anticoagulants, hemorrhagic conditions
- Neuropathic pain: tricyclic antidepressants, carbamazepine, gabapentin, phenytoin, pregabalin; muscle relaxants such as baclofen, metaxalone, or tizanidine may be helpful.
- Severe pain: Consider opiates for brachial plexus nerve block, steroid injections.

ISSUES FOR REFERRAL
- Referral is recommended after 4 to 6 months of failed conservative management (1).
- Sports medicine or PM&R can be considered for diagnostic and therapeutic injections.
- Vascular surgery (aTOS and vTOS), orthopedic surgery (nTOS), or neurosurgery (nTOS) can be considered for surgical evaluation.

SURGERY/OTHER PROCEDURES
- BTX-A injection therapy
  - Benefit from decreased muscular tension and pain
  - 64–69% of patients have relief for up to 3 months although with a risk for prolonged duration of symptoms (1).
- Alternative injection therapies show best efficacy when combined with physical therapy modalities (1).
  - Trigger point
  - Corticosteroid
  - Local anesthetic
- Surgical options can provide greater relief to symptoms than conservative management alone (9).
- Complete 1st rib resection and anterior scalenectomy are common combined surgical interventions to provide pressure relief to the thoracic outlet structures in all subtypes.
- Thrombolytic may be necessary for acute vTOS with consideration of venoplasty thereafter.

ADMISSION, INPATIENT, AND NURSING CONSIDERATIONS
Conservative outpatient treatment is reasonable first-line therapy except in cases of thromboembolic phenomena and acute ischemia, symptoms of chronic vascular occlusion, stenosis, arterial dilatation, or progressive neurologic deficit (8)[B].

 ONGOING CARE

FOLLOW-UP RECOMMENDATIONS
Practice proper posture, exercises to strengthen shoulder elevator and neck extensor muscles, stretching exercises for scalene muscles, support bra for women with pendulous breasts, breast reduction surgery in selected cases; sleep with arms below chest level; avoid/reduce prolonged hyperabduction.

Patient Monitoring
Office follow-up visits every 3 to 4 weeks

PATIENT EDUCATION
Physical therapy, postural exercises, ergonomic workstation

PROGNOSIS
Durable long-term functional outcomes can be achieved predicated on a highly selective approach to the surgical management of patients with TOS. A majority of operated patients will not require adjunctive procedures or chronic narcotic use (10)[C].

COMPLICATIONS
- Postoperative shoulder, arm, hand pain, and paresthesias in 10%
- Patients who will have symptomatic recurrences at 1 month to 7 years postoperatively (usually within 3 months): 1.5–2%
- Patients who will have brachial plexus injury, probably due to intraoperative traction: 0.5–1%
- Reoperation is indicated for symptomatic recurrence with long posterior remnant of 1st rib (posterior approach) or with disrupted fibrous adhesions (transaxillary approach).
- Venous obstruction or arterial emboli; usually responds to thrombolytics

REFERENCES
1. Li N, Dierks G, Vervaeke HE, et al. Thoracic outlet syndrome: a narrative review. *J Clin Med*. 2021;10(5):962.
2. Sanders RJ, Hammond SL, Rao NM. Diagnosis of thoracic outlet syndrome. *J Vasc Surg*. 2007;46(3):601–604.
3. Hussain MA, Aljabri B, Al-Omran M. Vascular thoracic outlet syndrome. *Semin Thorac Cardiovasc Surg*. 2016;28(1):151–157.
4. Zurkiya O, Ganguli S, Kalva SP, et al; for Expert Panels on Vascular Imaging, Thoracic Imaging, and Neurological Imaging. ACR Appropriateness Criteria® thoracic outlet syndrome. *J Am Coll Radiol*. 2020;17(5 Suppl):S323–S334.
5. Povlsen S, Povlsen B. Diagnosing thoracic outlet syndrome: current approaches and future directions. *Diagnostics (Basel)*. 2018;8(1):21.
6. Vanti C, Natalini L, Romeo A, et al. Conservative treatment of thoracic outlet syndrome. A review of the literature. *Eura Medicophys*. 2007;43(1):55–70.
7. Lee GW, Kwon YH, Jeong JH, et al. The efficacy of scalene injection in thoracic outlet syndrome. *J Korean Neurosurg Soc*. 2011;50(1):36–39.
8. Christo PJ, Christo DK, Carinci AJ, et al. Single CT-guided chemodenervation of the anterior scalene muscle with botulinum toxin for neurogenic thoracic outlet syndrome. *Pain Med*. 2010;11(4):504–511.
9. Balderman J, Abuirqeba AA, Eichaker L, et al. Physical therapy management, surgical treatment, and patient-reported outcomes measures in a prospective observational cohort of patients with neurogenic thoracic outlet syndrome. *J Vasc Surg*. 2019;70(3):832–841.
10. Scali S, Stone D, Bjerke A, et al. Long-term functional results for the surgical management of neurogenic thoracic outlet syndrome. *Vasc Endovascular Surg*. 2010;44(7):550–555.

 CODES

ICD10
G54.0 Brachial plexus disorders

CLINICAL PEARLS
- This syndrome is caused by compression of the neurovascular structures (brachial plexus and subclavian vessels) at the thoracic outlet, specifically in the area superior to the 1st rib and posterior to the clavicle.
- Three subtypes exist: neurogenic, arterial, venous.
- Physical therapy, activity modification, rest, and NSAIDs are the first-line treatment.
- Referral for injection therapy and/or surgical evaluation should be considered for those that fail conservative management.

THROMBOPHILIA AND HYPERCOAGULABLE STATES

Kirsten Vitrikas, MD • Brian C. Glaser, MD

 BASICS

DESCRIPTION

- An inherited or acquired disorder of the coagulation system predisposing an individual to thromboembolism (the formation of a venous, or less commonly, an arterial blood clot)
- Venous thrombosis typically manifests as deep venous thrombosis (DVT) of the lower extremity in the legs or pelvis and pulmonary embolism (PE).
- System(s) affected: cardiovascular, nervous, pulmonary, reproductive, hematologic
- Synonym(s): hypercoagulation syndrome; prothrombotic state

EPIDEMIOLOGY

- VTE incidence is higher in age 16 to 44 years; then, higher in men when >45 years of age (1)
- VTE incidence is higher in African American populations (1).
- Inherited thrombophilias
  - An inherited thrombophilic defect or risk can be detected in up to 50% of patients with VTE.
  - Factor V Leiden (FVL) is the most common inherited thrombophilia (1/2 of all currently characterizable inherited thrombophilia cases involve the FVL mutation), and it is present in its heterozygous form in up to ~20% of patients with a first VTE.
  - Heterozygous prothrombin G20210A mutation, the second most common inherited thrombophilia, is present in up to ~8% of patients with VTE.
- Acquired thrombophilias:
  - Pregnancy: ~1–2 /1000 pregnancies affected by VTE
  - Cancer: ~20% of all VTEs occur in setting of active cancer; ~6% of unprovoked VTEs have undiagnosed cancer.
  - Antiphospholipid antibodies are found in ~50% of patients with systemic lupus erythematosus (SLE) and up to 5% of the general population.
  - See "Risk Factors."

Incidence

First-time thromboembolism
- ~100/100,000/year among the general population
- <1/100,000/year in those age <15 years
- ~1,000/100,000/year in those age ≥85 years

Prevalence

- 40–80% of lower extremity orthopedic procedures can result in DVT if prophylaxis is not used.
- VTE accounts for ~1.2 to 4.7 deaths per 100,000 pregnancies.

ETIOLOGY AND PATHOPHYSIOLOGY

- Virchow triad as a cause of VTE includes blood stasis, vascular endothelial injury, and abnormalities in circulating blood constituents.
- An imbalance between the hemostatic and fibrinolytic pathways leads to thrombus formation.
- VTE is considered to be the result of genetic tendencies with other acquired risks.
- Upper extremity DVT: >60% are associated with venous catheters. Malignancy is an additional significant risk (2).

Genetics

- The most common genetic thrombophilias (FVL, prothrombin G20210A, proteins C and S defects, and antithrombin III deficiency) are inherited in an autosomal dominant pattern.
- Homozygous mutations have a higher risk of VTE.

- FVL/activated protein C (aPC) resistance:
  - Heterozygous FVL: 3–8% prevalence in Caucasians; 1.2% in African Americans
  - Heterozygous FVL carries 3- to 5-fold increase risk in first-time VTE; mild increase risk of recurrence.
  - Homozygous FVL carries 18-fold increase risk in first-time VTE compared to patients without FVL mutation.
  - Other acquired risks are synergistic (3).
- Prothrombin gene mutation G20210A:
  - Prevalence 6% among Caucasians, 2% of general U.S. population, 0.5% of African Americans
  - Heterozygous carriers have 3-fold increased risk in first-time VTE.
- Antithrombin deficiency: <0.2% among the general population; acquired deficiency in disseminated intravascular coagulation (DIC), sepsis, liver disease, nephrotic syndrome; RR of 8.1 for thrombosis
- Protein C and S deficiencies: 0.5% and 1% incidences, respectively, among the general population. Homozygotes and heterozygotes are hypercoagulable. Vitamin K–dependent, produced in the liver. Protein C inactivates Va and VIIIa. Protein C may become an acquired deficiency in liver disease, sepsis, DIC, acute respiratory distress syndrome, and after surgery. RR of 7.3 for thrombosis. Protein S is a cofactor for protein C, and it may become an acquired deficiency with oral contraceptive pill (OCP) use, pregnancy, liver disease, sepsis, DIC, HIV, and nephrosis; RR of 8.5 for thrombosis

RISK FACTORS

- Acquired risk factors
  - Previous thromboembolism
  - First-degree relative with VTE (2- to 4-fold increased risk; regardless of relative's test results)
  - Immobilization or prolonged travel (e.g., flight time >8 hours)
  - Trauma
  - Surgery, especially orthopedic
  - Malignancies (especially pancreatic, ovarian, brain, and lymphoma)
  - Pregnancy (5- to 10-fold fold increased relative risk [RR] compared to nonpregnant women)
  - Postpartum state (15- to 35-fold fold increased risk)
  - Acute medical illness
    ○ Pneumonia, particularly involving SARS-CoV, MERS-CoV, SARS-CoV-2
  - Exogenous female hormones/oral contraceptives
  - Androgen deprivation therapy
  - Obesity
  - Nephrotic syndrome, hypoalbuminemia
  - APS and lupus anticoagulant
  - Myeloproliferative disorders (polycythemia vera, essential thrombocythemia)
  - Hyperviscosity syndromes (sickle cell, paraproteinemias)
  - Hyperhomocysteinemia secondary to vitamin deficiencies (B_6, B_{12}, folic acid)
  - Tamoxifen, thalidomide, lenalidomide, bevacizumab, L-asparaginase, erythropoiesis-stimulating agents, pomalidomide, tranexamic acid
  - Dehydration
- Established genetic factors
  - FVL
  - Prothrombin G20210A mutation
  - Protein C deficiency
  - Protein S deficiency
  - Antithrombin III deficiency
- Rare genetic factors

  - Dysfibrinogenemia
  - Methylene tetrahydrofolate reductase mutation
- Indeterminate factors
  - Elevated factor VIII
- Age: >60 years
- Sex: male
- Race: See "Epidemiology."

GENERAL PREVENTION

- Consider medication prophylaxis in any hospitalized patient with VTE risk factors.
- Consider mechanical prophylaxis in patients at increased risk for VTE in whom anticoagulation may be contraindicated.
- Consider prophylaxis with low-molecular-weight heparin (LMWH) plus aspirin in pregnant patients with APS.
- Consider prophylaxis using direct oral anticoagulants (DOACs) (4) in patients with solid tumors who have additional risk factors for VTE.
- Prophylaxis with unfractionated heparin (UFH) or LMWH should be considered in patients with genetic or acquired risks of thrombosis and an anticipated additional risk, such as the immobilization associated with surgery.
- Use caution with procoagulant medicines (e.g., OCPs) in asymptomatic individuals who have a known hereditary predisposition.

COMMONLY ASSOCIATED CONDITIONS

Advanced age, cancer, pregnancy, obesity, prior history of thrombosis, surgery, immobilization

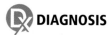 **DIAGNOSIS**

HISTORY

Consider prothrombotic assessment for the following:
- Thrombosis at an unusual anatomic site (e.g., cerebral, mesenteric, portal, hepatic) or recurrent thromboses
- Family history suggesting multiple individuals affected with VTE
- Purpura fulminans in children or neonates
- Skin necrosis associated with vitamin K antagonists
- Recurrent pregnancy loss
- See other scenarios under "Diagnostic Tests & Interpretation."

PHYSICAL EXAM

- DVT: swelling, pain, warmth, and redness, usually of one extremity
- PE: dyspnea, chest pain, hemoptysis, hypoxia, tachycardia
- Postthrombotic syndrome: pain, swelling, pigmentation, and/or ulceration

DIAGNOSTIC TESTS & INTERPRETATION

- Testing for thrombophilias is not recommended, unless it will affect management (2),(5)[B].
- Testing should be delayed until after the initial 3 months of anticoagulation (2),(5)[B].
- Rationale for screening
  - Inform patient of contributing factors.
  - Help predict VTE recurrence risk and guide duration of therapy or future risk management.
  - Help guide management of asymptomatic family members, especially in female patients seeking contraceptive counsel or who are planning pregnancy.

- Appropriate tests for unprovoked VTE, recurrent VTE, VTE at age <50 years, family history of VTE, unusual sites of VTE or VTE secondary to pregnancy, OCPs or HRT:
  - FVL (aPC), protein C and S, ATIII, G20210A assays if idiopathic VTE, younger patient and/or family history of VTE
  - Antiphospholipid antibody assays if idiopathic VTE or associated autoimmune disease or no family history of VTE
- Appropriate tests for arterial thrombosis, especially if younger patient or no atherosclerosis
  - Antiphospholipid antibody assays
  - Consider FVL, G20210A, protein C, and S, ATIII
  - Consider screening for vasculitides such as antineutrophil cytoplasmic antibody (ANCA)-associated vasculitis.
  - Do not test for FVL, G2021A, protein C and S, or ATIII if known atherosclerosis.

Initial Tests (lab, imaging)
- CBC
- aPC profile: ≤2.0 implies FVL mutation; 95–100% are FVL positive; false-positive finding in pregnancy or with use of OCPs, confirm with FVL mutation testing or consider FVL mutation testing up front.
  - aPC resistance may be unreliable while taking LMWH or UFH.
- Prothrombin G20210A genetic assay
- ATIII functional assay
  - Will be low with acute thrombosis and on heparin therapy; may be falsely high on dabigatran, apixaban, edoxaban, and rivaroxaban
- Protein C functional assay
  - May be low with acute thrombosis; will be lower on warfarin, dabigatran, apixaban, edoxaban, and rivaroxaban
- Protein S antigen and functional assay and free S
  - May be low with acute thrombosis; will be lower on warfarin, dabigatran, apixaban, edoxaban, and rivaroxaban
- Antiphospholipid antibodies: phospholipid-dependent tests and anticardiolipin antibodies, lupus anticoagulant
  - May be unreliable on heparin and DOACs; risk false-positive test.
- Consider evaluation for subclinical malignancy in an unprovoked thrombosis in those >40 years of age or at greater risk.
- Consider homocysteine level, although treatment of hyperhomocysteinemia (vitamins B_{12} and B_6, folate) does not alter the thrombophilic risk.
- Consider HIT antibody immunoassay or functional assay if clinical suspicion.

Follow-Up Tests & Special Considerations
Dysfibrinogenemia and plasminogen deficiency are very rare causes of thrombophilia.

Pregnancy Considerations
- Warfarin is teratogenic and should be avoided in pregnancy.
- LMWH or UFH are preferred for all prophylactic and treatment options.
- There is lack of safety data on DOACs in pregnancy.

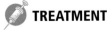 ## TREATMENT

- Assess VTE risk:
  - Low-risk inherited thrombophilias: heterozygous FVL, heterozygous prothrombin 20210 mutation
  - High-risk inherited thrombophilias: protein C deficiency, protein S deficiency, antithrombin deficiency

- Duration of treatment
  - Heterozygosity for FVL or prothrombin 20210 mutation, as isolated risk factors, should not affect decision.
  - Consider extended thromboprophylaxis post-discharge, up to 35 days, for medically ill patients with high VTE risk. A noteworthy example includes COVID-19 patients.
- For medication dosing and considerations, see VTE chapter

MEDICATION
First Line
- DOACs: Apixaban, dabigatran, edoxaban, and rivaroxaban are now recommended over vitamin K antagonists for initial and long-term oral anticoagulation (5)[B].
  - Use is supported for low-risk inherited thrombophilia (i.e., FVL or prothrombin 20210 mutation).
  - Few data available to support use in rare thrombophilias such as ATIII, protein C or protein S deficiencies
  - May consider DOACs for patients with active cancer, but data is lacking to recommend over LMWH
- Parenteral anticoagulation: LMWH has largely replaced UFH as first-line therapy for VTE.
  - Enoxaparin is preferred in patients with active cancer for a minimum of 6 months (can dose at 1.5 mg/kg SC daily), after which time the patient can be reevaluated to continue treatment.
- Vitamin K antagonist
  - Warfarin requires careful and frequent monitoring because of many drug–drug and drug–diet (e.g., vitamin K) interactions.
- Pregnancy: low-dose aspirin and/or LMWH or UFH; warfarin is contraindicated.
- APS: Warfarin and LMWH remain first-line agents for anticoagulation.

Second Line
Usually indicated when contraindication to heparin or LMWH, such as heparin-associated thrombosis and thrombocytopenia
- Factor Xa inhibitors (fonduparinux)
- Direct thrombin inhibtors (argatroban)

SURGERY/OTHER PROCEDURES
- Consider systemic thrombolysis for unstable cases.
- Inferior vena cava filter
  - Reduces short-term risk of PE in those with contraindications to anticoagulation
  - May increase long-term risk of recurrent DVT
  - Used for patients with multiple episodes of recurrent thromboembolism despite therapeutic anticoagulation and contraindication to anticoagulation

 ## ONGOING CARE

FOLLOW-UP RECOMMENDATIONS
Patient Monitoring
Monitor warfarin as frequently as needed to maintain an INR goal of 2 to 3.

DIET
- Vitamin K–stable diet if patient is taking warfarin
- Rivaroxaban should be taken with a large meal to aid absorption.

PATIENT EDUCATION
- Advise the use of medical alert bracelets.
- Caution against contact sports or other high-risk activities.

- Seek immediate medical attention with any trauma.
- Assume that any drug may enhance or attenuate the warfarin effect.
- Increase the frequency of monitoring following any medication change to ensure therapeutic anticoagulation and to avoid overanticoagulation.
- Many drugs may modulate warfarin effect: alcohol, antibiotics, aspirin, NSAIDs, acetaminophen.

PROGNOSIS
- Anticoagulation should be continued for 3 months with consideration for longer in those with unprovoked VTE.
- Patients with a provoked VTE (i.e., surgery, hospitalization) not receiving chronic anticoagulation have risks of recurrence of 7% (year 1), 16% (year 5), and 23% (year 10).
- Patients with an unprovoked VTE not receiving chronic anticoagulation have risks of recurrence of 15% (year 1), 41% (year 5), and 53% (year 10).
- Currently, there are no data from randomized, controlled trials or controlled clinical trials about the benefits of thrombophilia testing to decrease the risk of recurrent VTE (1).

COMPLICATIONS
Venous or arterial thrombosis; bleeding in anticoagulated patients

REFERENCES
1. Heit J. Epidemiology of venous thromboembolism. *Nat Rev Cardiol*. 2015;12(8):464–474.
2. Baglin T, Gray E, Greaves M, et al; for British Committee for Standards in Haematology. Clinical guidelines for testing for heritable thrombophilia. *Br J Haematol*. 2010;149(2):209–220.
3. Anderson JA, Weitz JI. Hypercoagulable states. *Clin Chest Med*. 2010;31(4):659–673.
4. Key NS, Khorana AA, Kuderer NM, et al. Venous thromboembolism prophylaxis and treatment in patients with cancer: ASCO clinical practice guideline update. *J Clin Oncol*. 2020;38(5):496–520.
5. Kearon C, Akl EA, Ornelas J, et al. Antithrombotic therapy for VTE disease: CHEST guideline and expert panel report. *Chest*. 2016;149(2):315–352.

ADDITIONAL READING
Stevens SM, Woller SC, Bauer KA, et al. Guidance for the evaluation and treatment of hereditary and acquired thrombophilia. *J Thromb Thrombolysis*. 2016;41(1):154–164.

CODES

ICD10
- D68.59 Other primary thrombophilia
- D68.51 Activated protein C resistance
- D68.2 Hereditary deficiency of other clotting factors

CLINICAL PEARLS
- FVL (resistance to aPC) is the most common inherited thrombophilia, with a prevalence of 3–8% in the U.S. Caucasian population.
- Test patients for thrombophilias only if it will affect management of the condition.
- Rule out malignancy, especially in those >50 years of age.

Theresa A. Townley, MD, MPH • Rutendo Jokomo-Nyakabau, MD

BASICS

DESCRIPTION

- An acute syndrome of microangiopathic hemolytic anemia (MAHA) and consumptive thrombocytopenia with deposition of hyaline thrombi in terminal arterioles and capillaries leading to ischemic multiorgan damage
- Thrombotic thrombocytopenic purpura (TTP) is characterized by MAHA (schistocytes on peripheral smear) and thrombocytopenia (generally <30,000), with or without the following signs and symptoms:
  - Neurologic symptoms, renal dysfunction, fever
  - Most patients do not show the historic pentad of MAHA, thrombocytopenia, renal dysfunction, neurologic abnormalities, and fever because treatment is initiated before the pentad can develop.

EPIDEMIOLOGY

Annual prevalence of ~10 cases per million people

Incidence

- First episode mostly in adulthood (~90%) and 10% in childhood to adolescence (1)
- Predominant sex: female > male (2:1) (1)
  - Higher relapse in females (1)
- Incidence ratio in blacks to whites is 7:1.
- Annual incidence of ~1 new case per million people (1)

ETIOLOGY AND PATHOPHYSIOLOGY

- In TTP, the aggregating agent responsible for platelet thrombi is unusually large von Willebrand factor (UL vWF) multimers, which are far larger than those found in normal plasma.
- A metalloprotease, ADAMTS13, which normally enzymatically cleaves UL vWF multimers to prevent clumping within vessels, is deficient, defective, or absent, allowing UL vWF to react with platelets. This leads to the endothelial cell damage and disseminated thrombi characteristic of TTP.
- Arterioles often affected: brain, kidney, pancreas, heart, adrenal glands. Lungs and liver are relatively spared.
- In familial TTP, patients have an inherited deficiency of ADAMTS13.
- In acquired idiopathic TTP, autoantibodies are directed against the metalloprotease ADAMTS13 (1).
- Endothelial injury, either directly from a drug/toxin or indirectly via platelet/neutrophil activation, has been proposed as a cause of secondary TTP especially in those without ADAMTS13 deficiency.

Genetics

- TTP is most often an acquired disorder. A congenital form of inherited TTP (Upshaw-Schulman syndrome) is due to a mutation at the ADAMTS13 metalloprotease gene locus on chromosome 9q34. This rare form of TTP has an autosomal recessive pattern of inheritance.
- USS typically presents in infancy and is rarely diagnosed after 10 years of age. It does not have the female predominance seen in idiopathic TTP, more often has notable renal impairment, and there is some heterogeneity among siblings, although parents who are carriers of a single heterozygous ADAMTS13 mutation are typically asymptomatic.

RISK FACTORS

- Pregnancy, oral contraceptives, AIDS and early HIV infection, bacterial infection/sepsis, acute pancreatitis
- Autoimmune disease—antiphospholipid antibody syndrome, systemic lupus erythematosus (especially increased in women of African ancestry between ages 30 and 50 years), scleroderma
- Cancer
- Hematopoietic stem cell transplantation and solid organ transplant
- Drugs of abuse: MDMA, cocaine, oxymorphone ER
- Drug toxicity
  - Antimicrobials—trimethoprim, ciprofloxacin, famciclovir
  - Cancer chemotherapy—mitomycin C and gemcitabine; pentostatin and vincristine; bleomycin and cisplatin; oxaliplatin; bevacizumab and sunitinib; adalimumab; bortezomib, carfilzomib, and ixazomib
  - Calcineurin inhibitors—tacrolimus and cyclosporine
  - Immune mediated—quinine and quinidine; ticlopidine and clopidogrel

COMMONLY ASSOCIATED CONDITIONS

- TTP/hemolytic uremic syndrome (HUS)/atypical HUS have similar presentations with MAHA and thrombocytopenia and multiorgan involvement.
- TTP generally presents with minimal renal involvement and may have neurologic abnormalities, whereas the opposite is more characteristic of HUS/atypical HUS. Creatinine of >2 to 3 is suggestive against TTP.
- However, patients with HUS and TTP may have both prominent renal and neurologic manifestations, often making the diagnosis unclear, hence the historical hybrid name "TTP-HUS."
- ADAMTS13 levels are diminished (generally <10%) in adults with familial or acquired idiopathic TTP but are normal in children diagnosed with HUS following infection with *Escherichia coli* (particularly type O157:H7), so-called Shiga toxin–HUS, and in "atypical HUS," also called complement-mediated thrombotic microangiopathy reflecting the pathophysiology which is related to complement dysregulation.

DIAGNOSIS

- Most common symptoms are nonspecific: nausea, vomiting, weakness, abdominal pain, fatigue, fever.
- Related to thrombocytopenia—easy bruising, purpura, or petechiae; epistaxis, menorrhagia, bleeding gums; GI bleeding; intracranial hemorrhage
  - Visual symptoms due to retinal hemorrhage
- Related to hemolytic anemia (MAHA): jaundice, fatigue; end-organ ischemia
  - Neurologic: CNS symptoms occur in ~60% of the patients (1)
    - A scoring system (PLASMIC) was devised to predict ADAMTS13 activity <10% in adults with unexplained thrombotic angiopathy (inferred from thrombocytopenia and MAHA).

It is used to support the diagnosis of TTP while ADAMTS13 lab test is pending; 1 point each for:
  - Platelet count <30,000/μL
  - Hemolysis (reticulocyte count >2.5%, undetectable haptoglobin, or indirect bilirubin >2 mg/dL)
  - No active cancer
  - No solid organ or stem cell transplant history
  - MCV <90 fL
  - INR <1.5
  - Creatinine <2.0 mg/dL
  - Score 6 to 7 predictive of ADAMTS13 activity of <10%. Score of 0 to 4 predictive of ADAMTS13 activity was not <10%.
  ○ ADAMTS13 activity level <10% defines severe deficiency and makes TTP more likely. Levels of 10–20% suggest possible TTP especially if drawn after plasma exchange (PEX) has been initiated. ADAMTS13 >20% make TTP less likely.
  ○ Cardiac: arrhythmia, myocardial infarction, heart failure
  ○ Renal: hematuria, proteinuria, oliguria, or anuria
  ○ Often fluctuating symptoms: headache, altered mental status: Spectrum runs from behavioral/personality changes—obtundation/stupor/coma; seizures, stroke

HISTORY

- Generally acute onset of symptoms but subacute in about 1/4 of patients
- In about 50% of cases, a trigger/risk factor of some kind is identified.

PHYSICAL EXAM

- Fever
- Mental status/neurologic: confusion, coma, stupor, weakness
- HEENT: retinal hemorrhage, scleral icterus, epistaxis
- Abdomen/GI: nonspecific tenderness
- Skin: jaundice, petechiae, purpura, ecchymoses

DIFFERENTIAL DIAGNOSIS

- HUS and atypical HUS
- Antiphospholipid antibody syndrome: prolonged partial thromboplastin time (PTT) and presence of lupus anticoagulant
- Systemic lupus erythematosus
- Malignant hypertension: diastolic >130 mm Hg, papilledema, retinal hemorrhages
- Pregnancy-associated preeclampsia/eclampsia or hemolysis, elevated liver enzyme levels, and low platelet HELLP levels: low ATIII levels
- Disseminated intravascular coagulation
  - Prolonged prothrombin time (PT)/PTT, low fibrinogen, low factors V and VIII
  - Secondary to sepsis/shock or widely disseminated malignancy
- Idiopathic thrombocytopenic purpura (ITP)
  - No hemolysis, normal lactate dehydrogenase (LDH) and bilirubin
  - Presence of antiplatelet antibodies
- Malignancy-associated microangiopathy
- Evan syndrome (autoimmune hemolytic anemia and thrombocytopenia): positive direct Coombs test
- Scleroderma kidney

DIAGNOSTIC TESTS & INTERPRETATION
Initial Tests (lab, imaging)
- CBC
  - Hemoglobin (decreased): Average is 8 to 10 g/dL.
  - Platelets decreased: in the 10 to 30,000/μL range
- High reticulocyte count ($>120 \times 10^9$/L)
- Undetectable haptoglobin (hemolysis)
- Peripheral smear
  - Schistocytes (prominent, $>1\%$ of RBCs)
  - Helmet cells, RBC fragments
  - Nucleated RBCs
  - Polychromasia (reticulocytosis)
- Coagulation studies
  - Normal in most; mild elevation in 15%
  - Fibrinogen normal
- Coombs test: negative direct Coombs test
- Electrolytes, BUN/creatinine: mild elevation of BUN and creatinine (creatinine <3 mg/dL)
- Liver function studies: increased indirect bilirubin (hemolysis)
- LDH: 5 to 10 times normal
- Urinalysis
  - Proteinuria, microscopic hematuria
  - Positive dipstick for large blood but minimal RBCs on microscopic exam
- ECG changes (10%): sinus tachycardia, heart block
- Stool for Shiga toxin
- Increased troponin in 60% cases (>0.1 μg/L)
- HIV, hepatitis A, B, C testing: Exclude underlying viral precipitant.
- Pregnancy test (women with inherited TTP often have their first episode during their pregnancy)
- Pretreatment ADAMTS13 activity level of $<10\%$ is useful in distinguishing acquired or familial TTP from other disorders.
- Head CT/MRI scan: in patients with mental status changes to rule out possible intracranial pathology

 ## TREATMENT

ALERT
- Prompt treatment of presumptive or confirmed TTP is necessary due to the high mortality (90%).
- Complete response to treatment is defined by a platelet count $>150 \times 10^9$/L for 2 consecutive days, together with normal or normalizing LDH and clinical recovery (1).
- In the absence of another apparent cause, the dyad of MAHA and thrombocytopenia is sufficient to begin treatment for TTP while the workup proceeds (1):
  - PEX transfusion is the cornerstone of treatment of TTP and should begin immediately.
  - PEX replaces deficient or defective metalloprotease (ADAMTS13) and removes UL vWF and antimetalloprotease antibodies.
  - Optimal PEX duration is variable. Continue for 2 days after platelet count is $\geq$150,000 and then consider tapering.
  - Fresh frozen plasma: temporary until PEX can be initiated; reserve for those with active bleeding

MEDICATION
First Line
- Glucocorticoids has adjunctive benefit in some patients. British guidelines recommend its use for all patients.
  - Steroids may work by suppressing the autoantibodies inhibiting ADAMTS13 activity.
  - May be used in patients with severe ADAMTS13 deficiency, in the setting of exacerbation when PEX is stopped or in relapse after remission
  - Little benefit of steroids when used as monotherapy
  - Doses: prednisone 1 to 2 mg/kg/day and taper once in remission or methylprednisolone 1 g/day IV for 3 days
- Rituximab, an anti-CD20 antibody that deletes B cells, may reduce relapse when given in conjunction with PEX and steroids.
  - Dose: 375 mg/m^2 IV once weekly for 4 weeks

Second Line
The following medications are used in refractory cases:
- Rituximab
- Vincristine, cyclophosphamide, cyclosporine
- Intravenous immunoglobulin (IVIG)
- Bortezomib
- Caplacizumab, a monoclonal antibody that inhibits vWF-glycoprotein 1b interaction
- Jehovah's witness patients can be treated with steroids plus rituximab.
- Splenectomy in the acute phase

ISSUES FOR REFERRAL
- Hematology or blood bank for PEX
- Nephrology for dialysis; cardiology for heart block or ischemia; neurosurgery for hemorrhage

SURGERY/OTHER PROCEDURES
Splenectomy is reserved for severe, refractory cases (1).

ADMISSION, INPATIENT, AND NURSING CONSIDERATIONS
- ABCs, oxygen, IV access, telemetry
- Volume resuscitation if hypotensive/actively bleeding
- Packed RBCs can be transfused safely.
- Platelet transfusion may be used for the treatment of hemorrhage.
- Discharge on normalization and stabilization of neurologic symptoms, LDH, platelets, and renal function

 ## ONGOING CARE

FOLLOW-UP RECOMMENDATIONS
Maintenance therapy is not required. After PEX is discontinued, blood counts should be monitored for months. If results remain normal, testing interval can be lengthened.

PATIENT EDUCATION
- Self-monitor for signs of relapse (e.g., fever, headache, bruising)
- Prolonged periods of fatigue following the acute phase
- See National Heart, Lung, and Blood Institute Web site: http://www.nhlbi.nih.gov/health/health-topics/topics/ttp

PROGNOSIS
- Most recover fully from idiopathic TTP when treated promptly:
  - 30-day mortality is 10% in those who receive PEX.
  - 70% respond within 14 days; 90% respond within 28 days.
  - 80% survival in idiopathic TTP treated with PEX (1)
- Prior to widespread PEX treatment, TTP carried up to a 90% mortality rate.
- Initial LDH and platelet counts are not predictive of response to treatment.
- Final platelet count and LDH or the length or intensity of treatment does not predict relapse.
- Low levels of ADAMTS13 activity during remission are associated with higher risk of relapse (1).
- In patients with severe ADAMTS13 deficiency, the risk of relapse is estimated to be 41% at 7.5 years, with the greatest risk being in the 1st year.
- In patients with autoimmune TTP, there is a 40% relapse rate.

COMPLICATIONS
- Mild cognitive impairments in attention, concentration, and memory following $\geq$1 episode of TTP
- Complications of PEX include the following:
  - Central line infections and hemorrhage; citrate toxicity; hypersensitivity reactions to frequent plasma exposure; electrolyte abnormalities

REFERENCE
1. Joly BS, Coppo P, Veyradier A. Thrombotic thrombocytopenic purpura. *Blood*. 2017;129(21):2836–2846.

ADDITIONAL READING
Joly BS, Coppo P, Veyradier A. An update on pathogenesis and diagnosis of thrombotic thrombocytopenic purpura. *Expert Rev Hematol*. 2019;12(6):383–395.

CODES

ICD10
- M31.1 Thrombotic microangiopathy
- D69.42 Congenital and hereditary thrombocytopenia purpura
- D69.3 Immune thrombocytopenic purpura

CLINICAL PEARLS
- The diagnosis of TTP is made clinically; symptoms are nonspecific: nausea; vomiting; weakness; abdominal pain; fatigue; fever; and easy bruising, purpura, or petechiae.
- The historical pentad of fever, neurologic symptoms, renal dysfunction, MAHA, and thrombocytopenia is not present in most patients.
- The dyad of MAHA (schistocytes on peripheral smear) and severe thrombocytopenia ($<30,000$) is sufficient to initiate treatment with PEX.
- Do not wait for results of ADAMTS13 determination to initiate therapy.

THYROID MALIGNANT NEOPLASIA

Hannan Qureshi, MD • Yousef Ahmed, MD • Matthew E. Herberg, MD

 BASICS

DESCRIPTION

Thyroid malignant neoplasia is an uncontrolled pro-liferation of cells within the thyroid gland. There are several different types:

- Papillary thyroid carcinoma (PTC)
  - Differentiated tumor with papillary cells with finger-like projections
  - Most common variety, 75–80% of thyroid cancers
  - Peak incidence in the 3rd or 4th decade of life
  - Associated with radiation exposure
  - Metastasizes by lymphatic route (15–30% have palpable lymphadenopathy at time of diagnosis)
  - Many subtypes: conventional, follicular variant, oxyphilic, cribriform-morular, and more aggressive forms such as tall cell or diffuse sclerosing
- Follicular carcinoma
  - Differentiated tumor with spherical follicular cells
  - Second most common variety, 10–20% of thyroid tumors
  - Peak incidence in 5th decade of life
  - Metastasizes by the hematogenous route
  - Can be divided into invasive and minimally invasive forms based on morphology
- Hürthle cell carcinoma (variant of follicular with poorer prognosis)
  - Often considered subtype of FTC with overall poorer prognosis
  - Also known as oncocytic or oxyphilic carcinoma
  - 2–3% of thyroid malignancies
  - Usually in patients >60 years old
- Medullary thyroid carcinoma (MTC)
  - Neuroendocrine tumor arising from parafollicular C cells
  - 3–4% of all thyroid carcinoma
  - 25–35% are associated with multiple endocrine neoplasia (MEN) syndromes.
  - MTC associated with MEN2B occur in childhood, those with MEN2A occur in young adults, and those with familial non-MEN medullary thyroid cancer (FMTC) occur in middle age.
  - Calcitonin is a serologic marker.
  - *RET* proto-oncogene mutation is used for screen-ing; family members who carry the *RET* gene should consider early prophylactic thyroidectomy.
- Anaplastic carcinoma
  - Undifferentiated tumor arising de novo or from dedifferentiation of preexisting differentiated thyroid carcinoma
  - 1–3% of thyroid tumors
  - Most aggressive form of thyroid neoplasia
  - Almost uniformly fatal (median survival 2 to 6 months)
  - More common in elderly patients
- Poorly differentiated thyroid carcinoma (PDTC)
  - Intermediate between differentiated (follicular and papillary carcinomas) and undifferentiated (anaplastic) carcinomas
  - Aggressive tumor similar to anaplastic carcinoma but may have better treatment response
- Other: lymphoma, sarcoma, or metastatic (renal, breast, or lung)

- System(s) affected: endocrine/metabolic
- Synonym(s): well-differentiated, poorly differentiated, and undifferentiated thyroid carcinoma

Geriatric Considerations
Risk of malignancy (ROM) increases, and prognosis is worse >60 years old.

Pediatric Considerations
- Thyroid nodules are more frequently malignant (22–25% in children vs. 5–10% in adults).
- <2% of thyroid malignancies occur in children and adolescents.
- Increased tumor size (>4 cm), extrathyroidal extension, and multifocal disease are independent factors associated with nodal metastases in pediatric differentiated thyroid cancer and require further evaluation with FNA for suspicious nodes to consider neck dissection (1)[C].

EPIDEMIOLOGY
- Incidence: 14.5/100,000 per year in the United States
- Deaths: 0.5/100,000 per year in the United States
- In 2018, estimated 53,990 new cases and 2,060 deaths from thyroid cancer in the United States
- Predominant age: usually >40 years old
- Predominant sex: female > male (3:1) prevalence
- Lifetime risk of developing thyroid cancer is 1.2%.

ETIOLOGY AND PATHOPHYSIOLOGY
- No established etiologic factors of pathogenesis; most cases arise spontaneously.
- Radiation exposure likely has a role in the develop-ment of thyroid malignancies.

Genetics
Gene mutations that activate the MAPK pathway (e.g., *BRAF*) and PI3K-AKT pathway (e.g., *PTEN*) have been implicated.

RISK FACTORS
- Family history (first-degree relative)
- Radiation exposure: papillary carcinoma
- Iodine deficiency: follicular carcinoma
- MEN2: medullary carcinoma; autosomal dominant inheritance; *RET* proto-oncogene
- Previous history of subtotal thyroidectomy for malignancy: anaplastic carcinoma

GENERAL PREVENTION
- Physical exam in high-risk group
- Calcitonin stimulation screening in high-risk MEN patients
- Screening for *RET* proto-oncogene in groups at risk for MTC

COMMONLY ASSOCIATED CONDITIONS
- Papillary carcinoma: Hashimoto thyroiditis
- Medullary carcinoma: pheochromocytoma, hyper-parathyroidism, ganglioneuroma of the GI tract, neuromata of mucosal membranes

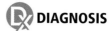 **DIAGNOSIS**

HISTORY
- Change in voice (dysphonia)
- Difficulty swallowing (dysphagia)
- Difficulty breathing (dyspnea)
- Stridor (in aggressive cancer)
- Growing neck mass
- Positive family history
- History of radiation exposure (environmental or radiation therapy for childhood cancer)

PHYSICAL EXAM
- Thyroid nodule/mass
- Fixation to surrounding tissues suggests malignancy.
- Cervical lymphadenopathy

DIFFERENTIAL DIAGNOSIS
- Multinodular goiter
- Thyroid adenoma
- Thyroglossal duct or dermoid cyst
- Thyroiditis
- Thyroid cyst
- Ectopic thyroid

DIAGNOSTIC TESTS & INTERPRETATION
Initial Tests (lab, imaging)
- Ultrasound (US): Nodule characteristics suggestive of malignancy include hypoechoic pattern, micro-calcifications, irregular margins, and shape taller than wide (2)[A].
- Thyroid-stimulating hormone (TSH): usually normal in the setting of malignancy but recommended for all nodule workup

Follow-Up Tests & Special Considerations
- CT and MRI neck: useful to evaluate large substernal masses, extent of invasion for fixed bulky tumors, if suspicion of MTC with neck disease or calcitonin >400 pg/mL, and to evaluate for recurrent disease
- Calcitonin levels: Measure in patients with FNA results or with personal or family history of MEN2 syndrome suggestive of MTC (consider IV pentagas-trin stimulation test to increase sensitivity).
- Thyroid scan: 12–15% of cold nodules are malig-nant; rate is higher in patients <40 years of age and those with microcalcifications on US. ^{18}F-FDG positron-emission tomographic scan can help if the cytology is indeterminant; also helpful with recurrent disease when patient has a negative ^{131}I scan and an elevated thyroglobulin (TG) level (3)[B]
- TG: not recommended in initial evaluation but used as postoperative tumor marker for recurrence

Diagnostic Procedures/Other
- Fine-needle aspiration biopsy (FNAB)
- Flexible fiberoptic laryngoscopy: if vocal cord paraly-sis is suspected and in high-risk disease

Test Interpretation
- FNAB: The 2017 Bethesda System for Reporting Thyroid Cytopathology classification of cytology
  - Nondiagnostic or unsatisfactory
  - Benign: 0–3% ROM

– Atypia of undetermined significance (AUS) or follicular lesion of undetermined significance (FLUS): 10–30% ROM
– Follicular neoplasm or suspicious for a follicular neoplasm: 25–40% ROM
– Suspicious for malignancy: 50–75% ROM
– Malignant: 97–99% ROM

- Papillary: psammoma bodies, anaplastic epithelial papillae
- Follicular: anaplastic epithelial cords with follicles
- Hürthle cell: large eosinophilic cells with granular cytoplasm
- Medullary: large amounts of amyloid stroma
- Anaplastic: small cell and giant cell undifferentiated tumors

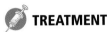 TREATMENT

GENERAL MEASURES
- Most cases of thyroid cancer are managed surgically and medically with a good prognosis (2)[A].
- Palliative support has a role in case of advanced thyroid malignancy (4)[C].
- Papillary and follicular: ^{131}I thyroid remnant ablation
- Medullary: Vandetanib and other tyrosine kinase inhibitors have been tried in patients with advanced disease (5)[B].
- Anaplastic: Doxorubicin and cisplatin have achieved partial remission in some patients.

MEDICATION
Postoperatively, will require thyroid hormone replacement after total thyroidectomy
- Thyroxine suppression therapy may reduce recurrence with goal to keep TSH <0.1 mU/L for high-risk patients, 0.1 to 0.5 mU/L for intermediate-risk patients, and 0.5 to 2.0 mU/L for low-risk patients (2)[A].
- Levothyroxine (T$_4$, Synthroid)
- Liothyronine (T$_3$, Cytomel)

ADDITIONAL THERAPIES
- External beam radiation or chemotherapy may be considered for radioactive iodine insensitive tumors, inoperable recurrence, and for palliative care.
- ^{131}I is used in high-risk patients with papillary and follicular tumors. The role is to ablate remnant thyroid tissue to improve specificity of future TG assays to monitor for recurrence.

SURGERY/OTHER PROCEDURES
- Papillary: total thyroidectomy with elective neck dissection for suspicious lymph nodes in central or lateral neck compartments or for large tumors (>4 cm in size). Lobectomy with isthmectomy can be considered if lesion <1 cm in low-risk patient (controversial).
- Follicular and Hürthle cell: similar management as papillary carcinoma
- Medullary: total thyroidectomy with central node dissection; unilateral or bilateral modified radical neck dissection if lateral nodes are suspicious
- Anaplastic: palliative care; no adequate treatment available and surgery is controversial. Consider tracheostomy (protect airway) and clinical trials utilizing chemotherapy/radiation.

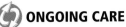 ONGOING CARE

FOLLOW-UP RECOMMENDATIONS
Patient Monitoring
- 10–30% of initially disease-free patients will develop recurrence and/or metastases. 80% recur in neck and 20% with distant metastases (lung).
- TSH, TG, and anti-TG antibodies at 6 months, 12 months, and then yearly after that for surveillance (6)[C].
- Periodic US to monitor for recurrence is recommended in intermediate- to high-risk patients and may also consider TSH-stimulated radioiodine whole body imaging in high-risk patients (6)[C].
- Medullary: Calcitonin level should be done yearly with pentagastrin stimulation.
- The thyroid scan and TG level should be done with the patient in the hypothyroid state induced by 6-week withdrawal of levothyroxine or 2- to 3-week withdrawal of liothyronine.

DIET
Low-iodine diet recommended in patients undergoing radioactive iodine therapy following surgery for thyroid cancer

PATIENT EDUCATION
- National Cancer Institute: https://www.cancer.gov/types/thyroid/patient/thyroid-treatment-pdq
- American Thyroid Association: https://www.thyroid.org/thyroid-information/
- National Comprehensive Cancer Network: https://www.nccn.org/professionals/physician_gls/pdf/thyroid.pdf

PROGNOSIS
- 5-year survival of thyroid cancer is 98.1%.
- Adverse factors: age >45 years, primary tumor >4 cm, extrathyroid extension, distant metastases
- Low risk: no extrathyroidal invasion, all macroscopic tumor resected, no local or distant metastases, no vascular invasion, and no aggressive tumor histology
- Intermediate risk: microscopic extrathyroidal invasion, cervical lymph node metastases on ^{131}I update outside of thyroid bed on first whole body after remnant ablation
- High risk: macroscopic extrathyroidal tumor invasion, incomplete tumor resection, distant metastases
- Papillary carcinoma: 10-year overall survival is 93%; 30-year cancer-related death rate of 6%
- Follicular carcinoma: 10-year overall survival is 85%; histologically, microinvasive tumors parallel papillary tumor results, whereas grossly invasive tumors do far worse; 30-year cancer-related death rate of 15%
- Hürthle cell carcinoma: 93% 5-year survival rate and 83% survival rate overall; grossly invasive tumor survival <25%
- Medullary carcinoma: negative nodes, 90% 5-year survival rate and 85% 10-year survival rate; with positive nodes, 65% 5-year survival rate and 40% 10-year survival rate. Prognosis worse for MEN2B compared to MEN2A. Overall, 10-year survival is 75%.
- Anaplastic carcinoma: survival unexpected. Long-term survivors should have original pathology reexamined.

COMPLICATIONS
- Hoarseness either from tumor invasion or iatrogenic injury to recurrent laryngeal nerve
- Hypocalcemia/hypoparathyroidism from devascularization of parathyroid glands during surgery (usually transient)

REFERENCES

1. Francis GL, Waguespack SG, Bauer AJ, et al; for American Thyroid Association Guidelines Task Force. Management guidelines for children with thyroid nodules and differentiated thyroid cancer. *Thyroid*. 2015;25(7):716–759.
2. Haugen BR, Alexander EK, Bible KC, et al. 2015 American Thyroid Association management guidelines for adult patients with thyroid nodules and differentiated thyroid cancer: the American Thyroid Association Guidelines Task Force on thyroid nodules and differentiated thyroid cancer. *Thyroid*. 2016;26(1):1–133.
3. de Koster EJ, de Geus-Oei LF, Dekkers OM, et al. Diagnostic utility of molecular and imaging biomarkers in cytological indeterminate thyroid nodules. *Endocr Rev*. 2018;39(2):154–191.
4. Goyal A, Gupta R, Mehmood S, et al. Palliative and end of life care issues of carcinoma thyroid patient. *Indian J Palliat Care*. 2012;18(2):134–137.
5. Wells SA Jr, Robinson BG, Gagel RF, et al. Vandetanib in patients with locally advanced or metastatic medullary thyroid cancer: a randomized, double-blind phase III trial. *J Clin Oncol*. 2012;30(2):134–141.
6. National Comprehensive Cancer Network. Thyroid carcinoma (Version 1.2018). https://www.nccn.org/professionals/physician_gls/pdf/thyroid.pdf. Accessed October 15, 2018.

SEE ALSO

Multiple Endocrine Neoplasia (MEN) Syndromes

CODES

ICD10
C73 Malignant neoplasm of thyroid gland

CLINICAL PEARLS
- Standard workup for a patient suspected of having a thyroid cancer is a physical exam, TSH level, neck US, and FNA.
- TG levels can be elevated in several thyroid disorders. Its usefulness comes once the diagnosis of cancer has been made. It serves as a better marker for recurrent disease.
- FNA results will be benign, malignant, indeterminate, or nondiagnostic. It is very helpful in guiding the initial surgical approach.

T

THYROIDITIS

Allegra Tenkman, MD • Tiffany Chen, DO

 BASICS

DESCRIPTION
Painful or painless inflammatory dysfunction of the thyroid gland

- Painful thyroiditis
  - Subacute granulomatous thyroiditis (nonsuppurative thyroiditis, de Quervain thyroiditis, giant cell thyroiditis): self-limited; viral URI prodrome, symptoms and signs of thyroid dysfunction (variable)
  - Infectious/suppurative thyroiditis is most commonly associated with *Streptococcus pyogenes*, *Staphylococcus aureus*, and *Streptococcus pneumoniae* but can be due to fungal, mycobacterial, or parasitic infections of the thyroid.
- Radiation-induced thyroiditis: from radioactive iodine therapy (1%) or external irradiation
- Painless thyroiditis
  - Hashimoto (autoimmune) thyroiditis (chronic lymphocytic thyroiditis): most common etiology of chronic hypothyroidism; 90% of patients with high-serum antithyroid peroxidase (TPO) antibodies
  - Postpartum thyroiditis: thyrotoxicosis followed by hypothyroidism in the 1st year postpartum or after spontaneous/induced abortion in women who were without clinically evident thyroid disease before pregnancy
  - Painless (silent) thyroiditis (subacute lymphocytic thyroiditis): mild hyperthyroidism, small painless goiter, and no Graves ophthalmopathy/pretibial myxedema
  - Riedel (fibrous) thyroiditis: rare inflammatory process involving the thyroid and surrounding cervical tissues; associated with various forms of systemic fibrosis; presents as a firm mass in the thyroid commonly associated with compressive symptoms (dyspnea, dysphagia, hoarseness, and aphonia) caused by local infiltration of the advancing fibrotic process with hypocalcemia and hypothyroidism
  - Drug-induced thyroiditis: interferon-α, interleukin-2, amiodarone, kinase inhibitors, or lithium

EPIDEMIOLOGY
- Subacute granulomatous thyroiditis: most common cause of thyroid pain; peaks during summer; incidence: 3/100,000/year; female > male (4:1); peak age: 40 to 50 years
- Hashimoto thyroiditis: peak onset 30 to 50 years; can occur in children; female > male (7:1)
- Postpartum thyroiditis: occurs within 12 months of pregnancy in 1–18% of pregnancies
- Painless (silent) thyroiditis: accounts for 1–5% of cases; female > male (4:1) with peak age 30 to 40 years; common in areas of iodine sufficiency
- Riedel thyroiditis: female > male (4:1); highest prevalence age 30 to 60 years. Rare with estimated incidence of 1.06 cases per 100,000 patients

ETIOLOGY AND PATHOPHYSIOLOGY
- Subacute granulomatous thyroiditis: probably viral
- Hashimoto disease: Antithyroid antibodies may be produced in response to an environmental antigen and cross-react with thyroid proteins (molecular mimicry). Precipitating factors include infection, stress, sex steroids, pregnancy, iodine intake, and radiation exposure.
- Postpartum thyroiditis: autoimmunity-induced discharge of preformed hormone from the thyroid
- Painless (silent) thyroiditis: autoimmune
- Riedel (fibrous) thyroiditis: rare inflammatory process involving the thyroid and surrounding cervical tissues; associated with various forms of systemic fibrosis

Genetics
Autoimmune thyroiditis is associated with the CT60 polymorphism of cytotoxic T-cell lymphocyte–associated antigen 4; also associated with HLA-DR4, HLA-DR5, and HLA-DR6 in whites

RISK FACTORS
- Subacute granulomatous thyroiditis: recent viral respiratory infection or HLA-B35
- Hashimoto disease: family/personal history of thyroid/autoimmune disease, high iodine intake, cigarette smoking, selenium deficiency

GENERAL PREVENTION
Insufficient evidence to justify the use of vitamin D or selenium supplementation (1),(2)

DIAGNOSIS

HISTORY
- Hypothyroid symptoms (e.g., constipation, heavy menstrual bleeding, fatigue, weakness, dry skin, hair loss, cold intolerance)
- Hyperthyroid symptoms (e.g., irritability, heat intolerance, increased sweating, palpitations, loose stools, disturbed sleep, and lid retraction)
- Subacute granulomatous thyroiditis: sudden/gradual onset, with preceding upper respiratory infection/viral illness (fever, fatigue, malaise, anorexia, and myalgia are common); pain may be limited to thyroid region or radiate to upper neck, jaw, throat, or ears.
- Classic triphasic course (thyrotoxic, hypothyroid, recovery) but variable in the following: subacute, silent, and postpartum thyroiditis

PHYSICAL EXAM
- Hashimoto disease: 90% have a symmetric, diffusely enlarged, painless thyroid gland, with a firm, pebbly texture; 10% have atrophy.
- Postpartum thyroiditis: painless, small, nontender, firm goiter (2 to 6 months after delivery)
- Reidel thyroiditis: rock-hard, wood-like, fixed, painless goiter, often accompanied by symptoms of esophageal/tracheal compression (stridor, dyspnea, a suffocating feeling, dysphagia, and hoarseness).

Should be considered when restrictive and infiltrative symptoms are out of proportion of the size of the mass on exam
- Signs of hypothyroid: delayed relaxation phase of deep tendon reflexes, nonpitting edema, dry skin, alopecia, bradycardia
- Signs of hyperthyroid: moist palms, hyperreflexia, tachycardia/atrial fibrillation

DIFFERENTIAL DIAGNOSIS
Simple goiter; iodine-deficient/lithium-induced goiter; Graves disease; lymphoma; oropharynx and trachea infections; thyroid cancer; amiodarone; contrast dye; amyloid

DIAGNOSTIC TESTS & INTERPRETATION
- Subacute granulomatous (de Quervain) thyroiditis
  - In the thyrotoxic phase, decreased TSH; elevated T_4, ESR, CRP, WBC count; mild anemia
  - 25% of patients have low concentrations of antithyroid antibodies.
  - ESR normalizes during hypothyroid phase.
  - Consider ultrasound to rule out thyroid cancer (3)[A].
- Suppurative (acute) thyroiditis (thyroid abscess)
  - Generally, patients are euthyroid. Occasionally presents with destructive thyrotoxicosis
  - US or CT is usually diagnostic. Fine needle aspiration can confirm diagnosis (4)[C].
- Hashimoto thyroiditis
  - Anti-TPO antibodies present in 95% of cases
  - Antithyroglobulin antibodies present in 60–80%
  - Ultrasonography may demonstrate decreased echogenicity and hypoechoic nodules with an echogenic rim (5)[C].
- Postpartum thyroiditis
  - Thyroid antibodies (TPOAb, TgAb) present
    - If Ab positive in the 1st trimester, higher risk of developing postpartum thyroiditis
    - Higher Ab titers, higher risk of postpartum thyroiditis
  - Must distinguish from thyrotoxicosis caused by Graves disease (which has a positive TSH receptor antibody), high radioiodine uptake, and specific physical findings (e.g., goiter, ophthalmopathy)
  - After the thyrotoxic phase, obtain a TSH level in 4 to 8 weeks (or if the patient develops new symptoms) to screen for the hypothyroid phase.
  - If patient has a history of postpartum thyroiditis, screen for permanent hypothyroidism with an annual TSH level (6)[C].
- Painless (silent) thyroiditis
  - 5–20% of patients undergo a thyrotoxic phase that lasts 3 to 4 months.
  - Thyroid function normalizes within 12 months.
  - ~50% of patients have anti-TPO antibodies.
  - Absence of TSH receptor antibodies distinguishes from Grave's disease (4)[C].
- Reidel thyroiditis
  - Thyroglobulin and TPO antibody titers are elevated (likely due to simultaneous Hashimoto disease).
  - 72% of individuals have elevated CRP and 97% have elevated ESR.

– Parathyroid involvement can cause hypocalcemia.
– Histology confirms diagnosis and reveals a fibroinflammatory process.
• Drug-induced thyroiditis
– Thyroid function test results vary and depend on the offending medication. Thyrotoxicosis is common. Lithium associated with hypothyroidism (4)[C].

Initial Tests (lab, imaging)
TSH, free T_4, T_3; antithyroid antibodies

Follow-Up Tests & Special Considerations
• US: shows variable heterogeneous texture, hypoechogenic in subacute, painless (silent), and postpartum thyroiditis
• Thyroid RAIU scan: decreased in all forms of thyroiditis but not helpful in establishing diagnosis of Hashimoto disease; high RAIU in hashitoxicosis, Graves disease
• Random urine iodine measurement may be helpful to distinguish from other causes of low RAIU.
– Urine iodine <500 μg/L (subacute granulomatous thyroiditis)
– Urine iodine >1,000 μg/L (in patients with exposure to excess exogenous iodine/radiocontrast material)

Diagnostic Procedures/Other
• Hashimoto with a dominant nodule should have FNA to rule out thyroid carcinoma.
• Open biopsy is necessary for a definitive diagnosis of Reidel thyroiditis.

Test Interpretation
• Subacute granulomatous thyroiditis: giant cells, mononuclear cell (granulomatous) infiltrate
• Hashimoto disease: lymphocytic infiltration with formation of Askanazy (Hürthle) cells, oxyphilic changes in follicular cells, fibrosis, thyroid atrophy
• Postpartum thyroiditis: lymphocytic infiltration, occasional germinal centers, disruption and collapse of thyroid follicles
• Painless (silent) thyroiditis: lymphocytic infiltration, but without fibrosis, Askanazy cells, and extensive lymphoid follicle formation

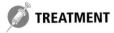 ## TREATMENT

GENERAL MEASURES
• If thyrotoxic and symptomatic: propylthiouracil and propranolol, except not used in postpartum thyroiditis or painless thyroiditis
• An elevated TSH level in a woman who is pregnant or attempting to become pregnant is an indication for thyroid replacement.

MEDICATION
• Subacute granulomatous thyroiditis
– β-blockers and NSAIDs may be used to treat mild symptomatic cases.
– Prednisone 40 mg qDay × 1 to 2 weeks, followed by 2- to 4-week taper in severe cases

– Levothyroxine may be used in the hypothyroid phase. Discontinue after 3 to 6 months with normalization of thyroid function (4)[C].
• Suppurative (acute) thyroiditis (thyroid abscess)
– Systemic antibiotics
– Abscess drainage or removal
– Excision or occlusion of the pyriform sinus (4)[C]
• Hashimoto thyroiditis
– Levothyroxine 1.6 to 1.8 μg/kg
• Postpartum thyroiditis
– Treatment is guided by stage.
– Metoprolol and propranolol for lactating women in the thyrotoxic state. Antithyroid medications are not recommended.
– If lactating or trying to conceive, treat symptomatic hypothyroidism.
– Levothyroxine may be tapered starting at 12 months postpartum. Monitor TSH every 6 to 8 weeks. Avoid tapering if a woman is trying to conceive or is pregnant (6)[C].
• Painless (silent) thyroiditis
– If symptomatic during hyperthyroid state, treat with β-blocker.
– Antithyroid medications are unnecessary.
– For severe cases, corticosteroids may reduce the severity and length of the hyperthyroid state (4)[C].
• Reidel thyroiditis (no management consensus)
– Medical therapy is first line in absence of obstructive symptoms. Neither meds are validated by RCTs due to rarity of the condition. Glucocorticoids is first line, and tamoxifen is second line.
– Treat hypothyroidism with levothyroxine and hypoparathyroidism with calcium and calcitriol.
– Debulking surgery if obstruction present
• Drug-induced thyroiditis
– Discontinue offending drug.

 ## ONGOING CARE

FOLLOW-UP RECOMMENDATIONS
Patient Monitoring
• Subacute granulomatous thyroiditis: Repeat thyroid function tests every 3 to 6 weeks until euthyroid and then every 6 to 12 months.
• Hashimoto disease: Repeat thyroid function tests every 3 to 12 months.
• Postpartum thyroiditis: Check TSH annually.
• Reidel thyroiditis: Consider CT if extrathyroidal disease is suspected.
• Check thyroid function before and after 3 months of starting amiodarone. Then monitor every 3 to 6 months.

Pregnancy Considerations
[131]I is contraindicated in breastfeeding women.

PROGNOSIS
• Subacute granulomatous thyroiditis: Most patients are euthyroid at 12 months. 5–15% have persistent hypothyroidism.
• Hashimoto disease: persistent goiter; eventual thyroid failure
• Postpartum thyroiditis: Thyroid function normalizes in 12 months. 10–20% of patients have persistent hypothyroidism.
• Painless (silent) thyroiditis: 5–20% of patients undergo a thyrotoxic phase that lasts 3 to 4 months.
• Reidel thyroiditis: 90% have improvement or resolution of symptoms within 12 months. It is unclear at this time what factors contribute to poor prognosis due to the rarity of the condition.

REFERENCES

1. Winther KH, Wichman JE, Bonnema SJ, et al. Insufficient documentation for clinical efficacy of selenium supplementation in chronic autoimmune thyroiditis, based on a systematic review and meta-analysis. *Endocrine.* 2017;55(2):376–385.
2. Behera KK, Saharia GK, Hota D, et al. Effect of vitamin D supplementation on thyroid autoimmunity among subjects of autoimmune thyroid disease in a coastal province of India: a randomized open-label trial. *Niger Med J.* 2020;61(5):237–240.
3. Stasiak M, Michalak R, Lewinski A. Thyroid primary and metastatic malignant tumours of poor prognosis may mimic subacute thyroiditis—time to change the diagnostic criteria: case reports and a review of the literature. *BMC Endocr Disord.* 2019;19(1):86.
4. Ross DS, Burch HB, Cooper DS, et al. 2016 American Thyroid Association guidelines for diagnosis and management of hyperthyroidism and other causes of thyrotoxicosis. *Thyroid.* 2016;26(10):1343–1421.
5. Massimo R, Angeletti D, Fiore M, et al. Hashimoto's thyroiditis: an update on pathogenic mechanisms, diagnostic protocols, therapeutic strategies, and potential malignant transformation. *Autoimmun Rev.* 2020;19(10):102649.
6. Alexander E, Pearce E, Brent G, et al. 2017 guidelines of the American Thyroid Association for the diagnosis and management of thyroid disease during pregnancy and the postpartum. *Thyroid.* 2017;27(3):315–389.

 ## CODES

ICD10
• E06.5 Other chronic thyroiditis
• E06.0 Acute thyroiditis
• E06 Thyroiditis

CLINICAL PEARLS

Hashimoto thyroiditis is the most common etiology of chronic hypothyroidism.

T

TINEA (CAPITIS, CORPORIS, CRURIS)

Elisabeth L. Backer, MD

BASICS

DESCRIPTION
- Superficial fungal infections of the skin/scalp; various forms of dermatophytosis; the names relate to the particular area affected (1).
  - Tinea cruris: infection of crural fold and gluteal cleft
  - Tinea corporis: infection involving the face, trunk, and/or extremities; often presents with ring-shaped lesions, hence the misnomer *ringworm*
  - Tinea capitis: infection of the scalp and hair; affected areas of the scalp can show characteristic black dots resulting from broken hairs.
- Dermatophytes have the ability to subsist on protein, namely keratin.
- They cause disease in keratin-rich structures such as skin, nails, and hair.
- Infections result from contact with infected persons/animals.
  - Zoophilic infections are acquired from animals.
  - Anthropophilic infections are acquired from personal contact (e.g., wrestling) or fomites.
  - Geophile infections are acquired from the soil.
- System(s) affected: skin, exocrine
- Synonym(s): jock itch; ringworm

EPIDEMIOLOGY
Incidence
- Tinea cruris
  - Predominant age: any age; rare in children
  - Predominant sex: male > female
- Tinea corporis
  - Predominant age: all ages
  - Predominant sex: male = female
- Tinea capitis
  - Predominant age: 3 to 9 years; almost always occurs in young children
  - Predominant sex: male = female

Prevalence
Common worldwide

Pediatric Considerations
- Tinea cruris is rare prior to puberty.
- Tinea capitis is common in young children.

Geriatric Considerations
Tinea cruris is more common in the geriatric population due to an increase in risk factors.

Pregnancy Considerations
Tinea cruris and capitis are rare in pregnancy.

ETIOLOGY AND PATHOPHYSIOLOGY
Superficial fungal infection of skin/scalp
- Tinea cruris: Source of infection is usually the patient's own tinea pedis, with agent being transferred from the foot to the groin via the underwear when dressing; most common causative dermatophyte is *Trichophyton rubrum*; rare cases caused by *Epidermophyton floccosum* and *Trichophyton mentagrophytes*
- Tinea corporis: most commonly caused by *T. rubrum*; *Trichophyton tonsurans* most often found in patients with tinea gladiatorum
- Tinea capitis: *T. tonsurans* found in 90% and *Microsporum* sp. in 10% of patients

Genetics
Evidence suggests a genetic susceptibility in certain individuals.

RISK FACTORS
- Warm climates; summer months and/or copious sweating; wearing wet clothing/multiple layers (tinea cruris)
- Daycare centers/schools/confined quarters (tinea corporis and capitis)
- Depression of cell-mediated immune response (e.g., individuals with atopy or AIDS)
- Obesity (tinea cruris and corporis)
- Direct contact with an active lesion on a human, an animal, or rarely, from soil; working with animals (tinea corporis)

GENERAL PREVENTION
- Avoidance of risk factors, such as contact with suspicious lesions
- Fluconazole or itraconazole may be useful in wrestlers to prevent outbreaks during competitive season.

COMMONLY ASSOCIATED CONDITIONS
Tinea pedis, tinea barbae, tinea manus

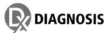

DIAGNOSIS

HISTORY
- Lesions range from asymptomatic to pruritic.
- In tinea cruris, acute inflammation may result from wearing occlusive clothing; chronic scratching may result in an eczematous appearance.
- Previous application of topical steroids, especially in tinea cruris and corporis, may alter the overall appearance causing a more extensive eruption with irregular borders and erythematous papules. This modified form is called *tinea incognito*.

PHYSICAL EXAM
- Tinea cruris: well-marginated, erythematous, half-moon–shaped plaques in crural folds that spread to medial thighs; advancing border is well defined, often with fine scaling and sometimes vesicular eruptions. Lesions are usually bilateral and do not include scrotum/penis (unlike with *Candida* infections) but may migrate to perineum, perianal area, and gluteal cleft and onto the buttocks in chronic/progressive cases. The area may be hyperpigmented on resolution.
- Tinea corporis: scaling, round or oval pruritic plaques characterized by a sharply defined annular pattern with peripheral activity and central clearing (ring-shaped lesions); papules and occasionally pustules/vesicles present at border and, less commonly, in center
- Tinea capitis: commonly begins with round patches of scale (alopecia less common). In its later stages, the infection frequently takes on patterns of chronic scaling with either little/marked inflammation or alopecia. Less often, patients will present with multiple patches of alopecia and the characteristic black-dot appearance of broken hairs. Extreme inflammation results in kerion formation (exudative, pustular nodulation).

DIFFERENTIAL DIAGNOSIS
- Tinea cruris
  - Intertrigo: inflammatory process of moist-opposed skin folds, often including infection with bacteria, yeast, and fungi; painful longitudinal fissures may occur in skin folds.
  - Erythrasma: diffuse brown, scaly, noninflammatory plaque with irregular borders, often involving groin; caused by bacterial infection with *Corynebacterium minutissimum*; fluoresces coral red with Wood lamp
  - Seborrheic dermatitis of groin
  - Psoriasis of groin ("inverse psoriasis")
  - Candidiasis of groin (typically involves the scrotum)
  - Acanthosis nigricans
- Tinea capitis
  - Psoriasis
  - Seborrheic dermatitis
  - Pyoderma
  - Alopecia areata and trichotillomania
  - Aplasia cutis congenital
- Tinea corporis
  - Pityriasis rosea
  - Eczema (nummular)
  - Contact dermatitis
  - Syphilis
  - Psoriasis
  - Seborrheic dermatitis
  - Subacute systemic lupus erythematosus (SLE)
  - Erythema annulare centrifugum
  - Erythema multiforme; erythema migrans
  - Impetigo circinatum
  - Granuloma annulare

DIAGNOSTIC TESTS & INTERPRETATION
Wood lamp exam reveals no fluorescence in most cases (*Trichophyton* sp.); 10% of infections, those caused by *T. rubrum*, will fluoresce with a green light.

Initial Tests (lab, imaging)
- Potassium hydroxide (KOH) preparation of skin scrapings from dermatophyte leading border shows characteristic translucent, branching, rod-shaped hyphae.
- Arthrospores can be visualized within hair shafts. Spores and/or hyphae may be seen on KOH exam.

Follow-Up Tests & Special Considerations
- Reevaluate to assess response, especially in resistant/extensive cases.
- Fungal culture using Sabouraud dextrose agar/dermatophyte test medium

Test Interpretation
- Skin scrapings show fungal hyphae in epidermis; best yield from scrapings from active border
- Arthrospores found in hair shafts; spores and/or hyphae seen on KOH exam

TREATMENT

GENERAL MEASURES
- Careful hand washing and personal hygiene; laundering of towels/clothing of affected individual; no sharing of towels/clothes/headgear/pillows
- Evaluate other family members, close contacts, or household pets (especially kittens and puppies).
- Use of prophylactic antifungal shampoo by all household members for 2 to 4 weeks in cases of tinea capitis
- Avoid predisposing conditions such as hot baths and tight-fitting clothing (boxer shorts are better than briefs).
- Keep area as dry as possible (talcum/powders may be beneficial).
- Itching can be alleviated by OTC preparations such as Sarna or Prax.
- Topical steroid preparations should be avoided, unless absolutely needed to control itching and only after definitive diagnosis and initiation of antifungal treatment.
- Nystatin should be avoided in tinea infections but is indicated for cutaneous candidal infections.
- Avoid contact sports (e.g., wrestling) temporarily while starting treatment.

MEDICATION
First Line
- Tinea cruris/corporis (2),(3)
  - Topical azole antifungal compounds
    - Terbinafine 1% (Lamisil): OTC inexpensive and effective compound; can be applied once or BID for 1 to 3 weeks
    - Econazole 1% (Spectazole), ketoconazole (Nizoral): usually applied BID for 2 to 3 weeks
    - Butenafine 1% (Mentax): applied once daily for 2 weeks; also very effective. To prevent relapse, use for 1 week after resolution.
- Tinea capitis (4)[A]
  - PO griseofulvin for *Trichophyton* and *Microsporum* sp.; microsized preparation available; dosage 10 to 20 mg/kg/day (max 1,000 mg); taken BID or as a single dose daily for 6 to 12 weeks
  - PO terbinafine can be used for *Trichophyton* sp. at 62.5 mg/day in patients weighing 10 to 20 kg; 125 mg/day if weight 20 to 40 kg; 250 mg/day if weight >40 kg; use for 4 to 6 weeks.
  - PO itraconazole can be used for *Microsporum* sp. and matches griseofulvin efficacy while being better tolerated; dosage of 3 to 5 mg/kg/day, but most studies have used 100 mg/day for 6 weeks in children >2 years of age

Second Line
Tinea cruris/corporis
- Oral antifungal agents are effective but not indicated in uncomplicated tinea cruris/corporis cases. They can be used for resistant and extensive infections or if the patient is immunocompromised. If topical therapy fails, consider possible oral therapy. Griseofulvin can be given 500 mg/day for 1 to 2 weeks.
- The following oral regimens have been reported in medical literature as being effective but currently are not specifically approved by FDA for tinea cruris:
  - PO terbinafine (Lamisil): 250 mg/day for 1 week
  - PO itraconazole (Sporanox): 100 mg BID once and repeated 1 week later
  - PO fluconazole (Diflucan): 150 mg once per week for 4 weeks
- Topical terbinafine 1% solution has been studied recently and appears effective as a once-daily application for 1 week.
- Oral antifungals have many interactions including warfarin, OCPs, and alcohol; advise checking for drug interactions prior to use; contraindicated in pregnancy. Monitor for liver toxicity when using oral antifungals.

ISSUES FOR REFERRAL
Refer if disease is nonresponsive/resistant, especially in immunocompromised host.

ADDITIONAL THERAPIES
Treatment of secondary bacterial infections

 ONGOING CARE

FOLLOW-UP RECOMMENDATIONS
Reevaluate response to treatment.

Patient Monitoring
Liver function testing prior to therapy and at regular intervals during course of therapy for patients requiring oral terbinafine, fluconazole, itraconazole, and griseofulvin

PATIENT EDUCATION
Explain the causative agents, predisposing factors, and prevention measures.

PROGNOSIS
- Excellent prognosis for cure with therapy in tinea cruris and corporis
- In tinea capitis, lesions will heal spontaneously in 6 months without treatment, but scarring is more likely.

COMPLICATIONS
- Secondary bacterial infection
- Generalized, invasive dermatophyte infection
- Secondary eruptions called dermatophytid reactions (which occur in association with primary/inflammatory skin disorders) may occur at distant sites.

REFERENCES
1. Ameen M. Epidemiology of superficial fungal infections. *Clin Dermatol*. 2010;28(2):197–201.
2. van Zuuren EJ, Fedorowicz Z, El-Gohary M. Evidence-based topical treatments for tinea cruris and tinea corporis: a summary of a Cochrane systematic review. *Br J Dermatol*. 2015;172(3):616–641.
3. El-Gohary M, van Zuuren EJ, Fedorowicz Z, et al. Topical antifungal treatments for tinea cruris and tinea corporis. *Cochrane Database Syst Rev*. 2014;(8):CD009992.
4. Gupta AK, Drummond-Main C. Meta-analysis of randomized, controlled trials comparing particular doses of griseofulvin and terbinafine for the treatment of tinea capitis. *Pediatr Dermatol*. 2013;30(1):1–6.

ADDITIONAL READING
- Bell-Syer SE, Khan SM, Torgerson DJ. Oral treatments for fungal infections of the skin of the foot. *Cochrane Database Syst Rev*. 2012;(10):CD003584.
- González U, Seaton T, Bergus G, et al. Systemic antifungal therapy for tinea capitis in children. *Cochrane Database Syst Rev*. 2007;(4):CD004685.
- Hawkins DM, Smidt AC. Superficial fungal infections in children. *Pediatr Clin North Am*. 2014;61(2):443–455.
- Mirmirani P, Tucker LY. Epidemiologic trends in pediatric tinea capitis: a population-based study from Kaiser Permanente Northern California. *J Am Acad Dermatol*. 2013;69(6):916–921.
- Seebacher C, Bouchara JP, Mignon B. Updates on the epidemiology of dermatophyte infections. *Mycopathologia*. 2008;166(5–6):335–352.
- Tey HL, Tan AS, Chan YC. Meta-analysis of randomized, controlled trials comparing griseofulvin and terbinafine in the treatment of tinea capitis. *J Am Acad Dermatol*. 2011;64(4):663–670.

 CODES

ICD10
- B35.0 Tinea barbae and tinea capitis
- B35.4 Tinea corporis
- B35.6 Tinea cruris

CLINICAL PEARLS
- Tinea corporis is characterized by scaly plaque, with peripheral activity and central clearing.
- Tinea cruris is characterized by erythematous plaque in crural folds usually sparing the scrotum. Treatment of concomitant tinea pedis is advised.
- Tinea capitis is a fungal infection of the scalp affecting hair growth. Topical therapy is ineffective for this infection.

TINEA PEDIS

Roland W. Newman II, DO • Bonnie A. Buechel, MD, MS

BASICS

DESCRIPTION
- Superficial infection of the feet caused by dermatophytes
- Most common dermatophyte infection encountered in clinical practice; contagious
- Often accompanied by tinea manuum, tinea unguium, and tinea cruris
- Clinical forms: interdigital (most common), hyperkeratotic (moccasin type), vesiculobullous (inflammatory), and rarely ulcerative
- System(s) affected: skin/exocrine
- Synonym(s): athlete's foot, foot ringworm

EPIDEMIOLOGY
- Predominant age: 20 to 50 years, although can occur at any age (1)
- Predominant gender: male > female

Prevalence
4–10% of population

Pediatric Considerations
Rare in younger children; common in adolescents

Geriatric Considerations
Elderly are more susceptible to outbreaks because of immunocompromised and impaired perfusion of distal extremities.

ETIOLOGY AND PATHOPHYSIOLOGY
Superficial infection caused by dermatophytes that release enzymes called keratinases to invade and thrive only in nonviable keratinized tissue
- *Trichophyton interdigitale* (previously *Trichophyton mentagrophytes*) (acute)
- *Trichophyton rubrum* (chronic): most common
- *Trichophyton tonsurans*
- *Epidermophyton floccosum*

Genetics
No known genetic pattern

RISK FACTORS
- Hot, humid weather
- Sweating
- Occlusive/tight-fitting footwear
- Immunosuppression
- Prolonged application of topical steroids

GENERAL PREVENTION
- Good personal hygiene

- Wearing rubber or wooden sandals in community showers, bathing places, locker rooms
- Careful drying between toes after showering or bathing; blow-drying feet with hair dryer may be more effective than drying with towel.
- Changing socks and shoes frequently
- Applying drying or dusting powder
- Applying topical antiperspirants
- Putting on socks before underwear to prevent infection from spreading to groin

COMMONLY ASSOCIATED CONDITIONS
- Hyperhidrosis
- Onychomycosis
- Tinea manuum/unguium/cruris/corporis

DIAGNOSIS

HISTORY
- Itchy, scaly rash on foot, usually between toes; may progress to fissuring/maceration in toe web spaces
- May be associated with onychomycosis and other tinea infections
- May be complicated by secondary bacterial infections

PHYSICAL EXAM
- Acute form: self-limited, intermittent, recurrent; scaling, thickening, and fissuring of sole and heel; silvery white scaling or fissuring of toe webs; or pruritic vesicular/bullous lesions between toes or on soles
- Chronic form: most common; slowly progressive, pruritic erythematous erosion/scales between toes, in digital interspaces; extension onto soles, sides/dorsum of feet (moccasin distribution); if untreated, may persist indefinitely
- Other features: strong odor, hyperkeratosis, maceration, ulceration
- Tinea pedis may occur unilaterally or bilaterally.
- Secondary presumably immune-mediated eruptions called dermatophytid reactions may occur at distant sites.

DIFFERENTIAL DIAGNOSIS
- Interdigital type: erythrasma, impetigo, pitted keratolysis, candidal intertrigo
- Moccasin type: psoriasis vulgaris, eczematous dermatitis, pitted keratolysis
- Inflammatory/bullous type: impetigo, allergic contact dermatitis, dyshidrotic eczema (negative potassium hydroxide examination of scrapings), bullous disease

DIAGNOSTIC TESTS & INTERPRETATION
Wood lamp exam will not fluoresce unless complicated by another fungus, which is uncommon: *Malassezia furfur* (yellow to white), *Corynebacterium* (red), or *Microsporum* (blue green).

Initial Tests (lab, imaging)
Testing is not needed in typical presentation.
- Direct microscopic exam (potassium hydroxide) of scrapings of the lesions
- Culture (Sabouraud medium)

Test Interpretation
- Potassium hydroxide preparation: septate and branched mycelia
- Culture: dermatophyte

TREATMENT

Treatment is generally with topical antifungal medications for up to 4 weeks and is more effective than placebo.
- Acute treatment
  - Aluminum acetate soak (Burow solution; Domeboro, 1 pack to 1 quart warm water) to decrease itching and acute eczematous reaction
  - Antifungal cream of choice BID after soaks (allylamines slightly more effective than azoles)
- Chronic treatment
  - Antifungal creams BID, continuing for 3 days after the rash is resolved: terbinafine 1% (possibly most effective topical), clotrimazole 1%, econazole 1%, ketoconazole 2%, tolnaftate 1%, etc. (2)[A]
  - May try systemic antifungal therapy (see below); consider if concomitant onychomycosis or after failed topical treatment.

GENERAL MEASURES
- Soak with aluminum chloride 30% or aluminum acetate for 20 minutes BID.
- Perform careful removal of dead/thickened skin after soaking or bathing.
- Treat shoes with antifungal powders.
- Avoid occlusive footwear.
- Chronic, extensive disease, or nail involvement requires oral antifungal medication for systemic therapy.

MEDICATION
For use when topical therapy has failed

First Line

- Systemic antifungals (3)[A]:
  - Itraconazole: 200 mg PO BID for 7 days (cure rate >90%)
  - Terbinafine: 250 mg PO daily for 14 days
- If concomitant onychomycosis:
  - Itraconazole: 200 mg PO BID for 1st week of month for 3 months (Liver function testing is recommended.)
  - Terbinafine: 250 mg PO daily for 12 weeks, or pulse dosing: 500 mg PO daily for 1st week of month for 3 months (not recommended if creatinine clearance <50 mL/min)
- Pediatric dosing options:
  - Griseofulvin: 10 to 15 mg/kg/day or divided
  - Terbinafine:
    - 10 to 20 kg: 62.5 mg/day
    - 20 to 40 kg: 125 mg/day
    - >40 kg: 250 mg/day
  - Itraconazole: 3 to 5 mg/kg/day
  - Fluconazole: 6 mg/kg/week
- Contraindications: itraconazole, pregnancy Category C
- Precautions: All systemic antifungal drugs may have potential hepatotoxicity.
- Significant possible interactions: Itraconazole requires gastric acid for absorption; effectiveness is reduced with antacids, H_2 blockers, proton pump inhibitors, etc. Take with acidic beverage, such as soda if on antacids.
- Side effects: itraconazole and terbinafine may lead to gastrointestinal distress including diarrhea; itraconazole may also lead to peripheral edema especially if used in conjunction with calcium channel blockers.

Second Line

- Systemic antifungals: griseofulvin V (griseofulvin microsize) 250 to 500 mg daily for 21 days
- Contraindications (griseofulvin):
  - Patients with porphyria, hepatocellular failure
  - Patients with history of hypersensitivity to griseofulvin
- Precautions (griseofulvin):
  - Should be used only in severe cases
  - Periodic monitoring of organ system functioning, including renal, hepatic, and hematopoietic
  - Possible photosensitivity reactions
  - Lupus erythematosus, lupus-like syndromes, or exacerbation of existing lupus erythematosus has been reported.
- Significant possible interactions (griseofulvin):
  - Decreases activity of warfarin-type anticoagulants
  - Barbiturates usually depress griseofulvin activity.
  - May potentiate effect of alcohol, producing tachycardia and flush

ISSUES FOR REFERRAL

Consider dermatology referral if extensive or resistant disease, especially in immunocompromised host.

ADDITIONAL THERAPIES

- Treatment of secondary bacterial infections
- Treatment of eczematoid changes

COMPLEMENTARY & ALTERNATIVE MEDICINE

- Baking soda soak (1/2 cup in 1 quart warm water) has been shown to provide antifungal activity (4).
- White vinegar soak (1:1 white vinegar to warm water) may be used to aid in gram-negative bacterial coinfection.

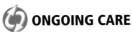 ONGOING CARE

FOLLOW-UP RECOMMENDATIONS

Avoid sweat buildup along feet.

Patient Monitoring

Evaluate for response, recognizing that infections may be chronic/recurrent.

DIET

No restrictions

PATIENT EDUCATION

See "General Prevention."

PROGNOSIS

- Often may obtain control but not completely cure
- Infections tend to be chronic with exacerbations (e.g., in hot, humid weather).
- Personal hygiene and preventive measures, such as open-toed sandals, careful drying, and frequent sock changes are essential.

COMPLICATIONS

- Secondary bacterial infections (common portal of entry for streptococcal infections, producing lymphangitis/cellulitis of lower extremity)
- Eczematoid changes

REFERENCES

1. Ameen M. Epidemiology of superficial fungal infections. *Clin Dermatol.* 2010;28(2):197–201.
2. Crawford F, Hollis S. Topical treatments for fungal infections of the skin and nails of the foot. *Cochrane Database Syst Rev.* 2007;(3):CD001434.
3. Bell-Syer SE, Khan SM, Torgerson DJ. Oral treatments for fungal infections of the skin of the foot. *Cochrane Database Syst Rev.* 2012;(10):CD003584.
4. Letscher-Bru V, Obszynski CM, Samsoen M, et al. Antifungal activity of sodium bicarbonate against fungal agents causing superficial infections. *Mycopathologia.* 2013;175(1–2):153–158.

ADDITIONAL READING

- Hawkins DM, Smidt AC. Superficial fungal infections in children. *Pediatr Clin North Am.* 2014;61(2):443–455.
- Rotta I, Sanchez A, Gonçalves PR, et al. Efficacy and safety of topical antifungals in the treatment of dermatomycosis: a systematic review. *Br J Dermatol.* 2012;166(5):927–933.
- Sahoo AK, Mahajan R. Management of tinea corporis, tinea cruris, and tinea pedis: a comprehensive review. *Indian Dermatol Online J.* 2016;7(2):77–86.

 SEE ALSO

Dermatitis, Contact; Dyshidrosis

 CODES

ICD10

B35.3 Tinea pedis

CLINICAL PEARLS

- Tinea pedis is often recurrent or chronic in nature.
- Careful drying between toes after showering or bathing helps prevent recurrences; blow-drying feet with hair dryer may be more effective than drying with towel.
- Socks should be changed frequently; put on socks before underwear to prevent infection from spreading to groin (tinea cruris).
- Treatment with topical antifungal medications for up to 4 weeks is usually sufficient.
- Dusting and desiccating powders (containing antifungal agents) may help prevent recurrences.

T

TINEA VERSICOLOR

Arabelle Abellard, MD, MSc

BASICS

DESCRIPTION
- Superficial fungal infection that interferes with normal skin pigmentation resulting in macules or patches that are hypopigmented, tan, brown, or salmon-colored. Tinea versicolor is usually well-demarcated, finely scaling, occurring primarily on the trunk and proximal upper extremities. Tinea versicolor is not a dermatophyte infection. It is caused by lipophilic (fat/oil-loving) *Malassezia* yeast organisms that normally inhabit the skin.
- System(s) affected: skin/exocrine
- Synonym(s): pityriasis versicolor

EPIDEMIOLOGY

Incidence
- Common, occurs worldwide, especially in tropical climates
- Predominant age: adolescents and young adults
- Predominant sex: male = female

Pediatric Considerations
Skin eruptions usually occur after puberty, when sebaceous glands are more active. However, tinea versicolor can also be seen in children, especially in tropical climates; facial lesions are more common in children.

Geriatric Considerations
Not common in the geriatric population

Prevalence
Prevalence can reach up to 50%, especially in warm climates.

ETIOLOGY AND PATHOPHYSIOLOGY
The inhibition of pigment synthesis in epidermal melanocytes leads to hypopigmented skin patches. In the hyperpigmented type, melanosomes increase in size resulting in brown or darker patches of skin of varying shades.
- Tinea versicolor is caused by saprophytic yeast: *Pityrosporum orbiculare* (also known as *Plasmodium ovale*, *Malassezia furfur*, or *Malassezia ovalis*), which is a known colonizer of all humans.
- Development of clinical disease is associated with transformation of *Malassezia* from yeast cells to pathogenic mycelial form. Several endogenous (host) and exogenous/external factors may play a role in the transformation to active disease.
- Tinea versicolor is not linked to poor hygiene.
- Tinea versicolor is generally not contagious.

Genetics
Genetic predisposition may exist.

RISK FACTORS
- Hot, humid weather
- Use of topical skin oils
- Hyperhidrosis
- HIV infection/immunosuppression
- High cortisol levels (Cushing syndrome/disease, prolonged steroid administration)
- Pregnancy
- Malnutrition
- Oral contraceptives

GENERAL PREVENTION
- Prophylaxis can be used in warm summer months and prior to tanning season in people with frequent recurrences.
- Avoiding skin oils may help.
- Tinea versicolor is not contagious.

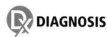

DIAGNOSIS

HISTORY
- Asymptomatic scaling macules typically affect the trunk and shoulders.
- Mild pruritus may occur.
- Skin eruptions are more prominent in summer months.
- Sun tanning accentuates lesions because affected areas usually do not tan.
- Periodic recurrences are common, especially in warm, summer months and in tropical regions.

PHYSICAL EXAM
- *Versicolor* refers to the variety and changing shades of colors. Color variations can exist between individuals and also between lesions.
- Sun exposure usually makes hypopigmented, light-colored patches more noticeable.
- In covered areas, lesions are often brown or salmon-colored.
- Usual distribution involves sebum-rich areas, the chest, shoulders, and back, and sometimes the face and intertriginous areas. In children, the face is more likely to be involved.
- Appearance: Tinea versicolor usually presents as small individual macules that frequently coalesce to form patches.
- Fine scales are present over the lesions and become more visible with scraping.

DIFFERENTIAL DIAGNOSIS
Other skin diseases with discolored macules and plaques or patches include the following:
- Pityriasis alba/rosea ("Christmas tree-like" distribution visible in *P. rosea*)
- Vitiligo (presents without scaling)
- Seborrheic dermatitis (more erythematous; thicker scales)
- Nummular eczema
- Secondary syphilis
- Erythrasma
- Mycosis fungoides

DIAGNOSTIC TESTS & INTERPRETATION
Visualization of affected skin under Wood's light often appears fluorescent yellow to yellow-green.

Initial Tests (lab, imaging)
- Direct microscopy of scales with 10% potassium hydroxide (KOH) preparation shows hyphae and spores ("spaghetti and meatballs" pattern).
- Routine lab tests are usually not necessary.
- Fungal culture is not useful.

Test Interpretation
- Short, stubby, or Y-shaped hyphae
- Small, round spores in clusters on hyphae

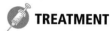

TREATMENT

GENERAL MEASURES
- Apply prescribed topical medications to the affected skin.
- Pigmentation/discoloration may take months to improve.
- In people with recurrences, repeat treatment each spring prior to sun exposure may be beneficial; consider monthly prophylaxis during the summer months.
- Patients who fail topical treatment can be treated with an oral/systemic medication.

MEDICATION
Topical antifungal therapy is the treatment of choice in limited disease and is safe and usually effective. Evidence is generally of poor quality, but data suggest that longer durations of treatment and higher concentrations of active agents produce greater cure rates (1)[A].

First Line

- Ketoconazole 2% shampoo applied to damp skin for 1 to 3 days and left on for 5 minutes (Ketoconazole is contraindicated in pregnancy.) *or*
- Ketoconazole 2% (Nizoral) cream applied twice daily for 2 to 4 weeks (Ketoconazole is contraindicated in pregnancy.) *or*
- Selenium sulfide shampoo 2.5% (Selsun):
  – Applied daily for 1 week to the affected areas and allowed to dry and remain on skin for 10 minutes prior to showering *or*
  – Allowed to remain on body once a week for 4 weeks for 12 to 24 hours prior to rinsing off *or*
- Clotrimazole 1% topical (Lotrimin) twice daily for 2 to 4 weeks *or*
- Miconazole 2% (Micatin, Monistat) twice daily for 2 to 4 weeks *or*
- Topical ciclopirox olamine 1% cream twice daily for 2 weeks *or*
- Terbinafine (Lamisil) 1% solution twice daily for 1 week *or*
- Terbinafine (Lamisil DermGel) once daily for 1 week
- Newer preparations include 2.25% selenium sulfide foam and ketoconazole 2% gel
- Cure rates of topical antiyeast preparations typically 70–80%; healing continues after active treatment. Even pigmentation may take months to return.

Second Line

- Can be used for extensive and recalcitrant disease (nonresponders)
- Oral fluconazole 300 mg once weekly for 2 weeks (2)[A]
- Itraconazole 200 mg/day PO for 1 week (7 days); cure rate >90% (2)[A]
- Oral ketoconazole is no longer recommended by the FDA due to risks of hepatotoxicity, adrenal insufficiency, and drug–drug interactions.
- Oral terbinafine or griseofulvin is not effective.

ISSUES FOR REFERRAL

- If resistant to treatment
- If extensive disease occurs in immunocompromised host

 ## ONGOING CARE

- Ketoconazole 2% or selenium sulfide 2.5% shampoo can be used weekly for maintenance or monthly for prophylaxis.
- Itraconazole 400 mg once monthly (in 2 divided dosages) during the warmer months of the year can also reduce recurrences.

FOLLOW-UP RECOMMENDATIONS

Inform patients that pigment changes/variations may remain for several months after treatment.

Patient Monitoring

- Prophylactic medication can be used in warm summer months and prior to tanning season in people with frequent recurrences.
- Failure to respond should prompt reassessment or dermatology referral.
- Resistance to treatment, frequent recurrences, or widespread disease may point to immunodeficiency.

DIET

There is no proven diet to treat and prevent recurrence of tinea versicolor.

PATIENT EDUCATION

For patient education materials on this topic, contact American Academy of Dermatology, 930 N. Meacham Road, P.O. Box 4014, Schaumburg, IL 60168-4014; (708) 330-0230.

PROGNOSIS

- Lesions may last for months to years.
- Lesions may recur periodically because *Malassezia* yeast organisms are known human colonizers and natural inhabitants of the skin.
- Pigment changes/variations may take months to resolve.

REFERENCES

1. Hald M, Arendrup M, Svejgaard E, et al; and Danish Society of Dermatology. Evidence-based Danish guidelines for the treatment of *Malassezia*-related skin diseases. *Acta Derm Venereol*. 2015;95(1):12–19.
2. Gupta AK, Lane D, Paquet M. Systematic review of systemic treatments for tinea versicolor and evidence-based dosing regimen recommendations. *J Cutan Med Surg*. 2014;18(2):79–90.

ADDITIONAL READING

- Bhogal CS, Singal A, Baruah MC. Comparative efficacy of ketoconazole and fluconazole in the treatment of pityriasis versicolor: a one year follow-up study. *J Dermatol*. 2001;28(10):535–539.
- Faergemann J, Todd G, Pather S, et al. A double-blind, randomized, placebo-controlled, dose-finding study of oral pramiconazole in the treatment of pityriasis versicolor. *J Am Acad Dermatol*. 2009;61(6):971–976.
- Gupta AK, Lyons DC. Pityriasis versicolor: an update on pharmacological treatment options. *Expert Opin Pharmacother*. 2014;15(12):1707–1713.
- Hawkins DM, Smidt AC. Superficial fungal infections in children. *Pediatr Clin North Am*. 2014;61(2):443–455.
- Köse O, Bülent Taştan H, Riza Gür A, et al. Comparison of a single 400 mg dose versus a 7-day 200 mg daily dose of itraconazole in the treatment of tinea versicolor. *J Dermatolog Treat*. 2002;13(2):77–79.

 ## CODES

ICD10

B36.0 Pityriasis versicolor

CLINICAL PEARLS

- Tinea versicolor, also called pityriasis versicolor, is characterized by noncontagious, finely scaling macules of varying colors.
- Recurrence is common in summer months.
- Lesions tend to become more apparent after tanning because they typically do not tan; hypopigmented patches become more visible.
- Inform patients that discoloration/pigment variations may remain for several months after treatment.

T

TINNITUS

Donna I. Meltzer, MD

 BASICS

DESCRIPTION

- Tinnitus is a perceived sensation of sound in the absence of an external acoustic stimulus; often described as a ringing, hissing, buzzing, clicking, or whooshing
- Derived from the Latin word *tinnire*, meaning "to ring"
- May be heard in one or both ears or centrally within the head
- Two types: subjective (most common) and objective tinnitus
  - Subjective tinnitus: perceived only by the patient; can be continuous, intermittent, or pulsatile
  - Objective tinnitus: audible to the examiner; rare
- Primary tinnitus: idiopathic with or without sensori-neural hearing loss (SNHL) (1)
- Secondary tinnitus: associated with a specific cause (other than SNHL)

EPIDEMIOLOGY

Incidence

- Incidence increasing in association with excessive noise exposure
- Higher rates of tinnitus in smokers, hypertensives, diabetics, and obese patients

Prevalence

- Tinnitus reported by 35 to 50 million adults in United States; although underreported, 12 million seek medical care.
- Affects 10–15% of adults (2)
- Prevalence increases with age and peaks in 6th decade.
- Prevalence of 13–53% in general pediatric population
- Ethnic: whites > blacks and Hispanics
- Gender: males > females

ETIOLOGY AND PATHOPHYSIOLOGY

- Precise pathophysiology is unknown; numerous theories have been proposed. Ototoxic agents or noise exposure damage hair cells so that there is abnormal neural activity in the auditory cortex.
- Causes of secondary tinnitus (2):
  - Otologic: cholesteatoma, cerumen impaction, foreign body, middle ear effusion, otosclerosis, Ménière disease, vestibular schwannoma, patulous eustachian tube
  - Medications: anti-inflammatory agents (aspirin, NSAIDs); antimalarial agents, antimicrobial drugs (aminoglycosides, macrolides); antineoplastic agents, loop diuretics, miscellaneous drugs (antiarrhythmics, antiulcer, anticonvulsants, antihypertensives); anesthetics
  - Somatic: temporomandibular joint (TMJ) dysfunction, head or neck injury

- Neurologic: multiple sclerosis, spontaneous intracranial hypertension, vestibular migraine, type I Chiari malformation, palatal myoclonus, idiopathic stapedial muscle spasm
- Infectious: viral, bacterial, fungal
- Metabolic: diabetes mellitus, dyslipidemia, vitamin B_{12} deficiency
- Vascular: aortic or carotid stenosis, venous hum, arteriovenous fistula or malformation, vascular tumors, high cardiac output state (anemia)

Genetics

Limited evidence to support a genetic component

RISK FACTORS

- Hearing loss (but can have tinnitus with normal hearing)
- High-level noise exposure
- Advanced age
- Use of ototoxic medications (some are irreversible)
- Otologic disease (otosclerosis, Ménière disease, cerumen impaction)
- Depression and anxiety associated with increased odds of tinnitus

GENERAL PREVENTION

- Avoid loud noise exposure and wear appropriate ear protection to prevent hearing loss.
- Monitor ototoxic medications and avoid prescribing more than one ototoxic agent concurrently.

COMMONLY ASSOCIATED CONDITIONS

- SNHL caused by presbycusis (age-associated hearing loss) or prolonged loud noise exposure
- Conductive hearing loss due to cerumen, otosclerosis, cholesteatoma
- Psychological disorders: depression, anxiety, insomnia, suicidal ideation
- Despair, frustration, interference with concentration and social interactions, work hindrance

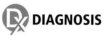 **DIAGNOSIS**

HISTORY

- Onset gradual (presbycusis) or abrupt (following loud noise exposure)
- Duration: acute versus chronic (<6 months)
- Timing: can be continuous (hearing loss) or intermittent (Ménière disease)
- Pattern: nonpulsatile > pulsatile (often vascular cause)
- Location: bilateral > unilateral (vestibular schwannoma, cerumen, Ménière disease)
- Pitch: high pitch (with SNHL) > low pitch (Ménière disease)
- Associated symptoms: hearing loss, headache, noise intolerance, vertigo, TMJ dysfunction, neck pain

- Exacerbating factors: loud noise; jaw, head, or neck movements
- Alleviating factors: hearing aid, position change, medications
- Medication use (prescription, OTC, supplements)
- Hearing and past noise exposure (occupational, military, recreational)
- Psychosocial history (depression, sleep habits)
- Impact of tinnitus: Tinnitus Handicap Inventory, Tinnitus Functional Index

PHYSICAL EXAM

- HEENT, neck, neurologic, and vascular examinations to help with etiology or guide next steps
- Ear: cerumen impaction, effusion, cholesteatoma
- Check hearing; air and bone conduction testing with 512- or 1,024-Hz tuning fork (Weber and Rinne tests)
- Eye: funduscopic exam for papilledema (intracranial hypertension) or visual field change (mass)
- TMJ: Palpate for tenderness and crepitus with movement.
- Cranial nerve, Romberg test (equilibrium), finger to nose, gait; assess for nystagmus.
- Auscultate for bruits or murmurs; compress jugular vein (suspect venous etiology if maneuver reduces tinnitus)

DIFFERENTIAL DIAGNOSIS

- Pulsatile tinnitus: carotid stenosis, aortic valve disease, arteriovenous malformation, high cardiac output state (anemia, hyperthyroidism), paraganglioma (glomus tumor)
- Nonpulsatile tinnitus: auditory hallucinations

DIAGNOSTIC TESTS & INTERPRETATION

- Tinnitus is a symptom; no objective test to confirm diagnosis
- Pure tone audiometry (air and bone conduction)
- Tympanometry
- Carotid Doppler ultrasonography (neck bruit)

Initial Tests (lab, imaging)

- Little evidence to support lab testing other than targeted lab studies based on history and physical exam. Use clinical judgment and consider the following:
  - CBC, BUN/creatinine, fasting glucose, lipid panel
- Newer guidelines advise against imaging studies unless have unilateral, pulsatile tinnitus; focal neurologic abnormality; or asymmetric hearing loss (1)[C].
  - CT of temporal bone is initial imaging study of middle ear, especially if conductive hearing loss
  - Pulsatile tinnitus: temporal bone CT without contrast, CTA/CTV with contrast, MRA without or with contrast, or MRI head and internal auditory canal (IAC) without and with contrast are usually appropriate (3)[C]; could also consider carotid artery duplex scan

- Unilateral nonpulsatile tinnitus: MRI head and IAC without and with contrast; might consider CT temporal bone without or with contrast or CTA head with contrast (3)[C]
- Bilateral nonpulsatile tinnitus: imaging not indicated if no hearing loss, neurologic deficit, or trauma (3)[C]

Follow-Up Tests & Special Considerations
Consider TSH, HIV, RPR, autoimmune panel, Lyme test, vitamin B$_{12}$ level; low quality evidence for these studies (2)

Diagnostic Procedures/Other
Electronystagmography (vestibular testing for Ménière disease)

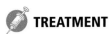 TREATMENT

GENERAL MEASURES
- Individualize treatment based on the severity of tinnitus and impact on function.
- Cognitive behavioral therapy (CBT), education, relaxation therapy
- Reassure patient.
- Manage treatable pathology.
- Hearing aids (corrects hearing and might mask tinnitus) can be tried if there is hearing loss and bothersome tinnitus (1)[C].
- Protect hearing against future loud noise.
- Masking sound devices or generators on discontinuation might have decreased tinnitus (residual inhibition).
- Discontinue ototoxic medications (some medications have reversible ototoxic effects).

MEDICATION
No pharmacologic agent has been shown to consistently alleviate tinnitus.

First Line
- Antidepressants (SSRIs or TCAs): probably help with psychological distress; insufficient evidence that antidepressant drug therapy improves tinnitus (2),(4)[A]
- Anxiolytics (benzodiazepines) do not provide consistent benefit and risk side effect of dependency (2).

Second Line
Anticonvulsants: potentially suppress central auditory hyperactivity but not recommended (1)[C]

ISSUES FOR REFERRAL
- Audiologist for comprehensive hearing evaluation and management
- Otolaryngologist, neurologist, or neurosurgeon depending on pathology
- Dental referral for TMJ treatment and dental orthotics (splint, night guard)
- Therapists for CBT, biofeedback, education, and relaxation techniques

ADDITIONAL THERAPIES
- CBT employs relaxation exercises, coping strategies, and deconditioning techniques to reduce arousal levels and reverse negative thoughts about tinnitus; might reduce negative impact of tinnitus on quality of life (5)[A]; recommended as beneficial based on randomized controlled trials (1)[C]
- Sound therapy (masking): Patients wear low-level noise generators to mask the tinnitus noise; optional therapy (1)[C]
- Tinnitus retraining therapy (TRT) combines counseling, education, and acoustic therapy (soft music, sound machine) to minimize bothersome nature of tinnitus. One randomized study reported reduction in tinnitus but no benefit over standard counseling with enriched sound (6).
- Internet-based technology or smartphone apps to mask tinnitus may hold promise, but high-quality studies are lacking.
- Transcranial magnetic stimulation (TMS): a noninvasive method to stimulate neurons in the brain by rapidly changing magnetic fields; not recommended as randomized trials were inconclusive (1)[C]
- Botulism toxin (for palatal myoclonus)
- Intratympanic steroid injections not recommended (1)[C]
- Cannabis: not enough evidence to recommend

SURGERY/OTHER PROCEDURES
- Cochlear implants (for severe SNHL)
- Ablation of cochlear nerve (destroys hearing)
- Otosclerosis: stapedectomy surgery with implantation of ossicular prosthesis
- Severe Ménière disease not alleviated by medications: installation of endolymphatic shunt, labyrinthectomy, or vestibular neurectomy
- Auditory neoplasms: surgical resection/radiation
- Pulsatile tinnitus due to atherosclerotic carotid artery disease: carotid endarterectomy

COMPLEMENTARY & ALTERNATIVE MEDICINE
- Acupuncture, Ginkgo biloba, melatonin, zinc, or antioxidants might alleviate tinnitus in some patients; however, many conflicting studies report no benefit with these methods (7)[B].
- Hypnosis (unknown effectiveness)

 ONGOING CARE

FOLLOW-UP RECOMMENDATIONS
- Audiologist: for hearing evaluation and therapy
- Counseling: as needed for psychological distress
- Family physician: as needed for support and guidance

PATIENT EDUCATION
- American Tinnitus Association: (800) 634-8978; https://www.ata.org/
- National Institute on Deafness and Other Communication Disorders: (800) 241-1044; https://www.nidcd.nih.gov/health/tinnitus

PROGNOSIS
- Tinnitus persisted in 80% of older patients and increased in severity in 50%.
- Focus on managing tinnitus and reducing severity, not curing.

REFERENCES
1. Tunkel DE, Bauer CA, Sun GH, et al. Clinical practice guideline: tinnitus executive summary. *Otolaryngol Head Neck Surg*. 2014;151(4):533–541.
2. Dalrymple SN, Lewis SH, Philman S. Tinnitus: diagnosis and management. *Am Fam Physician*. 2021;103(11):663–671.
3. Kessler MM, Moussa M, Bykowski J, et al. ACR Appropriateness Criteria® tinnitus. *J Am Coll Radiol*. 2017;14(11S):S584–S591.
4. Baldo P, Doree C, Molin P, et al. Antidepressants for patients with tinnitus. *Cochrane Database Syst Rev*. 2012;(9):CD003853.
5. Fuller T, Cima R, Langguth B, et al. Cognitive behavioural therapy for tinnitus. *Cochrane Database Syst Rev*. 2020;1(1):CD012614.
6. The Tinnitus Retraining Therapy Trial Research Group. Effect of tinnitus retraining vs standard of care on tinnitus-related quality of life: a randomized clinical trial. *JAMA Otolaryngol Head Neck Surg*. 2019;145(7):597–608.
7. Luetzenberg FS, Babu S, Seidman MD. Alternative treatments of tinnitus: alternative medicine. *Otolaryngol Clin North Am*. 2020;53(4):637–650.

CODES

ICD10
- H93.19 Tinnitus, unspecified ear
- H93.11 Tinnitus, right ear
- H93.12 Tinnitus, left ear

CLINICAL PEARLS
- People have different levels of tolerance to tinnitus. It may affect sleep, concentration, and emotional state. Many patients with chronic tinnitus have depression.
- To keep tinnitus from worsening, avoid loud noises and minimize stress.
- Optimal management may involve multiple strategies.

TOBACCO USE AND SMOKING CESSATION

Felix B. Chang, MD, DABMA, ABIHM, ABIM

BASICS

Use of tobacco of any form

DESCRIPTION
- Nicotine sources: cigars, pipes, water pipes, hookahs, cigarettes, and electronic cigarettes (e-cigarettes)
- Electronic nicotine delivery system (ENDS) use is on the rise.
- E-cigarettes are called e-cigs, vapes, ehookahs, vape pens, and electronic nicotine delivery systems.

EPIDEMIOLOGY
Smoking causes more deaths each year than alcohol use, motor vehicle accidents, illegal drug use, and firearm-related injuries combined.

Incidence
- 2.4 million new smokers annually in the United States
- 59% of new smokers are <18 years of age (6% initiation rate for teens).

Prevalence
- Age: highest among those ages 45 to 64 years (16%)
- Gender: male > female (15% vs. 12%)
- Cigarette smoking among adults has declined significantly since the 1960s.
- Cigarette smoking is responsible for >480,000 deaths per year in the United States, including >41,000 deaths from secondhand smoke exposure. This is about 1 in 5 deaths annually or 1,300 deaths every day.
- Each day, about 2,000 people <18 years smoke their first cigarette.
- Each day, about 1,600 youth try their first cigarette.
- In 2018, 21% of high school students reported current use of e-cigarettes.
- In 2019, 14% of all adults (34.1 million people) currently smoked cigarettes: 15.3% in men, 12.7% of women.
- 5% of middle school students report current e-cigarette use.

ETIOLOGY AND PATHOPHYSIOLOGY
- Addiction due to nicotine's rapid stimulation of the brain's dopamine system (teenage brain especially susceptible)
- Atherosclerotic risk due to adrenergic stimulation, endothelial damage, carbon monoxide, and adverse effects on lipids
- Direct airway damage from cigarette tar.
- Carcinogens in all tobacco products
- E-cigarettes produce an aerosol by heating liquid nicotine, flavoring, and chemicals.
- Potential adverse effects of e-cigarettes are related to exposure to nicotine as well as to other vapor components produced by the devices.
- If e-cigarette, or vaping product, use is suspected as a possible etiology of a patient's lung injury, obtain detailed history regarding:
  - Substance(s) used: nicotine, cannabinoids (e.g., marijuana, THC, THC concentrates, CBD, CBD oil, synthetic cannabinoids [e.g., K2 or spice], hash oil, Dank vapes), flavors, or other substances
  - Substance source(s): commercially available liquids, homemade liquids
  - Device(s) used: manufacturer; brand name; product name; model

- Vitamin E acetate is strongly linked to the EVALI outbreaks.
- Most product use-associated lung injury (EVALI) associated with products containing THC

RISK FACTORS
- Presence of a smoker in the household
- Easy access to cigarettes
- Comorbid stress and psychiatric disorders
- Low self-esteem/self-worth
- Poor academic performance
- Boys: high levels of aggression and rebelliousness
- Girls: preoccupation with weight and body image
- E-cigarette use has been associated with several cases of idiopathic acute eosinophilic pneumonia.

GENERAL PREVENTION
- Most first-time tobacco use occurs before high school graduation.
- Smoking bans in public areas and workplaces
- Restrict minors' access to tobacco
- Restrict tobacco advertisements
- Tobacco-free sports initiatives
- The net benefit of behavioral interventions and use of FDA-approved pharmacotherapy for tobacco smoking cessation, alone or combined, in adults who smoke is substantial (1)[A].
- The evidence on pharmacotherapy interventions for tobacco smoking cessation in pregnancy is insufficient.
- Current evidence is insufficient to recommend use e-cigarettes for tobacco cessation in adults.

COMMONLY ASSOCIATED CONDITIONS
- Coronary artery disease, cerebrovascular disease
- Peripheral vascular disease
- Abdominal aortic aneurysm (AAA)
- Chronic obstructive pulmonary disease (COPD)
- Cancer of the lip, oral cavity, pharynx, larynx, lung, esophagus, stomach, pancreas, kidney, urinary bladder, cervix, and blood
- Pneumonia, osteoporosis
- Periodontitis
- Alcohol use
- Depression and anxiety, reduced fertility

Pregnancy Considerations
Smoking during pregnancy can increase the risk of miscarriage, congenital anomalies, stillbirth, fetal growth restriction, preterm birth, placental abruption.

Pediatric Considerations
Secondhand smoke increases the risk for:
- Sudden infant death syndrome
- Acute upper and lower respiratory tract infections, exacerbations of asthma, otitis media
- Nicotine passes through breast milk.

DIAGNOSIS

HISTORY
- Ask about tobacco use and secondhand smoke exposure at every physician encounter.
- Type and quantity of tobacco used: "Heavy smoking" is 20 or more cigarettes per day or 20 or more pack-years.
  - Pack-years = packs/day × years
  - Assess for awareness of health risks and interest in quitting.

- Identify triggers for smoking: stress, habit, pleasure.
- Prior attempts to quit: method, duration of success, reason for relapse

PHYSICAL EXAM
- General: tobacco odor, staining of nails, hair
- Skin: premature wrinkling, especially the face
- Mouth: nicotine-stained teeth; inspect for mucosal changes, hypertrophy, fungating lesions.
- Lungs: crackles, wheezing, increased or decreased volume, chronic cough
- Vessels: carotid or abdominal bruits, abdominal aortic enlargement or aneurysm, weak peripheral pulses, stigmata of peripheral vascular disease

DIAGNOSTIC TESTS & INTERPRETATION
- The U.S. Preventive Services Task Force (USPSTF) recommends one-time screening abdominal ultrasound (US) for AAA in men ≥65 years of age who ever smoked (number needed to screen to prevent one AAA = 500).
- USPSTF recommends yearly screening for lung cancer with low-dose CT for individuals 55 to 80 years with a 30 pack-year history of smoking, current smokers, or those who have quit within past 15 years.

Diagnostic Procedures/Other
Pulmonary function tests (PFTs) for smokers with chronic pulmonary symptoms, such as wheezing, cough, or dyspnea.

TREATMENT

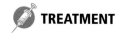

ALERT
Report cases of lung injury of unclear etiology and a history of e-cigarette or vaping product use within the past 90 days to state or local health department.

GENERAL MEASURES
- Behavioral counseling (5 As):
  - Ask about tobacco use at every office visit.
  - Advise all smokers to quit.
  - Assess the patient's willingness to quit.
  - Assist the patient in his or her attempt to quit and provide quit line number (1-800-QUIT-NOW).
  - Arrange follow-up and support.
- Patients ready to quit smoking should set a quit date within the next 2 weeks; no difference in success rates between patients who taper prior to their quit date and those who stop abruptly

MEDICATION
Varenicline and nicotine gum therapy may each reduce relapse in patients who had stopped smoking.

First Line
- Varenicline (Chantix): 0.5 mg/day PO for 3 days, then 0.5 mg BID for 4 days, and then 1 mg BID for 11 weeks:
  - Start 1 to 4 weeks prior to smoking cessation and continue for 12 to 24 weeks.
  - Superior versus placebo and bupropion; number needed to treat = 6 and 15, respectively
  - May be combined with nicotine replacement therapy (NRT) for those with cravings
  - Side effects: nausea, insomnia, headache, depression, suicidal ideation; safety not established in adolescents or patients with psychiatric or cardiovascular disease; pregnancy Category C

- Bupropion SR (Zyban): 150 mg PO for 3 days and then 150 mg BID (2)[A]:
  - Start 1 week prior to smoking cessation and continue for 7 to 12 weeks.
  - Twice as effective as placebo
  - Drug of choice for patients with depression or schizophrenia; additional benefit of weight loss
  - May be combined with varenicline and NRT in men who smoke >1 PPD
  - Side effects: tachycardia, headache, nausea, insomnia, dry mouth; contraindicated in patients who have seizure disorders or anorexia/bulimia; pregnancy Category C
- NRT (e.g., patch, gum, lozenge, inhaler, nasal spray) (3)[A]:
  - Improves quit rates by 50–70% versus placebo
  - Available over the counter
  - Patch (NicoDerm CQ 21, 14, and 7 mg):
    - 1 patch q24h. Start with 21 mg if smoking ≥10 cigarettes per day; otherwise, start with 14 mg.
    - 6 weeks on initial dose and then taper
    - 2 weeks each on subsequent doses
    - No proven benefit beyond 8 weeks
  - ENDS
    - Contain less nicotine than cigarette
    - Controversial if less "dangerous" than tobacco
    - Conflicting data on whether teen use increases or decreases risk to cigarette progression.
    - Insufficient evidence to recommend as adjunct for tobacco cessation
  - Gum (Nicorette, 2 and 4 mg):
    - Use 4 mg if smoking ≥25 cigarettes per day.
    - Chew 1 piece q1–2h for 6 weeks, then 1 piece q2–4h for 3 weeks, and then 1 piece q4–8h for 3 weeks.
    - May use in combination with bupropion; monitor for hypertension.
    - Side effects: headache, pharyngitis, cough, rhinitis, dyspepsia; all mainly with inhaler and spray forms
    - Pregnancy Category D
  - NRT is reasonable in hospitalized smokers because NRT products immediately treat nicotine withdrawal symptoms, whereas varenicline and bupropion take time to reach steady state.

Second Line
- Nortriptyline: 25 to 75 mg/day PO or in divided doses:
  - Start 10 to 14 days prior to smoking cessation and continue for at least 12 weeks.
  - Efficacy similar to bupropion, but side effects are more common; pregnancy Category D
  - The antidepressants bupropion and nortriptyline aid long-term smoking cessation.
- Clonidine: 0.1 mg PO BID or 0.1 mg/day transdermal patch weekly:
  - Side effects: hypotension, bradycardia, depression, fatigue; pregnancy Category C

ADDITIONAL THERAPIES
- Pharmacotherapy and behavior support increase success compared with minimal intervention or usual care.
- Naltrexone: no evidence

COMPLEMENTARY & ALTERNATIVE MEDICINE
Acupuncture may increase smoking cessation in short term.

ADMISSION, INPATIENT, AND NURSING CONSIDERATIONS
Intense counseling interventions in hospitalized patients combined with follow-up for >1 month after discharge showed significant improvement in smoking cessation rates at 6 months or more postdischarge.

 ONGOING CARE

35–40% of patients relapse between years 1 and 5 after quitting. 2/3 of smokers who relapse report wanting to quit again within 30 days.

FOLLOW-UP RECOMMENDATIONS
Follow up 3 to 7 days after scheduled quit date and at least monthly for 3 months thereafter. Refraining from tobacco products for first 2 weeks is critical to long-term abstinence. Inpatient counseling plus four postdischarge telephone calls effective for relapse prevention in hospitalized smokers

Patient Monitoring
- Short-term withdrawal symptoms include dysphoria, depressed mood, irritability, anxiety, insomnia, increased appetite, and poor concentration.
- Nicotine withdrawal syndrome: dysphoric or depressed mood, insomnia, irritability, frustration, or anger; anxiety, difficulty concentrating, restlessness, and increased appetite or weight gain. Within 2 to 5 years after quitting, risk for stroke ~ to that of a nonsmoker
- The risk for cancer of the mouth, throat, esophagus, and bladder drops by half within 5 years of quitting. Ten years after quitting, the risk of dying from lung cancer drops by 50%.

DIET
Healthy eating for limiting weight gain

PATIENT EDUCATION
1-800-QUIT-NOW. https://www.cdc.gov/tobacco/

PROGNOSIS
- Smoking increases the risk for coronary heart disease (2- to 4-fold), stroke (2- to 4-fold), and lung cancer (25-fold).
- Smokers are more likely to die from COPD than nonsmokers (12-fold increased risk).
- Tobacco cessation reduces the risk of coronary heart disease sharply in the first 2 years after quitting (more slowly after that).
- Tobacco cessation slows the progression of COPD and reduces the loss of lung function over time. Tobacco cessation also reduces the risk of acute myeloid leukemia, cancer of the lung, cervix, colon, rectum, bladder esophagus, kidney, liver, mouth and throat.
- The risk of developing diabetes is 30–40% higher for active smokers than nonsmokers.
- People who quit smoking after a heart attack or cardiac surgery reduce their risk of death by 1/3.
- Relapse rates initially >60% but decrease to 2–4% after 2 years of abstinence.
- The incidence of myocardial infarction (MI) is increased 6-fold in women and 3-fold in men who smoke at least 20 cigarettes per day, when compared with nonsmokers.
- Tobacco cessation reduces the risk of premature death and can add as much as 10 years of life expectancy.

COMPLICATIONS
- Disability and premature death due to heart attack, stroke, cancer, COPD
- Causation proven cancers associated with smoking: colorectal, head and neck, esophagus, kidney, liver, lower urinary tract, renal pelvis, ureter, and bladder, lung, mesothelioma, nasal cavity, paranasal sinuses, pancreas, penis, stomach, uterine, cervix; evidence equivocal: breast, skin
- Smoking more than doubles the risk of coronary artery disease and doubles the risk of stroke.

REFERENCES
1. U.S. Preventive Services Task Force. Tobacco smoking cessation in adults, including pregnant persons: interventions. https://www.uspreventive servicestaskforce.org/uspstf/recommendation /tobacco-use-in-adults-and-pregnant-women -counseling-and-interventions. Published January 19, 2021. Accessed November 3, 2021.
2. Howes S, Hartmann-Boyce J, Livingstone-Banks J, et al. Antidepressants for smoking cessation. *Cochrane Database Syst Rev.* 2020;(4):CD000031.
3. Lindson N, Chepkin SC, Ye W, et al. Different doses, durations and modes of delivery of nicotine replacement therapy for smoking cessation. *Cochrane Database Syst Rev.* 2019;(4):CD013308.

ADDITIONAL READING
U.S. Department of Health and Human Services. *Smoking Cessation: A Report of the Surgeon General.* Rockville, MD: U.S. Department of Health and Human Services, Centers for Disease Control and Prevention, National Center for Chronic Disease Prevention and Health Promotion, Office on Smoking and Health; 2020. https://www.cdc.gov/tobacco/data_statistics /sgr/2020-smoking-cessation/index.html. Accessed November 3, 2021.

 CODES

ICD10
- F17.210 Nicotine dependence, cigarettes, uncomplicated
- F17.213 Nicotine dependence, cigarettes, with withdrawal
- F17.211 Nicotine dependence, cigarettes, in remission

CLINICAL PEARLS
- Addressing tobacco cessation regularly improves patient satisfaction.
- Nicotine replacement improves cessation rates.
- Establish a quit date and provide resources to promote success (1-800-QUIT-NOW).

T

TOURETTE SYNDROME

Marvin H. Sineath Jr., MD, FAAFP, CAQSM • Chandler Brandenburg

BASICS

DESCRIPTION

Tourette syndrome (TS) is a childhood-onset neurobehavioral disorder characterized by the presence of multiple motor and at least one phonic tic.

- Tics are sudden, brief, repetitive, stereotyped motor movements (motor tics) or sounds (phonic tics) produced by moving air through the nose, mouth, or throat.
- Patients can suppress their tics, but this often causes inner tension that eventually results in more forceful tics.
- System(s) affected: nervous

EPIDEMIOLOGY

Incidence

- Average age of onset: 7 years with greatest tic severity between 10 and 12 years (1)
- Male > female (3:1); heterogeneous disorder but non-Hispanic whites (2:1) compared with Hispanics and/or blacks

Prevalence

0.77% overall in children (1.06% in boys, 0.25% in girls)

ETIOLOGY AND PATHOPHYSIOLOGY

Abnormalities of dopamine neurotransmission and receptor hypersensitivity, most likely in the ventral striatum, play a primary role in the pathophysiology. May involve dysfunction of basal ganglia–thalamocortical circuits, likely involving decreased inhibitory output from the basal ganglia, which results in an imbalance of inhibition and excitation in the motor cortex

- Thought to result from a complex interaction between social, environmental, and multiple genetic abnormalities
- Controversial pediatric autoimmune neuropsychiatric disorder associated with streptococcal infection (PANDAS); TS/OCD cases linked to immunologic response to previous group A β-hemolytic *Streptococcus* (GABHS)

Genetics

- Predisposition: frequent familial history of tic disorders and OCD
- Recent studies suggest polygenic inheritance with evidence for a locus on chromosome 17q; sequence variants in *SLITRK1* gene on chromosome 13q also are associated with TS.

RISK FACTORS

- Risk of TS among relatives: 9.8–15%
- Low birth weight, maternal stress, nausea/vomiting in 1st trimester, maternal smoking (2)

COMMONLY ASSOCIATED CONDITIONS

- OCD (28–67%), ADHD (50–60%), conduct disorder, learning disabilities (23%)
- Depression/anxiety including phobias, panic attacks, and stuttering; increased risk of contemplating suicide (1)
- Impairments of visual perception, sleep disorders, restless leg syndrome, and migraine headaches
- Cardiometabolic disorders, especially obesity, circulatory system diseases, type 2 diabetes (50%) (3)

DIAGNOSIS

HISTORY

Diagnosis of TS is based on history and clinical presentation (i.e., observation of tics with/without presence of coexisting disorders). Identify comorbid conditions.

PHYSICAL EXAM

- Typically, the physical exam is normal.
- Motor and vocal tics are the clinical hallmarks.
  - Tics fluctuate in type, frequency, and anatomic distribution over time.
  - Multiple motor tics include facial grimacing, blinking, head/neck jerking, tongue protruding, sniffing, touching, and burping.
  - Vocal tics include grunts, snorts, throat clearing, barking, yelling, hiccupping, sucking, and coughing.
  - Tics are exacerbated by anticipation, emotional upset, anxiety, or fatigue.
  - Tics subside when patient is concentrating/absorbed in activities but may persist during sleep.
- *Diagnostic and Statistical Manual of Mental Disorders*, 5th edition (*DSM-5*) criteria:
  - Both multiple motor and one or more vocal tics have been present at some time, although not necessarily concurrently.
  - Tics may wax and wane in frequency but have persisted for >1 year since onset.
  - Onset before age 18 years
  - Not attributable to the physiologic effects of a substance (e.g., cocaine) or another medical condition (e.g., Huntington disease, postviral encephalitis)

DIFFERENTIAL DIAGNOSIS

- Chorea/Huntington disease
- Myoclonus
- Seizure
- Ischemic or hemorrhagic stroke
- Essential tremor
- Posttraumatic/head injury
- Headache
- Dementia
- Wilson disease
- Sydenham chorea
- Multiple sclerosis
- Postviral encephalitis
- Toxin exposure (e.g., carbon monoxide, cocaine)
- Drug effects (e.g., dopamine agonists, fluoroquinolones)

DIAGNOSTIC TESTS & INTERPRETATION

Initial Tests (lab, imaging)

- No definitive lab tests diagnose TS; based on clinical features
- Measure thyroid-stimulating hormone (TSH) due to association of tics with hyperthyroidism.
- EEG shows nonspecific abnormalities; useful only to differentiate tics from epilepsy

Test Interpretation

Smaller caudate volumes and increased striatal dopaminergic terminals

TREATMENT

GENERAL MEASURES

- Goal of treatment should be to improve social functioning, self-esteem, and quality of life. Patients should play an active role in treatment decisions and be educated that tics are not voluntary or psychiatric.
- Watchful waiting is an acceptable approach to treatment in patients without functional impairments (1)[A].
- Valid, reliable, responsive tic severity scales for treatment assessment (4): Yale Global Tic Severity Scale (most extensively used and validated) (1); Shapiro Tourette Syndrome Severity Scale; Tourette's Disorder Scale
- Educate patient, family, teachers, and friends to identify and address psychosocial stressors and environmental triggers.
- No cure for tics: Treatment is purely symptomatic, and multimodal treatment usually is indicated.
- TS clusters with several comorbid conditions; each disorder must be evaluated for associated functional impairment because patients often are more disabled by their psychiatric conditions than by the tics; choice of initial treatment depends largely on worst symptoms (tics, obsessions, or impulsivity).
- Comprehensive Behavioral Intervention for Tics (CBIT) should be offered as an initial treatment before medications (1)[B].
  - Includes habit reversal training, relaxation training, and function intervention
  - Reduced tic severity with CBIT compared to psychoeducation and supportive therapy
- When pharmacotherapy is employed, monotherapy is preferred to polytherapy. Additionally, physicians should routinely reevaluate the necessity of pharmacotherapy (1)[A].

MEDICATION

First Line

- Recommendations should be individualized based on shared decision-making after considering benefits and harms along with treating comorbid conditions (1).
- Most of the data points to antipsychotics being most effective, but use is limited by side effects and other medications (i.e., α_2-agonists) are generally used first (5).

- Antipsychotics (5)
  - Haloperidol, risperidone, aripiprazole, tiapride are probably more likely than placebo to reduce tic severity (1).
  - Pimozide and ziprasidone are possibly more likely than placebo to reduce tic severity (1).
  - Prescribe the lowest effective dose to decrease risk of side effects (1)[A].
  - Atypical (risk of weight gain an other metabolic disturbances, EPS)
    - Risperidone: Initiate 0.25 mg BID; titrate up to 4 mg/day.
    - Olanzapine: Initiate 2.5 to 5.0 mg/day; titrate up to 20 mg/day.
    - Quetiapine: Initiate 12.5 to 25.0 mg/day; titrate to 300 to 400 mg/day.
    - Ziprasidone: Initiate 5 to 10 mg/day; titrate up to 10 to 40 mg/day.
      - Must be given under ECG monitoring (1)[A]
    - Aripiprazole: Initiate 2 mg/day; titrate up to 10 to 20 mg/day.
  - Typical (high risk for EPS)
    - Haloperidol: Initiate 0.5 mg/day; titrate up to 2 to 10 mg QHS.
      - FDA approved for treating tics but considered last option of typical antipsychotics due to lower efficacy and increased side effects
    - Pimozide: Initiate 0.05 mg/kg/dose; titrate up to 0.2 mg/kg/day QHS with a max of 10 mg/day
      - FDA approved for treating tics; good for long-term control of tics, not exacerbations
      - Risk of cardiac toxicity (prolonged QTc) so give under ECG monitoring
    - Fluphenazine: Initiate 0.5 to 1.0 mg/day; titrate up to 3 mg/day in kids and 10 mg/day in adults.
- α_2-Adrenergic receptor agonists (6)[B]
  - Historically first line due to favorable side-effects but suboptimal efficacy in limited clinical trials
  - Good choice in patients with comorbid ADHD due to efficacy in treating both conditions (1)
  - Side effects: bradycardia, sedation, and hypotension. Monitor heart rate and blood pressure (1)[A].
  - Clonidine 0.1 to 0.3 mg/day given BID–TID; maximum dose 0.5 mg/day
  - Guanfacine 1 to 3 mg/day given daily or BID
    - Less sedating and longer duration of action compared with clonidine
    - Monitor QTc interval in patients with a history of cardiac conditions, patients taking QT-prolonging drugs, or patients with family history of long QT syndrome (1)[A].
- Alternative treatments
  - Topiramate: 25 to 200 mg/day (6)[A]
  - Tetrabenazine
  - Baclofen: Initiate 10 mg/day; titrate up to 10 to 80 mg/day (5).
  - Preliminary data for deutetrabenazine and valbenazine (vesicular monoamine transporter 2 [VMAT2] inhibitors) and ecopipam (novel D1 receptor antagonist) (5)
- Comorbid ADHD:
  - Stimulants: methylphenidate: 2.5 to 30.0 mg/day; dextroamphetamine: 5 to 30 mg/day
  - α_2-Adrenergic agonists: guanfacine, clonidine
  - Other medications: atomoxetine, desipramine

- Comorbid OCD (7)[B]:
  - SSRIs: fluoxetine: 10 to 80 mg/day, fluvoxamine: 50 to 300 mg/day, or sertraline: 50 to 200 mg/day
    - First-line treatment of OCD; can be used in TS as well
    - Side effects: nausea, insomnia, sexual dysfunction, headache, agitation, suicidality
    - SSRIs are not as effective in treating OCD symptoms in children with tics compared to those without tics; however, cognitive-behavioral therapy was effective in both populations making this intervention first line for OCD in patients with tic disorders (1).
  - Tricyclic antidepressants: clomipramine: 25 to 200 mg/day
    - Can be used in patients refractory to SSRIs or to augment SSRIs in partial responders
    - Side effects: weight gain, dry mouth, lowered seizure threshold, and constipation; ECG changes, including QT prolongation and tachycardia

ADDITIONAL THERAPIES
- Botulinum toxin injections for localized simple motor tics and disabling vocal tics (1)
- Habit-reversal training for tic suppression treatment: works equally for motor and vocal tics

SURGERY/OTHER PROCEDURES
Thalamic ablation and deep brain stimulation have been used experimentally and can be considered for severe, self-injurious tics (1)[C]. Patients must have failed multiple classes of medications and behavioral therapy (1)[A].

COMPLEMENTARY & ALTERNATIVE MEDICINE
- Reassurance and environmental modification
- Identification and treatment of triggers
- CBIT, hypnotherapy, biofeedback, acupuncture
- Cannabinoids: insufficient evidence to recommend; small trials show small positive effects (8).
- Physical exercise (9)

 ONGOING CARE

FOLLOW-UP RECOMMENDATIONS
Patient Monitoring
Observe for associated psychiatric disorders and inquire about suicidal thoughts (1).

PATIENT EDUCATION
- Reassurance that many patients with tics do not need medication; simply education and/or therapy
- National Tourette Syndrome Association: http://www.tsa-usa.org

PROGNOSIS
- Symptoms will fluctuate throughout illness.
- Tic severity typically stabilizes by age 25 years.
- 60–75% of young adults show some improvement in symptoms; 10–40% of patients will exhibit full remission.

REFERENCES

1. Pringsheim T, Okun MS, Müller-Vahl K, et al. Practice guideline recommendations summary: treatment of tics in people with Tourette syndrome and chronic tic disorders. *Neurology.* 2019;92(19):896–906.
2. Ayubi E, Mansori K, Doosti-Irani A. Effect of maternal smoking during pregnancy on Tourette syndrome and chronic tic disorders among offspring: a systematic review and meta-analysis. *Obstet Gynecol Sci.* 2021;64(1):1–12.
3. Brander G, Isomura K, Chang Z, et al. Association of Tourette syndrome and chronic tic disorder with metabolic and cardiovascular disorders. *JAMA Neurol.* 2019;76(4):454–461.
4. Martino D, Pringsheim TM, Cavanna AE, et al. Systematic review of severity scales and screening instruments for tics: critique and recommendations. *Mov Disord.* 2017;32(3):467–473.
5. Quezada J, Coffman KA. Current approaches and new developments in the pharmacological management of Tourette syndrome. *CNS Drugs.* 2018;32(1):33–45.
6. Huys D, Hardenacke K, Poppe P, et al. Update on the role of antipsychotics in the treatment of Tourette syndrome. *Neuropsychiatr Dis Treat.* 2012;8:95–104.
7. Pringsheim T, Steeves T. Pharmacological treatment for attention deficit hyperactivity disorder (ADHD) in children with comorbid tic disorders. *Cochrane Database Syst Rev.* 2011;(4):CD007990.
8. Curtis A, Clarke CE, Rickards HE. Cannabinoids for Tourette's syndrome. *Cochrane Database Syst Rev.* 2009;(4):CD006565.
9. Reilly C, Grant M, Bennett S, et al. Review: physical exercise in Tourette syndrome—a systematic review. *Child Adolesc Ment Health.* 2019;24(1):3–11.

CODES

ICD10
F95.2 Tourette's disorder

CLINICAL PEARLS
- TS is diagnosed by history and witnessing tics; have parent video patient's tics if not present on exam.
- Many patients require no treatment; patient should play an active role in treatment decisions.
- Nearly 50% of children with tics also have ADHD. Stimulants may be used as first-line treatment for ADHD (tics are not a contraindication, as previously believed).

T

TOXOPLASMOSIS

Jonathan Edward MacClements, MD, FAAFP

BASICS

- *Toxoplasma gondii* is an obligate intracellular protozoan parasite.
- Most common latent protozoan infection
- Clinically significant disease typically manifests only in pregnancy or in an immunocompromised patient.

DESCRIPTION

- Acute self-limited infection in immunocompetent individuals
- Acute symptomatic or reactivated latent infection in immunocompromised patients
- Congenital toxoplasmosis (acute primary infection during pregnancy)
- Ocular toxoplasmosis

Pediatric Considerations

- The earlier a fetal infection occurs, the more severe the resulting disease.
- Risk of perinatal death is 5% if infected in 1st trimester.

Pregnancy Considerations

- Pregnant immunocompromised and HIV-infected women should undergo serologic testing.
- Counsel pregnant women regarding risks of toxoplasmosis.
- Serologic testing during pregnancy is controversial.

EPIDEMIOLOGY

Incidence

- Prevalence of congenital toxoplasmosis in the United States: 10 to 100/100,000 live births
- Predominant sex: male > female

Prevalence

- Present in every country with prevalence differing worldwide. Seropositivity rates range from <10% to >90% (1)[A] with overall seroprevalence declining (2).
- In the United States, 11% of individuals aged 6 to 49 years are seropositive.
- Age-adjusted prevalence in the United States is 10%.
- Seroprevalence among women in the United States is 9%.
- Increasing prevalence of IgG seropositivity with age as a result of cumulative seropositivity
- Toxoplasmosis is considered a neglected parasitic infection in the United States and has been targeted by CDC for public health action.

ETIOLOGY AND PATHOPHYSIOLOGY

- *T. gondii* has 2 life cycles. The sexual portion of the life cycle is exclusive to felines. The asexual cycle occurs in humans. Cats become infected by eating contaminated meat (birds, mice). Oocysts form within the tract of the cat and are shed in the stool.
- Transmission to humans
  - Ingestion of raw or undercooked meat, food, or water containing tissue cysts or oocytes that is usually from soil contaminated with feline feces
  - Transplacental passage from infected mother to fetus; risk of transmission is 30% on average.
  - Blood product transfusion or solid-organ transplantation
  - Ingested *T. gondii* oocysts enter host's gastrointestinal tract where bradyzoites/tachyzoites are released, penetrate contiguous cells, replicate, and are transported to susceptible tissues causing clinical disease.

Genetics

Human leukocyte antigen (HLA) DQ3 is a genetic marker for susceptibility in HIV/AIDS patients.

RISK FACTORS

- Immunocompromised states, including HIV infection with CD4 cell count <100/μL
- Primary infection during pregnancy; risk of fetal transmission increases with gestational age at seroconversion. Transmission in the 1st trimester is associated with more severe consequences.
- Chronically infected immunocompromised pregnant women are at increased risk for transmitting congenital toxoplasmosis.

GENERAL PREVENTION

- Avoid eating undercooked meat: Cook to 152°F (66°C) or freeze for 24 hours at ≤ −12°C.
- Avoid drinking unfiltered water.
- Wash produce thoroughly.
- Wear gloves and wash hands after gardening and handling soil
- Wear gloves and wash hands after handling raw meat or cat litter.
- Avoid shellfish (*Toxoplasma* cysts).

COMMONLY ASSOCIATED CONDITIONS

- Chorioretinitis; self-limiting, febrile lymphadenopathy; mononucleosis-like illness
- Potential association with schizophrenia

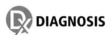

DIAGNOSIS

HISTORY

- Congenital toxoplasmosis
  - Clinical presentation varies widely; 80% of patients are asymptomatic at birth.
  - Classic triad (*uncommon*): chorioretinitis, hydrocephalus, cerebral calcifications
  - Manifestations may include prematurity, intrauterine growth retardation (IUGR).
  - Jaundice, rash with a mononucleosis-like illness
  - Mental retardation, seizures, visual defects, spasticity, sensorineural hearing loss
- Ocular toxoplasmosis
  - Chorioretinitis: focal necrotizing retinitis
  - Yellowish-white elevated cotton patch
  - Congenital disease usually bilateral; acquired is more often unilateral.
  - Symptoms include blurred vision, scotoma, pain, and photophobia.
- Acute toxoplasmosis (immunocompetent host)
  - ~90% of patients are asymptomatic.
  - Most common manifestation is bilateral, symmetric, nontender cervical lymphadenopathy.
  - Constitutional symptoms such as fever, chills, and sweats are usually mild.
  - Headaches, myalgias, pharyngitis, hepatosplenomegaly, and diffuse nonpruritic maculopapular rash may occur.
  - Pregnant women are often asymptomatic.
  - CNS: encephalitis
  - Headache; focal neurologic deficits and seizures
  - Fever usually present
  - Extracerebral toxoplasmosis: pneumonitis, chorioretinitis; rarely: GI system, liver, musculoskeletal system, heart, bone marrow, bladder, and orchitis

PHYSICAL EXAM

- In adults: fever, lymphadenopathy, nonpruritic maculopapular rash (spares palms and soles), hepatosplenomegaly, visual changes, funduscopic changes
- In newborns: hydrocephalus, neurologic abnormalities, hepatosplenomegaly, chorioretinitis, microcephaly, mental retardation

DIFFERENTIAL DIAGNOSIS

Syphilis, lymphoma, progressive multifocal leukoencephalopathy, cryptococcal meningitis, congenital TORCH infections, HIV; *Listeria* infection, tuberculosis (TB), tularemia; CMV infection; leukemia; erythroblastosis fetalis

DIAGNOSTIC TESTS & INTERPRETATION

- CBC: atypical lymphocytosis, anemia, thrombocytopenia
- Serology interpretation
  - IgM antibodies appear in the 1st week if acute infection
  - Initial test demonstrates positive IgM and negative IgG, with both tests being positive 2 weeks later.
  - If follow-up IgG is negative 2 to 4 weeks later and IgM is positive, this is likely a false positive.
  - Negative IgG rules out prior infection (IgG persists for life).
- Types of serologic tests
  - ELISA: most commonly used
  - Sabin-Feldman dye test: gold standard against which all other serologic assays are compared
  - IFA test: more available in commercial labs
  - ISAGA: widely available commercially; more sensitive and specific than IFA for detecting IgM
  - Avidity testing: confirmatory test to establish if positive IgM/IgG reflects recent or chronic infection
- PCR: *T. gondii* DNA amplification in blood or amniotic fluid; used for diagnosis of fetal infection
- Culture (rarely necessary): Organism can be isolated either by cell culture or by mouse inoculation.

Initial Tests (lab, imaging)

- Diagnosis of primary infection is typically based on history and confirmed by serology.
- Serum *Toxoplasma*-specific IgG and IgM are first step.
- According to IgM result, determine IgG avidity.
- Diagnosis of maternal infection and congenital toxoplasmosis
  - Test pregnant women who have mononucleosis-like illness but negative heterophile test for toxoplasmosis.
  - Diagnose maternal infection based on two blood samples at least 2 weeks to show seroconversion.
  - High avidity of IgG during 1st trimester argues against maternal primary infection.
  - Real-time PCR analysis of amniotic fluid predicts fetal infection and guides treatment.
  - Fetal ultrasound is useful for prognosis.
  - Routine screening for toxoplasmosis is not recommended in pregnancy.
- Neonatal diagnosis of congenital toxoplasmosis
  - Serology requires repeat testing for IgM and IgA.
  - Sample cord or peripheral blood within 2 weeks
  - Ophthalmologic, auditory, and neurologic examinations; lumbar puncture and head CT
- Diagnosis of toxoplasmic encephalitis
  - Serology for IgG
  - Imaging: MRI is more sensitive than CT scan to identify characteristic ring-enhancing lesions.
- SPECT and PET scans can help distinguish toxoplasmosis from CNS lymphoma.

Diagnostic Procedures/Other
- Lymph node biopsy
- Brain biopsy in CNS disease
- Amniocentesis with PCR (risk of false negatives and false positives)
- Placental isolation of *Toxoplasma* is diagnostic.

Test Interpretation
- Confirmatory, meningocerebritis ± abscesses with necrosis, Giemsa
- Lymph node histology shows triad of:
  - Reactive follicular hyperplasia
  - Irregular clusters of epithelioid histiocytes blurring margins of germinal centers
  - Distension of sinuses with monocytoid cells
- Sensitivity of triad 63%, specificity 91%

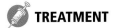 **TREATMENT**

GENERAL MEASURES
Immunocompetent patients usually require no treatment.

MEDICATION
First Line

> **ALERT**
>
> *Important*: All pyrimethamine-containing regimens should include leucovorin (folinic acid 10 to 25 mg/day PO) during and 1 week after completion of pyrimethamine to prevent drug-induced hematologic toxicity (3)[A].

- Treatment in immunocompromised hosts
  - Initial regimen of choice is pyrimethamine 200 mg loading dose PO, followed by 50 mg/day plus sulfadiazine 4 to 6 g/day PO in 4 divided doses; for those intolerant or allergic to sulfadiazine, clindamycin 600 to 1,200 mg IV or 450 mg PO QID can be used instead.
  - Alternative regimens for patients intolerant to sulfadiazine and clindamycin include the following:
    - Pyrimethamine: 200 mg loading dose PO, followed by 50 mg/day plus azithromycin 900 to 1,200 mg PO once daily
    - Pyrimethamine: 200 mg loading dose PO and then 50 mg/day plus atovaquone 1,500 mg PO BID
    - Sulfadiazine: 1,000 to 1,500 mg QID plus atovaquone 1,500 mg BID
    - Trimethoprim-sulfamethoxazole: 10/50 mg/kg/day PO or IV divided BID (for 30 days) may be a cost-effective alternative
  - Duration of therapy: typically 6 weeks, lower doses for secondary prophylaxis (3)[A]
  - Use adjunctive steroids in patients with signs of increased intracranial pressure.
  - Anticonvulsants, if there is a history of seizures
- Prophylaxis in immunocompromised patients
  - Primary prophylaxis: indicated for patients with HIV infection and CD4 count <100 cells/μL who are *T. gondii* IgG–positive
    - Trimethoprim-sulfamethoxazole-DS: 1 tablet PO daily. Alternative for sulfa allergy is dapsone 50 mg/day PO *plus* pyrimethamine 50 mg PO weekly *plus* leucovorin 25 mg PO weekly *or* atovaquone 1,500 mg PO daily.

- Secondary prophylaxis: Following 6 weeks of therapy, administer lower doses of drugs:
  - Sulfadiazine 2 to 4 g/day in 2 to 4 divided doses *plus* pyrimethamine 25 to 50 mg/day is the first choice.
  - Alternative regimens include clindamycin 600 mg PO q8h *plus* pyrimethamine 25 to 50 mg/day PO *or* atovaquone 750 mg PO BID to QID ± pyrimethamine 25 mg PO daily.
- Pregnant women (4)[A]
  - Although typically offered, it is unsure if antenatal treatment reduces congenital transmission.
  - <18 weeks' gestation: spiramycin 1 g PO q8h without food until delivery if amniotic fluid PCR is negative; does not treat infection in the fetus
  - >18 weeks' gestation: Pyrimethamine and sulfadiazine should be considered only if fetal infection is documented by positive amniotic fluid PCR (pyrimethamine is teratogenic):
    - Pyrimethamine: 50 mg PO q12h for 2 days, then 50 mg/day plus sulfadiazine 75 mg/kg PO × 1 dose and then 50 mg/kg q12h (max 4 g/day)
- Treat infected newborns regardless of clinical manifestations:
  - Pyrimethamine 2 mg/kg/day (max 50 mg) for 2 days, then 1 mg/kg/day (max 25 mg) for 2 to 6 months, and then 1 mg/kg (max 25 mg) on Monday, Wednesday, and Friday; sulfadiazine 100 mg/kg/day divided BID; and leucovorin 10 mg 3 times per week during pyrimethamine and 1 week after discontinuation
- Immunocompetent nonpregnant patients generally do not require treatment unless symptoms are severe or prolonged; one of two regimens can be used:
  - Pyrimethamine: 100 mg loading dose PO, followed by 25 to 50 mg/day *plus* sulfadiazine 2 to 4 g/day in 4 divided doses
  - Pyrimethamine: 100 mg loading dose PO, followed by 25 to 50 mg/day *plus* clindamycin 300 mg PO QID

Second Line
- Clindamycin: 900 to 1,200 mg TID IV used for ocular and CNS toxoplasmosis alone and in combination with pyrimethamine; as effective as the sulfadiazine-pyrimethamine with fewer adverse effects
- Corticosteroids (prednisone 1 to 2 mg/kg/day) are added for macular chorioretinitis or CNS infection.
- Alternatives: atovaquone (Mepron), azithromycin (Zithromax), clarithromycin (Biaxin), or dapsone *plus* pyrimethamine and leucovorin
- Trimethoprim-sulfamethoxazole appears to be equivalent to pyrimethamine-sulfadiazine in AIDS patients with CNS disease.

ADDITIONAL THERAPIES
For prevention of recurrent episode of chorioretinitis, trimethoprim-sulfamethoxazole-DS q 12 for 45 days (5)

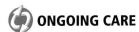 **ONGOING CARE**

FOLLOW-UP RECOMMENDATIONS
Patient Monitoring
Precautions
- Monitor for bone marrow, renal, or liver toxicity.
- Good hydration: Sulfadiazine is poorly soluble and may crystallize in the urine.

- Watch for antibiotic-associated diarrhea.
- Sulfonamides may alter phenytoin and warfarin levels or interfere with oral hypoglycemic agents.

PATIENT EDUCATION
- http://www.aafp.org/afp/2003/0515/p2145.html
- http://familydoctor.org/familydoctor/en/diseases-conditions/toxoplasmosis.html

PROGNOSIS
- Immunodeficient patients often relapse if treatment or suppression therapy is stopped.
- Treatment may prevent the development of untoward sequelae in infants with congenital toxoplasmosis.

REFERENCES

1. Torgerson PR, Mastroiacovo P. The global burden of congenital toxoplasmosis: a systematic review. *Bull World Health Organ*. 2013;91(7):501–508.
2. Jones JL, Kruszon-Moran D, Elder S, et al. *Toxoplasma gondii* Infection in the United States, 2011–2014. *Am J Trop Med Hyg*. 2018;98(2):551–557.
3. Dunay IR, Gajurel K, Dhakal R, et al. Treatment of toxoplasmosis: historical perspective, animal models and current clinical practice. *Clin Microbiol Rev*. 2018;31(4):e00057–17.
4. Paquet C, Yudin MH; and Society of Obstetricians and Gynaecologists of Canada. Toxoplasmosis in pregnancy: prevention, screening, and treatment. *J Obstet Gynaecol Can*. 2013;35(1):78–81.
5. Felix JPF, Lira RPC, Zacchia RS, et al. Trimethoprim-sulfamethoxazole versus placebo to reduce the risk of recurrences of *Toxoplasma gondii* retinochoroiditis: randomized controlled clinical trial. *Am J Ophthalmol*. 2014;157(4):762–766.e1.

 CODES

ICD10
- B58.9 Toxoplasmosis, unspecified
- P37.1 Congenital toxoplasmosis
- B58.2 Toxoplasma meningoencephalitis

CLINICAL PEARLS
- Toxoplasmosis is typically asymptomatic in immunocompetent patients.
- Primary prevention is important, particularly for pregnant women and immunodeficient patients.
- The most common manifestation of acute toxoplasmosis in immunocompetent host is bilateral, symmetric, nontender cervical lymphadenopathy.
- Universal screening for congenital toxoplasmosis is not currently recommended.
- Serologic testing should be performed at a reference laboratory. CDC recommends the reference laboratory at Palo Alto Medical Foundation Toxoplasma Serology Laboratory (http://www.pamf.org/serology/External).

T

TRACHEITIS, BACTERIAL

Mary E. Cataletto, MD, FAAP, FCCP • Margaret J. McCormick, MS, RN, CNE

 BASICS

DESCRIPTION
- Acute, life-threatening upper airway obstruction due to infraglottic bacterial infection following a primary viral infection (typically parainfluenza or influenza)
- Historically high mortality rates of up to 20% in children (1); more recent experience suggests changing epidemiology resulting in a more atypical presentation and variable course (2) but which can still result in severe, acute, upper airway obstruction
- Affects two major groups of patients in the pediatric age range (1)
  – Those with a native intact airway
  – Those with an artificial airway
- Often preceded by viral infection, such as influenza, parainfluenza, or respiratory syncytial virus (1)
- *Staphylococcus* is the most common bacteria identified (2).
- Diagnostic hallmarks on endoscopy: ulceration, pseudomembranes in the trachea with thick mucopurulent exudates and mucosal sloughing (1),(2)
- System(s) affected: pulmonary
- Synonym(s): laryngotracheobronchitis; bacterial croup; pseudomembranous croup

EPIDEMIOLOGY
Incidence
- Incidence: 4 to 8 per 1 million children (1)
- Approximately 0.1/100,000 children-years in United Kingdom
- Peak incidence in children: fall and winter (1)
- Mean age: 5 years (1),(3)
- Infections in adolescents and adults have been reported.

Prevalence
- Rare illness
- Methicillin-resistant *Staphylococcus aureus* (MRSA) may contribute to changing epidemiology and virulence.

ETIOLOGY AND PATHOPHYSIOLOGY
- Methicillin-sensitive *S. aureus* (MSSA) accounted for 50% cases in Casazza series (2019) (2).
- Mixed respiratory
- *Streptococcus pneumoniae*
- In children with artificial airway, most common organisms are *S. aureus*, *Haemophilus influenzae*, *S. pneumoniae*, *Pseudomonas aeruginosa*, and other gram-negative organisms (1).
- Viral-induced injury to the respiratory epithelium in conjunction with localized immune impairment can predispose individuals to bacterial superinfection.

Genetics
No known genetic predisposition

RISK FACTORS
- Periods of increased seasonal activity of respiratory viruses
- Reports following tonsillectomy, adenoidectomy, with chronic tracheal aspiration, and with evidence of other concurrent infections, including sinusitis, otitis, pneumonia, or pharyngitis

GENERAL PREVENTION
- Standard precautions, with scrupulous attention to hand washing
- Vaccination against viruses that may predispose to bacterial tracheitis
- In children with artificial airways, periodic surveillance of tracheal cultures can be helpful.

COMMONLY ASSOCIATED CONDITIONS
- Consider anatomic abnormalities, foreign bodies as well as recent pharyngeal or laryngeal surgery.
- Predisposing: Down syndrome, immunodeficiency, subglottic hemangioma, tracheoesophageal fistula repair, tracheobronchomalacia
- More common in children with tracheostomy
- Viral coinfection may occur.

DIAGNOSIS
- Careful history and physical exam are the best methods to help distinguish bacterial tracheitis from croup and other rare causes of upper airway obstruction.
- The diagnosis of bacterial tracheitis is confirmed by flexible laryngoscopy, operative bronchoscopy, and/or autopsy. Findings include mucopurulent exudates, ulcerations, and pseudomembranes within the subglottis and/or trachea (2).

HISTORY
- Presentation can be variable from mild to severe with high fever and systemic toxicity (2).
- Classic presentation (1):
  – Prodromal upper respiratory tract symptoms
  – Gradual progression of mild upper airway symptoms over 1 hour to 6 days to acute, febrile phase of rapid respiratory decompensation
  – Drooling usually absent
  – No response to aerosolized epinephrine and/or systemic corticosteroids
- Individuals with artificial airways may have a more indolent case and are also more likely to experience recurrence.

PHYSICAL EXAM
- Acute onset
- High fever
- Inspiratory stridor
- Respiratory distress
- Toxic appearance
- Voice and cry usually normal
- Drooling uncommon
- Atypical presentations can also occur and some may present with URI symptoms.
- Children with artificial airways can have more indolent onset (2).

DIFFERENTIAL DIAGNOSIS
- Severe croup (viral)
- Spasmodic croup
- Diphtheria in unimmunized individuals
- Retropharyngeal abscess
- Epiglottitis
- Bronchiolitis
- Bacterial pneumonia
- Foreign body aspiration
- Angioneurotic edema

DIAGNOSTIC TESTS & INTERPRETATION
- Tracheal endoscopy (rigid bronchoscopy in children with intact airway or tracheoscopy in those with artificial airway) provides a definitive diagnosis (1)[C].
- Diffuse inflammation of larynx, trachea, and bronchi
- Mucopurulent exudate; microabscesses may be present.
- Semiadherent membranes (containing numerous neutrophils and cellular debris) may be identified within the trachea.

Initial Tests (lab, imaging)
Obtain Gram stain and aerobic, anaerobic, and viral cultures of tracheal secretions during the tracheal endoscopy. Bacterial cultures of tracheal secretions are required for culture isolates and sensitivities.
- Tracheal biopsy is rarely indicated but may be considered in immunodeficient child or child with ulcerative colitis.
- Routine laboratory studies are not required to make the diagnosis and are rarely helpful.
- Rapid antigen or polymerase chain reaction (PCR)-based testing for respiratory viruses may be helpful.
- CBC results may vary.
  – WBC count may show marked leukocytosis or may be normal.
  – Increased band cell count
- Chest radiographs are neither definitive nor diagnostic of bacterial tracheitis but may be helpful in identifying associated pneumonia.

- Anteroposterior (AP) and lateral neck x-rays show subglottic and tracheal narrowing (i.e., steeple sign on AP film).

Follow-Up Tests & Special Considerations

- In patients with pneumonia, follow-up chest films may be required.
- Repeat bronchoscopies may be needed to remove pseudomembranes.
- Children with or at risk for acute airway obstruction should be carefully monitored in a setting and with personnel capable of securing a pediatric airway.

 TREATMENT

- Consider as a potentially life-threatening airway emergency.
- Children with suspected or actual bacterial tracheitis should be cared for in a pediatric ICU (3)[C].
- Assess and monitor respiratory status; supplemental oxygen may be necessary.
- Airway protection and support, as necessary (at least 50% require intubation; some studies report up to 100% [80% require intubation; 94% admitted to PICU])
- Ventilatory support may be required.

GENERAL MEASURES

- Consider bacterial tracheitis as a potentially life-threatening airway emergency.
- Support care and monitoring in PICU care often required (1)[C].
- Supplemental oxygen, endotracheal intubation, and/or mechanical ventilation may be required.

MEDICATION

- Empiric therapy should cover the most common pathogens until sensitivities are available: antistaphylococcal agent (vancomycin or clindamycin) and a 3rd-generation cephalosporin (e.g., ceftriaxone or cefotaxime) (1)[C].
- In the case of technology-dependent children with tracheostomy, make initial antibiotic choices based on previous tracheal culture.
- Narrow regimen when pathogens and sensitivities available (1)[C]
- Systemic or inhaled corticosteroids or racemic epinephrine have no proven efficacy in relieving airway obstruction in bacterial tracheitis (1).
- Contraindications: Refer to the manufacturer's literature for each drug.
- Precautions: Refer to the manufacturer's literature for each drug.
- Significant possible interactions: Refer to the manufacturer's literature for each medication.

- Complications:
  - Acute respiratory distress syndrome (1),(2)
  - Pneumonia
  - Pneumothorax
  - Toxic shock syndrome (2)
  - Septic shock (2)
  - Disseminated intravascular coagulation (2)
  - Tracheal stenosis, especially with prolonged intubation
  - Cardiopulmonary arrest

ISSUES FOR REFERRAL

- All children with suspected or actual bacterial tracheitis should be cared for in a pediatric ICU.
- Critical care teams may include ID, ENT, and pulmonary consultants in addition to the pediatric intensivist.

SURGERY/OTHER PROCEDURES

- Therapeutic bronchoscopy may be needed to facilitate the removal of inspissated secretions and accumulated debris (3).
- Tracheostomy is usually not necessary.

COMPLEMENTARY & ALTERNATIVE MEDICINE

No evidence to support use

ADMISSION, INPATIENT, AND NURSING CONSIDERATIONS

- Diagnostic endoscopic evaluation of the upper airway
- Airway stabilization and support
- Pediatric intensive care admission

Pediatric Considerations

- Suctioning and pulmonary toilet
- Hydration
- Antibiotics as described above
- Nursing
  - Provide a calm, quiet environment for child once endoscopy and cultures are done.
  - Airway monitoring
  - Frequent suctioning
  - Monitor fluid balance.
  - Establish and maintain open lines of communication with child and parent.

 ONGOING CARE

FOLLOW-UP RECOMMENDATIONS

Patient Monitoring

Children with artificial airway will require ongoing follow-up.

DIET

Varies with clinical situations

PATIENT EDUCATION

Keep immunizations up to date.

PROGNOSIS

- Intubation generally 3 to 11 days
- Usually requires 3 to 7 days of hospitalization
- With effective early recognition and management, complete recovery can be expected.
- Cardiopulmonary arrest and death have occurred.
- Higher recurrence rates in children with artificial airways

REFERENCES

1. Kuo CY, Parikh SR. Bacterial tracheitis. *Pediatr Rev.* 2014;35(11):497–499.
2. Casazza G, Graham ME, Nelson D, et al. Pediatric bacterial tracheitis—a variable entity: case series with literature review. *Otolaryngol Head Neck Surg.* 2019;160(3):546–549.
3. Blot M, Bonniaud-Blot P, Favrolt N, et al. Update on childhood and adult infectious tracheitis. *Med Mal Infect.* 2017;47(7):443–452.

ADDITIONAL READING

- Huang YL, Peng CC, Chiu NC, et al. Bacterial tracheitis in pediatrics: 12 year experience at a medical center in Taiwan. *Pediatr Int.* 2009;51(1):110–113.
- Russell CJ, Shiroishi MS, Siantz E, et al. The use of inhaled antibiotic therapy in the treatment of ventilator-associated pneumonia and tracheobronchitis: a systematic review. *BMC Pulm Med.* 2016;16:40.

CODES

ICD10

- J04.10 Acute tracheitis without obstruction
- J04.11 Acute tracheitis with obstruction
- J05.0 Acute obstructive laryngitis [croup]

CLINICAL PEARLS

- Bacterial tracheitis is an acute, potentially life-threatening, infraglottic bacterial infection which generally follows a primary viral infection.
- Bacterial tracheitis should be suspected in croup-like cases who fail to respond to oral or inhaled corticosteroids and racemic epinephrine.
- Bronchoscopy (or tracheoscopy in the child with an artificial airway) provides a definitive diagnosis.
- Initial treatment priorities include broad-spectrum antibiotic coverage, aggressive airway protection, and supportive care.

T

TRANSGENDER HEALTH
George W. Matar, MD • Michelle Caster, MD

BASICS

DESCRIPTION

- Lesbian, gay, bisexual, and transgender individuals continue to be medically underserved and subject to unique health care disparities, including higher rates of mental and physical comorbidities and a greater need for health care services. Better education of physicians and other providers is imperative to improve the health of the transgender population. Such education begins with teaching acceptance of all human beings into health care and ensuring a welcoming and safe office environment for transgender individuals to speak openly with knowledgeable and culturally competent clinicians.
  - As of 2015, estimates indicate 0.7% of youth (age 13 to 17 years), or some 150,000 people, and 0.6% of U.S. adults, or some 1.4 million people, identify themselves as transgender, a 2-fold increase since 2011 (1).
- Gender identity, the sense of one's self as male or female, and especially gender presentation, the outward expression of gender, may or may not reflect the self-identification of a transgender and gender nonbinary (TGNB) patient. Transgender status says nothing about an individual's sexual orientation. Transgender people may be sexually oriented toward men, women, other transgender people, or any combination of the above. TGNB patients are further defined by those who have undergone surgical procedures and/or medical treatment to better align gender identity, by those who plan such procedures in the future, and by others who do not.
- Ask transgender patients how they would describe themselves and to honor terminology acceptable to each patient, specifically preferred name, preferred pronoun, preferred gender identity, and sex assigned at birth, those attributes then entered in the electronic medical record (2).
- Transgender people have a unique set of mental and physical needs (3),(4).
  - Stigma and discrimination are barriers to health care.
  - 24% of transgender persons report unequal treatment in health care environments, 19% report refusal of care altogether, 33% do not seek preventive services, and 23% delay needed care (4).
  - 91% of transgender patients want counseling and/or hormones even though only 65% ever get any of these (2).
- Many U.S. insurance companies require a diagnosis of gender dysphoria (definition: distress and unease experienced if gender identity and designated gender are not completely congruent) for reimbursement of transgender medical and surgical interventions (5).
  - Despite the fact that being transgender is not a behavioral health condition, the codes for a transgender diagnosis are in the mental health section in the International Classification of Diseases, 10th revision (ICD-10).

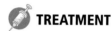

DIAGNOSIS

- Specific health concerns
  - Transition-related medical care, or gender-affirming therapy, including hormone therapy and surgical treatment, or gender-affirming surgery (GAS), helps patients align primary and secondary sexual characteristics with gender identity (3).
  - The World Professional Association for Transgender Health (WPATH) has published standards of care (SOCs) that include hormone therapy and GAS (3),(4).
    - Hormone therapy and surgery not only treat symptoms of gender dysphoria but also help transgender patients improve quality of life, self-esteem, and anxiety (4).
    - Hormone therapy does convey a greater risk of thromboembolic disease (venous thromboembolism [VTE]), erythrocytosis, hypertriglyceridemia, elevated liver enzymes, development of gallstones, cardiovascular (CV) disease, metabolic disease, and decreased fertility (3),(4).
    - Treatment is associated with a high degree of patient satisfaction, low prevalence of regrets, and significant relief of gender dysphoria.
- Specific diseases
  - HIV/AIDS
    - Among those respondents to the Transgender Discrimination Survey, 1.4% were living with HIV, which is 5 times higher than that of the general population in the U.S. Worldwide, the prevalence may be 50 times higher than the background rate (1),(3).
    - Requires increased vigilance on the part of the health care providers to counsel patients
- Psychosocial considerations
  - Transgender people are at risk of intimate partner violence; mental health issues, including depression and anxiety; and suicide.
    - 40% of transgender people have attempted suicide compared to 1.6% of the U.S. general population (3).
    - Transgender people are at greater risk of societal discrimination including housing and workforce discrimination, are more likely to be unemployed, homeless, be victims of truancy and bullying, and lacking in social support, owing to federal and state laws that inadequately protect transgender people from discrimination (3),(4).
  - Psychosocial assessment is recommended at baseline and at least annually (4).
  - Mental health and substance abuse screening are also indicated (4).

ALERT

- Transgender patients are at increased risk of suicidal ideation, suicide attempts, and suicide (3),(4).
- Transgender patients are often reluctant to disclose gender identity or expression, owing to the risk of stigma or discrimination.
- Improving access to care
  - Barriers to health care and the need for respectful, supportive and inclusive clinic environments by following transgender-friendly concepts

- Financial barriers
  - According to the 2015 transgender survey, 29% of respondents were currently living in poverty, compared with 14% of the general U.S. population. More than half (55%) of transgender participants who completed the survey had been denied coverage for transition-related surgery and 25% were denied coverage for hormone therapy.

HISTORY

- When assessing transgender patients for gender-affirming care, evaluate the magnitude, duration, and stability of any gender dysphoria or incongruence (3),(4).
- Evaluation of the support and safety of patients' social environment is ideally accomplished with multidisciplinary care (3),(4).

PHYSICAL EXAM

Transgender patients may experience discomfort during the physical examination because of ongoing dysphoria or negative past experiences (4). Examinations should be based on the patient's current anatomy and specific needs for the visit and should be explained, chaperoned, and stopped as indicated by the patient's comfort level.

TREATMENT

GENERAL MEASURES

- Care of transgender people, including hormone therapy, is within the scope of primary care providers.
- Education of health care providers, for physicians, and those beginning in medical school, is crucial to providing optimal care to transgender patients (1).

MEDICATION

First Line

- Gender-affirming hormone therapy (specific information on gender-affirming hormone therapy can be found in the Endocrine Society's Clinical Practice Guidelines) (6)
- Hormonal therapy for transgender adolescents (6)
  - Suppress pubertal development using reversible puberty blockers, such as gonadotropin-releasing hormone (GnRH) analogues, when adolescents first exhibit pubertal physical changes (Tanner stage 2).
  - Gender-affirming hormones at about age 16 years or with adolescents presenting for gender-affirming hormone therapy after initiation of puberty
  - Initiate treatment after persistent gender dysphoria has been confirmed by a multidisciplinary team of medical and mental health providers and the patient has the mental capacity to provide informed consent, generally by age 16 years.
- Hormonal therapy for transgender adults
  - The two major goals of hormonal therapy are to reduce endogenous sex hormone levels, and thus reduce the secondary sex characteristics of the individual's designated gender, and to replace endogenous sex hormone levels consistent with the individual's gender identity by using the principles of hormone replacement treatment of hypogonadal patients.

– Feminizing therapy
  ○ Treatment with physiologic doses of estrogen alone is insufficient to suppress testosterone levels into the normal range for females. Multiple adjunctive medications such as progestins with antiandrogen activity and GnRH agonists are needed.
  ○ Results in redistribution of body fat, decrease in muscle mass and strength, softening of skin/decreased oiliness, decreased sexual desire, decreased spontaneous erections, male sexual dysfunction, breast growth, decreased testicular volume, decreased sperm production, and possible scalp hair
– Masculinizing therapy
  ○ Regimens similar to the general principle of hormone replacement treatment with testosterone in male hypogonadism; results in skin oiliness/acne, facial/body hair growth, scalp hair loss, increased muscle mass/strength, fat redistribution, cessation of menses, clitoral enlargement, vaginal atrophy, deepening of voice

SURGERY/OTHER PROCEDURES

- Criteria for GAS per the WPATH includes persistent, well-documented gender dysphoria; capacity to make a fully informed decision and to consent for treatment; legal age of majority in the given country; and if significant medical or mental health concerns are present, they must be well controlled.
- 12 months of continuous hormone therapy are recommended or required for some procedures (e.g., genital surgery) but not for others (e.g., mastectomy) per WPATH.
- The rate of GAS is increasing, with some 25% of transgender patients having undergone some form of GAS (2).
- GAS has a positive impact on individual health in that it improves mental health, results in a higher quality of life, and results in a higher socioeconomic status. It also enhances public health by increasing cultural awareness and decreasing social stigma (5).

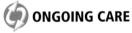 **ONGOING CARE**

FOLLOW-UP RECOMMENDATIONS
Interacting with the health care system
- Discrimination on the part of health care providers is a major barrier to care.

Patient Monitoring
- Transmasculine individuals (3)
  – Breast cancer screening for patients who have breast tissue with careful review of operative reports
  – Cervical cancer screening for those who have a cervix according to age-related guidelines
- Transfeminine individuals (3)
  – Prostate cancer screening should follow the recommendations for cisgender men.
  – Breast cancer screening should begin after 50 years of age and after a minimum of 5 years of feminizing hormone use, with a health care professional–patient discussion about the potential harms of over screening.

- Routine laboratory testing and physical exam should be completed per hormone use as indicated by the Endocrine Society's Clinical Practice Guidelines (6).
- Screening for HIV and sexually transmitted infections (STIs) based on patient's behaviors and present anatomy; pre- and post-exposure HIV prophylaxis should be considered for patients who meet criteria.
- Anal cancer screening with anal Pap smear. If performed, abnormal results should be followed with high-resolution anoscopy, which is not available in all settings.
- Evaluation of CV risk factors
- Bone mineral density tests, as indicated
- Age-appropriate and behavior-specific immunizations (e.g., human papillomavirus)
- Screening for intimate partner violence
- Fertility, pregnancy, contraception, and abortion (3)
  – Fertility and parenting desires should be discussed early in the process of transition, before the initiation of hormone therapy or gender affirmation surgery; patients should be informed of out-of-pocket costs, which vary by state and insurance coverage.
  – Transmasculine individuals
    ○ May safely achieve pregnancy after cessation of testosterone
    ○ Contraception can be underutilized in this population because of concerns of adverse effects or access to care.
  – Transfeminine individuals
    ○ If retaining gonads, may need to use assisted reproductive technologies to achieve pregnancy and others may have return of fertility within months of ceasing hormone therapy; it is best practice to encourage sperm banking.
  – Contraception
    ○ Gender-affirming hormone therapy is not effective contraception. Transmasculine individuals should be consulted that lack of menses does not mean they are unable to conceive. In addition, testosterone use is not a specific contraindication to using any form of contraception. All patients should be counseled on barrier use for prevention of STIs.
    ○ In adults, monitor physical changes and any adverse changes every 3 months during the 1st year of hormone therapy and then once or twice yearly. Transgender males: Check serum testosterone every 3 months until levels are in the normal physiologic male range; check hematocrit and hemoglobin at baseline and every 3 months in year 1 and then once or twice a year; monitor lipids as indicated. Transgender females: Check serum testosterone and estradiol every 3 months; if patient is on spironolactone, check serum electrolytes every 3 months in the 1st year of treatment and then annually.

PATIENT EDUCATION
- Hormone therapy and potential health risks
- Counseling for GAS
- Legal issues
  – Under the Affordable Care Act (ACA), denial of treatment of being transgender as a "preexisting condition" is banned.

– Since 2014, Centers for Medicare & Medicaid Services (CMS) has been providing transition-related coverage (7).
– The U.S. Department of Veterans Affairs (VA), although acknowledging the need to care for transgender veterans, denies coverage of gender-confirming surgery on the basis of a VA regulation that excludes gender alterations from the medical benefits package.

REFERENCES

1. Korpaisarn S, Safer JD. Gaps in transgender medical education among healthcare providers: a major barrier to care for transgender persons. *Rev Endocr Metab Disord*. 2018;19(3):271–275.
2. Nolan IT, Kuhner CJ, Dy GW. Demographic and temporal trends in transgender identities and gender confirming surgery. *Trans Androl Urol*. 2019;8(3):184–190.
3. Health care for transgender and gender diverse individuals: ACOG Committee Opinion, Number 823. *Obstet Gynecol*. 2021;137(3):e75–e88.
4. Klein D, Paradise SL, Goodwin E. Caring for transgender and gender-diverse persons: what clinicians should know. *Am Fam Physician*. 2018;98(11):645–653.
5. Safer JD, Tangpricha V. Care of transgender persons. *N Engl J Med*. 2019;381(25):2451–2460.
6. Hembree WC, Cohen-Kettenis PT, Gooren L, et al. Endocrine treatment of gender-dysphoric/gender-incongruent persons: an Endocrine Society clinical practice guideline. *J Clin Endocrinol Metab*. 2017;102(11):3869–3903.
7. Williams EA, Patete CL, Thaller SR. Gender affirmation surgery from public health perspective: advances, challenges, and areas of opportunity. *J Craniofac Surg*. 2019;30(5):1349–1351.

ADDITIONAL READING

HealthyPeople.gov. Lesbian, gay, bisexual, and transgender health. https://www.healthypeople.gov/2020/topics-objectives/topic/lesbian-gay-bisexual-and-transgender-health. Accessed September 14, 2020.

 CODES

ICD10
- F64.1 Gender identity disorder in adolescence and adulthood
- Z11.4 Encounter for screening for human immunodeficiency virus
- Z72.52 High risk homosexual behavior

CLINICAL PEARLS

- Health care providers must be sensitive to the unique needs of transgender patients; must be open to the care of such patients; and should, as with all patients, display an ethical, principled, and timely approach to care.
- Do use inclusive language in the care of transgender patients, assessing the individuals' preferences, and respect differences among transgender patients.

TRANSIENT ISCHEMIC ATTACK (TIA)

Samuel E. Mathis, MD • Haris Vakil, MD

 BASICS

DESCRIPTION

- A transient episode of neurologic dysfunction due to focal brain, retinal, or spinal cord ischemia without acute infarction
- Major predictor of stroke: 7.5–17.4% of patients with transient ischemic attack (TIA) experience a stroke within 3 months (1). 15% of patients with stroke report recent TIA.
- Synonym(s): ministroke

EPIDEMIOLOGY

Incidence
200,000 to 500,000 new TIA cases reported each year. Nearly 800,000 patients experience stroke per year in the United States, of which nearly 700,000 are acute ischemic stroke (1).

Prevalence
- Prevalence of TIA in general population: ~2.0%
- Predominant age: Risk increases >60 years; highest in 7th and 8th decades
- Predominant sex: male > female
- Predominant race/ethnicity: African Americans > Hispanics > Caucasians

ETIOLOGY AND PATHOPHYSIOLOGY
Temporary reduction/cessation of cerebral blood flow adversely affecting neuronal function

- Carotid/vertebral atherosclerotic disease
  - Artery-to-artery thromboembolism
  - Low-flow ischemia
- Small, deep vessel disease associated with hypertension (HTN) and diabetes
  - Lacunar infarcts
- Embolism secondary to the following:
  - Valvular (mitral valve) pathology
  - Mural hypokinesias/akinesias with thrombosis (acute anterior MI/congestive cardiomyopathies)
  - Cardiac arrhythmia (Atrial fibrillation accounts for 5–20% incidence.)
- Hypercoagulable states
  - Antiphospholipid antibodies
  - Increased estrogen (e.g., oral contraceptives)
  - Pregnancy and parturition
- Arteritis
  - Noninfectious necrotizing vasculitis
  - Drugs, irradiation, local trauma
- Sympathomimetic drugs (e.g., cocaine)
- Other causes: spontaneous and posttraumatic (e.g., chiropractic manipulation) arterial dissection
- Fibromuscular dysplasia

Genetics
Inheritance is polygenic, with tendency to clustering of risk factors within families.

RISK FACTORS
- Older age (i.e., >60 years old)
- HTN, cardiac diseases (atrial fibrillation, MI, valvular disease)
- Atherosclerotic disease (carotid/vertebral stenosis)
- Diabetes
- Hyperlipidemia
- Obesity
- Cigarette smoking
- Thrombophilias

GENERAL PREVENTION
- Lifestyle changes: smoking cessation, diet modification, weight loss, regular aerobic exercise, and limited alcohol intake
- Strict control of medical risk factors: *diabetes* (glycemic control), *HTN* (thiazide and/or ACE/ARB), *hyperlipidemia* (statins), anticoagulation when high risk of cardioembolism (e.g., atrial fibrillation, mechanical valves)
- Improved blood pressure control has been very useful, with antiplatelet therapy being key for preventing recurrence if previous TIA (2)

ALERT
- 1.5–3.5% risk of stroke in first 48 hours after TIA
- Up to 40% of patients with stroke have history of TIA

Geriatric Considerations
- Older patients have a higher mortality rate—highest in 7th and 8th decades.
- Atrial fibrillation is a frequent cause among the elderly.

Pediatric Considerations
- Congenital heart disease is a common cause among pediatric patients.
- Genetic: Marfan syndrome, moyamoya, or sickle cell disease

Pregnancy Considerations
- Preeclampsia, eclampsia, and HELLP syndrome
- TTP and hemolytic uremic syndrome
- Postpartum angiopathy
- Cerebral venous thrombosis
- Hypercoagulable states related to pregnancy

COMMONLY ASSOCIATED CONDITIONS
- Atrial fibrillation, uncontrolled HTN
- Carotid stenosis
- Some disease processes mimic TIA presentation (seizures, migraines, metabolic disturbances, syncope, multiple sclerosis)
  - Difference: gradual onset with nonspecific symptoms (headache, memory loss) vs acute onset with specific neurologic deficits (TIA)

DIAGNOSIS

HISTORY
- Emphasis on symptom onset, progression, and recovery
- Carotid circulation (hemispheric): monocular visual loss, hemiplegia, hemianesthesia, neglect, aphasia, visual field defects (amaurosis fugax); less often, headaches, seizures, amnesia, confusion
- Vertebrobasilar (brain stem/cerebellar): bilateral visual obscuration, diplopia, vertigo, ataxia, facial paresis, Horner syndrome, dysphagia, dysarthria; also headache, nausea, vomiting, and ataxia
- Past medical history, baseline functional status

- ABCD2 with imaging or ABCD3-I score: helps predict CVA risk after TIA (3)[B]
  - Score of 0 to 1: 0%; 2 to 3: 1.3%; 4 to 5: 4.1%; 6 to 7: 8.1%
    - **A**ge >65 years: 1 point
    - **B**P 140/90 mm Hg: 1 point
    - **C**linical presentation
      - Unilateral weakness: 2 points
      - Speech impaired without weakness: 1 point
    - **D**uration: 1 to 2 points based on time
    - **D**iabetes: 1 point
    - **D**ual TIA (within 7 days preceding): 2 points
    - **I**maging (new lesion or carotid stenosis): 2 points

PHYSICAL EXAM
- Vital signs, oxygen saturation
- Thorough neurologic and cardiac exams

DIFFERENTIAL DIAGNOSIS
- Evolving stroke
- Migraine (hemiplegic)
- Focal seizure (Todd paralysis)
- Bell palsy
- Neoplasm of brain, subarachnoid hemorrhage
- Intoxication
- Glucose or other electrolyte abnormalities
- Central nervous system infection
- Multiple sclerosis

DIAGNOSTIC TESTS & INTERPRETATION

Initial Tests (lab, imaging)
- Neuroimaging within 24 hours of symptom onset
- MRI, including diffusion-weighted imaging, is the preferred brain diagnostic modality to rule out stroke; if not available, then noncontrast head CT (1)
- Noninvasive imaging of the cervicocephalic vessels should be performed routinely in suspected TIA by carotid US/TCD, MRA, or CTA depending on availability and expertise and characteristics of the patient (4)[B].
- Routine blood tests (CBC, chemistry, PT/PTT, UPT, coagulation screen, fasting lipid panel, ECG) are reasonable in evaluation of patient with TIA (4)[B].

Follow-Up Tests & Special Considerations
- Transesophageal echo (TEE) is useful in identifying patent foramen ovale (PFO), aortic arch atherosclerosis, and valvular disease (4)[B].
- Prolonged cardiac monitoring is useful in patients with an unclear etiology after initial brain imaging and ECG (4)[B].
- EEG: if seizure suspected

Diagnostic Procedures/Other
- Computed tomography (CT) is typically the first neuroimaging test. Preferred variant is noncontrast, but probability of detecting acute tissue changes after ischemic symptoms resolve within 24 hours is 4% (1).
- Diffusion-weighted MRI can identify brain ischemia within minutes of onset and is highly sensitive (88% sensitivity within 24 hours) and specific (95% specificity) for acute infarction and will guide management (1).

TREATMENT

GENERAL MEASURES

- TIA is a neurologic emergency. Current evidence suggests that patients with high-risk TIAs require rapid referral and a 24-hour admission for observation and workup.
- Outpatient investigations may be considered based on patient's stroke risk, arrangement of follow-up, and social circumstances.
- Antiplatelet therapy to prevent recurrence or future CVA
- Treatment/control of underlying associated conditions

MEDICATION

- For patients with TIA, the use of antiplatelet agents rather than oral anticoagulation is recommended to reduce risk of recurrent stroke and other cardiovascular events, with the exception of cardioembolic etiologies (4)[A].
- Uncertain if switching agent in patients who have additional ischemic attacks while on antiplatelet therapy is beneficial (5)[C]

First Line

- Enteric-coated aspirin: 160 to 325 mg/day in the acute phase (5)[A] followed by long-term antiplatelet therapy for noncardioembolic TIA and anticoagulation for cardioembolic etiology
- Antiplatelet therapy
  – Aspirin 81 to 325 mg/day (5)[A]
    o Contraindications: active peptic ulcer disease and hypersensitivity to aspirin or NSAIDs
    o Precautions: may aggravate preexisting PUD; or worsen symptoms of asthma
    o Significant possible interactions: may potentiate effects of anticoagulants and sulfonylurea analogues
  – ER dipyridamole—aspirin (Aggrenox): 25/200 mg BID (5)[B]
    o Combined therapy with dipyridamole and aspirin not proven to have greater efficacy (4)
    o More expensive than aspirin alone and may have more associated side effects
  – Clopidogrel 75 mg/day (5)[B]
    o Can be used in patients who are allergic to aspirin (5)[B]
    o Precautions: Thrombotic thrombocytopenic purpura (TTP) can occur and increases risk of bleeding when combined with aspirin.
    o May be very slightly more effective than aspirin alone (5)[B]; more expensive and more side effects than aspirin
- Combined aspirin and clopidogrel therapy has shown to reduce the incidence of subsequent stroke for high-risk TIA patients by 21% without increased risk of bleeding when used for a duration of 1 month or less immediately following TIA or CVA (2)[A].
- Anticoagulation therapy
  – Direct thrombin inhibitor:
    o Dabigatran (Pradaxa)
    o Idarucizumab (Praxbind) reversal agent
  – Factor Xa inhibitors:
    o Apixaban (Eliquis)
    o Rivaroxaban (Xarelto)
    o Edoxaban (Savaysa)
  – Warfarin (INR-adjusted dose) (5)[A]

Second Line

- Aspirin 325 mg/day or aspirin 81 mg/day plus clopidogrel 75 mg/day (5)[A]
  – Reserved for patients who cannot take anticoagulation for reasons other than bleeding risk
- Ticlopidine (Ticlid): 250 mg PO BID
  – For patients unable to tolerate other agents
  – Contraindications: hypersensitivity, presence of hematopoietic/hemostatic disorders, conditions associated with bleeding, severe liver dysfunction
  – Precautions: neutropenia (0.8% severe), which is reversible with cessation of the drug. Monitor blood counts every 2 weeks for first 3 months. TTP can occur.
  – Significant possible interactions: Digoxin plasma levels decreased 15%; theophylline half-life increased from 8.6 to 12.2 hours.

ISSUES FOR REFERRAL

Vascular surgery if carotid endarterectomy appropriate

ADDITIONAL THERAPIES

- Secondary prevention of TIA should be initiated; venous thromboembolism (VTE) prophylaxis
- High-dose statin (4)
- BP should be reduced after 24 hours. Thiazides, ACE inhibitors, and ARBs have shown to be of benefit. β-Blockers have not shown benefit in reducing TIA recurrence or stroke.
- Patients with diabetes mellitus or pre-DM should be advised to follow ADA guidelines to maintain glycemic control.

SURGERY/OTHER PROCEDURES

- Consider carotid endarterectomy in patients with a high degree of carotid artery stenosis ≥70%.
- When carotid endarterectomy is indicated for patients with TIA, surgery within 2 weeks is reasonable if there are no contraindications to early revascularization.

ADMISSION, INPATIENT, AND NURSING CONSIDERATIONS

Symptoms <72 hours and the following:

- ABCD2-I score of >3
- ABCD2-I score of 0 to 3 and uncertainty that diagnostic workup can be completed within 2 days as outpatient. Alternatively: If urgent imaging not available through ED or urgent neurology follow-up not available, admit ABCD2-I score ≥3 with evidence of focal ischemia.

ONGOING CARE

FOLLOW-UP RECOMMENDATIONS

Patient Monitoring

- Follow-up with neurologic support every 3 months for 1st year and then annually
- Strict control of blood pressure

DIET

- DASH diet or as appropriate for medical problems
- Any level of physical activity is beneficial, but at least 30 minutes of moderate-intensity physical activity daily is preferred (150 minutes/week).

PROGNOSIS

- Patients with larger artery occlusion or cardioembolic etiology are at increased risk for recurrence.
- High mortality risk associated with TIA; up to 25% of patients will die within 1 year of TIA.

COMPLICATIONS

Stroke and functional impairment

REFERENCES

1. Kleindorfer DO, Towfighi A, Chaturvedi S, et al. 2021 Guideline for the prevention of stroke in patients with stroke and transient ischemic attack: a guideline from the American Heart Association/American Stroke Association. *Stroke*. 2021;52(7):e364–e467.
2. Pan Y, Elm JJ, Li H, et al. Outcomes Associated With Clopidogrel-Aspirin Use in Minor Stroke or Transient Ischemic Attack: A Pooled Analysis of Clopidogrel in High-Risk Patients With Acute Non-Disabling Cerebrovascular Events (CHANCE) and Platelet-Oriented Inhibition in New TIA and Minor Ischemic Stroke (POINT) Trials. *JAMA Neurol*. 2019;76(12):1466–1473.
3. Zhao M, Wang S, Zhang D, et al. Comparison of stroke prediction accuracy of ABCD2 and ABCD3-I in patients with transient ischemic attack: a meta-analysis. *J Stroke Cerebrovasc Dis*. 2017;26(10):2387–2395.
4. Coutts SB. Diagnosis and management of transient ischemic attack. *Continuum (Minneap Minn)*. 2017;23(1):82–92.
5. Lansberg MG, O'Donnell MJ, Khatri P, et al. Antithrombotic and thrombolytic therapy for ischemic stroke: Antithrombotic Therapy and Prevention of Thrombosis, 9th ed: American College of Chest Physicians Evidence-Based Clinical Practice Guidelines. *Chest*. 2012;141(Suppl 2):e601S–e636S.

ADDITIONAL READING

Amarenco P, Lavallée PC, Labreuche J, et al. One-year risk of stroke after transient ischemic attack or minor stroke. *N Engl J Med*. 2016;374(16):1533–1542.

SEE ALSO

Algorithms: Stroke; Transient Ischemic Attack and Transient Neurologic Defects

CODES

ICD10

- G45.9 Transient cerebral ischemic attack, unspecified
- G45.1 Carotid artery syndrome (hemispheric)
- G45.0 Vertebro-basilar artery syndrome

CLINICAL PEARLS

- Utilize the ABCD2-I or ABCD3-I scoring systems to help with risk stratification.
- Encourage smoking cessation, exercise, weight loss, limited ETOH intake, and control of HTN, hyperlipidemia, and diabetes.
- Antiplatelet therapy (e.g., aspirin, clopidogrel, or aspirin-clopidogrel) should be initiated.
- Anticoagulation therapy (e.g., warfarin, apixaban, etc.) should be initiated in patients with atrial fibrillation or cardioembolic risk factors.
- Strict control of blood pressure is essential.

T

TRANSIENT STRESS CARDIOMYOPATHY

Adedapo Iluyomade, MD, MBA • Ana De Diego, MD

BASICS

DESCRIPTION

- Transient stress cardiomyopathy (TSC) is a unique cause of reversible left ventricle (LV) dysfunction with a presentation indistinguishable from the acute coronary syndromes (ACS), particularly ST-segment elevation myocardial infarction (STEMI) (1).
- Typically, the patient is a postmenopausal woman who presents with acute chest pain, dyspnea, or syncope and an identifiable "trigger" (i.e., an acute emotional or physiologic stressor).
- First reported by authors from Japan as takotsubo cardiomyopathy, the Japanese word for octopus trap, due to the characteristic shape of the LV at the end of systole. It has been described under numerous names in the literature including "broken heart syndrome," "stress cardiomyopathy," and "apical ballooning syndrome."
- Presenting clinical features include the following:
  - Chest pain/pressure, dyspnea, and/or syncope
  - ECG changes, including ST-segment elevations or diffuse T-wave inversions
  - Mild elevation in cardiac biomarkers (creatine kinase [CK], troponin)
  - Transient wall motion abnormalities that may involve the base, midportion, and/or lateral walls of the LV
  - The apex of the right ventricle (RV) may be affected in up to 25% of cases (1)[B].
- Clinical features may vary on a case-by-case basis, and formal diagnostic criteria have not been established.
- Authors from the Mayo Clinic have proposed that three of the four following criteria establish the diagnosis (1)[A]:
  - Transient akinesis or dyskinesis of the LV apical and midventricular segments with regional wall motion abnormalities extending beyond a single epicardial vascular distribution
  - Absence of obstructive coronary artery disease (CAD) or angiographic evidence of acute plaque rupture
  - New ECG abnormalities, either ST-segment elevation or T-wave inversion
  - Absence of
    - Recent significant head trauma
    - Intracranial bleeding
    - Pheochromocytoma
    - Obstructive epicardial CAD
    - Myocarditis
    - Hypertrophic cardiomyopathy
- Synonym(s): takotsubo cardiomyopathy; apical ballooning syndrome; stress cardiomyopathy; broken heart syndrome; ampulla cardiomyopathy

EPIDEMIOLOGY

Incidence

- TSC accounts for an estimated 1–3% of all and 5–6% of female patients presenting with suspected STEMI.
- In a recent prospective evaluation of patients admitted to the ICU, as many as 28% had apical ballooning, often in association with sepsis.
- Predominant sex: 82–100% of cases occur in women.
- Predominant age: Mean age of patients is 62 to 75 years.

Prevalence

2.2% of patients presenting to a referral hospital with ST-segment MIs were found to have TSC.

ETIOLOGY AND PATHOPHYSIOLOGY

- The precise pathophysiologic mechanisms of TSC are not well understood.
- There is considerable evidence that sympathetic stimulation is central to its pathogenesis. A clear emotional or physiologic triggering event precipitates the syndrome in most cases, and TSC has been associated with conditions of catecholamine excess (e.g., pheochromocytoma, central nervous system disorders) and activated specific cerebral regions (1).
- Occurs primarily in subjects with increased susceptibility of the coronary microcirculation and of cardiac myocytes to stress hormones leading to temporary left ventricular dysfunction with secondary myocardial inflammation (1)
- A perturbation in the brain-heart axis, originating in the insular cortex, may be the inciting event (2).
- Subsequent overwhelming activation of the sympathetic nervous system initiates a cascade of events, including the following:
  - Catecholamine-induced LV dysfunction: "biased agonism" of epinephrine for β_2-adrenergic receptors, located predominantly at the cardiac apex
  - Endothelial dysfunction and vasospasm
  - Cellular metabolic injury
    - Myocardial norepinephrine release
    - Calcium overload
    - Contraction band necrosis

Genetics

No genetic associations have been described to date.

RISK FACTORS

- Female sex
- Postmenopausal state
- Emotional stress (i.e., argument, death of family member), more common in women
- Physiologic stress (i.e., acute medical illness), more common in men
- Chronic neurologic or psychiatric disease (2)

COMMONLY ASSOCIATED CONDITIONS

Death from TSC is rare, and most cases resolve rapidly, within 2 to 3 days. Reported complications include

- Left-sided heart failure
- Pulmonary edema
- Cardiogenic shock and hemodynamic compromise
- Dynamic LV outflow tract gradient complicated by hypotension
- Mitral regurgitation
- Ventricular arrhythmias
- LV thrombus formation
- LV free wall rupture
- Death (rare, 0–8%)

DIAGNOSIS

Because TSC often is indistinguishable from an ACS, it should be treated initially as such:

- Activate emergency medical services or report to emergency department.
- Oxygen if needed, IV access, and ECG monitoring
- Urgent cardiology consultation

HISTORY

- In 2/3 of patients, there is exposure to a "trigger event."
  - Emotional stress: argument, death of family member, divorce, public speaking, and so forth
  - Physiologic stress: acute medical condition such as head trauma, asthma attack, seizure, and so forth

- In 1/3 of patients, there is no identifiable trigger (2).
- Studies suggest preference for time of day, day of the week, and months/season of the year; summer and winter most commonly reported
- Acute onset of dyspnea or chest pain
- Palpitations
- Syncope

PHYSICAL EXAM

Exam may be unremarkable or may include any of the following:

- Tachypnea
- Tachycardia
- Hypotension
- Jugular venous distension
- Bibasilar rales
- S_3 gallop
- Systolic ejection murmur due to dynamic LV outflow tract gradient
- Holosystolic murmur of mitral regurgitation

DIFFERENTIAL DIAGNOSIS

- Acute ST-segment elevation MI
- Pulmonary embolism
- Myopericarditis
- Pheochromocytoma
- Hypertrophic cardiomyopathy
- Subarachnoid hemorrhage or stroke

DIAGNOSTIC TESTS & INTERPRETATION

- The InterTAK Diagnostic Score comprises seven parameters (female sex, emotional trigger, physical trigger, absence of ST-segment depression [except in lead aVR], psychiatric disorders, neurologic disorders, and QT prolongation) ranked by their diagnostic importance with a maximum attainable score of 100 points (1)[C].
- In patients with non–ST-segment elevation, the InterTAK Diagnostic Score can be considered. Patients with a low probability (InterTAK score ≤70 points) should undergo coronary angiography with left ventriculography, whereas in patients with a high score (score ≥70), transthoracic echocardiography should be considered (1)[C].

Initial Tests (lab, imaging)

- ECG should be done urgently and may show the following:
  - Diffuse ST-segment elevations
  - Diffuse and often dramatic T-wave inversions
  - QTc interval prolongation (3)[B]
  - Q waves
- Laboratory tests typically reveal a mild elevation in cardiac biomarkers such as
  - CK (rarely >500 U/mL)
  - Troponin I, troponin T, or high-sensitivity cardiac troponin
  - B-type natriuretic peptide (BNP)
  - Markers of high filling pressures (e.g., BNP) tend to be higher than markers of necrosis (e.g., CK, troponin).
  - TSC can be distinguished from AMI with 95% specificity using a BNP/TnT ratio ≥1,272 (sensitivity 52%) (4)[B].
- Chest radiograph
  - Cardiomegaly
  - Pulmonary edema
- Echocardiogram
  - Reduced LV systolic function
  - Abnormal diastolic function, including evidence of increased filling pressures

– Regional wall motion abnormalities in one of the following patterns:
  ○ Classic or "takotsubo-type" ballooning of the apex with a hypercontractile base
  ○ "Reverse takotsubo": apical hypercontractility with basal akinesis
  ○ "Midventricular" akinesis with apical and basal hypercontractility
  ○ Focal or localized akinesis of an isolated segment
– Dynamic intracavitary LV gradient
– Mitral regurgitation
– Variable involvement of the RV

Follow-Up Tests & Special Considerations
Cardiac MRI
- Reduced LV function
- Wall motion abnormalities as described for transthoracic echocardiography
- Absence of delayed hyperenhancement with gadolinium
- Allows for differentiation between reversible and irreversible changes

Diagnostic Procedures/Other
- The diagnosis of TSC is often challenging because its clinical phenotype may closely resemble STEMI regarding electrocardiographic abnormalities and biomarkers. Although a widely established noninvasive tool allowing a rapid and reliable diagnosis of TSC is currently lacking, coronary angiography with left ventriculography is considered the "gold standard" diagnostic tool to exclude or confirm TSC.
- Coronary angiography
  – Nonocclusive CAD
  – Rarely, epicardial coronary spasm
  – Endothelial dysfunction as measured by fractional flow reserve or TIMI frame counts
- Left-sided heart catheterization: increased LV end-diastolic pressure to a similar degree as AMI
- Ventriculography: wall motion abnormalities as described for transthoracic echocardiography
- Right-sided heart catheterization
  – Increased pulmonary capillary wedge pressure
  – Secondary pulmonary hypertension
  – Increased right ventricular filling pressures
  – Reduced cardiac output or cardiogenic shock (cardiac index <2 and mean arterial pressure [MAP] <60 mm Hg)

Test Interpretation
Characteristic pathologic findings of involved myocardium have not been described.

TREATMENT
- Guidelines regarding TSC management are lacking because no prospective randomized clinical trials have been performed in this patient population. Therapeutic strategies are therefore based on clinical experience and expert consensus (5)[C].
- Activation of emergency medical services
- Advanced cardiac life support therapies as needed
- Oxygen
- IV access
- ECG monitoring

MEDICATION
After diagnostic cardiac catheterization, empirical treatment goals are as follows:
- Management of hypotension: differentiation between cardiogenic shock and dynamic LV cavity gradient

- Management of increased filling pressures and congestive states
- Attenuation of sympathetic drive

First Line
- There are no evidence-based treatment recommendations for TSC.
- Although β-blockers are of theoretical benefit, their use has not been associated with improved outcomes in observational cohorts (2)[B].
- Due to the potential risk of pause-dependent torsade de pointes, β-blockers should be used cautiously, especially in patients with bradycardia and QTc >500 ms (5).
- If there is evidence of left ventricular systolic dysfunction or pulmonary edema, consider the following:
  – Furosemide: 20 to 40 mg IV/PO BID as needed to reduce LV filling pressures and dyspnea (6)
  – The use of angiotensin-converting enzyme (ACE) inhibitors or angiotensin receptor blockers was associated with improved survival at 1-year follow-up even after propensity matching (2),(5): Lisinopril 10 to 40 mg/day PO or equivalent or valsartan 80 to 160 mg PO BID has been associated with improved outcomes in observational cohorts (2)[B].

Second Line
Short-term anticoagulation should be considered in patients with severely reduced LV function to prevent LV thrombus formation; unfractionated heparin 80 U/kg IV bolus followed by 18 U/kg/hr IV or enoxaparin sodium (Lovenox) 1 mg/kg SC BID

ISSUES FOR REFERRAL
All patients with TSC generally should be comanaged with cardiology while inpatient and referred to cardiology as an outpatient.

ADDITIONAL THERAPIES
- Urgent cardiology consultation and consideration of cardiac catheterization
- Hypotension may require the following:
  – Vasopressors (e.g., dopamine or norepinephrine (Levophed)) if there is no LV outflow tract gradient (6)[C]
  – Phenylephrine and IV fluids to increase afterload in the presence of an LV outflow tract gradient (6)[C]
  – Cardiogenic shock that is not due to an LV outflow tract gradient may require placement of an intra-aortic balloon pump.

ADMISSION, INPATIENT, AND NURSING CONSIDERATIONS
- Admission criteria/initial stabilization
  – 12-lead ECG
  – Chest radiograph
  – Laboratory testing
  – Echocardiography
  – Patients with TSC usually are admitted for observation because the differential diagnosis includes ACS.
- Normal saline infusion to support BP, if necessary, and no evidence of heart failure
- Discharge criteria generally considered after exclusion of ACS and resolution of
  – Congestive state
  – Hypotension
  – Profound impairments of systolic function

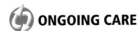

FOLLOW-UP RECOMMENDATIONS
- Impairments in systolic function typically resolve in 2 to 3 days but may last as long as 1 month.

- Patients should follow up with cardiology and serial echocardiography to document improved LV function.

PROGNOSIS
- Although TSC has generally been considered a benign disease, contemporary observations show that rates of cardiogenic shock and death are comparable to ACS patients treated according to current guidelines (5).
- Recurrence is rare; it also has been reported in 0–8% of patients.

REFERENCES
1. Ghadri JR, Wittstein IS, Prasad A, et al. International expert consensus document on takotsubo syndrome (part I): clinical characteristics, diagnostic criteria, and pathophysiology. *Eur Heart J.* 2018;39(22):2032–2046.
2. Templin C, Ghadri JR, Diekmann J, et al. Clinical features and outcomes of takotsubo (stress) cardiomyopathy. *N Engl J Med.* 2015;373(10):929–938.
3. Madias C, Fitzgibbons TP, Alsheikh-Ali AA, et al. Acquired long QT syndrome from stress cardiomyopathy is associated with ventricular arrhythmias and torsades de pointes. *Heart Rhythm.* 2011;8(4):555–561.
4. Randhawa MS, Dhillon AS, Taylor HC, et al. Diagnostic utility of cardiac biomarkers in discriminating takotsubo cardiomyopathy from acute myocardial infarction. *J Card Fail.* 2014;20(1):2–8.
5. Ghadri JR, Wittstein IS, Prasad A, et al. International expert consensus document on takotsubo syndrome (part II): diagnostic workup, outcome, and management. *Eur Heart J.* 2018;39(22):2047–2062.
6. Hunt SA, Abraham WT, Chin MH, et al. 2009 Focused update incorporated into the ACC/AHA 2005 guidelines for the diagnosis and management of heart failure in adults: a report of the American College of Cardiology Foundation/American Heart Association Task Force on Practice Guidelines developed in collaboration with the International Society for Heart and Lung Transplantation. *J Am Coll Cardiol.* 2009;53(15):e1–e90.

 SEE ALSO

Algorithm: Chest Pain/Acute Coronary Syndrome

 CODES

ICD10
I51.81 Takotsubo syndrome

CLINICAL PEARLS
- TSC is poorly recognized and often regarded as a benign condition. However, it may be associated with severe clinical complications including death, and its prevalence is likely underestimated.
- TSC is a cause of reversible LV dysfunction with a clinical presentation indistinguishable from the ACS, particularly ST-segment elevation MI.
- Echocardiography may strongly suggest the diagnosis.
- Treatment is supportive and should include diuretics and ACE inhibitors in patients with CHF.

TRICHOMONIASIS

Michael J. Arnold, MD

BASICS

DESCRIPTION

- Sexually transmitted urogenital infection caused by a pear-shaped, parasitic protozoan
- Causes vaginitis/urethritis in women, nongonococcal urethritis in men
- In pregnancy, increases risk of preterm labor, preterm premature rupture of membranes, small for gestational age infant, and possibly stillbirth
- Synonym(s): trich; trichomonal urethritis

EPIDEMIOLOGY

Incidence

- The most common curable sexually transmitted infection (STI); in 2008, >275 million new cases worldwide, over half of curable STIs (1)
- Estimated 1.1 million new cases annually in United States
  - 10–25% of vaginal infections
  - In males, up to 17% of nongonococcal urethritis; French study shows decreasing prevalence in men since 2007.
- Predominant age: middle-aged adults
  - Rare until onset of sexual activity
  - Common in postmenopausal women; age is not protective, and long-term carriage is common.

Pediatric Considerations

Rare in prepubertal children; diagnosis should raise concern of sexual abuse.

Prevalence

- 2.1% in United States women age 14 to 59 years
- 0.5% of U.S. men age 14 to 59 years
- Racial disparity demonstrated
  - 9.6% of black women versus 0.8% of other women
  - 3.4% of black men versus 0.03% of other men

ETIOLOGY AND PATHOPHYSIOLOGY

- *Trichomonas vaginalis*: pear-shaped, flagellated, parasitic protozoan
- Grows best at 35–37°C in anaerobic conditions with pH 5.5 to 6.0
- STI, but nonsexual transmission possible because it can survive several hours in moist environment

Genetics

No known genetic considerations

RISK FACTORS

- Multiple sexual partners
- Unprotected intercourse
- Lower socioeconomic status
- Other STIs
- Untreated partner with previous infection
- Use of douching or feminine powders

GENERAL PREVENTION

- Use of male or female condoms
- Limiting sexual partners
- Male circumcision may be protective.

COMMONLY ASSOCIATED CONDITIONS

- Other STIs, including HIV
- Bacterial vaginosis

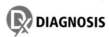

DIAGNOSIS

HISTORY

- Women—up to 80% may be asymptomatic.
  - Yellow-green, malodorous vaginal discharge
  - Vulvovaginal pruritus
  - Dysuria
  - Symptoms often worsen during menses.
- Men—80% are asymptomatic.
  - Dysuria
  - Urethral discharge, often scant
  - Pruritus or burning after intercourse

PHYSICAL EXAM

- Women
  - Vaginal erythema
  - Yellow-green, frothy, malodorous vaginal discharge
  - Cervical petechiae ("strawberry cervix"; seen in <5% of patients)
  - Pelvic exams do not improve STI diagnosis (2).
- Men: penile discharge, spontaneous and with expression

DIFFERENTIAL DIAGNOSIS

- Women (other vaginitides)
  - Bacterial vaginosis
  - Vaginal candidiasis
  - Chlamydial infection
  - Gonorrheal infection
- Men (other urethritis)
  - Chlamydial infection
  - Gonorrheal infection

DIAGNOSTIC TESTS & INTERPRETATION

Initial Tests (lab, imaging)

- Wet mounts of vaginal or urethral discharge: direct visualization of motile trichomonads; most common because inexpensive and available
  - Sensitivity: as low as 26%; declines rapidly within 1 hour from collection
  - Specificity: 99.8%
- Culture: sensitivity >95%, specificity >99%; takes 4 to 7 days for growth
- Nucleic acid amplification test (NAAT)
  - Gold standard for diagnosis (3)
  - Sensitivity and specificity 95–99% (3)
  - Vaginal, endocervical, or urine specimens

- British analysis shows that combined NAAT for *Trichomonas*, gonorrhea, *Chlamydia*, and *Mycoplasma genitalium* most cost-effective (3)[B].
- Antigen detection
  - ELISA and direct fluorescent antibody tests: sensitivity of 80–90%
  - Limited clinical availability

Follow-Up Tests & Special Considerations

Detection on cervical Papanicolaou smear

- Treat because highly specific (97–99%)
- Not effective for *Trichomonas* screening—sensitivity as low as 60%

Diagnostic Procedures/Other

In males, urethral meatal swab increases *Trichomonas* detection rate by 4 times over urine.

TREATMENT

- Symptomatic individuals require treatment.
- Sexual partners should be treated presumptively.
- Patients should abstain from sexual intercourse during treatment and until they are asymptomatic.

GENERAL MEASURES

The nitroimidazole class is only proven effective antimicrobial treatment. If metronidazole resistance is suspected, use tinidazole (4)[A].

MEDICATION

It is essential to treat partners to prevent reinfection.

First Line

- Metronidazole: 2 g PO, 1 dose (4)[A]
  - FDA pregnancy risk Category B
  - Cure rate: 84–98%
  - Increasing resistance—study of PID treatment showed that metronidazole did not improve *T. vaginalis* rate compared to control (5).
- Tinidazole: 2 g PO, 1 dose (4)[A]
  - FDA pregnancy risk Category C
  - Abstain from breastfeeding during treatment and for 3 days after the dose.
  - More expensive
  - Reaches higher levels in genitourinary tract
  - Cure rate: 92–100%

Second Line

- Metronidazole: 500 mg PO BID for 7 days
  - Number needed to treat of 13 for negative test of cure versus single-dose metronidazole (6)[B]
  - Considered first line in HIV-positive individuals
- Can dose with metronidazole or tinidazole 2 g daily for 7 days if infection persists
- Consider IV dosing of metronidazole based on case report demonstrating cure after multiple failed oral regimens.

- Recommendations for metronidazole resistance include tinidazole with intravaginal paromomycin, intravaginal boric acid, and intravaginal metronidazole with miconazole.

Pregnancy Considerations
Metronidazole is effective for trichomoniasis infection during pregnancy but may increase risk of preterm delivery and low-birth-weight babies.

- Studies showed risk in patients receiving 4 times the standard dosing.
- Trichomoniasis is also associated with prematurity.

ISSUES FOR REFERRAL
- Multidrug-resistant organism
- Patient allergy to metronidazole: Desensitization to metronidazole is recommended.

ADDITIONAL THERAPIES
- Limited clinical trials assessing effectiveness of alternative therapies
- Intravaginal metronidazole gel is only effective if adding miconazole (7).

COMPLEMENTARY & ALTERNATIVE MEDICINE
See "Additional Therapies."

 ONGOING CARE

FOLLOW-UP RECOMMENDATIONS
- If symptoms persist after initial treatment, repeat testing.
- Retest women for *T. vaginalis* recommended within 3 months of treatment; data insufficient for retesting men (6)
- HIV-positive patients should be screened for *Trichomonas* at time of HIV diagnosis and at least annually (6).

DIET
Abstain from alcohol during treatment and for 24 hours following last dose of metronidazole or 48 to 72 hours following last dose of tinidazole due to disulfiram-like reaction.

PATIENT EDUCATION
Educate about the sexually transmitted aspect.

- Advise patient to notify sexual partner to be treated.
- Discuss STI prevention—condom use can prevent recurrence.
- Abstain from intercourse while undergoing treatment; use condoms if abstention is not feasible.
- Avoid alcohol during treatment with metronidazole or tinidazole.

PROGNOSIS
- Excellent
- Usually eliminated after one course of antibiotics although resistance is increasing

COMPLICATIONS
Pregnancy Considerations
Linked to low birth weight, preterm premature rupture of membranes, and preterm birth; associations with infertility, but not proven

REFERENCES

1. Bouchemal K, Bories C, Loiseau PM. Strategies for prevention and treatment of *Trichomonas vaginalis* infections. *Clin Microbiol Rev*. 2017;30(3):811–825.
2. Farrukh S, Sivitz AB, Onogul B, et al. The additive value of pelvic examinations to history in predicting sexually transmitted infections for young female patients with suspected cervicitis or pelvic inflammatory disease. *Ann Emerg Med*. 2018;72(6):703.e1–712.e1.
3. Huntington SE, Burns RM, Harding-Esch E, et al. Modelling-based evaluation of the costs, benefits and cost-effectiveness of multipathogen point-of-care tests for sexually transmitted infections in symptomatic genitourinary medicine clinic attendees. *BMJ Open*. 2018;8(9):e020394.
4. Workowski KA, Bolan GA; for Centers for Disease Control and Prevention. Sexually transmitted diseases treatment guidelines, 2015. *MMWR Recomm Rep*. 2015;64(RR–03):1–137.
5. Trent M, Yusuf HE, Perin J, et al. Clearance of *Mycoplasma genitalium* and *Trichomonas vaginalis* among adolescents and young adults with pelvic inflammatory disease: results from the Tech-N study. *Sex Transm Dis*. 2020;47(11):e47–e50.
6. Kissinger P, Muzny CA, Mena LA, et al. Single-dose versus 7-day-dose metronidazole for the treatment of trichomoniasis in women: an open-label, randomised controlled trial. *Lancet Infect Dis*. 2018;18(11):1251–1259.
7. Alessio C, Nyirjesy P. Management of resistant trichomoniasis. *Curr Infect Dis Rep*. 2019;21(9):31.

ADDITIONAL READING

- Chernesky M, Jang D, Smieja M, et al. Urinary meatal swabbing detects more men infected with *Mycoplasma genitalium* and four other sexually transmitted infections than first catch urine. *Sex Transm Dis*. 2017;44(8):489–491.
- Daugherty M, Glynn K, Byler T. Prevalence of *Trichomonas vaginalis* infection among US males, 2013–2016. *Clin Infect Dis*. 2019;68(3):460–465
- Fastring DR, Amedee A, Gatski M, et al. Co-occurrence of *Trichomonas vaginalis* and bacterial vaginosis and vaginal shedding of HIV-1 RNA. *Sex Transm Dis*. 2014;41(3):173–179.
- Hawkins I, Carne C, Sonnex C, et al. Successful treatment of refractory *Trichomonas vaginalis* infection using intravenous metronidazole. *Int J STD AIDS*. 2015;26(9):676–678.
- Helms DJ, Mosure DJ, Secor WE, et al. Management of *Trichomonas vaginalis* in women with suspected metronidazole hypersensitivity. *Am J Obstet Gynecol*. 2008;198(4):370.e1–377.e1.
- Kirkcaldy RD, Augostini P, Asbel LE, et al. *Trichomonas vaginalis* antimicrobial drug resistance in 6 US cities, STD Surveillance Network, 2009–2010. *Emerg Infect Dis*. 2012;18(6):939–943.
- Meites E. Trichomoniasis: the "neglected" sexually transmitted disease. *Infect Dis Clin North Am*. 2013;27(4):755–764.
- Patel EU, Gaydos CA, Packman ZR, et al. Prevalence and correlates of *Trichomonas vaginalis* infection among men and women in the United States. *Clin Infect Dis*. 2018;67(2):211–217.
- Saperstein AK, Firnhaber GC. Clinical inquiries. Should you test or treat partners of patients with gonorrhea, chlamydia, or trichomoniasis? *J Fam Pract*. 2010;59(1):46–48.
- Seña AC, Bachmann LH, Hobbs MM. Persistent and recurrent *Trichomonas vaginalis* infections: epidemiology, treatment and management considerations. *Expert Rev Anti Infect Ther*. 2014;12(6):673–685.
- Silver BJ, Guy RJ, Kaldor JM, et al. *Trichomonas vaginalis* as a cause of perinatal morbidity: a systematic review and meta-analysis. *Sex Transm Dis*. 2014;41(6):369–376.
- Sobngwi-Tambekou J, Taljaard D, Nieuwoudt M, et al. Male circumcision and *Neisseria gonorrhoeae*, *Chlamydia trachomatis* and *Trichomonas vaginalis*: observations after a randomised controlled trial for HIV prevention. *Sex Transm Infect*. 2009;85(2):116–120.
- Wiese W, Patel SR, Patel SC, et al. A meta-analysis of the Papanicolaou smear and wet mount for the diagnosis of vaginal trichomoniasis. *Am J Med*. 2000;108(4):301–308.

 CODES

ICD10
- A59.02 Trichomonal prostatitis
- A59 Trichomoniasis
- A59.0 Urogenital trichomoniasis

CLINICAL PEARLS

- Both partners need to be treated for trichomoniasis.
- Retest women within 3 months of treatment.
- Avoid alcohol during treatment.
- Treatment in pregnancy does not reduce risk of adverse pregnancy outcomes.
- Annual screening recommended for HIV-positive patients
- Not a nationally notifiable condition

TRIGEMINAL NEURALGIA

Daniel R. Matta, MD • Sandya Gul Jiandani, MD

 BASICS

DESCRIPTION

- A painful disorder of the sensory nucleus of the 5th cranial (trigeminal) nerve that produces episodic, paroxysmal, severe, lancinating facial pain lasting seconds to minutes
- Often precipitated by stimulation of well-defined, ipsilateral trigger zones: usually perioral, perinasal, and occasionally intraoral (e.g., by talking, washing your face, shaving, or exposure to cold air)
- Subtypes:
  - Classical: secondary to neurovascular compression
  - Idiopathic: no abnormalities seen on neuroimaging
  - Secondary: cerebellopontine angle tumors (e.g., meningioma); tumors of cranial nerve (CN) V (e.g., neuroma, vascular malformations, trauma, demyelinating disease (e.g., multiple sclerosis [MS])
- System(s) affected: nervous
- Synonym(s): tic douloureux; Fothergill neuralgia; trifacial neuralgia; prosopalgia

EPIDEMIOLOGY

Incidence
- 4 to 13 per 100,000 per year
  - Women: 5.9/100,000 per year
  - Men: 3.4/100,000 per year
  - >70 years of age: ~25.6/100,000 per year
- Predominant age:
  - >50 years
  - Rare: <35 years of age (consider another primary disease, such as MS; see "Etiology and Pathophysiology."
- Predominant sex: female (~2:1)

Prevalence
16/100,000 with lifetime prevalence of 0.16–0.3%

Pediatric Considerations
Unusual during childhood

Pregnancy Considerations
Teratogenicity of medication therapy limits their use during 1st and 2nd trimesters

ETIOLOGY AND PATHOPHYSIOLOGY

- Compression of the trigeminal nerve root by an anomalous artery or vein usually within a few millimeters of entry of the nerve into the pons (accounts for up to 90% cases)
- Compression of trigeminal nerve by tumors such as meningioma, acoustic neuroma, or arteriovenous malformation
- Demyelination around the compression site seems to be the mechanism by which compression of nerves leads to symptoms.
- Demyelinated lesions may set up an ectopic impulse generation causing erratic responses such as hyperexcitability of damaged nerves and transmission of action potentials along adjacent, undamaged, and unstimulated sensory fibers.

Genetics
None confirmed, possible mutations in voltage-gated sodium channels

RISK FACTORS
Unknown

COMMONLY ASSOCIATED CONDITIONS
- Sjögren syndrome; rheumatoid arthritis
- Chronic meningitis
- Acute polyneuropathy
- MS
- Hemifacial spasm
- Charcot-Marie-Tooth neuropathy
- Glossopharyngeal neuralgia

 DIAGNOSIS

HISTORY
Paroxysms of pain in the distribution of the trigeminal nerve. The trigeminal nerve has three branches and innervates the entire side of the face. They are known as ophthalmologic (V1), maxillary (V2), and mandibular (V3) branches. Patients typically experience pain in the V2 and V3 dermatomes. Attacks are stereotyped in the individual patient.

PHYSICAL EXAM
Exam findings typically are negative due to the paroxysmal nature of the disorder.

DIFFERENTIAL DIAGNOSIS
Other forms of neuralgia usually have sensory loss. Presence of sensory loss nearly excludes the diagnosis of trigeminal neuralgia (TN) (if younger patient, frequently MS).
- Neoplasia in cerebellopontine angle
- Vascular malformation of brainstem
- Demyelinating lesion (MS is diagnosed in 2–4% of patients with TN.)
- Vascular insult
- Migraine, cluster headache
- Giant cell arteritis
- Postherpetic neuralgia
- Chronic meningitis
- Acute polyneuropathy
- Atypical odontalgia
- SUNCT syndrome (short-lasting, unilateral neuralgiform pain with conjunctival injection and tearing)

DIAGNOSTIC TESTS & INTERPRETATION
- The International Headache Society diagnostic criteria for classical and idiopathic TN requires all 3 of the following:
  - Pain has all of the following characteristics: (i) lasts from a fraction of a second to 2 minutes, affecting ≥ 1 branch of the trigeminal nerve; (ii) sharp in intensity; (iii) shock-like, stabbing, or shooting in nature
  - Precipitated from innocuous stimulus within the affected nerve distribution
  - Cannot be attributed to another disorder
- Additional criteria for classical: demonstration on MRI or surgical findings of neurovascular compression, with nerve root changes
- Subclassifications of TN with concomitant continuous pain: presence of background pain between episodes in the same distribution; typically burning, throbbing, or aching
- Secondary TN is characterized by pain that is indistinguishable from classic TN but is caused by a demonstrable structural lesion other than vascular compression.

Initial Tests (lab, imaging)
Imaging is indicated in patients with suspected TN or recurrent trigeminal pain attacks without obvious cause to rule out secondary causes.
- Routine head imaging identifies structural causes in up to 15%.
- MRI, with and without contrast, offers more detailed imaging and is preferred to CT, if not contraindicated.

Follow-Up Tests & Special Considerations
Dependent on treatment; no specific follow-up testing for primary condition after diagnosis is established.
- Labs (e.g., electrolytes, liver and kidney function) and EKG prior to initiating medications.

Test Interpretation
Imaging confirmation of morphologic changes associated with neurovascular compression:
- Trigeminal nerve: inflammatory changes, demyelination, displacement, and degenerative changes
- Trigeminal ganglion: hypermyelination and microneuromata

TREATMENT

GENERAL MEASURES
- Avoid stimulation (e.g., air, heat, cold) of trigger zones, including lips, cheeks, and gums.
- Medication treatment is first line.
- Invasive procedures are reserved for patients who cannot tolerate, fail to respond to, or relapse after chronic drug treatment.

MEDICATION

First Line
- Carbamazepine (Tegretol) (1)[A]: Start 100 to 200 mg BID; effective dose usually 200 mg QID; max dose 1,200 mg/day:
  - 70–90% of patients respond initially (number needed to treat [NNT] = 1.9) (1)[A].
  - By 3 years, 30% are no longer helped.
  - Common side effects: sedation, gastrointestinal (GI) upset, hyponatremia
  - Contraindications: AV block, concurrent use of monoamine oxidase inhibitors (MAOIs)
  - Precautions: Consider decreased dose in those with decreased liver function; be careful when using in combination with other anticholinergics in elderly and those with dementia.
  - Significant possible medication interactions: macrolide antibiotics, oral anticoagulants (such as warfarin), anticonvulsants, tricyclics, oral contraceptives, steroids, digitalis, isoniazid, MAOIs, methyprylon, nabilone, nizatidine, other H_2 blockers, phenytoin, propoxyphene, benzodiazepines, and calcium channel blockers
- Oxcarbazepine (Trileptal): Start 150 to 300 mg BID; effective dose usually 375 mg BID; max dose 1,800 mg/day:
  - Efficacy, side effects, and precautions similar to carbamazepine
  - Faster, with less drowsiness and fewer drug interactions than carbamazepine
  - Often causes hyponatremia
  - Common side effects: sedation, GI upset, and hyponatremia

Second Line

- Nonantiepileptic drugs: insufficient evidence from randomized controlled trials to show significant benefit (2)[A]
- Phenytoin (Dilantin): 300 to 400 mg/day (synergistic with carbamazepine):
  - Potent P450 inducer (enhanced metabolism of many drugs)
  - Various CNS side effects (sedation, ataxia)
- Baclofen (Lioresal): 10 to 80 mg/day; start 5 to 10 mg TID with food (as an adjunct to phenytoin or carbamazepine); side effects: drowsiness, weakness, nausea, vomiting
- Gabapentin (Neurontin): Start 100 mg TID or 300 mg at bedtime; can increase dose up to 300 to 600 mg TID–QID; can be used as monotherapy or in combination with other medications
- Lamotrigine: Titrate up to 200 mg BID over weeks; side effect: 10% experience rash.
- Antidepressants, including amitriptyline, fluoxetine, trazodone:
  - Used especially with anticonvulsants
  - Particularly effective for atypical forms of TN
- Clonazepam (Klonopin) frequently causes drowsiness and ataxia.
- Sumatriptan (Imitrex) 3 mg subcutaneous (SC) reduces acute symptoms and may be helpful after failure of conventional therapy.
- Capsaicin cream topically
- Botulinum toxin injection into zygomatic arch may be beneficial for patients who did not respond well to first-line therapy.
- Valproic acid (Depakene, Depakote)

ISSUES FOR REFERRAL
Initial treatment failure or positive findings on imaging studies; evaluation at pain clinic prior to surgical referral

ADDITIONAL THERAPIES
- Radiotherapy
- Stereotactic radiosurgery, such as Gamma Knife radiosurgery, has been shown to be effective after drug failure:
  - Produces lesions with focused Gamma Knife radiation, with therapy aimed at the proximal trigeminal root
  - Minimal clinically effective dose: 70 Gy
  - ~78–94% of patients achieve complete relief after 3 years; by 7 years, ~65–90% maintain complete relief (3)[B].
  - Most common side effect: sensory disturbance (facial numbness)
  - Failure rates are higher in patients with past TN-related invasive procedures.

SURGERY/OTHER PROCEDURES
- Microvascular decompression of CN V at its entrance to (or exit from) brainstem:
  - 98% of patients achieve initial pain relief; by 20 months, 86% maintain complete relief (NNT = 2) (4)[B].
  - Surgical mortality across studies was 0.3–0.4%.
  - Most common side effect: transient facial numbness and diplopia, headache, nausea, vomiting
  - Pain relief after procedure strongly correlates with the type of TN pain: paroxysmal results in better outcomes than concomitant continuous (aching pain between paroxysms).
- Peripheral nerve ablation (multiple methods):
  - Higher rates of failure and facial numbness than decompression surgery
  - Radiofrequency thermocoagulation
  - Neurectomy

- Cryotherapy: high relapse rate
- Partial sensory rhizotomy
- 4% tetracaine dissolved in 0.5% bupivacaine nerve block (only a few case reports); also, ropivacaine or lidocaine)
- Alcohol block or glycerol injection into trigeminal cistern: unpredictable side effects (dysesthesia and anesthesia dolorosa) and temporary relief
- Peripheral block or section of CN V proximal to gasserian ganglion
- Balloon compression of gasserian ganglion
- Evidence supporting destructive procedures for benign pain conditions remains limited (5)[A].

COMPLEMENTARY & ALTERNATIVE MEDICINE
- Acupuncture: evidence of analgesic effect in both idiopathic TN and associated secondary myofascial pain (6)[A]
- Moxibustion (herb): weak evidence for efficacy

ADMISSION, INPATIENT, AND NURSING CONSIDERATIONS
Severe acute exacerbations, with high attack frequency leading to dehydration or anorexia due to trigger avoidance, may benefit from in-hospital treatment for rehydration and titration of antiepileptic medication.

ONGOING CARE

FOLLOW-UP RECOMMENDATIONS
Follow up, every 3 to 6 months in initial few years, to monitor symptoms and treatment efficacy.

Patient Monitoring
- Carbamazepine and/or phenytoin serum levels
- Liver and renal function
- Sodium concentrations after 3 and 12 months
- If carbamazepine is prescribed: CBC and platelets at baseline, then weekly for a month, then monthly for 4 months, and then every 6 to 12 months if dose is stable (Regimens for monitoring vary.)
- Reduce drugs after 4 to 6 weeks to determine whether condition is in remission; resume at previous dose if pain recurs. Withdraw drugs slowly after several months, again to check for remission or if lower dose of drugs can be tolerated.

DIET
No special diet

PATIENT EDUCATION
- Instruct patient regarding medication dosage and side effects, risk-to-benefit ratios of surgery or radiation therapy.
- Support organizations:
  - Facial Pain Association (formerly the Trigeminal Neuralgia Association): https://www.facepain.org/
  - Living with Facial Pain: https://www.livingwithfacialpain.org/

PROGNOSIS
- 50–60% eventually fail pharmacologic treatment.
- Of those, relapse is seen in ~50% of stereotactic radiosurgeries and ~27% of surgical microvascular decompressions.

COMPLICATIONS
- Mental and physical sluggishness; dizziness with carbamazepine
- Paresthesias and corneal reflex loss with stereotactic radiosurgery

- Surgical mortality and morbidity associated with microvascular decompression

REFERENCES

1. Wiffen PJ, Derry S, Moore RA, et al. Carbamazepine for chronic neuropathic pain and fibromyalgia in adults. *Cochrane Database Syst Rev.* 2014;(4):CD005451.
2. Zhang J, Yang M, Zhou M, et al. Non-antiepileptic drugs for trigeminal neuralgia. *Cochrane Database Syst Rev.* 2013;(12):CD004029.
3. Martínez Moreno NE, Gutiérrez-Sárraga J, Rey-Portolés G, et al. Long-term outcomes in the treatment of classical trigeminal neuralgia by Gamma Knife radiosurgery: a retrospective study in patients with minimum 2-year follow-up. *Neurosurgery.* 2016;79(6):879–888.
4. Sekula RF Jr, Frederickson AM, Jannetta PJ, et al. Microvascular decompression for elderly patients with trigeminal neuralgia: a prospective study and systematic review with meta-analysis. *J Neurosurg.* 2011;114(1):172–179.
5. Zakrzewska JM, Akram H. Neurosurgical interventions for the treatment of classical trigeminal neuralgia. *Cochrane Database Syst Rev.* 2011;(9):CD007312.
6. Ichida MC, Zemuner M, Hosomi J, et al. Acupuncture treatment for idiopathic trigeminal neuralgia: a longitudinal case-control double blinded study. *Chin J Integr Med.* 2017;23(11):829–836.

ADDITIONAL READING

- Bendtsen L, Zakrzewska J, Abbott J, et al. Academy of Neurology guideline on trigeminal neuralgia. *Eur J Neurology.* 2019;26(6):831–849.
- Bendtsen L, Zakrzewska J, Heinskou T, et al. Advances in diagnosis, classification, pathophysiology, and management of trigeminal neuralgia. *Lancet Neurol.* 2020;19(9):784–796.
- Headache Classification Committee of the International Headache Society (IHS) The International Classification of Headache disorders, 3rd Edition. *Cephalalgia.* 2018;38(1):1–211.

CODES

ICD10
- B02.22 Postherpetic trigeminal neuralgia
- G50.0 Trigeminal neuralgia

CLINICAL PEARLS
- Patients with TN typically have a normal physical exam.
- Imaging, ideally MRI, should be obtained to rule out secondary causes in newly presenting patients with clinical suspicion of TN.
- The long-term efficacy of pharmacotherapy for TN is 40–50%.
- First-line treatment: carbamazepine or oxcarbazepine
- If pharmacotherapy fails, stereotactic radiosurgery or surgical microvascular decompression often is successful.

T

TRIGGER FINGER (DIGITAL STENOSING TENOSYNOVITIS)

Jill N. Tirabassi, MD, MPH

BASICS

DESCRIPTION
A clicking, snapping, or locking of a finger/thumb with extension ± associated pain

EPIDEMIOLOGY

Incidence
- Adult population: 2–3% of adults (1)
  - Rare in children
- 4 times increased risk in diabetics (2)[B]
- Thumb is predominant digit.
- Predominant age
  - Adult form typically presents in the 5th and 6th decades of life.
- Predominant sex
  - Children: female = male
  - Adults: female > male (6:1)

Prevalence
Lifetime prevalence in the general population is 2.6%.

Pediatric Considerations
- Surgery is often more complicated for children with a trigger finger (as opposed to a trigger thumb).
- Release of the A1 pulley alone is often insufficient; other procedures may be necessary.

ETIOLOGY AND PATHOPHYSIOLOGY
- Narrowing around the A1 pulley from inflammation, protein deposition, or thickening of the tendon itself. Prolonged inflammation leads to fibrocartilaginous metaplasia of the tendon sheath.
- If flexor tendon becomes nodular, the triggering phenomenon is worse because the nodule has difficulty passing under the A1 pulley.
- Because intrinsic flexor muscles are stronger than extensors, the finger can get stuck in the flexed position.
- No clear association with repetitive movements

RISK FACTORS
- Diabetes mellitus
- Rheumatoid arthritis
- Hypothyroidism
- Mucopolysaccharide disorders
- Amyloidosis

GENERAL PREVENTION
Most cases are idiopathic, and no known prevention exists; no clear association with repetitive movements

COMMONLY ASSOCIATED CONDITIONS
- De Quervain tenosynovitis
- Carpal tunnel syndrome
- Dupuytren contracture
- Diabetes mellitus
- Rheumatoid arthritis
- Hypothyroidism
- Amyloidosis

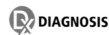

DIAGNOSIS

Diagnosis is based on clinical presentation.

HISTORY
- Clicking, catching, snapping, or locking of a digit while attempting to extend; with or without associated pain; usual progression is painless clicking, then painful triggering, then flexed and locked digit.
- Functional limitations tend to include difficulty with grasping and holding objects, manipulating coins, or buttoning (1).

PHYSICAL EXAM
- A1 pulley of finger is located at the metacarpal head.
- A palpable nodule may be present.
- Snapping/locking may be present, but neither is necessary for the diagnosis.
- Tenderness to palpation is variable.

DIFFERENTIAL DIAGNOSIS
- Osteoarthritis
- Suppurative tenosynovitis
- Ganglion of tendon sheath
- Dupuytren contracture (palmar fibromatosis; caused by progressive fibrous proliferation and tightening of the fascia of the palms, resulting in flexion deformities and loss of function)
- Rheumatoid arthritis

DIAGNOSTIC TESTS & INTERPRETATION

Diagnostic Procedures/Other
Generally, no need for imaging for diagnosis. If needed, musculoskeletal ultrasound or MRI is potentially useful.

Test Interpretation
On ultrasound or MRI:
- Thickening of the A1 pulley with fibrocartilaginous metaplasia
- Thickening/nodule formation of flexor tendon

TREATMENT

GENERAL MEASURES
- Generally, conservative treatment is recommended first line, which includes activity modification, NSAIDs, splinting ,or consideration of steroid injection.
- Activity modification can be helpful in early disease (3)[C].
- Splinting may be more effective in preventing recurrence than initial treatment choice (4)[B].
- Splinting the metacarpophalangeal (MCP) joint at 10 to 15 degrees of flexion for 6 weeks with the distal joints free to move:
  - Splinting is more effective for fingers than thumbs (70% vs. 50%).
  - Splinting is less effective with severe symptoms, symptoms >6 months, or if multiple digits are involved (2)[B].
- Most recommend attempting steroid injection prior to surgery (3)[C].
- Injection of long-acting corticosteroid may provide symptom relief. Subsequent injections are less likely to help (2)[B].
- Surgery often successful for patients unresponsive to splinting/corticosteroid injections or who suffered recurrence (3)[B]

MEDICATION

First Line
- Oral NSAIDs may reduce pain and discomfort but have not been shown to alter underlying disease. NSAIDs do not reduce symptoms of snapping/locking.
- Steroid injection of the tendon sheath/surrounding subcutaneous tissue has 57–90% success rate.

- Triamcinolone appears more effective than dexamethasone (3)[B].
- Injection in surrounding tissues is as efficacious as injecting into the tendon sheath (2),(3)[B]. Injection into the palmar surface at the midproximal phalanx is associated with less pain than injection of tendon sheath at MCP joint (5)[B].
- Corticosteroid injection has higher success rate than splinting (4)[B]; however, a recent systematic review quotes the efficacy of orthotic use as 47–93% effective (1)[A].

Second Line
- Injection with diclofenac may be an alternative to corticosteroid for patients with diabetes mellitus if increase in blood sugar is a concern (3)[A].
- Corticosteroids are more effective than diclofenac during the first 3 weeks postinjection. Efficacy is similar to other modalities by 3 months postinjection (3)[B].

ISSUES FOR REFERRAL
Refer to a hand surgeon for A1 pulley release if the patient is not responding to conservative treatment.

ADDITIONAL THERAPIES
Physiotherapy is helpful, particularly in children.

SURGERY/OTHER PROCEDURES
- Surgical release can be done as an open procedure or percutaneously.
- No apparent differences in success or rates of complications between surgical approaches (6)[A]
- Surgery has lower rate of recurrence than corticosteroid injection but has disadvantage of being more painful initially (6)[A].

ADMISSION, INPATIENT, AND NURSING CONSIDERATIONS
- Day surgery for trigger finger release
- Discharge criteria: absence of complications

 ONGOING CARE

FOLLOW-UP RECOMMENDATIONS
- Follow-up is needed only if symptoms persist or if complications develop after surgery.
- Splinting of the affected digit to minimize flexion/extension of the MCP joint helps symptom resolution (2)[B].

PROGNOSIS
Prognosis is excellent with conservative treatment or surgical intervention. Recurrence following corticosteroid injection is more likely for patients with type 1 diabetes mellitus, younger patients, involvement of multiple digits, and history of other upper extremity tendinopathies (3)[B].

COMPLICATIONS
- Diabetic patients may have increased blood sugar levels for up to 5 days following steroid injection.
- Other minor steroid injection complications include skin depigmentation and fat necrosis; tendon attrition or rupture is rare.
- Complications from surgery include infection, bleeding, digital nerve injury, persistent pain, and loss of range of motion of the affected finger. The rate of major complications is low (3%). The rate of minor complications (including loss of range of motion) is higher (up to 28%).
- Another surgical complication, injury to the A2 pulley, may result in bowstringing (bulging of the flexor tendon in the palm with flexion) and pain.

REFERENCES

1. Lundsford D, Valdes K, Hengy S. Conservative management of trigger finger: a systematic review. *J Hand Ther*. 2019;(32):212–221.
2. Akhtar S, Bradley MJ, Quinton DN, et al. Management and referral for trigger finger/thumb. *BMJ*. 2005;331(7507):30–33.
3. Giugale JM, Fowler JR. Trigger finger: adult and pediatric treatment strategies. *Orthop Clin North Am*. 2015;46(4):561–569.
4. Salim N, Abdullah S, Sapuan J, et al. Outcome of corticosteroid injection versus physiotherapy in the treatment of mild trigger fingers. *J Hand Surg Eur Vol*. 2012;37(1):27–34.
5. Cecen GS, Gulabi D, Saglam F, et al. Corticosteroid injection for trigger finger: blinded or ultrasound-guided injection? *Arch Orthop Trauma Surg*. 2015;135(1):125–131.
6. Fiorini HJ, Tamaoki MJ, Lenza M, et al. Surgery for trigger finger. *Cochrane Database Syst Rev*. 2018;(2):CD009860.

ADDITIONAL READING

- Amirfeyz R, McNinch R, Watts A, et al. Evidence-based management of adult trigger digits. *J Hand Surg Eur Vol*. 2017;42(5):473–480.
- Fleisch SB, Spindler KP, Lee DH. Corticosteroid injections in the treatment of trigger finger: a level I and II systematic review. *J Am Acad Orthop Surg*. 2007;15(3):166–171.
- Huisstede BM, Hoogvliet P, Coert JH, et al; for European HANDGUIDE Group. Multidisciplinary consensus guideline for managing trigger finger: results from the European HANDGUIDE Study. *Phys Ther*. 2014;94(10):1421–1433.
- Wang J, Zhao JG, Liang CC. Percutaneous release, open surgery, or corticosteroid injection, which is the best treatment method for trigger digits? *Clin Orthop Relat Res*. 2013;471(6):1879–1886.

 CODES

ICD10
- M65.30 Trigger finger, unspecified finger
- M65.319 Trigger thumb, unspecified thumb
- M65.329 Trigger finger, unspecified index finger

CLINICAL PEARLS
- Trigger finger is caused by narrowing of the A1 flexor tendon pulley.
- Diagnosis is based on clinical presentation.
- Initial conservative treatment can include NSAIDS, splinting, or corticosteroid injection.
- Long-acting corticosteroid injections are effective for treatment of trigger finger but have higher recurrence rate than surgery.
- Open and percutaneous surgical release have high success rates for patients not responsive to splinting or injections.

TROCHANTERIC BURSITIS (GREATER TROCHANTERIC PAIN SYNDROME)

Daniel L. Warden, MD • Nicholas Moore, MD, FAAFP, CAQSM • Kyle M. Samyn, DO, MS

 BASICS

Trochanteric bursitis is often used as a general term to describe lateral hip pain and tenderness over the greater trochanter. There may be inflammation at one of a number of bursa at the lateral hip, but more commonly, the pain is due to hip abductor tendon injury and external snapping hip. More recently, there has been a shift to describe this condition as greater trochanteric pain syndrome (GTPS) (1).

DESCRIPTION
- Bursae are fluid-filled sacs found primarily at tendon attachment sites with bony protuberances:
  - Multiple bursae are in the area of the greater trochanter of the femur.
  - These bursae are associated with the tendons of the gluteus muscles, iliotibial band (ITB), and tensor fasciae latae.
  - The subgluteus maximus bursa is implicated most commonly in lateral hip pain (1).
- Other structures of the lateral hip include the following:
  - ITB, tensor fasciae latae, gluteus maximus tendon, gluteus medius tendon, gluteus minimus tendon, quadratus femoris muscle, vastus latera-lis tendon, piriformis tendon
- *Bursitis* refers to bursal inflammation.
- *Tendinopathy* refers to any abnormality of a tendon, inflammatory or degenerative.
- *Enthesopathy* refers to abnormalities of the zones of attachment of ligaments and tendons to bones.

EPIDEMIOLOGY
Incidence
- 1.8/1,000 persons/year
- Peak incidence in 4th to 6th decades

Prevalence
- Predominant sex: female > male
- More common in running and contact athletes
  - Football, rugby, soccer

ETIOLOGY AND PATHOPHYSIOLOGY
- Acute: Abnormal gait or poor muscle flexibility and strength imbalances lead to bursal friction and secondary inflammation.
  - Tendon overuse and inflammation
  - Direct trauma from contact or frequently lying with body weight on hip can cause an inflammatory response.
- Chronic
  - Fibrosis and thickening of bursal sac due to chronic inflammatory process
  - Tendinopathy due to chronic overuse and degeneration: gluteus medius and minimus most commonly involved (1)

Genetics
No known genetic factors

RISK FACTORS
Multiple factors have been implicated (1):
- Female gender
- Obesity
- Tight hip musculature (including ITB)
- Direct trauma
- Total hip arthroplasty
- Abnormal gait or pelvic architecture
  - Leg length discrepancy
  - Sacroiliac (SI) joint dysfunction
  - Knee or hip osteoarthritis
  - Abnormal foot mechanics (e.g., pes planus, overpronation)
  - Neuromuscular disorder: Trendelenburg gait

GENERAL PREVENTION
- Maintain ITB, hip, and lower back flexibility and strength.
- Avoid direct trauma (use of appropriate padding in contact sports).
- Avoid prolonged running on banked or crowned surfaces.
- Wear appropriate shoes.
- Appropriate bedding and sleeping surface
- Maintain appropriate body weight loss.

COMMONLY ASSOCIATED CONDITIONS
- Biomechanical factors (1)
  - Tight ITBs, leg length discrepancy, SI joint dysfunction, pes planus
  - Width of greater trochanters greater than width of iliac wings
- Other associated pathology (1):
  - Low back pain
  - Knee and hip osteoarthritis
  - Obesity

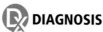 **DIAGNOSIS**

HISTORY
General history (1)
- Pain localized to the lateral hip or buttock
- Pain may radiate to groin or lateral thigh (pseudoradiculopathy).
- Pain exacerbated by:
  - Prolonged walking or standing
  - Rising after prolonged sitting
  - Sitting with legs crossed
  - Lying on affected side

- Other historical features:
  - Direct trauma to affected hip
  - Chronic low back pain
  - Chronic leg/knee/ankle/hip pain
  - Recent increase in running distance or intensity
  - Change in running surfaces

PHYSICAL EXAM
- Palpate for point tenderness with direct palpation over the lateral hip is characteristic of GTPS (1)[B].
- Other exam features have lower sensitivity (1)[B]:
  - Pain with extremes of passive rotation, abduction, or adduction
  - Pain with resisted hip abduction and external or internal rotation
  - Trendelenburg sign
- Other tests to rule out associated conditions:
  - Patrick-FABERE (flexion, abduction, external rotation, extension) test for SI joint dysfunction
  - Ober test for ITB pathology
  - Flexion and extension of hip for osteoarthritis
  - Leg length measurement
  - Foot inspection for pes planus or overpronation
  - Lower extremity neurologic assessment for lumbar radiculopathy or neuromuscular disorders
  - Hip lag sign

DIFFERENTIAL DIAGNOSIS
- ITB syndrome
- Piriformis syndrome
- Osteoarthritis or avascular necrosis of the hip
- Lumbosacral osteoarthritis/disc disease with nerve root compression
- Fracture or contusion of the hip or pelvis—particularly in setting of trauma
- Stress reaction/fracture of femoral neck—particularly in female runners
- Septic bursitis/arthritis

DIAGNOSTIC TESTS & INTERPRETATION
No routine lab testing is recommended.

Initial Tests (lab, imaging)
- Diagnosis can be made by history and exam (2).
- If imaging is ordered:
  - US can aid in diagnosis and guide aspiration and/or injection.
  - Anteroposterior and frog-leg views of affected hip to rule out specific bony pathology (OA, stress fracture, etc.)
  - Consider lumbar spine radiographs if back pain is thought to be a contributing factor.
  - MRI is image of choice in recalcitrant pain or to formally exclude stress fracture.

Follow-Up Tests & Special Considerations
- If there is a concern for a septic bursitis, then aspiration or incision and drainage may be necessary.
- Advanced imaging rarely necessary; detection of abnormalities on MRI is a poor predictor of GTPS.

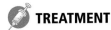 **TREATMENT**

GENERAL MEASURES
- Physical therapy to address underlying dysfunction and weakness
- Correct pelvic/hip instability.
- Correct lower limb biomechanics.
- Low-impact conditioning and aquatic therapy
- Gait training
- Weight loss (if applicable)
- Minimize aggravating activities such as prolonged walking or standing.
- Avoid lying on affected side.
- Runners
  – May need to decrease distance and/or intensity of runs during treatment. Some need to stop running. Amount of time is case specific but may range from 2 to 4 weeks.
  – Avoid banked tracks or roads with excessive tilt.

MEDICATION
First Line
- NSAIDs (1)[B]: Treat for 2 to 4 weeks.
  – Naproxen: 500 mg PO BID
  – Ibuprofen: 800 mg PO TID
- Corticosteroid injection is effective for pain relief (3)[C] and can be considered first-line therapy for selected cases:
  – Dexamethasone: 4 mg/mL or
  – Kenalog: 40 mg/mL; use 1 to 2 mL.
  – Consider adding a local anesthetic (short- and/or long-acting) for more immediate pain relief.
  – Can be repeated with similar effect if original treatment showed a strong response
  – Goal is pain relief.
  – Corticosteroid injections may not be effective for certain cases (4). A noninflammatory cause, such as a chronic tendinopathy or referred pain, should be considered and further explored in these cases.

ISSUES FOR REFERRAL
- Septic bursitis
- Recalcitrant bursitis
- Positive sag test concerning for gluteal tendon tear

ADDITIONAL THERAPIES
- Ice
- Low-energy shock wave therapy has been shown to be superior to other nonoperative modalities.
- Focus on achieving flexibility of hip musculature, particularly the ITB.
- Address contributing factors:
  – Low back flexibility
  – If leg length discrepancy, consider heel lift.
  – If pes planus or overpronation, consider arch supports or custom orthotics.

SURGERY/OTHER PROCEDURES
- Surgery rare but effective in refractory cases
- If surgery is indicated, potential options include:
  – Arthroscopic bursectomy
  – ITB release
  – Gluteus medius tendon repair
- Tenotomy

COMPLEMENTARY & ALTERNATIVE MEDICINE
- Acupuncture
- Prolotherapy
- Growth factor injection techniques
- Platelet-rich plasma injection

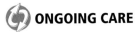 **ONGOING CARE**

FOLLOW-UP RECOMMENDATIONS
4 weeks posttreatment, sooner if significant worsening

PATIENT EDUCATION
- Maintain hip musculature flexibility, including ITB.
- Correct issues that may cause abnormal gait:
  – Low back pain
  – Knee pain
  – Leg length discrepancy (heel lift)
  – Foot mechanics (orthotics)
- Gradual return to physical activity

PROGNOSIS
Depends on chronicity and recurrence, with more acute cases having an excellent prognosis

COMPLICATIONS
Bursal thickening and fibrosis

REFERENCES
1. Williams BS, Cohen SP. Greater trochanteric pain syndrome: a review of anatomy, diagnosis and treatment. *Anesth Analg.* 2009;108(5):1662–1670.
2. Chowdhury R, Naaseri S, Lee J, et al. Imaging and management of greater trochanteric pain syndrome. *Postgrad Med J.* 2014;90(1068):576–581.
3. Stephens MB, Beutler AI, O'Connor FG. Musculoskeletal injections: a review of the evidence. *Am Fam Physician.* 2008;78(8):971–976.
4. Nissen MJ, Brulhart L, Faundez A, et al. Glucocorticoid injections for greater trochanteric pain syndrome: a randomised double-blind placebo-controlled (GLUTEAL) trial. *Clin Rheumatol.* 2019;38(3):647–655.

ADDITIONAL READING
- Barratt PA, Brookes N, Newson A. Conservative treatments for greater trochanteric pain syndrome: a systematic review. *Br J Sports Med.* 2017;51(2):97–104.
- Pretell J, Ortega J, García-Rayo R, et al. Distal fascia lata lengthening: an alternative surgical technique for recalcitrant trochanteric bursitis. *Int Orthop.* 2009;33(5):1223–1227.

 CODES

ICD10
- M70.60 Trochanteric bursitis, unspecified hip
- M70.62 Trochanteric bursitis, left hip
- M70.61 Trochanteric bursitis, right hip

CLINICAL PEARLS
- Patients with GTPS often present with an inability to lie on the affected side.
- Femoral neck stress fractures are a do-not-miss diagnosis, particularly in young female runners.
- Corticosteroid injection helps as an initial therapy, particularly for pain relief to allow for aggressive physical therapy.
- Physical therapy is treatment mainstay for correcting biomechanical imbalances and restoring proper function.

T

TUBERCULOSIS

Jorge Finke, MD

BASICS

DESCRIPTION
- Active tuberculosis (TB)
  - Primary infection or reactivation of latent infection
  - Risk increases with immunosuppression: highest risk first 2 years after infection. Reactivation risk increases with comorbid disease (e.g., HIV, diabetes).
  - Well-described forms: pulmonary (85% of cases), miliary (disseminated), meningeal, abdominal, lymphadenitis (scrofula)
- Usually acquired by inhalation of airborne bacilli from an individual with active TB. Bacilli multiply in alveoli and spread via macrophages, lymphatics, and blood. Three possible outcomes:
  - Eradication: Tissue hypersensitivity halts infection within 10 weeks.
  - Primary TB
  - Latent TB (see "Tuberculosis, Latent (LTBI)")

EPIDEMIOLOGY
Incidence
- Worldwide (2017): 10.4 million (133 cases per 100,000) population; highest incidence in Asia and Africa. Higher burden countries have approximately 150 cases/100,000 population.
- United States (2020): 7,163 (2.2/100,000); 71% of U.S. cases were in persons born outside of the United States. TB incidence has decreased by an average of 2–3% annually during the previous 10 years.

Prevalence
- Worldwide (2019): World Health Organization estimates 10 million new cases of TB in 2019.
- Mortality
  - Worldwide (2019): 1.4 million deaths due to TB. TB is one of the top 10 leading causes of death worldwide.

ETIOLOGY AND PATHOPHYSIOLOGY
- *Mycobacterium tuberculosis, Mycobacterium bovis,* or *Mycobacterium africanum* are causative organisms.
- Spread by aerosol droplets and reach alveolar space. Alveolar macrophages ingest and migrate.
- Cell-mediated response by activated T lymphocytes and macrophages forms a granuloma ("tubercle") that limits bacterial replication. If bacterial replication continues, the tubercle grows with spread to regional lymph nodes. An expanding tubercle within the lung parenchyma combined with regional lymph node enlargement is called a Ranke complex.
- As the infection is contained, destruction of the macrophages produces early "solid necrosis." In 2 to 3 weeks, "caseous necrosis" develops and LTBI ensues. In the immunocompetent, granuloma undergoes "fibrosis" and calcification. In the immunocompromised, primary progressive TB develops. Cavitary lesions may form.

RISK FACTORS
- For infection: homeless, correctional facilities, close contact with infected person, living in areas with high incidence of active TB, health care workers; medically underserved, low income, substance abuse
- For development of disease once infected: renal failure; lymphoma; silicosis; diabetes; cancer of head, neck, or lung; children <5 years old; malnutrition; systemic corticosteroids; HIV; immunosuppressive drugs; IV drug abuse, alcohol abuse, cigarette smokers; <2 years since infection with *M. tuberculosis;* <90% of ideal body weight

GENERAL PREVENTION
- Screen for and treat LTBI. Report active TB to health department; test and treat all close contacts.
- Bacillus Calmette-Guérin (BCG) vaccine: More commonly used in endemic countries. In the United States, BCG is generally not recommended and very rarely used for high-risk children with negative PPD and ongoing exposure from parents or close contacts.

COMMONLY ASSOCIATED CONDITIONS
Immunosuppression; HIV coinfection; malignancy

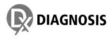

DIAGNOSIS

HISTORY
Signs and symptoms
- General: fever, night sweats, unintentional weight loss, malaise, painless lymph node swelling, arthralgias
- Pulmonary TB: unexplained cough >2 to 3 weeks, hemoptysis, pleuritic chest pain
- Abdominal TB: acutely as surgical abdomen; chronic abdominal TB varies (vague abdominal symptoms, abdominal mass, "doughy" abdomen).
- Meningitis (see "Tuberculosis, CNS")
- Miliary (see "Tuberculosis, Miliary")

PHYSICAL EXAM
- Often entirely normal. Specific findings depend on organs involved: hepatosplenomegaly, adenopathy, rales; poor weight gain in children
- Late findings: renal, bone, or CNS disease

DIFFERENTIAL DIAGNOSIS
- Pulmonary TB: pneumonia, malignancy, actinomycosis, coccidiomycosis, sarcoidosis, tularemia, etc.
- Extrapulmonary TB: other mycobacterial infections, syphilis, cat-scratch disease, leishmaniasis, erythema nodosum, rheumatic disease, erythema induratum

DIAGNOSTIC TESTS & INTERPRETATION
- For individuals >5 years old, interferon-γ release assay (IGRA) is generally preferred over tuberculin skin test (TST). For children <5 years old, TST is preferred over IGRA (1)[B]. However, the American Academy of Pediatrics now endorses IGRA in BCG-vaccinated children ≥2 years old.
- Persons at low risk for TB infection should not be tested. However, testing is often required by schools, employers, etc. In these cases, IGRA is preferred. If initial test is positive in low-risk patients, a second test is recommended which can be either an IGRA or TST. The patient is considered positive for TB infection only if both tests are positive (1)[C].

- TST (e.g., PPD): Measure induration at 48 to 72 hours:
  - PPD positive if induration
    - >5 mm PLUS HIV infection, recent TB contact, immunosuppressed, or positive x-ray
    - >10 mm PLUS age <5, moved to the US from high prevalence country in the last 5 years, IV drug users, or other risk factors
    - >15 mm PLUS age >4 years with no risk factors
  - Two-step test, 1 to 3 weeks apart: no recent PPD, age >55 years, nursing home resident, prison inmate, or health care workers
  - Context of PPD results:
    - False positive: BCG (unreliable, should not affect decision to treat)
    - False negative: HIV, steroids, gastrectomy, alcoholism, renal failure, sarcoidosis, recent viral vaccination, malnutrition, hematologic or lymphoreticular disorder, very recent exposure
    - If positive once, no need to repeat
- IGRAs measure interferon release after stimulation in vitro by *M. tuberculosis* antigens.
  - May be falsely negative in severely immunosuppressed patients (AIDS, chemotherapy)
- TST and IGRA cannot discern LTBI from active TB.
- Updated Centers for Disease Control (CDC) guidelines no longer recommend annual LTBI screening of health care workers without elevated risk profile once baseline testing complete.

Initial Tests (lab, imaging)
Active TB
- Three sputum samples for acid-fast bacilli (AFB) stain and mycobacterial culture by aerosol induction, gastric aspirate (children), or bronchoalveolar lavage (1)[B]
- Positive AFB: Treat immediately; culture and sensitivity guide treatment.
- Nucleic acid amplification test (NAAT): Use as an adjunct to culture and AFB smear (1)[C]. Positive result supports presumptive diagnosis of TB while culture pending. Negative NAAT does not rule out TB.
- Chest radiograph
  - Primary TB: infiltrate with or without atelectasis, effusion, or adenopathy
- CT chest: good sensitivity, tree-in-bud (centrilobular nodules with branching linear opacities)

Follow-Up Tests & Special Considerations
- Baseline CBC, creatinine, liver function tests, visual acuity, and red-green color discrimination (regimens involving ethambutol [EMB])
- HIV: If positive, get baseline CD4 count, viral load and genotype.
- Check hepatitis B and C if injection drug users, Africa or Asia born, HIV infected or otherwise high risk.
- Extrapulmonary: urine, CSF, bone marrow, and liver biopsy for culture as indicated; interferon-gamma (IFN-γ) and adenosine deaminase levels
- Nonspecific findings: anemia, thrombocytosis, SIADH, hypergammaglobulinemia, monocytosis, sterile pyuria

Diagnostic Procedures/Other
- Culture: takes several weeks for definitive results
- Xpert MTB/RIF (rapid molecular test): currently the only FDA-approved molecular assay for pulmonary TB diagnosis and detection of rifampicin resistance in areas with high prevalence of MDR TB

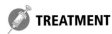 **TREATMENT**

GENERAL MEASURES
- If clinical suspicion, treat immediately. Prescribing physician is responsible for treatment completion.
- Respiratory and droplet precautions
- Not infectious if favorable clinical response after 2 to 3 weeks of therapy and each of three repeat AFB smears are negative

MEDICATION
Use ideal body weight for dosing; DOT recommended for all and required for children, institutionalized patients, nonadherent patients, and nondaily regimens

First Line
- LTBI (see "Tuberculosis, Latent (LTBI)")
- Active TB infection
  – Regimen 1 (preferred regimen for patients with newly diagnosed pulmonary TB)
    ○ Initial phase:
      ▪ Isoniazid, rifampin (RIF), pyrazinamide (PZA), and EMB for 8 weeks (2)[B] *or*
      ▪ INH/RIF/PZA/EMB 5 days/week for 8 weeks under directly observed therapy (DOT) (2)[C]
    ○ Continuation phase:
      ▪ INH/RIF daily for 18 weeks; or, if DOT, INH/RIF 5 days/week for 18 weeks (2)[B]
  – Regimen 2 (preferred when more frequent DOT in continuation phase is difficult to achieve)
    ○ Initial phase:
      ▪ INH/RIF/PZA/EMB daily for 8 weeks *or*
      ▪ INH/RIF/PZA/EMB 5 days/week for 8 weeks
    ○ Continuation phase:
      ▪ INH/RIF 3 times per week for 18 weeks (2)[C]
  – Regimen 3 (caution if HIV infected or with cavitary disease; missed doses can lead to treatment failure, relapse, and acquired drug resistance)
    ○ Initial phase: INH/RIF/PZA/EMB 3 times per week for 8 weeks
    ○ Continuation phase: INH/RIF 3 times per week for 18 weeks (2)[C]
  – Regimen 4 (do not use if HIV positive, smear positive, or cavitary disease)
    ○ Initial phase: INH/RIF/PZA/EMB daily for 14 doses and then twice a week for 12 doses
    ○ Continuation phase: INH/RIF twice a week for 18 weeks (2)[C]

Pregnancy Considerations
- Treatment for TB is initiated whenever the probability of maternal disease is moderate to high because of the risk of untreated TB to a pregnant woman and her fetus (2)[C].
- Although antituberculosis drugs cross the placenta, they do not appear to have teratogenic effects in humans. However, streptomycin should not be used in pregnancy.
- Treat TB in pregnancy with INH/RIF/EMB/PZA; add pyridoxine 25 to 50 mg/day.

- Congenital infection: from maternal miliary or endometrial TB. PPD, CXR, lumbar puncture, and culture placenta. Treat promptly if suspected.
- Breastfeeding: OK while taking TB drugs; supplement with pyridoxine 25 to 50 mg/day.

Pediatric Considerations
- Children may attend school if they are taking the appropriate medications.
- Children more commonly have severe disease and faster rate of progression to disease. However, most are asymptomatic.
- Pediatric TB treatment should be directly observed (DOT) using four drugs.

> **ALERT**
> - If patient does not receive PZA for all of the first 2 months, extend treatment to 9 months.
> - *M. bovis* is resistant to PZA; must be treated 9 months
> - Continue EMB until organism susceptibility to INH plus RIF is determined.
> - Initiation of ART therapy in HIV-positive patients infected with TB carries an increased risk of immune reconstitution inflammatory syndrome (IRIS) with pulmonary TB (2)[A].

Second Line
Fluoroquinolones and injectable aminoglycosides. Use when MDR is suspected or patient intolerance; pretomanid newly FDA approved for use in XDR-TB

ISSUES FOR REFERRAL

> **ALERT**
> Notify public health authorities for all cases of active TB. Consult infectious disease specialist for drug-resistant TB and HIV-positive patients on ART.

Case management referral is recommended.

ADDITIONAL THERAPIES
- Pyridoxine: 50 mg should be given to all persons at risk for INH neuropathy: pregnant women, diabetes, breastfed infants, HIV positive, alcoholism, chronic renal failure, malnutrition, or advanced age. Give 100 mg daily to patients with preexisting neuropathy.
- Steroids: recommended for TB meningitis; not recommended for TB pericarditis

SURGERY/OTHER PROCEDURES
For extrapulmonary complications (spinal cord compression, bowel obstruction, constrictive pericarditis)

ADMISSION, INPATIENT, AND NURSING CONSIDERATIONS
Negative pressure isolation with personal respirators and droplet precautions
- Three consecutive negative sputum AFB smears are necessary for release from isolation.

 ONGOING CARE

FOLLOW-UP RECOMMENDATIONS
Patient Monitoring
- Monthly sputum for AFB smear and culture until two consecutive cultures are negative; must confirm this prior to starting continuation phase
- Monthly visits to monitor medication adherence and adverse effects; CXR after 2 months of treatment

- Liver enzymes monthly for chronic liver disease, alcohol use, pregnant, or postpartum patients. Drug-induced liver injury is most common side effect of treatment. Temporarily halt medications for enzyme increase ≥5 × ULN if asymptomatic or ≥3 × ULN if symptomatic.
- Visual acuity and red-green color monthly if on EMB >2 months or doses >20 mg/kg/day
- If culture positive after 2 months of therapy, reassess drug sensitivity, initiate DOT, coordinate care with public health authorities, and consider infectious disease consultation. Persistent culture positive patients may warrant extended treatment.

PATIENT EDUCATION
- Emphasize medication adherence.
- Screen and treat close contacts.
- Alert patient that health authorities must be notified.

PROGNOSIS
Few complications and full resolution of infection if medications are taken for full course as prescribed

COMPLICATIONS
- Cavitary lesions can become secondarily infected.
- Risk for drug resistance increases with HIV positive, treatment nonadherence, or residence in area with high incidence of resistance.

REFERENCES
1. Lewinsohn DM, Leonard MK, LoBue PA, et al. Official American Thoracic Society/Infectious Diseases Society of America/Centers for Disease Control and Prevention clinical practice guidelines: diagnosis of tuberculosis in adults and children. *Clin Infect Dis.* 2017;64(2):111–115.
2. Nahid P, Dorman SE, Alipanah N, et al. Official American Thoracic Society/Centers for Disease Control and Prevention/Infectious Diseases Society of America clinical practice guidelines: treatment of drug-susceptible tuberculosis. *Clin Infect Dis.* 2016;63(7):e147–e195.

 SEE ALSO

Tuberculosis, CNS; Tuberculosis, Latent (LTBI); Tuberculosis, Miliary

CODES

ICD10
- A15.9 Respiratory tuberculosis, unspecified
- A15.0 Tuberculosis of lung
- A19.9 Miliary tuberculosis, unspecified

CLINICAL PEARLS
- TB is fully curable when treated appropriately.
- Children and elderly patients exhibit fewer classic clinical features of TB.
- TST and IGRA cannot discern active TB from LTBI.
- Notify public health authorities for all cases of active TB. Consult infectious disease for drug-resistant TB and HIV-positive patients on ART.

TUBERCULOSIS, LATENT (LTBI)

Laurel Banach, MD

BASICS

DESCRIPTION
- Latent tuberculosis infection (LTBI) is an asymptomatic, noninfectious condition following exposure to an active case of tuberculosis (TB). LTBI is usually detected by a screening skin or blood test.
- Active TB occurs in 5–10% of infected individuals who have not received preventive therapy. Chance of active TB increases with immunosuppression and is highest for all individuals within 2 years of infection; 85% of the cases are pulmonary, which can be spread person-to-person via aerosol route.
- Greater than 80% of active TB cases in United States result from untreated LTBI (1).
- LTBI treatment is a key component of the TB elimination strategy for the United States.

ALERT
- Nitrosamine particles have been isolated in rifampin and rifapentine products in 2020 and 2021. These nitrosamine particles are potential or probable carcinogens, and due to the life-threatening nature of TB, the FDA has approved ongoing production of these antimicrobials with close monitoring (2).
- The current pace of decline in TB incidence will not eliminate TB in the United States in the 21st century. Extra effort is needed to identify patients with LTBI (3).

EPIDEMIOLOGY
- In the United States, high-risk groups include immigrants from countries with a high TB rate (countries other than the United States, Canada, Australia, New Zealand, or a country in western or northern Europe); persons with a history of drug use or experiencing homelessness; HIV-infected or immunocompromised individuals; persons living or working in high-risk congregate settings such as nursing homes, carceral facilities, and health care workers (3)
- TB is a major cause of death in individuals infected with HIV (3).
- Newly exposed (particularly children) are also at high risk.
- In 2020, there were 7,163 TB cases reported in the United States (4).
- In 2020, of the 7,163 TB cases, 71% of them were in non–U.S.-born persons (4). Incidence decreased in both populations, U.S.-born decreased from 0.9 to 0.7 cases per 100,000, and non–U.S.-born decreased from 14.2 to 11.5 cases per 100,000.
- Among non–U.S.-born persons with TB, incidence in 2018 was highest among Asians, followed by Native Hawaiians/Pacific Islanders, non-Hispanic blacks (blacks), Hispanics, and American Indian/Alaska Natives and was lowest among non-Hispanic whites (whites) (1),(3).
- The highest TB incidence for U.S.-born persons occurred among Native Hawaiians/Pacific Islanders, followed by American Indians/Alaska Natives, blacks, Asians, and Hispanics and was lowest in whites (1).

Incidence
In 2018, a total of 9,029 new TB cases were reported in the United States (1).

Prevalence
- Globally, 10 million people were infected with TB in 2020. 1.1 million of these people were children (5).
- Globally, TB incidence fell about 2% per year between 2015 and 2020 (5).
- In the United States, there were 7,163 cases of TB reported in 2020 (4).

ETIOLOGY AND PATHOPHYSIOLOGY
Mycobacterium tuberculosis, Mycobacterium bovis, and *Mycobacterium africanum*

RISK FACTORS
- Immigrants from TB-endemic countries, which include most countries of Africa, Asia, and Eastern Europe
- Close contact with infected individual
- Living or working in a congregate setting (e.g., prison, nursing home)
- Use of illicit drugs
- Lower socioeconomic status or experiencing homelessness
- Health care workers
- Laboratory personnel working with mycobacteria

GENERAL PREVENTION
- Screen for LTBI and treat individuals with positive tests.
- If a person has fibrotic lung changes on imaging and no evidence of TB treatment, these patients should be screened for LTBI, regardless of their other risk factors.
- Special population: Organ donors should be screened. If donor is deceased, IGRA testing is still possible.

COMMONLY ASSOCIATED CONDITIONS
- HIV infection (see "Initial Tests (lab, imaging)")
- Immunosuppression
- IV drug use and substance use disorders

DIAGNOSIS

HISTORY
- Assess risk; history of immigration from a high-risk area including those with temporary visas for school or work (note: TB screening for this type of visa is not required, unlike regulations for those seeking permanent residence in the United States), history of IV drug use and/or drug treatment, HIV, recent incarceration or experience of homelessness, immunosuppression
  - If household contact has LTBI, test all household contacts.
- Assess for active TB cough for more than 2 to 3 weeks, fevers, night sweats, weight loss, hemoptysis.

PHYSICAL EXAM
- No active signs of infection on exam in patients with LTBI
- Assess for active TB by performing vital signs, weight, pulmonary, and lymph node exams.

DIFFERENTIAL DIAGNOSIS
- Fungal infections; atypical mycobacteria or *Nocardia*
- Immunosuppression from conditions such as HIV

DIAGNOSTIC TESTS & INTERPRETATION
Initial Tests (lab, imaging)
- Test for TB infection with tuberculin skin (PPD) or interferon-γ release assay (3).
- Chest X-ray to rule out active TB

- Only if concern for active disease, perform acid fast bacilli sputum smear and culture (3).
- Screen at-risk patients for HIV (3).
- Baseline lab testing prior to treatment is not required but recommended for patients at risk for liver disease including heavy alcohol use as hepatotoxicity is the primary side effect of treatment or patients that are HIV-infected.

Follow-Up Tests & Special Considerations
- Repeat liver transaminases are recommended during LTBI treatment, if symptoms develop concerning for hepatotoxicity.
- Discontinue treatment if ALT elevation is >5× the upper limit of normal or >3× the upper limit of normal with signs/symptoms consistent with hepatic damage.
- The CDC recently updated recommendations regarding LTBI surveillance of Health Care Workers. Without known exposure or evidence of TB transmission, health care workers in the United States do not need to serial TB screening at any interval after a baseline test (1).

Test Interpretation
- TST: PPD: 5 U (0.1 mL) intermediate-strength intradermal volar forearm. Measure induration at 48 to 72 hours:
  - Positive if induration is (3)
    - >5 mm and patient has HIV infection (or suspected), is immunosuppressed, had recent close TB contact, or has clinical evidence of active or old disease on CXR
    - >10 mm and patient age <4 years or has other risk factors noted earlier
    - >15 mm and patient age >4 years and has no risk factors
  - Negative if induration <5 mm on initial test and, if indicated, on second test
  - Use the two-step test (administer a second intradermal test 1 to 3 weeks after initial test; measure and interpret as usual) if patient has had no recent PPD and is age >55 years or is a nursing home resident, prison inmate, or health care worker.
  - Preferred for children <2 years
- The IGRA QuantiFERON-TB and QuantiFERON-TB GOLD; T-SPOT measures the release of interferon by sensitized lymphocytes when exposed to antigens of *M. tuberculosis*.
  - It is unaffected by prior BCG vaccination.
  - Requires only one visit for the lab draw
  - Improved sensitivity and specificity but is costly
- Special considerations
  - Measles vaccine: may suppress tuberculin activity; simultaneous PPD and measles vaccine recommended; if not simultaneous, defer PPD for 4 to 6 weeks after measles vaccine.
  - The history of BCG vaccination should not alter the management of a positive PPD test but consider IGRA test in persons who have received the BCG vaccination.
  - Situations that may give a false-negative skin test:
    - Recent viral infection
    - New (<10 weeks) infection
    - Severe malnutrition; HIV; anergy
    - Age <6 months
    - Active TB
    - Steroid use

TREATMENT

GENERAL MEASURES
- Must first exclude active TB by history, physical exam, and lung imaging
- Chest x-ray must be obtained within 2 months prior to starting LTBI treatment.
- Treatment for LTBI is critical for the control and elimination of TB disease. LTBI treatment decreases the risk of active TB and decreases risk of potential spread to others. Treat all persons with LTBI.
- Directly observed therapy (DOT) is recommended if patient adherence is not assured. Video DOT is an effective alternative.
- Treat LTBI during pregnancy if patient has recent infection or is HIV positive (use isoniazid [INH] with pyridoxine and monitor liver enzymes); otherwise, postpone treatment until after delivery.
- Consult public health or infectious disease specialist for suspected INH resistance in HIV patients.
- Consult public health or infectious disease specialist for complicated medication interactions, especially in the circumstance of nitrosamine products in rifampin and rifapentine.

MEDICATION
The CDC and National Tuberculosis Controllers Association (NTCA) recently convened in 2020 to complete a systemic review and update the treatment recommendations.

First Line
- Rifamycin-based antimicrobials (rifamycins) have many drug interactions (via CYP3A4 pathway), and a drug-interaction tool should be used before prescribing.
  - Rifamycins can reduce the effectiveness of hormonal contraception; persons using hormonal contraception should consider the copper IUD, switch to, or add a barrier method for the full duration of latent TB treatment.
  - Rifamycins can interact with warfarin—patients require increased monitoring.
  - Monitor for hypersensitivity reaction, hepatotoxicity.
  - Monitor for hypotensive or flulike reaction to weekly INH/rifapentine and discontinue if this occurs.
  - Rifamycins cause temporary red-orange discoloration of body fluids (urine, sweat, tears, saliva); this reverses on discontinuation of medication.
- INH should be closely monitored for hepatotoxicity, especially in patients with a history of alcohol use disorder, HBV, HCV, fatty liver, NASH, or other signs of liver dysfunction or injury.
  - Peripheral neuritis and hypersensitivity are possible. Consider concurrent pyridoxine (vitamin B_6) 25 to 50 mg/day
- Regimens:
  - Rifampin alone
    - 4 months duration, rifampin given daily
    - Rifampin: max daily dose 600 mg; adults 10 mg/kg and children 15 to 20 mg/kg
  - INH + rifampin daily
    - 3 months duration
    - INH: max daily dose 900 mg; adults 15 mg/kg and children (ages 2 to 11 years) 25 mg/kg
    - Rifampin dosing see above

- Once-weekly INH + rifapentine (3HP)
  - 3 months duration, weekly administration with DOT
  - INH dosing (see above)
  - Rifapentine dosing
    - 10 to 14.0 kg, 300 mg
    - 14.1 to 25.0 kg, 450 mg
    - 25.1 to 32.0 kg, 600 mg
    - 32.1 to 49.9 kg, 750 mg
    - >50.0 kg, 900 mg (max daily dose)

Second Line
Alternative options include INH daily for 6 or 9 months.
- Reduced adherence when compared to shorter-course regimens
- Longer duration could increase risk for hepatotoxicity.
- These two durations have not been directly compared.

ISSUES FOR REFERRAL
- Consult public health or infectious disease specialist for suspected INH resistance in HIV patients.
- Consult public health or infectious disease specialist for complicated medication interactions, especially in the circumstance of nitrosamine products in rifampin and rifapentine.
- Consult infectious disease specialists for concerns for multidrug-resistant cases.

ADDITIONAL THERAPIES
Pediatric Considerations
- Follow public health recommendations for assessing and treating newborns.
- If contact has abnormal CXR, separate infant until infectious status is known; if not contagious, monitor infant PPD.
- If mother has disease and is possibly contagious, evaluate infant for congenital TB and test for HIV; separate newborn until mother is noninfectious.
- Treat suspected congenital TB.

ADMISSION, INPATIENT, AND NURSING CONSIDERATIONS
Geriatric Considerations
- Before entering a chronic care setting, patients should have two-step PPD using facility protocols.
- INH side effects are more pronounced.
- No isolation required

 ONGOING CARE

FOLLOW-UP RECOMMENDATIONS
Patient Monitoring
- During treatment course for LTBI, monthly visits to assess adherence and monitor for signs and symptoms of active TP or signs of adverse treatment effects (hepatitis, hypersensitivity, neuropathy); consider partnering with local public health offices for DOT monitoring if appropriate.
- Check liver enzymes if patient is symptomatic, HIV positive, has chronic liver disease, uses alcohol, or is pregnant or postpartum. Modify drugs as needed.
- In a patient who has elected to defer LTBI treatment, there is no indication to repeat chest x-ray unless symptoms develop or the patient elects to initiate treatment.

DIET
Regular. In patients treated with INH, consider pyridoxine 10 to 50 mg/day.

PROGNOSIS
- Generally, there are few complications, and treatment is effective if medications are taken as prescribed.
- If LTBI treatment is erroneously offered to a patient with active TB, it can result in monotherapy of active disease.
- Nonadherence during LTBI treatment does not lead to drug resistance but does result in untreated LTBI.
- Retreatment is not necessary.

COMPLICATIONS
Recrudescent TB

REFERENCES
1. Sosa LE, Njie GJ, Lobato MN, et al. Tuberculosis screening, testing, and treatment of U.S. health care personnel: recommendations from the National Tuberculosis Controllers Association and CDC, 2019. *MMWR Morb Mortal Wkly Rep.* 2019;68(19):439–443.
2. Yanes-Lane M, Trajman A, Bastos ML, et al. Effects of programmatic interventions to improve the management of latent tuberculosis: a follow up study up to five months after implementation. *BMC Public Health.* 2021;21(1):177.
3. Centers for Disease Control and Prevention. Diagnosing latent TB infection & disease. https://www.cdc.gov/tb/topic/testing/diagnosingltbi.htm. Published April 18, 2016. Accessed September 3, 2021.
4. Deutsch-Feldman M, Pratt RH, Price SF, et al. Tuberculosis—United States, 2020. *MMWR Morb Mortal Wkly Rep.* 2021;70(12):409–414.
5. World Health Organization. Global tuberculosis report 2021. https://www.who.int/teams/global-tuberculosis-programme/tb-reports/global-tuberculosis-report-2021. Accessed December 3, 2021.

ADDITIONAL READING
Mehtani NJ, Puryear S, Pham P, et al. Infectious diseases learning unit: understanding advances in the treatment of latent tuberculosis infection among people with human immunodeficiency virus. *Open Forum Infect Dis.* 2021;8(8):ofab319.

 SEE ALSO

Tuberculosis; Tuberculosis, Miliary

CODES

ICD10
R76.11 Nonspecific reaction to skin test w/o active tuberculosis

CLINICAL PEARLS
- Treatment of LTBI is crucial to the control and elimination of TB disease in the United States.
- Screen persons from TB-endemic countries and treat those who are positive.
- Screen household contacts of patients who are LTBI positive.
- The interferon-γ (IGRA) blood test is unaffected by prior BCG vaccination.

TYPHOID FEVER

Douglas William MacPherson, MD, MSc(CTM), FRCPC

BASICS

- A common enteric bacterial disease transmitted by ingestion of contaminated food or water
- Most cases in the United States are imported from endemic areas of South or Southeast Asia and Latin America.
- Multiple drug-resistant (MDRO) salmonellae are increasingly common worldwide, particularly in Latin America and Asia.
- Extensively drug-resistant (XDR) salmonella infections have emerged in Asia with outbreaks originating in Pakistan in 2016. Importation via travel and secondary (non-travel) related cases occurred in United States (1).

DESCRIPTION

- Typhoid fever is an acute systemic illness in humans caused by *Salmonella typhi* (2).
  – Classic example of enteric fever caused by *Salmonella* bacterium
- Enteric fevers due to *Salmonella paratyphi* and other Salmonella spp. can present in a manner similar to classic typhoid fever.
- Typhoid is endemic in developing nations with poor sanitation. Most cases in North America and other developed nations are acquired after travel to disease-endemic areas.
- Travelers are at greater risk of typhoid.
- Mode of transmission is fecal–oral through ingestion of contaminated food (poultry or milk) or water.
- Incubation period varies from 7 to 21 days.
- System(s) affected: gastrointestinal; pulmonary; skin/exocrine
- Synonym(s): typhoid; typhus abdominalis; enteric fever; nervous fever; slow fever

Geriatric Considerations
Disease is more serious in the elderly.

Pediatric Considerations
Disease is more serious in infants and children.

EPIDEMIOLOGY
Although typhoid outbreaks have been described in the United States, most cases are reported in international travelers returning from endemic transmission areas.
- Predominant age: all ages
- Predominant sex: male = female

Incidence
In the United States, 300 to 500 new cases per year. Worldwide, typhoid fever infects over 21 million people/year with ~ 200,000 deaths.

ETIOLOGY AND PATHOPHYSIOLOGY
- Historically, typhoid fever (untreated) occurs in several week-long stages.
- The initial infection is transmitted via the fecal–oral route, with resultant bacteremia and sepsis. Involvement of the bowel wall (Peyer patch) rarely may be associated with bleeding from the bowel or bowel perforation.
- The first stage involves fluctuations in temperature with relative bradycardia (Faget sign). Other symptoms include headache, cough, malaise, epistaxis, and abdominal pain.

- The second stage involves higher fever (with persistent relative bradycardia). Mental status changes are possible (agitation—"nervous fever"). Rose spots appear on the chest and abdomen. In some patients, abdominal pain is common as is constipation or diarrhea (with characteristic malodorous "pea soup" appearance).
- The third week is when most complications occur due to intestinal hemorrhage or encephalitis.
- The final week is defervescence and recovery.
- A chronic carrier state may occur with *S. typhi* shedding in the stools. Potential person-to-person transmission may occur. In a chronic carrier state, *S. typhi* resides in the biliary tract and gallbladder. Chronic suppressive antimicrobials may clear the carrier state; in rare cases, cholecystectomy is performed to clear *S. typhi* carrier state.

RISK FACTORS
- Consider in patients presenting with fever after tropical travel or exposure to a chronic carrier.
- Small inocula of *S. typhi* (~100,000 organisms) cause disease in >50% of healthy individuals.

GENERAL PREVENTION
- Food and water precautions help prevent all enteric infections, including typhoid fever.
- Avoid tap water, salad/raw vegetables, unpeeled fruits, and dairy products in tropical travel.
- Avoid undercooked poultry or poultry products left unrefrigerated for prolonged periods.
- Wash hands before and after food preparation.
- For high-risk travel to an endemic area, consider typhoid vaccination (3).
  – Parenteral ViCPS or capsular polysaccharide typhoid vaccine (Typhim Vi) *or*
  – Ty21a or live oral typhoid vaccine (Vivotif Berna), particularly if prolonged risk (>4 weeks)
- Consider vaccination for workers exposed to *S. typhi* or those with close contact with a carrier of *S. typhi*.
- Occupational health and safety precautions. Consider screening of domestic and commercial food handlers.

DIAGNOSIS

Assess clinical presentation and exposure history, including travel and exposures to *S. typhi* carriers.

HISTORY
- Travel history to an endemic region and exposure to contaminated food or water
- Exposure to a chronic *S. typhi* carrier
- Fever, headache
- Malaise
- Abdominal discomfort/bloating/constipation
- Diarrhea (less common)
- Dry cough
- Confusion/lethargy

PHYSICAL EXAM
- Fever with relative bradycardia
- Cervical adenopathy
- Conjunctivitis
- Rose spot (transient erythematous maculopapular rash in anterior thorax or upper abdomen)
- Splenomegaly
- Hepatomegaly

DIFFERENTIAL DIAGNOSIS
- Enteric fever caused by nontyphoid *Salmonella* spp.
- "Enteric fever–like" syndrome caused by *Yersinia enterocolitica*, pseudotuberculosis, and *Campylobacter* spp.
- Infectious hepatitis
- Malaria, dengue
- Atypical pneumonia
- Infectious mononucleosis
- Subacute bacterial endocarditis
- Tuberculosis
- Brucellosis; Q fever; typhus
- Rickettsial diseases
- Toxoplasmosis
- Viral infections: Epstein-Barr virus (EBV), cytomegalovirus (CMV), viral hemorrhagic agents

DIAGNOSTIC TESTS & INTERPRETATION
Enteric fevers/typhoid syndromes are rare in the United States. Therefore, a high level of clinical suspicion is required.
- Definitive diagnosis is by culture of *S. typhi* from blood or other sterile body fluid.
- Isolation of *S. typhi* in sputum, urine, or stool leads to a presumptive diagnosis.
- Serology is nonspecific and typically not useful.
- If there are multiple negative blood cultures or patient has recent been on antibiotic therapy, diagnostic yield is better with bone marrow culture.
- Anemia, leukopenia (neutropenia), thrombocytopenia, or evidence of disseminated intravascular coagulopathy. Elevated liver enzymes are common.
- Suspect intestinal perforation (consider serial plain abdominal films looking for evidence of perforation) in ill patients complaining of persistent abdominal tenderness.

Diagnostic Procedures/Other
- Bone marrow aspirate for culture of *S. typhi* is more sensitive than blood cultures but rarely used as a primary investigation.
- Bone marrow aspiration may be done for evaluation of a fever of unknown origin.

Test Interpretation
Classically, bowel pathology shows mononuclear lymphoid proliferation, especially Peyer patches of the terminal ileum.

TREATMENT

- Treatment of typhoid disease and chronic carrier states must be determined on an individual basis. Factors to consider include age, public health and occupational health risk (e.g., food handler, chronic care facilities, medical personnel), intolerance to antibiotics, and evidence of biliary tract disease.
- Awareness of emerging drug-resistant *S. typhi* strains and the epidemiology of the patient's exposure help direct primary therapy. Knowledge of local resistance patterns for presumptive treatment or laboratory sensitivity also guides therapy. Fluoroquinolone-resistant *S. typhi* is common in Asia.

GENERAL MEASURES
- Fluid and electrolyte support
- Strict isolation of patient's linen, stool, and urine
- Consider serial plain abdominal films for evidence of perforation, usually in the 3rd to 4th week of illness.
- For hemorrhage: blood transfusion and management of shock

MEDICATION

First Line
- MDRO and XDR must be considered in all cases of typhoid fevers acquired during travel:
  - A carbapenem (with a travel history to Pakistan, Iraq, and other emerging XDR destinations) and/or azithromycin (depending on clinical severity)
  - Azithromycin (see dose below)
- Lower risk acquisition destinations:
  - Ceftriaxone: pediatric 100 mg/kg/day for 2 weeks; adult dose: 1 to 2 g IV once daily for 2 weeks *or*
  - Azithromycin: pediatric 10 to 20 mg/kg (max 1 g) PO daily for 5 to 7 days; adult dose: 1 g PO once followed by 500 mg PO daily for 5 to 7 days
  - The following agents have historical therapeutic relevance but due to MDRO and XDR salmonella infections should be considered only in specific situations (known sensitivity patterns) or in consultation with an infectious diseases expert.
  - Chloramphenicol: pediatric 50 mg/kg/day PO QID for 2 weeks; adult dose 2 to 3 g per day PO divided q6h for 2 weeks *or*
  - Ampicillin: pediatric 100 mg/kg/day (max 2 g) QID PO for 2 weeks; adults 500 mg q6h for 2 weeks *or*
  - Ciprofloxacin: 500 mg PO BID for 2 weeks, *indicated in multiple-drug–resistant typhoid*
    - Has been used safely in children; WHO recommends as first line in areas with drug resistance to older first-line antibiotics.
    - Fluoroquinolones may prevent clinical relapse better than chloramphenicol.
- Chronic carrier state—consult with an infectious diseases expert
  - Ampicillin: 4 to 5 g/day plus probenecid 2 g/day QID for 6 weeks (for patients with normal gallbladder function and no evidence of cholelithiasis)
  - Ciprofloxacin: 500 mg PO BID for 4 to 6 weeks is also efficacious. Chloramphenicol resistance has been reported in Mexico, South America, Central America, Southeast Asia, India, Pakistan, Middle East, and Africa.
- Contraindications: Refer to manufacturer's profile.
- Precautions: Rarely, Jarisch-Herxheimer reaction appears after antimicrobial therapy.
- Significant possible interactions: Refer to manufacturer's profile for each drug.

Second Line
- Trimethoprim–sulfamethoxazole one double-strength tablet twice a day for 10 days (Note: Drug resistance is common; local resistance patterns and expert consultation should guide treatment.)
- Furazolidone: 7.5 mg/kg/day PO for 10 days; in uncomplicated multidrug-resistant typhoid; safe in children; efficacy >85% cure

Pregnancy Considerations
Ciprofloxacin and sulfonamides are relatively contraindicated in children and in pregnant patients—seek consultation.

ISSUES FOR REFERRAL
Complications of sepsis, bowel perforation

SURGERY/OTHER PROCEDURES
- Complications: bowel perforation
- Cholecystectomy may be warranted in carriers with cholelithiasis, relapse after therapy, or intolerance to antimicrobial therapy.

ADMISSION, INPATIENT, AND NURSING CONSIDERATIONS
- Inpatient if acutely ill
- Outpatient for less ill patient or for carrier
- Observe enteric precautions.

 ONGOING CARE

FOLLOW-UP RECOMMENDATIONS
Bed rest initially and then activity as tolerated

Patient Monitoring
See "General Measures."

DIET
NPO if abdominal symptoms are severe. With improvement, begin normal low-residue diet, with high-calorie supplementation if malnourished.

PATIENT EDUCATION
- Discuss chronic carrier state and its complications.
- For family members, travelers, or workers at risk, educate about food/water hygiene and provide vaccination.
- Educate patients that the typhoid vaccines do not protect against *S. paratyphi* infection.
- Typhoid vaccines protect 50–80% of recipients (not 100%). Efficacy wanes over 2 to 4 years.
- CDC patient handout: http://www.cdc.gov/vaccines/hcp/vis/vis-statements/typhoid.html

PROGNOSIS
Overall prognosis is good; with appropriate treatment, <2% mortality rate, 15% relapse rate with some antibiotic treatments, and 3% bowel perforation.

COMPLICATIONS
- Intestinal hemorrhage and perforation in distal ileum
- Patients (up to 3%) may become chronic carriers-persistent stool excretor of *S. typhi* for >1 year.
- Seeding of the biliary tract may become a focus for relapse of typhoid fever; most common in females and older patients (>50 years of age).
- Osteomyelitis is more common in patients with sickle cell anemia, systemic lupus erythematosus, and hematologic neoplasms as well as in immunosuppressed hosts.
- Endovascular infection in the elderly and in patients with a history of bypass operation or aneurysm
- Rarely, endocarditis or meningitis

REFERENCES
1. Centers for Disease Control. CDC Health Advisory: extensively drug-resistant *Salmonella typhi* infections among U.S. residents without international travel. https://emergency.cdc.gov/han/pdf/CDC-HAN-439-XDR-Salmonella-Typhi-Infections-in-U.S.-Without-Intl-Travel-02.12.2021.pdf. Accessed August 25, 2021.
2. Appiah GD, Hughes MJ, Chatham-Stephens K. Typhoid & paratyphoid fever. In: Centers for Disease Control and Prevention, Brunette GW, Nemhauser JB, eds. *CDC Yellow Book 2020: Health Information for International Travel*. New York, NY: Oxford University Press; 2019. https://wwwnc.cdc.gov/travel/yellowbook/2020/travel-related-infectious-diseases/typhoid-and-paratyphoid-fever. Accessed August 25, 2021.
3. Centers for Disease Control. Typhoid and paratyphoid fever: vaccination. https://www.cdc.gov/typhoid-fever/typhoid-vaccination.html. Accessed August 25, 2021.

ADDITIONAL READING
- Date KA, Bentsi-Enchill A, Marks F, et al. Typhoid fever vaccination strategies. *Vaccine*. 2015;33(Suppl 3):C55–C61.
- Marchello CS, Hong CY, Crump JA. Global typhoid fever incidence: a systematic review and meta-analysis. *Clin Infect Dis*. 2019;68(Suppl 2): S105–S116.
- Newton AE, Routh JA, Mahon BE. Chapter 3. Infectious diseases related to travel. Typhoid and paratyphoid fever. http://wwwnc.cdc.gov/travel/yellowbook/2016/infectious-diseases-related-to-travel/typhoid-paratyphoid-fever. Accessed August 25, 2021.

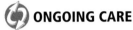 **CODES**

ICD10
- A01.00 Typhoid fever, unspecified
- Z22.0 Carrier of typhoid
- A01.03 Typhoid pneumonia

CLINICAL PEARLS
- Consider typhoid (along with malaria, dengue, and other travel-associated infections) in febrile travelers returning from endemic areas (Latin America, sub-Saharan Africa, South Asia). Individualize treatment based on patient characteristics and potential exposures.
- Routine blood cultures detect *S. typhi* but may be negative if antibiotics are administered prior to testing.
- A history or documentation of vaccination against *S. typhi* does not exclude the diagnosis of typhoid fever.

T

TYPHUS FEVERS

Douglas William MacPherson, MD, MSc(CTM), FRCPC

 BASICS

An infectious disease syndrome caused by several species of *Rickettsia* resulting in acute, chronic, and recurrent disease

DESCRIPTION
- Acute infection caused by three species of *Rickettsia* (1)
  - Epidemic typhus: human-to-human transmission by body louse; primarily in setting of refugee camps, war, famine, and disaster. Recurrent disease occurs years after initial infection and can be a source of human outbreak. Flying squirrels are a reservoir.
  - Endemic (murine) typhus: spread to humans by rat flea bite
  - Scrub typhus: infection and infestation of chiggers and of rodents to humans by the Trombiculidae mite "chigger"; primarily in Asia and western Pacific areas
- System(s) affected: endocrine/metabolic; hematologic/lymphatic/immunologic; pulmonary; skin/exocrine
- Synonym(s): louse-borne typhus; Brill-Zinsser disease; murine typhus

EPIDEMIOLOGY
- Epidemic and endemic typhus: rare in the United States (outside of South Texas)
- Scrub typhus: travelers returning from endemic areas

Incidence
Endemic typhus: <100 cases annually, primarily in states around the Gulf of Mexico, especially South Texas; underreporting suspected

ETIOLOGY AND PATHOPHYSIOLOGY
- Epidemic typhus by *Rickettsia prowazekii*
- Endemic typhus by *Rickettsia typhi* (2)[A]
- Scrub typhus by *Rickettsia tsutsugamushi*

RISK FACTORS
- Vector exposure
- Travel to endemic countries

Geriatric Considerations
Elderly may have more severe disease.

GENERAL PREVENTION
Vector control:
- Scrub typhus: protective clothing and insect repellents
- Endemic typhus: ectoparasite and rodent control
- Epidemic typhus: delousing and cleaning of clothing; vaccine for those at high risk of exposure (typhus vaccine production discontinued in the United States)

 DIAGNOSIS

Typhus syndromes are rare in the United States. A high level of clinical suspicion is necessary.

HISTORY
Travel or other risk exposure
- Fever, chills
- Intractable headache
- Myalgias, malaise
- Cough, rash, ocular pain

PHYSICAL EXAM
- General
  - Fever
  - Relative bradycardia (scrub typhus)
- Epidemic typhus
  - Incubation period ~1 week
  - Macular or maculopapular rash beginning on trunk ~5th day of illness
  - Nonproductive cough
  - Pulmonary infiltrates
- Endemic typhus
  - Incubation period 1 to 2 weeks
  - Macular or maculopapular rash beginning on trunk 3rd to 5th day of illness
- Scrub typhus
  - Incubation period 1 to 3 weeks
  - Eschar at bite site
  - Regional lymphadenopathy
  - Generalized lymphadenopathy
  - Splenomegaly
  - Macular or maculopapular rash beginning on trunk approximately 5th day of illness
  - Relative bradycardia early in disease
  - Ocular pain
  - Conjunctival injection

DIFFERENTIAL DIAGNOSIS
- Other rickettsial disease: Rocky Mountain spotted fever; ehrlichiosis; Mediterranean spotted fever (boutonneuse fever) (*Rickettsia conorii*)
- Bacterial meningitis; meningococcemia
- Measles, rubella
- Toxoplasmosis
- Leptospirosis
- Typhoid fever
- Dengue, malaria
- Relapsing fever
- Secondary syphilis
- Viral syndromes: mononucleosis, acute retroviral syndrome

DIAGNOSTIC TESTS & INTERPRETATION
- Specific serologies with rising antibody titer
- If suspected, isolate *Rickettsia* in qualified laboratory to minimize the risk of laboratory-acquired infection.
- CDC Rickettsial Zoonoses Branch 404-639-1075

Initial Tests (lab, imaging)
- CBC often normal
- Weil-Felix serologic reaction may be positive; test hampered by low sensitivity and nonspecificity; epidemic and endemic typhus, 4-fold titer rise or titer >1/320 to OX19; scrub typhus, 4-fold rise in titer to OXK
- Hyponatremia in severe cases
- Hypoalbuminemia in severe cases
- Recent antibiotic exposure may alter lab results.

Test Interpretation
Diffuse vasculitis on skin biopsy

 TREATMENT

Initiate treatment based on epidemiologic risk and clinical presentation.

GENERAL MEASURES
- Skin and mouth care
- Supportive care—directed at complications

MEDICATION

First Line

- Begin treatment when diagnosis is likely and continue until clinically improved and the patient is afebrile for at least 48 hours; usual course is 5 to 7 days.
- Children ≥8 years of age and adults
  - Doxycycline IV/PO: adults 100 mg q12h, children ≤45 kg: 5 mg/kg/day divided twice daily (max of 200 mg/day); >45 kg: adult dosing
  - Children ≤8 years of age: risk of dental staining from tetracyclines minimal with short courses
  - Tetracycline: 25 mg/kg PO initially and then 25 mg/kg/day in equally divided doses q6h
- Children ≤8 years of age, pregnant women, or if typhoid fever is suspected
  - Chloramphenicol: 50 mg/kg PO initially and then 50 mg/kg/day in equally divided doses q6h
  - If severely ill, chloramphenicol sodium succinate: 20 mg/kg IV initially, infused over 30 to 45 minutes and then 50 mg/kg/day infused in equally divided doses q6h until orally tolerable Azithromycin, fluoroquinolones, and rifampin alternatives depending on scenario
- Precautions and interactions: Refer to the manufacturer's profile for each specific drug.

Second Line

- Doxycycline: single oral dose of 100 or 200 mg PO for those in refugee camps, victims of disasters, or in the presence of limited medical services
- Isolated reports indicate that erythromycin and ciprofloxacin are effective.
- Azithromycin 1,000 mg PO once a day for 3-day course is effective for scrub typhus; better tolerated than doxycycline but more expensive
- Rifampin may be effective in areas where scrub typhus responds poorly to standard antirickettsial drugs.

ISSUES FOR REFERRAL

Infectious disease consultation is recommended. Contact CDC and local public health authorities.

ADMISSION, INPATIENT, AND NURSING CONSIDERATIONS

- Outpatient care unless severely ill
- Severely ill or constitutionally unstable (e.g., shock)

ONGOING CARE

FOLLOW-UP RECOMMENDATIONS

Patient Monitoring

- Admit severely ill patients.
- If treated as an outpatient, ensure regular follow-up to assess clinical improvement and resolution.

DIET

As tolerated

PATIENT EDUCATION

Travel advice (minimize exposure risks, vector avoidance, vaccination as appropriate)

PROGNOSIS

- Recovery is expected with prompt treatment.
- Relapses may follow treatment, especially if initiated within 48 hours of onset (this is *not* an indication to delay treatment). Treat relapses the same as primary disease.
- Without treatment, the mortality rate of typhus is 40–60% for epidemic, 1–2% for endemic, and up to 30% for scrub disease.
- Mortality is higher among the elderly.

COMPLICATIONS

Organ-specific complications (particularly in the 2nd week of illness): azotemia, meningoencephalitis, seizures, delirium, coma, myocardial failure, hyponatremia, hypoalbuminemia, hypovolemia, shock, and death

REFERENCES

1. Centers for Disease Control and Prevention. Typhus fevers. https://www.cdc.gov/typhus/index.html. Accessed February 2, 2021.
2. Afzal Z, Kallumadanda S, Wang F, et al. Acute febrile illness and complications due to murine typhus, Texas, USA1,2. *Emerg Infect Dis*. 2017;23(8):1268–1273.

ADDITIONAL READING

- Chikeka I, Dumler JS. Neglected bacterial zoonoses. *Clin Microbiol Infect*. 2015;21(5):404–415.
- Fang R, Blanton LS, Walker DH. Rickettsiae as emerging infectious agents. *Clin Lab Med*. 2017;37(2):383–400.

- Kispotta R, Kasinathan A, Kumar Kommu PP, et al. Analysis of 262 children with scrub typhus infection: a single-center experience [published online ahead of print November 9, 2020]. *Am J Trop Med Hyg*. 2020. doi:10.4269/ajtmh.20-1019
- Murray KO, Evert N, Mayes B, et al. Typhus group rickettsiosis, Texas, USA, 2003–2013. *Emerg Infect Dis*. 2017;23(4):645–648.
- Nelson K, Maina AN, Brisco A, et al. A 2015 outbreak of flea-borne rickettsiosis in San Gabriel Valley, Los Angeles County, California. *PLoS Negl Trop Dis*. 2018;12(4):e0006385.
- Panpanich R, Garner P. Antibiotics for treating scrub typhus. *Cochrane Database Syst Rev*. 2002;(3):CD002150.
- van Eekeren LE, de Vries SG, Wagenaar JFP, et al. Under-diagnosis of rickettsial disease in clinical practice: a systematic review. *Travel Med Infect Dis*. 2018;26:7–15. doi:10.1016/j.tmaid.2018.02.006.

CODES

ICD10

- A75.9 Typhus fever, unspecified
- A75.0 Epidemic louse-borne typhus fever d/t Rickettsia prowazekii
- A75.2 Typhus fever due to Rickettsia typhi

CLINICAL PEARLS

- Consider typhus (along with malaria and dengue) in febrile travelers returning from endemic areas.
- Rickettsial infections typically present within 2 to 14 days. Febrile illnesses presenting >18 days after travel are unlikely to be rickettsial.
- Doxycycline is the treatment of choice.
- Routine blood cultures do not detect *Rickettsia*.
- Prior vaccination does not exclude typhus.

ULCER, APHTHOUS

Cynthia Y. Ohata, MD • Leila N. Patterson, MD

 BASICS

Aphthous ulcers are the most common ulcerative disease of the oral mucosa.

DESCRIPTION

- Self-limited, painful ulcerations of the nonkeratinized oral mucosa, which are often recurrent
- Synonyms: canker sores; aphthae; aphthous stomatitis
  - Comes from *aphth* meaning "to set on fire" or "to inflame" in Greek; first used by Hippocrates to categorize oral disease (1)
- Classification based on severity (2)
  - Simple aphthosis
    ○ Common, episodic, infrequent (<7 episodes annually)
    ○ Prompt healing (resolution in 1 to 2 weeks), few ulcers
    ○ Minimal pain, little disability, limited to oral cavity
    ○ Self-limiting, responds well to local treatments
  - Complex aphthous ulcers
    ○ Uncommon, episodic or continuous, slow healing
    ○ Few to many ulcers, frequent or continuous ulceration
    ○ Short or nonexistent disease free intervals
    ○ Marked pain, major disability
    ○ Often need systemic treatments
    ○ May have genital aphthae
- Ulcer morphology (1),(2),(3),(4)
  - Minor aphthous ulcers,
    ○ Age of onset 5 to 19 years
    ○ Usually <10 mm in diameter
    ○ Number of ulcers: 1 to 5
    ○ Self-limited, healing within 4 to 14 days
    ○ Distribution: lips, cheeks, tongue, floor of mouth
    ○ Rarely affects the roof of the mouth
    ○ Nonscarring
    ○ Affects males and females equally
  - Major aphthous ulcers, 10% of all aphthae
    ○ Age of onset 10 to 19 years
    ○ Usually >10 mm in diameter
    ○ Number of ulcers: 1 to 10
    ○ Distribution: lips, soft palate, pharynx
    ○ May take weeks to months to heal
    ○ Generally more painful than minor aphthous ulcers
    ○ May cause scarring and be accompanied by fever and malaise
    ○ Affects males and females equally
  - Herpetiform ulcers, 5% of all aphthae
    ○ Age of onset 20 to 29 years
    ○ Usually 1 to 2 mm in diameter, form larger lesions when coalesced
    ○ No association with herpes simplex virus (HSV)
    ○ Occur in small clusters numbering 10s to 100s, lasting 1 to 4 weeks
    ○ Generally more painful than minor aphthous ulcers
    ○ Scarring unusual
    ○ May also affect the palate, gingiva, and pharynx
    ○ Affects more females than males

EPIDEMIOLOGY

- Recurrent aphthous stomatitis (RAS) is the most common ulcerative disease of the oral mucosa and accounts for 25% of recurrent ulcers in adults and 40% in children (1).
- More common in patients <40 years of age, Caucasians, nonsmokers, and those of higher socioeconomic status (2),(3)

Incidence
5–60% depending on ethnic and socioeconomic groups (2)

Prevalence
Lifetime prevalence of 5–85% (2)

ETIOLOGY AND PATHOPHYSIOLOGY
Associated with stress-induced rise in salivary cortisol, multiple HLA antigens, cell-mediated immunity, and inflammation (4)

Genetics
Associations with specific HLA subtypes

RISK FACTORS
- Local trauma: sharp teeth, dental treatments, or mucosal injury secondary to toothbrushing
- Sodium lauryl sulfate–containing toothpaste
- Increased stress and anxiety
- Nutritional deficiencies: iron, zinc, vitamin B complex, and folate
- Immunodeficiency
- Recent cessation of tobacco use
- Medications (numerous)
- Endocrine alterations (i.e., menstrual cycle)
- *Helicobacter pylori* infection
- Underlying medical disorders (e.g., celiac, inflammatory bowel disease [IBD], Behçet)

 DIAGNOSIS

The diagnosis of recurrent aphthous stomatitis is made by history (recurrent oral ulcers since childhood) and clinical presentation (characteristic lesion). Lab work is rarely contributory.

HISTORY
- Patients typically complain of oral ulcerations, which are painful and exacerbated by movement of the mouth. Exacerbation may also be reported with certain foods (hot, spicy, acidic, or carbonated foods or drinks).
- May experience prodrome of burning sensation of oral mucosa 2 to 48 hours prior to appearance of ulcers (4)[A], progressing to pain which peaks before ulceration (2)[A]
- Aphthae typically begin between the ages of 5 and 29 years and are recurrent (4)[A].
- Ask about ulcerative lesions of other anatomic areas, family history, prior history of aphthous ulcers, and new medications prior to onset of ulcers. Ask about the risk factors and take a comprehensive review of systems in order to prioritize the differential.

PHYSICAL EXAM
- Round or ovoid ulcerations generally <10 mm in size; covered with a grayish-white pseudomembrane surrounded by an erythematous halo (1)[A],(2)[A]
- Ulcers are typically found in the buccal or lip mucosa, ventral tongue, soft palate, or oral vestibule; rarely on the roof of the mouth or lips (1)[A],(2)[A],(4)[A]
- Evaluate for signs of secondary infection: elevated temperature, increased surrounding edema, or pus drainage.

DIFFERENTIAL DIAGNOSIS
- Oral trauma (biting, dentures) (1)[A]
- Infection (1)[A],(2)[A],(4)[A]
  - HSV (stomatitis): vesicular lesions on keratinized tissue (dorsal tongue, vermillion border); generally not present on mucosa, often with prodromal symptoms (fever, headache, malaise, etc.)
  - HIV: Ulcerations have lengthened healing time and tend to be more painful. May be seen in acute seroconversion syndrome or in advanced disease (low CD4 count)
  - Hand-foot-and-mouth disease: small vesicles within the oral cavity, along with lesions on the hands and feet
  - Association with *H. pylori* remains controversial
- Mucocutaneous syndromes (lichen planus, pemphigus); especially if chronic or nonhealing (3)[A]
- Medication induced (1)[A]
  - Fixed drug eruptions
  - Linear IgA bullous dermatosis: tense vesicles or bullae appearing 1 to 15 days after initiation of medication, most commonly caused by vancomycin
- Malignancy: Investigate nonhealing lesions, especially those with leukoplakia or ipsilateral cervical lymphadenopathy (3)[A].
- Systemic disease should be considered, causing aphthous-like ulcerations.
  - Particularly in adults with their first episode (late onset) or lesions elsewhere (atypical presentation)
  - Behçet syndrome (1)[A],(3)[A],(4)[A]: autoimmune systemic vasculitis usually involving mucous membranes
    ○ In 80% of Behçet syndrome, ulcers are the presenting sign.
    ○ Genital and oral ulceration, more likely major than minor aphthae
    ○ Signs and symptoms can include uveitis, arthritis, skin lesions, or central nervous system deficits.
  - Reiter syndrome (3)[A]: reactive arthritis, preceded by infection, usually of the genital tract, predominantly found in men
    ○ Uveitis, urethritis, HLA-B27–associated arthritis
  - Sweet syndrome (3)[A]
  - IBD (1)[A],(3)[A]: Crohn disease, ulcerative colitis
    ○ Persistent diarrhea
  - PFAPA syndrome: periodic fevers, aphthous ulcers, pharyngitis, adenitis, abdominal pain, and joint pain (1)[A]

– Cyclic neutropenia begins in infancy (recurrent fevers associated with painful oral and colonic ulcers, fevers, throat and abdominal pain) (1)[A]
– Systemic lupus erythematosus (SLE) (3)[A]: auto-immune vascular collagen disease
– Gluten-sensitive enteropathy (celiac disease) (3)[A]
– Herpangina and hand-foot-and-mouth disease (1)[A]

DIAGNOSTIC TESTS & INTERPRETATION

Lab work is rarely contributory in cases with a clear history consistent with RAS but useful for evaluation for other etiologies of aphthae.

Initial Tests (lab, imaging)

May consider complete blood count, zinc, folic acid, ferritin, B vitamins to evaluate for systemic causes in severe or recurrent cases (3)[A]

Follow-Up Tests & Special Considerations

- Biopsy and viral testing for nonhealing ulcers or atypical presentations (3)[A]
- Rheumatologic serology if underlying systemic disease is suspected (3)[A]
- Gastroenterology evaluation if gastroenterologic disease is suspected (3)[A]

 TREATMENT

GENERAL MEASURES

Management is symptomatic. Goal is to reduce inflammation, relieve pain, promote healing, and decrease frequency of recurrence (3)[A],(4)[A].

MEDICATION

In general, treatment is supportive. Topicals can be helpful and effective for minor aphthae, but systemic treatment may be needed for major aphthae.

First Line

- Topical corticosteroids (to improve healing time and symptoms) (1)[A],(3)[A],(4)[A]
  - Adverse effects: may increase risk of oral candidiasis (more likely with higher potency formulations)
  - Topical steroid preparations
    ○ Triamcinolone 1% dental paste
      ▪ Apply sparingly to ulcers 3 times daily for up to 2 weeks or until ulcer resolution.
    ○ Fluocinonide 0.05% gel or ointment
      ▪ Apply sparingly to ulcer 4 times daily for up to 2 weeks or until ulcer resolution.
- Topical anesthetics (to reduce symptoms only) (1)[A],(3)[A]
  - Preparations
    ○ Lidocaine 5% ointment or 10% spray
      ▪ Apply 4 times daily or prior to eating as needed for pain for up to 2 weeks or until ulcer resolution.
    ○ Hyaluronic acid 2.5% gel
      ▪ Apply 2 times per day for 2 weeks until ulcer resolution.
    ○ Benzocaine topical (OTC)
  - Adverse effects: may cause initial stinging; benzocaine rarely causes methemoglobinemia, especially in children age <2 years

- Antimicrobial/antiseptic mouth rinses (improve healing time, decrease pain, and may prevent recurrence) (1)[A],(3)[A]
  - Preparations
    ○ Chlorhexidine aqueous mouthwash 0.12% or 0.2%
      ▪ Use 3 times daily while lesions persist.
      ▪ May cause superficial tooth staining
    ○ Doxycycline
      ▪ 100 mg in 10 mL of water
      ▪ Use rinses for 2 to 3 minutes 4 times per day for 3 days.
    ○ May consider rinses of hydrogen peroxide with menthol
- Topical immunomodulators (improves healing time, reduces symptoms, and prevents recurrence when used in prodromal phase) (1)[A],(3)[A]
  - Adverse effects: may cause stinging sensation
  - Preparation
    ○ Amlexanox 5% oral paste
      ▪ Apply to ulcers 4 times daily for up to 2 weeks or until ulcer resolution.

Second Line

- Oral medications
  - Systemic corticosteroids (1)[A],(2)[A],(3)[A],(4)[A]—rescue therapy in acute, severe, recurrent outbreaks
    ○ Prednisone 0.75 mg/kg/day, tapered by 0.25 mg/kg/day every 2 weeks (1)[A]
  - Montelukast 10 mg daily can have similar efficacy to steroids (1)[A],(2)[A].
  - Colchicine, pentoxifylline, thalidomide, and dapsone have been used with variable success but should be used with caution due to side effects (1)[A],(2)[A],(3)[A],(4)[A].
  - Levamisole—immune modulator, typically well tolerated, pregnancy category C (2)[A]
  - Antibiotics—penicillin G potassium, 50 mg 4 times daily for 4 days (1)[A]

ISSUES FOR REFERRAL

Otolaryngology or dental referral if lesions have not resolved as expected

ADDITIONAL THERAPIES

- Vitamin B12 1,000 μg sublingual daily may be effective in decreasing the duration of outbreaks, number of ulcers, and level of pain (2)[A].
- Vitamin C 2,000 mg/day may also be an effective adjunctive therapy given its antiinflammatory properties (1)[A].
- *H. pylori* eradication has been associated with lower number of aphthous lesions (1)[A].

SURGERY/OTHER PROCEDURES

Low-level laser therapy at wavelength of 658 nm can improve pain and hasten healing (1)[A].

 ONGOING CARE

FOLLOW-UP RECOMMENDATIONS

Evaluation for infection, mucocutaneous or systemic disease, or malignancy should be pursued for non-healing lesions or lesions with lymphadenopathy or unusual presentation.

Patient Monitoring

Aphthous ulcers are often recurrent, so patients should be monitored for recurrence.

DIET

Deficiencies of iron, vitamin B12, and folic acid are significantly associated with recurrent aphthous ulcers (1)[A].

PATIENT EDUCATION

- Avoid (2)[A],(3)[A]
  - Acidic food or drink
  - Abrasive, hard foods
  - Sodium laurel sulfate–containing toothpaste
- Behavior modification to reduce dental trauma with toothbrush or bruxism (3)[A]

PROGNOSIS

Varies from single or infrequent recurrences of few, mild, self-resolving lesions to chronic, large, or deep painful lesions. Symptoms improve with age.

COMPLICATIONS

Aphthous ulcers can provide a site for infection and can leave scars.

REFERENCES

1. Edgar NR, Saleh D, Miller RA. Recurrent aphthous stomatitis: a review. *J Clin Aesthet Dermatol*. 2017;10(3):26–36.
2. Cui RZ, Bruce AJ, Rogers RS. Recurrent aphthous stomatitis. *Clin Dermatol*. 2016;34(4):475–481.
3. Scully C. Aphthous ulceration. *N Engl J Med*. 2006;355(2):165–172.
4. Akintoye SO, Greenberg MS. Recurrent aphthous stomatitis. *Dent Clin North Am*. 2014;58(2):281–297.

 CODES

ICD10

K12.0 Recurrent oral aphthae

CLINICAL PEARLS

- Aphthous ulcers are the most common chronic disease of the oral cavity.
- Most cases are mild, self-limited episodes.
- Appropriate treatment should be aimed at symptom control and promotion of healing.
- Nonhealing ulcers, extraoral involvement, and sudden onset in adulthood require additional workup.

U

ULCERATIVE COLITIS
Etny Raul Candelario, MD, MS • Maureen Alvarado, DO

BASICS

DESCRIPTION
- Ulcerative colitis (UC), one of the two inflammatory bowel disease, is a chronic disease characterized by diffuse mucosal inflammatory changes limited to the colon.
- Most cases involve the rectum or terminal colon and may extend proximally in a continuous fashion involving part or the entire large intestine (pan-ulcerative colitis) (1).
- Frequently manifested by recurrent episodes of bloody and mucoid diarrhea often associated with abdominal pain, rectal urgency, stool incontinence, fever, and weight loss
- Clinical course includes exacerbations and spontaneous or treatment-induced remissions.
- Colonic involvement is universal and may be accompanied by other systemic manifestations including large joint arthritis, ocular inflammation, skin lesions, biliary disease, liver disease, thromboembolic disease, and pulmonary complications.

EPIDEMIOLOGY
Prevalence
Because UC is commonly diagnosed in young people and has relatively low mortality, prevalence may continue to rise:
- North America: 249/100,000 persons
- Europe: 505/100,000 persons

ETIOLOGY AND PATHOPHYSIOLOGY
- Idiopathic inflammatory disorder; hypothesized to result from autoimmune dysfunction in response to colonic microbiome, genetic predisposition, and distinct risk factors
- Almost universally associated with inflammation of the terminal colon. >95% of patients have rectal involvement, 50% have disease limited to the rectum and sigmoid, and 20% have pancolitis. The absence of rectal involvement has been noted in <5% of adult patients and in up to 1/3 of pediatric patients.

Genetics
- Genetic factors contribute to IBD susceptibility.
- Several genetic syndromes have been associated with IBD (Turner syndrome, Hermansky-Pudlak syndrome, and glycogen storage disease type 1b).

RISK FACTORS
- Incidence rates were highest among persons 20 to 40 years old.
- Incidence rates of IBD are higher in white and Jewish people.
- Increasing incidence of UC in developing nations suggest that UC may be influenced by environmental factors.
- Having multiple family members with UC (2)
- Theorized risk factors include disruption of the colonic microbiome by enteric infection, dietary factors (Western diet in particular), antibiotic use, lack of breastfeeding in infant, obesity, and NSAID use.

GENERAL PREVENTION
Smoking may lower the risk of UC.

Pregnancy Considerations
- Patient should be advised to conceive during remission if planning a pregnancy.
  - Given the higher risk of thromboembolism in patients with UC, an estrogen-free contraceptive is preferred (2).
- Variable disease course in pregnancy seems to mirror disease state at conception; 3 to 6 months of remission before conceiving decreases the risks of an exacerbation during pregnancy (2).
- There is increased risk of preterm delivery and small for gestational age in women with active disease.
- Incidence rate of offspring from a UC mother of having UC is 3.7 (absolute rate of 1.6%).
- Ideally, pregnant women should be monitored by both gastroenterologist and maternal–fetal medicine specialist (2).

Pediatric Considerations
- Breastfeeding may protect against pediatric IBD.
- Pancolonic involvement is more likely at onset with shorter time from diagnosis to colectomy (median 11 years) than adults.

COMMONLY ASSOCIATED CONDITIONS
- Arthritis: large joint, sacroiliitis, ankylosing spondylitis (common)
- Aphthous ulcers (common)
- Erythema nodosum (common)
- Osteoporosis (common)
- Fatty liver (common)
- Episcleritis and uveitis (rare)
- Autoimmune liver disease (rare)
- Liver cirrhosis (rare)
- Primary sclerosing cholangitis (rare)
- Bile duct carcinoma (rare)
- Thromboembolic disease (rare)
- Pyoderma gangrenosum (rare)
- Colon cancer (rare)
- Anemia (rare)
- Pulmonary diseases (very rare)

DIAGNOSIS

HISTORY
- Symptoms may include:
  - Small frequent bloody or mucoid diarrhea associated with tenesmus, rectal urgency, fecal incontinence and abdominal pain; onset is gradual and progressive over weeks.
  - Weight loss, anorexia, fatigue, and anemia
  - Extraintestinal manifestation including joint, skin, ocular, oral, hepatobiliary-related symptoms
- Assess for potential precipitating factors:
  - Recent smoking cessation
  - NSAID use
  - Enteric infection like *Clostridium difficile* infection (may be a differential or superimposed with UC) (1)
- Assess for a family history of IBD.
- Predominant age of onset: 15 to 30 years; smaller peak in ages 50 to 80 years
- About 50% of all patient diagnosed with UC have a relapse or exacerbation in any year.

PHYSICAL EXAM
- Exam may often be normal.
- Weight loss
- Signs of fluid depletion (tachycardia, low blood pressure)
- Signs of anemia (pallor)
- Abdominal tenderness or tenderness
- Presence of blood on rectal exam
- Severe disease: fever, hypotension, tachycardia, pallor, loss of subcutaneous fat, muscle atrophy, peripheral edema, clubbing

DIFFERENTIAL DIAGNOSIS
- Crohn disease
- Infectious colitis: bacterial, parasitic, or viral (cytomegalovirus [CMV])
- Ischemic colitis
- Pseudomembranous colitis (*C. difficile* infection)
- Irritable bowel syndrome
- Diverticular colitis
- Diversion colitis in patients with prior bowel surgery
- Medication-induced colitis
- Radiation colitis
- Graft versus host disease
- Celiac disease

DIAGNOSTIC TESTS & INTERPRETATION
Initial Tests (lab, imaging)
- CBC: leukocytosis and anemia
- BMP: abnormal urea and electrolytes, especially hypokalemia
- LFTs: can be abnormal; low albumin indicates severe disease.
- ESR or CRP may be elevated, especially in more severe disease.
- Vitamin B_{12} and folate levels
- Fecal calprotectin (FC): elevated; (levels >782 μg/g differentiate acute severe colitis from mild to moderate UC). FC may also used to differentiate IBD from irritable bowel syndrome (1).
- Stool studies to rule out infectious cause: *C. difficile* (CDI in newly diagnosed or relapsing IBD ranges from 5% to 47%), stool cultures, Shiga toxin, ova and parasite microscopy, *Giardia* antigen (1)
- STI testing to rule out proctitis, particularly in men who have sexual with men
- Abdominal x-ray to exclude dangerous colonic dilation and assess disease severity

Follow-Up Tests & Special Considerations
FC can be used to monitor disease severity in relapsing UC in response to treatment (1).

Diagnostic Procedures/Other
Diagnosis of UC requires examination with lower gastrointestinal endoscopy with biopsies:
- Complete colonoscopy with at least two biopsies from each of five sites along the entire colon (unaffected and affected areas) (1)
- Complete colonoscopy in severe UC may be contraindicated due to risk of perforation or precipitation of toxic megacolon. In this case, a sigmoidoscopy with biopsy may be more appropriate (1).

Test Interpretation
- Endoscopic findings: mucosal engorgement with vascular markings, mucosal erythema, friability, erosions, and granularity. In severe UC, deep ulcerations and active bleeding may be found. Affected areas will most likely include the rectum and extend proximally and continuously (1).
- Histologic findings: mucosal separation, distortion, and atrophy of the crypts; chronic inflammatory cells in lamina propria; lymphocytes and plasma cells in crypt bases
- Rectal biopsy: Villous mucosal architecture and Paneth cells metaplasia support UC.

- Mild ileal inflammation ("backwash ileitis") may be present in UC.
- Characterize extent of disease according to Montreal classification: proctitis (within 18 cm of anal verge), left-sided colitis (sigmoid to splenic flexure), or extensive colitis (extension proximally from to the splenic flexure).

 ## TREATMENT

- Disease severity (see Table 1) and extent (i.e., proctitis, left-sided colitis vs. extensive colitis) dictate induction and maintenance treatment (1).
- Goals are to restore normal bowel function, reverse inflammatory changes, and to maintain a steroid-free remission without extraintestinal manifestations (1).

MEDICATION
First Line
- Induction of remission in mildly active UC:
  - Proctitis
    - Rectal 5-ASA 1 g/day (1)[A] or oral 5-ASA (1)[B]
    - If 5-ASA fails, add budesonide MMX 9 mg/day (1)[B].
    - If 5-ASA fails, use oral systemic corticosteroid (1)[C].
  - Left-sided colitis
    - Rectal 5-ASA 1 g/day (1)[A] and oral 5-ASA (1)[B]
    - If 5-ASA fails, use budesonide MMX 9 mg/day (1)[B].
    - If 5-ASA fails, use oral systemic corticosteroid (1)[C].
  - Extensive
    - Oral 5-ASA 2 g/day (1)[B]
    - If 5-ASA fails, use budesonide MMX 9 mg/day (1)[B].
    - If 5-ASA fails, use oral systemic corticosteroid (1)[C].
  - Reassess within 6 weeks to determine response to induction therapy.
- Maintenance of remission in patient with previously mild active UC:
  - Proctitis
    - Rectal 5-ASA 1 g/day (1)[B]
  - Left-side colitis
    - Oral 5-ASA (1)[B]
  - Extensive
    - Oral 5-ASA (1)[B]
- Induction of remission in moderate to severe active UC:
  - Moderate
    - Budesonide MMX (1)[B]
  - Moderate to severe

- Anti-TNF therapy (adalimumab, golimumab, infliximab) (1)[A]
  - If infliximab is used, use in addition with thiopurine (1)[B].
  - Vedolizumab (1)[B]
  - Tofacitinib 10 mg BID for 8 weeks (1)[B]
  - Oral systemic corticosteroid (1)[B]
  - If anti-TNF therapy fails, use vedolizumab or tofacitinib (1)[B].
- Maintenance of remission in patient with previously moderate to severe active UC:
  - Corticosteroid induction, use thiopurine (1)[C].
  - Anti-TNF induction, continue anti-TNF (1)[B].
  - Vedolizumab induction, continue vedolizumab (1)[B].
  - Tofacitinib induction, continue tofacitinib (1)[B].
- Maintenance of remission in patient with previously acute ulcerative colitis (ASUC):
  - Infliximab induction, continue infliximab (1)[B]
  - Cyclosporine induction, thiopurine (1)[C] or vedolizumab (1)[C]

Pediatric Considerations
- Pediatric growth and development can be affected due to malabsorption.
- Avoid live vaccines (rotavirus) in the first 6 months of life of infant born to mother with UC with exposure to biologic therapy (except certolizumab) (2).

Pregnancy Considerations
- Stop methotrexate at least 3 months prior to conceiving. It is contraindicated in pregnancy.
- In general, aminosalicylate, biologic, and immunomodulator therapies may be continued during pregnancy and lactation.

SURGERY/OTHER PROCEDURES
- Surgery is indicated for those who refractory or intolerant to medical therapy (high-dose steroids).
- Total colectomy with ileostomy is curative.

ADMISSION, INPATIENT, AND NURSING CONSIDERATIONS
Initiate IV corticosteroids and rule out infectious etiologies (C. difficile, CMV, Shigella/amoeba).

 ## ONGOING CARE

FOLLOW-UP RECOMMENDATIONS
Patient Monitoring
- UC patient should be screened for anxiety and depression (1).
- Assess for colorectal carcinoma (CRC) or dysplasia with surveillance colonoscopy

DIET
NPO during acute exacerbations

PATIENT EDUCATION
Crohn and Colitis Foundation of America (CCFA): http://www.ccfa.org/

PROGNOSIS
- Poor prognostic factors as measured by the likelihood of colectomy (1):
  - <40 years old at prognosis
  - Extensive UC
  - Severe endoscopic disease
  - Previous hospitalization for colitis
  - Elevated CRP
  - Low serum albumin
- Variable: Mortality for initial attack is ~5%; 75–85% experience relapse; up to 20% require colectomy.
- Colon cancer risk is the single most important factor affecting long-term prognosis.
- Left-sided colitis and ulcerative proctitis have favorable prognoses with probable normal lifespan.

COMPLICATIONS
- Perforation: Treat toxic megacolon with prompt surgery. Limit colonoscopies in severe disease.
- Obstruction
- Anemia
- Fulminant colitis
- Toxic megacolon
- Liver disease
- Stricture formation
- Osteoporosis
- Colorectal cancer

REFERENCES
1. Rubin DT, Ananthakrishnan AN, Siegel CA, et al. ACG clinical guideline: ulcerative colitis in adults. Am J Gastroenterol. 2019;114(3):384–413.
2. Mahadevan U, Robinson C, Bernasko N, et al. Inflammatory bowel disease in pregnancy clinical care pathway: a report from the American Gastroenterological Association IBD Parenthood Project Working Group. Gastroenterology. 2019;156(5):1508–1524.

 ### SEE ALSO

Algorithm: Hematemesis (Bleeding, Upper Gastrointestinal)

 ### CODES

ICD10
- K51.90 Ulcerative colitis, unspecified, without complications
- K51.919 Ulcerative colitis, unspecified with unspecified complications
- K51.80 Other ulcerative colitis without complications

CLINICAL PEARLS
- Diffuse, uninterrupted colonic mucosal inflammation
- The hallmark symptom is bloody diarrhea.
- Common medical treatments include 5-ASA, steroids, and anti–TNF-α therapy.
- Refractory disease or severe complications may require surgical intervention.
- Annual or biannual surveillance colonoscopy after 8 to 10 years of colitis due to increased risk of colorectal cancer (1)

Table 1. Activity index of UC (1)

Symptom/Labs	Remission	Mild	Moderate-Severe	Fulminant
Stools (no./d)	Formed stools	<4	>6	>10
Blood in stools	None	Intermittent	Frequent	Continuous
Urgency	None	Mild/occasional	Often	Continuous
Hemoglobin	Normal	Normal	<75% of normal	Transfusion required
ESR	<30	<30	>30	>30
CRP (mg/L)	Normal	Elevated	Elevated	Elevated
FC (μg/g)	<150–200	>150–200	>150–200	>150–200
Endoscopy (Mayo subscore)	0–1	1	2–3	3
UCEIS	0–1	2–4	5–8	7–8

Adapted from Rubin DT, Ananthakrishnan AN, Siegel CA, et al. ACG clinical guideline: ulcerative colitis in adults. Am J Gastroenterol. 2019;114(3):384–413.

URETHRITIS

Katherine L. Rotker, MD

BASICS

DESCRIPTION
- Inflammation of the urethra
- Common manifestation of sexually transmitted infection (STI)
- Frequently associated with dysuria, pruritus, and/or urethral discharge; classified as gonococcal (caused by *Neisseria gonorrhoeae*) and nongonococcal (caused by other bacteria, or less commonly autoimmune disorders [Reiter syndrome], trauma, or chemical irritation)

EPIDEMIOLOGY
Incidence
- In 2018, gonorrhea increased 5% to >580,000 cases—the highest number reported since 1991.
- In 2018, chlamydia increased 3% to >1.7 million cases—the most ever reported to CDC.
- Chlamydia is the most commonly reported STD (1).
- Rate of chlamydial infection in U.S. women was more than twice that of men, reflecting higher rates of screening (1).
- Highest incidences of gonorrhea and chlamydia among young men and women, ages 15 to 24 years (>50% of all cases) (1)
- Chlamydial infections are 5 times more likely in young adult women than gonococcal infections (1).
- In 2018, there were 115,000 reported cases of syphilis: the number of primary and secondary syphilis cases—the most infectious stages of syphilis—increased 14% to >35,000 cases, the highest number reported since 1991.

ETIOLOGY AND PATHOPHYSIOLOGY
- Most common cause is infection via sexual transmission of *N. gonorrhoeae*, a gram-negative diplococcus.
- *N. gonorrhoeae* is a gram-negative diplococcus which interacts with nonciliated epithelial cells → cellular invasion → inflammation, neutrophil production, bacterial cell phagocytosis (2).
- Sexually transmitted *C. trachomatis* infection is the most common cause of nongonococcal urethritis.
- Other established pathogens:
  - *Mycoplasma genitalium*
  - *Trichomonas vaginalis*
  - *Ureaplasma urealyticum*
  - Herpes simplex virus (rare)
  - Adenovirus (rare)
- Noninfectious causes (less common)
  - Chemical irritants (i.e., soaps, shampoos, douches, spermicides)
  - Foreign bodies
  - Urethral instrumentation

RISK FACTORS
- Age 15 to 24 years
- New sex partner
- One or more sex partner(s)
- History of or coexisting STI
- Sex partner with concurrent partner(s)
- Inconsistent condom use outside of a mutually monogamous relationship
- Exchanging sex for money or drugs
- Member of population with increased prevalence of infection, including incarcerated populations, military recruits, and economically disadvantaged populations

GENERAL PREVENTION
- Use of male condoms, female condoms, or cervical diaphragms
- Abstinence or reduction in the number of sex partners
- Behavioral counseling

COMMONLY ASSOCIATED CONDITIONS

> **ALERT**
> Annual chlamydia and gonorrhea screening is recommended for all sexually active women <25 years, women >25 years with risk factors, and all men who have sex with men. There is insufficient evidence to recommend testing all men <25 year (3)[A].

DIAGNOSIS

- Chief complaint
  - Urethral discharge (mucopurulent suggestive of *N. gonorrhoeae*)
  - Dysuria
  - Erythema of the urethral meatus
  - Symptom onset 2 to 8 days following exposure
- History
  - Sexual history, including condom use, number of partners, sexual behaviors
  - Previous STIs
  - Substance abuse
  - Recent travel
  - Symptoms indicative of complications or additional sites of infection (i.e., men: testicular pain and swelling, anal itching, rectal pain or bleeding; women: lower abdominal pain, dyspareunia, irregular vaginal bleeding)
- Male genitourinary (GU) exam (possible findings)
  - Urethral discharge
  - Meatal erythema
  - Testicular tenderness
  - Palpate scrotum to check for epididymitis or orchitis.
  - Assess for ulcers.
  - Assess for inguinal lymphadenopathy.
- Female GU exam (possible findings)
  - Vaginal discharge
  - Endocervical discharge, hyperemia, and/or friability

Pediatric Considerations
Pediatric infections with gonorrhea and chlamydia after the neonatal period strongly suggest sexual contact. If indicated, investigations should be initiated promptly (4).

DIFFERENTIAL DIAGNOSIS
- Other GU tract diseases
  - Cystitis/urinary tract infection
  - Epididymitis
  - Prostatitis
  - PID
  - Pyelonephritis
- Vaginal atrophy, especially in postmenopausal women
- Stevens-Johnson syndrome
- Reiter syndrome: uveitis, urethritis, arthritis
- Wegener granulomatosis
- Urethral syndrome (pain without infection or purulence), longstanding or intermittent symptoms

DIAGNOSTIC TESTS & INTERPRETATION

> **ALERT**
> Health care providers are required to report all gonorrhea and chlamydia infections in accordance with local and state requirements.

Initial Tests (lab, imaging)
- Gonorrhea
  - Nucleic acid amplification test (NAAT)
  - Sensitivity: 90–100%
  - Specificity: 97–100%
  - Preferred specimen collection in first void (men) and vaginal swab (women)
  - Tissue culture was the traditional gold standard but typically only used now in cases of suspected treatment resistance (4).
- Chlamydia
  - NAAT
  - Sensitivity: 85–95%
  - Specificity: 93–99%
  - Preferred specimen collection is same as for gonorrhea.
  - Tissue culture was the traditional gold standard but currently NOT recommended (4).
- Gram stain diagnosis criteria
  - Urethral secretions with ≥2 WBC per oil immersion
  - Mucopurulent or purulent discharge
  - First void urine sediment with ≥10 WBC per high-power field (4)
  - Symptom onset 2 to 8 days following exposure
- Methylene blue/gentian violet [MB/GV]
  - Alternative to Gram staining
  - Does not require heat fixation
  - Sensitivity: 97.3% (same as gram stain)
- If concern for *Trichomonas*: NAAT (urine, urethral, vaginal, or endocervical swab), wet mount, or culture
- There is no FDA-approved diagnostic test available for *M. genitalium*, an emerging pathogen with a greater prevalence than gonorrhea in many populations (5).

> **ALERT**
> Due to the similarity in clinical symptoms and high rates of coinfection, cotesting for gonorrhea and chlamydia infection is recommended. In addition, given that risk factors for gonorrhea and chlamydia indicate risks for other STIs, screening for HIV, RPR, hepatitis C, and hepatitis B may also be indicated.

Follow-Up Tests & Special Considerations
- Test of cure (TOC) for chlamydia and gonorrhea is recommended in pregnant women or when treatment noncompliance is suspected (4).
- Repeat testing in 3 months recommended due to rates of reinfection (4)
- HIV infection: Persons with HIV infection should receive the same treatment as patients without HIV infection (4).

Diagnostic Procedures/Other
Cystourethroscopy for cases with suspected foreign body, intraurethral warts, urethral stricture

Test Interpretation
Urethral strictures (untreated gonorrhea), intraurethral lesions (venereal warts, congenital anomalies), PID, or tubo-ovarian abscesses are possible.

TREATMENT

- Most cases can be treated in the outpatient setting.
- Single-dose regimens with direct observation preferred (4)

MEDICATION

CDC recommendations

- Chlamydia
  - First line
    - Azithromycin 1 g PO × 1 dose OR
    - Doxycycline 100 mg PO BID for 7 days (3)[A]
    - Alternate regimens (all for 7 days)
      - Erythromycin base 500 mg PO QID
      - Erythromycin ethylsuccinate 800 mg PO QID
      - Levofloxacin 500 mg daily
      - Ofloxacin 300 mg PO BID
  - Second line (all for a duration of 7 days)
    - Erythromycin base 500 mg PO QID
    - Erythromycin ethylsuccinate 800 mg PO QID
    - Levofloxacin 500 mg daily
    - Ofloxacin 300 mg PO BID
- Gonorrhea
  - First line
    - Ceftriaxone 250 mg IM plus either
    - Azithromycin 1 g PO × 1 dose (preferred) OR
    - Doxycycline 100 mg PO BID × 7 days (6)[C]
    - For children ≤45 kg
      - Ceftriaxone 25 to 50 mg/kg IM × 1 dose
    - For children >45 kg, use adult dosing.
  - Second line
    - Cefixime 400 mg IM plus either
    - Azithromycin 1 g PO × 1 dose (preferred) OR
    - Doxycycline 100 mg PO BID × 7 days
    - TOC in 1 week
- *Trichomonas*
  - Metronidazole 2 g PO × 1 dose
- Recurrent and persistent urethritis
  - If azithromycin was initially used, moxifloxacin 400 mg PO QD × 7 days
  - If doxycycline was initially used, azithromycin 1 g PO × 1 dose
- General considerations
  - Contraindications: sensitivity to any of the indicated medications
  - Precautions: Patients taking tetracyclines may have increased photosensitivity.
  - Significant possible interactions
    - Tetracyclines should not be taken with milk products or antacids.
    - Oral contraceptives may be rendered less effective by oral antibiotics. Patients and partners should use a back-up method of birth control for the remainder of the cycle.
      - QID × 7 days (7)

Pregnancy Considerations

- Chlamydia:
  - Screen all pregnant patients.
  - All pregnant women at increased risk should be screened for chlamydia at their prenatal visit and again in the 3rd trimester.
  - TOC 3 weeks after therapy to check for chlamydial eradication and retest in 3 months
  - Azithromycin 1 g PO × 1 dose (3)[A]
  - Alternative regimens:
    - Amoxicillin 500 mg TID × 7 days
    - OR
    - Erythromycin 500 mg QID × 7 days (3)[A]
- Gonorrhea:
  - Screen all pregnant patients.
  - All pregnant women at increased risk should be screened for chlamydia at their prenatal visit and again in the 3rd trimester.
  - TOC 3 weeks after therapy to check for gonococcal eradication and retest in 3 months
  - Tetracyclines and quinolones are contraindicated.

- Dual therapy treatment
  - Ceftriaxone 250 mg IM × 1 dose
  - Azithromycin 1 g PO × 1 dose
- If cephalosporin allergy and spectinomycin is not available, infectious disease consult is recommended.

ONGOING CARE

FOLLOW-UP RECOMMENDATIONS

- Sexual activity should be avoided for 7 days following administration of single-dose therapy or until completion of multiday regimen.
- All sexual partners who came in contact with the patient within 60 days should be referred for evaluation, testing, and presumptive treatment (4).
- Expedited partner therapy (EPT) is an acceptable alternative; EPT—the practice of treating the diagnosed patient's sex partner(s) for chlamydia or gonorrhea by providing medications to the partner(s) without clinical evaluation (4)

Patient Monitoring

- Instruct patients to return if symptoms persist or recur after completing treatment.
- Screen for reinfection in all patients at 3 months.

PATIENT EDUCATION

- Behavioral counseling interventions are recommended. Evidence of benefit increase with intensity of intervention (6),(8)[B].
- Successful approaches include basic information about STIs and transmission, assess risk for transmission, include training skills (i.e., condom use, communication about safe sex, problem solving, goal setting) (8).

PROGNOSIS

If the diagnosis is firmly established, appropriate medications are prescribed and the patient is compliant with treatment; relief of symptoms occurs within days, and the problem will resolve without sequela.

COMPLICATIONS

- Stricture formation
- Epididymitis
- Prostatitis
- PID in women
- Disseminated gonococcal infection
- Gonococcal meningitis
- Gonococcal endocarditis
- Perinatal transmission (chlamydial conjunctivitis, chlamydial pneumonia, ophthalmia neonatorum)
- Reiter syndrome
- Chronic cervical chlamydial infection has been proposed to increase risk of cervical cancer (9).

REFERENCES

1. Centers for Disease Control and Prevention. *Sexually Transmitted Disease Surveillance 2019*. Atlanta, GA: U.S. Department of Health and Human Services; 2021.
2. LeFevre ML; for U.S. Preventive Services Task Force. Screening for chlamydia and gonorrhea: U.S. Preventive Services Task Force recommendation statement. *Ann Intern Med*. 2014;161(12):902–910.
3. Mishori R, McClaskey EL, WinklerPrins VJ. *Chlamydia trachomatis* infections: screening, diagnosis, and management. *Am Fam Physician*. 2012;86(12):1127–1132.
4. Workowski KA, Bolan GA; for Centers for Disease Control and Prevention. Sexually transmitted diseases treatment guidelines, 2015. *MMWR Recomm Rep*. 2015;64(RR-03):1–137.
5. Munoz JL, Goje OJ. *Mycoplasma genitalium*: an emerging sexually transmitted infection. *Scientifica (Cairo)*. 2016;2016:7537318.
6. Mayor MT, Roett MA, Uduhiri KA. Diagnosis and management of gonococcal infections. *Am Fam Physician*. 2012;86(10):931–938.
7. Centers for Disease Control and Prevention. *Sexually Transmitted Disease Surveillance 2018*. Atlanta, GA: U.S. Department of Health and Human Services; 2019.
8. O'Connor EA, Lin JS, Burda BU, et al. Behavioral sexual risk-reduction counseling in primary care to prevent sexually transmitted infections: a systematic review for the U.S. Preventive Services Task Force. *Ann Intern Med*. 2014;161(12):874–883.
9. O'Connell CM, Ferone ME. *Chlamydia trachomatis* genital infections. *Microb Cell*. 2016;3(9):390–403.

ADDITIONAL READING

U.S. Preventive Services Task Force. Final recommendation statement. Chlamydia and gonorrhea: screening. http://www.uspreventiveservicestaskforce.org /Page/Document/RecommendationStatementFinal /chlamydia-and-gonorrhea-screening. Accessed December 17, 2018.

SEE ALSO

- Chlamydia Infection (Sexually Transmitted); Epididymitis; Gonococcal Infections; Pelvic Inflammatory Disease; Prostatitis; Urinary Tract Infection (UTI) in Females; Urinary Tract Infection (UTI) in Males; Vulvovaginitis, Estrogen Deficient; Vulvovaginitis, Prepubescent
- Algorithms: Dysuria; Genital Ulcers; Urethral Discharge

CODES

ICD10

- N34.2 Other urethritis
- A56.01 Chlamydial cystitis and urethritis
- A54.01 Gonococcal cystitis and urethritis, unspecified

CLINICAL PEARLS

- Inflammation of the urethra, frequently associated with dysuria, pruritus, and/or urethral discharge
- Common manifestation of STI
- Classified as gonococcal (caused by *N. gonorrhoeae*) and nongonococcal
- NAAT preferred method of diagnosis for men and women
- Single-dose regimens with direct observation preferred
- In cases of gonorrhea or chlamydia infection, in person or EPT recommended for all partners of patients within the last 60 days
- Given that risk factors for gonorrhea and chlamydia indicate risk for other STIs, screening for HIV, RPR, hepatitis C, and hepatitis B may also be indicated.
- Repeat testing for gonorrhea and chlamydia in 3 months recommended due to rates of reinfection
- Special considerations in pediatric and pregnant populations
- Treatment in persons with HIV infection is the same as in patients without HIV infection.
- Health care providers are required to report all gonorrhea and chlamydia infections in accordance with local and state requirements.

U

URINARY TRACT INFECTION (UTI) IN FEMALES
Akhil Das, MD, FACS • Radhika Ragam, MD

 BASICS

DESCRIPTION
- UTI is the presence of pathogenic microorganisms within the urinary tract and associated symptoms (dysuria, urinary urgency/frequency, hematuria, new or worsening incontinence).
- Uncomplicated UTI: infection in patients with an unobstructed and anatomically normal urinary tract, no predisposing risk factors and whose symptoms are confined to the lower urinary tract
- Complicated UTI: infection of the urinary tract in the presence of an anatomic or functional abnormality, immunocompromised host, or presence of a multi-drug resistant organism (see "Risk Factors")
- Recurrent UTI: symptomatic UTI that occurs following complete treatment and resolution of documented infection
  - Two or more culture-proven infections in 6 months or >3 in 12 months
  - Affects 20–40% of women with prior cystitis episodes (1)
- Asymptomatic bacteriuria (ASB): presence of bacteria in urine without reports of associated symptoms
- Synonym(s): cystitis

EPIDEMIOLOGY
Incidence
- Accounts for 10.5 million office visits and 2 to 3 million emergency room visits; contributes to >100,000 hospital admissions each year with a cost of over $2.6 billion annually (2)
- Primary affects young adults and older adults; predominantly female > male

Prevalence
- Up to 60% of females have at least one UTI in their lifetime, and 11% report having at least one per year (3).
- 1/4 of women with uncomplicated UTI experience a second UTI within 6 months and half at some time during their lifetime.

ETIOLOGY AND PATHOPHYSIOLOGY
- Ascension of bacteria into the bladder via the urethra is the most common etiology.
- Pathogenic organisms possess adherence factors (pili or fimbriae) and toxins that allow initiation and propagation of genitourinary infections.
- Most UTIs are caused by bacteria originating from bowel flora:
  - *Escherichia coli* is the causative organism in 80–85% of cases of uncomplicated cystitis.
  - *Staphylococcus saprophyticus* accounts for 10–15% of infections.
  - *Klebsiella pneumoniae* and *Proteus mirabilis* each account for approximately 4%.

Genetics
Women with human leukocyte antigen 3 (HLA-3) and nonsecretor Lewis antigen have an increased bacterial adherence, which may lead to an increased risk in UTI.

RISK FACTORS
- Biologic:
  - Urinary stasis/obstruction: pelvic organ prolapse, bladder diverticula, neurogenic bladder, voiding dysfunction, urethral stricture, anatomic anomalies of the lower urinary tract
  - Urinary calculi
  - Immunosuppression: diabetes, HIV, steroid use, malignancy, malnutrition
- Behavioral practices (promote colonization):
  - Sexual intercourse, spermicide, estrogen depletion, antimicrobial use, poor hygiene

GENERAL PREVENTION
- Mitigate urinary obstruction or stasis.
- Adequate hydration
- Women with frequent or intercourse-related UTI should empty bladder immediately before and following intercourse.
- Avoid feminine hygiene sprays, diaphragms, spermicidal agents, and douches.
- Wipe urethra from front to back.
- Vaginal estrogen in postmenopausal women may aid in preventing recurrent UTI.

COMMONLY ASSOCIATED CONDITIONS
See "Risk Factors."

Geriatric Considerations
- Elderly patients are more likely to have underlying urinary tract abnormality or voiding dysfunction.
  - Poor perineal hygiene, urinary or fecal incontinence, pelvic organ prolapse are common risk factors.
  - Decreased estrogen levels increase vaginal pH and alter microbial flora, leading to increased colonization.
- May present with atypical symptoms such as altered mental status or urinary incontinence
- Treatment of ASB does not improve outcomes and should be avoided due to associated morbidity.

Pediatric Considerations
Bowel bladder dysfunction or congenital urinary tract abnormalities such as vesicoureteral reflux (VUR) or duplicated collecting system are risk factors.

DIAGNOSIS

HISTORY
- Dysuria, urgency, frequency, sensation of incomplete bladder emptying, hematuria, suprapubic pain, malodorous urine, altered mental status, nocturia, sudden onset or worsening of urinary incontinence, dyspareunia
- Number of UTIs, recent sexual activity or new sexual partner(s)

PHYSICAL EXAM
- Suprapubic tenderness
- Urethral and/or vaginal tenderness; evaluate for diverticulum or other urethral masses.
- Fever or costovertebral angle tenderness indicates upper tract infection.

DIFFERENTIAL DIAGNOSIS
Vaginal infection, ASB, STDs causing urethritis or pyuria, neoplasm, calculi, interstitial cystitis

DIAGNOSTIC TESTS & INTERPRETATION
Initial Tests (lab, imaging)
- Clean catch midstream voided urine may be contaminated with either vaginal or perineal organisms. Suspect contamination when growth of normal vaginal flora (lactobacillus) or mixed cultures with more than one organism arise.
- Urinalysis (microscopic)
  - Pyuria (>10 neutrophils/high-power field [HPF])
  - Bacteriuria (any amount on unspun urine or five bacteria/HPF on centrifuged urine)
  - Hematuria (≥3 RBCs/HPF)
  - Squamous cells indicate poor collection/quality (>15 to 20 squamous cells/HPF is suggestive of contamination).
- Dipstick urinalysis
  - Leukocyte esterase (indicates presence of 5 to 15 WBC/HPF; 75–96% sensitivity, 94–98% specificity, when >100,000 colony-forming units [CFU])
  - Nitrite tests are specific, but not sensitive, if nitrite-reducing organisms (e.g., *E. coli, Klebsiella, Proteus*) are causative.
- Urine culture: not indicated in the setting of an uncomplicated UTI; necessary for patients with either unclear diagnosis, recurrent UTI or complicated UTI

Follow-Up Tests & Special Considerations
- Empiric antibiotics may be given without urine culture for uncomplicated UTI. Guidelines recommend urine culture for recurrent or complicated UTI.
- Imaging may be indicated for UTIs in infants, immunocompromised patients, febrile infections, signs of urinary obstruction, or recurrent UTI.
- CT or MR urogram provide detailed anatomic information but should generally only be considered in patients with recurrent UTIs or have known risk factors for anatomic abnormalities (4).

Pediatric Considerations
A renal bladder ultrasound or voiding cystourethrogram can evaluate pelvocaliectasis or ureteral dilatation or VUR.

Diagnostic Procedures/Other
- If the urine specimen is suspected to be contaminated, a catheterized specimen may be necessary.
- Suprapubic bladder aspiration or urethral catheterization can be used to obtain specimens from infants, although these methods are more invasive.
- Cystourethroscopy can be used to evaluate patients with recurrent UTIs, history of nephrolithiasis, previous anti-incontinence surgery, or hematuria in the absence of an active infection.

Test Interpretation
See "Initial Tests (lab, imaging)."

TREATMENT

GENERAL MEASURES
- ASB in a nonpregnant woman should not be treated with antibiotics (5).
- Maintain adequate hydration with at least 2L water daily.
- Many women with uncomplicated UTI have resolution without treatment and rarely progress to serious infections.

MEDICATION

First Line
- Phenazopyridine 100 to 200 mg TID is a urinary topical analgesic and should only be used for rapid symptom relief, not definitive treatment. This medication may mislead urinalysis interpretation (presents as nitrite positive and obscures interpretation of leukocyte esterase) but not the urine culture.
- Uncomplicated UTI:
  – Trimethoprim/sulfamethoxazole (TMP/SMX; Bactrim): 160/800 mg PO BID for 3 days, best where resistance of *E. coli* strains <20%. Rash may be higher than with other antibiotics; preferred 1st line
  – Nitrofurantoin (Macrobid): 100 mg PO BID for 5 days should be used in patients with allergy to TMP/SMX and in areas where *E. coli* resistance to TMP/SMX >20%. Macrobid does not penetrate renal parenchyma and thus is ineffective in treating upper UTI (6).
  – Fosfomycin (Monurol): 3 g PO single dose (expensive)
- Lower UTI in pregnancy:
  – Nitrofurantoin: 100 mg PO BID for 7 day. Discontinue at 35 weeks for risk of neonatal hemolytic anemia.
  – Cephalexin (Keflex): 500 mg PO BID for 7 days
  – TMP/SMX is avoided in pregnancy (especially in 1st and 3rd trimester) due to risk of kernicterus.
  – Fluoroquinolones are not safe during pregnancy and are avoided in treatment of children.
- Postcoital UTI: Single-dose TMP/SMX or cephalexin may reduce frequency of UTI in sexually active women.
- Complicated UTI: Extend course to 7 to 10 days; may begin with fluoroquinolone, TMP/SMX, or cephalosporin (Avoid using nitrofurantoin for complicated UTI due to lack of tissue penetration.)

Second Line
- Uncomplicated UTI
  – β-Lactams (amoxicillin/clavulanate, cefdinir, cefpodoxime) for 3 to 7 days
  – *Fluoroquinolones should not be used in uncomplicated UTI due to risk of potentially irreversible adverse reactions, which may occur even with single doses (see FDA black box warnings regarding hypoglycemia, tendon rupture risk, neuropathy).*
- Recurrent UTIs
  – Recurrent UTIs treatment aims at shortest antibiotic course with symptom resolution. Urine culture is required for these patients. Consider 3 to 6 months of daily suppressive antibiotic therapy, followed by observation for reinfection after discontinuing prophylaxis. Continuous antimicrobial prophylaxis involves daily low-dose TMP/SMX 80/400 mg or nitrofurantoin 50 to 100 mg.
  – Other options are patient-initiated treatment for early UTI symptoms (minimizes office visits, antibiotic use), postcoital prophylaxis, and intermittent-dosed prophylaxis (e.g., Monday-Wednesday-Friday).

Pediatric Considerations
Long-term antibiotics appear to reduce the risk of recurrent symptomatic UTI in susceptible children, but the benefit must be considered together with the increased risk of microbial resistance.

ISSUES FOR REFERRAL
Patients with recurrent or complicated UTIs should be referred to a urologist.

Pediatric Considerations
UTI in children, especially <1 year of age, should prompt referral to a pediatric urologist.

SURGERY/OTHER PROCEDURES
- Sepsis from urinary tract obstruction requires prompt drainage often in the setting of upper tract obstruction/dilation requiring ureteral stent or percutaneous nephrostomy tube.
- Emphysematous pyelonephritis presents with advanced and life-threatening infections that may need immediate surgical intervention or percutaneous drainage.
- Children with febrile UTIs and VUR may be appropriate for antirefluxing surgery such as ureteral reimplantation.

COMPLEMENTARY & ALTERNATIVE MEDICINE
- *Vaccinium macrocarpon* (cranberry, not cranberry juice cocktail) may help to prevent and treat UTIs by inhibiting bacterial adherence to the bladder epithelium.
- Probiotic use for UTI prophylaxis or methenamine (Hiprex) can be used for recurrent UTIs.
- Vaginal estrogen can prevent recurrent UTIs in peri- and postmenopausal women.

ADMISSION, INPATIENT, AND NURSING CONSIDERATIONS
Inpatient evaluation is reserved for patients with complicated UTIs. Majority of uncomplicated UTIs are managed in an outpatient setting.

 ONGOING CARE

FOLLOW-UP RECOMMENDATIONS
First UTI: Middle-age, nonpregnant females require no follow-up if UTI is clinically cured after 3-day therapy (5)[C]. Obtain urine culture if symptoms persist after 2 to 3 days of treatment.

Pregnancy Considerations
- UTI during pregnancy always requires culture and usually requires a 7- to 14-day treatment.
- Following the treatment of acute infection, pregnant women warrant surveillance urine cultures every trimester. They may receive prophylactic antibiotics for the remainder of pregnancy.

Patient Monitoring
- Repeat culture in asymptomatic patients after completing therapy for a UTI to document bacterial clearance is unnecessary and may promote overtreatment of ASB.
- Obtain repeat urine cultures in patients with persistent symptoms after treatment. An empiric course of alternate antibiotics can be started but preferably after a urine sample is obtained.

DIET
Proper dietary glucose control in diabetic patients can help reduce the frequency of UTIs.

PATIENT EDUCATION
Urology Care Foundation: https://www.urologyhealth.org/resources/urinary-tract-infection-prevention

PROGNOSIS
Symptoms resolve within 2 to 3 days of antibiotic treatment in almost all patients.

COMPLICATIONS
Pyelonephritis or sepsis, renal abscess, urinary outlet obstruction

Pregnancy Considerations
Pregnant females, infants, and young children with cystitis are at higher risk of pyelonephritis.

REFERENCES
1. Gupta K, Trautner BW. Diagnosis and management of recurrent urinary tract infections in non-pregnant women. *BMJ.* 2013;346:f3140.
2. Foxman B. Urinary tract infection syndromes: occurrence, recurrence, bacteriology, risk factors, and disease burden. *Infect Dis Clin North Am.* 2014;28(1):1–13.
3. Fihn SD. Clinical practice. Acute uncomplicated urinary tract infection in women. *N Engl J Med.* 2003;349(3):259–266.
4. Venkatesan AM, Oto A, Allen BC, et al; for Expert Panel on Urological Imaging. ACR Appropriateness Criteria® recurrent lower urinary tract infections in females. *J Am Coll Radiol.* 2020;17(Suppl 11):S487–S496.
5. Anger J, Lee U, Ackerman AL, et al. Recurrent uncomplicated urinary tract infections in women: AUA/CUA/SUFU guideline. *J Urol.* 2019;202(2):282–289.
6. Griebling TL. Urologic diseases in America project: trends in resource use for urinary tract infections in women. *J Urol.* 2005;173(4):1281–1287.

 SEE ALSO

Algorithm: Dysuria

CODES

ICD10
- N39.0 Urinary tract infection, site not specified
- N30.90 Cystitis, unspecified without hematuria
- N30.91 Cystitis, unspecified with hematuria

CLINICAL PEARLS
- Urine culture is generally not indicated for women with uncomplicated UTI.
- Uncomplicated UTIs should be treated for 3 days (TMP/SMX) or 5 days (nitrofurantoin). Pregnant women with bacteriuria should be treated due to risk of poor outcomes with incompletely or untreated UTI.
- Nonpregnant women with ASB should not be treated.
- Fluoroquinolones should be reserved for complicated UTI and not used as first-line agents due to adverse effects.

U

URINARY TRACT INFECTION (UTI) IN MALES

Suzanne Florczyk, PharmD • Laura Ross, MD

 BASICS

DESCRIPTION
- Cystitis is an infection of the lower urinary tract, usually resulting from a single gram-negative enteric bacteria (see also "Prostatitis," "Pyelonephritis," and "Urethritis").
- System(s) affected: renal/urologic
- Synonym(s): urinary tract infection (UTI); cystitis
- In otherwise healthy males ages 15 to 50 years, UTI is uncommon and considered uncomplicated.
- In male newborns, infants, and elderly men, UTI is considered complicated, with associated functional/structural mechanisms.

EPIDEMIOLOGY
Incidence
- Predominant age: increases with age
- Uncommon in men <50 years of age; 6 to 8 infections per 10,000 men aged 21 to 50 years (1)

Prevalence
Lifetime prevalence approximately 14%

ETIOLOGY AND PATHOPHYSIOLOGY
- *Escherichia coli* (majority of infections)
- *Klebsiella* spp.
- *Enterobacter*
- *Enterococcus*
- *Proteus*
- *Citrobacter*
- *Providencia*
- *Streptococcus faecalis* and *Staphylococcus* spp.
- *Pseudomonas* and *Morganella* (more common in elderly and catheterized patients)
- Pathogenesis—bacterial entry into urinary tract via ascension or bladder instrumentation

Genetics
Not applicable

RISK FACTORS
- Age
- Obesity
- History of prior UTI
- Outlet obstruction
  - Benign prostatic hypertrophy (BPH)—incidence of 33% of men with UTIs (2)
  - Urethral stricture
  - Calculi
- Fecal incontinence
- Urinary incontinence
- Recent urologic surgery
- Urinary tract instrumentation/catheterization
- Infection of the prostate/kidney
- Immunocompromised
- Diabetes
- Bladder diverticula
- Neurogenic bladder
- Cognitive impairment
- Institutionalization
- Uncircumcised
- Anal intercourse
- Intercourse with an infected female partner (1)

GENERAL PREVENTION
- Prompt treatment of predisposing factors
- Use a catheter only when necessary; if needed, use aseptic technique and closed system and remove as soon as possible.
- Cranberry products are not recommended for preventing UTI.

COMMONLY ASSOCIATED CONDITIONS
- Acute bacterial pyelonephritis
- Chronic bacterial pyelonephritis
- Urethritis
- Prostatitis
- Prostatic hypertrophy
- Prostate cancer

Geriatric Considerations
Bacteriuria is more common among the elderly, usually is transient, and may be related to functional status. Of men >65 years of age, 5–10% have asymptomatic bacteriuria (ASB). If ASB is noted, no treatment is needed (3),(4).

Pediatric Considerations
Can be associated with obstruction to normal flow of urine, such as vesicoureteral reflux. Unique diagnostic criteria and evaluation recommendations exist (see below).

 DIAGNOSIS

HISTORY
- Urinary frequency
- Urinary urgency
- Dysuria
- Hesitancy
- Slow urinary stream
- Dribbling of urine
- Nocturia
- Suprapubic discomfort or perineal pain
- Constipation
- Low back pain
- Hematuria
- Systemic symptoms (chills, fever) or flank pain, nausea, vomiting present with concomitant pyelonephritis or prostatitis

PHYSICAL EXAM
- Suprapubic tenderness
- Costovertebral angle (CVA) tenderness and/or fever may be present with concomitant pyelonephritis/prostatitis/epididymitis.
- Perform genital examination.
- Consider digital rectal exam, including palpation of the prostate gland, to rule out bacterial prostatitis.

DIFFERENTIAL DIAGNOSIS
- Anatomic/functional pathology of the urinary tract
- Urethritis/STIs
- Infections in other sites of the genitourinary tract (e.g., epididymis, prostatitis). >90% of men with febrile UTI have concomitant prostate infection (1)[A].

DIAGNOSTIC TESTS & INTERPRETATION
- Urine dipstick/manual microscopy of clean catch midstream void showing the following:
  - Pyuria (>10 WBCs)
  - Bacteriuria
  - Leukocyte esterase is more sensitive, and nitrite is more specific in detecting UTI (5).
  - Positive leukocyte esterase (in males: sensitivity, 78%; specificity, 59%; positive predictive value [PPV], 71%; negative predictive value [NPV], 67%)
  - Positive nitrite (in males: sensitivity, 47%; specificity, 98%; PPV, 96%; NPV, 59%)

ALERT
All patients presenting with dysuria should be tested for STIs, as gonorrhea, chlamydia, and syphilis are epidemic in the United States.

- Automated microscopy/flow cytometry that measures cell counts and bacterial counts can be used to improve screening characteristics (sensitivity, 92%; specificity, 55%; PPV, 47%; NPV, 97%). The high NPV of these screening tests allows for more judicious use of urine culture (5)[B].
- Urine culture: >100,000 colony-forming units (CFU; $>10^5$ CFU) of bacteria/mL of urine confirm diagnosis.
- Lower counts, such as $>10^3$ CFU, also may be indicative of infection, especially in the presence of pyuria.
- Diagnosis in infants and children <24 months made on the basis of both pyuria and 50,000 CFU on culture
- Renal and bladder ultrasound recommended in infants and young children after first confirmed UTI

Follow-Up Tests & Special Considerations
- Consider assessing for risk factors for STIs because chlamydial/gonococcal urethritis can mimic a UTI. If risk factors are present, use urine nucleic acid amplification tests to identify gonococcal and *Chlamydia* infections and treat as necessary.
- Further urologic evaluation is warranted to rule out other disorders in men with recurrent UTI, febrile UTI, or pyelonephritis. This may include the following:
  - Ultrasound
  - Cystoscopy
  - Urodynamics
  - IV pyelography
- Value of a urologic evaluation in a single uncomplicated UTI has not been determined.
- Antibiotics prior to culture or phenazopyridine prior to urine dipstick can alter results.
- Blood cultures are not routine; perform if concern for sepsis or bacteremia.

Test Interpretation
Depends on site of infection

TREATMENT

- Catheter management: In general, avoid unnecessary catheterization.
- Minimize the use of indwelling catheters. Those who require extended catheterization should be managed by intermittent catheterization, if possible. There is no benefit of using prophylactic antibiotics to reduce the risk of catheter-associated UTIs.
- Exchange the Foley for acute infections when initiating antibiotics.

GENERAL MEASURES
- Hydration
- Analgesia, if required
- Aggressive treatment to prevent constipation with both soluble (psyllium) and insoluble (wheat germ) fiber
- Patient with indwelling catheters
  - If ASB colonization, no need to treat (Sterilization of urine is not possible, and resistant organisms may take up residence.)
  - If symptomatic of acute infection, institute treatment.

MEDICATION
First Line
- Acute, uncomplicated cystitis
  - Treat empirically; strongly consider if nitrite positive, using local resistance patterns or based on culture and sensitivity results for 5 to 7 days.
  - For empirical therapy, a fluoroquinolone or trimethoprim-sulfamethoxazole DS usually used to treat the most likely pathogens. Fosfomycin, nitrofurantoin, and β-lactams do not achieve reliable tissue concentration in the prostate.
- Complicated, febrile, or recurrent infection
  - Prescribe a minimum of 2 weeks antibiotics based on antimicrobial sensitivities with repeat urine check after the treatment. In men with febrile UTI or pyelonephritis, prostatic involvement also must be considered. Total duration of antimicrobial therapy generally ranges from 10 to 14 days. 5- to 7-day regimens of fluoroquinolones are comparable to longer durations (6). Treatment of concomitant prostatitis requires antimicrobials with good prostatic tissue and fluid penetration (fluoroquinolones).

Second Line
According to culture and sensitivity results and patient's history

ISSUES FOR REFERRAL
Further urologic evaluation and referral are warranted to rule out other disorders in male infants and men with recurrent UTI, febrile UTI, or pyelonephritis.

ADDITIONAL THERAPIES
- Probiotics
- Polyethylene Glycol 3350 for constipation
- Phenazopyridine—limit use to 48 hours when used concomitantly with an antibacterial agent.

ADMISSION, INPATIENT, AND NURSING CONSIDERATIONS
- Inability to tolerate oral medications
- Acute renal failure
- Suspected sepsis

 ONGOING CARE

FOLLOW-UP RECOMMENDATIONS
Patient Monitoring
Any patient who have worsening symptoms following initiation of antimicrobials, persistent symptoms after 48 to 72 hours of appropriate therapy, or recurrent symptoms within a few week of treatment should have additional evaluation.

DIET
Encourage adequate fluid intake.

PATIENT EDUCATION
For patient education materials about this topic that have been reviewed favorably, contact the National Kidney Foundation, 30 E. 33rd Street, Suite 1100, New York, NY 10016; 212-889-2210.

PROGNOSIS
Clearing of infections with appropriate antibiotic treatment

COMPLICATIONS
- Pyelonephritis
- Ascending infection
- Recurrent infection
- Prostatitis

REFERENCES
1. Wagenlehner FM, Weidner W, Pilatz A, et al. Urinary tract infections and bacterial prostatitis in men. *Curr Opin Infect Dis*. 2014;27(1):97–101.
2. Drekonja DM, Rector TS, Cutting A, et al. Urinary tract infection in male veterans: treatment patterns and outcomes. *JAMA Intern Med*. 2013;173(1): 62–68.
3. Rowe TA, Juthani-Mehta M. Diagnosis and management of urinary tract infection in older adults. *Infect Dis Clin North Am*. 2014;28(1):75–89.
4. Matthews SJ, Lancaster JW. Urinary tract infections in the elderly population. *Am J Geriatr Pharmacother*. 2011;9(5):286–309.
5. Koeijers JJ, Kessels AG, Nys S, et al. Evaluation of the nitrite and leukocyte esterase activity tests for the diagnosis of acute symptomatic urinary tract infection in men. *Clin Infec Dis*. 2007;45(7): 894–896.
6. van Nieuwkoop C, van der Starre WE, Stalenhoef JE, et al. Treatment duration of febrile urinary tract infection: a pragmatic randomized, double-blind, placebo-controlled non-inferiority trial in men and women. *BMC Med*. 2017;15(1):70.

ADDITIONAL READING
- Coupat C, Pradier C, Degand N, et al. Selective reporting of antibiotic susceptibility data improves the appropriateness of intended antibiotic prescriptions in urinary tract infections: a case-vignette randomised study. *Eur J Clin Microbiol Infect Dis*. 2013;32(5):627–636.
- Foxman B. Urinary tract infection syndromes: occurrence, recurrence, bacteriology, risk factors, and disease burden. *Infect Dis Clin North Am*. 2014;28(1):1–13.
- Gerber GS, Brendler CB. Evaluation of the urologic patient: history, physical examination, and urinalysis. In: Walsh PC, Retik AB, Vaughn ED Jr, et al, eds. *Campbell-Walsh Urology*. 8th ed. Philadelphia, PA: Saunders; 2002:107.
- Koeijers JJ, Verbon A, Kessels AG, et al. Urinary tract infection in male general practice patients: uropathogens and antibiotic susceptibility. *Urology*. 2010;76(2):336–340.

 SEE ALSO

- Prostate Cancer; Prostatic Hyperplasia, Benign (BPH); Prostatitis; Pyelonephritis; Urethritis
- Algorithms: Dysuria; Urethral Discharge

 CODES

ICD10
- N39.0 Urinary tract infection, site not specified
- N30.90 Cystitis, unspecified without hematuria
- N30.91 Cystitis, unspecified with hematuria

CLINICAL PEARLS
- Cystitis is an infection of the lower urinary tract, usually resulting from a single gram-negative enteric bacteria.
- Risk factors/causes: age, obesity, history of UTI, BPH/outlet obstruction, incontinence, urinary tract instrumentation or catheterization, infection of the prostate/kidney, immunocompromised or diabetes, cognitive impairment, institutionalization, neurogenic bladder, uncircumcised, anal intercourse, intercourse with infected female partner
- Evaluation: urinalysis, urine culture, STI testing (e.g., gonorrhea, *Chlamydia* by culture/DNA probe)
- Treat empirically with fluoroquinolones or trimethoprim-sulfamethoxazole DS for 5 to 7 days.

U

UROLITHIASIS
Roland W. Newman II, DO • Jana W. Qiao, MD

 BASICS

DESCRIPTION
- Stone formation within the urinary tract: Urinary crystals bind to form a nidus, which grows to form a calculus (stone).
- Range of symptoms: asymptomatic to obstructive; febrile morbidity if result of infection

EPIDEMIOLOGY
- The worldwide epidemiology differs according to both geographic area (higher prevalence in hot, arid, or dry climates) and socioeconomic conditions (dietary intake and lifestyle). Radiolucent stones and stones secondary to infection are less influenced by environmental conditions.
- Vesical calculosis (bladder stones) due to malnutrition during early life is frequent in Middle East and Asian countries.
- Incidence in industrialized countries seems to be increasing, probably due to improved diagnostics as well as to increasingly rich diets.
- Increased incidence in patients with surgically induced absorption issues, such as Crohn disease and gastric bypass surgery (1)

Incidence
- In industrialized countries: 100 to 200/100,000 per year
- Predominant age: Mean age is 40 to 60 years.
- Predominant sex: male > female (~3:1)

Prevalence
- 10–15% in the United States
- Lifetime risk of >14% in men, >6% in women
  - Prevalence in women increasing

ETIOLOGY AND PATHOPHYSIOLOGY
- Supersaturation and dehydration lead to high salt content in urine which congregates.
- Stasis of urine
  - Renal malformation (e.g., horseshoe kidney, ureteropelvic junction obstruction)
  - Incomplete bladder emptying (e.g., neurogenic bladder, prostate enlargement, multiple sclerosis)
- Crystals may form in pure solutions (homogeneous) or on existing surfaces, such as other crystals or cellular debris (heterogeneous).
- Balance of promoters and inhibitors: organic (Tamm-Horsfall protein, glycosaminoglycan, uropontin, nephrocalcin) and inorganic (citrate, pyrophosphate)
- Calcium oxalate and/or phosphate stones (80%)
  - Hypercalciuria
    ○ Absorptive hypercalciuria: increased jejunal calcium absorption
    ○ Renal leak: increased calcium excretion from renal proximal tubule
    ○ Resorptive hypercalciuria: mild hyperparathyroidism
  - Hypercalcemia
    ○ Hyperparathyroidism
    ○ Sarcoidosis
    ○ Malignancy
    ○ Immobilization
    ○ Paget disease
- Hyperoxaluria
  - Enteric hyperoxaluria
    ○ Intestinal malabsorptive state associated with irritable bowel disease, celiac sprue, or intestinal resection
    ○ Bile salt malabsorption leads to formation of calcium soaps.
  - Primary hyperoxaluria: autosomal recessive, types I and II
  - Dietary hyperoxaluria: overindulgence in oxalate-rich food
- Hyperuricosuria
  - Seen in 10% of calcium stone formers
  - Caused by increased dietary purine intake, systemic acidosis, myeloproliferative diseases, gout, chemotherapy, Lesch-Nyhan syndrome
  - Thiazides, probenecid
- Hypocitraturia
  - Caused by acidosis: renal tubular acidosis, malabsorption, thiazides, enalapril, excessive dietary protein
- Uric acid stones (10–15%): hyperuricemia causes as discussed earlier
- Struvite stones (5–10%): infected urine with urease-producing organisms (most commonly *Proteus* sp.)
- Cystine stones (<1%): autosomal recessive disorder of renal tubular reabsorption of cystine
- Bladder stones: seen with chronic bladder catheterization and some medications (indinavir)
- In children: usually due to malnutrition

Genetics
- Up to 20% of patients have a family history. However, spouses of those who form stones have higher calcium excretion rates than controls, suggesting strong dietary–environmental factors.
- Autosomal dominant: idiopathic hypercalciuria
- Autosomal recessive
  - Cystinuria, Lesch-Nyhan syndrome, hyperoxaluria types I and II
  - Ehlers-Danlos syndrome, Marfan syndrome, Wilson disease, familial renal tubular acidosis

RISK FACTORS
- White > Asian > African American in regions with both populations
- Male sex
- Family history (increases risk by up to 2.5 times)
- Previous history of nephrolithiasis
- Diet rich in protein, refined carbohydrates, and sodium; carbonated drinks; low calcium diet, low fluid intake
- Occupations associated with a sedentary lifestyle or with a hot, dry workplace
- Incidence rates peak during summer secondary to dehydration, hot climates.
- Obesity
- Surgically/medically induced malabsorption (Crohn disease, gastric bypass, celiac, primary hyperparathyroidism)
- Medications that can increase risk of forming calcium, uric acid stones (1)

GENERAL PREVENTION
- Hydration (2)
- Decrease salt and meat intake.
- Avoid oxalate-rich foods.

Pediatric Considerations
- Increasing in prevalence due to obesity, diabetes, hypertensions
- Additional risk factor considerations include renal disease or immaturity, preterm birth, low birth weight.
- Ultrasound should be considered in children before CT imaging to reduce radiation exposure.
- Consider additional workup to evaluate for metabolic abnormality or hereditary etiology.

Pregnancy Considerations
- Pregnant women have the same incidence of renal colic as do nonpregnant women.
- Most symptomatic stones occur during the 2nd and 3rd trimesters, heralded by symptoms of flank pain/hematuria.
- Most common differential diagnosis is physiologic hydronephrosis of pregnancy. Use ultrasound to avoid irradiation. Noncontrast-enhanced CT scan also is diagnostic.
- 30% require intervention, such as stent placement.

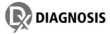 **DIAGNOSIS**

HISTORY
- Pain
  - Renal colic: acute onset of severe groin and/or flank pain
  - Distal stones may present with referred pain in labia, penile meatus, or testis.
- Microscopic/gross hematuria occurs in 95% of patients.
- Nonspecific symptoms of nausea, vomiting, tachycardia, diaphoresis
- Low-grade fever without signs of infection
- Infectious origin: associated with high-grade fevers require more urgent treatment (see the following text)
- Frequency and dysuria especially occur with stones at the vesicoureteric junction (VUJ).
- Asymptomatic: nonobstructing stones within the renal calyces

PHYSICAL EXAM
Tender costovertebral angle with palpation/percussion and/or iliac fossa

DIFFERENTIAL DIAGNOSIS
- Appendicitis
- Ruptured aortic aneurysm
- Musculoskeletal strain
- Pyelonephritis (upper UTI)
- Pyonephrosis (obstructed upper UTI; emergency)
- Perinephric abscess
- Pelvic or ovarian pathology: ectopic pregnancy, cyst, torsion
- Salpingitis
- Myocardial infarction
- Additional GI pathology: biliary colic, diverticulitis, obstruction, incarcerated hernia

DIAGNOSTIC TESTS & INTERPRETATION
- Urinalysis for RBCs, leukocytes, nitrates, pH (acidic urine <5.5 is associated with uric acid stones; alkaline >7 with struvite stones)
- Midstream urine for microscopy, culture, and sensitivity
- Blood: urea, creatinine, electrolytes, calcium, and urate; consider CBC.
- Parathyroid hormone only if calcium is elevated
- Stone analysis if/when stone passed

Initial Tests (lab, imaging)
- Noncontrast-enhanced helical CT scan of the abdomen and pelvis has replaced IV pyelogram.
  - Stone is found most commonly at levels of ureteric luminal narrowing: pelviureteric junction, pelvic brim, and VUJ.
  - Acute obstruction: Proximal ureter and renal pelvis are dilated to the level of obstruction, and perinephric stranding is possible on imaging.

- Renal ultrasound may be as effective with lower radiation at diagnosis as well as identifying obstruction.
- X-ray of kidneys, ureter, and bladder to determine if stone is radiopaque or lucent
  - Calcium oxalate/phosphate stones are radiopaque.
  - Uric acid stones are radiolucent.
  - Staghorn calculi (that fill the shape of the renal calyces) are usually struvite and opaque.
  - Cystine stones are faintly opaque (ground-glass appearance).
- Ultrasound has low sensitivity and specificity but is often the first choice for pregnant women and children.

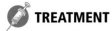 TREATMENT

GENERAL MEASURES

- 75% of patients are successfully treated conservatively and pass the stone spontaneously.
- Most stones <5 mm will pass spontaneously with conservative treatment.
- Stones between 5 and 10 mm may pass with medical expulsive therapy.
- Most stones >10 mm generally require surgical intervention.
- Stones that do not pass usually require surgical intervention.
- 30–50% of patients will have recurrent stones within 5 to 10 years.
- Increased fluid intake; eliminate carbonated drinks.

MEDICATION

- Medical expulsive therapy: α_1-Antagonists (e.g., tamsulosin) may improve likelihood of spontaneous stone passage. Calcium channel blockers (e.g., nifedipine) may not be as effective.
- Passage of larger stones (i.e., 5 to 10 mm) increased with tamsulosin.
- Category C in pregnancy
- Initiation of medical expulsive therapy should factor comorbidities, medication side effects, into consideration (e.g., hypotension, heart palpitations).
- Adequate pain control can be achieved with NSAIDs (anti-inflammatory effect decreases smooth muscle stimulation and spasms).

ISSUES FOR REFERRAL

- Urgent referral of patients with UTI, sepsis, acute renal failure, anuria
- Early referral of pregnant patients, children, adults >60 years, large stones (>8 mm), bilateral obstruction, solitary kidney, chronic renal failure
- Refer patients if no passage at 4 to 6 weeks or poorly controlled pain.

ADDITIONAL THERAPIES

- Uric acid stone dissolution therapy
  - Alkalinize urine with potassium citrate; keep pH >6.5.
  - Allopurinol 100 to 300 mg/day PO (for those who continue to form stones despite alkalinization of urine)
- Cystine stone dissolution/prevention
  - Alkalinize urine with potassium citrate; keep pH >6.5.
  - Chelating agents: captopril, α-mercaptopropionyl-glycine, D-penicillamine
- Consider altering medications that increase risk of stone formation: probenecid, loop diuretics, salicylic acid, salbutamol, indinavir, triamterene, acetazolamide.

- Vitamin D supplementation alone has not been proven to induce stone formation; recommend against taking calcium supplementation (or as antacid) with Vitamin D supplementation.
- Treat hypercalciuria with thiazides on an acute basis only.
- Treat hypocitraturia with potassium citrate and high-citrate juices (e.g., orange, lemon).
- Treat enteric hyperoxaluria with oral calcium/magnesium, cholestyramine, and potassium citrate.

SURGERY/OTHER PROCEDURES

- Immediate relief of obstruction is required for patients with the following conditions:
  - Sepsis
  - Renal failure (obstructed solitary kidney, bilateral obstruction)
  - Uncontrolled pain, despite adequate analgesia
- Emergency surgery for obstruction
  - Placement of a retrograde stent (i.e., endoscopic surgery, usually requires an anesthetic)
  - Radiologic placement of a percutaneous nephrostomy tube
- Elective surgery for stone treatment
  - Extracorporeal shock wave lithotripsy
  - Ureteroscopy with basket extraction/lithotripsy (laser/pneumatic)
  - Percutaneous nephrolithotomy
- Open surgery is uncommon.

ADMISSION, INPATIENT, AND NURSING CONSIDERATIONS

- Analgesia
  - Combination of NSAIDs (ketorolac 30 to 60 mg) and oral opiate
  - Parenteral opioid if vomiting or if preceding fails to control pain (morphine 5 to 10 mg IV or IM q4h)
  - Antiemetic if required or prophylactically with parenteral narcotics
- Septic patients with urosepsis or pyonephrosis may require IV antibiotics (once blood and urine cultures are taken), IV fluids, and in severe cases cardiorespiratory support in intensive care during recovery.

 ONGOING CARE

FOLLOW-UP RECOMMENDATIONS

- Patients with ureteric stones who are being treated conservatively should be followed until imaging is clear or stone is visibly passed.
  - Strain urine and send stone for composition.
  - Tamsulosin and nifedipine in selected patients to speed passage
  - Present to the hospital if pain worsens/signs of infection.
  - If pain management is suboptimal or stone does not progress or pass within 4 to 6 weeks, patient should be referred to a urologist and imaging should be repeated.
- Patients with recurrent stone formation should have follow-up with a urologist for metabolic workup: 24-hour urine for volume, pH, creatinine, calcium, cystine, phosphate, oxalate, uric acid, and magnesium.
  - PTH if serum calcium is found elevated
  - Ultrasonography to evaluate for renal anomaly if indicated

DIET

ALERT

- Increased fluid intake for life cannot be overemphasized for decreasing recurrence. Encourage intake of 2 to 3 L/day; advise patient to have clear urine rather than yellow.
- Decrease or eliminate carbonated drinks.
- Patients who form calcium stones should minimize high-oxalate foods such as green leafy vegetables, rhubarb, peanuts, chocolates, and beer.
- Decrease protein and salt intake.
- Lowering calcium intake is inadvisable and may even increase urine calcium excretion.
- Increase phytate-rich foods such as natural dietary bran, legumes and beans, and whole cereal.
- Avoid excessive vitamin C.

PROGNOSIS

- Spontaneous stone passage depends on stone location (proximal vs. distal) and stone size (<5 mm, 90% pass; >8 mm, 10% pass).
- Stone recurrence: 50% of patients at 10 years

REFERENCES

1. Corbo J, Wang J. Kidney and ureteral stones. *Emerg Med Clin North Am.* 2019;37(4):637–648.
2. Bao Y, Tu X, Wei Q. Water for preventing urinary stones. *Cochrane Database Syst Rev.* 2020;2(2):CD004292.

ADDITIONAL READING

Campschroer T, Zhu X, Vernooij RW, et al. Alpha-blockers as medical expulsive therapy for ureteral stones. *Cochrane Database Syst Rev.* 2018;4(4):CD008509.

 SEE ALSO

Algorithms: Dysuria; Renal Calculi; Urethral Discharge

CODES

ICD10

- N20.9 Urinary calculus, unspecified
- N20.0 Calculus of kidney
- N20.1 Calculus of ureter

CLINICAL PEARLS

- Incidence in industrialized countries seems to be increasing, probably due to improved diagnostics as well as to increasingly rich diets.
- Vesical calculosis (bladder stones) due to malnutrition during early life is frequent in Middle East and Asian countries.
- Medical expulsive therapy may improve likelihood of spontaneous stone passage.
- Increased fluid intake for life cannot be overemphasized for decreasing recurrence. Encourage 2 to 3 L/day intake; advise patient to have clear urine rather than yellow.
- Patients who form calcium stones should minimize high-oxalate foods such as green leafy vegetables, rhubarb, peanuts, chocolates, and beer.
- Decrease protein and salt intake.
- Lowering calcium intake is inadvisable and may even increase urine calcium excretion.

U

URTICARIA
Todd A. Wical, DO

 BASICS

DESCRIPTION
- A cutaneous lesion or lesions involving edema of the epidermis and/or dermis presenting with rapid onset and pruritus, returning to normal skin appearance within 24 hours
- Pathophysiology is primarily mast cell degranulation and subsequent histamine release.
- Angioedema may occur with urticaria, which is characterized by sudden pronounced erythematous nonpitting edema of the lower dermis and subcutis; may take up to 72 hours to remit
- Pruritus and burning are more commonly associated with urticaria; pain more often with angioedema
- Lesions can occur on any part of the body.
- Urticaria can be classified as acute or chronic.
  - Acute: if lesions recur within <6 weeks
  - Chronic: recurring lesions that persist for >6 weeks
- Three main causal categories of urticarial lesions
  - Immunoglobulin E (IgE) mediated
  - Non-IgE immunologically mediated
  - Nonimmunologically mediated
- Underlying etiology may be difficult to pinpoint, although in some cases possible.
- For those with chronic urticaria, 40% have concurrent angioedema
- Etiology of urticaria is either spontaneous or induced.
- System(s) affected: integumentary
- Synonym(s): hives; wheals

EPIDEMIOLOGY
Incidence
- Equally distributed across all ages: female > male (2:1 in chronic urticaria)
- In 20% of patients, chronic urticaria lasts >10 years.

Prevalence
- 5–25% of the population
- Of people with urticaria, 40% have no angioedema, 40% have urticaria and angioedema, and 20% have angioedema with no urticaria.
- Up to 3% of the population has chronic idiopathic urticaria.

ETIOLOGY AND PATHOPHYSIOLOGY
- Mast cell degranulation with release of inflammatory reactants, which leads to vascular leakage, inflammatory cell extravasation, and dermal (angioedema) and/or epidermal (wheals/hives) edema
- Histamine, cytokines, leukotrienes, and proteases are main active substances released.
- If release of histamine and other mediators occurs in the dermis, urticaria lesions result. If release occurs deep in the dermis, then angioedema develops.
- Acute spontaneous urticaria (ASU)
  - Bacterial infections: strep throat, sinusitis, otitis, urinary tract
  - Viral infections: rhinovirus, rotavirus, hepatitis B, mononucleosis, herpes

- Foods: peanuts, tree nuts, seafood, milk, soy, fish, wheat, and eggs; tend to be IgE-mediated; pseudoallergenic foods such as strawberries, tomatoes, preservatives, and coloring agents contain histamine.
  - Drugs: IgE-mediated (e.g., penicillin and other antibiotics), direct mast cell stimulation (e.g., aspirin, NSAIDs, opiates)
  - Inhalant, contact, ingestion, or occupational exposure (e.g., latex, cosmetics)
  - Parasitic infection; insect bite/sting
  - Transfusion reaction
- Chronic spontaneous urticaria (CSU)
  - Chronic subclinical allergic rhinitis, eczema, and other atopic disorders
  - Chronic indolent infections: *Helicobacter pylori*, fungal, parasitic (*Anisakis simplex*, strongyloidiasis), and chronic viral infections (hepatitis)
  - Collagen vascular disease (cutaneous vasculitis, serum sickness, lupus)
  - Thyroid autoimmunity, especially Hashimoto
  - Hormonal: pregnancy and progesterone
  - Autoimmune antibodies to the IgE receptor α chain on mast cells and to the IgE antibody
  - Chronic medications (e.g., NSAIDs, hormones, ACE inhibitors). NSAID sensitivity demonstrated almost in half of adults with chronic urticaria and presents with a worsening of symptoms 4 hours after ingestion.
  - Malignancy
  - Physical stimuli (cold, heat, vibration, pressure) in physical urticaria
- Chronic inducible urticaria (CIU)
  - Dermatographism: "skin writing" or the appearance of linear wheals at the site of any type of irritation. This is the most common physical induced urticaria.
  - Cold urticaria: Wheals occur within minutes of rewarming after cold exposure; 95% idiopathic but can be due to infections (mononucleosis, HIV), neoplasia, or autoimmune diseases.
  - Delayed pressure urticaria: Urticaria occurs 0.5 to 12 hours after pressure to skin (e.g., from elastic or shoes), may be pruritic and/or painful, and may not subside for several days.
  - Solar urticaria: from sunlight exposure, usually UV; onset in minutes; subsides within 2 hours
  - Heat urticaria: from direct contact with warm objects or air; rare
  - Vibratory urticaria/angioedema: very rare; secondary to vibrations (e.g., motorcycle)
  - Cholinergic urticaria: due to brief increase of core body temperature from exercise, baths, or emotional stress. This is the second most common induced urticaria.
  - Adrenergic urticaria: caused by stress; extremely rare; vasoconstricted, blanched skin around pink wheals as opposed to cholinergic's erythematous surrounding
  - Contact urticaria: wheals at sites where chemical substances contact the skin, may be either IgE-dependent (e.g., latex) or IgE-independent (e.g., stinging nettle)
  - Aquagenic and solar urticaria: small wheals after contact with water of any temperature or UV light, respectively; rare

Genetics
No consistent pattern known: Chronic urticaria has increased frequency of HLA-DR4 and HLA-D8Q MHC II alleles.

GENERAL PREVENTION
Avoidance of known triggers is the mainstay of prevention.

COMMONLY ASSOCIATED CONDITIONS
- Angioedema (common)
- Anaphylaxis (somewhat common)

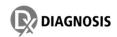 **DIAGNOSIS**

HISTORY
Rapid onset; individual lesions resolve in <24 hours, pruritus

> **ALERT**
> Important to rule out underlying anaphylaxis in those patients presenting with acute onset of urticaria (1)[C],(2)[C]

PHYSICAL EXAM
- Single/multiple raised, polymorphic indurated plaques with central pallor and edema with an erythematous flare
- Evaluate for underlying conditions including thyroid abnormalities (nodules), bacterial, viral, or fungal infection (e.g., fever).

DIFFERENTIAL DIAGNOSIS
- Anaphylaxis (may present with urticaria)
- Morbilliform or fixed drug eruptions
- Erythema multiforme
- Systemic lupus erythematosus (SLE), vasculitis, and polyarteritis
- Angioedema without urticaria
- Urticaria pigmentosa/systemic mastocytosis
- Bullous pemphigoid (urticarial stage)
- Arthropod bite
- Atopic/contact dermatitis
- Viral exanthem

DIAGNOSTIC TESTS & INTERPRETATION
- Diagnosis is usually clinical (1),(2).
- In general, only if the history or physical are suggestive of a specific underlying disease should targeted laboratory studies be utilized.

Initial Tests (lab, imaging)
- Acute: generally not indicated
- Chronic: directed by clinical suspicion of underlying cause
  - Allergy skin tests and radioallergosorbent test (RAST) for inhaled allergens, insects, drugs, or foods
  - Infection: Consider pharyngeal culture, LFTs, mononucleosis test, urinalysis in appropriate setting.

Follow-Up Tests & Special Considerations

Chronic urticaria (CIU/CSU): Extensive lab testing is not indicated and has not proven to improve outcome nor is it cost-effective. Limit lab testing according to clinical history and indication. Skin or IgE testing should be limited to specific history of provoking allergen (3)[C].

- CBC, ESR, and CRP are recommended by most guidelines.
- Thyroid function tests, LFTs, and urinalysis are recommended by several guidelines.
- Consider allergy skin tests and RAST for inhaled allergens, insects, drugs, or foods; total IgE level
- Autoimmune: ESR, ANA, RF, complement (e.g., CH50, C3, C4), cryoglobulins in urticarial vasculitis
- Tests for *H. pylori* (e.g., antibodies) in dyspeptic patients. Consider stool for ova and parasites in at-risk individuals.
- Autologous serum skin testing: injection of serum under skin to test for presence of IgE receptor–activating antibodies
- Consider malignancy workup, including serum protein electrophoresis and immunofixation in the proper setting.

Diagnostic Procedures/Other

- Food and drug reactions: elimination of (or challenges with) suspected agents
- Physical and special forms of urticaria challenge tests:
  - Dermatographism: stroke skin lightly with rounded object and observe for surrounding urticaria
  - Cold urticaria: ice cube test—place ice cube on skin for 5 minutes; observe for 10 to 15 minutes.
  - Cholinergic: exercise to the point of sweating/partial immersion in 42°C bath for 10 minutes
  - Solar: exposure to different wavelengths of light
  - Delayed pressure: Apply 5-lb sandbag to back for 20 minutes; observe 6 hours later.
  - Aquagenic: Apply water at various temperatures.
  - Vibratory: Apply vibration 4 to 5 minutes with a lab mixing device; observe.
- Skin biopsy with lesions lasting >24 hours or if concern for underlying vasculitis (1)[C],(2)[C]

 ## TREATMENT

GENERAL MEASURES
The mainstay of therapy for urticaria is the avoidance of identified triggers.

MEDICATION

First Line
2nd-generation antihistamine (H₁) blockers are the first-line treatment of any urticaria in which avoidance of stimulus is impossible or not feasible (1)[C],(2)[C]:

- Fexofenadine (Allegra): 180 mg/day
- Loratadine (Claritin): 10 mg/day, increasing to 30 mg/day if needed; only medication studied for safe use in pregnancy

- Desloratadine (Clarinex): 5 mg/day (4)[B]
- Cetirizine (Zyrtec): 10 mg/day, increasing to 30 mg per day if needed
- Levocetirizine (Xyzal): 5 mg/day; requires weight-based dosing in children (4)[B]
- Rupatadine: novel H₁ antagonist with antiplatelet-activating factor activity

Second Line
Doubling the typical 2nd-generation H₁ blocker dosages should be attempted before adding 1st-generation H₁ or H₂ blockers (1),(2)[C],(4)[B].

- H₂-specific antihistamines (beneficial as adjuvants): cimetidine, ranitidine, nizatidine, famotidine
- 1st-generation antihistamines (H₁; for patients with sleep disturbed by itching):
  - Older children and adults: hydroxyzine or diphenhydramine 25 to 50 mg q6h
  - Children <6 years of age: diphenhydramine 12.5 mg q6–8h (5 mg/kg/day) or hydroxyzine (10 mg/5 mL) 2 mg/kg/day divided q6–8h

Geriatric Considerations
1st-generation H₁ blockers may cause excessive drowsiness as well as dry mouth and eyes.

ISSUES FOR REFERRAL
Referral to an allergist, immunologist, or dermatologist for recalcitrant cases, especially if lesions consistently remain present for >24 hours

ADMISSION, INPATIENT, AND NURSING CONSIDERATIONS
Educating patient on use of EpiPen as pathophysiology is similar to anaphylaxis; if the airway is threatened, immediate consultation to evaluate for laryngeal edema and need for definitive airway management

 ## ONGOING CARE

FOLLOW-UP RECOMMENDATIONS
After initial diagnosis, follow-up is recommended within 6 weeks as nearly 1/3 of acute patient go on to have persistent urticaria.

Patient Monitoring
- Use the urticaria activity score (UAS7) for assessing CSU.
- Recently was developed urticaria control test (UCT)
  - The tool to assess disease control in patients with chronic urticaria (spontaneous and inducible) (5)[A]

PROGNOSIS
- Resolution of acute symptoms: 70% <72 hours
- Chronic urticaria: 35% symptom-free in a year; another 30% will see symptom reduction.

REFERENCES

1. Zuberbier T, Aberer W, Asero R, et al. The EAACI/GA²LEN/EDF/WAO guideline for the definition, classification, diagnosis and management of urticaria. *Allergy.* 2018;73(7):1393–1414.
2. Bernstein JA, Lang DM, Khan DA, et al. The diagnosis and management of acute and chronic urticaria: 2014 update. *J Allergy Clin Immunol.* 2014;133(5):1270–1277.
3. Choosing Wisely. American Academy of Allergy, Asthma & Immunology. Don't routinely do diagnostic testing in patients with chronic urticaria. http://www.choosingwisely.org/clinician-lists/american-academy-allergy-asthma-immunology-chronic-urticaria/. Accessed July 15, 2021.
4. Staevska M, Popov TA, Kralimarkova T, et al. The effectiveness of levocetirizine and desloratadine in up to 4 times conventional doses in difficult-to-treat urticaria. *J Allergy Clin Immunol.* 2010;125(3):676–682.
5. Weller K, Groffik A, Church MK, et al. Development and validation of the urticaria control test: a patient-reported outcome instrument for assessing urticaria control. *J Allergy Clin Immunol.* 2014;133(5):1365–1372.

ADDITIONAL READING

- Dressler C, Werner RN, Eisert L, et al. Chronic inducible urticaria: a systematic review of treatment options. *J Allergy Clin Immunol.* 2018;141(5):1726–1734. doi:10.1016/j.jaci.2018.01.031.
- Poonawalla T, Kelly B. Urticaria: a review. *Am J Clin Dermatol.* 2009;10(1):9–21.
- Powell R, Leech S, Till S, et al. BSACI guideline for the management of chronic urticaria and angioedema. *Clin Exp Allergy.* 2015;45(3):547–565.
- Zuberbier T, Balke M, Worm M, et al. Epidemiology of urticaria: a representative cross-sectional survey. *Clin Exp Dermatol.* 2010;35(8):869–873.

 ## CODES

ICD10
- L50.9 Urticaria, unspecified
- L50.1 Idiopathic urticaria
- L50.8 Other urticaria

CLINICAL PEARLS

- Urticaria occurs rapidly, and individual lesions resolve within 24 hours, although multiple crops of lesions can occur in stages.
- Mainstay of therapy is to avoid identified triggers.
- Antihistamines are the best studied and most efficacious therapy but may require higher-than-normal doses for efficacy.
- If individual lesions last >24 hours, patient should be evaluated for urticarial vasculitis and other more serious diagnoses.

U

UTERINE AND PELVIC ORGAN PROLAPSE

Deepali Maheshwari, DO, MPH • Michael P. Flynn, MD, MHS

 BASICS

DESCRIPTION

- Symptomatic descent of one or more of (1),(2)
  - The anterior vaginal wall (bladder or cystocele)
  - The posterior vaginal wall (rectum or rectocele)
  - The uterus and cervix
  - The vaginal apex (vault or cuff scar after hysterectomy)
- Prolapses above or to the level of the hymen are generally not symptomatic (2).
- Associated symptoms (2)
  - Feeling of vaginal or pelvic pressure
  - Heaviness
  - Bulging
  - Bowel or bladder symptoms
- Cost associated with treatment is >$1 billion annually (~200,000 surgeries per year) (2).

EPIDEMIOLOGY

Incidence
- The incidence of pelvic organ prolapse (POP) ranges from 1.5 to 1.8 per 1,000 woman-years and peaks in women aged 60 to 69 years (3).
- In the United States, there are approximately 300,000 surgeries for POP each year (3), and a woman's lifetime risk of undergoing surgery for pelvic floor prolapse ranges from 6% to 18% (3).

Prevalence
- A national survey of 7,924 women (>20 years of age) found a prevalence of 25% for one or more pelvic floor disorders (including urinary incontinence, fecal incontinence, and POP). Prevalence of POP was 3–6% (4).
- POP is common but not always symptomatic. It does not always progress. It is estimated that 50% of women will develop prolapse, but only 10–20% of those will seek care for their condition (3).

ETIOLOGY AND PATHOPHYSIOLOGY

- Pelvic organs are supported by attachments between pelvic floor muscles, connective tissue, and the bony pelvis. Defects in this support can lead to prolapse in one or multiple compartments (5).
- Symptomatic women typically have defects in more than one compartment as well as damage to the levator ani and its attachments to the pelvis (5).
- Gradual process that begins long before symptoms develop

RISK FACTORS

- Vaginal childbirth: Each additional vaginal birth increases risk (2),(4).
- Age
- Family history (2)
- Race: White and Hispanic women may be at higher risk than black or Asian women (1),(2).
- Obesity BMI >30 kg/m^2 (2),(4)
- Chronic straining (constipation, chronic cough from pulmonary disease, repeated heavy lifting) (2)
- History of hysterectomy (2),(4)

GENERAL PREVENTION

There is some evidence that pelvic floor muscle training ("Kegel exercises") may decrease the risk of symptomatic POP (5)[B]. Weight loss and proper management of conditions that cause increase in intra-abdominal pressure such as constipation may help prevent prolapse (5)[C]. Elective caesarean delivery has not been shown to prevent prolapse.

COMMONLY ASSOCIATED CONDITIONS

- Constipation
- Fecal incontinence
- Urinary incontinence or retention
- Other urinary symptoms
  - Urgency
  - Frequency

 DIAGNOSIS

Less than half of women discuss symptoms with PCP. Only 10–12% seek medical attention. Barriers include embarrassment, social stigma, ability to cope, belief that POP is part of the aging process, belief that treatment options are limited, and fear of surgery.

HISTORY

- Common symptoms include the following:
  - Feeling a bulge in vagina
  - Something "falling out" of vagina
  - Pelvic pressure with activity or prolonged standing
  - Difficulty with voiding or defecation
  - Splinting the bulge to evacuate
  - Urinary or fecal urgency
  - Urinary frequency
  - Urinary or fecal incontinence
  - Constipation

- Document the presence, duration, and severity of coexisting urinary or bowel symptom.
- Assess impact on sexual function and quality of life.
- Assess past medical and surgical history.
  - Gravidity and parity/obstetric history
  - Chronic constipation
  - Pulmonary disease
  - Prior pelvic procedures

PHYSICAL EXAM

- Abdominal examination to document any distention or masses
- Complete pelvic and rectal examination. Have patient cough or strain, particularly in an upright (standing) position while examining the distal vagina.
- The standard to measure prolapse is the validated Pelvic Organ Prolapse Quantification (POP-Q) scale.
  - Describes prolapse of each compartment in relationship to the vaginal hymen
  - Patient is supine with the head of the bed at 45 degrees, performing Valsalva.
    - Stage 1: prolapse in which the distal point is superior or equal to 1 cm above hymen
    - Stage 2: prolapse in which the distal point is between 1 cm above and 1 cm below hymen
    - Stage 3: prolapse in which the distal point is superior or equal to 1 cm below the hymen, but some vaginal mucosa is not everted
    - Stage 4: complete vaginal vault eversion ("procidentia"); entire vaginal mucosa everted (2)
- A split speculum should be used to observe apical, anterior, and posterior compartments successively.
- Patient can be evaluated in supine position. If prolapse is not well demonstrated, patient can stand and Valsalva to assess maximum descent.

DIFFERENTIAL DIAGNOSIS

- Rectal prolapse
- Hemorrhoids
- Bartholin cyst
- Vaginal cyst
- Urethral diverticulum
- Cervical elongation

DIAGNOSTIC TESTS & INTERPRETATION

Initial Tests (lab, imaging)
- Urinalysis if symptomatic POP (1)
- Postvoid residual (1)

Follow-Up Tests & Special Considerations

- Consider urodynamic testing if results would alter treatment plan.
- Selective use of upper urinary tract imaging if observation is planned or if evidence of obstruction (e.g., abnormal postvoid residual) (1)
- If fecal incontinence or significant change in bowel habits, selective use of lower GI tract imaging or endoscopy (1)
- Consider defecography if severity of symptoms is out of proportion with the extent of prolapse.

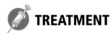 TREATMENT

GENERAL MEASURES

- Treatment is generally guided by degree of bother for the patient. It is important to document the patient's desire, goals, and expectations.
- Treatment should consider type and severity of symptoms, patient's age, other comorbid conditions, sexual function, infertility, and risk of recurrence.
- Treatment for asymptomatic patients:
  – Stage 1 or 2: clinical observation
  – Stage 3 or 4: regular follow-up and evaluation (every 3 to 6 months) (2)
- Expectant management is an acceptable option for patients without evidence of urinary or bowel obstruction.
- Treatment is indicated when there is urinary/bowel obstruction or hydronephrosis regardless of the degree of prolapse.
- A vaginal pessary should be considered in all women presenting with symptomatic prolapse.
  – There are >13 types of pessaries.
  – The most commonly used pessaries are the ring pessary and Gellhorn.
  – Most women can be successfully fitted with a pessary.
  – Satisfaction rate for patients using pessaries is very high (5).
- Minor complications such as vaginal discharge and odor can often be treated with vaginal estrogen.
- Vaginal erosion can be treated by removal of pessary and optional vaginal estrogen supplementation.
- Complications such as erosions, abrasions, ulcerations, vaginal bleeding, and fistulas may be seen with neglected pessaries.

MEDICATION

There are no data to support the use of vaginal estrogen or other medications for the prevention or treatment of POP.

ISSUES FOR REFERRAL

Referral when pessary or surgery is necessary

ADDITIONAL THERAPIES

Pelvic floor muscle training: may reduce the symptoms of POP. Pelvic floor muscle training does not affect the degree of prolapse, only the symptoms (5).

SURGERY/OTHER PROCEDURES

- Reconstructive procedures are performed with the goal of restoration of vaginal anatomy and resolution of symptoms.
- There are a variety of surgeries for repair of the anterior, apical, and posterior compartments. Surgical approaches include vaginal, abdominal, and laparoscopic (straight stick and robot assisted).
- Reconstructive surgery using native tissue is associated with an increased rate of failure (1 in 3 lifetime risk of repeat surgery). Procedures using surgical mesh and graft material have higher success rates.
- Surgical repair should focus on repairing all affected compartments in a single procedure.
- Coexisting stress incontinence should be addressed at the same time as the prolapse repair.
- For apical repairs:
  – Sacral colpopexy uses surgical mesh and has higher success rates and overall durability. It can be performed abdominally, laparoscopically, or robotically. The risk of recurrent prolapse is considered lower with sacral colpopexy than vaginal approaches; there may be an elevated risk of complications (6).
  – Concomitant hysterectomy is generally performed with prolapse repair. The risk of mesh extrusions appears to be decreased by retaining the cervix.
  – Uterine preservation via hysteropexy is also an option and may be offered by some surgeons. The risks and benefits of uterine preservation in prolapse repair remain unclear.

ONGOING CARE

PATIENT EDUCATION

- Patients should have POP explained to them with diagrams and descriptions of their anatomy.
- Important to emphasize that surgery is geared toward improving quality of life
- Patients should be educated about pessary complications and possible symptoms of POP if they are still asymptomatic.
- Using insoluble fibers may help patients with bowel complaints such as constipation.

COMPLICATIONS

- Recurrence rates are variable and quoted between 3.4% and 29.2% (3).
- There is a risk of dyspareunia and pelvic pain after any surgical repair. Those repairs using mesh may also be complicated by mesh erosion (6).
- Risk of complications with pessary includes vaginal erosion and fistula in patients that are lost to follow-up.
- Severe prolapse can lead to urinary retention and defecatory dysfunction that may go unrecognized in the elderly.

REFERENCES

1. Dumoulin C, Hunter KF, Moore K, et al. Conservative management for female urinary incontinence and pelvic organ prolapse review 2013: summary of the 5th International Consultation on Incontinence. *Neurourol Urodyn.* 2016;35(1):15–20.
2. Weber A, Richter H. Pelvic organ prolapse. *Obstet Gynecol.* 2005;106(3):615–634.
3. Barber MD, Maher C. Epidemiology and outcome assessment of pelvic organ prolapse. *Int Urogynecol J.* 2013;24(11):1783–1790.
4. Wu JM, Vaughan CP, Goode PS, et al. Prevalence and trends of symptomatic pelvic floor disorders in U.S. women. *Obstet Gynecol.* 2014;123(1):141–148.
5. Hagen S, Stark D. Conservative prevention and management of pelvic organ prolapse in women. *Cochrane Database Syst Rev.* 2011;(12):CD003882.
6. Maher C, Feiner B, Baessler K, et al. Surgical management of pelvic organ prolapse in women. *Cochrane Database Syst Rev.* 2013;(4):CD004014.

CODES

ICD10

- N81.9 Female genital prolapse, unspecified
- N81.10 Cystocele, unspecified
- N99.3 Prolapse of vaginal vault after hysterectomy

CLINICAL PEARLS

- Many women do not discuss POP with their doctor—ask routinely.
- Vaginal pessary should be considered in all patients with symptomatic prolapse.
- Treatment should be guided by degree of bother and impact on patient's quality of life.

U

UTERINE MYOMAS

Sareena Singh, MD, FACOG • Kimberly Resnick, MD

 BASICS

DESCRIPTION
- Uterine leiomyomas are well-circumscribed, pseudoencapsulated, benign monoclonal tumors composed mainly of smooth muscle with varying amounts of fibrous connective tissue (1).
- Three major subtypes
  - Subserous: common; external; may become pedunculated
  - Intramural: common; within myometrium; may cause marked uterine enlargement
  - Submucous: ~5% of all cases; internal, evoking abnormal uterine bleeding and infection; occasionally protruding from cervix
- Rare locations: broad, round, and uterosacral ligaments
- System affected: reproductive
- Synonym(s): fibroids; myoma; fibromyoma; myofibroma; fibroleiomyoma

EPIDEMIOLOGY
Incidence
- Cumulative incidence up to 80%
  - 60% in African American women by age 35 years; 80% by age 50 years
  - 40% in Caucasian women by age 35 years; 70% by age 50 years (1),(2)
- Incidence increases with each decade during reproductive years.
- Rarely seen in premenarchal females
- Predominant sex: females only

ETIOLOGY AND PATHOPHYSIOLOGY
- Enlargement of benign smooth muscle tumors that may lead to symptoms affecting the reproductive, GI, or genitourinary system
- Complex multifactorial process involving transition from normal myocyte to abnormal cells and then to visibly evident tumor (monoclonal expansion)
  - Hormones (1): Increases in estrogen and progesterone are correlated with myoma formation (i.e., rarely seen before menarche). Estrogen receptors in myomas bind more estradiol than normal myometrium.
  - Growth factors (1)
    ○ Increased smooth muscle proliferation (transforming growth factor β [TGF-β], basic fibroblast growth factor [bFGF])
    ○ Increase DNA synthesis (epidermal growth factor [EGF], platelet-derived growth factor [PDGF], activin, myostatin)
    ○ Stimulate synthesis of extracellular matrix (TGF-β)
    ○ Promote mitogenesis (TGF-β, EGF, insulin-like growth factor [IGF], prolactin)
    ○ Promote angiogenesis (bFGF, vascular endothelial growth factor [VEGF])
  - Vasoconstrictive hypoxia (1): proposed, but not confirmed, mechanism of myometrial injury during menstruation

Genetics
- A variety of somatic chromosomal rearrangements have been described in 40% of uterine myomas. Mutations in the gene encoding mediator complex subunit 12 (MED12) on the X chromosome were found in 70% of myomas in one study (3).
- Higher levels of aromatase and therefore estrogen have been found in myomas in African American women (3).

RISK FACTORS
- African American heritage: 2.9 times greater risk than Caucasian women; occur at a younger age, are more numerous, larger, and more symptomatic (1),(2)
- Early menarche (<10 years)
- Oral contraceptive use before 16 years old (2)
- Nulliparous
- Hypertension
- Familial predisposition: 2.5 times more likely in women with a first-degree relative with myomas (1)
- Obesity: Risk increases by 21% with each 10 kg of weight gain (1).
- Alcohol
- Risk decreased by parity, progesterone-only contraceptives, diet (fruits, veggies, low fat dairy) (2).

COMMONLY ASSOCIATED CONDITIONS
Endometrial and breast cancer also associated with high, unopposed estrogen stimulation

 DIAGNOSIS

HISTORY
- Usually asymptomatic; 30% present with abnormal symptoms—usually enlarged uterus or heavy bleeding (2).
- Symptoms include the following:
  - Abnormal uterine bleeding: usually heavy/prolonged menses
  - Pain: infrequent; usually associated with torsion of pedunculated myoma, degeneration, or cervical dilation by submucous myoma near cervical os
  - Pressure on bladder: suprapubic discomfort, urinary frequency/obstruction
  - Pressure on rectosigmoid: may cause low back pain, constipation
  - Infertility: rare, estimated 1–2.5%; usually from submucous myoma distorting the uterine cavity or interference with implantation

ALERT
Rapid growth, particularly in perimenopausal/postmenopausal patients; may indicate sarcoma; extremely rare, 0.1–0.3% of cases

PHYSICAL EXAM
- Usually incidental finding on abdominal and pelvic exam
- Firm, smooth nodules/masses arising from uterus
- Masses are mobile without tenderness.

DIFFERENTIAL DIAGNOSIS
Intrauterine pregnancy, cancer, including ovarian, uterine, or leiomyosarcoma; cecal/sigmoid tumor, appendiceal abscess, diverticulitis, pelvic kidney, urachal cyst

DIAGNOSTIC TESTS & INTERPRETATION
Initial Tests (lab, imaging)
- Pregnancy test
- Hemoglobin
- Pelvic ultrasound: standard confirmatory test; shows characteristic hypoechoic appearance (2)
- Saline infusion hysterosonography: helps to distinguish submucosal myomas

- Hysterosalpingogram: evaluates the contour of the endometrial cavity
- CT scan or MRI: provides info on degeneration and special relationships (2); may help to differentiate complex cases or used when uterine artery embolization is planned

Follow-Up Tests & Special Considerations
Consider cancer antigen 125 (CA-125): may be slightly elevated in some cases of uterine myoma but generally more useful in differentiating myomas from various gynecologic adenocarcinomas
- IV pyelogram: if suspect ureteral distortion
- Barium enema

Diagnostic Procedures/Other
- Fractional dilation and curettage: aids in ruling out cervical/uterine carcinomas when clinically suspicious
- Hysteroscopy: helps to diagnose submucosal/intracavitary myomas
- Laparoscopy: useful in complex cases and to rule out other pelvic diseases/disorders

Test Interpretation
- Myomas are usually multiple and vary in size and location; have been reported up to 100 lb
- Gross pathology: firm tumors with characteristic whorl-like trabeculated appearance; a thin pseudocapsular layer is present.
- Microscopic: bundles of smooth muscle mixed with varying amounts of connective tissue elements running in different directions
- Cellular variant has a preponderance of muscle cells. Mitoses are rare.
- May undergo various types of degeneration
  - Hyaline degeneration: very common
  - Calcification: late result of circulatory impairment to myomas
  - Infection and suppuration: most common with submucosal myomas
  - Necrosis: most common with pedunculated myomas secondary to torsion

TREATMENT
- Treatment must be individualized and based on symptoms, fertility desires, and time until menopause.
- Medical therapy may be of benefit.
- Patients with minimal symptoms may be treated with iron preparations and analgesics.
- Conservative management of asymptomatic myomas
  - Pelvic exams and ultrasounds at ≥3-month intervals if size remains stable
  - Substantial regression usually occurs after menopause.
- Surgical options should be considered if symptomatic or worrisome myomas are unresponsive to conservative/medical management.

GENERAL MEASURES

Patients not desiring pharmacologic therapy or surgery may consider the following:

- Uterine artery embolization: averages 50% shrinkage of myomas (4)[A]; painful and may cause ovarian failure (1–2%), amenorrhea, postembolization syndrome, or other complications; shorter hospital stay and quicker recovery but no difference in satisfaction compared with hysterectomy (2); high reintervention rate (15–32% by 2 years) compared to hysterectomy/myomectomy (7% by 2 years) (4)[A]
- MR-guided focused ultrasound (MRgFUS): noninvasive, ultrasound transducer passes through abdominal wall and causes coagulative necrosis of fibroid; up to 98% reduction in myoma volume and symptoms. Not appropriate for some types of myomas. Efficacy may be comparable with other hysterectomy-sparing procedures. Fertility has been shown to be preserved (2) although risks and outcomes data are limited (2).

MEDICATION

- Progestins may reduce overall uterine size.
  - Norethindrone 10 mg/day
  - Medroxyprogesterone 200 mg IM monthly
  - Levonorgestrel intrauterine device
- Combination oral contraceptives: may help prevent development of new fibroids and control bleeding
- Gonadotropin-releasing hormone agonists
  - Nafarelin (nasal spray), goserelin acetate, and leuprolide
  - Induces abrupt artificial menopause; may reduce myoma symptoms dramatically; induces atrophy of myomas by up to 40% in 2 to 3 months
  - May be valuable as preoperative adjunct to myomectomy/hysterectomy by allowing recovery of anemia, donation of autologous blood, and possibly converting abdominal to vaginal hysterectomy (2)[B]
  - Not recommended for use >6 months because of osteoporosis risk
  - Following discontinuation, myomas return within 60 days to pretherapy size.
- Antiprogesterones
  - Mifepristone
    - Shown to have similar reduction in myoma size as gonadotropin-releasing hormone agonists
    - Decreases heavy bleeding and increases quality of life (5)[A]
  - Selective progesterone receptor modulator (SPRM): ulipristal acetate: may be as effective as gonadotropin-releasing hormones with fewer side effects (2)[B]

ISSUES FOR REFERRAL

- Medical therapy may be initiated by a primary care physician/gynecologist after adequate pelvic examination.
- Surgical considerations may be pursued with gynecologic consultation.
- Uterine embolization may be discussed with an interventional radiologist.

SURGERY/OTHER PROCEDURES

- Surgical management is indicated in the following situations:
  - Excessive uterine size or excessive rate of growth (except during pregnancy)
  - Submucosal myomas when associated with hypermenorrhea
  - Pedunculated myomas that are painful or undergo torsion, necrosis, and hemorrhage
  - If a myoma causes symptoms from pressure on bladder/rectum
  - If differentiation from ovarian mass is not possible
  - If associated pelvic disease is present (endometriosis, pelvic inflammatory disease)
  - If infertility/habitual abortion is likely due to the anatomic location of the myoma
- Surgical procedures
  - Preliminary pelvic examination, Pap smear, and endometrial biopsy should be performed to rule out malignant/premalignant conditions.
  - Hysterectomy: may be performed vaginally, laparoscopically, robotically, or by laparotomy
    - Effective in relieving symptoms and improving quality of life (2)[B]
    - Similar fertility and live birth rates between laparoscopic and abdominal myomectomy
    - FDA discourages the use of laparoscopic power morcellation during hysterectomy or myomectomy for uterine fibroids given the risk of spreading an occult malignancy and all patients should be counseled preoperatively of risk (2).
  - Abdominal, laparoscopic, robotic, or hysteroscopic myomectomy may be performed in younger women who want to maintain fertility.
  - Hysteroscopic/laparoscopic cautery/laser myoma resection can be performed in selected patients.
  - Endometrial ablation: for small submucosal myomas

ADMISSION, INPATIENT, AND NURSING CONSIDERATIONS

- Usually outpatient
- Inpatient for some surgical procedures

ONGOING CARE

FOLLOW-UP RECOMMENDATIONS

Patient Monitoring

- Pelvic examination and ultrasound: every 2 to 3 months for newly diagnosed symptomatic/excessively large myomas
- Hemoglobin and hematocrit: if uterine bleeding is excessive
- Once uterine size and symptoms stabilize, monitor every 6 to 12 months, although no high-quality evidence exists (2).

DIET

No restrictions

PATIENT EDUCATION

- Society of Interventional Radiology: https://www.sirweb.org/patient-center/conditions-and-treatments/uterine-fibroids/
- U.S. Department of Health and Human Services: https://www.womenshealth.gov/a-z-topics/uterine-fibroids
- American Congress of Obstetricians and Gynecologists: http://www.acog.org

PROGNOSIS

- Resection of submucosal fibroids has been associated with increased fertility.
- At least 10% of myomas recur after myomectomy; however, only 25% require further treatment (2)[B].

COMPLICATIONS

- May mask other gynecologic malignancies (e.g., uterine sarcoma, ovarian cancer)
- Degenerating fibroids may cause pain and bleeding.
- May rarely prolapse through the cervix

Pregnancy Considerations

- Rapid growth of fibroids is common.
- Pregnant women may need additional fetal testing if placenta is located over or near fibroid.
- Complications during pregnancy: abortion, premature labor, 2nd-trimester rapid growth leading to degeneration/pain, 3rd-trimester fetal malpresentation, and dystocia during labor and delivery
- Cesarean section is recommended if the endometrial cavity was entered during myomectomy due to increased risk of uterine rupture.

Geriatric Considerations

Postmenopausal patients with newly diagnosed uterine myoma/enlarging uterine myomas have a high suspicion of uterine sarcoma/other gynecologic malignancy.

REFERENCES

1. Parker WH. Etiology, symptomatology, and diagnosis of uterine myomas. *Fertil Steril*. 2007; 87(4):725–736.
2. Stewart EA. Clinical practice. Uterine fibroids. *N Engl J Med*. 2015;372(17):1646–1655.
3. Bulun SE. Uterine fibroids. *N Engl J Med*. 2013;369(14):1344–1355.
4. Gupta JK, Sinha A, Lumsden MA, et al. Uterine artery embolization for symptomatic uterine fibroids. *Cochrane Database Syst Rev*. 2014;(12):CD005073.
5. Tristan M, Orozco LJ, Steed A, et al. Mifepristone for uterine fibroids. *Cochrane Database Syst Rev*. 2012;(8):CD007687.

CODES

ICD10

- D25.9 Leiomyoma of uterus, unspecified
- D25.2 Subserosal leiomyoma of uterus
- D25.1 Intramural leiomyoma of uterus

CLINICAL PEARLS

- Uterine myomas are benign smooth muscle tumors composed mainly of fibrous connective tissue.
- Usually incidental finding on pelvic exam or ultrasound but may cause pelvic pain and pressure, abnormal uterine bleeding, and/or infertility
- Management ranges from conservative to medical to surgical.

UVEITIS

Mikayla L. Spangler, PharmD • Laura K. Klug, PharmD • Michael Allen Greene, MD

 BASICS

DESCRIPTION
- A nonspecific term used to describe any intraocular inflammatory disorder
- The uvea is the middle layer of the eye between the sclera and retina. The anterior part of the uvea includes the iris and ciliary body. The posterior part of the uvea is the choroid.
  - Anterior uveitis: refers to ocular inflammation limited to the iris (iritis) alone or iris and ciliary body (iridocyclitis)
  - Intermediate uveitis: refers to inflammation of the structures just posterior to the lens (pars planitis or peripheral uveitis)
  - Posterior uveitis: refers to inflammation of the choroid (choroiditis), retina (retinitis), or vitreous near the optic nerve and macula
  - Panuveitis: refers to inflammation of all of the above areas of the uvea
- System(s) affected: nervous
- Synonym(s): iritis; iridocyclitis; choroiditis; retinochoroiditis; chorioretinitis; anterior uveitis; posterior uveitis; pars planitis; panuveitis. Synonyms are anatomic descriptions of the focus of the uveal inflammation.

Pediatric Considerations
- Infection should be the primary consideration.
- Allergies and psychological factors (depression, stress) may serve as a trigger.
- Trauma is also a common cause in this population.

EPIDEMIOLOGY
Predominant sex: male = female, except for human leukocyte antigen B27 (HLA-B27) anterior uveitis: male > female, autoimmune etiology: female > male

Incidence
Overall incidence is 17 to 52 cases/100,000 per year in the developed world.

Prevalence
- Overall prevalence is 38 to 714 cases/100,000 annual incidence.
- Anterior uveitis is the most common (80% of cases) with iritis being 4 times more prevalent than posterior uveitis.

ETIOLOGY AND PATHOPHYSIOLOGY
- Infectious: may result from viral, bacterial, parasitic, or fungal etiologies
- Suspected immune mediated: possible autoimmune or immune complex–mediated mechanism postulated in association with systemic (especially rheumatologic) disorders
  - Autoimmune uveitis (AIU) patients should be referred to an ophthalmologist for local treatment.
- Isolated eye disease
- Undifferentiated (~25%)

- Some medications may cause uveitis. The most causative medications include rifabutin, bisphosphonates, sulfonamides, metipranolol, brimonidine, prostaglandin analogs, immune checkpoint inhibitors, TNF-α inhibitors, protein kinase inhibitors (BRAF and MEK), anti–vascular endothelial growth factor (anti-VEGF) agents, bacillus Calmette-Guérin (BCG) vaccination, and systemic and intraocular cidofovir.
- Masquerade syndromes: diseases such as malignancies that may be mistaken for primary inflammation of the eye

Genetics
- Iritis: 50–70% are HLA-B27 positive.
- Predisposing gene for posterior uveitis associated with Behçet disease may include HLA-B51.

RISK FACTORS
No specific risk factors

COMMONLY ASSOCIATED CONDITIONS
- Viral infections: herpes simplex, herpes zoster, HIV, cytomegalovirus, congenital Zika virus
- Bacterial infections: brucellosis, leprosy, leptospirosis, Lyme disease, propionibacterium infection, syphilis, tuberculosis (TB), Whipple disease
- Parasitic infections: acanthamebiasis, cysticercosis, onchocerciasis, toxocariasis, toxoplasmosis
- Fungal infections: aspergillosis, blastomycosis, candidiasis, coccidioidomycosis, cryptococcosis, histoplasmosis, sporotrichosis
- Suspected immune mediated: ankylosing spondylitis, Behçet disease, Crohn disease, drug or hypersensitivity reaction, interstitial nephritis, juvenile rheumatoid arthritis, Kawasaki disease, multiple sclerosis, psoriatic arthritis, Reiter syndrome, relapsing polychondritis, sarcoidosis, Sjögren syndrome, systemic lupus erythematosus, ulcerative colitis, vasculitis, vitiligo, Vogt-Koyanagi (Harada) syndrome
- Isolated eye disease: acute multifocal placoid pigmentary epitheliopathy, acute retinal necrosis, birdshot choroidopathy, Fuchs heterochromic cyclitis, glaucomatocyclitic crisis, lens-induced uveitis, multifocal choroiditis, pars planitis, serpiginous choroiditis, sympathetic ophthalmia, trauma
- Masquerade syndromes: leukemia, lymphoma, retinitis pigmentosa, retinoblastoma

 DIAGNOSIS

HISTORY
- Decreased visual acuity
- Pain, photophobia, blurring of vision (1)[C]
  - Usually acute
- Anterior uveitis
  - Generally acute in onset
  - Deep eye pain
  - Photophobia (consensual)

- Intermediate and posterior uveitis
  - Unresolving floaters
  - Generally insidious in onset
  - More commonly bilateral

PHYSICAL EXAM
Slit-lamp exam and indirect ophthalmoscopy are necessary for precise diagnosis (1)[C].
- Anterior uveitis
  - Conjunctival vessel dilation
  - Perilimbal (circumcorneal) dilation of episcleral and scleral vessels (ciliary flush)
  - Small pupillary size of affected eye
  - Hypopyon or hyphema (WBCs or RBCs pooled in the anterior chamber)
  - Frequently unilateral (95% of HLA-B27–associated cases); if first occurrence and otherwise asymptomatic, no further diagnostic testing is needed (1)[C].
  - Bilateral involvement and systemic symptoms (fever, fatigue, abdominal pain) may be associated with interstitial nephritis (1)[C].
  - Systemic disease is most likely to be associated with anterior uveitis (in one study, 53% of patients were found to have systemic disease) (1)[C].
- Intermediate and posterior uveitis
  - More commonly bilateral
  - Posterior inflammation will generally cause minimal pain or redness unless associated with an iritis.

DIFFERENTIAL DIAGNOSIS
- Acute angle-closure glaucoma
- Conjunctivitis; episcleritis; keratitis; scleritis

DIAGNOSTIC TESTS & INTERPRETATION
No specific test for the diagnosis of uveitis. Tests for etiologic factors or associated conditions should be based on history and physical exam (1)[C].

Initial Tests (lab, imaging)
- CBC, BUN, creatinine (interstitial nephritis) (1)[C]
- HLA-B27 typing (ankylosing spondylitis, Reiter syndrome) (1)[C],(2)
- Antinuclear antibody, ESR (systemic lupus erythematosus, Sjögren syndrome) (1)[C],(2)
- Venereal disease research laboratory (VDRL) test, fluorescent titer antibody (syphilis) (1)[C],(2)
- Fluorescent treponemal antibody absorption (FTA-ABS) or microhemagglutination assay for antibodies to Treponema pallidum (MHA-TP) (1)[C]
- Purified protein derivative (PPD) tuberculin skin test (TB) (1)[C]
- Lyme serology (Lyme disease) (1)[C],(2)
- Chest x-ray (sarcoidosis, histoplasmosis, TB, lymphoma) (1)[C],(2)
- Sacroiliac radiograph (ankylosing spondylitis) (1)[C]

Diagnostic Procedures/Other
Slit-lamp exam (1)[C],(2)

Test Interpretation
- Keratic precipitates
- Inflammatory cells in anterior chamber or vitreous

- Synechiae (fibrous tissue scarring between iris and lens)
- Macular edema
- Perivasculitis of retinal vessels

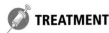 **TREATMENT**

GENERAL MEASURES
- Urgent ophthalmologic consultation
- Medical therapy is best initiated following full ophthalmologic evaluation.
- Treatment of underlying cause, if identified
- Anti-inflammatory therapy

MEDICATION

First Line
- The treatment depends on the etiology, location, and severity of the inflammation.
- Prednisolone acetate 1% ophthalmic suspension: 1 to 2 drops to the affected eye 2 to 4 times per day, during first 24 to 48 hours, dosing frequency may be increased OR dexamethasone 0.1% ophthalmic suspension: 1 to 2 drops to affected eye 4 to 6 times per day, may use hourly in severe disease. Other corticosteroid options include prednisolone sodium phosphate 1%, dexamethasone sodium phosphate 0.1%, and loteprednol etabonate 0.5% (Lotemax), difluprednate (Durezol) 0.05% (1),(2)[C].
  – Taper prior to discontinuation
  – Contraindications
    ○ Hypersensitivity to the medication or component of the preparation
    ○ Topical corticosteroid therapy is contraindicated in uveitis secondary to infectious etiologies, unless used in conjunction with appropriate anti-infectious agents.
  – Precautions
    ○ Topical corticosteroids may increase intraocular pressure, increase susceptibility to infections, impair corneal or scleral wound healing, or cause corneal epithelial toxicity or crystalline keratopathy. Prolonged use may cause cataract formation and exacerbate existing herpetic keratitis, which may masquerade as iritis.
    ○ Significant possible interactions
- Cycloplegic agents may be used to dilate the eye and relieve pain. Agents include scopolamine hydrobromide 0.25% (Isopto Hyoscine) or atropine 1% 1 to 2 drops up to QID or homatropine hydrobromide (Isopto) 2% or 5% 1 to 2 drops BID or as often as q3h if necessary (1)[C].
  – Contraindications
    ○ Cycloplegia is contraindicated in patients known to have, or be predisposed to, glaucoma.
  – Precautions
    ○ Use extreme caution in infants, young children, and elderly because of increased susceptibility to systemic effects.

Second Line
- Systemic corticosteroids are useful for maintenance therapy for patients with noninfectious posterior uveitis or for severe ocular inflammation. These should always be used with other immunosuppressive medications for steroid-sparing effects; prednisone ≤7.5 mg daily (2)[B]

- Intravitreal corticosteroid deposits may also be used for long-term maintenance; fluocinolone acetonide (Retisert [590 μg released over 30 months] and Yutiq [180 μg released over 36 months]), dexamethasone (Ozurdex) 0.7 mg released slowly >3 to 6 months (2),(3)[C]
  – Retisert has caused nearly all patients to develop cataracts and significant increases in intraocular pressure in just >75% of patients, whereas Ozurdex resulted in less occurrence of an increase in intraocular pressure and cataract development (2),(3)[C].
- Intravitreal triamcinolone acetonide injections can be given (2)[C].
- Immunosuppressive agents including antimetabolites (methotrexate, azathioprine, and mycophenolate mofetil), T-cell inhibitors (cyclosporine and tacrolimus), and alkylating agents (cyclophosphamide, chlorambucil) may be employed in cases resistant or intolerant to initial treatment, or used for their corticosteroid-sparing effect. Close monitoring is required (3),(4)[C].
- Advancing research suggests benefit of the biologic agents in refractory uveitis. Adalimumab has gained FDA approval for this indication. Some expert panels recommend adalimumab and infliximab as second-line therapy options. Other biologic agents, including golimumab, certolizumab-pegol, abatacept , and tocilizumab, have also been studied (2),(3),(4)[C].
  – Benefits of biologic therapy include glucocorticoid sparing effects, but limitations may include high cost and adverse effect potential.
- Systemic and ophthalmic preparations of NSAIDs may provide some symptom relief (1)[C].

ISSUES FOR REFERRAL
Caution when using empiric treatment; referral to an ophthalmologist is recommended in most cases.

SURGERY/OTHER PROCEDURES
Various surgical procedures may be used to manage complications associated with uveitis but do not reverse the underlying cause (4).

 ONGOING CARE

FOLLOW-UP RECOMMENDATIONS

Patient Monitoring
- Complete history and physical to evaluate for associated systemic disease
- Ophthalmologic follow-up as recommended by consultant

PATIENT EDUCATION
- Instruct on proper method for instilling eye drops.
- Wear dark glasses if photophobia is a problem.

PROGNOSIS
- Depends on the presence of causal diseases or associated conditions
- Uveitis resulting from infections (systemic or local) tends to resolve with eradication of the underlying infection.
- Uveitis associated with seronegative arthropathies tends to be acute (lasting <3 months) and frequently recurrent.

COMPLICATIONS
- Cycloplegia: paralysis of the ciliary muscle of the eye, resulting in a loss of accommodation
- Loss of vision as a result of the following:
  – Keratic precipitate deposition on the corneal or lens surfaces
  – Increased intraocular pressure, acute angle-closure glaucoma
  – Formation of synechiae
  – Cataract formation
  – Vasculitis with vascular occlusion, retinal infarction
  – Macular edema
  – Optic nerve damage

REFERENCES
1. Harthan JS, Optiz DL, Fromstein SR, et al. Diagnosis and treatment of anterior uveitis: optometric management. *Clin Optom (Auckl)*. 2016;8:23–35.
2. Burkholder BM, Jabs DA. Uveitis for the non-ophthalmologist. *BMJ*. 2021;372:m4989.
3. Pleyer U, Neri P, Deuter C. New pharmacotherapy options for noninfectious posterior uveitis. *Int Ophthalmol*. 2021;41(6):2265–2281.
4. Dick AD, Rosenbaum JT, Al-Dhibi HA, et al. Guidance on noncorticosteroid systemic immunomodulatory therapy in noninfectious uveitis: Fundamentals Of Care for UveitiS (FOCUS) initiative. *Ophthalmology*. 2018;125(5):757–773.

ADDITIONAL READING
- Abdalla Elsayed MEA, Kozak I. Pharmacologically induced uveitis. *Surv Ophthalmol*. 2021;66(5):781–801.
- Majumder PD, Biswas J. Pediatric uveitis: an update. *Oman J Ophthalmol*. 2013;6(3):140–150.

 SEE ALSO

Conjunctivitis, Acute; Glaucoma, Primary Closed-Angle; Scleritis

 CODES

ICD10
- H20.9 Unspecified iridocyclitis
- H30.90 Unspecified chorioretinal inflammation, unspecified eye
- H20.019 Primary iridocyclitis, unspecified eye

CLINICAL PEARLS
- Symptoms vary depending on depth of involvement and associated conditions but should be suspected when eye pain is associated with visual changes.
- Severe or unresponsive uveitis may require therapy, including periocular injection of corticosteroids, sustained-release corticosteroid implants, systemic corticosteroids, cytotoxic agents, immunosuppressive agents, immunomodulatory agents, or tumor necrosis factor inhibitors.

U

VAGINAL ADENOSIS

Sareena Singh, MD, FACOG • Kimberly Resnick, MD

BASICS

DESCRIPTION
- The normal vagina is lined with squamous epithelium. Adenosis is characterized by the presence of columnar epithelium or glandular tissue in the wall of the vagina.
- Around week 15 of embryologic development, the müllerian system, which forms the upper 2/3 of the vagina, fuses with the invaginating cloaca or urogenital sinus to form the lower 1/3 of the vagina. Squamous metaplasia from the cloacal region then produces squamous epithelium within the vagina (1).
- *Adenosis* occurs when this squamous epithelium fails to epithelialize the vagina completely.
- Three main types of adenosis epithelium:
  - Endocervical
  - Endometrial
  - Tubal
- System(s) affected: reproductive

Geriatric Considerations
- Adenosis is a disorder of the young female. By menopause, the vagina and cervix should be completely epithelialized.
- In a postmenopausal patient, the presence of glandular epithelium is an indication for excision and evaluation, given the risk of well-differentiated adenocarcinoma.

Pregnancy Considerations
Pregnancy produces a wide eversion of the transformation zone of the cervix. This can become so widely everted that it will extend onto the vaginal fornices, leading to the impression of adenosis. This will resolve after pregnancy.

EPIDEMIOLOGY
Incidence
- Although the cumulative incidence of vaginal adenosis is unknown, the incidence of cloacal malformations is 1/20,000 to 1/25,000 live births.
- Although spontaneous vaginal adenosis appears to be fairly common (10% of adult women), it is mostly an insignificant coincidental finding. Widespread symptomatic involvement is rare (2).

Prevalence
- In the United States, adenosis is common in young women, affecting 10–20%. As maturation progresses with puberty, epithelialization occurs.
- Predominant age
  - Age <1 month: 15%
  - Prepubertal: typically absent
  - Age 13 to 25 years: 13%
  - Age >25 years: decreasing prevalence, uncommon beyond age 30 years (2)

ETIOLOGY AND PATHOPHYSIOLOGY
- In most young females, the etiology is incomplete squamous metaplasia or epithelialization. This occurs as a natural phenomenon and resolves with age.
- Described as congenital or acquired:
  - Congenital: proliferation of the remnant müllerian epithelium in the vagina due to exposure to diethylstilbestrol (DES) in utero ("DES daughters"). DES is a synthetic, nonsteroidal estrogen used to prevent miscarriage or premature deliveries from 1938 to 1971 (3). An estimated 5 million women were prescribed DES during this period (4).
  - Transformation-related protein 63 (TRP63/p63) marks the cell fate of müllerian duct epithelium to become squamous epithelium in the cervix and vagina. DES disrupts the TRP63 expression and induces adenosis lesions (4). It has also been suggested that DES induces vaginal adenosis by inhibiting the BMP4/Activin A-regulated vaginal cell fate through a downregulation of RUNX1 (5).
  - Acquired: trauma and inflammation causing spontaneous de novo changes or changes in an acquired lesion in the vaginal epithelium
  - Additional reports documented adenosis subsequent to sulfonamide-induced Stevens–Johnson syndrome and after treatment of vaginal condylomas with 5-fluorouracil (6).

RISK FACTORS
Adenosis of the vagina/cervix may arise in up to 90% of DES daughters and has a 40-fold increased risk of developing into clear cell adenocarcinoma (3).

GENERAL PREVENTION
None: Last DES exposure was in the 1970s.

COMMONLY ASSOCIATED CONDITIONS
DES exposure
- Adenosis from DES exposure should lead to an evaluation of other DES-related abnormalities.
- Müllerian tract anomalies associated with DES exposure include cervical hood, cervical ridge, shortened cervix, incompetent cervix, and T-shaped uterine cavity.
- Patients with known DES exposure should have their reproductive tract evaluated prior to conception.
- Most patients with adenosis have not been DES-exposed and do not require evaluation of the reproductive system.
- The FDA issued a drug bulletin in 1971 advising physicians to stop prescribing DES to pregnant women because of its link to vaginal clear cell adenocarcinoma in DES daughters (3).

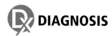

DIAGNOSIS

HISTORY
- Maternal DES exposure
- Complaints of
  - Profuse mucoid vaginal discharge from the glandular epithelium
  - Pruritus
  - Pain/soreness of the vaginal introitus
  - Postcoital bleeding
  - Dyspareunia

PHYSICAL EXAM
On pelvic exam, adenosis appearance is varied: patchy or diffuse red stippling, granularity or nodularity, single or multiple cysts, erosions, ulcers, or warty protuberances that may even extend to the vulva.

DIFFERENTIAL DIAGNOSIS
- Erosive lichen planus
- Fixed drug eruption
- Erythema multiforme
- Bullous skin disease
- Adenocarcinoma

DIAGNOSTIC TESTS & INTERPRETATION
Initial Tests (lab, imaging)
Four-quadrant Pap smear should be used liberally to isolate quadrants of the vagina that may contain abnormalities. No imaging is indicated, unless diagnosed with underlying malignancy.

Follow-Up Tests & Special Considerations

Pap smear can be followed by colposcopy and biopsy.

Diagnostic Procedures/Other

- Colposcopy should be used to outline areas of adenosis to ensure that no malignancy is present.
- A thorough evaluation for adenocarcinoma of the vagina arising in adenosis should be done.
- A biopsy may be necessary to ensure that the process represents only benign adenosis.

Test Interpretation

- Biopsy will show benign glandular epithelium.
- Biopsies may show areas of ongoing squamous metaplasia.

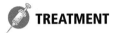 ## TREATMENT

GENERAL MEASURES

- Unless malignancy is present, treatment is conservative.
- In most young females with this condition, it will resolve with expectant management.
- Treatment is warranted in women with severe subjective symptoms that impair the quality of life.
- First-line treatment: If indicated in patients with focal lesions and no history of DES exposure, simple excision is an effective treatment (6).

ISSUES FOR REFERRAL

Malignancy found on biopsy warrants referral to gynecologic oncology specialist.

SURGERY/OTHER PROCEDURES

- Aggressive therapy, such as laser or surgical excision, is necessary if premalignant or malignant changes arise (5).
- Symptomatic treatment has been performed with carbon dioxide laser coagulation, unipolar coagulation, or vaginal resection.

ADMISSION, INPATIENT, AND NURSING CONSIDERATIONS

Outpatient management

 ## ONGOING CARE

FOLLOW-UP RECOMMENDATIONS

Patient Monitoring

If the initial colposcopy is normal, a yearly four-quadrant Pap smear of the vagina and of the cervix should be performed.

DIET

No special diet is recommended.

PATIENT EDUCATION

- No limitations
- It is not necessary to avoid intercourse or placing objects in the vagina.
- The patient should be educated to keep normal guideline-recommended pelvic and Pap smear appointments. In most situations, this is benign, and expectant management is all that is necessary.
- http://www.acog.org/

PROGNOSIS

- Most patients will have squamous metaplasia and epithelialization with complete resolution of the adenosis.
- The rare patient, 1/1,000 to 1/10,000, may develop adenocarcinoma in the adenosis and will require definitive therapy as for vaginal cancer.
  - Cumulative incidence of progression of adenosis to adenocarcinoma is 1.5/1,000 for DES daughters (3).

COMPLICATIONS

- Infertility with DES association
- Adverse pregnancy outcome with DES association
- Adenocarcinoma of vagina
- Clear cell adenocarcinoma with DES association

REFERENCES

1. Reich O, Fritsch H. The developmental origin of cervical and vaginal epithelium and their clinical consequences: a systematic review. *J Low Genit Tract Dis*. 2014;18(4):358–360.
2. Kranl C, Zelger B, Kofler H, et al. Vulval and vaginal adenosis. *Br J Dermatol*. 1998;139(1):128–131.
3. National Toxicology Program, Department of Health and Human Services. Diethylstilbestrol. In: *Report on Carcinogens*. 12th ed. Research Triangle Park, NC: National Toxicology Program, U.S. Department of Health and Human Services; 2011:159–161.
4. Laronda MM, Unno K, Butler LM, et al. The development of cervical and vaginal adenosis as a result of diethylstilbestrol exposure in utero. *Differentiation*. 2012;84(3):252–260.
5. Laronda M, Unno K, Ishi K, et al. Diethylstilbestrol induces vaginal adenosis by disrupting SMAD/RUNX1-mediated cell fate decision in the Müllerian duct epithelium. *Dev Biol*. 2013;381(1):5–16.
6. Martin AA, Atkins KA, Lonergan CL, et al. Vaginal adenosis as a dermatologic complaint. *J Am Acad Dermatol*. 2013;69(2):e92–e93.

ADDITIONAL READING

Bamigboye AA, Morris J. Oestrogen supplementation, mainly diethylstilbestrol, for preventing miscarriages and other adverse pregnancy outcomes. *Cochrane Database Syst Rev*. 2003;(3):CD004353.

 ## SEE ALSO

Vaginal Malignancy

 ## CODES

ICD10

- Q52.4 Other congenital malformations of vagina
- N89.8 Other specified noninflammatory disorders of vagina
- T38.5X5A Adverse effect of other estrogens and progestogens, initial encounter

CLINICAL PEARLS

- Adenosis is characterized by the presence of columnar epithelium or glandular tissue in the wall of the vagina.
- Adenosis is common among the daughters of women exposed to DES.
- Rarely, adenosis can be associated with an underlying vaginal malignancy.

V

VAGINAL BLEEDING DURING PREGNANCY

Virginia J. Van Duyne, MD

 BASICS

DESCRIPTION

- Vaginal bleeding during pregnancy has many causes and ranges in severity from benign with normal pregnancy outcome to life-threatening for both infant and mother.
- Etiology can be from the vagina, cervix, uterus, fetus, or placenta. The differential diagnosis is guided by the gestational age of the fetus.

EPIDEMIOLOGY

Prevalence

- In early pregnancy: 7–25% of patients
- In late pregnancy: 0.3–2% of patients

ETIOLOGY AND PATHOPHYSIOLOGY

- Many times the cause is unknown.
- Anytime in pregnancy:
  - Cervicitis (infectious or noninfectious)
  - Vaginal or cervical trauma (including postcoital)
  - Cervical lesion or neoplasia
  - Hyperemia of cervix (increased blood flow from pregnancy)
- Early pregnancy:
  - For up to 50% of early pregnancy bleeding, no cause is ever found.
  - Ectopic pregnancy: leading cause of 1st-trimester maternal death in the United States. Risk factors: previous ectopic, trauma to fallopian tubes (tubal surgery, infection, tumor), congenital anomaly of tubes, in utero diethylstilbestrol (DES) exposure, current use of IUD, history of infertility, tobacco use
  - Spontaneous abortion: risk factors: advanced maternal age (AMA), alcohol use, tobacco use, anesthetic gas, heavy caffeine use, cocaine use, chronic maternal diseases (poorly controlled diabetes mellitus [DM], celiac disease, autoimmune diseases such as antiphospholipid syndrome), short interconception time (3 to 6 months), current use of IUD, maternal infection (e.g., herpes simplex virus [HSV], gonorrhea, chlamydia, toxoplasmosis, listeriosis, HIV, syphilis, malaria), medications (e.g., retinoids, methotrexate, NSAIDs), multiple previous therapeutic abortions, previous spontaneous abortion, toxins (arsenic, lead, polyurethane), uterine abnormalities (congenital, adhesions, fibroids)
  - Implantation bleeding: benign, about 6 days after fertilization
  - Uterine fibroids
  - Subchorionic bleeding: in late 1st trimester
  - Low-lying placenta
  - Gestational trophoblastic disease: hydatidiform mole (most common), choriocarcinoma, or placental-site trophoblastic tumors
- Late pregnancy:
  - Bloody show of labor (mucus plug)
  - Placenta previa: painless bleeding; occurs in 0.4% deliveries in the United States. Risk factors: previous history of placenta previa, previous uterine surgery (cesarean section, D&C), chronic hypertension, multiparity, multiple gestation, tobacco use, AMA

- Placental abruption: (typically) painful bleeding; occurs in 1–2% deliveries in the United States. Risk factors: previous placental abruption, 1st-trimester bleeding, hypertension, preeclampsia, multiple gestation, tobacco, cocaine or methamphetamine use, unexplained elevated maternal α-fetoprotein, poly- or oligohydramnios, AMA, trauma to abdomen, premature rupture of membranes, thrombophilia, short umbilical cord, male fetus, chorioamnionitis, nutritional deficiency
- Vasa previa: minimal bleeding with fetal distress; rare (1:2,500 deliveries). Risk factors: in vitro fertilization, multiple gestations, placental abnormalities (low-lying position, bilobate, succenturiate lobe, velamentous insertion of umbilical cord)
- Placenta accreta, increta, percreta: risk factors: uterine scar (e.g., from cesarean section, endometrial ablation, or D&C), current placenta previa, AMA, tobacco use, multiparity, uterine anomalies, uterine fibroids, hypertension
- Uterine rupture: vaginal bleeding, abnormal fetal heart rate, and disordered or hypertonic uterine contractions with or without pain. Risk factors: previous cesarean section (most common), trauma, use of oxytocin or prostaglandins, multiparity, external cephalic version, placental abruption, shoulder dystocia, placenta percreta, müllerian duct anomalies, history of pelvic radiation

RISK FACTORS

See specific etiologies in earlier discussion.

GENERAL PREVENTION

- Address modifiable risk factors such as domestic violence and tobacco and drug use.
- If placenta or vasa previa, nothing per vagina

 DIAGNOSIS

HISTORY

- Anytime in pregnancy: quality of pregnancy dating, context (e.g., following bowel movement, during voiding, after intercourse, drug use, or trauma including domestic violence), amount of bleeding, obstetrical history, personal or family history of inherited bleeding disorders
- Early pregnancy: severe nausea/vomiting (can be associated with molar pregnancy); amount of bleeding, pelvic pain, or suprapubic cramping (e.g., spontaneous abortion, ectopic) complications in previous pregnancies (e.g., spontaneous abortion, abruption, 1st-trimester vaginal bleeding)
- Late pregnancy: contractions (labor), abdominal pain especially between contractions (abruption, uterine rupture), presence or absence of fetal movement, rupture of membranes
- See "Etiology and Pathophysiology" for additional pertinent history.

PHYSICAL EXAM

- Vital signs: When present, signs of hemodynamic instability are first tachycardia and tachypnea and then hypotension and thready pulse.

- Abdomen: uterine tenderness, fundal height (increasing fundal height may be associated with placental abruption)
- Speculum: Visualize cervix and identify source of bleeding (from cervical os or from within vagina).
- Cervix: Assess for dilation; required to assess for labor but should not be performed until placenta previa ruled out via ultrasound
- Fetal monitoring: Doppler heart tones in early pregnancy; external fetal monitoring for gestational age >26 weeks

DIFFERENTIAL DIAGNOSIS

- Hematuria (UTI, kidney stones)
- Rectal bleeding

DIAGNOSTIC TESTS & INTERPRETATION

Initial Tests (lab, imaging)

- CBC
- Blood type and screen; if significant hemorrhage, type and cross-match
- Quantitative β-human chorionic gonadotropin (β-hCG):
  - Prior to 12 weeks, levels can be followed serially every 2 days with following trends:
    - Doubles or at least 66% rise in 48 hours in normal pregnancy
    - Falls in spontaneous abortion
    - Extremely high in molar pregnancy
    - Rises gradually (<50% in 48 hours) or plateaus in ectopic pregnancy
- Transvaginal ultrasound should be used to confirm an intrauterine pregnancy (IUP) when the quantitative β-hCG >2,000 (1)[A].
- Other lab tests based on clinical scenario:
  - Wet mount, gonorrhea/chlamydia, Pap smear
  - Progesterone level occasionally used to determine viability in threatened abortion (<5 indicates not viable, >25 indicates viability, 5 to 25 is equivocal)
  - Bleeding time, fibrinogen, and fibrin split products: if suspect coagulopathy or abruption
  - Kleihauer-Betke: low sensitivity and specificity for abruption; helpful for dosing RhoGAM
- Ultrasound is the preferred imaging modality.
  - Early pregnancy:
    - Gestational sac seen at 5 to 6 weeks; fetal heartbeat observed by 8 to 9 weeks
    - Diagnostic of ectopic with nearly 100% sensitivity when β-hCG level 1,500 to 2,000 mIU/mL. If no IUP is present and ultrasound does not confirm ectopic pregnancy, serial quantitative β-hCG values should be followed (2)[C].
  - Late pregnancy:
    - Proceed to rule out placenta previa with ultrasound, labor with serial cervical exams, and abruption with external fetal monitoring.

ALERT

Confirm fetal presentation and placental position prior to cervical exam.

TREATMENT

MEDICATION

First Line

- Treat underlying cause of bleeding, if identified.
- If mother is Rh-negative, give RhoGAM to prevent autoimmunization. In late pregnancy, dose according to the amount of estimated fetomaternal hemorrhage.
- If cause of bleeding is preterm labor, consider betamethasone for fetal lung maturity if <36 weeks' gestation. Tocolytics may be used to prolong pregnancy to allow for course of steroids.
- If threatened abortion: Consider progesterone (relative risk 0.53) (3)[A].
- If mother has an inherited bleeding disorder or if bleeding is severe, consider recombinant or donor blood products.

SURGERY/OTHER PROCEDURES

- Cesarean section may be indicated for recurrent or uncontrolled bleeding with placenta or vasa previa.
- If ectopic is diagnosed, immediate surgical treatment may be needed. Some early ectopic pregnancies can be treated medically if certain criteria are met (2)[C].
- Surgical uterine evacuation is necessary for molar pregnancy due to malignant potential (4)[C].
- Incomplete or inevitable spontaneous abortion: Management is patient centered. In the absence of infection, patient may elect expectant, medical, or surgical management. If expectant management, typically wait 2 weeks for patient to complete abortion; most complete by 9 days. If at 2 weeks abortion is not completed or medical management has failed, surgical intervention (D&C or aspiration) is generally indicated (5)[A]; may send tissue to pathology to confirm

ADMISSION, INPATIENT, AND NURSING CONSIDERATIONS

- In early pregnancy: based on quantity of bleeding, need for surgical treatment for ectopic pregnancy, or presence of infection in case of spontaneous abortion
- In late pregnancy, if significant bleeding and/or presence of maternal or fetal compromise
- In late pregnancy with trauma, if ≥2 contractions per 10 minutes
- In late pregnancy, may discharge when bleeding has stopped; labor, previa, and abruption have been ruled out; and fetal heart tracing is normal.
- After trauma in late pregnancy, may discharge home if normal fetal heart tracing for ≥4 hours with <2 contractions per 10 minutes

 ONGOING CARE

FOLLOW-UP RECOMMENDATIONS

Patient Monitoring

- Patient should be instructed to report any increase in the amount or frequency of bleeding and to seek immediate care if experiencing fever, abdominal pain, or sudden increased bleeding. Patient should save any tissue passed vaginally for examination.
- Frequency of outpatient follow-up as indicated based on etiology of bleeding

PATIENT EDUCATION

- American Academy of Family Physicians (AAFP): http://www.familydoctor.org
- American College of Obstetricians and Gynecologists (ACOG): https://www.acog.org/

PROGNOSIS

- Prognosis depends on the etiology of vaginal bleeding, severity of bleeding, and rapidity of diagnosis.
- Maternal mortality is 31.9 deaths per 100,000 ectopic pregnancies.
- 1/2 of patients with early pregnancy bleeding miscarry; if fetal heart activity (ultrasound) present in 1st-trimester bleeding, <10% chance of pregnancy loss
- Heavy bleeding in early pregnancy, particularly when accompanied by pain, is associated with higher risk of spontaneous abortion. Spotting and light episodes are not, especially if lasting only 1 to 2 days.
- Subchorionic hemorrhage has about 2- to 3-fold increased risk of spontaneous abortion. Smaller hemorrhage and presence of viable fetal heart rate confer lower risk of loss; most resolve spontaneously.
- Women with early pregnancy bleeding have an increased risk of preterm delivery, premature rupture of membranes, manual removal of placenta, placental abruption, elective cesarean delivery, and term labor induction later in the same pregnancy. These women also have an increased risk of adverse pregnancy outcomes, including hyperbilirubinemia, congenital anomalies, NICU admission, and reduced neonatal birth weight. Finally, there is an increased risk in subsequent pregnancies of recurrence of early pregnancy bleeding.
- Bed rest has not been shown to affect the outcome of bleeding in early pregnancy but may be indicated for bleeding in late pregnancy with placenta or vasa previa or with maternal hypertension.

REFERENCES

1. Crochet JR, Bastian LA, Chireau MV. Does this woman have an ectopic pregnancy? The rational clinical examination systematic review. *JAMA*. 2013;309(16):1722–1729.
2. Deutchman M, Tubay AT, Turok D. First trimester bleeding. *Am Fam Physician*. 2009;79(11):985–994.
3. Wahabi HA, Fayed AA, Esmaeil SA, et al. Progestogen for treating threatened miscarriage. *Cochrane Database Syst Rev*. 2011;(12):CD005943.
4. Snell BJ. Assessment and management of bleeding in the first trimester of pregnancy. *J Midwifery Womens Health*. 2009;54(6):483–491.
5. Nanda K, Lopez LM, Grimes DA, et al. Expectant care versus surgical treatment for miscarriage. *Cochrane Database Syst Rev*. 2012;(3):CD003518.

ADDITIONAL READING

- ACOG Practice Bulletin No. 193: tubal ectopic pregnancy. *Obstet Gynecol*. 2018;131(3):e91–e103.
- Al-Ma'ani WI, Solomayer EF, Hammadeh M. Expectant versus surgical management of first-trimester miscarriage: a randomised controlled study. *Arch Gynecol Obstet*. 2014;289(5):1011–1015.
- Belfort MA; and Publications Committee, Society for Maternal-Fetal Medicine. Placenta accreta. *Am J Obstet Gynecol*. 2010;203(5):430–439.
- Bhandari S, Raja EA, Shetty A, et al. Maternal and perinatal consequences of antepartum haemorrhage of unknown origin. *BJOG*. 2014;121(1):44–52.
- Boisramé T, Sananès N, Fritz G, et al. Placental abruption: risk factors, management and maternal-fetal prognosis. Cohort study over 10 years. *Eur J Obstet Gynecol Reprod Biol*. 2014;179:100–104.
- Chi C, Kadir RA. Inherited bleeding disorders in pregnancy. *Best Pract Res Clin Obstet Gynaecol*. 2012;26(1):103–117.
- Dadkhah F, Kashanian M, Eliasi G. A comparison between the pregnancy outcome in women both with or without threatened abortion. *Early Hum Dev*. 2010;86(3):193–196.
- Lykke JA, Dideriksen KL, Lidegaard O, et al. First-trimester vaginal bleeding and complications later in pregnancy. *Obstet Gynecol*. 2010;115(5):935–944.
- Prine LW, MacNaughton H. Office management of early pregnancy loss. *Am Fam Physician*. 2011;84(1):75–82.

 SEE ALSO

Abnormal Pap and Cervical Dysplasia; Abruptio Placentae; Cervical Malignancy; Cervical Polyps; Cervicitis, Ectropion, and True Erosion; Chlamydia Infection (Sexually Transmitted); Ectopic Pregnancy; Miscarriage (Early Pregnancy Loss); Placenta Previa; Preterm Labor; Trichomoniasis; Vaginal Malignancy

 CODES

ICD10

- O20.9 Hemorrhage in early pregnancy, unspecified
- O46.90 Antepartum hemorrhage, unspecified, unspecified trimester
- O20.0 Threatened abortion

CLINICAL PEARLS

- Obtain blood type and screen all women presenting with vaginal bleeding in pregnancy and administer RhoGAM to all Rh-negative patients.
- For up to 50% of early pregnancy bleeding, no cause is ever found.
- Always consider ectopic pregnancy in 1st-trimester bleeding.
- Do not perform digital exam in late pregnancy bleeding until placenta has been located on ultrasound.

V

VAGINAL MALIGNANCY

Michael P. Hopkins, MD, MEd

 BASICS

DESCRIPTION
- Carcinomas of the vagina are uncommon: 2–3% of gynecologic malignancies, 2,300 new cases annually.
- Vaginal intraepithelial neoplasia (VAIN), defined by squamous cell atypia, is classified by the depth of epithelial involvement:
  - VAIN 1: 1/3 thickness
  - VAIN 2: 2/3 thickness
  - VAIN 3 and carcinoma in situ (CIS): >2/3
  - CIS, designating full-thickness neoplastic changes without invasion through the basement membrane
- Invasive malignancies: Vaginal malignancies include squamous cell carcinoma (85–90%), adenocarcinoma (5–10%), sarcoma (2–3%), and melanoma (2–3%). Clear cell carcinoma is a subtype of adenocarcinoma. Invasive squamous cell carcinoma has the potential for metastasis to the lungs and liver.
- To be classified as a vaginal malignancy, only the vagina can be involved. If the cervix or vulva is involved, then the tumor is classified as a primary cancer arising from the cervix or the vulva.
- Most vaginal malignancies are metastatic (e.g., cervix, vulva, endometrium, breast, ovary).
- Most common sites of metastases: lung, liver, bone

Pregnancy Considerations
This malignancy is not associated with pregnancy.

EPIDEMIOLOGY
Incidence
Predominant age
- CIS: mid-40 to 60 years
- Invasive squamous cell malignancy: mid-60 to 70 years
- Adenocarcinoma: any age; 50 years is the mean age. Peak incidence is between 17 and 21 years of age.
- Clear cell adenocarcinoma occurs most often in females <30 years with a history of exposure to diethylstilbestrol (DES) in utero.
- Mixed müllerian sarcomas and leiomyosarcomas in the adult population: mean age 60 years

Pediatric Considerations
Vaginal tumors are extremely rare. Rhabdomyosarcoma (botryoid and embryonal subtype) is the most common malignant neoplasm of the vagina. Less common entities are germ cell tumor and clear cell adenocarcinoma.

Prevalence
In the United States, it is one of the rarest of all gynecologic malignancies (3%).

ETIOLOGY AND PATHOPHYSIOLOGY
- Women with a history of cervical malignancy have a higher probability of developing squamous cell malignancy in the vagina even after hysterectomy.
- Human papillomavirus (HPV) is found in 80–93% of patients with vaginal CIS and 50–65% of the patients with invasive vaginal carcinoma.

- HPV-16 is the most common, found in 66% of CIS and 55% of invasive vaginal cancers.
- Smokers have a higher incidence.
- Clear cell adenocarcinoma of the vagina in young women has been associated with DES exposure. The incidence, however, is exceedingly rare, estimated at 1/1,000 to 1/10,000 exposed females.
- Metastatic lesions can involve the vagina, spreading from the other gynecologic organs.
- Although rare, renal cell carcinoma, lung adeno-carcinoma, GI cancer, pancreatic adenocarcinoma, ovarian germ cell cancer, trophoblastic neoplasm, and breast cancer can all metastasize to the vagina.

Genetics
No known genetic pattern

RISK FACTORS
- Similar risk factors as cervical cancer
- Age
- African American
- Smoking
- Multiple sex partners, early age of first sexual intercourse
- History of squamous cell cancer of the cervix or vulva
- HPV infection
- Vaginal adenosis
- Vaginal irritation
- DES exposure in utero
- Immunocompromised, HIV
- Prior pelvic radiation

COMMONLY ASSOCIATED CONDITIONS
Due to the field effect, patients with vaginal cancer are more likely to develop malignancy in the cervix or vulva and should be followed closely.

 DIAGNOSIS

HISTORY
- Abnormal bleeding is the most common symptom.
- Postcoital bleeding can result from direct trauma to the tumor.
- Vaginal discharge
- Dyspareunia
- Urinary symptoms, including hematuria and increased frequency
- Constipation
- Pain along with symptoms and signs of hydroureter are late findings when the tumor has spread into the paravaginal tissues and extends to the pelvic sidewall (1)[A].

Pediatric Considerations
In children, sarcomas can present either as a mass protruding from the vagina or as abnormal genital bleeding (1)[A].

PHYSICAL EXAM
Pelvic examination
- The vagina, uterus, adnexa (fallopian tubes and ovaries), bladder, and rectum should be evaluated for unusual changes.
- Vaginal malignancies are found most commonly on the posterior wall in the upper 1/3 of the vagina.

DIFFERENTIAL DIAGNOSIS
- Premalignant changes: VAIN 1, 2, 3, and CIS
- Adequate biopsies ensure that invasive lesions are not overlooked. Invasive lesions penetrate the basement membrane and cannot be treated conservatively.
- Other malignancies, such as endometrial, cervix, bladder, or colon cancer, can invade directly into the vagina or metastasize to the vagina.
- In the childbearing years, trophoblastic disease should be considered.
  - The vagina is a common site of metastases; however, biopsy should typically be avoided because the implants are very vascular and may hemorrhage if sampled.
  - The clinical presentation is typically obvious so histopathologic confirmation before treatment is not required.

DIAGNOSTIC TESTS & INTERPRETATION
Initial Tests (lab, imaging)
- Pap smear may incidentally detect asymptomatic lesions.
- Biopsy suspicious lesions
- Chest x-ray (CXR): to evaluate for metastatic disease
- CT scan and MRI: to evaluate the liver and retro-peritoneum, especially the lymph nodes in the pelvic and periaortic area
- PET scan detects primary and secondary metastatic lesions more often than CT scan.

ALERT
PET scan correlation with CT scan lesions strongly suggests malignancy.

Follow-Up Tests & Special Considerations
- Lymphoscintigraphy (sentinel lymph node mapping) as part of the pretreatment evaluation can result in a change in the radiation fields and improve comprehensive treatment planning in women with vaginal cancer.
- HPV vaccination: Implementation of prophylac-tic HPV vaccination could prevent ~2/3 of the intraepithelial lesions in the lower genital tract but is yet proven.

Diagnostic Procedures/Other
- Colposcopy with directed biopsies for small lesions
- Wide excision under anesthesia of superficial disease may be necessary to ensure that invasive cancer is not present.
- Cystoscopy to rule out bladder invasion
- Proctosigmoidoscopy to rule out rectal invasion

Test Interpretation
Tumors are staged clinically:
- Stage 0: VAIN and CIS
- Stage I: carcinoma limited to the vaginal wall (26%)
- Stage II: involves the subvaginal tissues but has not extended to the pelvic wall (37%)
- Stage III: extends to the pelvic wall (24%)
- Stage IV: extends beyond the true pelvis (13%)
  - IVa: Tumor invades bladder and/or rectal mucosa and/or direct extension beyond the true pelvis
  - IVb: spread to distant organs

TREATMENT

GENERAL MEASURES
Treatment methods for VAIN and CIS include the following:
- Wide local excision
- Partial or total vaginectomy
- Intravaginal chemotherapy with 5% fluorouracil cream
- Laser therapy
- Intracavitary radiation therapy

MEDICATION
- Imiquimod
  - In a review of the effectiveness of 5% imiquimod cream in the treatment of VAIN, the following results were reported (2)[C]:
    o 26–100% of patients had complete regression.
    o 0–60% of patients had partial regression.
    o 0–37% experienced recurrence.
- Contraindications
  - The diagnosis must be established with certainty prior to treatment.
  - If there is any doubt that a process beyond in situ disease exists, vaginectomy must be performed. These patients are often elderly, and aggressive therapy is limited by the patient's performance status and ability to tolerate radical surgery, chemotherapy, or radiation.

ISSUES FOR REFERRAL
Patients should be treated by a gynecologic oncologist and/or a radiation oncologist.

ADDITIONAL THERAPIES
- Treatment with radiotherapy depends on the stage of disease. This treatment option should be discussed with physicians experienced with this malignancy.
- It is common to use radiotherapy and chemotherapy (chemoradiation) for better cancer control.
- Early-stage primary squamous cell carcinoma treated with radiation alone has shown good results.
- Stage III vaginal cancer may benefit from combined radiation and hyperthermia (1)[C].
- Patients with advanced squamous cell carcinoma or adenocarcinoma receive concurrent irradiation and cisplatin-based chemotherapy.
- Neoadjuvant chemotherapy followed by radical surgery may benefit selected patients (3)[C].
- In most tumor types, metastatic disease from the vagina to other sites is only minimally responsive to chemotherapy.
- With one exception, no chemotherapeutic agents have shown a survival advantage. The exception is childhood sarcomas, which have been treated with combinations of the following:
  - Vincristine
  - Dactinomycin (actinomycin-D)
  - Cyclophosphamide (Cytoxan)
  - Cisplatin
  - Etoposide (VP-16)

SURGERY/OTHER PROCEDURES
- Whenever there is a doubt as to the presence or absence of invasive disease, vaginectomy must be performed.
- Invasive lesions usually are treated by radiation therapy, but stage I lesions can be treated with radical hysterectomy or radical vaginectomy with pelvic lymph node dissection (2)[A].
- If the lesion involves the lower vagina, inguinal node dissection also must be done because cancer involving the lower vagina can metastasize to the groin region (inguinal–femoral nodes).
- Premenopausal women who desire to retain ovarian function are better candidates for radical surgery for early-stage disease, with vaginal reconstruction possible afterward.
- Patients who have not completed their family can occasionally be treated with limited resection and localized radiation to the area (4)[A].
- Sarcomas are treated by radiation therapy followed by pelvic exenteration if persistent disease is present.

Pediatric Considerations
The treatment of vaginal tumors today mainly consists of neoadjuvant chemotherapy followed by local control with surgery or radiotherapy (1)[A].

Geriatric Considerations
Older patients, many with a long history of smoking, are at a higher risk for malignancies requiring surgical treatments.

ONGOING CARE

FOLLOW-UP RECOMMENDATIONS
- Patients are usually ambulatory and able to resume full activity by 6 weeks after surgery.
- Most patients are fully active while receiving chemotherapy and radiation therapy.

Patient Monitoring
- Pelvic examination and Pap smear every 3 months for 2 years, then every 6 months for the next 3 years, and then yearly thereafter
- Annual CXR

PATIENT EDUCATION
- Printed patient information available from American College of Obstetricians and Gynecologists, 409 12th St., SW, Washington, DC 20024-2188; 800-762-ACOG: http://www.acog.org
- American Cancer Society: http://www.cancer.gov
- Medline Plus: http://www.nlm.nih.gov/medlineplus/vaginalcancer.html

PROGNOSIS
Stage and 5-year survival (5)
- I: 77.6%
- II: 52.2%
- III: 42.5%
- IVA: 20.5%
- IVB: 12.9%
- Stage is the most important determinant of survival (4).
- Tumor size >2 cm, correlated with worse survival outcome

COMPLICATIONS
- Those typically associated with major abdominal surgery or radiation therapy
- Common complications of treatment include rectovaginal or vesicovaginal fistulas, rectal/vaginal strictures, radiation cystitis, and/or proctitis.
- Most recurrences occur within the first 2 years after initial diagnosis.

REFERENCES

1. Fernandez-Pineda I, Spunt SL, Parida L, et al. Vaginal tumors in childhood: the experience of St. Jude Children's Research Hospital. *J Pediatr Surg.* 2011;46(11):2071–2075.
2. Guerri S, Perrone AM, Buwenge M, et al. Definitive radiotherapy in invasive vaginal carcinoma: a systematic review [published online ahead of print August 23, 2018]. *Oncologist.* doi:10.1634/theoncologist.2017-0546.
3. Hacker NF, Eifel PJ, van der Velden J. Cancer of the vagina. *Int J Gynaecol Obstet.* 2015;131(Suppl 2): S84–S87.
4. Gadducci A, Fabrini MG, Lanfredini N, et al. Squamous cell carcinoma of the vagina: natural history, treatment modalities and prognostic factors. *Crit Rev Oncol Hematol.* 2015;93(3): 211–224.
5. Adams TS, Cuello MA. Cancer of the vagina. *Int J Gynaecol Obstet.* 2018;143(Suppl 2):14–21.

ADDITIONAL READING

- Gray HJ. Advances in vulvar and vaginal cancer treatment. *Gynecol Oncol.* 2010;118(1):3–5.
- Iavazzo C, Pitsouni E, Athanasiou S, et al. Imiquimod for treatment of vulvar and vaginal intraepithelial neoplasia. *Int J Gynaecol Obstet.* 2008;101(1):3–10.
- Wolfson AH, Reis IM, Portelance L, et al. Prognostic impact of clinical tumor size on overall survival for subclassifying stages I and II vaginal cancer: a SEER analysis. *Gynecol Oncol.* 2016;141(2):255–259.

 CODES

ICD10
- C52 Malignant neoplasm of vagina
- D07.2 Carcinoma in situ of vagina
- N89.3 Dysplasia of vagina, unspecified

CLINICAL PEARLS
- Vaginal cancer is rare; 85–90% of vaginal cancers are squamous cell.
- Vaginal malignancies are found most commonly on the posterior wall in the upper 1/3 of the vagina.
- Most vaginal malignancies are metastatic (from cervix, vulva, endometrium, breast, or ovary).

V

VAGINITIS AND VAGINOSIS

Brett Johnson, MD • Katherine E. Bouchard, DO

BASICS

DESCRIPTION
- "Vaginosis" and "vaginitis" are broad terms indicating any disease process of the vagina caused by or leading to infection, inflammation, or changes in the normal vaginal flora. The difference between vaginitis and vaginosis is the presence (vaginitis) or absence (vaginosis) of inflammation.
- Common symptoms of vaginitis/vaginosis are vaginal discharge, odor, itching, burning, or pain.
- The most common causes of vaginitis/vaginosis are bacterial vaginosis (BV), vulvovaginal candidiasis (VVC), and trichomoniasis. Noninfectious causes (<10%) can include atrophic, irritant, allergic and inflammatory vaginitis.
- Diagnosis of vaginitis relies on a thorough history, physical exam, and clinical assessment. Microscopy, cultures, and DNA probes can be helpful in confirming the diagnosis.
- Normal physiologic vaginal discharge is clear to white, not malodorous, not associated with pain or pruritus, and the quantity varies during the menstrual cycle.

EPIDEMIOLOGY
- Vaginal symptoms are typical and common in the general population and are one of the most frequent reasons women present to their medical care providers accounting for approximately 10 million office visits each year (1).
- BV is the most common cause of vaginal discharge in reproductive-aged women (2).
- VVC is the second most common cause of vaginitis in reproductive-aged women (2).

Incidence
An estimated 7.4 million cases of BV occur yearly in the United States (1).

Prevalence
- Prevalence rates of BV are in the range of 15% in pregnant women, 20–25% young females at student health clinics, and up to 30–40% among women seen at sexually transmitted disease (STD) clinics (1).
- The prevalence of BV in the United States is estimated to be 21.2 million among women ages 14 to 49 based on a nationally representative sample of women who participated in NHANES 2001 to 2004.
- Nonwhite women have higher rates of BV (African-American 51%, Mexican Americans 32%) than white women (23%).
- 29–40% of all females report at least one episode of VVC.
- VVC is uncommon in prepubescent girls and post-menopausal women and is often overdiagnosed in these populations.
- Recurrent VVC (four or more documented episodes in 1 year) occurs in <5% of the population.
- Vaginal trichomoniasis is a common STD with 3 to 5 million cases diagnosed in the United States yearly (2).
- African-American women are 10 times more commonly affected by vaginal trichomoniasis when compared to white and Hispanic women (2).
- Desquamative inflammatory vaginitis (DIV) is found in 2–20% of pregnant and nonpregnant women (1).

ETIOLOGY AND PATHOPHYSIOLOGY
- BV is caused by a change in the normal vaginal flora, it is neither a true infectious nor inflammatory state (2). Dominant lactobacilli responsible for maintaining the acidic vaginal pH are overcome with an overgrowth of facultative anaerobic organisms and lack of hydrogen peroxide producing lactobacilli (2).
  - Change in the vaginal environment leads to an increase in the pH, causing a malodorous, clear, white, or gray discharge and a fishy odor.
  - The organisms generally implicated in BV infections: *Gardnerella vaginalis*, *Prevotella* species, *Porphyromonas* species, *Bacteroides* species, *Peptostreptococcus* species, *Mycoplasma hominis*, *Ureaplasma urealyticum*, *Mobiluncus* species, *Fusobacterium* species, *Atopobium vaginae*
  - Not directly caused by the sexual transmission of a single pathogen
- VVC is caused by *Candida* species, particularly *Candida albicans* (80–92%) and *Candida glabrata* (<10%).
  - *Candida* organisms can be identified in the lower genital tract in healthy women, and it is thought to gain access via rectal and perianal colonization and migration.
  - *C. albicans* can be found in normal flora as a commensal agent in 10–25% of asymptomatic women.
  - Symptoms occur when candidal organisms overwhelm the normal vaginal flora and invade the superficial vaginal epithelial cells, causing inflammation, pruritus, and thick vaginal discharge.
  - Complicated VVC should be considered in pregnant patients, patients with diabetes, or immuno-compromising conditions. Patients who experience four or more episodes of VVC in a year or who have only budding yeast on wet mount may also be considered to have complicated VVC.
- Trichomoniasis caused by an infection via *Trichomonas vaginalis*, a flagellate protozoan. The organism infects the squamous epithelium of the vagina as well as the urethra and paraurethral glands. This infection is primarily transmitted during sexual intercourse.
- DIV—a chronic, purulent vaginitis occurring most commonly in the perimenopause with an uncertain etiology or pathogenesis. Inflammation is cardinal feature. The vagina is colonized with facultative bacteria, not the obligate anaerobic bacteria that colonize the vagina in BV (1). The microflora in DIV consist of *Escherichia coli*, *Staphylococcus aureus*, group B streptococcus, and *Enterococcus faecalis*.
- Atrophic vaginitis—genitourinary symptoms resulting from a lack of estrogen
- Irritant/allergic vaginitis—vaginal symptoms can result from mechanical, chemical, or allergic irritation.

Genetics
No genetic component known at this time

RISK FACTORS
- BV
  - Sexual activity; although BV is not considered an STD, studies show increased rates of BV in women with multiple sexual partners.
  - Women who have sex with women, smoking, vaginal douching, low socioeconomic status, the presence of STDs such as HSV-2, use of an IUD
  - Male circumcision decreases risk.
- VVC—diabetes, recent use of antibiotics, immunosuppression, higher estrogen levels, estrogen-containing contraceptives

- Trichomoniasis
  - Inconsistent use of barrier contraception, multiple sexual partners, limited education and low socio-economic status, illicit drug use, smoking, another coexistent STI, douching, incarceration (2)
- Other risk factors associated with vaginitis/vaginosis:
  - Decreased estrogen; smoking; use of vaginal douches, creams, gels, or lubricants; tight-fitting clothing; poor hygienic practice; changes in diet; condoms, sex toys, tampons

GENERAL PREVENTION
- Vulvar hygiene with warm water and unscented cleanser; advise patients not to douche. Wear cotton underwear.
- Except in cases of trichomoniasis, treatment of sexual partners generally is not recommended but may be considered in recurrent cases.

COMMONLY ASSOCIATED CONDITIONS
- STDs such as gonorrhea, chlamydia, HSV, or HIV
- Vaginal intraepithelial neoplasia and cancer can present with symptoms of vaginitis.

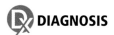DIAGNOSIS

HISTORY
- General principles:
  - The key to diagnosis is clarification of the presenting symptoms.
  - It is important to distinguish vulvar versus vaginal symptoms.
  - Onset, timing, severity, duration, and character of the vaginal symptoms are important questions to ask.
  - Symptomatic patients generally complain of itching, burning, irritation, dyspareunia, and abnormal discharge.
  - Other important topics to discuss include age, menstrual status and relation to cycle, discharge characteristics (color, consistency, amount, odor), recurrence of symptoms, sexual history (including risk factors for STDs, number of partners, gender identification, specific sexual practices), vulvovaginal hygiene practices (shaving, douching), self-treatment (OTC medications), and other underlying medical conditions (DM, HIV, IBD) (2).
- BV—thin homogenous discharge with characteristic "fishy" odor. Discharge may worsen after intercourse or menses. Pain and pruritus are uncommon.
- VVC
  - Symptomatic women report itching, burning, irritation, dyspareunia, dysuria, and a white thick discharge. Odor is uncommon.
- Trichomoniasis
  - A majority of patients will have minimal or no genitourinary symptoms (70–85%).
  - Symptomatic patients will complain of abnormal discharge, itching, burning, or postcoital bleeding (2).
- DIV
  - Purulent vaginal discharge with burning, dyspareunia, and/or introital pain. Homogenous and yellowish discharge with no fishy smell (1). Symptoms may last for long period of time and fluctuate (1).

PHYSICAL EXAM

- Because many patients with vaginitis have vulvar manifestations, the physical exam should begin with a thorough evaluation of the vulva and the skin surrounding the anus (2).
- BV—thin, watery discharge that can range from clear to gray or tan colored. An amine or "fishy" smell may be present on exam. The vaginal epithelium should appear normal and noninflamed; does not affect vulva
- VVC—erythema and swelling of the vulva and vaginal mucosa. Severely affected patients may have vulvar excoriations and fissures. Although described as typically cottage cheese–like, the discharge can vary from watery to homogenously thick; lack of odor
- Trichomoniasis—yellow or green frothy discharge with foul odor. Discharge can also appear purulent in some patients. Vulvar or vaginal erythema can be visualized. Rarely, punctate hemorrhages can be seen on the cervix ("strawberry cervix").
- DIV—purulent discharge and vaginal inflammation. Submucosal cervico-vaginal petechiae; no fishy smell

DIFFERENTIAL DIAGNOSIS

Physiologic discharge; leukorrhea of pregnancy; STDs; foreign body (retained tampon or condom); contact dermatitis; cervicitis; urinary tract infection (UTI); atrophic vaginitis; dermatoses: lichen sclerosus, lichen planus, seborrheic dermatitis, psoriasis; genitourinary syndrome of menopause (2)

DIAGNOSTIC TESTS & INTERPRETATION

Initial Tests (lab, imaging)

- BV
  - Symptomatic patients complain of an abnormal vaginal discharge and a fishy odor.
  - Clinical diagnosis is established with Amsel criteria. A positive diagnosis can be made if 3 out of 4 of the following criteria are present.
    - Thin, homogenous discharge that smoothly coats vaginal wall
    - Vaginal pH >4.5
    - A positive amine or "Whiff" test with use of KOH solution added to discharge
    - >20% of the epithelial cells identified as "clue cells" most reliable indicator of BV
- VVC
  - Visualization of blastospores or pseudohyphae on saline or 10% KOH microscopy
  - A positive culture in a symptomatic patient (2)
- Trichomoniasis
  - Visualization of motile trichomonads on saline microscopy
  - Nucleic acid amplification test (NAAT) is preferred as microscopy has limited sensitivity (50–60%) (2).
  - Several POC identification tests, including patient performed, are available with increased sensitivity compared to microscopy but are expensive.
- DIV
  - Wet mount with increase in inflammatory cells and parabasal (immature) squamous epithelial cells, with pH >4.5
  - Wet mount is preferred diagnostic method.

Follow-Up Tests & Special Considerations

BV/VVC/trichomoniasis

- New testing modalities such as oligonucleotide probes and NAATs may be used in some settings for patient comfort but outcomes are not clearly improved compared to more standard diagnostic methods and treatment, and the tests are expensive.

Diagnostic Procedures/Other

Microscopy and physical exam aid in diagnosis.

TREATMENT

GENERAL MEASURES

- Avoid douching and tight-fitting clothing.
- Regular use of condoms may help to prevent BV (2).
- Asymptomatic, pregnant women generally do not require treatment for BV.
- Consider avoiding use of tampons during intravaginal treatment to ensure adequate dispersion of medication.

MEDICATION

Medication recommendations based on CDC treatment guidelines and ACOG Practice Bulletin (2)[C],(3)

First Line

- BV
  - Metronidazole 500 mg orally BID for 7 days, 0.75% gel 1 full applicator (5 g) vaginally daily for 5 days, or clindamycin 2% cream vaginally daily for 5 to 7 days
  - Recurrent infection may require repeated treatment (e.g., 1 week monthly for 6 months). Advise patients to avoid alcohol during treatment with oral metronidazole and for 24 hours following or for 72 hours after treatment with tinidazole.
- VVC
  - Uncomplicated infections can be treated with a one-time dose of fluconazole 150 mg tab. Topical/vaginal suppository antifungal regimens such as butoconazole, clotrimazole, miconazole, terconazole, or nystatin creams. Treatment can range from 3 to 7 days. Recurrent infection fluconazole 150 mg 3 times in 1st week, then weekly for up to 6 months
  - Avoid oral azoles in pregnant women.
  - Advise patients that topical medications may weaken rubber or latex condoms.
- Trichomoniasis
  - Metronidazole 500 mg orally BID for 7 days
  - The patient's partner should be treated as well and counseled to abstain from sex until both patients have completed treatment and are asymptomatic.
  - Test of cure is not necessary, although retesting 3 months after initial treatment is indicated given increased rate of reinfection in sexually active women.
  - Advise patients to avoid alcohol during treatment with oral metronidazole and for 24 hours following or for 72 hours after treatment with tinidazole.
- DIV
  - Address estrogen deficiency.
  - Clindamycin 2% cream intravaginally at bedtime for 1 to 3 weeks
  - May need additional maintenance therapy

Second Line

- BV
  - Alternatively could consider use of secnidazole 2 g orally once or tinidazole/clindamycin orally ranging from 2 to 5 days
- VVC
  - Recurrent infections benefit from speciation to help determine treatment course.
  - Non-albican candidiasis may require longer duration of treatment with topical or oral azoles or boric acid.
- Trichomoniasis
  - One-time 2-g oral dose of either tinidazole or metronidazole
- DIV
  - Topical glucocorticoid such as hydrocortisone cream 300 to 500 mg intravaginally nightly for 3 weeks or clobetasol intravaginally nightly for 1 week

COMPLEMENTARY & ALTERNATIVE MEDICINE

It is unclear if probiotics are effective as treatment or preventive strategy.

ONGOING CARE

FOLLOW-UP RECOMMENDATIONS

- Delay sexual relations until symptoms clear/discomfort resolves.
- Use of condoms may reduce recurrence of BV.
- Consider suppressive therapy for recurrent infection.
- Monthly presumptive treatment may help reduce colonization of bacteria associated with BV (3)[C].

Patient Monitoring

No specific follow-up needed; if symptoms persist or recur within 2 months, repeat pelvic exam and culture.

PATIENT EDUCATION

American College of Obstetricians and Gynecologists (ACOG), 800-762-ACOG; www.acog.org

PROGNOSIS

VVC: 80–90% of uncomplicated cases cured with appropriate treatment; 30–50% of recurrent infections return after discontinuation of maintenance therapy; there is a relatively high spontaneous remission rate of untreated symptoms as well.

COMPLICATIONS

- BV has been associated with an increased risk of acquisition and transmission of HIV and other sexually transmitted infections, such as chlamydia and gonorrhea.
- BV has been associated with increased risk of preterm birth, chorioamnionitis, postpartum and postabortal endometritis, and pelvic inflammatory disease.
- VVC may occur following treatment of BV.

REFERENCES

1. Paavonen J, Brunham RC. Bacterial vaginosis and desquamative inflammatory vaginitis. *N Engl J Med*. 2018;379(23):2246–2254.
2. Committee on Practice Bulletins—Gynecology. Vaginitis in nonpregnant patients: ACOG Practice Bulletin, Number 215. *Obstet Gynecol*. 2020;135(1):e1–e17.
3. Balkus JE, Srinivasan S, Anzala O, et al. Impact of periodic presumptive treatment for bacterial vaginosis on the vaginal microbiome among women participating in the preventing vaginal infections trial. *J Infect Dis*. 2017;215(5):723–731.

SEE ALSO

Algorithm: Vaginal Discharge

CODES

ICD10

- N76.0 Acute vaginitis
- B37.3 Candidiasis of vulva and vagina
- N95.2 Postmenopausal atrophic vaginitis

CLINICAL PEARLS

- Most women experience relief of symptoms with therapy chosen without gold standard tests, even when the treatment does not correspond with the underlying infection.
- Vaginal pH is underused as a diagnostic tool for evaluation of vaginitis.

VARICOSE VEINS

Sibley Strader, MD

 BASICS

Varicose veins (VV), or varicosities, are dilated subcutaneous veins of at least 3 mm in diameter, measured with patient in upright position. They are part of a spectrum of chronic venous disorders ranging from telangiectasias to chronic venous insufficiency. Ovarian vein failure can also cause pelvic VV and subsequently pelvic congestion syndrome.

DESCRIPTION

- Lower extremities venous drainage is accomplished via a network of superficial veins > small perforator veins > deep veins; diseases in any of these systems may result in VV.
- VV usually form in the greater and lesser saphenous veins and sometimes their branches.

Geriatric Considerations

- Surgeries has low morbidity and mortality in patients >60, with significant self-reported improvement despite more advanced disease on presentation.
- >High-risk geriatric patients should avoid hybrid procedures and general anesthesia when possible.

Pregnancy Considerations

External compression is first-line treatment in pregnant female.

EPIDEMIOLOGY

Treatment of VV late complications such as chronic venous ulcerations results in an estimated 3 billion per year to treat in the United States (1).

Prevalence

- Approximately 23% of U.S. adult have VV.
- VV affect an estimate of 22 million women and 11 million men between 40 and 80 years old; of which, 2 million will develop symptom.

ETIOLOGY AND PATHOPHYSIOLOGY

Exact pathophysiology is debated, but it involves: venous hypertension, valves dysfunction, structural changes in the vessel wall, inflammation, alteration of shear wall stress, and genetic disposition (2).

- Venous hypertension is caused by reflux from valvular incompetence, outflow obstruction, calf muscle failure, or increased intra-abdominal pressure from pregnancy, obesity, chronic constipation, tumor, or other proximal obstruction.
- Valve dysfunction may be due to deformation, tearing, thinning or adhesion of the valve leaflets, the vein wall stiffening with failure of the leaflet to fit together, trauma, deep thrombophlebitis, and congenital valvular incompetence.
- Structural changes in the vein wall (disruption of smooth muscle cells and elastic fibers, etc.) lead to vessels weakening and dilation.
- Turbulent flow, reflux, and increases in shear stress promote inflammatory and prothrombotic changes that further contribute to the loss of wall and leaflet integrity.
- Deep venous insufficiency can lead to secondary VV via enlarging collaterals.

Genetics

VV is highly polygenic; a cohort study of >500,000 individuals has generated a list of genetic associations that include 30 new loci, with the strongest associations occurring in intron region CASZ1 (implicated in blood pressure) and 16q24 (contains genes that encode a vascular mechanosensory channel).

RISK FACTORS

- Inherited: tall height (>180 cm), congenital syndromes
- Acquired: age, DVT, pregnancy, decreased leg impedance
- Lifestyle: prolonged standing and/or sitting, tobacco use, obesity
- Hormonal: female gender (high estrogen state)
- Socioeconomical: lower education level

GENERAL PREVENTION

- Maintain a healthy body mass index.
- Avoid sitting or standing for prolonged periods of time.
- Wear compression stockings.

COMMONLY ASSOCIATED CONDITIONS

- Stasis dermatitis
- Lipodermatosclerosis
- Venous ulceration (usually near medial malleolus/gaiter area)

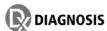 **DIAGNOSIS**

HISTORY

- Symptoms range from asymptomatic, minor annoyance/cosmetic concern to debilitating complaints
- Localized symptoms: pain/tingling, burning, itching
- Generalized symptoms: leg cramp, fatigue, swelling and heaviness
- Symptoms often worse at the end of the day and after prolonged standing
- Women are more prone to symptoms due to hormonal influences; symptom is usually worse during menses.

PHYSICAL EXAM

- Inspection
  - Performed while the patient is standing. VV in proximal femoral ring and distal legs may not be visible when the patient is supine.
  - Telangiectasias (spider veins) are small, dilated blood vessels (arteriole, venule, or capillary).
  - VV features:
    - Dilated, tortuous superficial veins, ≥3 mm in diameter
    - Dark purple/blue in color, raised above the surface of the skin
    - Often twisted, bulging, and can look like cords
    - Most commonly found on the posterior/medial lower extremity
  - Skin changes may include erythema, eczema, hemosiderosis, atrophie blanche, lipodermatosclerosis, ulcers (most often above the medial malleus).
  - Edema of the affected limb may be present.
  - Vulva, perineal, or groin VV may be a sign of pelvic vein issue.

- Palpation
  - Palpate saphenofemoral junction (SFJ)—~4 cm inferolateral to pubic tubercle—for any saphena varix.
- Beside tests, including tap and cough test, have limited value.
  - Tap test: Examiner places one finger on the SFJ and uses another hand to tap along the VV. A thrill will be felt on the SFJ if the examiner taps on a defective vein. A healthy valve will block the transmission of the thrill.
  - Cough test: Examiner palpates the SFJ for thrill when the patient cough.
- Duplex ultrasound has largely replaced the tourniquet tests.
  - Trendelenburg test locates the defective valves. Patient starts by lying spine and elevating the leg. Once the patient's venous blood is drained, the examiner ties a tourniquet on the leg and the patient stands up. If the VV remains flat, the defect is above the tourniquet level. If the VV fills back up, the problem is below the tourniquet level. The examiner repeats the test till the site of the defect is found.
  - Perthes test access the deep system. Patient starts by lying supine. The examiner ties a tourniquet around the patient's upper thigh. Patient then walk for 5 minutes. Persistent VV indicates deep vein pathology. VV disappears with competent deep venous system.

DIFFERENTIAL DIAGNOSIS

- For lower extremity pain:
  - Nerve root compression
  - Arthritis
  - Peripheral neuritis
  - Deep vein thrombosis
  - Superficial thrombophlebitis
  - Ischemia
  - Trauma
- For lower extremity ulcers:
  - Arterial/venous insufficiency
  - Neuropathy
  - Infection
  - Trauma
  - Vasculitides
  - Drugs (e.g., warfarin skin necrosis, heparin-induced thrombocytopenia)
  - Inflammatory disorders (e.g., pyoderma gangrenosum, panniculitis)

DIAGNOSTIC TESTS & INTERPRETATION

Initial Tests (lab, imaging)

Venous duplex ultrasonography is recommended for severe disease requiring intervention. It can determine saphenous junction competency, the junction diameter, the extend of the reflux, and the location and size of the affected vein. It can also assess for DVT and thrombophlebitis (2).

Follow-Up Tests & Special Considerations

- Lab tests are only needed to rule out other differentials.
- Magnetic resonance imaging, venography, and plethysmography are only used if venous ultrasound is inconclusive or for more complex surgical situations.

Test Interpretation

The CEAP (Clinical, Etiologic, Anatomic, Pathophysiologic) classification is the gold standard of classification of chronic venous disorders.

- Uncomplicated:
  - C0: no visible or palpable signs of venous disease
  - C1: telangiectasias or reticular veins
- Local symptoms and complication:
  - C2: VV; CV2r: recurrent VV
  - C3: edema
- Complex varicose disease:
  - C4a: pigmentation or eczema; C4b: lipodermatosclerosis or atrophie blanch, C4c: corona phlebectatica
  - C5: healed venous ulcer
  - C6: active venous ulcer; C6r: recurrent active venous ulcer

 TREATMENT

- VV is not curable because chronic venous insufficiency causes irreversible damages to the veins and valves.
- Indications for treatment include pain, aching, heaviness, fatigue, burning, edema, stasis dermatitis, recurrent superficial phlebitis or ulceration.
- Management options (most treatment involves multiple modalities and repetition): lifestyle modifications, compression therapy, local ablative therapies, surgery, and endovenous ablative therapies
- Lifestyle modification
  - Elevation of feet to at least heart level for 30 minutes 4 times daily
  - Avoid prolonged standing and sitting.
  - Weight loss, exercise such as walking and foot flexion exercises to improve calf muscle pump function
- Compression stockings while awake; nonadherence rate up to 60% due to difficulty with applying the stocking
- Local ablative therapy: for telangiectasias and reticular vein
  - Rely on chemical (sclerotherapy) or heat-based (thermoregulation, cutaneous laser) endothelial injury resulting in fibrosis of the veins
  - Liquid or foam sclerotherapy
    ○ Results in cosmetic improvement in 70% of patients and a patient satisfaction rate >70% (1)
    ○ Best result when compression stocking are worn 7 to 10 days after the procedure
    ○ Complications include allergic reactions to the sclerosants, hyperpigmentation, superficial thread-like capillaries causing a bluish discoloration (matting), cellulitis, and rarely ulceration or thromboembolism.
    ○ Ultrasound-guided sclerotherapy is useful in treating perforator vein reflux.
  - Limited efficacy studies with thermal or cutaneous laser but helpful in patients who prefer needleless procedure

- Surgery: for large branch, residual postablation VV and saphenous VV
  - CHIVA/stab phlebectomy:
    ○ French acronym for Conservatrice Hémodynamique de l'Insuffisance Veineuse en Ambulatoire (ambulatory conservative hemodynamic treatment venous insufficiency)—a procedure aim to alleviate signs and symptoms without destroying the vein
    ○ The surgeon maps the affected veins with ultrasound, makes a few small incisions, and ties off the veins.
    ○ Only requires local anesthesia and leaves minimal scar; reduces VV recurrence and produces fewer side effects than vein stripping
  - Surgical stripping
    ○ Less used with the development of less invasive procedures
    ○ Recurrence is up to 50% of the patients by 5 years
    ○ Complications include extensive ecchymosis, scarring, hematoma, lymphocele, infection, nerve damage, and DVT.
- Endovenous ablation—indicated for saphenous VV
- Radiofrequency ablation (RFA) uses thermal energy (85–120°C) to seal the incompetent vein via heat damage; endovenous laser ablation (EVLA) uses laser and fiber-optic catheter to generate thermal energy (up to 800°C).
  - 3 years estimated pooled success rates of 84% for RFA, 94% for EVLA compared to 78% in surgical stripping
  - Recommended by National Institute for Health and Care Excellence (NICE) as first-line treatment of truncal vein incompetence
  - RFA has a much lower subsequence incidence of thromboembolism and peripheral artery disease compared to other treatment.
- Mechanochemical endovenous ablation (MOCA) is a hybrid system composed of a rotating tip with simultaneous injection of liquid sclerosant.

GENERAL MEASURES

Sclerotherapy, surgery, and endovenous ablation are considered invasive.

- Indicated if noninvasive measures fail or if the patient has cosmetic concerns, recurrent hemorrhage and superficial thrombophlebitis
- Contraindicated in pregnancy, acute venous thromboembolism, peripheral artery disease (ankle-brachial index <0.9)

MEDICATION

- Low-dose diuretics have minimal effect.
- Topical steroid is helpful with stasis dermatitis.

ISSUES FOR REFERRAL

NICE recommends referral of patients with:

- Symptomatic primary (or recurrent) VV
- Skin changes
- Superficial venous thrombosis
- Active and healed leg ulcers

ADDITIONAL THERAPIES

- Activity modification
  - If standing is necessary, shift weight from side to side.
  - Never sit with legs hanging down.
- Physical therapy

COMPLEMENTARY & ALTERNATIVE MEDICINE

Phlebotonics including horse chestnut seed extract may ease symptoms, but long-term studies for safety and efficacy is lacking.

ADMISSION, INPATIENT, AND NURSING CONSIDERATIONS

- Compression stockings or sequential compression
- Encourage ambulation, VTE prevention

 ONGOING CARE

DIET

Weight-loss diet if obesity is a problem.

PATIENT EDUCATION

- Avoid long periods of standing and crossing legs.
- Exercise (walking, running) regularly to improve leg strength and circulation.
- Maintain a healthy weight.
- Wear elastic support stockings.
- Avoid clothing that constricts legs.

PROGNOSIS

- Will progress to advanced chronic venous diseases without treatment or correction to underlying cause
- Associated with a 7-fold increased risk of DVT (1)

COMPLICATIONS

- Chronic edema
- Petechial hemorrhages
- Venous stasis dermatitis, pigmentation, lipodermatosclerosis
- Venous ulcers +/− superimposed infection
- Recurrence after surgical treatment

REFERENCES

1. Piazza G. Varicose veins. *Circulation*. 2014;130(7):582–587.
2. Raetz J, Wilson M, Collins K. Varicose veins: diagnosis and treatment. *Am Fam Physician*. 2019;99(11):682–688.

 CODES

ICD10

- I83.90 Asymptomatic varicose veins of unspecified lower extremity
- I83.009 Varicose veins of unsp lower extremity w ulcer of unsp site
- I83.10 Varicose veins of unsp lower extremity with inflammation

CLINICAL PEARLS

RFA and EVLA have been demonstrated to be superior to open surgical techniques for VV treatment with similar improvement in quality of life.

V

VASCULITIS

Irene J. Tan, MD, FACR

BASICS

DESCRIPTION
An inflammatory disorder of blood vessels
- Clinical features result from the destruction of blood vessel walls with subsequent thrombosis, ischemia, bleeding, and/or aneurysm formation.
- Vasculitis is a large, heterogeneous group of diseases classified by the predominant size, type, and location of involved blood vessels.
  - Small-vessel vasculitis
    - Microscopic polyangiitis (MPA)
    - Granulomatosis with polyangiitis (GPA; formerly Wegener granulomatosis)
    - Eosinophilic granulomatosis with polyangiitis (EGPA; formerly Churg-Strauss syndrome)
    - Antiglomerular basement membrane disease (anti-GBM)
    - Cryoglobulinemic vasculitis
    - IgA vasculitis (formerly Henoch-Schönlein purpura)
    - Hypocomplementemic urticarial vasculitis
  - Medium-vessel vasculitis
    - Polyarteritis nodosa (PAN)
    - Kawasaki disease (KD)
  - Large-vessel vasculitis
    - Takayasu arteritis (TAK)
    - Giant cell arteritis (GCA)
- Vasculitis occurs as a primary disorder or secondary to infection, a drug reaction, malignancy, or connective tissue disease (CTD).
  - Variable vessel vasculitis
    - Behçet disease
    - Cogan syndrome
  - Single-organ vasculitis
    - Cutaneous leukocytoclastic angiitis
    - Cutaneous arteritis
    - Primary CNS vasculitis
  - Vasculitis associated with systemic disease
    - Lupus vasculitis
    - Rheumatoid vasculitis
    - Sarcoid vasculitis
  - Vasculitis associated with other etiology
    - Hepatitis C–associated cryoglobulinemic vasculitis
    - Hepatitis B–associated vasculitis
    - Syphilis-associated aortitis
    - Drug-induced immune complex vasculitis
    - Drug-associated antineutrophil cytoplasmic antibodies (ANCA)-associated vasculitis
    - Cancer-associated vasculitis
- Protean features often delay definitive diagnosis.

EPIDEMIOLOGY
Highly variable, depending on the particular syndrome
- Hypersensitivity vasculitis is most commonly encountered in clinical practice.
- KD, IgA vasculitis, and dermatomyositis are more common in children.
- TAK is most prevalent in young Asian women. GPA, MPA, and EGPA are more common in middle-aged males.
- GCA occurs exclusively in those >50 years of age and is rare in the African-American population.

Incidence
Annual incidence in adults (unless otherwise specified)
- IgA vasculitis: 200 to 700/1 million in children <17 years of age

- GCA: 100 to 170/1 million in Caucasians age >50 years
- KD: depends on race/age; ~200/1 million
- PAN: 2 to 33/1 million
- GPA: 4 to 15/1 million
- MPA: 1 to 24/1 million
- EGPA: 1 to 3/1 million
- TAK: 2/1 million
- Primary CNS vasculitis: 2/1 million in adults
- Hypersensitivity vasculitis: depends on drug exposure
- Viral-/retroviral-associated vasculitis: unknown; >90% of cases of cryoglobulinemic vasculitis are associated with hepatitis C.
- Connective tissue disorder–associated vasculitis: variable

ETIOLOGY AND PATHOPHYSIOLOGY
- Three major immunopathogenic mechanisms
  - Immune-complex formation: systemic lupus erythematosus (SLE), IgA vasculitis, and cryoglobulinemic vasculitis
  - ANCAs: GPA, MPA, and EGPA
  - Pathogenic T-lymphocyte response: GCA and TAK
- Pathophysiology best understood where known drug triggers have been identified (e.g., antibiotics, sulfonamides, and hydralazine)

Genetics
- Several vasculitides linked to candidate genes
- Mutation in CECR1 encoding adenosine deaminase 2 is associated with PAN.
- Angiotensin-converting enzyme insertion/deletion polymorphism is associated with susceptibility to vasculitis, especially in Behçet disease and IgA vasculitis.

RISK FACTORS
A combination of genetic susceptibility and environmental exposure likely triggers onset.

GENERAL PREVENTION
Early identification is the key to prevent irreversible organ damage in severe forms of systemic vasculitis.

COMMONLY ASSOCIATED CONDITIONS
Hepatitis C (cryoglobulinemic vasculitis), hepatitis B (PAN), cytomegalovirus (CMV), Epstein-Barr virus (EBV), HIV (viral-/retroviral-associated vasculitis), SLE, rheumatoid arthritis (RA), Sjögren syndrome, mixed connective tissue disease (MCTD), dermatomyositis, ankylosing spondylitis, Behçet disease, relapsing polychondritis (CTD-associated vasculitis), respiratory tract methicillin-resistant *Staphylococcus aureus* (MRSA) in GPA, levamisole-adulterated cocaine, medications: propylthiouracil, methimazole, hydralazine, minocycline; SARS-CoV2 infection

DIAGNOSIS

HISTORY
- Consider age, gender, and ethnicity.
- Comprehensive medication history
- Family history of vasculitis
- Constitutional symptoms: fever, weight loss, malaise, fatigue, diminished appetite, sweats
- CNS/PNS: mononeuritis multiplex, polyneuropathy, headaches, visual loss, tinnitus, stroke, seizure, encephalopathy

- Heart/lung: myocardial infarction, cardiomyopathy, pericarditis, cough, chest pain, hemoptysis, dyspnea
- Renal: hematuria, hypertension
- GI: abdominal pain, hematochezia, perforation
- Musculoskeletal: arthralgia, myalgia
- Miscellaneous: unexplained ischemic or hemorrhagic events, chronic sinusitis, and recurrent epistaxis
- Note the organs affected and estimate the size of blood vessels involved.
- Demographics, clinical features, and the predominant vessel size/organ involvement help identify specific type of vasculitis.
- Vasculitis is a presenting condition in SARS-CoV2/COVID-19 infection.

PHYSICAL EXAM
- Vital signs: blood pressure (hypertension) and pulse (regularity and rate)
- Skin: palpable purpura, livedo reticularis, nodules, ulcers, gangrene, nail bed capillary changes
- Neurologic: cranial nerve exam, sensorimotor exam
- Ocular exam: visual fields, scleritis, episcleritis
- Cardiopulmonary exam: rubs, murmurs, arrhythmias
- Abdominal exam: tenderness, organomegaly

DIFFERENTIAL DIAGNOSIS
- Fibromuscular dysplasia
- Embolic disease (atheroma, cholesterol emboli, atrial myxoma, mycotic aneurysm with embolization)
- Drug-induced vasospasm (cocaine, amphetamines, ergots)
- Thrombotic thrombocytopenic disorders (disseminated intravascular coagulation [DIC], thrombotic thrombocytopenic purpura [TTP], antiphospholipid syndrome, heparin- or warfarin-induced thrombosis), thromboangiitis obliterans
- Systemic infection (infective endocarditis, fungal infections, disseminated gonococcal infection, Lyme disease, syphilis, Rocky Mountain spotted fever [RMSF], bacteremia, ehrlichiosis, babesiosis)
- Malignancy (lymphomatoid granulomatosis, angioimmunoblastic T-cell lymphoma, intravascular lymphoma)
- Miscellaneous (Goodpasture syndrome, sarcoidosis, amyloidosis, Whipple disease, congenital coarctation of aorta)

DIAGNOSTIC TESTS & INTERPRETATION

ALERT
Renal involvement is often clinically silent. Routine serum creatinine and urinalysis with microscopy are needed to identify underlying glomerulonephritis.

- Initial tests exclude alternate diagnoses and guide therapy.
- Routine tests
  - CBC
  - Liver enzymes
  - Serum creatinine
  - Urinalysis with microscopy
- Specific serology
  - Antinuclear antibodies (ANA)
  - Rheumatoid factor (RF)
  - Rapid plasma reagin/venereal disease reaction level (RPR/VDRL)
  - RMSF titers; Lyme titers
  - Complement levels C3, C4
  - ANCA
  - Antiproteinase 3 (anti-PR3) antibodies

- Antimyeloperoxidase (anti-MPO) antibodies
- Hepatitis screen for B and C
- Cryoglobulin
- Anti-GBM titer
- HIV
- Serum and urine protein electrophoresis
- RT-PCR and antigen test for SARS-CoV-2
- Miscellaneous
  - Drug screen
  - ESR
  - C-reactive protein
  - Creatine kinase (CK)
  - Blood culture
  - ECG
- CXR, CT scan, MRI, and arteriography may be required to delineate extent of organs involved.

Diagnostic Procedures/Other
- Electromyography with nerve conduction can document neuropathy and target nerve for biopsy.
- Biopsy of affected site confirms diagnosis (e.g., temporal artery, sural nerve, renal biopsy).
- If biopsy is not practical, angiography may be diagnostic for large- and medium-vessel vasculitides.
- Bronchoscopy may be required to differentiate pulmonary infection from potentially life-threatening hemorrhagic vasculitis in patients with hemoptysis.

Test Interpretation
Blood vessel biopsy shows immune cell infiltration into vessel wall layers with varying degrees of necrosis and granuloma formation, depending on the type.

 TREATMENT

GENERAL MEASURES
- Discontinue offending drug (hypersensitivity vasculitis).
- Simple observation for mild cases of pediatric IgA vasculitis
- ANCA-associated vasculitis has two-phase treatment: initial induction followed by maintenance (steady tapering of corticosteroids with immunosuppressants or immunomodulators).

MEDICATION

First Line
Corticosteroids are initial anti-inflammatory of choice.

Second Line
Cytotoxic medications, immunomodulatory, or biologic agents, for example, cyclophosphamide (1)[B],(2)[A], methotrexate (3)[A], azathioprine (3)[A], leflunomide (3)[A], mycophenolate mofetil (1)[B], and rituximab (2)[A], are often required in combination with corticosteroids for rapidly progressive vasculitis with significant organ involvement or inadequate response to corticosteroids. Rituximab (2)[A] is the first FDA-approved treatment for GPA and MPA for both adults and children age 2 years or older. Tocilizumab (4)[A] is the first FDA-approved treatment for GCA. Mepolizumab (5)[A] is the first FDA-approved treatment for EGPA. Intravenous immunoglobulins (IVIg) is the FDA-approved treatment for KD in combination with aspirin. Apremilast is the FDA-approved treatment for oral ulcers in Behçet disease (6)[A].

ISSUES FOR REFERRAL
- Rheumatology referral for complicated cases where newer or more toxic treatments are required
- Nephrology referral for persistent hematuria or proteinuria, rising creatinine, or a positive ANCA titer
- Pulmonary referral for persistent pulmonary infiltrate unresponsive to antibiotic therapy or if gross hemoptysis

ADDITIONAL THERAPIES
Plasma exchange does not improve mortality or progression to ESRD in severe ANCA-associated vasculitis.

SURGERY/OTHER PROCEDURES
Rarely, corrective surgery is required to repair tissue damage as a result of aggressive vasculitis.

ADMISSION, INPATIENT, AND NURSING CONSIDERATIONS
- Hemoptysis, acute renal failure, intestinal ischemia, any organ-threatening symptoms or signs, and/or need for biopsy
- Initial therapy is guided by the organ system involved.
  - If pulmonary hemorrhage is present, life-saving measures may include mechanical ventilation, plasmapheresis, and immunosuppression.
  - If acute renal failure is present, attend to electrolyte and fluid balance and consider plasma exchange and immunosuppression.
  - If signs of intestinal ischemia are present, make NPO and consider plasmapheresis, immunosuppression, and parenteral nutrition.
- Discharge criteria: stabilization or resolution of potential life-threatening symptoms

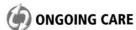 ONGOING CARE

FOLLOW-UP RECOMMENDATIONS
If significant coronary artery disease is involved in KD, moderate activity restriction may be of benefit.

Patient Monitoring
Frequent clinical follow-up supported by patient self-monitoring to identify disease relapse

DIET
Alter diets for patients with renal involvement or hyperglycemia/dyslipidemia.

PROGNOSIS
Prognosis is good for patients with vasculitis and limited organ involvement. Relapsing courses, renal, intestinal, or extensive lung involvement have a poorer prognosis.

COMPLICATIONS
- Persistent organ dysfunction may be the result of the disease, medications, or inflammation/scarring in the more serious forms of vasculitis.
- Early morbidity/mortality is due to active vasculitic disease; delayed morbidity/mortality may also be secondary to complications of chronic therapy with cytotoxic medications.

REFERENCES
1. Sunderkötter CH, Zelger B, Chen K-R, et al. Nomenclature of cutaneous vasculitis: dermatologic addendum to the 2012 Revised International Chapel Hill Consensus Conference nomenclature of vasculitides. *Arthritis Rheumatol*. 2018;70(2):171–184.
2. Stone JH, Merkel PA, Spiera R, et al; for RAVE-ITN Research Group. Rituximab versus cyclophosphamide for ANCA-associated vasculitis. *N Engl J Med*. 2010;363(3):221–232.
3. Walters GD, Willis NS, Craig JC. Interventions for renal vasculitis in adults. A systematic review. *BMC Nephrol*. 2010;11:12.
4. Villiger PM, Adler S, Kuchen S, et al. Tocilizumab for induction and maintenance of remission in giant cell arteritis: a phase 2, randomised, double-blind, placebo-controlled trial. *Lancet*. 2016;387(10031):1921–1927.
5. Wechsler ME, Akuthota P, Jayne D, et al; for EGPA Mepolizumab Study Team. Mepolizumab or placebo for eosinophilic granulomatosis with polyangiitis. *N Engl J Med*. 2017;376(20):1921–1932.
6. Hatemi G, Mahr A, Ishigatsubo Y, et al. Trial of apremilast for oral ulcers in Behçet's syndrome. *N Engl J Med*. 2019;381(20):1918.

ADDITIONAL READING
- Gatto M, Iaccarino L, Canova M, et al. Pregnancy and vasculitis: a systematic review of the literature. *Autoimmun Rev*. 2012;11(6–7):A447–A459.
- Iba T, Connors JM, Levy JH. The coagulopathy, endotheliopathy, and vasculitis of COVID-19. *Inflamm Res*. 2020;69(12):1181–1189.
- Walsh M, Merkel PA, Peh C-A, et al. Plasma exchange and glucocorticoids in severe ANCA-associated vasculitis. *N Engl J Med*. 2020;382:622–631.

 CODES

ICD10
- M31.7 Microscopic polyangiitis
- M31.30 Wegener's granulomatosis without renal involvement
- M31.9 Necrotizing vasculopathy, unspecified

CLINICAL PEARLS
- Suspect vasculitis in patients with a petechial rash, palpable purpura, glomerulonephritis, pulmonary–renal syndrome, intestinal ischemia, or mononeuritis multiplex.
- Exclude silent renal involvement by routinely obtaining serum creatinine and urinalysis with microscopy.
- Vasculitis has "skip" lesions, which may complicate diagnostic biopsy.
- In patients with vasculitis, look for an underlying inciting process such as medication, infection, thrombosis, or malignancy.

V

VENOUS INSUFFICIENCY ULCERS

Marcy R. Wiemers, MD • Hyunyoung G. Kim, MD, MPH • Rachel P. Walker, BA, MD

 BASICS

- Venous insufficiency is a condition that occurs when the venous wall and/or valves in the leg veins are not working effectively, making it difficult for blood to return to the heart and causing stasis.
- Signs of chronic venous insufficiency include edema, bulging veins, hyperpigmentation, dermatitis, woody fibrosis, lipodermatosclerosis, and ulcers.
- Venous stasis ulcers are the most serious consequence of chronic venous insufficiency.
- Venous stasis ulcers affect up to 3% of adults in developed countries at some point during their lives.
- The annual estimated treatment cost of chronic venous ulcers is $2.5 to $3.5 billion dollars per year.

DESCRIPTION
- Irregular and shallow skin defect with surrounding hyperpigmentation and well-defined borders
- Most frequently located in the lower leg or ankle over the bony prominences
- Present for >30 days and fails to heal spontaneously
- May only have mild pain unless infected

EPIDEMIOLOGY
80% of leg ulcers are caused by venous disease vs. 10–25% arterial disease

Incidence
- The overall incidence of venous ulcers is 18/100,000 persons; more common in women than in men (20.4 vs. 14.6/100,000), incidence increases with age in both men and women.
- >20,000 patients are newly diagnosed with venous ulcers in the United States yearly.

Prevalence
- Venous ulcers are seen in ~1% of the adult population and up to 4% in adults ≥80 years old in industrialized countries.
- 70% of ulcers recur within 5 years of closure.

ETIOLOGY AND PATHOPHYSIOLOGY
- In a diseased venous system, venous pressure in the deep system fails to fall with ambulation, causing venous hypertension.
- Venous hypertension comes from the following:
  - Venous obstruction
  - Incompetent venous valves in the deep or superficial system
  - Inadequate muscle contraction (e.g., arthritis, myopathies, neuropathies)
- Venous pressure transmitted to capillaries leads to venous hypertensive microangiopathy and extravasation of RBCs and proteins (especially fibrinogen).
- Increased RBC aggregation leads to reduced oxygen transport, slowed arteriolar circulation, and ischemia at the skin level, contributing to ulcers.
- Leukocytes aggregate to the hypoxic areas and increase local inflammation.
- Prolonged chronic inflammation and bacterial infection promote the persistence of ulcers.

RISK FACTORS
- History of leg injury
- Age >55 years
- High BMI
- Congestive heart failure (CHF)
- History of deep venous thrombosis (DVT)
- Failure of the calf muscle pump (e.g., ankle fusion, inactivity)
- Previous varicose vein surgery or ulcers
- Smoking
- Prolonged standing
- Pregnancy
- Family history

GENERAL PREVENTION
- Primary prevention after symptomatic DVT: Prescribe compression hose as soon as feasible, to be used for at least 2 years (≥20 to 30 mm Hg compression).
- Secondary prevention of recurrent ulceration includes compression, correction of the underlying problem, and surveillance.
- Encourage exercise to improve muscle pump function.

COMMONLY ASSOCIATED CONDITIONS
Up to 50% of patients have allergic reactions to topical agents commonly used for treatment.
- Avoid triple antibiotic ointment, including anything containing neomycin sulfate.

DIAGNOSIS

HISTORY
- Family history of venous insufficiency and ulcers
- Recent trauma
- Prevalent features: cramping, pruritus, prickling, and throbbing sensation
- Pain that may improve with leg elevation
- Wound drainage
- Duration of wound and over-the-counter (OTC) treatments already attempted
- History of DVTs (especially factor V Leiden mutation; strongly associated with ulceration)
- History of leg edema that improves overnight (Edema that does not improve overnight is more likely lymphedema.)

PHYSICAL EXAM
- Look for evidence of venous insufficiency:
  - Pitting edema
  - Hemosiderin staining (red and brown diffuse pigment changes)
  - Stasis dermatitis
  - Atrophie blanche, ivory-colored stellate scars
  - Lipodermatosclerosis ("bottle neck" narrowing in the lower leg from fibrosis and scarring)
- Look for evidence of significant lymphedema (i.e., dorsal foot or toe edema, edema that does not resolve overnight or with elevation). This may require referral for comprehensive lymph therapy.

- Examine for palpable pulses.
- Examine wound for the following:
  - Length, width, and depth to monitor wound healing rate
  - Presence of necrotic tissue
  - Presence of biofilms or infection: fever, chills, purulent material in the wound, increased amount of odorous exudate, and/or spreading cellulitis
- Get initial and interim girth measurements (ankle and midcalf) to monitor edema.
- Important to rule out poor arterial circulation because compression dressings cannot be used in patients with ankle-brachial index (ABI) <0.8

DIFFERENTIAL DIAGNOSIS
- Arterial insufficiency ulcer
- Neuropathic ulcer
- Lymphedema
- Cellulitis (unilateral, febrile, patient feels ill, area warm, erythema without hyperpigmentation)
- Malignancy
- Sickle cell ulcer
- Vasculitic ulcer
- Rare: cryoglobulinemia, leishmaniasis, cutaneous tuberculosis, calciphylaxis
- Pyoderma gangrenosum
- Collagen vascular disease

DIAGNOSTIC TESTS & INTERPRETATION
- Consider biopsy of leg ulcers that fail to heal or have atypical features (1)[C].
- Consider factor V Leiden mutation, which is strongly associated with venous ulcers.
- Screen for diabetes as necessary with a fasting glucose.
- Use duplex imaging to diagnose anatomic and hemodynamic abnormalities with venous insufficiency and also to screen for DVT.

Initial Tests (lab, imaging)
For any patient with suspected venous ulcer, arterial pulse examination and ankle-brachial indexes are recommended (1)[C].

Diagnostic Procedures/Other
- Check ankle-brachial index for evidence of arterial disease.
- Duplex imaging for evaluation of superficial and deep venous reflux and incompetent perforator veins
- Venography
- With concomitant severe arterial insufficiency, refer to a vascular surgeon for revascularization.
- Strongly consider biopsy on wounds with atypical locations, failure to heal, or any suspicion of malignancy.

TREATMENT

- Treatment options: conservative management, mechanical treatment, medications, and surgical options
- Goals: Reduce edema, improve ulcer healing, and prevent recurrence.

GENERAL MEASURES

- Compression therapy is the standard of care for venous ulcers and chronic venous insufficiency and should be started as early as possible (2)[C].
- Leg elevation above the level of the heart can reduce edema and improve microcirculation and oxygen delivery; it is most effective if performed for 30 minutes, 3 to 4 times a day.
- Dressings are used under compression bandages to promote faster healing and prevent adherence of the bandage to the ulcer; types include hydrocolloids, foams, hydrogels, paste, and simple nonadherent dressing.
- The choice of dressing can be guided by cost, ease of application, patient's, and physician's preference.
- A microorganism binding dressing is more effective than a silver containing hydrofiber dressing in controlling the bacterial load (2)[A].
- To prevent maceration of surrounding skin, use a barrier ointment/cream.
- Conservative management
  - Compression therapy methods: inelastic, elastic, and intermittent pneumatic compression
  - Outcome: reduces edema, improves venous reflux, enhances healing, and reduces pain
  - Barriers: pain, drainage, application difficulty, and physical limitations (obesity and contact dermatitis)
  - Contraindications: clinically significant arterial disease (ABI <0.8) and uncompensated heart failure
  - Inelastic compression therapy: provides pressure during ambulation and muscle contraction but no resting pressure; most common: Unna boot (zinc oxide moist bandage that hardens after application)
  - Elastic compression therapy: sustains compression during rest and activity. Compression stockings: Pressure should be at least 20 to 30 mm Hg and preferably 30 to 40 mm Hg. They should be removed at night and should be replaced every 6 months. Elastic bandages (i.e., Profore) are alternatives to compression stockings.
  - Intermittent pneumatic compression: generally reserved for bedridden patients because it is expensive and requires immobilization
  - Compression stockings reduce the risk of venous insufficiency ulcer reoccurrence.

MEDICATION

- Systemic therapy with pentoxifylline (400 mg PO TID) improves healing with or without adjuvant compression therapy. Adverse effects include prolonged bleeding time, GI upset, headaches, light headedness (1)[A].
- Evidence is inconsistent regarding the benefits of aspirin (1).
- Oral antibiotic therapy is indicated if infection is suspected (1)[C].

ALERT

Routine use of antibiotics for all venous ulcers is not recommended.

ISSUES FOR REFERRAL

- With prominent toe or foot edema, consider lymphedema. Refer to a certified lymphedema therapist (CLT).
- Refer to a wound clinic for complex, large, or poorly healing ulcers (>3 months or >10 cm).
- Refer to a vascular specialist for recurrent ulcers and/ or ABI <0.8.
- Use home health nurses to help with immobile patients needing frequent wrapping/dressing changes.

ADDITIONAL THERAPIES

- Edema management: Reduce venous hypertension and improve venous return.
- Exercise (e.g., activation of calf muscle pump with ankle flexion and extension) has a significant effect on venous leg ulcer healing, which may be enhanced in conjunction with leg compression and elevation.
- Infection control if likelihood is high (elevated WBC, unilateral, sudden onset, patient ill, etc.)
  - Débridement of necrotic tissue
  - Treat cellulitis (usually gram-positive bacteria) with bactericidal systemic antibiotics. Suspect local infection when there is pain or no improvement in the wound after 2 weeks of compression.
  - Treatment of critical colonization with topical antimicrobials, such as cadexomer iodine (Silver dressings and honey are widely used, but definitive data are lacking) (2).
- Due to lack of evidence, hyperbaric oxygen treatment is not currently recommended for treatment (1).

SURGERY/OTHER PROCEDURES

- Current evidence does not support the superiority of surgical interventions (open or endovascular) vs. compression alone for ulcer healing and recurrence.
- If necrotic tissue, consider sharp, enzymatic, mechanical, larval, or autolytic débridement (1)[A].
- Skin grafting generally is not effective if there is persistent edema and the underlying venous disease is not addressed.
- Allografts made of synthetic bilayered skin with living keratinocytes and fibroblasts are the only cellular tissue product (CTP) to improve healing at 6 months. There is insufficient evidence to support the use of autografts, xenografts.

ADMISSION, INPATIENT, AND NURSING CONSIDERATIONS

Consider for those with acute significant cellulitis or diabetic patients requiring IV antibiotics.

ONGOING CARE

FOLLOW-UP RECOMMENDATIONS

When ulcers are nearly healed and edema is controlled, switch from compression bandages to compression hose. (Consider referral for compression hose fitting early because insurance may not reimburse for the hose unless an ulcer is present.)

Patient Monitoring

- Monitor the ulcer for healing by measuring its size.
- Expect at least a 10% reduction every 2 weeks.
- Monitor for infection and rare malignant changes.

DIET

- Low-sodium diet is recommended for patients with fluid overload.
- Weight loss for patients with a high BMI

PATIENT EDUCATION

- Patient education on the underlying mechanism and appropriate wound care
- A long-term plan for edema management and the use of compression therapy is essential.

PROGNOSIS

- Venous insufficiency is a lifelong medical problem.
- Early identification and immediate treatment are essential.
- Ongoing diligence with edema control, avoiding infections, and avoiding trauma are important because ulcers recur frequently.
- Poor prognostic factors
  - Ulcer duration >3 months
  - Ulcer >10 cm
  - Presence of arterial disease in the lower limbs
  - Advanced age
  - Elevated BMI

COMPLICATIONS

- Venous insufficiency ulcers significantly reduce health-related quality of life, especially in younger cohorts.
- Venous insufficiency ulcers are associated with higher health-related expenditures and missed work (1)[B].
- Complications of venous insufficiency ulcers include infection and skin cancers (squamous cell carcinoma) (1).

REFERENCES

1. Bonkemeyer Millan S, Gan R, Townsend PE. Venous ulcers: diagnosis and treatment. *Am Fam Physician*. 2019;100(5):298–305.
2. Ren S-Y, Liu Y-S, Zhu G-J, et al. Strategies and challenges in the treatment of chronic venous leg ulcers. *World J Clin Cases*. 2020;8(21):5070–5085.

CODES

ICD10

- I87.2 Venous insufficiency (chronic) (peripheral)
- I83.009 Varicose veins of unsp lower extremity w ulcer of unsp site
- I89.0 Lymphedema, not elsewhere classified

CLINICAL PEARLS

- The diagnosis of venous ulcers is clinical; however, exams such as ABI and color duplex ultrasonography may be helpful if the diagnosis is unclear.
- Compression therapy is the standard of care for venous ulcers and chronic venous insufficiency but may be contraindicated if ABI <0.8.
- Treat critical colonization with topical antimicrobials (avoid neomycin).
- Refer patients with recurrent or venous ulcers failing to heal after 4 to 6 weeks of moist wound care and compression to a wound specialist.

V

VENTRICULAR SEPTAL DEFECT

Luay Sarsam, MD • Cherry Onaiwu, MD, MS

BASICS

DESCRIPTION
- Congenital (usually) or acquired defect in the inter-ventricular septum that allows communication of blood between the left and the right ventricles
- Second most common congenital heart malformation reported in infants and children. It can also occur as a late complication of acute myocardial infarction (MI)
- Severity of the defect is correlated with its size, with large defects being the most severe
- Blood flow across the defect typically is left to right, depending on defect size and pulmonary vascular resistance (PVR)
- Prolonged left to right shunting of blood can lead to pulmonary hypertension (HTN). This may eventually lead to a reversal of flow across the defect and cyanosis (Eisenmenger complex)

Geriatric Considerations
Almost entirely associated with late complication of MI

Pediatric Considerations
Congenital defect

ALERT
- Pregnancy may exacerbate symptoms and signs of a ventricular septal defect (VSD).
- Can be tolerated during pregnancy if VSD is small
- May be associated with an increased risk of pre-eclampsia in women with an unrepaired VSD

EPIDEMIOLOGY
Incidence
- Congenital defect: no gender predilection, occurs in ~2/1,000 live births and accounts for 30% of all congenital cardiac malformations
- Post-MI: Some studies suggest that gender may play a role

Prevalence
In the United States:
- Occurs in ~50% of all children with congenital heart disease
- Low prevalence in adults (~0.3 per 1,000) due to spontaneous closure
- Post-MI complication in ~0.2–3% of cases

ETIOLOGY AND PATHOPHYSIOLOGY
- Congenital
- In adults, late complication of MI
- Some reports of iatrogenic causes

Genetics
Multifactorial etiology; autosomal dominant and recessive transmissions have been reported.

RISK FACTORS
- Congenital VSD:
  - Risk of sibling being affected: 4.2%
  - Risk of offspring being affected: 4%
  - Prematurity
- Post-MI VSD:
  - Advanced age
  - Arterial HTN
  - First MI
  - Most frequent within 1st week after MI
  - Most commonly after anterior wall acute MI

GENERAL PREVENTION
Avoid prenatal exposure to known risk factors (ibuprofen cyclooxygenase [COX] inhibitors, marijuana, organic solvents, febrile illness). For adults, avoid risk factors for MI and obtain evaluation before pregnancy.

COMMONLY ASSOCIATED CONDITIONS
- Congenital:
  - Tetralogy of Fallot
  - Aortic valvular deformities, especially aortic insuf-ficiency and bicuspid aortic valve
  - Down syndrome (trisomy 21), endocardial cushion defect
  - Transposition of great arteries
  - Coarctation of aorta
  - Tricuspid atresia
  - Truncus arteriosus
  - Patent ductus arteriosus
  - Atrial septal defect
  - Pulmonic stenosis
  - Subaortic stenosis
- Adult: coronary artery disease

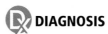 DIAGNOSIS

HISTORY
- Presentation depends on degree of shunting across the defect; may be completely asymptomatic with small defects
- Respiratory distress, tachypnea, tachycardia
- Diaphoresis with feeds, poor weight gain in infants

PHYSICAL EXAM
- Small defect:
  - Harsh holosystolic murmur loudest at left lower sternal border
  - Detected after PVR drops at 4 to 8 weeks of life
- Moderate defect:
  - Harsh holosystolic murmur at left lower sternal border associated with a thrill
  - Forceful apical impulse with lateral displacement
  - Increased intensity of P_2
  - Diastolic rumble at apex due to increased flow across the mitral valve
- Large defect:
  - Holosystolic murmur heard throughout the precor-dium with diastolic rumble at apex with precordial bulge and hyperactivity, although large defects may have little or no murmur initially
  - If congestive heart failure (CHF) exists: tachycardia, tachypnea, and hepatomegaly
  - If pulmonary HTN exists: cyanosis with exertion
  - If severe, irreversible pulmonary HTN (Eisenmenger complex) exists: cyanosis, clubbing, syncope, arrhythmias, and polycythemia

DIFFERENTIAL DIAGNOSIS
- Patent ductus arteriosus, atrial septal defect
- Children: tetralogy of Fallot
- Adults: mitral regurgitation

DIAGNOSTIC TESTS & INTERPRETATION
Initial Tests (lab, imaging)
- A 12-lead electrocardiogram may show left ventricu-lar hypertrophy and left atrial enlargement initially. As pulmonary HTN develops, right ventricular hyper-trophy and right atrial enlargement may be seen.
- A chest x-ray (CXR) may demonstrate increased pulmonary vascularity and/or cardiomegaly.

- A 2D echocardiogram using color Doppler and bubble study for visualization of location, size of defect, and shunt direction
- Color flow Doppler for direction and velocity of VSD jet; may be used to estimate right ventricular pressure
- Ventriculography in conjunction with above imaging modalities can aid in characterization of VSD but is invasive

Follow-Up Tests & Special Considerations
- Weight and hematocrit check
- Serial echocardiograms
- Cardiac catheterization performed occasionally for perioperative planning or to assess need for closure of defect

Diagnostic Procedures/Other
- Cardiac catheterization (left and right sides of heart) can confirm the diagnosis, document number of defects, quantify ratio of pulmonary blood flow to systemic blood flow (Qp/Qs), and determine PVR.
- Demonstration of an oxygen saturation step up from the right atrium to the distal pulmonary artery

Test Interpretation
- Congenital VSD (four major anatomic types)
  - Membranous (70%)
  - Muscular (20%)
  - Atrioventricular canal type (5%)
  - Supracristal (5%; higher in Asians)
- Post-MI VSD predominantly involves muscular septum.
- Right bundle branch block is common after surgical repair.

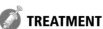 TREATMENT

- Small VSD tends to close spontaneously during childhood and has low risk for complications.
- Larger VSD tends to persist into adulthood and has more risk for complications.
- Start diuretic therapy if signs of fluid overload
- Minimize IV fluids.
- Consider angiotensin-converting enzyme inhibitor and/or digoxin.
- Nasogastric feeds for neonates
- Correct anemia via iron supplementation or a pos-sible red blood cell transfusion.

GENERAL MEASURES
- Appropriate health care maintenance
- Outpatient, until surgical repair is indicated
- Inpatient management in setting of acute MI
- Inpatient for treatment of severe CHF

MEDICATION
First Line
- Per the 2007 American Heart Association guidelines, endocarditis antibiotic prophylaxis is not recom-mended for most VSDs. It is recommended for VSDs associated with complex cyanotic heart disease, during the first 6 months after surgical repair, or for residual VSDs located near the patch following surgery (1)[A]
- Pediatric: Medications aim to control pulmonary edema, decrease work of breathing, and allow for growth:
  - Furosemide 1 to 2 mg/kg PO/IV once to twice a day
  - Spironolactone 1 to 2 mg/kg/day divided BID

– Captopril
  ○ Infants: oral: 0.3 to 2.5 mg/kg/day divided every 8 to 12 hours; max 2 mg/kg/day
  ○ Children and adolescents: oral: 0.3 to 6.0 mg/kg/day divided every 8 to 12 hours; maximum daily dose: 150 mg/day
– Digoxin: infants <2 years of age, 10 μg/kg/day PO divided BID; children, 2 to 10 years of age, 5 to 10 μg/kg/day PO divided BID; children >10 years of age, 2 to 5 μg/kg/day PO divided BID
- Adults: Digoxin and diuretics may be beneficial in some circumstances
- Side effects:
  – Drugs that increase systemic vascular resistance may increase left-to-right shunting and cause signs and symptoms of pulmonary overcirculation.
  – HTN

Second Line
- Surgical closure is indicated if the pulmonic-to-systemic flow is >2:1 or with poorly controlled pulmonary overcirculation despite maximal medical and dietary interventions.
- If an infant with a VSD has persistent pulmonary HTN or failure to grow, surgical repair is recommended prior to 6 months of age even if patient is otherwise asymptomatic.
- For post-MI VSDs, afterload reduction, inotropic support, intra-aortic balloon pump, and left ventricular assist device may be used to stabilize the patient prior to surgery. Surgical repair includes septal débridement and patch placement.

ISSUES FOR REFERRAL
Close follow-up of a congenital VSD is necessary until primary intracardiac repair is performed to ensure that significant pulmonary HTN does not develop.

ADDITIONAL THERAPIES
- Infant caloric requirements up to 150 kcal/kg/day or more for adequate weight gain
- Treatment of iron deficiency anemia to increase oxygen-carrying capacity

SURGERY/OTHER PROCEDURES
- Surgical correction with either a VSD patch or repair is commonly used. Postsurgical outcomes for isolated VSD are excellent. Complications are rare and include reoperation for residual VSD, extended hospital stay, arrhythmias, valve injury, depressed ventricular function, and heart block (2)[B]
- Percutaneous transcatheter device closure has become a safe and effective option for some children with small to moderate VSDs. Complications include valvular regurgitation, residual defects, and heart block. There is a greater risk of conduction abnormality with this technique compared to surgical closure. Recent studies have shown steroids may decrease this risk (3)[A]
- Perventricular device closure (hybrid technique) of some subtypes of isolated VSDs without cardiopulmonary bypass is feasible under transesophageal echocardiographic (TEE) guidance. Complications are similar to percutaneous closure (4)[A].

ADMISSION, INPATIENT, AND NURSING CONSIDERATIONS
- Failure to thrive
- Pulmonary overcirculation/CHF
- Stabilize airway
- Reduce temperature stress.
- Frequent vital sign monitoring; daily weight and calorie counts
- Discharge criteria: CHF stabilization, weight gain, or successful repair

 ## ONGOING CARE

FOLLOW-UP RECOMMENDATIONS
- Small VSDs without evidence of CHF or pulmonary HTN generally can be followed every 1 to 5 years after the neonatal period
- Moderate to large VSDs require more frequent follow-up
- Potential complications of VSDs include right ventricular outflow obstruction and aortic valve prolapse

Patient Monitoring
- Physical growth and development monitoring
- Influenza vaccine for children >6 months of age
- Palivizumab to children <12 months of age with hemodynamically significant lesions. Children with small VSDs do not need RSV prophylaxis (5)[A].

DIET
- Low sodium in heart failure
- High calorie in failure to thrive

PATIENT EDUCATION
- No activity restriction in absence of pulmonary HTN
- Parents need support and instructions for prevention of complications until the child is ready for surgery.

PROGNOSIS
- Congenital:
  – Course is variable depending on the size of the VSD
  – Small VSD: Many will close spontaneously by age 3 years. Muscular defects are more likely to close spontaneously.
  – Large VSD: CHF or failure to thrive in infancy necessitating surgical repair
  – 20-year cumulative survival rate after surgery for isolated VSD is 87%; 40 years is 78% (6)
  – Progressive pulmonary vascular disease and pulmonary HTN are the most feared complications of VSD caused by left-to-right shunting and may eventually lead to reversal of the shunt (Eisenmenger complex). Death usually occurs in the 4th decade of life if untreated.
- Post-MI:
  – With medical management alone, 80–90% mortality in the first 2 weeks
  – Prognosis worse with inferior MI compared with anterior MI

COMPLICATIONS
- CHF
- Aortic insufficiency
- Sudden death
- Hemoptysis
- Cerebral abscess
- Paradoxical emboli
- Cardiogenic shock
- Heart block rarely may accompany surgical closure
- Pulmonary HTN, particularly Eisenmenger complex

REFERENCES
1. Wilson W, Taubert KA, Gewitz M, et al. Prevention of infective endocarditis: guidelines from the American Heart Association: a guideline from the American Heart Association Rheumatic Fever, Endocarditis, and Kawasaki Disease Committee, Council on Cardiovascular Disease in the Young, and the Council on Clinical Cardiology, Council on Cardiovascular Surgery and Anesthesia, and the Quality of Care and Outcomes Research Interdisciplinary Working Group. *Circulation.* 2007;116(15):1736–1754.
2. Scully BB, Morales DL, Zafar F, et al. Current expectations for surgical repair of isolated ventricular septal defects. *Ann Thorac Surg.* 2010;89(2): 544–549.
3. Yang L, Tai BC, Khin LW, et al. A systematic review on the efficacy and safety of transcatheter device closure of ventricular septal defects (VSD). *J Interv Cardiol.* 2014;27(3):260–272.
4. Yin S, Zhu D, Lin K, et al. Perventricular device closure of congenital ventricular septal defects. *J Card Surg.* 2014;29(3):390–400.
5. American Academy of Pediatrics Committee on Infectious Diseases, American Academy of Pediatrics Bronchiolitis Guidelines Committee. Updated guidance for palivizumab prophylaxis among infants and young children at increased risk of hospitalization for respiratory syncytial virus infection. *Pediatrics.* 2014;134(2):415–420.
6. Menting ME, Cuypers JA, Opić P, et al. The unnatural history of the ventricular septal defect: outcome up to 40 years after surgical closure. *J Am Coll Cardiol.* 2015;65(18):1941–1951.

ADDITIONAL READING
Penny DJ, Vick GW III. Ventricular septal defect. *Lancet.* 2011;377(9771):1103–1112.

 ## SEE ALSO

Acute Coronary Syndromes: NSTE-ACS (Unstable Angina and NSTEMI); Down Syndrome; Tetralogy of Fallot

 ## CODES

ICD10
- Q21.0 Ventricular septal defect
- I23.2 Ventricular septal defect as current comp following AMI
- Q21.3 Tetralogy of Fallot

CLINICAL PEARLS
- A loud 2/6 to 3/6 low-pitched harsh holosystolic murmur at the left lower sternal border is typical.
- A diastolic rumble at the apex indicates moderate to large VSD or ratio of pulmonary to systemic blood flow (Qp/Qs) >2:1, which likely will require surgical or percutaneous closure.
- Disappearance of the murmur could be secondary to spontaneous closure of the defect or the development of pulmonary HTN.
- Development of a new murmur of semilunar valve insufficiency should be further evaluated. Pulmonary regurgitation may occur as PVR increases, and the development of aortic regurgitation usually will require early surgery.

V

VERTIGO

James J. Arnold, DO, FACOFP

 BASICS

DESCRIPTION

- A symptom, not a disease process. Causes can be peripheral or central, benign, or life-threatening.
- May be described as a sensation of movement ("room spinning") when no movement is actually occurring
- System(s) affected: nervous, cardiovascular, psych
- Synonym(s): dizziness

EPIDEMIOLOGY

Incidence

- Vertigo/dizziness accounts for >4 million ED visits a year in United States, of which 80–85% have no serious underlying condition (1).
- Predominant sex: female = male; women are 3 times more likely to experience vertiginous migraine (2).

Geriatric Considerations

- Keep a higher index of suspicion for cardiovascular disease, arrhythmias, and orthostatic hypotension.
- Benign paroxysmal positional vertigo (BPPV) is more common in ages 50 to 70 years (2), an important risk factor for falls but is often undiagnosed.
- Medications are implicated almost 1/4 of the time (2).

Prevalence

- Ranges from 5% to 10% within the general population
- Lifetime prevalence for BPPV is 2.4%.

ETIOLOGY AND PATHOPHYSIOLOGY

- Dysfunction of the rotational velocity sensors of the inner ear results in asymmetric central processing; combination of sensory disturbance of motion and malfunction of the central vestibular apparatus
- Peripheral causes: acute vestibular neuritis, BPPV (posterior canal 85–95%, lateral canal 5–15%), Ménière disease, otosclerosis, acute labyrinthitis, cholesteatoma, perilymphatic fistula, superior canal dehiscence syndrome, motion sickness (2). BPPV, vestibular neuritis, and Ménière disease account for majority of peripheral causes (2).
- Central causes: cerebellar tumor, stroke, migraine, vestibular ischemia (1),(2)
- Drug causes: psychotropic agents, anticonvulsants, aspirin, aminoglycosides, furosemide (diuretics), amiodarone, α-/β-blockers, nitrates, urologic medications, muscle relaxants, phosphodiesterase inhibitors (sildenafil), excessive insulin, ethanol, quinine, cocaine
- Other causes: orthostasis, arrhythmia, psychological

Genetics

Family history of CVD/migraines may indicate higher risk of central causes.

RISK FACTORS

- History of migraines
- History of CVD/risk factors for CVD
- Use of ototoxic medications
- Trauma/barotrauma
- Perilymphatic fistula
- Heavy weight-bearing
- Psychosocial stress/depression
- Exposure to toxins

GENERAL PREVENTION

If due to motion sickness, consider pretreatment with anticholinergics, such as scopolamine.

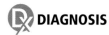 **DIAGNOSIS**

HISTORY

- Do not rely on symptom quality—often unreliable. Focus on timing and triggers (2).
  - TiTrATE is a clinically useful evaluation tool: **T**iming, **Tr**iggers, **A**nd a **T**argeted **E**valuation (1),(2).
  - Timing: episodic or continuous. Episodic may last seconds to a few days. Continuous lasts days to weeks.
    - If continuous, assess for trauma or toxins (including prescribed and recreational).
    - To further evaluate continuous, spontaneous vertigo, perform HINTS exam (1),(2),(3) (see "Physical Exam").
    - If episodic, assess for triggers.
  - **Tr**iggers: present or absent
    - If triggers, perform Dix-Hallpike maneuver (see "Physical Exam").
    - Do not confuse *worsening* of symptoms with motion to be the same as triggering. Many central vertigos are worse with movement (1),(2).
    - If no triggers, assess for hearing loss, migraines, or psych symptoms. Cardiovascular causes may also fall into this category.
  - **A**nd a **T**argeted **E**valuation: See "Physical Exam" for more details.
- Specific history items that suggest a diagnosis:
  - Unilateral hearing loss suggests Ménière disease (2). Further assess to determine if sensorineural versus conductive because the latter suggests otosclerosis.
  - Symptoms triggered by sudden change in head position suggest BPPV.
  - Symptoms triggered when going from sitting to standing suggests orthostatic hypotension.
  - History of migraines suggests vestibular migraine. Differentiate from nonmigrainous headaches, which can also be present with CNS tumors.
  - Depressed mood/anxiety with episodic vertigo that has since become continuous suggests psychiatric causes.
  - History of unilateral sensory or motor symptoms indicates a central cause such as TIA or CVA until proven otherwise.
  - Onset after decompression (diving, flying) suggests decompression sickness or barotrauma and warrants emergency evaluation.

PHYSICAL EXAM

- Cardiovascular: orthostatic blood pressure assessment on patients with episodic symptoms (1),(2)
- HEENT: may identify barotrauma, otosclerosis, cholesteatoma. Also check Rinne and Weber tests if hearing loss.
- Neurologic: Assess for nystagmus in all patients (2).
  - Vertical nystagmus is almost always of central origin.
  - Nystagmus of peripheral origin may be horizontal or rotational.
- Dix-Hallpike maneuver: for episodic, triggered vertigo (2),(4): Rapidly move the patient from a seated to supine position with the head turned 45 degrees to the right and held just over (below) the edge of the exam table. Observe for nystagmus and patient report of vertigo. Nystagmus/vertigo may not appear immediately. Wait until symptoms resolve and then return the patient to the sitting position. Repeat on the left.
  - The presence of extinguishing horizontal nystagmus is a positive test for BPPV. If induced nystagmus does not subside however, consider central causes and perform HINTS.
  - Vertical nystagmus always indicates a central cause even if triggered by Dix-Hallpike.
  - In primary care, PPV of 83% for BPPV and NPV of 52%
  - If Dix-Hallpike negative, check for lateral canal BPPV with a log roll test (4).
  - If duration and trigger of symptoms are not consistent with BPPV, do not perform Dix-Hallpike to avoid overlooking a central cause.
- HINTS exam: Perform for continuous, spontaneous vertigo with spontaneous nystagmus (1),(2),(3).
  - Horizontal **H**ead **I**mpulse: Rapidly and repeatedly bring patient's head to midline from 20 degrees. Patients with vestibular neuritis will show rapid saccades to refocus on a target. With normal peripheral nervous function, eyes stay on target, raising concern for central causes.
  - Direction changing **N**ystagmus: Having already assessed for presence and direction of nystagmus, now check for changing direction. Nystagmus that changes direction with eye motion indicates a central lesion.
  - **T**est of **S**kew: Vertical eye movement during cover-uncover test indicates a central lesion. A normal test has no movement.
  - A combination of these findings is 96.8% sensitive and 98.5% specific for CVA/other central cause (HINTS positive) (3)[C].
  - If a patient meets criteria for HINTS exam, do not perform Dix-Hallpike.
- Perform a full neuro exam if diagnosis not already clear, paying attention to sensation, gait, and Romberg testing.

DIFFERENTIAL DIAGNOSIS

Causes (1),(2):

- BPPV (episodic, triggered, positive Dix-Hallpike)
- Orthostatic hypotension (episodic, triggered, positive orthostatic blood pressure drop)
- Ménière disease (episodic, spontaneous, associated with unilateral sensorineural hearing loss)
- Otosclerosis (spontaneous, duration varies, unilateral conductive hearing loss)
- Vestibular migraine (episodic, associated with migraine HA)
- CVD (continuous, spontaneous; HINTS exam shows normal horizontal head impulse, direction-changing nystagmus, or vertical skew on cover-uncover)
- Posterior fossa tumor (continuous, spontaneous)
- Psychiatric (associated psych symptoms)
- Medication/toxin (continuous, medication/substance history, evaluation otherwise negative)
- Other cardiovascular such as arrhythmia (episodic, often no triggers or triggered by exertion)

- Hypoglycemia (episodic, associated medications or comorbidities)
- Perilymphatic fistula, canal dehiscence (trauma including suspicion of barotrauma from history)
- Decompression sickness (acute, recent dive or flight)
- Degenerative neurologic disease (often progressive by history, associated neurologic findings)
- Peripheral neuropathy

DIAGNOSTIC TESTS & INTERPRETATION
Initial Tests (lab, imaging)
- Labs not routinely necessary unless abnormal neuro exam and identify a cause in <1% of patients (2)[C]
- Obtain STAT MRI if a central cause is suspected to rule out stroke. CT cannot reliably see the posterior fossa and will not show changes in the early stages of an infarct. Vertigo may be the only symptom of acute stroke (3)[C].
- ENT/audiology referral if Ménière disease suspected for electronystagmography (2)[C]
- If acoustic neuroma is suspected, either CT or MRI to evaluate internal auditory canal (2)[C]

Diagnostic Procedures/Other
Audiometry if acoustic neuroma or Ménière disease is suspected

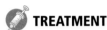 **TREATMENT**

GENERAL MEASURES
Treatments depend on cause.
- If medication is likely cause: Stop medication and reassess (2).
- BPPV: Epley maneuver and modified Epley maneuver (2)[A] (Epley maneuver–YouTube) (5)[B]
- Vestibular neuritis and labyrinthitis
  – Vestibular-suppressant medications (2)[C]
  – Vestibular rehabilitation exercises (2)[B]
  – No evidence to support improvement of symptoms with corticosteroid use (6)[B]
- Ménière disease (see separate topic) (2)[B]:
  – Low-salt diet (<1 to 2 g/day)
  – Diuretics such as hydrochlorothiazide
- Perilymphatic fistula, canal dehiscence—consult ENT (2).
- Vascular ischemia: prevention of future events through blood pressure reduction, lipid lowering, smoking cessation, antiplatelet therapy, and anticoagulation, if necessary (2),(3)[C]; MRI or CT if suspected
- Vertiginous migraines: dietary and lifestyle modifications, vestibular rehab, prophylactic and abortive medications (2)[C]
- Psychological: SSRIs are better than benzodiazepines for anxiety-related vertigo. Use slow titration to avoid worsening symptoms (7)[B].

MEDICATION
Avoid use of medication in mild cases. Use for a few days only because longer use may impair adaptation/compensation by the brain (2); medications not recommended for BPPV (4)[C]
- Meclizine: 12.5 to 50.0 mg PO q4–8h (2)
- Dimenhydrinate: 50 mg PO q6h (2)
  – Precautions: prostatic hyperplasia, glaucoma
  – Adverse effects: sedation, xerostomia

- Prochlorperazine: 5 to 10 mg PO or IM q6–8h; 25 mg rectally q12h; 5 to 10 mg by slow IV over 2 minutes (2)
  – Contraindications: blood dyscrasias, age <2 years, hypotension
  – Precautions: acutely ill children, glaucoma, breast cancer history, impaired cardiac function, prostatic hyperplasia
  – Adverse effects: sedation, extrapyramidal effects
- Metoclopramide: 5 to 10 mg PO q6h, 5 to 10 mg slow IV q6h (2)
  – Contraindications: concomitant use of drugs with extrapyramidal effects, seizure disorders
  – Precautions: history of depression, Parkinson disease, hypertension
  – Adverse effects: sedation, fluid retention, constipation
- Psychiatric causes
  – SSRIs preferred for frequent vertigo related to depression/anxiety (6)[B]
  – Lorazepam (Ativan) 0.5 to 2.0 mg PO, IM, or IV q4–8h for short-term relief of more severe anxiety-related vertigo
  – Diazepam (Valium) 2 to 10 mg PO or IV q4–8h for short-term relief of more severe symptoms

Geriatric Considerations
Use vestibular-suppressant medications with caution due to increased risk of falls and urinary retention.

Pregnancy Considerations
Meclizine and dimenhydrinate are pregnancy Category B.

ISSUES FOR REFERRAL
Consider referral to otolaryngologist, ENT specialist, vestibular rehabilitation therapist, or neurologist if patient requires further care.

ADDITIONAL THERAPIES
- Epley maneuver/modified Epley maneuver for BPPV to displace calcium deposits in the semicircular canals (4)[A]
  – Effective for short-term symptomatic improvement and for converting patient from positive to negative Dix-Hallpike maneuver. Some studies suggest long-term relief (4)[C].
- Lateral canal BPPV may respond to barbecue roll maneuver (4)[C].
- Vestibular rehabilitation exercises: ball toss, lying-to-standing, target-change, thumb-tracking, tightrope, walking turns (7)[B]

 ONGOING CARE

FOLLOW-UP RECOMMENDATIONS
Balance exercises should be adhered to for symptom reduction and return to normal activities of daily living (ADLs).

Patient Monitoring
After 1 to 2 weeks, assess for the following:
- Recurrence or new symptoms
- Medication-related adverse effects

DIET
- Restricted salt intake for Ménière disease
- Dietary modifications for vertiginous migraine

PATIENT EDUCATION
Avoid triggers such as caffeine/alcohol (vertiginous migraine).

PROGNOSIS
Depends on diagnosis and response to treatment

COMPLICATIONS
- Anxiety, depression
- Disability, injuries from falls

REFERENCES
1. Newman-Toker DE, Edlow JA. TiTrATE: a novel, evidence-based approach to diagnosing acute dizziness and vertigo. *Neurol Clin.* 2015;33(3):577–599.
2. Muncie H, Sirmans S, James E. Dizziness: approach to evaluation and management. *Am Fam Physician.* 2017;95(3):154–162.
3. Yew KS, Cheng EM. Diagnosis of acute stroke. *Am Fam Physician.* 2015;91(8):528–536.
4. Bhattacharyya N, Baugh RF, Orvidas L, et al; for American Academy of Otolaryngology-Head and Neck Surgery Foundation. Clinical practice guideline: benign paroxysmal positional vertigo. *Otolaryngol Head Neck Surg.* 2008;139(5 Suppl 4):S47–S81.
5. Hilton M, Pinder D. The Epley (canalith repositioning) manoeuvre for benign paroxysmal positional vertigo. *Cochrane Database Syst Rev.* 2014;(12):CD003162.
6. Fishman JM, Burgess C, Waddell A. Corticosteroids for the treatment of idiopathic acute vestibular dysfunction (vestibular neuritis). *Cochrane Database Syst Rev.* 2011;(5):CD008607.
7. Swartz R, Longwell P. Treatment of vertigo. *Am Fam Physician.* 2005;71(6):1115–1122.

 SEE ALSO

- Ménière Disease; Motion Sickness; Vertigo, Benign Paroxysmal Positional (BPPV)
- Algorithm: Dizziness

CODES

ICD10
- R42 Dizziness and giddiness
- H81.10 Benign paroxysmal vertigo, unspecified ear
- H81.49 Vertigo of central origin, unspecified ear

CLINICAL PEARLS
- TiTrATE your assessment.
- Acute, spontaneous, continuous vertigo with a normal horizontal head impulse, direction-changing nystagmus, and skew deviation (HINTS positive) is highly sensitive and specific for CVA.
- Episodic, triggered vertigo with positive Dix-Hallpike test is consistent with BPPV.
- If patient warrants a HINTS exam, do not perform Dix-Hallpike because central cause can also produce a positive Dix-Hallpike.
- The Epley maneuver is recommended for the treatment of BPPV.
- Medications are not recommended for BPPV.

V

Chirag N. Shah, MD • Kyung In Yoon, MD

 BASICS

DESCRIPTION

- Benign paroxysmal positional vertigo (BPPV) is a mechanical disorder of the inner ear characterized by a brief period of vertigo experienced when the position of the patient's head is changed relative to gravity.
- Vertigo results from the mismatch of the perception of movement by the visual, vestibular, and proprioceptive symptoms when none exist.
- The brief period of vertigo is caused by abnormal stimulation of ≥1 of the 3 semicircular canals of the inner ear, with the posterior canal most commonly affected.
- BPPV is the single most common cause of vertigo.

EPIDEMIOLOGY

- Lifetime prevalence is 2.4%, and 1-year incidence is 0.6%.
- Age of onset is most commonly between the 5th and 7th decades of life.
- Incidence increases with each decade of life.
- Prevalent sex: female > male
- BPPV affects the quality of life of elderly patients and is associated with reduced activities of daily living scores, falls, and depression.

Incidence
1-year incidence 0.6%

Prevalence
Lifetime prevalence 2.4%

ETIOLOGY AND PATHOPHYSIOLOGY

- In BPPV, calcite particles (otoconia) that normally weigh the sensory membrane of the maculae become dislodged and settle into the semicircular canal, changing the dynamics of the canal. Reorientation of the canal relative to gravity causes the otoconia to move to the lowest part of the canal, causing displacement of the endolymph, deflection of the cupula, and activation of the primary afferent. This results in the generation of nystagmus and the associated sensation of vertigo.
- BPPV may be idiopathic, posttraumatic, or associated with viral neurolabyrinthitis.

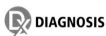 **DIAGNOSIS**

- The diagnosis is established based on history and findings on positional testing, clarified by Dix and Hallpike in 1952 (1),(2)[A].
- Positional tests place the plane of the canal being tested into the plane parallel with gravity.
- Systematic approach to prevent misdiagnosis or failure to recognize a stroke, notably posterior stroke (3)[C]

HISTORY

- Most common form of triggered episodic vestibular syndrome. Brief in duration with head motion intolerance.
- Patients present with usual chief complaint of dizziness, light-headedness, and/or feeling "off balance."
- Brief episodes of vertigo (sensation that the room is spinning) are associated with
  - Rolling over in bed
  - Getting out of bed
  - Looking up (referred to as "top-shelf syndrome")
  - Bending forward
  - Quick head movements
- Frequently, patients complain of nausea and, if severe enough, vomiting.

PHYSICAL EXAM

- The Dix-Hallpike test (DHT) is used to diagnose BPPV (1)[A]. The test provokes the characteristic nystagmus associated with the symptoms of vertigo, with an estimated sensitivity of 79% (95% CI 65–94) and specificity of 75% (95% CI 33–100) (2)[B].
  - To perform the DHT, rapidly move the patient from seated to the supine position with the head turned 45 degrees to the right and held just over (below) the edge of the exam table. The position is maintained for 45 to 60 seconds. Observe for nystagmus and patient report of vertigo. Nystagmus/vertigo may not appear immediately. Wait until symptoms resolve and then return the patient to the sitting position. Repeated on the left. The position is maintained for 45 to 60 seconds.
- The direction of the fast phase of the nystagmus, along with any latency period before onset and duration of the nystagmus, before it ceases is recorded.
- BPPV is consistent with a latency period of <30 seconds between lowering the head and the subsequent onset of nystagmus; the eye movements peak then slowly resolve within 40 seconds. The direction of the nystagmus reverses when the patient's head is brought back upright and to the neutral position. Repeated testing results in diminished vertiginous symptoms and nystagmus fatigue.
- DHT followed by canalith repositioning movement (CRM) for treatment; it aims to reduce CT utilization and LOS.
- The following characteristics help to distinguish a peripheral etiology for the patient with vertigo versus a central cause:
  - Triggered nystagmus (vs. spontaneous or gaze)
  - Onset is sudden (vs. sudden or slow).
  - Severity is intense spinning (vs. less intense).
  - Pattern is paroxysmal (vs. constant).
  - Symptoms are aggravated by movement (vs. variable).
  - Nausea or diaphoresis is frequent (vs. variable).

- Nystagmus has rotatory-vertical, horizontal eye movements (vs. vertical).
- Symptoms fatigue (vs. ongoing)
- Hearing loss or tinnitus may occur (vs. not typically an associated symptom).
- An abnormal TM may be seen (vs. this is not an associated finding).
- CNS symptoms are not associated (vs. CNS findings usually present).
- Red flags in vertigo
  - Neurologic deficit, ipsilateral hearing loss, gait abnormality, direction-changing nystagmus (nystagmus that changes its direction with different body and head positions)
- Head Impulse Nystagmus Test of Skew (HINTS) + no hearing loss
  - Head impulse test of vestibulo-ocular reflex function
    ○ Normally, eye movement will correct with rapid head movement so that the center of the vision remains on a target. This reflex fails in peripheral causes of vertigo.
    ○ Have patient fix their eyes on your nose and move their head in the horizontal plane to the left and then to the right.
    ○ When the head is turned toward the normal side, the vestibulo-ocular reflex remains intact and eyes are fixated on the examiner's nose.
    ○ When the head is turned toward the affected side, the vestibulo-ocular reflex fails and the eyes make a corrective saccade to refixate on the examiner's nose.
    ○ It is reassuring if the reflex is *abnormal* (due to dysfunction of the peripheral nerve).
  - Unidirectional gaze-evoked nystagmus
  - Test for skew deviation "vertical dysconjugate gaze."
    ○ Skew deviation is a fairly specific predictor of central lesion in patients with acute vestibular syndrome.
    ○ The presence of skew may help identify stroke when a positive head impulse test falsely suggests a peripheral lesion.
    ○ Have patient look at your nose with their eyes and start by covering one eye and then rapidly move to cover the other eye; do this rapidly back and forth.
    ○ When each eye is uncovered, quickly look to see if the eye has movement or refixation. Horizontal is normal; vertical is not.
  - In the setting of dizziness and vertigo, HINTS substantially outperforms ABCD2 for stroke diagnosis and outperforms MRI obtained within the first 2 days after symptom onset (4)[B].
  - Use of HINTS is limited in evaluation in the ED to specifically rule out a stroke in those presenting with acute vestibular syndromes (5).

DIFFERENTIAL DIAGNOSIS

- Orthostatic hypotension and other disorders that cause low BP; symptoms usually occur when the patient stands up.
- Damage to the brainstem or cerebellum can cause positional vertigo but is accompanied by other neurologic signs and usually has a different pattern of nystagmus.
- Low spinal fluid pressure may cause positional symptoms that are better when the patient lies down.
- Migraine-associated vertigo
- Traumatic brain injury
- Brain tumors, hemorrhage or infarction
- Vestibular neuronitis

DIAGNOSTIC TESTS & INTERPRETATION

Systematic approach: triage, TiTrATE, then treatment

- TiTrATE approach: Timing, Triggers, and Targeted examinations (3)[C]
  - Timing classifies the disease processes into episodic versus continuous.
  - Triggers further seeks to find underlying causes by looking at exam findings (e.g., Dix-Hallpike).
  - Targeted examination and ancillary tests are based on findings.
- Combination of all this information allows the clinician to further evaluate with CT or MRI.

TREATMENT

- The CRP or Epley maneuver is effective in the treatment of posterior canal BPPV (6)[A]. Using a particle repositioning maneuver, the clinician moves the patient through a series of positions. In randomized controlled trials, the average short-term success rate of the CRP following one treatment session is 80% ± 9% (6)[A].
- The clinician moves the patient through a series of four provoking positions:
  - Placement of the right posterior canal (involved canal) in the right head-hanging position of the DHT
  - The head is then rotated a total of 90 degrees toward the left (uninvolved side) into 45 degrees of left head rotation.
  - Maintaining 45 degrees of left head rotation, the patient is rolled onto the left side (uninvolved side) with the head slightly elevated from the supporting surface.
  - The patient then sits up and flexes the neck 36 degrees. Each position is maintained for a minimum of 45 seconds or as long as the nystagmus lasts. The procedure is repeated 3 times.
- CRP is the best maneuver for posterior BPPV and should be offered to all age groups (3)[A].
- Semont maneuver is also another maneuver, less superior when performed alone (3)[A].
- Lempert roll maneuver (3)[C]

- Contraindications are carotid stenosis, unstable cardiac disease, and severe neck disease. If the CRP is ineffective, self-administered CRP is performed at home (1)[A]. The patient performs the CRP on the bed with the head extended over the edge of a pillow. Better outcomes are achieved with a combination of CRP with self-administered CRP.
- CRP and Semont are ineffective for horizontal BPPV; variations of the Lempert maneuver, barbecue roll, or Gufoni maneuver are widely used treatment methods for horizontal BPPV.
- Postmaneuver activity restrictions were previously advocated, but in controlled trials, it did not differ in clinical outcomes (1)[A],(3)[A].

MEDICATION

- Vestibular suppressant medications are not recommended for the treatment of BPPV, other than for the short-term management of vegetative symptoms (2)[A].
- Antiemetics such as ondansetron (Zofran) may be considered for prophylaxis for patients who have had severe nausea or vomiting with the DHT.
- Vestibular suppressants such as benzodiazepines and antihistamine anticholinergics such as meclizine should be avoided because they may suppress nystagmus during the DHT and treatment.

ISSUES FOR REFERRAL

Consider a referral to a specialist if BPPV is unresponsive to treatment or if the patient is diagnosed with atypical BPPV involving the anterior or lateral canal. Consider referring to a physical therapist, a neurologist, or an otolaryngologist.

ADDITIONAL THERAPIES

- Brandt-Daroff exercises and habituation exercises are not as effective as self-administered CRP. At 1 week, the average success rate for the Brandt-Daroff exercise is 23–24% compared with 90% for self-administered CRP (1)[A].
- Surgical intervention is rarely indicated, except for refractory BPPV, and includes posterior canal occlusion and singular neurectomy.

ONGOING CARE

FOLLOW-UP RECOMMENDATIONS
The patient should follow up within a week after treatment to ensure resolution.

PATIENT EDUCATION
A number of illustrative YouTube videos are available for education and self CRP maneuvers.

PROGNOSIS
80% cure rate with CRP maneuvers, with a 30% recurrence rate at 1 year, and 44% redevelop BPPV within 2 years

COMPLICATIONS
During the maneuvers, a canal conversion may occur. The debris from the canal being treated may reflux into another canal.

REFERENCES

1. Devaiah AK, Andreoli S. Postmaneuver restrictions in benign paroxysmal positional vertigo: an individual patient data meta-analysis. *Otolaryngol Head Neck Surg*. 2010;142(2):155–159.
2. Halker RB, Barrs DM, Wellik KE, et al. Establishing a diagnosis of benign paroxysmal positional vertigo through the Dix-Hallpike and side-lying maneuvers: a critically appraised topic. *Neurologist*. 2008;14(3):201–204.
3. Bhattacharyya N, Gubbels SP, Schwartz SR, et al. Clinical practice guideline: benign paroxysmal positional vertigo (update). *Otolaryngol Head Neck Surg*. 2017;156(3 Suppl):S1–S47.
4. Newman-Toker DE, Kerber KA, Hsieh YH, et al. HINTS outperforms ABCD2 to screen for stroke in acute continuous vertigo and dizziness. *Acad Emerg Med*. 2013;20(10):986–996.
5. Kattah JC, Talkad AV, Wang DZ, et al. HINTS to diagnose stroke in the acute vestibular syndrome: three-step bedside oculomotor examination more sensitive than early MRI diffusion-weighted imaging. *Stroke*. 2009;40(11):3504–3510.
6. Hilton MP, Pinder DK. The Epley (canalith repositioning) manoeuvre for benign paroxysmal positional vertigo. *Cochrane Database Syst Rev*. 2014;(12):CD003162.

ADDITIONAL READING

Epley JM. The canalith repositioning procedure: for treatment of benign paroxysmal positional vertigo. *Otolaryngol Head Neck Surg*. 1992;107(3):399–404.

CODES

ICD10
- H81.10 Benign paroxysmal vertigo, unspecified ear
- H81.12 Benign paroxysmal vertigo, left ear
- H81.11 Benign paroxysmal vertigo, right ear

CLINICAL PEARLS

- The diagnosis of BPPV is based on history and findings on positional testing.
- The typical presentation is a report of transient episodes of vertigo (sensation that the room is spinning) associated with a change in position of the head relative to gravity.
- BPPV may be treated effectively with particle-repositioning maneuvers in the office and at home.
- Vestibular suppressant medications and antiemetics are not recommended for treatment of BPPV, other than for the short-term management of symptoms.
- Patients should always be ambulated in order to verify normal gait prior to discharge.

V

VINCENT STOMATITIS

Daniel V. Girzadas Jr., MD • Edward N. Northrup, MD

BASICS

DESCRIPTION
- A distinct form of periodontal disease due to inflammatory infection of the gingiva, characterized by pain, ulcerations, and necrotizing damage to interdental papillae
- Caused by an imbalance of oral flora, resulting in a predominance of invasive anaerobic bacteria, such as *Fusobacterium*, *Prevotella intermedia*, and spirochetes
- Concomitant infection with Epstein-Barr virus, herpes simplex virus, and type 1 human cytomegalovirus is common.
- Organisms invade gingiva and interdental papillae and form a gray pseudomembranous exudate.
- Clinical presentation includes pain, fetid breath, gingival ulcerations, bleeding, and interdental papillary necrosis. It is differentiated from other periodontal diseases by rapid onset, pain, ulcerated gingival mucosa, and "punched out" interdental papillary necrosis.
- Synonym(s): Vincent angina; Vincent's disease; trench mouth; fusospirochetal gingivitis; acute necrotizing ulcerative gingivitis (ANUG); necrotizing ulcerative gingivitis (NUG)
- Necrotizing gingivitis, necrotizing periodontitis, and necrotizing stomatitis are classified together under the umbrella term necrotizing periodontal disease (NPD).

EPIDEMIOLOGY
Incidence
- Predominant age: 18 to 30 years in developed countries
- Malnourished children ages 3 to 14 years
- Affects both genders with similar frequency
- Historically, incidence increased in military personnel exposed to battlefield conditions (1)

Prevalence
- True prevalence is unknown, but probable overall prevalence <1% (1).
- Rare disease in developed countries; however, in recent data prevalence rate was 6.7% in Chilean students between 12 and 21 years and approaching 25% in children in sub-Saharan African countries (2),(3).
- Prevalence is low in healthy children up to age 18 years and more common in persons aged 18 to 30 years. Increased prevalence with malnutrition, immunocompromise, poor oral hygiene, and smoking

ETIOLOGY AND PATHOPHYSIOLOGY
- Impaired host immunologic response due to immunocompromised state or malnutrition
- Disruption of normal oral flora with predominance of invasive anaerobic bacteria (*Treponema* spp., *Selenomonas* spp., *Fusobacterium* spp., and *Prevotella intermedia*) (2)
- Loss of integrity and necrosis of the gingival mucosa and interdental papillae
- Increased bacterial attachment with active herpesvirus infection

RISK FACTORS
- Malnutrition
- Immunosuppression (HIV, cancer and chemotherapy)
- Diabetes
- Lower socioeconomic status
- Tobacco use
- Poor oral hygiene, infrequent or absent dental care
- Orthodontics
- Herpesvirus infection
- Psychological stress

GENERAL PREVENTION
- Appropriate nutrition
- Proper oral hygiene
- Regular dental care
- Prompt recognition and institution of therapy
- Management of medical problems such as cancer and HIV infection
- Smoking cessation
- Stress management

COMMONLY ASSOCIATED CONDITIONS
- Seen most commonly in malnourished patients, patients undergoing cancer treatment, or those from underdeveloped countries
- HIV infection
- Vitamin deficiencies
- Bacteremia
- Osteomyelitis
- Tooth loss
- Chronic gingivitis
- Dehydration
- Noma (cancrum oris), which can be life-threatening
- Aspiration pneumonia

DIAGNOSIS

HISTORY
- Acute onset of oral pain
- Gingival ulcerations
- Fetid odor of breath
- Bleeding and necrosis of interdental papillae
- Cervical adenopathy
- Fever
- Malaise
- Immunosuppression
- Chemotherapy
- Active herpesvirus infection or HIV

PHYSICAL EXAM
- Fetid odor of breath
- Ulceration of gingival mucosa
- Inflamed, erythematous gingiva
- Necrosis of interdental papillae
- Gingival bleeding
- Formation of gray, pseudomembranous exudate
- Cervical and submandibular lymphadenopathy
- Fever

DIFFERENTIAL DIAGNOSIS
- Herpes simplex virus
- Periodontitis
- Recurrent aphthous stomatitis
- Medication side effects
- Oral malignancy
- Xerostomia
- Diphtheria
- Lymphoma/leukemia
- Primary syphilis
- Ascorbic acid deficiency
- Gingivitis
- Behçet disease
- Granulomatosis with polyangiitis
- Oral mucositis
- Erosive lichen planus
- Oral histoplasmosis

DIAGNOSTIC TESTS & INTERPRETATION
Initial Tests (lab, imaging)
Diagnosis is primarily based on clinical exam, but if systemic illness or invasive spread to deeper tissue or bone is suspected, the following studies should be considered:
- Aerobic and anaerobic cultures of inflamed or debrided tissue
- Group A strep rapid antigen detection assay or throat culture
- Blood cultures if systemic involvement
- Dental radiographs
- CT imaging of the face and neck if infection has progressed

Diagnostic Procedures/Other
Although biopsy could be performed for histopathology, the diagnosis is largely clinical in nature. Microbiology testing often does not add relevant diagnostic information given many of these bacterial pathogens are typical of healthy gingiva and other nonspecific cases of gingivitis and periodontitis (1).

TREATMENT

GENERAL MEASURES
- Multimodal treatment approach with superficial débridement, oral hygiene, antimicrobial mouthwash, and consideration for oral antibiotics in those with poor response to débridement or those with symptoms of systemic involvement (fever, malaise, vomiting).
- Débridement can be accomplished by cotton-topped swab soaked with hydrogen peroxide for gentle local débridement, rinse with hydrogen peroxide or chlorhexidine, ultrasonic débridement with a dental specialist, or surgical débridement under local anesthesia.
- Elimination of tobacco, improved nutritional status, and improved immunologic status will increase rate of healing and reduce risk of future gingival disease.

MEDICATION

Most cases are treatable on outpatient basis. Severe disease with systemic effects and/or neck involvement requires inpatient treatment. Other than chlorhexidine, there is no role for topical antibiotics, given they cannot effectively penetrate the periodontal tissue (2).

First Line

- Chlorhexidine gluconate 0.12% 15 mL 30 seconds rinse/spit twice daily (1)[C] *plus*
- Penicillin V potassium 250 to 500 mg PO q6h PO for 5 to 7 days for adults and children >12 years of age *or*
- Metronidazole 250 to 500 mg PO or IV q8h for 7 to 10 days (1)[C],(2)[C],(4)[C]; pediatric dosing: 30 to 50 mg/kg/day divided q8h (3)[A] *or*
- Amoxicillin 250 to 500 mg PO q8h PO for 7 days (4)[C]; pediatric dosing: 25 to 45 mg/kg/day divided q12h *or*
- Amoxicillin-clavulanate 875 mg PO q12h for 7 to 10 days; pediatric dosing: 25 to 45 mg/kg/day divided q12h (based on amoxicillin component) *or*
- Clindamycin 450 mg PO or 600 mg IV q8h for 7 to 10 days; pediatric dosing: 8 to 25 mg/kg/day divided q6–8h
- Some historical data suggests combination therapy of metronidazole with either amoxicillin or penicillin V potassium

Second Line

- Tetracycline 250 to 500 mg QID PO for 10 days (do not use for children <8 years of age); pediatric dosing: 25 to 50 mg/kg/day divided q6h *or*
- Erythromycin 250 to 500 mg q6–12h PO for 10 days; pediatric dosing: 30 to 50 mg/kg/day divided q6–8h

Pediatric Considerations

- Chlorhexidine and alcohol mouth rinses are generally avoided due to risk of ingestion, but chlorhexidine may be prescribed in gel form for topical application.
- Alternatively, can consider 3% hydrogen peroxide diluted by half with water as a safer mouthwash in children to help remove pseudomembranous coating and decrease bleeding (3).
- In addition to amoxicillin or amoxicillin-clavulanate, metronidazole may be considered as first-line oral therapy (refer to dosing above) (3)[A].

ISSUES FOR REFERRAL

Severe disease requires débridement by consultant dentist, oral surgeon, or ENT specialist.

ADDITIONAL THERAPIES

- Warm saline rinses q2h
- Sodium bicarbonate toothpaste, brush q2h
- Viscous lidocaine 2% 1 tbsp rinse/spit q6–8h
- NSAID medications q4–12h
- Opioid analgesics q4–6h (severe pain)
- Treatment of underlying immunodeficiency (if present)

SURGERY/OTHER PROCEDURES

- Débridement of inflamed/necrotic gingival tissue
- Dental extraction
- Gingival restoration
- Adjuvant therapies
  - Low-level laser therapy (LLLT) has been shown in one case series to decrease pain and accelerate healing.
  - Photochemotherapy has been shown to reduce bleeding ulcers and bacterial counts compared to conventional therapy alone (5)[B].

COMPLEMENTARY & ALTERNATIVE MEDICINE

3% hydrogen peroxide and warm sterile saline in a 1:1 ratio q2–3h as an oral rinse (1)[C]

ADMISSION, INPATIENT, AND NURSING CONSIDERATIONS

- Severe disease, failure of oral antibiotics, or ongoing comorbidities
- Parenteral antibiotics and/or analgesia requirement
- Inability to tolerate PO

 ONGOING CARE

FOLLOW-UP RECOMMENDATIONS

- Close dental follow-up
- Primary care follow-up
- Specialty follow-up (if underlying immunodeficiency)

DIET

- Soft diet until healed
- Balanced nutritional diet
- Multivitamin supplementation

PATIENT EDUCATION

- Proper nutrition
- Oral hygiene
- Tobacco cessation

PROGNOSIS

- With appropriate treatment, including chlorhexidine rinse, systemic antibiotics, débridement if necessary, and smoking cessation, infection usually completely resolves in 5 to 7 days.
- Maintenance of adequate oral hygiene is needed to prevent recurrence.

COMPLICATIONS

- Pain
- Malnutrition
- Gingival/tooth loss
- Deep infection of neck
- Systemic infection
- Cancrum oris (Noma), an often fatal gangrenous orofacial lesion particularly in resource-scarce environments

REFERENCES

1. Dufty J, Gkranias N, Donos N. Necrotising gingivitis: a literature review. *Oral Health Prev Dent*. 2017;15(4):321–327.
2. Malek R, Gharibi A, Khlil N, et al. Necrotizing ulcerative gingivitis. *Contemp Clin Dent*. 2017;8(3):496–500.
3. Marty M, Palmieri J, Noirrit-Esclassan E, et al. Necrotizing periodontal diseases in children: a literature review and adjustment of treatment. *J Trop Pediatr*. 2016;62(4):331–337.
4. Atout RN, Todescan S. Managing patients with necrotizing ulcerative gingivitis. *J Can Dent Assoc*. 2013;79:d46.
5. Siddiqui AZ, Vellappally S, Fouad H, et al. Bactericidal and clinical efficacy of photochemotherapy in acute necrotizing ulcerative gingivitis. *Photodiagnosis Photodyn Ther*. 2020;29:101668.

ADDITIONAL READING

- Hegde S, Madhurkar JG, Sruthi G, et al. Conservative management of necrotizing gingival disease—a case report. *IOSR J Dent Med Sci*. 2020;19(8):019–022.
- Herrera D, Retamal-Valdes B, Alonso B, et al. Acute periodontal lesions (periodontal abscesses and necrotizing periodontal diseases) and endo-periodontal lesions. *J Clin Periodontol*. 2018;45(Suppl 20):S78–S94.
- Hu J, Kent P, Lennon JM, et al. Acute necrotising ulcerative gingivitis in an immunocompromised young adult. *BMJ Case Rep*. 2015;2015:bcr2015211092.
- Sangani I, Watt E, Cross D. Necrotizing ulcerative gingivitis and the orthodontic patient: a case series. *J Orthod*. 2013;40:77–80.

CODES

ICD10

A69.1 Other Vincent's infections

CLINICAL PEARLS

- Immunosuppression, malnourishment, smoking, and poor oral hygiene are key risk factors for necrotizing ulcerative gingivitis.
- Diagnosis is largely clinical based on symptoms of oral pain, fetid breath, gingival ulcerations, interdental papillary necrosis, and grayish exudate on the gingival surface.
- Most patients experience rapid improvement following appropriate treatment with gentle débridement, chlorhexidine rinses, improved oral hygiene, and oral antibiotics.
- Smoking cessation and treatment of malnutrition or underlying illness are additional important treatment considerations.
- Severe disease requires extensive débridement of necrotic gingival tissue and close follow-up with a periodontal specialist or oral surgeon to limit recurrence and prevent rapid destruction of the periodontium.

V

VITAMIN B₁₂ DEFICIENCY

Sahil Mullick, MD • Maisam T. Begum, MD

BASICS

- Vitamin deficiency related to inadequate intake or absorption of cobalamin (vitamin B_{12})
- Cobalamin is critical for central nervous system myelination, red blood cell production, and DNA synthesis.
- Deficiency can cause megaloblastic anemia, bone marrow dysfunction, and diverse and potentially irreversible neuropsychiatric changes.
- Neuropsychiatric disorders are due to demyelination of cervical, thoracic dorsal, and lateral spinal cords; demyelination of white matter; and demyelination of cranial and peripheral nerves.
- Elevated MMA and homocysteine levels may be early markers of vitamin B_{12} deficiency (1).

DESCRIPTION
Normal vitamin B_{12} absorption

- Vitamin B_{12} is a water-soluble vitamin present in animal-source foods and foods fortified with vitamin B_{12}.
- Dietary vitamin B_{12} (cobalamin) bound to food is cleaved by acids in stomach and bound to haptocorrin (commonly known as R-factor).
- Duodenal proteases cleave vitamin B_{12} from haptocorrin.
- In duodenum, vitamin B_{12} uptake depends on binding to intrinsic factor (IF) secreted by gastric parietal cells.
- Vitamin B_{12}–IF complex is absorbed by terminal ileum into portal circulation.
- Body's vitamin B_{12} stored in liver = 50–90%
  - Vitamin B_{12} secreted into bile from liver recycled via enterohepatic circulation
  - Delay 5 to 10 years from onset of vitamin B_{12} deficiency to clinical symptoms due to hepatic stores and enterohepatic circulation
- Typical Western diet: 5 to 30 mg/day; however, only 1 to 5 mg/day is effectively absorbed.
  - Recommend 2.4 mg/day for adults and 2.6 mg/day during pregnancy and 2.8 mg/day during lactation (most prenatal vitamins contain vitamin B_{12}).

EPIDEMIOLOGY
Prevalence
- Endemic area: Northern Europe, including Scandinavia; more common in those of African ancestry
- Increasing recognition in breastfed-only infant populations with vitamin B_{12}–deficient mothers (2)
- Prevalence 5–20% in developed countries
- Prevalence in those <60 years old is 6%, and in those >60 years old, it is 20%.

ETIOLOGY AND PATHOPHYSIOLOGY
- Decreased oral intake
  - Vegetarians and vegans: Vitamin B_{12} is found in animal source foods.
- Decreased IF
  - Pernicious anemia (PA): can be associated with autoantibodies directed against gastric parietal cells and/or IF
  - Chronic atrophic gastritis: autoimmune attack on gastric parietal cells causing autoimmune gastritis and leading to decreased IF production
  - Gastrectomy: removal of entire or part of stomach

- Decreased absorption
  - Crohn disease: Terminal ileal inflammation decreases body's ability to absorb vitamin B_{12}.
  - Chronic alcoholism: decreases body's ability to absorb vitamin B_{12}
  - Gluten hypersensitivity (celiac disease) intestinal villi atrophy and subsequent malabsorption
  - Ileal resection
  - Pancreatic insufficiency: Pancreatic proteases are required to cleave the vitamin B_{12}–haptocorrin bond to allow vitamin B_{12} to bind to IF.
  - *Helicobacter pylori* infection: impairs release of vitamin B_{12} from bound proteins
- Medications:
  - Proton pump inhibitors (PPIs), H_2 antagonists, and antacids decrease gastric acidity, inhibiting vitamin B_{12} release from dietary protein; metformin
  - Metformin usage can cause calcium-dependent membrane inhibition, interfering with vitamin B_{12}–IF absorption
- Hereditary (rare)
- Causes:
  - Food-cobalamin malabsorption syndrome
    ○ As many as 60–70% of cases
    ○ Primary cause in elderly
    ○ Pathophysiology: inability to release cobalamin from food or binding protein, especially if in the setting of hypochlorhydria
    ○ Seen in atrophic gastritis, long-term ingestion of antacids and biguanides, possible relationship to *H. pylori* infection
  - PA
    ○ 15–30% of all cases; most frequent cause of severe disease. Neurologic disorders are common presenting complaints.
    ○ Common in elderly, as high as 20%, with mild atrophic gastritis, hypochlorhydria, and impaired release of dietary vitamin B_{12}
    ○ Antigastric parietal cell antibodies: sensitivity >90%, specificity 50%; use for screening test.
  - Insufficient dietary intake: 2% of cases; vegans or long-standing vegetarians
  - Infants born to vitamin B_{12}–deficient mothers may develop it if breastfed exclusively.
  - Intestinal causes:
    ○ 1% of cases; prevalence depends on risk factors, such as surgical conditions.
    ○ Gastrectomy: due to decreased production of IF
    ○ Gastric bypass: appears 1 to 9 years after surgery, prevalence 12–33%
    ○ Ileal resection or disease
    ○ Fish tapeworm
    ○ Severe pancreatic insufficiency
  - Undetermined etiology

Genetics
Imerslund-Gräsbeck disease (juvenile megaloblastic anemia) caused by mutations in the amnionless (AMN) or cubilin (CUBN) genes with autosomal recessive pattern of inheritance; inadequate ileal uptake of vitamin B_{12}-IF complex and vitamin B_{12} renal protein reabsorption

GENERAL PREVENTION
Eating a diet with foods that contain vitamin B_{12} such as meat, fish, poultry, and dairy

COMMONLY ASSOCIATED CONDITIONS
- Gastric abnormalities: PA, gastritis, gastrectomy/bariatric surgery
- Small bowel disease: malabsorption syndrome, ileal resection, IBD, celiac disease
- Pancreatitis: pancreatic insufficiency
- Diet: breastfed infant in vitamin B_{12}–deficient mother, strict vegan diet
- Medications: neomycin, metformin, PPI, histamine 2 receptor antagonists, nitrous oxide (NO) abuse (3)

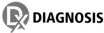

DIAGNOSIS
Symptoms and physical exam findings:

- Asymptomatic patients may be diagnosed by the incidental finding of anemia or an elevated mean corpuscular volume (MCV) during routine testing or evaluation of unassociated disorders.
- Neuropsychiatric
  - Frequent: sensory polyneuritis, paresthesias, positive Babinski sign, weakness, gait unsteadiness, loss of proprioception (impaired vibratory sensation, positive Romberg, ataxia, hyperreflexia)
  - Classic but uncommon: subacute combined degeneration of spinal cord associated with PA; areflexia, ataxia, proprioception and vibration loss, bowel and bladder incontinence, orthostatic hypotension, decreased memory, mania, delirium, psychosis, depression
- Digestive
  - Classic: Hunter glossitis, jaundice, and high lactate dehydrogenase and bilirubin
  - Possible: abdominal pain, dyspepsia, nausea, vomiting, diarrhea
  - Rare: mucocutaneous ulcers
- Other
  - Frequent: fatigue with exertion, skin pallor, palpitations, edema, jaundice
  - Under investigation: chronic vaginal and urinary infections, atrophy of vaginal mucosa, hypofertility, venous thromboembolism, angina, miscarriages

HISTORY
- Underlying disease associated with vitamin B_{12} deficiency
- Fatigue, anorexia
- Depression
- Falls (due to diminished proprioception), loss of sensation in "stocking-glove" distribution
- Glossitis/loss of sense of taste

PHYSICAL EXAM
- Lymphadenopathy, hepatosplenomegaly, enlarged tongue (glossitis)
- Neurologic exam: impaired vibratory sense, altered proprioception possible ataxia, diminished sensations in light touch, and/or weakness

DIFFERENTIAL DIAGNOSIS
Folate deficiency, copper deficiency, hypothyroidism

DIAGNOSTIC TESTS & INTERPRETATION

- Measurement of vitamin B$_{12}$, complete blood count (MCV)
- Measurement of vitamin B$_{12}$ may be low or low normal depending on institution's cutoff value.
  - 95–97% sensitive levels <200 pg/mL
  - May need additional tests such as MMA and homocysteine if vitamin B$_{12}$ level is low normal (<350 pg/mL)
- MCV often increased
- Measurement of MMA
  - More sensitive and specific than homocysteine
  - Levels increased in renal failure and volume depletion.
- Measurement of homocysteine
  - Levels increased in folate deficiency, renal failure, homocystinuria; vitamin B$_6$ deficiency and hypothyroidism (1)
- MMA and homocysteine levels only reliable in an untreated patient because levels fall with supplementation
- Other tests: folate and other markers of anemia (iron studies)
- MCV may be normal, decreased, or increased if vitamin B$_{12}$ deficiency coexists with other forms of anemia, such as iron deficiency or hemolysis. Thus, RBCs may be normochromic, normocytic, or hypochromic microcytic.
- Holotranscobalamin (holo-TC) accounts for approximately 10% of the circulating vitamin B$_{12}$ and is the earliest marker showing vitamin B$_{12}$ depletion. It is also known as active vitamin B$_{12}$ which is the only form of vitamin B$_{12}$ that is taken up and used by the cells in the body.

ALERT
- Low levels of vitamin B$_{12}$ are seen in folate deficiency, HIV, and multiple myeloma.
- Elevated levels of vitamin B$_{12}$ are seen in renal disease, occult malignancy, and alcoholic liver disease and as a result of technical error.
- Macrocytosis may be due to folate deficiency, reticulocytosis, medications, bone marrow dysplasia, and hypothyroidism or be masked by concomitant microcytic anemia.
- In asymptomatic individuals, vitamin B$_{12}$ deficiency associated with reductions in the binding protein haptocorrin. However, this condition may be difficult to discriminate from true vitamin B$_{12}$ deficiency in the presence of symptoms.
- Check antibody to IF; positive test is confirmatory for PA, but sensitivity is only 50–70%.
- For antibody positive patients, consider screening for autoimmune thyroid disease.
- For patients with negative anti-IF result and high suspicion for PA, check serum gastrin level (elevated level is consistent with diagnosis of PA).

Pregnancy Considerations
- Pregnant women with low vitamin B$_{12}$ have higher risk of having children with neural tube defects, developmental delay, failure to thrive, hypotonia, ataxia, and anemia.
- Exclusively breastfed infants of mothers who are vitamin B$_{12}$ deficient are at risk of developing vitamin B$_{12}$ deficiency. Infants might not show signs or symptoms until 4 to 6 months of age, which may include developmental regression, feeding difficulties, lethargy, or hypotonia.

ALERT
Children born to mothers with normal to high folate levels and low serum vitamin B$_{12}$ values have higher truncal adiposity and insulin resistance which may influence long-term risk of development of type 2 diabetes and cardiovascular disease.

- Low vitamin B$_{12}$ has a negative influence on children's development and cognitive functioning; may cause growth and motor retardation (2)
- Untreated severe vitamin B$_{12}$ deficiency during pregnancy can lead to severe anemia, peripheral neuropathy, cognitive decline, and a variety of neuropsychiatric manifestations.
- May also manifest with microangiopathic hemolytic anemia and thrombocytopenia, mimicking other thrombotic microangiopathy disorders such as atypical hemolytic uremic syndrome, HELLP syndrome, and thrombotic thrombocytopenic purpura

Initial Tests (lab, imaging)
Vitamin B$_{12}$ level, MMA level, homocysteine level

Diagnostic Procedures/Other
Bone marrow exam is usually unnecessary.

Test Interpretation
- If vitamin B$_{12}$ level is:
  - >400 pg/mL, no deficiency
  - Between 150 and 399 pg/mL, obtain MMA level and homocysteine level.
  - <150 pg/mL deficiency is present.
- If MMA and homocysteine level testing is warranted
  - If MMA levels and homocysteine levels are high, vitamin B$_{12}$ deficiency is confirmed.
  - If MMA levels are normal but homocysteine levels are high, folate deficiency is confirmed.
  - If both are normal, vitamin B$_{12}$ deficiency is unlikely.

 TREATMENT

All individuals with documented vitamin B$_{12}$ deficiency should be treated, unless there's a strong reason not to such as patient refusal or palliative care setting.

GENERAL MEASURES
Repleting deficiency can be done over weeks; must be done urgently in symptomatic patients

MEDICATION
- Parenteral cyanocobalamin replacement recommended in patients with severe neurologic symptoms or severe anemia: IM cyanocobalamin (4)
  - 1,000 μg injected every other day for 1 to 2 weeks, then
  - 1,000 μg every week for 1 month, then
  - 1,000 μg once a month for life
- Can also use high-dose, daily oral cyanocobalamin at doses of 1,000 to 2,000 μg (5)

ALERT
Folic acid without vitamin B$_{12}$ in patients with PA is contraindicated; it will not correct neurologic abnormalities.

ADMISSION, INPATIENT, AND NURSING CONSIDERATIONS
Consider blood transfusion for severe anemia.

 ## ONGOING CARE

FOLLOW-UP RECOMMENDATIONS
Patient Monitoring
- Hematologic
  - Reticulocytosis in 1 week
  - Hemoglobin will usually return to normal in 6 to 8 weeks
  - Monitor potassium in profoundly anemic patients (hypokalemia due to potassium use).
- Neurologic: improvement within 6 weeks to 3 months of treatment; however, maximum improvement noticed at 6 to 12 months. Some symptoms may be irreversible.

DIET
Meat, animal protein, foods fortified with B$_{12}$ unless contraindicated

REFERENCES

1. Lee SM, Oh J, Chun MR, et al. Methylmalonic acid and homocysteine as indicators of Vitamin B$_{12}$ deficiency in patients with gastric cancer after gastrectomy. *Nutrients.* 2019;11(2):450.
2. Honzik T, Adamovicova M, Smolka V, et al. Clinical presentation and metabolic consequences in 40 breastfed infants with nutritional vitamin B$_{12}$ deficiency—what have we learned? *Eur J Paediatr Neurol.* 2010;14(6):488–495.
3. Stabler SP. Clinical practice. Vitamin B$_{12}$ deficiency. *N Engl J Med.* 2013;368(2):149–160.
4. Devalia V, Hamilton MS, Molloy AM; for British Committee for Standards in Haematology. Guidelines for the diagnosis and treatment of cobalamin and folate disorders. *Br J Haematol.* 2014;166(4):496–513.
5. Green R. Vitamin B$_{12}$ deficiency from the perspective of a practicing hematologist. *Blood.* 2017;129(19):2603–2611.

 ## CODES

ICD10
- D51 Vitamin B$_{12}$ deficiency anemia
- D51.3 Other dietary vitamin B$_{12}$ deficiency anemia
- D51.8 Other vitamin B$_{12}$ deficiency anemias

CLINICAL PEARLS

- Vitamin B$_{12}$ deficiency can coexist with other anemia; thus, MCV can be normal, decreased, or increased.
- For PA, cyanocobalamin must be lifelong.

V

VITAMIN D DEFICIENCY

Frank J. Domino, MD

BASICS

This topic covers the commonly acquired vitamin D deficiency and not type II vitamin D–resistant rickets/type I pseudovitamin D–resistant rickets (both rare autosomal recessive disorders).

DESCRIPTION
- Vitamin D is a hormone and a vitamin.
- Cholecalciferol (D_3) is synthesized in the skin by exposure to ultraviolet B (UV-B) radiation. Ergocalciferol (D_2) and D_3 are present in foods.
- D_2 and D_3 are hydroxylated in the liver to 25 vitamin D (calcidiol), the major circulating form.
- Calcidiol is further hydroxylated in the kidney to the active metabolite 1,25 vitamin D (calcitriol).
- Hypocalcemia stimulates parathyroid hormone (PTH) secretion, which prompts increased conversion of 25 vitamin D to 1,25 vitamin D.
  - 1,25 vitamin D decreases renal calcium and phosphorus excretion, increases intestinal calcium and phosphorus absorption, and increases osteoclast activity. The net result is an increase in serum calcium.

EPIDEMIOLOGY
The overall prevalence rate of vitamin D deficiency has been reported to be around 40%. Rates are highest rate in blacks (82%), followed by Hispanics (69%). Vitamin D deficiency was more common among individuals who were obese, had no college education, were in poor overall health, had hypertension, low HDL, and did not consume milk regularly (1).

Pediatric Considerations
NHANES data suggest 70% of children do not have sufficient 25-OH vitamin D serum levels (9% deficient and 61% insufficient); deficiency has been associated with an increase in BP and decrease in high-density lipoprotein (HDL) cholesterol.

ETIOLOGY AND PATHOPHYSIOLOGY
- Insufficient dietary intake of vitamin D and/or lack of UV-B exposure (in sunlight) results in low levels of vitamin D.
  - This limits calcium absorption, causing excess PTH release.
- PTH stimulates osteoclast activity, which helps to normalize calcium and phosphorous but results in osteomalacia.
- Dietary deficiency
  - Inadequate vitamin D intake
- Inadequate sunlight exposure
  - Institutionalized/hospitalized patients
- Chronic illness: liver/kidney disease
- Malabsorptive states (including inflammatory bowel diseases)

Genetics
Vitamin D–dependent rickets type 1 occurs due to inactivating mutation of the 1α-hydroxylase gene; as a result, calcidiol is not hydroxylated to calcitriol.

RISK FACTORS
- Inadequate sun exposure; dark skin
- Female; elderly; obesity
- Low socioeconomic status; immigrant populations; rates higher in Blacks and Hispanics.
- Latitudes higher than 38 degrees
- Institutionalized; depression
- Medications (phenobarbital, phenytoin); gastric bypass surgery/malabsorption syndromes

GENERAL PREVENTION
- Adequate exposure to sunlight and dietary sources of vitamin D (plants, fish); many foods are fortified with vitamin D_2 and D_3.
- Recommended minimum daily requirement is 600 IU/day from age 1 to 70 years and 800 IU/day for those >70 years. Up to 4,000 IU/day is safe in healthy adults without risk of toxicity.
- For ages 51 to 70 years, minimally recommended supplementation is 800 IU/day to prevent nonvertebral fractures.

Pediatric Considerations

ALERT
- The American Academy of Pediatrics recommends all breastfed babies receive 400 IU/day of vitamin D beginning "within the first few days of life."
- 2016 Global Consensus Recommendations suggest all infants, regardless of feeding method, begin vitamin D 400 IU within a few days of birth (1).

- Midgestational vitamin D deficiency doubled risk of autism spectrum disorder in European cohort (2).

Pregnancy Considerations
Insufficient data to recommend routine screening of all pregnancies; only "at risk" should be screened; it is safe to take 1,000 to 2,000 IU/day during pregnancy (3)[B].

COMMONLY ASSOCIATED CONDITIONS
- Osteomalacia, osteoporosis
- Premenstrual syndrome
- Rickets
- Celiac disease; gastric bypass
- Chronic renal disease
- Bacterial vaginosis in pregnant women
- Hypertension
- Cohort study found that vitamin D deficiency is correlated with increased risk of all-cause mortality.

ALERT
Vitamin D deficiency is associated with risk of myocardial infarction (MI) and all-cause mortality (4)[A].

DIAGNOSIS

- Nonspecific musculoskeletal complaints
- Weak antigravity muscles
- Fracture with minimal trauma

HISTORY
- Senior citizens at risk for falling
- Renal disease
- GI (malabsorption) disorders; liver dysfunction
- Immigration from tropical to colder climates
- Dark-skinned/veiled individuals
- Housebound patients
- Women at perimenopause

PHYSICAL EXAM
- Vague neurologic signs: numbness, proximal myopathy, paresthesias, muscle cramps, laryngospasm
- Chvostek sign: contraction of the facial muscles by tapping along the facial nerve
- Trousseau phenomenon: carpal spasms and paresthesia produced by pressure on nerves and vessels of the upper arm, by inflation of a BP cuff
- Tetany, seizures
- Bowed legs

DIFFERENTIAL DIAGNOSIS
- Malabsorptive disease (e.g., IBD, gastric bypass, celiac disease)
- Malnutrition

DIAGNOSTIC TESTS & INTERPRETATION
Initial Tests (lab, imaging)
- Only test those at increased risk for deficiency (those lacking dietary exposure, sun exposure, etc.).
- 25-OH vitamin D (most sensitive measure of vitamin D status)
- Vitamin D deficiency
  - <20 ng/mL
- PTH elevation: not routinely obtained unless severe deficiency
- Low-normal/low calcium and phosphorous
- Elevated alkaline phosphatase (in later disease)
- Plain radiographs: If atypical fracture, radiographs may show osteomalacia (pseudofractures/looser zones) in pelvis, femur, and fibula.
- Osteoporosis screen
  - Women ≥65 years with no risk factors
  - Women ≥60 years at risk: body weight <70 kg (best predictor)
  - Less evidence: smoking, low body mass index, family history, decreased activity, alcohol, or caffeine use
  - African American women have higher bone density than Caucasians.

TREATMENT

- Treatment goals remain unclear, but current "normal" 25-OH vitamin D levels are based on suppression of PTH.
- Obesity: Treatment of VDD in obesity, especially those who are obese and depressed, improves depressive symptoms and may improve weight loss.

ALERT
All-cause mortality: Cochrane Systematic Review found vitamin D supplementation lowers all-cause mortality (5)[A]. Recent long-term data show treatment to 25 vitamin D levels >30 ng/mL lowered both MI and all-cause mortality risk (6).

Geriatric Considerations
In senior citizens, serum 25-OH vitamin D of 20 ng/mL resulted in improved physical performance scores; recent data suggest supplementation may not improve fracture risk and remains unclear about a true benefit.

MEDICATION
- Vitamin D sufficient (25-OH vitamin D $\geq$20 ng/mL)
  - Vitamin D 800 to 2,000 IU/day D_2/D_3
  - D_3 (animal derived) may be slightly more effective than D_2 (plant derived)
  - Calcium supplementation: unclear benefit and may increase some CHD risk in patients; no supplementation currently required (see below)
- Vitamin D deficiency (25-OH vitamin D <20 ng/mL)
  - D_2 50,000 IU/week for 8 to 12 weeks, followed by 1,000 to 2,000 IU/day of vitamin D_3
- Calcium: meta-analysis data support
  - Dietary intake of ~700 mg/day leads to best outcomes; higher doses did NOT decrease risk of osteoporotic fractures.
  - Dietary calcium may be more beneficial than calcium supplementation.
  - Supplementary calcium associated with an increased risk of MI, especially in women, but this data remain controversial.
  - Supplementation of both vitamin D and calcium may increase risk of renal stone formation.

ISSUES FOR REFERRAL
Endocrinology if no response to treatment

ADDITIONAL THERAPIES
Aggressive calcium in ICU patients with ionized calcium <3.2 mg/dL or if symptomatic (tetany, seizures, QT prolongation, bradycardia, or hypotension or ventilated patient with decreased diaphragmatic function)

ADMISSION, INPATIENT, AND NURSING CONSIDERATIONS
- Symptoms of severe hypocalcemia
- Malabsorption syndromes

 ONGOING CARE

FOLLOW-UP RECOMMENDATIONS
Follow-up of abnormal 25-OH vitamin D not required

DIET
- Cod liver oil is most potent source of vitamin D and has ~1,300 IU vitamin D/tablet/tablespoon.
- Fatty fish (tuna, salmon)
- Fortified milk (100 IU/8 oz), cereal, and foods

PROGNOSIS
- Cancer
  - Systematic review of 63 observational studies found adequate 25-OH vitamin D levels correlate with lower rates of colon, breast, and prostate cancer.
  - Observational data show inverse relationship between serum 25-OH vitamin D levels and breast cancer.
  - Serum level >30 ng/mL lowered risk of bladder cancer (7).
  - Vitamin D supplementation lowers cancer mortality all-cause mortality (8).
- Cardiovascular disease: A serum 25 vitamin D level >30 ng/mL lowers MI risk (6) and CV mortality.
- Vitamin D supplementation reduces adverse events in asthma (9).
- Upper respiratory infections: Vitamin D supplementation lowers risk of upper respiratory infections (10).
- Other outcomes: Adequate vitamin D levels may lower pain scores in osteoarthritis of the knee, decrease PMS symptoms, lower risk of metabolic syndrome in women, lower dementia risk, and improve depression symptoms.

REFERENCES
1. Forrest KY, Stuhldreher WL. Prevalence and correlates of vitamin D deficiency in US adults. *Nutr Res*. 2011;31(1):48–54.
2. Vinkhuyzen AAE, Eyles DW, Burne THJ, et al. Gestational vitamin D deficiency and autism spectrum disorder. *BJPsych Open*. 2017;3(2):85–90.
3. American College of Obstetricians and Gynecologists Committee on Obstetric Practice. ACOG Committee Opinion No. 495: vitamin D: screening and supplementation during pregnancy. *Obstet Gynecol*. 2011;118(1):197–198.
4. Correia LC, Sodré F, Garcia G, et al. Relation of severe deficiency of vitamin D to cardiovascular mortality during acute coronary syndromes. *Am J Cardiol*. 2013;111(3):324–327.
5. Bjelakovic G, Gluud LL, Nikolova D, et al. Vitamin D supplementation for prevention of mortality in adults. *Cochrane Database Syst Rev*. 2011;(7):CD007470.
6. Acharya P, Dalia T, Ranka S, et al. The effects of vitamin D supplementation and 25-hydroxyvitamin D levels on the risk of myocardial infarction and mortality. *J Endocr Soc*. 2021;5(10):bvab124.
7. Zhao Y, Chen C, Pan W, et al. Comparative efficacy of vitamin D status in reducing the risk of bladder cancer: systematic review and meta-analysis. *Nutrition*. 2016;5:515–523.
8. Zhang Y, Fang F, Tang J, et al. Association between vitamin D supplementation and mortality: systematic review and meta-analysis. *BMJ*. 2019;366:l4673.
9. Jolliffe DA, Greenberg L, Hooper RL, et al. Vitamin D supplementation to prevent asthma exacerbations: a systematic review and meta-analysis of individual participant data [published correction appears in Lancet Respir Med. 2018 Jun;6(6):e27]. *Lancet Respir Med*. 2017;5(11):881–890.
10. Martineau AR, Jolliffe DA, Hooper RL, et al. Vitamin D supplementation to prevent acute respiratory tract infections: systematic review and meta-analysis of individual participant data. *BMJ*. 2017;356:i6583.

 CODES

ICD10
- E55 Vitamin D deficiency
- E55.0 Rickets, active
- E55.9 Vitamin D deficiency, unspecified

CLINICAL PEARLS
- Common risk factors for vitamin D deficiency include inadequate sun exposure or dietary intake, black or Hispanic ethnicity, and obesity.
- 25-OH vitamin D (most sensitive measure of vitamin D status) is the most sensitive laboratory test for diagnosis.
- Vitamin D deficiency is defined by serum levels <20 ng/mL.
- Up to 2,000 IU/day of supplemental vitamin D is safe in healthy adults without risk of toxicity.
- The American Academy of Pediatrics recommends all breastfed babies receive 400 IU/day of vitamin D beginning within a few days of birth.

V

VITAMIN DEFICIENCY

Tricia Bautista, MD • Jyothi R. Patri, MD, MHA, FAAFP, HMDC

 BASICS

DESCRIPTION
- Vitamins are essential micronutrients required for normal metabolism, growth, and development.
- Vitamin supplementation in food products, adequate food security, and availability of supplements make vitamin deficiencies less common in developed countries. Certain populations are at increased risk.
- Toxicity is rare for water-soluble vitamins, whereas possible with fat-soluble vitamins (A, D, E, K).

EPIDEMIOLOGY
Incidence
- Higher incidence seen in geriatric patients, pregnant women, exclusively breastfed infants, individuals with highly restricted diets or certain chronic disease states
- Increased risk among individuals from Africa and Southeast Asia
- True incidence is unknown because most vitamin deficiencies are asymptomatic.

Prevalence
- Varies by age groups, comorbid conditions, geography, and setting (i.e., urban, rural)
- The prevalence of vitamin B_{12} deficiency is ~6% in patients <60 years old and increases to ~20% after age 60 (1).
- Vitamin D deficiency prevalence is increased in individuals with darker skin pigmentation, obesity, low dietary intake of vitamin D, or low sunlight exposure. This deficiency is seen in ~5% of the general population, with non-Hispanic blacks having the highest prevalence.

ETIOLOGY AND PATHOPHYSIOLOGY
- Deficiency usually develops from one of five mechanisms: reduced intake, diminished absorption, increased use, increased demand, or increased excretion
- Chronic disease states: HIV, malabsorption (i.e., celiac sprue, short bowel syndrome), chronic liver and kidney disease, alcoholism, malignancies, pernicious anemia, inborn errors of metabolism
- Bariatric surgeries: gastric bypass, gastrectomy, small or large bowel resection
- Related to certain drugs: prednisone, phenytoin, isoniazid, protease inhibitors, methotrexate, phenobarbital, alcohol, nitrous oxide, H_2 receptor antagonists, metformin, colchicine, cholestyramine, 5-fluorouracil, 6-mercaptopurine, azathioprine, chloramphenicol, proton pump inhibitors, chronically used antibiotics, penicillamine, hydralazine
- Malnutrition, imbalanced nutrition, obesity, fad diets, extreme vegetarianism, total parenteral nutrition, bulimia/anorexia, other eating disorders, parasitic infection

Genetics
- Cystic fibrosis
- Hartnup disease, A-β-lipoproteinemia
- Rare genetic predisposition
  - Autoimmune disease (i.e., pernicious anemia)
  - Congenital enzyme deficiencies (i.e., biotinidase or holocarboxylase synthetase deficiency)
  - Transcobalamin II deficiency
  - Ataxia with vitamin E deficiency (AVED)

RISK FACTORS
Poverty, malnutrition, chronic excessive alcohol intake, chronic disease states, advanced age, dietary restrictions, bariatric surgery, certain medications, and exclusively breastfed infants

GENERAL PREVENTION
- Ingesting large and varied amounts of vitamin supplements increases risk of toxicity and drug–drug interactions and is not recommended.
- Antioxidant supplements have not been shown to impact cancer incidence; *increased* mortality risk seen in some studies (2)
- Avoid restrictive diets.
- USPSTF recommends against low-dose supplementation with vitamin D (<400 IU) and calcium (<1,000 mg) to reduce fracture risk in community-dwelling postmenopausal women (3).
- USPSTF concludes insufficient evidence of benefits and harms of daily supplementation with doses >400 IU of vitamin D and >1,000 mg of calcium for primary prevention of fractures in community-dwelling, postmenopausal women (3).
- USPSTF also concludes that current evidence is insufficient to assess the balance of the benefits and harms of vitamin D and calcium supplementation, for primary prevention of fractures in men and premenopausal women (3).
- USPSTF recommends all women planning or capable of pregnancy take a daily supplement containing 0.4 to 0.8 mg of folic acid (4)[A].
- USPSTF recommends against using β-carotene or vitamin E supplements for the prevention of cardiovascular disease or cancer (2).
- All infants should receive 400 IU/day of vitamin D soon after birth if exclusively or partially breastfed (5).

COMMONLY ASSOCIATED CONDITIONS
Anemia, neuropathies, dermatitis, visual disturbances

 DIAGNOSIS

HISTORY
- Review dietary intake and supplement use.
- Decreased visual acuity, night blindness
- Poor wound healing, easy bruising
- Skin changes, new rash
- Neuropathy
- Abnormal food cravings (pica)
- Osteomalacia, history of pathologic fracture
- Birth of a child with spina bifida
- Previous GI or bariatric surgery (1)
- Recurrent or persistent vomiting or diarrhea
- Prior or current medical conditions
  - Tuberculosis (TB), HIV infection, hepatitis, cancer
  - Hypermetabolic state: thyrotoxicosis, 2nd- or 3rd-degree burns, extensive or chronic wound, any systemic infection
- Chronic disease requiring steroids, disease-modifying antirheumatic drugs (DMARDs), or immunosuppressants
- Malabsorptive or chronic GI disorder: celiac disease, sprue, Crohn disease, ulcerative colitis, GERD

- Parenteral or enteral nutrition via tube feeding
- Pregnancy
- Amenorrhea or infertility issues
- Medications, supplements
- Food allergies or intolerances, fad or restrictive diet

PHYSICAL EXAM
- Neurologic exam: gait, memory/cognitive impairment, reflexes, sensory or motor impairment, peripheral neuropathy (1)
- Oropharyngeal exam: glossitis, bleeding gums, hyperemic pharynx, stomatitis, cheilitis (1)
- Skin exam: maculosquamous dermatitis, photosensitive pigmented dermatitis, ecchymosis, petechiae
- Visual assessment

DIFFERENTIAL DIAGNOSIS
Multiple conditions mimic signs and symptoms of vitamin deficiencies.
- Diabetes mellitus, thyroid disorders, hyperparathyroidism, heart failure, Alzheimer disease, multiple sclerosis, substance abuse, toxic ingestions, hematologic disorders/malignancies

DIAGNOSTIC TESTS & INTERPRETATION
Initial Tests (lab, imaging)
- No routine screening indicated
- Test if symptomatic, history indicates high risk, or clinical characteristics are present:
  - 25-OH vitamin D
    - Sufficient levels are >20 ng/mL (20 to 50 ng/mL is a level that is safe and sufficient for skeletal health).
    - Vitamin D insufficiency is 12 to 20 ng/mL.
    - Vitamin D deficiency is <12 ng/mL (increased risk of rickets and osteomalacia) (6).
  - Prothrombin time (PT)/partial thromboplastin time (PTT)
  - Vitamin B_{12} and folate levels (1)
  - Serum homocysteine and methylmalonic acid (if high suspicion of vitamin B_{12} deficiency with normal B_{12} level)
  - Retinol serum level, retinol-binding protein
- Cyanocobalamin, thiamine, vitamin A
- Ancillary tests:
  - BUN, calcium, phosphorus, magnesium
  - Albumin, liver function tests
  - CBC
  - Parathyroid hormone
- Bone densitometry for:
  - Women ≥65 years old without previous fractures or risk factors
  - Women <65 years old whose 10-year fracture risk is equal to a 65-year-old white woman without additional risk factors
- Disease states from vitamin deficiency
  - Vitamin A (retinol): night blindness, complete blindness, xerophthalmia
  - Vitamin B_1 (thiamine)
    - Wernicke encephalopathy: acute syndrome with memory disturbance, truncal ataxia, nystagmus, ophthalmoplegia
    - Korsakoff syndrome: anterograde and retrograde amnesia, confabulation

○ Dry beriberi: symmetric motor and sensory peripheral neuropathy, paresthesias, loss of reflexes
○ Wet beriberi: neuropathy with cardiovascular symptoms of peripheral vasodilation, high-output failure, dyspnea, and tachycardia
○ Infantile beriberi: loud piercing cry, cyanosis, tachycardia, cardiomegaly, dyspnea, vomiting, seizures
– Vitamin B_2 (riboflavin): glossitis, stomatitis, cheilitis, hyperemia of the pharyngeal mucosal membranes, normocytic-normochromic anemia
– Vitamin B_3 (niacin): pellagra = photosensitive pigmented dermatitis, dementia, and diarrhea
– Vitamin B_5 (pantothenic acid): paresthesias and dysesthesias ("burning feet syndrome"), anemia
– Vitamin B_6 (pyridoxine): dermatitis, cheilosis, atrophic glossitis, stomatitis, neuropathy
– Vitamin B_9 (folate): megaloblastic anemia, rarely manifest neurologic symptoms
– Vitamin B_{12} (cobalamin): pernicious anemia, leukopenia, pancytopenia, shuffling broad-based gait, atrophic glossitis, loss of vibration and position sense, cognitive impairment, areflexia, olfactory impairment, peripheral neuropathy, hyperpigmentation, jaundice, vitiligo
– Vitamin C (ascorbic acid): scurvy = ecchymoses, bleeding gums and petechiae; hyperkeratosis, arthralgias, impaired wound healing
– Vitamin D (calciferol): rickets, osteomalacia
– Vitamin E: neuromuscular disorders and hemolysis
– Vitamin K: easy bruising, mucosal bleeding, melena, hematuria
– Biotin: changes in mental status, dysesthesias, nausea, maculosquamous dermatitis of the extremities

 TREATMENT

MEDICATION
- Ask patients about supplement use; encourage patients to bring vitamin and supplement bottles for review.
- Assess for potential adverse drug effects/reactions. Patients with alcohol use disorders should receive thiamine, folic acid, and MVI.
- Give patients with suspected thiamine deficiency 100 mg thiamine prior to IV fluids containing glucose to prevent precipitating Korsakoff psychosis.
- Treat vitamin D deficiency with weekly 50,000 IU of oral ergocalciferol for 6 to 8 weeks. Recommended daily supplementation for children, adolescents and adults up to age 70 is 600 IU/day. Those aged >71 years old is 800 IU/day.
- If there is concomitant B_{12} and folate deficiency, start vitamin B_{12} first to avoid precipitating subacute combined degeneration of the spinal cord (1).
- Consider obtaining prealbumin/albumin levels and a dietary consult for malnourished patients.
- Bariatric surgery patients will need lifelong vitamin supplementation; there are no consensus practice guidelines for supplement dosing regimens.

Geriatric Considerations
- Vitamin B_{12} deficiency exists in ~20% of patients age >60 years. Treat symptomatic or severe deficiency with an IM injection of cyanocobalamin 1,000 μg/day 3 times a week for 2 weeks. For neurologic symptoms, give same dose every other day for 3 weeks or until symptom resolution. To prevent recurrence or treat mild deficiency, take daily oral vitamin B_{12} 1,000 μg or monthly IM vitamin B_{12} 1,000 μg. High-dose (1,000 to 2,000 μg/day) oral treatment is as effective as monthly IM injections, but use caution with malabsorption or compliance issues (1)[C].
- Vitamin D deficiency target level of >30 ng/mL minimizes risk of falls and fractures in the elderly.

Pediatric Considerations
- Vitamin K deficiency increases bleeding risk.
  - More common in neonates because they lack intestinal flora that produces vitamin K during the 1st week of life.
  - Condition peaks 2 to 10 days after birth: bleeding from the umbilical stump and/or circumcision site, generalized bruising, and GI hemorrhage.
  - Infrequent in developed countries due to routine injection of newborns with vitamin K (1 mg)
- Vitamin D deficiency increases risk of rickets.
  - Vitamin D supplementation (400 IU/day) is recommended for all infants starting in the first few days of life.
  - 600 IU/day of vitamin D is recommended for children >12 months and adults either through diet or supplementation.
  - Morbidly obese and minority children are at increased risk for vitamin D deficiency.
- In children age >6 months in developing countries, vitamin A supplementation has been shown to decrease mortality.

Pregnancy Considerations
All pregnant women and women of childbearing age considering pregnancy are strongly encouraged to take a multivitamin containing at least 0.4 mg folic acid daily to prevent neural tube defects (4)[A].

 ONGOING CARE

DIET
Vitamins are best used by the body from food intake. Supplements should be used where it is not feasible to ingest the recommended amount of a particular vitamin.

PATIENT EDUCATION
- Drug–drug interactions may occur between vitamins and medications. Patients should report all supplements and medications to their health care provider.
- Risk of vitamin toxicity is most common with fat-soluble vitamins (A, D, E, K).

PROGNOSIS
Most vitamin deficiencies are fully reversible if treated without undue delay.

COMPLICATIONS
- Vitamin toxicities
- Liver failure (vitamins A, D, E, K)
- Desquamation of skin (vitamin A)
- Neuropathy (vitamin B_6)
- Kidney stones (vitamin C, vitamin D)
- Hypercoagulability (vitamin K)
- Pseudohyperparathyroidism (vitamin D)
- Masking of pernicious anemia (folic acid)

REFERENCES
1. Langan RC, Goodbred AJ. Vitamin B_{12} deficiency: recognition and management. *Am Fam Physician.* 2017;96(6):384–389.
2. Moyer VA; for U.S. Preventive Services Task Force. Vitamin, mineral, and multivitamin supplements for the primary prevention of cardiovascular disease and cancer: U.S. Preventive Services Task Force recommendation statement. *Ann Intern Med.* 2014;160(8):558–564.
3. Kahwati LC, Weber RP, Pan H, et al. Vitamin D, calcium, or combined supplementation for the primary prevention of fractures in community-dwelling adults: evidence report and systematic review for the US Preventive Services Task Force. *JAMA.* 2018;319(15):1600–1612.
4. Bibbins-Domingo K, Grossman DC, Curry SJ, et al; for U.S. Preventive Services Task Force. Folic acid supplementation for the prevention of neural tube defects: US Preventive Services Task Force recommendation statement. *JAMA.* 2017;317(2):183–189.
5. Wagner CL, Greer FR; and American Academy of Pediatrics Section on Breastfeeding, American Academy of Pediatrics Committee on Nutrition. Prevention of rickets and vitamin D deficiency in infants, children, and adolescents. *Pediatrics.* 2008;122(5):1142–1152.
6. Giustina A, Adler RA, Binkley N, et al. Controversies in vitamin D: summary statement from an international conference. *J Clin Endocrinol Metab.* 2019;104(2):234–240.

ADDITIONAL READING
- Herrick KA, Storandt RJ, Afful J, et al. Vitamin D status in the United States, 2011–2014. *Am J Clin Nutr.* 2019;110(1):150–157.
- Tack J, Deloose E. Complications of bariatric surgery: dumping syndrome, reflux and vitamin deficiencies. *Best Pract Res Clin Gastroenterol.* 2014;28(4):741–749.
- U.S. Department of Agriculture and U.S. Department of Health and Human Services. *Dietary Guidelines for Americans, 2020–2025.* 9th edition. Washington, DC: U.S. Department of Agriculture and U.S. Department of Health and Human Services; 2020.

 CODES

ICD10
- E56.9 Vitamin deficiency, unspecified
- E56.0 Deficiency of vitamin E
- E55.9 Vitamin D deficiency, unspecified

CLINICAL PEARLS
- In healthy adults, multivitamins have no value if dietary intake is adequate.
- Vitamin D supplementation (400 IU/day) is recommended for all infants.
- No routine screening for Vitamin D deficiency is indicated.

V

VITILIGO

Sonia Rivera-Martinez, DO, FACOFP • Karen Sheflin, DO

 BASICS

DESCRIPTION

- An acquired depigmentation of the skin, which correlates with a loss of epidermal melanocytes. There are three clinical variants, each with subtypes.
- Localized: often in childhood, rapid onset then stabilizes. Involvement of hair is common early in the course; lacks associated autoimmune diseases
  - Focal: few lesions, random distribution
  - Segmental: Lesions occur within a dermatome (mostly trigeminal) or may follow Blaschko lines. Lesions usually stop abruptly at the midline.
  - Mucosal: only mucosal surfaces involved
- Generalized/nonsegmental (most common variant): progressive, with flares, commonly associated with autoimmunity. Common locations are acral, periorificial, and in sites sensitive to pressure/friction (Koebner phenomenon).
  - Vulgaris: most common subtype; scattered macules; often symmetric, wide distribution; mostly hands, axillae, and groin
  - Acrofacial: on distal extremities and face
  - Mixed: coexistence of above
- Universal: involves >80% of the body surface area (BSA). Most likely to have family history; comorbidities are common and associated with poorest quality-of-life (QOL) scores.
- Other rare variants
  - Ponctué: discrete, confetti-like macules
  - Inflammatory: peripheral erythematous rim
  - Trichrome: Tan zone is present between normal and depigmented skin.
  - Quadrichrome: as above but with marginal/perifollicular hyperpigmentation
  - Blue: Dermal melanophages give blue hue in areas affected by prior postinflammatory hyperpigmentation.
- System(s) affected: skin, mucous membranes
- Synonym(s): leukoderma

EPIDEMIOLOGY

- 50% begin before age 20 years, peak in females: 1st decade; males: 5th decade. Onset earlier with positive family history; can appear as early as 6 weeks
- Predominance: male = female; however, females are more likely to seek treatment.
- No race or socioeconomic predilection

Prevalence
~1% in the United States and Europe (1); 0.1–8% in the world; highest in Gujarat, India at 8.8% (1),(2)

ETIOLOGY AND PATHOPHYSIOLOGY
Most likely a spectrum of disorders with a common phenotype and multiple mechanisms contribute to the pathology (convergence theory).
- Genetic: See "Genetics."
- Autoimmune: humoral autoantibodies and skin-homing T cells
- Neural: local or systemic dysregulation leading to excess neurotransmitters
- Viral: direct melanocyte toxicity, cytomegalovirus (CMV), hepatitis C, and Epstein-Barr virus (EBV) found in lesional biopsies
- Oxidative stress from elevated H_2O_2 and NO and decreased catalase and erythrocyte glutathione

Genetics
- Polygenic/multifactorial inheritance
- 20% of patients report affected relative, but monozygotic twins have only 23% concordance.

- HLA haplotypes, small nucleotide polymorphisms, and specific genes are all possible contributors.

RISK FACTORS
- Family history of vitiligo/autoimmune disorders
- Personal history of associated conditions

COMMONLY ASSOCIATED CONDITIONS
- Most common
  - Endocrine: thyroid disease (hypo-/hyperthyroidism), hypoparathyroidism, Addison disease, insulin-dependent diabetes
  - Dermatologic: psoriasis, atopic dermatitis, alopecia areata, chronic urticaria, halo nevi, ichthyosis
  - Pernicious anemia
  - Hypoacusis, rheumatoid arthritis
  - Ocular abnormalities in up to 40%
  - Elevated antinuclear antibodies in up to 40%
  - Elevated thyroperoxidase antibodies in 50%
- Less common
  - Systemic lupus erythematosus
  - Inflammatory bowel disease
  - Melanoma (may be a sign of positive outcome of melanoma) and other skin cancers
  - Syndromes: Alezzandrini; mitochondrial encephalomyopathy, lactic acidosis, and stroke-like episodes (MELAS); Schmidt; and autoimmune polyendocrinopathy-candidiasis-ectodermal dystrophy (APECED)
- Age >50 years at onset should prompt investigation for associated conditions.

Pediatric Considerations
Associated with Hashimoto thyroiditis in a significant portion of children. Screening at onset and possibly annually may be beneficial.

 DIAGNOSIS

HISTORY
- Inquire about recent history of sunburns, pregnancy, skin trauma, or emotional stress.
- Family history of premature graying, vitiligo, and autoimmune disorders
- Review of systems for related associated conditions
- Ascertain psychological impact on QOL, Dermatology Life Quality Index (DLQI).

PHYSICAL EXAM
- Full-body skin exam with Wood lamp to accentuate lesions and distinguish depigmentation from hypopigmentation
- Lesions are well-demarcated, uniform, white macules and patches.
- Look for evidence of repigmentation (most commonly around hair follicles).

DIFFERENTIAL DIAGNOSIS
- Infectious: tinea versicolor, leprosy, leishmaniasis, onchocerciasis, treponematoses (pinta/syphilis)
- Postinflammatory hypopigmentation: psoriasis, atopic dermatitis, pityriasis alba, systemic lupus erythematosus, scleroderma
- Inherited hypomelanoses: piebaldism, tuberous sclerosis, Waardenburg, hypomelanosis of Ito, Vogt-Koyanagi-Harada
- Malformations: nevus anemicus, nevus depigmentosus
- Paraneoplastic: mycosis fungoides, melanoma-associated leukoderma
- Occupational and chemical induced
  - Occupational: phenolic/catechol derivatives and arsenic-containing compounds

- Chemical: numerous, including cosmetics, cleansers, insecticides, and even medications (imatinib, potent topical corticosteroids [TCS])
- Melasma: Normal skin may be confused as vitiligo in the setting of surrounding hyperpigmentation.
- Halo nevi
- Lichen sclerosus et atrophicus
- Idiopathic guttate hypomelanosis
- Progressive-acquired macular hypomelanosis

DIAGNOSTIC TESTS & INTERPRETATION

Initial Tests (lab, imaging)
- TSH, CBC, ANA
- Consider antithyroid peroxidase, antithyroglobulin antibodies, hemoglobin, vitamin B_{12} levels if family/patient history of autoimmune disease.

Follow-Up Tests & Special Considerations
- Monitor for disease progression/flares.
- Monitor for symptoms of related conditions.

Diagnostic Procedures/Other
- Skin biopsy is rarely needed. Highest yield is with comparison of lesional/perilesional biopsies.
- Consider ophthalmologic and audiologic evaluation.

Test Interpretation
Few or no epidermal melanocytes. At margins, melanocytes may be larger, vacuolated, and dendritic. Early lesions show inflammation and later, degeneration, including of adnexa and nerves.

 TREATMENT

The variant of vitiligo may affect response.
- If untreated, progression is the natural course for those with mucosal involvement, family history, koebnerization, and nonsegmental variants.
- Lesions that respond best are on the face, of recent onset, in darker skin type, and in younger patients.

GENERAL MEASURES
- Sunscreen to decrease sunburn and prevent accentuation of uninvolved skin
- Corrective camouflage as cover-up (Cover FX, Dermablend)

MEDICATION
- Individualize therapy depending on age, extent, distribution, and rate of progression.
- Many therapies are considered "off-label" and not FDA-approved for vitiligo, although they are often considered first-line therapy.
- Corticosteroids: Midpotency TCS (mometasone furoate, fluticasone propionate) applied daily as monotherapy are considered first-line treatments. Do not use on face/axilla/groin; do not occlude except under close monitoring. Pediatric: as above, for children >12 years of age. Consider decreased potency. Local side effects including atrophy, telangiectasia, hypertrichosis, acneiform eruptions, and striae limit treatment; regular steroid holidays are recommended (1). The combination of light therapy and TCS is the most effective treatment overall (2). Most efficacious on sun-exposed areas: face/neck, dark-skinned patients, newer lesion (1). Addition of tretinoin 0.025–0.05% BID is effective and can decrease potential skin atrophy (2),(3). Systemic corticosteroids can be helpful, but dosage and safety parameters have not been fully evaluated for long-term treatment (2),(4)[A].

- Topical calcineurin inhibitors: slightly inferior to TCS as monotherapy but better side effect profile (2),(5),(6)[B]; can be used as adjunctive to light therapy; carries a controversial black box warning for a theoretical risk of lymphoma or skin cancer. Extensive safety profiling has not revealed any evidence for this in children or adults using topical calcineurin inhibitors. Local reactions include burning sensation, pruritus, erythema, and rare transient hyperpigmentation (4).
  - Tacrolimus 0.03% or 0.1% ointment BID (2); pediatric: 0.03% ointment BID, for children >2 years of age (6)
  - Pimecrolimus 1% cream BID (2); pediatric: as adults, for children >2 years of age (6)
- Topical vitamin D_3 analogs: less effective than TCS alone but in combination with TCS or phototherapy can shorten time until, and improve stability of, repigmentation (4),(5)[B]
  - Calcipotriene ointment 1 to 2 times per day; pediatric: not defined
  - Available as a combination formulation, betamethasone dipropionate 0.064%/calcipotriene 0.005% ointment daily, max dose of 100 g/week for 4 weeks, not for >30% BSA, and not for face/axilla/groin; pediatric: not defined
- Oral vitamin D_3: reported to induce repigmentation. Oral vitamin D_3 35,000 IU once daily plus low-calcium diet for 6 months; pediatric: not defined
- Phototherapy: Narrow band UVB (NBUVB) is superior to UVA and indicated for lesions involving >15–20% BSA (3),(5),(6)[A]. Psoralen and khellin enhance the effect of light. Psoralen plus UVA (PUVA) may increase the incidence of skin cancers. Khellin may have reduced cross-linking of DNA and may be less carcinogenic; however, it is associated with increased liver toxicity (6). L-phenylalanine can be used topically and orally as a photosensitizer for natural or artificial light. Pediatric: Oral PUVA is contraindicated.
- Laser therapy: Excimer laser (308 nm) is superior to other light therapy. Helium–neon laser works for segmental vitiligo (5)[A].
- Antioxidants: may have protective role in preventing melanocyte degradation from reactive oxygen species. Options include vitamin C, vitamin E, Vitix, Polypodium leucotomos extracts, and *Ginkgo biloba* (5)[B].
- Surgical therapy: See later discussion.
- New concepts: Tumor necrosis factor-α inhibitors, cyclosporine, cyclophosphamide, azathioprine, minocycline, and immunosuppressants are currently being evaluated (6).

First Line
- Recommended: avoidance of triggering factors plus TCS alone or in combination with NBUVB
- Alternatively
  - Topical calcineurin inhibitors (preferred for face, neck, axilla, and groin)
  - NBUVB
  - PUVA in adults
  - Camouflage and psychotherapy should be offered to all patients at any stage (6).

Second Line
- Recommended: photochemotherapy with psoralens or vitamin D analogues
- Alternatively
  - Topical vitamin D analogues
  - Targeted phototherapy
  - 308-nm laser in combination with topical steroids, topical calcineurin inhibitors, or vitamin D analogues

- Oral corticosteroids (pulse therapy)
- Surgical treatments indicated for stable 2- to 3-cm lesions, refractory to other treatments
  - Mini-punch graft (pretreat with cryotherapy/ dermabrasion or posttreat with phototherapy) (6)[B]
  - Suction blister graft (6)[B]
  - Autologous melanocyte suspension transplant (5)[B]

ISSUES FOR REFERRAL
- Dermatologist: for facial/widespread vitiligo or when advanced therapy is necessary
- Ophthalmologist: for ocular symptoms or monitoring of TCS near eyes
- Endocrinologist: evaluation/management of associated conditions
- Psychologist: for severe distress
- Medical geneticist for associated conditions

ADDITIONAL THERAPIES
- Depigmentation therapy with monobenzone, hydroquinone, or Q-switched ruby laser: for extensive vitiligo recalcitrant to therapy (6)
- Pseudocatalase with addition of NBUVB (1)[B]
- Prostaglandin E for short-duration disease and localization to face and scalp (2)[B]
- Cosmetic tattooing for localized stable vitiligo

SURGERY/OTHER PROCEDURES
- Goal is to transport melanocytes from other areas of the skin. Methods include punch, blister, or split-thickness skin grafting, or transplantation of autologous melanocytes.
- Dermabrasion and curettage alone or in combination with 5-fluorouracil may induce follicular melanocyte reservoirs (5)[A].
- Patients who koebnerize or form keloids may be worse, and permanent scarring is a risk for all patients.

COMPLEMENTARY & ALTERNATIVE MEDICINE
Ginkgo biloba 60 mg PO daily may significantly improve extension and spreading of lesions (4)[B].
- Polypodium leucotomos may help with repigmentation with NBUVB and aid in reducing phototoxic reactions (5)[B].

 ONGOING CARE

FOLLOW-UP RECOMMENDATIONS
- Monitor for symptoms of related conditions.
- With topical steroids, follow at regular intervals to avoid steroid atrophy, telangiectasia, and striae distensae.

DIET
No restrictions

PATIENT EDUCATION
- Discussion of disease course, progression, and cosmesis
- Education regarding trauma/friction and Koebner phenomenon

PROGNOSIS
- Vitiligo may remain stable or slowly or rapidly progress.
- Spontaneous repigmentation is uncommon.
- Generalized vitiligo is often progressive, with flares. Focal vitiligo often has rapid onset and then stabilizes.

COMPLICATIONS
- Adverse effects of each treatment modality
- Psychiatric morbidity: depression, adjustment disorder, low self-esteem, sexual dysfunction, and embarrassment in relationships (1),(2)
  - Different cultures may have different perceptions/ social stigmas about vitiligo. Some believe it to be contagious or related to infection. Women with vitiligo may have difficulty finding a marriage partner and have low self-esteem.

REFERENCES
1. Ezzedine K, Eleftheriadou V, Whitton M, et al. Vitiligo. *Lancet*. 2015;386(9988):74–84.
2. Colucci R, Lotti T, Moretti S. Vitiligo: an update on current pharmacotherapy and future directions. *Expert Opin Pharmacother*. 2012;13(13): 1885–1899.
3. Felsten LM, Alikhan A, Petronic-Rosic V. Vitiligo: a comprehensive overview part II: treatment options and approach to treatment. *J Am Acad Dermatol*. 2011;65(3):493–514.
4. Bacigalupi RM, Postolova A, Davis RS. Evidence-based, non-surgical treatments for vitiligo: a review. *Am J Clin Dermatol*. 2012;13(4):217–237.
5. Whitton ME, Pinart M, Batchelor J, et al. Interventions for vitiligo. *Cochrane Database Syst Rev*. 2015;(2):CD003263.
6. Patel NS, Paghdal KV, Cohen GF. Advanced treatment modalities for vitiligo. *Dermatol Surg*. 2012;38(3):381–391.

ADDITIONAL READING
- Alikhan A, Felsten LM, Daly M, et al. Vitiligo: a comprehensive overview part I. Introduction, epidemiology, quality of life, diagnosis, differential diagnosis, associations, histopathology, etiology, and work-up. *J Am Acad Dermatol*. 2011;65(3): 473–491.
- Silverberg NB. The epidemiology of vitiligo. *Curr Derm Rep*. 2015;4(1):36–43.
- Taieb A, Alomar A, Böhm M, et al; for Vitiligo European Task Force, European Academy of Dermatology and Venereology, Union Européenne des Médecins Spécialistes. Guidelines for the management of vitiligo: the European Dermatology Forum consensus. *Br J Dermatol*. 2013;168(1):5–19.

CODES

ICD10
L80 Vitiligo

CLINICAL PEARLS
- Vitiligo can be a psychologically devastating skin disease.
- Screen for associated diseases, particularly if onset occurs later in life.
- Treatment should be individualized based on BSA, skin type, and patient goals.
- Dermatology consultation when extensive disease, facial involvement, and when advanced treatments are considered

V

VON WILLEBRAND DISEASE

Jennifer M. Shoemaker, MD, MPH

BASICS

DESCRIPTION

- von Willebrand disease (vWD) is an inherited bleeding disorder resulting from either a quantitative or qualitative defect in *von Willebrand factor* (vWF) protein.
- vWF plays an essential role in primary hemostasis, which facilitates the adherence of platelets to the injured blood vessel; it also serves as a carrier for factor VIII (FVIII) in the circulation.
- The most common clinical consequences of vWD are mucocutaneous bleeding, bleeding during childbirth and dental procedures, easy bruising, and menorrhagia (signs of platelet type bleeding).
- vWD is most commonly diagnosed as an autosomal inherited condition but rarely can also be acquired (AvWD).

EPIDEMIOLOGY

Prevalence

- vWD is the most common inherited bleeding disorder.
- Prevalence of the inherited forms of vWD is 1 in 100 to 10,000 of the general population with more females being diagnosed than males.
- Exact prevalence of the acquired forms of vWD (AvWD) is unknown but is estimated to be up to 0.1% of the general population (1).

ETIOLOGY AND PATHOPHYSIOLOGY

- vWF is a large, multimeric glycoprotein that is released from endothelial cells and stored within the α-granules of platelets (2).
- vWF binds to subendothelial collagen at sites of vascular injury and facilitates platelet adhesion to these sites via its interaction with the platelet GP1b receptor. A platelet plug is formed, allowing for the initial arrest of bleeding (primary hemostasis). The formation of a fibrin clot follows the creating of the platelet plug, which requires normal amounts of and function of coagulation factors (secondary hemostasis).
- vWF acts as a carrier for FVIII in the circulation, protecting it from degradation. A deficiency in vWF may result in decreased FVIII levels.
- When vWF is deficient or dysfunctional, primary hemostasis is compromised, resulting in the clinical symptoms described above.
- There are three distinct types of inherited vWD. Within this classification scheme, type 2 vWD has several subtypes, described below (2). Whereas type 1 and type 3 are associated with quantitative deficiencies in vWF (decreased in type 1, absent in type 3), type 2 vWD results from functional defects in the glycoprotein.
  - Type 1, the most common and mildest form, represents 70–80% of cases.
  - Type 2, caused by qualitative defects in vWF, accounts for 10–15% of cases. The various subtypes are described below:
    - Type 2A results from the absence of high- and intermediate-molecular weight multimers of vWF.

- Type 2B occurs due to a gain-of-function mutation in vWF, which increases its affinity for the platelet GP1b receptor. Complexes of platelet and vWF form as result and are subsequently removed from the circulation. Removal of these aggregates results in loss of the high-molecular-weight multimers on vWF as well as thrombocytopenia.
    - Type 2M results from a defect in the platelet binding domain of vWF; however, in contrast to types 2A and 2B, the entire vWF multimer remains intact.
    - Type 2N results from a mutation in the FVIII binding domain of vWF, resulting in low FVIII levels with an intact multimer.
  - Type 3 represents 1–5% of cases, the least common and most severe form.
    - Most severe form with markedly decreased-to-undetectable levels of vWF and FVIII
  - Platelet-type vWD (PT-vWD), also known as pseudo vWD, results from a hyperaffinity mutation in the platelet GP1b receptor, causing increased binding to vWF. Consequently, many platelet-vWF complexes form, which are then cleared from the circulation. Similar to vWD type 2B, these patients will demonstrate loss of high-molecular-weight multimers of vWF in addition to thrombocytopenia.
  - AvWD may be due to cardiovascular, hematologic, or autoimmune conditions as well as tumors and medications. The pathophysiology of AvWD is related to the underlying cause and may result from shear-induced cleaving of vWF in cardiovascular conditions, increased adsorption of vWF by certain tumor cells or activated platelets, or presence of anti-vWF autoantibodies in hematologic disorders.

Genetics

- The 175-kb gene for vWF is located on short arm of chromosome 12.
- Type 1 follows an autosomal dominant inheritance pattern, with variable expressivity.
- Type 2 follows both autosomal dominant and autosomal recessive inheritance patterns.
- Type 3 follows an autosomal recessive inheritance pattern.

RISK FACTORS

- Inherited (vWD): Risk factors include personal and/or family history of bleeding disorders.
- Acquired (AvWD): Risk factors include lymphoproliferative disorders, myeloproliferative disorders, autoimmune disorders, states of high vascular flow (e.g., aortic stenosis, presence of LVAD or ventricular septal defect).

COMMONLY ASSOCIATED CONDITIONS

Individuals with type O blood have accelerated clearance of vWF leading to vWF levels that are 25–30% lower than other those with blood type A, B, or AB. Type 1 disease is diagnosed more frequently in individuals with type O blood.

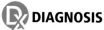

DIAGNOSIS

- For patients with low probability of vWD: Utilize a validated Bleeding Assessment Tool (BAT) as first-line screening assessment prior to ordering laboratory studies (http://www1.wfh.org/docs/en/Resources/Assessment_Tools_ISTHBAT.pdf).
- For patients with moderate to high probability of vWD (family history of bleeding disorders, personal history of unusual bleeding diathesis, abnormal initial laboratory tests): do not only rely on the BAT only but also order:
  - vWF antigen (vWF:Ag), platelet-dependent vWF activity (e.g., vWF:GPIbM), and FVIII:C lab studies
  - vWF is an acute-phase reactant that increases as a result of a variety of stimuli (e.g., bleed, trauma, pregnancy). vWD diagnostic testing should be performed when patients are at a baseline state of health (3).

HISTORY

- A positive family history of a bleeding disorder; however, patients with mild forms of vWD and their families may be unaware of their disease.
- Common symptoms include mucocutaneous (recurrent epistaxis, menorrhagia, ecchymosis) or postprocedural bleeding.
- vWD should be in the differential for heavy menstrual bleeding, at any age, but especially adolescents, when bleeding disorders may be overlooked and incorrectly attributed to an immature hypothalamic-pituitary axis.

PHYSICAL EXAM

Physical exam may be entirely normal but may demonstrate ecchymoses and/or petechiae.

DIFFERENTIAL DIAGNOSIS

Congenital thrombocytopenia, qualitative platelet defects, coagulation factor deficiencies, hemophilia, dysfibrinogenemias, fibrinolytic disorders, liver disease, uremia, connective tissue disorders, coagulation factor inhibitors

DIAGNOSTIC TESTS & INTERPRETATION

- Initial evaluation of a suspected bleeding abnormality (2)
  - Complete blood count (platelet count)
  - Prothrombin time
  - Partial thromboplastin time
  - Fibrinogen level
  - Peripheral blood smear
- Initial evaluation of suspected inherited vWD (2)
  - vWF:Ag: determines total amount of vWF present
  - vWF activity (vWF:RCo): functional assay tests vWF function by assessing its ability to agglutinate platelets in the presence of the antibiotic ristocetin
  - FVIII:C level
  - Of note, multimeric analysis is not recommended in the initial evaluation of vWD laboratory values for vWD.

Condition	Description	vWF:RCo (IU/dL)	vWF:Ag (IU/dL)	FVIII	vWF:RCo/ VWF:Ag
Type 1	Partial quantitative vWF deficiency (75% of symptomatic vWD patients)	<30*	<30*	↓ or Normal	>0.5–0.7
Type 2A	↓ vWF-dependent platelet adhesion with selective deficiency of high-molecular-weight multimers	<30*	<30–200*†	↓ or Normal	<0.5–0.7
Type 2B	increased affinity for platelet GPIb	<30*	<30–200*†	↓ or Normal	Usually <0.5–0.7
Type 2M	↓ vWF-dependent platelet adhesion without selective deficiency of high-molecular-weight multimers	<30*	<30–200*†	↓ or Normal	<0.5–0.7
Type 2N	Markedly decreased binding affinity for FVIII	30–200	30–200	↓↓	>0.5–0.7
Type 3	Virtually complete deficiency of vWF (Severe, rare)	<3	<3	↓↓↓ (<10 IU/dL)	Not applicable
"Low vWF"**		30–50	30–50	Normal	>0.5–0.7
Normal		50–200	50–200	Normal	>0.5–0.7

↓ refers to a decrease in the test result compared to the laboratory reference range.

* <30 IU/dL is designated as the level for a definitive diagnosis of vWD; some patients with type 1 or type 2 vWD have levels of vWF:RCo and/or vWF:Ag of 30–50 IU/dL.

† The vWF:Ag in the majority of individuals with type 2A, 2B, or 2M vWD is <50 IU/dL.

** This does not preclude the diagnosis of vWD in patients with vWF:RCo of 30–50 IU/dL if there is supporting clinical and/or family evidence for vWD, nor does this preclude the use of agents to increase vWF levels in those who have vWF:RCo of 30–50 IU/dL and who may be at risk for bleeding.

Follow-Up Tests & Special Considerations
vWF is an acute-phase reactant, so elevations may be seen in inflammatory conditions, liver disease, pregnancy (which may correct mild deficits), or with estrogen use. Levels also increase with age; however, it is unclear if this decreases bleeding risk.

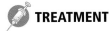

TREATMENT

GENERAL MEASURES
- Minor bleeding episodes generally do not require therapeutic intervention. Most commonly, these individuals receive treatment prior to receiving surgeries, dental procedures, and following injury.
- In patients with mild disease, trauma-related and spontaneous bleeding events may be managed with desmopressin acetate (DDAVP), which releases endogenous vWF stored in the patient's endothelial cells.
- Chronic menorrhagia can be managed with hormonal contraception (oral contraceptives or hormone-containing intrauterine device [IUD]), endometrial ablation (for women no longer desiring future pregnancy), DDAVP, or antifibrinolytic agents.

MEDICATION

First Line
- Desmopressin (DDAVP)
  - Enhances release of vWF from endothelial cells
  - Primarily effective for type 1 vWD; not indicated in type 2B. Trial of DDAVP should initially be measured in nonbleeding state to determine response.
  - Not effective in vWD type 3

- Replacement therapy with vWF and/or FVIII concentrates are the most effective treatment for patients with type 2 and type 3 vWD. However, in cases of PT-vWD, administration of exogenous platelets is the treatment of choice.
  - Dose of vWF concentrate may be adjusted for FVIII levels and ristocetin cofactor activity.
  - FVIII levels should be monitored to avoid supranormal levels and possible venous thromboembolism (VTE).
  - Contraindicated if patient develops alloantibodies to vWF
  - In patients with severe bleeding phenotype, prophylactic treatment is used.
- Antifibrinolytics (aminocaproic acid, tranexamic acid)
  - Contraindicated in patients with hematuria due to risk of retention of large blood clots in the renal collecting system
  - Given as adjunct to DDAVP
- Recombinant FVIIa (NovoSeven)
  - Used for patients who develop alloantibodies to vWF
  - Used effectively in the treatment of patients with type 3 vWD

Second Line
- Combined oral contraceptives or the levonorgestrel-releasing intrauterine system raise vWF/FVIII levels in the blood and also have a role in the treatment of chronic menorrhagia.
- Platelets may be given as an adjunct to factor concentrates if hemostasis has not been achieved.
- Intravenous immunoglobulin has been useful in some patients with AvWD associated with monoclonal gammopathy.

ONGOING CARE

FOLLOW-UP RECOMMENDATIONS
Patients should be seen by a hematologist prior to invasive procedures.

Patient Monitoring
Patients with mild disease do not require monitoring.

DIET
No dietary restrictions are recommended. However, aspirin and other NSAIDs should be avoided.

PATIENT EDUCATION
National Hemophilia Foundation: https://www.hemophilia.org/NHFWeb/MainPgs/MainNHF.aspx?menuid=182&contentid=47&rptname=bleeding

PROGNOSIS
Most patients with vWD have normal life expectancy.

COMPLICATIONS
- Significant perioperative bleeding may occur.
- Patients with type 3 vWD and type 2N can have bleeding complications similar to patients with hemophilia A, such as hemarthrosis and intracranial hemorrhage.
- Multiple transfusions may result in alloantibodies against vWF.
- VTE may result from supranormal levels of FVIII.

REFERENCES
1. Leebeek FW, Eikenboom JC. Von Willebrand's disease. *N Engl J Med*. 2016;375(21):2067–2080.
2. Baronciani L, Peyvandi F. How we make an accurate diagnosis of von Willebrand disease. *Thromb Res*. 2020;196:579–589.
3. James PD, Connell NT, Ameer B, et al. ASH ISTH NHF WFH 2021 guidelines on the diagnosis of von Willebrand disease. *Blood Adv*. 2021;5(1):280–300.

SEE ALSO

Algorithms: Bleeding Gums; Ecchymosis

CODES

ICD10
D68.0 Von Willebrand's disease

CLINICAL PEARLS
- vWD is the most common inherited bleeding disorder in American women, and its manifestations vary from minor to severe bleeding episodes.
- Treatment should be administered for recurrent bleeding episodes in all types of vWD, but prophylaxis is not required for minor bleeding events.

V

VULVAR MALIGNANCY

Jessica C. Nazzaro, DO • Michael P. Hopkins, MD, MEd

 BASICS

DESCRIPTION

- Premalignant lesions of the vulva are collectively known as vulvar intraepithelial neoplasia (VIN).
- Exposure to human papillomavirus (HPV) has been linked to >70% of VIN.
- Invasive squamous cell carcinoma is the most common malignancy involving the vulva (90% of patients); can be well, moderately, or poorly differentiated and derives from keratinized skin covering the vulva and perineum
- Melanoma is the second most common type of vulvar malignancy (8%) and sarcoma is the third.
- Other invasive cell types include basal cell carcinoma, Paget disease, adenocarcinoma arising from Bartholin gland or apocrine sweat glands, adenoid cystic carcinoma, small cell carcinoma, verrucous carcinoma, and sarcomas.
- Sarcomas are usually leiomyosarcoma and probably arise at the insertion of the round ligament in the labium major; however, sarcoma can arise from any structure of the vulva, including blood vessels, skeletal muscle, and fat.
- Rarely, breast carcinoma has been reported in the vulva and is thought to arise from ectopic breast tissue.
- System(s) affected: reproductive

Geriatric Considerations
- Older patients with associated medical problems are at high risk from radical surgery. The surgery, however, is usually well tolerated.
- Patients who are not surgical candidates can be treated with combination chemotherapy and/or radiation.
- In the very elderly, palliative vulvectomy provides relief of symptoms for ulcerating symptomatic advanced disease.

EPIDEMIOLOGY

Incidence
- In 2015, 5,150 women were diagnosed with vulvar cancer and 1,080 women died from vulvar cancer in the United States (1); accounting for approximately 4% of all gynecologic malignancies
- Estimated 6,020 new cases and 1,150 deaths in 2017
- Surveillance, epidemiology, and end result (SEER) data showed that the incidence of in situ vulvar carcinoma increased by >400% between 1973 and 2000.
- Mean age at diagnosis 65 years; in situ disease: mean age 40 years; invasive malignancy: mean age 60 years
- 30–35% of vulvar cancer cases are diagnosed at FIGO stages III and IV.
- Ethnic distribution: more common in Caucasian women than in any other race

ETIOLOGY AND PATHOPHYSIOLOGY
- Patients with cervical cancer are more likely to develop vulvar cancer later in life, secondary to "field effect" phenomenon with a carcinogen involving the lower genital tract.
- HPV has been associated with squamous cell abnormalities of the cervix, vagina, and vulva; 55% of vulvar cancers are attributable to oncogenic HPV, predominantly HPV 16 and 33; vaginal intraepithelial neoplasia (VAIN) 2/3 and anal intraepithelial neoplasia (AIN) are attributable to HPV.

- Squamous cell carcinoma
  - There are two etiologic pathways for developing vulvar squamous cell carcinoma: lichen sclerosus and HPV.
  - The International Society for the Study of Vulvovaginal Disease (ISSVD) proposed a revised terminology in 2015: low-grade squamous intraepithelial lesion (LSIL), which includes flat condyloma and HPV effect, high-grade squamous intraepithelial lesion (HSIL), and VIN differentiated type (dVIN). The ISSVD previously used a three level system grading VIN as 1, 2, 3, which has been abandoned.
  - Differentiated type occurs in older age groups, is associated with lichen sclerosus and chronic venereal diseases, and is not related to HPV. It carries a higher risk of progression to malignancy.
- The warty basaloid type, also known as bowenoid type, is related to HPV infection and occurs in younger women. Melanoma, second most common histology, often identified in postmenopausal women; often pigmented but can be amelanotic, arising de novo, often found on clitoris or labia minora. Prognosis is poor, 5-year survival <50%.
- Smoking is associated with squamous cell disease of the vulva, possibly from direct irritation of the vulva by the transfer of tars and nicotine on the patient's hands or from systemic absorption of carcinogen.

Genetics
No known genetic pattern

RISK FACTORS
- VIN or cervical intraepithelial neoplasia (CIN)
- Smoking
- Lichen sclerosus (vulvar dystrophy)
- HPV infection, condylomata, or sexually transmitted diseases (STD) in the past
- Low economic status
- Autoimmune processes
- Immunodeficiency syndromes or immunosuppression
- Northern European ancestry
- Risk factors for recurrence: age >50 years, positive excision margins, concurrent VAIN

GENERAL PREVENTION
- HPV vaccination has the potential to decrease vulvar cancer by 60%.
- Abstinence from smoking/smoking cessation counseling

COMMONLY ASSOCIATED CONDITIONS
- Patients with invasive vulvar cancer are often elderly and have associated medical conditions.
- High rate of other gynecologic malignancies

DIAGNOSIS

HISTORY
Complaints of pruritus or raised lesion in the vaginal area, vaginal bleeding, discharge

PHYSICAL EXAM
- In situ disease: a small raised area associated with pruritus, single vulvar plaque, ulcer, or mass on labia majora, perineum, clitoris; most commonly found on labia majora
- Vulvar bleeding, dysuria, enlarged lymph nodes less common symptomatology
- Invasive malignancy: an ulcerated, nonhealing area; as lesions become large, bleeding occurs with associated pain and foul-smelling discharge; enlarged inguinal lymph nodes indicative of advanced disease

DIFFERENTIAL DIAGNOSIS
- Infectious processes can present as ulcerative lesions and include syphilis, lymphogranuloma venereum, and granuloma inguinale.
- Disorder of Bartholin gland, seborrheic keratosis, hidradenomas, lichen sclerosus, epidermal inclusion cysts
- Crohn disease can present as an ulcerative area on the vulva.
- Rarely, lesions can metastasize to the vulva.

DIAGNOSTIC TESTS & INTERPRETATION

Initial Tests (lab, imaging)
- Hypercalcemia can occur when metastatic disease is present.
- Squamous cell antigen can be elevated with invasive disease.

Follow-Up Tests & Special Considerations
- Upon examination, any suspicious lesions should be biopsied.
- Diagnosis based on histologic findings following vulvar biopsy (2)
- The vulva can be washed with 3% acetic acid to highlight areas and visualized with a colposcope, allows for visualization of acetowhite lesions and vascular lesions (2).
- For patients with new onset of pruritus, the area of pruritus should be biopsied.
- Liberal biopsies must be used to diagnose in situ disease prior to invasion and to diagnose early invasive disease.
- The patient should not be treated for presumed benign conditions of the vulva without full exam and biopsy, including Pap smear and colposcopy of cervix, vagina, and vulva.
- When symptoms persist, reexamine and rebiopsy.
- Treatment of benign condyloma of the vulva has not been shown to decrease the eventual incidence of in situ or invasive disease of the vulva.
- CT scan to evaluate pelvic and periaortic lymph node status if tumor >2 cm or if suspicion of metastatic disease (2)[A]

Diagnostic Procedures/Other
Office vulvar biopsy is done to establish the diagnosis.

Test Interpretation
A surgical staging system is used for vulvar cancer (International Federation of Obstetrics and Gynecology Classification).
- Stage I: tumor confined to the vulva
  - Stage IA: lesions ≤2 cm in size, confined to the vulva or perineum and with stromal invasion ≤1 mm, no node metastasis
  - Stage IB: lesions >2 cm in size or with stromal invasion >1 mm, confined to the vulva or perineum, with negative nodes
- Stage II: tumor of any size with extension to adjacent perineal structures (lower 1/3 urethra, lower 1/3 vagina, anus) with negative nodes
- Stage III: tumor of any size with or without extension to adjacent perineal structures (lower 1/3 urethra, lower 1/3 vagina, anus) with positive inguinofemoral lymph nodes
- Stage IIIA
  - With 1 lymph node metastasis (≥5 mm), or
  - 1 to 2 lymph node metastases (<5 mm)

- Stage IIIB
  - With ≥2 lymph node metastases (≥5 mm), or
  - ≥3 lymph node metastases (<5 mm)
- Stage IIIC: with positive nodes with extracapsular spread
- Stage IV: Tumor invades other regional (upper 2/3 urethra, upper 2/3 vagina) or distant structures.
- Stage IVA: Tumor invades any of the following:
  - Upper urethral and/or vaginal mucosa, bladder mucosa, rectal mucosa, or fixed to pelvic bone
  - Fixed or ulcerated inguinofemoral lymph nodes
- Stage IVB: any distant metastasis, including pelvic lymph nodes

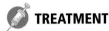

TREATMENT

GENERAL MEASURES
- Wide excision can be performed for carcinoma in situ, and any suspicious lesion should be excised for definitive diagnosis.
- Cystoscopy and sigmoidoscopy should be performed if there is a question of invasion into the urethra, bladder, or rectum.

MEDICATION
- Neoadjuvant therapy is being investigated with bleomycin-cisplatin and paclitaxel-based regimens showing high-response rates and tolerable side effects (3)[A].
- As an adjuvant therapy, fluorouracil (Efudex) cream for in situ disease can produce occasional results but is not well tolerated because of irritation of the vulva (4)[A].
- Chemoradiotherapy with cisplatin and 5-fluorouracil (5-FU) has been successful in advanced or recurrent disease, although local morbidity is increased (4)[A].
- Contraindications: elderly patients: If chemotherapeutic agents are used, pay close attention to the patient's performance status and ability to tolerate aggressive chemotherapy.

ISSUES FOR REFERRAL
Patients may need care from a gynecologic oncologist and/or a radiation oncologist.

ADDITIONAL THERAPIES
- Preoperative radiation therapy can be used in those with advanced vulvar cancer (2)[B].
- Adjuvant radiation should be considered with tumor size >4 cm, evidence of lymphovascular invasion, positive surgical margins, or lymph node involvement.
- Preoperative chemoradiation allows for a less radical surgical procedure in patients who are not surgical candidates (4)[A].
- Postoperative radiation decreases recurrence frequency and may improve survival (4)[A].
- Radiation is contraindicated with verrucous carcinoma because it induces anaplastic transformation and increases metastases.

SURGERY/OTHER PROCEDURES
- In situ disease can be treated with wide excision or laser vaporization of the affected area. Laser vaporization is preferable in the younger patient, whereas wide excision is preferable in the elderly patient, in whom the risk of invasive disease is also higher (2)[A].
- If tumor extension within <1 cm from structures that will not be removed, preoperative radiation to prevent inadequate surgical margins prior to excision 1-cm tumor-free margin is required because smaller margin would increase risk of recurrence (4)[A].

- Inguinofemoral lymphadenectomy: removal of superficial inguinal and deep femoral lymph nodes
- Targeted dissection of grossly involved nodes, termed nodal debulking, is being investigated due to high rates of complication after full inguinofemoral lymphadenectomy.
- Stage IA: radical local excision without lymph node dissection
- Stage IB: radical local excision with either sentinel lymph node biopsy (SLNB) or ipsilateral inguinofemoral lymph node dissection because the risk of metastases is >8%
- Stage II: modified radical vulvectomy and/or chemoradiation and groin node dissection
- Stages III and IV: neoadjuvant chemoradiation and less radical surgery
- Pelvic exenteration after radiation provides effective therapy for advanced or recurrent malignancies involving the bladder or rectum.
- More limited surgery has been undertaken for early invasive lesions, especially in young patients, to preserve the clitoris and sexual function.
- SLNB also has been advocated for early invasive lesion (stage IB or higher). It has shown to accurately diagnose groin metastases in women with early vulval cancer and unknown groin node status. This will limit the surgical morbidity associated with inguinofemoral lymphadenectomy in those with early stage disease.
- Radical vulvectomy with bilateral groin node dissection through separate incisions provides better cosmetic results than en bloc technique.
- Unilateral lymphadenectomy should be considered when lesion <2 cm, lateral lesion >2 cm from vulvar midline, or no palpable groin nodes.

ADMISSION, INPATIENT, AND NURSING CONSIDERATIONS
- Typically inpatient for treatment
- Concurrent chemotherapy with radiation is considered standard of care if the patient can tolerate it, based on extrapolation from squamous cell cancers of the cervix and anus (4)[B].
- In advanced malignancy involving the urethra and rectum, concomitant cisplatin/5-FU chemotherapy with radiation produces a significant decrease in size of the primary tumor, usually obviating the need for pelvic exenteration.

ONGOING CARE

FOLLOW-UP RECOMMENDATIONS
Patient Monitoring
- Early stage, treated with surgery alone: clinical exam of the groin nodes and vulvar area every 6 months for 2 years and then annually
- Following chemoradiation, assessment for further treatment within 6 to 12 weeks of therapy completion
- Advance stage, clinical exam of the groin nodes and vulvar area every 3 months for 2 years, then every 6 months for 3 years, and then annually
- Cervical and/or vaginal cytology annually
- Majority of relapses occur within 1st year.

DIET
As tolerated and according to comorbid conditions

PATIENT EDUCATION
- American College of Obstetricians and Gynecologists (ACOG), 409 12th St. SW, Washington, DC 20024-2188; (800) 762-ACOG; http://www.acog.org/
- American Cancer Society: http://www.cancer.org/

PROGNOSIS
The 5-year survival is based on stage:
- Stage I: 78.5%
- Stage II: 58.8%
- Stage III: 43.2%
- Stage IV: 13.0%
- Inguinal and/or femoral node involvement is the most important determinant of survival.

COMPLICATIONS
- The major complications from radical vulvectomy and groin node dissection are wound breakdown, lymphedema, urinary stress incontinence, and psychosexual consequences.
- In the immediate postoperative period, ~50% of patients experience breakdown of the wound. This requires aggressive wound care by visiting nurses as often as twice a day. The wounds usually granulate and heal over a period of 6 to 10 weeks.
- ~15–20% of patients experience some form of mild to moderate lymphedema after the groin node dissection. These patients should be instructed in the use of leg elevation and support hose. <1% of patients experience severe, debilitating lymphedema.

REFERENCES
1. Siegel RL, Miller KD, Jemal A. Cancer statistics, 2015. *CA Cancer J Clin*. 2015;65(1):5–29.
2. de Hullu JA, van der Zee AG. Surgery and radiotherapy in vulvar cancer. *Crit Rev Oncol Hematol*. 2006;60(1):38–58.
3. Niu Y, Yin R, Wang D, et al. Clinical analysis of neoadjuvant chemotherapy in patients with advanced vulvar cancer: a STROBE-compliant article. *Medicine (Baltimore)*. 2018;97(34):e11786.
4. Shylasree TS, Bryant A, Howells RE. Chemoradiation for advanced primary vulval cancer. *Cochrane Database Syst Rev*. 2011;(4):CD003752.

ADDITIONAL READING
- Hinten F, Molijn A, Eckhardt L, et al. Vulvar cancer: two pathways with different localization and prognosis. *Gynecol Oncol*. 2018;149(2):310–317.
- Stecklein SR, Frumovitz M, Klopp AH, et al. Effectiveness of definitive radiotherapy for squamous cell carcinoma of the vulva with gross inguinal lymphadenopathy. *Gynecol Oncol*. 2018;148(3):474–479.

CODES

ICD10
- C51.9 Malignant neoplasm of vulva, unspecified
- D07.1 Carcinoma in situ of vulva
- C51.0 Malignant neoplasm of labium majus

CLINICAL PEARLS
- 55% of vulvar cancers are attributable to oncogenic HPV. VAIN 2/3 and AIN are attributable to HPV. Therefore, HPV vaccination has the potential to decrease vulvar cancer by 1/3.
- Biopsy all suspicious or nonhealing vulvar lesions.

V

VULVODYNIA

Jessica Johnson, MD, MPH • Amy L. Wiser, MD

 BASICS

DESCRIPTION

- Vulvar pain lasting 3 months or more; occurs in the absence of relevant visible findings, relevant lab abnormalities, or a clinically identifiable neurologic disorder
- 2015 ISSVD (International Society for the Study of Vulvovaginal Disease) classification is based on whether vulvar pain is caused by a specific disorder or has no clear identifiable cause (1).
- Specific disorders (differential diagnosis) include infectious, inflammatory, neoplastic, neurologic, trauma, iatrogenic, or hormonal deficiency.
- Descriptors for unclear etiology include localized versus generalized versus mixed, provoked versus spontaneous versus mixed, primary versus secondary onset, and temporal.

EPIDEMIOLOGY

- Can occur at any age, but most women diagnosed between age 20 and 40 years (2)
- Nearly half of women opt not to seek treatment (3).
- Patients are psychologically comparable with asymptomatic controls and have similar marital satisfaction, but poorer overall sexual satisfaction.

Incidence

- Recent retrospective study estimates annual rate of new onset vulvodynia to be 1.8%.
- Evidence indicates lifetime cumulative incidence approaches 15%, suggesting nearly 14 million U.S. women will experience persistent vulvar discomfort at some point in their lives (4).

Prevalence

- Reports between 8.3% and 16%; non–clinical-based studies approximate a prevalence of 7% with validation by exam (3).
- Studies show Hispanics are 80% more likely to present with vulvar pain compared with Caucasians and African Americans.

ETIOLOGY AND PATHOPHYSIOLOGY

- Vulvodynia is likely neuropathically mediated:
  - Hypothesized that neurogenic inflammation sensitizes afferent nerves, and transmits impulses to the central nervous system (CNS), where reinforcing signals sustain pain loop
  - In recent investigations of vulvar biopsy specimens, increased neuronal proliferation and branching in vulvar tissue are evident when compared with tissue of asymptomatic women.
- Pelvic floor pathology also should be considered: In one study, the vulvodynia group showed an increase in pelvic floor hypertonicity at the superficial muscle layer, less vaginal muscle strength with contraction, and decreased relaxation of pelvic floor muscles after contraction (4).
- No cause of vulvodynia has been established. It is most likely a neuropathic pain caused by a combination of the following:
  - Recurrent vulvovaginal candidiasis or other infections
  - Immune-mediated chronic neuroinflammatory process within vulvar tissues
  - Chemical exposure (trichloroacetic acid) or physical trauma
  - Reduced estrogen receptor expression/changes in estrogen concentration
  - CNS etiology, similar to other regional pain syndromes

Genetics

Proposed genetic deficiency impairing one's ability to stop the inflammatory response triggered by infection or chemicals; homozygosity of the two alleles of the interleukin (IL)-1 receptor antagonist occurs in 25–50% of vestibulodynia patients, compared with <10% in controls.

RISK FACTORS

- Vulvovaginal infections, specifically candidiasis. Unclear if infection, treatment, or underlying hypersensitivity is the cause (3). Multiple infections compound this risk.
- Hormonal factors: Controversial evidence proposes increased risk with use of oral contraceptive pills (OCPs); pain onset or increased severity may be associated with menopause. Symptoms may flare before menses.
- Pelvic floor dysfunction: Increased instability of pelvic floor muscles may perpetuate vulvar tissue inflammation, leading to vascular changes and histamine release.
- Comorbid interstitial cystitis and painful bladder syndrome; potentially related to common embryologic origin of structures
- Abuse: increased risk of vulvodynia if childhood had physical or sexual abuse by a primary family member; causal relationship remains unclear (4).
- Depression and anxiety (3)
- Other neuropathic and chronic pain disorders, including regional pain syndrome

GENERAL PREVENTION

- Wear 100% cotton underwear in the daytime and no underwear to sleep.
- Avoid douching and other vulvar irritants such as perfumes, dyes, and detergents.
- Avoid abrasive activities and tight, synthetic clothing.
- Avoid panty liners.
- Clean the vulva with water only and pat area dry after bathing.
- Avoid use of hair dryers in the vulvar area.

COMMONLY ASSOCIATED CONDITIONS

Higher incidence of chronic pain syndromes associated with vulvodynia, including chronic cystitis, irritable bowel syndrome, fibromyalgia, migraines, depression, endometriosis, low back pain. Women with vulvodynia have a higher incidence of depression and anxiety both preceding and resulting from their symptoms (3).

DIAGNOSIS

- Vulvodynia is a clinical diagnosis and it should be suspected in any women with chronic pain at the introitus and vulva.
- Pain should be characterized using a standard measure such as the McGill Pain Questionnaire; duration and nature of the pain should be established.
- Use physical exam to rule out other causes of vulvovaginal pain. Negative fungal culture, along with relevant history and positive cotton swab test, confirms diagnosis.

HISTORY

Adequate sexual, social, and pain history should be taken to assess degree of symptoms. Visual pain scales and pain diaries may be helpful (5)[B]:

- Onset of vulvodynia often sudden and without precedents
- Pain often described as generalized, unprovoked
- Quality of pain is burning, stinging, irritating, or rawness (3).
- Specifically ask about bowel and bladder habits, history of trauma or abuse, history of infections including herpes and personal hygiene.
- Specific skin complaints may suggest alternate diagnosis; a history of allergies may suggest vulvar dermatitis.

- Assess for precipitants of vulvar pain: tight garments, bicycle riding, tampon use, prolonged sitting, perfumed or deodorant soaps, douching (3).
- Assess for complaints of dyspareunia:
  - Presence of vaginismus (involuntary vaginal muscle spasm), adequate lubrication, anorgasmia, partner problems, abuse
  - Psychosexual morbidity significantly higher in patients with vulvodynia; counseling may complement medical interventions.

PHYSICAL EXAM

- Ask patient to show where pain is localized or most painful.
- Mouth and skin exams to assess for lesions suggestive of lichen planus or lichen sclerosus
- Vaginal exam should be done to exclude other causes of vulvovaginal pain, including external inspection; palpation; and single digit, speculum, and bimanual exams:
  - The vulva may be erythematous, especially at the vestibule. Discomfort with separation of the labia minora is common.
  - Spontaneous or elicited pain at the lower 1/2 of anterior vaginal wall suggests bladder etiology.
- Bulbocavernosus and anal wink reflexes should be checked to assess for peripheral neuropathy.

DIFFERENTIAL DIAGNOSIS

- Infections: candidiasis, herpes, human papillomavirus (HPV), bacterial vaginosis, trichomoniasis, dermatophytes
- Inflammation: lichen planus, immunobullous disorder, allergic vulvitis, lichen sclerosus, atrophic vaginitis
- Neoplasia: Paget disease, vulvar or vaginal intraepithelial neoplasia, squamous cell carcinoma
- Neurologic/muscular: herpes neuralgia, spinal nerve compression, vaginismus

DIAGNOSTIC TESTS & INTERPRETATION

- Tampon test: reproduces pain in real-life settings
- Cotton swab or Q-tip test: Vulva tested for localized areas of pain, beginning at thighs and continuing medially toward vestibule, using the soft end and broken sharp end of the cotton swab. Five distinct positions (2, 4, 6, 8, and 10 o'clock) surveyed using light palpation. Pain rated on a scale from 0 (none) to 10 (most severe); posterior introitus and posterior hymenal remnants most common sites of increased sensitivity
- Test for concurrent vaginismus: Apply pressure with a gloved finger to levator ani and obturator internus muscles to assess for tenderness, pain, or contracture.

Initial Tests (lab, imaging)

- Vaginal pH, wet mount, and yeast culture are recommended to rule out vaginitis.
- Gonorrhea and chlamydia testing done at physician's discretion
- HPV screening is unnecessary; association is controversial between HPV and vulvodynia.

Follow-up Tests & Special Considerations

- Varicella-zoster and herpes simplex virus should be considered if ulcers or vesicular eruptions are present.
- Consider biopsy if concerned for neoplasm or dermatophyte infection or if the patient is resistant to treatment.

Diagnostic Procedures/Other

Colposcopy can be helpful if epidermal abnormalities are present. This should be done with caution because acetic acid worsens vulvar pain.

Test Interpretation

No specific histologic features are associated with vulvodynia, although reactive squamous atypia has been observed. Biopsies are unnecessary for diagnosis. Presence of rash/altered mucosa is not consistent with vulvodynia; this requires further evaluation (5)[C].

 ## TREATMENT

Treatment is mostly based on expert opinion; high-quality research is limited by lack of standardized treatment outcome measures (6). Some experts prioritize non-pharmacologic therapies as evidence is stronger. For pharmacologic treatment, a trial of several medications for at least 3 months is usually needed to see effect.

GENERAL MEASURES

Combining treatments should be encouraged when treating women with vulvodynia (5)[C]. Various reports on use of a combination of medical treatments, and psychotherapy, reveal women on these combinations do significantly better compared with those who receive medication only.

MEDICATION
- Oral therapies
  - Tricyclic antidepressants (TCAs): first-line treatment for unprovoked vulvodynia (5)[B]; do not stop use abruptly; contraindicated in patients with cardiac abnormalities and those taking MAOIs; fatigue, constipation, sweating, palpitations, and weight gain are most common side effects.
    - Amitriptyline, nortriptyline: most widely studied; start at 10 mg daily; dose titrated to pain control. Average effective dose is 60 mg daily. In one study, a 47% complete response rate was recorded (7)[B]. Nortriptyline may be preferred due to less anticholinergic adverse effects.
  - Anticonvulsant therapies:
    - Gabapentin: started at 300 mg daily at HS and increased by 300 mg every 3 days. Maximum recommended dose is 3,600 mg daily divided into 3 doses. 2018 randomized controlled trial showed no improvement in tampon test pain compared to placebo.
    - Topiramate and lamotrigine have been recommended if other therapies are not effective.
  - Selective serotonin reuptake inhibitor/serotonin norepinephrine reuptake inhibitors: not commonly used; but there is some benefit for generalized vulvodynia (6) and can be helpful in those who cannot tolerate TCAs.
  - Opioids/nonsteroidal anti-inflammatory drugs: not consistently helpful in relieving vulvar pain; not appropriate for maintenance
- Topical therapies
  - Generally, these are preferred in those with provoked vulvodynia (6).
  - A trial of local anesthetics may be recommended for all patients who present with vulvodynia. Use judiciously to avoid increased irritation (5)[C].
  - Lidocaine 5% ointment: for provoked vestibulodynia; application advised 15 to 20 minutes prior to intercourse. Penile numbness and possible toxicity with ingestion can occur.
    - In one study, lidocaine 5% ointment was left in vestibule overnight (average of 8 hours) for a period of 6 to 8 weeks; at follow-up, up to 76% of women reported no discomfort with intercourse (4)[C].
  - Cromolyn 4% cream: decreases mast cell degranulation in vulvar tissue; recommended application TID (3)[C]
  - Capsaicin 0.025%: decreases in discomfort and increases in frequency of intercourse with 20-minute daily application (4)[B]

  - Topical amitriptyline 2% combined with baclofen 2% is helpful in patients with comorbid vaginismus.
  - Topical corticosteroids and testosterone creams have not been shown to alleviate symptoms of vulvodynia.
  - Gabapentin 3–6% ointment (must be compounded)
  - Topical nitroglycerin may be helpful but may cause headaches.
  - Topical estrogen
- Injectable therapies
  - Triamcinolone acetonide: maximum of 40 mg should be injected monthly; is best when combined with 0.25–0.50% bupivacaine
  - Submucosal methylprednisone and lidocaine: reports of up to 68% response rate with weekly injections (5)[B]
  - Interferon-α: useful in treatment of vestibulodynia. Side effects (myalgias, fever, malaise) limit its use.
  - Botulinum toxin A injectable is being studied.

ISSUES FOR REFERRAL

A team approach is recommended for most effective management. Referral to psychosexual medicine, psychology, partner therapy, and pain management teams should be strongly considered (5)[B].

ADDITIONAL THERAPIES
- Cognitive-behavioral therapy (CBT): One randomized trial revealed that CBT is associated with a 30% decrease in vulvar discomfort with sexual intercourse. CBT is the recommended treatment for patients who present with dyspareunia as a main complaint (8)[B].
- Biofeedback/pelvic floor physical therapy: useful with concomitant vaginismus. Treats both generalized and localized vulvar pain; treatment value for unprovoked pain remains unclear. Most studies report an average of 12- to 16-week treatment time.
- Vaginal dilators
- Surface electromyography (sEMG): effective for pelvic floor rehabilitation. Patients are more likely to experience pain-free sexual intercourse after sEMG; significant reductions seen on pain measures at long-term follow-up

SURGERY/OTHER PROCEDURES
- Surgery may be considered for patients with localized/provoked symptoms who have failed to respond to other measures; not recommended for generalized vulvodynia (5)[B]
- 60–80% of women who undergo surgery report a significant reduction in pain symptoms; however, when surveyed, patients prefer behavioral therapies than surgical intervention.
- All patients who are considering surgical intervention should be tested and treated for vaginismus. Vestibulectomy is less successful in this subgroup, and also in those with generalized symptoms (6).
- Surgical approaches
  - Local excision: precise localization of painful areas; tissue closed in elliptical fashion
  - Total vestibulectomy: Tissue is removed from Skene ducts to perineum. The vagina is then brought down to cover defect.
  - Perineoplasty: vestibulectomy plus removal of perineal tissue; incision usually terminated above the anal orifice; reserved for severe cases (3)[B]

COMPLEMENTARY & ALTERNATIVE MEDICINE

Acupuncture: Small studies of women with unprovoked vulvodynia who did not respond to conventional treatment reported significant decreases in pain severity with acupuncture; treatment value with provoked pain is unknown (5)[C].

 ## ONGOING CARE

PATIENT EDUCATION

Patients should be reassured that this condition is neither infectious, nor does it predispose to cancer (5)[C]. Counsel that condition is manageable, but likely not curable, and may require multiple therapeutic trials before remission is achieved. Emphasize self-hygiene. Encourage treatment with home remedies, including ice packs, sitz baths with baking soda, olive oil, and barrier cream to preserve moisture after bathing.

PROGNOSIS

Traditionally viewed as a chronic pain disorder, new evidence of remission has been documented; recent 2-year follow-up study revealed 1 in 10 vulvodynia patients reported remission regardless of treatment.

REFERENCES

1. Bornstein J, Goldstein AT, Stockdale CK, et al. 2015 ISSVD, ISSWSH and IPPS consensus terminology and classification of persistent vulvar pain and vulvodynia. *Obstet Gynecol*. 2016;127(4):745–751.
2. Sadownik LA. Etiology, diagnosis, and clinical management of vulvodynia. *Int J Womens Health*. 2014;6:437–449.
3. Shah M, Hoffstetter S. Vulvodynia. *Obstet Gynecol Clin N Am*. 2014;41(3):453–464.
4. Boardman LA, Stockdale CK. Sexual pain. *Clin Obstet Gynecol*. 2009;52(4):682–690.
5. Nunns D, Mandal D, Byrne M, et al; for British Society for the Study of Vulval Disease Guideline Group. Guidelines for the management of vulvodynia. *Br J Dermatol*. 2010;162(6):1180–1185.
6. Stenson AL. Vulvodynia: diagnosis and management. *Obstet Gynecol Clin N Am*. 2017;44(3):493–508.
7. Stockdale CK, Lawson HW. 2013 vulvodynia guideline update. *J Low Genit Tract Dis*. 2014;18(2):93–100.
8. De Andres J, Sanchis-Lopez N, Asensio-Samper JM, et al. Vulvodynia: an evidence-based literature review and proposed treatment algorithm. *Pain Pract*. 2016;16(2):204–236.

ADDITIONAL READING

Goldstein AT, Pukall CF, Brown C, et al. Vulvodynia: assessment and treatment. *J Sexual Med*. 2016;13(4):572–590.

 ## CODES

ICD10
- N94.819 Vulvodynia, unspecified
- N94.818 Other vulvodynia
- N94.810 Vulvar vestibulitis

CLINICAL PEARLS
- Vulvodynia is a clinical diagnosis; it should be suspected in any woman with chronic pain at the introitus and vulva.
- A decrease in pain may take weeks to months and may not be complete.
- No single treatment is proven in all women; improvement over time is common even without treatment.

V

VULVOVAGINITIS, ESTROGEN DEFICIENT

Karla M. Alba, MD • Michelle Rodriguez, MD • Mark T. Nadeau, MD, MBA

 BASICS

DESCRIPTION
- Estrogen-deficient vulvovaginitis is a hypoestrogenic state with external genital, urologic, and sexual sequelae.
- Estrogen deficiency affects all tissues in the female body; however, the genital tissues are especially hormone responsive and are most affected.
- Decreased estrogen leads to decreased blood flow to vaginal tissues and thinning of vaginal tissues, dryness, and atrophy. Patients with estrogen-deficient vulvovaginitis may present with urinary incontinence, vaginal burning and itching, dyspareunia, increased urinary frequency, recurrent UTIs, or various other symptoms.
- This condition is also referred to as genitourinary syndrome of menopause when associated with the postmenopausal state, although this condition may occur in women of all ages.
- System(s) affected: reproductive

EPIDEMIOLOGY
Incidence
Predominant age: postmenopausal females. The average age of menopause in the United States is 51.3 years but ranges from 45 to 55 years old.

Prevalence
- Approximately 40–54% of postmenopausal women are affected.
- Approximately 15% of premenopausal women are also affected.
- This condition is likely underdiagnosed because patients may be reluctant to report symptoms because of embarrassment or the misconception that symptoms should be accepted as a natural part of aging (1).

ETIOLOGY AND PATHOPHYSIOLOGY
- Estrogen is vasoactive, increasing blood flow to target tissues, lubrication, and elasticity.
- Decreased estrogen levels in the vagina and vulva result in decreased blood flow and decreased lubrication and elasticity of vaginal and vulvar tissues as well as thinning of these tissues.
- Decreased cellular maturation results in decreased glycogen stores, which affects the normal vaginal flora and consequently the pH.
- The resulting increased pH impairs the viability of the normal flora, permitting the proliferation of fecal and other flora, resulting in UTIs and vaginal infections (1)[C].
- Estrogen deficiency is caused by the following:
  - Menopause (surgical or natural)
  - Premature ovarian failure (chemotherapy, radiation, autoimmune, anorexia, genetic)
  - Postpartum estrogen deficiency in lactating women
  - Medications that alter hormonal concentration, such as gonadotropin-releasing hormone agonists, tamoxifen, danazol, medroxyprogesterone, and aromatase inhibitors
  - Elevated prolactin from hypothalamic–pituitary disorders

Genetics
No known pattern

RISK FACTORS
- Estrogen-deficient states, including lactation
- Smoking
- Alcohol abuse
- Sexual abstinence or decreased frequency of coital activity
- Lack of exercise
- Absence of vaginal childbirth
- Chemotherapy
- Radiation therapy

COMMONLY ASSOCIATED CONDITIONS
- Urge and stress urinary incontinence
- Pelvic organ prolapse
- Frequent UTIs
- Bacterial or fungal vulvovaginitis
- Vaginal stenosis
- Loss of libido
- Dyspareunia

 DIAGNOSIS

HISTORY
- All female patients should be asked about symptoms because many women are embarrassed to discuss these issues with their health care providers (1).
  - Vaginal dryness
  - Dyspareunia
  - Pruritus
  - Burning
  - Pressure
  - Tenderness
  - Malodorous discharge
  - Urinary symptoms: dysuria, hematuria, frequency, infections, stress, and urge urinary incontinence
- Ask about exposure to radiation therapy and medications.
- Ask about self-treatment and products used.
- Determine exposure to irritants (e.g., soaps, feminine sprays, lotions, lubricants, constant pad use).

PHYSICAL EXAM
Evidence for the diagnosis includes the following:
- Loss of pubic hair
- Decreased vulvar and vaginal fullness
- Fusion of labia minora
- Vulvar erythema or ecchymosis
- Decreased vulvar subcuticular fat and moisture
- Pale-appearing, shiny, smooth vaginal and urethral epithelium
- Vaginal shortening, intolerance to speculum exams
- Loss of vaginal rugation
- Pelvic organ prolapse
- Urethral atrophy
- Atrophy of Bartholin glands
- Cervical atrophy and stenosis of os

DIFFERENTIAL DIAGNOSIS
- Malignancy
- Sexual trauma
- Infection secondary to foreign bodies (e.g., piercings)
- Dermatologic conditions of vulva and vagina:
  - Dermatitis
  - Lichen sclerosis
  - Lichen planus
- Bacterial or fungal vulvovaginitis

DIAGNOSTIC TESTS & INTERPRETATION
Because vulvovaginitis is a clinical diagnosis, labs are not always necessary, but if a dermatologic or oncologic condition is suspected, biopsy is recommended (2)[C].

Initial Tests (lab, imaging)
Lab tests are generally unnecessary to make the diagnosis. However, the following labs and imaging may be obtained as corroborative of clinical impression:
- Follicle-stimulating hormone (FSH) and estrogen levels. FSH rises and estrogen drops with menopause.
- Evaluate for infections via wet preparation and vaginal pH (usually >5).
- Urinalysis if suspected concomitant UTI
- Cytology for maturation index: Higher proportion of parabasal cells and lower proportion of intermediate and superficial cells indicate decreased maturation index.
- Transvaginal ultrasound: Endometrial stripe <5 mm indicates loss of estrogen stimulation.

Follow-Up Tests & Special Considerations
Drugs that may alter lab results:
- Estrogen therapy will alter the maturation index but may improve symptoms.
- Digoxin has estrogen-like properties.
- Tamoxifen may produce menopausal-type symptoms but also may act on genital tissues as a weak estrogen agonist.
- Progestins, danazol, and gonadotropin-releasing hormone agonists may produce a reversible pseudomenopausal state.

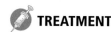 **TREATMENT**

GENERAL MEASURES
- Wear loose-fitting, undyed cotton underwear.
- Avoid prolonged pad use, especially scented pads.
- Avoid feminine deodorant sprays and douching.
- Symptomatic relief, if needed (e.g., cool baths or compresses)
- Increase coital activity.
- Smoking cessation

MEDICATION

- Nonhormonal vaginal moisturizers and lubricants are generally regarded as first-line therapy for mildly symptomatic estrogen-deficient vulvovaginitis (1)[C], although one recent study has shown that neither nonhormonal vaginal moisturizers nor lubricants and vaginal estrogen provided greater benefit than placebo gel or tablet (3)[A].
  - Estrogen therapy is preferred for moderate to severe symptoms: Local hormonal therapy (vaginal estrogen) is the first-line hormonal treatment and can reverse atrophic changes and alleviate symptoms (1)[C].
    - Vaginal cream: Insert via applicator 2 to 4 g daily for 1 to 2 weeks, then 1 to 2 g daily for 1 to 2 weeks and then 1 g 1 to 3 times a week.
    - Vaginal estradiol 10-μg tablet: Insert via preloaded applicator each night for 14 days and then twice weekly.
    - Estradiol-containing vaginal ring 2 mg: Insert into vagina and replace every 3 months.
  - Systemic hormonal therapy is typically reserved for patients wanting treatment for vasomotor symptoms associated with estrogen deficiency in addition to atrophic vulvovaginitis.
  - Transdermal preparations may be safer from a cardiovascular standpoint than oral preparations. Systemic estrogen therapy should be used in the lowest possible dose for the shortest duration of time (4)[B].
  - Long-term therapy may be necessary due to the chronic nature of estrogen-deficient vulvovaginitis (5)[A].
  - Contraindications:
    - Breast or estrogen-dependent cancers
    - Undiagnosed vaginal bleeding
    - Thromboembolic disorders
    - Endometrial hyperplasia or cancer
    - Hypertension
    - Hyperlipidemia
    - Liver disease
    - History of stroke
    - Coronary heart disease
    - Smoking in ages >35 years
    - Migraines with neurologic symptoms
    - Acute cholecystitis/cholangitis
    - Pregnancy
- Nonestrogen therapy: ospemifene (Osphena) 60-mg tablet daily; recommended for women with estrogen-deficient vulvovaginitis not responsive to nonpharmacologic therapies and who cannot or prefer not to use a vaginal estrogen (1)[C],(6)[B]
  - Contraindications:
    - Breast or estrogen-dependent carcinoma
    - Undiagnosed vaginal bleeding
    - Thromboembolic disorders
    - Thrombophlebitis
    - Hepatic impairment
- Precautions: Any abnormal vaginal bleeding must be evaluated. Monitor for DVT and stroke.

ISSUES FOR REFERRAL

- Refer to urogynecologist for evaluation if symptomatic due to pelvic organ prolapse and/or refractory stress and urge urinary incontinence.
- Recurrent UTIs should be further evaluated and may require a referral to urogynecology and/or urology.

ADDITIONAL THERAPIES

- Laser therapy with fractional CO_2 has demonstrated promise in initial studies; however, randomized controlled trials with long-term follow-up are still needed (1)[C].
- Lasofoxifene (Fablyn, Oporia) and oxytocin vaginal gel (Vagitocin) are under development but not yet approved (1)[C].

ADMISSION, INPATIENT, AND NURSING CONSIDERATIONS

Management of this condition occurs primarily in the outpatient setting.

 ## ONGOING CARE

FOLLOW-UP RECOMMENDATIONS

Follow up as needed to determine response to treatment and for adjustment of treatment regimen.

Patient Monitoring

Instruct the patient that symptoms should improve within 30 to 60 days. If they do not, reevaluate and reexamine for other causes.

DIET

Increased consumption of cranberry juice or extract to prevent recurrent UTIs has been recommended but not well supported by evidence.

PATIENT EDUCATION

- American College of Obstetricians and Gynecologists (ACOG), 409 12th St., SW, Washington, DC 20024-2188; 800-762-ACOG: http://www.acog.org/
- Lactating postpartum women with high levels of prolactin are in a hypoestrogenic state. These women should be instructed to use lubrication for symptoms of dyspareunia and reassured that the symptoms will resolve when they are no longer breastfeeding.

PROGNOSIS

The prognosis is good. Most symptoms will be alleviated with vaginal estrogen replacement therapy.

COMPLICATIONS

- Recurrent UTIs may occur in women with vaginal atrophy.
- Vaginal atrophy predisposes patients to vaginal infections.

REFERENCES

1. Gandhi J, Chen A, Dagur G, et al. Genitourinary syndrome of menopause: an overview of clinical manifestations, pathophysiology, etiology, evaluation, and management. *Am J Obstet Gynecol*. 2016;215(6):704–711.
2. Johnston SL, Farrell SA, Bouchard C, et al; for SOGC Joint Committee-Clinical Practice Gynaecology and Urogynaecology. The detection and management of vaginal atrophy. *J Obstet Gynaecol Can*. 2004; 26(5):503–515.
3. Mitchell CM, Reed SD, Diem S, et al. Efficacy of vaginal estradiol or vaginal moisturizer vs placebo for treating postmenopausal vulvovaginal symptoms: a randomized clinical trial. *JAMA Intern Med*. 2018;178(5):681–690.
4. Ibe C, Simon JA. Vulvovaginal atrophy: current and future therapies (CME). *J Sex Med*. 2010;7(3):1042–1051.
5. Suckling J, Lethaby A, Kennedy R. Local oestrogen for vaginal atrophy in postmenopausal women. *Cochrane Database Syst Rev*. 2006;(4):CD001500.
6. Constantine G, Graham S, Portman DJ, et al. Female sexual function improved with ospemifene in postmenopausal women with vulvar and vaginal atrophy: results of a randomized, placebo-controlled trial. *Climacteric*. 2015;18(2):226–232.

ADDITIONAL READING

- Pitsouni E, Grigoriadis T, Falagas M, et al. Laser therapy for the genitourinary syndrome of menopause. A systematic review and meta-analysis. *Maturitas*. 2017;103:78–88.
- Ruan X, Mueck A. Impact of smoking on estrogenic efficacy. *Climacteric*. 2015;18(1):38–46.

 ## CODES

ICD10

- N95.2 Postmenopausal atrophic vaginitis
- E28.39 Other primary ovarian failure

CLINICAL PEARLS

- Estrogen-deficient vulvovaginitis affects virtually all postmenopausal women to some degree as well as some premenopausal women.
- This disorder is associated with genital, urologic, and sexual symptoms including vaginal itching, vaginal dryness, urinary incontinence, increased urinary frequency, recurrent UTIs, and dyspareunia.
- Estrogen-deficient vulvovaginitis is a clinical diagnosis; lab tests are generally unnecessary.
- Vaginal moisturizers and lubricants are first-line therapy for mild symptoms, and vaginal estrogen preparations, rather than systemic preparations, are the preferred hormonal therapy for women with moderate to severe symptoms of estrogen-deficient vulvovaginitis.

VULVOVAGINITIS, PREPUBESCENT

Simon B. Griesbach, MD • Erin M. Glembocki, MD

BASICS

DESCRIPTION

- Vulvitis is inflammation of the external genitalia.
- Vaginitis is inflammation involving the vaginal mucosa and can be characterized with or without odor or bleeding.
- In premenarchal girls, vulvitis is usually primary with secondary extension into the vagina.
- Vulvovaginitis can be classified as either nonspecific (not likely infectious but rather hygienic/behavioral cause) or specific (likely infectious cause).
- Systems affected: reproductive, integumentary
- Clinical features: vaginal/vulvar itching, soreness, dysuria, redness, discharge, bleeding, odor, and pain

EPIDEMIOLOGY

Incidence
Unknown

Prevalence
Most common gynecologic problem in prepubertal girls

ETIOLOGY AND PATHOPHYSIOLOGY

- In the prepubertal child, levels of estrogen are low, leading to thin, immature and fragile vaginal epithelium.
- Anatomically, underdeveloped labia minora, absence of pubic hair, minimal adiposity of the labia majora, and close proximity of the introitus to the anus make contamination more likely (1).
- The prepubertal child also has an alkaline vaginal pH due to a relative deficiency of lactobacilli (which is lactic acid forming) as compared to adolescent and adult females (1).
- Infectious organisms causing vulvovaginitis are typically respiratory, enteric, or rarely sexually transmitted.
- Most cases (~75%) of pediatric vulvovaginitis are classified as nonspecific vulvovaginitis and do not have an infectious etiology.
- Nonspecific vulvovaginitis causes include:
  – Poor perineal hygiene (wiping back to front) (2)
  – Chemical irritants (bubble baths, scented soaps, wipes, laundry detergents)
  – Tight-fitting clothing or underwear made of synthetic materials
- Specific vulvovaginitis causes include:
  – Bacterial:
    ○ The most common respiratory pathogen is *Streptococcus pyogenes* (3). Vulvitis may occur in the absence of respiratory symptoms.
    ○ *Escherichia coli* is the most common fecal pathogen.
    ○ *Shigella* vaginitis is associated with mucopurulent bloody discharge and is not always accompanied by a history of diarrhea.

ALERT
Presence of *Neisseria gonorrhoeae* or *Chlamydia trachomatis* strongly suggests sexual transmission and should prompt consideration of sexual abuse.

- *Enterobius vermicularis* (pinworms)
  – Most common symptom is nocturnal perineal itching.
  – Should be considered in children with vaginal itching and irritation
  – Very common in young children and certain populations
- Considerations for recurrent/chronic vulvovaginitis:
  – Anatomic abnormalities could include double vagina with fistula, ectopic ureter, and urethral prolapse.
  – Systemic inflammatory diseases
  – Other conditions, such as lichen sclerosus, vitiligo, psoriasis, and atopic dermatitis are possible.
  – Foreign body
    ○ Presents with foul-smelling, bloody, or brown discharge from the vagina
    ○ Should be considered in patients with recurrent vulvovaginitis after other causes are ruled out.
    ○ Most common objects: toilet paper, small toys, hair clips
    ○ If there is gray watery discharge, consider possibility of battery as foreign body (1).

RISK FACTORS

- Inadequate hand washing or perineal cleansing after urination and defecation (2)
- Wearing of tight-fitting clothing
- Obesity
- Immunosuppression
  – Diabetes
  – Recent antibiotic use
- Anatomic abnormalities

GENERAL PREVENTION

- Good perineal hygiene (including wiping from front to back)
- Urination with legs spread apart and labia separated
- Avoidance of tight-fitting clothing and nonabsorbent underwear
- Avoidance of irritants such as harsh/perfumed soaps and bubble baths

COMMONLY ASSOCIATED CONDITIONS

- Urinary tract infections are common in children with vulvovaginitis.
- Constipation predisposes to vulvovaginitis and vice versa.

DIAGNOSIS

HISTORY

- In taking the history from pediatric patient, develop good rapport with the patient and family as both the history and physical exam are sensitive to discuss.
- Symptoms may include:
  – Vaginal discharge
  – Vaginal or anal itching, burning, or discomfort
  – Vulvar redness
  – Dysuria or perineal pain during urination
  – Prepubertal vaginal bleeding
  – Enuresis or encopresis
- Obtain careful history addressing any recent respiratory or enteric infections in the patient or close contacts.
- Ask questions to determine character of any vaginal discharge, if present.
- Determine exposure to irritants that may predispose to vulvovaginitis.

- Question when symptoms most often occur/worsen.
- Inquire about patient's toileting habits:
  – Wiping technique
  – Position of legs while urinating
  – If rushing to the bathroom and inadequate voiding
  – If not voiding/stooling while away at school

PHYSICAL EXAM

- Inform patients and family that exam may be embarrassing and uncomfortable but not painful (4).
- Explain physical exam thoroughly to the patient and her caregivers prior to beginning, giving opportunities to ask questions.
- If exam provokes significant anxiety, consider deferring exam or, for urgent/emergent concerns, performing exam under anesthesia.
- Examine pediatric patients in two positions for best visualization:
  – Supine in frog-leg position: provides view of external anatomy; Valsalva brings distal vagina into view
  – Prone in knee–chest position: Taking deep breath separates vaginal walls and provides view of internal vagina and cervix; foreign body can be seen in this position.
- Look for excoriation, erythema, swelling of the introitus, discharge, foreign body, lichenification of external skin and evaluate degree of estrogenized tissue.
- Perform rectovaginal exam if vaginal bleeding, abdominal pain, or in cases concerning for tumor or foreign body.
- Perform culture collection if necessary.

DIFFERENTIAL DIAGNOSIS

- Lichen sclerosus
- Contact dermatitis
- Eczema
- Psoriasis

DIAGNOSTIC TESTS & INTERPRETATION
Diagnosis is often clinical with testing only necessary in patients with history or exam concerning for an infectious cause.

Initial Tests (lab, imaging)
- Definitive diagnosis of bacterial vulvovaginitis requires a culture of vulvar and vaginal secretions.
  – Collect this specimen with a moistened small-diameter collection swab.
- Perform polymerase chain reaction (PCR) for sexually transmitted infection (STI) or herpes virus if suspected.
- Potassium hydroxide and saline smears of vaginal discharge, if present, can aid in diagnoses of fungal or certain bacterial causes. They have limited sensitivity and specificity.
- Urinalysis and urine culture can be considered evaluate for concurrent urinary infection.
- Tape test can be considered to evaluate for pinworm; some treat based on history and exam alone due to low sensitivity of testing.

Follow-Up Tests & Special Considerations
Consider consultation with a provider with specific training/experience to determine the most appropriate imaging study.

Diagnostic Procedures/Other
- Exploration of the vagina for a foreign body may be necessary in cases of persistent, recurrent symptoms.
- If an anatomic abnormality is suspected, imaging may be necessary to confirm.
- If available, consider referral to a pediatric or adult gynecologist provider with specific training/experience to determine next steps.

Test Interpretation
Culture often reveals organisms identical to those cultured in asymptomatic individuals.

TREATMENT

- Treatment is appropriate in the outpatient health care setting, except where systemic illness requires hospital care.
- Approximately 75% of the time, no specific infectious cause is identified. In this case, general hygiene/behavioral changes should always be recommended as first-line treatment, with recommendations tailored to patient's history.
- A known concomitant respiratory illness or visualized purulent vaginal discharge suggests infection. A culture should be obtained and antibiotic use should be directed against the species with the highest colony count.

GENERAL MEASURES
- Avoid irritants, including scented soaps, wipes, and bubble baths.
- Soak the vulva/perineum in a small amount of clear, warm water for 15 minutes 1 to 4 times per day.
- Advise the patient to avoid wearing underwear to bed or to instead wear loose-fitting boxer-shorts bottoms with loose pajamas.

MEDICATION
- Nonantibiotic options
  - To break the itching–scratching–infection cycle, consider clobetasol propionate 0.05% as initial treatment and hydrocortisone cream 1% to follow for short-term maintenance.
  - For estrogen deficiency with labial adhesion/agglutination or urethral prolapse: estrogen cream 0.625 mg to fused area nightly for 2 weeks
  - Emollients or barrier creams (unscented) may offer symptomatic relief.
- Antibiotic options
  - Antibiotic use should be restricted to cases of bacterial infection only (5) and directed toward highest colony count bacteria.
    - *S. pyogenes*:
      - Amoxicillin, 50 mg/kg/day PO divided into 3 doses/day for 10 days
    - Group A *Streptococcus*, *Streptococcus pneumoniae*:
      - Penicillin V, 250 mg PO BID–TID for 10 days
    - *Haemophilus influenzae*:
      - Amoxicillin, 20 to 40 mg/kg/day PO divided TID for 7 days
    - *Staphylococcus aureus*:
      - Cephalexin, 25 to 50 mg/kg/day PO divided QID for 7 to 10 days *or*
      - Dicloxacillin, 25 mg/kg/day divided QID for 7 to 10 days *or*
      - Amoxicillin-clavulanate, 20 to 40 mg/kg/day PO divided BID for 7 to 10 days

  - *Candida* spp.:
    - Topical nystatin, miconazole, clotrimazole, or terconazole
  - *Shigella*:
    - Trimethoprim/sulfamethoxazole or ampicillin for 5 days
  - *E. coli*:
    - Base treatment on your local resistance pattern.
  - Pinworms:
    - Mebendazole, 100 mg PO once, repeated in 2 weeks
  - *C. trachomatis*:
    - ≤45 kg: erythromycin base, 50 mg/kg/day QID for 14 days
    - ≥45 kg and <8 years old: azithromycin, 1 g PO single dose
    - ≥45 kg and ≥8 years old: azithromycin, 1 g PO single dose or doxycycline 100 mg BID for 7 days
  - *N. gonorrhoeae*:
    - ≤45 kg: ceftriaxone, 25–50 mg/kg up to 250 mg IM or IV once
    - >45 kg: ceftriaxone, 250 mg IM or IV once
    - Consider treatment for chlamydia if not excluded.
  - *Trichomonas*:
    - Metronidazole, 15 mg/kg/day PO divided TID (max 250 mg TID) for 7 days

ISSUES FOR REFERRAL
- Suspected sexual abuse
- Suspected anatomic abnormality (except minor labial agglutination)
- Persistent, severe, or recurrent infections
- Inability to tolerate physical exam with serious cause suspected

COMPLEMENTARY & ALTERNATIVE MEDICINE
Consider the need for further psychological support for both parent (most often mother) and child (4):
- Parents play a large role in trial and error process of hygiene changes for their child which adds stress. Normalize this is not something the parent did wrong.
- Often, this can feel a "taboo" subject. Offer psychological support if there have been lifestyle changes that have affected socialization of the child (e.g., scared to go to sleep overs without parental support overnight).
- Delays in diagnosis may result in traumatic experiences and cause sequelae such as vaginismus.

ONGOING CARE

FOLLOW-UP RECOMMENDATIONS
Patient Monitoring
Monitor for fever, pruritus, and vaginal discharge.

DIET
- Healthy balanced diet, high in fiber to prevent constipation
- Adequate fluid intake

PATIENT EDUCATION
Hygiene
- Urinate with legs apart, sitting forward to decrease likelihood urine will collect in the vagina.
  - Consider facing "backward" on toilet seat to facilitate this.
- Wipe front to back after elimination and avoid reuse of toilet paper.
- Avoid bubble baths and other irritating products, including all scented products.
- Clean daily with mild soap and water and dry gently with soft towel or cool hair dryer.
- Defer hair shampooing to the end of bath time; consider washing hair while standing up.
- Apply unscented ointments or barrier creams for skin protection.
- Avoid tight clothing, underwear made of synthetic materials, sitting in wet swimsuits, or wearing full body sleeper pajamas.

COMPLICATIONS
- If an STI is identified and not treated effectively, the patient is at risk for pelvic inflammatory disease (PID).
- Untreated vulvovaginitis can cause labial adhesions
- Vaginismus

REFERENCES
1. Romano ME. Prepubertal Vulvovaginitis. *Clin Obstet Gynecol*. 2020;63(3):479–485.
2. Cemek F, Odabaş D, Şenel Ü, et al. Personal hygiene and vulvovaginitis in prepubertal children. *J Pediatr Adolesc Gynecol*. 2016;29(3):223–227.
3. Gorbachinsky I, Sherertz R, Russell G, et al. Altered perineal microbiome is associated with vulvovaginitis and urinary tract infection in preadolescent girls. *Ther Adv Urol*. 2014;6(6):224–229.
4. McKenna J, Bray L, Doyle S. Parental experiences of their child's vulvovaginitis: a qualitative interview study. *J Pediatr Urol*. 2019;15(6):659.e1–659.e5.
5. Dei M, Di Maggio F, Di Paolo G, et al. Vulvovaginitis in childhood. *Best Pract Res Clin Obstet Gynaecol*. 2010;24(2):129–137.

CODES

ICD10
- N76.0 Acute vaginitis
- N77.1 Vaginitis, vulvitis and vulvovaginitis in dis classd elswhr

CLINICAL PEARLS
- Vulvovaginitis is the most common gynecologic problem in prepubescent girls.
- The hypoestrogenic state and prepubescent anatomy may increase susceptibility to vulvar and vaginal infection.
- Treatment is typically supportive (avoid scratching, warm soaks) but may require antibiotics if a bacterial infection is suspected.
- Isolating an infection with known sexual transmission should prompt further investigation.
- Recurrent or persistent vulvovaginitis, especially with foul-smelling discharge, should prompt a skilled exam of the vagina for a retained foreign body (most common toilet paper).
- Good perineal hygiene will limit this condition.

V

WARKS

Karl T. Clebak, MD, MHA, FAAFP • Rensa Chen, DO

BASICS

- Warts (verrucae) are benign growths that are confined to the epidermis. All warts are caused by the human papillomavirus (HPV). Warts can appear on any area of the skin or mucous membranes. Common warts are predominantly seen in children and young adults.
- Clinically, warts are described as follows:
  – Common warts (verrucae vulgaris)
  – Plantar warts (verrucae plantaris)
  – Flat warts (verruca plana)
  – Genital warts (condyloma acuminatum)
  – Epidermodysplasia verruciformis is a rare, lifelong hereditary disorder characterized by chronic infection with HPV.
- System(s) affected: skin/exocrine

DESCRIPTION
- Common warts are most often found at sites subject to frequent trauma, such as the hands and feet. Because warts often vary widely in shape, size, and appearance, the various descriptive names for them generally reflect their clinical appearance, location, or both.
- For example: Filiform (fingerlike) warts are thread-like, planar warts are flat, and plantar warts are located on the plantar surfaces (soles) of the feet.
- Genital warts, or condyloma acuminata, may be large and cauliflower-like, or they may consist of small papules.
- Warts on mucous membranes (mucosal papillomas), such as those in the mouth or vagina, tend to be white in color due to moisture retention.

EPIDEMIOLOGY
Incidence
- Predominant age: young adults and children
- No sex predominance: female = male

Prevalence
- ~7–10% of the U.S. population
- ~10% of all school children and young adults experience common warts
- Common warts appear 2 times as frequently in whites compared with blacks or Asians.

ETIOLOGY AND PATHOPHYSIOLOGY
- HPV is a double-stranded, circular, nonenveloped, supercoiled DNA virus.
- The virus infects epidermal keratinocytes, stimulating cell proliferation.
- Various strains of DNA HPV: To date, >200 different subtypes have been identified.
- The virus is passed primarily through skin-to-skin contact or from the recently shed virus kept intact in a moist, warm environment.

RISK FACTORS
- HIV/AIDS and other immunosuppressive diseases (e.g., lymphomas)
- Immunosuppressive drugs that decrease cell-mediated immunity (e.g., prednisone, cyclosporine, and chemotherapeutic agents)
- Pregnancy
- Handling raw meat, fish, or other types of animal matter in one's occupation (e.g., butchers)
- Previous wart infection
- Use of communal shower room
- Close contact recreational activities
- Close contact with affected person
- Trauma

GENERAL PREVENTION
- Avoid sharing shoes, socks, towels, tools (nail file, razors).
- Maintain personal hygiene, keep feet clean and dry.
- Wear breathable footwear.
- Wear footwear in communal shower room.
- Avoid scratching or manipulating warts.

COMMONLY ASSOCIATED CONDITIONS
Warts, hypogammaglobulinemia, infections, myelo-kathexis (WHIM) syndrome, warts, immunodeficiency, lymphedema, dysplasia (WILD) syndrome, hyper-IgE recurrent infection syndrome

DIAGNOSIS

Most often made on clinical appearance

HISTORY
History of a growing skin lesion. Usually asymptomatic; however, warts on soles of feet or around nails may cause discomfort.

PHYSICAL EXAM
- Distribution of warts is generally asymmetric, and lesions are often clustered or may appear in a linear configuration due to scratching (autoinoculation).
- Common wart: rough-surfaced, hyperkeratotic, papillomatous, raised, skin-colored to tan papules, 5 to 10 mm in diameter; several may coalesce into a larger cluster (mosaic wart); most frequently seen on hands, knees, and elbows; usually asymptomatic but may cause cosmetic disfigurement or tenderness
- Filiform warts: These are long, slender, delicate, fingerlike growths, usually seen on the face around the lips, eyelids, or nares.
- Plantar warts often have a rough surface and appear on the plantar surface of the feet in children and young adults.
  – Can be tender and painful; extensive involvement on the sole of the foot may impair ambulation, particularly when present on a weight-bearing surface.
  – Most often seen on the metatarsal area, heels, and toes in an asymmetric distribution (pressure points)
  – Pathognomonic "black dots" (thrombosed dermal capillaries); punctate bleeding becomes more evident after paring with a no. 15 blade.
  – Both common and plantar warts generally demonstrate the following clinical findings:
    ○ A loss of normal skin markings (dermatoglyphics) such as finger, foot, and hand prints
    ○ Lesions may be solitary or multiple, or they may appear in clusters (mosaic warts).
- Flat warts: slightly elevated, smooth, numerous, flat-topped, skin-colored or tan papules, small (1 to 3 mm) in diameter
  – Commonly found on the face, arms, dorsa of hands, knees, and shins (women)
  – Sometimes exhibit a linear configuration caused by autoinoculation
  – In men, shaving spreads flat warts.
  – In women, they often occur on the shins where leg shaving spreads lesions.
- Epidermodysplasia verruciformis (rare): Widespread flat, reddish brown pigmented papules and plaques that present in childhood with lifelong persistence on the trunk, hands, upper and lower extremities, and face are characteristics.
- Focal epithelial hyperplasia (rare): multiple painless, 1- to 5-mm whitish painless, soft, sessile papules or plaques on the oral mucosa, gingiva, tongue or lips

DIFFERENTIAL DIAGNOSIS
- Molluscum contagiosum, seborrheic keratosis, epidermal nevus, acrochordon (skin tag), solar keratosis and cutaneous horn, acquired digital fibrokeratoma, squamous cell carcinoma (SCC), keratoacanthoma, subungual SCC can easily be misdiagnosed as a subungual wart or onychomycosis, lichen planus, lichen nitidus, talon noir (black heel)
- Corns/calluses
  – Corns (clavi) are sometimes difficult to distinguish from plantar warts. Like calluses, corns are thickened areas of the skin and most commonly develop at sites subjected to repeated friction and pressure, such as the tops and the tips of toes and along the sides of the feet.
    ○ Corns are usually hard and circular, with a polished or central translucent core, like the kernel of corn from which they take their name.
    ○ Corns do not have "black dots," and skin markings are retained, except for the area of the central core.

ALERT
- A melanoma on the plantar surface of the foot can mimic a plantar wart.
- Verrucous carcinoma, a slow-growing, locally invasive, well-differentiated SCC, also may be easily mistaken for a common or plantar wart.

DIAGNOSTIC TESTS & INTERPRETATION
Initial Tests (lab, imaging)
Diagnosis
- HPV cannot be cultured, and lab testing is rarely necessary.
- Definitive HPV diagnosis can be achieved by the following:
  – Electron microscopy
  – Viral DNA identification employing Southern blot hybridization is used to identify the specific HPV type present in tissue.
  – Polymerase chain reaction may be used to amplify viral DNA for testing.

Follow-Up Tests & Special Considerations
Skin biopsy if suspicious for malignancy or if the diagnosis is unclear

Test Interpretation
In the granular layer, HPV-infected cells may have coarse keratohyalin granules and vacuoles surrounding wrinkled-appearing nuclei. These koilocytic (vacuolated) cells are pathognomonic for warts.

TREATMENT

- The abundance of therapeutic modalities described below is a reflection of the fact that none of them is uniformly or even clearly effective in trials. Placebo treatment response rate is significant, and quality of evidence in general is poor. Beyond topical salicylates, there is no clear evidence-based rationale for choosing one method over another (1)[A].
- The choice of method of treatment depends on the following:
  – Age of the patient
  – Cosmetic and psychological considerations
  – Relief of symptoms
  – Patient's pain threshold
  – Type of wart
  – Location of the wart
  – Experience of the physician

GENERAL MEASURES
- There is no ideal treatment.
- In children and immunocompetent adults, most warts regress spontaneously.
- In many adults and immunocompromised patients, warts are often difficult to eradicate.
- Painful, aggressive therapy should be avoided unless there is a need to eliminate the wart(s).
- For surgical procedures, especially in anxious children, pretreat with anesthetic cream such as EMLA (emulsion of lidocaine and prilocaine).

MEDICATION
First Line
- Self-administered topical therapy
  - Keratolytic (peeling) agents: The affected area(s) should be hydrated first by soaking in warm water for 5 minutes before application. Apply daily for 12 weeks. Most over-the-counter agents contain salicylic acid and/or lactic acid: agents such as Duofilm, Occlusal-HP, Trans-Ver-Sal, and Mediplast. Avoid use on face due to hyper- and hypopigmentation.
- Office based:
  - Cantharidin 0.7%, an extract of the blister beetle that causes epidermal necrosis and blistering but may be difficult to obtain as a solution in the United States. It may be compounded in compounding pharmacies.
  - Plantar warts had high rates of clearance with combination cantharidin 1%, salicylic acid 20–30%, and podophyllin resin 5% in flexible collodion even after single treatment. Warts were thoroughly débrided, applied a thin topical coat, occluded for several hours and then washed off (2).
  - Generally well-tolerated and effective
  - Potential adverse effects: pain, blistering, scarring, hyper-/hypopigmentation

Second Line
- Home based:
  - Imiquimod 5% (Aldara) cream, a local inducer of interferon, is applied at home by the patient. It is approved for external genital and perianal warts and is used off-label and may be applied to warts under duct tape occlusion. It is applied at bedtime and washed off after 6 to 10 hours; applied to flat warts without occlusion. Use 5 times a week up to 16 weeks.
  - Topical retinoids (e.g., tretinoin 0.025–0.1% cream or gel) for flat warts
- Office based:
  - Cryotherapy is effective and can be used as a second-line treatment.
  - Immunotherapy: induction of delayed-type hypersensitivity with the following:
    - Diphenylcyclopropenone (DPCP) or diphencyprone (DCP): cure rate 44–88% (3); mutagenic effects in vitro
    - Dinitrochlorobenzene (DNCB): cure rate 66–95% (3). Its mutagenicity limits its use.
    - Squaric acid dibutylester (SADBE): cure rate 58–86% (3). There is possible mutagenicity; side effects: erythema, edema, itching, burning (4)
    - Efficacy compared to other treatment modalities requires further research. Contact immunotherapy requires sensitization before rechallenge (3).
  - Intralesional injections using mumps, *Candida* antigen. Bleomycin, interferon, and MTB antigen used occasionally.

- Oral therapy
  - Oral high-dose cimetidine: possibly works better in children (40 mg/kg/day; max 1,600 mg)
  - Acitretin or isotretinoin (oral retinoids)
- Other treatments (All have all been used with varying results.)
  - Dichloroacetic acid, trichloroacetic acid, podophyllin, formic acid, aminolevulinic acid in combination with blue light, 5-fluorouracil, silver nitrate, formaldehyde, levamisole, topical cidofovir or IV cidofovir for recalcitrant warts in the setting of HIV, and glutaraldehyde
- The quadrivalent HPV vaccine has cleared recalcitrant, chronic oral, and cutaneous warts.

ISSUES FOR REFERRAL
Consider referral to dermatology immunocompromised patients who do not respond to initial treatments.

SURGERY/OTHER PROCEDURES
- Cryotherapy with liquid nitrogen (LN_2) may be applied with a cotton swab or with a cryotherapy gun (Cryogun). Aggressive cryotherapy may be more effective than salicylic acid (5)[A], but it is associated with increased adverse effects (blistering and scarring):
  - Typically combined with salicylic acid to augment efficacy
  - Best for warts on hands; also during pregnancy and breastfeeding
  - Fast; can treat many lesions per visit
  - Painful; not tolerated well by young children
  - Freezing periungual warts may result in nail deformation.
  - In darkly pigmented skin, treatment can result in hypo- or hyperpigmentation.
  - Uneven uptake of LN^2 can result in a larger ring wart.
  - Adverse effects: erythema, blistering, pain, tenderness; heals within 4 to 7 days
- Light electrocautery with or without curettage
  - Best for warts on the knees, elbows, and dorsa of hands, also good for filiform warts, tolerable in most adults, requires local anesthesia, may cause scarring
- Photodynamic therapy: Topical 5-aminolevulinic acid is applied to warts followed by photoactivation; better cosmetic outcome for recalcitrant facial flat warts
- CO_2 laser ablation: expensive; clearance rate 50–200%; adverse effects: postprocedure pain, delayed wound healing, scarring, pigment changes (4)
- Pulse-dye laser: expensive; clearance rate 32–92%. Adverse effects: mild pain, dyspigmentation, mild scaring; safe for children and adults (4)
- For filiform warts: Dip hemostat into LN_2 for 10 seconds, then gently grasp the wart for 10 seconds and repeat. Wart sheds in 7 to 10 days.

COMPLEMENTARY & ALTERNATIVE MEDICINE
- Duct tape: Cover wart with waterproof tape (e.g., duct tape). Leave the tape on for 6 days and then soak, pare with emery board, and leave uncovered overnight; then, reapply tape cyclically for eight cycles; unclear efficacy as single agent
- Hyperthermia: safe and inexpensive approach; immerse affected area into 45°C water bath for 30 minutes 3 times per week.
- Oral daily zinc therapy at a maximum dose of 600 mg/day increased clearance rates compared to placebo.

Pregnancy Considerations
The use of some topical chemical approaches may be contraindicated during pregnancy or in women who are likely to become pregnant during the treatment period.

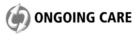 ONGOING CARE

FOLLOW-UP RECOMMENDATIONS
Patient Monitoring
1/3 of the warts of epidermodysplasia may become malignant.

PATIENT EDUCATION
- The HPV types causing common, plantar, or flat warts are usually different from HPV causing genital warts.
- Vaccine is available to protect against those causing genital warts.

PROGNOSIS
More often than not (especially in children), warts tend to "cure" themselves over time. In many adults and immunocompromised patients, warts often prove difficult to eradicate.

COMPLICATIONS
- Autoinoculation (pseudo-Koebner reaction)
- Scar formation
- Chronic pain after plantar wart removal or scar formation
- Nail deformity after injury to nail matrix

REFERENCES
1. Kwok CS, Gibbs S, Bennett C, et al. Topical treatments for cutaneous warts. *Cochrane Database Syst Rev.* 2012;(9):CD001781.
2. Vakharia PP, Chopra R, Silverberg NB, et al. Efficacy and safety of topical cantharidin treatment for molluscum contagiosum and warts: a systematic review. *Am J Clin Dermatol.* 2018;19(6):791–803.
3. Word AP, Nezafati KA, Cruz PD Jr. Treatment of warts with contact allergens. *Dermatitis.* 2015;26(1):32–37.
4. Leerunyakul K, Thammarucha S, Suchonwanit P, et al. A comprehensive review of treatment options for recalcitrant nongenital cutaneous warts [published online ahead of print March 11, 2020]. *J Dermatolog Treat.* 2020:1–18.
5. Kwok CS, Holland R, Gibbs S. Efficacy of topical treatments for cutaneous warts: a meta-analysis and pooled analysis of randomized controlled trials. *Br J Dermatol.* 2011;165(2):233–246.

 CODES

ICD10
- A63.0 Anogenital (venereal) warts
- B07 Viral warts
- B07.9 Viral wart, unspecified

CLINICAL PEARLS
- No single therapy for warts is uniformly effective or superior; thus, treatment involves a certain amount of trial and error.
- Because most warts in children tend to regress spontaneously within 2 years, benign neglect is often a prudent option.
- Conservative, nonscarring, least painful, least expensive treatments are preferred.

W

WILMS TUMOR
Chad Hamner, MD

 BASICS

DESCRIPTION
- The most common renal tumor in children; fifth most common pediatric malignancy
- An embryonal renal neoplasm containing blastemal, stromal, or epithelial cell types
- System(s) affected: renal/urologic
- Synonym(s): nephroblastoma

Pediatric Considerations
Occurs predominately in children; rare incidence in late adolescence and adults

EPIDEMIOLOGY
Incidence
- WT represents 6–7% of all childhood cancers and comprises 95% of renal cancers in children <15 years (1).
- 650 cases diagnosed annually; incidence of 8.2 cases per 1 million children (1)
- Median age of diagnosis is 36.5 months (1).

ETIOLOGY AND PATHOPHYSIOLOGY
Genetics
- Tumors display recurrent gene mutations involved in either early renal development or epigenetic regulation (e.g., chromatin modification, transcription regulation, miRNA) (1).
- 1/3 of tumors involve mutations of WT1, CTNNB1, or WTX genes (1).
- Majority occur sporadically; familial inheritance <2% (1)

RISK FACTORS
More frequent in black children; rare in Asian (1)

GENERAL PREVENTION
Genetic counseling recommended for WT and one major abnormality: overgrowth syndromes, hemihyperplasia, aniridia, mental disability, diffuse mesangial sclerosis; or two minor malformations—inguinal or umbilical hernia, hypospadias, renal abnormalities, ectopic testis (1)

COMMONLY ASSOCIATED CONDITIONS
- Overgrowth syndromes: Beckwith-Wiedemann syndrome, isolated hemihyperplasia, Perlman syndrome, Simpson-Golabi-Behmel syndrome, CLOVES syndrome, and Sotos syndrome (1)
- Nonovergrowth syndromes: Denys-Drash and Frasier, WAGR, sporadic, familial WT, Bohring-Opitz syndrome, Bloom syndrome, Li-Fraumeni syndrome, Fanconi anemia, Alagille syndrome, trisomy 18, and genitourinary anomalies (1)

 DIAGNOSIS

HISTORY
- Abdominal mass (>90%), abdominal pain (40%), hypertension (25%), gross hematuria (18%) (1)
- Associated symptoms (10%): fever, weight loss, anorexia, malaise (1)
- History of increasing abdominal size

PHYSICAL EXAM
Palpable upper abdominal mass, hypertension, fever, hepatosplenomegaly, ascites, prominent abdominal wall veins, varicocele, or cardiac murmur

DIFFERENTIAL DIAGNOSIS
Neuroblastoma, hepatic tumor, sarcoma, rhabdoid tumor, cystic nephroma, clear cell renal sarcoma, renal cell carcinoma, mesoblastic nephroma, nephroblastomatosis, pheochromocytoma

DIAGNOSTIC TESTS & INTERPRETATION
Initial Tests (lab, imaging)
- Urinalysis (occasional hematuria, proteinuria), CBC (anemia), renal function studies, liver function studies, coagulation factors (association with acquired von Willebrand factor deficiency), lactate dehydrogenase, urine catecholamines (present with neuroblastoma)
- Chest radiograph
- Abdominal US: best initial test; provides information about tumor thrombus extension into inferior vena cava (IVC) (6–10% of tumors)
- CT scan (IV and oral contrast) of chest and abdomen provides anatomic visualization for surgical planning and staging information.
- MRI may be used as alternative to CT; routine use limited by need for sedation

Diagnostic Procedures/Other
- Tumor biopsy should be avoided as violation of the tumor capsule upstages the local disease (stage III).
- Surgical resection with aortocaval lymph node sampling is recommended for unilateral tumors.
- Contraindications to upfront resection:
  - High risk of renal failure: solitary kidney, bilateral WT, genetic risk for bilateral tumors
  - Presence of lung metastases does not typically influence indication for tumor resection (2).
- Tumor molecular analysis has prognostic and treatment implications.

Test Interpretation
- Histologic features grouped into favorable and unfavorable categories (1):
  - Favorable histology, present in 90% of tumors (survival rate >90%):
    ○ Triphasic pattern of blastemal, stromal, and epithelial elements
    ○ Predominance of blastemal elements indicates more aggressive tumors.
  - Unfavorable histology (anaplasia, focal or diffuse), survival rate 33–85% (1):
    ○ Anaplasia defined as hyperchromatic, markedly enlarged pleomorphic nuclei with multipolar polypoid mitotic figures
    ○ Single most important histologic predictor of survival and response to treatment; diffuse pattern worse prognosis than focal pattern
- COG stage (incidence) (1):
  - I: completely excised tumor limited to kidney; negative lymph nodes (43%)
  - II: completely excised tumor (includes capsular invasion; tumor in renal sinus vessels; atriocaval thrombus removed en bloc with tumor); (−) lymph nodes (20%)
  - III: residual tumor confined to abdomen (tumor spillage or biopsy, peritoneal implants, extension beyond resection region, atriocaval thrombus not removed en bloc with tumor); (+) lymph nodes (21%)
  - IV: metastases (lung most common, liver, brain, or bones) or (+) lymph nodes outside the abdomen/pelvis (11%)
  - V: bilateral WT (5%)

- Molecular features associated with worse prognosis (1):
  - Loss of heterozygosity (LOH) on chromosomes 16q and 1p is associated with higher risk of recurrence.
  - Chromosome 1q gain is present in 30% tumors; single most powerful predictor of outcome

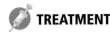

TREATMENT

GENERAL MEASURES

- Surgical resection with varying regimens of combination chemotherapy and radiation therapy dependent on stage of disease
- Risk stratification is used to determine appropriate treatment protocols.
- Neoadjuvant chemotherapy following biopsy (percutaneous or open) indicated in COG protocols for following situations: tumor in solitary kidney, synchronous bilateral WT, extensive IVC thrombus, locally invasive tumor involving contiguous organs other than adrenal gland, inoperable tumors, or pulmonary compromise due to extensive metastases (1),(2)
- Radiation therapy reserved for advanced stage disease (stages III and IV) and anaplastic tumors (1),(2)
- Nephrectomy alone may be offered to select children (<2 years) with small (<550 g), stage I, favorable histology tumors (1),(2).

MEDICATION

First Line

Multiagent chemotherapy regimens are used as standard therapy (1):

- EE-4A: vincristine and dactinomycin; 18 weeks duration after nephrectomy
- DD-4A: vincristine, dactinomycin, and doxorubicin; 24 weeks duration after nephrectomy or biopsy with subsequent nephrectomy
- I: vincristine, doxorubicin, cyclophosphamide, and etoposide; 24 weeks after nephrectomy
- M: DD-4A plus cyclophosphamide and etoposide; time frame variable
- UH1: vincristine, doxorubicin, cyclophosphamide, carboplatin, and etoposide; 30 weeks plus radiation therapy
- UH2: UH1 plus additional vincristine and irinotecan; 36 weeks plus radiation therapy

ISSUES FOR REFERRAL

Clinical trials and referred to a multidisciplinary pediatric cancer team

ADDITIONAL THERAPIES

High-dose chemotherapy plus autologous hemopoietic stem cell rescue has been utilized for relapsed disease.

SURGERY/OTHER PROCEDURES

- Unilateral WT (1):
  - Radical nephroureterectomy with renal hilar and aortocaval lymph node sampling
  - Renal vein and IVC palpation should be performed to asses for tumor thrombus.
  - Lung metastases does not preclude local tumor resection.
  - Resection of contiguous organs except adrenal gland and hepatic metastectomy is not recommended.
  - Nephron-sparing partial nephrectomy remains controversial for unilateral WT.
- Bilateral WT: Surgery goal is eradicate all tumor while preserving renal function (risk of end-stage renal failure 12%) (1):
  - Tissue diagnosis is not necessary prior to neoadjuvant chemotherapy in appropriate age children (<10 years) and typical imaging features.
  - Neoadjuvant chemotherapy recommended with reevaluation by CT or MRI after 4 to 8 weeks
  - Tissue biopsy (if tumors unresectable) or bilateral nephron-sparing partial nephrectomy should be undertaken no later than 12 weeks from diagnosis.

 ONGOING CARE

FOLLOW-UP RECOMMENDATIONS

Patient Monitoring

- Monitoring for toxic effects of therapy should be performed throughout treatment and long-term: liver function tests; serum creatinine; CBC; echocardiogram
- Surveillance imaging (CT or MRI) varies by risk stratification.
- Reduced sexual development and fertility (1)
- Survivors demonstrate lower neurocognitive function (1).
- Secondary malignancies occur in 4% of survivors by age 30 years, median 12.5 years to onset, especially GI and breast (breast cancer incidence 15% by age 40 years following whole lung XRT) (1),(2).

PROGNOSIS

Outcomes are reported as 4-year event-free survival (EFS) or relapse-free survival (RFS) and 4-year overall survival (OS) and depend on staging.

COMPLICATIONS

- Surgical complications include intestinal obstruction (5%), extensive hemorrhage (2%), wound infection (2%), and vascular injury (1.5%).
- Cumulative incidence of severe chronic health condition 25 years after surgery is 65%.
- Premature mortality: 5–23% cumulative mortality 30 to 50 years after diagnosis; excess death due to secondary malignancy (50%) and CHF (25%) (1)
- Radiation therapy is major risk factor for premature death; also associated with impaired lung function, kyphosis, and osteoporosis (2)
- Recurrent WT typically occurs in the lungs within 2 years of diagnosis.

REFERENCES

1. National Cancer Institute. Wilms tumor and other childhood kidney tumors treatment (PDQ®)—health professional version. https://www.cancer.gov/types/kidney/hp/wilms-treatment-pdq#link/_1203. Updated October 8, 2021. Accessed December 5, 2021.
2. Aldrink JH, Heaton TE, Dasgupta R, et al. Update on Wilms tumor. *J Pediatr Surg*. 2019;54(3):390–397.

 CODES

ICD10

- C64.9 Malignant neoplasm of unsp kidney, except renal pelvis
- C64.1 Malignant neoplasm of right kidney, except renal pelvis
- C64.2 Malignant neoplasm of left kidney, except renal pelvis

CLINICAL PEARLS

- WT is the most common renal tumor in children; usually affecting children <5 years
- Overall survival 30–100%.
- Outcomes worse with anaplasia, older age, advanced stage, chromosome gain 1q, and LOH 1p/16q

W

ZOLLINGER-ELLISON SYNDROME

Douglas S. Parks, MD

 BASICS

DESCRIPTION

- Zollinger-Ellison syndrome (ZES) triad
  - Markedly elevated gastric acid secretion
  - Peptic ulcer disease
  - A gastrinoma or non-β islet cell tumor of the pancreas or duodenal wall that produces gastrin (hypergastrinemia)
    - Gastrinomas (at the time of diagnosis) may be single or multiple (1/2 to 2/3), large or small, benign or malignant (2/3), sporadic (70–75%), or associated with *multiple endocrine neoplasia type 1* (MEN1) (25–30%).
- System(s) affected: endocrine/metabolic, gastrointestinal
- Synonym(s): Z-E syndrome; pancreatic ulcerogenic tumor syndrome; multiple endocrine neoplasia, partial; ulcerogenic islet cell tumor

EPIDEMIOLOGY

Incidence

- 1 to 3 per million per year in the United States
- Predominant age: middle age (30 to 65 years). Mean age of onset is 43 years; presents a decade earlier in patients with ZES/MEN1
- Predominant sex: male > female (1.3:1)

Pediatric Considerations

Aggressive cases have been reported in teenagers.

Pregnancy Considerations

Rare, pregnancy alters medication choices and surgical timing.

ETIOLOGY AND PATHOPHYSIOLOGY

- Gastrinoma is found the head of the pancreas (20–30%) and the first or second portion of the duodenum (70–80%); if in the pancreas, the lesion is more likely to metastasize to the liver (1).
- Hypergastrinemia results in gastric mucosal hypertrophy and increased acid production. Increased acid production causes mucosal ulceration. Diarrhea (60%) and malabsorption are also common in ZES (1).
- Increasing number found in stomach wall, up to 8%; may be due to increased surveillance and/or increased PPI use masking symptoms
- Also may be found rarely in the mesentery, peritoneum, spleen, skin, or mediastinum (possibly metastasis with primary not identified)

Genetics

- ~25–30% of cases occur in association with the autosomal dominant MEN1 syndrome—tumors of pancreas, pituitary, and parathyroid.
- Can occur sporadically as well

RISK FACTORS

- MEN1
- Family history of ulcer disease

GENERAL PREVENTION

Screen first-degree relatives of patients with MEN1.

COMMONLY ASSOCIATED CONDITIONS

- MEN1
- Insulinoma
- Carcinoid tumors

 DIAGNOSIS

HISTORY

Average of 5 years of symptoms (including recurrent ulcers) before diagnosis is made

- Abdominal pain is the most common symptom (80%).
- Diarrhea (postprandial and fasting) (70%)
- Heartburn (60%)
- Nausea (30%)
- Reflux esophagitis
- Vomiting that is unresponsive to standard therapy
- Weight loss

PHYSICAL EXAM

- Hepatomegaly with metastasis
- Conjunctival pallor if anemic
- Jaundice (tumor compressing common bile duct)
- Epigastric tenderness
- Dental erosions
- Heme + stools on rectal exam
- Complications of severe peptic ulcer disease, including hemorrhage, perforation, and obstruction
- Signs of MEN1 are hypercalcemia, hyperparathyroidism, and Cushing syndrome.

Geriatric Considerations

Consider the diagnosis in a patient with persistent or recurring peptic ulcer disease; it is a less aggressive disease if it appears after 65 years.

DIFFERENTIAL DIAGNOSIS

- Elevated serum gastrin with hypochlorhydria/achlorhydria
  - Atrophic gastritis
  - Drug-induced (associated with proton pump inhibitors [PPIs])
  - Gastric cancer
  - Pernicious anemia
  - Postvagotomy
- Elevated serum gastrin with normal or increased gastric acid
  - Antral G-cell hyperfunction
  - Chronic renal failure
  - *Helicobacter pylori* infection
  - Gastric outlet obstruction
  - Retained gastric antrum
- Consider gastrinoma in all patients with:
  - Recurrent or refractory ulcer disease
  - Gastric hypertrophy and ulcers
  - Duodenal and jejunal ulcers
  - Ulcers and diarrhea
  - Ulcers and kidney stones
  - Hypercalcemia and ulcers
  - Pituitary disease
  - Family history of ulcer disease or endocrine tumors suggestive of MEN1

DIAGNOSTIC TESTS & INTERPRETATION

- Secretin stimulation test is preferred: gastrin level >120 pg/mL (>120 ng/L); may be difficult to find lab that can do this (1),(2)
- Some gastrin assays undermeasure serum gastrin; if have strong index of suspicion but gastrin levels low, may need to repeat with a different lab (1)
- Gastric secretory studies: basal acid output
- Elevated fasting serum gastrin: >1,000 pg/mL with ulcers diagnostic; >200 pg/mL with ulcers is suggestive.

- Elevated basal gastric acid output: >15 mEq/hr (>15 mmol/hr)
- Gastric pH <2 with elevated gastrin
- Check serum calcium, phosphorus, cortisol, and prolactin to rule out MEN1.
- Drugs may alter lab results:
  - Histamine (H_2) blockers and PPIs may increase gastric pH and serum gastrin.
  - Hold PPIs 7 days and H_2 blockers 2 days prior to drawing gastrin level.
- Endoscopic US: finds 24–38% of primary tumors in pancreas, much less effective in duodenum
- Endoscopic findings include esophagitis, duodenal ulceration with multiple ulcers, and prominent gastric and duodenal folds.
- Used to localize tumor for possible resection
- Much more likely to find tumors >3 cm (95%) than <1 cm (<15%)
- Abdominal CT scan: most useful for pancreatic tumors and metastasis >3 cm
- Abdominal US, MRI, and angiography are not typically useful except in large tumors.
- Somatostatin receptor scintigraphy (SRS): more sensitive than radiologic studies; still only finds 30% of small tumors.
- Newest modality is ^{68}Gallium labeled somatostatin PET/CT scanning, which is showing excellent sensitivity and specificity (1),(2).
- Portal venous sampling and selective venous sampling for gastrin can localize the area of tumor and metastasis (80–90% sensitivity) for surgical intervention (3).
- Brain imaging (MRI) and serum calcium are useful if MEN1 is suspected.
- Because pancreatic tumors are most likely to be large and to metastasize to the liver (worse prognosis), SRS and an abdominal CT scan are suggested to look for resectable tumors. Resection improves prognosis.

Initial Tests (lab, imaging)

- Diagnosis is based on elevated fasting plasma gastrin levels and Gastric pH <2 in the absence of PPI or H_2 blockers.
- Radiologic studies help locate and identify tumors for resection (1),(2),(3).

Follow-Up Tests & Special Considerations

Annual radiologic studies to look for recurrent or growing tumors and liver metastasis that may require reoperation (4)

Diagnostic Procedures/Other

Endoscopy may reveal tumors in the duodenal or stomach wall; multiple ulcers, including jejunal ulcers; and prominent gastric and duodenal folds.

Test Interpretation

- 90% of gastrinomas are found in the gastric triangle (bordered by the bile duct, the junction of second and third portions of the duodenum, and the junction of the head and body of pancreas).
- ~30% of gastrinomas are in the head of the pancreas (more likely >3 cm, metastasis to liver).
- ~70% of gastrinomas are in the wall of the first or second portion of duodenum (more likely small and solitary) (2).
- 2/3 of gastrinomas are malignant.

- 50% of gastrinomas stain positive for adrenocorticotropic hormone (ACTH), vasoactive intestinal polypeptide, insulin, or neurotensin.
- 1/3 of patients have metastasis on presentation: regional nodes > liver > bone, > peritoneum, spleen, skin, and mediastinum.
- Biopsy shows hyperplasia of antral gastrin-producing cells; histology appears similar to carcinoid.

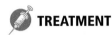 **TREATMENT**

GENERAL MEASURES
- Goals are to control acid hypersecretion and resect the tumor.
- Advanced imaging initially to evaluate for resection
- Surgical removal when primary tumor can be identified and as adjunct to control symptoms. Surgical resection of primary may enable stopping acid secretion and need for medical treatment (3).
- Medical treatment for symptom control when primary tumor is not found or metastasis on initial diagnosis

MEDICATION
- PPIs are the first-line treatment; add H_2 blockers if PPI not tolerated or insufficient.
- Medications heal 80–85% of ulcers, most of which recur. Lifelong medication use should be anticipated.
- 4- to 8-fold higher H_2 dose often necessary; may need up to double dose of PPI (3)
  - Start at a lower dose and titrate to symptoms (or maximum recommended dosage).
- If hyperparathyroidism is present (MEN1), correct hypercalcemia.

First Line
- PPIs
  - Omeprazole 60 to 120 mg/day
  - Lansoprazole 60 to 180 mg/day (doses >120 mg need to be divided BID)
  - Rabeprazole 60 to 100 mg/day up to 60 mg BID
  - Pantoprazole 40 to 240 mg/day PO; 80 to 120 mg q12h IV
- H_2 blockers
  - Cimetidine 300 mg q6h up to 2.4 g/day
  - Ranitidine 150 mg q12h up to 6 g/day
  - Famotidine 20 mg q6h; up to 640 mg/day
- Contraindications
  - Known hypersensitivity to the drug
  - H_2 blockers: antiandrogen effects, drug interactions due to cytochrome P450 inhibition
  - PPIs: none
- Precautions
  - Adjust doses for geriatric patients and patients with renal insufficiency.
  - Gynecomastia has been reported with high-dose cimetidine (>2.4 g/day).
  - PPIs may induce a profound and long-lasting effect on gastric acid secretion, thereby affecting the bioavailability of drugs depending on low gastric pH (e.g., ketoconazole, ampicillin, iron).
- Significant possible interactions: Consider drug–drug interactions and consult prescribing materials accordingly.

Second Line
- Octreotide may slow growth of liver metastases or (occasionally) promote regression. Octreotide LAR can be given every 28 days.
- Chemotherapy regimens using streptozocin, 5-fluorouracil, and doxorubicin shows limited response.
- Interferon shows a limited response but may be useful in combination with octreotide.

SURGERY/OTHER PROCEDURES
- Laparotomy to search for resectable tumors unless patient has liver metastasis on presentation or MEN1; surgery improves outcomes.
- Definitive therapy: removal of identifiable gastrinomas (95% of tumors are found at the time of surgery; 5-year cure is 40% when all are removed.) Second surgeries are worth considering if there is radiologic evidence of new or growing tumors and resection may prolong life span (4).
- Total gastrectomy is rarely indicated.
- In MEN1, parathyroidectomy, by lowering calcium, may also decrease acid production and decrease antisecretory drug use. Gastrinomas in MEN1 are generally small, benign, and multiple, and surgery is not usually curative in this situation.

ADMISSION, INPATIENT, AND NURSING CONSIDERATIONS
- Titrate medication to symptom control.
- Appropriate surveillance postoperatively to look for metastasis

 ONGOING CARE

FOLLOW-UP RECOMMENDATIONS
Patient Monitoring
- Longitudinal follow-up to evaluate for metastases. Reoperation may be considered (4).
- Titrate medical therapy to control symptoms.
- Advise patients of potential danger of stopping antisecretory treatment. Rare cases have been reported of severe adverse outcomes within 2 days of stopping PPIs (5)[B]. Gastric acid analysis can help guide medical therapy to maintain basal gastric acid output at <10 mEq/hr (<2 mEq/hr if patient has complications such as perforation or esophagitis).

DIET
Restrict foods that aggravate symptoms.

PATIENT EDUCATION
Inform patients as to the nature of disease and prognosis.

PROGNOSIS
- Overall survival rate: 5 to 10 years: 69–94%
- The prognosis improves with complete surgical removal of the tumor.
- If liver metastasis is present on initial surgery, 5-year survival is 30–40%; 10-year survival is 25%.
- Mortality is directly related to liver metastasis, tumor size, and presence of pancreatic tumors.

COMPLICATIONS
- Complications of peptic ulcer disease (bleeding, perforation, obstruction)
- 2/3 of gastrinomas are malignant with metastasis.
- Paraneoplastic phenomena (e.g., production of ACTH with resulting Cushing syndrome) is possible.
- Decrease in vitamin B_{12} levels is possible with long-term PPI use.

REFERENCES

1. Metz DC, Cadiot G, Poitras P, et al. Diagnosis of Zollinger-Ellison syndrome in the era of PPIs, faulty Gastrin assays, sensitive imaging and limited access to acid secretory testing. *Int J Edocr Oncol.* 2017;4(4):167–185.
2. Mendelson AH, Donowitz M. Catching the zebra: clinical pearls and pitfalls for the successful diagnosis of Zollinger-Ellison syndrome. *Dig Dis Sci.* 2017;62:2258–2265.
3. Norton JA, Foster DS, Ito T, et al. Gastrinomas medical or surgical treatment. *Endocrinol Metab Clin N Am.* 2018;37:577–601.
4. Norton JA, Krampitz GW, Poultsides GA, et al. Prospective evaluation of results of reoperation in Zollinger-Ellison syndrome. *Ann Surg.* 2018;267(4):782–788.
5. Poitras P, Gingras MH, Rehfeld JF. The Zollinger-Ellison syndrome: dangers and consequences of interrupting antisecretory treatment. *Clin Gastroenterol Hepatol.* 2012;10(2):199–202.

ADDITIONAL READING

- De Angelis C, Corgegoso-Valdivia P, Venezia L, et al. Diagnosis and management of Zollinger-Ellison syndrome in 2018. *Minerva Endocrinol.* 2018;43(2):212–220.
- Smallfield GB, Allison J, Wilcox CM. Prospective evaluation of quality of life in patients with Zollinger-Ellison syndrome. *Dig Dis Sci.* 2010;55(11):3108–3112.

 CODES

ICD10
E16.4 Increased secretion of gastrin

CLINICAL PEARLS
- Consider Zollinger-Ellison syndrome if peptic ulcers recur or if unusually high doses of PPI are needed to control symptoms.
- Abdominal pain and diarrhea should be totally controllable with adequate medical treatment.
- ~25–30% of cases of ZES occur in association with MEN1.
- Once ZES is diagnosed, search for gastrinomas in the head of the pancreas and the first or second portion of the duodenum.
- PPIs heal ZES ulcers. Patients should anticipate lifelong therapy.

Z

INDEX

NOTE: Page numbers preceded by A- indicate Algorithms.

peripheral, 700–701
posterior tibial nerve (tarsal tunnel syndrome), 972–973
Neurosyphilis, 970–971
Neutropenia, A-83
Neutropenia, in myelodysplastic syndromes, 686–687
Nevus
  abnormal, 96–97, 636–637
  dysplastic, 96–97, 636–637
  giant congenital, 636
Nexplanon, 223
Niacin deficiency, 1081
Nicotine addiction, 606–607, 702–703, 958–959, 1004–1005
Nightmares, in children, 114
Night terrors, in children, 114
Night waking, in children, 114
Nipple, Paget disease of, 134
Nipple (breast) discharge, 384–385, 508
Nociceptive pain, 196
Nocturnal enuresis, 114–115, 338–339
Nocturnal hypoglycemia, 522, 523
Nocturnal myoclonus. See Periodic limb movement disorder
Nocturnal polyuria, 546
Nocturnal upper airway occlusion. See Obstructive sleep apnea
Nodular episcleritis, 344–345
Nodular lymphangitis, 614–615
Nodular melanoma, 636, 637
Nonalcoholic fatty liver disease (NAFLD), 198, 199, 704–705
Nonalcoholic steatohepatitis (NASH), 198, 704–705
Nonallergic rhinitis, 892
Nonallergic rhinitis with eosinophilia syndrome (NARES), 892
Nonbinary, 1012–1013
Nonbullous impetigo, 540–541
Noncommunicating hydrocele, 492
Noncompliance, behavioral, 114–115
Nondiabetic hypoglycemia, 524–525
Nonexertional (classic) heat stroke, 444
Nonfatal drowning, 706–707
Nonhistaminergic acquired angioedema, idiopathic (INH-AAE), 52–53
Nonimmune heparin-associated thrombocytopenia, 456–457
Nonmonosymptomatic NE (NMNE), 338–339
Nonobstructive atelectasis, 86–87
Nonorganic dyspepsia. See Functional dyspepsia
Nonpalpable cryptorchidism, 240–241
Nonpulsatile tinnitus, 1002–1003
Nonscarring (noncicatricial) alopecia, 32–33
Nonseminomatous germ cell tumors, 978–979
Non–small cell lung cancer (NSCLC), 606–607
Nonspecific interstitial pneumonia (NSIP), 298–299
Nonsteroidal anti-inflammatory drugs (NSAIDs)
  nephritis induced by, 564–565
  ulcers induced by, 760–761

Non–ST-segment elevation myocardial infarction (NSTEMI), 12–13, 230–231, A-22
Nonulcer dyspepsia. See Functional dyspepsia
Noonan syndrome, 90, 888
Normal consciousness delirium, 256
Normal pressure hydrocephalus (NPH), 494–495, A-38
Normative sexual behaviors, 114–115
Norovirus, 294
Nosebleed (epistaxis), 346–347
Nosocomial infections
  MRSA, 210–211
  pneumonia, 784–785
NRDS. See Neonatal respiratory distress syndrome
NSAIDs. See Nonsteroidal anti-inflammatory drugs
NSCLC. See Non–small cell lung cancer
NSTEMI (non–ST-segment elevation myocardial infarction), 12–13, 230–231, A-22
Nut allergy, 376–377
NuvaRing, 222
Nystagmus, labyrinthitis and, 578

O

OA. See Osteoarthritis
Obesity, 708–709
  and asthma, 84
  and diabetes mellitus type 2, 288
  and hypertension, 514, 516–517
  lesbian health, 588
  and metabolic syndrome, 654–655
  and obstructive sleep apnea, 936–937
  and polycystic ovary syndrome, 794–795
  surgery for (See Bariatric surgery)
  and vitamin D deficiency, 1078, 1079
  and vitamin deficiency, 1080, 1081
Objective tinnitus, 1002–1003
Obsessive-compulsive disorder (OCD), 710–711
  PTSD and, 808, 809
  Tourette syndrome and, 1006–1007
Obstetric emergency, in-flight, 26–27
Obstipation. See Constipation
Obstructive atelectasis, 86–87
Obstructive sleep apnea (OSA), 936–937
  pediatric, 114–115
Obstructive uropathy, 496
Occupational allergic rhinitis, 892
OCD. See Obsessive-compulsive disorder
Ocular chemical burns, 712–713
Ocular herpes, 468–473
Ocular migraine, 434
Ocular myasthenia gravis, 684–685
Ocular rosacea, 8–9
Ocular toxoplasmosis, 1008–1009
Oculopharyngeal muscular dystrophy (OPMD), 680–681
Oculosympathetic deficiency. See Horner syndrome
Oculosympathetic paralysis. See Horner syndrome
Oculosympathetic paresis. See Horner syndrome

Oculosympathetic syndrome. See Horner syndrome
Odontoid fractures, 179
OME. See Otitis media with effusion
Onychocryptosis. See Ingrown toenail
Onychomycosis, 714–715
Open-angle glaucoma, primary, 406–407
Ophthalmia neonatorum, 218, 414–415
Opioid abuse, 196–197, 306–307, 557, 716–717, 958–959
Opioid detoxification, 307, 557
Opioid poisoning/overdose, 557
Opioid therapy, for pain, 196–197
Opioid use disorder (OUD), 307, 557, 716–717, 958–959
Opioid withdrawal, 716–717
OPMD. See Oculopharyngeal muscular dystrophy
Optic neuritis, 468–469, 676–677, 718–719
Oral contraceptives, 222–223
Oral leukoplakia, 598–599
Oral rehydration (ORT), 254–255, 295, A-36
Orbital cellulitis, 170, 172–173, 174
Orchidopexy (orchiopexy), 241
Orchitis
  epididymo-orchitis, 342
  Henoch-Schönlein purpura and, 454, 455
  mumps, 678–679
Organic brain syndrome. See Delirium
Orgasm
  female, disorders in, 928–929
  male, disorders in (ejaculatory disorders), 324–325
Orofacial pain. See Temporomandibular joint disorder
Oropharyngeal candidiasis, 152–153
Oropharyngeal dysphagia, 320–321
ORT. See Oral rehydration
Ortho Evra, 222
Orthostatic hypotension, 396, 964–967, 1070
Orthostatic intolerance, 682
OSA. See Obstructive sleep apnea
Osgood-Schlatter disease (OSD), 720–721
Osler phenomenon, 516
Osmotic diarrhea, 296–297
Osteoarthritis (OA), 722–723, A-24
Osteoarthritis of knee, 576–577, 722–723
Osteoarthritis of shoulder, 930–931
Osteoarthrosis. See Osteoarthritis
Osteomyelitis, 210–211, 724–725
Osteopathic manipulation, 212
Osteopenia, 726–727
  in menopause, 648, A-79
Osteoporosis, 726–727, 952
  in female athlete triad, 366–367
  in menopause, 648–649, 726–727, A-79
Ostium primum defect, 90
Ostium secundum defect, 90
Otitis externa, 728–729
Otitis media, 730–733
  acute, 730–731
  chronic, 730–731
  eustachian tube dysfunction with, 360–361
  mastoiditis with, 626–627
  measles and, 629
Otitis media with effusion (OME), 730–733